Lexicomp®
Drug Information Handbook for Oncology

An Extensive Guide to Combination
Chemotherapy Regimens

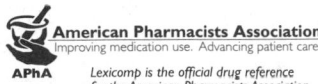

American Pharmacists Association
Improving medication use. Advancing patient care.

APhA   *Lexicomp is the official drug reference
for the American Pharmacists Association*

SENIOR EDITORS
Diedra L. Bragalone, PharmD, MBA, BCOP, BCPS

Stephanie S. Minich, PharmD, BCOP

15th Edition

ers Kluwer

Lexicomp®
Drug Information Handbook for Oncology

An Extensive Guide to Combination Chemotherapy Regimens

Diedra L. Bragalone, PharmD, MBA, BCOP, BCPS
Pharmacotherapy Specialist
Wolters Kluwer Health

Stephanie S. Minich, PharmD, BCOP
Senior Clinical Content Specialist
Wolters Kluwer

Lexicomp®

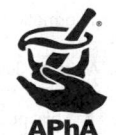

APhA

NOTICE

This data is intended to serve the user as a handy reference and not as a complete drug information resource. It does not include information on every therapeutic agent available. The publication covers over 300 commonly used drugs. In addition, it does not include all potentially relevant information about any particular drug. Instead, it is intended to present important aspects of drug data in a more concise and accessible format than is typically found in medical literature or product material supplied by manufacturers.

The nature of drug information is that it is constantly evolving because of ongoing research and clinical experience and is often subject to interpretation. While Wolters Kluwer Clinical Drug Information makes reasonable efforts to publish accurate information, users are advised that the authors, editors, reviewers, contributors, and publishers cannot be responsible for the continued currency of the information or for any errors, omissions, or the application of this information, or for any consequences arising therefrom. Therefore, the authors, editors, reviewers, contributors, and publishers shall have no liability to any person or entity with regard to claims, loss, or damage caused, or alleged to be caused, directly or indirectly, by the use of information contained herein. Because of the dynamic nature of drug information and the characteristics and needs unique to individual patients, readers are advised that decisions regarding drug therapy must be based on the independent judgment of the clinician. Users must regularly consult multiple sources (eg, medical literature and a manufacturer's most current product information) to remain aware of changing information about a drug and medical practices regarding its use. Therefore, this data is intended to be used in conjunction with other necessary information and is not intended to be solely relied upon by any user. The user of this data hereby and forever releases the authors, editors, reviewers, contributors, and publishers of this data from any and all liability of any kind that might arise out of the use of this data. The authors, editors, reviewers, contributors, and publishers are not responsible for any inaccurate source materials developed by third-parties or for any user misunderstandings that may arise from the data.

Certain of the authors, editors, reviewers, and contributors have written portions of this book in their individual capacities. The inclusion of content is not intended to indicate that it has been reviewed or endorsed by any federal or state agency, pharmaceutical company, or regulatory body.

The publishers have made reasonable efforts to avoid reproducing without permission, any content that may be subject to third-party copyright claims. Any questions regarding content that may be subject to such claims will be addressed at the first opportunity.

If you have any suggestions or questions regarding any information presented in this data, please contact our drug information pharmacists at (855) 633-0577. Book revisions are available at our website at http://www.wolterskluwercdi.com/clinical-notices/revisions/.

This manual was produced using LIMS — A complete publishing service of Wolters Kluwer Clinical Drug Information, Inc.

Lexicomp®

Wolters Kluwer

ISBN 978-1-59195-368-5

TABLE OF CONTENTS

ONCOLOGY EDITORIAL ADVISORY PANEL

ONCOLOGY OFF-LABEL REVIEW PANEL MEMBERS

Diedra L. Bragalone, PharmD, MBA, BCOP, BCPS
Senior Clinical Content Specialist
Wolters Kluwer

Stephanie S. Minich, PharmD, BCOP
Senior Clinical Content Specialist
Wolters Kluwer

Corey A. Carter, MD
Chief of Thoracic Oncology
John P. Murtha Cancer Center, Walter Reed National Military Medical Center

Mark T. Holdsworth, PharmD
Associate Professor of Pharmacy & Pediatrics and Pharmacy Practice Area Head
College of Pharmacy,
The University of New Mexico

Polly E. Kintzel, PharmD, BCPS, BCOP
Clinical Pharmacy Specialist – Oncology
Spectrum Health

Omer N. Koc, MD
Staff Physician
Hematology and Medical Oncology Department, Cleveland Clinic

Nicholas A. Link, PharmD, BCOP
Clinical Specialist, Oncology
Hillcrest Hospital

Heidi Trinkman, PharmD
Pediatric Hematology/Oncology Clinical Pharmacy Specialist
Cook Children's Medical Center

DRUG INTERACTIONS EDITORIAL ADVISORY PANEL

EDITORIAL ADVISORY PANEL

Angela Clark, PharmD, BCPS
Clinical Pharmacy Specialist,
Cardiothoracic Intensive Care Unit and
Cardiology Team Lead
University of Michigan Health System

M. Petrea Cober, PharmD, BCNSP
Clinical Pharmacy Coordinator
Neonatal Intensive Care Unit,
Children's Hospital of Akron
Assistant Professor of Pharmacy
Practice
Northeast Ohio Medical University
(NEOMED)

Adam Cochrane, PharmD, BCPS
Organ Transplant Clinical Specialist
Inova Fairfax Hospital
Adjunct Assistant Professor
Butler University

Christine M. Cohn, PharmD, BCPS
Senior Clinical Content Specialist
Wolters Kluwer

Jessica Connell, RN, BSN
Pharmacotherapy Contributor
Tifton, Georgia

Kim Connell, PharmD
Pharmacotherapy Contributor
Thomasville, Georgia

Ann P. Conrad, ANP-BC, RN, ACRN
Advanced Practice Nurse
Community Hospitalists

Amanda H. Corbett, PharmD,
BCPS, FCCP, AAHIVE
Clinical Assistant Professor
Eshelman School of Pharmacy,
University of North Carolina

Susan Cornell, PharmD, CDE,
FAPhA, FAADE
Associate Professor
Department of Pharmacy Practice
Assistant Director of Experimental
Education
Midwestern University, Chicago
College of Pharmacy

Marilyn Cortell, RDH, MS, FAADH
Associate Professor
New York City College of Technology,
City University of New York

Harold L. Crossley, DDS, MS, PhD
Professor Emeritus
Baltimore College of Dental Surgery,
University of Maryland Baltimore

Melanie W. Cucchi, BS, PharmD,
RPh
Clinical Manager, Pediatric & Neonatal
Content
Wolters Kluwer

Lacey Davis, PharmD, BCPS
Clinical Pharmacist, Hospice,
Palliative Care, and Post-Acute Care
Aultman Hospital

Beth Deen, PharmD, BDNSP
Senior Pediatric Clinical Pharmacy
Specialist
Cook Children's Medical Center

Renee K. Dixon, MD
Attending Physician, Critical and
Pulmonary Care
University of Maryland Medical Center,
UMMC Midtown Campus, and
Baltimore Veterans Affairs Hospital

Jodi Dreiling, PharmD, BCPS
Pharmacotherapy Specialist in
Critical Care
Cleveland Clinic Akron General

Kim S. Dufner, PharmD
Clinical Content Specialist
Wolters Kluwer

Mary Eche, PharmD, BCPS, BCCCP
Clinical Pharmacist II
Beth Israel Deaconess Medical Center

Michael S. Edwards, PharmD, MBA,
BCOP
Pharmacotherapy Contributor
Chevy Chase, Maryland

Vicki L. Ellingrod, PharmD, BCPP
Head, Clinical Pharmacogenomics
Laboratory and *Associate Professor*
Department of Psychiatry, Colleges of
Pharmacy and Medicine, University of
Michigan

John Grabenstein, RPh, PhD, FAPhA
Pharmacotherapy Contributor
West Point, Pennsylvania

Tracy Hagemann, PharmD
Associate Dean and *Professor of Clinical Pharmacy*
University of Tennessee
College of Pharmacy

Kat Hall, MPharm, IPresc, PGCertClinEd, PGDipGPP, MFRPSII, MRPharmS, FHEA
Director of Centre for Inter-Professional Postgraduate Education and Training
University of Reading

Martin D. Higbee, PharmD
Retired Associate Professor
Department of Pharmacy Practice and Science, The University of Arizona

Mark T. Holdsworth, PharmD
Associate Professor of Pharmacy & Pediatrics and *Pharmacy Practice Area Head*
College of Pharmacy,
The University of New Mexico

Edward Horn, PharmD, BCPS
Clinical Specialist, Transplant/Cardiothoracic Surgery
Allegheny General Hospital

Collin A. Hovinga, PharmD, MS, FCCP
Director of Research Support Services
Seton Healthcare Family, Dell Children's Medical Center
Clinical Associate Professor of Pharmacy
UT Austin School of Pharmacy

Jane Hurlburt Hodding, PharmD
Executive Director, Inpatient Pharmacy Services and Clinical Nutrition Services
Long Beach Memorial Medical Center and Miller Children's Hospital

Makiko Iwasawa, PharmD, BCPS
Chief Pharmacist, Drug Information Center
National Cerebral and Cardiovascular Center

Adam B. Jackson, PharmD, BCPS
Clinical Pharmacy Specialist in Infectious Diseases
Kaiser Permanente

Anna M. Wodlinger Jackson, PharmD, BCPS-AQ Cardiology
Pharmacotherapy Contributor
Fort Lauderdale, Florida

Douglas L. Jennings, PharmD, AACC, BCPS-AQ Cardiology, FCCP
Clinical Pharmacy Manager, Heart Transplant and Mechanical Circulatory Support
New York Presbyterian Columbia Medical Center

Sallie Johnson, PharmD, BCPS, AQ Cardiology
Clinical Pharmacy Specialist, Cardiology
Penn State Milton S. Hershey Medical Center

Michael A. Kahn, DDS
Professor and Chairman
Department of Oral and Maxillofacial Pathology, Tufts University School of Dental Medicine

Julie J. Kelsey, PharmD
Clinical Specialist
Women's Health and Family Medicine, Department of Pharmacy Services, University of Virginia Health System

Patrick J. Kiel, PharmD, BCPS, BCOP
Clinical Pharmacy Specialist
Hematology and Stem Cell Transplant, Indiana University Simon Cancer Center

Jooran Kim, PharmD
Pharmacotherapy Contributor
Vancouver, Canada

10

Sherry Luedtke, PharmD
Associate Professor
Department of Pharmacy Practice, Texas Tech University HSC School of Pharmacy

Viki Lui, BPharm, MPH, MSHP
Lead Education Pharmacist for Pharmacy Department
The Royal Melbourne Hospital

Shannon N. Lukez, RN, MSN, ANP-BC
Adult Nurse Practitioner – Orthopedics
Mountaineer Orthopedic Specialists

Tracy Macaulay, PharmD, AACC, BCPS (AQ-CV)
Clinical Pharmacy Specialist
UKHealthcare Pharmacy Services

Janis MacKichan, PharmD, FAPhA
Professor Emeritus
Department of Pharmacy Practice, Northeast Ohio Medical University (NEOMED)

Jason Makii, PharmD, BCPS
Clinical Pharmacy Specialist, Neurosciences Critical Care
University Hospitals Case Medical Center

Melissa Makii, PharmD, BCPS
Clinical Pharmacy Specialist
Pediatric Oncology, Rainbow Babies & Children's Hospital

Vincent F. Mauro, BS, PharmD, FCCP
Professor of Clinical Pharmacy and *Adjunct Professor of Medicine*
Colleges of Pharmacy and Medicine, The University of Toledo

Shawn Mazur, PharmD
Clinical Pharmacy Manager, Infectious Diseases
New York-Presbyterian/Weill Cornell Medical Center

Debra McDonald, RN
Oncology Staff Nurse
St. Louis University Cancer Center

Joseph McGraw, PharmD, MPH, PhD, BCPS
Assistant Professor of Pharmaceutical Science and *Metabolism Laboratory Director*
Concordia University Wisconsin, School of Pharmacy

Ann Marie McMullin, MD
Associate Staff
Emergency Services Institute, Cleveland Clinic

Christopher McPherson, PharmD
Clinical Pharmacist
Neonatal Intensive Care Unit, St. Louis Children's Hospital
Assistant Professor
Department of Pediatrics, Washington University School of Medicine

Timothy F. Meiller, DDS, PhD
Professor
Oncology and Diagnostic Sciences, Baltimore College of Dental Surgery
Professor of Oncology
Marlene and Stewart Greenebaum Cancer Center, University of Maryland Medical System

Micheline Meiners, MSc, PhD
Pharmacotherapy Contributor
Lago Norte, Brazil

Cathy A. Meives, PharmD
Clinical Manager, Core Pharmacology
Wolters Kluwer

Megan Menon, PharmD, BCOP
Clinical Pharmacy Specialist
Roswell Park Cancer Institute

Julie Miller, PharmD
Pharmacy Clinical Specialist, Cardiology
Nationwide Children's Hospital

Stacy E. Miller, PharmD, BCPS, BCPP
Senior Clinical Content Specialist
Wolters Kluwer

Katherine Mills, PharmD
Pharmacotherapy Contributor
Bristow, Virginia

Rebecca Pettit, PharmD, MBA, BCPS
Pediatric Pulmonary Clinical Pharmacy Specialist
Riley Hospital for Children, Indiana University Health,
Department of Pharmacy

Cameron Phillips, BPharm, MClin Pharm
Clinical Pharmacist
Flinders Medical Center

Jennifer L. Placencia, PharmD
Neonatal Clinical Pharmacy Specialist
Texas Children's Hospital

Sacha R. Pollard, PharmD, BCPS
Pharmacotherapy Contributor
Fort Mill, South Carolina

Amy L. Potts, PharmD, BCPS
Assistant Director
Department of Pharmacy
PGY1 & PGY2 Residency Program Director
Monroe Carell Jr. Children's Hospital at Vanderbilt

Saira Rab, PharmD, BCPS (AQ-ID), AAHIVP
Infectious Diseases/HIV Clinical Pharmacist Specialist
Grady Health System

Sally Rafie, PharmD, BCPS
Medical Safety Pharmacist
UC San Diego Health System

Melissa Ray, PharmD, BCPS, BCPPS
Clinical Pharmacist III
UnitedHealth Group — Optum

Esta Razavi, PharmD
Clinical Content Specialist
Wolters Kluwer

James Reissig, PharmD, BCPS
Assistant Director, Clinical Services
Cleveland Clinic Akron General

A.J. (Fred) Remillard, PharmD
Assistant Dean, Research and Graduate Affairs
College of Pharmacy and Nutrition, University of Saskatchewan

Neil Reynolds, BPharm, MSc
Senior Pharmacist
Fiona Stanley Hospital

Amy Rybarczyk, PharmD, BCPS
Pharmacotherapy Specialist, Internal Medicine
Cleveland Clinic Akron General

Rikki L. Rychel, PharmD, BCPS, CDE
Clinical Pharmacy Specialist, Ambulatory Care
Louis Stokes Cleveland Department of Veterans Affairs Medical Center

Shannon Saldana, PharmD, MS, BCPP
Psychiatry Advanced Clinical Pharmacist
Primary Children's Hospital

Reem Santos, BPharm, MSc
Specialist Antimicrobial Pharmacist
Cambridge University Hospitals

Cheryl Sargel, PharmD
Advanced Patient Care Pharmacist
Nationwide Children's Hospital

Todd P. Semla, MS, PharmD, BCPS, FCCP, AGSF
National PBM Clinical Program Manager – Mental Health & Geriatrics
Department of Veterans Affairs, Pharmacy Benefits Management Services
Associate Professor, Clinical
Department of Medicine, Psychiatry and Behavioral Health, Feinberg School of Medicine, Northwestern University

Chasity M. Shelton, PharmD, BCPS, BCNSP
Assistant Professor of Clinical Pharmacy
Department of Clinical Pharmacy, University of Tennessee Health Science Center
Clinical Pharmacy Specialist
Pediatric Infectious Diseases and Antimicrobial Stewardship,
Le Bonheur Children's Hospital

Kelan Thomas, PharmD, MS, BCPS, BCPP
Assistant Professor of Pharmacy Practice
Touro University California, College of Pharmacy
Clinical Pharmacist
St. Helena Hospital Center for Behavioral Health Office

Kristina M. Thurber, PharmD, BCPS
Internal Medicine Clinical Pharmacist
Mayo Clinic Hospital

Elizabeth A. Tomsik, PharmD, BCPS
Senior Clinical Director, Drug Content
Wolters Kluwer

Leslye Trachte, PharmD
Pharmacotherapy Contributor
Lawton, Oklahoma

Dana Travis, RPh
Clnical Content Specialist
Wolters Kluwer

Heidi Trinkman, PharmD
Pediatric Hematology/Oncology Clinical Pharmacy Specialist
Cook Children's Medical Center

Jennifer Trofe-Clark, PharmD, FAST, FCCP, BCPS
Clinical Transplant Pharmacist
Hospital of The University of Pennsylvania

Andriette van Jaarsveld, BPharm, MScMed
Clinical Pharmacy Specialist
Mediclinic Southern Africa (Stellenbosch)

Amy Van Orman, PharmD, BCPS
Senior Clinical Content Specialist
Wolters Kluwer

Carlos Vidotti
Pharmacotherapy Contributor
Brasilia DF, Brazil

Geoffrey Wall, RPh, PharmD, FCCP, BCPS, CGP
Professor of Clinical Sciences and Associate Professor of Pharmacy Practice
Drake University

Kristin Watson, PharmD, BCPS
Assistant Professor, Cardiology and Clinical Pharmacist, Cardiology Service
Heart Failure Clinic, University of Maryland Medical Center

JoEllen L. Weilnau, PharmD
Clinical Coordinator
Department of Hematology/Oncology/Bone Marrow Transplant, Children's Hospital of Akron

David M. Weinstein, PhD, RPh
Senior Director, Clinical Content
Wolters Kluwer

Regine L. White, PharmD, RPh
Clinical Pharmacist
University of Michigan Health System

Greg Wiggers, PharmD, PhD
Clinical Content Specialist
Wolters Kluwer

Sherri J. Willard Argyres, MA, PharmD
Senior Clinical Content Specialist
Wolters Kluwer

Andrea Williams, RPh
Clinical Content Specialist
Wolters Kluwer

Nathan Wirick, PharmD, BCPS
Clinical Specialist in Infectious Diseases and Antibiotic Management
Hillcrest Hospital

Adrian Wong, PharmD, BCPS, BCCCP
Senior Pharmacist, Fellow, Outcomes Research and Pharmacy Informatics
Brigham and Women's Hospital

PREFACE

The *Drug Information Handbook for Oncology* was designed to meet the needs of all oncology professionals involved in prescribing, preparing, and administering therapy. Presented in a concise and uniform format, this book contains monographs with information pertaining to both antineoplastic agents and ancillary or supportive care medications. This handbook serves as a portable quick reference while providing comprehensive oncology-related drug information. Organized like a dictionary for ease-of-use, a drug monograph can be quickly located by generic name.

The Chemotherapy Regimen section provides a comprehensive presentation of combination cancer chemotherapy regimens. The regimens are listed alphabetically by regimen name (acronym). An index lists regimens by indication. In addition, a special Combination Chemotherapy Regimen field in each drug monograph will refer you to the page(s) for the applicable regimens.

A special topics section addresses issues regarding Cancer Treatment-Related Complications (eg, management of drug extravasations, management of chemotherapy-induced nausea and vomiting (adults), common toxicity criteria, chemotherapy-induced peripheral neuropathy, mucositis and stomatitis, tumor lysis syndrome); Cancer-Related Topics (eg, chronic pain management, hospice (end of life) care, hypercalcemia of malignancy, malignant pleural effusions, palliative care management (cancer), venous thromboembolism in the cancer patient); and Safe Handling of Hazardous Drugs.

The appendix section includes information related to conversions, renal function, comparative drug charts, and laboratory reference values for adults. A pharmacologic category index provides a practical approach to categorizing drugs by their respective therapeutic classification.

We know you will find this handbook to be a valuable source of information and we welcome comments or suggestions to further improve future editions.

DESCRIPTION OF SECTIONS AND FIELDS USED IN THIS HANDBOOK

The *Drug Information Handbook for Oncology* is divided into six sections.

The first section is a compilation of introductory text pertinent to the use of this book.

The drug information section of the handbook, in which all drugs are listed alphabetically, details information pertinent to each drug. Extensive cross-referencing is provided by US brand names, Canadian brand names, and index terms.

The Chemotherapy Regimen section provides a comprehensive presentation of cancer chemotherapy regimens. The regimens are listed alphabetically by regimen name (acronym). An index at the beginning of this section lists regimens by indications. In addition, a special Combination Chemotherapy Regimen field in each drug monograph will link you to the applicable regimens.

The Special Topics section contains important cancer-related issues (ie, chemotherapy-induced peripheral neurophathy, management of chemotherapy-induced nausea and vomiting in adults, palliative care medicine (cancer), and safe handling of hazardous drugs). These issues are discussed in detail.

The fifth section is an appendix section.

The last section of this handbook is an index listing drugs in their unique pharmacologic category.

Alphabetical Listing of Drugs

Drug information is presented in a consistent format and provides the following:

Generic Name	US adopted name
Pronunciation Guide	Phonetic pronunciation
Related Information	Cross-reference to other pertinent drug information found elsewhere in this handbook
Brand Names: US	Trade names found in the United States (manufacturer-specific). The symbol [DSC] appears after trade names that have been recently discontinued.
Brand Names: Canada	Trade names found in Canada
Index Terms	Other names or accepted abbreviations of the generic drug. May also include common brand names no longer available; this field is used to create cross-references to monographs.
Pharmacologic Category	Unique systematic classification of medications
Use	Information pertaining to FDA- or Canadian-approved indications for the drug
Labeled Contraindications	Information pertaining to inappropriate use of the drug as dictated by approved labeling

Pregnancy Risk Factor	Five categories established by the FDA to indicate the potential of a systemically absorbed drug for causing risk to fetus
Pregnancy Considerations	A summary of human and/or animal information pertinent to or associated with the use of the drug as it relates to clinical effects on the fetus, newborn, or pregnant woman
Breastfeeding Considerations	Information pertinent to or associated with the human use of the drug as it relates to clinical effects on the breastfeeding infant or postpartum woman
Warnings/Precautions	Precautionary considerations, hazardous conditions related to use of the drug, and disease states or patient populations in which the drug should be cautiously used. Boxed warnings, when present, are clearly identified and are adapted from the FDA approved labeling. Consult the product labeling for the exact black box warning through the manufacturer's or the FDA website.
Adverse Reactions	Side effects are grouped by percentage of incidence (if known) and/or body system; <1% effects are grouped only by percentage (**Note:** Includes postmarketing and/or case report information if available)

Drug Interactions

Metabolism/Transport Effects	If a drug has demonstrated involvement with cytochrome P450 enzymes, or other metabolism or transport proteins, this field will identify the drug as an inhibitor, inducer, or substrate of the specific enzyme(s) (eg, CYP1A2 or UGT1A1). CYP450 isoenzymes are identified as substrates (minor or major), inhibitors (weak, moderate, or strong), and inducers (weak or strong).
Avoid Concomitant Use	Designates drug combinations which should not be used concomitantly, due to an unacceptable risk:benefit assessment. Frequently, the concurrent use of the agents is explicitly prohibited or contraindicated by the product labeling.
Increased Effect/Toxicity	Drug combinations that result in a increased or toxic therapeutic effect between the drug listed in the monograph and other drugs or drug classes
Decreased Effect	Drug combinations that result in a decreased therapeutic effect between the drug listed in the monograph and other drugs or drug classes
Food Interactions	Possible important interactions between the drug listed in the monograph and food, alcohol, or other beverages
Hazardous Drugs Handling Considerations	Indicates whether a drug is considered to be hazardous and provides handling recommendations for hazardous drugs
Storage/Stability	Information regarding storage and stability of commercially available products and products that have been reconstituted, diluted, or otherwise prepared. Provides the time and conditions for which a solution or mixture will maintain potency.
Preparation for Administration	Provides information regarding the preparation of drug products prior to administration, including dilution, reconstitution, etc.
Mechanism of Action	How the drug works in the body to elicit a response

◀ Pharmacodynamics/ Kinetics

The magnitude of a drug's effect depends on the drug concentration at the site of action. The pharmacodynamics are expressed in terms of onset of action and duration of action. Pharmacokinetics are expressed in terms of absorption, distribution, protein binding, metabolism, bioavailability, half-life, time to peak serum concentration, and elimination.

Dosing

The amount of drug to be typically given or taken during therapy; may include the following:

Adult

The recommended amount of drug to be given to adult patients

Adult & Geriatric

This combined field is only used to indicate that no specific adjustments for elderly patients were identified. However, other issues should be considered (eg, renal or hepatic impairment).

Geriatric

A suggested amount of drug to be given to elderly patients; may include adjustments from adult dosing (lack of information in the monograph may imply that the drug is not used in the elderly patient or no specific adjustments could be identified)

Pediatric

Suggested amount of drug to be given to neonates, infants, and children. The following age group definitions are utilized to characterize age-related dosing unless otherwise specified in the monograph: Neonate (0 to 28 days of age), infant (>28 days to 1 year of age), children (1 to 12 years of age), and adolescent (13 to 18 years of age).

Renal Impairment

Suggested dosage adjustments based on compromised renal function; may include dosing instructions for patients on dialysis

Hepatic Impairment

Suggested dosage adjustments based on compromised liver function

Obesity

Dosing adjustment or dosing considerations for the obese adult patient. Obesity is defined as a BMI ≥ 30 kg/m^2 (based on the World Health Organization [WHO]).

Adjustment for Toxicity

Suggested dosage adjustments in the event specific toxicities related to therapy are noted, such as hematologic toxicities related to cancer chemotherapy

Combination Regimens

List of combination chemotherapy regimens in which the drug is a component

Usual Infusion Concentrations

Information describing the usual concentrations of drugs for continuous infusion administration in the pediatric and adult populations as appropriate. Concentrations are derived from the literature, manufacturer's recommendation, or organizational recommendations (eg, the Institute for Safe Medication Practices [ISMP]) and are universally established. Institution-specific standard concentrations may differ from those listed.

Administration

Information regarding the recommended final concentrations, rates of administration for parenteral drugs, or other guidelines or relevant information to properly administer medications

Vesicant/Extravasation Risk

Indicates whether the drug is considered to be a vesicant and likely to cause significant morbidity if the infusion infiltrates soft tissues

Emetic Potential

Likelihood that the drug will cause nausea or vomiting

Extemporaneous Preparations	Directions for preparing liquid formulations from solid drug products. May include stability information and references.
Monitoring Parameters	Laboratory tests and patient physical parameters that should be monitored for safety and efficacy of drug therapy
Test Interactions	Listing of assay interferences when relevant; (B) = Blood; (S) = Serum; (U) = Urine
Dietary Considerations	Specific dietary modifications and/or restrictions (eg, information about sodium content)
Additional Information	Pertinent information about specific brands
Product Availability	Provides availability information on products that have been approved by the FDA but are not yet available for use. Estimates for when a product may be available are included, when this information is known. May also provide any unique or critical drug availability issues.
Prescribing and Access Restrictions	Provides information on any special requirements regarding the prescribing, obtaining, or dispensing of drugs, including access restrictions.
Medication Guide Available	Identifies drugs that have an FDA-approved Medication Guide
Dosage Forms Considerations	More specific Information regarding product concentrations, ingredients, package sizes, amount of doses per container, and other important details pertaining to various formulations of medications
Dosage Forms	Information with regard to form, strength, and availability of the drug in the United States. **Note:** Additional formulation information (eg, excipients, preservatives) is included when available. Please consult product labeling for further information.
Dosage Forms: Canada	Information with regard to form, strength, and availability of products that are uniquely available in Canada but currently are not available in the United States
Controlled Substance	Contains controlled substance schedule information as assigned by the United States Drug Enforcement Administration (DEA) or Canadian Controlled Substance Act (CDSA). CDSA information is only provided for drugs available in Canada and not available in the US

Chemotherapy Regimens

The Chemotherapy Regimen section provides a comprehensive presentation of cancer chemotherapy regimens. The regimens are listed alphabetically by regimen name (acronym). An index lists regimens by indications. In addition, a special Combination Chemotherapy Regimen field in each drug monograph will guide you to the applicable regimens.

Special Topics

Important cancer-related issues (ie, chemotherapy-induced peripheral neuro-pathy, management of chemotherapy-induced nausea and vomiting in adults, prevention of chemotherapy-induced nausea and vomiting in children, mucositis and stomatitis, chronic pain management [cancer], hospice [end of life] care, malignant pleural effusions, hypercalcemia of malignancy, palliative care medicine [cancer], hematopoietic stem cell transplantation, safe handling of hazard-ous drugs, venous thromboembolism in the cancer patient) are discussed in detail.

Appendix

The appendix offers a compilation of tables, guidelines, nomograms, algorithms, and conversion information which can often be helpful when considering patient care.

Pharmacologic Category Index

This index provides a useful listing of drugs by their pharmacologic classification.

PREGNANCY CATEGORIES

Pregnancy Categories (sometimes referred to as pregnancy risk factors) are a letter system presented under the *Teratogenic Effects* subsection of the product labeling. The system was initiated in 1979. The categories were required to be part of the package insert for prescription drugs that are systemically absorbed. The Food and Drug Administration (FDA) has updated prescribing labeling requirements and as of June 2015, the pregnancy categories will no longer be part of new product labeling. Prescription products which currently have a pregnancy category letter will be phasing this out of their product information.

The categories are defined as follows:

A   Adequate and well-controlled studies in pregnant women have not shown that the drug increases the risk of fetal abnormalities.

B   Animal reproduction studies show no evidence of impaired fertility or harm to the fetus; however, no adequate and well-controlled studies have been conducted in pregnant women.
or
Animal reproduction studies have shown adverse events; however, studies in pregnant women have not shown that the drug increases the risk of abnormalities.

C   Animal reproduction studies have shown an adverse effect on the fetus. There are no adequate and well-controlled studies in humans and the benefits from the use of the drug in pregnant women may be acceptable, despite its potential risks.
or
Animal reproduction studies have not been conducted.

D   Based on human data, the drug can cause fetal harm when administered to pregnant women, but the potential benefits from the use of the drug may be acceptable, despite its potential risks.

X   Studies in animals or humans have demonstrated fetal abnormalities (or there is positive evidence of fetal risk based on reports and/or marketing experience) and the risk of using the drug in pregnant women clearly outweighs any possible benefit (for example, safer drugs or other forms of therapy are available).

In 2008, the Food and Drug Administration (FDA) proposed new labeling requirements which would eliminate the use of the pregnancy category system and replace it with scientific data and other information specific to the use of the drug in pregnant women. These proposed changes were suggested because the current category system may be misleading. For instance, some practitioners may believe that risk increases from category A to B to C to D to X, which is not the intent. In addition, practitioners may not be aware that some medications are categorized based on animal data, while others are based on human data. The new labeling requirements will contain pregnancy and lactation subsections, each describing a risk summary, clinical considerations, and section for specific data.

For full descriptions of the final rule, refer to the following website: http://www.fda.gov/Drugs/DevelopmentApprovalProcess/DevelopmentResources/Labeling/ucm093307.htm

REDUCING ONCOLOGY MEDICATION ERRORS

Medication errors occurring in patients receiving treatment and supportive care for cancer remain a serious problem. Risk factors are numerous and include the multiple numbers and cycles of medication, the various routes of administration, the various locations of administration (which can progress from inpatient to ambulatory care to home administration), and the fact that patients from the very young to the elderly are frequently administered these agents. Many of the antineoplastic agents have a narrow therapeutic index and can produce unexpected toxicities with the slightest alteration in dosage. Subtherapeutic dosing may also be detrimental, producing less toxicity, but possibly resulting in decreased efficacy and affecting patient outcomes.

The incidence of medication errors in oncology patients noted in the published literature range from 3% to 4% in adult and pediatric inpatient and ambulatory settings, and from 10% to 20% for patients receiving oral antineoplastic therapy at home. Although the numbers appear small in some settings and many of the published medication errors are caught before reaching the patient ("near misses"), the impact can be disastrous. Published literature indicates that antineoplastic agents rank second only to central nervous system medications in causing fatal medication errors.

Medication errors involving chemotherapy and supportive care have been documented in all stages of the drug therapy process, from prescribing to compounding, dispensing, and administration, including patient self-medication at home. Various risk factors for medication errors have been identified at each stage. Accordingly, institutions and health care organizations have developed and continue to refine various standards, consensus documents, policies/procedures, and other safeguards to minimize the safety risk. Examples are noted in the following paragraphs.

Anticancer therapy should be based on standard regimens and modalities selected according to the patient's diagnosis and ability to tolerate treatment. Investigational therapy must be administered by way of an institutional review board-approved clinical trial or single patient Investigational New Drug (IND) license (compassionate use).

Facilities providing chemotherapy should establish and ensure that members of the oncology team have appropriate credentials to care for patients receiving antineoplastic therapy as well as have processes in place for creating a safe environment.

The American Society of Clinical Oncology (ASCO) and the Oncology Nursing Society (ONS) have developed comprehensive safety standards for facilities caring for oncology patients which include the following elements (ASCO/ONS [Neuss 2016]):

General Safety Competencies

- A facility must have a policy to document the qualifications of clinical staff who order, prepare, and administer chemotherapy. Requirements include:

    – Documentation of initial educational requirements and description of annual (at a minimum) ongoing continuing education requirements

    – Description of credentialing processes (licensed independent practitioners) and how credentialing is documented

    – Description of competency demonstration and how competency is documented

- Utilization of a comprehensive education program for initial and ongoing educational requirements for all staff who prepare and administer chemotherapy

- At least one clinical staff member who maintains current certification in (age-appropriate) basic life support who is present during chemotherapy administration

- A licensed independent practitioner is on-site and immediately available to staff who administer chemotherapy in the health care setting.

- Prior to the initial administration of a new chemotherapy regimen, chart documentation is available that includes a minimum of these 8 elements: Pathologic confirmation or verification of initial diagnosis, initial cancer stage or current cancer status, complete medical history and physical exam (including pregnancy status if applicable), allergies information and hypersensitivity reactions history, assessment of the patient/caregiver disease and treatment plan comprehension, initial psychosocial assessment (with action taken when indicated), chemotherapy treatment plan (including diagnosis, medications, doses, treatment duration, and goals of therapy), and planned frequency of office visits and patient monitoring (as appropriate for individual chemotherapy agents).

- On each clinical encounter or treatment day, staff should perform (and document) a patient assessment that includes these 8 elements and appropriate actions if indicated: Functional and/or performance status, vital signs, weight (at least weekly when present in a health care setting), height (at least weekly when present in a health care setting and when appropriate to the treatment population), age (as appropriate to the treatment population), allergies and previous treatment-related reactions, treatment toxicities, and pain assessment.

- Staff assesses/documents psychosocial concerns and support needs at each cycle (more frequently if indicated) and action taken (when indicated).

- Facility provides information and financial resources and/or refers for psychosocial and other cancer support services.

- Update patient's medications at every visit and review changes.

- Facility has a policy for documentation/follow-up of patients who miss or cancel scheduled visits and/or treatments.

- Facility has a policy that addresses mandates and processes for pediatric patients to account for legal requirements.

- Facility has a policy to identify a process to provide 24/7 triage to a practitioner (eg, on-call practitioners, emergency department) to manage treatment-related toxicities and emergencies; if the patient's initial contact is not a practitioner from the treating facility, the patient's contact person must have continuous access to consultation with an experienced oncology practitioner and the opportunity to transfer the patient to a facility with dedicated oncology services.

- The facility has a policy for standardized documentation/communication of toxicities, dosage/schedule modifications, or treatment discontinuation.

- Standardized and clearly defined systems are in place to promote a safe handoff between all sites of care, including provision of timely, accurate information about a patient's care plan, treatment (including a schedule for chemotherapy administration), safety concerns (including critical lab values), current condition, and any recent or anticipated changes.

- Adverse events and near-miss reporting system and a formal process to collect and evaluate data at a defined frequency

Treatment Planning, Patient Consent/Education

- Facility has a policy documenting a standardized process to obtain and document chemotherapy consent (or assent).

- Informed consent and assent (optional) for chemotherapy treatment (as appropriate to the treatment population) are documented prior to initiation of a chemotherapy regimen.

- Provide patients with verbal and written or electronic information as part of an education process prior to initial administration of each treatment plan; the content of the educational material is documented and at least the following:

  - Patient diagnosis

  - Treatment goals (eg, curative treatment, life-prolongation, symptom reduction)

  - Planned treatment duration, treatment administration schedule, medication names, supportive medications, drug-drug/drug-food interactions, and a plan for missed doses

  - Potential adverse effects of therapy (long-term and short-term), including infertility risks, if applicable

  - Symptoms or adverse effects that require the patient to contact the health care provider or to seek immediate medical attention

  - Symptoms or events that require immediate discontinuation of oral or other self-administered treatments

  - Procedures for handling medications in the home (including storage, safe handling, and management of unused medication)

  - Procedures for handling body secretions and waste at home

  - Follow-up plans, including lab and health care provider visits

- – Contact information for the facility, including availability and instructions on when and who to call

- – Missed appointment policy and expectations for rescheduling or cancelling

- Education (including family, caregivers, or others) based on the patient's ability to assume responsibility for therapy management and need-based educational activities (based on the patient's learning needs, abilities, preferences, and readiness to learn)

Medication Prescribing, Preparation, Dispensing, and Administration

- Facilities define standard chemotherapy regimens by diagnosis and include references.

- Institutional review board approval should be verified for research regimens.

- Chemotherapy orders are signed manually or electronically by licensed independent practitioners who are determined to be qualified by the facility.

- The facility has a policy to manage chemotherapy orders which vary from standard regimens; the policy requires supporting reference(s) and/or authorization by a second licensed independent practitioner (and the rationale for the exception order is documented in the medical record).

- The facility has a policy for chemotherapy orders that ensure that verbal orders are not allowed except to hold or stop chemotherapy administration and that new orders or change orders (including oral chemotherapy regimen changes such as dose adjustments) are communicated directly to patients and are documented in the medical record.

- The facility uses a standardized, regimen-level, preprinted or electronic form for injectable chemotherapy. Chemotherapy orders are to include at least the following elements:

  - – The patient's full name

  - – A second patient identifier

  - – The date the order is written

  - – Regimen or protocol name and number

  - – Cycle number and day, when applicable

  - – List all medications within the order set by full generic names.

  - – Drug dose is written following standards for abbreviations with no trailing zeros and with no leading zeros

  - – The dose calculation, including calculation methodology, variables used to calculate the dose, the frequency at which variables are reevaluated, and changes in the values that prompt dosing confirmation

  - – Date of administration

- Route of administration
- Allergies
- Appropriate supportive care treatments for the regimen, including premedications, hydration, growth factors, and hypersensitivity medications
- Parameters that would require dose interruption or modification (eg, lab values, diagnostic test results, patient clinical status)
- Sequence of drug administration (when applicable)
- Rate of medication administration (when applicable)
- Explanation of time limitation, such as the number of cycles for which the order is valid

- Prescriptions for oral chemotherapy (whether dispensed by the health care setting or another facility) include the following elements:
  - The patient's full name
  - A second patient identifier
  - Full generic name of medicine
  - The date of order
  - Drug dose (following standards for abbreviations, symbols, and dose designations)
  - Calculation methodology
  - Route of administration and special instructions (if applicable)
  - Quantity to be dispensed
  - Administration schedule
  - Duration of therapy with an explanation of time limitation (eg, number of cycles)
  - Number of refills (zero is the acceptable default value)

- Chemotherapy is prepared by a licensed pharmacist, pharmacy techni-cian, physician, or registered nurse with documented chemotherapy preparation education, training, and annual competency validation.

- A licensed pharmacist verifies all orders prior to administration or dis-pensing chemotherapy in a facility that treats pediatric patients under 18 years of age.

- A second person (a practitioner or other personnel approved by the facility to prepare or administer chemotherapy) performs three independent verifications:

- Prior to preparation, a second person independently verifies:
  - Two patient identifiers
  - The drug name
  - The drug dose

- – Route of administration
- – Rate of administration
- – Dosing calculation (including variables used in the calculation)
- – Treatment cycle and day of cycle

- Upon preparation, a second person (approved by the facility health care setting to prepare parenteral chemotherapy) verifies:

  - – The drug vial(s)
  - – Concentration
  - – Drug volume or weight
  - – Diluent type and volume (when applicable)
  - – Administration fluid type, volume, and tubing

- Prior to chemotherapy administration, at least two practitioners (approved by the facility to administer or prepare chemotherapy) verify and document the accuracy of the following elements:

  - – Drug name
  - – Drug dose
  - – Infusion volume or drug volume when prepared in a syringe
  - – Rate of administration
  - – Route of administration
  - – Expiration dates and/or times
  - – Drug appearance and physical integrity
  - – Rate set on infusion pump, when used

- Chemotherapy drugs are labeled immediately upon preparation and labels include at least the following 10 elements:

  - – Patient's full name
  - – A second patient identifier
  - – Full generic drug name
  - – Drug dose
  - – Drug administration route
  - – Total volume required to administer
  - – Date the medication is to be administered
  - – Expiration dates and/or times

- Sequencing of drug administration (when applicable) and total number of products to be given when medication is provided in divided doses (each product should be labeled with the total number of products to be administered and the individual products sequence within that total grouping (eg, 1 of 5 or 2 of 2)

- A warning or precautionary label or sticker, as applicable, to storage and handling; may be included within the label or on an auxiliary label

- Labels for medications dispensed from the facility and to be taken at home include:

  - Patient's full name

  - A second patient identifier

  - Date of preparation and expiration

  - Full generic drug name

  - Dosage form and strength

  - Quantity dispensed within each container

  - Number of pills per dose when the container holds more than one dose

  - Administration schedule, including number of times per day and days on and off treatment (when applicable)

  - Administration instructions related to food ingestion and to other medications

  - A warning or precaution statement, as applicable, to storage and handling

  - Caution statement label attached to the prepared product (eg, "caution: chemotherapy" or "hazardous drug")

  - Storage conditions

  - Prescriber name

- Facilities where intrathecal medication is administered maintains a policy that specifies that intrathecal medication is:

  - Prepared separately

  - Stored in an isolated container or location after preparation

  - Labeled with a uniquely identifiable intrathecal medication label

  - Delivered to the patient only with other medication intended for CNS administration

  - Administered immediately after a time-out, double-check procedure that involves two licensed practitioners or other personnel approved the facility to prepare or administer chemotherapy.

- Facilities that administer intrathecal chemotherapy have a policy that specifies that intravenous vinca alkaloids are administered only by infusion (eg, mini-bags)

- If the facility administers chemotherapy that is prepared (mixed) off-site, the facility maintains a policy for quality control of that chemotherapy, including documentation that the offsite pharmacy complies with all applicable regulatory requirements

- If a facility maintains its own pharmacy, there is policy regarding the safe storage of chemotherapy, including separation of look-alike products, sound-alike products, investigational agents, and agents available in multiple strengths

- Chemotherapy is administered by a qualified physician, physician assistant, registered nurse, or advanced practice nurse as defined in the general safety competencies.

- Before initiation of each chemotherapy cycle, the practitioner administering the chemotherapy confirms the treatment with the patient, including (at a minimum) the drug name, infusion time, route of administration, and infusion-related symptoms to report (eg, hypersensitivity symptoms, pain during infusion).

- At least two individuals (in the presence of the patient) verify the patient identification by using at least two identifiers.

- When chemotherapy is administered in a non-health care setting by a health care provider, a second identifier, such as a driver's license, is used to verify the patient's or parent's identify.

- Documentation of chemotherapy administration confirms the verification of the eight elements of chemotherapy administration and also includes the patient's clinical status during and upon completion of treatment.

- Extravasation management procedures are defined and align with current literature and guidelines; antidote order sets and antidotes are accessible within the appropriate timeframe.

Monitoring for Adherence, Toxicity, and/or Complications After Administration

- The facility uses standard, disease-specific processes to monitor treatment response and has a policy that determines the appropriate time interval for regimen-specific lab and organ function tests that are based on evidence and national guidelines (when available).

- The facility has a policy for emergent treatment that aligns with current literature and guidelines and addresses availability of appropriate treatment agents and procedures to follow and a plan for care escalation (when required) for life-threatening emergencies.

- The facility outlines a procedure to monitor an initial assessment of patients' adherence to chemotherapy administered outside of the health care setting.

- The facility has a policy requiring assessment of each patient's ongoing chemotherapy adherence and toxicity at each clinical encounter to address any identified issues.

- The facility has policy that requires evaluation and documentation of treatment-related toxicities, dose modification related to toxicities, and how these are communicated prior to subsequent administration.

- Cumulative chemotherapy doses are tracked for agents associated with cumulative toxicity.

Additional Medication Safety Pearls

Chemotherapy agents are highly susceptible to sound-alike/look-alike confusion (eg, fluorouracil/flucytosine/fluocinonide, leucovorin/Leukine/Alkeran/Leukeran) so particular precaution should be heeded to ensure correct drug identified by those interpreting the order.

- Use full generic names including descriptive terms, (eg, liposomal). Brand names should be reserved for products when they assist in further identifying the correct product (eg, combination product or liposomal vs nonliposomal formulation).

- Use full study name and/or protocol number with investigational antineoplastic treatments.

- Avoid abbreviated medication names, (eg, CTX, HN$_2$, MTX, VCR, or generalized generic terms [eg, "platinum" which can create confusion between CISplatin, CARBOplatin, and oxaliplatin]).

- Avoid investigational names for medications **with FDA approval** (eg, VP-16, FK-506, CBDCA).

- Utilize TALLman lettering (eg, DAUNOrubicin/DOXOrubicin, VinBLAStine/VinCRIStine).

- Omit the use of numbers within a medication name (eg, fluorouracil is correct, 5-fluorouracil is **incorrect**; mercaptopurine is correct, 6-mercaptopurine is **incorrect**).

- Avoid abbreviated names or acronyms for multidrug regimens, (eg, MOPP, ICE, ProMACE).

- Avoid or minimize look-alike drug product containers in the procurement process.

- Use guideline-based and/or manufacturer's recommendations for adjustment of dose based on body size. As an example, use of actual body weight for dose calculation in obese patients receiving treatment with curative intent is recommended. In comparison, the manufacturer of ixabepilone recommends capping the calculated dose amount at 88 mg for patients who are larger than 2.2 m^2 (40 mg/m^2/dose).

- Use guideline-based and/or manufacturer's recommendations for adjustment of dose based on organ function. As an example, for carboplatin dose calculation using the Calvert formula, the Food and Drug Administration recommends capping the calculated creatinine clearance (representing glomerular filtration rate) at a value of 125 mL/min.

- Provide supporting references and/or rationale when doses vary from a standard regimen or are prescribed as flat doses to allow for necessary double-checks.

- Provide complete dosing information including calculated dose with reduction noted with rationale, total volume and solution to administer dose (if applicable), route of administration, rate or number of hours or days that dose is to be administered, which specific days dose is to be administered and total dose per treatment course, cycle or cumulative lifetime (if applicable). In some situations, clearly defining when to initiate therapy (Day 0 or Day 1) may be necessary for clarity.
  Example: Patient = 1.8 m^2
  Drug "X" 50 mg/m^2/day IV push for 3 days = 90 mg IV push on Days 3, 4, and 5
  (Total Dose Drug "X" per cycle = 150 mg/m^2 = 270 mg)

- For doses that are greater than 1,000 dosing units, use properly placed commas to prevent 10-fold errors (100,000 units is correct and 100000 units is **incorrect**).

- Avoid dangerous, error-prone abbreviations (eg, regardless of letter-case: U, IU, QD, QOD, μg, cc, @, MS, MS04, MgS04). Regarding the example above, the terminology "IV push" is commonly used and accepted. However, consider using the complete term "intravenous push," and stating the rate of infusion for the "push" dose to minimize confusion.

- Establish dosing and administration constraints including maximum single doses, maximum doses within specified time limits and acceptable routes and rates of administration.

VINCA ALKALOID ADMINISTRATION

The vinca alkaloids vinblastine, vincristine, vincristine liposomal, and vinorelbine are for intravenous administration only. Inadvertent intrathecal administration of a vinca alkaloid can cause serious neurologic toxicity and is usually fatal. The Institute for Safe Medication Practices (ISMP) recommends admixture of vinca alkaloids in a minibag with volume of compatible fluid that is too large for intrathecal administration (adult patients, 50 mL; pediatric patients, 25 mL) in order to prevent inadvertent intrathecal administration.

ORAL CHEMOTHERAPY

Medication errors involving oral chemotherapy in both adult and pediatric patients are being increasingly reported and like other routes of administration, the origin of the error ranges from prescribing to dispensing to patient self-administration. Oral chemotherapy should go through the same double-check system in which parenteral chemotherapy is processed.

The following additional recommendations should also be adhered to for oral chemotherapy (Goldspiel 2015):

- Drug doses and schedules should be described as the amount to be taken per dose (not as a total daily dose divided).

- Medication orders, instructions, and patient instructions should be clearly documented in the treatment plan and the number of doses to be administered should be clearly identified.

- Doses with solid dosage forms should specify if and how doses are to be rounded to the nearest tablet/capsule size.

33

- Only the quantity necessary to cover the administration period until the next clinical evaluation should be ordered.

- Oral chemotherapy medications ordered should be provided with parenteral chemotherapy orders to allow for appropriate medication screening/ review.

- Oral chemotherapy medications ordered should be included on the patient's home medication list to allow for appropriate medication screening/review.

- Oral chemotherapy medications ordered should be communicated to the pharmacist to allow for appropriate medication screening/review.

- Discourage refills on oral chemotherapy (if feasible).

- Patients should be educated as appropriate on access and cost of the intended oral chemotherapy.

THE ROLE OF TECHNOLOGY

Computerized provider order entry (CPOE) and bar-code technology have been adopted by some institutions and practices in an effort to improve safety and efficiency and enhance communication between health care providers. Both technology tools have been shown to be useful, but certainly do not replace the need for continued surveillance and safety checks in all stages of the chemotherapy order process. For example, CPOE has been shown to decrease prescribing errors, but has little or no impact on dispensing and administration mistakes.

Medication errors are inevitable in all health care scenarios, including oncology. When such events occur, the issues of appropriate disclosure and follow-up are first priorities. The published literature has provided some insight to disclosure and to the support required by the patient and the health care team in such events. References addressing this issue are among the list at the end of the chapter.

ON-GOING INSTITUTIONAL REVIEW TO INCREASE ONCOLOGY MEDICATION SAFETY

Institutions and oncology practices should constantly review the chemotherapy order process and look for opportunities to promote a culture of safety:

- Consistent education to the health care team on all aspects of chemotherapy management

- Re-engineer processes if needed, as per the following examples:

  - Centralize the pharmaceutical chemotherapy compound process

  - Observe work flow: Minimize nursing interruptions during the administration of oncology medications, which has been shown to affect the incidence and severity of errors with high-risk medications

  - Restrict certain high-risk medications from specific hospital or clinic locations, such as keeping vinca alkaloids away from certain procedure areas to minimize risk of wrong route administration

- Special packaging and warning labels for high-alert medications

- Computer pop-up alerts

- Document, review, and discuss all oncology medication errors, including the "near misses"; not for punitive measures, but as teaching tools to improve the oncology medication process.

- Enhance communication among all health care team members (ie, utilize or improve the medication reconciliation process).

Selected Readings

Bartel SB. Safe practices and financial considerations in using oral chemotherapeutic agents. *Am J Health Syst Pharm.* 2007;64(9 Suppl 5):S8-S14.

Brunetti L, Santell JP, Hicks RW. The impact of abbreviations on patient safety. *Jt Comm J Qual Patient Saf.* 2007;33(9):576-583.

Crossno CL, Cartwright JA, Hargrove FR. Using CPOE to improve communication, safety, and policy compliance when ordering pediatric chemotherapy. *Hosp Pharm.* 2007;42(4):368–373.

DuBeshter B, Griggs J, Angel C, et al. Chemotherapy dose limits set by users of a computer order entry system. *Hosp Pharm.* 2006;41(2):136-142.

Goldspiel B, Hoffman JM, Griffith NL, et al. ASHP guidelines on preventing medication errors with chemotherapy and biotherapy. *Am J Health Syst Pharm.* 2015;72(8):e6-e35.

Griggs JJ, Mangu PB, Anderson H, et al. Appropriate chemotherapy dosing for obese adult patients with cancer: American Society of Clinical Oncology clinical practice guideline. *J Clin Oncol.* 2012;30(13):1553-1561.

Institute for Safe Medication Practices. 2014-2015 targeted medication safety best practices for hospitals. Available at http://www.ismp.org/tools/bestpractices/TMSBP-for-Hospitals.pdf. Accessed October 14, 2014.

Neuss MN, Gilmore TR, Belderson KM, et al. 2016 updated American Society of Clinical Oncology/Oncology Nursing Society chemotherapy administration safety standards, including standards for pediatric oncology. *J Oncol Pract.* 2016;12(12):1262-1271.

Neuss MN, Polovich M, McNiff K, et al. 2013 updated American Society of Clinical Oncology/Oncology Nursing Society chemotherapy administration safety standards including standards for the safe administration and management of oral chemotherapy. *J Oncol Pract* 2013;9(2 Suppl):5s-13s.

Poon EG, Keohane CA, Yoon CS, et al. Effect of bar-code technology on the safety of medication administration. *N Engl J Med.* 2010;362(18):1698-1707.

Weingart SN, Toro J, Spencer J, et al. Medication errors involving oral chemotherapy. *Cancer.* 2010;116(10):2455-2464.

Westbrook JI, Woods A, Rob MI, Dunsmuir WT, Day RO. Association of interruptions with an increased risk and severity of medication administration errors. *Arch Intern Med.* 2010;170(8):683-690.

FDA NAME DIFFERENTIATION PROJECT: THE USE OF TALL-MAN LETTERS

Confusion between similar drug names is an important cause of medication errors. For years, The Institute For Safe Medication Practices (ISMP), has urged generic manufacturers to use a combination of large and small letters as well as bolding (ie, chlorpro**MAZINE** and chlorpro**PAMIDE**) to help distinguish drugs with look-alike names, especially when they share similar strengths. Recently the FDA's Division of Generic Drugs began to issue recommendation letters to manufacturers suggesting this novel way to label their products to help reduce this drug name confusion. Although this project has had marginal success, the method has successfully eliminated problems with products such as diphenhydr-**AMINE** and dimenhy**DRINATE**. Hospitals should also follow suit by making similar changes in their own labels, preprinted order forms, computer screens and printouts, and drug storage location labels.

Lexi-Comp, Inc. Medical Publishing will use "Tall-Man" letters for the drugs suggested by the FDA or recommended by ISMP.

The following is a list of generic and brand name product names and recommended revisions.

Drug Product	Recommended Revision
acetazolamide	aceta**ZOLAMIDE**
alprazolam	**ALPRAZ**olam
amiloride	a**MIL**oride
amlodipine	am**LODIP**ine
aripiprazole	**ARIP**iprazole
atomoxetine	ato**MOX**etine
atorvastatin	atorva**STAT**in
Avinza	**AVIN**za
azacitidine	aza**CITID**ine
azathioprine	aza**THIO**prine
bupropion	bu**PROP**ion
buspirone	bus**PIR**one
carbamazepine	car**BAM**azepine
carboplatin	**CARBO**platin
cefazolin	ce**FAZ**olin
cefotetan	cefo**TE**tan
cefoxitin	cef**OX**itin

Drug Product	Recommended Revision
ceftazidime	cefTAZidime
ceftriaxone	cefTRIAXone
Celebrex	CeleBREX
Celexa	CeleXA
chlordiazepoxide	chlordiazePOXIDE
chlorpromazine	chlorproMAZINE
chlorpropamide	chlorproPAMIDE
cisplatin	CISplatin
clobazam	cloBAZam
clomiphene	clomiPHENE
clomipramine	clomiPRAMINE
clonazepam	clonazePAM
clonidine	cloNIDine
clozapine	cloZAPine
cycloserine	cycloSERINE
cyclosporine	cycloSPORINE
dactinomycin	DACTINomycin
daptomycin	DAPTOmycin
daunorubicin	DAUNOrubicin
Depo-Medrol	DEPO-Medrol
diazepam	diazePAM
diltiazem	dilTIAZem
dimenhydrinate	dimenhyDRINATE
diphenhydramine	diphenhydrAMINE
dobutamine	DOBUTamine
docetaxel	DOCEtaxel
dopamine	DOPamine
doxorubicin	DOXOrubicin
duloxetine	DULoxetine
ephedrine	ePHEDrine
epinephrine	EPINEPHrine
epirubicin	epiRUBicin
eribulin	eriBULin
fentanyl	fentaNYL

Drug Product	Recommended Revision
flavoxate	flavox**ATE**
fluoxetine	**FLU**oxetine
fluphenazine	flu**PHENAZ**ine
fluvoxamine	fluvoxa**MINE**
glipizide	glipi**ZIDE**
glyburide	gly**BURIDE**
guaifenesin	guai**FEN**esin
guanfacine	guan**FACINE**
Humalog	Huma**LOG**
Humulin	Humu**LIN**
hydralazine	hydr**ALAZINE**
hydrochlorothiazide	hydro**CHLORO**thiazide
hydrocodone	**HYDRO**codone
hydromorphone	**HYDRO**morphone
hydroxyprogesterone	**HYDROXY**progesterone
hydroxyzine	hydr**OXY**zine
idarubicin	**IDA**rubicin
idarucizumab	idaru**CIZU**mab
infliximab	in**FLIX**imab
Invanz	**INV**anz
isotretinoin	**ISO**tretinoin
Klonopin	Klono**PIN**
Lamictal	La**MIC**tal
Lamisil	Lam**ISIL**
lamivudine	lami**VUD**ine
lamotrigine	lamo**TRI**gine
levetiracetam	Lev**ETIRA**cetam
levocarnitine	lev**OCARN**itine
levofloxacin	levo**FLOX**acin
levoleucovorin	**LEVO**leucovorin
lorazepam	**LOR**azepam
medroxyprogesterone	medroxy**PROGESTER**one
metformin	met**FORMIN**
methazolamide	methazol**AMIDE**

Drug Product	Recommended Revision
methimazole	methIMAzole
methylprednisolone	methylPREDNISolone
methyltestosterone	methylTESTOSTERone
metolazone	metOLazone
metronidazole	metroNIDAZOLE
metyrapone	metyraPONE
metyrosine	metyroSINE
mifepristone	miFEPRIStone
misoprostol	miSOPROStol
mitomycin	mitoMYcin
mitoxantrone	MitoXANTRONE
Nexavar	NexAVAR
Nexium	NexIUM
nicardipine	niCARdipine
nifedipine	NIFEdipine
nimodipine	niMODipine
Novolin	NovoLIN
Novolog	NovoLOG
olanzapine	OLANZapine
oxcarbazepine	OXcarbazepine
oxycodone	oxyCODONE
Oxycontin	OxyCONTIN
oxymorphone	oxyMORphone
paclitaxel	PACLitaxel
paroxetine	PARoxetine
pazopanib	PAZOPanib
pemetrexed	PEMEtrexed
penicillamine	penicillAMINE
pentobarbital	PENTobarbital
phenobarbital	PHENobarbital
ponatinib	PONATinib
pralatrexate	PRALAtrexate
prednisolone	prednisoLONE
prednisone	predniSONE

▶

Drug Product	Recommended Revision
Prilosec	PriLOSEC
Prozac	PROzac
quetiapine	QUEtiapine
quinidine	quiNIDine
quinine	quiNINE
rabeprazole	RABEprazole
ranitidine	raNITIdine
rifampin	rifAMPin
rifaximin	rifAXIMin
rimantadine	riMANTAdine
Risperdal	RisperDAL
risperidone	risperiDONE
rituximab	riTUXimab
romidepsin	romiDEPsin
romiplostim	romiPLOStim
ropinirole	rOPINIRole
Sandimmune	sandIMMUNE
Sandostatin	SandoSTATIN
saxagliptin	SAXagliptin
Seroquel	SEROquel
Sinequan	SINEquan
sitagliptin	SITagliptin
Solu-Cortef	Solu-CORTEF
Solu-Medrol	SOLU-Medrol
sorafenib	SORAfenib
sufentanil	SUFentanil
sulfadiazine	sulfADIAZINE
sulfasalazine	sulfaSALAzine
sumatriptan	SUMAtriptan
sunitinib	SUNItinib
Tegretol	TEGretol
tiagabine	tiaGABine
tizanidine	tiZANidine
tolazamide	TOLAZamide

Drug Product	Recommended Revision
tolbutamide	**TOLBUT**amide
tramadol	tra**MAD**ol
trazodone	tra**ZOD**one
Trental	**TREN**tal
valacyclovir	val**ACY**clovir
valganciclovir	val**GAN**ciclovir
vinblastine	vin**BLAS**tine
vincristine	vin**CRIS**tine
zolmitriptan	**ZOLM**itriptan
Zyprexa	Zy**PREXA**
Zyrtec	Zyr**TEC**

FDA and ISMP lists of look-alike drug names with recommended tall man letter. http://www.ismp.org/tools/tallmanletters.pdf. Accessed January 6, 2011.

Name differentiation project. http://www.fda.gov/Drugs/DrugSafety/MedicationErrors/ucm164587.htm. Accessed January 6, 2011.

U.S. Pharmacopeia. USP quality review: use caution – avoid confusion. March 2001, No. 76. http://www.usp.org

ALPHABETICAL LISTING OF DRUGS

- ◆ **Abbott-43818** *see* Leuprolide *on page 1131*
- ◆ **Abelcet** *see* Amphotericin B (Lipid Complex) *on page 119*
- ◆ **ABI-007** *see* PACLitaxel (Protein Bound) *on page 1411*
- ◆ **Abiraterone** *see* Abiraterone Acetate *on page 44*

Abiraterone Acetate (a bir A ter one AS e tate)

Related Information
Palliative Care Medicine (Cancer) *on page 2352*

Brand Names: US Zytiga

Brand Names: Canada Zytiga

Index Terms Abiraterone; CB7630

Pharmacologic Category Antiandrogen; Antineoplastic Agent, Antiandrogen

Use Prostate cancer: Treatment of metastatic, castration-resistant prostate cancer (in combination with prednisone)

Labeled Contraindications
Women who are or may become pregnant

Canadian labeling: Additional contraindication (not in the US labeling): Hypersensitivity to abiraterone acetate or any component of the formulation or container

Pregnancy Considerations Adverse effects were observed in animal reproduction studies at doses resulting in less systemic exposure than in humans. Adverse effects were also observed in the reproductive system of animals during toxicology and pharmacology studies. Based on the mechanism of action, abiraterone may cause fetal harm or fetal loss if administered during pregnancy. Abiraterone is not indicated for use in women and is specifically contraindicated in women who are or may become pregnant. It is not known if abiraterone is excreted in semen, therefore, men should use a condom and another method of birth control during treatment and for 1 week following therapy if having intercourse with a woman of reproductive age. Women who are or may become pregnant should wear gloves if contact with tablets may occur.

Breastfeeding Considerations Not indicated for use in women

Warnings/Precautions Severe hepatotoxicity (eg, fulminant hepatitis, acute liver failure, and death) has been reported. Significant increases in liver enzymes have also been observed (higher likelihood in patients with baseline elevations), generally occurring in the first 3 months of treatment. May require dosage reduction, treatment interruption, and/ or discontinuation. ALT, AST, and bilirubin should be monitored prior to treatment, every 2 weeks for 3 months and monthly thereafter; patients with hepatic impairment, elevations in liver function tests, or experiencing hepatotoxicity require more frequent monitoring (see Dosing: Hepatic Impairment and Monitoring Parameters). Evaluate liver function promptly with signs or symptoms of hepatotoxicity. The safety of retreatment after significant elevations (ALT or AST ≥20 times the upper limit of normal [ULN] and/or total bilirubin ≥10 times ULN) has not been evaluated. Do not use in patients with preexisting severe hepatic impairment (Child-Pugh class C); dosage reduction is recommended in patients with baseline moderate impairment.

Concurrent infection, stress, or interruption of daily corticosteroids is associated with reports of adrenocortical insufficiency. Monitor closely for signs and symptoms of adrenocorticoid insufficiency, which could be masked by adverse events associated with mineralocorticoid excess. Diagnostic testing for adrenal insufficiency may be clinically indicated. Increased corticosteroid doses may be required before, during, and after stress. May cause increased mineralocorticoid levels, which may result in hypertension, hypokalemia and fluid retention (including grades 3 and 4 events). Concomitant administration with corticosteroids reduces the incidence and severity of these adverse events. Control hypertension and correct hypokalemia prior to and during treatment. Use with caution in patients with cardiovascular disease (particularly heart failure, recent MI, or ventricular arrhythmia); patients with left ventricular ejection fraction (LVEF) <50% or NYHA class II, III, or IV heart failure were excluded from clinical trials. Monitor at least monthly for hypertension, hypokalemia, and fluid retention.

Abiraterone must be administered on an empty stomach (administer at least 1 hour before and 2 hours after any food); abiraterone AUC (exposure) may be increased up to 10-fold if administered with a meal. Potentially significant drug-drug interactions may exist, requiring dose or frequency adjustment, additional monitoring, and/or selection of alternative therapy.

Adverse Reactions Adverse reactions reported for use in combination with prednisone.

>10%:

Cardiovascular: Edema (25% to 27%; includes anasarca, peripheral edema, pitting edema), hypertension (9% to 22%)

Central nervous system: Fatigue (39%), insomnia (14%)

Dermatologic: Bruise (13%)

Endocrine & metabolic: Hypertriglyceridemia (63%), hyperglycemia (57%), hypernatremia (33%), hypokalemia (17% to 28%), hypophosphatemia (24%; grades 3/4: 7%), hot flash (19% to 22%)

Gastrointestinal: Constipation (23%), diarrhea (18% to 22%), dyspepsia (6% to 11%)

Genitourinary: Urinary tract infection (12%)

Hematologic & oncologic: Lymphocytopenia (38%; grades 3/4: 9%)

Hepatic: Increased serum ALT (11% to 42%; grades 3/4: 1% to 6%), increased serum AST (37%; grades 3/4: 3%)

Neuromuscular & skeletal: Joint swelling (30%, includes arthralgia, arthritis, joint discomfort, joint stiffness), myalgia (26%; includes muscle rigidity, muscle spasm, musculoskeletal discomfort, musculoskeletal pain)

Respiratory: Cough (11% to 17%), upper respiratory infection (5% to 13%), dyspnea (12%), nasopharyngitis (11%)

1% to 10%:

Cardiovascular: Cardiac arrhythmia (7%; includes atrial fibrillation, atrial tachycardia, bradycardia, cardiac conduction disturbance, complete atrioventricular block, supraventricular tachycardia, tachycardia), chest pain (4%, includes angina pectoris, chest discomfort, unstable angina pectoris), cardiac failure (2%; includes cardiogenic shock, cardiomegaly, cardiomyopathy, congestive heart failure, left ventricular dysfunction, reduced ejection fraction)

Central nervous system: Falling (6%)

Dermatologic: Skin rash (8%)

Genitourinary: Hematuria (10%), groin pain (7%), urinary frequency (7%), nocturia (6%)

Hepatic: Increased serum bilirubin (7%; grades 3/4: <1%)

Neuromuscular & skeletal: Bone fracture (6%)

Miscellaneous: Fever (9%)

<1%, postmarketing, and/or case reports: Acute hepatic failure, adrenocortical insufficiency, fulminant hepatitis, myopathy (includes rhabdomyolysis), pneumonia

Drug Interactions

Metabolism/Transport Effects Substrate of CYP3A4 (major); **Note:** Assignment of Major/Minor substrate status based on clinically relevant drug interaction potential; **Inhibits** CYP2C8 (weak), CYP2C9 (moderate), CYP2D6 (moderate), SLCO1B1

Avoid Concomitant Use

Avoid concomitant use of Abiraterone Acetate with any of the following: Amodiaquine; CYP3A4 Inducers (Strong); Indium 111 Capromab Pendetide; Thioridazine

Increased Effect/Toxicity

Abiraterone Acetate may increase the levels/effects of: Amodiaquine; Bosentan; Cannabis; CloZAPine; CYP1A2 Substrates; CYP2C8 Substrates; CYP2C9 Substrates; CYP2D6 Substrates; DOXOrubicin (Conventional); Dronabinol; Eliglustat; Fesoterodine; Metoprolol; Nebivolol; Perhexiline; Tetrahydrocannabinol; Thioridazine

Decreased Effect

Abiraterone Acetate may decrease the levels/effects of: Choline C 11; Codeine; Indium 111 Capromab Pendetide; Tamoxifen; TraMADol

The levels/effects of Abiraterone Acetate may be decreased by: Bosentan; CYP3A4 Inducers (Moderate); CYP3A4 Inducers (Strong); Dabrafenib; Deferasirox; Sarilumab; Siltuximab; Spironolactone; St John's Wort; Tocilizumab

Food Interactions Taking abiraterone with food will increase systemic exposure (up to 10-fold). Management: Do not administer with food. Abiraterone must be taken on an empty stomach, at least 1 hour before and 2 hours after food.

Hazardous Drugs Handling Considerations

Hazardous agent (NIOSH 2016 [group 1]).

Use appropriate precautions for receiving, handling, administration, and disposal. Gloves (single) should be worn during receiving, unpacking, and placing in storage. NIOSH recommends single gloving for administration of intact tablets or capsules (NIOSH 2016).

Storage/Stability Store at 20°C to 25°C (68°F to 77°F); excursions are permitted between 15°C and 30°C (59°F and 86°F).

Mechanism of Action Selectively and irreversibly inhibits CYP17 (17 alpha-hydroxylase/C17,20-lyase), an enzyme required for androgen biosynthesis which is expressed in testicular, adrenal, and prostatic tumor tissues. Inhibits the formation of the testosterone precursors dehydroepiandrosterone (DHEA) and androstenedione.

Pharmacodynamics/Kinetics

Distribution: V_{dss}: 19,669 ± 13,358 L

Protein binding: >99%; to albumin and alpha$_1$-acid glycoprotein

Metabolism: Abiraterone acetate is hydrolyzed to the active metabolite abiraterone; further metabolized to inactive metabolites abiraterone sulphate and N-oxide abiraterone sulphate via CYP3A4 and SULT2A1

Bioavailability: Systemic exposure is increased by food

Half-life elimination: 14.4 to 16.5 hours (Acharya 2012); prolonged in patients with mild and moderate hepatic impairment, ~18 and ~19 hours, respectively

Time to peak: 2 hours (Acharya 2012)

Excretion: Feces (~88%); urine (~5%)

Dosing

Adult & Geriatric

Prostate cancer, metastatic, castration-resistant: Oral: 1,000 mg once daily (in combination with prednisone 5 mg twice daily)

Prostate cancer, metastatic or high-risk locally advanced, castration-sensitive (off-label use): Oral: 1,000 mg once daily (in combination with prednisone 5 mg once daily and androgen-deprivation therapy; Fizazi 2017) **or** 1,000 mg once daily (in combination with prednisolone 5 mg once daily and androgen-deprivation therapy; James 2017)

Dosage adjustment for concomitant strong CYP3A4 inducers: Avoid concomitant strong CYP3A4 inducers; if a strong CYP3A4 inducer must be administered concurrently, increase the abiraterone frequency to twice daily (eg, from 1,000 mg once daily to 1,000 mg twice daily). Upon discontinuation of the strong CYP3A4 inducer, reduce abiraterone back to the prior dose and frequency.

Renal Impairment No dosage adjustment necessary.

Hepatic Impairment

Hepatic impairment *prior to* treatment initiation:

Mild (Child-Pugh class A): No dosage adjustment necessary.

Moderate (Child-Pugh class B): 250 mg once daily. Permanently discontinue if ALT and/or AST >5 times the upper limit of normal (ULN) or total bilirubin >3 times ULN occur during treatment in patients with baseline moderate hepatic impairment.

Severe (Child-Pugh class C): Do not use.

Hepatotoxicity *during* treatment:

ALT and/or AST >5 times ULN **or** total bilirubin >3 times ULN: Withhold treatment until liver function tests return to baseline or ALT and AST ≤2.5 times ULN and total bilirubin ≤1.5 times ULN, then reinitiate at 750 mg once daily.

Recurrent hepatotoxicity on 750 mg/day: Withhold treatment until liver function tests return to baseline or ALT and AST ≤2.5 times ULN and total bilirubin ≤1.5 times ULN, then reinitiate at 500 mg once daily.

Recurrent hepatotoxicity on 500 mg once daily: Discontinue treatment

ALT >3 times ULN **and** total bilirubin >2 times ULN (in the absence of biliary obstruction or other contributing cause responsible for concurrent elevation): Permanently discontinue treatment

Adjustment for Toxicity Hepatotoxicity: Refer to Dosing: Hepatic Impairment.

Combination Regimens

Prostate cancer: Abiraterone-Prednisone (Prostate) on page 1974

Administration Administer abiraterone orally on an empty stomach, at least 1 hour before and 2 hours after food. **Note:** The prescribing information describes when to give food with respect to abiraterone; no food should be consumed for at least 2 hours before or for at least 1 hour after the abiraterone dose. Swallow tablets whole with water. Do not crush or chew.

Monitoring Parameters ALT, AST, and bilirubin prior to treatment, every 2 weeks for 3 months and monthly thereafter; if baseline moderate hepatic impairment (Child-Pugh class B), monitor ALT, AST, and bilirubin prior to treatment, weekly for the first month, every 2 weeks for 2 months then monthly thereafter. If hepatotoxicity develops during treatment (and only after therapy is interrupted and liver function tests have returned to safe levels), monitor ALT, AST, and bilirubin every 2 weeks for 3 months and monthly thereafter.

Monitoring of testosterone levels is not necessary. Serum potassium (prior to treatment and at least monthly).

Monitor for signs and symptoms of adrenocorticoid insufficiency; if clinically indicated, consider appropriate diagnostics to confirm adrenal insufficiency. Monitor blood pressure and for fluid retention (prior to treatment and at least monthly). Monitor adherence.

Dosage Forms Excipient information presented when available (limited, particularly for generics); consult specific product labeling.

Tablet, Oral:

Zytiga: 250 mg, 500 mg

Dosage Forms: Canada Information with regard to form, strength, and availability of products uniquely available in Canada but currently not available in the US. Refer also to Dosage Forms.

Excipient information presented when available (limited, particularly for generics); consult specific product labeling.

Tablet, Oral:

Zytiga: 250mg, 500 mg [film-coated]

- **Actinomycin CI** *see* DACTINomycin *on page 499*
- **Activase** *see* Alteplase *on page 97*
- **Activase rt-PA (Can)** *see* Alteplase *on page 97*
- **Activated Factor XIII** *see* Factor XIII Concentrate (Human) *on page 782*
- **Active Injection D** *see* Dexamethasone (Systemic) *on page 579*
- **ACT Levofloxacin (Can)** *see* LevoFLOXacin (Systemic) *on page 1140*
- **ACT Nabilone (Can)** *see* Nabilone *on page 1293*
- **ACT Olanzapine (Can)** *see* OLANZapine *on page 1364*
- **ACT Olanzapine ODT (Can)** *see* OLANZapine *on page 1364*
- **ACT Ondansetron (Can)** *see* Ondansetron *on page 1380*
- **ACT Raloxifene (Can)** *see* Raloxifene *on page 1568*
- **ACT Temozolomide (Can)** *see* Temozolomide *on page 1746*
- **ACV** *see* Acyclovir (Systemic) *on page 49*
- **ACV** *see* Acyclovir (Topical) *on page 56*
- **Acycloguanosine** *see* Acyclovir (Systemic) *on page 49*
- **Acycloguanosine** *see* Acyclovir (Topical) *on page 56*

Acyclovir (Systemic) (ay SYE kloe veer)

Brand Names: US Zovirax

Brand Names: Canada Acyclovir Sodium Injection; Apo-Acyclovir; Mylan-Acyclovir; ratio-Acyclovir; Teva-Acyclovir; Zovirax

Index Terms Aciclovir; ACV; Acycloguanosine; Acyclovir Sodium; Zovirax

Pharmacologic Category Antiviral Agent

Use

Oral:

Herpes zoster (shingles): Acute treatment of herpes zoster (shingles).

Herpes simplex virus (HSV), genital: Treatment of initial episodes and the management of recurrent episodes of genital herpes.

Varicella (chickenpox): Treatment of varicella (chickenpox).

Injection:

Herpes simplex virus (HSV), mucocutaneous infection in immunocompromised patients: Treatment of initial and recurrent mucosal and cutaneous herpes simplex (HSV-1 and HSV-2) in immunocompromised patients.

Herpes simplex virus (HSV), genital infection (severe): Treatment of severe initial clinical episodes of genital herpes in immunocompetent patients.

Herpes simplex encephalitis: Treatment of herpes simplex encephalitis.

Herpes simplex virus (HSV), neonatal: Treatment of neonatal herpes infections.

Herpes zoster (shingles) in immunocompromised patients: Treatment of herpes zoster (shingles) in immunocompromised patients.

Pregnancy Risk Factor B

Dosing

Adult & Geriatric

Bell's palsy (off-label use; alternate therapy): Oral: 2,000 mg/day in divided doses for 10 days in combination with corticosteroids (Gronseth 2012)

Herpes simplex virus (HSV), genital infection:
Immunocompetent:
IV: Initial episode, severe:
Manufacturer's labeling: 5 mg/kg/dose every 8 hours for 5 to 7 days
Alternate recommendation: 5 to 10 mg/kg/dose every 8 hours for 2 to 7 days, follow with oral therapy to complete at least 10 days of therapy (CDC [Workowski 2015])
Oral:
Initial episode:
Manufacturer's labeling: 200 mg 5 times daily while awake for 10 days
Alternate recommendation: 200 mg 5 times daily for 7 to 10 days **or** 400 mg 3 times daily for 7 to 10 days (CDC [Workowski 2015])
Recurrence: **Note:** Begin at earliest signs of disease
Manufacturer's labeling: 200 mg 5 times daily while awake for 5 days
Alternate recommendation: 400 mg 3 times daily for 5 days **or** 800 mg twice daily for 5 days **or** 800 mg 3 times daily for 2 days (CDC [Workowski 2015])
Chronic suppression: 400 mg twice daily for up to 12 months (followed by re-evaluation); **Note:** Safety and efficacy have been documented in patients receiving daily therapy with acyclovir for up to 6 years (CDC [Workowski 2015])
HIV-infected patients (off-label use):
Initial or recurrent episodes: 400 mg 3 times daily for 5 to 14 days (HHS [OI adult 2015]) **or** 400 mg 3 times daily for 5 to 10 days (CDC [Workowski 2015])
Chronic suppressive therapy: 400 mg twice daily; continue indefinitely regardless of CD4 count in patients with severe recurrences of genital herpes or in patients who want to minimize frequency of recurrences (HHS [OI adult 2015]) **or** 400 to 800 mg 2 to 3 times daily (CDC [Workowski 2015])

HSV encephalitis: IV: Independent of HIV status:
Manufacturer's labeling: 10 mg/kg/dose every 8 hours for 10 days
Alternate recommendation: 10 mg/kg/dose every 8 hours for 14 to 21 days (*Red Book* [AAP 2012])

HSV, mucocutaneous treatment:
Immunocompromised:
IV:
Manufacturer's labeling: 5 mg/kg/dose every 8 hours for 7 days
Alternate recommendations: 5 to 10 mg/kg/dose every 8 hours for 7 days (Leflore 2000)
Oral (off-label use): 400 mg 5 times daily for 7 days (Leflore 2000)
HIV-infected patients: (off-label use)
IV: 5 mg/kg/dose every 8 hours; may switch to oral after lesions begin to heal (HHS [OI adult 2015])
Oral: After initial IV therapy, may switch to 400 mg 3 times daily; continue until lesions are completely healed (HHS [OI adult 2015])

HSV, orolabial (cold sores) (off-label use): Oral:
Immunocompetent:
Treatment: (episodic/recurrent): 200 to 400 mg 5 times daily for 5 days (Cernik 2008; Leflore 2000; Spruance 1990).
Chronic suppression: 400 mg 2 times daily (has been clinically evaluated for up to 1 year) (Cernik 2008; Rooney 1993)

HIV-infected patients: Treatment: 400 mg 3 times daily for 5 to 10 days (HHS [OI adult 2015])

Herpes zoster (shingles), treatment:
Manufacturer's labeling:
IV: Immunocompromised: 10 mg/kg/dose every 8 hours for 7 days
Oral: Immunocompetent: 800 mg 5 times daily for 7 to 10 day
Alternate recommendations: HIV-infected patients (HHS [OI adult 2015]):
IV: *Extensive cutaneous lesions or visceral involvement:* 10 to 15 mg/kg/dose every 8 hours until clinical improvement; switch to oral famciclovir or valacyclovir (preferred) or acyclovir (alternative) to complete a 10 to 14 day course when formation of new lesions has ceased and signs/symptoms of visceral infection are improving
Oral (off-label use): *Acute localized infection (as an alternative to valacyclovir or famciclovir):* 800 mg 5 times daily for 7 to 10 days; consider longer duration if lesions resolve slowly

Prevention of early HSV reactivation in seropositive hematopoietic stem cell transplant (HSCT) recipients (off-label use): Note: Start at the beginning of conditioning therapy and continue until engraftment or until mucositis resolves (~30 days) (Tomblyn 2009)
Adults ≥40 kg:
Oral: 400 to 800 mg twice daily
IV: 250 mg/m^2 every 12 hours

Prevention of late HSV reactivation in seropositive HSCT recipients (off-label use): Adults ≥40 kg: Oral: 800 mg twice daily; continue therapy for 1 year after HSCT (Tomblyn 2009).

Prevention of HSV reactivation in seropositive patients undergoing acute myeloid leukemia induction or reinduction (off-label use): Adults ≥40 kg: Oral: 400 mg twice daily; continue during active therapy and throughout periods of neutropenia (Bergmann 1995; Freifeld 2011)

Prevention of VZV reactivation in HSCT recipients (off-label use): Oral: 800 mg twice daily; continue therapy for 1 year after HSCT (Tomblyn 2009).

Prophylaxis of CMV in low risk allogeneic HSCT (off-label use; alternate therapy): Note: Begin at engraftment and continue to day 100; requires close monitoring for CMV reactivation (due to weak activity); not for use in patients at high risk for CMV disease (Tomblyn 2009)
Oral: 800 mg 4 times daily
IV: 500 mg/m^2 every 8 hours

Varicella (chickenpox), treatment: Begin treatment within the first 24 hours of rash onset:
Oral:
Immunocompetent (>40 kg): 800 mg 4 times daily for 5 days
HIV-infected patients (off-label use): *Uncomplicated cases (as an alternative to valacyclovir or famciclovir):* 800 mg 5 times daily for 5 to 7 days (HHS [OI adult 2015])
IV: HIV- infected patients (off-label use): Severe or complicated cases: 10 to 15 mg/kg/dose every 8 hours for 7 to 10 days; may switch to oral famciclovir or valacyclovir (preferred) or acyclovir (alternative) after defervescence if no evidence of visceral involvement (HHS [OI adult 2015])

◀ **Varicella-zoster virus acute retinal necrosis (ARN) in HIV-infected patients (off-label use):** IV: 10 to 15 mg/kg/dose every 8 hours for 10 to 14 days, followed by valacyclovir for 6 weeks plus intravitreal ganciclovir twice weekly for 1 to 2 doses (HHS [OI adult 2015])

Pediatric

Herpes simplex virus (HSV), genital infection:

IV: Children ≥12 years and Adolescents: Immunocompetent: Initial episode, severe: *Manufacturer's labeling:* 5 mg/kg/dose every 8 hours for 5 to 7 days

Oral:

Infants and Children <12 years: Immunocompetent (off-label use):

Initial episode: 40 to 80 mg/kg/day divided into 3 to 4 doses for 5-10 days (maximum: 1,000 mg daily) (*Red Book* [AAP 2012])

Chronic suppression: 40 to 80 mg/kg/day in 3 divided doses for ≤12 months; (maximum: 1,000 mg daily) (*Red Book* [AAP 2009])

Children ≥12 years and Adolescents: Immunocompetent (off-label use):

Initial episode: 200 mg every 4 hours while awake (5 times daily) **or** 400 mg 3 times daily for 7 to 10 days; treatment can be extended beyond 10 days if healing is not complete (*Red Book* [AAP 2012])

Chronic suppression: 800 mg daily in 2 divided doses for ≤12 continuous months (*Red Book* [AAP 2012])

Children: HIV-exposed/-positive (off-label use):

Children <45 kg:

Initial episode: 60 mg/kg/day divided into 3 doses daily for 5 to 14 days (maximum: 1,200 mg daily) (CDC 2009)

Chronic suppression: 20 mg/kg/dose twice daily (maximum dose: 400 mg) (CDC 2009)

Children ≥45 kg:

Initial episode: 400 mg twice daily for 5 to 14 days (CDC 2009)

Chronic suppression: 20 mg/kg/dose twice daily (maximum dose: 400 mg) (CDC 2009)

Children <12 years: Recurrence: Immunocompetent: Oral: 20 to 25 mg/kg/dose twice daily; maximum dose: 400 mg (Bradley 2011)

Children ≥12 years: Recurrence: Immunocompetent:

Manufacturer's labeling: 200 mg every 4 hours while awake (5 times daily) for 5 days

Alternate recommendation: 400 mg 3 times daily for 5 days **or** 800 mg twice daily for 5 days **or** 800 mg 3 times daily for 2 days (CDC [Workowski 2015]; *Red Book* [AAP 2015])

Adolescents: HIV-positive patients: (off-label use): Refer to adult dosing.

HSV encephalitis: IV:

Infants and Children 3 months to <12 years:

Immunocompetent:

Manufacturer's labeling: 20 mg/kg/dose every 8 hours for 10 days. **Note:** Doses ≥20 mg/kg may be associated with a higher incidence of nephrotoxicity (*Red Book* [AAP 2012])

Alternate recommendation: 10 to 15 mg/kg/dose every 8 hours for 14 to 21 days (*Red Book* [AAP 2012])

HIV-exposed/-positive: 10 mg/kg/dose every 8 hours for 21 days; do not discontinue therapy until a repeat HSV DNA PCR assay of the cerebrospinal fluid is negative (CDC 2009)

Children ≥12 years and Adolescents: Independent of HIV status:

Manufacturer's labeling: 10 mg/kg/dose every 8 hours for 10 days

Alternate recommendation: 10 mg/kg/dose every 8 hours for 14 to 21 days (*Red Book* [AAP 2012])

HSV gingivostomatitis (off-label use): HIV-exposed/-positive:
  Mild, symptomatic: Oral: Infants and Children: 20 mg/kg/dose 3 times daily for 5 to 10 days (maximum dose: 400 mg) (CDC 2009)
  Moderate to severe, symptomatic: IV: Infants and Children: 5 to 10 mg/kg/dose every 8 hours; **Note:** switch to oral therapy once lesions begin to regress (CDC 2009)

HSV, mucocutaneous treatment:
  Immunocompromised:
    IV:
      Infants, Children, and Adolescents: 10 mg/kg/dose every 8 hours for 7 to 14 days (*Red Book* [AAP 2012])
    Oral (off-label use):
      Children ≥2 years and Adolescents: 1,000 mg daily in 3 to 5 divided doses for 7 to 14 days; some suggest the maximum daily dose should not exceed 80 mg/kg/day (*Red Book* [AAP 2009]; Red Book [AAP 2012])
  HIV-infected patients (off-label use): Adolescents: IV, Oral: Refer to adult dosing.
  Suppression, chronic (cutaneous, ocular) episodes: Immunocompromised:
    Oral:
      Infants and Children (HIV-exposed/-positive): 20 mg/kg/dose twice daily for 5 to 14 days; maximum dose: 400 mg (CDC 2009)
      Children and Adolescents ≥12 years (independent of HIV status): 400 mg twice daily for up to 12 months (*Red Book* [AAP 2012])

HSV, neonatal: IV: Infants: Birth to 3 months: Treatment:
  Manufacturer's labeling: 10 mg/kg/dose every 8 hours for 10 days
  Alternate recommendations: 20 mg/kg/dose every 8 hours for 14 days (skin and mucous membrane disease) to 21 days (disseminated disease and CNS disease) (CDC [Workowski 2015]; Kimberlin 2013; *Red Book* [AAP 2012])

HSV, orolabial (cold sores) (off-label use): Oral:
  Immunocompetent: Chronic suppression: Children: 30 mg/kg/day in 3 divided doses for up to 12 months (maximum: 1,000 mg/day). **Note:** Re-evaluate after 12 months (*Red Book* [AAP 2012])
  HIV-infected patients: Treatment: Adolescents: Refer to adult dosing.

Herpes zoster (shingles), treatment:
  IV:
    Immunocompetent (off-label use):
      Infants: 10 mg/kg/dose every 8 hours for 7 to 10 days (*Red Book* [AAP 2012])
      Children ≥1 year and Adolescents: 500 mg/m^2/dose every 8 hours for 7 to 10 days; some experts recommend 10 mg/kg/dose every 8 hours (*Red Book* [AAP 2012])
    Immunocompromised:
      Children <12 years: (off-label dose): 10 mg/kg/dose every 8 hours for 7 to 10 days (*Red Book* [AAP 2012])
      Children ≥12 years and Adolescents: Manufacturer's labeling: Refer to adult dosing.

HIV-infected patients: Adolescents (off-label dose): *Extensive cutaneous lesions or visceral involvement:* Refer to adult dosing.

Oral:

Immunocompetent:

Children ≥12 years and Adolescents (off-label dose): 800 mg 5 times daily for 5 to 7 days (*Red Book* [AAP 2012])

Immunocompromised: HIV-infected patients (off-label use): *Acute localized infection (as an alternative to valacyclovir or famciclovir):* Adolescents: Refer to adult dosing.

Prevention of HSV reactivation in HIV-exposed/-positive patients (off-label use): Oral: Children: 20 mg/kg/dose twice daily (maximum: 400 mg per dose) (CDC 2009)

Prevention of early HSV reactivation in seropositive hematopoietic stem cell transplant (HSCT) recipients (off-label use): Note: Start at the beginning of conditioning therapy and continue until engraftment or until mucositis resolves (~30 days) (Tomblyn 2009):

Oral:

Children and Adolescents <40 kg (alternate therapy): 60 to 90 mg/kg/day in 2 to 3 divided doses

Children and Adolescents ≥40 kg: Refer to adult dosing.

IV:

Children and Adolescents <40 kg: 250 mg/m^2 every 8 hours or 125 mg/m^2 every 6 hours (maximum daily dose: 80 mg/kg/day)

Children and Adolescents ≥40 kg: Refer to adult dosing.

Prevention of late HSV reactivation in seropositive HSCT recipients (off-label use): Note: Continue therapy for 1 year after HSCT (Tomblyn 2009).

Children and Adolescents <40 kg: Oral: 60 to 90 mg/kg/day in 2 to 3 divided doses (maximum dose: 800 mg twice daily)

Children and Adolescents ≥40 kg: Refer to adult dosing.

Prevention of VZV reactivation in HSCT recipients (off-label use): Note: Continue therapy for 1 year after HSCT (Tomblyn 2009)

Children and Adolescents <40 kg: Oral: 60 to 80 mg/kg/day in 2 to 3 divided doses

Children and Adolescents ≥40 kg: Refer to adult dosing.

Prophylaxis of CMV in low-risk allogeneic HSCT (off-label use; alternate therapy): Note: Begin at engraftment and continue to day 100; requires close monitoring for CMV reactivation (due to weak activity); not for use in patients at high risk for CMV disease (Tomblyn 2009)

Oral:

Infants, Children, and Adolescents <40 kg: 600 mg/m^2 4 times daily

Children and Adolescents ≥40 kg: 800 mg 4 times daily

IV: Infants, Children, and Adolescents: 500 mg/m^2 every 8 hours

Varicella (chickenpox), treatment: Begin treatment within the first 24 hours of rash onset:

Oral:

Immunocompetent:

Children ≥2 years and ≤40 kg: 20 mg/kg/dose (maximum: 800 mg per dose) 4 times daily for 5 days

Children >40 kg: Refer to adult dosing.

HIV-infected patients (off-label use):

Infants and Children: Mild, uncomplicated disease and no or moderate immune suppression: 20 mg/kg/dose (maximum dose: 800 mg) 4 times daily for 7 to 10 days or until no new lesions for 48 hours (CDC 2009)

Adolescents: Uncomplicated cases (as an alternative to valacyclovir or famciclovir): Refer to adult dosing.

IV:

Immunocompetent (off-label use): Children ≥2 years: 10 mg/kg/dose or 500 mg/m^2/dose every 8 hours for 7 to 10 days (CDC 2009; *Red Book* [AAP 2012])

Immunocompromised (off-label use):

Infants (off-label dose): 10 mg/kg/dose every 8 hours for 7 to 10 days (*Red Book* [AAP 2012])

Children and Adolescents (off-label dose): 500 mg/m^2/dose every 8 hours for 7 to 10 days; some experts recommend 10 mg/kg/dose every 8 hours (*Red Book* [AAP 2012])

HIV-exposed/-positive (off-label use):

Infants: 10 mg/kg/dose every 8 hours for 7 to 10 days or until no new lesions for 48 hours (CDC 2009)

Children ≥1 year: 10 mg/kg/dose or 500 mg/m^2/dose every 8 hours for 7 to 10 days or until no new lesions for 48 hours (CDC 2009)

Adolescents: Refer to adult dosing.

Varicella-zoster virus acute retinal necrosis in HIV-exposed/-positive patients (off-label use): IV:

Infants and Children: 10 to 15 mg/kg/dose every 8 hours for 10 to 14 days, followed by oral acyclovir or valacyclovir for 4 to 6 weeks (CDC 2009)

Adolescents: Refer to adult dosing.

Renal Impairment Note: Monitor closely for neurotoxicity (Chowdhury 2016)

Oral:

CrCl 10 to 25 mL/minute/1.73 m^2: Normal dosing regimen 800 mg 5 times daily: Administer 800 mg every 8 hours

CrCl <10 mL/minute/1.73 m^2:

Normal dosing regimen 200 mg 5 times daily or 400 mg every 12 hours: Administer 200 mg every 12 hours

Normal dosing regimen 800 mg 5 times daily: Administer 200 mg every 12 hours (IDSA [Gupta 2005])

Intermittent hemodialysis (IHD): Dialyzable (60% reduction following a 6-hour session):

Normal dosing regimen 200 mg 5 times daily or 400 mg every 12 hours: Administer 200 mg every 12 hours; administer after hemodialysis on dialysis days

Normal dosing regimen 800 mg 5 times daily: Administer a loading dose of 400 mg and a maintenance dose of 200 mg twice daily plus a single 400 mg dose after each dialysis (Almond 1995). **Note:** Dose based on pharmacokinetic data and computer modeling.

Continuous ambulatory peritoneal dialysis (CAPD): 600 to 800 mg daily (Stathoulopoulou 1996)

IV:

CrCl 25 to 50 mL/minute/1.73 m^2: Administer recommended dose every 12 hours

CrCl 10 to 25 mL/minute/1.73 m²: Administer recommended dose every 24 hours

CrCl <10 mL/minute/1.73 m²: Administer 50% of recommended dose every 24 hours

Intermittent hemodialysis (IHD) (administer after hemodialysis on dialysis days): Dialyzable (60% reduction following a 6-hour session): 2.5-5 mg/kg every 24 hours (Heintz 2009). **Note:** Dosing dependent on the assumption of 3 times weekly, complete IHD sessions.

Peritoneal dialysis (PD): Administer 50% of normal dose once daily; no supplemental dose needed (Aronoff 2007)

Continuous renal replacement therapy (CRRT) (Heintz 2009; Trotman 2005): Drug clearance is highly dependent on the method of renal replacement, filter type, and flow rate. Appropriate dosing requires close monitoring of pharmacologic response, signs of adverse reactions due to drug accumulation, as well as drug concentrations in relation to target trough (if appropriate). The following are general recommendations only (based on dialysate flow/ultrafiltration rates of 1 to 2 L/hour and minimal residual renal function) and should not supersede clinical judgment:

CVVH: 5 to 10 mg/kg every 24 hours

CVVHD/CVVHDF: 5 to 10 mg/kg every 12 to 24 hours

Note: The higher end of dosage range (eg, 10 mg/kg every 12 hours for CVVHDF) is recommended for viral meningoencephalitis and varicella-zoster virus infections.

Hepatic Impairment Oral, IV: There are no dosage adjustments provided in the manufacturer's labeling; use caution in patients with severe impairment.

Obesity Obese patients should be dosed using ideal body weight.

Additional Information Complete prescribing information should be consulted for additional detail.

Dosage Forms Excipient information presented when available (limited, particularly for generics); consult specific product labeling. [DSC] = Discontinued product

Capsule, Oral:
Zovirax: 200 mg [contains fd&c blue #2 (indigotine), parabens]
Generic: 200 mg

Solution, Intravenous, as sodium [strength expressed as base]:
Generic: 50 mg/mL (10 mL, 20 mL)

Solution Reconstituted, Intravenous, as sodium [strength expressed as base]:
Generic: 500 mg (1 ea); 1000 mg (1 ea [DSC])

Suspension, Oral:
Zovirax: 200 mg/5 mL (473 mL) [contains methylparaben, propylparaben; banana flavor]
Generic: 200 mg/5 mL (473 mL)

Tablet, Oral:
Zovirax: 400 mg
Zovirax: 800 mg [contains fd&c blue #2 (indigotine)]
Generic: 400 mg, 800 mg

Acyclovir (Topical) (ay SYE kloe veer)

Brand Names: US Sitavig; Zovirax
Brand Names: Canada Zovirax
Index Terms Aciclovir; ACV; Acycloguanosine
Pharmacologic Category Antiviral Agent, Topical

Use Herpes virus:
Buccal tablet: Treatment of recurrent herpes labialis (cold sores) in immuno-competent adults.
Cream: Treatment of recurrent herpes labialis (cold sores) in immunocompetent children ≥12 years of age, adolescents, and adults.
Ointment: Management of initial genital herpes and in limited non-life-threatening mucocutaneous herpes simplex virus infections in immunocompromised patients.

Pregnancy Risk Factor B

Dosing

Adult & Geriatric

Genital HSV: Topical ointment: Initial episode: 1/2" ribbon of ointment for a 4" square surface area every 3 hours (6 times daily) for 7 days

Herpes labialis (cold sores):
Topical cream: Apply 5 times daily for 4 days
Buccal tablet: Apply one 50 mg tablet as a single dose to the upper gum region (canine fossa).

Mucocutaneous HSV (non-life-threatening, immunocompromised): Topical ointment: 1/2" ribbon of ointment for a 4" square surface area every 3 hours (6 times daily) for 7 days

Pediatric Herpes labialis (cold sores): Children ≥12 years and Adolescents: Topical cream: Refer to adult dosing.

Renal Impairment There are no dosage adjustments provided in the manufacturer's labeling. However, dosage adjustment is unlikely due to low systemic absorption.

Hepatic Impairment There are no dosage adjustments provided in the manufacturer's labeling. However, dosage adjustment is unlikely due to low systemic absorption.

Additional Information Complete prescribing information should be consulted for additional detail.

Dosage Forms Excipient information presented when available (limited, particularly for generics); consult specific product labeling.
Cream, External:
Zovirax: 5% (5 g) [contains cetostearyl alcohol, propylene glycol]
Ointment, External:
Zovirax: 5% (30 g)
Generic: 5% (5 g, 15 g, 30 g)
Tablet, Buccal:
Sitavig: 50 mg [contains milk protein concentrate]

◆ **Acyclovir Sodium** *see* Acyclovir (Systemic) *on page 49*

◆ **Acyclovir Sodium Injection (Can)** *see* Acyclovir (Systemic) *on page 49*

◆ **AD32** *see* Valrubicin *on page 1858*

◆ **Adcetris** *see* Brentuximab Vedotin *on page 285*

◆ **Ado Trastuzumab** *see* Ado-Trastuzumab Emtansine *on page 57*

Ado-Trastuzumab Emtansine (a do tras TU zoo mab em TAN seen)

Related Information
Common Toxicity Criteria *on page 2242*
Management of Drug Extravasations *on page 2271*
Safe Handling of Hazardous Drugs *on page 2379*

Brand Names: US Kadcyla

◀ **Brand Names: Canada** Kadcyla

Index Terms Ado Trastuzumab; Adotrastuzumab; T-DM1; Trastuzumab Emtansine; Trastuzumab-DM1; Trastuzumab-MCC-DM1

Pharmacologic Category Antineoplastic Agent, Anti-HER2; Antineoplastic Agent, Antibody Drug Conjugate; Antineoplastic Agent, Antimicrotubular; Antineoplastic Agent, Monoclonal Antibody

Use Breast cancer, metastatic: Treatment (single-agent) of HER2-positive, metastatic breast cancer in patients who previously received trastuzumab and a taxane, separately or in combination, and have either received prior therapy for metastatic disease or developed disease recurrence during or within 6 months of completing adjuvant therapy.

Labeled Contraindications

US labeling: There are no contraindications in the manufacturer's labeling.

Canadian labeling: Hypersensitivity to trastuzumab emtansine or any component of the formulation.

Pregnancy Considerations Animal reproduction studies have not been conducted. **[US Boxed Warning]: Exposure to ado-trastuzumab emtansine during pregnancy may cause embryo-fetal harm. Effective contraception must be used in women of reproductive potential.** Oligohydramnios and oligohydramnios sequence (manifested as pulmonary hypoplasia, skeletal malformations and neonatal death) were observed following trastuzumab exposure during pregnancy (trastuzumab is the antibody component of ado-trastuzumab emtansine). Monitor for oligohydramnios if trastuzumab exposure occurs during pregnancy or within 7 months prior to conception; conduct appropriate fetal testing if oligohydramnios occurs. Based on the mechanism of action, the DM1 component of the ado-trastuzumab emtansine formulation may also cause fetal harm if administered during pregnancy. Verify pregnancy status (in females of reproductive potential) prior to therapy. Effective contraception is recommended during therapy and for 7 months after the last dose for women of childbearing potential. Males with female partners of reproductive potential should use effective contraception during therapy and for 4 months after the last dose. Ado-trastuzumab emtansine may impair fertility in females and males.

If ado-trastuzumab emtansine exposure occurs during pregnancy or within 7 months prior to conception, healthcare providers should report the exposure to the Genentech Adverse Event Line (888-835-2555). Women exposed to ado-trastuzumab emtansine during pregnancy or within 7 months prior to conception are encouraged to enroll in MotHER Pregnancy Registry (1-800-690-6720).

European Society for Medical Oncology (ESMO) guidelines for cancer during pregnancy recommend delaying treatment with HER-2 targeted agents until after delivery in pregnant patients with HER-2 positive disease (Peccatori 2013).

Breastfeeding Considerations It is not known if ado-trastuzumab emtansine is present in breast milk. Endogenous immunoglobulins are found in breast milk. Due to the potential for serious adverse reactions in the breastfed infant, women should not breastfeed during treatment and for 7 months following the last dose.

Warnings/Precautions [US Boxed Warning]: May result in left ventricular ejection fraction (LVEF) reductions. Evaluate left ventricular function (in all patients) prior to and at least every 3 months during treatment; withhold for clinically significant left ventricular function decreases.

Treatment interruption or dosage reductions are required inpatients who develop decreased LVEF. Use has not been studied in patients with LVEF <50% at baseline, with a history of symptomatic CHF, serious arrhythmia, or recent history (within 6 months) of MI or unstable angina.

[US Boxed Warning]: Serious hepatotoxicity, including liver failure and death, has been reported. Monitor transaminases and bilirubin at baseline and prior to each dose. Increases (transaminases or total bilirubin) may require dose reductions or discontinuation. Hepatotoxicity is typically manifested by asymptomatic and transient increases in transaminases, although fatal cases of drug induced liver injury and hepatic encephalopathy have occurred; may be confounded by comorbidities or concomitant hepatotoxic medications. Use with caution in patients with hepatic impairment (has not been studied in patients with baseline serum transaminases >2.5 times ULN or bilirubin >1.5 times ULN, or in patients with active hepatitis B or C virus). Cases of idiopathic noncirrhotic portal hypertension (including nodular regenerative hyperplasia), a rare liver disorder characterized by widespread benign transformation of hepatic parenchyma into small regenerative nodules, have been observed (by biopsy). Idiopathic noncirrhotic portal hypertension (including nodular regenerative hyperplasia) may develop into noncirrhotic portal hypertension. Consider idiopathic noncirrhotic portal hypertension (including nodular regenerative hyperplasia) in patients with clinical symptoms of portal hypertension and/or cirrhosis-like pattern seen on liver CT scan, although without associated transaminase elevations or other manifestations of cirrhosis. Diagnosis of idiopathic noncirrhotic portal hypertension (including nodular regenerative hyperplasia) is confirmed by histopathology; permanently discontinue if histopathology confirms idiopathic noncirrhotic portal hypertension (including nodular regenerative hyperplasia).

[US Boxed Warning]: Exposure to ado-trastuzumab emtansine during pregnancy may cause embryo-fetal harm. Effective contraception must be used in women of reproductive potential. Pregnancy status should be verified prior to therapy; effective contraception is recommended during therapy and for 7 months after the last dose for women of childbearing potential and for 4 months after the last dose in males with female partners of reproductive potential.

Infusion reactions (flushing, chills, fever, bronchospasm, dyspnea, wheezing, hypotension, and/or tachycardia) have been reported. After termination of infusion, these reactions generally resolved within several hours to a day. Medications for the treatment of reactions should be available for immediate use. Monitor closely for infusion reactions, especially during initial infusion. If reaction occurs, decrease infusion rate; for severe infusion reactions, interrupt infusion; permanently discontinue for life-threatening reactions. Serious allergic/anaphylactic reaction was observed (rare). Use is not recommended in patients who had trastuzumab permanently discontinued due to infusion reaction or hypersensitivity (has not been evaluated). May be a vesicant. Local reactions (erythema, irritation, pain, swelling, or tenderness) secondary to extravasation have been noted; these were generally mild and typically occurred within 24 hours of infusion. There is a case report of skin necrosis (delayed) following extravasation (Shafaee 2017). Monitor infusion site during infusion for possible infiltration.

◀ Thrombocytopenia may occur (nadir achieved: by day 8; generally resolves to ≤ grade 1 by the next scheduled dose); the incidence of thrombocytopenia may be higher in patients of Asian ancestry; monitor platelet count at baseline and prior to each dose; may require treatment interruption or dose reduction. Monitor closely if at bleeding risk due to thrombocytopenia and/or concomitant anticoagulant use. Has not been studied in patients with platelets <100,000/mm³ at treatment initiation. Neutropenia and anemia have also occurred. Hemorrhagic events, including central nervous system, respiratory, and gastrointestinal hemorrhage, have been observed; some hemorrhages were fatal. Some events occurred in patients who were receiving anticoagulation or antiplatelet therapy, or in patients with thrombocytopenia, although bleeding also occurred in patients without additional risk factors. Use caution when administering with antiplatelet agents or anticoagulants; consider additional monitoring when indicated. Sensory peripheral neuropathy has been reported, usually grade 1, although grade 3 peripheral neuropathy was also described; monitor for signs and symptoms of neuropathy; may require treatment interruption and/or dose reduction. Interstitial lung disease (ILD), including pneumonitis has been reported; some cases resulted in acute respiratory distress syndrome and/or fatalities; permanently discontinue with diagnosis of ILD or pneumonitis. Signs and symptoms of pneumonitis include dyspnea, cough, fatigue, and pulmonary infiltrates; may or may not occur in correlation with infusion reaction. Patients with dyspnea at rest (due to advance malignancy complications or comorbidity) may be at increased risk for pulmonary toxicity.

[US Boxed Warning]: Ado-trastuzumab emtansine and conventional trastuzumab are NOT interchangeable. Do not substitute. In Canada, the generic name for Kadcyla is trastuzumab emtansine (ie, lacks Ado- prefix) and may be confused with conventional trastuzumab. Verify product label prior to reconstitution and administration to prevent medication errors. Potentially significant drug-drug or drug-food interactions may exist, requiring dose or frequency adjustment, additional monitoring, and/or selection of alternative therapy. Establish HER2 overexpression or gene amplification status prior to treatment; has only been studied in patients with evidence of HER2 overexpression, either as 3+ IHC (Dako Herceptest) or FISH amplification ratio ≥2 (Dako HER2 FISH pharmDx test); there is only limited data on patients with breast cancer positive by FISH and 0 or 1+ by IHC.

Adverse Reactions

>10%:

Central nervous system: Fatigue (36%), headache (28%), peripheral neuropathy (21%; grades 3/4: 2%), insomnia (12%)

Dermatologic: Skin rash (12%)

Endocrine & metabolic: Decreased serum potassium (33%; grade 3: 3%)

Gastrointestinal: Nausea (40%), constipation (27%), diarrhea (24%), abdominal pain (19%), vomiting (19%), xerostomia (17%), stomatitis (14%)

Hematologic & oncologic: Decreased platelet count (83% [nadir by day 8]; grade 3: 14%; grade 4: 3%), decreased hemoglobin (60%; grade 3: 4%; grade 4: 1%), decreased neutrophils (39%; grade 3: 3%; grade 4: <1%), hemorrhage (32%; grades 3/4: 2%), thrombocytopenia (31%; grades 3/4: 15%; Asians grades 3/4: 45%), anemia (14%; grades 3/4: 4%)

Hepatic: Increased serum AST (98%; grades 3/4: <8%), increased serum ALT (82%; grades 3/4: <6%), increased serum transaminases (29%), increased serum bilirubin (17%)

Neuromuscular & skeletal: Musculoskeletal pain (36%), arthralgia (19%), weakness (18%), myalgia (14%)
Respiratory: Epistaxis (23%), cough (18%), dyspnea (12%)
Miscellaneous: Fever (19%)

1% to 10%:
Cardiovascular: Peripheral edema (7%), hypertension (5%; grades 3/4: 1%), left ventricular dysfunction (2%; grades 3/4: <1%)
Central nervous system: Dizziness (10%), chills (8%)
Dermatologic: Pruritus (6%)
Endocrine & metabolic: Hypokalemia (10%; grades 3/4: 3%)
Gastrointestinal: Dyspepsia (9%), dysgeusia (8%)
Genitourinary: Urinary tract infection (9%)
Hematologic & oncologic: Neutropenia (7%; grades 3/4: 2%)
Hepatic: Increased serum alkaline phosphatase (5%)
Hypersensitivity: Hypersensitivity (2%)
Immunologic: Antibody development (5%)
Ophthalmic: Blurred vision (5%), conjunctivitis (4%), dry eye syndrome (4%), increased lacrimation (3%)
Respiratory: Pneumonitis (≤1%)
Miscellaneous: Infusion related reaction (1%)

<1%: Anaphylactoid reaction, hepatic encephalopathy, hepatotoxicity, idiopathic noncirrhotic portal hypertension (including nodular regenerative hyperplasia), portal hypertension

Drug Interactions

Metabolism/Transport Effects Substrate of CYP3A4 (major); **Note:** Assignment of Major/Minor substrate status based on clinically relevant drug interaction potential

Avoid Concomitant Use

Avoid concomitant use of Ado-Trastuzumab Emtansine with any of the following: BCG (Intravesical); Belimumab; Conivaptan; CYP3A4 Inhibitors (Strong); Deferiprone; Dipyrone; Fusidic Acid (Systemic); Idelalisib; Natalizumab; Pimecrolimus (Topical); Vaccines (Live)

Increased Effect/Toxicity

Ado-Trastuzumab Emtansine may increase the levels/effects of: Antineoplastic Agents (Anthracycline, Systemic); Belimumab; CloZAPine; Deferiprone; Fingolimod; Leflunomide; Natalizumab; Tofacitinib; Vaccines (Live)

The levels/effects of Ado-Trastuzumab Emtansine may be increased by: Aprepitant; Conivaptan; CYP3A4 Inhibitors (Moderate); CYP3A4 Inhibitors (Strong); Dasatinib; Denosumab; Dipyrone; Fosaprepitant; Fusidic Acid (Systemic); Idelalisib; Netupitant; Ocrelizumab; Palbociclib; Pimecrolimus; Promazine; Roflumilast; Simeprevir; Stiripentol; Tacrolimus (Topical); Trastuzumab

Decreased Effect

Ado-Trastuzumab Emtansine may decrease the levels/effects of: BCG (Intravesical); Coccidioides immitis Skin Test; Nivolumab; Sipuleucel-T; Tertomotide; Vaccines (Inactivated); Vaccines (Live)

The levels/effects of Ado-Trastuzumab Emtansine may be decreased by: Echinacea

Hazardous Drugs Handling Considerations

Hazardous agent (NIOSH 2016 [group 1]).

Use appropriate precautions for receiving, handling, administration, and disposal. Gloves (single) should be worn during receiving, unpacking, and placing in storage.

NIOSH recommends double gloving, a protective gown, ventilated engineering controls (a class II biological safety cabinet or a compounding aseptic containment isolator), and closed system transfer devices (CSTDs) for preparation. Double gloving, a gown, and (if dosage form allows) CSTDs are required during administration (NIOSH 2016).

Storage/Stability Store intact vials at 2°C to 8°C (36°F to 46°F). Do not freeze or shake intact vials, reconstituted solution, or solutions diluted for infusion. Reconstituted vials do not contain preservative and should be used immediately, although may be stored for up to 24 hours at 2°C to 8°C (36°F to 46°F). Solutions diluted for infusion in NS should be used immediately, although may be stored at 2°C to 8°C (36°F to 46°F) for up to 24 hours prior to use. This storage time is additional to the time allowed for the reconstituted vials.

Preparation for Administration Check vial labels to assure appropriate product is being reconstituted (ado-trastuzumab emtansine and conventional trastuzumab are different products and are **NOT** interchangeable).

Slowly inject sterile water for injection into the vial (5 mL for 100 mg vial or 8 mL for 160 mg vial) to a reconstituted concentration of 20 mg/mL. Gently swirl vial until completely dissolved. Reconstituted solution will be clear or slightly opalescent (there should be no visible particles) and colorless to pale brown. Dilute for infusion by adding to 250 mL sodium chloride 0.9%; gently invert bag to mix (do not shake).

Mechanism of Action Ado-trastuzumab emtansine is a HER2-antibody drug conjugate which incorporates the HER2 targeted actions of trastuzumab with the microtubule inhibitor DM1 (a maytansine derivative). The conjugate, which is linked via a stable thioether linker, allows for selective delivery into HER2 overexpressing cells, resulting in cell cycle arrest and apoptosis.

Pharmacodynamics/Kinetics

Distribution: V_d: 3.13 L
Protein binding: DM1: 93%
Metabolism: DM1 undergoes hepatic metabolism via CYP3A4/5
Half-life elimination: ~4 days
Time to peak: Near the end of the infusion

Dosing

Adult & Geriatric Note: Do not substitute ado-trastuzumab emtansine (US) or trastuzumab emtansine (Canada) for or with conventional trastuzumab; products are different and are **NOT** interchangeable.

Breast cancer, metastatic, HER2+: IV: 3.6 mg/kg every 3 weeks until disease progression or unacceptable toxicity; Maximum dose: 3.6 mg/kg
Missed or delayed doses: If a planned dose is missed or delayed, administer as soon as possible (at the dose and rate most recently tolerated), do not wait until the next planned cycle. Then adjust schedule to maintain a 3-week interval between doses.

Renal Impairment
CrCl ≥30 mL/minute: No dosage adjustment necessary.

CrCl <30 mL/minute: There are no dosage adjustments provided in the manufacturer's labeling (has not been studied).

Hepatic Impairment
Hepatic impairment prior to treatment initiation:

Mild to moderate impairment (Child-Pugh class A or B): No dosage adjustment necessary; use with caution.

Severe impairment (Child-Pugh class C): There are no dosage adjustments provided in the manufacturer's labeling (has not been studied).

Hepatotoxicity during treatment: Refer to Dosing: Adjustment for Toxicity for dose level reductions:

Grade 2 ALT, AST elevations (>2.5 to ≤5 times ULN): Continue at same dose level.

Grade 3 ALT, AST elevations (>5 to ≤20 times ULN): Withhold until ALT, AST recover to ≤ grade 2, then resume with one dose level reduction.

Grade 4 ALT, AST elevations (>20 times ULN): Permanently discontinue treatment.

Grade 2 hyperbilirubinemia (>1.5 to ≤3 times ULN): Withhold until bilirubin recovers to ≤ grade 1 (≤1.5 times ULN), then resume at the same dose level.

Grade 3 hyperbilirubinemia (>3 to ≤10 times ULN): Withhold until bilirubin recovers to ≤ grade 1, then resume with one dose level reduction.

Grade 4 hyperbilirubinemia (>10 times ULN): Permanently discontinue treatment.

Concomitant ALT, AST >3 times ULN and total bilirubin >2 times ULN: Permanently discontinue treatment.

Idiopathic noncirrhotic portal hypertension (including nodular regenerative hyperplasia): Permanently discontinue treatment.

Adjustment for Toxicity Note: After a dose reduction is implemented, do not re-escalate dose.

Infusion-related reaction: Slow infusion rate or interrupt infusion. Permanently discontinue if life-threatening infusion reactions occur.

Dose levels for dosage reductions and/or discontinuation:

Starting dose: 3.6 mg/kg

First dose reduction: Reduce dose to 3 mg/kg

Second dose reduction: Reduce dose to 2.4 mg/kg

Further reductions necessary: Discontinue treatment.

Hematologic toxicity:

Grade 3 thrombocytopenia (platelets 25,000/mm^3 to <50,000/mm^3): Withhold treatment until platelet count recovers to ≤ grade 1 (platelets ≥75,000/mm^3), then resume treatment at the same dose level.

Grade 4 thrombocytopenia (platelets <25,000/mm^3): Withhold treatment until platelet count recovers to ≤ grade 1 (platelets ≥75,000/mm^3), then resume treatment with one dose level reduction.

Cardiotoxicity:

LVEF >45%: Continue treatment.

LVEF 40% to ≤45% and decrease is <10% points from baseline: Continue treatment and repeat LVEF assessment within 3 weeks.

LVEF 40% to ≤45% and decrease is ≥10% points from baseline: Withhold treatment and repeat LVEF assessment within 3 weeks; if repeat LVEF has not recovered to within 10% points from baseline, discontinue treatment.

LVEF <40%: Withhold treatment and repeat LVEF assessment within 3 weeks; if repeat LVEF is confirmed <40%, discontinue treatment.

HF (symptomatic): Discontinue treatment.

Peripheral neuropathy, grade 3 or 4: Temporarily discontinue until resolves to ≤ grade 2.

Pulmonary toxicity: Interstitial lung disease or pneumonitis: Permanently discontinue.

Administration Check label to ensure appropriate product is being administered (ado-trastuzumab emtansine [US] or trastuzumab emtansine [Canada] and conventional trastuzumab are different products and are **NOT** interchangeable).

Infuse over 90 minutes (first infusion) or over 30 minutes (subsequent infusions if prior infusions were well tolerated) through a 0.2 or 0.22 micron inline nonprotein adsorptive polyethersulfone filter. Do not administer IV push or bolus. Do not administer with other medications.

Monitor patient during infusion for signs of infusion-related reactions (eg, fever, chills); monitor for at least 90 minutes following initial infusion and (if tolerated) for at least 30 minutes following subsequent infusions.

May be a vesicant; avoid extravasation. Ensure proper needle or catheter position prior to administration. Closely monitor infusion site during administration.

Extravasation management: If extravasation occurs, stop infusion immediately and disconnect (leave cannula/needle in place); gently aspirate extravasated solution (do **NOT** flush the line); remove needle/cannula; elevate extremity.

Vesicant/Extravasation Risk May be a vesicant; skin necrosis (delayed) has been observed (case report) following extravasation (Shafaee 2017).

Emetic Potential Low (10% to 30%)

Monitoring Parameters Platelet count (at baseline and prior to each dose), transaminases and bilirubin (at baseline and prior to each dose); verify pregnancy status prior to treatment initiation; HER2 expression status. Evaluate left ventricular function (prior to and at least every 3 months during treatment; for LVEF <40% or 40% to 45% with ≥10% absolute decrease below baseline value, reassess within 3 weeks). Monitor infusion site during infusion for possible infiltration; monitor for infusion reactions (during infusion and for 90 minutes after initial infusion and for 30 minutes after subsequent infusions); signs and symptoms of bleeding, neuropathy, and/or pulmonary toxicity

Dosage Forms Excipient information presented when available (limited, particularly for generics); consult specific product labeling.

Solution Reconstituted, Intravenous [preservative free]:

Kadcyla: 100 mg (1 ea); 160 mg (1 ea) [contains mouse (murine) and/or hamster protein]

◆ **Advagraf (Can)** *see* Tacrolimus (Systemic) *on page 1715*

◆ **Advate** *see* Antihemophilic Factor (Recombinant) *on page 143*

◆ **Adynovate** *see* Antihemophilic Factor (Recombinant [Pegylated]) *on page 149*

◆ **AF802** *see* Alectinib *on page 78*

Afatinib (a FA ti nib)

Related Information

Common Toxicity Criteria *on page 2242*

Management of Chemotherapy-Induced Nausea and Vomiting in Adults *on page 2253*

Management of EGFR Inhibitor Toxicities: Dermatologic, Ocular, and Gastrointestinal *on page 2291*

Safe Handling of Hazardous Drugs *on page 2379*

Brand Names: US Gilotrif

Brand Names: Canada Giotrif

Index Terms Afatinib Dimaleate; BIBW 2992

Pharmacologic Category Antineoplastic Agent, Epidermal Growth Factor Receptor (EGFR) Inhibitor; Antineoplastic Agent, Tyrosine Kinase Inhibitor

Use

Non-small cell lung cancer, metastatic, EGFR mutation-positive: First-line treatment of metastatic non-small cell lung cancer (NSCLC) in patients whose tumors have epidermal growth factor receptor (EGFR) exon 19 deletions or exon 21 (L858R) substitution mutations as detected by an approved test.

Limitations of use: Safety and efficacy have not been established in patients whose tumors express EGFR mutations other than exon 19 deletion or exon 21 (L858R) substitution.

Non-small cell lung cancer, metastatic squamous: Treatment of previously treated metastatic squamous cell NSCLC which has progressed following platinum-based chemotherapy.

Labeled Contraindications

US labeling: There are no contraindications listed in the manufacturer's labeling.

Canadian labeling: Hypersensitivity to afatinib or any component of the formulation.

Pregnancy Considerations Based on animal reproduction studies and on the mechanism of action, afatinib may cause fetal harm if used during pregnancy. Women of reproductive potential should use highly-effective contraception during therapy and for at least 2 weeks after treatment has been discontinued.

Breastfeeding Considerations It is not known if afatinib is excreted into breast milk. Due to the potential for serious adverse reactions in the breastfeeding infant, the manufacturer recommends against breastfeeding during therapy and for at least 2 weeks after treatment has been discontinued.

Warnings/Precautions Cutaneous reactions (eg, acneiform rash, erythema, and rash) are common; grade 3 reactions (characterized by bullous, blistering, and exfoliating lesions) and palmar-plantar erythrodysesthesia syndrome were also seen in clinical trials. Cases of skin reactions consistent with Stevens Johnson syndrome (SJS) and toxic epidermal necrolysis (TEN) have been reported; SJS and TEN result from a mechanism which is distinct and separate from the bullous skin toxicity typically observed with EGFR inhibitor therapy. Dermatologic toxicity may require therapy interruption and dosage reduction; discontinue if life-threatening bullous, blistering, or exfoliating lesions occur or for suspected SJS or TEN. Patients should be cautioned to avoid sun exposure and/or utilize adequate sun protection. Paronychia requiring dose reduction and discontinuation of therapy has been observed. In clinical trials, diarrhea (including grade 3 and 4 events) and stomatitis frequently occurred in patients treated with afatinib; diarrhea was observed in the majority of patients and typically appeared within the first 6 weeks of therapy. Dehydration and renal impairment may occur as a consequence of diarrhea; monitor closely. Patients may require antidiarrheal therapy (eg, loperamide); initiate at the onset of diarrhea and continue until free of loose bowel movements for 12 hours. May necessitate therapy interruption and dosage reduction.

Decreases from baseline in left ventricular ejection fraction (LVEF) were noted in some patients receiving afatinib. Patients with abnormal LVEF or a significant cardiac history were excluded from clinical trials; use with caution in patients with cardiac risk factors and/or decreased LVEF. Keratitis (including rare grade 3 events) was reported rarely in clinical trials; monitor for signs/symptoms of keratitis (eg, acute or worsening eye inflammation, blurred vision, eye pain, lacrimation, light sensitivity, red eye). Interrupt therapy in patients with suspected keratitis and consider discontinuation if diagnosis of ulcerative keratitis is confirmed (permanently discontinue for persistent ulcerative keratitis). Use with caution in patients with a history of keratitis, severe dry eye, ulcerative keratitis, or who wear contact lens (risk factor for keratitis and ulceration). Interstitial lung disease (ILD) or ILD-like reactions occurred in a small percentage of patients treated with afatinib (some fatal). ILD incidence appeared to be higher in Asian as compared to non-Asian patients. Monitor closely for signs/symptoms of ILD (eg, acute respiratory distress syndrome, allergic alveolitis, lung infiltration, pneumonitis). Interrupt therapy for suspected ILD; discontinue therapy with confirmed diagnosis.

Hepatic function test abnormalities (some fatal) were observed in clinical trials. Monitor liver function tests periodically; may require therapy interruption and dosage reduction. Discontinue if severe hepatic impairment occurs during therapy. Dosage reduction is recommended in patients with severe renal impairment (estimated glomerular filtration rate [eGFR] 15 to 29 mL/minute/ 1.73 m^2). Potentially significant drug-drug interactions may exist, requiring dose or frequency adjustment, additional monitoring, and/or selection of alternative therapy. Safety and efficacy have not been established in patients with non-small cell lung cancer whose tumors express EGFR mutations other than exon 19 deletion or exon 21 (L858R) substitution. Increased mortality has been observed in a clinical trial evaluating afatinib in combination with vinorelbine for HER2-positive metastatic breast cancer (not an approved use). This combination was also associated with a higher incidence of adverse events (eg, diarrhea, rash), as well as fatalities due to infection and cancer progression. Afatinib should not be used in combination with vinorelbine for the treatment of HER2-positive metastatic breast cancer. Formulation may contain lactose.

Adverse Reactions
>10%:
  Dermatologic: Acneiform eruption (≤70% to 90%; grade 3: ≤16%), skin rash (≤70% to 90%; grade 3: ≤16%), paronychia (11% to 58%), xeroderma (31%), pruritus (10% to 21%), cheilitis (12%)

Endocrine & metabolic: Decreased serum potassium (11% to 30%), weight loss (17%), hypokalemia (11%)

Gastrointestinal: Diarrhea (75% to 96%; grade 3: 15%; grades 3/4: 11% to 16%), stomatitis (30% to 71%), decreased appetite (25% to 29%), nausea (21% to 25%), vomiting (13% to 23%)

Genitourinary: Cystitis (13%)

Hematologic & oncologic: Abnormal lymphocytes (decreased: 38%; grades 3/4: 9%), decreased white blood cell count (12%; grades 3/4: 1%)

Hepatic: Increased serum ALT (10% to 54%; grades 3/4: 1% to 2%), increased serum alkaline phosphatase (34% to 51%; grades 3/4: 2% to 3%), increased serum AST (7% to 46%; grades 3/4: 1% to 3%), abnormal hepatic function tests (6% to 18%; grades 3/4: ≤4%), increased serum bilirubin (3% to 16%; grades 3/4: ≤1%)

Ophthalmic: Conjunctivitis (11%)

Renal: Decreased creatinine clearance (49%; grades 3/4: 2%)

Respiratory: Epistaxis (17%), rhinorrhea (11%)

Miscellaneous: Fever (12%)

1% to 10%:

Central nervous system: Fatigue (<2%)

Dermatologic: Palmar-plantar erythrodysesthesia (2% to 7%)

Ophthalmic: Keratitis (≤2%; grade 3: <1%)

Renal: Renal insufficiency (0%; grade 3: >1%)

Respiratory: Interstitial pulmonary disease (2%; grades 3/4: ≤1%), dyspnea (<2%)

Frequency not defined:

Endocrine & metabolic: Dehydration

Infection: Sepsis

Renal: Acute renal failure

Respiratory: Pneumonia

Miscellaneous: Physical health deterioration

<1%, postmarketing, and/or case reports: Pancreatitis, Stevens-Johnson syndrome, toxic epidermal necrolysis

Drug Interactions

Metabolism/Transport Effects Substrate of BCRP, P-glycoprotein; **Inhibits** BCRP

Avoid Concomitant Use

Avoid concomitant use of Afatinib with any of the following: Aminolevulinic Acid (Systemic)

Increased Effect/Toxicity

Afatinib may increase the levels/effects of: Aminolevulinic Acid (Systemic); Aminolevulinic Acid (Topical); Porfimer; Verteporfin

The levels/effects of Afatinib may be increased by: Lumacaftor; Nelfinavir; P-glycoprotein/ABCB1 Inhibitors; Saquinavir; Tacrolimus (Systemic)

Decreased Effect

The levels/effects of Afatinib may be decreased by: CarBAMazepine; Lumacaftor; P-glycoprotein/ABCB1 Inducers; PHENobarbital; Primidone

Food Interactions Administration with a high-fat meal decreases C_{max} by 50% and AUC by 39% as compared to the fasted state. Management: Take at least 1 hour before or 2 hours after a meal.

◀ **Hazardous Drugs Handling Considerations**
Hazardous agent (NIOSH 2016 [group 1]).

Use appropriate precautions for receiving, handling, administration, and disposal. Gloves (single) should be worn during receiving, unpacking, and placing in storage. NIOSH recommends single gloving for administration of intact tablets or capsules (NIOSH 2016).

Storage/Stability Store at 25°C (77°F); excursions are permitted between 15°C and 30°C (59°F and 86°F). Dispense in original bottle; protect from high humidity and light.

Mechanism of Action Highly selective blocker of the ErbB family, including EGFR (ErbB1), HER2 (ErbB2), and HER4 (ErbB4); covalently and irreversibly binds to the intracellular tyrosine kinase domain, resulting in tumor growth inhibition and tumor regression. Inhibits autophosphorylation and proliferation (in vitro) in cell lines expressing both wild-type EGFR and selected EGFR mutations.

Pharmacodynamics/Kinetics
Absorption: Decreased with high-fat meals
Protein binding: ~95%
Metabolism: Covalently adducted to proteins and nucleophilic small molecules (minimal enzymatic metabolism) (Wind, 2013)
Bioavailability: Tablets: 92% (as compared to an oral solution)
Half-life elimination: 37 hours
Time to peak: 2 to 5 hours
Excretion: Feces (85%); urine (4%); primarily as unchanged drug

Dosing

Adult & Geriatric

Non-small cell lung cancer (NSCLC), metastatic, with EGFR exon 19 deletions or exon 21 (L858R) substitution mutations: Oral: 40 mg once daily until disease progression or unacceptable toxicity

NSCLC, metastatic squamous: Oral: 40 mg once daily until disease progression or unacceptable toxicity

Missed doses: Do not take a missed dose within 12 hours of next dose

Dosage adjustment for concomitant therapy:
P-gp inhibitors: If concomitant therapy is not tolerated, reduce afatinib daily dose by 10 mg. Upon discontinuation of the P-gp inhibitor, resume previous dose as tolerated.
P-gp inducers: Increase afatinib daily dose by 10 mg as tolerated if on chronic concomitant therapy with a P-gp inducer. Resume previous dose 2 to 3 days after discontinuation of P-gp inducer.

Renal Impairment Note: The manufacturer recommends using the Modification of Diet in Renal Disease (MDRD) formula to estimate the glomerular filtration rate (eGFR).

Preexisting impairment:
eGFR >30 mL/minute/1.73 m^2: No dosage adjustment is necessary.
eGFR 15 to 29 mL/minute/1.73 m^2: Reduce dose to 30 mg once daily.
eGFR <15 mL/minute/1.73 m^2 and hemodialysis: There are no dosage adjustments provided in the manufacturer's labeling (has not been studied).

Renal toxicity during treatment: If ≥ grade 2 renal toxicity occurs, withhold therapy. Upon improvement to baseline or ≤ grade 1, resume therapy at 10 mg per day less than previous dose.

Hepatic Impairment

Preexisting mild to moderate impairment (Child-Pugh class A or B): No dosage adjustment is necessary.

Preexisting severe impairment (Child-Pugh class C): There are no dosage adjustments provided in the manufacturer's labeling (has not been studied); closely monitor and adjust dose if necessary.

Hepatotoxicity during treatment: Withhold therapy for ≥ grade 3 hepatic dysfunction. Upon improvement to baseline or ≤ grade 1, resume therapy at 10 mg per day less than previous dose. Permanently discontinue for severe afatinib-induced hepatic impairment.

Adjustment for Toxicity Note: Permanently discontinue for intolerability or severe reaction occurring at a dose of 20 mg daily.

Cardiovascular: Permanently discontinue for symptomatic left ventricular dysfunction.

Dermatologic: Withhold therapy for prolonged (>7 days) or intolerable grade 2 or higher cutaneous reactions. Upon improvement to baseline or ≤ grade 1, resume therapy at 10 mg per day less than previous dose. Discontinue permanently for life-threatening bullous, blistering, or exfoliative skin lesions, as well as for suspected toxic epidermal necrolysis (TEN) or Stevens Johnson syndrome (SJS).

Gastrointestinal:

Diarrhea: Grade 2 or higher diarrhea that persists for ≥2 consecutive days despite antidiarrheal therapy: Interrupt therapy until resolution to ≤ grade 1, then resume at 10 mg per day less than previous dose.

Nausea/vomiting: For intolerable grade 2 or persistent (≥7 days) nausea/vomiting despite antiemetic therapy, the following recommendations have been made: Interrupt therapy for up to 14 days until resolution to ≤ grade 1, then resume at 10 mg per day less than previous dose; if symptoms do not resolve within 14 days, discontinue permanently (Giotrif Canadian product labeling 2016).

Ocular: Interrupt therapy for suspected keratitis; consider discontinuation if diagnosis of ulcerative keratitis is confirmed. Permanently discontinue for persistent ulcerative keratitis.

Pulmonary: Interrupt therapy for suspected interstitial lung disease (ILD); permanently discontinue if diagnosis is confirmed.

Other toxicity: Grade 3 or higher adverse reactions: Withhold therapy for ≥ grade 3 adverse reactions. Upon improvement to baseline or ≤ grade 1, resume therapy at 10 mg per day less than previous dose.

Administration Administer orally at least 1 hour before or 2 hours after a meal. Do not take a missed dose within 12 hours of the next dose.

Emetic Potential Low (10% to 30%)

Monitoring Parameters EGFR mutation status; liver and renal function (periodically); monitor for skin toxicity, diarrhea, signs/symptoms of dehydration; monitor for signs/symptoms of interstitial lung disease (eg, acute respiratory distress syndrome, allergic alveolitis, lung infiltration, pneumonitis) and keratitis (eg, acute or worsening eye inflammation, blurred vision, eye pain, lacrimation, light sensitivity, red eye). Consider left ventricular ejection fraction assessment prior to and during therapy in patients with cardiac risk factors or conditions that may impair left ventricular function.

◀ **Dosage Forms** Excipient information presented when available (limited, particularly for generics); consult specific product labeling.
Tablet, Oral:
  Gilotrif: 20 mg
  Gilotrif: 30 mg, 40 mg [contains fd&c blue #2 (indigotine)]
Dosage Forms: Canada Information with regard to form, strength, and availability of products uniquely available in Canada but currently not available in the US. Refer also to Dosage Forms.

  Excipient information presented when available (limited, particularly for generics); consult specific product labeling.
  Tablet, Oral:
    Giotrif: 20 mg, 30 mg, 40 mg

- ◆ **Afatinib Dimaleate** *see* Afatinib *on page 65*
- ◆ **Afinitor** *see* Everolimus *on page 744*
- ◆ **Afinitor Disperz** *see* Everolimus *on page 744*
- ◆ **Aflibercept I.V.** *see* Ziv-Aflibercept (Systemic) *on page 1940*
- ◆ **Afstyla** *see* Antihemophilic Factor (Recombinant) *on page 143*
- ◆ **AG-221** *see* Enasidenib *on page 676*
- ◆ **AG-013736** *see* Axitinib *on page 201*
- ◆ **AG014699** *see* Rucaparib *on page 1641*
- ◆ **AG-Ondansetron (Can)** *see* Ondansetron *on page 1380*
- ◆ **AgonEaze** *see* Lidocaine and Prilocaine *on page 1150*
- ◆ **Agrylin** *see* Anagrelide *on page 131*
- ◆ **AHF (Human)** *see* Antihemophilic Factor (Human) *on page 140*
- ◆ **AHF (Recombinant [Fc Fusion Protein])** *see* Antihemophilic Factor (Recombinant [Fc Fusion Protein]) *on page 147*
- ◆ **AHF (Recombinant [Pegylated])** *see* Antihemophilic Factor (Recombinant [Pegylated]) *on page 149*
- ◆ **AHF (Recombinant [Porcine Sequence])** *see* Antihemophilic Factor (Recombinant [Porcine Sequence]) *on page 151*
- ◆ **AHF (Recombinant)** *see* Antihemophilic Factor (Recombinant) *on page 143*
- ◆ **A-hydroCort** *see* Hydrocortisone (Systemic) *on page 921*
- ◆ **A-Hydrocort [DSC]** *see* Hydrocortisone (Systemic) *on page 921*
- ◆ **AJ-PIP/TAZ (Can)** *see* Piperacillin and Tazobactam *on page 1513*
- ◆ **Akynzeo** *see* Netupitant and Palonosetron *on page 1311*
- ◆ **ALA** *see* Aminolevulinic Acid (Topical) *on page 114*
- ◆ **5-ALA** *see* Aminolevulinic Acid (Systemic) *on page 114*
- ◆ **5-ALA** *see* Aminolevulinic Acid (Topical) *on page 114*
- ◆ **ALA HCl** *see* Aminolevulinic Acid (Systemic) *on page 114*
- ◆ **Albumin-Bound Paclitaxel** *see* PACLitaxel (Protein Bound) *on page 1411*
- ◆ **Albumin-Stabilized Nanoparticle Paclitaxel** *see* PACLitaxel (Protein Bound) *on page 1411*
- ◆ **Aldara** *see* Imiquimod *on page 987*
- ◆ **Aldara P (Can)** *see* Imiquimod *on page 987*

Aldesleukin (al des LOO kin)

Related Information

Management of Chemotherapy-Induced Nausea and Vomiting in Adults *on page 2253*

Prevention of Chemotherapy-Induced Nausea and Vomiting in Children *on page 2310*

Brand Names: US Proleukin

Brand Names: Canada Proleukin

Index Terms IL-2; Interleukin 2; Interleukin-2; Lymphocyte Mitogenic Factor; Recombinant Human Interleukin-2; T-Cell Growth Factor; TCGF; Thymocyte Stimulating Factor

Pharmacologic Category Antineoplastic Agent, Biological Response Modulator; Antineoplastic Agent, Miscellaneous

Use

Melanoma, metastatic: Treatment of metastatic melanoma

Renal cell cancer, metastatic: Treatment of metastatic renal cell cancer

Limitations of use: Careful patient selection is necessary. Assess performance status (PS); patients with a more favorable PS (Eastern Cooperative Oncology Group [ECOG] PS 0) at treatment initiation respond better to aldesleukin (higher response rate and lower toxicity). Experience in patients with ECOG PS >1 is limited.

Labeled Contraindications Hypersensitivity to aldesleukin or any component of the formulation; patients with abnormal thallium stress or pulmonary function tests; patients who have had an organ allograft. **Re-treatment is contraindicated** in patients who have experienced sustained ventricular tachycardia (≥5 beats), uncontrolled or unresponsive cardiac arrhythmias, chest pain with ECG changes consistent with angina or MI, cardiac tamponade, intubation >72 hours, renal failure requiring dialysis for >72 hours, coma or toxic psychosis lasting >48 hours, repetitive or refractory seizures, bowel ischemia/perforation, or GI bleeding requiring surgery.

Pregnancy Considerations Adverse events were observed in animal reproduction studies. Use during pregnancy only if benefits to the mother outweigh potential risk to the fetus. Effective contraception is recommended for fertile males and/or females using this medication.

Breastfeeding Considerations It is not known if aldesleukin is excreted in breast milk. Due to the potential for serious adverse reactions in the breast-feeding infant, a decision should be made to discontinue breastfeeding or to discontinue the drug, taking into account the importance of treatment to the mother.

Warnings/Precautions [US Boxed Warning]: Aldesleukin therapy has been associated with capillary leak syndrome (CLS), characterized by vascular tone loss and extravasation of plasma proteins and fluid into extravascular space. CLS results in hypotension and reduced organ perfusion, which may be severe and can result in death. Cardiac arrhythmia, angina, myocardial infarction, respiratory insufficiency (requiring intubation), gastrointestinal bleeding or infarction, renal insufficiency, edema and mental status changes are also associated with CLS. CLS onset is immediately after treatment initiation. Monitor fluid status and organ perfusion status carefully; consider fluids and/or pressor agents to maintain organ perfusion. **[US Boxed Warning]: Therapy should be restricted to patients with normal cardiac and pulmonary functions as defined by thallium stress and formal pulmonary function testing.** ▶

◄ Extreme caution should be used in patients with a history of prior cardiac or pulmonary disease and in patients who are fluid-restricted or where edema may be poorly tolerated. In a scientific statement from the American Heart Association, interleukin-2 has been determined to be an agent that may either cause direct myocardial toxicity (rare) or exacerbate underlying myocardial dysfunction (magnitude: major) (AHA [Page 2016]). Withhold treatment for signs of organ hypoperfusion, including altered mental status, reduced urine output, systolic BP <90 mm Hg or cardiac arrhythmia. Once blood pressure is normalized, may consider diuretics for excessive weight gain/edema. Recovery from CLS generally begins soon after treatment cessation. Perform a thorough clinical evaluation prior to treatment initiation; exclude patients with significant cardiac, pulmonary, renal, hepatic, or central nervous system impairment from treatment. Patients with a more favorable performance status prior to treatment initiation are more likely to respond to aldesleukin treatment, with a higher response rate and generally lower toxicity.

[US Boxed Warning]: Should be administered under the supervision of an experienced cancer chemotherapy physician in a facility with cardiopulmonary or intensive specialists and intensive care facilities available. Adverse effects are frequent and sometimes fatal. May exacerbate preexisting or initial presentation of autoimmune diseases and inflammatory disorders; exacerbation and/or new onset have been reported with aldesleukin and interferon alfa combination therapy. Thyroid disease (hypothyroidism, biphasic thyroiditis, and thyrotoxicosis) may occur; the onset of hypothyroidism is usually 4 to 17 weeks after treatment initiation; may be reversible upon treatment discontinuation (Hamnvik, 2011). Patients should be evaluated and treated for CNS metastases and have a negative scan prior to treatment; new neurologic symptoms and lesions have been reported in patients without preexisting evidence of CNS metastases (symptoms generally improve upon discontinuation, however, cases with permanent damage have been reported). Mental status changes (irritability, confusion, depression) can occur and may indicate bacteremia, sepsis, hypoperfusion, CNS malignancy, or CNS toxicity. May cause seizure; use with caution in patients with seizure disorder. Ethanol use may increase CNS adverse effects.

[US Boxed Warning]: Impaired neutrophil function is associated with treatment; patients are at risk for disseminated infection (including sepsis and bacterial endocarditis), and central line-related gram-positive infections. Treat preexisting bacterial infection appropriately prior to treatment initiation. Antibiotic prophylaxis that has been associated with a reduced incidence of staphylococcal infections in aldesleukin studies includes the use of oxacillin, nafcillin, ciprofloxacin, or vancomycin. Monitor for signs of infection or sepsis during treatment.

[US Boxed Warning]: Withhold treatment for patients developing moderate-to-severe lethargy or somnolence; continued treatment may result in coma. Standard prophylactic supportive care during high-dose aldesleukin treatment includes acetaminophen to relieve constitutional symptoms and an H_2 antagonist to reduce the risk of GI ulceration and/or bleeding. May impair renal or hepatic function; patients must have a serum creatinine ≤1.5 mg/dL prior to treatment. Concomitant nephrotoxic or hepatotoxic agents may increase the risk of renal or hepatic toxicity. Potentially significant drug-drug interactions may exist, requiring dose or frequency adjustment, additional monitoring, and/or selection of alternative therapy. Enhancement of cellular immune function may increase the risk of allograft rejection in transplant patients. An acute array of symptoms resembling aldesleukin adverse reactions (fever, chills, nausea, rash, pruritus, diarrhea, hypotension, edema, and oliguria) were observed within 1 to 4 hours after iodinated contrast media administration, usually when given within 4 weeks after aldesleukin treatment, although has been reported several months after aldesleukin treatment. The incidence of dyspnea and severe urogenital toxicities is potentially increased in elderly patients. Aldesleukin doses >12 to 15 million units/m^2 are associated with a moderate emetic potential; antiemetics are recommended to prevent nausea and vomiting (Dupuis, 2011).

Adverse Reactions

>10%:

Cardiovascular: Hypotension (71%, grade 4: 3%), peripheral edema (28%), tachycardia (23%), edema (15%), vasodilatation (13%), supraventricular tachycardia (12%, grade 4: 1%), cardiac disease (11%; includes blood pressure changes, HF and ECG changes)

Central nervous system: Chills (52%), confusion (34%, grade 4: 1%), malaise (27%), drowsiness (22%), anxiety (12%), pain (12%), dizziness (11%)

Dermatologic: Skin rash (42%), pruritus (24%), exfoliative dermatitis (18%)

Endocrine & metabolic: Weight gain (16%), acidosis (12%, grade 4: 1%), hypomagnesemia (12%), hypocalcemia (11%)

Gastrointestinal: Diarrhea (67%, grade 4: 2%), vomiting (19% to 50%, grade 4: 1%), nausea (19% to 35%), stomatitis (22%), anorexia (20%), abdominal pain (11%)

Genitourinary: Oliguria (63%, grade 4: 6%)

Hematologic & oncologic: Thrombocytopenia (37%, grade 4: 1%), anemia (29%), leukopenia (16%)

Hepatic: Hyperbilirubinemia (40%, grade 4: 2%), increased serum AST (23%, grade 4: 1%)

Immunologic: Antibody development (66% to 74%)

Infection: Infection (13%, grade 4: 1%)

Miscellaneous: Fever (29%, grade 4: 1%)

Neuromuscular & skeletal: Weakness (23%)

Renal: Increased serum creatinine (33%, grade 4: 1%)

Respiratory: Dyspnea (43%, grade 4: 1%), pulmonary disease (24%; includes pulmonary congestion, rales, rhonchi), cough (11%), respiratory tract disease (11%; includes acute respiratory distress syndrome, pulmonary infiltrates, and pulmonary changes)

1% to 10%:

Cardiovascular: Cardiac arrhythmia (10%), cardiac arrest (grade 4: 1%), myocardial infarction (grade 4: 1%), ventricular tachycardia (grade 4: 1%)

Central nervous system: Coma (grade 4: 2%), psychosis (grade 4: 1%), stupor (grade 4: 1%)

Gastrointestinal: Enlargement of abdomen (10%)

Genitourinary: Anuria (grade 4: 5%)

Hematologic & oncologic: Blood coagulation disorder (grade 4: 1%; includes intravascular coagulopathy)

Hepatic: Increased serum alkaline phosphatase (10%)

Infection: Sepsis (grade 4: 1%)

Renal: Acute renal failure (grade 4: 1%)

Respiratory: Rhinitis (10%), apnea (grade 4: 1%)

◄ <1%, postmarketing, and/or case reports: Agitation, allergic interstitial nephritis, anaphylaxis, angioedema, asthma, atrial arrhythmia, atrioventricular block, blindness (transient or permanent), bowel infarction, bradycardia, brain disease, bullous pemphigoid, capillary leak syndrome, cardiomyopathy, cellulitis, cerebral edema, cerebral lesion, cerebral vasculitis, cerebrovascular accident, cholecystitis, colitis, delirium, depression (severe; leading to suicide), diabetes mellitus, duodenal ulcer, endocarditis, eosinophilia, exacerbation of Crohn's disease, extrapyramidal reaction, gastritis, hematemesis, hemoptysis, hemorrhage (including cerebral, gastrointestinal, retroperitoneal, subarachnoid, subdural), hepatic failure, hepatitis, hepatosplenomegaly, hypertension, hyperthyroidism, hyperuricemia, hyperventilation, hypothermia, hypoventilation, hypoxia, IgA glomerulonephritis (crescentic), increased blood urea nitrogen, increased nonprotein nitrogen, inflammatory arthritis, insomnia, intestinal necrosis, intestinal obstruction, intestinal perforation, ischemic heart disease, leukocytosis, lymphocytopenia, malignant hyperthermia, meningitis, myasthenia gravis (oculo-bulbar), mydriasis, myocarditis, myopathy, myositis, neuralgia, neuritis, neuropathy, neutropenia, optic neuritis, pancreatitis, paranoia, pericardial effusion, pericarditis, peripheral gangrene, phlebitis, pneumonia, pneumothorax, pulmonary edema, pulmonary embolism, renal tubular necrosis, respiratory acidosis, respiratory arrest, respiratory failure, restricted systemic blood flow, rhabdomyolysis, scleroderma, seizure, shock, Stevens-Johnson syndrome, syncope, thrombosis, thyroiditis, tissue necrosis at injection site, tracheoesophageal fistula, transient ischemic attacks, urticaria, ventricular premature contractions

Drug Interactions
Metabolism/Transport Effects None known.
Avoid Concomitant Use
Avoid concomitant use of Aldesleukin with any of the following: BCG (Intravesical); Corticosteroids; Deferiprone; Dipyrone

Increased Effect/Toxicity
Aldesleukin may increase the levels/effects of: Amifostine; Antipsychotic Agents (Second Generation [Atypical]); CloZAPine; Deferiprone; DULoxetine; Iodinated Contrast Agents; Levodopa; Nitroprusside; Pholcodine

The levels/effects of Aldesleukin may be increased by: Alfuzosin; Barbiturates; Benperidol; Blood Pressure Lowering Agents; Brimonidine (Topical); Diazoxide; Dipyrone; Herbs (Hypotensive Properties); Interferons (Alfa); Lormetazepam; Molsidomine; Naftopidil; Nicergoline; Nicorandil; Obinutuzumab; Pentoxifylline; Phosphodiesterase 5 Inhibitors; Promazine; Prostacyclin Analogues; Quinagolide

Decreased Effect
Aldesleukin may decrease the levels/effects of: BCG (Intravesical)

The levels/effects of Aldesleukin may be decreased by: Corticosteroids

Storage/Stability Store intact vials under refrigeration at 2°C to 8°C (36°F to 46°F). Protect from light. Plastic (polyvinyl chloride) bags result in more consistent drug delivery and are recommended. According to the manufacturer, reconstituted vials and solutions diluted in D5W for infusion are stable for 48 hours at room temperature or refrigerated although refrigeration is preferred because they do not contain preservatives. Do not freeze.

Preparation for Administration Reconstitute vials with 1.2 mL SWFI (preservative free) to a concentration of 18 million units (1.1 mg)/1 mL (sterile water should be injected towards the side of the vial). Gently swirl; do not

shake. Further dilute with 50 mL of D5W. Smaller volumes of D5W should be used for doses ≤1.5 mg; avoid concentrations <30 **mcg**/mL and >70 **mcg**/mL (an increased variability in drug delivery has been seen). Plastic (polyvinyl chloride) bags result in more consistent drug delivery and are recommended. Filtration may result in loss of bioactivity. Addition of 0.1% albumin has been used to increase stability and decrease the extent of sorption if low final concentrations cannot be avoided.

Avoid bacteriostatic water for injection and NS for reconstitution or dilution; increased aggregation may occur.

Mechanism of Action Aldesleukin is a human recombinant interleukin-2 product which promotes proliferation, differentiation, and recruitment of T and B cells, natural killer (NK) cells, and thymocytes; causes cytolytic activity in a subset of lymphocytes and subsequent interactions between the immune system and malignant cells; can stimulate lymphokine-activated killer (LAK) cells and tumor-infiltrating lymphocytes (TIL) cells.

Pharmacodynamics/Kinetics

Absorption: Oral: Not absorbed

Distribution: Primarily into plasma, lymphocytes, lungs, liver, kidney, and spleen; V_d: 6.3 to 7.9 L (Whittington 1993)

Metabolism: Renal (metabolized to amino acids in the cells lining the proximal convoluted tubules of the kidney)

Half-life elimination: IV:

Children: Distribution: 14 ± 6 minutes; Elimination: 51 ± 11 minutes

Adults: Distribution: 13 minutes; Terminal: 85 minutes

Excretion: Urine (primarily as metabolites)

Dosing

Adult & Geriatric Consider premedication with an antipyretic to reduce fever, an H_2 antagonist for prophylaxis of gastrointestinal irritation/bleeding, antiemetics, and antidiarrheals; continue for 12 hours after the last aldesleukin dose. Antibiotic prophylaxis is recommended to reduce the incidence of infection. Aldesleukin doses >12 to 15 million units/m^2 are associated with a moderate emetic potential; antiemetics are recommended to prevent nausea and vomiting

Renal cell carcinoma, metastatic: IV: 600,000 units/kg every 8 hours for a maximum of 14 doses; repeat after 9 days for a total of 28 doses per course; re-treat if tumor shrinkage observed (and if no contraindications) at least 7 weeks after hospital discharge date

   or

Off-label dosing: 720,000 units/kg every 8 hours for up to 12 doses; repeat with a second cycle 10 to 15 days later (Klapper, 2008)

Melanoma, metastatic: IV:

Single-agent use: 600,000 units/kg every 8 hours for a maximum of 14 doses; repeat after 9 days for a total of 28 doses per course; re-treat if tumor shrinkage observed (and if no contraindications) at least 7 weeks after hospital discharge date

   or

Off-label dosing: 720,000 units/kg every 8 hours for 12 to 15 doses; repeat with a second cycle ~14 days after the first dose of the initial cycle (Smith, 2008)

Combination biochemotherapy (off-label use): 9 million units/m^2/day continuous infusion over 24 hours for 4 days every 3 weeks for up to 4 cycles (Atkins, 2008) **or** 9 million units/m^2/day continuous infusion over 24 hours days 5 to 8, 17 to 20, and 26 to 29 every 42 days for up to 5 cycles (Eton, 2002) **or** 9 million units/m^2/day continuous infusion over 24 hours for 4 days every 3 weeks for 6 cycles (Legha, 1998)

Pediatric Consider premedication with an antipyretic to reduce fever, an H$_2$ antagonist for prophylaxis of gastrointestinal irritation/bleeding, antiemetics, and antidiarrheals; continue for 12 hours after the last aldesleukin dose. Antibiotic prophylaxis is recommended to reduce the incidence of infection. Aldesleukin doses >12 to 15 million units/m^2 are associated with a moderate emetic potential; antiemetics are recommended to prevent nausea and vomiting (Dupuis, 2011).

Neuroblastoma (off-label use): IV: 3 million units/m^2/day continuous infusion over 24 hours daily for 4 days during week 1 and 4.5 million units/m^2/day continuous infusion over 24 hours daily for 4 days during week 2 of cycles 2 and 4 (regimen also includes isotretinoin, dinutuximab, and sargramostim) (Yu, 2010).

Renal Impairment Adults:

Renal impairment prior to treatment initiation:
Serum creatinine ≤1.5 mg/dL: There are no dosage adjustments provided in the manufacturer's labeling.
Serum creatinine >1.5 mg/dL: Do not initiate treatment.

Renal toxicity during treatment:
Serum creatinine >4.5 mg/dL (or ≥4 mg/dL with severe volume overload, acidosis, or hyperkalemia): Withhold dose; may resume when <4 mg/dL and fluid/electrolyte status is stable.
Persistent oliguria or urine output <10 mL/hour for 16 to 24 hours with rising serum creatinine: Withhold dose; may resume when urine output >10 mL/hour with serum creatinine decrease of >1.5 mg/dL or normalization.
Hemodialysis: Re-treatment is contraindicated in patients with renal failure requiring dialysis for >72 hours.

Hepatic Impairment Adults:

Hepatic impairment prior to treatment initiation: There are no dosage adjustments provided in the manufacturer's labeling.
Hepatotoxicity during treatment: Signs of hepatic failure (encephalopathy, increasing ascites, liver pain, hypoglycemia): Withhold dose and discontinue treatment for balance of cycle; may initiate a new course if indicated only after at least 7 weeks past resolution of all signs of hepatic failure (including hospital discharge).

Adjustment for Toxicity Withhold or interrupt a dose for toxicity; do not reduce the dose.

Cardiovascular toxicity:
Atrial fibrillation, supraventricular tachycardia, or bradycardia that is persistent, recurrent, or requires treatment: Withhold dose; may resume when asymptomatic with full recovery to normal sinus rhythm.
Systolic BP <90 mm Hg (with increasing pressor requirements): Withhold dose; may resume treatment when systolic BP ≥90 mm Hg and stable or pressor requirements improve.
Any ECG change consistent with MI, ischemia or myocarditis (with or without chest pain), or suspected cardiac ischemia: Withhold dose; may resume when asymptomatic, MI/myocarditis have been ruled out, suspicion of angina is low, or there is no evidence of ventricular hypokinesia.

CNS toxicity: Mental status change, including moderate confusion or agitation: Withhold dose; may resume when resolved completely.

Dermatologic toxicity: Bullous dermatitis or marked worsening of preexisting skin condition: Withhold dose; may treat with antihistamines or topical products (do not use topical steroids); may resume with resolution of all signs of bullous dermatitis.

Gastrointestinal: Stool guaiac repeatedly >3-4+: Withhold dose; may resume with negative stool guaiac.

Infection: Sepsis syndrome, clinically unstable: Withhold dose; may resume when sepsis syndrome has resolved, patient is clinically stable, and infection is under treatment.

Respiratory toxicity: Oxygen saturation <90%: Withhold dose; may resume when >90%.

Re-treatment with aldesleukin is contraindicated with the following toxicities: Sustained ventricular tachycardia (≥5 beats), uncontrolled or unresponsive cardiac arrhythmias, chest pain with ECG changes consistent with angina or MI, cardiac tamponade, intubation >72 hours, renal failure requiring dialysis for >72 hours, coma or toxic psychosis lasting >48 hours, repetitive or refractory seizures, bowel ischemia/perforation, or GI bleeding requiring surgery

Combination Regimens

Melanoma: CVD-Interleukin-Interferon (Melanoma) on page 2075

Renal cell cancer: Interleukin 2-Interferon Alfa-2 (RCC) on page 2156

Administration Aldesleukin doses >12 to 15 million units/m^2 are associated with a moderate emetic potential; antiemetics are recommended to prevent nausea and vomiting (Dupuis, 2011).

Administer as IV infusion over 15 minutes (do not administer with an inline filter). Allow solution to reach room temperature prior to administration. Flush before and after with D5W, particularly if maintenance IV line contains sodium chloride. Some off-label uses/doses are infused as a continuous infusion (Legha, 1998; Yu, 2010). Has also been administered by SubQ injection (off-label route).

Emetic Potential Children and Adults:

>12 million units/m^2: Moderate (30% to 90%)

≤12 million units/m^2: Low (10% to 30%)

Monitoring Parameters

Baseline and periodic: CBC with differential and platelets, blood chemistries including electrolytes, renal and hepatic function tests, and chest x-ray; pulmonary function tests and arterial blood gases (baseline), thallium stress test (prior to treatment). Monitor thyroid function tests (TSH at baseline then every 2-3 months during aldesleukin treatment [Hamnvik, 2011]).

Monitoring during therapy should include daily (hourly if hypotensive) vital signs (temperature, pulse, blood pressure, and respiration rate), weight and fluid intake and output; in a patient with a decreased blood pressure, especially systolic BP <90 mm Hg, cardiac monitoring for rhythm should be conducted. If an abnormal complex or rhythm is seen, an ECG should be performed; vital signs in these hypotension patients should be taken hourly and central venous pressure (CVP) checked; monitor for change in mental status, and for signs of infection.

Additional Information 18 x 10^6 units = 1.1 mg protein

◄ **Dosage Forms** Excipient information presented when available (limited, particularly for generics); consult specific product labeling.
Solution Reconstituted, Intravenous [preservative free]:
  Proleukin: 22,000,000 units (1 ea)

♦ **Alecensa** see Alectinib on page 78
♦ **Alecensaro (Can)** see Alectinib on page 78

Alectinib (al EK ti nib)

Related Information
Common Toxicity Criteria on page 2242
Management of Chemotherapy-Induced Nausea and Vomiting in Adults on page 2253
Safe Handling of Hazardous Drugs on page 2379

Brand Names: US Alecensa

Brand Names: Canada Alecensaro

Index Terms AF802; Alectinib Hydrochloride; CH5424802; RG7853; RO5424802; UNII-LIJ4CT1Z3Y

Pharmacologic Category Antineoplastic Agent, Anaplastic Lymphoma Kinase Inhibitor; Antineoplastic Agent, Tyrosine Kinase Inhibitor

Use Non-small cell lung cancer, metastatic: Treatment of patients with anaplastic lymphoma kinase (ALK)-positive, metastatic non-small cell lung cancer (NSCLC) who have progressed on or are intolerant to crizotinib.

Labeled Contraindications There are no contraindications listed in the manufacturer's US labeling.
Canadian labeling: Known hypersensitivity to alectinib or any component of the formulation.

Pregnancy Considerations Based on data from animal reproduction studies and its mechanism of action, alectinib may be expected to cause fetal harm if administered during pregnancy. Women of reproductive potential should use effective contraception during therapy and for 1 week after the final dose. Males with female partners of reproductive potential should use effective contraception during therapy and for 3 months after the last dose.

Breastfeeding Considerations It is not known if alectinib is excreted in breast milk. Due to the potential for serious adverse reactions in the nursing infant, the manufacturer does not recommend breastfeeding during therapy or for 1 week after the final dose.

Warnings/Precautions Liver function test abnormalities have been reported, including elevations of AST/ALT >5 times ULN and bilirubin >3 times ULN; most abnormalities occurred during the first 3 months of therapy. Concurrent ALT/AST elevations ≥3 times ULN and total bilirubin ≥2 times ULN with normal alkaline phosphatase occurred rarely. Liver biopsy demonstrated drug induced liver injury in some patients with grade 3 to 4 AST or ALT elevations. Monitor liver function tests (ALT, AST, and total bilirubin) every 2 weeks during the first 3 months of therapy and then once a month and as clinically necessary; monitor more frequently in patients who develop transaminase and bilirubin elevations. May require therapy interruption, dose reduction, or permanent discontinuation. Severe interstitial lung disease (ILD) has been reported rarely. Monitor for ILD/pneumonitis; evaluate promptly in patients who present with worsening of respiratory symptoms or who have signs/symptoms suggestive of ILD/pneumonitis (eg, cough, dyspnea, fever). Immediately interrupt therapy for confirmed ILD/pneumonitis; permanently discontinue if alectinib is determined to be the causative factor.

Symptomatic bradycardia may occur; heart rate <50 beats per minute has been reported in ~20% of patients treated with alectinib. Monitor heart rate and blood pressure regularly. If symptomatic bradycardia (non-life-threatening) occurs, withhold treatment until recovery to asymptomatic bradycardia or to a heart rate of ≥60 beats per minute, evaluate concurrent medications, and potentially reduce alectinib dose. Permanently discontinue for life-threatening bradycardia due to alectinib if no contributing concomitant medication is identified and for recurrent bradycardia. If life-threatening bradycardia occurs and concurrent medications associated with bradycardia can be discontinued or dose adjusted, restart alectinib at a reduced dose (with frequent monitoring). Myalgia or musculoskeletal pain occurred in over one-quarter of patients treated with alectinib (including grade 3 toxicity). Elevations of creatine phosphokinase (CPK) were reported in close to half of patients in clinical trials. The median time to grade 3 CPK elevations was 14 days. Monitor; advise patients to report unexplained muscle pain, tenderness, or weakness. Assess CPK every 2 weeks for the first month of therapy and then as clinically necessary. May require therapy interruption and/or dose reduction.

Photosensitivity occurred in some patients. Patients should avoid sun exposure (during treatment and for 7 days after the final dose) and use a broad spectrum sunscreen and lip balm (SPF ≥50). Approved for use only in patients with metastatic non-small cell lung cancer (NSCLC) who test positive for the abnormal anaplastic lymphoma kinase (ALK) gene. Potentially significant interactions may exist, requiring dose or frequency adjustment, additional monitoring, and/or selection of alternative therapy.

Adverse Reactions

>10%:

Cardiovascular: Edema (30%), bradycardia (8% to 20%)

Central nervous system: Fatigue (≤41%), headache (17%)

Dermatologic: Skin rash (18%)

Endocrine & metabolic: Hyperglycemia (36%), hypocalcemia (32%), hypokalemia (29%), hypophosphatemia (21%), hyponatremia (20%), weight gain (11%)

Gastrointestinal: Constipation (34%), nausea (18%), diarrhea (16%), vomiting (12%)

Hematologic & oncologic: Anemia (56%, grades 3/4: 2%), lymphocytopenia (22%, grades 3/4: 5%)

Hepatic: Increased serum AST (51%, grades 3/4: 4%), increased serum alkaline phosphatase (47%), hyperbilirubinemia (39%, grades 3/4: 2% to 3%), increased serum ALT (34%, grades 3/4: 5%)

Neuromuscular & skeletal: Increased creatine phosphokinase (43%, grades 3/4: 5%), weakness (≤41%), musculoskeletal pain (≤29%), myalgia (≤29%), back pain (12%)

Renal: Increased serum creatinine (28%)

Respiratory: Cough (19%), dyspnea (16%)

1% to 10%:

Cardiovascular: Pulmonary embolism (1%)

Dermatologic: Photosensitivity dermatitis (10%)

Ophthalmic: Visual disturbances (10%)

<1%, postmarketing, and/or case reports: Interstitial pulmonary disease, pneumonitis

◀ **Drug Interactions**

Metabolism/Transport Effects Substrate of CYP3A4 (minor); **Note:** Assignment of Major/Minor substrate status based on clinically relevant drug interaction potential

Avoid Concomitant Use

Avoid concomitant use of Alectinib with any of the following: Ceritinib

Increased Effect/Toxicity

Alectinib may increase the levels/effects of: Bradycardia-Causing Agents; Ceritinib; Ivabradine; Lacosamide

The levels/effects of Alectinib may be increased by: Bretylium; Ruxolitinib; Tofacitinib

Decreased Effect There are no known significant interactions involving a decrease in effect.

Hazardous Drugs Handling Considerations

Hazardous agent (meets NIOSH 2016 criteria). This medication is not on the NIOSH (2016) list; however, it meets the criteria for a hazardous drug. Drugs are classified as hazardous based on their properties; the properties of a hazardous drug include one or more of the following characteristics: carcinogenic, teratogenic (or other developmental toxicity), reproductive toxicity, organotoxic at low doses, genotoxic, and/or new agents with structural or toxicity profiles similar to existing hazardous agents.

Use appropriate precautions for receiving, handling, administration, and disposal. Gloves (single) should be worn during receiving, unpacking, and placing in storage. NIOSH recommends single gloving for administration of intact tablets or capsules (NIOSH 2016).

Storage/Stability Store at ≤30°C (86°F); store in original container to protect from light and moisture.

Mechanism of Action Alectinib is a tyrosine kinase receptor inhibitor which inhibits anaplastic lymphoma kinase (ALK) and RET (with similar potency to ALK; Ou 2016). ALK gene abnormalities due to mutations or translocations may result in expression of oncogenic fusion proteins (eg, ALK fusion protein) which alter signaling and expression and result in increased cellular proliferation and survival in tumors which express these fusion proteins. Inhibition of ALK phosphorylation and ALK-mediated activation of downstream signaling results in decreased tumor cell viability. Alectinib is more potent than crizotinib against ALK, and can inhibit most of the clinically observed acquired ALK resistance mutations to crizotinib (Ou 2016).

Pharmacodynamics/Kinetics

Absorption: A high-fat, high-calorie meal increased the combined exposure of alectinib plus its active metabolite M4 by 3.1-fold

Distribution: Parent drug: 4,016 L; M4 (active metabolite): 10,093 L; distributes in the CSF at approximately the free concentrations in plasma

Protein binding: >99% to plasma proteins

Metabolism: Hepatic via CYP3A4 to major active metabolite M4; M4 is also metabolized by CYP3A4

Bioavailability: 37% (under fed conditions)

Half-life elimination: Parent drug: 33 hours; M4: 31 hours

Time to peak: 4 hours

Excretion: Feces (98%; 84% as unchanged parent drug and 6% as M4); urine (<0.5%)

Dosing

Adult & Geriatric

Non-small cell lung cancer (NSCLC), metastatic (ALK-positive): Oral: 600 mg twice daily; continue until disease progression or unacceptable toxicity (Ou 2016)

Missed doses: If a dose is missed or if vomiting occurs, take the next dose at the regularly scheduled time.

Renal Impairment

CrCl ≥30 mL/minute: No dosage adjustment is necessary.

CrCl <30 mL/minute or ESRD: There are no dosage adjustments provided in the manufacturer's labeling (has not been studied).

Hepatic Impairment

Preexisting hepatic impairment:

Mild impairment (total bilirubin ≤ULN and AST >ULN **or** total bilirubin >1 to 1.5 times ULN and any AST): No dosage adjustment is necessary.

Moderate or severe impairment: There are no dosage adjustments provided in the manufacturer's labeling (has not been studied).

Hepatotoxicity during treatment:

ALT or AST >5 times ULN **and** total bilirubin ≤2 times ULN: Withhold alectinib; upon recovery to baseline or to ALT/AST ≤3 times ULN, may resume at a reduced dose.

ALT or AST >3 times ULN **and** total bilirubin >2 times ULN (in the absence of cholestasis or hemolysis): Permanently discontinue.

Total bilirubin >3 times ULN: Withhold alectinib; upon recovery to baseline or to total bilirubin ≤1.5 times ULN, may resume at a reduced dose.

Adjustment for Toxicity

Recommended alectinib dosage reductions for toxicity:

Initial starting dose: 600 mg twice daily

First dose reduction: 450 mg twice daily

Second dose reduction: 300 mg twice daily

If unable to tolerate 300 mg twice daily, discontinue alectinib

Cardiac toxicity:

Symptomatic bradycardia: Withhold alectinib until recovery to asymptomatic bradycardia or until the heart rate is ≥60 beats per minutes (bpm). If a contributing concomitant medication is identified and discontinued (or dose adjusted), resume alectinib at the previous dose upon recovery (to asymptomatic bradycardia or heart rate ≥60 bpm). If no contributing concomitant medication is identified (or cannot be discontinued or dose adjusted), resume alectinib at a reduced dose upon recovery (to asymptomatic bradycardia or heart rate ≥60 bpm).

Life-threatening bradycardia/heart rate <60 bpm (urgent intervention required): Permanently discontinue alectinib if no contributing concomitant medication is identified. If a contributing concomitant medication is identified and discontinued (or dose adjusted), resume alectinib (with frequent monitoring) at a reduced dose upon recovery to asymptomatic bradycardia or to a heart rate ≥60 bpm. Permanently discontinue for recurrent life-threatening bradycardia.

CPK elevation:

CPK >5 times ULN: Withhold alectinib; upon recovery to baseline or to ≤2.5 times ULN, may resume alectinib at the same dose.

CPK >10 times ULN or 2nd occurrence of CPK >5 times ULN: Withhold alectinib; upon recovery to baseline or to ≤2.5 times ULN, may resume alectinib at a reduced dose.

◀ *Pulmonary toxicity:* Interstitial lung disease (ILD)/pneumonitis, any grade (treatment-related): Permanently discontinue

Administration Administer with food. Swallow capsule whole; do not open or dissolve the contents of the capsule. If vomiting occurs after taking the dose, do not administer an extra dose; administer the next dose at the regularly scheduled time.

Emetic Potential Minimal (<10%)

Monitoring Parameters Test for ALK positivity. Liver function tests (ALT, AST, total bilirubin) every 2 weeks during the first 3 months of therapy, then monthly and as clinically necessary (monitor more frequently in patients who develop transaminase and bilirubin elevations; CPK levels every 2 weeks for the first month of therapy, then as clinically necessary; monitor heart rate and blood pressure regularly; monitor for signs/symptoms of interstitial lung disease/pneumonitis and myalgia.

Prescribing and Access Restrictions Available through specialty pharmacies and distributors. Further information may be obtained from the manufacturer, Genentech, at 1-888-249-4918 or at https://www.alecensa. com/.

Dosage Forms Excipient information presented when available (limited, particularly for generics); consult specific product labeling.
Capsule, Oral:
Alecensa: 150 mg

Dosage Forms: Canada Information with regard to form, strength, and availability of products uniquely available in Canada but currently not available in the US. Refer also to Dosage Forms.

Excipient information presented when available (limited, particularly for generics); consult specific product labeling.
Capsule, Oral:
Alecensaro: 150 mg

◆ **Alectinib Hydrochloride** *see* Alectinib *on page 78*

Alemtuzumab (ay lem TU zoo mab)

Related Information
Common Toxicity Criteria *on page 2242*
Hematopoietic Cell Transplantation *on page 2365*
Management of Chemotherapy-Induced Nausea and Vomiting in Adults *on page 2253*
Prevention of Chemotherapy-Induced Nausea and Vomiting in Children *on page 2310*

Brand Names: US Campath; Lemtrada

Brand Names: Canada Lemtrada; MabCampath

Index Terms Anti-CD52 Monoclonal Antibody; Campath-1H; Humanized IgG1 Anti-CD52 Monoclonal Antibody; MoAb CD52; Monoclonal Antibody Campath-1H; Monoclonal Antibody CD52

Pharmacologic Category Antineoplastic Agent, Anti-CD52; Antineoplastic Agent, Monoclonal Antibody; Monoclonal Antibody

Use
B-cell chronic lymphocytic leukemia: Campath or MabCampath [Canadian product]: Treatment (as a single agent) of B-cell chronic lymphocytic leukemia (B-CLL)

Multiple sclerosis, relapsing: Lemtrada: Treatment of patients with relapsing forms of multiple sclerosis (MS), generally who have had an inadequate response to 2 or more medications indicated for the treatment of MS.

Labeled Contraindications

US labeling: Lemtrada is contraindicated in patients infected with HIV (due to prolonged reduction in CD4+ lymphocytes). There are no contraindications listed in the manufacturer's Campath labeling.

Canadian labeling:

Lemtrada: Hypersensitivity to alemtuzumab or any component of the formulation; HIV infection; active or latent tuberculosis; severe active infections; active malignancies; concurrent antineoplastic or immunosuppressive therapy; history of progressive multifocal leukoencephalopathy (PML)

MabCampath: Known type 1 hypersensitivity or anaphylactic reactions to alemtuzumab or any component of the formulation; active infections; underlying immunodeficiency (eg, seropositive for HIV); active secondary malignancies; current or history of progressive multifocal leukoencephalopathy (PML)

Pregnancy Considerations Adverse events were observed in animal reproduction studies. Human IgG is known to cross the placental barrier; therefore, alemtuzumab may also cross the barrier and cause fetal B- and T-lymphocyte depletion. Use during pregnancy only if the benefit to the mother outweighs the potential risk to the fetus. Effective contraception is recommended during and for at least 6 months (Campath) or 4 months (Lemtrada) after treatment for women of childbearing potential and men of reproductive potential.

Breastfeeding Considerations Human IgG is excreted in breast milk; therefore, alemtuzumab may also be excreted in milk. Due to the potential for serious adverse reactions in the nursing infant, the decision to discontinue alemtuzumab or to discontinue breastfeeding should take into account the importance of treatment to the mother and the half-life of alemtuzumab. The Canadian labeling recommends discontinuing nursing during treatment and for at least 3 months (MabCampath) or 4 months (Lemtrada) after completing treatment course.

Warnings/Precautions [US Boxed Warning (Lemtrada)]: Alemtuzumab causes serious, sometimes fatal, autoimmune conditions, such as immune thrombocytopenia and antiglomerular basement membrane disease, in patients receiving alemtuzumab for the treatment of multiple sclerosis (MS). Monitor complete blood counts with differential, serum creatinine levels, and urinalysis with urine cell counts at periodic intervals for 48 months after the last dose of alemtuzumab. Monitor for symptoms of immune thrombocytopenia (easy bruising, petechiae, spontaneous mucocutaneous bleeding, heavy menstrual bleeding) in patients receiving alemtuzumab for MS. Monitor for nephropathy symptoms (eg, elevated serum creatinine, hematuria, proteinuria). Alveolar hemorrhage manifesting as hemoptysis may be present in antiglomerular basement membrane disease. Glomerular nephropathies require urgent evaluation; may lead to renal failure if not treated. Prompt intervention is necessary for autoimmune cytopenias. Immune thrombocytopenia (formerly known as idiopathic thrombocytopenic purpura), thyroid disorders, autoimmune hemolytic anemia, autoimmune pancytopenia, undifferentiated connective tissue disorders, acquired hemophilia A, rheumatoid arthritis, vitiligo, retinal pigment epitheliopathy have been reported in patients receiving alemtuzumab for MS. Guillain-Barre syndrome and chronic inflammatory demyelinating polyradiculoneuropathy have been reported in patients receiving alemtuzumab for other uses. Alemtuzumab may increase the risk for other autoimmune conditions. Autoimmune thyroid disorders occurred in over one-third of patients receiving alemtuzumab for MS. In a trial evaluating alemtuzumab versus interferon beta-1a in patients with MS, thyroid dysfunction occurred more frequently in patients taking alemtuzumab (34% versus 6.5%) (Daniels, 2014). The incidence of the first episode of thyroid dysfunction increased annually the first 3 years (year 1: 4.6%; year 2: 13.3%; year 3: 16.1%) then gradually decreased thereafter. Among patients with alemtuzumab-related thyroid dysfunction, Graves' hyperthyroidism occurred most commonly (23%), followed by hypothyroidism and subacute thyroiditis (7% and 4%, respectively). Thyroid dysfunction (thyroiditis, Graves' disease) has also been reported with alemtuzumab use for the treatment of other conditions. For B-CLL treatment, TSH monitoring is recommended; monitor TSH at baseline and every 2 to 3 months during alemtuzumab treatment (Hamnvik, 2011). For MS, monitor TSH at baseline and every 3 months until 48 months after last infusion or longer or at any time during therapy if clinically indicated.

[US Boxed Warning]: Serious and potentially fatal infusion-related reactions may occur; monitor for infusion reaction; carefully monitor during infusion; withhold treatment for serious or grade 3 or 4 infusion reactions. For B-cell chronic lymphocytic leukemia (B-CLL), gradual escalation to the recommended maintenance dose is required at initiation and with treatment interruptions (for ≥7 days) to minimize infusion-related reactions. For multiple sclerosis, must be administered in a setting with appropriate equipment and personnel to manage anaphylaxis or serious infusion reaction; monitor for 2 hours after each infusion; inform patients that serious infusion reactions may also occur after the 2-hour monitoring period. Infusion reactions have been reported more than 24 hours after infusion. In patients treated for B-CLL, infusion reaction symptoms may include acute respiratory distress syndrome, anaphylactic shock, angioedema, bronchospasm, cardiac arrest, cardiac arrhythmias, chills, dyspnea, fever, hypotension, myocardial infarction, pulmonary infiltrates, rash, rigors, syncope, or urticaria. The incidence of infusion reaction is highest during the first week of B-CLL treatment. Premedicate with acetaminophen and an oral antihistamine. Medications for the treatment of reactions should be available for immediate use. Use caution and carefully monitor blood pressure in patients with ischemic heart disease and patients on antihypertensive therapy. For B-CLL, reinitiate with gradual dose escalation if treatment is withheld ≥7 days. Similar infusion reactions have been observed with use in the treatment of multiple sclerosis; premedication with corticosteroids for initial 3 days of each treatment course is recommended. Antihistamines and/or antipyretics may also be considered. Consider additional monitoring in patients with existing cardiovascular or respiratory compromise (the Canadian labeling recommends obtaining an ECG prior to each treatment course). Observe for infusion-related reactions; advise patients to monitor for signs/symptoms of infusion reaction, particularly during the 24 hours following infusion.

[US Boxed Warning (Campath)]: Serious and fatal cytopenias (including pancytopenia, bone marrow hypoplasia, autoimmune hemolytic anemia, and autoimmune idiopathic thrombocytopenia) have occurred. Single doses >30 mg or cumulative weekly doses >90 mg are associated with an increased incidence of pancytopenia. Severe prolonged myelosuppression, hemolytic anemia, pure red cell aplasia, bone marrow aplasia, and bone marrow hypoplasia have also been reported with use at the normal dose for the treatment of B-CLL. Discontinue for serious hematologic or other serious toxicity (except lymphopenia) until the event resolves. Permanently discontinue if autoimmune anemia or autoimmune thrombocytopenia occurs. Patients receiving blood products should only receive irradiated blood products due to the potential for transfusion-associated GVHD during lymphopenia.

[US Boxed Warning (Campath)]: Serious and potentially fatal infections (bacterial, viral, fungal, and protozoan) have been reported. Administer prophylactic medications against PCP pneumonia and herpes viral infections during treatment and for at least 2 months following last dose or until CD4+ counts are ≥200 cells/mm^3 (whichever is later). Severe and prolonged lymphopenia may occur; CD4+ counts usually return to ≥200 cells/mm^3 within 2 to 6 months; however, CD4+ and CD8+ lymphocyte counts may not return to baseline levels for more than 1 year. Withhold treatment during serious infections; may be reinitiated upon resolution of infection. Monitor for CMV infection (during and for at least 2 months after completion of therapy); initiate appropriate antiviral treatment and withhold alemtuzumab for CMV infection or confirmed CMV viremia (withhold alemtuzumab during CMV antiviral treatment). For patients being treated for MS, initiate antiviral prophylaxis (for herpetic viral infections) beginning on the first day of treatment and continue for at least 2 months or until CD4+ lymphocyte count is ≥200/mm^3. In clinical trials for MS, infections seen more commonly in alemtuzumab-treated patients included nasopharyngitis, urinary tract infection, upper respiratory tract infection, sinusitis, herpetic infections, influenza, and bronchitis; serious cases of appendicitis, gastroenteritis, pneumonia, herpes zoster, and tooth infection also occurred. Consider delaying treatment in patients with active infection until infection is controlled. Patients should be screened for human papilloma virus (HPV) and tuberculosis as clinically necessary. Progressive multifocal leukoencephalopathy (PML) been reported with use (rarely); withhold therapy immediately for signs/symptoms suggestive of PML. According to the Canadian labeling, alemtuzumab is contraindicated in patients with a history of PML.

[US Boxed Warning (Lemtrada)]: Alemtuzumab may cause an increased risk of malignancies, including thyroid cancer, melanoma, and lymphoproliferative disorders, Perform baseline and yearly skin exams. Other malignant neoplasm (breast cancer or basal cell carcinoma) has been observed (rarely) in patients receiving treatment for MS. Use of Lemtrada in patients with active malignancies is contraindicated; use caution if initiating treatment in patients with preexisting malignancy (Canadian labeling).

Pneumonitis (hypersensitivity or fibrosis) has been reported. Monitor for symptoms (dyspnea, cough, wheezing, hemoptysis, chest pain/tightness). Alemtuzumab is associated with a moderate emetic potential in the oncology setting; antiemetics may be recommended to prevent nausea and vomiting (Basch, 2011; Roila, 2010). Potentially significant drug-drug interactions may exist, requiring dose or frequency adjustment, additional monitoring, and/or selection of alternative therapy. If considering Lemtrada treatment for use in a patient who has previously received Campath/MabCampath, consider the additive and long-lasting immune system effects. Patients should not be immunized with live, viral vaccines during or recently after treatment. The ability to respond to any vaccine following therapy is unknown. Testing for antibodies to varicella zoster virus (VZV) is recommended prior to initiation of Lemtrada if history of chickenpox or VZV vaccination status is unknown. When using for the treatment of multiple sclerosis, complete necessary immunizations at least 6 weeks prior to initiating alemtuzumab. Determine if patient has a history varicella or vaccination for VZV; if not, test for VZV antibodies and consider vaccinations for antibody-negative patients; postpone alemtuzumab treatment for 6 weeks following VZV vaccination.

Alemtuzumab is not recommended for use in MS patients with inactive disease or who are stable on other treatment. Patients should commit to at least 48 months of follow-up after the last infusion. Alemtuzumab has not been studied in MS patients infected with HBV or HCV; consider screening patients at increased risk of infection prior to initiating treatment. Use with caution in HBV or HCV carriers; patients may be at risk for viral reactivation. **[US Boxed Warning (Lemtrada)]: Due to the risk of autoimmunity, infusion reactions, and malignancies, alemtuzumab is available only through restricted distribution under a Risk Evaluation Mitigation Strategy (REMS) Program when used for the treatment of MS. Contact 1-855-676-6326 to enroll in the Lemtrada REMS program.** Prescribers and pharmacies must be certified with the REMS program, and patients and healthcare facilities must be enrolled and comply with ongoing monitoring.

Adverse Reactions

>10%:

Central nervous system: Headache (44% to 52%), fatigue (8% to 21%), insomnia (11% to 17%), paresthesia (10% to 12%)

Dermatologic: Skin rash (43% to 53%), urticaria (15% to 17%), pruritus (13% to 17%)

Endocrine & metabolic: Thyroid disease (13% to 34%)

Gastrointestinal: Nausea (16% to 22%), diarrhea (12%), oral candidiasis (3% to 12%)

Genitourinary: Urinary tract infection (18% to 19%), vulvovaginal candidiasis (3% to 12%)

Hematologic & oncologic: Lymphocytopenia (6% to 100%)

Immunologic: Antibody development (8% to 85%; no effect on drug efficacy; anti-alemtuzumab: 2%)

Infection: Infection (71%), herpes virus infection (16%), fungal infection (12% to 13%)

Local: Infusion related reaction (92%)

Neuromuscular & skeletal: Arthralgia (12% to 13%), limb pain (13%), back pain (12%)

Respiratory: Nasopharyngitis (24% to 25%), upper respiratory tract infection (15% to 16%), oropharyngeal pain (11%), sinusitis (11%)

Miscellaneous: Fever (26% to 30%)

1% to 10%:

Cardiovascular: Flushing (10%), chest discomfort (7% to 8%), tachycardia (6% to 8%), peripheral edema (5%), palpitations (4%), bradycardia (3%), hypotension (3%), chest pain (2%), cold extremities (1%)

Central nervous system: Chills (9% to 10%), dizziness (10%), anxiety (7%), pain (5% to 7%), vertigo (4%), equilibrium disturbance (3%), hyperthermia (3%), increased body temperature (3%), drowsiness (2%), facial hypoesthesia (2%), hypertonia (2%)

Dermatologic: Skin rash (generalized; 7% to 8%), erythema (6%), acne vulgaris (3%), allergic dermatitis (3%), alopecia (3%), erythematous rash (3%), hyperhidrosis (3%), pruritic rash (3%), papular rash (2%), pruritus (generalized; 2%), skin blister (1%), xeroderma (1%)

Endocrine & metabolic: Hypothyroidism (5%), hypermenorrhea (4%), hyperthyroidism (4%), chronic lymphocytic thyroiditis (2%), Graves' disease (2%), thyroid stimulating hormone suppression (2%), goiter (1%)

Gastrointestinal: Vomiting (10%), abdominal pain (5% to 10%), oral herpes (9%), dyspepsia (6% to 9%), dysgeusia (8%), gastroenteritis (4%), upper abdominal pain (4%), abdominal distention (2%), oral mucosa ulcer (1%)

Genitourinary: Occult blood in urine (4% to 8%), uterine hemorrhage (5%), hematuria (3%), cystitis (2%), fungal vaginosis (2%), increase in urinary protein (2%), irregular menses (2%), proteinuria (2%), abnormal urinalysis (1%), herpes genitalis (1%), vaginal hemorrhage (1%)

Hematologic & oncologic: Bruise (10%), decreased CD-4 cell count (5% to 6%), decreased CD-8 cell counts (5% to 6%), decreased absolute lymphocyte count (4% to 5%), decreased T cell lymphocytes (4%), reduction of B-cells (4%), abnormal white blood cell differential (lymphocyte percentage decreased: 3%; lymphocyte percentage increased: 2%), immune thrombocytopenia (2%), nonthrombocytopenic purpura (2%), hematoma (1%), petechia (1%)

Hypersensitivity: Cytokine release syndrome (2%)

Infection: Influenza (8%), herpes zoster (4%), bacterial infection (3%), herpes simplex infection (2%), human papilloma virus infection (2%)

Local: Catheter pain (1%)

Neuromuscular & skeletal: Myalgia (6% to 7%), myasthenia (7%), muscle spasm (6%), weakness (5% to 6%), neck pain (5%), joint sprain (2%), joint swelling (2%), musculoskeletal chest pain (2%)

Ophthalmic: Blurred vision (5%), conjunctivitis (2%), Graves' ophthalmopathy (1%)

Otic: Otalgia (3%), otic infection (3%)

Respiratory: Cough (9%), dyspnea (8% to 9%), bronchitis (7%), epistaxis (5%), pharyngitis (4%), rhinitis (4%), sinus congestion (3%), nasal congestion (2%), wheezing (2%), bronchospasm (1%)

<1%, postmarketing, and/or case reports: Abnormal gait, abnormal hepatic function tests, acquired blood coagulation disorder, agitation, allodynia, altered blood pressure, amenorrhea, anaphylactic shock, anaphylaxis, anemia, angina pectoris, angioedema, anti-GBM disease, antithyroid antibody positive, aphthous stomatitis, aplastic anemia, asthma, ataxia, atrial fibrillation, autoimmune hemolytic anemia, autoimmune thrombocytopenia, bacterial vaginosis, bacteriuria, bacteriuria (asymptomatic), burning sensation, candidiasis, cardiac failure, cardiomyopathy, casts in urine, catheter-site erythema, catheter-site reaction (rash), cellulitis, cervical dysplasia, cervicitis, choking sensation, chronic inflammatory demyelinating polyradiculoneuropathy, connective tissue disease (undifferentiated), constipation, constriction of the pharynx, crystalluria, cutaneous papilloma, decreased appetite, decreased free T4, decreased hematocrit, decreased hemoglobin, decreased monocytes, decreased neutrophils, decreased T3 level, dehydration, depression, desquamation, diaphoresis, disturbance in attention, dry eye syndrome, dysesthesia, dysmenorrhea, dysphagia, dyssomnia, dysuria, ecchymoses, eczema, edema, eosinopenia, eosinophilia, Epstein-Barr-associated lymphoproliferative disorder, Epstein-Barr infection, esophageal candidiasis, esophagitis, eye pain, eyelid edema, facial edema, facial pain, facial swelling, feeling of heaviness, flatulence, fungal skin infection,

furuncle, gastritis, gastroesophageal reflux disease, gastrointestinal disease, gingival hemorrhage, gingival pain, gingivitis, glossalgia, glycosuria, graft versus host disease (transfusion associated), Guillain-Barre syndrome, hematochezia, hemiparesis, hemolytic anemia, hemophilia A (acquired [anti-Factor VIII antibodies]), hemoptysis, hiccups, hyperemia, hyperesthesia, hypersensitivity reaction, hypopigmentation, increased blood pressure, increased free T4, increased heart rate, increased monocytes, increased serum alkaline phosphatase, increased serum ALT, increased serum AST, increased serum bilirubin, increased T3 level, infusion site reaction, iron deficiency anemia, irritability, joint stiffness, labyrinthitis, laryngitis, leukocytosis, leukocyturia, limb pain, local alterations in temperature sensations, lower respiratory tract infection, lymphoproliferative disorder, macular eruption, maculopapular rash, major hemorrhage, malignant lymphoma, malignant melanoma, malignant neoplasm of thyroid, membranous glomerulonephritis, memory impairment, meningitis due to listeria monocytogenes, meningitis (herpes), menstrual disease, microcytic anemia, migraine, mucosal inflammation, multiple sclerosis, muscle spasticity, musculoskeletal pain, natural killer cell count increased, neutropenia, night sweats, noncardiac chest pain, onychomycosis, optic neuropathy, oropharyngeal blistering, ostealgia, ovarian cyst, pain at injection site, painful respiration, pallor, pancytopenia, papule, periorbital edema, peripheral neuropathy, pharyngeal erythema, photophobia, pityriasis rosea, pleurisy, pneumonia, pneumonitis, pollakiuria, positive direct Coombs test, postherpetic neuralgia, presyncope, progressive multifocal leukoencephalopathy, protozoal infection, prurigo, pruritus of ear, psychomotor agitation, pyelonephritis, reactivation of disease, reduced ejection fraction, respiratory congestion (upper), respiratory tract infection, restless leg syndrome, restlessness, retinal pigment changes (epitheliopathy), rheumatoid arthritis, rhinorrhea, seasonal allergy, sensation of cold, sensory disturbance, serum sickness, skin hyperpigmentation, skin infection, skin irritation, skin lesion, stiffness, streptococcal pharyngitis, subacute thyroiditis, suicidal ideation, suicidal tendencies, syncope, tachypnea, throat irritation, thrombocytopenia, thyroiditis, tinea, tinea pedis, tinea versicolor, tinnitus, tongue discoloration, tonsillitis, tooth abscess, tooth infection, toothache, tracheobronchitis, tuberculosis, tumor lysis syndrome, type 1 diabetes mellitus, upper airway symptoms (cough syndrome), urethritis, urinary incontinence, urinary urgency, urine abnormality, vaginal infection, varicella, viral infection, viral respiratory tract infection, visual disturbance, vitiligo, voice disorder, weight gain, weight loss, xerostomia

Drug Interactions

Metabolism/Transport Effects None known.

Avoid Concomitant Use

Avoid concomitant use of Alemtuzumab with any of the following: BCG (Intravesical); Belimumab; Deferiprone; Dipyrone; Natalizumab; Pimecrolimus; Tacrolimus (Topical); Vaccines (Live)

Increased Effect/Toxicity

Alemtuzumab may increase the levels/effects of: Belimumab; CloZAPine; Deferiprone; Fingolimod; Leflunomide; Natalizumab; Tofacitinib; Vaccines (Live)

The levels/effects of Alemtuzumab may be increased by: Denosumab; Dipyrone; Ocrelizumab; Pimecrolimus; Promazine; Roflumilast; Tacrolimus (Topical); Trastuzumab

Decreased Effect

Alemtuzumab may decrease the levels/effects of: BCG (Intravesical); Coccidioides immitis Skin Test; Nivolumab; Sipuleucel-T; Tertomotide; Vaccines (Inactivated); Vaccines (Live)

The levels/effects of Alemtuzumab may be decreased by: Echinacea

Storage/Stability

Campath: Prior to dilution in NS or D5W, store intact (30 mg/1 mL) vials at 2°C to 8°C (36°F to 46°F); do not freeze (if accidentally frozen, thaw in refrigerator prior to administration). Do not shake; protect from light. Following dilution, store at room temperature or refrigerate; protect from light; use within 8 hours. Discard unused portion in the vial.

Lemtrada: Prior to dilution in NS or D5W, store intact vials at 2°C to 8°C (36°F to 46°F). Do not freeze. Do not shake; protect from light. Following dilution, store at room temperature or refrigerate; use within 8 hours.

MabCampath [Canadian product]: Prior to dilution in NS or D5W, store vials at 2°C to 8°C (36°F to 46°F). Do not freeze (discard vial if frozen). Do not shake. Protect from light. Following dilution, store at room temperature or refrigerate; use within 8 hours.

Preparation for Administration

Campath, MabCampath [Canadian product]: Dilute for infusion in 100 mL NS or D5W. Compatible in polyvinylchloride (PVC) bags. Gently invert the bag to mix the solution. Do not shake prior to use.

Lemtrada: Withdraw 12 mg (1.2 mL) from vial and add to 100 mL bag of NS or D5W. Gently invert the bag to mix the solution.

Mechanism of Action

Binds to CD52, a nonmodulating antigen present on the surface of B and T lymphocytes, a majority of monocytes, macrophages, NK cells, and a subpopulation of granulocytes. After binding to $CD52^+$ cells, an antibody-dependent lysis of malignant cells occurs. In multiple sclerosis, alemtuzumab immunomodulatory effects may include alteration in the number, proportions, and properties of some lymphocyte subsets following treatment.

Pharmacodynamics/Kinetics

Distribution: V_d: IV: Campath: 0.18 L/kg (range: 0.1 to 0.4 L/kg); Lemtrada: 14.1 L

Metabolism: Campath: Clearance decreases with repeated dosing (due to loss of CD52 receptors in periphery), resulting in a sevenfold increase in AUC after 12 weeks of therapy.

Half-life elimination: IV: Campath: 11 hours (following first 30 mg dose; range: 2 to 32 hours); 6 days (following the last 30 mg dose; range: 1 to 14 days); Lemtrada: ~2 weeks

Dosing

Adult & Geriatric

B-cell chronic lymphocytic leukemia (B-CLL): Campath: IV: Gradually escalate to a maintenance of 30 mg per dose 3 times weekly on alternate days for a total duration of therapy of up to 12 weeks (Hillmen 2007; Keating 2002)

Note: Dose escalation is required; usually accomplished in 3 to 7 days. Single doses >30 mg or cumulative doses >90 mg/week increase the incidence of pancytopenia. Pretreatment (with acetaminophen 500 to 1,000 mg and diphenhydramine 50 mg) is recommended prior to the first dose, with dose escalations, and as clinically indicated; IV glucocorticoids may be used for severe infusion-related reactions. Administer antiviral prophylaxis (for herpetic viral infections) and *Pneumocystis jirovecii* pneumonia (PCP) prophylaxis; continue for at least 2 months after completion of alemtuzumab and until CD4+ lymphocyte count is ≥200/mm^3. Reinitiate with gradual dose escalation if treatment is withheld ≥7 days. Alemtuzumab is associated with a moderate emetic potential in the oncology setting; antiemetics may be recommended to prevent nausea and vomiting (Basch 2011; Roila 2010).

Dose escalation: Initial: 3 mg daily beginning on day 1; if tolerated (infusion reaction ≤ grade 2), increase to 10 mg daily; if tolerated (infusion reaction ≤ grade 2), may increase to maintenance of 30 mg per dose 3 times weekly if required.

B-CLL (off-label route): SubQ: Initial: 3 mg on day 1; if tolerated 10 mg on day 3; if tolerated increase to 30 mg on day 5; maintenance: 30 mg per dose 3 times weekly for a maximum of 18 weeks (Lundin 2002) **or** 3 mg on day 1; if tolerated 10 mg on day 2; if tolerated 30 mg on day 3, followed by 30 mg per dose 3 times weekly for 4 to 12 weeks (Stilgenbauer 2009)

Multiple sclerosis, relapsing: Lemtrada: IV: 12 mg daily for 5 consecutive days (total 60 mg), followed 12 months later by 12 mg daily for 3 consecutive days (total 36 mg); total duration of therapy: 24 months.

Note: Premedicate with corticosteroids (methylprednisolone 1,000 mg or equivalent) immediately prior to alemtuzumab for the first 3 days of each treatment course. Antihistamines and/or antipyretics may also be considered. Administer antiviral prophylaxis (for herpetic viral infections) beginning on the first day of treatment and continue for at least 2 months after completion of alemtuzumab and until CD4+ lymphocyte count is ≥200/mm^3. In some clinical trials patients received an additional 12 mg daily for 3 consecutive days 12 months later (total duration of 36 months) (CAMMS223 2008; Coles 2012).

Autoimmune cytopenias, CLL-induced, refractory (off-label use): IV, SubQ: Gradually escalate to a maintenance of 10 to 30 mg per dose 3 times weekly for 4 to 12 weeks (Karlsson 2007; Osterborg 2009)

Graft versus host disease (GVHD), acute, steroid refractory, treatment (off-label use): IV: 10 mg daily for 5 consecutive days, then 10 mg weekly on days 8, 15, and 22 if CR not achieved (Martinez 2009) **or** 10 mg weekly until symptom resolution (Schnitzler 2009)

Solid organ transplantation:

Heart transplant, induction (off-label use): IV: 30 mg once intra-operatively at the time of transplant followed by minimized maintenance immunosuppression (Teuteberg 2010). Additional data may be necessary to further define the role of alemtuzumab in this condition.

Lung transplant, induction (off-label use): IV, SubQ: 30 mg once either immediately before allograft reperfusion or immediately following transplant; followed by minimized maintenance immunosuppression (Jaksch 2014; Shyu 2011; Whited 2015). Additional data may be necessary to further define the role of alemtuzumab in this condition.

Renal transplant, induction (off-label use): IV: 30 mg as a single dose at the time of transplant (immediately following reperfusion) followed by a second 30 mg dose 24 hours later (the second dose was omitted in patients >60 years of age); followed by minimized maintenance immunosuppression (Haynes 2014).

Stem cell transplant (allogeneic) conditioning regimen (off-label use): IV: 20 mg daily for 5 days (in combination with fludarabine and melphalan) beginning 8 days prior to transplant (Mead 2010) **or** beginning 7 days prior to transplant (Van Besien 2009)

T-cell prolymphocytic leukemia (T-PLL; off-label use): IV: Initial test dose 3 mg or 10 mg, followed by dose escalation to 30 mg per dose 3 times weekly as tolerated until maximum response (Dearden 2001) **or** Initial dose: 3 mg day 1, if tolerated increase to 10 mg day 2, if tolerated increase to 30 mg on day 3 (days 1, 2, and 3 are consecutive days), followed by 30 mg per dose every Monday, Wednesday, Friday for a total of 4 to 12 weeks (Keating 2002)

Renal Impairment There are no dosage adjustments provided in the manufacturer's labeling (has not been studied).

Hepatic Impairment There are no dosage adjustments provided in the manufacturer's labeling (has not been studied).

Obesity *American Society for Blood and Marrow Transplantation (ASBMT) practice guideline committee position statement on chemotherapy dosing in obesity:* Utilize a flat dose based on the regimen selected for hematopoietic stem cell transplant conditioning in adults (Bubalo 2014).

Adjustment for Toxicity

Dosage adjustment for nonhematologic toxicity:

Treatment of B-CLL: Campath:

Note: If treatment is withheld ≥7 days, reinitiate at 3 mg with re-escalation to 10 mg and then 30 mg.

Grade 3 or 4 infusion reaction: Withhold infusion

Serious infection or other serious adverse reaction: Withhold alemtuzumab until resolution

Autoimmune anemia or autoimmune thrombocytopenia: Discontinue alemtuzumab

Treatment of MS: Lemtrada: Serious infusion reaction: Consider immediate discontinuation

Dosage adjustment for hematologic toxicity (severe neutropenia or thrombocytopenia, not autoimmune): Treatment of B-CLL: Campath:

Note: If treatment is withheld ≥7 days, reinitiate at 3 mg with re-escalation to 10 mg and then 30 mg.

ANC <250/mm^3 and/or platelet count ≤25,000/mm^3:

First occurrence: Withhold treatment; resume at 30 mg per dose when ANC ≥500/mm^3 and platelet count ≥50,000/mm^3

Second occurrence: Withhold treatment; resume at 10 mg per dose when ANC ≥500/mm^3 and platelet count ≥50,000/mm^3

Third occurrence: Discontinue alemtuzumab.

Patients with a baseline ANC ≤250/mm^3 and/or a baseline platelet count ≤25,000/mm^3 at initiation of therapy: If ANC and/or platelet counts decrease to ≤50% of the baseline value:

First occurrence: Withhold treatment; resume at 30 mg per dose upon return to baseline values

Second occurrence: Withhold treatment; resume at 10 mg per dose upon return to baseline values

Third occurrence: Discontinue alemtuzumab.

Administration

Campath or MabCampath [Canadian product]: Administer by IV infusion over 2 hours. Premedicate with diphenhydramine 50 mg and acetaminophen 500 to 1000 mg 30 minutes before each infusion. IV glucocorticoids have been effective in decreasing severe infusion-related events. Start anti-infective prophylaxis. Other drugs should not be added to or simultaneously infused through the same IV line. Do not give IV push or bolus. Compatible in polyvinylchloride (PVC) or polyethylene lined administration sets or low protein binding filters. May be given through peripheral IV.

Campath: SubQ (off-label route): SubQ administration has been studied (Lundin 2002; Stilgenbauer 2009); an increased rate of injection site reactions has been observed, with only rare incidences of chills or infusion-like reactions typically observed with IV infusion. A longer dose escalation time (1 to 2 weeks) may be needed due to injection site reactions (Lundin 2002). Premedicate with diphenhydramine 50 mg and acetaminophen 500 to 1000 mg 30 minutes before dose. The subQ route should **NOT** be used for the treatment of T-PLL (Deardon 2011).

Alemtuzumab is associated with a moderate emetic potential in the oncology setting; antiemetics may be recommended to prevent nausea and vomiting (Basch 2011; Roila 2010).

Lemtrada: Administer by IV infusion over 4 hours (beginning within 8 hours after dilution); do not administer by IV push or IV bolus. Do not infuse other medications through the same IV line. Premedicate with corticosteroids (methylprednisolone 1,000 mg or equivalent) for first 3 days of each treatment course. Administer in a setting with personnel and equipment appropriate to manage infusion reactions. Monitor vital signs prior to and periodically during the infusion. Infusion reactions should be managed symptomatically; consider discontinuing immediately for severe infusion reaction. Observe for at least 2 hours after each infusion, longer if clinically indicated.

Emetic Potential

Children: Minimal (<10%)

Adults: Moderate (30% to 90%)

Monitoring Parameters Campath: CBC with differential and platelets (weekly, more frequent if worsening); signs and symptoms of infection; CD4+ lymphocyte counts (after treatment until recovery); CMV antigen (routinely during and for 2 months after treatment); consider TSH at baseline and then every 2 to 3 months during alemtuzumab treatment (Hamnvik 2011). Monitor closely for infusion reactions (including hypotension, rigors, fever, shortness of breath, bronchospasm, chills, and/or rash); vital signs (prior to and during infusion); carefully monitor BP especially in patients with ischemic heart disease or on antihypertensive medications;

Lemtrada: CBC with differential prior to initiation then monthly until 48 months after last infusion; serum creatinine prior to initiation then monthly until 48 months after last infusion or at any time during therapy if clinically indicated; urinalysis with urine cell counts (prior to initiation then monthly); signs/symptoms of infection; TSH at baseline and every 3 months until 48 months after last infusion or longer or at any time during therapy if clinically indicated; observe for at least 2 hours after each infusion, longer if clinically indicated; ECG prior to each treatment course; annual HPV screening; signs/symptoms of PML; baseline and annual skin exams (for melanoma).

Test Interactions May interfere with diagnostic serum tests that utilize antibodies.

Prescribing and Access Restrictions As of September 4, 2012, alemtuzumab (Campath) is no longer commercially available in the United States (or Europe); a restricted distribution program will allow access (free of charge) for appropriate patients. Information on necessary documentation and requirements is available at Campath Distribution Program (1-877-422-6728) or Genzyme Medical Information (1-800-745-4447, option 2).

Medication Guide Available Yes

Dosage Forms Excipient information presented when available (limited, particularly for generics); consult specific product labeling.

Solution, Intravenous [preservative free]:

Campath: 30 mg/mL (1 mL) [contains edetate disodium dihydrate, mouse (murine) and/or hamster protein, polysorbate 80]

Lemtrada: 12 mg/1.2 mL (1.2 mL) [contains edetate disodium dihydrate, mouse (murine) and/or hamster protein, polysorbate 80]

Dosage Forms: Canada Information with regard to form, strength, and availability of products uniquely available in Canada but currently not available in the US. Refer also to Dosage Forms.

Excipient information presented when available (limited, particularly for generics); consult specific product labeling.

Injection, solution [preservative free]:

MabCampath: 30 mg/mL (1 mL) [contains edetate disodium, polysorbate 80]

Injection, solution [preservative free]:

Lemtrada: 10 mg/mL (1.2 mL) [contains edetate disodium, polysorbate 80]

◆ **Alimta** see PEMEtrexed on page 1494

Alitretinoin (Topical) (a li TRET i noyn)

Brand Names: US Panretin

Pharmacologic Category Antineoplastic Agent, Retinoic Acid Derivative

Use Topical treatment of cutaneous lesions in AIDS-related Kaposi's sarcoma. Not indicated when systemic therapy is necessary (eg, >10 new lesions in previous month, symptomatic visceral involvement, symptomatic pulmonary Kaposi's sarcoma, symptomatic lymphedema)

Pregnancy Risk Factor D

Hazardous Drugs Handling Considerations

Hazardous agent (NIOSH 2016 [group 3]).

Use appropriate precautions for receiving, handling, administration, and disposal. Gloves (single) should be worn during receiving, unpacking, and placing in storage.

NIOSH recommends double gloving, a protective gown, and (if liquid that could splash) eye/face protection for administration of a topical product; if there is potential for inhalation, respiratory protection is recommended (NIOSH 2016).

Dosing

Adult Kaposi's sarcoma: Topical: Initial: Apply gel twice daily to cutaneous lesions; may gradually increase application frequency to 3-4 times daily based on lesion tolerance. Response may be observed within 2 weeks of initiation, but typically a longer period is required (some patients have required >14 weeks). Continue therapy for as long as patients derives benefit (in clinical trials, therapy lasted up to 96 weeks).

Renal Impairment No dosage adjustment provided in manufacturer's labeling; however, systemic absorption is not extensive making the need for a dose adjustment appear unlikely.

Hepatic Impairment No dosage adjustment provided in manufacturer's labeling; however, systemic absorption is not extensive making the need for a dose adjustment appear unlikely.

◀ **Adjustment for Toxicity** Reduce application frequency for application site toxicity; for severe reactions, temporarily discontinue therapy until symptoms resolve.

Additional Information Complete prescribing information should be consulted for additional detail.

Dosage Forms Information with regard to form, strength, and availability of products uniquely available in Canada but currently not available in the US.

Excipient information presented when available (limited, particularly for generics); consult specific product labeling.

Gel, External:

Panretin: 0.1% (60 g)

◆ **Alkeran** see Melphalan on page 1182

◆ **Alloprin (Can)** see Allopurinol on page 94

Allopurinol (al oh PURE i nole)

Brand Names: US Aloprim; Zyloprim

Brand Names: Canada Alloprin; Apo-Allopurinol; JAMP-Allopurinol; Mar-Allopurinol; Novo-Purol; Zyloprim

Index Terms Allopurinol Sodium

Pharmacologic Category Antigout Agent; Xanthine Oxidase Inhibitor

Use

Oral:

Calcium oxalate calculi (recurrent): Management of recurrent calcium oxalate calculi (with uric acid excretion >800 mg/day in men and >750 mg/day in women)

Cancer therapy-induced hyperuricemia: Management of hyperuricemia associated with cancer treatment for leukemia, lymphoma, and other malignancies

Gout: Management of primary or secondary gout (acute attack, tophi, joint destruction, uric acid lithiasis, and/or nephropathy)

Limitations of use: Allopurinol is not recommended for the treatment of asymptomatic hyperuricemia. Allopurinol reduces serum and urinary uric acid concentrations; its use should be individualized for each patient and requires an understanding of its mode of action and pharmacokinetics.

IV: **Cancer therapy-induced hyperuricemia:** Management of hyperuricemia associated with cancer treatment for leukemia, lymphoma, or solid tumor malignancies in patients who cannot tolerate oral therapy.

Pregnancy Risk Factor C

Dosing

Adult & Geriatric Note: Oral doses >300 mg should be given in divided doses.

Gout: Oral:

Manufacturer's labeling: Initial: 100 mg once daily; increase at weekly intervals in increments of 100 mg/day as needed to achieve desired serum uric acid level. Usual dosage range: 200 to 300 mg/day in mild gout; 400 to 600 mg/day in moderate to severe tophaceous gout. Maximum daily dose: 800 mg/day.

Off-label dosing: Initial: 100 mg/day, increasing the dose gradually in increments of 100 mg/day every 2 to 5 weeks as needed to achieve desired serum uric acid level of ≤6 mg/dL (ACR guidelines [Khanna 2012]; EULAR guidelines [Zhang 2006]; McGill 2010). Some patients may require therapy targeted at a serum uric acid level <5 mg/dL to control symptoms. Allopurinol may be initiated during an acute gout attack so long as anti-inflammatory therapy has been initiated as well (ACR guidelines [Khanna 2012]).

Cancer therapy-induced hyperuricemia:

Oral: 600 to 800 mg daily in divided doses for ~2 to 3 days

Off-label dosing: Intermediate risk for tumor lysis syndrome: 10 mg/kg daily divided every 8 hours (maximum: 800 mg/day) **or** 50 to 100 mg/m^2 every 8 hours (maximum: 300 mg/m^2/day), begin 1 to 2 days before initiation of induction chemotherapy; may continue for 3 to 7 days after chemotherapy (Coiffier 2008)

IV: **Note:** Intravenous daily dose can be given as a single infusion or in equally divided doses at 6-, 8-, or 12-hour intervals.

Manufacturer's labeling: 200 to 400 mg/m^2 daily (maximum: 600 mg daily) beginning 1 to 2 days before chemotherapy

Off-label dosing: Intermediate risk for tumor lysis syndrome: 200 to 400 mg/m^2 daily (maximum: 600 mg/day) in 1 to 3 divided doses beginning 1 to 2 days before the start of induction chemotherapy; may continue for 3 to 7 days after chemotherapy (Coiffier 2008)

Calcium oxalate stones (recurrent): Oral: 200 to 300 mg daily in single or divided doses; may adjust dose as needed to control hyperuricosuria

Pediatric

Cancer therapy-induced hyperuricemia:

Oral: **Note:** Oral doses >300 mg should be given in divided doses. Adjust dose as necessary after 48 hours.

Children <6 years: 150 mg daily

Children 6 to 10 years: 300 mg daily

Children >10 years: Refer to adult dosing.

Off-label dosing: Intermediate risk for tumor lysis syndrome: 10 mg/kg daily divided every 8 hours (maximum dose: 800 mg daily) **or** 50 to 100 mg/m^2 every 8 hours (maximum: 300 mg/m^2/day), begin 12 to 24 hours before initiation of induction chemotherapy; may continue for 3 to 7 days after chemotherapy (Coiffier 2008)

IV: **Note:** Intravenous daily dose can be given as a single infusion or in equally divided doses at 6-, 8-, or 12-hour intervals.

Manufacturer's labeling: Starting dose: 200 mg/m^2 daily beginning 1 to 2 days before chemotherapy

Off-label dosing: Intermediate risk for tumor lysis syndrome: 200 to 400 mg/m^2 daily (maximum: 600 mg/day) in 1 to 3 divided doses beginning 12 to 24 hours before the start of induction chemotherapy; may continue for 3 to 7 days after chemotherapy (Coiffier 2008)

Lesch-Nyhan syndrome-associated hyperuricemia (off-label use): Infants, Children, and Adolescents: Oral: Initial: 5 to 10 mg/kg daily in 1 or 2 divided doses; adjust dose as necessary to maintain high-normal serum uric acid levels and a urinary uric acid/creatinine ration <1; doses ranged from 50 to 600 mg/day (Torres 2007a; Torres 2007b). Additional data may be necessary to further define the role of allopurinol in the management of this condition.

Renal Impairment

Manufacturer's labeling: Oral, IV: Lower doses are required in renal impairment due to potential for accumulation of allopurinol and metabolites.

CrCl 10 to 20 mL/minute: 200 mg/day

CrCl 3 to 10 mL/minute: Do not exceed 100 mg/day.

CrCl <3 mL/minute: The dosing interval may need to be extended; do not exceed 100 mg/day.

Allopurinol and oxypurinol are dialyzable.

Indication-specific renal dosing (off-label):

Cancer therapy-induced hyperuricemia: Dosage reduction of 50% is recommended in renal impairment (Coiffier 2008)

Gout: Oral:

Initiate therapy with 50 to 100 mg daily, and gradually increase to a maintenance dose to achieve a serum uric acid level of ≤6 mg/dL (with close monitoring of serum uric acid levels and for hypersensitivity) (Dalbeth 2007).

or

In patients with stage 4 CKD or worse, initiate therapy at 50 mg/day, increasing the dose every 2 to 5 weeks to achieve desired uric acid levels of <6 mg/dL; doses >300 mg/day are permitted so long as they are accompanied by appropriate patient education and monitoring for toxicity (eg, pruritus, rash, elevated hepatic transaminases). Some patients may require therapy targeted at a serum uric acid level <5 mg/dL to control symptoms (ACR [Khanna 2012]).

Hemodialysis: Initial: 100 mg alternate days given postdialysis, increase cautiously to 300 mg based on response. If dialysis is on a daily basis, an additional 50% of the dose may be required postdialysis (Dalbeth 2007)

Hepatic Impairment There are no dosage adjustments provided in the manufacturer's labeling.

Additional Information Complete prescribing information should be consulted for additional detail.

Dosage Forms Excipient information presented when available (limited, particularly for generics); consult specific product labeling.

Solution Reconstituted, Intravenous, as sodium [strength expressed as base]:
Generic: 500 mg (1 ea)

Solution Reconstituted, Intravenous, as sodium [strength expressed as base, preservative free]:
Aloprim: 500 mg (1 ea)

Tablet, Oral:
Zyloprim: 100 mg, 300 mg [scored]
Generic: 100 mg, 300 mg

Dosage Forms: Canada Information with regard to form, strength, and availability of products uniquely available in Canada but currently not available in the US. Refer also to Dosage Forms.

Excipient information presented when available (limited, particularly for generics); consult specific product labeling.

Tablet, Oral, as sodium:
Zyloprim: 200 mg [scored]

♦ **Alpharadin** *see* Radium Ra 223 Dichloride *on page 1566*

♦ **Alprolix** *see* Factor IX (Recombinant [Fc Fusion Protein]) *on page 778*

Alteplase (AL te plase)

Brand Names: US Activase; Cathflo Activase

Brand Names: Canada Activase rt-PA; Cathflo Activase

Index Terms Alteplase Recombinant; Alteplase, Tissue Plasminogen Activator, Recombinant; tPA

Pharmacologic Category Thrombolytic Agent

Use

Activase:

Acute ischemic stroke: Treatment of acute ischemic stroke (AIS) as soon as possible but within 3 hours of symptom onset.

Pulmonary embolism: Management of acute massive pulmonary embolism (PE)

ST-elevation myocardial infarction: Management of ST-elevation myocardial infarction (STEMI) for the lysis of thrombi in coronary arteries.

Limitations of use: The risk of stroke may outweigh the benefit produced by thrombolytic therapy in patients whose acute myocardial infarction (MI) puts them at low risk for death or heart failure.

Recommended criteria for treatment:

STEMI (ACCF/AHA [O'Gara 2013]): Ischemic symptoms within 12 hours of treatment or evidence of ongoing ischemia 12 to 24 hours after symptom onset with a large area of myocardium at risk or hemodynamic instability.

STEMI ECG definition: New ST-segment elevation at the J point in at least 2 contiguous leads of ≥2 mm (0.2 mV) in men or ≥1.5 mm (0.15 mV) in women in leads V_2-V_3 and/or of ≥1 mm (0.1 mV) in other contiguous precordial leads or limb leads. New or presumably new left bundle branch block (LBBB) may interfere with ST-elevation analysis and should not be considered diagnostic in isolation.

At non-PCI-capable hospitals, the ACCF/AHA recommends thrombolytic therapy administration when the anticipated first medical contact (FMC)-to-device time at a PCI-capable hospital is >120 minutes due to unavoidable delays.

AIS: Onset of stroke symptoms within 3 hours of treatment

Acute PE: Age ≤75 years: Documented massive PE (defined as acute PE with sustained hypotension [SBP <90 mm Hg for ≤15 minutes or requiring inotropic support], persistent profound bradycardia [HR <40 bpm with signs or symptoms of shock], or pulselessness); alteplase may be considered for submassive PE with clinical evidence of adverse prognosis (eg, new hemodynamic instability, worsening respiratory insufficiency, severe right ventricular (RV) dysfunction, or major myocardial necrosis) and low risk of bleeding complications. **Note:** Not recommended for patients with low-risk PE (eg, normotensive, no RV dysfunction, normal biomarkers) or submassive acute PE with minor RV dysfunction, minor myocardial necrosis, and no clinical worsening (AHA [Jaff 2011]).

Cathflo Activase: Restoration of function to central venous access device

Pregnancy Risk Factor C

Dosing

Adult & Geriatric

Acute ischemic stroke: Activase: IV: Within 3 hours of the onset of symptom onset (labeled use) **or** within 3 to 4.5 hours of symptom onset (off-label use; Hacke 2008; Jauch 2013; Powers 2015): **Note:** Perform ▶

noncontrast-enhanced CT or MRI prior to administration. Initiation of anti-coagulants (eg, heparin) or antiplatelet agents (eg, aspirin) within 24 hours after starting alteplase is not recommended; however, initiation of aspirin within 24 to 48 hours after stroke onset is recommended (Jauch 2013). Initiation of SubQ heparin (≤10,000 units) or equivalent doses of low molecular weight heparin for prevention of DVT during the first 24 hours of the 3 to 4.5 hour window trial did not increase incidence of intracerebral hemorrhage (Hacke 2008).

Recommended total dose: 0.9 mg/kg (maximum total dose: 90 mg)

Patients ≤100 kg: Load with 0.09 mg/kg (10% of 0.9 mg/kg dose) as an IV bolus over 1 minute, followed by 0.81 mg/kg (90% of 0.9 mg/kg dose) as a continuous infusion over 60 minutes.

Patients >100 kg: Load with 9 mg (10% of 90 mg) as an IV bolus over 1 minute, followed by 81 mg (90% of 90 mg) as a continuous infusion over 60 minutes.

Central venous catheter clearance: Cathflo Activase (1 mg/mL): Intra-catheter:

Patients <30 kg: 110% of the internal lumen volume of the catheter, not to exceed 2 mg/2 mL; retain in catheter for 0.5 to 2 hours; may instill a second dose if catheter remains occluded

Patients ≥30 kg: 2 mg/2 mL; retain in catheter for 0.5 to 2 hours; may instill a second dose if catheter remains occluded

Pulmonary embolism (PE) (acute massive): Activase: IV: 100 mg over 2 hours; may be administered as a 10 mg bolus followed by 90 mg over 2 hours as was done in patients with submassive PE (Konstantinides 2002). Institute or resume parenteral anticoagulation near the end of or immediately following the alteplase infusion when the partial thromboplastin time or thrombin time returns to twice normal or less. **Note:** Use in submassive PE is off-label.

ST-elevation myocardial infarction (STEMI): Activase: IV: **Note:** Manufacturer's labeling recommends 3-hour infusion regimen; however, accelerated regimen preferred by the ACCF/AHA (O'Gara 2013).

Accelerated regimen (weight-based):

Patients >67 kg: Total dose: 100 mg over 1.5 hours; administered as a 15 mg IV bolus over 1 to 2 minutes followed by infusions of 50 mg over 30 minutes, then 35 mg over 1 hour. Maximum total dose: 100 mg

Patients ≤67 kg: Infuse 15 mg IV bolus over 1 to 2 minutes followed by infusions of 0.75 mg/kg (not to exceed 50 mg) over 30 minutes then 0.5 mg/kg (not to exceed 35 mg) over 1 hour. Maximum total dose: 100 mg

Note: Thrombolytic should be administered within 30 minutes of hospital arrival. Generally, there is only a small trend for benefit of therapy after a delay of 12 to 24 hours from symptom onset, but thrombolysis may be considered for selected patients with ongoing ischemic pain and extensive ST elevation; however, primary PCI is preferred in these patients. Administer concurrent aspirin, clopidogrel, and anticoagulant therapy (ie, unfractionated heparin, enoxaparin, or fondaparinux) with alteplase (O'Gara 2013).

Acute peripheral arterial occlusion (off-label use): Intra-arterial:

Weight-based regimen: 0.001 to 0.02 mg/kg/hour (maximum dose: 2 mg/hour) (Semba 2000)

or

Fixed-dose regimen: 0.12 to 2 mg/hour (Semba 2000)

Note: The ACC/AHA guidelines state that thrombolysis is an effective and beneficial therapy for those with acute limb ischemia (Rutherford categories I and IIa) of <14 days duration (Hirsch 2006). The optimal dosage and concentration has not been established; a number of intra-arterial delivery techniques are employed with continuous infusion being the most common (Ouriel 2004). The Advisory Panel to the Society for Cardiovascular and Interventional Radiology on Thrombolytic Therapy recommends dosing of ≤2 mg/hour and concomitant administration of subtherapeutic heparin (aPTT 1.25 to 1.5 times baseline) (Semba 2000). Duration of alteplase infusion dependent upon size and location of the thrombus; typically between 6 to 48 hours (Disini 2008).

Frostbite (off-label use): Note: For use in patients with deep frostbite injury with potential significant morbidity (eg, extending proximally to the proximal interphalangeal joints of digits), without contraindications to the use of alteplase, who present within 24 hours of injury. Use of alteplase in the field is not recommended; administer treatment in a facility capable of intensive-care monitoring (WMS [McIntosh 2014]). Additional data may be necessary to further define the role of alteplase in the treatment of frostbite.

Intra-arterial: 2 to 4 mg bolus followed by a continuous intra-arterial infusion of 0.5 to 1 mg/hour (total dose if bilateral extremity involvement) via femoral or brachial artery; administer with continuous infusion heparin via an intra-arterial catheter. Discontinue alteplase if fibrinogen levels decrease to <150 mg/dL, if reperfusion is complete (as evidenced by angiography), or after a period of 48 hours whether or not reperfusion is achieved (Bruen 2007; Ibrahim 2015).

Parapneumonic effusions and empyema (off-label use): Intrapleural: 10 mg (diluted in 30 mL of normal saline) administered twice daily for a total of 3 days; each alteplase dose was followed >2 hours later by an intrapleural dornase alfa dose (with a 1-hour dwell time for each drug) (Rahman 2011). Some clinicians suggest consideration of fibrinolytic use in patients in whom treatment with at least 24 hours of chest tube drainage has failed and who are poor surgical candidates (Hamblin 2010). Dosing for this indication has not been established. Alteplase monotherapy dosing regimens have varied (range: 10 to 100 mg) and produced conflicting results in small trials and case series. These regimens have also included variations in chest tube sizes, number of doses, patient positions (still vs rotation), and clamping durations (Thommi 2007; Thommi 2012).

Prosthetic valve thrombosis, right-sided (any size thrombus) or left-sided (thrombus area <0.8 cm², recent onset [<14 days] of NYHA class I to II symptoms), or left-sided (thrombus area ≥0.8 cm²) when contraindications to surgery exist (off-label use) (ACCP [Guyatt 2012]; AHA/ACC [Nishimura 2014]; Alpert 2003; Roudaut 2003): IV:

High-dose regimen: Load with 10 mg, followed by 90 mg over 90 to 180 minutes (without heparin during infusion)

Low-dose regimen (preferred for very small adults): Load with 20 mg, followed by 10 mg/hour for 3 hours (without heparin during infusion)

Note: After successful administration of alteplase, heparin infusion should be introduced until warfarin achieves therapeutic INR (aortic: 3.0 to 4.0; mitral: 3.5 to 4.5) (Bonow 2008). The 2012 ACCP guidelines for antithrombotic therapy make no recommendation regarding INR range after prosthetic valve thrombosis.

Pulmonary embolism (PE) (submassive) (off-label use): Activase: IV: 100 mg over 2 hours; administered as a 10 mg bolus followed by 90 mg over 2 hours (Konstantinides 2002). Institute or resume parenteral anticoagulation near the end of or immediately following the alteplase infusion when the partial thromboplastin time or thrombin time returns to twice normal or less. **Note:** Not recommended for submassive PE with minor RV dysfunction, minor myocardial necrosis, and no clinical worsening or low-risk PE (ie, normotensive, no RV dysfunction, normal biomarkers) (AHA [Jaff 2011]).

Pediatric

Central venous catheter clearance: Intracatheter:

Patients <30 kg: 110% of the internal lumen volume of the catheter, not to exceed 2 mg/2 mL; retain in catheter for 0.5 to 2 hours; may instill a second dose if catheter remains occluded

Patients ≥30 kg: 2 mg/2 mL; retain in catheter for 0.5 to 2 hours; may instill a second dose if catheter remains occluded

Parapneumonic effusions and empyema (off-label use): Infants >3 months, Children, and Adolescents: Intrapleural: 4 mg (diluted in 40 mL of normal saline), with the first dose administered at time of chest tube placement (with a 1-hour dwell time); repeat every 24 hours for a total of 3 doses; or 0.1 mg/kg (maximum: 3 mg) (diluted in 10 to 30 mL of normal saline), with the first dose administered after pigtail catheter (chest tube) placement (45- to 60-minute dwell time) and repeat doses administered every 8 hours for 3 days (total of 9 doses) (Bradley 2011; Hawkins 2004; St Peter 2009). Dosing for this indication has not been established. Several intrapleural dosage regimens have been evaluated and have included variations in chest tube sizes, number of doses, patient positions (still vs rotation), and clamping durations.

Renal Impairment

There are no dosage adjustments provided in the manufacturer's labeling. Plasma clearance is rapid and mediated primarily by the liver; therefore, degree of renal impairment is unlikely to influence elimination of alteplase. Hemostatic defects due to severe renal disease may increase the risk for bleeding.

Hemodialysis: Dialyzable: Unknown, but unlikely (NCS/SCCM [Frontera 2016])

Hepatic Impairment There are no dosage adjustments provided in the manufacturer's labeling. Plasma clearance is rapid and mediated primarily by the liver. Significant hepatic impairment and hemostatic defects due to severe hepatic disease may increase the risk for bleeding.

Additional Information Complete prescribing information should be consulted for additional detail.

Dosage Forms Excipient information presented when available (limited, particularly for generics); consult specific product labeling.

Solution Reconstituted, Injection:

Cathflo Activase: 2 mg (1 ea)

Solution Reconstituted, Intravenous:

Activase: 50 mg (1 ea); 100 mg (1 ea)

◆ **Alteplase Recombinant** *see* Alteplase *on page* 97

◆ **Alteplase, Tissue Plasminogen Activator, Recombinant** *see* Alteplase *on page* 97

◆ **Alti-MPA (Can)** *see* MedroxyPROGESTERone *on page* 1175

Altretamine (al TRET a meen)

Related Information

Management of Chemotherapy-Induced Nausea and Vomiting in Adults *on page 2253*

Prevention of Chemotherapy-Induced Nausea and Vomiting in Children *on page 2310*

Safe Handling of Hazardous Drugs *on page 2379*

Brand Names: US Hexalen

Brand Names: Canada Hexalen

Index Terms Hexamethylmelamine; HMM; HXM

Pharmacologic Category Antineoplastic Agent, Alkylating Agent

Use Ovarian cancer (persistent or recurrent): Palliative treatment (single agent) of persistent or recurrent ovarian cancer after first-line treatment with a cisplatin and/or alkylating agent-based combination.

Labeled Contraindications Hypersensitivity to altretamine or any component of the formulation; preexisting severe bone marrow suppression or severe neurologic toxicity

Pregnancy Considerations Adverse effects were observed in animal reproduction studies. Altretamine may cause fetal harm if administered during pregnancy. Women of childbearing potential should avoid becoming pregnant while on therapy.

Breastfeeding Considerations It is not known if altretamine is excreted in breast milk. Due to the potential for toxicity in the nursing infant, breastfeeding should be discontinued during altretamine treatment.

Warnings/Precautions [US Boxed Warning]: Peripheral blood counts should be monitored at least monthly, prior to each cycle, and as clinically indicated. Mild to moderate dose-related hematological toxicity has been reported; may require dosage modification. With an intermittent dosing schedule, WBC and platelet nadirs occur at 3 to 4 weeks, with recovery by 6 weeks. **[US Boxed Warning]: Due to the potential for altretamine-associated neurologic toxicity, neurologic examinations should be done regularly during altretamine treatment.** Mild to moderate neurotoxicity, including peripheral neuropathy and CNS symptoms (ataxia, dizziness, vertigo, mood disorders, and disorders of consciousness) have been reported; may require dosage modification. Neurotoxicity is generally reversible upon discontinuation. Peripheral neuropathy and CNS symptoms are more common in patients receiving a continuous high-dose daily schedule (compared to an intermittent schedule). Altretamine has been administered safely in patients with preexisting cisplatin-associated neuropathy; close monitoring is required. Altretamine is associated with a high emetic potential; antiemetics are recommended to prevent nausea and vomiting (Dupuis 2011; Roila 2010). Concurrent use of altretamine and MAO inhibitors may cause severe orthostatic hypotension; symptomatic orthostatic hypotension has been reported 4 to 7 days after concurrent administration. **[US Boxed Warning]: Should be administered under the supervision of an experienced cancer chemotherapy physician.** Potentially significant drug-drug interactions may exist, requiring dose or frequency adjustment, additional monitoring, and/or selection of alternative therapy.

Adverse Reactions

>10%:

Central nervous system: Peripheral sensory neuropathy (31%; mild: 9%; moderate-to-severe: 9%)

Gastrointestinal: Nausea and vomiting (33%; severe 1%)

Hematologic & oncologic: Anemia (33%), leukopenia (5% to 15%, grade 4: <1%):

1% to 10%:

Central nervous system: Fatigue, seizure

Gastrointestinal: Anorexia

Hematologic & oncologic: Thrombocytopenia

Hepatic: Increased serum alkaline phosphatase

Renal: Increased blood urea nitrogen, increased serum creatinine

<1%, postmarketing, and/or case reports: Alopecia, ataxia, depression, dizziness, hepatotoxicity, mood disorder, neurotoxicity, pruritus, skin rash, vertigo

Drug Interactions

Metabolism/Transport Effects None known.

Avoid Concomitant Use

Avoid concomitant use of Altretamine with any of the following: BCG (Intravesical); Deferiprone; Dipyrone; Natalizumab; Pimecrolimus; Tacrolimus (Topical); Vaccines (Live)

Increased Effect/Toxicity

Altretamine may increase the levels/effects of: CloZAPine; Deferiprone; Fingolimod; Leflunomide; MAO Inhibitors; Natalizumab; Tofacitinib; Tricyclic Antidepressants; Vaccines (Live)

The levels/effects of Altretamine may be increased by: Denosumab; Dipyrone; Ocrelizumab; Palifermin; Pimecrolimus; Promazine; Roflumilast; Tacrolimus (Topical); Trastuzumab

Decreased Effect

Altretamine may decrease the levels/effects of: BCG (Intravesical); Coccidioides immitis Skin Test; Lenograstim; Nivolumab; Sipuleucel-T; Tertomotide; Vaccines (Inactivated); Vaccines (Live)

The levels/effects of Altretamine may be decreased by: Echinacea; Multivitamins/Fluoride (with ADE); Multivitamins/Minerals (with ADEK, Folate, Iron); Multivitamins/Minerals (with AE, No Iron); Pyridoxine

Hazardous Drugs Handling Considerations

Hazardous agent (NIOSH 2016 [group 1]).

Use appropriate precautions for receiving, handling, administration, and disposal. Gloves (single) should be worn during receiving, unpacking, and placing in storage. NIOSH recommends single gloving for administration of intact tablets or capsules (NIOSH 2016).

Storage/Stability Store at 25°C (77°F); excursions permitted to 15°C to 30°C (59°F to 86°F).

Mechanism of Action Altretamine structurally resembles alkylating agents, although has demonstrated activity in tumors resistant to classic alkylating agents. Cytotoxic effect not fully characterized, however it is likely that after activation, metabolites form crosslinks with DNA and RNA and inhibit DNA and RNA synthesis (Perry 2012). Altretamine has demonstrated more activity in platinum-sensitive ovarian cancers than platinum-resistant disease (Alberts 2004).

Pharmacodynamics/Kinetics

Absorption: Well absorbed

Distribution: Distributed into tissues high in lipid content and into tumor tissue (Damia 1995)

Metabolism: Hepatic; rapid and extensive demethylation to active metabolites (pentamethylmelamine and tetramethylmelamine)

Half-life elimination: 4.7 to 10.2 hours

Time to peak, plasma: 0.5 to 3 hours

Excretion: Urine (90% [at 72 hours], <1% as unchanged drug)

Dosing

Adult & Geriatric Note: Altretamine is associated with a high emetic potential; antiemetics are recommended to prevent nausea and vomiting (Roila 2010)

Ovarian cancer (persistent or recurrent): Oral: 260 mg/m^2/day in 4 divided doses for 14 or 21 days of a 28-day cycle

Renal Impairment There are no dosage adjustments provided in the manufacturer's labeling (has not been studied).

Hepatic Impairment There are no dosage adjustments provided in the manufacturer's labeling (has not been studied).

Obesity *ASCO Guidelines for appropriate chemotherapy dosing in obese adults with cancer:* Utilize patient's actual body weight (full weight) for calculation of body surface area- or weight-based dosing, particularly when the intent of therapy is curative; manage regimen-related toxicities in the same manner as for nonobese patients; if a dose reduction is utilized due to toxicity, consider resumption of full weight-based dosing with subsequent cycles, especially if cause of toxicity (eg, hepatic or renal impairment) is resolved (Griggs, 2012).

Adjustment for Toxicity Temporarily withhold for 14 days or longer, and resume dose at 200 mg/m^2/day for any of the following:

Platelet count <75,000/mm^3

White blood cell count <2000/mm^3 or granulocyte count <1000/mm^3

Progressive neurotoxicity

Gastrointestinal intolerance not responsive to antiemetic regimens

Discontinue if neurotoxicity does not stabilize at 200 mg/m^2/day.

Administration Altretamine is associated with a high emetic potential; antiemetics are recommended to prevent nausea and vomiting (Dupuis, 2011; Roila, 2010)

Administer total daily dose orally as 4 divided doses after meals and at bedtime.

Emetic Potential Children and Adults: High (>90%)

Monitoring Parameters CBC with differential (prior to treatment initiation, before each cycle, and regularly during treatment), neurologic examination (before each cycle and regularly during treatment)

Dosage Forms Excipient information presented when available (limited, particularly for generics); consult specific product labeling.

Capsule, Oral:

Hexalen: 50 mg

- ◆ **AMG 073** *see* Cinacalcet *on page 392*
- ◆ **AMG-162** *see* Denosumab *on page 566*
- ◆ **AMG 531** *see* RomiPLOStim *on page 1638*
- ◆ **Amicar** *see* Aminocaproic Acid *on page 111*

Amifostine (am i FOS teen)

Related Information

Chemotherapy-Induced Peripheral Neuropathy *on page 2236*

Management of Chemotherapy-Induced Nausea and Vomiting in Adults *on page 2253*

Prevention of Chemotherapy-Induced Nausea and Vomiting in Children *on page 2310*

Brand Names: US Ethyol

Brand Names: Canada Ethyol

Index Terms Ethiofos; Gammaphos; WR-2721; YM-08310

Pharmacologic Category Antidote; Chemoprotective Agent

Use

Renal toxicity (cisplatin-induced): Reduce the cumulative renal toxicity associated with repeated administration of cisplatin in patients with advanced ovarian cancer.

Xerostomia due to radiation therapy for head and neck cancer: Reduce the incidence of moderate-to-severe xerostomia in patients undergoing postoperative radiation treatment for head and neck cancer, where the radiation port includes a substantial portion of the parotid glands.

Limitations of use: The clinical data do not suggest the efficacy of cisplatin-based chemotherapy or radiation therapy for the approved indications is altered by amifostine. Data on the effects of amifostine on the efficacy of chemotherapy or radiotherapy in other settings is limited. Do not administer amifostine in other settings where chemotherapy can produce a significant survival benefit or cure, or in patients receiving definitive radiotherapy, unless within the context of a clinical study.

Labeled Contraindications Hypersensitivity to amifostine, aminothiol compounds, or any component of the formulation

Pregnancy Considerations Adverse events have been observed in animal reproduction studies.

Breastfeeding Considerations It is not known if amifostine is present in breast milk. Due to the potential for adverse reactions in the breastfed infant, the manufacturer recommends discontinuing breastfeeding during amifostine treatment.

Warnings/Precautions Hypotension may occur during or shortly after infusion. Short term (reversible) syncope (loss of consciousness) has been rarely reported. Patients who are hypotensive or dehydrated should not receive amifostine. Interrupt antihypertensive therapy for 24 hours before treatment; patients who cannot safely stop their antihypertensives 24 hours before should not receive amifostine. Adequately hydrate prior to treatment and keep in a supine position during infusion. Monitor blood pressure every 5 minutes during the infusion. If hypotension requiring interruption of therapy occurs, patients should be placed in the Trendelenburg position and given an infusion of normal saline using a separate IV line; subsequent infusions may require a dose reduction. Infusions >15 minutes are associated with a higher incidence of adverse effects. Use caution in patients with cardiovascular and cerebrovascular disease and any other patients in whom the adverse effects of hypotension may have serious adverse events.

Serious cutaneous reactions (some fatal), including erythema multiforme, Stevens-Johnson syndrome, toxic epidermal necrolysis, toxicoderma, exfoliative dermatitis, and drug reaction with biopsy-proven eosinophilia and system symptoms (DRESS) have been reported with amifostine. May be delayed, developing up to weeks after treatment initiation. Cutaneous reactions have been reported more frequently when used as a radioprotectant. Evaluate for dermatologic reactions prior to each dose, during therapy and after treatment discontinuation. Discontinue treatment for severe/serious cutaneous reactions or mucosal lesions which appear outside of the radiation port and for bullous, edematous or erythematous lesions on the palms or soles.

Amifostine doses >300 mg/m^2 are associated with a moderate emetic potential (Dupuis 2011). It is recommended that antiemetic medication, including dexamethasone 20 mg IV and a serotonin 5-HT$_3$ receptor antagonist be administered prior to and in conjunction with amifostine. Rare hypersensitivity reactions, including anaphylaxis and allergic reaction, have been reported; discontinue if severe acute allergic reaction occurs; do not rechallenge. Medications for the treatment of hypersensitivity reactions should be available.

Reports of clinically-relevant hypocalcemia are rare, but serum calcium levels should be monitored in patients at risk of hypocalcemia, such as those with nephrotic syndrome; may require calcium supplementation. According to the manufacturer, amifostine should not be used (in patients receiving chemotherapy for malignancies other than ovarian cancer) where chemotherapy is expected to provide significant survival benefit or in patients receiving definitive radiotherapy, unless within the context of a clinical trial. The American Society of Clinical Oncology (ASCO) has published guidelines for the use of protectants for chemotherapy and radiation (Hensley 2009). According to the ASCO guidelines, amifostine may be considered for prevention of nephrotoxicity in patients receiving cisplatin-based therapy. While amifostine may be considered to reduce the incidence of grade 3 or 4 neutropenia associated with chemotherapy, the guidelines suggest that alternative strategies (eg, growth factors) may be utilized in this situation. The guidelines recommend against the use of amifostine to reduce the incidence of thrombocytopenia associated with chemotherapy or radiation therapy. Data is insufficient to recommend amifostine for prevention of neurotoxicity or ototoxicity associated with platinum-based chemotherapy, for prevention of neurotoxicity associated with paclitaxel, for prevention of radiation therapy-induced mucositis associated with head and neck cancer, or for prevention of esophagitis due to chemotherapy in patients with non-small cell lung cancer. Additionally, amifostine may be considered to decrease the incidence of acute and late xerostomia in patients undergoing radiation therapy alone (for head and neck cancer); however, the guidelines do not support the use of amifostine in patients with head and neck cancer receiving concurrent platinum-based chemotherapy.

Adverse Reactions

>10%:

Cardiovascular: Hypotension (ovarian cancer: 61% to 62%; head and neck cancer: 15%; generally transient)

◄ Gastrointestinal: Nausea and vomiting (ovarian cancer: 96%; head and neck cancer: 53%), severe nausea and vomiting (ovarian cancer: 19%; head and neck cancer: 8%)

1% to 10%: Endocrine & metabolic: Hypocalcemia (head and neck cancer: 1%; clinically significant)

Frequency not defined:

Cardiovascular: Bradycardia, chest pain, extrasystoles, flushing, ischemic heart disease, tachycardia

Central nervous system: Chills, dizziness, drowsiness, malaise, sensation of cold

Dermatologic: Erythema multiforme, skin rash

Gastrointestinal: Diarrhea, hiccups

Hypersensitivity: Anaphylaxis

Local: Injection site reaction (includes bruising at injection site, erythema at injection site, inflammation at injection site, injection site pruritus, pain at injection site, rash at injection site, swelling at injection site, urticaria at injection site)

Ophthalmic: Blurred vision, diplopia

Respiratory: Apnea, dyspnea, hypoxia, sneezing

Miscellaneous: Fever

<1%, postmarketing, and/or case reports: Anaphylactoid reaction, atrial fibrillation, atrial flutter, cardiac arrhythmia, DRESS syndrome, hypersensitivity reaction (includes chest discomfort, laryngeal edema, pruritus, rigors, urticaria), myocardial infarction, renal failure, seizure, Stevens-Johnson syndrome, supraventricular tachycardia, syncope, toxic epidermal necrolysis, transient hypertension

Drug Interactions

Metabolism/Transport Effects None known.

Avoid Concomitant Use There are no known interactions where it is recommended to avoid concomitant use.

Increased Effect/Toxicity

Amifostine may increase the levels/effects of: Antipsychotic Agents (Second Generation [Atypical]); DULoxetine; Pholcodine

The levels/effects of Amifostine may be increased by: Alfuzosin; Barbiturates; Benperidol; Blood Pressure Lowering Agents; Brimonidine (Topical); Diazoxide; Herbs (Hypotensive Properties); Lormetazepam; Molsidomine; Naftopidil; Nicergoline; Nicorandil; Obinutuzumab; Pentoxifylline; Phosphodiesterase 5 Inhibitors; Prostacyclin Analogues; Quinagolide

Decreased Effect There are no known significant interactions involving a decrease in effect.

Storage/Stability Store intact vials at 20°C to 25°C (68°F to 77°F). Reconstituted solutions (500 mg/10 mL) and solutions diluted in NS (in polyvinyl chloride [PVC] bags) for infusion are chemically stable for up to 5 hours at room temperature (~25°C [~77°F]) or up to 24 hours under refrigeration (2°C to 8°C [36°F to 46°F]).

Preparation for Administration For IV infusion, reconstitute intact vials with 9.7 mL NS injection and dilute in NS to a final concentration of 5 mg/mL to 40 mg/mL.

Mechanism of Action Amifostine is a prodrug that is dephosphorylated by alkaline phosphatase in tissues to a pharmacologically-active free thiol metabolite. The free thiol is available to bind to, and detoxify, reactive metabolites of cisplatin; and can also act as a scavenger of free radicals that may be generated (by cisplatin or radiation therapy) in tissues.

Pharmacodynamics/Kinetics

Metabolism: Hepatic dephosphorylation to two metabolites (active-free thiol and disulfide)

Half-life elimination: Children: 9.3 minutes (Fouladi 2001); Adults: ~8 minutes

Excretion: Urine (minimal; as amifostine and metabolites)

Dosing

Adult & Geriatric Note: Amifostine doses >300 mg/m^2 are associated with a moderate emetic potential. Antiemetic medication, including dexamethasone (20 mg IV when used for cisplatin-induced renal toxicity) and a serotonin 5-HT$_3$ receptor antagonist, is recommended prior to and in conjunction with amifostine.

Renal toxicity (cisplatin-induced): IV: 910 mg/m^2 once daily over 15 minutes 30 minutes prior to cytotoxic therapy

For 910 mg/m^2 doses, the manufacturer suggests the following blood pressure-based adjustment schedule:

The infusion of amifostine should be interrupted if the systolic blood pressure decreases significantly from baseline, as defined below:
Decrease of 20 mm Hg if baseline systolic blood pressure <100
Decrease of 25 mm Hg if baseline systolic blood pressure 100 to 119
Decrease of 30 mm Hg if baseline systolic blood pressure 120 to 139
Decrease of 40 mm Hg if baseline systolic blood pressure 140 to 179
Decrease of 50 mm Hg if baseline systolic blood pressure ≥180

If blood pressure returns to normal within 5 minutes (assisted by fluid administration and postural management) and the patient is asymptomatic, the infusion may be restarted so that the full dose of amifostine may be administered. If the full dose of amifostine cannot be administered, the dose of amifostine for subsequent cycles should be 740 mg/m^2.

Xerostomia due to radiation therapy for head and neck cancer: IV: 200 mg/m^2 over 3 minutes once daily 15 to 30 minutes prior to radiation therapy

Radiation proctitis in rectal cancer, prevention (off-label use): IV: 340 mg/m^2 once daily prior to radiation therapy (Lalla 2014; Peterson 2015)

Renal Impairment There are no dosage adjustments provided in the manufacturer's labeling.

Hepatic Impairment There are no dosage adjustments provided in the manufacturer's labeling.

Adjustment for Toxicity

Dermatologic toxicity:
Cutaneous reactions or mucosal lesions appearing outside of the injection site or radiation port: Discontinue.
Bullous, edematous or erythematous lesions on the palms or soles: Discontinue.

Severe acute allergic reaction: Discontinue permanently.

Administration Amifostine doses >300 mg/m^2 are associated with a moderate emetic potential; antiemetics are recommended to prevent nausea/vomiting (Dupuis 2011)

IV: Administer over 3 minutes (15 to 30 minutes prior to radiation therapy) or over 15 minutes (30 minutes prior to cisplatin); administration as a longer infusion is associated with a higher incidence of side effects. Patients should be adequately hydrated and kept in supine position during infusion.

Emetic Potential Children and Adults:
>300 mg/m^2: Moderate (30% to 90%)
≤300 mg/m^2: Low (10% to 30%)

Monitoring Parameters Blood pressure (monitor every 5 minutes during the infusion and after administration if clinically indicated); serum calcium levels (in patients at risk for hypocalcemia). Evaluate for cutaneous reactions prior to each dose, during therapy, and after treatment discontinuation. Monitor hydration status.

Dosage Forms Excipient information presented when available (limited, particularly for generics); consult specific product labeling. [DSC] = Discontinued product

Solution Reconstituted, Intravenous:
  Ethyol: 500 mg (1 ea)
  Generic: 500 mg (1 ea [DSC])
Solution Reconstituted, Intravenous [preservative free]:
  Generic: 500 mg (1 ea [DSC])

Amikacin (am i KAY sin)

Brand Names: Canada Amikacin Sulfate Injection, USP; Amikin
Index Terms Amikacin Sulfate
Pharmacologic Category Antibiotic, Aminoglycoside
Use Serious infections: Treatment of serious infections (eg, bone infections, respiratory tract infections, endocarditis, septicemia) due to gram-negative organisms, including *Pseudomonas*, *Escherichia coli*, *Proteus*, *Providencia*, *Klebsiella*, *Enterobacter*, *Serratia*, and *Acinetobacter*
Pregnancy Risk Factor D
Dosing

Adult & Geriatric Individualization is critical because of the low therapeutic index

In underweight and nonobese patients, use of total body weight (TBW) instead of ideal body weight for determining the initial mg/kg/dose is widely accepted (Nicolau, 1995). Ideal body weight (IBW) also may be used to determine doses for patients who are neither underweight nor obese (Gilbert 2009).

Initial and periodic peak and trough plasma drug levels should be determined, particularly in critically-ill patients with serious infections or in disease states known to significantly alter aminoglycoside pharmacokinetics (eg, cystic fibrosis, burns, or major surgery). Manufacturer recommends a maximum daily dose of 15 mg/kg/day (or 1.5 g/day in heavier patients). Higher doses may be warranted based on therapeutic drug monitoring or susceptibility information.

Usual dosage range:

IM, IV: 5 to 7.5 mg/kg/dose every 8 hours; **Note:** Some clinicians suggest a daily dose of 15 to 20 mg/kg/day for all patients with normal renal function. This dose is at least as efficacious with similar, if not less, toxicity than conventional dosing.

Intrathecal/intraventricular (off-label route): Meningitis (susceptible gram-negative organisms): 5 to 50 mg/day (Gilbert, 1986; Guardado 2008; IDSA 2004; Kasiakou 2005)

Indication-specific dosing:
Cystic fibrosis exacerbation (off-label use/route): Inhalation for nebulization:
Monotherapy: 500 mg twice daily (Le 2010)
Adjunctive therapy: 100 mg twice daily with concomitant IV amikacin and ceftazidime (Schaad 1987)
Endophthalmitis, bacterial (off-label use): Intravitreal: 0.4 mg/0.1 mL NS in combination with vancomycin
Meningitis (susceptible gram-negative organisms):
IV: 5 mg/kg every 8 hours (administered with another bactericidal drug) (IDSA 2004)
Intrathecal/intraventricular (off-label route): Usual dose: 30 mg/day (IDSA 2004); Range: 5 to 50 mg/day (with concurrent systemic antimicrobial therapy) (Gilbert, 1986; Guardado 2008; IDSA 2004; Kasiakou 2005)
Mycobacterium avium **complex (MAC) (off-label use):** IV: Adjunct therapy (with macrolide, rifamycin, and ethambutol): 8 to 25 mg/kg 2 to 3 times weekly for first 2 to 3 months for severe disease (maximum single dose for age >50 years: 500 mg) (Griffith 2007)
Mycobacterium fortuitum, M. chelonae, **or** *M. abscessus:* IV: 10 to 15 mg/kg daily for at least 2 weeks with high dose cefoxitin
Pneumonia, hospital-acquired (HAP) or ventilator-associated (VAP) (alternative therapy) (off-label dose): IV: 15 to 20 mg/kg/dose once every 24 hours for 7 days; may consider shorter or longer durations depending on rate of clinical improvement. When used as empiric therapy, use in combination with an agent active against *S. aureus* and an additional antipseudomonal agent. **Note:** Aminoglycosides are not recommended as monotherapy in patients with HAP or VAP due to *P. aeruginosa* (Kalil 2016).
Pediatric General dosing, severe, susceptible infections: Infants, Children, and Adolescents: IM, IV: 15 to 22.5 mg/kg/**day** divided every 8 hours **or** 15 to 20 mg/kg/**dose** every 24 hours (*Red Book* [AAP 2015])
Dosage should be based on an estimate of ideal body weight. In morbidly obese children and adolescents, dosage requirement may best be estimated using a dosing weight of IBW + 0.4 (TBW - IBW). Initial dosing recommendation presented; dosage should be individualized based upon serum concentration monitoring. Initial and periodic plasma drug concentrations (eg, peak and trough with conventional dosing, post dose level at a prespecified time with extended-interval dosing) should be determined, particularly in critically ill patients with serious infections or in disease states known to significantly alter aminoglycoside pharmacokinetics (eg, cystic fibrosis, burns, or major surgery).
Indication-specific dosing:
CNS infections (off-label dose):
Meningitis (Tunkel 2004):
Infants and Children: IV: 20 to 30 mg/kg/**day** divided every 8 hours
Adolescents: IV: 15 mg/kg/**day** divided every 8 hours
VP-shunt infection, ventriculitis: Limited data available: Intraventricular/ intrathecal **(use a preservative free preparation):** Infants, Children, and Adolescents: 5 to 50 mg/**day**; usual dose: 30 mg/**day**
Cystic fibrosis, pulmonary infection (systemic use) (off-label use):
Infants, Children, and Adolescents:
Traditional dosing: IV, IM: 10 mg/kg/dose every 8 hours (Wallace 1993)

Extended-interval dosing: IV: 30 mg/kg/dose every 24 hours (Flume 2009); **Note:** The CF Foundation recommends extended-interval dosing as preferred over traditional dosing.

Cystic fibrosis, pulmonary infection (inhalational use; off-label use/route): Inhalation for nebulization:

Adolescents ≥14 years: Monotherapy: Refer to adult dosing

Children ≥3 years and Adolescents: Adjunctive therapy: Refer to adult dosing

Endocarditis, treatment (off-label dose): Children and Adolescents: IV: 15 mg/kg/**day** divided every 8 to 12 hours; use in combination with other antibiotics dependent upon organism and source of infection (ie, valve-type) (AHA [Baltimore 2015])

Intra-abdominal infection, complicated (off-label dose): Infants, Children and Adolescents: IV: 15 to 22.5 mg/kg/day divided every 8 to 24 hours (Solomkin 2010)

Mycobacterium, avium complex infection (MAC) (off-label use): HIV-exposed/-positive:

Infants and Children: IV: 15 to 30 mg/kg/**day** divided every 12 to 24 hours as part of a multiple drug regimen; maximum daily dose: 1,500 mg/**day** (HHS [pediatric] 2013)

Adolescents: IV: 10 to 15 mg/kg/**day** every 24 hours as part of a multiple drug regimen (HHS [adult] 2015; HHS [pediatric] 2013)

Peritonitis (CAPD): Infants, Children, and Adolescents: Intraperitoneal: Continuous: Loading dose: 25 mg per liter of dialysate; maintenance dose: 12 mg per liter (Warady 2012)

Tuberculosis, drug-resistant (off-label use):

Infants, Children, and Adolescents ≤14 years: IM, IV: 15 to 30 mg/kg/dose once daily as part of a multiple drug regimen; maximum daily dose: 1,000 mg/**day** (ATS/CDC/IDSA 2003; HHS [pediatric] 2013)

Adolescents ≥15 years, HIV-exposed/-positive: IM, IV: 15 mg/kg/dose once daily as part of a multiple drug regimen for the first 2 to 3 months; maximum daily dose: 1,000 mg/**day** (ATS/CDC/IDSA 2003)

Renal Impairment Some patients may require larger or more frequent doses if serum levels document the need (ie, cystic fibrosis or febrile granulocytopenic patients).

Adults: The following adjustments have been recommended: **Note:** Renally adjusted dose recommendations are based on a dose of 7.5 mg/kg every 12 hours (Aronoff 2007).

GFR >50 mL/minute: No dosage adjustment necessary.

GFR 10 to 50 mL/minute: Administer every 24 to 72 hours based on serum concentrations

GFR <10 mL/minute: Administer every 48 to 72 hours based on serum concentrations

Intermittent hemodialysis (IHD) (administer after hemodialysis on dialysis days): Dialyzable (20%; variable; dependent on filter, duration, and type of HD): 5 to 7.5 mg/kg every 48 to 72 hours. Follow levels. Redose when pre-HD concentration <10 mg/L; redose when post-HD concentration <6 to 8 mg/L (Heintz 2009). **Note:** Dosing dependent on the assumption of 3 times/week, complete IHD sessions.

Peritoneal dialysis (PD) (Li 2010):

Intermittent dosing: 2 mg/kg per exchange once daily; allow to dwell ≥6 hours

Continuous dosing (all exchanges): Loading dose: 25 mg/L; maintenance dose: 12 mg/L

Continuous renal replacement therapy (CRRT) (Heintz 2009; Trotman 2005): Drug clearance is highly dependent on the method of renal replacement, filter type, and flow rate. Appropriate dosing requires close monitoring of pharmacologic response, signs of adverse reactions due to drug accumulation, as well as drug concentrations in relation to target trough (if appropriate). The following are general recommendations only (based on dialysate flow/ultrafiltration rates of 1 to 2 L/hour and minimal residual renal function) and should not supersede clinical judgment:

CVVH/CVVHD/CVVHDF: Loading dose of 10 mg/kg followed by maintenance dose of 7.5 mg/kg every 24 to 48 hours

Note: For severe gram-negative rod infections, target peak concentration of 15 to 30 mg/L; redose when concentration <10 mg/L (Heintz 2009).

Infants, Children, and Adolescents: There are no dosage adjustments provided in the manufacturer's labeling; however, the following adjustments have been recommended (Aronoff 2007):

Renally adjusted dose recommendations are based on doses of 5 to 7.5 mg/kg/dose every 8 hours.

GFR >50 mL/minute/1.73 m^2: No dosage adjustment necessary

GFR 30 to 50 mL/minute/1.73 m^2: Administer every 12 to 18 hours

GFR 10 to 29 mL/minute/1.73 m^2: Administer every 18 to 24 hours

GFR <10 mL/minute/1.73 m^2: Administer every 48 to 72 hours

Intermittent hemodialysis: 5 mg/kg/dose; redose as indicated by serum concentrations

Peritoneal dialysis (PD): 5 mg/kg/dose; redose as indicated by serum concentrations

Continuous renal replacement therapy (CRRT): 7.5 mg/kg/dose every 12 hours, monitor serum concentrations

Hepatic Impairment There are no dosage adjustments provided in the manufacturer's labeling.

Obesity In moderate obesity (TBW/IBW ≥1.25) or greater (eg, morbid obesity [TBW/IBW >2]), initial dosage requirement may be estimated using a dosing weight of IBW + 0.4 (TBW - IBW) (Traynor 1995).

Additional Information Complete prescribing information should be consulted for additional detail.

Dosage Forms Excipient information presented when available (limited, particularly for generics); consult specific product labeling.

Solution, Injection, as sulfate:

Generic: 500 mg/2 mL (2 mL); 1 g/4 mL (4 mL)

Solution, Injection, as sulfate [preservative free]:

Generic: 500 mg/2 mL (2 mL); 1 g/4 mL (4 mL)

◆ **Amikacin Sulfate** *see* Amikacin *on page 108*

◆ **Amikacin Sulfate Injection, USP (Can)** *see* Amikacin *on page 108*

◆ **Amikin (Can)** *see* Amikacin *on page 108*

◆ **2-Amino-6-Mercaptopurine** *see* Thioguanine *on page 1774*

◆ **2-Amino-6-Methoxypurine Arabinoside** *see* Nelarabine *on page 1302*

Aminocaproic Acid (a mee noe ka PROE ik AS id)

Brand Names: US Amicar

Index Terms EACA; Epsilon Aminocaproic Acid

◀

Pharmacologic Category Antifibrinolytic Agent; Antihemophilic Agent; Hemostatic Agent; Lysine Analog

Use To enhance hemostasis when fibrinolysis contributes to bleeding (causes may include cardiac surgery, hematologic disorders, neoplastic disorders, abruptio placentae, hepatic cirrhosis, and urinary fibrinolysis)

Pregnancy Risk Factor C

Dosing

Adult & Geriatric

Acute bleeding: Oral, IV: Loading dose: 4 to 5 g during the first hour, followed by 1 g/hour for 8 hours (or 1.25 g/hour using oral solution) or until bleeding controlled (maximum daily dose: 30 g)

Control of bleeding with severe thrombocytopenia (off-label use) (Bartholomew 1989, Gardner 1980):

Initial: IV: 100 mg/kg (maximum dose: 5 g) over 30 to 60 minutes

Maintenance: Oral, IV: 1 to 4 g every 4 to 8 hours or 1 g/hour (maximum daily dose: 24 g). Additional data may be necessary to further define the role of aminocaproic acid in the treatment of this condition.

Control of oral bleeding in congenital and acquired coagulation disorder (off-label use): Oral: 50 to 60 mg/kg every 4 hours (Mannucci 1998). Additional data may be necessary to further define the role of aminocaproic acid in the treatment of this condition.

Control of refractory bleeding associated with extracorporeal membrane oxygenation (off-label use): IV: 4 to 5 g loading dose; follow with an infusion of 1 to 1.25 g/hour until bleeding controlled (Buckley 2016). Additional data may be necessary to further define the role of aminocaproic acid in the treatment of this condition.

Intracranial hemorrhage associated with thrombolytics (plasminogen-activator) (eg, alteplase, reteplase, tenecteplase) (off-label use): IV: 4 to 5 g (as an alternative to cryoprecipitate); check fibrinogen levels after administration, if fibrinogen <150 mg/dL, cryoprecipitate is recommended (NCS/SCCM [Frontera 2016]).

Prevention of dental procedure bleeding in patients on oral anticoagulant therapy (off-label use): Oral rinse: Hold 4 g/10 mL in mouth for 2 minutes then spit out. Repeat every 6 hours for 2 days after procedure (Souto 1996). Concentration and frequency may vary by institution and product availability. Additional data may be necessary to further define the role of aminocaproic acid in the treatment of this condition.

Prevention of perioperative bleeding associated with cardiac surgery (off-label use): IV: Loading dose of 75 to 150 mg/kg (typically 5 to 10 g), followed by 10 to 15 mg/kg/hour (typically 1 g/hour); may add 2 to 2.5 g/L of cardiopulmonary bypass circuit priming solution (Gravlee 2008)

or

Loading dose of 10 g followed by 2 g/hour during surgery; no medication added to the bypass circuit (Fergusson 2008)

or

10 g over 20 to 30 minutes prior to skin incision, followed by 10 g after heparin administration then 10 g at discontinuation of cardiopulmonary bypass (Vander Salm1996)

Subarachnoid hemorrhage (off-label use): IV: Loading dose of 4 g followed by 1 g/hour infusion for up to 72 hours after SAH onset. **Note:** Discontinue infusion 4 hours prior to angiography or 2 hours prior to endovascular ablation of aneurysm (Diringer 2011; Starke 2008). Additional data may be necessary to further define the role of aminocaproic acid in the treatment of this condition.

Traumatic hyphema (off-label use): Oral: 50 mg/kg/dose every 4 hours (maximum daily dose: 30 g) for 5 days (Brandt 2001; Crouch 1999)

Pediatric

Prevention of perioperative bleeding associated with cardiac surgery (off-label use): IV: 100 mg/kg given over 20-30 minutes after induction and prior to incision, 100 mg/kg during cardiopulmonary bypass, and 100 mg/kg after heparin reversal over 3 hours (Chauhan, 2004)

Prevention of bleeding associated with extracorporeal membrane oxygenation (ECMO) (off-label use): IV: 100 mg/kg prior to or immediately after cannulation, followed by 25-30 mg/kg/hour for up to 72 hours (Download, 2003; Horwitz, 1998; Wilson, 1993)

Prevention of perioperative bleeding associated with spinal surgery (eg, idiopathic scoliosis) (off-label use): Children and Adolescents: IV: 100 mg/kg given over 15-20 minutes after induction, followed by 10 mg/kg/hour for the remainder of the surgery; discontinue at time of wound closure (Florentino-Pineda, 2001; Florentino-Pineda, 2004)

Traumatic hyphema (off-label use): Oral: Refer to adult dosing.

Renal Impairment May accumulate in patients with decreased renal function. When used during cardiopulmonary bypass in anephric patients, a normal or slightly reduced loading dose and a continuous infusion rate of 5 mg/kg/hour has been recommended (Gravlee, 2008).

Hepatic Impairment No dosage adjustment provided in the manufacturer's labeling.

Additional Information Complete prescribing information should be consulted for additional detail.

Dosage Forms Excipient information presented when available (limited, particularly for generics); consult specific product labeling. [DSC] = Discontinued product

Solution, Intravenous:
  Generic: 250 mg/mL (20 mL)
Solution, Oral:
  Amicar: 25% (236.5 mL) [contains edetate disodium, methylparaben, propylparaben, saccharin sodium; raspberry flavor]
Syrup, Oral:
  Amicar: 25% (473 mL [DSC])
  Generic: 25% (237 mL [DSC], 473 mL [DSC])
Tablet, Oral:
  Amicar: 500 mg [DSC]
  Amicar: 500 mg [scored]
  Amicar: 1000 mg [DSC]
  Amicar: 1000 mg [scored]
  Generic: 500 mg [DSC], 1000 mg [DSC]

◆ **Amino Levulinic Acid** see Aminolevulinic Acid (Topical) on page 114

◆ **5-Aminolevulinic Acid** see Aminolevulinic Acid (Systemic) on page 114

◆ **5-Aminolevulinic Acid** see Aminolevulinic Acid (Topical) on page 114

Aminolevulinic Acid (Systemic) (a MEE noh lev yoo lin ik AS id)

Index Terms 5-ALA; 5-Aminolevulinic Acid; ALA HCl; Aminolevulinic Acid HCl; Aminolevulinic Acid Hydrochloride; Delta-Aminolevulinic Acid Hydrochloride

Pharmacologic Category Diagnostic Agent

Use Glioma (optical imaging agent): Adjunct for visualization of malignant tissue during surgery in patients with glioma (suspected WHO grades III or IV on preoperative imaging)

Dosing

Adult & Geriatric Glioma (optical imaging agent): Oral: 20 mg/kg administered 3 hours (range: 2 to 4 hours) prior to the start of anesthesia.

Renal Impairment There are no dosage adjustments provided in the manufacturer's labeling. Clearance may be reduced in patients with renal impairment; approximately one-third of a dose is excreted unchanged in the urine, however, it is not known if dosage adjustment is necessary.

Hepatic Impairment There are no dosage adjustments provided in the manufacturer's labeling. Clearance may be reduced in patients with hepatic impairment, however, it is not known if dosage adjustment is necessary.

Additional Information Complete prescribing information should be consulted for additional detail.

Product Availability Gleolan: FDA approved June 2017; anticipated availability is currently undetermined

Aminolevulinic Acid (Topical) (a MEE noh lev yoo lin ik AS id)

Brand Names: US Ameluz; Levulan Kerastick

Brand Names: Canada Levulan Kerastick

Index Terms 5-ALA; 5-Aminolevulinic Acid; ALA; Amino Levulinic Acid; Aminolevulinic Acid HCl; Aminolevulinic Acid Hydrochloride; Delta-Aminolevulinic Acid Hydrochloride

Pharmacologic Category Photosensitizing Agent, Topical; Topical Skin Product

Use

Actinic keratoses:

Gel (Ameluz): Lesion-directed and field-directed topical treatment of mild to moderate actinic keratosis of the face and scalp; to be used in conjunction with photodynamic therapy with narrowband red light illumination (using BF-RhodoLED lamp).

Solution (Levulan Kerastick): Topical treatment of minimally to moderately thick actinic keratoses of the face or scalp; to be used in conjunction with photodynamic therapy with blue light illumination (using BLU-U blue light).

Pregnancy Risk Factor C

Dosing

Adult & Geriatric Note: Should only be applied by qualified medical personnel (not intended for application by patients).

Actinic keratoses: Topical:

Gel (Ameluz): Apply ~1 mm thick to actinic keratosis and to ~5 mm of surrounding skin; application area should not exceed 20 cm^2 and a maximum of 2 g at one time. Cover with an light-blocking occlusive dressing and leave on for 3 hours. After 3 hours of occlusion, remove dressing, wipe off remaining gel, and follow with red light illumination. Lesions that have not completely resolved after 3 months following the initial treatment may be retreated.

Solution (Levulan Kerastick): Apply to actinic keratoses (**not** perilesional skin) followed 14 to 18 hours later by blue light illumination. Application/treatment may be repeated at a treatment site (once) after 8 weeks.

Actinic cheilitis (off-label use): Topical: Apply solution (20%) to lip lesion followed 2 to 3 hours later by photodynamic therapy. Application/treatment may be repeated as necessary once every 4 weeks or until complete clearing, for up to 3 treatment sessions (Alexiades-Armenakas 2004). Additional data may be necessary to further define the role of aminolevulinic acid in the treatment of this condition.

Renal Impairment There are no dosage adjustments provided in the manufacturer's labeling.

Hepatic Impairment There are no dosage adjustments provided in the manufacturer's labeling.

Additional Information Complete prescribing information should be consulted for additional detail.

Dosage Forms Excipient information presented when available (limited, particularly for generics); consult specific product labeling.

Gel, External, as hydrochloride:

Ameluz: 10% (2 g) [contains isopropyl alcohol, phosphatidylcholine, soy, polysorbate 80, propylene glycol, sodium benzoate]

Solution Reconstituted, External, as hydrochloride:

Levulan Kerastick: 20% (1 ea) [contains alcohol, usp, isopropyl alcohol, laureth, polyethylene glycol]

◆ **Aminolevulinic Acid HCl** *see* Aminolevulinic Acid (Systemic) *on page 114*

◆ **Aminolevulinic Acid HCl** *see* Aminolevulinic Acid (Topical) *on page 114*

◆ **Aminolevulinic Acid Hydrochloride** *see* Aminolevulinic Acid (Systemic) *on page 114*

◆ **Aminolevulinic Acid Hydrochloride** *see* Aminolevulinic Acid (Topical) *on page 114*

◆ **AMJ 9701** *see* Palifermin *on page 1425*

◆ **AMN107** *see* Nilotinib *on page 1314*

◆ **Amnesteem** *see* ISOtretinoin *on page 1063*

◆ **Amphadase** *see* Hyaluronidase *on page 917*

Amphotericin B (Conventional)
(am foe TER i sin bee con VEN sha nal)

Brand Names: Canada Fungizone

Index Terms Amphotericin B Deoxycholate; Amphotericin B Desoxycholate; Conventional Amphotericin B

Pharmacologic Category Antifungal Agent, Parenteral

Use

Life-threatening fungal infections: Treatment of patients with progressive, potentially life-threatening fungal infections: Aspergillosis, cryptococcosis (torulosis), North American blastomycosis, systemic candidiasis, coccidioidomycosis, histoplasmosis, zygomycosis (including mucormycosis due to susceptible species of the genera *Absidia, Mucor,* and *Rhizopus*), and infections due to related susceptible species of *Conidiobolus, Basidiobolus,* and sporotrichosis.

Leishmaniasis: May be useful in the treatment of American mucocutaneous leishmaniasis, but it is not the drug of choice as primary therapy.

Pregnancy Risk Factor B

◀ **Dosing**

Adult & Geriatric Note: Conventional amphotericin formulations (desoxycholate [Amphocin, Fungizone]) may be confused with lipid-based formulations (AmBisome, Abelcet, Amphotec). Lipid-based and conventional formulations are **not** interchangeable and have different dosage recommendations. Overdoses have occurred when conventional formulations were dispensed inadvertently for lipid-based products.

Note: Premedication: For patients who experience infusion-related immediate reactions, premedicate with the following drugs 30 to 60 minutes prior to drug administration: NSAID and/or diphenhydramine **or** acetaminophen with diphenhydramine **or** hydrocortisone. If the patient experiences rigors during the infusion, meperidine may be administered.

Test dose: IV: 1 mg infused over 20 to 30 minutes. Many clinicians believe a test dose is unnecessary.

Susceptible fungal infections: IV: Adults: 0.3 to 1.5 mg/kg/day; 1 to 1.5 mg/kg over 4 to 6 hours every other day may be given once therapy is established; aspergillosis, rhinocerebral mucormycosis, often require 1 to 1.5 mg/kg/day; do not exceed 1.5 mg/kg/day

Aspergillosis, disseminated: IV: 0.6 to 0.7 mg/kg/day for 3 to 6 months.
Note: IDSA recommends amphotericin B (conventional) be reserved for use in resource limited settings when no alternatives are available; voriconazole is preferred therapy for invasive *Aspergillus* infections (IDSA [Patterson 2016]).

Aspergillosis (ocular) (off-label use): Ophthalmic:
Intraocular: Inject 5 to 10 mcg in a 0.1 mL volume as a single dose intravitreally or intracamerally to the affected eye; may be repeated in 4 to 7 days as clinically indicated (Kaushik 2001; Patterson 2016). Guidelines recommend concomitant vitrectomy and use in combination with systemic voriconazole (Patterson 2016).

Topical (0.1% to 0.2% solution): Apply to affected eye every 30 to 60 minutes until symptoms resolve (may take weeks) (Kaushik 2001; Ritterband 2002; Tamcelik 2002). **Note:** Ophthalmic natamycin is the preferred treatment (Patterson 2016)

Blastomycosis: Moderately severe to severe pulmonary disease, disseminated extrapulmonary disease or immunosuppressed patients: IV: 0.7 to 1 mg/kg/day for 1 to 2 weeks or until improvement is noted, followed by oral itraconazole for 6 to 12 months (IDSA [Chapman 2008])

Candidiasis, esophageal (alternative therapy) (off-label use): IV: 0.3 to 0.7 mg/kg/day. Consider step down to an oral antifungal once patient is able to tolerate oral intake. In fluconazole-refractory disease, continue amphotericin B (conventional) for 21 days (IDSA [Pappas 2016])

Candidiasis, esophageal, in HIV-infected patients (alternative therapy) (off-label use): IV: 0.6 mg/kg/day for 14 to 21 days (HHS [OI adult 2016])

Candidiasis, oropharyngeal (fluconazole-refractory) (alternative therapy) (off-label use): Oral: 100 mg of an extemporaneously compounded 100 mg/mL suspension 4 times daily (IDSA [Pappas 2016])

Coccidioidomycosis in HIV-infected patients with severe, non-meningeal infection (ie, diffuse pulmonary or severely ill with extrathoracic disseminated disease) (off-label use): IV: 0.7 to 1 mg/kg/day until clinical improvement, then initiate triazole therapy (eg, fluconazole or itraconazole) (HHS [OI adult 2015])

Endophthalmitis due to *Candida* **(off-label use):** Patients with vitritis or with macular involvement (with or without vitritis): Intravitreal: 5 to 10 mcg/ 0.1 mL of an extemporaneously prepared solution in sterile water; administer with concomitant systemic antifungal therapy (IDSA [Pappas 2016])

Histoplasmosis: Moderately severe to severe pulmonary or disseminated disease: IV: 0.7 to 1 mg/kg/day for 1 to 2 weeks, followed by oral itraconazole for 12 weeks (pulmonary disease) or 12 months (disseminated disease) (IDSA [Wheat 2007])

Meningitis:

Candidal (ventricular device cannot be removed) (off-label route): Intraventricular: 0.01 to 0.5 mg/2 mL of an extemporaneously prepared solution in D5W (IDSA [Pappas 2016])

Cryptococcal or Coccidioides: Intrathecal: Initial: 0.01 to 0.05 mg as single daily dose; may increase daily in increments of 0.025 to 0.1 mg as tolerated (maximum: 1.5 mg/day; most patients will tolerate a maximum dose of ~0.5 mg/treatment). Once titration to a maximum tolerated dose is achieved, that dose is administered daily. Once CSF improvement noted, may decrease frequency on a weekly basis (eg, 5 times/ week, then 3 times/week, then 2 times/week, then once weekly, then once every other week, then once every 2 weeks, etc) until administration occurs once every 6 weeks. Typically, concurrent oral azole therapy is maintained (Stevens 2001). **Note:** IDSA notes that the use of intrathecal amphotericin for cryptococcal meningitis is generally discouraged and rarely necessary (Perfect 2010).

Histoplasma: IV: 0.5 to 1 mg/kg/day for 7 days, then 0.8 mg/kg every other day (or 3 times/week) for 3 months total duration; follow with fluconazole suppressive therapy for up to 12 months

Meningoencephalitis, cryptococcal: IV:

HIV-infected: Induction: 0.7 to 1 mg/kg/day (with our without flucytosine or fluconazole) for 2 weeks, then change to oral fluconazole consolidation therapy for at least 8 weeks; maintenance: Oral fluconazole for at least 1 year (HHS [OI adult] 2016)

HIV negative: Induction: 0.7 to 1 mg/kg/day (plus flucytosine 100 mg/kg/ day) for 2 weeks (low-risk patients), ≥4 weeks (non-low-risk, but without neurologic complication, immunosuppression, underlying disease, and negative CSF culture at 2 weeks), >6 weeks (neurologic complication or patients intolerant of flucytosine) Follow with azole consolidation/maintenance treatment (Perfect 2010)

Sporotrichosis: Pulmonary, meningeal, osteoarticular, or disseminated: IV: 0.7 to 1 mg/kg/day; after the patient has shown a favorable response, can change to oral itraconazole for suppressive therapy for a total duration of therapy of ≥12 months (IDSA [Kauffman 2007])

Urinary tract candidiasis (off-label use) (IDSA [Pappas 2016]):

Asymptomatic candiduria in patients undergoing urologic procedures: IV: 0.3 to 0.6 mg/kg daily for several days before and after the procedure

Fungus balls: Irrigation via nephrostomy tubes (off-label route): Irrigate with an extemporaneously prepared solution of 25 to 50 mg in 200 to 500 mL sterile water (final concentration range: 0.05 to 0.25 mg/mL)

Pyelonephritis: C. krusei or fluconazole-resistant C. glabrata: IV: 0.3 to 0.6 mg/kg/day for 1 to 7 days (with or without flucytosine for fluconazole-resistant *C. glabrata*)

Symptomatic cystitis:
   C. krusei or fluconazole-resistant C. glabrata: IV: 0.3 to 0.6 mg/kg/day for 1 to 7 days
   Fluconazole-resistant species (eg, C. krusei, C. glabrata) Bladder irrigation (off-label route): Irrigate with a 0.05 mg/mL (50 mg/L) sterile water solution instilled for 5 to 7 days or until cultures are clear. **Note:** Recommended for use in conjunction with other treatment modalities (Fisher 2011).

Pediatric Note: Conventional amphotericin formulations (desoxycholate [Amphocin, Fungizone]) may be confused with lipid-based formulations (AmBisome, Abelcet, Amphotec). Lipid-based and conventional formulations are **not** interchangeable and have different dosage recommendations. Overdoses have occurred when conventional formulations were dispensed inadvertently for lipid-based products.

Note: Premedication: For patients who experience infusion-related immediate reactions, premedicate with the following drugs 30 to 60 minutes prior to drug administration: NSAID and/or diphenhydramine **or** acetaminophen with diphenhydramine **or** hydrocortisone. If the patient experiences rigors during the infusion, meperidine may be administered.

Test dose: IV: Infants and Children: 0.1 mg/kg/dose to a maximum of 1 mg; infuse over 30 to 60 minutes. Many clinicians believe a test dose is unnecessary.

Susceptible fungal infections: IV: Infants and Children: Maintenance dose: 0.25 to 1 mg/kg/day given once daily; infuse over 2 to 6 hours. Once therapy has been established, amphotericin B can be administered on an every-other-day basis at 1 to 1.5 mg/kg/dose; cumulative dose: 1.5 to 2 g over 6 to 10 weeks

Note: Duration of therapy varies with nature of infection: Usual duration is 4 to 12 weeks or cumulative dose of 1 to 4 g.

Indication-specific dosing:
Infants and Children:
   Candidiasis (HIV-exposed/-positive):
      Invasive: IV: 0.5 to 1.5 mg/kg/day once daily (CDC 2009)
      Esophageal: IV: 0.3 to 0.5 mg/kg/day once daily (CDC 2009)
      Oropharyngeal, refractory: IV: 0.3 to 0.5 mg/kg/day (CDC 2009)
   Coccidioidomycosis (HIV-exposed/-positive): IV: 0.5 to 1 mg/kg/day (CDC 2009)
   ***Cryptococcus,* CNS disease (HIV-exposed/-positive):** IV: 0.7 to 1 mg/kg/day plus flucytosine; **Note:** Minimum 2 week induction followed by consolidation and chronic suppressive therapy; may increase amphotericin dose to 1.5 mg/kg/day if flucytosine is not tolerated.
   ***Cryptococcus,* disseminated (non-CNS disease) or severe pulmonary disease (HIV-exposed/-positive):** IV: 0.7 to 1 mg/kg/day once daily with or without flucytosine
   Histoplasma, CNS or severe disseminated: IV: 1 mg/kg/day once daily (CDC 2009)
Adolescents:
   Coccidioidomycosis in HIV-infected patients with severe, non-meningeal infection (ie, diffuse pulmonary or severely ill with extrathoracic disseminated disease) (off-label use): IV: Refer to adult dosing.

Renal Impairment

If renal dysfunction is due to the drug, the daily total can be decreased by 50% or the dose can be given every other day. IV therapy may take several months.

Renal replacement therapy: Poorly dialyzed; no supplemental dose or dosage adjustment necessary, including patients on intermittent hemodialysis or CRRT.

Hepatic Impairment No dosage adjustment provided in manufacturer's labeling.

Additional Information Complete prescribing information should be consulted for additional detail.

Dosage Forms Excipient information presented when available (limited, particularly for generics); consult specific product labeling.

Solution Reconstituted, Injection, as desoxycholate:

Generic: 50 mg (1 ea)

♦ **Amphotericin B Deoxycholate** *see* Amphotericin B (Conventional) *on page 115*

♦ **Amphotericin B Desoxycholate** *see* Amphotericin B (Conventional) *on page 115*

Amphotericin B (Lipid Complex)
(am foe TER i sin bee LIP id KOM pleks)

Brand Names: US Abelcet

Brand Names: Canada Abelcet

Index Terms ABLC

Pharmacologic Category Antifungal Agent, Parenteral

Use Fungal infection (invasive): Treatment of invasive fungal infection in patients who are refractory to or intolerant of conventional amphotericin B (amphotericin B deoxycholate) therapy

Pregnancy Risk Factor B

Dosing

Adult & Geriatric

Note: Lipid-based amphotericin formulations (Abelcet) may be confused with conventional formulations (desoxycholate [Amphocin, Fungizone]) or with other lipid-based amphotericin formulations (amphotericin B liposomal [AmBisome]; amphotericin B cholesteryl sulfate complex [Amphotec]). Lipid-based and conventional formulations are **not** interchangeable and have different dosing recommendations. Overdoses have occurred when conventional formulations were dispensed inadvertently for lipid-based products.

Note: Premedication: For patients who experience infusion-related immediate reactions, premedicate with the following drugs 30 to 60 minutes prior to drug administration: A nonsteroidal anti-inflammatory agent ± diphenhydramine **or** acetaminophen with diphenhydramine **or** hydrocortisone. If the patient experiences rigors during the infusion, meperidine may be administered.

Usual dose: IV: 5 mg/kg once daily

Manufacturer's labeling: Invasive fungal infections (when patients are intolerant or refractory to conventional amphotericin B): IV: 5 mg/kg/day

119

Indication-specific dosing:

Aspergillosis, invasive (salvage therapy): IV: 5 mg/kg/day; minimum duration of treatment is 6 to 12 weeks and depends on site of infection, extent of disease, and level/duration of immunosuppression (IDSA [Patterson 2016]). **Note:** Amphotericin B lipid complex should be reserved as salvage therapy for those intolerant of or refractory to voriconazole, isavuconazole, or liposomal amphotericin B (IDSA [Patterson 2016]).

Blastomycosis, moderately severe to severe, non-CNS disease (off-label dose): IV: 3 to 5 mg/kg/day for 1 to 2 weeks or until improvement, followed by oral itraconazole (Chapman 2008).

Candidiasis (alternative agent) (IDSA [Pappas 2016]): IV:

Candidemia (non-neutropenic patients) (off-label dose): 3 to 5 mg/kg/day; may transition to fluconazole (usually after 5 to 7 days) in clinically stable patients, with fluconazole-susceptible isolates and negative repeat cultures. Total duration of antifungal therapy is at least 2 weeks *after* the documented clearance of *Candida* from the bloodstream and resolution of candidemia-associated symptoms in patients without metastatic complications. **Note:** An amphotericin B lipid formation is considered a reasonable alternative agent if there is intolerance, limited availability, or resistance to other antifungals. In patients with suspected azole- and echinocandin-resistant infections, an amphotericin B lipid formulation is recommended.

Candidemia (neutropenic patients) (off-label dose): 3 to 5 mg/kg/day; may transition to fluconazole during persistent neutropenia in clinically stable patients, with fluconazole-susceptible isolates and negative repeat cultures. Total duration of antifungal therapy is at least 2 weeks *after* the documented clearance of *Candida* from the bloodstream and resolution of neutropenia and candidemia-associated symptoms in patients without metastatic complications. **Note:** An amphotericin B lipid formation is considered a potential alternative agent, but less attractive option due to its potential for toxicity. However, for infections due to *C. krusei*, an amphotericin B lipid formulation is a recommended agent.

Chronic disseminated (hepatosplenic) (off-label dose): 3 to 5 mg/kg/day for several weeks; transition to oral fluconazole in clinically stable patients unlikely to have a fluconazole-resistant isolate.

Empiric therapy (non-neutropenic ICU patients) (off-label use): 3 to 5 mg/kg/day; treatment should continue for 14 days in patients with clinical improvement. Consider discontinuing after 4 to 5 days in patients with no clinical response.

Endocarditis (native or prosthetic valve) or infected implantable cardiac devices (eg, pacemaker, ICD, VAD) (off-label dose): 3 to 5 mg/kg/day (with or without flucytosine); for native or prosthetic valve endocarditis, therapy should continue for at least 6 weeks after valve replacement surgery (longer durations in patients with abscesses or other complications); for patients with implantable cardiac devices, therapy should continue for 4 to 6 weeks after surgery (4 weeks for infections limited to generator pockets and at least 6 weeks for infections involving the wires). **Note:** May transition to fluconazole if patient clinically stable with fluconazole-susceptible isolates in whom *Candida* has cleared from the bloodstream.

Intra-abdominal candidiasis (off-label dose): 3 to 5 mg/kg/day; duration of therapy determined by clinical response and source control.

Osteomyelitis or septic arthritis (alternative therapy) (off-label dose): 3 to 5 mg/kg/day for at least 2 weeks, followed by fluconazole.

Suppurative thrombophlebitis (off-label dose): 3 to 5 mg/kg/day; continue for at least 2 weeks after candidemia has cleared; consider transition to fluconazole in clinically stable patients with a fluconazole-susceptible isolate.

Coccidioidomycosis, progressive, disseminated (alternative agent) (off-label dose): IV: 2 to 5 mg/kg/day (Galgiani 2005)

Coccidioidomycosis in HIV-infected patients with severe, nonmeningeal infection (ie, diffuse pulmonary or severely ill with extrathoracic disseminated disease) (off-label use): 3 to 5 mg/kg/day until clinical improvement, then switch to fluconazole or itraconazole (HHS [OI adult 2017]).

Cryptococcosis: IV:

Cryptococcal meningitis in HIV-infected patients (alternative agent) (off-label use): Induction therapy: 5 mg/kg/day with flucytosine for at least 2 weeks, followed by fluconazole for consolidation therapy (HHS [OI adult 2017]; IDSA [Perfect 2010]). **Note:** If flucytosine is not given due to intolerance, duration of amphotericin B lipid complex therapy should be 4 to 6 weeks (IDSA [Perfect 2010]).

Cryptococcal meningoencephalitis in HIV-negative patients and non-transplant patients (alternative agent): Induction therapy: 5 mg/kg/day (with flucytosine) for ≥4 weeks followed by oral fluconazole. **Note:** If flucytosine is not given or treatment is interrupted, consider prolonging induction therapy for an additional 2 weeks (IDSA [Perfect 2010]).

Cryptococcal meningoencephalitis in transplant recipients: Induction therapy: 5 mg/kg/day (with flucytosine) for at least 2 weeks, followed by oral fluconazole **Note:** If flucytosine is not given, duration of amphotericin B lipid complex therapy should be 4 to 6 weeks (IDSA [Perfect 2010]).

Nonmeningeal cryptococcosis: Induction therapy: 5 mg/kg/day (with flucytosine) for ≥4 weeks may be used for severe pulmonary cryptococcosis or for cryptococcemia with evidence of high fungal burden, followed by oral fluconazole. Note: If flucytosine is not given or treatment is interrupted, consider prolonging induction therapy for an additional 2 weeks (IDSA [Perfect 2010]).

Empiric antifungal therapy (neutropenic fever) (alternative agent) (off-label use): IV: 5 mg/kg/day once daily (Wingard 2000). **Note:** Guidelines recommend amphotericin B lipid formulations be considered for invasive aspergillosis only when triazoles, specifically voriconazole, are contraindicated or not tolerated (IDSA [Patterson 2016]).

Histoplasmosis: IV:

Acute pulmonary (moderately severe to severe): 5 mg/kg/day for 1 to 2 weeks, followed by oral itraconazole (Wheat 2007)

Moderate to severe disseminated disease in HIV-infected patients (alternative agent) (off-label use): 3 mg/kg/day for at least 2 weeks, followed by itraconazole maintenance therapy (HHS [OI adult 2017])

Progressive disseminated, non-CNS disease (alternative agent): 5 mg/kg/day for 1 to 2 weeks, followed by oral itraconazole (Wheat 2007)

Leishmaniasis (visceral) in HIV-infected patients (off-label use): IV:

Chronic maintenance therapy (for patients with a CD4 count <200 cells/mm^3): 3 mg/kg every 21 days (HHS [OI adult 2017])

Sporotrichosis (off-label dose): IV:

Meningeal: 5 mg/kg/day for 4 to 6 weeks, followed by oral itraconazole (Kauffman 2007)

Pulmonary, osteoarticular, and disseminated: 3 to 5 mg/kg/day, followed by oral itraconazole after a favorable response is seen with amphotericin initial therapy (Kauffman 2007)

Pediatric

Note: Lipid-based amphotericin formulations (Abelcet) may be confused with conventional formulations (desoxycholate [Amphocin, Fungizone]) or with other lipid-based amphotericin formulations (amphotericin B liposomal [AmBisome]; amphotericin B cholesteryl sulfate complex [Amphotec]). Lipid-based and conventional formulations are **not** interchangeable and have different dosing recommendations. Overdoses have occurred when conventional formulations were dispensed inadvertently for lipid-based products.

Note: Premedication: For patients who experience infusion-related immediate reactions, premedicate with the following drugs 30 to 60 minutes prior to drug administration: A nonsteroidal anti-inflammatory agent ± diphenhydramine **or** acetaminophen with diphenhydramine **or** hydrocortisone. If the patient experiences rigors during the infusion, meperidine may be administered.

Usual dose: 5 mg/kg once daily

Manufacturer's labeling: Invasive fungal infections (when patients are intolerant or refractory to conventional amphotericin B): Children: IV: 5 mg/kg/day

Indication-specific dosing:

Candidiasis, invasive (HIV-positive patients) (alternative to preferred therapy): Infants and Children: IV: 5 mg/kg/day; treatment duration based on clinical response, treat until 2 to 3 weeks after last positive blood culture (CDC [pediatric 2009])

Coccidioidomycosis in HIV-infected patients with severe, nonmeningeal infection (ie, diffuse pulmonary or severely ill with extrathoracic disseminated disease) (off-label use): Adolescents: Refer to adult dosing.

Cryptococcosis:

Cryptococcus neoformans, disseminated disease (non-CNS disease) (HIV-positive patients): Infants and Children: IV: 5 mg/kg/day (with or without flucytosine); treatment duration of non-CNS disease varies by clinical response and site/severity of infection (CDC [pediatric 2009])

Cryptococcal meningitis in HIV-infected patients (alternative agent) (off-label use): Adolescents: Refer to adult dosing.

Histoplasmosis in HIV-infected patients with moderate to severe disseminated disease (alternative agent): Adolescents: Refer to adult dosing.

Leishmaniasis (visceral), chronic maintenance therapy in HIV-infected patients (off-label use): Adolescents: Refer to adult dosing.

Renal Impairment

Manufacturer's labeling: No dosage adjustment provided in manufacturer's labeling (has not been studied).

Alternate recommendations (Aronoff 2007):

Intermittent hemodialysis: Not hemodialyzable; no supplemental dosage necessary.

Peritoneal dialysis: No supplemental dosage necessary.

Continuous renal replacement therapy (CRRT): No supplemental dosage necessary.

Hepatic Impairment No dosage adjustment provided in manufacturer's labeling (has not been studied).

Additional Information Complete prescribing information should be consulted for additional detail.

Dosage Forms Excipient information presented when available (limited, particularly for generics); consult specific product labeling.

Suspension, Intravenous:

Abelcet: 5 mg/mL (20 mL)

Amphotericin B (Liposomal) (am foe TER i sin bee lye po SO mal)

Brand Names: US AmBisome

Brand Names: Canada AmBisome

Index Terms Amphotericin B Liposome; L-AmB; Liposomal Amphotericin; Liposomal Amphotericin B

Pharmacologic Category Antifungal Agent, Parenteral

Use

Cryptococcal meningitis in HIV-infected patients: Treatment of cryptococcal meningitis in HIV-infected patients.

Fungal infections, empiric therapy: Empiric treatment in febrile neutropenic patients with presumed fungal infection.

Fungal infections, systemic therapy: Treatment of systemic infections caused by *Aspergillus* sp, *Candida* sp, and/or *Cryptococcus* sp in patients refractory to conventional amphotericin B deoxycholate therapy or when renal impairment or unacceptable toxicity precludes the use of the deoxycholate formulation.

Leishmaniasis (visceral): Treatment of visceral leishmaniasis.

Pregnancy Risk Factor B

Dosing

Adult & Geriatric Note: Lipid-based amphotericin formulations (AmBisome) may be confused with conventional formulations (desoxycholate [Amphocin, Fungizone]) or with other lipid-based amphotericin formulations (amphotericin B lipid complex [Abelcet], amphotericin B cholesteryl sulfate complex [Amphotec]). Lipid-based and conventional formulations are **not** interchangeable and have different dosing recommendations. Overdoses have occurred when conventional formulations were dispensed inadvertently for lipid-based products.

Usual dosage range: IV: 3 to 6 mg/kg/day

Note: Premedication: For patients who experience nonanaphylactic immediate infusion-related reactions, premedicate with the following drugs 30 to 60 minutes prior to drug administration: A nonsteroidal anti-inflammatory agent ± diphenhydramine; **or** acetaminophen with diphenhydramine; **or** hydrocortisone. If the patient experiences rigors during the infusion, meperidine may be administered.

Indication-specific dosing: IV:

Aspergillus (systemic infection) (alternative therapy) (off-label dose): 3 to 5 mg/kg/day; minimum duration of treatment is 6 to 12 weeks and depends on site of infection, extent of disease and level/duration of immunosuppression (IDSA [Patterson 2016]). **Note:** Guidelines recommend amphotericin B lipid formulations be considered for invasive aspergillosis only when triazoles, specifically voriconazole, are contraindicated or not tolerated (IDSA [Patterson 2016]).

◄ **Aspergillosis, empiric therapy (off-label dose):** 3 mg/kg/day. **Note:** Guidelines recommend amphotericin B lipid formulations be considered for invasive aspergillosis only when triazoles, specifically voriconazole, are contraindicated or not tolerated (IDSA [Patterson 2016]).

Candidiasis:

Manufacturer's labeling:

Empiric therapy: 3 mg/kg/day

Invasive infection: 3 to 5 mg/kg/day

Alternate recommendations (IDSA [Pappas 2016]):

Candidemia (non-neutropenic patients): 3 to 5 mg/kg/day; may transition to fluconazole (usually after 5 to 7 days) in clinically stable patients, with fluconazole-susceptible isolates and negative repeat cultures. Total duration of antifungal therapy is at least 2 weeks *after* the documented clearance of *Candida* from the bloodstream and resolution of candidemia-associated symptoms in patients without metastatic complications. **Note:** An amphotericin B lipid formation is considered a reasonable alternative agent if there is intolerance, limited availability, or resistance to other antifungals. In patients with suspected azole- and echinocandin-resistant infections, an amphotericin B lipid formulation is preferred.

Candidemia (neutropenic patients): 3 to 5 mg/kg/day; may transition to fluconazole during persistent neutropenia in clinically stable patients, with fluconazole-susceptible isolates and negative repeat cultures. Total duration of antifungal therapy is at least 2 weeks *after* the documented clearance of *Candida* from the bloodstream and resolution of neutropenia and candidemia-associated symptoms in patients without metastatic complications. **Note:** An amphotericin B lipid formation is considered a potential alternative agent, but less attractive option due to its potential for toxicity. However, for infections due to *C. krusei*, an amphotericin B lipid formulation is a preferred agent.

Central nervous system (eg, meningitis): 5 mg/kg/day (with or without oral flucytosine); step-down to fluconazole therapy is recommended after initial response to treatment

Chronic disseminated (hepatosplenic): 3 to 5 mg/kg/day; after several weeks, transition to oral fluconazole in clinically stable, fluconazole-susceptible patients

Empiric therapy, suspected invasive candidiasis (non-neutropenic ICU patients) (off-label use): 3 to 5 mg/kg/day; treatment should continue for 14 days in patients with clinical improvement. Consider discontinuing after 4 to 5 days in patients with no clinical response. **Note:** considered an alternative to echinocandins.

Endocarditis (native or prosthetic valve) or infected implantable cardiac devices (eg, pacemaker, ICD, VAD): 3 to 5 mg/kg/day (with or without flucytosine); for native or prosthetic valve endocarditis, therapy should continue for at least 6 weeks after valve replacement surgery (longer durations in patients with abscesses or other complications); for patients with implantable cardiac devices, therapy should continue for 4 to 6 weeks after surgery (4 for infections limited to generator pockets and at least 6 weeks for infections involving the wires). **Note:** May transition to fluconazole if patient clinically stable with fluconazole-susceptible isolates in whom *Candida* has cleared from the bloodstream; chronic or long-term suppression with fluconazole may be required (eg, prosthetic valve, valve-replacement not possible).

Endophthalmitis (with or without vitritis): Fluconazole- or voriconazole-resistant isolates: 3 to 5 mg/kg/day (with or without flucytosine) for at least 4 to 6 weeks until examination indicates resolution; for patients with vitritis or with macular involvement (with or without vitritis), an intravitreal injection of voriconazole or amphotericin B deoxycholate is also recommended.

Intra-abdominal candidiasis: 3 to 5 mg/kg/day; duration of therapy determined by clinical response and source control

Osteomyelitis or septic arthritis due to Candida (alternative therapy): 3 to 5 mg/kg/day for at least 2 weeks, followed by fluconazole

Coccidioidomycosis in HIV-infected patients with severe, non-meningeal infection (ie, diffuse pulmonary or severely ill with extrathoracic, disseminated disease) (off-label use): 4 to 6 mg/kg/day until clinical improvement, then initiate triazole therapy (eg, fluconazole or itraconazole) (HHS [OI adult 2015])

***Cryptococcus* (systemic infection):** 3 to 5 mg/kg/day

Cryptococcal meningitis in HIV-infected patients:

Manufacturer's labeling: 6 mg/kg/day

Alternate recommendations: 3 to 4 mg/kg/day, with (preferred) or without oral flucytosine (HHS [OI adult 2015])

Fungal sinusitis: Limited data in immunocompromised patients have shown efficacy with 3 to 10 mg/kg/day (Barron 2005; Pagano 2004; Rokicka 2006). **Note:** An azole antifungal is recommended if causative organism is *Aspergillus* spp or *Pseudallescheria boydii* (*Scedosporium* sp).

Histoplasmosis in HIV-infected patients (off-label use; HHS [OI adult 2015]):

Moderately severe to severe disseminated disease: Induction therapy: 3 mg/kg/day for at least 2 weeks, followed by oral itraconazole for maintenance therapy

Histoplasma meningitis: Induction therapy: 5 mg/kg/day for 4 to 6 weeks, followed by oral itraconazole for maintenance therapy

Leishmaniasis (cutaneous) in HIV-infected patients (off-label use): 2 to 4 mg/kg/day for 10 days or an interrupted schedule (eg, 4 mg/kg on days 1 through 5, and then on days 10, 17, 24, 31, 38). Total dose administered should be 20 to 60 mg/kg (HHS [OI adult 2015])

Leishmaniasis (visceral):

Immunocompetent: 3 mg/kg/day on days 1 through 5, and 3 mg/kg/day on days 14 and 21; a repeat course may be given in patients who do not achieve parasitic clearance

Immunocompromised: 4 mg/kg/day on days 1 through 5, and 4 mg/kg/day on days 10, 17, 24, 31, and 38

Leishmaniasis (visceral) in HIV-infected patients (off-label use; HHS [OI adult 2015]):

Treatment: 2 to 4 mg/kg/day **or** an interrupted schedule (eg, 4 mg/kg on days 1 through 5, and then on days 10, 17, 24, 31, and 38). Total dose administered: 20 to 60 mg/kg

Chronic maintenance therapy (for patients with a CD4 count <200 cells/mm^3): 4 mg/kg every 2 to 4 weeks

Meningitis (secondary to contaminated [eg, *Exserohilum rostratum*] steroid products), severe or in patients not improving with voriconazole monotherapy (off-label use) (CDC 2013; Kauffman 2012): IV: 5 to 6 mg/kg/day in combination with voriconazole for ≥3 months; a higher dose (7.5 mg/kg/day) may be considered in patients who are not improving. **Note:** Consult an infectious disease specialist and current CDC guidelines for specific treatment recommendations.

Osteoarticular infection (secondary to contaminated [eg, *Exserohilum rostratum*] steroid products), severe or in patients with clinical instability (off-label use) (CDC 2013; Kauffman 2012): IV: 5 mg/kg/day in combination with voriconazole for ≥3 months. **Note:** Consult an infectious disease specialist and current CDC guidelines for specific treatment recommendations.

***Talaromyces marneffei* infection in HIV-infected patients (off-label use):** 3 to 5 mg/kg/day for 2 weeks, followed by oral itraconazole for 10 weeks, followed by chronic maintenance therapy (HHS [OI adult 2015])

Pediatric Note: Lipid-based amphotericin formulations (AmBisome) may be confused with conventional formulations (desoxycholate [Amphocin, Fungizone]) or with other lipid-based amphotericin formulations (amphotericin B lipid complex [Abelcet], amphotericin B cholesteryl sulfate complex [Amphotec]). Lipid-based and conventional formulations are **not** interchangeable and have different dosing recommendations. Overdoses have occurred when conventional formulations were dispensed inadvertently for lipid-based products.

Usual dosage range: Infants, Children, and Adolescents: IV: 3 to 6 mg/kg/day

Note: Premedication: For patients who experience nonanaphylactic immediate infusion-related reactions, premedicate with the following drugs 30 to 60 minutes prior to drug administration: A nonsteroidal antiinflammatory agent ± diphenhydramine; **or** acetaminophen with diphenhydramine; **or** hydrocortisone. If the patient experiences rigors during the infusion, meperidine may be administered.

Indication-specific dosing:

Infants, Children, and Adolescents: IV:

Empiric therapy: 3 mg/kg/day

Cryptococcal meningitis in HIV-exposed/infected patients:

Infants and Children: 6 mg/kg/dose once daily with flucytosine; if flucytosine is unavailable or not tolerated, may administer amphotericin B liposomal alone or in combination with high-dose fluconazole (HHS [OI pediatric 2013]; off-label combination)

Adolescents: Refer to adult dosing.

Systemic fungal infections *(Aspergillus, Candida, Cryptococcus)*; non-HIV-exposed/-infected: 3 to 5 mg/kg/day

Systemic fungal infections (HIV-exposed/-infected [HHS (OI pediatric 2013; OI adult 2015)]); off-label use):

Infants and Children:

Candidiasis, invasive: 5 mg/kg/dose once daily

Coccidioidomycosis (severe illness with respiratory compromise due to diffuse pulmonary or disseminated non-meningitic disease): 5 mg/kg/dose once daily until clinical improvement, then initiate triazole therapy (eg, fluconazole or itraconazole); dosage may be increased to 10 mg/kg/dose once daily for life-threatening infection.

Cryptococcus, disseminated (non-CNS): 3 to 5 mg/kg/dose once daily (may consider addition of oral flucytosine)

Histoplasmosis:

CNS infection: 5 mg/kg/dose once daily

Disseminated: 3 to 5 mg/kg/day once daily

Adolescents: Refer to adult dosing.

Leishmaniasis (cutaneous) in HIV-infected patients (off-label use): Adolescents: Refer to adult dosing.

Leishmaniasis (visceral):

Immunocompetent: 3 mg/kg/day on days 1 to 5, and 3 mg/kg/day on days 14 and 21; a repeat course may be given in patients who do not achieve parasitic clearance

Immunocompromised: 4 mg/kg/day on days 1 to 5, and 4 mg/kg/day on days 10, 17, 24, 31, and 38

Leishmaniasis (visceral) in HIV-infected patients (off-label use): Adolescents: Refer to adult dosing.

***Talaromyces marneffei* infection in HIV-infected patients (off-label use):** Adolescents: Refer to adult dosing.

Renal Impairment

There are no dosage adjustments provided in the manufacturer's labeling; has been successfully administered to patients with preexisting renal impairment.

End-stage renal disease (ESRD) on intermittent hemodialysis (IHD) (administer after hemodialysis on dialysis days): Poorly dialyzed; no dosage adjustment necessary (Heintz 2009)

CVVH/CVVHD/CVVHDF: No dosage adjustment necessary (Heintz 2009)

Hepatic Impairment There are no dosage adjustments provided in the manufacturer's labeling (has not been studied).

Additional Information Complete prescribing information should be consulted for additional detail.

Dosage Forms Excipient information presented when available (limited, particularly for generics); consult specific product labeling.

Suspension Reconstituted, Intravenous:

AmBisome: 50 mg (1 ea) [contains cholesterol, distearoyl phosphatidylglycerol, hydrogenated soy phosphatidylcholine, sodium succinate hexahydrate, sucrose, tocopherol, dl-alpha]

◆ **Amphotericin B Liposome** *see* Amphotericin B (Liposomal) *on page 123*

◆ **AMSA** *see* Amsacrine *on page 127*

◆ **Amsacrin** *see* Amsacrine *on page 127*

Amsacrine (AM sah kreen)

Related Information

Management of Drug Extravasations *on page 2271*

Safe Handling of Hazardous Drugs *on page 2379*

Brand Names: Canada AMSA PD

Index Terms 4-(9-Acridinylamino) Methanesulfon-m-Anisidide; Acridinyl Anisidide; AMSA; Amsacrin; m-AMSA

Pharmacologic Category Antineoplastic Agent, Miscellaneous

Use Note: Not approved in the US.

Acute leukemia: Remission induction in refractory acute leukemia in adults

Labeled Contraindications Hypersensitivity to amsacrine, acridine derivatives (eg, acriflavine), or any component of the formulation; preexisting drug-induced or radiation therapy-induced bone marrow suppression

Pregnancy Considerations Animal reproduction studies have not been conducted. Women of childbearing potential should avoid becoming pregnant while receiving treatment.

◄ **Breastfeeding Considerations** It is not known if amsacrine is excreted in breast milk. Breastfeeding should be discontinued prior to treatment.

Warnings/Precautions Amsacrine is a potent bone marrow suppressant; effects may be prolonged and may require supportive therapy. Monitor CBC with differential during induction therapy. Leukopenia is generally transient. The WBC nadir usually occurs at 11 to 13 days after treatment; recovery usually occurs by days 17 to 25. Anemia and thrombocytopenia may also occur. Monitor for infection (due to neutropenia) and bleeding (due to thrombocytopenia). Hematologic toxicity may require dose reduction, therapy interruption or treatment delay. Doses higher than recommended may result in severe and prolonged marrow suppression.

Arrhythmia, heart failure, bradycardia, and tachycardia have been reported. Risk factors for arrhythmia may include hypokalemia and a history of anthracycline therapy. Correct fluid and electrolyte imbalance prior to treatment initiation. Serum potassium should be >4 mEq/L prior to administration (Arlin, 1988). The risk for arrhythmia is decreased by ensuring normal potassium levels. Monitor ECG during and after infusion.

Vesicant; ensure proper needle or catheter placement prior to and during infusion. Avoid extravasation. Extravasation may result in severe irritation or necrosis. Tumor lysis syndrome may occur; adequate hydration and prophylactic uric acid reduction should be considered prior to or during treatment; monitor closely.

Use with caution in patients with significant hepatic impairment (bilirubin >2 mg/dL); toxicity may be increased. Hepatic metabolism and biliary excretion are major routes of elimination. Dosage reductions may be recommended. Evaluate hepatic function prior to and during treatment. Use with caution in patients with significant renal impairment (BUN >20 mg/dL; serum creatinine >1.2 mg/dL); toxicity may be increased. Dosage reductions may be recommended. Evaluate renal function prior to and during treatment. Potentially significant drug-drug interactions may exist, requiring dose or frequency adjustment, additional monitoring, and/or selection of alternative therapy. Avoid vaccination with live virus vaccines during treatment. Amsacrine contains N,N-dimethylacetamide, which is incompatible with many closed system transfer devices (CSTDs); the plastic components of CSTDs may dissolve and result in subsequent leakage and potential infusion of dissolved plastic into the patient (ISMP [Smetzer 2015]). The manufacturer reports a low risk of microbial contamination and infection exists with use of AMSA PD injection (50 mg/mL); risk may be further minimized with the use of Sartorius sterile filters (Minisart SRP [PTFE] 0.2 micrometer, 15 mm; provided by the manufacturer) prior to transferring AMSA PD to the diluent. Monitor for signs/symptoms of infection during therapy (Health Canada 2014).

Adverse Reactions Frequency not always defined.

Cardiovascular: Atrial fibrillation, atrial tachycardia, bradycardia, cardiomyopathy (rare), cardiorespiratory arrest, congestive heart failure (rare), ECG changes (prolonged QT interval on ECG, nonspecific ST or T wave changes on ECG), hypotension, phlebitis, reduced ejection fraction, sinus tachycardia, tachycardia, ventricular arrhythmia, ventricular fibrillation, ventricular premature contractions, ventricular tachyarrhythmia

Central nervous system: Confusion, dizziness, emotional lability, headache, hypoesthesia, lethargy, paresthesia, seizure

Dermatologic: Allergic dermatitis, alopecia, dermatological reaction, maculopapular rash, urticaria

Endocrine & metabolic: Weight changes

Gastrointestinal: Abdominal pain (>10%), diarrhea (>10%), nausea (>10%), stomatitis (>10%), vomiting (>10%), anorexia, dysphagia, gingival hemorrhage, gingivitis, hematemesis

Genitourinary: Perirectal abscess (>10%), hematuria, proteinuria, urine abnormality (orange-red discoloration)

Hematologic & oncologic: Bone marrow depression (>10%), leukopenia (>10%; nadir: 11-13 days; recovery: days 17-25), anemia, granulocytopenia, hemorrhage, pancytopenia, purpura, purpuric rash, thrombocytopenia

Hepatic: Hepatic failure (progressive), hepatic insufficiency, hepatitis, hepatotoxicity, increased serum alkaline phosphatase, increased serum AST, increased serum bilirubin, jaundice

Hypersensitivity: Hypersensitivity reaction

Infection: Infection

Local: Inflammation at injection site

Neuromuscular & skeletal: Musculoskeletal pain, weakness

Renal: Increased blood urea nitrogen, increased serum creatinine, renal failure

Respiratory: Dyspnea

Miscellaneous: Fever

Drug Interactions

Metabolism/Transport Effects None known.

Avoid Concomitant Use

Avoid concomitant use of Amsacrine with any of the following: BCG (Intravesical); Deferiprone; Dipyrone; Natalizumab; Pimecrolimus; Tacrolimus (Topical); Vaccines (Live)

Increased Effect/Toxicity

Amsacrine may increase the levels/effects of: CloZAPine; Deferiprone; Fingolimod; Leflunomide; Natalizumab; Tofacitinib; Vaccines (Live)

The levels/effects of Amsacrine may be increased by: Denosumab; Dipyrone; Ocrelizumab; Palifermin; Pimecrolimus; Promazine; Roflumilast; Tacrolimus (Topical); Trastuzumab

Decreased Effect

Amsacrine may decrease the levels/effects of: BCG (Intravesical); Coccidioides immitis Skin Test; Lenograstim; Nivolumab; Sipuleucel-T; Tertomotide; Vaccines (Inactivated); Vaccines (Live)

The levels/effects of Amsacrine may be decreased by: Echinacea

Hazardous Drugs Handling Considerations

Hazardous agent (NIOSH 2016 [group 1]).

Use appropriate precautions for receiving, handling, administration, and disposal. Gloves (single) should be worn during receiving, unpacking, and placing in storage.

NIOSH recommends double gloving, a protective gown, ventilated engineering controls (a class II biological safety cabinet or a compounding aseptic containment isolator), and (if compatible) closed system transfer devices (CSTDs) for preparation. Double gloving, a gown and (if compatible and dosage form allows) CSTDs are required during administration (NIOSH 2016).

Storage/Stability Store intact ampuls and diluent vials at controlled room temperature of 15°C to 25°C (59°F to 77°F). Concentrated amsacrine should not be stored in plastic syringes for >15 minutes. Reconstituted vials may be stored at room temperature for up to 24 hours, under ambient light conditions.

Solutions diluted in D5W for administration are stable for up to 7 days in glass or Abbott plastic containers, however, the manufacturer recommends use within 24 hours when stored at room temperature and 72 hours if refrigerated.

Preparation for Administration Note: A low risk of microbial contamination exists with use of AMSA PD injection (50 mg/mL); risk may be further minimized with the use of Sartorius sterile filters (Minisart SRP [PTFE] 0.2 micrometer, 15 mm; provided by the manufacturer) prior to transferring AMSA PD to the diluent (Health Canada 2014).

Reconstitute by adding 1.5 mL amsacrine to diluent vial (containing 13.5 mL L-lactic acid), resulting in a 5 mg/mL reconstituted solution. Glass syringes should be used, however if using plastic syringes, do not allow concentrated amsacrine to remain in plastic syringe for >15 minutes. Further dilute appropriate dose in 500 mL D5W (the solution may be mixed in plastic bags when diluted for infusion). Amsacrine contains N,N-dimethylacetamide, which is incompatible with many closed system transfer devices (CSTDs); the plastic components of CSTDs may dissolve and result in subsequent leakage and potential infusion of dissolved plastic into the patient (ISMP [Smetzer 2015]).

Mechanism of Action Amsacrine has been shown to inhibit DNA synthesis by binding to, and intercalating with, DNA; inhibits topoisomerase II activity.

Pharmacodynamics/Kinetics

Protein binding: 85% to 95% (Hall, 1983)

Metabolism: Hepatic

Half-life elimination: Terminal: Mean 7.4 hours; range: 6 to 10 hours (Hall, 1983)

Excretion: Bile (primarily); urine (35%; 20% as unchanged drug)

Dosing

Adult & Geriatric

Acute leukemia: IV:

Induction: 75 to 125 mg/m^2/day for 5 days every 3 to 4 weeks (125 mg/m^2/day is preferred; two courses may be necessary to achieve induction; increase dose by 20% in second and subsequent cycles if marrow hypoplasia not achieved and in absence of significant toxicity in previous course.)

Maintenance: Once remission has been achieved, maintenance dose should be ~50% of induction dose, administered every 4 to 8 weeks, depending on blood cell counts and marrow recovery

Acute myeloid leukemia (off-label dosing): IV: 120 mg/m^2 over 60 minutes on days 3, 5, and 7 of induction cycle 2 (in combination with cytarabine) (Löwenberg, 2011) **or** 120 mg/m^2 over 60 minutes on days 4, 5, and 6 of induction cycle 2 (in combination with cytarabine ± G-CSF) (Löwenberg, 2003)

Renal Impairment BUN >20 mg/dL and/or serum creatinine >1.2 mg/dL: Dosage reduction is recommended; however there are no specific adjustments provided in the manufacturer's labeling. The following adjustments have been reported:

Hall, 1983:

Serum creatinine 1.2 to 1.8 mg/dL: No dosage adjustment necessary.

Serum creatinine 2 to 3 mg/dL, oliguric patients: Reduce dose by 30% to 40%; may increase subsequent dose based on toxicity.

Hepatic Impairment Bilirubin >2 mg/dL: Dosage reduction is recommended; however, there are no specific adjustments provided in the manufacturer's labeling. The following adjustments have been reported:

Hall, 1983: Bilirubin >2 mg/dL: Reduce dose by 30% to 40%; may increase subsequent dose based on toxicity.

Koren, 1992: Severe hepatic dysfunction: Reduce dose by at least 50%

Adjustment for Toxicity Consider decreasing dose by 20% if life-threatening infection or hemorrhage occurred in previous cycle; delay second and subsequent cycles until recovery from myelosuppression or evidence of leukemic infiltrate is evident.

Administration IV: Infuse over 60 to 90 minutes.

Amsacrine contains N,N-dimethylacetamide, which is incompatible with many closed system transfer devices (CSTDs); the plastic components of CSTDs may dissolve and result in subsequent leakage and potential infusion of dissolved plastic into the patient (ISMP [Smetzer 2015]).

Vesicant; ensure proper needle or catheter placement prior to and during infusion; avoid extravasation.

Extravasation management: If extravasation occurs, stop infusion immediately and disconnect (leave cannula/needle in place); gently aspirate extravasated solution (do **NOT** flush the line); remove needle/cannula; elevate extremity.

Vesicant/Extravasation Risk Vesicant

Monitoring Parameters CBC with differential, bone marrow studies, electrolytes (serum potassium), hepatic function, renal function; ECG (during and after infusion); monitor for infection, bleeding, monitor fluid status, signs/symptoms of tumor lysis syndrome; monitor infusion site during infusion.

Product Availability Not available in the US

Dosage Forms: Canada Information with regard to form, strength, and availability of products uniquely available in Canada but currently not available in the US.

Excipient information presented when available (limited, particularly for generics); consult specific product labeling.

Injection, solution [preservative free]:

AMSA PD: 50 mg/mL (1.5 mL) [supplied with L-lactic acid 0.0353 M 13.5 mL]

◆ **AMSA PD (Can)** see Amsacrine on page 127

Anagrelide (an AG gre lide)

Brand Names: US Agrylin

Brand Names: Canada Agrylin; Dom-Anagrelide; Mylan-Anagrelide; PMS-Anagrelide; Sandoz-Anagrelide

Index Terms Anagrelide Hydrochloride; BL4162A

Pharmacologic Category Antiplatelet Agent; Phosphodiesterase-3 Enzyme Inhibitor

Use Thrombocythemia: Treatment of thrombocythemia associated with myeloproliferative disorders to reduce the risk of thrombosis and reduce associated symptoms (including thrombohemorrhagic events)

Labeled Contraindications There are no contraindications listed in the manufacturer's labeling.

Pregnancy Considerations Adverse events were observed in some animal reproduction studies. Data regarding use of anagrelide during pregnancy is limited. The manufacturer recommends effective contraception in women of childbearing potential.

Breastfeeding Considerations It is not known if anagrelide is excreted in breast milk. Due to the potential for serious adverse reactions in the nursing infant, a decision should be made whether to discontinue nursing or to discontinue the drug, taking into account the importance of treatment to the mother.

Warnings/Precautions Major hemorrhagic events have occurred when used concomitantly with aspirin. Monitor closely for bleeding, particularly when used concurrently with other agents known to increase bleeding risk (eg, anticoagulants, NSAIDs, antiplatelet agents, other phosphodiesterase 3 (PDE3) inhibitors, and selective serotonin reuptake inhibitors). Ventricular tachycardia and torsades de pointes have been reported. As with other PDE3 inhibitors, anagrelide may cause vasodilation, tachycardia, palpitations and heart failure. PDE3 inhibitors are associated with decreased survival (compared to placebo) in patients with class III or IV heart failure. In a scientific statement from the American Heart Association, anagrelide has been determined to be an agent that may cause direct myocardial toxicity (magnitude: major) (AHA [Page 2016]). Dose-related increases in heart rate and mean QTc interval have been observed in a clinical trial. The maximum change in mean heart rate was ~8 beats per minute (bpm) at a dose of 0.5 mg and ~29 bpm with a 2.5 mg dose. The maximum mean change in QTc I (individual subject correlation) from placebo was 7 ms and 13 ms with doses of 0.5 mg and 2.5 mg, respectively. Use is not recommended in patients with hypokalemia, congenital long QT syndrome, a known history of acquired QTc prolongation, or when using concomitant therapy which may prolong the QTc interval. Hypotension accompanied by dizziness may occur, particularly with higher doses. Use with caution in patients with cardiovascular disease (eg, heart failure, bradyarrhythmias, electrolyte abnormalities); consider periodic ECGs; benefits should outweigh risks. Pretreatment cardiovascular evaluation (including ECG) and careful monitoring during treatment is recommended. Interstitial lung disease (including allergic alveolitis, eosinophilic pneumonia, and interstitial pneumonitis) has been associated with use; onset is from 1 week to several years, usually presenting with progressive dyspnea with lung infiltrations; symptoms usually improve after discontinuation. Use caution in patients with mild to moderate hepatic dysfunction; dosage reduction and careful monitoring are required for moderate hepatic impairment; use has not been studied in patients with severe impairment. Hepatic impairment increases anagrelide exposure and may increase the risk of QTc prolongation. Monitor liver function prior to and during treatment. Renal abnormalities (including renal failure) have been observed with anagrelide use; may be associated with preexisting renal impairment, although dosage adjustment due to renal insufficiency was not required; monitor closely in patients with renal insufficiency. Potentially significant drug-drug interactions may exist, requiring dose or frequency adjustment, additional monitoring, and/or selection of alternative therapy.

Adverse Reactions Frequency not always defined; reactions similar in adult and pediatric patients unless otherwise noted.

Cardiovascular: Palpitations (26%), edema (21%), peripheral edema (9%), chest pain (8%), tachycardia (8%), angina pectoris (1% to <5%), cardiac arrhythmia (1% to <5%), cardiac failure (1% to <5%), hypertension (1% to <5%), orthostatic hypotension (1% to <5%), syncope (1% to <5%), vasodilatation (1% to <5%), atrial fibrillation, cardiomegaly, cardiomyopathy, cerebrovascular accident, complete atrioventricular block, decreased diastolic pressure (pediatric patients), increased heart rate (pediatric patients), myocardial infarction, pericardial effusion, systolic hypotension (pediatric patients)

Central nervous system: Headache (44%), dizziness (15%), pain (15%), malaise (6%), paresthesia (6%), amnesia (1% to <5%), chills (1% to <5%), confusion (1% to <5%), depression (1% to <5%), drowsiness (1% to <5%), insomnia (1% to <5%), migraine (1% to <5%), nervousness (1% to <5%), fatigue (pediatric patients)

Dermatologic: Skin rash (8%), pruritus (6%), alopecia (1% to <5%)

Gastrointestinal: Diarrhea (26%), nausea (17%), abdominal pain (16%), flatulence (10%), vomiting (10%), anorexia (8%), dyspepsia (5%), constipation (1% to <5%), gastritis (1% to <5%), gastrointestinal hemorrhage (1% to <5%), pancreatitis

Hematologic & oncologic: Anemia (1% to <5%), bruise (1% to <5%), hemorrhage (1% to <5%), thrombocytopenia (1% to <5%)

Hepatic: Increased liver enzymes (1% to <5%)

Neuromuscular & skeletal: Weakness (23%), back pain (6%), arthralgia (1% to <5%), myalgia (1% to <5%), muscle cramps (pediatric patients)

Ophthalmic: Diplopia (1% to <5%), visual field defect (1% to <5%)

Otic: Tinnitus (1% to <5%)

Renal: Hematuria (1% to <5%), renal failure (1%)

Respiratory: Dyspnea (12%), cough (6%), epistaxis (1% to <5%), flu-like symptoms (1% to <5%), pneumonia (1% to <5%), pleural effusion, pulmonary hypertension, pulmonary fibrosis, pulmonary infiltrates

Miscellaneous: Fever (9%)

<1%, postmarketing, and/or case reports: Eosinophilic pneumonitis, hepatotoxicity, hypersensitivity pneumonitis, increased serum ALT (>3 x ULN), increased serum AST (>3 x ULN), interstitial nephritis, interstitial pneumonitis, leukocytosis, prolonged Q-T interval on ECG, skin photosensitivity (pediatric patients), torsades de pointes, ventricular tachycardia

Drug Interactions

Metabolism/Transport Effects None known.

Avoid Concomitant Use

Avoid concomitant use of Anagrelide with any of the following: Amifampridine; Cilostazol; Enoximone; Highest Risk QTc-Prolonging Agents; Hydroxychloroquine; MiFEPRIStone; Milrinone; Mizolastine; Moderate Risk QTc-Prolonging Agents; Probucol; Promazine; Urokinase; Vinflunine

Increased Effect/Toxicity

Anagrelide may increase the levels/effects of: Agents with Antiplatelet Properties; Anticoagulants; Apixaban; Cephalothin; Cilostazol; Collagenase (Systemic); Dabigatran Etexilate; Deoxycholic Acid; Edoxaban; Highest Risk QTc-Prolonging Agents; Ibritumomab; Milrinone; Obinutuzumab; Riociguat; Rivaroxaban; Salicylates; Thrombolytic Agents; Tositumomab and Iodine I 131 Tositumomab; Urokinase

The levels/effects of Anagrelide may be increased by: Amifampridine; Bilastine; Buprenorphine; Enoximone; Glucosamine; Herbs (Anticoagulant/Antiplatelet Properties); Hydroxychloroquine; Ibrutinib; Indapamide; Limaprost; MiFEPRIStone; Mizolastine; Moderate Risk QTc-Prolonging Agents; Multivitamins/Fluoride (with ADE); Multivitamins/Minerals (with ADEK, Folate, Iron); Multivitamins/Minerals (with AE, No Iron); Omega-3 Fatty Acids; Pentosan Polysulfate Sodium; Pentoxifylline; Probucol; Promazine; Prostacyclin Analogues; QTc-Prolonging Agents (Indeterminate Risk and Risk Modifying); Teneligliptin; Tipranavir; Vinflunine; Vitamin E (Systemic); Xipamide

Decreased Effect There are no known significant interactions involving a decrease in effect.

Storage/Stability Store at 25°C (77°F); excursions permitted to 15°C to 30°C (59°F to 86°F). Protect from light.

Mechanism of Action Anagrelide appears to inhibit cyclic nucleotide phosphodiesterase and the release of arachidonic acid from phospholipase, possibly by inhibiting phospholipase A_2. It also causes a dose-related reduction in platelet production, which results from decreased megakaryocyte hypermaturation (disrupts the postmitotic phase of maturation).

Pharmacodynamics/Kinetics Note: In pediatric patients 7-14 years; data has shown a decreased maximum serum concentration (48%) and AUC (55%) compared to adults when normalized to dose and bodyweight.

Onset of action: Initial: Within 7 to 14 days; complete response (platelets ≤600,000/mm^3): 4 to 12 weeks

Duration: 6 to 24 hours; upon discontinuation, platelet count begins to rise within 4 days

Metabolism: Hepatic, partially via CYP1A2; to two major metabolites, RL603 and 3-hydroxy anagrelide

Bioavailability: Food has no clinically significant effect

Half-life elimination: Anagrelide: 1.5 hours, similar data reported in pediatric patients 7-14 years; 3-hydroxy anagrelide: 2.5 hours

Time to peak, serum: 1 hour, similar data reported in pediatric patients 7-14 years

Excretion: Urine (<1% as unchanged drug)

Dosing

Adult & Geriatric

Thrombocythemia: Oral: Initial: 0.5 mg 4 times daily or 1 mg twice daily (most patients will experience adequate response at dose ranges of 1.5 to 3 mg per day)

Note: Maintain initial dose for ≥1 week, then adjust to the lowest effective dose to reduce and maintain platelet count <600,000/mm^3 ideally to the normal range; the dose must not be increased by >0.5 mg per day in any 1 week; maximum single dose: 2.5 mg; maximum daily dose: 10 mg

Thrombocythemia, essential (off-label dosing): Oral: 0.5 mg twice daily for 1 week, then adjust dose to maintain platelet counts at normal (≤450,000/mm^3) or near normal (450,000/mm^3 to 600,000/mm^3) levels (Gisslinger, 2013).

Pediatric Thrombocythemia: Oral: Initial: 0.5 mg once daily (range: 0.5 mg 1 to 4 times daily)

Note: Maintain initial dose for ≥1 week, then adjust to the lowest effective dose to reduce and maintain platelet count <600,000/mm^3 ideally to the normal range; the dose must not be increased by >0.5 mg per day in any 1 week; maximum single dose: 2.5 mg; maximum daily dose: 10 mg

Renal Impairment

No dosage adjustment necessary; monitor closely.

Hemodialysis: Not dialyzable (NCS/SCCM [Frontera 2016])

Hepatic Impairment

Moderate impairment (Child-Pugh score 7 to 9): Initial: 0.5 mg once daily; maintain for at least 1 week with careful monitoring of cardiovascular status; the dose must not be increased by >0.5 mg per day in any 1 week.

Severe impairment (Child-Pugh score ≥10): Avoid use.

Administration May be administered without regard to food.

Monitoring Parameters Platelet count (every 2 days during the first week of treatment and at least weekly until the maintenance dose is reached); continue to monitor after cessation of treatment); CBC with differential (monitor closely during first 2 weeks of treatment), liver function (ALT and AST; baseline and during treatment), BUN, and serum creatinine (monitor closely during first weeks of treatment); serum electrolytes; blood pressure; heart rate; cardiovascular exam, including ECG (pretreatment; monitor during therapy); signs/ symptoms of interstitial lung disease; monitor for thrombosis or bleeding

Dosage Forms Excipient information presented when available (limited, particularly for generics); consult specific product labeling.

Capsule, Oral:

Agrylin: 0.5 mg

Generic: 0.5 mg, 1 mg

◆ **Anagrelide Hydrochloride** see Anagrelide on page 131

◆ **Anandron (Can)** see Nilutamide on page 1321

Anastrozole (an AS troe zole)

Brand Names: US Arimidex

Brand Names: Canada ACH-Anastrozole; ACT-Anastrozole; Apo-Anastrozole; Arimidex; Auro-Anastrozole; Bio-Anastrozole; JAMP-Anastrozole; Mar-Anastrozole; Med-Anastrozole; Mint-Anastrozole; Mylan-Anastrozole; Nat-Anastrozole; PMS-Anastrozole; RAN-Anastrozole; Riva-Anastrozole; Sandoz-Anastrozole; Taro-Anastrozole; Teva-Anastrozole; Zinda-Anastrozole

Index Terms ICI-D1033; ZD1033

Pharmacologic Category Antineoplastic Agent, Aromatase Inhibitor

Use Breast cancer:

First-line treatment of locally-advanced or metastatic breast cancer (hormone receptor-positive or unknown) in postmenopausal women

Adjuvant treatment of early hormone receptor-positive breast cancer in postmenopausal women

Treatment of advanced breast cancer in postmenopausal women with disease progression following tamoxifen therapy

Labeled Contraindications Hypersensitivity to anastrozole or any component of the formulation; use in women who are or may become pregnant

Canadian labeling: Additional contraindications (not in US labeling): Lactating women

Pregnancy Considerations Adverse events were observed in animal reproduction studies. Anastrozole is contraindicated in women who are or may become pregnant (may cause fetal harm if administered during pregnancy). Use in premenopausal women with breast cancer does not provide any clinical benefit.

◄ **Breastfeeding Considerations** It is not known if anastrozole is excreted in breast milk. Due to the potential for serious adverse reactions in the nursing infant, a decision should be made whether to discontinue nursing or to discontinue the drug, taking into account the importance of treatment to the mother.

Warnings/Precautions Use is contraindicated in women who are or may become pregnant. Anastrozole offers no clinical benefit in premenopausal women with breast cancer. Patients with preexisting ischemic cardiac disease have an increased risk for ischemic cardiovascular events.

Due to decreased circulating estrogen levels, anastrozole is associated with a reduction in bone mineral density (BMD); decreases (from baseline) in total hip and lumbar spine BMD have been reported. Patients with preexisting osteopenia are at higher risk for developing osteoporosis (Eastell 2008). When initiating anastrozole treatment, follow available guidelines for bone mineral density management in postmenopausal women with similar fracture risk; concurrent use of bisphosphonates may be useful in patients at risk for fractures.

Elevated total cholesterol levels (contributed to by LDL cholesterol increases) have been reported in patients receiving anastrozole; use with caution in patients with hyperlipidemias; cholesterol levels should be monitored/managed in accordance with current guidelines for patients with LDL elevations. Plasma concentrations in patients with stable hepatic cirrhosis were within the range of concentrations seen in normal subjects across all clinical trials; use has not been studied in patients with severe hepatic impairment.

Adverse Reactions

>10%:

Cardiovascular: Vasodilatation (25% to 36%), ischemic heart disease (4%; 17% in patients with preexisting ischemic heart disease), hypertension (2% to 13%), angina pectoris (2%; 12% in patients with preexisting ischemic heart disease), edema (7% to 11%)

Central nervous system: Fatigue (19%), mood disorder (19%), headache (9% to 18%), pain (11% to 17%), depression (2% to 13%)

Dermatologic: Skin rash (6% to 11%)

Endocrine & metabolic: Hot flash (12% to 36%)

Gastrointestinal: Gastrointestinal distress (29% to 34%), nausea (11% to 20%), vomiting (8% to 13%)

Neuromuscular & skeletal: Weakness (13% to 19%), arthritis (17%), arthralgia (2% to 15%), back pain (10% to 12%), ostealgia (6% to 12%), osteoporosis (11%)

Respiratory: Pharyngitis (6% to 14%), dyspnea (8% to 11%), increased cough (7% to 11%)

1% to 10%:

Cardiovascular: Peripheral edema (5% to 10%), chest pain (5% to 7%), venous thrombosis (2% to 4%; including pulmonary embolism, thrombophlebitis, retinal vein thrombosis), myocardial infarction (1%)

Central nervous system: Insomnia (2% to 10%), dizziness (5% to 8%), paresthesia (5% to 7%), anxiety (2% to 6%), confusion (2% to 5%), drowsiness (2% to 5%), malaise (2% to 5%), nervousness (2% to 5%), carpal tunnel syndrome (3%), hypertonia (3%), cerebrovascular insufficiency (2%), lethargy (1%)

Dermatologic: Alopecia (2% to 5%), pruritus (2% to 5%), diaphoresis (1% to 5%)

Endocrine & metabolic: Hypercholesterolemia (9%), increased serum cholesterolemia (9%), weight gain (2% to 9%), increased gamma-glutamyl transferase (2% to 5%), weight loss (2% to 5%)

Gastrointestinal: Constipation (7% to 9%), diarrhea (7% to 9%), abdominal pain (6% to 9%), anorexia (5% to 8%), dyspepsia (7%), gastrointestinal disease (7%), xerostomia (4% to 6%)

Genitourinary: Mastalgia (2% to 8%), urinary tract infection (2% to 8%), pelvic pain (5% to 7%), vulvovaginitis (6%), vaginal dryness (1% to 5%), vaginal hemorrhage (1% to 5%), vaginal discharge (4%), vaginitis (4%), leukorrhea (2% to 3%)

Hematologic & oncologic: Lymphedema (10%), breast neoplasm (5%), neoplasm (5%), anemia (2% to 5%), leukopenia (2% to 5%), tumor flare (3%)

Hepatic: Increased serum alkaline phosphatase (2% to 5%), increased serum ALT (2% to 5%), increased serum AST (2% to 5%)

Infection: Infection (2% to 9%)

Neuromuscular & skeletal: Bone fracture (1% to 10%), arthrosis (7%), myalgia (2% to 6%), neck pain (2% to 5%), pathological fracture (2% to 5%)

Ophthalmic: Cataract (6%)

Respiratory: Flu-like symptoms (2% to 7%), sinusitis (2% to 6%), bronchitis (2% to 5%), rhinitis (2% to 5%)

Miscellaneous: Accidental injury (2% to 10%), cyst (5%), fever (2% to 5%)

<1%, postmarketing, and/or case reports: Anaphylaxis, angioedema, cerebral infarction, cerebral ischemia, decreased bone mineral density, dermal ulcer, endometrial carcinoma, erythema multiforme, hepatitis, hepatomegaly, hypercalcemia, hypersensitivity angiitis (including anaphylactoid purpura [IgA vasculitis]), increased serum bilirubin, jaundice, joint stiffness, pulmonary embolism, retinal thrombosis, skin blister, skin lesion, Stevens-Johnson syndrome, tenosynovitis (stenosing), urticaria

Drug Interactions

Metabolism/Transport Effects Inhibits CYP2C8 (weak), CYP2C9 (weak)

Avoid Concomitant Use

Avoid concomitant use of Anastrozole with any of the following: Amodiaquine; Estrogen Derivatives

Increased Effect/Toxicity

Anastrozole may increase the levels/effects of: Amodiaquine; Methadono

Decreased Effect

The levels/effects of Anastrozole may be decreased by: Estrogen Derivatives; Tamoxifen

Hazardous Drugs Handling Considerations

Hazardous agent (NIOSH 2016 [group 1]).

Use appropriate precautions for receiving, handling, administration, and disposal. Gloves (single) should be worn during receiving, unpacking, and placing in storage. NIOSH recommends single gloving for administration of intact tablets or capsules (NIOSH 2016).

Storage/Stability Store at 20°C to 25°C (68°F to 77°F).

Mechanism of Action Potent and selective nonsteroidal aromatase inhibitor. By inhibiting aromatase, the conversion of androstenedione to estrone, and testosterone to estradiol, is prevented, thereby decreasing tumor mass or delaying progression in patients with tumors responsive to hormones. Anastrozole causes an 85% decrease in estrone sulfate levels.

◄ **Pharmacodynamics/Kinetics**

Onset of estradiol reduction: 70% reduction after 24 hours; 80% after 2 weeks of therapy

Duration of estradiol reduction: 6 days

Absorption: Well absorbed; extent of absorption not affected by food

Protein binding, plasma: 40%

Metabolism: Extensively hepatic (~85%) via N-dealkylation, hydroxylation, and glucuronidation; primary metabolite (triazole) inactive

Half-life elimination: ~50 hours

Time to peak, plasma: ~2 hours without food; 5 hours with food

Excretion: Feces; urine (urinary excretion accounts for ~10% of total elimination, mostly as metabolites)

Dosing

Adult & Geriatric

Breast cancer, advanced: Postmenopausal females: Oral: 1 mg once daily; continue until tumor progression

Breast cancer, early (adjuvant treatment): Postmenopausal females: Oral: 1 mg once daily.

Duration of therapy: The American Society of Clinical Oncology (ASCO) guidelines for Adjuvant Endocrine Therapy of Hormone-Receptor Positive Breast Cancer (Focused Update) recommend a maximum duration of 5 years of aromatase inhibitor (AI) therapy for postmenopausal women; AIs may be combined with tamoxifen for a total duration of up to 10 years of endocrine therapy. Refer to the guidelines for specific recommendations based on menopausal status and tolerability (Burstein 2014). In a phase III study with another AI (letrozole), treatment with an additional 5 years of AI therapy (for a total of 10 years of AI therapy) demonstrated a significantly improved rate of disease-free survival and a decreased risk of disease recurrence and contralateral breast cancer (when compared to placebo), although overall survival was not significantly different between groups and bone-related adverse events occurred more frequently with letrozole versus placebo (Goss 2016).

Breast cancer, risk reduction (off-label use): Postmenopausal females ≥40 years: Oral: 1 mg once daily for 5 years (Cuzick 2014)

Endometrial or uterine cancer, recurrent or metastatic (off-label use): Oral: 1 mg once daily (Rose 2000)

Ovarian cancer, recurrent (off-label use): Oral: 1 mg once daily until disease progression or unacceptable toxicity (del Carmen 2003)

Renal Impairment No dosage adjustment necessary.

Hepatic Impairment

Mild to moderate impairment or stable hepatic cirrhosis: No dosage adjustment necessary.

Severe hepatic impairment: There are no dosage adjustments provided in the manufacturer's labeling (has not been studied).

Administration May be administered with or without food.

Monitoring Parameters

Bone mineral density; total cholesterol and LDL

Breast cancer risk reduction (off-label use): Bone mineral density at baseline, mammograms, and clinical breast exam at baseline and at least every 2 years (Cuzick, 2014)

Dosage Forms Excipient information presented when available (limited, particularly for generics); consult specific product labeling.
Tablet, Oral:
Arimidex: 1 mg
Generic: 1 mg

◆ **Ancobon** *see* Flucytosine *on page 815*

◆ **Androcur (Can)** *see* Cyproterone *on page 468*

◆ **Androcur Depot (Can)** *see* Cyproterone *on page 468*

◆ **Androxy** *see* Fluoxymesterone *on page 838*

Anidulafungin (ay nid yoo la FUN jin)

Brand Names: US Eraxis
Brand Names: Canada Eraxis
Index Terms LY303366
Pharmacologic Category Antifungal Agent, Parenteral; Echinocandin
Use Treatment of candidemia and other forms of *Candida* infections (including those of intra-abdominal, peritoneal, and esophageal locus)
Pregnancy Risk Factor B
Dosing
Adult & Geriatric
Candidemia, intra-abdominal or peritoneal candidiasis: IV: Initial dose: 200 mg on day 1; subsequent dosing: 100 mg daily; treatment should continue until 14 days after last positive culture. **Note:** IDSA Candidiasis guidelines recommend transition to fluconazole (eg, after 5 to 7 days in nonneutropenic patients) in clinically stable patients with fluconazole-susceptible isolates and negative repeat cultures (IDSA [Pappas 2016])
Candidiasis, chronic disseminated (hepatosplenic) (off-label use): IV: 200 mg on day 1; subsequent dosing: 100 mg daily for several weeks, followed by oral fluconazole therapy (IDSA [Pappas 2016])
Candidiasis, empiric therapy (suspected invasive candidiasis in non-neutropenic ICU patients) (off-label use): IV: 200 mg on day 1; subsequent dosing: 100 mg daily; treatment should continue in patients with clinical improvement. Consider discontinuing after 4 to 5 days in patients with no clinical response (IDSA [Pappas 2016])
Candidiasis, intravascular infections (native or prosthetic valve endocarditis, infection of implantable cardiac devices, suppurative thrombophlebitis) (off-label use): IV: 200 mg daily. For native or prosthetic valve endocarditis, therapy should continue for at least 6 weeks after valve replacement surgery (longer durations in patients with abscesses or other complications); for patients with implantable cardiac devices, therapy should continue for 4 to 6 weeks after surgery (4 weeks for infections limited to generator pockets and at least 6 weeks for infections involving the wires); for suppurative thrombophlebitis, continue for at least 2 weeks after candidemia has cleared. **Note:** Step-down to fluconazole therapy is recommended in clinically stable patients with fluconazole-susceptible isolates and negative repeat cultures (IDSA [Pappas 2016])
Candidiasis, osteoarticular infections (osteomyelitis or septic arthritis) (alternative therapy) (off-label use): IV: 100 mg daily for at least 14 days, followed by fluconazole (IDSA [Pappas 2016])

Candidiasis, prophylaxis against invasive candidiasis (high-risk ICU patients in units with a high incidence of invasive candidiasis) (alternative therapy; off-label use): IV: Initial dose: 200 mg on day 1; subsequent doses: 100 mg daily (IDSA [Pappas 2016])

Candidiasis, esophageal: IV:

Manufacturer's labeling: Initial dose: 100 mg on day 1; subsequent dosing: 50 mg daily; treatment should continue for a minimum of 14 days and for at least 7 days after symptom resolution

Alternate recommendations: 200 mg daily; may transition to oral fluconazole therapy once oral intake tolerable. In patients with fluconazole-refractory disease, continue anidulafungin for 14 to 21 days (IDSA [Pappas 2016])

Candidiasis, oropharyngeal (refractory disease) (alternative therapy) (off-label use): IV: Initial dose: 200 mg on day 1; subsequent dosing: 100 mg daily (IDSA [Pappas 2016])

Renal Impairment No dosage adjustment necessary, including dialysis patients.

Hepatic Impairment No dosage adjustment necessary.

Additional Information Complete prescribing information should be consulted for additional detail.

Dosage Forms Excipient information presented when available (limited, particularly for generics); consult specific product labeling.

Solution Reconstituted, Intravenous [preservative free]:

Eraxis: 50 mg (1 ea); 100 mg (1 ea) [contains polysorbate 80]

♦ **Anodyne LPT** *see* Lidocaine and Prilocaine *on page 1150*

♦ **Anti-D Immunoglobulin** *see* Rh₀(D) Immune Globulin *on page 1591*

♦ **131 I Anti-B1 Antibody** *see* Tositumomab and Iodine I 131 Tositumomab *on page 1801*

♦ **131 I-Anti-B1 Monoclonal Antibody** *see* Tositumomab and Iodine I 131 Tositumomab *on page 1801*

♦ **Antibody-Drug Conjugate SGN-35** *see* Brentuximab Vedotin *on page 285*

♦ **Anti-CD20 Monoclonal Antibody** *see* RiTUXimab *on page 1610*

♦ **Anti-CD20 Monoclonal Antibody** *see* Rituximab and Hyaluronidase *on page 1623*

♦ **Anti-CD20-Murine Monoclonal Antibody I-131** *see* Tositumomab and Iodine I 131 Tositumomab *on page 1801*

♦ **Anti-CD30 ADC SGN-35** *see* Brentuximab Vedotin *on page 285*

♦ **Anti-CD30 Antibody-Drug Conjugate SGN-35** *see* Brentuximab Vedotin *on page 285*

♦ **Anti-CD52 Monoclonal Antibody** *see* Alemtuzumab *on page 82*

♦ **anti-c-erB-2** *see* Trastuzumab *on page 1822*

♦ **Anti-EGFR Monoclonal Antibody IMC-11F8** *see* Necitumumab *on page 1298*

♦ **anti-ERB-2** *see* Trastuzumab *on page 1822*

Antihemophilic Factor (Human)

(an tee hee moe FIL ik FAK tor HYU man)

Brand Names: US Hemofil M; Koate; Koate-DVI; Monoclate-P

Brand Names: Canada Hemofil M

Index Terms AHF (Human); Factor VIII (Human); Koate DVI

Pharmacologic Category Antihemophilic Agent; Blood Product Derivative

Use Hemophilia A: Control and prevention of bleeding episodes in patients with hemophilia A (classic hemophilia); perioperative management of hemophilia A.

Limitations of use: Not indicated for the treatment of von Willebrand disease.

Pregnancy Risk Factor C

Dosing

Adult & Geriatric Hemophilia A: IV: Individualize dosage based on coagulation studies performed prior to treatment and at regular intervals during treatment. In general, administration of factor VIII 1 unit/kg will increase circulating factor VIII levels by ~2 units/dL. **Refer to product information for specific manufacturer recommended dosing.** Alternatively, the World Federation of Hemophilia (WFH) has recommended general dosing for factor VIII products.

Dosage based on desired factor VIII increase (%):
To calculate dosage needed based on desired factor VIII increase (%):
Body weight (kg) x 0.5 units/kg x desired factor VIII increase (%) = units factor VIII required
For example:
50 kg x 0.5 units/kg x 30 (% increase) = 750 units factor VIII

Dosage based on expected factor VIII increase (%):
It is also possible to calculate the **expected** % factor VIII increase:
(# units administered x 2%/units/kg) divided by body weight (kg) = expected % factor VIII increase
For example:
(1400 units x 2%/units/kg) divided by 70 kg = 40%

World Federation of Hemophilia (WFH) treatment recommendations when no significant resource constraint exists (WFH [Srivastava 2013]):

2013 World Federation of Hemophilia Treatment Recommendations (When No Significant Resource Constraint Exists)

Site of Hemorrhage/ Clinical Situation	Desired Factor VIII Level to Maintain	Duration
Joint	40 to 60 units/dL	1 to 2 days, may be longer if response is inadequate
Superficial muscle/no neurovascular compromise	40 to 60 units/dL	2 to 3 days, sometimes longer if response is inadequate
Iliopsoas and deep muscle with neurovascular injury, or substantial blood loss	*Initial:* 80 to 100 units/dL	*Initial:* 1 to 2 days
	Maintenance: 30 to 60 units/dL	*Maintenance:* 3 to 5 days, sometimes longer as secondary prophylaxis during physiotherapy
CNS/Head	*Initial:* 80 to 100 units/dL	*Initial:* 1 to 7 days
	Maintenance: 50 units/dL	*Maintenance:* 8 to 21 days
Throat and neck	*Initial:* 80 to 100 units/dL	*Initial:* 1 to 7 days
	Maintenance: 50 units/dL	*Maintenance:* 8 to 14 days

(continued) ▶

◀ **2013 World Federation of Hemophilia Treatment Recommendations (When No Significant Resource Constraint Exists)** (continued)

Site of Hemorrhage/ Clinical Situation	Desired Factor VIII Level to Maintain	Duration
Gastrointestinal	*Initial:* 80 to 100 units/dL	*Initial:* 7 to 14 days
	Maintenance: 50 units/dL	*Maintenance:* Not specified
Renal	50 units/dL	3 to 5 days
Deep laceration	50 units/dL	5 to 7 days
Surgery (major)	*Preop:* 80 to 100 units/dL	
	Postop: 60 to 80 units/dL	*Postop:* 1 to 3 days
	Postop: 40 to 60 units/dL	*Postop:* 4 to 6 days
	Postop: 30 to 50 units/dL	*Postop:* 7 to 14 days
Surgery (minor)	*Preop:* 50 to 80 units/dL	
	Postop: 30 to 80 units/dL	*Postop:* 1 to 5 days depending on procedure type

Note: Factor VIII level may either be expressed as units/dL or as %. Dosing frequency most commonly corresponds to the half-life of factor VIII but should be determined based on an assessment of factor VIII levels before the next dose.

> *Continuous infusion (for patients who require prolonged periods of treatment [eg, intracranial hemorrhage or surgery] to avoid peaks and troughs associated with intermittent infusions) (Batorova 2002; Batorova 2012; Poon 2012; Rickard 1995; WFH [Srivastava 2013]):* Following initial bolus to achieve the desired factor VIII level, initiate 2 to 4 units/kg/hour; adjust dose based on frequent factor assays and calculation of factor VIII clearance at steady-state using the following equations:
> Factor VIII clearance (mL/kg/hour) = (current infusion rate in units/kg/hour) divided by (plasma level in units/mL)
> New infusion rate (units/kg/hour) = (factor VIII clearance in mL/kg/hour) x (desired plasma level in units/mL)

Pediatric Hemophilia A: Children and Adolescents: Refer to adult dosing.

Renal Impairment There are no dosage adjustments provided in the manufacturer's labeling.

Hepatic Impairment There are no dosage adjustments provided in the manufacturer's labeling.

Additional Information Complete prescribing information should be consulted for additional detail.

Dosage Forms Considerations

Strengths expressed with approximate values. Consult individual vial labels for exact potency within each vial.

Hemofil M packaged contents may contain natural rubber latex.

Dosage Forms Excipient information presented when available (limited, particularly for generics); consult specific product labeling. [DSC] = Discontinued product

Kit, Intravenous:

Monoclate-P: ~250 units [DSC], ~500 units [DSC], ~1000 units, ~1500 units [contains mouse (murine) and/or hamster protein]

Solution Reconstituted, Intravenous:

Koate: ~250 units (1 ea); ~500 units (1 ea); ~1000 units (1 ea) [contains albumin human, polyethylene glycol, polysorbate 80]

Solution Reconstituted, Intravenous [preservative free]:
　Hemofil M: ~250 units (1 ea) [contains albumin human, mouse (murine) and/
　　or hamster protein, polyethylene glycol]
　Hemofil M: ~250 units (1 ea [DSC]) [contains mouse (murine) and/or
　　hamster protein, polyethylene glycol]
　Hemofil M: ~500 units (1 ea) [contains albumin human, mouse (murine) and/
　　or hamster protein, polyethylene glycol]
　Hemofil M: ~500 units (1 ea [DSC]) [contains mouse (murine) and/or
　　hamster protein, polyethylene glycol]
　Hemofil M: ~1000 units (1 ea); ~1700 units (1 ea) [contains albumin human,
　　mouse (murine) and/or hamster protein, polyethylene glycol]
　Koate-DVI: ~250 units (1 ea); ~500 units (1 ea); ~1000 units (1 ea) [contains
　　albumin human, polyethylene glycol, polysorbate 80]

Antihemophilic Factor (Recombinant)
(an tee hee moe FIL ik FAK tor ree KOM be nant)

Brand Names: US Advate; Afstyla; Helixate FS; Kogenate FS; Kogenate FS
Bio-Set; Kovaltry; Novoeight; Nuwiq; Recombinate; Xyntha; Xyntha Solofuse

Brand Names: Canada Advate; Helixate FS; Kogenate FS; Kovaltry; Nuwiq;
Xyntha; Xyntha Solofuse

Index Terms AHF (Recombinant); Antihemophilic Factor (Recombinant),
Single Chain; Efraloctocog Alfa; Factor VIII (Recombinant); Moroctocog Alfa;
Octacog Alfa; rAHF

Pharmacologic Category Antihemophilic Agent

Use

Hemophilia A:

Control and prevention of bleeding episodes: Prevention and control of
bleeding episodes in adults and children with hemophilia A.

Perioperative management: Surgical prophylaxis in adults and children
with hemophilia A.

Routine prophylaxis to prevent or reduce the frequency of bleeding:
Routine prophylactic treatment to prevent or reduce the frequency of
bleeding episodes in adults and children with hemophilia A.

**Routine prophylaxis to prevent bleeding episodes and joint damage
(Helixate FS, Kogenate FS):** Routine prophylactic treatment to reduce the
frequency of bleeding episodes and the risk of joint damage in children
without preexisting joint damage.

Limitations of use: Not indicated for the treatment of von Willebrand disease.

Pregnancy Risk Factor C

Dosing

Adult & Geriatric Hemophilia A: IV: Individualize dosage based on
coagulation studies performed prior to treatment and at regular intervals
during treatment. In general, administration of factor VIII 1 unit/kg will
increase circulating factor VIII levels by ~2 units/dL.

**Control and prevention of bleeding episodes or perioperative manage-
ment:**

Manufacturer's labeling: Refer to manufacturer's labeling for specific recommendations; varies by product.

◀

Alternate recommendations (WFH [Srivastava 2013]):
Dosage based on desired factor VIII increase (%):
To calculate dosage needed based on desired factor VIII increase (%):
[Body weight (kg) x desired factor VIII increase (%)] divided by 2
(%/units/kg) = units factor VIII required
For example:
50 kg x 30 (% increase) divided by 2 = 750 units factor VIII
Dosage based on expected factor VIII increase (%):
It is also possible to calculate the **expected** % factor VIII increase:
[# units administered x 2 (%/units/kg)] divided by body weight (kg) =
expected % factor VIII increase
For example:
[1,400 units x 2] divided by 70 kg = 40%
World Federation of Hemophilia (WFH) treatment recommendations when no significant resource constraint exists (WFH [Srivastava 2013]):

2013 World Federation of Hemophilia Treatment Recommendations (When No Significant Resource Constraint Exists)

Site of Hemorrhage/ Clinical Situation	Desired Factor VIII Level to Maintain	Duration
Joint	40 to 60 units/dL	1 to 2 days, may be longer if response is inadequate
Superficial muscle/no neurovascular compromise	40 to 60 units/dL	2 to 3 days, sometimes longer if response is inadequate
Iliopsoas and deep muscle with neurovascular injury, or substantial blood loss	*Initial:* 80 to 100 units/dL	*Initial:* 1 to 2 days
	Maintenance: 30 to 60 units/dL	*Maintenance:* 3 to 5 days, sometimes longer as secondary prophylaxis during physiotherapy
CNS/Head	*Initial:* 80 to 100 units/dL	*Initial:* 1 to 7 days
	Maintenance: 50 units/dL	*Maintenance:* 8 to 21 days
Throat and neck	*Initial:* 80 to 100 units/dL	*Initial:* 1 to 7 days
	Maintenance: 50 units/dL	*Maintenance:* 8 to 14 days
Gastrointestinal	*Initial:* 80 to 100 units/dL	*Initial:* 7 to 14 days
	Maintenance: 50 units/dL	*Maintenance:* Not specified
Renal	50 units/dL	3 to 5 days
Deep laceration	50 units/dL	5 to 7 days
Surgery (major)	*Preop:* 80 to 100 units/dL	
	Postop: 60 to 80 units/dL	*Postop:* 1 to 3 days
	Postop: 40 to 60 units/dL	*Postop:* 4 to 6 days
	Postop: 30 to 50 units/dL	*Postop:* 7 to 14 days
Surgery (minor)	*Preop:* 50 to 80 units/dL	
	Postop: 30 to 80 units/dL	*Postop:* 1 to 5 days depending on procedure type

Note: Factor VIII level may either be expressed as units/dL or as %. Dosing frequency most commonly corresponds to the half-life of factor VIII but should be determined based on an assessment of factor VIII levels before the next dose.

Continuous infusion (for patients who require prolonged periods of treatment [eg, intracranial hemorrhage or surgery] to avoid peaks and troughs associated with intermittent infusions) (Batorova 2002; Batorova 2012; Poon 2012; Rickard 1995; WFH [Srivastava 2013]): Following initial bolus to achieve the desired factor VIII level, initiate 2 to 4 units/kg/hour; adjust dose based on frequent factor assays and calculation of factor VIII clearance at steady-state using the following equations:

Factor VIII clearance (mL/kg/hour) = (current infusion rate in units/kg/hour) divided by (plasma level in units/mL)

New infusion rate (units/kg/hour) = (factor VIII clearance in mL/kg/hour) x (desired plasma level in units/mL)

Routine prophylaxis to prevent or reduce the frequency of bleeding episodes: Note: Maintain factor VIII trough levels between 1% and 5% as clinically indicated (Collins 2011; Rossbach 2010).

Advate: 20 to 40 units/kg every other day (3 to 4 times weekly). Alternatively, an every-third-day dosing regimen may be used to target factor VIII trough levels of ≥1%.

Afstyla: 20 to 50 units/kg 2 to 3 times weekly

Helixate FS: 25 units/kg 3 times weekly

Kogenate FS: 25 units/kg 3 times weekly

Kovaltry: 20 to 40 units/kg 2 or 3 times weekly

Novoeight: 20 to 50 units/kg 3 times weekly **or** 20 to 40 units/kg every other day

Nuwiq: 30 to 40 units/kg every other day

Pediatric Hemophilia A: Children and Adolescents: IV: Individualize dosage based on coagulation studies performed prior to treatment and at regular intervals during treatment. In general, administration of factor VIII 1 unit/kg will increase circulating factor VIII levels by ~2 units/dL. Children <6 years may require higher doses and/or more frequent administration.

Control and prevention of bleeding episodes or perioperative management: Refer to adult dosing.

Routine prophylaxis to prevent bleeding episodes: Note: Maintain factor VIII trough levels between 1% and 5% as clinically indicated (Collins 2011; Rossbach 2010).

Advate: Refer to adult dosing.

Afstyla:

Children <12 years: 30 to 50 units/kg 2 to 3 times weekly.

Children ≥12 years and Adolescents: Refer to adult dosing.

Kovaltry:

Children ≤12 years: 25 to 50 units/kg twice weekly, 3 times weekly, or every other day according to individual requirements.

Children >12 years and Adolescents: Refer to adult dosing.

Novoeight:

Children <12 years: 25 to 60 units per kg 3 times weekly **or** 25 to 50 units/kg every other day.

Children ≥12 years and Adolescents: Refer to adult dosing.

Nuwiq:

Children 2 to 11 years: 30 to 50 units/kg every other day or 3 times weekly.

Children ≥12 years and Adolescents: Refer to adult dosing.

◄ **Routine prophylaxis to prevent bleeding episodes and joint damage (in patients without preexisting joint damage):**
Helixate FS, Kogenate FS: Infants, Children, and Adolescents: 25 units/kg every other day.

Renal Impairment There are no dosage adjustments provided in the manufacturer's labeling.

Hepatic Impairment There are no dosage adjustments provided in the manufacturer's labeling.

Additional Information Complete prescribing information should be consulted for additional detail.

Dosage Forms Considerations Strengths expressed with approximate values. Consult individual vial labels for exact potency within each vial.

Dosage Forms Excipient information presented when available (limited, particularly for generics); consult specific product labeling.

Kit, Intravenous:

Kogenate FS: 250 units, 500 units, 1000 units [contains mouse (murine) and/or hamster protein]

Kit, Intravenous [preservative free]:

Afstyla: 250 units, 500 units, 1000 units, 1500 units, 2000 units, 2500 units, 3000 units [contains polysorbate 80]

Helixate FS: 250 units, 500 units, 1000 units, 2000 units, 3000 units [contains polysorbate 80]

Kogenate FS: 2000 units, 3000 units [contains mouse (murine) and/or hamster protein]

Kogenate FS Bio-Set: 250 units, 500 units, 1000 units, 2000 units, 3000 units [contains mouse (murine) and/or hamster protein]

Nuwiq: 250 units, 500 units, 1000 units, 2000 units, 2500 units, 3000 units, 4000 units

Xyntha: 250 units, 500 units, 1000 units, 2000 units [albumin free; contains mouse (murine) and/or hamster protein, polysorbate 80]

Xyntha Solofuse: 250 units, 500 units, 1000 units, 2000 units, 3000 units [albumin free; contains mouse (murine) and/or hamster protein, polysorbate 80]

Solution Reconstituted, Intravenous:

Kovaltry: 250 units (1 ea); 500 units (1 ea); 1000 units (1 ea); 2000 units (1 ea); 3000 units (1 ea) [contains mouse (murine) and/or hamster protein, polysorbate 80]

Solution Reconstituted, Intravenous [preservative free]:

Advate: 250 units (1 ea); 500 units (1 ea); 1000 units (1 ea); 1500 units (1 ea); 2000 units (1 ea); 3000 units (1 ea); 4000 units (1 ea) [albumin free; contains polysorbate 80]

Novoeight: 250 units (1 ea); 500 units (1 ea); 1000 units (1 ea); 1500 units (1 ea); 2000 units (1 ea); 3000 units (1 ea) [contains mouse (murine) and/or hamster protein, polysorbate 80]

Nuwiq: 250 units (1 ea); 500 units (1 ea); 1000 units (1 ea); 2000 units (1 ea); 2500 units (1 ea); 3000 units (1 ea); 4000 units (1 ea)

Recombinate: 220-400 units (1 ea); 401-800 units (1 ea); 801-1240 units (1 ea); 1241-1800 units (1 ea); 1801-2400 units (1 ea) [contains albumin human, polyethylene glycol, polysorbate 80]

Antihemophilic Factor (Recombinant [Fc Fusion Protein])

(an tee hee moe FIL ik FAK tor ree KOM be nant eff see FYOO zhun PRO teen)

Brand Names: US Eloctate

Brand Names: Canada Eloctate

Index Terms AHF (Recombinant [Fc Fusion Protein]); Efmoroctocog Alfa; Factor VIII (Recombinant [Fc Fusion Protein]); rAHF (Fc Fusion Protein)

Pharmacologic Category Antihemophilic Agent

Use Hemophilia A:

Control and prevention of bleeding episodes: For the prevention and control of bleeding episodes in adults and children with hemophilia A.

Perioperative management: For surgical prophylaxis in adults and children with hemophilia A.

Routine prophylaxis to prevent or reduce the frequency of bleeding: For routine prophylactic treatment to prevent or reduce the frequency of bleeding episodes in adults and children with hemophilia A.

Limitation of use: Not indicated for the treatment of von Willebrand disease.

Dosing

Adult & Geriatric

Hemophilia A: IV: Individualize dosage based on coagulation studies performed prior to treatment and at regular intervals during treatment. In general, administration of factor VIII 1 unit/kg will increase circulating factor VIII levels by ~2 units/dL.

Control and prevention of bleeding episodes or perioperative management:

Manufacturer's labeling: Refer to manufacturer's labeling for specific recommendations.

Alternate recommendations (WFH [Srivastava 2013]):

Dosage based on desired factor VIII increase (%):

To calculate dosage needed based on desired factor VIII increase (%):

[Body weight (kg) x desired factor VIII increase (%)] divided by 2 (%/units/kg) = units factor VIII required

For example:

50 kg x 30 (% increase) divided by 2 = 750 units factor VIII

Dosage based on expected factor VIII increase (%):

It is also possible to calculate the **expected** % factor VIII increase:

[# units administered x 2 (%/units/kg)] divided by body weight (kg) = expected % factor VIII increase

For example:

[1,400 units x 2] divided by 70 kg = 40%

World Federation of Hemophilia (WFH) treatment recommendations when no significant resource constraint exists (WFH [Srivastava 2013]):

2013 World Federation of Hemophilia Treatment Recommendations (When No Significant Resource Constraint Exists)

Site of Hemorrhage/ Clinical Situation	Desired Factor VIII Level to Maintain	Duration
Joint	40 to 60 units/dL	1 to 2 days, may be longer if response is inadequate
Superficial muscle/no neurovascular compromise	40 to 60 units/dL	2 to 3 days, sometimes longer if response is inadequate
Iliopsoas and deep muscle with neurovascular injury, or substantial blood loss	Initial: 80 to 100 units/dL	Initial: 1 to 2 days
	Maintenance: 30 to 60 units/dL	Maintenance: 3 to 5 days, sometimes longer as secondary prophylaxis during physiotherapy
CNS/Head	Initial: 80 to 100 units/dL	Initial: 1 to 7 days
	Maintenance: 50 units/dL	Maintenance: 8 to 21 days
Throat and neck	Initial: 80 to 100 units/dL	Initial: 1 to 7 days
	Maintenance: 50 units/dL	Maintenance: 8 to 14 days
Gastrointestinal	Initial: 80 to 100 units/dL	Initial: 7 to 14 days
	Maintenance: 50 units/dL	Maintenance: Not specified
Renal	50 units/dL	3 to 5 days
Deep laceration	50 units/dL	5 to 7 days
Surgery (major)	Preop: 80 to 100 units/dL	
	Postop: 60 to 80 units/dL	Postop: 1 to 3 days
	Postop: 40 to 60 units/dL	Postop: 4 to 6 days
	Postop: 30 to 50 units/dL	Postop: 7 to 14 days
Surgery (minor)	Preop: 50 to 80 units/dL	
	Postop: 30 to 80 units/dL	Postop: 1 to 5 days depending on procedure type

Note: Factor VIII level may either be expressed as units/dL or as %. Dosing frequency most commonly corresponds to the half-life of factor VIII but should be determined based on an assessment of factor VIII levels before the next dose.

Routine prophylaxis to prevent or reduce the frequency of bleeding episodes: IV: 50 units/kg every 4 days; at 3- to 5-day intervals, may adjust dose within the range of 25 to 65 units/kg based on patient response. Maintain trough levels between 1% and 3% above baseline, or higher, as clinically indicated.

Pediatric

Hemophilia A: Children and Adolescents: IV: Individualize dosage based on coagulation studies performed prior to treatment and at regular intervals during treatment. In general, administration of factor VIII 1 unit/kg will increase circulating factor VIII levels by ~2 units/dL. Children <6 years may require higher doses and/or more frequent administration.

Control and prevention of bleeding episodes or perioperative management: *Refer to adult dosing.*

Routine prophylaxis to prevent bleeding episodes:

Children <6 years: 50 units/kg twice weekly; at 3- to 5-day intervals, may adjust dose within the range of 25 to 65 units/kg based on patient response. More frequent or higher doses (up to 80 units/kg) may be required.

Children ≥6 years and Adolescents: Refer to adult dosing.

Renal Impairment There are no dosage adjustments provided in the manufacturer's labeling; however, renal impairment has no bearing.

Hepatic Impairment There are no dosage adjustments provided in the manufacturer's labeling.

Additional Information Complete prescribing information should be consulted for additional detail.

Dosage Forms Considerations Strengths expressed with approximate values. Consult individual vial labels for exact potency within each vial.

Dosage Forms Excipient information presented when available (limited, particularly for generics); consult specific product labeling.

Solution Reconstituted, Intravenous [preservative free]:

Eloctate: 250 units (1 ea); 500 units (1 ea); 750 units (1 ea); 1000 units (1 ea); 1500 units (1 ea); 2000 units (1 ea); 3000 units (1 ea); 4000 units (1 ea); 5000 units (1 ea); 6000 units (1 ea)

Antihemophilic Factor (Recombinant [Pegylated])

(an tee hee moe FIL ik FAK tor ree KOM be nant PEG i late ed)

Brand Names: US Adynovate

Index Terms AHF (Recombinant [Pegylated]); Factor VIII (Recombinant [Pegylated])

Pharmacologic Category Antihemophilic Agent

Use Hemophilia A:

Perioperative management: Surgical prophylaxis in adults and children with hemophilia A.

Treatment and control of bleeding episodes: On-demand treatment and control of bleeding episodes in adults and children with hemophilia A.

Routine prophylaxis to reduce the frequency of bleeding: Routine prophylaxis to reduce the frequency of bleeding episodes in adults and children with hemophilia A.

Limitations of use: Not indicated for the treatment of von Willebrand disease.

Dosing

Adult & Geriatric

Hemophilia A: IV: Dose, dosing frequency, and duration based on location and severity of bleeding, target factor VIII levels, and clinical condition of the patient. Individualize dosage based on coagulation studies performed prior to treatment and at regular intervals during treatment. In general, administration of factor VIII 1 unit/kg will increase circulating factor VIII levels by ~2 units/dL.

Treatment and control of bleeding episodes:

Dosage based on desired factor VIII increase (%):

To calculate dosage needed based on desired factor VIII increase (%).
[Body weight (kg) x desired factor VIII increase (%)] divided by 2 (%/units/kg) = units factor VIII required

For example:

50 kg x 30 (% increase) divided by 2 = 750 units factor VIII

◀

Dosage based on expected factor VIII increase (%):
It is also possible to calculate the **expected** % factor VIII increase:
[# units administered x 2(%/units/kg)] divided by body weight (kg) = expected % factor VIII increase
For example:
[1,400 units x 2] divided by 70 kg = 40%

General Antihemophilic Factor Dosing for On-demand Treatment and Control of Bleeding Episodes

Type of Bleeding	Target Factor VIII Level (Units/dL or % of normal)	Dose (Units/kg)	Frequency of Dosing (hours)	Duration of therapy
Minor early hemarthrosis, mild muscle bleeding, or mild oral bleeding episode.	20 to 40	10 to 20	12 to 24	Until bleeding is resolved
Moderate muscle bleeding, moderate bleeding into the oral cavity, definite hemarthroses, and known trauma.	30 to 60	15 to 30	12 to 24	Until bleeding is resolved
Major significant gastrointestinal bleeding, intracranial, intra-abdominal or intrathoracic bleeding, central nervous system bleeding, bleeding in the retropharyngeal or retroperitoneal spaces or iliopsoas sheath, fractures, head trauma.	60 to 100	30 to 50	8 to 24	Until bleeding is resolved

Note: Factor VIII level may either be expressed as units/dL or as %. Dosing frequency most commonly corresponds to the half-life of factor VIII but should be determined based on an assessment of factor VIII levels before the next dose.

Perioperative management:
Minor (including tooth extraction): Initial: 30 to 50 units/kg/dose beginning 1 hour before surgery to achieve factor VIII level of 60% to 100% of normal; repeat after 24 hours if necessary until bleeding is resolved.
Major (intracranial, intra-abdominal, or intrathoracic surgery, joint replacement surgery): Initial: 40 to 60 units/kg/dose beginning 1 hour before surgery to achieve factor VIII level of 80% to 120% of normal pre- and postoperatively. Verify 100% activity has been achieved prior to surgery. Maintenance: 40 to 60 units/kg/dose every 8 to 24 hours until adequate wound healing.
Routine prophylaxis to reduce the frequency of bleeding episodes: 40 to 50 units/kg/dose twice weekly; adjust dose based on clinical response.
Pediatric Hemophilia A:
Perioperative management:
Children 1 to <12 years: IV:
Minor (including tooth extraction): Refer to adult dosing.
Major (intracranial, intra-abdominal, or intrathoracic surgery, joint replacement surgery): Initial: 40 to 60 units/kg/dose beginning 1 hour before surgery to achieve factor VIII level of 80% to 120% of normal pre- and postoperatively. Verify 100% activity has been achieved prior to surgery. Maintenance: 40 to 60 units/kg/dose every 6 to 24 hours until adequate wound healing.

Children ≥12 years and Adolescents: IV: Refer to adult dosing.

Treatment and control of bleeding episodes: Children ≥1 years and Adolescents: IV: Refer to adult dosing.

Routine prophylaxis to reduce the frequency of bleeding episodes:
Children 1 to <12 years: IV: 55 units/kg/dose twice weekly (maximum dose: 70 units/kg/dose); adjust dose based on clinical response.

Children ≥12 years and Adolescents: IV: Refer to adult dosing.

Renal Impairment There are no dosage adjustments provided in the manufacturer's labeling.

Hepatic Impairment There are no dosage adjustments provided in the manufacturer's labeling.

Additional Information Complete prescribing information should be consulted for additional detail.

Dosage Forms Excipient information presented when available (limited, particularly for generics); consult specific product labeling.
Solution Reconstituted, Intravenous:
Adynovate: 250 units (1 ea); 500 units (1 ea); 750 units (1 ea); 1000 units (1 ea); 1500 units (1 ea); 2000 units (1 ea) [contains mouse (murine) and/or hamster protein, polysorbate 80]
Adynovate: 3000 units (1 ea) [contains polysorbate 80]

Antihemophilic Factor (Recombinant [Porcine Sequence]) (an tee hee moe FIL ik FAK tor ree KOM be nant POR sine SEE kwens)

Brand Names: US Obizur

Brand Names: Canada Obizur

Index Terms AHF (Recombinant [Porcine Sequence]); Factor VIII (Recombinant [Porcine Sequence]); pFVIII; rAHF; rpFVIII

Pharmacologic Category Antihemophilic Agent

Use

Acquired hemophilia A: Treatment of bleeding episodes in adults with acquired hemophilia A

Limitations of use: Not indicated for the treatment of congenital hemophilia A or von Willebrand disease; safely and efficacy of has not been established in patients with baseline anti- porcine factor VIII inhibitor titer >20 BU.

Pregnancy Risk Factor C

Dosing

Adult & Geriatric

Acquired hemophilia A: IV: **Note:** Dose, dosing frequency, and duration based on location and severity of bleeding, target factor VIII levels, and clinical condition of the patient. Plasma levels of factor VIII should not exceed 200% of normal or 200 units/dL.

Minor to moderate hemorrhage: 200 units/kg initially to achieve factor VIII plasma level 50% to 100% of normal; titrate subsequent doses to maintain recommended factor VIII trough levels and individual clinical response; dose every 4 to 12 hours (frequency may be adjusted based on clinical response/factor VIII levels).

Major hemorrhage: 200 units/kg initially to achieve factor VIII plasma level 100% to 200% (for acute bleed) or 50% to 100% (after acute bleed is controlled, if required) of normal; titrate subsequent doses to maintain recommended factor VIII trough levels and individual clinical response; dose every 4 to 12 hours (frequency may be adjusted based on clinical response/factor VIII levels).

▶

◄ **Renal Impairment** There are no dosage adjustments provided in the manufacturer's labeling.

Hepatic Impairment There are no dosage adjustments provided in the manufacturer's labeling.

Additional Information Complete prescribing information should be consulted for additional detail.

Dosage Forms Excipient information presented when available (limited, particularly for generics); consult specific product labeling.

Solution Reconstituted, Intravenous:

Obizur: 500 units (1 ea) [contains mouse (murine) and/or hamster protein, polysorbate 80]

◆ **Antihemophilic Factor (Recombinant), Single Chain** *see* Antihemophilic Factor (Recombinant) *on page 143*

◆ **Anti-PD-1 Human Monoclonal Antibody MDX-1106** *see* Nivolumab *on page 1328*

◆ **Anti-PD-1 Monoclonal Antibody MK-3475** *see* Pembrolizumab *on page 1486*

◆ **Anti-PDGFR Alpha Monoclonal Antibody IMC-3G3** *see* Olaratumab *on page 1372*

◆ **Anti-PD-L1 Monoclonal Antibody MPDL3280A** *see* Atezolizumab *on page 188*

◆ **Anti-PD-L1 Monoclonal Antibody MSB0010718C** *see* Avelumab *on page 195*

Antithrombin (an tee THROM bin)

Brand Names: US ATryn; Thrombate III

Brand Names: Canada Antithrombin III NF; Thrombate III®

Index Terms Antithrombin Alfa; Antithrombin III; AT; AT-III; hpAT; rhAT; rhATIII

Pharmacologic Category Anticoagulant; Blood Product Derivative

Use

Treatment and prevention of antithrombin deficiency: Thrombate III: Treatment and prevention of thromboembolism and prevention of perioperative and peri-partum thromboembolism in patients with hereditary antithrombin (AT) deficiency.

Prevention of thromboembolic events: ATryn: Prevention of perioperative and peripartum thromboembolic events in patients with hereditary antithrombin deficiency.

Limitations of use: Not indicated for treatment of thromboembolic events in patients with hereditary antithrombin deficiency.

Pregnancy Risk Factor B (Thrombate III); C (ATryn)

Dosing

Adult & Geriatric Antithrombin deficiency: IV:

ATryn: Prophylaxis of thrombosis during perioperative and peripartum procedures:

Dosing is individualized based on pretherapy antithrombin (AT) activity levels. Therapy should begin before delivery or ~24 hours prior to surgery to obtain target AT activity levels. Dosing should be targeted to keep levels between 80% to 120% of normal. Loading dose should be given as a 15-minute infusion, followed by maintenance dose as a continuous infusion. Doses may be calculated based on the following formulas:

Surgical patients (nonpregnant):

Loading dose: [(100 - baseline AT activity level) **divided** by 2.3] x body weight (kg) = units of antithrombin required

Maintenance infusion: [(100 - baseline AT activity level) **divided** by 10.2] x body weight (kg) = units of antithrombin required/hour

Pregnant patients: **Note:** Pregnant women undergoing surgical procedures (other than a Cesarean section) should also be dosed according to the formula below.

Loading dose: [(100 - baseline AT activity level) **divided** by 1.3] x body weight (kg) = units of antithrombin required

Maintenance infusion: [(100 - baseline AT activity level) **divided** by 5.4] x body weight (kg) = units of antithrombin required/hour

Dosing adjustments: Adjustments should be made based on AT activity levels to maintain levels between 80% to 120% of normal. Surgery or delivery may rapidly decrease AT levels; check AT level just after surgery or delivery. The first AT level should be obtained 2 hours after initiation and adjusted as follows:

AT activity level <80%: Increase dose by 30%; recheck AT level 2 hours after adjustment. Alternatively, an additional bolus dose (using loading dose formula) may be needed to rapidly restore AT levels. Calculate the additional bolus/loading dose using the last available AT activity result. After additional loading/bolus dose given, resume maintenance infusion at the same rate prior to bolus administration.

AT activity level 80% to 120%: No dosage adjustment needed; recheck AT level in 6 hours

AT activity level >120%: Decrease dose by 30%; recheck AT level 2 hours after adjustment

Thrombate III: Prophylaxis of thrombosis during surgical or obstetrical procedures or treatment of thromboembolism:

Initial loading dose: Dosing is individualized based on pretherapy antithrombin (AT) levels. The initial dose should raise AT levels to 120% and may be calculated based on the following formula:

[(desired AT level % - baseline AT level %) x body weight (kg)] **divided** by 1.4 = units of antithrombin required

For example, if a 70 kg adult patient had a baseline AT level of 57%, the initial dose would be:

[(120% - 57%) x 70] divided by 1.4 = 3150 units

◀ Maintenance dose: In general, subsequent dosing should be targeted to keep levels between 80% to 120% which may be achieved by administering 60% of the initial loading dose every 24 hours. Adjustments may be made by adjusting dose or interval. Maintain level within normal range for 2-8 days depending on type of procedure/situation.

Renal Impairment There are no dosage adjustments provided in the manufacturer's labeling.

Hepatic Impairment There are no dosage adjustments provided in the manufacturer's labeling.

Additional Information Complete prescribing information should be consulted for additional detail.

Dosage Forms Excipient information presented when available (limited, particularly for generics); consult specific product labeling.

Injection, powder for reconstitution [human, preservative free]:
Thrombate III: 500 units, 1000 units [contains heparin; exact potency labeled on each vial]

Injection, powder for reconstitution [recombinant, preservative free]:
ATryn: 525 units, 1750 units [contains goat protein; exact potency labeled on each vial]

◆ **Antithrombin III** see Antithrombin on page 152

◆ **Antithrombin III NF (Can)** see Antithrombin on page 152

◆ **Antithrombin Alfa** see Antithrombin on page 152

Antithymocyte Globulin (Equine)

(an te THY moe site GLOB yu lin, E kwine)

Related Information
Hematopoietic Cell Transplantation on page 2365

Brand Names: US Atgam

Brand Names: Canada Atgam

Index Terms Anti-Thymocyte Globulin (Equine); Antithymocyte Immunoglobulin; ATG; Horse Antihuman Thymocyte Gamma Globulin; Lymphocyte Immune Globulin

Pharmacologic Category Immune Globulin; Immunosuppressant Agent; Polyclonal Antibody

Use
Aplastic anemia: Treatment of moderate-to-severe aplastic anemia in patients not considered suitable candidates for bone marrow transplantation
Limitations of use: The usefulness of antithymocyte globulin (equine) has not been demonstrated in patients with aplastic anemia who are suitable candidates for transplantation, or in aplastic anemia secondary to neoplastic disease, storage disease, myelofibrosis, Fanconi syndrome, or in patients with known prior treatment with myelotoxic agents or radiation therapy

Labeled Contraindications History of systemic reaction (eg, anaphylactic reaction) to prior administration of antithymocyte globulin or any other equine gamma globulin preparation

Pregnancy Considerations Adverse events were observed in some animal reproduction studies.

The National Transplantation Pregnancy Registry (NTPR) is a registry which follows pregnancies which occur in maternal transplant recipients or those fathered by male transplant recipients. The NTPR encourages reporting of pregnancies following solid organ transplant by contacting them at 877-955-6877 or NTPR@giftoflifeinstitute.org.

Breastfeeding Considerations It is not known if antithymocyte globulin (equine) is excreted into breast milk. Due to the potential for serious adverse reactions in the nursing infant, the manufacturer recommends a decision be made to discontinue nursing or to discontinue the drug, taking into account the importance of treatment to the mother.

Warnings/Precautions [US Boxed Warning]: Antithymocyte globulins may cause anaphylaxis when injected intravenously. Although antithymocyte globulin (equine) is processed to reduce the level of antibodies that will react to non-T cells, health care providers should be prepared for the potential risk of anaphylaxis and monitor for signs/symptoms during infusion. Hypersensitivity and anaphylactic reactions may occur; discontinue for symptoms of anaphylaxis; immediate treatment (including epinephrine 1 mg/mL) should be available. Systemic reaction (rash, dyspnea, hypotension, tachycardia, or anaphylaxis) precludes further administration of antithymocyte globulin (equine; ATG). Respiratory distress, hypotension, or pain (chest, flank, or back) may indicate an anaphylactoid/anaphylactic reaction. Serious immune-mediated reactions have been reported (rare), including anaphylaxis, infusion reactions, and serum sickness. Skin testing is recommended prior to administration of the initial ATG dose. A positive skin test is suggestive of an increased risk for systemic allergic reactions with an infusion, although anaphylaxis may occur in patients who display negative skin tests. If ATG treatment is deemed appropriate following a positive skin test, the first infusion should be administered in a controlled environment with intensive life support immediately available. Also observe for signs/symptoms of allergic reactions during repeat courses of administration. Skin testing is not predictive for later development of serum sickness.

Thrombocytopenia may occur; may require platelets transfusion support. Discontinue if severe and unremitting thrombocytopenia and/or leukopenia occur in solid organ transplant patients. Clinically significant hemolysis has been reported (rarely); severe and unremitting hemolysis may require treatment discontinuation; chest, flank or back pain may indicate hemolysis. Abnormal hepatic function tests have been observed in patients with aplastic anemia and other hematologic disorders receiving ATG. ATG is an immunosuppressant; monitor closely for signs of infection. An increased incidence of cytomegalovirus (CMV) infection has been reported in studies. Administer via central line due to chemical phlebitis that may occur with a peripheral vein. Dose must be administered over at least 4 hours. Patient may need to be pretreated with an antipyretic, antihistamine, and/or corticosteroid. Intradermal skin testing is recommended prior to first-dose administration. Product of equine and human plasma; may have a risk of transmitting disease, including a theoretical risk of Creutzfeldt-Jakob disease (CJD). Product potency and activity may vary from lot to lot. Potentially significant drug-drug interactions may exist, requiring dose or frequency adjustment, additional monitoring, and/or selection of alternative therapy. Live viral vaccines may not replicate and antibody response may be reduced if administered during ATG treatment. Patients should not be immunized with attenuated live viral vaccines prior to planned ATG treatment, during, and after treatment.

Adverse Reactions

>10%:

Central nervous system: Chills, headache

◀

Dermatologic: Dermatological reaction (wheal/flare), pruritus, skin rash, urticaria

Hematologic & oncologic: Leukopenia, thrombocytopenia

Neuromuscular & skeletal: Arthralgia

Miscellaneous: Fever

1% to 10%:

Cardiovascular: Bradycardia, cardiac disease, cardiac failure, chest pain, edema, hypertension, hypotension, myocarditis, phlebitis, thrombophlebitis

Central nervous system: Agitation, brain disease (viral), burning sensation (burning of soles and burning of palms), dizziness, encephalitis, generalized ache, lethargy, seizure

Dermatologic: Diaphoresis, night sweats

Gastrointestinal: Diarrhea, nausea, stomatitis, vomiting

Genitourinary: Proteinuria

Hematologic & oncologic: Lymphadenopathy

Hepatic: Abnormal hepatic function tests, hepatosplenomegaly

Hypersensitivity: Anaphylaxis, serum sickness

Infection: Viral infection

Local: Injection site reaction (pain, redness, swelling)

Neuromuscular & skeletal: Back pain, joint stiffness, myalgia

Ophthalmic: Periorbital edema

Renal: Renal function test abnormality

Respiratory: Dyspnea, pleural effusion, respiratory distress

<1%, postmarketing, and/or case reports: Abdominal pain, acute renal failure, anaphylactoid reaction, anemia, apnea, confusion, cough, deep vein thrombosis, disorientation, dizziness, eosinophilia, epigastric pain, epistaxis, erythema, flank pain, gastrointestinal hemorrhage, gastrointestinal perforation, granulocytopenia, hemolysis, hemolytic anemia, herpes simplex infection (reactivation), hiccups, hyperglycemia, infection, involuntary body movements, laryngospasm, malaise, muscle rigidity, neutropenia, pancytopenia, paresthesia, pulmonary edema, pure red cell aplasia, renal artery thrombosis, sore mouth, sore throat, tachycardia, thrombosis of vein (iliac), toxic epidermal necrolysis, tremor, vasculitis, viral hepatitis, weakness, wound dehiscence

Drug Interactions

Metabolism/Transport Effects None known.

Avoid Concomitant Use

Avoid concomitant use of Antithymocyte Globulin (Equine) with any of the following: BCG (Intravesical); Natalizumab; Pimecrolimus; Tacrolimus (Topical); Vaccines (Live)

Increased Effect/Toxicity

Antithymocyte Globulin (Equine) may increase the levels/effects of: Fingolimod; Leflunomide; Natalizumab; Tofacitinib; Vaccines (Live)

The levels/effects of Antithymocyte Globulin (Equine) may be increased by: Denosumab; Ocrelizumab; Pimecrolimus; Roflumilast; Tacrolimus (Topical); Trastuzumab

Decreased Effect

Antithymocyte Globulin (Equine) may decrease the levels/effects of: BCG (Intravesical); Coccidioides immitis Skin Test; Nivolumab; Sipuleucel-T; Tertomotide; Vaccines (Inactivated); Vaccines (Live)

The levels/effects of Antithymocyte Globulin (Equine) may be decreased by: Echinacea

Storage/Stability Store ampules at 2°C to 8°C (36°F to 46°F). Do not freeze. Do not shake. Solutions diluted for infusion NS, D5¼NS, or D5½NS to a concentration of up to 4 mg/mL are stable for 24 hours (including infusion time) under refrigeration. Allow infusion solution to reach room temperature prior to administration.

Preparation for Administration Dilute into inverted container of sterile infusion solution to ensure that undiluted lymphocyte immune globulin does not contact air. Gently rotate or swirl to mix; do not shake (to avoid excessive foaming and/or denaturation of the protein). Final concentration should not exceed 4 mg/mL. May be diluted in NS, D5¼NS, or D5½NS **(do not use D5W; low salt concentrations may result in precipitation)**. Inspect for particulate matter or discoloration prior to administration (solution may be transparent to slightly opalescent, colorless to faintly pink or brown, and may develop a slight granular or flaky deposit during storage).

Mechanism of Action Immunosuppressant involved in the elimination of antigen-reactive T lymphocytes (killer cells) in peripheral blood or alteration in the function of T-lymphocytes, which are involved in humoral immunity and partly in cell-mediated immunity; induces complete or partial hematologic response in aplastic anemia

Pharmacodynamics/Kinetics

Distribution: Poor into lymphoid tissues; binds to circulating lymphocytes, granulocytes, platelets, bone marrow cells

Half-life elimination: 5.7 ± 3 days

Excretion: Urine (~1%)

Dosing

Adult Note: Test dose: A skin test is recommended prior to administration of the initial dose. Test initially with an epicutaneous prick of undiluted antithymocyte globulin (ATG); if no wheal in 10 minutes, then use 0.02 mL intradermally of a 1:1000 dilution of ATG in normal saline along with a separate saline control of 0.02 mL; observe in 10 minutes. A positive skin reaction consists of a wheal with the initial prick test (undiluted) or ≥3 mm in diameter larger than the saline control with the diluted intradermal test. Alternatively, a 0.1 mL test dose (5 mg/mL concentration) may be administered intradermally along with a separate saline control; erythema larger than 5 mm in diameter (compared to the control) is considered a positive test (Molldrem 2002). A positive skin test is suggestive of an increased risk for systemic allergic reactions with an infusion, although anaphylaxis may occur in patients who display negative skin tests. If ATG treatment is deemed appropriate following a positive skin test, the first infusion should be administered in a controlled environment with intensive life support immediately available. A systemic reaction precludes further administration.

Consider premedication with an antihistamine, corticosteroids, and/or an antipyretic. Concomitant immunosuppressants should also be administered.

Aplastic anemia: IV: 10 to 20 mg/kg once daily for 8 to 14 days, then if needed, may administer every other day for 7 more doses for a total of 21 doses in 28 days **or**
  Off-label dosing: 40 mg/kg once daily for 4 days in combination with cyclosporine (Rosenfeld 1995; Scheinberg 2011)

Acute graft-versus-host disease (GVHD) treatment (off-label use): IV: 30 mg/kg every other day for 6 doses (MacMillan 2007) **or** 15 mg/kg twice daily for 10 doses (MacMillan 2002)

Lung transplant, induction therapy (off- label use): IV: 5 to 15 mg/kg daily for the first 3 days after transplant (Hachem 2005). Additional data may be necessary to further define the role of antithymocyte globulin (equine) in this condition.

Myelodysplastic syndromes, refractory, lower-risk disease (off-label use): IV: 40 mg/kg once daily for 4 days; an intradermal test dose was administered prior to treatment (Molldrem 2002)

Geriatric Refer to adult dosing. Begin at the lower end of dosing ranges.

Pediatric Note: Test dose: A skin test is recommended prior to administration of the initial dose. Test initially with an epicutaneous prick of undiluted antithymocyte globulin (ATG); if no wheal in 10 minutes, then use 0.02 mL intradermally of a 1:1000 dilution of ATG in normal saline along with a separate saline control of 0.02 mL; observe in 10 minutes. A positive skin reaction consists of a wheal with the initial prick test (undiluted) or ≥3 mm in diameter larger than the saline control with the diluted intradermal test. A positive skin test is suggestive of an increased risk for systemic allergic reactions with an infusion, although anaphylaxis may occur in patients who display negative skin tests. If ATG treatment is deemed appropriate following a positive skin test, the first infusion should be administered in a controlled environment with intensive life support immediately available. A systemic reaction precludes further administration.

Consider premedication with an antihistamine, corticosteroids, and/or an antipyretic. Concomitant immunosuppressants should also be administered.

Aplastic anemia, moderate to severe when no HLA-matched sibling donor: IV: 10 to 20 mg/kg once daily for 8 to 14 days; then if needed, may administer every other day for 7 more doses for up to a total of 21 doses in 28 days **or**

Off-label dosing (in combination with cyclosporine): Children ≥2 years and Adolescents: IV: 40 mg/kg/day once daily for 4 days (Afable 2011; Rosenfeld 1995; Scheinberg 2009; Scheinberg 2011).

Acute graft-versus-host disease (GVHD) treatment (off-label use): Children and Adolescents: IV: 30 mg/kg every other day for 6 doses (MacMillan 2007) **or** 15 mg/kg twice daily for 10 doses (MacMillan 2002)

Renal Impairment There are no dosage adjustments provided in the manufacturer's labeling.

Hepatic Impairment There are no dosage adjustments provided in the manufacturer's labeling.

Obesity *American Society for Blood and Marrow Transplantation (ASBMT) practice guideline committee position statement on chemotherapy dosing in obesity:* Utilize actual body weight (full weight) to calculate mg/kg dosing for hematopoietic stem cell transplant conditioning regimens (Bubalo, 2014).

Adjustment for Toxicity

Anaphylaxis: Discontinue infusion immediately; administer epinephrine. May require corticosteroids, respiration assistance, and/or other resuscitative measures. Do not resume infusion.

Hemolysis (severe and unremitting): May require discontinuation of treatment.

Administration For IV use only. Infuse over at least 4 hours through a 0.2 to 1 micron inline filter. Allow solution to reach room temperature prior to infusion. Infusion must be completed with 24 hours of preparation. Administration through a central line is recommended; high flow veins are preferred to reduce phlebitis (infuse into vascular shunt, arterial venous fistula, or high-flow central vein). May cause vein irritation (chemical phlebitis) if administered peripherally (peripheral administration is not recommended).

Monitor closely throughout the infusion for allergic reactions. Appropriate resuscitative equipment should be nearby during administration. May require premedication with an antipyretic, antihistamine, and/or a corticosteroid to prevent reactions. Discontinue infusion for anaphylaxis or respiratory distress. Administer epinephrine, corticosteroids, antihistamines, and/or antipyretics as indicated to manage reactions.

Due to possible infusion-related reactions, it may be preferable to avoid initiating treatment late in the day or on weekends; consider withholding beta-blockers prior to administration to avoid suppressing compensatory responses to anaphylaxis (Scheinberg, 2012).

Monitoring Parameters Complete blood count with differential and platelet count, monitor vital signs during administration; monitor for infusion reactions; monitor for signs/symptoms of infection.

Solid organ transplant: Absolute CD3 count (cells/µL) monitoring and CD3 based-dosing has been considered in renal and heart transplant recipients. It may be beneficial in certain patient populations but is not routinely recommended or utilized. Dose adjustments have been recommended based on the CD3 count (Krasinska 2002).

Dosage Forms Excipient information presented when available (limited, particularly for generics); consult specific product labeling.
Injectable, Intravenous:
Atgam: 50 mg/mL (5 mL) [thimerosal free]

◆ **Anti-Thymocyte Globulin (Equine)** *see* Antithymocyte Globulin (Equine) on page 154

Antithymocyte Globulin (Rabbit)
(an te THY moe site GLOB yu lin RAB bit)

Related Information
Hematopoietic Cell Transplantation *on page* 2365

Brand Names: US Thymoglobulin

Brand Names: Canada Thymoglobulin

Index Terms Antithymocyte Immunoglobulin; rATG

Pharmacologic Category Immune Globulin; Immunosuppressant Agent; Polyclonal Antibody

Use

Renal transplant rejection: Prophylaxis and treatment of acute rejection in renal transplantation (in conjunction with concomitant immunosuppression)

Note: In a multicenter, double-blind, randomized trial, antithymocyte globulin (rabbit) was shown to be superior to antithymocyte globulin (equine) in reversing acute rejection and preventing subsequent episodes (Gaber 1998). Based on data from studies (including 10 years follow up) comparing ATG (rabbit) to ATG (equine) for induction, ATG (rabbit) has emerged as the T-cell lymphocyte depleting induction therapy of choice over ATG (equine) in adult kidney transplantation due to its improved efficacy and lower incidence of acute rejection (Brennan 1999; Hardinger 2008).

◀ **Labeled Contraindications**
Hypersensitivity (allergy or anaphylaxis) to rabbit proteins or any component of the formulation; active acute or chronic infection which contraindicate additional immunosuppression

Documentation of allergenic cross-reactivity for drugs in this class is limited. However, because of similarities in chemical structure and/or pharmacologic actions, the possibility of cross-sensitivity cannot be ruled out with certainty.

Pregnancy Considerations Animal reproduction studies have not been conducted. Females of reproductive potential should use effective contraception during and for at least 3 months following treatment.

The National Transplantation Pregnancy Registry (NTPR) is a registry which follows pregnancies which occur in maternal transplant recipients or those fathered by male transplant recipients. The NTPR encourages reporting of pregnancies following solid organ transplant by contacting them at 877-955-6877 or NTPR@giftoflifeinstitute.org.

Breastfeeding Considerations This product has not been evaluated in breastfeeding women and it is not known if antithymocyte globulin (rabbit) is present in breast milk. Because other immunoglobulins are present in breast milk, the manufacturer recommends that breastfeeding be discontinued during antithymocyte globulin (rabbit) therapy.

Warnings/Precautions [US Boxed Warning]: Should only be used by physicians experienced in immunosuppressive therapy in transplantation. Maintenance immunosuppression may require dosage reduction. Medical surveillance is required during the infusion. Should be administered in combination with other immunosuppressants. Antithymocyte globulin (ATG) (rabbit) is available (based on region) in different product formulations, ATG-Thymoglobulin and ATG-Fresenius; the dosing differs among the formulations. Dosing of antithymocyte globulin (rabbit) also differs from dosing of other antithymocyte globulin products (eg, ATG [equine]); protein compositions and concentrations are different. Use caution to ensure dose prescribed is intended for product being administered. Initial dose must be administered over at least 6 hours into a high flow vein. Reducing the infusion rate (and prolonging the administration time) may minimize infusion reactions. May pretreat with an antipyretic, antihistamine, and/or corticosteroid.

Hypersensitivity and fatal anaphylactic reactions have been reported. Stop infusion immediately if anaphylactic reaction occurs. Immediate treatment (including subcutaneous epinephrine and corticosteroids) should be available during infusion for management of hypersensitivity. Release of cytokines by activated monocytes and lymphocytes may lead to cytokine release syndrome (CRS) during infusion; may cause serious cardiopulmonary events (sometimes fatal). Rapid infusion rates have been associated with CRS (case reports). Other infusion reaction symptoms, including flu-like symptoms (fever, chills, nausea, muscle/joint pain) may also occur. Local infusion site reactions (pain, swelling, skin redness) have been reported.

Severe infections (bacterial, fungal, viral and/or protozoal) may develop following concomitant use of immunosuppressants with antithymocyte globulin. Reactivation of infections (particularly CMV) and sepsis have been reported. Appropriate antiviral, antibacterial, antiprotozoal, and/or antifungal prophylaxis is recommended. Monitor closely for infection. Immunosuppressants, including antithymocyte globulins may increase the incidence of malignancies, including lymphoma, post-transplant lymphoproliferative disease (PTLD) or other malignancies; may be fatal. Reversible leukopenia, neutropenia, thrombocytopenia, and lymphopenia may occur. Monitor blood counts; leukopenia or thrombocytopenia may require dosage adjustment. Antithymocyte globulin (rabbit) has been associated with increased adverse effects when used for induction in liver transplantation and should be used cautiously in this population (Boillot 2009). Patients should not be immunized with attenuated live viral vaccines during or shortly after treatment; safety of immunization following therapy has not been studied. Potentially significant drug-drug interactions may exist, requiring dose or frequency adjustment, additional monitoring, and/or selection of alternative therapy.

Adverse Reactions

>10%:

Cardiovascular: Hypertension (27% to 37%), tachycardia (23%), peripheral edema (20%), hypotension (10% to 16%)

Central nervous system: Chills (55% to 57%), headache (27% to 40%), pain (26%), insomnia (12% to 20%), malaise (9% to 13%), acne vulgaris (12%)

Dermatologic: Skin rash (7% to 13%), diaphoresis (6% to 13%), acne vulgaris (12%)

Endocrine & metabolic: Hyperkalemia (17% to 27%), hypokalemia (12%)

Gastrointestinal: Abdominal pain (17% to 38%), nausea (29% to 37%), diarrhea (20%), vomiting (20%), constipation (15%)

Hematologic & oncologic: Leukopenia (49% to 57%; including lymphopenia and neutropenia), thrombocytopenia (29% to 37%), leukocytosis (13%), anemia (12%)

Infection: Infection (31%), cytomegalovirus disease (13%), sepsis (12%)

Neuromuscular & skeletal: Myalgia (11% to 20%), arthralgia (15%), weakness (13%), back pain (12%)

Respiratory: Dyspnea (15% to 28%), pulmonary disease (12%)

Miscellaneous: Fever (46%)

1% to 10%:

Cardiovascular: Chest pain (9%), edema (6%)

Central nervous system: Anxiety (7%)

Dermatologic: Pruritus (6%)

Endocrine & metabolic: Acidosis (9%), hypophosphatemia (6%)

Gastrointestinal: Dyspepsia (10%), anorexia (6%), intestinal candidiasis (5%), gastritis (1%)

Hematologic & oncologic: Malignant neoplasm (2%)

Hypersensitivity: Serum sickness (2%)

Infection: Herpes simplex infection (5%)

Respiratory: Increased cough (7%)

Miscellaneous: Drug overdose (6%)

<1%, postmarketing, and/or case reports: Anaphylaxis, blood coagulation disorder, cytokine release syndrome, decreased oxygen saturation, increased liver enzymes, infusion related reaction, lymphadenopathy, lymphoproliferative disorder (post-transplant), malignant lymphoma, proteinuria, solid tumor

Drug Interactions

Metabolism/Transport Effects None known.

Avoid Concomitant Use

Avoid concomitant use of Antithymocyte Globulin (Rabbit) with any of the following: BCG (Intravesical); Natalizumab; Pimecrolimus; Tacrolimus (Topical); Vaccines (Live)

◀ **Increased Effect/Toxicity**
Antithymocyte Globulin (Rabbit) may increase the levels/effects of: Fingolimod; Leflunomide; Natalizumab; Tofacitinib; Vaccines (Live)

The levels/effects of Antithymocyte Globulin (Rabbit) may be increased by: Denosumab; Ocrelizumab; Pimecrolimus; Roflumilast; Tacrolimus (Topical); Trastuzumab

Decreased Effect
Antithymocyte Globulin (Rabbit) may decrease the levels/effects of: BCG (Intravesical); Coccidioides immitis Skin Test; Nivolumab; Sipuleucel-T; Tertomotide; Vaccines (Inactivated); Vaccines (Live)

The levels/effects of Antithymocyte Globulin (Rabbit) may be decreased by: Echinacea

Storage/Stability Store intact vial at 2°C to 8°C (36°F to 46°F); do not freeze. Protect from light. Reconstituted product is stable for up to 24 hours at room temperature; however, the product contains no preservative and room temperature storage is not recommended; the manufacturer recommends use immediately after reconstitution and preparation for infusion in D5W or NS.

Preparation for Administration Allow vials to reach room temperature, then reconstitute each vial with SWFI 5 mL to a concentration of 5 mg/mL. Rotate vial gently until completely dissolved. Prior to administration, further dilute for infusion, each 25 mg vial should be diluted in 50 mL NS or D5W (total volume is usually 50 to 500 mL depending on total number of vials needed per dose). Mix by gently inverting infusion bag only once or twice. For peripheral administration, dilution in 500 mL NS (only) with the addition of 1,000 units heparin and 20 mg hydrocortisone has been reported (Trofe-Clark 2012).

Mechanism of Action Antithymocyte globulin (rabbit) is a polyclonal antibody which appears to cause immunosuppression by acting on T-cell surface antigens and depleting CD4 lymphocytes

Pharmacodynamics/Kinetics
Onset of action (T-cell depletion): Within 24 hours (Hardinger 2006)
Duration: Lymphopenia may persist for up to 1 year (Hardinger 2006)
Half-life elimination: 2 to 3 days

Dosing
Adult & Geriatric Note: Premedicate with corticosteroids, acetaminophen, and/or an antihistamine 1 hour prior to infusion to reduce the incidence and severity of infusion-related reactions. Administer antifungal and antibacterial prophylaxis therapy if clinically indicated. Antiviral prophylaxis is recommended in patients who are CMV-seropositive at the time of transplant and for CMV-seronegative patients scheduled to receive a kidney from a CMV-seropositive donor.

Renal transplant (acute rejection treatment): IV: 1.5 mg/kg/day for 7 to 14 days
Renal transplant (induction therapy): IV: 1.5 mg/kg/day for 4 to 7 days; the first dose should be administered prior to reperfusion of the donor kidney

Off-label induction dosing: IV: 1.5 mg/kg once daily for 5 to 7 days (Brennan 1999; Brennan 2006; Hardinger 2008) **or** 1 mg/kg once daily for 3 to 6 days (Goggins 2003); alternative dosing strategies with higher doses for shorter durations such as 2 mg/kg once daily for 3 days have also been recommended (Hardinger 2010); dosing based on peripheral blood CD3+ lymphocyte counts has also been described with an initial dose of 1.5 mg/kg followed by repeat doses when CD3+ count is >20 cells/mm^3 (Peddi 2002)

Chronic graft-versus-host disease (prevention) (off-label use): IV: 0.5 mg/kg administered 2 days prior to transplant and 2 mg/kg administered 1 day before and 1 day after transplant (Walker 2016) **or** 2.5 mg/kg once daily for 3 days beginning 3 days prior to transplant (Ruutu 2013)

Heart transplant (induction therapy in high risk patients) (off-label use): IV: 1 to 1.5 mg/kg once daily for up to 7 days (Zuckermann 2015)

Heart transplant (acute cellular rejection, treatment) (off-label use): IV: 0.75 to 1.5 mg/kg/day for 5 to 14 days (ISHLT [Costanzo 2010])

Intestinal and multivisceral transplantation (induction therapy) (off-label use): IV: 2 mg/kg/day on postoperative days 0, 2, 4, 6, and 8 (in combination with rituximab) (Vianna 2008). Additional trials data may be necessary to further define the role of antithymocyte globulin (rabbit) in this condition.

Lung transplant (induction therapy) (off-label use): IV: 1.5 mg/kg/day for 3 days; the first dose was administered within 24 hours of transplantation (Palmer 1999; Hartwig 2008). Additional trails may be necessary to further define the role of antithymocyte globulin (rabbit) for prevention of rejection after lung transplant.

Lung transplant (persistent acute cellular rejection, treatment) (off-label use): IV: Pulse treatments have been used to manage persistent acute cellular rejection (Martinu 2000). Additional data may be necessary to further define the role of antithymocyte globulin (rabbit) in treatment of acute cellular rejection after lung transplantation.

Pediatric Renal transplant (induction therapy and acute rejection treatment): Refer to adult dosing.

Renal Impairment There are no dosage adjustments provided in the manufacturer's labeling.

Hepatic Impairment There are no dosage adjustments provided in the manufacturer's labeling.

Obesity *American Society for Blood and Marrow Transplantation (ASBMT) practice guideline committee position statement on chemotherapy dosing in obesity:* Utilize actual body weight (full weight) to calculate mg/kg dosing for hematopoietic stem cell transplant conditioning regimens (Bubalo 2014).

Adjustment for Toxicity

Renal transplantation:

WBC count 2,000 to 3,000 cells/mm^3 or platelet count 50,000 to 75,000 cells/mm^3: Reduce dose by 50%.

WBC count <2,000 cells/mm^3 or platelet count <50,000 cells/mm^3: Consider discontinuing treatment.

Administration

Infuse the first dose over at least 6 hours; subsequent doses may be infused over at least 4 hours. Infuse through a high-flow vein (central line). Administer through an in-line 0.22 micron filter. Premedication with corticosteroids, acetaminophen, and/or an antihistamine 1 hour prior to infusion may reduce the incidence and severity of infusion-related reactions. Reducing the infusion rate may minimize infusion reactions. Infusion rate may vary for off-label uses; refer to specific protocol.

In renal transplantation, administration through a peripheral vein has been reported with the addition of 1,000 units heparin and 20 mg hydrocortisone (in 500 mL NS only) to decrease the risk of thrombosis and phlebitis (Marvin 2003; Trofe-Clark 2012). The first 2 doses were infused over 6 hours and subsequent doses were infused over 4 hours (Trofe-Clark 2012).

Monitoring Parameters

Lymphocyte count (total lymphocyte and/or T-cell subset), CBC with differential and platelet count; vital signs during administration; signs and symptoms of infection

Solid organ transplant: Absolute CD3 count (cells/µL) monitoring and CD3 based dosing has been considered in renal and heart transplant recipients. It may be beneficial in certain patient populations but is not routinely recommended or utilized. Dose adjustments have been recommended based on the CD3 count (Krasinska 2002).

Test Interactions Potential interference with rabbit antibody-based immunoassays and with cross-match or panel-reactive antibody cytotoxicity assays. Has not been shown to interfere with routine clinical laboratory tests which do not use immunoglobulins.

Dosage Forms Excipient information presented when available (limited, particularly for generics); consult specific product labeling.

Solution Reconstituted, Intravenous:

Thymoglobulin: 25 mg (1 ea) [contains glycine, mannitol, sodium chloride]

Aprepitant (ap RE pi tant)

Related Information

Management of Chemotherapy-Induced Nausea and Vomiting in Adults *on page 2253*

Palliative Care Medicine (Cancer) *on page 2352*

Prevention of Chemotherapy-Induced Nausea and Vomiting in Children *on page 2310*

Brand Names: US Emend; Emend Tri-Pack

Brand Names: Canada Emend

Index Terms L 754030; MK 869

Pharmacologic Category Antiemetic; Substance P/Neurokinin 1 Receptor Antagonist

Use

Prevention of chemotherapy-induced nausea and vomiting:

Prevention of acute and delayed nausea and vomiting associated with **highly** emetogenic chemotherapy (initial and repeat courses; in combination with other antiemetics) in patients ≥12 years (capsules) and in patients ≥6 months (oral suspension).

Prevention of nausea and vomiting associated with **moderately** emetogenic chemotherapy (initial and repeat courses; in combination with other antiemetics) in patients ≥12 years (capsules) and in patients ≥6 months (oral suspension).

Postoperative nausea and vomiting: Prevention of postoperative nausea and vomiting (PONV) in adults.

Limitations of use: Aprepitant has not been studied for the management of existing nausea and vomiting. Chronic, continuous administration is not recommended (has not been studied and chronic use may alter aprepitant's drug interaction profile).

Labeled Contraindications Hypersensitivity to aprepitant or any component of the formulation; concurrent use with pimozide
Canadian labeling: Additional contraindications (not in the US labeling): Concurrent use with astemizole, cisapride, or terfenadine.

Pregnancy Considerations Adverse events were not observed in animal reproduction studies. Efficacy of hormonal contraceptive may be reduced during and for 28 days following the last aprepitant dose; alternative or additional effective methods of contraception should be used both during treatment with fosaprepitant or aprepitant and for at least 1 month following the last fosaprepitant/aprepitant dose.

Breastfeeding Considerations It is not known if aprepitant is present in breast milk. According to the manufacturer, the decision to breastfeed during therapy should take into account the risk of exposure to the infant and the benefits of treatment to the mother.

Warnings/Precautions Potentially significant drug-drug interactions may exist, requiring dose or frequency adjustment, additional monitoring, and/or selection of alternative therapy. Use caution with severe hepatic impairment (Child-Pugh class C); has not been studied. Due to a risk of significantly increased pimozide plasma concentrations and potential for QT prolongation, concurrent use with pimozide is contraindicated. Other CYP3A4-mediated drug interactions may occur. In patients receiving concurrent warfarin, a clinically significant decrease in INR or prothrombin time (PT) may occur; monitor INR/PT for 2 weeks (particularly at 7 to 10 days) following aprepitant administration. Hypersensitivity reactions, including anaphylactic reactions have been reported. For prevention of chemotherapy-induced nausea and vomiting, use is not recommended in pediatric patients weighing <6 kg. Not approved for prevention of postoperative nausea and vomiting in children.

Adverse Reactions Adverse reactions may be reported in combination with other antiemetic agents. As reported for highly emetogenic cancer chemotherapy or moderately emetogenic cancer chemotherapy, unless otherwise noted as reported for postoperative nausea and vomiting (PONV).

>10%:

Central nervous system: Fatigue (adults: 13%; children & adolescents: 5%)

Hematologic & oncologic: Neutropenia (children & adolescents: 13%; adults: <3%)

0.5% to 10%:

Cardiovascular: Hypotension (PONV: 6%), bradycardia (PONV: <3%), flushing (<3%), palpitations (<3%), peripheral edema (<3%), syncope (PONV: <3%)

Central nervous system: Headache (children & adolescents: 9%), dizziness (<3% to 5%), anxiety (<3%), hypoesthesia (PONV: <3%), hypothermia (PONV: <3%), malaise (<3%), peripheral neuropathy (<3%), abnormal behavior (children & adolescents: 2%), agitation (children & adolescents: 2%)

Dermatologic: Alopecia (<3%), hyperhidrosis (<3%), skin rash (<3%), urticaria (<3%)

Endocrine & metabolic: Dehydration (≤3%), decreased serum albumin (PONV: <3%), decreased serum potassium (PONV: <3%), decreased serum sodium (<3%), hot flash (<3), hypokalemia (<3%), hypovolemia (PONV: <3%), increased serum glucose (PONV: <3%), weight loss (<3%)

Gastrointestinal: Constipation (PONV: 9%), diarrhea (6% to 9%), dyspepsia (≤7%), abdominal pain (≤6%), hiccups (4% to 5%), decreased appetite (<3% to 5%), dysgeusia (<3%), eructation (<3%), flatulence (<3%), gastritis (<3%), gastroesophageal reflux disease (<3%), nausea (<3%), vomiting (<3%), xerostomia (<3%)

Genitourinary: Proteinuria (<3%)

Hematologic & oncologic: Decreased hemoglobin (children & adolescents: 5%), decreased white blood cell count (≤4%), anemia (<3%), febrile neutropenia (<3%), hematoma (PONV: <3%), thrombocytopenia (<3%)

Hepatic: Increased serum ALT (3%), increased serum alkaline phosphatase (<3%), increased serum AST (<3%), increased serum bilirubin (PONV: <3%)

Infection: Candidiasis (<3%), postoperative infection (PONV: <3%)

Neuromuscular & skeletal: Weakness (≤7%), musculoskeletal pain (<3%)

Renal: Increased blood urea nitrogen (<3%)

Respiratory: Cough (<3% to 5%), dyspnea (<3%), hypoxia (PONV: <3%), oropharyngeal pain (<3%), pharyngitis (<3%), respiratory depression (PONV: <3%)

Miscellaneous: Wound dehiscence (PONV: <3%)

<0.5%, postmarketing, and/or case reports: Anaphylaxis, angioedema, hypersensitivity reaction, pruritus, Stevens-Johnson syndrome, toxic epidermal necrolysis

Drug Interactions

Metabolism/Transport Effects Substrate of CYP1A2 (minor), CYP2C19 (minor), CYP3A4 (major); Note: Assignment of Major/Minor substrate status based on clinically relevant drug interaction potential; **Inhibits** CYP2C9 (weak), CYP3A4 (moderate); **Induces** CYP2C9 (strong)

Avoid Concomitant Use

Avoid concomitant use of Aprepitant with any of the following: Astemizole; Asunaprevir; Bosutinib; Budesonide (Systemic); Cisapride; Cobimetinib; Conivaptan; CYP3A4 Inducers (Strong); CYP3A4 Inhibitors (Moderate); CYP3A4 Inhibitors (Strong); Domperidone; Flibanserin; Fusidic Acid (Systemic); Idelalisib; Ivabradine; Lomitapide; Naloxegol; Neratinib; Olaparib; Pimozide; Simeprevir; Terfenadine; Tolvaptan; Trabectedin; Ulipristal

Increased Effect/Toxicity

Aprepitant may increase the levels/effects of: AmLODIPine; Apixaban; ARIPiprazole; Astemizole; Asunaprevir; Avanafil; Blonanserin; Bosentan; Bosutinib; Brexpiprazole; Bromocriptine; Budesonide (Systemic); Budesonide (Topical); Cannabis; Cilostazol; Cisapride; Cobimetinib; Colchicine; Corticosteroids (Systemic); CYP3A4 Substrates; Dapoxetine; Deflazacort; Dofetilide; Domperidone; DOXOrubicin (Conventional); Dronabinol; Eletriptan; Eliglustat; Eplerenone; Everolimus; FentaNYL; Flibanserin;

GuanFACINE; Halofantrine; HYDROcodone; HydrOXYzine; Ibrutinib; Ifosfa-mide; Ivabradine; Ivacaftor; Lomitapide; Lurasidone; Manidipine; Mirodenafil; Naldemedine; Naloxegol; Neratinib; NiMODipine; Olaparib; OxyCODONE; Pimecrolimus; Pimozide; Propafenone; Ranolazine; Rupatadine; Salmeterol; SAXagliptin; Sildenafil; Simeprevir; Sirolimus; Sonidegib; Suvorexant; Terfe-nadine; Tetrahydrocannabinol; Ticagrelor; Tolvaptan; Trabectedin; Udenafil; Uliprital; Venetoclax; Vilazodone; Vindesine; Zopiclone; Zuclopenthixol

The levels/effects of Aprepitant may be increased by: Conivaptan; CYP3A4 Inhibitors (Moderate); CYP3A4 Inhibitors (Strong); Dasatinib; Fosaprepitant; Fusidic Acid (Systemic); Idelalisib; Palbociclib; Stiripentol

Decreased Effect

Aprepitant may decrease the levels/effects of: Contraceptives (Estrogens); Contraceptives (Progestins); CYP2C9 Substrates; Diclofenac (Systemic); PARoxetine; TOLBUTamide; Warfarin

The levels/effects of Aprepitant may be decreased by: Bosentan; CYP3A4 Inducers (Moderate); CYP3A4 Inducers (Strong); Dabrafenib; Deferasirox; PARoxetine; Sarilumab; Siltuximab; St John's Wort; Tocilizumab

Food Interactions Aprepitant serum concentration may be increased when taken with grapefruit juice. Management: Avoid concurrent use.

Storage/Stability

Capsules: Store at room temperature of 20°C to 25°C (68°F to 77°F).

Oral suspension: Store unopened pouch at 20°C to 25°C (68°F to 77°F); excursions permitted between 15°C to 30°C (59°F to 86°F). Store in the original container. Do not open pouch until ready to use. Once prepared, if suspension is not used immediately, store refrigerated (between [2°C to 8°C/ 36°F to 46°F]) for up to 72 hours. When ready to use, the mixture may be kept at room temperature (between [20°C to 25°C/68°F to 77°F]) for up to 3 hours.

Preparation for Administration Suspension: Aprepitant for oral suspension is packaged as a kit, with a 1 mL and a 5 mL oral dosing dispenser, one cap, one mixing cup, and the aprepitant pouch. Fill mixing cup with room temper-ature drinking water, using the 5 mL dosing dispenser, measure 4.6 mL of water from the mixing cup and discard unused water from cup. Make sure no air is in the dispenser. Add the 4.6 mL water back to the empty cup. Shake content of aprepitant pouch to bottom of pouch and pour entire contents of pouch into mixing cup, add lid and snap shut. Mix suspension by gently swirling 20 times, then gently invert cup 5 times (to avoid foaming, do not shake vigorously). This results in a 25 mg/mL cloudy pink to light pink suspension. If clumps are present, repeat mixing by gently swirling 20 times and gently inverting 5 times. If foam is present, wait for foam to disappear. Measure calculated dose into oral dosing dispenser (use the 1 mL dispenser if dose is ≤1 mL and the 5 mL dispenser if dose is >1 mL). If dose is <1 mL, round to nearest 0.1 mL; if dose is >1 mL, round to the nearest 0.2 mL. Make sure all air is removed from dispenser and dispenser contains the prescribed dose. Place cap on dispenser until it clicks. Discard mixing cup and any suspension remaining in cup. Refer to manufacturer's instructions for further preparation details.

Mechanism of Action Aprepitant prevents acute and delayed vomiting by inhibiting the substance P/neurokinin 1 (NK_1) receptor; augments the antie-metic activity of $5-HT_3$ receptor antagonists and corticosteroids to inhibit acute and delayed phases of chemotherapy-induced emesis.

Pharmacodynamics/Kinetics

Distribution: V_d: ~70 L; crosses the blood-brain barrier

Protein binding: >95%

Metabolism: Extensively hepatic via CYP3A4 (major); CYP1A2 and CYP2C19 (minor); forms 7 metabolites (weakly active)

Bioavailability: ~60% to 65%

Half-life elimination: Terminal: ~9 to 13 hours

Time to peak, plasma: Pediatric: Capsule: ~4 hours; Suspension ~6 hours; Adults: 40 mg: ~3 hours; 125 mg followed by 80 mg for 2 days: ~4 hours

Excretion: Primarily via metabolism

Dosing

Adult & Geriatric

Prevention of chemotherapy-induced nausea and vomiting:

Manufacturer's labeling:

Prevention of acute and delayed nausea/vomiting associated with highly-emetogenic chemotherapy:

Capsules: Oral: 125 mg 1 hour prior to chemotherapy on day 1, followed by 80 mg once daily on days 2 and 3 (in combination with a 5-HT$_3$ antagonist antiemetic on day 1 and dexamethasone on days 1 to 4)

Suspension: Adults unable to swallow capsules: Oral: 3 mg/kg (maximum: 125 mg/dose) 1 hour prior to chemotherapy on day 1, followed by 2 mg/kg (maximum: 80 mg/dose) once daily on days 2 and 3 (in combination with a 5-HT$_3$ antagonist antiemetic on day 1 and dexamethasone on days 1 to 4)

Prevention of nausea/vomiting associated with moderately-emetogenic chemotherapy:

Capsules: Oral: 125 mg 1 hour prior to chemotherapy on day 1, followed by 80 mg once daily on days 2 and 3 (in combination with a 5-HT$_3$ antagonist antiemetic and dexamethasone on day 1)

Suspension: Adults unable to swallow capsules: Oral: 3 mg/kg (maximum: 125 mg/dose) 1 hour prior to chemotherapy on day 1, followed by 2 mg/kg (maximum: 80 mg/dose) once daily on days 2 and 3 (in combination with a 5-HT$_3$ antagonist antiemetic and dexamethasone on day 1)

Guideline recommendations:

Prevention of nausea/vomiting associated with highly-emetogenic chemotherapy (including anthracycline and cyclophosphamide [AC] regimens): Oral:

American Society of Clinical Oncology (ASCO [Basch 2011]): 125 mg prior to chemotherapy on day 1, followed by 80 mg once daily on days 2 and 3 (in combination with a 5-HT$_3$ antagonist antiemetic on day 1 and dexamethasone on days 1 to 4 or days 1 to 3)

Multinational Association of Supportive Care in Cancer and European Society of Medical Oncology (MASCC/ESMO [Roila 2016]): 125 mg prior to chemotherapy on day 1, followed by 80 mg once daily on days 2 and 3 (in combination with dexamethasone and a 5-HT$_3$ antagonist antiemetic on day 1, followed by dexamethasone for 3 to 4 more days

Prevention of postoperative nausea and vomiting (PONV): Oral: 40 mg within 3 hours prior to anesthesia induction

◄ **Pediatric**
   Manufacturer's labeling:
   Prevention of acute and delayed nausea and vomiting associated with highly-emetogenic chemotherapy:
      Capsules: Children ≥12 years, and Adolescents: Oral: 125 mg 1 hour prior to chemotherapy on day 1, followed by 80 mg once daily on days 2 and 3 (in combination with a 5-HT$_3$ antagonist antiemetic on day 1 and dexamethasone on days 1 to 4 [reduce dexamethasone dose to 50% of recommended dose])
      Suspension: Infants ≥6 months (and ≥6 kg), Children <12 years (and ≥6 kg) and patients (any age and ≥6 kg) unable to swallow capsules: Oral: 3 mg/kg (maximum: 125 mg/dose) 1 hour prior to chemotherapy on day 1, followed by 2 mg/kg (maximum: 80 mg/dose) once daily on days 2 and 3 (in combination with a 5-HT$_3$ antagonist antiemetic on day 1 and dexamethasone on days 1 to 4 [reduce dexamethasone dose to 50% of recommended dose])
   Prevention of nausea and vomiting associated with moderately-emetogenic chemotherapy:
      Capsules: Children ≥12 years, and Adolescents: Oral: 125 mg 1 hour prior to chemotherapy on day 1, followed by 80 mg once daily on days 2 and 3 (in combination with a 5-HT$_3$ antagonist antiemetic and dexamethasone on day 1 [reduce dexamethasone dose to 50% of recommended dose])
      Suspension: Infants ≥6 months (and ≥6 kg), Children <12 years (and ≥6 kg) and patients (any age and ≥6 kg) unable to swallow capsules: Oral: 3 mg/kg (maximum: 125 mg/dose) 1 hour prior to chemotherapy on day 1, followed by 2 mg/kg (maximum: 80 mg/dose) once daily on days 2 and 3 (in combination with a 5-HT$_3$ antagonist antiemetic and dexamethasone on day 1 [reduce dexamethasone dose to 50% of recommended dose])
   Pediatric Oncology Group of Ontario (POGO) guidelines: Recommended antiemetic regimen combinations in pediatric patients ≥6 months receiving chemotherapy agents that do **not** potentially interact with aprepitant (Dupuis 2013; Patel 2017):
      High emetogenic risk: Aprepitant, plus ondansetron or granisetron or palonosetron, plus dexamethasone.
      High emetogenic risk **and** cannot receive corticosteroids (due to contraindications): Aprepitant plus palonosetron.
      Moderate emetogenic risk **and** cannot receive corticosteroids (due to contraindications): Aprepitant plus ondansetron or granisetron or palonosetron.
      Infants ≥6 months, Children, and Adolescents: Oral: 3 mg/kg (maximum dose: 125 mg) on day 1 prior to chemotherapy, followed by 2 mg/kg (maximum dose: 80 mg) once daily on days 2 and 3.

Renal Impairment
   No dosage adjustment necessary.
   ESRD undergoing dialysis: No dosage adjustment necessary. Aprepitant is not removed by hemodialysis.

Hepatic Impairment
   Mild-to-moderate impairment (Child-Pugh class A or B): No dosage adjustment necessary.
   Severe impairment (Child-Pugh class C): Use with caution; no data available; may require additional monitoring for adverse reactions.

Administration

Capsules: Swallow whole.

Prevention of chemotherapy-induced nausea/vomiting: Administer with or without food. First dose should be given 1 hour prior to chemotherapy; subsequent doses should be given 1 hour prior to chemotherapy or in the morning (if no chemotherapy is administered on days 2 and 3).

Oral suspension: Dose should be prepared by a health care provider and dispensed to patient or caregiver in an oral dispenser. Administer by placing the dispenser in the patient's mouth along the inner cheek and slowly dispensing the medicine.

Prevention of postoperative nausea/vomiting: Administer within 3 hours prior to induction; follow health care provider instructions about food/drink restrictions prior to surgery.

Extemporaneous Preparations A suspension for oral administration is commercially available.

A 20 mg/mL oral aprepitant suspension may be prepared with capsules and a 1:1 combination of Ora-Sweet and Ora-Plus (or Ora-Blend). Empty the contents of four 125 mg capsules into a mortar and reduce to a fine powder (process will take 10-15 minutes). Add small portions of vehicle and mix to a uniform paste. Add sufficient vehicle to form a liquid; transfer to a graduated cylinder, rinse mortar with vehicle, and add quantity of vehicle sufficient to make 25 mL. Label "shake well" and "refrigerate". Stable for 90 days refrigerated.

Dupuis LL, Lingertat-Walsh K, and Walker SE, "Stability of an Extemporaneous Oral Liquid Aprepitant Formulation," *Support Care Cancer*, 2009, 17(6):701-6.

Monitoring Parameters In patients receiving concurrent warfarin, monitor INR/PT for 2 weeks (particularly at 7 to 10 days) following aprepitant administration; signs/symptoms of hypersensitivity reaction.

Dosage Forms Excipient information presented when available (limited, particularly for generics); consult specific product labeling.

Capsule, Oral:
  Emend: 40 mg, 80 mg, 125 mg
  Emend Tri-Pack: 80 mg & 125 mg
  Generic: 40 mg, 80 mg, 125 mg, 80 mg & 125 mg
Suspension Reconstituted, Oral:
  Emend: 125 mg (1 ea)

Arsenic Trioxide (AR se nik tri OKS id)

Related Information

Common Toxicity Criteria *on page 2242*
Management of Chemotherapy-Induced Nausea and Vomiting in Adults *on page 2253*
Management of Drug Extravasations *on page 2271*
Prevention of Chemotherapy-Induced Nausea and Vomiting in Children *on page 2310*
Safe Handling of Hazardous Drugs *on page 2379*

Brand Names: US Trisenox

Brand Names: Canada Trisenox

Index Terms Arsenic (III) Oxide; As_2O_3; ATO

Pharmacologic Category Antineoplastic Agent, Miscellaneous

Use Acute promyelocytic leukemia: Remission induction and consolidation in patients with acute promyelocytic leukemia (APL) who are refractory to, or have relapsed from, retinoid and anthracycline chemotherapy, and whose APL is characterized by the presence of the t(15;17) translocation or PML/RAR-alpha gene expression

Labeled Contraindications

Hypersensitivity to arsenic or any component of the formulation

Canadian labeling: Additional contraindications (not in US labeling): Pregnancy; breastfeeding

Pregnancy Considerations Adverse events have been observed in animal reproduction studies. Arsenic crosses the human placenta. In studies of women exposed to high levels of arsenic from drinking water, cord blood levels were similar to maternal serum levels. Dimethylarsinic acid (DMA) was the form of arsenic found in the fetus. An increased risk of low birth weight and still births were observed in women who ingested high levels of dietary arsenic. Women of childbearing potential should avoid pregnancy; effective contraception should be used during and after therapy. The Canadian labeling contraindicates use in pregnant women. It also recommends that women of childbearing potential avoid pregnancy, and male patients wear condoms during intercourse with women who are pregnant or of childbearing potential during therapy and for 3 months following therapy discontinuation.

Breastfeeding Considerations Arsenic is naturally found in breast milk; concentrations range from 0.2 to 6 mcg/kg. In studies of women exposed to high levels of arsenic from drinking water, breast milk concentrations were low (~3.1 mcg/kg) and did not correlate with maternal serum levels. The possible effect of maternal arsenic trioxide therapy on breast milk concentrations is not known. Due to the potential for serious adverse reactions in a nursing infant, the manufacturer recommends discontinuing breastfeeding during therapy. The Canadian labeling contraindicates use in nursing women and recommends avoiding nursing during treatment and for 3 months after therapy discontinuation.

Warnings/Precautions [US Boxed Warnings]: May prolong the QT interval and lead to torsade de pointes or complete AV block, which may be fatal. Risk factors for torsade de pointes include extent of prolongation, HF, a history of torsade de pointes, preexisting QT interval prolongation, patients taking medications known to prolong the QT interval or potassium-wasting diuretics, and conditions which cause hypokalemia or hypomagnesemia. If possible, discontinue all medications known to prolong the QT interval. [US Boxed Warning]: A baseline 12-lead ECG,

serum electrolytes (potassium, calcium, magnesium), and creatinine should be obtained prior to treatment. QT prolongation was observed 1 to 5 weeks after infusion, and returned to baseline by 8 weeks after infusion. Monitor ECG at baseline and then weekly; more frequently if clinically indicated. If baseline QT_c >500 msec, correct prior to treatment. If QT_c >500 msec during treatment, reassess, correct contributing factors, and consider temporarily withholding treatment. If syncope or irregular heartbeat develop during therapy, hospitalize patient for monitoring; assess electrolytes and do not reinitiate until QT_c <460 msec, electrolyte abnormalities are corrected and syncope/irregular heartbeat has resolved.

[US Boxed Warning]: May cause APL differentiation syndrome (formerly called retinoic-acid-APL [RA-APL] syndrome), which is characterized by dyspnea, fever, weight gain, pulmonary infiltrates, and pleural or pericardial effusions, with or without leukocytosis. May be fatal. High-dose steroids (dexamethasone 10 mg IV twice daily for at least 3 days or until signs/symptoms subside; initiate immediately if APL differentiation syndrome is suspected) have been used for treatment; in general, most patients may continue arsenic trioxide during treatment of APL differentiation syndrome. May lead to the development of hyperleukocytosis (leukocytes ≥10,000/mm³); did not correlate with baseline WBC counts and generally was not as high during consolidation as observed during induction treatment. Use with caution in patients with hepatic impairment; in patients with severe hepatic impairment, monitor closely for toxicity. Use with caution in patients with severe renal impairment (dose reduction may be warranted); systemic exposure to metabolites may be higher; has not been studied in dialysis patients. Monitor electrolytes, CBC with differential, and coagulation parameters at least twice a week during induction and weekly during consolidation; more frequently if clinically indicated. Arsenic trioxide is associated with a moderate emetic potential; antiemetics are recommended to prevent nausea and vomiting (Dupuis 2011). Potentially significant interactions may exist, requiring dose or frequency adjustment, additional monitoring, and/or selection of alternative therapy.

Adverse Reactions

>10%:

Cardiovascular: Tachycardia (55%), edema (40%), prolonged Q-T interval on ECG (40%; >500 msec), chest pain (25%; grades 3/4: 5%), hypotension (25%; grades 3/4: 5%)

Central nervous system: Fatigue (63%), headache (60%), insomnia (43%), rigors (38%), paresthesia (33%), anxiety (30%), dizziness (23%), depression (20%), pain (15%)

Dermatologic: Dermatitis (43%), pruritus (33%), xeroderma (15%), diaphoresis (13%), erythema (13%)

Endocrine & metabolic: Hypokalemia (50%; grades 3/4: 13%), hyperglycemia (45%; grades 3/4: 13%), hypomagnesemia (45%; grades 3/4: 13%), hyperkalemia (18%; grades 3/4: 5%), weight gain (13%)

Gastrointestinal: Nausea (75%), abdominal pain (58%), vomiting (58%), diarrhea (53%), sore throat (35%), constipation (28%), anorexia (23%), decreased appetite (15%)

Genitourinary: Vaginal hemorrhage (13%)

Hematologic & oncologic: Leukocytosis (50%; grades 3/4: 3%), APL differentiation syndrome (23%; grades 3/4: 8%), anemia (20%; grades 3/4: 5%), bruise (20%), thrombocytopenia (18%; grades 3/4: 13%), febrile neutropenia (13%; grades 3/4: 8%)

Hepatic: Increased serum ALT (20%; grades 3/4: 5%), increased serum AST (13%; grades 3/4: 3%)

Infection: Herpes simplex infection (13%)

Local: Pain at injection site (20%), erythema at injection site (13%)

Neuromuscular & skeletal: Arthralgia (33%), myalgia (25%), ostealgia (23%), back pain (18%), limb pain (13%), neck pain (13%), tremor (13%)

Respiratory: Cough (65%), dyspnea (53%; grades 3/4: 10%), epistaxis (25%), hypoxia (23%), pleural effusion (20%), sinusitis (20%), post nasal drip (13%), upper respiratory tract infection (13%), wheezing (13%)

Miscellaneous: Fever (63%)

1% to 10%:

Cardiovascular: Hypertension (10%), flushing (10%), palpitations (10%), ECG abnormality (8%; non-QT prolongation), facial edema (8%), atrial arrhythmia (5%), torsades de pointes (3%)

Central nervous system: Drowsiness (8%), seizure (8%; grades 3/4: 5%), agitation (5%), coma (5%), confusion (5%)

Dermatologic: Pallor (10%), hyperpigmentation (8%), night sweats (8%), skin lesion (8%), urticaria (8%)

Endocrine & metabolic: Hypocalcemia (10%), hypoglycemia (8%), intermenstrual bleeding (8%), acidosis (5%)

Gastrointestinal: Dyspepsia (10%), loose stools (10%), abdominal distension (8%), abdominal tenderness (8%), bloody diarrhea (8%), fecal incontinence (8%), gastrointestinal hemorrhage (8%), oral bullae (8%), typhlitis (children: 8%), weight loss (8%), xerostomia (8%), oral candidiasis (5%)

Genitourinary: Oliguria (5%), urinary incontinence (5%)

Hematologic & oncologic: Neutropenia (10%; grades 3/4: 10%), disseminated intravascular coagulation (8%), hemorrhage (8%), lymphadenopathy (8%), petechia (8%)

Hypersensitivity: Hypersensitivity (5%)

Infection: Bacterial infection (8%), herpes zoster (8%), sepsis (5%; grades 3/4: 5%)

Local: Swelling at injection site (10%), local skin exfoliation (5%)

Neuromuscular & skeletal: Weakness (10%)

Ophthalmic: Blurred vision (10%), eye irritation (10%), xerophthalmia (8%), eye redness (with pain: 5%), eyelid edema (5%)

Otic: Otalgia (8%), tinnitus (5%)

Renal: Renal failure (8%; grades 3/4: 3%), renal insufficiency (8%)

Respiratory: Abnormal breath sounds (decreased: 10%), rales (10%), hemoptysis (8%), pulmonary edema (children: 8%), rhonchi (8%), tachypnea (8%), nasopharyngitis (5%)

<1%, postmarketing, and/or case reports: Acute respiratory distress, atrioventricular block, capillary leak syndrome, cardiac failure, dysphagia, heart block, hypoalbuminemia, hyponatremia, hypophosphatemia, increased serum lipase, mucosal inflammation, neuralgia, oropharyngeal pain, pancytopenia, peripheral neuropathy, pneumonitis, pulmonary infiltrates, respiratory distress, stomatitis, urinary incontinence, ventricular premature contractions, ventricular tachycardia

Drug Interactions

Metabolism/Transport Effects None known.

Avoid Concomitant Use

Avoid concomitant use of Arsenic Trioxide with any of the following: Amifampridine; BCG (Intravesical); Deferiprone; Dipyrone; Highest Risk

QTc-Prolonging Agents; Hydroxychloroquine; MiFEPRIStone; Mizolastine; Moderate Risk QTc-Prolonging Agents; Probucol; Promazine; Vinflunine

Increased Effect/Toxicity

Arsenic Trioxide may increase the levels/effects of: Amifostine; Antipsychotic Agents (Second Generation [Atypical]); Deferiprone; DULoxetine; Highest Risk QTc-Prolonging Agents; Hypotension-Associated Agents; Levodopa; Nitroprusside; Pholcodine

The levels/effects of Arsenic Trioxide may be increased by: Amifampridine; Barbiturates; Bilastine; Blood Pressure Lowering Agents; Brimonidine (Topical); Buprenorphine; Diazoxide; Dipyrone; Herbs (Hypotensive Properties); Hydroxychloroquine; Indapamide; Lormetazepam; MiFEPRIStone; Mizolastine; Moderate Risk QTc-Prolonging Agents; Molsidomine; Naftopidil; Nicergoline; Nicorandil; Obinutuzumab; Pentoxifylline; Phosphodiesterase 5 Inhibitors; Probucol; Promazine; Prostacyclin Analogues; QTc-Prolonging Agents (Indeterminate Risk and Risk Modifying); Quinagolide; Teneligliptin; Vinflunine; Xipamide

Decreased Effect

Arsenic Trioxide may decrease the levels/effects of: Antidiabetic Agents; BCG (Intravesical)

Hazardous Drugs Handling Considerations

Hazardous agent (NIOSH 2016 [group 1]).

Use appropriate precautions for receiving, handling, administration, and disposal. Gloves (single) should be worn during receiving, unpacking, and placing in storage.

NIOSH recommends double gloving, a protective gown, ventilated engineering controls (a class II biological safety cabinet or a compounding aseptic containment isolator), and closed system transfer devices (CSTDs) for preparation. Double gloving, a gown, and (if dosage form allows) CSTDs are required during administration (NIOSH 2016).

Storage/Stability Store at 25°C (77°F); excursions permitted to 15°C to 30°C (59°F to 86°F); do not freeze. Following dilution in D5W or NS, solution for infusion is stable for 24 hours at room temperature or 48 hours when refrigerated.

Preparation for Administration Dilute with 100 to 250 mL D5W or NS. Discard unused portion of ampule.

Mechanism of Action Induces apoptosis in APL cells via morphological changes and DNA fragmentation; also damages or degrades the fusion protein promyelocytic leukemia (PML)-retinoic acid receptor (RAR) alpha

Pharmacodynamics/Kinetics

Distribution: V_{dss}: Arsenious acid (As^{III}): 562 L; widely distributed throughout body tissues; dependent on body weight and increases as body weight increases; orally administered arsenic trioxide distributes into the CNS

Metabolism: Arsenic trioxide is immediately hydrolyzed to the active form, arsenious acid (As^{III}) which is methylated (hepatically) to the less active pentavalent metabolites, monomethylarsonic acid (MMA^V) and dimethylarsinic acid (DMA^V) by methyltransferases; As^{III} is also oxidized to the minor metabolite, arsenic acid (As^V)

Half-life elimination: As^{III}: 10 to 14 hours; MMA^V: ~32 hours; DMA^V: ~72 hours

Time to peak: As^{III}: At the end of infusion (2 hours); MMA^V and DMA^V: ~10 to 24 hours

Excretion: Urine (MMA^V, DMA^V, and 15% of a dose as unchanged As^{III})

◄ **Dosing**

Adult Note: Arsenic trioxide is associated with a moderate emetic potential; antiemetics are recommended to prevent nausea and vomiting.

Acute promyelocytic leukemia (APL), relapsed or refractory: IV:

Induction: 0.15 mg/kg once daily until bone marrow remission; maximum: 60 doses for induction

Consolidation: 0.15 mg/kg once daily starting 3 to 6 weeks after completion of induction therapy; maximum: 25 doses over a period of up to 5 weeks for consolidation

APL, newly diagnosed (off-label use): IV:

Low/intermediate risk (Lo-Coco 2013):

Induction: 0.15 mg/kg/day; administer daily until bone marrow remission (in combination with tretinoin)

Consolidation: 0.15 mg/kg/day; administer 5 days/week for 4 weeks every 8 weeks for a total of 4 cycles (in combination with tretinoin)

High-risk:

Consolidation therapy after remission induction with tretinoin, daunorubicin and cytarabine (Powell 2010): Two consolidation courses (2 weeks apart): 0.15 mg/kg/day 5 days/week for 5 weeks

In combination with tretinoin in patients unable to tolerate anthracycline-based therapy (Estey 2006; Ravandi 2009):

Induction (beginning 10 days after initiation of tretinoin): 0.15 mg/kg/day until bone marrow remission; maximum: 75 doses for induction

Consolidation: 0.15 mg/kg/day Monday through Friday for 4 weeks every 8 weeks for 4 cycles (weeks 1 to 4, 9 to 12, 17 to 20, and 25 to 28)

APML 4 protocol (Iland 2012):

Induction: 0.15 mg/kg/day over 2 hours on days 9 to 36 (in combination with tretinoin and age-adjusted idarubicin)

Consolidation (2 cycles): 0.15 mg/kg/day on days 1 to 28 of consolidation cycle 1 (in combination with tretinoin); 0.15 mg/kg/day on days 1 to 5, 8 to 12, 15 to 19, 22 to 26, and 29 to 33 of consolidation cycle 2 (in combination with tretinoin)

Pediatric Note: Arsenic trioxide is associated with a moderate emetic potential; antiemetics are recommended to prevent nausea and vomiting (Dupuis 2011).

Acute promyelocytic leukemia (APL), relapsed or refractory: Children ≥4 years (US labeling) or ≥5 years (Canadian labeling): IV: Refer to adult dosing. **Note:** The Canadian labeling recommends dosing obese pediatric patients based on ideal body weight.

APL, newly diagnosed (off-label use): IV:

Induction, consolidation, and maintenance (Mathews 2006):

Induction: 0.15 mg/kg/day (maximum dose: 10 mg); administer daily until bone marrow remission; maximum: 60 doses for induction

Consolidation: 0.15 mg/kg/day (maximum dose: 10 mg) for 4 weeks, starting 4 weeks after completion of induction therapy

Maintenance: 0.15 mg/kg/dose (maximum dose: 10 mg) administered 10 days per month for 6 months, starting 4 weeks after completion of consolidation therapy

Children >1 year and Adolescents (APML 4 protocol; Iland 2012):

Induction: 0.15 mg/kg/day over 2 hours on days 9 to 36 (in combination with tretinoin and idarubicin)

Consolidation (2 cycles): 0.15 mg/kg/day on days 1 to 28 of consolidation cycle 1 (in combination with tretinoin); 0.15 mg/kg/day on days 1 to 5, 8 to 12, 15 to 19, 22 to 26, and 29 to 33 of consolidation cycle 2 (in combination with tretinoin)

Renal Impairment

Mild-to-moderate impairment (CrCl ≥30 mL/minute): There are no dosage adjustments provided in the manufacturer's labeling.

Severe renal impairment (CrCl <30 mL/minute): Use with caution (systemic exposure to metabolites may be higher); may require dosage reduction; monitor closely for toxicity.

Dialysis patients: There are no dosage adjustments provided in the manufacturer's labeling (has not been studied).

Hepatic Impairment There are no dosage adjustments provided in the manufacturer's labeling; use with caution. Patients with severe impairment (Child-Pugh class C) should be monitored closely for toxicity.

Adjustment for Toxicity Consider delaying infusion if a severe nonhematologic reaction occurs (eg, neurologic or dermatologic toxicity) until the toxicity has improved to ≤ grade 1.

Combination Regimens

Leukemia, acute promyelocytic:

Tretinoin-Arsenic Trioxide (APL) on page 2218

Tretinoin-Daunorubicin-Cytarabine Induction, Consolidation, Maintenance (APL) on page 2218

Administration Arsenic trioxide is associated with a moderate emetic potential; antiemetics are recommended to prevent nausea and vomiting (Dupuis 2011). For relapsed/refractory APL, administer as an IV infusion over 1 to 2 hours. For newly diagnosed APL (off-label use), infusion rate may vary; refer to specific protocol. If acute vasomotor reactions occur, the infusion duration may be extended to up to 4 hours. Does not require administration via a central venous catheter.

Vesicant/Extravasation Risk May be an irritant

Emetic Potential Children and Adults: Moderate (30% to 90%)

Monitoring Parameters Monitor electrolytes (potassium, calcium, and magnesium), CBC with differential, serum creatinine, hepatic function, blood glucose, and coagulation parameters at baseline then at least twice weekly during induction and at least weekly during consolidation; more frequent monitoring may be necessary in unstable patients; baseline then weekly 12-lead ECG; signs/symptoms of APL differentiation syndrome (unexplained fever, dyspnea and/or weight gain, abnormal chest auscultatory findings or radiographic abnormalities)

Dosage Forms Excipient information presented when available (limited, particularly for generics); consult specific product labeling.

Solution, Intravenous:

Trisenox: 10 mg/10 mL (10 mL)

Asparaginase (E. coli) (a SPEAR a ji nase e ko lye)

Related Information

Common Toxicity Criteria on page 2242

Management of Chemotherapy-Induced Nausea and Vomiting in Adults on page 2253

Prevention of Chemotherapy-Induced Nausea and Vomiting in Children on page 2310

Brand Names: US Elspar [DSC]

Brand Names: Canada Kidrolase

Index Terms E. coli Asparaginase; ASNase; Asparaginase; Elspar; L-ASP; L-asparaginase (E. coli)

Pharmacologic Category Antineoplastic Agent, Enzyme; Antineoplastic Agent, Miscellaneous

Use Acute lymphoblastic leukemia: Treatment of acute lymphoblastic leukemia (ALL) (in combination with other chemotherapy)

Labeled Contraindications Known hypersensitivity to asparaginase (E. coli-derived) or any component of the formulation; hepatic insufficiency; pancreatitis, pregnancy, breastfeeding, recent yellow fever vaccination, concurrent administration with phenytoin

Pregnancy Considerations Use is contraindicated.

Warnings/Precautions [Canadian Boxed Warning]: Allergic reactions may occur during therapy, particularly in patients with known hypersensitivity to other forms of L-asparaginase. Observe for reactions following administration; reactions generally occur 30 to 60 minutes following administration (although may also occur beyond that time). Immediate treatment for hypersensitivity reactions should be available during administration. Discontinue if serious allergic reaction occurs. Prior exposure to asparaginase is a risk factor for allergic reactions; IV administration (compared to IM or SubQ administration) and younger age also may be associated with hypersensitivity reactions (Stock 2011; Woo 2000). Patients who have an allergic reaction to E. coli asparaginase may also react to asparaginase (Erwinia) or to pegaspargase.

[Canadian Boxed Warning]: Should be administered under the supervision of an experienced cancer chemotherapy physician in a setting where full resuscitative facilities are immediately available.

[Canadian Boxed Warning]: Adverse effects on liver function may be observed including exacerbation of preexisting liver impairment (due to prior therapy or underlying disease). Physicians should carefully consider therapeutic benefits versus toxicity risks. Altered liver function tests (eg, increased AST, ALT, alkaline phosphatase, bilirubin, and decreased serum albumin, plasma fibrinogen) may occur; fulminant hepatic failure has also occurred. Fatty liver may be observed on biopsy. Use with caution and monitor liver function tests at least weekly during therapy; discontinue therapy for any significant changes. May induce excessive ammonia production; monitor for signs of metabolic encephalopathy (confusion, stupor, coma).

Serious thrombosis, including sagittal sinus thrombosis may occur; discontinue with serious thrombotic events. Anticoagulation prophylaxis during therapy may be considered in some patients (Farge 2013). The risk for thrombosis may be higher in adult patients (Stock 2011). Increased prothrombin time, partial thromboplastin time and hypofibrinogenemia may occur; cerebrovascular thrombosis and hemorrhage have been reported; monitor coagulation parameters at baseline and periodically during and after therapy; use cautiously in patients with an underlying coagulopathy. Replacement therapy should be instituted if fibrinogen <1g/L or ATIII <60%; if ineffective, treatment should preferably be suspended and resumed only when the laboratory parameters have normalized.

May cause hyperglycemia/glucose intolerance (possibly irreversible). Cases of diabetic ketoacidosis have been observed; monitor blood glucose as clinically necessary. May cause serious and possibly fulminant or fatal pancreatitis; promptly evaluate patients with abdominal pain. May consider continuing therapy for asymptomatic chemical pancreatitis (amylase or lipase >3 times ULN) or only radiologic abnormalities; monitor closely for rising amylase and/or lipase levels (Stock 2011). Discontinue permanently for clinical pancreatitis (eg, vomiting, severe abdominal pain) with amylase/lipase elevation >3 times ULN for >3 days and/or development of a pancreatic pseudocyst. Avoid alcohol use (Stock 2011).

Posterior reversible encephalopathy syndrome (PRES) has been observed in patients treated with asparaginase (in combination with other chemotherapy agents). Monitor for signs/symptoms of PRES (eg, altered mental status, headache, hypertension, seizures, visual disturbances); interrupt therapy for suspected PRES. Control blood pressure and closely monitor for seizure activity. Appropriate measures must be taken to prevent tumor lysis syndrome and subsequent hyperuricemia and uric acid nephropathy; monitor, consider antihyperuricemic therapy, hydration and urinary alkalization.

Do not interchange *E. coli* asparaginase for *Erwinia* asparaginase or pegaspargase; ensure the proper formulation, route of administration, and dose prior to administration. The *E. coli* and the *Erwinia* strains of asparaginase differ slightly in their gene sequencing, and have slight differences in their enzyme characteristics. Both are highly specific for asparagine and have <10% activity for the D-isomer.

Adverse Reactions Frequency not defined.

Cardiovascular: Cerebrovascular accident (hemorrhagic stroke and thrombotic stroke [Morgan 2011]), thrombosis (including cerebral thrombosis)

Central nervous system: Central nervous system disease (adults; includes delusion, disorientation, mild depression, Parkinsonian-like syndrome, personality disorder, seizure), cerebral hemorrhage, cerebrovascular hemorrhage (Morgan 2011)

Endocrine & metabolic: Amenorrhea, decreased glucose tolerance, hyperammonemia (with clinical signs of metabolic encephalopathy [eg, impaired consciousness with coma, confusion, and stupor]), hypercholesterolemia, hyperglycemia, hypertriglyceridemia, hypoalbuminemia, hypocholesterolemia, increased uric acid, weight loss

Gastrointestinal: Abdominal pain (infrequent), acute pancreatitis (may be fatal), cholestatic injury, diarrhea (infrequent), intestinal perforation (rare), nausea (frequent, but rarely severe; may be secondary to increased blood urea nitrogen and increased uric acid), vomiting (frequent, but rarely severe; may be secondary to increased blood urea nitrogen and increased uric acid)

Genitourinary: Azoospermia

Hematologic: Antithrombin III deficiency, blood coagulation disorder (change in hemostatic function), bone marrow depression, decreased clotting factors (factors VII, VIII, IX, and X), decreased plasminogen, hypofibrinogenemia, prolonged partial thromboplastin time, prolonged prothrombin time

Hepatic: Hepatic injury, hepatotoxicity (usually mild and regressive, but may be fatal rarely), hyperbilirubinemia, increased serum alkaline phosphatase, increased serum ALT, increased serum AST (mild), jaundice, liver steatosis

Hypersensitivity: Allergic reactions (includes anaphylactic shock, anaphylaxis, bronchospasm, edema, hypotension, laryngeal edema, skin rash, urticaria; onset usually within 1 hour of administration and risk increasing with increasing number of exposures)

Immunologic: Increased serum globulins (beta and gamma)

Infection: Septicemia (during bone marrow depression)

Renal: Increased blood urea nitrogen, renal failure

Respiratory: Respiratory distress (with retrosternal pressure)

Miscellaneous: Fever

Drug Interactions

Metabolism/Transport Effects None known.

Avoid Concomitant Use There are no known interactions where it is recommended to avoid concomitant use.

Increased Effect/Toxicity

Asparaginase (E. coli) may increase the levels/effects of: Dexamethasone (Systemic)

Decreased Effect There are no known significant interactions involving a decrease in effect.

Storage/Stability Intact vials of powder should be refrigerated at 2°C to 8°C (36°F to 48°F). Reconstituted solution should be used immediately after preparation, although is stable for 3 hours at room temperature or 72 hours refrigerated.

Preparation for Administration Reconstitute each vial with 4 mL sterile water for injection; rotate gently, do not shake. For IM administration, the US manufacturer recommended reconstitution of the lyophilized powder with 2 mL NS to a concentration of 5000 units/mL; however, some institutions reconstitute with 1 mL NS for IM use, resulting in a concentration of 10,000 units/mL. Shake well, but not too vigorously. A 5 micron filter may be used to remove fiber-like particles in the solution (do not use a 0.2 micron filter; has been associated with loss of potency).

Standard IM dilution: 5,000 units/mL (10,000 units/mL has been used by some institutions)

Standard IV dilution: Dilute in 50 to 250 mL NS or D5W

Mechanism of Action In leukemic cells, asparaginase hydrolyzes L-asparagine to ammonia and L-aspartic acid, leading to depletion of asparagine. Leukemia cells, especially lymphoblasts, require exogenous asparagine; normal cells can synthesize asparagine. Asparagine depletion in leukemic cells leads to inhibition of protein synthesis and apoptosis. Asparaginase is cycle-specific for the G_1 phase.

Pharmacodynamics/Kinetics

Distribution: IV: Slightly higher than plasma volume; <1% CSF penetration

Metabolism: Systemically degraded

Half-life elimination: IM: 34 to 49 hours; IV: 8 to 30 hours

Time to peak, plasma: IM: 14 to 24 hours

Dosing

Adult & Geriatric Note: Dose, frequency, number of doses, and start date may vary by protocol and treatment phase.

Acute lymphoblastic leukemia (ALL; Canadian labeling): IM, IV:

Daily administration: 200 to 1,000 units/kg/day for 28 consecutive days; continue induction therapy for an additional 14 days if not in remission or begin maintenance therapy if in remission

Intermittent administration: 400 units/kg on Monday and Wednesday and 600 units/kg on Friday; repeat for 4 weeks; continue induction therapy for an additional 2 weeks if not in remission or begin maintenance therapy if in remission

Hyper-CVAD regimen (off-label dosing): IV 20,000 units weekly for 4 doses (starting on day 2) during either months 7 and 19 or months 7 and 11 of intensification phase (Thomas 2010)

Larson regimen (off-label dosing): SubQ: 6000 units/m^2/dose on days 5, 8, 11, 15, 18, and 22 (induction phase) and on days 15, 18, 22, and 25 (early intensification phase) (Larson, 1995)

Linker regimen (off-label dosing): IM:

Remission induction: 6000 units/m^2/dose on days 17-28; if bone marrow on day 28 is positive for residual leukemia: 6000 units/m^2/dose on days 29-35 (Linker, 1991)

Consolidation (Treatment A; cycles 1, 3, 5, and 7): 12,000 units/m^2/dose on days 2, 4, 7, 9, 11, and 14 (Linker, 1991)

Lymphoblastic lymphoma (off-label use): Hyper-CVAD regimen: IV: 20,000 units weekly for 4 doses (starting on day 2) for 2 cycles (months 7 and 11) during maintenance phase (Thomas 2004)

Pediatric Note: Dose, frequency, number of doses, and start date may vary by protocol and treatment phase.

Acute lymphoblastic leukemia (ALL): Children and Adolescents: Refer to adult dosing.

CCG 1922 protocol (off-label dosing): IM: 6,000 units/m^2/dose 3 times weekly for 9 doses beginning either on day 2, 3, or 4 (induction phase) and 6,000 units/m^2/dose on Monday, Wednesday, and Friday for 6 doses beginning day 3 (delayed intensification phase) (Bostrom 2004)

DFCI-ALL Consortium protocol 00-01 (off-label dosing): IM: 25,000 units/m^2 for 1 dose (induction phase) and 25,000 units/m^2/dose weekly for 30 weeks (intensification phase) (Vrooman 2013)

DFCI-ALL Consortium protocol 95-01 (off-label dosing): IM: 25,000 units/m^2 for 1 dose on day 4 (induction phase) and 25,000 units/m^2/dose weekly for 20 weeks (intensification phase) (Moghrabi 2007)

Hyper-CVAD regimen (off-label dosing): Adolescents ≥13 years: Refer to adult dosing.

Lymphoblastic lymphoma (off-label use): Adolescents >15 years: Refer to adult dosing.

Renal Impairment There are no dosage adjustments provided in the manufacturer's labeling.

Hepatic Impairment Use is contraindicated in patients with hepatic insufficiency. The following adjustments have been recommended for hepatotoxicity during treatment (Stock 2011):

ALT/AST 3 to 5 times ULN: Continue therapy.

ALT/AST >5 to 20 times ULN: Delay next dose until transaminases <5 times ULN.

ALT/AST >20 times ULN: Discontinue therapy if takes longer than 1 week for transaminases to return to <3 times ULN.

Direct bilirubin <3 mg/dL: Continue therapy.

Direct bilirubin 3.1 to 5 mg/dL: Hold asparaginase and resume when direct bilirubin <2 mg/dL; consider switching to alternate asparaginase product. Direct bilirubin >5 mg/dL: Discontinue asparaginase; do not substitute other asparaginase products; do not make up for missed doses.

Adjustment for Toxicity

Allergic reaction/hypersensitivity: Discontinue for severe reactions.

Neurotoxicity (posterior reversible encephalopathy syndrome; PRES): Interrupt therapy for suspected PRES; control blood pressure and closely monitor for seizure activity.

Pancreatitis: Discontinue permanently (per manufacturer).

Thrombotic event: Discontinue for serious reactions.

The following adjustments have also been recommended (Stock 2011):

Hyperammonemia-related fatigue: Continue therapy for grade 2 toxicity. If grade 3 toxicity occurs, reduce dose by 25%; resume full dose when toxicity ≤ grade 2 (make up for missed doses). If grade 4 toxicity occurs, reduce dose by 50%; resume full dose when toxicity ≤ grade 2 (make up for missed doses).

Hyperglycemia: Continue therapy for uncomplicated hyperglycemia. If hyperglycemia requires insulin therapy, hold asparaginase (and any concomitant corticosteroids) until blood glucose controlled; resume dosing at prior dose level. For life-threatening hyperglycemia or toxicity requiring urgent intervention, hold asparaginase (and corticosteroids) until blood glucose is controlled with insulin; resume asparaginase and do not make up for missed doses.

Hypersensitivity reactions: May continue dosing for urticaria without bronchospasm, hypotension, edema, or need for parenteral intervention. If wheezing or other symptomatic bronchospasm with or without urticaria, angioedema, hypotension, and/or life-threatening hypersensitivity reactions occur, discontinue asparaginase.

Hypertriglyceridemia: If serum triglyceride level <1,000 mg/dL, continue asparaginase but monitor closely for pancreatitis. If triglyceride level >1,000 mg/dL, hold asparaginase and monitor; resume therapy at prior dose level after triglyceride level returns to baseline.

Pancreatitis:

Asymptomatic amylase or lipase >3 times ULN (chemical pancreatitis) or radiologic abnormalities only: Continue asparaginase and monitor levels closely.

Symptomatic amylase or lipase >3 times ULN: Hold asparaginase until enzyme levels stabilize or are declining.

Symptomatic pancreatitis or clinical pancreatitis (abdominal pain with amylase or lipase >3 times ULN for >3 days and/or development of pancreatic pseudocyst): Permanently discontinue asparaginase.

Thrombosis and bleeding, CNS:

Thrombosis: Continue therapy for abnormal laboratory findings without a clinical correlate. If grade 3 toxicity occurs, discontinue therapy; if CNS signs/symptoms are fully resolved and further asparaginase doses are required, may resume therapy at a lower dose and/or longer intervals between doses. Discontinue therapy for grade 4 toxicity.

Hemorrhage: Discontinue therapy; do not withhold therapy for abnormal laboratory findings without a clinical correlate. If grade 3 toxicity occurs, discontinue therapy; if CNS signs/symptoms are fully resolved and further asparaginase doses are required, may resume therapy at a lower dose and/or longer intervals between doses. Discontinue therapy for grade 4 toxicity.

Thrombosis and bleeding, non-CNS:

Thrombosis: Continue therapy for abnormal laboratory findings without a clinical correlate. If grade 3 or 4 toxicity occurs, withhold therapy until acute toxicity and clinical signs resolve and anticoagulant therapy is stable or completed. Do not withhold therapy for abnormal laboratory findings without clinical correlate.

Hemorrhage: If grade 2 bleeding in conjunction with hypofibrinogenemia occurs, withhold therapy until bleeding ≤ grade 1. Do not withhold therapy for abnormal laboratory findings without clinical correlate. For grade 3 or 4 bleeding, withhold therapy until bleeding ≤ grade 1 and until acute toxicity and clinical signs resolve and coagulant replacement therapy is stable or completed.

Combination Regimens

Leukemia, acute lymphocytic:

CALGB 8811 Regimen (ALL) on page 2003
CALGB 9111 Regimen (ALL) on page 2004
Hyper-CVAD (Leukemia, Acute Lymphocytic) on page 2146
Linker Protocol (ALL) on page 2167
PVA (POG 8602) on page 2197
PVDA on page 2199

Administration May be administered IM (preferred for intermittent administration) or IV; has been administered SubQ (off-label route; Larson, 1995) in specific protocols. May administer corticosteroids 1 to 2 days prior to initiating reinduction therapy (to prevent hypersensitivity reaction). Observe patients for 1 hour after administration; have epinephrine, diphenhydramine, and hydrocortisone at the bedside. A physician should be readily accessible.

IM: Doses should be given as a deep intramuscular injection into a large muscle; volumes >2 mL should be divided and administered in 2 separate sites.

IV: Infuse over at least 30 minutes through the side arm of a NS or D5W infusion.

Emetic Potential Children and Adults: Minimal (<10%)

Monitoring Parameters CBC with differential, amylase, lipase, triglycerides, liver function prior to and weekly during therapy, coagulation parameters (baseline and prior to each injection), blood glucose, uric acid. Monitor for allergic reaction; monitor for onset of abdominal pain and mental status changes. Monitor vital signs during administration.

Product Availability US product, Elspar, was discontinued more than 1 year ago.

Dosage Forms Excipient information presented when available (limited, particularly for generics); consult specific product labeling. [DSC] = Discontinued product

Solution Reconstituted, Injection:

Elspar: 10,000 units (1 ea [DSC])

Dosage Forms: Canada Information with regard to form, strength, and availability of products uniquely available in Canada but currently not available in the US. Refer also to Dosage Forms.

Excipient information presented when available (limited, particularly for generics); consult specific product labeling.

Solution Reconstituted, Injection:

Kidrolase: 10,000 units (1 ea)

Asparaginase (*Erwinia*) (a SPEAR a ji nase er WIN i ah)

Related Information

Common Toxicity Criteria *on page 2242*

Management of Chemotherapy-Induced Nausea and Vomiting in Adults *on page 2253*

Prevention of Chemotherapy-Induced Nausea and Vomiting in Children *on page 2310*

Brand Names: US Erwinaze

Brand Names: Canada Erwinase

Index Terms *Erwinia chrysanthemi*; Asparaginase *Erwinia chrysanthemi*; Crisantaspase; L-asparaginase (*Erwinia*)

Pharmacologic Category Antineoplastic Agent, Enzyme; Antineoplastic Agent, Miscellaneous

Use Acute lymphoblastic leukemia: Treatment (in combination with other chemotherapy) of acute lymphoblastic leukemia (ALL) in patients with hypersensitivity to *E. coli*-derived asparaginase

Labeled Contraindications

History of serious hypersensitivity reactions, including anaphylaxis to asparaginase (*Erwinia*) or any component of the formulation; history of serious pancreatitis, serious thrombosis, or serious hemorrhagic events with prior asparaginase treatment

Canadian labeling: Additional contraindications (not in the US labeling): Women who are or may become pregnant

Pregnancy Considerations Adverse events were observed in animal reproduction studies.

Breastfeeding Considerations It is not known if asparaginase *Erwinia chrysanthemi* is excreted in breast milk. Due to the potential for serious adverse reactions in the nursing infant, the manufacturer recommends a decision be made to discontinue nursing or to discontinue the drug, taking into account the importance of treatment to the mother.

Warnings/Precautions Serious hypersensitivity reactions (grade 3 and 4), including anaphylaxis, have occurred in 5% of patients in clinical trials. Immediate treatment for hypersensitivity reactions should be available during treatment; discontinue for serious hypersensitivity reactions (and administer appropriate treatment).

Pancreatitis has been reported in 5% of patients in clinical trials; promptly evaluate with symptoms suggestive of pancreatitis. For mild pancreatitis, withhold treatment until signs and symptoms subside and amylase levels return to normal; may resume after resolution. Discontinue for severe or hemorrhagic pancreatitis characterized by abdominal pain >72 hours and amylase $\geq 2 \times$ ULN. Further use is contraindicated if severe pancreatitis is diagnosed.

Serious thrombotic events, including sagittal sinus thrombosis and pulmonary embolism, have been reported with asparaginase formulations. Decreases in fibrinogen, protein C activity, protein S activity, and antithrombin III have been noted following a 2-week treatment course administered intramuscularly. Discontinue for hemorrhagic or thrombotic events; may resume treatment after resolution (contraindicated with history of serious thrombosis or hemorrhagic event with prior asparaginase treatment).

In clinical trials, 4% of patients experienced glucose intolerance; may be irreversible; monitor glucose levels (baseline and periodic) during treatment; may require insulin administration.

Do not interchange *Erwinia* asparaginase for *E. coli* asparaginase or pegaspargase; ensure the proper formulation, route of administration, and dose prior to administration.

Adverse Reactions Frequency of adverse reactions is for both IM and IV routes unless specified.

>10%: Hypersensitivity: Hypersensitivity reaction (14% [IV: ≤37%]; grades 3/4: 4%; includes anaphylaxis, urticaria)

1% to 10%:

Cardiovascular: Thrombosis (2% [IV: ≤7%]; grades 3/4: ≤1%; includes pulmonary embolism and cerebrovascular accident)

Endocrine & metabolic: Hyperglycemia (4% [IV: ≤17%]; grades 3/4: 4%), abnormal transaminase (4%), decreased glucose tolerance (4%)

Gastrointestinal: Nausea (3% [IV: ≤20%]), vomiting (3% [IV: ≤17%]), pancreatitis (4%; grades 3/4: <1%), abdominal pain (1%), diarrhea (1%), mucositis (1%)

Local: Injection site reaction (3%)

Miscellaneous: Fever (4%)

<1%, postmarketing, and/or case reports: Acute renal failure, anorexia, azotemia, bone marrow depression (rare), changes in serum lipids, chills, decreased serum albumin, decreased serum cholesterol, disseminated intravascular coagulation, headache, hemorrhage, hepatomegaly, hyperammonemia, hyperbilirubinemia, irritability, malabsorption syndrome, proteinuria, seizure, transient ischemic attacks, weight loss

Drug Interactions

Metabolism/Transport Effects None known.

Avoid Concomitant Use There are no known interactions where it is recommended to avoid concomitant use.

Increased Effect/Toxicity

Asparaginase (Erwinia) may increase the levels/effects of: Dexamethasone (Systemic)

Decreased Effect There are no known significant interactions involving a decrease in effect.

Storage/Stability Store intact vials refrigerated at 2°C to 8°C (36°F to 46°F). Protect from light. Within 15 minutes of reconstitution, withdraw appropriate volume for dose into a polypropylene syringe. Do not freeze or refrigerate reconstituted solution; discard if not administered within 4 hours.

Preparation for Administration

Reconstitute each vial with 1 mL of preservative free sodium chloride 0.9% (NS) to obtain a concentration of 10,000 units/mL, or with 2 mL preservative free NS to obtain a concentration of 5,000 units/mL. Gently direct the NS down the wall of the vial (do not inject forcefully into or onto the powder). Dissolve by gently swirling or mixing; do not shake or invert the vial. Resulting reconstituted solution should be clear and colorless and free of visible particles or protein aggregates. Within 15 minutes of reconstitution, withdraw appropriate volume for dose into a polypropylene syringe. If administering intravenously, slowly inject the appropriate volume of reconstituted solution into a NS 100 mL infusion bag; do not shake or squeeze the bag. Administer within 4 hours of reconstitution.

Additional special preparation instructions may be required for select Aspar-aginase (*Erwinia*) batches. Asparaginase (*Erwinia*) vials from certain US batches should be **only** be administered intramuscularly.

Refer to the following for batch-specific information:

Erwinaze [US product]: http://erwinazesupply.com/product-updates/

Erwinase [Canadian product]: http://healthycanadians.gc.ca/recall-alert-rap-pel-avis/hc-sc/2017/63916a-eng.php

Mechanism of Action Asparaginase catalyzes the deamidation of aspar-agine to aspartic acid and ammonia, reducing circulating levels of asparagine. Leukemia cells lack asparagine synthetase and are unable to synthesize asparagine. Asparaginase reduces the exogenous asparagine source for the leukemic cells, resulting in cytotoxicity specific to leukemic cells.

Pharmacodynamics/Kinetics Half-life elimination: IM: ~16 hours (Asselin 1993; Avramis 2005); IV: ~7.5 hours

Dosing

Adult Note: If administering IV, consider monitoring nadir serum asparagi-nase activity (NSAA) levels; if desired levels are not achieved, change to IM administration.

Acute lymphoblastic leukemia (ALL): IM, IV:

As a substitute for pegaspargase: 25,000 units/m^2 3 times weekly (Mon, Wed, Fri) for 6 doses for each planned pegaspargase dose

As a substitute for asparaginase (E. coli): 25,000 units/m^2 for each scheduled asparaginase (*E. coli*) dose

Pediatric Note: If administering IV, consider monitoring nadir serum aspar-aginase activity (NSAA) levels; if desired levels are not achieved, change to IM administration.

Acute lymphoblastic leukemia (ALL): Children ≥1 year and Adolescents: IM, IV: Refer to adult dosing.

ALL induction: *Canadian labeling (not in the US labeling):* Children <14 years: IM: 6,000 units/m^2 3 times weekly for 9 doses beginning day 4 of week 1 (in combination with vincristine, prednisone, methotrexate, and daunorubicin)

Renal Impairment There are no dosage adjustments provided in the manufacturer's labeling.

Hepatic Impairment There are no dosage adjustments provided in the manufacturer's labeling; however, the following adjustments have been recommended for other asparaginase products for hepatotoxicity during treatment (Stock 2011):

ALT/AST >3 to 5 times ULN: Continue therapy

ALT/AST >5 to 20 times ULN: Delay next dose until transaminases <3 times ULN

ALT/AST >20 times ULN: Discontinue therapy if takes longer than 1 week for transaminases to return to <3 times ULN.

Direct bilirubin <3 mg/dL: Continue therapy

Direct bilirubin 3.1 to 5 mg/dL: Hold asparaginase and resume when direct bilirubin <2 mg/dL; consider switching to alternate asparaginase product.

Direct bilirubin >5 mg/dL: Discontinue asparaginase; do not substitute other asparaginase products; do not make up for missed doses.

Adjustment for Toxicity

Hemorrhagic or thrombotic event: Discontinue treatment; may resume treatment upon symptom resolution.

Pancreatitis:

Mild pancreatitis: Withhold treatment until signs and symptoms subside and amylase levels return to normal; may resume after resolution.

Severe or hemorrhagic pancreatitis (abdominal pain >72 hours and amylase ≥2 x ULN): Discontinue treatment; further use is contraindicated.

Serious hypersensitivity reaction: Discontinue treatment.

The following adjustments have also been recommended for asparaginase products (Stock 2011):

Hyperammonemia-related fatigue: Continue therapy for grade 2 toxicity. If grade 3 toxicity occurs, reduce dose by 25%; resume full dose when toxicity ≤ grade 2 (make up for missed doses). If grade 4 toxicity occurs, reduce dose by 50%; resume full dose when toxicity ≤ grade 2 (make up for missed doses).

Hyperglycemia: Continue therapy for uncomplicated hyperglycemia. If hyperglycemia requires insulin therapy, hold asparaginase (and any concomitant corticosteroids) until blood glucose controlled; resume dosing at prior dose level. For life-threatening hyperglycemia or toxicity requiring urgent intervention, hold asparaginase (and corticosteroids) until blood glucose is controlled with insulin; resume asparaginase and do not make up for missed doses.

Hypersensitivity reactions: May continue dosing for urticaria without bronchospasm, hypotension, edema, or need for parenteral intervention. If wheezing or other symptomatic bronchospasm with or without urticaria, angioedema, hypotension, and/or life-threatening hypersensitivity reactions occur, discontinue asparaginase.

Hypertriglyceridemia: If serum triglyceride level <1000 mg/dL, continue asparaginase but monitor closely for pancreatitis. If triglyceride level >1,000 mg/dL, hold asparaginase and monitor; resume therapy at prior dose level after triglyceride level returns to baseline.

Pancreatitis:

Asymptomatic amylase or lipase >3 times ULN (chemical pancreatitis) or radiologic abnormalities only: Continue asparaginase and monitor levels closely.

Symptomatic amylase or lipase >3 times ULN: Hold asparaginase until enzyme levels stabilize or are declining.

Symptomatic pancreatitis or clinical pancreatitis (abdominal pain with amylase or lipase >3 times ULN for >3 days and/or development of pancreatic pseudocyst): Permanently discontinue asparaginase.

Thrombosis and bleeding, CNS:

Thrombosis: Continue therapy for abnormal laboratory findings without a clinical correlate. If grade 3 toxicity occurs, discontinue therapy; if CNS signs/symptoms are fully resolved and further asparaginase doses are required, may resume therapy at a lower dose and/or longer intervals between doses. Discontinue therapy for grade 4 toxicity.

Hemorrhage: Discontinue therapy; do not withhold therapy for abnormal laboratory findings without a clinical correlate. If grade 3 toxicity occurs, discontinue therapy; if CNS signs/symptoms are fully resolved and further asparaginase doses are required, may resume therapy at a lower dose and/or longer intervals between doses. Discontinue therapy for grade 4 toxicity.

Thrombosis and bleeding, non-CNS:

Thrombosis: Continue therapy for abnormal laboratory findings without a clinical correlate. If grade 3 or 4 toxicity occurs, withhold therapy until acute toxicity and clinical signs resolve and anticoagulant therapy is

◀ stable or completed. Do not withhold therapy for abnormal laboratory findings without clinical correlate.

Hemorrhage: If grade 2 bleeding in conjunction with hypofibrinogenemia occurs, withhold therapy until bleeding ≤ grade 1. Do not withhold therapy for abnormal laboratory findings without clinical correlate. For grade 3 or 4 bleeding, withhold therapy until bleeding ≤ grade 1 and until acute toxicity and clinical signs resolve and coagulant replacement therapy is stable or completed.

Administration

IM: The volume of each single injection site should be limited to 2 mL; use multiple injections for volumes >2 mL.

IV: Infuse over 1 to 2 hours; do not infuse other medications through the same IV line.

Emetic Potential Children and Adults: Minimal (<10%)

Monitoring Parameters CBC with differential, amylase, lipase, triglycerides, liver enzymes, blood glucose (baseline and periodically during treatment), coagulation parameters; for IV administration, consider monitoring nadir serum asparaginase activity (NSAA) levels. Monitor for symptoms of hypersensitivity, symptoms of pancreatitis, thrombosis, or hemorrhage.

Prescribing and Access Restrictions For order information contact 877-625-2566 or visit http://erwinaze.com/healthcare-professionals/order-erwinaze/

Dosage Forms Excipient information presented when available (limited, particularly for generics); consult specific product labeling.

Solution Reconstituted, Intramuscular:

Erwinaze: 10,000 units (1 ea)

♦ Asparaginase *Erwinia chrysanthemi* see Asparaginase (*Erwinia*) *on page 184*

♦ Astagraf XL *see* Tacrolimus (Systemic) *on page 1715*

♦ AT *see* Antithrombin *on page 152*

♦ AT-III *see* Antithrombin *on page 152*

Atezolizumab (a te zoe LIZ ue mab)

Related Information

Common Toxicity Criteria *on page 2242*

Management of Chemotherapy-Induced Nausea and Vomiting in Adults *on page 2253*

Safe Handling of Hazardous Drugs *on page 2379*

Brand Names: US Tecentriq

Index Terms Anti-PD-L1 Monoclonal Antibody MPDL3280A; MPDL3280A; RG7446; RO5541267

Pharmacologic Category Antineoplastic Agent, Anti-PD-L1 Monoclonal Antibody; Antineoplastic Agent, Monoclonal Antibody

Use

Non-small cell lung cancer, metastatic: Treatment of metastatic non-small cell lung cancer (NSCLC) in patients with disease progression during or following platinum-containing chemotherapy. Patients should have disease progression on approved therapy for EGFR or ALK genomic tumor mutations (if present) prior to receiving atezolizumab.

Urothelial carcinoma, locally advanced or metastatic: Treatment of locally advanced or metastatic urothelial carcinoma in patients who are not eligible for cisplatin-containing chemotherapy, have disease progression during or following platinum-containing chemotherapy, or have disease progression within 12 months of neoadjuvant or adjuvant treatment with platinum-containing chemotherapy

Labeled Contraindications There are no contraindications listed in the manufacturer's labeling.

Pregnancy Considerations Adverse events were observed in animal reproduction studies. Based on the mechanism of action, atezolizumab is expected to cause fetal harm if used during pregnancy. Women of reproductive potential should use effective contraception during therapy and for at least 5 months after the last dose.

Breastfeeding Considerations It is not known if atezolizumab is present in breast milk; however, IgG immunoglobulins are found in milk. Due to the potential for serious adverse reactions in the breastfed infant, breastfeeding is not recommended by the manufacturer during therapy or for at least 5 months after the last dose.

Warnings/Precautions Immune-mediated pneumonitis and interstitial lung disease (defined as requiring corticosteroids and with no clear alternative etiology), including fatal cases, have been reported in patients receiving atezolizumab. The median time to onset was 2.6 to 3.3 months (range: 3 days to 18.7 months) and the median duration was 15 days to 1.4 months (range: up to 12.6 months or longer). Monitor for signs (with radiographic imaging) and symptoms of pneumonitis. Administer systemic corticosteroids (1 to 2 mg/kg/day prednisone or equivalent) followed by a taper for grade 2 or higher pneumonitis. Withhold treatment until resolution for grade 2 pneumonitis; permanently discontinue for grade 3 or 4 pneumonitis.

Immune-mediated hepatitis (defined as requiring corticosteroids and with no clear alternative etiology), including fatal cases, has occurred with atezolizumab. Liver test abnormalities have been reported, including grade 3 and 4 events. The median time to onset was ~1 month (range: 0.4 to 7.7 months). Monitor for signs/symptoms of hepatitis; monitor liver function tests (AST, ALT, and bilirubin) prior to treatment initiation and periodically throughout therapy. Administer systemic corticosteroids (1 to 2 mg/kg/day prednisone or equivalent) followed by a taper for grade 2 or higher transaminase elevations (with or without elevated bilirubin). Withhold treatment until resolution for grade 2 and permanently discontinue for grade 3 or 4 immune-mediated hepatitis. Patients with treatment interruption for immune-mediated hepatitis did not have recurrence upon resuming treatment.

Immune-mediated colitis or diarrhea (defined as requiring corticosteroids and with no clear alternative etiology) has occurred in nearly one-fifth of patients receiving atezolizumab, some events included grade 3 and 4 diarrhea. The median onset for some patients was 21 days to 1.7 months (range: 12 days to 3.4 months). Monitor for signs/symptoms of colitis and diarrhea. Withhold treatment for grade 2 or 3 diarrhea or colitis. For grade 2 diarrhea or colitis, if symptoms persist for >5 days or recur, administer systemic corticosteroids (1 to 2 mg/kg/day prednisone equivalent). For grade 3 diarrhea or colitis, administer IV methylprednisolone 1 to 2 mg/kg/day and convert to oral corticosteroids upon improvement in symptoms. If grade 2 and 3 symptoms improve to grade 0 or 1, taper corticosteroids over at least 1 month. Resume atezolizumab treatment if improves to grade 0 or 1 within 12 weeks and corticosteroids have been reduced to oral prednisone ≤10 mg/day. Discontinue permanently for grade 4 diarrhea or colitis. Pancreatitis, increases in amylase and lipase levels, and symptomatic pancreatitis (without other etiology) have occurred with atezolizumab. Monitor for signs/symptoms of acute pancreatitis. Discontinue permanently for grade 4 or any grade recurrent pancreatitis. Withhold treatment for grade 3 or higher serum amylase or lipase increases, or for grade 2 or 3 pancreatitis. Administer IV methylprednisolone 1 to 2 mg/kg/day and convert to oral corticosteroids (prednisone 1 to 2 mg/kg/day or equivalent) upon improvement in symptoms. Resume atezolizumab if amylase and lipase levels improve to grade 1 or lower within 12 weeks, pancreatitis symptoms have resolved, and corticosteroids have been reduced to oral prednisone ≤10 mg/day.

Hypophysitis has occurred in patients receiving atezolizumab (rare). Monitor for signs/symptoms of hypophysitis. Administer corticosteroids and hormone replacement as indicated. Withhold treatment for grade 2 or 3 hypophysitis; discontinue permanently for grade 4 hypophysitis. Hypothyroidism occurred in patients who received atezolizumab (including grades 1, 2, and 3 events), with a median time to first onset of 4.8 to 5.4 months (range: 15 days to 31 months). Hyperthyroidism was also reported, including grades 1 and 2 events, with a median onset of 3.2 to 4.9 months (range: 21 days to 31 months). Monitor thyroid function prior to and periodically during treatment. Patients with abnormal thyroid function tests who are asymptomatic can receive atezolizumab treatment. For symptomatic hypothyroidism, withhold atezolizumab treatment and initiate thyroid replacement therapy as needed. Isolated hypothyroidism should be managed with replacement therapy and without corticosteroids. For symptomatic hyperthyroidism, withhold atezolizumab and initiate antithyroid medications as needed. Resume atezolizumab treatment when symptoms of hypo- or hyperthyroidism are controlled and thyroid function is improving. Grades 1 to 3 adrenal insufficiency have been reported. For symptomatic adrenal insufficiency, withhold atezolizumab treatment and administer IV methylprednisolone 1 to 2 mg/kg/day and convert to oral prednisone 1 to 2 mg/kg/day or equivalent upon improvement in symptoms. When symptoms improve to grade 1 or lower, begin to taper steroids over at least 1 month. Resume atezolizumab treatment if symptoms improve to grade 0 or 1 within 12 weeks and corticosteroids have been reduced to oral prednisone ≤10 mg/day and patient is stable on adrenal replacement therapy (if needed). New-onset diabetes with ketoacidosis has been observed with atezolizumab. For type 1 diabetes, initiate insulin treatment. For grade 3 or higher hyperglycemia (fasting blood glucose >250 to 500 mg/dL), withhold atezolizumab; resume when metabolic control is achieved on insulin therapy.

Myocarditis has been reported with atezolizumab (case reports); may be related to the mechanism of action and/or may be immune-mediated. Discontinue atezolizumab for any grade myocarditis; may require systemic corticosteroids and/or other immunosuppressive therapy (Perez 2017).

Other immune-mediated adverse events have occurred, including meningoencephalitis, myasthenic syndrome/myasthenia gravis, Guillain-Barre syndrome, and ocular inflammatory toxicity. Monitor for clinical signs/symptoms of meningitis and encephalitis; discontinue permanently for any grade meningitis or encephalitis; administer IV corticosteroids (methylprednisolone 1 to 2 mg/kg/day) and convert to oral therapy (prednisone 60 mg/day or equivalent) upon improvement; when symptoms improve to grade 1 or lower, taper corticosteroids over at least 1 month. Monitor for neuropathy (motor and sensory);

permanently discontinue for any grade myasthenic syndrome/myasthenia gravis or Guillain-Barre syndrome and begin appropriate medical management; consider systemic corticosteroids (prednisone 1 to 2 mg/kg/day).

Infections occurred in over 1/3 of patients receiving atezolizumab. Grade 3 and 4 infections have occurred, with urinary tract infection and pneumonia being the most common cause of grade 3 or higher infection in patients with urothelial carcinoma and non-small cell lung cancer, respectively. There have been case reports of fatal infections. Serious infections, including sepsis, herpes encephalitis, and mycobacterial infection leading to retroperitoneal hemorrhage have been reported. Monitor for signs/symptoms of infection. Manage suspected and confirmed bacterial infections with antibiotics. Withhold treatment for grade 3 or higher infections. Severe infusion reactions have been reported in clinical trials; interrupt or slow the infusion rate in patients with mild to moderate infusion reactions; permanently discontinue for grade 3 or 4 infusion reactions. Potentially significant drug-drug interactions may exist, requiring dose or frequency adjustment, additional monitoring, and/or selection of alternative therapy.

Adverse Reactions

>10%:

Cardiovascular: Peripheral edema (18%)

Central nervous system: Fatigue (52%), insomnia (NSCLC: 14%)

Dermatologic: Skin rash (15%), pruritus (13%)

Endocrine & metabolic: Hypoalbuminemia (NSCLC: 48%), hyponatremia (NSCLC: 48%), hypokalemia (NSCLC: 18%), hypercalcemia (NSCLC: 13%)

Gastrointestinal: Decreased appetite (26%), nausea (25%), constipation (21%), colitis (19% to 20%), diarrhea (18% to 20%), abdominal pain (17%), vomiting (17%)

Genitourinary: Urinary tract infection (22%), hematuria (14%)

Hematologic & oncologic: Lymphocytopenia

Hepatic: Increased serum alkaline phosphatase (NSCLC: 42%), increased serum AST (NSCLC: 33%), increased serum ALT (NSCLC: 31%), increased serum bilirubin (NSCLC: 11%)

Immunologic: Antibody development (42%; no clinically significant impact on pharmacokinetics, safety, or efficacy)

Infection: Infection (38%)

Neuromuscular & skeletal: Musculoskeletal pain (NSCLC: 22%), back pain (≤15%), neck pain (≤15%), arthralgia (14%)

Renal: Increased serum creatinine (NSCLC: 19%)

Respiratory: Pneumonia (NSCLC: 18%), dyspnea (16%), cough (14%)

Miscellaneous: Fever (21%)

1% to 10%:

Cardiovascular: Venous thromboembolism

Central nervous system: Guillain-Barre syndrome (≤1%), meningoencephalitis (≤1%), myasthenia (≤1%), myasthenia gravis (≤1%), confusion

Endocrine & metabolic: Hypothyroidism (3% to 4%), hyperthyroidism (≤1%), hyperglycemia

Gastrointestinal: Increased serum amylase (≤1%), increased serum lipase (≤1%), pancreatitis (≤1%), dysphagia (NSCLC), intestinal obstruction

Genitourinary: Urinary tract obstruction

Hematologic & oncologic: Anemia

Hepatic: Hepatitis (≤1%)

Infection: Sepsis

◄ Ophthalmic: Intraocular inflammation (≤1%)

Renal: Acute renal failure

Respiratory: Pneumonitis (≤4%), pleural effusion (NSCLC: >2%), hypoxia (NSCLC)

Miscellaneous: Infusion related reaction (severe: 1% to 2%)

<1%, postmarketing, and/or case reports: Adrenocortical insufficiency, diabetes mellitus (with ketoacidosis), hypophysitis, myocarditis

Drug Interactions

Metabolism/Transport Effects None known.

Avoid Concomitant Use

Avoid concomitant use of Atezolizumab with any of the following: Belimumab

Increased Effect/Toxicity

Atezolizumab may increase the levels/effects of: Belimumab

Decreased Effect There are no known significant interactions involving a decrease in effect.

Storage/Stability Store intact vials at 2°C to 8°C (36°F to 46°F). Do not freeze. Do not shake. Store in original carton to protect from light. Solutions diluted in NS for infusion should be used immediately after preparation; if not used immediately, may be stored for up to 6 hours (including administration time) at room temperature or 24 hours refrigerated at 2°C to 8°C (36°F to 46°F). Do not freeze.

Preparation for Administration Withdraw 1,200 mg (20 mL) from vial and dilute into 250 mL of NS in a polyvinyl chloride (PVC), polyethylene (PE), or polyolefin (PO) infusion bag. Dilute only with NS. Mix by gently inverting; do not shake.

Mechanism of Action Atezolizumab is a humanized monoclonal antibody immune checkpoint inhibitor that binds to programmed death ligand 1 (PD-L1) to selectively prevent the interaction between the programmed cell death-1 (PD-1) and B7.1 (also known as CD80) receptors, while still allowing interaction between PD-L2 and PD-1. PD-L1 is an immune check point protein expressed on tumor cells and tumor infiltrating cells and down regulates antitumor t-cell function by binding to PD-1 and B7.1; blocking PD-1 and B7.1 interactions restores antitumor t-cell function (Fehrenbacher 2016, Rosenberg 2016).

Pharmacodynamics/Kinetics

Distribution: V_{dss}: 6.9 L

Half-life, elimination: 27 days

Excretion: Clearance: 0.2 L/day

Dosing

Adult & Geriatric

Non-small cell lung cancer, metastatic: IV: 1,200 mg every 3 weeks (Fehrenbacher 2016; Rittmeyer 2017); continue until disease progression or unacceptable toxicity

Urothelial carcinoma, locally advanced or metastatic: IV: 1,200 mg every 3 weeks (Balar 2017; Rosenberg 2016); continue until disease progression or unacceptable toxicity

Renal Impairment No dosage adjustment is necessary (the effect on atezolizumab pharmacokinetics in patients with estimated glomerular filtration rate 15 to 29 mL/minute has not been studied and is unknown).

Hepatic Impairment

Hepatic impairment prior to treatment:

Mild impairment (bilirubin ≤ upper limit of normal (ULN) and AST > ULN or bilirubin <1 times ULN and any AST): No dosage adjustment is necessary.

Moderate to severe impairment (bilirubin > ULN and AST > ULN or bilirubin ≥1 to 1.5 times ULN and any AST): There are no dosage adjustments provided in the manufacturer's labeling (has not been studied).

Hepatotoxicity during treatment:

AST or ALT >3 to 5 times ULN or total bilirubin >1.5 to 3 times ULN: Withhold treatment.

AST or ALT >5 times ULN or total bilirubin >3 times ULN: Discontinue permanently.

Immune-mediated hepatitis:

Grade 2 or greater transaminase elevations (with or without total bilirubin elevations): Withhold treatment and initiate high-dose systemic corticosteroids (prednisone 1 to 2 mg/kg daily or equivalent, followed by a taper)

Severe (grade 3) or life-threatening (grade 4): Permanently discontinue treatment and initiate high-dose systemic corticosteroids (prednisone 1 to 2 mg/kg daily or equivalent, followed by a taper)

Adjustment for Toxicity Dosage reductions are not recommended for toxicities. Treatment is withheld or permanently discontinued. If therapy is withheld, may resume if toxicity recovers to grade 0 or 1.

Dermatologic toxicity:

Rash, grade 3: Withhold treatment.

Rash, grade 4: Discontinue permanently.

Endocrinopathies:

Adrenal insufficiency (symptomatic): Withhold treatment. Administer IV methylprednisolone 1 to 2 mg/kg/day and convert to oral prednisone 1 to 2 mg/kg/day or equivalent upon improvement in symptoms. When symptoms improve to grade 1 or lower, begin to taper steroids over at least 1 month. Resume atezolizumab treatment if symptoms improve to grade 0 or 1 within 12 weeks, and corticosteroids have been reduced to oral prednisone ≤10 mg/day (or equivalent) and patient is stable on adrenal replacement therapy (if needed).

Hyperglycemia, grade 3 or 4: Withhold treatment. May require insulin treatment.

Hyperthyroidism or hypothyroidism: Withhold treatment. May require additional treatment for symptomatic hypo- or hyperthyroidism.

Hypophysitis (symptomatic): Withhold treatment. Administer corticosteroids and hormone replacement as clinically necessary.

Hypophysitis, grade 4: Discontinue permanently. Administer corticosteroids and hormone replacement as clinically necessary.

Gastrointestinal toxicity:

Amylase or lipase elevations, grade 3 or 4 (>2 times ULN): Withhold treatment. Administer IV methylprednisolone 1 to 2 mg/kg/day and convert to oral corticosteroids (prednisone 1 to 2 mg/kg/day or equivalent) upon improvement in symptoms. Resume atezolizumab if amylase and lipase levels improve to grade 1 or lower within 12 weeks and corticosteroids have been reduced to oral prednisone ≤10 mg/day (or equivalent).

Diarrhea or colitis, grade 2 or 3: Withhold treatment. For grade 2 diarrhea or colitis, if symptoms persist for >5 days or recur, administer systemic corticosteroids (1 to 2 mg/kg/day prednisone or equivalent). For grade 3 diarrhea or colitis, administer IV methylprednisolone 1 to 2 mg/kg/day and convert to oral corticosteroids upon improvement in symptoms. If grade 2 and 3 symptoms improve to grade 0 or 1, taper corticosteroids over at least 1 month. Resume atezolizumab treatment if improves to grade 0 or 1 within 12 weeks and corticosteroids have been reduced to oral prednisone ≤10 mg/day (or equivalent).

Diarrhea or colitis, grade 4: Discontinue permanently. Administer IV methylprednisolone 1 to 2 mg/kg/day and convert to oral corticosteroids upon improvement in symptoms.

Pancreatitis, grade 2 or 3: Withhold treatment. Administer IV methylprednisolone 1 to 2 mg/kg/day and convert to oral corticosteroids (prednisone 1 to 2 mg/kg/day or equivalent) upon improvement in symptoms. Resume atezolizumab if pancreatitis symptoms have resolved and corticosteroids have been reduced to oral prednisone ≤10 mg/day (or equivalent).

Pancreatitis, grade 4: Discontinue permanently. Administer IV methylprednisolone 1 to 2 mg/kg/day and convert to oral corticosteroids (prednisone 1 to 2 mg/kg/day or equivalent) upon improvement in symptoms.

Pancreatitis, recurrent (any grade): Discontinue permanently. Administer IV methylprednisolone 1 to 2 mg/kg/day and convert to oral corticosteroids (prednisone 1 to 2 mg/kg/day or equivalent) upon improvement in symptoms.

Myocarditis (any grade): Discontinue permanently; may require systemic corticosteroids and/or other immunosuppressant therapy as clinically indicated (Perez 2017).

Ophthalmic disorders:

Ocular inflammatory toxicity, grade 2: Withhold treatment.

Ocular inflammatory toxicity, grade 3 or 4: Discontinue permanently.

Pulmonary toxicities:

Pneumonitis, grade 2: Withhold treatment. Administer high-dose systemic corticosteroids (prednisone 1 to 2 mg/kg daily or equivalent) followed by a corticosteroid taper.

Pneumonitis, grade 3 or 4: Discontinue permanently. Administer high-dose systemic corticosteroids (prednisone 1 to 2 mg/kg daily or equivalent) followed by a corticosteroid taper.

Other/miscellaneous toxicities:

Guillain-Barre, any grade: Discontinue permanently.

Infection, grade 3 or 4: Withhold treatment.

Infusion-related reactions, grade 2 or mild to moderate: Withhold treatment or slow the rate of infusion.

Infusion-related reactions, grade 3 or 4: Discontinue permanently.

Meningoencephalitis, any grade: Discontinue permanently. Administer IV corticosteroids (methylprednisolone 1 to 2 mg/kg/day) and convert to oral therapy (prednisone 60 mg/day or equivalent) upon improvement; when symptoms improve to grade 1 or lower, taper corticosteroids over at least 1 month.

Myasthenic syndrome/myasthenia gravis: Discontinue permanently. Consider systemic corticosteroids (prednisone 1 to 2 mg/kg/day).

Administration IV: Infuse the initial dose over 60 minutes, if tolerated, may infuse subsequent doses over 30 minutes. May be infused with or without a 0.2- to 0.22-micron sterile, non-pyrogenic, low-protein binding in-line filter. Do not administer as an IV push or bolus. Do not administer other medications at the same time through the same IV line. Monitor for infusion reactions.

Emetic Potential Low (10% to 30%)

Monitoring Parameters Monitor liver function tests (AST, ALT, and bilirubin; at baseline and periodically during treatment), thyroid function (prior to and periodically during treatment), serum glucose. Monitor for signs/symptoms of colitis, diarrhea, endocrinopathies, hepatitis, hypophysitis, infection, infusion reactions, meningitis and encephalitis, myocarditis, neuropathy (motor and sensory), pancreatitis (acute), rash, and pneumonitis.

Medication Guide Available Yes

Dosage Forms Excipient information presented when available (limited, particularly for generics); consult specific product labeling.

Solution, Intravenous [preservative free]:

Tecentriq: 1200 mg/20 mL (20 mL)

* **ATG** see Antithymocyte Globulin (Equine) on page 154
* **Atgam** see Antithymocyte Globulin (Equine) on page 154
* **Ativan** see LORazepam on page 1164
* **ATO** see Arsenic Trioxide on page 172
* **ATRA** see Tretinoin (Systemic) on page 1830
* **Atriance (Can)** see Nelarabine on page 1302
* **ATryn** see Antithrombin on page 152
* **Auro-Anastrozole (Can)** see Anastrozole on page 135
* **Auro-Ciprofloxacin (Can)** see Ciprofloxacin (Systemic) on page 393
* **Auro-Letrozole (Can)** see Letrozole on page 1119
* **Auro-Olanzapine ODT (Can)** see OLANZapine on page 1364
* **Auro-Valacyclovir (Can)** see ValACYclovir on page 1852
* **Ava-Famciclovir (Can)** see Famciclovir on page 783
* **Avakine** see InFLIXimab on page 1002
* **Avastin** see Bevacizumab on page 237

Avelumab (a VEL ue mab)

Related Information

Common Toxicity Criteria on page 2242

Brand Names: US Bavencio

Index Terms Anti-PD-L1 Monoclonal Antibody MSB0010718C; Bavencio; MSB0010718C

Pharmacologic Category Antineoplastic Agent, Anti-PD-L1 Monoclonal Antibody; Antineoplastic Agent, Monoclonal Antibody

Use

Merkel cell carcinoma, metastatic: Treatment of metastatic Merkel cell carcinoma (MCC) in adults and children ≥12 years of age.

Urothelial carcinoma, locally advanced or metastatic: Treatment of locally advanced or metastatic urothelial carcinoma in patients who have disease progression during or following platinum-containing chemotherapy or have disease progression within 12 months of neoadjuvant or adjuvant treatment with platinum-containing chemotherapy

Labeled Contraindications There are no contraindications listed in the manufacturer's labeling.

Pregnancy Considerations Immunoglobulins are known to cross the placenta and fetal exposure to avelumab is expected. Based on the mechanism of action, avelumab may cause fetal harm. Immune-mediated fetal rejection causing increased abortion or stillbirth was observed in animal reproduction studies. Women of reproductive potential should use effective contraception during therapy and for at least 1 month after treatment is complete.

◀ **Breastfeeding Considerations** It is not known if avelumab is present in breast milk. According to the manufacturer, lactating women should not breastfeed during therapy and for at least 1 month after treatment is complete.

Warnings/Precautions Adrenal insufficiency may occur. The median time to onset was 2.5 months (range: 1 day to 8 months). In clinical studies, all patients received corticosteroid therapy for adrenal insufficiency; in patients who received high-dose corticosteroids, the median duration of high-dose systemic corticosteroid therapy was 1 day (range: 1 day to 24 days). Monitor for signs/symptoms of adrenal insufficiency both during and after treatment. Administer corticosteroids as appropriate. Withhold avelumab for severe (grade 3) or life-threatening (grade 4) toxicity. Type 1 diabetes mellitus has occurred (including diabetic ketoacidosis). Monitor closely for hyperglycemia and other signs/symptoms of diabetes. Insulin or other anti-hyperglycemic therapy may be required; if severe hyperglycemia is observed, administer antihyperglycemics or insulin and withhold avelumab treatment until glucose control has been accomplished. Immune-mediated hyperthyroidism, hypothyroidism, and thyroiditis have occurred; and may develop at any time during avelumab treatment. The median onset for immune-mediated thyroid disorders was 2.8 months (range: 2 weeks to 13 months). Monitor for changes in thyroid function (at baseline, periodically during treatment, and as clinically indicated) and for signs/symptoms of thyroid disorders. Administer medical management for hyperthyroidism as appropriate; may require treatment interruption and/or permanent discontinuation. Manage hypothyroidism with replacement therapy. Immune-mediated thyroid disorders may require treatment interruption.

Immune-mediated pneumonitis has been observed, including fatal cases. The median time to development was 2.5 months (range: 3 days to 11 months) and the median duration was 7 weeks (range: 4 days to over 4 months). Pneumonitis was managed with systemic corticosteroids; the median duration of initial corticosteroid therapy was 8 days (range: 1 day to 2.3 months) followed by a corticosteroid taper. Pneumonitis resolved in approximately half of the affected patients. May require treatment interruption, corticosteroid therapy (prednisone initial dose of 1 to 2 mg/kg/day [or equivalent] followed by a taper, for grade 2 or higher pneumonitis), and/or permanent discontinuation. Monitor for signs and symptoms of pneumonitis; if pneumonitis is suspected, evaluate with radiographic imaging; administer systemic corticosteroids for grade 2 or higher pneumonitis. Immune-mediated nephritis has occurred. Grade 2 or higher nephritis should be managed with systemic corticosteroids (prednisone initial dose of 1 to 2 mg/kg/day [or equivalent], followed by a taper). Monitor serum creatinine at baseline and periodically during therapy. May require treatment interruption, systemic corticosteroids (for grade 2 or higher toxicity), and/or permanent discontinuation.

Immune-mediated colitis has occurred. The median time to onset of colitis was 2.1 months (range: 2 days to 11 months) and the median duration was 6 weeks (range: 1 day to over 14 months). In many patients, colitis was managed with high-dose systemic corticosteroids for a median duration of 19 days (range: 1 day to 2.3 months), followed by a corticosteroid taper. More than two-thirds of patients with colitis experienced resolution. May require treatment interruption, systemic corticosteroid therapy, and/or permanent discontinuation. Monitor for signs and symptoms of colitis; administer systemic corticosteroids (prednisone initial dose of 1 to 2 mg/kg/day [or equivalent] followed by a taper) for grade 2 or higher colitis. Immune-mediated hepatitis has occurred, including fatal cases. The median onset for hepatitis was 3.2 months (range: 7 days to 15 months); the median duration was 2.5 months (range: 1 day to over 7 months). Hepatitis resolved in approximately half of the patients. Administer corticosteroids (prednisone initial dose of 1 to 2 mg/kg/day [or equivalent] followed by a taper for grade 2 or higher hepatitis), and withhold or discontinue therapy based on the severity of liver enzyme elevations. Systemic corticosteroids were used to manage immune-mediated hepatitis; the median duration of high-dose corticosteroid therapy was 14 days (range: 1 day to 2.5 months). Monitor for liver function changes. May require treatment interruption, systemic corticosteroids (for grade 2 or higher toxicity), and/or permanent discontinuation.

Other clinically relevant immune-mediated disorders have been observed rarely with avelumab use and may affect any organ system (may be fatal), including myocarditis, myositis, psoriasis, arthritis, exfoliative dermatitis, erythema multiforme, pemphigoid, hypopituitarism, uveitis, Guillain-Barré syndrome, and systemic inflammatory response. May occur during treatment or following discontinuation. Other immune-mediated disorders have been observed with other similar medications (same class), including bullous dermatitis, Stevens Johnson syndrome/toxic epidermal necrolysis, pancreatitis, rhabdomyolysis, myasthenia gravis, histiocytic necrotizing lymphadenitis, demyelination, vasculitis, hemolytic anemia, hypophysitis, iritis, and encephalitis. If an Immune-mediated adverse event is suspected, evaluate appropriately to confirm or exclude other causes; based on severity of reaction, withhold treatment and administer systemic corticosteroids and (if appropriate) hormone replacement therapy. Upon resolution to grade 0 or 1, initiate corticosteroid taper. When reaction remains at grade 1 or less during taper may reinitiate avelumab. Discontinue permanently for severe grade 3 immune-mediated adverse event that is recurrent or for life-threatening reactions.

Infusion-related reactions (including severe and life-threatening cases) have occurred. Prior to the initial four infusions, premedicate with an antihistamine and acetaminophen. Monitor for signs/symptoms of a reaction (eg, pyrexia, chills, wheezing, flushing, hypotension, dyspnea, back pain, abdominal pain, urticaria). Some infusion-related reactions occurred after completion of the infusion. Interrupt or slow the rate of infusion for mild or moderate infusion-related reactions. Stop infusion and permanently discontinue for severe (grade 3) or life-threatening (grade 4) infusion-related reactions. Potentially significant interactions may exist, requiring dose or frequency adjustment, additional monitoring, and/or selection of alternative therapy. Consult drug interactions database for more detailed information.

Adverse Reactions

>10%:

   Cardiovascular: Peripheral edema (20%), hypertension (13%)
   Central nervous system: Fatigue (50%), dizziness (14%)
   Dermatologic: Skin rash (22%)
   Endocrine & metabolic: Weight loss (15%)
   Gastrointestinal: Diarrhea (23%), nausea (22%), decreased appetite (20%), constipation (17%), abdominal pain (16%), increased serum lipase (14%), vomiting (13%)

◀ Hematologic & oncologic: Lymphocytopenia (49%; grades 3/4: 19%), anemia (35%; grades 3/4: 9%), thrombocytopenia (27%; grades 3/4: 1%)
Hepatic: Increased serum AST (34%), increased serum ALT (20%)
Neuromuscular & skeletal: Musculoskeletal pain (32%), arthralgia (16%)
Respiratory: Cough (18%), dyspnea (11%)
Miscellaneous: Infusion-related reaction (22% to 25%)
1% to 10%:
Central nervous system: Headache (10%)
Dermatologic: Pruritus (10%), cellulitis (>1%)
Endocrine & metabolic: Increased amylase (8%), hypothyroidism (immune-mediated: 5%)
Gastrointestinal: Colitis (immune-mediated: 2%), intestinal obstruction (>1%)
Hematologic & oncologic: Neutropenia (6%; grades 3/4: 1%)
Hepatic: Increased serum bilirubin (6%)
Immunologic: Antibody development (4%)
Neuromuscular & skeletal: Weakness (>1%)
Renal: Acute renal failure (>1%)
Respiratory: Pneumonitis (immune-mediated: 1%)
Frequency not defined:
Cardiovascular: Pericardial effusion
Neuromuscular & skeletal: Increased creatine phosphokinase
<1%, postmarketing, and/or case reports: Adrenocortical insufficiency (immune-mediated), arthritis (immune-mediated), erythema multiforme (immune-mediated), exfoliative dermatitis (immune-mediated), Guillain-Barré syndrome (immune-mediated), hepatitis (immune-mediated), hyperthyroidism (immune-mediated), myocarditis (immune-mediated), myositis (immune-mediated), nephritis (immune-mediated), pemphigoid (immune-mediated), pituitary insufficiency (immune-mediated), psoriasis (immune-mediated), sepsis (systemic inflammatory response; immune-mediated), thyroiditis (immune-mediated), type 1 diabetes mellitus (immune-mediated), uveitis (immune-mediated)

Drug Interactions

Metabolism/Transport Effects None known.

Avoid Concomitant Use

Avoid concomitant use of Avelumab with any of the following: Belimumab

Increased Effect/Toxicity

Avelumab may increase the levels/effects of: Belimumab

Decreased Effect There are no known significant interactions involving a decrease in effect.

Storage/Stability Store intact vials at 2°C to 8°C (36°F to 46°F); do not freeze. Protect vials from light (store in original packaging). Do not shake. Solutions diluted for infusion should be protected from light and may be stored at room temperature for up to 4 hours or refrigerated at 2°C to 8°C (36°F to 46°F) for no more than 24 hours from the time of dilution. Do not freeze or shake diluted solution. If refrigerated, allow to reach room temperature prior to administration.

Preparation for Administration Withdraw appropriate volume from vial and transfer to IV bag containing 250 mL NS or ½ NS. Mix by gently inverting bag (do not shake); avoid foaming or excessive shearing. Discard unused portion of the vial.

Mechanism of Action Avelumab is a fully human monoclonal antibody that binds to programmed death ligand 1 (PD-L1) to selectively prevent the interaction between the programmed cell death-1 (PD-1) and B7.1 receptors, while still allowing interaction between PD-L2 and PD-1 (Kaufman 2016). PD-L1 is an immune check point protein expressed on tumor cells and tumor infiltrating cells and down regulates anti-tumor t-cell function by binding to PD-1 and B7.1; blocking PD-1 and B7.1 interactions restores antitumor t-cell function (Fehrenbacher 2016, Rosenberg 2016).

Pharmacodynamics/Kinetics

Distribution: V_{dss}: 4.72 L (10 mg/kg dose)

Half-life elimination: 6.1 days

Excretion: Total systemic clearance was 0.59 L/day in patients receiving a 10 mg/kg dose.

Dosing

Adult & Geriatric Note: Premedicate with an antihistamine and acetaminophen prior to the first 4 infusions; consider premedication for subsequent infusions based on clinical judgment and the presence and/or severity of infusion-related reactions with previous infusions.

Merkel cell carcinoma, metastatic: IV: 10 mg/kg once every 2 weeks until disease progression or unacceptable toxicity (Kaufman 2016).

Urothelial carcinoma, locally advanced or metastatic: IV: 10 mg/kg once every 2 weeks until disease progression or unacceptable toxicity.

Pediatric Note: Premedicate with an antihistamine and acetaminophen prior to the first 4 infusions; consider premedication for subsequent infusions based on clinical judgment and the presence and/or severity of infusion-related reactions with previous infusions.

Merkel cell carcinoma, metastatic: Children ≥12 years and Adolescents: IV: 10 mg/kg once every 2 weeks until disease progression or unacceptable toxicity.

Renal Impairment

Renal impairment prior to treatment initiation: There are no dosage adjustments provided in the manufacturer's labeling; however, no clinically meaningful differences were observed in a population pharmacokinetic analysis in patients with CrCl 15 to 89 mL/minute.

Renal toxicity during treatment (nephritis and renal dysfunction):

Serum creatinine >1.5 to 6 times ULN: Withhold treatment. Administer high-dose systemic corticosteroids (prednisone initial dose of 1 to 2 mg/kg daily or equivalent, followed by a taper). Resume avelumab treatment if symptoms improve to grade 0 or 1 after corticosteroid taper.

Serum creatinine >6 times ULN: Discontinue permanently. Administer high-dose systemic corticosteroids (prednisone initial dose of 1 to 2 mg/kg daily or equivalent) followed by a corticosteroid taper.

Hepatic Impairment

Hepatic impairment prior to treatment: There are no dosage adjustments provided in the manufacturer's labeling; however, no clinically meaningful differences were observed in a population pharmacokinetic analysis in patients with mild (bilirubin ≤ ULN and AST > ULN **or** bilirubin between 1 to 1.5 times ULN) or moderate (bilirubin between 1.5 to 3 times ULN) impairment. Limited data is available in patients with severe (bilirubin >3 times ULN) impairment.

Hepatotoxicity during treatment:

AST or ALT >3 to 5 times ULN or total bilirubin >1.5 to 3 times ULN: Withhold treatment. Administer high-dose systemic corticosteroids (prednisone initial dose of 1 to 2 mg/kg daily or equivalent, followed by a taper). Resume avelumab treatment if hepatitis symptoms improve to grade 0 or 1 after corticosteroid taper.

◄   AST or ALT >5 times ULN or total bilirubin >3 times ULN: Discontinue permanently. Administer high-dose systemic corticosteroids (prednisone initial dose of 1 to 2 mg/kg daily or equivalent) followed by a corticosteroid taper.

Adjustment for Toxicity

Endocrinopathies:

Adrenal insufficiency, grade 3 or 4: Withhold treatment; administer corticosteroids as appropriate. Resume avelumab treatment if symptoms improve to grade 0 or 1 after corticosteroid taper.

Hyperglycemia, grade 3 or 4: Withhold treatment. May require insulin or other anti-hyperglycemic treatment. Resume avelumab once metabolic control has been achieved.

Hyperthyroidism or hypothyroidism, grade 3 or 4: Withhold treatment. Initiate medical management for hyperthyroidism; manage hypothyroidism with hormone replacement therapy.

Other endocrinopathies, grade 3 or 4: Withhold treatment; administer corticosteroids as appropriate. Resume avelumab treatment if symptoms improve to grade 0 or 1 after corticosteroid taper.

Gastrointestinal toxicity:

Diarrhea or colitis, grade 2 or 3: Withhold treatment. Administer high-dose systemic corticosteroids (prednisone initial dose of 1 to 2 mg/kg daily or equivalent) followed by a corticosteroid taper. May resume avelumab treatment if symptoms improve to grade 0 or 1 after corticosteroid taper.

Diarrhea or colitis, grade 4 or recurrent grade 3: Discontinue permanently. Administer high-dose systemic corticosteroids (prednisone initial dose of 1 to 2 mg/kg daily or equivalent) followed by a corticosteroid taper.

Infusion-related reaction:

Grade 1 or 2: Interrupt or slow the rate of infusion.

Grade 3 or 4: Permanently discontinue.

Pulmonary toxicities:

Pneumonitis, grade 2: Withhold treatment. Administer high-dose systemic corticosteroids (prednisone initial dose of 1 to 2 mg/kg daily or equivalent) followed by a corticosteroid taper. May resume avelumab treatment if symptoms improve to grade 0 or 1 after corticosteroid taper.

Pneumonitis, grade 3 or 4, or recurrent grade 2: Discontinue permanently. Administer high-dose systemic corticosteroids (prednisone initial dose of 1 to 2 mg/kg daily or equivalent) followed by a corticosteroid taper.

Other immune-mediated toxicities (eg, arthritis, bullous dermatitis, demyelination, encephalitis, erythema multiforme, exfoliative dermatitis, Guillain-Barré syndrome, hemolytic anemia, histiocytic necrotizing lymphadenitis, hypophysitis, hypopituitarism, iritis, myasthenia gravis, myocarditis, myositis, pancreatitis, pemphigoid, psoriasis, rhabdomyolysis, Stevens Johnson Syndrome (SJS)/toxic epidermal necrolysis (TEN), uveitis, vasculitis):

Immune-mediated toxicities, moderate or severe (not described previously): Withhold treatment and evaluate. Administer high-dose systemic corticosteroids, and if appropriate, initiate hormone replacement therapy. When toxicity improves to grade 1 or less, initiate a corticosteroid taper. May resume avelumab treatment if symptoms improve to grade 0 or 1 after corticosteroid taper.

Life-threatening reactions (excluding endocrinopathies), recurrent severe immune-mediated reactions, or persistent grade 2 or 3 immune-mediated reactions lasting 12 weeks or longer, or requirement for ≥10 mg/day prednisone (or equivalent) for >12 weeks: Discontinue permanently. If appropriate, administer high-dose systemic corticosteroids followed by a corticosteroid taper.

Administration IV: Infuse over 60 minutes through a 0.2 micron sterile, nonpyrogenic, low-protein binding inline filter. Do not infuse other medications through the same infusion line.

Monitoring Parameters Liver (AST, ALT, and total bilirubin), renal, and thyroid function tests (at baseline, periodically during treatment and as clinically indicated); blood glucose; signs/symptoms of colitis, thyroid disorders, pneumonitis, adrenal insufficiency, hepatitis, hyperglycemia, monitor for infusion reactions.

Medication Guide Available Yes

Dosage Forms Excipient information presented when available (limited, particularly for generics); consult specific product labeling.

Solution, Intravenous [preservative free]:

Bavencio: 200 mg/10 mL (10 mL)

Axitinib (ax I ti nib)

Related Information

Management of Chemotherapy-Induced Nausea and Vomiting in Adults *on page 2253*

Safe Handling of Hazardous Drugs *on page 2379*

Brand Names: US Inlyta

Brand Names: Canada Inlyta

Index Terms AG-013736

Pharmacologic Category Antineoplastic Agent, Tyrosine Kinase Inhibitor; Antineoplastic Agent, Vascular Endothelial Growth Factor (VEGF) Inhibitor

Use Renal cell carcinoma, advanced: Treatment of advanced renal cell carcinoma after failure of one prior systemic therapy.

Labeled Contraindications

There are no contraindications listed within the manufacturer's US labeling.

Canadian labeling: Hypersensitivity to axitinib or any component of the formulation.

Pregnancy Considerations Teratogenic, embryotoxic, and fetotoxic events were observed in animal reproduction studies when administered in doses less than the normal human dose. Based on its mechanism of action and because axitinib inhibits angiogenesis (a critical component of fetal development), adverse effects on pregnancy would be expected. Women of childbearing potential should be advised to avoid pregnancy during therapy.

Breastfeeding Considerations It is not known if axitinib is excreted in breast milk. Due to the potential for serious adverse reactions in the nursing infant, the manufacturer recommends a decision be made to discontinue nursing or to discontinue the drug, taking into account the importance of treatment to the mother.

Warnings/Precautions May cause hypertension; the median onset is within the first month, and has been observed as early as 4 days after treatment initiation. Hypertensive crisis has been reported. Blood pressure should be well-controlled prior to treatment initiation. Monitor blood pressure and treat with standard antihypertensive therapy. Persistent hypertension (despite antihypertensive therapy) may require dose reduction; discontinue if severe and persistent despite concomitant antihypertensives (or dose reduction), or with evidence of hypertensive crisis. Monitor for hypotension if on antihypertensive therapy and axitinib is withheld or discontinued. Cardiac failure,

201

◄ including fatal events, has been observed rarely. Monitor for signs/symptoms of cardiac failure throughout therapy; management may require permanent therapy discontinuation.

Gastrointestinal perforation and fistulas (including a fatality) have been reported. Monitor for signs/symptoms throughout treatment. Has not been studied in patients with recent active gastrointestinal bleeding; use is not recommended.

Arterial thrombotic events (cerebrovascular accident, MI, retinal artery occlusion, and transient ischemic attack), with fatalities, have been reported. Venous thrombotic events, including pulmonary embolism, deep vein thrombosis, retinal vein occlusion and retinal vein thrombosis, have been observed (with some fatalities). Use with caution in patients with a history of or risks for arterial or venous thrombotic events; has not been studied in patients within 12 months of an arterial thrombotic event or within 6 months of a venous thrombotic event. Hemorrhagic events (cerebral hemorrhage, gastrointestinal hemorrhage, hematuria, hemoptysis, and melena) have been reported (with some fatalities). Temporarily interrupt treatment with any hemorrhage requiring medical intervention.

Cases of reversible posterior leukoencephalopathy syndrome (RPLS) have been reported. Symptoms of RPLS include confusion, headache, hypertension (mild-to-severe), lethargy, seizure, blindness and/or other vision, or neurologic disturbances; interrupt treatment and manage hypertension. MRI is recommended to confirm RPLS diagnosis. Discontinue axitinib if RPLS is confirmed. The safety of reinitiating axitinib in patients previously experiencing RPLS is unknown.

Hypothyroidism occurs commonly with tyrosine kinase inhibitors, including axitinib. Hyperthyroidism has also been reported. Monitor thyroid function at baseline and periodically throughout therapy. Thyroid disorders should be treated according to standard practice to achieve/maintain euthyroid state. Proteinuria is associated with use. Monitor for proteinuria at baseline and periodically throughout therapy. If moderate or severe proteinuria occurs, reduce dose or temporarily withhold treatment. Although the effect on wound healing has not been studied with axitinib, vascular endothelial growth factor (VEGF) receptor inhibitors are associated with impaired wound healing. Discontinue treatment at least 24 hours prior to scheduled surgery; treatment reinitiation should be guided by clinical judgment and wound assessment. Has not been studied in patients with evidence of untreated brain metastases; use is not recommended. Systemic exposure to axitinib is increased in patients with moderate hepatic impairment; dose reductions are recommended. Has not been studied in patients with severe hepatic impairment. Increases in ALT have been observed during treatment; monitor liver function tests. Potentially significant drug-drug interactions may exist, requiring dose or frequency adjustment, additional monitoring, and/or selection of alternative therapy.

Adverse Reactions

>10%:

  Cardiovascular: Hypertension (40%; grades 3/4: 16%)

  Central nervous system: Fatigue (39%), voice disorder (31%), headache (14%)

  Dermatologic: Palmar-plantar erythrodysesthesia (27%; grades 3/4: 5%), skin rash (13%; grades 3/4: <1%)

Endocrine & metabolic: Decreased serum bicarbonate (44%), hypocalcemia (39%), hyperglycemia (28%), weight loss (25%), hypothyroidism (19%; grades 3/4: <1%), hypernatremia (17%), hyperkalemia (15%), hypoalbuminemia (15%), hyponatremia (13%), hypophosphatemia (13%), hypoglycemia (11%)

Gastrointestinal: Diarrhea (55%; grades 3/4: 11%), decreased appetite (34%), nausea (32%; grades 3/4: 3%), increased serum lipase (3% to 27%), increased serum amylase (25%), vomiting (24%; grades 3/4: 3%), constipation (20%), mucosal inflammation (15%), stomatitis (15%), abdominal pain (8% to 14%), dysgeusia (11%)

Genitourinary: Proteinuria (11%; grade 3: 3%)

Hematologic and oncologic: Anemia (4% to 35%; grades 3/4: <1%), lymphocytopenia (33%; grades 3/4: 3%), hemorrhage (16%; grades 3/4 1%), thrombocytopenia (15%; grades 3/4: <1%), leukopenia (11%)

Hepatic: Increased serum alkaline phosphatase (30%), increased serum ALT (22%; grades 3/4: <1%), increased serum AST (20%; grades 3/4: <1%)

Neuromuscular & skeletal: Weakness (21%), arthralgia (15%), limb pain (13%)

Renal: Increased serum creatinine (55%)

Respiratory: Cough (15%), dyspnea (15%)

1% to 10%:

Cardiovascular: Venous thrombosis (grades 3/4: 3%), arterial thrombosis (2%; grade 3/4: 1%), pulmonary embolism (2%) deep vein thrombosis (1%), transient ischemic attack (1%), retinal vein occlusion (≤1%), retinal thrombosis (≤1%)

Central nervous system: Dizziness (9%)

Dermatologic: Xeroderma (10%), pruritus (7%), alopecia (4%), erythema (2%)

Endocrine & metabolic: Dehydration (6%), hyperthyroidism (1%)

Gastrointestinal: Dyspepsia (10%), hemorrhoids (4%), gastrointestinal fistula (1%), gastrointestinal perforation (≤1%)

Genitourinary: Hematuria (3%)

Hematologic and Oncologic: Increased hemoglobin (9%), rectal hemorrhage (2%), polycythemia (1%)

Neuromuscular & skeletal: Myalgia (7%)

Otic: Tinnitus (3%)

Respiratory: Epistaxis (6%), hemoptysis (2%)

<1%, postmarketing, and/or case reports: Cardiac failure, cerebral hemorrhage, cerebrovascular accident, fever, hypertensive crisis, neutropenia, reversible posterior leukoencephalopathy syndrome

Drug Interactions

Metabolism/Transport Effects Substrate of CYP1A2 (minor), CYP2C19 (minor), CYP3A4 (major), UGT1A1; **Note:** Assignment of Major/Minor substrate status based on clinically relevant drug interaction potential

Avoid Concomitant Use

Avoid concomitant use of Axitinib with any of the following: Conivaptan; CYP3A4 Inducers (Moderate); CYP3A4 Inducers (Strong); CYP3A4 Inhibitors (Strong); Fusidic Acid (Systemic); Grapefruit Juice; Idelalisib; St John's Wort

◄ **Increased Effect/Toxicity**
Axitinib may increase the levels/effects of: Bisphosphonate Derivatives

The levels/effects of Axitinib may be increased by: Aprepitant; Conivaptan; CYP3A4 Inhibitors (Moderate); CYP3A4 Inhibitors (Strong); Dasatinib; Fosaprepitant; Fusidic Acid (Systemic); Grapefruit Juice; Idelalisib; Netupitant; Palbociclib; Simeprevir; Stiripentol

Decreased Effect
The levels/effects of Axitinib may be decreased by: CYP3A4 Inducers (Moderate); CYP3A4 Inducers (Strong); Deferasirox; Sarilumab; Siltuximab; St John's Wort; Tocilizumab

Food Interactions Axitinib serum concentrations may be increased when taken with grapefruit or grapefruit juice. Management: Avoid concurrent use.

Hazardous Drugs Handling Considerations
Hazardous agent (NIOSH 2016 [group 1]).

Use appropriate precautions for receiving, handling, administration, and disposal. Gloves (single) should be worn during receiving, unpacking, and placing in storage.

NIOSH recommends single gloving for administration of intact tablets or capsules. If manipulating tablets/capsules (eg, to prepare an oral suspension), NIOSH recommends double gloving, a protective gown, and preparation in a controlled device; if not prepared in a controlled device, respiratory and eye/face protection as well as ventilated engineering controls are recommended. NIOSH recommends double gloving, a protective gown, and (if there is a potential for vomit or spit up) eye/face protection for administration of an oral liquid/feeding tube administration (NIOSH 2016).

Storage/Stability Store at 20°C to 25°C (68°F to 77°F); excursions permitted to 15°C to 30°C (59°F to 86°F).

Mechanism of Action Axitinib is a selective second generation tyrosine kinase inhibitor which blocks angiogenesis and tumor growth by inhibiting vascular endothelial growth factor receptors (VEGFR-1, VEGFR-2, and VEGFR-3).

Pharmacodynamics/Kinetics
Absorption: Rapid (Rugo 2005)
Distribution: V_d: 160 L
Protein binding: >99%; to albumin (primarily) and to alpha$_1$ acid glycoprotein (AAG)
Metabolism: Hepatic; primarily via CYP3A4/5 and to a lesser extend via CYP1A2, CYP2C19 and UGT1A1
Bioavailability: 58%
Half-life elimination: 2.5 to 6.1 hours
Time to peak: 2.5 to 4 hours
Excretion: Feces (~41%; 12% as unchanged drug); urine (~23%; as metabolites)

Dosing
Adult

Renal cell cancer, advanced: Oral: Initial: 5 mg twice daily (approximately every 12 hours)
Dose increases: If dose is tolerated (no adverse events above grade 2, blood pressure is normal and no antihypertensive use) for at least 2 consecutive weeks, may increase the dose to 7 mg twice daily, and then further increase (using the same tolerance criteria) to 10 mg twice daily.

Dose decreases: For adverse events, reduce dose from 5 mg twice daily to 3 mg twice daily; further reduce to 2 mg twice daily if adverse events persist.

Dosage adjustment for strong CYP3A4 inhibitors: Avoid concomitant administration with strong CYP3A4 inhibitors (eg, clarithromycin, itraconazole, ketoconazole, nefazodone, protease inhibitors, telithromycin, voriconazole, grapefruit juice); if concomitant administration with a strong CYP3A4 inhibitor cannot be avoided, ~50% dosage reduction is recommended; adjust dose based on individual tolerance and safety. When the strong CYP3A4 inhibitor is discontinued, resume previous axitinib dose after 3 to 5 half-lives of the inhibitor have passed.

Thyroid cancer, differentiated, advanced (off-label use): Oral: Initial: 5 mg twice daily on an empty stomach; increase or decrease dose in 20% increments based on response or toxicity; continue until disease progression or unacceptable toxicity (Cohen 2014) **or** Initial: 5 mg twice daily with food; if tolerated for 2 consecutive weeks, may increase to 7 mg twice daily, and then to 10 mg twice daily (unless receiving antihypertensive medication or blood pressure >150/90 mm Hg); for grade 3 or higher toxicity, interrupt therapy and/or reduce dose to 3 mg twice daily, if further dose reduction necessary, reduce to 2 mg twice daily; continue until disease progression or unacceptable toxicity (Locati 2014).

Geriatric Refer to adult dosing. No adjustment necessary.

Renal Impairment

Mild to severe renal impairment (CrCl 15 to <89 mL/minute): No initial dosage adjustment necessary.

End-stage renal disease (ESRD): There are no dosage adjustments provided in the manufacturer's labeling; use with caution.

Hepatic Impairment

Mild impairment (Child-Pugh class A): No starting dosage adjustment necessary.

Moderate impairment (Child-Pugh class B): Reduce starting dose by ~50%; increase or decrease based on individual tolerance.

Severe impairment (Child-Pugh class C): There are no dosage adjustments provided in the manufacturer's labeling (has not been studied).

Adjustment for Toxicity

Adverse events: May require temporary interruption, dose decreases (reduce dose from 5 mg twice daily to 3 mg twice daily; further reduce to 2 mg twice daily) or discontinuation

Cardiac failure: May require permanent discontinuation

Hypertension: Treat with standard antihypertensive therapy.

Persistent hypertension: May require dose reduction

Severe, persistent (despite antihypertensives and dose reduction), or evidence of hypertensive crisis: Discontinue treatment

Hemorrhage: Any bleeding requiring medical intervention: Temporarily interrupt treatment.

Proteinuria (moderate-to-severe): Reduce dose or temporarily interrupt treatment.

Administration Oral: Swallow tablet whole with a glass of water. May be taken with or without food. If a dose is missed or vomited, do not make up; resume dosing with the next scheduled dose. A suspension may be prepared for nasogastric administration (refer to Extemporaneous Preparations information).

Emetic Potential Low (10% to 30%)

◀ **Extemporaneous Preparations** For patients unable to swallow tablets whole, a suspension may be prepared for nasogastric tube administration (for doses of 2 to 10 mg). Place a 20 mL tightly capped amber syringe in a small drinking glass, with the open end of the syringe pointing up. Place the appropriate axitinib dose in the open syringe barrel; add 15 mL of USP grade water (do not use tap water or bottled water) to the syringe. Allow at least 10 minutes to dissolve the tablets; avoid direct light. Place the plunger of the syringe into the barrel, invert the syringe so the tip is pointing upward and remove the cap. Expel excess air; replace the cap until ready for use (keep syringe tip facing up). Prior to administration, gently invert the syringe several times to ensure a uniform suspension. Flush the nasogastric feeding tube with 15 mL of USP grade water before administration. After administering the dose, draw up 10 mL of USP grade water (into the same syringe which contained the dose) and flush the feeding tube; repeat this step 5 additional times to ensure the entire dose has been administered. Lastly, flush the feeding tube with a separate syringe containing 15 mL of USP grade water. Administer within 15 minutes of preparation.

Borst DL, Arruda LS, MacLean E, Pithavala YK, Morgado JE. Common questions regarding clinical use of axitinib in advanced renal cell carcinoma. *Am J Health Syst Pharm*. 2014;71 (13):1092-1096.

Monitoring Parameters Hepatic function (ALT, AST, and bilirubin; baseline and periodic), thyroid function (baseline and periodic), urinalysis (for proteinuria; baseline and periodically); blood pressure, signs/symptoms of RPLS, gastrointestinal bleeding/perforation/fistula, signs/symptoms cardiac failure

Thyroid function testing recommendations (Hamnvik, 2011):
   Preexisting levothyroxine therapy: Obtain baseline TSH levels, then monitor every 4 weeks until levels and levothyroxine dose are stable, then monitor every 2 months
   Without preexisting thyroid hormone replacement: TSH at baseline, then monthly for 4 months, then every 2-3 months

Dietary Considerations Avoid grapefruit and grapefruit juice.

Prescribing and Access Restrictions Available from select specialty pharmacies. Further information may be obtained at 877-744-5675 or www.-inlytahcp.com.

Dosage Forms Excipient information presented when available (limited, particularly for generics); consult specific product labeling.
   Tablet, Oral:
      Inlyta: 1 mg, 5 mg

◆ **Axumin** *see* Fluciclovine F 18 *on page 807*

◆ **AY-25650** *see* Triptorelin *on page 1841*

◆ **5-Aza-2'-deoxycytidine** *see* Decitabine *on page 548*

AzaCITIDine (ay za SYE ti deen)

Related Information

Management of Chemotherapy-Induced Nausea and Vomiting in Adults *on page 2253*

Prevention of Chemotherapy-Induced Nausea and Vomiting in Children *on page 2310*

Safe Handling of Hazardous Drugs *on page 2379*

Brand Names: US Vidaza

Brand Names: Canada Vidaza

Index Terms 5-Azacytidine; 5-AZC; AZA-CR; Azacytidine; Ladakamycin

Pharmacologic Category Antineoplastic Agent, Antimetabolite; Antineoplastic Agent, DNA Methylation Inhibitor

Use Myelodysplastic syndromes: Treatment of myelodysplastic syndromes (MDS) in patients with the following French-American-British (FAB) classification subtypes: Refractory anemia or refractory anemia with ringed sideroblasts (if accompanied by neutropenia or thrombocytopenia or requiring transfusions), refractory anemia with excess blasts, refractory anemia with excess blasts in transformation, and chronic myelomonocytic leukemia.

Labeled Contraindications Hypersensitivity to azacitidine, mannitol, or any component of the formulation; advanced malignant hepatic tumors

Pregnancy Considerations Adverse events were observed in animal reproduction studies. Based on its mechanism of action, azacitidine may cause fetal harm if administered during pregnancy. Women of childbearing potential should be advised to avoid pregnancy during treatment; verify pregnancy status prior to therapy initiation. In addition, males should be advised to avoid fathering a child while on azacitidine therapy and should use effective contraception during therapy.

Breastfeeding Considerations It is not known if azacitidine is excreted in breast milk. Due to the potential for serious adverse reactions in the nursing infant, breastfeeding is not recommended by the manufacturer.

Warnings/Precautions May cause hepatotoxicity in patients with preexisting hepatic impairment. Progressive hepatic coma leading to death has been reported in patients with extensive tumor burden due to metastatic disease, especially those with a baseline albumin <30 g/L. Patients with hepatic impairment were excluded from clinical studies for myelodysplastic syndrome (MDS). Use is contraindicated in patients with advanced malignant hepatic tumors. Monitor liver function tests prior to therapy initiation and before each cycle. Renal toxicities, including serum creatinine elevations, renal tubular acidosis (serum bicarbonate decrease to <20 mEq/L associated with alkaline urine and serum potassium <3 mEq/L), and renal failure (some fatal), have been reported with intravenous azacitidine when used in combination with other chemotherapy agents. Monitor serum creatinine and electrolytes prior to therapy initiation and before each cycle. Withhold or reduce the dose with unexplained decreases in serum bicarbonate <20 mEq/L or if elevations in BUN or serum creatinine occur. Patients with renal impairment may be at increased risk for renal toxicity. Monitor closely for toxicity in patients with severe renal impairment (azacitidine and metabolites are excreted renally).

Neutropenia, thrombocytopenia, and anemia are common; may cause therapy delays and/or dosage reductions; monitor blood counts prior to each cycle (at a minimum), and as clinically indicated. Adjust dose in subsequent cycles based on nadir counts and hematologic response. Azacitidine is associated with a moderate emetic potential (Basch 2011; Dupuis 2011; Roila 2010); antiemetics are recommended to prevent nausea and vomiting. Injection site reactions commonly occurred with subcutaneous administration. Potentially significant drug-drug interactions may exist, requiring dose or frequency adjustment, additional monitoring, and/or selection of alternative therapy.

Some dosage forms may contain polysorbate 80 (also known as Tweens). Hypersensitivity reactions, usually a delayed reaction, have been reported following exposure to pharmaceutical products containing polysorbate 80 in certain individuals (Isaksson 2002; Lucente 2000; Shelley 1995). Thrombocytopenia, ascites, pulmonary deterioration, and renal and hepatic failure have been reported in premature neonates after receiving parenteral products

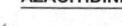 containing polysorbate 80 (Alade 1986; CDC 1984). See manufacturer's labeling.

Adverse Reactions

>10%:

Cardiovascular: Peripheral edema (7% to 19%), chest pain (16%)

Central nervous system: Fatigue (13% to 36%), rigors (26%), headache (22%), dizziness (19%), anxiety (5% to 13%), depression (12%), malaise (11%), pain (11%), insomnia (9% to 11%)

Dermatologic: Erythema (7% to 17%), pallor (16%), skin lesion (15%), skin rash (10% to 14%), pruritus (12%), diaphoresis (11%)

Endocrine & metabolic: Weight loss (≤16%), pitting edema (15%), hypokalemia (6% to 13%)

Gastrointestinal: Nausea (48% to 71%), vomiting (27% to 54%), constipation (34% to 50%), diarrhea (36%), anorexia (13% to 21%), abdominal pain (11% to 16%), abdominal tenderness (12%)

Hematologic & oncologic: Thrombocytopenia (66% to 70%; grades 3/4: 58%), anemia (51% to 70%; grades 3/4: 14%), neutropenia (32% to 66%; grades 3/4: 61%), leukopenia (18% to 48%; grades 3/4: 15%), bruise (19% to 31%), petechia (11% to 24%), febrile neutropenia (14% to 16%; grades 3/4: 13%), bone marrow depression (nadir: days 10 to 17; recovery: days 28 to 31)

Local: Injection site reactions (14% to 29%): Erythema (35% to 43%; more common with IV administration), pain (19% to 23%; more common with IV administration), bruising (5% to 14%)

Neuromuscular & skeletal: Weakness (29%), arthralgia (22%), limb pain (20%), back pain (19%), myalgia (16%)

Respiratory: Cough (11% to 30%), dyspnea (5% to 29%), pharyngitis (20%), epistaxis (16%), nasopharyngitis (15%), upper respiratory infection (9% to 13%), pneumonia (11%), rales (9% to 11%)

Miscellaneous: Fever (30% to 52%)

5% to 10%:

Cardiovascular: Heart murmur (10%), tachycardia (9%), hypertension (≤9%), hypotension (7%), syncope (6%), chest wall pain (5%)

Central nervous system: Lethargy (7% to 8%), hypoesthesia (5%), postoperative pain (5%)

Dermatologic: Night sweats (9%), cellulitis (8%), rash at injection site (6%), urticaria (6%), skin nodules (5%), xeroderma (5%)

Gastrointestinal: Gingival hemorrhage (10%), stomatitis (8%), hemorrhoids (7%), dyspepsia (6% to 7%), abdominal distention (6%), loose stools (6%), dysphagia (5%), tongue ulcer (5%)

Genitourinary: Urinary tract infection (8% to 9%), dysuria (8%), hematuria (≤6%)

Hematologic & oncologic: Lymphadenopathy (10%), hematoma (9%), oral mucosal petechiae (8%), postprocedural hemorrhage (6%), oral hemorrhage (5%)

Hypersensitivity: Transfusion reaction (7%)

Infection: Herpes simplex infection (9%)

Local: Itching at injection site (7%), hematoma at injection site (6%), induration at injection site (5%), injection site granuloma (5%), skin discoloration at injection site (5%), swelling at injection site (5%)

Neuromuscular & skeletal: Muscle cramps (6%)

Respiratory: Rhinorrhea (10%), wheezing (9%), abnormal breath sounds (8%), nasal congestion (6%), pharyngolaryngeal pain (6%), pleural effusion (6%), post nasal drip (6%), rhinitis (6%), rhonchi (6%), atelectasis (5%), sinusitis (5%)

Miscellaneous: Lymphadenopathy (10%), herpes simplex (9%), night sweats (9%), transfusion reaction (7%), mouth hemorrhage (5%)

<5%, postmarketing, and/or case reports: Abscess (limb, perirectal), aggravated bone pain, agranulocytosis, anaphylactic shock, atrial fibrillation, azotemia, bacterial infection, blastomycosis, bone marrow failure, cardiac failure, catheter site hemorrhage, cellulitis, cerebral hemorrhage, cholecystectomy, cholecystitis, congestive cardiomyopathy, decreased serum bicarbonate, dehydration, diverticulitis, fibrosis (interstitial and alveolar), gastrointestinal hemorrhage, glycosuria, hemophthalmos, hemoptysis, hepatic coma, hypersensitivity reaction, hypophosphatemia, increased serum creatinine, injection site infection, interstitial pulmonary disease, intracranial hemorrhage, leukemia cutis, melena, necrotizing fasciitis, neutropenic sepsis, orthostatic hypotension, pancytopenia, pneumonitis, polyuria, pulmonary infiltrates, pyoderma gangrenosum, renal failure, renal tubular acidosis, respiratory distress, seizure, sepsis, sepsis syndrome, septic shock, splenomegaly, Sweet's syndrome, tissue necrosis at injection site, toxoplasmosis, tumor lysis syndrome

Drug Interactions

Metabolism/Transport Effects None known.

Avoid Concomitant Use

Avoid concomitant use of AzaCITIDine with any of the following: BCG (Intravesical); Deferiprone; Dipyrone; Natalizumab; Pimecrolimus; Tacrolimus (Topical); Vaccines (Live)

Increased Effect/Toxicity

AzaCITIDine may increase the levels/effects of: CloZAPine; Deferiprone; Fingolimod; Leflunomide; Natalizumab; Tofacitinib; Vaccines (Live)

The levels/effects of AzaCITIDine may be increased by: Denosumab; Dipyrone; Ocrelizumab; Palifermin; Pimecrolimus; Promazine; Roflumilast; Tacrolimus (Topical); Trastuzumab

Decreased Effect

AzaCITIDine may decrease the levels/effects of: BCG (Intravesical); Coccidioides immitis Skin Test; Lenograstim; Nivolumab; Sipuleucel-T; Tertomotide; Vaccines (Inactivated); Vaccines (Live)

The levels/effects of AzaCITIDine may be decreased by: Echinacea

Hazardous Drugs Handling Considerations

Hazardous agent (NIOSH 2016 [group 1]).

Use appropriate precautions for receiving, handling, administration, and disposal. Gloves (single) should be worn during receiving, unpacking, and placing in storage.

NIOSH recommends double gloving, a protective gown, ventilated engineering controls (a class II biological safety cabinet or a compounding aseptic containment isolator), and closed system transfer devices (CSTDs) for preparation. Double gloving, a gown, and (if dosage form allows) CSTDs are required during administration (NIOSH 2016).

Storage/Stability

Prior to reconstitution, store intact vials at room temperature of 25°C (77°F); excursions permitted to 15°C to 30°C (59°F to 86°F).

◀ IV solution: **Solutions for IV administration have very limited stability and must be prepared immediately prior to each dose.** Administration must be completed within 1 hour of (vial) reconstitution.

SubQ suspension: Following reconstitution, suspension may be stored at room temperature for up to 1 hour prior to immediate administration (administer within 1 hour of reconstitution). If administration is delayed, refrigerate reconstituted suspension immediately (either in vial or syringe); may be stored for up to 8 hours (if reconstituted with room temperature SWFI) or up to 22 hours (if reconstituted with refrigerated SWFI). After removal from refrigerator, may be allowed up to 30 minutes to reach room temperature prior to immediate administration.

Preparation for Administration If reconstituted solution comes in contact with skin, wash immediately and thoroughly with soap and water; if comes in contact with mucous membranes, flush thoroughly with water.

IV: Reconstitute vial with 10 mL SWFI to form a 10 mg/mL solution; vigorously shake or roll vial until solution is dissolved and clear. Mix in 50 to 100 mL of NS or lactated Ringer's injection for infusion.

SubQ: Slowly add 4 mL SWFI to each vial, resulting in a concentration of 25 mg/mL. Vigorously shake or roll vial until a suspension is formed (suspension will be cloudy). The manufacturer recommends dividing doses >4 mL equally into 2 syringes. Do not filter after reconstitution (may remove active drug). Resuspend contents of syringe by vigorously rolling between palms immediately prior to administration.

Discard unused portion (does not contain preservatives); do not save unused portions for later administration.

Mechanism of Action Antineoplastic effects may be a result of azacitidine's ability to promote hypomethylation of DNA, restoring normal gene differentiation and proliferation. Azacitidine also exerts direct toxicity to abnormal hematopoietic cells in the bone marrow.

Pharmacodynamics/Kinetics

Absorption: SubQ: Rapid and complete

Distribution: V_d: IV: 76 ± 26 L; does not cross blood-brain barrier

Metabolism: Hepatic; hydrolysis to several metabolites

Bioavailability: SubQ: ~89%

Half-life elimination: IV, SubQ: ~4 hours

Time to peak, plasma: SubQ: 30 minutes

Excretion: Urine (50% to 85%); feces (<1%)

Dosing

Adult Note: Azacitidine is associated with a moderate emetic potential (Basch 2011; Roila 2010); antiemetics are recommended to prevent nausea and vomiting.

Myelodysplastic syndromes (MDS): IV, SubQ: Initial cycle: 75 mg/m^2/day for 7 days. Subsequent cycles: 75 mg/m^2/day for 7 days every 4 weeks; dose may be increased to 100 mg/m^2/day if no benefit is observed after 2 cycles and no toxicity other than nausea and vomiting have occurred. Patients should be treated for a minimum of 4 to 6 cycles; treatment may be continued as long as patient continues to benefit.

Note: Alternate (off-label) schedules (which have produced hematologic response) have been used for convenience in community oncology centers (Lyons 2009): SubQ:

75 mg/m^2/day for 5 days (Mon-Fri), 2 days rest (Sat, Sun), then 75 mg/m^2/day for 2 days (Mon, Tues); repeat cycle every 28 days **or**

50 mg/m^2/day for 5 days (Mon-Fri), 2 days rest (Sat, Sun), then 50 mg/m^2/day for 5 days (Mon-Fri); repeat cycle every 28 days **or**

75 mg/m^2/day for 5 days (Mon-Fri), repeat cycle every 28 days

Acute myeloid leukemia (AML) (off-label use): SubQ: 75 mg/m^2/day for 7 days every 4 weeks for at least 6 cycles; treatment may be continued as long as patient continues to benefit or until disease progression or unacceptable toxicity (Fenaux 2010). Dose reductions and/or therapy interruption may be required for hematologic toxicity.

Dosage adjustment based on serum electrolytes: If serum bicarbonate falls to <20 mEq/L (unexplained decrease): Reduce dose by 50% for next treatment course.

Geriatric Refer to adult dosing. Due to the potential for decreased renal function in the elderly, select dose carefully and closely monitor renal function.

Renal Impairment

Renal impairment at *baseline:*

Mild to moderate impairment (CrCl ≥30 mL/minute): No dosage adjustment necessary (Douvali 2012).

Severe impairment (CrCl <30 mL/minute): No dosage adjustment necessary for cycle 1; azacitidine and its metabolites are excreted renally, monitor closely for toxicity.

Renal toxicity *during* treatment: Unexplained increases in BUN or serum creatinine: Delay next cycle until values reach baseline or normal, then reduce dose by 50% for next treatment course.

Hepatic Impairment No dosage adjustment provided in the manufacturer's labeling (has not been studied). Use is contraindicated in patients with advanced malignant hepatic tumors.

Adjustment for Toxicity:

Hematologic toxicity: MDS:

For baseline WBC ≥3,000/mm^3, ANC ≥1,500/mm^3, and platelets ≥75,000/mm^3:

Nadir count: ANC <500/mm^3 or platelets <25,000/mm^3: Administer 50% of dose during next treatment course

Nadir count: ANC 500/mm^3 to 1,500/mm^3 or platelets 25,000 to 50,000/mm^3: Administer 67% of dose during next treatment course

Nadir count: ANC >1,500/mm^3 or platelets >50,000/mm^3: Administer 100% of dose during next treatment course

For baseline WBC <3,000/mm^3, ANC <1,500/mm^3, or platelets <75,000/mm^3: Adjust dose as follows based on nadir counts and bone marrow biopsy cellularity at the time of nadir, unless clear improvement in differentiation at the time of the next cycle:

WBC or platelet nadir decreased 50% to 75% from baseline and bone marrow biopsy cellularity at time of nadir 30% to 60%: Administer 100% of dose during next treatment course

WBC or platelet nadir decreased 50% to 75% from baseline and bone marrow biopsy cellularity at time of nadir 15% to 30%: Administer 50% of dose during next treatment course

WBC or platelet nadir decreased 50% to 75% from baseline and bone marrow biopsy cellularity at time of nadir <15%: Administer 33% of dose during next treatment course

WBC or platelet nadir decreased >75% from baseline and bone marrow biopsy cellularity at time of nadir 30% to 60%: Administer 75% of dose during next treatment course

WBC or platelet nadir decreased >75% from baseline and bone marrow biopsy cellularity at time of nadir 15% to 30%: Administer 50% of dose during next treatment course

WBC or platelet nadir decreased >75% from baseline and bone marrow biopsy cellularity at time of nadir <15%: Administer 33% of dose during next treatment course

Note: If a nadir defined above occurs, administer the next treatment course 28 days after the start of the preceding course as long as WBC and platelet counts are >25% above the nadir and rising. If a >25% increase above the nadir is not seen by day 28, reassess counts every 7 days. If a 25% increase is not seen by day 42, administer 50% of the scheduled dose.

Administration Azacitidine is associated with a moderate emetic potential (Basch 2011; Dupuis 2011; Roila 2010); antiemetics are recommended to prevent nausea and vomiting.

SubQ: The manufacturer recommends equally dividing volumes >4 mL into 2 syringes and injecting into 2 separate sites; however, policies for maximum SubQ administration volume may vary by institution; interpatient variations may also apply. Rotate sites for each injection (thigh, abdomen, or upper arm). Administer subsequent injections at least 1 inch from previous injection sites; do not inject into tender, bruised, red, or hard areas. Allow refrigerated suspensions to come to room temperature (up to 30 minutes) prior to administration. Resuspend by inverting the syringe 2 to 3 times and then rolling the syringe between the palms for 30 seconds.

IV: Infuse over 10 to 40 minutes; infusion must be completed within 1 hour of (vial) reconstitution.

If azacitidine suspension comes in contact with the skin, immediately wash with soap and water. If it comes into contact with mucous membranes, flush thoroughly with water.

Emetic Potential Children and Adults: Moderate (30% to 90%)

Monitoring Parameters Monitor liver function tests, electrolytes, CBC with differential and platelets, renal function (BUN and serum creatinine) at baseline, prior to each cycle, and more frequently if indicated. Also monitor for hematologic response, nausea/vomiting, and for injection site reactions.

Dosage Forms Excipient information presented when available (limited, particularly for generics); consult specific product labeling.

Suspension Reconstituted, Injection:
  Generic: 100 mg (1 ea)
Suspension Reconstituted, Injection [preservative free]:
  Vidaza: 100 mg (1 ea)
  Generic: 100 mg (1 ea)

◆ **AZA-CR** *see* AzaCITIDine *on page 206*

◆ **Azactam** *see* Aztreonam (Systemic) *on page 213*

◆ **Azactam in Dextrose** *see* Aztreonam (Systemic) *on page 213*

◆ **Azacytidine** *see* AzaCITIDine *on page 206*

Aztreonam (Systemic) (AZ tree oh nam)

Brand Names: US Azactam; Azactam in Dextrose

Index Terms Azthreonam

Pharmacologic Category Antibiotic, Monobactam

Use Treatment of patients with urinary tract infections, lower respiratory tract infections, septicemia, skin/skin structure infections, intra-abdominal infections, and gynecological infections caused by susceptible gram-negative bacilli

Pregnancy Risk Factor B

Dosing

Adult & Geriatric

Urinary tract infection: IM, IV: 500 mg to 1 g every 8 to 12 hours

Moderately severe systemic infections: 1 g IV or IM or 2 g IV every 8 to 12 hours. **Note:** IV route preferred for septicemia, intra-abdominal abscess, or peritonitis; higher doses (8 to 12 g daily) may be needed for patients with cystic fibrosis (Zobell 2013) or other infections (Solomkin 2010).

Osteomyelitis, native vertebral due to *P. aeruginosa* **(off-label use):** IV: 2 g every 8 hours for 6 weeks **Note:** Double coverage may be considered (ie, aztreonam plus an aminoglycoside) (IDSA [Berbari 2015])

Severe systemic or life-threatening infections (eg, *Pseudomonas aeruginosa***):** IV: 2 g every 6 to 8 hours; maximum: 8 g daily. **Note:** Higher doses (8 to 12 g daily) may be needed for patients with cystic fibrosis (Zobell 2013) or other infections (Solomkin 2010).

Pneumonia, hospital-acquired or ventilator-associated (alternative therapy) (off-label dose): IV: 2 g every 8 hours for 7 days; may consider shorter or longer durations depending on rate of clinical improvement. When used as empiric therapy, use in combination with an agent active against *Staphylococcus aureus* with or without an additional antipseudomonal agent (dependent on patient and institution-specific risk factors) (Kalil 2016).

Surgical (perioperative) prophylaxis (off-label use): IV: 2 g within 60 minutes prior to surgery. Doses may be repeated in 4 hours if procedure is lengthy or if there is excessive blood loss (Bratzler 2013).

Pediatric

Mild-to-moderate infections: Infants ≥9 months, Children, and Adolescents: IV: 30 mg/kg/dose every 8 hours; maximum: 120 mg/kg/day (8 g daily)

Moderate-to-severe infections: Infants ≥9 months, Children, and Adolescents: IV: 30 mg/kg/dose every 6 to 8 hours; maximum: 120 mg/kg/day (8 g daily)

Cystic fibrosis: Infants ≥9 months, Children, and Adolescents: IV: 50 mg/kg/dose every 6 to 8 hours (ie, up to 200 mg/kg/day); maximum: 8 g daily. **Note:** Higher doses (8 to 12 g daily) may be needed for patients with cystic fibrosis (Zobell 2013).

Surgical (perioperative) prophylaxis (off-label use): Children ≥1 year and Adolescents: IV: 30 mg/kg within 60 minutes prior to surgery (maximum: 2,000 mg per dose). Doses may be repeated in 4 hours if procedure is lengthy or if there is excessive blood loss (Bratzler 2013).

Renal Impairment

IM, IV: Adults: Following initial dose, maintenance doses should be given as follows:

CrCl 10 to 30 mL/minute: 50% of usual dose at the usual interval

CrCl <10 mL/minute: 25% of usual dosage at the usual interval

Intermittent hemodialysis (IHD): Dialyzable (20% to 50%): Loading dose of 500 mg, 1 g, or 2 g, followed by 25% of initial dose at usual interval; for serious/life-threatening infections, administer 12.5% of initial dose after each hemodialysis session (given in addition to the maintenance doses). Alternatively, may administer 500 mg every 12 hours (Heintz, 2009). **Note:** Dosing dependent on the assumption of 3 times/week, complete IHD sessions.

Peritoneal dialysis (PD): Administer as for CrCl <10 mL/minute (Aronoff, 2007)

Continuous renal replacement therapy (CRRT) (Heintz, 2009; Trotman, 2005): Drug clearance is highly dependent on the method of renal replacement, filter type, and flow rate. Appropriate dosing requires close monitoring of pharmacologic response, signs of adverse reactions due to drug accumulation, as well as drug concentrations in relation to target trough (if appropriate). The following are general recommendations only (based on dialysate flow/ultrafiltration rates of 1 to 2 L/hour and minimal residual renal function) and should not supersede clinical judgment:

CVVH: Loading dose of 2 g followed by 1 to 2 g every 12 hours

CVVHD/CVVHDF: Loading dose of 2 g followed by either 1 g every 8 hours **or** 2 g every 12 hours (Heintz, 2009)

Hepatic Impairment No dosage adjustment provided in manufacturer's labeling. Use with caution (minor hepatic elimination occurs).

Additional Information Complete prescribing information should be consulted for additional detail.

Dosage Forms Excipient information presented when available (limited, particularly for generics); consult specific product labeling.

Solution, Intravenous:

Azactam in Dextrose: 1 g (50 mL); 2 g (50 mL) [sodium free]

Solution Reconstituted, Injection:

Azactam: 1 g (1 ea); 2 g (1 ea) [sodium free]

Generic: 1 g (1 ea); 2 g (1 ea)

◆ **B1939** see EriBULin on page 712

◆ **Bacillus Calmette-Guérin (BCG) Live** see BCG (Intravesical) on page 219

◆ **Bactrim** see Sulfamethoxazole and Trimethoprim on page 1698

◆ **Bactrim DS** see Sulfamethoxazole and Trimethoprim on page 1698

◆ **BAL8557** see Isavuconazonium Sulfate on page 1061

Basiliximab (ba si LIK si mab)

Related Information

Hematopoietic Cell Transplantation *on page 2365*

Brand Names: US Simulect

Brand Names: Canada Simulect

Pharmacologic Category Immunosuppressant Agent; Monoclonal Antibody

Use

Renal transplant (prophylaxis of acute rejection): Prophylaxis of acute organ rejection in renal transplantation in combination with cyclosporine (modified) and corticosteroids

Guideline recommendations: While basiliximab is FDA-approved for prophylaxis of acute organ rejection in renal transplantation in combination with cyclosporine (modified) and corticosteroids, cyclosporine is no longer recommended as the first line agent of choice. The Kidney Disease: Improving Global Outcomes (KDIGO) clinical practice guidelines for care of kidney transplant recipients recommend induction as part of the initial immunosuppressive regimen for all kidney transplants to reduce the risk of acute rejection. KDIGO recommends an interleukin 2 receptor antagonist (eg, basiliximab) as the first line induction agent for acute rejection prophylaxis except in those patients at high immunologic risk. (KDIGO [Kasiske 2009]).

Labeled Contraindications Known hypersensitivity to basiliximab or any component of the formulation

Pregnancy Considerations Adverse effects were not observed in animal reproduction studies. Basiliximab is a monoclonal IgG antibody which targets IL-2 receptors. IgG is known to cross the placenta; IL-2 receptors play an important role in the development of the immune system.

Women of childbearing potential should use effective contraceptive measures before beginning treatment, during, and for 4 months after completion of basiliximab treatment.

The National Transplantation Pregnancy Registry (NTPR) is a registry which follows pregnancies which occur in maternal transplant recipients or those fathered by male transplant recipients. The NTPR encourages reporting of pregnancies following solid organ transplant by contacting them at 877-955-6877 or NTPR@giftoflifeinstitute.org.

Breastfeeding Considerations It is not known if basiliximab is excreted in human milk. Because many immunoglobulins are secreted in milk and the potential for serious adverse reactions exists, a decision should be made to discontinue breastfeeding or discontinue the drug, taking into account the importance of the drug to the mother.

Warnings/Precautions To be used as a component of an immunosuppressive regimen which includes cyclosporine and corticosteroids. The incidence of lymphoproliferative disorders and/or opportunistic infections may be increased by immunosuppressive therapy. Severe hypersensitivity reactions, occurring within 24 hours, have been reported. Reactions, including anaphylaxis, have occurred both with the initial exposure and/or following re-exposure after several months. Use caution during re-exposure to a subsequent course of therapy in a patient who has previously received basiliximab; patients in whom concomitant immunosuppression was prematurely discontinued due to abandoned transplantation or early graft loss are at increased risk for developing a severe hypersensitivity reaction upon re-exposure. Discontinue permanently if a severe reaction occurs. Medications for the treatment of hypersensitivity reactions should be available for immediate use. Treatment may result in the development of human antimurine antibodies (HAMA); however, limited evidence suggesting the use of muromonab-CD3 or other murine products is not precluded. **[U.S. Boxed Warning]: Should be administered under the supervision of a physician experienced in immunosuppression therapy and organ transplant management.** In renal transplant patients receiving basiliximab plus prednisone, cyclosporine, and mycophenolate, new-onset diabetes, glucose intolerance, and impaired fasting glucose were observed at rates significantly higher than observed in patients receiving prednisone, cyclosporine, and mycophenolate without basiliximab (Aasebo, 2010). Potentially significant drug-drug interactions may exist, requiring dose or frequency adjustment, additional monitoring, and/or selection of alternative therapy.

Adverse Reactions Frequency not defined. Administration of basiliximab did not appear to increase the incidence or severity of adverse effects in clinical trials. Adverse events were reported in 96% of both the placebo and basiliximab groups.

>10%:
  Cardiovascular: Hypertension, peripheral edema
  Central nervous system: Headache, insomnia, pain
  Dermatologic: Acne vulgaris
  Endocrine & metabolic: Hypercholesterolemia, hyperglycemia, hyperkalemia, hyperuricemia, hypokalemia, hypophosphatemia
  Gastrointestinal: Abdominal pain, constipation, diarrhea, dyspepsia, nausea, vomiting
  Genitourinary: Urinary tract infection
  Hematologic & oncologic: Anemia
  Infection: Viral infection
  Neuromuscular & skeletal: Tremor
  Respiratory: Dyspnea, upper respiratory infection
  Miscellaneous: Fever, postoperative wound complication
3% to 10%:
  Cardiovascular: Abnormal heart sounds, angina pectoris, atrial fibrillation, cardiac arrhythmia, cardiac failure, chest pain, hypotension, tachycardia, thrombosis
  Central nervous system: Agitation, anxiety, depression, dizziness, fatigue, hypoesthesia, malaise, rigors
  Dermatologic: Dermal ulcer, dermatological disease, hypertrichosis, pruritus, skin rash
  Endocrine & metabolic: Acidosis, albuminuria, anasarca, dehydration, diabetes mellitus, hypercalcemia, hyperlipidemia, hypertriglyceridemia, hypervolemia, hypocalcemia, hypoglycemia, hypomagnesemia, hyponatremia, increased nonprotein nitrogen, increased serum glucocorticoids, weight gain
  Gastrointestinal: Enlargement of abdomen, esophagitis, flatulence, gastroenteritis, gastrointestinal hemorrhage, GI moniliasis, gingival hyperplasia, hernia, melena, stomatitis (including ulcerative)
  Genitourinary: Bladder dysfunction, dysuria, genital edema (male), hematuria, impotence, oliguria, ureteral disease, urinary frequency, urinary retention
  Hematologic & oncologic: Hematoma, hemorrhage, hypoproteinemia, leukopenia, polycythemia, purpura, thrombocytopenia

Infection: Cytomegalovirus disease, herpes virus infection (simplex and zoster), infection, sepsis

Neuromuscular & skeletal: Arthralgia, arthropathy, back pain, bone fracture, leg pain, muscle cramps, myalgia, neuropathy, paresthesia, weakness

Ophthalmic: Cataract, conjunctivitis, visual disturbance

Renal: Renal insufficiency, renal tubular necrosis

Respiratory: Bronchitis, bronchospasm, cough, pharyngitis, pneumonia, pulmonary edema, rhinitis, sinusitis

Miscellaneous: Accidental injury, cyst

<1%, postmarketing, and/or case reports: Anaphylaxis, capillary leak syndrome, cytokine release syndrome, diabetes (new onset), hypersensitivity reaction (includes bronchospasm, cardiac failure, dyspnea, hypotension, pruritus, pulmonary edema, respiratory failure, skin rash, sneezing, tachycardia, urticaria), impaired glucose tolerance, increase in fasting plasma glucose, lymphoproliferative disorder

Drug Interactions

Metabolism/Transport Effects None known.

Avoid Concomitant Use

Avoid concomitant use of Basiliximab with any of the following: BCG (Intravesical); Belimumab; Natalizumab; Pimecrolimus; Tacrolimus (Topical); Vaccines (Live)

Increased Effect/Toxicity

Basiliximab may increase the levels/effects of: Belimumab; Fingolimod; Leflunomide; Natalizumab; Tofacitinib; Vaccines (Live)

The levels/effects of Basiliximab may be increased by: Denosumab; Ocrelizumab; Pimecrolimus; Roflumilast; Tacrolimus (Topical); Trastuzumab

Decreased Effect

Basiliximab may decrease the levels/effects of: BCG (Intravesical); Coccidioides immitis Skin Test; Nivolumab; Sipuleucel-T; Tertomotide; Vaccines (Inactivated); Vaccines (Live)

The levels/effects of Basiliximab may be decreased by: Echinacea

Storage/Stability Store intact vials refrigerated at 2°C to 8°C (36°F to 46°F). Should be used immediately after reconstitution; however, if not used immediately, reconstituted solution may be stored at 2°C to 8°C for up to 24 hours or at room temperature for up to 4 hours. Discard the reconstituted solution if not used within 24 hours.

Preparation for Administration Reconstitute with preservative-free sterile water for injection (reconstitute 10 mg vial with 2.5 mL, 20 mg vial with 5 mL). Shake gently to dissolve. May further dilute reconstituted solution with 25 mL (10 mg) or 50 mL (20 mg) 0.9% sodium chloride or dextrose 5% in water. When mixing the solution, gently invert the bag to avoid foaming. Do not shake solutions diluted for infusion.

Mechanism of Action Chimeric (murine/human) immunosuppressant monoclonal antibody which blocks the alpha-chain of the interleukin-2 (IL-2) receptor complex; this receptor is expressed on activated T lymphocytes and is a critical pathway for activating cell mediated allograft rejection

Pharmacodynamics/Kinetics

Duration: Mean: 36 days ± 14 days (determined by IL-2R alpha saturation in patients also on cyclosporine and corticosteroids)

Distribution: Mean: V_d: Children 1 to 11 years: 4.8 ± 2.1 L; Adolescents 12 to 16 years: 7.8 ± 5.1 L; Adults: 8.6 ± 4.1 L

◀ Half-life elimination: Children 1 to 11 years: 9.5 ± 4.5 days; Adolescents 12 to 16 years: 9.1 ± 3.9 days; Adults: Mean: 7.2 ± 3.2 days

Excretion: Clearance:

Children 1 to 11 years: 17 ± 6 mL/hour; in pediatric liver transplant patients, significant basiliximab loss through ascites fluid can increase total body clearance and reduce IL-2R (CD25) saturation duration; dosage adjustments may be necessary (Cintorino 2006; Kovarik 2002; Spada 2006)

Adolescents 12 to 16 years: 31 ±19 mL/hour

Adults: 41 ± 19 mL/hour

Dosing

Adult & Geriatric Note: Patients previously administered basiliximab should only be re-exposed to a subsequent course of therapy with extreme caution.

Renal transplant (prophylaxis of acute rejection): IV: 20 mg within 2 hours prior to transplant surgery, followed by a second 20 mg dose 4 days after transplantation (in combination with other immunosuppressants). The second dose should be withheld if complications occur (including severe hypersensitivity reactions or graft loss). Timing of basiliximab dosing may vary based on clinical and institutional factors; refer to institutional protocol for specific information.

Acute graft-versus-host disease (aGVHD), refractory (treatment) (off-label use): IV: 20 mg on days 1 and 4; may repeat for recurrent acute GVHD (Schmidt-Hieber 2005). Additional data may be necessary to further define the role of basiliximab in this condition.

Heart transplant (prophylaxis of acute rejection) (off-label use): IV: 20 mg on the day of transplant, followed by a second 20 mg dose on day 4 post-transplantation (in combination with other immunosuppressants) (Mehra 2005). The first dose is usually administered immediately prior to transplant or within the first hours postoperatively.

Liver transplant (prophylaxis of acute rejection) (off-label use): IV: 20 mg on the day of transplant (day 0), followed by a second 20 mg dose on day 4 post-transplantation (in combination with other immunosuppressants) (Neuhaus 2002; Trunecka 2015). In clinical trials, the first dose was administered during the procedure once hemostasis was achieved or immediately post-transplant, or within 6 hours of organ reperfusion.

Lung transplant (prophylaxis of acute rejection) (off-label use): IV: 20 mg prior to transplantation, followed by a second 20 mg dose 4 days after transplantation (in combination with other immunosuppressants) (Clinckart 2009; Swarup 2011). Additional trials may be necessary to further define the role of basiliximab in this condition.

Pediatric Note: Patients previously administered basiliximab should only be re-exposed to a subsequent course of therapy with extreme caution.

Renal transplant (prophylaxis of acute rejection): IV:

Children <35 kg: 10 mg within 2 hours prior to transplant surgery, followed by a second 10 mg dose 4 days after transplantation; the second dose should be withheld if complications occur (including severe hypersensitivity reactions or graft loss). Timing of basiliximab dosing may vary based on clinical and institutional factors; refer to institutional protocol for specific information.

Children and Adolescents ≥35 kg: Refer to adult dosing

Renal Impairment There are no dosage adjustments provided in the manufacturer's labeling.

Hepatic Impairment There are no dosage adjustments provided in the manufacturer's labeling.

Administration For intravenous administration only. Infuse as a bolus or IV infusion over 20 to 30 minutes (bolus dosing is associated with nausea, vomiting, and local pain at the injection site); may be administered through either a peripheral or central line. For the treatment of acute GVHD (off-label use), the dose was diluted in 250 mL NS and administered over 30 minutes (Schmidt-Hieber 2005).

Monitoring Parameters Signs and symptoms of acute rejection; hypersensitivity, infection

Dosage Forms Excipient information presented when available (limited, particularly for generics); consult specific product labeling.

Solution Reconstituted, Intravenous [preservative free]:

Simulect: 10 mg (1 ea); 20 mg (1 ea)

♦ **Bavencio** *see* Avelumab *on page* 195

♦ **BAY 43-9006** *see* SORAfenib *on page* 1685

♦ **BAY 73-4506** *see* Regorafenib *on page* 1585

♦ **BAY88-8223** *see* Radium Ra 223 Dichloride *on page* 1566

♦ **Baycadron [DSC]** *see* Dexamethasone (Systemic) *on page* 579

BCG (Intravesical) (bee see jee)

Related Information

Safe Handling of Hazardous Drugs *on page* 2379

Brand Names: US TheraCys; Tice BCG

Brand Names: Canada ImmuCyst; Oncotice

Index Terms Bacillus Calmette-Guérin (BCG) Live; BCG, Live

Pharmacologic Category Antineoplastic Agent, Biological Response Modulator

Use

Bladder cancer: Treatment and prophylaxis of carcinoma in situ of the urinary bladder; prophylaxis of primary or recurrent superficial or minimally invasive (stage Ta and/or T1) papillary tumors following transurethral resection

Limitations of use: BCG (intravesical) is not recommended for stage Ta low-grade papillary tumors unless judged to be at high risk for recurrence. BCG (intravesical) is not recommended for immunization against tuberculosis.

Labeled Contraindications Known hypersensitivity to BCG (intravesical) or any component of the formulations, hypersensitivity after a previous administration of BCG (intravesical) or after a previous administration of a medicinal product containing the same substances; immunosuppressed patients or persons with congenital or acquired immune deficiencies (eg, HIV infection, leukemia, lymphoma, cancer therapy, immunosuppressive therapy such as corticosteroids); active tuberculosis; concurrent febrile illness, urinary tract infection, or gross hematuria; current symptoms or previous history of a systemic BCG reaction; recent (TheraCys; <14 days; TICE BCG: <7 to 14 days) biopsy, transurethral resection (TUR), or traumatic catheterization

Pregnancy Considerations Animal reproduction studies have not been conducted. BCG (intravesical) is not recommended for use in pregnant women. Women of childbearing potential should be advised to avoid pregnancy while on BCG (intravesical) therapy.

Breastfeeding Considerations It is not known if BCG (intravesical) is excreted in breast milk. Due to the potential for serious adverse reactions in the nursing infant, a decision should be made to discontinue breastfeeding or avoid use of BCG (intravesical), taking into account the importance of BCG (intravesical) to the mother.

Warnings/Precautions [US Boxed Warning]: **Contains live, attenuated mycobacteria. Use appropriate precautions for handling and disposal. BCG is a biohazard; proper preparation technique, handling, and disposal of all equipment in contact with BCG as a biohazard material is recommended.** BCG infections have been reported in health care workers due to accidental exposure (needle stick, skin laceration); nosocomial infections have been reported in patients (including immunosuppressed patients) receiving parenteral medications prepared in areas where BCG was prepared. To avoid cross contamination, do not prepare parenteral medications in an area where BCG has been prepared. Determine PPD status prior to use (rule out active tuberculosis prior to treatment initiation). Prior to intravesical instillation, patients with a positive PPD test should be further assessed for signs and/or symptoms of active or latent tuberculosis. BCG may persist in the urinary tract for several months after treatment; delayed manifestations of disseminated BCG infection may develop months to years after BCG therapy. Patients who receive immunosuppressive therapy after BCG therapy may be at higher risk for disseminated infection. Monitor for signs/symptoms of infection/toxicity after each treatment. Discontinue for persistent fever or acute febrile illness consistent with BCG infection. Some male genitourinary tract infections (orchitis or epididymitis) have been refractory to multiple antituberculosis drug therapies and have required orchiectomy.

[US Boxed Warning]: **May cause disseminated (including fatal) infections following intravesical administration.** Instillation to actively bleeding mucosa may promote systemic BCG infection or sepsis. To prevent serious infections, avoid trauma and/or introduction of contaminants into the urinary tract; postpone treatment for at least 1 to 2 weeks (depending on product) following TUR, biopsy, traumatic catheterization (may resume original schedule after 14 days), or gross hematuria. Do not use in patients with concurrent infections. Use caution in patients with aneurysms and prosthetic devices; ectopic BCG infection may occur at these sites. If signs and symptoms of a systemic BCG infection occur, permanently discontinue BCG treatment and begin therapy with 2 or more antimycobacterial agents (do not use single-agent therapy) while conducting a diagnostic evaluation. Infection from BCG (intravesical) is not sensitive to pyrazinamide. Do not use prophylactic antimycobacterial therapy to prevent local adverse events during treatment (there is no data to support use and may alter efficacy). If a bacterial urinary tract infection occurs, withhold therapy until complete resolution.

A systemic granulomatous illness occurring following exposure to BCG is referred to as a systemic BCG reaction when any of the following are present without another detectable etiology: Fever ≥39.5°C for ≥12 hours or ≥38.5°C for ≥48 hours; pneumonitis; hepatitis; organ dysfunction outside of the GU tract with granulomatous inflammation; clinical signs of sepsis. It may be difficult to determine if reaction is due to infection process or inflammatory hypersensitivity. A systemic BCG reaction is more likely to occur with intravesical administration <14 days after a biopsy, transurethral resection (TUR), or traumatic catheterization. Fatalities have been reported with systemic BCG reactions.

Intravesical instillations should be postponed during antibiotic therapy; antibiotics may reduce the efficacy of therapy. BCG (intravesical) may cause symptoms of bladder irritability which usually begin 4 to 6 hours after instillation and may last 24 to 72 hours; symptoms may increase in severity following each instillation. Intravesical instillation may be associated with increased risk of severe local reactions in the presence of small bladder capacity; use with caution. Packaging may contain natural latex rubber. BCG (intravesical) is not a vaccine for the prevention of cancer. Information is not available for interchanging products used for intravesical administration. Potentially significant drug-drug interactions may exist, requiring dose or frequency adjustment, additional monitoring, and/or selection of alternative therapy.

Adverse Reactions

>10%:

Central nervous system: Malaise (≤40%), chills (9% to 34%), pain (≤17%)

Gastrointestinal: Nausea (≤16%), vomiting (≤16%), anorexia (≤11%)

Genitourinary: Dysuria (52% to 60%), irritable bladder (50% to 60%), urinary frequency (40% to ≤50%), urinary urgency (6% to ≤50%), hematuria (26% to 39%), cystitis (6% to 30%), urinary tract infection (2% to 18%)

Hematologic & oncologic: Anemia (≤21%)

Respiratory: Flu-like symptoms (24% to 33%)

Miscellaneous: Fever (17% to 38%)

1% to 10%:

Central nervous system: Fatigue (≤7%), dizziness (≤2%), headache (≤2%)

Dermatologic: Diaphoresis (3%), skin rash (≤3%)

Endocrine & metabolic: Weight loss (≤2%)

Gastrointestinal: Diarrhea (≤6%), abdominal pain (2% to 3%)

Genitourinary: Genital pain (10%), nephrotoxicity (10%), hemorrhagic cystitis (9%), bladder spasm (≤8%; including contracted bladder), bladder pain (≤6%), urinary incontinence (2% to 6%), nocturia (5%), bladder contraction (≤5%), urine sedimentation abnormality (debris and tissue; ≤2%), epididymitis (≤1%), orchitis (≤1%), prostatitis (≤1%), pyuria (≤1%), urethritis (≤1%), urinary tract obstruction (≤1%)

Hematologic & oncologic: Leukopenia (≤5%), blood coagulation disorder (≤1%); thrombocytopenia (≤1%)

Hepatic: Granulomatous hepatitis (≤1%), hepatitis (≤1%)

Hypersensitivity: Hypersensitivity (2%)

Infection: Sepsis (3%; BCG sepsis: ≤1%), abscess (genital; ≤2%)

Neuromuscular & skeletal: Arthritis (≤7%), arthralgia (≤7%), myalgia (≤7%), muscle cramps (≤4%), rigors (3%)

Respiratory: Pulmonary infection (3%), pneumonitis (≤1%)

Miscellaneous: Inflammation (genital; ≤2%)

<1%, postmarketing, and/or case reports: Arthritis (reactive), chorioretinitis (granulomatous), conjunctivitis, constipation, erythema nodosum, flank pain, increased blood urea nitrogen, increased serum creatinine, infection (including systemic mycobacterium bovis infection of bone, bone marrow, kidney, lung, liver, lymph nodes, prostate), interstitial pulmonary disease, iritis, keratitis, localized infection (renal abscess), nephritis (includes glomerulonephritis, interstitial nephritis, renal tubulo-interstitial nephritis), pneumonia, pyelonephritis, renal failure, urinary retention (includes bladder tamponade and increased post-void residual urine volume), uveitis

◄ **Drug Interactions**

Metabolism/Transport Effects None known.

Avoid Concomitant Use

Avoid concomitant use of BCG (Intravesical) with any of the following: Antibiotics; Hexaminolevulinate; Immunosuppressants; Myelosuppressive Agents

Increased Effect/Toxicity There are no known significant interactions involving an increase in effect.

Decreased Effect

BCG (Intravesical) may decrease the levels/effects of: Hexaminolevulinate

The levels/effects of BCG (Intravesical) may be decreased by: Antibiotics; Immunosuppressants; Myelosuppressive Agents

Hazardous Drugs Handling Considerations

Hazardous agent (NIOSH 2016 [group 1]).

Use appropriate precautions for receiving, handling, administration, and disposal. Gloves (single) should be worn during receiving, unpacking, and placing in storage.

NIOSH recommends double gloving, a protective gown, and preparation in a controlled device or use of ventilated engineering controls (a class II biological safety cabinet or a compounding aseptic containment isolator); if not prepared in a controlled device, respiratory and eye/face protection as well as ventilated engineering controls are recommended. NIOSH recommends double gloving, a protective gown, and eye/face and respiratory protection for intravesical administration (NIOSH 2016).

Storage/Stability Store intact vials at 2°C to 8°C (36°F to 46°F). Protect from sunlight (direct or indirect); minimize exposure to artificial light. Use TheraCys immediately after reconstitution if possible, and do not exceed 2 hours stored at 2°C to 25°C (35°F to 77°F). Store TICE BCG at 2°C to 8°C (36°F to 46°F) and use within 2 hours of reconstitution.

Preparation for Administration

TheraCys: Reconstitute with 3 mL of sterile preservative free saline and shake gently to create a fine, even suspension (avoid foaming). Do not use if flocculation or clumping (that is not dispersed with gentle shaking) occurs after reconstitution. Withdraw contents (~3 mL) and further dilute with sterile preservative free saline to a final volume of 50 mL.

TICE BCG: Reconstitute with 1 mL sterile preservative free saline using a 3 mL syringe. Add to vial and swirl gently to form a homogenous suspension (forceful agitation may cause clumping). Dispense into a catheter tip syringe containing 49 mL of sterile preservative free saline. Mix by gently rotating the syringe.

Mechanism of Action BCG (intravesical) is an attenuated strain of bacillus Calmette-Guérin (*Mycobacterium bovis*) used as a biological response modi-fier. BCG, when used intravesicularly for treatment of bladder carcinoma *in situ*, is thought to cause a local, chronic inflammatory response involving macrophage and leukocyte infiltration of the bladder. BCG (intravesical) is active immunotherapy which stimulates the host's immune mechanism to reject the tumor.

Dosing

Adult & Geriatric

Bladder cancer: Intravesicular:

TheraCys: Induction: One dose (81 mg or one vial) instilled into bladder (retain for up to 2 hours) once weekly for 6 weeks beginning at least 14 days after biopsy or transurethral resection, followed by maintenance therapy of 81 mg (one vial) at 3, 6, 12, 18, and 24 months after initial dose.

TICE BCG: Induction: One dose (~50 mg or one vial) instilled into the bladder (retain for 2 hours) once weekly for 6 weeks beginning 7 to 14 days after biopsy (may repeat cycle 1 time if tumor remission not achieved), followed by maintenance therapy of ~50 mg (one vial) approximately once a month for at least 6 to 12 months.

Renal Impairment There are no dosage adjustments provided in the manufacturer's labeling.

Hepatic Impairment There are no dosage adjustments provided in the manufacturer's labeling.

Adjustment for Toxicity

Bacterial urinary tract infection: Withhold treatment until complete resolution. Persistent fever or acute febrile illness consistent with BCG infection: Discontinue treatment.

Administration For intravesicular (bladder instillation) administration only; **do not administer IV, SubQ, IM, or intradermally**.

Intravesicular: Patients should not drink fluids for 4 hours prior to instillation. Empty or drain bladder. Instill BCG (intravesical) by gravity; retain for as long as possible, up to 2 hours. Patient should lie prone for at least 15 minutes, then rotate positions (lie on right side, left side, abdomen, and back) every 15 minutes to maximize bladder surface exposure (TICE BCG); for TheraCys, patient may be in an upright position after the first 15 minutes. Following bladder instillation, patients should be instructed to void in a seated position in order to avoid the splashing of urine; burning may occur with the first void following therapy. Prior to flushing, disinfect the urine for 15 minutes with an equal amount of household bleach (this should be done for the first 6 hours after therapy). After administration, patients should drink plenty of water in order to flush the bladder.

Monitoring Parameters

PPD test prior to treatment

Intravesical treatment: Monitor for signs/symptoms of toxicity/infection following every treatment. Signs that antituberculous therapy may be needed: Flu-like symptoms ≥72 hours, fever ≥101.3°F, systemic symptoms which worsen with each treatment, persistently abnormal liver function tests, prostatitis, epididymitis or orchitis of >2 to 3 day duration

Test Interactions Use of BCG (intravesical) may result in tuberculin sensitivity. Determine the tuberculin reactivity of patients receiving BCG by PPD skin testing PRIOR to treatment initiation.

Dosage Forms Excipient information presented when available (limited, particularly for generics); consult specific product labeling.

Suspension Reconstituted, Intravesical:

Tice BCG: 50 mg (1 ea)

Suspension Reconstituted, Intravesical [preservative free]:

TheraCys: 81 mg (1 ea) [contains monosodium glutamate (sodium glutamate)]

- ◆ **BCG, Live** *see* BCG (Intravesical) *on page* 219
- ◆ **BCL-2 Inhibitor GDC-0199** *see* Venetoclax *on page* 1883
- ◆ **BCNU** *see* Carmustine *on page* 346
- ◆ **Bebulin** *see* Factor IX Complex (Human) [(Factors II, IX, X)] *on page* 767
- ◆ **Becenum** *see* Carmustine *on page* 346
- ◆ **Beleodaq** *see* Belinostat *on page* 224

Belinostat (be LIN oh stat)

Related Information

Safe Handling of Hazardous Drugs *on page* 2379

Brand Names: US Beleodaq

Index Terms PXD101

Pharmacologic Category Antineoplastic Agent, Histone Deacetylase (HDAC) Inhibitor

Use Peripheral T-cell lymphoma, relapsed or refractory: Treatment of relapsed or refractory peripheral T-cell lymphoma (PTCL).

Labeled Contraindications There are no contraindications listed in the manufacturer's labeling.

Pregnancy Considerations Animal reproduction studies have not been conducted. Belinostat is a genotoxic drug that targets dividing cells; embryofetal toxicity is expected if exposure occurs during pregnancy. Based on animal data, belinostat may also impair male fertility. Women of reproductive potential should avoid pregnancy during treatment with belinostat.

Breastfeeding Considerations It is not known if belinostat is present in breast milk. Due to the potential for serious adverse reactions in the breastfeeding infant, the manufacturer recommends that a decision be made whether to discontinue breastfeeding or to discontinue the drug, taking into account the importance of treatment to the mother.

Warnings/Precautions May cause thrombocytopenia, leukopenia (neutropenia and lymphopenia), and/or anemia. Monitor blood counts at baseline and weekly during treatment. May require dosage reduction, treatment delay, or discontinuation. Serious infections (occasionally fatal), including pneumonia and sepsis, have occurred with treatment. Do not administer in patients with an active infection. Heavily pretreated patients (history of extensive or intensive prior chemotherapy) may be at higher risk for life-threatening infections.

May cause liver function test abnormalities and fatal hepatotoxicity. Monitor liver function tests at baseline and prior to each cycle. May require dosage reduction, treatment delay, or permanent discontinuation (based on the severity of the hepatotoxicity). Belinostat is metabolized hepatically and increased exposure is expected to occur in patients with hepatic impairment. Patients with moderate to severe hepatic impairment (total bilirubin >1.5 times ULN) were excluded from clinical studies. Tumor lysis syndrome (TLS) has been observed; closely monitor patients with advanced disease and/or high tumor burden. If TLS occurs, initiate appropriate treatment. Nausea, vomiting, and diarrhea occur with belinostat; may require management with antiemetic and antidiarrheal medications. In a phase 1 study, nausea/vomiting generally occurred at the end of the infusion each day (rarely persisting beyond day 5 each cycle) and was managed with standard antiemetics (Steele 2011).

Belinostat is primarily metabolized by UGT1A1; the initial dose should be reduced in patients known to be homozygous for UGT1A1*28 allele. Potentially significant drug-drug interactions may exist, requiring dose or frequency adjustment, additional monitoring, and/or selection of alternative therapy.

Adverse Reactions

>10%:

Cardiovascular: Peripheral edema (20%), prolonged Q-T interval on ECG (11%; grades 3/4: 4%)

Central nervous system: Fatigue (37%; grades 3/4: 5%), chills (16%; grades 3/4: 1%), headache (15%)

Dermatologic: Skin rash (20%; grades 3/4: 1%), pruritus (16%; grades 3/4: 3%)

Endocrine & metabolic: Increased lactate dehydrogenase (16%; grades 3/4: 2%), hypokalemia (12%; grades 3/4: 4%)

Gastrointestinal: Nausea (42%; grades 3/4: 1%), vomiting (29%; grades 3/4: 1%), constipation (23%; grades 3/4: 1%), diarrhea (23%; grades 3/4: 2%), decreased appetite (15%; grades 3/4: 2%), abdominal pain (11%; grades 3/4: 1%)

Hematologic & oncologic: Anemia (32%; grades 3/4: 11%), thrombocytopenia (16%; grades 3/4: 7%)

Local: Pain at injection site (14%)

Respiratory: Dyspnea (22%, grades 3/4: 6%), cough (19%)

Miscellaneous: Fever (35%; grades 3/4: 2%)

1% to 10%:

Cardiovascular: Hypotension (10%; grades 3/4: 3%), phlebitis (10%; grades 3/4: 1%)

Central nervous system: Dizziness (10%)

Infection: Infection (>2%)

Renal: Increased serum creatinine (>2%)

Respiratory: Pneumonia (>2%)

Miscellaneous: Multi-organ failure (>2%)

<1%, postmarketing, and/or case reports: Abnormal hepatic function tests, febrile neutropenia, hepatic failure, hepatotoxicity, leukopenia, sepsis, tumor lysis syndrome, ventricular fibrillation

Drug Interactions

Metabolism/Transport Effects Substrate of CYP2A6 (minor), CYP2C9 (minor), CYP3A4 (minor), P-glycoprotein, UGT1A1; **Note:** Assignment of Major/Minor substrate status based on clinically relevant drug interaction potential; **Inhibits** CYP2C8 (weak), CYP2C9 (weak)

Avoid Concomitant Use

Avoid concomitant use of Belinostat with any of the following: Amodiaquine; Atazanavir; BCG (Intravesical); Deferiprone; Dipyrone

Increased Effect/Toxicity

Belinostat may increase the levels/effects of: Amodiaquine; CloZAPine; Deferiprone

The levels/effects of Belinostat may be increased by: Atazanavir; Dipyrone; Promazine

Decreased Effect

Belinostat may decrease the levels/effects of: BCG (Intravesical)

◄ **Hazardous Drugs Handling Considerations**
Hazardous agent (NIOSH 2016 [group 1]).

Use appropriate precautions for receiving, handling, administration, and disposal. Gloves (single) should be worn during receiving, unpacking, and placing in storage.

NIOSH recommends double gloving, a protective gown, and ventilated engineering controls (a class II biological safety cabinet or a compounding aseptic containment isolator), and closed system transfer devices (CSTDs) for preparation. Double gloving, a gown, and (if dosage form allows) CSTDs are required during administration (NIOSH 2016).

Storage/Stability Store intact vials at 20°C to 25°C (68°F to 77°F); excursions are permitted between 15°C and 30°C (59°F and 86°F). Retain in original package until use. The reconstituted solution may be stored for 12 hours at 15°C to 25°C (59°F to 77°F). Solutions diluted for infusion in NS may be stored for up to 36 hours (including infusion time) at 15°C to 25°C (59°F to 77°F).

Preparation for Administration Reconstitute each 500 mg vial with SWFI 9 mL to a concentration of 50 mg/mL. Swirl vial contents until there are no visible particles in the reconstituted solution. Further dilute the appropriate dose in NS 250 mL; do not use if cloudy or precipitate is present.

Mechanism of Action Belinostat is a histone deacetylase (HDAC) inhibitor which catalyzes acetyl group removal from protein lysine residues (of histone and some nonhistone proteins). Inhibition of histone deacetylase results in accumulation of acetyl groups, leading to cell cycle arrest and apoptosis. Belinostat has preferential cytotoxicity toward tumor cells versus normal cells.

Pharmacodynamics/Kinetics
Distribution: ~114 L/m^2 (Steele 2011); mean volume of distribution approaches total body water

Protein binding: ~93% to 96%

Metabolism: Hepatic; predominantly via UGT1A1, also by CYP2A6, CYP2C9, and CYP3A4 to the amide and acid metabolites

Half-life elimination: 1.1 hours

Time to peak: At end of infusion (Steele 2011)

Excretion: Urine (84.8% ± 9.8% over 168 hours, predominantly as metabolites; <2% as unchanged drug); feces (9.7% ± 6.5% over 168 hours)

Dosing
Adult & Geriatric Note: ANC should be ≥1,000/mm^3 and platelets should be ≥50,000/mm^3 prior to each cycle

Peripheral T-cell lymphoma, relapsed or refractory: IV: 1,000 mg/m^2 daily on days 1 to 5 every 21 days until disease progression or unacceptable toxicity (O'Connor 2013)

Dosage adjustment for patients with reduced UGT1A1 activity: Reduce initial dose to 750 mg/m^2 for patients known to be homozygous for UGT1A1*28 allele.

Renal Impairment
CrCl >39 mL/minute: There are no dosage adjustments provided in the manufacturer's labeling. However, exposure is not altered; dosage adjustment is not likely necessary.

CrCl ≤39 mL/minute: There are no dosage adjustments provided in the manufacturer's labeling (data is insufficient to recommend a dose).

Hepatic Impairment

Mild hepatic impairment: There are no dosage adjustments provided in the manufacturer's labeling (exposure is expected to be increased in hepatic impairment).

Moderate to severe hepatic impairment (total bilirubin >1.5 times ULN): There are no dosage adjustments provided in the manufacturer's labeling (data is insufficient to recommend a dose).

Obesity *ASCO Guidelines for appropriate chemotherapy dosing in obese adults with cancer:* Utilize patient's actual body weight (full weight) for calculation of body surface area- or weight-based dosing, particularly when the intent of therapy is curative; manage regimen-related toxicities in the same manner as for nonobese patients; if a dose reduction is utilized due to toxicity, consider resumption of full weight-based dosing with subsequent cycles, especially if cause of toxicity (eg, hepatic or renal impairment) is resolved (Griggs, 2012).

Adjustment for Toxicity

Hematologic toxicity: ANC should be ≥1000/mm^3 and platelets should be ≥50,000/mm^3 prior to each cycle and prior to resuming treatment following a delay due to toxicity. Resume subsequent treatment according to the following parameters:

Platelets ≥25,000/mm^3 and nadir ANC ≥500/mm^3: No dosage adjustment necessary (continue treatment without modification).

Nadir ANC <500/mm^3 and any platelet count: Reduce dose to 75% of the usual dose (to 750 mg/m^2).

Platelets <25,000/mm^3 and any nadir ANC: Reduce dose to 75% of the usual dose (to 750 mg/m^2).

Recurrent nadir ANC <500/mm^3 and/or recurrent nadir platelets <25,000/mm^3 following 2 dosage reductions: Discontinue treatment.

Nonhematologic toxicity: Nonhematologic toxicities should be grade 2 or lower prior to retreatment. Resume subsequent treatment according to the following parameters:

Any grade 3 or 4 toxicity (except nausea, vomiting, or diarrhea): Reduce dose to 75% of the usual dose (to 750 mg/m^2).

Recurrent grade 3 or 4 toxicity following 2 dosage reductions: Discontinue treatment.

Grade 3 or 4 nausea, vomiting, or diarrhea: Manage with supportive care; reduce the dose only if duration is >7 days with supportive management.

Administration IV: Infuse over 30 minutes using a 0.22-micron inline filter; if infusion site pain or other symptoms associated with infusion occur, may increase infusion time to 45 minutes.

Emetic Potential Low (10% to 30%)

Monitoring Parameters Monitor CBC with platelets and differential at baseline and weekly; serum chemistries (including renal and hepatic functions tests) at baseline and before each cycle; monitor for signs/symptoms of gastrointestinal toxicity (eg, nausea, vomiting, diarrhea), tumor lysis syndrome, and infection.

Dosage Forms Excipient information presented when available (limited, particularly for generics); consult specific product labeling.

Solution Reconstituted, Intravenous:

Beleodaq: 500 mg (1 ea)

Bendamustine (ben da MUS teen)

Related Information

Common Toxicity Criteria *on page 2242*

Management of Chemotherapy-Induced Nausea and Vomiting in Adults *on page 2253*

Management of Drug Extravasations *on page 2271*

Prevention of Chemotherapy-Induced Nausea and Vomiting in Children *on page 2310*

Safe Handling of Hazardous Drugs *on page 2379*

Brand Names: US Bendeka; Treanda

Brand Names: Canada Treanda

Index Terms Bendamustine HCl; Bendamustine Hydrochloride; Cytostasan; SDX-105

Pharmacologic Category Antineoplastic Agent, Alkylating Agent; Antineoplastic Agent, Alkylating Agent (Nitrogen Mustard)

Use

Chronic lymphocytic leukemia: Treatment of chronic lymphocytic leukemia (CLL)

Non-Hodgkin lymphoma: Treatment of indolent B-cell non-Hodgkin lymphoma (NHL) which has progressed during or within 6 months of rituximab treatment or a rituximab-containing regimen

Labeled Contraindications Known hypersensitivity (eg, anaphylactic or anaphylactoid reactions) to bendamustine or any component of the formulation. Bendeka is also contraindicated in patients with hypersensitivity to polyethylene glycol 400, propylene glycol, or monothioglycerol.

Pregnancy Considerations Adverse events were observed in animal reproduction studies. May cause fetal harm if administered during pregnancy. For women and men of reproductive potential, effective contraception should be used during and for 3 months after treatment.

Breastfeeding Considerations It is not known if bendamustine is excreted in breast milk. Due to the potential for serious adverse reactions in the nursing infant, a decision should be made to discontinue bendamustine or discontinue breastfeeding, taking into account the benefits of treatment to the mother.

Warnings/Precautions Myelosuppression (neutropenia, thrombocytopenia, and anemia) is a common toxicity; may require therapy delay and/or dose reduction; monitor blood counts frequently (nadirs typically occurred in the third week of treatment). Complications due to febrile neutropenia and severe thrombocytopenia have been reported (some fatal). ANC should recover to ≥1000/mm^3 and platelets to ≥75,000/mm^3 prior to cycle initiation. Pneumonia, hepatitis, sepsis, and septic shock have been reported; fatalities due to infection have occurred; patients with myelosuppression are more susceptible to infection; monitor closely. Reactivation of hepatitis B, cytomegalovirus, Mycobacterium tuberculosis, and herpes zoster infection may occur in patients receiving bendamustine. Monitor; may require infection prophylaxis and/or treatment prior to bendamustine administration.

Infusion reactions, including chills, fever, pruritus, and rash are common; rarely, anaphylactic and anaphylactoid reactions have occurred, particularly with the second or subsequent cycle(s). Patients who experienced grade 3 or higher allergic reactions should not be rechallenged. Consider premedication with antihistamines, antipyretics, and corticosteroids for patients with a history of grade 1 or 2 infusion reaction. Discontinue for severe allergic reaction or grade 4 infusion reaction; consider discontinuation with grade 3 infusion reaction. Serious and fatal dermatologic toxicities, including Stevens-Johnson syndrome (SJS) and toxic epidermal necrolysis (TEN), drug reaction with eosinophilia and systemic symptoms (DRESS), bullous exanthema, and rash have been reported. Skin reactions have been reported with monotherapy and in combination with other antineoplastic agents or allopurinol and may be progressive or worsen with continued treatment. The risk for severe skin toxicity is increased with concurrent use of allopurinol and other medications known to cause skin toxicity. Monitor closely for dermatologic toxicity. Withhold or discontinue treatment for severe or progressive skin reaction. Bendamustine is an irritant with vesicant-like properties; ensure proper needle or catheter placement prior to and during infusion; avoid extravasation; erythema, marked swelling, and pain have been reported with extravasation. Bendamustine is associated with a moderate emetic potential (Basch 2011; Dupuis 2011; Roila 2016); antiemetics are recommended to prevent nausea and vomiting.

Tumor lysis syndrome (usually occurring in the first treatment cycle) may occur as a consequence of antineoplastic treatment, including treatment with bendamustine. May lead to life-threatening acute renal failure (without intervention); vigorous hydration and prophylactic measures (eg, antihyperuricemic therapy) should be instituted prior to treatment in high-risk patients; monitor closely. **Note:** Allopurinol may increase the risk for bendamustine skin toxicity. May cause hypokalemia; monitor potassium closely during therapy, particularly in patients with cardiac disease.

Serious and fatal cases of liver injury have been reported, usually within the first 3 months of treatment initiation. Confounding factors in some patients included combination therapy, progressive disease, and/or hepatitis B reactivation. Monitor liver function tests. Use with caution in patients with mild hepatic impairment. A pharmacokinetic study showed only slight differences in bendamustine AUC and C_{max} in patients with mild hepatic impairment (defined in the study as total bilirubin 1 to 1.5 times ULN or AST greater than ULN), as compared to patients with normal hepatic function (Owen 2010). Use is not recommended in patients with moderate (AST or ALT 2.5 to 10 times ULN and total bilirubin 1.5 to 3 times ULN) or severe (total bilirubin >3 times ULN) hepatic impairment.

Use with caution in patients with mild to moderate renal impairment. According to the manufacturer, use is not recommended in patients with CrCl <40 mL/minute. A pharmacokinetic study illustrated only slight differences in bendamustine AUC and C_{max} in patients with mild (CrCl >50 to ≤80 mL/minute) and moderate (CrCl >30 to ≤50 mL/minute) renal dysfunction, compared to patients with normal renal function (Owen 2010). A retrospective safety study found no significant difference in lab toxicities between CLL patients with renal impairment (CrCl <40 mL/minute) compared to those without renal impairment, although an increase in grades 3/4 thrombocytopenia and grades 3/4 BUN increases were detected in patients with renal impairment (Nordstrom 2012); monitor blood counts and renal function. **Note:** UK labeling (Levact prescribing information, October 2010) recommends no dosage adjustment for patients with CrCl >10 mL/minute. Secondary malignancies (including myelodysplastic syndrome, myeloproliferative disorders, acute myeloid leukemia and bronchial cancer) and premalignant diseases have been reported in patients who have received bendamustine. Potentially significant drug-drug interactions may exist, requiring dose or frequency adjustment, additional monitoring, and/or selection of alternative therapy.

Several formulations of bendamustine are available: a liquid solution formulation (45 mg/0.5 mL and 180 mg/2 mL [Treanda] and 100 mg/4 mL [Bendeka]) and a powder for reconstitution (5 mg/mL after reconstitution [Treanda]). Concentrations, storage, and compatibility differ between formulations. Use caution when selecting bendamustine formulation for preparation and administration. Do not mix or combine the formulations. Bendamustine solution (Treanda: 45 mg/0.5 mL and 180 mg/2 mL) contains N,N-dimethylacetamide, which is incompatible with closed-system transfer devices (CSTDs), adapters, and syringes containing polycarbonate or acrylonitrile-butadiene-styrene (ABS). When used to prepare or transfer the concentrated bendamustine solution into the infusion bag, the plastic components of these devices may dissolve, resulting in subsequent leakage and potential infusion of dissolved plastic into the patient (ISMP [Smetzer 2015]). Do not use the liquid solution formulation if CSTDs, adapters, and syringes containing polycarbonate or ABS are used **prior** to dilution in the infusion bag; according to the Treanda manufacturer, after dilution into the infusion bag, devices containing polycarbonate or ABS (including infusion sets) may be used. Some dosage forms may contain propylene glycol; large amounts are potentially toxic and have been associated with hyperosmolality, lactic acidosis, seizures and respiratory depression; use caution (AAP 1997; Zar 2007). See manufacturer's labeling.

Adverse Reactions

>10%:

Cardiovascular: Peripheral edema (13%)

Central nervous system: Fatigue (9% to 57%), headache (21%), dizziness (14%), chills (6% to 14%), insomnia (13%)

Dermatologic: Skin rash (8% to 16%)

Endocrine & metabolic: Weight loss (7% to 18%), dehydration (14%)

Gastrointestinal: Nausea (20% to 75%), vomiting (16% to 40%), diarrhea (9% to 37%), constipation (29%), anorexia (23%), stomatitis (15%), abdominal pain (13%), decreased appetite (13%), dyspepsia (11%)

Hematologic & oncologic: Lymphocytopenia (68% to 99%; grades 3/4: 47% to 94%), bone marrow depression (grades 3/4: 98%; nadir: in week 3), leukopenia (61% to 94%; grades 3/4: 28% to 56%), decreased hemoglobin (88% to 89%; grades 3/4: 11% to 13%), decreased neutrophils (75% to 86%; grades 3/4: 43% to 60%), thrombocytopenia (77% to 86%; grades 3/4: 11% to 25%)

Hepatic: Increased serum bilirubin (34%)

Neuromuscular & skeletal: Back pain (14%), weakness (8% to 11%)

Respiratory: Cough (4% to 22%), dyspnea (16%)

Miscellaneous: Fever (24% to 34%)

1% to 10%:

Cardiovascular: Tachycardia (7%), chest pain (6%), hypotension (6%), exacerbation of hypertension (3%)

Central nervous system: Anxiety (8%), depression (6%), pain (6%)

Dermatologic: Pruritus (5% to 6%), hyperhidrosis (5%), night sweats (5%), xeroderma (5%)

Endocrine & metabolic: Hypokalemia (9%), hyperuricemia (7%), hyperglycemia (grades 3/4: 3%), hypocalcemia (grades 3/4: 2%), hyponatremia (grades 3/4: 2%)

Gastrointestinal: Gastroesophageal reflux disease (10%), xerostomia (9%), dysgeusia (7%), oral candidiasis (6%), abdominal distention (5%), upper abdominal pain (5%)

Genitourinary: Urinary tract infection (10%)

Hematologic & oncologic: Febrile neutropenia (grades 3/4: 6%)

Hepatic: Increased serum ALT (grades 3/4: 3%), increased serum AST (grades 3/4: 1%)

Hypersensitivity: Hypersensitivity (5%)

Infection: Herpes zoster (10%), infection (6%), herpes simplex infection (3%)

Local: Infusion site pain (6%), catheter pain (5%)

Neuromuscular & skeletal: Arthralgia (6%), limb pain (5%), ostealgia (5%)

Renal: Increased serum creatinine (grades 3/4: 2%)

Respiratory: Upper respiratory tract infection (10%), sinusitis (9%), pharyngolaryngeal pain (8%), pneumonia (8%), nasopharyngitis (6% to 7%), nasal congestion (5%), wheezing (5%)

Frequency not defined:

Central nervous system: Drowsiness, malaise

Dermatologic: Dermatitis, skin necrosis

Gastrointestinal: Mucositis

Hematologic & oncologic: Hemolysis

<1%, postmarketing, and/or case reports: Acute renal failure, anaphylactoid reaction, anaphylaxis, atrial fibrillation, bronchogenic carcinoma, bullous rash, cardiac failure, dermatological reaction (toxic), DRESS syndrome, erythema, extravasation injury, hepatitis, hepatotoxicity, injection site reaction (including irritation, pain, phlebitis, pruritus, swelling), myelodysplastic syndrome, myeloid leukemia (acute), myocardial infarction, neutropenic sepsis, palpitations, pancytopenia, pneumonia (*Pneumocystis jirovecii*), pneumonitis, pulmonary alveolar hemorrhage (with grade 3 thrombocytopenia), pulmonary fibrosis, reactivation of disease (including, but not limited to hepatitis B, cytomegalovirus, *Mycobacterium tuberculosis*, herpes zoster), sepsis, septic shock, Stevens-Johnson syndrome, toxic epidermal necrolysis, tumor lysis syndrome

Drug Interactions

Metabolism/Transport Effects Substrate of BCRP, CYP1A2 (minor), P-glycoprotein; **Note:** Assignment of Major/Minor substrate status based on clinically relevant drug interaction potential

Avoid Concomitant Use

Avoid concomitant use of Bendamustine with any of the following: BCG (Intravesical); Deferiprone; Dipyrone

Increased Effect/Toxicity

Bendamustine may increase the levels/effects of: CloZAPine; Deferiprone

The levels/effects of Bendamustine may be increased by: Allopurinol; Ciprofloxacin (Systemic); CYP1A2 Inhibitors (Strong); Dipyrone; Palifermin; Promazine

Decreased Effect

Bendamustine may decrease the levels/effects of: BCG (Intravesical); Lenograstim

The levels/effects of Bendamustine may be decreased by: CYP1A2 Inducers (Moderate)

Hazardous Drugs Handling Considerations

Hazardous agent (NIOSH 2016 [group 1]).

Use appropriate precautions for receiving, handling, administration, and disposal. Gloves (single) should be worn during receiving, unpacking, and placing in storage.

NIOSH recommends double gloving, a protective gown, ventilated engineering controls (a class II biological safety cabinet or a compounding aseptic containment isolator), and (if compatible) closed system transfer devices (CSTDs) for preparation. Double gloving, a gown, and (if compatible and dosage form allows) CSTDs are required during administration (NIOSH 2016).

Storage/Stability

Bendeka:

Solution: Store intact vials between 2°C to 8°C (36°F to 46°F); protect from light. Refrigerated vials may partially freeze at the recommended storage temperature; allow to come to room temperature prior to use. Solutions for infusion should be prepared as close as possible to administration. Solutions diluted with NS or D2.5½NS are stable for up to 24 hours when stored at 2°C to 8°C (36°F to 46°F) or for up to 6 hours when stored at 15°C to 30°C (59°F to 86°F) and room light. Solutions diluted with D5W are stable for up to 24 hours when stored at 2°C to 8°C (36°F to 46°F) or for up to 3 hours when stored at 15°C to 30°C (59°F to 86°F) and room light. Infusion must be completed within these time frames. Bendeka is a multiple-dose vial; after the first use, partially used vials are stable for up to 28 days when stored in the original carton at 2°C to 8°C (36°F to 46°F). Do not withdraw more than 6 doses from each vial.

Treanda:

Powder for solution: Prior to reconstitution, store intact vials up to 25°C (77°F); excursions are permitted up to 30°C (86°F). Protect from light. The solution in the vial (reconstituted with SWFI) is stable for 30 minutes (transfer to 500 mL infusion bag within that 30 minutes). The solution diluted in 500 mL of NS or D2.5½NS for infusion is stable for 24 hours refrigerated (2°C to 8°C [36°F to 46°F]) or 3 hours at room temperature (15°C to 30°C [59°F to 86°F]) and room light. Infusion must be completed within these time frames.

Solution: Store intact vials between 2°C to 8°C (36°F to 46°F); protect from light. Solutions diluted for infusion in NS or D2.5½NS are stable for up to 24 hours when stored at 2°C to 8°C (36°F to 46°F) or for up to 2 hours when stored at 15°C to 30°C (59°F to 86°F) and room light. Infusion must be completed within these time frames.

Preparation for Administration

Several formulations of bendamustine are available: A liquid solution formulation (45 mg/0.5 mL and 180 mg/2 mL [Treanda] and 100 mg/4 mL [Bendeka]) and the powder for reconstitution (5 mg/mL after reconstitution [Treanda]). Concentrations, storage, and compatibility differ between formulations. Use caution when selecting bendamustine formulation for preparation and administration. Do not mix or combine the formulations.

Bendeka: Prior to administration, allow vial(s) to reach room temperature. Refrigerated vials may partially freeze while under refrigeration; do not use if particles are observed after reaching room temperature. Dilute appropriate dose in 50 mL of NS, D2.5½NS, or D5W to a final concentration of 1.85 to 5.6 mg/mL; thoroughly mix. The resulting solution should be clear and colorless to yellow.

Treanda:

Powder for solution (for reconstitution): Reconstitute 25 mg vial with 5 mL and 100 mg vial with 20 mL of sterile water for injection to a concentration of 5 mg/mL; powder usually dissolves within 5 minutes (do not use if particulates are visible). Within 30 minutes of reconstitution, dilute appropriate dose for infusion in 500 mL NS (or D2.5½NS) to a final concentration of 0.2 to 0.6 mg/mL; mix thoroughly. Closed-system transfer devices (CSTDs) or adaptors containing polycarbonate or acrylonitrile-butadiene-styrene (ABS) are safe to use with the lyophilized powder formulation.

Solution: Prior to administration, dilute appropriate dose (using polypropylene syringes with a metal needle and polypropylene hub) in 500 mL NS (or D2.5^1/$_2$NS) to a final concentration of 0.2 to 0.7 mg/mL; resulting solution should be colorless to yellow. Bendamustine contains N,N-dimethylacetamide, which is incompatible with CSTDs, adapters, and syringes containing polycarbonate or ABS. When used to prepare or transfer the concentrated bendamustine solution into the infusion bag, the plastic components of these devices may dissolve, resulting in subsequent leakage and potential infusion of dissolved plastic into the patient (ISMP [Smetzer 2015]). If using a syringe to withdraw and transfer bendamustine solution from the vial into the infusion bag, only use polypropylene syringes (translucent in appearance) with a metal needle and polypropylene hub. **After** dilution into the infusion bag, devices containing polycarbonate or ABS (including infusion sets) may be used.

Mechanism of Action Bendamustine is an alkylating agent (nitrogen mustard derivative) with a benzimidazole ring (purine analog) which demonstrates only partial cross-resistance (*in vitro*) with other alkylating agents. It leads to cell death via single and double strand DNA cross-linking. Bendamustine is active against quiescent and dividing cells. The primary cytotoxic activity is due to bendamustine (as compared to metabolites).

Pharmacodynamics/Kinetics

Distribution: V_{ss}: ~20 to 25 L

Protein binding: 94% to 96%

Metabolism: Hepatic (extensive), via CYP1A2 to active (minor) metabolites gamma-hydroxy bendamustine (M3) and N-desmethyl-bendamustine (M4); also via hydrolysis to low cytotoxic metabolites, monohydroxy bendamustine (HP1) and dihydroxy bendamustine (HP2)

Half-life elimination: Bendamustine: ~40 minutes; M3: ~3 hours; M4: ~30 minutes

Time to peak, serum: At end of infusion

Excretion: Feces (~25%); urine (~50%; ~3% as active parent drug)

Pharmacokinetic note: In a pharmacokinetic study, a 10 minute infusion of Bendeka (120 mg/m^2) resulted in higher maximum plasma concentrations and equivalent systemic exposure as the same dose of Treanda infused over 60 minutes.

Dosing

Adult & Geriatric Note: Treanda liquid solution formulation (45 mg/0.5 mL and 180 mg/2 mL) has been discontinued in the US for more than 1 year.

Note: Bendamustine is associated with a moderate emetic potential (Basch 2011; Roila 2016); antiemetics are recommended to prevent nausea and vomiting.

Chronic lymphocytic leukemia (CLL): IV: 100 mg/m^2 on days 1 and 2 of a 28-day treatment cycle (as a single agent) for up to 6 cycles (Knauf 2009; Knauf 2012)

CLL, first-line treatment (off-label dosing): IV: 90 mg/m^2 on days 1 and 2 of a 28-day treatment cycle (in combination with rituximab) for up to 6 cycles (Fischer 2012)

CLL, relapsed/refractory (off-label dosing): IV: 70 mg/m^2 on days 1 and 2 of a 28-day treatment cycle (in combination with rituximab) for up to 6 cycles (Fischer 2011)

◀ **Non-Hodgkin lymphomas:** IV:

Lymphoma, indolent B-cell, refractory: 120 mg/m^2 on days 1 and 2 of a 21-day treatment cycle (as a single agent) for up to 8 cycles (Kahl 2010)

Lymphoma, indolent B-cell, follicular, or mantle cell, first-line (off-label use): 90 mg/m^2 over 30 to 60 minutes on days 1 and 2 of a 28-day treatment cycle (in combination with rituximab) for up to 6 cycles (Rummel 2013) **or** 90 mg/m^2 over 30 minutes on days 1 and 2 of a 28-day treatment cycle (in combination with rituximab) for 6 to 8 cycles (Flinn, 2014)

Lymphoma, follicular, relapsed or refractory (off-label use): 90 mg/m^2 over 60 minutes on days 1 and 2 of a 35-day treatment cycle (in combination with bortezomib and rituximab) for 5 cycles (Fowler 2011) **or** 90 mg/m^2 on days 1 and 2 of a 28-day treatment cycle for 6 cycles (in combination with obinutuzumab, then followed by obinutuzumab monotherapy in patients with stable disease, complete response, or partial response after 6 cycles of combination therapy) (Sehn 2016)

Lymphoma, mantle cell, relapsed or refractory (off-label use): 90 mg/m^2 over 30 minutes on days 2 and 3 of a 28-day treatment cycle (in combination with rituximab) for up to 4 cycles (Rummel 2005)

Hodgkin lymphoma, relapsed or refractory (off-label use): IV: 120 mg/m^2 over 30 minutes on days 1 and 2 of a 28-day treatment cycle for up to 6 cycles (Moskowitz 2013)

Multiple myeloma, salvage therapy (off-label use): IV: 90 to 100 mg/m^2 on days 1 and 2 of a 28-day treatment cycle for at least 2 cycles (Knop, 2005) **or** 75 mg/m^2 on days 1 and 2 of a 28-day treatment cycle (in combination with lenalidomide and dexamethasone) for up to 8 cycles (Lentzsch 2012)

Waldenström macroglobulinemia, refractory (off-label use): IV: 90 mg/m^2 on days 1 and 2 of a 28-day treatment cycle (in combination with rituximab) for 6 cycles (Treon 2011) **or** 90 mg/m^2 over 30 minutes on days 2 and 3 of a 28-day treatment cycle (in combination with rituximab) for 4 cycles (Rummel 2005)

Renal Impairment

CrCl <40 mL/minute: Use is not recommended (according to the manufacturer's labeling).

Study data suggest minor changes in systemic exposure may occur with mild-to-moderate renal impairment. Based on a pharmacokinetic study (patients receiving 120 mg/m^2 for 2 days every 21 days), only slight differences in bendamustine AUC and C$_{max}$ were demonstrated in patients with mild (CrCl >50 to ≤80 mL/minute) and moderate (CrCl >30 to ≤50 mL/minute) renal dysfunction, compared to patients with normal renal function (Owen 2010). A retrospective study of bendamustine in CLL and NHL patients with renal impairment (CrCl <40 mL/minute) compared to those without (CrCl ≥60 mL/minute) found no significant difference in lab toxicities in CLL patients with renal impairment compared to those without renal impairment, although an increase in grades 3/4 thrombocytopenia was noted in NHL patients and grades 3/4 BUN increases were higher when combining data for CLL and NHL (Nordstrom 2012).

Note: UK manufacturer's labeling (Levact [prescribing information], October 2010) recommends no dosage adjustment is necessary for patients with CrCl >10 mL/minute.

Hepatic Impairment

Mild impairment: Use with caution. However, a pharmacokinetic study showed only slight differences in bendamustine AUC and C$_{max}$ in patients with mild hepatic impairment (defined in the study as total bilirubin 1 to 1.5 times ULN or AST greater than ULN), compared to patients with normal hepatic function (Owen 2010).

Moderate impairment (AST or ALT 2.5 to 10 times ULN and total bilirubin 1.5 to 3 times ULN): Use is not recommended.

Severe impairment (total bilirubin >3 times ULN): Use is not recommended.

Obesity *American Society of Clinical Oncology (ASCO) Guidelines for appropriate chemotherapy dosing in obese adults with cancer:* Utilize patient's actual body weight (full weight) for calculation of body surface area- or weight-based dosing, particularly when the intent of therapy is curative; manage regimen-related toxicities in the same manner as for nonobese patients; if a dose reduction is utilized due to toxicity, consider resumption of full weight-based dosing with subsequent cycles, especially if cause of toxicity (eg, hepatic or renal impairment) is resolved (Griggs 2012).

Adjustment for Toxicity

Infusion reactions:

Grade 1 or 2: Consider premedication with antihistamines, antipyretics, and corticosteroids in subsequent cycles

Grade 3: Consider discontinuing treatment

Grade 4: Discontinue treatment

Skin reaction, severe or progressive: Withhold or discontinue treatment

Treatment delay:

Hematologic toxicity ≥ grade 4: Delay treatment until resolves (ANC ≥1000/mm^3, platelets ≥75,000/mm^3)

Nonhematologic toxicity ≥ grade 2 (clinically significant): Delay treatment until resolves to ≤ grade 1

Dose modification CLL:

Hematologic toxicity ≥ grade 3: Reduce dose to 50 mg/m^2 on days 1 and 2 of each treatment cycle. For recurrent hematologic toxicity (≥ grade 3), further reduce dose to 25 mg/m^2 on days 1 and 2 of the treatment cycle. May cautiously re-escalate dose in subsequent cycles.

Nonhematologic toxicity ≥ grade 3 (clinically significant): Reduce dose to 50 mg/m^2 on days 1 and 2 of the treatment cycle with discretion. May cautiously re-escalate dose in subsequent cycles.

Dose modification in NHL:

Hematologic toxicity grade 4: Reduce dose to 90 mg/m^2 on days 1 and 2 of each treatment cycle. For recurrent hematologic toxicity (grade 4), further reduce dose to 60 mg/m^2 on days 1 and 2 of each treatment cycle.

Nonhematologic toxicity ≥ grade 3: Reduce dose to 90 mg/m^2 on days 1 and 2 of the treatment cycle with discretion. For recurrent toxicity ≥ grade 3, further reduce dose to 60 mg/m^2 on days 1 and 2 of each treatment cycle.

Combination Regimens

Leukemia, chronic lymphocytic:

Bendamustine-Rituximab (CLL) on page 1986

Ibrutinib-Bendamustine-Rituximab (CLL) on page 2152

Lymphoma, non-Hodgkin (Follicular):

Bendamustine-Bortezomib-Rituximab (NHL-Follicular) on page 1985

Bendamustine-Obinutuzumab (NHL-Follicular) on page 1986

Bendamustine-Rituximab (NHL-Follicular) on page 1987

Lymphoma, non-Hodgkin (Mantle cell): Bendamustine-Rituximab (NHL-Mantle Cell) on page 1987

Multiple myeloma: Bendamustine-Lenalidomide-Dexamethasone (Multiple Myeloma) on page 1986

Waldenstrom Macroglobulinemia: Bendamustine-Rituximab (Waldenstrom Macroglobulinemia) on page 1988

Administration

For chronic lymphocytic leukemia, infuse over 30 minutes (Treanda) or 10 minutes (Bendeka). For non-Hodgkin lymphoma, infuse over 60 minutes (Treanda) or 10 minutes (Bendeka). Administration times for off-label uses/doses vary by protocol.

Bendamustine solution (45 mg/0.5 mL and 180 mg/2 mL [Treanda]) contains N, N-dimethylacetamide, which is incompatible with closed-system transfer devices (CSTDs), adapters, and syringes containing polycarbonate or acrylonitrile-butadiene-styrene (ABS). After dilution of bendamustine solution (Treanda) into the infusion bag, devices containing polycarbonate or ABS (including infusion sets) may be used.

Consider premedication with antihistamines, antipyretics, and corticosteroids for patients with a previous grade 1 or 2 infusion reaction to bendamustine. Bendamustine is associated with a moderate emetic potential (Basch 2011; Dupuis 2011; Roila 2016); antiemetics are recommended to prevent nausea and vomiting.

Irritant with vesicant-like properties; ensure proper needle or catheter placement prior to and during infusion. Avoid extravasation; monitor IV site for redness, swelling, or pain.

Extravasation management: If extravasation occurs, stop infusion immediately and disconnect (leave cannula/needle in place); gently aspirate extravasated solution (do **NOT** flush the line); remove needle/cannula; elevate extremity. Apply dry cold compresses for 20 minutes 4 times daily (Perez Fildago 2012). May be managed with sodium thiosulfate in the same manner as mechlorethamine extravasation (Schulmeister 2011).

Sodium thiosulfate 1/6 M solution (instructions for mechlorethamine): Inject subcutaneously into extravasation area using 2 mL for each mg of drug suspected to have extravasated (Perez Fidalgo 2012; Polovich 2009).

Vesicant/Extravasation Risk Irritant with vesicant-like properties; there are case reports of erythema, swelling, and pain from extravasation

Emetic Potential Children and Adults: Moderate (30% to 90%)

Monitoring Parameters CBC with differential and platelets (monitored weekly [initially] in clinical trials); serum creatinine; liver function tests (ALT, AST, and total bilirubin; prior to and during treatment); monitor potassium and uric acid levels in patients at risk for tumor lysis syndrome; monitor for infusion reactions anaphylaxis, infection (including reactivations), and dermatologic toxicity; monitor IV site during and after infusion.

Product Availability Treanda liquid solution formulation (45 mg/0.5 mL and 180 mg/2 mL has been discontinued in the US for more than 1 year.

Dosage Forms Excipient information presented when available (limited, particularly for generics); consult specific product labeling. [DSC] = Discontinued product

Solution, Intravenous, as hydrochloride:

Bendeka: 100 mg/4 mL (4 mL) [contains polyethylene glycol, propylene glycol]

Treanda: 45 mg/0.5 mL (0.5 mL [DSC]); 180 mg/2 mL (2 mL [DSC]) [contains propylene glycol]

Solution Reconstituted, Intravenous, as hydrochloride:

Treanda: 25 mg (1 ea); 100 mg (1 ea)

- **Bendamustine HCl** *see* Bendamustine *on page* 228
- **Bendamustine Hydrochloride** *see* Bendamustine *on page* 228
- **Bendeka** *see* Bendamustine *on page* 228
- **BeneFIX** *see* Factor IX (Recombinant) *on page* 773
- **BeneFix (Can)** *see* Factor IX (Recombinant) *on page* 773
- **Benzmethyzin** *see* Procarbazine *on page* 1557
- **Benzoyl Metronidazole** *see* MetroNIDAZOLE (Systemic) *on page* 1249
- **Besponsa** *see* Inotuzumab Ozogamicin *on page* 1011

Bevacizumab (be vuh SIZ uh mab)

Related Information

Chemotherapy-Induced Peripheral Neuropathy *on page* 2236

Common Toxicity Criteria *on page* 2242

Management of Chemotherapy-Induced Nausea and Vomiting in Adults *on page* 2253

Prevention of Chemotherapy-Induced Nausea and Vomiting in Children *on page* 2310

Brand Names: US Avastin

Brand Names: Canada Avastin

Index Terms Anti-VEGF Monoclonal Antibody; Anti-VEGF rhuMAb; Bevacizumab, inj; rhuMAb-VEGF

Pharmacologic Category Antineoplastic Agent, Monoclonal Antibody; Antineoplastic Agent, Vascular Endothelial Growth Factor (VEGF) Inhibitor; Vascular Endothelial Growth Factor (VEGF) Inhibitor

Use

Cervical cancer, persistent/recurrent/metastatic: Treatment of persistent, recurrent, or metastatic cervical cancer (in combination with paclitaxel and either cisplatin or topotecan).

Colorectal cancer, metastatic: First- or second-line treatment of metastatic colorectal cancer (CRC) (in combination with fluorouracil-based chemotherapy); second-line treatment of metastatic CRC (in combination with fluoropyrimidine-irinotecan- or fluoropyrimidine-oxaliplatin-based chemotherapy) after progression on a first line treatment containing bevacizumab.

Limitations of use: Not indicated for the adjuvant treatment of colon cancer.

Glioblastoma: Treatment of progressive glioblastoma (as a single agent).

Non-small cell lung cancer, nonsquamous: First-line treatment of unresectable, locally advanced, recurrent or metastatic nonsquamous non-small cell lung cancer (NSCLC) (in combination with carboplatin and paclitaxel).

Ovarian (epithelial), fallopian tube, or primary peritoneal cancer (platinum-resistant recurrent): Treatment of platinum-resistant recurrent epithelial ovarian, fallopian tube, or primary peritoneal cancer (in combination with paclitaxel, doxorubicin [liposomal], or topotecan) in patients who received no more than 2 prior chemotherapy regimens.

Ovarian (epithelial), fallopian tube, or primary peritoneal cancer (platinum-sensitive recurrent): Treatment of platinum-sensitive recurrent epithelial ovarian, fallopian tube, or primary peritoneal cancer (in combination with carboplatin and paclitaxel or with carboplatin and gemcitabine and then followed by single-agent bevacizumab).

Renal cell carcinoma, metastatic: Treatment of metastatic renal cell carcinoma (RCC) (in combination with interferon alfa).

◄ **Labeled Contraindications**

There are no contraindications listed in the manufacturer's labeling.

Canadian labeling: Hypersensitivity to bevacizumab, any component of the formulation, Chinese hamster ovary cell products or other recombinant human or humanized antibodies; untreated CNS metastases

Pregnancy Considerations Based on its mechanism of action, bevacizumab would be expected to cause fetal harm if administered to a pregnant woman. Information from postmarketing reports following exposure in pregnancy is limited. Women of reproductive potential should use effective contraception during therapy and for 6 months following the last dose (due to the long half-life of bevacizumab). Bevacizumab treatment may also increase the risk of ovarian failure and impair fertility; long term effects on fertility are not known.

Breastfeeding Considerations It is not known if bevacizumab is excreted in breast milk. Immunoglobulins are excreted in breast milk, and it is assumed that bevacizumab may appear in breast milk. Because of the potential for serious adverse reactions in the nursing infant, breastfeeding is not recommended. The half-life of bevacizumab is up to 50 days (average 20 days), and this should be considered when decisions are made concerning breastfeeding resumption.

Warnings/Precautions [US Boxed Warning]: Gastrointestinal (GI) perforation (sometimes fatal) has occurred in 0.3 to 3.2% of clinical study patients receiving bevacizumab; discontinue (permanently) if GI perforation occurs. All cervical cancer patients with GI perforation had a history of prior pelvic radiation. GI perforation was observed in patients with platinum-resistant ovarian cancer, although patients with evidence of recto-sigmoid involvement (by pelvic exam), bowel involvement (on CT scan), or clinical symptoms of bowel obstruction were excluded from the study; avoid bevacizumab use in these ovarian cancer patient populations. Most cases occur within 50 days of treatment initiation; monitor patients for signs/symptoms (eg, fever, abdominal pain with constipation and/or nausea/vomiting). GI fistula (including enterocutaneous, esophageal, duodenal, and rectal fistulas), and intra-abdominal abscess have been reported in patients receiving bevacizumab for colorectal cancer, ovarian cancer, and other cancers (not related to treatment duration). Non-GI fistula formation (including tracheoesophageal, bronchopleural, biliary, vaginal, vesical, renal, bladder, and female tract fistulas) has been observed (rarely fatal), most commonly within the first 6 months of treatment. Gastrointestinal-vaginal fistulas have been reported in cervical cancer patients, all of whom had received prior pelvic radiation; patients may also have bowel obstructions requiring surgical intervention and diverting ostomies. Permanently discontinue in patients who develop internal organ fistulas, tracheoesophageal (TE) fistula, or any grade 4 fistula.

[US Boxed Warning]: The incidence of wound healing and surgical complications, including serious and fatal events, is increased in patients who have received bevacizumab; discontinue with wound dehiscence. Although the appropriate interval between withholding bevacizumab and elective surgery has not been defined, bevacizumab should be discontinued at least 28 days prior to surgery and should not be reinitiated for at least 28 days after surgery and until wound is fully healed. In a retrospective review of central venous access device placements (a minor procedure), a greater risk of wound dehiscence was observed when port placement and bevacizumab administration were separated by <14 days (Erinjeri 2011). If possible, it may be more appropriate to wait until at least 6 to 8 weeks after bevacizumab discontinuation for major surgical procedures (Cortes 2012; Gordon 2009).

[US Boxed Warning]: Severe or fatal hemorrhage, including hemoptysis, gastrointestinal bleeding, central nervous system hemorrhage, epistaxis, and vaginal bleeding have been reported (up to 5 times more frequently if receiving bevacizumab). Avoid use in patients with serious hemorrhage or recent hemoptysis (≥2.5 mL blood). Serious or fatal pulmonary hemorrhage has been reported in patients receiving bevacizumab (primarily in patients with non-small cell lung cancer with squamous cell histology [not an FDA-approved indication]). Intracranial hemorrhage, including cases of grade 3 or 4 hemorrhage, has occurred in patients with previously treated glioblastoma. Treatment discontinuation is recommended in all patients with intracranial or other serious hemorrhage. Use with caution in patients with CNS metastases; once case of CNS hemorrhage was observed in an ongoing study of NSCLC patients with CNS metastases. Use with caution in patients at risk for thrombocytopenia.

Bevacizumab is associated with an increased risk for arterial thromboembolic events (ATE), including cerebral infarction, stroke, MI, TIA, angina, and other ATEs, when used in combination with chemotherapy. History of ATE, diabetes, or ≥65 years of age may present an even greater risk. Although patients with cancer are already at risk for venous thromboembolism (VTE), a meta-analysis of 15 controlled trials has demonstrated an increased risk for VTE in patients who received bevacizumab (Nalluri 2008). Cervical cancer patients receiving bevacizumab plus chemotherapy may be at increased risk of grade 3 or higher VTE compared to those patients who received chemotherapy alone. Permanently discontinue therapy in patients with severe ATE or life-threatening (grade 4) VTE, including pulmonary embolism; the safety of treatment reinitiation after ATE has not been studied.

Use with caution in patients with cardiovascular disease. Among approved and nonapproved uses evaluated thus far, the incidence of heart failure (HF) and/or left ventricular dysfunction (including LVEF decline), is higher in patients receiving bevacizumab plus chemotherapy when compared to chemotherapy alone. Bevacizumab may potentiate the cardiotoxic effects of anthracyclines. HF is more common with prior anthracycline exposure and/or left chest wall irradiation. The safety of therapy resumption or continuation in patients with cardiac dysfunction has not been studied. In studies of patients with metastatic breast cancer (an off-label use), the incidence of grades 3 or 4 HF was increased in patients receiving bevacizumab plus paclitaxel, compared to the control arm. Patients with metastatic breast cancer who received prior anthracycline therapy had a higher rate of HF compared to those receiving paclitaxel alone (3.8% vs 0.6% respectively). A meta-analysis of 5 studies which enrolled patients with metastatic breast cancer who received bevacizumab suggested an association with an increased risk of heart failure; all trials included in the analysis enrolled patients who either received prior or were receiving concurrent anthracycline therapy (Choueiri 2011). In a scientific statement from the American Heart Association, bevacizumab has been determined to be an agent that may either cause reversible direct myocardial toxicity or exacerbate underlying myocardial dysfunction (magnitude: moderate/major) (AHA [Page 2016]).

Bevacizumab may cause and/or worsen hypertension; the incidence of severe hypertension in increased with bevacizumab. Use caution in patients with preexisting hypertension and monitor BP closely (every 2 to 3 weeks during treatment; regularly after discontinuation if bevacizumab-induced hypertension occurs or worsens). Permanent discontinuation is recommended in patients who experience a hypertensive crisis or hypertensive encephalopathy. Temporarily discontinue in patients who develop uncontrolled hypertension. An increase in diastolic and systolic blood pressures were noted in a retrospective review of patients with renal insufficiency (CrCl ≤60 mL/minute) who received bevacizumab for renal cell cancer (Gupta 2011). Cases of posterior reversible encephalopathy syndrome (PRES) have been reported. Symptoms (which include headache, seizure, confusion, lethargy, blindness and/or other vision, or neurologic disturbances) may occur from 16 hours to 1 year after treatment initiation. Resolution of symptoms usually occurs within days after discontinuation; however, neurologic sequelae may remain. PRES may be associated with hypertension; discontinue bevacizumab and begin management of hypertension, if present. The safety of treatment reinitiation after PRES is not known.

Infusion reactions (eg, hypertension, hypertensive crisis, wheezing, oxygen desaturation, hypersensitivity [including anaphylactic/anaphylactoid reactions], chest pain, rigors, headache, diaphoresis) may occur with the first infusion (uncommon); interrupt therapy in patients experiencing severe infusion reactions and administer appropriate therapy; there are no data to address routine premedication use or reinstitution of therapy in patients who experience severe infusion reactions. Cases of necrotizing fasciitis, including fatalities, have been reported (rarely); usually secondary to wound healing complications, GI perforation or fistula formation. Discontinue in patients who develop necrotizing fasciitis. Proteinuria and/or nephrotic syndrome have been associated with bevacizumab; risk may be increased in patients with a history of hypertension; thrombotic microangiopathy has been associated with bevacizumab-induced proteinuria. Withhold treatment for ≥2 g proteinuria/24 hours and resume when proteinuria is <2 g/24 hours; discontinue in patients with nephrotic syndrome. Elderly patients (≥65 years of age) are at higher risk for adverse events, including thromboembolic events and proteinuria; serious adverse events occurring more frequently in the elderly also include weakness, deep thrombophlebitis, sepsis, hyper-/hypotension, MI, CHF, diarrhea, constipation, anorexia, leukopenia, anemia, dehydration, hypokalemia, and hyponatremia. Potentially significant drug-drug interactions may exist, requiring dose or frequency adjustment, additional monitoring, and/or selection of alternative therapy. Microangiopathic hemolytic anemia (MAHA) has been reported when bevacizumab has been used in combination with sunitinib. Concurrent therapy with sunitinib and bevacizumab is also associated with dose-limiting hypertension in patients with metastatic renal cell cancer. The incidence of hand-foot syndrome is increased in patients treated with bevacizumab plus sorafenib in comparison to those treated with sorafenib monotherapy. When used in combination with myelosuppressive chemotherapy, increased rates of severe or febrile neutropenia and neutropenic infection were reported. Bevacizumab, in combination with chemotherapy (or biologic therapy), is associated with an increased risk of treatment-related mortality; a higher risk of fatal adverse events was identified in a meta-analysis of 16 trials in which bevacizumab was used for the treatment of various cancers (breast cancer, colorectal cancer, non-small cell lung cancer, pancreatic cancer, prostate cancer, and renal cell cancer) and compared to chemotherapy alone (Ranpura 2011). When bevacizumab is used in combination with myelosuppressive chemotherapy, increased rates of severe or febrile neutropenia and neutropenic infection have been reported. In premenopausal women receiving bevacizumab in combination with mFOLFOX (fluorouracil/oxaliplatin based chemotherapy) the incidence of ovarian failure (amenorrhea ≥3 months) was higher (34%) compared to women who received mFOLFOX alone (2%); ovarian function recovered in some patients after treatment was discontinued; premenopausal women should be informed of the potential risk of ovarian failure.

Medication-related osteonecrosis of the jaw (MRONJ) has been associated with bisphosphonates and other antiresorptive agents (denosumab), and antiangiogenic agents (eg, bevacizumab, sunitinib) used for the treatment of osteoporosis or malignancy according to a position paper by the American Association of Maxillofacial Surgeons (AAOMS). Antiangiogenic agents, when given concomitantly with antiresorptive agents, are associated with an increased risk of ONJ. Other risk factors for MRONJ include dentoalveolar surgery (eg, tooth extraction, dental implants), preexisting inflammatory dental disease, and concomitant corticosteroid use. The AAOMS suggests that if medically permissible, initiation of antiangiogenic agents for cancer therapy should be delayed until optimal dental health is attained (if extractions are required, antiangiogenesis therapy should delayed until the extraction site has mucosalized or until after adequate osseous healing). Once antiangiogenic therapy for oncologic disease is initiated, procedures that involve direct osseous injury and placement of dental implants should be avoided. Patients developing ONJ during therapy should receive care by an oral surgeon (AAOMS [Ruggiero 2014]). Cases of non-mandibular ONJ has also been reported in pediatric patients who have received bevacizumab (bevacizumab is not approved for use in pediatric patients).

Serious eye infections and vision loss due to endophthalmitis have been reported from intravitreal administration (off-label use/route).

Adverse Reactions Percentages reported as monotherapy and as part of combination chemotherapy regimens. Some studies only reported hematologic toxicities grades ≥4 and nonhematologic toxicities grades ≥3.

>10%:

Cardiovascular: Hypertension (19% to 42%), venous thromboembolism (secondary: 21%; with oral anticoagulants), peripheral edema (15%), hypotension (7% to 15%), venous thromboembolism (8% to 14%), arterial thrombosis (6%)

Central nervous system: Fatigue (33% to 82%), pain (8% to 62%), headache (22% to 49%), dizziness (13% to 26%), insomnia (21%), taste disorder (14% to 21%), peripheral sensory neuropathy (17% to 18%), anxiety (17%), myasthenia (13%)

Dermatologic: Alopecia (6% to 32%), exfoliative dermatitis (23%), palmar-plantar erythrodysesthesia (11%), xeroderma (7%)

Endocrine & metabolic: Ovarian failure (34%), hyperglycemia (26% to 31%), hypomagnesemia (24% to 27%), weight loss (15% to 21%), hyponatremia (17% to 19%), hypoalbuminemia (11% to 16%), hypooaloomia (12%)

Gastrointestinal: Nausea (72%), abdominal pain (33% to 61%), vomiting (33% to 52%), anorexia (35% to 43%), constipation (40%), diarrhea (21% to 39%), decreased appetite (34% to 35%), stomatitis (15% to 33%), gastrointestinal hemorrhage (19% to 24%), dyspepsia (17% to 24%), mucosal inflammation (13% to 15%)

◄ Genitourinary: Proteinuria (4% to 36%; median onset: 5.6 months; median time to resolution: 6.1 months), urinary tract infection (22%), pelvic pain (14%)

Hematologic & oncologic: Thrombocytopenia (5% to 58%; grade 3/4: 40%), hemorrhage (40%; grades 3/4: ≤7%), leukopenia (40%; grade 3/4: 37%), pulmonary hemorrhage (4% to 31%), neutropenia (12%; grades ≥3: 8% to 27%, grade 4: 27%), bruise (17%), lymphocytopenia (12%; grades 3/4: 6%)

Infection: Infection (55%; serious: 7% to 14%; pneumonia, catheter infection, or wound infection)

Neuromuscular & skeletal: Arthralgia (28% to 45%), myalgia (19% to 29%), limb pain (25%), back pain (12% to 21%), dysarthria (8% to 14%)

Renal: Increased serum creatinine (13% to 16%)

Respiratory: Epistaxis (17% to 55%), upper respiratory tract infection (40% to 47%), cough (26% to 30%), dyspnea (25% to 30%), allergic rhinitis (17%), oropharyngeal pain (16%), sinusitis (7% to 15%), nasal sign & symptoms (mucosal disorder: 14%), rhinitis (3% to >10%)

Miscellaneous: Postoperative wound complication (including dehiscence, 1% to 15%)

1% to 10%:

Cardiovascular: Thrombosis (8% to 10%), deep vein thrombosis (6% to 9%), chest pain (8%), intra-abdominal thrombosis (venous, grades 3/4: 3%), syncope (grades 3/4: 3%), left ventricular dysfunction (grades 3/4: 1%), pulmonary embolism (1%)

Central nervous system: Voice disorder (5% to 13%)

Dermatologic: Nail disease (10%), dermal ulcer (6%), cellulitis (grades 3/4: 3%), acne vulgaris (1%)

Endocrine & metabolic: Dehydration (grades 3/4: 4% to 10%), hyperkalemia (9%), hypokalemia (grades 3/4: 7%)

Gastrointestinal: Hemorrhoids (8%), xerostomia (4% to 7%), gingival hemorrhage (minor, 2% to 7%), rectal pain (6%), colitis (1% to 6%), intestinal obstruction (grades 3/4: 4%), gastrointestinal perforation (≤3%), gastroesophageal reflux disease (2%), gingivitis (2%), oral mucosa ulcer (2%), gastrointestinal fistula (≤2%), gastritis (1%), gingival pain (1%)

Genitourinary: Vaginal hemorrhage (4%)

Hematologic & oncologic: Febrile neutropenia (5%), neutropenic infection (grades 3/4: 5%), hemorrhage (CNS; 5%)

Hepatic: Increased serum AST (15%)

Infection: Abscess (tooth, 2%)

Neuromuscular & skeletal: Weakness (grades 3/4: 10%), neck pain (9%)

Ophthalmic: Blurred vision (2%)

Otic: Tinnitus (2%), deafness (1%)

Respiratory: Rhinorrhea (10%), nasal congestion (8%), pneumonitis (grades 3/4: 5%)

Miscellaneous: Fistula (gastrointestinal-vaginal; 8%), fistula (anal; 6%), infusion related reaction (<3%), fistula (≤2%)

<1%, postmarketing, and/or case reports: Anaphylaxis, anastomotic ulcer, angina pectoris, antibody development (anti-bevacizumab and neutralizing), bladder fistula, bronchopleural fistula, cerebral infarction, conjunctival hemorrhage, endophthalmitis (infectious and sterile), eye discomfort, eye pain, fistula of bile duct, fulminant necrotizing fasciitis, gallbladder perforation, gastrointestinal ulcer, hemolytic anemia (microangiopathic; when used in combination with sunitinib), hemoptysis, hemorrhagic stroke, hypersensitivity, hypertensive crisis, hypertensive encephalopathy, increased intraocular

pressure, inflammation of anterior segment of eye (toxic anterior segment syndrome) (Sato 2010), intestinal necrosis, intraocular inflammation (iritis, vitritis), mesenteric thrombosis, myocardial infarction, nasal septum perforation, nephrotic syndrome, ocular hyperemia, osteonecrosis of the jaw, pancytopenia, permanent vision loss, polyserositis, pulmonary hypertension, rectal fistula, renal failure, renal fistula, renal thrombotic microangiopathy, retinal detachment, retinal hemorrhage, reversible posterior leukoencephalopathy syndrome, sepsis, tracheoesophageal fistula, transient ischemic attacks, vaginal fistula, visual disturbance, vitreous hemorrhage, vitreous opacity

Drug Interactions

Metabolism/Transport Effects None known.

Avoid Concomitant Use

Avoid concomitant use of Bevacizumab with any of the following: BCG (Intravesical); Belimumab; Deferiprone; Dipyrone; SUNItinib

Increased Effect/Toxicity

Bevacizumab may increase the levels/effects of: Antineoplastic Agents (Anthracycline, Systemic); Belimumab; Bisphosphonate Derivatives; CloZAPine; Deferiprone; SORAfenib; SUNItinib

The levels/effects of Bevacizumab may be increased by: Dipyrone; Promazine; SUNItinib

Decreased Effect

Bevacizumab may decrease the levels/effects of: BCG (Intravesical)

Storage/Stability Store intact vials at 2°C to 8°C (36°F to 46°F) in original carton; do not freeze. Protect from light; do not shake. Solutions diluted in NS are stable for up to 8 hours under refrigeration. Discard unused portion of vial.

Preparation for Administration Dilute in 100 mL NS prior to infusion (the manufacturer recommends a total volume of 100 mL). Do not mix with dextrose-containing solutions.

Mechanism of Action Bevacizumab is a recombinant, humanized monoclonal antibody which binds to, and neutralizes, vascular endothelial growth factor (VEGF), preventing its association with endothelial receptors, Flt-1 and KDR. VEGF binding initiates angiogenesis (endothelial proliferation and the formation of new blood vessels). The inhibition of microvascular growth is believed to retard the growth of all tissues (including metastatic tissue).

Pharmacodynamics/Kinetics

Distribution: V_d: 46 mL/kg

Half-life elimination:

IV:

Pediatric patients (age: 1 to 21 years): Median: 11.8 days (range: 4.4 to 14.6 days) (Glade Bender 2008)

Adults: ~20 days (range: 11 to 50 days)

Intravitreal: ~5 to 10 days (Bakri 2007; Krohne 2008)

Dosing

Adult & Geriatric

Cervical cancer, persistent/recurrent/metastatic: IV: 15 mg/kg every 3 weeks (in combination with paclitaxel and either cisplatin or topotecan) until disease progression or unacceptable toxicity (Tewari 2014)

Colorectal cancer, metastatic, in combination with fluorouracil-based chemotherapy: IV: 5 mg/kg every 2 weeks (in combination with bolus-IFL) **or** 10 mg/kg every 2 weeks (in combination with FOLFOX4)

◄

Colorectal cancer, metastatic, following first-line therapy containing bevacizumab: IV: 5 mg/kg every 2 weeks **or** 7.5 mg/kg every 3 weeks (in combination with fluoropyrimidine-irinotecan or fluoropyrimidine-oxaliplatin based regimen)

Glioblastoma: IV: 10 mg/kg every 2 weeks as monotherapy **or** (off-label dosing) 10 mg/kg every 2 weeks (in combination with irinotecan) (Vredenburgh 2007)

Non-small cell lung cancer (nonsquamous cell histology): IV: 15 mg/kg every 3 weeks (in combination with carboplatin and paclitaxel) for 6 cycles followed by maintenance treatment (off-label use) of bevacizumab 15 mg/kg every 3 weeks as monotherapy until disease progression or unacceptable toxicity (Sandler 2006)

Ovarian (epithelial), fallopian tube, or primary peritoneal cancer (platinum-resistant recurrent): IV: 10 mg/kg every 2 weeks (in combination with weekly paclitaxel, every 4 week doxorubicin [liposomal], or days 1, 8, and 15 topotecan) **or** 15 mg/kg every 3 weeks (in combination with every 3 week topotecan) (Pujade-Lauraine 2014)

Ovarian (epithelial), fallopian tube, or primary peritoneal cancer (platinum-sensitive recurrent): IV: 15 mg/kg every 3 weeks (in combination with carboplatin and gemcitabine for 6 to 10 cycles or with carboplatin and paclitaxel for 6 to 8 cycles) then continue with bevacizumab (monotherapy) until disease progression or unacceptable toxicity (Aghajanian 2012; Aghajanian 2015; Coleman 2015).

Renal cell cancer, metastatic: IV: 10 mg/kg every 2 weeks (in combination with interferon alfa) **or** (off-label dosing) 10 mg/kg every 2 weeks as monotherapy (Yang 2003)

Age-related macular degeneration (off-label use/route): Intravitreal: 1.25 mg (0.05 mL) monthly for 3 months, then may be given scheduled (monthly) or as needed based on monthly ophthalmologic assessment (Chakravarthy 2013; Martin 2012)

Breast cancer, metastatic (off-label use): IV: 10 mg/kg every 2 weeks (in combination with paclitaxel) (Miller 2007)

Endometrial cancer, recurrent or persistent (off-label use): IV: 15 mg/kg every 3 weeks (as monotherapy) until disease progression or unacceptable toxicity (Aghajanian 2011)

Hereditary hemorrhagic telangiectasia (off-label use): IV: 5 mg/kg every 2 weeks for 6 doses (Dupuis-Girod 2012). Additional data may be necessary to further define the role of bevacizumab in this condition.

Malignant pleural mesothelioma, unresectable (off-label use): IV: 15 mg/kg every 3 weeks (in combination with pemetrexed and cisplatin) for up to 6 cycles, followed by bevacizumab maintenance therapy at 15 mg/kg once every 3 weeks until disease progression or unacceptable toxicity (Zalcman 2016)

Soft tissue sarcoma, angiosarcoma, metastatic or locally advanced (off-label use): IV: 15 mg/kg every 3 weeks until disease progression or unacceptable toxicity (Agulnik 2013). Additional data may be necessary to further define the role of bevacizumab in this condition.

Renal Impairment There are no dosage adjustments provided in the manufacturer's labeling.

Hepatic Impairment There are no dosage adjustments provided in the manufacturer's labeling.

Adjustment for Toxicity IV administration (systemic): There are no recommended dosage reductions. Temporary suspension is recommended for severe infusion reactions, at least 4 weeks prior to (and after) elective surgery, in moderate-to-severe proteinuria (in most studies, treatment was withheld for ≥2 g proteinuria/24 hours), or in patients with severe hypertension which is not controlled with medical management. Permanent discontinuation is recommended (by the manufacturer) in patients who develop wound dehiscence and wound healing complications requiring intervention, necrotizing fasciitis, fistula (gastrointestinal and nongastrointestinal), gastrointestinal perforation, intra-abdominal abscess, hypertensive crisis, hypertensive encephalopathy, serious bleeding/hemorrhage, severe arterial thromboembolic event, life-threatening (grade 4) venous thromboembolic events (including pulmonary embolism), nephrotic syndrome, or PRES.

Combination Regimens

Brain tumors: Bevacizumab-Irinotecan (Glioblastoma) on page 1994
Breast cancer: Bevacizumab-Paclitaxel (Breast) on page 1994
Cervical cancer:
  Bevacizumab-Cisplatin-Paclitaxel (Cervical) on page 1991
  Bevacizumab-Paclitaxel-Topotecan (Cervical) on page 1995
Colorectal cancer:
  Bevacizumab-Fluorouracil-Leucovorin (Colorectal) on page 1992
  Bevacizumab + FOLFIRI (Colorectal) on page 1992
  Bevacizumab FOLFOX (Colorectal) on page 1993
  Bevacizumab + XELOX (Colorectal) on page 1996
Lung cancer (non-small cell):
  Bevacizumab-Carboplatin-Paclitaxel (NSCLC) on page 1990
  Bevacizumab-Carboplatin-Pemetrexed (NSCLC) on page 1990
  Bevacizumab-Cisplatin-Gemcitabine (NSCLC) on page 1991
Ovarian cancer:
  Bevacizumab-Carboplatin-Gemcitabine (Ovarian) on page 1990
  Bevacizumab-Doxorubicin (Liposomal) (Ovarian) on page 1992
  Bevacizumab-Paclitaxel (Ovarian) on page 1995
  Bevacizumab-Topotecan Daily (Ovarian) on page 1995
  Bevacizumab-Topotecan Weekly (Ovarian) on page 1996
Renal cell cancer: Bevacizumab-Interferon Alfa (RCC) on page 1994

Administration

IV: Infuse the initial dose over 90 minutes. The second infusion may be shortened to 60 minutes if the initial infusion is well tolerated. The third and subsequent infusions may be shortened to 30 minutes if the 60-minute infusion is well tolerated. Monitor closely during the infusion for signs/symptoms of an infusion reaction. After tolerance at the 90-, 60-, and 30-minute infusion rates has been established, some institutions use an off-label 10-minute infusion rate (0.5 mg/kg/minute) for bevacizumab dosed at 5 mg/kg (Reidy 2007). In a study evaluating the safety of the 0.5 mg/kg/minute infusion rate, proteinuria and hypertension incidences were not increased with the shorter infusion time (Shah 2013). Do not administer IV push. Do not administer with dextrose solutions. Temporarily withhold bevacizumab for 4 weeks prior to elective surgery and for at least 4 weeks (and until the surgical incision is fully healed) after surgery.

Intravitreal injection (off-label use/route): Adequate local anesthesia and a topical broad-spectrum antimicrobial agent should be administered prior to the procedure.

Emetic Potential Children and Adults: Minimal <10%

◀ **Monitoring Parameters** Monitor closely during the infusion for signs/symptoms of an infusion reaction. Monitor CBC with differential; signs/symptoms of gastrointestinal perforation, fistula, or abscess (including abdominal pain, constipation, vomiting, and fever); signs/symptoms of bleeding, including hemoptysis, gastrointestinal, and/or CNS bleeding, and/or epistaxis. Monitor blood pressure every 2 to 3 weeks; more frequently if hypertension develops during therapy. Continue to monitor blood pressure after discontinuing due to bevacizumab-induced hypertension. Monitor for proteinuria/nephrotic syndrome with urine dipstick; collect 24-hour urine in patients with ≥2+ reading. Monitor for signs/symptoms of thromboembolism (arterial and venous).

AMD (off-label use): Monitor intraocular pressure and retinal artery perfusion

Hereditary hemorrhagic telangiectasia (off-label use): Cardiac output measurements and liver radiologic response (via ultrasound and hepatic CT exams) prior to initial treatment and at 3 and 6 months following the first dose.

Dosage Forms Excipient information presented when available (limited, particularly for generics); consult specific product labeling.

Solution, Intravenous [preservative free]:

Avastin: 100 mg/4 mL (4 mL); 400 mg/16 mL (16 mL)

◆ **Bevacizumab, inj** see Bevacizumab on page 237

Bexarotene (Systemic) (beks AIR oh teen)

Related Information

Common Toxicity Criteria on page 2242

Management of Chemotherapy-Induced Nausea and Vomiting in Adults on page 2253

Prevention of Chemotherapy-Induced Nausea and Vomiting in Children on page 2310

Safe Handling of Hazardous Drugs on page 2379

Brand Names: US Targretin

Index Terms 3-methyl TTNEB

Pharmacologic Category Antineoplastic Agent, Retinoic Acid Derivative

Use Cutaneous T-cell lymphoma, refractory: Treatment of cutaneous manifestations of cutaneous T-cell lymphoma in patients who are refractory to at least one prior systemic therapy

Labeled Contraindications

Known hypersensitivity to bexarotene or any component of the formulation; pregnancy

Documentation of allergenic cross-reactivity for retinoids is limited. However, because of similarities in chemical structure and/or pharmacologic actions, the possibility of cross-sensitivity cannot be ruled out with certainty.

Pregnancy Considerations [U.S. Boxed Warning]: Bexarotene is a retinoid, a drug class associated with birth defects in humans; do not administer during pregnancy. Bexarotene caused birth defects when administered orally to pregnant rats. It must not be given to a pregnant woman or a woman who intends to become pregnant. If a woman becomes pregnant while taking the drug, it must be stopped immediately and appropriate counseling be given. In women of childbearing potential, therapy should be started on the second or third day of a normal menstrual period. Either abstinence or 2 forms of reliable contraception (one should be nonhormonal) must be used for at least 1 month before initiating therapy, during therapy, and for 1 month following discontinuation of bexarotene. A negative pregnancy test (sensitivity of at least 50 milliunits/mL) within 1 week prior to beginning therapy, and monthly thereafter is required for women of childbearing potential. A maximum 1 month supply is recommended so that pregnancy tests may be evaluated. Male patients must use a condom during any sexual contact with women of childbearing age during therapy, and for at least 1 month following discontinuation of bexarotene.

Breastfeeding Considerations It is not known if bexarotene is excreted into breast milk. Due to the potential for serious adverse reactions in a nursing infant, breastfeeding is not recommended by the manufacturer.

Warnings/Precautions [U.S. Boxed Warning]: Bexarotene is a retinoid, a drug class associated with birth defects in humans; do not administer during pregnancy. Bexarotene caused birth defects when administered orally to pregnant rats. Pregnancy test needed within 1 week before initiation and every month thereafter. Effective contraception must be in place 1 month before initiation, during therapy, and for at least 1 month after discontinuation. Male patients with sexual partners who are pregnant, possibly pregnant, or who could become pregnant, must use condoms during sexual intercourse during treatment and for at least 1 month after last dose.

Bexarotene induces significant lipid abnormalities in a majority of patients (elevated triglycerides and total cholesterol, and decreased high-density lipoprotein [HDL]) and usually occur within 2 to 4 weeks; effects are reversible on discontinuation or generally mitigated by dose reduction and/or antilipemic therapy. Monitor fasting lipid panel; may require dose reduction, treatment interruption, and/or concomitant antilipemic therapy. Fasting triglycerides should be normal (or normalized with appropriate therapy) prior to initiation; triglycerides should be maintained <400 mg/dL. In studies, HMG-CoA reductase inhibitors were used to manage lipids; gemfibrozil is not recommended due to potential for drug interactions. Pancreatitis associated with hypertriglyceridemia has been reported. Interrupt treatment and evaluate if pancreatitis is suspected. Cutaneous T-cell lymphoma patients with risk factors for pancreatitis (eg, prior pancreatitis, uncontrolled hyperlipidemia, excessive ethanol consumption, uncontrolled diabetes, biliary tract disease, concomitant medications causing hyperlipidemia or concomitant medications associated with pancreatic toxicity) may be at increased risk for bexarotene-associated pancreatitis. Dose-related elevations in ALT, AST, and bilirubin have been reported; cases of cholestasis and liver failure (fatal) have occurred. Monitor for liver function test abnormalities and temporarily withhold or discontinue if ALT, AST, or bilirubin are >3 times the upper limit of normal (ULN). Liver function test elevations resolved within 1 month in most patients following dose reduction or discontinuation. Bexarotene rapidly suppresses thyroid-stimulating hormone (TSH) levels by directly inhibiting TSH secretion and also affects thyroid hormone metabolism (Hamnvik, 2011). Reductions in total thyroxine (T_4) and thyroid-stimulating hormone (TSH) are reversible. Hypothyroidism commonly occur. Monitor thyroid functions tests, including free T_4 levels at baseline and during treatment Thyroid supplementation is usually required; patients already receiving thyroid hormone therapy may require increased thyroid hormone doses to achieve therapeutic levels (Hamnvik, 2011). Grade 1 to 3 leukopenia has occurred (predominantly as neutropenia); the incidence is higher with doses >300 mg/m²/day. The onset of leukopenia was generally 4 to 8 weeks. Grade 3 and 4 neutropenia have occurred. Leukopenia and neutropenia typically resolved within 30 days after discontinuation or dose reduction. Monitor complete blood cell count (CBC) with differential at baseline and periodically during treatment. Leukopenia and neutropenia were rarely associated with severe conditions or serious adverse events. Any new visual abnormalities experienced by the patient should be evaluated by an ophthalmologist (cataracts may develop or worsen, especially in the geriatric population).

Retinoids are associated with photosensitivity; phototoxicity (sunburn, sunlight sensitivity) has occurred with bexarotene when patients were exposed to direct sunlight; advise patients to minimize exposure to sunlight and artificial ultraviolet light during treatment. Use with extreme caution in patients with hepatic impairment; bexarotene undergoes extensive hepatic elimination. Due to the potential for additive toxicities, patients should be advised to limit additional vitamin A intake (in studies, additional vitamin A was limited to ≤15,000 units/day). Use caution with diabetic patients; may enhance the actions of insulin, sulfonylureas or thiazolidinediones, resulting in hypoglycemia in patients receiving these agents (hypoglycemia has not been observed with bexarotene monotherapy). Monitor blood glucose as necessary. Potentially significant drug-drug interactions may exist, requiring dose or frequency adjustment, additional monitoring, and/or selection of alternative therapy.

Adverse Reactions Frequency not always defined.

>10%:
Cardiovascular: Peripheral edema (11% to 13%)
Central nervous system: Headache (30% to 42%), chills (10% to 13%), insomnia (5% to 11%)
Dermatologic: Exfoliative dermatitis (10% to 28%), skin rash (17% to 23%), xeroderma (9% to 11%), alopecia (4% to 11%)
Endocrine & metabolic: Hyperlipidemia (79%), hypercholesterolemia (32% to 62%), hypothyroidism (29% to 53%), increased lactate dehydrogenase (7% to 13%)
Gastrointestinal: Diarrhea (7% to 42%), anorexia (2% to 23%), nausea (8% to 16%), vomiting (4% to 13%), abdominal pain (4% to 11%)
Hematologic & oncologic: Leukopenia (17% to 47%), anemia (6% to 25%), hypochromic anemia (4% to 13%)
Infection: Infection (13% to 23%; bacterial infection: 1% to 13%)
Neuromuscular & skeletal: Weakness (20% to 45%), back pain (2% to 11%)
Respiratory: Flu-like symptoms (4% to 13%)
Miscellaneous: Fever (5% to 17%)
1% to 10%:
Cardiovascular: Angina pectoris, cardiac failure (right), cerebrovascular accident, chest pain, hypertension, subdural hematoma, syncope, tachycardia
Central nervous system: Agitation, ataxia, confusion, depression, dizziness, hyperesthesia, myasthenia, neuropathy
Dermatologic: Acne vulgaris, allergic skin reaction, cellulitis, cheilitis, cutaneous nodule, maculopapular rash, skin photosensitivity, pustular rash, skin rash, sunburn, vesiculobullous dermatitis
Endocrine & metabolic: Albuminuria, hyperglycemia, weight gain, weight loss
Gastrointestinal: Colitis, constipation, dyspepsia, flatulence, gastroenteritis, gingivitis, increased serum amylase, melena, pancreatitis, xerostomia
Genitourinary: Dysuria, hematuria, mastalgia, urinary incontinence, urinary tract infection, urinary urgency
Hematologic & oncologic: Acquired blood coagulation disorder, eosinophilia, hemorrhage, hypoproteinemia, lymphocytosis, thrombocythemia, thrombocytopenia

Hepatic: Hepatic failure, increased serum ALT, increased serum AST, increased serum bilirubin

Infection: Candidiasis, sepsis

Neuromuscular & skeletal: Arthralgia, arthrosis, myalgia, ostealgia

Ophthalmic: Blepharitis, cataract (new and worsening), conjunctivitis, corneal lesion, keratitis, visual field defect, xerophthalmia

Otic: Otalgia, otitis externa

Renal: Increased serum creatinine, renal function abnormality

Respiratory: Bronchitis, cough, dyspnea, hemoptysis, hypoxia, pharyngitis, pleural effusion, pneumonia, pulmonary edema, rhinitis

Miscellaneous: Serous drainage

Drug Interactions

Metabolism/Transport Effects Substrate of CYP3A4 (minor); **Note:** Assignment of Major/Minor substrate status based on clinically relevant drug interaction potential; **Induces** CYP3A4 (moderate)

Avoid Concomitant Use

Avoid concomitant use of Bexarotene (Systemic) with any of the following: Aminolevulinic Acid (Systemic); Antihepaciviral Combination Products; Asunaprevir; Axitinib; BCG (Intravesical); Bedaquiline; Bosutinib; Cobimetinib; Dasabuvir; Deferiprone; Deflazacort; Dipyrone; Elbasvir; Flibanserin; Gemfibrozil; Grazoprevir; Multivitamins/Fluoride (with ADE); Multivitamins/Minerals (with ADEK, Folate, Iron); Multivitamins/Minerals (with AE, No Iron); Neratinib; Nisoldipine; Olaparib; Ranolazine; Simeprevir; Sonidegib; Tetracycline Derivatives; Velpatasvir; Venetoclax; Vitamin A

Increased Effect/Toxicity

Bexarotene (Systemic) may increase the levels/effects of: Aminolevulinic Acid (Systemic); Aminolevulinic Acid (Topical); Clarithromycin; CloZAPine; Deferiprone; Ifosfamide; Porfimer; Verteporfin

The levels/effects of Bexarotene (Systemic) may be increased by: CARBOplatin; Dipyrone; Gemfibrozil; Multivitamins/Fluoride (with ADE); Multivitamins/Minerals (with ADEK, Folate, Iron); Multivitamins/Minerals (with AE, No Iron); PACLitaxel (Conventional); Promazine; Tetracycline Derivatives; Vitamin A

Decreased Effect

Bexarotene (Systemic) may decrease the levels/effects of: Antihepaciviral Combination Products; Asunaprevir; AtorvaSTATin; Axitinib; BCG (Intravesical); Bedaquiline; Bosutinib; Clarithromycin; CloZAPine; Cobimetinib; Contraceptives (Estrogens); Contraceptives (Progestins); CYP3A4 Substrates; Daclatasvir; Dasabuvir; Deflazacort; Elbasvir; Estriol (Systemic); Estriol (Topical); FentaNYL; Flibanserin; Glecaprevir and Pibrentasvir; Grazoprevir; GuanFACINE; HYDROcodone; Ibrutinib; Ifosfamide; Lurasidone; Mirodenafil; Naldemedine; Neratinib; NiMODipine; Nisoldipine; Olaparib; PACLitaxel (Conventional); Palbociclib; Perampanel; Ranolazine; Rolapitant; Simeprevir; Sonidegib; Tamoxifen; Velpatasvir; Venetoclax; Zolpidem

Food Interactions Bioavailability is increased when administered with a fat-containing meal. Management: Administer with food.

Hazardous Drugs Handling Considerations

Hazardous agent (NIOSH 2016 [group 1]).

Use appropriate precautions for receiving, handling, administration, and disposal. Gloves (single) should be worn during receiving, unpacking, and placing in storage.

NIOSH recommends single gloving for administration of intact tablets or capsules. If manipulating tablets/capsules (eg, to prepare an oral suspension), NIOSH recommends double gloving, a protective gown, and preparation in a controlled device; if not prepared in a controlled device, respiratory and eye/face protection as well as ventilated engineering controls are recommended. NIOSH recommends double gloving, a protective gown, and (if there is a potential for vomit or spit up) eye/face protection for administration of an oral liquid/feeding tube administration (NIOSH 2016).

Storage/Stability Store at 2°C to 25°C (36°F to 77°F). Protect from light. Avoid humidity and high temperatures after opening bottle.

Mechanism of Action Selectively binds to and activates retinoid X receptors (RXRs). Once activated, RXRs function as transcription factors to regulate the expression of genes which control cellular differentiation and proliferation. Bexarotene inhibits the growth *in vitro* of some tumor cell lines of hematopoietic and squamous cell origin and induces tumor regression *in vivo* in some animal models.

Pharmacodynamics/Kinetics

Absorption: Improved 48% by a fat-containing meal

Protein binding: >99% to plasma proteins

Metabolism: Hepatic via CYP3A4 isoenzyme to four metabolites; further metabolized by glucuronidation

Half-life elimination: ~7 hours

Time to peak: ~2 hours

Excretion: Feces (primarily); urine (minimal, <1%)

Dosing

Adult & Geriatric

Cutaneous T-cell lymphoma, refractory: Oral: Initial: 300 mg/m^2 once daily taken as a single daily dose; if well tolerated, but no tumor response after 8 weeks, may increase to 400 mg/m^2 once daily; continue as long as clinical benefit is demonstrated (bexarotene was administered in studies for up to 97 weeks).

Mycosis fungoides/Sezary syndrome, refractory/resistant (off-label dose): Oral: 75 to 150 mg daily in combination with PUVA; maximum dose: 300 mg daily (Rupoli, 2010; Singh, 2004)

Renal Impairment There are no dosage adjustments provided in the manufacturer's labeling (has not been studied); however, although renal elimination is a minor excretion pathway, renal insufficiency may result in significant protein binding changes and alter pharmacokinetics of bexarotene.

Hepatic Impairment There are no dosage adjustments provided in the manufacturer's labeling (has not been studied); however, hepatic impairment would be expected to result in decreased clearance of bexarotene due to the extensive hepatic contribution to elimination.

Obesity *ASCO Guidelines for appropriate chemotherapy dosing in obese adults with cancer:* Utilize patient's actual body weight (full weight) for calculation of body surface area- or weight-based dosing, particularly when the intent of therapy is curative; manage regimen-related toxicities in the same manner as for nonobese patients; if a dose reduction is utilized due to toxicity, consider resumption of full weight-based dosing with subsequent cycles, especially if cause of toxicity (eg, hepatic or renal impairment) is resolved (Griggs, 2012).

Adjustment for Toxicity If necessitated by toxicity, may decrease dose from 300 mg/m²/day to 200 mg/m²/day, then to 100 mg/m²/day, or temporarily hold. Upon recovery, may titrate dose upward with careful monitoring.
Hepatotoxicity: If AST, ALT, or bilirubin >3 times ULN, consider withholding or discontinuing therapy.
Hypertriglyceridemia: Consider dose reduction, treatment interruption, and or antilipemic therapy.
Leukopenia and neutropenia: Leukopenia and neutropenia resolved after dose reduction or discontinuation.

Administration Administer with a meal.

Emetic Potential Children and Adults: Low (10% to 30%)

Extemporaneous Preparations A 1 mg/mL oral suspension may be prepared with capsules. Cut one 75 mg capsule in half, rinse the interior contents of the capsule, and suspend with 75 mL sterile water. Administer immediately after preparation. To ensure administration of full dose, rinse empty glass with half a glass of water and administer residue.
Targretin data on file, Eisai Inc.

Monitoring Parameters If female, pregnancy test within 1 week before initiation then monthly while on bexarotene; fasting lipid panel (before initiation, then weekly until lipid response established [usually 2 to 4 weeks] and then at 8-week intervals thereafter); liver function tests (baseline, then at 1, 2, and 4 weeks after initiation, then at 8-week intervals thereafter if stable); monitor thyroid function tests (including free T_4) at baseline and weekly for the first 5 to 7 weeks, then every 1 to 2 months (Hamnvık, 2011); CBC with differential (baseline and periodic); blood glucose (in diabetic patients); ophthalmic exam (if visual abnormalities occur)

Test Interactions Treatment with bexarotene may interfere with CA125 assay values in patients with ovarian cancer (per manufacturer's labeling).

Dietary Considerations Avoid grapefruit juice.

Dosage Forms Excipient information presented when available (limited, particularly for generics); consult specific product labeling.
Capsule, Oral:
Targretin: 75 mg
Generic: 75 mg

Bexarotene (Topical) (beks AIR oh teen)

Brand Names: US Targretin

Pharmacologic Category Antineoplastic Agent, Retinoic Acid Derivative

Use Cutaneous T-cell lymphoma: Topical treatment of cutaneous lesions in patients with refractory or persistent cutaneous T-cell lymphoma (stage 1A and 1B) or who have not tolerated other therapies

Pregnancy Risk Factor X

Hazardous Drugs Handling Considerations
Hazardous agent (NIOSH 2016 [group 1]).

Use appropriate precautions for receiving, handling, administration, and disposal. Gloves (single) should be worn during receiving, unpacking, and placing into storage.

NIOSH recommends double gloving and a protective gown for administration of a topical product; if there is potential for inhalation, respiratory protection is recommended (NIOSH 2016).

◀ **Dosing**

Adult & Geriatric Cutaneous T-cell lymphoma: Topical: Apply to lesions once every other day for first week, then increase on a weekly basis to once daily, 2 times daily, 3 times daily, and finally 4 times daily, according to individual lesion tolerance. Continue as long as deriving benefit. Response is usually observed with application at 2 to 4 times daily. May decrease frequency if local toxicity occurs; for severe irritation, temporarily withhold for a few days until symptoms subside.

Renal Impairment There are no dosage adjustments provided in the manufacturer's labeling (has not been studied); however, although renal elimination is a minor excretion pathway, renal insufficiency may result in significant protein binding changes and altered pharmacokinetics of bexarotene.

Hepatic Impairment There are no dosage adjustments provided in the manufacturer's labeling (has not been studied); however, hepatic impairment would be expected to result in decreased clearance of bexarotene due to the extensive hepatic contribution to elimination.

Additional Information Complete prescribing information should be consulted for additional detail.

Dosage Forms Excipient information presented when available (limited, particularly for generics); consult specific product labeling.
Gel, External:
Targretin: 1% (60 g) [contains alcohol, usp]

◆ **Bexxar [DSC]** *see* Tositumomab and Iodine I 131 Tositumomab *on page 1801*

◆ **Bexxar (Can)** *see* Tositumomab and Iodine I 131 Tositumomab *on page 1801*

◆ **BIBW 2992** *see* Afatinib *on page 65*

Bicalutamide (bye ka LOO ta mide)

Related Information
Safe Handling of Hazardous Drugs *on page 2379*

Brand Names: US Casodex

Brand Names: Canada ACH-Bicalutamide; ACT Bicalutamide; Apo-Bicalutamide; Casodex; Dom-Bicalutamide; JAMP-Bicalutamide; Mylan-Bicalutamide; PHL-Bicalutamide; PMS-Bicalutamide; PRO-Bicalutamide; RAN-Bicalutamide; Sandoz-Bicalutamide; Teva-Bicalutamide

Index Terms CDX; ICI-176334

Pharmacologic Category Antineoplastic Agent, Antiandrogen

Use

Prostate cancer, metastatic: Treatment of stage D_2 metastatic prostate cancer (in combination with an LHRH agonist)
Limitation of use: Bicalutamide 150 mg daily is not approved for use alone or with other treatments

Labeled Contraindications
Hypersensitivity to bicalutamide or any component of the formulation; use in women.
Canadian labeling: Additional contraindications (not in the US labeling): Patients with localized prostate cancer undergoing watchful waiting; children

Pregnancy Considerations Bicalutamide is contraindicated in women. Androgen receptor inhibition during pregnancy may affect fetal development.

In addition, male fertility may be impaired. Males with female partners of reproductive potential should use effective contraception during therapy and for 130 days after the last dose.

Breastfeeding Considerations It is not known if bicalutamide is present in breast milk. Use is contraindicated in women.

Warnings/Precautions Rare cases of death or hospitalization due to severe liver injury have been reported (postmarketing). Use with caution in moderate-to-severe hepatic dysfunction. Hepatotoxicity generally occurs within the first 3 to 4 months of use. Monitor transaminases (baseline and periodically); if clinical signs/symptoms suggestive of liver dysfunction occur, promptly monitor liver function tests; discontinue if patients have jaundice or ALT is >2 times the upper limit of normal. Androgen-deprivation therapy may increase the risk for cardiovascular disease (Levine 2010). Androgen deprivation therapy may cause prolongation of the QT/QTc interval (Garnick 2004); evaluate risk versus benefit in patients with congenital long QT syndrome, heart failure, frequent electrolyte abnormalities, and in patients taking medication known to prolong the QT interval. Correct electrolytes prior to initiation and consider periodic electrolyte and ECG monitoring.

Anemia may occur with testosterone suppression; monitor CBC periodically as indicated. Interstitial lung disease has been reported rarely (including fatalities) although mostly at dosages greater than what is recommended; promptly evaluate any worsening of respiratory symptoms (eg, dyspnea, cough and fever). Prolonged use of antiandrogen therapy is associated with decreased bone mineral density and an increased risk of osteoporosis and fracture (Smith 2003); alcohol abuse, familial history of osteoporosis, and/or chronic use of drugs capable of decreasing bone mass (eg, corticosteroids) may increase risk. Evaluate risk carefully before initiating therapy.

May cause gynecomastia, breast pain, or lead to spermatogenesis inhibition. When used in combination with LHRH agonists, a loss of glycemic control and decrease in glucose tolerance has been reported in patients with diabetes; monitor. May cause gynecomastia or breast pain (at higher, off-label doses), or lead to spermatogenesis inhibition. Angioneurotic edema and urticaria have been reported. Potentially significant drug-drug interactions may exist, requiring dose or frequency adjustment, additional monitoring, and/or selection of alternative therapy. Discontinue use immediately if disease worsens; decreased prostate specific antigen (PSA) levels and/or clinical improvement may be observed in some patients when antiandrogen therapy is held due to worsening of disease.

Adverse Reactions Adverse reaction percentages reported as part of combination regimen with an LHRH analogue unless otherwise noted.

>10%:
  Cardiovascular: Peripheral edema (13%)
  Central nervous system: Pain (35%)
  Endocrine & metabolic: Hot flash (53%), gynecomastia (9%; monotherapy [150 mg]: 38% to 73% [McLeod 2006])
  Gastrointestinal: Constipation (22%), nausea (15%), diarrhea (12%), abdominal pain (11%)
  Genitourinary: Mastalgia (6%; monotherapy [150 mg]: 39% to 85% [McLeod 2006]), pelvic pain (21%), hematuria (12%), nocturia (12%)
  Hematologic & oncologic: Anemia (11%)
  Infection: Infection (18%)
  Neuromuscular & skeletal: Back pain (25%), weakness (22%)

Respiratory: Dyspnea (13%)

≥2% to 10%:

Cardiovascular: Chest pain (8%), hypertension (8%), angina pectoris (2% to <5%), cardiac arrest (2% to <5%), cardiac failure (2% to <5%), coronary artery disease (2% to <5%), edema (2% to <5%), myocardial infarction (2% to <5%), syncope (2% to <5%)

Central nervous system: Dizziness (10%), paresthesia (8%), headache (7%), insomnia (7%), myasthenia (7%), anxiety (5%), chills (2% to <5%), confusion (2% to <5%), drowsiness (2% to <5%), hypertonia (2% to <5%), nervousness (2% to <5%), neuropathy (2% to <5%), depression (4%)

Dermatologic: Skin rash (9%), diaphoresis (6%), alopecia (2% to <5%), pruritus (2% to <5%), xeroderma (2% to <5%)

Endocrine & metabolic: Weight loss (7%), hyperglycemia (6%), weight gain (5%), decreased libido (2% to <5%), dehydration (2% to <5%), gout (2% to <5%), hypercholesterolemia (2% to <5%)

Gastrointestinal: Dyspepsia (7%), anorexia (6%), flatulence (6%), vomiting (6%), dysphagia (2% to <5%), hernia (2% to <5%), melena (2% to <5%), periodontal abscess (2% to <5%), xerostomia (2% to <5%)

Genitourinary: Urinary tract infection (9%), impotence (7%), difficulty in micturition (5%), urinary retention (5%), dysuria (2% to <5%), urinary urgency (2% to <5%), urinary incontinence (4%)

Hematologic & oncologic: Gastrointestinal carcinoma (2% to <5%), rectal hemorrhage (2% to <5%), skin carcinoma (2% to <5%)

Hepatic: Increased liver enzymes (7%), increased serum alkaline phosphatase (5%)

Infection: Herpes zoster (2% to <5%), sepsis (2% to <5%)

Neuromuscular & skeletal: Ostealgia (9%), arthritis (5%), leg cramps (2% to <5%), myalgia (2% to <5%), neck pain (2% to <5%), pathological fracture (4%)

Ophthalmic: Cataract (2% to <5%)

Renal: Polyuria (6%), hydronephrosis (2% to <5%), increased blood urea nitrogen (2% to <5%), increased serum creatinine (2% to <5%)

Respiratory: Cough (8%), pharyngitis (8%), flu-like symptoms (7%), bronchitis (6%), asthma (2% to <5%), epistaxis (2% to <5%), sinusitis (2% to <5%), pneumonia (4%), rhinitis (4%)

Miscellaneous: Cyst (2% to <5%), fever (2% to <5%)

<1%, postmarketing, and/or case reports: Decreased glucose tolerance, decreased hemoglobin, decreased white blood cell count, hepatic failure, hepatitis, hepatotoxicity, hypersensitivity (including angioedema and urticaria), increased serum ALT, increased serum AST, increased serum bilirubin, interstitial pneumonitis, interstitial pulmonary disease (most often at doses >50 mg), pulmonary fibrosis, skin photosensitivity

Drug Interactions

Metabolism/Transport Effects Inhibits CYP3A4 (weak)

Avoid Concomitant Use

Avoid concomitant use of Bicalutamide with any of the following: Aminolevulinic Acid (Systemic); Astemizole; Cisapride; Indium 111 Capromab Pendetide; Pimozide; Terfenadine

Increased Effect/Toxicity

Bicalutamide may increase the levels/effects of: Aminolevulinic Acid (Systemic); Aminolevulinic Acid (Topical); ARIPiprazole; Astemizole; Cisapride; Dofetilide; Flibanserin; HYDROcodone; Lomitapide; NiMODipine; Pimozide; Porfimer; Terfenadine; Verteporfin; Vitamin K Antagonists

Decreased Effect

Bicalutamide may decrease the levels/effects of: Choline C 11; Indium 111 Capromab Pendetide

Hazardous Drugs Handling Considerations

Hazardous agent (NIOSH 2016 [group 1]).

Use appropriate precautions for receiving, handling, administration, and disposal. Gloves (single) should be worn during receiving, unpacking, and placing in storage. NIOSH recommends single gloving for administration of intact tablets or capsules (NIOSH 2016).

Storage/Stability Store at room temperature of 20°C to 25°C (68°F to 77°F).

Mechanism of Action Androgen receptor inhibitor; pure nonsteroidal anti-androgen that binds to androgen receptors; specifically a competitive inhibitor for the binding of dihydrotestosterone and testosterone; prevents testosterone stimulation of cell growth in prostate cancer

Pharmacodynamics/Kinetics

Absorption: Well absorbed; unaffected by food

Protein binding: 96%

Metabolism: Extensively hepatic; glucuronidation and oxidation of the R (active) enantiomer to inactive metabolites; the S enantiomer is inactive

Half-life elimination: Active enantiomer: ~6 days (~10 days in severe hepatic impairment)

Time to peak, plasma: Active enantiomer: ~31 hours

Excretion: Urine and feces

Dosing

Adult & Geriatric

Prostate cancer, metastatic: Oral: 50 mg once daily (in combination with an LHRH analogue)

Prostate cancer, locally-advanced, high recurrence risk (off-label use): Oral: 150 mg once daily (as monotherapy) (McLeod 2006). Additional trials may be necessary to further define the role of bicalutamide in this condition.

Renal Impairment No dosage adjustment necessary.

Hepatic Impairment

Hepatic impairment at treatment initiation: Mild, moderate, or severe impairment: No dosage adjustment is necessary. Use with caution in patients with moderate-to-severe impairment; clearance may be delayed in severe impairment (based on a limited number of patients).

Hepatic impairment during treatment: ALT >2 times ULN or development of jaundice: Discontinue immediately.

Administration Dose should be taken at the same time each day, either in the morning or in the evening. May be administered with or without food. Treatment for metastatic cancer should be started concomitantly with an LHRH analogue.

Monitoring Parameters Periodically monitor CBC, ECG, echocardiograms, serum testosterone, luteinizing hormone, and prostate specific antigen (PSA). Liver function tests should be obtained at baseline and repeated regularly during the first 4 months of treatment, and periodically thereafter; monitor for signs and symptoms of liver dysfunction. Monitor blood glucose in patients with diabetes. If initiating bicalutamide in patients who are on warfarin, closely monitor prothrombin time.

◀ **Dosage Forms** Excipient information presented when available (limited, particularly for generics); consult specific product labeling.
Tablet, Oral:
Casodex: 50 mg
Generic: 50 mg

◆ **BiCNU** *see* Carmustine *on page 346*

◆ **Bio-Anastrozole (Can)** *see* Anastrozole *on page 135*

◆ **Bio-Letrozole (Can)** *see* Letrozole *on page 1119*

◆ **Bio-Ondansetron (Can)** *see* Ondansetron *on page 1380*

◆ **Bio-Statin** *see* Nystatin (Oral) *on page 1339*

◆ **Biotene Moisturizing Mouth Spray [OTC]** *see* Saliva Substitute *on page 1653*

◆ **Biotene Oral Balance [OTC]** *see* Saliva Substitute *on page 1653*

◆ **bis(chloroethyl) nitrosourea** *see* Carmustine *on page 346*

◆ **bis-chloronitrosourea** *see* Carmustine *on page 346*

◆ **Bivigam** *see* Immune Globulin *on page 992*

◆ **BL4162A** *see* Anagrelide *on page 131*

◆ **Blenoxane** *see* Bleomycin *on page 256*

◆ **Bleo** *see* Bleomycin *on page 256*

Bleomycin (blee oh MYE sin)

Related Information

Malignant Pleural Effusions *on page 2346*
Management of Chemotherapy-Induced Nausea and Vomiting in Adults *on page 2253*
Management of Drug Extravasations *on page 2271*
Prevention of Chemotherapy-Induced Nausea and Vomiting in Children *on page 2310*
Safe Handling of Hazardous Drugs *on page 2379*

Brand Names: Canada Blenoxane; Bleomycin Injection, USP

Index Terms Blenoxane; Bleo; Bleomycin Sulfate; BLM

Pharmacologic Category Antineoplastic Agent, Antibiotic

Use

Head and neck cancers: Treatment of squamous cell carcinomas of the head and neck

Hodgkin lymphoma: Treatment of Hodgkin lymphoma

Malignant pleural effusion: Sclerosing agent for malignant pleural effusion

Testicular cancer: Treatment of testicular cancer

Labeled Contraindications Hypersensitivity to bleomycin or any component of the formulation

Pregnancy Considerations Adverse effects were observed in animal reproduction studies. According to the manufacturer, women of childbearing potential should avoid becoming pregnant during bleomycin treatment. The European Society for Medical Oncology has published guidelines for diagnosis, treatment, and follow-up of cancer during pregnancy; the guidelines recommend referral to a facility with expertise in cancer during pregnancy and encourage a multidisciplinary team (obstetrician, neonatologist, oncology team). In general, if chemotherapy is indicated, it should be avoided in the first trimester and there should be a 3-week time period between the last chemotherapy dose and anticipated delivery, and chemotherapy should not be administered beyond week 33 of gestation (Peccatori 2013). When multiagent therapy is needed to treat Hodgkin lymphoma during pregnancy, bleomycin (as a component of the ABVD [doxorubicin, bleomycin, vinblastine, and dacarbazine] regimen) may be used, starting with the second trimester (Follows 2014; Peccatori 2013).

Breastfeeding Considerations It is not known if bleomycin is present in breast milk. Due to the potential for serious adverse reactions in the breastfed infant, breastfeeding is not recommended by the manufacturer.

Warnings/Precautions [US Boxed Warning]: Occurrence of pulmonary fibrosis (commonly presenting as pneumonitis; occasionally progressing to pulmonary fibrosis) is the most severe toxicity. Risk is higher in elderly patients or patients receiving >400 units total lifetime dose; other possible risk factors include smoking and patients with prior radiation therapy or receiving concurrent oxygen (especially high inspired oxygen doses). A review of patients receiving bleomycin for the treatment of germ cell tumors suggests risk for pulmonary toxicity is increased in patients >40 years of age, with glomerular filtration rate <80 mL/minute, advanced disease, and cumulative doses >300 units (O'Sullivan 2003). Pulmonary toxicity may include bronchiolitis obliterans and organizing pneumonia (BOOP), eosinophilic hypersensitivity, and interstitial pneumonitis, progressing to pulmonary fibrosis (Sleijfer 2001); pulmonary toxicity may be due to a lack of the enzyme which inactivates bleomycin (bleomycin hydrolase) in the lungs (Morgan 2011; Sleijfer 2001). If pulmonary changes occur, withhold treatment and investigate if drug-related. In a study of patients with testicular cancer receiving bleomycin as part of the BEP regimen, pulmonary function testing (including forced vital capacity [FVC], forced expiratory volume in 1 second [FEV_1], and diffusing capacity of the lungs for carbon monoxide [DLCO]) was performed prior to treatment, before each chemotherapy cycle, and then repeated at 1 year, 3 years, and 5 years during follow up; if the carbon monoxide diffusing capacity corrected for hemoglobin content [DLCOc] decreased more than 25% during therapy (compared with baseline), bleomycin was discontinued to avoid further pulmonary toxicity (Lauritsen 2016). In children, a younger age at treatment, cumulative dose $\geq$400 units/m^2 (combined with chest irradiation), and renal impairment are associated with a higher incidence of pulmonary toxicity (Huang 2011). Positron emission tomography/computed tomography (PET/CT) may have a role in determining early response to therapy in patients with Hodgkin lymphoma; a negative interim PET/CT result after 2 cycles may indicate that bleomycin can be safely omitted from the ABVD treatment regimen (Johnson 2016). Longer follow-up is necessary to determine the effect of bleomycin omission on long-term morbidity and mortality in these patients.

A severe idiosyncratic reaction consisting of hypotension, mental confusion, fever, chills, and wheezing (similar to anaphylaxis) has been reported in 1% of lymphoma patients treated with bleomycin. Since these reactions usually occur after the first or second dose, careful monitoring is essential after these doses. Use caution when administering O_2 during surgery to patients who have received bleomycin; the risk of bleomycin-related pulmonary toxicity is increased. Use caution with renal impairment (CrCl <50 mL/minute), may require dose adjustment. May cause renal or hepatic toxicity. **[US Boxed Warning]: Should be administered under the supervision of an experienced cancer chemotherapy physician.** Potentially significant drug-drug interactions may exist, requiring dose or frequency adjustment, additional monitoring, and/or selection of alternative therapy. Some products available internationally may have vial strength and dosing expressed as international units or milligrams (instead of units or USP units). During shortages within the US, temporary importation of international products may be allowed by the FDA. The imported bleomycin vial and product labeling may express strength and dosing as international units instead of USP units. One USP unit of bleomycin = 1 mg (by potency) = 1,000 international units (Stefanou 2001). Refer to prescribing information for specific dosing information.

Adverse Reactions Frequency not always defined. The pathogenesis of respiratory adverse effects is not certain, but may be due to damage of pulmonary, vascular, or connective tissue. Response to steroid therapy is variable and somewhat controversial.

>10%:

Cardiovascular: Phlebitis

Central nervous system: Tumor pain

Dermatologic: Hyperpigmentation (50%), atrophic striae (≤50%), erythema (≤50%), exfoliation of the skin (≤50%; particularly on the palmar and plantar surfaces of the hands and feet), hyperkeratosis (≤50%), localized vesiculation (≤50%), skin rash (≤50%), skin sclerosis (≤50%), alopecia (may be dose-related and reversible with discontinuation), nailbed changes (may be dose-related and reversible with discontinuation)

Endocrine & metabolic: Weight loss

Gastrointestinal: Stomatitis (≤30%), mucositis (≤30%), anorexia

Miscellaneous: Febrile reaction (25% to 50%; acute)

1% to 10%:

Dermatologic: Onycholysis, pruritus, thickening of skin

Hypersensitivity: Anaphylactoid reaction (including chills, confusion, fever, hypotension, wheezing; onset may be immediate or delayed for several hours; includes idiosyncratic reaction in 1% of lymphoma patients)

Neuromuscular & skeletal: Scleroderma (diffuse)

Respiratory: Tachypnea (≤5% to 10%), rales (≤5% to 10%), interstitial pneumonitis (acute or chronic: ≤5% to 10%), pulmonary fibrosis (≤5% to 10%), hypoxia (1%)

<1%, postmarketing, and/or case reports: Angioedema, bone marrow depression (rare), cerebrovascular accident, cerebral arteritis, chest pain, coronary artery disease, hepatotoxicity, hyperpigmentation (flagellate), ischemic heart disease, malaise, myocardial infarction, nausea, nephrotoxicity, pericarditis, Raynaud's phenomenon, scleroderma (scleroderma-like skin changes), Stevens-Johnson syndrome, thrombotic thrombocytopenic purpura, toxic epidermal necrolysis, vomiting

Drug Interactions

Metabolism/Transport Effects None known.

Avoid Concomitant Use

Avoid concomitant use of Bleomycin with any of the following: BCG (Intravesical); Brentuximab Vedotin; Natalizumab; Pimecrolimus; Tacrolimus (Topical); Vaccines (Live)

Increased Effect/Toxicity

Bleomycin may increase the levels/effects of: Fingolimod; Leflunomide; Natalizumab; Tofacitinib; Vaccines (Live)

The levels/effects of Bleomycin may be increased by: Brentuximab Vedotin; Denosumab; Filgrastim; Gemcitabine; Lenograstim; Ocrelizumab; Palifermin; Pimecrolimus; Roflumilast; Sargramostim; Tacrolimus (Topical); Trastuzumab

Decreased Effect

Bleomycin may decrease the levels/effects of: BCG (Intravesical); Coccidioides immitis Skin Test; Lenograstim; Nivolumab; Phenytoin; Sipuleucel-T; Tertomotide; Vaccines (Inactivated); Vaccines (Live)

The levels/effects of Bleomycin may be decreased by: Echinacea

Hazardous Drugs Handling Considerations

Hazardous agent (NIOSH 2016 [group 1]).

Use appropriate precautions for receiving, handling, administration, and disposal. Gloves (single) should be worn during receiving, unpacking, and placing in storage.

NIOSH recommends double gloving, a protective gown, ventilated engineering controls (a class II biological safety cabinet or a compounding aseptic containment isolator), and closed system transfer devices (CSTDs) for preparation. Double gloving, a gown, and (if dosage form allows) CSTDs are required during administration (NIOSH 2016).

Storage/Stability Store intact vials at 2°C to 8°C (36°F to 46°F). Stable for 24 hours in NS at room temperature.

Preparation for Administration Note: During shortages within the US, temporary importation of international products may be allowed by the FDA. Refer to specific product labeling for reconstitution and preparation information.

For IV use, reconstitute 15-unit vial with 5 mL with NS and the 30-unit vial with 10 mL NS; for IM or SubQ use, reconstitute 15-unit vial with 1 to 5 mL of SWFI, BWFI, or NS and the 30-unit vial with 2 to 10 mL of SWFI, BWFI, or NS. For intrapleural use, mix in 50 to 100 mL of NS.

Mechanism of Action Bleomycin inhibits synthesis of DNA; binds to DNA leading to single- and double-strand breaks; also inhibits (to a lesser degree) RNA and protein synthesis

Pharmacodynamics/Kinetics

Absorption: IM, SubQ, and intrapleural administration: 100%, 70%, and 45%, respectively, of IV serum concentrations

Distribution: V_d: IV: 17.5 L/m^2

Protein binding: 1%

Metabolism: Enzymatic inactivation by bleomycin hydrolase, a cytosolic cysteine proteinase enzyme; bleomycin hydrolase is widely distributed in normal tissues (except for the skin and lungs)

Half-life elimination: Terminal: IV: 2 hours

Time to peak, serum: IM, SubQ, Intrapleural: 30 to 60 minutes

Excretion: Urine (~65% [IV], 40% [Intrapleural])

Dosing

Adult Note: The risk for pulmonary toxicity increases with age >70 years and cumulative lifetime dose of >400 units. **International considerations:** Dosages below expressed as USP units; 1 USP unit = 1 mg (by potency) = 1,000 international units (Stefanou 2001). During shortages within the US, temporary importation of international products may be allowed by the FDA. The imported bleomycin vial and product labeling may express strength and dosing as international units instead of USP units.

◄ **Hodgkin lymphoma (off-label dosing):** IV:

ABVD regimen: 10 units/m^2 days 1 and 15 of a 28-day treatment cycle (in combination with doxorubicin, vinblastine, and dacarbazine) (Straus 2004)

BEACOPP regimen: 10 units/m^2 day 8 of a 21-day treatment cycle (in combination with etoposide, doxorubicin, cyclophosphamide, vincristine, procarbazine, and prednisone) (Dann 2007, Diehl 2003)

Stanford V regimen: 5 units/m^2/dose in weeks 2, 4, 6, 8, 10 and 12 (in combination with mechlorethamine, vinblastine, vincristine, doxorubicin, etoposide, and prednisone) (Horning 2002; Horning 2000)

Test dose for lymphoma patients: IM, IV, SubQ: Due to the possibility of an anaphylactoid reaction, the manufacturer recommends administering bleomycin 2 units or less before the first 2 doses; if no acute reaction occurs, then the regular dosage schedule may be followed. Monitor carefully, particularly following the first 2 doses. **Note:** Test doses may not be predictive of a reaction (Lam 2005) and/or may produce false-negative results.

Testicular cancer (off-label dosing): IV: BEP regimen: 30 units/dose days 1, 8, and 15 of a 21-day treatment cycle for 4 cycles (in combination with etoposide and cisplatin) (Culine 2008; Nichols 1998)

Malignant pleural effusion: Intrapleural: 60 units as a single instillation; mix in 50 to 100 mL of NS

Ovarian germ cell cancer (off-label use): BEP regimen: IV: 30 units/dose days 1, 8, and 15 of a 21-day treatment cycle for 3 cycles (in combination with etoposide and cisplatin) (Williams 1994) **or** 15 units/m^2 day 1 of a 21-day treatment cycle for 4 cycles (in combination with etoposide and cisplatin) (Cushing 2004)

Geriatric Refer to adult dosing. The incidence of pulmonary toxicity is higher in patients >70 years of age.

Pediatric Note: The risk for pulmonary toxicity increases with cumulative lifetime dose of >400 units. **International considerations:** Dosages below expressed as USP units; 1 USP unit = 1 mg (by potency) = 1,000 international units (Stefanou 2001). During shortages within the US, temporary importation of international products may be allowed by the FDA. The imported bleomycin vial and product labeling may express strength and dosing as international units instead of USP units.

Hodgkin lymphoma (off-label use):

ABVD regimen (high-risk disease): Children and Adolescents: IV: 10 units/m^2 days 1 and 15 of a 28-day treatment cycle (in combination with doxorubicin, vinblastine, and dacarbazine) for up to 6 cycles (Hutchinson 1998).

ABVE-PC (intermediate-risk or high-risk disease): Children and Adolescents: IV or SubQ: 5 units/m^2 on day 1 and 10 units/m^2 on day 8 of a 21-day cycle (in combination with doxorubicin, vincristine, etoposide, prednisone, and cyclophosphamide) for 2 to 4 cycles, (Dharmarajan 2015; Friedman 2014; Schwartz 2009).

BEACOPP (high-risk disease): Children and Adolescents: IV: 10 units/m^2 on day 7 of a 21-day treatment cycle (in combination with etoposide, doxorubicin, cyclophosphamide, vincristine, procarbazine, and prednisone) for 4 cycles (Kelly 2002).

Stanford V (high-risk disease): Adolescent ≥16 years: IV: 5 units/m^2 in weeks 2, 4, 6, 8, 10, and 12 of a single 12-week treatment cycle (in combination with mechlorethamine, vinblastine, vincristine, doxorubicin, etoposide, and prednisone) (Gordon 2013; Horning 2000; Horning 2002).

Test dose for lymphoma patients: IM, IV, SubQ: Due to the possibility of an anaphylactoid reaction, the manufacturer recommends administering bleomycin 2 units or less before the first 2 doses; if no acute reaction occurs, then the regular dosage schedule may be followed. Monitor carefully, particularly following the first 2 doses.

Note: Test doses may not be predictive of a reaction (Lam 2005) and/or may produce false-negative results.

Germ cell tumors, malignant, high risk (off-label use): BEP regimen (Cushing 2004):

Infants: IV: 0.5 **mg**/kg on day 1 of a 21-day treatment cycle (in combination with cisplatin and etoposide) for 4 cycles.

Children ≥1 year and Adolescents: IV: 15 units/m^2 on day 1 of a 21-day treatment cycle (in combination with etoposide and cisplatin) for 4 cycles.

Renal Impairment

Manufacturer's labeling (creatinine clearance should be estimated using the Cockcroft-Gault formula):

CrCl ≥50 mL/minute: No dosage adjustment necessary.

CrCl 40 to 50 mL/minute: Reduce dose to 70% of normal dose

CrCl 30 to 40 mL/minute: Reduce dose to 60% of normal dose

CrCl 20 to 30 mL/minute: Reduce dose to 55% of normal dose

CrCl 10 to 20 mL/minute: Reduce dose to 45% of normal dose

CrCl 5 to 10 mL/minute: Reduce dose to 40% of normal dose

The following adjustments have also been recommended:

Aronoff 2007: Adults: Continuous renal replacement therapy (CRRT): Reduce dose to 75% of normal dose

Kintzel 1995: Adults:

CrCl 46 to 60 mL/minute: Reduce dose to 70% of normal dose

CrCl 31 to 45 mL/minute: Reduce dose to 60% of normal dose

CrCl <30 mL/minute: Consider use of alternative drug

Hepatic Impairment There are no dosage adjustments provided in the manufacturer's labeling (has not been studied); however, adjustment for hepatic impairment is not necessary (King 2001).

Obesity *ASCO Guidelines for appropriate chemotherapy dosing in obese adults with cancer:* Fixed doses (dosing which is independent of body weight or BSA), are used in some protocols (eg, testicular cancer); due to toxicity concerns, the same fixed dose should also be considered for obese patients (Griggs 2012).

Adjustment for Toxicity

Pulmonary toxicity: Discontinue until determined not to be drug-related.

Pulmonary diffusion capacity for carbon monoxide (DL$_{CO}$) <30% to 35% of baseline: Discontinue treatment.

Pulmonary diffusing capacity for carbon monoxide corrected for hemoglobin content [DLCOc] decrease of more than 25% during therapy (compared with baseline): Consider discontinuing bleomycin to avoid further pulmonary toxicity (Lauritsen 2016).

Combination Regimens
Lymphoma, Hodgkin:

Administration
IV doses should be administered slowly over 10 minutes (according to the manufacturer's labeling).

IM or SubQ: May cause pain at injection site

Intrapleural: 60 units in 50 to 100 mL NS; use of topical anesthetics or opioid analgesia is usually not necessary

Monitor for hypersensitivity, particularly following the first 2 doses in patients with lymphoma.

Vesicant/Extravasation Risk May be an irritant

Emetic Potential Children and Adults: Minimal (<10%)

Monitoring Parameters Pulmonary function tests, including total lung volume, forced vital capacity, diffusion capacity for carbon monoxide; vital capacity, total lung capacity and pulmonary capillary blood volume may be better indicators of changes induced by bleomycin (Sleijfer 2001); forced vital capacity [FVC], forced expiratory volume in 1 second [FEV_1], and diffusing capacity of the lungs for carbon monoxide [DLCO]) were performed prior to treatment, before each chemotherapy cycle, and then repeated at 1 year, 3 years, and 5 years during follow up for testicular cancer patients receiving bleomycin (Lauritsen 2016); chest x-ray, renal function, liver function; monitor for signs/symptoms of hypersensitivity; temperature initially; check body weight at regular intervals.

Dosage Forms Considerations During shortages within the US, temporary importation of international products may be allowed by the FDA. The imported bleomycin vial and product labeling may express strength and dosing as international units instead of USP units (1,000 international units = 1 USP unit).

Dosage Forms Excipient information presented when available (limited, particularly for generics); consult specific product labeling.
Solution Reconstituted, Injection:
Generic: 15 units (1 ea); 30 units (1 ea)
Solution Reconstituted, Injection [preservative free]:
Generic: 15 units (1 ea); 30 units (1 ea)

♦ **Bleomycin Injection, USP (Can)** *see* Bleomycin *on page* 256
♦ **Bleomycin Sulfate** *see* Bleomycin *on page* 256

Blinatumomab (blin a TOOM oh mab)

Related Information

Common Toxicity Criteria *on page 2242*

Management of Chemotherapy-Induced Nausea and Vomiting in Adults *on page 2253*

Brand Names: US Blincyto

Brand Names: Canada Blincyto

Index Terms MT103

Pharmacologic Category Antineoplastic Agent, Anti-CD19/CD3; Antineoplastic Agent, Monoclonal Antibody

Use Acute lymphoblastic leukemia: Treatment of relapsed or refractory B-cell precursor acute lymphoblastic leukemia (ALL)

Labeled Contraindications Known hypersensitivity to blinatumomab or any component of the formulation

Pregnancy Considerations Animal reproductions studies have not been conducted. Based on the mechanism of action, blinatumomab may cause fetal harm when administered to a pregnant woman. Newborns exposed in utero may develop B-cell lymphocytopenia; monitor B-lymphocytes prior to administering live virus vaccines. Verify pregnancy status of women of reproductive potential prior to initiating treatment; effective contraception should be used during treatment and for at least 48 hours after the last dose.

Breastfeeding Considerations It is not known if blinatumomab is present in breast milk. Due to the potential for serious adverse reactions in the breastfeeding infant, breastfeeding is not recommended by the manufacturer during treatment and for at least 48 hours after the last dose.

Warnings/Precautions [US Boxed Warning]: Cytokine release syndrome (CRS), which may be life-threatening or fatal, has occurred. Interrupt or discontinue therapy as recommended. Infusion reactions have also occurred, and may be difficult to distinguish from CRS. CRS symptoms may include pyrexia, headache, nausea, weakness, hypotension, increased transaminases, and elevated total bilirubin. In some patients, disseminated intravascular coagulation (DIC), capillary leak syndrome (CLS), and hemophagocytic histiocytosis/macrophage activation syndrome (MAS) have been reported in the setting of CRS. Monitor closely for signs/symptoms of these conditions; may require therapy interruption or discontinuation. CRS which was life-threatening or fatal occurred rarely. The highest cytokine elevation was observed in the first 2 days following the start of infusion. In 1 study, patients with a high tumor burden (≥50% leukemic blasts or >15,000/mm^3 peripheral blood leukemic blast counts), or elevated lactate dehydrogenase were pre-treated with dexamethasone (10 to 24 mg/m^2/day for up to 5 days and concluding 3 days prior to initiating blinatumomab) to reduce the incidence of severe CRS (Topp 2015). **[US Boxed Warning]: Neurological toxicities, which may be severe, life-threatening, or fatal, have occurred. Interrupt or discontinue therapy as recommended.** Neurotoxicity has occurred in almost two-thirds of patients with ALL in clinical trials. The median time to onset was within the first 2 weeks of therapy. Common neurological symptoms include headache and tremor (symptoms may differ in children <2 years, and elderly patients have a higher incidence of neurotoxicity). Grade 3 or higher neurotoxicity (eg, encephalopathy, convulsions, speech disorders, disturbances in consciousness, confusion and disorientation, and coordination and balance disorders) has also been observed. Neurotoxicity may be managed with dexamethasone (Topp 2015). Patients are at risk for loss of consciousness due to neurologic events while taking blinatumomab; advise patients to avoid driving, participating in hazardous occupations, or operating heavy or dangerous machinery during treatment. Patients with a history of (or current) clinically relevant CNS pathology were excluded from clinical trials. Monitor patients for signs/symptoms of neurotoxicity; may require therapy interruption or discontinuation. The majority of symptoms resolved after interrupting therapy. Leukoencephalopathy (as seen on MRI) has been reported, particularly in those patients who received prior treatment with cranial irradiation and antileukemia chemotherapy (eg, high-dose methotrexate, intrathecal cytarabine).

Neutropenia and neutropenic fever, including life-threatening episodes, have been reported. Monitor blood counts throughout therapy; may require therapy interruption if prolonged neutropenia occurs. Anemia and thrombocytopenia may also occur. Serious infections such as sepsis, pneumonia, bacteremia, opportunistic infections, and catheter-related infections have been reported in approximately one-fourth of patients with ALL in clinical trials (may be life-threatening or fatal). Consider prophylactic antibiotics if appropriate, and monitor closely for signs/symptoms of infection. Treat promptly if infection occurs. Transient increases in liver enzymes (associated both with and without CRS) may occur during therapy. In patients with ALL, the median time to enzyme elevation was 3 to 19 days; grade 3 or higher elevations were observed in a small percentage of patients. Monitor ALT, AST, GGT, and total bilirubin at baseline and during treatment. Interrupt therapy if transaminases are >5 times ULN or if bilirubin is >3 times ULN. Fatal cases of pancreatitis in patients receiving blinatumomab plus dexamethasone have been reported in the postmarketing setting. Monitor for signs/symptoms of pancreatitis; may require therapy interruption or discontinuation. Life-threatening or fatal tumor lysis syndrome (TLS) has been observed. Administer measures to prevent TLS (eg, pretreatment nontoxic cytoreduction, and hydration during treatment). Monitor for signs/symptoms of TLS (eg, acute renal failure, hyperkalemia, hypocalcemia, hyperuricemia, and/or hyperphosphatemia); may require treatment interruption or discontinuation. Pediatric patients experienced an increased rate of anemia, thrombocytopenia, vomiting, pyrexia, and hypertension as compared to adult patients. While the incidence of neurologic toxicities in patients <2 years of age did not differ from other age groups, the manifestations were different; reported toxicities were agitation, headache, insomnia, somnolence, and irritability. Elderly patients experienced an increased rate of neurotoxicity (including cognitive disorder), encephalopathy, confusion, and serious infections as compared to patients <65 years.

Preparation and administration errors have occurred. Do not flush infusion line, particularly when changing infusion bags or at completion of infusion; may result in overdose and complications. IV bag contains overfill and volume will be more than the volume administered to the patient to account for IV line priming and to ensure that the full dose is administered. Follow preparation and administration instructions carefully. Refer to manufacturer labeling for further information. Potentially significant drug-drug interactions may exist, requiring dose or frequency adjustment, additional monitoring, and/or selection of alternative therapy. Vaccination with live virus vaccines is not recommended for at least 2 weeks prior to blinatumomab initiation, during treatment, and until immune system recovery following the last cycle of therapy.

Diluent may contain benzyl alcohol; large amounts of benzyl alcohol (≥99 mg/kg/day) have been associated with a potentially fatal toxicity ("gasping syndrome") in neonates; the "gasping syndrome" consists of metabolic acidosis, respiratory distress, gasping respirations, CNS dysfunction (including convulsions, intracranial hemorrhage), hypotension and cardiovascular collapse (AAP ["Inactive" 1997]; CDC 1982); some data suggests that benzoate displaces bilirubin from protein binding sites (Ahlfors 2001); avoid or use dosage forms containing benzyl alcohol with caution in neonates. See manufacturer's labeling. Due to the addition of bacteriostatic saline, the 7-day infusion bags of blinatumomab contain benzyl alcohol and are not recommended for use in patients weighing <22 kg. Some dosage forms may contain polysorbate 80 (also known as Tweens). Hypersensitivity reactions, usually a delayed reaction, have been reported following exposure to pharmaceutical products containing polysorbate 80 in certain individuals (Isaksson 2002; Lucente 2000; Shelley 1995). Thrombocytopenia, ascites, pulmonary deterioration, and renal and hepatic failure have been reported in premature neonates after receiving parenteral products containing polysorbate 80 (Alade 1986; CDC 1984). See manufacturer's labeling.

Adverse Reactions Incidences are reported for all patient populations unless otherwise specified.

>10%:

Cardiovascular: Edema (patients ≥45 kg: 30%; patients <45 kg: 11%), hypertension (patients <45 kg: 25%; patients ≥45 kg: 9%), cardiac arrhythmia (11% to 19%), hypotension (12% to 13%)

Central nervous system: Neurotoxicity (64%; incidence increased in older adults), headache (28% to 36%), fatigue (9% to 16%), chills (patients ≥45 kg: 15%; patients <45 kg: 2%), insomnia (5% to 14%), dizziness (5% to 13%)

Dermatologic: Skin rash (patients ≥45 kg: 21%; patients <45 kg: 11%)

Endocrine & metabolic: Hypokalemia (21% to 27%; incidence increased in infants), weight gain (11% to 18%), hypophosphatemia (patients <45 kg: 16%; patients ≥45 kg: 6%), hyperglycemia (11% to 12%), hypomagnesemia (9% to 12%), hypocalcemia (5% to 11%)

Gastrointestinal: Nausea (26% to 30%), vomiting (patients <45 kg: 26%; patients ≥45 kg: 13%), abdominal pain (19% to 23%), constipation (patients ≥45 kg: 20%; patients <45 kg: 9%), diarrhea (19%)

Hematologic & oncologic: Anemia (patients <45 kg: 42%; ≥ grade 3: 35%; patients ≥45 kg: 21%; ≥ grade 3: 16%), thrombocytopenia (patients <45 kg: 35%; patients ≥45 kg: 16%; all patients, ≥ grade 3: 12% to 35%), neutropenia (patients <45 kg: 32%; ≥ grade 3: 32%; patients ≥45 kg: 19%; ≥ grade 3: 18%), leukopenia (patients <45 kg: 26%; patients ≥45 kg: 14%; ≥ grade 3: 12% to 21%), febrile neutropenia (19% to 25%; ≥ grade 3: 18% to 23%), decreased serum immunoglobulins (5% to 12%; grades 3/4, patients ≥45 kg: 2%)

Hepatic: Increased serum ALT (patients <45 kg: 36%; patients ≥45 kg: 21%), increased serum AST (11% to 18%), increased serum bilirubin (5% to 13%)

Hypersensitivity: Cytokine release syndrome (11% to 13%; including cytokine storms)

Infection: Infection (42% to 45%), serious infection (25%; including bacteremia, opportunistic infections, catheter-site infections), bacterial infection (11% to 19%), fungal infection (7% to 14%), viral infection (9% to 13%)

Neuromuscular & skeletal: Tremor (patients ≥45 kg: 19%; patients <45 kg: 7%), back pain (15% to 16%), limb pain (11% to 12%), ostealgia (9% to 11%)

◄ Respiratory: Cough (18% to 20%), dyspnea (patients ≥45 kg: 15%; patients <45 kg: 4%)

Miscellaneous: Fever (patients <45 kg: 75%; patients ≥45 kg: 64%), infusion related reaction (patients <45 kg: 44%; patients ≥45 kg: 34%)

1% to 10%:

Cardiovascular: Chest pain (4% to 10%)

Central nervous system: Impaired consciousness (7% to 10%), confusion (patients ≥45 kg: 7%), brain disease (2% to 5%), paresthesia (2% to 5%), aphasia (patients ≥45 kg: 4%), disorientation (patients ≥45 kg: 3%), memory impairment (patients ≥45 kg: 2%), cognitive dysfunction (patients ≥45 kg: 1%)

Endocrine & metabolic: Hypoalbuminemia (4% to 7%), increased gamma-glutamyl transferase (patients ≥45 kg: 6%; patients <45 kg: 2%)

Gastrointestinal: Decreased appetite (4% to 10%)

Hematologic & oncologic: Tumor lysis syndrome (patients ≥45 kg: 4%), leukocytosis (2% to 4%), lymphocytopenia (1% to 2%)

Hypersensitivity: Hypersensitivity reaction (1%)

Infection: Sepsis (≥2%)

Neuromuscular & skeletal: Arthralgia (4% to 10%)

Respiratory: Epistaxis (9% to 10%), pneumonia (≥45 kg: ≥2%)

<1%, postmarketing, and/or case reports: Antibody development, bronchospasm, leukoencephalopathy, pancreatitis, speech disturbance

Drug Interactions

Metabolism/Transport Effects None known.

Avoid Concomitant Use

Avoid concomitant use of Blinatumomab with any of the following: BCG (Intravesical); Deferiprone; Dipyrone; Natalizumab; Pimecrolimus; Tacrolimus (Topical); Vaccines (Live)

Increased Effect/Toxicity

Blinatumomab may increase the levels/effects of: CloZAPine; Deferiprone; Fingolimod; Leflunomide; Natalizumab; Tofacitinib; Vaccines (Live)

The levels/effects of Blinatumomab may be increased by: Denosumab; Dipyrone; Ocrelizumab; Pimecrolimus; Promazine; Roflumilast; Tacrolimus (Topical); Trastuzumab

Decreased Effect

Blinatumomab may decrease the levels/effects of: BCG (Intravesical); Coccidioides immitis Skin Test; Nivolumab; Sipuleucel-T; Tertomotide; Vaccines (Inactivated); Vaccines (Live)

The levels/effects of Blinatumomab may be decreased by: Echinacea

Storage/Stability Store intact vials (drug and solution stabilizer) in the original package at 2°C to 8°C (36°F to 46°F); protect from light. Do not freeze. Intact vials of both drug and stabilizer may be stored for up to 8 hours at room temperature. Reconstituted solution is stable for up to 4 hours at 23°C to 27°C (73°F to 81°F) or up to 24 hours at 2°C to 8°C (36°F to 46°F). Solutions diluted for infusion **(preservative free)** are stable in NS for up to 48 hours at 23°C to 27°C (73°F to 81°F) or up to 8 days at 2°C to 8°C (36°F to 46°F). Solutions diluted for infusion **(with preservative)** are stable in NS for up to 7 days at 23°C to 27°C (73°F to 81°F) or up to 14 days at 2°C to 8°C (36°F to 46°F). Infusion should be completed within these time frames; if IV bag of solution for infusion is not administered within the time frames and temperatures indicated, discard; do not refrigerate again.

Preparation for Administration Note: Preparation and administration errors have occurred; follow preparation instructions carefully. Refer to manufacturer labeling for further information.

Reconstitute each vial of lyophilized powder with 3 mL of preservative-free SWFI (do **not** reconstitute vials with the IV solution stabilizer); direct stream toward the side of the vial and gently swirl to avoid excess foaming. Do not shake; final reconstituted concentration is 12.5 **mcg**/mL. Reconstituted solution should be clear to slightly opalescent, colorless to slightly yellow; do not use if cloudy or if precipitation occurs. **Note:** Some doses may require reconstitution of more than 1 vial of lyophilized powder.

24- or 48-hour infusion: Add 270 mL NS to an empty IV bag; use only polyolefin, non-DEHP PVC (non-di-ethylhexylphthalate PVC), or ethyl vinyl acetate (EVA) infusion bags or pump cassettes. Transfer 5.5 mL of IV solution stabilizer to the IV bag; gently mix to avoid foaming. Transfer the appropriate volume of reconstituted blinatumomab solution to the IV bag and gently mix; refer to manufacturer labeling for the specific volume of reconstituted drug to be added. Attach the IV tubing (use only polyolefin, non-DEHP PVC, or EVA tubing) to the bag with a sterile, non-pyrogenic, low protein-binding 0.2 micron in-line filter. Remove air from the IV bag. **Prime the IV tubing only with the prepared infusion solution**; do **not** prime with NS. If not used immediately, store at 2°C to 8°C (36°F to 46°F) for up to 8 days (infusion must be completed within this time frame).

*7-day infusion (**not** recommended for patients weighing <22 kg):* Add 90 mL **bacteriostatic** NS to an empty IV bag; use only polyolefin, non-DEHP PVC, or ethyl vinyl acetate (EVA) infusion bags or pump cassettes. Transfer 2.2 mL of IV solution stabilizer to the IV bag; gently mix to avoid foaming. Transfer the appropriate volume of reconstituted blinatumomab solution to the IV bag and gently mix; refer to manufacturer labeling for the specific volume of reconstituted drug to be added. Add NS to the IV bag to a final volume of 110 mL (resulting in 0.74% benzyl alcohol); gently mix (avoid foaming). Attach the IV tubing (use only polyolefin, non-DEHP PVC, or EVA tubing) to the bag; an in-line filter is not required for the 7-day infusion bag. Remove air from the IV bag. **Prime the IV tubing only with the prepared infusion solution**; do **not** prime with NS. If not used immediately, store at 2°C to 8°C (36°F to 46°F) for up to 14 days (infusion must be completed within this time frame).

Mechanism of Action Blinatumomab is a bispecific T-cell engager (BiTE) which binds to CD19 expressed on B-cells and CD3 expressed on T-cells. It activates endogenous T cells by connecting CD3 in the T-cell receptor complex with CD19 on B-cells (malignant and benign), thus forming a cytolytic synapse between a cytotoxic T-cell and the cancer target B-cell (Topp 2014). Blinatumomab mediates the production of cytolytic proteins, release of inflammatory cytokines, and proliferation of T cells, which result in lysis of CD19-positive cells.

Pharmacodynamics/Kinetics

Distribution: Pediatric patients 0 to 17 years: 3.14 ± 2.97 L/m^2; Adults: 4.35 L

Half-life elimination: Pediatric patients 0 to 17 years: 2.04 ± 1.35 hours; Adults: 2.1 hours

Excretion: Urine (negligible amounts)

Dosing

Adult & Geriatric Note: Hospitalization is recommended for the first 9 days of cycle 1, and the first 2 days of cycle 2. Close observation by a healthcare professional (or hospitalization) is recommended for initiation of all subsequent cycles or for therapy reinitiation (eg, treatment is interrupted for 4 or more hours). Do **not** flush infusion line, particularly when changing infusion bags or at completion of infusion; may result in overdose.

Premedicate with dexamethasone 20 mg one hour prior to the first dose of each cycle, prior to a step dose (eg, Cycle 1 day 8), or when restarting therapy after an interruption of ≥4 hours.

Acute lymphoblastic leukemia (B-cell precursor), relapsed/refractory:
IV: Each induction and consolidation treatment cycle consists of 4 weeks of continuous infusion followed by a 2-week treatment-free interval (allow at least 2 weeks treatment-free between cycles). Each continued therapy cycle consists of 4 weeks of continuous infusion followed by an 8-week treatment-free interval. Therapy involves up to 2 induction cycles followed by 3 additional cycles for consolidation and up to 4 additional cycles of continued therapy (total of up to 9 cycles).

Patients ≥45 kg (fixed dose):

Cycle 1: 9 **mcg** daily administered as a continuous infusion on days 1 to 7, followed by 28 **mcg** daily as a continuous infusion on days 8 to 28 of a 6-week treatment cycle

Cycles 2 through 5: 28 **mcg** daily administered as a continuous infusion on days 1 to 28 of a 6-week treatment cycle

Cycles 6 through 9: 28 **mcg** daily administered as a continuous infusion on days 1 to 28 of a 12-week treatment cycle

Patients <45 kg (dose based on BSA):

Cycle 1: 5 **mcg**/m^2/day (maximum: 9 **mcg**/day) administered as a continuous infusion on days 1 to 7, followed by 15 **mcg**/m^2/day (maximum: 28 **mcg**/day) as a continuous infusion on days 8 to 28 of a 6-week treatment cycle

Cycles 2 through 5: 15 **mcg**/m^2/day (maximum: 28 **mcg**/day) administered as a continuous infusion on days 1 to 28 of a 6-week treatment cycle

Cycles 6 through 9: 15 **mcg**/m^2/day (maximum: 28 **mcg**/day) administered as a continuous infusion on days 1 to 28 of a 12-week treatment cycle

Pediatric Note: Hospitalization is recommended for the first 9 days of cycle 1, and the first 2 days of cycle 2. Close observation by a healthcare professional (or hospitalization) is recommended for initiation of all subsequent cycles or for therapy reinitiation (eg, treatment is interrupted for 4 or more hours). Do **not** flush infusion line, particularly when changing infusion bags or at completion of infusion; may result in overdose.

Premedicate with dexamethasone 5 mg/m^2 (maximum: 20 mg) one hour prior to the first dose of the first cycle, prior to a step dose (eg, Cycle 1 day 8), or when restarting therapy after an interruption of ≥4 hours in the first cycle.

Acute lymphoblastic leukemia (B-cell precursor), relapsed/refractory:
IV: Each induction or consolidation treatment cycle consists of 4 weeks of continuous infusion followed by a 2-week treatment-free interval (allow at least 2 weeks treatment-free between cycles). Each continued therapy cycle consists of 4 weeks of continuous infusion followed by an 8-week treatment-free interval. Therapy involves 2 induction cycles followed by 3 additional cycles for consolidation and up to 4 additional cycles of continued therapy (total of up to 9 cycles).

Patients ≥45 kg (fixed dose):

Cycle 1: 9 **mcg** daily administered as a continuous infusion on days 1 to 7, followed by 28 **mcg** daily as a continuous infusion on days 8 to 28 of a 6-week treatment cycle

Cycles 2 through 5: 28 **mcg** daily administered as a continuous infusion on days 1 to 28 of a 6-week treatment cycle

Cycles 6 through 9: 28 **mcg** daily administered as a continuous infusion on days 1 to 28 of a 12-week treatment cycle

Patients <45 kg (dose based on BSA):

Cycle 1: 5 **mcg**/m^2/day (maximum: 9 **mcg**/day) administered as a continuous infusion on days 1 to 7, followed by 15 **mcg**/m^2/day (maximum: 28 **mcg**/day) as a continuous infusion on days 8 to 28 of a 6-week treatment cycle

Cycles 2 through 5: 15 **mcg**/m^2/day (maximum: 28 **mcg**/day) administered as a continuous infusion on days 1 to 28 of a 6-week treatment cycle

Cycles 6 through 9: 15 **mcg**/m^2/day (maximum: 28 **mcg**/day) administered as a continuous infusion on days 1 to 28 of a 12-week treatment cycle

Renal Impairment

CrCl ≥30 mL/minute: There are no dosage adjustments provided in the manufacturer's labeling; however, a pharmacokinetic analysis showed that clearance values in patients with CrCl 30 to 59 mL/minute were similar to the range observed in patients with normal renal function.

CrCl <30 mL/minute: There are no dosage adjustments provided in the manufacturer's labeling (has not been studied).

Hemodialysis: There are no dosage adjustments provided in the manufacturer's labeling (has not been studied).

Hepatic Impairment

There are no dosage adjustments provided in the manufacturer's labeling (has not been studied).

Hepatotoxicity during treatment: Interrupt therapy if transaminases are >5 times ULN or if bilirubin is >3 times ULN.

Adjustment for Toxicity If the interruption after an adverse event is no longer than 7 days, continue the same cycle to a total of 28 days of infusion inclusive of days before and after the interruption in that cycle. If an interruption due to an adverse event is longer than 7 days, start a new cycle.

Cytokine release syndrome (CRS):

Grade 3: Interrupt therapy until resolved, then resume dosing at 9 **mcg** daily (or 5 **mcg**/m^2/day if <45 kg). Increase dose to 28 **mcg** daily (or 15 **mcg**/m^2/day if <45 kg) after 7 days if toxicity does not recur.

Grade 4: Discontinue permanently

Neurologic toxicity:

Grade 3: Interrupt therapy for at least 3 days and until toxicity is ≤ grade 1 (mild), then resume dosing at 9 **mcg** daily (or 5 **mcg**/m^2/day if <45 kg). Increase dose to 28 **mcg** daily (or 15 **mcg**/m^2/day if <45 kg) after 7 days if toxicity does not recur. If toxicity occurred at the 9 **mcg** daily dose (or 5 **mcg**/m^2/day dose if <45 kg), or if it takes more than 7 days to resolve, discontinue permanently.

Grade 4: Discontinue permanently

Seizure: Discontinue permanently if more than 1 seizure occurs.

◀

Other clinically relevant toxicity:

Grade 3: Interrupt therapy until toxicity is ≤ grade 1 (mild), then resume dosing at 9 **mcg** daily (or 5 **mcg**/m^2/day if <45 kg). Increase dose to 28 **mcg** daily (or 15 **mcg**/m^2/day if <45 kg) after 7 days if toxicity does not recur. If toxicity takes more than 14 days to resolve, discontinue permanently.

Grade 4: Consider discontinuing permanently.

Administration Note: Preparation and administration errors have occurred; carefully follow administration instructions.

IV:

24- or 48-hour infusion: Administer 240 mL as a continuous IV infusion at a constant flow rate of 10 mL/hour for 24 hours or 5 mL/hour for 48 hours (depending on dose, duration, and/or concentration) through a dedicated lumen. Use a programmable, lockable, non-elastomeric infusion pump with an alarm; IV tubing should include a sterile, nonpyrogenic, low protein-binding, 0.2 micron in-line filter.

*7-day infusion (**not** recommended in patients weighing <22 kg):* Administer 100 mL as a continuous IV infusion at a constant flow rate of 0.6 mL/hour for 7 days through a dedicated lumen. Use a programmable, lockable, non-elastomeric infusion pump with an alarm; an in-line filter is not required for the 7-day infusion bag.

Only use polyolefin, non-DEHP PVC (non-di-ethylhexylphthalate PVC), or ethyl vinyl acetate (EVA) infusion bags, pump cassettes and IV tubing. IV tubing should be primed with prepared infusion solution, not NS. For adults, premedicate with dexamethasone 20 mg one hour prior to the first dose of each cycle, prior to a step dose (such as cycle 1 day 8), or when restarting therapy after an interruption of ≥4 hours. For pediatric patients, premedicate with dexamethasone 5 mg/m^2 (maximum: 20 mg) one hour prior to the first dose of the first cycle, prior to a step dose (eg, Cycle 1 day 8), or when restarting therapy after an interruption of ≥4 hours in the first cycle.

Infuse bag contains overfill (to account for tubing priming volume). Do **not** flush infusion line, particularly when changing infusion bags or at completion of infusion; may result in excess dosage and complications. Do not infuse other medications through the same line.

Emetic Potential Low (10% to 30%)

Monitoring Parameters CBC with differential, liver function tests (ALT, AST, GGT, and total bilirubin) at baseline and throughout therapy; monitor for signs/symptoms of cytokine release syndrome, infusion reactions, neurotoxicity, infection, pancreatitis, and tumor lysis syndrome

Medication Guide Available Yes

Dosage Forms Considerations Provided with IV solution stabilizer to coat the prefilled NS bag prior to addition of reconstituted blinatumomab (do NOT use IV solution stabilizer for reconstitution of blinatumomab).

Dosage Forms Excipient information presented when available (limited, particularly for generics); consult specific product labeling.

Solution Reconstituted, Intravenous [preservative free]:

Blincyto: 35 mcg (1 ea) [contains polysorbate 80]

Dosage Forms: Canada Information with regard to form, strength, and availability of products uniquely available in Canada but currently not available in the US. Refer also to Dosage Forms.

Excipient information presented when available (limited, particularly for generics); consult specific product labeling.

Solution Reconstituted, Intravenous [preservative free]:

Blincyto: 38.5 mcg (1 ea) [contains polysorbate 80]

◆ **Blincyto** see Blinatumomab on page 263
◆ **BLM** see Bleomycin on page 256
◆ **BMS-247550** see Ixabepilone on page 1078
◆ **BMS-354825** see Dasatinib on page 523
◆ **BMS-901608** see Elotuzumab on page 663
◆ **BMS-907351** see Cabozantinib on page 311
◆ **BMS-936558** see Nivolumab on page 1328
◆ **BocaSal** see Saliva Substitute on page 1653
◆ **Bondronate** see Ibandronate on page 933
◆ **Bonefos (Can)** see Clodronate on page 416
◆ **Boniva** see Ibandronate on page 933

Bortezomib (bore TEZ oh mib)

Related Information

Chemotherapy-Induced Peripheral Neuropathy on page 2236
Common Toxicity Criteria on page 2242
Hematopoietic Cell Transplantation on page 2365
Hypercalcemia of Malignancy on page 2341
Management of Chemotherapy-Induced Nausea and Vomiting in Adults on page 2253
Management of Drug Extravasations on page 2271
Prevention of Chemotherapy-Induced Nausea and Vomiting in Children on page 2310
Safe Handling of Hazardous Drugs on page 2379

Brand Names: US Velcade

Brand Names: Canada Bortezomib For Injection; Velcade

Index Terms LDP-341; MLN341; PS-341

Pharmacologic Category Antineoplastic Agent, Proteasome Inhibitor

Use

Mantle cell lymphoma: Treatment of mantle cell lymphoma.

Multiple myeloma: Treatment of multiple myeloma.

Labeled Contraindications Hypersensitivity (excluding local reactions) to bortezomib, boron, mannitol, or any component of the formulation; administration via the intrathecal route

Pregnancy Considerations Based on the mechanism of action and on findings in animal reproduction studies, bortezomib may cause fetal harm if administered during pregnancy. Verify pregnancy status in women of reproductive potential prior to initiating therapy; women of reproductive potential should avoid becoming pregnant during bortezomib treatment. Females and males of reproductive potential should use effective contraception during and

◄ for at least 2 months following bortezomib treatment. Bortezomib may potentially affect male or female fertility (based on the mechanism of action).

Breastfeeding Considerations It is not known if bortezomib is present in breast milk. The manufacturer recommends lactating women avoid breastfeeding during and for 2 months following bortezomib treatment.

Warnings/Precautions Bortezomib may cause or worsen peripheral neuropathy (usually sensory but may be mixed sensorimotor); risk may be increased with previous use of neurotoxic agents or preexisting peripheral neuropathy (patients with preexisting neuropathy should use only after risk versus benefit assessment); monitor for signs and symptoms; adjustment of dose and/or schedule may be required. The incidence of grades 2 and 3 peripheral neuropathy may be lower with SubQ route (compared to IV); consider subQ administration in patients with preexisting or at high risk for peripheral neuropathy; the majority of patients with ≥ grade 2 peripheral neuropathy have improvement in or resolution of symptoms with dose adjustments or discontinuation; in a study of elderly patients receiving a weekly bortezomib schedule with combination chemotherapy, the incidence of peripheral neuropathy was significantly reduced without an effect on outcome (Boccadoro 2010; Palumbo 2009). May cause hypotension (including postural and orthostatic); use caution with dehydration, history of syncope, or medications associated with hypotension (may require adjustment of antihypertensive medication, hydration, and mineralocorticoids and/or sympathomimetics). Acute development or exacerbation of heart failure (HF) and new onset decreased left ventricular ejection fraction (LVEF) have been reported with bortezomib; some cases have occurred in patients without risk factors for HF and/or decreased LVEF. Monitor closely in patients with risk factors for HF or existing heart disease. Isolated case of QT_c prolongation have been reported with bortezomib.

Pulmonary disorders (some fatal) including pneumonitis, interstitial pneumonia, lung infiltrates, and acute respiratory distress syndrome (ARDS) have been reported. Pulmonary hypertension (without left heart failure or significant pulmonary disease has been reported rarely). Promptly evaluate with new or worsening cardiopulmonary symptoms; therapy interruption may be required. Tumor lysis syndrome has been reported; risk is increased in patients with high tumor burden prior to treatment. Posterior reversible leukoencephalopathy syndrome (PRES, formerly RPLS) has been reported (rarely). Symptoms of PRES include confusion, headache, hypertension, lethargy, seizure, blindness and/or other vision, or neurologic disturbances; discontinue bortezomib if PRES occurs. MRI is recommended to confirm PRES diagnosis. The safety of reinitiating bortezomib in patients previously experiencing PRES is unknown. Progressive multifocal leukoencephalopathy (PML) has been rarely observed; monitor closely and evaluate promptly. Herpes (zoster and simplex) reactivation has been reported with bortezomib; consider antiviral prophylaxis during therapy. Hematologic toxicity, including grade 3 and 4 neutropenia and severe thrombocytopenia, may occur (nadirs generally occur following the last dose of a cycle and recover prior to the next cycle); risk is increased in patients with pretreatment platelet counts <75,000/mm³. Monitor frequently throughout treatment; may require dosage or schedule adjustments; withhold treatment for platelets <30,000/mm³. Management with platelet transfusions, supportive care, and/or myeloid growth factors may be necessary. Nadirs generally occur following the last dose of a cycle and recover prior to the next cycle. Hemorrhage (gastrointestinal and intracerebral) due to low platelet count has been observed. Neutropenic fever has been observed. Acute liver failure has been reported (rarely) in patients receiving multiple concomitant medications and with serious underlying conditions. Hepatitis, transaminase increases, and hyperbilirubinemia have also been reported; interrupt therapy to assess reversibility. Use caution in patients with hepatic dysfunction; reduced initial doses are recommended for moderate and severe hepatic impairment (exposure is increased); closely monitor for toxicities. Hyper- and hypoglycemia may occur in diabetic patients receiving oral hypoglycemics; may require adjustment of diabetes medications. Nausea, vomiting, diarrhea or constipation may occur; may require antiemetics or antidiarrheals; ileus may occur; administer fluid and electrolytes to prevent dehydration (monitor closely); interrupt therapy for severe symptoms.

Anaphylactic reaction, drug hypersensitivity, immune complex mediated hypersensitivity, angioedema, and laryngeal edema have been reported with bortezomib. Potentially significant drug-drug/drug-food interactions may exist, requiring dose or frequency adjustment, additional monitoring, and/or selection of alternative therapy. Coadministration of strong CYP3A4 inhibitors may increase bortezomib exposure; monitor for toxicity and consider dose reduction if concurrent therapy cannot be avoided. Efficacy may be reduced when administered with strong CYP3A4 inducers; concomitant use is not recommended.

For IV or SubQ administration only. Intrathecal administration is contraindicated; inadvertent intrathecal administration has resulted in death. Bortezomib should **NOT** be prepared during the preparation of any intrathecal medications. After preparation, keep bortezomib in a location **away** from the separate storage location recommended for intrathecal medications. Bortezomib should **NOT** be delivered to the patient at the same time with any medications intended for central nervous system administration. The reconstituted concentrations for IV and SubQ administration are different; use caution when calculating the volume for each route and dose. The manufacturer provides stickers to facilitate identification of the route for reconstituted vials.

Adverse Reactions Incidences reported are associated with monotherapy. Additional adverse reactions reported with mono- or combination therapy; frequency not defined.

Cardiovascular: Hypotension (8% to 9%; grades 3/4: ≤2%), cardiac disease (treatment emergent; 8%), acute pulmonary edema (≤1%), cardiac failure (≤1%), cardiogenic shock (≤1%), pulmonary edema (≤1%), aggravated atrial fibrillation, angina pectoris, atrial flutter, atrioventricular block, bradycardia, cerebrovascular accident, deep vein thrombosis, edema, embolism (peripheral), facial edema, hemorrhagic stroke, hypertension, ischemic heart disease, myocardial infarction, pericardial effusion, pericarditis, peripheral edema, phlebitis, portal vein thrombosis, pulmonary embolism, septic shock, sinoatrial arrest, subdural hematoma, torsades de pointes, transient ischemic attacks, ventricular tachycardia

Central nervous system: Peripheral neuropathy (IV: 35% to 54%; SubQ: 37%; grade ≥2: 24% to 39%; grade ≥3: SubQ: 5% to 6%; IV: 7% to 15%; grade 4: <1%), fatigue (7% to 52%), neuralgia (23%), headache (10% to 19%), paresthesia (7% to 19%), dizziness (10% to 18%; excludes vertigo), agitation, anxiety, ataxia, brain disease, cerebral hemorrhage, chills, coma, confusion, cranial nerve palsy, dysarthria, dysautonomia, dysesthesia, insomnia, malaise, mental status changes, motor dysfunction, paralysis, psychosis, seizure, spinal cord compression, suicidal ideation, vertigo

Dermatologic: Skin rash (12% to 23%), pruritus, urticaria

Endocrine & metabolic: Dehydration (2%), amyloid heart disease, hyperglycemia (diabetic patients), hyperkalemia, hypernatremia, hyperuricemia, hypocalcemia, hypoglycemia (diabetic patients), hypokalemia, hyponatremia, weight loss

Gastrointestinal: Diarrhea (19% to 52%), nausea (14% to 52%), constipation (24% to 34%), vomiting (9% to 29%), anorexia (14% to 21%), abdominal pain (11%), decreased appetite (11%), cholestasis, duodenitis (hemorrhagic), dysphagia, fecal impaction, gastritis (hemorrhagic), gastroenteritis, gastroesophageal reflux disease, hematemesis, intestinal obstruction, intestinal perforation, melena, oral candidiasis, pancreatitis, paralytic ileus, peritonitis, stomatitis

Genitourinary: Bladder spasm, hematuria, hemorrhagic cystitis, urinary incontinence, urinary retention, urinary tract infection

Hematologic & oncologic: Thrombocytopenia (16% to 52%; grade 3: 5% to 24%; grade 4: 3% to 7%; nadir: Day 11; recovery: By day 21), neutropenia (5% to 27%; grade 3: 8% to 18%; grade 4: 2% to 4%; nadir: Day 11; recovery: By day 21), anemia (12% to 23%; grade 3: 4% to 6%; grade 4: <1%). leukopenia (18% to 20%; grade 3: 5%; grade 4: ≤1%), hemorrhage (≥ grade 3: 2%), disseminated intravascular coagulation, febrile neutropenia, lymphocytopenia, oral mucosal petechiae

Hepatic: Ascites, hepatic failure, hepatic hemorrhage, hepatitis, hyperbilirubinemia

Hypersensitivity: Anaphylaxis, angioedema, hypersensitivity, hypersensitivity angiitis

Infection: Herpes zoster (reactivation; 6% to 11%), herpes simplex infection (1% to 3%), herpes zoster (1% to 2%), aspergillosis, bacteremia, listeriosis, toxoplasmosis

Local: Injection site reaction (mostly redness; SubQ: 6%), irritation at injection site (IV 5%), catheter infection

Neuromuscular & skeletal: Weakness (7% to 16%), arthralgia, back pain, bone fracture, limb pain, myalgia, ostealgia

Ophthalmic: Blurred vision, conjunctival infection, conjunctival irritation, diplopia

Otic: Auditory impairment

Renal: Bilateral hydronephrosis, nephrolithiasis, proliferative glomerulonephritis, renal failure

Respiratory: Dyspnea (11%), pneumonia (1% to 3%), adult respiratory distress syndrome, aspiration pneumonia, atelectasis, bronchitis, chronic obstructive pulmonary disease (exacerbation), cough, epistaxis, hemoptysis, hypoxia, laryngeal edema, nasopharyngitis, pleural effusion, pneumonitis, pulmonary hypertension, pulmonary infiltrates (including diffuse), respiratory tract infection, sinusitis

Miscellaneous: Fever (8% to 23%)

<1%, postmarketing, and/or case reports: Acute ischemic stroke, amyloidosis, autonomic neuropathy, blindness, cardiac tamponade, chalazion (Fraunfelder 2016), deafness (bilateral), decreased left ventricular ejection fraction, dysgeusia, dyspepsia, hemolytic-uremic syndrome, herpes meningoencephalitis, increased gamma-glutamyl transferase, increased serum alkaline phosphatase, increased serum transaminases, interstitial pneumonitis, intestinal obstruction, ischemic colitis, ocular herpes simplex, optic neuritis, optic neuropathy, progressive multifocal leukoencephalopathy, prolonged Q-T interval on ECG, pulmonary disease, respiratory insufficiency, reversible posterior leukoencephalopathy syndrome, sepsis, SIADH, Stevens-Johnson

syndrome, subarachnoid hemorrhage, Sweet syndrome, syncope, tachycardia, toxic epidermal necrolysis, tumor lysis syndrome

Drug Interactions

Metabolism/Transport Effects Substrate of CYP1A2 (minor), CYP2C19 (major), CYP2C9 (minor), CYP2D6 (minor), CYP3A4 (major); **Note:** Assignment of Major/Minor substrate status based on clinically relevant drug interaction potential; **Inhibits** CYP2C9 (weak)

Avoid Concomitant Use

Avoid concomitant use of Bortezomib with any of the following: BCG (Intravesical); CYP3A4 Inducers (Strong); Deferiprone; Dipyrone; Green Tea; St John's Wort

Increased Effect/Toxicity

Bortezomib may increase the levels/effects of: Amifostine; Antipsychotic Agents (Second Generation [Atypical]); CloZAPine; Deferiprone; DULoxetine; Highest Risk QTc-Prolonging Agents; Hypotension-Associated Agents; Levodopa; Moderate Risk QTc-Prolonging Agents; Nitroprusside; Pholcodine

The levels/effects of Bortezomib may be increased by: Alfuzosin; Barbiturates; Benperidol; Blood Pressure Lowering Agents; Brimonidine (Topical); CYP3A4 Inhibitors (Strong); Diazoxide; Dipyrone; Herbs (Hypotensive Properties); Lormetazepam; MiFEPRIStone; Molsidomine; Naftopidil; Nicergoline; Nicorandil; Obinutuzumab; Pentoxifylline; Phosphodiesterase 5 Inhibitors; Promazine; Prostacyclin Analogues; Quinagolide

Decreased Effect

Bortezomib may decrease the levels/effects of: BCG (Intravesical)

The levels/effects of Bortezomib may be decreased by: Ascorbic Acid; Bosentan; CYP3A4 Inducers (Moderate); CYP3A4 Inducers (Strong); Dabrafenib; Deferasirox; Green Tea; Multivitamins/Fluoride (with ADE); Multivitamins/Minerals (with ADEK, Folate, Iron); Multivitamins/Minerals (with AE, No Iron); Sarilumab; Siltuximab; St John's Wort; Tocilizumab

Hazardous Drugs Handling Considerations

Hazardous agent (NIOSH 2016 [group 1]).

Use appropriate precautions for receiving, handling, administration, and disposal. Gloves (single) should be worn during receiving, unpacking, and placing in storage.

NIOSH recommends double gloving, a protective gown, ventilated engineering controls (a class II biological safety cabinet or a compounding aseptic containment isolator), and closed system transfer devices (CSTDs) for preparation. Double gloving, a gown, and (if dosage form allows) CSTDs are required during administration (NIOSH 2016).

Storage/Stability Prior to reconstitution, store intact vials at 25°C (77°F); excursions are permitted between 15°C and 30°C (59°F and 86°F). Once reconstituted, the manufacturer recommends use within 8 hours of reconstitution. However, stability studies have demonstrated solutions of 1 mg/mL (vial or syringe) may be stored at room temperature for up to 3 days, or under refrigeration for up to 5 days (Andre 2005); or refrigerated in the original vial for up to 15 days (Vanderloo 2010). Protect from light. After preparation, keep bortezomib in a location away from the separate storage location recommended for intrathecal medications.

◀ **Preparation for Administration Note:** The reconstituted concentrations for IV and SubQ administration are different; the manufacturer provides stickers to facilitate identification of the route for reconstituted vials. The amount contained in each vial may exceed the prescribed dose; use care with dosage and volume calculations.

Reconstitute only with normal saline (NS). Reconstituted solutions should be clear and colorless.

IV: Reconstitute each 3.5 mg vial with 3.5 mL NS to a concentration of 1 mg/mL.

SubQ: Reconstitute each 3.5 mg vial with 1.4 mL NS to a concentration of 2.5 mg/mL (Moreau 2011). If injection site reaction occurs, the more dilute 1 mg/mL concentration may be used SubQ.

Mechanism of Action Bortezomib inhibits proteasomes, enzyme complexes which regulate protein homeostasis within the cell. Specifically, it reversibly inhibits chymotrypsin-like activity at the 26S proteasome, leading to activation of signaling cascades, cell-cycle arrest, and apoptosis.

Pharmacodynamics/Kinetics

Distribution: 498 to 1884 L/m^2; distributes widely to peripheral tissues

Protein binding: ~83%

Metabolism: Hepatic primarily via CYP2C19 and 3A4 and to a lesser extent CYP1A2; forms metabolites (inactive) via deboronization followed by hydroxylation

Half-life elimination: Single dose: IV: 9 to 15 hours; Multiple dosing: 1 mg/m^2: 40 to 193 hours; 1.3 mg/m^2: 76 to 108 hours

Dosing

Adult & Geriatric Note: Consecutive doses should be separated by at least 72 hours.

Multiple myeloma (first-line therapy; in combination with melphalan and prednisone): IV, SubQ: 1.3 mg/m^2 days 1, 4, 8, 11, 22, 25, 29, and 32 of a 42-day treatment cycle for 4 cycles, followed by 1.3 mg/m^2 days 1, 8, 22, and 29 of a 42-day treatment cycle for 5 cycles.

Retreatment may be considered for multiple myeloma patients who had previously responded to bortezomib (either as monotherapy or in combination) and who have relapsed at least 6 months after completing prior bortezomib therapy; initiate at the last tolerated dose.

Alternative first-line therapy (off-label dosing/combinations):

CyBorD regimen: IV: 1.5 mg/m^2 days 1, 8, 15, and 22 of a 28-day treatment cycle for 4 cycles (may continue beyond 4 cycles) in combination with cyclophosphamide and dexamethasone (Khan 2012)

PAD regimen: IV: Induction: 1.3 mg/m^2 days 1, 4, 8, and 11 of a 28-day treatment cycle for 3 cycles (in combination with doxorubicin and dexamethasone), followed by conditioning/stem cell transplantation, and then maintenance bortezomib 1.3 mg/m^2 once every 2 weeks for 2 years (Sonneveld 2012)

VD regimen: IV: Induction: 1.3 mg/m^2 days 1, 4, 8, and 11 of a 21-day treatment cycle (in combination with dexamethasone) for 4 cycles, followed by autologous stem cell transplantation (Harousseau 2010)

VRd regimen: IV: 1.3 mg/m^2 days 1, 4, 8, and 11 of a 21-day treatment cycle for 8 cycles (in combination with lenalidomide and dexamethasone) (Durie 2017)

VTd regimen: IV: 1.3 mg/m^2 days 1, 4, 8, and 11 of a 21-day treatment cycle for 3 induction cycles (in combination with thalidomide and dexamethasone), followed by tandem transplant, then (3 months after second transplant) 1.3 mg/m^2 days 1, 8, 15, and 22 every 35 days for 2 consolidation cycles (in combination with thalidomide and dexamethasone) (Cavo 2010)

Patients ≥65 years: IV: 1.3 mg/m^2 days 1, 8, 15, and 22 of a 35-day treatment cycle, in combination with **either** melphalan and prednisone or melphalan, prednisone, and thalidomide (Boccadoro 2010; Bringhen 2010; Palumbo 2009)

Multiple myeloma (relapsed): IV, SubQ: 1.3 mg/m^2 on days 1, 4, 8, and 11 of a 21-day treatment cycle. Therapy extending beyond 8 cycles may be administered by the standard schedule or may be given once weekly for 4 weeks (days 1, 8, 15, and 22), followed by a 13-day rest (days 23 through 35).

Retreatment may be considered for multiple myeloma patients who had previously responded to bortezomib (either as monotherapy or in combination) and who have relapsed at least 6 months after completing prior bortezomib therapy; initiate at the last tolerated dose. Administer twice weekly for 2 weeks on days 1, 4, 8, and 11 of a 21-day treatment cycle (either as a single-agent or in combination with dexamethasone) for a maximum of 8 cycles.

Alternative relapsed therapy (off-label dosing):
IV: 1.3 mg/m^2 days 1, 4, 8, and 11 of a 21-day treatment cycle for at least 8 cycles or until disease progression or unacceptable toxicity (in combination with liposomal doxorubicin) (Orlowski 2007) **or**

SubQ: 1.3 mg/m^2 days 1, 4, 8, and 11 every 21 days (in combination with daratumumab and dexamethasone) for 8 cycles (Palumbo 2016)

Mantle cell lymphoma (first-line therapy; in combination with rituximab, cyclophosphamide, doxorubicin, and prednisone [VcR-CAP]): IV: 1.3 mg/m^2 on days 1, 4, 8, 11 of a 21-day treatment cycle for 6 cycles. If response first documented at cycle 6, treatment for an additional 2 cycles is recommended.

Mantle cell lymphoma (relapsed): IV, SubQ: 1.3 mg/m^2 on days 1, 4, 8, and 11 of a 21-day treatment cycle.

Antibody-mediated rejection in cardiac transplantation, treatment (off-label use): IV: 1.3 to 1.5 mg/m^2 typically given on days 1, 4, 8, and 11 (treatment frequency varies) for a total of 4 doses (treatment duration may vary) (AHA [Colvin 2015]).

Cutaneous or peripheral T-cell lymphoma, relapsed/refractory (off-label use): IV: 1.3 mg/m^2 on days 1, 4, 8, and 11 of a 21-day treatment cycle for up to 6 cycles (Zinzani 2007). Additional data may be necessary to further define the role of bortezomib in this condition.

Follicular lymphoma, relapsed/refractory (off-label use): IV: 1.3 mg/m^2 days 1, 4, 8, and 11 of a 28-day treatment cycle, in combination with bendamustine and rituximab for 6 cycles (Friedberg 2011) **or** 1.6 mg/m^2 days 1, 8, 15, and 22 of a 35-day treatment cycle, in combination with bendamustine and rituximab for 5 cycles (Fowler 2011)

Systemic light-chain amyloidosis (off-label use): IV: 1.3 mg/m^2 days 1, 4, 8, and 11 of a 21-day treatment cycle (with or without dexamethasone) (Kastritis 2010)

◀

Waldenström's macroglobulinemia, relapsed/refractory (off-label use):

IV: 1.3 mg/m^2 days 1, 4, 8, and 11 of a 21-day treatment cycle; continue until disease progression or until 2 cycles after achieving a complete response (Chen 2007) or 1.3 mg/m^2 days 1, 4, 8, and 11 of a 21-day treatment cycle (in combination with dexamethasone and rituximab) (Treon 2009) **or** 1.6 mg/m^2 days 1, 8, and 15 of a 28-day treatment cycle for 6 cycles (in combination with rituximab) (Ghobrial 2010)

Renal Impairment No dosage adjustment is necessary. The International Myeloma Working Group (IMWG) recommendations suggest that bortezomib may be safely administered to patients with renal impairment, including those on dialysis (Dimopoulos 2016). The IMWG recommends the use of the Chronic Kidney Disease Epidemiology Collaboration (CKD-EPI) equation (preferred) or the Modification of Diet in Renal Disease (MDRD) formula to evaluate renal function estimation in multiple myeloma patients with a stable serum creatinine. Dialysis may reduce bortezomib concentrations; administer postdialysis (Leal 2011).

Hepatic Impairment

Mild impairment (bilirubin ≤1 times ULN and AST >ULN or bilirubin >1 to 1.5 times ULN): No initial dose adjustment is necessary (LoRusso, 2012).

Moderate (bilirubin >1.5 to 3 times ULN) and severe impairment (bilirubin >3 times ULN): Reduce initial dose to 0.7 mg/m^2 in the first cycle; based on patient tolerance, may consider dose escalation to 1 mg/m^2 (LoRusso 2012) or further dose reduction to 0.5 mg/m^2 in subsequent cycles

Obesity *ASCO Guidelines for appropriate chemotherapy dosing in obese adults with cancer:* Utilize patient's actual body weight (full weight) for calculation of body surface area- or weight-based dosing, particularly when the intent of therapy is curative; manage regimen-related toxicities in the same manner as for nonobese patients; if a dose reduction is utilized due to toxicity, consider resumption of full weight-based dosing with subsequent cycles, especially if cause of toxicity (eg, hepatic or renal impairment) is resolved (Griggs 2012).

Adjustment for Toxicity

Myeloma (first-line therapy):

Platelets should be ≥70,000/mm^3, ANC should be ≥1000/mm^3, and nonhematologic toxicities should resolve to grade 1 or baseline prior to therapy initiation.

Platelets ≤30,000/mm^3 or ANC ≤750/mm^3 on bortezomib day(s) (except day 1): Withhold bortezomib; if several bortezomib doses in consecutive cycles are withheld, reduce dose 1 level (1.3 mg/m^2/dose reduced to 1 mg/m^2/dose; 1 mg/m^2/dose reduced to 0.7 mg/m^2/dose).

Grade ≥3 nonhematological toxicity (other than neuropathy): Withhold bortezomib until toxicity resolves to grade 1 or baseline. May reinitiate bortezomib at 1 dose level reduction (1.3 mg/m^2/dose reduced to 1 mg/m^2/dose; 1 mg/m^2/dose reduced to 0.7 mg/m^2/dose).

Neuropathic pain and/or peripheral sensory or motor neuropathy: See "Neuropathic pain and/or peripheral sensory or motor neuropathy" toxicity adjustment guidelines below.

Mantle cell lymphoma (first-line therapy):

Platelets should be ≥100,000/mm^3, ANC should be ≥1,500/mm^3, hemoglobin should be ≥8 g/dL, and nonhematologic toxicities should resolve to grade 1 or baseline prior to each cycle (cycle 2 and beyond).

Platelets <25,000/mm^3 or ≥ grade 3 neutropenia on bortezomib day(s) (except day 1): Withhold bortezomib for up to 2 weeks until platelets are ≥25,000/mm^3 and/or ANC ≥750/mm^3, then reduce dose 1 level (1.3 mg/m^2/dose reduced to 1 mg/m^2/dose; 1 mg/m^2/dose reduced to 0.7 mg/m^2/dose). If hematologic toxicity does not resolve after withholding therapy, discontinue bortezomib.

Grade ≥3 nonhematological toxicity (other than neuropathy): Withhold bortezomib until toxicity resolves to ≤ grade 2. May reinitiate bortezomib at 1 dose level reduction (1.3 mg/m^2/dose reduced to 1 mg/m^2/dose; 1 mg/m^2/dose reduced to 0.7 mg/m^2/dose).

Neuropathic pain and/or peripheral sensory or motor neuropathy: See "Neuropathic pain and/or peripheral sensory or motor neuropathy" toxicity adjustment guidelines below.

Relapsed multiple myeloma and mantle cell lymphoma:

Grade 3 nonhematological (excluding neuropathy) or grade 4 hematolog-ical toxicity: Withhold until toxicity resolved; may reinitiate with a 25% dose reduction (1.3 mg/m^2/dose reduced to 1 mg/m^2/dose; 1 mg/m^2/dose reduced to 0.7 mg/m^2/dose)

Neuropathic pain and/or peripheral sensory, motor, or autonomic neuropathy:

Note: Consider subQ administration in patients with preexisting or at high risk for peripheral neuropathy.

Grade 1 (asymptomatic; deep tendon reflex loss or paresthesia) without pain or loss of function: No action needed

Grade 1 with pain or grade 2 (moderate symptoms; limiting instrumental activities of daily living): Reduce dose to 1 mg/m^2

Grade 2 with pain or grade 3 (severe symptoms; limiting self-care activities of daily living): Withhold until toxicity resolved, may reinitiate at 0.7 mg/m^2 once weekly

Grade 4 (life-threatening consequences with urgent intervention indicated) and/or severe autonomic neuropathy: Discontinue therapy.

Combination Regimens

◀ Waldenstrom Macroglobulinemia:

Bortezomib-Dexamethasone-Rituximab (Waldenstrom Macroglobulinemia) on page 1998

Bortezomib-Rituximab (Waldenstrom Macroglobulinemia) on page 2000

Administration Note: The reconstituted concentrations for IV and SubQ administration are different; use caution when calculating the volume for each route and dose. Consider SubQ administration in patients with preexisting or at high risk for peripheral neuropathy.

IV: Administer via rapid IV push (3 to 5 seconds). When administering in combination with rituximab for first-line therapy of mantle cell lymphoma, administer bortezomib prior to rituximab.

SubQ: Subcutaneous administration of bortezomib 1.3 mg/m² days 1, 4, 8, and 11 of a 21-day treatment cycle has been studied in a limited number of patients with relapsed multiple myeloma; doses were administered subcutaneously (concentration of 2.5 mg/mL) into the thigh or abdomen, rotating the injection site with each dose; injections at the same site within a single cycle were avoided (Moreau 2010; Moreau 2011). Response rates were similar to IV administration; decreased incidence of grade 3 or higher adverse events were observed with SubQ administration. Administer at least 1 inch from an old site and never administer to tender, bruised, erythematous, or indurated sites. If injection site reaction occurs, the more dilute 1 mg/mL concentration may be used SubQ (or IV administration of 1 mg/mL concentration may be considered).

For IV or SubQ administration only; fatalities have been reported with inadvertent intrathecal administration. Bortezomib should **NOT** be delivered to the patient at the same time with any medications intended for central nervous system administration.

Vesicant/Extravasation Risk May be an irritant; extravasation has not been associated with tissue damage

Emetic Potential

Children: Minimal (<10%)

Adults: Low (10% to 30%)

Monitoring Parameters CBC with differential and platelets (monitor frequently throughout therapy); liver function tests (in patients with existing hepatic impairment); verify pregnancy status in women of reproductive potential prior to therapy initiation; signs/symptoms of peripheral neuropathy, dehydration, hypotension, PRES, or PML; renal function, baseline chest x-ray and then periodic pulmonary function testing (with new or worsening pulmonary symptoms)

Dietary Considerations Green tea and green tea extracts may diminish the therapeutic effect of bortezomib and should be avoided (Golden 2009). Avoid grapefruit juice. Avoid additional, nondietary sources of ascorbic acid supplements, including multivitamins containing ascorbic acid (may diminish bortezomib activity) during treatment, especially 12 hours before and after bortezomib treatment (Perrone 2009).

Dosage Forms Excipient information presented when available (limited, particularly for generics); consult specific product labeling.

Solution Reconstituted, Injection:

Velcade: 3.5 mg (1 ea)

◆ **Bortezomib For Injection (Can)** see Bortezomib on page 271

◆ **Bosulif** see Bosutinib on page 281

Bosutinib (boe SUE ti nib)

Related Information

Common Toxicity Criteria *on page 2242*

Management of Chemotherapy-Induced Nausea and Vomiting in Adults *on page 2253*

Safe Handling of Hazardous Drugs *on page 2379*

Brand Names: US Bosulif

Brand Names: Canada Bosulif

Index Terms Bosutinib Monohydrate; SKI-606

Pharmacologic Category Antineoplastic Agent, BCR-ABL Tyrosine Kinase Inhibitor; Antineoplastic Agent, Tyrosine Kinase Inhibitor

Use Chronic myelogenous leukemia: Treatment of chronic, accelerated, or blast phase Philadelphia chromosome-positive (Ph+) chronic myelogenous leukemia (CML) in patients resistant or intolerant to prior therapy

Labeled Contraindications

Hypersensitivity to bosutinib or any component of the formulation

Canadian labeling: Additional contraindications (not in the US labeling): History of long QT syndrome or with persistent QT interval >480 milliseconds; uncorrected hypokalemia or hypomagnesemia; hepatic impairment

Pregnancy Considerations Adverse events were observed in animal reproduction studies. Based on the mechanism of action, bosutinib may cause fetal harm if administered in pregnancy. Females of reproductive potential should use effective contraception during bosutinib treatment and for at least 30 days after completion of treatment.

Breastfeeding Considerations It is not known if bosutinib is present in breast milk. Due to the potential for serious adverse reactions in the breastfed infant, a decision should be made to discontinue breastfeeding or to discontinue bosutinib, taking into account the benefits of treatment to the mother.

Warnings/Precautions Diarrhea, nausea, vomiting, and abdominal pain may occur. Monitor; may require treatment interruption, dose reduction, or discontinuation. For patients experiencing diarrhea (all grades), the median time to onset was 2 days; median duration (per event) was 2 days and the median number of diarrhea episodes per patient was 3 (range: 1 to 200); manage diarrhea with antidiarrheals and/or fluid replacement. Bosutinib is associated with a moderate emetic potential (Roila 2016); nausea and vomiting may be managed with antiemetics and fluid replacement. GI hemorrhages have also been reported. Acute pancreatitis has been reported (rare); use caution in patients with a prior history of pancreatitis.

Anemia, neutropenia, and thrombocytopenia may also occur. May require treatment interruption, dose reduction, or discontinuation. Monitor blood counts weekly during first month, then monthly thereafter (or as clinically indicated). Fluid retention, manifesting as pericardial effusion, pleural effusion, pulmonary edema and/or peripheral edema may occur; may be severe. Monitor for fluid retention (eg, weight gain) and manage appropriately; may require treatment interruption, dose reduction, or discontinuation. QTcF >500 milliseconds was observed rarely in clinical trials (Cortes 2012); patients with significant or uncontrolled cardiovascular disease (including prolonged QT interval at baseline) were not studied.

Bosutinib exposure is increased in patients with hepatic impairment; dose reduction is recommended. Hepatotoxicity has been reported during treatment; dose reductions may be necessary. Monitor liver function. ALT and AST elevations may occur, usually with an onset in the first 3 months of treatment (median onset was ~33 to 35 days; median duration was 21 days). One case of drug-induced liver injury has been reported; full recovery occurred after discontinuation. Bosutinib exposure is increased in patients with moderate or severe renal impairment. Declines in glomerular filtration rates throughout bosutinib treatment have been observed in clinical studies; monitor renal function at baseline and during therapy, particularly in patients with preexisting impairment or other risk factors for renal dysfunction. Consider dosage adjustment in patients with renal dysfunction at baseline or with treatment emergent impairment. Hypersensitivity reactions have been reported, including anaphylaxis and anaphylactic shock (rare).

Potentially significant drug-drug interactions may exist, requiring dose or frequency adjustment, additional monitoring, and/or selection of alternative therapy. Proton pump inhibitors (PPIs) may decrease bosutinib effects; consider using short acting antacids or H_2 antagonists instead of PPIs; separate administration of antacids or H_2 antagonists from bosutinib by at least 2 hours.

Adverse Reactions

>10%:

Cardiovascular: Edema (17% to 20%), chest pain (7% to 12%)

Central nervous system: Fatigue (21% to 26%), headache (17% to 21%), dizziness (11% to 13%)

Dermatologic: Skin rash (38% to 42%), pruritus (7% to 12%)

Endocrine & metabolic: Hypophosphatemia (50% [Gambacorti-Passerini 2014]), hypokalemia (18% [Gambacorti-Passerini 2014])

Gastrointestinal: Diarrhea (76% to 85%), nausea (47% to 48%), vomiting (37% to 43%), abdominal pain (31% to 42%), increased serum lipase (15% to 38% [Cortes 2012; Gambacorti-Passerini 2014]), decreased appetite (13% to 14%)

Hematologic & oncologic: Thrombocytopenia (40% to 45%; grades 3/4: 26% to 39%), anemia (27% to 38%; grades 3/4: 11% to 27%), neutropenia (18% to 22%; grades 3/4: 12% to 20%), leukopenia (10% to 15%; grades 3/4: 4% to 12%)

Hepatic: Abnormal hepatic function tests (20% to 26%), increased serum ALT (18%), increased serum AST (15%)

Neuromuscular & skeletal: Arthralgia (14% to 17%), weakness (10% to 13%), back pain (8% to 13%)

Renal: Renal insufficiency (13%)

Respiratory: Respiratory tract infection (38% to 39%), cough (22%), dyspnea (12% to 20%), pleural effusion (9% to 12%)

Miscellaneous: Fever (23% to 37%)

1% to 10%:

Cardiovascular: Hypertension, pericardial effusion, prolonged Q-T interval on ECG

Central nervous system: Pain

Dermatologic: Urticaria

Endocrine & metabolic: Fluid retention (grade 3/4: 5%), dehydration, hyperkalemia

Gastrointestinal: Dysgeusia, gastritis, gastrointestinal hemorrhage, increased serum amylase

Hematologic & oncologic: Febrile neutropenia

Hepatic: Hepatic insufficiency, hepatotoxicity, increased serum bilirubin (grades ≥3: 1% to 3%)

Hypersensitivity: Hypersensitivity reaction

Neuromuscular & skeletal: Increased creatine phosphokinase, myalgia

Otic: Tinnitus

Frequency not defined: Genitourinary: Decreased estimated GFR (eGFR)

<1%, postmarketing, and/or case reports: Acute pancreatitis, anaphylactic shock, erythema multiforme, exfoliative dermatitis, fixed drug eruption, granulocytopenia, hepatic injury, pericarditis, pulmonary hypertension, respiratory failure, Stevens-Johnson syndrome

Drug Interactions

Metabolism/Transport Effects Substrate of CYP3A4 (major); **Note:** Assignment of Major/Minor substrate status based on clinically relevant drug interaction potential

Avoid Concomitant Use

Avoid concomitant use of Bosutinib with any of the following: BCG (Intravesical); Bitter Orange; Conivaptan; CYP3A4 Inducers (Moderate); CYP3A4 Inducers (Strong); CYP3A4 Inhibitors (Moderate); CYP3A4 Inhibitors (Strong); Deferiprone; Dipyrone; Fusidic Acid (Systemic); Idelalisib; Pomegranate; St John's Wort; Star Fruit

Increased Effect/Toxicity

Bosutinib may increase the levels/effects of: CloZAPine; Deferiprone; Highest Risk QTc-Prolonging Agents; Moderate Risk QTc-Prolonging Agents

The levels/effects of Bosutinib may be increased by: Bitter Orange; Conivaptan; CYP3A4 Inhibitors (Moderate); CYP3A4 Inhibitors (Strong); Dasatinib; Dipyrone; Fosaprepitant; Fusidic Acid (Systemic); Idelalisib; Palbociclib; Pomegranate; Promazine; Simeprevir; Star Fruit; Stiripentol

Decreased Effect

Bosutinib may decrease the levels/effects of: BCG (Intravesical)

The levels/effects of Bosutinib may be decreased by: Antacids; CYP3A4 Inducers (Moderate); CYP3A4 Inducers (Strong); Deferasirox; H2-Antagonists; Proton Pump Inhibitors; Sarilumab; Siltuximab; St John's Wort; Tocilizumab

Food Interactions Grapefruit juice may increase bosutinib plasma concentration. Management: Avoid grapefruit juice during bosutinib therapy.

Hazardous Drugs Handling Considerations

Hazardous agent (NIOSH 2016 [group 1]).

Use appropriate precautions for receiving, handling, administration, and disposal. Gloves (single) should be worn during receiving, unpacking, and placing in storage. NIOSH recommends single gloving for administration of intact tablets or capsules (NIOSH 2016).

Storage/Stability Store at 20°C to 25°C (68°F to 77°F); excursions permitted to 15°C to 30°C (59°F to 86°F).

Mechanism of Action BCR-ABL tyrosine kinase inhibitor (TKI); inhibits BCR-ABL kinase that promotes CML. Also inhibits SRC family (including SRC, LYN, and HCK). Bosutinib has minimal activity against c-KIT and platelet-derived growth factor receptor (PDGFR), which are nonspecific targets associated with toxicity in other TKIs (Cortes 2012). Bosutinib has activity in 16 of 18 imatinib-resistant BCR-ABL mutations, with the exceptions of the T315I and V299L mutants (Cortes 2011).

◀ **Pharmacodynamics/Kinetics**

Onset:

Median time to complete hematologic response (in responders): 2 weeks (Cortes 2011)

Median time to major cytogenetic response (in responders): 12.3 weeks (Cortes 2011)

Median time to first complete cytogenic response: 12.9 weeks (Cortes 2012)

Absorption: Slow (Abbas 2012)

Distribution: V_d: 6,080 ± 1,230 L

Protein binding: 94% to plasma proteins

Metabolism: Hepatic via CYP3A4, primarily to inactive metabolites oxydech-lorinated (M2) bosutinib and N-desmethylated (M5) bosutinib, also to bosu-tinib N-oxide (M6)

Bioavailability: 34% when administered with food

Half-life elimination: 22 to 27 hours (Cortes 2011)

Time to peak: 4 to 6 hours

Excretion: Feces (~91%); urine (3%)

Dosing

Adult & Geriatric Note: Bosutinib is associated with a moderate emetic potential (Roila 2016); nausea and vomiting may be managed with antie-metics and fluid replacement.

Philadelphia chromosome-positive chronic myelogenous leukemia (Ph+CML): Oral: 500 mg once daily; continue until disease progression or unacceptable toxicity. **Note:** If complete hematologic response is not achieved by week 8 or complete cytogenetic response is not achieved by week 12, in the absence of grade 3 or higher adverse reactions, consider increasing the dose from 500 mg once daily to 600 mg once daily.

Missed doses: If a dose is missed beyond 12 hours, skip the dose and resume the usual dose the following day

Renal Impairment

Preexisting impairment:

CrCl >50 to 80 mL/minute: There are no dosage adjustments provided in manufacturer's labeling, however, based on the pharmacokinetics, expo-sure is not altered and the need for dosage adjustment is not likely.

CrCl 30 to 50 mL/minute: Initial: 400 mg once daily.

CrCl <30 mL/minute: Reduce dose to 300 mg once daily (this dose is predicted to result in an AUC similar to that of patients with normal renal function, however, there is no efficacy data for this dose in CML patients with renal impairment).

Renal toxicity during treatment: If unable to tolerate initial dose, reduce dose per adjustment recommendations for toxicity (withhold treatment until resolved, then consider resuming at 400 mg once daily; if clinically appro-priate, may re-escalate dose to 500 mg once daily).

Hemodialysis: There are no dosage adjustments provided in the manufac-turer's labeling (has not been studied).

Hepatic Impairment

Preexisting impairment (mild, moderate, or severe): Child-Pugh class A, B, or C: Reduce initial dose to 200 mg once daily (this dose is predicted to result in an AUC similar to that of patients with normal hepatic function, however, there is no efficacy data for this dose in CML patients with hepatic impairment).

Hepatotoxicity during treatment:
ALT or AST >5 times ULN: Withhold treatment until recovery to ≤2.5 times ULN and resume at 400 mg once daily thereafter. If recovery to ≤2.5 times ULN takes >4 weeks: Discontinue bosutinib.

ALT or AST ≥3 times ULN in conjunction with bilirubin elevation >2 times ULN and alkaline phosphatase <2 times ULN: Discontinue bosutinib.

Adjustment for Toxicity

Hematologic toxicity: ANC <1000/mm^3 or platelets <50,000/mm^3: Withhold treatment until ANC ≥1000/mm^3 **and** platelets ≥50,000/mm^3; if recovery occurs within 2 weeks, resume treatment at the same dose. If ANC and platelets remain low for >2 weeks, upon recovery, resume treatment with the dose reduced by 100 mg. If cytopenia recurs, withhold until recovery and resume treatment with the dose reduced by an additional 100 mg. Doses <300 mg daily have not been evaluated.

Nonhematologic toxicity:

Diarrhea: Grade 3 or 4 (≥7 stools/day increase over baseline/pretreatment): Withhold treatment until recovery to ≤ grade 1; may resume at 400 mg once daily.

Other clinically significant nonhematologic toxicity, moderate or severe: Withhold treatment until resolved, then consider resuming at 400 mg once daily; may re-escalate dose to 500 mg once daily if clinically appropriate.

Administration
Bosutinib is associated with a moderate emetic potential (Roila 2016); nausea and vomiting may be managed with antiemetics and hydration.

Administer with food. Swallow tablet whole; do not crush or break.

Emetic Potential Moderate (30% to 90%)

Monitoring Parameters CBC with differential and platelets (weekly during first month, then monthly thereafter, or as clinically indicated); hepatic enzymes (monthly for first 3 months and as clinically indicated; monitor more frequently with transaminase elevations); renal function (at baseline and throughout therapy); diarrhea episodes; fluid/edema status (eg, weight gain)

Dosage Forms Excipient information presented when available (limited, particularly for generics); consult specific product labeling.

Tablet, Oral:
Bosulif: 100 mg, 500 mg

◆ **Bosutinib Monohydrate** *see* Bosutinib *on page 281*

◆ **BRAF(V600E) Kinase Inhibitor RO5185426** *see* Vemurafenib *on page 1876*

◆ **Brentuximab** *see* Brentuximab Vedotin *on page 285*

Brentuximab Vedotin (bren TUX i mab ve DOE tin)

Related Information
Management of Chemotherapy-Induced Nausea and Vomiting in Adults *on page 2253*

Safe Handling of Hazardous Drugs *on page 2379*

Brand Names: US Adcetris

Brand Names: Canada Adcetris

Index Terms Anti-CD30 ADC SGN-35; Anti-CD30 Antibody-Drug Conjugate SGN-35; Antibody-Drug Conjugate SGN-35; Brentuximab; SGN-35

Pharmacologic Category Antineoplastic Agent, Anti-CD30; Antineoplastic Agent, Antibody Drug Conjugate; Antineoplastic Agent, Monoclonal Antibody

◀ **Use**

Anaplastic large cell lymphoma (systemic): Treatment of systemic anaplastic large cell lymphoma after failure of at least 1 prior multiagent chemotherapy regimen

Hodgkin lymphoma, relapsed or refractory: Treatment of classical Hodgkin lymphoma after failure of at least 2 prior multiagent chemotherapy regimens (in patients who are not autologous hematopoietic stem cell transplant [HSCT] candidates) or after failure of autologous HSCT

Hodgkin lymphoma (post-autologous hematopoietic stem cell transplantation): Treatment of classical Hodgkin lymphoma in patients at high risk of relapse or progression as post-autologous HSCT consolidation

Labeled Contraindications

US labeling: Concurrent use with bleomycin

Canadian labeling: Hypersensitivity to brentuximab or any component of the formulation; concurrent use with bleomycin; patients who have or have had progressive multifocal leukoencephalopathy

Pregnancy Considerations Adverse events were observed in animal reproduction studies. Based on the mechanism of action and on animal data, brentuximab vedotin may cause fetal harm if administered to a pregnant woman. In women of reproductive potential, verify pregnancy prior to treatment initiation. Women of reproductive potential and men with female partners of reproductive potential should avoid pregnancy during treatment and for at least 6 months after the final dose. Brentuximab vedotin treatment may compromise fertility in males.

Breastfeeding Considerations It is not known if brentuximab vedotin is excreted in breast milk. Due to the potential for serious adverse reactions in the nursing infant, the manufacturer does not recommend breastfeeding during treatment.

Warnings/Precautions [US Boxed Warning]: Cases of progressive multifocal leukoencephalopathy (PML) and death due to JC virus infection have been reported. Immunosuppression due to prior chemotherapy treatments or underlying disease may also contribute to PML development. New-onset signs/symptoms of central nervous system abnormalities (eg, changes in mood, memory, cognition, motor incoordination and/or weakness, speech and/or visual disturbances) should receive prompt evaluation with neurology consultation, brain MRI, and lumbar puncture or brain biopsy. The time to initial symptom onset varies from treatment initiation, with some cases occurring within 3 months of initial drug exposure. Withhold treatment with new-onset symptoms suggestive of PML; discontinue if diagnosis of PML is confirmed.

Peripheral neuropathy is common and is generally cumulative; usually sensory neuropathy, although motor neuropathy has also been observed; neuropathy completely resolved in nearly half of patients; almost one-third had partial improvement. Monitor for symptoms of neuropathy (hypoesthesia, hyperesthesia, paresthesia, discomfort, burning sensation, neuropathic pain, or weakness); dose interruption, reduction or discontinuation may be recommended for new or worsening neuropathy.

Grade 3 or 4 neutropenia, thrombocytopenia, and anemia may occur; neutropenia may be severe and/or prolonged (≥1 week); neutropenic fever also has been reported; monitor blood counts prior to each dose and consider more frequent monitoring for patients with Grade 3 or 4 neutropenia; may require growth factor support, dose interruption, reduction or discontinuation.

Serious infections, including opportunistic infections (eg, pneumonia, bacteremia, sepsis/septic shock) have been reported (some fatal); monitor for signs or symptoms of bacterial, fungal, or viral infections. Infusion reactions, including anaphylaxis have been reported; monitor during infusion. For anaphylaxis, immediately and permanently discontinue and administer appropriate medical intervention. For infusion-related reaction, interrupt infusion and administer appropriate medical intervention; premedicate for subsequent infusions (with acetaminophen, an antihistamine, and/or a corticosteroid).

Noninfectious pulmonary toxicity (eg, pneumonitis, interstitial lung disease, acute respiratory distress syndrome), some fatal, has been reported in patients receiving brentuximab vedotin. Monitor for signs/symptoms of pulmonary toxicity (eg, cough, dyspnea). Withhold treatment and perform prompt diagnostic evaluation and management for new or worsening pulmonary symptoms. Due to the risk for pulmonary injury, concurrent use with bleomycin is contraindicated. In a study comparing brentuximab combined with ABVD (doxorubicin, bleomycin, vinblastine, and dacarbazine) to brentuximab combined with AVD (doxorubicin, vinblastine, and dacarbazine), the occurrence of pulmonary toxicity was higher in the brentuximab/ABVD group. Pulmonary symptoms/toxicities reported with brentuximab in combination with ABVD consisted of cough, dyspnea, and interstitial infiltration/inflammation; most patients responded to corticosteroids. Potentially significant drug-drug interactions may exist, requiring dose or frequency adjustment, additional monitoring, and/or selection of alternative therapy. Serious and fatal GI complications (including hemorrhage, obstruction, perforation, erosion, ulcer, enterocolitis, neutropenic colitis, and ileus) have been reported. The risk for GI complications may be increased in patients with lymphoma with preexisting GI involvement. Prompt diagnostic evaluation and management should be performed if new or worsening GI symptoms occur.

Serious hepatotoxicity, including fatalities, has occurred; cases were consistent with hepatocellular injury, with elevations of transaminases and/or bilirubin. Some have occurred after the initial dose or after rechallenge. The risk for hepatotoxicity may be increased with preexisting liver disease, elevated baseline liver enzymes, and concurrent medications. Monitor liver enzymes and bilirubin. Treatment delay, dose reduction or discontinuation may be required for new, worsening, or recurrent hepatotoxicity. Avoid use in patients with moderate to severe hepatic impairment (Child-Pugh classes B and C). The frequency of grade 3/4 toxicities (and deaths) was increased in patients with moderate or severe impairment (compared to patients with normal hepatic function). A component of brentuximab vedotin, the microtubule-disrupting agent monomethylauristatin E (MMAE) is excreted hepatically. MMAE exposure is increased ~2.2-fold in patients with hepatic impairment.

Avoid use in patients with severe renal impairment (CrCl <30 mL/minute). The frequency of grade 3/4 toxicities (and deaths) was increased in patients with severe impairment (compared to patients with normal renal function). A component of brentuximab vedotin, the microtubule-disrupting agent MMAE is excreted renally; MMAE exposure is increased in patients with severe impairment. Stevens-Johnson syndrome (SJS) and toxic epidermal necrolysis (TEN) have been reported (some fatal). Discontinue (and begin appropriate management) if SJS or TEN occur. Tumor lysis syndrome (TLS) may occur; risk of TLS is higher in patients with a high tumor burden or with rapid tumor proliferation; monitor closely.

◀ **Adverse Reactions**

>10%:

Cardiovascular: Peripheral edema (4% to 16%)

Central nervous system: Peripheral neuropathy (54% to 67%), peripheral sensory neuropathy (2% to 56%; grade 3: 8% to 10%), fatigue (24% to 49%), pain (7% to 28%), peripheral motor neuropathy (4% to 23%; grade 3: 3% to 6%), headache (11% to 19%), insomnia (14% to 16%), dizziness (11% to 16%), chills (10% to 13%), anxiety (7% to 11%)

Dermatologic: Skin rash (27% to 31%), pruritus (12% to 19%), alopecia (13% to 14%), night sweats (9% to 12%)

Endocrine & metabolic: Weight loss (6% to 19%)

Gastrointestinal: Nausea (2% to 42%), diarrhea (20% to 36%), abdominal pain (3% to 25%), vomiting (3% to 22%), constipation (13% to 19%), decreased appetite (11% to 16%)

Hematologic & oncologic: Neutropenia (54% to 78%; grade 3: 12% to 30%; grade 4: 6% to 9%), anemia (27% to 52%; grade 3: 2% to 8%; grade 4: 4%), thrombocytopenia (16% to 41%; grade 3: 5% to 7%; grade 4: 2% to 5%), lymphadenopathy (10% to 11%)

Immunologic: Antibody development (antibrentuximab; transient: 30%; persistent: 7%)

Neuromuscular & skeletal: Arthralgia (9% to 19%), myalgia (11% to 17%), back pain (10% to 14%), muscle spasm (9% to 11%)

Respiratory: Upper respiratory tract infection (12% to 47%), cough (17% to 25%), dyspnea (13% to 19%), oropharyngeal pain (9% to 11%)

Miscellaneous: Fever (2% to 38%), infusion related reaction (12% to 15%)

1% to 10%:

Cardiovascular: Septic shock (3%), supraventricular cardiac arrhythmia (3%), pulmonary embolism (2%)

Dermatologic: Xeroderma (4% to 10%)

Genitourinary: Urinary tract infection (3%)

Hepatic: Hepatotoxicity (2%)

Neuromuscular & skeletal: Limb pain (3% to 10%)

Renal: Pyelonephritis (2%)

Respiratory: Pulmonary toxicity (5%, noninfectious; including interstitial pulmonary disease, adult respiratory distress syndrome), pneumonia (4%), pneumonitis (2%), pneumothorax (2%)

Frequency not defined: Progressive multifocal leukoencephalopathy, Stevens-Johnson syndrome, tumor lysis syndrome

<1%, postmarketing, and/or case reports: Anaphylaxis, enterocolitis, febrile neutropenia, gastrointestinal erosion, gastrointestinal perforation, gastrointestinal ulcer, hyperglycemia, intestinal obstruction, JC virus infection, neutropenic enterocolitis, opportunistic infection, pancreatitis, serious infection, toxic epidermal necrolysis

Drug Interactions

Metabolism/Transport Effects Substrate of CYP3A4 (minor), P-glycoprotein; **Note:** Assignment of Major/Minor substrate status based on clinically relevant drug interaction potential

Avoid Concomitant Use

Avoid concomitant use of Brentuximab Vedotin with any of the following: BCG (Intravesical); Belimumab; Bleomycin; Natalizumab; Pimecrolimus; Tacrolimus (Topical); Vaccines (Live)

Increased Effect/Toxicity

Brentuximab Vedotin may increase the levels/effects of: Belimumab; Bleomycin; Fingolimod; Leflunomide; Natalizumab; Tofacitinib; Vaccines (Live)

The levels/effects of Brentuximab Vedotin may be increased by: CYP3A4 Inhibitors (Strong); Denosumab; Lumacaftor; Ocrelizumab; P-glycoprotein/ABCB1 Inhibitors; Pimecrolimus, Ranolazine; Roflumilast; Tacrolimus (Topical); Trastuzumab

Decreased Effect

Brentuximab Vedotin may decrease the levels/effects of: BCG (Intravesical); Coccidioides immitis Skin Test; Nivolumab; Sipuleucel-T; Tertomotide; Vaccines (Inactivated); Vaccines (Live)

The levels/effects of Brentuximab Vedotin may be decreased by: CYP3A4 Inducers (Strong); Echinacea; Lumacaftor; P-glycoprotein/ABCB1 Inducers

Hazardous Drugs Handling Considerations

Hazardous agent (NIOSH 2016 [group 1]).

Use appropriate precautions for receiving, handling, administration, and disposal. Gloves (single) should be worn during receiving, unpacking, and placing in storage.

NIOSH recommends double gloving, a protective gown, ventilated engineering controls (a class II biological safety cabinet or a compounding aseptic containment isolator), and closed system transfer devices (CSTDs) for preparation. Double gloving, a gown, and (if dosage form allows) CSTDs are required during administration (NIOSH 2016).

Storage/Stability Store intact vials refrigerated at 2°C to 8°C (36°F to 46°F) in the original carton. Protect from light. Reconstituted solution should be diluted immediately in NS, D5W, or LR; however, may be stored refrigerated for up to 24 hours; do not freeze. Solutions diluted for infusion should be used immediately after preparation; however, may be stored for 24 hours refrigerated (do not freeze); use within 24 hours of initial reconstitution.

Preparation for Administration Reconstitute each 50 mg vial with 10.5 mL sterile water for injection (SWFI), resulting in a concentration of 5 mg/mL. Direct SWFI toward the vial wall; do not direct toward the cake or powder. Swirl gently to dissolve, do not shake. Reconstituted solution should be clear to slightly opalescent without visible particles. Further dilute in at least 100 mL of either NS, D5W, or LR to a final concentration of 0.4 to 1.8 mg/mL; gently invert bag to mix. Do not mix with other medications. Use within 24 hours of initial reconstitution.

Mechanism of Action Brentuximab vedotin is an antibody drug conjugate (ADC) directed at CD30 consisting of 3 components: 1) a CD30-specific chimeric IgG1 antibody cAC10; 2) a microtubule-disrupting agent, monomethylauristatin E (MMAE); and 3) a protease cleavable dipeptide linker (which covalently conjugates MMAE to cAC10). The conjugate binds to cells which express CD30, and forms a complex which is internalized within the cell and releases MMAE. MMAE binds to the tubules and disrupts the cellular microtubule network, inducing cell cycle arrest (G2/M phase) and apoptosis.

Pharmacodynamics/Kinetics

Distribution: V_{dss}: ADC: ~6 to 10 L

Protein binding: MMAE: 68% to 82%

Metabolism: MMAE: Minimal, primarily via oxidation by CYP3A4/5

Half-life elimination: Terminal: ADC: ~4 to 6 days

Time to peak: ADC: At end of infusion; MMAE: ~1 to 3 days

Excretion: MMAE: Feces (~72% [of recovered MMAE], primarily unchanged); urine

Dosing

Adult & Geriatric

Hodgkin lymphoma, relapsed or refractory: IV: 1.8 mg/kg (maximum dose: 180 mg) every 3 weeks, continue until disease progression or unacceptable toxicities

Hodgkin lymphoma, consolidation therapy after autologous hematopoietic stem cell transplantation (HSCT): IV: 1.8 mg/kg (maximum dose: 180 mg) every 3 weeks, continue until a maximum of 16 cycles, disease progression, or unacceptable toxicity. Begin therapy within 4 to 6 weeks post HSCT or upon recovery from HSCT.

Systemic anaplastic large cell lymphoma (sALCL), refractory: IV: 1.8 mg/kg (maximum dose: 180 mg) every 3 weeks, continue until disease progression or unacceptable toxicities

Renal Impairment

CrCl ≥30 mL/minute: Initial: No dosage adjustment necessary.

CrCl <30 mL/minute: Avoid use.

Hepatic Impairment

Mild impairment (Child-Pugh class A): Initial: 1.2 mg/kg (maximum dose: 120 mg) every 3 weeks.

Moderate to severe impairment (Child-Pugh class B or C): Avoid use.

Adjustment for Toxicity

Hematologic toxicity:

Grade 3 or 4 neutropenia: Withhold treatment until resolves to baseline or ≤ grade 2, consider growth factor support in subsequent cycles.

Recurrent grade 4 neutropenia (despite the use of growth factor support): Consider reducing the dose to 1.2 mg/kg or discontinuing treatment

Nonhematologic toxicities:

Anaphylaxis: Discontinue immediately and permanently

Infusion reaction: Interrupt infusion and administer appropriate medical intervention. Premedicate subsequent infusions with acetaminophen, an antihistamine, and/or a corticosteroid.

Peripheral neuropathy, new or worsening grade 2 or 3: Withhold treatment until improves or returns to grade 1 or baseline; then resume with dose reduced to 1.2 mg/kg

Peripheral neuropathy, grade 4: Discontinue treatment

Progressive multifocal leukoencephalopathy (PML): Withhold treatment with new-onset symptoms suggestive of PML; discontinue if PML diagnosis confirmed

Pulmonary toxicity: Withhold treatment with new-onset or worsening pulmonary symptoms during evaluation and until symptomatic improvement

Stevens-Johnson syndrome or toxic epidermal necrolysis: Discontinue and administer appropriate medical intervention

Administration Infuse over 30 minutes. Do not administer as IV push or bolus; do not mix or infuse with other medications.

Emetic Potential Low (10% to 30%)

Monitoring Parameters CBC with differential prior to each dose (more frequently if clinically indicated); liver and renal function tests. Pregnancy test (in women of reproductive potential) prior to treatment initiation. Monitor for infusion reaction, tumor lysis syndrome, signs/symptoms of progressive multifocal leukoencephalopathy (PML), and for signs of neuropathy (hypoesthesia, hyperesthesia, paresthesia, discomfort, burning sensation, or neuropathic pain or weakness), dermatologic toxicity, pulmonary toxicity, GI toxicity, or infection.

Dosage Forms Excipient information presented when available (limited, particularly for generics); consult specific product labeling.

Solution Reconstituted, Intravenous [preservative free]:

Adcetris: 50 mg (1 ea) [contains polysorbate 80]

Brigatinib (bri GA ti nib)

Related Information

Common Toxicity Criteria *on page 2242*

Safe Handling of Hazardous Drugs *on page 2379*

Brand Names: US Alunbrig

Index Terms AP26113

Pharmacologic Category Antineoplastic Agent, Anaplastic Lymphoma Kinase Inhibitor; Antineoplastic Agent, Tyrosine Kinase Inhibitor

Use Non-small cell lung cancer, metastatic: Treatment of anaplastic lymphoma kinase (ALK)-positive metastatic non-small cell lung cancer (NSCLC) in patients who have progressed on or are intolerant to crizotinib

Labeled Contraindications There are no contraindications listed in the manufacturer's labeling.

Pregnancy Considerations Adverse events were observed in animal reproduction studies. Based on the mechanism of action, brigatinib may be expected to cause fetal harm if used in pregnant women.

Women of reproductive potential should use an effective nonhormonal contraceptive during therapy and for at least 4 months after the last dose. Males with female partners of reproductive potential should use effective contraception during therapy and for at least 3 months after the last dose. Based on animal data, fertility in males may be reduced.

Breastfeeding Considerations It is not known if brigatinib is present in breast milk. Due to the potential for serious adverse reactions in the breastfed infant, breastfeeding is not recommended by the manufacturer during therapy or for 1 week after the last dose.

Warnings/Precautions Approved for use only in patients with metastatic non-small cell lung cancer (NSCLC) who test positive for the abnormal anaplastic lymphoma kinase (ALK) gene. Severe, life-threatening, and fatal cases of pulmonary toxicity consistent with interstitial lung disease (ILD)/pneumonitis have been reported. ILD/pneumonitis occurred early (within 9 days of brigatinib initiation; median onset: 2 days) in some patients. A higher incidence was associated with the 180 mg/day dose (compared to 90 mg/day). Monitor for new or worsening pulmonary symptoms (eg, dyspnea, cough), particularly in the first week of therapy. Interrupt brigatinib in any patient with new or worsening respiratory symptoms; promptly evaluate for ILD/pneumonitis or other potential cause of toxicity (eg, pulmonary embolism, tumor progression, or infectious etiology). May require dose reduction or permanent discontinuation. Hypertension was reported in ~10% to 20% of patients receiving brigatinib (including grade 3 hypertension). Blood pressure should be controlled prior to initiating brigatinib therapy. Monitor blood pressure after 2 weeks and at least monthly subsequently. May require brigatinib therapy interruption, dose reduction, or permanent discontinuation; may also require antihypertensive therapy. Bradycardia has also occurred with brigatinib therapy; monitor heart rate (more frequently if on concomitant bradycardia-inducing medication). Symptomatic bradycardia may require therapy interruption or dose reduction. Permanently discontinue for life-threatening bradycardia that is not associated with a concomitant medication. Use caution when administering brigatinib in combination with antihypertensive medications that cause bradycardia.

CPK elevations have been reported in up to 50% of patients receiving brigatinib (including grade 3 or 4 elevations). A higher incidence was associated with the 180 mg/day dose (compared to 90 mg/day). Monitor CPK levels during treatment; advise patients to report unexplained muscle pain, tenderness, or weakness. Elevated CPK levels may require therapy interruption or dose reduction. Pancreatic enzyme elevations (lipase and amylase) have been reported, including grade 3 or 4 elevations. A higher incidence was associated with the 180 mg/day dose (compared to 90 mg/day). Monitor amylase/lipase during treatment. May require therapy interruption or dose reduction. Nausea, vomiting, diarrhea, constipation, and abdominal pain have also been observed with brigatinib therapy. More than 40% of patients receiving brigatinib experienced new or worsening hyperglycemia, including grade 3 toxicity. Some patients with diabetes or glucose intolerance (at baseline) required insulin therapy while receiving brigatinib. Monitor fasting serum glucose at baseline and periodically during treatment. Initiate or optimize antihyperglycemic therapy; if adequate serum glucose control cannot be achieved with optimal medical management, interrupt brigatinib until metabolic control is achieved. Dose reduction or permanent discontinuation may be necessary.

Visual disturbances such as blurred vision, diplopia, and reduced visual acuity have been reported. Grade 3 macular edema and cataract also occurred (rare). Advise patients to report visual symptoms. Interrupt brigatinib therapy and obtain an ophthalmologic evaluation in patients with new or worsening ≥ grade 2 visual symptoms. May require dose reduction or permanent discontinuation. Potentially significant interactions may exist, requiring dose or frequency adjustment, additional monitoring, and/or selection of alternative therapy.

Adverse Reactions

>10%:

Cardiovascular: Hypertension (11% to 21%)

Central nervous system: Fatigue (29% to 36%), headache (27% to 28%), peripheral neuropathy (13%, grades 3/4: ≤2%), insomnia (7% to 11%)

Dermatologic: Skin rash (15% to 24%)

Endocrine & metabolic: Increased serum AST (38% to 65%), hyperglycemia (38% to 49%; including exacerbations), increased serum ALT (34% to 40%), increased amylase (27% to 39%)

Gastrointestinal: Increased serum lipase (21% to 45%), nausea (33% to 40%), diarrhea (19% to 38%), vomiting (23% to 24%), decreased appetite (15% to 22%), constipation (15% to 19%), abdominal pain (10% to 17%)

Hematologic & oncologic: Anemia (23% to 40%; grades 3/4: <1%), lymphocytopenia (19% to 27%; grades 3/4: 3% to 5%), abnormal phosphorus levels (decreased; 15% to 23%; grades 3/4: <1%), prolonged partial thromboplastin time (20% to 22%; grades 3/4: ≤2%)

Hepatic: Increased serum alkaline phosphatase (15% to 29%)

Neuromuscular & skeletal: Increased creatine phosphokinase (27% to 48%), muscle spasm (12% to 17%), back pain (10% to 15%), myalgia (9% to 15%), arthralgia (14%), limb pain (4% to 11%)

Respiratory: Cough (18% to 34%), dyspnea (21% to 27%)

Miscellaneous: Fever (6% to 14%)

1% to 10%:

Cardiovascular: Bradycardia (6% to 8%)

Ophthalmic: Visual disturbance (7% to 10%; including blurred vision, diplopia, and reduced visual acuity)

Respiratory: Interstitial pneumonitis (≤9%), pneumonitis (≤9%), hypoxia (≤3%), pneumonia (5% to 10%)

Drug Interactions

Metabolism/Transport Effects Substrate of BCRP, CYP2C8 (minor), CYP3A4 (major), P-glycoprotein; **Note:** Assignment of Major/Minor substrate status based on clinically relevant drug interaction potential

Avoid Concomitant Use

Avoid concomitant use of Brigatinib with any of the following: Ceritinib; Conivaptan; CYP3A4 Inducers (Strong); Fusidic Acid (Systemic); Grapefruit Juice; Idelalisib; St John's Wort

Increased Effect/Toxicity

Brigatinib may increase the levels/effects of: Antihypertensive Agents; Bradycardia-Causing Agents; Ceritinib; Ivabradine; Lacosamide

The levels/effects of Brigatinib may be increased by: Aprepitant; Bretylium; Conivaptan; CYP3A4 Inhibitors (Moderate); CYP3A4 Inhibitors (Strong); Dasatinib; Fosaprepitant; Fusidic Acid (Systemic); Grapefruit Juice; Idelalisib; MiFEPRIStone; Netupitant; Palbociclib; Ruxolitinib; Simeprevir; Stiripentol; Tofacitinib

Decreased Effect

Brigatinib may decrease the levels/effects of: Antidiabetic Agents; Antihypertensive Agents; Contraceptives (Estrogens); Contraceptives (Progestins)

The levels/effects of Brigatinib may be decreased by: Bosentan; CYP3A4 Inducers (Moderate); CYP3A4 Inducers (Strong); Dabrafenib; Deferasirox; Sarilumab; Siltuximab; St John's Wort; Tocilizumab

Food Interactions Grapefruit juice may increase serum brigatinib levels. Management: Avoid grapefruit and grapefruit juice.

Hazardous Drugs Handling Considerations

Hazardous agent (meets NIOSH 2016 criteria). This medication is not on the NIOSH (2016) list; however, it meets the criteria for a hazardous drug. Drugs are classified as hazardous based on their properties; the properties of a hazardous drug include one or more of the following characteristics: carcinogenic, teratogenic (or other developmental toxicity), reproductive toxicity, organotoxic at low doses, genotoxic, and/or new agents with structural or toxicity profiles similar to existing hazardous agents.

Use appropriate precautions for receiving, handling, administration, and disposal. Gloves (single) should be worn during receiving, unpacking, and placing in storage. NIOSH recommends single gloving for administration of intact tablets or capsules (NIOSH 2016).

Storage/Stability Store at 20°C to 25°C (68°F to 77°F); excursions permitted between 15°C to 30°C (59°F to 86°F).

◀ **Mechanism of Action** Brigatinib is a broad spectrum multikinase inhibitor with activity against anaplastic lymphoma kinase (ALK), ROS1, insulin-like growth factor-1 receptor (IGF-1R), and FLT-3, as well as EGFR deletion and point mutations. ALK autophosphorylation and ALK-mediated phosphorylation of downstream signaling proteins STAT3, AKT, ERK1/2, and S6 are inhibited by brigatinib. In vitro, brigatinib also inhibited proliferation of cell lines expressing EML4-ALK and NPM-ALK fusion proteins. Brigatinib has activity against cells expressing EML4-ALK and 17 mutant forms associated with ALK inhibitor resistance, as well as EGFR-Del (E746-A750), ROS1-L2026M, FLT3-F691L, and FLT3-D835Y. Clinically, brigatinib showed anti-tumor activity against EML4-ALK mutant forms (including G1202R and L1196M) which were identified in NSCLC cells in patients who progressed on crizotinib.

Pharmacodynamics/Kinetics

Distribution: 153 L

Protein binding: 66% bound to plasma proteins (not concentration dependent)

Metabolism: Primarily hepatic via CYP2C8 and CYP3A4; N-demethylation and cysteine conjugation are the two major metabolic pathways; metabolite AP26123 inhibits ALK with ~3-fold lower potency than brigatinib (in vitro)

Half-life elimination: 25 hours

Time to peak: 1 to 4 hours

Excretion: Feces (65%; 41% as unchanged drug); urine (25%; 86% as unchanged drug)

Dosing

Adult & Geriatric

Non-small cell lung cancer, metastatic (ALK-positive): Oral: 90 mg once daily for 7 days; if tolerated, increase dose to 180 mg once daily; continue until disease progression or unacceptable toxicity (Kim 2017). **Note:** If therapy is interrupted for ≥14 days due to reasons other than toxicity, resume treatment at 90 mg once daily for 7 days before escalating dose to the previously tolerated dose.

Missed dose: If a dose is missed or vomited, do not administer an additional dose; take the next dose at the regularly scheduled time.

Dosage adjustment for concomitant strong CYP3A inhibitors: Avoid concomitant use of strong CYP3A inhibitors; if concurrent therapy cannot be avoided, reduce the brigatinib dose by approximately 50% (eg, from 180 mg once daily to 90 mg once daily, or from 90 mg once daily to 60 mg once daily). After the strong CYP3A inhibitor is discontinued, resume brigatinib dose that was tolerated prior to initiation of the strong CYP3A inhibitor.

Renal Impairment

CrCl 30 to 89 mL/minute: No dosage adjustment is necessary.

CrCl <30 mL/minute: There are no dosage adjustments provided in the manufacturer's labeling (has not been studied).

Hepatic Impairment

Mild (total bilirubin within ULN and AST > ULN **or** total bilirubin >1 to 1.5 times ULN and any AST) impairment: No dosage adjustment is necessary.

Moderate (total bilirubin >1.5 to 3 times ULN and any AST) or severe (total bilirubin >3 times ULN and any AST) impairment: There are no dosage adjustments provided in the manufacturer's labeling (has not been studied).

Adjustment for Toxicity Note: Once the dose is reduced for toxicity, do not subsequently escalate the dose.

Recommended brigatinib dosage adjustment levels:
If the dose received was 90 mg once daily:
  First dose reduction: 60 mg once daily.
  Second dose reduction: Permanently discontinue.
If the dose received was 180 mg once daily:
  First dose reduction: 120 mg once daily.
  Second dose reduction: 90 mg once daily.
  Third dose reduction: 60 mg once daily.
  Permanently discontinue if unable to tolerate the 60 mg once daily dose.

Cardiac toxicity:
Hypertension:
  Grade 3 (systolic blood pressure [SBP] ≥160 mm Hg or diastolic blood pressure [DBP] ≥100 mm Hg, medical intervention indicated, >1 anti-hypertensive medication necessary, or more intensive therapy than previously used): Interrupt brigatinib until hypertension improves to ≤ grade 1 (SBP <140 mm Hg and DBP <90 mm Hg), then resume at the next lower dose. If grade 3 hypertension recurs, interrupt brigatinib until improvement to ≤ grade 1 and resume at the next lower dose **or** permanently discontinue.
  Grade 4 (life-threatening, urgent intervention required): Interrupt brigatinib until improvement to ≤ grade 1, then resume at the next lower dose **or** permanently discontinue. If grade 4 hypertension recurs, permanently discontinue.
Bradycardia (heart rate <60 bpm):
  Symptomatic bradycardia: Interrupt brigatinib until recovery to asymptomatic bradycardia or to a resting heart rate of ≥60 bpm. If a concomitant bradycardia-inducing medication is identified and discontinued (or dose-adjusted), upon recovery to asymptomatic bradycardia or to a resting heart rate of ≥60 bpm, resume brigatinib at the previous dose. If no concomitant medication is identified (or cannot be discontinued or dose-adjusted), upon recovery to asymptomatic bradycardia or to a resting heart rate of ≥60 bpm, resume brigatinib at the next lower dose.
  Life-threatening bradycardia (urgent intervention required): Permanently discontinue brigatinib if no contributing concomitant medication is identified. If contributing concomitant medication is present and discontinued (or dose-adjusted), upon recovery to asymptomatic bradycardia or to a resting heart rate of ≥60 bpm, resume brigatinib at the next lower dose (with frequent monitoring). If life-threatening bradycardia recurs, permanently discontinue.

Creatine phosphokinase (CPK) elevation:
  Grade 3 (CPK >5 times ULN): Interrupt brigatinib therapy until improvement to ≤ grade 1 (≤2.5 times ULN) or to baseline, then resume at the previous dose.
  Grade 4 (CPK >10 times ULN) or recurrent grade 3 toxicity: Interrupt brigatinib therapy until improvement to ≤ grade 1 (≤2.5 times ULN) or to baseline, then resume at the next lower dose.
Hyperglycemia: Grade 3 or higher (glucose ≥250 mg/dL or 13.9 mmol/L): Interrupt brigatinib therapy if adequate hyperglycemic control cannot be achieved with optimal medical management. Once hyperglycemic control is achieved, consider dose reduction to the next lower dose or permanently discontinue.

Lipase/amylase elevation:

Grade 3 (>2 times ULN): Interrupt brigatinib until improvement to ≤ grade 1 (≤1.5 times ULN) or to baseline, then resume at the previous dose.

Grade 4 (>5 times ULN) or recurrent grade 3 toxicity: Interrupt brigatinib therapy until improvement to ≤ grade 1 (≤1.5 times ULN) or to baseline, then resume at the next lower dose.

Ocular toxicity:

Grade 2 or 3 visual disturbance: Interrupt brigatinib therapy until improvement to grade 1 or baseline, then resume at the next lower dose.

Grade 4 visual disturbance: Permanently discontinue.

Pulmonary toxicity (interstitial lung disease [ILD]/pneumonitis):

Grade 1: If new pulmonary symptoms develop during the first 7 days of therapy, interrupt brigatinib until improvement to baseline, then resume treatment at the same dose; do not escalate to 180 mg once daily if ILD/pneumonitis is suspected. If new pulmonary symptoms occur after the first 7 days of therapy, interrupt brigatinib until improvement to baseline, then resume at the previous dose. If ILD/pneumonitis recurs, permanently discontinue.

Grade 2: If new pulmonary symptoms develop during the first 7 days of therapy, interrupt brigatinib until improvement to baseline, then resume treatment at the next lower dose; do not escalate to 180 mg once daily if ILD/pneumonitis is suspected. If new pulmonary symptoms occur after the first 7 days of therapy, interrupt brigatinib until improvement to baseline. If ILD/pneumonitis is suspected, resume at the next lower dose; otherwise, resume at the previous dose. If ILD/pneumonitis recurs, permanently discontinue.

Grade 3 or 4: Permanently discontinue.

Other toxicities:

Grade 3: Interrupt brigatinib therapy until improvement to baseline, then resume at the previous dose. If grade 3 toxicity recurs, interrupt brigatinib until improvement to baseline and then resume at the next lower dose **or** discontinue.

Grade 4: First occurrence: Interrupt brigatinib therapy until recovery to baseline and resume at the next lower dose **or** permanently discontinue. If grade 4 toxicity recurs, permanently discontinue.

Administration Administer orally with or without food. Swallow tablets whole; do not crush or chew.

Monitoring Parameters ALK positivity; monitor creatine phosphokinase (CPK) and amylase/lipase levels periodically throughout therapy; fasting serum glucose at baseline and periodically thereafter; monitor heart rate and blood pressure (after 2 weeks and at least monthly thereafter); monitor for signs/symptoms of interstitial lung disease (ILD)/pneumonitis (new or worsening pulmonary symptoms), muscular symptoms of CPK elevations, and visual disturbances (obtain ophthalmologic evaluation in patients with new or worsening ≥ grade 2 visual symptoms).

Dietary Considerations Avoid grapefruit and grapefruit juice.

Dosage Forms Excipient information presented when available (limited, particularly for generics); consult specific product labeling.

Tablet, Oral:

Alunbrig: 30 mg

◆ **BRL 43694** see Granisetron on page 895

◆ **BTK Inhibitor PCI-32765** see Ibrutinib on page 944

◆ **Bussulfam** *see* Busulfan *on page 297*

Busulfan (byoo SUL fan)

Related Information

Hematopoietic Cell Transplantation *on page 2365*

Management of Chemotherapy-Induced Nausea and Vomiting in Adults *on page 2253*

Management of Drug Extravasations *on page 2271*

Prevention of Chemotherapy-Induced Nausea and Vomiting in Children *on page 2310*

Safe Handling of Hazardous Drugs *on page 2379*

Brand Names: US Busulfex; Myleran

Brand Names: Canada Busulfex; Myleran

Index Terms Bussulfam; Busulfanum; Busulphan

Pharmacologic Category Antineoplastic Agent, Alkylating Agent

Use

Chronic myeloid leukemia (CML):

Injection: Conditioning regimen prior to allogeneic hematopoietic progenitor cell transplantation for CML (in combination with cyclophosphamide)

Tablets: Palliative treatment of CML

Labeled Contraindications

Hypersensitivity to busulfan or any component of the formulation; oral busulfan is contraindicated in patients without a definitive diagnosis of CML

Canadian labeling: Additional contraindications (not in US labeling): Oral busulfan: Neutropenia or thrombocytopenia; disease that has demonstrated resistance to busulfan

Pregnancy Considerations Adverse events were observed in animal reproduction studies. May cause fetal harm if administered during pregnancy. The solvent in IV busulfan, DMA, is also associated with teratogenic effects and may impair fertility. Women and men of childbearing potential should use effective contraception to avoid pregnancy during and after busulfan treatment.

Breastfeeding Considerations It is not known if busulfan is excreted in breast milk. According to the manufacturer, the decision to discontinue breastfeeding during therapy or to discontinue busulfan should take into account the benefits of treatment to the mother; breastfeeding should be discontinued during IV busulfan treatment.

Warnings/Precautions [US Boxed Warning]: Severe and prolonged bone marrow suppression commonly occurs; reduce dose or discontinue oral busulfan for unusual suppression; may require bone marrow biopsy. Hematopoietic progenitor cell transplantation is required to prevent potentially fatal complications from prolonged myelosuppression due to IV busulfan. May result in severe neutropenia, thrombocytopenia, anemia, bone marrow failure, and/or severe pancytopenia; pancytopenia may be prolonged (1 month up to 2 years) and may be reversible. When used for transplantation, monitor CBC with differential daily during treatment and until engraftment. The onset of neutropenia is a median of 4 days post-transplant; recovery is within a median of 13 days following allogeneic transplant (with prophylactic G-CSF use in most patients). Thrombocytopenia occurred at a median of 5 to 6 days. Use with caution in patients with compromised bone marrow reserve (due to prior treatment or radiation therapy). Monitor closely for signs of infection (due to neutropenia) or bleeding ▶

(due to thrombocytopenia). May require antibiotic therapy and platelet and red blood cell support.

Seizures have been reported with IV busulfan and with high-dose oral busulfan. When using as a conditioning regimen for transplant, initiate prophylactic anticonvulsant therapy (eg, phenytoin, levetiracetam, benzodiazepines, or valproic acid) prior to treatment. Use with caution in patients predisposed to seizures, with a history of seizures, head trauma, or with other medications associated with inducing seizures. Phenytoin increases busulfan clearance by ≥15%; busulfan kinetics and dosing recommendations for high-dose HSCT conditioning were studied with concomitant phenytoin. If alternate anticonvulsants are used, busulfan clearance may be decreased and dosing should be monitored accordingly.

Bronchopulmonary dysplasia with pulmonary fibrosis ("busulfan lung") is associated with chronic busulfan use; onset is delayed with symptoms occurring at an average of 4 years (range: 4 months to 10 years) after treatment; may be fatal. Symptoms generally include a slow onset of cough, dyspnea, and fever (low-grade), although acute symptomatic onset may also occur. Diminished diffusion capacity and decreased pulmonary compliance have been noted with pulmonary function testing. Differential diagnosis should rule out opportunistic pulmonary infection or leukemic pulmonary infiltrates; may require lung biopsy. Discontinue busulfan if toxicity develops. Pulmonary toxicity may be additive if administered with other cytotoxic agents also associated with pulmonary toxicity. Cardiac tamponade as been reported in children with thalassemia treated with high-dose oral busulfan in combination with cyclophosphamide. Abdominal pain and vomiting preceded tamponade in most children. Monitor for signs/symptoms and evaluate/treat promptly if cardiac tamponade is suspected. Busulfan has been causally related to the development of secondary malignancies (tumors and acute leukemias); chromosomal alterations may also occur. Chronic low-dose busulfan has been associated with ovarian failure (including failure to achieve puberty). Busulfan is associated with a moderate emetic potential (depending on dose and/or administration route); antiemetics may be recommended to prevent nausea and vomiting (Dupuis 2011).

High busulfan area under the concentration versus time curve (AUC) values (>1500 micromolar•minute) are associated with increased risk of hepatic sinusoidal obstruction syndrome (SOS; formerly called veno-occlusive disease [VOD]) due to conditioning for allogenic HSCT; patients with a history of radiation therapy, prior chemotherapy (≥3 cycles), or prior stem cell transplantation are at increased risk; monitor liver function tests (serum transaminases, alkaline phosphatase, and bilirubin) daily until 28 days posttransplant to detect hepatotoxicity (which may preclude hepatic SOS). Oral busulfan doses above 16 mg/kg (based on IBW) and concurrent use with alkylating agents may also increase the risk for hepatic SOS. The solvent in IV busulfan, dimethylacetamide (DMA), may impair fertility. N,N-dimethylacetamide is incompatible with many closed-system transfer devices (CSTDs) used for preparing injectable antineoplastics (ISMP [Smetzer 2015]). DMA may also be associated with hepatotoxicity, hallucinations, somnolence, lethargy, and confusion. **[US Boxed Warning]: According to the manufacturer, oral busulfan should not be used until CML diagnosis has been established. The responsible health care provider should be experienced in assessing response to chemotherapy.** Cellular dysplasia in many organs has been observed (in addition to lung dysplasia); giant hyperchromatic nuclei have been noted in adrenal glands, liver, lymph nodes, pancreas, thyroid, and bone marrow. May obscure routine diagnostic cytologic exams (eg, cervical smear). Potentially significant drug-drug interactions may exist, requiring dose or frequency adjustment, additional monitoring, and/or selection of alternative therapy.

Adverse Reactions

Intravenous:

>10%:

Cardiovascular: Edema (28% to 36%), tachycardia (44%), hypertension (36%), thrombosis (33%), chest pain (26%), vasodilatation (25%), hepatic sinusoidal obstruction syndrome (formerly known as hepatic veno-occlusive disease; children: 21%; adults: 8% to 12%)

Central nervous system: Insomnia (84%), anxiety (72%), headache (69%), chills (46%), pain (44%), dizziness (30%), depression (23%)

Dermatologic: Skin rash (57%), pruritus (28%)

Endocrine & metabolic: Hypomagnesemia (77%), hyperglycemia (66%), hypokalemia (64%), hypocalcemia (49%)

Gastrointestinal: Vomiting (95% to 100%), nausea (adults 98%; children 83%), mucositis (≤97%), stomatitis (adults ≤97%; children 79%), anorexia (85%), diarrhea (84%; grades 3/4: 5%), abdominal pain (72%), dyspepsia (44%), constipation (38%), xerostomia (26%), rectal disease (25%), gastrointestinal fullness (23%)

Hematologic & oncologic: Neutropenia (100%; onset: 4 days; median recovery: 13 days [with G-CSF support]), bone marrow depression (≤100%), thrombocytopenia (98%; median onset: 5 to 6 days), lymphocytopenia (children: 79%), anemia (69%)

Hepatic: Hyperbilirubinemia (49%), increased serum ALT (31%)

Hypersensitivity: Hypersensitivity reaction (26%)

Immunologic: Graft versus host disease (children: 25%)

Local: Inflammation at injection site (25%)

Neuromuscular & skeletal: Weakness (51%), back pain (23%)

Renal: Increased serum creatinine (21%)

Respiratory: Rhinitis (44%), pulmonary disease (34%), cough (28%), dyspnea (25%), epistaxis (25%), pneumonia (children: 21%)

Miscellaneous: Fever (80%)

1% to 10%: Cardiovascular: Cardiac tamponade (children with thalassemia: 2%)

Frequency not defined:

Cardiovascular: Atrial fibrillation, cardiac arrhythmia, cardiomegaly, catheter site thrombosis (central venous catheter), complete atrioventricular block, ECG abnormality, flushing, hypotension, left heart failure, pericardial effusion, ventricular premature contractions

Central nervous system: Agitation, brain disease, cerebral hemorrhage, coma, confusion, delirium, drowsiness, hallucination, lethargy

Dermatologic: Acne vulgaris, alopecia, erythema nodosum, exfoliative dermatitis, maculopapular rash, skin discoloration, vesicular eruption, vesiculobullous dermatitis

Endocrine & metabolic: Hot flash, hypervolemia, hyponatremia, hypophosphatemia, weight gain

Gastrointestinal: Esophagitis, hematemesis, hiccups, intestinal obstruction, pancreatitis, rectal pain

Genitourinary: Dysuria, hematuria, hemorrhagic cystitis, oliguria

Hematologic & oncologic: Prolonged prothrombin time

Hepatic: Hepatomegaly, increased serum alkaline phosphatase, jaundice

Immunologic: Graft versus host disease (adults)

Infection: Infection

Local: Pain at injection site

Neuromuscular & skeletal: Arthralgia, myalgia

Otic: Ear disease

Renal: Increased blood urea nitrogen

Respiratory: Asthma, atelectasis, hemoptysis, hyperventilation, hypoxia, pharyngitis, pleural effusion, pulmonary alveolar hemorrhage, pulmonary interstitial fibrosis, sinusitis

Oral:

1% to 10%:

Central nervous system: Seizure (2%; despite prophylactic seizure therapy)

Dermatologic: Skin hyperpigmentation (5% to 10%)

Frequency not defined:

Endocrine & metabolic: Amenorrhea, ovarian failure

Hematologic & oncologic: Bone marrow depression (including anemia, leukopenia, thrombocytopenia), pancytopenia

Respiratory: Pulmonary interstitial fibrosis

IV and/or Oral: <1%, postmarketing, and/or case reports: Acute leukemia, adrenocortical insufficiency, alopecia (permanent), anhidrosis, aplastic anemia (may be irreversible), azoospermia, capillary leak syndrome, cardiomyopathy (endocardial fibrosis), cataract (rare), cheilosis, cholestatic jaundice, corneal thinning, dry mucous membranes, enamel hypoplasia, erythema multiforme, esophageal varices (with continuous busulfan and thioguanine therapy), febrile neutropenia, fragile skin, gynecomastia, hepatic fibrosis (centrilobular sinus), hepatic necrosis, hepatic sinusoidal obstruction syndrome (formerly known as hepatic veno-occlusive disease) (oral), lens disease (including particulate matter deposition), malignant neoplasm, myasthenia gravis, porphyria cutanea tarda, pulmonary fibrosis (with bronchopulmonary dysplasia), recall skin sensitization (skin rash), sepsis, sterility, testicular atrophy, thrombotic thrombocytopenic purpura, tumor lysis syndrome, urticaria, xeroderma

Drug Interactions

Metabolism/Transport Effects None known.

Avoid Concomitant Use

Avoid concomitant use of Busulfan with any of the following: BCG (Intravesical); Deferiprone; Dipyrone; Natalizumab; Pimecrolimus; Tacrolimus (Topical); Vaccines (Live)

Increased Effect/Toxicity

Busulfan may increase the levels/effects of: CloZAPine; Deferiprone; Fingolimod; Ifosfamide; Leflunomide; Natalizumab; Tofacitinib; Vaccines (Live)

The levels/effects of Busulfan may be increased by: Acetaminophen; Antifungal Agents (Azole Derivatives, Systemic); Denosumab; Dipyrone; MetroNIDAZOLE (Systemic); Ocrelizumab; Palifermin; Pimecrolimus; Promazine; Propacetamol; Roflumilast; Tacrolimus (Topical); Trastuzumab

Decreased Effect

Busulfan may decrease the levels/effects of: BCG (Intravesical); Coccidioides immitis Skin Test; Lenograstim; Nivolumab; Sipuleucel-T; Tertomotide; Vaccines (Inactivated); Vaccines (Live)

The levels/effects of Busulfan may be decreased by: Echinacea; Fospheny-toin; Phenytoin

Hazardous Drugs Handling Considerations

Hazardous agent (NIOSH 2016 [group 1]).

Use appropriate precautions for receiving, handling, administration, and disposal. Gloves (single) should be worn during receiving, unpacking, and placing in storage.

NIOSH recommends single gloving for administration of intact tablets or capsules. If manipulating tablets/capsules (eg, to prepare an oral suspension), NIOSH recommends double gloving, a protective gown, and preparation in a controlled device; if not prepared in a controlled device, respiratory and eye/face protection as well as ventilated engineering controls are recommended. NIOSH recommends double gloving, a protective gown, and (if there is a potential for vomit or spit up) eye/face protection for administration of an oral liquid/feeding tube administration. For IV preparation, NIOSH recommends double gloving, a protective gown, ventilated engineering controls (a class II biological safety cabinet or a compounding aseptic containment isolator), and (if compatible) closed system transfer devices (CSTDs). Double gloving, a gown, and (if compatible and dosage form allows) CSTDs are required during IV administration (NIOSH 2016).

Storage/Stability

Injection: Store intact vials under refrigeration at 2°C to 8°C (36°F to 46°F). Solutions diluted in sodium chloride (NS) injection or dextrose 5% in water (D5W) for infusion are stable for up to 8 hours at room temperature (25°C [77°F]); the infusion must also be completed within that 8-hour timeframe. Dilution of busulfan injection in NS is stable for up to 12 hours refrigerated (2°C to 8°C); the infusion must be completed within that 12-hour timeframe. Tablet: Store at 25°C (77°F); excursions permitted to 15°C to 30°C (59°F to 86°F).

Preparation for Administration

Injection: Dilute in NS or D5W. The dilution volume should be 10 times the volume of busulfan injection, ensuring that the final concentration of busulfan is 0.5 mg/mL. Always add busulfan to the diluent, and not the diluent to the busulfan. Mix with several inversions. Do not use polycarbonate syringes or filters for preparation or administration. Busulfan for injection contains N,N-dimethylacetamide, which is incompatible with many closed-system transfer devices (CSTDs); the plastic components of CSTDs may dissolve and result in subsequent leakage and potential infusion of dissolved plastic into the patient (ISMP [Smetzer 2015]).

Mechanism of Action

Busulfan is an alkylating agent which reacts with the N-7 position of guanosine and interferes with DNA replication and transcription of RNA. Busulfan has a more marked effect on myeloid cells than on lymphoid cells and is also very toxic to hematopoietic stem cells. Busulfan exhibits little immunosuppressive activity. Interferes with the normal function of DNA by alkylation and cross-linking the strands of DNA.

Pharmacodynamics/Kinetics

Absorption: Rapid and complete

Distribution: V_d: Pediatric (IV): ~0.64 L/kg; crosses blood brain barrier and distributes into CSF with levels equal to plasma

Protein binding: ~32% to plasma proteins and 47% to red blood cells

Metabolism: Extensively hepatic (may increase with multiple doses); gluta-thione conjugation followed by oxidation

◄ Bioavailability: Oral: Children ≥13 years and adults: 80% (range: 47% to 103%); Children 1.5 to 6 years: 68% (range: 22% to 120%)

Half-life elimination: 2 to 3 hours

Time to peak, serum: Oral: ~1 hour; IV: Within 5 minutes

Excretion: Urine (25% to 60% predominantly as metabolites; <2% as unchanged drug)

Clearance: Children: 3.37 mL/minute/kg; Adults: 2.52 mL/minute/kg (range: 1.49 to 4.31 mL/minute/kg)

Dosing

Adult Note: Premedicate with prophylactic anticonvulsant therapy (eg, phenytoin, levetiracetam, benzodiazepines, or valproic acid) beginning 12 hours prior to high-dose busulfan treatment and continuing for 24 hours after the last busulfan dose. Busulfan is associated with a moderate emetic potential (depending on dose and/or administration route); antiemetics may be recommended to prevent nausea and vomiting (Dupuis 2011). Antiemetics are recommended when used for transplantation.

Chronic myelogenous leukemia (CML), palliation (manufacturer's labeling): *Oral:*

Remission induction: 60 mcg/kg/day or 1.8 mg/m^2/day; usual range: 4 to 8 mg/day; titrate dose (or withhold) to maintain leukocyte counts ≥15,000/mm^3 (doses >4 mg/day should be reserved for patients with the most compelling symptoms)

Maintenance: When leukocyte count ≥50,000/mm^3: Resume induction dose **or** (if remission <3 months) 1 to 3 mg/day (to control hematologic status and prevent relapse)

Hematopoietic stem cell (HSCT) conditioning regimen:

IV: 0.8 mg/kg/dose (ideal or actual body weight, whichever is lower) every 6 hours for 4 days (a total of 16 doses) beginning 7 days prior to transplant (followed by cyclophosphamide).

Obesity: For obese or severely-obese patients, use of an adjusted body weight [IBW + 0.25 x (actual − IBW)] is recommended (by the manufacturer).

Reduced intensity conditioning regimen (off-label dosing): 0.8 mg/kg/day for 4 days starting 5 days prior to transplant (in combinations with fludarabine) (Ho 2009)

Oral (off-label use): 1 mg/kg/dose every 6 hours for 16 doses (in combination with cyclophosphamide) (Socié 2001) **or** 1 mg/kg/dose every 6 hours for 16 doses beginning 9 days prior to transplant (in combination with cyclophosphamide) (Cassileth 1993) **or** 0.44 mg/kg/dose every 6 hours for 16 doses (in combination with cyclophosphamide) (Anderson 1996) **or** 1 mg/kg/dose every 6 hours for 16 doses beginning 6 days prior to transplant (in combination with melphalan) (Fermand 2005)

Essential thrombocythemia (off-label use): Oral: 2 to 4 mg daily (Fabris 2009; Tefferi 2011)

Polycythemia vera, refractory (off-label use): Oral: 2 to 4 mg daily (Tefferi 2011)

Geriatric Oral (refer to individual protocols): Start with lowest recommended doses for adults.

Pediatric Note: Premedicate with prophylactic anticonvulsant therapy (eg, phenytoin, levetiracetam, benzodiazepines, or valproic acid) beginning 12 hours prior to high-dose busulfan treatment and continuing for 24 hours after the last busulfan dose. Busulfan is associated with a moderate emetic potential (depending on dose and/or administration route); antiemetics may be recommended to prevent nausea and vomiting (Dupuis 2011). Antiemetics are recommended when used for transplantation.

Chronic myelogenous leukemia (CML), palliation (manufacturer's labeling): *Oral:*

Remission induction: 60 mcg/kg/day or 1.8 mg/m^2/day; titrate dose (or withhold) to maintain leukocyte counts ≥15,000/mm^3 (doses >4 mg/day should be reserved for patients with the most compelling symptoms)

Maintenance: When leukocyte count ≥50,000/mm^3: Resume induction dose **or** (if remission <3 months) 1 to 3 mg/day (to control hematologic status and prevent relapse)

Hematopoietic stem cell transplant (HSCT) conditioning regimens: *IV:*

≤12 kg: 1.1 mg/kg/dose (actual body weight) every 6 hours for 16 doses (over 4 days) (followed by cyclophosphamide)

>12 kg: 0.8 mg/kg/dose (actual body weight) every 6 hours for 16 doses (over 4 days) (followed by cyclophosphamide)

Adjust dose to desired AUC (900 to 1,350 micromolar•minute) at the completion of dose 1 using the following formula:

Adjusted dose (mg) = Actual dose (mg) x [target AUC (micromolar•minute) / actual AUC (micromolar•minute)]

Reduced intensity conditioning regimen (off-label dosing): 0.8 mg/kg/dose for 1 dose 7 to 10 days prior to transplant, followed by ~0.8 mg/kg/dose (busulfan kinetics calculated after initial dose) every 6 hours for 7 doses beginning 3 to 6 days prior to transplant (in combination with fludarabine and antithymocyte globulin) (Pulsipher 2009)

Oral (off-label use): 1 mg/kg/dose every 6 hours for 16 doses beginning 9 days prior to transplant (in combination with cyclophosphamide) (Cassileth 1998)

Renal Impairment

IV: There are no dosage adjustments provided in the manufacturer's labeling (has not been studied).

Oral: There are no dosage adjustments provided in the manufacturer's labeling (elimination appears to be independent of renal function); however, it has been suggested that adjustment is not necessary (Aronoff 2007).

Hepatic Impairment

IV: There are no dosage adjustments provided in the manufacturer's labeling (has not been studied).

Oral: There are no dosage adjustments provided in the manufacturer's labeling.

Obesity *American Society for Blood and Marrow Transplantation (ASBMT) practice guideline committee position statement on chemotherapy dosing in obesity (Bubalo 2014):*

Busulfan (oral): **Note:** For doses over 12 mg/kg, utilize pharmacokinetically targeted dosage (as appropriate for disease state). When busulfan and cyclophosphamide are used in combination for HSCT conditioning, the maximum tolerated busulfan dose is 4 mg/kg/day for 4 days. The maximum tolerated busulfan dose has not been determined when used in combination with other agents.

Body surface area (BSA) dosing: Adults and pediatrics: Utilize actual body weight (ABW) to calculate BSA

Weight based dosing (mg/kg): Adults: Utilize ABW25 for obese and non-obese patients; Pediatric: Utilize actual body weight (ABW)

◀ ABW25: Adjusted wt (kg) = Ideal body weight (kg) + 0.25 [actual wt (kg) - ideal body weight (kg)]

Administration Busulfan is associated with a moderate emetic potential (depending on dose and/or administration route); antiemetics may be recommended to prevent nausea and vomiting (Dupuis 2011). Antiemetics are recommended when used for transplantation.

Intravenous busulfan should be infused over 2 hours via central line. Use an administration set with a minimal residual priming volume (2 to 5 mL for adults and 1 to 3 mL for pediatrics). Flush line before and after each infusion with 5 mL D5W or NS. Do not use polycarbonate syringes or filters for preparation or administration. Busulfan injection contains N,N-dimethylacetamide, which is incompatible with many closed-system transfer devices (CSTDs); the plastic components of CSTDs may dissolve and result in subsequent leakage and potential infusion of dissolved plastic into the patient (ISMP [Smetzer 2015]).

HSCT only: To facilitate ingestion of high oral doses, may insert multiple tablets into gelatin capsules.

Vesicant/Extravasation Risk May be an irritant

Emetic Potential

Children:
  IV: Moderate (30% to 90%)
  Oral: Minimal (<10%) to Low (10% to 30%)
Adults:
  IV: Moderate (30% to 90%)
  Oral ≥4 mg/day: Moderate (30% to 90%)
  Oral <4 mg/day: Minimal (<10%)

Extemporaneous Preparations A 2 mg/mL oral suspension can be prepared in a vertical flow hood with tablets and simple syrup. Crush one-hundred-twenty 2 mg tablets in a mortar and reduce to a fine powder. Add small portions of simple syrup and mix to a uniform paste; mix while adding the simple syrup in incremental proportions to **almost** 120 mL; transfer to a graduated cylinder, rinse mortar and pestle with simple syrup, and add quantity of vehicle sufficient to make 120 mL. Transfer contents of the graduated cylinder into an amber prescription bottle. Label "shake well", "refrigerate", and "caution chemotherapy". Stable for 30 days.
Allen LV, "Busulfan Oral Suspension," *US Pharm*, 1990, 15:94-5.

Monitoring Parameters

CBC with differential and platelet count (weekly for palliative treatment; daily until engraftment for HSCT); liver function tests (evaluate transaminases, alkaline phosphatase, and bilirubin daily for at least 28 days post transplant) and signs/symptoms of sinusoidal obstruction syndrome. Monitor for signs/symptoms of cardiac tamponade.

If conducting therapeutic drug monitoring for AUC calculations in HSCT, monitor blood samples at appropriate collections times (record collection times). Do not collect blood sample during busulfan infusion; collect blood sample from a different port than that used for infusion. Blood samples should be placed on wet ice immediately after collection and should be centrifuged (at 4°C [39.2°F]) within 1 hour. The plasma, harvested into appropriate cryovial storage tubes, should be frozen immediately at −20°C (−4°F). All plasma samples should be sent frozen (on dry ice) to the assay laboratory for the determination of plasma busulfan concentrations.

Dosage Forms Excipient information presented when available (limited, particularly for generics); consult specific product labeling.
Solution, Intravenous:
  Busulfex: 6 mg/mL (10 mL)
  Generic: 6 mg/mL (10 mL)
Solution, Intravenous [preservative free]:
  Generic: 6 mg/mL (10 mL)
Tablet, Oral:
  Myleran: 2 mg

- ◆ **Busulfanum** *see* Busulfan *on page 297*
- ◆ **Busulfex** *see* Busulfan *on page 297*
- ◆ **Busulphan** *see* Busulfan *on page 297*
- ◆ **C2B8 Monoclonal Antibody** *see* RiTUXimab *on page 1610*
- ◆ **2C4 Antibody** *see* Pertuzumab *on page 1506*
- ◆ **C225** *see* Cetuximab *on page 377*

Cabazitaxel (ca baz i TAKS el)

Related Information
Common Toxicity Criteria *on page 2242*
Management of Chemotherapy-Induced Nausea and Vomiting in Adults *on page 2253*
Safe Handling of Hazardous Drugs *on page 2379*

Brand Names: US Jevtana
Brand Names: Canada Jevtana
Index Terms RPR-116258A; XRP6258
Pharmacologic Category Antineoplastic Agent, Antimicrotubular; Antineoplastic Agent, Taxane Derivative
Use Prostate cancer, metastatic: Treatment of hormone-refractory metastatic prostate cancer (in combination with prednisone) in patients previously treated with a docetaxel-containing regimen
Labeled Contraindications
Severe hypersensitivity to cabazitaxel or any component of the formulation, or to other medications formulated with polysorbate 80; neutrophil count ≤1,500/mm³; severe hepatic impairment (total bilirubin >3 times ULN)

Canadian labeling: Additional contraindications (not in the US labeling): Concomitant vaccination with yellow fever vaccine
Pregnancy Considerations Adverse events have been observed in animal reproduction studies. Cabazitaxel is not indicated for use in women. May cause fetal harm if administered during pregnancy. Pregnant women should avoid exposure to cabazitaxel.
Breastfeeding Considerations It is not known if cabazitaxel is excreted in breast milk. Cabazitaxel is not indicated for use in women. Due to the potential for serious adverse reactions in the nursing infant, the manufacturer recommends a decision be made to discontinue nursing or to discontinue the drug, taking into account the importance of treatment to the mother.
Warnings/Precautions [US Boxed Warning]: Severe hypersensitivity reactions, including generalized rash, erythema, hypotension, and bronchospasm may occur; immediate discontinuation is required if hypersensitivity is severe; administer appropriate supportive medications. Premedicate with an IV antihistamine, corticosteroid and H₂ antagonist

prior to infusion. **Use in patients with history of severe hypersensitivity to cabazitaxel or other medications formulated with polysorbate 80 is contraindicated.** Observe closely during infusion, especially during the first and second infusions; reaction may occur within minutes. Do not rechallenge after severe hypersensitivity reactions.

[US Boxed Warning]: Deaths due to neutropenia have been reported. Cabazitaxel is contraindicated in patients with neutrophil count ≤1,500/mm³; monitor blood counts frequently. Neutropenia, anemia, thrombocytopenia, and/or pancytopenia may occur with use; grade 3 and 4 neutropenia was observed in over 80% of patients treated with cabazitaxel in a clinical trial. Dose reductions are recommended following neutropenic fever or prolonged neutropenia. Administration of WBC growth factors may reduce the risk of complications due to neutropenia; consider primary WBC growth factor prophylaxis in high-risk patients (eg, >65 years of age, poor performance status, history of neutropenic fever, extensive prior radiation, poor nutrition status, or other serious comorbidities); secondary prophylaxis and therapeutic WBC growth factors should be considered in all patients with increased risk for neutropenic complications. Use cautiously in patients with hemoglobin <10 g/dL. Monitor complete blood counts weekly during cycle 1 and prior to subsequent treatment cycles, or as clinically indicated. Patients ≥65 years of age are more likely to experience certain adverse reactions, including grade 3 and 4 neutropenia and neutropenic fever. Fatigue, asthenia, pyrexia, dizziness, urinary tract infection, and dehydration also occurred more frequently in elderly patients compared to younger patients. Death due to causes other than disease progression (within 30 days of the last cabazitaxel dose) was higher in elderly patients versus younger patients.

Use is contraindicated in patients with severe hepatic impairment (total bilirubin >3 times ULN). Dose reduction is necessary in patients with mild impairment (total bilirubin >1 to ≤1.5 times ULN or AST >1.5 times ULN) and moderate impairment (total bilirubin >1.5 to ≤3 times ULN); use with caution and monitor closely. Due to extensive hepatic metabolism, cabazitaxel exposure is increased in patients with hepatic impairment. Renal failure (including rare fatalities) has been reported from clinical trials; generally associated with dehydration, sepsis, or obstructive uropathy; use with caution in patients with severe renal impairment (CrCl <30 mL/minute) and end-stage renal disease. Nausea, vomiting, and diarrhea may occur. Diarrhea may be severe and may result in dehydration and electrolyte imbalance; fatalities have been reported. Per the manufacturer, antiemetic prophylaxis is recommended. Antidiarrheal medication and fluid and electrolyte replacement may be necessary. Diarrhea ≥ grade 3 may require treatment delay and or dosage reduction. Gastrointestinal hemorrhage and perforation, enterocolitis, neutropenic enterocolitis, and ileus (some fatal) have also been observed. Use with caution in patients at risk of developing gastrointestinal complications (eg, elderly patients, those with neutropenia or a prior history of pelvic radiation, adhesions, GI ulceration or bleeding, concomitant use of steroids, NSAIDs, antiplatelet or anticoagulant medications). Evaluate promptly if symptoms such as abdominal pain and tenderness, fever, persistent constipation, and diarrhea (with or without neutropenia) occur. May require treatment interruption and/or therapy discontinuation. Interstitial pneumonia/pneumonitis, interstitial lung disease, and acute respiratory distress syndrome have been observed; may be fatal. Patients with underlying pulmonary disease may be at higher risk for these events. Acute respiratory distress syndrome may occur in the setting of infection. If new or worsening pulmonary symptoms develop, interrupt cabazitaxel treatment, monitor closely and promptly investigate and manage symptoms. May require discontinuation (carefully evaluate the potential benefits of treatment resumption).

Failure to properly reconstitute the concentrated vial of cabazitaxel with the correct amount of diluent may lead to higher dosage being administered and increased risk of toxicity. Follow manufacturer instructions carefully. Potentially significant drug-drug interactions may exist, requiring dose or frequency adjustment, additional monitoring, and/or selection of alternative therapy.

Some dosage forms may contain polysorbate 80 (also known as Tweens). Hypersensitivity reactions, usually a delayed reaction, have been reported following exposure to pharmaceutical products containing polysorbate 80 in certain individuals (Isaksson 2002; Lucente 2000; Shelley 1995). Thrombocytopenia, ascites, pulmonary deterioration, and renal and hepatic failure have been reported in premature neonates after receiving parenteral products containing polysorbate 80 (Alade 1986; CDC 1984). See manufacturer's labeling.

Adverse Reactions Adverse reactions reported for combination therapy with prednisone.

>10%:
  Central nervous system: Fatigue (37%), peripheral neuropathy (13%; grades 3/4: <1%)
  Gastrointestinal: Diarrhea (47%), nausea (34%), vomiting (22%), constipation (20%), abdominal pain (17%), anorexia (16%), dysgeusia (11%)
  Genitourinary: Hematuria (17%)
  Hematologic & oncologic: Anemia (98%; grades 3/4: 11%), leukopenia (96%; grades 3/4: 69%), neutropenia (94%; grades 3/4: 82%), thrombocytopenia (48%; grades 3/4: 4%)
  Neuromuscular & skeletal: Weakness (20%), back pain (16%), arthralgia (11%)
  Respiratory: Dyspnea (12%), cough (11%)
  Miscellaneous: Fever (12%)
1% to 10%:
  Cardiovascular: Peripheral edema (9%), cardiac arrhythmia (5%), hypotension (5%)
  Central nervous system: Dizziness (8%), headache (8%), pain (5%)
  Dermatologic: Alopecia (10%)
  Endocrine & metabolic: Weight loss (9%), dehydration (5%)
  Gastrointestinal: Dyspepsia (10%), mucosal inflammation (6%)
  Genitourinary: Urinary tract infection (8%), dysuria (7%)
  Hematologic & oncologic: Febrile neutropenia (7%; grades 3/4: 7%)
  Hepatic: Increased serum ALT, increased serum AST, increased serum bilirubin
  Neuromuscular & skeletal: Muscle spasm (7%)
  Renal: Renal failure (4%)
Frequency not defined:
  Endocrine & metabolic: Electrolyte disturbance
<1%, postmarketing, and/or case reports: Adult respiratory distress syndrome, enterocolitis, gastritis, gastrointestinal hemorrhage, gastrointestinal perforation, hypersensitivity reaction (includes bronchospasm, erythema, hypotension, skin rash), interstitial pneumonitis, interstitial pulmonary disease, intestinal obstruction, neutropenic enterocolitis, sepsis, septic shock

◀ **Drug Interactions**

Metabolism/Transport Effects Substrate of CYP2C8 (minor), CYP3A4 (major); **Note:** Assignment of Major/Minor substrate status based on clinically relevant drug interaction potential

Avoid Concomitant Use

Avoid concomitant use of Cabazitaxel with any of the following: BCG (Intravesical); Conivaptan; Deferiprone; Dipyrone; Fusidic Acid (Systemic); Idelalisib; Natalizumab; Pimecrolimus; Tacrolimus (Topical); Vaccines (Live)

Increased Effect/Toxicity

Cabazitaxel may increase the levels/effects of: Antineoplastic Agents (Anthracycline, Systemic); CloZAPine; Deferiprone; DOXOrubicin (Conventional); Fingolimod; Leflunomide; Natalizumab; Tofacitinib; Vaccines (Live)

The levels/effects of Cabazitaxel may be increased by: Aprepitant; Conivaptan; CYP3A4 Inhibitors (Moderate); CYP3A4 Inhibitors (Strong); Dasatinib; Denosumab; Dipyrone; Fosaprepitant; Fusidic Acid (Systemic); Idelalisib; MiFEPRIStone; Netupitant; Ocrelizumab; Palbociclib; Palifermin; Pimecrolimus; Platinum Derivatives; Promazine; Roflumilast; Simeprevir; Stiripentol; Tacrolimus (Topical); Trastuzumab

Decreased Effect

Cabazitaxel may decrease the levels/effects of: BCG (Intravesical); Coccidioides immitis Skin Test; Lenograstim; Nivolumab; Sipuleucel-T; Tertomotide; Vaccines (Inactivated); Vaccines (Live)

The levels/effects of Cabazitaxel may be decreased by: Bosentan; CYP3A4 Inducers (Moderate); CYP3A4 Inducers (Strong); Dabrafenib; Deferasirox; Echinacea; Enzalutamide; Mitotane; Sarilumab; Siltuximab; St John's Wort; Tocilizumab

Food Interactions Grapefruit juice may increase the levels/effects of cabazitaxel. Management: Avoid grapefruit juice.

Hazardous Drugs Handling Considerations

Hazardous agent (NIOSH 2016 [group 1]).

Use appropriate precautions for receiving, handling, administration, and disposal. Gloves (single) should be worn during receiving, unpacking, and placing in storage.

NIOSH recommends double gloving, a protective gown, ventilated engineering controls (a class II biological safety cabinet or a compounding aseptic containment isolator), and closed system transfer devices (CSTDs) for preparation. Double gloving, a gown, and (if dosage form allows) CSTDs are required during administration (NIOSH 2016).

Storage/Stability Store intact vials at 25°C (77°F); excursions permitted between 15°C and 30°C (59°F and 86°F). Do not refrigerate. Do not prepare or administer in PVC-containing infusion containers or polyurethane infusion sets. The initial reconstituted solution (at 10 mg/mL) is stable for 30 minutes in the vial and solutions for infusion are stable for up to 8 hours at room temperature (includes the 1 hour infusion) or 24 hours refrigerated (includes the 1 hour infusion).

Preparation for Administration Do not prepare or administer in PVC-containing infusion containers or polyurethane infusion sets. Cabazitaxel and diluent vials contain overfill. **Preparation requires 2 steps.** Slowly inject the **entire contents** of the provided diluent vial into the cabazitaxel 60 mg/1.5 mL vial, directing the diluent down the vial wall. Mix gently by inverting the vial for at least 45 seconds; do not shake. Allow vial to sit so that foam dissipates and solution appears homogeneous. This results in an intermediate reconstituted concentration of 10 mg/mL. Further dilute within 30 minutes into a 250 mL D5W or NS non-PVC infusion container to final concentration of 0.1 to 0.26 mg/mL (total doses >65 mg will require a larger infusion volume; final concentration should not exceed 0.26 mg/mL). Gently invert container to mix. Do not use infusion solutions if crystals or precipitate appear; discard if this occurs. Infusion should be completed within 8 hours if stored at room temperature. For infusion solutions stored under refrigeration, the infusion should be completed within 24 hours.

Mechanism of Action Cabazitaxel is a taxane derivative which is a microtubule inhibitor; it binds to tubulin promoting assembly into microtubules and inhibiting disassembly which stabilizes microtubules. This inhibits microtubule depolymerization and cell division, arresting the cell cycle and inhibiting tumor proliferation. Unlike other taxanes, cabazitaxel has a poor affinity for multidrug resistance (MDR) proteins, therefore conferring activity in resistant tumors.

Pharmacodynamics/Kinetics

Distribution: V_{dss}: 4,864 L; has greater CNS penetration than other taxanes

Protein binding: 89% to 92%; primarily to serum albumin and lipoproteins

Metabolism: Extensively hepatic; primarily via CYP3A4 and 3A5; also via CYP2C8 (minor)

Half-life elimination: Terminal: 95 hours

Excretion: Feces (76% as metabolites); Urine (~4%)

Dosing

Adult Note: Premedicate at least 30 minutes prior to each dose of cabazitaxel with an antihistamine (eg, diphenhydramine IV 25 mg or equivalent), a corticosteroid (eg, dexamethasone 8 mg IV or equivalent), and an H_2 antagonist (eg, ranitidine 50 mg IV or equivalent). Per the manufacturer, antiemetic prophylaxis (oral or IV) is also recommended.

Prostate cancer, metastatic: IV: 25 mg/m^2 once every 3 weeks (in combination with prednisone) (de Bono 2010).

Off-label dosing: IV: A lower dose of 20 mg/m^2 once every 3 weeks (in combination with prednisone) has been studied and was found to be non-inferior to the 25 mg/m^2 dose. The lower dose also had a decreased incidence of grade 3 and 4 toxicities compared to the 25 mg/m^2 dose (de Bono 2016).

Dosage adjustment for concomitant medications.

Strong CYP3A inhibitors: Concomitant use with strong CYP3A inhibitors (eg, ketoconazole, itraconazole, clarithromycin, protease inhibitors, nefazodone, telithromycin, voriconazole) may increase cabazitaxel plasma concentrations; avoid concurrent use. If concomitant use cannot be avoided, consider reducing cabazitaxel dose by 25%.

Renal Impairment

Mild to moderate renal impairment (CrCl ≥30 mL/minute): No dosage adjustment necessary.

Severe renal impairment (CrCl <30 mL/minute) or end-stage renal disease: Use with caution; monitor closely.

Hepatic Impairment

Mild impairment (total bilirubin >1 to ≤1.5 times ULN or AST >1.5 times ULN): Reduce dose to 20 mg/m^2; use with caution and monitor closely.

Moderate impairment (total bilirubin >1.5 to ≤3 times ULN with any AST): Reduce dose to 15 mg/m^2 (based on tolerability; efficacy of this dose is not known); use with caution and monitor closely.

Severe impairment (total bilirubin >3 times ULN): Use is contraindicated.

◄ **Obesity** ASCO Guidelines for appropriate chemotherapy dosing in obese adults with cancer: Utilize patient's actual body weight (full weight) for calculation of body surface area- or weight-based dosing, particularly when the intent of therapy is curative; manage regimen-related toxicities in the same manner as for nonobese patients; if a dose reduction is utilized due to toxicity, consider resumption of full weight-based dosing with subsequent cycles, especially if cause of toxicity (eg, hepatic or renal impairment) is resolved (Griggs 2012).

Adjustment for Toxicity

Hematologic toxicity:

Neutropenia ≥ grade 3 for >1 week despite WBC growth factors: Delay treatment until ANC >1,500/mm^3 and then reduce dose to 20 mg/m^2 with continued WBC growth factor secondary prophylaxis.

Neutropenic fever or neutropenic infection: Delay treatment until improvement/resolution and ANC >1,500/mm^3 and then reduce dose to 20 mg/m^2 with continued WBC growth factor secondary prophylaxis.

Persistent hematologic toxicity (despite dosage reduction): Discontinue treatment.

Nonhematologic toxicity:

Severe hypersensitivity: Discontinue immediately.

Diarrhea ≥ grade 3 or persistent despite appropriate medication, fluids, and electrolyte replacement: Delay treatment until improves or resolves and then reduce dose to 20 mg/m^2.

Persistent diarrhea (despite dosage reduction): Discontinue treatment.

Peripheral neuropathy (grade 2): Delay treatment until improves or resolves and then reduce dose to 20 mg/m^2

Persistent peripheral neuropathy (despite dosage reduction) or ≥ grade 3 peripheral neuropathy: Discontinue treatment

Pulmonary symptoms (new or worsening): Interrupt cabazitaxel treatment, monitor closely and promptly investigate and manage symptoms. May require discontinuation (carefully evaluate the potential benefits of treatment resumption).

Combination Regimens

Prostate cancer: Cabazitaxel-Prednisone (Prostate) on page 2002

Administration IV: Infuse over 1 hour using a 0.22-micron inline filter. Do not use polyurethane-containing infusion sets for administration. Allow to reach room temperature prior to infusion. Premedicate with an antihistamine, a corticosteroid, and an H$_2$ antagonist at least 30 minutes prior to infusion. Observe closely during infusion (for hypersensitivity). Per the manufacturer, antiemetic prophylaxis (oral or IV) is also recommended.

Emetic Potential Low (10% to 30%)

Monitoring Parameters CBC with differential and platelets (weekly during first cycle, then prior to each treatment cycle and as clinically indicated); hepatic/renal function. Monitor for hypersensitivity reactions (especially during the first and second infusions). Monitor for signs/symptoms of gastrointestinal disorders (eg, nausea, vomiting, diarrhea, gastrointestinal hemorrhage and perforation, ileus, colitis, abdominal pain/tenderness). Monitor for new or worsening pulmonary symptoms.

Dietary Considerations Avoid grapefruit juice.

Dosage Forms Excipient information presented when available (limited, particularly for generics); consult specific product labeling.

Solution, Intravenous:

Jevtana: 60 mg/1.5 mL (1.5 mL) [contains alcohol, usp, polysorbate 80]

◆ **Cabometyx** *see* Cabozantinib *on page 311*

Cabozantinib (ka boe ZAN ti nib)

Related Information

Common Toxicity Criteria *on page 2242*

Management of Chemotherapy-Induced Nausea and Vomiting in Adults *on page 2253*

Safe Handling of Hazardous Drugs *on page 2379*

Brand Names: US Cabometyx; Cometriq

Index Terms BMS-907351; Cabozantinib (S)-malate; Cabozantinib s-Malate; Cabozantinib s-malate; XL184

Pharmacologic Category Antineoplastic Agent, Tyrosine Kinase Inhibitor; Antineoplastic Agent, Vascular Endothelial Growth Factor (VEGF) Inhibitor

Use

Renal cell carcinoma, advanced (Cabometyx): Treatment of advanced renal cell carcinoma (RCC) in patients who have received prior anti-angiogenic therapy

Thyroid cancer, medullary (Cometriq): Treatment of progressive, metastatic medullary thyroid cancer (MTC)

Labeled Contraindications There are no contraindications listed in the manufacturer's labeling.

Pregnancy Considerations Adverse events have been observed in animal reproduction studies. Based on its mechanism of action, adverse effects on pregnancy would be expected. Patients (male and female) should use effective contraception during therapy and for 4 months after therapy completion. Cabozantinib may impair fertility in females and males.

Breastfeeding Considerations It is not known if cabozantinib is excreted into breast milk. Due to the potential for serious adverse reactions in the nursing infant, the manufacturer recommends discontinuing breastfeeding during treatment and for 4 months after the last dose.

Warnings/Precautions Palmar-plantar erythrodysesthesia syndrome (PPES) was commonly observed in clinical trials; severe PPES (≥ grade 3) also occurred frequently. May require dosage reduction and/or discontinuation. Cabozantinib inhibits vascular endothelial growth factor receptors 1, 2, and 3; wound complications have been reported with therapy. Hold treatment at least 28 days prior to scheduled surgery (including dental surgery); resume based on judgment of adequate wound healing post surgery. Withhold treatment in patients with dehiscence or other wound healing complications requiring intervention. **[US Boxed Warning]: Cometriq: Serious and occasionally fatal hemorrhage (including hemoptysis and gastrointestinal) has occurred with cabozantinib when used for medullary thyroid cancer. Monitor for signs/symptoms of bleeding and do not administer to patients with severe hemorrhage** or a recent history of hemorrhage or hemoptysis. Severe hemorrhage has also been reported in patients with renal cell cancer, including grade 3 or higher events. Do not administer to patients with or at risk for severe hemorrhage.

Treatment emergent hypertension was commonly seen in clinical trials (including grade 3 or higher toxicity). Monitor blood pressure prior to therapy initiation and regularly thereafter; withhold for hypertension that is uncontrolled with appropriate medical management. May require cabozantinib dosage reduction and/or therapy discontinuation. An increased incidence of thrombotic events (venous thromboembolism, including pulmonary embolism and arterial thromboembolism) was seen in cabozantinib-treated patients in clinical trials; discontinue therapy in patients who develop an acute myocardial infarction, cerebral infarction, or other clinically significant arterial thromboembolic event. Proteinuria occurred in a small number of patients receiving cabozantinib in clinical trials; nephrotic syndrome was also reported (rare). Monitor urine protein regularly and discontinue therapy if nephrotic syndrome develops.

[US Boxed Warning]: Cometriq: Serious gastrointestinal (GI) perforations and fistulas have been reported when used for medullary thyroid cancer; discontinue for GI perforation or fistula formation. May be fatal. Tracheal/esophageal fistulas were also noted; some cases were fatal. Monitor for signs/symptoms of perforations and fistulas; if observed, discontinue therapy. Diarrhea was commonly observed in cabozantinib-treated patients in clinical trials. May require therapy interruption and/or dosage reduction. Reversible posterior leukoencephalopathy syndrome (RPLS), also referred to as posterior reversible leukoencephalopathy syndrome (PRES), occurred rarely in clinical studies. Monitor for signs/symptoms of RPLS (seizures, headache, visual disturbances, confusion or altered mental function); if diagnosis confirmed, discontinue therapy.

Osteonecrosis of the jaw (ONJ) occurred rarely; oral examinations should be performed prior to and periodically throughout therapy. Patients should maintain proper oral hygiene practices; if possible, withhold therapy for at least 28 days prior to scheduled invasive dental procedures. Discontinue cabozantinib if ONJ develops. Cabozantinib exposure is increased in patients with hepatic impairment. Reduced initial doses are recommended for patients with mild or moderate impairment; use is not recommended in patients with severe impairment. Potentially significant interactions may exist, requiring dose or frequency adjustment, additional monitoring, and/or selection of alternative therapy. Cabozantinib is available in tablets (Cabometyx) and capsules (Cometriq) which are NOT interchangeable; do NOT substitute.

Adverse Reactions

>10%:

Cardiovascular: Elevated blood pressure (≤39% to 96%), hypertension (33% to 61%; grades 3/4: 8% to ≤16%)

Central nervous system: Fatigue (41% to 56%), mouth pain (36%), voice disorder (20%), headache (11% to 18%), dizziness (11% to 14%)

Dermatologic: Palmar-plantar erythrodysesthesia (42% to 50%; grades 3/4: 8% to 13%), hair discoloration (34%), skin rash (19% to 23%), xeroderma (11% to 19%), alopecia (16%), erythema (11%)

Endocrine & metabolic: Increased serum triglycerides (53%), hypocalcemia (52%), weight loss (31% to 48%), hypophosphatemia (28% to 48%), hyperglycemia (37%), hypoalbuminemia (36%), hypomagnesemia (19% to 31%), hyponatremia (10% to 30%), increased gamma-glutamyl transferase (27%), hypothyroidism (21%), hypokalemia (18%)

Gastrointestinal: Diarrhea (63% to 74%; grade ≥3: 11% to 16%), stomatitis (22% to 51%), decreased appetite (46%), nausea (43% to 50%), dysgeusia (24% to 34%), abdominal pain (23% to 27%), constipation (25% to 27%), vomiting (24% to 32%), mucosal inflammation (19%), dysphagia (13%), dyspepsia (11% to 12%)

Hematologic & oncologic: Lymphocytopenia (53%; grades 3/4: 16%), thrombocytopenia (35%), neutropenia (35%; grades 3/4: 3%), decreased white blood cell count (35%; grades 3/4: <1%), decreased hemoglobin (31%; grades 3/4: 4%), decrease in absolute neutrophil count (31%; grades 3/4: 2%), anemia (17%; grades 3/4: 5%)

Hepatic: Increased serum ALT (68% to 86%), increased serum AST (74% to 86%), increased serum alkaline phosphatase (35% to 52%), hyperbilirubinemia (25%)

Neuromuscular & skeletal: Weakness (19% to 21%), arthralgia (11% to 14%), limb pain (14%), muscle spasm (12% to 13%)

Renal: Increased serum creatinine (58%)

Respiratory: Dyspnea (19%), cough (18%)

1% to 10%:

Cardiovascular: Hypotension (7%), venous thromboembolism (6% to 7%), pulmonary embolism (4%), arterial thromboembolism (≤2%)

Central nervous system: Anxiety (9%), paresthesia (7%), peripheral sensory neuropathy (7%), peripheral neuropathy (5%)

Dermatologic: Hyperkeratosis (7%)

Endocrine & metabolic: Dehydration (7%)

Gastrointestinal: Hemorrhoids (9%), gastrointestinal perforation (≤3%), gastrointestinal fistula (1%)

Genitourinary: Proteinuria (2%)

Hematologic & oncologic: Hemorrhage (≥ grade 3: 2% to 3%)

Neuromuscular & skeletal: Musculoskeletal chest pain (9%), osteonecrosis of the jaw (1%)

Miscellaneous: Fistula (nongastrointestinal: 4%)

<1%, postmarketing, and/or case reports: Reversible posterior leukoencephalopathy syndrome, wound healing impaired

Drug Interactions

Metabolism/Transport Effects Substrate of CYP2C9 (minor), CYP3A4 (major); **Note:** Assignment of Major/Minor substrate status based on clinically relevant drug interaction potential

Avoid Concomitant Use

Avoid concomitant use of Cabozantinib with any of the following: Conivaptan; Fusidic Acid (Systemic); Grapefruit Juice; Idelalisib; St John's Wort

Increased Effect/Toxicity

Cabozantinib may increase the levels/effects of: Bisphosphonate Derivatives

The levels/effects of Cabozantinib may be increased by: Aprepitant; Conivaptan; CYP3A4 Inhibitors (Moderate); CYP3A4 Inhibitors (Strong); Dasatinib; Fosaprepitant; Fusidic Acid (Systemic); Grapefruit Juice; Idelalisib; MiFEPRIStone; MRP2 Inhibitors; Netupitant; Palbociclib; Simeprevir; Stiripentol

Decreased Effect

The levels/effects of Cabozantinib may be decreased by: Bosentan; CYP3A4 Inducers (Moderate); CYP3A4 Inducers (Strong); Dabrafenib; Deferasirox; Enzalutamide; Mitotane; Sarilumab; Siltuximab; St John's Wort; Tocilizumab

Food Interactions A high-fat meal increased C_{max} and AUC by 41% and 57%, respectively compared to the fasted state. Cabozantinib serum concentrations may be increased when taken with grapefruit or grapefruit juice. Management: Must be taken on an empty stomach, at least 1 hour before and 2 hours after food. Avoid concurrent use with grapefruit or grapefruit juice.

Hazardous Drugs Handling Considerations

Hazardous agent (NIOSH 2016 [group 1]).

Use appropriate precautions for receiving, handling, administration, and disposal. Gloves (single) should be worn during receiving, unpacking, and placing in storage. NIOSH recommends single gloving for administration of intact tablets or capsules (NIOSH 2016).

Storage/Stability Store at 20°C to 25°C (68°F to 77°F); excursions permitted from 15°C to 30°C (59°F to 86°F).

Mechanism of Action Cabozantinib is a potent inhibitor of proinvasive receptor tyrosine kinases (RTKs), including AXL, FLT-3, KIT, MER, MET, RET, ROS1, TIE-2, TRKB, TYRO3, and VEGFR-1, -2, and -3; induces apoptosis of cancer cells and suppresses tumor growth, metastasis, and angiogenesis (Yakes, 2011).

Pharmacodynamics/Kinetics

Distribution: V_d: ~319 to 349 L

Bioavailability: Following a single 140 mg dose, a 19% increase in the C_{max} was observed with the tablet (compared to the capsule), although the difference in AUC was <10%.

Protein binding: ≥99.7% to plasma proteins

Metabolism: Hepatic via CYP3A4

Half-life elimination: ~55 hours (Cometriq); ~99 hours (Cabometyx)

Time to peak: 2 to 5 hours

Excretion: Feces (~54%; 43% as unchanged drug); urine (~27%)

Dosing

Adult Note: Do not substitute cabozantinib tablets and capsules.

Renal cell carcinoma, advanced: Cabometyx: Oral: 60 mg once daily, continue as long as benefiting clinically or until unacceptable toxicity occurs (Choueiri 2015)

Thyroid cancer, medullary, metastatic: Cometriq: Oral: 140 mg once daily until disease progression or unacceptable toxicity occurs; do not exceed 180 mg daily

Missed doses: Do not take a missed dose within 12 hours of the next dose.

Dosage adjustment for concomitant CYP3A4 inhibitors/inducers:

Strong CYP3A4 inhibitors:

Cabometyx: Reduce the daily dose of cabozantinib by 20 mg (from 60 mg to 40 mg daily or from 40 mg to 20 mg daily). If the strong inhibitor is discontinued, allow ~2 to 3 days to elapse prior to adjusting the cabozantinib dose upwards to the dose used prior to the initiation of the strong inhibitor.

Cometriq: Avoid concomitant use; if concomitant use is required, **reduce** the daily dose of cabozantinib by 40 mg (ie, from 140 mg to 100 mg daily or from 100 mg to 60 mg daily). If the strong inhibitor is discontinued, allow ~2 to 3 days to elapse prior to adjusting the cabozantinib dose upwards to the dose used prior to the initiation of the strong inhibitor.

Strong CYP3A4 inducers:

Cabometyx: Increase the daily dose of cabozantinib by 20 mg (from 60 mg to 80 mg daily or from 40 mg to 60 mg daily) as tolerated; do not exceed 80 mg daily. If the strong inducer is discontinued, allow ~2 to 3 days to elapse prior to reducing the cabozantinib dose to the dose used prior to the initiation of the strong inducer.

Cometriq: Avoid concomitant use; if concomitant use is required, **increase** the daily dose of cabozantinib by 40 mg (ie, from 140 mg to 180 mg daily or from 100 mg to 140 mg daily). If the strong inducer is discontinued, allow ~2 to 3 days to elapse prior to reducing the cabozantinib dose to the dose used prior to the initiation of the strong inducer.

Dosage adjustment for surgery: Withhold treatment for at least 28 days prior to scheduled surgery (including dental surgery). Resume therapy based on clinical judgment of adequate wound healing.

Renal Impairment Note: The estimated glomerular filtration rate (eGFR) is estimated using MDRD (modification of diet in renal disease) equation.

eGFR ≥30 mL/minute/1.73 m²: No dosage adjustment necessary.

eGFR <30 mL/minute/1.73 m² or dialysis: There are no dosage adjustments provided in the manufacturer's labeling (has not been studied).

Hepatic Impairment

Mild or moderate impairment (Child-Pugh classes A and B):

Cabometyx: Reduce the initial dose to 40 mg once daily.

Cometriq: Reduce the initial dose to 80 mg once daily.

Severe impairment (Child-Pugh class C): Use is not recommended (has not been studied).

Adjustment for Toxicity

Cabometyx: Withhold therapy for grade 4 adverse reactions, and for grade 3 or intolerable grade 2 reactions that cannot be managed with dosage reduction or supportive care. Upon return to baseline or improvement to grade 1, resume therapy with a reduction in dose. If previously receiving 60 mg daily, resume therapy at 40 mg daily. If previously receiving 40 mg daily, resume therapy at 20 mg daily. If previously receiving 20 mg daily, resume at 20 mg daily if tolerated; if not tolerated, discontinue therapy.

Permanently discontinue for:

Development of unmanageable fistula or gastrointestinal perforation

Hypertensive crisis, severe uncontrolled hypertension despite optimal therapy

Nephrotic syndrome

Reversible posterior leukoencephalopathy syndrome (RPLS)

Serious arterial thromboembolic event (eg, MI or cerebral infarction)

Severe hemorrhage

Cometriq:

Hematologic: Withhold therapy for grade 4 hematologic adverse reactions. Upon return to baseline or improvement to grade 1, reduce the dose to 100 mg daily. If previously receiving 100 mg daily, resume therapy at 60 mg daily. If previously receiving 60 mg daily, resume at 60 mg daily if tolerated; otherwise, discontinue therapy.

Other toxicity: Grade 3 or higher nonhematologic toxicity or intolerable grade 2 toxicity: Upon return to baseline or improvement to grade 1, reduce the dose to 100 mg daily. If previously receiving 100 mg daily, resume therapy at 60 mg daily. If previously receiving 60 mg daily, resume at 60 mg daily if tolerated; otherwise, discontinue therapy.

Permanently discontinue for:

Malignant hypertension, hypertensive crisis, persistent uncontrolled hypertension despite optimal therapy

Nephrotic syndrome

Osteonecrosis of the jaw

Reversible posterior leukoencephalopathy syndrome (RPLS)

Serious arterial thromboembolic event (eg, MI or cerebral infarction)
Severe hemorrhage
Visceral perforation or fistula formation

Administration Administer orally on an empty stomach (1 hour before or 2 hours after eating). **Note:** The prescribing information describe when to give food with respect to cabozantinib; no food should be consumed for at least 2 hours before or for at least 1 hour after the cabozantinib dose. Swallow whole; do not open capsules or crush tablets.

Emetic Potential Minimal (<10%)

Monitoring Parameters Renal function, liver function, CBC with differential and platelets, serum electrolytes; blood pressure (prior to initiation and regularly during therapy); monitor for perforations, fistulas, signs/symptoms of bleeding, palmar-plantar erythrodysesthesia syndrome (PPES), reversible posterior leukoencephalopathy syndrome (RPLS), proteinuria (regularly during therapy), osteonecrosis of the jaw (perform oral examination prior to initiation and periodically during therapy), wound healing complications, diarrhea, stomatitis

Dietary Considerations Avoid grapefruit and grapefruit juice throughout therapy.

Prescribing and Access Restrictions Contact Exelixus Access Services for information on obtaining cabozantinib (855-253-3273).

Dosage Forms Excipient information presented when available (limited, particularly for generics); consult specific product labeling.
Capsule, oral [each package contains four blister cards; each card contains the following]:
Cometriq: 60 mg daily-dose: 20 mg (21s)
Cometriq: 100 mg daily-dose: 80 mg (7s) and 20 mg (7s)
Cometriq: 140 mg daily-dose: 80 mg (7s) and 20 mg (21s)
Tablet, oral:
Cabometyx: 20 mg, 40 mg, 60 mg

◆ **Cabozantinib (S)-malate** *see* Cabozantinib *on page* 311

◆ **Caelyx (Can)** *see* DOXOrubicin (Liposomal) *on page* 636

◆ **CAFdA** *see* Clofarabine *on page* 417

◆ **CAL-101** *see* Idelalisib *on page* 956

◆ **Calcimar (Can)** *see* Calcitonin *on page* 316

Calcitonin (kal si TOE nin)

Brand Names: US Fortical [DSC]; Miacalcin
Brand Names: Canada Calcimar
Index Terms Calcitonin (Salmon); Salcatonin
Pharmacologic Category Antidote; Hormone
Use
Injection:
Hypercalcemia: Adjunctive therapy for hypercalcemia
Paget disease: Treatment of symptomatic Paget disease of bone (osteitis deformans) in patients who are nonresponsive or intolerant to alternative therapy
Postmenopausal osteoporosis: Treatment of osteoporosis in women more than 5 years postmenopause

Intranasal:
  Postmenopausal osteoporosis: Treatment of postmenopausal osteoporosis in women more than 5 years postmenopause
Pregnancy Risk Factor C
Dosing
  Adult & Geriatric
    Paget's disease, symptomatic: IM, SubQ: 100 units daily. Lower maintenance dosages (eg, 50 units 3 times/week) may be sufficient (DeRose 1974)
    Hypercalcemia: Initial: IM, SubQ: 4 units/kg every 12 hours; may increase up to 8 units/kg every 6 to 12 hours; hypocalcemic effect of calcitonin diminishes after 24 to 48 hours (Bilezikian 1993; Nilsson 1978; Stevenson 1988)
    Postmenopausal osteoporosis:
    IM, SubQ: 100 units daily
    Intranasal: 200 units (1 spray) in one nostril once daily
  Renal Impairment There are no dosage adjustments provided in the manufacturer's labeling.
  Hepatic Impairment There are no dosage adjustments provided in the manufacturer's labeling.
  Additional Information Complete prescribing information should be consulted for additional detail.
  Dosage Forms Excipient information presented when available (limited, particularly for generics); consult specific product labeling. [DSC] = Discontinued product
  Solution, Injection:
    Miacalcin: 200 units/mL (2 mL) [contains phenol]
  Solution, Nasal:
    Fortical: 200 units/actuation (3.7 mL [DSC])
    Miacalcin: 200 units/actuation (3.7 mL [DSC])
    Generic: 200 units/actuation (3.7 mL)
  Dosage Forms: Canada Information with regard to form, strength, and availability of products uniquely available in Canada but currently not available in the US. Refer also to Dosage Forms.

  Excipient information presented when available (limited, particularly for generics); consult specific product labeling.
  Solution, Injection:
    Calcimar: 200 units/mL (2 mL) [contains phenol]

◆ **Calcitonin (Salmon)** see Calcitonin on page 316
◆ **Calcium Folinate** see Leucovorin Calcium on page 1124
◆ **Calcium Leucovorin** see Leucovorin Calcium on page 1124
◆ **Calcium Levoleucovorin** see LEVOleucovorin on page 1145
◆ **Campath** see Alemtuzumab on page 82
◆ **Campath-1H** see Alemtuzumab on page 82
◆ **Camptosar** see Irinotecan (Conventional) on page 1037
◆ **Camptothecin-11** see Irinotecan (Conventional) on page 1037
◆ **Cancidas** see Caspofungin on page 354
◆ **CanesOral (Can)** see Fluconazole on page 807
◆ **CAPE** see Capecitabine on page 318

Capecitabine (ka pe SITE a been)

Related Information

Common Toxicity Criteria *on page 2242*

Management of Chemotherapy-Induced Nausea and Vomiting in Adults *on page 2253*

Management of EGFR Inhibitor Toxicities: Dermatologic, Ocular, and Gastrointestinal *on page 2291*

Mucositis and Stomatitis *on page 2299*

Prevention of Chemotherapy-Induced Nausea and Vomiting in Children *on page 2310*

Safe Handling of Hazardous Drugs *on page 2379*

Brand Names: US Xeloda

Brand Names: Canada Teva-Capecitabine; Xeloda

Index Terms CAPE

Pharmacologic Category Antineoplastic Agent, Antimetabolite; Antineoplastic Agent, Antimetabolite (Pyrimidine Analog)

Use

Breast cancer (metastatic):

Monotherapy: Treatment of metastatic breast cancer resistant to both paclitaxel and an anthracycline-containing regimen or resistant to paclitaxel in patients for whom further anthracycline therapy is not indicated

Combination therapy: Treatment of metastatic breast cancer (in combination with docetaxel) after failure of a prior anthracycline-containing regimen

Colorectal cancer: First-line treatment of metastatic colorectal cancer when treatment with a fluoropyrimidine alone is preferred; adjuvant therapy of Dukes' C colon cancer after complete resection of the primary tumor when fluoropyrimidine therapy alone is preferred

Labeled Contraindications

Known hypersensitivity to capecitabine, fluorouracil, or any component of the formulation; severe renal impairment (CrCl <30 mL/minute)

Canadian labeling: Additional contraindications (not in the US labeling): Known complete absence of dihydropyrimidine dehydrogenase (DPD) activity; concomitant administration with sorivudine or chemically related analogues (eg, brivudine)

Pregnancy Considerations Based on animal reproduction studies and its mechanism of action, fetal harm may occur if capecitabine is administered during pregnancy. Pregnancy testing is recommended prior to therapy initiation. Women of reproductive potential should use effective contraception during treatment and for 6 months after the last dose. Males with female partners of reproductive potential should use effective contraception during treatment and for 3 months after the last dose.

Breastfeeding Considerations It is not known if capecitabine is present in breast milk. Due to the potential for serious adverse reactions in the breastfed infant, breastfeeding is not recommended by the manufacturer during treatment and for 2 weeks after the last dose.

Warnings/Precautions Bone marrow suppression may occur, hematologic toxicity is more common when used in combination therapy; use with caution; dosage adjustments may be required. Product labeling recommends that patients with baseline platelets <100,000/mm^3 and/or neutrophils <1,500/mm^3 not receive capecitabine therapy and also to withhold for grade 3 or 4 hematologic toxicity during treatment. Patients with certain homozygous or heterozygous mutations of the dihydropyrimidine dehydrogenase (DPD) enzyme are at increased risk for acute early-onset (potentially severe, life-threatening, or fatal) toxicity due to total or near total absence of DPD activity. Toxicity may include mucositis/stomatitis, diarrhea, neutropenia, and neurotoxicity. Patients with partial DPD activity are also at risk for severe, life-threatening, or fatal toxicity. May require therapy interruption or permanent discontinuation, depending on the onset, duration, and severity of toxicity observed. No capecitabine dose has been shown to be safe in patients with complete DPD deficiency; data is insufficient to recommend a dose in patients with partial DPD activity.

Capecitabine may cause diarrhea (may be severe); median time to first occurrence of grade 2 to 4 diarrhea was 34 days; median duration of grades 3 or 4 diarrhea was 5 days. Withhold treatment for grades 2 to 4 diarrhea; subsequent doses should be reduced after grade 3 or 4 diarrhea or recurrence of grade 2 diarrhea. Antidiarrheal therapy (eg, loperamide) is recommended. Necrotizing enterocolitis (typhlitis) has been reported. Dehydration may occur rapidly in patients with diarrhea, nausea, vomiting, anorexia, and/or weakness; adequately hydrate prior to treatment initiation. Elderly patients may be a higher risk for dehydration. Interrupt treatment for grade 2 or higher dehydration; correct precipitating factors and ensure rehydration prior to resuming therapy; may require dose modification (based on precipitating factor).

Hand-and-foot syndrome is characterized by numbness, dysesthesia/paresthesia, tingling, painless or painful swelling, erythema, desquamation, blistering, and severe pain; median onset is 79 days (range: 11 to 360 days). Persistent hand-and foot syndrome (grade 2 and higher) could eventually lead to fingerprint loss. If grade 2 or 3 hand-and-foot syndrome occurs, interrupt administration of capecitabine until decreases to grade 1. Following grade 3 hand-and-foot syndrome, decrease subsequent doses of capecitabine. Stevens-Johnson syndrome and toxic epidermal necrolysis (TEN) have been reported (some fatal); permanently discontinue capecitabine if a severe dermatologic or mucocutaneous reaction occurs. In patients with colorectal cancer, treatment with capecitabine immediately following 6 weeks of fluorouracil/leucovorin (FU/LV) therapy has been associated with an increased incidence of grade ≥3 toxicity, when compared to patients receiving the reverse sequence, capecitabine (two 3-week courses) followed by FU/LV (Hennig 2008).

Grade 3 and 4 hyperbilirubinemia have been observed in patients with and without hepatic metastases at baseline (median onset: 64 days). Transaminase and alkaline phosphatase elevations have also been reported. If capecitabine-related grade 3 or 4 hyperbilirubinemia occurs, Interrupt treatment until bilirubin ≤3 times ULN. Bilirubin elevations may also require dose reductions. Use with caution in patients with mild to moderate hepatic impairment due to liver metastases; effect of severe hepatic impairment has not been studied. Dehydration may occur, resulting in acute renal failure (may be fatal); concomitant use with nephrotoxic agents and baseline renal dysfunction may increase the risk. Use with caution in patients with mild to moderate renal impairment; reduce dose with moderate impairment (exposure to capecitabine and metabolites is increased) and carefully monitor and reduce subsequent dose (with any grade 2 or higher adverse effect) with mild to moderate impairment; use is contraindicated in severe impairment. Use with caution in patients ≥60 years of age, the incidence of treatment-related adverse events may be higher.

Cardiotoxicity has been observed with capecitabine, including myocardial infarction, ischemia, angina, dysrhythmias, cardiac arrest, cardiac failure, sudden death, ECG changes, and cardiomyopathy; may be more common in patients with a history of coronary artery disease. In a scientific statement from the American Heart Association, capecitabine has been determined to be an agent that may either cause reversible direct myocardial toxicity or exacerbate underlying myocardial dysfunction (magnitude: moderate/major) (AHA [Page 2016]). **[US Boxed Warning]: Capecitabine may increase the anticoagulant effects of warfarin; bleeding events, including death, have occurred with concomitant use. Clinically significant increases in pro-thrombin time (PT) and INR have occurred within several days to months after capecitabine initiation (in patients previously stabilized on anti-coagulants), and may continue up to 1 month after capecitabine discontinuation; may occur in patients with or without liver metastases. Monitor PT and INR frequently and adjust anticoagulation dosing accordingly. An increased risk of coagulopathy is correlated with a cancer diagnosis and age >60 years.** Other potentially significant drug-drug interactions may exist, requiring dose or frequency adjustment, additional monitoring, and/or selection of alternative therapy. Concomitant use of proton pump inhibitors and capecitabine may alter capecitabine dissolution and absorption due to higher gastric pH levels. Secondary analysis of a large phase III study comparing capecitabine and oxaliplatin with or without lapatinib for the treatment of gastroesophageal cancer showed decreased overall survival in patients who received concurrent proton pump inhibitors (Chu 2017). Consider avoiding proton pump inhibitors (if possible) in patients receiving capecitabine.

Uridine triacetate (formerly called vistonuridine), has been studied in cases of fluoropyrimidine overdose. In a clinical study of 98 patients who received uridine triacetate for fluorouracil toxicity (due to overdose, accidental capecitabine ingestion, or possible DPD deficiency), 96 patients recovered fully (Bamat 2013). Of 17 patients receiving uridine triacetate beginning within 8 to 96 hours after fluorouracil overdose, all patients fully recovered (von Borstel 2009). An additional case report describes accidental capecitabine ingestion by a 22-month-old child; uridine triacetate was initiated approximately 7 hours after exposure. The patient received uridine triacetate every 6 hours for a total of 20 doses through nasogastric tube administration; he was asymptomatic throughout his course and was discharged with normal laboratory values (Kanie 2011). Refer to Uridine Triacetate monograph.

Adverse Reactions Frequency listed derived from monotherapy trials. Incidence reported for all indications and usage, unless otherwise noted. Frequency not always defined.

>10%:

Cardiovascular: Edema (≤15%)

Central nervous system: Fatigue (≤42%), paresthesia (stage IV breast cancer: 21%; grades 3/4: 1%), pain (≤12%)

Dermatologic: Palmar-plantar erythrodysesthesia (54% to 60%; grades ≥3: 11% to 17%), dermatitis (27% to 37%, grades ≥3: 1%)

Gastrointestinal: Diarrhea (47% to 57%, grades 3/4: 2% to 13%), nausea (34% to 43%; stage IV breast cancer: 53%), vomiting (metastatic colorectal cancer, stage IV breast cancer: 27% to 37%; Dukes' C colon cancer: 15%), abdominal pain (metastatic colorectal cancer: 35%; stage IV breast cancer: 20%; Dukes' C colon cancer: 14%), decreased appetite (26%), stomatitis

(22% to 25%), anorexia (stage IV breast cancer: 23%; Dukes' C colon cancer: 9%), constipation (9% to 15%)

Hematologic & oncologic: Lymphocytopenia (stage IV breast cancer: 94%; stage IV breast cancer, grades 3/4: 15% to 44%), anemia (72% to 80%, grades 3/4: ≤3%), neutropenia (≤26%, grades 3/4: ≤3%), thrombocytopenia (stage IV breast cancer: 24%; all: grades 3/4: 1% to 3%)

Hepatic: Hyperbilirubinemia (Metastatic colorectal cancer: 48%; stage IV breast cancer: 22%; all: grades 3/4: 2% to 23%)

Neuromuscular & skeletal: Weakness (≤42%)

Ophthalmic: Eye irritation (13% to 15%)

Miscellaneous: Fever (7% to 18%)

1% to 10%:

Cardiovascular: Venous thrombosis (8%), chest pain (≤6%), atrial fibrillation (<5%), bradycardia (<5%), collapse (<5%), extrasystoles (<5%), pericardial effusion (<5%), ventricular premature contractions (<5%), angina pectoris, cardiac arrest, cardiac arrhythmia, cardiac failure, cardiomyopathy, ECG changes, ischemic heart disease, myocardial infarction

Central nervous system: Lethargy (10%), peripheral sensory neuropathy (10%), headache (5% to 10%), insomnia (≤8%), dizziness (6% to 8%), ataxia (<5%), depression (≤5%), mood changes (5%), abnormal gait (<5%), brain disease (<5%), dysarthria (<5%), dysphasia (<5%), equilibrium disturbance (<5%), irritability (<5%), myasthenia (<5%), sedation (<5%), vertigo (<5%)

Dermatologic: Nail disease (≤7%), skin discoloration (7%), skin rash (7%), alopecia (6%), erythema (6%), dermal ulcer (<5%), pruritus (<5%)

Endocrine & metabolic: Dehydration (7%), hot flash (<5%), hypokalemia (<5%), hypomagnesemia (<5%), Increased thirst (<5%), weight gain (<5%), decreased serum calcium (Dukes' C colon cancer: grades 3/4: 2%), increased serum calcium (Dukes' C colon cancer: grades 3/4: 1%)

Gastrointestinal: Gastrointestinal motility disorder (10%), GI inflammation (upper: 8%), oral discomfort (grades 3/4: 10%), dyspepsia (6% to 8%), upper abdominal pain (7%), intestinal obstruction (≤6%), dysgeusia (6%), gastrointestinal hemorrhage (6%), abdominal distention (<5%), dysphagia (<5%), rectal pain (<5%), toxic dilation of intestine (<5%), sore throat (2%), necrotizing enterocolitis

Hematologic & oncologic: Hemorrhage (<5%), lymphedema (<5%), granulocytopenia (Dukes' C colon cancer: grades 3/4: 3%), immune thrombocytopenia (1%)

Hepatic: Abnormal hepatic function tests (<5%), increased serum ALT (Dukes' C colon cancer: grades 3/4: 2%)

Hypersensitivity: Drug-induced hypersensitivity (<5%)

Infection: Viral infection (metastatic colorectal cancer: 5%)

Neuromuscular & skeletal: Back pain (10%), myalgia (≤9%), arthralgia (8%), limb pain (stage IV breast cancer: 6%), tremor (<5%)

Ophthalmic: Visual disturbance (metastatic colorectal cancer: 5%), conjunctivitis (≤5%), keratoconjunctivitis (<5%)

Respiratory: Cough (≤7%), chest mass (<5%), dyspnea (<5%), flu-like symptoms (<5%), hemoptysis (<5%), hoarseness (<5%), pharyngeal disease (metastatic colorectal cancer: 5%), epistaxis (≤3%), laryngitis (1%)

<1%, postmarketing, and/or case reports (limited to important or life-threatening): Acute renal failure, arthritis, ascites, asthma, blood coagulation disorder, bone marrow depression, bronchitis, bronchopneumonia, bronchospasm, cachexia, cerebrovascular accident, cholestatic hepatitis, confusion, cutaneous lupus erythematosus, diaphoresis, ecchymoses, esophagitis,

fibrosis, flu-like symptoms, fungal infection, gastric ulcer, gastroenteritis, gastrointestinal perforation, hepatic failure, hepatic fibrosis, hepatitis, hypersensitivity, hypertension, hypertriglyceridemia, hypotension, jaundice, keratitis, lacrimal stenosis, leukoencephalopathy, leukopenia, loss of consciousness, myocarditis, nocturia, ostealgia, pancytopenia, phlebitis (venous), photophobia, pneumonia, pulmonary embolism, radiation recall phenomenon, renal insufficiency, respiratory distress, sepsis, Stevens-Johnson syndrome, syncope, tachycardia, toxic epidermal necrolysis

Drug Interactions

Metabolism/Transport Effects Inhibits CYP2C9 (strong)

Avoid Concomitant Use

Avoid concomitant use of Capecitabine with any of the following: BCG (Intravesical); Deferiprone; Dipyrone; Gimeracil; Natalizumab; Pimecrolimus; Tacrolimus (Topical); Vaccines (Live)

Increased Effect/Toxicity

Capecitabine may increase the levels/effects of: Alitretinoin (Systemic); Bosentan; Cannabis; Carvedilol; CloZAPine; CYP2C9 Substrates; Deferiprone; Diclofenac (Systemic); Dronabinol; Fingolimod; Fosphenytoin; Highest Risk QTc-Prolonging Agents; Lacosamide; Leflunomide; Moderate Risk QTc-Prolonging Agents; Natalizumab; Ospemifene; Parecoxib; Phenytoin; Ramelteon; Tetrahydrocannabinol; Tofacitinib; Vaccines (Live); Vitamin K Antagonists

The levels/effects of Capecitabine may be increased by: Cimetidine; Denosumab; Dipyrone; Gimeracil; Leucovorin Calcium-Levoleucovorin; MetroNIDAZOLE (Systemic); MiFEPRIStone; Ocrelizumab; Palifermin; Pimecrolimus; Promazine; Roflumilast; Tacrolimus (Topical); Trastuzumab

Decreased Effect

Capecitabine may decrease the levels/effects of: BCG (Intravesical); Coccidioides immitis Skin Test; Lenograstim; Nivolumab; Sipuleucel-T; Vaccines (Inactivated); Vaccines (Live)

The levels/effects of Capecitabine may be decreased by: Echinacea; Proton Pump Inhibitors

Food Interactions Food reduced the rate and extent of absorption of capecitabine. Management: Administer within 30 minutes after a meal.

Hazardous Drugs Handling Considerations

Hazardous agent (NIOSH 2016 [group 1]).

Use appropriate precautions for receiving, handling, administration, and disposal. Gloves (single) should be worn during receiving, unpacking, and placing in storage.

NIOSH recommends single gloving for administration of intact tablets or capsules. If manipulating tablets/capsules (eg, to prepare an oral suspension), NIOSH recommends double gloving, a protective gown, and preparation in a controlled device; if not prepared in a controlled device, respiratory and eye/face protection as well as ventilated engineering controls are recommended. NIOSH recommends double gloving, a protective gown, and (if there is a potential for vomit or spit up) eye/face protection for administration of an oral liquid/feeding tube administration (NIOSH 2016).

Storage/Stability Store at 25°C (77°F); excursions are permitted between 15°C and 30°C (59°F and 86°F). Keep bottle tightly closed.

Mechanism of Action Capecitabine is a prodrug of fluorouracil. It undergoes hydrolysis in the liver and tissues to form fluorouracil which is the active moiety. Fluorouracil is a fluorinated pyrimidine antimetabolite that inhibits thymidylate synthetase, blocking the methylation of deoxyuridylic acid to thymidylic acid, interfering with DNA, and to a lesser degree, RNA synthesis. Fluorouracil appears to be phase specific for the G_1 and S phases of the cell cycle.

Pharmacodynamics/Kinetics

Absorption: Rapid and extensive (rate and extent reduced by food)

Protein binding: <60%; ~35% to albumin

Metabolism:

Hepatic: Inactive metabolites: 5′-deoxy-5-fluorocytidine, 5′-deoxy-5-fluorouridine

Tissue: Enzymatically metabolized to fluorouracil, which is then metabolized to active metabolites, 5-fluoroxyuridine monophosphate (F-UMP) and 5-5-fluoro-2′-deoxyuridine-5′-O-monophosphate (F-dUMP)

Half-life elimination: ~0.75 hour

Time to peak: 1.5 hours; Fluorouracil: 2 hours

Excretion: Urine (96%, 57% as α-fluoro-β-alanine; <3% as unchanged drug); feces (<3%)

Dosing

Adult

Breast cancer, metastatic: Oral: 1,250 mg/m² twice daily for 2 weeks, every 21 days (as either monotherapy or in combination with docetaxel)

Breast cancer, metastatic (off-label dosing): Adults ≥65 years: Oral: 1,000 mg/m² twice daily on days 1 to 14 of a 21-day treatment cycle for at least 2 and up to 6 cycles or longer (Bajetta 2005).

Breast cancer, metastatic (off-label combination): Oral: 1,000 mg/m² twice daily (in combination with ixabepilone) on days 1 to 14 of a 3-week cycle until disease progression or unacceptable toxicity (Thomas 2007)

Breast cancer, metastatic, HER2+ (off-label combinations): Oral: 1,000 mg/m² twice daily (in combination with lapatinib) on days 1 to 14 of a 3-week cycle until disease progression or unacceptable toxicity (Coyor 2006) or 1,250 mg/m² twice daily (in combination with trastuzumab) on days 1 to 14 of a 3-week cycle (Bartsch 2007)

Breast cancer, metastatic, HER2+ with brain metastases, first-line therapy (off-label combination): Oral: 1,000 mg/m² twice daily (in combination with lapatinib) on days 1 to 14 of a 3-week cycle until disease progression or unacceptable toxicity (Bachelot 2012)

Breast cancer, adjuvant therapy (off-label; in HER2-negative patients with residual disease after neoadjuvant therapy and surgery): Oral: 1,250 mg/m² twice daily on days 1 to 14 of a 21-day treatment cycle for 6 to 8 cycles (Masuda 2017).

Colorectal cancer, metastatic: Oral: 1,250 mg/m² twice daily for 2 weeks, every 21 days. **Note:** Capecitabine toxicities, particularly hand-foot syndrome, may be higher in North American populations; therapy initiation at doses of 1,000 mg/m² twice daily (for 2 weeks every 21 days) may be considered (Haller 2008).

Colorectal cancer (off-label combination): Oral: 1,000 mg/m² twice daily (in combination with oxaliplatin) on days 1 to 14 of a 3-week cycle for 8 or 16 cycles (Cassidy 2008; Haller 2011; Schmoll 2007)

Dukes' C colon cancer, adjuvant therapy: Oral: 1,250 mg/m^2 twice daily for 2 weeks, every 21 days, for a recommended total duration of 24 weeks (8 cycles of 2 weeks of drug administration and 1 week rest period).

Anal carcinoma (off-label use): Oral: 825 mg/m^2 twice daily 5 days/week (Monday through Friday) (in combination with mitomycin [on day 1 only]) during radiation therapy; radiation therapy occurred over 5 to 6 weeks (Oliveria 2016) **or** 825 mg/m^2 twice daily on radiation therapy days (in combination with mitomycin [on day 1 only] and radiation therapy) (Meulendijks 2014; Thind 2014)

Esophageal and gastric cancers (off-label uses): Oral:

Preoperative or definitive chemoradiation: 800 mg/m^2 twice daily (in combination with cisplatin and radiation) on days 1 to 5 weekly for 5 weeks (Lee 2007) **or** 625 mg/m^2 twice daily (in combination with oxaliplatin and radiation) on days 1 to 5 weekly for 5 weeks (Javle 2009)

Postoperative chemoradiation: 625 to 825 mg/m^2 twice daily during radiation therapy (Lee 2006)

Locally advanced or metastatic (chemoradiation not indicated): 1,000 to 1,250 mg/m^2 twice daily (monotherapy or in combination with cisplatin with or without trastuzumab) on days 1 to 14 of a 3-week cycle (Bang 2010; Hong 2004; Kang 2009) **or** 625 mg/m^2 twice daily (in combination with epirubicin and cisplatin or oxaliplatin) on days 1 to 21 of a 3-week cycle for up to 8 cycles (Cunningham 2008; Sumpter 2005)

Hepatobiliary cancer, adjuvant therapy (off-label use): Oral: 1,250 mg/m^2 twice daily on days 1 to 14 of a 21-day treatment cycle for 8 cycles (Primrose 2017).

Hepatobiliary cancers, advanced (off-label use): Oral: 650 mg/m^2 twice daily (in combination with gemcitabine) on days 1 to 14 of a 3-week cycle (Knox 2005) **or** 1,000 mg/m^2 twice daily (in combination with oxaliplatin) on days 1 to 14 of a 3-week cycle (Nehls 2008) **or** 1,250 mg/m^2 twice daily (in combination with cisplatin) on days 1 to 14 of a 3-week cycle (Kim 2003); all regimens continued until disease progression or unacceptable toxicity

Neuroendocrine (pancreatic/islet cell) tumors, metastatic or unresectable (off label use): Oral: 750 mg/m^2 twice daily (in combination with temozolomide) on days 1 to 14 of a 4-week cycle (Strosberg 2011)

Ovarian, fallopian tube, or peritoneal cancer, platinum-refractory (off label use): Oral: 1,000 mg/m^2 twice daily on days 1 to 14 of a 3-week cycle until disease progression or unacceptable toxicity (Wolf 2006)

Pancreatic cancer (adjuvant therapy) (off-label use): Oral: 1,660 mg/m^2/day (in 2 divided doses) days 1 to 21 every 28 days (in combination with gemcitabine) for 6 cycles beginning within 12 weeks of resection (Neoptolemos 2017). American Society of Clinical Oncology guidelines recommend initiating within 8 weeks of resection (ASCO [Khorana 2017]).

Pancreatic cancer, metastatic (off-label use): Oral: 1,250 mg/m^2 twice daily on days 1 to 14 of a 3-week cycle (Cartwright 2002) **or** 830 mg/m^2 twice daily (in combination with gemcitabine) on days 1 to 21 of a 4-week cycle until disease progression or unacceptable toxicity (Cunningham 2009)

Unknown primary cancer (off-label use): Oral: 1,000 mg/m^2 twice daily (in combination with oxaliplatin) on days 1 to 14 of a 3-week cycle for up to 6 cycles or until disease progression (Hainsworth 2010) **or** 800 mg/m^2 twice daily (in combination with carboplatin and gemcitabine) on days 1 to 14 of a 3-week cycle for up to 8 cycles or until disease progression or unacceptable toxicity (Schneider 2007)

Geriatric The elderly may be more sensitive to the toxic effects of fluorouracil. Insufficient data are available to provide dosage modifications.

Renal Impairment Note: Renal function may be estimated using the Cockcroft-Gault formula for dosage adjustment purposes.

Renal impairment at treatment initiation:

CrCl ≥51 mL/minute: Initial: No dosage adjustment necessary.

CrCl 30 to 50 mL/minute: Initial: Reduce dose to 75% of usual dose (Cassidy 2002; Poole 2002; Xeloda prescribing information 2016)

CrCl <30 mL/minute: Use is contraindicated (Poole 2002; Xeloda prescribing information 2016)

Renal toxicity during treatment: Refer to Dosing: Adjustment for Toxicity.

Hepatic Impairment

Hepatic impairment at treatment initiation:

Mild to moderate impairment: No starting dose adjustment necessary (Ecklund 2005; Superfin 2007); however, carefully monitor patients.

Severe hepatic impairment: There are no dosage adjustments provided in the manufacturer's labeling (has not been studied).

Hepatotoxicity during treatment: Hyperbilirubinemia, grade 3 or 4: Interrupt treatment until bilirubin ≤3 times ULN; refer to Dosing: Adjustment for Toxicity for dosage recommendations.

Obesity *ASCO Guidelines for appropriate chemotherapy dosing in obese adults with cancer:* Utilize patient's actual body weight (full weight) for calculation of body surface area- or weight-based dosing, particularly when the intent of therapy is curative; manage regimen-related toxicities in the same manner as for nonobese patients; if a dose reduction is utilized due to toxicity, consider resumption of full weight-based dosing with subsequent cycles, especially if cause of toxicity (eg, hepatic or renal impairment) is resolved (Griggs 2012). The manufacturer recommends capping the dose (at a maximum of 5,600 mg/day) in patients with a body surface area of 2.18 m^2 or higher (refer to product labeling for details).

Adjustment for Toxicity See table (**Note:** Capecitabine dosing recommendations apply to both monotherapy and when used in combination therapy with docetaxel).

Monitor carefully for toxicity and adjust dose as necessary. Doses reduced for toxicity should not be increased at a later time. For combination therapy, also refer to docetaxel product labeling for docetaxel dose modifications. If treatment delay is required for either capecitabine or docetaxel, withhold both agents until appropriate to resume combination treatment.

Recommended Capecitabine Dose Modifications

Toxicity Grades	During a Course of Therapy	Dose Adjustment for Next Cycle (% of starting dose)
Grade 1	Maintain dose level	Maintain dose level
Grade 2 1st appearance	Interrupt until resolved to grade 0 to 1	100%
2nd appearance	Interrupt until resolved to grade 0 to 1	75%
3rd appearance	Interrupt until resolved to grade 0 to 1	50%
4th appearance	Discontinue treatment permanently	

(continued)

Recommended Capecitabine Dose Modifications *(continued)*

Toxicity Grades	During a Course of Therapy	Dose Adjustment for Next Cycle (% of starting dose)
Grade 3		
1st appearance	Interrupt until resolved to grade 0 to 1	75%
2nd appearance	Interrupt until resolved to grade 0 to 1	50%
3rd appearance	Discontinue treatment permanently	
Grade 4		
1st appearance	Discontinue permanently	
	or	
	If in the patient's best interest to continue, interrupt until resolved to grade 0 to 1	50%

Dosage adjustments for hematologic toxicity in combination therapy with ixabepilone:

Neutrophils <500/mm^3 for ≥7 days or neutropenic fever: Hold for concurrent diarrhea or stomatitis until neutrophils recover to >1000/mm^3, then continue at same dose

Platelets <25,000/mm^3 (or <50,000/mm^3 with bleeding): Hold for concurrent diarrhea or stomatitis until platelets recover to >50,000/mm^3, then continue at same dose

Combination Regimens

Biliary adenocarcinoma: Gemcitabine-Capecitabine (Biliary Cancer) on page 2134

Breast cancer:
  Capecitabine-Docetaxel (Breast) on page 2006
  Capecitabine-Ixabepilone (Breast) on page 2008
  Capecitabine + Lapatinib (Breast) on page 2008
  Capecitabine-Trastuzumab (Breast) on page 2010

Colorectal cancer:
  Bevacizumab + XELOX (Colorectal) on page 1996
  XELOX (Colorectal) on page 2233

Esophageal cancer:
  Cisplatin-Capecitabine (Esophageal Cancer) on page 2036
  Epirubicin-Cisplatin-Capecitabine (Gastric/Esophageal) on page 2103
  Epirubicin-Oxaliplatin-Capecitabine (Gastric/Esophageal) on page 2104
  Irinotecan-Capecitabine (Esophageal Cancer) on page 2157

Gastric cancer:
  Capecitabine-Docetaxel (Gastric Cancer) on page 2006
  Capecitabine-Oxaliplatin (Gastric) on page 2009
  Cisplatin-Capecitabine (Gastric Cancer) on page 2036
  Epirubicin-Cisplatin-Capecitabine (Gastric/Esophageal) on page 2103
  Epirubicin-Oxaliplatin-Capecitabine (Gastric/Esophageal) on page 2104
  Irinotecan-Capecitabine (Gastric Cancer) on page 2158
  Trastuzumab-Cisplatin-Capecitabine (Gastric Cancer) on page 2215

Gastrointestinal cancer: CAPOX (Biliary Cancer) on page 2010

Pancreatic cancer:
Capecitabine-Gemcitabine (Pancreatic) on page 2007
CAPOX (Pancreatic) on page 2011
GTX (Pancreatic) on page 2142
Unknown primary, adenocarcinoma: Capecitabine-Oxaliplatin (Unknown Primary, Adenocarcinoma) on page 2009

Administration Usually administered in 2 divided doses taken 12 hours apart. Doses should be taken with water within 30 minutes after a meal. Swallow tablets whole. Avoid cutting or crushing tablets.

Emetic Potential Children and Adults: Low (10% to 30%)

Extemporaneous Preparations A 10 mg/mL oral solution may be made with tablets. Crush four 500 mg tablets in a mortar and reduce to a fine powder; add to 200 mL water. Capecitabine tablets are water soluble (data on file from Roche). Administer immediately after preparation, 30 minutes after a meal.

Judson IR, Beale PJ, Trigo JM, et al, "A Human Capecitabine Excretion Balance and Pharmacokinetic Study After Administration of a Single Oral Dose of ^{14}C-Labelled Drug," *Invest New Drugs*, 1999, 17(1):49-56.

Monitoring Parameters Renal function should be estimated at baseline to determine initial dose. During therapy, CBC with differential, hepatic function, and renal function should be monitored. Monitor INR closely if receiving concomitant warfarin. Pregnancy test prior to treatment initiation (in females of reproductive potential). Monitor for diarrhea, dehydration, hand-foot syndrome, Stevens-Johnson syndrome, toxic epidermal necrolysis, stomatitis, and cardiotoxicity. Monitor adherence.

Dosage Forms Excipient information presented when available (limited, particularly for generics); consult specific product labeling.

Tablet, Oral:
Xeloda: 150 mg, 500 mg
Generic: 150 mg, 500 mg

◆ **Caphosol** see Saliva Substitute on page 1653

◆ **Caprelsa** see Vandetanib on page 1871

◆ **Carac** 300 Fluorouracil (Topical) on page 835

◆ **Carbon-11 Choline** see Choline C 11 on page 391

CARBOplatin (KAR boe pla tin)

Related Information

Chemotherapy-Induced Peripheral Neuropathy on page 2236
Hematopoietic Cell Transplantation on page 2365
Management of Chemotherapy-Induced Nausea and Vomiting in Adults on page 2253
Management of Drug Extravasations on page 2271
Prevention of Chemotherapy-Induced Nausea and Vomiting in Children on page 2310
Safe Handling of Hazardous Drugs on page 2379

Brand Names: Canada Carboplatin Injection; Carboplatin Injection BP

Index Terms CBDCA; Paraplatin

Pharmacologic Category Antineoplastic Agent, Alkylating Agent; Antineoplastic Agent, Platinum Analog

Use Ovarian cancer, advanced: Initial treatment of advanced ovarian cancer in combination with other established chemotherapy agents; palliative treatment of recurrent ovarian cancer after prior chemotherapy, including cisplatin-based treatment

Labeled Contraindications History of severe allergic reaction to carboplatin, cisplatin, other platinum-containing formulations, mannitol, or any component of the formulation; should not be used in patients with severe bone marrow depression or significant bleeding

Pregnancy Considerations Adverse events have been observed in animal reproduction studies. May cause fetal harm if administered during pregnancy. Women of childbearing potential should avoid becoming pregnant during treatment.

Breastfeeding Considerations It is not known if carboplatin is present in breast milk. Due to the potential for toxicity in breastfeeding infants, the manufacturer recommends discontinuing breastfeeding during carboplatin treatment.

Warnings/Precautions [US Boxed Warning]: Bone marrow suppression, which may be severe, is dose related; may result in infection (due to neutropenia) or bleeding (due to thrombocytopenia); anemia may require blood transfusion. Reduce dosage in patients with bone marrow suppression; cycles should be delayed until WBC and platelet counts have recovered. In patients receiving single agent carboplatin, the median nadir typically occurs at day 21. Patients who have received prior myelosuppressive therapy and patients with renal dysfunction are at increased risk for bone marrow suppression. Anemia is cumulative. Monitor blood counts closely. High doses (>4 times the recommended dose) have resulted in severe abnormalities of liver function tests.

When calculating the carboplatin dose using the Calvert formula and an eGFR, the laboratory method used to measure serum creatinine may impact dosing. Compared to other methods, standardized isotope dilution mass spectrometry (IDMS) may underestimate serum creatinine values in patients with low creatinine values (eg, ≤0.7 mg/dL) and may overestimate GFR in patients with normal renal function. This may result in higher calculated carboplatin doses and increased toxicities. If using IDMS, the FDA recommends that clinicians consider capping estimated GFR at a maximum of 125 mL/minute to avoid potential toxicity.

[US Boxed Warning]: Anaphylactic-like reactions have been reported with carboplatin; may occur within minutes of administration. Epinephrine, corticosteroids, and antihistamines have been used to treat symptoms. The risk of allergic reactions (including anaphylaxis) is increased in patients previously exposed to platinum therapy. Skin testing and desensitization protocols have been reported (Confina-Cohen 2005; Lee 2004; Markman 2003). When administered as sequential infusions, taxane derivatives (docetaxel, paclitaxel) should be administered before the platinum derivatives (carboplatin, cisplatin) to limit myelosuppression and to enhance efficacy. Ototoxicity may occur when administered concomitantly with aminoglycosides. Clinically significant hearing loss has been reported to occur in pediatric patients when carboplatin was administered at higher-than-recommended doses in combination with other ototoxic agents (eg, aminoglycosides). In a study of children receiving carboplatin for the treatment of retinoblastoma, those <6 months at treatment initiation were more likely to experience ototoxicity; long-term audiology monitoring is recommended (Qaddoumi

2012). Loss of vision (usually reversible within weeks of discontinuing) has been reported with higher-than-recommended doses.

Peripheral neuropathy occurs infrequently, the incidence of peripheral neuropathy is increased in patients >65 years of age and those who have previously received cisplatin treatment. Patients >65 years of age are more likely to develop severe thrombocytopenia.

Carboplatin has a limited potential for nephrotoxicity unless administered concomitantly with aminoglycosides. Use caution with concomitant administration with aminoglycosides or other nephrotoxic medications. **[US Boxed Warning]: Vomiting may occur.** Carboplatin is associated with a moderate to high emetic potential in adult patients (dose dependent) and a high emetic potential in pediatric patients; antiemetics are recommended to prevent nausea and vomiting (Basch 2011; Dupuis 2011; Roila 2016). Nausea and vomiting may be more severe in patients who have received prior emetogenic therapy. **[US Boxed Warning]: Should be administered under the supervision of an experienced cancer chemotherapy physician.** Potentially significant interactions may exist, requiring dose or frequency adjustment, additional monitoring, and/or selection of alternative therapy.

Adverse Reactions Percentages reported with single-agent therapy.

>10%:

Central nervous system: Pain (23%)

Endocrine & metabolic: Hyponatremia (29% to 47%), hypomagnesemia (29% to 43%), hypocalcemia (22% to 31%), hypokalemia (20% to 28%)

Gastrointestinal: Vomiting (65% to 81%), abdominal pain (17%), nausea (without vomiting: 10% to 15%)

Hematologic & oncologic: Bone marrow depression (dose related and dose limiting; nadir at ~21 days with single-agent therapy), anemia (71% to 90%; grades 3/4: 21%), leukopenia (85%; grades 3/4: 15% to 26%), neutropenia (67%; grades 3/4: 16% to 21%), thrombocytopenia (62%; grades 3/4: 25% to 35%)

Hepatic: Increased serum alkaline phosphatase (24% to 37%), increased serum AST (15% to 19%)

Hypersensitivity: Hypersensitivity (2% to 16%)

Neuromuscular & skeletal: Weakness (11%)

Renal: Decreased creatinine clearance (27%), increased blood urea nitrogen (14% to 22%)

1% to 10%:

Central nervous system: Peripheral neuropathy (4% to 6%), neurotoxicity (5%)

Dermatologic: Alopecia (2% to 3%)

Gastrointestinal: Constipation (6%), diarrhea (6%), dysgeusia (1%), mucositis (≤1%), stomatitis (≤1%)

Hematologic & oncologic: Bleeding complications (5%), hemorrhage (5%)

Hepatic: Increased serum bilirubin (5%)

Infection: Infection (5%)

Ophthalmic: Visual disturbance (1%)

Otic: Ototoxicity (1%)

Renal: Increased serum creatinine (6% to 10%)

<1%, postmarketing, and/or case reports (Limited to important or life-threatening): Anaphylaxis, anorexia, bronchospasm, cardiac failure, cerebrovascular accident, dehydration, embolism, erythema, febrile neutropenia, hemolytic anemia (acute), hemolytic-uremic syndrome, hypertension,

hypotension, injection site reaction (pain, redness, swelling), limb ischemia (acute), malaise, metastases, pruritus, skin rash, tissue necrosis (associated with extravasation), urticaria, vision loss

Drug Interactions

Metabolism/Transport Effects None known.

Avoid Concomitant Use

Avoid concomitant use of CARBOplatin with any of the following: BCG (Intravesical); Deferiprone; Dipyrone; Natalizumab; Pimecrolimus; SORAfenib; Tacrolimus (Topical); Vaccines (Live)

Increased Effect/Toxicity

CARBOplatin may increase the levels/effects of: Bexarotene (Systemic); CloZAPine; Deferiprone; Fingolimod; Leflunomide; Natalizumab; Taxane Derivatives; Tofacitinib; Topotecan; Vaccines (Live)

The levels/effects of CARBOplatin may be increased by: Aminoglycosides; Denosumab; Dipyrone; Ocrelizumab; Palifermin; Pimecrolimus; Promazine; Roflumilast; SORAfenib; Tacrolimus (Topical); Trastuzumab

Decreased Effect

CARBOplatin may decrease the levels/effects of: BCG (Intravesical); Coccidioides immitis Skin Test; Fosphenytoin-Phenytoin; Lenograstim; Nivolumab; Sipuleucel-T; Tertomotide; Vaccines (Inactivated); Vaccines (Live)

The levels/effects of CARBOplatin may be decreased by: Echinacea

Hazardous Drugs Handling Considerations

Hazardous agent (NIOSH 2016 [group 1]).

Use appropriate precautions for receiving, handling, administration, and disposal. Gloves (single) should be worn during receiving, unpacking, and placing in storage.

NIOSH recommends double gloving, a protective gown, ventilated engineering controls (a class II biological safety cabinet or a compounding aseptic containment isolator), and closed system transfer devices (CSTDs) for preparation. Double gloving, a gown, and (if dosage form allows) CSTDs are required during administration (NIOSH 2016).

Storage/Stability Store intact vials at room temperature at 25°C (77°F); excursions permitted to 15°C to 30°C (59°F to 86°F). Protect from light. Further dilution to a concentration as low as 0.5 mg/mL is stable at room temperature (25°C) for 8 hours in NS or D5W. Stability has also been demonstrated for dilutions in D5W in PVC bags at room temperature for 9 days (Benaji 1994); however, the manufacturer recommends use within 8 hours due to lack of preservative. Multidose vials are stable for up to 14 or 15 days after opening when stored at 25°C (77°F) following multiple needle entries (refer to specific product labeling for stability information).

Preparation for Administration

Solution for injection: Manufacturer's labeling states solution can be further diluted to concentrations as low as 0.5 mg/mL in NS or D5W; however, most clinicians generally dilute dose in either 100 mL or 250 mL of NS or D5W.

Concentrations used for desensitization vary based on protocol.

Needles or IV administration sets that contain aluminum should not be used in the preparation or administration of carboplatin; aluminum can react with carboplatin resulting in precipitate formation and loss of potency.

Mechanism of Action Carboplatin is a platinum compound alkylating agent which covalently binds to DNA; interferes with the function of DNA by producing interstrand DNA cross-links. Carboplatin is apparently not cell-cycle specific.

Pharmacodynamics/Kinetics

Distribution: V_d: 16 L (based on a dose of 300 to 500 mg/m^2); into liver, kidney, skin, and tumor tissue

Protein binding: Carboplatin: 0%; Platinum (from carboplatin): Irreversibly binds to plasma proteins

Metabolism: Minimally hepatic to aquated and hydroxylated compounds

Half-life elimination: CrCl >60 mL/minute: Carboplatin: 2.6 to 5.9 hours (based on a dose of 300 to 500 mg/m^2); Platinum (from carboplatin): ≥5 days

Excretion: Urine (~70% as carboplatin within 24 hours; 3% to 5% as platinum within 1 to 4 days)

Dosing

Adult Note: Doses for adults are commonly calculated by the target AUC using the Calvert formula, where **Total dose (mg) = Target AUC x (GFR + 25)**. If estimating GFR instead of a measured GFR, the FDA recommends that clinicians consider capping estimated GFR at a maximum of 125 mL/minute to avoid potential toxicity. Carboplatin is associated with a moderate to high emetic potential in adult patients (dose/AUC dependent); antiemetics are recommended to prevent nausea and vomiting.

Ovarian cancer, advanced: *Manufacturer's labeling:* IV: 360 mg/m^2 every 4 weeks (as a single agent) **or** 300 mg/m^2 every 4 weeks (in combination with cyclophosphamide) for 6 cycles **or** Target AUC 4 to 6 (single agent; in previously treated patients)

Off-label dosing for advanced ovarian cancer: IV: Target AUC 5 to 7.5 every 3 weeks (in combination with paclitaxel) (Ozols 2003; Parmar 2003) **or** Target AUC 2 once weekly (in combination with weekly paclitaxel) for 18 consecutive weeks (Pignata 2014) **or** Target AUC 5 every 3 weeks (in combination with docetaxel) (Vasey 2004)

Off-label dosing for malignant germ cell tumor: IV: 400 mg/m^2 on day 1 (in combination with etoposide) every 4 weeks for 3 cycles (Williams 2004)

Anal cancer, advanced (off-label use): IV: Target AUC 6 on days 1 and 22 every 6 weeks for up to 4 cycles (in combination with paclitaxel and fluorouracil) (Hainsworth 2001) **or** Target AUC 5 or 6 every 3 weeks (in combination with paclitaxel) (Kim 2014). Additional data may be necessary to further define the role of carboplatin in the treatment of this condition.

Bladder cancer (off-label use): IV: Target AUC 5 every 3 weeks (in combination with gemcitabine) (Bamias 2006) **or** Target AUC 6 every 3 weeks (in combination with paclitaxel) (Vaughn 2002)

Breast cancer, metastatic (off-label use): IV: Target AUC 6 every 3 weeks (in combination with trastuzumab and paclitaxel) (Robert 2006) **or** Target AUC 6 every 3 weeks (in combination with trastuzumab and docetaxel) (Pegram 2004; Valero 2011)

Cervical cancer, recurrent or metastatic (off-label use): IV: Target AUC 5 every 3 weeks (in combination with paclitaxel) (Pectasides 2009) **or** Target AUC 5 to 6 every 4 weeks (in combination with paclitaxel) (Tinker 2005) **or** 400 mg/m^2 every 28 days (as a single agent) (Weiss 1990)

Endometrial cancer (off-label use): IV: Target AUC 5 every 3 weeks (in combination with paclitaxel) (Pectasides 2008) **or** Target AUC 2 on days 1, 8, and 15 every 28 days (in combination with paclitaxel) (Secord 2007)

Esophageal cancer (off-label use): IV: Target AUC 2 once weekly for 5 weeks (in combination with paclitaxel and radiation therapy) prior to surgery (van Hagen 2012; van Meerten 2006) **or** Target AUC 5 every 3 weeks (in combination with paclitaxel) (El-Rayes 2004)

Gastric cancer (off-label use): IV: Target AUC 2 once weekly for 5 weeks (in combination with paclitaxel and concurrent radiation) prior to surgery (van Hagen 2012) **or** Target AUC 5 to 6 every 3 weeks (in combination with paclitaxel) (Gadgeel 2003)

Head and neck cancer (off-label use): IV: Target AUC 5 every 3 weeks (in combination with cetuximab) (Chan 2005) **or** Target AUC 5 every 3 weeks (in combination with cetuximab and fluorouracil) (Vermorken 2008) **or** 300 mg/m^2 every 4 weeks (in combination with fluorouracil) (Forastiere 1992) **or** Target AUC 6 every 3 weeks (in combination with paclitaxel) (Clark 2001) **or** Target AUC 1.5 weekly for 7 weeks (in combination with radiation, following 3 cycles of docetaxel, cisplatin, and fluorouracil [TPF] induction therapy [begin carboplatin/radiation therapy 3 to 8 weeks after the start of TPF cycle 3]) (Haddad 2013; Posner 2007)

Hematopoietic stem cell transplant (HSCT) for metastatic germ cell tumors: IV: 700 mg/m^2/day for 3 days beginning 5 days prior to peripheral stem cell infusion (in combination with etoposide) for 2 cycles (Einhorn 2007). Additional data may be necessary to further define the role of carboplatin in the treatment of this condition.

Hodgkin lymphoma, relapsed or refractory (off-label use): IV: Target AUC 5 (maximum dose: 800 mg) for 2 cycles (in combination with ifosfamide and etoposide) (Moskowitz 2001)

Malignant pleural mesothelioma (off-label use): IV: Target AUC 5 every 3 weeks (in combination with pemetrexed) (Castagneto 2008; Ceresoli 2006)

Melanoma, advanced or metastatic (off-label use): IV: Target AUC 2 days on 1, 8, and 15 every 4 weeks (in combination with paclitaxel) (Rao 2006). Additional data may be necessary to further define the role of carboplatin in the treatment of this condition.

Merkel cell carcinoma (off-label use): IV: Target AUC 4.5 on day 1 of weeks 1, 4, 7, and 10 (in combination with etoposide and synchronous radiation therapy) (Poulsen 2003) **or** Target AUC 2 on day 1 weekly for up to 5 doses (administered concurrently with radiation), followed (beginning 3 weeks after radiation therapy) by carboplatin with a target AUC of 4.5 on day 1 (in combination with etoposide) every 3 weeks for 3 cycles (Poulsen 2008)

Neuroendocrine tumors, advanced, atypical or poorly differentiated (nonpulmonary) (off-label use): IV: Target AUC 6 every 3 weeks (in combination with etoposide) for 4 to 6 cycles (Skarlos 2001; Strosberg 2010).

Non-Hodgkin lymphomas, relapsed or refractory (off-label use): IV: Target AUC 5 (maximum dose: 800 mg) per cycle for 3 cycles (in combination with rituximab, ifosfamide and etoposide) (Kewalramani 2004)

Non-small cell lung cancer (off-label use): IV: Target AUC 6 every 3 to 4 weeks (in combination with paclitaxel) (Ramalingam 2008; Schiller 2002; Strauss 2008) **or** Target AUC 6 every 3 weeks (in combination with bevacizumab and paclitaxel) (Sandler 2006) **or** Target AUC 5 every 3 weeks (in combination with pemetrexed) (Gronberg 2009) **or** Target AUC 6 every 3 weeks (in combination with pemetrexed and bevacizumab) for up to 4 cycles followed by maintenance therapy (Patel 2013) **or** in combination with radiation therapy and paclitaxel (Belani 2005):

Target AUC 6 every 3 weeks for 2 cycles **or**

Target AUC 6 every 3 weeks for 2 cycles; then target AUC 2 weekly for 7 weeks **or**

Target AUC 2 every week for 7 weeks; then target AUC 6 every 3 weeks for 2 cycles

Sarcomas: Ewing sarcoma, osteosarcoma (off-label uses): IV: 400 mg/m^2/day for 2 days every 21 days (in combination with ifosfamide and etoposide) (van Winkle 2005)

Small cell lung cancer (off-label use): IV: Target AUC 6 every 3 weeks (in combination with etoposide) (Skarlos 2001) **or** Target AUC 5 every 3 weeks (in combination with irinotecan) (Hermes 2008) **or** Target AUC 5 every 28 days (in combination with irinotecan) (Schmittel 2006)

Testicular cancer (off-label use): IV: Target AUC 7 as a one-time dose (Oliver 2011) **or** 700 mg/m^2/day for 3 days beginning 5 days prior to peripheral stem cell infusion (in combination with etoposide) for 2 cycles (Einhorn 2007)

Thymic malignancies (off-label use): IV: Target AUC 5 every 3 weeks (in combination with paclitaxel) (Lemma 2008)

Thyroid cancer (anaplastic), advanced: IV: Target AUC 6 on day 1 every 3 weeks (in combination with paclitaxel) for 6 cycles (Smallridge 2012; Sosa 2014) **or** Target AUC 2 once weekly (in combination with weekly paclitaxel) (Smallridge 2012)

Unknown primary adenocarcinoma (off-label use): IV: Target AUC 6 every 3 weeks (in combination with paclitaxel) (Briasoulis 2000) **or** Target AUC 6 every 3 weeks (in combination with docetaxel) (Greco 2000) **or** Target AUC 6 every 3 weeks (in combination with paclitaxel and etoposide) (Hainsworth 2006)

Geriatric The Calvert formula should be used to calculate dosing for elderly patients. Refer to adult dosing.

Pediatric Carboplatin is associated with a high emetic potential in pediatric patients; antiemetics are recommended to prevent nausea and vomiting (Dupuis 2011).

Central nervous system tumors (off-label use):

    Glioma: Infants ≥3 months, Children, and Adolescents: IV:

      Induction: 175 mg/m^2 weekly for 4 weeks every 6 weeks for 2 cycles, with a 2-week recovery period between courses (in combination with vincristine) (Packer 1997)

      Maintenance: 175 mg/m^2 weekly for 4 weeks (in combination with vincristine) for up to 12 cycles, with a 3-week recovery period between cycles (Packer 1997)

Neuroblastoma, localized and unresectable: IV: Children ≥10 kg: 200 mg/m^2/day days 1, 2, and 3 every 21 days for 2 cycles (in combination with etoposide for 2 cycles then followed by cyclophosphamide, doxorubicin and vincristine) (Rubie 1998) **or** Children <1 year: 6.6 mg/kg/day days 1, 2, and 3 (in combination with etoposide for 2 cycles, then followed by cyclophosphamide, doxorubicin, and vincristine) (Rubie 2001)

Hematopoietic stem cell transplant (HSCT) (off-label use): IV:

Infants ≥6 months and Children ≤3 years: Consolidation regimen: 17 mg/kg over 2 hours on days 0 and 1 of a 21-day cycle for 3 cycles (in combination with thiotepa), followed by stem cell infusion at least 48 hours after the last thiotepa dose (Cohen 2015)

Children and Adolescents: Conditioning regimen: ~500 mg/m^2/day for 3 consecutive days; dosing utilized pediatric Calvert formula with a target AUC 7 (in combination with thiotepa and topotecan) (Gilheeny 2010; Kushner 2001)

Retinoblastoma (off-label use):

Rodriguez-Galindo 2003: Infants and Children: IV:

GFR ≥50 mL/minute/m^2: 560 mg/m^2 in combination with vincristine every 21 days for 8 cycles

GFR <50 mL/minute/m^2: Dosing utilized modified Calvert formula with a target AUC 6.5 in combination with vincristine every 21 days for 8 cycles

Friedman 2000:

Infants and Children ≤3 years: IV: 18.6 mg/kg on day 0 every 28 days in combination with etoposide and vincristine for 6 cycles (VEC regimen)

Children >3 years: IV: 560 mg/m^2 on day 0 every 28 days in combination with etoposide and vincristine for 6 cycles (VEC regimen)

Sarcomas: Ewing sarcoma, osteosarcoma (off-label uses): IV: 400 mg/m^2/day for 2 days every 21 days (in combination with ifosfamide and etoposide) (van Winkle 2005)

Wilms tumor (off-label use): Children and Adolescents: IV: 160 mg/m^2/day for 5 consecutive days every 21 days (in combination with etoposide) for 2 cycles (Pein 1994) **or** 400 mg/m^2/day for 2 days (in combination with ifosfamide and etoposide) every 21 days (ICE regimen) (Abu-Ghosh 2002) **or** modified Calvert formula with a target AUC 6 for 1 day (in combination with ifosfamide and etoposide) every 21 days (ICE regimen) for 2 cycles, followed by vincristine, dactinomycin and doxorubicin (VAD regimen), surgery, radiation therapy, the VAD regimen and one more cycle of ICE for a total of 36 weeks of treatment (Daw 2009). Additional data may be necessary to further define the role of carboplatin in the treatment of this condition.

Renal Impairment Note: Dose determination with Calvert formula uses GFR and, therefore, inherently adjusts for renal dysfunction.

The manufacturer's labeling recommends the following dosage adjustments for single-agent therapy: Adults:

Baseline CrCl 41 to 59 mL/minute: Initiate at 250 mg/m^2 and adjust subsequent doses based on bone marrow toxicity

Baseline CrCl 16 to 40 mL/minute: Initiate at 200 mg/m^2 and adjust subsequent doses based on bone marrow toxicity

Baseline CrCl ≤15 mL/minute: There are no dosage adjustments provided in the manufacturer's labeling.

The following dosage adjustments have also been recommended:

Aronoff 2007:

Adults (**Note:** For dosing based on **mg/m^2**):

GFR >50 mL/minute: No dosage adjustment is necessary

GFR 10 to 50 mL/minute: Administer 50% of the usual dose

GFR <10 mL/minute: Administer 25% of the usual dose

Hemodialysis: Administer 50% of the usual dose

Continuous ambulatory peritoneal dialysis (CAPD): Administer 25% of the usual dose

Continuous renal replacement therapy (CRRT): 200 mg/m^2

Children:

GFR <50 mL/minute: Use Calvert formula incorporating patient's GFR

Hemodialysis, peritoneal dialysis, continuous renal replacement therapy (CRRT): Use Calvert formula incorporating patient's GFR

Janus 2010: Hemodialysis: Carboplatin dose (mg) = Target AUC x 25; administer on a nondialysis day, hemodialysis should occur between 12 to 24 hours after carboplatin dose

Hepatic Impairment There are no dosage adjustments provided in the manufacturer's labeling; however, carboplatin undergoes minimal hepatic metabolism therefore dosage adjustment may not be needed.

Obesity

American Society of Clinical Oncology (ASCO) Guidelines for appropriate chemotherapy dosing in obese adults with cancer (excludes HSCT dosing): Dosing based on GFR should be considered in obese patients; GFR should not exceed 125 mL/minute (Griggs 2012).

American Society for Blood and Marrow Transplantation (ASBMT) practice guideline committee position statement on chemotherapy dosing in obesity: Utilize actual body weight (full weight) for calculation of body surface area (when applicable) in carboplatin dosing for hematopoietic stem cell transplant conditioning regimens in adults. Based on the literature, there is no consensus for carboplatin dosing based on AUC in transplant conditioning regimens or dosing adjustments during transplant for obese patients (Bubalo 2014).

Adjustment for Toxicity Platelets <50,000 cells/mm^3 or ANC <500 cells/mm^3: Administer 75% of the usual dose

Combination Regimens

Bladder cancer: Carboplatin-Gemcitabine (Bladder) on page 2017

Bone sarcoma (Ewing sarcoma): Ifosfamide-Carboplatin-Etoposide (Ewing Sarcoma) on page 2154

Bone sarcoma (osteosarcoma): Ifosfamide-Carboplatin-Etoposide (Osteosarcoma) on page 2154

Breast cancer:

Carboplatin-Docetaxel-Trastuzumab (Breast) on page 2012

Carboplatin-Paclitaxel-Trastuzumab (Breast) on page 2022

Cervical cancer: Carboplatin-Paclitaxel (Cervical Cancer) on page 2018

Endometrial cancer: Carboplatin-Paclitaxel (Endometrial) on page 2019

Esophageal cancer: Paclitaxel-Carboplatin (Esophageal Cancer) on page 2183

Head and neck cancer:

Carboplatin-Cetuximab (Head and Neck Cancer) on page 2011

Cetuximab-Carboplatin-Fluorouracil (Head and Neck Cancer) on page 2030

Docetaxel-Cisplatin-Fluorouracil (Head and Neck) on page 2089

Fluorouracil-Carboplatin (Head and Neck Cancer) on page 2123

◀

Administration Carboplatin is associated with a moderate to high emetic potential in adult patients (dose dependent) and a high emetic potential in pediatric patients; antiemetics are recommended to prevent nausea and vomiting (Basch 2011; Dupuis 2011; Roila 2016).

Infuse over at least 15 minutes; usually infused over 15 to 60 minutes, although some protocols may require infusions up to 24 hours. When administered as a part of a combination chemotherapy regimen, sequence of administration may vary by regimen; refer to specific protocol for sequence recommendation.

Needles or IV administration sets that contain aluminum should not be used in the preparation or administration of carboplatin; aluminum can react with carboplatin resulting in precipitate formation and loss of potency.

Vesicant/Extravasation Risk May be an irritant

Emetic Potential
Children: High (>90%)
Adults:
AUC ≥4: High (>90%)
AUC <4: Moderate (30% to 90%)

Monitoring Parameters CBC (with differential and platelet count), serum electrolytes, serum creatinine and BUN, creatinine clearance, liver function tests; audiology evaluations (children <6 months); signs/symptoms of hypersensitivity reactions

Dosage Forms Excipient information presented when available (limited, particularly for generics); consult specific product labeling.
Solution, Intravenous:
Generic: 50 mg/5 mL (5 mL); 150 mg/15 mL (15 mL); 450 mg/45 mL (45 mL); 600 mg/60 mL (60 mL)
Solution, Intravenous [preservative free]:
Generic: 50 mg/5 mL (5 mL); 150 mg/15 mL (15 mL); 450 mg/45 mL (45 mL); 600 mg/60 mL (60 mL)

◆ **Carboplatin Injection (Can)** see CARBOplatin on page 327
◆ **Carboplatin Injection BP (Can)** see CARBOplatin on page 327
◆ **Carboxypeptidase-G2** see Glucarpidase on page 883
◆ **Cardiolite** see Technetium Tc 99m Sestamibi on page 1741

Carfilzomib (kar FILZ oh mib)

Related Information
Common Toxicity Criteria on page 2242
Management of Chemotherapy-Induced Nausea and Vomiting in Adults on page 2253
Safe Handling of Hazardous Drugs on page 2379
Brand Names: US Kyprolis
Brand Names: Canada Kyprolis
Index Terms CFZ; PR-171
Pharmacologic Category Antineoplastic Agent, Proteasome Inhibitor
Use Multiple myeloma, relapsed/refractory: Treatment (monotherapy) of relapsed or refractory multiple myeloma in patients who have received 1 or more lines of therapy; treatment of relapsed or refractory multiple myeloma (in combination with dexamethasone or lenalidomide plus dexamethasone) in patients who have received 1 to 3 prior lines of therapy

Labeled Contraindications
There are no contraindications listed in the manufacturer's US labeling
Canadian labeling: Hypersensitivity to carfilzomib or any component of the formulation

Pregnancy Considerations Adverse events were observed in animal reproduction studies. Based on the mechanism of action, adverse fetal events would be expected to occur with use in pregnant women. Females and males of reproductive potential are advised to avoid pregnancy during therapy; women of reproductive potential should abstain from sexual activity or use effective contraception during treatment and for at least 30 days following therapy completion. Male patients of reproductive potential should abstain from sexual activity or use effective contraception during treatment and for at least 90 days following therapy completion.

Breastfeeding Considerations It is not known if carfilzomib is present in breast milk. Due to the potential for serious adverse reactions in the breastfed infant, the manufacturer recommends a decision be made to discontinue breastfeeding or to discontinue the drug, taking into account the importance of treatment to the mother and the health benefits of breastfeeding. The appropriate timing to restart breastfeeding after treatment discontinuation should be determined with the health care provider.

Warnings/Precautions Thrombocytopenia (including grade 4) was observed in patients receiving carfilzomib, with platelet nadirs occurring between day 8 and day 15 of each 28-day treatment cycle, and recovery to baseline by the start of the next cycle. Monitor platelets closely and adjust dose or withhold therapy if necessary. Hemorrhage due to thrombocytopenia may occur. Anemia, lymphopenia, leukopenia, and neutropenia were also observed. Death caused by cardiac arrest has occurred within 24 hours of drug administration. Carfilzomib has been associated with new-onset or worsening of heart failure (HF), pulmonary edema, decreased left ventricular ejection fraction (LVEF), restrictive cardiomyopathy, myocardial ischemia, and myocardial infarction (including fatalities). Some events occurred in patients with normal ventricular function at baseline. Cardiac events typically were observed throughout the course of therapy. Patients 75 years of age or older have an increased risk of heart failure. Monitor closely for cardiac complications and for volume overload (due to pretreatment hydration), particularly in patients at risk for heart failure; withhold carfilzomib therapy for grade 3 or 4 cardiac events until recovery. Patients with New York Heart Association Class III and IV heart failure, recent myocardial infarction (within 3 to 6 months), and conduction abnormalities, angina, or arrhythmias not managed by medication were excluded from clinical trials and may be at increased risk for cardiac complications; evaluate with a comprehensive medical assessment prior to initiation and closely monitor. Hypertension has occurred with use; hypertensive crisis and hypertensive emergency have also been reported (some events were fatal). Monitor blood pressure throughout therapy; if hypertension cannot be adequately controlled, interrupt carfilzomib therapy and evaluate; assess risks versus benefits when determining to restart treatment.

Acute respiratory distress syndrome (ARDS), acute respiratory failure, and acute diffuse-infiltrative pulmonary disease (eg, pneumonitis and interstitial lung disease) have occurred in a small number of patients (some events were fatal); discontinue therapy if any of these drug-induced pulmonary toxicities occur. Pulmonary arterial hypertension (PAH) was observed (including grade 3 or higher events) in studies; perform cardiac imaging or other testing as appropriate, and withhold carfilzomib until PAH is resolved or returns to baseline. Dyspnea (including grade 3 or higher events) has been reported; monitor closely. Withhold carfilzomib for grade 3 or 4 dyspnea until pulmonary symptom resolution or return to baseline. Renal toxicity (eg, renal insufficiency, acute renal failure, renal failure) has been reported with carfilzomib. Acute renal failure was observed more frequently in patients receiving carfilzomib monotherapy for advanced relapsed/refractory multiple myeloma; renal failure risk is greater when patients have a baseline reduced creatinine clearance. Monitor renal function closely; may require therapy interruption or dose reduction.

Thrombotic microangiopathy, including cases of thrombocytopenic thrombotic purpura/hemolytic uremic syndrome (TTP/HUS) has been reported (some fatal); monitor for signs/symptoms. Interrupt therapy if TTP/HUS diagnosis is suspected and manage appropriately (eg, plasma exchange as clinically necessary). If TTP/HUS diagnosis is excluded, may consider reinitiating therapy; the safety of restarting carfilzomib after a TTP/HUS diagnosis is not known. Posterior reversible encephalopathy syndrome (PRES) has been reported rarely with use; symptoms include seizure, headache, lethargy, confusion, blindness, altered consciousness, hypertension, and other visual/neurological disturbances. Discontinue therapy if PRES diagnosis is suspected; the safety of reinitiating therapy after PRES diagnosis is not known. Venous thromboembolism (eg, deep vein thrombosis and pulmonary embolism) has been observed, particularly when used as part of combination therapy with dexamethasone or with lenalidomide plus dexamethasone. Thromboprophylaxis is recommended with combination therapy, and should be based on patients' underlying risk factors, treatment regimen, and clinical status. Due to risk of thrombosis with hormonal contraception, consider an alternative method of effective contraception during combination treatment of carfilzomib with dexamethasone or lenalidomide plus dexamethasone.

Infusion reactions such as chills, fever, arthralgia, myalgia, shortness of breath, hypotension, facial flushing, facial edema, vomiting, weakness, syncope, chest tightness, or angina may occur immediately following or within 24 hours of carfilzomib infusion (may be life-threatening). To lessen the incidence and intensity of infusion reactions, administer dexamethasone prior to drug administration. Tumor lysis syndrome (TLS), including fatalities has been observed. TLS risk is increased in multiple myeloma patients with a high tumor burden. Adequately hydrate patients prior to carfilzomib therapy and monitor closely for signs and symptoms of TLS; consider use of antihyperuricemic agents. If TLS occurs, interrupt treatment until resolved.

Hepatic failure, including fatal cases, has been reported rarely (<1%). Increased transaminases and hyperbilirubinemia have also been observed. Interrupt carfilzomib therapy in patients with grade 3 or higher hepatic toxicity until resolved or recovered to baseline (may require dose reduction if appropriate to reinitiate); monitor liver enzymes regularly. Serious or fatal cases of hemorrhage have been reported, including gastrointestinal, intracranial and pulmonary hemorrhage and epistaxis. Bleeding may be spontaneous; Intracranial hemorrhage has occurred without trauma. Hemorrhage has been reported in patients with and without low platelets and has also been reported in patients who were not receiving anticoagulation or antiplatelet therapy. Monitor for signs/symptoms of hemorrhage and promptly evaluate symptoms of blood loss. Reduce dose or withhold treatment as clinically indicated.

An increased incidence of serious and fatal adverse events was observed in a clinical trial comparing the combination of carfilzomib, melphalan, and prednisone (KMP) to bortezomib, melphalan, and prednisone (VMP) for the treatment of newly diagnosed multiple myeloma (MM) in transplant-ineligible patients. Cardiac failure, hypertension, acute renal failure, and dyspnea were observed more frequently in the KMP arm. KMP is not an approved carfilzomib combination regimen. Potentially significant interactions may exist, requiring dose or frequency adjustment, additional monitoring, and/or selection of alternative therapy. Vials contain the excipient cyclodextrin (sulfobutyl ether beta-cyclodextrin), which may accumulate in patients with renal insufficiency, although the clinical significance of this finding is uncertain (Luke 2010).

Adverse Reactions

≥10%:

Cardiovascular: Hypertension (15% to 42%), peripheral edema (20% to 21%), chest pain (3% to 21%)

Central nervous system: Fatigue (40% to 58%), chills (12% to 38%), headache (24% to 33%), insomnia (13% to 29%), dizziness (11% to 29%), hypoesthesia (Siegel 2013), peripheral neuropathy (Siegel 2012)

Gastrointestinal: Nausea (35% to 54%), vomiting (17% to 33%), diarrhea (25% to 27%), anorexia (15% to 21%), constipation (Siegel 2013)

Hematologic & oncologic: Thrombocytopenia (37% to 54%; ≥ grade 3: 25% to 54%), anemia (42% to 49%; ≥ grade 3: 24% to 29%), lymphocytopenia (14% to 33%; ≥ grade 3: 12% to 33%), leukopenia (Siegel 2013), neutropenia (Siegel 2013)

Neuromuscular & skeletal: Back pain (19% to 21%), muscle spasm (10% to 21%)

Renal: Increased serum creatinine (17% to 25%)

Respiratory: Dyspnea (28% to 58%), cough (22% to 33%), upper respiratory tract infection (19% to 21%), pneumonia (Siegel 2013)

Miscellaneous: Fever (30% to 58%)

1% to 10%:

Cardiovascular: Deep vein thrombosis (≤2%), pulmonary embolism (≤2%), pulmonary hypertension (1%), ischemic heart disease (Siegel 2013)

Central nervous system: Paresthesia (Siegel 2013), peripheral sensory neuropathy (Siegel 2013)

Endocrine & metabolic: Hypercalcemia (Siegel 2013), hyponatremia (Siegel 2012), hypophosphatemia (Siegel 2012)

Hematologic & oncologic: Febrile neutropenia

Renal: Renal insufficiency (10%), acute renal failure (more common in patients with advanced relapsed and refractory multiple myeloma [Siegel 2013]), renal failure (Siegel 2013)

Frequency not defined:

Cardiovascular: Hypotension, thromboembolic complications

Central nervous system: Anxiety, intracranial hemorrhage, pain, voice disorder

Dermatologic: Erythema, hyperhidrosis, pruritus, skin rash

Endocrine & metabolic: Hyperglycemia, hyperkalemia, hyperuricemia, hypoalbuminemia, hypocalcemia, hypokalemia, hypomagnesemia

Gastrointestinal: Abdominal pain, dyspepsia, gastrointestinal hemorrhage, toothache, upper abdominal pain

Genitourinary: Urinary tract infection

Hematologic & oncologic: Hemorrhage, pulmonary hemorrhage

Hepatic: Hepatic failure

Infection: Influenza, sepsis

Local: Infusion site reaction

Neuromuscular & skeletal: Arthralgia, limb pain, musculoskeletal chest pain, musculoskeletal pain, myalgia, weakness

Ophthalmic: Blurred vision, cataract

Respiratory: Bronchitis, bronchopneumonia, epistaxis, nasopharyngitis, oropharyngeal pain, pulmonary edema, pulmonary infection, respiratory tract infection, rhinitis

Miscellaneous: Multiorgan failure

<1%, postmarketing, and/or case reports: Cardiomyopathy (restrictive), gastrointestinal perforation, hemolytic-uremic syndrome, interstitial pulmonary disease, myocardial infarction (Siegel 2012), pericarditis, peripheral motor neuropathy (Siegel 2013), pneumonitis, pulmonary disease, respiratory distress syndrome (acute), reversible posterior leukoencephalopathy syndrome, tumor lysis syndrome (Siegel 2012)

Drug Interactions

Metabolism/Transport Effects Substrate of P-glycoprotein

Avoid Concomitant Use

Avoid concomitant use of Carfilzomib with any of the following: BCG (Intravesical); Deferiprone; Dipyrone

Increased Effect/Toxicity

Carfilzomib may increase the levels/effects of: CloZAPine; Contraceptives (Estrogens); Contraceptives (Progestins); Deferiprone

The levels/effects of Carfilzomib may be increased by: Dipyrone; Lumacaftor; P-glycoprotein/ABCB1 Inhibitors; Promazine; Ranolazine

Decreased Effect

Carfilzomib may decrease the levels/effects of: BCG (Intravesical)

The levels/effects of Carfilzomib may be decreased by: Lumacaftor; P-glycoprotein/ABCB1 Inducers

Hazardous Drugs Handling Considerations

Hazardous agent (NIOSH 2016 [group 1]).

Use appropriate precautions for receiving, handling, administration, and disposal. Gloves (single) should be worn during receiving, unpacking, and placing in storage.

NIOSH recommends double gloving, a protective gown, ventilated engineering controls (a class II biological safety cabinet or a compounding aseptic containment isolator), and closed system transfer devices (CSTDs) for preparation. Double gloving, a gown, and (if dosage form allows) CSTDs are required during administration (NIOSH 2016).

Storage/Stability Store intact vials at 2°C to 8°C (36°F to 46°F). Store in original carton until use to protect from light. Reconstituted drug (in the vial or in a syringe) and preparations diluted for infusion in D5W are stable for 4 hours at room temperature or for 24 hours refrigerated at 2°C to 8°C (36°F to 46°F).

Preparation for Administration Reconstitute the 60 mg vial with 29 mL, the 30 mg vial with 15 mL, and the 10 mg vial [Canadian product] with 5 mL of sterile water for injection using a 21-gauge or larger needle (0.8 mm or smaller external diameter needle), to a concentration of 2 mg/mL (directing solution onto the inside wall of the vial to avoid foaming). Gently invert and/or swirl vial slowly for ~1 minute to mix; do not shake. If foaming results, allow solution to sit for ~5 minutes until foaming resolves. Reconstituted solution should be clear and colorless. May further dilute dose by using a 21-gauge or larger needle (0.8 mm or smaller external diameter needle) to transfer the reconstituted solution into 50 or 100 mL (depending on dose and infusion duration) of D5W. Discard unused portion of the vial (do not pool unused solution from the vials).

Mechanism of Action Carfilzomib inhibits proteasomes, which are responsible for intracellular protein homeostasis. Specifically, it is a potent, selective, and irreversible inhibitor of chymotrypsin-like activity of the 20S proteasome, leading to cell cycle arrest and apoptosis.

◄ **Pharmacodynamics/Kinetics**

Distribution: V_{dss}: 28 L; penetrates all tissues extensively except the brain (Kortuem 2013)

Protein binding: 97%

Metabolism: Rapid and extensive; peptidase cleavage and epoxide hydrolysis; minimal metabolism through cytochrome P450-mediated mechanisms

Half-life elimination: Doses ≥15 mg/m^2: ≤1 hour on day 1 of cycle 1

Excretion: Urine (~25%, primarily as metabolites)

Dosing

Adult & Geriatric Note: Hydrate with oral fluids (30 mL/kg) at least 48 hours prior to initiating cycle 1, as well as with 250 to 500 mL normal saline (or other appropriate IV fluid) before dosing (recommended) and after (if needed) administration during cycle 1 (continue oral and/or IV hydration in subsequent cycles if necessary); monitor for evidence of volume overload and adjust hydration based on individual needs. Consider antiviral prophylaxis for patients with a history of herpes zoster infection. Thromboprophylaxis is recommended when administering in combination with dexamethasone or lenalidomide plus dexamethasone.

Premedication: When administering as monotherapy, premedicate with dexamethasone 4 mg orally or IV when infusing carfilzomib over 10 minutes or with dexamethasone 8 mg orally or IV when infusing carfilzomib over 30 minutes. When using combination therapy, administer the recommended dexamethasone dose (refer to prescribing information). Premedicate 30 minutes to 4 hours prior to all doses in cycle 1, and as needed with future cycles to reduce the incidence and severity of infusion reaction.

Note: Calculate dose using actual body surface area (BSA) at baseline. Patients with a BSA >2.2 m^2 should be dosed based upon a maximum BSA of 2.2 m^2. Dose adjustments for weight changes of ≤20% are not necessary, per manufacturer labeling. Continue until disease progression or unacceptable toxicity.

Multiple myeloma, relapsed/refractory (single-agent; 20/27 mg/m^2 regimen): IV:

Cycle 1: 20 mg/m^2 over 10 minutes on days 1 and 2; if tolerated, increase dose to 27 mg/m^2 over 10 minutes on days 8, 9, 15, and 16 of a 28-day treatment cycle

Cycles 2 to 12: 27 mg/m^2 over 10 minutes on days 1, 2, 8, 9, 15, and 16 of a 28-day treatment cycle

Cycle 13 and beyond: 27 mg/m^2 over 10 minutes on days 1, 2, 15, and 16 of a 28-day treatment cycle; continue until disease progression or unacceptable toxicity

Multiple myeloma, relapsed/refractory (single-agent; 20/56 mg/m^2 regimen): IV:

Cycle 1: 20 mg/m^2 over 30 minutes on days 1 and 2; if tolerated, increase dose to 56 mg/m^2 over 30 minutes on days 8, 9, 15, and 16 of a 28-day treatment cycle.

Cycles 2 to 12: 56 mg/m^2 over 30 minutes on days 1, 2, 8, 9, 15, and 16 of a 28-day treatment cycle.

Cycle 13 and beyond: 56 mg/m^2 over 30 minutes on days 1, 2, 15, and 16 of a 28-day treatment cycle; continue until disease progression or unacceptable toxicity.

Multiple myeloma, relapsed/refractory (in combination with lenalidomide and dexamethasone) (Stewart 2015): IV:

Cycle 1: 20 mg/m² over 10 minutes on days 1 and 2; if tolerated, increase dose to 27 mg/m² over 10 minutes on days 8, 9, 15, and 16 of a 28-day treatment cycle.

Cycles 2 to 12: 27 mg/m² over 10 minutes on days 1, 2, 8, 9, 15, and 16 of a 28-day treatment cycle.

Cycles 13 to 18: 27 mg/m² over 10 minutes on days 1, 2, 15, and 16 of a 28-day treatment cycle; beginning with cycle 19, lenalidomide and dexamethasone may be continued (until disease progression or unacceptable toxicity) without carfilzomib.

Multiple myeloma, relapsed/refractory (in combination with dexamethasone): IV:

Cycle 1: 20 mg/m² over 30 minutes on days 1 and 2; if tolerated, increase dose to 56 mg/m² over 30 minutes on days 8, 9, 15, and 16 of a 28-day treatment cycle.

Cycle 2 and beyond: 56 mg/m² over 30 minutes on days 1, 2, 8, 9, 15, and 16 of a 28-day treatment cycle; continue until disease progression or unacceptable toxicity.

Waldenström macroglobulinemia (off-label use): IV:

Induction (Treon 2014):

Cycle 1: 20 mg/m² over 20 minutes on days 1, 2, 8, and 9 of a 21-day treatment cycle (in combination with dexamethasone and rituximab)

Cycles 2 to 6: 36 mg/m² over 30 minutes on days 1, 2, 8, and 9 of a 21-day treatment cycle (in combination with dexamethasone and rituximab)

Maintenance (started 8 weeks after completion of induction therapy in patients with stable disease or better response): 36 mg/m² on days 1 and 2 every 8 weeks for 8 cycles (in combination with dexamethasone and rituximab) (Treon 2014).

Renal Impairment The International Myeloma Working Group recommends the use of the Chronic Kidney Disease Epidemiology Collaboration (CKD-EPI) equation (preferred) or the Modification of Diet in Renal Disease (MDRD) formula to evaluate renal function estimation in multiple myeloma patients with a stable serum creatinine (Dimopoulos 2016).

Preexisting renal impairment: No initial dosage adjustment necessary (Badros 2013; Quach 2017).

Hemodialysis: No initial dosage adjustment necessary (Quach 2017). Administer after dialysis.

The International Myeloma Working Group Recommendations suggest that (based on evaluating the 20/27 mg/m² dose), carfilzomib may be safely administered to patients with a CrCl ≥15 mL/minute; although there is less data, carfilzomib may also be administered to patients with CrCl <15 mL/minute (Dimopoulos 2016).

Renal toxicity during treatment: Serum creatinine ≥2 times baseline, CrCl <15 mL/minute or CrCl decreases to ≤50% of baseline, or patient requires dialysis: Withhold dose and monitor renal function. If renal toxicity is due to carfilzomib, resume dosing when renal function has improved to within 25% of baseline; resume with a reduced dose by 1 dose level (see Dosing: Adjustment for Toxicity for dose level reductions). If toxicity is not due to carfilzomib, restart at the discretion of the prescriber.

◀ **Hepatic Impairment**
Preexisting hepatic impairment:
Mild (bilirubin >1 to 1.5 times ULN or AST > ULN) or moderate (bilirubin >1.5 to 3 times ULN) impairment: Reduce dose to 75% of recommended dose.

Severe (bilirubin >3 times ULN) impairment: There are no dosage adjustments provided in the manufacturer's labeling (the pharmacokinetics of carfilzomib have not been evaluated in patients with bilirubin >3 times ULN and any AST).

Hepatotoxicity during treatment: Grade 3 or 4 elevation of bilirubin, transaminases, or other liver abnormalities: Withhold dose until resolved or at baseline. After resolution, if appropriate to reinitiate, consider restarting at 1 dose level reduction (see Dosing: Adjustment for Toxicity for dose level reductions) with frequent monitoring of hepatic function.

Obesity *ASCO Guidelines for appropriate chemotherapy dosing in obese adults with cancer:* In general, utilize patient's actual body weight (full weight) for calculation of body surface area- or weight-based dosing, particularly when the intent of therapy is curative; manage regimen-related toxicities in the same manner as for nonobese patients; if a dose reduction is utilized due to toxicity, consider resumption of full weight-based dosing with subsequent cycles, especially if cause of toxicity (eg, hepatic or renal impairment) is resolved (Griggs 2012). **Note:** According to the manufacturer, patients with a body surface area (BSA) >2.2 m^2 should be dosed based upon a maximum BSA of 2.2 m^2; dose adjustments for weight changes of ≤20% are not necessary.

Adjustment for Toxicity
Carfilzomib dose level reductions for toxicity:
If initial dose is **27** mg/m^2:
First dose reduction: 20 mg/m^2
Second dose reduction: 15 mg/m^2; if toxicity persists on 15 mg/m^2 dose, discontinue carfilzomib
If initial dose is **56** mg/m^2:
First dose reduction: 45 mg/m^2
Second dose reduction: 36 mg/m^2
Third dose reduction: 27 mg/m^2; if toxicity persists on 27 mg/m^2 dose, discontinue carfilzomib

Hematologic toxicity:
ANC <500/mm^3: Withhold dose; continue at same dose level if ANC recovers to ≥500/mm^3. For subsequent ANC levels <500/mm^3, withhold dose and consider reducing dose by 1 dose level when ANC ≥500/mm^3.
Neutropenic fever (ANC <500/mm^3 with an oral temperature >38.5°C or 2 consecutive readings of >38°C for 2 hours): Withhold dose; if ANC recovers to baseline and fever resolves, resume at the same dose level.
Platelets: <10,000/mm^3 or evidence of bleeding with thrombocytopenia: Withhold dose; continue at same dose level if platelets recover to ≥10,000/mm^3 and bleeding is controlled. For subsequent platelet levels <10,000/mm^3, withhold dose and consider reducing dose by 1 dose level when platelets ≥10,000/mm^3.

Nonhematologic toxicity:
Grade 3 or 4 nonhematologic toxicities: Withhold dose until resolved or at baseline. After resolution, consider restarting the next scheduled treatment at 1 dose level reduction.

Cardiac: Grade 3 or 4, new-onset or worsening of heart failure, decreased left ventricular function, or myocardial ischemia: Withhold dose until resolved or at baseline. After resolution, if considered appropriate to reinitiate, consider restarting at 1 dose level reduction.

Hemorrhage or symptoms of blood loss: Reduce dose or withhold treatment as clinically appropriate.

Hypertension, severe or life-threatening: If hypertension cannot be adequately controlled, withhold dose and evaluate. After resolution, consider if appropriate to reinitiate based on risk versus benefit.

Pulmonary toxicity

Acute respiratory distress syndrome, acute respiratory failure, and acute diffuse infiltrative pulmonary disease (drug-induced): Discontinue therapy.

Pulmonary hypertension: Withhold dose until resolved or at baseline. After resolution, consider if appropriate to reinitiate based on risk versus benefit.

Grade 3 or 4 dyspnea: Withhold dose until resolved or at baseline. After resolution, consider if appropriate to reinitiate based on risk versus benefit.

Tumor lysis syndrome: Interrupt treatment until resolved.

Combination Regimens

Multiple myeloma:
Carfilzomib-Dexamethasone (Multiple Myeloma) on page 2025
Carfilzomib, Lenalidomide, Dexamethasone (Multiple Myeloma) on page 2026

Administration

IV: Administer over 10 or 30 minutes depending on the carfilzomib dose regimen (see Dosing). Do not administer as an IV bolus. Hydrate with oral fluids (30 mL/kg) at least 48 hours prior to initiating cycle 1, as well as with 250 to 500 mL NS (or other appropriate IV fluid) prior to (recommended) and after (if needed) each dose in cycle 1; continue oral and/or IV hydration in subsequent cycles (if necessary). Flush line immediately before and after carfilzomib with NS or D5W. Do not administer with other medications.

When administering as monotherapy, premedicate with dexamethasone 4 mg orally or IV when infusing carfilzomib over 10 minutes or with dexamethasone 8 mg orally or IV when infusing carfilzomib over 30 minutes. When using combination therapy, administer the recommended dexamethasone dose (refer to prescribing information). Premedicate 30 minutes to 4 hours prior to all doses in cycle 1, and as needed with future cycles to reduce the incidence and severity of infusion reaction.

Emetic Potential Low (10% to 30%)

Monitoring Parameters CBC with differential and platelets (monitor frequently throughout therapy), serum potassium levels regularly during treatment, renal function, pulmonary function (with new or worsening pulmonary symptoms), liver function tests, blood pressure. Signs/symptoms of infusion-related reactions, congestive heart failure, tumor lysis syndrome, peripheral neuropathy, posterior reversible encephalopathy syndrome, thrombocytopenic thrombotic purpura/hemolytic uremic syndrome, and venous thromboembolic events. Monitor for evidence of volume overload due to pre- and posthydration.

◀ **Dosage Forms** Excipient information presented when available (limited, particularly for generics); consult specific product labeling.
Solution Reconstituted, Intravenous:
Kyprolis: 30 mg (1 ea); 60 mg (1 ea)
Dosage Forms: Canada Information with regard to form, strength, and availability of products uniquely available in Canada but currently not available in the US. Refer also to Dosage Forms.
Excipient information presented when available (limited, particularly for generics); consult specific product labeling.
Solution Reconstituted, Intravenous:
Kyprolis: 10 mg (1 ea)

◆ **Carimune NF** *see* Immune Globulin *on page 992*

Carmustine (kar MUS teen)
Related Information
Hematopoietic Cell Transplantation *on page 2365*
Management of Chemotherapy-Induced Nausea and Vomiting in Adults *on page 2253*
Management of Drug Extravasations *on page 2271*
Prevention of Chemotherapy-Induced Nausea and Vomiting in Children *on page 2310*
Safe Handling of Hazardous Drugs *on page 2379*
Brand Names: US BiCNU; Gliadel Wafer
Brand Names: Canada BiCNU; Gliadel Wafer
Index Terms BCNU; Becenum; bis(chloroethyl) nitrosourea; bis-chloronitrosourea; Carmustine Polymer Wafer; Carmustine Sustained-Release Implant Wafer; Carmustinum; WR-139021
Pharmacologic Category Antineoplastic Agent, Alkylating Agent; Antineoplastic Agent, Alkylating Agent (Nitrosourea)
Use
Brain tumors:
Injection: Palliative treatment of brain tumors including glioblastoma, brainstem glioma, medulloblastoma, astrocytoma, ependymoma, and metastatic brain tumors
Wafer (implant): Treatment of newly-diagnosed high-grade malignant glioma (as an adjunct to surgery and radiation); treatment of recurrent glioblastoma multiforme (as adjunct to surgery)
Hodgkin lymphoma, relapsed/refractory: Injection: Palliative treatment (secondary) of Hodgkin lymphoma (in combination with other antineoplastics) that has relapsed with or was refractory to primary therapy
Multiple myeloma: Injection: Palliative treatment of multiple myeloma (in combination with prednisone)
Non-Hodgkin lymphomas, relapsed/refractory: Injection: Palliative treatment (secondary) of non-Hodgkin lymphoma (in combination with other antineoplastics) that has relapsed with or was refractory to primary therapy
Labeled Contraindications
IV: Hypersensitivity to carmustine or any component of the formulation
Implant: There are no contraindications listed in the manufacturer's labeling.
Pregnancy Considerations Adverse events have been observed in animal reproduction studies. Based on the mechanism of action, carmustine may cause fetal harm if administered to a pregnant woman. Females of reproductive potential should use highly effective contraceptives during and for at least

6 months following treatment. Males of reproductive potential should use highly effective contraceptives during and for at least 3 months following treatment. May impair male fertility. Advise males of potential risk of infertility and to seek fertility/family planning counseling prior to receiving carmustine wafer implants.

Breastfeeding Considerations It is not known if carmustine is present in breast milk. Due to the potential for serious adverse reactions in the breastfed infant, the manufacturer recommends breastfeeding be discontinued during treatment.

Warnings/Precautions

Injection:

[US Boxed Warning]: Carmustine IV causes bone marrow suppression, primarily thrombocytopenia (which may lead to bleeding) and leukopenia (which may cause infection). Monitor blood counts weekly for at least 6 weeks following each dose. Adjust dosage based on nadir blood counts from prior dose for dosage adjustment. Do not administer a repeat course until blood counts recover. Hematologic toxicity is dose-limiting, may be severe, and is generally delayed and cumulative; thrombocytopenia is usually more severe than leukopenia. Myelosuppression generally occurs 4 to 6 weeks after administration; thrombocytopenia occurs at ~4 weeks and persists for 1 to 2 weeks; leukopenia occurs at 5 to 6 weeks and persists for 1 to 2 weeks. Anemia may occur (less common and less severe than leukopenia or thrombocytopenia). Platelet counts should be >100,000/mm^3 and leukocytes should be >4,000/mm^3 prior to a repeat course (repeat courses should not be administered more frequently than every 6 weeks). Long-term IV use is associated with the development of secondary malignancies (acute leukemias and bone marrow dysplasias).

[US Boxed Warning]: Carmustine IV is associated with dose-related pulmonary toxicity; patients receiving cumulative doses >1,400 mg/m^2 are at significantly higher risk. Delayed onset of pulmonary fibrosis may occur years after treatment (may be fatal), particularly in children. Pulmonary toxicity has occurred in children and adolescents up to 17 years after treatment; this occurred in ages 1 to 16 for the treatment of intracranial tumors; cumulative doses ranged from 770 to 1,800 mg/m^2 (in combination with cranial radiotherapy). Pulmonary toxicity is characterized by pulmonary infiltrates and/or fibrosis and has been reported from 9 days to 43 months after nitrosourea treatment (including carmustine). Although pulmonary toxicity generally occurs in patients who have received prolonged treatment, pulmonary fibrosis has been reported with cumulative doses below 1,400 mg/m^2. Interstitial fibrosis at lower doses has occurred (rare). In addition to high cumulative doses, other risk factors for pulmonary toxicity include history of lung disease and baseline predicted forced vital capacity (FVC) or carbon monoxide diffusing capacity (DLCO) <70%. Baseline and periodic pulmonary function tests are recommended. For high-dose treatment (transplant; off-label dose), acute lung injury may occur ~1 to 3 months post transplant; advise patients to contact their transplant physician for dyspnea, cough, or fever; interstitial pneumonia may be managed with a course of corticosteroids. Children are at higher risk of delayed pulmonary toxicity with IV carmustine.

Reversible increases in transaminases, bilirubin, and alkaline phosphatase have been reported (rare) with the IV formulation. Monitor liver function tests periodically during treatment. May require dosage adjustment or ▶

discontinuation in patients with renal impairment. Do not administer carmustine IV in patients with compromised renal function Renal failure, progressive azotemia, and decreased kidney size have been reported in patients who have received large cumulative doses or prolonged treatment. Renal toxicity has also been reported in patients who have received lower cumulative doses. Monitor renal function tests periodically during treatment.

Carmustine IV is associated with a moderate to high emetic potential (dose-related); antiemetics are recommended to prevent nausea and vomiting (Basch 2011; Dupuis 2011). Rapid infusions are associated with skin flushing and suffusion of the conjunctiva (onset: <2 hours; duration ~4 hours). Carmustine is also associated with injection site burning and local tissue reactions, including swelling, pain, erythema, and necrosis have been reported. Monitor infusion site closely for infiltration or injection site reactions. Avoid extravasation. Investigational administration (intraarterial intracarotid route [not an approved route]) has been associated with ocular toxicity. The diluent for IV carmustine contains ethanol.

Wafer implant:
Seizures occurred in patients who received carmustine wafer implants, including new or worsening seizures and treatment-emergent seizures. Just over half of treatment-emergent seizures occurred within 5 days of surgery; the median onset of first new or worsened post-operative seizure was 4 days. Optimal anti-seizure therapy should be initiated prior to surgery. Monitor (postoperatively) for seizures. Brain edema has been reported in patients with newly diagnosed glioma, including one report of intracranial mass effect unresponsive to corticosteroids which led to brain herniation. Monitor closely for intracranial hypertension related to brain edema, inflammation, or necrosis of brain tissue surrounding resection. Re-operation to remove wafers (or remnants) may be necessary for refractory cases. Cases of meningitis have occurred in patients with recurrent glioma receiving wafer implants. Two cases were bacterial (one patient required removal of implants 4 days after implantation and the other developed meningitis following reoperation for recurrent tumor). Another case was determined to be chemical meningitis and resolved with corticosteroids. Monitor postoperatively for signs/symptoms of meningitis and CNS infection.

Monitor closely for known craniotomy-related complications (seizure, intracranial infection, abnormal wound healing, brain edema). Wafer migration may occur; avoid communication between the resection cavity and the ventricular system to prevent wafer migration; communications larger than the wafer should be closed prior to implantation; wafer migration into the ventricular system may cause obstructive hydrocephalus. Monitor for signs/symptoms of obstructive hydrocephalus.

Impaired neurosurgical wound healing, including would dehiscence, delayed healing, and subdural, subgleal or wound effusions may occur with carmustine wafer implant treatment; cerebrospinal fluid leaks have also been reported. Monitor post-operatively for impaired neurosurgical wound healing.

Potentially significant drug-drug interactions may exist, requiring dose or frequency adjustment, additional monitoring, and/or selection of alternative therapy.

Adverse Reactions
Implant:
>10%:
Central nervous system: Seizure (37%; new or worsening: 20%), cerebral edema (4% to 23%), depression (16%)
Dermatologic: Skin rash (5% to 12%)
Gastrointestinal: Nausea (22%), vomiting (21%), constipation (19%)
Genitourinary: Urinary tract infection (21%)
Neuromuscular & skeletal: Weakness (22%)
Miscellaneous: Wound healing impairment (14% to 16%), fever (12%)
1% to 10%:
Cardiovascular: Chest pain (5%)
Central nervous system: Intracranial hypertension (9%), cerebral hemorrhage (6%), meningitis (4%)
Gastrointestinal: Abdominal pain (8%)
Infection: Abscess (local 6%)
Neuromuscular & skeletal: Back pain (7%)
IV: Frequency not defined:
Cardiovascular: Chest pain, flushing (with rapid infusion), occlusive arterial disease, tachycardia
Central nervous system: Brain disease, headache, seizure
Dermatologic: Alopecia, burning sensation of skin, hyperpigmentation
Gastrointestinal: Anorexia, diarrhea, nausea, vomiting
Genitourinary: Gynecomastia
Hematologic & oncologic: Acute leukemia, anemia, bone marrow dysplasia, leukemia, leukopenia (common; onset: 5 to 6 weeks; recovery: after 1 to 2 weeks), thrombocytopenia (common: onset: ~4 weeks; recovery: after 1 to 2 weeks)
Hepatic: Increased serum alkaline phosphatase, increased serum bilirubin, increased serum transaminases
Hypersensitivity: Hypersensitivity reaction
Infection: Opportunistic infection
Local: Burning sensation at injection site, erythema at injection site, pain at injection site, swelling at injection site, tissue necrosis at injection site
Ophthalmic: Blurred vision, conjunctival edema, conjunctival hemorrhage, ophthalmic signs and symptoms (loss of depth perception), suffusion of the conjunctiva (with rapid infusion)
Renal: Azotemia (progressive), nephron atrophy, renal failure
Respiratory: Interstitial pulmonary disease, pneumonitis, pulmonary fibrosis (occurring up to 17 years after treatment), pulmonary infiltrates
<1%, postmarketing, and/or case reports: Febrile neutropenia (Chopra 1993), sepsis (implant), venous thrombosis at injection site (IV)

Drug Interactions
Metabolism/Transport Effects None known.
Avoid Concomitant Use
Avoid concomitant use of Carmustine with any of the following: BCG (Intravesical); Deferiprone; Dipyrone; Natalizumab; Pimecrolimus; Tacrolimus (Topical); Vaccines (Live)
Increased Effect/Toxicity
Carmustine may increase the levels/effects of: CloZAPine; Deferiprone; Fingolimod; Leflunomide; Natalizumab; Tofacitinib; Vaccines (Live)

The levels/effects of Carmustine may be increased by: Cimetidine; Denosumab; Dipyrone; Melphalan; Ocrelizumab; Palifermin; Pimecrolimus; Promazine; Roflumilast; Tacrolimus (Topical); Trastuzumab

Decreased Effect

Carmustine may decrease the levels/effects of: BCG (Intravesical); Coccidioides immitis Skin Test; Lenograstim; Nivolumab; Sipuleucel-T; Tertomotide; Vaccines (Inactivated); Vaccines (Live)

The levels/effects of Carmustine may be decreased by: Echinacea

Hazardous Drugs Handling Considerations

Hazardous agent (NIOSH 2016 [group 1]).

Use appropriate precautions for receiving, handling, administration, and disposal. Gloves (single) should be worn during receiving, unpacking, and placing in storage.

NIOSH recommends double gloving, a protective gown, ventilated engineering controls (a class II biological safety cabinet or a compounding aseptic containment isolator), and (if applicable) closed system transfer devices (CSTDs) for preparation. Double gloving, a gown, and (if dosage form allows) CSTDs are required during administration (NIOSH 2016).

Storage/Stability

Injection: Store intact vials and provided diluent at 2°C to 8°C (36°F to 46°F). Carmustine has a low melting point (30.5°C to 32°C [86.9°F to 89.6°F]); exposure to temperature at or above the melting point will cause the drug to liquefy and appear as an oil film on the vials; if drug liquefies, discard the vials as this is a sign of decomposition. If there is a question of proper refrigeration upon receipt of product, inspect vials; a small amount of dry flakes or dry congealed mass is acceptable and the vial should be refrigerated immediately.

Reconstituted solutions are stable for 24 hours refrigerated (2°C to 8°C) and protected from light. Examine reconstituted vials for crystal formation prior to use. If crystals are observed, they may be redissolved by warming the vial to room temperature with agitation.

Solutions diluted for infusion to a concentration of 0.2 mg/mL in D5W or NS in glass or polypropylene containers and protected from light should be used within 8 hours when stored at room temperature (25°C); infusion solutions are also stable for 24 hours refrigerated followed by an additional 6 hours at room temperature. Although the manufacturer recommends glass or polypropylene containers be used, stability of a 1 mg/mL solution in D5W has also been demonstrated for up to 6 hours (with a 6% to 7% loss of potency) in polyolefin containers (Trissel 2006).

Wafer: Store at or below -20°C (-4°F). Unopened outer foil pouches may be kept at room temperature for up to 6 hours at a time for up to 3 cycles within a 30-day period.

Preparation for Administration

Injection: Reconstitute initially with 3 mL of supplied diluent (dehydrated alcohol injection, USP); then further dilute with SWFI (27 mL), this provides a concentration of 3.3 mg/mL in ethanol 10%; protect from light; further dilute for infusion with 500 mL D5W or NS using a non-PVC container (eg, glass, polypropylene or polyolefin) to a concentration of 0.2 mg/mL.

Implant: Each wafer is packaged within 2 nested aluminum foil pouches; the inner pouch is sterile and is designed to maintain sterility and protect from moisture; the outer wrap is not sterile. Deliver to the operating room in the unopened outer aluminum foil pouch. Do not open until the wafers are ready to be implanted. Follow manufacturer's instructions for opening the pouch, being careful not to apply pressure to the wafer.

Mechanism of Action Carmustine interferes with the normal function of DNA and RNA by alkylation and cross-linking the strands of DNA and RNA, and by possible protein modification; may also inhibit enzyme processes by carbamylation of amino acids in protein.

Pharmacodynamics/Kinetics

Distribution: IV: 3.3 L/kg; readily crosses blood-brain barrier producing CSF levels ≥50% of blood plasma levels; highly lipid soluble

Metabolism: Rapidly hepatic; forms active metabolites

Half-life elimination: IV: 15 to 75 minutes

Excretion: IV: Urine (~60% to 70%) within 96 hours; lungs (~10% as CO_2)

Dosing

Adult & Geriatric Note: Carmustine (IV) is associated with a moderate to high emetic potential (dose-related); antiemetics are recommended to prevent nausea and vomiting (Basch 2011; Dupuis 2011).

Brain tumors, Hodgkin lymphoma, multiple myeloma, non-Hodgkin lymphoma: *Manufacturer's labeling:* IV: 150 to 200 mg/m² every 6 weeks or 75 to 100 mg/m²/day for 2 days every 6 weeks (as a single agent in previously untreated patients; lower doses are used in combination with other chemotherapy agents)

Glioblastoma multiforme (recurrent), glioma (malignant, newly-diagnosed high-grade): Implantation (wafer): 8 wafers (7.7 mg each) implanted intracranially into in the resection cavity (total dose 61.6 mg); should the size and shape not accommodate 8 wafers, the maximum number of wafers feasible (up to 8) should be placed

Indication-specific dosing:

Brain tumor, primary (off-label doses): IV:

80 mg/m²/day for 3 days every 8 weeks for 6 cycles (Brandes 2004)

200 mg/m² every 8 weeks [maximum cumulative dose: 1,500 mg/m²] (Selker 2002)

Hodgkin lymphoma, relapsed or refractory (off-label dose): IV: Mini-BEAM regimen: 60 mg/m² day 1 every 4 to 6 weeks (in combination with etoposide, cytarabine, and melphalan) (Colwill 1995; Martin 2001)

Multiple myeloma, relapsed, refractory (off-label dose). IV: VBMCP regimen: 20 mg/m² day 1 every 35 days (in combination with vincristine, melphalan, cyclophosphamide, and prednisone) (Kyle 2006; Oken 1997)

Mycosis fungoides, early stage (off-label use) (Zackheim 2003): Topical:

Ointment (10 mg/100 grams petrolatum): Apply (with gloves) once daily to affected areas. Additional data may be necessary to further define the role of carmustine in this condition.

Solution (0.2% solution in alcohol; dilute 5 mL in 60 mL water): Apply (with gloves) once daily to affected areas. Additional data may be necessary to further define the role of carmustine in this condition.

Stem cell or bone marrow (autologous) transplant conditioning regimen (off-label use): IV:

BEAM regimen: 300 mg/m² as a single dose 6 days prior to transplant (in combination with etoposide, cytarabine, and melphalan) (Chopra 1993; Linch 2010)

CBV regimen: 600 mg/m² as a single dose 3 days prior to transplant (in combination with cyclophosphamide and etoposide) (Reece 1991)

▶

Pediatric Note: Carmustine (IV) is associated with a moderate to high emetic potential (dose-related); antiemetics are recommended to prevent nausea and vomiting (Basch 2011; Dupuis 2011).

Stem cell or bone marrow transplant (autologous) myeloablative conditioning regimen for relapsed or refractory Hodgkin or non-Hodgkin lymphoma (off-label use):

BEAM regimen: Adolescents ≥15 years: IV: 300 mg/m^2 as a single dose 6 days prior to transplant (in combination with etoposide, cytarabine, and melphalan) (Chopra 1993; Mills 1995). Additional data may be necessary to further define the role of carmustine in this condition.

CBV regimen: Children and Adolescents: IV: 100 mg/m^2 once daily for 3 days beginning 8 days prior to transplant (in combination with cyclophosphamide and etoposide) (Harris 2011). Additional data may be necessary to further define the role of carmustine in this condition.

Renal Impairment

IV: Manufacturer's labeling: CrCl <10 mL/minute: Discontinue treatment.

The following dosage adjustments have also been reported (Kintzel 1995):

CrCl 46 to 60 mL/minute: Reduce dose to 80% of the usual dose

CrCl 31 to 45 mL/minute: Reduce dose to 75% of the usual dose

CrCl ≤30 mL/minute: Consider use of alternative drug.

Wafer implant: There are no dosage adjustments provided in the manufacturer's labeling.

Hepatic Impairment IV and wafer implant: There are no dosage adjustments provided in the manufacturer's labeling.

Obesity

*American Society of Clinical Oncology (ASCO) Guidelines for appropriate chemotherapy dosing in obese adults with cancer (**Note:** Excludes HSCT dosing):* Utilize patient's actual body weight (full weight) for calculation of body surface area- or weight-based dosing, particularly when the intent of therapy is curative; manage regimen-related toxicities in the same manner as for nonobese patients; if a dose reduction is utilized due to toxicity, consider resumption of full weight-based dosing with subsequent cycles, especially if cause of toxicity (eg, hepatic or renal impairment) is resolved (Griggs 2012).

American Society for Blood and Marrow Transplantation (ASBMT) practice guideline committee position statement on chemotherapy dosing in obesity: Utilize actual body weight (full weight) for calculation of body surface area in carmustine dosing for hematopoietic stem cell transplant conditioning regimens in adult patients weighing ≤120% of their ideal body weight (IBW). In patients weighing >120% IBW, utilize adjusted body weight 25% (ABW25) to calculate BSA (Bubalo 2014).

ABW25: Adjusted wt (kg) = Ideal body weight (kg) + 0.25 [actual wt (kg) - ideal body weight (kg)]

Adjustment for Toxicity Hematologic toxicity: Based on nadir counts with previous dose (manufacturer's labeling). IV:

If leukocytes ≥3,000/mm^3 and platelets ≥75,000/mm^3: Administer 100% of dose

If leukocytes 2,000 to 2,999/mm^3 or platelets 25,000 to 74,999/mm^3: Reduce dose to 70% of usual dose

If leukocytes <2,000/mm^3 or platelets <25,000/mm^3: Reduce dose to 50% of usual dose

Combination Regimens

Lymphoma, Hodgkin:

Administration

Carmustine (IV) is associated with a moderate to high emetic potential (dose-related); antiemetics are recommended to prevent nausea and vomiting (Basch 2011; Dupuis 2011).

Injection: Infuse slowly over at least 2 hours (infusions <2 hours may lead to injection site pain or burning); infuse through a free-flowing saline or dextrose infusion, or administer through a central catheter to alleviate venous pain/irritation. Do not exceed a rate of 1.66 mg/m^2/minute.

Irritant; infiltration may result in local pain, erythema, swelling, burning and skin necrosis; the alcohol-based diluent may be an irritant, especially with high doses. Avoid extravasation. Monitor infusion site.

High-dose carmustine (transplant dose; off-label use): Infuse over a least 2 hours to avoid excessive flushing, agitation, and hypotension; was infused over 1 hour in some trials (Chopra 1993). **High-dose carmustine may be fatal if not followed by stem cell rescue.** Monitor vital signs frequently during infusion; patients should be supine during infusion and may require the Trendelenburg position, fluid support, and vasopressor support.

Implant: Double glove before handling; outer gloves should be discarded as chemotherapy waste after handling wafers. Any wafer or remnant that is removed upon repeat surgery should be discarded as chemotherapy waste. The outer surface of the external foil pouch is not sterile. Open pouch gently; avoid pressure on the wafers to prevent breakage. Wafers that are broken in half may be used, however, wafers broken into more than 2 pieces should be discarded in a biohazard container. Slight overlapping of wafers during placement is acceptable. Oxidized regenerated cellulose (Surgicel) may be placed over the wafer to secure; irrigate cavity prior to closure.

Topical (off-label use): Apply solution with brush or gauze pads; ointment and solution should be applied while wearing gloves to involved areas only; avoid contact with eyes or mouth (Zackheim 2003).

Vesicant/Extravasation Risk Irritant; infiltration may result in local pain, erythema, swelling, burning and skin necrosis; the alcohol-based diluent may be an irritant, especially with high doses.

Emetic Potential Children and Adults:
>250 mg/m^2: High (>90%)
≤250 mg/m^2: Moderate (30% to 90%)

Monitoring Parameters

Injection: CBC with differential and platelet count (weekly for at least 6 weeks after a dose), pulmonary function tests (FVC, DL$_{CO}$; at baseline and frequently during treatment), liver function (periodically), renal function tests (periodically); monitor blood pressure and vital signs during administration, monitor infusion site for possible infiltration; monitor for signs/symptoms of pulmonary toxicity

Wafer: Monitor postoperatively for seizures, impaired neurosurgical wound healing, and signs/symptoms of meningitis, CNS infection, and obstructive hydrocephalus; monitor closely for intracranial hypertension related to brain edema, inflammation, or necrosis of brain tissue surrounding resection.

◀ **Dosage Forms** Excipient information presented when available (limited, particularly for generics); consult specific product labeling.
Solution Reconstituted, Intravenous:
  BiCNU: 100 mg (1 ea) [contains alcohol, usp]
Wafer, Implant:
  Gliadel Wafer: 7.7 mg (8 ea) [contains polifeprosan 20]

- ◆ **Carmustine Polymer Wafer** *see* Carmustine *on page 346*
- ◆ **Carmustine Sustained-Release Implant Wafer** *see* Carmustine *on page 346*
- ◆ **Carmustinum** *see* Carmustine *on page 346*
- ◆ **Casodex** *see* Bicalutamide *on page 252*

Caspofungin (kas poe FUN jin)

Brand Names: US Cancidas
Brand Names: Canada Cancidas
Index Terms Caspofungin Acetate
Pharmacologic Category Antifungal Agent, Parenteral; Echinocandin

Use

Aspergillosis, invasive: Treatment of invasive aspergillosis in patients 3 months and older who are refractory to or intolerant of other therapies (eg, amphotericin B, lipid formulations of amphotericin B, itraconazole).

Candidemia and other *Candida* infections: Treatment of candidemia and the following *Candida* infections in patients 3 months and older: intraabdominal abscesses, peritonitis, and pleural space infections.

Candidiasis, esophageal: Treatment of esophageal candidiasis in patents 3 months and older.

Fungal infections, empiric therapy (neutropenic patients): Empiric therapy for presumed fungal infections in febrile, neutropenic patients 3 months and older.

Pregnancy Risk Factor C

Dosing

Adult & Geriatric Note: Duration of caspofungin treatment should be determined by patient status and clinical response.

Aspergillosis, invasive (salvage therapy): IV: Initial dose: 70 mg on day 1; subsequent dosing: 50 mg once daily. Duration of therapy should be a minimum of 6 to 12 weeks and depends on site of infection, extent of disease, and level/duration of immunosuppression (IDSA [Patterson 2016]).

Candidemia and other *Candida* infections: IV: Initial dose: 70 mg on day 1; subsequent dosing: 50 mg once daily; generally continue for at least 14 days after the last positive culture or longer if neutropenia warrants. Higher doses (150 mg once daily infused over ~2 hours) compared to the standard adult dosing regimen (50 mg once daily) have not demonstrated additional benefit or toxicity in patients with invasive candidiasis (Betts 2009). **Note:** IDSA Candidiasis guidelines recommend transition to fluconazole (usually after 5 to 7 days in non-neutropenic patients) in clinically stable patients with fluconazole-susceptible isolates and negative repeat cultures (IDSA [Pappas 2016]).

***Candida* infection, prophylaxis in neutropenic cancer patients at substantial risk (off-label use):** IV: 50 mg once daily (Mattiuzzi 2006).

Candidiasis, chronic disseminated (hepatosplenic) (off-label use): IV: Initial dose: 70 mg on day 1; subsequent dosing: 50 mg daily for several weeks, followed by oral fluconazole therapy (IDSA [Pappas 2016])

Candidiasis, empiric therapy (non-neutropenic ICU patients) (off-label use): IV: Initial dose: 70 mg on day 1; subsequent dosing: 50 mg once daily. Consider discontinuing after 4 to 5 days in patients with no clinical response; continue treatment for 2 weeks in patients who improve on antifungal therapy (IDSA [Pappas 2016]).

Candidiasis, esophageal: IV:

Manufacturer's labeling: 50 mg once daily; continue for 7 to 14 days after symptom resolution. **Note:** The majority of patients studied for this indication also had oropharyngeal involvement.

Alternate recommendations: Initial dose: 70 mg on day 1; subsequent dosing: 50 mg daily; may transition to oral fluconazole therapy once oral intake tolerable. In patients with fluconazole-refractory disease, continue caspofungin for 14 to 21 days (Pappas [IDSA 2016])

Candidiasis, esophageal, in HIV-infected patients (off-label use): IV: 50 mg once daily; continue for 14 to 21 days (HHS [OI adult 2015]).

Candidiasis, intravascular infections (native or prosthetic valve endocarditis, infection of implantable cardiac devices, suppurative thrombophlebitis) (off-label use): IV: 150 mg daily. For native or prosthetic valve endocarditis, therapy should continue for at least 6 weeks after valve replacement surgery (longer durations in patients with abscesses or other complications); for patients with implantable cardiac devices, therapy should continue for 4 to 6 weeks after surgery (4 weeks for infections limited to generator pockets and at least 6 weeks for infections involving the wires); for suppurative thrombophlebitis, continue for at least 2 weeks after candidemia has cleared. **Note:** Step-down to fluconazole therapy is recommended in clinically stable patients with fluconazole-susceptible isolates and negative repeat cultures (IDSA [Pappas 2016]).

Candidiasis, osteoarticular infections (osteomyelitis or septic arthritis) (alternative therapy) (off-label use): IV: 50 to 70 mg daily for at least 14 days, followed by fluconazole (IDSA [Pappas 2016])

Candidiasis, prophylaxis against invasive candidiasis (high-risk ICU patients in units with a high rate of invasive candidiasis) (alternative therapy; off-label use): IV: Loading dose: 70 mg on day 1, then 50 mg daily (IDSA [Pappas 2016])

Candidiasis, oropharyngeal (refractory disease) (alternative therapy) (off-label use): IV: Initial dose: 70 mg on day 1; subsequent doses: 50 mg once daily (Pappas [IDSA 2016])

Fungal infections, empiric therapy (neutropenic patients): IV: Initial dose: 70 mg on day 1; subsequent dosing: 50 mg once daily; continue until resolution of neutropenia; if fungal infection confirmed, continue for a minimum of 14 days (continue for at least 7 days after resolution of both neutropenia and clinical symptoms); if clinical response inadequate, may increase up to 70 mg once daily if tolerated

Dosage adjustment with concomitant use of an enzyme inducer:

Patients receiving rifampin: 70 mg caspofungin once daily

Patients receiving carbamazepine, dexamethasone, efavirenz, nevirapine, or phenytoin (and possibly other enzyme inducers): May require an increased dose of caspofungin 70 mg once daily.

◀ **Pediatric**

Aspergillosis (invasive), candidemia, esophageal candidiasis, and fungal infections (empiric therapy, neutropenic patients): Infants ≥3 months, Children, and Adolescents ≤17 years: IV: Initial dose: 70 mg/m^2 on day 1, subsequent dosing: 50 mg/m^2 once daily, if clinical response inadequate, may increase to 70 mg/m^2 once daily if tolerated (maximum daily dose, loading or maintenance: 70 mg). Duration of caspofungin treatment should be determined by patient status and clinical response; refer to adult dosing for indication-specific recommended durations.

Candidiasis, esophageal, in HIV-infected patients (off-label use): Adolescents: IV: Refer to adult dosing.

Dosage adjustment with concomitant use of an enzyme inducer: *Patients receiving carbamazepine, dexamethasone, efavirenz, nevirapine, phenytoin, or rifampin (and possibly other enzyme inducers):* Consider 70 mg/m^2 once daily (maximum daily dose: 70 mg/day)

Renal Impairment No dosage adjustment necessary.

End-stage renal disease (ESRD) requiring dialysis: Poorly dialyzed; no supplemental dose or dosage adjustment necessary in patients on intermittent hemodialysis (IHD). No supplemental dose or dosage adjustment needed in peritoneal dialysis or continuous renal replacement therapy (eg, CVVHD) (Aronoff 2007, Heintz 2009).

Hepatic Impairment

Adults:

Mild insufficiency (Child-Pugh class A): No dosage adjustment necessary.

Moderate insufficiency (Child-Pugh class B): 70 mg on day 1 (where recommended), followed by 35 mg once daily

Severe insufficiency (Child-Pugh class C): No dosage adjustment provided in manufacturer's labeling (has not been studied)

Children: Mild-to-severe insufficiency (Child-Pugh classes A, B, or C): No dosage adjustment provided in manufacturer's labeling (has not been studied).

Additional Information Complete prescribing information should be consulted for additional detail.

Dosage Forms Excipient information presented when available (limited, particularly for generics); consult specific product labeling.

Solution Reconstituted, Intravenous, as acetate [preservative free]:

Cancidas: 50 mg (1 ea); 70 mg (1 ea)

Generic: 50 mg (1 ea); 70 mg (1 ea)

♦ **2-CdA** see Cladribine *on page 411*

♦ **CDDP** see CISplatin *on page 400*

♦ **CDX** see Bicalutamide *on page 252*

♦ **CeeNU** see Lomustine *on page 1159*

Cefepime (SEF e pim)

Brand Names: US Maxipime

Brand Names: Canada Maxipime

Index Terms Cefepime HCl; Cefepime HCl/D5W; Cefepime Hydrochloride

Pharmacologic Category Antibiotic, Cephalosporin (Fourth Generation)

Use

Febrile neutropenia: Empiric treatment of febrile neutropenic patients.

Intra-abdominal infections: Treatment of complicated intra-abdominal infections, in combination with metronidazole, caused by *Escherichia coli*, viridans group streptococci, *Pseudomonas aeruginosa*, *Klebsiella pneumoniae*, *Enterobacter* species, or *Bacteroides fragilis*.

Pneumonia (moderate to severe): Treatment of moderate to severe pneumonia caused by *Streptococcus pneumoniae*, including cases associated with concurrent bacteremia, *P. aeruginosa*, *K. pneumoniae*, or *Enterobacter* species.

Skin and skin structure infections: Treatment of moderate to severe uncomplicated skin and skin structure infections caused by *Staphylococcus aureus* (methicillin-susceptible isolates only) or *Streptococcus pyogenes*.

Urinary tract infections (including pyelonephritis): Treatment of complicated and uncomplicated urinary tract infections, including pyelonephritis, caused by *E. coli* or *K. pneumoniae*, when the infection is severe, or caused by *E. coli*, *K. pneumoniae*, or *Proteus mirabilis*, when the infection is mild to moderate, including cases associated with concurrent bacteremia with these microorganisms.

Pregnancy Risk Factor B

Dosing

Adult & Geriatric

Febrile neutropenia: IV: 2 g every 8 hours

Intra-abdominal infections, complicated, severe (in combination with metronidazole): IV: **Note:** 2010 IDSA guidelines recommend a duration of 4 to 7 days (provided source controlled). Not recommended for hospital-acquired intra-abdominal infections (IAI) associated with multidrug-resistant gram negative organisms or in mild-to-moderate community-acquired IAIs due to risk of toxicity and the development of resistant organisms (Solomkin [IDSA] 2010).

Due to *P. aeruginosa:* 2 g every 8 hours for 7 to 10 days

Not due to *P. aeruginosa:* 2 g every 8 to 12 hours for 7 to 10 days

Pneumonia: IV:

Manufacturer's labeling:

Due to *P. aeruginosa:* 2 g every 8 hours for 10 days

Not due to *P. aeruginosa:* 1 to 2 g every 8 to 12 hours for 10 days

Alternate dosing: Hospital-acquired or ventilator-associated: 2 g every 8 hours for 7 days; may consider shorter or longer duration depending on rate of clinical improvement. Administration as an extended infusion may be considered. When used as empiric therapy, use in combination with an agent active against MRSA (unless coverage of MSSA only is appropriate) with or without an additional antipseudomonal agent (dependent on patient and institution-specific risk factors) (Kalil 2016)

Skin and skin structure infection, uncomplicated (moderate to severe): IV: 2 g every 12 hours for 10 days

Urinary tract infections, complicated and uncomplicated:
Mild-to-moderate: IM, IV: 0.5 to 1 g every 12 hours for 7 to 10 days
Severe: IV: 2 g every 12 hours for 10 days

Bacterial meningitis (off-label use): IV: 2 g every 8 hours duration of therapy varies depending on pathogen (IDSA [Tunkel 2004])

Osteomyelitis, native vertebral (off-label use) (IDSA [Berbari 2015]): IV:
P. aeruginosa: 2 g every 8 to 12 hours for 6 weeks. **Note:** Double coverage may be considered (ie, cefepime plus an aminoglycoside or ciprofloxacin). Enterobacteriaceae: 2 g every 12 hours for 6 weeks

Prosthetic joint infection, *Enterobacter spp.* or *Pseudomonas aeruginosa* (off-label use): IV: 2 g every 12 hours for 4 to 6 weeks. **Note:** When treating *P. aeruginosa*, consider addition of an aminoglycoside (Osmon 2013).

Pediatric

General dosing, susceptible infection (*Red Book* [AAP 2015]): Infants, Children, and Adolescents: IM, IV:
Mild to moderate infection: 50 mg/kg/dose every 12 hours; maximum dose: 2,000 mg/dose
Severe infection: 50 mg/kg/dose every 8 to 12 hours; maximum dose: 2,000 mg/dose

Febrile neutropenia: Infants, Children, and Adolescents: IV: 50 mg/kg/dose every 8 hours (maximum dose: 2,000 mg/dose) (*Red Book* [AAP 2015])

Pneumonia: Infants ≥2 months, Children, and Adolescents: IV:
Due to *P. aeruginosa:* 50 mg/kg/dose every 8 hours for 10 days (maximum dose: 2,000 mg/dose)
Not due to *P. aeruginosa:* 50 mg/kg/dose every 12 hours for 10 days (maximum dose: 2,000 mg/dose)

Skin and skin structure infections (uncomplicated): Infants ≥2 months, Children, and Adolescents: IV: 50 mg/kg/dose every 12 hours for 10 days (maximum dose: 2,000 mg/dose)

Urinary tract infections, complicated and uncomplicated: Infants ≥2 months, Children, and Adolescents: IV, IM: **Note:** IM may be considered for mild to moderate infection only.
Mild to moderate infection: IV, IM: 50 mg/kg/dose every 12 hours for 7 to 10 days (maximum dose: 1,000 mg/dose)
Severe infection: IV: 50 mg/kg/dose every 12 hours for 10 days (maximum dose: 2,000 mg/dose)

Intra-abdominal infection, complicated (off-label): Infants, Children, and Adolescents: IV: 50 mg/kg/dose every 12 hours in combination with metronidazole (maximum dose: 2,000 mg/dose). **Note:** IDSA 2010 guidelines recommend duration of 4 to 7 days (provided source controlled) (Solomkin [IDSA] 2010).

Renal Impairment Adults: Recommended maintenance schedule based on creatinine clearance (may be estimated using the Cockcroft-Gault formula), compared to normal dosing schedule: See table.

Cefepime Hydrochloride

Creatinine Clearance (mL/minute)	Recommended Maintenance Schedule			
>60 (normal recommended dosing schedule)	500 mg every 12 hours	1 g every 12 hours	2 g every 12 hours	2 g every 8 hours
30-60	500 mg every 24 hours	1 g every 24 hours	2 g every 24 hours	2 g every 12 hours
11-29	500 mg every 24 hours	500 mg every 24 hours	1 g every 24 hours	2 g every 24 hours
<11	250 mg every 24 hours	250 mg every 24 hours	500 mg every 24 hours	1 g every 24 hours

Intermittent hemodialysis (IHD) (administer after hemodialysis on dialysis days): IV: Initial: 1 g (single dose) on day 1. Maintenance: 0.5-1 g every 24 hours **or** 1-2 g every 48-72 hours (Heintz 2009) **or** 2 g 3 times weekly after dialysis (Perez 2012). **Note:** Dosing dependent on the assumption of 3 times weekly, complete IHD sessions.

Peritoneal dialysis (PD): Removed to a lesser extent than hemodialysis; administer normal recommended dose every 48 hours

Continuous renal replacement therapy (CRRT) (Heintz 2009; Trotman 2005): Drug clearance is highly dependent on the method of renal replacement, filter type, and flow rate. Appropriate dosing requires close monitoring of pharmacologic response, signs of adverse reactions due to drug accumulation, as well as drug concentrations in relation to target trough (if appropriate). The following are general recommendations only (based on dialysate flow/ultrafiltration rates of 1-2 L/hour and minimal residual renal function) and should not supersede clinical judgment:

CVVH: Loading dose of 2 g followed by 1-2 g every 12 hours

CVVHD/CVVHDF: Loading dose of 2 g followed by either 1 g every 8 hours **or** 2 g every 12 hours. **Note:** Dosage of 1 g every 8 hours results in similar steady-state concentrations as 2 g every 12 hours and is more cost effective (Heintz 2009).

Note: Consider higher dosage of 4 g/day if treating *Pseudomonas* or life-threatening infections in order to maximize time above MIC (Trotman 2005). Dosage of 2 g every 8 hours may be needed for gram-negative rods with MIC ≥4 mg/L (Heintz 2009).

Infants ≥2 months, Children, and Adolescents: There are no dosage adjustments provided in the manufacturer's labeling; however, similar dosage adjustments to adults would be anticipated based on comparable pharmacokinetics between children and adults.

Hepatic Impairment No dosage adjustment necessary.

Additional Information Complete prescribing information should be consulted for additional detail.

Dosage Forms Excipient information presented when available (limited, particularly for generics); consult specific product labeling.

Solution, Intravenous, as hydrochloride:

Generic: 1 g/50 mL (50 mL); 2 g/100 mL (100 mL)

Solution Reconstituted, Injection, as hydrochloride:
  Maxipime: 1 g (1 ea); 2 g (1 ea)
  Generic: 1 g (1 ea); 2 g (1 ea)
Solution Reconstituted, Injection, as hydrochloride [preservative free]:
  Generic: 2 g (1 ea)
Solution Reconstituted, Intravenous, as hydrochloride:
  Maxipime: 1 g (1 ea); 2 g (1 ea)
  Generic: 1 g/50 mL (1 ea); 2 g/50 mL (1 ea)

◆ **Cefepime HCl** see Cefepime on page 357
◆ **Cefepime HCl/D5W** see Cefepime on page 357
◆ **Cefepime Hydrochloride** see Cefepime on page 357

CefTAZidime (SEF tay zi deem)

Brand Names: US Fortaz; Fortaz in D5W; Tazicef
Brand Names: Canada Ceftazidime For Injection; Fortaz
Index Terms Tazidime
Pharmacologic Category Antibiotic, Cephalosporin (Third Generation)
Use

Bacterial septicemia: Treatment of septicemia caused by *Pseudomonas aeruginosa*, *Klebsiella* spp., *Haemophilus influenzae*, *Escherichia coli*, *Serratia* spp., *Streptococcus pneumoniae*, and *Staphylococcus aureus* (methicillin-susceptible strains).

Bone and joint infections: Treatment of bone and joint infections caused by *Pseudomonas aeruginosa*, *Klebsiella* spp., *Enterobacter* spp., and *Staphylococcus aureus* (methicillin-susceptible strains).

CNS infections: Treatment of meningitis caused by *Haemophilus influenzae* and *Neisseria meningitidis*. Ceftazidime has also been used successfully in cases of meningitis due to *Pseudomonas aeruginosa* and *Streptococcus pneumoniae*.

Empiric therapy in the immunocompromised patient: Empiric treatment of infections in immunocompromised patients.

Gynecologic infections: Treatment of endometritis, pelvic cellulitis, and other infections of the female genital tract caused by *Escherichia coli*.

Intra-abdominal infections: Treatment of peritonitis caused by *Escherichia coli*, *Klebsiella* spp., and *Staphylococcus aureus* (methicillin-susceptible strains) and polymicrobial intra-abdominal infections caused by aerobic and anaerobic organisms and some *Bacteroides* spp. (many strains of *Bacteroides fragilis* are resistant).

Lower respiratory tract infections: Treatment of lower respiratory tract infections, including pneumonia, caused by *Pseudomonas aeruginosa* and other *Pseudomonas* spp.; *Haemophilus influenzae*, including ampicillin-resistant strains; *Klebsiella* spp.; *Enterobacter* spp.; *Proteus mirabilis*; *Escherichia coli*; *Serratia* spp.; *Citrobacter* spp.; *Streptococcus pneumoniae*; and *Staphylococcus aureus* (methicillin-susceptible strains).

Skin and skin-structure infections: Treatment of skin and skin-structure infections caused by *Pseudomonas aeruginosa*; *Klebsiella* spp.; *Escherichia coli*; *Proteus* spp.; including *Proteus mirabilis* and indole-positive *Proteus*; *Enterobacter* spp.; *Serratia* spp.; *Staphylococcus aureus* (methicillin-susceptible strains); and *Streptococcus pyogenes* (group A beta-hemolytic streptococci).

Urinary tract infections (UTI): Treatment of complicated and uncomplicated UTIs caused by *Pseudomonas aeruginosa*; *Enterobacter* spp.; *Proteus* spp., including *Proteus mirabilis* and indole-positive *Proteus*; *Klebsiella* spp.; and *Escherichia coli*.

Pregnancy Risk Factor B

Dosing

Adult & Geriatric

Cystic fibrosis: IV:

Manufacturer's labeling: 90 to 150 mg/kg/day every 8 hours (maximum: 6 g daily)

Alternative recommendations: Intermittent IV infusion: 200 to 400 mg/kg/day divided every 6 to 8 hours (maximum: 8 to 12 g daily); **or** by continuous IV infusion: 100 to 200 mg/kg/day (maximum: 12 g daily) (Zobell, 2013)

Empiric therapy in immunocompromised patients: IV: 2 g every 8 hours

Endophthalmitis, bacterial (off-label use): Intravitreal: 2 to 2.25 mg/0.1 mL NS in combination with vancomycin (Jackson, 2003; Roth, 1997)

Intra-abdominal infection, severe (in combination with metronidazole): IV: 2 g every 8 hours for 4 to 7 days (provided source controlled). Not recommended for hospital-acquired intra-abdominal infections (IAI) associated with multidrug-resistant gram negative organisms or in mild-to-moderate community-acquired IAIs due to risk of toxicity and the development of resistant organisms (Solomkin, 2010).

Melioidosis (off-label use): IV: Note: Switching to meropenem therapy is indicated if patient condition worsens (eg, organ failure, new infection focus development, repeat blood cultures remained positive). Oral eradication therapy is recommended after the intensive (acute) phase treatment is complete (Lipsitz, 2012).

Severe, acute phase: 50 mg/kg/dose every 8 hours (maximum dose: 2 g) or 2 g for one dose, followed by 6 g daily by continuous infusion for ≥10 days with or without TMP/SMX (Lipsitz, 2012).

Non-cystic fibrosis bronchiectasis (off-label use/route): Inhalation for nebulization: 250 to 1,000 mg every 12 hours or 500 mg every 6 hours for up to 12 months (Le 2010, Orriols 1999)

Osteomyelitis, native vertebral due to P. aeruginosa (alternative therapy) (off-label dose): IV: 2 g every 8 hours for 6 weeks **Note:** Double coverage may be considered (ie, ceftazidime plus an aminoglycoside or ciprofloxacin) (IDSA [Berbari 2015])

Peritonitis (CAPD) (off-label route; Li, 2010): Intraperitoneal:

Intermittent: 1 to 1.5 g every 24 hours per exchange in the long dwell (≥6 hours)

Continuous (per liter exchange): Loading dose: 500 mg; maintenance dose: 125 mg. **Note:** If patient has residual renal function (eg, >100 mL/day urine output), empirically increase each dose by 25%.

Pneumonia:

Uncomplicated: IM, IV: 500 mg to 1 g every 8 hours

Hospital-acquired or ventilator-associated (off-label): IV: 2 g every 8 hours for 7 days; may consider shorter or longer duration depending on rate of clinical improvement. When used as empiric therapy, use in combination with an agent active against *S. aureus* with or without an additional antipseudomonal agent (dependent on patient and institution-specific risk factors) (Kalil 2016)

◀ **Prosthetic joint infection, *Pseudomonas aeruginosa* (alternative to cefepime or meropenem):** IV: 2 g every 8 hours for 4 to 6 weeks (consider addition of an aminoglycoside) (Osmon, 2013)

Skin and soft tissue infections: IV, IM: 500 mg to 1 g every 8 hours

Severe infections, including meningitis, CNS infection, osteomyelitis, gynecological: IV: 2 g every 8 hours

Urinary tract infections:

Manufacturer's labeling: IV, IM:

Uncomplicated: 250 mg every 12 hours

Complicated: 500 mg every 8 to 12 hours

Alternative recommendations: IV: Complicated: 1 to 2 g every 8 to 12 hours (Hoepelman 1993; Norrby 1992).

Pediatric

General dosing, susceptible infections: IM, IV:

Manufacturer's labeling: Infants and Children: 30 to 50 mg/kg/dose every 8 hours; maximum daily dose: 6 g/**day**; higher doses reserved for immunocompromised patients, cystic fibrosis, or meningitis

Alternate dosing (Red Book [AAP 2015]): Infants, Children, and Adolescents:

Mild to moderate infections: 90 to 150 mg/kg/day divided every 8 hours; maximum daily dose: 3,000 mg/**day**

Severe infections: 200 mg/kg/day divided every 8 hours; maximum daily dose: 6 g/**day**; higher doses (300 mg/kg/**day**) have been recommended for cystic fibrosis patients

Indication-specific dosing:

Catheter-related blood stream infections (off-label use): Infants and Children ≤12 years: IV: 100 to 150 mg/kg/day in divided doses every 8 hours for 7 to 14 days (Maximum daily dose: 6 g daily) (Mermel 2009)

Cystic fibrosis, lung infection caused by *Pseudomonas* spp: Infants, Children, and Adolescents: IV: 150 to 200 mg/kg/day divided every 6 to 8 hours, maximum daily dose: 6 g/**day**; higher doses have been used: 200 to 400 mg/kg/day divided every 6 to 8 hours; maximum daily dose: 12 g/**day** (Zobell 2013)

Melioidosis (off-label use): Note: Switching to meropenem therapy is indicated if patient condition worsens (eg, organ failure, new infection focus development, repeat blood cultures remained positive). Oral eradication therapy is recommended after the intensive (acute) phase treatment is complete (Lipsitz 2012).

Severe, acute phase: Infants ≥3 months, Children, and Adolescents: IV: 50 mg/kg/dose every 8 hours for ≥10 days with or without TMP/SMX (maximum dose: 2,000 mg/dose) (Lipsitz 2012). **Note:** Depending on infection severity, the dose for patients ≥3 months can be ≤40 mg/kg (maximum dose: 2,000 mg/dose) (Lipsitz 2012).

Renal Impairment Note: If the dose recommended in the dosing section is lower than that recommended for patients with renal insufficiency as outlined below, the lower dose should be used. In severe infections, when the usual dose would be ceftazidime 6 g/day in patients without renal impairment, consider increasing the doses below by 50% or increase the dosing frequency. Further dosage adjustments should be determined by infection severity, susceptibility and patient response to therapy.

CrCl 31 to 50 mL/minute: 1 g every 12 hours

CrCl 16 to 30 mL/minute: 1 g every 24 hours

CrCl 6 to 15 mL/minute: 500 mg every 24 hours

CrCl <5 mL/minute: 500 mg every 48 hours

Intermittent hemodialysis (IHD) (administer after hemodialysis on dialysis days): Dialyzable (50% to 100%): 500 mg to 1 g every 24 hours **or** 1 to 2 g every 48 to 72 hours (Heintz, 2009). **Note:** Dosing dependent on the assumption of 3 times per week, complete IHD sessions.

Peritoneal dialysis (PD): IV:

Intermittent: Loading dose of 1 g, followed by 500 mg every 24 hours

Continuous: Loading dose of 1 g, followed by 500 mg every 24 hours. **Note:** an additional 125 mg per liter of exchange fluid may be added to the dialysate if clinically warranted.

Continuous renal replacement therapy (CRRT) (Heintz, 2009; Trotman, 2005): Drug clearance is highly dependent on the method of renal replacement, filter type, and flow rate. Appropriate dosing requires close monitoring of pharmacologic response, signs of adverse reactions due to drug accumulation, as well as drug concentrations in relation to target trough (if appropriate). The following are general recommendations only (based on dialysate flow/ultrafiltration rates of 1 to 2 L/hour and minimal residual renal function) and should not supersede clinical judgment:

CVVH: Loading dose of 2 g followed by 1 to 2 g every 12 hours

CVVHD/CVVHDF: Loading dose of 2 g followed by either 1 g every 8 hours **or** 2 g every 12 hours. **Note:** Dosage of 1 g every 8 hours results in similar steady-state concentrations as 2 g every 12 hours and is more cost effective. Dosage of 2 g every 8 hours may be needed for gram-negative rods with MIC ≥4 mg/L (Heintz, 2009).

Note: For patients receiving CVVHDF, some recommend giving a loading dose of 2 g followed by 3 g over 24 hours as a continuous IV infusion to maintain concentrations ≥4 times the MIC for susceptible pathogens (Heintz, 2009).

Hepatic Impairment No dosage adjustment necessary.

Additional Information Complete prescribing information should be consulted for additional detail.

Dosage Forms Excipient information presented when available (limited, particularly for generics); consult specific product labeling.

Solution, Intravenous, as sodium [strength expressed as base]:
Fortaz in D5W: 1 g (50 mL); 2 g (50 mL)
Tazicef: 1 g/50 mL (50 mL)

Solution Reconstituted, Injection:
Fortaz: 500 mg (1 ea); 1 g (1 ea); 2 g (1 ea); 6 g (1 ea)
Tazicef: 1 g (1 ea); 2 g (1 ea); 6 g (1 ea)
Generic: 1 g (1 ea); 2 g (1 ea); 6 g (1 ea); 100 g (1 ea)

Solution Reconstituted, Injection [preservative free]:
Generic: 1 g (1 ea); 2 g (1 ea); 6 g (1 ea)

Solution Reconstituted, Intravenous:
Fortaz: 1 g (1 ea); 2 g (1 ea)
Tazicef: 1 g (1 ea); 2 g (1 ea)
Generic: 1 g/50 mL (1 ea); 2 g/50 mL (1 ea)

◆ **Ceftazidime For Injection (Can)** see CefTAZidime on page 360

CefTRIAXone (sef trye AKS one)

Brand Names: US Rocephin [DSC]
Brand Names: Canada Ceftriaxone for Injection; Ceftriaxone for Injection USP; Ceftriaxone Sodium for Injection; Ceftriaxone Sodium for Injection BP
Index Terms Ceftriaxone Sodium

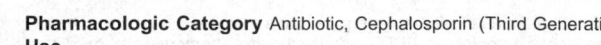

Pharmacologic Category Antibiotic, Cephalosporin (Third Generation)
Use

Acute bacterial otitis media: Caused by *Streptococcus pneumoniae*, *Haemophilus influenzae* (including beta-lactamase-producing strains), or *Moraxella catarrhalis* (including beta-lactamase-producing strains).

Bacterial septicemia: Caused by *Staphylococcus aureus*, *S. pneumoniae*, *Escherichia coli*, *H. influenzae*, or *Klebsiella pneumoniae*.

Bone and joint infections: Caused by *S. aureus*, *S. pneumoniae*, *E. coli*, *Proteus mirabilis*, *K. pneumoniae*, or *Enterobacter* spp.

Intra-abdominal infections: Caused by *E. coli*, *K. pneumoniae*, *Bacteroides fragilis*, *Clostridium* spp., or *Peptostreptococcus* spp.

Lower respiratory tract infections: Caused by *S. pneumoniae*, *S. aureus*, *H. influenzae*, *Haemophilus parainfluenzae*, *K. pneumoniae*, *E. coli*, *Enterobacter aerogenes*, *P. mirabilis*, or *Serratia marcescens*.

Meningitis: Caused by *H. influenzae*, *Neisseria meningitidis*, or *S. pneumoniae*. Ceftriaxone has also been used successfully in a limited number of cases of meningitis and shunt infection caused by *Staphylococcus epidermidis* and *E. coli* (efficacy for these 2 organisms in this organ system was studied in fewer than 10 infections).

Pelvic inflammatory disease: Caused by *N. gonorrhoeae*. Ceftriaxone, like other cephalosporins, has no activity against *Chlamydia trachomatis*. Therefore, when cephalosporins are used in the treatment of patients with pelvic inflammatory disease and *C. trachomatis* is one of the suspected pathogens, appropriate antichlamydial coverage should be added.

Skin and skin structure infections: Caused by *S. aureus*, *S. epidermidis*, *Streptococcus pyogenes*, viridans group streptococci, *E. coli*, *Enterobacter cloacae*, *Klebsiella oxytoca*, *K. pneumoniae*, *P. mirabilis*, *Morganella morganii* (efficacy for this organism in this organ system was studied in fewer than 10 infections), *Pseudomonas aeruginosa*, *S. marcescens*, *Acinetobacter calcoaceticus*, or *B. fragilis* (efficacy for this organism in this organ system was studied in fewer than 10 infections), or *Peptostreptococcus* spp.

Surgical prophylaxis: Reduce the incidence of postoperative infections in patients undergoing surgical procedures classified as contaminated or potentially contaminated (eg, vaginal or abdominal hysterectomy or cholecystectomy for chronic calculous cholecystitis in high-risk patients, such as those older than 70 years, with acute cholecystitis not requiring therapeutic antimicrobials, obstructive jaundice, or common duct bile stones) and in surgical patients for whom infection at the operative site would present serious risk (eg, during coronary artery bypass surgery).

Uncomplicated gonorrhea (cervical/urethral and rectal): Caused by *N. gonorrhoeae*, including both penicillinase- and nonpenicillinase-producing strains, and pharyngeal gonorrhea caused by nonpenicillinase-producing strains of *N. gonorrhoeae*.

Urinary tract infections (complicated and uncomplicated): Caused by *E. coli*, *P. mirabilis*, *Proteus vulgaris*, *M. morganii*, or *K. pneumoniae*.

Pregnancy Risk Factor B
Dosing

Adult & Geriatric

Dosage range: IM, IV: Usual dose: 1 to 2 g every 12 to 24 hours, depending on the type and severity of infection

Acute bacterial rhinosinusitis, severe infection requiring hospitalization (off-label use): IV: 1 to 2 g every 12 to 24 hours (Chow 2012)

Arthritis, septic (off-label use): IV: 1 to 2 g once daily (Coiffier 2014; Dalla Vestra 2008; Harwood 2008; Raad 2004). Additional data may be necessary to further define the role of ceftriaxone in this condition.

Bacterial enteric infections in HIV-infected patients (empiric treatment) (off-label use): IV: 1 g every 24 hours (HHS [OI adult 2016])

Bite wounds (animal) (off-label use): IV: 1 g every 12 hours in combination with clindamycin or metronidazole for anaerobic coverage (IDSA [Stevens 2014])

Brain abscess (off-label use): IV: 2 g every 12 hours in combination with other antibiotics (Brouwer 2014; Louvois 2000). Additional data may be necessary to further define the role of ceftriaxone in this condition.

Chancroid (off-label use): IM: 250 mg as single dose (CDC [Workowski 2015])

Cholecystitis, mild-to-moderate: IV: 1 to 2 g every 12 to 24 hours for 4 to 7 days (provided source controlled) (Solomkin 2010). **Note:** The addition of anaerobic therapy is recommended if biliary-enteric anastomosis is present.

Cystitis (acute, complicated): IV: 1 to 2 g once daily (Stamm 1993)

Epididymitis, acute (off-label use) (CDC [Workowski 2015]):
Likely caused by sexually transmitted chlamydia and gonorrhea: IM: 250 mg in a single dose plus doxycycline
Likely caused by sexually transmitted chlamydia and gonorrhea and enteric organisms in men who practice insertive anal sex: IM: 250 mg in a single dose plus oral levofloxacin or oral ofloxacin

Gonococcal infections:
Conjunctivitis (off-label use): IM: 1 g in a single dose plus oral azithromycin; additionally, consider a one-time saline lavage of the infected eye. Data on treatment in adults are limited, consultation with an infectious-disease specialist should be considered (CDC [Workowski 2015])
Disseminated gonococcal infection (arthritis and arthritis-dermatitis syndrome) (off-label use): IM, IV: 1 g once daily plus single dose oral azithromycin; continue for 24 to 48 hours after clinical improvement, then may switch to an oral agent guided by antimicrobial susceptibility to complete a total of at least 7 days of therapy (CDC [Workowski 2015])
Endocarditis (off-label use): IV: 1 to 2 g every 12 to 24 hours plus oral azithromycin; continue ceftriaxone for at least 28 days (CDC [Workowski 2015])
Meningitis (off-label use): IV: 1 to 2 g every 12 to 24 hours plus oral azithromycin; continue ceftriaxone for 10 to 14 days (CDC [Workowski 2015])
Uncomplicated gonorrhea:
  Cervicitis, proctitis, urethritis (off-label regimen): IM: 250 mg in a single dose plus oral azithromycin (CDC [Workowski 2015])
  Pharyngitis (off-label use): IM: 250 mg in a single dose plus oral azithromycin (CDC [Workowski 2015])

Infective endocarditis, treatment (off-label use) (AHA [Baddour 2015]):
Enterococcus, native or prosthetic valve (penicillin-susceptible/gentamicin-susceptible or penicillin-susceptible/aminoglycoside resistant): IV: 2 g every 12 hours for 6 weeks with concomitant ampicillin
HACEK organisms, native or prosthetic valve: IV, IM: 2 g once daily for 4 weeks (native valve) or 6 weeks (prosthetic valve)
Viridans group Streptococcus (VGS) and S. bovis: IV, IM:
  Native valve: Highly penicillin-susceptible (MIC ≤0.12 mcg/mL): 2 g once daily for 4 weeks **or** for 2 weeks with concomitant gentamicin

Prosthetic valve: Highly penicillin-susceptible (MIC ≤0.12 mcg/mL): 2 g once daily for 6 weeks (with or without concomitant gentamicin for the first 2 weeks)

Prosthetic valve: Relatively or fully penicillin-resistant (MIC >0.12 mcg/mL): 2 g once daily with concomitant gentamicin for 6 weeks

Infective endocarditis, prophylaxis (off-label use): IM, IV: 1 g 30 to 60 minutes before procedure (Wilson 2007). Intramuscular injections should be avoided in patients who are receiving anticoagulant therapy. In these circumstances, orally administered regimens should be given whenever possible. Intravenously administered antibiotics should be used for patients who are unable to tolerate or absorb oral medications.

Note: American Heart Association (AHA) guidelines now recommend prophylaxis only in patients undergoing invasive procedures and in whom underlying cardiac conditions may predispose to a higher risk of adverse outcomes should infection occur. As of April 2007, routine prophylaxis for GI/GU procedures is no longer recommended by the AHA.

Intra-abdominal infection, complicated, community-acquired, mild-to-moderate (in combination with metronidazole): IV: 1 to 2 g every 12 to 24 hours for 4 to 7 days (provided source controlled) (IDSA [Solomkin 2010])

Lyme disease (off-label use): IV: 2 g once daily for 14 days (neurologic), or 21 to 28 days (carditis), or 28 days (arthritis with neurologic manifestations) (AAN [Halperin 2007]; IDSA [Wormser 2006])

Meningitis, community-acquired (empiric treatment): IV: 2 g every 12 hours for 7 to 14 days (longer courses may be necessary for selected organisms) in combination with other agents (eg, vancomycin) (IDSA [Tunkel 2004]).

Meningococcal disease, invasive, high-risk patient contacts (chemo-prophylaxis) (off-label use): IM: 250 mg in a single dose (CDC 2005; *Red Book* [AAP 2015])

Osteomyelitis, native vertebral: IV:

Staphylococci, oxacillin-susceptible (off-label dose): 2 g every 24 hours for 6 weeks (IDSA [Berbari 2015]).

Streptococci (beta-hemolytic), *Cutibacterium acnes* or *Salmonella* spp (off-label use): IV: 2 g every 24 hours for 6 weeks. **Note:** In the treatment of *Salmonella* spp, a 6- to 8-week duration is recommended (IDSA [Berbari 2015]).

Pelvic inflammatory disease (mild to moderately severe): IM: 250 mg in a single dose plus oral doxycycline (with or without oral metronidazole) (CDC [Workowski 2015])

Pneumonia, community-acquired (in combination with other antibiotics):

Manufacturer's labeling: IM, IV: 1 to 2 g/day in 1 or 2 divided doses.

Alternate dosing: IV: 1 g once daily (Roson 2001; Segev 1995)

Proctitis, proctocolitis, enteritis (off-label use): IM: 250 mg in a single dose plus oral doxycycline (CDC [Workowski 2015])

Prophylaxis against sexually transmitted diseases following sexual assault (off-label use): IM: 250 mg as a single dose in combination with azithromycin plus metronidazole (or tinidazole) (CDC [Workowski 2015])

Prosthetic joint infection: IV: *Streptococci, beta-hemolytic:* 2 g every 24 hours for 4 to 6 weeks (Osmon 2013)

Pyelonephritis (acute, uncomplicated): IV: 1 to 2 g once daily; after improvement, may be switched to an oral regimen to complete a 1- to 2-week treatment course (Grabe 2015). In females, some clinicians administer a single dose of 1 g before initiating oral outpatient empiric therapy (IDSA [Gupta 2011]).

Salmonellosis in HIV-infected patients (off-label use): IV: 1 g every 24 hours. Duration of therapy in patients with CD4 count ≥200 cells/mm^3 is 7 to 14 days (without concurrent bacteremia) or ≥14 days (patients with concurrent bacteremia); patients with CD4 count <200 cells/mm^3 should be treated for 2 to 6 weeks (regardless of presence of bacteremia) (HHS [OI adult 2016]).

Skin and soft tissue necrotizing infection (off-label use) (IDSA [Stevens 2014]): Note: Continue until further debridement is not necessary, patient has clinically improved, and patient is afebrile for 48 to 72 hours.

Due to *Aeromonas hydrophilia:* IV: 1 to 2 g once daily in combination with doxycycline

Due to *Vibrio vulnificus:* IV: 1 g once daily in combination with doxycycline

Spontaneous bacterial peritonitis (prevention) (off-label use): IV: 1 g once daily during active gastrointestinal bleeding (may be transitioned to an oral antibiotic after oral intake is resumed) for total duration of antibiotic therapy of 7 days (AASLD [Runyon 2012]).

Surgical (perioperative) prophylaxis: IV: 1 g 30 minutes to 2 hours before surgery

Manufacturer's labeling: 1 g 30 minutes to 2 hours before surgery

Alternate dosing: 1 to 2 g within 60 minutes prior to surgery (Bratzler 2013)

Alternate dosing for colorectal procedures: 2 g within 60 minutes prior to surgery with concomitant metronidazole (Bratzler 2013)

Cholecystectomy: 1 to 2 g every 12 to 24 hours, discontinue within 24 hours unless infection outside gallbladder suspected (Solomkin 2010)

Surgical site infections (intestinal or genitourinary tract surgery, surgery of axilla, or perineum) (off-label use): IV: 1 g every 24 hours, in combination with metronidazole (IDSA [Stevens 2014])

Syphilis in penicillin allergic patients (off-label use) (CDC [Workowski 2015]): IM, IV:

Primary or secondary: 1 to 2 g once daily for 10 to 14 days (limited study data; optimal dose and duration have not been defined)

Neurosyphilis: 2 g once daily for 10 to 14 days (limited study data)

Typhoid fever (off-label use): IV: 2 g every 12 to 24 hours for 10 to 14 days; Note: Usually reserved for fluoroquinolone resistant disease (WHO 2003).

Whipple disease (off-label use): IV: Initial: 2 g once daily for 10 to 14 days, then oral therapy (sulfamethoxazole and trimethoprim preferred) (Feurle 2010; Feurle 2013)

Pediatric

Dosage range: Infants, Children, and Adolescents: Usual dose: IM, IV:

Mild to moderate infections: 50 to 75 mg/kg/day in 1 to 2 divided doses every 12 to 24 hours (maximum: 2,000 mg daily); continue until at least 2 days after signs and symptoms of infection have resolved

Serious infections: 80 to 100 mg/kg/day in 1 to 2 divided doses (maximum: 4,000 mg daily)

Acute bacterial rhinosinusitis, severe infection requiring hospitalization (off-label use): IV: 50 mg/kg/day divided every 12 hours for 10 to 14 days (Chow 2012)

Bacterial enteric infections in HIV-infected patients (empiric treatment) (off-label use): Adolescents: IV: Refer to adult dosing.

Community-acquired pneumonia (CAP) (IDSA/PIDS [Bradley 2011]) (off-label dose): Infants >3 months and Children: IV: 50 to 100 mg/kg/day once daily or divided every 12 hours (maximum: 2,000 mg daily). **Note:** May consider addition of vancomycin or clindamycin to empiric therapy if community-acquired MRSA suspected. Use the higher end of the range for penicillin-resistant *S. pneumoniae*; in children ≥5 years, a macrolide antibiotic should be added if atypical pneumonia cannot be ruled out; preferred in patients not fully immunized for *H. influenzae* type b and *S. pneumoniae*, or significant local resistance to penicillin in invasive pneumococcal strains.

Epiglottis (off-label use): IV: 100 mg/kg/day as a single dose on day 1, then 50 mg/kg as a single dose on day 2 (Sawyer 1994) or 75 mg/kg once daily for 10 to 14 days (Low 2003). Additional data may be necessary to further define the role of ceftriaxone in this condition.

Gonococcal infections:

Bacteremia (off-label use) (CDC [Workowski 2015]): IM, IV:

Children ≤45 kg: 50 mg/kg/dose once daily (maximum: 1,000 mg) for 7 days

Children >45 kg: 1,000 mg once daily for 7 days

Conjunctivitis (off-label use): IM, IV:

Neonates and Infants: 25 to 50 mg/kg/dose as a single dose (maximum dose: 125 mg) (CDC [Workowski 2015]). **Note:** Use contraindicated in hyperbilirubinemic neonates.

Adolescents: Refer to adult dosing.

Disseminated gonococcal infection (DGI) in infants including scalp abscess (off-label use): IM, IV:

Infants: 25 to 50 mg/kg/dose once daily for 7 days (10 to 14 days for meningitis) (CDC [Workowski 2015]); **Note:** Use contraindicated in hyperbilirubinemic neonates.

Disseminated gonococcal infection (arthritis, arthritis-dermatitis syndrome) (off-label use): IM, IV:

Children ≤45 kg: Arthritis: 50 mg/kg/dose once daily (maximum dose: 1,000 mg) for 7 days (CDC [Workowski 2015])

Children >45 kg: Arthritis: 1,000 mg once daily for 7 days (CDC [Workowski 2015])

Adolescents: Refer to adult dosing.

Endocarditis (off-label use):

Children ≤45 kg: IM, IV: 50 mg/kg/day divided every 12 or 24 hours (maximum: 2,000 mg daily) for at least 28 days (*Red Book* [AAP 2015])

Children >45 kg and Adolescents: Refer to adult dosing.

Meningitis (off-label use): IV, IM:

Infants: 25 to 50 mg/kg/day in a single daily dose for 10 to 14 days (CDC [Workowski 2015]); **Note:** Use contraindicated in hyperbilirubinemic neonates.

Children ≤45 kg: 50 mg/kg/day divided every 12 or 24 hours (maximum: 2,000 mg daily); usual duration of treatment is 10 to 14 days (*Red Book* [AAP 2015])

Children >45 kg and Adolescents: Refer to adult dosing.

Prophylactic treatment in neonates due to untreated maternal gonococcal infection (off-label use): Neonates: IM, IV: 25 to 50 mg/kg as a single dose (maximum: 125 mg) (CDC [Workowski 2015]). **Note:** Use contraindicated in hyperbilirubinemic neonates.

Uncomplicated gonorrhea (cervicitis, proctitis, or urethritis) (off-label population) CDC [Workowski 2015]):
Infants and Children ≤45 kg: IM, IV: 25 to 50 mg/kg/dose as a single dose (maximum dose: 125 mg IM)
Children >45 kg and Adolescents: Refer to adult dosing.
Uncomplicated gonorrhea: Pharyngitis or vulvovaginitis (off-label use) (CDC [Workowski 2015]):
Infants and Children ≤45 kg: IM, IV: 25 to 50 mg/kg/dose as a single dose (maximum dose: 125 mg IM)
Children >45 kg and Adolescents: IM: 250 mg in a single dose plus oral azithromycin

Infective endocarditis (off-label use): IM, IV:
Native valve: 100 mg/kg once daily (maximum: 2,000 mg daily) for 2 to 4 weeks; **Note:** If using 2-week regimen or for relatively penicillin-resistant streptococcus, concurrent gentamicin is recommended; for HACEK organisms, duration of therapy is 4 weeks (Baddour 2005)
Prosthetic valve: 100 mg/kg once daily (maximum: 2,000 mg daily) for 6 weeks (with or without gentamicin [dependent on penicillin MIC]); for HACEK organisms, duration of therapy is 4 weeks (Baddour 2005)
Enterococcus faecalis (resistant to penicillin, aminoglycoside, and vancomycin), native or prosthetic valve: 100 mg/kg/day divided every 12 hours for ≥8 weeks administered concurrently with ampicillin (Baddour 2005)
Prophylaxis: 50 mg/kg 30 to 60 minutes before procedure; maximum dose: 1,000 mg (*Red Book* [AAP 2015]; Wilson 2007). Intramuscular injections should be avoided in patients who are receiving anticoagulant therapy. In these circumstances, orally administered regimens should be given whenever possible. Intravenously administered antibiotics should be used for patients who are unable to tolerate or absorb oral medications.
Note: American Heart Association (AHA) guidelines now recommend prophylaxis only in patients undergoing invasive procedures and in whom underlying cardiac conditions may predispose to a higher risk of adverse outcomes should infection occur. As of April 2007, routine prophylaxis for GI/GU procedures is no longer recommended by the AHA.

Lyme disease (off-label use): IM, IV:
Atrioventricular heart block or carditis: 50 to 75 mg/kg once daily (maximum: 2,000 mg) for 14 to 21 days (*Red Book* [AAP 2015])
Encephalitis or other late neurologic disease: 50 to 75 mg/kg once daily (maximum: 2,000 mg) for 14 to 28 days (*Red Book* [AAP 2015])
Neurologic: 50 to 75 mg/kg once daily (maximum: 2,000 mg) for 14 days (Halperin 2007)
Meningitis: 50 to 75 mg/kg once daily (maximum: 2,000 mg) for 14 to 21 days (*Red Book* [AAP 2015])
Recurrent arthritis: 50 to 75 mg/kg once daily (maximum: 2,000 mg) for 14 to 28 days (*Red Book* [AAP 2015])

Meningitis (empiric treatment): IM, IV: Loading dose of 100 mg/kg (maximum: 4,000 mg), followed by:
Manufacturer's labeling: 100 mg/kg/day divided every 12 to 24 hours (maximum: 4,000 mg daily); usual duration of treatment is 7 to 14 days
Alternate dosing: 80 to 100 mg/kg/day divided every 12 to 24 hours (maximum: 4,000 mg daily) (Tunkel 2004)

Meningococcal disease, invasive, high-risk patient contacts (chemoprophylaxis) (off-label use):
Children and Adolescents <15 years: IM: 125 mg in a single dose (CDC 2005; *Red Book* [AAP 2015]).

◄ Adolescents ≥15 years: Refer to adult dosing.

Otitis media: IM:

Acute: 50 mg/kg in a single dose (maximum: 1,000 mg)

Persistent or relapsing (off-label dose): 50 mg/kg once daily for 3 days (AAP 2014; Lieberthal 2013)

Prophylaxis against sexually transmitted diseases following sexual assault (off-label use): Adolescents: Refer to adult dosing.

Salmonellosis in HIV-infected patients (off-label use): Adolescents: IV: Refer to adult dosing.

Shigella dysentery type 1 (off-label dose): IM: 50 to 100 mg/kg/day for 2 to 5 days (WHO 2005)

Skin/skin structure infections: IM, IV: 50 to 75 mg/kg/day in 1 to 2 divided doses (maximum: 2,000 mg daily)

Surgical (perioperative) prophylaxis (off-label dose): Children ≥1 year: IV: 50 to 75 mg/kg within 60 minutes prior to surgery (maximum: 2,000 mg) (Bratzler 2013)

Typhoid fever (off-label use): IV: 80 mg/kg once daily for 14 days (Stephens 2002)

Renal Impairment There are no dosage adjustments provided in the manufacturer's labeling; however, in patients with concurrent renal and hepatic impairment, maximum daily dose should not exceed 2 g.

ESRD requiring dialysis: Poorly dialyzed; no supplemental dose or dosage adjustment necessary, including patients on intermittent hemodialysis, peritoneal dialysis, or continuous renal replacement therapy (eg, CVVHD) (Aronoff 2007).

Hepatic Impairment There are no dosage adjustments provided in the manufacturer's labeling; however, in patients with concurrent renal and hepatic impairment, maximum daily dose should not exceed 2 g.

Additional Information Complete prescribing information should be consulted for additional detail.

Dosage Forms Excipient information presented when available (limited, particularly for generics); consult specific product labeling. [DSC] = Discontinued product

Solution, Intravenous:

Generic: 20 mg/mL (50 mL); 40 mg/mL (50 mL)

Solution Reconstituted, Injection:

Rocephin: 500 mg (1 ea [DSC]); 1 g (1 ea [DSC])

Generic: 250 mg (1 ea); 500 mg (1 ea); 1 g (1 ea); 2 g (1 ea); 100 g (1 ea)

Solution Reconstituted, Intravenous:

Generic: 1 g (1 ea); 2 g (1 ea); 10 g (1 ea)

♦ **Ceftriaxone for Injection (Can)** *see* CefTRIAXone *on page 363*

♦ **Ceftriaxone for Injection USP (Can)** *see* CefTRIAXone *on page 363*

♦ **Ceftriaxone Sodium** *see* CefTRIAXone *on page 363*

♦ **Ceftriaxone Sodium for Injection (Can)** *see* CefTRIAXone *on page 363*

♦ **Ceftriaxone Sodium for Injection BP (Can)** *see* CefTRIAXone *on page 363*

♦ **CellCept** *see* Mycophenolate *on page 1283*

♦ **CellCept Intravenous** *see* Mycophenolate *on page 1283*

♦ **CellCept I.V. (Can)** *see* Mycophenolate *on page 1283*

Ceritinib (se RI ti nib)

Related Information
Safe Handling of Hazardous Drugs *on page* 2379
Brand Names: US Zykadia
Brand Names: Canada Zykadia
Index Terms LDK378
Pharmacologic Category Antineoplastic Agent, Anaplastic Lymphoma Kinase Inhibitor; Antineoplastic Agent, Tyrosine Kinase Inhibitor
Use Non-small cell lung cancer, metastatic: Treatment of anaplastic lymphoma kinase (ALK)-positive (as detected by an approved test) metastatic non-small cell lung cancer (NSCLC).

Labeled Contraindications
There are no contraindications listed in the manufacturer's US labeling.
Canadian labeling: Known hypersensitivity to ceritinib or any component of the formulation; congenital long QT syndrome or persistent Fridericia-corrected electrocardiogram interval (QTcF) of >500 msec.

Pregnancy Considerations Based on findings in animal reproduction studies and its mechanism of action, ceritinib may cause fetal harm if administered to a pregnant woman. Women of reproductive potential should use effective contraception during treatment and for 6 months following therapy discontinuation. Based on the potential for genotoxicity, males with female partners of reproductive potential should use condoms during treatment and for 3 months following completion of therapy.

Breastfeeding Considerations It is not known if ceritinib is present in breast milk. Due to the potential for serious adverse reactions (gastrointestinal toxicity, pneumonitis, bradycardia, and pancreatitis) in the breastfed infant, breastfeeding is not recommended during treatment and for 2 weeks following completion of therapy.

Warnings/Precautions Symptomatic bradycardia has been reported; heart rate <50 beats/minute has occurred. If possible, avoid concurrent use with other agents known to cause bradycardia (eg, beta blockers, nondihydropyridine calcium channel blockers, clonidine, digoxin). Monitor heart rate and blood pressure regularly. If symptomatic bradycardia (not life-threatening) occurs, withhold treatment until recovery to asymptomatic bradycardia or to a heart rate of ≥60 beats/minute, evaluate concurrent medications, and adjust ceritinib dose. Permanently discontinue for life-threatening bradycardia due to ceritinib; if life-threatening bradycardia occurs and concurrent medications associated with bradycardia can be discontinued or dose adjusted, restart ceritinib at a reduced dose (with frequent monitoring). QTc interval prolongation has occurred in clinical studies, and may be concentration-dependent. Based on post-baseline ECG assessment, a QTc interval increase of >60 msec over baseline was observed in a small percentage of patients; some patients experienced a QTc >500 msec. QT prolongation may lead to an increased risk for ventricular tachyarrhythmias (eg, torsades de pointes) or sudden death. Avoid use in patients with congenital long QTc syndrome. Correct electrolyte abnormalities prior to initiating therapy. Periodically monitor ECG and electrolytes in patients with heart failure, bradyarrhythmias, electrolyte abnormalities, or who are taking medications known to prolong the QTc interval. QT prolongation may require treatment interruption, dosage reduction, or discontinuation. Permanently discontinue in patients who develop QTc interval prolongation in combination with torsades de pointes or polymorphic ventricular tachycardia or signs/symptoms of serious arrhythmia.

Severe and/or persistent gastrointestinal toxicity has occurred with ceritinib. Diarrhea, nausea, vomiting, or abdominal pain occurred in the majority of patients in clinical trials (including some grade 3 and 4 events); over one-third of patients required treatment interruptions or dose reductions due to severe or persistent gastrointestinal toxicity. Manage symptoms medically with appropriate therapy (eg, antidiarrheals, antiemetics, fluid replacement) as indicated. May require therapy interruption and dosage reduction. Ceritinib is associated with a moderate emetic potential (Roila 2016); antiemetics may be needed to prevent nausea and vomiting. If vomiting occurs, do not administer an additional dose; continue with the next scheduled dose. Hepatotoxicity has been observed in patients treated with ceritinib in clinical trials, including ALT levels >5 times ULN in over one-quarter of patients and AST elevations in nearly one-fifth of patients. Concurrent ALT elevations >3 times ULN with total bilirubin >2 times ULN (with normal alkaline phosphatase) occurred rarely. Monitor liver function tests (eg, ALT, AST, total bilirubin) monthly and as clinically necessary, more frequently in patients who develop transaminase abnormalities. May require therapy interruption, dosage reduction, and/or permanent discontinuation. Use with caution in patients with hepatic impairment (has not been studied in patients with moderate or severe impairment). Ceritinib is metabolized and eliminated hepatically; systemic exposure and toxicities may be increased in patients with hepatic dysfunction. Although rare, pancreatitis (with fatality) has been reported. Grade 3 to 4 lipase and amylase elevations occurred in clinical trials. Monitor lipase and amylase prior to treatment and periodically during treatment as clinically necessary. May require treatment interruption and dose reduction.

Hyperglycemia, including grade 3 and 4 toxicity, has been observed in ceritinib-treated patients. Monitor fasting blood glucose levels at baseline and as clinically necessary. May require initiation or optimization of antihyperglycemic therapy. Temporarily interrupt therapy for hyperglycemia until adequately controlled; reduce dose upon recovery. If adequate glycemic control is not possible with medical management, permanently discontinue ceritinib. Severe and life-threatening interstitial lung disease (ILD)/pneumonitis have been reported, including grade 3 or 4 events and fatalities. Monitor for signs/symptoms of pulmonary toxicity; permanently discontinue in patients diagnosed with treatment-related ILD/pneumonitis. Potentially significant interactions may exist, requiring dose or frequency adjustment, additional monitoring, and/or selection of alternative therapy. In vitro studies indicate that ceritinib solubility and bioavailability may be decreased at higher pH; concurrent use with proton pump inhibitors, H_2-receptor antagonists, or antacids has not been evaluated. Approved for use only in patients with metastatic non-small cell lung cancer (NSCLC) who test positive for the abnormal anaplastic lymphoma kinase (ALK) gene.

Adverse Reactions

>10%:

Central nervous system: Fatigue (52%), neuropathy (17%; including paresthesia, muscular weakness, gait disturbance, peripheral neuropathy, hypoesthesia, peripheral sensory neuropathy, dysesthesia, neuralgia, peripheral motor neuropathy, hypotonia, polyneuropathy)

Dermatologic: Skin rash (16%; including maculopapular rash, acneiform dermatitis)

Endocrine & metabolic: Increased serum glucose (49%; grades 3/4: 13%), decreased serum phosphate (36%)

Gastrointestinal: Diarrhea (86%; grades 3/4: 6%), nausea (80%; grades 3/4: 4%), vomiting (60%; grades 3/4: 4%), abdominal pain (54%), decreased appetite (34%), constipation (29%), increased serum lipase (28%), disease of esophagus (16%; including dyspepsia, gastroesophageal reflux disease, dysphagia)

Hematologic & oncologic: Decreased hemoglobin (84%)

Hepatic: Increased serum ALT (80%; grades 3/4: 27%), increased serum AST (75%; grades 3/4: 13%), increased serum bilirubin (15%; grades 3/4: 1%)

Renal: Increased serum creatinine (58%)

1% to 10%:

Cardiovascular: Prolonged Q-T interval on ECG (4%; >60 msec increase from baseline: 3%; >500 msec: <1%), bradycardia (3%), sinus bradycardia (1%)

Ophthalmic: Visual disturbance (9%; including vision impairment, blurred vision, photopsia, accommodation disorder, presbyopia, reduced visual acuity)

Respiratory: Interstitial pulmonary disease (4%; grades 3/4: 3%)

Drug Interactions

Metabolism/Transport Effects Substrate of CYP3A4 (major), P-glycoprotein; **Note:** Assignment of Major/Minor substrate status based on clinically relevant drug interaction potential; **Inhibits** CYP2C9 (moderate), CYP3A4 (strong)

Avoid Concomitant Use

Avoid concomitant use of Ceritinib with any of the following: Ado-Trastuzumab Emtansine; Alfuzosin; Aprepitant; Astemizole; Asunaprevir; Avanafil; Axitinib; Barnidipine; Blonanserin; Bosutinib; Bradycardia-Causing Agents; Bromocriptine; Budesonide (Systemic); Cobimetinib; Conivaptan; Crizotinib; CYP3A4 Inducers (Strong); CYP3A4 Inhibitors (Strong); Dabrafenib; Dapoxetine; Domperidone; Dronedarone; Eletriptan; Eplerenone; Everolimus; Flibanserin; Fluticasone (Nasal); Fusidic Acid (Systemic); Grapefruit Juice; Halofantrine; Highest Risk QTc-Prolonging Agents; Hydroxychloroquine; Ibrutinib; Idelalisib; Irinotecan Products; Isavuconazonium Sulfate; Ivabradine; Lapatinib; Lercanidipine; Lomitapide; Lovastatin; Lurasidone; Macitentan; MiFEPRIStone; Naloxegol; Neratinib; Nilotinib; NiMODipine; Nisoldipine; Olaparib; Palbociclib; Pimozide; Probucol; Promazine; Radotinib; Ranolazine; Red Yeast Rice; Regorafenib; Rupatadine; Salmeterol; Silodosin; Simeprevir; Simvastatin; Sonidegib; St John's Wort; Suvorexant; Tamsulosin; Terfenadine; Ticagrelor; Tolvaptan; Toremifene; Trabectedin; Udenafil; Ulipristal; Vemurafenib; VinCRIStine (Liposomal); Vinflunine; Vorapaxar

Increased Effect/Toxicity

Ceritinib may increase the levels/effects of: Ado-Trastuzumab Emtansine; Alfuzosin; Alitretinoin (Systemic); Almotriptan; Alosetron; AmLODIPine; Apixaban; Aprepitant; ARIPiprazole; ARIPiprazole Lauroxil; Astemizole; Asunaprevir; Avanafil; Axitinib; Barnidipine; Bedaquiline; Blonanserin; Bortezomib; Bosentan; Bosutinib; Brentuximab Vedotin; Brexpiprazole; Brinzolamide; Bromocriptine; Budesonide (Nasal); Budesonide (Oral Inhalation); Budesonide (Systemic); Budesonide (Topical); Buprenorphine; Cabazitaxel; Cabozantinib; Calcifediol; Cannabidiol; Cannabis; Cariprazine; Cilostazol; Cobimetinib; Colchicine; Conivaptan; Corticosteroids (Systemic); Crizotinib; CycloSPORINE (Systemic); CYP2C9 Substrates; CYP3A4 Substrates; Dabrafenib; Daclatasvir; Dapoxetine; Dasatinib; Deflazacort; Delamanid;

Dexamethasone (Ophthalmic); Dienogest; DOCEtaxel; Domperidone; DOX-Orubicin (Conventional); Dronabinol; Dronedarone; Drospirenone; Dutasteride; Eletriptan; Eplerenone; Erlotinib; Estazolam; Eszopiclone; Etizolam; Everolimus; Evogliptin; FentaNYL; Fesoterodine; Flibanserin; Fluticasone (Nasal); Fluticasone (Oral Inhalation); Gefitinib; Halofantrine; Highest Risk QTc-Prolonging Agents; HYDROcodone; HydrOXYzine; Ibrutinib; Imatinib; Imidafenacin; Irinotecan Products; Isavuconazonium Sulfate; Ivabradine; Ivacaftor; Ixabepilone; Lacosamide; Lapatinib; Lercanidipine; Levobupivacaine; Levomilnacipran; Lomitapide; Lovastatin; Lurasidone; Macitentan; Manidipine; Maraviroc; MedroxyPROGESTERone; MethylPREDNISolone; Midostaurin; Mirodenafil; Moderate Risk QTc-Prolonging Agents; Naldemedine; Naloxegol; Neratinib; Nilotinib; NiMODipine; Nisoldipine; Olaparib; Ospemifene; Oxybutynin; OxyCODONE; Palbociclib; Panobinostat; Parecoxib; Paricalcitol; PAZOPanib; Pimecrolimus; Pimozide; PONATinib; Pranlukast; Praziquantel; PrednisoLONE (Systemic); PredniSONE; Radotinib; Ramelteon; Ranolazine; Reboxetine; Red Yeast Rice; Regorafenib; Repaglinide; Retapamulin; Rilpivirine; RomiDEPsin; Rupatadine; Ruxolitinib; Salmeterol; SAXagliptin; Sildenafil; Silodosin; Simeprevir; Simvastatin; Sonidegib; SORAfenib; Suvorexant; Tacrolimus (Systemic); Tadalafil; Tamsulosin; Tasimelteon; Temsirolimus; Terfenadine; Tetrahydrocannabinol; Ticagrelor; Tofacitinib; Tolterodine; Tolvaptan; Toremifene; Trabectedin; TraMADol; Udenafil; Ulipristal; Valbenazine; Vardenafil; Vemurafenib; Venetoclax; Vilazodone; VinCRIStine (Liposomal); Vindesine; Vinflunine; Vinorelbine; Vorapaxar; Zolpidem; Zopiclone

The levels/effects of Ceritinib may be increased by: Bradycardia-Causing Agents; Bretylium; Conivaptan; Corticosteroids; CYP3A4 Inhibitors (Moderate); CYP3A4 Inhibitors (Strong); Fusidic Acid (Systemic); Grapefruit Juice; Hydroxychloroquine; Idelalisib; MiFEPRIStone; Netupitant; P-glycoprotein/ABCB1 Inhibitors; Probucol; Promazine; QTc-Prolonging Agents (Indeterminate Risk and Risk Modifying); Stiripentol; Vinflunine; Xipamide

Decreased Effect

Ceritinib may decrease the levels/effects of: Antidiabetic Agents; Doxercalciferol; Ifosfamide; Prasugrel; Ticagrelor

The levels/effects of Ceritinib may be decreased by: Bosentan; CYP3A4 Inducers (Moderate); CYP3A4 Inducers (Strong); Deferasirox; Sarilumab; Siltuximab; St John's Wort; Tocilizumab

Food Interactions

A high-fat meal increases AUC and C_{max} by 73% and 41%, respectively and a low-fat meal increases AUC and C_{max} by 58% and 43%, respectively; systemic exposure when administered with a meal may exceed that of a typical dose, and may result in increased toxicity. Management: Administer on an empty stomach, at least 1 hour before or 2 hours after a meal.

Grapefruit and grapefruit juice may inhibit the metabolism of ceritinib and increase its systemic exposure. Management: Avoid grapefruit juice during therapy.

Hazardous Drugs Handling Considerations

Hazardous agent (meets NIOSH 2016 criteria). This medication is not on the NIOSH (2016) list; however, it meets the criteria for a hazardous drug. Drugs are classified as hazardous based on their properties; the properties of a hazardous drug include one or more of the following characteristics: carcinogenic, teratogenic (or other developmental toxicity), reproductive toxicity, organotoxic at low doses, genotoxic, and/or new agents with structural or toxicity profiles similar to existing hazardous agents.

Use appropriate precautions for receiving, handling, administration, and disposal. Gloves (single) should be worn during receiving, unpacking, and placing in storage. NIOSH recommends single gloving for administration of intact tablets or capsules (NIOSH 2016).

Storage/Stability Store at 25°C (77°F); excursions are permitted between 15°C and 30°C (59°F and 86°F).

Mechanism of Action Ceritinib is a potent inhibitor of anaplastic lymphoma kinase (ALK), a tyrosine kinase involved in the pathogenesis of non-small cell lung cancer. ALK gene abnormalities due to mutations or translocations may result in expression of oncogenic fusion proteins (eg, ALK fusion protein) which alter signaling and expression and result in increased cellular proliferation and survival in tumors which express these fusion proteins. ALK inhibition reduces proliferation of cells expressing the genetic alteration. Ceritinib also inhibits insulin-like growth factor 1 receptor (IGF-1R), insulin receptor (InsR), and ROS1. Ceritinib has demonstrated activity in crizotinib-resistant tumors in NSCLC xenograft models.

Pharmacodynamics/Kinetics

Absorption: AUC and C_{max} increased 73% and 41%, respectively, when administered with a high-fat meal, and 58% and 43%, respectively when taken with a low-fat meal (when compared to fasting)

Distribution: 4,230 L (following a single dose), with a small preferential distribution to red blood cells versus plasma

Protein binding: 97% to human plasma proteins

Metabolism: Primarily hepatic via CYP3A

Half-life elimination: 41 hours

Time to peak: ~4 to 6 hours

Excretion: Feces (~92% with 68% as unchanged drug); urine (~1%)

Dosing

Adult & Geriatric Note: Ceritinib is associated with a moderate emetic potential (Roila 2016); antiemetics may be needed to prevent nausea and vomiting.

Non-small cell lung cancer (ALK-positive), metastatic: Oral: 750 mg once daily; continue until disease progression or unacceptable toxicity.

Missed doses: If a dose is missed, take the missed dose unless the next dose is due within 12 hours. If vomiting occurs, do not administer an additional dose, patients should continue with the next scheduled dose.

Dosage adjustment for concomitant therapy:

Strong CYP3A4 inhibitors: Avoid concomitant use of strong CYP3A inhibitors; if concurrent administration cannot be avoided, reduce ceritinib dose by approximately one-third (rounded to the nearest multiple of the 150 mg strength). After discontinuation of the strong CYP3A inhibitor, resume ceritinib therapy at the dose used prior to initiation of the CYP3A4 inhibitor.

Strong CYP3A4 inducers: Avoid concurrent use of strong CYP3A inducers (eg, carbamazepine, phenytoin, rifampin, and St John's wort) during treatment with ceritinib.

Renal Impairment

CrCl ≥30 to 90 mL/minute: No dosage adjustment is necessary.

CrCl <30 mL/minute: There are no dosage adjustments provided in the manufacturer's labeling (has not been studied).

Hepatic Impairment

Preexisting mild impairment (total bilirubin ≤ULN and AST >ULN **or** total bilirubin >1 to 1.5 times ULN and any AST): No dosage adjustment is necessary.

Preexisting moderate or severe impairment: There are no dosage adjustments provided in the manufacturer's labeling (has not been studied). Ceritinib is primarily metabolized and eliminated hepatically; exposure is likely increased in patients with hepatic impairment.

Hepatotoxicity during treatment:

ALT or AST >5 times ULN **with** total bilirubin ≤2 times ULN: Interrupt therapy until recovery to baseline or ALT/AST ≤3 times ULN, then resume with a 150 mg dose reduction.

ALT or AST >3 times ULN **with** total bilirubin >2 times ULN in the absence of cholestasis or hemolysis: Permanently discontinue therapy.

Adjustment for Toxicity

Recommended ceritinib dosage adjustment levels:

Initial starting dose: 750 mg once daily

First dose reduction: 600 mg once daily

Second dose reduction: 450 mg once daily

Third dose reduction: 300 mg once daily

Discontinue if patients are unable to tolerate 300 mg daily.

Cardiac:

Bradycardia:

Symptomatic bradycardia (not life-threatening): Interrupt therapy and evaluate concomitant medications known to cause bradycardia.

Upon recovery to asymptomatic bradycardia or to a heart rate ≥60 beats per minute, adjust the dose.

Alternatively, the following recommendations have been made: Upon recovery to asymptomatic bradycardia or to a heart rate ≥60 beats per minute. If concomitant medication is identified and discontinued or its dose adjusted, reinitiate ceritinib at its previous dose. If no concomitant medication is identified or if it is identified but not discontinued or not dose-adjusted, reinitiate ceritinib with the dose reduced by 150 mg (Zykadia Canadian product labeling 2016).

Symptomatic bradycardia (life-threatening or requiring intervention) in patients taking concomitant medications known to cause bradycardia/hypotension: Interrupt therapy until recovery to asymptomatic bradycardia or to a heart rate ≥60 beats per minute.

If the concomitant medication can be adjusted or discontinued, resume ceritinib therapy with the dose reduced by 150 mg.

Alternatively, the following recommendations have been made: If concomitant medication can be discontinued or its dose adjusted, resume ceritinib with the dose reduced by 300 mg; monitor frequently; permanently discontinue ceritinib for recurrence (Zykadia Canadian product labeling 2016).

Symptomatic bradycardia (life-threatening) in patients not taking concomitant medications known to cause bradycardia/hypotension: Permanently discontinue therapy.

QTc prolongation:

QTc interval >500 msec on at least 2 separate ECGs: Interrupt therapy until QTc interval is <481 msec or recovers to baseline if baseline QTc is ≥481 msec, then resume therapy with a 150 mg dose reduction.

QTc prolongation in combination with torsades de pointes, polymorphic ventricular tachycardia, or signs/symptoms of serious arrhythmia: Permanently discontinue therapy.

Gastrointestinal:
Severe or intolerable nausea, vomiting, or diarrhea (despite appropriate management): Interrupt therapy until improved, then resume treatment with a 150 mg dose reduction.

Lipase or amylase elevation >2 times ULN: Interrupt therapy and monitor serum lipase and amylase; upon recovery to <1.5 times ULN, resume treatment with a 150 mg dose reduction.

Metabolic: Persistent hyperglycemia >250 mg/dL (despite optimal antihyperglycemic therapy): Interrupt therapy until hyperglycemia is adequately controlled, then resume therapy with a 150 mg dose reduction. If hyperglycemia cannot be controlled (with optimal medical management), discontinue ceritinib.

Pulmonary: Treatment-related interstitial lung disease/pneumonitis (any grade): Permanently discontinue therapy.

Administration
Ceritinib is associated with a moderate emetic potential (Roila 2016); antiemetics may be needed to prevent nausea and vomiting.

Administer orally on an empty stomach (at least 1 hour before or 2 hours after a meal).

Emetic Potential Moderate (30% to 90%).

Monitoring Parameters ALK positivity; renal function, liver function (ALT, AST, total bilirubin monthly and as clinically necessary, more frequently in patients who develop transaminase abnormalities), fasting blood glucose (baseline and as clinically necessary); lipase and amylase (baseline and periodically as clinically necessary); electrolytes (baseline and periodically thereafter); cardiac monitoring (heart rate and QTc interval; ECG in patients with heart failure, bradyarrhythmias, electrolyte abnormalities, or on concomitant medications known to prolong the QTc interval); blood pressure; signs/symptoms of gastrointestinal, pulmonary toxicity, and/or pancreatitis.

Dietary Considerations Avoid grapefruit and grapefruit juice.

Dosage Forms Excipient information presented when available (limited, particularly for generics); consult specific product labeling.
Capsule, Oral:
Zykadia: 150 mg [contains fd&c blue #2 (indigotine)]

♦ **Cerubidine** see DAUNOrubicin (Conventional) on page 530

♦ **Cesamet** see Nabilone on page 1293

Cetuximab (se TUK see mab)
Related Information
Common Toxicity Criteria on page 2242

Management of Chemotherapy-Induced Nausea and Vomiting in Adults on page 2253

Management of EGFR Inhibitor Toxicities: Dermatologic, Ocular, and Gastrointestinal on page 2291

Prevention of Chemotherapy-Induced Nausea and Vomiting in Children on page 2310

Brand Names: US Erbitux
Brand Names: Canada Erbitux
Index Terms C225; IMC-C225; MOAB C225

Pharmacologic Category Antineoplastic Agent, Epidermal Growth Factor Receptor (EGFR) Inhibitor; Antineoplastic Agent, Monoclonal Antibody

Use

Colorectal cancer, metastatic: Treatment of *KRAS* wild-type (without mutation), epidermal growth factor receptor (EGFR)-expressing metastatic colorectal cancer as determined by approved tests (in combination with FOLFIRI [irinotecan, fluorouracil, and leucovorin] as first-line treatment, in combination with irinotecan [in patients refractory to irinotecan-based chemotherapy], or as a single agent in patients who have failed irinotecan- and oxaliplatin-based chemotherapy or who are intolerant to irinotecan).

Limitation of use: Cetuximab is not indicated for the treatment of *RAS*-mutant colorectal cancer or when results of the *RAS* mutation tests are unknown.

Head and neck cancer, squamous cell: Treatment of squamous cell cancer of the head and neck (as a single agent for recurrent or metastatic disease after platinum-based chemotherapy failure; in combination with radiation therapy as initial treatment of locally or regionally advanced disease; in combination with platinum and fluorouracil-based chemotherapy as first-line treatment of locoregional or metastatic disease).

Labeled Contraindications

There are no contraindications listed in the manufacturer's US labeling.

Canadian labeling: Known severe hypersensitivity to cetuximab or any component of the formulation

Pregnancy Considerations Adverse events were observed in animal reproduction studies. Human IgG is known to cross the placenta. Because cetuximab inhibits epidermal growth factor (EGF), a component of fetal development, adverse effects on pregnancy would be expected. The manufacturer recommends that males and females use effective contraception during therapy and for 6 months following the last dose of cetuximab.

Breastfeeding Considerations It is not known if cetuximab is excreted in breast milk. IgG antibodies can be detected in breast milk. Due to the potential for serious adverse reactions in the nursing infant, the manufacturer recommends that the decision to discontinue cetuximab or discontinue breastfeeding should take into account the benefits of treatment to the mother. If breastfeeding is interrupted for cetuximab treatment, based on the half-life, breastfeeding should not be resumed for at least 60 days following the last cetuximab dose.

Warnings/Precautions [US Boxed Warning]: In clinical trials, serious infusion reactions have been reported in approximately 3% of patients; fatal outcome has been reported rarely (less than 1 in 1,000); interrupt infusion promptly and permanently discontinue for serious infusion reactions. Reactions have included airway obstruction (bronchospasm, stridor, hoarseness), hypotension, loss of consciousness, shock, myocardial infarction (MI), and/or cardiac arrest. Premedicate with an intravenous (IV) H_1 antagonist 30 to 60 minutes prior to the first dose; premedication for subsequent doses is based on clinical judgment and with consideration of prior reaction to the initial infusion. The use of nebulized albuterol-based premedication to prevent infusion reaction has been reported (Tra, 2008). Approximately 90% of reactions occur with the first infusion despite the use of prophylactic antihistamines. Immediate treatment for anaphylactic/anaphylactoid reactions should be available during administration. The manufacturer recommends monitoring patients for at least 1 hour following completion of infusion, or longer if a reaction occurs. Mild to moderate infusion reactions are managed by slowing the infusion rate (by 50%) and administering antihistamines. Patients with preexisting IgE antibody against cetuximab (specific for galactose-α-1,3-galactose) are reported to have a higher incidence of severe hypersensitivity reaction. Severe hypersensitivity reaction has been reported more frequently in patients living in the middle south area of the United States, including North Carolina and Tennessee (Chung, 2008; O'Neil, 2007).

[US Boxed Warning]: In patients with squamous cell head and neck cancer, cardiopulmonary arrest and/or sudden death has occurred in 2% of patients receiving radiation therapy in combination with cetuximab and in 3% of patients receiving combination chemotherapy (platinum and fluorouracil-based) with cetuximab. Closely monitor serum electrolytes (magnesium, potassium, calcium) during and after cetuximab treatment (monitor for at least 8 weeks after treatment). Use with caution in patients with history of coronary artery disease, heart failure, and arrhythmias; fatalities have been reported. Interstitial lung disease has been reported; use with caution in patients with preexisting lung disease; interrupt treatment for acute onset or worsening of pulmonary symptoms; permanently discontinue with confirmed interstitial lung disease.

Acneiform rash has been reported in 76% to 88% of patients (severe in 1% to 17%), usually developing within the first 2 weeks of therapy; may require dose modification; generally resolved after discontinuation in most patients, although persisted beyond 28 days in some patients. Acneiform rash should be treated with topical and/or oral antibiotics; topical corticosteroids are not recommended. In colorectal cancer, the presence of acneiform rash correlates with treatment response and prolonged survival (Cunningham, 2004). Life-threatening and fatal bullous mucocutaneous disease (with blisters, erosions, and skin sloughing) has been observed with cetuximab; etiology is not determined; may be due to EGFR inhibition or to idiosyncratic immune-related effects (eg, Stevens-Johnson syndrome, toxic epidermal necrolysis). Other dermatologic toxicities, including dry skin, fissures, hypertrichosis, paronychial inflammation, and skin infections, have been reported; related ocular toxicities (blepharitis, conjunctivitis, keratitis, ulcerative keratitis with decreased visual acuity) may also occur. Monitor closely for dermatologic toxicities and potential infectious sequelae. Sunlight may exacerbate skin reactions (limit sun exposure).

Hypomagnesemia is common (may be severe); the onset of electrolyte disturbance may occur within days to months after initiation of treatment; monitor magnesium, calcium, and potassium during treatment and for at least 8 weeks after completion; may require electrolyte replacement. Non-neutralizing anti-cetuximab antibodies were detected in 5% of evaluable patients. In a study of radiation therapy **and** cisplatin with or without cetuximab in patients with squamous cell head and neck cancer, an increase in the incidence of adverse reactions (eg, grade 3/4 mucositis, radiation recall, acneiform rash, electrolyte abnormalities, cardiac events including ischemia) was noted in patients receiving cetuximab, including fatal reactions; there was no improvement in the primary end point of progression-free survival.

In patients with colorectal cancer, cetuximab is only indicated for EGFR-expressing metastatic colorectal cancer without *RAS* (*KRAS* or *NRAS*) mutations. Determine *RAS* mutation status prior to treatment (with an approved test). Patients with a codon 12 and 13 (exon 2), codon 59 and 61 (exon 3), and codon 117 and 146 (exon 4) *RAS* mutation are unlikely to benefit from EGFR inhibitor therapy (while experiencing toxicities) and should not receive cetuximab treatment; cetuximab is not effective for colorectal cancer with RAS mutations. Cetuximab is also reported to be ineffective in patients with *BRAF* V600E mutation (Di Nicolantonio, 2008). The American Society of Clinical Oncology (ASCO) provisional clinical opinion (Allegra 2009) recommends genotyping tumor tissue for KRAS mutation in all patients with metastatic colorectal cancer (genotyping may be done on archived specimens). In trials for colorectal cancer, evidence of EGFR expression was required, although the response rate did not correlate with either the percentage of cells positive for EGFR or the intensity of expression. EGFR expression has been detected in nearly all patients with head and neck cancer; therefore laboratory evidence of EGFR expression is not necessary for head and neck cancers.

Adverse Reactions

>10%:

Central nervous system: Fatigue (91%), malaise (≤73%), pain (59%), peripheral sensory neuropathy (45%; grades 3/4: 1%), headache (19% to 38%), insomnia (27%), confusion (18%), chills (≤16%), rigors (≤16%), anxiety (14%), depression (14%)

Dermatologic: Desquamation (95%), acneiform eruption (15% to 88%; grades 3/4: 1% to 18%), radiodermatitis (86%), xeroderma (14% to 57%), pruritus (14% to 47%), skin rash (28% to 44%), changes in nails (31%), acne vulgaris (14% to 22%), paronychia (20%), palmar-plantar erythrodysesthesia (19%), skin fissure (19%), alopecia (12%)

Endocrine & metabolic: Weight loss (15% to 84%), hypomagnesemia (6% to 55%), dehydration (13% to 25%), hypocalcemia (12%), hypokalemia (12%)

Gastrointestinal: Diarrhea (19% to 72%), nausea (49% to 64%), abdominal pain (59%), constipation (53%), vomiting (40%), stomatitis (31% to 32%), anorexia (25% to 30%), dyspepsia (14% to 16%), xerostomia (12%)

Hematologic & oncologic: Neutropenia (49%; grades 3/4: 31%), leukopenia (grades 3/4: 17%)

Hepatic: Increased serum ALT (43%), increased serum AST (38%), increased serum alkaline phosphatase (33%)

Infection: Infection (13% to 44%), infection without neutropenia (38%)

Local: Application site reaction (18%)

Neuromuscular & skeletal: Weakness (≤73%), ostealgia (15%), arthralgia (14%)

Ophthalmic: Conjunctivitis (10% to 18%)

Respiratory: Dyspnea (49%), cough (30%), pharyngitis (26%)

Miscellaneous: Fever (22% to 29%), infusion related reaction (10% to 18%; grades 3/4: 2% to 5%)

1% to 10%:

Cardiovascular: Cardiorespiratory arrest (2% to 3%), ischemic heart disease (2%)

Dermatologic: Hypertrichosis

Gastrointestinal: Dysgeusia (10%)

Immunologic: Antibody development (5%)

Infection: Sepsis (1% to 4%)

Renal: Renal failure (1%: colorectal cancer patients; frequency not defined in other populations)

<1%, postmarketing, and/or case reports: Abscess, aseptic meningitis, blepharitis, bronchospasm, bullous pemphigoid, cardiac arrhythmia, cellulitis, cheilitis, corneal ulcer, electrolyte disturbance, hoarseness, hypotension,

interstitial pulmonary disease, keratitis, loss of consciousness, mucosal inflammation, myocardial infarction, pulmonary embolism, shock, skin infection, Stevens-Johnson syndrome, stridor, toxic epidermal necrolysis

Drug Interactions

Metabolism/Transport Effects None known.

Avoid Concomitant Use There are no known interactions where it is recommended to avoid concomitant use.

Increased Effect/Toxicity There are no known significant interactions involving an increase in effect.

Decreased Effect There are no known significant interactions involving a decrease in effect.

Storage/Stability Store intact vials refrigerated at 2°C to 8°C (36°F to 46°F); do not freeze. Preparations in infusion containers are stable for up to 12 hours refrigerated at 2°C to 8°C (36°F to 46°F) and up to 8 hours at room temperature of 20°C to 25°C (68°F to 77°F).

Preparation for Administration Reconstitution is not required. Appropriate dose should be added to empty sterile container (may contain a small amount of visible white, amorphous cetuximab particles); do not shake or dilute. Discard unused portion of the vial; discard any remaining solution in infusion container after 8 hours at room temperature or after 12 hours refrigerated.

Mechanism of Action Recombinant human/mouse chimeric monoclonal antibody which binds specifically to the epidermal growth factor receptor (EGFR, HER1, c-ErbB-1) and competitively inhibits the binding of epidermal growth factor (EGF) and other ligands. Binding to the EGFR blocks phosphorylation and activation of receptor-associated kinases, resulting in inhibition of cell growth, induction of apoptosis, and decreased matrix metalloproteinase and vascular endothelial growth factor production. EGFR signal transduction results in *RAS* wild-type activation; cells with *RAS* mutations appear to be unaffected by EGFR inhibition.

Pharmacodynamics/Kinetics

Distribution: V_d: ~2 to 3 L/m^2

Half-life elimination: ~112 hours (range: 63 to 230 hours)

Dosing

Adult & Geriatric Note: Premedicate with an H_1 antagonist (eg, diphenhydramine) IV 30 to 60 minutes prior to the first dose; premedication for subsequent doses is based on clinical judgment.

Colorectal cancer, metastatic, KRAS wild-type (without mutation): IV:

Initial loading dose: 400 mg/m^2 infused over 120 minutes

Maintenance dose: 250 mg/m^2 infused over 60 minutes weekly until disease progression or unacceptable toxicity

Note: If given in combination with FOLFIRI (irinotecan, fluorouracil, and leucovorin), complete cetuximab infusion 1 hour prior to FOLFIRI.

Head and neck cancer (squamous cell): IV:

Initial loading dose: 400 mg/m^2 infused over 120 minutes

Maintenance dose: 250 mg/m^2 infused over 60 minutes weekly

Note: If given in combination with radiation therapy, administer loading dose 1 week prior to initiation of radiation course; weekly maintenance dose should be completed 1 hour prior to radiation for the duration of radiation therapy (6 to 7 weeks). If given in combination with chemotherapy, administer loading dose on the day of initiation of platinum and fluorouracil-based chemotherapy, cetuximab infusion should be completed 1 hour prior to initiation of chemotherapy; weekly maintenance dose should be completed 1 hour prior to chemotherapy; continue until disease progression or unacceptable toxicity. Monotherapy weekly doses should be continued until disease progression or unacceptable toxicity

Colorectal cancer, advanced, biweekly administration (off-label dosing): IV: 500 mg/m^2 every 2 weeks (initial dose infused over 120 minutes, subsequent doses infused over 60 minutes) in combination with irinotecan (Pfeiffer 2008)

Non-small cell lung cancer (NSCLC), EGFR-expressing, advanced (off-label use): IV: Initial loading dose: 400 mg/m^2, followed by maintenance dose: 250 mg/m^2 weekly in combination with cisplatin and vinorelbine for up to 6 cycles, then as monotherapy until disease progression or unacceptable toxicity (Pirker 2009; Pirker 2012)

Squamous cell skin cancer, unresectable (off-label use): IV: Initial loading dose: 400 mg/m^2, followed by maintenance dose: 250 mg/m^2 weekly until disease progression (Maubec 2011)

Renal Impairment There are no dosage adjustments provided in the manufacturer's labeling.

Hepatic Impairment There are no dosage adjustments provided in the manufacturer's labeling.

Adjustment for Toxicity

Infusion reactions, grade 1 or 2 and nonserious grade 3: Reduce the infusion rate by 50% and continue to use prophylactic antihistamines

Infusion reactions, severe: Immediately and permanently discontinue treatment

Pulmonary toxicity:

Acute onset or worsening pulmonary symptoms: Hold treatment

Interstitial lung disease: Permanently discontinue

Skin toxicity, mild to moderate: No dosage modification required

Acneiform rash, severe (grade 3 or 4):

First occurrence: Delay cetuximab infusion 1 to 2 weeks

If improvement, continue at 250 mg/m^2

If no improvement, discontinue therapy

Second occurrence: Delay cetuximab infusion 1 to 2 weeks

If improvement, continue at reduced dose of 200 mg/m^2

If no improvement, discontinue therapy

Third occurrence: Delay cetuximab infusion 1 to 2 weeks

If improvement, continue at reduced dose of 150 mg/m^2

If no improvement, discontinue therapy

Fourth occurrence: Discontinue therapy

Combination Regimens

Colorectal cancer:

Cetuximab (Biweekly)-Irinotecan (Colorectal) on page 2029

Cetuximab + FOLFIRI (Colorectal) on page 2031

Cetuximab-Irinotecan (Colorectal) on page 2032

Head and neck cancer:

Carboplatin-Cetuximab (Head and Neck Cancer) on page 2011

Cetuximab-Carboplatin-Fluorouracil (Head and Neck Cancer) on page 2030

Cetuximab-Cisplatin-Fluorouracil (Head and Neck Cancer) on page 2030

Cisplatin-Cetuximab (Head and Neck Cancer) on page 2037

Paclitaxel-Cetuximab on page 2183

Lung cancer, non-small cell: Cetuximab-Cisplatin-Vinorelbine (NSCLC) on page 2031

Administration Administer via IV infusion; loading dose over 2 hours, weekly maintenance dose over 1 hour. Do not administer as IV push or bolus. Do not shake or dilute. Administer via infusion pump or syringe pump. Following the infusion, an observation period (1 hour) is recommended; longer observation time (following an infusion reaction) may be required. Premedication with an H_1 antagonist prior to the initial dose is recommended. The maximum infusion rate is 10 mg/minute. Administer through a low protein-binding 0.22 micrometer in-line filter.

For biweekly administration (off-label frequency and dose), the initial dose was infused over 120 minutes and subsequent doses infused over 60 minutes (Pfeiffer 2007; Pfeiffer 2008).

Emetic Potential Children and Adults: Minimal (<10%)

Monitoring Parameters Vital signs during infusion and observe for at least 1 hour postinfusion. Patients developing dermatologic toxicities should be monitored for the development of complications. Periodic monitoring of serum magnesium, calcium, and potassium are recommended to continue over an interval consistent with the half-life (8 weeks); monitor closely (during and after treatment) for cetuximab plus radiation therapy. *KRAS* genotyping of tumor tissue in patients with colorectal cancer

Dosage Forms Excipient information presented when available (limited, particularly for generics); consult specific product labeling.

Solution, Intravenous [preservative free]:

Erbitux: 100 mg/50 mL (50 mL); 200 mg/100 mL (100 mL) [contains galactose-alpha-1,3-galactose]

Chlorambucil (klor AM byoo sil)

Related Information

Management of Chemotherapy-Induced Nausea and Vomiting in Adults *on page 2253*

Prevention of Chemotherapy-Induced Nausea and Vomiting in Children *on page 2310*

Safe Handling of Hazardous Drugs *on page 2379*

Brand Names: US Leukeran

Brand Names: Canada Leukeran

Index Terms CB-1348; Chlorambucilum; Chloraminophene; Chlorbutinum; WR-139013

Pharmacologic Category Antineoplastic Agent, Alkylating Agent; Antineoplastic Agent, Alkylating Agent (Nitrogen Mustard)

Use

Chronic lymphocytic leukemia: Management of chronic lymphocytic leukemia (CLL)

Lymphomas: Management of Hodgkin lymphoma (HL) and non-Hodgkin lymphomas (NHL)

Labeled Contraindications Hypersensitivity to chlorambucil or any component of the formulation; hypersensitivity to other alkylating agents (may have cross-hypersensitivity); prior (demonstrated) resistance to chlorambucil

Canadian labeling: Additional contraindications (not in US labeling): Use within 4 weeks of a full course of radiation or chemotherapy

Pregnancy Considerations Animal reproduction studies have demonstrated teratogenicity. Chlorambucil crosses the human placenta. Following exposure during the first trimester, case reports have noted adverse renal effects (unilateral agenesis). Women of childbearing potential should avoid becoming pregnant while receiving treatment. **[U.S. Boxed Warning]: Affects human fertility; probably mutagenic and teratogenic as well;** chromosomal damage has been documented. Reversible and irreversible sterility (when administered to prepubertal and pubertal males), azoospermia (in adult males) and amenorrhea (in females) have been observed. Fibrosis, vasculitis and depletion of primordial follicles have been noted on autopsy of the ovaries.

Breastfeeding Considerations It is not known if chlorambucil is excreted in breast milk. Due to the potential for serious adverse reactions in the nursing infant, the decision to discontinue chlorambucil or to discontinue breastfeeding should take into account the benefits of treatment to the mother.

Warnings/Precautions Seizures have been observed; use with caution in patients with seizure disorder or head trauma; history of nephrotic syndrome and high pulse doses are at higher risk of seizures. **[U.S. Boxed Warning]: May cause severe bone marrow suppression;** neutropenia may be severe. Reduce initial dosage if patient has received myelosuppressive or radiation therapy within the previous 4 weeks, or has a depressed baseline leukocyte or platelet count. Irreversible bone marrow damage may occur with total doses approaching 6.5 mg/kg. Progressive lymphopenia may develop (recovery is generally rapid after discontinuation). Avoid administration of live vaccines to immunocompromised patients. Rare instances of severe skin reactions (eg, erythema multiforme, Stevens-Johnson syndrome, toxic epidermal necrolysis) have been reported; discontinue promptly if skin reaction occurs.

Chlorambucil is primarily metabolized in the liver. Dosage reductions should be considered in patients with hepatic impairment. **[U.S. Boxed Warning]: Affects human fertility; carcinogenic in humans and probably mutagenic and teratogenic as well;** chromosomal damage has been documented. Reversible and irreversible sterility (when administered to prepubertal and pubertal males), azoospermia (in adult males) and amenorrhea (in females) have been observed. **[U.S. Boxed Warning]: Carcinogenic;** acute myelocytic leukemia and secondary malignancies may be associated with chronic therapy. Duration of treatment and higher cumulative doses are associated with a higher risk for development of leukemia. Potentially significant drug-drug interactions may exist, requiring dose or frequency adjustment, additional monitoring, and/or selection of alternative therapy.

Adverse Reactions Frequency not defined.

Central nervous system: Drug fever, peripheral neuropathy

Dermatologic: Allergic skin reaction, skin rash, urticaria

Endocrine & metabolic: Amenorrhea

Gastrointestinal: Diarrhea (infrequent), nausea (infrequent), oral mucosa ulcer (infrequent), vomiting (infrequent)

Genitourinary: Azoospermia, cystitis (sterile), infertility

Hematologic & oncologic: Anemia, bone marrow depression, bone marrow failure (irreversible), leukemia (secondary), leukopenia, lymphocytopenia, malignant neoplasm (secondary), neutropenia (onset: 3 weeks; recovery: 10 days after last dose), pancytopenia, thrombocytopenia

Hepatic: Hepatotoxicity, jaundice

Hypersensitivity: Angioedema, hypersensitivity reaction

Respiratory: Interstitial pneumonitis, pulmonary fibrosis

Miscellaneous: Fever

1%, postmarketing, and/or case reports: Agitation, ataxia, confusion, erythema multiforme, flaccid paralysis, seizure (focal/generalized), hallucination, muscle twitching, myoclonus, SIADH (syndrome of inappropriate antidiuretic hormone secretion), Stevens-Johnson syndrome, toxic epidermal necrolysis, tremor

Drug Interactions

Metabolism/Transport Effects None known.

Avoid Concomitant Use

Avoid concomitant use of Chlorambucil with any of the following: BCG (Intravesical); Deferiprone; Dipyrone; Natalizumab; Pimecrolimus; Tacrolimus (Topical); Vaccines (Live)

Increased Effect/Toxicity

Chlorambucil may increase the levels/effects of: CloZAPine; Deferiprone; Fingolimod; Leflunomide; Natalizumab; Tofacitinib; Vaccines (Live)

The levels/effects of Chlorambucil may be increased by: Denosumab; Dipyrone; Ocrelizumab; Palifermin; Pimecrolimus; Promazine; Roflumilast; Tacrolimus (Topical); Trastuzumab

Decreased Effect

Chlorambucil may decrease the levels/effects of: BCG (Intravesical); Coccidioides immitis Skin Test; Lenograstim; Nivolumab; Sipuleucel-T; Tertomotide; Vaccines (Inactivated); Vaccines (Live)

The levels/effects of Chlorambucil may be decreased by: Echinacea

Food Interactions Absorption is decreased when administered with food. Management: Administer preferably on an empty stomach.

Hazardous Drugs Handling Considerations

Hazardous agent (NIOSH 2016 [group 1]).

Use appropriate precautions for receiving, handling, administration, and disposal. Gloves (single) should be worn during receiving, unpacking, and placing in storage.

NIOSH recommends single gloving for administration of intact tablets or capsules. If manipulating tablets/capsules (eg, to prepare an oral suspension), NIOSH recommends double gloving, a protective gown, and preparation in a controlled device; if not prepared in a controlled device, respiratory and eye/face protection as well as ventilated engineering controls are recommended. NIOSH recommends double gloving, a protective gown, and (if there is a potential for vomit or spit up) eye/face protection for administration of an oral liquid/feeding tube administration (NIOSH 2016).

Storage/Stability Store in refrigerator at 2°C to 8°C (36°F to 46°F).

Mechanism of Action Alkylating agent; interferes with DNA replication and RNA transcription by alkylation and cross-linking the strands of DNA

◄ **Pharmacodynamics/Kinetics**
Absorption: Rapid and complete (>70%) from GI tract; reduced with food
Distribution: V_d: ~0.3 L/kg
Protein binding: ~99%; primarily to albumin
Metabolism: Hepatic (extensively); primarily to active metabolite, phenylacetic acid mustard
Half-life elimination: ~1.5 hours; Phenylacetic acid mustard: ~1.8 hours
Time to peak, plasma: Within 1 hour; Phenylacetic acid mustard: Within 1.9 ± 0.7 hours
Excretion: Urine (~20% to 60% within 24 hours, primarily as inactive metabolites, <1% as unchanged drug or phenylacetic acid mustard)

Dosing
Adult Note: Reduce initial dose if full-dose radiation or myelotoxic drugs have been administered within the last month. With bone marrow lymphocytic infiltration involvement (in CLL, Hodgkin lymphoma, or NHL), the maximum dose is 0.1 mg/kg/day. While short treatment courses are preferred, if maintenance therapy is required, the maximum dose is 0.1 mg/kg/day.
Chronic lymphocytic leukemia (CLL): Oral: 0.1 mg/kg/day for 3 to 6 weeks **or** 0.4 mg/kg pulsed doses administered intermittently, biweekly, or monthly (increased by 0.1 mg/kg/dose until response/toxicity observed)
CLL (off-label dosing): 0.4 mg/kg day 1 every 2 weeks; if tolerated may increase by 0.1 mg/kg with each treatment course to a maximum dose of 0.8 mg/kg and maximum of 24 cycles (Eichhorst 2009) **or** 30 mg/m² day 1 every 2 weeks (in combination with prednisone) (Raphael 1991) **or** 40 mg/m² day 1 every 4 weeks until disease progression or complete remission or response plateau for up to a maximum of 12 cycles (Rai 2000)
CLL in previously untreated patients (off-label combinations): Oral:
In combination with obinutuzumab: 0.5 mg/kg on days 1 and 15 every 28 days for 6 cycles (Goede 2014)
In combination with ofatumumab: 10 mg/m² once daily for 7 days (days 1 to 7) every 28 days for a minimum of 3 cycles and up to 12 cycles or best response (clinical response that did not improve after 3 additional cycles); if necessary, reduce dose to 7.5 mg/m²/day and then to 5 mg/m²/day for hematologic toxicity (Hillmen 2015)
Hodgkin lymphoma: Oral: 0.2 mg/kg/day for 3 to 6 weeks
Non-Hodgkin lymphomas (NHL): Oral: 0.1 mg/kg/day for 3 to 6 weeks
Waldenström macroglobulinemia (off-label use): Oral: 0.1 mg/kg/day (continuously) for at least 6 months **or** 0.3 mg/kg/day for 7 days every 6 weeks for at least 6 months (Kyle 2000)
Geriatric Refer to adult dosing. Begin at the lower end of dosing range(s)
Pediatric Nephrotic syndrome, steroid sensitive (off-label use): Oral: 0.2 mg/kg once daily for ~8 weeks (Hodson 2010)
Renal Impairment There are no dosage adjustments provided in the manufacturer's labeling; however, renal elimination of unchanged chlorambucil and active metabolite (phenylacetic acid mustard) is minimal and renal impairment is not likely to affect elimination. The following adjustments have been recommended: Adults:
Aronoff 2007:
CrCl >50 mL/minute: No adjustment necessary.
CrCl 10 to 50 mL/minute: Administer 75% of dose.
CrCl <10 mL/minute: Administer 50% of dose.
Peritoneal dialysis (PD): Administer 50% of dose.

Kintzel 1995: Based on the pharmacokinetics, dosage adjustment is not indicated

Hepatic Impairment Chlorambucil undergoes extensive hepatic metabolism. Although dosage reduction should be considered in patients with hepatic impairment, there are no dosage adjustments provided in the manufacturer's labeling (data is insufficient).

Obesity *ASCO Guidelines for appropriate chemotherapy dosing in obese adults with cancer:* Utilize patient's actual body weight (full weight) for calculation of body surface area- or weight-based dosing, particularly when the intent of therapy is curative; manage regimen-related toxicities in the same manner as for nonobese patients; if a dose reduction is utilized due to toxicity, consider resumption of full weight-based dosing with subsequent cycles, especially if cause of toxicity (eg, hepatic or renal impairment) is resolved (Griggs, 2012). **Note:** The manufacturer recommends the maximum dose should not exceed 0.1 mg/kg/day if maintenance therapy is required and with bone marrow infiltration.

Adjustment for Toxicity
Skin reactions: Discontinue treatment
Hematologic:
WBC or platelets below normal: Reduce dose.
Severely depressed WBC or platelet counts: Discontinue.
Persistently low neutrophil or platelet counts or peripheral lymphocytosis: May be suggestive of bone marrow infiltration; if infiltration confirmed, do not exceed 0.1 mg/kg/day.
Concurrent or within 4 weeks (before or after) of chemotherapy/radiotherapy: Initiate treatment cautiously; reduce dose; monitor closely.

Combination Regimens
Leukemia, chronic lymphocytic:
Chlorambucil-Obinutuzumab (CLL) on page 2034
Chlorambucil-Ofatumumab (CLL) on page 2034
Chlorambucil-Prednisone (CLL) on page 2035
Lymphoma, Hodgkin: ChIVPP (Hodgkin) on page 2033

Administration Oral: May be administered as a single daily dose.

Emetic Potential Children and Adults: Minimal (<10%)

Extemporaneous Preparations A 2 mg/mL oral suspension may be prepared with tablets. Crush sixty 2 mg tablets in a mortar and reduce to a fine powder. Add small portions of methylcellulose 1% and mix to a uniform paste (total methylcellulose: 30 mL); mix while adding simple syrup in incremental proportions to **almost** 60 mL; transfer to a graduated cylinder, rinse mortar and pestle with simple syrup, and add quantity of vehicle sufficient to make 60 mL. Transfer contents of graduated cylinder to an amber prescription bottle. Label "shake well", "refrigerate", and "protect from light". Stable for 7 days refrigerated.

Dressman JB and Poust RI. Stability of Allopurinol and of Five Antineoplastics in Suspension. *Am J Hosp Pharm.* 1983;40(4):616-618.

Nahata MC, Pai VB, and Hipple TF. *Pediatric Drug Formulations,* 5th ed, Cincinnati, OH: Harvey Whitney Books Co, 2004.

Monitoring Parameters Liver function tests, CBC with differential (weekly, with WBC monitored twice weekly during the first 3 to 6 weeks of treatment)

Dosage Forms Excipient information presented when available (limited, particularly for generics); consult specific product labeling.
Tablet, Oral:
Leukeran: 2 mg

- ◆ **Chlorambucilum** *see* Chlorambucil *on page 383*
- ◆ **Chloraminophene** *see* Chlorambucil *on page 383*
- ◆ **Chlorbutinum** *see* Chlorambucil *on page 383*
- ◆ **Chlorethazine** *see* Mechlorethamine (Systemic) *on page 1168*
- ◆ **Chlorethazine Mustard** *see* Mechlorethamine (Systemic) *on page 1168*
- ◆ **Chlormeprazine** *see* Prochlorperazine *on page 1563*
- ◆ **2-Chlorodeoxyadenosine** *see* Cladribine *on page 411*

ChlorproMAZINE (klor PROE ma zeen)

Brand Names: Canada Chlorpromazine Hydrochloride Inj; Teva-Chlorpromazine

Index Terms Chlorpromazine HCl; Chlorpromazine Hydrochloride; CPZ; Thorazine

Pharmacologic Category Antimanic Agent; First Generation (Typical) Antipsychotic; Phenothiazine Derivative

Use

Behavioral problems: Treatment of severe behavioral problems in children 1 to 12 years of age marked by combativeness and/or explosive hyperexcitable behavior (out of proportion to immediate provocations).

Bipolar disorder: Treatment of manic episodes associated with bipolar disorder.

Hiccups: Treatment of intractable hiccups.

Hyperactivity: Short-term treatment of hyperactive children who show excessive motor activity with accompanying conduct disorders consisting of some or all of the following symptoms: impulsivity, difficulty sustaining attention, aggressiveness, mood lability, and poor frustration tolerance.

Nausea/Vomiting: Management of nausea and vomiting.

Porphyria, acute intermittent: Treatment of acute intermittent porphyria.

Schizophrenia/Psychotic disorders: Treatment of schizophrenia and psychotic disorders.

Surgery: Management of restlessness and apprehension prior to surgery.

Tetanus: Adjunctive therapy in the treatment of tetanus.

Dosing

Adult

Bipolar disorder/psychotic disorders/schizophrenia:

Oral: Range: 30 to 800 mg daily in 2 to 4 divided doses, initiate at lower doses and titrate as needed; usual dose: 200 to 800 mg daily; some patients may require 1 to 2 g daily, however, therapeutic gain is limited at doses >1 g daily

IM: Initial: 25 mg, may repeat (25 to 50 mg) in 1 hour, gradually increase to a maximum of 400 mg/dose every 4 to 6 hours until symptoms are controlled; usual dose: 200 to 800 mg daily

Intractable hiccups:

Oral: 25 to 50 mg 3 to 4 times daily

IM (refractory to oral treatment): 25 to 50 mg; **Note:** If symptoms persist after one dose, administer IV dose.

IV (refractory to oral or IM treatment): 25 to 50 mg via slow IV infusion

Nausea and vomiting:

Oral: 10 to 25 mg every 4 to 6 hours as needed

IM: Initial: 25 mg; if no hypotension occurs, can administer 25 to 50 mg every 3 to 4 hours as needed until vomiting stops

During surgery: Initial: 12.5 mg; repeat in 30 minutes if necessary and if no hypotension occurs

IV (during surgery): 2 mg per fractional injection at 2 minute intervals using a 1 mg/mL solution; do not exceed 25 mg

Porphyria, acute intermittent:

Oral: 25 to 50 mg 3 to 4 times daily; usually may be discontinued after several weeks although maintenance therapy may be necessary

IM: 25 mg 3 or 4 times daily (until patient can tolerate oral administration)

Presurgical apprehension:

Oral: 25 to 50 mg 2 to 3 hours prior to surgery

IM: 12.5 to 25 mg 1 to 2 hours prior to surgery

Tetanus:

IM: 25 to 50 mg 3 or 4 times daily; titrate to response

IV: 25 to 50 mg

Discontinuation of therapy: The manufacturer and American Psychiatric Association (APA), Canadian Psychiatric Association (CPA), and World Federation of Societies of Biological Psychiatry (WFSBP) guidelines recommend gradually tapering antipsychotics to avoid withdrawal symptoms and minimize the risk of relapse (APA [Lehman 2004]; Cerovecki 2013; CPA [Addington 2005]; WFSBP [Hasan 2012]); risk for withdrawal symptoms may be highest with highly anti-cholinergic or dopaminergic antipsychotics (Cerovecki 2013). When stopping antipsychotic therapy in patients with schizophrenia, the CPA guidelines recommend a gradual taper over 6 to 24 months, and the APA guidelines recommend reducing the dose by 10% each month (APA [Lehman 2004]; CPA [Addington 2005]). Continuing anti-parkinsonism agents for a brief period after discontinuation may prevent withdrawal symptoms (Cerovecki 2013). When switching antipsychotics, three strategies have been suggested: Cross-titration (gradually discontinuing the first antipsychotic while gradually increasing the new antipsychotic), overlap and taper (maintaining the dose of the first antipsychotic while gradually increasing the new antipsychotic, then tapering the first antipsychotic), and abrupt change (abruptly discontinuing the first antipsychotic and either increasing the new antipsychotic gradually or starting it at a treatment dose). Evidence supporting ideal switch strategies and taper rates is limited, and results are conflicting (Cerovecki 2013; Remington 2005).

Geriatric

Manufacturer's labeling: Oral, IM, IV: Dosages in the lower range of recommended adult dosing are generally sufficient. Titrate dosage slowly and monitor carefully.

Alternate dosing: Psychotic disorders: Oral: Routine use is not recommended; however, if used, the following doses have been used: Initial: 10 to 25 mg 3 times daily (Denham 1980; Gareri 2003; Salzman 2005); titrate dose slowly. Usual dosage range: 50 to 200 mg daily in divided doses (Salzman 2005). Mean dosage range: 25 to 75 mg daily in divided doses (Gareri 2003). Doses greater than 300 to 400 mg/day are rarely necessary (Denham 1980). **Note:** IM administration may be used in the very acutely disturbed patient (Denham 1980). IM doses are approximately 4 times more potent than comparable oral doses (ie, 25 mg IM is approximately equivalent to 100 mg oral) (Salzman 2005).

Psychosis/agitation associated with dementia (off-label use): Oral: Initial: One-third to one-half the usual dose to treat psychosis in younger adults or the smallest available dosage. In patients without a clinically significant response after 4 weeks, taper and withdraw therapy. In patients with an adequate response, attempt to taper and withdraw therapy within 4 months, unless symptoms recurred with a previous taper attempt. Assess symptoms at least monthly during taper and for at least 4 months after withdrawal of therapy (APA [Reus 2016]).

Pediatric

Behavior problems; severe: Note: Begin with low doses and gradually titrate as needed to lowest effective dose; route of administration should be determined by severity of symptoms.

Infants ≥6 months, Children, and Adolescents weighing ≤45.5 kg:

Oral: Initial: 0.55 mg/kg/dose every 4 to 6 hours as needed; may titrate as required; in severe cases, higher doses may be required (50 to 100 mg daily); in older children, higher daily doses (200 mg daily or higher) may be necessary; maximum daily dose: 500 mg/**day**; daily doses >500 mg have not been shown to further improve behavior in pediatric patients with severe mental impairment

IM, IV (off-label): Initial: 0.55 mg/kg/dose every 6 to 8 hours as needed; may titrate as required in severe cases (Kliegman, 2007)

Maximum recommended daily doses:

Children <5 years or weighing <22.7 kg: 40 mg/**day**

Children ≥5 years and Adolescents or weighing 22.7 to 45.5 kg: 75 mg/**day**

Adolescents weighing >45.5 kg:

Oral: Range: 30 to 800 mg daily in 2 to 4 divided doses, initiate at lower doses and titrate as needed; usual dose is 200 mg daily

IM, IV (off-label): 25 mg initially, may repeat (25 to 50 mg) in 1 to 4 hours, gradually increase to a maximum of 400 mg/dose every 4 to 6 hours until symptoms are controlled; usual dose 200 to 800 mg daily (Kliegman 2007)

Nausea and vomiting, treatment (non-CINV):

Infants ≥6 months, Children, and Adolescents weighing ≤45.5 kg: Oral, IM, IV: 0.55 mg/kg/dose every 6 to 8 hours as needed; in severe cases, higher doses may be needed; usual maximum daily dose: IM, IV:

Children <5 years or weighing <22.7 kg: 40 mg/**day**

Children ≥5 years or weighing 22.7 to 45.5 kg: 75 mg/**day**

Adolescents weighing >45.5 kg:

Oral: 10 to 25 mg every 4 to 6 hours as needed

IM, IV: Initial: 25 mg; if tolerated (no hypotension), then may give 25 to 50 mg every 4 to 6 hours as needed

Prevention of chemotherapy-associated nausea and vomiting (Pediatric Oncology Group of Ontario [POGO] dosing recommendation): Highly or moderately emetogenic chemotherapy (patients who cannot receive corticosteroids): Infants ≥6 months, Children, and Adolescents: IV: 0.5 mg/kg/dose every 6 hours (in combination with ondansetron or granisetron); if not controlled, may increase up to 1 mg/kg/dose; monitor for sedation, maximum dose: 50 mg (Dupuis, 2013)

Presurgical apprehension: Infants ≥6 months, Children, and Adolescents: Oral: 0.55 mg/kg 2 to 3 hours prior to surgery; maximum dose 50 mg

IM: 0.55 mg/kg/dose 1 to 2 hours prior to surgery; maximum dose 25 mg

Tetanus:
Infants ≥6 months, Children, and Adolescents weighing ≤45.5 kg: IM, IV: 0.55 mg/kg/dose every 6 to 8 hours; in severe cases higher doses may be needed:
Usual maximum daily dose:
Weight <22.7 kg: 40 mg/**day**
Weight 22.7 to 45.5 kg: 75 mg/**day**, except in severe cases
Adolescents weighing ≥45.5 kg: IM, IV: 25 to 50 mg given 3 or 4 times daily; begin with low dose titrate to response

Renal Impairment There are no dosage adjustments provided in the manufacturer's labeling; use with caution. Not dialyzable (0% to 5%)

Hepatic Impairment There are no dosage adjustments provided in the manufacturer's labeling; use with caution.

Additional Information Complete prescribing information should be consulted for additional detail.

Dosage Forms Excipient information presented when available (limited, particularly for generics); consult specific product labeling.
Solution, Injection, as hydrochloride:
Generic: 25 mg/mL (1 mL); 50 mg/2 mL (2 mL)
Tablet, Oral, as hydrochloride:
Generic: 10 mg, 25 mg, 50 mg, 100 mg, 200 mg

◆ **Chlorpromazine HCl** see ChlorproMAZINE on page 388

◆ **Chlorpromazine Hydrochloride** see ChlorproMAZINE on page 388

◆ **Chlorpromazine Hydrochloride Inj (Can)** see ChlorproMAZINE on page 388

Choline C 11 (KOH leen see E lev en)

Index Terms 11 C-Choline; Carbon-11 Choline

Pharmacologic Category Radiopharmaceutical

Use Prostate imaging: Radiopharmaceutical imaging agent used in conjunction with positron emission tomography (PET) for patients with suspected prostate cancer recurrence and noninformative bone scintigraphy, computerized tomography (CT), or magnetic resonance imaging (MRI).

Pregnancy Risk Factor C

Dosing
Adult & Geriatric Note: Total injection volume per patient will vary based on patient body dimensions and the characteristics of the image acquisition system.
Prostate imaging: IV: 10 to 20 mCi (370 to 740 MBq)

Renal Impairment There are no dosage adjustments provided in the manufacturer's labeling.

Hepatic Impairment There are no dosage adjustments provided in the manufacturer's labeling.

Additional Information Complete prescribing information should be consulted for additional detail.

Dosage Forms Excipient information presented when available (limited, particularly for generics); consult specific product labeling.
Injection, solution: 148 to 1225 megabecquerels (4 to 33.1 mCi) per 1 mL (10 mL)

◆ **Ciclosporin** see CycloSPORINE (Systemic) on page 452

♦ **Cilastatin and Imipenem** *see* Imipenem and Cilastatin *on page 983*

Cinacalcet (sin a KAL cet)

Brand Names: US Sensipar
Brand Names: Canada Sensipar
Index Terms AMG 073; Cinacalcet Hydrochloride
Pharmacologic Category Calcimimetic
Use
Hyperparathyroidism, primary: Treatment of hypercalcemia in adults with primary hyperparathyroidism for whom parathyroidectomy would be indicated on the basis of serum calcium levels, but who are unable to undergo parathyroidectomy.

Hyperparathyroidism, secondary: Treatment of secondary hyperparathyroidism in adults with chronic kidney disease (CKD) on dialysis.

Parathyroid carcinoma: Treatment of hypercalcemia in adults with parathyroid carcinoma.

Dosing
Adult & Geriatric
Hyperparathyroidism, primary: Oral: Initial: 30 mg twice daily; increase dose incrementally every 2 to 4 weeks (to 60 mg twice daily, 90 mg twice daily, and 90 mg 3 or 4 times daily) as necessary to normalize serum calcium levels.

Hyperparathyroidism, secondary: Oral: Initial: 30 mg once daily; increase dose incrementally every 2 to 4 weeks (to 60 mg once daily, 90 mg once daily, 120 mg once daily, and 180 mg once daily) as necessary to maintain intact parathyroid hormone (iPTH) level between 150 to 300 pg/mL. May be used alone or in combination with vitamin D and/or phosphate binders.

Parathyroid carcinoma: Oral: Initial: 30 mg twice daily; increase dose incrementally every 2 to 4 weeks (to 60 mg twice daily, 90 mg twice daily, and 90 mg 3 to 4 times daily) as necessary to normalize serum calcium levels.

Renal Impairment No dosage adjustment necessary.

Hepatic Impairment
Mild impairment (Child-Pugh class A): No dosage adjustment necessary.

Moderate to severe impairment (Child-Pugh class B or C): There are no specific dosage adjustments provided in the manufacturer's labeling; exposure and half-life of cinacalcet is increased. Dosage adjustments may be necessary based on serum calcium, serum phosphorus, and/or intact parathyroid hormone (iPTH).

Adjustment for Toxicity Dosage adjustment for hypocalcemia:
If iPTH <150 pg/mL: Reduce dose or discontinue cinacalcet and/or vitamin D.

Hyperparathyroidism, secondary:
If serum calcium >7.5 mg/dL but <8.4 mg/dL **or** if hypocalcemia symptoms occur: Use calcium-containing phosphate binders and/or vitamin D to raise calcium levels.

If serum calcium <7.5 mg/dL **or** if hypocalcemia symptoms persist and the dose of vitamin D cannot be increased: Withhold cinacalcet until serum calcium ≥8 mg/dL and/or symptoms of hypocalcemia resolve. Reinitiate cinacalcet at the next lowest dose.

Additional Information Complete prescribing information should be consulted for additional detail.

Dosage Forms Excipient information presented when available (limited, particularly for generics); consult specific product labeling.
Tablet, Oral:
Sensipar: 30 mg, 60 mg, 90 mg

◆ **Cinacalcet Hydrochloride** *see* Cinacalcet *on page 392*
◆ **Cipro** *see* Ciprofloxacin (Systemic) *on page 393*
◆ **Cipro XL (Can)** *see* Ciprofloxacin (Systemic) *on page 393*

Ciprofloxacin (Systemic) (sip roe FLOKS a sin)

Brand Names: US Cipro; Cipro in D5W; Cipro XR
Brand Names: Canada ACT Ciprofloxacin; Apo-Ciproflox; Auro-Ciprofloxacin; Cipro; Cipro XL; Ciprofloxacin Injection; Ciprofloxacin Injection USP; Ciprofloxacin Intravenous Infusion; Ciprofloxacin Intravenous Infusion BP; Dom-Ciprofloxacin; JAMP-Ciprofloxacin; Mar-Ciprofloxacin; Mint-Ciproflox; Mint-Ciprofloxacin; Mylan-Ciprofloxacin; PHL-Ciprofloxacin; PMS-Ciprofloxacin; PMS-Ciprofloxacin XL; PRO-Ciprofloxacin; RAN-Ciproflox; ratio-Ciprofloxacin; Riva-Ciprofloxacin; Sandoz-Ciprofloxacin; Septa-Ciprofloxacin; Taro-Ciprofloxacin; Teva-Ciprofloxacin
Index Terms Ciprofloxacin HCl; Ciprofloxacin Hydrochloride; Proquin XR
Pharmacologic Category Antibiotic, Fluoroquinolone
Use
Children and Adolescents: Treatment of complicated urinary tract infections and pyelonephritis due to *E. coli*. **Note:** Although effective, ciprofloxacin is not the drug of first choice in children.
Infants, Children, Adolescents, and Adults: Prophylaxis to reduce incidence or progression of disease following inhalation exposure to *Bacillus anthracis*; prophylaxis and treatment of plague (*Yersinia pestis*).
Adults: Treatment of the following infections when caused by susceptible bacteria: Urinary tract infections; acute uncomplicated cystitis in females, chronic bacterial prostatitis, bone and joint infections, complicated intra-abdominal infections (in combination with metronidazole), infectious diarrhea, typhoid fever (*Salmonella typhi*), hospital-acquired (nosocomial) pneumonia.
Limitations of use: Because fluoroquinolones have been associated with disabling and potentially irreversible serious adverse reactions (eg, tendinitis and tendon rupture, peripheral neuropathy, CNS effects), reserve ciprofloxacin for use in patients who have no alternative treatment options for acute uncomplicated cystitis.
Pregnancy Risk Factor C
Dosing
Adult & Geriatric Note: Extended-release tablets and immediate-release formulations are not interchangeable. Unless otherwise specified, oral dosing reflects the use of immediate-release formulations.

Anthrax: Note: Consult public health officials for event-specific recommendations.
Inhalational exposure (postexposure prophylaxis):
Oral: 500 mg every 12 hours for 60 days
IV: 400 mg every 12 hours for 60 days

Cutaneous (without systemic involvement), empiric therapy (off-label use): Oral: 500 mg every 12 hours for 7 to 10 days after naturally acquired infection; 60 days following biological weapon-related event (Hendricks 2014). **Note**: Patients with cutaneous lesions of the head or neck or extensive edema should be treated for systemic involvement.

Systemic (meningitis excluded) (off-label use): IV: 400 mg every 8 hours in combination with other appropriate agents for 2 weeks until clinically stable (Hendricks 2014)

Meningitis (off-label use): IV: 400 mg every 8 hours in combination with other appropriate agents for 2 to 3 weeks until clinically stable (Hendricks 2014)

Note: Following the course of IV combination therapy for systemic anthrax infection (including meningitis), patients exposed to aerosolized spores require oral monotherapy to complete a total antimicrobial course of 60 days.

Bite wound infection, prophylaxis or treatment (animal and human bites; alternative agent) (off-label use) (IDSA [Stevens 2014]): Note: Use in combination with an appropriate agent for anaerobes.
Oral: 500 to 750 mg twice daily
IV: 400 mg every 12 hours
Duration of therapy: 3 to 5 days for prophylaxis; duration of treatment for established infection varies based on patient-specific factors

Cat scratch disease lymphadenitis (non-disseminated; alternative agent) (off-label use): Oral: 500 mg twice daily (Holley 1991). Additional data may be necessary to further define the role of ciprofloxacin in this condition.

Chancroid (alternative agent) (off-label use): Oral: 500 mg twice daily for 3 days (CDC [Workowski 2015])

Cholera (*Vibrio cholerae*) (off-label use; alternative agent): Oral: 1 g as a single dose (IDSA [Guerrant 2001]; Khan 1996)

Diabetic foot infections (off-label use) (IDSA [Lipsky 2012]; Weintrob 2017): Note: When used as empiric therapy, must be used in combination with other appropriate agents.
Mild to moderate: Oral: 750 mg every 12 hours
Moderate to severe: IV: 400 mg every 8 to 12 hours

Endocarditis due to HACEK organisms (alternative agent) (off-label use) (AHA [Baddour 2015]):
Oral: 500 mg every 12 hours for 4 weeks (native valve) or 6 weeks (prosthetic valve)
IV: 400 mg every 12 hours for 4 weeks (native valve) or 6 weeks (prosthetic valve)

Febrile neutropenia, low-risk cancer patients (empiric) (off-label use): Oral: 750 mg every 12 hours until afebrile and neutropenia has resolved; use in combination with amoxicillin and clavulanate. **Note**: Avoid in patients who have received fluoroquinolone prophylaxis (ASCO [Flowers 2013]; IDSA [Freifeld 2011]; Kern 1999)

Granuloma inguinale (Donovanosis) (alternative agent) (off-label use): Oral: 750 mg twice daily for at least 3 weeks (and until lesions have healed) (CDC [Workowski 2015]). **Note:** If symptoms do not improve within the first few days of therapy, another agent (eg, aminoglycoside) can be added (CDC [Workowski 2015]).

Hematopoietic cell transplant (HCT) antibacterial prophylaxis (off-label use): Oral: 500 mg twice daily; begin at the time of stem cell infusion and continue until recovery of neutropenia or until initiation of empiric antibiotic therapy for febrile neutropenia (Tomblyn 2009)

Intra-abdominal infections (including perforated appendix, appendiceal abscess, acute diverticulitis, acute cholecystitis), community-acquired: Note: For empiric therapy, use in combination with metronidazole.

Oral: 500 mg every 12 hours

IV: 400 mg every 12 hours

Duration of therapy: Duration depends on whether source of infection has been controlled. Guidelines recommend treatment duration of 4 to 7 days (provided source controlled) (IDSA [Solomkin 2010])

Meningitis, bacterial (community-acquired or health care-associated; alternative agent) (off-label use): IV: 400 mg every 8 to 12 hours; for empiric therapy, must be used in combination with other appropriate agents (IDSA [Tunkel 2004, 2017])

Meningococcal meningitis prophylaxis (off-label use): Oral: 500 mg as a single dose (CDC 2005)

Neutropenia (chemotherapy-induced), antibacterial prophylaxis in high-risk patients anticipated to have an ANC ≤100 cells/mm^3 for >7 days (off-label use): Oral: 500 mg twice daily (IDSA [Freifeld 2011]; Wingard 2017); some clinicians will provide antibacterial prophylaxis if ANC is anticipated to be <500 cells/mm^3 for >7 days (Wingard 2017)

Osteomyelitis:

IV: 400 mg every 12 hours; when treating *P. aeruginosa*, 400 mg every 8 hours (Calhoun 2005; IDSA [Berbari 2015])

Oral:

Treatment: 500 to 750 mg every 12 hours; when treating *P. aeruginosa*, 750 mg every 12 hours (Calhoun 2005; IDSA [Berbari 2015])

Chronic suppression in presence of retained infected orthopedic hardware: 250 to 500 mg every 12 hours (IDSA [Osmon 2013])

Peritoneal dialysis catheter, exit site or tunnel infection (off-label use): Oral: 250 mg twice daily. When used for empiric therapy, must be used in combination with other appropriate agents. (ISPD [Szeto 2017])

Plague (*Yersinia pestis*) infection (alternative agent) (CDC [plague] 2015): Note: Consult public health officials for event-specific recommendations:

Postexposure prophylaxis: Oral: 500 mg twice daily for 7 days

*Treatment: **Note:** Duration of therapy is 10 to 14 days*

Oral: 500 to 750 mg every 12 hours

IV: 400 mg every 8 to 12 hours

Pneumonia, community-acquired, as a component of empiric therapy for *P. aeruginosa* coverage (hospitalized patient) (off-label use) (File 2017a; IDSA/ATS [Mandell 2007]): Note: For empiric therapy, must be used in combination with other appropriate agents.

IV: 400 mg every 8 hours for 5 to 7 days

Oral: 750 mg every 12 hours for 5 to 7 days

Pneumonia, hospital-acquired (nosocomial) including ventilator-associated, as a component of empiric therapy for *P. aeruginosa* coverage (File 2017b; IDSA [Kalil 2016]): Note: For empiric therapy, must be used in combination with other appropriate agents.

IV: 400 mg every 8 hours for 7 days

Oral: 750 mg every 12 hours for 7 days

Prostatitis (acute, bacterial) (off-label use): Note: When used for empiric therapy, must be used in combination with other appropriate agents.
Oral: 500 mg every 12 hours (Meyrier 2017a)
IV: 400 mg every 12 hours (Meyrier 2017a)
Duration of therapy: 6 weeks (Meyrier 2017a; Yoon 2013)

Prostatitis (chronic, bacterial) (Meyrier 2017b):
Oral: 500 mg every 12 hours for ≥6 weeks
IV: 400 mg every 12 hours for ≥6 weeks

Prosthetic joint infection (off-label use): Note: Alternative agent for certain pathogens.
Treatment:
  Gram-negative bacilli (IDSA [Osmon 2013]):
    Oral: 750 mg twice daily
    IV: 400 mg every 12 hours
  Staphylococci: Oral: 750 mg twice daily (Zimmerli 1998). **Note:** For use in combination with rifampin, following pathogen-specific IV therapy in patients undergoing 1-stage exchanges or debridement with retention of prosthesis (IDSA [Osmon 2013]).
Chronic suppressive therapy (for P. aeruginosa): Oral: 250 to 500 mg twice daily (IDSA [Osmon 2013])

***Salmonella* species, GI infection:**
Nontyphoidal, severe (non-bacteremic) illness or any severity in patients at high risk for invasive disease: Oral: 500 mg twice daily for 3 to 7 days. **Note:** Immunosuppressed patients require longer duration of treatment (eg, weeks to months) (Hohmann 2017; IDSA [Guerrant 2001]).
Typhoid fever (Salmonella typhi and paratyphi): Severe disease or mild to moderate infection in patients at high-risk of developing invasive disease (Ryan 2017)
Oral: 500 mg every 12 hours for 7 to 10 days
IV: 400 mg every 12 hours for 7 to 10 days

Septic arthritis (without prosthetic material; alternative agent): Note: Use in combination with an aminoglycoside for initial treatment if *P. aeruginosa* suspected (Goldenberg 2017).
Oral: 500 to 750 mg twice daily
IV: 400 mg every 12 hours

***Shigella* GI infection (off-label dose):** Oral: 500 mg twice daily or 750 mg once daily for 3 days; the duration should be extended to 5 to 7 days for those with *S. dysenteriae* type 1 infection or HIV coinfection (Agha 2017; IDSA [Guerrant 2001])

Spontaneous bacterial peritonitis (SBP) (prevention), high risk patients (eg, hospitalized patients with Child-Pugh class B or C cirrhosis and active GI bleeding) (alternative agent) (off-label use) (Runyon 2017):
Oral: 500 mg every 12 hours for total duration of 7 days (oral and IV)
IV (alternative for nonfunctional GI tract): 400 mg every 12 hours for total duration of 7 days (oral and IV)
Long-term secondary SBP prophylaxis: Oral: 500 mg once daily

Surgical (preoperative) prophylaxis (alternative agent) (off-label use): Note: Use in combination with other appropriate agents may be warranted (procedure-dependent). IV: 400 mg within 120 minutes prior to surgical incision (Bratzler 2013)

Surgical site infection (intestinal or GU tract, perineum, or axilla) (off-label use) (IDSA [Stevens 2014]):
Oral: 750 mg every 12 hours, in combination with metronidazole
IV: 400 mg every 12 hours, in combination with metronidazole

Traveler's diarrhea, uncomplicated (empiric therapy) (off-label dose):
Oral: 500 mg twice daily for 1 to 3 days (IDSA [Hill 2006])

Tularemia (*Francisella tularensis*) (off-label use): Note: Consult public health officials for event-specific recommendations.

Mild disease or postexposure prophylaxis: Oral: 500 or 750 mg twice daily (Bossi [tularemia] 2004; Dennis 2001).

Urinary tract infection:

Cystitis, acute uncomplicated: **Note:** Use for uncomplicated urinary tract infections is discouraged due to significant *E. coli* resistance and safety issues; reserve for clinical situations where other appropriate treatment options cannot be used (Bidell 2016; IDSA [Gupta 2011]).

Oral, immediate release: 250 mg every 12 hours for 3 days

Oral, extended release: 500 mg every 24 hours for 3 days

Cystitis, acute complicated (Hooton 2017):

Oral, immediate release: 250 mg every 12 hours for 5 to 7 days

Oral, extended release: 1,000 mg every 24 hours for 5 to 7 days

Pyelonephritis, uncomplicated (outpatient): Oral: 500 mg every 12 hours for 7days (IDSA [Gupta 2010])

Pyelonephritis, complicated (inpatient): IV: 400 mg every 12 hours for a total of 7 to 14 days (Hooton 2017)

Pediatric

Note: In pediatric patients, ciprofloxacin is not routinely first-line therapy, but after assessment of risks and benefits, can be considered a reasonable alternative for some situations [eg, anthrax, resistance (cystic fibrosis)] or in situations where the only alternative is parenteral therapy and ciprofloxacin offers an oral therapy option (Bradley 2011b).

Note: Extended release tablets and immediate release formulations are not interchangeable. Unless otherwise specified, oral dosing reflects the use of immediate release formulations.

Usual dosage range (*Red Book* [AAP 2015]): Infants, Children, and Adolescents:

Mild to moderate infections: Oral: 10 mg/kg/dose twice daily (maximum dose: 500 mg/dose)

Severe infections:

Oral: 15 to 20 mg/kg/dose twice daily (maximum dose: 750 mg/dose)

IV: 10 mg/kg/dose every 8 to 12 hours (maximum dose: 400 mg/dose)

Anthrax: Infants, Children, and Adolescents: **Note:** Consult public health officials for event-specific recommendations:

Inhalational exposure (postexposure prophylaxis):

Oral: 15 mg/kg/dose every 12 hours for 60 days (maximum dose: 500 mg/dose)

IV: 10 mg/kg/dose every 12 hours for 60 days; do **not** exceed 400 mg/dose (800 mg/day)

Cutaneous, treatment (without systemic involvement) (off-label use) (AAP [Bradley 2014]): Oral: 15 mg/kg/dose every 12 hours (maximum dose: 500 mg/dose). Duration: 7 to 10 days for naturally acquired infection, up to 60 days for biological weapon-related event.

Systemic, treatment (including meningitis) (off-label use) (AAP [Bradley 2014]): IV: Initial: 10 mg/kg/dose every 8 hours (maximum dose: 400 mg/dose) as part of combination therapy; continue until clinical criteria for stability are met, then may switch to oral therapy (15 mg/kg/dose orally twice daily) to complete a 60-day course

Chancroid (off-label use): Adolescents: Oral: 500 mg twice daily for 3 days (*Red Book* [AAP 2015])

Endocarditis, culture negative, empiric therapy (off-label use): Note: Administer in combination with other antibiotics: Children and Adolescents (AHA [Baltimore 2015]):

Oral: 10 to 15 mg/kg/dose twice daily for 4 to 6 weeks; maximum dose: 750 mg/dose

IV: 10 to 15 mg/kg/dose twice daily for 4 to 6 weeks; maximum dose: 400 mg/dose

Intra-abdominal infection, complicated (off-label use): Infants, Children, and Adolescents: IV: 10 to 15 mg/kg/dose every 12 hours; maximum dose: 400 mg/dose (IDSA [Solomkin 2010])

Meningococcal invasive disease prophylaxis, high-risk contacts (off-label use): Infants, Children, and Adolescents: Oral: 20 mg/kg as a single dose; maximum dose: 500 mg/dose (*Red Book* [AAP 2015])

Mycobacterium avium **complex, severe or disseminated disease, HIV-exposed/-infected (off-label use):** Infants and Children: Oral: 10 to 15 mg/kg/dose twice daily in addition to other antibiotics; maximum dose: 750 mg/dose (HHS [pediatric] 2013)

Peritoneal dialysis catheter, exit site or tunnel infection (off-label use): Infants, Children, and Adolescents: 10 to 15 mg/kg/dose once daily (maximum dose: 500 mg/dose) (Warady [ISPD 2012])

Plague:

Manufacturer's labeling: Infants, Children, and Adolescents:

Oral: 15 mg/kg/dose every 8 to 12 hours for 10 to 21 days; maximum: 500 mg/dose

IV: 10 mg/kg/dose every 8 to 12 hours for 10 to 21 days; maximum: 400 mg/dose

Alternate dosing (CDC [plague] 2015)*:* Children and Adolescents:

Treatment:

Initial treatment: IV: 15 mg/kg/dose every 12 hours; maximum dose: 400 mg/dose; continue until 2 days after fever subsides, then may change to oral therapy.

Oral step down to complete a 10 to 14 day course: Oral: 20 mg/kg/dose twice daily; maximum dose: 500 mg/dose.

Postexposure prophylaxis: Oral: 20 mg/kg/dose twice daily for 7 days; maximum dose: 500 mg/dose)

Pneumonia, community-acquired (*H. influenzae*) **(off-label use):** Infants >3 months and Children: IV: 15 mg/kg/dose every 12 hours (IDSA/PIDS [Bradley 2011a])

Surgical (preoperative) prophylaxis (off-label use): Children and Adolescents: IV: 10 mg/kg/dose within 120 minutes prior to surgical incision (maximum dose: 400 mg/dose) (Bratzler 2013)

Urinary tract infection:

Cystitis, acute uncomplicated: Adolescents ≥18 years: Oral, extended release: Refer to adult dosing

Complicated, including pyelonephritis:

Oral, immediate release: Children and Adolescents ≤17 years: 10 to 20 mg/kg/dose every 12 hours for 10 to 21 days; maximum dose: 750 mg/dose.

Oral, extended release: Adolescents ≥18 years: Refer to adult dosing

IV: 6 to 10 mg/kg/dose every 8 hours for 10 to 21 days (maximum dose: 400 mg/dose)

Renal Impairment Adults:

Manufacturer's labeling:

Oral, immediate release:

CrCl >50 mL/minute: No dosage adjustment necessary.

CrCl 30 to 50 mL/minute: 250 to 500 mg every 12 hours

CrCl 5 to 29 mL/minute: 250 to 500 mg every 18 hours

ESRD on intermittent hemodialysis (IHD)/peritoneal dialysis (PD) (administer after dialysis on dialysis days): 250 to 500 mg every 24 hours

Oral, extended release:

CrCl ≥30 mL/minute: No dosage adjustment necessary.

CrCl <30 mL/minute: 500 mg every 24 hours

ESRD on intermittent hemodialysis (IHD)/peritoneal dialysis (PD) (administer after dialysis on dialysis days): 500 mg every 24 hours

IV:

CrCl ≥30 mL/minute: No dosage adjustment necessary.

CrCl 5 to 29 mL/minute: 200 to 400 mg every 18 to 24 hours

Alternate recommendations: Oral (immediate release), IV:

CrCl >50 mL/minute: No dosage adjustment necessary (Aronoff 2007).

CrCl 10 to 50 mL/minute: Administer 50% to 75% of usual dose every 12 hours (Aronoff 2007).

CrCl <10 mL/minute: Administer 50% of usual dose every 12 hours (Aronoff 2007).

Intermittent hemodialysis (IHD) (administer after hemodialysis on dialysis days): Minimally dialyzable (<10%): Oral: 250 to 500 mg every 24 hours **or** IV: 200 to 400 mg every 24 hours (Heintz 2009). **Note:** Dosing dependent on the assumption of 3 times weekly, complete IHD sessions.

Continuous renal replacement therapy (CRRT) (Heintz 2009; Trotman 2005): Drug clearance is highly dependent on the method of renal replacement, filter type, and flow rate. Appropriate dosing requires close monitoring of pharmacologic response, signs of adverse reactions due to drug accumulation, as well as drug concentrations in relation to target trough (if appropriate). The following are general recommendations only (based on dialysate flow/ultrafiltration rates of 1 to 2 L/hour and minimal residual renal function) and should not supersede clinical judgment:

CVVH/CVVHD/CVVHDF: IV: 200 to 400 mg every 12 to 24 hours

Hepatic Impairment There are no dosage adjustments provided in manufacturer's labeling. Use with caution in severe impairment.

Additional Information Complete prescribing information should be consulted for additional detail.

Medication Guide Available Yes

Dosage Forms Excipient information presented when available (limited, particularly for generics); consult specific product labeling. [DSC] = Discontinued product

Solution, Intravenous:

Cipro in D5W: 200 mg/100 mL (100 mL [DSC]) [latex free]

Generic: 200 mg/100 mL (100 mL); 400 mg/200 mL (200 mL); 200 mg/20 mL (20 mL [DSC]); 400 mg/40 mL (40 mL [DSC])

Solution, Intravenous [preservative free]:

Cipro in D5W: 200 mg/100 mL (100 mL [DSC]); 400 mg/200 mL (200 mL) [latex free]

Generic: 200 mg/100 mL (100 mL); 400 mg/200 mL (200 mL); 200 mg/20 mL (20 mL); 400 mg/40 mL (40 mL)

◄

Suspension Reconstituted, Oral:
   Cipro: 250 mg/5 mL (100 mL); 500 mg/5 mL (100 mL) [strawberry flavor]
   Generic: 250 mg/5 mL (100 mL); 500 mg/5 mL (100 mL)
Tablet, Oral, as hydrochloride [strength expressed as base]:
   Cipro: 250 mg, 500 mg
   Generic: 100 mg, 250 mg, 500 mg, 750 mg
Tablet Extended Release 24 Hour, Oral, as base and hydrochloride [strength expressed as base]:
   Cipro XR: 500 mg, 1000 mg
   Generic: 500 mg, 1000 mg

◆ **Ciprofloxacin HCl** *see* Ciprofloxacin (Systemic) *on page 393*

◆ **Ciprofloxacin Hydrochloride** *see* Ciprofloxacin (Systemic) *on page 393*

◆ **Ciprofloxacin Injection (Can)** *see* Ciprofloxacin (Systemic) *on page 393*

◆ **Ciprofloxacin Injection USP (Can)** *see* Ciprofloxacin (Systemic) *on page 393*

◆ **Ciprofloxacin Intravenous Infusion (Can)** *see* Ciprofloxacin (Systemic) *on page 393*

◆ **Ciprofloxacin Intravenous Infusion BP (Can)** *see* Ciprofloxacin (Systemic) *on page 393*

◆ **Cipro in D5W** *see* Ciprofloxacin (Systemic) *on page 393*

◆ **Cipro XR** *see* Ciprofloxacin (Systemic) *on page 393*

◆ **cis-DDP** *see* CISplatin *on page 400*

◆ **cis-Diamminedichloroplatinum** *see* CISplatin *on page 400*

CISplatin (SIS pla tin)

Related Information

Chemotherapy-Induced Peripheral Neuropathy *on page 2236*
Hematopoietic Cell Transplantation *on page 2365*
Management of Chemotherapy-Induced Nausea and Vomiting in Adults *on page 2253*
Management of Drug Extravasations *on page 2271*
Prevention of Chemotherapy-Induced Nausea and Vomiting in Children *on page 2310*
Safe Handling of Hazardous Drugs *on page 2379*

Brand Names: Canada Cisplatin Injection; Cisplatin Injection BP; Cisplatin Injection, Mylan STD

Index Terms CDDP; cis-DDP; cis-Diamminedichloroplatinum; cis-platinum; DDP; Platinol; Platinol-AQ

Pharmacologic Category Antineoplastic Agent, Alkylating Agent; Antineoplastic Agent, Platinum Analog

Use

Bladder cancer, advanced: Treatment (as a single agent) of advanced bladder cancer (transitional cell) in patients who are no longer candidates for local therapy including surgery and/or radiation therapy

Ovarian cancer, metastatic: Treatment of metastatic ovarian cancer (in combination with other chemotherapy agents) in patients who have previously received appropriate surgery and/or radiation therapy, or as a single agent for refractory tumors in patients who have not previously received cisplatin

Testicular cancer, metastatic: Treatment of metastatic testicular cancer (in combination with other chemotherapy agents) in patients who have previously received appropriate surgery and/or radiation therapy

Labeled Contraindications History of allergic reactions to cisplatin, other platinum-containing compounds, or any component of the formulation; preexisting renal impairment; myelosuppressed patients; hearing impairment

Pregnancy Considerations Adverse effects have been observed in animal reproduction studies. Women of childbearing potential should be advised to avoid pregnancy during treatment. May case fetal harm if administered during pregnancy.

Breastfeeding Considerations Cisplatin is excreted in breast milk. Breastfeeding is not recommended by the manufacturer.

Warnings/Precautions [US Boxed Warning]: Doses >100 mg/m²/cycle (once every 3 to 4 weeks) are rare; verify with the prescriber. Exercise caution to avoid inadvertent overdose due to potential sound-alike/look-alike confusion between CISplatin and CARBOplatin or prescribing practices that fail to differentiate daily doses from the total dose per cycle. At the approved dose, cisplatin should not be administered more frequently than once every 3 to 4 weeks. Patients should receive adequate hydration, with or without diuretics, prior to and for 24 hours after cisplatin administration. **[US Boxed Warning]: Cumulative renal toxicity associated with cisplatin is severe.** Monitor serum creatinine, blood urea nitrogen, creatinine clearance, and serum electrolytes (calcium, magnesium, potassium, and sodium) closely. According to the manufacturer's labeling, use is contraindicated in patients with preexisting renal impairment and renal function must return to normal prior to administering subsequent cycles; some literature recommends reduced doses with renal impairment. Nephrotoxicity may be potentiated by aminoglycosides.

Elderly patients may be more susceptible to nephrotoxicity and peripheral neuropathy; select dose cautiously and monitor closely.

[US Boxed Warning]: Dose-related toxicities include myelosuppression, nausea, and vomiting. Cisplatin is associated with a high emetic potential; antiemetics are recommended to prevent nausea and vomiting (Basch 2011; Dupuis 2011; Roila 2016). Nausea and vomiting are dose-related and may be immediate and/or delayed. Diarrhea may also occur. **[US Boxed Warning]: Ototoxicity, which may be more pronounced in children, is manifested by tinnitus and/or loss of high frequency hearing and occasionally, deafness; may be significant.** Ototoxicity is cumulative and may be severe. Audiometric testing should be performed at baseline and prior to each dose. Certain genetic variations in the thiopurine S-methyltransferase (TPMT) gene may be associated with an increased risk of ototoxicity in children administered conventional cisplatin doses (Pussegoda 2013). Controversy may exist regarding the role of TPMT variants in cisplatin ototoxicity (Ratain 2013; Yang 2013); the association has not been consistent across populations and studies. Children without the TPMT gene variants may still be at risk for ototoxicity. Cumulative dose, prior or concurrent exposure to other ototoxic agents (eg, aminoglycosides, carboplatin), prior cranial radiation, younger age, and type of cancer may also increase the risk for ototoxicity in children (Knight 2005; Landier 2014). Pediatric patients should receive audiometric testing at baseline, prior to each dose, and for several years after discontinuing therapy. An international grading scale (SIOP Boston scale) has been developed to assess ototoxicity in children (Brock 2012). Severe (and possibly ▶

◀ irreversible) neuropathies (including stocking-glove paresthesias, areflexia, and loss of proprioception/vibratory sensation) may occur with higher than recommended doses or more frequent administration; may require therapy discontinuation. Seizures, loss of motor function, loss of taste, leukoencephalopathy, and posterior reversible leukoencephalopathy syndrome (PRES [formerly RPLS]) have also been described. Serum electrolytes, particularly magnesium and potassium, should be monitored and replaced as needed during and after cisplatin therapy.

[US Boxed Warning]: Anaphylactic-like reactions have been reported; may include facial edema, bronchoconstriction, tachycardia, and hypotension and may occur within minutes of administration; symptoms may be managed with epinephrine, corticosteroids, and/or antihistamines. Hyperuricemia has been reported with cisplatin use, and is more pronounced with doses >50 mg/mm^2; consider antihyperuricemic therapy to reduce uric acid levels. Local infusion site reactions may occur; monitor infusion site during administration; avoid extravasation. Secondary malignancies have been reported with cisplatin in combination with other chemotherapy agents. Potentially significant drug-drug interactions may exist, requiring dose or frequency adjustment, additional monitoring, and/or selection of alternative therapy. **[US Boxed Warning]: Should be administered under the supervision of an experienced cancer chemotherapy physician. Adequate diagnostic and treatment facilities and appropriate management of potential complications should be readily available.** Cisplatin is a vesicant at higher concentrations, and an irritant at lower concentrations; ensure proper needle or catheter placement prior to and during infusion; avoid extravasation. Local infusion site reactions may occur; monitor infusion site during administration.

Adverse Reactions

>10%:

Central nervous system: Neurotoxicity (peripheral neuropathy is dose and duration dependent)

Gastrointestinal: Nausea and vomiting (76% to 100%)

Genitourinary: Nephrotoxicity (28% to 36%; acute renal failure and chronic renal insufficiency)

Hematologic & oncologic: Anemia (≤40%), leukopenia (25% to 30%; nadir: Day 18 to 23; recovery: By day 39; dose related), thrombocytopenia (25% to 30%; nadir: Day 18 to 23; recovery: By day 39; dose related)

Hepatic: Increased liver enzymes

Otic: Ototoxicity (children 40% to 60%; adults 10% to 31%; as tinnitus, high frequency hearing loss)

1% to 10%: Local: Local irritation

<1%, postmarketing, and/or case reports: Alopecia (mild), ageusia, anaphylaxis, autonomic neuropathy, bradycardia (Schlumbrecht 2015), bronchoconstriction, cardiac arrhythmia, cardiac failure, cerebral arteritis, cerebrovascular accident, dehydration, diarrhea, dysgeusia (Rehwaldt 2009), extravasation, heart block, hemolytic anemia (acute), hemolytic-uremic syndrome, hiccups, hypercholesterolemia, hyperuricemia, hypocalcemia, hypokalemia, hypomagnesemia, hyponatremia, hypophosphatemia, hypotension, increased serum amylase, ischemic heart disease, leukoencephalopathy, Lhermitte's sign, mesenteric ischemia (acute; Morgan 2011), myocardial infarction, neutropenic enterocolitis (Furonaka 2005), optic neuritis, pancreatitis (Trivedi 2005), papilledema, peripheral ischemia (acute), phlebitis (Tokuda 2014), reversible posterior leukoencephalopathy

syndrome, seizure, SIADH, skin rash, tachycardia, tetany, thrombosis (aortic; Fernandes 2011), thrombotic thrombocytopenic purpura, vasospasm (acute arterial; Morgan 2011), vision color changes, vision loss

Drug Interactions

Metabolism/Transport Effects None known.

Avoid Concomitant Use

Avoid concomitant use of CISplatin with any of the following: BCG (Intravesical); Deferiprone; Dipyrone; Natalizumab; Pimecrolimus; Tacrolimus (Topical); Vaccines (Live)

Increased Effect/Toxicity

CISplatin may increase the levels/effects of: Aminoglycosides; CloZAPine; Deferiprone; Fingolimod; Leflunomide; Natalizumab; Taxane Derivatives; Tofacitinib; Topotecan; Vaccines (Live); Vinorelbine

The levels/effects of CISplatin may be increased by: Denosumab; Dipyrone; Loop Diuretics; Ocrelizumab; Palifermin; Pimecrolimus; Promazine; Roflumilast; Tacrolimus (Topical); Trastuzumab

Decreased Effect

CISplatin may decrease the levels/effects of: BCG (Intravesical); Coccidioides immitis Skin Test; Fosphenytoin-Phenytoin; Lenograstim; Nivolumab; Sipuleucel-T; Tertomotide; Vaccines (Inactivated); Vaccines (Live)

The levels/effects of CISplatin may be decreased by: Alpha-Lipoic Acid; Echinacea

Hazardous Drugs Handling Considerations
Hazardous agent (NIOSH 2016 [group 1]).

Use appropriate precautions for receiving, handling, administration, and disposal. Gloves (single) should be worn during receiving, unpacking, and placing in storage.

NIOSH recommends double gloving, a protective gown, ventilated engineering controls (a class II biological safety cabinet or a compounding aseptic containment isolator), and closed system transfer devices (CSTDs) for preparation. Double gloving, a gown, and (if dosage form allows) CSTDs are required during administration (NIOSH 2016).

Storage/Stability Store intact vials at 20°C to 25°C (68°F to 77°F). Protect from light. Do not refrigerate solution (precipitate may form). According to the manufacturer, after initial entry into the vial, solution is stable for 28 days protected from light or for at least 7 days under fluorescent room light at room temperature. When diluted for administration in D5¼NS, D5½NS, D5NS, ¼NS, ⅓NS, ½NS, or NS, stability is dependent on the chloride ion concentration.

Preparation for Administration Prior to infusion, dilute in NS, D5½NS or D5NS. Do **NOT** dilute in D5W. The manufacturer recommends dilution in up to 2 liters. Needles or IV administration sets that contain aluminum should not be used in the preparation or administration; aluminum can react with cisplatin resulting in precipitate formation and loss of potency.

Mechanism of Action Inhibits DNA synthesis by the formation of DNA cross-links; denatures the double helix; covalently binds to DNA bases and disrupts DNA function; may also bind to proteins; the *cis*-isomer is 14 times more cytotoxic than the *trans*-isomer; both forms cross-link DNA but cis-platinum is less easily recognized by cell enzymes and, therefore, not repaired. Cisplatin can also bind two adjacent guanines on the same strand of DNA producing intrastrand cross-linking and breakage.

◀ **Pharmacodynamics/Kinetics**

Distribution: IV: Rapidly into tissue; high concentrations in kidneys, liver, ovaries, uterus, and lungs

Protein binding: >90% (O'Dwyer 2000)

Metabolism: Nonenzymatic; inactivated (in both cell and bloodstream) by sulfhydryl groups; covalently binds to glutathione and thiosulfate

Half-life elimination:

Children: Free drug: 1.3 hours; Total platinum: 44 hours

Adults: Initial: 14 to 49 minutes; Beta: 0.7 to 4.6 hours; Gamma: 24 to 127 hours (O'Dwyer 2000)

Excretion: Urine (>90%); feces (minimal)

Dosing

Adult VERIFY ANY CISPLATIN DOSE EXCEEDING 100 mg/m² PER COURSE. Pretreatment hydration with 1 to 2 L of IV fluid is recommended. Cisplatin is associated with a high emetic potential; antiemetics are recommended to prevent nausea and vomiting (Basch 2011; Roila 2016).

Bladder cancer, advanced: IV: 50 to 70 mg/m² every 3 to 4 weeks; heavily pretreated patients: 50 mg/m² every 4 weeks

Ovarian cancer, metastatic: IV:

Single agent: 100 mg/m² every 4 weeks

Combination therapy: 75 to 100 mg/m² every 4 weeks or (off-label dosing) 75 mg/m² every 3 weeks (Ozols 2003)

Intraperitoneal (off-label route): 100 mg/m² on day 2 of a 21-day treatment cycle (in combination with IV and intraperitoneal paclitaxel) for 6 cycles (Armstrong 2006)

Testicular cancer, metastatic: IV: 20 mg/m²/day for 5 days repeated every 3 weeks (in combination with bleomycin and etoposide) (Cushing 2004; Saxman 1998)

Testicular germ cell tumor, malignant (off-label dosing): IV: 25 mg/m² on days 2 to 5 every 3 weeks (in combination with paclitaxel and ifosfamide) for 4 cycles (Kondagunta 2005) **or** 20 mg/m² on days 1 to 5 every 3 weeks (in combination with bleomycin and etoposide) for 4 cycles (Nichols 1998) **or** 20 mg/m² on days 1 to 5 every 3 weeks (in combination with etoposide and ifosfamide) for 4 cycles (Nichols 1998)

Breast cancer, triple-negative (off-label use): IV: Neoadjuvant therapy (single agent): 75 mg/m² on day 1 every 3 weeks for 4 cycles (Silver 2010). Additional data may be necessary to further define the role of cisplatin in this setting.

Cervical cancer (off-label use): IV: 75 mg/m² on day 1 every 3 weeks (in combination with fluorouracil and radiation) for 3 cycles (Morris 1999) **or** 70 mg/m² on day 1 every 3 weeks for 4 cycles (in combination with fluorouracil; cycles 1 and 2 given concurrently with radiation) (Peters 2000) **or** 50 mg/m² on day 1 every 4 weeks (in combination with radiation and fluorouracil) for 2 cycles (Whitney 1999)

Endometrial carcinoma, recurrent, metastatic, or high-risk (off-label use): IV: 50 mg/m² on day 1 every 3 weeks (in combination with doxorubicin ± paclitaxel) for 7 cycles or until disease progression or unacceptable toxicity (Fleming 2004)

Esophageal and gastric cancers (off-label uses): IV:
CF regimen: 100 mg/m^2 over 30 minutes on days 1 and 29 (preoperative chemoradiation; in combination with fluorouracil) (Tepper 2008)

ECF, ECX regimens: 60 mg/m^2 on day 1 every 21 days for up to 8 cycles in combination with epirubicin (E) and either fluorouracil (F) or capecitabine (X) (Cunningham 2008) **or**

ECF regimen: 60 mg/m^2 on day 1 every 21 days for 3 preoperative and 3 postoperative cycles in combination with epirubicin and fluorouracil (Cunningham 2006)

TCF or DCF regimen: 75 mg/m^2 on day 1 every 3 weeks (in combination with docetaxel and fluorouracil) until disease progression or unacceptable toxicity (Ajani 2007; Van Cutsem 2006)

Head and neck cancer (off-label use): IV:
Locally-advanced disease: 100 mg/m^2 every 3 weeks for 3 doses (with concurrent radiation) (Bernier 2004; Cooper 2004) **or** 75 mg/m^2 every 3 weeks (in combination with docetaxel and fluorouracil) for 4 cycles or until disease progression or unacceptable toxicity (if no disease progression after 4 cycles, chemotherapy was followed by radiation) (Vermorken 2007) **or** 100 mg/m^2 every 3 weeks (in combination with docetaxel and fluorouracil) for 3 cycles or until disease progression or unacceptable toxicity (chemotherapy was followed by chemoradiation) (Posner 2007)

Metastatic disease: 100 mg/m^2 every 3 weeks (in combination with fluorouracil and cetuximab) until disease progression or unacceptable toxicity or a maximum of 6 cycles (Vermorken 2008)

Hodgkin lymphoma, relapsed/refractory (off-label use): IV:
DHAP regimen: 100 mg/m^2 continuous infusion over 24 hours on day 1 for 2 cycles; median duration between cycle 1 and 2 was 16 days (in combination with dexamethasone and cytarabine) (Josting 2002)

ESHAP regimen: 25 mg/m^2/day on days 1 to 4 (in combination with etoposide, methylprednisolone, and cytarabine) every 3 to 4 weeks for 3 or 6 cycles (Aparicio 1999)

Malignant pleural mesothelioma (off-label use): IV: 75 mg/m^2 on day 1 of each 21-day cycle (in combination with pemetrexed) (Vogelzang 2003) **or** 100 mg/m^2 on day 1 of a 28-day cycle (in combination with gemcitabine) (Nowak 2002) **or** 80 mg/m^2 on day 1 of a 21-day cycle (in combination with gemcitabine) (van Haarst 2002)

Multiple myeloma (off-label use): IV: VDT-PACE regimen: 10 mg/m^2/day administered as a continuous infusion on days 1 to 4 of each cycle; repeat every 4 to 6 weeks (in combination with bortezomib, dexamethasone, thalidomide, doxorubicin, cyclophosphamide, and etoposide) (Lee 2003; Pineda-Roman 2008)

Non-Hodgkin lymphoma, relapsed/refractory: IV:
DHAP regimen: 100 mg/m^2 continuous infusion over 24 hours on day 1 every 3 to 4 weeks for 6 to 10 cycles (in combination with dexamethasone and cytarabine) (Velasquez 1988)

ESHAP regimen: 25 mg/m^2/day continuous infusion over 24 hours on days 1 to 4 every 3 to 4 weeks for 6 to 8 cycles (in combination with etoposide, methylprednisolone, and cytarabine) (Velasquez 1994)

◀ **Non-small cell lung cancer (NSCLC; off-label use):** IV: **Note:** There are multiple cisplatin-containing regimens for the treatment of NSCLC. Listed below are several commonly used regimens:

100 mg/m^2 on day 1 every 4 weeks (in combination with etoposide) for 3 to 4 cycles; (Arriagada 2004), or

100 mg/m^2 on day 1 every 4 weeks (in combination with vinorelbine) (Kelly 2001; Wozniak 1998), or

100 mg/m^2 on day 1 every 4 weeks (in combination with gemcitabine) (Comella 2000), or

80 mg/m^2 on day 1 every 3 weeks (in combination with gemcitabine) (Ohe 2007), or

75 mg/m^2 on day 1 every 3 weeks (in combination with pemetrexed) for up to 6 cycles or until disease progression or unacceptable toxicity (Scagliotti 2008)

Osteosarcoma (off-label use; combination chemotherapy): Adults <30 years: IV: 60 mg/m^2/day for 2 days on weeks 2, 7, 25, and 28 (neoadjuvant) or weeks 5, 10, 25, and 28 (adjuvant) in combination with methotrexate, leucovorin, doxorubicin, cyclophosphamide, bleomycin, and dactinomycin (Goorin 2003)

Penile cancer, metastatic (off-label use): IV: 25 mg/m^2 over 2 hours on days 1, 2, and 3 every 3 to 4 weeks (in combination with paclitaxel and ifosfamide) for 4 cycles (Pagliaro 2010)

Small cell lung cancer (off-label use): IV:

Limited-stage disease: 60 mg/m^2 on day 1 every 3 weeks for 4 cycles (in combination with etoposide and concurrent radiation) (Turrisi 1999)

Extensive-stage disease: 80 mg/m^2 on day 1 every 3 weeks (in combination with etoposide) for 4 cycles (Lara 2009) or a maximum of 8 cycles (Ihde 1994) **or** 60 mg/m^2 on day 1 every 4 weeks for 4 cycles (in combination with irinotecan) (Lara 2009)

Geriatric Refer to adult dosing. Select dose cautiously and monitor closely in the elderly; may be more susceptible to nephrotoxicity and peripheral neuropathy.

Pediatric VERIFY ANY CISPLATIN DOSE EXCEEDING 100 mg/m^2 PER COURSE. Pretreatment hydration is recommended. Cisplatin is associated with a high emetic potential; antiemetics are recommended to prevent nausea and vomiting (Dupuis 2011).

Germ cell tumors (off-label use; combination chemotherapy): IV: 20 mg/m^2/day on days 1 to 5 or 100 mg/m^2 on day 1 of a 21-day treatment cycle (Pinkerton 1986)

Hepatoblastoma (off-label use; combination chemotherapy): IV: 80 mg/m^2 continuous infusion over 24 hours on day 1 of a 21-day treatment cycle (Pritchard 2000)

Medulloblastoma (off-label use; combination chemotherapy): IV: 75 mg/m^2 on either day 0 or day 1 of each chemotherapy cycle (Packer 2006)

Neuroblastoma, high-risk (off-label use; combination chemotherapy): IV: 50 mg/m^2/day on days 0 to 3 of a 21-day cycle (cycles 3 and 5) (Naranjo 2011) **or** 50 mg/m^2/day on days 1 to 4 (cycles 3, 5, and 7) (Kushner 1994)

Osteosarcoma (off-label use; combination chemotherapy): IV: 60 mg/m^2/day for 2 days on weeks 2, 7, 25, and 28 (neoadjuvant) or weeks 5, 10, 25, and 28 (adjuvant) in combination with methotrexate, leucovorin, doxorubicin, cyclophosphamide, bleomycin, and dactinomycin (Goorin 2003)

Renal Impairment Note: The manufacturer(s) recommend that repeat courses of cisplatin should not be given until serum creatinine is <1.5 mg/dL and/or BUN is <25 mg/dL and use is contraindicated in preexisting renal impairment. The following adjustments have been recommended.

Aronoff 2007:

CrCl 10 to 50 mL/minute: Administer 75% of dose

CrCl <10 mL/minute: Administer 50% of dose

Hemodialysis: Partially cleared by hemodialysis

Administer 50% of dose posthemodialysis

Continuous ambulatory peritoneal dialysis (CAPD): Administer 50% of dose

Continuous renal replacement therapy (CRRT): Administer 75% of dose

Janus 2010: Hemodialysis: Reduce initial dose by 50%; administer post hemodialysis or on nondialysis days.

Kintzel 1995:

CrCl 46 to 60 mL/minute: Administer 75% of dose

CrCl 31 to 45 mL/minute: Administer 50% of dose

CrCl <30 mL/minute: Consider use of alternative drug

Hepatic Impairment There are no dosage adjustments provided in the manufacturer's labeling. However, cisplatin undergoes nonenzymatic metabolism and predominantly renal elimination; therefore, dosage adjustment is likely not necessary.

Obesity *ASCO Guidelines for appropriate chemotherapy dosing in obese adults with cancer:* Utilize patient's actual body weight (full weight) for calculation of body surface area- or weight-based dosing, particularly when the intent of therapy is curative; manage regimen-related toxicities in the same manner as for nonobese patients; if a dose reduction is utilized due to toxicity, consider resumption of full weight-based dosing with subsequent cycles, especially if cause of toxicity (eg, hepatic or renal impairment) is resolved (Griggs 2012).

Combination Regimens

Biliary adenocarcinoma: Gemcitabine-Cisplatin (Biliary Cancer) on page 2135

Bladder cancer:

Cisplatin-Docetaxel-Gemcitabine (Bladder) on page 2038

Cisplatin-Fluorouracil (Bladder Cancer) on page 2044

Cisplatin-Gemcitabine (Bladder) on page 2051

CMV (Bladder) on page 2068

Dose Dense MVAC (Bladder Cancer) on page 2096

MVAC (Bladder) on page 2179

PCG (Bladder) on page 2191

Bone sarcoma (osteosarcoma):

Ifosfamide-Cisplatin-Epirubicin (Osteosarcoma) on page 2155

MAP (Osteosarcoma) on page 2170

Brain tumors:

CDDP/VP-16 on page 2028

COPE on page 2074

Cervical cancer:

Bevacizumab-Cisplatin-Paclitaxel (Cervical) on page 1991

Cisplatin-Fluorouracil (Cervical Cancer) on page 2044

Cisplatin-Gemcitabine (Cervical) on page 2052

Cisplatin-Paclitaxel (Cervical Cancer) on page 2057

Cisplatin-Topotecan (Cervical Cancer) on page 2060

Cisplatin-Vinorelbine (Cervical Cancer) on page 2063

Administration Cisplatin is associated with a high emetic potential; antiemetics are recommended to prevent nausea and vomiting (Basch 2011; Dupuis 2011; Roila 2016). Pretreatment hydration with 1 to 2 L of fluid is recommended prior to cisplatin administration; adequate post hydration and urinary output (>100 mL/hour) should be maintained for 24 hours after administration.

◄ IV: Infuse over 6 to 8 hours (according to the manufacturer's labeling); has also been infused (off-label rates) over 30 minutes to 3 hours, at a rate of 1 mg/minute, or as a continuous infusion; infusion rate varies by protocol (refer to specific protocol for infusion details). Do not administer as a rapid IV injection. Also refer to specific protocol for information regarding recommended concomitant hydration and diuretics.

Intraperitoneal (off-label route): Solution was prepared in warmed saline and infused as rapidly as possible through an implantable intraperitoneal catheter (Armstrong 2006).

Needles or IV administration sets that contain aluminum should not be used in the preparation or administration; aluminum may react with cisplatin resulting in precipitate formation and loss of potency.

Vesicant (at higher concentrations); ensure proper needle or catheter placement prior to and during infusion; avoid extravasation.

Extravasation management: If extravasation occurs, stop infusion immediately and disconnect (leave cannula/needle in place); gently aspirate extravasated solution (do **NOT** flush the line); initiate sodium thiosulfate antidote; elevate extremity.

Sodium thiosulfate 1/6 M solution: Inject 2 mL into existing IV line for each 100 mg of cisplatin extravasated; then consider also injecting 1 mL as 0.1 mL subcutaneous injections (clockwise) around the area of extravasation, may repeat subcutaneous injections several times over the next 3 to 4 hours (Ener 2004).

Dimethyl sulfoxide (DMSO) may also be considered an option: Apply to a region covering twice the affected area every 8 hours for 7 days; begin within 10 minutes of extravasation; do not cover with a dressing (Perez Fidalgo 2012).

Vesicant/Extravasation Risk Vesicant (>0.4 mg/mL); Irritant (≤0.4 mg/mL)

Emetic Potential Children and Adults: High (>90%)

Monitoring Parameters Renal function (serum creatinine, BUN, CrCl [baseline and before each cycle]); electrolytes (particularly calcium, magnesium, potassium, and sodium [baseline and before each cycle]); CBC with differential and platelet count (weekly); liver function tests (periodic); urine output, urinalysis; audiography (baseline and prior to each subsequent dose, and following treatment in children), neurologic exam (with high dose); monitor infusion site during infusion

Dietary Considerations Some products may contain sodium.

Dosage Forms Excipient information presented when available (limited, particularly for generics); consult specific product labeling.

Solution, Intravenous:
Generic: 50 mg/50 mL (50 mL); 100 mg/100 mL (100 mL); 200 mg/200 mL (200 mL)

Solution, Intravenous [preservative free]:
Generic: 50 mg/50 mL (50 mL); 100 mg/100 mL (100 mL); 200 mg/200 mL (200 mL)

- **13-*cis*-Vitamin A Acid** *see* ISOtretinoin *on page 1063*
- **Citrovorum Factor** *see* Leucovorin Calcium *on page 1124*
- **CL-118,532** *see* Triptorelin *on page 1841*
- **CL-184116** *see* Porfimer *on page 1535*
- **CL-232315** *see* MitoXANTRONE *on page 1271*

Cladribine (KLA dri been)

Related Information

Common Toxicity Criteria *on page 2242*
Management of Chemotherapy-Induced Nausea and Vomiting in Adults *on page 2253*
Management of Drug Extravasations *on page 2271*
Prevention of Chemotherapy-Induced Nausea and Vomiting in Children *on page 2310*
Safe Handling of Hazardous Drugs *on page 2379*

Brand Names: Canada Cladribine Injection

Index Terms 2-CdA; 2-Chlorodeoxyadenosine; Leustatin

Pharmacologic Category Antineoplastic Agent, Antimetabolite; Antineoplastic Agent, Antimetabolite (Purine Analog)

Use Treatment of active hairy cell leukemia

Labeled Contraindications Hypersensitivity to cladribine or any component of the formulation

Pregnancy Considerations Teratogenic effects and fetal mortality were observed in animal reproduction studies. May cause fetal harm if administered during pregnancy. Women of reproductive potential should use highly effective contraception during treatment.

Breastfeeding Considerations Due to the potential for serious adverse reactions in the nursing infant, the decision to discontinue cladribine or to discontinue breastfeeding should take into account the importance of treatment to the mother.

Warnings/Precautions [U.S. Boxed Warning]: Dose-dependent, reversible myelosuppression (neutropenia, anemia, and thrombocytopenia) is common and generally reversible; use with caution in patients with preexisting hematologic or immunologic abnormalities; monitor blood counts, especially during the first 4-8 weeks after treatment. **[U.S. Boxed Warning]: Serious, dose-related neurologic toxicity (including irreversible paraparesis and quadriparesis) has been reported with continuous infusions of higher doses (4-9 times the FDA-approved dose); may also occur at approved doses (rare).** Neurotoxicity may be delayed and may present as progressive, irreversible weakness; diagnostics with electromyography and nerve conduction studies were consistent with demyelinating disease. **[U.S. Boxed Warning]: Acute nephrotoxicity (eg, acidosis, anuria, increased serum creatinine), possibly requiring dialysis, has been reported with high doses (4-9 times the FDA-approved dose), particularly when administered with other nephrotoxic agents.** Use with caution in patients with renal or hepatic impairment. Fever (>100°F) may occur, with or without neutropenia, observed more commonly in the first month of treatment. Infections (bacterial, viral, and fungal) were reported more commonly in the first month after treatment (generally mild or moderate in severity, although serious infections including sepsis have been reported); the incidence is reduced in the second month; due to neutropenia and T-cell depletion, risk versus benefit of treatment should be evaluated in patients with active infections. Administration of live vaccines is not recommended during treatment with cladribine (may increase the risk of infection due to immunosuppression). Use caution in patients with high tumor burden; tumor lysis syndrome may occur (rare). **[U.S. Boxed Warning]: Should be administered under the supervision of an experienced cancer chemotherapy physician.**

Benzyl alcohol and derivatives: Weekly (7-day) infusion preparation recommends further dilution with bacteriostatic normal saline which contains benzyl alcohol; large amounts of benzyl alcohol (≥99 mg/kg/day) have been associated with a potentially fatal toxicity ("gasping syndrome") in neonates; the "gasping syndrome" consists of metabolic acidosis, respiratory distress, gasping respirations, CNS dysfunction (including convulsions, intracranial hemorrhage), hypotension, and cardiovascular collapse (AAP ["Inactive" 1997]; CDC, 1982); some data suggests that benzoate displaces bilirubin from protein binding sites (Ahlfors, 2001); avoid or use dosage forms containing benzyl alcohol with caution in neonates. See manufacturer's labeling.

Adverse Reactions

>10%:

Central nervous system: Fatigue (11% to 45%), headache (7% to 22%)

Dermatologic: Skin rash (10% to 27%)

Gastrointestinal: Nausea (22% to 28%), decreased appetite (8% to 17%), vomiting (9% to 13%)

Hematologic & oncologic: Neutropenia (grade 4: 70%; recovery by week 5), febrile neutropenia (8% to 47%; severe: 32%), anemia (1% to 37%; recovery by week 8), bone marrow depression (34%; prolonged), thrombocytopenia (grade 4: 12%; recovery by day 12)

Infection: Infection (month 1: 28% [serious: 6%]; month 2: 6%)

Local: Injection site reaction (9% to 19%)

Respiratory: Abnormal breath sounds (4% to 11%)

Miscellaneous: Fever (33% to 69%; ≥100°F: 67%; ≥104°F: 11%)

1% to 10%:

Cardiovascular: Edema (2% to 6%), tachycardia (2% to 6%), phlebitis (2%), thrombosis (2%)

Central nervous system: Dizziness (6% to 9%), chills (2% to 9%), malaise (5% to 7%), insomnia (3% to 7%), pain (6%), anxiety (1%), myasthenia (1%)

Dermatologic: Diaphoresis (9%), erythema (6%), pruritus (2% to 6%), hyperhidrosis (3%)

Gastrointestinal: Diarrhea (7% to 10%), constipation (4% to 9%), abdominal pain (4% to 6%), flatulence (1%)

Hematologic & oncologic: Purpura (10%), petechia (2% to 8%), bruise (1% to 2%)

Neuromuscular & skeletal: Weakness (6% to 9%), myalgia (6% to 7%), arthralgia (3% to 5%)

Respiratory: Cough (7% to 10%), dyspnea (5% to 7%), epistaxis (5%), rales (1%)

<1%, postmarketing, and/or case reports: Aplastic anemia, bacteremia, cellulitis, cerebrovascular accident, confusion, conjunctivitis, decreased CD-4 cell count (nadir: 4 to 6 months), eosinophilia (hypereosinophilia or persistent), hemolytic anemia, hypersensitivity reaction, impaired consciousness, increased serum bilirubin, increased serum transaminases, lower extremity weakness, myelodysplastic syndrome, opportunistic infection

(cytomegalovirus disease, fungal infection, herpes virus infection, listeriosis, *Pneumocystis jirovecii*), pancytopenia (prolonged), paresis (at high doses; paraparesis/quadriparesis), pneumonia, polyneuropathy (with high doses), progressive multifocal leukoencephalopathy, pulmonary infiltrates (interstitial), reactivated tuberculosis, renal failure, renal insufficiency (with high doses), septic shock, Stevens-Johnson syndrome, toxic epidermal necrolysis, tumor lysis syndrome, urticaria

Drug Interactions

Metabolism/Transport Effects None known.

Avoid Concomitant Use

Avoid concomitant use of Cladribine with any of the following: BCG (Intravesical); Deferiprone; Dipyrone; Natalizumab; Pimecrolimus; Tacrolimus (Topical); Vaccines (Live)

Increased Effect/Toxicity

Cladribine may increase the levels/effects of: CloZAPine; Deferiprone; Fingolimod; Leflunomide; Natalizumab; Tofacitinib; Vaccines (Live)

The levels/effects of Cladribine may be increased by: Denosumab; Dipyrone; Ocrelizumab; Palifermin; Pimecrolimus; Promazine; Roflumilast; Tacrolimus (Topical); Trastuzumab

Decreased Effect

Cladribine may decrease the levels/effects of: BCG (Intravesical); Coccidioides immitis Skin Test; Lenograstim; Nivolumab; Sipuleucel-T; Tertomotide; Vaccines (Inactivated); Vaccines (Live)

The levels/effects of Cladribine may be decreased by: Echinacea

Hazardous Drugs Handling Considerations

Hazardous agent (NIOSH 2016 [group 1]).

Use appropriate precautions for receiving, handling, administration, and disposal. Gloves (single) should be worn during receiving, unpacking, and placing in storage.

NIOSH recommends double gloving, a protective gown, ventilated engineering controls (a class II biological safety cabinet or a compounding aseptic containment isolator), and closed system transfer devices (CSTDs) for preparation. Double gloving, a gown, and (if dosage form allows) CSTDs are required during administration (NIOSH 2016).

Storage/Stability

Store intact vials refrigerated at 2°C to 8°C (36°F to 46°F). Protect from light. A precipitate may develop at low temperatures and may be resolubilized at room temperature or by shaking the solution vigorously. Inadvertent freezing does not affect the solution; if freezing occurs prior to dilution, allow to thaw naturally prior to reconstitution; do not heat or microwave; do not refreeze.

24-hour continuous infusion: Dilutions in NS for infusion should be used promptly; if not used promptly, the 24-hour infusion may be stored refrigerated for up to 8 hours prior to administration.

7-day continuous infusion: Dilutions in NS for infusion should be used promptly; if not used promptly, the 7-day infusion may be stored refrigerated for up to 8 hours prior to administration. Reconstituted solution is stable for 7 days (when diluted in bacteriostatic NS) in a CADD® medication cassette reservoir. For patients weighing >85 kg, the effectiveness of the preservative in the bacteriostatic diluent may be reduced (due to dilution).

◀ **Preparation for Administration**

A precipitate may develop at low temperatures and may be resolubilized at room temperature or by shaking the solution vigorously. Inadvertent freezing does not affect the solution; if freezing occurs prior to dilution, allow to thaw naturally; do not heat or microwave; do not refreeze.

To prepare a 24-hour continuous infusion: Dilute in 500 mL NS. The manufacturer recommends filtering with a 0.22 micron hydrophilic syringe filter prior to adding to infusion bag.

To prepare a 7-day continuous infusion: Dilute to a total volume of 100 mL in a CADD medication cassette reservoir using bacteriostatic NS. Filter diluent and cladribine with a 0.22 micron hydrophilic filter prior to adding to cassette/reservoir.

Mechanism of Action A purine nucleoside analogue; prodrug which is activated via phosphorylation by deoxycytidine kinase to a 5'-triphosphate derivative (2-CdAMP). This active form incorporates into DNA to result in the breakage of DNA strand and shutdown of DNA synthesis and repair. This also results in a depletion of nicotinamide adenine dinucleotide and adenosine triphosphate (ATP). Cladribine is cell-cycle nonspecific.

Pharmacodynamics/Kinetics

Distribution: V_d:

Children 8 months to 18 years: 12.7 ± 8.5 L/kg; penetrates CSF (CSF concentrations are ~18% of plasma concentration) (Kearns 1994)

Adults: ~9 L/kg; penetrates CSF (CSF concentrations are ~25% of plasma concentrations)

Protein binding: ~20%

Half-life elimination:

Children 8 months to 18 years: 19.7 ± 3.4 hours (Kearns 1994)

Adults: After a 2-hour infusion (with normal renal function): 5.4 hours

Excretion: Urine (18%)

Dosing

Adult & Geriatric Details concerning dosing in combination regimens should also be consulted.

Hairy cell leukemia: IV: 0.09 mg/kg/day continuous infusion for 7 days for 1 cycle **or** (off-label dosing) 0.1 mg/kg/day continuous infusion for 7 days for 1 cycle (Goodman, 2003; Saven, 1998)

Acute myeloid leukemia, induction (off-label use): IV: CLAG or CLAG-M regimen: 5 mg/m²/day over 2 hours for 5 days; a second induction may be administered if needed (Robak, 2000; Wierzbowska, 2008; Wrzesień-Kuś, 2003)

Chronic lymphocytic leukemia (off-label use): IV: 0.1 mg/kg/day continuous infusion for 7 days every 4-5 weeks (Saven, 1995) **or** 0.14 mg/kg/day over 2 hours for 5 days every 28 days for 3-6 cycles (Byrd, 2003)

Mantle cell lymphoma (off-label use): IV: 5 mg/m²/day over 2 hours for 5 days every 4 weeks for 2-6 cycles (Inwards, 2008; Rummel, 1999) **or** 5 mg/m²/day over 2 hours for 5 days every 4 weeks for 2-6 cycles (in combination with rituximab) (Inwards, 2008)

Waldenström's macroglobulinemia (off-label use):

IV: 0.1 mg/kg/day continuous infusion for 7 days every 4 weeks for 2 cycles (Dimopoulos, 1994)

SubQ: 0.1 mg/kg/day for 5 consecutive days every month for 4 cycles (in combination with rituximab) (Laszlo, 2010)

Pediatric

Acute myeloid leukemia (off-label use): IV: 8.9 mg/m^2/day continuous infusion for 5 days for 1 or 2 courses (Krance, 2001) **or** 9 mg/m^2/day over 30 minutes for 5 days for 1 course (in combination with cytarabine) (Crews, 2002; Rubnitz, 2009)

Langerhans cell histiocytosis, refractory (off-label use): IV: 5 mg/m^2/day over 2 hours for 5 days every 21 days for up to 6 cycles (Weitzman, 2009)

Renal Impairment No dosage adjustment provided in the manufacturer's labeling (due to inadequate data); use with caution. The following adjustments have been used (Aronoff, 2007):

Adults:

CrCl 10-50 mL/minute: Administer 75% of dose

CrCl <10 mL/minute: Administer 50% of dose

Continuous ambulatory peritoneal dialysis (CAPD): Administer 50% of dose

Children:

CrCl 10-50 mL/minute: Administer 50% of dose

CrCl <10 mL/minute: Administer 30% of dose

Hemodialysis: Administer 30% of dose

Continuous renal replacement therapy (CRRT): Administer 50% of dose

Hepatic Impairment No dosage adjustment provided in the manufacturer's labeling (due to inadequate data); use with caution.

Obesity ASCO Guidelines for appropriate chemotherapy dosing in obese adults with cancer: Utilize patient's actual body weight (full weight) for calculation of body surface area- or weight-based dosing, particularly when the intent of therapy is curative; manage regimen-related toxicities in the same manner as for nonobese patients; if a dose reduction is utilized due to toxicity, consider resumption of full weight-based dosing with subsequent cycles, especially if cause of toxicity (eg, hepatic or renal impairment) is resolved (Griggs, 2012).

Combination Regimens

Leukemia, acute myeloid:

CLAG (AML Induction) on page 2065

CLAG-M (AML Induction) on page 2065

Lymphoma, non-Hodgkin (Mantle Cell): Cladribine-Rituximab (NHL-Mantle Cell) on page 2064

Waldenstrom Macroglobulinemia: Cladribine-Rituximab (Waldenstrom Macroglobulinemia) on page 2064

Administration

IV: Administer as a continuous infusion. May also be administered over 30 minutes or over 2 hours (off-label administration rates) depending on indication and/or protocol.

SubQ (off-label route): May also be administered SubQ (Laszlo, 2010)

Vesicant/Extravasation Risk May be an irritant.

Emetic Potential Children and Adults: Minimal (<10%)

Monitoring Parameters CBC with differential (particularly during the first 4-8 weeks post-treatment), renal and hepatic function; bone marrow biopsy (after CBC has normalized, to confirm treatment response); monitor for fever; monitor for signs/symptoms of neurotoxicity

Dosage Forms Excipient information presented when available (limited, particularly for generics); consult specific product labeling.

Solution, Intravenous [preservative free]:

Generic: 10 mg/10 mL (10 mL)

Clodronate (KLOE droh nate)

Brand Names: Canada Bonefos; Clasteon

Index Terms Clodronate Disodium

Pharmacologic Category Bisphosphonate Derivative

Use Note: Not approved in the US

Hypercalcemia of malignancy: Management of hypercalcemia of malignancy

Osteolytic bone metastases: Adjunct in the management of osteolysis due to bone metastases of malignant tumors

Dosing

Adult & Geriatric

Hypercalcemia of malignancy:

IV:

Clasteon:

Single infusion: 1,500 mg over at least 4 hours as a single dose

Multiple infusions: 300 mg over 2 to 6 hours once daily; treatment duration should not exceed 10 days

Note: Regardless of infusion method, plasma calcium levels usually normalize within 2 to 5 days

Bonefos: Multiple infusions: 300 mg over at least 2 hours once daily; continue until plasma calcium levels return to normal (usually 2 to 5 days); treatment duration should not exceed 7 days

Oral: Recommended daily maintenance dose following calcium normalization with IV therapy:

Clasteon: Range: 1,600 mg to 2,400 mg given in a single dose or in 2 divided doses; maximum recommended daily dose: 3,200 mg.

Bonefos: Range: 1,600 mg to 2,400 mg given in a single dose or in 2 divided doses; maximum recommended daily dose: 3,200 mg.

Note: Re-treatment: Limited data suggest that patients who develop hypercalcemia following discontinuation of therapy or during oral therapy may be retreated with Bonefos or Clasteon at a higher oral dosage (up to 3,200 mg/day) or by IV infusion with Clasteon (1,500 mg as single dose or 300 mg once daily) or Bonefos (300 mg once daily).

Osteolytic bone metastases:

IV:

Clasteon:

Single infusion: 1,500 mg over at least 4 hours as a single dose

Multiple infusions: 300 mg over 2 to 6 hours once daily; treatment duration should not exceed 10 days

Bonefos: Multiple infusions: 300 mg over at least 2 hours once daily; treatment duration should not exceed 7 days

Oral:

Clasteon: Recommended daily maintenance dose following IV therapy: Range: 1,600 mg to 2,400 mg given in a single dose or in 2 divided doses; maximum recommended daily dose: 3,200 mg.

Bonefos: Initial: 1,600 mg/day; may be increased to a maximum of 3,200 mg/day

Breast cancer, adjuvant therapy (off-label use): Oral: 1,600 mg daily for 2 to 3 years (CCO/ASCO [Dhesy-Thind 2017).

Renal Impairment

Deterioration of renal function during IV therapy: Stop treatment.

Clasteon:

Serum creatinine (S_{cr}) >5 mg/dL: Use is contraindicated.

S_{cr} ≥2.5 to 5 mg/dL: There are no specific dosage adjustments provided in manufacturer's labeling; however, the manufacturer recommends considering a dose reduction or withholding therapy.

Bonefos:

S_{cr} >5 mg/dL: Use is contraindicated.

IV:

CrCl >50 to 80 mL/minute: Administer 75% to 100% of normal dose.

CrC: 12 to 50 mL/minute: Administer 50% to 75% of normal dose.

CrCl <12 mL/minute: Administer 50% of normal dose.

Oral: **Note:** Daily doses >1,600 mg should not be used continuously.

CrCl >50 mL/minute: No dosage adjustment necessary.

CrCl 30 to 50 mL/minute: Administer 75% of normal dose.

CrCl <30 mL/minute: Administer 50% of normal dose.

Hepatic Impairment There are no dosage adjustments provided in the manufacturer's labeling; however, elimination is predominantly renal.

Additional Information Complete prescribing information should be consulted for additional detail.

Product Availability Not available in the US

Dosage Forms: Canada Information with regard to form, strength, and availability of products uniquely available in Canada but currently not available in the US.

Excipient information presented when available (limited, particularly for generics); consult specific product labeling.

Capsule, Oral:

Bonefos, Clasteon: 400 mg

Solution, Intravenous:

Bonefos: 60 mg/mL (5 mL)

Clasteon: 30 mg/mL (10 mL)

◆ **Clodronate Disodium** see Clodronate on page 416

Clofarabine (klo FARE a been)

Related Information

Common Toxicity Criteria on page 2242

Management of Chemotherapy-Induced Nausea and Vomiting in Adults on page 2253

Prevention of Chemotherapy-Induced Nausea and Vomiting in Children on page 2310

Safe Handling of Hazardous Drugs on page 2379

Brand Names: US Clolar

Brand Names: Canada Clolar

Index Terms CAFdA; Clofarex

Pharmacologic Category Antineoplastic Agent, Antimetabolite; Antineoplastic Agent, Antimetabolite (Purine Analog)

◀ **Use Acute lymphoblastic leukemia, relapsed or refractory:** Treatment of relapsed or refractory acute lymphoblastic leukemia (ALL) in patients 1 to 21 years of age (after at least 2 prior regimens)

Labeled Contraindications

There are no contraindications listed in the manufacturer's US labeling.

Canadian labeling: Hypersensitivity to clofarabine or any component of the formulation; symptomatic CNS involvement; history of serious heart, liver, kidney, or pancreas disease; severe hepatic impairment (AST and/or ALT >5 x ULN, and/or bilirubin >3 x ULN); severe renal impairment (CrCl <30 mL/ minute)

Pregnancy Considerations Adverse events were observed in animal reproduction studies. May cause fetal harm if administered to a pregnant woman. Women of childbearing potential should avoid becoming pregnant during therapy. All patients should use effective contraception to prevent pregnancy during treatment.

Breastfeeding Considerations It is not known if clofarabine is excreted in breast milk. Due to the potential for serious adverse reactions in the nursing infant, breastfeeding is not recommended by the manufacturer.

Warnings/Precautions Cytokine release syndrome (eg, tachypnea, tachy-cardia, hypotension, pulmonary edema) may develop into capillary leak syndrome, systemic inflammatory response syndrome (SIRS), and organ dysfunction; immediately discontinue with signs/symptoms of SIRS or capillary leak syndrome (rapid onset respiratory distress, hypotension, pleural/ pericardial effusion, and multiorgan failure) and manage appropriately. Consider supportive treatment with diuretics, corticosteroids, and/or albumin. Prophylactic corticosteroids may prevent or diminish the signs/symptoms of cytokine release. May require dosage reduction. Monitor blood pressure during 5 days of treatment; discontinue if hypotension develops. Monitor if on concurrent medications known to affect blood pressure. Dose-dependent, reversible myelosuppression (neutropenia, thrombocytopenia, and anemia) is common; may be severe and prolonged. Monitor blood counts and platelets. May be at increased risk for infection due to neutropenia; opportunistic infection or sepsis (may be severe or fatal), is increased due to prolonged neutropenia and immunocompromised state; monitor for signs and symptoms of infection and treat promptly if infection develops. May require therapy discontinuation. Serious and fatal hemorrhages (including cerebral, gastro-intestinal, and pulmonary hemorrhage) have occurred, usually associated with thrombocytopenia. Monitor and manage coagulation parameters.

Serious and fatal cases of Stevens-Johnson syndrome (SJS) and toxic epidermal necrolysis (TEN) have been reported. Discontinue clofarabine for exfoliative or bullous rash, or if SJS or TEN are suspected. Clofarabine is associated with a moderate emetic potential; antiemetics are recommended to prevent nausea and vomiting (Basch 2011; Dupuis 2011; Roila 2016). Serious and fatal enterocolitis (including neutropenic colitis, cecitis, and *C. difficile* colitis) has been reported, usually occurring within 30 days of treatment, and when used in combination with other chemotherapy. May lead to necrosis, perforation, hemorrhage or sepsis complications. Monitor for signs/symptoms of enterocolitis and manage promptly.

Transaminases and bilirubin may be increased during treatment; hepatitis and hepatic failure have been reported. Transaminase elevations generally occur within 10 days of administration and persist for ≤15 days. In some cases, hepatotoxicity was severe and fatal. The risk for hepatotoxicity, including hepatic sinusoidal obstruction syndrome (SOS; formerly called veno-occlusive disease), is increased in patients who have previously undergone a hematopoietic stem cell transplant. Monitor liver function closely; discontinue immediately for grade ≥3 elevations in hepatic enzymes and/or bilirubin. Discontinue if SOS is suspected. Elevated creatinine, acute renal failure, and hematuria were observed in clinical studies. Infection, sepsis, or tumor lysis syndrome may cause an increased risk of renal toxicity in patients receiving clofarabine. Monitor renal function closely; may require dosage reduction or therapy discontinuation. A pharmacokinetic study demonstrated that systemic exposure increases as creatinine clearance decreases (CrCl <60 mL/minute) (Bonate 2011). Dosage reduction required for CrCl 30 to 60 mL/minute; use with caution in patients with CrCl <30 mL/minute (has not been studied). Minimize the use of drugs known to cause renal toxicity during the 5-day treatment period; avoid concomitant hepatotoxic medications. Tumor lysis syndrome/hyperuricemia may occur as a consequence of leukemia treatment, including treatment with clofarabine, usually occurring in the first treatment cycle. May lead to life-threatening acute renal failure; adequate hydration and prophylactic antihyperuricemic therapy throughout treatment will reduce the risk/effects of tumor lysis syndrome; monitor closely. Potentially significant drug-drug interactions may exist, requiring dose or frequency adjustment, additional monitoring, and/or selection of alternative therapy.

Adverse Reactions Incidences include off-label use in the treatment of AML.

>10%:

Cardiovascular: Tachycardia (35%), hypotension (29%), flushing (19%), hypertension (13%), edema (12%)

Central nervous system: Headache (43%), chills (34%), fatigue (34%), anxiety (21%), pain (15%)

Dermatologic: Pruritus (43%), skin rash (38%), palmar-plantar erythrodysesthesia (16%), erythema (11%)

Gastrointestinal: Vomiting (78%), nausea (73%), diarrhea (56%), abdominal pain (35%), anorexia (30%), gingival bleeding (17%), mucosal inflammation (16%), oral candidiasis (11%)

Genitourinary: Hematuria (13%)

Hematologic & oncologic: Leukopenia (88%; grades 3/4: 88%), anemia (83%; grades 3/4: 75%), lymphocytopenia (82%; grades 3/4: 82%), thrombocytopenia (81%; grades 3/4: 80%), neutropenia (10% to 64%; grades 3/4: 64%; grade 4: 7%), febrile neutropenia (55%; grade 3: 51%; grade 4: 3%), petechia (26%; grade 3: 6%)

Hepatic: Increased serum ALT (81%), increased serum AST (74%), increased bilirubin (45%)

Infection: Infection (83%; includes bacterial, fungal, and viral), sepsis (including septic shock; 17%)

Local: Catheter infection (12%)

Neuromuscular & skeletal: Limb pain (30%), myalgia (14%)

Renal: Increased serum creatinine (50%)

Respiratory: Epistaxis (27%), dyspnea (13%), pleural effusion (12%)

Miscellaneous: Fever (39%)

1% to 10%:

Cardiovascular: Pericardial effusion (8%), capillary leak syndrome (4%), hepatic sinusoidal obstruction syndrome (formerly known as hepatic veno-occlusive disease) (2%)

Central nervous system: Drowsiness (10%), irritability (10%), lethargy (10%), agitation (5%), mental status changes (1% to 4%)

◀ Dermatologic: Cellulitis (8%), pruritic rash (8%)

Gastrointestinal: Rectal pain (8%), upper abdominal pain (8%), pseudomembranous colitis (7%), stomatitis (7%), pancreatitis (1% to 4%), typhlitis (1% to 4%)

Hematologic & oncologic: Tumor lysis syndrome (6%; grade 3: 6%), oral mucosal petechiae (5%; grade 3: 4%)

Hepatic: Jaundice (8%), hyperbilirubinemia (1% to 4%)

Hypersensitivity: Hypersensitivity (1% to 4%)

Infection: Herpes simplex infection (10%), bacteremia (9%), candidiasis (7%), herpes zoster (7%), staphylococcal bacteremia (6%), staphylococcal sepsis (5%), influenza (1% to 4%), sepsis syndrome (2%)

Neuromuscular & skeletal: Back pain (10%), ostealgia (10%), weakness (10%), arthralgia (9%)

Renal: Acute renal failure

Respiratory: Pneumonia (10%), respiratory distress (10%), tachypnea (9%), upper respiratory tract infection (5%), pulmonary edema (1% to 4%), sinusitis (1% to 4%)

<1%, postmarketing, and/or case reports: Enterocolitis (occurs more frequently within 30 days of treatment and with combination chemotherapy), exfoliative dermatitis, gastrointestinal hemorrhage, hallucination (Jeha 2006), hepatic failure, hepatitis, hepatomegaly (Jeha 2006), hypokalemia (Jeha 2006), hyponatremia, hypophosphatemia, increased right ventricular pressure (Jeha 2006), left ventricular systolic dysfunction (Jeha 2006), major hemorrhage (including cerebral and pulmonary; majority of cases associated with thrombocytopenia), Stevens-Johnson syndrome, toxic epidermal necrolysis

Drug Interactions

Metabolism/Transport Effects None known.

Avoid Concomitant Use

Avoid concomitant use of Clofarabine with any of the following: BCG (Intravesical); Deferiprone; Dipyrone; Natalizumab; Pimecrolimus; Tacrolimus (Topical); Vaccines (Live)

Increased Effect/Toxicity

Clofarabine may increase the levels/effects of: Amifostine; Antipsychotic Agents (Second Generation [Atypical]); CloZAPine; Deferiprone; DULoxetine; Fingolimod; Hypotension-Associated Agents; Leflunomide; Levodopa; Natalizumab; Nitroprusside; Pholcodine; Tofacitinib; Vaccines (Live)

The levels/effects of Clofarabine may be increased by: Alfuzosin; Barbiturates; Benperidol; Blood Pressure Lowering Agents; Brimonidine (Topical); Denosumab; Diazoxide; Dipyrone; Herbs (Hypotensive Properties); Lormetazepam; Molsidomine; Naftopidil; Nicergoline; Nicorandil; Obinutuzumab; Ocrelizumab; Palifermin; Pentoxifylline; Phosphodiesterase 5 Inhibitors; Pimecrolimus; Promazine; Prostacyclin Analogues; Quinagolide; Roflumilast; Tacrolimus (Topical); Trastuzumab

Decreased Effect

Clofarabine may decrease the levels/effects of: BCG (Intravesical); Coccidioides immitis Skin Test; Lenograstim; Nivolumab; Sipuleucel-T; Tertomotide; Vaccines (Inactivated); Vaccines (Live)

The levels/effects of Clofarabine may be decreased by: Echinacea

Hazardous Drugs Handling Considerations
Hazardous agent (NIOSH 2016 [group 1]).

Use appropriate precautions for receiving, handling, administration, and disposal. Gloves (single) should be worn during receiving, unpacking, and placing in storage.

NIOSH recommends double gloving, a protective gown, ventilated engineering controls (a class II biological safety cabinet or a compounding aseptic containment isolator), and closed system transfer devices (CSTDs) for preparation. Double gloving, a gown, and (if dosage form allows) CSTDs are required during administration (NIOSH 2016).

Storage/Stability Store intact vials at 25°C (77°F); excursions permitted to 15°C to 30°C (59°F to 86°F). Solutions diluted for infusion in D5W or NS may be stored for up to 24 hours at room temperature (use within 24 hours of preparation).

Preparation for Administration Clofarabine should be diluted with NS or D5W to a final concentration of 0.15 to 0.4 mg/mL. Manufacturer recommends the product be filtered through a 0.2 micron filter prior to dilution.

Mechanism of Action Clofarabine, a purine (deoxyadenosine) nucleoside analog, is metabolized to clofarabine 5'-triphosphate. Clofarabine 5'-triphosphate decreases cell replication and repair as well as causing cell death. To decrease cell replication and repair, clofarabine 5'-triphosphate competes with deoxyadenosine triphosphate for the enzymes ribonucleotide reductase and DNA polymerase. Cell replication is decreased when clofarabine 5'-triphosphate inhibits ribonucleotide reductase from reacting with deoxyadenosine triphosphate to produce deoxynucleotide triphosphate which is needed for DNA synthesis. Cell replication is also decreased when clofarabine 5'-triphosphate competes with DNA polymerase for incorporation into the DNA chain; when done during the repair process, cell repair is affected. To cause cell death, clofarabine 5'-triphosphate alters the mitochondrial membrane by releasing proteins, an inducing factor and cytochrome C.

Pharmacodynamics/Kinetics

Distribution: V_d: Decreased with increasing age, based on pharmacokinetic simulations: 5.8 L/kg (3 years old); 3.1 L/kg (30 years old); 2.7 L/kg (82 years old) (Bonate 2011); Children and Adolescents 2 to 19 years: 172 L/m^2

Protein binding: 47%, primarily to albumin

Metabolism: Intracellular by deoxycytidine kinase and mono- and diphosphokinases to active metabolite clofarabine 5'-triphosphate; limited hepatic metabolism (0.2%)

Half-life elimination: Children and Adolescents 2 to 19 years: 5.2 hours; Children and Adults: 7 hours; may be prolonged in in the elderly and in patients with renal impairment (Bonate, 2011)

Excretion: Urine (49% to 60%, as unchanged drug)

Dosing

Adult Note: Calculate body surface area (BSA) prior to each cycle, utilizing actual body weight.

Premedications: Clofarabine is associated with a moderate emetic potential; antiemetics are recommended to prevent nausea and vomiting (Basch 2011; Roila 2016). Consider prophylactic corticosteroids (hydrocortisone 100 mg/m^2 on days 1 to 3) to prevent signs/symptoms of capillary leak syndrome or systemic inflammatory response syndrome (SIRS), and hydration and antihyperuricemic therapy (to reduce the risk of tumor lysis syndrome/hyperuricemia).

◀ **Acute lymphoblastic leukemia (ALL), relapsed or refractory:** Adults ≤21 years: IV: 52 mg/m²/day days 1 through 5; repeat every 2 to 6 weeks; subsequent cycles should begin no sooner than 14 days from day 1 of the previous cycle (subsequent cycles may be administered when ANC ≥750/mm³)

Off-label dosing: IV: 20 to 30 mg/m² once daily on days 1 through 5 (in combination with cyclophosphamide and etoposide [CLOVE regimen]) as a bridging regimen to hematopoietic stem cell transplant in patients with relapsed or very high risk disease (Gossai 2014)

Acute lymphoblastic leukemia, relapsed/refractory (ALL; off-label population): IV:

Induction: 40 mg/m² once daily for 5 days; may repeat induction cycle once in 3 to 6 weeks if needed (depending on marrow response and recovery) (Kantarjian 2003)

Consolidation: 30 mg/m² once daily for 5 days (or last tolerated induction dose, whichever is lower); repeat every 4 weeks for up to a maximum of 6 consolidation cycles (Kantarjian 2003)

Acute myeloid leukemia (AML), refractory (off-label use): Adults <70 years: IV:

Induction: 25 mg/m²/day for 5 days (in combination with cytarabine and filgrastim) may repeat one time after 21 days if needed (Becker 2011)

Consolidation: 20 mg/m²/day for 5 days (in combination with cytarabine and filgrastim) for 1 or 2 cycles (Becker 2011)

Pediatric Note: Calculate body surface area (BSA) prior to each cycle, utilizing actual body weight.

Premedications: Clofarabine is associated with a moderate emetic potential; antiemetics are recommended to prevent nausea and vomiting (Dupuis 2011). Consider prophylactic corticosteroids (hydrocortisone 100 mg/m² on days 1 to 3) to prevent signs/symptoms of capillary leak syndrome or systemic inflammatory response syndrome (SIRS), and hydration and antihyperuricemic therapy (to reduce the risk of tumor lysis syndrome/hyperuricemia).

Acute lymphoblastic leukemia (ALL), relapsed or refractory: Children ≥1 year and Adolescents: IV: 52 mg/m²/day days 1 through 5; repeat every 2 to 6 weeks; subsequent cycles should begin no sooner than 14 days from day 1 of the previous cycle (subsequent cycles may be administered when ANC ≥750/mm³)

Off-label dosing: IV: 20 to 30 mg/m² once daily on days 1 through 5 (in combination with cyclophosphamide and etoposide [CLOVE regimen]) as a bridging regimen to hematopoietic stem cell transplant in patients with relapsed or very high risk disease (Gossai 2014)

Langerhans cell histiocytosis, refractory (off-label use): Children 1 to 18 years: IV: 25 mg/m²/day days 1 through 5; repeat every 28 days for 2 to 8 cycles (Simko 2014). Additional data may be necessary to further define the role of clofarabine in this condition.

Renal Impairment Clofarabine undergoes renal elimination and exposure is increased as creatinine clearance decreases (Bonate 2011).

Renal impairment at baseline:

CrCl >60 mL/minute: No dosage adjustment necessary.

CrCl 30 to 60 mL/minute: Reduce dose to 50% of the usual dose

CrCl <30 mL/minute: There are no dosage adjustments provided in the manufacturer's labeling; use with caution (has not been studied).

Dialysis: There are no dosage adjustments provided in the manufacturer's labeling (has not been studied).

Renal toxicity during treatment: Grade 3 or higher increase in serum creatinine: Discontinue clofarabine; may reinitiate with a 25% dose reduction after patient is stable and organ function recovers to baseline

Hepatic Impairment

Hepatic impairment at baseline: There are no dosage adjustments provided in the manufacturer's labeling; use with caution (has not been studied).

Hepatotoxicity during treatment: Grade 3 or higher increase in hepatic enzymes/bilirubin: Discontinue clofarabine; may reinitiate with a 25% dose reduction after patient is stable and organ function recovers to baseline.

Obesity *American Society for Blood and Marrow Transplantation (ASBMT) practice guideline committee position statement on chemotherapy dosing in obesity:* Utilize actual body weight (full weight) for calculation of body surface area in clofarabine dosing for hematopoietic stem cell transplant conditioning regimens in pediatrics and adults (Bubalo, 2014).

Adjustment for Toxicity

Hematologic toxicity: ANC <500/mm^3 lasting ≥4 weeks: Reduce dose by 25% for next cycle

Nonhematologic toxicity:

Clinically significant infection: Withhold treatment until infection is under control, then restart at full dose

Grade 3 toxicity excluding infection, nausea and vomiting controlled by antiemetics, or transient elevations in transaminases and bilirubin: Withhold treatment; may reinitiate with a 25% dose reduction with resolution or return to baseline

Grade 4 toxicity (noninfectious): Discontinue clofarabine.

Capillary leak or systemic inflammatory response syndrome (SIRS) early signs/symptoms (eg, hypotension, tachycardia, tachypnea, pulmonary edema): Discontinue clofarabine; institute supportive measures. May consider reinitiating with a 25% dose reduction after patient is stable and organ function recovers to baseline.

Dermatologic toxicity: Exfoliative or bullous rash, or suspected Stevens-Johnson syndrome or toxic epidermal necrolysis: Discontinue clofarabine.

Hypotension (during the 5 days of infusion): Discontinue clofarabine.

Combination Regimens

Leukemia, acute lymphocytic: Clofarabine-Cyclophosphamide-Etoposide (ALL) on page 2065

Leukemia, acute myeloid: Clofarabine-Cytarabine (AML) on page 2066

Administration

Clofarabine is associated with a moderate emetic potential; antiemetics are recommended to prevent nausea and vomiting (Basch 2011; Dupuis 2011; Roila 2016).

IV infusion: Infuse over 2 hours for relapsed/refractory ALL. May be infused over 1 hour for some off-label protocols (Becker 2011; Kantarjian 2003). Continuous IV fluids are encouraged to decrease adverse events and tumor lysis effects. Hypotension may be a sign of capillary leak syndrome or systemic inflammatory response syndrome (SIRS). Discontinue if the patient becomes hypotensive during administration; may consider therapy reinitiation with a 25% dose reduction after return to baseline. Do not administer any other medications through the same intravenous line.

Emetic Potential Children and Adults: Moderate (30% to 90%)

◀ **Monitoring Parameters** CBC with differential and platelets (daily during treatment, then 1 to 2 times weekly or as necessary); liver and kidney function (during 5 days of clofarabine administration); coagulation parameters, blood pressure, cardiac function, and respiratory status during infusion; signs and symptoms of tumor lysis syndrome, infection, hepatic sinusoidal obstruction syndrome, enterocolitis, and cytokine release syndrome (tachypnea, tachycardia, hypotension, pulmonary edema); hydration status

Dosage Forms Excipient information presented when available (limited, particularly for generics); consult specific product labeling.
Solution, Intravenous [preservative free]:
  Clolar: 1 mg/mL (20 mL)
  Generic: 1 mg/mL (20 mL)

◆ **Clofarex** see Clofarabine on page 417
◆ **Clolar** see Clofarabine on page 417

Clotrimazole (Oral) (kloe TRIM a zole)

Index Terms Mycelex
Pharmacologic Category Antifungal Agent, Imidazole Derivative; Antifungal Agent, Oral Nonabsorbed
Use
Oropharyngeal candidiasis (treatment): Local treatment of oropharyngeal candidiasis.
Oropharyngeal candidiasis (prophylaxis): To reduce the incidence of oropharyngeal candidiasis in immunocompromised patients undergoing chemotherapy, radiotherapy, or steroid therapy utilized in the treatment of leukemia, solid tumors, or renal transplantation.
Pregnancy Risk Factor C
Dosing
Adult & Geriatric
Oropharyngeal candidiasis (prophylaxis): Oral: 10 mg dissolved slowly 3 times daily for the duration of chemotherapy or until steroids are reduced to maintenance levels.
Oropharyngeal candidiasis (treatment): Oral: 10 mg dissolved slowly 5 times daily for 14 consecutive days. Note: When used for initial treatment in patients with HIV-1, duration of therapy is 7 to 14 days (DHHS [adult] 2014; DHHS [pediatric] 2013).
Pediatric Oropharyngeal candidiasis (treatment): Children ≥3 years and Adolescents: Refer to adult dosing.
Renal Impairment There are no dosage adjustments provided in the manufacturer's labeling.
Hepatic Impairment There are no dosage adjustments provided in the manufacturer's labeling.
Additional Information Complete prescribing information should be consulted for additional detail.
Dosage Forms Excipient information presented when available (limited, particularly for generics); consult specific product labeling.
Lozenge, Mouth/Throat:
  Generic: 10 mg (70 ea, 140 ea)
Troche, Mouth/Throat:
  Generic: 10 mg

◆ **CMA-676** see Gemtuzumab Ozogamicin on page 874

◆ **CMC-544** *see* Inotuzumab Ozogamicin *on page 1011*

◆ **C-Met/Hepatocyte Growth Factor Receptor Tyrosine Kinase Inhibitor PF-02341066** *see* Crizotinib *on page 432*

◆ **C-Met/HGFR Tyrosine Kinase Inhibitor PF-02341066** *see* Crizotinib *on page 432*

◆ **CMV Hyperimmune Globulin** *see* Cytomegalovirus Immune Globulin (Intravenous-Human) *on page 485*

◆ **CMV-IGIV** *see* Cytomegalovirus Immune Globulin (Intravenous-Human) *on page 485*

◆ **CNTO 328** *see* Siltuximab *on page 1663*

◆ **CO-338** *see* Rucaparib *on page 1641*

◆ **Coagulation Factor I** *see* Fibrinogen Concentrate (Human) *on page 791*

◆ **Coagulation Factor VIIa** *see* Factor VIIa (Recombinant) *on page 765*

Cobimetinib (koe bi ME ti nib)

Related Information

Common Toxicity Criteria *on page 2242*

Management of Chemotherapy-Induced Nausea and Vomiting in Adults *on page 2253*

Safe Handling of Hazardous Drugs *on page 2379*

Brand Names: US Cotellic

Brand Names: Canada Cotellic

Index Terms Cobimetinib Fumarate; Cotellic; GDC-0973; XL518

Pharmacologic Category Antineoplastic Agent, MEK Inhibitor

Use Melanoma, unresectable or metastatic: Treatment of unresectable or metastatic melanoma in patients with a BRAF V600E or V600K mutation (in combination with vemurafenib)

Labeled Contraindications

There are no contraindications listed in the US manufacturer's labeling.

Canadian labeling: Known hypersensitivity to cobimetinib or any component of the formulation

Pregnancy Considerations Adverse events were observed in animal reproduction studies. Based on the mechanism of action, cobimetinib would be expected to cause fetal harm. Women of reproductive potential should use effective contraception during therapy and for 2 weeks after the final dose. The study protocol recommended the use of two forms of effective contraception during therapy and for at least 6 months following discontinuation for women of reproductive potential and for males with partners of reproductive potential (Larkin 2013 [Protocol GO28141]).

Breastfeeding Considerations It is not known if cobimetinib is excreted in breast milk. The manufacturer does not recommend breastfeeding during therapy and for 2 weeks after the final dose.

Warnings/Precautions New primary cutaneous malignancies may occur. Malignancies included cutaneous squamous cell carcinoma (cuSCC) or keratoacanthoma (KA), basal cell carcinoma (BCC), and second primary melanoma. The median time to detection of first cuSCC or KA was 4 months (range: 2 to 11 months); the median time to first detection of BCC was 4 months (range: 1 to 13 months). Dermatologic exams should be performed prior to initiation, every 2 months during treatment, and for 6 months following discontinuation of cobimetinib/vemurafenib combination therapy. Suspicious lesions should be managed with excision and dermatopathologic evaluation. Dosage adjustment is not recommended for new cutaneous malignancies. Vemurafenib may be associated with the development of noncutaneous malignancy; monitor for signs/symptoms of noncutaneous malignancy during combination treatment.

Hemorrhage, including major symptomatic bleeding in a critical area/organ, may occur with cobimetinib. Grade 3 to 4 bleeding has occurred. Cerebral hemorrhage, gastrointestinal bleeding, reproductive system hemorrhage, and hematuria have been reported. May require treatment interruption, dose reduction, and/or discontinuation. Symptomatic or asymptomatic declines in left ventricular ejection fraction (LVEF) may occur with cobimetinib. Safety has not been established in patients with baseline LVEF below the institutional lower limit of normal (LLN) or below 50%. Assess LVEF (by echocardiogram or MUGA scan) prior to therapy initiation, 1 month after initiation, and every 3 months thereafter until cobimetinib is discontinued. May require treatment interruption, dose reduction and/or discontinuation. Also assess LVEF at ~2 weeks, 4 weeks, 10 weeks, 16 weeks, and then as clinically indicated after a dose reduction or treatment interruption. The median time to first onset of LVEF decline was 4 months (range: 23 days to 13 months). Decreased LVEF resolved to >LLN or within 10% of baseline at nearly two-thirds of patients with a median time to resolution of 3 months (range: 4 days to 12 months). Hypertension has been observed with cobimetinib in combination with vemur-afenib, including grades 3 or 4 hypertension.

Severe rash and other skin reactions (including grades 3 and 4 toxicity) may occur; some events required hospitalization. The median time to onset of grade 3 and 4 rash events was 11 days (range: 3 days to ~3 months); most patients with grades 3 and 4 rash experienced complete resolution at a median time of 21 days (range: 4 days to 17 months). May require treatment interruption, dose reduction and/or discontinuation. Photosensitivity was reported in nearly one-half of patients (may be severe). The median time to first onset of photosensitivity was 2 months (range: 1 day to 14 months); the median duration was 3 months (range: 2 days to 14 months). Photosensitivity resolved in nearly two-thirds of patients. Advise patients to avoid sun exposure, wear protective clothing, and use a broad-spectrum UVA/UVB sunscreen and lip balm (SPF 30 or higher) when outdoors. Photosensitivity may require treatment interruption, dose reduction, and/or discontinuation. Ocular toxicities may occur, including serous retinopathy (fluid accumulation under retina layers). Chorioretinopathy and retinal detachment have been reported; retinal vein occlusion has also been reported (case reports); permanently discontinue if retinal vein occlusion occurs. The time to first onset of serous retinopathy ranged between 2 days to 9 months with a duration of 1 day to 15 months. Perform ophthalmic examinations regularly during treatment, and with reports of new or worsening visual disturbances. If serous retinopathy is diagnosed, interrupt treatment until visual symptoms improve; may require treatment interruption, dose reduction, and/or discontin-uation.

Hepatotoxicity (including grades 3 or 4 transaminase, total bilirubin, or alkaline phosphatase elevations) may occur with cobimetinib. Monitor liver function test at baseline and monthly during treatment, or as clinically necessary. Grade 3 and 4 elevations may require treatment interruption, dose reduction, and/or discontinuation. Rhabdomyolysis and creatine phosphokinase (CPK) elevations may occur with cobimetinib. The median time to first occurrence of grade 3 or 4 CPK elevations was 16 days (range: 12 days to 11 months), with a median time to resolution of 15 days (range: 9 days to 11 months).

Obtain baseline serum CPK and creatinine levels at baseline, periodically during treatment and as clinically indicated. If CPK is elevated, evaluate for signs/symptoms of rhabdomyolysis or other etiology. Depending on severity, may require treatment interruption, dose reduction, and/or discontinuation.

Prior to initiating therapy, confirm BRAF V600K or V600E mutation status with an approved test; approved for use in patients with BRAF V600K and BRAF V600E mutations. Not indicated for use in patients with wild-type BRAF melanoma. Potentially significant drug-drug interactions may exist, requiring dose or frequency adjustment, additional monitoring, and/or selection of alternative therapy.

Adverse Reactions Percentages reported as part of combination chemotherapy regimens.

>10%:

Cardiovascular: Decreased left ventricular ejection fraction (grades 2/3: 26%), hypertension (15%)

Dermatologic: Skin photosensitivity (46% to 47%, grades 3/4: 4%; includes solar dermatitis and sunburn), acneiform eruption (16%, grades 3/4: 2%)

Endocrine & metabolic: Hypophosphatemia (68%), increased gamma-glutamyl transferase (65%; grades 3/4: 21%), hypoalbuminemia (42%), hyponatremia (38%), hyperkalemia (26%), hypokalemia (25%), hypocalcemia (24%)

Gastrointestinal: Diarrhea (60%), nausea (41%), vomiting (24%), stomatitis (14%; includes aphthous stomatitis, mucositis, and oral mucosa ulcer)

Hematologic & oncologic: Lymphocytopenia (73%, grades 3/4: 10%), anemia (69%; grades 3/4: 3%), thrombocytopenia (18%), hemorrhage (13%, grades 3/4: 1%; includes bruise, ecchymoses, epistaxis, gingival hemorrhage, hematemesis, hematochezia, hemoptysis, hemorrhoidal bleeding, hypermenorrhea, melena, menometrorrhagia, nail bed bleeding, pulmonary hemorrhage, purpura, rectal hemorrhage, rupture of ovarian cyst, subarachnoid hemorrhage, subgaleal hematoma, traumatic hematoma, uterine hemorrhage, and vaginal hemorrhage)

Hepatic: Increased serum AST (73%, grades 3/4: 7% to 8%), increased serum alkaline phosphatase (71%, grades 3/4: 7%), increased serum ALT (68%, grades 3/4: 11%)

Neuromuscular & skeletal: Increased creatine phosphokinase (79%, grades 3/4: 12% to 14%)

Ophthalmic: Visual impairment (15%, grades 3/4: <1%; includes blurred vision, decreased visual acuity), chorioretinopathy (13%, grades 3/4: <1%), retinal detachment (12%, grades 3/4: 2%; includes detachment of macular retinal pigment epithelium and retinal pigment epithelium detachment)

Renal: Increased serum creatinine (100%; grades 3/4: 3%)

Miscellaneous: Fever (28%)

1% to 10%:

Central nervous system: Chills (10%)

Dermatologic: Skin rash (grades 3/4: 16%; grade 4: 2%; rash resulting in hospitalization: 3%)

Gastrointestinal: Gastrointestinal hemorrhage (4%)

Genitourinary: Genitourinary tract hemorrhage (2%), hematuria (2%)

◀ Hematologic & oncologic: Keratoacanthoma (≤6%), squamous cell carcinoma of skin (≤6%), basal cell carcinoma (5%)

Hepatic: Abnormal bilirubin levels (grades 3/4: 2%)

<1%, postmarketing, and/or case reports: Cerebral hemorrhage, malignant melanoma (second primary), malignant neoplasm (noncutaneous)

Drug Interactions

Metabolism/Transport Effects Substrate of CYP3A4 (major), P-glycoprotein; **Note:** Assignment of Major/Minor substrate status based on clinically relevant drug interaction potential

Avoid Concomitant Use

Avoid concomitant use of Cobimetinib with any of the following: Aminolevulinic Acid (Systemic); Conivaptan; CYP3A4 Inducers (Moderate); CYP3A4 Inducers (Strong); CYP3A4 Inhibitors (Moderate); CYP3A4 Inhibitors (Strong); Fusidic Acid (Systemic); Idelalisib

Increased Effect/Toxicity

Cobimetinib may increase the levels/effects of: Aminolevulinic Acid (Systemic); Aminolevulinic Acid (Topical); Porfimer; Verteporfin

The levels/effects of Cobimetinib may be increased by: Conivaptan; CYP3A4 Inhibitors (Moderate); CYP3A4 Inhibitors (Strong); Dasatinib; Fosaprepitant; Fusidic Acid (Systemic); Idelalisib; Palbociclib; Simeprevir; Stiripentol

Decreased Effect

The levels/effects of Cobimetinib may be decreased by: CYP3A4 Inducers (Moderate); CYP3A4 Inducers (Strong); Deferasirox; Sarilumab; Siltuximab; Tocilizumab

Hazardous Drugs Handling Considerations

Hazardous agent (meets NIOSH 2016 criteria). This medication is not on the NIOSH (2016) list; however, it meets the criteria for a hazardous drug. Drugs are classified as hazardous based on their properties; the properties of a hazardous drug include one or more of the following characteristics: carcinogenic, teratogenic (or other developmental toxicity), reproductive toxicity, organotoxic at low doses, genotoxic, and/or new agents with structural or toxicity profiles similar to existing hazardous agents.

Use appropriate precautions for receiving, handling, administration, and disposal. Gloves (single) should be worn during receiving, unpacking, and placing in storage. NIOSH recommends single gloving for administration of intact tablets or capsules (NIOSH 2016).

Storage/Stability Store below 30°C (86°F).

Mechanism of Action Cobimetinib is a potent and selective inhibitor of the mitogen-activated extracellular kinase (MEK) pathway (Larkin 2014); it reversibly inhibits MEK1 and MEK2, which are upstream regulators of the extracellular signal-related kinase (ERK) pathway. The ERK pathway promotes cellular proliferation. MEK1 and MEK2 are part of the BRAF pathway, which is activated by BRAF V600E and K mutations. Vemurafenib targets a different kinase in the RAS/RAF/MEK/ERK pathway; when cobimetinib and vemurafenib are used in combination, increased apoptosis and reduced tumor growth occurs.

Pharmacodynamics/Kinetics

Distribution: 806 L

Protein binding: 95%; to plasma proteins

Metabolism: Hepatic; via CYP3A4 oxidation and UGT2B7 glucuronidation

Bioavailability, absolute: 46%

Half-life elimination, mean: 44 hours (range: 23 to 70 hours)

Time to peak, median: 2.4 hours (range: 1 to 24 hours)

Excretion: Feces (76%; ~7 as unchanged drug); Urine (~18%; ~2% as unchanged drug)

Dosing

Adult & Geriatric

Melanoma, unresectable or metastatic (with BRAF V600E or V600K mutations): Oral: 60 mg once daily days 1 to 21 of each 28-day treatment cycle (in combination with vemurafenib); continue until disease progression or unacceptable toxicity (Larkin 2014).

Missed doses: If a dose is missed or if vomiting occurs after a dose is taken, resume with the next scheduled dose (do not take an additional dose). In the clinical trial, a dose was considered missed if not taken within 4 hours of the scheduled time (Larkin 2013 [Protocol GO28141]).

Dosage adjustment for concurrent CYP3A4 inhibitors: Avoid concurrent use of strong or moderate CYP3A4 inhibitors with cobimetinib. If concurrent short-term use (≤14 days) of a moderate CYP3A4 inhibitor cannot be avoided, reduce the cobimetinib dose from 60 mg to 20 mg; after the moderate CYP3A4 inhibitor is discontinued, resume the previous dose of 60 mg. If the current dose is 40 or 20 mg daily, alternatives to the strong or moderate CYP3A4 inhibitor should be used.

Renal Impairment

CrCl ≥30 mL/minute: No dosage adjustment is necessary.

CrCl <30 mL/minute: There is no dosage adjustment provided in the manufacturer's labeling (has not been studied).

Hepatic Impairment

Hepatic impairment prior to treatment: Mild, moderate, or severe impairment (Child Pugh class A, B, or C): No initial dosage adjustment is necessary.

Hepatotoxicity during treatment:

First occurrence of grade 4 lab abnormality (ALT, AST, or alkaline phosphatase >20 times ULN or total bilirubin >10 times ULN) or hepatotoxicity: Withhold cobimetinib for up to 4 weeks; if improves to grades 0 or 1, resume at the next lower dose level. Permanently discontinue if not improved to grade 0 or 1 within 4 weeks.

Recurrent grade 4 lab abnormality or hepatotoxicity: Permanently discontinue.

Adjustment for Toxicity

Recommended cobimetinib dose reductions for toxicity (vemurafenib may also require dosage adjustment):

First dose reduction: 40 mg once daily

Second dose reduction: 20 mg once daily

Subsequent modification (if unable to tolerate 20 mg once daily): Permanently discontinue

Cardiotoxicity:

Asymptomatic cardiomyopathy (absolute decrease in LVEF >10% [from baseline] and less than the institutional lower limit of normal [LLN]): Withhold cobimetinib for 2 weeks and repeat LVEF. If LVEF ≥ LLN **and** absolute decrease from baseline is ≤10%, resume at the next lower dose level. Permanently discontinue if LVEF < LLN **or** absolute decrease from baseline is >10%.

Symptomatic cardiomyopathy (symptomatic LVEF decrease from baseline): Withhold cobimetinib for up to 4 weeks and repeat LVEF. If symptoms resolve **and** LVEF ≥ LLN **and** absolute decrease from baseline is ≤10%, resume at the next lower dose level. Permanently discontinue if

◀ symptoms persist **or** LVEF < LLN **or** absolute decrease from baseline is >10%.

CPK elevation or rhabdomyolysis:

Grade 4 CPK elevation (>10 times ULN) or any CPK elevation with myalgia: Withhold cobimetinib for up to 4 weeks; if improves to grade 3 or lower, resume at the next lower dose level. Permanently discontinue if not improved within 4 weeks.

Dermatologic toxicity:

Grade 2 or lower (tolerable): Manage with supportive care.

Grade 2 (intolerable) or grade 3 or 4: Withhold or reduce dose.

New primary cutaneous or noncutaneous malignancies: No cobimetinib dosage modification is necessary.

Hemorrhage:

Grade 3: Withhold cobimetinib for up to 4 weeks; if improves to grades 0 or 1, resume at the next lower dose level. Permanently discontinue if not improved within 4 weeks.

Grade 4: Permanently discontinue.

Ocular:

Serous retinopathy: Withhold cobimetinib for up to 4 weeks; if signs/symptoms improve, resume at the next lower dose level. Permanently discontinue if not improved or symptoms recur within 4 weeks at the lower dose.

Retinal vein occlusion: Permanently discontinue.

Photosensitivity:

Grade 2 or lower (tolerable): Manage with supportive care.

Grade 2 (intolerable), grade 3 or 4: Withhold cobimetinib for up to 4 weeks; if improves to grades 0 or 1, resume at the next lower dose level. Permanently discontinue if not improved within 4 weeks.

Other toxicities:

Grade 2 (intolerable), or any grade 3: Withhold cobimetinib for up to 4 weeks; if improves to grades 0 or 1, resume at the next lower dose level. Permanently discontinue if not improved within 4 weeks.

Grade 4, first occurrence: Withhold cobimetinib until adverse reaction improves to grade 0 or 1 and then resume at the next lower dose level or permanently discontinue.

Grade 4, recurrent: Permanently discontinue.

Combination Regimens

Melanoma: Cobimetinib-Vemurafenib (Melanoma) on page 2068

Administration Oral: May be administered with or without food. In the clinical trial, cobimetinib tablets were administered whole with water; tablets should not be chewed, cut, or crushed (Larkin 2013 [Protocol GO28141]).

Emetic Potential Minimal (<10%)

Monitoring Parameters

BRAF V600K or V600E mutation status (prior to treatment); liver function tests (baseline and monthly during treatment, more frequently if clinically indicated); creatine phosphokinase (CPK) and serum creatinine (baseline and periodically during treatment, more frequently if clinically indicated); electrolytes (prior to and routinely during treatment). Assess left ventricular ejection fraction (LVEF) by echocardiogram or MUGA scan prior to therapy initiation, 1 month after initiation, and every 3 months thereafter until cobimetinib is discontinued; also assess LVEF at ~2 weeks, 4 weeks, 10 weeks, 16 weeks, and then as clinically indicated after a dose reduction or treatment interruption. Monitor ECG prior to and routinely during treatment.

Dermatologic exams (baseline, every 2 months during treatment, and for 6 months following discontinuation); ophthalmic examinations (baseline, regularly during treatment and with reports of new or worsening visual disturbances); monitor for signs/symptoms of dermatologic toxicity, hemorrhage, noncutaneous malignancy, photosensitivity, and rhabdomyolysis.

Prescribing and Access Restrictions Available through specialty pharmacies. Further information may be obtained from the manufacturer, Genentech, at 1-888-249-4918, or at http://www.cotellic.com.

Dosage Forms Excipient information presented when available (limited, particularly for generics); consult specific product labeling.

Tablet, Oral:

Cotellic: 20 mg

- **CPX-351** *see* Daunorubicin and Cytarabine (Liposomal) *on page 537*
- **CPZ** *see* ChlorproMAZINE *on page 388*
- **13-CRA** *see* ISOtretinoin *on page 1063*
- **CRA-032765** *see* Ibrutinib *on page 944*
- **Cresemba** *see* Isavuconazonium Sulfate *on page 1061*
- **Crisantaspase** *see* Asparaginase (*Erwinia*) *on page 184*

Crizotinib (kriz OH ti nib)

Related Information

Common Toxicity Criteria *on page 2242*

Management of Chemotherapy-Induced Nausea and Vomiting in Adults *on page 2253*

Safe Handling of Hazardous Drugs *on page 2379*

Brand Names: US Xalkori

Brand Names: Canada Xalkori

Index Terms C-Met/Hepatocyte Growth Factor Receptor Tyrosine Kinase Inhibitor PF-02341066; C-Met/HGFR Tyrosine Kinase Inhibitor PF-02341066; MET Tyrosine Kinase Inhibitor PF-02341066; PF-02341066

Pharmacologic Category Antineoplastic Agent, Anaplastic Lymphoma Kinase Inhibitor; Antineoplastic Agent, Tyrosine Kinase Inhibitor

Use Non-small cell lung cancer, metastatic: Treatment of patients with metastatic non-small cell lung cancer (NSCLC) whose tumors are anaplastic lymphoma kinase (ALK)-positive or are ROS1-positive (as detected by an approved test)

Labeled Contraindications

There are no contraindications listed in the manufacturer's US labeling.

Canadian labeling: Known hypersensitivity to crizotinib or any component of the formulation; congenital long QT syndrome or with persistent Fridericia-corrected QT interval (QTcF) ≥500 msec

Pregnancy Considerations Adverse events have been observed in animal reproduction studies. Based on the mechanism of action, crizotinib may cause fetal harm if administered during pregnancy. Women of childbearing potential should use adequate contraception during treatment and for at least 45 days after the last crizotinib dose; males with female partners of reproductive potential should use condoms during treatment and for at least 90 days after the final dose. The Canadian labeling recommends adequate contraception during treatment and for at least 90 days after the last dose for both males and females.

Breastfeeding Considerations It is not known if crizotinib is present in breast milk. Due to the potential for serious adverse reactions in the breastfeeding infant, the manufacturer recommends against breastfeeding during treatment and for 45 days after the final dose.

Warnings/Precautions Approved for use only in patients with metastatic non-small cell lung cancer (NSCLC) who test positive for the abnormal anaplastic lymphoma kinase (ALK) gene or ROS1 rearrangements. The Vysis ALK break-apart FISH probe kit is approved to test for the ALK gene abnormality. An approved test is not currently available for detection of ROS1 rearrangements; in clinical trials, ROS1 positivity was determined by laboratory-developed break-apart FISH or RT-PCR.

Fatalities due to crizotinib-induced hepatotoxicity have occurred. Grade 3 or 4 ALT increases (usually asymptomatic and reversible) have been observed in clinical trials. May require dosage interruption and/or reduction; permanent discontinuation was necessary in some cases; elevations in ALT or AST >5 × ULN were observed; concurrent ALT or AST elevations ≥3 × ULN and total bilirubin elevations ≥2 × ULN (without alkaline phosphatase elevations) occurred rarely. Transaminase elevation onset generally was within 2 months of treatment initiation. Monitor liver function tests, including ALT, AST, and total bilirubin every 2 weeks during the first 2 months of therapy, then monthly and as clinically necessary. Use with caution in patients with hepatic impairment (has not been studied); crizotinib is extensively metabolized in the liver and liver impairment is likely to increase crizotinib levels.

Severe, life-threatening, and potentially fatal interstitial lung disease (ILD)/ pneumonitis has been associated with crizotinib. Onset was generally within 3 months of treatment initiation. Monitor for pulmonary symptoms which may indicate ILD/pneumonitis; exclude other potential causes (eg, disease progression, infection, other pulmonary disease, or radiation therapy). Permanently discontinue if treatment-related ILD/pneumonitis is confirmed.

Symptomatic bradycardia may occur; heart rate <50 beats/minute has occurred. If possible, avoid concurrent use with other agents known to cause bradycardia (eg, beta blockers, nondihydropyridine calcium channel blockers, clonidine, digoxin). Monitor heart rate and blood pressure regularly. If symptomatic bradycardia (not life-threatening) occurs, withhold treatment until recovery to asymptomatic bradycardia or to a heart rate of ≥60 beats/minute, evaluate concurrent medications, and potentially reduce crizotinib dose. Permanently discontinue for life-threatening bradycardia due to crizotinib; if life-threatening bradycardia occurs and concurrent medications associated with bradycardia can be discontinued or dose adjusted, restart crizotinib at a reduced dose (with frequent monitoring). QTc prolongation has been observed; monitor ECG and electrolytes in patients with heart failure, bradyarrhythmias, electrolyte abnormalities, or who are taking medications known to prolong the QT interval. May require treatment interruption, dosage reduction, or discontinuation. Avoid use in patients with congenital long QT syndrome.

Ocular toxicities (eg, blurred vision, diplopia, photophobia, photopsia, visual acuity decreased, visual brightness, visual field defect, visual impairment, and/or vitreous floaters) commonly occur. Onset is generally within 1 week of treatment initiation. Grade 4 visual field defect with vision loss had been reported (rare); optic atrophy and optic nerve disorder have been reported as potential causes of vision loss. Discontinue with new onset of severe visual loss (best corrected vision less than 20/200 in one or both eyes). Obtain ophthalmic evaluation (including best corrected visual acuity, retinal photographs, visual fields, optical coherence tomography, and other evaluations as appropriate). The risks of re-starting crizotinib after severe vision loss have not been evaluated; the decision to resume therapy should consider the potential benefits of treatment. Reduce initial dose in patients with severe renal impairment not requiring dialysis. Potentially significant drug-drug and drug-food interactions may exist, requiring dose or frequency adjustment, additional monitoring, and/or selection of alternative therapy. Avoid concomitant use with strong CYP3A4 inhibitors and inducers and with CYP3A4 substrates. Crizotinib is associated with a moderate emetic potential (Hesketh 2017); antiemetics may be needed to prevent nausea and vomiting.

◄ **Adverse Reactions**
>10%:
Cardiovascular: Edema (31% to 49%), bradycardia (5% to 14%)
Central nervous system: Fatigue (27% to 29%), neuropathy (19% to 25%; includes dysesthesia, gait disturbance, hypoesthesia, muscular weakness, neuralgia, peripheral neuropathy, parasthesia, peripheral sensory neuropathy, polyneuropathy, burning sensation in skin), headache (22%), dizziness (18% to 22%)
Dermatologic: Skin rash (9% to 11%)
Endocrine & metabolic: Hypophosphatemia (28% to 32%), hypokalemia (18%)
Gastrointestinal: Diarrhea (60% to 61%), nausea (55% to 56%), vomiting (46% to 47%), constipation (42% to 43%), decreased appetite (30%), abdominal pain (26%), dysgeusia (26%), dyspepsia (8% to 14%)
Genitourinary: Decreased estimated GFR (eGFR) (<90 mL/min/1.73 m^2: 76%; <60 mL/min/1.73 m^2: 38%; <30 mL/min/1.73 m^2: 4%)
Hematologic & oncologic: Neutropenia (49% to 52%; grades 3/4: 11% to 12%), lymphocytopenia (48% to 51%; grades 3/4: 7% to 9%)
Hepatic: Increased serum ALT (76% to 79%), increased serum AST (61% to 66%)
Neuromuscular & skeletal: Limb pain (16%)
Ophthalmic: Visual disturbance (60% to 71%; onset: <2 weeks; includes blurred vision, diplopia, photophobia, photopsia, visual acuity decreased, visual brightness, visual field defect, visual impairment, vitreous floaters)
Respiratory: Upper respiratory tract infection (26% to 32%)
Miscellaneous: Fever (19%)
1% to 10%:
Cardiovascular: Pulmonary embolism (6%), prolonged Q-T interval on ECG (5% to 6%), syncope (1% to 3%)
Endocrine & metabolic: Weight loss (10%), weight gain (8%), diabetic ketoacidosis (≤2%), decreased plasma testosterone (1%; hypogonadism)
Gastrointestinal: Dysphagia (10%), esophagitis (2% to 6%)
Hepatic: Hepatic failure (1%)
Infection: Sepsis (≤5%)
Neuromuscular & skeletal: Muscle spasm (8%)
Renal: Renal cyst (3% to 5%)
Respiratory: Adult respiratory distress syndrome (≤5%), interstitial pulmonary disease (≤5%; grades 3/4: 1%; includes acute respiratory distress syndrome, pneumonitis), pneumonia (≤5%), respiratory failure (≤5%), dyspnea (2%)
Frequency not defined:
Cardiovascular: Cardiac arrhythmia, septic shock
<1%, postmarketing, and/or case reports: Hepatotoxicity

Drug Interactions
Metabolism/Transport Effects Substrate of CYP3A4 (major), P-glycoprotein; **Note:** Assignment of Major/Minor substrate status based on clinically relevant drug interaction potential; **Inhibits** CYP3A4 (moderate), OCT1, OCT2

Avoid Concomitant Use
Avoid concomitant use of Crizotinib with any of the following: Alfentanil; Aprepitant; Asunaprevir; Bosutinib; Budesonide (Systemic); Ceritinib; Cobimetinib; Conivaptan; CycloSPORINE (Systemic); CYP3A4 Inducers (Strong); CYP3A4 Inhibitors (Strong); Dihydroergotamine; Domperidone;

Ergotamine; FentaNYL; Flibanserin; Fusidic Acid (Systemic); Grapefruit Juice; Highest Risk QTc-Prolonging Agents; Hydroxychloroquine; Idelalisib; Ivabradine; Lomitapide; MiFEPRIStone; Naloxegol; Neratinib; Olaparib; Pimozide; Probucol; Promazine; QuiNIDine; Simeprevir; Sirolimus; St John's Wort; Tacrolimus (Systemic); Tolvaptan; Trabectedin; Ulipristal; Vinflunine

Increased Effect/Toxicity

Crizotinib may increase the levels/effects of: Alfentanil; AmLODIPine; Apixaban; Aprepitant; ARIPiprazole; Asunaprevir; Avanafil; Blonanserin; Bosentan; Bosutinib; Bradycardia-Causing Agents; Brexpiprazole; Bromocriptine; Budesonide (Systemic); Budesonide (Topical); Cannabis; Ceritinib; Cilostazol; Cobimetinib; Colchicine; CycloSPORINE (Systemic); CYP3A4 Substrates; Dapoxetine; Deflazacort; Dihydroergotamine; Domperidone; DOXOrubicin (Conventional); Dronabinol; Eletriptan; Eplerenone; Ergotamine; Everolimus; FentaNYL; Flibanserin; GuanFACINE; Highest Risk QTc-Prolonging Agents; HYDROcodone; HydrOXYzine; Ibrutinib; Imatinib; Ivabradine; Ivacaftor; Lacosamide; Lomitapide; Lurasidone; Manidipine; Mirodenafil; Moderate Risk QTc-Prolonging Agents; Naldemedine; Naloxegol; Neratinib; NiMODipine; Olaparib; OxyCODONE; Pimecrolimus; Pimozide; QuiNIDine; Ranolazine; Rupatadine; Salmeterol; SAXagliptin; Sildenafil; Simeprevir; Sirolimus; Sonidegib; Suvorexant; Tacrolimus (Systemic); Tetrahydrocannabinol; Ticagrelor; Tolvaptan; Trabectedin; Udenafil; Ulipristal; Venetoclax; Vilazodone; Vindesine; Zopiclone

The levels/effects of Crizotinib may be increased by: Bretylium; Conivaptan; CYP3A4 Inhibitors (Moderate); CYP3A4 Inhibitors (Strong); Dasatinib; Fosaprepitant; Fusidic Acid (Systemic); Grapefruit Juice; Hydroxychloroquine; Idelalisib; MiFEPRIStone; Netupitant; Palbociclib; P-glycoprotein/ABCB1 Inhibitors; Probucol; Promazine; QTc-Prolonging Agents (Indeterminate Risk and Risk Modifying); Ruxolitinib; Stiripentol; Tofacitinib; Vinflunine; Xipamide

Decreased Effect

Crizotinib may decrease the levels/effects of: Ifosfamide

The levels/effects of Crizotinib may be decreased by: Bosentan; CYP3A4 Inducers (Moderate); CYP3A4 Inducers (Strong); Dabrafenib; Deferasirox; Sarilumab; Siltuximab; St John's Wort; Tocilizumab

Food Interactions Grapefruit juice may increase serum crizotinib levels. Management: Avoid grapefruit and grapefruit juice.

Hazardous Drugs Handling Considerations

Hazardous agent (NIOSH 2016 [group 1]).

Use appropriate precautions for receiving, handling, administration, and disposal. Gloves (single) should be worn during receiving, unpacking, and placing in storage. NIOSH recommends single gloving for administration of intact tablets or capsules (NIOSH 2016).

Storage/Stability Store between 20°C and 25°C (68°F and 77°F); excursions are permitted between 15°C and 30°C (59°F and 86°F).

Mechanism of Action Tyrosine kinase receptor inhibitor, which inhibits anaplastic lymphoma kinase (ALK), Hepatocyte Growth Factor Receptor (HGFR, c-MET), ROS1 (c-ros), and Recepteur d'Origine Nantais (RON). ALK gene abnormalities due to mutations or translocations may result in expression of oncogenic fusion proteins (eg, ALK fusion protein) which alter signaling and expression and result in increased cellular proliferation and survival in tumors which express these fusion proteins. Approximately 2% to 7% of patients with NSCLC have the abnormal echinoderm microtubule-associated protein-like 4, or EML4-ALK gene (which has a higher prevalence in never smokers or light smokers and in patients with adenocarcinoma). Inhibition of ALK, ROS1, and c-Met phosphorylation is concentration-dependent. Crizotinib selectively inhibits ALK tyrosine kinase, which reduces proliferation of cells expressing the genetic alteration.

Pharmacodynamics/Kinetics

Distribution: V_{ss}: 1772 L

Protein binding: 91%

Metabolism: Hepatic, via CYP3A4/5 (oxidation and dealkylation)

Bioavailability: 43% (range: 32% to 66%); bioavailability is reduced 14% with a high-fat meal

Half-life elimination: Terminal: 42 hours

Time to peak: 4 to 6 hours

Excretion: Feces (63%; 53% as unchanged drug); urine (22%; 2% as unchanged drug)

Dosing

Adult & Geriatric Note: Crizotinib is associated with a moderate emetic potential (Hesketh 2017); antiemetics may be needed to prevent nausea and vomiting.

Non-small cell lung cancer (NSCLC), metastatic (ALK- or ROS1-positive): Oral: 250 mg twice daily, continue treatment until disease progression or unacceptable toxicity

Missed doses: If a dose is missed, take as soon as remembered unless it is <6 hours prior to the next scheduled dose (skip the dose if <6 hours before the next dose); do not take 2 doses at the same time to make up for a missed dose. If vomiting occurs after dose, administer the next dose at the regularly scheduled time.

Renal Impairment

CrCl 30 to 89 mL/minute: No dosage adjustment necessary.

CrCl <30 mL/minute not requiring dialysis: Initial: 250 mg once daily.

Hepatic Impairment

Hepatotoxicity **prior to** treatment: There are no dosage adjustments provided in the manufacturer's labeling (has not been studied); crizotinib undergoes extensive hepatic metabolism and systemic exposure may be increased with impairment; use with caution.

Hepatotoxicity **during** treatment:

Grade 3 or 4 ALT or AST elevation (ALT or AST >5 x ULN) with ≤ grade 1 total bilirubin elevation (total bilirubin ≤1.5 x ULN): Withhold treatment until recovery to baseline or ≤ grade 1 (<3 x ULN), then resume at a reduced dose (200 mg twice daily).

Recurrent grade 3 or 4 ALT or AST elevation with ≤ grade 1 total bilirubin elevation: Withhold treatment until recovery to baseline or ≤ grade 1, then resume at the next lower reduced dose (250 mg once daily).

Recurrent grade 3 or 4 ALT or AST elevation on 250 mg once daily: Permanently discontinue.

Grade 2, 3, or 4 ALT or AST elevation (ALT or AST >3 x ULN) with concurrent grade 2, 3, or 4 total bilirubin elevation (>1.5 x ULN) in the absence of cholestasis or hemolysis: Permanently discontinue.

Adjustment for Toxicity Note: If dose reduction is necessary, reduce dose to 200 mg orally twice daily; if necessary, further reduce to 250 mg once daily. If unable to tolerate 250 mg once daily, permanently discontinue therapy.

Hematologic toxicity (except lymphopenia, unless lymphopenia is associated with clinical events such as opportunistic infection):

Grade 3 toxicity (WBC 1,000 to 2,000/mm^3, ANC 500 to 1,000/mm^3, platelets 25,000 to 50,000/mm^3), grade 3 anemia: Withhold treatment until recovery to $\leq$ grade 2, then resume at the same dose and schedule.

Grade 4 toxicity (WBC <1,000/mm^3, ANC <500/mm^3, platelets <25,000/mm^3), grade 4 anemia: Withhold treatment until recovery to $\leq$ grade 2, then resume at 200 mg twice daily.

Recurrent grade 4 toxicity on 200 mg twice daily: Withhold treatment until recovery to $\leq$ grade 2, then resume at 250 mg once daily.

Recurrent grade 4 toxicity on 250 mg once daily: Permanently discontinue.

Nonhematologic toxicities:

Cardiovascular toxicities:

QTc prolongation:

Grade 3 QTc prolongation (QTc >500 msec without life-threatening signs or symptoms) on at least 2 separate ECGs: Withhold treatment until recovery to baseline or to $\leq$ grade 1 (QTc <481 msec), then resume at 200 mg twice daily.

Recurrent grade 3 QTc prolongation at 200 mg twice daily: Withhold treatment until recovery to baseline or to $\leq$ grade 1, then resume at 250 mg once daily.

Recurrent grade 3 QTc prolongation at 250 mg once daily: Permanently discontinue.

Grade 4 QTc prolongation: QTc >500 msec or $\geq$60 msec change from baseline with life-threatening symptoms: Permanently discontinue.

Bradycardia:

Grade 2 bradycardia (symptomatic with medical intervention indicated) or grade 3 bradycardia (severe/medically significant with intervention indicated): Withhold until recovery to asymptomatic bradycardia or to a heart rate of $\geq$60 beats/minute and evaluate concomitant medications. If contributing concomitant medication is identified and discontinued (or dose adjusted), then resume crizotinib at the previous dose. If no contributing concomitant medication is identified (or cannot be discontinued or dose adjusted), resume crizotinib at a reduced dose.

Grade 4 bradycardia (life-threatening with urgent intervention indicated): Withhold until recovery to asymptomatic bradycardia or to a heart rate of $\geq$60 beats/minute and evaluate concomitant medications. If contributing concomitant medication is identified and discontinued (or dose adjusted), then resume crizotinib at 250 mg once daily with frequent monitoring. If no contributing concomitant medication is identified, permanently discontinue crizotinib. Permanently discontinue for recurrence.

Hepatotoxicity: Refer to dosage adjustment in hepatic impairment.

Ocular toxicity: Visual loss (grade 4 visual disorder) or new onset of severe visual loss (best corrected vision less than 20/200 in one or both eyes): Discontinue during evaluation of severe vision loss.

Pulmonary toxicity: Interstitial lung disease (ILD)/pneumonitis (any grade; not attributable to disease progression, infection, other pulmonary disease or radiation therapy): Permanently discontinue.

◀ **Administration**
   Crizotinib is associated with a moderate emetic potential (Hesketh 2017); antiemetics may be needed to prevent nausea and vomiting.
   Swallow capsules whole (do not crush, dissolve, or open capsules). Administer with or without food. If vomiting occurs after dose, administer the next dose at the regularly scheduled time.

Emetic Potential Moderate (30% to 90%)

Monitoring Parameters ALK or ROS1 positivity; CBC with differential monthly and as clinically appropriate (monitor more frequently if grades 3 or 4 abnormalities observed or with fever or infection); liver function tests every 2 weeks for the first 2 months, then monthly and as clinically appropriate (monitor more frequently if grades 2, 3, or 4 abnormalities observed); renal function (baseline and periodic). Monitor pulmonary symptoms (for interstitial lung disease [ILD]/pneumonitis). Monitor heart rate and blood pressure; monitoring ECG and electrolytes in patients with heart failure, bradycardia, bradyarrhythmias, electrolyte abnormalities, or who are taking medications known to prolong the QT interval. Obtain ophthalmic evaluation (including best corrected visual acuity, retinal photographs, visual fields, optical coherence tomography, and other evaluations as appropriate) if severe visual loss occurs. Monitor adherence.

Dietary Considerations Avoid grapefruit and grapefruit juice.

Prescribing and Access Restrictions Available through specialty pharmacies. Further information may be obtained from the manufacturer, Pfizer, at 1-877-744-5675, or at http://www.pfizerpro.com

Dosage Forms Excipient information presented when available (limited, particularly for generics); consult specific product labeling.
   Capsule, Oral:
      Xalkori: 200 mg, 250 mg

◆ **CsA** see CycloSPORINE (Systemic) on page 452

◆ **CTL019** see Tisagenlecleucel on page 1787

◆ **CTX** see Cyclophosphamide on page 438

◆ **Cuvitru** see Immune Globulin on page 992

◆ **CyA** see CycloSPORINE (Systemic) on page 452

Cyclophosphamide (sye kloe FOS fa mide)

Related Information
   Hematopoietic Cell Transplantation on page 2365
   Management of Chemotherapy-Induced Nausea and Vomiting in Adults on page 2253
   Management of Drug Extravasations on page 2271
   Mucositis and Stomatitis on page 2299
   Prevention of Chemotherapy-Induced Nausea and Vomiting in Children on page 2310
   Safe Handling of Hazardous Drugs on page 2379

Brand Names: Canada Procytox

Index Terms CPM; CTX; CYT; Cytoxan; Neosar

Pharmacologic Category Antineoplastic Agent, Alkylating Agent; Antineoplastic Agent, Alkylating Agent (Nitrogen Mustard); Antirheumatic Miscellaneous; Immunosuppressant Agent

Use

Oncology uses: Treatment of acute lymphoblastic leukemia (ALL), acute myelocytic leukemia (AML), breast cancer, chronic lymphocytic leukemia (CLL), chronic myeloid leukemia (CML), Hodgkin lymphoma, mycosis fungoides, multiple myeloma, neuroblastoma, non-Hodgkin lymphomas (including Burkitt lymphoma), ovarian adenocarcinoma, and retinoblastoma

Limitations of use: Although potentially effective as a single-agent in susceptible malignancies, cyclophosphamide is more frequently used in combination with other chemotherapy drugs

Nononcology uses: Nephrotic syndrome: Treatment of minimal change nephrotic syndrome (biopsy proven) in children who are unresponsive or intolerant to corticosteroid therapy

Limitations of use: The safety and efficacy for the treatment of nephrotic syndrome in adults or in other renal diseases has not been established.

Labeled Contraindications

US labeling: Hypersensitivity to cyclophosphamide or any component of the formulation; urinary outflow obstruction

Canadian labeling: Hypersensitivity to cyclophosphamide or its metabolites, urinary outflow obstructions, severe myelosuppression, severe renal or hepatic impairment, active infection (especially varicella zoster), severe immunosuppression

Pregnancy Considerations Cyclophosphamide crosses the placenta and can be detected in amniotic fluid (D'Incalci 1982). Based on the mechanism of action, cyclophosphamide may cause fetal harm if administered during pregnancy. Adverse events (including ectrodactylia) were observed in human studies following exposure to cyclophosphamide. Women of childbearing potential should avoid pregnancy while receiving cyclophosphamide and for up to 1 year after completion of treatment. Males with female partners who are or may become pregnant should use a condom during and for at least 4 months after cyclophosphamide treatment. Cyclophosphamide may cause sterility in males and females (may be irreversible) and amenorrhea in females. When treatment is needed for lupus nephritis, cyclophosphamide should be avoided in women who are pregnant or those who wish to preserve their fertility (Hahn 2012).

Chemotherapy, if indicated, may be administered to pregnant women with breast cancer as part of a combination chemotherapy regimen (common regimens administered during pregnancy include doxorubicin (or epirubicin), cyclophosphamide, and fluorouracil); chemotherapy should not be administered during the first trimester, after 35 weeks gestation, or within 3 weeks of planned delivery (Amant 2010; Loibl 2006). The European Society for Medical Oncology has published guidelines for diagnosis, treatment, and follow-up of cancer during pregnancy. The guidelines recommend referral to a facility with expertise in cancer during pregnancy and encourage a multidisciplinary team (obstetrician, neonatologist, oncology team). In general, if chemotherapy is indicated, it should be avoided during in the first trimester, there should be a 3-week time period between the last chemotherapy dose and anticipated delivery, and chemotherapy should not be administered beyond week 33 of gestation (Peccatori 2013).

Breastfeeding Considerations Cyclophosphamide is excreted into breast milk. Leukopenia and thrombocytopenia were noted in an infant exposed to cyclophosphamide while nursing. The mother was treated with one course of cyclophosphamide 6 weeks prior to delivery then cyclophosphamide IV 6 mg/kg (300 mg) once daily for 3 days beginning 20 days postpartum.

Complete blood counts were obtained in the breastfeeding infant on each day of therapy; WBC and platelets decreased by day 3 (Durodola 1979). Due to the potential for serious adverse effects in the nursing infant, a decision should be made to discontinue cyclophosphamide or to discontinue breastfeeding, taking into account the importance of treatment to the mother.

Warnings/Precautions Cyclophosphamide is associated with the development of hemorrhagic cystitis, pyelitis, ureteritis, and hematuria. Hemorrhagic cystitis may rarely be severe or fatal. Bladder fibrosis may also occur, either with or without cystitis. Urotoxicity is due to excretion of cyclophosphamide metabolites in the urine and appears to be dose- and treatment duration-dependent, although may occur with short-term use. Increased hydration and frequent voiding is recommended to help prevent cystitis; some protocols utilize mesna to protect against hemorrhagic cystitis. Monitor urinalysis for hematuria or other signs of urotoxicity. Severe or prolonged hemorrhagic cystitis may require medical or surgical treatment. While hematuria generally resolves within a few days after treatment is withheld, it may persist in some cases. Discontinue cyclophosphamide with severe hemorrhagic cystitis. Exclude or correct any urinary tract obstructions prior to treatment initiation (use is contraindicated with bladder outlet obstruction). Use with caution (if at all) in patients with active urinary tract infection. Use with caution in patients with renal impairment; dosage adjustment may be needed. Decreased renal excretion and increased serum levels (cyclophosphamide and metabolites) may occur in patients with severe renal impairment (CrCl 10 to 24 mL/minute); monitor for signs/symptoms of toxicity. Cyclophosphamide and metabolites are dialyzable; differences in amount dialyzed may occur due to dialysis system used. If dialysis is required, maintain a consistent interval between administration and dialysis.

Leukopenia, neutropenia, thrombocytopenia, and anemia may commonly occur; may be dose related. Bone marrow failure has been reported. Bone marrow failure and severe immunosuppression may lead to serious (and fatal) infections, including sepsis and septic shock, or may reactive latent infections. Antimicrobial prophylaxis may be considered in appropriate patients. Initiate antibiotics for neutropenic fever; antifungal and antiviral medications may also be necessary. Monitor blood counts during treatment. Avoid use if neutrophils are ≤1,500/mm^3 and platelets are <50,000/mm^3. Consider growth factors (primary or secondary prophylaxis) in patients at increased risk for complications due to neutropenia. Platelet and neutrophil nadirs are usually at weeks 1 and 2 of treatment and recovery is expected after ~20 days. Severe myelosuppression may be more prevalent in heavily pretreated patients or in patients receiving concomitant chemotherapy and/or radiation therapy. Monitor for infections; immunosuppression and serious infections may occur; serious infections may require dose reduction, or interruption or discontinuation of treatment.

Cardiotoxicity has been reported (some fatal), usually with high doses associated with transplant conditioning regimens, although may rarely occur with lower doses. Cardiac abnormalities do not appear to persist. Cardiotoxicities reported have included arrhythmias (supraventricular and ventricular [some with QT prolongation]), congestive heart failure, heart block, hemopericardium (secondary to hemorrhagic myocarditis and myocardial necrosis), myocarditis (including hemorrhagic), pericarditis, pericardial effusion including cardiac tamponade, and tachyarrhythmias. Cardiotoxicity is related to endothelial capillary damage; symptoms may be managed with diuretics, ACE inhibitors, beta-blockers, or inotropics (Floyd 2005). The risk for cardiotoxicity may be increased with higher doses, advanced age, and in patients with prior radiation to the cardiac region, and in patients who have received prior or concurrent cardiotoxic medication. Use with caution in patients with preexisting cardiovascular disease or those at risk for cardiotoxicity. For patients with cardiac risk factors or preexisting cardiac disease, monitor during treatment. In a scientific statement from the American Heart Association, cyclophosphamide has been determined to be an agent that may either cause reversible direct myocardial toxicity or exacerbate underlying myocardial dysfunction (magnitude: moderate/major) (AHA [Page 2016]).

Pulmonary toxicities, including pneumonitis, pulmonary fibrosis, pulmonary veno-occlusive disease, and acute respiratory distress syndrome, have been reported. Monitor for signs/symptoms of pulmonary toxicity. Consider pulmonary function testing to assess the severity of pneumonitis (Morgan 2011). Cyclophosphamide-induced pneumonitis is rare and may present as early (within 1 to 6 months) or late onset (several months to years). Early onset may be reversible with discontinuation; late onset is associated with pleural thickening and may persist chronically (Malik 1996). In addition, late onset pneumonitis (>6 months after therapy initiation) may be associated with increased mortality.

Hepatic sinusoidal obstruction syndrome (SOS), formerly called veno-occlusive liver disease (VOD), has been reported in patients receiving chemotherapy regimens containing cyclophosphamide. A major risk factor for SOS is cytoreductive conditioning transplantation regimens with cyclophosphamide used in combination with total body irradiation or busulfan (or other agents). Other risk factors include preexisting hepatic dysfunction, prior radiation to the abdominal area, and low performance status. Children <3 years of age are reported to be at increased risk for hepatic SOS; monitor for signs or symptoms of hepatic SOS, including bilirubin >1.4 mg/dL, unexplained weight gain, ascites, hepatomegaly, or unexplained right upper quadrant pain (Arndt 2004). SOS has also been reported in patients receiving long-term lower doses for immunosuppressive indications. Use with caution in patients with hepatic impairment; dosage adjustment may be needed. The conversion between cyclophosphamide to the active metabolite may be reduced in patients with severe hepatic impairment, potentially reducing efficacy.

Nausea and vomiting commonly occur. Cyclophosphamide is associated with a moderate to high emetic potential (depending on dose, regimen, or administration route); antiemetics are recommended to prevent nausea and vomiting (Basch 2011; Dupuis 2011; Roila 2016). Stomatitis/mucositis may also occur. Anaphylactic reactions have been reported; cross-sensitivity with other alkylating agents may occur. Hyponatremia associated with increased total body water, acute water intoxication, and a syndrome resembling SIADH (syndrome of inappropriate secretion of antidiuretic hormone) has been reported; some have been fatal. May interfere with wound healing. May impair fertility; interferes with oogenesis and spermatogenesis. Effect on fertility is generally dependent on dose and duration of treatment and may be irreversible. The age at treatment initiation and cumulative dose were determined to be risk factors for ovarian failure in cyclophosphamide use for the treatment of systemic lupus erythematosus (SLE) (Mok 1998). Potentially significant drug-drug interactions may exist, requiring dose or frequency adjustment, additional monitoring, and/or selection of alternative therapy. Secondary malignancies (bladder cancer, myelodysplasia, acute leukemias, lymphomas, thyroid cancer, and sarcomas) have been reported with both single-agent and with combination chemotherapy regimens; onset may be delayed (up to several years after treatment). Bladder cancer usually occurs in patients previously experiencing hemorrhagic cystitis; risk may be reduced by preventing hemorrhagic cystitis.

Adverse Reactions Frequency not defined.

Dermatologic: Alopecia (reversible; onset: 3 to 6 weeks after start of treatment)

Endocrine & metabolic: Altered hormone level (increased gonadotropin secretion), amenorrhea

Gastrointestinal: Abdominal pain, anorexia, diarrhea, mucositis, nausea and vomiting (dose-related), stomatitis

Genitourinary: Azoospermia, defective oogenesis, hemorrhagic cystitis, oligospermia, sterility

Hematologic & oncologic: Anemia, bone marrow depression, febrile neutropenia, leukopenia (dose-related; recovery: 7 to 10 days after cessation), neutropenia, thrombocytopenia

Infection: Infection

<1%, postmarketing, and/or case reports: Acute respiratory distress, anaphylaxis, auditory disturbance, blurred vision, cardiac arrhythmia (with high-dose [HSCT] therapy), cardiac failure (with high-dose [HSCT] therapy), cardiac tamponade (with high-dose [HSCT] therapy), cardiotoxicity, confusion, C-reactive protein increased, dizziness, dyschromia (skin/fingernails), dyspnea, erythema multiforme, gastrointestinal hemorrhage, heart block, hematuria, hemopericardium, hemorrhagic colitis, hemorrhagic myocarditis (with high-dose [HSCT] therapy), hemorrhagic ureteritis, hepatic sinusoidal obstruction syndrome (formerly known as hepatic veno-occlusive disease), hepatitis, hepatotoxicity, hypersensitivity reaction, hyperuricemia, hypokalemia, hyponatremia, increased lactate dehydrogenase, interstitial pneumonitis, jaundice, malaise, mesenteric ischemia (acute), methemoglobinemia (with high-dose [HSCT] therapy), multi-organ failure, myocardial necrosis (with high-dose [HSCT] therapy), neurotoxicity, neutrophilic eccrine hidradenitis, ovarian fibrosis, pancreatitis, pericarditis, pneumonia, pulmonary hypertension, pulmonary infiltrates, pulmonary interstitial fibrosis (with high doses), pulmonary veno-occlusive disease, pyelonephritis, radiation recall phenomenon, reactivation of disease, reduced ejection fraction, renal tubular necrosis, reversible posterior leukoencephalopathy syndrome, rhabdomyolysis, sepsis, septic shock, SIADH, skin rash, Stevens-Johnson syndrome, testicular atrophy, thrombocytopenia (immune-mediated), thrombosis (arterial and venous), toxic epidermal necrolysis, toxic megacolon, tumor lysis syndrome, urinary fibrosis, weakness, wound healing impairment

Drug Interactions

Metabolism/Transport Effects Substrate of CYP2A6 (minor), CYP2B6 (major), CYP2C19 (minor), CYP2C9 (minor), CYP3A4 (minor); **Note:** Assignment of Major/Minor substrate status based on clinically relevant drug interaction potential; **Induces** CYP2C9 (weak/moderate)

Avoid Concomitant Use

Avoid concomitant use of Cyclophosphamide with any of the following: BCG (Intravesical); Belimumab; Deferiprone; Dipyrone; Etanercept; Natalizumab; Pimecrolimus; Tacrolimus (Topical); Vaccines (Live)

Increased Effect/Toxicity

Cyclophosphamide may increase the levels/effects of: Amiodarone; Antineoplastic Agents (Anthracycline, Systemic); CloZAPine; CycloSPORINE (Systemic); Deferiprone; Fingolimod; Leflunomide; Mivacurium; Natalizumab; Sargramostim; Succinylcholine; Tofacitinib; Vaccines (Live)

The levels/effects of Cyclophosphamide may be increased by: Allopurinol; AzaTHIOprine; Belimumab; Denosumab; Dipyrone; Etanercept; Filgrastim; Lenograstim; MiFEPRIStone; Ocrelizumab; Palifermin; Pentostatin; Pimecrolimus; Promazine; Protease Inhibitors; Roflumilast; Tacrolimus (Topical); Thiazide and Thiazide-Like Diuretics; Thiotepa; Trastuzumab

Decreased Effect

Cyclophosphamide may decrease the levels/effects of: BCG (Intravesical); Coccidioides immitis Skin Test; CycloSPORINE (Systemic); Lenograstim; Nivolumab; Sipuleucel-T; Tertomotide; Vaccines (Inactivated); Vaccines (Live)

The levels/effects of Cyclophosphamide may be decreased by: CYP2B6 Inducers (Moderate); Dabrafenib; Echinacea; Lumacaftor; Nilotinib

Hazardous Drugs Handling Considerations

Hazardous agent (NIOSH 2016 [group 1]).

Use appropriate precautions for receiving, handling, administration, and disposal. Gloves (single) should be worn during receiving, unpacking, and placing in storage.

NIOSH recommends single gloving for administration of intact tablets or capsules. If manipulating tablets/capsules (eg, to prepare an oral suspension), NIOSH recommends double gloving, a protective gown, and preparation in a controlled device; if not prepared in a controlled device, respiratory and eye/face protection as well as ventilated engineering controls are recommended. NIOSH recommends double gloving, a protective gown, and (if there is a potential for vomit or spit up) eye/face protection for administration of an oral liquid/feeding tube administration. For IV preparation, NIOSH recommends double gloving, a protective gown, ventilated engineering controls (a class II biological safety cabinet or a compounding aseptic containment isolator), and closed system transfer devices (CSTDs). Double gloving, a gown, and (if dosage form allows) CSTDs are required during IV administration (NIOSH 2016).

Storage/Stability

Injection powder for reconstitution: Store intact vials of powder at ≤25°C (77°F). Exposure to excessive temperatures during transport or storage may cause active ingredient to melt (vials with melting may have a clear to yellow viscous liquid which may appear as droplets); do not use vials with signs of melting. Solutions reconstituted in sterile water for injection should be further diluted immediately. According to the manufacturer, reconstituted solutions in normal saline (NS) are stable for 24 hours at room temperature and for 6 days refrigerated at 2°C to 8°C (36°F to 46°F). Solutions diluted for infusion in ½NS are stable for 24 hours at room temperature and for 6 days refrigerated and solutions diluted in D5W or D5NS are stable for 24 hours at room temperature and for 36 hours refrigerated (according to product labeling).

Capsules: Store at 20°C to 25°C (68°F to 77°F); excursions are permitted between 15°C and 30°C (59°F and 86°F).

Tablets: Store tablets at ≤25°C (77°F); brief excursions are permitted up to 30°C (86°F); protect from temperatures >30°C (86°F).

Preparation for Administration

Injection powder for reconstitution: Reconstitute with 25 mL for a 500 mg vial, 50 mL for a 1,000 mg vial, or 100 mL for a 2,000 mg vial to a concentration of 20 mg/mL using NS or SWFI. Solutions reconstituted in SWFI are hypotonic and should not be used for direct IV push administration. May reconstitute with NS or SWFI for solutions that will be further diluted for IV infusion. Swirl gently to mix. For IV infusion, further dilute for infusion in D5W, ½NS, or D5NS, to a minimum concentration of 2 mg/mL.

Mechanism of Action Cyclophosphamide is an alkylating agent that prevents cell division by cross-linking DNA strands and decreasing DNA synthesis. It is a cell cycle phase nonspecific agent. Cyclophosphamide also possesses potent immunosuppressive activity. Cyclophosphamide is a prodrug that must be metabolized to active metabolites in the liver.

Pharmacodynamics/Kinetics

Absorption: Oral: Well absorbed

Distribution: V_d: 30 to 50 L (approximates total body water); crosses into CSF (not in high enough concentrations to treat meningeal leukemia)

Protein binding: ~20%; some metabolites are bound at >60%

Metabolism: Hepatic to active metabolites acrolein, 4-aldophosphamide, 4-hydroperoxycyclophosphamide, and nor-nitrogen mustard

Bioavailability: >75%

Half-life elimination: IV: 3 to 12 hours; Children: 4 hours; Adults: 6 to 8 hours

Time to peak: Oral: ~1 hour; IV: Metabolites: 2 to 3 hours

Excretion: Urine (10 to 20% as unchanged drug); feces (4%)

Dosing

Adult Cyclophosphamide is associated with a moderate to high emetic potential (depending on dose, regimen, or administration route); antiemetics are recommended to prevent nausea and vomiting (Basch 2011; Roila 2016).

Malignancy:

IV: 40 to 50 mg/kg in divided doses over 2 to 5 days **or** 10 to 15 mg/kg every 7 to 10 days **or** 3 to 5 mg/kg twice weekly

Oral: 1 to 5 mg/kg/day (initial and maintenance dosing)

Indication specific and/or off-label uses/dosing:

Acute lymphoblastic leukemia (off-label dosing): Multiple-agent regimens:

Hyper-CVAD regimen: IV: 300 mg/m² over 3 hours (with mesna) every 12 hours for 6 doses on days 1, 2, and 3 during odd-numbered cycles (cycles 1, 3, 5, 7) of an 8-cycle phase (Kantarjian 2004)

CALGB8811 regimen: IV:

Adults <60 years: Induction phase: 1,200 mg/m² on day 1 of a 4-week cycle; Early intensification phase: 1,000 mg/m² on day 1 of a 4-week cycle (repeat once); Late intensification phase: 1,000 mg/m² on day 29 of an 8-week cycle (Larson 1995)

Adults ≥60 years: Induction phase: 800 mg/m² on day 1 of a 4-week cycle; Early intensification phase: 1,000 mg/m² on day 1 of a 4-week cycle (repeat once); Late intensification phase: 1,000 mg/m² on day 29 of an 8-week cycle (Larson 1995)

Breast cancer (off-label dosing):

AC regimen: IV: 600 mg/m² on day 1 every 21 days (in combination with doxorubicin) for 4 cycles (Fisher 1990)

CEF regimen: Oral: 75 mg/m²/day days 1 to 14 every 28 days (in combination with epirubicin and fluorouracil) for 6 cycles (Levine 1998)

CMF regimen: Oral: 100 mg/m²/day days 1 to 14 every 28 days (in combination with methotrexate and fluorouracil) for 6 cycles (Levine 1998) **or** IV: 600 mg/m² on day 1 every 21 days (in combination with methotrexate and fluorouracil); Goldhirsch 1998)

Chronic lymphocytic leukemia (off-label dosing): IV: R-FC regimen: 250 mg/m²/day for 3 days every 28 days (in combination with rituximab and fludarabine) for 6 cycles (Robak 2010)

Ewing sarcoma (off-label use): IV: VAC/IE regimen: VAC: 1,200 mg/m² (plus mesna) on day 1 of a 21-day treatment cycle (in combination with vincristine and doxorubicin [then dactinomycin when maximum doxorubicin dose reached]), alternates with IE (ifosfamide and etoposide) for a total of 17 cycles (Grier 2003)

Gestational trophoblastic tumors, high-risk (off-label use): IV: EMA/CO regimen: 600 mg/m² on day 8 of 2-week treatment cycle (in combination with etoposide, methotrexate, dactinomycin, and vincristine), continue for at least 2 treatment cycles after a normal hCG level (Escobar 2003; Lurain 2006)

Granulomatosis with polyangiitis (GPA; Wegener granulomatosis) (off-label use; in combination with glucocorticoids):

Low-dose: Oral: 1.5 to 2 mg/kg/day (Jayne 2003; Stone 2010) or 2 mg/kg/day until remission, followed by 1.5 mg/kg/day for 3 additional months (de Groot 2009; Harper 2012)

Pulse: IV: 15 mg/kg (maximum dose: 1,200 mg) every 2 weeks for 3 doses, followed by maintenance pulses of either 15 mg/kg IV (maximum dose: 1,200 mg) every 3 weeks or 2.5 to 5 mg/kg/day orally on days 1, 2, and 3 every 3 weeks for 3 months after remission achieved (de Groot 2009; Harper 2012)

Hodgkin lymphoma (off-label dosing): IV:

BEACOPP regimen: 650 mg/m² on day 1 every 3 weeks (in combination with bleomycin, etoposide, doxorubicin, vincristine, procarbazine, and prednisone) for 8 cycles (Diehl 2003)

BEACOPP escalated regimen: 1,200 mg/m² on day 1 every 3 weeks (in combination with bleomycin, etoposide, doxorubicin, vincristine, procarbazine, and prednisone) for 8 cycles (Diehl 2003)

Multiple myeloma (off-label dosing): Oral: CyBorD regimen: 300 mg/m² on days 1, 8, 15, and 22 every 4 weeks (in combination with bortezomib and dexamethasone) for 4 cycles; may continue beyond 4 cycles (Khan 2012) **or** 500 mg/m² on days 1, 8, and 15 every 3 weeks (in combination with bortezomib and dexamethasone) for 8 cycles (Kumar 2012)

Non-Hodgkin lymphoma (off-label dosing): IV:

R-CHOP regimen: 750 mg/m² on day 1 every 3 weeks (in combination with rituximab, doxorubicin, vincristine, and prednisone) for 8 cycles (Coiffier 2002)

R-EPOCH (dose adjusted) regimen: 750 mg/m² on day 5 every 3 weeks (in combination with rituximab, etoposide, prednisone, vincristine, and doxorubicin) for 6 to 8 cycles (Garcia-Suarez 2007)

CODOX-M/IVAC (Burkitt lymphoma): Cycles 1 and 3 (CODOX-M): 800 mg/m² on day 1, followed by 200 mg/m² on days 2 to 5 (Magrath 1996) **or** 800 mg/m² on days 1 and 2 (Lacasce 2004), in combination with vincristine, doxorubicin, and methotrexate; CODOX-M alternates with IVAC (etoposide, ifosfamide, and cytarabine) for a total of 4 cycles

◄ **Immune thrombocytopenia, refractory (off-label use; Provan 2010):**
Oral: 1 to 2 mg/kg/day for at least 16 weeks
IV: 300 to 1,000 mg/m^2 for 1 to 3 doses every 2 to 4 weeks

Lupus nephritis (off-label use): IV: 500 mg once every 2 weeks for 6 doses or 500 to 1,000 mg/m^2 once every month for 6 doses (Hahn 2012) **or** 500 to 1,000 mg/m^2 every month for 6 months, then every 3 months for a total of at least 2.5 years (Austin 1986; Gourley 1996)

Ovarian germ cell tumors (malignant; off-label use): IV: 150 mg/m^2 on days 1 to 5 every 28 days (in combination with dactinomycin and vincristine) for at least 10 cycles (Slayton 1985)

Pericarditis, recurrent (off-label use):
Oral: 100 to 150 mg daily for 2 to 3 months (Marcolongo 1995). Based on very limited data (case report); additional data may be necessary to further define the role of cyclophosphamide in the treatment of this condition.

IV: 600 mg/m^2 once every month (Agard 2007). Based on very limited data (case report); additional data may be necessary to further define the role of cyclophosphamide in the treatment of this condition.

Pheochromocytoma, malignant (off-label use): IV: 750 mg/m^2 on day 1 every 3 or 4 weeks (in combination with dacarbazine and vincristine) (Huang 2008). Additional data may be necessary to further define the role of dacarbazine in this condition.

Small cell lung cancer (SCLC), refractory (off-label use): IV: 1,000 mg/m^2 (maximum: 2,000 mg) on day 1 every 3 weeks (in combination with doxorubicin and vincristine) until disease progression or unacceptable toxicity (von Pawel 1999)

Stem cell transplant conditioning (off-label use): IV:
Nonmyeloablative transplant (allogeneic): 750 mg/m^2/day for 3 days beginning 5 days prior to transplant (in combination with fludarabine) (Khouri 2008)

Myeloablative transplant:
100 mg/kg (based on IBW, unless actual weight <95% of IBW) as a single dose 2 days prior to transplant (in combination with total body irradiation and etoposide) (Thompson 2008)

50 mg/kg/day for 4 days beginning 5 days before transplant (with or without antithymocyte globulin [equine]) (Champlin 2007)

50 mg/kg/day for 4 days beginning 5 days prior to transplant (in combination with busulfan) (Cassileth 1993)

60 mg/kg/day for 2 days (in combination with busulfan and total body irradiation) (Anderson 1996)

1,800 mg/m^2/day for 4 days beginning 7 days prior to transplant (in combination with etoposide and carmustine) (Reece 1991)

Uveitis (off-label use):
Oral: 20 to 100 mg daily (Diaz-Llopis 2009) **or** 100 to 150 mg daily (Purjari 2010) **or** 1 to 3 mg/kg/day (Jabs 2000); adjust dose based on response or toxicity. May use IV dosing for more resistant cases (Diaz-Llopis 2009).

IV: 750 to 1,000 mg every 4 weeks (Diaz-Llopis 2009)

Geriatric Refer to adult dosing; adjust for renal clearance.

Pediatric Cyclophosphamide is associated with a moderate to high emetic potential (depending on dose, regimen, or administration route); antiemetics are recommended to prevent nausea and vomiting (Dupuis 2011).

Malignancy:
IV: 40 to 50 mg/kg in divided doses over 2 to 5 days **or** 10 to 15 mg/kg every 7 to 10 days **or** 3 to 5 mg/kg twice weekly

Oral: 1 to 5 mg/kg/day (initial and maintenance dosing)

Nephrotic syndrome, corticosteroid refractory or intolerant, or corticosteroid sparing: Oral: Initial: 2 mg/kg once daily for 8 to 12 weeks (maximum cumulative dose: 168 mg/kg); treatment beyond 90 days may increase the potential for sterility in males; treatment beyond 1 course is not recommended (Lombel 2013)

Indication specific and/or off-label uses/dosing:

Ewing sarcoma (off-label use): IV: VAC/IE regimen: VAC: 1200 mg/m^2 (plus mesna) on day 1 of a 21-day treatment cycle (in combination with vincristine and doxorubicin [then dactinomycin when maximum doxorubicin dose reached]), alternates with IE (ifosfamide and etoposide) for a total of 17 cycles (Grier 2003)

Hodgkin lymphoma (off-label dosing): IV: BEACOPP escalated regimen: 1200 mg/m^2 on day 0 of a 21-day treatment cycle (in combination with bleomycin, etoposide, doxorubicin, vincristine, prednisone, and procarbazine) for 4 cycles (Kelly 2011)

Lupus nephritis (off-label use): IV: 500 to 1000 mg/m^2 every month for 6 months, then every 3 months for a total of 2.5 to 3 years (Austin 1986; Gourley 1996; Lehman 2000)

Ovarian germ cell tumors (malignant; off-label use): IV: 150 mg/m^2 on days 1 to 5 every 28 days (in combination with dactinomycin and vincristine) for at least 10 cycles (Slayton 1985)

Neuroblastoma (off-label dosing): IV: CE-CAdO regimen, courses 3 and 4: 300 mg/m^2 days 1 to 5 every 21 days for 2 cycles (Rubie 1998) **or** 10 mg/kg days 1 to 5 every 21 days for 2 cycles (Rubie 2001). **Note:** Decreased doses may be recommended for newborns or children <10 kg.

Stem cell transplant conditioning (off-label use): Myeloablative transplant: IV: 50 mg/kg/day for 4 days beginning 5 days before transplant (with or without antithymocyte globulin [equine]) (Champlin 2007)

Wilms tumor, relapsed (off-label use): Infants, Children, and Adolescents: IV (in combination with vincristine, doxorubicin, mesna, etoposide, filgrastim, and radiation therapy) (Green 2007):
Pediatrics ≤30 kg: 14.7 mg/kg days 1 to 5 of weeks 3, 9, 15, and 21 and 14.7 mg/kg days 1 to 3 of weeks 6, 12, 18, and 24
Pediatrics >30 kg: 440 mg/m^2 days 1 to 5 of weeks 3, 9, 15, and 21 and 440 mg/m^2 days 1 to 3 of weeks 6, 12, 18, and 24

Renal Impairment There are no dosage adjustments provided in the manufacturer's labeling (use with caution; elevated levels of metabolites may occur).

The following adjustments have also been recommended:

Aronoff 2007: Children and Adults:

CrCl ≥10 mL/minute: No dosage adjustment required.

CrCl <10 mL/minute: Administer 75% of normal dose.

Hemodialysis: Moderately dialyzable (20% to 50%); administer 50% of normal dose; administer after hemodialysis

Continuous ambulatory peritoneal dialysis (CAPD): Administer 75% of normal dose.

Continuous renal replacement therapy (CRRT): Administer 100% of normal dose.

◄ Janus 2010: Hemodialysis: Administer 75% of normal dose; administer after hemodialysis

Hematopoietic stem cell transplantation (Bodge 2014):
Moderate impairment: No dosage adjustment necessary.
Moderate to severe impairment: Consider dosage reduction.
Hemodialysis: Administer after hemodialysis. Cyclophosphamide is 20% to 50% dialyzed.

International Myeloma Working Group (IMWG) Recommendations: The International Myeloma Working Group (IMWG) recommendations suggest that cyclophosphamide may be administered without dosage adjustment in multiple myeloma patients with renal impairment, including those on dialysis. The IMWG recommends the use of the Chronic Kidney Disease Epidemiology Collaboration (CKD-EPI) equation (preferred) or the Modification of Diet in Renal Disease (MDRD) formula to evaluate renal function estimation in multiple myeloma patients with a stable serum creatinine (Dimopoulos 2016).

Hepatic Impairment The conversion between cyclophosphamide to the active metabolite may be reduced in patients with severe hepatic impairment, potentially reducing efficacy.

There are no dosage adjustments provided in the manufacturer's labeling.

The following adjustments have been recommended (Floyd 2006):
Serum bilirubin 3.1 to 5 mg/dL or transaminases >3 times ULN: Administer 75% of dose.
Serum bilirubin >5 mg/dL: Avoid use.

Obesity
American Society of Clinical Oncology (ASCO) Guidelines for appropriate chemotherapy dosing in obese adults with cancer (Note: Excludes HSCT dosing): Utilize patient's actual body weight (full weight) for calculation of body surface area- or weight-based dosing, particularly when the intent of therapy is curative; manage regimen-related toxicities in the same manner as for nonobese patients; if a dose reduction is utilized due to toxicity, consider resumption of full weight-based dosing with subsequent cycles, especially if cause of toxicity (eg, hepatic or renal impairment) is resolved (Griggs 2012).

American Society for Blood and Marrow Transplantation (ASBMT) practice guideline committee position statement on chemotherapy dosing in obesity (Bubalo 2014):
Cy200 (cyclophosphamide total dose of 200 mg/kg): Use the lesser of IBW or actual body weight (ABW).
Cy120 (cyclophosphamide total dose of 120 mg/kg): Use either IBW or ABW for patients ≤120% IBW (preferred method for adults of all body sizes); use ABW25 for patients >120% IBW (preferred for pediatric patients).
ABW25: Adjusted wt (kg) = Ideal body weight (kg) + 0.25 [actual wt (kg) - ideal body weight (kg)]

Adjustment for Toxicity
Hematologic toxicity: May require dose reduction or treatment interruption
Hemorrhagic cystitis, severe: Discontinue treatment

Combination Regimens
Bone sarcoma (Ewing sarcoma):
Cyclophosphamide-Topotecan (Ewing Sarcoma) on page 2078
VAC Alternating With IE (Ewing Sarcoma) on page 2224
Brain tumor: COPE on page 2074

◀ Lymphoma, non-Hodgkin (Burkitt):

Lymphoma, non-Hodgkin (DLBCL):

Lymphoma, non-Hodgkin (Follicular):

Lymphoma, non-Hodgkin (Mantle cell):

Multiple myeloma:

Neuroblastoma:

Soft tissue sarcoma (rhabdomyosarcoma):

Administration

Cyclophosphamide is associated with a moderate to high emetic potential (depending on dose, regimen, or administration route); antiemetics are recommended to prevent nausea and vomiting (Basch 2011; Dupuis 2011; Roila 2016).

IV: Infusion rate may vary based on protocol (refer to specific protocol for infusion rate). Administer by direct IV injection (if reconstituted in NS), IVPB, or continuous IV infusion

Bladder toxicity: To minimize bladder toxicity, increase normal fluid intake during and for 1 to 2 days after cyclophosphamide dose. Most adult patients will require a fluid intake of at least 2 L/day. High-dose regimens should be accompanied by vigorous hydration with or without mesna therapy. Morning administration may be preferred to ensure adequate hydration throughout the day.

Hematopoietic stem cell transplant: Approaches to reduction of hemorrhagic cystitis include infusion of 0.9% NaCl 3 L/m^2/24 hours, infusion of 0.9% NaCl 3 L/m^2/24 hours with continuous 0.9% NaCl bladder irrigation 300 to 1000 mL/hour, and infusion of 0.9% NaCl 1.5 to 3 L/m^2/24 hours with intravenous mesna. Hydration should begin at least 4 hours before cyclophosphamide and continue at least 24 hours after completion of cyclophosphamide. The daily mesna dose (as a percentage of cyclophosphamide dose) may vary; refer to protocol and/or primary literature for mesna dose. Mesna can be administered as a continuous 24-hour intravenous infusion or be given in divided doses every 4 hours. Mesna should begin at the start of treatment, and continue at least 24 hours following the last dose of cyclophosphamide.

Oral: Tablets are not scored and should not be cut, chewed, or crushed. Swallow capsules whole; do not open, crush, or chew. To minimize bladder toxicity, increase normal fluid intake. Morning administration may be preferred to ensure adequate hydration throughout the day; do not administer tablets/capsules at bedtime. Avoid exposure to broken capsules; if contact occurs, wash hands immediately and thoroughly.

Vesicant/Extravasation Risk May be an irritant

Emetic Potential

Children:

IV:

≥1,000 mg/m^2: High (>90%)

<1,000 mg/m^2: Moderate (30% to 90%)

Oral: Moderate (30% to 90%)

Adults:

IV:

≥1,500 mg/m^2: High (>90%)

<1,500 mg/m^2: Moderate (30% to 90%)

Oral: Moderate (30% to 90%)

Extemporaneous Preparations Liquid solutions for oral administration may be prepared by dissolving cyclophosphamide injection in Aromatic Elixir, N F Store refrigerated (in glass container) for up to 14 days.

Cyclophosphamide Prescribing Information, Baxter Healthcare Corporation, Deerfield, Il, May, 2013.

A 10 mg/mL oral suspension may be prepared by reconstituting one 2 g vial for injection with 100 mL of NaCl 0.9%, providing an initial concentration of 20 mg/mL. Mix this solution in a 1:1 ratio with either Simple Syrup, NF or Ora-Plus® to obtain a final concentration of 10 mg/mL. Label "shake well" and "refrigerate". Stable for 56 days refrigerated.

Kennedy R, Groepper D, Tagen M, et al, "Stability of Cyclophosphamide in Extemporaneous Oral Suspensions," *Ann Pharmacother*, 2010, 44(2):295-301.

Monitoring Parameters CBC with differential and platelets, BUN, UA, serum electrolytes, serum creatinine; monitor for signs/symptoms of hemorrhagic cystitis or other urinary/renal toxicity, pulmonary, cardiac, and/or hepatic toxicity

Additional Information In patients with CYP2B6 G516T variant allele, cyclophosphamide metabolism is markedly increased; metabolism is not influenced by CYP2C9 and CYP2C19 isotypes (Xie 2006).

◀ **Dosage Forms** Excipient information presented when available (limited, particularly for generics); consult specific product labeling. [DSC] = Discontinued product

Capsule, Oral:

Generic: 25 mg, 50 mg

Solution Reconstituted, Injection:

Generic: 500 mg (1 ea); 1 g (1 ea); 2 g (1 ea)

Tablet, Oral:

Generic: 25 mg [DSC], 50 mg [DSC]

Dosage Forms: Canada Information with regard to form, strength, and availability of products uniquely available in Canada but currently not available in the US. Refer also to Dosage Forms.

Excipient information presented when available (limited, particularly for generics); consult specific product labeling.

Injection, powder for reconstitution: 200 mg

◆ **Cyclosporin A** see CycloSPORINE (Systemic) on page 452

CycloSPORINE (Systemic) (SYE kloe spor een)

Related Information

Hematopoietic Cell Transplantation on page 2365

Safe Handling of Hazardous Drugs on page 2379

Brand Names: US Gengraf; Neoral; SandIMMUNE

Brand Names: Canada Apo-Cyclosporine; Neoral; Sandimmune I.V.; Sandoz-Cyclosporine

Index Terms Ciclosporin; CsA; CyA; Cyclosporin A

Pharmacologic Category Calcineurin Inhibitor; Immunosuppressant Agent

Use

Cyclosporine modified:

Transplant rejection prophylaxis: Prophylaxis of organ rejection in kidney, liver, and heart transplants (commonly used in combination with an antiproliferative immunosuppressive agent and corticosteroid).

Rheumatoid arthritis: Treatment of severe, active rheumatoid arthritis (RA) not responsive to methotrexate alone

Psoriasis: Treatment of severe, recalcitrant plaque psoriasis in non-immunocompromised adults unresponsive to or unable to tolerate other systemic therapy

Cyclosporine non-modified:

Transplant rejection (prophylaxis): Prophylaxis of organ rejection in kidney, liver, and heart transplants (commonly used in combination with an antiproliferative agent and a corticosteroid)

Transplant rejection, chronic (treatment): May be used for the treatment of chronic rejection (kidney, liver, and heart) in patients previously treated with other immunosuppressive agents. **Note:** While approved for the treatment of chronic organ rejection, other therapies are clinically preferred in this setting.

Labeled Contraindications

Hypersensitivity to cyclosporine or any component of the formulation. IV cyclosporine is contraindicated in hypersensitivity to polyoxyethylated castor oil (Cremophor EL).

Rheumatoid arthritis and psoriasis patients with abnormal renal function, uncontrolled hypertension, or malignancies. Concomitant treatment with PUVA or UVB therapy, methotrexate, other immunosuppressive agents, coal tar, or radiation therapy are also contraindications for use in patients with psoriasis.

Canadian labeling: Additional contraindications (not in the US labeling): Concurrent use with bosentan; rheumatoid arthritis and psoriasis patients with primary or secondary immunodeficiency excluding autoimmune disease, uncontrolled infection, or malignancy (excluding non-melanoma skin cancer).

Pregnancy Considerations Adverse events were not observed following the use of oral cyclosporine in animal reproduction studies (using doses that were not maternally toxic). In humans, cyclosporine crosses the placenta; maternal concentrations do not correlate with those found in the umbilical cord. Cyclosporine may be detected in the serum of newborns for several days after birth (Claris 1993). Based on clinical use, premature births and low birth weight were consistently observed in pregnant transplant patients (additional pregnancy complications also present). Formulations may contain alcohol; the alcohol content should be taken into consideration in pregnant women.

The pharmacokinetics of cyclosporine may be influenced by pregnancy (Grimer 2007). Cyclosporine may be used in pregnant renal, liver, or heart transplant patients (Cowan 2012; EBPG Expert Group on Renal Transplantation 2002; McGuire 2009; Parhar 2012). If therapy is needed for psoriasis, other agents are preferred; however, cyclosporine may be used as an alternative agent along with close clinical monitoring; use should be avoided during the first trimester if possible (Bae 2012). If treatment is needed for lupus nephritis, other agents are recommended to be used in pregnant women (Hahn 2012).

Following transplant, normal menstruation and fertility may be restored within months; however, appropriate contraception is recommended to prevent pregnancy until 1-2 years following the transplant to improve pregnancy outcomes (Cowan 2012; EBPG Expert Group on Renal Transplantation 2002; McGuire 2009; Parhar 2012).

The National Transplantation Pregnancy Registry (NTPR) is a registry which follows pregnancies which occur in maternal transplant recipients or those fathered by male transplant recipients. The NTPR encourages reporting of pregnancies following solid organ transplant by contacting them at 877-955-6877 or NTPR@giftoflifeinstitute.org.

Breastfeeding Considerations Cyclosporine is excreted in breast milk. Concentrations of cyclosporine in milk vary widely and breastfeeding during therapy is generally not recommended (Bae 2012; Cowan 2012). Due to the potential for serious adverse in the breastfeeding infant, a decision should be made to discontinue cyclosporine or to discontinue breastfeeding, taking into account the importance of treatment to the mother. Formulations may contain alcohol which may be present in breast milk and could be absorbed orally by the breastfeeding infant.

Warnings/Precautions [US Boxed Warning]: Increased risk of lymphomas and other malignancies (including fatal outcomes), **particularly skin cancers;** risk is related to intensity/duration of therapy and the use of more than one immunosuppressive agent; all patients should avoid excessive sun/ UV light exposure. **[US Boxed Warning]: May cause hypertension; risk is**

◀ **increased with increasing doses/duration.** Use caution when changing dosage forms.

[US Boxed Warning]: Renal impairment, including structural kidney damage has occurred (when used at high doses); risk is increased with increasing doses/duration; monitor renal function closely. Elevations in serum creatinine and BUN generally respond to dosage reductions. Use caution with other potentially nephrotoxic drugs (eg, acyclovir, aminoglycoside antibiotics, amphotericin B, ciprofloxacin); monitor renal function closely with concomitant use. If significant renal impairment occurs, reduce the dose of the coadministered medication or consider alternative treatment. Elevations in serum creatinine and BUN associated with nephrotoxicity generally respond to dosage reductions. In renal transplant patients with rapidly rising BUN and creatinine, carefully evaluate to differentiate between cyclosporine-associated nephrotoxicity and renal rejection episodes. In cases of severe rejection that fail to respond to pulse steroids and monoclonal antibodies, switching to an alternative immunosuppressant agent may be preferred to increasing cyclosporine to excessive blood concentrations.

[US Boxed Warning]: Increased risk of infection with use; serious and fatal infections have been reported. Bacterial, viral, fungal, and protozoal infections (including opportunistic infections) have occurred. Polyoma virus infections, such as the JC virus and BK virus, may result in serious and sometimes fatal outcomes. The JC virus is associated with progressive multifocal leukoencephalopathy (PML), and PML has been reported in patients receiving cyclosporine. PML may be fatal and presents with hemiparesis, apathy, confusion, cognitive deficiencies, and ataxia; consider neurologic consultation as indicated. The BK virus is associated with nephropathy, and polyoma virus-associated nephropathy (PVAN) has been reported in patients receiving cyclosporine. PVAN is associated with serious adverse effects including renal dysfunction and renal graft loss. If PML or PVAN occur in transplant patients, consider reducing immunosuppression therapy as well as the risk that reduced immunosuppression poses to grafts.

Hepatotoxicity (transaminase and bilirubin elevations) and liver injury, including cholestasis, jaundice, hepatitis, and liver failure, has been reported. These events were mainly in patients with confounding factors including infections, coadministration with other potentially hepatotoxic medications, underlying conditions, and significant comorbidities. Fatalities have also been reported rarely, primarily in transplant patients. Increased hepatic enzymes and bilirubin have occurred, usually in the first month and when used at high doses; improvement is usually seen with dosage reduction.

Should be used initially with corticosteroids in transplant patients. Significant hyperkalemia (with or without hyperchloremic metabolic acidosis) and hyperuricemia have occurred with therapy. Syndromes of microangiopathic hemolytic anemia and thrombocytopenia have occurred and may result in graft failure; it is accompanied by platelet consumption within the graft. Syndrome may occur without graft rejection. Although management of the syndrome is unclear, discontinuation or reduction of cyclosporine, in addition to streptokinase and heparin administration or plasmapheresis, has been associated with syndrome resolution. However, resolution seems to be dependent upon early detection of the syndrome via indium 111 labeled platelet scans.

May cause seizures, particularly if used with high-dose corticosteroids. Encephalopathy (including posterior reversible encephalopathy syndrome [PRES]) has also been reported; predisposing factors include hypertension, hypomagnesemia, hypocholesterolemia, high-dose corticosteroids, high cyclosporine serum concentration, and graft-versus-host disease (GVHD). Encephalopathy may be more common in patients with liver transplant compared to kidney transplant. Other neurotoxic events, such as optic disc edema (including papilloedema and potential visual impairment), have been rarely reported primarily in transplant patients.

[US Boxed Warning]: The modified/non-modified formulations are not bioequivalent; cyclosporine (modified) has increased bioavailability as compared to cyclosporine (non-modified) and the products cannot be used interchangeably without close monitoring. Cyclosporine (modified) refers to the oral solution and capsule dosage formulations of cyclosporine in an aqueous dispersion (previously referred to as "microemulsion"). Potentially significant drug-drug/drug-food interactions may exist, requiring dose or frequency adjustment, additional monitoring, and/or selection of alternative therapy. Gingival hyperplasia may occur; avoid concomitant nifedipine in patients who develop gingival hyperplasia (may increase frequency of hyperplasia). Monitor cyclosporine concentrations closely following the addition, modification, or deletion of other medication. Live, attenuated vaccines may be less effective; vaccination should be avoided. Make dose adjustments based on cyclosporine blood concentrations. **[US Boxed Warning]: Cyclosporine non-modified absorption is erratic; monitor blood concentrations closely. [US Boxed Warning]: Prescribing and dosage adjustment should only be under the direct supervision of an experienced physician. Adequate laboratory/medical resources and follow-up are necessary.** Anaphylaxis has been reported with IV use; reserve for patients who cannot take oral form. **[US Boxed Warning]: Risk of skin cancer may be increased in transplant patients.** Due to the increased risk for nephrotoxicity in renal transplantation, avoid using standard doses of cyclosporine in combination with everolimus; reduced cyclosporine doses are recommended; monitor cyclosporine concentrations closely. Cyclosporine and everolimus combination therapy may increase the risk for proteinuria. Cyclosporine combined with either everolimus or sirolimus may increase the risk for thrombotic microangiopathy/thrombotic thrombocytopenic purpura/hemolytic uremic syndrome (TMA/TTP/HUS). Cyclosporine has extensive hepatic metabolism and exposure is increased in patients with severe hepatic impairment; may require dose reduction.

Patients with psoriasis should avoid excessive sun exposure. **[US Boxed Warning]: Risk of skin cancer may be increased with a history of PUVA and possibly methotrexate or other immunosuppressants, UVB, coal tar, or radiation.**

Psoriasis: If receiving other immunosuppressive agents, radiation or UV therapy, concurrent use of cyclosporine is not recommended.

Products may contain corn oil, ethanol (consider alcohol content in certain patient populations, including pregnant or breastfeeding women, patients with liver disease, seizure disorders, alcohol dependency, or pediatrics), or propylene glycol; injection also contains the vehicle Cremophor EL (polyoxyethylated castor oil), which has been associated with hypersensitivity (anaphylactic) reactions. Due to the risk for anaphylaxis, IV cyclosporine should be reserved for use in patients unable to take an oral formulation. Some dosage forms may contain propylene glycol; large amounts are potentially toxic and have been associated hyperosmolality, lactic acidosis, seizures, and respiratory depression; use caution (AAP 1997; Zar 2007).

Adverse Reactions Adverse reactions reported with systemic use, including rheumatoid arthritis, psoriasis, and transplantation (kidney, liver, and heart). Percentages noted include the highest frequency regardless of indication/ dosage. Frequencies may vary for specific conditions or formulation.

>10%:
  Cardiovascular: Hypertension (8% to 53%), edema (5% to 14%)
  Central nervous system: Headache (2% to 25%), paresthesia (1% to 11%)
  Dermatologic: Hypertrichosis (5% to 19%)
  Endocrine & metabolic: Hirsutism (21% to 45%), increased serum triglycerides (15%), female genital tract disease (9% to 11%)
  Gastrointestinal: Nausea (2% to 23%), diarrhea (3% to 13%), gingival hyperplasia (2% to 16%), abdominal distress (<1% to 15%), dyspepsia (2% to 12%)
  Genitourinary: Urinary tract infection (kidney transplant: 21%)
  Infection: Increased susceptibility to infection (3% to 25%), viral infection (kidney transplant: 16%)
  Neuromuscular & skeletal: Tremor (7% to 55%), leg cramps (2% to 12%)
  Renal: Increased serum creatinine (16% to ≥50%), renal insufficiency (10% to 38%)
  Respiratory: Upper respiratory tract infection (1% to 14%)

Kidney, liver, and heart transplant only (≤2% unless otherwise noted):
  Cardiovascular: Chest pain (≤4%), flushing (<1% to 4%), glomerular capillary thrombosis, myocardial infarction
  Central nervous system: Convulsions (1% to 5%), anxiety, confusion, lethargy, tingling sensation
  Dermatologic: Skin infection (7%), acne vulgaris (1% to 6%), nail disease (brittle fingernails), hair breakage, night sweats, pruritus
  Endocrine & metabolic: Gynecomastia (<1% to 4%), hyperglycemia, hypomagnesemia, weight loss
  Gastrointestinal: Vomiting (2% to 10%), anorexia, aphthous stomatitis, constipation, dysphagia, gastritis, hiccups, pancreatitis
  Genitourinary: Hematuria
  Hematologic & oncologic: Leukopenia (<1% to 6%), lymphoma (<1% to 6%), anemia, thrombocytopenia, upper gastrointestinal hemorrhage
  Hepatic: Hepatotoxicity (<1% to 7%)
  Infection: Localized fungal infection (8%), cytomegalovirus disease (5%), septicemia (5%), abscess (4%), fungal infection (systemic: 2%)
  Neuromuscular & skeletal: Arthralgia, myalgia, weakness
  Ophthalmic: Conjunctivitis, visual disturbance
  Otic: Hearing loss, tinnitus
  Respiratory: Sinusitis (<1% to 7%), pneumonia (6%)
  Miscellaneous: Fever

Rheumatoid arthritis only (1% to <3% unless otherwise noted):
  Cardiovascular: Chest pain (4%), cardiac arrhythmia (2%), abnormal heart sounds, cardiac failure, myocardial infarction, peripheral ischemia

Central nervous system: Dizziness (8%), pain (6%), insomnia (4%), depression (3%), migraine (2% to 3%), anxiety, drowsiness, emotional lability, hypoesthesia, lack of concentration, malaise, neuropathy, nervousness, paranoia, vertigo

Dermatologic: Cellulitis, dermatological reaction, dermatitis, diaphoresis, dyschromia, eczema, enanthema, folliculitis, nail disease, pruritus, urticaria, xeroderma

Endocrine & metabolic: Menstrual disease (3%), decreased libido, diabetes mellitus, goiter, hot flash, hyperkalemia, hyperuricemia, hypoglycemia, increased libido, weight gain, weight loss

Gastrointestinal: Vomiting (9%), flatulence (5%), gingivitis (4%), constipation, dysgeusia, dysphagia, enlargement of salivary glands, eructation, esophagitis, gastric ulcer, gastritis, gastroenteritis, gingival hemorrhage, glossitis, peptic ulcer, tongue disease, xerostomia

Genitourinary: Leukorrhea (1%), breast fibroadenosis, hematuria, mastalgia, nocturia, urine abnormality, urinary incontinence, urinary urgency, uterine hemorrhage

Hematologic & oncologic: Purpura (3% to 4%), anemia, carcinoma, leukopenia, lymphadenopathy

Hepatic: Hyperbilirubinemia

Infection: Abscess (including renal), bacterial infection, candidiasis, fungal infection, herpes simplex infection, herpes zoster, viral infection

Neuromuscular & skeletal: Arthralgia, bone fracture, dislocation, myalgia, stiffness, synovial cyst, tendon disease, weakness

Ophthalmic: Cataract, conjunctivitis, eye pain, visual disturbance

Otic: Tinnitus, deafness, vestibular disturbance

Renal: Abscess (renal), increased blood urea nitrogen, polyuria, pyelonephritis

Respiratory: Cough (5%), dyspnea (5%), sinusitis (4%), abnormal breath sounds, bronchospasm, epistaxis, tonsillitis

Psoriasis only (1% to <3% unless otherwise noted):

Cardiovascular: Chest pain, flushing

Central nervous system: Psychiatric disturbance (4% to 5%), pain (3% to 4%), dizziness, insomnia, nervousness, vertigo

Dermatologic: Acne vulgaris, folliculitis, hyperkeratosis, pruritus, skin rash, xeroderma

Endocrine & metabolic: Hot flash

Gastrointestinal: Abdominal distention, constipation, gingival hemorrhage, increased appetite

Genitourinary: Urinary frequency

Hematologic & oncologic: Abnormal erythrocytes, altered platelet function, blood coagulation disorder, carcinoma, hemorrhagic diathesis

Hepatic: Hyperbilirubinemia

Neuromuscular & skeletal: Arthralgia (1% to 6%)

Ophthalmic: Visual disturbance

Respiratory: Flu-like symptoms (8% to 10%), bronchospasm (5%), cough (5%), dyspnea (5%), rhinitis (5%), respiratory tract infection

Miscellaneous: Fever

Postmarketing and/or case reports (any indication): Anaphylaxis/anaphylactoid reaction (possibly associated with Cremophor EL vehicle in injection formulation), brain disease, central nervous system toxicity, cholestasis, cholesterol increased, exacerbation of psoriasis (transformation to erythrodermic or pustular psoriasis), fatigue, gout, haemolytic uremic syndrome, hepatic insufficiency, hepatitis, hyperbilirubinemia, hyperkalemia, hyperlipidemia, hypertrichosis, hyperuricemia, hypomagnesemia, impaired consciousness, increased susceptibility to infection (including JC virus and BK virus), jaundice, leg pain (possibly a manifestation of Calcineurin-Inhibitor Induced Pain Syndrome), malignant lymphoma, migraine, myalgia, myopathy, myositis, papilledema, progressive multifocal leukoencephalopathy, pseudotumor cerebri, pulmonary edema (noncardiogenic), renal disease (polyoma virus-associated), reversible posterior leukoencephalopathy syndrome, rhabdomyolysis, thrombotic microangiopathy

Drug Interactions

Metabolism/Transport Effects Substrate of CYP3A4 (major), P-glycoprotein; **Note:** Assignment of Major/Minor substrate status based on clinically relevant drug interaction potential; **Inhibits** BCRP, BSEP, CYP2C9 (weak), CYP3A4 (weak), P-glycoprotein, SLCO1B1

Avoid Concomitant Use

Avoid concomitant use of CycloSPORINE (Systemic) with any of the following: Aliskiren; Asunaprevir; AtorvaSTATin; BCG (Intravesical); Bosentan; Cholic Acid; Conivaptan; Crizotinib; Dronedarone; Enzalutamide; Eplerenone; Foscarnet; Fusidic Acid (Systemic); Glecaprevir and Pibrentasvir; Grazoprevir; Idelalisib; Lercanidipine; Lovastatin; MiFEPRIStone; Natalizumab; PAZOPanib; Pimecrolimus; Pimozide; Pitavastatin; Potassium-Sparing Diuretics; Silodosin; Simeprevir; Simvastatin; Tacrolimus (Systemic); Tacrolimus (Topical); Topotecan; Vaccines (Live); VinCRIStine (Liposomal); Voxilaprevir

Increased Effect/Toxicity

CycloSPORINE (Systemic) may increase the levels/effects of: Afatinib; Aliskiren; Ambrisentan; ARIPiprazole; Asunaprevir; AtorvaSTATin; Betrixaban; Bilastine; Boceprevir; Bosentan; Brentuximab Vedotin; Calcium Channel Blockers (Dihydropyridine); Calcium Channel Blockers (Nondihydropyridine); Caspofungin; Celiprolol; Cholic Acid; Colchicine; Dabigatran Etexilate; Dexamethasone (Systemic); Digoxin; Dofetilide; DOXOrubicin (Conventional); Dronedarone; Edoxaban; Eluxadoline; Etoposide; Etoposide Phosphate; Everolimus; Ezetimibe; Fibric Acid Derivatives; Fimasartan; Fingolimod; Flibanserin; Fluvastatin; Glecaprevir and Pibrentasvir; Grazoprevir; HYDROcodone; Ibrutinib; Imipenem; Leflunomide; Lercanidipine; Lomitapide; Loop Diuretics; Lovastatin; Methotrexate; MethylPREDNISolone; Minoxidil (Systemic); Minoxidil (Topical); MitoXANTRONE; Naldemedine; Naloxegol; Natalizumab; Neratinib; Neuromuscular-Blocking Agents; NiMODipine; Nonsteroidal Anti-Inflammatory Agents; PAZOPanib; P-glycoprotein/ABCB1 Substrates; Pimozide; Pitavastatin; Pravastatin; PrednisoLONE; PredniSONE; Protease Inhibitors; Prucalopride; Ranolazine; Repaglinide; RifAXIMin; Rosuvastatin; Silodosin; Simeprevir; Simvastatin; Sirolimus; Tacrolimus (Systemic); Tacrolimus (Topical); Ticagrelor; Tofacitinib; Topotecan; Vaccines (Live); Venetoclax; VinCRIStine (Liposomal); Voxilaprevir

The levels/effects of CycloSPORINE (Systemic) may be increased by: AcetaZOLAMIDE; Aminoglycosides; Amiodarone; Amphotericin B; Androgens; Angiotensin II Receptor Blockers; Antifungal Agents (Azole Derivatives, Systemic); Aprepitant; Azithromycin (Systemic); Boceprevir; Bromocriptine; Calcium Channel Blockers (Dihydropyridine); Calcium Channel Blockers (Nondihydropyridine); Carvedilol; Chloramphenicol; Clarithromycin; Conivaptan; Crizotinib; Cyclophosphamide; CYP3A4 Inhibitors

(Moderate); CYP3A4 Inhibitors (Strong); Dasatinib; Denosumab; Dexamethasone (Systemic); Dronabinol; Eplerenone; Erythromycin (Systemic); Ezetimibe; Fluconazole; Fosaprepitant; Foscarnet; Fusidic Acid (Systemic); Ganciclovir-Valganciclovir; GlyBURIDE; Grapefruit Juice; Idelalisib; Imatinib; Imipenem; Isavuconazonium Sulfate; Lercanidipine; Melphalan; Methotrexate; MethylPREDNISolone; Metoclopramide; Metreleptin; MiFEPRIStone; Netupitant; Nonsteroidal Anti-Inflammatory Agents; Norfloxacin; Ocrelizumab; Ombitasvir, Paritaprevir, and Ritonavir; Ombitasvir, Paritaprevir, Ritonavir, and Dasabuvir; Omeprazole; Palbociclib; P-glycoprotein/ABCB1 Inhibitors; Pimecrolimus; Potassium-Sparing Diuretics; Pravastatin; PrednisoLONE (Systemic); PredniSONE; Protease Inhibitors; Quinupristin; Ranolazine; Ritonavir; Roflumilast; Simeprevir; Sirolimus; Stiripentol; Sulfonamide Derivatives; Tacrolimus (Systemic); Tacrolimus (Topical); Telaprevir; Telithromycin; Temsirolimus; Trastuzumab

Decreased Effect

CycloSPORINE (Systemic) may decrease the levels/effects of: BCG (Intravesical); Coccidioides immitis Skin Test; Eltrombopag; GlyBURIDE; Mycophenolate; Nivolumab; Sipuleucel-T; Tertomotide; Vaccines (Inactivated); Vaccines (Live)

The levels/effects of CycloSPORINE (Systemic) may be decreased by: Adalimumab; Armodafinil; Ascorbic Acid; Barbiturates; Bosentan; CarBAMazepine; Colesevelam; Cyclophosphamide; CYP3A4 Inducers (Moderate); CYP3A4 Inducers (Strong); Dabrafenib; Deferasirox; Dexamethasone (Systemic); Echinacea; Efavirenz; Enzalutamide; Fibric Acid Derivatives; Fosphenytoin; Griseofulvin; Imipenem; MethylPREDNISolone; Metreleptin; Mitotane; Modafinil; Multivitamins/Fluoride (with ADE); Multivitamins/Minerals (with ADEK, Folate, Iron); Multivitamins/Minerals (with AE, No Iron); Nafcillin; Orlistat; Phenytoin; PrednisoLONE (Systemic); PredniSONE; Probucol; Pyrazinamide; Rifamycin Derivatives; Sarilumab; Sevelamer; Siltuximab; Somatostatin Analogs; St John's Wort; Sulfinpyrazone; Sulfonamide Derivatives; Tocilizumab; Vitamin E (Systemic)

Food Interactions Grapefruit juice increases cyclosporine serum concentrations. Management: Avoid grapefruit juice.

Hazardous Drugs Handling Considerations

Hazardous agent (NIOSH 2016 [group 2]).

Use appropriate precautions for receiving, handling, administration, and disposal. Gloves (single) should be worn during receiving, unpacking, and placing in storage.

NIOSH recommends single gloving for administration of intact tablets or capsules. NIOSH recommends double gloving, a protective gown, and (if there is a potential for vomit or spit up) eye/face protection for administration of an oral liquid/feeding tube administration. For IV preparation, when compounding, double gloves, a protective gown, ventilated engineering controls (a class II biological safety cabinet or a compounding aseptic containment isolator), and closed system transfer devices (CSTDs) are recommended. Double gloving and a gown are required during IV administration (NIOSH 2016). Assess risk to determine appropriate containment strategy (USP-NF 2017).

Storage/Stability

Capsules (modified): Store in the original unit-dose container at 20°C to 25°C (68°F to 77°F).

◄ Capsules (non-modified): Store at 25°C (77°F); excursions are permitted between 15°C and 30°C (59°F and 86°F). An odor may be detected upon opening the unit-dose container, which will dissipate shortly thereafter. This odor does not affect the quality of the product.

Injection: Store below 30°C (86°F) or at controlled room temperature (product dependent). Protect from light. The manufacturer recommends discarding diluted infusion solutions in D5W or NS after 24 hours.

Oral solution (modified): Store in the original container at 20°C to 25°C (68°F to 77°F). Do not store in the refrigerator. Once opened, use within 2 months. At temperatures below 20°C (68°F), the solution may gel; light flocculation or the formation of a light sediment also may occur. There is no impact on product performance or dosing using the syringe provided. Allow to warm to room temperature (25°C [77°F]) to reverse these changes.

Oral solution (non-modified): Store in the original container at temperatures below 30°C (86°F). Do not store in the refrigerator. Protect from freezing. Once opened, use within 2 months.

Preparation for Administration

Injection: To minimize leaching of DEHP, non-PVC containers and sets should be used for preparation and administration.

Sandimmune injection: Injection should be further diluted (1 mL [50 mg] of concentrate in 20-100 mL of D5W or NS) for administration by intravenous infusion.

Oral solution: Should be mixed in glass containers (not in plastic).

Mechanism of Action Inhibition of production and release of interleukin II and inhibits interleukin II-induced activation of resting T-lymphocytes.

Pharmacodynamics/Kinetics

Absorption: Oral:

Cyclosporine (non-modified): Erratic and incomplete; dependent on presence of food, bile acids, and GI motility; larger oral doses are needed in pediatrics due to shorter bowel length and limited intestinal absorption

Cyclosporine (modified): Erratic and incomplete; increased absorption, up to 30% when compared to cyclosporine (non-modified); less dependent on food, bile acids, or GI motility when compared to cyclosporine (non-modified)

Distribution: Widely in tissues and body fluids including the liver, pancreas, and lungs

V_{dss}: 4-6 L/kg in renal, liver, and marrow transplant recipients (slightly lower values in cardiac transplant patients; children <10 years have higher values); ESRD: 3.49 L/kg

Protein binding: 90% to 98% to lipoproteins

Metabolism: Extensively hepatic via CYP3A4; forms at least 25 metabolites; extensive first-pass effect following oral administration

Bioavailability: Oral:

Cyclosporine (non-modified): Dependent on patient population and transplant type (<10% in adult liver transplant patients and as high as 89% in renal transplant patients); bioavailability of Sandimmune capsules and oral solution are equivalent; bioavailability of oral solution is ~30% of the IV solution

Children: 28% (range: 17% to 42%); gut dysfunction common in BMT patients and oral bioavailability is further reduced

Cyclosporine (modified): Bioavailability of Neoral capsules and oral solution are equivalent:

Children: 43% (range: 30% to 68%)

Adults: 23% greater than with cyclosporine (non-modified) in renal transplant patients; 50% greater in liver transplant patients

Half-life elimination: Oral: May be prolonged in patients with hepatic impairment and shorter in pediatric patients due to the higher metabolism rate

Cyclosporine (non-modified): Biphasic: Alpha: 1.4 hours; Terminal: 19 hours (range: 10-27 hours)

Cyclosporine (modified): Biphasic: Terminal: 8.4 hours (range: 5-18 hours)

Time to peak, serum: Oral:

Cyclosporine (non-modified): 2-6 hours; some patients have a second peak at 5-6 hours

Cyclosporine (modified): Renal transplant: 1.5-2 hours

Excretion: Primarily feces; urine (6%, 0.1% as unchanged drug and metabolites); clearance is more rapid in pediatric patients than in adults

Dosing

Adult & Geriatric Neoral/Gengraf (cyclosporine modified) and Sandimmune (cyclosporine non-modified) are not bioequivalent and cannot be used interchangeably. Use caution when selecting, dispensing, and administrating cyclosporine products; in general, cyclosporine (modified) is more commonly used clinically.

Psoriasis: Oral: Cyclosporine (modified): Initial dose: 2.5 mg/kg/day in 2 divided doses

Titration:

Increase by 0.5 mg/kg/day if insufficient response is seen after 4 weeks of treatment. Additional dosage increases may be made every 2 weeks if needed (maximum dose: 4 mg/kg/day)

Guideline recommended dosing: 2.5 to 5 mg/kg/day in 2 divided doses, adjust dose downward in 0.5 to 1 mg/kg increments when clearance of psoriasis is achieved or if hypertension or decreased renal function occur; interval therapy is preferred (Menter 2009).

Discontinue if no benefit is seen by 6 weeks of therapy at the maximum dose. Once patients are adequately controlled, the dose should be decreased to the lowest effective dose. Doses lower than 2.5 mg/kg/day may be effective. Treatment longer than 1 year is not recommended.

Note: Increase the frequency of blood pressure monitoring after each alteration in dosage of cyclosporine. Cyclosporine dosage should be decreased by 25% to 50% in patients with no history of hypertension who develop sustained hypertension during therapy and, if hypertension persists, treatment with cyclosporine should be discontinued.

Rheumatoid arthritis: Oral: Cyclosporine (modified): Initial dose: 2.5 mg/kg/day in 2 divided doses; salicylates, NSAIDs, and oral glucocorticoids may be continued (refer to Drug Interactions)

Titration: Dose may be increased by 0.5 to 0.75 mg/kg/day if insufficient response is seen after 8 weeks of treatment; additional dosage increases may be made again at 12 weeks (maximum dose: 4 mg/kg daily). Discontinue if no benefit is seen by 16 weeks of therapy.

Note: Increase the frequency of blood pressure monitoring after each alteration in dosage of cyclosporine. Cyclosporine dosage should be decreased by 25% to 50% in patients with no history of hypertension who develop sustained hypertension during therapy and, if hypertension persists, treatment with cyclosporine should be discontinued.

Solid organ transplant (newly transplanted patients): Cyclosporine is commonly used in combination with an antiproliferative immunosuppressive agent and a corticosteroid. Although cyclosporine may be initiated preoperatively, it is more frequently started postoperatively (depending on concomitant renal function); adjust dose to achieve desired plasma concentration.

Oral: Dose is dependent upon type of transplant and formulation; refer to institutional protocol for specific dosing:

Cyclosporine (modified): Manufacturer's labeling:

Renal: 9 ± 3 mg/kg/day in 2 divided doses

Liver: 8 ± 4 mg/kg/day in 2 divided doses

Heart: 7 ± 3 mg/kg/day in 2 divided doses

Cyclosporine (non-modified): Refer to institutional protocol for specific dosing; dosing in clinical practice may differ greatly compared to the manufacturer's labeling.

Note: When using the non-modified formulation, cyclosporine levels may increase in liver transplant patients when the T-tube is closed; dose may need decreased

IV: Cyclosporine (non-modified): Manufacturer's labeling: Initial dose: 5 to 6 mg/kg/day or one-third of the oral dose as a single dose, infused over 2 to 6 hours; use should be limited to patients unable to take capsules or oral solution; patients should be switched to an oral dosage form as soon as possible.

Note: Many transplant centers administer cyclosporine as "divided dose" infusions (in 2 doses daily) or as a continuous (24-hour) infusion; dosages range from 3 to 7.5 mg/kg/day. Specific institutional protocols should be consulted.

Note: Conversion to cyclosporine (modified) from cyclosporine (non-modified): Start with daily dose previously used and adjust to obtain preconversion cyclosporine trough concentration. Plasma concentrations should be monitored every 4 to 7 days and dose adjusted as necessary, until desired trough level is obtained. When transferring patients with previously poor absorption of cyclosporine (non-modified), monitor trough levels at least twice weekly (especially if initial dose exceeds 10 mg/kg daily); high plasma levels are likely to occur.

Acute graft versus host disease (aGVHD), prevention (off-label use): IV followed by oral:

Initial: IV: 3 mg/kg/day 1 day prior to transplant; may convert to oral therapy when tolerated; titrate dose to appropriate cyclosporine trough concentration (in combination with methotrexate); taper per protocol (refer to specific references and institutional protocols for tapering and target trough details); discontinue 6 months post-transplant in the absence of acute GVHD (Ratanatharathorn 1998; Ruutu 2014; Storb 1986a; Storb 1986b)

or

Initial: IV: 5 mg/kg/day (as a continuous infusion over 20 hours) for 6 days (loading dose) starting 2 days prior to transplant, then 3 mg/kg/day over 20 hours for 11 days starting on post-transplant day 4, then 3.75 mg/kg/day over 20 hours for 21 days starting on day 15, then **oral** (in 2 divided daily doses): 10 mg/kg/day days 36 to 83, then 8 mg/kg/day days 84 to 97, then 6 mg/kg/day days 98 to 119, then 4 mg/kg/day days 120 to 180, then discontinue (in combination with methotrexate +/- corticosteroid) (Chao 1993; Chao 2000)

Focal segmental glomerulosclerosis (off-label use): Oral: Initial: 3.5 to 5 mg/kg/day in 2 divided doses (every 12 hours; in combination with oral prednisone) (Braun 2008; Cattran 1999)

Immune thrombocytopenia, refractory (off-label use): Oral: 5 mg/kg/day in 2 divided doses (every 12 hours) for 6 days, followed by 2.5 to 3 mg/kg/day (titrate to serum levels of 100 to 200 ng/mL); time to response in clinical trials was ~3 to 4 weeks (Provan 2010). Additional studies have used initial doses of 2.5 to 5 mg/kg/day in 2 divided doses; maintenance doses were adjusted to maintain serum levels between 150 and 400 ng/mL (Choudhary 2008; Emilia 2002; Zver 2006).

Interstitial cystitis (bladder pain syndrome) (off-label use): Oral: Initial: 2 to 3 mg/kg/day in 2 divided doses (maximum of 300 mg daily). Once symptom relief is established, the dose can be tapered as tolerated (to as low as 1 mg/kg as a single daily dose) and in some cases can be stopped with continued benefit. Treatment duration was at least 6 months to more than 1 year in some patients (Forrest 2012; Sairanen 2004; Sairanen 2005; Sairanen 2008).

Lung transplant (prevention of acute rejection) (off-label use): IV followed by oral: Initial: 1 mg/kg/day IV beginning immediately after transplantation (in combination with other transplant immunosuppressants); convert to oral cyclosporine as soon as possible post extubation. Target cyclosporine levels were maintained between 250 and 350 ng/mL during the first month, and around 200 ng/mL thereafter (Zuckermann 2003).

Nephrotic syndrome *(Canadian labeling):* Oral: Cyclosporine (modified):
Initial: 3.5 mg/kg/day in 2 divided doses (every 12 hours); titrate for induction of remission and renal function. Adjunct therapy with low-dose oral corticosteroids is recommended for patients with an inadequate response to cyclosporine (particularly if steroid-resistant).
Maintenance: Dose is individualized based on proteinuria, serum creatinine, and tolerability but should be maintained at lowest effective dose; maximum dose: 5 mg/kg daily. Discontinue if no improvement is observed after 3 months.

Lupus nephritis (off-label use): Oral: Cyclosporine (modified): Initial: 4 mg/kg/day for 1 month (reduce dose if trough concentrations >200 ng/mL); reduce dose by 0.5 mg/kg every 2 weeks to a maintenance dose of 2.5 to 3 mg/kg/day (Moroni 2006)

Ulcerative colitis, severe (steroid-refractory) (off-label use):
IV: Cyclosporine (non-modified): 2 to 4 mg/kg/day, infused continuously over 24 hours. (Lichtiger 1994; Van Assche 2003). **Note:** Some studies suggest no therapeutic difference between low-dose (2 mg/kg) and high-dose (4 mg/kg) cyclosporine regimens (Van Assche 2003).
Oral: Cyclosporine (modified): 2.3 to 3 mg/kg every 12 hours (De Saussure 2005; Weber 2006)
Note: Patients responsive to IV therapy should be switched to oral therapy when possible.

Uveitis (off-label dose): Oral: 2.5 to 5 mg/kg/day in 2 divided doses; gradually decrease to maintenance dose; used alone or in conjunction with other corticosteroids (Isnard Bagnis 2002; Matthews 2010; Murphy 2005; Ozdal 2002; Zaghetto 2010). An expert panel recommends initial dose of 3 to 5 mg/kg/day; reducing dose, once inflammation was under control, to 2 to 3 mg/kg/day until a maintenance dose of 1 mg/kg/day is achieved (Diaz-Llopis 2009).

Pediatric Neoral/Gengraf (cyclosporine modified) and Sandimmune (cyclosporine non-modified) are not bioequivalent and cannot be used interchangeably. Use caution when selecting, dispensing, and

administrating cyclosporine products; in general, cyclosporine (modified) is more commonly used clinically.

Acute graft versus host disease (aGVHD), prevention (off-label use): Infants, Children, and Adolescents: IV followed by oral: Initial: 3 to 5 mg/kg/day in 2 divided doses (every 12 hours) administered over 2 hours or as a single daily dose administered over 8 hours (Lanino 2009; Martin 2003; Storb 1986a) or 3 mg/kg/day as a continuous infusion (Nash 2000) beginning one day prior to transplant; may be given with or without methotrexate. May convert to oral therapy when tolerating oral intake; titrate dose to appropriate cyclosporine trough concentration (reported doses ranged from 6 to 12.5 mg/kg/day in divided doses every 12 hours); taper per protocol (refer to specific references for tapering and target trough details). Discontinue 6 months post-transplant in the absence of acute GVHD; refer to specific references for discontinuation details (Lanino 2009; Martin 2003; Storb 1986a).

Nephrotic syndrome (off-label use): Children and Adolescents: Oral: Initial: 4 to 5 mg/kg/day in 2 divided doses for at least 12 months **or** 150 mg/m^2/day in 2 divided doses; adjust doses based on trough levels (Gellermann 2013; KDIGO 2012).

Solid organ transplant: Refer to adult dosing. Children may require, and are able to tolerate, higher doses than adults.

Renal Impairment

Psoriasis (severe):

Abnormal renal function prior to treatment: Use is contraindicated.

Abnormal renal function during treatment:

Serum creatinine levels ≥25% above pretreatment levels: Take another sample within 2 weeks; if the level remains ≥25% above pretreatment levels, decrease dosage of cyclosporine (modified) by 25% to 50%. If two dosage adjustments do not reverse the increase in serum creatinine levels, treatment should be discontinued.

Serum creatinine levels ≥50% above pretreatment levels: Decrease cyclosporine dosage by 25% to 50%. If two dosage adjustments do not reverse the increase in serum creatinine levels, treatment should be discontinued.

Rheumatoid arthritis:

Abnormal renal function prior to treatment: Use is contraindicated.

Abnormal renal function during treatment: Serum creatinine levels >30% above pretreatment levels: Decrease cyclosporine dosage by 25% to 50%; discontinue if dose reduction is ineffective in controlling serum creatinine elevation or if serum creatinine is severe.

Nephrotic syndrome: *Canadian labeling:* Initial: 2.5 mg/kg daily

Serum creatinine levels >30% above pretreatment levels: Take another sample within 2 weeks; if the level remains >30% above pretreatment levels, decrease dosage of cyclosporine (modified) by 25% to 50%.

Hemodialysis: Adults: Supplemental dose is not necessary (Aronoff 2007). Dialysis does not significantly alter cyclosporine clearance.

Peritoneal dialysis: Adults: Supplemental dose is not necessary (Aronoff 2007).

Hepatic Impairment

Mild-to-moderate impairment: There are no dosage adjustments provided in the manufacturer's labeling; monitor blood concentrations.

Severe impairment: There are no dosage adjustments provided in the manufacturer's labeling; however, metabolism is extensively hepatic (exposure is increased). Monitor blood concentrations; may require dose reduction.

Administration

Oral solution: Do not administer liquid from plastic or styrofoam cup. May dilute Neoral oral solution with room temperature orange juice or apple juice. May dilute Sandimmune oral solution with milk, chocolate milk, or orange juice. Avoid changing diluents frequently. Mix thoroughly and drink at once. Use syringe provided to measure dose. Mix in a glass container and rinse container with more diluent to ensure total dose is taken. Do not rinse syringe before or after use (may cause dose variation).

Administer this medication consistently with relation to time of day and meals. Combination therapy with renal or heart transplantation:

Everolimus: May administer cyclosporine at the same time as everolimus

Sirolimus: Must administer cyclosporine 4 hours separate from sirolimus

IV: The manufacturer recommends that following dilution, intravenous admixture be administered over 2 to 6 hours. However, many transplant centers administer as divided doses (2 doses/day) or as a 24-hour continuous infusion. Anaphylaxis has been reported with IV use; reserve for patients who cannot take oral form. Patients should be under continuous observation for at least the first 30 minutes of the infusion, and should be monitored frequently thereafter. Maintain patent airway; other supportive measures and agents for treating anaphylaxis should be present when IV drug is given. To minimize leaching of DEHP, non-PVC sets should be used for administration.

Monitoring Parameters

Monitor plasma concentrations, renal function (serum creatinine and BUN), and blood pressure periodically and following the addition, modification, or deletion of other medications. Monitor for hypersensitivity reactions (IV cyclosporine). Monitor for signs/symptoms of hepatotoxicity, secondary malignancy, diabetes mellitus, infection. Monitor for progressive cognitive or motor deficits; magnetic resonance imaging may be required for diagnosis of posterior reversible encephalopathy syndrome (PRES).

Nephrotic syndrome (Canadian labeling): Baseline blood pressure (2 readings within 2 weeks), fasting serum creatinine (at least 3 levels within 2 weeks), creatinine clearance, urinalysis, CBC, liver function, serum uric acid, serum potassium, and malignancy screening (eg, skin, mouth, lymph nodes). Biweekly monitoring of blood pressure for initial 3 months and then monthly thereafter, frequent monitoring of renal function and periodic cyclosporine trough levels are recommended during therapy. Consider renal biopsy in patients with steroid-dependent minimal change neuropathy who have been maintained on therapy >1 year.

Transplant patients: Cyclosporine trough levels, serum electrolytes, renal function, hepatic function, blood pressure, lipid profile, blood sugar, and HbA1c

Psoriasis therapy: Baseline blood pressure, serum creatinine (2 levels each), BUN, CBC, serum magnesium, potassium, uric acid, lipid profile. Every other week monitoring of blood pressure, complete blood count, serum creatinine, and levels of BUN, uric acid, potassium, lipids, and magnesium during the first 3 months of treatment for psoriasis. Monthly monitoring is recommended after this initial period. (**Note:** The Canadian labeling recommends bimonthly monitoring of serum creatinine after the initial period if serum creatinine remains stable and cyclosporine dose is ≤2.5 mg/kg daily, and monthly monitoring for higher doses). Also evaluate any atypical skin lesions prior to therapy. Increase the frequency of blood pressure monitoring after each alteration in dosage of cyclosporine.

Rheumatoid arthritis: Baseline blood pressure, and serum creatinine (2 levels each); serum creatinine every 2 weeks for first 3 months, then monthly if patient is stable. Increase the frequency of blood pressure monitoring after each alteration in dosage of cyclosporine. Additional Canadian labeling recommendations include CBC, hepatic function, urinalysis, serum potassium and uric acid (baseline and periodic thereafter).

Test Interactions Specific whole blood assay for cyclosporine may be falsely elevated if sample is drawn from the same central venous line through which dose was administered (even if flush has been administered and/or dose was given hours before); cyclosporine metabolites cross-react with radioimmunoassay and fluorescence polarization immunoassay

Dietary Considerations Avoid grapefruit juice with oral cyclosporine use.

Dosage Forms Considerations
Cyclosporine (modified): Gengraf and Neoral
Cyclosporine (non-modified): SandIMMUNE
Cyclosporine injection contains polyoxyethylated castor oil (Cremophor EL)

Dosage Forms Excipient information presented when available (limited, particularly for generics); consult specific product labeling.
Capsule, Oral:
Gengraf: 25 mg [contains cremophor el, fd&c blue #2 (indigotine)]
Gengraf: 50 mg [contains alcohol, usp, fd&c blue #2 aluminum lake]
Gengraf: 100 mg [contains cremophor el, fd&c blue #2 (indigotine)]
Neoral: 25 mg, 100 mg [contains alcohol, usp]
SandIMMUNE: 25 mg, 100 mg
Generic: 25 mg, 50 mg, 100 mg
Solution, Intravenous:
SandIMMUNE: 50 mg/mL (5 mL) [contains alcohol, usp, cremophor el]
Generic: 50 mg/mL (5 mL)
Solution, Oral:
Gengraf: 100 mg/mL (50 mL) [contains propylene glycol]
Neoral: 100 mg/mL (50 mL) [contains alcohol, usp]
SandIMMUNE: 100 mg/mL (50 mL) [contains alcohol, usp]
Generic: 100 mg/mL (50 mL)

Dosage Forms: Canada Information with regard to form, strength, and availability of products uniquely available in Canada but currently not available in the US. Refer also to Dosage Forms.

Excipient information presented when available (limited, particularly for generics); consult specific product labeling.
Capsule, Oral:
Neoral: 10 mg, 25 mg, 50 mg, 100 mg [contains alcohol]
Solution, Intravenous:
SandIMMUNE IV: 50 mg/mL (1 mL, 5 mL) [contains alcohol, cremophor el]
Solution, Oral:
Neoral: 100 mg/mL (50 mL) [contains alcohol, propylene glycol]

◆ **Cyklokapron** *see* Tranexamic Acid *on page 1816*

Cyproheptadine (si proe HEP ta deen)

Brand Names: Canada Euro-Cyproheptadine; PMS-Cyproheptadine

Index Terms Cyproheptadine HCl; Cyproheptadine Hydrochloride; Periactin

Pharmacologic Category Histamine H_1 Antagonist; Histamine H_1 Antagonist, First Generation; Piperidine Derivative

Use Allergic conditions: Perennial and seasonal allergic rhinitis; vasomotor rhinitis; allergic conjunctivitis caused by inhalant allergens and foods; mild, uncomplicated allergic skin manifestations of urticaria and angioedema; amelioration of allergic reactions to blood or plasma; cold urticaria; dermatographism; adjunctive anaphylactic therapy.

Pregnancy Risk Factor B

Dosing

Adult

Allergic conditions: Oral: Initial: 4 mg 3 times daily; maintenance: 4 to 20 mg daily in divided doses; maximum: 0.5 mg/kg/day; some patients may require up to 32 mg/day for adequate control of symptoms

Decreased appetite secondary to chronic disease (off-label use): Oral: Initial: 2 mg 4 times per day for one week, then 4 mg 4 times per day (Homnick 2004; Homnick 2005)

Serotonin syndrome (off-label use): Oral: Initial: 12 mg followed by 2 mg every 2 hours or 4 to 8 mg every 6 hours as needed for symptom control (Boyer 2005; Sun-Edelstein 2008)

Spasticity associated with spinal cord damage (off-label use): Oral: Initial: 2 to 4 mg every 8 hours; maximum: 8 mg every 8 hours (Barbeau 1982; Wainberg 1990)

Geriatric Refer to adult dosing. Initiate therapy at the lower end of the dosage range.

Pediatric

Allergic conditions:

Children 2 to 6 years: Oral: Usual dose: 0.25 mg/kg/day **or** 8 mg/m^2/day in 2 to 3 divided doses **or** 2 mg 2 or 3 times daily; maximum: 12 mg/day

Children ≥7 years and Adolescents ≤14 years: Oral: Usual dose: 4 mg 2 or 3 times daily; maximum: 16 mg/day

Adolescents >14 years: Oral: Refer to adult dosing

Episodic migraine preventions (off-label use): Children ≥3 years and Adolescents: Oral: Usual dose: 0.2 to 0.4 mg/kg/day divided twice daily; maximum: 0.5 mg/kg/day (Lewis 2004a; Lewis 2004b)

Renal Impairment No dosage adjustment provided in manufacturer's labeling. However, elimination is diminished in renal insufficiency.

Hepatic Impairment No dosage adjustment provided in manufacturer's labeling.

Additional Information Complete prescribing information should be consulted for additional detail.

Dosage Forms Excipient information presented when available (limited, particularly for generics); consult specific product labeling. [DSC] = Discontinued product

Syrup, Oral, as hydrochloride:

Generic: 2 mg/5 mL (10 mL [DSC], 473 mL)

Tablet, Oral, as hydrochloride:

Generic: 4 mg

◆ **Cyproheptadine HCl** see Cyproheptadine on page 467

◆ **Cyproheptadine Hydrochloride** *see* Cyproheptadine *on page* 467

Cyproterone (sye PROE ter one)

Brand Names: Canada Androcur; Androcur Depot; Med-Cyproterone; Riva-Cyproterone

Index Terms Cyproterone Acetate; SH 714

Pharmacologic Category Antiandrogen; Antineoplastic Agent, Antiandrogen

Use Note: Not approved in the US

Prostate cancer: Palliative treatment of advanced prostate cancer

Hazardous Drugs Handling Considerations

Hazardous agent (meets NIOSH 2016 criteria). This medication is not on the NIOSH (2016) list; however, it meets the criteria for a hazardous drug. Drugs are classified as hazardous based on their properties; the properties of a hazardous drug include one or more of the following characteristics: carcinogenic, teratogenic (or other developmental toxicity), reproductive toxicity, organotoxic at low doses, genotoxic, and/or new agents with structural or toxicity profiles similar to existing hazardous agents.

Use appropriate precautions for receiving, handling, administration, and disposal. Gloves (single) should be worn during receiving, unpacking, and placing in storage. NIOSH recommends single gloving for administration of intact tablets or capsules. For IM preparation, NIOSH recommends double gloving, a protective gown, and preparation in a controlled device or the use of ventilated engineering controls (a class II biological safety cabinet or a compounding aseptic containment isolator); if not prepared in a controlled device, respiratory and eye/face protection are recommended. Double gloving and a protective gown are recommended during IM administration (NIOSH 2016).

Dosing

Adult & Geriatric

Prostate cancer, advanced (palliative treatment): Males:

Oral: 200 to 300 mg daily in 2 to 3 divided doses (maximum: 300 mg daily); following orchiectomy, reduce dose to 100 to 200 mg daily

IM: 300 mg (3 mL) once weekly; reduce dose in orchiectomized patients to 300 mg (3 mL) every 2 weeks

Note: May interchange between oral and IM administration during chronic therapy; dosages should remain within usual ranges (oral: 100 to 300 mg daily; IM: 300 mg weekly or every 2 weeks).

Treatment of paraphilia/hypersexuality (off-label use) (Guay 2009; Reilly 2000): Males (**Note:** Avoid use if active pituitary pathology, hepatic failure, or thromboembolic disease):

Oral: 50 to 600 mg daily

IM: 300 to 600 mg weekly or every other week

Renal Impairment There are no dosage adjustments provided in the manufacturer's labeling (has not been studied); use with caution

Hepatic Impairment Use is contraindicated with hepatic impairment or liver disease.

Additional Information Complete prescribing information should be consulted for additional detail.

Product Availability Not available in the US

Dosage Forms: Canada Information with regard to form, strength, and availability of products uniquely available in Canada but currently not available in the US.

Excipient information presented when available (limited, particularly for generics); consult specific product labeling.
Injection, solution, as acetate: 100 mg/mL (3 mL)
  Androcur Depot: 100 mg/mL (3 mL) [contains benzyl benzoate and castor oil]
Tablet, as acetate: 50 mg
  Androcur: 50 mg

◆ **Cyproterone Acetate** *see* Cyproterone *on page 468*

◆ **Cyramza** *see* Ramucirumab *on page 1576*

◆ **Cysview** *see* Hexaminolevulinate *on page 911*

◆ **CYT** *see* Cyclophosphamide *on page 438*

◆ **Cytarabine** *see* Cytarabine (Conventional) *on page 469*

Cytarabine (Conventional) (sye TARE a been con VEN sha nal)
Related Information
Hematopoietic Cell Transplantation *on page 2365*
Management of Chemotherapy-Induced Nausea and Vomiting in Adults *on page 2253*
Prevention of Chemotherapy-Induced Nausea and Vomiting in Children *on page 2310*
Safe Handling of Hazardous Drugs *on page 2379*
Brand Names: Canada Cytarabine Injection; Cytosar
Index Terms Ara-C; Arabinosylcytosine; Conventional Cytarabine; Cytarabine; Cytarabine Hydrochloride; Cytosar-U; Cytosine Arabinosine Hydrochloride
Pharmacologic Category Antineoplastic Agent, Antimetabolite; Antineoplastic Agent, Antimetabolite (Pyrimidine Analog)
Use
  Acute myeloid leukemia: Remission induction (in combination with other chemotherapy medications) in acute myeloid leukemia (AML)
  Acute lymphocytic leukemia: Treatment of acute lymphocytic leukemia (ALL)
  Chronic myeloid leukemia: Treatment of chronic myeloid leukemia (CML; blast phase)
  Meningeal leukemia: Prophylaxis and treatment of meningeal leukemia
Labeled Contraindications Hypersensitivity to cytarabine or any component of the formulation
Pregnancy Considerations Adverse effects were demonstrated in animal reproduction studies. Limb and ear defects have been noted in case reports of cytarabine exposure during the first trimester of pregnancy. The following have also been noted in the neonate: Pancytopenia, WBC depression, electrolyte abnormalities, prematurity, low birth weight, decreased hematocrit or platelets. Risk to the fetus is decreased if treatment can be avoided during the first trimester; however, women of childbearing potential should be advised of the potential risks.

▶

◄ **Breastfeeding Considerations** It is not known if cytarabine is excreted in breast milk. Due to the potential for serious adverse reactions in the nursing infant, the decision to discontinue cytarabine or to discontinue breastfeeding should take into account the importance of treatment to the mother.

Warnings/Precautions [U.S. Boxed Warning]: Myelosuppression (leukopenia, thrombocytopenia and anemia) is the major toxicity of cytarabine. Use with caution in patients with prior drug-induced bone marrow suppression. Monitor blood counts frequently; once blasts are no longer apparent in the peripheral blood, bone marrow should be monitored frequently. Monitor for signs of infection or neutropenic fever due to neutropenia or bleeding due to thrombocytopenia. **[U.S. Boxed Warning]: Toxicities (less serious) include nausea, vomiting, diarrhea, abdominal pain, oral ulcerations and hepatic dysfunction.** In adults, doses >1000 mg/m^2 are associated with a moderate emetic potential (Basch, 2011; Roila, 2010). In pediatrics, doses >200 mg/m^2 are associated with a moderate emetic potential and 3000 mg/m^2 is associated with a high emetic potential (Dupuis, 2011); antiemetics are recommended to prevent nausea and vomiting.

High-dose regimens are associated with CNS, gastrointestinal, ocular (reversible corneal toxicity and hemorrhagic conjunctivitis; prophylaxis with ophthalmic corticosteroid drops is recommended), pulmonary toxicities and cardiomyopathy. Neurotoxicity associated with high-dose treatment may present as acute cerebellar toxicity (with or without cerebral impairment), personality changes, or may be severe with seizure and/or coma; may be delayed, occurring up to 3 to 8 days after treatment has begun. Risk factors for neurotoxicity include cumulative cytarabine dose, prior CNS disease and renal impairment; high-dose therapy (>18 g/m^2 per cycle) and age >50 years also increase the risk for cerebellar toxicity (Herzig, 1987). Tumor lysis syndrome and subsequent hyperuricemia may occur; monitor, consider antihyperuricemic therapy and hydrate accordingly. Potentially significant drug-drug interactions may exist, requiring dose or frequency adjustment, additional monitoring, and/or selection of alternative therapy. There have been case reports of fatal cardiomyopathy when high dose cytarabine was used in combination with cyclophosphamide as a preparation regimen for transplantation.

Use with caution in patients with impaired renal and hepatic function; may be at higher risk for CNS toxicities; dosage adjustments may be necessary. Sudden respiratory distress, rapidly progressing to pulmonary edema and cardiomegaly has been reported with high dose cytarabine. May present as severe dyspnea with a rapid onset and refractory hypoxia with diffuse pulmonary infiltrates, leading to respiratory failure; may be fatal (Morgan, 2011). Cytarabine (ARA-C) syndrome is characterized by fever, myalgia, bone pain, chest pain (occasionally), maculopapular rash, conjunctivitis, and malaise; generally occurs 6 to 12 hours following administration; may be managed with corticosteroids. Anaphylaxis resulting in acute cardiopulmonary arrest has been reported (rare). There have been reports of acute pancreatitis in patients receiving continuous infusion cytarabine and in patients receiving cytarabine who were previously treated with L-asparaginase. **[U.S. Boxed Warning]: Should be administered under the supervision of an experienced cancer chemotherapy physician. Due to the potential toxicities, induction treatment with cytarabine should be in a facility with sufficient laboratory and supportive resources.** Some products may contain benzyl alcohol; do not use products containing benzyl alcohol or products reconstituted with bacteriostatic diluent intrathecally or for high-dose cytarabine regimens. Benzyl alcohol is associated with gasping syndrome in premature infants. Delayed progressive ascending paralysis has been reported in two children who received combination chemotherapy with IV and intrathecal cytarabine at conventional doses for the treatment of acute myeloid leukemia (was fatal in one patient). When used for intrathecal administration, should not be prepared during the preparation of any other agents; after preparation, store intrathecal medications in an isolated location or container clearly marked with a label identifying as "intrathecal" use only; delivery of intrathecal medications to the patient should only be with other medications also intended for administration into the central nervous system (Jacobson, 2009).

Adverse Reactions Frequency not always defined. CNS, gastrointestinal, ophthalmic, and pulmonary toxicities are more common with high-dose regimens.

Cardiovascular: Angina pectoris, chest pain, hepatic sinusoidal obstruction syndrome (formerly known as hepatic veno-occlusive disease), local thrombophlebitis, pericarditis

Central nervous system: Aseptic meningitis, cerebral dysfunction, dizziness, headache, neuritis, neurotoxicity, paralysis (intrathecal and IV combination therapy), reversible posterior leukoencephalopathy syndrome

Dermatologic: Acute generalized exanthematous pustulosis, alopecia, dermal ulcer, ephelis, pruritus, skin rash, urticaria

Endocrine & metabolic: Hyperuricemia

Gastrointestinal: Abdominal pain, anal fissure, anorexia, diarrhea, esophageal ulcer, esophagitis, increased serum amylase, increased serum lipase, intestinal necrosis, mucositis, nausea, pancreatitis, sore throat, toxic megacolon, vomiting

Genitourinary: Urinary retention

Hematologic & oncologic: Anemia, bone marrow depression, hemorrhage, leukopenia, megaloblastic anemia, neutropenia (onset: 1 to 7 days; nadir [biphasic]: 7 to 9 days and at 15 to 24 days; recovery [biphasic]: 9 to 12 days and at 24 to 34 days), reticulocytopenia, thrombocytopenia (onset: 5 days; nadir: 12 to 15 days; recovery 15 to 25 days)

Hepatic: Hepatic insufficiency, increased serum transaminases (acute), jaundice

Hypersensitivity: Allergic edema, anaphylaxis

Infection: Sepsis

Local: Cellulitis at injection site, inflammation at injection site (SC injection), local inflammation (anus), pain at injection site (SC injection)

Neuromuscular & skeletal: Rhabdomyolysis

Ophthalmic: Conjunctivitis

Renal: Renal insufficiency

Respiratory: Acute respiratory distress, dyspnea, interstitial pneumonitis

Miscellaneous: Drug toxicity (cytarabine syndrome; chest pain, conjunctivitis, fever, maculopapular rash, malaise, myalgia, ostealgia), fever

Adverse events associated with high-dose cytarabine

Cardiovascular: Cardiomegaly, cardiomyopathy (in combination with cyclophosphamide)

Central nervous system: Neurotoxicity (patients with renal impairment: ≤55%), coma, drowsiness, neurocerebellar toxicity, peripheral neuropathy (motor and sensory), personality changes

Dermatologic: Alopecia (complete), desquamation, skin rash (severe)

Gastrointestinal: Gastrointestinal ulcer, necrotizing enterocolitis, pancreatitis, peritonitis, pneumatosis cystoides intestinalis

Hepatic: Hepatic abscess, hepatic injury, hyperbilirubinemia

Infection: Sepsis

Ophthalmic: Corneal toxicity, hemorrhagic conjunctivitis

Respiratory: Acute respiratory distress, pulmonary edema

Adverse events associated with intrathecal cytarabine administration

Central nervous system: Aphonia, leukoencephalopathy (necrotizing; with concurrent cranial irradiation, intrathecal methotrexate, and intrathecal hydrocortisone), nerve palsy (accessory nerve), neurotoxicity, paraplegia

Gastrointestinal: Dysphagia, nausea, vomiting

Ophthalmic: Blindness (with concurrent systemic chemotherapy and cranial irradiation), diplopia

Respiratory: Cough, hoarseness

Miscellaneous: Fever

Drug Interactions

Metabolism/Transport Effects None known.

Avoid Concomitant Use

Avoid concomitant use of Cytarabine (Conventional) with any of the following: BCG (Intravesical); Deferiprone; Dipyrone; Natalizumab; Pimecrolimus; Tacrolimus (Topical); Vaccines (Live)

Increased Effect/Toxicity

Cytarabine (Conventional) may increase the levels/effects of: CloZAPine; Deferiprone; Fingolimod; Leflunomide; Natalizumab; Tofacitinib; Vaccines (Live)

The levels/effects of Cytarabine (Conventional) may be increased by: Denosumab; Dipyrone; Ocrelizumab; Palifermin; Pimecrolimus; Promazine; Roflumilast; Tacrolimus (Topical); Trastuzumab

Decreased Effect

Cytarabine (Conventional) may decrease the levels/effects of: BCG (Intravesical); Coccidioides immitis Skin Test; Flucytosine; Lenograstim; Nivolumab; Sipuleucel-T; Tertomotide; Vaccines (Inactivated); Vaccines (Live)

The levels/effects of Cytarabine (Conventional) may be decreased by: Echinacea

Hazardous Drugs Handling Considerations

Hazardous agent (NIOSH 2016 [group 1]).

Use appropriate precautions for receiving, handling, administration, and disposal. Gloves (single) should be worn during receiving, unpacking, and placing in storage.

NIOSH recommends double gloving, a protective gown, ventilated engineering controls (a class II biological safety cabinet or a compounding aseptic containment isolator), and closed system transfer devices (CSTDs) for preparation. Double gloving, a gown, and (if dosage form allows) CSTDs are required during administration (NIOSH 2016).

Storage/Stability Store intact vials of powder for reconstitution at 20°C to 25°C (68°F to 77°F); store intact vials of solution at 15°C to 30°C (59°F to 86°F).

IV:

Powder for reconstitution: Reconstituted solutions should be stored at room temperature and used within 48 hours.

For IV infusion: Solutions for IV infusion diluted in D5W or NS are stable for 8 days at room temperature, although the manufacturer recommends administration as soon as possible after preparation.

Intrathecal: Administer as soon as possible after preparation. After preparation, store intrathecal medications in an isolated location or container clearly marked with a label identifying as "intrathecal" use only.

Preparation for Administration Note: Solutions containing bacteriostatic agents may be used for SubQ and standard-dose (100 to 200 mg/m^2) IV cytarabine preparations, but should not be used for the preparation of either intrathecal doses or high-dose IV therapies.

IV:

Powder for reconstitution: Reconstitute with bacteriostatic water for injection (for standard-dose).

For IV infusion: Further dilute in 250 to 1000 mL 0.9% NaCl or D5W.

Intrathecal: Powder for reconstitution: Reconstitute with preservative free sodium chloride 0.9%; may further dilute to preferred final volume (volume generally based on institution or practitioner preference; may be up to 12 mL) with Elliott's B solution, sodium chloride 0.9% or lactated Ringer's. Intrathecal medications should not be prepared during the preparation of any other agents.

Triple intrathecal therapy (TIT): Cytarabine 30 to 50 mg with hydrocortisone sodium succinate 15 to 25 mg and methotrexate 12 mg are reported to be compatible together in a syringe (Cheung, 1984) and cytarabine 18 to 36 mg with hydrocortisone 12 to 24 mg and methotrexate 6 to 12 mg, prepared to a final volume of 6 to 12 mL, is reported compatible as well (Lin, 2008).

Intrathecal preparations should be administered as soon as possible after preparation because intrathecal preparations are preservative free.

Mechanism of Action Inhibits DNA synthesis. Cytarabine gains entry into cells by a carrier process, and then must be converted to its active compound, aracytidine triphosphate. Cytarabine is a pyrimidine analog and is incorporated into DNA; however, the primary action is inhibition of DNA polymerase resulting in decreased DNA synthesis and repair. The degree of cytotoxicity correlates linearly with incorporation into DNA; therefore, incorporation into the DNA is responsible for drug activity and toxicity. Cytarabine is specific for the S phase of the cell cycle (blocks progression from the G_1 to the S phase).

Pharmacodynamics/Kinetics

Absorption: Not effective when administered orally; less than 20% absorbed orally

Distribution: V_d: 3 ± 11.9 L/kg; total body water; widely and rapidly since it enters the cells readily; crosses blood-brain barrier with CSF levels of 40% to 50% of plasma level

Protein binding: 13%

Metabolism: Primarily hepatic; metabolized by deoxycytidine kinase and other nucleotide kinases to aracytidine triphosphate (active); about 86% to 96% of dose is metabolized to inactive uracil arabinoside (ARA-U); intrathecal administration results in little conversion to ARA-U due to the low levels of deaminase in the cerebral spinal fluid

Half-life elimination: IV: Initial: 7 to 20 minutes; Terminal: 1 to 3 hours; Intrathecal: 2 to 6 hours

Time to peak, plasma: SubQ: 20 to 60 minutes

Excretion: Urine (~80%; 90% as metabolite ARA-U) within 24 hours

◀ **Dosing**

Adult & Geriatric Note: Doses >1000 mg/m^2 are associated with a moderate emetic potential in adults (Basch, 2011; Roila, 2010); antiemetics are recommended to prevent nausea and vomiting.

Acute myeloid leukemia (AML) remission induction: IV: Standard-dose (manufacturer's labeling; in combination with other chemotherapy agents): 100 mg/m^2/day continuous infusion for 7 days **or** 200 mg/m^2/day continuous infusion (as 100 mg/m^2 over 12 hours every 12 hours) for 7 days

Indication-specific dosing:

AML induction: IV:

7 + 3 regimens (a second induction course may be administered if needed; refer to specific references): 100 mg/m^2/day continuous infusion for 7 days (in combination with daunorubicin **or** idarubicin **or** mitoxantrone) (Arlin, 1990; Dillman, 1991; Fernandez, 2009; Vogler, 1992; Wiernik, 1992) **or** (Adults <60 years) 200 mg/m^2/day continuous infusion for 7 days (in combination with daunorubicin) (Dillman, 1991)

Low intensity therapy (off-label dosing): Adults ≥65 years: SubQ: 20 mg/m^2/day for 14 days out of every 28-day cycle for at least 4 cycles (Fenaux, 2010) **or** 10 mg/m^2 every 12 hours for 21 days; if complete response not achieved, may repeat a second course after 15 days (Tilly, 1990)

AML consolidation (off-label use): IV:

5 + 2 regimens: 100 mg/m^2/day continuous infusion for 5 days (in combination with daunorubicin **or** idarubicin **or** mitoxantrone) (Arlin, 1990; Wiernik, 1992)

5 + 2 + 5 regimen: 100 mg/m^2/day continuous infusion for 5 days (in combination with daunorubicin **and** etoposide) (Bishop, 1996)

Single-agent: Adults ≤60 years: 3000 mg/m^2 over 3 hours every 12 hours on days 1, 3, and 5 (total of 6 doses); repeat every 28 to 35 days for 4 courses (Mayer, 1994)

AML salvage treatment (off-label use): IV:

CLAG regimen: 2000 mg/m^2/day over 4 hours for 5 days (in combination with cladribine and G-CSF); may repeat once if needed (Wrzesień-Kuś, 2003)

CLAG-M regimen: 2000 mg/m^2/day over 4 hours for 5 days (in combination with cladribine, G-CSF, and mitoxantrone); may repeat once if needed (Wierzbowska, 2008)

FLAG regimen: 2000 mg/m^2/day over 4 hours for 5 days (in combination with fludarabine and G-CSF); may repeat once if needed (Montillo, 1998)

GCLAC regimen: Adults 18 to 70 years (Becker, 2011):

Induction: 2,000 mg/m^2 over 2 hours once daily for 5 days (in combination with clofarabine and filgrastim; administer 4 hours after initiation of clofarabine); may repeat induction once if needed.

Consolidation: 1,000 mg/m^2 over 2 hours once daily for 5 days (in combination with clofarabine and filgrastim; administer 4 hours after initiation of clofarabine) for 1 or 2 cycles

HiDAC (high-dose cytarabine) ± an anthracycline: 3000 mg/m^2 over 1 hour every 12 hours for 6 days (total of 12 doses) (Herzig, 1985)

MEC regimen: 1000 mg/m^2/day over 6 hours for 6 days (in combination with mitoxantrone and etoposide) (Amadori, 1991) **or**

Adults <60 years: 500 mg/m^2/day continuous infusion days 1, 2, and 3 and days 8, 9, and 10 (in combination with mitoxantrone and etoposide); may administer a second course if needed (Archimbaud, 1991; Archimbaud, 1995)

Acute promyelocytic leukemia (APL) induction (off-label dosing): IV: 200 mg/m^2/day continuous infusion for 7 days beginning on day 3 of treatment (in combination with tretinoin and daunorubicin) (Ades, 2006; Ades, 2008; Powell, 2010)

APL consolidation (off-label use): IV:

In combination with idarubicin and tretinoin: High-risk patients (WBC ≥10,000/mm^3) (Sanz, 2010): Adults ≤60 years:

First consolidation course: 1000 mg/m^2/day for 4 days

Third consolidation course: 150 mg/m^2 every 8 hours for 4 days

In combination with idarubicin, tretinoin, and thioguanine: High-risk patients (WBC >10,000/mm^3) (Lo Coco, 2010): Adults ≤61 years:

First consolidation course: 1000 mg/m^2/day for 4 days

Third consolidation course: 150 mg/m^2 every 8 hours for 5 days

In combination with daunorubicin (Ades, 2006; Ades, 2008):

First consolidation course: 200 mg/m^2/day for 7 days

Second consolidation course:

Age ≤60 years and low risk (WBC <10,000/mm^3): 1000 mg/m^2 every 12 hours for 4 days (8 doses)

Age <50 years and high risk (WBC ≥10,000/mm^3): 2000 mg/m^2 every 12 hours for 5 days (10 doses)

Age 50 to 60 years and high risk (WBC ≥10,000/mm^3): 1500 mg/m^2 every 12 hours for 5 days (10 doses) (Ades, 2008)

Age >60 years and high risk (WBC ≥10,000/mm^3): 1000 mg/m^2 every 12 hours for 4 days (8 doses)

Acute lymphocytic leukemia (ALL; off-label dosing):

Induction regimen, relapsed or refractory: IV: 3000 mg/m^2 over 3 hours daily for 5 days (in combination with idarubicin [day 3]) (Weiss, 2002)

Dose-intensive regimen: IV: 3000 mg/m^2 over 2 hours every 12 hours days 2 and 3 (4 doses/cycle) of even numbered cycles (in combination with methotrexate; alternates with Hyper-CVAD) (Kantarjian, 2000)

CALGB 8811 regimen (Larson, 1995): SubQ

Early intensification phase: 75 mg/m^2/dose days 1 to 4 and 8 to 11 (4-week cycle; repeat once)

Late intensification phase: 75 mg/m^2/dose days 29 to 32 and 36 to 39

Linker protocol: Adults <50 years: IV: 300 mg/m^2/day days 1, 4, 8, and 11 of even numbered consolidation cycles (in combination with teniposide) (Linker, 1991)

Chronic lymphocytic leukemia (CLL; off-label use): *OFAR regimen:* IV: 1000 mg/m^2/dose over 2 hours days 2 and 3 every 4 weeks for up to 6 cycles (in combination with oxaliplatin, fludarabine, and rituximab) (Tsimberidou, 2008)

Primary central nervous system (CNS) lymphoma (off-label use): IV: 2000 mg/m^2 over 1 hour every 12 hours days 2 and 3 (total of 4 doses) every 3 weeks (in combination with methotrexate and followed by whole brain irradiation) for a total of 4 courses (Ferreri, 2009)

◀ **Hodgkin lymphoma, relapsed or refractory (off-label use):** IV:

DHAP regimen: 2000 mg/m^2 over 3 hours every 12 hours day 2 (total of 2 doses/cycle) for 2 cycles (in combination with dexamethasone and cisplatin) (Josting, 2002)

ESHAP regimen: 2000 mg/m^2 day 5 (in combination with etoposide, methylprednisolone, and cisplatin) every 3 to 4 weeks for 3 or 6 cycles (Aparicio, 1999)

Mini-BEAM regimen: 100 mg/m^2 every 12 hours days 2 to 5 (total of 8 doses) every 4 to 6 weeks (in combination with carmustine, etoposide, and melphalan) (Colwill, 1995; Martin, 2001)

BEAM regimen (transplant preparative regimen): 200 mg/m^2 twice daily for 4 days beginning 5 days prior to transplant (in combination with carmustine, etoposide, and melphalan) (Chopra, 1993)

Non-Hodgkin lymphomas (off-label use): IV:

CALGB 9251 regimen: Cycles 2, 4, and 6: 150 mg/m^2/day continuous infusion days 4 and 5 (Lee, 2001; Rizzieri, 2004)

CODOX-M/IVAC regimen:

Adults ≤60 years: Cycles 2 and 4 (IVAC): 2000 mg/m^2 every 12 hours days 1 and 2 (total of 4 doses/cycle) (IVAC is combination with ifosfamide, mesna, and etoposide; IVAC alternates with CODOX-M) (Magrath, 1996)

Adults ≤65 years: Cycles 2 and 4 (IVAC): 2000 mg/m^2 over 3 hours every 12 hours days 1 and 2 (total of 4 doses/cycle) (IVAC is combination with ifosfamide, mesna, and etoposide; IVAC alternates with CODOX-M) (Mead, 2008)

Adults >65 years: Cycles 2 and 4 (IVAC): 1000 mg/m^2 over 3 hours every 12 hours days 1 and 2 (total of 4 doses/cycle) (IVAC is combination with ifosfamide, mesna, and etoposide; IVAC alternates with CODOX-M) (Mead, 2008)

DHAP regimen:

Adults ≤70 years: 2000 mg/m^2 over 3 hours every 12 hours day 2 (total of 2 doses/cycle) every 3 to 4 weeks for 6 to 10 cycles (in combination with dexamethasone and cisplatin) (Velasquez, 1988)

Adults >70 years: 1000 mg/m^2 over 3 hours every 12 hours day 2 (total of 2 doses/cycle) every 3 to 4 weeks for 6 to 10 cycles (in combination with dexamethasone and cisplatin) (Velasquez, 1988)

ESHAP regimen: 2000 mg/m^2 over 2 hours day 5 every 3 to 4 weeks for 6 to 8 cycles (in combination with etoposide, methylprednisolone, and cisplatin) (Velasquez, 1994)

BEAM regimen (transplant preparative regimen): 200 mg/m^2 twice daily for 3 days beginning 4 days prior to transplant (in combination with carmustine, etoposide, and melphalan) (Linch, 2010) **or** 100 mg/m^2 over 1 hour every 12 hours for 4 days beginning 5 days prior to transplant (in combination with carmustine, etoposide, and melphalan) (van Imhoff, 2005)

Meningeal leukemia: Intrathecal: **Note:** Optimal intrathecal chemotherapy dosing should be based on age rather than on body surface area (BSA); CSF volume correlates with age and not to BSA (Bleyer, 1983; Kerr, 2001). Dosing provided in the manufacturer's labeling is BSA-based (usual dose 30 mg/m^2 every 4 days; range: 5 to 75 mg/m^2 once daily for 4 days or once every 4 days until CNS findings normalize, followed by 1 additional treatment).

Off-label uses or doses for intrathecal therapy: Intrathecal:

CNS prophylaxis (ALL): 100 mg weekly for 8 doses, then every 2 weeks for 8 doses, then monthly for 6 doses (high-risk patients) **or** 100 mg on day 7 or 8 with each chemotherapy cycle for 4 doses (low risk patients) **or** 16 doses (high-risk patients) (Cortes, 1995)

or as part of intrathecal triple therapy (TIT): 40 mg days 0 and 14 during induction, days 1, 4, 8, and 11 during CNS therapy phase, every 18 weeks during intensification and maintenance phases (Storring, 2009)

CNS prophylaxis (APL, as part of TIT): 50 mg per dose; administer 1 dose prior to consolidation and 2 doses during each of 2 consolidation phases (total of 5 doses) (Ades, 2006; Ades, 2008)

CNS leukemia treatment (ALL, as part of TIT): 40 mg twice weekly until CSF cleared (Storring, 2009)

CNS lymphoma treatment: 50 mg twice a week for 4 weeks, then weekly for 4-8 weeks, then every other week for 4 weeks, then every 4 weeks for 4 doses (Glantz, 1999)

Leptomeningeal metastases treatment: 25 to 100 mg twice weekly for 4 weeks, then once weekly for 4 weeks, then a maintenance regimen of once a month (Chamberlain, 2010) **or** 40 to 60 mg per dose (DeAngelis, 2005)

Pediatric Note: Doses >200 mg/m^2 are associated with a moderate emetic potential and 3000 mg/m^2 is associated with a high emetic potential (Dupuis, 2011); antiemetics are recommended to prevent nausea and vomiting.

Acute myeloid leukemia (AML) remission induction: IV: Standard-dose (manufacturer's labeling labeling; in combination with other chemotherapy agents). 100 mg/m^2/day continuous infusion for 7 days **or** 200 mg/m^2/day continuous infusion (as 100 mg/m^2 over 12 hours every 12 hours) for 7 days

Indication-specific dosing:

AML induction: *7 + 3 regimen:* IV:

Children <3 years (off-label dosing): 3.3 mg/kg/day continuous infusion for 7 days; minimum of 2 courses (in combination with daunorubicin) (Woods, 1990)

Children ≥3 years: 100 mg/m^2/day continuous infusion for 7 days; minimum of 2 courses (in combination with daunorubicin) (Woods, 1990)

AML consolidation (off-label use): *5 + 2 + 5 regimen:* IV: Adolescents ≥15 years: 100 mg/m^2/day continuous infusion for 5 days for 2 consolidation courses (in combination with daunorubicin and etoposide) (Bishop, 1996)

AML salvage treatment (off-label use):

Clofarabine/Cytarabine regimen: Induction: IV: Children ≥1 year and Adolescents: 1,000 mg/m^2/day over 2 hours for 5 days (in combination with clofarabine; cytarabine is administered 4 hours after initiation of clofarabine) for up to 2 induction cycles (Cooper, 2014)

FLAG regimen: IV: Children ≥11 years: 2,000 mg/m^2/day over 4 hours for 5 days (in combination with fludarabine and G-CSF); may repeat once if needed (Montillo, 1998)

MEC regimen: IV:

Children ≥5 years: 1,000 mg/m^2/day over 6 hours for 6 days (in combination with etoposide and mitoxantrone) (Amadori, 1991)

Adolescents ≥15 years: 500 mg/m^2/day continuous infusion days 1, 2, and 3 and days 8, 9, and 10 (in combination with mitoxantrone and etoposide); may administer a second course if needed (Archimbaud, 1991; Archimbaud, 1995)

◄ **Acute lymphocytic leukemia (ALL; off-label dosing):** *POG 8602/PVA regimen, intensification phase:* IV: Children ≥1 year: 1,000 mg/m² continuous infusion over 24 hours day 1 (beginning 12 hours after start of methotrexate) every 3 weeks or every 12 weeks for 6 cycles (Land, 1994)

Non-Hodgkin lymphomas (off-label use):

CODOX-M/IVAC regimen: IV: Children ≥3 years: Cycles 2 and 4 (IVAC): 2,000 mg/m² every 12 hours days 1 and 2 (total of 4 doses/cycle) (IVAC is combination with ifosfamide, mesna and etoposide; IVAC alternates with CODOX-M) (Magrath, 1996)

High-dose cytarabine: IV: Children >1 year and Adolescents: 3,000 mg/m² over 3 hours every 12 hours on days 2 and 3 (secondary phase; total of 4 doses) in combination with methotrexate and intrathecal methotrexate/cytarabine (Bowman, 1996)

Meningeal leukemia: Intrathecal: **Note:** Optimal intrathecal chemotherapy dosing should be based on age rather than on body surface area (BSA); CSF volume correlates with age and not to BSA (Bleyer, 1983; Kerr, 2001). Dosing provided in the manufacturer's labeling is BSA-based (usual dose 30 mg/m² every 4 days; range: 5 to 75 mg/m² once daily for 4 days or once every 4 days until CNS findings normalize, followed by 1 additional treatment).

Age-based intrathecal dosing (off-label; Woods, 1990): Intrathecal:

CNS prophylaxis:
<1 year: 20 mg per dose
1 to 1.99 years: 30 mg per dose
2 to 2.99 years: 50 mg per dose
≥3 years: 70 mg per dose

ALL CNS prophylaxis, age-specific doses from literature:
Administer on day 0 of induction therapy (Gaynon, 1993):
1 to <2 years: 30 mg per dose
2 to <3 years: 50 mg per dose
≥3 years: 70 mg per dose

Administer as part of triple intrathecal therapy (TIT) on days 1 and 15 of induction therapy; days 1, 15, 50, and 64 (standard risk patients) or days 1, 15, 29, and 43 (high-risk patients) during consolidation therapy; day 1 of reinduction therapy, and during maintenance therapy (very high-risk patients receive on days 1, 22, 45, and 59 of induction, days 8, 22, 36, and 50 of consolidation therapy, days 8 and 38 of reinduction therapy, and during maintenance) (Lin, 2007):
<1 year: 18 mg per dose
1 to 2 years: 24 mg per dose
2 to 3 years: 30 mg per dose
≥3 years: 36 mg per dose

Administer on day 0 of induction therapy, then as part of TIT on days 7, 14, and 21 during consolidation therapy; as part of TIT on days 0, 28, and 35 for 2 cycles of delayed intensification therapy, and then maintenance treatment as part of TIT on day 0 every 12 weeks for 38 months (boys) or 26 months (girls) from initial induction treatment (Matloub, 2006):
1 to <2 years: 16 mg per dose
2 to <3 years: 20 mg per dose
≥3 years: 24 to 30 mg per dose

Administer on day 15 of induction therapy, days 1 and 15 of reinduction phase; and day 1 of cycle 2 of maintenance 1A phase (Pieters, 2007):
<1 year: 15 mg per dose
≥1 year: 20 mg per dose

Treatment, CNS leukemia (ALL): Intrathecal: Administer as part of TIT weekly until CSF remission, then every 4 weeks throughout continuation treatment (Lin, 2007):

<1 year: 18 mg per dose
1 to 2 years: 24 mg per dose
2 to 3 years: 30 mg per dose
≥3 years: 36 mg per dose

Renal Impairment There are no dosage adjustments provided in the manufacturer's labeling; however, the following adjustments have been recommended:

Aronoff, 2007 (cytarabine 100 to 200 mg/m^2): Children and Adults: No adjustment necessary

Kintzel, 1995 (high-dose cytarabine 1 to 3 g/m^2):

CrCl 46 to 60 mL/minute: Administer 60% of dose
CrCl 31 to 45 mL/minute: Administer 50% of dose
CrCl <30 mL/minute: Consider use of alternative drug

Smith, 1997 (high-dose cytarabine; ≥2 g/m^2/dose):

Serum creatinine 1.5 to 1.9 mg/dL or increase (from baseline) of 0.5 to 1.2 mg/dL: Reduce dose to 1 g/m^2/dose

Serum creatinine ≥2 mg/dL or increase (from baseline) of >1.2 mg/dL: Reduce dose to 0.1 g/m^2/day as a continuous infusion

Hemodialysis: In 4 hour dialysis sessions (with high flow polysulfone membrane) 6 hours after cytarabine 1 g/m^2 over 2 hours, 63% of the metabolite ARA-U was extracted from plasma (based on a single adult case report) (Radeski, 2011)

Hepatic Impairment Dose may need to be adjusted in patients with liver failure since cytarabine is partially detoxified in the liver. There are no dosage adjustments provided in the manufacturer's labeling; however, the following adjustments have been recommended:

Floyd, 2006: Transaminases (any elevation): Administer 50% of dose; may increase subsequent doses in the absence of toxicities

Koren, 1992 (dose level not specified): Bilirubin >2 mg/dL: Administer 50% of dose; may increase subsequent doses in the absence of toxicities

Obesity

American Society of Clinical Oncology (ASCO) Guidelines for appropriate chemotherapy dosing in obese adults with cancer. Utilize patient's actual body weight (full weight) for calculation of body surface area- or weight-based dosing, particularly when the intent of therapy is curative; manage regimen-related toxicities in the same manner as for nonobese patients; if a dose reduction is utilized due to toxicity, consider resumption of full weight-based dosing with subsequent cycles, especially if cause of toxicity (eg, hepatic or renal impairment) is resolved (Griggs, 2012).

American Society for Blood and Marrow Transplantation (ASBMT) practice guideline committee position statement on chemotherapy dosing in obesity: Utilize actual body weight (full weight) for calculation of body surface area in cytarabine dosing for hematopoietic stem cell transplant conditioning regimens in pediatrics and adults (Bubalo, 2014).

Combination Regimens

Leukemia, acute lymphocytic:

CALGB 8811 Regimen (ALL) on page 2003
CALGB 9111 Regimen (ALL) on page 2004
Hyper-CVAD + Imatinib on page 2145
Hyper-CVAD (Leukemia, Acute Lymphocytic) on page 2146

Administration

IV: Infuse standard dose therapy for AML (100 to 200 mg/m^2/day) as a continuous infusion. Infuse high-dose therapy (off-label) over 1 to 3 hours (usually). Other rates have been used, refer to specific reference.

In adults, doses >1000 mg/m^2 are associated with a moderate emetic potential (Basch, 2011; Roila, 2010). In pediatrics, doses >200 mg/m^2 are associated with a moderate emetic potential and 3000 mg/m^2 is associated with a high emetic potential (Dupuis, 2011); antiemetics are recommended to prevent nausea and vomiting.

Intrathecal: Intrathecal doses should be administered as soon as possible after preparation.

May also be administered SubQ.

Emetic Potential

Children:
3000 mg/m^2: High (>90%)
>200 mg/m^2 to <3000 mg/m^2: Moderate (30% to 90%)
≤200 mg/m^2: Low (10% to 30%)

Adults:
>1000 mg/m^2: Moderate (30% to 90%)
≤1000 mg/m^2: Low (10% to 30%)

Monitoring Parameters Liver function tests, CBC with differential and platelet count, serum creatinine, BUN, serum uric acid

Dosage Forms Excipient information presented when available (limited, particularly for generics); consult specific product labeling.

Solution, Injection:
Generic: 20 mg/mL (25 mL)
Solution, Injection [preservative free]:
Generic: 20 mg/mL (5 mL, 50 mL); 100 mg/mL (20 mL)
Solution Reconstituted, Injection:
Generic: 100 mg (1 ea); 500 mg (1 ea); 1 g (1 ea)

Cytarabine (Liposomal) (sye TARE a been lye po SO mal)

Related Information

Common Toxicity Criteria on page 2242

Management of Chemotherapy-Induced Nausea and Vomiting in Adults on page 2253

Safe Handling of Hazardous Drugs on page 2379

Brand Names: US DepoCyt [DSC]

Brand Names: Canada DepoCyt

Index Terms Cytarabine Lipid Complex; Cytarabine Liposome; DepoFoam-Encapsulated Cytarabine; DTC 101; Liposomal Cytarabine

Pharmacologic Category Antineoplastic Agent, Antimetabolite; Antineoplastic Agent, Antimetabolite (Pyrimidine Analog)

Use Lymphomatous meningitis: Intrathecal treatment of lymphomatous meningitis

Labeled Contraindications Hypersensitivity to cytarabine or any component of the formulation; active meningeal infection

Pregnancy Considerations Adverse effects were observed in animal reproductive studies with conventional cytarabine. Conventional cytarabine has been associated with fetal malformations when given as a component of systemic combination chemotherapy during the first trimester. Systemic exposure following intrathecal administration of cytarabine liposomal is negligible; however, women of childbearing potential should avoid becoming pregnant during treatment.

Breastfeeding Considerations It is not known if cytarabine (liposomal) is excreted in breast milk; the systemic exposure following intrathecal administration of cytarabine (liposomal) is negligible. Due to the potential for serious adverse reactions in the nursing infant, a decision should be made to discontinue cytarabine (liposomal) or to discontinue breastfeeding, taking into account the importance of treatment to the mother.

Warnings/Precautions [US Boxed Warning]: Chemical arachnoiditis (nausea, vomiting, headache, fever) occurs commonly; may be fatal if untreated. Dexamethasone should be administered concomitantly with cytarabine (liposomal) to diminish chemical arachnoid symptoms; the incidence and severity of chemical arachnoiditis is reduced with dexamethasone. If chemical arachnoiditis is suspected, exclude other possible inflammatory, infectious, or neoplastic conditions. Toxic effects may be related to a single dose or to cumulative administration and usually occur within 5 days, although may occur at any time during treatment. Monitor continuously for development of neurotoxicity; dose reduction or discontinuation may be necessary. Hydrocephalus has been reported and may be precipitated by chemical arachnoiditis.

May cause neurotoxicity (including myelopathy), which may lead to permanent neurologic deficit (rare). The risk for neurotoxicity is increased when administered with other antineoplastic agents or with cranial/spinal irradiation. CSF flow blockage may lead to increased free cytarabine concentrations in the CSF and increases the risk for neurotoxicity; consider assessing CSF flow prior to administration. Persistent (extreme) somnolence, hemiplegia, visual disturbances (including blindness; may be total and permanent), deafness, cranial nerve palsies have been reported. Signs/symptoms of peripheral neuropathy (eg, pain, numbness, paresthesia, weakness, impaired bowel/bladder control) have also been reported. Combined neurologic features (cauda equina syndrome) have been reported in some cases. If neurotoxicity develops, reduce subsequent doses or discontinue treatment. Headache, nausea, and fever are early signs of neurotoxicity. Transient elevations in CSF protein and CSF white blood cell counts have been observed following administration.

For intrathecal use only. Intrathecal medications should not be prepared during the preparation of any other agents. After preparation, store intrathecal medications in an isolated location or container clearly marked with a label identifying as "intrathecal" use only. Delivery of intrathecal medications to the patient should only be with other medications intended for administration into the central nervous system (Jacobson, 2009).

Adverse Reactions

>10%:

Cardiovascular: Peripheral edema (11%)

Central nervous system: Chemical arachnoiditis (without dexamethasone premedication: 100%; with dexamethasone premedication: 33% to 42%; grade 4: 19% to 30%; onset: ≤5 days), headache (56%), confusion (33%), fatigue (25%), abnormal gait (23%), seizure (20% to 22%), dizziness (18%), lethargy (16%), insomnia (14%), memory impairment (14%), pain (14%)

Endocrine & metabolic: Dehydration (13%)

Gastrointestinal: Nausea (46%), vomiting (44%), constipation (25%), diarrhea (12%), decreased appetite (11%)

Genitourinary: Urinary tract infection (14%)

Hematologic & oncologic: Anemia (12%), thrombocytopenia (3% to 11%)

Neuromuscular & skeletal: Weakness (40%), back pain (24%), limb pain (15%), neck pain (14%), arthralgia (11%), neck stiffness (11%)

Ophthalmic: Blurred vision (11%)

Miscellaneous: Fever (32%)

1% to 10%:

Cardiovascular: Tachycardia (9%), hypotension (8%), hypertension (6%), syncope (3%), edema (2%)

Central nervous system: Agitation (10%), hypoesthesia (10%), myasthenia (10%), depression (8%), anxiety (7%), peripheral neuropathy (3% to 4%), abnormal reflexes (3%), sensorimotor neuropathy (3%)

Dermatologic: Diaphoresis (2%), pruritus (2%)

Endocrine & metabolic: Hypokalemia (7%), hyponatremia (7%), hyperglycemia (6%)

Gastrointestinal: Abdominal pain (9%), dysphagia (8%), anorexia (5%), hemorrhoids (3%), mucosal inflammation (3%)

Genitourinary: Urinary incontinence (7%), urinary retention (5%)

Hematologic & oncologic: Neutropenia (10%), bruise (2%)

Neuromuscular & skeletal: Tremor (9%)

Otic: Hypoacusis (6%)

Respiratory: Dyspnea (10%), cough (7%), pneumonia (6%)

<1%, postmarketing, and/or case reports: Anaphylaxis, bladder disease (bladder control impaired), blindness, brain disease, cauda equina syndrome, cranial nerve palsy, deafness, drowsiness, fecal incontinence, hemiplegia, hydrocephalus, increased intracranial pressure, leukocytosis (in CSF), meningitis (infectious), myelopathy, nervous system disease (neurologic deficit), numbness, papilledema, visual disturbance

Drug Interactions

Metabolism/Transport Effects None known.

Avoid Concomitant Use

Avoid concomitant use of Cytarabine (Liposomal) with any of the following: BCG (Intravesical)

Increased Effect/Toxicity

Cytarabine (Liposomal) may increase the levels/effects of: Fingolimod; Tofacitinib

The levels/effects of Cytarabine (Liposomal) may be increased by: Ocrelizumab

Decreased Effect

Cytarabine (Liposomal) may decrease the levels/effects of: BCG (Intravesical); Nivolumab; Tertomotide

Hazardous Drugs Handling Considerations

Hazardous agent (NIOSH 2016 [group 1]).

Use appropriate precautions for receiving, handling, administration, and disposal. Gloves (single) should be worn during receiving, unpacking, and placing in storage.

NIOSH recommends double gloving, a protective gown, ventilated engineering controls (a class II biological safety cabinet or a compounding aseptic containment isolator), and closed system transfer devices (CSTDs) for preparation. Double gloving, a gown, and (if dosage form allows) CSTDs are required during administration (NIOSH 2016).

Storage/Stability

Store intact vial at 2°C to 8°C (36°F to 46°F); protect from freezing. Avoid aggressive agitation. Withdraw from the vial immediately prior to administration; solutions should be used within 4 hours of withdrawal from the vial.

After preparation, store intrathecal medications in an isolated location or container clearly marked with a label identifying as "intrathecal" use only (Jacobson, 2009).

Preparation for Administration Gloves should be worn during preparation and administration. Allow vial to warm to room temperature. Particles may settle in diluent over time, and may be resuspended with gentle agitation or inversion immediately prior to withdrawing from the vial. Do not agitate aggressively. Withdraw from the vial immediately prior to administration. No further reconstitution or dilution is required. Do not mix with any other medications. Intrathecal medications should not be prepared during the preparation of any other agents (Jacobson, 2009).

Mechanism of Action Cytarabine liposomal is a sustained-release formulation of the active ingredient cytarabine, an antimetabolite which acts through inhibition of DNA synthesis and is cell cycle-specific for the S phase of cell division. Cytarabine is converted intracellularly to its active metabolite cytarabine-5'-triphosphate (ara-CTP). Ara-CTP also appears to be incorporated into DNA and RNA; however, the primary action is inhibition of DNA polymerase, resulting in decreased DNA synthesis and repair. The liposomal formulation allows for gradual release, resulting in prolonged exposure.

Pharmacodynamics/Kinetics

Absorption: Systemic exposure following intrathecal administration is negligible since transfer rate from CSF to plasma is slow

Half-life elimination, CSF: 6 to 82 hours

Time to peak, CSF: Intrathecal: <1 hour

Dosing

Adult & Geriatric Note: Initiate dexamethasone 4 mg twice daily (oral or IV) for 5 days, beginning on the day of cytarabine liposomal administration.

Lymphomatous meningitis: Intrathecal:
Induction: 50 mg every 14 days for a total of 2 doses (weeks 1 and 3)
Consolidation: 50 mg every 14 days for 3 doses (weeks 5, 7, and 9), followed by an additional dose at week 13
Maintenance: 50 mg every 28 days for 4 doses (weeks 17, 21, 25, and 29)

Renal Impairment There are no dosage adjustments provided in the manufacturer's labeling (has not been studied).

Hepatic Impairment There are no dosage adjustments provided in the manufacturer's labeling (has not been studied).

Adjustment for Toxicity If drug-related neurotoxicity develops, reduce dose to 25 mg. If toxicity persists, discontinue treatment.

Administration For intrathecal use only. Dose should be removed from vial immediately before administration (must be administered within 4 hours of removal from the vial). An in-line filter should **NOT** be used. Administer directly into the CSF via an intraventricular reservoir or by direct injection into the lumbar sac. Injection should be made slowly (over 1 to 5 minutes). Patients should lie flat for 1 hour after lumbar puncture. After administration, observe for immediate toxic reactions. Gloves should be worn during preparation and administration. If contact with skin occurs, immediately wash with soap and water; if contact with mucous membranes occurs, flush thoroughly with water.

Monitoring Parameters Monitor closely for signs of an immediate reaction; chemical arachnoiditis; neurotoxicity

Dosage Forms Excipient information presented when available (limited, particularly for generics); consult specific product labeling. [DSC] = Discontinued product

Suspension, Intrathecal [preservative free]:

DepoCyt: 50 mg/5 mL (5 mL [DSC]) [contains cholesterol, dioleoylphosphatidylcholine (dopc), dipalmitoylphosphatidylglycerol (dppg), triolein]

◆ **Cytarabine and Daunorubicin (Liposomal)** see Daunorubicin and Cytarabine (Liposomal) on page 537

◆ **Cytarabine Hydrochloride** see Cytarabine (Conventional) on page 469

◆ **Cytarabine Injection (Can)** see Cytarabine (Conventional) on page 469

◆ **Cytarabine Lipid Complex** see Cytarabine (Liposomal) on page 481

◆ **Cytarabine (Liposomal) and Daunorubicin (Liposomal)** see Daunorubicin and Cytarabine (Liposomal) on page 537

◆ **Cytarabine Liposome** see Cytarabine (Liposomal) on page 481

◆ **Cytarabine Liposome and Daunorubicin Liposome** see Daunorubicin and Cytarabine (Liposomal) on page 537

◆ **CytoGam** see Cytomegalovirus Immune Globulin (Intravenous-Human) on page 485

Cytomegalovirus Immune Globulin (Intravenous-Human) (sye toe meg a low VYE rus i MYUN GLOB yoo lin in tra VEE nus HYU man)

Brand Names: US CytoGam

Brand Names: Canada CytoGam

Index Terms CMV Hyperimmune Globulin; CMV-IGIV

Pharmacologic Category Blood Product Derivative; Immune Globulin

Use Prophylaxis of cytomegalovirus (CMV) disease associated with kidney, lung, liver, pancreas, and heart transplants; concomitant use with ganciclovir should be considered in organ transplants (other than kidney) from CMV seropositive donors to CMV seronegative recipients

Pregnancy Risk Factor C

Dosing

Adult & Geriatric

Prophylaxis of CMV disease in kidney transplant: IV:

Initial dose (within 72 hours of transplant): 150 mg/kg/dose

2-, 4-, 6-, and 8 weeks after transplant: 100 mg/kg/dose

12- and 16 weeks after transplant: 50 mg/kg/dose

Prophylaxis of CMV disease in liver, lung, pancreas, or heart transplant: IV:

Initial dose (within 72 hours of transplant): 150 mg/kg/dose

2-, 4-, 6-, and 8 weeks after transplant: 150 mg/kg/dose

12- and 16 weeks after transplant: 100 mg/kg/dose

Treatment of severe CMV pneumonitis in hematopoietic stem cell transplant (off-label use; in combination with ganciclovir): IV: 400 mg/kg on days 1, 2, and 7, followed by 200 mg/kg on day 14; if still symptomatic, may administer an additional 200 mg/kg on day 21 (Reed, 1988) **or** 150 mg/kg twice weekly (Alexander, 2010)

Pediatric Prophylaxis of CMV disease in kidney, liver, lung, pancreas, or heart transplant: Children and Adolescents: IV: Refer to adult dosing.

Renal Impairment There are no dosage adjustments provided in the manufacturer's labeling; use with caution. Infuse at minimum rate possible.

Hepatic Impairment There are no dosage adjustments provided in the manufacturer's labeling.

Additional Information Complete prescribing information should be consulted for additional detail.

Dosage Forms Excipient information presented when available (limited, particularly for generics); consult specific product labeling.

Injection, solution [preservative free]:

CytoGam®: 50 mg (± 10 mg)/mL (50 mL) [contains sodium 20-30 mEq/L, human albumin, and sucrose 50 mg/mL]

♦ **Cytosar (Can)** *see* Cytarabine (Conventional) *on page 469*

♦ **Cytosar-U** *see* Cytarabine (Conventional) *on page 469*

♦ **Cytosine Arabinosine Hydrochloride** *see* Cytarabine (Conventional) *on page 469*

♦ **Cytostasan** *see* Bendamustine *on page 228*

♦ **Cytovene** *see* Ganciclovir (Systemic) *on page 855*

♦ **Cytoxan** *see* Cyclophosphamide *on page 438*

♦ **D1694** *see* Raltitrexed *on page 1572*

Dabrafenib (da BRAF e nib)

Brand Names: US Tafinlar
Brand Names: Canada Tafinlar
Index Terms GSK2118436
Pharmacologic Category Antineoplastic Agent, BRAF Kinase Inhibitor
Use

Melanoma (metastatic or unresectable): Treatment of unresectable or metastatic melanoma in patients with a BRAF V600E mutation (single agent therapy) or in patients with BRAF V600E or BRAF V600K mutations (in combination with trametinib); confirm BRAF V600E or BRAF V600K mutation status with an approved test prior to treatment.

Non-small cell lung cancer (metastatic): Treatment of metastatic non-small cell lung cancer (NSCLC) in patients with BRAF V600E mutation as detected by an approved test (in combination with trametinib).

Limitations of use: Not indicated for treatment of patients with wild-type BRAF melanoma or wild-type BRAF NSCLC.

Labeled Contraindications

There are no contraindications listed in the manufacturer's US labeling.

Canadian labeling: Hypersensitivity to dabrafenib or any component of the formulation.

Pregnancy Considerations Adverse effects were observed in animal reproduction studies. Based on its mechanism of action, dabrafenib would be expected to cause fetal harm if administered to a pregnant woman. Females of reproductive potential should use a highly effective nonhormonal contraceptive during therapy and for at least 2 weeks for single-agent therapy or 4 months for combination therapy with trametinib after treatment is complete; hormonal contraceptives may not be effective. Spermatogenesis may be impaired in males (observed in animal studies); family planning and fertility counseling should be considered prior to therapy.

Breastfeeding Considerations It is not known if dabrafenib is present in breast milk. Due to the potential for serious adverse reactions in the breastfed infant, breastfeeding is not recommended by the manufacturer during treatment and for 2 weeks (single agent therapy) or 4 months (combination therapy with trametinib) after the last dose.

Warnings/Precautions Serious adverse reactions (retinal vein occlusion, interstitial lung disease) that occur with single-agent trametinib may also occur when dabrafenib is administered in combination with trametinib. Cardiomyopathy may be observed when used as a single agent or in combination with trametinib. The median time to onset of cardiomyopathy in patients with melanoma was ~8 months (range: 28 days to ~25 months) when used in combination with trametinib, and ~4 months (range: 28 days to ~19 months) for single agent therapy. The median time of onset of cardiomyopathy in patients with NSCLC was 6.7 months (range: 1.4 to 14.1 months). Assess LVEF (by echocardiogram or MUGA scan) prior to combination therapy initiation, at 1 month, and then at 2- to 3-month intervals while on therapy. Cardiac dysfunction may require dabrafenib treatment interruption (see trametinib monograph for dosage modifications). Cardiomyopathy resolved in some patients following dose adjustments, treatment interruption or permanent discontinuation. QTcF prolongation >60 msec above baseline or to >500 msec was reported (rare), both as a single agent or when used in combination with trametinib. Hemorrhage, including symptomatic bleeding in a critical area/organ, may occur with dabrafenib either as a single agent or in combination with trametinib. Major bleeding events (some fatal) included intracranial or gastrointestinal hemorrhage. May require treatment interruption and dosage reduction; permanently discontinue dabrafenib (and trametinib) for all grade 4 hemorrhagic events and any grade 3 event that does not improve with therapy interruption. Venous thromboembolism events (some fatal) may occur when dabrafenib is used in combination with trametinib. DVT and PE occurred at an increased incidence with combination therapy. Patients should seek immediate medical attention with symptoms of DVT or PE (shortness of breath, chest pain, arm/leg swelling). Dabrafenib therapy may be continued for uncomplicated DVT or PE; permanently discontinue trametinib for life-threatening PE.

Serious febrile reactions and fever (any severity) complicated by hypotension, rigors or chills, dehydration, or renal failure were observed in melanoma studies during dabrafenib single-agent therapy and when used in combination with trametinib. The median time to initial fever (single-agent therapy) was 11 days (range: 1 day to 6.6 months); median duration was 3 days (range: 1 day to 4.2 months). In patients treated with combination therapy, the median time to onset of fever was 1 month (range 1 day to 23.5 months) and the median duration was 3 days (range: 1 day to 11.3 months). Interrupt dabrafenib therapy for fever ≥38.5°C (101.3°F) or for any other serious febrile reaction complicated by hypotension, rigors/chills, dehydration, or renal failure; evaluate promptly for signs/symptoms of infection. Dosage reduction (or discontinuation) may be required; when resuming therapy after a febrile reaction, may require administration of antipyretics as secondary prophylaxis. Administer corticosteroids (eg, prednisone 10 mg daily or equivalent) for at least 5 days for second or subsequent episodes of pyrexia if temperature does not return to baseline within 3 days of fever onset, or for pyrexia associated with complications (eg, dehydration, hypotension, severe chills/rigors with no evidence of active infection). Hyperglycemia may occur while on therapy (either as a single agent or in combination with trametinib); may require initiation of insulin or oral hypoglycemic agent therapy (or an increased dose if already taking). Monitor serum glucose at baseline and as clinically necessary in patients with preexisting diabetes or hyperglycemia. Instruct patients to report symptoms of severe hyperglycemia (eg, polydipsia, polyuria).

Serious dermatologic toxicity (eg, rash, dermatitis, acneiform rash, palmar-plantar erythrodysesthesia syndrome, erythema) may occur when used in combination with trametinib (known complication of single-agent trametinib therapy); some patients required hospitalization for severe toxicity or for secondary skin infections. In melanoma studies, the median time to onset and resolution of skin toxicity for combination therapy was 2 months (range: 1 day to 22 months) and 1.2 months (range: 1 day to ~24 months), respectively. Monitor for dermatologic toxicity and signs/symptoms of secondary infections. Treatment interruption, dose reduction, and/or therapy discontinuation may be necessary. Cutaneous squamous cell carcinoma and keratoacanthoma (cuSCC) and new primary melanoma were observed during single agent dabrafenib therapy at an increased incidence compared with control therapy in clinical trials. In melanoma, the median time to the first occurrence of cuSCC was 2.1 months (range: 1 to 53 weeks); approximately one-third of patients who developed cuSCC had more than one occurrence (with continued treatment). The median time between diagnosis of the first and second lesions was 6 weeks. When used in combination with trametinib for the treatment of melanoma, cuSCC occurred less frequently than with single-agent dabrafenib therapy; time to diagnosis ranged from 1.8 to 16.8 months after the initiation of combination treatment, and from 9 days to ~21 months for single-agent therapy. Cases of cuSCC also occurred in patients with NSCLC, with a first occurrence onset ranging from 25 days to ~12 months. Basal cell carcinoma (BCC) may also occur with combination or single-agent therapy; the incidence of BCC is ~3% for combination therapy versus 6% for single-agent dabrafenib. The time to BCC diagnosis ranged from ~3 to ~24 months for melanoma patients receiving combination therapy. Dermatologic evaluations should be performed prior to initiating therapy, every 2 months during therapy, and for up to 6 months post discontinuation. There are case reports of noncutaneous malignancies, including pancreatic cancer (KRAS mutation-positive), colorectal cancer (recurrent NRAS mutation-positive), hand and neck cancer, and glioblastoma, with combination therapy; monitor for signs/symptoms of noncutaneous malignancies. Dabrafenib should be permanently discontinued if RAS mutation-positive noncutaneous malignancies develop (no trametinib dosage reduction is required).

Retinal pigment epithelial detachments (RPED) were seen in melanoma clinical trials when used in combination with trametinib (a known complication of trametinib single-agent therapy). Detachments were typically bilateral and multifocal and occurred in the central macular area of the retina. Promptly (within 24 hours) refer patients for ophthalmological evaluations if loss of vision or other visual disturbances occur; dabrafenib dosage modification is not necessary for RPED (trametinib therapy modification may be required). Ophthalmic exams (including retinal evaluation) should be performed periodically during treatment with combination therapy. Uveitis, including iritis and iridocyclitis, has been reported with dabrafenib single-agent therapy and when used in combination with trametinib; manage symptomatically with local ophthalmic steroid and mydriatic drops. May require dabrafenib treatment interruption or permanent discontinuation (does not require alteration in trametinib therapy). Monitor for signs/symptoms of uveitis (eg, eye pain, photophobia, vision changes).

Potentially significant drug-drug interactions may exist, requiring dose or frequency adjustment, additional monitoring, and/or selection of alternative therapy. Drugs affecting gastric pH (eg, proton pump inhibitors, H2-receptor antagonists, antacids) may alter dabrafenib solubility, resulting in decreased bioavailability. Clinical trials have not been performed to evaluate concomitant administration and its effect on dabrafenib efficacy. Patients with glucose-6-phosphate dehydrogenase (G6PD) deficiency may be at risk for hemolytic anemia when administered dabrafenib; use with caution and closely observe for signs/symptoms of hemolytic anemia. Not indicated for treatment of patients with wild-type BRAF melanoma or wild-type BRAF NSCLC. Exposing wild-type cells to BRAF inhibitors such as dabrafenib may result in paradoxical activation of MAP-kinase signaling and increased cell proliferation. Prior to initiating therapy, confirm BRAF V600E or BRAF V600K mutation status with an approved test. Data regarding single-agent use for melanoma in patients with BRAF V600K mutation is limited; compared to BRAF V600E mutation, lower response rates have been observed with BRAF V600K mutation. Data regarding other less common BRAF V600 mutations in melanoma is lacking.

Adverse Reactions

Monotherapy:

>10%:

Cardiovascular: Peripheral edema (17%)

Central nervous system: Fatigue (40%), headache (28% to 32%), chills (17%)

Dermatologic: Dermatological reaction (68%), skin rash (17% to 53%), hyperkeratosis (37%), alopecia (22%), palmar-plantar erythrodysesthesia (20%), pruritus (13%)

Endocrine & metabolic: Hyperglycemia (49% to 50%; grades 3/4: 2% to 6%), hypophosphatemia (37% to 40%), increased gamma-glutamyl transferase (38%), hyponatremia (8% to 36%), hypoalbuminemia (23%), hypokalemia (23%), hyperkalemia (15%)

Gastrointestinal: Diarrhea (28%), abdominal pain (21%), nausea (21%), decreased appetite (19%), vomiting (15%), constipation (11%)

Hematologic & oncologic: Lymphocytopenia (40%; grades 3/4: 6%), anemia (28%), papilloma (27%), leukopenia (21%), malignant neoplasm of skin (keratoacanthoma and squamous cell carcinoma; 7% to 19%; grades 3/4: 4%)

Hepatic: Increased serum alkaline phosphatase (19% to 26%), increased serum AST (15%), increased serum ALT (11%)

Neuromuscular & skeletal: Arthralgia (27% to 34%), myalgia (11% to 23%), limb pain (19%), back pain (11% to 12%)

Respiratory: Cough (12% to 21%)

Miscellaneous: Fever (26% to 28%; grades 3/4: ≤4%)

1% to 10%:

Cardiovascular: Prolonged Q-T interval on ECG (>60 msec from baseline: 2%; >500 msec: 2%)

Central nervous system: Dizziness (9%), insomnia (8%)

Dermatologic: Actinic keratosis (9%), night sweats (6%), xeroderma (6%), acneiform eruption (4%), erythema (2%)

Endocrine & metabolic: Hypocalcemia (9%), hypomagnesemia (6%), hypercalcemia (4%), dehydration (2%)

Gastrointestinal: Pancreatitis (<10%), xerostomia (6%)

Genitourinary: Urinary tract infection (9%)

Hematologic & oncologic: Neutropenia (9%; grades 3/4: 2%), thrombocy-topenia (8%), basal cell carcinoma (2%), hemorrhage (2%), malignant melanoma (2%)

Hypersensitivity: Hypersensitivity (bullous rash, <10%)

Neuromuscular & skeletal: Muscle spasm (4%)

Ophthalmic: Uveitis (including iritis, 1%)

Renal: Interstitial nephritis (<10%), increased serum creatinine (9%)

Respiratory: Nasopharyngitis (10%)

Miscellaneous: Febrile reaction (2%)

Combination therapy with trametanib:

>10%:

Cardiovascular: Peripheral edema (28% to 31%), prolonged Q-T interval on ECG (>60 msec from baseline: 13%; >500 msec: 4%)

Central nervous system: Chills (50% to 58%), fatigue (53% to 57%), headache (29% to 37%), insomnia (11% to 18%), dizziness (13% to 16%)

Dermatologic: Dermatological reaction (65%; 3% required hospitalization), skin rash (43% to 45%), night sweats (15% to 24%), xeroderma (9% to 18%), acneiform eruption (11% to 16%), actinic keratosis (7% to 15%), erythema (6% to 15%), pruritus (11%)

Endocrine & metabolic: Hyperglycemia (58% to 67%; grades 3/4: 5% to 6%), increased gamma-glutamyl transferase (54% to 56%), hyponatremia (48% to 55%), hypoalbuminemia (43% to 53%), hypophosphatemia (41% to 47%), hypokalemia (15% to 29%), hyperkalemia (18% to 22%), hypocalcemia (13% to 20%), hypercalcemia (15% to 19%), hypomagne-semia (2% to 18%), dehydration (6% to 11%)

Gastrointestinal: Nausea (44% to 46%), vomiting (40% to 43%), diarrhea (26% to 36%), abdominal pain (24% to 33%), decreased appetite (22% to 30%), constipation (17% to 22%), xerostomia (11%)

Genitourinary: Urinary tract infection (6% to 13%)

Hematologic & oncologic: Leukopenia (46% to 62%; grades 3/4: 4% to 5%), lymphocytopenia (55% to 59%; grades 3/4: 19% to 22%), anemia (46% to 55%; grades 3/4: 4% to 7%), neutropenia (37% to 55%; grades 3/4: 2% to 13%), thrombocytopenia (31%; grades 3/4: 2% to 4%), hemorrhage (11% to 16%; major hemorrhage [intracranial or gastric]: 5%)

Hepatic: Increased serum alkaline phosphatase (60% to 67%), increased serum AST (54% to 60%), increased serum ALT (35% to 42%), hyper-bilirubinemia (7% to 15%)

Neuromuscular & skeletal: Arthralgia (27% to 44%), myalgia (22% to 24%), back pain (11% to 18%), limb pain (11% to 16%), muscle spasm (2% to 16%)

Renal: Increased serum creatinine (20% to 24%)

Respiratory: Cough (11% to 29%), oropharyngeal pain (7% to 13%)

Miscellaneous: Fever (57% to 71%; grades 3/4: 5% to 9%), febrile reac-tion (25%)

1% to 10%:

Cardiovascular: Hypertension (<10%), cardiomyopathy (≤9%), venous thromboembolism (deep vein thrombosis or pulmonary embolism; 7%)

Dermatologic: Cellulitis (<10%), folliculitis (<10%), hyperhidrosis (<10%), hyperkeratosis (<10%), palmar-plantar erythrodysesthesia (<10%), paro-nychia (<10%), pustular rash (<10%), secondary skin infection (3%)

Endocrine & metabolic: Hyperglycemia (grade 3: 5% to 6%)

Gastrointestinal: Pancreatitis (<10%), stomatitis (<10%)

Hematologic & oncologic: Cutaneous papilloma (<10%), basal cell carcinoma (9%), malignant neoplasm of skin (keratoacanthoma and squamous cell carcinoma; 7%)

Neuromuscular & skeletal: Weakness (<10%)

Ophthalmic: Blindness (transient; <10%), blurred vision (<10%), retinal detachment (pigment epithelium; 1%), uveitis (1%)

Renal: Renal failure (2% to 7%)

<1%: Glioblastoma, Kaposi sarcoma, malignant neoplasm of colon and rectum (recurrent NRAS mutation-positive), malignant neoplasm of head and neck, pancreatic adenocarcinoma (KRAS mutation-positive)

Drug Interactions

Metabolism/Transport Effects Substrate of BCRP, CYP2C8 (major), CYP3A4 (major), P-glycoprotein; **Note:** Assignment of Major/Minor substrate status based on clinically relevant drug interaction potential; **Inhibits** BCRP, SLCO1B1; **Induces** CYP2C8 (weak/moderate), CYP2C9 (weak/moderate), CYP3A4 (moderate)

Avoid Concomitant Use

Avoid concomitant use of Dabrafenib with any of the following: Asunaprevir; Axitinib; Bedaquiline; Bosutinib; Cobimetinib; Conivaptan; CYP2C8 Inhibitors (Strong); CYP3A4 Inhibitors (Strong); Dasabuvir; Deflazacort; Elbasvir; Flibanserin; Fusidic Acid (Systemic); Grazoprevir; Idelalisib; Neratinib; Nisoldipine; Olaparib; Ranolazine; Simeprevir; Sonidegib; Velpatasvir; Venetoclax

Increased Effect/Toxicity

Dabrafenib may increase the levels/effects of: Highest Risk QTc-Prolonging Agents; Ifosfamide; Moderate Risk QTc-Prolonging Agents

The levels/effects of Dabrafenib may be increased by: Conivaptan; CYP2C8 Inhibitors (Moderate); CYP2C8 Inhibitors (Strong); CYP3A4 Inhibitors (Moderate); CYP3A4 Inhibitors (Strong); Deferasirox; Fusidic Acid (Systemic); Idelalisib; Lumacaftor; Trametinib

Decreased Effect

Dabrafenib may decrease the levels/effects of: Antidiabetic Agents; Asunaprevir; Axitinib; Bedaquiline; Bosutinib; CloZAPine; Cobimetinib; Contraceptives (Estrogens); Contraceptives (Progestins); CYP2B6 Substrates; CYP2C19 Substrates; CYP2C8 Substrates; CYP2C9 Substrates; CYP3A4 Substrates; Daclatasvir; Dasabuvir; Deflazacort; Elbasvir; Estriol (Systemic); Estriol (Topical); FentaNYL; Flibanserin; Glecaprevir and Pibrentasvir; Grazoprevir; GuanFACINE; Ifosfamide; Lurasidone; Neratinib; Nisoldipine; Olaparib; Palbociclib; Perampanel; Proton Pump Inhibitors; Ranolazine; Simeprevir; Sonidegib; Velpatasvir; Venetoclax

The levels/effects of Dabrafenib may be decreased by: Antacids; CYP2C8 Inducers (Strong); CYP3A4 Inducers (Strong); H2-Antagonists; Lumacaftor; Proton Pump Inhibitors; St John's Wort

Food Interactions Administration with a high-fat meal decreased C_{max} and AUC by 51% and 31%, respectively, and delayed median T_{max} by ~4 hours. Management: Administer 1 hour before or 2 hours after a meal.

Hazardous Drugs Handling Considerations

Hazardous agent (NIOSH 2016 [group 1]).

Use appropriate precautions for receiving, handling, administration, and disposal. Gloves (single) should be worn during receiving, unpacking, and placing in storage. NIOSH recommends single gloving for administration of intact tablets or capsules (NIOSH 2016).

◄ **Storage/Stability** Store at 25°C (77°F); excursions permitted to 15°C to 30°C (59°F to 86°F).

Mechanism of Action Dabrafenib selectively inhibits some mutated forms of the protein kinase B-raf (BRAF). BRAF V600 mutations result in constitutive activation of the BRAF pathway; through BRAF inhibition, dabrafenib inhibits tumor cell growth. The combination of dabrafenib and trametinib allows for greater inhibition of the MAPK pathway, resulting in BRAF V600 melanoma cell death (Flaherty 2012). Dabrafenib plus trametinib has been reported to synergistically inhibit cell growth in lung cancer cell lines which are BRAF V600E-mutant (Planchard 2016)

Pharmacodynamics/Kinetics

Absorption: Decreased with a high-fat meal

Distribution: 70.3 L

Protein binding: 99.7% to plasma proteins

Metabolism: Hepatic via CYP2C8 and CYP3A4 to hydroxy-dabrafenib (active) which is further metabolized via CYP3A4 oxidation to desmethyl-dabrafenib (active)

Bioavailability: 95%

Half-life elimination: Parent drug: 8 hours; Hydroxy-dabrafenib (active metabolite): 10 hours; Desmethyl-dabrafenib (active metabolite): 21 to 22 hours

Time to peak: 2 hours; delayed with a high-fat meal

Excretion: Feces (71%); urine (23%; metabolites only)

Dosing

Adult & Geriatric Note: Confirm BRAF V600 mutation status prior to treatment initiation.

Melanoma (metastatic or unresectable) (with BRAF V600E mutation): Oral: 150 mg twice daily (approximately every 12 hours) (single-agent therapy); continue until disease progression or unacceptable toxicity

Melanoma (metastatic or unresectable) (with BRAF V600E or BRAF V600K mutation): Oral: 150 mg twice daily (approximately every 12 hours (in combination with trametinib); continue until disease progression or unacceptable toxicity

Non-small cell lung cancer (metastatic) (with BRAF V600E mutation): Oral: 150 mg twice daily, approximately every 12 hours (in combination with trametinib); continue until disease progression or unacceptable toxicity (Planchard 2016)

Missed doses: A missed dose may be administered up to 6 hours prior to the next dose; do not administer if <6 hours until the next dose.

Renal Impairment

Mild to moderate impairment (GFR ≥30 mL/minute/1.73 m^2): No dosage adjustment necessary.

Severe impairment (GFR <30 mL/minute/1.73 m^2): There are no dosage adjustments provided in the manufacturer's labeling (has not been studied)

Hepatic Impairment

Mild impairment: No dosage adjustment necessary.

Moderate to severe impairment: There are no dosage adjustments provided in the manufacturer's labeling (has not been studied); however, metabolism is primarily hepatic and exposure may be increased in patients with moderate to severe impairment.

Adjustment for Toxicity
Recommended dabrafenib dose reductions for toxicity:
First dose reduction: 100 mg twice daily
Second dose reduction: 75 mg twice daily
Third dose reduction: 50 mg twice daily
Subsequent modifications (if unable to tolerate 50 mg twice daily): Permanently discontinue.

Note: If using combination therapy, refer to Trametinib monograph for recommended trametinib dose reductions.

Cardiac:
>20% absolute decrease in LVEF from baseline and LVEF is below institutional LLN: Interrupt dabrafenib therapy; if improved, may resume at the same dose.

Symptomatic heart failure: Interrupt dabrafenib therapy; if improved, may resume at the same dose.

Dermatologic:
Intolerable grade 2 skin toxicity or grade 3 or 4 skin toxicity: Interrupt dabrafenib therapy for up to 3 weeks. If toxicity improves within 3 weeks, resume at a lower dose level. If toxicity does not improve within 3 weeks following therapy interruption, permanently discontinue dabrafenib.

New primary cutaneous malignancy: No dabrafenib dosage modification is necessary.

Fever:
Fever of 38.5°C to 40°C (101.3°F to 104°F): Interrupt dabrafenib therapy until temperature normalizes. Resume at the same or lower dose level.

Fever >40°C (104°F) and/or fever complicated by rigors, hypotension, dehydration, or renal failure: Interrupt dabrafenib therapy until temperature normalizes. Resume at a lower dose level or permanently discontinue. May require prophylactic antipyretics (secondary prophylaxis) upon resumption. Administer corticosteroids (eg, prednisone 10 mg daily or equivalent) for at least 5 days for second or subsequent pyrexia if temperature does not return to baseline within 3 days of onset of fever, or for fever associated with complications (eg, dehydration, renal failure, hypotension, or severe chills/rigors with no evidence of active infection).

Hemorrhage:
Grade 3 hemorrhage: Interrupt dabrafenib therapy. If hemorrhage improves, resume at a lower dose level. If hemorrhage does not improve following therapy interruption, permanently discontinue dabrafenib.

Grade 4 hemorrhage: Permanently discontinue dabrafenib.

Ocular:
Uveitis including iritis and iridocyclitis: If mild or moderate uveitis does not respond to local ocular therapy (or for severe uveitis), interrupt dabrafenib therapy for up to 6 weeks. If improves to ≤ grade 1 within 6 weeks following therapy interruption, resume at the same dose or a lower dose. If does not improve, or for persistent grade 2 or higher uveitis of >6 week duration, permanently discontinue dabrafenib.

Grade 2 or 3 retinal pigment epithelial detachments (RPED): No dabrafenib dosage modification is necessary.

Retinal vein occlusion: No dabrafenib dosage modification is necessary.

Pulmonary: Interstitial lung disease or pneumonitis: No dabrafenib dosage modification is necessary.

Venous thromboembolism: Uncomplicated DVT or PE: No dabrafenib dosage modification is necessary.

◀ **Other toxicity:**
Intolerable grade 2 or any grade 3 toxicity: Interrupt dabrafenib therapy until resolution to ≤ grade 1; resume at a lower dose level. If toxicity does not improve following therapy interruption, permanently discontinue dabrafenib.

Grade 4 toxicity (first occurrence): Interrupt dabrafenib therapy until resolution to ≤ grade 1; consider resuming at a lower dose level or permanently discontinue.

Grade 4 toxicity (recurrent after dosage reduction): Permanently discontinue dabrafenib.

New primary noncutaneous malignancy (RAS mutation-positive): Permanently discontinue dabrafenib.

Combination Regimens
Lung cancer (non-small cell): Dabrafenib-Trametinib (NSCLC) on page 2083
Melanoma: Dabrafenib-Trametinib (Melanoma) on page 2082

Administration Administer orally at least 1 hour before or 2 hours after a meal; doses should be ~12 hours apart. Do not open, crush, or break capsules. A missed dose may be administered up to 6 hours prior to the next dose. When administered in combination with trametinib, take the once-daily dose of trametinib at the same time each day with either the morning or evening dose of dabrafenib.

Emetic Potential Low (10% to 30%)

Monitoring Parameters BRAFV600 mutation status (prior to treatment); serum glucose (particularly in patients with preexisting diabetes mellitus or hyperglycemia); electrolytes; renal function; dermatologic evaluations prior to initiation, every 2 months during therapy, and for up to 6 months following discontinuation to assess for new cutaneous malignancies; monitor for febrile drug reactions and signs/symptoms of infections; signs/symptoms of uveitis (eg, eye pain, photophobia, vision changes), monitor for signs/symptoms of hemolytic anemia.

For patients receiving combination therapy with trametinib: Hepatic function; CBC (baseline and periodically during therapy); assess LVEF (by echocardiogram or MUGA scan) at baseline, 1 month after therapy initiation, and then at 2- to 3-month intervals; monitor for signs/symptoms of hemorrhage, venous thromboembolism, interstitial lung disease, and RPED, or retinal vein occlusion.

Monitor adherence.

Medication Guide Available Yes

Dosage Forms Excipient information presented when available (limited, particularly for generics); consult specific product labeling.
Capsule, Oral:
Tafinlar: 50 mg, 75 mg

Dacarbazine (da KAR ba zeen)
Related Information
Management of Chemotherapy-Induced Nausea and Vomiting in Adults on page 2253
Prevention of Chemotherapy-Induced Nausea and Vomiting in Children on page 2310
Safe Handling of Hazardous Drugs on page 2379
Brand Names: Canada Dacarbazine for Injection, BP

Index Terms DIC; Dimethyl Triazeno Imidazole Carboxamide; DTIC; DTIC-Dome; Imidazole Carboxamide; Imidazole Carboxamide Dimethyltriazene; WR-139007

Pharmacologic Category Antineoplastic Agent, Alkylating Agent (Triazene)

Use

Hodgkin lymphoma: Treatment of Hodgkin lymphoma (in combination with other chemotherapy agents)

Metastatic malignant melanoma: Treatment of metastatic malignant melanoma

Labeled Contraindications

Hypersensitivity to dacarbazine or any component of the formulation

Canadian labeling: Additional contraindications (not in the US labeling): Prior severe myelosuppression

Pregnancy Considerations [US Boxed Warning]: Studies have demonstrated this agent to be carcinogenic and/or teratogenic when used in animals; adverse effects have been observed in animal reproduction studies. Women of reproductive potential should avoid becoming pregnant during treatment. The European Society for Medical Oncology has published guidelines for diagnosis, treatment, and follow-up of cancer during pregnancy. The guidelines recommend referral to a facility with expertise in cancer during pregnancy and encourage a multidisciplinary team (obstetrician, neonatologist, oncology team). In general, if chemotherapy is indicated, it should be avoided during in the first trimester, there should be a 3-week time period between the last chemotherapy dose and anticipated delivery, and chemotherapy should not be administered beyond week 33 of gestation (Peccatori 2013). An international consensus panel has published guidelines for hematologic malignancies during pregnancy. Dacarbazine is a component of the ABVD regimen, which is used for the treatment of Hodgkin lymphoma. If treatment cannot be deferred until after delivery in patients with early stage Hodgkin lymphoma, ABVD may be administered safely and effectively in the latter phase of pregnancy (based on limited data); for patients with advanced-stage disease, ABVD can be administered in the second and third trimesters (Lishner 2016).

Breastfeeding Considerations It is not known if dacarbazine is excreted in breast milk. Due to the potential for serious adverse reactions in the breastfeeding infant, a decision should be made to discontinue dacarbazine or to discontinue breastfeeding, taking into account the benefits of treatment to the mother.

Warnings/Precautions [US Boxed Warning]: Bone marrow suppression is the most common toxicity; leukopenia and thrombocytopenia may be severe; may result in treatment delays or discontinuation; anemia may also occur. Monitor CBC with differential. The onset for leukopenia is ~14 days (range: 10 to 30 days) and the duration is ~1 to 3 weeks. The onset for thrombocytopenia is ~18 days (range: 12 to 30 days) and the duration is ~1 to 3 weeks. **[US Boxed Warning]: Hepatic necrosis has been reported.** Hepatotoxicity may be accompanied with hepatic vein thrombosis and hepatocellular necrosis; may be fatal. Hepatotoxicity usually occurs with combination chemotherapy, but may occur with dacarbazine alone. Use with caution in patients with hepatic or renal impairment; half-life is increased, monitor for toxicity and consider dosage reduction. Dacarbazine is associated with a high emetic potential; antiemetics are recommended to prevent nausea and vomiting (Basch 2011; Dupuis 2011; Roila 2010). Anaphylaxis may occur following dacarbazine administration. Dacarbazine is an irritant; local ▶

reactions may occur (Perez Fidalgo 2012); according to the manufacturer, extravasation may result in tissue damage and severe pain.

Potentially significant drug-drug interactions may exist, requiring dose or frequency adjustment, additional monitoring, and/or selection of alternative therapy. **[US Boxed Warning]: Studies have demonstrated this agent to be carcinogenic and/or teratogenic when used in animals. [US Boxed Warning]: Should be administered under the supervision of an experienced cancer chemotherapy physician.** Carefully evaluate the potential benefits of therapy against the risk for toxicity. Adequate laboratory facilities should be available for appropriate monitoring.

Adverse Reactions Frequency not always defined.

Central nervous system: Infusion-site pain

Dermatologic: Alopecia

Gastrointestinal: Nausea and vomiting (>90%), anorexia

Hematologic & oncologic: Bone marrow depression (onset: 5 to 7 days; nadir: 7 to 10 days; recovery: 21 to 28 days), leukopenia, thrombocytopenia

<1%, postmarketing, and/or case reports: Anaphylaxis, anemia, diarrhea, dysgeusia, eosinophilia, erythema, facial flushing, facial paresthesia, flu-like symptoms (fever, myalgia, malaise), hepatic necrosis, increased liver enzymes (transient), paresthesia, renal function test abnormality, skin photosensitivity, skin rash, urticaria, venous obstruction (hepatic vein)

Drug Interactions

Metabolism/Transport Effects Substrate of CYP1A2 (major), CYP2E1 (major); **Note:** Assignment of Major/Minor substrate status based on clinically relevant drug interaction potential

Avoid Concomitant Use

Avoid concomitant use of Dacarbazine with any of the following: BCG (Intravesical); Deferiprone; Dipyrone; Natalizumab; Pimecrolimus; Tacrolimus (Topical); Vaccines (Live)

Increased Effect/Toxicity

Dacarbazine may increase the levels/effects of: CloZAPine; Deferiprone; Fingolimod; Leflunomide; Natalizumab; Tofacitinib; Vaccines (Live)

The levels/effects of Dacarbazine may be increased by: Abiraterone Acetate; CYP1A2 Inhibitors (Moderate); CYP1A2 Inhibitors (Strong); CYP2E1 Inhibitors (Moderate); CYP2E1 Inhibitors (Strong); Deferasirox; Denosumab; Dipyrone; Obeticholic Acid; Ocrelizumab; Palifermin; Peginterferon Alfa-2b; Pimecrolimus; Promazine; Roflumilast; Tacrolimus (Topical); Trastuzumab; Vemurafenib

Decreased Effect

Dacarbazine may decrease the levels/effects of: BCG (Intravesical); Coccidioides immitis Skin Test; Lenograstim; Nivolumab; Sipuleucel-T; Tertomotide; Vaccines (Inactivated); Vaccines (Live)

The levels/effects of Dacarbazine may be decreased by: Cannabis; Cyproterone; Echinacea; SORAfenib; Teriflunomide

Hazardous Drugs Handling Considerations

Hazardous agent (NIOSH 2016 [group 1]).

Use appropriate precautions for receiving, handling, administration, and disposal. Gloves (single) should be worn during receiving, unpacking, and placing in storage.

NIOSH recommends double gloving, a protective gown, ventilated engineering controls (a class II biological safety cabinet or a compounding aseptic containment isolator), and closed system transfer devices (CSTDs) for preparation. Double gloving, a gown, and (if dosage form allows) CSTDs are required during administration (NIOSH 2016).

Storage/Stability Store intact vials at 2°C to 8°C (36°F to 46°F). Protect from light. Extended stability of intact vials outside of the refrigerator has been reported; intact vials are stable for 3 months at room temperature (Cohen 2007). According to the manufacturer, the reconstituted solution (in the vial) should be used within 72 hours if refrigerated and 8 hours if at room temperature; however, additional stability data indicates the reconstituted solution may be stable for 24 hours at room temperature (20°C) and 96 hours refrigerated (4°C) when protected from light (El Aatmani 2002). Following dilution for infusion (in D5W or NS), solutions may be stored for up to 24 hours refrigerated (4°C) or for up to 8 hours at normal room conditions (dacarbazine is light sensitive).

Preparation for Administration

The manufacturer recommends reconstituting 100 mg and 200 mg vials with 9.9 mL and 19.7 mL SWFI, respectively, to a concentration of 10 mg/mL; some institutions may use different standard dilutions (eg, 20 mg/mL). Further dilute for infusion in D5W or NS.

Canadian labeling: Reconstitute the 600 mg vial with 59.1 mL SWFI; further dilute with 150 or 250 mL D5W or NS.

Mechanism of Action Alkylating agent which is converted to the active alkylating metabolite MTIC [(methyl-triazene-1-yl)-imidazole-4-carboxamide] via the cytochrome P450 system. The cytotoxic effects of MTIC are manifested through alkylation (methylation) of DNA at the O^6, N^7 guanine positions which lead to DNA double strand breaks and apoptosis. Dacarbazine is non-cell cycle specific (Marchesi 2007).

Pharmacodynamics/Kinetics

Distribution: Exceeds total body water; suggesting binding to some tissue (probably liver) (Perry 2012)

Metabolism: Extensively hepatic to the active metabolite MTIC [(methyl-triazene-1-yl)-imidazole-4-carboxamide]

Half-life elimination: Biphasic: Initial: 19 minutes, Terminal: 5 hours

Excretion: Urine (40%; as unchanged drug)

Dosing

Adult & Geriatric Note: Dacarbazine is associated with a high emetic potential; antiemetics are recommended to prevent nausea and vomiting (Basch 2011; Roila 2010).

Hodgkin lymphoma: ABVD regimen: IV: 375 mg/m² on days 1 and 15 every 4 weeks (in combination with doxorubicin, bleomycin, and vinblastine)

Metastatic malignant melanoma: IV: 250 mg/m² over 30 minutes once daily on days 1 to 5 every 3 weeks (Middleton 2000)

Metastatic melanoma (off-label dosing/combinations): IV:

CVD regimen: 800 mg/m² over 60 minutes on day 1 every 3 weeks (in combination with cisplatin and vinblastine) (Atkins 2008; Eton 2002)

Biochemotherapy regimen: 800 mg/m² over 60 minutes on day 1 every 3 weeks (in combination with cisplatin, vinblastine, interleukin-2 and interferon alfa-2b) (Flaherty 2014) Medullary thyroid cancer, advanced (off-label use): IV: 200 mg/m² once daily for 5 days every 6 weeks (in combination with fluorouracil and streptozocin) or 600 mg/m² once daily for 2 days every 3 or 4 weeks (in combination with cyclophosphamide and vincristine) or 250 mg/m^2 over 15 to 30 minutes once daily for 5 days every 4 weeks (in combination with fluorouracil) (Orlandi 1994; Schlumberger 1995; Wu 1994). Additional data may be necessary to further define the role of dacarbazine in this condition.

Pancreatic neuroendocrine tumors, advanced (off-label use): IV: 850 mg/m^2 over 60 to 90 minutes on day 1 every 4 weeks (Ramanathan 2001).

Pheochromocytoma, malignant (off-label use): IV: 600 mg/m^2 once daily for 2 days every 3 or 4 weeks (in combination with cyclophosphamide and vincristine) (Huang 2008). Additional data may be necessary to further define the role of dacarbazine in this condition.

Soft tissue sarcoma, advanced (off-label use): MAID regimen: IV: 250 mg/m^2/day as a continuous infusion for 4 days every 3 weeks (total of 1,000 mg/m^2/cycle) (in combination with mesna, doxorubicin, and ifosfamide) (Antman 1993; Antman 1998).

Pediatric Note: Dacarbazine is associated with a high emetic potential; antiemetics are recommended to prevent nausea and vomiting (Dupuis 2011).

Hodgkin lymphoma: Children and Adolescents: ABVD regimen: IV: 375 mg/m^2 over 30 to 60 minutes on days 1 and 15 every 4 weeks (in combination with doxorubicin, bleomycin, and vinblastine) (Hutchinson 1998)

Renal Impairment There are no dosage adjustments provided in the manufacturer's labeling. The following adjustments have been recommended (Kintzel 1995):

CrCl 46 to 60 mL/minute: Reduce dose to 80% of usual dose

CrCl 31 to 45 mL/minute: Reduce dose to 75% of usual dose

CrCl ≤30 mL/minute: Reduce dose to 70% of usual dose

Hepatic Impairment There are no dosage adjustments provided in the manufacturer's labeling. May cause hepatotoxicity; monitor closely for signs of toxicity.

Obesity *ASCO Guidelines for appropriate chemotherapy dosing in obese adults with cancer:* Utilize patient's actual body weight (full weight) for calculation of body surface area- or weight-based dosing, particularly when the intent of therapy is curative; manage regimen-related toxicities in the same manner as for nonobese patients; if a dose reduction is utilized due to toxicity, consider resumption of full weight-based dosing with subsequent cycles, especially if cause of toxicity (eg, hepatic or renal impairment) is resolved (Griggs, 2012).

Combination Regimens

Lymphoma, Hodgkin:

Melanoma:

Soft tissue sarcoma:

Administration Dacarbazine is associated with a high emetic potential; antiemetics are recommended to prevent nausea and vomiting (Basch 2011; Dupuis 2011; Roila 2010).

Infuse over 15 to 60 minutes; rapid infusion may cause severe venous irritation. Other infusion durations have been reported; refer to literature and/or regimen for infusion details (may vary by protocol).

Dacarbazine is an irritant; local reactions may occur (Perez Fidalgo 2012). Monitor infusion site.

Vesicant/Extravasation Risk Irritant

Emetic Potential Children and Adults: High (>90%)

Monitoring Parameters CBC with differential, liver function

Dosage Forms Excipient information presented when available (limited, particularly for generics); consult specific product labeling.

Solution Reconstituted, Intravenous:

Generic: 100 mg (1 ea); 200 mg (1 ea)

Solution Reconstituted, Intravenous [preservative free]:

Generic: 200 mg (1 ea)

Dosage Forms: Canada Information with regard to form, strength, and availability of products uniquely available in Canada but currently not available in the US. Refer also to Dosage Forms.

Excipient information presented when available (limited, particularly for generics); consult specific product labeling.

Solution Reconstituted, Intravenous:

Dacarbazine for injection, BP: 600 mg

◆ **Dacarbazine for Injection, BP (Can)** see Dacarbazine on page 494

◆ **Dacogen** see Decitabine on page 548

◆ **DACT** see DACTINomycin on page 499

DACTINomycin (dak ti noe MYE sin)

Related Information

Management of Chemotherapy-Induced Nausea and Vomiting in Adults on page 2253

Management of Drug Extravasations on page 2271

Safe Handling of Hazardous Drugs on page 2379

Brand Names: US Cosmegen

Brand Names: Canada Cosmegen

Index Terms ACT-D; Actinomycin; Actinomycin Cl; Actinomycin D; DACT

Pharmacologic Category Antineoplastic Agent, Antibiotic

Use

Ewing sarcoma: Treatment of Ewing sarcoma (as part of a combination chemotherapy and/or multimodality treatment regimen)

Gestational trophoblastic neoplasia: Treatment of gestational trophoblastic neoplasia (as a single agent or in combination with other chemotherapy agents)

Rhabdosarcoma: Treatment of childhood rhabdosarcoma (as part of a combination chemotherapy and/or multimodality treatment regimen)

Solid tumors: Palliative and/or adjunctive treatment of locally recurrent or locoregional solid malignancies (as a component of regional perfusion)

Testicular cancer, metastatic (nonseminomatous): Treatment of metastatic nonseminomatous testicular cancer

◀ **Wilms tumor:** Treatment of Wilms tumor (as part of a combination chemotherapy and/or multimodality treatment regimen)

Labeled Contraindications Hypersensitivity to dactinomycin or any component of the formulation; patients with concurrent or recent infection with chickenpox or herpes zoster

Pregnancy Considerations [US Boxed Warning]: Avoid exposure during pregnancy. Adverse effects have been observed in animal reproduction studies. Women of childbearing potential are advised not to become pregnant. When used for gestational trophoblastic neoplasm, unfavorable outcomes have been reported when subsequent pregnancies occur within 6 months of treatment. It is recommended to use effective contraception for 6 months to 1 year after therapy (Matsui 2004; Seckl 2013)

Breastfeeding Considerations It is not known if dactinomycin is excreted in human breast milk. According to the manufacturer labeling, due to the potential for serious adverse reactions in the nursing infant, the decision to discontinue dactinomycin or to discontinue breastfeeding during therapy should take into account the benefits of treatment to the mother.

Warnings/Precautions [US Boxed Warning]: Avoid inhalation of vapors or contact with skin, mucous membrane, or eyes; use caution for handling and administration. If accidental exposure occurs, immediately irrigate copiously for at least 15 minutes with water, saline, or balanced ophthalmic irrigation solution (eye exposure) and at least 15 minutes with water (skin exposure); prompt ophthalmic or medical consultation is also recommended. Contaminated clothing should be destroyed and shoes thoroughly cleaned prior to reuse.

Vesicant; ensure proper needle or catheter placement prior to and during infusion; avoid extravasation. **[US Boxed Warning]: Extremely corrosive to soft tissues; if extravasation occurs during IV use, severe damage to soft tissues will occur; has led to contracture of the arm (rare). Avoid exposure during pregnancy.** Recommended for IV administration only.

Leukopenia, thrombocytopenia, and anemia may occur. Onset may occur at 2 to 4 days following treatment course and may require 1 to 2 weeks to reach maximum severity. Discontinue treatment with severe myelosuppression. May cause hepatic sinusoidal obstruction syndrome (SOS; formerly called veno-occlusive liver disease); use with caution in hepatobiliary dysfunction. Monitor for signs or symptoms of hepatic SOS, including bilirubin >1.4 mg/dL, unexplained weight gain, ascites, hepatomegaly, or unexplained right upper quadrant pain (Arndt, 2004). The risk of fatal SOS is increased in children <4 years of age.

Dactinomycin potentiates the effects of radiation therapy; use with caution in patients who have received radiation therapy; reduce dosages in patients who are receiving dactinomycin and radiation therapy simultaneously; combination with radiation therapy may result in increased toxicity (eg, GI toxicity, myelosuppression, severe oropharyngeal mucositis). Avoid dactinomycin use within 2 months of radiation treatment for right-sided Wilms' tumor, may increase the risk of hepatotoxicity.

Dactinomycin is associated with a high emetic potential; antiemetics are recommended to prevent nausea and vomiting (Basch, 2011; Dupuis, 2011). Discontinue treatment if diarrhea or stomatitis occur. Long-term observation of cancer survivors is recommended due to the increased risk of second primary tumors following treatment with radiation and antineoplastic agents. Regional perfusion therapy may result in local limb edema, soft tissue damage, and possible venous thrombosis; leakage of dactinomycin into systemic circulation may result in hematologic toxicity, infection, impaired wound healing, and mucositis. Dosage is usually expressed in **MICRO**grams and should be calculated on the basis of body surface area (BSA) in obese or edematous adult patients (to relate dose to lean body mass). Avoid administration of live vaccines during dactinomycin treatment. Avoid use in infants <6 months of age (toxic effects may occur more frequently). May be associated with an increased risk of myelosuppression in the elderly; use with caution. **[US Boxed Warning]: Should be administered under the supervision of an experienced cancer chemotherapy physician.** Potentially significant drug-drug interactions may exist, requiring dose or frequency adjustment, additional monitoring, and/or selection of alternative therapy.

Adverse Reactions Frequency not defined.

Cardiovascular: Hepatic sinusoidal obstruction syndrome (formerly known as hepatic veno-occlusive disease)

Central nervous system: Fatigue, lethargy, malaise

Dermatologic: Acne vulgaris, alopecia (reversible), cheilitis, dermal ulcer (following extravasation), epidermolysis, erythema (of previously irradiated skin), erythema multiforme, exfoliation of skin, localized erythema, skin pigmentation (of previously irradiated skin), skin rash, Stevens-Johnson syndrome, toxic epidermal necrolysis

Endocrine & metabolic: Growth suppression, hyperuricemia, hypocalcemia

Gastrointestinal: Abdominal pain, anorexia, diarrhea, dysphagia, esophagitis, gastrointestinal ulcer, mucositis, nausea, proctitis, stomatitis, vomiting

Hematologic & oncologic: Agranulocytosis, anemia, aplastic anemia, bone marrow depression (onset: 7 days; nadir: 14 to 21 days; recovery: 21 to 28 days), febrile neutropenia, leukopenia, neutropenia, pancytopenia, reticulocytopenia, thrombocytopenia, thrombocytopenia (immune-mediated)

Hepatic: Abnormal hepatic function tests, ascites, hepatic failure, hepatitis, hepatomegaly, hepatopathy thrombocytopenia syndrome, hepatotoxicity, increased serum bilirubin

Hypersensitivity: Anaphylactoid reaction

Infection: Infection, sepsis (including neutropenic sepsis)

Local: Localized edema, local pain

Neuromuscular & skeletal: Myalgia

Renal: Renal function abnormality

Respiratory: Pharyngitis, pneumonitis

Miscellaneous: Fever, tissue necrosis

Drug Interactions

Metabolism/Transport Effects None known.

Avoid Concomitant Use

Avoid concomitant use of DACTINomycin with any of the following: BCG (Intravesical); Deferiprone; Dipyrone; Natalizumab; Pimecrolimus; Tacrolimus (Topical); Vaccines (Live)

Increased Effect/Toxicity

DACTINomycin may increase the levels/effects of: CloZAPine; Deferiprone; Fingolimod; Leflunomide; Natalizumab; Tofacitinib; Vaccines (Live)

The levels/effects of DACTINomycin may be increased by: Denosumab; Dipyrone; Ocrelizumab; Palifermin; Pimecrolimus; Promazine; Roflumilast; Tacrolimus (Topical); Trastuzumab

Decreased Effect

DACTINomycin may decrease the levels/effects of: BCG (Intravesical); Coccidioides immitis Skin Test; Lenograstim; Nivolumab; Sipuleucel-T; Tertomotide; Vaccines (Inactivated); Vaccines (Live)

The levels/effects of DACTINomycin may be decreased by: Echinacea

Hazardous Drugs Handling Considerations

Hazardous agent (NIOSH 2016 [group 1]).

Use appropriate precautions for receiving, handling, administration, and disposal. Gloves (single) should be worn during receiving, unpacking, and placing in storage.

NIOSH recommends double gloving, a protective gown, ventilated engineering controls (a class II biological safety cabinet or a compounding aseptic containment isolator), and closed system transfer devices (CSTDs) for preparation. Double gloving, a gown, and (if dosage form allows) CSTDs are required during administration (NIOSH 2016).

Storage/Stability Store at 20°C to 25°C (68°F to 77°F). Protect from light and humidity. According to the manufacturer's labeling, recommended final concentrations (≥10 mcg/mL) in D5W or NS are stable for 10 hours at room temperature but should be administered within 4 hours due to the lack of preservative.

Preparation for Administration Reconstitute initially with 1.1 mL of preservative-free SWFI to yield a concentration of 500 mcg/mL (diluent containing preservatives will cause precipitation). May further dilute in D5W or NS in glass or polyvinyl chloride (PVC) containers to a recommended concentration of ≥10 mcg/mL; final concentrations <10 mcg/mL are not recommended. Cellulose ester membrane filters may partially remove dactinomycin from solution and should not be used during preparation or administration.

Mechanism of Action Binds to the guanine portion of DNA intercalating between guanine and cytosine base pairs inhibiting DNA and RNA synthesis and protein synthesis

Pharmacodynamics/Kinetics

Distribution: Children: Extensive extravascular distribution (59 to 714 L) (Veal 2005); does not penetrate blood-brain barrier

Metabolism: Minimal

Half-life elimination: ~36 hours; Children: Range: 14 to 43 hours (Veal 2005)

Excretion: ~30% in urine and feces within 1 week

Dosing

Adult Note: Medication orders for dactinomycin are commonly written in MICROgrams (eg, 150 mcg) although many regimens list the dose in MILLIgrams (eg, mg/kg or mg/m²). The dose intensity per 2-week cycle should not exceed 15 mcg/kg/day for 5 days or 400 to 600 mcg/m²/day for 5 days. The manufacturer recommends calculation of the dosage for obese or edematous adult patients on the basis of body surface area in an effort to relate dosage to lean body mass. Dactinomycin is associated with a high emetic potential; antiemetics are recommended to prevent nausea and vomiting (Basch, 2011).

Ewing sarcoma: IV: 15 mcg/kg/day for 5 days (in various combination regimens and schedules)

Off-label dosing: VAIA regimen: Adults ≤35 years: IV: 500 mcg/m²/dose for 3 days (dactinomycin alternates with doxorubicin) every 3 weeks for 14 cycles (in combination with vincristine, ifosfamide, and mesna) (Paulussen 2008)

Gestational trophoblastic neoplasm: IV: 12 mcg/kg/day for 5 days (as a single agent) **or** 500 mcg/dose on days 1 and 2 (in combination with etoposide, methotrexate, leucovorin, vincristine, cyclophosphamide, and cisplatin) **or** (off-label dosing for low-risk disease) 1.25 **mg**/m² every 2 weeks as a single agent (Osborne 2011)

Rhabdomyosarcoma: IV: 15 mcg/kg/day for 5 days (in various combination regimens and schedules)

Testicular cancer, metastatic (nonseminomatous): IV: 1,000 mcg/m² on day 1 (in combination with cyclophosphamide, bleomycin, cisplatin, and vinblastine)

Wilms tumor: IV: 15 mcg/kg/day for 5 days (in various combination regimens and schedules)

Regional perfusion in solid tumors (dosages and techniques may vary by institution; obese patients and patients with prior chemotherapy or radiation therapy may require lower doses): Lower extremity or pelvis: 50 mcg/kg; Upper extremity: 35 mcg/kg

Osteosarcoma (off-label use): IV: 600 mcg/m² on days 1, 2, and 3 of weeks 15, 31, 34, 39, and 42 (as part of a combination chemotherapy regimen including cyclophosphamide, bleomycin, methotrexate [high dose], leucovorin, doxorubicin, and cisplatin; refer to protocol for specific details) (Goorin 2003)

Ovarian germ cell tumors, malignant (off-label use): IV: 500 mcg daily for 5 days every 4 weeks (in combination with vincristine and cyclophosphamide) (Gershenson 1985) **or** 300 mcg/m²/day for 5 days every 4 weeks (in combination with vincristine and cyclophosphamide) (Slayton 1985)

Soft tissue sarcoma of the extremities, locally advanced/unresectable (off-label use): Isolated limb infusion (ILI) protocol: 50 to 100 mcg/L of tissue in 400 mL warmed, heparinized NS (in combination with melphalan) over 20 to 30 minutes (Moncrieff 2008). Additional data may be necessary to further define the role of dactinomycin in the treatment of this condition.

Geriatric Refer to adult dosing. Elderly patients are at increased risk of myelosuppression; dosing should begin at the low end of the dosing range.

Pediatric Note: Medication orders for dactinomycin are commonly written in MICROgrams (eg, 150 mcg) although many regimens list the dose in MILLIgrams (eg, mg/kg or mg/m²). The dose intensity per 2-week cycle should not exceed 15 mcg/kg/day for 5 days or 400 to 600 mcg/m²/day for 5 days. Dactinomycin is associated with a high emetic potential; antiemetics are recommended to prevent nausea and vomiting (Dupuis 2011).

Ewing sarcoma: Children >6 months: IV: 15 mcg/kg/day for 5 days (in various combination regimens and schedules)

Off-label dosing: VAIA regimen: IV: 500 mcg/m²/dose for 3 days (dactinomycin alternates with doxorubicin) every 3 weeks for 14 cycles (in combination with vincristine, ifosfamide, and mesna) (Paulussen 2008)

Rhabdomyosarcoma: Children >6 months: IV: 15 mcg/kg/day for 5 days (in various combination regimens and schedules)

◀

Off-label dosing: IV:
  VAC regimen:
    Children <1 year: 25 mcg/kg every 3 weeks, weeks 0 to 45 (in combination with vincristine and cyclophosphamide, and mesna); dose omission required following radiation therapy (Raney 2011)
    Children ≥1 year: 45 mcg/kg (maximum dose: 2,500 mcg) every 3 weeks, weeks 0 to 45 (in combination with vincristine and cyclophosphamide, and mesna); dose omission required following radiation therapy (Raney 2011)
Wilms tumor: Children >6 months: IV: 15 mcg/kg/day for 5 days (in various combination regimens and schedules)
Off-label dosing: IV:
  DD-4A regimen: 45 mcg/kg on day 1 every 6 weeks for 54 weeks (in combination with doxorubicin and vincristine) (Green 1998)
  EE-4A regimen: 45 mcg/kg on day 1 every 3 weeks for 18 weeks (in combination with vincristine) (Green 1998)
  VAD regimen:
    Children <1 year: 750 mcg/m^2 every 6 weeks for 1 year (stage III disease) (in combination with vincristine and doxorubicin) (Pritchard 1995)
    Children ≥1 year: 1500 mcg/m^2 every 6 weeks for 1 year (stage III disease) (in combination with vincristine and doxorubicin) (Pritchard 1995)
Osteosarcoma (off-label use): IV: 600 mcg/m^2 on days 1, 2, and 3 of weeks 15, 31, 34, 39, and 42 (as part of a combination chemotherapy regimen including cyclophosphamide, bleomycin, methotrexate [high dose], leucovorin, doxorubicin, and cisplatin; refer to protocol for specific details) (Goorin 2003)

Renal Impairment There are no dosage adjustments provided in the manufacturer's labeling; however, based on the amount of urinary excretion, dosage adjustments may not be necessary.

Hepatic Impairment
  There are no dosage adjustments provided in manufacturer's labeling.
  The following adjustments have also been recommended: Any transaminase increase: Reduce dose by 50%; may increase by monitoring toxicities (Floyd 2006).

Obesity *ASCO Guidelines for appropriate chemotherapy dosing in obese adults with cancer:* Utilize patient's actual body weight (full weight) for calculation of body surface area- or weight-based dosing, particularly when the intent of therapy is curative; manage regimen-related toxicities in the same manner as for nonobese patients; if a dose reduction is utilized due to toxicity, consider resumption of full weight-based dosing with subsequent cycles, especially if cause of toxicity (eg, hepatic or renal impairment) is resolved (Griggs 2012).

Adjustment for Toxicity Severe myelosuppression, stomatitis, or diarrhea: Interrupt therapy until toxicity has resolved.

Combination Regimens
  Bone sarcoma (Ewing sarcoma): VAC Alternating With IE (Ewing Sarcoma) on page 2224
  Gestational trophoblastic tumor:
    EMA/CO (Gestational Trophoblastic Tumor) on page 2101
    EMA/EP (Gestational Trophoblastic Tumor) on page 2101
    EMA (Gestational Trophoblastic Tumor) on page 2102

Administration Dactinomycin is associated with a high emetic potential; antiemetics are recommended to prevent nausea and vomiting (Basch 2011, Dupuis 2011).

For IV administration; do not administer IM or SubQ. Administer by slow IV push or infuse over 10 to 15 minutes. Do not filter with cellulose ester membrane filters.

Regional perfusion: Technique may vary by institution; consult protocol for details. Local reactions including epidermolysis, erythema, and edema have been reported (may be severe).

Vesicant; ensure proper needle or catheter placement prior to and during infusion; avoid extravasation.

Extravasation management: If extravasation occurs, stop infusion immediately and disconnect (leave cannula/needle in place); gently aspirate extravasated solution (do **NOT** flush the line); remove needle/cannula; elevate extremity. Apply dry cold compresses for 20 minutes 4 times a day for 1-2 days (Perez Fildago 2012).

Vesicant/Extravasation Risk Vesicant

Emetic Potential Children and Adults: High (>90%)

Monitoring Parameters CBC with differential and platelet count, liver function tests, and renal function tests; monitor for signs/symptoms of hepatic SOS, including unexplained weight gain, ascites, hepatomegaly, or unexplained right upper quadrant pain (Arndt, 2004)

Test Interactions May interfere with bioassays of antibacterial drug levels

Dosage Forms Excipient information presented when available (limited, particularly for generics); consult specific product labeling.
Solution Reconstituted, Intravenous:
Cosmegen: 0.5 mg (1 ea)

Dalteparin (dal TE pa rin)

Brand Names: US Fragmin
Brand Names: Canada Fragmin
Index Terms Dalteparin Sodium
Pharmacologic Category Anticoagulant; Anticoagulant, Low Molecular Weight Heparin
Use

Deep vein thrombosis prophylaxis: Prevention of deep vein thrombosis (DVT) which may lead to pulmonary embolism (PE), in patients requiring abdominal surgery who are at risk for thromboembolism complications (eg, >40 years, obesity, malignancy, history of DVT or PE, surgical procedures requiring general anesthesia lasting >30 minutes); patients undergoing hip-replacement surgery; or in patients who are at risk for thromboembolism complications due to severe immobility during an acute illness.

Unstable angina/non-Q-wave myocardial infarction: Prevention of ischemic complications in patients with unstable angina or non-Q-wave myocardial infarction on concurrent aspirin therapy.

Venous thromboembolism, extended treatment in cancer patients: Extended treatment (6 months) of acute symptomatic venous thromboembolism (DVT and/or PE) to reduce the recurrence of venous thromboembolism in cancer patients.

Dosing

Adult & Geriatric Note: Each 2,500 units of anti-Xa activity is equal to dalteparin 16 mg.

DVT prophylaxis: Note: In morbidly obese patients (BMI ≥40 kg/m^2), increasing the prophylactic dose by 30% may be appropriate (Nutescu 2009):

Abdominal surgery:

Low-to-moderate DVT risk: SubQ: 2,500 units 1 to 2 hours prior to surgery, then 2,500 units once daily for 5 to 10 days postoperatively.

High DVT risk: SubQ: 5,000 units the evening prior to surgery and then 5,000 units once daily for 5 to 10 days postoperatively. Alternatively in patients with malignancy: 2,500 units 1 to 2 hours prior to surgery, 2,500 units 12 hours later, then 5,000 units once daily for 5 to 10 days postoperatively.

Total hip replacement surgery: SubQ: **Note:** Three treatment options are currently available. Dose is usually given for 5 to 10 days, although up to 14 days of treatment have been tolerated in clinical trials. The American College of Chest Physicians (ACCP) recommends a minimum duration of at least 10 to 14 days; extended duration of up to 35 days is suggested (Guyatt 2012).

Postoperative regimen:

Initial: 2,500 units 4 to 8 hours after surgery (or later if hemostasis not achieved). The ACCP recommends initiation ≥12 hours after surgery if postoperative regimen chosen (Guyatt 2012).

Maintenance: 5,000 units once daily; allow at least 6 hours to elapse after initial postsurgical dose (adjust administration time accordingly).

Preoperative regimen (starting day of surgery):

Initial: 2,500 units within 2 hours **before** surgery. The ACCP recommends initiation ≥12 hours before surgery if preoperative regimen chosen (Guyatt 2012). At 4 to 8 hours **after** surgery (or later if hemostasis not achieved), administer 2,500 units.

Maintenance: 5,000 units once daily; allow at least 6 hours to elapse after initial postsurgical dose (adjust administration time accordingly).

Preoperative regimen (starting evening prior to surgery):

Initial: 5,000 units 10 to 14 hours **before** surgery. The ACCP recommends initiation ≥12 hours before surgery if preoperative regimen chosen (Guyatt 2012). At 4 to 8 hours **after** surgery (or later if hemostasis not achieved), administer 5,000 units.

Maintenance: 5,000 units once daily, allowing 24 hours between doses.

Immobility during acute illness: SubQ: 5,000 units once daily; in clinical trials, the usual duration of therapy was 12 to 14 days.

Unstable angina or non-Q-wave myocardial infarction: SubQ: 120 units/ kg (maximum dose: 10,000 units) every 12 hours with concurrent aspirin therapy. Discontinue dalteparin once patient is clinically stable; usual duration of therapy is 5 to 8 days.

Obesity: Use actual body weight to calculate dose; dose capping at 10,000 units recommended (Nutescu 2009)

Venous thromboembolism, extended treatment in cancer patients: SubQ:

Initial (month 1): 200 units/kg (maximum dose: 18,000 units) once daily for 30 days.

Maintenance (months 2 to 6): ~150 units/kg (maximum dose: 18,000 units) once daily. If platelet count between 50,000 to 100,000/mm^3, reduce dose by 2,500 units until platelet count recovers to ≥100,000/mm^3. If platelet count <50,000/mm^3, discontinue dalteparin until platelet count recover to >50,000/mm^3.

Obesity: Use actual body weight to calculate dose; dose capping is not recommended (Nutescu 2009). However, the manufacturer recommends a maximum dose of 18,000 units per day for the treatment of VTE in cancer patients.

Acute pulmonary embolism (noncancer-related) (off-label use): SubQ: 200 units/kg once daily (Kovacs 2000). **Note:** Start warfarin on the first treatment day and continue dalteparin until INR is ≥2 for at least 24 hours (usually 5 to 7 days) (ACCP [Guyatt 2012]).

Anticoagulant for hemodialysis and hemofiltration (off-label use): IV: (Fragmin Canadian product labeling 2016):

Chronic renal failure with no other bleeding risks:

Hemodialysis/filtration ≤4 hours: IV bolus: 5,000 units

Hemodialysis/filtration >4 hours: IV bolus: 30 to 40 units/kg, followed by an infusion of 10 to 15 units/kg/hour (typically produces plasma concentrations of 0.5 to 1 units anti-Xa/mL)

Acute renal failure and high bleeding risk: IV bolus: 5 to 10 units/kg, followed by an infusion of 4 to 5 units/kg/hour (typically produces plasma concentrations of 0.2 to 0.4 units anti-Xa/mL)

DVT (with or without PE; noncancer-related) treatment (off-label use): SubQ: 200 units/kg once daily (AHA [Jaff 2011]; Feissinger 1996; Wells 2005) or 100 units/kg twice daily (AHA [Jaff 2011]). **Note:** Use of once daily dalteparin dosing regimen is suggested. Start warfarin on the first treatment day and continue dalteparin until INR is ≥2 for at least 24 hours (usually 5 to 7 days) (ACCP [Guyatt 2012]).

Alternative recommendations (Fragmin Canadian product labeling 2016):

SubQ: 200 units/kg once daily (maximum dose: 18,000 units/day) **or** alternatively, may adapt dose as follows (SubQ):

46 to 56 kg: 10,000 units once daily

57 to 68 kg: 12,500 units once daily

69 to 82 kg: 15,000 units once daily

≥83 kg: 18,000 units once daily

IV (patients with increased bleeding risk): 100 units/kg as continuous infusion over 12 hours may be considered.

Obesity: Use actual body weight to calculate dose; dose capping is not recommended (Nutescu 2009). One study demonstrated similar anti-Xa levels after 3 days of therapy in obese patients (>40% above IBW; range: 82 to 190 kg) compared to those ≤20% above IBW or between 20% to 40% above IBW (Wilson 2001).

Pregnant women (off-label use): 200 units/kg/dose once daily or 100 units/kg/dose every 12 hours. Discontinue ≥24 hours prior to the induction of labor or cesarean section. Dalteparin therapy may be substituted with heparin near term. Continue anticoagulation therapy for ≥6 weeks postpartum (minimum duration of therapy: 3 months). LMWH or heparin therapy is preferred over warfarin during pregnancy (Bates 2012).

General surgery with risk factors for VTE (off-label use): SubQ: 2,500 units 1 to 2 hours preoperatively followed by 2,500 to 5,000 units every morning (may administer 2,500 units no sooner than 4 hours after surgery and 8 hours after previous dose provided hemostasis has been achieved) or if other risk factors are present (eg, malignancy, heart failure), then may administer 5,000 units the evening prior to surgery followed by 5,000 units every evening postoperatively; continue treatment until patient is mobilized (approximately ≥5 to 7 days) (Fragmin Canadian product labeling 2016).

Mechanical heart valve (aortic or mitral position) to bridge anticoagulation (off-label use): SubQ: 100 units/kg/dose every 12 hours (ACCP [Douketis 2012]). **Note:** If used in pregnant patients, target anti-Xa level of 0.8 to 1.2 units/mL, 4 to 6 hours postdose (AHA/ACC [Nishimura 2014]).

Prevention of recurrent venous thromboembolism in pregnancy (off-label use): SubQ: 5,000 units once daily. Therapy should continue for 6 weeks postpartum in high-risk women (Bates 2012).

Conversion:

Conversion from IV unfractionated heparin (UFH) infusion to SubQ dalteparin (Nutescu 2007): Calculate specific dose for dalteparin based on indication, discontinue UFH and begin dalteparin within 1 hour

Conversion from SubQ dalteparin (therapeutically dosed) to IV UFH infusion (Nutescu 2007): **Note:** The following recommendations are based on use of therapeutic doses of dalteparin (eg, 100 units/kg twice daily). If converting from a prophylactic dalteparin dose (eg, 5,000 units once daily) to a therapeutic IV UFH dose, there should not be any delay in starting the IV UFH infusion and may include an UFH bolus/loading dose, when indicated.

Discontinue dalteparin, calculate specific dose for IV UFH infusion based on indication, omit UFH bolus/loading dose

Converting from SubQ dalteparin dosed every 12 hours: Start IV UFH infusion 10 to 11 hours after last dose of dalteparin

Converting from SubQ dalteparin dosed every 24 hours: Start IV UFH infusion 22 to 23 hours after last dose of dalteparin

Renal Impairment

There are no dosage adjustments provided in the manufacturer's labeling. Use with caution in severe renal impairment; accumulation may occur with repeated dosing, increasing the risk for bleeding. Accumulation was not observed in critically ill patients with severe renal insufficiency (CrCl <30 mL/minute) receiving prophylactic doses (5,000 units/day) for a median of 7 days (Douketis 2008). In cancer patients, receiving treatment for venous thromboembolism, if CrCl <30 mL/minute, manufacturer recommends monitoring anti-Xa levels to determine appropriate dose.

Hemodialysis: Not dialyzable (NCS/SCCM [Frontera 2016])

Hepatic Impairment There are no dosage adjustments provided in the manufacturer's labeling. Use with caution in patients with severe hepatic impairment; accumulation may occur with repeated dosing, increasing the risk for bleeding.

Obesity Refer to indication-specific dosing for obesity-related information (may not be available for all indications).

Additional Information Complete prescribing information should be consulted for additional detail.

Dosage Forms Excipient information presented when available (limited, particularly for generics); consult specific product labeling. [DSC] = Discontinued product

Solution, Subcutaneous:
  Fragmin: 25,000 units/mL (3.8 mL [DSC]); 95,000 units/3.8 mL (3.8 mL) [contains benzyl alcohol]

Solution, Subcutaneous [preservative free]:
  Fragmin: 10,000 units/mL (1 mL); 2500 units/0.2 mL (0.2 mL); 5000 units/0.2 mL (0.2 mL); 7500 units/0.3 mL (0.3 mL); 12,500 units/0.5 mL (0.5 mL); 15,000 units/0.6 mL (0.6 mL); 18,000 units/0.72 mL (0.72 mL)

◆ **Dalteparin Sodium** see Dalteparin on page 505

Daratumumab (dar a TOOM ue mab)

Brand Names: US Darzalex
Brand Names: Canada Darzalex
Index Terms JNJ-54767414
Pharmacologic Category Antineoplastic Agent, Anti-CD38; Antineoplastic Agent, Monoclonal Antibody

Use Multiple myeloma, relapsed/refractory:
  Treatment of multiple myeloma (in combination with dexamethasone and either lenalidomide or bortezomib) in patients who have received at least one prior therapy.
  Treatment of multiple myeloma (in combination with dexamethasone and pomalidomide) in patients who have received at least two prior therapies, including lenalidomide and a proteasome inhibitor.
  Treatment of multiple myeloma (as monotherapy) in patients who have received at least 3 prior lines of therapy, including a proteasome inhibitor and an immunomodulatory agent or who are double refractory to a proteasome inhibitor and an immunomodulatory agent.

Labeled Contraindications
  There are no contraindications listed in the manufacturer's US labeling.
  Canadian labeling: Hypersensitivity to daratumumab or any component of the formulation

Pregnancy Considerations Animal reproduction studies have not been conducted. Daratumumab is a monoclonal antibody; monoclonal antibodies are known to cross the placenta. Based on the mechanism of action, daratumumab may cause myeloid or lymphoid cell depletion and decreased bone density in the fetus. Females of reproduction potential should use effective contraception during therapy and for 3 months after treatment is complete. The administration of live vaccines should be deferred for neonates and infants exposed to daratumumab in utero until a hematology evaluation can be completed.

Breastfeeding Considerations It is not known if daratumumab is present in breast milk. Daratumumab is a monoclonal antibody; monoclonal antibodies can be detected in breast milk and are not expected to enter the neonatal or infant circulation in substantial amounts. According to the manufacturer, the decision to breastfeed during therapy should take into account the risk of exposure to the infant and the benefits of treatment to the mother.

◀ **Warnings/Precautions** Severe infusion reactions may occur (including bronchospasm, hypoxia, dyspnea, hypertension, laryngeal edema, and pulmonary edema), mostly during the first infusion. Signs and symptoms include cough, throat irritation, and nasal congestion, as well as chills, vomiting, and nausea. Less commonly reported symptoms include wheezing, allergic rhinitis, pyrexia, chest discomfort, pruritus, and hypotension. Infusion reactions were reported in approximately 50% of patients in clinical trials. Reactions may also be seen during subsequent infusions, and generally occur either during the infusion or within 4 hours of completion; some reactions occurred up to 48 hours after the infusion. Premedication with antihistamines, antipyretics, and corticosteroids is required; interrupt infusion for any reaction and manage as appropriate. Reduce the infusion rate for grade 1, 2, or 3 reaction; permanently discontinue therapy for grade 4 infusion reaction. Administer in a facility with immediate access to resuscitative measures (eg, glucocorticoids, epinephrine, bronchodilators, and/or oxygen). Administer oral corticosteroids to all patients after daratumumab infusion to reduce the risk of delayed infusion reactions. Also consider short- and long-acting bronchodilators and inhaled corticosteroids for patients with chronic obstructive pulmonary disease; monitor closely.

Daratumumab may increase neutropenia and thrombocytopenia when used in combination with other chemotherapy agents for the treatment of multiple myeloma. Lymphopenia, neutropenia, thrombocytopenia, and anemia (including grade 3 and 4 toxicity) were commonly reported as treatment emergent adverse reactions in clinical trials. Monitor for signs/symptoms of infection and bleeding. Monitor complete blood counts periodically; may require delay of daratumumab infusion to allow for neutrophil and/or platelet recovery. Supportive care with growth factors and/or platelet transfusions may be necessary. Daratumumab (a human IgG kappa monoclonal antibody) may be detected on serum protein electrophoresis and immunofixation assays which monitor for endogenous M-protein. Interference with these assays by daratumumab may affect the determination of complete response and disease progression in some patients with IgG kappa myeloma protein. Through binding to CD38 on red blood cells, daratumumab use may result in a positive indirect antiglobulin test (indirect Coombs test). Daratumumab-mediated Coombs test positivity may persist for up to 6 months after the last infusion. In addition, daratumumab (bound to red blood cells) masks antibody detection to minor antigens in the patient's serum; ABO and Rh blood type determination are not affected. Notify blood transfusion centers and blood banks that a patient has received daratumumab, and type and screen patients prior to therapy initiation. Potentially significant interactions may exist, requiring dose or frequency adjustment, additional monitoring, and/or selection of alternative therapy.

Adverse Reactions

>10%:

Central nervous system: Fatigue (39%), headache (12%)

Gastrointestinal: Nausea (27%), diarrhea (16%), constipation (15%), decreased appetite (15%), vomiting (14%)

Hematologic & oncologic: Lymphocytopenia (72%; grade: 3: 30%; grade 4: 10%), neutropenia (60%; grade 3: 17%; grade 4: 3%), thrombocytopenia (48%; grade 3: 10%; grade 4: 8%), anemia (45%; grade 3: 19%)

Neuromuscular & skeletal: Back pain (23%), arthralgia (17%), limb pain (15%), musculoskeletal chest pain (12%)

Respiratory: Cough (21%), upper respiratory tract infection (20%), nasal congestion (17%), dyspnea (15%), nasopharyngitis (15%), pneumonia (6% to 11%)

Miscellaneous: Infusion related reaction (48%), fever (3% to 21%)

1% to 10%:

Cardiovascular: Hypertension (10%)

Central nervous system: Chills (10%)

Infection: Herpes zoster (3%)

Miscellaneous: Physical health deterioration (3%)

Drug Interactions

Metabolism/Transport Effects None known.

Avoid Concomitant Use

Avoid concomitant use of Daratumumab with any of the following: BCG (Intravesical); Deferiprone; Dipyrone

Increased Effect/Toxicity

Daratumumab may increase the levels/effects of: CloZAPine; Deferiprone

The levels/effects of Daratumumab may be increased by: Dipyrone; Promazine

Decreased Effect

Daratumumab may decrease the levels/effects of: BCG (Intravesical)

Storage/Stability
Store intact vials at 2°C to 8°C (36°F to 46°F). Do not freeze or shake; protect from light. Solutions diluted for infusion should be administered immediately at room temperature and in room light; diluted solution may be kept at room temperature for a maximum of 15 hours (including infusion time). If not used immediately, solutions diluted for infusion may be stored for up to 24 hours at 2°C to 8°C (36°F to 46°F) and protected from light; do not freeze. Discard any unused portion of the solution.

Preparation for Administration
Determine the appropriate dose and volume of daratumumab required (based on patient's actual body weight); daratumumab should be colorless to pale yellow (do not use if opaque particles, discoloration, or other foreign particles are observed). Remove the volume of 0.9% sodium chloride injection from the infusion bag that is equal to the required volume of the daratumumab dose. Add the appropriate daratumumab volume to a 1,000 mL (first infusion) or 500 mL (subsequent infusions) 0.9% sodium chloride bag; gently invert to mix (do not shake). Infusion bags/containers must be made of polyvinylchloride (PVC), polypropylene (PP), polyethylene (PE), or polyolefin blend (PP+PE). If the diluted solution is refrigerated prior to use, allow to come to room temperature before administration. After dilution, may develop very small translucent to white proteinaceous particles; do not use if discolored or if visibly opaque or foreign particles are observed.

Mechanism of Action
Daratumumab is an IgG1κ human monoclonal antibody directed against CD38. CD38 is a cell surface glycoprotein which is highly expressed on myeloma cells, yet is expressed at low levels on normal lymphoid and myeloid cells (Lokhorst 2015). By binding to CD38, daratumumab inhibits the growth of CD38 expressing tumor cells by inducing apoptosis directly through Fc mediated cross linking as well as by immune-mediated tumor cell lysis through complement dependent cytotoxicity, antibody dependent cell mediated cytotoxicity, and antibody dependent cellular phagocytosis.

Pharmacodynamics/Kinetics

Distribution: Central: Monotherapy: 4.7 ± 1.3 L; Combination therapy: 4.4 ± 1.5 L

◀ Half-life elimination: Monotherapy: 18 ± 9 days; Combination therapy: 23 ± 12 days

Dosing

Adult & Geriatric Note: Premedicate approximately 1 to 3 hours prior to infusion with a corticosteroid, an oral antipyretic, and an oral or IV antihistamine (see Premedications below). Post-infusion, administer an oral corticosteroid to all patients to reduce the risk of delayed infusion reactions (see Post-infusion medications below). To prevent herpes zoster reactivation, initiate antiviral prophylaxis within 1 week after starting daratumumab and continue for 3 months following completion of treatment. Per the manufacturer, daratumumab dosing should be based on actual body weight.

Multiple myeloma, relapsed/refractory: Adults: IV: **Note:** Refer to specific protocol or to dexamethasone and lenalidomide, bortezomib, or pomalidomide monographs for dosing when used in combination with daratumumab.
Monotherapy:
  Weeks 1 to 8: 16 mg/kg once weekly for 8 doses
  Weeks 9 to 24: 16 mg/kg once every 2 weeks for 8 doses
  Weeks 25 and beyond: 16 mg/kg once every 4 weeks until disease progression
In combination with lenalidomide and low-dose dexamethasone (Dimopoulos 2016):
  Weeks 1 to 8: 16 mg/kg once weekly for 8 doses
  Weeks 9 to 24: 16 mg/kg once every 2 weeks for 8 doses
  Weeks 25 and beyond: 16 mg/kg once every 4 weeks until disease progression
In combination with pomalidomide and low-dose dexamethasone (Chari 2017):
  Weeks 1 to 8: 16 mg/kg once weekly for 8 doses
  Weeks 9 to 24: 16 mg/kg once every 2 weeks for 8 doses
  Weeks 25 and beyond: 16 mg/kg once every 4 weeks until disease progression
In combination with bortezomib and dexamethasone (Palumbo 2016):
  Weeks 1 to 9: 16 mg/kg once weekly for 9 doses
  Weeks 10 to 24: 16 mg/kg once every 3 weeks for 5 doses
  Weeks 25 and beyond: 16 mg/kg once every 4 weeks until disease progression
Missed dose: If a dose is missed, administer as soon as possible and adjust the schedule accordingly (maintain the treatment interval).

Premedications: Administer 1 to 3 hours prior to each infusion
Corticosteroid:
  Monotherapy: Methylprednisolone 100 mg IV or equivalent intermediate- or long-acting corticosteroid; following the second infusion, the dose may be decreased (eg, methylprednisolone 60 mg [IV or oral] or equivalent)
  Combination therapy: Dexamethasone 20 mg prior to each infusion; administer IV prior to the first infusion; oral administration may be considered prior to subsequent infusions **plus**
Antipyretic: Oral: Acetaminophen 650 to 1,000 mg **plus**
Antihistamine: IV or Oral: Diphenhydramine 25 to 50 mg or equivalent

The following premedication regimen has also been reported (Hofmeister 2016):

First infusion: Acetaminophen 325 mg orally, diphenhydramine 25 mg orally or IV, dexamethasone 20 mg IV, montelukast 10 mg orally, and famotidine 20 mg IV.

Subsequent infusions: Acetaminophen 325 mg orally, diphenhydramine 25 mg IV, and dexamethasone 20 mg IV.

Post-infusion medication:

Monotherapy: Administer an oral intermediate- or long-acting corticosteroid (eg, methylprednisolone 20 mg or equivalent) on the first and second day after all infusions.

Combination therapy: Consider administering low-dose oral methylprednisolone (20 mg or less) or equivalent on the first day after the infusion. If dexamethasone is administered the day after the infusion as part of combination chemotherapy, additional post-infusion corticosteroid therapy may not be necessary.

In patients with a history of chronic obstructive pulmonary disease, also consider short- and long-acting bronchodilators and inhaled corticosteroids post-infusion. If no major infusion reactions occur during the first 4 infusions, these additional inhaled post-infusion medications may be discontinued.

Renal Impairment CrCl 15 to 89 mL/minute: There are no dosage adjustments provided in the manufacturer's labeling; however, CrCl between 15 to 89 mL/minute did not have any meaningful effect on daratumumab pharmacokinetics.

Hepatic Impairment

Mild (total bilirubin 1 to 1.5 times ULN and any ALT) or moderate (total bilirubin 1.5 to 3 times ULN and any ALT) impairment: There are no dosage adjustments provided in the manufacturer's labeling, however, mild or moderate impairment did not have any meaningful effect on daratumumab pharmacokinetics.

Severe impairment (total bilirubin >3 times ULN and any ALT): There are no dosage adjustments provided in the manufacturer's labeling (has not been studied).

Adjustment for Toxicity Note: Refer to specific protocol or to dexamethasone and lenalidomide, bortezomib, or pomalidomide monographs for dosing adjustment for toxicity when used in combination with daratumumab.

Hematologic toxicity: No dose reductions of daratumumab are recommended; delay of daratumumab infusion may be required to allow for neutrophil and/or platelet recovery. Supportive care with growth factors and/or platelet transfusions may be necessary.

Infusion reactions: Immediately interrupt infusion for reaction of any severity. Manage symptoms as clinically appropriate.

Grade 1 or 2 (mild to moderate) infusion reaction: Once symptoms resolve, resume the infusion at no more than 50% of the rate at which the reaction occurred. If no further reactions are observed, may escalate the infusion rate as appropriate up to the maximum rate of 200 mL/hour (see Administration).

Grade 3 (severe) infusion reaction: Once symptoms resolve, consider resuming the infusion at no more than 50% of the rate at which the reaction occurred. If no further reactions are observed, may escalate the infusion rate as appropriate (see Administration). If a grade 3 reaction recurs, repeat

◀ the steps above. Permanently discontinue if a grade 3 infusion reaction occurs for the third time.

Grade 4 (life-threatening) infusion reaction: Permanently discontinue.

Combination Regimens

Multiple myeloma:

Daratumumab-Bortezomib-Dexamethasone (Multiple Myeloma) on page 2083

Daratumumab-Lenalidomide-Dexamethasone (Multiple Myeloma) on page 2084

Daratumumab-Pomalidomide-Dexamethasone (Multiple Myeloma) on page 2085

Administration

For IV infusion only. Do not administer IV push or as a bolus. Premedicate with a corticosteroid, acetaminophen, and an IV or oral antihistamine (see Dosing) approximately 1 to 3 hours prior to administration. Infuse in an environment equipped to monitor for and manage infusion reactions. Administer with an infusion set fitted with a flow regulator and with an inline, sterile, non-pyrogenic, low protein-binding polyethersulfone filter (0.22 or 0.2 micrometer). Polyurethane, polybutadiene, polyvinylchloride, polypropylene, or polyethylene administration sets are required. Do not mix with or infuse with other medications.

Do not exceed infusion rates below. Begin infusion immediately after infusion bag reaches room temperature (if refrigerated). Infusion should be completed within 15 hours. Interrupt infusion for any severity of infusion reaction; if the reaction resolves, may resume infusion (see Dosing: Adjustment for Toxicity). If infusion cannot be completed, do not save unused portion for reuse. Post-infusion, administer an oral corticosteroid to all patients to reduce the risk of delayed infusion reactions (see Dosing). In patients with a history of obstructive pulmonary disorder, consider short- and long-acting bronchodilators and inhaled corticosteroids post-infusion.

Infusion rate:

First infusion (1,000 mL volume): Infuse at 50 mL/hour for the first hour. If no infusion reactions occur, may increase the rate by 50 mL/hour every hour (maximum rate: 200 mL/hour).

Second infusion (500 mL volume): Use a dilution volume of 500 mL only if there were no grade 1 or greater infusion reactions during the first 3 hours of the first infusion. Otherwise, continue to use a dilution volume of 1,000 mL and instructions for the first infusion. Infuse at 50 mL/hour for the first hour. If no infusion reactions occur, may increase the rate by 50 mL/hour every hour (maximum rate: 200 mL/hour).

Subsequent infusions (500 mL volume): Use a modified initial rate for subsequent infusions (ie, third infusion onwards) only if there were no grade 1 or greater infusion reactions during a final infusion rate of ≥100 mL/hour in the first 2 infusions. Otherwise, continue to use instructions for the second infusion. Infuse at 100 mL/hour for the first hour. If no infusion reactions occur, may increase the rate by 50 mL/hour every hour (maximum rate: 200 mL/hour).

Emetic Potential Minimal (<10%)

Monitoring Parameters

Complete blood cell counts periodically; type and screen (blood type) prior to initiating therapy; signs/symptoms of infusion reactions.

Test Interactions Daratumumab binds to CD38 on red blood cells and results in a positive indirect antiglobulin test (Coombs test), which may persist for up to 6 months after the last infusion. Daratumumab may also mask antibody detection to minor antigens in the patient's serum. Mitigation methods include treating reagent red blood cells with dithiothreitol (DTT) to disrupt daratumumab binding or genotyping. As the Kell blood group system is also sensitive to DTT, K-negative units should be supplied after ruling out or identifying alloantibodies using DTT-treated red blood cells.

Daratumumab may be detected on both serum protein electrophoresis and immunofixation assays used for multiple myeloma endogenous M-protein monitoring, and may affect the determination of complete response and disease progression of some patients with IgG kappa myeloma protein. In patients with persistent very good partial response, consider other methods to evaluate the depth of treatment response.

Dosage Forms Excipient information presented when available (limited, particularly for generics); consult specific product labeling.

Solution, Intravenous [preservative free]:

Darzalex: 100 mg/5 mL (5 mL); 400 mg/20 mL (20 mL) [contains mouse (murine) and/or hamster protein]

Darbepoetin Alfa (dar be POE e tin AL fa)

Related Information

Palliative Care Medicine (Cancer) *on page 2352*

Brand Names: US Aranesp (Albumin Free)

Brand Names: Canada Aranesp

Index Terms Darbepoetin Alfa Polysorbate; Erythropoiesis-Stimulating Agent (ESA); Erythropoiesis-Stimulating Protein; NESP; Novel Erythropoiesis-Stimulating Protein

Pharmacologic Category Colony Stimulating Factor; Erythropoiesis-Stimulating Agent (ESA); Hematopoietic Agent

Use

Anemia due to chemotherapy in patients with cancer: Treatment of anemia in patients with nonmyeloid malignancies when anemia is due to the effect of concomitant myelosuppressive chemotherapy, and upon initiation, there is a minimum of 2 additional months of planned chemotherapy.

Anemia due to chronic kidney disease: Treatment of anemia due to chronic kidney disease, including patients on dialysis and patients not on dialysis.

Limitations of use: Darbepoetin alfa has not demonstrated improved quality of life, fatigue, or well-being. Darbepoetin alfa is **not** indicated for use under the following conditions:

- Cancer patients receiving hormonal therapy, therapeutic biologic products, or radiation therapy unless also receiving concurrent myelosuppressive chemotherapy
- Cancer patients receiving myelosuppressive chemotherapy when the expected outcome is curative

 Cancer patients receiving myelosuppressive chemotherapy when anemia can be managed by transfusion
- As a substitute for red blood cell (RBC) transfusion in patients requiring immediate correction of anemia

◀ **Labeled Contraindications**
Serious allergic reaction to darbepoetin alfa or any component of the formulation; uncontrolled hypertension; pure red cell aplasia (PRCA) that begins after treatment with darbepoetin alfa or other erythropoietin protein drugs
Canadian labeling: Additional contraindications (not in the US labeling): Sensitivity to mammalian cell-derived products

Pregnancy Considerations Adverse events were observed in animal reproduction studies. Women who become pregnant during treatment with darbepoetin alfa are encouraged to enroll in Amgen's Pregnancy Surveillance Program (800-772-6436).

Breastfeeding Considerations It is not known if darbepoetin alfa is present in breast milk. The manufacturer recommends that caution be exercised when administering darbepoetin alfa to breastfeeding women.

Warnings/Precautions [US Boxed Warning]: Erythropoiesis-stimulating agents (ESAs) increased the risk of serious cardiovascular events, myocardial infarction, stroke, venous thromboembolism, vascular access thrombosis, and/or tumor progression in clinical studies when administered to target hemoglobin levels >11 g/dL (and provide no additional benefit); a rapid rise in hemoglobin (>1 g/dL over 2 weeks) may also contribute to these risks. **[US Boxed Warning]: A shortened overall survival and/or increased risk of tumor progression or recurrence has been reported in studies with breast, cervical, head and neck, lymphoid, and non-small cell lung cancer patients.** It is of note that in most of these studies, patients received ESAs to a target hemoglobin of ≥12 g/dL; although risk has not been excluded when dosed to achieve a target hemoglobin of <12 g/dL. **[US Boxed Warnings]: To decrease these risks, and risk of cardio- and thrombovascular events, use ESAs in cancer patients only for the treatment of anemia related to concurrent myelosuppressive chemotherapy and use the lowest dose needed to avoid red blood cell transfusions. Discontinue ESA following completion of the chemotherapy course. ESAs are <u>not</u> indicated for patients receiving myelosuppressive therapy when the anticipated outcome is curative.** A dosage modification is appropriate if hemoglobin levels rise >1 g/dL per 2-week time period during treatment (Rizzo 2010). Use of ESAs has been associated with an increased risk of venous thromboembolism (VTE) without a reduction in transfusions in patients >65 years of age with cancer (Hershman 2009). Improved anemia symptoms, quality of life, fatigue, or well-being have not been demonstrated in controlled clinical trials.

[US Boxed Warning]: An increased risk of death, serious cardiovascular events, and stroke was reported in patients with chronic kidney disease (CKD) administered ESAs to target hemoglobin levels >11 g/dL; use the lowest dose sufficient to reduce the need for RBC transfusions. An optimal target hemoglobin level, dose or dosing strategy to reduce these risks has not been identified in clinical trials. Hemoglobin rising >1 g/dL in a 2-week period may contribute to the risk (dosage reduction recommended). The American College of Physicians recommends against the use of ESAs in patients with mild to moderate anemia and heart failure or coronary heart disease (ACP [Qaseem 2013]). The American College of Cardiology Foundation/American Heart Association (ACCF/AHA) 2013 Heart Failure Guidelines do not provide a clear recommendation on the use of ESAs in anemic heart failure patients. The effects of ESAs on quality of life measures, morbidity, and mortality are potentially modest and still unclear. The authors declined to provide an official recommendation regarding the use of ESAs pending the completion of ongoing randomized trials (ACCF/AHA [Yancy 2013]).

CKD patients who exhibit an inadequate hemoglobin response to ESA therapy may be at a higher risk for cardiovascular events and mortality compared to other patients. ESA therapy may reduce dialysis efficacy (due to increase in red blood cells and decrease in plasma volume); adjustments in dialysis parameters may be needed. Patients treated with epoetin may require increased heparinization during dialysis to prevent clotting of the extracorporeal circuit. CKD patients not requiring dialysis may have a better response to darbepoetin alfa and may require lower doses. Increased mortality was observed in patients undergoing coronary artery bypass surgery who received epoetin; these deaths were associated with thrombotic events. An increased risk of deep vein thrombosis (DVT) has been observed in patients treated with epoetin undergoing surgical orthopedic procedures. Darbepoetin alfa is **not** approved for reduction in allogeneic red blood cell transfusions in patients scheduled for surgical procedures. The risk for seizures is increased with darbepoetin alfa use in patients with CKD; use with caution in patients with a history of seizures. Monitor closely for neurologic symptoms during the first several months of therapy. Use with caution in patients with hypertension; hypertensive encephalopathy has been reported. Use is contraindicated in patients with uncontrolled hypertension. If hypertension is difficult to control, reduce or hold darbepoetin alfa. Due to the delayed onset of erythropoiesis, darbepoetin alfa is **not** recommended for acute correction of severe anemia or as a substitute for emergency transfusion.

Prior to treatment, correct or exclude deficiencies of iron, vitamin B_{12}, and/or folate, as well as other factors that may impair erythropoiesis (inflammatory conditions, infections, bleeding). Prior to and during therapy, iron stores must be evaluated. Supplemental iron is recommended if serum ferritin <100 mcg/L or serum transferrin saturation <20%; most patients with CKD will require iron supplementation. Poor response should prompt evaluation of these potential factors, as well as possible malignant processes and hematologic disease (thalassemia, refractory anemia, myelodysplastic disorder), occult blood loss, hemolysis, osteitis fibrosa cystic, and/or bone marrow fibrosis. Severe anemia and pure red cell aplasia (PRCA) with associated neutralizing antibodies to erythropoietin has been reported, predominantly in patients with CKD receiving SubQ darbepoetin alfa (the intravenous (IV) route is preferred for hemodialysis patients). Cases have also been reported in patients with hepatitis C who were receiving ESAs, interferon, and ribavirin. Patients with a sudden loss of response to darbepoetin alfa (with severe anemia and a low reticulocyte count) should be evaluated for PRCA with associated neutralizing antibodies to erythropoietin; discontinue treatment (permanently) in patients with PRCA secondary to neutralizing antibodies to erythropoietin. Antibodies may cross-react; do not switch to another ESA in patients who develop antibody-mediated anemia.

The American Society of Clinical Oncology (ASCO) and American Society of Hematology (ASH) 2010 updates to the clinical practice guidelines for the use of ESAs in patients with cancer indicate that ESAs are appropriate when used according to the parameters identified within the Food and Drug Administration (FDA)-approved labeling for epoetin and darbepoetin alfa (Rizzo 2010). ESAs are an option for chemotherapy-associated anemia when the hemoglobin has fallen to <10 g/dL to decrease the need for RBC transfusions. ESAs should only be used in conjunction with concurrent chemotherapy. Although the FDA label now limits ESA use to the palliative setting, the ASCO/ASH guidelines suggest using clinical judgment in weighing risks versus benefits as formal outcomes studies of ESA use defined by intent of chemotherapy treatment have not been conducted.

Potentially serious allergic reactions have been reported (rarely), including anaphylactic reactions, angioedema, bronchospasm, rash, and urticaria. Discontinue immediately (and permanently) in patients who experience serious allergic/anaphylactic reactions. Some products may contain latex. Some dosage forms may contain polysorbate 80 (also known as Tweens). Hypersensitivity reactions, usually a delayed reaction, have been reported following exposure to pharmaceutical products containing polysorbate 80 in certain individuals (Isaksson 2002; Lucente 2000; Shelley 1995). Thrombocytopenia, ascites, pulmonary deterioration, and renal and hepatic failure have been reported in premature neonates after receiving parenteral products containing polysorbate 80 (Alade 1986; CDC 1984). See manufacturer's labeling.

Adverse Reactions

>10%:
  Cardiovascular: Hypertension (31%), peripheral edema (17%), edema (6% to 13%)
  Gastrointestinal: Abdominal pain (10% to 13%)
  Respiratory: Dyspnea (17%), cough (12%)
1% to 10%:
  Cardiovascular: Angina pectoris, hypotension, myocardial infarction, pulmonary embolism, thromboembolism, thrombosis of hemodialysis vascular access, thrombosis of vascular graft (arteriovenous)
  Central nervous system: Cerebrovascular disease
  Dermatologic: Erythema, skin rash
  Endocrine & metabolic: Hypervolemia
<1%, postmarketing, and/or case reports: Anaphylaxis, anemia (associated with neutralizing antibodies; severe; with or without other cytopenias), angioedema, bronchospasm, cerebrovascular accident, hypersensitivity reaction, hypertensive encephalopathy, pure red cell aplasia, seizure, tumor growth (progression/recurrence; cancer patients), urticaria

Drug Interactions

Metabolism/Transport Effects None known.

Avoid Concomitant Use There are no known interactions where it is recommended to avoid concomitant use.

Increased Effect/Toxicity
  Darbepoetin Alfa may increase the levels/effects of: Lenalidomide; Pomalidomide; Thalidomide

  The levels/effects of Darbepoetin Alfa may be increased by: Nandrolone

Decreased Effect There are no known significant interactions involving a decrease in effect.

Storage/Stability Store at 2°C to 8°C (36°F to 46°F); do not freeze. Do not shake. Protect from light. Store in original carton until use. The following stability information has also been reported: May be stored at room temperature for up to 7 days (Cohen 2007).

Mechanism of Action Darbepoetin alfa induces erythropoiesis by stimulating the division and differentiation of committed erythroid progenitor cells; induces the release of reticulocytes from the bone marrow into the bloodstream, where they mature to erythrocytes. There is a dose-response relationship with this effect. This results in an increase in reticulocyte counts followed by a rise in hematocrit and hemoglobin levels. When administered SubQ or IV, darbepoe-tin alfa's half-life is ~3 times that of epoetin alfa concentrations.

Pharmacodynamics/Kinetics

Onset of action: Increased hemoglobin levels not generally observed until 2 to 6 weeks after initiating treatment

Absorption: SubQ: Slow

Distribution: V_d:

Children: Initial dose: 51.6 ± 13.7 mL/kg (Lerner 2002); Steady state: 80.9 ± 32.5 mL/kg (Lerner 2002)

Adults: 52.4 ± 2 mL/kg (Macdougall 1999)

Bioavailability: CKD: SubQ: Adults: ~37% (range: 30% to 50%); Children: 54% (range: 32% to 70%)

Half-life elimination:

Children:

IV: Terminal: 22.1 hours (range: 12 to 30 hours)

SubQ: Terminal: 42.8 hours (range: 16 to 86 hours); Children with cancer: 49.4 hours

Adults:

CKD: IV: 21 hours; SubQ: Nondialysis patients: 70 hours (range: 35 to 139 hours), Dialysis patients: 46 hours (range: 12 to 89 hours)

Cancer: SubQ: 74 hours (range: 24 to 144 hours)

Note: Darbepoetin alfa half-life is approximately 3-fold longer than epoetin alfa following IV administration

Time to peak: SubQ:

CKD: Adults: 48 hours (range: 12 to 72 hours; independent of dialysis); Children: 36 hours (range: 10 to 58 hours)

Cancer: Adults: 71 to 90 hours (range: 28 to 123 hours); Children: 71 hours (range: 21 to 143 hours)

Excretion: Clearance: IV:

Children: 2.29 mL/hour/kg (range: 1.6 to 3.5 mL/hour/kg)

Adults: 1.6 ± 1.0 mL/hour/kg

Dosing

Adult & Geriatric Note: Evaluate iron status in all patients before and during treatment and maintain iron repletion.

Anemia due to chronic kidney disease (CKD): Individualize dosing and use the lowest dose necessary to reduce the need for red blood cell (RBC) transfusions.

*Chronic kidney disease patients **ON dialysis*** (IV route is preferred for hemodialysis patients; initiate treatment when hemoglobin is <10 g/dL; reduce dose or interrupt treatment if hemoglobin approaches or exceeds 11 g/dL): IV, SubQ: Initial: 0.45 mcg/kg once weekly **or** 0.75 mcg/kg once every 2 weeks **or** conversion from epoetin alfa: Epoetin alfa doses of <1,500 to ≥90,000 units per week may be converted to darbepoetin alfa doses ranging from 6.25 to 200 mcg per week (see adult column in conversion table).

*Chronic kidney disease patients **NOT on dialysis*** (consider initiating treatment when hemoglobin is <10 g/dL; use only if rate of hemoglobin decline would likely result in RBC transfusion and desire is to reduce risk of alloimmunization or other RBC transfusion-related risks; reduce dose or interrupt treatment if hemoglobin exceeds 10 g/dL): IV, SubQ: Initial: 0.45 mcg/kg once every 4 weeks

Dosage adjustments for chronic kidney disease patients (either on dialysis or not on dialysis): Do not increase dose more frequently than every 4 weeks (dose decreases may occur more frequently).

If hemoglobin increases >1 g/dL in any 2-week period: Decrease dose by ≥25%

If hemoglobin does not increase by >1 g/dL after 4 weeks: Increase dose by 25%

Inadequate or lack of response: If adequate response is not achieved over 12 weeks, further increases are unlikely to be of benefit and may increase the risk for adverse events; use the minimum effective dose that will maintain a hemoglobin level sufficient to avoid RBC transfusions **and** evaluate patient for other causes of anemia; discontinue treatment if responsiveness does not improve

Anemia due to chemotherapy in cancer patients: Initiate treatment only if hemoglobin <10 g/dL and anticipated duration of myelosuppressive chemotherapy is at least 2 additional months. Titrate dosage to use the minimum effective dose that will maintain a hemoglobin level sufficient to avoid RBC transfusions. Discontinue darbepoetin alfa following completion of chemotherapy.

SubQ: Initial: 2.25 mcg/kg once weekly **or** 500 mcg once every 3 weeks until completion of a chemotherapy course

Dosage adjustments:

Increase dose: If hemoglobin does not increase by 1 g/dL **and** remains below 10 g/dL after initial 6 weeks (for patients receiving weekly therapy only), increase dose to 4.5 mcg/kg once weekly (no dosage adjustment if using every-3-week dosing).

Reduce dose by 40% if hemoglobin increases >1 g/dL in any 2-week period **or** hemoglobin reaches a level sufficient to avoid RBC transfusion.

Withhold dose if hemoglobin exceeds a level needed to avoid RBC transfusion. Resume treatment with a 40% dose reduction when hemoglobin approaches a level where transfusions may be required.

Discontinue: On completion of chemotherapy or if after 8 weeks of therapy there is no hemoglobin response or RBC transfusions still required

Symptomatic anemia in myelodysplastic syndromes (off-label use): SubQ: 150 to 300 mcg once weekly (Giraldo 2006; Stasi 2005) **or** 500 mcg once every 2 to 3 weeks (Gabrilove 2008)

Conversion from epoetin alfa to darbepoetin alfa in CKD (on dialysis): See table

Conversion From Epoetin Alfa to Darbepoetin Alfa in Chronic Kidney Disease (Estimated Initial Dose)

Previous Dosage of Epoetin Alfa (units/week)	Children Darbepoetin Alfa Dosage (mcg/week)	Adults Darbepoetin Alfa Dosage (mcg/week)
<1,500	Not established	6.25
1,500 to 2,499	6.25	6.25
2,500 to 4,999	10	12.5
5,000 to 10,999	20	25
11,000 to 17,999	40	40
18,000 to 33,999	60	60
34,000 to 89,999	100	100
≥90,000	200	200

Note: In patients receiving epoetin alfa 2 to 3 times per week, darbepoetin alfa is administered once weekly. In patients receiving epoetin alfa once weekly, darbepoetin alfa is administered once every 2 weeks. The darbepoetin alfa dose to be administered every 2 weeks is derived by adding together 2 weekly epoetin alfa doses and then converting to the appropriate darbepoetin alfa dose. Titrate dose to hemoglobin response thereafter. The dose conversion in this table does not accurately estimate the once-monthly dose in chronic kidney disease (CKD) patients not on dialysis.

Pediatric Note: Evaluate iron status in all patients before and during treatment and maintain iron repletion.

Anemia due to chronic kidney disease (CKD): Individualize dosing and use the lowest dose necessary to reduce the need for red blood cell (RBC) transfusions.

Chronic kidney disease patients **ON dialysis** (IV route is preferred for hemodialysis patients; initiate treatment when hemoglobin is <10 g/dL; reduce dose or interrupt treatment if hemoglobin approaches or exceeds 12 g/dL): IV, SubQ: Initial: 0.45 mcg/kg once weekly or conversion from epoetin alfa: Initial dose: Epoetin alfa doses of 1,500 to ≥90,000 units per week may be converted to darbepoetin alfa doses ranging from 6.25 to 200 mcg per week (see conversion table in adult dosing).

Chronic kidney disease patients **NOT on dialysis** (consider initiating treatment when hemoglobin is <10 g/dL; use only if rate of hemoglobin decline would likely result in RBC transfusion and desire is to reduce risk of alloimmunization or other RBC transfusion-related risks; reduce dose or interrupt treatment if hemoglobin exceeds 12 g/dL): IV, SubQ: Initial: 0.45 mcg/kg once weekly or 0.75 mcg/kg once every 2 weeks

Dosage adjustments for chronic kidney disease patients: Do not increase dose more frequently than every 4 weeks (dose decreases may occur more frequently).

If hemoglobin increases >1 g/dL in any 2-week period: Decrease dose by ≥25%

If hemoglobin does not increase by >1 g/dL after 4 weeks: Increase dose by 25%

Inadequate or lack of response: If adequate response is not achieved over 12 weeks, further increases are unlikely to be of benefit and may increase the risk for adverse events; use the minimum effective dose that will maintain a hemoglobin level sufficient to avoid RBC transfusions **and** evaluate patient for other causes of anemia; discontinue treatment if responsiveness does not improve

Renal Impairment No dosage adjustment necessary.

Hepatic Impairment There are no dosage adjustments provided in the manufacturer's labeling.

Administration May be administered by SubQ or IV injection. The IV route is recommended in hemodialysis patients. Do not shake; vigorous shaking may denature darbepoetin alfa, rendering it biologically inactive. Do not dilute or administer in conjunction with other drug solutions. Discard any unused portion of the vial; do not pool unused portions.

Monitoring Parameters Hemoglobin (at least once per week until maintenance dose established and after dosage changes; monitor less frequently once hemoglobin is stabilized); CKD patients should be also be monitored at least monthly following hemoglobin stability); iron stores (transferrin saturation and ferritin) prior to and during therapy; serum chemistry (CKD patients); blood pressure; fluid balance (CKD patients); monitor for signs of seizures (CKD patients following initiation for first few months; includes new-onset or change in seizure frequency or premonitory symptoms)

Cancer patients: Examinations recommended by the ASCO/ASH guidelines (Rizzo 2010) prior to treatment include peripheral blood smear (in some situations a bone marrow exam may be necessary), assessment for iron, folate, or vitamin B_{12} deficiency, reticulocyte count, renal function status, and occult blood loss; during ESA treatment, assess baseline and periodic iron, total iron-binding capacity, and transferrin saturation or ferritin levels.

Dietary Considerations Supplemental iron intake may be required in patients with low iron stores.

Medication Guide Available Yes

Dosage Forms Excipient information presented when available (limited, particularly for generics); consult specific product labeling. [DSC] = Discontinued product

Solution, Injection [preservative free]:
Aranesp (Albumin Free): 25 mcg/mL (1 mL); 40 mcg/mL (1 mL); 60 mcg/mL (1 mL); 100 mcg/mL (1 mL); 150 mcg/0.75 mL (0.75 mL [DSC]); 200 mcg/mL (1 mL); 300 mcg/mL (1 mL) [albumin free; contains mouse (murine) and/or hamster protein, polysorbate 80]

Solution Prefilled Syringe, Injection [preservative free]:
Aranesp (Albumin Free): 10 mcg/0.4 mL (0.4 mL); 25 mcg/0.42 mL (0.42 mL); 40 mcg/0.4 mL (0.4 mL); 60 mcg/0.3 mL (0.3 mL); 100 mcg/0.5 mL (0.5 mL); 150 mcg/0.3 mL (0.3 mL); 200 mcg/0.4 mL (0.4 mL); 300 mcg/0.6 mL (0.6 mL); 500 mcg/mL (1 mL) [albumin free; contains mouse (murine) and/or hamster protein, polysorbate 80]

◆ **Darbepoetin Alfa Polysorbate** see Darbepoetin Alfa on page 515
◆ **Darzalex** see Daratumumab on page 509

Dasatinib (da SA ti nib)

Related Information

Common Toxicity Criteria *on page 2242*

Management of Chemotherapy-Induced Nausea and Vomiting in Adults *on page 2253*

Prevention of Chemotherapy-Induced Nausea and Vomiting in Children *on page 2310*

Safe Handling of Hazardous Drugs *on page 2379*

Brand Names: US Sprycel

Brand Names: Canada Sprycel

Index Terms BMS-354825

Pharmacologic Category Antineoplastic Agent, BCR-ABL Tyrosine Kinase Inhibitor; Antineoplastic Agent, Tyrosine Kinase Inhibitor

Use

Acute lymphoblastic leukemia: Treatment of Philadelphia chromosome-positive (Ph+) acute lymphoblastic leukemia (ALL) with resistance or intolerance to prior therapy.

Chronic myeloid leukemia: Treatment of newly diagnosed Ph+ chronic myeloid leukemia (CML) in chronic phase; treatment of chronic, accelerated, or myeloid or lymphoid blast phase Ph+ CML with resistance or intolerance to prior therapy, including imatinib.

Labeled Contraindications

There are no contraindications listed in the manufacturer's US labeling.

Canadian labeling: Hypersensitivity to dasatinib or any other component of the formulation; breastfeeding

Pregnancy Considerations Dasatinib crosses the placenta, with fetal plasma and amniotic concentrations comparable to maternal concentrations. Adverse effects, including hydrops fetalis and fetal leukopenia and thrombocytopenia have been reported following maternal exposure to dasatinib. Women of reproductive potential should use effective contraception during and for 30 days after the final dose to avoid becoming pregnant. Pregnant women are advised to avoid contact with crushed or broken tablets.

Breastfeeding Considerations It is not known if dasatinib is excreted in breast milk. According to the manufacturer, due to the potential for serious adverse reactions in the nursing infant, breastfeeding is not recommended during treatment and for 2 weeks following the final dose.

Warnings/Precautions Severe dose-related bone marrow suppression (thrombocytopenia, neutropenia, anemia) is associated with treatment (usually reversible); dosage adjustment and/or temporary interruption may be required for severe myelosuppression; the incidence of myelosuppression is higher in patients with advanced chronic myeloid leukemia (CML) and Ph+ acute lymphoblastic leukemia (ALL). Monitor blood counts every 2 weeks for 12 weeks and then every 3 months thereafter or as clinically indicated (for chronic phase CML) or weekly for the first 2 months, then monthly thereafter or as clinically necessary (for accelerated or blast phase CML or for ALL). Fatal intracranial and GI hemorrhage have been reported in association with dasatinib use. Severe hemorrhage (including CNS, GI) may occur due to thrombocytopenia; in addition to thrombocytopenia, dasatinib may also cause platelet dysfunction. Concomitant medications that inhibit platelet function or anticoagulants may increase the risk of bleeding. Potentially significant drug-drug interactions may exist, requiring dose or frequency adjustment, additional monitoring, and/or selection of alternative therapy. Use caution with ▶

◀ patients taking anticoagulants or medications interfering with platelet function; not studied in clinical trials. Avoid concomitant use with CYP3A4 inducers and inhibitors; if concomitant use cannot be avoided, consider dasatinib dosage adjustments. Elevated gastric pH may reduce dasatinib bioavailability; avoid concomitant use with proton pump inhibitors and H_2 blockers. If needed, may consider antacid administration at least 2 hours before or 2 hours after the dasatinib dose.

Cardiomyopathy, diastolic dysfunction, heart failure (congestive), left ventricular dysfunction, and MI have been reported; monitor for signs and symptoms of cardiac dysfunction. Dasatinib may cause fluid retention, including pleural and pericardial effusions, pulmonary hypertension, and generalized or superficial edema. A prompt chest x-ray (or other appropriate diagnostic imaging) is recommended for symptoms suggestive of effusion (new or worsening dyspnea on exertion or at rest, pleuritic chest pain, or dry cough). Fluid retention may be managed with supportive care (diuretics or corticosteroids); thoracentesis and oxygen therapy may be necessary for severe fluid retention; consider dose reduction or treatment interruption. Utilizing once-daily dosing is associated with a decreased frequency of fluid retention. The risk for pleural effusion is increased in patients with hypertension, prior cardiac history and a twice a day administration schedule; interrupt treatment for grade ≥2 effusion; may consider reinitiating at a reduced dose after resolution (Quintás-Cardama 2007). Use caution in patients where fluid accumulation may be poorly tolerated, such as in cardiovascular disease (HF or hypertension) and pulmonary disease. Patients 65 years of age and older are more likely to experience toxicity (compared with younger patients). Dasatinib may increase the risk for pulmonary arterial hypertension (PAH). PAH may occur at any time after starting treatment, including after >12 months of treatment. Evaluate for underlying cardiopulmonary disease prior to therapy initiation and during therapy; evaluate and rule out alternative etiologies in patients with symptoms suggestive of PAH (eg, dyspnea, fatigue, hypoxia, fluid retention) and interrupt therapy if symptoms are severe. Discontinue permanently with confirmed PAH diagnosis (may be reversible upon discontinuation).

May prolong QT interval; there are reports of patients with QTcF >500 msec. Use caution in patients at risk for QT prolongation, including patients with long QT syndrome, patients taking antiarrhythmic medications or other medications that lead to QT prolongation or potassium-wasting diuretics, patients with cumulative high-dose anthracycline therapy, and conditions which cause hypokalemia or hypomagnesemia. Correct hypokalemia and hypomagnesemia prior to and during dasatinib therapy. Cases of severe mucocutaneous dermatologic reactions (including Stevens-Johnson syndrome and erythema multiforme) have been reported with dasatinib. Discontinue dasatinib if severe mucocutaneous reaction occurs and other etiologies have been ruled out. Use caution with hepatic impairment due to extensive hepatic metabolism. Tumor lysis syndrome (TLS) has been reported in patients with resistance to imatinib therapy, usually in patients with advanced phase disease. Risk for TLS is higher in patients with advanced stage disease and/or a high tumor burden; monitor patients at risk more frequently. Maintain adequate hydration and correct uric acid levels prior to treatment; monitor electrolyte levels.

Adverse Reactions

≥10%:

Cardiovascular: Facial edema, peripheral edema

Central nervous system: Headache (12% to 33%), fatigue (8% to 26%), pain (11%)

Dermatologic: Skin rash (11% to 21%; includes drug eruption, erythema, erythema multiforme, erythematous rash, erythrosis, exfoliative rash, follicular rash, heat rash, macular rash, maculopapular rash, milia, papular rash, pruritic rash, pustular rash, skin exfoliation, skin irritation, urticaria vesiculosa, vesicular rash), pruritus (12%)

Endocrine & metabolic: Fluid retention (19% to 48%; grades 3/4: 1% to 8%; cardiac-related: 9%)

Gastrointestinal: Diarrhea (17% to 31%), nausea (8% to 24%), vomiting (5% to 16%), abdominal pain (7% to 12%)

Hematologic & oncologic: Thrombocytopenia (grades 3/4: 22% to 85%), neutropenia (grades 3/4: 29% to 79%), anemia (grades 3/4: 13% to 74%), hemorrhage (8% to 26%; grades 3/4: 1% to 9%), febrile neutropenia (4% to 12%; grades 3/4: 4% to 12%)

Infection: Infection (9% to 14%; includes bacterial, fungal, viral)

Local: Localized edema (3% to 22%; grades 3/4: ≤1%; superficial)

Neuromuscular & skeletal: Musculoskeletal pain (<22%), myalgia (7% to 13%), arthralgia (≤13%)

Respiratory: Pleural effusion (5% to 28%; grades 3/4: ≤7%), dyspnea (3% to 24%)

Miscellaneous: Fever (6% to 18%)

1% to <10%:

Cardiovascular: Cardiac conduction disturbance (7%), ischemic heart disease (4%), cardiac disease (≤4%; includes cardiac failure, cardiomyopathy, diastolic dysfunction, ejection fraction decreased, left ventricular dysfunction, ventricular failure), edema (≤4%; generalized), pericardial effusion (≤4%; grades 3/4: ≤1%), prolonged Q-T interval on ECG (≤1%), cardiac arrhythmia, chest pain, flushing, hypertension, palpitations, tachycardia

Central nervous system: Intracranial hemorrhage (≤3%; grades 3/4: ≤3%), chills, depression, dizziness, drowsiness, insomnia, myasthenia, neuropathy, peripheral neuropathy

Dermatologic: Acne vulgaris, alopecia, dermatitis, eczema, hyperhidrosis, urticaria, xeroderma

Endocrine & metabolic: Hyperuricemia, weight gain, weight loss

Gastrointestinal: Constipation (10%), gastrointestinal hemorrhage (2% to 9%; grades 3/4: 1% to 7%), abdominal distention, change in appetite, colitis (including neutropenic colitis), dysgeusia, dyspepsia, enterocolitis, gastritis, mucositis, stomatitis

Hematologic & oncologic: Bruise

Hepatic: Increased serum bilirubin (grades 3/4: ≤6%), increased serum ALT (grades 3/4: ≤5%), increased serum AST (grades 3/4: ≤4%), ascites (≤1%)

Infection: Herpes virus infection, sepsis

Neuromuscular & skeletal: Muscle spasm (5%), stiffness, weakness

Ophthalmic: Blurred vision, decreased visual acuity, dry eye syndrome, visual disturbance

Otic: Tinnitus

Renal: Increased serum creatinine (grades 3/4: ≤8%)

Respiratory: Pulmonary hypertension (≤5%; grades 3/4: ≤1%), pulmonary edema (≤4%; grades 3/4: ≤3%), cough, pneumonia (bacterial, viral, or fungal), pneumonitis, pulmonary infiltrates, upper respiratory tract infection

Miscellaneous: Soft tissue injury (oral)

<1%, postmarketing, and/or case reports: Abnormal gait, abnormal platelet aggregation, abnormal T waves on ECG, acute coronary syndrome, acute pancreatitis, acute respiratory distress, amnesia, anal fissure, angina pectoris, anxiety, arthritis, asthma, ataxia, atrial fibrillation, atrial flutter, bronchospasm, bullous skin disease, cardiomegaly, cerebrovascular accident, cholecystitis, cholestasis, confusion, conjunctivitis, coronary artery disease, cor pulmonale, cranial nerve palsy (facial), decreased libido, deep vein thrombosis, dehydration, dementia, dermal ulcer, diabetes mellitus, dyschromia, dysphagia, embolism, emotional lability, epistaxis, equilibrium disturbance, erythema nodosum, esophagitis, fibrosis (dermal), fistula (anal), gastroesophageal reflux disease, gastrointestinal disease (protein wasting), gingival hemorrhage, gynecomastia, hearing loss, hematoma, hematuria, hemoptysis, hemorrhage (ocular), hepatitis, hypercholesterolemia, hypersensitivity reaction, hypersensitivity angiitis, hyperthyroidism, hypoalbuminemia, hypotension, hypothyroidism, increased creatine phosphokinase, increased gamma-glutamyl transferase, increased lacrimation, increased pulmonary artery pressure, increased troponin, inflammation (panniculitis), interstitial pulmonary disease, intestinal obstruction, livedo reticularis, lymphadenopathy, lymphocytopenia, malaise, menstrual disease, myocarditis, nail disease, nephrotic syndrome, optic neuritis, osteonecrosis, ototoxicity (hemorrhage), palmar-plantar erythrodysesthesia, pancreatitis, pericarditis, petechia, photophobia, pleuropericarditis, prolongation P-R interval on ECG, proteinuria, pulmonary embolism, pure red cell aplasia, reactivation of HBV, renal failure, renal insufficiency, rhabdomyolysis, seizure, skin photosensitivity, Stevens-Johnson syndrome, Sweet syndrome, syncope, tendonitis, thrombophlebitis, thrombosis, thyroiditis, transient ischemic attacks, tremor, tumor lysis syndrome, upper gastrointestinal tract ulcer, urinary frequency, uterine hemorrhage, vaginal hemorrhage, ventricular arrhythmia, ventricular tachycardia, vertigo, voice disorder

Drug Interactions

Metabolism/Transport Effects Substrate of CYP3A4 (major); **Note:** Assignment of Major/Minor substrate status based on clinically relevant drug interaction potential; **Inhibits** CYP3A4 (weak)

Avoid Concomitant Use

Avoid concomitant use of Dasatinib with any of the following: BCG (Intravesical); Conivaptan; Deferiprone; Dipyrone; Fusidic Acid (Systemic); H2-Antagonists; Idelalisib; Natalizumab; Pimecrolimus; Pimozide; Proton Pump Inhibitors; St John's Wort; Tacrolimus (Topical); Vaccines (Live)

Increased Effect/Toxicity

Dasatinib may increase the levels/effects of: Acetaminophen; Agents with Antiplatelet Properties; Anticoagulants; ARIPiprazole; CloZAPine; CYP3A4 Substrates; Deferiprone; Fingolimod; Flibanserin; Highest Risk QTc-Prolonging Agents; HYDROcodone; Leflunomide; Lomitapide; Moderate Risk QTc-Prolonging Agents; Natalizumab; NiMODipine; Pimozide; Propacetamol; Tofacitinib; Vaccines (Live)

The levels/effects of Dasatinib may be increased by: Acetaminophen; Aprepitant; Conivaptan; CYP3A4 Inhibitors (Moderate); CYP3A4 Inhibitors (Strong); Denosumab; Dipyrone; Fosaprepitant; Fusidic Acid (Systemic); Idelalisib; MiFEPRIStone; Netupitant; Ocrelizumab; Palbociclib;

Pimecrolimus; Promazine; Roflumilast; Simeprevir; Stiripentol; Tacrolimus (Topical); Trastuzumab; Voriconazole

Decreased Effect

Dasatinib may decrease the levels/effects of: BCG (Intravesical); Coccidioides immitis Skin Test; Nivolumab; Sipuleucel-T; Tertomotide; Vaccines (Inactivated); Vaccines (Live)

The levels/effects of Dasatinib may be decreased by: Antacids; Bosentan; CYP3A4 Inducers (Moderate); CYP3A4 Inducers (Strong); Dabrafenib; Deferasirox; Dexamethasone (Systemic); Echinacea; Enzalutamide; H2-Antagonists; Mitotane; Proton Pump Inhibitors; Sarilumab; Siltuximab; St John's Wort; Tocilizumab

Food Interactions Dasatinib serum concentrations may be increased when taken with grapefruit or grapefruit juice. Management: Avoid concurrent use.

Hazardous Drugs Handling Considerations

Hazardous agent (NIOSH 2016 [group 1]).

Use appropriate precautions for receiving, handling, administration, and disposal. Gloves (single) should be worn during receiving, unpacking, and placing in storage.

NIOSH recommends single gloving for administration of intact tablets or capsules. If manipulating tablets/capsules (eg, to prepare an oral suspension), NIOSH recommends double gloving, a protective gown, and preparation in a controlled device; if not prepared in a controlled device, respiratory and eye/face protection as well as ventilated engineering controls are recommended. NIOSH recommends double gloving, a protective gown, and (if there is a potential for vomit or spit up) eye/face protection for administration of an oral liquid/feeding tube administration (NIOSH 2016).

Storage/Stability Store at 20°C to 25°C (68°F to 77°F); excursions permitted to 15°C to 30°C (59°F to 86°F).

Mechanism of Action BCR-ABL tyrosine kinase inhibitor; targets most imatinib-resistant BCR-ABL mutations (except the T315I and F317V mutants) by distinctly binding to active and inactive ABL-kinase. Kinase inhibition halts proliferation of leukemia cells. Also inhibits SRC family (including SRC, LKC, YES, FYN); c-KIT, EPHA2 and platelet derived growth factor receptor (PDGFRβ)

Pharmacodynamics/Kinetics

Distribution: 2505 L

Protein binding: Dasatinib: 96%; metabolite (active): 93%

Metabolism: Hepatic (extensive); metabolized by CYP3A4 (primarily), flavin-containing mono-oxygenase-3 (FOM-3) and uridine diphosphate-glucuronosyltransferase (UGT) to an active metabolite and other inactive metabolites (the active metabolite plays only a minor role in the pharmacology of dasatinib)

Half-life elimination: Terminal: 3 to 5 hours

Time to peak, plasma: 0.5 to 6 hours

Excretion: Feces (~85%, 19% as unchanged drug); urine (~4%, 0.1% as unchanged drug)

Dosing

Adult & Geriatric Note: The effect of discontinuation on long-term disease outcome after achieving cytogenetic response (including complete cytogenetic response) or major molecular response is not known.

◀ **Chronic myelogenous leukemia (CML), Philadelphia chromosome-positive (Ph+), newly diagnosed in chronic phase:** Oral: 100 mg once daily until disease progression or unacceptable toxicity. In clinical studies, a dose escalation to 140 mg once daily was allowed in patients not achieving hematologic or cytogenetic response at recommended initial dosage.

CML, Ph+, resistant or intolerant: Oral:

Chronic phase: 100 mg once daily until disease progression or unacceptable toxicity. In clinical studies, a dose escalation to 140 mg once daily was allowed in patients not achieving hematologic or cytogenetic response at recommended initial dosage.

Accelerated or blast phase: 140 mg once daily until disease progression or unacceptable toxicity. In clinical studies, a dose escalation to 180 mg once daily was allowed in patients not achieving hematologic or cytogenetic response at recommended initial dosage.

Acute lymphoblastic leukemia (ALL), Ph+: Oral: 140 mg once daily until disease progression or unacceptable toxicity. In clinical studies, a dose escalation to 180 mg once daily was allowed in patients not achieving hematologic or cytogenetic response at recommended initial dosage.

Gastrointestinal stromal tumors (GIST; off-label use): Oral: 70 mg twice daily (Montemurro 2012; Trent 2011).

Missed doses: If a dose is missed, take the next regularly scheduled dose; 2 doses should not be taken at the same time.

Dosage adjustment for concomitant CYP3A4 inhibitors: Avoid concomitant administration with strong CYP3A4 inhibitors (eg, clarithromycin, itraconazole, ketoconazole, nefazodone, protease inhibitors, telithromycin, voriconazole, grapefruit juice); if concomitant administration with a strong CYP3A4 inhibitor cannot be avoided, consider reducing dasatinib from 100 mg once daily to 20 mg once daily **or** from 140 mg once daily to 40 mg once daily, with careful monitoring. If reduced dose is not tolerated, the strong CYP3A4 inhibitor must be discontinued or dasatinib therapy temporarily held until concomitant inhibitor use has ceased. When a strong CYP3A4 inhibitor is discontinued, allow a washout period (~1 week) prior to adjusting dasatinib dose upward.

Dosage adjustment for concomitant CYP3A4 inducers: Avoid concomitant administration with strong CYP3A4 inducers (eg, carbamazepine, dexamethasone, phenobarbital, phenytoin, rifabutin, rifampin, St John's wort); if concomitant administration with a strong CYP3A4 inducer cannot be avoided, consider increasing the dasatinib dose with careful monitoring.

Renal Impairment There are no dosage adjustments provided in the manufacturer's labeling. However, <4% of dasatinib and metabolites are renally excreted.

Hepatic Impairment No initial dosage adjustment is necessary; use with caution. Transaminase or bilirubin elevations during treatment may be managed with treatment interruption or dose reduction.

Adjustment for Toxicity

Hematologic toxicity: Note: Growth factor support may be considered in patients with resistant myelosuppression.

Chronic phase CML (100 mg daily starting dose): For ANC <500/mm^3 or platelets <50,000/mm^3, withhold treatment until ANC ≥1000/mm^3 and platelets ≥50,000/mm^3; then resume treatment at the original starting dose if recovery occurs in ≤7 days. If platelets <25,000/mm^3 or recurrence of ANC <500/mm^3 for >7 days, withhold treatment until ANC ≥1000/mm^3 and platelets ≥50,000/mm^3; then resume treatment at 80 mg once daily (second episode). For third episode, further reduce dose to 50 mg once daily (for newly diagnosed patients) or discontinue (for patients resistant or intolerant to prior therapy)

Accelerated or blast phase CML and Ph+ ALL (140 mg once daily starting dose): For ANC <500/mm^3 or platelets <10,000/mm^3, if cytopenia unrelated to leukemia, withhold treatment until ANC ≥1000/mm^3 and platelets ≥20,000/mm^3; then resume treatment at the original starting dose. If cytopenia recurs, withhold treatment until ANC ≥1000/mm^3 and platelets ≥20,000/mm^3; then resume treatment at 100 mg once daily (second episode) or 80 mg once daily (third episode). For cytopenias related to leukemia (confirm with marrow aspirate or biopsy), consider dose escalation to 180 mg once daily.

Nonhematologic toxicity: Withhold treatment until toxicity improvement or resolution; if appropriate, resume treatment at a reduced dose based on the event severity and recurrence.

Dermatologic toxicities: Manage rash with antihistamines or topical or systemic steroids (Khoury 2009), or treatment interruption, dose reduction, or discontinuation. Discontinue if dasatinib-related severe mucocutaneous reaction occurs.

Fluid retention: Manage with diuretics, short courses of corticosteroids, and/or supportive care. Severe pleural effusions may require thoracentesis and oxygen therapy; consider dose reduction or treatment interruption. For grade 3 pleural effusion, withhold treatment until resolves to grade 1 or lower and consider corticosteroids (eg, prednisone 20 to 40 mg/day for 3 to 4 days), diuretics, thoracentesis and/or pleurodesis; may resume dasatinib at a decreased dose when effusion resolves (Khoury 2009).

Pulmonary arterial hypertension: Discontinue with confirmed pulmonary arterial hypertension.

Administration Administer once daily (morning or evening). May be taken without regard to food. Swallow whole; do not break, crush, or chew tablets. Take with a meal if GI upset occurs (Khoury 2009).

Emetic Potential

Children: Minimal (<10%)

Adults: Low (10% to 30%)

Extemporaneous Preparations An oral suspension may be prepared by dissolving dasatinib tablet(s) for one dose in 30 mL chilled orange or apple juice (without preservatives). After 5 minutes, swirl the contents for 3 seconds and repeat the process every 5 minutes for a total of 20 minutes following addition of tablet(s). Minimize time between end of 20 minutes and administration since suspension will taste more bitter if allowed to stand longer. Swirl contents of container one last time, then administer immediately. To ensure the full dose is administered, rinse container with 15 mL juice and administer residue. May be administered orally (or by nasogastric tube). Discard any unused portion after 60 minutes.

Sprycel data on file, Bristol-Myers Squibb

Monitoring Parameters CBC with differential every 2 weeks for 12 weeks and then every 3 months thereafter or as clinically indicated (for chronic phase chronic myeloid leukemia [CML]) **or** weekly for 2 months, then monthly or as clinically necessary (for accelerated or blast phase CML or for acute lymphoblastic leukemia [ALL]); bone marrow biopsy; liver function tests, electrolytes including calcium, phosphorus, magnesium; monitor for fluid retention; monitor for signs/symptoms of cardiac dysfunction; ECG monitoring if at risk for

QT$_c$ prolongation; chest x-ray is recommended for symptoms suggestive of pleural effusion (eg, cough, dyspnea); signs/symptoms of tumor lysis syndrome and dermatologic reactions.

Thyroid function testing recommendations (Hamnvik 2011):
Preexisting levothyroxine therapy: Obtain baseline TSH levels, then monitor every 4 weeks until levels and levothyroxine dose are stable, then monitor every 2 months
Without preexisting thyroid hormone replacement: TSH at baseline, then monthly for 4 months, then every 2 to 3 months

Dietary Considerations Avoid grapefruit juice.

Dosage Forms Excipient information presented when available (limited, particularly for generics); consult specific product labeling.
Tablet, Oral:
Sprycel: 20 mg, 50 mg, 70 mg, 80 mg, 100 mg, 140 mg

◆ **Daunomycin** see DAUNOrubicin (Conventional) on page 530

◆ **Daunorubicin and Cytarabine Liposome** see Daunorubicin and Cytarabine (Liposomal) on page 537

◆ **DAUNOrubicin Citrate** see DAUNOrubicin (Liposomal) on page 544

◆ **DAUNOrubicin Citrate (Liposomal)** see DAUNOrubicin (Liposomal) on page 544

◆ **DAUNOrubicin Citrate Liposome** see DAUNOrubicin (Liposomal) on page 544

DAUNOrubicin (Conventional) (daw noe ROO bi sin con VEN sha nal)

Related Information
Management of Chemotherapy-Induced Nausea and Vomiting in Adults on page 2253
Management of Drug Extravasations on page 2271
Prevention of Chemotherapy-Induced Nausea and Vomiting in Children on page 2310
Safe Handling of Hazardous Drugs on page 2379

Brand Names: Canada Cerubidine; Daunorubicin Hydrochloride for Injection

Index Terms Cerubidine; Conventional Daunomycin; Daunomycin; DAUNOrubicin Hydrochloride; Rubidomycin Hydrochloride

Pharmacologic Category Antineoplastic Agent, Anthracycline; Antineoplastic Agent, Topoisomerase II Inhibitor

Use
Acute lymphocytic leukemia: Treatment (remission induction) of acute lymphocytic leukemia (ALL) in children and adults (in combination with other chemotherapy)

Acute myeloid leukemia: Treatment (remission induction) of acute myeloid leukemia (AML) in adults (in combination with other chemotherapy)

Labeled Contraindications Hypersensitivity to daunorubicin or any component of the formulation

Pregnancy Considerations Adverse events have been observed in animal reproduction studies. Daunorubicin crosses the placenta. Women of reproductive potential should avoid pregnancy.

Breastfeeding Considerations It is not known if daunorubicin is excreted into breast milk. Due to the potential for serious adverse reactions in the nursing infant, the manufacturer recommends a decision be made whether to discontinue nursing or to discontinue the drug, taking into account the importance of treatment to the mother.

Warnings/Precautions [U.S. Boxed Warning]: Potent vesicant; if extravasation occurs, severe local tissue damage leading to ulceration and necrosis, and pain may occur. For IV administration only. NOT for IM or SubQ administration. Administer through a rapidly flowing IV line. Ensure proper needle or catheter placement prior to and during infusion. Avoid extravasation. **[U.S. Boxed Warning]: Severe bone marrow suppression may occur when used at therapeutic doses; may lead to infection or hemorrhage.** Use with caution in patients with drug-induced bone marrow suppression (preexisting), unless the therapy benefit outweighs the toxicity risk. Monitor blood counts at baseline and frequently during therapy.

[U.S. Boxed Warning]: May cause cumulative, dose-related myocardial toxicity; may lead to heart failure. May occur either during treatment or may be delayed (months to years after cessations of treatment). The incidence of irreversible myocardial toxicity increases as the total cumulative (lifetime) dosages approach 550 mg/m^2 in adults, 400 mg/m^2 in adults receiving chest radiation, 300 mg/m^2 in children >2 years of age, or 10 mg/kg in children <2 years of age. Total cumulative dose should take into account prior treatment with other anthracyclines or anthracenediones, previous or concomitant treatment with cardiotoxic agents or irradiation of chest. Although the risk increases with cumulative dose, irreversible cardiotoxicity may occur at any dose level. Patients with preexisting heart disease, hypertension, concurrent administration of other antineoplastic agents, prior or concurrent chest irradiation, advanced age; and infants and children are at increased risk. Monitor left ventricular (LV) function (baseline and periodic) with ECHO or MUGA scan; monitor ECG. Cardiotoxicity may occur more frequently in elderly patients. Use with caution in patients with impaired renal function and/or poor marrow reserve due to advanced age; dosage adjustment may be necessary. Infants and children are at increased risk for developing delayed cardiotoxicity; long-term periodic cardiac function monitoring is recommended.

[U.S. Boxed Warning]: Dosage reductions are recommended in patients with renal or hepatic impairment; significant impairment may result in increased toxicities. May cause tumor lysis syndrome and hyperuricemia. Urinary alkalinization and prophylaxis with an antihyperuricemic agent may be necessary. Monitor electrolytes, renal function, and hydration status. Use with caution in patients who have received radiation therapy; reduce dosage in patients who are receiving radiation therapy simultaneously. Secondary leukemias may occur when used with combination chemotherapy or radiation therapy. **[U.S. Boxed Warning]: Should be administered under the supervision of an experienced cancer chemotherapy physician.** Use caution when selecting product for preparation and dispensing; indications, dosages, and adverse event profiles differ between conventional daunorubicin hydrochloride solution and daunorubicin liposomal. Potentially significant drug-drug interactions may exist, requiring dose or frequency adjustment, additional monitoring, and/or selection of alternative therapy.

Adverse Reactions Frequency not defined.
>10%:
Cardiovascular: Cardiac failure (dose-related, may be delayed for 7 to 8 years after treatment), ECG abnormality (transient, generally asymptomatic and self-limiting; includes atrial premature contractions, ST segment changes on ECG, supraventricular tachycardia, ventricular premature contractions)
Dermatologic: Alopecia (reversible)
Gastrointestinal: Nausea (mild), stomatitis, vomiting (mild)
Genitourinary: Red urine discoloration
Hematologic & oncologic: Bone marrow depression (onset: 7 days; nadir: 10 to 14 days; recovery: 21 to 28 days; primarily leukopenia; anemia, thrombocytopenia)
Miscellaneous: Radiation recall phenomenon
1% to 10%:
Dermatologic: Discoloration of sweat
Endocrine & metabolic: Hyperuricemia
Gastrointestinal: Abdominal pain, diarrhea, discoloration of saliva, gastrointestinal ulcer
Local: Post-injection flare
Ophthalmic: Discoloration of tears
<1%, postmarketing, and/or case reports: Anaphylactoid reaction, cardiac arrhythmia, cardiomyopathy, hepatitis, hypersensitivity reaction (systemic; includes angioedema, dysphagia, dyspnea, pruritus, urticaria), increased serum bilirubin, increased serum transaminases, infertility, injection site reaction (includes injection site cellulitis, local thrombophlebitis, pain at injection site), leukemia (secondary), myocardial infarction, myocarditis, nail bed changes (pigmentation), nail disease (banding), onycholysis, pericarditis, skin rash, sterility, typhlitis (neutropenic)

Drug Interactions
Metabolism/Transport Effects Substrate of P-glycoprotein
Avoid Concomitant Use
Avoid concomitant use of DAUNOrubicin (Conventional) with any of the following: BCG (Intravesical); Deferiprone; Dipyrone; Natalizumab; Pimecrolimus; Tacrolimus (Topical); Vaccines (Live)
Increased Effect/Toxicity
DAUNOrubicin (Conventional) may increase the levels/effects of: CloZAPine; Deferiprone; Fingolimod; Leflunomide; Natalizumab; Tofacitinib; Vaccines (Live)

The levels/effects of DAUNOrubicin (Conventional) may be increased by: Ado-Trastuzumab Emtansine; Bevacizumab; Cyclophosphamide; Denosumab; Dipyrone; Lumacaftor; Ocrelizumab; Palifermin; P-glycoprotein/ABCB1 Inhibitors; Pimecrolimus; Promazine; Ranolazine; Roflumilast; Tacrolimus (Topical); Taxane Derivatives; Trastuzumab
Decreased Effect
DAUNOrubicin (Conventional) may decrease the levels/effects of: BCG (Intravesical); Cardiac Glycosides; Coccidioides immitis Skin Test; Lenograstim; Nivolumab; Sipuleucel-T; Tertomotide; Vaccines (Inactivated); Vaccines (Live)

The levels/effects of DAUNOrubicin (Conventional) may be decreased by: Cardiac Glycosides; Echinacea; Lumacaftor; P-glycoprotein/ABCB1 Inducers

Hazardous Drugs Handling Considerations

Hazardous agent (NIOSH 2016 [group 1]).

Use appropriate precautions for receiving, handling, administration, and disposal. Gloves (single) should be worn during receiving, unpacking, and placing in storage.

NIOSH recommends double gloving, a protective gown, ventilated engineering controls (a class II biological safety cabinet or a compounding aseptic containment isolator), and closed system transfer devices (CSTDs) for preparation. Double gloving, a gown, and (if dosage form allows) CSTDs are required during administration (NIOSH 2016).

Storage/Stability

Solution: Store intact vials at 2°C to 8°C (36°F to 46°F). Protect from light. Retain in carton until time of use. Solution prepared for infusion in D5W or NS may be stored at 20°C to 25°C (68°F to 77°F) for up to 24 hours. Discard unused portion.

Lyophilized powder [Canadian product]: Store intact vials of powder at 15°C to 30°C (59°F to 86°F). Protect from light. Retain in carton until time of use. Reconstituted daunorubicin is stable for 24 hours at room temperature or 48 hours when refrigerated at 2°C to 8°C (36°F to 46°F). Protect reconstituted solution from light.

Preparation for Administration

Dilute vials of powder for injection [Canadian product] with 4 mL SWFI for a final concentration of 5 mg/mL. May further dilute solution or reconstituted daunorubicin solution in D5W or NS for infusion.

Mechanism of Action

Inhibits DNA and RNA synthesis by intercalation between DNA base pairs and by steric obstruction. Daunomycin intercalates at points of local uncoiling of the double helix. Although the exact mechanism is unclear, it appears that direct binding to DNA (intercalation) and inhibition of DNA repair (topoisomerase II inhibition) result in blockade of DNA and RNA synthesis and fragmentation of DNA.

Pharmacodynamics/Kinetics

Distribution: Distributes widely into tissues, particularly the liver, kidneys, lung, spleen, and heart; does not distribute into the CNS

Metabolism: Primarily hepatic to daunorubicinol (active), then to inactive aglycones, conjugated sulfates, and glucuronides

Half-life elimination: Initial: 45 minutes; Terminal: 18.5 hours; Daunorubicinol plasma half-life: ~27 hours

Excretion: Feces (40%); urine (~25% as unchanged drug and metabolites)

Dosing

Adult & Geriatric Daunorubicin is associated with a moderate emetic potential; antiemetics are recommended to prevent nausea and vomiting (Basch, 2011; Roila, 2010).

Manufacturer's labeling: **Note:** Cumulative doses above 550 mg/m^2 in adults without risk factors for cardiotoxicity and above 400 mg/m^2 in adults receiving chest irradiation are associated with an increased risk of cardiomyopathy.

Acute lymphocytic leukemia (ALL):

IV: 45 mg/m^2 on days 1, 2, and 3 (in combination with vincristine, prednisone, and asparaginase)

◄

Acute myeloid leukemia (AML):

Adults <60 years: Induction: IV: 45 mg/m^2 on days 1, 2, and 3 of the first course of induction therapy; subsequent courses: 45 mg/m^2 on days 1 and 2 (in combination with cytarabine)

Adults ≥60 years: Induction: IV: 30 mg/m^2 on days 1, 2, and 3 of the first course of induction therapy; subsequent courses: 30 mg/m^2 on days 1 and 2 (in combination with cytarabine)

Indication-specific dosing (off-label dosing):
ALL:

CALGB 8811 regimen: IV: 45 mg/m^2 (in patients <60 years) or 30 mg/m^2 (in patients ≥60 years) on days 1, 2, and 3 of induction (Course I; 4 week cycle), in combination with cyclophosphamide, prednisone, vincristine, and asparaginase (Larson, 1995)

CCG 1961: Adults ≤21 years: IV: Induction: 25 mg/m^2 once weekly for 4 weeks (in combination with vincristine, prednisone, and asparaginase) (Nachman, 2009)

GRAALL-2003: Adults ≤60 years: IV:

Induction: 50 mg/m^2 on days 1, 2, and 3 **and** 30 mg/m^2 on days 15 and 16 (in combination with prednisone, vincristine, asparaginase, cyclophosphamide, and G-CSF support) (Huguet, 2009)

Late intensification: 30 mg/m^2 on days 1, 2, and 3 (in combination with prednisone, vincristine, asparaginase, cyclophosphamide, and G-CSF support) (Huguet, 2009)

MRC UKALLXII/ECOG E2993: Adults <60 years: IV: Induction (Phase I): 60 mg/m^2 on days 1, 8, 15, and 22 (in combination with vincristine, asparaginase, and prednisone) (Rowe, 2005)

PETHEMA ALL-96: Adults ≤30 years: IV:

Induction: 30 mg/m^2 on days 1, 8, 15, and 22 (in combination with vincristine, prednisone, asparaginase, and cyclophosphamide) (Ribera, 2008)

Consolidation-2/Reinduction: 30 mg/m^2 on days 1, 2, 8, and 9 (in combination with vincristine, dexamethasone, asparaginase, and cyclophosphamide) (Ribera, 2008)

Protocol 8707: Adults ≤60 years: IV: Induction and Consolidation 2A cycles: 60 mg/m^2 on days 1, 2, and 3 (in combination with vincristine, prednisone, and asparaginase). An additional 60 mg/m^2 daunorubicin dose may be administered on day 15 of induction if bone marrow biopsy on day 14 shows residual disease (Linker, 2002).

AML: Induction:

CCG 2891: Adults <21 years: IV: 20 mg/m^2/day continuous infusion on days 0 to 4 and 10 to 14 (in combination with dexamethasone, cytarabine, thioguanine, and etoposide) (Woods, 1996)

Adults <60 years: IV: 90 mg/m^2 on days 1, 2, and 3 (in combination with cytarabine). If residual disease was observed on day 12 to day 14 bone marrow biopsy, 45 mg/m^2 for 3 days was administered (in combination with cytarabine) (Fernandez, 2009).

Adults <60 years: IV: 60 mg/m^2 on days 1, 2, and 3 (in combination with cytarabine and cladribine); may repeat if partial remission occurs (Holowiecki, 2012).

Adults ≥60 years: IV: 45 or 90 mg/m^2 on days 1, 2, and 3 (in combination with cytarabine); the escalated 90 mg/m^2 dose was associated with increased remission rates and overall survival in the subgroup of patients 60 to 65 years of age as compared to patients >65 years (Lowenberg, 2009)

Acute promyelocytic leukemia (APL):

Induction: Adults: IV: 50 mg/m^2 on days 3, 4, 5, and 6 (in combination with ATRA and cytarabine) (Powell, 2010) **or** 60 mg/m^2 on days 1, 2, and 3 (in combination with ATRA and cytarabine) (Ades, 2008)

Consolidation: Adults: IV: 50 mg/m^2 on days 1, 2, and 3 for 2 cycles (in combination with ATRA; arsenic trioxide was administered for 2 cycles prior to daunorubicin and ATRA) (Powell, 2010) **or** 60 mg/m^2 on days 1, 2, and 3 during cycle 1 of consolidation (in combination with cytarabine), followed by 45 mg/m^2 on days 1, 2, and 3 during cycle 2 of consolidation (in combination with cytarabine) (Ades, 2008)

Pediatric Daunorubicin is associated with a moderate emetic potential; antiemetics are recommended to prevent nausea and vomiting (Dupuis, 2011).

Manufacturer's labeling: **Note:** Cumulative doses above 300 mg/m^2 in children >2 years or 10 mg/kg in children <2 years of age are associated with an increased risk of cardiomyopathy.

Acute lymphocytic leukemia (ALL):

Children <2 years or BSA <0.5 m^2: Remission induction: IV: 1 mg/kg/dose on day 1 every week for up to 4 to 6 cycles (in combination with vincristine and prednisone)

Children ≥2 years and BSA ≥0.5 m^2: Remission induction: IV: 25 mg/m^2 on day 1 every week for up to 4 to 6 cycles (in combination with vincristine and prednisone)

Indication-specific dosing (off-label dosing):

ALL:

CCG 1961: Children ≥10 years and Adolescents: IV: Induction: 25 mg/m^2 once weekly for 4 weeks (in combination with vincristine, prednisone, and asparaginase) (Nachman, 2009)

GRAALL-2003: Adolescents ≥15 years: IV:

Induction: 50 mg/m^2 on days 1, 2, and 3 **and** 30 mg/m^2 on days 15 and 16 (in combination with prednisone, vincristine, asparaginase, cyclophosphamide, and G-CSF support) (Huguet, 2009)

Late intensification: 30 mg/m^2 on days 1, 2, and 3 (in combination with prednisone, vincristine, asparaginase, cyclophosphamide, and G-CSF support) (Huguet, 2009)

MRC UKALLXII/ECOG E2993: Adolescents ≥15 years: IV: Induction (Phase I): 60 mg/m^2 on days 1, 8, 15, and 22 (in combination with vincristine, asparaginase, and prednisone) (Rowe, 2005)

PETHEMA ALL-96: Adolescents ≥15 years: IV:

Induction: 30 mg/m^2 on days 1, 8, 15, and 22 (in combination with vincristine, prednisone, asparaginase, and cyclophosphamide) (Ribera, 2008)

Consolidation-2/Reinduction: 30 mg/m^2 on days 1, 2, 8, and 9 (in combination with vincristine, dexamethasone, asparaginase, and cyclophosphamide) (Ribera, 2008)

Acute myeloid leukemia (AML): Induction:
CCG 2891:
Children <3 years: IV: 0.67 mg/kg/day continuous infusion on days 0 to 4 and 10 to 14 (in combination with dexamethasone, cytarabine, thioguanine, and etoposide) (Woods, 1996)
Children ≥3 years and Adolescents: IV: 20 mg/m^2/day continuous infusion on days 0 to 4 and 10 to 14 (in combination with dexamethasone, cytarabine, thioguanine, and etoposide) (Woods, 1996)
MRC AML 10/12: Children ≤14 years: IV: 50 mg/m^2 on days 1, 3, and 5 for 2 cycles (in combination with cytarabine and etoposide) (Gibson, 2005)

Renal Impairment The manufacturer's labeling recommends the following adjustment: S_{cr} >3 mg/dL: Administer 50% of normal dose
The following adjustments have also been recommended (Aronoff, 2007):
Adults: No dosage adjustment necessary.
Children:
CrCl <30 mL/minute: Administer 50% of dose
Hemodialysis/continuous ambulatory peritoneal dialysis (CAPD): Administer 50% of dose

Hepatic Impairment
The manufacturer's labeling recommends the following adjustments:
Serum bilirubin 1.2 to 3 mg/dL: Administer 75% of dose
Serum bilirubin >3 mg/dL: Administer 50% of dose
The following adjustments have also been recommended (Floyd, 2006):
Serum bilirubin 1.2 to 3 mg/dL: Administer 75% of dose
Serum bilirubin 3.1 to 5 mg/dL: Administer 50% of dose
Serum bilirubin >5 mg/dL: Avoid use

Combination Regimens
Leukemia, acute lymphocytic:
CALGB 8811 Regimen (ALL) on page 2003
CALGB 9111 Regimen (ALL) on page 2004
DVP on page 2099
Linker Protocol (ALL) on page 2167
PVDA on page 2199
Leukemia, acute myeloid:
5 + 2 (Cytarabine-Daunorubicin) (AML Induction) on page 1970
5 + 2 (Cytarabine-Daunorubicin) (AML Postremission) on page 1970
5 + 2 + 5 (Cytarabine-Daunorubicin-Etoposide) (AML Consolidation) on page 1971
7 + 3 (Cytarabine-Daunorubicin) (AML Induction) on page 1971
7 + 3 + 7 (Cytarabine-Daunorubicin-Etoposide) (AML Induction) on page 1973
Cytarabine (High Dose)-Daunorubicin (AML Induction) on page 2080
Cytarabine (High Dose)-Daunorubicin-Etoposide (AML Induction) on page 2080
Leukemia, acute promyelocytic: Tretinoin-Daunorubicin-Cytarabine Induction, Consolidation, Maintenance (APL) on page 2218

Administration Daunorubicin is associated with a moderate emetic potential; antiemetics are recommended to prevent nausea and vomiting (Basch, 2011; Dupuis, 2011; Roila, 2010).

For IV administration only. Do not administer IM or SubQ. Administer as slow IV push over 1 to 5 minutes into the tubing of a rapidly infusing IV solution of D5W or NS or may dilute further and infuse over 15 to 30 minutes.

Vesicant; ensure proper needle or catheter placement prior to and during infusion; avoid extravasation.

Extravasation management: If extravasation occurs, stop infusion immediately and disconnect (leave cannula/needle in place); gently aspirate extravasated solution (do **NOT** flush the line); remove needle/cannula; elevate extremity. Initiate antidote (dexrazoxane or dimethyl sulfate [DMSO]). Apply dry cold compresses for 20 minutes 4 times daily for 1 to 2 days (Perez Fidalgo, 2012); withhold cooling beginning 15 minutes before dexrazoxane infusion; continue withholding cooling until 15 minutes after infusion is completed. Topical DMSO should not be administered in combination with dexrazoxane; may lessen dexrazoxane efficacy.

Dexrazoxane: Adults: 1000 mg/m^2 (maximum dose: 2000 mg) IV (administer in a large vein remote from site of extravasation) over 1 to 2 hours days 1 and 2, then 500 mg/m^2 (maximum dose: 1000 mg) IV over 1-2 hours day 3; begin within 6 hours of extravasation. Day 2 and day 3 doses should be administered at approximately the same time (± 3 hours) as the dose on day 1 (Mouridsen, 2007; Perez Fidalgo, 2012). **Note:** Reduce dexrazoxane dose by 50% in patients with moderate to severe renal impairment (CrCl <40 mL/minute).

DMSO: Children and Adults: Apply topically to a region covering twice the affected area every 8 hours for 7 days; begin within 10 minutes of extravasation; do not cover with a dressing (Perez Fidalgo, 2012).

Vesicant/Extravasation Risk Vesicant

Emetic Potential Children and Adults: Moderate (30% to 90%)

Monitoring Parameters CBC with differential and platelet count, liver function test, ECG, left ventricular ejection function (echocardiography [ECHO] or multigated radionuclide angiography [MUGA] scan), renal function test, signs/symptoms of extravasation

Dosage Forms Excipient information presented when available (limited, particularly for generics); consult specific product labeling.

Injectable, Intravenous:
  Generic: 5 mg/mL (4 mL)
Injectable, Intravenous [preservative free]:
  Generic: 5 mg/mL (4 mL, 10 mL)

Daunorubicin and Cytarabine (Liposomal)
(daw noe ROO bi sin & sye TARE a been lye po SO mal)

Related Information

Common Toxicity Criteria *on page 2242*

Management of Chemotherapy-Induced Nausea and Vomiting in Adults *on page 2253*

Management of Drug Extravasations *on page 2271*

Safe Handling of Hazardous Drugs *on page 2379*

Brand Names: US Vyxeos

Index Terms CPX-351; Cytarabine (Liposomal) and Daunorubicin (Liposomal); Cytarabine and Daunorubicin (Liposomal); Cytarabine Liposome and Daunorubicin Liposome; Daunorubicin (Liposomal) and Cytarabine (Liposomal); Daunorubicin and Cytarabine Liposome; Liposomal Cytarabine and Daunorubicin; Liposomal Cytarabine-Daunorubicin; Liposomal Daunorubicin and Cytarabine; Liposome-Encapsulated Daunorubicin-Cytarabine; Vyxeos

Pharmacologic Category Antineoplastic Agent, Anthracycline; Antineoplastic Agent, Antimetabolite; Antineoplastic Agent, Antimetabolite (Pyrimidine Analog); Antineoplastic Agent, Topoisomerase II Inhibitor

Use Acute myeloid leukemia: Treatment of adults with newly-diagnosed therapy-related acute myeloid leukemia (t-AML) or AML with myelodysplasia-related changes (AML-MRC)

Labeled Contraindications Serious hypersensitivity to daunorubicin, cytarabine, or any component of the formulation

Pregnancy Considerations Based on the mechanism of action, anecdotal data of cytarabine use in pregnant women, and data from animal reproduction studies, use of daunorubicin and cytarabine (liposomal) in pregnancy may cause fetal harm. Women of reproductive potential should have a pregnancy test prior to treatment; effective contraception should be used during therapy and for at least 6 months after the last dose. Male patients with female partners of reproductive potential should also use effective contraception during therapy and for at least 6 months after the last dose. Based on animal data, treatment with daunorubicin and cytarabine (liposomal) may impair fertility in males.

Also refer to individual monographs.

Breastfeeding Considerations It is not known if daunorubicin, cytarabine, or their metabolites are present in breast milk. According to the manufacturer, breastfeeding is not recommended during therapy or for at least 2 weeks after the last dose.

Also refer to individual monographs.

Warnings/Precautions [US Boxed Warning]: Daunorubicin and cytarabine (liposomal) has different dosage recommendations than daunorubicin (conventional), cytarabine (conventional), daunorubicin (liposomal), and cytarabine (liposomal). Verify drug name and dose prior to preparation and administration to avoid dosing errors. The schedule and pharmacokinetics also vary among the formulations. Do not substitute other daunorubicin- or cytarabine-containing products for daunorubicin and cytarabine (liposomal). Neutropenia, thrombocytopenia, and anemia occurred in all patients in a clinical study comparing daunorubicin and cytarabine (liposomal) to conventional 7 + 3 therapy; prolonged thrombocytopenia and neutropenia were also observed more frequently with the daunorubicin and cytarabine (liposomal) arm. Neutropenic fever has also been reported. Monitor blood counts frequently. Do not initiate a new cycle until ANC recovers to >500/mm^3 and platelets recover to >50,000/mm^3. Serious hemorrhage events (associated with prolonged severe thrombocytopenia), including grade 3 and higher events have occurred; fatal CNS hemorrhages have also been reported. In a clinical study, epistaxis was the most frequently reported hemorrhagic event. Monitor blood counts frequently; may require platelet transfusion support.

Cardiotoxicity may occur due to the anthracycline component (daunorubicin) of the formulation. Risk factors for cardiotoxicity include prior exposure to anthracyclines, preexisting cardiac disease, previous mediastinal radiotherapy, or concomitant use of cardiotoxic medications. Other risk factors for anthracycline-induced cardiotoxicity include age 60 and older at time of treatment and 2 or more cardiovascular risk factors (smoking, hypertension, diabetes, dyslipidemia, or obesity) during or after treatment (Armenian 2017). Prior to therapy initiation, obtain an electrocardiogram (ECG), a multi-gated radionuclide angiography (MUGA) scan, or echocardiography (ECHO) to assess cardiac function. Repeat cardiac assessment via MUGA or ECHO prior to consolidation therapy with daunorubicin and cytarabine (liposomal) and as clinically necessary. Therapy is not recommended in patients with left ventricular ejection fraction (LVEF) less than normal; discontinue in patients with abnormal cardiac function unless benefit of treatment outweighs the risks. A total cumulative dose of daunorubicin (conventional) 550 mg/m^2 (400 mg/m^2 in patients with prior mediastinal radiation) has been associated with an increased incidence of heart failure; calculate the total lifetime cumulative anthracycline dose prior to each cycle of daunorubicin and cytarabine (liposomal). Treatment is not recommended in patients whose exposure has reached the maximum cumulative threshold.

Serious or fatal hypersensitivity reactions (including anaphylactic reactions) have been reported with daunorubicin and cytarabine; monitor closely. The infusion rate of daunorubicin and cytarabine (liposomal) may be interrupted or slowed for mild or moderate hypersensitivity reactions; manage symptoms as appropriate. If a severe or life-threatening reaction occurs, discontinue daunorubicin and cytarabine (liposomal) permanently and manage symptoms as clinically necessary. Premedication with antihistamines and or corticosteroids may be required. Reconstituted daunorubicin and cytarabine (liposomal) contains copper gluconate (14% elemental copper). The maximum (theoretical) total copper exposure during daunorubicin and cytarabine (liposomal) therapy is 106 mg/m^2. There is no clinical experience with use of this medication in patients with Wilson disease or other copper-related metabolic disorders; monitor total serum copper, serum non-ceruloplasmin bound copper, 24-hour urine copper levels and serial neuropsychological exams in these patient populations (use daunorubicin and cytarabine [liposomal] only if the benefits outweigh the risks). May require consultation with a hepatologist and nephrologist for management of acute copper toxicity; discontinue therapy if acute copper toxicity occurs.

Daunorubicin (conventional) is a potent vesicant; extravasation of conventional daunorubicin has been associated with severe local tissue necrosis. The daunorubicin (liposomal) component of the formulation may be an irritant (injection site reactions have been reported). Daunorubicin and cytarabine (liposomal) is for IV administration only; do not administer IM or SubQ. Ensure proper needle or catheter placement prior to and during infusion. Avoid extravasation. Nausea, vomiting, diarrhea/colitis, constipation, and decreased appetite have been reported with daunorubicin and cytarabine (liposomal). Administer antiemetics prior to treatment to prevent nausea and vomiting. Bleeding events occurred more frequently in patients 65 years and older compared to younger patients. Potentially significant drug-drug interactions may exist, requiring dose or frequency adjustment, additional monitoring, and/or selection of alternative therapy.

Adverse Reactions

>10%:

Cardiovascular: Edema (51%), cardiac arrhythmia (30%), cardiotoxicity (20%), hypotension (20%), hypertension (18%), chest pain (17%)

Central nervous system: Headache (33%), fatigue (32%), sleep disorder (25%), chills (23%), dizziness (18%), delirium (16%), anxiety (14%)

Dermatologic: Skin rash (54%), pruritus (15%)

Endocrine & metabolic: Hyponatremia (grades 3/4: 6% to 14%)

Gastrointestinal: Diarrhea (≤66%), nausea (47%), colitis (≤45%), mucositis (44%), constipation (40%), abdominal pain (33%), decreased appetite (29%), vomiting (24%), hemorrhoids (11%)

Hematologic & oncologic: Anemia (100%), neutropenia (100%; grade 4 [prolonged]: 10% to 17%), thrombocytopenia (100%; grade 3 [prolonged]: 25% to 28%), hemorrhage (70%; grades 3 to 5: 10%), febrile neutropenia (68%; grades 3 to 5: 66%), petechia (11%)

Hypersensitivity: Transfusion reaction (11%)

Infection: Bacteremia (24%), fungal infection (18%), sepsis (11%)

Local: Injection site reaction (16%; includes catheter and device site)

Neuromuscular & skeletal: Musculoskeletal pain (38%)

Ophthalmic: Visual impairment (11%)

Renal: Renal insufficiency (11%)

Respiratory: Cough (33%), dyspnea (32%), pneumonia (26%), hypoxia (18%), upper respiratory tract infection (18%), pleural effusion (16%)

Miscellaneous: Fever (17%)

1% to 10%:

Central nervous system: Hallucination (<10%)

Endocrine & metabolic: Hypokalemia (grades 3/4: 6% to 9%), hypoalbuminemia (grades 3/4: 2% to 7%), abnormal alanine aminotransferase (grades 3/4: ≤5%)

Gastrointestinal: Dyspepsia (<10%)

Hepatic: Hyperbilirubinemia (grades 3/4: 2% to 6%)

Ophthalmic: Conjunctivitis (<10%), dry eye syndrome (<10%), eye irritation (<10%), eye pain (<10%), injected sclera (<10%), ocular hyperemia (<10%), periorbital edema (<10%), swelling of eye (<10%)

Otic: Deafness (<10%)

Respiratory: Pneumonitis (<10%)

Drug Interactions

Metabolism/Transport Effects Refer to individual components.

Avoid Concomitant Use

Avoid concomitant use of Daunorubicin and Cytarabine (Liposomal) with any of the following: BCG (Intravesical); Deferiprone; Dipyrone; Natalizumab; Pimecrolimus; Tacrolimus (Topical); Vaccines (Live)

Increased Effect/Toxicity

Daunorubicin and Cytarabine (Liposomal) may increase the levels/effects of: CloZAPine; Deferiprone; Fingolimod; Leflunomide; Natalizumab; Tofacitinib; Vaccines (Live)

The levels/effects of Daunorubicin and Cytarabine (Liposomal) may be increased by: Ado-Trastuzumab Emtansine; Bevacizumab; Cyclophosphamide; Denosumab; Dipyrone; Lumacaftor; Ocrelizumab; Palifermin; P-glycoprotein/ABCB1 Inhibitors; Pimecrolimus; Promazine; Ranolazine; Roflumilast; Tacrolimus (Topical); Taxane Derivatives; Trastuzumab

Decreased Effect

Daunorubicin and Cytarabine (Liposomal) may decrease the levels/effects of: BCG (Intravesical); Cardiac Glycosides; Coccidioides immitis Skin Test; Flucytosine; Lenograstim; Nivolumab; Sipuleucel-T; Tertomotide; Vaccines (Inactivated); Vaccines (Live)

The levels/effects of Daunorubicin and Cytarabine (Liposomal) may be decreased by: Cardiac Glycosides; Echinacea; Lumacaftor; P-glycoprotein/ABCB1 Inducers

Hazardous Drugs Handling Considerations

Hazardous agent (NIOSH 2016 [group 1]).

Use appropriate precautions for receiving, handling, administration, and disposal. Gloves (single) should be worn during receiving, unpacking, and placing in storage.

NIOSH recommends double gloving, a protective gown, ventilated engineering controls (a class II biological safety cabinet or a compounding aseptic containment isolator), and closed system transfer devices (CSTDs) for preparation. Double gloving, a gown, and (if dosage form allows) CSTDs are required during administration (NIOSH 2016).

Storage/Stability Store intact vials 2°C to 8°C (36°F to 46°F) in an upright position. Protect from light (retain in original container). Reconstituted solution and solutions further diluted for infusion (if not used immediately) are stable for up to 4 hours when refrigerated.

Preparation for Administration Allow vials to come to room temperature for 30 minutes prior to reconstitution. Reconstitute each vial with 19 mL sterile water for injection (using a sterile syringe) to a concentration of 2.2 mg/mL; swirl the vial contents for 5 minutes (using a timer) while gently inverting the vial every 30 seconds. Do not heat, vortex, or shake the vials vigorously. Allow reconstituted vials to rest for 15 minutes (product should be opaque, purple, with homogenous dispersion and essentially free of visible particulates). Gently invert each vial 5 times prior to withdrawing dose for further dilution. Transfer appropriate dose volume (dose is calculated based on the daunorubicin component) to an infusion bag containing 500 mL of NS or D5W (discard unused residual solution in the vial). Mix bag by gentle inversion; the final solution will be deep purple, translucent, with homogeneous dispersion and free from visible particulates.

Mechanism of Action

Daunorubicin and cytarabine (liposomal) is a combination product with a fixed 1:5 (daunorubicin:cytarabine) molar ratio; this ratio has been shown to have synergistic effects in killing leukemia cells in vitro and in animal models.

Daunorubicin (conventional) inhibits DNA and RNA synthesis by intercalation between DNA base pairs and by steric obstruction. Daunomycin intercalates at points of local uncoiling of the double helix. Although the exact mechanism is unclear, it appears that direct binding to DNA (intercalation) and inhibition of DNA repair (topoisomerase II inhibition) result in blockade of DNA and RNA synthesis and fragmentation of DNA. Cytarabine (conventional) is a pyrimidine analog and is incorporated into DNA; however, the primary action is inhibition of DNA polymerase resulting in decreased DNA synthesis and repair. The degree of cytotoxicity correlates linearly with incorporation into DNA; therefore, incorporation into the DNA is responsible for drug activity and toxicity. Cytarabine is specific for the S phase of the cell cycle (blocks progression from the G1 to the S phase).

Per animal data, liposomes are taken up intact by bone marrow cells (to a greater degree in leukemia cells versus normal bone marrow cells) and are degraded following cellular internalization, thus releasing cytarabine and daunorubicin within the cells.

◀ **Pharmacodynamics/Kinetics**

Distribution: Daunorubicin 6.6 L; Cytarabine 7.1 L

Metabolism: Upon release from the liposomes, daunorubicin is catalyzed by aldoketo reductase and carbonyl reductase to daunorubicinol (active metabolite); cytarabine is metabolized by cytidine deaminase to Ara-U (inactive metabolite).

Half-life elimination: 31.5 hours (daunorubicin); 40.4 hours (cytarabine) with >99% of drug(s) remaining encapsulated in the liposomes

Excretion: Urine (9% daunorubicin; 71% cytarabine and Ara-U)

Dosing

Adult & Geriatric Note: Calculate dose based on the daunorubicin component. Prior to each dose, calculate the cumulative anthracycline exposure. Assess cardiac function, liver, and renal function prior to therapy initiation; also evaluate complete blood counts in addition to cardiac function and liver/renal function prior to each consolidation cycle. Therapy consists of 1 to 2 induction cycles followed by up to 2 consolidation cycles. Administer antiemetics prior to treatment to prevent nausea and vomiting.

Acute myeloid leukemia (newly diagnosed for therapy-related AML [t-AML] or AML with myelodysplasia-related changes [AML-MRC]): IV:

Induction (first cycle): Daunorubicin 44 mg/m^2 and cytarabine 100 mg/m^2 (liposomal) on days 1, 3, and 5

Induction (second cycle in patients who do not achieve remission with first cycle): Daunorubicin 44 mg/m^2 and cytarabine 100 mg/m^2 (liposomal) on days 1 and 3; the second induction cycle may be administered 2 to 5 weeks after the first induction cycle (if no unacceptable toxicity with previous cycle).

Consolidation: Daunorubicin 29 mg/m^2 and cytarabine 65 mg/m^2 (liposomal) on days 1 and 3; administer the first consolidation cycle 5 to 8 weeks after the start of the last induction; administer the second consolidation cycle 5 to 8 weeks after the start of the first consolidation cycle.

Missed dose: If a planned dose is missed, administer the dose as soon as possible and adjust the schedule accordingly (maintain the treatment interval).

Renal Impairment

CrCl 30 to 89 mL/minute: No dosage adjustment necessary.

CrCl <30 mL/minute: There are no dosage adjustments provided in the manufacturer's labeling (has not been studied).

ESRD: There are no dosage adjustments provided in the manufacturer's labeling (has not been studied).

Hepatic Impairment

Total bilirubin ≤3 mg/dL: No dosage adjustment necessary.

Total bilirubin >3 mg/dL: There are no dosage adjustments provided in the manufacturer's labeling (has not been studied).

Adjustment for Toxicity

Cardiotoxicity: Discontinue daunorubicin and cytarabine (liposomal) in patients with impaired cardiac function unless the benefits of continued treatment outweigh the toxicity risks.

Hematologic toxicity: Do not initiate a new cycle until ANC recovers to >500/mm^3 and platelets recover to >50,000/mm^3. Hematologic toxicity may require platelet transfusion support.

Hypersensitivity reactions:

Mild symptoms: Interrupt infusion immediately and manage symptoms as clinically appropriate. Upon symptom resolution, reinitiate infusion at 50% of the previous infusion rate; consider premedication with antihistamines and/or corticosteroids with subsequent daunorubicin and cytarabine (liposomal) doses.

Moderate symptoms: Interrupt infusion immediately and manage symptoms as clinically appropriate. Do not reinitiate infusion. Premedicate with antihistamines and/or corticosteroids with subsequent daunorubicin and cytarabine (liposomal) doses prior to initiating infusion at the same rate.

Severe or life-threatening symptoms: Interrupt infusion immediately and manage symptoms as clinically appropriate; monitor until symptom resolution. Permanently discontinue daunorubicin and cytarabine (liposomal).

Administration

Administer prophylactic antiemetics prior to infusion.

For IV administration only; do not administer IM or SubQ. Administer over 90 minutes (for induction and consolidation cycles) via an infusion pump through a central venous or peripherally inserted central catheter. Do not use an in-line filter. Flush the line with NS or D5W after infusion. Do not mix with or administer with any other medications. If infusion-related reactions occur, premedication with antihistamines and/or corticosteroids may be necessary.

The daunorubicin (liposomal) component may be an irritant; avoid extravasation.

Vesicant/Extravasation Risk The daunorubicin (liposomal) component may be an irritant

Emetic Potential Moderate (30% to 90%)

Monitoring Parameters Complete blood counts (prior to treatment and each consolidation cycle), liver and renal function tests (prior to treatment and each consolidation cycle), pregnancy test prior to treatment initiation (in women of reproductive potential); total serum copper, serum non ceruloplasmin bound copper, 24-hour urine copper levels (in patients with Wilson disease or other copper-related metabolic disorders); assess cardiac function via ECG, MUGA, or ECHO prior to treatment initiation, consolidation therapy, and as clinically necessary; monitor infusion site (for extravasation), nausea/vomiting, and signs/symptoms of hemorrhage and hypersensitivity reactions

Dosage Forms Excipient information presented when available (limited, particularly for generics); consult specific product labeling.

Suspension Reconstituted, Intravenous [preservative free]:

Vyxeos: Daunorubicin 44 mg and cytarabine 100 mg (1 ea) [contains trolamine (triethanolamine)]

◆ **DAUNOrubicin Hydrochloride** *see* DAUNOrubicin (Conventional) *on page* 530

◆ **Daunorubicin Hydrochloride for Injection (Can)** *see* DAUNOrubicin (Conventional) *on page* 530

DAUNOrubicin (Liposomal) (daw noe ROO bi sin lye po SO mal)

Related Information

Common Toxicity Criteria *on page 2242*
Management of Chemotherapy-Induced Nausea and Vomiting in Adults *on page 2253*
Management of Drug Extravasations *on page 2271*
Safe Handling of Hazardous Drugs *on page 2379*

Brand Names: US DaunoXome [DSC]

Index Terms DAUNOrubicin Citrate; DAUNOrubicin Citrate (Liposomal); DAUNOrubicin Citrate Liposome; Liposomal DAUNOrubicin

Pharmacologic Category Antineoplastic Agent, Anthracycline; Antineoplastic Agent, Topoisomerase II Inhibitor

Use

Kaposi sarcoma: First-line treatment of advanced HIV-associated Kaposi sarcoma

Limitation of use: Daunorubicin (liposomal) is not recommended in HIV-related Kaposi sarcoma which is less than advanced.

Labeled Contraindications

Hypersensitivity to daunorubicin (liposomal) or any component of the formulation

Documentation of allergenic cross-reactivity for drugs in this class is limited. However, because of similarities in chemical structure and/or pharmacologic actions, the possibility of cross-sensitivity cannot be ruled out with certainty.

Pregnancy Considerations Adverse events were observed in animal reproduction studies. May cause fetal harm if administered during pregnancy. Women of childbearing potential should avoid becoming pregnant while receiving treatment.

Breastfeeding Considerations Based on information from daunorubicin (conventional), it is not known if daunorubicin (liposomal) is excreted into breast milk. Daunorubicin (liposomal) is indicated for advanced HIV-associated Kaposi sarcoma. In the United States, where formula is accessible, affordable, safe, and sustainable, and the risk of infant mortality due to diarrhea and respiratory infections is low, complete avoidance of breastfeeding by HIV-infected women is recommended to decrease potential transmission of HIV (DHHS [perinatal], 2012).

Warnings/Precautions [US Boxed Warning]: Due to the potential for cardiac toxicity and heart failure, monitor cardiac function regularly, especially in patients with previous therapy with anthracyclines, thoracic radiation, or who have preexisting cardiac disease. Cardiomyopathy is usually associated with a decrease left in ventricular ejection fraction (LVEF). Although the risk increases with cumulative dose, irreversible cardiotoxicity may occur with anthracycline treatment at any dose level. Patients who have received prior anthracycline therapy (DOXOrubicin >300 mg/m^2 or equivalent), with preexisting heart disease, hypertension, concurrent administration of other antineoplastic agents, prior or concurrent chest irradiation, and advanced age are at increased risk. Evaluate LVEF prior to treatment and periodically during treatment (at cumulative doses of daunorubicin liposomal 320 mg/m^2 and every 160 mg/m^2 thereafter or every 160 mg/m^2 in patients at higher risk).

[US Boxed Warning]: May cause bone marrow suppression, particularly neutropenia (may be severe). Monitor blood counts. Monitor closely for infections (including opportunistic infections). **[US Boxed Warning]: Reduce**

dosage in patients with hepatic impairment. Use caution with renal impairment; may require dose adjustment. **[US Boxed Warning]: The lipid component is associated with infusion-related reactions (back pain, flushing, chest tightness) usually within the first 5 minutes of infusion and subsides with interruption of the infusion, and generally does not recur if the infusion is resumed at a lower rate.** Monitor for infusion reactions; interrupt infusion if reaction occurs, and resume at reduced infusion rate.

Although not reported with daunorubicin (liposomal), daunorubicin (conventional) is associated with local tissue necrosis if extravasated. Potentially significant drug-drug interactions may exist, requiring dose or frequency adjustment, additional monitoring, and/or selection of alternative therapy. **[US Boxed Warning]: Should be administered under the supervision of an experienced cancer chemotherapy physician.**

Adverse Reactions Frequency not always defined.

Cardiovascular: Edema (11%), chest pain (10%), angina pectoris (≤5%), atrial fibrillation (≤5%), cardiac arrest (≤5%), cardiac tamponade (≤5%), hypertension (≤5%), myocardial infarction (≤5%), palpitations (≤5%), pericardial effusion (≤5%), pulmonary hypertension (≤5%), sinus tachycardia (≤5%), supraventricular tachycardia (≤5%), syncope (≤5%), tachycardia (≤5%), ventricular premature contractions (≤5%), decreased left ventricular ejection fraction (3%; reduction of 20% to 25%), cardiomyopathy (cumulative, dose-related; total dose above 300 mg/m^2)

Central nervous system: Fatigue (49%), headache (25%), rigors (19%), neuropathy (13%), depression (10%), malaise (10%), dizziness (8%), insomnia (6%), abnormality in thinking (≤5%), amnesia (≤5%), anxiety (≤5%), ataxia (≤5%), confusion (≤5%), drowsiness (≤5%), emotional lability (≤5%), hallucination (≤5%), hypertonia (≤5%), meningitis (≤5%), seizure (≤5%)

Dermatologic: Diaphoresis (14%), alopecia (8%), pruritus (7%), folliculitis (≤5%), seborrhea (≤5%), xeroderma (≤5%)

Endocrine & metabolic: Dehydration (≤5%), hot flash (≤5%), increased thirst (≤5%)

Gastrointestinal: Nausea (54%), diarrhea (38%), abdominal pain (23%), anorexia (23%), vomiting (23%), stomatitis (10%), constipation (7%), tenesmus (5%), dental caries (≤5%), dysgeusia (≤5%), dysphagia (≤5%), gastritis (≤5%), gastrointestinal hemorrhage (≤5%), gingival hemorrhage (≤5%), hemorrhoids (≤5%), hiccups (≤5%), increased appetite (≤5%), melena (≤5%), xerostomia (≤5%)

Genitourinary: Dysuria (≤5%), nocturia (≤5%)

Hematologic & oncologic: Neutropenia (<1,000 cells/mm^3: 36%; grade 4: 15%), lymphadenopathy (≤5%), splenomegaly (≤5%), bone marrow depression (especially granulocytes; platelets and erythrocytes less effected), severe granulocytopenia (may be associated with fever and result in infection)

Hepatic: Hepatomegaly (≤5%)

Hypersensitivity: Hypersensitivity reaction (24%)

Infection: Opportunistic infection (40%; median time to first infection/illness: 214 days)

Local: Inflammation at injection site (≤5%)

Neuromuscular & skeletal: Back pain (16%), arthralgia (7%), myalgia (7%), abnormal gait (≤5%), hyperkinesia (≤5%), tremor (≤5%)

Ophthalmic: Visual disturbance (5%), conjunctivitis (≤5%), eye pain (≤5%)

Otic: Deafness (≤5%), otalgia (≤5%), tinnitus (≤5%)

Renal: Polyuria (≤5%)

Respiratory: Cough (28%), dyspnea (26%), rhinitis (12%), sinusitis (8%), flu-like symptoms (5%), hemoptysis (≤5%), increased bronchial secretions (≤5%), pulmonary infiltrates (≤5%)

Miscellaneous: Fever (47%), infusion-related reaction (14%; includes back pain, flushing, chest tightness)

Drug Interactions

Metabolism/Transport Effects Substrate of P-glycoprotein

Avoid Concomitant Use

Avoid concomitant use of DAUNOrubicin (Liposomal) with any of the following: BCG (Intravesical); Deferiprone; Dipyrone; Natalizumab; Pimecrolimus; Tacrolimus (Topical); Vaccines (Live)

Increased Effect/Toxicity

DAUNOrubicin (Liposomal) may increase the levels/effects of: CloZAPine; Deferiprone; Fingolimod; Leflunomide; Natalizumab; Tofacitinib; Vaccines (Live)

The levels/effects of DAUNOrubicin (Liposomal) may be increased by: Ado-Trastuzumab Emtansine; Bevacizumab; Cyclophosphamide; Denosumab; Dipyrone; Lumacaftor; Ocrelizumab; Palifermin; P-glycoprotein/ABCB1 Inhibitors; Pimecrolimus; Promazine; Ranolazine; Roflumilast; Tacrolimus (Topical); Taxane Derivatives; Trastuzumab

Decreased Effect

DAUNOrubicin (Liposomal) may decrease the levels/effects of: BCG (Intravesical); Cardiac Glycosides; Coccidioides immitis Skin Test; Lenograstim; Nivolumab; Sipuleucel-T; Tertomotide; Vaccines (Inactivated); Vaccines (Live)

The levels/effects of DAUNOrubicin (Liposomal) may be decreased by: Cardiac Glycosides; Echinacea; Lumacaftor; P-glycoprotein/ABCB1 Inducers

Hazardous Drugs Handling Considerations

Hazardous agent (NIOSH 2016 [group1]).

Use appropriate precautions for receiving, handling, administration, and disposal. Gloves (single) should be worn during receiving, unpacking, and placing in storage.

NIOSH recommends double gloving, a protective gown, ventilated engineering controls (a class II biological safety cabinet or a compounding aseptic containment isolator), and closed system transfer devices (CSTDs) for preparation. Double gloving, a gown, and (if dosage form allows) CSTDs are required during administration (NIOSH 2016).

Storage/Stability Store intact vials at 2°C to 8°C (36°F to 46°F); do not freeze. Protect from light. Diluted daunorubicin liposomal for infusion in D5W may be refrigerated at 2°C to 8°C (36°F to 46°F) for a maximum of 6 hours (if not used immediately).

Preparation for Administration The only fluid that may be mixed with daunorubicin (liposomal) is D5W. Dilute with an equivalent volume of D5W to a 1:1 solution (to a concentration of 1 mg daunorubicin liposomal/mL). Must **not** be mixed with saline, bacteriostatic agents (such as benzyl alcohol), or any other solution. Do not mix with other medications.

Mechanism of Action Liposomal preparation of daunorubicin; liposomes have been shown to penetrate solid tumors more effectively, possibly because of their small size and longer circulation time. Once in tissues, daunorubicin is released (over time). Daunorubicin inhibits DNA and RNA synthesis by intercalation between DNA base pairs and by steric obstruction; and intercalates at points of local uncoiling of the double helix. Although the exact mechanism is unclear, it appears that direct binding to DNA (intercalation) and inhibition of DNA repair (topoisomerase II inhibition) result in blockade of DNA and RNA synthesis and fragmentation of DNA.

Pharmacodynamics/Kinetics

Distribution: V_d: ~5 to 8 L

Metabolism: Daunorubicinol (major active metabolite) is detected at low levels in plasma

Half-life elimination: Distribution: 4.4 hours

Excretion: Primarily feces; some urine

Dosing

Adult & Geriatric Note: DAUNOrubicin (liposomal) is different from the conventional DAUNOrubicin formulation; do **NOT** substitute (indications and doses are different).

Kaposi sarcoma: IV: 40 mg/m² once every 2 weeks; continue until disease progression.

Renal Impairment Serum creatinine >3 mg/dL: Administer 50% of normal dose.

Hepatic Impairment

Bilirubin 1.2 to 3 mg/dL: Administer 75% of normal dose.

Bilirubin >3 mg/dL: Administer 50% of normal dose.

Obesity *ASCO Guidelines for appropriate chemotherapy dosing in obese adults with cancer:* Utilize patient's actual body weight (full weight) for calculation of body surface area- or weight-based dosing, particularly when the intent of therapy is curative; manage regimen-related toxicities in the same manner as for nonobese patients; if a dose reduction is utilized due to toxicity, consider resumption of full weight-based dosing with subsequent cycles, especially if cause of toxicity (eg, hepatic or renal impairment) is resolved (Griggs 2012).

Adjustment for Toxicity

ANC <750/mm³: Withhold treatment.

Infusion reactions (back pain, flushing, chest tightness): Temporarily interrupt infusion; may resume at a slower rate.

Combination Regimens

Leukemia, acute lymphocytic: Hyper-CVAD (Leukemia, Acute Lymphocytic) on page 2146

Administration Infuse over 1 hour; do not mix with other drugs. Do NOT administer with an in-line filter. Avoid extravasation.

Vesicant/Extravasation Risk May be an irritant

Emetic Potential Low (10% to 30%).

Monitoring Parameters CBC with differential and platelets (prior to each dose), liver function tests, renal function tests; evaluate cardiac function (baseline left ventricular ejection fraction [LVEF] prior to treatment initiation; repeat LVEF at total cumulative doses of 320 mg/m², and every 160 mg/m² thereafter; patients with preexisting cardiac disease, history of prior chest irradiation, or history of prior anthracycline treatment should have baseline LVEF and every 160 mg/m² thereafter); signs and symptoms of infection or disease progression; monitor closely for infusion reactions

◀ **Dosage Forms Considerations** Daunorubicin (liposomal) injection contains sucrose 2,125 mg/25 mL

Dosage Forms Excipient information presented when available (limited, particularly for generics); consult specific product labeling. [DSC] = Discontinued product

Injectable, Intravenous [preservative free]:

DaunoXome: 2 mg/mL (25 mL [DSC]) [pyrogen free]

Decitabine (de SYE ta been)

Related Information

Brand Names: US Dacogen

Index Terms 5-Aza-2'-deoxycytidine; 5-Aza-dCyd; Deoxyazacytidine; Dezocitidine

Pharmacologic Category Antineoplastic Agent, Antimetabolite; Antineoplastic Agent, DNA Methylation Inhibitor

Use Myelodysplastic syndromes: Treatment of myelodysplastic syndromes (MDS), including previously treated and untreated, de novo and secondary MDS of all French-American-British (FAB) subtypes (refractory anemia, refractory anemia with ringed sideroblasts, refractory anemia with excess blasts, refractory anemia with excess blasts in transformation, and chronic myelomonocytic leukemia) and intermediate-1, intermediate-2, and high-risk International Prognostic Scoring System (IPSS) groups

Labeled Contraindications There are no contraindications listed in the manufacturer's labeling.

Pregnancy Considerations Adverse events were observed in animal reproduction studies. Based on the mechanism of action, decitabine may cause fetal harm if administered during pregnancy. Women of childbearing potential should be advised to use effective contraception to avoid pregnancy during treatment and for 1 month after treatment. In addition, males should be advised to avoid fathering a child while on decitabine therapy and for 2 months after treatment.

Breastfeeding Considerations Because of the potential for serious adverse reactions in the nursing infant, a decision should be made to discontinue breastfeeding or the drug, taking into account the importance of treatment to the mother.

Warnings/Precautions Neutropenia and thrombocytopenia commonly occur; anemia and neutropenic fever have also been reported. Myelosuppression and worsening neutropenia are more common in first two treatment cycles and may not correlate with progression of underlying MDS. Hematologic toxicity may require dosage adjustment (after the first cycle), growth factor support, and/or antimicrobial agents. Monitor for infection. Potentially significant drug-drug interactions may exist, requiring dose or frequency adjustment, additional monitoring, and/or selection of alternative therapy.

Adverse Reactions

>10%:

Cardiovascular: Peripheral edema (25% to 27%), edema (5% to 18%), heart murmur (16%), hypotension (6% to 11%)

Central nervous system: Fatigue (46%), headache (23% to 28%), insomnia (14% to 28%), rigors (22%), dizziness (18% to 21%), chills (16%), pain (5% to 13%), confusion (8% to 12%), lethargy (12%), hypoesthesia (11%), anxiety (9% to 11%)

Dermatologic: Pallor (23%), skin rash (11% to 19%), erythema (5% to 14%), cellulitis (9% to 12%), pruritus (9% to 11%)

Endocrine & metabolic: Hyperglycemia (6% to 33%), hypoalbuminemia (7% to 24%), hypomagnesemia (5% to 24%), hypokalemia (12% to 22%), hyponatremia (19%), hyperkalemia (13%)

Gastrointestinal: Nausea (40% to 42%), constipation (30% to 35%), diarrhea (28% to 34%), vomiting (16% to 25%), anorexia (≤8% to 23%), decreased appetite (≤8% to 23%), abdominal pain (5% to 14%), stomatitis (11% to 12%), dyspepsia (10% to 12%)

Hematologic & oncologic: Neutropenia (38% to 90%; grades 3/4: 37% to 87%; recovery 28 to 50 days), thrombocytopenia (27% to 89%; grades 3/4: 24% to 85%), anemia (31% to 82%; grades 3/4: 22%), petechia (12% to 39%), febrile neutropenia (20% to 29%; grades 3/4: 23%), leukopenia (6% to 28%; grades 3/4: 22%), bruise (9% to 22%), oral mucosal petechiae (13%), lymphadenopathy (12%)

Hepatic: Hyperbilirubinemia (6% to 14%), increased serum alkaline phosphatase (11%)

Local: Localized tenderness (11%)

Neuromuscular & skeletal: Arthralgia (17% to 20%), limb pain (18% to 19%), back pain (17% to 18%), weakness (15%)

Respiratory: Cough (27% to 40%), dyspnea (29%), pneumonia (20% to 22%), pharyngitis (16%), rales (8% to 14%), epistaxis (13%)

Miscellaneous: Fever (6% to 53%), lesion (5% to 11%)

5% to 10%:

Cardiovascular: Tachycardia (8%), chest wall pain (7%), chest pain (≤6% to 7%), chest discomfort (≤6% to 7%), facial edema (6%), hypertension (6%), cardiac failure (5%)

Central nervous system: Depression (9%), falling (8%), malaise (5%), mouth pain (5%)

Dermatologic: Alopecia (8%), xeroderma (8%), urticaria (6%), catheter site erythema (5%), night sweats (5%)

◀

Endocrine & metabolic: Hyperuricemia (10%), weight loss (9%), increased lactate dehydrogenase (8%), dehydration (6% to 8%), hypochloremia (6%), increased serum bicarbonate (6%), decreased serum bicarbonate (5%), hypoproteinemia (5%)

Gastrointestinal: Mucosal inflammation (9%), gingival hemorrhage (8%), hemorrhoids (8%), loose stools (7%), tongue ulcer (7%), oral candidiasis (6%), toothache (6%), dysphagia (5% to 6%), abdominal distention (5%), gastroesophageal reflux disease (5%), glossalgia (5%), oral mucosa ulcer (lip: 5%)

Genitourinary: Urinary tract infection (7%), dysuria (6%)

Hematologic & oncologic: Hematoma (5%), pancytopenia (5%), thrombocythemia (5%)

Hepatic: Ascites (10%), increased serum AST (10%), decreased serum bilirubin (5%)

Hypersensitivity: Transfusion reaction (7%)

Infection: Candidiasis (10%), bacteremia (5% to 8%), staphylococcal infection (7%), tooth abscess (5%)

Local: Catheter infection (8%), catheter pain (5%), swelling at injection site (5%)

Neuromuscular & skeletal: Myalgia (5% to 9%), muscle spasm (7%), ostealgia (6%), musculoskeletal pain (≤6%; includes discomfort)

Ophthalmic: Blurred vision (6%)

Otic: Otalgia (6%)

Renal: Polyuria (5%)

Respiratory: Hypoxia (10%), upper respiratory tract infection (10%), abnormal breath sounds (5% to 10%), pharyngolaryngeal pain (8%), pulmonary edema (6%), sinusitis (5% to 6%), pleural effusion (5%), post nasal drip (5%), pulmonary signs and symptoms (crepitations: 5%), sinus congestion (5%)

<5%, postmarketing, and/or case reports: Abscess (peridiverticular), acute cardiorespiratory failure, anaphylaxis, atrial fibrillation, cardiomyopathy, catheter site hemorrhage, cholecystitis, fungal infection, gastrointestinal hemorrhage, gingival pain, hemoptysis, hypersensitivity reaction, intracranial hemorrhage, mental status change, myocardial infarction, mycobacterium avium complex, nodule (pulmonary), pulmonary aspergillosis, pulmonary embolism, pulmonary infection (pseudomonas), pulmonary infiltrates, renal failure, sepsis, splenomegaly, supraventricular tachycardia, Sweet's syndrome (acute febrile neutrophilic dermatosis), urethral bleeding

Drug Interactions

Metabolism/Transport Effects None known.

Avoid Concomitant Use

Avoid concomitant use of Decitabine with any of the following: BCG (Intravesical); Deferiprone; Dipyrone

Increased Effect/Toxicity

Decitabine may increase the levels/effects of: CloZAPine; Deferiprone

The levels/effects of Decitabine may be increased by: Dipyrone; Palifermin; Promazine

Decreased Effect

Decitabine may decrease the levels/effects of: BCG (Intravesical); Lenograstim

Hazardous Drugs Handling Considerations

Hazardous agent (NIOSH 2016 [group 1]).

Use appropriate precautions for receiving, handling, administration, and disposal. Gloves (single) should be worn during receiving, unpacking, and placing in storage.

NIOSH recommends double gloving, a protective gown, ventilated engineering controls (a class II biological safety cabinet or a compounding aseptic containment isolator), and closed system transfer devices (CSTDs) for preparation. Double gloving, a gown, and (if dosage form allows) CSTDs are required during administration (NIOSH 2016).

Storage/Stability Store intact vials at 25°C (77°F); excursions permitted to 15°C to 30°C (59°F to 86°F). Solutions diluted for infusion in NS or D5W may be stored for up to 4 hours prior to infusion refrigerated at 2°C to 8°C (36°F to 46°F) **if** prepared with cold infusion fluids. Infusion should begin within 15 minutes of preparation if room temperature infusion solutions are utilized.

Preparation for Administration Vials should be reconstituted with 10 mL SWFI to a concentration of 5 mg/mL. Immediately further dilute with NS or D5W to a final concentration of 0.1 to 1 mg/mL. Use appropriate precautions for handling and disposal. Solutions not administered within 15 minutes of preparation should be prepared with cold (2°C to 8°C [36°F to 46°F]) infusion solutions.

Mechanism of Action After phosphorylation, decitabine is incorporated into DNA and inhibits DNA methyltransferase causing hypomethylation and subsequent cell death (within the S-phase of the cell cycle).

Pharmacodynamics/Kinetics

Distribution: ~63 to 89 L/m^2 (Cashen 2008)

Metabolism: Possibly via deamination by cytidine deaminase

Half-life elimination: ~30 to 35 minutes

Dosing

Adult & Geriatric

Myelodysplastic syndromes (MDS): IV:

15 mg/m^2 over 3 hours every 8 hours (45 mg/m^2/day) for 3 days (135 mg/m^2/cycle) every 6 weeks; treatment is recommended for at least 4 cycles and may continue until the patient no longer benefits.

Adjustment for prolonged hematologic toxicity (ANC <1,000/mm^3 and platelets <50,000/mm^3):

>6 weeks but <8 weeks: Delay dose for up to 2 weeks and temporarily reduce dose to 11 mg/m^2 every 8 hours (33 mg/m^2/day) for 3 days (99 mg/m^2/cycle)

>8 weeks but <10 weeks: Assess for disease progression; if no disease progression, delay dose for up to 2 weeks and reduce dose to 11 mg/m^2 every 8 hours (33 mg/m^2/day) for 3 days (99 mg/m^2/cycle); maintain or increase dose with subsequent cycles if clinically indicated

or

20 mg/m^2 over 1 hour daily for 5 days every 28 days (delay subsequent treatment cycles until hematologic recovery [ANC ≥1,000/mm^3 and platelets ≥50,000/mm^3]); treatment is recommended for at least 4 cycles and may continue until the patient no longer benefits.

Acute myeloid leukemia (AML) (off-label use): Adults ≥60 years: IV: 20 mg/m^2 over 1 hour daily for 5 days every 28 days until relapse, disease progression, or unacceptable toxicity (Cashen 2010; Kantarjian 2012)

◀ **Renal Impairment**

Preexisting impairment: There are no dosage adjustments provided in the manufacturer's labeling (has not been studied); use with caution.

Renal toxicity during treatment: Serum creatinine ≥2 mg/dL: Temporarily hold treatment until resolution.

Hepatic Impairment

Preexisting impairment: There are no dosage adjustments provided in the manufacturer's labeling (has not been studied); use with caution.

Hepatotoxicity during treatment: ALT and/or bilirubin ≥2 times ULN: Temporarily hold treatment until resolution.

Adjustment for Toxicity

Hematologic toxicity (ANC <1,000/mm^3 and platelets <50,000/mm^3): Delay and/or reduce dose; refer to adult dosing for recommendations specific to each MDS dosing regimen

Nonhematologic toxicity: Temporarily hold treatment until resolution for any of the following toxicities:

Serum creatinine ≥2 mg/dL

ALT, bilirubin ≥2 times ULN

Active or uncontrolled infection

Administration Infuse over 1 to 3 hours. For the treatment of myelodysplastic syndromes, administer by IV infusion over 3 hours (15 mg/m^2 dose) or over 1 hour (20 mg/m^2 dose). For the treatment of acute myeloid leukemia (off-label use), administer by IV infusion over 1 hour (Cashen 2010; Kantarjian 2012). Premedication with antiemetics is recommended according to the manufacturer.

Emetic Potential Children and Adults: Minimal (<10%)

Monitoring Parameters CBC with differential and platelets (with each cycle and more frequently if needed); liver enzymes (prior to treatment initiation and periodically); serum creatinine (prior to treatment initiation and periodically)

Dosage Forms Excipient information presented when available (limited, particularly for generics); consult specific product labeling.

Solution Reconstituted, Intravenous:

Dacogen: 50 mg (1 ea)

Generic: 50 mg (1 ea)

Deferasirox (de FER a sir ox)

Brand Names: US Exjade; Jadenu; Jadenu Sprinkle

Brand Names: Canada Exjade; Jadenu

Index Terms ICL670

Pharmacologic Category Chelating Agent

Use

Chronic iron overload due to transfusions: Treatment of chronic iron overload caused by blood transfusions (transfusional hemosiderosis) in patients 2 years and older.

Chronic iron overload in nontransfusion-dependent thalassemia syndromes: Treatment of chronic iron overload in patients 10 years and older with nontransfusion-dependent thalassemia syndromes and with a liver iron concentration (LIC) of at least 5 mg of iron per gram of liver dry weight (mg Fe/g dw) and a serum ferritin greater than 300 mcg/L.

Limitations of use: Safety and efficacy of deferasirox in combination with other iron chelation therapies have not been established. Controlled studies of deferasirox in myelodysplastic syndromes and chronic iron overload due to transfusions have not been conducted.

Pregnancy Risk Factor C

Dosing

Adult & Geriatric Note: Calculate dose to the nearest whole tablet size or nearest whole granules packet.

Chronic iron overload due to transfusions: Oral: **Note:** Treatment should only be initiated with evidence of chronic iron overload (ie, transfusion of ≥100 mL/kg of packed red blood cells [eg, ≥20 units for a 40 kg individual] and serum ferritin consistently >1,000 mcg/L).

Exjade:

Initial: 20 mg/kg once daily

Maintenance: Adjust dose every 3 to 6 months based on serum ferritin trends; adjust by 5 or 10 mg/kg/day; titrate to individual response and treatment goals. In patients not adequately controlled with 30 mg/kg/day, doses up to 40 mg/kg/day may be considered for serum ferritin levels persistently >2,500 mcg/L and not decreasing over time (doses >40 mg/kg/day are not recommended). Consider interrupting therapy for serum ferritin consistently <500 mcg/L.

Jadenu:

Initial: 14 mg/kg once daily

Maintenance: Adjust dose every 3 to 6 months based on serum ferritin trends; adjust by 3.5 or 7 mg/kg/day; titrate to individual response and treatment goals. In patients not adequately controlled with 21 mg/kg/day, doses up to 28 mg/kg/day may be considered for serum ferritin levels persistently >2,500 mcg/L and not decreasing over time (doses >28 mg/kg/day are not recommended). Consider interrupting therapy for serum ferritin consistently <500 mcg/L.

Chronic iron overload in non-transfusion-dependent thalassemia syndromes: Oral: **Note:** Treatment should only be initiated with evidence of chronic iron overload (hepatic iron concentration ≥5 mg Fe/g dry weight and serum ferritin >300 mcg/L).

Exjade:

Initial: 10 mg/kg once daily. Consider increasing to 20 mg/kg once daily after 4 weeks if baseline hepatic iron concentration is >15 mg Fe/g dry weight.

Maintenance: Dependent upon serum ferritin measurements (monthly) and hepatic iron concentrations (every 6 months):

If serum ferritin is <300 mcg/L: Interrupt therapy and obtain hepatic iron concentration

If hepatic iron concentration:

<3 mg Fe/g dry weight: Interrupt therapy; resume treatment when hepatic iron concentration is >5 mg Fe/g dry weight

3 to 7 mg Fe/g dry weight: Continue treatment at a dose ≤10 mg/kg/day

>7 mg Fe/g dry weight: Increase dose to 20 mg/kg/day; Maximum dose: 20 mg/kg/day

Jadenu:

Initial: 7 mg/kg once daily. Consider increasing to 14 mg/kg once daily after 4 weeks if baseline hepatic iron concentration is >15 mg Fe/g dry weight.

Maintenance: Dependent upon serum ferritin measurements (monthly) and hepatic iron concentrations (every 6 months):

If serum ferritin is <300 mcg/L: Interrupt therapy and obtain hepatic iron concentration

◄

If hepatic iron concentration:

<3 mg Fe/g dry weight: Interrupt therapy; resume treatment when hepatic iron concentration is >5 mg Fe/g dry weight

3 to 7 mg Fe/g dry weight: Continue treatment at a dose ≤7 mg/kg/day

>7 mg Fe/g dry weight: Increase dose to 14 mg/kg/day; Maximum dose: 14 mg/kg/day

Dosage adjustment with concomitant medications: Bile acid sequestrants (eg, cholestyramine, colesevelam, colestipol) or potent UGT inducers (eg, rifampin, phenytoin, phenobarbital, ritonavir): Avoid concomitant use; if coadministration is necessary, consider increasing the initial dose of deferasirox dose by 50%; monitor serum ferritin and clinical response.

Conversion from Exjade to Jadenu: The dose for Jadenu should be ~30% lower

Pediatric Note: Calculate dose to the nearest whole tablet size or nearest whole granules packet. When calculating dose, consider changes in weight over time.

Chronic iron overload due to transfusions: Children ≥2 years and Adolescents: Refer to adult dosing.

Chronic iron overload in non-transfusion-dependent thalassemia syndromes: Children ≥10 years and Adolescents: Refer to adult dosing.

Conversion from Exjade to Jadenu: Children ≥2 years and Adolescents: Refer to adult dosing.

Renal Impairment CrCl should be estimated using the Cockcroft-Gault formula.

Renal impairment at treatment initiation:

CrCl >60 mL/minute: No dosage adjustment necessary.

CrCl 40 to 60 mL/minute: Initial: Reduce dose by 50%.

CrCl <40 mL/minute or serum creatinine >2 times age-appropriate ULN: Use is contraindicated.

Renal toxicity during treatment:

Transfusional iron overload:

Adolescents ≥16 years and Adults: For increase in serum creatinine ≥33% above the average baseline, repeat within 1 week; if still elevated by ≥33%: Reduce daily dose by 10 mg/kg (for Exjade) **or** 7 mg/kg (for Jadenu)

Children ≥2 years to Adolescents 15 years: For increase in serum creatinine >33% above the average baseline level and above the age-appropriate ULN: Reduce daily dose by 10 mg/kg (for Exjade) **or** 7 mg/kg (for Jadenu)

All patients: CrCl <40 mL/minute or serum creatinine >2 times age-appropriate ULN: Discontinue treatment.

Non-transfusion-dependent thalassemia syndromes:

Adolescents ≥16 years and Adults: For increase in serum creatinine ≥33% above the average baseline, repeat within 1 week; if still elevated by ≥33%:

Exjade: Interrupt therapy if the dose is 5 mg/kg; reduce dose by 50% if the dose is 10 or 20 mg/kg

Jadenu: Interrupt therapy if the dose is 3.5 mg/kg; reduce dose by 50% if the dose is 7 or 14 mg/kg

Children ≥10 years to Adolescents 15 years: For increase in serum creatinine >33% above the average baseline level and above the age-appropriate ULN: Reduce daily dose by 5 mg/kg (for Exjade) **or** 3.5 mg/kg (for Jadenu).

All patients: CrCl <40 mL/minute or serum creatinine >2 times age-appropriate ULN: Discontinue treatment.

Hepatic Impairment

Hepatic impairment at treatment initiation:

Mild impairment (Child-Pugh class A): No dosage adjustment necessary; monitor closely for efficacy and for adverse reactions requiring dosage reduction.

Moderate impairment (Child-Pugh class B): Initial: Reduce dose by 50%; monitor closely for efficacy and for adverse reactions requiring dosage reduction.

Severe impairment (Child-Pugh class C): Avoid use.

Hepatic toxicity during treatment: Severe or persistent increases in trans-aminases/bilirubin: Reduce dose or temporarily interrupt treatment.

Adjustment for Toxicity

Bone marrow suppression: Interrupt treatment; may reinitiate once cause of cytopenia has been determined; use contraindicated if platelet count <50,000/mm^3

Dermatologic toxicity:

Rash (severe): Interrupt treatment; may reintroduce at a lower dose (with future dose escalation) and short-term oral corticosteroids.

Severe skin reaction (Stevens-Johnson syndrome, toxic epidermal necrolysis, erythema multiforme): Discontinue and evaluate.

Gastrointestinal: Discontinue treatment for suspected GI ulceration or hemorrhage.

Hearing loss or visual disturbance: Consider dose reduction or treatment interruption.

Additional Information Complete prescribing information should be consulted for additional detail.

Dosage Forms Excipient information presented when available (limited, particularly for generics); consult specific product labeling.

Packet, Oral:

Jadenu Sprinkle: 90 mg (30 ea); 180 mg (30 ea); 360 mg (30 ea)

Tablet, Oral:

Jadenu: 90 mg, 180 mg, 360 mg

Tablet Soluble, Oral:

Exjade: 125 mg, 250 mg, 500 mg

Deferiprone (de FER i prone)

Brand Names: US Ferriprox

Index Terms APO-066

Pharmacologic Category Chelating Agent

Use

Transfusional iron overload: Treatment of transfusional iron overload due to thalassemia syndromes with inadequate response to other chelation therapy.

Limitation of use: Safety and effectiveness have not been established for the treatment of transfusional iron overload in patients with other chronic anemias.

Pregnancy Risk Factor D

◄ **Hazardous Drugs Handling Considerations**
Hazardous agent (NIOSH 2016 [group 2]).

Use appropriate precautions for receiving, handling, administration, and disposal. Gloves (single) should be worn during receiving, unpacking, and placing in storage. NIOSH recommends single gloving for administration of intact tablets or capsules. NIOSH recommends double gloving, a protective gown, and (if there is a potential for vomit or spit up) eye/face protection for administration of an oral liquid/feeding tube administration (NIOSH 2016).

Dosing

Adult Note: Round dose to the nearest 250 mg (or $1/2$ tablet) or 2.5 mL (oral solution). If serum ferritin falls consistently below 500 mcg/L, consider temporary treatment interruption.

Transfusional iron overload: Oral: Initial: 25 mg/kg 3 times/day (75 mg/kg/day); individualize dose based on response and therapeutic goal; maximum dose: 33 mg/kg 3 times/day (99 mg/kg/day)

Geriatric Refer to adult dosing. Begin at the low end of dosing range.

Renal Impairment There are no dosage adjustments provided in the manufacturer's labeling.

Hepatic Impairment There are no dosage adjustments provided in the manufacturer's labeling (has not been studied in patients with severe impairment).

Adjustment for Toxicity

ANC <1,500/mm^3 and >500/mm^3: Interrupt treatment immediately and monitor until recovery; do not rechallenge unless the potential benefit outweighs the risk.

ANC <500/mm^3: In addition to treatment interruption, consider hospitalization (and other clinically-appropriate management); do not resume unless the potential benefits outweigh potential risks

Infection: Interrupt treatment; monitor ANC more frequently

Additional Information Complete prescribing information should be consulted for additional detail.

Medication Guide Available Yes

Dosage Forms Excipient information presented when available (limited, particularly for generics); consult specific product labeling.

Solution, Oral:

Ferriprox: 100 mg/mL (500 mL) [contains fd&c yellow #6 (sunset yellow); cherry-peppermint flavor]

Tablet, Oral:

Ferriprox: 500 mg [scored]

Deferoxamine (de fer OKS a meen)

Brand Names: US Desferal

Brand Names: Canada Deferoxamine Mesylate for Injection; Desferal; PMS-Deferoxamine

Index Terms Deferoxamine Mesylate; Desferrioxamine; Desferrioxamine Methanesulphonate; DFM

Pharmacologic Category Antidote; Chelating Agent

Use

Acute iron toxicity: Adjunct in the treatment of acute iron intoxication

Chronic iron overload: Treatment of chronic iron overload secondary to multiple transfusions (often due to the presence of thalassemia major or sickle cell disease [Borgna-Pignatti 2015; Marsella 2015])

Pregnancy Risk Factor C

Dosing

Adult

Acute iron toxicity: Note: The IV route is preferred and is used when severe toxicity is evidenced by cardiovascular collapse or systemic symptoms (coma, shock, metabolic acidosis, or gastrointestinal bleeding) or potentially severe intoxications (peak serum iron level >500 mcg/dL) (Perrone 2015). The IM route may be used (per the manufacturer) but is not preferred and rarely indicated. The use of deferoxamine in situations in which the peak serum iron concentration is <500 mcg/dL or when severe toxicity is not evident is a subject of clinical debate (Howland 2015; Perrone 2015).

IM, IV: Initial: 1,000 mg, may be followed by 500 mg every 4 hours for 2 doses; subsequent doses of 500 mg have been administered every 4 to 12 hours based on clinical response (maximum recommended dose: 6,000 mg/day [per manufacturer])

Chronic iron overload:

IM: 500 to 1,000 mg/day (maximum: 1000 mg/day)

IV: 40 to 50 mg/kg/day (maximum: 60 mg/kg/day) over 8 to 12 hours for 5 to 7 days per week

SubQ: 1,000 to 2,000 mg/day or 20 to 40 mg/kg/day over 8 to 24 hours

Off-label dosing: IV, SubQ: 25 to 50 mg/kg over 8 to 10 hours 5 to 7 days per week (Brittenham, 2011)

Diagnosis of aluminum-induced toxicity with CKD (off-label use) (K/DOQI guidelines 2003): IV: Test dose: 5 mg/kg during the last hour of dialysis if baseline serum aluminum concentrations are 60 to 200 mcg/L, or clinical signs/symptoms of toxicity, or aluminum exposure prior to parathyroid surgery. Measure aluminum just prior to deferoxamine; remeasure 2 days later (test is positive if serum aluminum increases by ≥50 mcg/L). Do not use if unstimulated aluminum serum concentrations are >200 mcg/L to avoid deferoxamine-induced neurotoxicity.

Treatment of aluminum toxicity with CKD (off-label use) (K/DOQI guideline, 2003): IV:

Administer after diagnostic deferoxamine test dose. **Note:** The risk for deferoxamine-associated neurotoxicity is increased if unstimulated aluminum serum concentrations are >200 mcg/L; do not perform the deferoxamine-stimulation test and administer intensive dialysis until <200 mcg/L.

*If the serum aluminum concentration rises to ≥300 mcg/L two days after the deferoxamine test dose **or** there are side effects after the deferoxamine-stimulation test:* 5 mg/kg once a week 5 hours before dialysis for 4 months. Then discontinue deferoxamine for one month and perform the deferoxamine-stimulation test again.

*If the serum aluminum concentration is <300 mcg/L two days after the deferoxamine test dose **and** there are no side effects after the deferoxamine-stimulation test:* 5 mg/kg once a week during the last hour of dialysis for 2 months. The discontinue deferoxamine for one month and perform the deferoxamine-stimulation test again.

Geriatric Refer to adult dosing. May initiate at the lower end of the dosing range.

Pediatric

Acute iron toxicity: Children and Adolescents: **Note:** The IV route is preferred and is used when severe toxicity is evidenced by cardiovascular collapse or systemic symptoms (coma, shock, metabolic acidosis, or gastrointestinal bleeding) or potentially severe intoxications (peak serum iron level >500 mcg/dL) (Perrone 2015). The IM route may be used (per the manufacturer) but is not preferred and rarely indicated. The use of deferoxamine in situations in which the peak serum iron concentration is <500 mcg/dL or when severe toxicity is not evident is a subject of clinical debate (Howland 2015; Perrone 2015).

IM: 90 mg/kg/dose every 8 hours (maximum: 6,000 mg/24 hours)

IV: 15 mg/kg/hour (maximum: 6,000 mg/24 hours)

Chronic iron overload: Children ≥3 years and Adolescents:

IV: 20 to 40 mg/kg/day over 8 to 12 hours for 5 to 7 days per week; dose should not exceed 40 mg/kg/day until growth has ceased

SubQ: 20 to 40 mg/kg/day over 8 to 12 hours (maximum: 1,000 to 2,000 mg/day)

Off-label dosing: IV, SubQ: 25 to 30 mg/kg over 8 to 10 hours 5 to 7 days per week (Brittenham, 2011)

Diagnosis of aluminum induced toxicity with CKD (off-label use) (K/DOQI guidelines 2003): Children and Adolescents: IV: Test dose: 5 mg/kg during the last hour of dialysis if baseline serum aluminum concentrations are 60 to 200 mcg/L, or clinical signs/symptoms of toxicity, or aluminum exposure prior to parathyroid surgery. Measure aluminum just prior to deferoxamine; remeasure 2 days later (test is positive if serum aluminum increases by ≥50 mcg/L). Do not use if unstimulated aluminum serum concentrations are >200 mcg/L to avoid deferoxamine-induced neurotoxicity.

Treatment of aluminum toxicity with CKD (off-label use) (K/DOQI guidelines 2003): Children and Adolescents: IV: Administer after diagnostic deferoxamine test dose. **Note:** The risk for deferoxamine-associated neurotoxicity is increased if unstimulated aluminum serum concentrations are >200 mcg/L; do not perform the deferoxamine-stimulation test and administer intensive dialysis until <200 mcg/L.

If the serum aluminum concentration rises to ≥300 mcg/L two days after the deferoxamine test dose **or** *there are side effects after the deferoxamine-stimulation test:* 5 mg/kg once a week 5 hours before dialysis for 4 months. Then discontinue deferoxamine for one month and perform the deferoxamine-stimulation test again.

If the serum aluminum concentration is <300 mcg/L two days after the deferoxamine test dose **and** *there are no side effects after the deferoxamine-stimulation test:* 5 mg/kg once a week during the last hour of dialysis for 2 months. The discontinue deferoxamine for one month and perform the deferoxamine-stimulation test again.

Renal Impairment Severe renal disease or anuria: Use is contraindicated in the manufacturer's US labeling.

The following adjustments have been used by some clinicians (Aronoff 2007): Adults:

CrCl >50 mL/minute: No adjustment required

CrCl 10 to 50 mL/minute, CRRT: Administer 25% to 50% of normal dose

CrCl<10 mL/minute, hemodialysis, peritoneal dialysis: Avoid use

Hepatic Impairment There are no dosage adjustments provided in the manufacturer's labeling (has not been studied).

Additional Information Complete prescribing information should be consulted for additional detail.

Dosage Forms Excipient information presented when available (limited, particularly for generics); consult specific product labeling. [DSC] = Discontinued product

Solution Reconstituted, Injection, as mesylate:
  Desferal: 500 mg (1 ea); 2 g (1 ea [DSC])
  Generic: 500 mg (1 ea); 2 g (1 ea)

◆ **Deferoxamine Mesylate** *see* Deferoxamine *on page 556*

◆ **Deferoxamine Mesylate for Injection (Can)** *see* Deferoxamine *on page 556*

Defibrotide (DE fib ro tide)

Related Information

Hematopoietic Cell Transplantation *on page 2365*

Brand Names: US Defitelio

Index Terms Defibrotide Sodium; DF; Polydeoxyribonucleotide; Prociclide

Pharmacologic Category Antiplatelet Agent; Thrombolytic Agent

Use Hepatic sinusoidal obstruction syndrome (treatment): Treatment of hepatic sinusoidal obstruction syndrome (SOS; formerly called veno-occlusive disease [VOD]) with renal or pulmonary dysfunction following hematopoietic stem cell transplant (HSCT).

Labeled Contraindications Known hypersensitivity to defibrotide or any component of the formulation; concomitant administration with systemic anticoagulant or fibrinolytic therapy

Pregnancy Considerations Adverse effects have been observed in animal reproduction studies.

Breastfeeding Considerations It is not known if defibrotide is excreted in breast milk. Due to the potential for serious adverse reactions in the nursing infant, breastfeeding is not recommended by the manufacturer.

Warnings/Precautions Defibrotide may increase the risk of bleeding (based on increased activity of fibrinolytic enzymes *in vitro*). Do not initiate therapy in patients with active bleeding; monitor closely for signs of bleeding. If bleeding develops while on therapy, discontinue defibrotide, evaluate/treat the underlying cause, and provide supportive care until bleeding resolves. Concomitant use with systemic anticoagulant or fibrinolytic therapy is contraindicated; may increase the risk of bleeding (not including agents [anticoagulant or fibrinolytic] used to maintain or clear central lines). Discontinue anticoagulants and fibrinolytic medications prior to initiating defibrotide; consider delaying defibrotide until anticoagulant effects have subsided. Patients were excluded from studies if on concurrent medication which increased the risk of hemorrhage (except heparin flushes when used for central line management or dialysis) (Richardson 2016). There is no known reversal agent for defibrotide. Discontinue infusion at least 2 hours prior to an invasive procedure; may resume infusion post-procedure once the risk of procedure-related bleeding is resolved.

Hypersensitivity reactions (eg, rash, urticaria, and angioedema) have been reported (rare). One patient with a history of previous defibrotide exposure experienced an anaphylactic reaction. Monitor closely for hypersensitivity reactions, particularly in patients who have received defibrotide previously. Discontinue therapy for severe hypersensitivity reactions and treat accordingly; monitor until symptoms resolve.

Predominant exclusion criteria from phase III studies were preexisting liver cirrhosis, prior solid organ transplant, dialysis dependence (at the time of transplant), oxygen dependence during conditioning, clinically significant bleeding, and hemodynamic instability (>1 pressor agent to maintain blood pressure) (Richardson 2011; Richardson 2016). Defibrotide is derived from porcine tissue. Potentially significant interactions may exist, requiring dose or frequency adjustment, additional monitoring, and/or selection of alternative therapy.

Adverse Reactions

>10%:
  Cardiovascular: Hypotension (11% to 37%)
  Gastrointestinal: Diarrhea (24%), vomiting (18%), nausea (16%)
  Hematologic & oncologic: Hemorrhage (59%; any type)
  Respiratory: Epistaxis (14%)

1% to 10%:
  Central nervous system: Intracranial hemorrhage (3%), cerebral hemorrhage (2%)
  Endocrine & metabolic: Hyperuricemia (2%)
  Gastrointestinal: Gastrointestinal hemorrhage (9%)
  Hematologic & oncologic: Pulmonary hemorrhage (4%)
  Hypersensitivity: Hypersensitivity reaction (<2%)
  Immunologic: Graft versus host disease (6%)
  Infection: Sepsis (7%), infection (3%)
  Respiratory: Pulmonary alveolar hemorrhage (7% to 9%), pulmonary infiltrates (6%), pneumonia (5%)

Frequency not defined:
  Cardiovascular: Thrombophlebitis
  Endocrine & metabolic: Hot flash
  Gastrointestinal: Abdominal cramps, abdominal pain, bloody diarrhea, hematemesis
  Genitourinary: Hematuria
  Hematologic & oncologic: Oral hemorrhage
  Renal: Renal failure
  Miscellaneous: Fever

Drug Interactions

Metabolism/Transport Effects None known.

Avoid Concomitant Use
  Avoid concomitant use of Defibrotide with any of the following: Urokinase

Increased Effect/Toxicity
  Defibrotide may increase the levels/effects of: Agents with Antiplatelet Properties; Anticoagulants; Apixaban; Cephalothin; Collagenase (Systemic); Dabigatran Etexilate; Deoxycholic Acid; Desirudin; Edoxaban; Ibritumomab; Obinutuzumab; Prostacyclin Analogues; Rivaroxaban; Salicylates; Thrombolytic Agents; Tositumomab and Iodine I 131 Tositumomab; Urokinase

  The levels/effects of Defibrotide may be increased by: Agents with Antiplatelet Properties; Dasatinib; Glucosamine; Herbs (Anticoagulant/Antiplatelet Properties); Ibrutinib; Limaprost; Multivitamins/Fluoride (with ADE); Multivitamins/Minerals (with ADEK, Folate, Iron); Multivitamins/Minerals (with AE, No Iron); Omega-3 Fatty Acids; Pentosan Polysulfate Sodium; Pentoxifylline; Prostacyclin Analogues; Salicylates; Tipranavir; Vitamin E (Systemic)

Decreased Effect

The levels/effects of Defibrotide may be decreased by: Aprotinin

Storage/Stability Store intact vials at 20°C to 25°C (68°F to 77°F); excursions permitted between 15°C to 30°C (59°F to 86°F). Solutions diluted for infusion in D5W or NS should be used within 4 hours if stored at room temperature or within 24 hours if refrigerated. Discard partially used vials.

Preparation for Administration Withdraw the calculated dose from the vial(s) and add to an infusion bag containing NS or D5W to a final concentration of 4 to 20 mg/mL; gently mix.

Mechanism of Action Defibrotide augments plasmin enzymatic activity to hydrolyze fibrin clots. It reduces endothelial cell (EC) activation and increases EC-mediated fibrinolysis by increasing tissue plasminogen activator and thrombomodulin expression, as well as by decreasing von Willebrand factor and plasminogen activator inhibitor-1 expression.

Pharmacodynamics/Kinetics

Distribution: V_d: 8.1 to 9.1 L

Protein binding: 93% to human plasma proteins

Metabolism: Polynucleotides are metabolized via nucleases, nucleotidases, nucleosidases, deaminases, and phosphorylases to oligonucleotides, nucleotides, nucleosides, and then to the free 2'-deoxyribose sugar, purine and pyrimidine bases

Half-life elimination: <2 hours

Excretion: Urine (5% to 15% of total dose)

Dosing

Adult & Geriatric Note: Utilize baseline body weight (prior to the preparative hematopoietic stem cell transplantation regimen) to calculate the defibrotide dose. Ensure that patients are hemodynamically stable (on no more than 1 vasopressor agent) and are not experiencing clinically significant bleeding prior to defibrotide administration.

Hepatic sinusoidal obstruction syndrome (SOS; formerly called veno-occlusive disease [VOD]), treatment: IV: 6.25 mg/kg every 6 hours for at least 21 days and up to a maximum of 60 days (until SOS resolution or hospital discharge) (Richardson 2016)

Pediatric Note: Utilize baseline body weight (prior to the preparative hematopoietic stem cell transplantation regimen) to calculate the defibrotide dose. Ensure that patients are hemodynamically stable (on no more than 1 vasopressor agent) and are not experiencing clinically significant bleeding prior to defibrotide administration.

Hepatic sinusoidal obstruction syndrome (SOS; formerly called veno-occlusive disease [VOD]), treatment: Infants >1 month, Children, and Adolescents: IV: 6.25 mg/kg every 6 hours for at least 21 days and up to a maximum of 60 days (until SOS resolution or hospital discharge) (Richardson 2016)

Hepatic sinusoidal obstruction syndrome (SOS; formerly called VOD), prevention (off-label use): Infants >1 month, Children, and Adolescents: IV: 6.25 mg/kg every 6 hours beginning the same day as the conditioning regimen and continuing for at least 14 and up to 30 days post-transplant (Corbacioglu 2012).

Renal Impairment There are no dosage adjustments provided in the manufacturer's labeling. Defibrotide is not removed by hemodialysis.

Hepatic Impairment There are no dosage adjustments provided in the manufacturer's labeling.

◄ **Adjustment for Toxicity**
Bleeding:
Persistent, severe or potentially life-threatening: Withhold defibrotide; treat underlying cause of bleeding and provide supportive care. Consider reinitiating treatment (at the same dose and volume) when bleeding has resolved and the patient is hemodynamically stable.
Recurrent significant bleeding: Discontinue permanently (do not resume).
Hypersensitivity reactions, severe or life-threatening (eg, anaphylaxis): Discontinue permanently (do not resume).
Invasive procedures: Discontinue defibrotide at least 2 hours prior to procedure. May resume treatment post-procedure once any risk of bleeding (related to procedure) is resolved.
Administration IV: Infuse over 2 hours using a 0.2 micron in-line filter. Flush the IV line with D5W or NS immediately before and after administration. Do not administer with other medications.
Monitoring Parameters Monitor for signs and symptoms of hepatic SOS and hypersensitivity reactions; monitor for bleeding
Product Availability Defitelio: FDA approved March 2016; anticipated availability is currently unknown.
Dosage Forms Excipient information presented when available (limited, particularly for generics); consult specific product labeling.
Solution, Intravenous, as sodium [preservative free]:
Defitelio: 200 mg/2.5 mL (2.5 mL)

◆ **Defibrotide Sodium** see Defibrotide on page 559
◆ **Defitelio** see Defibrotide on page 559

Degarelix (deg a REL ix)
Related Information
Safe Handling of Hazardous Drugs on page 2379
Brand Names: US Firmagon
Brand Names: Canada Firmagon
Index Terms Degarelix Acetate; FE200486
Pharmacologic Category Antineoplastic Agent, Gonadotropin-Releasing Hormone Antagonist; Gonadotropin Releasing Hormone Antagonist
Use Prostate cancer, advanced: Treatment of advanced prostate cancer
Labeled Contraindications
Known hypersensitivity to degarelix or any component of the formulation; women who are or may become pregnant.
Documentation of allergenic cross-reactivity for drugs in this class is limited. However, because of similarities in chemical structure and/or pharmacologic actions, the possibility of cross-sensitivity can not be ruled out with certainty.
Pregnancy Considerations Use is contraindicated in women who are or may become pregnant.
Adverse events were observed in animal reproduction studies.
Breastfeeding Considerations It is not known if degarelix is excreted in breast milk. This product is not indicated for use in women.
Warnings/Precautions Hypersensitivity reactions (including anaphylaxis, urticaria, and angioedema) have been reported. Discontinue for serious hypersensitivity reaction (immediately if dose not fully injected); manage hypersensitivity as clinically indicated. Do not rechallenge after serious hypersensitivity reaction.

Androgen deprivation therapy may prolong the QT interval; use with caution in patients with congenital long QT syndrome, a known history of QT prolongation or other risk factors for QT prolongation (eg, concomitant use of medications known to prolong QT interval, heart failure, and/or electrolyte abnormalities). Consider periodic electrolyte and ECG monitoring. Androgen-deprivation therapy may increase the risk for cardiovascular disease (Levine 2010) and decreased bone mineral density. Androgen deprivation therapy may be associated with an increased risk for insulin resistance and diabetes (Keating 2006). Testosterone suppression is associated with the development of anemia.

Degarelix exposure is decreased in patients with hepatic impairment, dosage adjustment is not recommended in patients with mild to moderate hepatic impairment, although testosterone levels should be monitored. Has not been studied in patients with severe hepatic impairment; use with caution. Mild transient increases in transaminases have been observed; monitor liver function in patients with known or suspected hepatic disorder. Data for use in patients with moderate to severe renal impairment (CrCl <50 mL/minute) is limited; use with caution. Potentially significant drug-drug interactions may exist, requiring dose or frequency adjustment, additional monitoring, and/or selection of alternative therapy.

Adverse Reactions

>10%:

Central nervous system: Fatigue (3% to >10%)

Endocrine & metabolic: Hot flash (26%), increased gamma-glutamyl transferase (≥10%), weight loss (≥10%), weight gain (9% to ≥10%)

Hepatic: Increased serum transaminases (47%)

Local: Injection site reactions (35%, grade 3: ≤2%; pain at injection site [28%], erythema at injection site [17%], swelling at injection site [6%], induration at injection site [4%], injection site nodule [3%], injection site infection [including abscess, 1%])

Miscellaneous: Fever (1% to ≥10%)

1% to 10%:

Cardiovascular: Hypertension (6%)

Central nervous system: Chills (5%), dizziness (1% to 5%), headache (1% to 5%), insomnia (1% to 5%)

Dermatologic: Diaphoresis

Endocrine & metabolic: Hypercholesterolemia (3%), gynecomastia

Gastrointestinal: Constipation (5%), nausea (1% to 5%), diarrhea

Genitourinary: Urinary tract infection (5%), erectile dysfunction, testicular atrophy

Hepatic: Increased serum ALT (10%; grade 3: <1%), increased serum AST (5%; grade 3: <1%)

Immunologic: Antibody development (antidegarelix: 10%)

Neuromuscular & skeletal: Back pain (6%), arthralgia (5%), weakness (1% to 5%)

Miscellaneous: Night sweats (1% to 5%)

<1%, postmarketing, and/or case reports: Bone metastases (worsening), cerebrovascular accident, depression, hypersensitivity reaction (including anaphylaxis, urticaria, and angioedema), itching at injection site, local soreness/soreness at injection site, malignant lymphoma, mental status changes, myocardial infarction, osteoarthritis, prolonged Q-T interval on ECG, squamous cell carcinoma, unstable angina pectoris

◄ **Drug Interactions**
Metabolism/Transport Effects None known.
Avoid Concomitant Use
Avoid concomitant use of Degarelix with any of the following: Indium 111 Capromab Pendetide
Increased Effect/Toxicity
Degarelix may increase the levels/effects of: Highest Risk QTc-Prolonging Agents; Moderate Risk QTc-Prolonging Agents

The levels/effects of Degarelix may be increased by: MiFEPRIStone
Decreased Effect
Degarelix may decrease the levels/effects of: Indium 111 Capromab Pendetide

Hazardous Drugs Handling Considerations
Hazardous agent (NIOSH 2016 [group 1]).

Use appropriate precautions for receiving, handling, administration, and disposal. Gloves (single) should be worn during receiving, unpacking, and placing in storage.

NIOSH recommends double gloving, a protective gown, ventilated engineering controls (a class II biological safety cabinet or a compounding aseptic containment isolator), and closed system transfer devices (CSTDs) for preparation. Double gloves and a protective gown are required during administration (NIOSH 2016).

Storage/Stability Store at 25°C (77°F); excursions permitted to 15°C to 30°C (59°F to 86°F). Use within 1 hour of reconstitution (US labeling). The Canadian labeling recommends immediate administration following reconstitution (preferred); stability has been demonstrated for 2 hours following reconstitution. Do not shake the vials.

Preparation for Administration Wear gloves for preparation and administration. Reconstitute with provided prefilled syringe containing preservative free sterile water for injection (reconstitute each 120 mg vial with 3 mL; reconstitute the 80 mg vial with 4.2 mL). Swirl gently; do NOT shake (to prevent foaming). Dissolution usually takes a few minutes, although may take up to 15 minutes. May tilt the vial slightly if the powder adheres to the side of the vial. To withdraw for administration, turn the vial completely upside down and pull down on the plunger to withdraw all of the reconstituted solution from the vial to the syringe; expel all air bubbles. Administer within 1 hour (US labeling) or 2 hours (Canadian labeling, although immediate administration is preferred) of reconstitution. Use of concentrations other than those described in the manufacturer's labeling is not recommended.

Mechanism of Action Gonadotropin-releasing hormone (GnRH) antagonist which reversibly binds to GnRH receptors in the anterior pituitary gland, blocking the receptor and decreasing secretion of luteinizing hormone (LH) and follicle stimulation hormone (FSH), resulting in rapid androgen deprivation by decreasing testosterone production, thereby decreasing testosterone levels. Testosterone levels do not exhibit an initial surge, or flare, as is typical with GnRH agonists (Crawford 2011).

Pharmacodynamics/Kinetics
Onset of action: Rapid; ~96% of patients had testosterone levels ≤50 ng/dL within 3 days (Klotz 2008)
Distribution: V_d: >1000 L
Protein binding: ~90%

Metabolism: Hepatobiliary, via peptide hydrolysis

Bioavailability: Biphasic release: Rapid release initially, then slow release from depot formed after subcutaneous injection administration (Tornoe 2007). Bioavailability is decreased in patients with mild-to-moderate hepatic impairment.

Half-life elimination: Loading dose: SubQ: ~53 days; Maintenance dose: SubQ: ~31 days (Canadian labeling)

Time to peak, plasma: Loading dose: SubQ: Within 2 days

Excretion: Feces (~70% to 80%, primarily as peptide fragments); urine (~20% to 30%)

Dosing

Adult & Geriatric Prostate cancer, advanced: SubQ:

Loading dose: 240 mg administered as two 120 mg (3 mL) injections

Maintenance dose: 80 mg administered as one 4 mL injection every 28 days (beginning 28 days after initial loading dose)

Renal Impairment

CrCl 50 to 80 mL/minute: No dosage adjustment necessary.

CrCl <50 mL/minute: There are no dosage adjustments provided in the manufacturer's labeling; use with caution.

Hepatic Impairment

Mild to moderate hepatic impairment (Child Pugh classes A and B): No dosage adjustment necessary; monitor serum testosterone levels.

Severe hepatic impairment (Child Pugh class C): There are no dosage adjustments provided in the manufacturer's labeling (has not been studied); use with caution.

Administration Administer (deep) SubQ in the abdominal area by pinching skin and elevating SubQ tissue; insert needle at a 45 degree angle. Gently pull plunger back to check for aspiration (if blood is aspirated into syringe, do not inject; discard and reconstitute a new dose); slowly inject over 30 seconds, remove needle and then release skin. For SubQ administration only; do not inject into a vein or into muscle. Avoid exposed areas (eg, waistband, belt, or near ribs). Rotate injection site. Inject loading dose as two 3 mL injections (40 mg/mL) in different sites; maintenance dose should be administered as a single 4 mL injection (20 mg/mL); begin maintenance dose 28 days after initial loading dose.

Monitoring Parameters Prostate-specific antigon (PSA) periodically, serum testosterone levels (if PSA increases; in patients with hepatic impairment: monitor testosterone levels monthly until achieve castration levels, then consider monitoring every other month), liver function tests (at baseline); consider baseline and periodic monitoring of serum electrolytes (calcium, magnesium, potassium, sodium); bone mineral density; consider baseline and periodic ECG monitoring.

Screen for diabetes and cardiovascular risk (blood pressure, lipid profile, serum glucose) prior to initiating treatment and 3 to 6 months after initiation (Levine 2010).

Test Interactions Suppression of pituitary-gonadal function may affect diagnostic tests of pituitary gonadotropic and gonadal functions.

Dosage Forms Excipient information presented when available (limited, particularly for generics); consult specific product labeling.

Solution Reconstituted, Subcutaneous, as acetate:

Firmagon: 80 mg (1 ea); 120 mg (1 ea)

◆ **Degarelix Acetate** see Degarelix on page 562

- **Delta-9-tetrahydro-cannabinol** *see* Dronabinol *on page 647*
- **Delta-9 THC** *see* Dronabinol *on page 647*
- **Delta-Aminolevulinic Acid Hydrochloride** *see* Aminolevulinic Acid (Systemic) *on page 114*
- **Delta-Aminolevulinic Acid Hydrochloride** *see* Aminolevulinic Acid (Topical) *on page 114*
- **Deltacortisone** *see* PredniSONE *on page 1545*
- **Deltadehydrocortisone** *see* PredniSONE *on page 1545*
- **Deltasone** *see* PredniSONE *on page 1545*
- **4-Demethoxydaunorubicin** *see* IDArubicin *on page 951*

Denosumab (den OH sue mab)

Related Information
Hypercalcemia of Malignancy *on page 2341*

Brand Names: US Prolia; Xgeva

Brand Names: Canada Prolia; Xgeva

Index Terms AMG-162

Pharmacologic Category Bone-Modifying Agent; Monoclonal Antibody

Use
Bone metastases from solid tumors (Xgeva): Prevention of skeletal-related events (eg, fracture, spinal cord compression, bone pain requiring surgery/radiation therapy) in patients with bone metastases from solid tumors.
Limitation of use: Denosumab is NOT indicated for prevention of skeletal-related events in patients with multiple myeloma

Giant cell tumor of bone (Xgeva): Treatment of giant cell tumor of bone (in adults and skeletally mature adolescents) that is unresectable or where surgical resection is likely to result in severe morbidity.

Hypercalcemia of malignancy (Xgeva): Treatment of hypercalcemia of malignancy refractory to bisphosphonate therapy

Osteoporosis/bone loss (Prolia): Treatment of osteoporosis in postmenopausal women at high risk of fracture; treatment of osteoporosis (to increase bone mass) in men at high risk of fracture; treatment of bone loss in men receiving androgen-deprivation therapy (ADT) for nonmetastatic prostate cancer; treatment of bone loss in women receiving aromatase inhibitor (AI) therapy for breast cancer

Labeled Contraindications
Prolia: Hypersensitivity (systemic) to denosumab or any component of the formulation; preexisting hypocalcemia; pregnancy

Xgeva: Known clinically significant hypersensitivity to denosumab or any component of the formulation; preexisting hypocalcemia

Pregnancy Considerations Use of Prolia is contraindicated in pregnant women. Based on data from animal reproduction studies and the mechanism of action, denosumab may cause fetal harm if administered to a pregnant woman. In females of reproductive potential, pregnancy status should be verified prior to treatment initiation. Denosumab is a human IgG monoclonal antibody; fetal exposure to monoclonal antibodies is expected to increase as pregnancy progresses. Women of reproductive potential should be advised to use effective contraception during denosumab treatment and for at least 5 months following the last dose. Studies of denosumab when used for osteoporosis/bone loss in men demonstrated that denosumab is present in the semen in low concentrations (~2% of serum exposure) and therefore unlikely that a female partner or fetus would be exposed during unprotected sex to pharmacologically relevant denosumab concentrations via seminal fluid; however, exposure from seminal fluid of men receiving denosumab for other indications and higher doses is unknown and; therefore, their pregnant partners should be counseled regarding this potential risk.

Women exposed to denosumab during pregnancy should contact the Amgen Pregnancy Surveillance Program (800-772-6436).

Breastfeeding Considerations It is not known if denosumab is present in breast milk. According to the manufacturer, the decision to discontinue denosumab or discontinue breastfeeding should take into account the benefits of treatment to the mother as well as the potential adverse effects on the breastfed infant. In some animal studies, mammary gland development was impaired following exposure to denosumab during pregnancy, resulting in impaired lactation postpartum; although development and lactation effects were not fully studied, mammary gland histopathology in female offspring exposed to denosumab in utero was normal at 6 months.

Warnings/Precautions Clinically significant hypersensitivity (including anaphylaxis) has been reported. May include throat tightness, facial edema, upper airway edema, lip swelling, dyspnea, pruritus, rash, urticaria, and hypotension. If anaphylaxis or clinically significant hypersensitivity occurs, initiate appropriate management and permanently discontinue. Denosumab may cause or exacerbate hypocalcemia; severe symptomatic cases (including fatalities) have been reported. An increased risk has been observed with increasing renal dysfunction, most commonly severe dysfunction (creatinine clearance <30 mL/minute and/or on dialysis), and with inadequate/no calcium supplementation. Monitor calcium levels; correct preexisting hypocalcemia prior to therapy. Monitor levels more frequently when denosumab is administered with other drugs that can also lower calcium levels. Use caution in patients with a history of hypoparathyroidism, thyroid surgery, parathyroid surgery, malabsorption syndromes, excision of small intestine, severe renal impairment/dialysis, or other conditions which would predispose the patient to hypocalcemia; monitor calcium, phosphorus, and magnesium closely during therapy (the manufacturer recommends monitoring within 14 days of injection [Prolia] or during the first weeks of therapy initiation [Xgeva]). Hypocalcemia lasting weeks to months (and requiring frequent monitoring) has been reported in postmarketing analyses. Administer calcium, vitamin D, and magnesium as necessary. Patients with severe renal impairment (CrCl <30 mL/minute) or those on dialysis may also develop marked elevations of serum parathyroid hormone (PTH). Hypercalcemia (clinically significant) may occur in patients with growing skeletons weeks to months following discontinuation of denosumab therapy. Monitor for signs/symptoms of hypercalcemia (eg, nausea, vomiting, headache, decreased alertness) and treat accordingly. Incidence of infections may be increased, including serious skin infections, abdominal, urinary, ear, or periodontal infections. Endocarditis has also been reported following use. Patients should be advised to contact their healthcare provider if signs or symptoms of severe infection or cellulitis develop. Use with caution in patients with impaired immune systems or using concomitant immunosuppressive therapy; may be at increased risk for serious infections. Evaluate the need for continued treatment with serious infection.

Atypical femur fractures have been reported in patients receiving denosumab. The fractures may occur anywhere along the femoral shaft (may be bilateral) and commonly occur with minimal to no trauma to the area. Some patients experience prodromal pain weeks or months before the fracture occurs. Because these fractures also occur in osteoporosis patients not treated with denosumab, it is unclear if denosumab therapy is the cause for the fractures; concomitant glucocorticoids may contribute to fracture risk. Advise patients to report new/unusual hip, thigh, or groin pain; and if so, evaluate for atypical/incomplete fracture. Contralateral limb should be assessed if atypical fracture occurs. Consider interrupting therapy in patients who develop an atypical femoral fracture. Following treatment discontinuation (in patients being treated for osteoporosis), the fracture risk increases, including risk of multiple vertebral fractures; vertebral fractures occurred as early as 7 months (average: 19 months) after the last dose of denosumab. Evaluate benefit/risk before initiating denosumab treatment for osteoporosis, especially in patients with prior vertebral fracture. If denosumab is discontinued, consider transitioning to an alternative osteoporosis therapy.

Osteonecrosis of the jaw (ONJ), also referred to as medication-related osteonecrosis of the jaw (MRONJ), has been reported in patients receiving denosumab. ONJ may manifest as jaw pain, osteomyelitis, osteitis, bone erosion, tooth/periodontal infection, toothache, gingival ulceration/erosion. Risk factors include invasive dental procedures (eg, tooth extraction, dental implants, oral surgery), cancer diagnosis, immunosuppressive therapy, angiogenesis inhibitor therapy, chemotherapy, systemic corticosteroids, poor oral hygiene, use of a dental appliance, ill-fitting dentures, periodontal and/or other preexisting dental disease, diabetes and gingival infections, local infection with delayed healing, anemia, and/or coagulopathy. In studies of patients with osseous metastasis, a longer duration of denosumab exposure was associated with a higher incidence of ONJ, although a majority of patients had predisposing factors, including a history of poor oral hygiene, tooth extraction, or the use of a dental appliance. Patients should maintain good oral hygiene during treatment. A dental exam and appropriate preventive dentistry should be performed prior to therapy. The manufacturer's labeling recommends avoiding invasive dental procedures in patients with bone metastases receiving denosumab for prevention of skeletal-related events and to consider temporary discontinuation of therapy in these patients if invasive dental procedure is required. According to a position paper by the American Association of Maxillofacial Surgeons (AAOMS), MRONJ has been associated with bisphosphonates and other antiresorptive agents (denosumab), and antiangiogenic agents (eg, bevacizumab, sunitinib) used for the treatment of osteoporosis or malignancy; risk is significantly higher in cancer patients receiving antiresorptive therapy compared to patients receiving osteoporosis treatment (regardless of medication used or dosing schedule). MRONJ risk is increased with intravenous antiresorptive therapy compared to the minimal risk associated with oral bisphosphonate use, although risk appears to increase with oral bisphosphonates when duration of therapy exceeds 4 years. The AAOMS suggests that if medically permissible, initiation of denosumab for cancer therapy should be delayed until optimal dental health is attained (if extractions are required, antiresorptive therapy should delayed until the extraction site has mucosalized or until after adequate osseous healing). Once denosumab is initiated for oncologic disease, procedures that involve direct osseous injury and placement of dental implants should be avoided. Patients developing ONJ during therapy should receive care by an oral surgeon (AAOMS [Ruggiero 2014]). According to the manufacturer, discontinuation of denosumab should be considered (based on risk/benefit evaluation) in patients who develop ONJ.

Postmenopausal osteoporosis: For use in women at high risk for fracture which is defined as a history of osteoporotic fracture or multiple risk factors for fracture. May also be used in women who failed or did not tolerate other therapies.

Bone metastases: Denosumab is not indicated for the prevention of skeletal-related events in patients with multiple myeloma. In trials of with multiple myeloma patients, denosumab was noninferior to zoledronic acid in delaying time to first skeletal-related event and mortality was increased in a subset of the denosumab-treated group.

Breast cancer: The American Society of Clinical Oncology (ASCO) updated guidelines on the role of bone-modifying agents (BMAs) in the prevention and treatment of skeletal-related events for metastatic breast cancer patients (Van Poznak 2011). The guidelines recommend initiating a BMA (denosumab, pamidronate, zoledronic acid) in patients with metastatic breast cancer to the bone. There is currently no literature indicating the superiority of one particular BMA. Optimal duration is not defined; however, the guidelines recommend continuing therapy until substantial decline in patient's performance status. The ASCO guidelines are in alignment with package insert guidelines for dosing, renal dose adjustments, infusion times, prevention and management of osteonecrosis of the jaw, and monitoring of laboratory parameter recommendations. BMAs are not the first-line therapy for pain. RMAs are to be used as adjunctive therapy for cancer-related bone pain associated with bone metastasis, demonstrating a modest pain control benefit. BMAs should be used in conjunction with agents such as NSAIDs, opioid and nonopioid analgesics, corticosteroids, radiation/surgery, and interventional procedures.

Denosumab therapy results in significant suppression of bone turnover; the long term effects of treatment are not known but may contribute to adverse outcomes such as ONJ, atypical fractures, or delayed fracture healing; monitor. Use with caution in patients with renal impairment (CrCl <30 mL/minute) or patients on dialysis; risk of hypocalcemia is increased. Dose adjustment is not needed when administered at 60 mg every 6 months (Prolia); once-monthly dosing has not been evaluated in patients with renal impairment (Xgeva). Dermatitis, eczema, and rash (which are not necessarily specific to the injection site) have been reported; consider discontinuing if severe symptoms occur. Packaging may contain natural latex rubber. May impair bone growth in children with open growth plates or inhibit eruption of dentition. In pediatrics, indicated only for the treatment of giant cell tumor of bone in adolescents who are skeletally mature. Do not administer Prolia and Xgeva to the same patient for different indications. Denosumab is intended for subcutaneous route only and should not be administered intravenously, intramuscularly, or intradermally. Potentially significant interactions may exist, requiring dose or frequency adjustment, additional monitoring, and/or selection of alternative therapy.

Adverse Reactions A postmarketing safety program for Prolia is available to collect information on adverse events; more information is available at http://www.proliasafety.com. To report adverse events for either Prolia or Xgeva, prescribers may also call Amgen at 800-772-6436 or FDA at 800-332-1088.

Percentages noted with Prolia (60 mg every 6 months) unless specified as Xgeva (120 mg every 4 weeks):

>10%:

Cardiovascular: Hypertension (11%, Lewiecki 2007)

Central nervous system: Fatigue (Xgeva: ≤45%), headache (Xgeva: 13% to 24%), peripheral edema (5%; Xgeva: 24%)

Dermatologic: Dermatitis (4% to 11%), eczema (4% to 11%), skin rash (3% to 11%)

Endocrine & metabolic: Hypophosphatemia (Xgeva: 32%; grade 3: 10% to 15%), hypocalcemia (2%; Xgeva: 3% to 18%; grade 3: 3%)

Gastrointestinal: Nausea (Xgeva: 31%), decreased appetite (Xgeva: 24%), vomiting (Xgeva: 24%), constipation (Xgeva: 21%), diarrhea (Xgeva: 20%)

Hematologic & oncologic: Anemia (Xgeva: 21%)

Infection: Influenza (11%, Lewiecki 2007)

Neuromuscular & skeletal: Weakness (Xgeva: ≤45%), arthralgia (7% to 14%), limb pain (10% to 12%), back pain (8% to 12%)

Respiratory: Dyspnea (Xgeva: 21% to 27%), cough (Xgeva: 15%)

1% to 10%:

Cardiovascular: Angina pectoris (3%)

Central nervous system: Sciatica (5%)

Endocrine & metabolic: Hypercholesterolemia (7%)

Gastrointestinal: Flatulence (2%)

Hematologic & oncologic: Malignant neoplasm (new; 3% to 5%)

Infection: Serious infection (4%)

Neuromuscular & skeletal: Musculoskeletal pain (6%), ostealgia (4%), myalgia (3%), osteonecrosis (jaw; ≤2%; Xgeva ≤2%)

Ophthalmic: Cataract (≤5%)

Respiratory: Nasopharyngitis (7%), upper respiratory tract infection (5%)

<1%, postmarketing, and/or case reports: Anaphylaxis (both formulations), antibody development (both formulations), endocarditis, erythema, facial swelling, femur fracture (both formulations; diaphyseal, subtrochanteric), hearing loss (FDA Safety Alert June 6, 2016), hypercalcemia (Xgeva, following discontinuation), hypersensitivity (both formulations), hypotension, pancreatitis, severe hypocalcemia (symptomatic; both formulations), urticaria

Drug Interactions

Metabolism/Transport Effects None known.

Avoid Concomitant Use

Avoid concomitant use of Denosumab with any of the following: Belimumab

Increased Effect/Toxicity

Denosumab may increase the levels/effects of: Belimumab; Immunosuppressants

Decreased Effect There are no known significant interactions involving a decrease in effect.

Storage/Stability Store in original carton at 2°C to 8°C (36°F to 46°F). Do not freeze. Prior to use, bring to room temperature of 25°C (77°F) in original container (usually takes 15 to 30 minutes); do not use any other methods for warming. Use within 14 days once at room temperature. Protect from direct heat and light; do not expose to temperatures >25°C (77°F). Avoid vigorous shaking.

Mechanism of Action Denosumab is a monoclonal antibody with affinity for nuclear factor-kappa ligand (RANKL). Osteoblasts secrete RANKL; RANKL activates osteoclast precursors and subsequent osteolysis which promotes release of bone-derived growth factors, such as insulin-like growth factor-1 (IGF1) and transforming growth factor-beta (TGF-beta), and increases serum calcium levels. Denosumab binds to RANKL, blocks the interaction between RANKL and RANK (a receptor located on osteoclast surfaces), and prevents osteoclast formation, leading to decreased bone resorption and increased bone mass in osteoporosis. In solid tumors with bony metastases, RANKL inhibition decreases osteoclastic activity leading to decreased skeletal related events and tumor-induced bone destruction. In giant cell tumors of the bone (which express RANK and RANKL), denosumab inhibits tumor growth by preventing RANKL from activating its receptor (RANK) on the osteoclast surface, osteoclast precursors, and osteoclast-like giant cells.

Pharmacodynamics/Kinetics

Onset of action: Decreases markers of bone resorption by ~85% within 3 days; maximal reductions observed within 1 month

Hypercalcemia of malignancy: Time to response (median): 9 days; Time to complete response (median): 23 days (Hu 2014)

Duration: Markers of bone resorption return to baseline within 12 months of discontinuing therapy

Hypercalcemia of malignancy: Duration of response (median): 104 days; Duration of complete response (median): 34 days (Hu 2014)

Bioavailability: SubQ: 62%

Half-life elimination: ~25 to 28 days

Time to peak, serum: 10 days (range: 3 to 21 days)

Dosing

Adult & Geriatric Note: Administer calcium and vitamin D as necessary to prevent or treat hypocalcemia

Bone metastases from solid tumors (prevention of skeletal-related events; Xgeva): SubQ: 120 mg every 4 weeks (Fizazi 2011; Henry 2011; Stopeck 2010)

Giant cell tumor of bone (Xgeva): SubQ: 120 mg once every 4 weeks; during the first month, give an additional 120 mg on days 8 and 15 (Blay 2011; Thomas 2010)

Hypercalcemia of malignancy (Xgeva): SubQ: 120 mg every 4 weeks; during the first month, give an additional 120 mg on days 8 and 15 (Hu 2014)

Osteoporosis/bone loss (Prolia):

Treatment of androgen deprivation-induced bone loss in men with prostate cancer: SubQ: 60 mg as a single dose, once every 6 months (Smith 2009)

Treatment of aromatase inhibitor-induced bone loss in women with breast cancer: SubQ: 60 mg as a single dose, once every 6 months (Ellis 2008)

Treatment of osteoporosis in men or in postmenopausal women: SubQ: 60 mg as a single dose, once every 6 months

Bone destruction caused by rheumatoid arthritis (off-label use): SubQ: 60 mg or 180 mg as a single one time dose and repeated at 6 months (in combination with continued methotrexate); a total of 2 doses was administered in the study (Cohen 2008). Additional data may be necessary to further define the role of denosumab in this condition.

◄ **Pediatric Note:** Administer calcium and vitamin D as necessary to prevent or treat hypocalcemia

Giant cell tumor of bone (Xgeva): Adolescents (skeletally mature) 13 to 17 years: SubQ: 120 mg once every 4 weeks; during the first month, give an additional 120 mg on days 8 and 15

Renal Impairment Monitor patients with severe impairment (CrCl <30 mL/minute or on dialysis) closely due to increased risk of hypocalcemia.

Prolia: No dosage adjustment necessary.

Xgeva: There are no dosage adjustments provided in the manufacturer's labeling. Guidelines suggest dosage adjustment is not necessary; close monitoring for hypocalcemia is recommended (Gravalos 2016; Van Poznak 2011).

Hepatic Impairment There are no dosage adjustments provided in the manufacturer's labeling (has not been studied).

Administration SubQ: Denosumab is intended for subcutaneous route only and should not be administered intravenously, intramuscularly, or intradermally. Prior to administration, bring to room temperature in original container (allow to stand ~15 to 30 minutes); do not warm by any other method. Solution may contain trace amounts of translucent to white protein particles; do not use if cloudy, discolored (normal solution should be clear and colorless to pale yellow), or contains excessive particles or foreign matter. Avoid vigorous shaking. Administer via SubQ injection in the upper arm, upper thigh, or abdomen.

Prolia: If a dose is missed, administer as soon as possible, then continue dosing every 6 months from the date of the last injection.

Monitoring Parameters

Recommend monitoring of serum creatinine, serum calcium, phosphorus and magnesium (especially within the first 14 days of therapy [Prolia] or during the first weeks of therapy initiation [Xgeva]), pregnancy test (to verify pregnancy status in females of reproductive potential); signs and symptoms of hypocalcemia, especially in patients predisposed to hypocalcemia (severe renal impairment, thyroid/parathyroid surgery, malabsorption syndromes, hypoparathyroidism); signs/symptoms of hypercalcemia (following discontinuation in patients with growing skeletons); infection, or dermatologic reactions; routine oral exam (prior to treatment); dental exam if risk factors for ONJ; monitor for sings/symptoms of hypersensitivity

Osteoporosis: Bone mineral density (BMD) should be re-evaluated every 2 years (or more frequently) after initiating therapy (NOF 2014); annual measurements of height and weight, assessment of chronic back pain; serum calcium and 25(OH)D; may consider monitoring biochemical markers of bone turnover

Dietary Considerations Ensure adequate calcium and vitamin D intake to prevent or treat hypocalcemia. Calcium 1000 mg/day and vitamin D ≥400 units/day is recommended in product labeling (Prolia). If dietary intake is inadequate, dietary supplementation is recommended. Women and men should consume:

Calcium: 1000 mg/day (men: 50 to 70 years) **or** 1200 mg/day (women ≥51 years and men ≥71 years) (IOM 2011; NOF 2014)

Vitamin D: 800 to 1000 units/day (men and women ≥50 years) (NOF 2014). Recommended Dietary Allowance (RDA): 600 units/day (men and women ≤70 years) **or** 800 units/day (men and women ≥71 years) (IOM 2011).

Medication Guide Available Yes

Dosage Forms Excipient information presented when available (limited, particularly for generics); consult specific product labeling.
Solution, Subcutaneous [preservative free]:
Prolia: 60 mg/mL (1 mL) [contains mouse (murine) and/or hamster protein]
Xgeva: 120 mg/1.7 mL (1.7 mL)

Desmopressin (des moe PRES in)

Brand Names: US DDAVP; DDAVP Rhinal Tube; Stimate
Brand Names: Canada Apo-Desmopressin; DDAVP; DDAVP Melt; DDAVP Rhinyle; Nocdurna; Octostim; PMS-Desmopressin; Teva-Desmopressin
Index Terms 1-Deamino-8-D-Arginine Vasopressin; Desmopressin Acetate; Noctiva
Pharmacologic Category Antihemophilic Agent; Hemostatic Agent; Hormone, Posterior Pituitary; Vasopressin Analog, Synthetic
Use
Injection:
Diabetes insipidus: Antidiuretic replacement therapy in the management of central (cranial) diabetes insipidus; management of the temporary polyuria and polydipsia following head trauma or surgery in the pituitary region.
Limitations of use: Desmopressin is ineffective for the treatment of nephrogenic diabetes insipidus.
Hemophilia A: For use in patients with hemophilia A with factor VIII coagulant activity levels >5% to maintain hemostasis during surgical procedures and postoperatively when administered 30 minutes prior to the scheduled procedure and to also stop bleeding due to spontaneous or trauma-induced injuries, such as hemarthroses, intramuscular hematomas, or mucosal bleeding.

◄ Limitations of use: Not indicated for the treatment of hemophilia A with factor VIII coagulant activity levels ≤5%, for the treatment of hemophilia B, or in patients who have factor VIII antibodies. In certain clinical situations, it may be justified to try desmopressin with careful monitoring in patients with factor VIII levels between 2% and 5%.

Nocturia (Noctiva): Treatment of nocturia due to nocturnal polyuria in adults who awaken at least 2 times per night to void.

Limitations of use: Has not been studied in patients <50 years of age.

Von Willebrand disease (type 1): For use in patients with mild to moderate classic von Willebrand disease (type 1) with factor VIII coagulant activity levels >5% to maintain hemostasis during surgical procedures and post-operatively when administered 30 minutes prior to the scheduled procedure and to stop bleeding due to spontaneous or trauma-induced injuries, such as hemarthroses, intramuscular hematomas, or mucosal bleeding.

Limitations of use: Patients with von Willebrand disease who are least likely to respond are those with severe homozygous von Willebrand disease with factor VIII coagulant activity and factor VIII von Willebrand factor antigen levels <1%; other patients may respond (variable) depending on the type of molecular defect they have. Check bleeding time and factor VIII coagulant activity, ristocetin cofactor activity, and von Willebrand factor antigen during administration of desmopressin to ensure that adequate levels are being achieved. Not indicated for the treatment of severe classic von Willebrand disease (type I) or when there is evidence of an abnormal molecular form of factor VIII antigen.

Uremic bleeding (Octostim [Canadian product]): Prevention or treatment of bleeding in patients with uremia.

Intranasal:

Diabetes insipidus (DDAVP Rhinal tube): Antidiuretic replacement therapy in the management of central (cranial) diabetes insipidus; management of the temporary polyuria and polydipsia following head trauma or surgery in the pituitary region.

Limitation of use: Desmopressin is ineffective for the treatment of nephrogenic diabetes insipidus.

Hemophilia A (Stimate; Octostim [Canadian product]): For use in patients with hemophilia A with factor VIII coagulant activity levels >5% and to stop bleeding due to spontaneous or trauma-induced injuries, such as hemarthroses, intramuscular hematomas, or mucosal bleeding.

Limitations of use: Not indicated for the treatment of hemophilia A with factor VIII coagulant activity levels ≤5%, for the treatment of hemophilia B, or in patients who have factor VIII antibodies.

von Willebrand disease (type 1) (Stimate; Octostim [Canadian product]): For use in patients with mild to moderate classic von Willebrand disease (type 1) with factor VIII coagulant activity levels >5% and to stop bleeding due to spontaneous or trauma-induced injuries, such as hemarthroses, intramuscular hematomas, mucosal bleeding, or menorrhagia.

Limitations of use: Not indicated for the treatment of severe classic von Willebrand disease (type 1) or when there is evidence of an abnormal molecular form of factor VIII antigen.

Tablets:

Diabetes insipidus: Antidiuretic replacement therapy in the management of central diabetes insipidus; management of the temporary polyuria and polydipsia following head trauma or surgery in the pituitary region.

Limitation of use: Desmopressin is ineffective for the treatment of nephrogenic diabetes insipidus.

Nocturia (Nocdurna [Canadian product] only): Treatment of nocturia in adults with four or less nocturnal voids.

Primary nocturnal enuresis: Management of primary nocturnal enuresis, either alone or as an adjunct to behavioral conditioning or other non-pharmacologic intervention.

Pregnancy Risk Factor B
Dosing
Adult & Geriatric

Diabetes insipidus: Note: Fluid restriction should be observed. Dosing should be individualized to response.

IV, SubQ: US labeling: 2 to 4 mcg daily (0.5 to 1 mL) in 2 divided doses or one-tenth ($^1/_{10}$) of the maintenance intranasal dose. Fluid restriction should be observed.

IM, IV, SubQ: Canadian labeling (DDAVP Injection only): 1 to 4 mcg (0.25 to 1 mL) once daily or one-tenth ($^1/_{10}$) of the maintenance intranasal dose. Fluid restriction should be observed.

Intranasal (100 mcg/mL nasal solution): Usual dose range: 10 to 40 mcg daily (0.1 to 0.4 mL) as a single dose or divided 2 to 3 times daily; adjust morning and evening doses separately for an adequate diurnal rhythm of water turnover. Most adults require 10 mcg (0.1 mL) twice daily. **Note:** The nasal spray pump can only deliver doses of 10 mcg (0.1 mL) or multiples of 10 mcg (0.1 mL); if doses other than this are needed, the rhinal tube delivery system is preferred. Fluid restriction should be observed.

Oral:

US labeling: Initial: 0.05 mg twice daily; total daily dose should be increased or decreased as needed to obtain adequate antidiuresis (range: 0.1 to 1.2 mg divided 2 to 3 times daily). Fluid restriction should be observed.

Canadian labeling: Initial: 0.1 mg 3 times daily; total daily dose should be increased or decreased as needed to obtain adequate antidiuresis (maximum: 1.2 mg/day in 3 divided doses). Fluid restriction should be observed.

Sublingual formulation [Canadian product]: DDAVP Melt: Initial: 60 mcg 3 times daily; total daily dose should be increased or decreased as needed to obtain adequate antidiuresis. Usual maintenance: 120 to 720 mcg equally divided 2 or 3 times daily. Fluid restriction should be observed.

Intracranial hemorrhage associated with certain antiplatelet agents (aspirin, clopidogrel, prasugrel, ticlopidine, ticagrelor, cangrelor) (off-label use): *IV:* 0.4 mcg/kg once (NCS/SCCM [Frontera 2016]).

Nocturia:

Intranasal (0.83 mcg/0.1 mL and 1.66 mcg/0.1 mL nasal solution):

Not at risk for hyponatremia: 1.66 mcg in either the left or right nostril ~30 minutes before bed.

At risk for hyponatremia: 0.83 mcg in either the left or right nostril ~30 minutes before bedtime. After ≥7 days, may increase to 1.66 mcg, if needed (provided the serum sodium is within the normal range during treatment with the 0.83 mcg dose). **Note:** The 0.83 mcg dose did not meet all prespecified efficacy endpoints in clinical trials but may have a lower risk of hyponatremia.

Sublingual formulation [Canadian product]: Nocdurna:

Females: 25 mcg once daily at bedtime. Fluid intake should be limited 1 hour prior to dose until the next morning, or at least 8 hours after administration.

Males: 50 mcg once daily at bedtime; **Note:** In males ≥65 years, evaluate serum sodium within 4 to 8 days after initiation and at 1 month of treatment; discontinue therapy if sodium falls below normal range. Fluid intake should be limited 1 hour prior to dose until the next morning, or at least 8 hours after administration.

Primary nocturnal enuresis:

Oral: Initial: 0.2 mg at bedtime; dose may be titrated up to 0.6 mg to achieve desired response.

Sublingual formulation [Canadian product]: DDAVP Melt: Initial: 120 mcg administered 1 hour before bedtime; if bedwetting occurs after 3 days increase dose by 120 mcg/day. Dose may be further titrated up to a maximum of 360 mcg/day to achieve desired response. Fluid intake should be limited 1 hour prior to dose until the next morning, or at least 8 hours after administration. Treatment period is up to 3 months and then reassess with 1 week off treatment; if additional therapy is necessary, resume at same dosage prior to discontinuation.

Hemophilia A and von Willebrand disease (type 1):

IV: 0.3 mcg/kg by slow infusion; may repeat dose if needed (based on clinical response and laboratory results); if used preoperatively, administer 30 minutes before procedure. The Canadian labeling recommends a maximum IV dose of 20 mcg.

Intranasal (using high concentration spray [1.5 mg/mL]): <50 kg: 150 mcg (1 spray in a single nostril); ≥50 kg: 300 mcg (1 spray each nostril); repeat use is determined by the patient's clinical condition and laboratory work. If using preoperatively, administer 2 hours before surgery.

Uremic bleeding: Octostim [Canadian product]: *IV:* 0.3 mcg/kg over 20 to 30 minutes (maximum dose: 20 mcg)

Uremic bleeding associated with acute or chronic renal failure (off-label use in US): *IV:* 0.4 mcg/kg over 10 minutes (Watson 1984)

Prevention of surgical bleeding in patients with uremia (off-label use in US): *IV:* 0.3 mcg/kg over 30 minutes (Mannucci 1983)

Pediatric

Diabetes insipidus: Note: Fluid restriction should be observed in these patients; younger patients more susceptible to plasma osmolality shifts and possible hyponatremia. Dosing should be individualized to response.

Parenteral:

US labeling: Children ≥12 years and Adolescents: IV, SubQ: Refer to adult dosing.

Alternative recommendations (off-label): Infants and Children <12 years: IV, SubQ: No definitive dosing available. Adult dosing should **not** be used in this age group; adverse events such as hyponatremia-induced seizures may occur. Dose should be reduced. Some have suggested an initial dosage range of 0.1 to 1 mcg daily in 1 or 2 divided doses (Cheetham 2002). Initiate at low dose and increase as necessary. Closely monitor serum sodium levels and urine output; fluid restriction is recommended.

Canadian labeling (DDAVP Injection only): IM, IV, SubQ: Children and Adolescents: 0.4 mcg (0.1 mL) once daily or one-tenth ($^1/_{10}$) of the maintenance intranasal dose. Fluid restriction should be observed.

Intranasal (using 100 mcg/mL nasal solution:

Infants ≥3 months and Children ≤12 years: Usual dose range: 5 to 30 mcg daily (0.05 to 0.3 mL daily) as a single dose or divided 2 times daily; adjust morning and evening doses separately for an adequate diurnal rhythm of water turnover. **Note:** The nasal spray pump can only deliver doses of 10 mcg (0.1 mL) or multiples of 10 mcg (0.1 mL); if doses other than this are needed, the rhinal tube delivery system is preferred. Fluid restriction should be observed.

Adolescents: Refer to adult dosing.

Oral:

US labeling: Children ≥4 years and Adolescents: Refer to adult dosing.

Canadian labeling:

Children: Initial: 0.1 mg 3 times daily; total daily dose should be increased or decreased as needed to obtain adequate antidiuresis (maximum: 1.2 mg/day in 3 divided doses). Divide daily doses so that the evening dose is 2 times higher than the morning or afternoon dose to ensure adequate antidiuresis during the night. Fluid restriction should be observed.

Adolescents: Refer to adult dosing.

Sublingual formulation [Canadian product]: DDAVP Melt:

Children: Initial: 60 mcg 3 times daily; total daily dose should be increased or decreased as needed to obtain adequate antidiuresis. Usual maintenance: 120 to 720 mcg equally divided 2 to 3 times daily; divide daily doses so that the evening dose is 2 times higher than the morning or afternoon dose to ensure adequate antidiuresis during the night. Fluid restriction should be observed.

Adolescents: Refer to adult dosing.

Hemophilia A and von Willebrand disease (type 1):

IV: Infants ≥3 months, Children, and Adolescents: Refer to adult dosing.

Note: Adverse events such as hyponatremia-induced seizures have been reported especially in young children using this dosing regimen (Das 2005; Molnar 2005; Smith 1989; Thumfart 2005; Weinstein 1989). Fluid restriction and careful monitoring of serum sodium levels and urine output are necessary.

Intranasal (using high concentration spray [1.5 mg/mL]): Infants ≥11 months, Children, and Adolescents: Refer to adult dosing.

SubQ: Infants ≥3 months, Children, and Adolescents: Octostim [Canadian product]: Refer to adult dosing.

Primary nocturnal enuresis:

Oral:

US labeling: Children ≥6 years and Adolescents: Initial: 0.2 mg at bedtime. Dose may be titrated up to 0.6 mg to achieve desired response. Fluid intake should be limited 1 hour prior to dose until the next morning, or at least 8 hours after administration.

Canadian labeling: Children ≥5 years and Adolescents: Initial: 0.2 mg at bedtime; if bedwetting occurs after 3 days may increase dose by 0.2 mg/day up to a maximum of 0.6 mg/day. Fluid intake should be limited 1 hour prior to dose until the next morning, or at least 8 hours after administration. Treatment period is up to 3 months and then reassess with 1 week off treatment; if additional therapy is necessary, resume at same dosage prior to discontinuation.

◄   *Sublingual [Canadian product]:* DDAVP Melt: Children ≥5 years and Adolescents: Refer to adult dosing.

Renal Impairment

CrCl ≥50 mL/minute: There are no dosage adjustments provided in the manufacturer's labeling.

CrCl <50 mL/minute: Use is contraindicated according to the manufacturer's labeling (except 1.5 mg/mL nasal spray); however, has been used in acute and chronic renal failure patients experiencing uremic bleeding or for prevention of surgical bleeding (off-label uses in US) (Mannucci 1983; Watson 1984).

Hepatic Impairment There are no dosage adjustments provided in the manufacturer's labeling.

Additional Information Complete prescribing information should be consulted for additional detail.

Product Availability Noctiva nasal spray: FDA approved March 2017; anticipated availability is currently undetermined.

Dosage Forms Considerations

DDAVP and Minirin 5 mL bottles contain 50 sprays.

Stimate 2.5 mL bottles contain 25 sprays.

Dosage Forms Excipient information presented when available (limited, particularly for generics); consult specific product labeling. [DSC] = Discontinued product

Solution, Injection, as acetate:

  DDAVP: 4 mcg/mL (1 mL)

  DDAVP: 4 mcg/mL (10 mL) [contains chlorobutanol (chlorobutol)]

  Generic: 4 mcg/mL (1 mL, 10 mL)

Solution, Injection, as acetate [preservative free]:

  Generic: 4 mcg/mL (1 mL)

Solution, Nasal, as acetate:

  DDAVP: 0.01% (5 mL) [contains benzalkonium chloride]

  DDAVP Rhinal Tube: 0.01% (2.5 mL) [contains chlorobutanol (chlorobutol)]

  Stimate: 1.5 mg/mL (2.5 mL) [contains benzalkonium chloride]

  Generic: 0.01% (2.5 mL, 5 mL)

Tablet, Oral, as acetate:

  DDAVP: 0.1 mg

  DDAVP: 0.1 mg [DSC], 0.2 mg [scored]

  Generic: 0.1 mg, 0.2 mg

Dosage Forms: Canada Information with regard to form, strength, and availability of products uniquely available in Canada but currently not available in the US. Refer also to Dosage Forms.

Excipient information presented when available (limited, particularly for generics); consult specific product labeling.

Solution, Injection, as acetate [preservative free]:

  Octostim: 15 mcg/mL (1 mL)

Solution, Nasal, as acetate:

  Octostim: 1.5 mg/mL (2.5 mL) [contains benzalkonium chloride]

Tablet, Sublingual, as acetate:

  DDAVP Melt: 60 mcg, 120 mcg, 240 mcg

  Nocdurna: 25 mcg, 50 mcg

◆ **Desmopressin Acetate** see Desmopressin *on page 573*

◆ **Detryptoreline** see Triptorelin *on page 1841*

Dexamethasone (Systemic) (deks a METH a sone)

Related Information

Corticosteroids Systemic Equivalencies *on page 2417*

Management of Chemotherapy-Induced Nausea and Vomiting in Adults *on page 2253*

Palliative Care Medicine (Cancer) *on page 2352*

Brand Names: US Active Injection D; Baycadron [DSC]; Dexamethasone Intensol; DexPak 10 Day; DexPak 13 Day; DexPak 6 Day; DoubleDex; LoCort 11-Day; LoCort 7-Day; ReadySharp Dexamethasone; ZonaCort 11 Day; ZonaCort 7 Day

Brand Names: Canada Apo-Dexamethasone; Dexasone; Dom-Dexamethasone; PHL-Dexamethasone; PMS-Dexamethasone; PRO-Dexamethasone; ratio-Dexamethasone

Index Terms Decadron; Dexamethasone Sod Phosphate; Dexamethasone Sodium Phosphate

Pharmacologic Category Anti-inflammatory Agent; Antiemetic; Corticosteroid, Systemic

Use Note: Treatment guidelines recommend the use of high dose IV or oral methylprednisolone for acute exacerbations of multiple sclerosis (AAN [Scott 2011], NICE 2014).

Oral, IV or IM injection:

Allergic states: Control of severe or incapacitating allergic conditions intractable to adequate trials of conventional treatment: seasonal or perennial allergic rhinitis, bronchial asthma, contact dermatitis, atopic dermatitis, serum sickness, drug hypersensitivity reactions; acute noninfectious laryngeal edema, urticarial transfusion reactions (injection only).

Collagen diseases: During an exacerbation or as maintenance therapy in selected cases of systemic lupus erythematosus or acute rheumatic carditis.

Dermatologic diseases: Pemphigus; bullous dermatitis herpetiformis; severe erythema multiforme (Stevens-Johnson syndrome); exfoliative dermatitis; exfoliative erythroderma; mycosis fungoides; severe psoriasis; severe seborrheic dermatitis.

Diagnostic testing: Diagnostic testing of adrenocortical hyperfunction.

Edematous states: To induce a diuresis or remission of proteinuria in idiopathic nephrotic syndrome or that because of systemic lupus erythematosus.

Endocrine disorders: Primary, secondary, or acute (injection only) adrenocortical insufficiency (hydrocortisone or cortisone is the first choice); preoperatively, and in the event of serious trauma or illness, in adrenal insufficiency or when adrenocortical reserve is doubtful (injection only); shock unresponsive to conventional therapy if adrenocortical insufficiency exists or is suspected (injection only); congenital adrenal hyperplasia; nonsuppurative thyroiditis; hypercalcemia associated with cancer.

GI diseases: To tide the patient over a critical period of the disease in ulcerative colitis or regional enteritis.

Hematologic disorders: Immune thrombocytopenia (formerly known as idiopathic thrombocytopenic purpura) in adults (not IM); secondary thrombocytopenia in adults (select cases); acquired (autoimmune) hemolytic anemia; pure red cell aplasia; congenital (erythroid) hypoplastic anemia (Diamond Blackfan anemia).

◄ **Neoplastic diseases:** Palliative management of leukemias and lymphomas in adults and acute leukemia of childhood.

Nervous system: Acute exacerbations of multiple sclerosis; cerebral edema associated with primary or metastatic brain tumor or craniotomy.

Ophthalmic diseases: Severe acute and chronic allergic and inflammatory processes involving the eye and its adnexa such as allergic conjunctivitis; keratitis; allergic corneal marginal ulcers; herpes zoster ophthalmicus; iritis and iridocyclitis; chorioretinitis; anterior segment inflammation; diffuse posterior uveitis and choroiditis; optic neuritis; sympathetic ophthalmia; temporal arteritis; uveitis; ocular inflammatory conditions unresponsive to topical corticosteroids.

Respiratory diseases: Symptomatic sarcoidosis; Loeffler syndrome not manageable by other means; berylliosis; fulminating or disseminated pulmonary tuberculosis when used concurrently with appropriate antituberculous chemotherapy; aspiration pneumonitis; idiopathic eosinophilic pneumonias.

Rheumatic disorders: As adjunctive therapy for short-term administration in psoriatic arthritis, rheumatoid arthritis (RA), juvenile RA, ankylosing spondylitis, acute and subacute bursitis, acute nonspecific tenosynovitis, acute gouty arthritis, posttraumatic osteoarthritis, synovitis of osteoarthritis, epicondylitis; treatment of dermatomyositis, polymyositis, and systemic lupus erythematosus.

Miscellaneous: Tuberculous meningitis with subarachnoid block or impending block when used with appropriate antituberculous chemotherapy; trichinosis with neurologic or myocardial involvement.

Intraarticular or soft tissue injection: As adjunctive therapy for short-term administration in synovitis of osteoarthritis, RA, acute and subacute bursitis, acute gouty arthritis, epicondylitis, acute nonspecific tenosynovitis, posttraumatic osteoarthritis

Intralesional injection: Keloids; localized hypertrophic, infiltrated, inflammatory lesions of lichen planus, psoriatic plaques, granuloma annulare, and lichen simplex chronicus (neurodermatitis); discoid lupus erythematosus; necrobiosis lipoidica diabeticorum; alopecia areata; cystic tumors of an aponeurosis or tendon (ganglia)

Labeled Contraindications

Hypersensitivity to dexamethasone or any component of the formulation; systemic fungal infections

Documentation of allergenic cross-reactivity for corticosteroids is limited. However, because of similarities in chemical structure and/or pharmacologic actions, the possibility of cross-sensitivity cannot be ruled out with certainty.

Pregnancy Considerations Adverse events have been observed with corticosteroids in animal reproduction studies. Dexamethasone crosses the placenta (Brownfoot 2013); and is partially metabolized by placental enzymes to an inactive metabolite (Murphy 2007). Some studies have shown an association between first trimester systemic corticosteroid use and oral clefts (Park-Wyllie 2000; Pradat 2003). Systemic corticosteroids may have an effect on fetal growth (decreased birth weight); however, information is conflicting (Lunghi 2010). Hypoadrenalism may occur in newborns following maternal use of corticosteroids during pregnancy; monitor.

Because antenatal corticosteroid administration may reduce the incidence of intraventricular hemorrhage, necrotizing enterocolitis, neonatal mortality, and respiratory distress syndrome, the injection is often used for antenatal fetal lung maturation in patients with preterm premature rupture of membranes or preterm labor who are at risk of preterm delivery (most data is available for betamethasone). A single course of corticosteroids is recommended for women between 24 and 34 weeks gestation who are at risk of delivering within 7 days, including those with ruptured membranes or multiple gestations. A single course of corticosteroids may be considered for women beginning at 23 weeks gestation, who are at risk of delivering within 7 days, in consultation with the family. In addition, a single course of corticosteroids may be given to women between 34 0/7 weeks and 36 6/7 weeks who are at risk of preterm delivery within 7 days and who have not previously received corticosteroids; use of concomitant tocolytics is not currently recommended and administration of late preterm corticosteroids has not been evaluated in women with intrauterine infection, multiple gestations, pregestational diabetes, or women who delivered previously by cesarean section at term. Multiple repeat courses are not recommended. However, in women with pregnancies less than 34 weeks gestation at risk for delivery within 7 days and who had a course of antenatal corticosteroids >14 days prior, a single repeat course may be considered; use of a repeat course in women with premature rupture of membranes is controversial (ACOG 171 2016; ACOG 172 2016; ACOG 677 2016).

When systemic corticosteroids are needed in pregnancy, it is generally recommended to use the lowest effective dose for the shortest duration of time, avoiding high doses during the first trimester (Leachman 2006; Lunghi 2010; Makol 2011; Østensen 2009). Dexamethasone should not be used to treat primary adrenal insufficiency in pregnant women (Bornstein 2016).

Breastfeeding Considerations Corticosteroids are excreted in breast milk; information specific to dexamethasone has not been located. The manufacturer notes that when used systemically, maternal use of corticosteroids have the potential to cause adverse events in a nursing infant (eg, growth suppression, interfere with endogenous corticosteroid production). Due to the potential for serious adverse reactions in the nursing infant, the manufacturer recommends a decision be made whether to discontinue nursing or to discontinue the drug, taking into account the importance of treatment to the mother. If there is concern about exposure to the infant, some guidelines recommend waiting 4 hours after the maternal dose of an oral systemic corticosteroid before breastfeeding in order to decrease potential exposure to the nursing infant (based on a study using prednisolone) (Bae 2011; Leachman 2006; Makol 2011; Ost 1985).

Warnings/Precautions Corticosteroids are not approved for epidural injection. Serious neurologic events (eg, spinal cord infarction, paraplegia, quadriplegia, cortical blindness, stroke), some resulting in death, have been reported with epidural injection of corticosteroids, with and without use of fluoroscopy. Intra-articular injection may produce systemic as well as local effects. Appropriate examination of any joint fluid present is necessary to exclude a septic process. Avoid injection into an infected site. Do not inject into unstable joints. Patients should not overuse joints in which symptomatic benefit has been obtained as long as the inflammatory process remains active. Frequent intra-articular injection may result in damage to joint tissues.

Use with caution in patients with thyroid disease, hepatic impairment, renal impairment, cardiovascular disease, diabetes, glaucoma, cataracts, myasthenia gravis, osteoporosis, seizures, or GI diseases (diverticulitis, fresh intestinal anastomoses, active or latent peptic ulcer, ulcerative colitis, abscess or other pyogenic infection) due to perforation risk. Use caution following acute MI (corticosteroids have been associated with myocardial rupture). Use with caution in patients with a history of ocular herpes simplex; corneal perforation has occurred; do not use in active ocular herpes simplex. Not recommended for the treatment of optic neuritis; may increase frequency of new episodes. Use with caution in the elderly with the smallest possible effective dose for the shortest duration. May affect growth velocity; growth should be routinely monitored in pediatric patients. Withdraw therapy with gradual tapering of dose.

May cause hypercortisolism or suppression of hypothalamic-pituitary-adrenal (HPA) axis, particularly in younger children or in patients receiving high doses for prolonged periods. HPA axis suppression may lead to adrenal crisis. Withdrawal and discontinuation of a corticosteroid should be done slowly and carefully. Particular care is required when patients are transferred from systemic corticosteroids to inhaled products due to possible adrenal insufficiency or withdrawal from steroids, including an increase in allergic symptoms. Adult patients receiving >20 mg per day of prednisone (or equivalent) may be most susceptible. Fatalities have occurred due to adrenal insufficiency in asthmatic patients during and after transfer from systemic corticosteroids to aerosol steroids; aerosol steroids do not provide the systemic steroid needed to treat patients having trauma, surgery, or infections. Dexamethasone does not provide adequate mineralocorticoid activity in adrenal insufficiency (may be employed as a single dose while cortisol assays are performed). In the management/prevention of adrenal crisis in patients with known primary adrenal insufficiency, the Endocrine Society practice guidelines state dexamethasone (intravenous) is the least preferred alternative agent and should be used only if no other glucocorticoid is available. For the treatment of chronic primary adrenal insufficiency (ie, physiologic replacement), dexamethasone (oral) is not recommended due to the risk of Cushingoid side effects (ES [Bornstein 2016]). Rare cases of anaphylactoid reactions have been observed in patients receiving corticosteroids. Patients may require higher doses when subject to stress (ie, trauma, surgery, severe infection).

Acute myopathy has been reported with high dose corticosteroids, usually in patients with neuromuscular transmission disorders; may involve ocular and/or respiratory muscles; monitor creatine kinase; recovery may be delayed. Perineal burning, tingling, pain and pruritus have been reported with IV administration. May occur more commonly in females, with higher doses, and with rapid administration. Symptom onset is sudden and usually resolves in <1 minute (Allan 1986; Neff 2002; Perron 2003; Singh 2011). Corticosteroid use may cause psychiatric disturbances, including depression, euphoria, insomnia, mood swings, severe depression to psychotic manifestations. Preexisting psychiatric conditions may be exacerbated by corticosteroid use. Prolonged use of corticosteroids may increase the incidence of secondary infection, cause activation of latent infections, mask acute infection (including fungal infections), prolong or exacerbate viral infections, or limit response to killed or inactivated vaccines. Exposure to chickenpox or measles should be avoided; corticosteroids should not be used to treat ocular herpes simplex. Corticosteroids should not be used for cerebral malaria, fungal infections, or viral hepatitis. Close observation is required in patients with latent tuberculosis and/or TB reactivity; restrict use in active TB (only fulminating or disseminated TB in conjunction with antituberculosis treatment). Amebiasis should be ruled out in any patient with recent travel to tropic climates or unexplained diarrhea prior to initiation of corticosteroids. Use with extreme caution in patients with Strongyloides infections; hyperinfection, dissemination and fatalities have occurred.

Prolonged treatment with corticosteroids has been associated with the development of Kaposi sarcoma (case reports); if noted, discontinuation of therapy should be considered (Goedert 2002). High-dose corticosteroids should not be used to manage acute head injury (BTF [Carney 2016]). Some products may contain sodium sulfite, a sulfite that may cause allergic-type reactions including anaphylaxis and life-threatening or less severe asthmatic episodes in susceptible patients. Potentially significant drug-drug interactions may exist, requiring dose or frequency adjustment, additional monitoring, and/or selection of alternative therapy. Some dosage forms may contain propylene glycol; large amounts are potentially toxic and have been associated hyperosmolality, lactic acidosis, seizures, and respiratory depression; use caution (AAP ["Inactive" 1997]; Zar 2007).

Benzyl alcohol and derivatives: Some dosage forms may contain sodium benzoate/benzoic acid; benzoic acid (benzoate) is a metabolite of benzyl alcohol; large amounts of benzyl alcohol (≥99 mg/kg/day) have been associated with a potentially fatal toxicity ("gasping syndrome") in neonates; the "gasping syndrome" consists of metabolic acidosis, respiratory distress, gasping respirations, CNS dysfunction (including convulsions, intracranial hemorrhage), hypotension, and cardiovascular collapse (AAP ["Inactive" 1997]; CDC 1982); some data suggests that benzoate displaces bilirubin from protein binding sites (Ahlfors 2001); avoid or use dosage forms containing benzyl alcohol derivative with caution in neonates. See manufacturer's labeling.

Adverse Reactions Some reactions listed are based on reports for other agents in this same pharmacologic class and may not be specifically reported for dexamethasone.

Frequency not defined:

Cardiovascular: Bradycardia, cardiac arrhythmia, cardiac failure, cardiomegaly, circulatory shock, edema, embolism (fat), hypertension, hypertrophic cardiomyopathy (premature infants), myocardial rupture (post-MI), syncope, tachycardia, thromboembolism, thrombophlebitis, vasculitis

Central nervous system: Depression, emotional lability, euphoria, headache, increased intracranial pressure, insomnia, malaise, myasthenia, neuritis, neuropathy, paresthesia, personality changes, pseudotumor cerebri (usually following discontinuation), psychic disorder, seizure, vertigo

Dermatologic: Acne vulgaris, allergic dermatitis, alopecia, atrophic striae, diaphoresis, ecchymoses, erythema, facial erythema, fragile skin, hyperpigmentation, hypertrichosis, hypopigmentation, perianal skin irritation (itching, burning, tingling; following IV injection), petechiae, skin atrophy, skin rash, subcutaneous atrophy, suppression of skin test reaction, urticaria, xeroderma

Endocrine & metabolic: Adrenal suppression, carbohydrate intolerance, Cushing syndrome, decreased glucose tolerance, decreased serum potassium, diabetes mellitus, fluid retention, glycosuria, growth suppression (children), hirsutism, HPA-axis suppression, hyperglycemia, hypokalemic alkalosis, menstrual disease, moon face, negative nitrogen balance, protein catabolism, redistribution of body fat, sodium retention, weight gain

Gastrointestinal: Abdominal distention, gastrointestinal hemorrhage, gastrointestinal perforation, hiccups, increased appetite, nausea, pancreatitis, peptic ulcer, pruritus ani (following IV injection), ulcerative esophagitis

Genitourinary: Defective (increased or decreased) spermatogenesis

Hematologic & oncologic: Kaposi sarcoma, petechial, tumor lysis syndrome

Hepatic: Hepatomegaly, increased serum transaminases

Hypersensitivity: Anaphylactoid reaction, anaphylaxis, angioedema, hypersensitivity

Infection: Infection, sterile abscess

Local: Postinjection flare (intra-articular use)

Neuromuscular & skeletal: Amyotrophy, aseptic necrosis of bones (femoral and humoral heads), bone fractures, Charcot-like arthropathy, myasthenia, myopathy (particularly in conjunction with neuromuscular disease or neuromuscular-blocking agents), osteoporosis, rupture of tendon, steroid myopathy, vertebral compression fracture

Ophthalmic: Exophthalmos, glaucoma, increased intraocular pressure, subcapsular posterior cataract

Respiratory: Pulmonary edema

Miscellaneous: Wound healing impairment

Drug Interactions

Metabolism/Transport Effects Substrate of CYP3A4 (major), P-glycoprotein; **Note:** Assignment of Major/Minor substrate status based on clinically relevant drug interaction potential; **Induces** CYP2A6 (weak/moderate), CYP2C9 (weak/moderate), CYP3A4 (weak), UGT1A1

Avoid Concomitant Use

Avoid concomitant use of Dexamethasone (Systemic) with any of the following: Aldesleukin; BCG (Intravesical); Conivaptan; Desmopressin; Fusidic Acid (Systemic); Idelalisib; Indium 111 Capromab Pendetide; Lapatinib; MiFEPRIStone; Natalizumab; Nilotinib; Pimecrolimus; Rilpivirine; RomiDEPsin; Simeprevir; Tacrolimus (Topical); VinCRIStine (Liposomal)

Increased Effect/Toxicity

Dexamethasone (Systemic) may increase the levels/effects of: Acetylcholinesterase Inhibitors; Amphotericin B; Androgens; CycloSPORINE (Systemic); Deferasirox; Desirudin; Desmopressin; Fingolimod; Fosphenytoin; Leflunomide; Lenalidomide; Loop Diuretics; Natalizumab; Nicorandil; NSAID (COX-2 Inhibitor); NSAID (Nonselective); Phenytoin; Quinolone Antibiotics; Thalidomide; Thiazide and Thiazide-Like Diuretics; Tofacitinib; Vaccines (Live); Warfarin

The levels/effects of Dexamethasone (Systemic) may be increased by: Aprepitant; Asparaginase (E. coli); Asparaginase (Erwinia); Conivaptan; CycloSPORINE (Systemic); CYP3A4 Inhibitors (Moderate); CYP3A4 Inhibitors (Strong); Denosumab; DilTIAZem; Estrogen Derivatives; Fosamprenavir; Fosaprepitant; Fusidic Acid (Systemic); Idelalisib; Indacaterol; MiFEPRIStone; Netupitant; Neuromuscular-Blocking Agents (Nondepolarizing); Ocrelizumab; Palbociclib; P-glycoprotein/ABCB1 Inhibitors; Pimecrolimus; Ranolazine; Roflumilast; Salicylates; Stiripentol; Tacrolimus (Topical); Telaprevir; Trastuzumab

Decreased Effect

Dexamethasone (Systemic) may decrease the levels/effects of: Aldesleukin; Antidiabetic Agents; BCG (Intravesical); Calcitriol (Systemic); Caspofungin; CloZAPine; Cobicistat; Coccidioides immitis Skin Test; Corticorelin; CycloSPORINE (Systemic); Daclatasvir; Dasatinib; Elvitegravir; Fosamprenavir; Fosphenytoin; Hyaluronidase; HYDROcodone; Imatinib; Indium 111 Capromab Pendetide; Isoniazid; Ixabepilone; Lapatinib; Nalmefene; Nilotinib; NiMODipine; Nivolumab; Phenytoin; Rilpivirine; RomiDEPsin; Salicylates; Simeprevir; Sipuleucel-T; SUNITinib; Telaprevir; Temsirolimus; Tertomotide;

Triazolam; Urea Cycle Disorder Agents; Vaccines (Inactivated); Vaccines (Live); VinCRIStine (Liposomal); Voriconazole

The levels/effects of Dexamethasone (Systemic) may be decreased by: Antacids; Bile Acid Sequestrants; Bosentan; CYP3A4 Inducers (Moderate); CYP3A4 Inducers (Strong); Dabrafenib; Deferasirox; Echinacea; Enzalutamide; Fosphenytoin; MiFEPRIStone; Mitotane; Phenytoin; Sarilumab; Siltuximab; St John's Wort; Tocilizumab

Storage/Stability

Elixir: Store at 15°C to 30°C (59°F to 86°F); avoid freezing.

Injection: Store intact vials at 20°C to 25°C (68°F to 77°F). Protect from light, heat, and freezing. Do not autoclave. Diluted solutions should be used within 24 hours.

Oral concentrated solution (Intensol): Store at 20°C to 25°C (68°F to 77°F); do not freeze; do not use if precipitate is present; dispense only in original bottle and only with manufacturer-supplied calibrated dropper; discard open bottle after 90 days.

Oral solution, tablets: Store at 20°C to 25°C (68°F to 77°F); protect from moisture.

Preparation for Administration

Oral: Oral administration of dexamethasone for croup may be prepared using a parenteral dexamethasone formulation and mixing it with an oral flavored syrup (Bjornson 2004).

IV: May be given undiluted or further diluted in NS or D5W. Use the preservative-free product in neonates, especially premature infants.

Mechanism of Action A long acting corticosteroid with minimal sodium-retaining potential. Decreases inflammation by suppression of neutrophil migration, decreased production of inflammatory mediators, and reversal of increased capillary permeability; suppresses normal immune response. Dexamethasone's mechanism of antiemetic activity is unknown.

Pharmacodynamics/Kinetics

Onset of action: IV: Rapid

Immune thrombocytopenia: Oral: Initial response: 2 to 14 days; Peak response: 4 to 28 days (Neunert 2011)

Duration: IV: Short

Absorption: Oral: 61% to 86% (Czock 2005)

Metabolism: Hepatic

Half-life elimination:

Extremely low birth-weight infants with BPD: 9.26 ± 3.34 hours (range: 5.85 to 16.1 hours) (Charles 1993)

Children 4 months to 16 years: 4.34 ± 4.14 hours (range: 2.33 to 9.54 hours) (Richter 1983)

Adults: Oral: 4 ± 0.9 hours (Czock 2005); IV: ~1 to 5 hours (Hochhaus 2001; Miyabo 1991; Rohdewald 1987; Toth 1999)

Time to peak, serum: Oral: 1 to 2 hours (Czock 2005); IM: ~30 to 120 minutes (Egerman 1997; Hochhaus 2001); IV: 5 to 10 minutes (free dexamethasone) (Miyabo 1991; Rohdewald 1987)

Excretion: Urine (~10%) (Duggan 1975; Miyabo 1991)

Dosing

Adult

Adrenal crisis (shock due to adrenal insufficiency and unresponsive to conventional therapy) (off-label dose): IV: 4 to 10 mg as a single dose, which may be repeated if necessary. **Note:** Hydrocortisone is the preferred agent in this setting (ES [Bornstein 2016]).

◄ **Anti-inflammatory/immunosuppressive/endocrine disorders:**
Oral, IM, IV: 0.5 to 9 mg/day in divided doses every 6 to 12 hours; dose depends upon condition being treated and response of patient.

Intra-articular, intralesional, or soft tissue injection: Dosage and frequency depend on the condition and the site of injection; frequency range: once every 3 to 5 days to once every 2 to 3 weeks

Large joints (eg, knee): Single dose: 2 to 4 mg

Small joints (eg, interphalangeal, temporomandibular): Single dose: 0.8 to 1 mg

Bursae: Single dose: 2 to 4 mg

Tendon Sheaths: Single dose: 0.4 to 1 mg

Soft tissue infiltration: Single dose: 2 to 6 mg

Ganglia: 1 to 2 mg

Brain tumor (palliative management of cerebral edema or neurological deficits associated with recurrent or inoperable brain tumors): Oral, IV: 2 mg 2 to 3 times daily may be effective; individualize dose based on disease response and patient tolerance.

Cerebral edema (associated with brain tumor or craniotomy): IM, IV: 10 mg IV immediately, followed by 4 mg IM every 6 hours until cerebral edema subsides, then switch to oral regimen; dosage may be reduced after 2 or 4 days and gradually discontinued over 5 to 7 days

Cushing syndrome, diagnostic (low dose): Oral: 1 mg at 11 PM, draw blood at 8 AM; greater accuracy for Cushing syndrome may be achieved with 0.5 mg every 6 hours for 48 hours (with 24-hour urine collection for 17-hydroxycorticosteroid excretion)

Differentiation of Cushing syndrome due to ACTH excess from Cushing due to other causes: Oral: 2 mg every 6 hours for 48 hours (with 24-hour urine collection for 17-hydroxycorticosteroid excretion)

Immune thrombocytopenia (primary), initial therapy: Oral: 40 mg once daily for 4 consecutive days; if platelet count continues to remain <30,000/mm^3 or bleeding symptoms occur by day 10, may administer an additional 4-day course of 40 mg once daily (Wei 2016) **or** 40 mg once daily for 4 consecutive days, if platelets fall below 30,000/mm^3 within 6 months a second course may be administered, followed by a prednisone taper (Cheng 2003). Pulsed dexamethasone dosing of 40 mg once daily for 4 days every 14 or 28 days for 4 to 6 cycles has also been used (Mazzucconi 2007; Provan 2010).

Multiple sclerosis (acute exacerbation):

Note: Treatment guidelines recommend the use of high dose IV or oral methylprednisolone for acute exacerbations of multiple sclerosis (AAN [Scott 2011], NICE 2014).

Oral: 30 mg/day for 1 week, followed by 4 to 12 mg every other day for 1 month

Acute mountain sickness (AMS)/high altitude cerebral edema (HACE) (off-label use):

Prevention: Oral: 2 mg every 6 hours **or** 4 mg every 12 hours starting on the day of ascent; may be discontinued after staying at the same elevation for 2 to 3 days or if descent is initiated; do not exceed a 10 day duration (Luks 2010). **Note:** In situations of rapid ascent to altitudes >3500 meters (such as rescue or military operations), 4 mg every 6 hours may be considered (Luks 2010).

Treatment: Oral, IM, IV:

AMS: 4 mg every 6 hours (Luks 2010)

HACE: Initial: 8 mg as a single dose; Maintenance: 4 mg every 6 hours until symptoms resolve (Luks 2010)

Accelerated fetal lung maturation (off-label use): IM: 6 mg every 12 hours for a total of 4 doses (ACOG 171 2016). A single course is recommended for women between 24 and 34 weeks of gestation, including those with ruptured membranes or multiple gestations, who are at risk of delivering within 7 days. A single course may be appropriate in some women beginning at 23 weeks gestation or late preterm (between 34 0/7 weeks and 36 6/7 weeks gestation). A single repeat course may be considered in some women with pregnancies less than 34 weeks gestation at risk for delivery within 7 days and who had a course of antenatal corticosteroids >14 days prior (ACOG 171 2016; ACOG 172 2016; ACOG 677 2016).

Airway edema or extubation (off-label use): IV: 0.5 mg/kg/dose (maximum dose: 10 mg/dose) 6 to 12 hours prior to extubation then every 6 hours for 5 doses (Khemani 2009) **or** 5 mg every 6 hours for 4 doses with extubation performed 24 hours after last injection (Lee 2007).

Chemotherapy-associated nausea and vomiting, prevention (off-label use):

High emetic potential chemotherapy: Oral, IV: 12 mg on day 1 prior to chemotherapy (in combination with aprepitant or fosaprepitant and a $5HT_3$ antagonist on day 1) followed by 8 mg on days 2 to 3 or days 2 to 4 (with aprepitant on days 2 and 3 if aprepitant used on day 1) (Basch 2011; Roila 2016) **or** (if aprepitant/fosaprepitant not used): 20 mg day 1 (in combination with a $5HT_3$ antagonist on day 1) followed by 8 mg twice daily for 3 to 4 days (Roila 2016)

Moderate emetic potential chemotherapy: Oral, IV: 8 mg on day 1 prior to chemotherapy (in combination with a $5HT_3$ antagonist on day 1) and 8 mg on days 2 and 3; may be administered as 4 mg twice daily (Basch 2011; Roila 2016)

Low emetic potential chemotherapy: Oral, IV: 4 to 8 mg prior to chemotherapy (Basch 2011; Roila 2016)

Dosing when used in combination with extended-release granisetron (Raftopoulos 2015):

Day 1: IV: 20 mg (for highly emetic chemotherapy) **or** 8 mg (for moderately emetic chemotherapy)

Days 2, 3, and 4: Oral: 8 mg twice daily (for highly emetic chemotherapy)

Dexamethasone suppression test (depression/suicide indicator) (off-label use): Oral: 1 mg at 11 PM, draw blood at 8 AM the following day for plasma cortisol determination

Glucocorticoid remediable aldosteronism, treatment (off-label use): Oral: Initial: 0.125 to 0.25 mg once daily, preferably at bedtime to suppress early morning ACTH surge (Funder 2016)

Multiple myeloma (off-label use): Note: Multiple dexamethasone-containing regimens are available for the treatment of multiple myeloma. Refer to appropriate literature/guidelines for additional details.

Oral: 40 mg once daily on days 1 to 4, 9 to 12, and 17 to 20 (as induction therapy) in combination with bortezomib and doxorubicin for 3 cycles (Sonneveld 2012) **or** 40 mg once weekly on days 1, 8, 15, and 22 every 28 days (in combination with lenalidomide) until disease progression (Rajkumar 2010) or 40 mg once weekly on days 1, 8, 15, and 22 every 28 days (in combination with pomalidomide) until disease progression or unacceptable toxicity (San Miguel 2013) **or** 40 mg once weekly on days 1, 8, 15, and 22 every 28 days (in combination with ixazomib and lenalidomide) until disease progression or unacceptable toxicity (Moreau 2015) **or** 28 mg orally plus 8 mg IV (prior to elotuzumab) on days 1, 8, 15, and 22 every 28 days for 2 cycles, followed by 28 mg orally plus 8 mg IV (prior to elotuzumab) on days 1 and 15 and 40 mg orally on days 8 and 22 every 28 days thereafter until disease progression or unacceptable toxicity (in combination with elotuzumab and lenalidomide) (Lonial 2015).

Oral or IV: 20 mg once daily days 1, 2, 4, 5, 8, 9, 11, and 12 every 21 days (in combination with daratumumab and bortezomib) for 8 cycles (Palumbo 2016) **or** 20 mg on days 1 (prior to daratumumab infusion) and 2 each week (in combination with daratumumab and lenalidomide) until disease progression or unacceptable toxicity (Dimopoulos 2016a); for patients >75 years of age, BMI <18.5, poorly controlled diabetes, or corticosteroid intolerance a reduced dexamethasone dose of 20 mg once a week was used (Dimopoulous 2016a; Palumbo 2016).

Geriatric Refer to adult dosing. Use cautiously in the elderly in the smallest possible dose.

Pediatric

Anti-inflammatory/immunosuppressive/endocrine disorders: Infants, Children, and Adolescents: Oral, IM, IV: Initial dose range: 0.02 to 0.3 mg/kg/**day** (0.6 to 9 mg/m^2/**day**) in divided doses every 6 to 12 hours; dose depends upon condition being treated and response of patient; dosage for infants and children should be based on disease severity and patient response

Asthma exacerbation: Limited data available: Infants, Children, and Adolescents: Oral, IM, IV: 0.6 mg/kg once daily as a single dose or once daily for 2 days; maximum dose: 16 mg/dose (Hegenbarth 2008; Keeney 2014; Quereshi 2001; single dose regimens as low as 0.3 mg/kg/dose and as high as 1.7 mg/kg/dose have also been reported (Keeney 2014; Qureshi 2001; Shefrin 2009). **Note:** Duration greater than 2 days is not recommended due to increased risk of metabolic effects (GINA 2014).

Cerebral edema: Infants, Children, and Adolescents: Oral, IM, IV: Loading dose: 1 to 2 mg/kg/dose as a single dose; maintenance: 1 to 1.5 mg/kg/**day** in divided doses every 4 to 6 hours; maximum: 16 mg/**day** (Kleigman 2007).

Congenital adrenal hyperplasia: Adolescents (fully grown): Oral: 0.25 to 0.5 mg once daily (AAP 2010; Speiser 2010). **Note:** For younger patients who are still growing, hydrocortisone or fludrocortisone are preferred.

Physiologic replacement: Infants, Children, and Adolescents: Oral, IM, IV: 0.03 to 0.15 mg/kg/**day** in divided doses every 6 to 12 hours (Kleigman 2007) or 0.2 to 0.25 mg/m^2/**day** once daily; some patients may require 0.3 mg/m^2/**day** (Gupta 2008)

Acute mountain sickness (AMS) (moderate)/high altitude cerebral edema (HACE) (off-label use): Limited data available: Infants, Children, and Adolescents: Oral, IM, IV: 0.15 mg/kg/dose every 6 hours; maximum dose: 4 mg/dose; consider using for high altitude pulmonary edema because of associated HACE with this condition (Luks 2010; Pollard 2001)

Airway edema or extubation (off-label use): Limited data available: Infants, Children, and Adolescents: IV: 0.5 mg/kg/dose (maximum dose: 10 mg/dose) 6 to 12 hours prior to extubation then every 6 hours for 5 doses (total dexamethasone dose: 3 mg/kg) (Anene 1996; Khemani 2009; Tellez 1991)

Bacterial meningitis (*H. influenzae* type b) (off-label use): Limited data available: Infants >6 weeks and Children: IV: 0.15 mg/kg/dose every 6 hours for the first 2 to 4 days of antibiotic treatment; start dexamethasone 10 to 20 minutes before or with the first dose of antibiotic; if antibiotics have already been administered, dexamethasone use has not been shown to improve patient outcome and is not recommended (Tunkel 2004).

Chemotherapy-associated nausea and vomiting, prevention (off-label use): Pediatric Oncology Group of Ontario guideline recommendations (Dupuis 2013): Infants, Children, and Adolescents:

High emetic potential chemotherapy: Oral, IV: 6 mg/m^2/dose every 6 hours (in combination with a $5HT_3$ antagonist and aprepitant [if no interaction with aprepitant and if ≥12 years]); reduce dexamethasone dose by 50% if administered concomitantly with aprepitant

Moderate emetic potential chemotherapy: Oral, IV:

BSA ≤0.6 m^2: 2 mg every 12 hours (in combination with a $5HT_3$ antagonist)

BSA >0.6 m^2: 4 mg every 12 hours (in combination with a $5HT_3$ antagonist)

Croup (laryngotracheobronchitis) (off-label use): Limited data available: Infants and Children: Oral, IM, IV: 0.6 mg/kg once; usual maximum dose: 16 mg (doses as high as 20 mg have been used) (Bjornson 2004; Hegenbarth 2008; Rittichier 2000). **Note:** a single oral dose of 0.15 mg/kg has been shown effective in children with mild to moderate croup (Russell 2004; Sparrow 2006).

Immune thrombocytopenia (primary), second-line treatment (off-label use): Children and Adolescents: Oral: 0.6 mg/kg/**day** for 4 days every 4 weeks up to 6 cycles (Neunert 2011). Consider a maximum daily dose cap (eg, 24 mg or 40 mg) based on response, individual tolerance and/or institutional policy.

Immune thrombocytopenia, chronic (refractory) (off-label use): Children and Adolescents: Oral: 0.6 mg/kg/**day** for 4 days every 4 weeks for 6 cycles (Hedlund-Treutiger 2003; Neunert 2011) **or** 28 to 40 mg/m^2/**day** for 4 days every 4 weeks for 6 cycles (response usually observed within 3 days); maximum dose: 40 mg/**day** (Chen 1997; Khune 1997; Provan 2010]). Consider a maximum daily dose cap (eg, 24 mg or 40 mg) based on response, individual tolerance and/or institutional policy.

Renal Impairment There are no dosage adjustments provided in the manufacturer's labeling; use with caution.

Hemodialysis: Supplemental dose is not necessary (Aronoff 2007).

Peritoneal dialysis: Supplemental dose is not necessary (Aronoff 2007).

International Myeloma Working Group (IMWG) Recommendations: The International Myeloma Working Group (IMWG) recommendations suggest that dexamethasone may be administered without dosage adjustment in multiple myeloma patients with renal impairment, including those on dialysis. The IMWG recommends the use of the Chronic Kidney Disease Epidemiology Collaboration (CKD-EPI) equation (preferred) or the Modification of Diet in Renal Disease (MDRD) formula to evaluate renal function estimation in multiple myeloma patients with a stable serum creatinine (Dimopoulos 2016b).

Hepatic Impairment There are no dosage adjustments provided in the manufacturer's labeling.

◀ **Combination Regimens**

Administration

Oral: Administer with meals to help prevent GI upset. May administer antacids between meals to help prevent peptic ulcers.

Oral concentrate: Use only the calibrated dropper provided. Draw dose into dropper; squeeze dropper contents into a liquid or semi-solid food (water, juice, soda or soda-like beverage, applesauce, pudding). Gently stir for a few seconds. Administer the entire mixture immediately. Do not store for future use.

IV: Use preservative-free dosage forms in neonates. May administer 4 mg/mL or 10 mg/mL concentration undiluted over ≤1 minute (Gahart 2015). Rapid administration may be associated with perineal irritation (especially with higher doses); consider further dilution and administration by IV intermittent infusion over 5 to 15 minutes (Allan 1986; Neff 2002; Perron 2003; Singh 2011).

IM: Administer 4 mg/mL or 10 mg/mL concentration by deep IM injection.

Intra-articular: Administer into affected joint using the 4 mg/mL concentration only.

Intralesional injection: Administer into affected area using the 4 mg/mL concentration only.

Soft tissue injection: Administer into affected tissue using the 4 mg/mL concentration only.

Monitoring Parameters Hemoglobin, occult blood loss, blood pressure, serum potassium, glucose, bone mineral density; IOP with systemic use >6 weeks; weight and height in children; HPA axis suppression

Test Interactions May suppress the wheal and flare reactions to skin test antigens

Dietary Considerations May be taken with meals to decrease GI upset. May need diet with increased potassium, pyridoxine, vitamin C, vitamin D, folate, calcium, and phosphorus.

Additional Information Effects of inhaled/intranasal steroids on growth have been observed in the absence of laboratory evidence of HPA axis suppression, suggesting that growth velocity is a more sensitive indicator of systemic corticosteroid exposure in pediatric patients than some commonly used tests of HPA axis function. The long-term effects of this reduction in growth velocity associated with orally-inhaled and intranasal corticosteroids, including the impact on final adult height, are unknown. The potential for "catch up" growth following discontinuation of treatment with inhaled corticosteroids has not been adequately studied.

◄ **Withdrawal/tapering of therapy:** Corticosteroid tapering following short-term use is limited primarily by the need to control the underlying disease state; tapering may be accomplished over a period of days. Following longer-term use, tapering over weeks to months may be necessary to avoid signs and symptoms of adrenal insufficiency and to allow recovery of the HPA axis. Testing of HPA axis responsiveness may be of value in selected patients. Subtle deficits in HPA response may persist for months after discontinuation of therapy, and may require supplemental dosing during periods of acute illness or surgical stress.

Dosage Forms Excipient information presented when available (limited, particularly for generics); consult specific product labeling. [DSC] = Discontinued product

Concentrate, Oral:
  Dexamethasone Intensol: 1 mg/mL (30 mL) [contains alcohol, usp; unflavored flavor]

Elixir, Oral:
  Baycadron: 0.5 mg/5 mL (237 mL [DSC]) [contains alcohol, usp, benzoic acid, fd&c red #40, propylene glycol; raspberry flavor]
  Generic: 0.5 mg/5 mL (237 mL)

Kit, Injection, as sodium phosphate:
  ReadySharp Dexamethasone: 10 mg/mL [contains benzyl alcohol, sodium sulfite]

Kit, Injection, as sodium phosphate [preservative free]:
  Active Injection D: 10 mg/mL
  DoubleDex: 10 mg/mL

Solution, Oral:
  Generic: 0.5 mg/5 mL (240 mL, 500 mL)

Solution, Injection, as sodium phosphate:
  Generic: 4 mg/mL (1 mL); 20 mg/5 mL (5 mL); 120 mg/30 mL (30 mL); 10 mg/mL (1 mL); 100 mg/10 mL (10 mL)

Solution, Injection, as sodium phosphate [preservative free]:
  Generic: 4 mg/mL (1 mL); 10 mg/mL (1 mL)

Solution, Intravenous, as sodium phosphate:
  Generic: 10 mg/50 mL in NaCl 0.9% (50 mL)

Solution Prefilled Syringe, Intravenous, as sodium phosphate:
  Generic: 10 mg/2.5 mL (2.5 mL); 12 mg/3 mL (3 mL)

Tablet, Oral:
  DexPak 10 Day: 1.5 mg [scored; contains fd&c red #40 aluminum lake]
  DexPak 13 Day: 1.5 mg [scored; contains fd&c red #40 aluminum lake]
  DexPak 6 Day: 1.5 mg [scored; contains fd&c red #40 aluminum lake]
  Generic: 0.5 mg, 0.75 mg, 1 mg, 1.5 mg, 2 mg, 4 mg, 6 mg

Tablet Therapy Pack, Oral:
  LoCort 11-Day: 1.5 mg (41 ea) [scored; contains fd&c red #40]
  LoCort 7-Day: 1.5 mg (27 ea) [scored; contains fd&c red #40]
  ZonaCort 11 Day: 1.5 mg (41 ea) [scored; contains fd&c red #40]
  ZonaCort 7 Day: 1.5 mg (27 ea) [scored; contains fd&c red #40]

◆ **Dexamethasone Intensol** *see* Dexamethasone (Systemic) *on page 579*

◆ **Dexamethasone Sodium Phosphate** *see* Dexamethasone (Systemic) *on page 579*

◆ **Dexamethasone Sod Phosphate** *see* Dexamethasone (Systemic) *on page 579*

◆ **Dexasone (Can)** *see* Dexamethasone (Systemic) *on page 579*

◆ **Dexferrum [DSC]** *see* Iron Dextran Complex *on page 1053*

◆ **Dexiron (Can)** *see* Iron Dextran Complex *on page 1053*

◆ **DexPak 6 Day** *see* Dexamethasone (Systemic) *on page 579*

◆ **DexPak 10 Day** *see* Dexamethasone (Systemic) *on page 579*

◆ **DexPak 13 Day** *see* Dexamethasone (Systemic) *on page 579*

Dexrazoxane (deks ray ZOKS ane)

Related Information

Management of Chemotherapy-Induced Nausea and Vomiting in Adults *on page 2253*

Management of Drug Extravasations *on page 2271*

Prevention of Chemotherapy-Induced Nausea and Vomiting in Children *on page 2310*

Safe Handling of Hazardous Drugs *on page 2379*

Brand Names: US Totect; Zinecard

Brand Names: Canada Zinecard

Index Terms Dexrazoxane HCl; ICRF-187

Pharmacologic Category Antidote; Antidote, Extravasation; Chemoprotective Agent

Use

Prevention of cardiomyopathy associated with doxorubicin (Zinecard, generic products): To reduce the incidence and severity of cardiomyopathy associated with doxorubicin administration in women with metastatic breast cancer who have received a cumulative doxorubicin dose of 300 mg/m² and will benefit from continuing doxorubicin therapy to maintain tumor control. Not recommended for use with initial doxorubicin therapy.

Extravasation of anthracyclines (Totect): Treatment of extravasation resulting from intravenous anthracycline chemotherapy.

Labeled Contraindications

Zinecard:

US labeling: Use with chemotherapy regimens that do not contain an anthracycline

Canadian labeling: Hypersensitivity to dexrazoxane or any component of the formulation; use with chemotherapy regimens that do not contain an anthracycline; use as a chemotherapeutic agent

Totect: There are no contraindications listed in the manufacturer's labeling.

Pregnancy Considerations Adverse events were observed in animal reproduction studies using doses less than the equivalent human dose (based on BSA). Based on the mechanism of action, dexrazoxane may cause fetal harm if administered during pregnancy. Women of reproductive potential should use highly effective contraception to prevent pregnancy during treatment.

Breastfeeding Considerations It is not known if dexrazoxane is present in breast milk. Due to the potential for serious adverse reactions in the breastfed infant, a decision should be made to discontinue breastfeeding or to discontinue dexrazoxane, taking into account the importance of treatment to the mother.

Warnings/Precautions Dexrazoxane may cause mild myelosuppression (leukopenia, neutropenia, and thrombocytopenia); myelosuppression may be additive with concurrently administered chemotherapeutic agents. Dexrazoxane does not eliminate the potential for anthracycline-induced cardiac toxicity; carefully monitor cardiac function (left ventricular ejection fraction [LVEF]) prior to and periodically during treatment. Potentially significant drug-drug interactions may exist, requiring dose or frequency adjustment, additional monitoring, and/or selection of alternative therapy. May interfere with the antitumor effect of chemotherapy when given concurrently with fluorouracil, doxorubicin and cyclophosphamide (FAC). Acute myeloid leukemia (AML) and myelodysplastic syndrome (MDS) have been reported in pediatric patients and some adult patients receiving dexrazoxane in combination with chemotherapy. When used for the prevention of cardiomyopathy, doxorubicin should be administered within 30 minutes after the completion of the dexrazoxane infusion (do not administer doxorubicin before dexrazoxane). Dosage adjustment required for moderate or severe renal insufficiency (clearance is reduced). Due to dosage adjustments for doxorubicin in hepatic impairment, a proportional dose reduction in dexrazoxane is recommended to maintain the dosage ratio of 10:1. Do not use DMSO in patients receiving dexrazoxane for anthracycline extravasation; may diminish dexrazoxane efficacy. For IV administration; not for local infiltration into extravasation site.

Adverse Reactions Note: Most adverse reactions are thought to be attributed to chemotherapy, except for increased myelosuppression, pain at injection site, and phlebitis.

Prevention of doxorubicin cardiomyopathy (reactions listed are those which were greater in the dexrazoxane arm in a comparison of chemotherapy plus dexrazoxane vs chemotherapy alone):
Cardiovascular: Phlebitis (6%)
Central nervous system: Fatigue (61%), neurotoxicity (17%)
Dermatologic: Erythema (5%)
Hematologic & oncologic: Bone marrow depression, granulocytopenia, leukopenia, thrombocytopenia
Infection: Infection (23%), sepsis (17%)
Local: Pain at injection site pain (12%)
Miscellaneous: Fever (34%)
Postmarketing, and/or case reports: Metastases (including acute myeloid leukemia, myelodysplastic syndrome)

Anthracycline extravasation:
Cardiovascular: Peripheral edema (10%), localized phlebitis (6%)
Central nervous system: Fatigue (13%), dizziness (11%), depression (8%), headache (6%), insomnia (5%)
Dermatologic: Alopecia (14%)
Endocrine & metabolic: Hypercalcemia (7%), hyponatremia (6%), increased lactate dehydrogenase (5%)
Gastrointestinal: Nausea (43%), vomiting (19%), diarrhea (11%), abdominal pain (6%), constipation (6%), anorexia (5%)
Hematologic & oncologic: Decreased white blood cell count (73%; grade 3: 25%; grade 4: 20%), decreased neutrophils (61%; grade 3: 22%; grade 4: 24%), decreased hemoglobin (43%; grade 3: 3%), anemia (6%), febrile neutropenia (3%), neutropenia (3%), leukopenia, thrombocytopenia
Hepatic: Increased serum AST (28%), increased serum ALT (22%), increased serum bilirubin (11%), increased serum alkaline phosphatase (4%)
Infection: Postoperative infection (16%)
Local: Pain at injection site (16%)
Renal: Increased serum creatinine (14%)

Respiratory: Dyspnea (8%), pneumonia (6%), cough (5%)

Miscellaneous: Fever (21%)

Drug Interactions

Metabolism/Transport Effects None known.

Avoid Concomitant Use

Avoid concomitant use of Dexrazoxane with any of the following: BCG (Intravesical); Deferiprone; Dimethyl Sulfoxide; Dipyrone

Increased Effect/Toxicity

Dexrazoxane may increase the levels/effects of: CloZAPine; Deferiprone

The levels/effects of Dexrazoxane may be increased by: Dipyrone; Promazine

Decreased Effect

Dexrazoxane may decrease the levels/effects of: BCG (Intravesical); DOXOrubicin (Conventional)

The levels/effects of Dexrazoxane may be decreased by: Dimethyl Sulfoxide

Hazardous Drugs Handling Considerations

Hazardous agent (NIOSH 2016 [group 2]).

Use appropriate precautions for receiving, handling, administration, and disposal. Gloves (single) should be worn during receiving, unpacking, and placing in storage.

NIOSH recommends double gloving, a protective gown, ventilated engineering controls (a class II biological safety cabinet or a compounding aseptic containment isolator), and closed system transfer devices (CSTDs) if compounding. Double gloving and a gown are required during administration (NIOSH 2016). Assess risk to determine appropriate containment strategy (USP-NF 2017).

Storage/Stability Note: Preparation and storage are product specific; refer to individual product labeling for further details. Discard unused solutions.

Totect: Store intact vials at 25°C (77°F); excursions permitted to 15°C to 30°C (59°F to 86°F). Protect from light. Reconstituted solution (10 mg/mL) is stable for 2 hours (must be further diluted within 2 hours). Solutions diluted for infusion in NS are stable for 4 hours when stored at <25°C (77°F).

Zinecard: Store intact vials at 25°C (77°F); excursions permitted to 15°C to 30°C (59°F to 86°F). When reconstituted with SWFI, the reconstituted solution is stable for 30 minutes at room temperature or 3 hours refrigerated at 2°C to 8°C (36°F to 46°F). Solutions diluted for infusion in LR are stable for 1 hour when stored at room temperature or 4 hours refrigerated.

Dexrazoxane generic formulation (Mylan): Store intact vials at 20°C to 25°C (68°F to 77°F). Reconstituted solutions and solutions diluted for infusion in NS or D5W are stable for 6 hours when stored at room temperature or refrigerated at 2°C to 8°C (36°F to 46°F).

Additional stability information: When studied as a 24-hour continuous infusion for the prevention of cardiomyopathy, solutions prepared with sodium lactate diluent and diluted to a final concentration of 0.1 or 0.5 mg/mL in D5W were found to retain ≥90% of their initial concentration when stored at room temperature (ambient light conditions) for ≤24 hours (Tetef, 2001).

Preparation for Administration Note: Preparation and storage are product specific; refer to individual product labeling for further details. Discard unused solutions. Do not mix in the same container with other medications. ▶

Totect: Reconstitute 500 mg vial with 50 mL of 0.167 Molar sodium lactate injection solution to a reconstituted concentration of 10 mg/mL. To prepare the diluent, add 1.67 mL of 5 mEq/mL sodium lactate injection to 50 mL SWFI to make 50 mL of 0.167 Molar sodium lactate injection. Prior to infusion, further dilute reconstituted dexrazoxane solution in NS 1,000 mL.

Zinecard: Reconstitute vial with sterile water for injection to a reconstituted concentration of dexrazoxane 10 mg/mL. Prior to infusion, further dilute reconstituted dexrazoxane solution in LR injection to a final concentration of 1.3 to 3 mg/mL.

Dexrazoxane generic formulation (Mylan): Reconstitute with the supplied diluent (0.167 Molar sodium lactate injection) to a reconstituted concentration of 10 mg/mL. Prior to infusion, further dilute reconstituted dexrazoxane solution with D5W or NS to a final concentration of 1.3 to 5 mg/mL.

Mechanism of Action Dexrazoxane is a derivative of ethylenediaminetetraacetic acid (EDTA); a potent intracellular chelating agent. As a cardioprotectant, dexrazoxane appears to be converted intracellularly to a ring-opened chelating agent that interferes with iron-mediated oxygen free radical generation thought to be responsible, in part, for anthracycline-induced cardiomyopathy. In the management of anthracycline extravasation, dexrazoxane may act by reversibly inhibiting topoisomerase II, protecting tissue from anthracycline cytotoxicity, thereby decreasing tissue damage.

Pharmacodynamics/Kinetics

Distribution: Distributes to heart, liver, and kidneys; V_d: Children: 0.96 L/kg; Adults: 22 to 25 L/m^2

Protein binding: None

Metabolism: Hydrolyzed by dihydropyrimidine aminohydrolase and dihydroorotase

Half-life elimination: 2.1 to 2.5 hours

Excretion: Urine (42%)

Dosing

Adult & Geriatric

Prevention of doxorubicin cardiomyopathy: IV: A 10:1 ratio of dexrazoxane:doxorubicin (dexrazoxane 500 mg/m^2:doxorubicin 50 mg/m^2). **Note:** Cardiac monitoring should continue during dexrazoxane therapy; doxorubicin/dexrazoxane should be discontinued in patients who develop a decline in LVEF or clinical CHF.

Treatment of anthracycline extravasation: IV: 1000 mg/m^2 on days 1 and 2 (maximum dose: 2000 mg), followed by 500 mg/m^2 on day 3 (maximum dose: 1000 mg); begin treatment as soon as possible, within 6 hours of extravasation

Pediatric Prevention of doxorubicin cardiomyopathy associated with acute lymphoblastic leukemia treatment (high-risk patients; off-label use): IV: A 10:1 ratio of dexrazoxane:doxorubicin (eg, dexrazoxane 300 mg/m^2:doxorubicin 30 mg/m^2) was used in patients with high-risk acute lymphoblastic leukemia; dexrazoxane is administered immediately prior to the doxorubicin dose (Lipshultz 2010; Moghrabi 2007; Silverman 2010)

Renal Impairment Note: Renal function may be estimated using the Cockcroft-Gault formula.

Mild (CrCl ≥40 mL/minute) impairment: No dosage adjustment necessary.

Moderate-to-severe (CrCl <40 mL/minute) impairment:

Prevention of cardiomyopathy: Reduce dose to 50% of the usual dose, using a 5:1 dexrazoxane:doxorubicin ratio (eg, dexrazoxane 250 mg/m^2: doxorubicin 50 mg/m^2)

Anthracycline extravasation: Reduce dose to 50% of the usual dose

Hepatic Impairment

Prevention of cardiomyopathy: Since doxorubicin dosage is reduced in hyperbilirubinemia, a proportional reduction in dexrazoxane dosage is recommended (maintain a 10:1 ratio of dexrazoxane:doxorubicin)

Anthracycline extravasation: There are no dosage adjustments provided in the manufacturer's labeling (has not been studied).

Administration

Prevention of doxorubicin cardiomyopathy: Administer doxorubicin within 30 minutes after completion of the dexrazoxane infusion (do not administer doxorubicin before dexrazoxane).

Zinecard: Administer by rapid drip infusion over 15 minutes; do **not** administer by IV push

Dexrazoxane generic formulation (Mylan): Administer by slow IV push or rapid drip infusion

Treatment of anthracycline extravasation: Stop vesicant infusion immediately and disconnect IV line (leave needle/cannula in place); gently aspirate extravasated solution from the IV line (do **NOT** flush the line); remove needle/cannula; elevate extremity. Administer dexrazoxane IV over 1 to 2 hours; begin infusion as soon as possible, within 6 hours of extravasation. Day 2 and 3 doses should be administered at approximately the same time (± 3 hours) as the dose on day 1. Infusion solution should be at room temperature prior to administration. Infuse in a large vein in an area remote from the extravasation. For IV administration only; not for local infiltration into extravasation.

Apply dry cold compresses for 20 minutes 4 times daily for 1 to 2 days (Pérez Fidalgo 2012); withhold cooling beginning 15 minutes before dexrazoxane infusion; continue withholding cooling until 15 minutes after infusion is completed. Do not use DMSO in combination with dexrazoxane; may lessen efficacy.

Emetic Potential Children and Adults: Minimal (<10%)

Monitoring Parameters CBC with differential (frequent); liver function; serum creatinine; cardiac function (repeat monitoring at 400 mg/m^2, 500 mg/m^2 and with every 50 mg/m^2 of doxorubicin thereafter); monitor site of extravasation

Dosage Forms Excipient information presented when available (limited, particularly for generics); consult specific product labeling.

Solution Reconstituted, Intravenous:

Totect: 500 mg (1 ea) [pyrogen free]

Zinecard: 250 mg (1 ea); 500 mg (1 ea) [pyrogen free]

Generic: 250 mg (1 ea); 500 mg (1 ea)

- ◆ **Diaminocyclohexane Oxalatoplatinum** *see* Oxaliplatin *on page* 1394
- ◆ **DIC** *see* Dacarbazine *on page* 494
- ◆ **Diflucan** *see* Fluconazole *on page* 807
- ◆ **Diflucan injection (Can)** *see* Fluconazole *on page* 807
- ◆ **Diflucan One (Can)** *see* Fluconazole *on page* 807
- ◆ **Diflucan PWS (Can)** *see* Fluconazole *on page* 807
- ◆ **Difluorodeoxycytidine Hydrochlorothiazide** *see* Gemcitabine *on page* 864
- ◆ **Dihematoporphyrin Ether** *see* Porfimer *on page* 1535
- ◆ **Dihydroxyanthracenedione** *see* MitoXANTRONE *on page* 1271
- ◆ **Dihydroxyanthracenedione Dihydrochloride** *see* MitoXANTRONE *on page* 1271
- ◆ **Dihydroxydeoxynorvinkaleukoblastine** *see* Vinorelbine *on page* 1915

Dimethyl Sulfoxide (dye meth il sul FOKS ide)

Related Information
Management of Drug Extravasations *on page* 2271

Brand Names: US Rimso-50

Brand Names: Canada Dimethyl Sulfoxide Irrigation, USP; Kemsol; Rimso-50

Index Terms Dimethylsulfoxide; DMSO

Pharmacologic Category Antidote, Extravasation; Urinary Tract Product

Use

Interstitial cystitis: Symptomatic relief of interstitial cystitis.

Limitation of use: There is no clinical evidence of effectiveness of dimethyl sulfoxide in the treatment of bacterial urinary tract infections.

Labeled Contraindications There are no contraindications listed in the manufacturer's labeling.

Pregnancy Considerations Adverse events have been observed in some animal reproduction studies.

Breastfeeding Considerations It is not known if dimethyl sulfoxide is excreted in breast milk. The manufacturer recommends that caution be exercised when administering dimethyl sulfoxide to nursing women.

Warnings/Precautions For bladder instillation or topical administration for extravasation management (off-label use) only; not for IV or IM administration. Do not use in patients receiving dexrazoxane for anthracycline extravasation (Mourdisen, 2007); dimethyl sulfoxide (DMSO) may diminish dexrazoxane efficacy. Hypersensitivity reactions with intravesical administration have been reported rarely; hypersensitivity has also occurred with topical administration. If anaphylactoid symptoms occur, manage appropriately. Use with caution in patients with urinary tract malignancy; may be harmful due to vasodilatory effects. Lens changes and opacities have been observed in animal studies; full eye exams (including slit lamp) are recommended prior to use and periodically during treatment. A garlic-like taste may occur, beginning a few minutes after instillation and lasting for several hours. Garlic odor on the breath and skin may also occur and persist for up to 3 days. Bladder discomfort may occur; generally diminishes with repeated administration.

Adverse Reactions Frequency not defined.

Dermatologic: Body odor (garlic; duration: Up to 72 hours)

Gastrointestinal: Halitosis/unpleasant taste (garlic; onset: Within a few minutes after instillation; duration: Up to 72 hours)

Genitourinary: Bladder pain, cystitis (transient)

Local: Localized erythema (topical application; Perez Fidalgo, 2012)

Hypersensitivity: Hypersensitivity

Postmarketing and/or case reports: Contact dermatitis, cystitis (eosinophilic), pigment deposits on lens

Drug Interactions

Metabolism/Transport Effects Inhibits CYP2C9 (weak)

Avoid Concomitant Use

Avoid concomitant use of Dimethyl Sulfoxide with any of the following: Dexrazoxane

Increased Effect/Toxicity

Dimethyl Sulfoxide may increase the levels/effects of: Sulindac

Decreased Effect

Dimethyl Sulfoxide may decrease the levels/effects of: Dexrazoxane

Storage/Stability Store at 20°C to 25°C (68°F to 77°F). Protect from strong light.

Mechanism of Action For management of cystitis, dimethyl sulfoxide (DMSO) has anti-inflammatory, analgesic, mast cell inhibition, and muscle relaxing effects (Chancellor, 2004). DMSO also has free-radical scavenger properties, which increases removal of vesicant drugs from tissues to minimize tissue damage in extravasation management (Perez Fidalgo, 2012).

Pharmacodynamics/Kinetics

Absorption: Topical: Well absorbed from application site

Distribution: Topical: Rapidly penetrates tissues (Bertelli 1995)

Metabolism: Oxidation to dimethyl sulfone; reduction to dimethyl sulfide

Excretion: Urine and feces (as unchanged drug and dimethyl sulfone); some elimination via skin and lungs (dimethyl sulfide)

Dosing

Adult & Geriatric

Interstitial cystitis: Bladder instillation: Instill 50 mL directly into bladder and retain for 15 minutes; repeat every 2 weeks until symptoms are relieved, then increase intervals between treatments **or** 50 mL directly into bladder and retain for 15 to 20 minutes every 1 to 2 weeks for 4 to 8 treatments (Chancellor, 2004)

Extravasation management (anthracyclines, mitomycin, or mitoxantrone; off-label use): Topical DMSO: Apply to a region covering twice the affected area every 8 hours for 7 days; begin within 10 minutes of extravasation; do not cover with a dressing (Perez Fidalgo, 2012)

Pediatric Extravasation management (anthracyclines, mitomycin, or mitoxantrone; off-label use): Children and Adolescents: Refer to adult dosing.

Administration

Intravesical: Instill directly into the bladder via catheter or syringe. To reduce bladder spasm, apply an analgesic lubricant (eg, lidocaine jelly) to urethra prior to catheter insertion; oral analgesics or belladonna and opium suppositories prior to administration may be of benefit. **Not for IV or IM use.**

◄ Extravasation management (off-label use): Stop vesicant infusion immediately and disconnect IV line (leave needle/cannula in place); gently aspirate extravasated solution from the IV line (do **NOT** flush the line); remove needle/cannula; elevate extremity. Apply DMSO topically (within 10 minutes of extravasation) to extravasation site, covering an area twice the size of extravasation; allow to air dry; do not cover with a dressing (Perez Fidalgo, 2012). **Not for IV or IM use.**

Monitoring Parameters CBC, chemistry panel, liver and renal function tests about every 6 months; eye examinations and slit lamp examinations (baseline and periodically during treatment). For extravasation management, monitor and document extravasation site.

Dosage Forms Excipient information presented when available (limited, particularly for generics); consult specific product labeling.
Solution, Intravesical:
Rimso-50: 50% (50 mL)

♦ **Dimethylsulfoxide** see Dimethyl Sulfoxide on page 598

♦ **Dimethyl Sulfoxide Irrigation, USP (Can)** see Dimethyl Sulfoxide on page 598

♦ **Dimethyl Triazeno Imidazole Carboxamide** see Dacarbazine on page 494

Dinutuximab (din ue TUX i mab)

Related Information
Chemotherapy-Induced Peripheral Neuropathy on page 2236
Common Toxicity Criteria on page 2242
Management of Chemotherapy-Induced Nausea and Vomiting in Adults on page 2253
Prevention of Chemotherapy-Induced Nausea and Vomiting in Children on page 2310

Brand Names: US Unituxin

Index Terms ch14.18; MOAB Ch14.18

Pharmacologic Category Antineoplastic Agent, Anti-GD2; Antineoplastic Agent, Monoclonal Antibody

Use Neuroblastoma: Treatment of high-risk neuroblastoma (in combination with granulocyte-macrophage colony-stimulating factor [GM-CSF; sargramostim], interleukin-2 [IL-2; aldesleukin] and 13-cis-retinoic acid [RA; isotretinoin]) in pediatric patients who achieve at least a partial response to prior first-line multiagent, multimodality therapy.

Labeled Contraindications History of anaphylaxis to dinutuximab

Pregnancy Considerations Reproduction studies have not been completed with dinutuximab. Monoclonal antibodies cross the placenta, the largest amount during the third trimester of pregnancy. Based on the mechanism of action, dinutuximab may cause fetal harm. Women of reproductive potential should use effective contraception during therapy and for 2 months after the last dose.

Breastfeeding Considerations It is not known if dinutuximab is present in breast milk. IgG molecules are excreted in breast milk. Due to the potential for serious adverse reactions in the breastfed infant, breastfeeding is not recommended by the manufacturer.

Warnings/Precautions [US Boxed Warning]: Serious and potentially life-threatening infusion reactions occurred in approximately one-fourth of patients treated with dinutuximab. Administer required prehydration and

premedication, including antihistamines, prior to each dinutuximab infusion. Monitor patients closely for signs and symptoms of an infusion reaction during and for at least 4 hours following completion of each dinutuximab infusion. Immediately interrupt dinutuximab for severe infusion reactions and permanently discontinue dinutuximab for anaphylaxis. Infusion reactions typically occurred during infusion or within 24 hours of completion and may include facial and upper airway edema, dyspnea, bronchospasm, stridor, urticaria, and hypotension. Infusion reactions may require blood pressure support, bronchodilator therapy, corticosteroids, infusion rate interruption and/or reduction, or permanent therapy discontinuation. Infusion should be in a facility with cardiopulmonary medication/equipment available. Severe capillary leak syndrome was reported in close to one-fourth of patients receiving dinutuximab. Immediately interrupt infusion if capillary leak syndrome develops; infusion rate reduction and/or therapy discontinuation may be necessary. Initiate appropriate management in patients with symptomatic or severe capillary leak syndrome. Severe hypotension occurred more frequently in patients receiving dinutuximab. Intravenous hydration is required prior to each infusion; closely monitor blood pressure during infusion. May require therapy interruption or discontinuation; initiate appropriate medical management in patients with a systolic blood pressure (SBP) less than lower limit of normal for age, or SBP that is decreased by more than 15% compared to baseline. Electrolyte abnormalities (such as hyponatremia, hypokalemia, and hypocalcemia) were reported in at least one-fourth of patients who received dinutuximab, Including grade 3 or 4 events. In a study of a related anti-GD2 antibody, syndrome of inappropriate antidiuretic hormone secretion (SIADH) resulting in severe hyponatremia was reported. Monitor electrolytes closely during therapy.

[US Boxed Warning]: Dinutuximab causes serious neurologic adverse reactions including severe neuropathic pain and peripheral neuropathy; severe neuropathic pain occurs in the majority of patients. Administer intravenous opioids prior to, during, and for 2 hours following completion of the dinutuximab infusion. In clinical studies of patients with high-risk neuroblastoma, grade 3 peripheral sensory neuropathy occurred in 2% to 9% of patients. In clinical studies of dinutuximab and related GD2-binding antibodies, severe motor neuropathy has occurred. Resolution of motor neuropathy did not occur in all cases. Discontinue dinutuximab for severe unresponsive pain, severe sensory neuropathy, or moderate to severe peripheral motor neuropathy. Discontinue permanently for grade 2 or higher peripheral motor neuropathy, grade 3 sensory neuropathy that interferes with activities of daily living for more than 2 weeks, or grade 4 sensory neuropathy. In patients who experienced peripheral sensory neuropathy of any grade, the median duration was 9 days (range: 3 to 163 days). Most patients experienced pain; severe pain was observed in over 50% of patients treated with dinutuximab; pain may occur despite analgesic/opioid therapy. Pain typically occurred during infusion and included abdominal, generalized, extremity, or back pain, neuralgia, musculoskeletal chest pain, and arthralgia. Premedication with analgesics, including opioids, is required prior to each dose, during the infusion, and for 2 hours following the infusion. Severe pain may require reduction of the infusion rate or therapy discontinuation.

Severe (grade 3 or 4) anemia, neutropenia, thrombocytopenia, and neutropenic fever were observed in dinutuximab-treated patients. Monitor complete blood counts closely during treatment. Severe (grade 3 or 4) bacteremia was reported more frequently in dinutuximab-treated patients, and required intravenous antibiotics or other urgent interventions. Sepsis was also observed in patients receiving dinutuximab. Monitor closely for signs/symptoms of systemic infection; may require therapy interruption until resolution of infection. Hemolytic uremic syndrome (without documented infection) resulted in renal insufficiency, electrolyte abnormalities, anemia, and hypertension in a small number of patients. Atypical hemolytic uremic syndrome recurred in one patient upon rechallenge. Permanently discontinue if hemolytic uremic syndrome develops; manage supportively. Neurological ocular toxicity such as blurred vision, photophobia, mydriasis, fixed or unequal pupils, optic nerve disorder, eyelid ptosis, and papilledema were reported in clinical trials. In patients who experienced complete resolution of ocular toxicity, the median duration of toxicity was 4 days (range: 0 to 221 days). May require therapy interruption, dosage reduction, and/or treatment discontinuation.

Reversible posterior leukoencephalopathy syndrome (RPLS) has been reported; symptoms of RPLS include severe headache, hypertension, visual changes, seizures or lethargy; begin appropriate management and discontinue dinutuximab in patients with RPLS signs/symptoms. Transverse myelitis has occurred in patients receiving dinutuximab; signs/symptoms (weakness, paresthesia, sensory loss or incontinence) should be evaluated promptly; discontinue permanently in patients who develop transverse myelitis. Prolonged urinary retention that persists for weeks to months after opioid discontinuation has occurred in patients receiving dinutuximab; discontinue permanently if urinary retention does not resolve following opioid discontinuation. Potentially significant interactions may exist, requiring dose or frequency adjustment, additional monitoring, and/or selection of alternative therapy. Dinutuximab is associated with a moderate emetic potential; antiemetics are recommended to prevent nausea and vomiting.

Adverse Reactions

>10%:

Cardiovascular: Hypotension (60%), capillary leak syndrome (40%), tachycardia (19%), edema (17%), hypertension (14%)

Central nervous system: Pain (85%), peripheral neuropathy (13%; grades 3/4: 6%)

Dermatologic: Urticaria (37%)

Endocrine & metabolic: Hyponatremia (58%), hypokalemia (43%), hypoalbuminemia (33%), hypocalcemia (27%), hypophosphatemia (20%), hyperglycemia (18%), hypertriglyceridemia (16%), hypomagnesemia (12%)

Gastrointestinal: Increased serum ALT (56%), vomiting (46%), diarrhea (43%), increased serum AST (28%), decreased appetite (15%)

Genitourinary: Proteinuria (16%)

Hematologic & oncologic: Thrombocytopenia (66%; grades 3/4: 39%), lymphocytopenia (62%; grades 3/4: 51%), anemia (51%; grades 3/4: 34%), neutropenia (39%; grades 3/4: 34%), hemorrhage (17%; grades 3/4: 6%)

Hypersensitivity: Severe infusion-related reaction (26%)

Infection: Sepsis (18%), infection (device-related: 16%), bacteremia (grades 3/4: 13%)

Renal: Increased serum creatinine (15%)

Respiratory: Hypoxia (24%)

Miscellaneous: Fever (72%), infusion-related reaction (60%)

1% to 10%:

Central nervous system: Peripheral sensory neuropathy (9%; grade 3: 1%), peripheral motor neuropathy (grade 3: 1%)

Dermatologic: Anaphylaxis (1%)

Endocrine & metabolic: Weight gain (10%)

Gastrointestinal: Nausea (10%)

Hematologic & oncologic: Febrile neutropenia (grades 3/4: 4%), hemolytic-uremic syndrome (2%)

Ophthalmic: Blurred vision (2%)

Frequency not defined: Ophthalmic: Blepharoptosis, optic nerve damage, papilledema, photophobia

<1%, postmarketing, and/or case reports: Diplopia, fixation of pupils, mydriasis, reversible posterior leukoencephalopathy syndrome, transverse myelitis, urinary retention (prolonged)

Drug Interactions

Metabolism/Transport Effects None known.

Avoid Concomitant Use

Avoid concomitant use of Dinutuximab with any of the following: BCG (Intravesical); Belimumab; Deferiprone; Dipyrone; Natalizumab; Pimecrolimus; Tacrolimus (Topical); Vaccines (Live)

Increased Effect/Toxicity

Dinutuximab may increase the levels/effects of: Amifostine; Antipsychotic Agents (Second Generation [Atypical]); Belimumab; CloZAPine; Deferiprone; DULoxetine; Fingolimod; Hypotension-Associated Agents; Leflunomide; Levodopa; Natalizumab; Nitroprusside; Pholcodine; Tofacitinib; Vaccines (Live)

The levels/effects of Dinutuximab may be increased by: Alfuzosin; Barbiturates; Benperidol; Blood Pressure Lowering Agents; Brimonidine (Topical); Denosumab; Diazoxide; Dipyrone; Herbs (Hypotensive Properties); Lormetazepam; Molsidomine; Naftopidil; Nicergoline; Nicorandil; Obinutuzumab; Ocrelizumab; Pentoxifylline; Phosphodiesterase 5 Inhibitors; Pimecrolimus; Promazine; Prostacyclin Analogues; Quinagolide; Roflumilast; Tacrolimus (Topical); Trastuzumab

Decreased Effect

Dinutuximab may decrease the levels/effects of: BCG (Intravesical); Coccidioides immitis Skin Test; Nivolumab; Sipuleucel-T; Tertomotide; Vaccines (Inactivated); Vaccines (Live)

The levels/effects of Dinutuximab may be decreased by: Echinacea

Storage/Stability Store intact vials at 2°C to 8°C (36°F to 46°F); do not freeze. Do not shake. Keep the vial in the outer carton to protect from light. Solutions diluted for infusion in NS should be stored at 2°C to 8°C (36°F to 46°F). Initiate infusion within 4 hours of preparation. Discard diluted solution 24 hours after preparation.

Preparation for Administration Must be diluted prior to infusion. Withdraw the required dinutuximab volume and inject into a 100 mL bag of NS. Mix by gentle inversion; do not shake. Discard unused vial contents. Initiate infusion within 4 hours of preparation. Do not use if cloudy, discolored (pronounced), or contains particulates.

Mechanism of Action Dinutuximab binds to the disialoganglioside GD2, which is highly expressed in neuroblastoma, most melanomas, and other tumors, as well as on normal tissues such as neurons, skin melanocytes, and

◀ peripheral sensory nerve fibers (Yu 2010). By binding to cell surface GD2, dinutuximab induces cell lysis (of GD2-expressing cells) through antibody-dependent cell-mediated cytotoxicity (ADCC) and complement-dependent cytotoxicity (CDC).

Pharmacodynamics/Kinetics

Distribution: Pediatric patients (age: 3.9 ± 1.9 years): V_{dss}: 5.4 L

Half-life elimination, terminal: 10 days

Excretion: Clearance: Pediatric patients (age: 3.9 ± 1.9 years): 0.21 L/day; increased with body size

Dosing

Pediatric

Neuroblastoma, high-risk: IV: 17.5 mg/m^2/day for 4 consecutive days for a maximum of 5 cycles (in combination with GM-CSF [sargramostim], IL-2 [aldesleukin] and 13-cis-retinoic acid [isotretinoin]). Infuse on days 4, 5, 6, and 7 during cycles 1, 3, and 5 (cycles 1, 3, and 5 are 24 days in duration); infuse on days 8, 9, 10, and 11 during cycles 2 and 4 (cycles 2 and 4 are 32 days in duration).

Premedications:

Analgesics: Administer morphine 50 mcg/kg IV immediately prior to dinutuximab infusion initiation; continue as a morphine drip at an infusion rate of 20 to 50 mcg/kg/hour during and for 2 hours following completion of infusion. May administer additional doses of 25 to 50 mcg/kg IV as needed up to once every 2 hours followed by an increase in the drip rate in clinically stable patients. Consider conversion to fentanyl or hydromorphone if morphine is not tolerated; if pain is inadequately controlled with opioids, consider adjunct therapy with gabapentin or lidocaine.

Antiemetics: Dinutuximab is associated with a moderate emetic potential; antiemetics are recommended to prevent nausea and vomiting.

Antihistamine: Administer an antihistamine (eg, diphenhydramine 0.5 to 1 mg/kg/dose; maximum dose 50 mg) IV over 10 to 15 minutes starting 20 minutes prior to dinutuximab infusion and every 4 to 6 hours as tolerated during the infusion.

Antipyretics: Administer acetaminophen (10 to 15 mg/kg/dose; maximum dose 650 mg) 20 minutes prior to each infusion and every 4 to 6 hours as needed for fever and pain. May administer ibuprofen (5 to 10 mg/kg/dose) every 6 hours as needed for control of persistent fever or pain.

IV hydration: Administer NS 10 mL/kg IV over 1 hour just prior to each dinutuximab infusion.

Renal Impairment There are no dosage adjustments provided in the manufacturer's labeling (has not been studied).

Hepatic Impairment There are no dosage adjustments provided in the manufacturer's labeling (has not been studied).

Adjustment for Toxicity

Anaphylaxis, grade 3 or 4: Permanently discontinue therapy.

Capillary leak syndrome:

Moderate to severe, but not life-threatening: Immediately interrupt infusion; upon resolution, resume infusion at 50% of the previous rate.

Life-threatening: Discontinue infusion for the current cycle; in subsequent cycles, infuse at 50% of the previous rate. If life-threatening capillary leak syndrome recurs, permanently discontinue therapy.

Hemolytic uremic syndrome: Permanently discontinue therapy and administer supportive management.

Hyponatremia, grade 4 (despite appropriate fluid management): Permanently discontinue therapy.

Hypotension (symptomatic hypotension, systolic blood pressure [SBP] less than lower limit of normal for age, or SBP decreased by more than 15% compared to baseline): Interrupt infusion; upon resolution, resume infusion at 50% of the previous rate. If blood pressure remains stable for ≥2 hours, increase infusion rate as tolerated up to a maximum rate of 1.75 mg/m²/hour.

Infection (systemic)/sepsis, severe: Discontinue therapy until infection resolves; may resume therapy with subsequent cycles.

Infusion-related reaction:

Mild to moderate reaction (eg, transient rash, fever, rigors, and localized urticaria that respond promptly to symptomatic treatment): Reduce infusion rate by 50%; monitor closely. Upon resolution, gradually increase infusion rate up to a maximum of 1.75 mg/m²/hour.

Severe or prolonged reaction (eg, mild bronchospasm without other symptoms, angioedema that does not affect the airway): Immediately interrupt infusion; if symptoms resolve rapidly, resume infusion at 50% of the previous rate and monitor closely. If reaction recurs, discontinue therapy until the following day. If symptoms resolve and further treatment is warranted, premedicate with IV hydrocortisone 1 mg/kg (maximum: 50 mg) and infuse at a rate of 0.875 mg/m²/hour in an intensive care unit. If reaction recurs again, permanently discontinue therapy.

Life-threatening reaction: Permanently discontinue therapy and administer supportive management.

Neuropathy:

Grade 4 sensory neuropathy or grade 3 sensory neuropathy that interferes with daily activities for more than 2 weeks: Permanently discontinue therapy.

Grade 2 or higher peripheral motor neuropathy: Permanently discontinue therapy.

Ocular neurological disorders (eg, blurred vision, photophobia, mydriasis, fixed or unequal pupils, optic nerve disorder, eyelid ptosis, and/or papilledema): Discontinue infusion until symptom resolution; upon resolution, reduce **dose** by 50%. If reaction recurs, or if reaction is accompanied by visual impairment (eg, subtotal or total vision loss), permanently discontinue therapy.

Pain, severe (grade 3): Decrease the infusion rate to 0.875 mg/m²/hour. If pain is not adequately controlled despite rate reduction and use of maximum supportive measures, permanently discontinue therapy.

Reversible posterior leukoencephalopathy syndrome: Permanently discontinue therapy.

Serum sickness, grade 3 or 4: Permanently discontinue therapy.

Transverse myelitis: Permanently discontinue therapy.

Urinary retention (persistent after opioid discontinuation): Permanently discontinue therapy.

Administration Dinutuximab is associated with a moderate emetic potential; antiemetics are recommended to prevent nausea and vomiting.

Administer as an IV infusion only; **do not administer as an IV push or bolus.** Administer NS 10 mL/kg IV over 1 hour just prior to each dinutuximab infusion. Premedicate with analgesics, an antihistamine, and an antipyretic prior to administration (see Dosing). Infuse in an environment equipped to monitor for

◀ and manage infusion reactions. Interrupt infusion for toxicity (see Dosing: Adjustment for Toxicity).

Initiate infusion at a rate of 0.875 mg/m^2/hour for 30 minutes. Increase infusion rate gradually as tolerated to a maximum rate of 1.75 mg/m^2/hour to infuse over 10 to 20 hours each day. Monitor patients closely for signs and symptoms of an infusion reaction during and for at least 4 hours following completion of each dinutuximab infusion.

Emetic Potential Moderate (30% to 90%)

Monitoring Parameters CBC with differential, serum electrolytes, renal function, blood pressure; monitor for signs/symptoms of infusion reactions (during and for at least 4 hours after infusion), pain, peripheral neuropathy, capillary leak syndrome, infection/sepsis, hemolytic uremic syndrome, ocular toxicity, urinary retention, transverse myelitis, and/or reversible posterior leukoencephalopathy syndrome.

Dosage Forms Excipient information presented when available (limited, particularly for generics); consult specific product labeling.

Solution, Intravenous [preservative free]:

Unituxin: 17.5 mg/5 mL (5 mL) [contains mouse (murine) and/or hamster protein]

◆ **Disodium Thiosulfate Pentahydrate** see Sodium Thiosulfate on page 1678

◆ **5071-1DL(6)** see Megestrol on page 1178

◆ **4-DMDR** see IDArubicin on page 951

◆ **DMSO** see Dimethyl Sulfoxide on page 598

◆ **Docefrez [DSC]** see DOCEtaxel on page 606

DOCEtaxel (doe se TAKS el)

Related Information

Common Toxicity Criteria on page 2242

Management of Chemotherapy-Induced Nausea and Vomiting in Adults on page 2253

Management of Drug Extravasations on page 2271

Mucositis and Stomatitis on page 2299

Prevention of Chemotherapy-Induced Nausea and Vomiting in Children on page 2310

Safe Handling of Hazardous Drugs on page 2379

Brand Names: US Docefrez [DSC]; Taxotere

Brand Names: Canada Docetaxel for Injection; Docetaxel Injection; Taxotere

Index Terms RP-6976

Pharmacologic Category Antineoplastic Agent, Antimicrotubular; Antineoplastic Agent, Taxane Derivative

Use

Docefrez:

Breast cancer: Treatment of breast cancer (locally advanced/metastatic) after prior chemotherapy failure

Non-small cell lung cancer: Treatment of locally advanced or metastatic non-small cell lung cancer (NSCLC) after prior platinum-based chemotherapy failure; treatment of previously untreated unresectable locally advanced or metastatic NSCLC (in combination with cisplatin)

Prostate cancer: Treatment of hormone-refractory metastatic prostate cancer (in combination with prednisone)

Taxotere (and various generic brands):

Breast cancer: Treatment of breast cancer (locally advanced/metastatic) after prior chemotherapy failure; adjuvant treatment (in combination with doxorubicin and cyclophosphamide) of operable node-positive breast cancer

Gastric cancer: Treatment of advanced gastric adenocarcinoma, including gastroesophageal junction adenocarcinoma (in combination with cisplatin and fluorouracil) in patients who have not received prior chemotherapy for advanced disease

Head and neck cancer: Treatment (induction) of locally advanced squamous cell head and neck cancer (in combination with cisplatin and fluorouracil)

NSCLC: Treatment of locally advanced or metastatic NSCLC after failure of prior platinum-based chemotherapy; treatment of previously untreated unresectable locally advanced or metastatic NSCLC (in combination with cisplatin)

Prostate cancer: Treatment of androgen-independent (hormone refractory) metastatic prostate cancer (in combination with prednisone)

Labeled Contraindications

Severe hypersensitivity to docetaxel or any component of the formulation; severe hypersensitivity to other medications containing polysorbate 80; neutrophil count <1,500/mm^3

Canadian labeling: Additional contraindications (not in the US labeling): Severe hepatic impairment; pregnancy; breastfeeding

Pregnancy Considerations Adverse events have been observed in animal reproduction studies. An *ex vivo* human placenta perfusion model illustrated that docetaxel crossed the placenta at term. Placental transfer was low and affected by the presence of albumin; higher albumin concentrations resulted in lower docetaxel placental transfer (Berveiller, 2012). Some pharmacokinetic properties of docetaxel may be altered in pregnant women (van Hasselt 2014). Women of childbearing potential should avoid becoming pregnant during therapy. A pregnancy registry is available for all cancers diagnosed during pregnancy at Cooper Health (877-635-4499).

Breastfeeding Considerations It is not known if docetaxel is excreted into breast milk. Due to the potential for serious adverse reactions in breastfeeding the infant, the US labeling recommends a decision be made to discontinue breastfeeding or the drug, taking into account the importance of treatment to the mother.

Warnings/Precautions [US Boxed Warning]: Avoid use in patients with bilirubin exceeding upper limit of normal (ULN) or AST and/or ALT >1.5 times ULN in conjunction with alkaline phosphatase >2.5 times ULN. Patients with bilirubin elevations or abnormal transaminases (with concurrent abnormal alkaline phosphatase) are at increased risk for grade 4 neutropenia, neutropenic fever, infections, severe thrombocytopenia, severe stomatitis, severe skin toxicity, and toxic death. Patients with isolated transaminase elevations >1.5 times ULN also had a higher rate of grade 4 neutropenic fever, although no increased incidence of toxic death. Monitor bilirubin, AST or ALT, and alkaline phosphatase prior to each docetaxel cycle. The alcohol content of the docetaxel formulation should be taken into account when administering to patients with hepatic impairment. **[US Boxed Warnings]: Severe hypersensitivity reactions, characterized by generalized rash/erythema, hypotension, bronchospasms, or rare anaphylaxis may occur (may be fatal; has occurred**

in patients receiving 3-day corticosteroid premedication). **Hypersensitivity reactions require immediate discontinuation of the docetaxel infusion and administration of appropriate therapy. Do not administer to patients with a history of severe hypersensitivity to docetaxel or polysorbate 80 (component of formulation). Severe fluid retention, characterized by pleural effusion (requiring immediate drainage, ascites with pronounced abdominal distention, peripheral edema (poorly tolerated), dyspnea at rest, cardiac tamponade, generalized edema, and weight gain, has been reported (despite the use of premedication with 3 days of dexamethasone).** Fluid retention may begin as lower extremity peripheral edema and become generalized with a median weight gain of 2 kg. In patients with breast cancer, the median cumulative dose to onset of moderate or severe fluid retention was 819 mg/m^2; fluid retention resolves in a median of 16 weeks after discontinuation. In a scientific statement from the American Heart Association, docetaxel has been determined to be an agent that may either cause direct myocardial toxicity or exacerbate underlying myocardial dysfunction (magnitude: moderate) (AHA [Page 2016]). Minor reactions including flushing or localized skin reactions may also occur. Observe for hypersensitivity, especially with the first two infusions. Discontinue for severe reactions; do not rechallenge if severe. Patients should be premedicated with a corticosteroid (starting one day prior to administration) to reduce the incidence and severity of hypersensitivity reactions and fluid retention; severity is reduced with dexamethasone premedication starting one day prior to docetaxel administration. Premedication with oral corticosteroids is recommended to decrease the incidence and severity of fluid retention and severity of hypersensitivity reactions. The manufacturer recommends dexamethasone 16 mg/day (8 mg twice daily) orally for 3 days, starting the day before docetaxel administration; for prostate cancer, when prednisone is part of the antineoplastic regimen, dexamethasone 8 mg orally is administered at 12 hours, 3 hours, and 1 hour prior to docetaxel.

[US Boxed Warning]: Patients with abnormal liver function, those receiving higher doses, and patients with non-small cell lung cancer and a history of prior treatment with platinum derivatives who receive single-agent docetaxel at a dose of 100 mg/m^2 are at higher risk for treatment-related mortality.

Neutropenia is the dose-limiting toxicity. Patients with increased liver function tests experienced more episodes of neutropenia with a greater number of severe infections. **[US Boxed Warning]: Patients with an absolute neutrophil count <1,500/mm^3 should not receive docetaxel. Monitor blood counts frequently to monitor for neutropenia (which may be severe and result in infection).** The dose-limiting toxicity is neutropenia. Platelets should recover to >100,000/mm^3 prior to treatment. Monitor liver function tests frequently. Hematologic toxicity may require dose reduction or therapy discontinuation.

Cutaneous reactions including erythema (with edema) and desquamation have been reported; may require dose reduction. Cystoid macular edema (CME) has been reported; if vision impairment occurs, a prompt comprehensive ophthalmic exam is recommended. If CME is diagnosed, initiate appropriate CME management and discontinue docetaxel (consider non-taxane treatments). In a study of patients receiving docetaxel for the adjuvant treatment of breast cancer, a majority of patients experienced tearing, which occurred in patients with and without lacrimal duct obstruction at baseline;

onset was generally after cycle 1, but subsided in most patients within 4 months after therapy completion (Chan 2013). Dosage adjustment is recommended with severe neurosensory symptoms (paresthesia, dysesthesia, pain); persistent symptoms may require discontinuation; reversal of symptoms may be delayed after discontinuation. Some docetaxel formulations contain alcohol (content varies by formulation), which may affect the central nervous system and cause symptoms of alcohol intoxication. Consider alcohol content and use with caution in patients for whom alcohol intake should be avoided or minimized. Patients should avoid driving or operating machinery immediately after the infusion. An FDA-approved non-alcohol generic formulation (20 mg/mL) is available. Treatment-related acute myeloid leukemia or myelodysplasia occurred in patients receiving docetaxel in combination with anthracyclines and/or cyclophosphamide. Fatigue and weakness (may be severe) have been reported; symptoms may last a few days up to several weeks; in patients with progressive disease, weakness may be associated with a decrease in performance status. Potentially significant drug-drug interactions may exist, requiring dose or frequency adjustment, additional monitoring, and/or selection of alternative therapy. Docetaxel is an irritant with vesicant-like properties; ensure proper needle or catheter placement prior to and during infusion; avoid extravasation.

Some dosage forms may contain polysorbate 80 (also known as Tweens). Hypersensitivity reactions, usually a delayed reaction, have been reported following exposure to pharmaceutical products containing polysorbate 80 in certain individuals (Isaksson 2002; Lucente 2000; Shelley 1995). Thrombocytopenia, ascites, pulmonary deterioration, and renal and hepatic failure have been reported in premature neonates after receiving parenteral products containing polysorbate 80 (Alade 1986; CDC 1984). See manufacturer's labeling.

Adverse Reactions Percentages reported for docetaxel monotherapy; frequency may vary depending on diagnosis, dose, liver function, prior treatment, and premedication.

>10%:

Central nervous system: Central nervous system toxicity (20% to 58%; severe: ≤6%; including neuropathy)

Dermatologic: Alopecia (56% to 76%), dermatological reaction (20% to 48%; severe: ≤5%), nail disease (11% to 41%)

Endocrine & metabolic: Fluid retention (includes edema and effusion; 13% to 60%; severe: 7% to 9%; dose dependent)

Gastrointestinal: Stomatitis (19% to 53%; severe 1% to 8%), diarrhea (23% to 43%; severe: 5% to 6%), nausea (34% to 42%), vomiting (22% to 23%)

Hematologic & oncologic: Neutropenia (84% to 99%; grade 4: 75% to 86%; nadir [median]: 7 days, duration [severe neutropenia]: 7 days; dose dependent), leukopenia (84% to 99%; grade 4: 32% to 44%), anemia (65% to 97%; dose dependent; grades 3/4: 8% to 9%), thrombocytopenia (8% to 14%; grade 4: 1%; dose dependent), febrile neutropenia (≤14%; dose dependent)

Hepatic: Increased serum transaminases (4% to 19%)

Hypersensitivity: Hypersensitivity (1% to 21%; with premedication 15%)

Infection: Infection (1% to 34%; dose dependent)

◀

Neuromuscular & skeletal: Weakness (53% to 66%; severe: ≤18%), myalgia (3% to 23%), neuromuscular reaction (16%)

Respiratory: Pulmonary reaction (41%)

Miscellaneous: Fever (31% to 35%)

1% to 10%:

Cardiovascular: Decreased left ventricular ejection fraction (8%), hypotension (3%)

Central nervous system: Peripheral motor neuropathy (4%; severe; mainly distal extremity weakness)

Gastrointestinal: Dysgeusia (6%)

Hepatic: Increased serum bilirubin (9%), increased serum alkaline phosphatase (4% to 7%)

Infection: Severe infection (6%)

Local: Infusion site reactions (4%, including hyperpigmentation, inflammation, redness, dryness, phlebitis, extravasation, swelling of the vein)

Neuromuscular and skeletal: Arthralgia (3% to 9%)

<1%, postmarketing, and/or case reports: Abdominal pain, acute hepatic failure (Morgan 2011), acute myelocytic leukemia, acute respiratory distress, alopecia (permanent), anaphylactic shock, anorexia, ascites, atrial fibrillation, atrial flutter, back pain, bronchospasm, cardiac arrhythmia, cardiac tamponade, chest pain, chest tightness, chills, colitis, confusion, conjunctivitis, constipation, cystoid macular edema, deep vein thrombosis, dehydration, disease of the lacrimal apparatus (duct obstruction), disseminated intravascular coagulation, drug fever, duodenal ulcer, dyspnea, ECG abnormality, epiphora (more common with weekly administration [Kintzel 2006]), erythema multiforme, esophagitis, flushing, gastrointestinal hemorrhage, gastrointestinal obstruction, gastrointestinal perforation, hearing loss, hemorrhagic diathesis, hepatitis, hypertension, hyponatremia, intestinal obstruction, interstitial pulmonary disease, ischemic colitis, lacrimation, localized erythema of the extremities, loss of consciousness (transient), lymphedema (peripheral), multiorgan failure, myelodysplastic syndrome, myocardial infarction, neutropenic enterocolitis, ototoxicity, pain, palmar-plantar erythrodysesthesia, pneumonia, pneumonitis, pruritus, pulmonary edema, pulmonary embolism, pulmonary fibrosis, radiation pneumonitis, radiation recall phenomenon, renal failure, renal insufficiency, respiratory failure, skin changes (scleroderma-like), seizure, sepsis, sinus tachycardia, skin rash, Stevens-Johnson syndrome, subacute cutaneous lupus erythematosus, syncope, tachycardia, thrombophlebitis, toxic epidermal necrolysis, unstable angina pectoris, visual disturbance (transient)

Drug Interactions

Metabolism/Transport Effects Substrate of CYP3A4 (major), P-glycoprotein; **Note:** Assignment of Major/Minor substrate status based on clinically relevant drug interaction potential

Avoid Concomitant Use

Avoid concomitant use of DOCEtaxel with any of the following: BCG (Intravesical); Conivaptan; Deferiprone; Dipyrone; Fusidic Acid (Systemic); Idelalisib; Natalizumab; Pimecrolimus; Tacrolimus (Topical); Vaccines (Live)

Increased Effect/Toxicity

DOCEtaxel may increase the levels/effects of: Antineoplastic Agents (Anthracycline, Systemic); CloZAPine; Deferiprone; Fingolimod; Leflunomide; Natalizumab; Tofacitinib; Vaccines (Live)

The levels/effects of DOCEtaxel may be increased by: Conivaptan; CYP3A4 Inhibitors (Moderate); CYP3A4 Inhibitors (Strong); Dasatinib; Denosumab; Dipyrone; Dronedarone; Fusidic Acid (Systemic); Idelalisib; MiFEPRIStone; Netupitant; Ocrelizumab; Palbociclib; Palifermin; P-glycoprotein/ABCB1 Inhibitors; Pimecrolimus; Platinum Derivatives; Promazine; Ranolazine; Roflumilast; Simeprevir; SORAfenib; Stiripentol; Tacrolimus (Topical); Trastuzumab

Decreased Effect

DOCEtaxel may decrease the levels/effects of: BCG (Intravesical); Coccidioides immitis Skin Test; Lenograstim; Nivolumab; Sipuleucel-T; Vaccines (Inactivated); Vaccines (Live)

The levels/effects of DOCEtaxel may be decreased by: Bosentan; CYP3A4 Inducers (Moderate); CYP3A4 Inducers (Strong); Dabrafenib; Deferasirox; Echinacea; Enzalutamide; Mitotane; Sarilumab; Siltuximab; St John's Wort; Tocilizumab

Hazardous Drugs Handling Considerations

Hazardous agent (NIOSH 2016 [group 1]).

Use appropriate precautions for receiving, handling, administration, and disposal. Gloves (single) should be worn during receiving, unpacking, and placing in storage.

NIOSH recommends double gloving, a protective gown, ventilated engineering controls (a class II biological safety cabinet or a compounding aseptic containment isolator), and closed system transfer devices (CSTDs) for preparation. Double gloving, a gown, and (if dosage form allows) CSTDs are required during administration (NIOSH 2016).

Storage/Stability Storage and stability may vary by manufacturer, refer to specific prescribing information.

Docetaxel 10 mg/mL: Store intact vials between 2°C to 25°C (36°F to 77°F) (actual recommendations may vary by generic manufacturer; consult manufacturer's labeling). Protect from bright light. Freezing does not adversely affect the product. Multi-use vials (80 mg/8 mL and 160 mg/16 mL) are stable for up to 28 days after first entry when stored between 2°C to 8°C (36°F to 46°F) and protected from light. Solutions diluted for infusion should be used within 4 hours of preparation, including infusion time.

Docetaxel 20 mg/mL concentrate/solution:

Taxotere: Store intact vials between 2°C to 25°C (36°F to 77°F). Protect from bright light. Freezing does not adversely affect the product. Solutions diluted for infusion in D5W or NS in non-PVC containers should be used within 6 hours of preparation, including infusion time, when stored between 2°C to 25°C (36°F to 77°F) or within 48 hours when stored between 2°C to 8°C (36°F to 46°F).

Generic formulations: Store intact vials at 25°C (77°F); excursions permitted between 15°C to 30°C (59°F to 86°F). Protect from light. Solutions diluted for infusion in D5W or NS should be used within 4 hours of preparation, including infusion time.

Non-alcohol formulation: Store intact vials at 20°C to 25°C (68°F to 77°F). Protect from light. After the first use and following multiple needle entries and withdrawals, multi-use vials (80 mg/4 mL and 160 mg/8 mL) are stable for up to 28 days when stored between 2°C to 8°C (36°F to 46°F) and protected from light. Solutions diluted for infusion in NS or D5W are stable for 24 hours when stored between 2°C to 8°C (36°F to 46°F).

Docetaxel lyophilized powder (Docefrez): Store intact vials between 2°C to 8°C (36°F to 46°F). Protect from light. Allow vials (and provided diluent) to stand at room temperature for 5 minutes prior to reconstitution. After reconstitution, may be stored refrigerated or at room temperature for up to 8 hours. Solutions diluted for infusion in D5W or NS should be used within 6 hours of preparation, including infusion time. According to the manufacturer, physical and chemical in-use stability of the infusion solution (prepared as recommended) has been demonstrated in non-PVC bags up to 48 hours when stored between 2°C and 8°C (36°F and 46°F).

Two-vial formulation *(generic; concentrate plus diluent formulation):* Reconstituted solutions of the two-vial formulation are stable in the vial for 8 hours at room temperature or under refrigeration. Solutions diluted for infusion in NS or D5W in polyolefin containers should be used within 4 hours of preparation, including infusion time.

Preparation for Administration

Preparation instructions may vary by manufacturer, refer to specific prescribing information. **Note:** Some formulations contain overfill.

Note: Multiple concentrations: Docetaxel is available as a one-vial formulation at concentrations of 10 mg/mL (generic formulation) and 20 mg/mL (concentrate/solution; Taxotere, generic [including a non-alcohol generic formulation]), and as a lyophilized powder (Docefrez) which is reconstituted (with provided diluent) to 20 mg/0.8 mL (20 mg vial) or 24 mg/0.8 mL (80 mg vial). Admixture errors have occurred due to the availability of various concentrations. Docetaxel was previously available as a two-vial formulation which included two vials (a concentrated docetaxel vial and a diluent vial), resulting in a reconstituted concentration of 10 mg/mL; the two-vial formulation has been discontinued by the Taxotere manufacturer (available generically).

One-vial formulations: Further dilute for infusion in 250 to 500 mL of NS or D5W in a non-DEHP container (eg, glass, polypropylene, polyolefin) to a final concentration of 0.3 to 0.74 mg/mL. Gently rotate and invert manually to mix thoroughly; avoid shaking or vigorous agitation.

Non-alcohol formulation: Use a 20 gauge needle to withdraw docetaxel from the vial; dilute in 250 mL of NS or D5W to a final concentration of 0.3 to 0.74 mg/mL. If docetaxel dose is >200 mg, use a larger volume of infusion fluid to maintain a final concentration of 0.3 to 0.74 mg/mL. Mix by gentle manual rotation.

Taxotere: Use **only** a 21 gauge needle to withdraw docetaxel from the vial (larger bore needles, such as 18 gauge or 19 gauge needles, may cause stopper coring and rubber precipitates). If intact vials were stored refrigerated, allow to stand at room temperature for 5 minutes prior to dilution. Inspect vials prior to dilution; solution is supersaturated and may crystalize over time; do not use if crystalized.

Lyophilized powder: Dilute with the provided diluent (contains ethanol in polysorbate 80); add 1 mL to each 20 mg vial (resulting concentration is 20 mg/0.8 mL) and 4 mL to each 80 mg vial (resulting concentration is 24 mg/mL). Shake well to dissolve completely. Reconstituted solution is supersaturated and could crystallize over time; if crystals appear, discard the solution (should no longer be used). If air bubbles are present, allow to stand for a few minutes while air bubbles dissipate. Further dilute in 250 mL of NS or D5W in a non-DEHP container (eg, glass, polypropylene, polyolefin) to a final concentration of 0.3 to 0.74 mg/mL (for doses >200 mg, use a larger volume of NS or D5W, not to exceed a final concentration of 0.74 mg/mL). Mix thoroughly by manual agitation.

Two-vial formulation *(generic; concentrate plus diluent formulation):* Vials should be diluted with 13% (w/w) polyethylene glycol 400/water (provided with the drug) to a final concentration of 10 mg/mL. Do not shake. Further dilute for infusion in 250 to 500 mL of NS or D5W in a non-DEHP container (eg, glass, polypropylene, polyolefin) to a final concentration of 0.3 to 0.74 mg/mL. Gently rotate to mix thoroughly. Do not use the two-vial formulation with the one-vial formulation for the same admixture product.

Mechanism of Action Docetaxel promotes the assembly of microtubules from tubulin dimers, and inhibits the depolymerization of tubulin which stabilizes microtubules in the cell. This results in inhibition of DNA, RNA, and protein synthesis. Most activity occurs during the M phase of the cell cycle.

Pharmacodynamics/Kinetics Exhibits linear pharmacokinetics at the recommended dosage range

Distribution: Extensive extravascular distribution and/or tissue binding; V_{dss}: 113 L (mean steady state)

Protein binding: ~94% to 97%, primarily to alpha$_1$-acid glycoprotein, albumin, and lipoproteins

Metabolism: Hepatic; oxidation via CYP3A4 to metabolites

Half-life elimination: Terminal: ~11 hours

Excretion: Feces (~75%, <8% as unchanged drug); urine (~6%)

Dosing

Adult & Geriatric Note: Premedicate with corticosteroids for 3 days, beginning one day prior to docetaxel administration, to reduce the severity of hypersensitivity reactions and fluid retention. Patients being treated for prostate cancer with concurrent prednisone should be premedicated with oral dexamethasone at 12 hours, 3 hours, and 1 hour prior to docetaxel administration.

Breast cancer: IV:

Locally advanced or metastatic: 60 to 100 mg/m^2 every 3 weeks (as a single agent)

Operable, node-positive (adjuvant treatment): TAC regimen: 75 mg/m^2 every 3 weeks for 6 courses (in combination with doxorubicin and cyclophosphamide) (Mackey 2013; Martin 2005)

Adjuvant treatment (off-label dosing): 75 mg/m^2 every 21 days (in combination with cyclophosphamide) for 4 cycles (Jones 2006) **or** 75 mg/m^2 every 21 days (in combination with carboplatin and trastuzumab) for 6 cycles (Slamon 2011)

Neoadjuvant treatment (off-label dosing): 75 mg/m^2 (cycle 1; if tolerated, may increase to 100 mg/m^2 in subsequent cycles) every 21 days for a total of 4 cycles (in combination with trastuzumab and pertuzumab) (Gianni 2012)

Metastatic treatment (off-label dosing):

Every-3-week administration: 75 mg/m^2 (cycle 1; may increase to 100 mg/m^2 in subsequent cycles) every 21 days for at least 6 cycles (in combination with trastuzumab and pertuzumab) (Baselga 2012; Swain 2013) **or** 100 mg/m^2 every 21 days (in combination with trastuzumab) for at least 6 cycles (Marty 2005) **or** 75 mg/m^2 every 21 days (in combination with capecitabine) until disease progression or

◄   unacceptable toxicity (O'Shaughnessy 2002) **or** 60 mg/m^2, 75 mg/m^2, or 100 mg/m^2 every 21 days for at least 6 cycles until disease progression, unacceptable toxicity, or discontinuation (Harvey 2006)

Weekly administration: 40 mg/m^2/dose once a week (as a single agent) for 6 weeks followed by a 2-week rest, repeat until disease progression or unacceptable toxicity (Burstein 2000) **or** 35 mg/m^2/dose once weekly for 3 weeks, followed by a 1-week rest, may increase to 40 mg/m^2 once weekly for 3 weeks followed by a 1-week rest with cycle 2 (Rivera 2008) **or** 35 mg/m^2/dose once weekly (in combination with trastuzumab) for 3 weeks followed by a 1-week rest; repeat until disease progression or unacceptable toxicity (Esteva 2002)

Gastric adenocarcinoma: IV: 75 mg/m^2 every 3 weeks (in combination with cisplatin and fluorouracil)

Sequential chemotherapy and chemoradiation (off-label dosing): Induction: 75 mg/m^2 on days 1 and 22 (in combination with cisplatin) for 2 cycles, followed by chemoradiation: 20 mg/m^2 weekly for 5 weeks (in combination with cisplatin and radiation) (Ruhstaller 2009)

Locally advanced or metastatic disease (off-label dosing): 50 mg/m^2 on day 1 every 2 weeks (in combination with fluorouracil, leucovorin, and oxaliplatin) until disease progression or unacceptable toxicity up to a maximum of 8 cycles (Al-Batran 2008)

Head and neck cancer: IV: 75 mg/m^2 every 3 weeks (in combination with cisplatin and fluorouracil) for 3 or 4 cycles, followed by radiation therapy

Non-small cell lung cancer: IV: 75 mg/m^2 every 3 weeks (as a single agent or in combination with cisplatin)

Prostate cancer: IV: 75 mg/m^2 every 3 weeks (in combination with prednisone)

Bladder cancer, metastatic (off-label use): IV: 100 mg/m^2 every 3 weeks (as a single agent) (McCaffrey 1997) **or** 35 mg/m^2 on days 1 and 8 of a 21-day cycle (in combination with gemcitabine and cisplatin) for at least 6 cycles or until disease progression or unacceptable toxicity (Pectasides 2002)

Esophageal cancer (off-label use): IV:

Sequential chemotherapy and chemoradiation: Induction: 75 mg/m^2 on days 1 and 22 (in combination with cisplatin) for 2 cycles, followed by chemoradiation: 20 mg/m^2 weekly for 5 weeks (in combination with cisplatin and radiation) (Ruhstaller 2009)

Definitive chemoradiation: 60 mg/m^2 on days 1 and 22 (in combination with cisplatin and radiation) for 1 cycle (Li 2010)

Locally advanced or metastatic disease: 75 mg/m^2 on day 1 every 3 weeks (in combination with cisplatin and fluorouracil) (Ajani 2007; Van Cutsem 2006) **or** 50 mg/m^2 on day 1 every 2 weeks (in combination with fluorouracil, leucovorin, and oxaliplatin) until disease progression or unacceptable toxicity up to a maximum of 8 cycles (Al-Batran 2008) **or** 35 mg/m^2 on days 1, 8, 15, 29, 36, 43, 50, and 57 (in combination with cisplatin, fluorouracil, and radiotherapy; neoadjuvant setting) (Pasini 2013)

Ewing sarcoma or osteosarcoma (recurrent or progressive; off-label uses): IV: 100 mg/m^2 on day 8 of a 21-day cycle (in combination with gemcitabine) (Navid 2008)

Ovarian cancer (off-label use): IV: 60 mg/m^2 every 3 weeks (in combination with carboplatin) for up to 6 cycles (Markman 2001) **or** 75 mg/m^2 every 3 weeks (in combination with carboplatin) for 6 cycles (Vasey 2004) **or** 35 mg/m^2 (maximum dose: 70 mg) weekly for 3 weeks followed by a 1-week rest (in combination with carboplatin) (Kushner 2007)

Prostate cancer, metastatic, hormone-sensitive (off-label use): 75 mg/m^2 on day 1 every 3 weeks (in combination with androgen deprivation therapy and prednisolone) for 6 cycles (James 2016) **or** 75 mg/m^2 on day 1 every 3 weeks (in combination with androgen deprivation therapy; daily prednisone not required) for 6 cycles (Sweeney 2015).

Small cell lung cancer, relapsed (off-label use): IV: 100 mg/m^2 every 3 weeks (Smyth 1994)

Soft tissue sarcoma (off-label use): IV: 100 mg/m^2 on day 8 of a 3-week treatment cycle (in combination with gemcitabine and filgrastim or pegfilgrastim) (Leu 2004; Maki 2007)

Unknown-primary, adenocarcinoma (off-label use): IV: 65 mg/m^2 every 3 weeks (in combination with carboplatin) (Greco 2000) **or** 75 mg/m^2 on day 8 of a 3-week treatment cycle (in combination with gemcitabine) for up to 6 cycles (Pouessel 2004) **or** 60 mg/m^2 on day 1 of a 3-week treatment cycle (in combination with cisplatin) (Mukai 2010)

Dosing adjustment for concomitant CYP3A4 inhibitors: Avoid the concomitant use of strong CYP3A4 inhibitors with docetaxel. If concomitant use of a strong CYP3A4 inhibitor cannot be avoided, consider reducing the docetaxel dose by 50% (based on limited pharmacokinetic data).

Pediatric Note: Premedicate with corticosteroids for 3 days, beginning one day prior to docetaxel administration, to reduce the severity of hypersensitivity reactions and fluid retention. Dexamethasone (dose not specified) was administered for 3 to 4 days, starting the day before or the day of docetaxel administration and continuing for 2 days afterward in the bone sarcoma study (Navid 2008).

Ewing sarcoma or osteosarcoma (recurrent or progressive; off-label uses): Children ≥8 years and Adolescents: IV: 100 mg/m^2 on day 8 of a 21-day cycle (in combination with gemcitabine) (Navid 2008)

Renal Impairment Renal excretion is minimal (~6%), therefore, the need for dosage adjustments for renal dysfunction is unlikely (Janus 2010; Li 2007). Not removed by hemodialysis, may be administered before or after hemodialysis (Janus 2010).

Hepatic Impairment

Total bilirubin greater than the ULN, or AST and/or ALT >1.5 times ULN concomitant with alkaline phosphatase >2.5 times ULN: Use is not recommended.

Hepatic impairment dosing adjustment specific for gastric or head and neck cancer:

AST/ALT >2.5 to ≤5 times ULN and alkaline phosphatase ≤2.5 times ULN: Administer 80% of dose

AST/ALT >1.5 to ≤5 times ULN and alkaline phosphatase >2.5 to ≤5 times ULN: Administer 80% of dose

AST/ALT >5 times ULN and /or alkaline phosphatase >5 times ULN: Discontinue docetaxel

The following adjustments have also been used (Floyd 2006):

Transaminases 1.6 to 6 times ULN: Administer 75% of dose.

Transaminases >6 times ULN: Use clinical judgment.

◀ **Obesity** *ASCO Guidelines for appropriate chemotherapy dosing in obese adults with cancer:* Utilize patient's actual body weight (full weight) for calculation of body surface area- or weight-based dosing, particularly when the intent of therapy is curative; manage regimen-related toxicities in the same manner as for nonobese patients; if a dose reduction is utilized due to toxicity, consider resumption of full weight-based dosing with subsequent cycles, especially if cause of toxicity (eg, hepatic or renal impairment) is resolved (Griggs 2012).

Adjustment for Toxicity Note: Toxicity includes febrile neutropenia, neutrophils <500/mm^3 for >1 week, severe or cumulative cutaneous reactions; in non-small cell lung cancer, this may also include platelet nadir <25,000/mm^3 and other grade 3/4 nonhematologic toxicities. Refer to specific reference/protocol for dosage adjustments for off-label uses or combinations.

Breast cancer (single agent): Patients dosed initially at 100 mg/m^2; reduce dose to 75 mg/m^2; **Note:** If the patient continues to experience these adverse reactions, the dosage should be reduced to 55 mg/m^2 or therapy should be discontinued; discontinue for peripheral neuropathy ≥ grade 3. Patients initiated at 60 mg/m^2 who do not develop toxicity may tolerate higher doses.

Breast cancer, adjuvant treatment (combination chemotherapy): TAC regimen should be administered when neutrophils are ≥1,500/mm^3. Patients experiencing febrile neutropenia should receive G-CSF in all subsequent cycles. Patients with persistent febrile neutropenia (while on G-CSF), patients experiencing severe/cumulative cutaneous reactions, moderate neurosensory effects (signs/symptoms) or grade 3 or 4 stomatitis should receive a reduced dose (60 mg/m^2) of docetaxel. Discontinue therapy with persistent toxicities after dosage reduction.

Non-small cell lung cancer:

Monotherapy: Patients dosed initially at 75 mg/m^2 should have dose held until toxicity is resolved, then resume at 55 mg/m^2; discontinue for peripheral neuropathy ≥ grade 3.

Combination therapy (with cisplatin): Patients dosed initially at 75 mg/m^2 should have the docetaxel dosage reduced to 65 mg/m^2 in subsequent cycles; if further adjustment is required, dosage may be reduced to 50 mg/m^2.

Prostate cancer: Reduce dose to 60 mg/m^2; discontinue therapy if toxicities persist at lower dose.

Gastric cancer, head and neck cancer: Note: Cisplatin may require dose reductions/therapy delays for peripheral neuropathy, ototoxicity, and/or nephrotoxicity. Patients experiencing febrile neutropenia, documented infection with neutropenia or neutropenia >7 days should receive G-CSF in all subsequent cycles. For neutropenic complications despite G-CSF use, further reduce dose to 60 mg/m^2. Dosing with neutropenic complications in subsequent cycles should be further reduced to 45 mg/m^2. Patients who experience grade 4 thrombocytopenia should receive a dose reduction from 75 mg/m^2 to 60 mg/m^2. Discontinue therapy for persistent toxicities.

Gastrointestinal toxicity for docetaxel in combination with cisplatin and fluorouracil for treatment of gastric cancer or head and neck cancer:

Diarrhea, grade 3:

First episode: Reduce fluorouracil dose by 20%

Second episode: Reduce docetaxel dose by 20%

Diarrhea, grade 4:
First episode: Reduce fluorouracil and docetaxel doses by 20%
Second episode: Discontinue treatment
Stomatitis, grade 3:
First episode: Reduce fluorouracil dose by 20%
Second episode: Discontinue fluorouracil for all subsequent cycles
Third episode: Reduce docetaxel dose by 20%
Stomatitis, grade 4:
First episode: Discontinue fluorouracil for all subsequent cycles
Second episode: Reduce docetaxel dose by 20%

Combination Regimens

Unknown primary, squamous cell:

Administration Administer IV infusion over 1-hour through nonsorbing polyethylene lined (non-DEHP) tubing. **Note:** Premedication with corticosteroids for 3 days, beginning the day before docetaxel administration, is recommended to reduce the incidence and severity of hypersensitivity reactions and fluid retention. Some docetaxel formulations contain alcohol (content varies by formulation); use with caution in patients for whom alcohol intake should be avoided or minimized (a non-alcohol generic formulation [20 mg/mL] is also available).

The use of an in-line filter is not necessary during Taxotere administration; according to the manufacturer, studies have not been performed to determine the compatibility of IV filters for administration and filters are not recommended for use with docetaxel (data on file [Sanofi Aventis 2016]). The use of an inline filter is also not recommended for administration of the non-alcohol docetaxel formulation (data on file [Eagle Pharmaceuticals 2016]).

Irritant with vesicant-like properties; avoid extravasation. Assure proper needle or catheter position prior to administration.

Extravasation management: If extravasation occurs, stop infusion immediately and disconnect (leave cannula/needle in place); gently aspirate extravasated solution (do **NOT** flush the line); remove needle/cannula; elevate extremity. Information conflicts regarding the use of warm or cold compresses (Perez Fidalgo 2012; Polovich 2009).

Vesicant/Extravasation Risk Irritant with vesicant-like properties

Emetic Potential Children and Adults: Low (10% to 30%)

Monitoring Parameters CBC with differential, liver function tests, bilirubin, alkaline phosphatase, renal function; monitor for hypersensitivity reactions, neurosensory symptoms, gastrointestinal toxicity (eg, diarrhea, stomatitis), cutaneous reactions, visual impairment, fluid retention, epiphora, and canalicular stenosis

Dosage Forms Considerations Non-alcohol formulation (Eagle/Teikuku pharmaceuticals): Solution, Intravenous [alcohol-free]: Generic: 20 mg/mL (1 mL; single-dose vial); 80 mg/4 mL (4 mL multi-dose vial); 160 mg/8 mL (8 mL; multi-dose vial)

Dosage Forms Excipient information presented when available (limited, particularly for generics); consult specific product labeling. [DSC] = Discontinued product
Concentrate, Intravenous:
Taxotere: 20 mg/mL (1 mL); 80 mg/4 mL (4 mL) [contains alcohol, usp, polysorbate 80]
Generic: 20 mg/mL (1 mL); 80 mg/4 mL (4 mL); 160 mg/8 mL (8 mL); 200 mg/10 mL (10 mL); 20 mg/0.5 mL (0.5 mL); 80 mg/2 mL (2 mL)
Concentrate, Intravenous [preservative free]:
Generic: 20 mg/mL (1 mL); 80 mg/4 mL (4 mL); 140 mg/7 mL (7 mL [DSC]); 160 mg/8 mL (8 mL)

Solution, Intravenous:
Generic: 20 mg/2 mL (2 mL); 80 mg/8 mL (8 mL); 160 mg/16 mL (16 mL); 200 mg/20 mL (20 mL [DSC]); 20 mg/mL (1 mL); 80 mg/4 mL (4 mL); 160 mg/8 mL (8 mL)
Solution Reconstituted, Intravenous:
Docefrez: 20 mg (1 ea [DSC]); 80 mg (1 ea [DSC]) [contains alcohol, usp, polysorbate 80]

◆ **Docetaxel for Injection (Can)** *see* DOCEtaxel *on page 606*
◆ **Docetaxel Injection (Can)** *see* DOCEtaxel *on page 606*

Dolasetron (dol A se tron)

Related Information
Management of Chemotherapy-Induced Nausea and Vomiting in Adults *on page 2253*

Brand Names: US Anzemet
Index Terms Dolasetron Mesylate; MDL 73,147EF
Pharmacologic Category Antiemetic; Selective 5-HT$_3$ Receptor Antagonist

Use
Injection: Prevention and treatment of postoperative nausea and vomiting in adults and children ≥2 years
Oral: Prevention of nausea and vomiting associated with moderately emetogenic cancer chemotherapy (initial and repeat courses) in adults and children ≥2 years

Labeled Contraindications
Injection: Hypersensitivity to dolasetron or any component of the formulation; intravenous administration is contraindicated when used for prevention of chemotherapy-associated nausea and vomiting
Tablet: Hypersensitivity to dolasetron or any component of the formulation

Pregnancy Considerations Adverse events have not been observed in animal reproduction studies.

Breastfeeding Considerations It is not known if dolasetron is excreted in breast milk. The manufacturer recommends that caution be exercised when administering dolasetron to nursing women.

Warnings/Precautions Dolasetron is associated with a number of dose-dependent increases in ECG intervals (eg, PR, QRS duration, QT/QTc, JT), usually occurring 1-2 hours after IV administration and usually lasting 6-8 hours; however, may last ≥24 hours and rarely lead to heart block or arrhythmia. Clinically relevant QT-interval prolongation may occur resulting in torsade de pointes, when used in conjunction with other agents that prolong the QT interval (eg, Class I and III antiarrhythmics). Avoid use in patients at greater risk for QT prolongation (eg, patients with congenital long QT syndrome, medications known to prolong QT interval, electrolyte abnormalities, and cumulative high-dose anthracycline therapy) and/or ventricular arrhythmia. Correct potassium or magnesium abnormalities prior to initiating therapy. IV formulations of 5-HT$_3$ antagonists have more association with ECG interval changes, compared to oral formulations. Reduction in heart rate may also occur with the 5-HT$_3$ antagonists. Use with caution in children and adolescents who have or may develop QTc prolongation; rare cases of supraventricular and ventricular arrhythmias, cardiac arrest, and MI have been reported in this population. ECG monitoring is recommended in patients with renal impairment and in the elderly.

Serotonin syndrome has been reported with 5-HT$_3$ receptor antagonists, predominantly when used in combination with other serotonergic agents (eg, SSRIs, SNRIs, MAOIs, mirtazapine, fentanyl, lithium, tramadol, and/or methylene blue). Some of the cases have been fatal. The majority of serotonin syndrome reports due to 5-HT$_3$ receptor antagonist have occurred in a post-anesthesia setting or in an infusion center. Serotonin syndrome has also been reported following overdose of another 5-HT$_3$ receptor antagonist. Monitor patients for signs of serotonin syndrome, including mental status changes (eg, agitation, hallucinations, delirium, coma); autonomic instability (eg, tachycardia, labile blood pressure, diaphoresis, dizziness, flushing, hyperthermia); neuromuscular changes (eg, tremor, rigidity, myoclonus, hyperreflexia, incoordination); gastrointestinal symptoms (eg, nausea, vomiting, diarrhea); and/or seizures. If serotonin syndrome occurs, discontinue 5-HT$_3$ receptor antagonist treatment and begin supportive management.

Use with caution in patients allergic to other 5-HT$_3$ receptor antagonists; cross-reactivity has been reported with other 5-HT$_3$ receptor antagonists. **For chemotherapy-associated nausea and vomiting, should be used on a scheduled basis, not on an "as needed" (PRN) basis,** since data support the use of this drug only in the prevention of nausea and vomiting (due to antineoplastic therapy) and not in the rescue of nausea and vomiting. Not intended for treatment of nausea and vomiting or for chronic continuous therapy. If the prophylaxis dolasetron dose for postoperative nausea and vomiting has failed, a repeat dose should not be administered as rescue or treatment for postoperative nausea and vomiting. Potentially significant drug-drug interactions may exist, requiring dose or frequency adjustment, additional monitoring, and/or selection of alternative therapy.

Some dosage forms may contain polysorbate 80 (also known as Tweens). Hypersensitivity reactions, usually a delayed reaction, have been reported following exposure to pharmaceutical products containing polysorbate 80 in certain individuals (Isaksson, 2002; Lucente 2000; Shelley, 1995). Thrombocytopenia, ascites, pulmonary deterioration, and renal and hepatic failure have been reported in premature neonates after receiving parenteral products containing polysorbate 80 (Alade, 1986; CDC, 1984). See manufacturer's labeling.

Adverse Reactions Adverse events may vary according to indication and route of administration.

>10%: Central nervous system: Headache (oral: 18% to 23%; IV: 9%)

1% to 10%:

Cardiovascular: Bradycardia (4% to 5%; may be severe after IV administration), tachycardia (≤3%), edema (<2%), facial edema (<2%), flushing (<2%), hypotension (<2%; may be severe after IV administration), orthostatic hypotension (<2%), peripheral edema (<2%), peripheral ischemia (<2%), phlebitis (<2%), sinus arrhythmia (<2%), thrombophlebitis (<2%)

Central nervous system: Fatigue (oral: 3% to 6%), dizziness (1% to 6%), pain (≤3%), abnormal dreams (<2%), agitation (<2%), anxiety (<2%), ataxia (<2%), chills (≤2%), confusion (<2%), depersonalization (<2%), paresthesia (<2%), shivering (≤2%), sleep disorder (<2%), twitching (<2%), vertigo (<2%)

Dermatologic: Diaphoresis (<2%), skin rash (<2%), urticaria (<2%)

Endocrine & metabolic: Increased gamma-glutamyl transferase (<2%)

Gastrointestinal: Diarrhea (oral: 2% to 5%), dyspepsia (≤3%), abdominal pain (<2%), anorexia (<2%), constipation (<2%), dysgeusia (<2%), pancreatitis (<2%)

Genitourinary: Dysuria (<2%), hematuria (<2%)

Hematologic and oncologic: Anemia (<2%), hematoma (<2%), prolonged prothrombin time (<2%), prolonged partial thromboplastin time (<2%), purpura (<2%), thrombocytopenia (<2%)

Hepatic: Hyperbilirubinemia (<2%), increased serum alkaline phosphatase (<2%)

Hypersensitivity: Anaphylaxis (<2%)

Local: Burning sensation at injection site (IV: <2%), pain at injection site (IV: <2%)

Neuromuscular & skeletal: Arthralgia (<2%), myalgia (<2%), tremor (<2%)

Ophthalmic: Photophobia (<2%), visual disturbance (<2%)

Otic: Tinnitus (<2%)

Renal: Acute renal failure (<2%), polyuria (<2%)

Respiratory: Bronchospasm (<2%), dyspnea (<2%), epistaxis (<2%)

<1%, postmarketing, and/or case reports: Abnormal T waves on ECG, appearance of U waves on ECG, atrial fibrillation, atrial flutter, atrioventricular block, bundle branch block (left and right), cardiac arrest, chest pain, extrasystoles (APCs or VPCs), increased serum ALT (transient), increased serum AST (transient), ischemic heart disease, nodal arrhythmia, palpitations, prolongation P-R interval on ECG (dose dependent), prolonged Q-T interval on ECG, serotonin syndrome, slow R wave progression, ST segment changes on ECG, syncope (may be severe after IV administration), torsades de pointes, ventricular arrhythmia, ventricular fibrillation cardiac arrest (IV), ventricular tachycardia (IV), wide complex tachycardia (IV), widened QRS complex on ECG (dose-dependent)

Drug Interactions

Metabolism/Transport Effects Substrate of CYP2C9 (minor), CYP3A4 (minor); **Note:** Assignment of Major/Minor substrate status based on clinically relevant drug interaction potential

Avoid Concomitant Use

Avoid concomitant use of Dolasetron with any of the following: Apomorphine; Highest Risk QTc-Prolonging Agents; Hydroxychloroquine; Mequitazine; MiFEPRIStone; Probucol; Promazine; Vinflunine

Increased Effect/Toxicity

Dolasetron may increase the levels/effects of: Apomorphine; Highest Risk QTc-Prolonging Agents; Mequitazine; Moderate Risk QTc-Prolonging Agents; Panobinostat; Serotonin Modulators

The levels/effects of Dolasetron may be increased by: Hydroxychloroquine; MiFEPRIStone; Probucol; Promazine; QTc-Prolonging Agents (Indeterminate Risk and Risk Modifying); Vinflunine; Xipamide

Decreased Effect

Dolasetron may decrease the levels/effects of: Tapentadol; TraMADol

Food Interactions Food does not affect the bioavailability of oral doses.

Storage/Stability

Injection: Store intact vials at 20°C to 25°C (68°F to 77°F); excursions are permitted to 15°C to 30°C (59°F to 86°F). Protect from light. Solutions diluted for infusion in NS, D5W, D5½NS, D5LR, LR, or mannitol 10% are stable under normal lighting conditions at room temperature for 24 hours or under refrigeration for 48 hours.

◄ Tablets: Store at 20°C to 25°C (68°F to 77°F). Protect from light.

Preparation for Administration May be administered undiluted, or diluted in 50 mL of a compatible solution (ie, NS, D5W, D5$\frac{1}{2}$NS, D5LR, LR, and 10% mannitol injection).

Mechanism of Action Selective serotonin receptor (5-HT$_3$) antagonist, blocking serotonin both peripherally (primary site of action) and centrally at the chemoreceptor trigger zone

Pharmacodynamics/Kinetics

Absorption: Oral: Rapid and complete

Distribution: Hydrodolasetron: Children: 5.9 to 7.4 L/kg; Adults: 5.8 L/kg

Protein binding: Hydrodolasetron: 69% to 77% (50% bound to alpha$_1$-acid glycoprotein)

Metabolism: Hepatic; rapid reduction by carbonyl reductase to hydrodolasetron (active metabolite); further metabolized by CYP2D6, CYP3A, and flavin monooxygenase

Bioavailability: Oral: Not affected by food; Children: 59% (formulation not specified); Adults: ~75%

Half-life elimination:

Dolasetron: IV: ≤10 minutes

Hydrodolasetron:

Oral: Children: 5.5 hours; Adolescents: 6.4 hours; Adults: 8.1 hours

IV: Children: 4.8 hours; Adults: 7.3 hours

Severe renal impairment: 11 hours

Severe hepatic impairment: 11 hours

Time to peak, plasma: Hydrodolasetron: IV: 0.6 hours; Oral: ~1 hour

Excretion: Urine ~67% (dolasetron: <1% excreted unchanged in urine; hydro-dolasetron: 53% to 61% of the total dose); Feces ~33%

Dosing

Adult & Geriatric Note: Use of intravenous dolasetron is contraindicated for the prevention of chemotherapy induced nausea and vomiting.

Prevention of chemotherapy-associated nausea and vomiting (including initial and repeat courses): Oral: 100 mg within 1 hour before chemotherapy

Postoperative nausea and vomiting:

Prevention: IV: 12.5 mg ~15 minutes before cessation of anesthesia (do not exceed the recommended dose)

Treatment: IV: 12.5 mg as soon as nausea or vomiting present (do not exceed the recommended dose)

Pediatric

Prevention of chemotherapy-associated nausea and vomiting (including initial and repeat courses): Children 2-16 years: Oral: 1.8 mg/kg within 1 hour before chemotherapy; maximum: 100 mg/dose

Postoperative nausea and vomiting: Children 2-16 years:

Prevention:

Oral: 1.2 mg/kg within 2 hours before surgery; maximum: 100 mg/dose

IV: 0.35 mg/kg ~15 minutes before cessation of anesthesia; maximum: 12.5 mg/dose

Treatment:

IV: 0.35 mg/kg as soon as nausea or vomiting present; maximum: 12.5 mg/dose

Renal Impairment No dosage adjustment necessary; however, ECG monitoring is recommended in patients with renal impairment.

Hepatic Impairment No dosage adjustment necessary.

Administration

IV injection may be given either undiluted as an IV push over 30 seconds or diluted in 50 mL of compatible fluid and infused over 15 minutes. Flush line before and after dolasetron administration.

Oral: When unable to administer in tablet form, dolasetron injection may be diluted in apple or apple-grape juice and taken orally; this dilution is stable for 2 hours at room temperature (Anzemet prescribing information, 2013).

Extemporaneous Preparations Dolasetron injection may be diluted in apple or apple-grape juice and taken orally; this dilution is stable for 2 hours at room temperature (Anzemet prescribing information, 2013).

A 10 mg/mL oral suspension may be prepared with tablets and either a 1:1 mixture of Ora-Plus and Ora-Sweet SF or a 1:1 mixture of strawberry syrup and Ora-Plus. Crush twelve 50 mg tablets in a mortar and reduce to a fine powder. Slowly add chosen vehicle to **almost** 60 mL; transfer to a calibrated bottle, rinse mortar with vehicle, and add quantity of vehicle sufficient to make 60 mL. Label "shake well" and "refrigerate". Stable for 90 days refrigerated.

Anzemet® prescribing information, sanofi-aventis U.S. LLC, Bridgewater, NJ, 2013.

Johnson CE, Wagner DS, and Bussard WE, "Stability of Dolasetron in Two Oral Liquid Vehicles," *Am J Health Syst Pharm*, 2003, 60(21):2242-4.

Monitoring Parameters ECG (in patients with cardiovascular disease, elderly, renally impaired, those at risk of developing hypokalemia and/or hypomagnesemia); potassium, magnesium

Additional Information Efficacy of dolasetron, for chemotherapy treatment, is enhanced with concomitant administration of dexamethasone 20 mg (increases complete response by 10% to 20%). Oral administration of the intravenous solution is equivalent to tablets.

Dosage Forms Excipient information presented when available (limited, particularly for generics); consult specific product labeling. [DSC] = Discontinued product

Solution, Intravenous, as mesylate:
  Anzemet: 20 mg/mL (0.625 mL [DSC], 5 mL [DSC], 25 mL [DSC])
Tablet, Oral, as mesylate:
  Anzemet: 50 mg, 100 mg

◆ **Dolasetron Mesylate** see Dolasetron on page 619

◆ **Dolotranz** see Lidocaine and Prilocaine on page 1150

◆ **Dom-Anagrelide (Can)** see Anagrelide on page 131

◆ **Dom-Bicalutamide (Can)** see Bicalutamide on page 252

◆ **Dom-Ciprofloxacin (Can)** see Ciprofloxacin (Systemic) on page 393

◆ **Dom-Dexamethasone (Can)** see Dexamethasone (Systemic) on page 579

◆ **Dom-Fluconazole (Can)** see Fluconazole on page 807

◆ **Dom-Lorazepam (Can)** see LORazepam on page 1164

◆ **Dom-Medroxyprogesterone (Can)** see MedroxyPROGESTERone on page 1175

◆ **Dom-Ondansetron (Can)** see Ondansetron on page 1380

◆ **DOM-Valacyclovir (Can)** see ValACYclovir on page 1852

◆ **DoubleDex** see Dexamethasone (Systemic) on page 579

◆ **Doxil** see DOXOrubicin (Liposomal) on page 636

DOXOrubicin (Conventional) (doks oh ROO bi sin con VEN sha nal)

Related Information

Management of Chemotherapy-Induced Nausea and Vomiting in Adults *on page 2253*

Management of Drug Extravasations *on page 2271*

Prevention of Chemotherapy-Induced Nausea and Vomiting in Children *on page 2310*

Safe Handling of Hazardous Drugs *on page 2379*

Brand Names: US Adriamycin

Brand Names: Canada Adriamycin PFS; Doxorubicin Hydrochloride For Injection, USP; Doxorubicin Hydrochloride Injection

Index Terms ADR (error-prone abbreviation); Adria; Conventional Doxorubicin; Doxorubicin HCl; Doxorubicin Hydrochloride; Hydroxydaunomycin Hydrochloride; Hydroxyldaunorubicin Hydrochloride

Pharmacologic Category Antineoplastic Agent, Anthracycline; Antineoplastic Agent, Topoisomerase II Inhibitor

Use

Breast cancer: Treatment component of adjuvant therapy in women with evidence of axillary lymph node involvement following resection of primary breast cancer

Metastatic cancers or disseminated neoplastic conditions: Treatment of acute lymphoblastic leukemia, acute myeloid leukemia, Wilms tumor, neuroblastoma, soft tissue and bone sarcomas, breast cancer, ovarian cancer, transitional cell bladder carcinoma, thyroid carcinoma, gastric carcinoma, Hodgkin lymphoma, non-Hodgkin lymphoma, and bronchogenic carcinoma in which the small cell histologic type is the most responsive compared with other cell types

Labeled Contraindications Hypersensitivity (including anaphylaxis) to doxorubicin, any component of the formulation, or to other anthracyclines or anthracenediones; recent MI (within past 4 to 6 weeks), severe myocardial insufficiency, severe arrhythmia; previous therapy with high cumulative doses of doxorubicin, daunorubicin, idarubicin, or other anthracycline and anthracenediones; severe persistent drug-induced myelosuppression or baseline neutrophil count <1500/mm^3; severe hepatic impairment (Child-Pugh class C or bilirubin >5 mg/dL)

Pregnancy Considerations Adverse events have been observed in animal reproduction studies. Based on the mechanism of action, doxorubicin may cause fetal harm if administered during pregnancy (according to the manufacturer's labeling). Advise patients (females of reproductive potential and males with female partners of reproductive potential) to use effective nonhormonal contraception during and for 6 months following therapy. Limited information is available from a retrospective study of women who received doxorubicin (in combination with cyclophosphamide) during the second or third (prior to week 35) trimester for the treatment of pregnancy-associated breast cancer (Ring 2005). Some pharmacokinetic properties of doxorubicin may be altered in pregnant women (van Hasselt 2014). The European Society for Medical Oncology (ESMO) has published guidelines for diagnosis, treatment, and follow-up of cancer during pregnancy (Peccatori 2013); the guidelines recommend referral to a facility with expertise in cancer during pregnancy and encourage a multidisciplinary team (obstetrician, neonatologist, oncology team). If chemotherapy is indicated, it should **not** be administered in the first trimester, but may begin in the second trimester. There should be a 3-week time period between the last chemotherapy dose and anticipated delivery, and chemotherapy should not be administered beyond week 33 of gestation.

A pregnancy registry is available for all cancers diagnosed during pregnancy at Cooper Health (877-635-4499).

Breastfeeding Considerations Doxorubicin and its metabolites are excreted in breast milk. Due to the potential for serious adverse reactions in the nursing infant, the manufacturer recommends a decision be made whether to discontinue nursing or to discontinue the drug, taking into account the importance of treatment to the mother.

Warnings/Precautions [U.S. Boxed Warning]: May cause cumulative, dose-related, myocardial toxicity (early or delayed, including acute left ventricular failure and HF). The risk of cardiomyopathy increases with cumulative exposure and with concomitant cardiotoxic therapy; the incidence of irreversible myocardial toxicity increases as the total cumulative (lifetime) dosages approach 300 to 500 mg/m^2. Assess left ventricular ejection fraction (LVEF) with either an echocardiogram or MUGA scan before, during, and after therapy; increase the frequency of assessments as the cumulative dose exceeds 300 mg/m^2. Cardiotoxicity is dose-limiting. Delayed cardiotoxicity may occur late in treatment or within months to years after completion of therapy, and is typically manifested by LVEF reduction and/or heart failure (may be life threatening). Subacute effects such as pericarditis and myocarditis may also occur. Early toxicity may consist of tachyarrhythmias, including sinus tachycardia, premature ventricular contractions, and ventricular tachycardia, as well as bradycardia. Electrocardiographic changes including ST-T wave changes, atrioventricular and bundle-branch block have also been reported. These effects are not necessarily predictive of subsequent delayed cardiotoxicity. Total cumulative dose should take into account prior treatment with other anthracyclines or anthracenediones, previous or concomitant treatment with other cardiotoxic agents or irradiation of chest. Although the risk increases with cumulative dose, irreversible cardiotoxicity may occur at any dose level. Patients with active or dominant cardiovascular disease, concurrent administration of cardiotoxic drugs, prior therapy with other anthracyclines or anthracenediones, prior or concurrent chest irradiation, advanced age, and infants and children are at increased risk. Alternative administration schedules (weekly or continuous infusions) have are associated with less cardiotoxicity.

[US Boxed Warning]: Vesicant; if extravasation occurs, severe local tissue damage leading to tissue injury, blistering, ulceration, and necrosis may occur. Discontinue infusion immediately and apply ice to the affected area. For IV administration only. Do not administer IM or SubQ. Ensure proper needle or catheter placement prior to and during infusion. Avoid extravasation.

[US Boxed Warning]: May cause severe myelosuppression, which may result in serious infection, septic shock, transfusion requirements, hospitalization, and death. Myelosuppression may be dose-limiting and primarily manifests as leukopenia and neutropenia; anemia and thrombocytopenia may also occur. The nadir typically occurs 10 to 14 days after administration with cell count recovery around day 21. Monitor blood counts at baseline and regularly during therapy.

◀ **[US Boxed Warning]: Secondary acute myelogenous leukemia (AML) and myelodysplastic syndrome (MDS) have been reported following treatment.** AML and MDS typically occur within one to three years of treatment; risk factors for development of secondary AML or MDS include treatment with anthracyclines in combination with DNA-damaging antineoplastics (eg, alkylating agents) and/or radiation therapy, heavily pretreated patients, and escalated anthracycline doses. May cause tumor lysis syndrome and hyperuricemia (in patients with rapidly growing tumors). Urinary alkalinization and prophylaxis with an antihyperuricemic agent may be necessary. Monitor electrolytes, renal function, and hydration status. **[US Boxed Warning]: Dosage modification is recommended in patients with impaired hepatic function;** toxicities may be increased in patients with hepatic impairment. Use is contraindicated in patients with severe impairment (Child-Pugh class C or bilirubin >5 mg/dL). Monitor hepatic function tests (eg, transaminases, alkaline phosphatase, and bilirubin) closely. Use with caution in patients who have received radiation therapy; radiation recall may occur. May increase radiation-induced toxicity to the myocardium, mucosa, skin, and liver. Doxorubicin is associated with a moderate or high emetic potential (depending on dose or regimen); antiemetics are recommended to prevent nausea and vomiting (Basch 2011; Dupuis 2011; Roila 2016). Potentially significant drug-drug interactions may exist, requiring dose or frequency adjustment, additional monitoring, and/or selection of alternative therapy.

In men, doxorubicin may damage spermatozoa and testicular tissue, resulting in possible genetic fetal abnormalities; may also result in oligospermia, azoospermia, and permanent loss of fertility (sperm counts have been reported to return to normal levels in some men, occurring several years after the end of therapy). In females of reproductive potential, doxorubicin may cause infertility and result in amenorrhea; premature menopause can occur. Children are at increased risk for developing delayed cardiotoxicity; long-term cardiac function monitoring is recommended. Doxorubicin may contribute to prepubertal growth failure in children; may also contribute to gonadal impairment (usually temporary). Radiation recall pneumonitis has been reported in children receiving concomitant dactinomycin and doxorubicin. **[US Boxed Warning]: Should be administered under the supervision of an experienced cancer chemotherapy physician.** Use caution when selecting product for preparation and dispensing; indications, dosages and adverse event profiles differ between conventional doxorubicin hydrochloride solution and doxorubicin liposomal. Both formulations are the same concentration. As a result, serious errors have occurred.

Adverse Reactions Frequency not always defined.

Cardiovascular:

Acute cardiotoxicity: Atrioventricular block, bradycardia, bundle branch block, ECG abnormality, extrasystoles (atrial or ventricular), nonspecific ST or T wave changes on ECG, sinus tachycardia, supraventricular tachycardia, tachyarrhythmia, ventricular tachycardia

Delayed cardiotoxicity: Cardiac failure (manifestations include ascites, cardiomegaly, dyspnea, edema, gallop rhythm, hepatomegaly, oliguria, pleural effusion, pulmonary edema, tachycardia), decreased left ventricular ejection fraction, myocarditis, pericarditis

Central nervous system: Malaise

Dermatologic: Alopecia, discoloration of sweat, pruritus, skin photosensitivity, skin rash; urticaria

Endocrine & metabolic: Amenorrhea, dehydration, hyperuricemia

Gastrointestinal: Abdominal pain, anorexia, diarrhea, discoloration of saliva, gastrointestinal ulcer, mucositis, nausea, vomiting

Genitourinary: Urine discoloration, infertility (may be temporary)

Hematologic & oncologic: Leukopenia (≤75%; nadir: 10 to 14 days; recovery: by day 21), neutropenia (≤75%; nadir: 10 to 14 days; recovery: by day 21), anemia, thrombocytopenia

Local: Post-injection flare

Neuromuscular & skeletal: Weakness

Ophthalmic: Discoloration of tears

Miscellaneous: Necrosis (colon), radiation recall phenomenon

<1%, postmarketing, and/or case reports: Acute myelocytic leukemia (secondary), anaphylaxis, azoospermia, chills, coma (when in combination with cisplatin or vincristine), conjunctivitis, dysgeusia (Rehwaldt 2009), febrile neutropenia, fever, gonadal disease (gonadal impairment; children), growth suppression (prepubertal), hepatitis, hyperpigmentation (nail, oral mucosa, skin), hypersensitivity reaction (systemic; including angioedema, dysphagia, and dyspnea, pruritus, urticaria), increased serum bilirubin, increased serum transaminases, infection, keratitis, lacrimation, myelodysplastic syndrome, oligospermia, onycholysis, peripheral neurotoxicity (with intra-arterial doxorubicin), phlebosclerosis, pneumonitis (radiation recall; children), seizure (when in combination with cisplatin or vincristine), sepsis, shock, Stevens-Johnson syndrome, toxic epidermal necrolysis, typhlitis (neutropenic)

Drug Interactions

Metabolism/Transport Effects Substrate of CYP2D6 (major), CYP3A4 (major), P-glycoprotein; **Note:** Assignment of Major/Minor substrate status based on clinically relevant drug interaction potential

Avoid Concomitant Use

Avoid concomitant use of DOXOrubicin (Conventional) with any of the following: BCG (Intravesical); Conivaptan; Deferiprone; Dipyrone; Fusidic Acid (Systemic); Idelalisib; Natalizumab; Pimecrolimus; Tacrolimus (Topical); Vaccines (Live)

Increased Effect/Toxicity

DOXOrubicin (Conventional) may increase the levels/effects of: CloZAPine; Deferiprone; Fingolimod; Leflunomide; Mercaptopurine; Natalizumab; Tofacitinib; Vaccines (Live); Vinflunine; Zidovudine

The levels/effects of DOXOrubicin (Conventional) may be increased by: Abiraterone Acetate; Ado-Trastuzumab Emtansine; Ajmaline; Asunaprevir; Bevacizumab; Conivaptan; Cyclophosphamide; CycloSPORINE (Systemic); CYP2D6 Inhibitors (Moderate); CYP2D6 Inhibitors (Strong); CYP3A4 Inhibitors (Moderate); CYP3A4 Inhibitors (Strong); Dasatinib; Denosumab; Dipyrone; Fosaprepitant; Fusidic Acid (Systemic); Idelalisib; Lumefantrine; MiFEPRIStone; Ocrelizumab; Palbociclib; Palifermin; Panobinostat; Peginterferon Alfa-2b; P-glycoprotein/ABCB1 Inhibitors; Pimecrolimus; Promazine; Roflumilast; SORAfenib; Stiripentol; Tacrolimus (Topical); Taxane Derivatives; Trastuzumab

Decreased Effect

DOXOrubicin (Conventional) may decrease the levels/effects of: BCG (Intravesical); Cardiac Glycosides; Coccidioides immitis Skin Test; Lenograstim; Nivolumab; Sipuleucel-T; Stavudine; Tertomotide; Vaccines (Inactivated); Vaccines (Live); Zidovudine

The levels/effects of DOXOrubicin (Conventional) may be decreased by:
Bosentan; Cardiac Glycosides; CYP3A4 Inducers (Moderate); CYP3A4 Inducers (Strong); Dabrafenib; Deferasirox; Dexrazoxane; Echinacea; Enzalutamide; Mitotane; Peginterferon Alfa-2b; P-glycoprotein/ABCB1 Inducers; Sarilumab; Siltuximab; St John's Wort; Tocilizumab

Hazardous Drugs Handling Considerations

Hazardous agent (NIOSH 2016 [group 1]).

Use appropriate precautions for receiving, handling, administration, and disposal. Gloves (single) should be worn during receiving, unpacking, and placing in storage.

NIOSH recommends double gloving, a protective gown, ventilated engineering controls (a class II biological safety cabinet or a compounding aseptic containment isolator), and closed system transfer devices (CSTDs) for preparation. Double gloving, a gown, and (if dosage form allows) CSTDs are required during administration (NIOSH 2016).

Storage/Stability

Lyophilized powder: Store powder at 20°C to 25°C (68°F to 77°F). Protect from light. Retain in carton until time of use. Discard unused portion from single-dose vials. Reconstituted doxorubicin is stable for 7 days at room temperature under normal room lighting and for 15 days when refrigerated at 2°C to 8°C (36°F to 46°F). Protect reconstituted solution from light.

Solution: Store refrigerated at 2°C to 8°C (36°F to 46°F). Protect from light. Retain in carton until time of use. Discard unused portion. Storage of vials of solution under refrigeration may result in formation of a gelled product; if gelling occurs, place vials at room temperature for 2 to 4 hours to return the product to a slightly viscous, mobile solution.

Preparation for Administration Reconstitute lyophilized powder with NS (using 5 mL for the 10 mg vial; 10 mL for the 20 mg vial; or 25 mL for the 50 mg vial) to a final concentration of 2 mg/mL; gently shake until contents are dissolved. May further dilute doxorubicin solution or reconstituted doxorubicin solution in 50 to 1000 mL D5W or NS for infusion. Unstable in solutions with a pH <3 or >7.

Mechanism of Action Inhibition of DNA and RNA synthesis by intercalation between DNA base pairs by inhibition of topoisomerase II and by steric obstruction. Doxorubicin intercalates at points of local uncoiling of the double helix. Although the exact mechanism is unclear, it appears that direct binding to DNA (intercalation) and inhibition of DNA repair (topoisomerase II inhibition) result in blockade of DNA and RNA synthesis and fragmentation of DNA. Doxorubicin is also a powerful iron chelator; the iron-doxorubicin complex can bind DNA and cell membranes and produce free radicals that immediately cleave the DNA and cell membranes.

Pharmacodynamics/Kinetics

Distribution: V_d: 809 to 1,214 L/m^2; does not cross the blood-brain barrier

Protein binding, plasma: ~75%

Metabolism: Primarily hepatic to doxorubicinol (active), then to inactive aglycones, conjugated sulfates, and glucuronides

Half-life elimination:

Distribution: ~5 minutes

Terminal: 20 to 48 hours

Male: 54 hours; Female: 35 hours

Excretion: Feces (~40% as unchanged drug); urine (5% to 12% as unchanged drug and metabolites)

Clearance:
Infants and Children <2 years: 813 mL/minute/m^2
Children and Adolescents >2 years: 1,540 mL/minute/m^2
Adults: 324 to 809 mL/minutes/m^2 (appears to be higher in men than women)

Dosing

Adult & Geriatric Doxorubicin is associated with a moderate to high emetic potential (depending on dose or regimen); antiemetics are recommended to prevent nausea and vomiting (Basch 2011; Roila 2016).

Manufacturer's labeling: **Note:** Lower dosages should be considered for patients with inadequate marrow reserve (due to advanced age, prior treatment, or neoplastic marrow infiltration). Cumulative doses above 550 mg/m^2 are associated with an increased risk of cardiomyopathy.

Breast cancer: IV: 60 mg/m^2 on day 1 of a 21-day cycle (in combination with cyclophosphamide) for 4 cycles

Metastatic solid tumors, leukemia, or lymphoma: IV:
Single-agent therapy: 60 to 75 mg/m^2 every 21 days
Combination therapy: 40 to 75 mg/m^2 every 21 to 28 days

Indication-specific dosing (off-label dosing):
Acute lymphoblastic leukemia: IV:
Hyper-CVAD regimen: 50 mg/m^2 on day 4 of Courses 1, 3, 5, and 7 (in combination with cyclophosphamide, vincristine, and dexamethasone); alternating cycles with high-dose methotrexate and cytarabine (Kantarjian 2004)
CALGB 8811 regimen: 30 mg/m^2 on days 1, 8 and 15 of late intensification (Course IV; 8-week cycle); in combination with vincristine, dexamethasone, cyclophosphamide, thioguanine, and cytarabine (Larson1995)
Bladder cancer, transitional cell: IV: *Dose-dense MVAC regimen:* 30 mg/m^2 on day 2 every 14 days (in combination with methotrexate, vinblastine, and cisplatin) (Sternberg 2001)
Breast cancer: IV:
CAF regimen: 30 mg/m^2 on days 1 and 8 every 28 days for 6 cycles (in combination with cyclophosphamide and fluorouracil) (Bull 1978)
FAC regimen: 50 mg/m^2 on day 1 (or administered as a 72-hour continuous infusion) every 21 days for 6 cycles (in combination with fluorouracil and cyclophosphamide) (Assikis 2003)
TAC regimen: 50 mg/m^2 on day 1 every 21 days for 6 cycles (in combination with docetaxel and cyclophosphamide) (Martin 2005)
Ewing sarcoma: IV:
VAC/IE regimen: Adults ≤30 years: 75 mg/m^2 on day 1 every 21 days for 5 cycles (in combination with vincristine and cyclophosphamide; after 5 cycles, dactinomycin replaced doxorubicin), alternating cycles with ifosfamide and etoposide for a total of 17 cycles (Grier 2003)
VAIA regimen: Adults <35 years: 30 mg/m^2/day on days 1 and 2 every 21 days (doxorubicin alternates with dactinomycin; in combination with vincristine and ifosfamide) for14 cycles (Paulussen 2008)
VIDE regimen: 20 mg/m^2/day over 4 hours on days 1 to 3 every 21 days for 6 cycles (in combination with vincristine, ifosfamide, and etoposide) (Juergens 2006)

◄ **Hodgkin lymphoma:** IV:

ABVD regimen: 25 mg/m^2 on days 1 and 15 every 28 days (in combination with bleomycin, vinblastine, and dacarbazine) for 2 to 4 cycles (Bonadonna 2004; Engert 2010)

BEACOPP and escalated BEACOPP regimens: 25 mg/m^2 (BEACOPP) or 35 mg/m^2 (escalated BEACOPP) on day 1 every 21 days (in combination with bleomycin, etoposide, cyclophosphamide, vincristine, procarbazine, and prednisone) (Engert 2009)

Stanford V regimen: 25 mg/m^2 on weeks 1, 3, 5, 7, 9, and 11 of a 12-week cycle (in combination with mechlorethamine, vinblastine, vincristine, bleomycin, etoposide, and prednisone) (Horning 2002)

Non-Hodgkin lymphoma: IV:

CHOP or RCHOP regimen: 50 mg/m^2 on day 1 every 21 days (in combination with cyclophosphamide, vincristine, and prednisone +/- rituximab) (Coiffier 2010; McKelvey 1976)

Hyper-CVAD + rituximab regimen: 50 mg/m^2 administered as a continuous infusion over 24 hours on day 4 of Courses 1, 3, 5, and 7 (21-day treatment cycles; in combination with cyclophosphamide, vincristine, dexamethasone, and rituximab); alternating cycles with high-dose methotrexate and cytarabine (Thomas 2006)

Dose-adjusted EPOCH or REPOCH regimen: 10 mg/m^2/day administered as a continuous infusion on days 1 to 4 every 21 days (in combination with etoposide, vincristine, cyclophosphamide, and prednisone +/- rituximab) (Garcia-Suarez 2007; Wilson 2002)

Nordic regimen (Maxi-CHOP): 75 mg/m^2 on day 1 every 21 days (in combination with cyclophosphamide, vincristine, prednisone, and rituximab), alternating cycles with high-dose cytarabine (Geisler 2008)

Osteosarcoma: IV:

Cisplatin/doxorubicin regimen: Adults ≤40 years: 25 mg/m^2 (bolus infusion) on days 1 to 3 every 21 days (in combination with cisplatin) (Bramwell 1992)

High-dose methotrexate/cisplatin/doxorubicin/ifosfamide regimen: Adults <40 years:

Preoperative: 75 mg/m^2 administered as a continuous infusion over 24 hours on day 3 of weeks 1 and 7 (in combination with methotrexate, cisplatin, and ifosfamide) (Bacci 2003)

Postoperative: 90 mg/m^2 administered as a continuous infusion over 24 hours on weeks 13, 22, and 31 (in combination with methotrexate, cisplatin, and ifosfamide) (Bacci 2003)

High-dose methotrexate/cisplatin/doxorubicin regimen: Adults <40 years:

Preoperative: 60 mg/m^2 over 8 hours on days 9 and 36 (in combination with methotrexate and cisplatin) (Bacci 2000)

Postoperative: 45 mg/m^2/day over 4 hours for 2 consecutive days (in combination with methotrexate, cisplatin +/- ifosfamide, +/- etoposide; refer to protocol for criteria, frequency, and other specific information) (Bacci 2000)

Small cell lung cancer, recurrent: IV: *CAV regimen:* 45 mg/m^2 (maximum dose: 100 mg) on day 1 every 21 days (in combination with cyclophosphamide and vincristine) until disease progression or unacceptable toxicity or for at least 4 or 6 cycles past maximum response (von Pawel 1999)

Soft tissue sarcoma: IV:
Nonspecific histologies:

AD regimen: 60 mg/m^2 on day 1 every 21 days (either as a bolus infusion or administered continuously over 96 hours; in combination with dacarbazine) (Zalupski 1991)

AIM regimen: 30 mg/m^2 on days 1 and 2 every 21 days (in combination with ifosfamide and mesna) (Edmonson, 1993)

MAID regimen: 20 mg/m^2/day as a continuous infusion on days 1 to 3 every 21 days (in combination with ifosfamide, mesna, and dacarbazine) (Elias 1989)

Single-agent regimen: 75 mg/m^2 on day 1 every 21 days until disease progression or unacceptable toxicity (Santoro 1995)

Rhabdomyosarcoma:

VAC/IE regimen: Adults <21 years: 37.5 mg/m^2 on days 1 and 2 (administered over 18 hours each day) every 6 weeks (in combination with vincristine and cyclophosphamide), alternating cycles with ifosfamide and etoposide (Arndt 1998)

VAI regimen (based on a limited number of patients): Adults: 25 mg/m^2/day on days 1 to 3 every 21 days (in combination with vincristine and ifosfamide) (Ogilvie 2010)

Off-label uses:

Endometrial carcinoma, advanced: IV: 60 mg/m^2 on day 1 every 21 days for 8 cycles; maximum cumulative dose: 420 mg/m^2 (in combination with cisplatin) (Randall 2006)

Multiple myeloma: IV:

PAD regimen: Induction: 9 mg/m^2/day on days 1 to 4 for 3 cycles (in combination with bortezomib and dexamethasone) (Sonneveld 2012)

VDT-PACE regimen: 10 mg/m^2/day administered as a continuous infusion on days 1 to 4 of each cycle (in combination with bortezomib, dexamethasone, thalidomide, cisplatin, cyclophosphamide, and etoposide) (Lee 2003; Pineda-Roman 2008)

Thymomas and thymic malignancies: IV:

CAP regimen: 50 mg/m^2 on day 1 every 21 days for up to 8 cycles (in combination with cisplatin and cyclophosphamide) (Loehrer 1994)

ADOC regimen: 40 mg/m^2 on day 1 every 21 days (in combination with cisplatin, vincristine, and cyclophosphamide) (Fornasiero 1991)

Uterine sarcoma: IV: 60 mg/m^2 on day 1 every 21 days; maximum cumulative dose: 480 mg/m^2 (Omura, 1983) **or** 50 mg/m^2 (over 15 minutes) on day 1 every 21 days; maximum cumulative dose: 450 mg/m^2 (in combination with ifosfamide/mesna) (Sutton 1996)

Waldenstrom macroglobulinemia: IV: *R-CHOP regimen:* 50 mg/m^2 on day 1 every 21 days for 4 to 8 cycles (in combination with cyclophosphamide, vincristine, prednisone, and rituximab) (Buske 2009)

Pediatric Doxorubicin is associated with a moderate to high emetic potential (depending on dose or regimen); antiemetics are recommended to prevent nausea and vomiting (Dupuis 2011).

Manufacturer's labeling: Note: Lower dosages should be considered for patients with inadequate marrow reserve (due to advanced age, prior treatment, or neoplastic marrow infiltration). Cumulative doses above 550 mg/m^2 are associated with an increased risk of cardiomyopathy.

◀

Metastatic solid tumors, leukemia, or lymphoma: Children and Adolescents: IV:

Single-agent therapy: 60 to 75 mg/m^2 every 21 days

Combination therapy: 40 to 75 mg/m^2 every 21 to 28 days

Indication-specific dosing (off-label dosing):

Acute lymphoblastic leukemia: IV:

DFCI Consortium Protocol 00-01: Children ≥1 year and Adolescents:

Induction: 30 mg/m^2/dose on days 0 and 1 of a 4-week cycle (Vrooman 2013)

CNS therapy: High-risk patients: 30 mg/m^2 on day 1 of a 3-week cycle (with dexrazoxane) (Vrooman 2013)

Intensification: High-risk patients: 30 mg/m^2 on day 1 of every 3-week cycle (with dexrazoxane; cumulative doxorubicin dose: 300 mg/m^2) (Vrooman 2013)

Ewing sarcoma: Children and Adolescents: IV:

VAC/IE regimen: 75 mg/m^2 on day 1 every 21 days for 5 cycles (in combination with vincristine and cyclophosphamide; after 5 cycles, dactinomycin replaced doxorubicin), alternating cycles with ifosfamide and etoposide for a total of 17 cycles (Grier 2003)

VAIA regimen: 30 mg/m^2/day on days 1 and 2 every 21 days (doxorubicin alternates with dactinomycin; in combination with vincristine and ifosfamide) for 14 cycles (Paulussen 2008)

VIDE regimen: 20 mg/m^2/day over 4 hours on days 1 to 3 every 21 days for 6 cycles (in combination with vincristine, ifosfamide, and etoposide) (Juergens 2006)

Osteosarcoma: Children and Adolescents: IV:

Cisplatin/doxorubicin regimen: 25 mg/m^2 (bolus infusion) on days 1 to 3 every 21 days (in combination with cisplatin) (Bramwell, 1992)

High-dose methotrexate/cisplatin/doxorubicin/ifosfamide regimen:

Preoperative: 75 mg/m^2 administered as a continuous infusion over 24 hours on day 3 of weeks 1 and 7 (in combination with methotrexate, cisplatin, and ifosfamide) (Bacci 2003)

Postoperative: 90 mg/m^2 administered as a continuous infusion over 24 hours on weeks 13, 22, and 31 (in combination with methotrexate, cisplatin, and ifosfamide) (Bacci 2003)

High-dose methotrexate/cisplatin/doxorubicin regimen:

Preoperative: 60 mg/m^2 over 8 hours on days 9 and 36 (in combination with methotrexate and cisplatin) (Bacci 2000)

Postoperative: 45 mg/m^2/day over 4 hours for 2 consecutive days (in combination with methotrexate, cisplatin +/- ifosfamide, +/- etoposide; refer to protocol for criteria, frequency, and other specific information) (Bacci 2000)

Rhabdomyosarcoma: Children and Adolescents: IV:

VAC/IE regimen: 37.5 mg/m^2 on days 1 and 2 (administered over 18 hours each day) every 6 weeks (in combination with vincristine and cyclophosphamide), alternating cycles with ifosfamide and etoposide (Arndt, 1998)

Renal Impairment

Mild, moderate, or severe impairment: No dosage adjustment provided in the manufacturers' labeling; however, adjustments are likely not necessary given limited renal excretion.

The following adjustments have also been recommended:

CrCl <50 mL/minute: No dosage adjustment necessary (Aronoff 2007).

Hemodialysis: Supplemental dose is not necessary (Aronoff 2007).

Renal insufficiency or hemodialysis: While the AUC of doxorubicin and doxorubicinol (active metabolite) are higher in patients with renal insufficiency, the half-lives are similar to those in patients without renal impairment. Dosage adjustment does not appear necessary in renal insufficiency or in patients on hemodialysis; administer after dialysis or on a non-dialysis day (Janus 2010).

International Myeloma Working Group Recommendations: The International Myeloma Working Group (IMWG) recommendations suggest that doxorubicin may be administered without dosage adjustment in multiple myeloma patients with renal impairment, including those on dialysis. The IMWG recommends the use of the Chronic Kidney Disease Epidemiology Collaboration (CKD-EPI) equation (preferred) or the Modification of Diet in Renal Disease (MDRD) formula to evaluate renal function estimation in multiple myeloma patients with a stable serum creatinine (Dimopoulos 2016).

Hepatic Impairment

The manufacturers' labeling recommends the following adjustments:

Serum bilirubin 1.2 to 3 mg/dL: Administer 50% of dose.

Serum bilirubin 3.1 to 5 mg/dL: Administer 25% of dose.

Severe hepatic impairment (Child-Pugh class C or bilirubin >5 mg/dL): Use is contraindicated.

The following adjustments have also been recommended (Floyd 2006):

Transaminases 2 to 3 times ULN: Administer 75% of dose.

Transaminases >3 times ULN: Administer 50% of dose.

Obesity *ASCO Guidelines for appropriate chemotherapy dosing in obese adults with cancer:* Utilize patient's actual body weight (full weight) for calculation of body surface area- or weight-based dosing, particularly when the intent of therapy is curative; manage regimen-related toxicities in the same manner as for nonobese patients; if a dose reduction is utilized due to toxicity, consider resumption of full weight-based dosing with subsequent cycles, especially if cause of toxicity (eg, hepatic or renal impairment) is resolved (Griggs 2012).

Adjustment for Toxicity Cardiotoxicity: Discontinue in patients who develop signs/symptoms of cardiomyopathy.

Combination Regimens

Bladder cancer:

Dose Dense MVAC (Bladder Cancer) on page 2096

MVAC (Bladder) on page 2179

Bone sarcoma (Ewing sarcoma): VAC Alternating With IE (Ewing Sarcoma) on page 2224

Bone sarcoma (osteosarcoma): MAP (Osteosarcoma) on page 2170

Breast cancer:

AC (Breast) on page 1976

AC (Dose-Dense) followed by Paclitaxel (Dose-Dense) (Breast) on page 1976

AC (Dose-Dense) followed by Paclitaxel (Dose-Dense)-Trastuzumab (Breast) on page 1977

AC (Dose-Dense) followed by Paclitaxel Weekly (Breast) on page 1978

AC followed by Docetaxel Every 3 Weeks (Breast) on page 1978

AC followed by Paclitaxel-Trastuzumab (Breast) on page 1979

Neuroblastoma:
Soft tissue sarcoma:
Wilms' tumor:

Administration Doxorubicin is associated with a moderate to high emetic potential (depending on dose or regimen); antiemetics are recommended to prevent nausea and vomiting (Basch 2011; Dupuis 2011; Roila 2016).

Administer IV push over at least 3 to 10 minutes or by continuous infusion (infusion via central venous line recommended). Do not administer IM or SubQ. Rate of administration varies by protocol, refer to individual protocol for details. Protect from light until completion of infusion. Avoid contact with alkaline solutions. Monitor for local erythematous streaking along vein and/or facial flushing (may indicate rapid infusion rate); decrease the rate if occurs.

Vesicant; ensure proper needle or catheter placement prior to and during infusion; avoid extravasation.

Extravasation management: If extravasation occurs, stop infusion immediately and disconnect (leave cannula/needle in place); gently aspirate extravasated solution (do **NOT** flush the line); remove needle/cannula; elevate extremity. Initiate antidote (dexrazoxane or dimethyl sulfate [DMSO]). Apply dry cold compresses for 20 minutes 4 times daily for 1 to 2 days (Perez Fidalgo 2012); withhold cooling beginning 15 minutes before dexrazoxane infusion; continue withholding cooling until 15 minutes after infusion is completed. Topical DMSO should not be administered in combination with dexrazoxane; may lessen dexrazoxane efficacy.
Dexrazoxane: Adults: 1000 mg/m^2 (maximum dose: 2000 mg) IV (administer in a large vein remote from site of extravasation) over 1 to 2 hours days 1 and 2, then 500 mg/m^2 (maximum dose: 1000 mg) IV over 1 to 2 hours day 3; begin within 6 hours of extravasation. Day 2 and day 3 doses should be administered at approximately the same time (± 3 hours) as the dose on day 1 (Mouridsen 2007; Perez Fidalgo 2012). **Note:** Reduce dexrazoxane dose by 50% in patients with moderate to severe renal impairment (CrCl <40 mL/minute).
DMSO: Children and Adults: Apply topically to a region covering twice the affected area every 8 hours for 7 days; begin within 10 minutes of extravasation; do not cover with a dressing (Perez Fidalgo 2012).

Vesicant/Extravasation Risk Vesicant; see Management of Drug Extravasations in Special Topics

◄ **Emetic Potential**
Children: Moderate (30% to 90%)
Adults:
≥60 mg/m^2 or when used in combination with cyclophosphamide: High (>90%)
<60 mg/m^2: Moderate (30% to 90%)

Monitoring Parameters CBC with differential and platelet count; liver function tests (bilirubin, ALT/AST, alkaline phosphatase); serum uric acid, calcium, potassium, phosphate and creatinine; hydration status; cardiac function (baseline, periodic, and followup): ECG, left ventricular ejection fraction (echocardiography [ECHO] or multigated radionuclide angiography [MUGA]); monitor infusion site

Dosage Forms Excipient information presented when available (limited, particularly for generics); consult specific product labeling. [DSC] = Discontinued product
Solution, Intravenous, as hydrochloride:
  Adriamycin: 2 mg/mL (5 mL, 10 mL, 25 mL, 100 mL)
  Generic: 2 mg/mL (5 mL, 10 mL, 25 mL, 100 mL)
Solution, Intravenous, as hydrochloride [preservative free]:
  Generic: 2 mg/mL (5 mL, 10 mL, 25 mL, 75 mL, 100 mL)
Solution Reconstituted, Intravenous, as hydrochloride:
  Adriamycin: 10 mg (1 ea); 20 mg (1 ea); 50 mg (1 ea)
  Generic: 50 mg (1 ea)
Solution Reconstituted, Intravenous, as hydrochloride [preservative free]:
  Generic: 10 mg (1 ea); 50 mg (1 ea [DSC])

DOXOrubicin (Liposomal) (doks oh ROO bi sin lye po SO mal)
Related Information
Common Toxicity Criteria *on page 2242*
Management of Chemotherapy-Induced Nausea and Vomiting in Adults *on page 2253*
Management of Drug Extravasations *on page 2271*
Prevention of Chemotherapy-Induced Nausea and Vomiting in Children *on page 2310*
Safe Handling of Hazardous Drugs *on page 2379*

Brand Names: US Doxil; Lipodox 50; Lipodox [DSC]
Brand Names: Canada Caelyx
Index Terms DOXOrubicin HCl Peg-Liposomal; DOXOrubicin Hydrochloride (Liposomal); DOXOrubicin Hydrochloride Liposome; Lipodox; Liposomal DOXOrubicin; Pegylated DOXOrubicin Liposomal; Pegylated Liposomal DOXOrubicin; Pegylated Liposomal DOXOrubicin Hydrochloride (Doxil, Caelyx)
Pharmacologic Category Antineoplastic Agent, Anthracycline; Antineoplastic Agent, Topoisomerase II Inhibitor
Use
AIDS-related Kaposi sarcoma: Treatment of AIDS-related Kaposi sarcoma (after failure of or intolerance to prior systemic therapy)
Multiple myeloma: Treatment of multiple myeloma (in combination with bortezomib) in patients who are bortezomib-naïve and have received at least 1 prior therapy
Ovarian cancer, advanced: Treatment of progressive or recurrent ovarian cancer (after platinum-based treatment)

Labeled Contraindications

Severe hypersensitivity (including anaphylaxis) to doxorubicin liposomal, conventional doxorubicin, or any component of the formulation

Canadian labeling: Additional contraindications (not in the US labeling): Breastfeeding

Pregnancy Considerations Adverse events were observed in animal reproduction studies. May cause fetal harm if administered during pregnancy. Women and men of reproductive potential should use effective contraception during therapy and for 6 months after treatment. Doxorubicin liposomal may damage spermatozoa and testicular tissue in males and may result in oligospermia, azoospermia, and permanent loss of fertility. May cause amenorrhea, infertility, and premature menopause in females.

Breastfeeding Considerations It is not known if doxorubicin liposomal is excreted in breast milk. Due to the potential for serious adverse reactions in the nursing infant, breastfeeding should be discontinued during treatment.

Warnings/Precautions [US Boxed Warning]: Doxorubicin liposomal may cause myocardial damage (including congestive heart failure) as the total cumulative dose of doxorubicin approaches 550 mg/m^2. In a clinical study of 250 patients with advanced cancer who were treated with doxorubicin liposomal, the risk of cardiotoxicity was 11% when the cumulative anthracycline dose was between 450 to 550 mg/m^2. Prior use of other anthracyclines or anthracenediones should be included in calculations of total cumulative dosage. The risk of cardiomyopathy may be increased at lower cumulative doses in patients with prior mediastinal irradiation. Myocardial damage may manifest as acute left ventricular failure; cardiotoxicity is defined as a >20% decrease in resting left ventricular ejection fraction (LVEF) from baseline (if LVEF remained in the normal range) or a >10% decrease from baseline (where LVEF was less than the institutional lower limit of normal). Some patients developed signs/symptoms of heart failure without documented evidence of cardiotoxicity. The risk of cardiomyopathy with doxorubicin is generally proportional to the cumulative exposure, although the relationship between cumulative doxorubicin liposomal dose and the risk of cardiotoxicity is not known. Anthracycline-induced cardiotoxicity may be delayed (after discontinuation of anthracycline treatment). Assess left ventricular function with echocardiogram or MUGA prior to and during treatment to detect acute changes; monitor after treatment to detect delayed cardiotoxicity. Use in patients with a history of cardiovascular disease only if potential benefits outweigh cardiovascular risk.

[US Boxed Warning]: Acute infusion-related reactions consisting of, but not limited to, flushing, shortness of breath, facial swelling, headache, chills, back pain, tightness in the chest or throat, and/or hypotension occurred in 11% of patients with solid tumors treated with doxorubicin liposomal. Serious, life-threatening and fatal infusion reactions have been reported. Infusion reactions have also included chest pain, pruritus, rash, cyanosis, syncope, tachycardia, bronchospasm, asthma, and apnea. Most reactions occurred during the first infusion. Some reactions have resulted in dose interruption. Medication and equipment to manage infusion reactions should be immediately available during infusion. Initiate infusion at a rate of 1 mg/minute, with the rate increased (to complete infusion over 60 minutes) as tolerated. If an infusion reaction occurs, temporarily interrupt infusion until resolved and resume at a reduced rate. Discontinue for serious or life-threatening infusion reactions.

Neutropenia, anemia, and thrombocytopenia may occur. Monitor blood counts. Treatment delay, dosage modification, or discontinuation may be required. Hematologic toxicity may occur at a higher frequency and severity with combination chemotherapy. Palmar-plantar erythrodysesthesia (hand-foot syndrome) has been reported in patients receiving doxorubicin liposomal; it is usually seen after 2 to 3 treatment cycles, although may also occur earlier; dosage modification may be required; in severe or debilitating cases, treatment discontinuation may be required. Pharmacokinetics in patients with hepatic impairment has not been adequately studied. Doxorubicin is predominantly eliminated hepatically; reduce doxorubicin liposomal dose in patients with serum bilirubin ≥1.2 mg/dL.

Cases of secondary oral cancers (primarily squamous cell carcinoma) have been reported with long-term (>1 year) doxorubicin liposomal exposure; these secondary oral malignancies have occurred during treatment and up to 6 years after treatment. The development of oral ulceration or discomfort should be monitored and further evaluated in patients with past or present use of doxorubicin liposomal. Tissue distribution of the liposomal doxorubicin compared to free doxorubicin may play a role in the development of oral secondary malignancies associated with long-term use.

Liposomal vs conventional formulation dosing: Liposomal formulations of doxorubicin should **NOT** be substituted for conventional doxorubicin hydrochloride on a mg-per-mg basis. Potentially significant drug-drug interactions may exist, requiring dose or frequency adjustment, additional monitoring, and/or selection of alternative therapy. Use in splenectomized patients with AIDS-related Kaposi sarcoma has not been studied and is not recommended (Canadian labeling [Caelyx] 2016).

Adverse Reactions Frequency not always defined.

>10%:

Cardiovascular: Cardiomyopathy (dose related: 11%; Kaposi sarcoma: <1%), cardiotoxicity (11%), chest tightness (11%), flushing (11%), hypotension (1% to 11%)

Central nervous system: Fatigue (>20%), headache (≤11%)

Dermatologic: Palmar-plantar erythrodysesthesia (ovarian cancer: ≤51%; grades 3/4: 24%), skin rash (grades 3/4: 29%, Kaposi sarcoma: 1% to 5%), alopecia (9% to 19%), facial swelling (11%)

Gastrointestinal: Nausea (ovarian cancer: 46%; Kaposi sarcoma: 17% to 18%; grades 3/4: 5%), stomatitis (grades 3/4: 41%, Kaposi sarcoma: 5% to 8%), vomiting (grades 3/4: 33%; Kaposi sarcoma: 8%), constipation (>20%), diarrhea (grades 3/4: 21%; Kaposi sarcoma: 3% to 8%), anorexia (20%; Kaposi sarcoma: 1% to 5%), mucous membrane disease (14%; grades 3/4: 4%), dyspepsia 12%; grades 3/4: <1%)

Hematologic & oncologic: Thrombocytopenia (dose related, Kaposi sarcoma: 1% to 61%), neutropenia (dose related: 4% to 49%), leukopenia (37%), anemia (16% to 58%; dose related <1% to 5%)

Neuromuscular & skeletal: Weakness (grades 3/4: 40%; Kaposi sarcoma: 7% to 10%), back pain (grades 3/4: 11% to 12%; Kaposi sarcoma: 1% to 5%)

Respiratory: Pharyngitis (16%; Kaposi sarcoma <1%), dyspnea (1% to 15%)

Miscellaneous: Fever (21%; Kaposi sarcoma: 8% to 9%; grades 3/4: <1%), infusion related reaction (7% to 11%)

1% to 10%:

Cardiovascular: Cardiac arrest (≤10%), chest pain (Kaposi sarcoma: 1% to 5%), deep thrombophlebitis (ovarian cancer: 1% to 10%), tachycardia (1% to 10%), vasodilation (ovarian cancer: 1% to 10%)

Central nervous system: Depression (ovarian cancer: 1% to 10%), dizziness (1% to 10%), drowsiness (1% to 10%), chills (Kaposi sarcoma: 1% to 5%)

Dermatologic: Acne vulgaris (ovarian cancer: 1% to 10%), ecchymoses (ovarian cancer: 1% to 10%), exfoliative dermatitis (ovarian cancer: 1% to 10%), fungal dermatitis (ovarian cancer: 1% to 10%), furunculosis (ovarian cancer: 1% to 10%), herpes simplex dermatitis (1% to 10%), pruritus (1% to 10%), skin discoloration (ovarian cancer: 1% to 10%), vesiculobullous dermatitis (ovarian cancer: 1% to 10%), xeroderma (ovarian cancer: 1% to 10%), maculopapular rash (≤10%)

Endocrine & metabolic: Hypercalcemia (ovarian cancer: 1% to 10%), hypokalemia (ovarian cancer: 1% to 10%), hyponatremia (ovarian cancer: 1% to 10%), weight loss (1% to 10%), dehydration (≤10%), hyperglycemia (1% to 5%)

Gastrointestinal: Dysphagia (1% to 10%), esophagitis (ovarian cancer: 1% to 10%), intestinal obstruction (ovarian cancer: 1% to 10%), oral candidiasis (1% to 10%), oral mucosa ulcer (1% to 10%), dysgeusia (1% to ≤10%), abdomen enlarged (ovarian cancer 1% to 5%), glossitis (1% to 5%), cachexia

Genitourinary: Hematuria (ovarian cancer: 1% to 10%), hemorrhagic cystitis, urinary tract infection (ovarian cancer: 1% to 10%), vulvovaginal candidiasis (ovarian cancer 1% to 10%)

Hematologic & oncologic: Rectal hemorrhage (ovarian cancer: 1% to 10%), hemolysis (1% to 5%), prolonged prothrombin time (1% to 5%), bone marrow depression (Kaposi sarcoma), progression of cancer (Kaposi sarcoma)

Hepatic: Hyperbilirubinemia (1% to 10%), increased serum alkaline phosphatase (Kaposi sarcoma 1% to 8%), increased serum ALT (Kaposi sarcoma 1% to 5%)

Hypersensitivity: Hypersensitivity reaction (Kaposi sarcoma 1% to 5%)

Infection: Infection (1% to 12%), herpes zoster (≤10%), paresthesia (5%), myalgia (ovarian cancer: 1% to 5%), neuropathy (ovarian cancer 1% to 5%), toxoplasmosis (Kaposi sarcoma)

Ophthalmic: Dry eye syndrome (ovarian cancer: 1% to 10%), conjunctivitis (≤10%), retinitis (Kaposi sarcoma 1% to 5%) optic neuritis (Kaposi sarcoma)

Respiratory: Epistaxis (ovarian cancer: 1% to 10%), pneumonia (1% to 10%), rhinitis (ovarian cancer: 1% to 10%), sinusitis (ovarian cancer: 1% to 10%), increased cough (≤10%), cough (Kaposi sarcoma)

<1%, postmarketing, and/or case reports (Limited to important or life-threatening): Abnormal vision, abscess, acute brain syndrome, albuminuria, alkaline phosphatase increased anaphylactic reaction, anxiety, arthralgia, asthma, balanitis, blindness, bone pain, bronchitis, bundle branch block (Kaposi sarcoma), BUN increased, candidiasis (Kaposi sarcoma), cardiomegaly, cardiomyopathy, cellulitis, CHF, colitis, confusion, congestive heart failure (Kaposi sarcoma), creatinine increased, cryptococcosis, cryptococcosis (Kaposi sarcoma), diabetes mellitus, dysuria, edema, emotional lability, erythema multiforme, erythema nodosum, fecal impaction, flatulence, flu-like syndrome, gastritis, hemorrhage, hepatic failure, hepatitis (Kaposi sarcoma), hepatosplenomegaly, hyperkalemia, hyperlipidemia, hypernatremia, hyperuricemia, hyperventilation, hypoglycemia,

hypomagnesemia, hypophosphatemia, hypoproteinemia, hypothermia, injection site hemorrhage, injection site pain, insomnia, jaundice, ketosis, lactic dehydrogenase increased, lymphadenopathy, lymphangitis, migraine, myositis, muscle spasm, optic neuritis, pain, pallor, palpitations (Kaposi sarcoma), pancreatitis, pericardial effusion, petechia, pneumothorax, peripheral edema, pleural effusion, pulmonary embolism, radiation injury, sclerosing cholangitis, seizure, secondary acute myelocytic leukemia, sepsis (Kaposi sarcoma), skin necrosis, skin ulcer, syncope, squamous cell carcinoma, Stevens-Johnson syndrome, tenesmus, thrombophlebitis (Kaposi sarcoma), thromboplastin decreased, thrombosis (Kaposi sarcoma), tinnitus, toxic epidermal necrolysis, urticaria, vertigo (Kaposi sarcoma), ventricular arrhythmia (Kaposi sarcoma)

Drug Interactions

Metabolism/Transport Effects Substrate of CYP2D6 (major), CYP3A4 (major); **Note:** Assignment of Major/Minor substrate status based on clinically relevant drug interaction potential

Avoid Concomitant Use

Avoid concomitant use of DOXOrubicin (Liposomal) with any of the following: BCG (Intravesical); Conivaptan; Deferiprone; Dipyrone; Fusidic Acid (Systemic); Idelalisib; Natalizumab; Pimecrolimus; Tacrolimus (Topical); Vaccines (Live)

Increased Effect/Toxicity

DOXOrubicin (Liposomal) may increase the levels/effects of: CloZAPine; Deferiprone; Fingolimod; Leflunomide; Natalizumab; Tofacitinib; Vaccines (Live); Vinflunine; Zidovudine

The levels/effects of DOXOrubicin (Liposomal) may be increased by: Abiraterone Acetate; Ado-Trastuzumab Emtansine; Ajmaline; Aprepitant; Asunaprevir; Bevacizumab; Conivaptan; Cyclophosphamide; CYP2D6 Inhibitors (Moderate); CYP2D6 Inhibitors (Strong); CYP3A4 Inhibitors (Moderate); CYP3A4 Inhibitors (Strong); Dasatinib; Denosumab; Dipyrone; Fosaprepitant; Fusidic Acid (Systemic); Idelalisib; Imatinib; Lumefantrine; MiFEPRIStone; Netupitant; Ocrelizumab; Palbociclib; Palifermin; Panobinostat; Peginterferon Alfa-2b; Pimecrolimus; Promazine; QuiNINE; Roflumilast; Simeprevir; Stiripentol; Tacrolimus (Topical); Taxane Derivatives; Trastuzumab

Decreased Effect

DOXOrubicin (Liposomal) may decrease the levels/effects of: BCG (Intravesical); Cardiac Glycosides; Coccidioides immitis Skin Test; Lenograstim; Nivolumab; Sipuleucel-T; Stavudine; Tertomotide; Vaccines (Inactivated); Vaccines (Live); Zidovudine

The levels/effects of DOXOrubicin (Liposomal) may be decreased by: Bosentan; Cardiac Glycosides; CYP3A4 Inducers (Moderate); CYP3A4 Inducers (Strong); Dabrafenib; Deferasirox; Echinacea; Enzalutamide; Mitotane; Peginterferon Alfa-2b; Sarilumab; Siltuximab; St John's Wort; Tocilizumab; Vinflunine

Hazardous Drugs Handling Considerations

Hazardous agent (NIOSH 2016 [group 1]).

Use appropriate precautions for receiving, handling, administration, and disposal. Gloves (single) should be worn during receiving, unpacking, and placing in storage.

NIOSH recommends double gloving, a protective gown, ventilated engineering controls (a class II biological safety cabinet or a compounding aseptic containment isolator), and closed system transfer devices (CSTDs) for preparation. Double gloving, a gown, and (if dosage form allows) CSTDs are required during administration (NIOSH 2016).

Storage/Stability Store intact vials refrigerated at 2°C to 8°C (36°F to 46°F); avoid freezing. Solutions diluted for infusion in D5W should be refrigerated at 2°C to 8°C (36°F to 46°F); administer within 24 hours.

Preparation for Administration Dilute doses ≤90 in D5W 250 mL prior to administration. Dilute doses >90 mg in D5W 500 mL. Solution is not clear, but has a red, translucent appearance due to the liposomal dispersion. Dilute ONLY in D5W; do not use bacteriostatic agents; do not mix with other medications.

Mechanism of Action Doxorubicin inhibits DNA and RNA synthesis by intercalating between DNA base pairs causing steric obstruction and inhibits topoisomerase-II at the point of DNA cleavage. Doxorubicin is also a powerful iron chelator. The iron-doxorubicin complex can bind DNA and cell membranes, producing free hydroxyl (OH) radicals that cleave DNA and cell membranes. Active throughout entire cell cycle. Doxorubicin liposomal is a pegylated formulation which protects the liposomes, and thereby increases blood circulation time.

Pharmacodynamics/Kinetics

Distribution: V_{dss}: ~2.7 to 2.8 L/m^2; largely confined to vascular fluid

Protein binding, plasma: Unknown; nonliposomal (conventional) doxorubicin: ~70%

Half-life elimination: Terminal: Distribution: ~4.7 to 5.2 hours, Elimination: ~52 to 55 hours

Metabolism: Hepatic and in plasma to doxorubicinol and the sulfate and glucuronide conjugates of 4-demethyl,7-deoxyaglycones

Dosing

Adult & Geriatric Liposomal formulations of doxorubicin should NOT be substituted for conventional doxorubicin hydrochloride on a mg-per-mg basis.

AIDS-related Kaposi sarcoma: IV: 20 mg/m^2 once every 21 days until disease progression or unacceptable toxicity

Multiple myeloma: IV: 30 mg/m^2 on day 4 every 21 days (in combination with bortezomib) for 8 cycles or until disease progression or unacceptable toxicity (Orlowski 2007)

Multiple myeloma, newly diagnosed (off-label dosing): IV: 40 mg/m^2 on day 1 every 4 weeks (in combination with vincristine and dexamethasone) for at least 4 cycles (Rifkin 2006).

Ovarian cancer, advanced: IV: 50 mg/m^2 once every 28 days until disease progression or unacceptable toxicity

Ovarian cancer, advanced, recurrent (off- label dosing): IV: 40 mg/m^2 once every 28 days (as a single agent) until disease progression or unacceptable toxicity (Ferrandina 2008; Rose 2001) or 30 mg/m^2 once every 28 days (in combination with carboplatin) for at least 6 cycles (Pujade-Lauraine 2010) or 40 mg/m^2 once every 28 days (in combination with bevacizumab) until disease progression or unacceptable toxicity (Pujade-Lauraine 2014).

Breast cancer, metastatic (off-label use): IV: 50 mg/m^2 every 4 weeks (Keller 2004)

◄ **Cutaneous T-cell lymphomas (off-label use):** IV: 20 mg/m^2 days 1 and 15 every 4 weeks for 6 cycles (Dummer 2012) **or** 20 mg/m^2 every 4 weeks (Wollina 2003)

Hodgkin lymphoma, salvage treatment (off-label use): IV: GVD regimen: 10 mg/m^2 (post-transplant patients) or 15 mg/m^2 (transplant-naive patients) days 1 and 8 every 3 weeks (in combination with gemcitabine and vinorelbine) for 2 to 6 cycles (Bartlett 2007)

Soft tissue sarcoma, advanced (off-label use): IV: 50 mg/m^2 every 4 weeks for 6 cycles (Judson 2001)

Uterine sarcoma, advanced or recurrent (off-label use): IV: 50 mg/m^2 every 4 weeks until disease progression or unacceptable toxicity (Sutton 2005)

Renal Impairment There are no dosage adjustments provided in the manufacturer's labeling (has not been studied).

Hepatic Impairment

US labeling: There are no dosage adjustments provided in the manufacturer's labeling. However, doxorubicin is predominantly hepatically eliminated and reduced doxorubicin liposomal doses are recommended in patients with serum bilirubin ≥1.2 mg/dL.

Canadian labeling:

AIDS-related Kaposi sarcoma:

Bilirubin 1.2 to 3 mg/dL: Reduce dose to 50% of normal dose

Bilirubin >3 mg/dL: Reduce dose to 25% of normal dose

Breast cancer and ovarian cancer:

Bilirubin 1.2 to 3 mg/dL: Initial dose: Reduce dose to 75% of normal dose; if tolerated and no change in bilirubin/hepatic enzymes, may increase to full dose with cycle 2

Bilirubin >3 mg/dL: Initial dose: Reduce dose to 50% of normal dose; if tolerated and no change in bilirubin/hepatic enzymes, may increase dose to 75% of normal dose for cycle 2; if cycle 2 dose tolerated, may increase to full dose for subsequent cycles.

Obesity *ASCO Guidelines for appropriate chemotherapy dosing in obese adults with cancer:* Utilize patient's actual body weight (full weight) for calculation of body surface area- or weight-based dosing, particularly when the intent of therapy is curative; manage regimen-related toxicities in the same manner as for nonobese patients; if a dose reduction is utilized due to toxicity, consider resumption of full weight-based dosing with subsequent cycles, especially if cause of toxicity (eg, hepatic or renal impairment) is resolved (Griggs 2012).

Adjustment for Toxicity

US labeling: **Note:** Once a dosage reduction due to toxicity has been implemented, the dose should not be increased at a later time.

Hematologic toxicity:

AIDS-related Kaposi sarcoma and ovarian cancer:

*Grade 1 (ANC 1,500 to 1,900/mm^3 **or platelets** 75,000 to 150,000/mm^3):* No dosage adjustment necessary.

*Grade 2 (ANC 1,000 to <1,500/mm^3 **or platelets** 50,000 to <75,000/mm^3):* Delay treatment until ANC ≥1,500/mm^3 and platelets ≥75,000/mm^3; resume treatment at previous dose.

Grade 3 (ANC 500 to 999/mm^3 or platelets 25,000 to <50,000/mm^3): Delay treatment until ANC ≥1,500/mm^3 and platelets ≥75,000/mm^3; resume treatment at previous dose.

Grade 4 (ANC <500/mm³ or platelets <25,000/mm³): Delay treatment until ANC ≥1,500/mm³ and platelets ≥75,000/mm³; then resume at 25% dose reduction or continue at previous dose with granulocyte growth factor support.

Multiple myeloma (in combination with Bortezomib) (see Bortezomib monograph for bortezomib dosage reduction with toxicity guidelines):

Fever ≥38°C and ANC <1,000/mm³: If prior to doxorubicin liposomal treatment (day 4), do not administer (withhold); if after doxorubicin liposomal administered, reduce dose by 25% in next cycle.

ANC <500/mm³, platelets <25,000/mm³, hemoglobin <8 g/dL: If prior to doxorubicin liposomal treatment (day 4); do not administer (withhold); if after doxorubicin liposomal administered and if bortezomib dose reduction occurred for hematologic toxicity, reduce dose by 25% in next cycle

Nonhematologic toxicity:

Hand-foot syndrome (HFS):

Grade 1 (mild erythema, swelling, or desquamation not interfering with daily activities): If no prior grade 3 or 4 HFS toxicity, no dosage adjustment is necessary. If prior grade 3 or 4 HFS toxicity, delay dose up to 2 weeks and decrease dose by 25%.

Grade 2 (erythema, desquamation, or swelling interfering with, but not precluding, normal physical activities; small blisters or ulcerations <2 cm in diameter): Delay dosing up to 2 weeks or until resolved to grade 0 or 1. If after 2 weeks there is no resolution, discontinue liposomal doxorubicin. If resolved to grade 0 or 1 within 2 weeks and no prior grade 3 or 4 HFS, continue treatment at previous dose. If a prior grade 3 or 4 HFS has occurred, decrease dose by 25%.

Grade 3 (blistering, ulceration, or swelling interfering with walking or normal daily activities; cannot wear regular clothing): Delay dosing up to 2 weeks or until resolved to grade 0 or 1, then decrease dose by 25%. If no resolution after 2 weeks, discontinue liposomal doxorubicin.

Grade 4 (diffuse or local process causing infectious complications, or a bedridden state or hospitalization): Delay dosing up to 2 weeks or until resolved to grade 0 or 1, then decrease dose by 25%. If no resolution after 2 weeks, discontinue liposomal doxorubicin.

Infusion reaction: Temporarily stop infusion until resolution and then resume at a reduced rate. For serious or life threatening reaction, discontinue infusion.

Stomatitis:

Grade 1 (painless ulcers, erythema, or mild soreness): If no prior grade 3 or 4 toxicity, no dosage adjustment is necessary. If prior grade 3 or 4 toxicity, delay dose up to 2 weeks and decrease dose by 25%.

Grade 2 (painful erythema, edema, or ulcers, but can eat): Delay dosing up to 2 weeks or until resolved to grade 0 or 1. If after 2 weeks there is no resolution, discontinue liposomal doxorubicin. If resolved to grade 0 or 1 within 2 weeks and no prior grade 3 or 4 stomatitis, continue treatment at previous dose. If prior grade 3 or 4 stomatitis, decrease dose by 25%.

Grade 3 (painful erythema, edema, or ulcers, and cannot eat): Delay dosing up to 2 weeks or until resolved to grade 0 or 1. Decrease dose by 25% and return to original dosing interval. If after 2 weeks there is no resolution, discontinue liposomal doxorubicin.

◀

Grade 4 (requires parenteral or enteral support): Delay dosing up to 2 weeks or until resolved to grade 0 or 1. Decrease dose by 25% and return to original dosing interval. If after 2 weeks there is no resolution, discontinue liposomal doxorubicin.

Multiple myeloma (in combination with Bortezomib) (see Bortezomib monograph for bortezomib dosage reduction with toxicity guidelines):

Grade 3 or 4 nonhematologic toxicity: Delay dose until resolved to grade <2 and then reduce dose by 25%

Neuropathic pain or peripheral neuropathy: No dose reductions needed for doxorubicin liposomal, refer to Bortezomib monograph for bortezomib dosing adjustment.

Canadian labeling:
Hematologic toxicity:
Breast cancer, ovarian cancer: Refer to US dosage adjustment for hematologic toxicity section.

AIDS-related Kaposi sarcoma:

Grade 1 or grade 2 (ANC 1,500 to 1,900/mm^3 or platelets 75,000 to 150,000/mm^3 or ANC 1,000 to <1,500/mm^3 or platelets 50,000 to <75,000/mm^3): No dosage adjustment necessary.

Grade 3 (ANC 500 to 999/mm^3 and platelets 25,000 to <50,000/mm^3): Delay treatment until ANC ≥1,000/mm^3 and/or platelets ≥50,000/mm^3 and then resume with a 25% dose reduction.

Grade 4 (ANC <500/mm^3 and platelets <25,000/mm^3): Delay treatment until ANC ≥1,000/mm^3 and/or platelets ≥50,000/mm^3 and then resume with a 50% dose reduction.

Nonhematologic toxicity:
Breast cancer, ovarian cancer:
Hand-foot syndrome (HFS; palmar-plantar erythrodysesthesia):

Grade 1 (mild erythema, swelling, or desquamation not interfering with daily activities): If at weeks 4 and 5 following prior dose, resume unless patients has experienced prior grade 3 or 4 HFS toxicity (if so, wait an additional week). If at week 6, decrease dose by 25%; return to 4-week interval.

Grade 2 (erythema, desquamation, or swelling interfering with, but not precluding, normal physical activities; small blisters or ulcerations <2 cm in diameter): If at weeks 4 and 5 following prior dose, wait an additional week. If at week 6, decrease dose by 25%; return to 4-week interval.

Grade 3 or grade 4 (blistering, ulceration, or swelling interfering with walking or normal daily activities; cannot wear regular clothing or diffuse or local process causing infectious complications, or a bed-ridden state or hospitalization): If at weeks 4 and 5 following prior dose, wait an additional week. If at week 6, discontinue therapy.

Stomatitis:

Grade 1 (painless ulcers, erythema, or mild soreness): If at weeks 4 and 5 following prior dose, resume unless patients has experienced prior grade 3 or 4 HFS toxicity (if so, wait an additional week). If at week 6, decrease dose by 25%; return to 4-week interval or discontinue therapy (based on physical assessment).

Grade 2 (painful erythema, edema, or ulcers, but can eat): If at weeks 4 and 5 following prior dose, wait an additional week. If at week 6, decrease dose by 25%; return to 4-week interval or discontinue therapy (based on physical assessment).

Grade 3 or grade 4 (painful erythema, edema, or ulcers, and cannot eat or requires parenteral or enteral support): If at weeks 4 and 5 following prior dose, wait an additional week. If at week 6, discontinue therapy.

Aids-related Kaposi sarcoma:

Hand-foot syndrome (HFS; palmar-plantar erythrodysesthesia):

Grade 0 (no symptoms): If at week 3 or 4 following prior dose, redose at a 2-to 3-week interval.

Grade 1 (mild erythema, swelling, or desquamation not interfering with daily activities): If at week 3 following prior dose, resume unless patients has experienced prior grade 3 or 4 HFS toxicity (if so, wait an additional week). If at week 4 following prior dose, decrease dose by 25% and return to 3-week interval.

Grade 2 (erythema, desquamation, or swelling interfering with, but not precluding, normal physical activities; small blisters or ulcerations <2 cm in diameter): If at week 3 following prior dose, wait an additional week. If at week 4 following prior dose, decrease dose by 50% and return to 3-week interval.

Grade 3 or grade 4 (blistering, ulceration, or swelling interfering with walking or normal daily activities; cannot wear regular clothing, diffuse or local process causing infectious complications, or a bedridden state or hospitalization): If at week 3 following prior dose, wait an additional week. If at week 4, discontinue therapy.

Stomatitis:

Grade 1 (painless ulcers, erythema, or mild soreness): No dosage adjustment necessary.

Grade 2 (painful erythema, edema, or ulcers, but can eat): Wait 1 week and if symptoms improve, resume at 100% dose.

Grade 3 (painful erythema, edema, or ulcers, and cannot eat): Wait 1 week and if symptoms improve, resume with a 25% dose reduction.

Grade 4 (requires parenteral or enteral support): Wait 1 week and if symptoms improve, resume with a 50% dose reduction.

Combination Regimens

Lymphoma, Hodgkin: GVD (Hodgkin) on page 2143

Multiple myeloma:

Bortezomib-Doxorubicin (Liposomal) (Multiple Myeloma) on page 1999
Doxorubicin (Liposomal)-Vincristine-Dexamethasone (Multiple Myeloma) on page 2098

Ovarian cancer:

Bevacizumab-Doxorubicin (Liposomal) (Ovarian) on page 1992
Carboplatin-Doxorubicin (Liposomal) (Ovarian) on page 2014
Trabectedin-Doxorubicin (Liposomal) (Ovarian) on page 2215

Administration Monitor for infusion reaction. For IV infusion only; do not administer IV push. If contact with skin/mucosa occurs, wash immediately with soap and water.

Administer IVPB over 60 minutes; the manufacturer recommends infusing the first dose at initial rate of 1 mg/minute to minimize risk of infusion reactions; if no infusion-related reactions are observed, then increase the infusion rate for completion over 1 hour. Do **NOT** administer undiluted. Do **NOT** infuse with in-line filters. Do not mix with other medications. Monitor for local erythematous streaking along vein and/or facial flushing (may indicate rapid infusion rate).

For multiple myeloma, administer doxorubicin liposomal after bortezomib on day 4 of each cycle.

Irritant (Perez Fidalgo 2012); monitor infusion site; avoid extravasation. Assure proper needle or catheter position prior to administration.

Extravasation management: If extravasation, infiltration, or burning/stinging sensation occurs, stop infusion immediately and disconnect (leave cannula/needle in place); gently aspirate extravasated solution (do **NOT** flush the line); remove needle/cannula; elevate extremity (Perez Fidalgo 2012; Polovich 2009). Do not apply pressure to the site. Apply ice to the site for 15 minutes 4 times a day for 3 days.

Vesicant/Extravasation Risk Irritant

Emetic Potential Children and Adults: Low (10% to 30%)

Monitoring Parameters CBC with differential and platelet count, liver function tests (ALT/AST, bilirubin, alkaline phosphatase); monitor infusion site, monitor for infusion reactions, hand-foot syndrome, stomatitis, and oral ulceration/discomfort suggestive of secondary oral malignancy

Cardiac function (left ventricular ejection fraction [LVEF]; baseline and periodic); echocardiography, or MUGA scan may be used.

Dosage Forms Considerations

Doxil, Lipodox, generic doxorubicin HCl liposomal (Sun Pharma), and Caclyx (Canadian product) are pegalyated liposomal formulations of doxorubicin hydrochloride.

Myocet (Canadian product) is encapsulated liposomes of doxorubicin hydrochloride.

Dosage Forms Excipient information presented when available (limited, particularly for generics); consult specific product labeling. [DSC] = Discontinued product

Injectable, Intravenous, as hydrochloride:
Doxil: 2 mg/mL (10 mL, 25 mL)
Lipodox: 2 mg/mL (10 mL [DSC])
Lipodox 50: 2 mg/mL (25 mL)
Generic: 2 mg/mL (10 mL, 25 mL)

Dosage Forms: Canada Information with regard to form, strength, and availability of products uniquely available in Canada but currently not available in the US. Refer also to Dosage Forms.

Excipient information presented when available (limited, particularly for generics); consult specific product labeling.
Injection, solution, as hydrochloride, pegylated:
Caelyx: 2 mg/mL (10 mL, 25 mL)

◆ **Doxorubicin HCl** see DOXOrubicin (Conventional) on page 624

◆ **DOXOrubicin HCl Peg-Liposomal** see DOXOrubicin (Liposomal) on page 636

◆ **Doxorubicin Hydrochloride** see DOXOrubicin (Conventional) on page 624

◆ **Doxorubicin Hydrochloride For Injection, USP (Can)** see DOXOrubicin (Conventional) on page 624

◆ **Doxorubicin Hydrochloride Injection (Can)** see DOXOrubicin (Conventional) on page 624

◆ **DOXOrubicin Hydrochloride (Liposomal)** see DOXOrubicin (Liposomal) on page 636

◆ **DOXOrubicin Hydrochloride Liposome** see DOXOrubicin (Liposomal) on page 636

Dronabinol (droe NAB i nol)

Related Information

Management of Chemotherapy-Induced Nausea and Vomiting in Adults on page 2253

Brand Names: US Marinol; Syndros

Index Terms Delta-9 THC; Delta-9-tetrahydro-cannabinol; Syndros; Tetrahydrocannabinol; THC

Pharmacologic Category Antiemetic; Appetite Stimulant

Use

Appetite stimulation in AIDS patients: Treatment of anorexia associated with weight loss in patients with AIDS.

Chemotherapy-induced nausea and vomiting: Treatment of nausea and vomiting associated with cancer chemotherapy in patients who have failed to respond adequately to conventional antiemetic treatments.

Labeled Contraindications Hypersensitivity to dronabinol, cannabinoids, sesame oil (capsules), alcohol (oral solution) or any component of the formulation; receiving, or have recently received, disulfiram- or metronidazole-containing products within 14 days (oral solution).

Pregnancy Considerations Adverse events have been observed in animal reproduction studies. Although information related to the use of synthetic cannabinoids during pregnancy is limited, cannabinoids cross the placenta. Maternal use may increase the risk of adverse fetal/neonatal outcomes including growth restriction, low birth weight, preterm birth, and stillbirth. Some dosage forms also contain a significant amount of alcohol.

Breastfeeding Considerations Dronabinol is excreted in breast milk. When used for chemotherapy-induced nausea and vomiting, the manufacturer recommends not to breastfeed during treatment and for 9 days after the last dose. When used to treat anorexia in women with AIDS, complete avoidance of breastfeeding is recommended to decrease potential transmission of HIV.

Warnings/Precautions Dronabinol has been associated with seizures and seizure-like activity. Assess potential risks versus benefits in patient with a history of seizure disorder, those receiving anti-epileptic medications, or with other factors that may lower the seizure threshold. Monitor patients with a history of seizure disorder for worsened control. Discontinue dronabinol immediately in patients who develop seizures. Monitor for CNS adverse effects; may require dosage modification. Dronabinol has been reported to exacerbate depression, mania, or schizophrenia; screen patients for history of these conditions prior to treatment initiation. Avoid use in patients with a psychiatric history; if use cannot be avoided, monitor for new or worsening psychiatric symptoms. Avoid concomitant use with other medications associated with similar psychiatric adverse effects. May cause cognitive impairment, altered mental state, or CNS depression, which may impair physical or mental abilities; patients must be cautioned about performing tasks that require mental alertness (eg, operating machinery, driving). Elderly and pediatric patients may be more sensitive to neurologic and psychiatric effects of dronabinol; may require dose reduction or discontinuation. Consider reduced initial doses in elderly patients. May cause occasional hypotension, possible hypertension, syncope, or tachycardia; patients with cardiac disorders may be at higher risk for hemodynamic instability. Monitor for changes in heart rate, blood pressure and for signs/symptoms of syncope after initiating treatment and with dosage increases. Avoid concomitant use with other medications associated with similar cardiovascular adverse effects. New or worsening paradoxical nausea, vomiting, and/or abdominal pain may occur with synthetic cannabinoids; may be severe and require dose reduction or discontinuation. Symptoms are similar to cannabinoid hyperemesis syndrome, which is a cyclical syndrome with the same symptoms occurring with long-term use of cannabinoid products. Hypersensitivity reactions, including disseminated rash, lip swelling, oral lesions, skin burning, flushing, and throat tightness have been reported.

Administration with phenothiazines (eg, prochlorperazine) for the management of chemotherapy-induced nausea and vomiting may result in improved efficacy (compared to either drug alone) without additional toxicity. Use with caution in patients with a history of substance abuse, including marijuana or alcohol abuse or dependence; potential for drug dependency exists. Assess risk for abuse or misuse prior to treatment and monitor patients with a history of substance abuse throughout treatment. Tolerance, psychological, and physical dependence may occur with prolonged use. May cause withdrawal symptoms upon abrupt discontinuation. EEG changes consistent with withdrawal have been reported upon abrupt dechallenge of dronabinol. Sleep disturbances have been observed for several weeks after discontinuing treatment with high dronabinol doses. Use with caution in patients with mania, depression, or schizophrenia; careful psychiatric monitoring is recommended.

Dronabinol oral solution contains dehydrated alcohol, which may cause a disulfiram-like reaction (abdominal cramps, nausea, vomiting, headache, and flushing) in patients receiving disulfiram or other medications associated with this reaction (eg, metronidazole). Medications containing disulfiram or metronidazole should be discontinued at least 14 days prior to initiation of dronabinol oral solution and do not administer until 7 days following completion of dronabinol oral solution. Clearance may be reduced and systemic effects increased in patients with CYP2C9 genetic polymorphism. Monitor for increased adverse effects in patients known to carry genetic variants associated with diminished CYP2C9 function. Safety and efficacy of dronabinol oral solution have not been established in pediatric patients. Dronabinol oral solution contains dehydrated alcohol and propylene glycol, which should be avoided in preterm neonates and in the immediate postnatal period due to possible toxicities associated with propylene glycol. Pediatric patients may be more sensitive to CNS adverse effects. Some dosage forms may contain propylene glycol; large amounts are potentially toxic and have been associated with hyperosmolality, lactic acidosis, seizures, and respiratory depression; use caution (AAP 1997; Zar 2007). See manufacturer's labeling.

Adverse Reactions Frequency not always defined.

>1%:

Cardiovascular: Facial flushing, palpitations, tachycardia, vasodilatation

Central nervous system: Euphoria (antimetic: 24%; appetite stimulant: 8%), abnormality in thinking (3% to 10%), dizziness (3% to 10%), drowsiness (3% to 10%), paranoia (3% to 10%), amnesia, anxiety, ataxia, confusion, depersonalization, hallucination, nervousness

Gastrointestinal: Abdominal pain (3% to 10%), nausea (3% to 10%), vomiting (3% to 10%)

Neuromuscular & skeletal: Weakness

<1%, postmarketing, and/or case reports: Anorexia, burning sensation of skin, chills, conjunctival injection, conjunctivitis, cough, delirium, depression, diaphoresis, diarrhea, disorientation, exacerbation of depression, falling, fatigue, fecal incontinence, flushing, headache, hypotension, increased liver

enzymes, insomnia, loss of consciousness, malaise, mental status change (exacerbation of mania or schizophrenia), movement disorder, myalgia, nightmares, oral lesion, panic attack, pharyngeal edema, rhinitis, seizure, sinusitis, skin rash, speech disturbance, swelling of lips, syncope, tinnitus, urticaria, visual disturbance

Drug Interactions

Metabolism/Transport Effects Substrate of CYP2C9 (minor), CYP3A4 (minor); **Note:** Assignment of Major/Minor substrate status based on clinically relevant drug interaction potential

Avoid Concomitant Use There are no known interactions where it is recommended to avoid concomitant use.

Increased Effect/Toxicity

Dronabinol may increase the levels/effects of: Alcohol (Ethyl); Amphotericin B; CNS Depressants; CycloSPORINE (Systemic); Sympathomimetics; Warfarin

The levels/effects of Dronabinol may be increased by: Anticholinergic Agents; Cocaine; CYP2C9 Inhibitors (Moderate); CYP2C9 Inhibitors (Strong); CYP3A4 Inhibitors (Moderate); CYP3A4 Inhibitors (Strong); Disulfiram; MetroNIDAZOLE (Systemic); Ritonavir

Decreased Effect

The levels/effects of Dronabinol may be decreased by: CYP3A4 Inducers (Strong)

Food Interactions *Oral solution:* A high-fat meal (59 g of fat) or high-calorie meal (~950 calories) resulted in a 2.5-fold increase in AUC and a 5-hour delay in the median time to peak; food also decreased the C_{max} by ~20%.

Storage/Stability

Capsules: Store in a cool environment between 8°C and 15°C (46°F and 59°F) or refrigerated; protect from freezing. Capsules should be stored in a well-closed container.

Oral solution: Store in a refrigerator between 2°C and 8°C (36°F and 46°F); excursions permitted to 15°C and 25°C (59°F and 77°F). The opened bottle may be stored at 25°C (77°F). Discard unused portion 28 days after first opening. Keep in original carton (keep calibrated dosing syringe in original carton, too).

Mechanism of Action Dronabinol (synthetic delta-9-tetrahydrocannabinol [delta-9-THC]), an active cannabinoid and natural occurring component of *Cannabis sativa L.* (marijuana), activates cannabinoid receptors CB_1 and CB_2. Activation of the CB_1 receptor produces marijuana-like effects on psyche and circulation, whereas activation of the CB_2 receptor does not. Dronabinol has approximately equal affinity for the CB_1 and CB_2 receptors; however, efficacy is less at CB_2 receptors. Activation of the cannabinoid system with dronabinol causes psychological effects that can be divided into 4 groups: affective (euphoria and easy laughter); sensory (increased perception of external stimuli and of the person's own body); somatic (feeling of the body floating or sinking in the bed); and cognitive (distortion of time perception, memory lapses, difficulty in concentration). Most effects (eg, analgesia, appetite enhancement, muscle relaxation, hormonal actions) are mediated by central cannabinoid receptors (CB_1), their distribution reflecting many of the medicinal benefits and adverse effects (Grotenhermen 2003).

Pharmacodynamics/Kinetics

Onset of action: ~0.5 to 1 hour

Peak effect: 2 to 4 hours

Duration: 4 to 6 hours (psychoactive effects); ≥24 hours (appetite stimulation)

Absorption: Oral: 90% to 95%; 10% to 20% of dose reaches systemic circulation

Distribution: V_d: ~10 L/kg; dronabinol is highly lipophilic

Protein binding: ~97%

Metabolism: Extensive first-pass hepatic primarily via microsomal hydroxylation to metabolites, some of which are active; 11-hydroxy-delta-9-tetrahydrocannabinol (11-OH-THC) is the major active metabolite

Half-life elimination: Biphasic: Alpha: 4 to 5 hours; Terminal: 25 to 36 hours

Time to peak, serum: 0.5 to 4 hours

Excretion: Feces (50%, <5% as unchanged drug); Urine (10% to 15%)

Dosing

Adult Note: Use caution when increasing the dose of dronabinol because of the increased frequency of dose-related adverse reactions at higher dosages.

Appetite stimulation in AIDS patients: Oral:

Capsules: Initial: 2.5 mg twice daily (before lunch and dinner); for patients unable to tolerate this dosage, may reduce to 2.5 mg once daily (in the evening or at bedtime). May increase dose gradually based on response and tolerability (maximum: 20 mg per day [in divided doses]).

Oral solution: Initial: 2.1 mg twice daily (1 hour before lunch and dinner); although most patients respond to this dose, if further therapeutic effect is desired and if tolerated, may gradually increase to 2.1 mg 1 hour before lunch and 4.2 mg 1 hour before dinner, and then (if needed) to 4.2 mg twice daily (1 hour before lunch and dinner). Maximum: 16.8 mg per day [in 2 divided doses]. In patients unable to tolerate 2.1 mg twice daily, consider 2.1 mg once daily (1 hour before dinner or at bedtime) to reduce the risk of CNS effects.

Chemotherapy-induced nausea and vomiting (manufacturer's labeling): Oral:

Capsules: 5 mg/m^2 administered 1 to 3 hours before chemotherapy, then give 5 mg/m^2/dose every 2 to 4 hours after chemotherapy for a total of 4 to 6 doses/day; increase doses in increments of 2.5 mg/m^2 based on response and tolerability (maximum: 15 mg/m^2/dose). **Note:** Initiate with the lowest recommended dose and titrate to response; most patients respond to 5 mg 3 to 4 times daily; based on initial results, the dose may be escalated during a chemotherapy cycle or with subsequent cycles.

Oral solution: Initial: 4.2 mg/m^2 (rounded to the nearest 0.1 mg increment [or to the nearest 0.1 mL measurable increment on the calibrated oral dosing syringe]) 1 to 3 hours prior to chemotherapy and then every 2 to 4 hours after chemotherapy for a total of 4 to 6 doses/day. Titrate dose in 2.1 mg/m^2 increments (during a cycle or in subsequent cycles) to clinical response. Maximum: 12.6 mg/m^2/dose and 4 to 6 doses/day.

Chemotherapy-induced nausea and vomiting, refractory (off-label dosing): Oral: Capsules: 2.5 to 10 mg 3 or 4 times daily (Lohr 2008)

Geriatric

Capsules: Refer to adult dosing.

Oral solution:

Appetite stimulation in AIDS patients: Initial: Consider 2.1 mg once daily (1 hour before dinner or at bedtime) to reduce the risk of central nervous system effects.

Chemotherapy-induced nausea and vomiting: Initial: Consider 2.1 mg/m^2 1 to 3 hours prior to chemotherapy to reduce the risk of central nervous system effects.

Pediatric Chemotherapy-induced nausea and vomiting: Oral: Capsules: Refer to adult dosing. Use caution when increasing the dose because of the increased frequency of dose-related adverse reactions at higher dosages.

Renal Impairment There are no dosage adjustments provided in the manufacturer's labeling.

Hepatic Impairment There are no dosage adjustments provided in the manufacturer's labeling.

Adjustment for Toxicity

Appetite stimulation in AIDS patients:

CNS adverse reactions: Reduce dose if needed. **Note:** Administering the dose later in the day may reduce the frequency of CNS adverse effects.

Dizziness, somnolence, confusion, or euphoria: Adverse effects typically resolve within 1 to 3 days and usually do not require dose reduction.

Severe or persistent CNS adverse effects: Reduce dose to 2.1 mg once daily 1 hour before dinner or in the evening at bedtime.

In patients unable to tolerate 2.1 mg twice daily, consider 2.1 mg once daily (1 hour before dinner or at bedtime) to reduce the risk of CNS effects.

Chemotherapy-induced nausea and vomiting:

CNS adverse reactions: Consider decreasing the dose to 2.1 mg once daily 1 to 3 hours prior to chemotherapy to reduce the risk of CNS adverse reactions.

Administration

Capsules: For appetite stimulation, administer twice-daily doses before lunch and dinner; administer single doses in the evening or at bedtime.

Oral solution: Always use the provided calibrated oral dosing syringe when administering to ensure dose is measured and administered accurately. If the prescribed dose is >5 mg, the total dose will need to be divided and drawn up in 2 or more portions using the oral syringe. Administer orally directly from oral dosing syringe; immediately follow with a full glass of water (180 to 240 mL).

Appetite stimulation in AIDS patients: Administer 1 hour before lunch and 1 hour before dinner initially; if persistent or severe CNS adverse effects occur, administering later in the day (1 hour before dinner and at bedtime) may reduce the frequency of CNS adverse effects.

Chemotherapy-induced nausea and vomiting: The first dose should be administered on an empty stomach at least 30 minutes prior to eating; subsequent doses within a chemotherapy cycle may be administered without regard to meals. Once a dose has been titrated, the timing of doses with regard to food in subsequent cycles should maintain consistency with prior cycles.

Monitoring Parameters Monitor heart rate and blood pressure. Monitor for CNS adverse effects, seizures, and substance abuse behavioral profile.

Dietary Considerations Capsules contain sesame oil.

Dosage Forms Excipient information presented when available (limited, particularly for generics); consult specific product labeling.

Capsule, Oral:

Marinol: 2.5 mg, 5 mg, 10 mg [contains sesame oil]

Generic: 2.5 mg, 5 mg, 10 mg

Solution, Oral:
Syndros: 5 mg/mL (30 mL) [contains alcohol, usp, methylparaben, polyethylene glycol, propylene glycol, propylparaben]
Controlled Substance Marinol: C-III; Syndros: C-II

◆ **Droxia** see Hydroxyurea on page 925

◆ **DTC 101** see Cytarabine (Liposomal) on page 481

◆ **DTIC** see Dacarbazine on page 494

◆ **DTIC-Dome** see Dacarbazine on page 494

◆ **D-Trp(6)-LHRH** see Triptorelin on page 1841

Durvalumab (dur VAL ue mab)

Brand Names: US Imfinzi
Index Terms MEDI4736
Pharmacologic Category Antineoplastic Agent, Anti-PD-L1 Monoclonal Antibody; Antineoplastic Agent, Monoclonal Antibody
Use Urothelial carcinoma, locally advanced or metastatic: Treatment of locally advanced or metastatic urothelial carcinoma in patients who have disease progression during or following platinum-containing chemotherapy, or disease progression within 12 months of neoadjuvant or adjuvant treatment with platinum-containing chemotherapy.
Labeled Contraindications There are no contraindications listed in the manufacturer's labeling.
Pregnancy Considerations Adverse events were observed in animal reproduction studies. Immunoglobulins are known to cross the placenta and fetal exposure to durvalumab may be expected. Based on the mechanism of action, durvalumab may cause fetal harm if administered to pregnant women. Women of reproductive potential should use effective contraception during therapy and for at least 3 months after the last dose.
Breastfeeding Considerations It is not known if durvalumab is present in breast milk; however, endogenous immunoglobulins are excreted in breast milk. Due to the potential for adverse events in a breastfed infant, breastfeeding is not recommended by the manufacturer during therapy or for at least 3 months after the last dose.
Warnings/Precautions Immune-mediated pneumonitis or interstitial lung disease has occurred in patients receiving durvalumab (including fatal cases). The median time to onset was ~56 days (range: 24 to 423 days). Monitor for signs/symptoms of pneumonitis; evaluate suspected pneumonitis with radiographic imaging and manage with systemic corticosteroids and treatment interruption or discontinuation. In one study, recovery occurred in approximately half of patients experiencing immune-mediated pneumonitis.

Immune-mediated hepatitis has occurred in patients receiving durvalumab (some fatal). The median time to onset was ~52 days (range: 15 to 312 days). Monitor for abnormal liver function tests each cycle during durvalumab treatment. Manage immune-mediated hepatitis with systemic corticosteroids and treatment interruption or discontinuation. In one study most patients experiencing immune-mediated hepatitis received high-dose corticosteroids; one patient also received mycophenolate. Recovery occurred in approximately half of patients experiencing immune-mediated hepatitis. Grade 3 or 4 ALT, AST, and/or total bilirubin elevations have been reported.

Immune-mediated colitis or diarrhea occurred in patients receiving durvalumab. Grades 3 and 4 diarrhea or colitis has been reported. The median time to onset is 73 days (range: 13 to 345 days). Monitor for signs/symptoms of colitis or diarrhea and manage with treatment interruption or discontinuation, antidiarrheal agents, and systemic corticosteroids. Resolution occurred in approximately half of patients who experienced immune-mediated diarrhea/colitis.

Immune-related thyroid disorders have occurred in patients receiving durvalumab. Monitor thyroid function at baseline and periodically during treatment; monitor for clinical signs and symptoms of thyroid disorders. Patients with abnormal thyroid function tests who are asymptomatic can receive durvalumab. Hypothyroid events included thyroiditis leading to hypothyroidism, grades 1 and 2 hypothyroidism, and elevated (above baseline) thyroid stimulating hormone (TSH). Manage hypothyroidism with hormone replacement (if indicated). The median time to first onset of hypothyroidism was 42 days (range: 15 to 239 days). Hyperthyroidism (grades 1 or 2) or thyroiditis leading to hyperthyroidism, and decreased or below baseline TSH also occurred. The median time to first onset of hyperthyroidism was 43 days (range: 14 to 71 days). Withhold durvalumab and manage symptomatically for hyperthyroidism. Treatment with a beta-blocker and/or thioamide was administered for hyperthyroidism in some patients. In several patients with thyroiditis, transient hyperthyroidism preceded hypothyroidism. Treatment with a beta-blocker and/or thioamide was administered for hyperthyroidism in five of these patients.

Immune-related adrenal insufficiency has been reported with durvalumab; monitor for clinical signs and symptoms of adrenal insufficiency. If adrenal insufficiency occurs, interrupt durvalumab treatment and if clinically indicated, administer systemic corticosteroids and hormone replacement. Immune-related type 1 diabetes mellitus has occurred in patients receiving durvalumab; monitor glucose and monitor for clinical signs and symptoms of diabetes; initiate insulin for type 1 diabetes mellitus and interrupt durvalumab treatment until clinically stable. Immune-related hypophysitis/hypopituitarism has occurred in patients receiving durvalumab. Monitor for clinical signs and symptoms of hypophysitis or hypopituitarism. If hypophysitis/hypopituitarism occurs, interrupt durvalumab until clinically stable and administer corticosteroids and hormone replacement as indicated. Hypopituitarism leading to adrenal insufficiency and diabetes insipidus has occurred (rarely).

Durvalumab has caused immune-mediated rash, including grade 3 rash and vitiligo. Monitor for signs and symptoms of dermatologic toxicity; may require treatment interruption or discontinuation; consider systemic corticosteroids if indicated. Durvalumab has caused immune thrombocytopenia (formerly known as immune thrombocytopenic purpura) (ITP). Monitor for signs and symptoms of ITP; may require treatment interruption or discontinuation and systemic corticosteroids with or without immunoglobulin or rituximab. Durvalumab has caused immune-mediated nephritis; monitor renal function prior to initiating treatment and before each cycle of durvalumab treatment. Nephritis may require systemic corticosteroids and treatment interruption or discontinuation; nephritis typically resolved following treatment with systemic corticosteroids. Other immune-related adverse reactions associated with durvalumab (rarely) include aseptic meningitis, hemolytic anemia, myocarditis, myositis, and ocular inflammatory toxicity including uveitis and keratitis.

Infections occurred in approximately one-third of patients receiving durvalumab. Severe infections, including sepsis, necrotizing fasciitis, and osteomyelitis have been reported. The most common grade 3 or 4 infections were urinary tract infections. Monitor for signs/symptoms of infection; if infection is suspected or confirmed, manage with anti-infectives. Withhold treatment for grade 3 or 4 infection.

Infusion reactions have been observed with durvalumab, including severe infusion-related reactions. Monitor for signs/symptoms of an infusion reactions. Interrupt or slow the infusion rate for mild or moderate infusion reactions (consider premedications with subsequent infusions). Discontinue durvalumab permanently for grade 3 or 4 infusion reactions. Urticaria developed (rarely), usually within 48 hours of durvalumab administration.

Potentially significant drug-drug interactions may exist, requiring dose or frequency adjustment, additional monitoring, and/or selection of alternative therapy. Some dosage forms may contain polysorbate 80 (also known as Tweens). Hypersensitivity reactions, usually a delayed reaction, have been reported following exposure to pharmaceutical products containing polysorbate 80 in certain individuals (Isaksson 2002; Lucente 2000; Shelley 1995). Thrombocytopenia, ascites, pulmonary deterioration, and renal and hepatic failure have been reported in premature neonates after receiving parenteral products containing polysorbate 80 (Alade 1986; CDC 1984). See manufacturer's labeling.

Adverse Reactions

>10%:

Cardiovascular: Peripheral edema (15%)

Central nervous system: Fatigue (39%)

Dermatologic: Skin rash (11% to 16%; including immune-mediated rashes)

Endocrine & metabolic: Hyponatremia (grades 3/4: 12%)

Gastrointestinal: Constipation (21%), decreased appetite (19%), nausea (16%), abdominal pain (14%), colitis (≤13%), diarrhea (≤13%)

Genitourinary: Urinary tract infection (4% to 15%)

Hematologic & oncologic: Lymphocytopenia (grades 3/4: 11%)

Infection: Infection (30% to 38%)

Neuromuscular & skeletal: Musculoskeletal pain (24%)

Respiratory: Dyspnea (≤13%), dyspnea on exertion (≤13%)

Miscellaneous: Fever (14%; including tumor-associated fever)

1% to 10%:

Cardiovascular: Myocarditis (≤1%; immune-mediated)

Central nervous system: Aseptic meningitis (≤1%; immune-mediated)

Endocrine & metabolic: Hypothyroidism (6% to 10%), hyperthyroidism (5% to 6%), hypermagnesemia (grades 3/4: 4%), dehydration (grades 3/4: ≥3%), hypercalcemia (grades 3/4: 3%), hyperglycemia (grades 3/4: 3%), hyperkalemia (grades 3/4: 1%), hypoalbuminemia (grades 3/4: 1%), hypokalemia (grades 3/4: 1%)

Hematologic & oncologic: Anemia (grades 3/4: 8%), neutropenia (grades 3/4: 1%), hemolytic anemia (≤1%; immune-mediated), immune thrombocytopenia (≤1%)

Hepatic: Increased serum alkaline phosphatase (grades 3/4: 4%), increased serum bilirubin (grades 3/4: 3%), increased serum AST (grades 3/4: 2%), hepatitis (1%), hyperbilirubinemia (grades 3/4: 1%), increased serum ALT (grades 3/4: 1%)

Immunologic: Antibody development (3%)

Neuromuscular & skeletal: Myositis (≤1%; immune-mediated)

Ophthalmic: Ocular toxicity (≤1%, immune-mediated; including uveitis and keratitis)

Renal: Increased serum creatinine (grades 3/4: 1%), nephritis (≤1%; immune-mediated)

Respiratory: Cough (≤10%), productive cough (≤10%), pneumonitis (2%)

Miscellaneous: Infusion-related reaction (2%)

Frequency not defined:

Endocrine & metabolic: Hypophysitis

Hepatic: Hepatic injury

Renal: Acute renal failure

<1%, postmarketing, and/or case reports: Adrenocortical insufficiency, pituitary insufficiency, type 1 diabetes mellitus, urticaria, vitiligo

Drug Interactions

Metabolism/Transport Effects None known.

Avoid Concomitant Use

Avoid concomitant use of Durvalumab with any of the following: Belimumab

Increased Effect/Toxicity

Durvalumab may increase the levels/effects of: Belimumab

Decreased Effect There are no known significant interactions involving a decrease in effect.

Storage/Stability Store intact vials at 2°C to 8°C (36°F to 46°F); do not freeze. Protect vials from light (store in original packaging). Do not shake. Solutions diluted for infusion should be used immediately after preparation. If not administered immediately, may be stored (from the time of vial puncture to the start of administration) for up to 24 hours refrigerated at 2°C to 8°C (36°F to 46°F) or for up to 4 hours at room temperature of 25°C (77°F). Do not freeze or shake diluted solution.

Preparation for Administration Withdraw appropriate volume from vial (solution should be clear to opalescent and colorless to slightly yellow and free of visible particles; do not use if cloudy, discolored or if visible particulates are present) and transfer to IV bag containing NS or D5W. Mix by gently inverting bag (do not shake). The final concentration of the diluted solution should be between 1 and 15 mg/mL. Discard unused portion of the vial.

Mechanism of Action Durvalumab is a human immunoglobulin G1 kappa monoclonal antibody which blocks programmed cell death ligand 1 (PD-L1) binding to PD-1 and CD80 (B7.1); PD-L1 blockade leads to increased T-cell activation, allowing T-cells to kill tumor cells (Massard 2016). PD-L1 is an immune check point protein expressed on tumor cells and tumor infiltrating cells and down regulates anti-tumor t-cell function by binding to PD-1 and B7.1; blocking PD-1 and B7.1 interactions restores antitumor t-cell function (Fehrenbacher 2016; Rosenberg 2016).

Pharmacodynamics/Kinetics

Distribution: V_{dss}: 5.6 L

Half-life, elimination: Terminal half-life: ~17 days

Excretion: Steady-state clearance: 8.24 mL/hour

Dosing

Adult & Geriatric Urothelial carcinoma, locally advanced or metastatic: IV: 10 mg/kg once every 2 weeks until disease progression or unacceptable toxicity.

◄ **Renal Impairment**

Renal impairment prior to treatment initiation:

CrCl 30 to 89 mL/minute: There are no dosage adjustments provided in the manufacturer's labeling; however, there is no clinically relevant effect on pharmacokinetics.

CrCl 15 to 29 mL/minute: There are no dosage adjustments provided in the manufacturer's labeling (has not been studied).

Renal toxicity during treatment (nephritis): **Note:** Based on the nephritis severity, withhold durvalumab and administer systemic corticosteroids (See **"Note"** in Dosing: Adjustment for Toxicity).

Nephritis, grade 2 (creatinine >1.5 to 3 times ULN): Withhold dose. Administer systemic corticosteroids (prednisone initial dose of 1 to 2 mg/kg daily or equivalent) followed by a taper.

Nephritis, grade 3 (creatinine >3 to 6 times ULN): Discontinue permanently. Administer systemic corticosteroids (prednisone initial dose of 1 to 2 mg/kg daily or equivalent) followed by a taper.

Nephritis, grade 4 (creatinine >6 times ULN): Discontinue permanently. Administer systemic corticosteroids (prednisone initial dose of 1 to 2 mg/kg daily or equivalent) followed by a taper.

Hepatic Impairment

Hepatic impairment prior to treatment initiation:

Mild impairment (bilirubin ≤ ULN and AST > ULN **or** bilirubin >1 to 1.5 times ULN and any AST): There are no dosage adjustments provided in the manufacturer's labeling; however, there is no clinically relevant effect on pharmacokinetics.

Moderate impairment (bilirubin >1.5 to 3 times ULN and any AST) or severe (bilirubin >3 times ULN and any AST): There are no dosage adjustments provided in the manufacturer's labeling (has not been studied).

Hepatotoxicity during treatment: **Note:** Based on the hepatitis severity, withhold durvalumab and administer systemic corticosteroids (see **"Note"** in Dosing: Adjustment for Toxicity).

Hepatitis, grade 2 (ALT or AST >3 to 5 times ULN or total bilirubin >1.5 to 3 times ULN): Withhold dose. Administer systemic corticosteroids (prednisone initial dose of 1 to 2 mg/kg daily or equivalent) followed by a taper.

Hepatitis, grade 3 (ALT or AST ≤8 times ULN or total bilirubin ≤5 times ULN): Withhold dose. Administer systemic corticosteroids (prednisone initial dose of 1 to 2 mg/kg daily or equivalent) followed by a taper.

Hepatitis, grade 3 (ALT or AST >8 times ULN or total bilirubin >5 times ULN): Discontinue permanently. Administer systemic corticosteroids (prednisone initial dose of 1 to 2 mg/kg daily or equivalent) followed by a taper.

Hepatitis, concurrent ALT or AST >3 times ULN and total bilirubin >2 times ULN with no other cause: Discontinue permanently. Administer systemic corticosteroids (prednisone initial dose of 1 to 2 mg/kg daily or equivalent) followed by a taper.

Adjustment for Toxicity

Withhold and/or discontinue durvalumab to manage adverse reactions (no dosage reductions are recommended). **Note:** Based on the severity of the adverse reaction, withhold durvalumab and administer systemic corticosteroids. Consider increasing the corticosteroid dose (and/or other immunosuppressants) if there is no improvement or if toxicity worsens. Begin corticosteroid taper when adverse reaction improves to below grade 1 and continue taper over at least 1 month. For adverse reactions that do not result in permanent discontinuation, when improved to grade 1 or lower and the corticosteroid dose is reduced to <10 mg/day prednisone (or equivalent), resume durvalumab.

Dermatologic toxicity:

Rash or dermatitis, grade 2 for >1 week or grade 3: Withhold dose. Consider systemic corticosteroids (prednisone initial dose of 1 to 2 mg/kg daily or equivalent) followed by a taper.

Rash or dermatitis, grade 4: Discontinue permanently. Consider systemic corticosteroids (prednisone initial dose of 1 to 2 mg/kg daily or equivalent) followed by a taper.

Endocrinopathies:

Adrenal insufficiency, hypophysitis/hypopituitarism, grades 2, 3, or 4: Withhold dose until clinically stable. Administer systemic corticosteroids (prednisone initial dose of 1 to 2 mg/kg daily or equivalent) followed by a taper. Administer hormone replacement therapy as clinically indicated.

Diabetes mellitus type 1, grades 2, 3, or 4: Withhold dose until clinically stable. Initiate insulin treatment as clinically indicated.

Hyperthyroidism, grades 2, 3, or 4: Withhold dose until clinically stable. Initiate symptomatic management.

Hypothyroidism, grades 2, 3, or 4: Initiate thyroid replacement therapy as clinically indicated.

GI toxicity:

Colitis or diarrhea, grade 2: Withhold dose. Administer systemic corticosteroids (prednisone initial dose of 1 to 2 mg/kg daily or equivalent) followed by a taper.

Colitis or diarrhea, grade 3 or 4: Discontinue permanently. Administer systemic corticosteroids (prednisone initial dose of 1 to 2 mg/kg daily or equivalent) followed by a taper.

Infection: Grade 3 or 4: Withhold dose. Initiate symptomatic management with anti-infectives for suspected or confirmed infections.

Infusion-related reactions:

Grade 1 or 2: Interrupt or slow infusion. Consider premedications with subsequent doses.

Grade 3 or 4: Discontinue permanently.

Pulmonary toxicity:

Pneumonitis, grade 2: Withhold dose. Administer systemic corticosteroids (prednisone initial dose of 1 to 2 mg/kg daily or equivalent) followed by a taper.

Pneumonitis, grade 3 or 4: Discontinue permanently. Administer systemic corticosteroids (prednisone initial dose of 1 to 4 mg/kg daily or equivalent) followed by a taper.

Other toxicities:

Grade 3: Withhold dose. Manage symptomatically.

Grade 4: Discontinue permanently. Consider systemic corticosteroids (prednisone initial dose of 1 to 4 mg/kg daily or equivalent) followed by a taper.

Administration

IV: Infuse over 60 minutes through an IV line containing a sterile, low-protein binding 0.2 or 0.22 micron in-line filter. Do not administer other medications through the same IV line.

Monitor for infusion reactions. Interrupt or slow the infusion for grade 1 or 2 infusion-related reactions (consider premedications with subsequent infusions); discontinue permanently for grade 3 or 4 reactions.

Monitoring Parameters Monitor liver function (during each cycle); renal function tests (prior to treatment and each cycle); thyroid function tests (at baseline, periodically during treatment); blood glucose. Monitor for clinical signs/symptoms of adrenal insufficiency, colitis/diarrhea, dermatologic toxicity, diabetes/hyperglycemia, hepatitis/hepatotoxicity, hypophysitis or hypopituitarism, immune thrombocytopenia purpura, infection, pneumonitis (evaluate suspected pneumonitis with radiographic imaging), thyroid disorders; monitor for infusion reactions.

Product Availability Imfinzi: FDA approved May 2017; anticipated availability is currently undetermined

Medication Guide Available Yes

Dosage Forms Excipient information presented when available (limited, particularly for generics); consult specific product labeling.

Solution, Intravenous [preservative free]:

Imfinzi: 120 mg/2.4 mL (2.4 mL); 500 mg/10 mL (10 mL) [contains polysorbate 80]

- ◆ **DVA** *see* Vindesine *on page 1910*
- ◆ **E7080** *see* Lenvatinib *on page 1112*
- ◆ **E7389** *see* EriBULin *on page 712*
- ◆ **EACA** *see* Aminocaproic Acid *on page 111*
- ◆ **E. coli Asparaginase** *see* Asparaginase (*E. coli*) *on page 178*
- ◆ **Econopred** *see* PrednisoLONE (Ophthalmic) *on page 1544*
- ◆ **Ecteinascidin** *see* Trabectedin *on page 1803*
- ◆ **Ecteinascidin 743** *see* Trabectedin *on page 1803*

Eculizumab (e kue LIZ oo mab)

Brand Names: US Soliris

Brand Names: Canada Soliris

Index Terms h5G1.1; Monoclonal Antibody 5G1.1; Monoclonal Antibody Anti-C5

Pharmacologic Category Monoclonal Antibody; Monoclonal Antibody, Complement Inhibitor

Use

Atypical hemolytic uremic syndrome: Treatment of atypical hemolytic uremic syndrome (aHUS) to inhibit complement-mediated thrombotic microangiopathy.

Limitation of use: Eculizumab is not indicated for the treatment of patients with Shiga toxin *Escherichia coli*-related hemolytic uremic syndrome.

Paroxysmal nocturnal hemoglobinuria: Treatment of paroxysmal nocturnal hemoglobinuria (PNH) to reduce hemolysis.

Labeled Contraindications

US labeling: Unresolved serious *Neisseria meningitidis* infection; patients not currently vaccinated against *Neisseria meningitidis* (unless risks of treatment delay outweigh risk of developing a meningococcal infection)

Canadian labeling: Hypersensitivity to eculizumab, murine proteins, or any component of the formulation; unresolved *Neisseria meningitidis* infection; patients not currently vaccinated against *Neisseria meningitidis* (unless receiving appropriate prophylactic antibiotic treatment until 2 weeks after vaccination)

Pregnancy Considerations Adverse events were observed in animal reproduction studies. Eculizumab crosses the placenta and can be detected in cord blood. Pregnant women with PNH and their fetuses have high rates of morbidity and mortality during pregnancy and the postpartum period. Treatment of PNH with eculizumab has been shown to increase fetal survival and decrease maternal complications (Kelly 2015). Use of eculizumab for the treatment of a HUS in pregnancy has also been described (Ardissino 2013).

Breastfeeding Considerations Excretion of eculizumab into breast milk was not noted in breast milk samples from 10 women. In a separate case report, eculizumab was detected in the initial breast milk sample of a woman, but not subsequent samples (Kelly 2015). The manufacturer recommends that caution be used if administered to nursing women.

Warnings/Precautions [US Boxed Warning]: Meningococcal *(Neisseria meningitidis)* **infections have occurred in patients receiving eculizumab; may be fatal or life-threatening if not detected and treated promptly. Monitor closely for early signs of meningococcal infection; evaluate and treat promptly if suspected. Follow current meningococcal immunization recommendations for patients with complement deficiencies. Vaccinate with meningococcal vaccines at least 2 weeks prior to initiation of treatment (unless the risks of delaying eculizumab outweigh the risk of developing meningococcal infection);** revaccinate according to current guidelines, considering the eculizumab duration of therapy. If urgent treatment is necessary in an unvaccinated patient, administer meningococcal vaccine(s) as soon as possible. Although the risk/benefits of prophylactic meningococcal antibiotic therapy have not been determined, prophylactic antibiotics were administered in clinical studies until at least 2 weeks after vaccination. Meningococcal infections developed in some patients despite vaccination. Discontinue eculizumab during the treatment of serious meningococcal infections. In addition to meningitis, the risk of other infections, especially encapsulated bacteria (eg, *Streptococcus pneumoniae, H. influenzae*) is increased with eculizumab treatment (because eculizumab blocks terminal complement activation). Aspergillus infections have occurred in immunocompromised and neutropenic patients. Children should receive vaccination for prevention of *S. pneumoniae, H. influenzae* according to current ACIP guidelines. Use with caution in patients with any systemic infection. Patients should be up to date with all immunizations before initiating therapy. **[US Boxed Warning]: Access is restricted through a REMS program. Prescribers must be enrolled in the program; enrollment and additional information is available at 1-888-765-4747 or solirisrems.com.** Counsel patients on the risk of meningococcal infection; ensure patients are vaccinated and provide educational materials.

Infusion reactions, including anaphylaxis or hypersensitivity, may occur; interrupt infusion for severe reaction (eg, cardiovascular instability, respiratory compromise). Continue monitoring for 1 hour after completion of infusion. Patients with PNH who discontinue treatment may be at increased risk for serious hemolysis; monitor closely for at least 8 weeks after treatment discontinuation. When used for aHUS, monitor for at least 12 weeks after treatment discontinuation for signs/symptoms of thrombotic microangiopathy (TMA) complications (angina, dyspnea, mental status changes, seizure, or thrombosis; occurrence of two or repeated measurement of any one of the following: Serum creatinine elevation (≥25% from baseline or nadir), serum LDH elevation (≥25% from baseline or nadir), thrombocytopenia (platelet decrease by ≥25% compared to baseline or peak). If TMA complications occur after stopping eculizumab, consider reinitiation of treatment, plasmapheresis, plasma exchange, fresh frozen plasma infusion, and/or appropriate organ-specific measures. In clinical trials, anticoagulant therapy was continued in patients who were receiving these agents (due to history of or risk for thromboembolism) prior to initiation of eculizumab. Potentially significant drug-drug interactions may exist, requiring dose or frequency adjustment, additional monitoring, and/or selection of alternative therapy. The effect of anticoagulant therapy withdrawal is unknown; treatment with eculizumab should not alter anticoagulation management

Adverse Reactions Frequency reported for adolescent and adult patients ≥13 years unless otherwise noted.

>10%:

Cardiovascular: Hypertension (aHUS: 17% to 59%; infants, children, and adolescents 5 months through 17 years: 18%), peripheral edema (20% to 29%), tachycardia (aHUS: children 21%), hypotension (12% to 20%)

Central nervous system: Headache (37% to 50%; serious: 2%; infants, children, and adolescents 5 months through 17 years: 18%), insomnia (10% to 24%), fatigue (7% to 20%)

Dermatologic: Skin rash (infants ≥5 months, children, adolescents, and adults: 12% to 18%), pruritus (6% to 15%)

Endocrine & metabolic: Hypokalemia (10% to 18%)

Gastrointestinal: Diarrhea (32% to 47%; infants, children, and adolescents 2 months through 17 years: 32%), vomiting (15% to 47%; infants, children, and adolescents 2 months through 17 years: 21% to 27%), nausea (12% to 40%), abdominal pain (15% to 30%), gastroenteritis (5% to 18%), dyspepsia (infants, children, and adolescents 5 months through 17 years: 14%)

Genitourinary: Urinary tract infection (15% to 35%; infants, children, and adolescents 5 months through 17 years: 18%), uropathy (infants, children, and adolescents 5 months through 17 years: 18%), proteinuria (5% to 12%)

Hematologic & oncologic: Anemia (17% to 35%; serious: 2%), neoplasm (6% to 30%), leukopenia (16% to 24%)

Local: Catheter infection (infants, children, and adolescents 5 months through 17 years: 14%)

Neuromuscular & skeletal: Weakness (15% to 20%), back pain (5% to 19%), arthralgia (6% to 17%), muscle spasm (infants, children, and adolescents 5 months through 17 years: 14%), limb pain (7% to 11%)

Ophthalmic: Eye disease (10% to 29%; infants, children, and adolescents 5 months through 17 years: 14%)

Renal: Renal insufficiency (15% to 29%)

Respiratory: Nasopharyngitis (18% to 55%; infants, children, and adolescents 5 months through 17 years: 27%), upper respiratory tract infection (infants ≥2 months, children, adolescents, and adults 5% to 40%), cough (infants ≥5 months, children, adolescents, and adults 12% to 36%), nasal congestion (aHUS: children 21%), rhinitis (infants, children, and adolescents 5 months through 17 years: 18%), bronchitis (10% to 18%), oropharyngeal pain (infants, children, and adolescents 5 months through 17 years: 14%)

Miscellaneous: Fever (infants, children, and adolescents 2 months through 17 years: 47% to 50%; adults 17% to 25%)

1% to 10%:

Gastrointestinal: Constipation (7%)

Immunologic: Antibody development (2% to 3%; neutralizing: 1%)

Infection: Herpes virus infection (7%), viral infection (serious: 2%), meningococcal infection (≤1%)

Neuromuscular & skeletal: Myalgia (7%)

Respiratory: Respiratory tract infection (7%), sinusitis (7%), flu-like symptoms (5%)

<1%, postmarketing, and/or case reports: Abdominal distention, anxiety,
aspergillosis, cholangitis, dizziness, dysgeusia, endometritis, hematoma
(mild), infusion related reaction, pyelonephritis

Drug Interactions

Metabolism/Transport Effects None known.

Avoid Concomitant Use

Avoid concomitant use of Eculizumab with any of the following: BCG (Intravesical); Belimumab; Natalizumab; Pimecrolimus; Tacrolimus (Topical); Vaccines (Live)

Increased Effect/Toxicity

Eculizumab may increase the levels/effects of: Belimumab; Fingolimod;
Leflunomide; Natalizumab; Tofacitinib; Vaccines (Live)

The levels/effects of Eculizumab may be increased by: Denosumab; Ocrelizumab; Pimecrolimus; Roflumilast; Tacrolimus (Topical); Trastuzumab

Decreased Effect

Eculizumab may decrease the levels/effects of: BCG (Intravesical); Coccidioides immitis Skin Test; Meningococcal Group B Vaccine; Nivolumab;
Sipuleucel-T; Tertomotide; Vaccines (Inactivated); Vaccines (Live)

The levels/effects of Eculizumab may be decreased by: Echinacea; Meningococcal Group B Vaccine

Storage/Stability Prior to dilution, store intact vials at 2°C to 8°C (36°F to
46°F); do not freeze. Vials may be held in the original carton at not more than
25°C (77°F) for only a single period up to 3 days. Protect from light; do not
shake. Following dilution, store at room temperature or refrigerate; use within
24 hours. If refrigerated, allow admixture to reach room temperature prior to
administration (do not use a heat source for warming).

Preparation for Administration Add eculizumab to an empty infusion bag
and dilute with an equal volume of D5W, sodium chloride 0.9%, sodium
chloride 0.45%, or Ringer's injection to a final concentration of 5 mg/mL
(eg, 300 mg to a total volume of 60 mL, 600 mg in a total volume of 120
mL, 900 mg in a total volume of 180 mL, or 1,200 mg to a total volume of 240
mL). Gently invert bag to mix thoroughly; do not shake.

Mechanism of Action Terminal complement-mediated intravascular hemolysis is a key clinical feature of paroxysmal nocturnal hemoglobinuria (PNH);
blocking the formation of membrane attack complex (MAC) results in stabilization of hemoglobin and a reduction in the need for RBC transfusions.
Impairment of complement activity regulation leads to uncontrolled complement activation in atypical hemolytic uremic syndrome (aHUS). Eculizumab is
a humanized monoclonal IgG antibody that binds to complement protein C5,
preventing cleavage into C5a and C5b. Blocking the formation of C5b inhibits
the subsequent formation of terminal complex C5b-9 or MAC.

Pharmacodynamics/Kinetics

Onset of action: PNH: Reduced hemolysis: ≤1 week

Distribution: PNH: 7.7 L; aHUS: 6.14 L

Half-life elimination: PNH: ~11 days (range: ~8 to 15 days); aHUS: ~12 days
(during plasma exchange the half-life is reduced to 1.26 hours)

◄ **Dosing**

Adult & Geriatric Note: Patients must receive meningococcal vaccine at least 2 weeks prior to treatment initiation; revaccinate according to current guidelines. Administer eculizumab at the recommended time interval or within 2 days of the interval.

Atypical hemolytic uremic syndrome (aHUS): IV: Induction: 900 mg weekly for 4 doses; Maintenance: 1,200 mg at week 5, then 1,200 mg every 2 weeks thereafter

Supplemental dosing for patients receiving plasmapheresis or plasma exchange: If most recent dose was ≥600 mg, administer 600 mg within 60 minutes after each plasmapheresis or plasma exchange

Supplemental dosing for patients receiving fresh frozen plasma infusion: If most recent dose was ≥300 mg, administer 300 mg within 60 minutes prior to each infusion of fresh frozen plasma

Paroxysmal nocturnal hemoglobinuria (PNH): IV: Induction: 600 mg weekly for 4 doses; Maintenance: 900 mg at week 5; then 900 mg every 2 weeks thereafter

Pediatric Note: Patients must receive meningococcal vaccine at least 2 weeks prior to treatment initiation; revaccinate according to current guidelines. Administer eculizumab at the recommended time interval or within 2 days of the interval.

Atypical hemolytic uremic syndrome (aHUS): IV:

Infants ≥2 months, Children, and Adolescents:

5 kg to <10 kg: Induction: 300 mg weekly for 1 dose; Maintenance: 300 mg at week 2, then 300 mg every 3 weeks

10 kg to <20 kg: Induction: 600 mg weekly for 1 dose; Maintenance: 300 mg at week 2, then 300 mg every 2 weeks

20 kg to <30 kg: Induction: 600 mg weekly for 2 doses; Maintenance: 600 mg at week 3, then 600 mg every 2 weeks

30 kg to <40 kg: Induction: 600 mg weekly for 2 doses; Maintenance: 900 mg at week 3, then 900 mg every 2 weeks

≥40 kg: Induction: 900 mg weekly for 4 doses; Maintenance: 1200 mg at week 5, then 1200 mg every 2 weeks

Supplemental dosing for patients receiving plasmapheresis or plasma exchange:

If most recent dose was 300 mg, administer 300 mg within 60 minutes after each plasmapheresis or plasma exchange

If most recent dose was ≥600 mg, administer 600 mg within 60 minutes after each plasmapheresis or plasma exchange

Supplemental dosing for patients receiving fresh frozen plasma infusion: If most recent dose was ≥300 mg, administer 300 mg within 60 minutes prior to each infusion of fresh frozen plasma

Renal Impairment There are no dosage adjustments provided in the manufacturer's labeling (has not been studied).

Hepatic Impairment There are no dosage adjustments provided in the manufacturer's labeling (has not been studied).

Administration IV: Allow to reach room temperature prior to administration. Infuse over 35 minutes in adults and over 1 to 4 hours in pediatric patients; do not administer as an IV push or bolus. Decrease infusion rate or discontinue for infusion reactions; do not exceed a maximum 2-hour duration of infusion in adults. Monitor for at least 1 hour following completion of infusion (for signs/symptoms of infusion reaction).

Monitoring Parameters CBC with differential, lactic dehydrogenase (LDH), serum creatinine, AST, urinalysis; early signs/symptoms of meningococcal infection; signs and symptoms of infusion reaction (during infusion and for 1 hour after infusion complete).

After discontinuation:
aHUS: Signs/symptoms of thrombotic microangiopathy (TMA) complications (monitor for at least 12 weeks after treatment discontinuation), including angina, dyspnea, mental status changes, seizure, or thrombosis; occurrence of two or repeated measurement of any one of the following: Serum creatinine elevation (≥25% from baseline or nadir), serum LDH elevation (≥25% from baseline or nadir), thrombocytopenia (platelet decrease by ≥25% compared to baseline or peak).
PNH: Signs and symptoms of intravascular hemolysis (monitor for at least 8 weeks after discontinuation), including anemia, fatigue, pain, dark urine, dyspnea, or thrombosis.

Medication Guide Available Yes

Dosage Forms Excipient information presented when available (limited, particularly for generics); consult specific product labeling.
Solution, Intravenous [preservative free]:
Soliris: 10 mg/mL (30 mL)

♦ **Efmoroctocog Alfa** *see* Antihemophilic Factor (Recombinant [Fc Fusion Protein]) *on page 147*

♦ **Efraloctocog Alfa** *see* Antihemophilic Factor (Recombinant) *on page 143*

♦ **Efudex** *see* Fluorouracil (Topical) *on page 835*

♦ **Eldisine** *see* Vindesine *on page 1910*

♦ **Eligard** *see* Leuprolide *on page 1131*

♦ **Elitek** *see* Rasburicase *on page 1581*

♦ **Ellence** *see* EpiRUBicin *on page 694*

♦ **Eloctate** *see* Antihemophilic Factor (Recombinant [Fc Fusion Protein]) *on page 147*

Elotuzumab (el oh TOOZ ue mab)

Related Information
Management of Chemotherapy-Induced Nausea and Vomiting in Adults *on page 2253*

Brand Names: US Empliciti
Brand Names: Canada Empliciti
Index Terms BMS-901608; HuLuc63; PDL-063
Pharmacologic Category Antineoplastic Agent, Anti-SLAMF7; Antineoplastic Agent, Monoclonal Antibody
Use Multiple myeloma, relapsed/refractory: Treatment of multiple myeloma (in combination with lenalidomide and dexamethasone) in patients who have received 1 to 3 prior therapies
Labeled Contraindications There are no contraindications listed in the manufacturer's US labeling.
Canadian labeling: Hypersensitivity to elotuzumab or any component of the formulation.
Pregnancy Considerations Animal reproduction studies have not been conducted. Elotuzumab is indicated for use in combination with lenalidomide. Due to its potential to cause fetal harm, lenalidomide is only available through ▶

◄ a REMS program. Males and females of reproductive potential using this combination must be able to comply with pregnancy testing and contraception requirements for lenalidomide. Refer to the Lenalidomide monograph for additional information.

Breastfeeding Considerations It is not known if elotuzumab is present in breast milk. Due to the potential for serious adverse reactions in the breastfed infant, breastfeeding is not recommended by the manufacturer.

Warnings/Precautions Infusion reactions (eg, fever, chills, hypertension) have been reported; all reactions were grade 3 or lower. Bradycardia and hypotension have also occurred during infusion. The majority of infusion reactions (~70%) occurred during the first dose. Premedicate with dexamethasone, H_1- and H_2-blockers, and acetaminophen prior to each dose. Administer in a facility with immediate access to resuscitative measures (eg, glucocorticoids, epinephrine, bronchodilators, and/or oxygen). May require treatment interruption, infusion rate modification, and/or discontinuation.

Infections were reported in the majority of multiple myeloma patients treated in the clinical trial, including fatal infections. Monitor for opportunistic, fungal, herpes zoster, and other infections during therapy; treat promptly if infections occur. Invasive second primary malignancies have been reported. The rate of hematologic malignancies was the same between the elotuzumab/lenalidomide/dexamethasone group versus the lenalidomide/dexamethasone group. Solid tumors and skin cancer were reported more frequently in the elotuzumab arm versus the control group. Monitor for the development of secondary malignancies.

Liver enzyme elevations (AST/ALT more than 3 times ULN, total bilirubin more than 2 times ULN, and alkaline phosphatase less than 2 times ULN) have occurred. Monitor liver function tests periodically; may require treatment interruption and/or discontinuation. Elotuzumab (a human IgG kappa monoclonal antibody) may be detected on serum protein electrophoresis and immunofixation assays which monitor for endogenous M-protein. Interference with these assays by elotuzumab may affect the determination of complete response and disease progression in some patients with IgG kappa myeloma protein. Potentially significant interactions may exist, requiring dose or frequency adjustment, additional monitoring, and/or selection of alternative therapy. Some dosage forms may contain polysorbate 80 (also known as Tweens). Hypersensitivity reactions, usually a delayed reaction, have been reported following exposure to pharmaceutical products containing polysorbate 80 in certain individuals (Isaksson 2002; Lucente 2000; Shelley 1995). Thrombocytopenia, ascites, pulmonary deterioration, and renal and hepatic failure have been reported in premature neonates after receiving parenteral products containing polysorbate 80 (Alade 1986; CDC 1984). See manufacturer's labeling.

Adverse Reactions

All incidences reported in combination with lenalidomide and dexamethasone.
>10%:

  Cardiovascular: Decreased heart rate (66%; <60 bpm), increased heart rate (48%; ≥100 bpm), altered blood pressure (systolic ≥160 mmHg: 33%; systolic <90 mmHg: 29%; diastolic ≥100 mmHg: 17%)

  Central nervous system: Fatigue (62%), peripheral neuropathy (27%; grades 3/4: 4%), headache (15%)

Endocrine & metabolic: Hyperglycemia (89%), hypocalcemia (78%), hypo-albuminemia (73%), decreased serum bicarbonate (63%), hyperkalemia (32%), weight loss (14%)

Gastrointestinal: Diarrhea (47%), constipation (36%), decreased appetite (21%), vomiting (15%)

Hematologic & oncologic: Lymphocytopenia (13% to 99%; grades 3/4: 9% to 77%), leukopenia (91%; grades 3/4: 32%), thrombocytopenia (84%; grades 3/4: 19%)

Hepatic: Increased serum alkaline phosphatase (39%; grades 3/4: 1%)

Immunologic: Immunogenicity (19%; neutralizing: 6%)

Infection: Infection (81%; grades 3/4: 28%), opportunistic infection (22%), herpes zoster (14%), fungal infection (10%)

Neuromuscular & skeletal: Limb pain (16%)

Ophthalmic: Cataract (12%)

Respiratory: Cough (34%), nasopharyngitis (25%), upper respiratory tract infection (23%), pneumonia (15% to 20%), oropharyngeal pain (10%)

Miscellaneous: Fever (7% to 37%), infusion related reaction (10%; grade 3: 1%)

1% to 10%:

Cardiovascular: Chest pain (≥5%), pulmonary embolism (3%)

Central nervous system: Hypoesthesia (≥5%), mood changes (≥5%)

Dermatologic: Night sweats (≥5%)

Hematologic & oncologic: Second primary malignant neoplasm (9%), malignant neoplasm of skin (4%), solid tumor (4%), anemia (3%), malignant neoplasm (hematologic: 2%)

Hepatic: Hepatotoxicity (3%)

Hypersensitivity: Hypersensitivity (≥5%)

Renal: Acute renal failure (3%)

Respiratory: Respiratory tract infection (3%)

Drug Interactions

Metabolism/Transport Effects None known.

Avoid Concomitant Use

Avoid concomitant use of Elotuzumab with any of the following: BCG (Intravesical); Belimumab; Natalizumab; Pimecrolimus; Tacrolimus (Topical); Vaccines (Live)

Increased Effect/Toxicity

Elotuzumab may increase the levels/effects of: Belimumab; Fingolimod; Leflunomide; Natalizumab; Tofacitinib; Vaccines (Live)

The levels/effects of Elotuzumab may be increased by: Denosumab; Ocrelizumab; Pimecrolimus; Roflumilast; Tacrolimus (Topical); Trastuzumab

Decreased Effect

Elotuzumab may decrease the levels/effects of: BCG (Intravesical); Coccidioides immitis Skin Test; Nivolumab; Sipuleucel-T; Tertomotide; Vaccines (Inactivated); Vaccines (Live)

The levels/effects of Elotuzumab may be decreased by: Echinacea

Storage/Stability Store intact vials at 2°C to 8°C (36°F to 46°F). Protect from light (store in the original packaging until use); do not freeze or shake. Solutions diluted for infusion in NS or D5W may be stored at 2°C to 8°C (36°F to 46°F) for up to 24 hours (protected from light). A maximum of 8 hours of the 24 hour storage time may be at room temperature and room light. Infusion must be completed within 24 hours of lyophilized powder reconstitution

◄ **Preparation for Administration** Reconstitute the 300 mg vial with 13 mL of SWFI, and the 400 mg vial with 17 mL of SWFI (to a concentration of 25 mg/mL) with an 18-gauge or lower (eg, 17-gauge) needle. Slight back pressure may occur during reconstitution. Rotate the vial to dissolve the lyophilized powder (holding the vial upright). To dissolve any powder on the stopper or top of the vial, invert the vial several times; avoid vigorous agitation. **Do not shake.** The powder should dissolve in <10 minutes. After dissolution, allow the reconstituted vials to stand for 5 to 10 minutes (solution should be colorless to slightly yellow, clear to slightly opalescent). Discard if any particulate matter or discoloration is observed.

Each vial contains overfill to allow for withdrawal of 12 mL (300 mg vial) and 16 mL (400 mg vial), respectively. Withdraw appropriate dose from each vial (maximum of 12 mL from the 300 mg vial and 16 mL from the 400 mg vial). Further dilute with 230 mL of NS or D5W in a polyvinyl chloride or polyolefin infusion bag; the volume of diluent may be adjusted in order to not exceed 5 mL/kg of body weight. Do not mix with other medications.

To minimize manipulation and preparation steps, dilution in 250 mL NS or D5W (instead of 230 mL) has been reported; dilution in 500 mL NS or D5W was used if the concentration exceeded 6 mg/mL. Infusion rates followed the manufacturer's product labeling (Hofmeister 2016).

Mechanism of Action Elotuzumab is a humanized IgG1 immunostimulatory monoclonal antibody directed against signaling lymphocytic activation molecule family member 7 (SLAMF7, also called CS1 [cell surface glycoprotein CD2 subset 1). SLAMF7 is expressed on most myeloma and natural killer cells, but not on normal tissues; more than 95% of bone marrow myeloma cells express SLAMF7 (Lonial 2015). Elotuzumab directly activates natural killer cells through both the SLAMF7 pathway and Fc receptors. It also targets SLAMF7 on myeloma cells and mediates antibody-dependent cellular cytotoxicity (ADCC) through the CD16 pathway (Lonial 2015). This immunostimulatory activity, through the increased activation of natural killer cells, increases anti-tumor activity.

Pharmacodynamics/Kinetics Half-life elimination: ~97% of the maximum steady-state concentration is expected to be eliminated with a geometric mean (CV%) of 82.4 days.

Dosing

Adult & Geriatric Note: Premedicate with dexamethasone, an H_1-blocker (eg, diphenhydramine), an H_2-blocker (eg, ranitidine), and acetaminophen ~45 to 90 minutes prior to infusion (see Premedications below). Refer to the Lenalidomide and Dexamethasone (Systemic) monographs for dosing information.

Multiple myeloma, relapsed/refractory: IV: Continue until disease progression or unacceptable toxicity (Lonial 2015)

Cycles 1 and 2: 10 mg/kg once weekly on days 1, 8, 15, and 22 of a 28-day treatment cycle (in combination with lenalidomide and dexamethasone)

Cycle 3 and beyond: 10 mg/kg once every 2 weeks on days 1 and 15 of a 28-day treatment cycle (in combination with lenalidomide and dexamethasone)

Premedications:

Dexamethasone: Oral and IV: On days that elotuzumab is administered, give dexamethasone 28 mg **orally** 3 to 24 hours before elotuzumab infusion **plus** dexamethasone 8 mg **IV** 45 to 90 minutes prior to infusion. On days that elotuzumab is **not** administered but dexamethasone is due (eg, days 8 and 22 of cycle 3 and beyond), administer the standard dexamethasone dose (40 mg orally).

Due to compliance concerns on days that elotuzumab is administered, a one-time dexamethasone dose of 20 to 40 mg IV has been reported (in lieu of administering both oral and IV dexamethasone) (Hofmeister 2016).

Antipyretic: Oral: Acetaminophen 650 to 1,000 mg

H₁-blocker: IV or Oral: Diphenhydramine 25 to 50 mg or equivalent

H_1-blocker: IV or Oral: Diphenhydramine 25 to 50 mg or equivalent

H_2-blocker: Ranitidine: 50 mg IV or 150 mg orally or equivalent. The use of famotidine 20 mg IV has also been reported (Hofmeister 2016).

Renal Impairment CrCl ≤89 mL/minute: There are no dosage adjustments provided in the manufacturer's labeling; however, based on pharmacokinetics, dosage adjustment is not likely necessary.

Hepatic Impairment

Hepatic impairment prior to treatment:

Mild (total bilirubin ≤ULN and AST >ULN **or** total bilirubin 1 to 1.5 times ULN and any AST) impairment: There are no dosage adjustments provided in the manufacturer's labeling; however, based on pharmacokinetics, dosage adjustment is not likely necessary.

Moderate (total bilirubin >1.5 to 3 times ULN and any AST) to severe (total bilirubin >3 times ULN and any AST) impairment: There are no dosage adjustments provided in the manufacturer's labeling (has not been studied).

Hepatotoxicity during treatment: Grade 3 or higher transaminase elevations: Withhold treatment; may consider continuing treatment after liver enzymes return to baseline.

Adjustment for Toxicity

Refer to Lenalidomide monograph for dosage modifications for toxicity. If dosing of one drug in the regimen is delayed, interrupted, or discontinued, treatment with the other medications may continue as scheduled. However, if dexamethasone is delayed or discontinued, administer elotuzumab based on clinical judgment (due to hypersensitivity risk).

Infusion reactions: Grade 2 or greater: Interrupt infusion and manage symptoms as clinically appropriate. When symptoms improve to ≤ grade 1, restart elotuzumab infusion at a rate of 0.5 mL/minute and gradually increase the rate by 0.5 mL/minute every 30 minutes as tolerated to the rate at which the infusion reaction occurred. May continue to escalate the rate if there is no recurrence of the infusion reaction (see Administration). Monitor vital signs every 30 minutes during and for 2 hours after the end of the infusion in patients who experience an infusion reaction. If the reaction recurs, discontinue the elotuzumab infusion and do not restart on that day. Severe infusion reactions may require therapy discontinuation and emergency management.

Combination Regimens

Multiple Myeloma: Elotuzumab-Lenalidomide-Dexamethasone (Multiple Myeloma) on page 2100

Administration For IV infusion only. Do not administer IV push or as a bolus. Premedicate with dexamethasone, acetaminophen, and an H_1- and H_2-blocker (see Dosing) approximately 45 to 90 minutes prior to administration. Infuse in an environment equipped to monitor for and manage infusion reactions. Administer with an infusion set and a sterile, non-pyrogenic, low protein-binding filter (0.2 to 1.2 micrometer) using an automated infusion pump. Do not mix with or infuse with other medications. Infusion should be completed within 24 hours of reconstitution. Monitor for infusion reaction. Interrupt infusion for grade 2 or higher infusion reactions; if the reaction resolves or improves to ≤ grade 1, may resume infusion (see Dosing: Adjustment for Toxicity). Monitor vital signs every 30 minutes during and for 2 hours after the end of the infusion in patients who experience an infusion reaction.

Infusion rate:
First infusion (Cycle 1, Dose 1): Infuse at 0.5 mL/minute for the first 30 minutes. If no infusion reactions occur, may increase the rate to 1 mL/minute for the next 30 minutes. If tolerated, may then increase the rate to 2 mL/minute until infusion completion (maximum rate: 2 mL/minute).
Second infusion (Cycle 1, Dose 2): If no infusion reactions occurred during the prior infusion, initiate at 3 mL/minute for the first 30 minutes. If tolerated, may then increase the rate to 4 mL/minute until infusion completion (maximum rate: 4 mL/minute).
Subsequent infusions (Cycle 1, Doses 3 and 4 and all subsequent infusions): If no infusion reactions occurred during the prior infusion, initiate and infuse at 5 mL/minute until completion (maximum rate: 5 mL/minute).

Emetic Potential Minimal (<10%)

Monitoring Parameters Liver function tests (periodically); signs/symptoms of infusion reactions (monitor vital signs every 30 minutes during and for 2 hours after the end of the infusion in patients who experience an infusion reaction), infections, and second primary malignancies

Test Interactions Elotuzumab may be detected on both serum protein electrophoresis (SPEP) and serum immunofixation assays used for multiple myeloma endogenous M-protein monitoring, and may affect the determination of complete response and disease progression of some patients with IgG kappa myeloma protein. A small peak in the early gamma region on SPEP that is IgG kappa on serum immunofixation may potentially be attributed to elotuzumab (especially when endogenous myeloma protein is IgA, IgM, IgD, or lambda light chain restricted).

Dosage Forms Excipient information presented when available (limited, particularly for generics); consult specific product labeling.
Solution Reconstituted, Intravenous:
Empliciti: 300 mg (1 ea); 400 mg (1 ea) [contains mouse (murine) and/or hamster protein, polysorbate 80]

♦ **Eloxatin** see Oxaliplatin on page 1394
♦ **Eloxatin [DSC]** see Oxaliplatin on page 1394
♦ **Elspar** see Asparaginase (E. coli) on page 178
♦ **Elspar [DSC]** see Asparaginase (E. coli) on page 178

Eltrombopag (el TROM boe pag)

Brand Names: US Promacta
Brand Names: Canada Revolade
Index Terms Eltrombopag Olamine; Revolade; SB-497115; SB-497115-GR
Pharmacologic Category Colony Stimulating Factor; Hematopoietic Agent; Thrombopoietic Agent
Use
Aplastic anemia, severe: Treatment of severe aplastic anemia in patients who have had an insufficient response to immunosuppressive therapy.

Chronic hepatitis C infection-associated thrombocytopenia: Treatment of thrombocytopenia in patients with chronic hepatitis C (CHC) to allow the initiation and maintenance of interferon-based therapy.

Chronic immune (idiopathic) thrombocytopenia: Treatment of thrombocytopenia in adult and pediatric patients ≥1 year of age with chronic immune (idiopathic) thrombocytopenia (ITP) who have had insufficient response to corticosteroids, immune globulin, or splenectomy.

Limitations of use: For ITP, eltrombopag should only be used if the degree of thrombocytopenia and clinical condition increase the risk for bleeding. For chronic hepatitis C (CHC), eltrombopag should only be used if the degree of thrombocytopenia prevents initiation of or limits the ability to maintain interferon-based therapy. For CHC, safety and efficacy have not been established when used in combination with direct-acting antiviral agents without interferon for treatment of CHC infection.

Labeled Contraindications
There are no contraindications listed in the manufacturer's US labeling.
Canadian labeling: Hypersensitivity to eltrombopag or any component of the formulation; severe hepatic impairment (Child-Pugh class C)

Pregnancy Considerations Adverse effects were observed in animal reproduction studies. A Promacta pregnancy registry has been established to monitor outcomes of women exposed to eltrombopag during pregnancy (1-888-825-5249).

Breastfeeding Considerations It is not known if eltrombopag is excreted in breast milk. Due to the potential for serious adverse effects in the nursing infant, a decision should be made to discontinue therapy or to discontinue breastfeeding, taking into account the importance of treatment to the mother.

Warnings/Precautions [US Boxed Warning]: Eltrombopag may increase the risk of severe and potentially life-threatening hepatotoxicity. Monitor hepatic function and discontinue dosing as recommended. Liver enzyme elevations may occur; obtain ALT, AST, and bilirubin prior to treatment initiation, every 2 weeks during adjustment phase, then monthly (after stable dose established). Eltrombopag inhibits UGT1A1 and OATP1B1, which may lead to indirect hyperbilirubinemia; obtain fractionation for elevated bilirubin levels. Repeat abnormal liver function tests within 3 to 5 days; if confirmed abnormal, monitor weekly until resolves, stabilizes, or returns to baseline. Discontinue treatment for ALT levels ≥3 times the upper limit of normal (ULN) in patients with normal hepatic function, or ≥3 times baseline (or >5 times ULN; whichever is lower) in those with preexisting transaminase elevations and which are progressively increasing, or persistent (≥4 weeks), or accompanied by increased direct bilirubin, or accompanied by clinical signs of liver injury or evidence of hepatic decompensation. Hepatotoxicity may reoccur with re-treatment after therapy interruption; however, if the benefit of treatment outweighs the hepatotoxicity risk, initiate carefully, and monitor liver function tests weekly during the dose adjustment phase; permanently discontinue if liver abnormalities persist, worsen, or recur with rechallenge. In clinical trials, isolated cases of severe liver injury occurred, liver function test abnormalities usually occurred ~3 months after initiation of eltrombopag and resolved with discontinuation. Use with caution in patients with preexisting hepatic impairment (clearance may be reduced); dosage reductions are recommended in patients with ITP (except children 1 to 5 years) and severe aplastic anemia who have hepatic dysfunction (no initial dose reductions are necessary in patients with chronic hepatitis C-related thrombocytopenia); monitor closely.

▶

◄ **[US Boxed Warning]: May increase risk of hepatic decompensation when used in combination with interferon and ribavirin in patients with chronic hepatitis C.** In clinical trials, patients with low albumin (<3.5 g/dL) or a Model for End-Stage Liver Disease (MELD) score ≥10 at baseline had an increased risk of hepatic decompensation; closely monitor these patients during therapy. If antiviral therapy is discontinued for hepatic decompensation according to interferon/ribavirin recommendations, eltrombopag should also be discontinued. Indirect hyperbilirubinemia is commonly observed with eltrombopag when used in combination with peginterferon and ribavirin. In addition, ascites, encephalopathy, and thrombotic events were reported more frequently than placebo in chronic hepatitis C trials.

Monitor peripheral blood smear for cellular morphologic abnormalities; analyze CBC monthly; discontinue treatment with onset of new or worsening abnormalities (eg, teardrop and nucleated RBC, immature WBC) or cytopenias and consider bone marrow biopsy (with staining for fibrosis).

Thromboembolism may occur with excessive increases in platelet levels. Use with caution in patients with known risk factors for thromboembolism (eg, Factor V Leiden, ATIII deficiency, antiphospholipid syndrome, chronic liver disease). Thrombotic events, primarily involving the portal venous system, were more commonly seen in eltrombopag-treated chronic hepatitis C patients with thrombocytopenia (when compared to placebo). Thrombotic events (including portal venous thrombosis) were also reported in a study of non-ITP thrombocytopenic patients with chronic liver disease undergoing elective invasive procedures receiving eltrombopag 75 mg once daily. Symptoms of portal vein thrombosis include abdominal pain, nausea, vomiting, and diarrhea. The risk for portal venous thrombosis is increased in thrombocytopenic patients with chronic liver disease receiving 75 mg once daily for 2 weeks as preparation for invasive procedures.

Cataract formation or worsening was observed in clinical trials. Monitor regularly for signs and symptoms of cataracts; obtain ophthalmic exam at baseline and during therapy. Use with caution in patients at risk for cataracts (eg, advanced age, long-term glucocorticoid use). Potentially significant drug-drug interactions may exist, requiring dose or frequency adjustment, additional monitoring, and/or selection of alternative therapy. Patients of East-Asian ethnicity (eg, Chinese, Japanese, Korean, Taiwanese) may have greater drug exposure (compared to non-East Asians); therapy should be initiated with lower starting doses in ITP and severe aplastic anemia patients. Use with caution in renal impairment (any degree) and monitor closely; initial dosage adjustment is not necessary.

Do not use to normalize platelet counts. *ITP:* Indicated only when the degree of thrombocytopenia and clinical conditions increase the risk for bleeding in patients with chronic immune ITP; use the lowest dose necessary to achieve and maintain platelet count ≥50,000/mm^3. Discontinue if platelet count does not respond to a level to avoid clinically important bleeding after 4 weeks at the maximum recommended dose. *Chronic hepatitis C-associated thrombocytopenia:* Use only when thrombocytopenia prevents the initiation and maintenance of interferon-based therapy; discontinue if antiviral therapy is discontinued. Safety and efficacy have not been established when combined with direct acting antiviral medications approved for chronic hepatitis C genotype 1 infection therapy. *Severe aplastic anemia:* Use the lowest dose to achieve and maintain hematologic response. Discontinue if no hematologic response has occurred after 16 weeks of therapy, excessive platelet count responses or important liver test abnormalities. Consider discontinuation if new cytogenetic abnormalities are observed.

Adverse Reactions Adverse reactions and incidences reported are associated with adults unless otherwise indicated.

>10%:

Central nervous system: Fatigue (ITP: 5%; chronic hepatitis C: 28%; aplastic anemia: 28%), headache (ITP: 10%; chronic hepatitis C: 21%; aplastic anemia 21%), insomnia (chronic hepatitis C: 16%), chills (chronic hepatitis C: 14%), dizziness (aplastic anemia: 14%)

Dermatologic: Pruritus (chronic hepatitis C: 15%), ecchymosis (aplastic anemia: 12%)

Gastrointestinal: Nausea (ITP: 4% to 9%; chronic hepatitis C: 19%; aplastic anemia 33%), diarrhea (aplastic anemia: 21%; chronic hepatitis C: 19%; ITP: 3% to 9%; children and adolescents: 9%), appetite decreased (chronic hepatitis C: 18%), abdominal pain (aplastic anemia 12%; children and adolescents: 8%)

Hematologic & oncologic: Anemia (chronic hepatitis C: 40%), febrile neutropenia (aplastic anemia: 14%)

Hepatic: Hyperbilirubinemia (total bilirubin ≥1.5 x ULN: 76%; ITP and chronic hepatitis C: 3% to 8%), increased serum transaminases (aplastic anemia: 12%), abnormal hepatic function (ITP: 11%), increased serum ALT (children and adolescents: 6%; ITP: 6%), increased serum AST (ITP: 5%; children and adolescents: 4%)

Neuromuscular & skeletal: Limb pain (aplastic anemia: 19%), weakness (chronic hepatitis C: 16%), arthralgia (aplastic anemia: 12%), muscle spasm (aplastic anemia: 12%), myalgia (ITP and chronic hepatitis C: 5% to 12%)

Respiratory: Cough (aplastic anemia: 23%; chronic hepatitis C: 15%; children and adolescents: 9%), flu-like syndrome (chronic hepatitis C: 18%), upper respiratory infection (children and adolescents: 17%; ITP: 7%), dyspnea (aplastic anemia: 14%), oropharyngeal pain (aplastic anemia: 14%; children and adolescents: 8%; ITP: 4%), nasopharyngitis (children and adolescents: 12%), rhinorrhea (aplastic anemia: 12%, children and adolescents: 4%)

Miscellaneous: Fever (chronic hepatitis C: 30%; aplastic anemia: 14%; children and adolescents: 9%)

1% to 10%:

Cardiovascular: Peripheral edema (chronic hepatitis C: 10%), thrombosis (chronic hepatitis C: 3%)

Dermatologic: Alopecia (ITP: 2%; chronic hepatitis C: 10%), skin rash (chronic hepatitis C: 9%; aplastic anemia: 7%; children and adolescents: 5%; ITP: 3%)

Gastrointestinal: Toothache (children and adolescents: 6%), vomiting (ITP: 6%), xerostomia (ITP: 2%)

Genitourinary: Urinary tract infection (ITP: 5%)

Hematologic & oncologic: Thrombocytopenia (chronic hepatitis C: 3%)

Hepatic: Alkaline phosphatase increased (ITP: 2%)

Infection: Influenza (ITP: 3%)

Neuromuscular & skeletal: Back pain (ITP: 3%), paresthesia (ITP: 3%), musculoskeletal pain (ITP: 2%)

Ophthalmic: Cataract (ITP and chronic hepatitis C: 4% to 8%)

Respiratory: Rhinitis (children and adolescents: 9%), pharyngitis (ITP: 4%)

▶

◄ <1%, postmarketing, and/or case reports: Abdominal distension, constipation, decreased visual acuity, deep vein thrombosis, desquamation, drowsiness, dry eye syndrome, dysesthesia, dysgeusia, dyspepsia, eye pain, facial swelling, fecal discoloration, foreign body sensation, glossalgia, hemorrhage, hemorrhoids, hot flash, hyperhidrosis, hypoesthesia, hypokalemia, increased hemoglobin, increased lacrimation, increased serum albumin, increased serum creatinine, increased serum total protein, lesion (hepatic), local inflammation (wound), malaise, malignant neoplasm (rectosigmoid), night sweats, oral herpes, oropharyngeal blistering, ostealgia, portal vein thrombosis, pulmonary embolism, pulmonary infarct, retinal hemorrhage, retinal pigment changes, sinus tachycardia, skin discoloration (including hyperpigmentation and skin yellowing), sleep disorder, superficial thrombophlebitis, tachycardia, thromboembolic complications, thrombotic microangiopathy (with acute renal failure), upper abdominal pain, urticaria, vertigo

Drug Interactions

Metabolism/Transport Effects Substrate of BCRP, CYP1A2 (minor), CYP2C8 (minor), UGT1A1, UGT1A3; **Note:** Assignment of Major/Minor substrate status based on clinically relevant drug interaction potential; **Inhibits** BCRP, SLCO1B1, UGT1A1, UGT1A3, UGT1A4, UGT1A6, UGT1A9, UGT2B15, UGT2B7

Avoid Concomitant Use

Avoid concomitant use of Eltrombopag with any of the following: Asunaprevir; Grazoprevir; Irinotecan Products; PAZOPanib; Voxilaprevir

Increased Effect/Toxicity

Eltrombopag may increase the levels/effects of: Asunaprevir; BCRP/ABCG2 Substrates; Deferiprone; Eluxadoline; Grazoprevir; Irinotecan Products; OATP1B1/SLCO1B1 Substrates; PAZOPanib; Rosuvastatin; Topotecan; Voxilaprevir

Decreased Effect

The levels/effects of Eltrombopag may be decreased by: Aluminum Hydroxide; Calcium Salts; CycloSPORINE (Systemic); Iron Salts; Magnesium Salts; Multivitamins/Minerals (with ADEK, Folate, Iron); Multivitamins/Minerals (with AE, No Iron); Selenium; Sucralfate; Zinc Salts

Food Interactions Food, especially dairy products, may decrease the absorption of eltrombopag. Management: Take on an empty stomach at least 1 hour before or 2 hours after a meal. Take eltrombopag at least 2 hours before and 4 hours after foods high in calcium.

Storage/Stability

Oral suspension: Store at 20°C to 25°C (68°F to 77°F); excursions permitted to 15°C to 30°C (59°F to 86°F). Once reconstituted (if not used immediately), the suspension may be stored for a maximum of 30 minutes between 20°C and 25°C (68°F to 77°F); excursions permitted to 15°C to 30°C (59°F to 86°F). Discard the mixture if not used within 30 minutes.

Tablets: Store at 20°C to 25°C (68°F to 77°F); excursions are permitted between 15°C and 30°C (59°F and 86°F). If present, do not remove desiccant. Dispense in original bottle.

Preparation for Administration The oral suspension must be reconstituted with cool or cold water only (do not use hot water). Fill the provided oral syringe with 20 mL of drinking water and empty into the mixing bottle. Add the appropriate eltrombopag dose to the mixing bottle; gently and slowly shake the bottle for at least 20 seconds to mix. If not used immediately, suspension may be stored for up to 30 minutes at room temperature; discard any solution if not used within 30 minutes. Following administration, discard suspension remaining in bottle in trash (do not dispose of in drain); clean supplies by removing plunger from oral syringe, rinse bottle, lid, syringe, and plunger under running water and air-dry (bottle may stain, this is normal); wash hands with soap and water. If powder or suspension spills during preparation or administration, consider wearing disposable gloves during spill clean-up to avoid staining skin.

Mechanism of Action Thrombopoietin (TPO) nonpeptide agonist which increases platelet counts by binding to and activating the human TPO receptor. Activates intracellular signal transduction pathways to increase proliferation and differentiation of marrow progenitor cells.

Pharmacodynamics/Kinetics

Onset of action: Platelet count increase: Within 1 to 2 weeks

Duration: Platelets return to baseline: 1 to 2 weeks after last dose

Protein binding: >99%

Metabolism: Extensive hepatic metabolism; via CYP 1A2, 2C8 oxidation and UGT 1A1, 1A3 glucuronidation

Bioavailability: At least 52%; in adults, plasma AUC was increased by 22% with the oral suspension versus tablets

Half-life elimination: ~21 to 32 hours in healthy individuals; ~26 to 35 hours in patients with ITP

Time to peak, plasma: 2 to 6 hours

Excretion: Feces (~59%, 20% as unchanged drug); urine (31%, as metabolites)

Dosing

Adult & Geriatric Note: Do not use eltrombopag to normalize platelet counts.

Chronic Immune (idiopathic) thrombocytopenia (ITP): Oral: **Note:** Use the lowest dose to achieve and maintain platelet count ≥50,000/mm³ as needed to reduce the risk of bleeding. Discontinue if platelet count does not respond to a level that avoids clinically important bleeding after 4 weeks at the maximum of 75 mg/day.

Initial: 50 mg once daily (25 mg once daily for patients of East-Asian ethnicity [eg, Chinese, Japanese, Korean, Taiwanese]); dose should be titrated based on platelet response. Maximum dose: 75 mg/day.

Dosage adjustment based on platelet response:

Platelet count <50,000/mm³ (≥2 weeks after treatment initiation or a dose increase): Increase daily dose by 25 mg (if taking 12.5 mg once daily, increase dose to 25 mg once daily prior to increasing the dose amount by 25 mg daily); maximum: 75 mg/day

Platelet count ≥200,000/mm³ and ≤400,000/mm³ (at any time): Reduce daily dose by 25 mg (if taking 25 mg once daily, decrease dose to 12.5 mg once daily); reassess in 2 weeks

Platelet count >400,000/mm³: Withhold dose; assess platelet count twice weekly; when platelet count <150,000/mm³, resume with the daily dose reduced by 25 mg (if taking 25 mg once daily, resume with 12.5 mg once daily)

Platelet count >400,000/mm³ after 2 weeks at the lowest dose: Discontinue treatment

Chronic hepatitis C-associated thrombocytopenia: Oral: **Note:** Use the lowest dose to achieve the target platelet count necessary to initiate antiviral therapy (peginterferon and ribavirin) or to avoid dose reductions of peginterferon during antiviral therapy. Discontinue when antiviral therapy is stopped.

Initial: 25 mg once daily; dose should be titrated based on platelet response. Maximum dose: 100 mg/day

Dosage adjustment based on platelet response:

Platelet count <50,000/mm^3 (after at least 2 weeks): Increase daily dose by 25 mg every 2 weeks; maximum dose: 100 mg/day

Platelet count ≥200,000/mm^3 and ≤400,000/mm^3 (at any time): Reduce daily dose by 25 mg; reassess in 2 weeks

Platelet count >400,000/mm^3: Withhold dose; assess platelet count twice weekly; when platelet count <150,000/mm^3, resume with the daily dose reduced by 25 mg (if taking 25 mg once daily, resume with 12.5 mg once daily)

Platelet count >400,000/mm^3 after 2 weeks at the lowest dose: Discontinue treatment

Severe aplastic anemia: Oral: **Note:** Use the lowest dose to achieve and maintain hematologic response. Hematologic response may take up to 16 weeks and requires dose titration. Discontinue therapy if hematologic response is not achieved after 16 weeks of treatment, for excessive platelet responses or for liver function abnormalities. Consider discontinuing if new cytogenetic abnormalities are observed.

Initial: 50 mg once daily (25 mg once daily for patients of East-Asian ethnicity); dose should be titrated based on platelet response. Maximum dose: 150 mg/day.

Dosage adjustment based on platelet response:

Platelet count <50,000/mm^3 (≥2 weeks after treatment initiation or a dose increase): Increase daily dose by 50 mg (if taking 25 mg once daily, increase dose to 50 mg once daily prior to increasing the dose amount by 50 mg daily); maximum: 150 mg/day

Platelet count ≥200,000/mm^3 and ≤400,000/mm^3 (at any time): Reduce daily dose by 50 mg; reassess in 2 weeks

Platelet count >400,000/mm^3: Withhold dose for 1 week; when platelet count <150,000/mm^3, resume with the daily dose reduced by 50 mg

Platelet count >400,000/mm^3 after 2 weeks at the lowest dose: Discontinue treatment

For patients who achieve tri-lineage response, including transfusion independence, lasting 8 weeks, may reduce the dose by 50%. If counts remain stable after 8 weeks at the reduced dose, discontinue and monitor blood counts. If platelets counts drop to <30,000/mm^3, hemoglobin to <9 g/dL, or ANC to <500/mm^3, may reinitiate at the prior effective dose.

Pediatric Note: Do not use eltrombopag to normalize platelet counts.

Chronic immune (idiopathic) thrombocytopenia (ITP): Note: Use the lowest dose to achieve and maintain platelet count ≥50,000/mm^3 as needed to reduce the risk of bleeding. Discontinue if platelet count does not respond to a level that avoids clinically important bleeding after 4 weeks at the maximum of 75 mg/day.

Children 1 to 5 years: Oral: Initial: 25 mg once daily; dose should be titrated based on platelet response (no dosage adjustment required for patients of East Asian ancestry). Maximum dose: 75 mg/day.

Children ≥6 years and Adolescents: Oral: Refer to adult dosing

Renal Impairment No dosage adjustment is necessary.

Hepatic Impairment

Adjustment for hepatic impairment prior to initiating treatment:

Chronic ITP: **Note:** In patients with ITP and hepatic impairment, wait 3 weeks (instead of 2 weeks) after therapy initiation or subsequent dosage changes prior to increasing dose.

Mild, moderate, or severe impairment (Child-Pugh classes A, B, or C): Initial: 25 mg once daily

Patients of East-Asian ethnicity with hepatic impairment (Child-Pugh classes A, B, or C): Initial: Consider 12.5 mg once daily

Chronic hepatitis C-associated thrombocytopenia:

Initial: No dosage adjustment is necessary

Severe aplastic anemia:

Mild, moderate, or severe impairment (Child-Pugh classes A, B, or C): Initial: 25 mg once daily

Adjustment for hepatic impairment during treatment:

ALT levels ≥3 times the upper limit of normal (ULN) in patients with normal hepatic function or ≥3 times baseline in those with preexisting trans-aminase elevations **and** which are progressive, persistent (≥4 weeks), accompanied by increased direct bilirubin, or accompanied by clinical signs of liver injury or evidence of hepatic decompensation: Discontinue treatment. Hepatotoxicity may recur with re-treatment after therapy inter-ruption, but if determined to be clinically beneficial, may cautiously resume treatment; monitor ALT weekly during dosage titration; perma-nently discontinue if liver function test elevations persist, worsen, or recur.

Administration Administer on an empty stomach, 1 hour before or 2 hours after a meal. Swallow tablets whole; do not crush and mix with food or liquids. Prepare the suspension with cool or cold water only (do not use hot water); discard any suspension not administered within 30 minutes after reconstitu-tion. If powder or suspension spills during preparation or administration, consider wearing disposable gloves during spill clean-up to avoid staining skin. Do not administer concurrently with antacids, foods high in calcium, or minerals (eg, iron, calcium, aluminum, magnesium, selenium, zinc); adminis-ter eltrombopag at least 2 hours before and 4 hours after. Do not administer more than one dose within 24 hours.

Monitoring Parameters

Monitor liver function tests, including ALT, AST, and bilirubin (baseline, every 2 weeks during dosage titration, then monthly after a stable dose is achieved; evaluate abnormal liver function tests within 3 to 5 days; monitor weekly until abnormalities resolve, stabilize, or return to baseline or if re-treating [not recommended] after therapy interruption for hepatotoxicity); bilirubin fractio-nation (for elevated bilirubin); ophthalmic exam (baseline and during treat-ment).

Thrombocytopenia due to CHC and chronic ITP: CBC with differential and platelet count (weekly at initiation and during dosage titration, then monthly when stable; after cessation, monitor weekly for ≥4 weeks; when switching between the oral suspension and tablet, monitor platelet counts weekly for 2 weeks, then monthly when stable);

Severe aplastic anemia: CBC with differential and platelets (regularly through-out therapy)

Dietary Considerations Food, especially dairy products, may decrease the absorption of eltrombopag.

Product Availability Promacta oral suspension: FDA approved August 2015; anticipated availability is currently unknown.

◀ **Medication Guide Available** Yes

Dosage Forms Excipient information presented when available (limited, particularly for generics); consult specific product labeling.

Tablet, Oral:

Promacta: 12.5 mg

Promacta: 25 mg [contains fd&c yellow #6 aluminum lake]

Promacta: 50 mg [contains fd&c blue #2 aluminum lake]

Promacta: 75 mg

Dosage Forms: Canada Information with regard to form, strength, and availability of products uniquely available in Canada but currently not available in the US. Refer also to Dosage Forms.

Excipient information presented when available (limited, particularly for generics); consult specific product labeling.

Tablet, Oral:

Revolade: 25 mg, 50 mg

- **Eltrombopag Olamine** see Eltrombopag on page 668
- **Emcyt** see Estramustine on page 724
- **Emend** see Aprepitant on page 165
- **Emend** see Fosaprepitant on page 844
- **Emend IV (Can)** see Fosaprepitant on page 844
- **Emend Tri-Pack** see Aprepitant on page 165
- **EMLA [DSC]** see Lidocaine and Prilocaine on page 1150
- **EMLA (Can)** see Lidocaine and Prilocaine on page 1150
- **Empliciti** see Elotuzumab on page 663

Enasidenib (en a SID a nib)

Related Information

Common Toxicity Criteria on page 2242

Safe Handling of Hazardous Drugs on page 2379

Brand Names: US IDHIFA

Index Terms AG-221; CC-90007; Enasidenib Mesylate; IDH2 inhibitor; Idhifa

Pharmacologic Category Antineoplastic Agent, IDH2 Inhibitor

Use Acute myeloid leukemia (relapsed/refractory): Treatment of relapsed or refractory acute myeloid leukemia (AML) in patients with an isocitrate dehydrogenase-2 (IDH2) mutation as detected by an approved test

Labeled Contraindications There are no contraindications listed in the manufacturer's labeling.

Pregnancy Considerations Based on the mechanism of action and data from animal reproduction studies, the use of enasidenib in pregnancy may cause fetal harm. Women of reproductive potential should have a pregnancy test prior to treatment initiation; effective contraception should be used during therapy and for at least 1 month after the last dose. Male patients with female partners of reproductive potential should also use effective contraception during therapy and for at least 1 month after the last dose. Based on animal data, treatment with enasidenib may impair fertility in females and males.

Breastfeeding Considerations It is not known if enasidenib is present in breast milk. According to the manufacturer, breastfeeding is not recommended during therapy or for at least 1 month after the last dose.

Warnings/Precautions [US Boxed Warning]: Patients treated with ena-sidenib have experienced symptoms of differentiation syndrome, which can be fatal if not treated. Symptoms may include fever, dyspnea, acute respiratory distress, pulmonary infiltrates, pleural or pericardial effu-sions, rapid weight gain or peripheral edema, lymphadenopathy, bone pain, and hepatic, renal, or multi-organ dysfunction. If differentiation syndrome is suspected, initiate corticosteroid therapy and hemody-namic monitoring until symptom resolution. Differentiation syndrome, which is associated with rapid proliferation and differentiation of myeloid cells, has occurred (with and without concomitant hyperleukocytosis) as early as 10 days and up to 5 months after initiating enasidenib. If differentiation syndrome is suspected, initiate IV or oral corticosteroids (eg, dexamethasone 10 mg twice daily); taper corticosteroids only after symptom resolution (symptoms may recur if steroid therapy is stopped early). Interrupt enasidenib therapy for severe pulmonary symptoms requiring intubation or ventilator support and/or renal dysfunction that continues for more than 48 hours after corticosteroid initiation; may resume therapy when signs/symptoms have improved. Hospi-talization is recommended for patients with pulmonary and/or renal toxicity for close monitoring.

Noninfectious leukocytosis may occur due to myeloid proliferation leading to a rapid rise in white blood cell count. May require treatment with hydroxyurea (per institutional practice) and therapy interruption. Hyperbilirubinemia has been commonly reported; the majority of patients did not have concomitant transaminase elevation or other severe toxicity due to other liver disorders. Enasidenib may interfere with bilirubin metabolism through UGT1A1 inhibition. Persistent hyperbilirubinemia may require dosage reduction. Hypocalcemia, hypokalemia, and hypophosphatemia have also been reported. Tumor lysis syndrome may occur; monitor electrolytes and renal function. Nausea, vomit-ing, diarrhea, decreased appetite, and taste disturbances have been reported.

Confirm IDH2 mutation status prior to therapy initiation. Information on tests approved to detect IDH2 mutation in AML may be found at http://www.FDA. gov/CompanionDiagnostics. Potentially significant drug-drug interactions may exist, requiring dose or frequency adjustment, additional monitoring, and/or selection of alternative therapy.

Adverse Reactions

>10%:

Endocrine & metabolic: Decreased serum calcium (74%), decreased serum potassium (41%)

Gastrointestinal: Nausea (50%), diarrhea (43%), decreased appetite (34%), vomiting (34%), dysgeusia (12%)

Hematologic & oncologic: Abnormal phosphorus levels (27%; ≥3 grade: 8%; decreased), leukocytosis (12%; ≥3 grade: 6%; noninfectious)

Hepatic: Increased serum bilirubin (81%)

Miscellaneous: Cytokine release syndrome (14%)

1% to 10%:

Hematologic & oncologic: Tumor lysis syndrome (6%)

Respiratory: Acute respiratory distress (≤10%), pulmonary edema (≤10%)

Drug Interactions

Metabolism/Transport Effects Substrate of CYP1A2 (minor), CYP2B6 (minor), CYP2C19 (minor), CYP2C8 (minor), CYP2C9 (minor), CYP2D6 (minor), CYP3A4 (minor), UGT1A1, UGT1A3, UGT1A4, UGT1A9,

◄ UGT2B15, UGT2B7; **Note:** Assignment of Major/Minor substrate status based on clinically relevant drug interaction potential

Avoid Concomitant Use There are no known interactions where it is recommended to avoid concomitant use.

Increased Effect/Toxicity There are no known significant interactions involving an increase in effect.

Decreased Effect There are no known significant interactions involving a decrease in effect.

Hazardous Drugs Handling Considerations

Hazardous agent (meets NIOSH 2016 criteria). This medication is not on the NIOSH (2016) list; however, it meets the criteria for a hazardous drug. Drugs are classified as hazardous based on their properties; the properties of a hazardous drug include one or more of the following characteristics: carcinogenic, teratogenic (or other developmental toxicity), reproductive toxicity, organotoxic at low doses, genotoxic, and/or new agents with structural or toxicity profiles similar to existing hazardous agents.

Use appropriate precautions for receiving, handling, administration, and disposal. Gloves (single) should be worn during receiving, unpacking, and placing in storage. NIOSH recommends single gloving for administration of intact tablets or capsules (NIOSH 2016).

Storage/Stability Store at 20°C to 25°C (68°F to 77°F); excursions permitted between 15°C and 30°C (59°F and 86°F). Keep bottle tightly closed. Protect from moisture; store in original bottle (with desiccant canister).

Mechanism of Action Enasidenib is a small molecule inhibitor of the enzyme isocitrate dehydrogenase 2 (IDH2); it targets the mutant IDH2 variants R140Q, R172S, and R172K at ~40-fold lower concentrations than the wild-type enzyme. Mutant IDH2 inhibition results in decreased 2-hydroxyglutarate (2-HG) levels, reduced abnormal histone hypermethylation, and restored myeloid differentiation (Stein 2017). Additionally, enasidenib reduces blast counts and increases percentages of mature myeloid cells.

Pharmacodynamics/Kinetics

Distribution: 55.8 L

Protein binding: Parent drug: 98.5%; AGI-16903 (metabolite): 96.6%

Metabolism: In vitro data suggests that metabolism of parent drug is hepatic through multiple CYP enzymes (eg, CYP1A2, CYP2B6, CYP2C8, CYP2C9, CYP2C19, CYP2D6, and CYP3A4), and by multiple UGTs (UGT1A1, UGT1A3, UGT1A4, UGT1A9, UGT2B7, and UGT2B15). The metabolite AGI-16903 is further metabolized by CYP1A2, CYP2C19, CYP3A4, UGT1A1, UGT1A3, and UGT1A9.

Bioavailability: ~57% (100 mg dose)

Half-life elimination: 137 hours

Time to peak: 4 hours

Excretion: Feces (89%; 34% as unchanged drug); urine (11%; <1% as unchanged drug)

Dosing

Adult & Geriatric Note: Confirm IDH2 mutation status in the blood or bone marrow prior to treatment initiation.

Acute myeloid leukemia (relapsed/refractory): Oral: 100 mg once daily until disease progression or unacceptable toxicity; treat for a minimum of 6 months in patients without disease progression or unacceptable toxicity to allow time for clinical response.

Missed dose: If a dose is vomited, missed, or delayed, administer the dose as soon as possible on the same day; return to the normal administration schedule the following day.

Renal Impairment

CrCl ≥30 mL/minute: There are no dosage adjustments provided in the manufacturer's labeling; however, this level of renal function does not have a clinically significant effect on enasidenib pharmacokinetics.

CrCl <30 mL/minute: There are no dosage adjustments provided in the manufacturer's labeling.

Hepatic Impairment

Hepatic impairment prior to treatment initiation:

Mild (total bilirubin within ULN and AST > ULN or total bilirubin 1 to 1.5 times ULN and any AST) impairment: There are no dosage adjustments provided in the manufacturer's labeling; however, mild hepatic impairment does not have a clinically significant effect on enasidenib pharmacokinetics.

Moderate (total bilirubin >1.5 to 3 times ULN and any AST) to severe (total bilirubin >3 times ULN and any AST) impairment: There are no dosage adjustments provided in the manufacturer's labeling.

Hepatotoxicity during treatment: Bilirubin >3 times ULN for ≥2 weeks without elevated transaminases or other hepatic disorders: Reduce dose to 50 mg once daily. Resume enasidenib at 100 mg once daily if bilirubin elevation resolves to <2 times ULN.

Adjustment for Toxicity

Differentiation syndrome: If differentiation syndrome is suspected, initiate systemic corticosteroids (eg, dexamethasone IV or oral 10 mg twice daily) and monitor hemodynamics. Interrupt enasidenib for severe pulmonary symptoms requiring intubation or ventilator support and/or renal dysfunction persisting for more than 48 hours after systemic corticosteroid initiation. Resume enasidenib when signs/symptoms improve to ≤ grade 2. Taper systemic corticosteroids only after symptom resolution.

Noninfectious leukocytosis (WBC >30,000/mm³): Initiate hydroxyurea (per standard institutional practice); interrupt enasidenib if leukocytosis is not improved with hydroxyurea therapy, then resume enasidenib at 100 mg once daily when WBC <30,000/mm³.

Other toxicity: Grade 3 or higher (attributed to enasidenib [including tumor lysis syndrome]): Interrupt enasidenib until toxicity improves to ≤ grade 2. Resume enasidenib at 50 mg once daily; may increase to 100 mg once daily if toxicity resolves to ≤ grade 1. If ≥ grade 3 toxicity recurs, discontinue enasidenib.

Administration Administer orally once daily with or without food at approximately the same time each day. Swallow whole with a glass of water. Do not split or crush tablets.

Monitoring Parameters IDH2 mutation status (prior to treatment initiation); blood counts and blood chemistries prior to therapy initiation and every 2 weeks for at least the first 3 months; liver function tests; renal function; pregnancy test (prior to treatment in in females of reproductive potential); monitor for signs/symptoms of differentiation syndrome (eg, fever, cough, dyspnea, bone pain, rapid weight gain, edema, lymphadenopathy) and tumor lysis syndrome. Monitor adherence.

Prescribing and Access Restrictions Enasidenib is available through select specialty pharmacies and authorized distributors. Refer to http://www.idhifa.com for further information.

◀ **Medication Guide Available** Yes

Dosage Forms Excipient information presented when available (limited, particularly for generics); consult specific product labeling.

Tablet, Oral:

IDHIFA: 50 mg, 100 mg

◆ **Enasidenib Mesylate** see Enasidenib on page 676

◆ **Endari** see Glutamine on page 886

Enoxaparin (ee noks a PA rin)

Related Information

Venous Thromboembolism in the Cancer Patient on page 2360

Brand Names: US Lovenox

Brand Names: Canada Lovenox; Lovenox HP; Lovenox With Preservative

Index Terms Enoxaparin Sodium

Pharmacologic Category Anticoagulant; Anticoagulant, Low Molecular Weight Heparin

Use

Acute coronary syndromes: Unstable angina (UA), non-ST-elevation (NSTEMI), and ST-elevation myocardial infarction (STEMI)

DVT prophylaxis: Following hip or knee replacement surgery, abdominal surgery, or in medical patients with severely-restricted mobility during acute illness who are at risk for thromboembolic complications. **Note:** Patients at risk of thromboembolic complications who undergo abdominal surgery include those with one or more of the following risk factors: >40 years of age, obesity, general anesthesia lasting >30 minutes, malignancy, history of deep vein thrombosis or pulmonary embolism

DVT treatment (acute): Inpatient treatment (patients with or without pulmonary embolism) and outpatient treatment (patients without pulmonary embolism)

Labeled Contraindications

Hypersensitivity to enoxaparin, heparin, pork products, or any component of the formulation (including benzyl alcohol in multiple-dose vials); thrombocytopenia associated with a positive in vitro test for antiplatelet antibodies in the presence of enoxaparin; active major bleeding

Canadian labeling: Additional contraindications (not in U.S. labeling): Use of multiple-dose vials in newborns or premature neonates; history of confirmed or suspected immunologically-mediated heparin-induced thrombocytopenia; acute or subacute bacterial endocarditis; major blood clotting disorders; active gastric or duodenal ulcer; hemorrhagic cerebrovascular accident (except if there are systemic emboli); severe uncontrolled hypertension; diabetic or hemorrhagic retinopathy; other conditions or diseases involving an increased risk of hemorrhage; injuries to and operations on the brain, spinal cord, eyes, and ears; spinal/epidural anesthesia when repeated dosing of enoxaparin (1 mg/kg every 12 hours or 1.5 mg/kg daily) is required, due to increased risk of bleeding.

Note: Use of enoxaparin in patients with current heparin-induced thrombocytopenia (HIT) or HIT with thrombosis is **not** recommended and considered contraindicated due to high cross-reactivity to heparin-platelet factor-4 antibody (Guyatt [ACCP], 2012; Warkentin, 1999).

Pregnancy Considerations Adverse events were not observed in animal reproduction studies. Low molecular weight heparin (LMWH) does not cross the placenta; increased risks of fetal bleeding or teratogenic effects have not been reported (Bates 2012).

LMWH is recommended over unfractionated heparin for the treatment of acute venous thromboembolism (VTE) in pregnant women. LMWH is also recommended over unfractionated heparin for VTE prophylaxis in pregnant women with certain risk factors (eg, homozygous factor V Leiden, antiphospholipid antibody syndrome with ≥3 previous pregnancy losses). Prophylaxis is not routinely recommended for women undergoing assisted reproduction therapy; however, LMWH therapy is recommended for women who develop severe ovarian hyperstimulation syndrome. LMWH should be discontinued at least 24 hours prior to induction of labor or a planned cesarean delivery. For women undergoing cesarean section and who have additional risk factors for developing VTE, the prophylactic use of LMWH may be considered (Bates 2012).

LMWH may also be used in women with mechanical heart valves (consult current guidelines for details) (Bates 2012; Nishimura 2014). Women who require long-term anticoagulation with warfarin and who are considering pregnancy, LMWH substitution should be done prior to conception when possible. When choosing therapy, fetal outcomes (ie, pregnancy loss, malformations), maternal outcomes (ie, VTE, hemorrhage), burden of therapy, and maternal preference should be considered (Bates 2012). Monitoring antifactor Xa levels is recommended (Bates 2012; Nishimura 2014).

Multiple-dose vials contain benzyl alcohol (avoid in pregnant women due to association with gasping syndrome in premature infants); use of preservative-free formulations is recommended.

Breastfeeding Considerations It is not known if enoxaparin is present in breast milk. Small amounts of another LMWH have been detected in breast milk; however, because they have a low oral bioavailability, LMWHs are unlikely to cause adverse events in a breastfeeding infant. According to the manufacturer, the decision to continue or discontinue breastfeeding during therapy should take into account the risk of infant exposure, the benefits of breastfeeding to the infant, and benefits of treatment to the mother. However, antithrombotic guidelines state that use of LMWH may be continued in breastfeeding women (Bates 2012).

Warnings/Precautions **[US Boxed Warning]: Spinal or epidural hematomas, including subsequent long-term or permanent paralysis, may occur with recent or anticipated neuraxial anesthesia (epidural or spinal anesthesia) or spinal puncture in patients anticoagulated with LMWH or heparinoids. Consider risk versus benefit prior to spinal procedures; risk is increased by the use of concomitant agents which may alter hemostasis, the use of indwelling epidural catheters, a history of spinal deformity or spinal surgery, as well as a history of traumatic or repeated epidural or spinal punctures. Optimal timing between neuraxial procedures and enoxaparin administration is not known.** Delay placement or removal of catheter for at least 12 hours after administration of low-dose enoxaparin (eg, 30 to 60 mg/day) and at least 24 hours after high-dose enoxaparin (eg, 0.75 to 1 mg/kg twice daily or 1.5 mg/kg once daily) and consider doubling these times in patients with creatinine clearance <30 mL/minute; risk of neuraxial hematoma may still exist since antifactor Xa levels are still detectable at these time points. Patients receiving twice daily high-dose enoxaparin should have the second dose withheld to allow a longer time period prior to catheter placement or removal. Upon removal of catheter, consider withholding enoxaparin for at least 4 hours. **Patient should be observed closely for bleeding and signs and symptoms of neurological impairment if therapy is administered during or immediately following diagnostic lumbar puncture, epidural anesthesia, or spinal anesthesia. If neurological compromise is noted, urgent treatment is necessary.** If spinal hematoma is suspected, diagnose and treat immediately; spinal cord decompression may be considered although it may not prevent or reverse neurological sequelae.

Do not administer intramuscularly. In surgical patients receiving bridging anticoagulation with therapeutic dose enoxaparin, the American College of Chest Physicians suggests that the last preoperative dose of enoxaparin be administered ~24 hours prior to surgery (ACCP [Douketis 2012]). Not recommended for thromboprophylaxis in patients with prosthetic heart valves (especially pregnant women). Not to be used interchangeably (unit for unit) with heparin or any other low molecular weight heparins. Monitor patient closely for signs or symptoms of bleeding. Certain patients are at increased risk of bleeding. Risk factors include bacterial endocarditis; congenital or acquired bleeding disorders; active ulcerative or angiodysplastic GI diseases; severe uncontrolled hypertension; hemorrhagic stroke; use shortly after brain, spinal, or ophthalmic surgery; patients treated concomitantly with platelet inhibitors; recent GI bleeding or ulceration; renal dysfunction and hemorrhage; thrombocytopenia or platelet defects or history of heparin-induced thrombocytopenia; severe liver disease; hypertensive or diabetic retinopathy; or in patients undergoing invasive procedures. Protamine may be considered as a partial reversal agent in overdose situations (consult Protamine monograph for dosing recommendations). To minimize risk of bleeding following PCI, achieve hemostasis at the puncture site after PCI. If a closure device is used, sheath can be removed immediately. If manual compression is used, remove sheath 6 hours after the last IV/SubQ dose of enoxaparin. Do not administer further doses until 6 to 8 hours after sheath removal; observe for signs of bleeding/hematoma formation. Cases of enoxaparin-induced thrombocytopenia and thrombosis (similar to heparin-induced thrombocytopenia or [HIT]), some complicated by organ infarction, limb ischemia, or death, have been observed. Use with extreme caution or avoid in patients with history of HIT, especially if administered within 100 days of HIT episode (Warkentin, 2001); monitor platelet count closely. Use is contraindicated in patients with thrombocytopenia associated with a positive *in vitro* test for antiplatelet antibodies in the presence of enoxaparin. Discontinue therapy and consider alternative treatment if platelets are <100,000/mm³ and/or thrombosis develops. Use caution in patients with congenital or drug-induced thrombocytopenia or platelet defects. Risk of bleeding may be increased in women <45 kg and in men <57 kg. Use caution in patients with renal failure; dosage adjustment needed if CrCl <30 mL/minute. Use with caution in the elderly (delayed elimination may occur); dosage alteration/adjustment may be required (eg, omission of IV bolus in acute STEMI in patients ≥75 years of age). Monitor for hyperkalemia; can cause hyperkalemia possibly by suppressing aldosterone production.

Benzyl alcohol and derivatives: Some dosage forms may contain benzyl alcohol and should not be used in pregnant women. In neonates, large amounts of benzyl alcohol (≥99 mg/kg/day) have been associated with a potentially fatal toxicity ("gasping syndrome"); the "gasping syndrome" consists of metabolic acidosis, respiratory distress, gasping respirations, CNS dysfunction (including convulsions, intracranial hemorrhage), hypotension, and cardiovascular collapse (AAP ["Inactive" 1997]; CDC, 1982); some data suggests that benzoate displaces bilirubin from protein binding sites (Ahlfors, 2001); avoid or use dosage forms containing benzyl alcohol with caution in neonates. See manufacturer's labeling.

Safety and efficacy of prophylactic dosing of enoxaparin has not been established in patients who are obese (>30 kg/m^2) nor is there a consensus regarding dosage adjustments. The American College of Chest Physicians Practice Guidelines suggest consulting with a pharmacist regarding dosing in bariatric surgery patients and other obese patients who may require higher doses of LMWH (ACCP [Gould, 2012]).

Adverse Reactions As with all anticoagulants, bleeding is the major adverse effect of enoxaparin. Hemorrhage may occur at virtually any site. Risk is dependent on multiple variables. At the recommended doses, single injections of enoxaparin do not significantly influence platelet aggregation or affect global clotting time (ie, PT or aPTT).

>10%: Hematologic & oncologic: Anemia (≤16%), hemorrhage (4% to 13%)

1% to 10%:

Cardiovascular: Peripheral edema (6%)

Central nervous system: Confusion (2%)

Gastrointestinal: Nausea (3%)

Hematologic & oncologic: Major hemorrhage (<1% to 4%; includes cases of intracranial [up to 0.8%], retroperitoneal, or intraocular hemorrhage; incidence varies with indication/population), ecchymoses (3%), thrombocytopenia (1% to 2%)

Hepatic: Increased serum ALT (>3 x ULN: 6%), increased serum AST (>3 x ULN: 6%)

Local: Hematoma at injection site (9%), bleeding at injection site (3% to 5%), pain at injection site (2%)

Renal: Hematuria (≤2%)

Miscellaneous: Fever (≤8%)

<1%, postmarketing, and/or case reports: Acute posthemorrhagic anemia, alopecia, anaphylactoid reaction, anaphylaxis, atrial fibrillation, bruising at injection site, eosinophilia, epidural hematoma (spinal; after neuroaxial anesthesia or spinal puncture; risk may be increased with indwelling epidural catheter or concomitant use of other drugs affecting hemostasis), erythema at injection site, headache, hepatic injury (hepatocellular and cholestatic), hyperkalemia, hyperlipidemia (very rare), hypersensitivity angiitis, hypersensitivity reaction, hypertriglyceridemia, injection site reactions (including nodules, inflammation, oozing), irritation at injection site, osteoporosis (following long-term therapy), pneumonia, pruritus, pulmonary edema, purpura, shock, skin necrosis, thrombocythemia, thrombosis in heparin-induced thrombocytopenia, thrombosis (prosthetic value [in pregnant females] or associated with enoxaparin-induced thrombocytopenia; can cause limb ischemia or organ infarction), urticaria, vesicobullous rash

Drug Interactions

Metabolism/Transport Effects None known.

Avoid Concomitant Use

Avoid concomitant use of Enoxaparin with any of the following: Apixaban; Dabigatran Etexilate; Edoxaban; Hemin; MiFEPRIStone; Omacetaxine; Rivaroxaban; Urokinase; Vorapaxar

◀ **Increased Effect/Toxicity**

Enoxaparin may increase the levels/effects of: ACE Inhibitors; Aliskiren; Angiotensin II Receptor Blockers; Canagliflozin; Collagenase (Systemic); Deferasirox; Deoxycholic Acid; Desirudin; Eplerenone; Ibritumomab; Nintedanib; Obinutuzumab; Omacetaxine; Palifermin; Potassium Salts; Potassium-Sparing Diuretics; Rivaroxaban; Tositumomab and Iodine I 131 Tositumomab; Vitamin K Antagonists

The levels/effects of Enoxaparin may be increased by: 5-ASA Derivatives; Agents with Antiplatelet Properties; Antithrombin; Apixaban; Dabigatran Etexilate; Dasatinib; Edoxaban; Hemin; Herbs (Anticoagulant/Antiplatelet Properties); Ibrutinib; Limaprost; MiFEPRIStone; Nonsteroidal Anti-Inflammatory Agents; Omega-3 Fatty Acids; Pentosan Polysulfate Sodium; Pentoxifylline; Prostacyclin Analogues; Salicylates; Sugammadex; Thrombolytic Agents; Tibolone; Tipranavir; Urokinase; Vitamin E (Systemic); Vorapaxar

Decreased Effect

Enoxaparin may decrease the levels/effects of: Factor X (Human)

The levels/effects of Enoxaparin may be decreased by: Estrogen Derivatives; Progestins

Storage/Stability Store at 25°C (77°F); excursions permitted to 15°C to 30°C (59°F to 86°F); do not freeze. Do not store multiple-dose vials for >28 days after first use.

Mechanism of Action Standard heparin consists of components with molecular weights ranging from 4000 to 30,000 daltons with a mean of 16,000 daltons. Heparin acts as an anticoagulant by enhancing the inhibition rate of clotting proteases by antithrombin III impairing normal hemostasis and inhibition of factor Xa. Low molecular weight heparins have a small effect on the activated partial thromboplastin time and strongly inhibit factor Xa. Enoxaparin is derived from porcine heparin that undergoes benzylation followed by alkaline depolymerization. The average molecular weight of enoxaparin is 4500 daltons which is distributed as (≤20%) 2000 daltons (≥68%) 2000 to 8000 daltons, and (≤18%) >8000 daltons. Enoxaparin has a higher ratio of antifactor Xa to antifactor IIa activity than unfractionated heparin.

Pharmacodynamics/Kinetics

Onset of action: Peak effect: SubQ: Antifactor Xa and antithrombin (antifactor IIa): 3 to 5 hours

Duration: 40 mg dose: Antifactor Xa activity: ~12 hours

Distribution: 4.3 L (based on antifactor Xa activity)

Protein binding: Does not bind to heparin binding proteins

Metabolism: Hepatic, via desulfation and depolymerization to lower molecular weight molecules with very low biological activity

Bioavailability: Adults: SubQ: ~100%

Half-life elimination, plasma: 2 to 4 times longer than standard heparin, independent of dose; based on anti-Xa activity: 4.5 to 7 hours

Excretion: Urine (40% of dose as active and inactive fragments; 10% as active fragments; 8% to 20% of antifactor Xa activity is recovered within 24 hours)

Clearance: Decreased by 30% in patients with CrCl <30 mL/minute

Dosing

Adult Note: One mg of enoxaparin is equal to 100 units of anti-Xa activity (World Health Organization First International Low Molecular Weight Heparin Reference Standard). Weight-based doses (eg, 1 mg/kg) are commonly rounded to the nearest 10 mg; also see institution-specific rounding protocols if available. Most available prefilled syringes are graduated in 10 mg increments.

DVT prophylaxis: SubQ:

Obesity: **Note:** In morbidly-obese patients (BMI ≥40 kg/m^2), increasing the prophylactic dose by 30% may be appropriate for some indications (Nutescu, 2009). For bariatric surgery, dose increases may be >30% based on clinical trial data.

Abdominal surgery: 40 mg once daily, with initial dose given 2 hours prior to surgery; continue until risk of DVT has diminished (usually 7 to 10 days).

Hip replacement surgery:

Twice-daily dosing: 30 mg every 12 hours, with initial dose within 12 to 24 hours after surgery, and every 12 hours for at least 10 days or until risk of DVT has diminished or the patient is adequately anticoagulated on warfarin. The American College of Chest Physicians recommends initiation ≥12 hours preoperatively **or** ≥12 hours postoperatively; extended duration of up to 35 days suggested (Guyatt, 2012).

Once-daily dosing: 40 mg once daily, with initial dose within 9 to 15 hours before surgery, and daily for at least 10 days (or up to 35 days postoperatively) or until risk of DVT has diminished or the patient is adequately anticoagulated on warfarin. The American College of Chest Physicians recommends initiation ≥12 hours preoperatively **or** ≥12 hours postoperatively; extended duration of up to 35 days suggested (Guyatt, 2012).

Knee replacement surgery: 30 mg every 12 hours, with initial dose within 12 to 24 hours after surgery, and every 12 hours for at least 10 days or until risk of DVT has diminished or the patient is adequately anticoagulated on warfarin. The American College of Chest Physicians recommends initiation ≥12 hours preoperatively **or** ≥12 hours postoperatively; extended duration of up to 35 days suggested (Guyatt, 2012).

Medical patients with severely-restricted mobility during acute illness: 40 mg once daily; continue until risk of DVT has diminished (usually 6 to 11 days).

Bariatric surgery (off-label use): Roux-en-Y gastric bypass: Appropriate dosing strategies have not been clearly defined (Borkgren-Okonek, 2008; Scholten, 2002):

BMI ≤50 kg/m^2: 40 mg every 12 hours

BMI >50 kg/m^2: 60 mg every 12 hours

Note: The 2013 AACE/TOS/ASMBS bariatric surgery guidelines recommend, along with early ambulation, both sequential compression devices and subcutaneous LMWH or unfractionated heparin administered within 24 hours after surgery with consideration of extended prophylaxis for those who are at high risk for VTE (eg, history of DVT) (AACE/TOS/ASMBS [Mechanick, 2013]).

Prevention of recurrent venous thromboembolism in pregnancy (off-label use): 40 mg once daily. Therapy should continue for 6 weeks postpartum in high-risk women (Bates, 2012).

DVT treatment (acute): SubQ: **Note:** Start warfarin on the first or second treatment day and continue enoxaparin until INR is ≥2 for at least 24 hours (usually 5 to 7 days) (Guyatt, 2012).

Inpatient treatment (with or without pulmonary embolism): 1 mg/kg/dose every 12 hours or 1.5 mg/kg once daily.

Outpatient treatment (without pulmonary embolism): 1 mg/kg/dose every 12 hours.

Obesity: Use actual body weight to calculate dose; dose capping not recommended; use of twice daily dosing preferred (Nutescu, 2009)

Pregnant women (off-label use): 1 mg/kg/dose every 12 hours. Discontinue ≥24 hours prior to the induction of labor or cesarean section. Enoxaparin therapy may be substituted with heparin near term. Continue anticoagulation therapy for ≥6 weeks postpartum (minimum duration of therapy: 3 months). LMWH or heparin therapy is preferred over warfarin during pregnancy (Bates, 2012).

Percutaneous coronary intervention (PCI), adjunctive therapy (off-label dosing) (ACCF/AHA/SCAI [Levine, 2011]): IV:

If patient undergoing PCI has been treated with multiple doses of enoxaparin and PCI occurs within 8 hours after the last SubQ enoxaparin dose: No additional enoxaparin is needed.

If PCI occurs 8 to 12 hours after the last SubQ enoxaparin dose or the patient received only 1 therapeutic SubQ dose (eg, 1 mg/kg): Administer a single IV dose of 0.3 mg/kg.

If PCI occurs >12 hours after the last SubQ dose: May use an established anticoagulation regimen (eg, full-dose unfractionated heparin or bivalirudin).

If patient has not received prior anticoagulant therapy: 0.5 to 0.75 mg/kg IV bolus dose

ST-elevation MI (STEMI):

Patients <75 years of age: Initial: 30 mg IV single bolus plus 1 mg/kg (maximum: 100 mg for the first 2 doses only) SubQ every 12 hours. The first SubQ dose should be administered with the IV bolus. Maintenance: After first 2 doses, administer 1 mg/kg SubQ every 12 hours.

Patients ≥75 years of age: Initial: SubQ: 0.75 mg/kg every 12 hours (**Note:** No IV bolus is administered in this population); a maximum dose of 75 mg is recommended for the first 2 doses. Maintenance: After first 2 doses, administer 0.75 mg/kg SubQ every 12 hours

Obesity: Use weight-based dosing; a maximum dose of 100 mg is recommended for the first 2 doses (Nutescu, 2009)

Additional notes on STEMI treatment: Therapy may be continued for up to 8 days or until revascularization. Unless contraindicated, all patients should receive aspirin (indefinitely) and clopidogrel (ACCF/AHA [O'Gara, 2013]). In patients with STEMI receiving thrombolytics, initiate enoxaparin dosing between 15 minutes before and 30 minutes after fibrinolytic therapy.

Mechanical heart valve (aortic or mitral position) to bridge anticoagulation (off-label use): SubQ: 1 mg/kg every 12 hours (ACCP [Douketis, 2012]). **Note:** If used in pregnant patients, target anti-Xa level of 0.8 to 1.2 units/mL, 4 to 6 hours postdose (AHA/ACC [Nishimura, 2014]).

Unstable angina or non-ST-elevation MI (NSTEMI) (also referred to as NSTE-ACS): SubQ: 1 mg/kg every 12 hours in conjunction with oral aspirin therapy; continue for the duration of hospitalization or until PCI is performed; in select patients, an initial 30 mg IV loading dose has been used (ACC/AHA [Amsterdam 2014]).

Obesity: Use actual body weight to calculate dose; dose capping not recommended (Nutescu, 2009)

Conversion:

Conversion from IV unfractionated heparin (UFH) infusion to SubQ enoxaparin (Nutescu, 2007): Calculate specific dose for enoxaparin based on indication, discontinue UFH and begin enoxaparin within 1 hour.

Conversion from SubQ enoxaparin (therapeutically dosed) to IV UFH infusion (Nutescu, 2007): **Note:** The following recommendations are based on use of therapeutic doses of enoxaparin (eg, 1 mg/kg every 12 hours).If converting from a prophylactic enoxaparin dose (eg, 30 mg twice daily) to a therapeutic IV UFH dose, there should not be any delay in starting the IV UFH infusion and may include an UFH bolus/loading dose, when indicated.

Discontinue enoxaparin, calculate specific dose for IV UFH infusion based on indication, omit UFH bolus/loading dose:

Converting from SubQ enoxaparin dosed every 12 hours: Start IV UFH infusion 10 to 11 hours after last dose of enoxaparin

Converting from SubQ enoxaparin dosed every 24 hours: Start IV UFH infusion 22 to 23 hours after last dose of enoxaparin

Geriatric SubQ: Refer to adult dosing. Increased incidence of bleeding with doses of 1.5 mg/kg/day or 1 mg/kg every 12 hours; injection-associated bleeding and serious adverse reactions are also increased in the elderly. Careful attention should be paid to elderly patients, particularly those <45 kg. **Note:** Dosage alteration/adjustment may be required.

Pediatric Note: One mg of enoxaparin is equal to 100 units of anti-Xa activity (World Health Organization First International Low Molecular Weight Heparin Reference Standard).

Thromboembolism (off-label use; Monagle 2012): SubQ:

Infants <2 months: Initial:

Prophylaxis: 0.75 mg/kg every 12 hours

Treatment: 1.5 mg/kg every 12 hours

Infants >2 months and Children ≤18 years: Initial:

Prophylaxis: 0.5 mg/kg every 12 hours

Treatment: 1 mg/kg every 12 hours

Maintenance: See **Dosage Titration** table:

Enoxaparin Pediatric Dosage Titration[1]

Anti-Xa Result	Dose Titration	Time to Repeat Anti-Xa Measurement
<0.35 units/mL	Increase dose by 25%	4 h after next dose
0.35-0.49 units/mL	Increase dose by 10%	4 h after next dose
0.5-1 unit/mL	Keep same dosage	Next day, then 1 wk later, then monthly (4 h after dose)
1.1-1.5 units/mL	Decrease dose by 20%	Before next dose
1.6-2 units/mL	Hold dose for 3 h and decrease dose by 30%	Before next dose, then 4 h after next dose
>2 units/mL	Hold all doses until anti-Xa is 0.5 units/mL, then decrease dose by 40%	Before next dose and every 12 h until anti-Xa <0.5 units/mL

[1]Nomogram to be used for treatment dosing.

Modified from Duplaga BA, et al, "Dosing and Monitoring of Low-Molecular-Weight Heparins in Special Populations," *Pharmacotherapy*, 2001, 21(2):218-34; Monagle P, Michelson AD, Bovill E, et al. Antithrombotic therapy in children. *Chest*, 2001;119:344S-370S.

Renal Impairment

CrCl ≥30 mL/minute: No specific adjustment recommended (per manufacturer); monitor closely for bleeding.

CrCl <30 mL/minute:

DVT prophylaxis in abdominal surgery, hip replacement, knee replacement, or in medical patients during acute illness: SubQ: 30 mg once daily. **Note:** The Canadian labeling recommends 20 to 30 mg once daily (based on risk/benefit assessment) for prophylaxis in abdominal or colorectal surgery or in medical patients during acute illness.

DVT treatment: SubQ: 1 mg/kg once daily

STEMI:

<75 years: Initial: IV: 30 mg as a single dose with the first dose of the SubQ maintenance regimen administered at the same time as the IV bolus; Maintenance: SubQ: 1 mg/kg once daily. **Note:** Canadian labeling recommends a maximum dose of 100 mg for the first SubQ dose.

≥75 years of age: Omit IV bolus; Maintenance: SubQ: 1 mg/kg once daily. **Note:** Canadian labeling recommends a maximum dose of 100 mg for the first SubQ dose.

Unstable angina, NSTEMI: SubQ: 1 mg/kg once daily

Dialysis: Enoxaparin has not been FDA approved for use in dialysis patients. Its elimination is primarily via the renal route. Serious bleeding complications have been reported with use in patients who are dialysis dependent or have severe renal failure. LMWH administration at fixed doses without monitoring has greater unpredictable anticoagulant effects in patients with chronic kidney disease. If used, dosages should be reduced and anti-Xa levels frequently monitored, as accumulation may occur with repeated doses. Many clinicians would not use enoxaparin in this population especially without timely anti-Xa levels.

Hemodialysis: Not dialyzable (NCS/SCCM [Frontera 2016]). Supplemental dose is not necessary.

Peritoneal dialysis: Significant drug removal is unlikely based on physiochemical characteristics.

Hepatic Impairment There are no dosage adjustments provided in the manufacturer's labeling (has not been studied); use with caution.

Obesity Refer to indication-specific dosing for obesity-related information (may not be available for all indications).

Administration Note: Enoxaparin is available in 100 mg/mL and 150 mg/mL concentrations.

SubQ: Administer by deep SubQ injection alternating between the left or right anterolateral and left or right posterolateral abdominal wall. Do not mix with other infusions or injections. In order to minimize bruising, do not rub injection site. To avoid loss of drug from the 30 mg and 40 mg prefilled syringes, do not expel the air bubble from the syringe prior to injection.

IV: STEMI and PCI only: The U.S. labeling recommends using the multipledose vial to prepare IV doses. The Canadian labeling recommends either the multiple-dose vial or a prefilled syringe. Do not mix or coadminister with other medications; may be administered with NS or D5W. Flush IV access site with a sufficient amount of NS or D5W prior to and following IV bolus administration. When used prior to percutaneous coronary intervention or as part of treatment for ST-elevation myocardial infarction (STEMI), a single dose may be administered IV except when the patient is ≥75 years of age and is experiencing STEMI then only administer by SubQ injection.

Monitoring Parameters Platelets, occult blood, anti-Xa levels, serum creatinine; monitoring of PT and/or aPTT is not necessary. Routine monitoring of anti-Xa levels is not required, but has been utilized in patients with obesity and/or renal insufficiency. Monitoring anti-Xa levels is recommended in pregnant women receiving therapeutic doses of enoxaparin or when receiving enoxaparin for the prevention of thromboembolism with mechanical heart valves (Guyatt, 2012). For patients >190 kg, if anti-Xa monitoring is available, adjusting dose based on anti-Xa levels is recommended; if anti-Xa monitoring is unavailable, reduce dose if bleeding occurs (Nutescu, 2009). Monitor obese patients closely for signs/symptoms of thromboembolism.

Dosage Forms Excipient information presented when available (limited, particularly for generics); consult specific product labeling.

Solution, Injection, as sodium:

Lovenox: 300 mg/3 mL (3 mL) [contains benzyl alcohol, pork (porcine) protein]

Generic: 300 mg/3 mL (3 mL)

Solution, Subcutaneous, as sodium [preservative free]:

Lovenox: 30 mg/0.3 mL (0.3 mL); 40 mg/0.4 mL (0.4 mL); 60 mg/0.6 mL (0.6 mL); 80 mg/0.8 mL (0.8 mL); 100 mg/mL (1 mL); 120 mg/0.8 mL (0.8 mL); 150 mg/mL (1 mL) [contains pork (porcine) protein]

Generic: 30 mg/0.3 mL (0.3 mL); 40 mg/0.4 mL (0.4 mL); 60 mg/0.6 mL (0.6 mL); 80 mg/0.8 mL (0.8 mL); 100 mg/mL (1 mL); 120 mg/0.8 mL (0.8 mL); 150 mg/mL (1 mL)

◆ **Enoxaparin Sodium** see Enoxaparin on page 680

◆ **Entertainer's Secret [OTC]** see Saliva Substitute on page 1653

◆ **Envarsus XR** see Tacrolimus (Systemic) on page 1715

Enzalutamide (en za LOO ta mide)

Related Information

Safe Handling of Hazardous Drugs on page 2379

Brand Names: US Xtandi

Brand Names: Canada Xtandi

Index Terms MDV3100

Pharmacologic Category Antineoplastic Agent, Antiandrogen

Use Prostate cancer, metastatic: Treatment of metastatic, castration-resistant prostate cancer

Labeled Contraindications Pregnancy

Canadian labeling: Additional contraindications (not in the US labeling): Hypersensitivity to enzalutamide or any component of the formulation; women who are lactating

Pregnancy Considerations Enzalutamide is contraindicated in pregnant women and is not indicated for use in women. Adverse effects were observed in animal reproduction studies. Enzalutamide is an androgen receptor inhibitor; based on the mechanism of action, fetal harm and potential loss of pregnancy would be expected. Male patients with female partners of reproductive potential should use effective contraception during treatment and for 3 months after the last enzalutamide dose and should use a condom if having intercourse with a pregnant woman. May impair male fertility.

Breastfeeding Considerations Enzalutamide is not indicated for use in women.

Warnings/Precautions Seizures were observed in clinical trials; patients with predisposing risk factors for seizures were generally excluded from these studies. The onset of seizure ranged from ~1 to 20 months after treatment initiation. Enzalutamide was permanently discontinued in patients experiencing seizures; seizures resolved upon therapy cessation. In a study designed to assess seizure risk in patients with predisposing factors, 2.2% of patients who received enzalutamide experienced a seizure; after the first seizure resolved, a few of those patients experienced a second seizure with continued enzalutamide treatment. It is not known if antiepileptic medications can prevent enzalutamide-related seizures. Patients in the study had one or more predisposing factors, including the use of concomitant medications that may lower the seizure threshold, history of traumatic brain or head injury, history of cerebrovascular accident/transient ischemic attack, and Alzheimer disease, meningioma, or leptomeningeal disease from prostate cancer, unexplained loss of consciousness within the last 12 months, prior seizure history, presence of a space occupying brain lesion, history of arteriovenous malformation, or history of brain infection; some patients had more than one risk factor. Advise patients of the risk of seizures during enzalutamide treatment and of the risk of engaging in activities where sudden loss of consciousness could cause serious harm to themselves or others. Discontinue enzalutamide permanently if seizures develop during treatment. Posterior reversible encephalopathy syndrome (PRES) has been reported in patients receiving enzalutamide. PRES is a neurological disorder which may present with rapidly evolving symptoms (headache, seizure, lethargy, confusion, blindness, and other visual/neurologic disturbances) with or without associated hypertension. PRES diagnosis may be confirmed with magnetic resonance imagining (MRI). Discontinue enzalutamide in patients who develop PRES.

Enzalutamide may cause hypospermatogenesis and may impair male fertility. Androgen-deprivation therapy may increase the risk of cardiovascular disease (Levine 2010). An increase in systolic and diastolic blood pressures has been observed (Scher 2012); may worsen preexisting hypertension.

Potentially significant drug-drug interactions may exist, requiring dose or frequency adjustment, additional monitoring, and/or selection of alternative therapy. May contain sorbitol.

Adverse Reactions

>10%:
  Cardiovascular: Peripheral edema (12% to 15%), hypertension (6% to 14%)
  Central nervous system: Fatigue (≤51%), falling (5% to 13%), headache (11% to 12%), dizziness (10% to 11%)
  Endocrine & metabolic: Hot flash (15% to 20%), weight loss (11% to 12%)
  Gastrointestinal: Constipation (13% to 23%), diarrhea (12% to 22%), decreased appetite (19%), nausea (14%)
  Hematologic & oncologic: Neutropenia (15%; grades 3/4: 1%)
  Neuromuscular & skeletal: Weakness (≤51%), back pain (19% to 29%), arthralgia (21%), musculoskeletal pain (15% to 16%)
  Respiratory: Upper respiratory tract infection (11% to 16%), dyspnea (11%)
1% to 10%:
  Central nervous system: Myasthenia (10%), insomnia (8% to 9%), anxiety (7%), paresthesia (7%), cauda equina syndrome (≤7%), spinal cord compression (≤7%), altered mental status (4% to 6%), hypoesthesia (4%), hallucination (2%), restless leg syndrome (2%)
  Dermatologic: Pruritus (4%), xeroderma (4%)

Endocrine & metabolic: Gynecomastia (3%)
Gastrointestinal: Dysgeusia (8%)
Genitourinary: Hematuria (7% to 9%), pollakiuria (5%)
Hematologic & oncologic: Thrombocytopenia (6%)
Hepatic: Increased serum bilirubin (3%)
Infection: Infection (≤6%; including sepsis)
Neuromuscular & skeletal: Bone fracture (4% to 9%), stiffness (3%)
Respiratory: Lower respiratory tract infection (8% to 9%), epistaxis (3%)
<1%, postmarketing, and/or case reports: Hypersensitivity reaction (including lip edema, pharyngeal edema, tongue edema), reversible posterior leukoencephalopathy syndrome, seizure, skin rash, vomiting

Drug Interactions

Metabolism/Transport Effects Substrate of CYP2C8 (major), CYP3A4 (major); **Note:** Assignment of Major/Minor substrate status based on clinically relevant drug interaction potential; **Inhibits** BCRP, MRP2; **Induces** CYP2C19 (moderate), CYP2C9 (weak/moderate), CYP3A4 (strong)

Avoid Concomitant Use

Avoid concomitant use of Enzalutamide with any of the following: Abiraterone Acetate; Alfentanil; Antihepaciviral Combination Products; Apixaban; Apremilast; Aprepitant; Artemether; Asunaprevir; Axitinib; Bedaquiline; Boceprevir; Bortezomib; Bosutinib; Brigatinib; Cariprazine; Ceritinib; CloZAPine; Cobimetinib; Crizotinib; CycloSPORINE (Systemic); CYP2C8 Inducers (Strong); CYP2C8 Inhibitors (Strong); CYP3A4 Inducers (Strong); Daclatasvir; Dasabuvir; Deflazacort; Delamanid; Dienogest; Dihydroergotamine; Dronedarone; Eliglustat; Ergotamine; Everolimus; FentaNYL; Flibanserin; Fosphenytoin Phenytoin; Gemigliptin; Grazoprevir; Ibrutinib; Idelalisib; Indium 111 Capromab Pendetide; Irinotecan Products; Isavuconazonium Sulfate; Itraconazole; Ivabradine; Ivacaftor; Ixazomib; Lapatinib; Lumefantrine; Lurasidone; Macitentan; Midostaurin; MiFEPRIStone; Naldemedine; Naloxegol; Neratinib; Netupitant; NIFEdipine; Nilotinib; NiMODipine; Nisoldipine; Olaparib; Palbociclib; Panobinostat; PAZOPanib; Pimozide; PONATinib; Praziquantel; QuiNIDine; Ranolazine; Regorafenib; Ribociclib; Rivaroxaban; Roflumilast; RomiDEPsin; Simeprevir; Sirolimus; Sonidegib; SORAfenib; St John's Wort; Suvorexant; Tacrolimus (Systemic); Tasimelteon; Telaprevir; Ticagrelor; Tofacitinib; Tolvaptan; Toremifene; Trabectedin; Ulipristal; Valbenazine; Vandetanib; Velpatasvir; Venetoclax; VinCRIStine (Liposomal); Vinflunine; Vorapaxar; Voxilaprevir

Increased Effect/Toxicity

Enzalutamide may increase the levels/effects of: Clarithromycin; Doxercalciferol; Ifosfamide

The levels/effects of Enzalutamide may be increased by: Clarithromycin; CYP2C8 Inhibitors (Moderate); CYP2C8 Inhibitors (Strong); CYP3A4 Inhibitors (Strong); Deferasirox

Decreased Effect

Enzalutamide may decrease the levels/effects of: Abiraterone Acetate; Alfentanil; Antihepaciviral Combination Products; Apixaban; Apremilast; Aprepitant; ARIPiprazole; ARIPiprazole Lauroxil; Artemether; Asunaprevir; Axitinib; Bedaquiline; Benperidol; Boceprevir; Bortezomib; Brentuximab Vedotin; Brexpiprazole; Brigatinib; Cabozantinib; Calcifediol; Cannabidiol; Cannabis; Cariprazine; Ceritinib; Choline C 11; Clarithromycin; Clindamycin (Systemic); CloZAPine; Cobimetinib; Corticosteroids (Systemic); Crizotinib; CycloSPORINE (Systemic); CYP2C19 Substrates; CYP2C9 Substrates; CYP3A4 Substrates; Daclatasvir; Dasabuvir;

Dasatinib; Deflazacort; Delamanid; Dexamethasone (Systemic); Dienogest; Diethylstilbestrol; Dihydroergotamine; DOXOrubicin (Conventional); Dronabinol; Dronedarone; Eliglustat; Ergotamine; Erlotinib; Estriol (Systemic); Estriol (Topical); Etoposide; Etoposide Phosphate; Everolimus; Evogliptin; Exemestane; FentaNYL; Flibanserin; Fosphenytoin-Phenytoin; Gefitinib; Gemigliptin; Glecaprevir and Pibrentasvir; Grazoprevir; GuanFACINE; Hydrocortisone (Systemic); Ibrutinib; Idelalisib; Ifosfamide; Imatinib; Indium 111 Capromab Pendetide; Irinotecan Products; Isavuconazonium Sulfate; Itraconazole; Ivabradine; Ivacaftor; Ixabepilone; Ixazomib; Lapatinib; Linagliptin; Lumefantrine; Lurasidone; Macitentan; Manidipine; Maraviroc; MethylPREDNISolone; Midostaurin; MiFEPRIStone; Mirodenafil; Naldemedine; Naloxegol; Neratinib; Netupitant; NIFEdipine; Nilotinib; NiMODipine; Nisoldipine; Olaparib; Osimertinib; Palbociclib; Panobinostat; PAZOPanib; Perampanel; Pimavanserin; Pimozide; PONATinib; Praziquantel; PrednisoLONE (Systemic); PredniSONE; Propafenone; QUEtiapine; QuiNIDine; Radotinib; Ramelteon; Ranolazine; Reboxetine; Regorafenib; Ribociclib; Rivaroxaban; Roflumilast; Rolapitant; RomiDEPsin; SAXagliptin; Sertraline; Simeprevir; Sirolimus; Sonidegib; SORAfenib; SUFentanil; SUNItinib; Suvorexant; Tacrolimus (Systemic); Tadalafil; Tasimelteon; Telaprevir; Temsirolimus; Tetrahydrocannabinol; TiaGABine; Ticagrelor; Tofacitinib; Tolvaptan; Toremifene; Trabectedin; Tropisetron; Udenafil; Ulipristal; Valbenazine; Vandetanib; Velpatasvir; Vemurafenib; Venetoclax; Vilazodone; VinCRIStine (Liposomal); Vinflunine; Vorapaxar; Vortioxetine; Voxilaprevir; Warfarin; Zaleplon; Zuclopenthixol

The levels/effects of Enzalutamide may be decreased by: Bosentan; CYP2C8 Inducers (Strong); CYP3A4 Inducers (Moderate); CYP3A4 Inducers (Strong); Dabrafenib; Deferasirox; Sarilumab; Siltuximab; St John's Wort; Tocilizumab

Hazardous Drugs Handling Considerations
Hazardous agent (NIOSH 2016 [group 1]).

Use appropriate precautions for receiving, handling, administration, and disposal. Gloves (single) should be worn during receiving, unpacking, and placing in storage. NIOSH recommends single gloving for administration of intact tablets or capsules (NIOSH 2016).

Storage/Stability Store at 20°C to 25°C (68°F to 77°F); excursions permitted to 15°C to 30°C (59°F to 86°F). Protect from moisture; keep bottle tightly closed.

Mechanism of Action Enzalutamide is a pure androgen receptor signaling inhibitor; unlike other antiandrogen therapies, it has no known agonistic properties. It inhibits androgen receptor nuclear translocation, DNA binding, and coactivator mobilization, leading to cellular apoptosis and decreased prostate tumor volume.

Pharmacodynamics/Kinetics
Absorption: Rapid

Distribution: 110 L

Protein binding: Parent drug: 97% to 98% to primarily albumin; active metabolite: 95% to plasma proteins

Metabolism: Primarily hepatic via CYP2C8 (responsible for formation of active metabolite N-desmethyl enzalutamide) and CYP3A4; carboxylesterase 1 metabolizes N-desmethyl enzalutamide and enzalutamide to the inactive carboxylic acid metabolite.

Half-life elimination: Parent drug: 5.8 days (range: 2.8 to 10.2 days); N-desmethyl enzalutamide: 7.8 to 8.6 days

Time to peak: 1 hour (range: 0.5 to 3 hours)

Excretion: Urine (71%); feces (14%); primarily as inactive metabolite

Dosing

Adult & Geriatric

Prostate cancer, metastatic, castration-resistant: Oral: 160 mg once daily

Dosage adjustment for concomitant strong CYP2C8 inhibitors: Avoid concomitant use if possible. If coadministration is necessary, reduce enzalutamide dose to 80 mg once daily. If the strong CYP2C8 inhibitor is discontinued, adjust the enzalutamide dose back up to the dose used prior to the initiation of the strong CYP2C8 inhibitor.

Dosage adjustment for concomitant strong CYP3A4 inducers: Avoid concomitant use if possible. If coadministration is necessary, increase the enzalutamide dose to 240 mg once daily. If the strong CYP3A4 inducer is discontinued, adjust the enzalutamide dose back to the dose used prior to the initiation of the strong CYP3A4 inducer.

Renal Impairment

Preexisting mild-to-moderate impairment (CrCl 30 to 89 mL/minute): No initial dosage adjustment necessary.

Preexisting severe impairment (CrCl <30 mL/minute), including end-stage renal disease (ESRD): There are no dosage adjustments provided in the manufacturer's labeling (has not been studied).

Hepatic Impairment Preexisting mild, moderate, or severe impairment (Child-Pugh class A, B, or C): No dosage adjustment necessary.

Adjustment for Toxicity If ≥ grade 3 toxicity or intolerable side effects occur, withhold treatment for 1 week or until symptom(s) improve to ≤ grade 2, then resume at same dose, or reduce dose to 120 mg or 80 mg once daily, if necessary.

Seizures: Permanently discontinue treatment.

Administration Administer at the same time each day, either with or without food. Swallow capsules whole; do not chew, dissolve, or open the capsules.

Monitoring Parameters Monitor for signs/symptoms of seizure, loss of consciousness, dizziness, and hallucinations; CBC with differential and liver function tests (baseline and periodic); additional INR monitoring (if on warfarin); blood pressure (baseline and periodic), signs/symptoms of posterior reversible encephalopathy syndrome. Monitor adherence.

Dosage Forms Excipient information presented when available (limited, particularly for generics); consult specific product labeling.

Capsule, Oral:

Xtandi: 40 mg

♦ **EPEG** see Etoposide on page 729
♦ **EPEG** see Etoposide on page 729

♦ **Epidoxorubicin** see EpiRUBicin on page 694
♦ **Epidoxorubicin** see EpiRUBicin on page 694

♦ **Epipodophyllotoxin** see Etoposide on page 729
♦ **Epipodophyllotoxin** see Etoposide on page 729

♦ **Epipodophyllotoxin** see Etoposide Phosphate on page 740
♦ **Epipodophyllotoxin** see Etoposide Phosphate on page 740

EpiRUBicin (ep i ROO bi sin)

Related Information

Management of Chemotherapy-Induced Nausea and Vomiting in Adults *on page 2253*

Management of Drug Extravasations *on page 2271*

Prevention of Chemotherapy-Induced Nausea and Vomiting in Children *on page 2310*

Safe Handling of Hazardous Drugs *on page 2379*

Brand Names: US Ellence

Brand Names: Canada Ellence; Epirubicin for Injection; Epirubicin Hydrochloride Injection; Pharmorubicin

Index Terms Epidoxorubicin; Epirubicin HCl; Epirubicin Hydrochloride; Pidorubicin; Pidorubicin Hydrochloride

Pharmacologic Category Antineoplastic Agent, Anthracycline; Antineoplastic Agent, Topoisomerase II Inhibitor

Use Breast cancer, adjuvant treatment: Adjuvant therapy component for primary breast cancer in patients with evidence of axillary node involvement following tumor resection

Labeled Contraindications

Hypersensitivity to epirubicin, other anthracyclines, anthracenediones, or any component of the formulation; cardiomyopathy and/or heart failure, recent myocardial infarction, severe arrhythmias; previous treatment with anthracyclines up to the maximum cumulative dose

Canadian labeling: Additional contraindications (not in the US labeling): Marked persistent myelosuppression induced by prior treatment with other chemotherapy agents or by radiotherapy; severe hepatic impairment.

Pregnancy Considerations Adverse events were observed in animal reproduction studies. Women of childbearing potential should be advised to use effective contraception and avoid becoming pregnant during treatment. Men undergoing treatment should use effective contraception. Epirubicin may cause irreversible amenorrhea in premenopausal women.

Limited information is available from a retrospective study of women who received epirubicin (in combination with cyclophosphamide or weekly as a single-agent) during the second or third (prior to week 35) trimester for the treatment of pregnancy-associated breast cancer (Ring 2005) and from a study of women who received epirubicin (weekly as a single-agent) at gestational weeks 16 through 30 for the treatment of pregnancy-associated breast cancer (Peccatori 2009). Some pharmacokinetic properties of epirubicin may be altered in pregnant women (van Hasselt 2014). The European Society for Medical Oncology (ESMO) has published guidelines for diagnosis, treatment, and follow-up of cancer during pregnancy (Peccatori 2013); the guidelines recommend referral to a facility with expertise in cancer during pregnancy and encourage a multidisciplinary team (obstetrician, neonatologist, oncology team). If chemotherapy is indicated, it should not be administered in the first trimester, but may begin in the second trimester. There should be a 3-week time period between the last chemotherapy dose and anticipated delivery, and chemotherapy should not be administered beyond week 33 of gestation.

A pregnancy registry is available for all cancers diagnosed during pregnancy at Cooper Health (877-635-4499).

Breastfeeding Considerations It is not known if epirubicin is present in human breast milk; however, other anthracyclines are excreted in breast milk.

Due to the potential for serious adverse reactions in the breastfed infant, the manufacturer recommends a decision be made to discontinue breastfeeding or to discontinue the drug, taking into account the importance of treatment to the mother.

Warnings/Precautions [US Boxed Warning]: Myocardial toxicity, including fatal heart failure (HF) may occur, particularly in patients who have received prior anthracyclines (or anthracenediones), prior or concomitant radiotherapy to the mediastinal/pericardial area, who have preexisting cardiac disease (active or dormant), or with concomitant cardiotoxic medications. Cardiotoxicity may be concurrent or delayed (months to years after treatment). The risk of HF is ~0.9% at a cumulative dose of 550 mg/m^2, ~1.6% at a cumulative dose of 700 mg/m^2, and ~3.3% at a cumulative dose of 900 mg/m^2. Cardiotoxicity may also occur at lower cumulative doses or without risk factors. The risk of delayed cardiotoxicity increases more steeply with cumulative doses >900 mg/m^2 and this dose should be exceeded only with extreme caution. The maximum cumulative dose used in adjuvant studies was 720 mg/m^2. Cardiotoxicity is dose-limiting. Early toxicity may consist of tachyarrhythmias, including sinus tachycardia, premature ventricular contractions, and ventricular tachycardia, as well as bradycardia. Electrocardiographic changes including ST-T wave changes, atrioventricular and bundle-branch block have also been reported. These effects are not necessarily predictive of subsequent delayed cardiotoxicity. Delayed toxicity is typically caused by cardiomyopathy which presents as decreased left ventricular ejection fraction (LVEF) and/or signs/symptoms of HF (eg, tachycardia, dyspnea, pulmonary edema, edema, hepatomegaly, ascites, pleural effusion, gallop rhythm). Total cumulative dose should take into account prior treatment with other anthracyclines or anthracenediones, previous or concomitant treatment with other cardiotoxic agents or irradiation of chest. Although the risk increases with cumulative dose, irreversible cardiotoxicity may occur at any dose level. Patients with active or dormant cardiovascular disease, concurrent administration of cardiotoxic drugs, prior therapy with other anthracyclines or anthracenediones, prior or concurrent chest irradiation, advanced age, and infants and children are at increased risk. Children are at increased risk for developing delayed cardiotoxicity. Regular monitoring of LVEF and discontinuation at the first sign of impairment is recommended especially in patients with cardiac risk factors or impaired cardiac function. Discontinue treatment with signs of decreased LVEF. The half-life of other cardiotoxic agents (eg, trastuzumab) must be considered in sequential therapy.

[US Boxed Warning]: May cause severe myelosuppression, including leukopenia, thrombocytopenia, and anemia. Myelosuppression is the dose-limiting toxicity. Obtain baseline and periodic blood counts. Patients should recover from myelosuppression due to prior chemotherapy treatment before beginning treatments. Severe neutropenia and severe infections may require supportive care. Thrombophlebitis and thromboembolic phenomena (including pulmonary embolism) have occurred.

[US Boxed Warning]: Dosage reduction is recommended in patients with mild-to-moderate hepatic impairment. Use is not recommended in severe hepatic impairment; predominantly hepatically eliminated; impaired hepatic function may lead to increased exposure and toxicity and in patients with serum creatinine >5 mg/dL (has not been studied in patients on dialysis). Monitor hepatic and renal function at baseline and during treatment. May

◄ cause tumor lysis syndrome (TLS), although generally does not occur in patients with breast cancer; if TLS risk is suspected, consider monitoring serum uric acid, potassium, calcium, phosphate, and serum creatinine after initial administration; hydration and antihyperuricemic prophylaxis may minimize potential TLS complications. Radiation recall (inflammatory) has been reported; epirubicin may have radiosensitizing activity. **[US Boxed Warning]: Treatment with anthracyclines (including epirubicin) may increase the risk of secondary acute myeloid leukemia (AML). AML is more common when given in combination with other antineoplastic agents, in patients who have received multiple courses of previous chemotherapy, or with escalated anthracycline doses. In breast cancer patients, the risk for treatment-related AML or myelodysplastic syndrome (MDS) was estimated at 0.27% at 3 years, 0.46% at 5 years, and 0.55% at 8 years after treatment.** The latency period for secondary leukemias may be short (1 to 3 years).

[US Boxed Warning]: For IV administration only. Vesicant; if extravasation occurs, severe local tissue damage and necrosis may occur; not for IM or SubQ use. Injection in to a small vein or repeated administration in the same vein may result in venous sclerosis. Ensure proper needle or catheter placement prior to and during infusion. Avoid extravasation. If perivenous infiltration occurs, immediately discontinue infusion and restart in another vein. Women ≥70 years of age should be closely monitored for toxicity. Children may be at increased risk for developing acute and delayed cardiotoxicity; long-term periodic cardiac function monitoring is recommended. **[US Boxed Warning]: Should be administered under the supervision of an experienced cancer chemotherapy physician.** Epirubicin is associated with a moderate to high emetic potential (depending on dose or regimen); antiemetics are recommended to prevent nausea and vomiting (Basch 2011; Dupuis 2011; Roila 2016). Patients should recover from acute toxicities (stomatitis, myelosuppression, infections) prior to initiating treatment. Assess baseline labs (blood counts, bilirubin, ALT, AST, serum creatinine) and cardiac function (with LVEF). Prophylactic antibiotics should be administered with the CDF-120 regimen. Patients should not be immunized with live viral vaccines during or shortly after treatment. Inactivated vaccines may be administered (response may be diminished). Potentially significant interactions may exist, requiring dose or frequency adjustment, additional monitoring, and/or selection of alternative therapy.

Adverse Reactions Frequency not always defined. Percentages reported as part of combination chemotherapy regimens.

Cardiovascular: Decreased left ventricular ejection fraction (asymptomatic; delayed: 1% to 2%), cardiac failure (≤2%), atrioventricular block, bradycardia, bundle branch block, cardiac arrhythmia, cardiomyopathy, ECG abnormality, myocarditis, non-specific T wave on ECG, sinus tachycardia, ST segment changes on ECG, tachyarrhythmia, thromboembolism, ventricular premature contractions, ventricular tachycardia

Central nervous system: Lethargy (1% to 46%)

Dermatologic: Alopecia (70% to 96%), skin rash (1% to 9%), skin changes (1% to 5%)

Endocrine & metabolic: Amenorrhea (69% to 72%), hot flash (5% to 39%)

Gastrointestinal: Nausea and vomiting (83% to 92%; grades 3/4: 22% to 25%), mucositis (9% to 59%; grades 3/4: ≤9%), diarrhea (7% to 25%), anorexia (2% to 3%), abdominal pain, esophagitis, neutropenic enterocolitis, stomatitis, toxic megacolon

Genitourinary: Menopause (premature or early)

Hematologic & oncologic: Neutropenia (54% to 80%; grades 3/4: 11% to 67%; nadir: 10 to 14 days; recovery: by day 21), leukopenia (50% to 80%; grades 3/4: 2% to 59%), anemia (13% to 72%; grades 3/4: ≤6%), thrombocytopenia (5% to 49%; grades 3/4: ≤5%), febrile neutropenia (grades 3/4: ≤6%), acute lymphocytic leukemia, acute myelocytic leukemia, myelodysplastic syndrome

Hepatic: Ascites, hepatomegaly, increased serum transaminases

Hypersensitivity: Hypersensitivity reaction

Infection: Infection (15% to 22%; grades 3/4: ≤2%)

Local: Injection site reaction (3% to 20%; grades 3/4: <1%)

Ophthalmic: Conjunctivitis (1% to 15%)

Respiratory: Dyspnea, pulmonary edema

Miscellaneous: Fever (1% to 5%)

<1%, postmarketing, case reports: Anaphylaxis, arterial embolism, burning sensation of gastrointestinal tract, chills, dehydration, erythema, flushing, gastrointestinal erosion, gastrointestinal hemorrhage, gastrointestinal pain, gastrointestinal ulcer, hyperuricemia, nail hyperpigmentation, oral mucosa hyperpigmentation, phlebitis, pneumonia, pulmonary embolism, radiation recall phenomenon, red urine discoloration, sepsis, shock, skin hyperpigmentation, skin photosensitivity, thrombophlebitis, urticaria

Drug Interactions

Metabolism/Transport Effects None known.

Avoid Concomitant Use

Avoid concomitant use of EpiRUBicin with any of the following: BCG (Intravesical); Cimetidine; Deferiprone; Dipyrone; Natalizumab; Pimecrolimus; Tacrolimus (Topical); Vaccines (Live)

Increased Effect/Toxicity

EpiRUBicin may increase the levels/effects of: CloZAPine; Deferiprone; Fingolimod; Leflunomide; Natalizumab; Tofacitinib; Vaccines (Live)

The levels/effects of EpiRUBicin may be increased by: Ado-Trastuzumab Emtansine; Bevacizumab; Cimetidine; Cyclophosphamide; Denosumab; Dipyrone; Ocrelizumab; Palifermin; Pimecrolimus; Promazine; Roflumilast; Tacrolimus (Topical); Taxane Derivatives; Trastuzumab

Decreased Effect

EpiRUBicin may decrease the levels/effects of: BCG (Intravesical); Cardiac Glycosides; Coccidioides immitis Skin Test; Lenograstim; Nivolumab; Sipuleucel-T; Tertomotide; Vaccines (Inactivated); Vaccines (Live)

The levels/effects of EpiRUBicin may be decreased by: Cardiac Glycosides; Echinacea

Hazardous Drugs Handling Considerations

Hazardous agent (NIOSH 2016 [group 1]).

Use appropriate precautions for receiving, handling, administration, and disposal. Gloves (single) should be worn during receiving, unpacking, and placing in storage.

NIOSH recommends double gloving, a protective gown, ventilated engineering controls (a class II biological safety cabinet or a compounding aseptic containment isolator), and closed system transfer devices (CSTDs) for preparation. Double gloving, a gown, and (if dosage form allows) CSTDs are required during administration (NIOSH 2016).

Storage/Stability Protect from light.

Solution: Store intact vials at 2°C to 8°C (36°F to 46°F); do not freeze. Protect from light. Product may "gel" at refrigerated temperatures; will return to slightly viscous solution after 2 to 4 hours at room temperature (15°C to 25°C). Discard unused solution from single dose vials within 24 hours of entry.

Lyophilized powder: Store at room temperature of 25°C (77°F); excursions permitted to 15°C to 30°C (59°F to 86°F). Reconstituted solutions are stable for 24 hours when stored at 2°C to 8°C (36°F to 46°F) or at room temperature.

Preparation for Administration Reconstitute lyophilized powder with sterile water for injection (25 mL for the 50 mg vial) to a final concentration of 2 mg/mL. Shake vigorously; may take several minutes for dissolution. May be further diluted with sterile water for injection.

Mechanism of Action Epirubicin is an anthracycline antineoplastic agent; known to inhibit DNA and RNA synthesis by steric obstruction after intercalating between DNA base pairs; active throughout entire cell cycle. Intercalation triggers DNA cleavage by topoisomerase II, resulting in cytocidal activity. Also inhibits DNA helicase, and generates cytotoxic free radicals.

Pharmacodynamics/Kinetics

Distribution: V_{dss}: 21 to 27 L/kg

Protein binding: ~77% to albumin

Metabolism: Extensively via hepatic and extrahepatic (including RBCs) routes

Half-life elimination: Triphasic; Mean terminal: 33 hours

Excretion: Feces (34% to 35%); urine (20% to 27%)

Dosing

Adult Note: Patients receiving 120 mg/m^2/cycle as part of combination therapy (CEF-120 regimen) should also receive prophylactic antibiotic therapy with sulfamethoxazole/trimethoprim or a fluoroquinolone. Lower starting doses may be necessary for heavily pretreated patients, patients with preexisting myelosuppression, or with bone marrow involvement. If clinically reasonable, delay epirubicin therapy until other cardiotoxic agents with long half-lives (eg, trastuzumab) have been cleared. The recommended lifetime maximum dose is 900 mg/m^2. Epirubicin is associated with a moderate to high emetic potential (depending on dose or regimen); antiemetics are recommended to prevent nausea and vomiting (Basch 2011; Dupuis 2011; Roila 2016).

Breast cancer, adjuvant treatment: IV: Usual dose: 100 to 120 mg/m² per 3- or 4-week treatment cycle as follows:

60 mg/m² on days 1 and 8 every 28 days for 6 cycles in combination with cyclophosphamide and fluorouracil (CEF-120 regimen; Levine 2005) **or**

100 mg/m² on day 1 every 21 days for 6 cycles in combination with cyclophosphamide and fluorouracil (FEC-100 regimen; Bonneterre 2005) **or**

Breast cancer (off-label regimens): IV:

EC regimen: 100 mg/m² on day 1 every 21 days for 8 cycles in combination with cyclophosphamide (Piccart 2001) **or**

EP or EC regimen: 75 mg/m² on day 1 every 21 days for up to 6 cycles in combination with either paclitaxel or cyclophosphamide (Langley 2005) **or**

FEC regimen ± paclitaxel: 90 mg/m² on day 1 every 21 days for 6 cycles in combination with fluorouracil and cyclophosphamide or for 4 cycles in combination with fluorouracil and cyclophosphamide followed by paclitaxel (Martin 2008) **or**

FEC regimen followed by pertuzumab + trastuzumab + docetaxel: 100 mg/m² on day 1 every 21 days for 3 cycles in combination with fluorouracil and cyclophosphamide, followed by 3 cycles of pertuzumab, trastuzumab, and docetaxel (Schneeweiss 2013) **or**

CEF regimen: 50 mg/m² on days 1 and 8 every 21 or 28 days for 6 to 9 cycles in combination with cyclophosphamide and fluorouracil (Ackland 2001)

Esophageal cancer (off-label use): IV:

ECF, ECX, EOF, and EOX regimens: 50 mg/m² on day 1 every 21 days for up to 8 cycles in combination with cisplatin (C), oxaliplatin (O), fluorouracil (F), and/or capecitabine (X) (Cunningham 2008) **or**

ECF regimen: 50 mg/m² on day 1 every 21 days for 3 preoperative and 3 postoperative cycles in combination with cisplatin and fluorouracil (Cunningham 2006)

Gastric cancer (off-label use): IV:

ECF, ECX, EOF, and EOX regimens: 50 mg/m² on day 1 every 21 days for up to 8 cycles in combination with cisplatin (C), oxaliplatin (O), fluorouracil (F), and/or capecitabine (X) (Cunningham 2008; Waters 1999) **or**

ECF regimen: 50 mg/m² on day 1 every 21 days for 3 preoperative and 3 postoperative cycles in combination with cisplatin and fluorouracil (Cunningham 2006)

Osteosarcoma (off-label use): IV: 90 mg/m² on day 1 every 21 days for 3 cycles before surgery and 90 mg/m² on day 1 every 28 days for 3 cycles after surgery (in combination with cisplatin, ifosfamide and mesna) (Basaran 2007)

Soft tissue sarcoma (off-label use): IV: 25 mg/m² on days 1, 2, and 3 every 28 days for 4 cycles (in combination with ifosfamide and mesna) (Petrioli 2002) **or** 60 mg/m² on days 1 and 2 every 21 days for 5 cycles (in combination with ifosfamide, mesna, and filgrastim) (Frustaci 2001)

Dosage adjustment for toxicity (breast cancer; labeled dosing):

Note: Heavily-treated patients, patients with preexisting bone marrow depression or neoplastic bone marrow infiltration: Lower starting doses (75 to 90 mg/m²) should be considered.

Delay day 1 dose of subsequent cycles until platelets are ≥100,000/mm³, ANC ≥1500/mm³, and nonhematologic toxicities have recovered to ≤ grade 1

◀

Reduce day 1 dose in subsequent cycles to 75% of previous day 1 dose if patient experiences nadir platelet counts <50,000/mm^3, ANC <250/mm^3, neutropenic fever, or grade 3/4 nonhematologic toxicity during the previous cycle

For CEF-120 regimen, reduce day 8 dose to 75% of day 1 dose if platelet counts are 75,000 to 100,000/mm^3 and ANC is 1000 to 1499/mm^3; omit day 8 dose if platelets are <75,000/mm^3, ANC <1000/mm^3, or grade 3/4 nonhematologic toxicity

Geriatric Plasma clearance of epirubicin in elderly female patients was noted to be reduced by 35%. Although no initial dosage reduction is specifically recommended, particular care should be exercised in monitoring toxicity and adjusting subsequent dosage in elderly patients (particularly females >70 years of age).

Renal Impairment The manufacturer's labeling recommends lower doses (dose not specified) in patients with severe renal impairment (serum creatinine >5 mg/dL). Other sources (Aronoff 2007) suggest no dosage adjustment is needed for CrCl <50 mL/minute.

Hepatic Impairment The manufacturer's labeling recommends the following adjustments (based on clinical trial information):

Bilirubin 1.2 to 3 mg/dL or AST 2 to 4 times the upper limit of normal: Administer 50% of recommended starting dose

Bilirubin >3 mg/dL or AST >4 times the upper limit of normal: Administer 25% of recommended starting dose

Severe hepatic impairment: Use is not recommended (has not been studied).

Obesity *ASCO Guidelines for appropriate chemotherapy dosing in obese adults with cancer:* Utilize patient's actual body weight (full weight) for calculation of body surface area- or weight-based dosing, particularly when the intent of therapy is curative; manage regimen-related toxicities in the same manner as for nonobese patients; if a dose reduction is utilized due to toxicity, consider resumption of full weight-based dosing with subsequent cycles, especially if cause of toxicity (eg, hepatic or renal impairment) is resolved (Griggs 2012).

Combination Regimens

Bone sarcoma (osteosarcoma): Ifosfamide-Cisplatin-Epirubicin (Osteosarcoma) on page 2155

Breast cancer:

Cyclophosphamide-Epirubicin (Breast) on page 2077

Docetaxel-Trastuzumab followed by FEC (Breast) on page 2095

FEC followed by Docetaxel Every 3 Weeks (Breast) on page 2112

FEC followed by Paclitaxel Weekly (Breast) on page 2112

FEC IV (Breast) on page 2112

FEC Oral (Breast) on page 2113

Esophageal cancer:

Epirubicin-Cisplatin-Capecitabine (Gastric/Esophageal) on page 2103

Epirubicin-Cisplatin-Fluorouracil (Gastric/Esophageal) on page 2103

Epirubicin-Oxaliplatin-Capecitabine (Gastric/Esophageal) on page 2104

Epirubicin-Oxaliplatin-Fluorouracil (Gastric/Esophageal) on page 2105

Gastric cancer:

Epirubicin-Cisplatin-Capecitabine (Gastric/Esophageal) on page 2103

Epirubicin-Cisplatin-Fluorouracil (Gastric/Esophageal) on page 2103

Epirubicin-Oxaliplatin-Capecitabine (Gastric/Esophageal) on page 2104

Epirubicin-Oxaliplatin-Fluorouracil (Gastric/Esophageal) on page 2105

Soft tissue sarcoma: Epirubicin-Ifosfamide (Soft Tissue Sarcoma) on page 2103

Administration Epirubicin is associated with a moderate to high emetic potential (depending on dose or regimen); antiemetics are recommended to prevent nausea and vomiting (Basch 2011; Dupuis 2011; Roila 2016).

IV: Infuse over 15 to 20 minutes or slow IV push; if lower doses due to dose reduction are administered, may reduce infusion time proportionally. Do not infuse over <3 minutes. Infuse into a free-flowing IV solution (NS or D5W). Avoid the use of veins over joints or in extremities with compromised venous or lymphatic drainage.

Vesicant; ensure proper needle or catheter placement prior to and during infusion; avoid extravasation.

Extravasation management: If extravasation occurs, stop infusion immediately and disconnect (leave cannula/needle in place); gently aspirate extravasated solution (do **NOT** flush the line); remove needle/cannula; elevate extremity. Initiate antidote (dexrazoxane or dimethyl sulfate [DMSO]). Apply dry cold compresses for 20 minutes 4 times daily for 1 to 2 days (Perez Fidalgo 2012); withhold cooling beginning 15 minutes before dexrazoxane infusion; continue withholding cooling until 15 minutes after infusion is completed. Topical DMSO should not be administered in combination with dexrazoxane; may lessen dexrazoxane efficacy.

Dexrazoxane: Adults: 1,000 mg/m^2 (maximum dose: 2,000 mg) IV (administer in a large vein remote from site of extravasation) over 1 to 2 hours days 1 and 2, then 500 mg/m^2 (maximum dose: 1,000 mg) IV over 1 to 2 hours day 3; begin within 6 hours of extravasation. Day 2 and day 3 doses should be administered at approximately the same time (± 3 hours) as the dose on day 1 (Mouridsen 2007; Perez Fidalgo 2012). **Note:** Reduce dexrazoxane dose by 50% in patients with moderate to severe renal impairment (CrCl <40 mL/minute).

DMSO: Children and Adults: Apply topically to a region covering twice the affected area every 8 hours for 7 days; begin within 10 minutes of extravasation; do not cover with a dressing (Perez Fidalgo 2012).

Vesicant/Extravasation Risk Vesicant

Emetic Potential

Children: Moderate (30% to 90%)

Adults:

>90 mg/m^2 or when used in combination with cyclophosphamide: High (>90%)

≤90 mg/m^2: Moderate (30% to 90%)

Monitoring Parameters Baseline and repeated measurements of CBC with differential, liver function tests, serum creatinine, electrolytes, ECG, and LVEF. The method used for assessment of LVEF (echocardiogram or MUGA) should be consistent during routine monitoring. Monitor injection site during infusion for possible extravasation or local reactions.

Dosage Forms Excipient information presented when available (limited, particularly for generics); consult specific product labeling. [DSC] = Discontinued product

Solution, Intravenous, as hydrochloride [preservative free]:

Ellence: 50 mg/25 mL (25 mL); 200 mg/100 mL (100 mL)

Generic: 50 mg/25 mL (25 mL); 200 mg/100 mL (100 mL)

Solution Reconstituted, Intravenous, as hydrochloride:

Generic: 50 mg (1 ea [DSC])

Epoetin Alfa (e POE e tin AL fa)

Related Information

Palliative Care Medicine (Cancer) *on page 2352*

Brand Names: US Epogen; Procrit

Brand Names: Canada Eprex

Index Terms rHuEPO; rHuEPO-α; EPO; Epoetin Alfa, Recombinant; Erythropoiesis-Stimulating Agent (ESA); Erythropoietin

Pharmacologic Category Colony Stimulating Factor; Erythropoiesis-Stimulating Agent (ESA); Hematopoietic Agent

Use

Anemia due to chemotherapy in patients with cancer: Treatment of anemia in patients with nonmyeloid malignancies in which anemia is due to the effect of concomitant myelosuppressive chemotherapy, and upon initiation, there is a minimum of 2 additional months of planned chemotherapy.

Anemia due to chronic kidney disease: Treatment of anemia due to chronic kidney disease, including patients on dialysis and not on dialysis, to decrease the need for RBC transfusion.

Anemia due to zidovudine in HIV-infected patients: Treatment of anemia due to zidovudine administered at ≤4,200 mg/week in HIV-infected patients with endogenous serum erythropoietin levels of ≤500 milliunits/mL.

Reduction of allogeneic RBC transfusion in patients undergoing elective, noncardiac, nonvascular surgery: To reduce the need for allogeneic RBC transfusions among patients with perioperative hemoglobin >10 to ≤13 g/dL who are at high risk of perioperative blood loss from elective, noncardiac, nonvascular surgery. Epoetin alfa is not indicated for patients who are willing to donate autologous blood preoperatively.

Limitations of use: Epoetin alfa has not been shown to improve quality of life, fatigue, or patient well-being. Epoetin alfa is **not** indicated for use under the following conditions:
- Cancer patients receiving hormonal therapy, therapeutic biologic products, or radiation therapy unless also receiving concurrent myelosuppressive chemotherapy
- Cancer patients receiving myelosuppressive chemotherapy when the expected outcome is curative
- Cancer patients receiving myelosuppressive chemotherapy when anemia can be managed by transfusion
- Surgery patients who are willing to donate autologous blood
- Surgery patients undergoing cardiac or vascular surgery
- As a substitute for RBC transfusion in patients requiring immediate correction of anemia

Labeled Contraindications Serious allergic reactions to epoetin alfa or any component of the formulation; uncontrolled hypertension; pure red cell aplasia (PRCA) that begins after treatment with epoetin alfa or other epoetin protein drugs; multidose vials contain benzyl alcohol and are contraindicated in neonates, infants, pregnant women, and nursing women

Pregnancy Considerations Adverse events were observed in animal reproduction studies. In vitro studies suggest that recombinant erythropoietin does not cross the human placenta (Reisenberger 1997). Polyhydramnios and intrauterine growth retardation have been reported with use in women with chronic kidney disease (adverse effects also associated with maternal disease). Hypospadias and pectus excavatum have been reported with first trimester exposure (case report).

Recombinant erythropoietin alfa has been evaluated as adjunctive treatment for severe pregnancy associated iron deficiency anemia (Breymann 2001; Krafft 2009) and has been used in pregnant women with iron-deficiency anemia associated with chronic kidney disease (CKD) (Furaz-Czerpak 2012; Josephson 2007).

Amenorrheic premenopausal women should be cautioned that menstruation may resume following treatment with recombinant erythropoietin (Furaz-Czerpak 2012). Multidose formulations containing benzyl alcohol are contra-indicated for use in pregnant women; if treatment during pregnancy is needed, single dose preparations should be used.

Women who become pregnant during treatment with epoetin alfa are encouraged to enroll In Amgen's Pregnancy Surveillance Program (1-800-772-6436).

Breastfeeding Considerations Endogenous erythropoietin is found in breast milk (Semba 2002). It is not known if recombinant erythropoietin alfa is present in breast milk. The manufacturer recommends caution be used if the single dose vial preparation is administered to breastfeeding women; use of the multiple dose vials containing benzyl alcohol is contraindicated in breastfeeding women. When administered enterally to neonates (mixed with human milk or infant formula), recombinant erythropoietin did not significantly increase serum EPO concentrations. If passage via breast milk does occur, risk to a breastfed infant appears low (Juul 2003).

Warnings/Precautions [US Boxed Warning]: Erythropoiesis-stimulating agents (ESAs) increased the risk of serious cardiovascular events, MI, stroke, venous thromboembolism, vascular access thrombosis, mortality, and/or tumor progression in clinical studies when administered to target hemoglobin levels >11 g/dL (and provide no additional benefit); a rapid rise in hemoglobin (>1 g/dL over 2 weeks) may also contribute to these risks. **[US Boxed Warning]: A shortened overall survival and/or increased risk of tumor progression or recurrence has been reported in studies with breast, cervical, head and neck, lymphoid, and non-small cell lung cancer patients.** It is of note that in most of these studies, patients received ESAs to a target hemoglobin of ≥12 g/dL; although risk has not been excluded when dosed to achieve a target hemoglobin of <12 g/dL. **[US Boxed Warnings]: To decrease these risks, and risk of cardio- and thrombovascular events, use the lowest dose needed to avoid red blood cell transfusions. Use ESAs in cancer patients only for the treatment of anemia related to concurrent myelosuppressive chemotherapy; discontinue ESA following completion of the chemotherapy course. ESAs are not indicated for patients receiving myelosuppressive therapy when the anticipated outcome is curative.** A dosage modification is appropriate if hemoglobin levels ▶

rise >1 g/dL per 2-week time period during treatment (Rizzo 2010). Use of ESAs has been associated with an increased risk of VTE without a reduction in transfusions in patients with cancer (Hershman 2009). Improved anemia symptoms, quality of life, fatigue, or well-being have not been demonstrated in controlled clinical trials.

[US Boxed Warning]: An increased risk of death, serious cardiovascular events, and stroke was reported in chronic kidney disease (CKD) patients administered ESAs to target hemoglobin levels >11 g/dL; use the lowest dose sufficient to reduce the need for RBC transfusions. An optimal target hemoglobin level, dose or dosing strategy to reduce these risks has not been identified in clinical trials. Hemoglobin rising >1 g/dL in a 2-week period may contribute to the risk (dosage reduction recommended). The American College of Physicians recommends against the use of ESAs in patients with mild to moderate anemia and heart failure or coronary heart disease (ACP [Qaseem 2013]). The ACCF/AHA 2013 Heart Failure Guidelines do not provide a clear recommendation on the use of erythropoiesis-stimulating agents (ESA) in anemic heart failure patients. The effects of ESAs on quality of life measures, morbidity, and mortality are potentially modest and still unclear. Additionally, the safety of epoetin alfa has not been well studied in this population. The authors declined to provide an official recommendation regarding the use of ESAs pending the completion of ongoing randomized trials (ACCF/AHA [Yancy 2013]).

Chronic kidney disease patients who exhibit an inadequate hemoglobin response to ESA therapy may be at a higher risk for cardiovascular events and mortality compared to other patients. ESA therapy may reduce dialysis efficacy (due to increase in red blood cells and decrease in plasma volume); adjustments in dialysis parameters may be needed. Patients treated with epoetin may require increased heparinization during dialysis to prevent clotting of the extracorporeal circuit. **[US Boxed Warning]: DVT prophylaxis is recommended in perisurgery patients due to the risk of DVT.** Increased mortality was also observed in patients undergoing coronary artery bypass surgery who received epoetin alfa; these deaths were associated with thrombotic events. Epoetin alfa is **not** approved for reduction of red blood cell transfusion in patients undergoing cardiac or vascular surgery and is **not** indicated for surgical patients willing to donate autologous blood.

Use with caution in patients with hypertension (contraindicated in uncontrolled hypertension) or with a history of seizures; hypertensive encephalopathy and seizures have been reported. If hypertension is difficult to control, reduce or hold epoetin alfa. An excessive rate of rise of hemoglobin is associated with hypertension or exacerbation of hypertension; decrease the epoetin alfa dose if the hemoglobin increase exceeds 1 g/dL in any 2-week period. Blood pressure should be controlled prior to start of therapy and monitored closely throughout treatment. The risk for seizures is increased with epoetin alfa use in patients with CKD; monitor closely for neurologic symptoms during the first several months of therapy. Due to the delayed onset of erythropoiesis, epoetin alfa is **not** recommended for acute correction of severe anemia or as a substitute for emergency transfusion.

Prior to treatment, correct or exclude deficiencies of iron, vitamin B_{12}, and/or folate, as well as other factors which may impair erythropoiesis (inflammatory conditions, infections, bleeding). Prior to and periodically during therapy, iron stores must be evaluated. Supplemental iron is recommended if serum ferritin

<100 mcg/L or serum transferrin saturation <20%; most patients with chronic kidney disease will require iron supplementation. Poor response should prompt evaluation of these potential factors, as well as possible malignant processes and hematologic disease (thalassemia, refractory anemia, myelo-dysplastic disorder), occult blood loss, hemolysis, osteitis fibrosa cystic, and/or bone marrow fibrosis. Severe anemia and pure red cell aplasia (PRCA) with associated neutralizing antibodies to erythropoietin has been reported, pre-dominantly in patients with CKD receiving SubQ epoetin alfa (the IV route is preferred for hemodialysis patients). Cases have also been reported in patients with hepatitis C who were receiving ESAs, interferon, and ribavirin. Patients with a sudden loss of response to epoetin alfa (with severe anemia and a low reticulocyte count) should be evaluated for PRCA with associated neutralizing antibodies to erythropoietin; discontinue treatment (permanently) in patients with PRCA secondary to neutralizing antibodies to epoetin alfa. Antibodies may cross-react; do not switch to another ESA in patients who develop antibody-mediated anemia.

The American Society of Clinical Oncology (ASCO) and American Society of Hematology (ASH) 2010 updates to the clinical practice guidelines for the use of ESAs in patients with cancer indicate that ESAs are appropriate when used according to the parameters identified within the FDA-approved labeling for epoetin and darbepoetin alfa (Rizzo 2010). ESAs are an option for chemo-therapy associated anemia when the hemoglobin has fallen to <10 g/dL to decrease the need for RBC transfusions. ESAs should only be used in conjunction with concurrent chemotherapy. Although the FDA label now limits ESA use to the palliative setting, the ASCO/ASH guidelines suggest using clinical judgment in weighing risks versus benefits as formal outcomes studies of ESA use defined by intent of chemotherapy treatment have not been conducted.

Potentially serious allergic reactions have been reported (rarely), including anaphylactic reactions, angioedema, bronchospasm, rash, and urticaria. Discontinue immediately (and permanently) in patients who experience seri-ous allergic/anaphylactic reactions. Some products may contain albumin. Some dosage forms may contain polysorbate 80 (also known as Tweens). Hypersensitivity reactions, usually a delayed reaction, have been reported following exposure to pharmaceutical products containing polysorbate 80 in certain individuals (Isaksson 2002; Lucente 2000; Shelley 1995). Thrombo-cytopenia, ascites, pulmonary deterioration, and renal and hepatic failure have been reported in premature neonates after receiving parenteral products containing polysorbate 80 (Alade 1986; CDC 1984). See manufacturer's labeling. Benzyl alcohol and derivatives: Some dosage forms may contain benzyl alcohol; large amounts of benzyl alcohol (≥99 mg/kg/day) have been associated with a potentially fatal toxicity ("gasping syndrome") in neonates; the "gasping syndrome" consists of metabolic acidosis, respiratory distress, gasping respirations, CNS dysfunction (including convulsions, intracranial hemorrhage), hypotension and cardiovascular collapse (AAP ["Inactive" 1997]; CDC 1982); some data suggests that benzoate displaces bilirubin from protein binding sites (Ahlfors 2001); avoid or use dosage forms containing benzyl alcohol with caution in neonates. See manufacturer's labeling.

Adverse Reactions

>10%:

Cardiovascular: Hypertension (3% to 28%)

Central nervous system: Headache (5% to 18%)

Dermatologic: Pruritus (12% to 21%), skin rash (2% to 19%)
Gastrointestinal: Nausea (35% to 56%), vomiting (12% to 28%)
Local: Injection site reaction (7% to 13%)
Neuromuscular & skeletal: Arthralgia (10% to 16%)
Respiratory: Cough (4% to 26%)
Miscellaneous: Fever (10% to 42%)
1% to 10%:
Cardiovascular: Deep vein thrombosis, edema, pulmonary embolism, thrombosis, thrombosis of hemodialysis vascular access
Central nervous system: Chills, depression, dizziness, insomnia
Dermatologic: Urticaria
Endocrine & metabolic: Hyperglycemia, hypokalemia, weight loss
Gastrointestinal: Dysphagia, stomatitis
Hematologic & oncologic: Leukopenia
Neuromuscular & skeletal: Muscle spasm, myalgia, ostealgia
Respiratory: Respiratory congestion, upper respiratory tract infection
<1%, postmarketing, and/or case reports: Anaphylaxis, angioedema, antibody development (neutralizing), bronchospasm, cerebrovascular accident, erythema, hypersensitivity reaction, hypertensive encephalopathy, myocardial infarction, porphyria, pure red cell aplasia, retinal thrombosis (arterial), seizure, tachycardia, thrombophlebitis, thrombosis (includes microvascular and temporal), transient ischemic attacks, tumor growth, venous thrombosis

Drug Interactions

Metabolism/Transport Effects None known.

Avoid Concomitant Use There are no known interactions where it is recommended to avoid concomitant use.

Increased Effect/Toxicity

Epoetin Alfa may increase the levels/effects of: Lenalidomide; Pomalidomide; Thalidomide

The levels/effects of Epoetin Alfa may be increased by: Nandrolone

Decreased Effect There are no known significant interactions involving a decrease in effect.

Storage/Stability Vials should be stored at 2°C to 8°C (36°F to 46°F). **Do not freeze. Do not shake.** Protect from light.

Single-dose 1 mL vial contains no preservative. Use one dose per vial. Do not re-enter vial; discard unused portions.

Single-dose vials (except 40,000 units/mL vial) are stable for 2 weeks at room temperature (Cohen 2007). Single-dose 40,000 units/mL vial is stable for 1 week at room temperature.

Multidose 1 mL or 2 mL vial contains preservative. Store at 2°C to 8°C after initial entry and between doses. Discard 21 days after initial entry.

Multidose vials (with preservative) are stable for 1 week at room temperature (Cohen 2007).

Prefilled syringes containing the 20,000 units/mL formulation with preservative are stable for 6 weeks refrigerated (2°C to 8°C) (Naughton 2003).

Dilutions of 1:10 and 1:20 (1 part epoetin alfa:19 parts sodium chloride) are stable for 18 hours at room temperature (Ohls 1996).

Prior to SubQ administration, preservative free solutions may be mixed with bacteriostatic NS containing benzyl alcohol 0.9% in a 1:1 ratio (Corbo 1992).

Dilutions of 1:10 in D10W with human albumin 0.05% or 0.1% are stable for 24 hours.

Preparation for Administration Prior to SubQ administration, preservative free solutions may be mixed with bacteriostatic NS containing benzyl alcohol 0.9% in a 1:1 ratio.

Mechanism of Action Epoetin alfa induces erythropoiesis by stimulating the division and differentiation of committed erythroid progenitor cells; induces the release of reticulocytes from the bone marrow into the bloodstream, where they mature to erythrocytes. There is a dose response relationship with this effect. This results in an increase in reticulocyte counts followed by a rise in hematocrit and hemoglobin levels.

Pharmacodynamics/Kinetics Note: While a much higher peak plasma concentration is achieved after IV bolus administration, it declines at a more rapid rate than after subcutaneous administration (McMahon 1990; Salmonson 1990)

Onset of action: Reticulocyte count increase: Within 10 days.

Peak effect: Hemoglobin level: 2 to 6 weeks

Absorption: SubQ: Slow (McMahon 1990; Salmonson 1990)

Distribution: V_d: 9 L; rapid in the plasma compartment; concentrated in liver, kidneys, and bone marrow; similar to extracellular plasma volume in adults (McMahon 1990; Salmonson 1990); reported to be higher in premature neonates on body weight basis (Brown 1993)

Metabolism: Some degradation does occur

Bioavailability: SubQ: Premature neonates: 42% (Brown 1993); Adults: 36% (Salmonson 1990); intraperitoneal epoetin alfa: 3% (Macdougall 1989)

Half-life elimination:

Neonates: With high doses, nonlinear kinetics have been observed (Wu 2012)

Anemia of prematurity:

Post menstrual age (PMA) <32 week (weight: 800 ± 206 grams): IV: 8.1 ± 2.7 hours; SubQ: 7.1 ± 4.1 hours (Brown 1993)

PMA ≥32 weeks (weight range: 1,330 to 1,740 g): SubQ: Median: 7.9 hours (range: 5.6 to 19.4 hours) (Krishnan 1996)

Neuroprotective/hypoxic ischemia encephalopathy (HIE) (Wu 2012): ≥36 weeks GA; IV:

250 units/kg: 7.6 ± 6.9 hours

500 units/kg: 7.2 ± 1.9 hours

1,000 units/kg: 15 ± 4.5 hours

2,500 units/kg: 18.7 ± 4.7 hours

Infants, Children, and Adolescents: Chronic kidney disease: IV: 4 to 13 hours

Adults: Cancer: SubQ: 16 to 67 hours; Chronic kidney disease: IV: 4 to 13 hours

Time to peak, serum: Pediatric patients >1 month and Adults: Chronic kidney disease: SubQ: 5 to 24 hours

Dosing

Adult & Geriatric Note: Evaluate iron status in all patients before and during treatment and maintain iron repletion.

Anemia due to chronic kidney disease (CKD): Individualize dosing and use the lowest dose necessary to reduce the need for RBC transfusions.

*Chronic kidney disease patients **ON dialysis*** (IV route is preferred for hemodialysis patients; initiate treatment when hemoglobin is <10 g/dL; reduce dose or interrupt treatment if hemoglobin approaches or exceeds 11 g/dL): IV, SubQ: Initial dose: 50 to 100 units/kg 3 times a week

*Chronic kidney disease patients **NOT on dialysis*** (consider initiating treatment when hemoglobin is <10 g/dL; use only if rate of hemoglobin decline would likely result in RBC transfusion and desire is to reduce risk of alloimmunization and/or other RBC transfusion-related risks; reduce dose or interrupt treatment if hemoglobin exceeds 10 g/dL): IV, SubQ: Initial dose: 50 to 100 units/kg 3 times a week

Dosage adjustments for chronic kidney disease patients (either on dialysis or not on dialysis): Do not increase dose more frequently than every 4 weeks (dose decreases may occur more frequently); avoid frequent dosage adjustments.

If hemoglobin does not increase by >1 g/dL after 4 weeks: Increase dose by 25%

If hemoglobin increases >1 g/dL in any 2-week period: Reduce dose by ≥25%

Inadequate or lack of response over a 12-week escalation period: Further increases are unlikely to improve response and may increase risks; use the minimum effective dose that will maintain a hemoglobin level sufficient to avoid RBC transfusions and evaluate patient for other causes of anemia. Discontinue therapy if responsiveness does not improve.

Anemia due to chemotherapy in cancer patients: Initiate treatment only if hemoglobin <10 g/dL and anticipated duration of myelosuppressive chemotherapy is at least 2 additional months. Titrate dosage to use the minimum effective dose that will maintain a hemoglobin level sufficient to avoid red blood cell transfusions. Discontinue erythropoietin following completion of chemotherapy. SubQ: Initial dose: 150 units/kg 3 times a week or 40,000 units once weekly until completion of chemotherapy

Dosage adjustments:

If hemoglobin does not increase by ≥1 g/dL **and** remains below 10 g/dL after initial 4 weeks: Increase to 300 units/kg 3 times a week or 60,000 units weekly; discontinue after 8 weeks of treatment if RBC transfusions are still required or there is no hemoglobin response

If hemoglobin exceeds a level needed to avoid red blood cell transfusion: Withhold dose; resume treatment with a 25% dose reduction when hemoglobin approaches a level where transfusions may be required.

If hemoglobin increases >1 g/dL in any 2-week period **or** hemoglobin reaches a level sufficient to avoid red blood cell transfusion: Reduce dose by 25%.

Anemia due to zidovudine in HIV-infected patients: Titrate dosage to use the minimum effective dose that will maintain a hemoglobin level sufficient to avoid red blood cell transfusions. Hemoglobin levels should not exceed 12 g/dL.

Serum erythropoietin levels ≤500 milliunits/mL and zidovudine doses ≤4200 mg/week): IV, SubQ: Initial: 100 units/kg 3 times a week; if hemoglobin does not increase after 8 weeks, increase dose by ~50 to 100 units/kg at 4 to 8 week intervals until hemoglobin reaches a level sufficient to avoid RBC transfusion; maximum dose: 300 units/kg. Withhold dose if hemoglobin exceeds 12 g/dL, may resume treatment with a 25% dose reduction once hemoglobin <11 g/dL. Discontinue if hemoglobin increase is not achieved with 300 units/kg for 8 weeks.

Reduction of allogeneic RBC transfusion in patients undergoing elective, noncardiac, nonvascular surgery (perioperative hemoglobin should be >10 g/dL and ≤13 g/dL; DVT prophylactic anticoagulation is recommended): SubQ: Initial dose:

300 units/kg/day for 15 days total, beginning 10 days before surgery, on the day of surgery, and for 4 days after surgery **or**

600 units/kg once weekly for 4 doses, given 21-, 14-, and 7 days before surgery, and on the day of surgery

Red blood cell transfusion refusal (substitute) (off-label use): Note: Concomitantly administer iron (with or without vitamin B_{12} and folic acid supplementation) with epoetin alfa and use in conjunction with other blood conservation techniques.

Spinal (elective) surgery: SubQ: 40,000 units weekly for 4 weeks prior to surgery (Joseph 2008).

Cardiac (elective) surgery:

One protocol based on timing of elective surgery and preoperative hemoglobin (Hgb) used the following (McCartney 2014):

>21 days until surgery:

Hgb <10 g/dL: Delay surgery; identify cause of anemia.

Hgb 10 to 12 g/dL: SubQ: 40,000 units (if <65 kg, use 600 units/**kg**/dose) weekly starting 21 days before surgery.

Hgb >12 to <13 g/dL: SubQ: 40,000 units (if <65 kg, use 600 units/**kg**/dose) weekly starting 10 days before surgery and repeat 3 days before surgery or on the morning of surgery.

<21 days until surgery:

Hgb <10 g/dL: Delay surgery; identify cause of anemia.

Hgb 10 to 12 g/dL: SubQ: 20,000 units (if <65 kg, use 300 units/**kg**/dose) daily starting up to 10 days before surgery, on the day of surgery, and 4 days postoperatively if necessary.

Hgb >12 to <13 g/dL: SubQ: 20,000 units (if <65 kg, use 300 units/**kg**/dose) daily starting up to 10 days before surgery, on the day of surgery, and 4 days postoperatively if necessary.

Another protocol utilized weight-based dosing (Tanaka 2015):

Preoperative:

IV: 200 units/kg every 24 hours.

SubQ: 250 to 500 units/kg every 48 hours.

Note: Timing prior to surgery was not described; target Hgb of 12 g/dL.

Postoperative:

IV: 200 to 300 units/kg every 24 hours.

SubQ: 250 to 500 units/kg every 48 hours.

Note: Target Hgb >10 g/dL.

Symptomatic anemia in myelodysplastic syndromes (off-label use): SubQ: 150 to 300 units/kg once daily (Greenburg 2009) or 450 to 1000 units/kg/week in divided doses, 3 to 7 times a week (Hellström-Lindberg 1995) or 60,000 units once weekly (Park 2008)

Pediatric Note: Evaluate iron status in all patients before and during treatment and maintain iron repletion.

Anemia due to chemotherapy in cancer patients: Initiate treatment only if hemoglobin <10 g/dL and anticipated duration of myelosuppressive chemotherapy is at least 2 additional months. Titrate dosage to use the minimum effective dose that will maintain a hemoglobin level sufficient to avoid red blood cell transfusions. Discontinue erythropoietin following completion of chemotherapy.

Children ≥5 years and Adolescents: IV: Initial dose: 600 units/kg once weekly until completion of chemotherapy.

Dosage adjustments:

If hemoglobin does not increase by ≥1 g/dL **and** remains <10 g/dL after initial 4 weeks: Increase to 900 units/kg (maximum dose: 60,000 units); discontinue after 8 weeks of treatment if RBC transfusions are still required or there is no hemoglobin response.

If hemoglobin exceeds a level needed to avoid red blood cell transfusion: Withhold dose; resume treatment with a 25% dose reduction when hemoglobin approaches a level where transfusions may be required.

If hemoglobin increases >1 g/dL in any 2-week period **or** hemoglobin reaches a level sufficient to avoid red blood cell transfusion: Reduce dose by 25%.

Anemia due to chronic kidney disease (CKD): Individualize dosing and use the lowest dose necessary to reduce the need for RBC transfusions.

Chronic kidney disease patients ON dialysis (IV route is preferred for hemodialysis patients; initiate treatment when hemoglobin is <10 g/dL; reduce dose or interrupt treatment if hemoglobin approaches or exceeds 11 g/dL):

Pediatrics 1 month to 16 years: IV, SubQ: Initial dose: 50 units/kg 3 times a week

Dosage adjustments for chronic kidney disease patients: Do not increase dose more frequently than every 4 weeks (dose decreases may occur more frequently); avoid frequent dosage adjustments

If hemoglobin does not increase by >1 g/dL after 4 weeks: Increase dose by 25%

If hemoglobin increases >1 g/dL in any 2-week period: Reduce dose by ≥25%

Inadequate or lack of response over a 12-week escalation period: Further increases are unlikely to improve response and may increase risks; use the minimum effective dose that will maintain a hemoglobin level sufficient to avoid RBC transfusions and evaluate patient for other causes of anemia. Discontinue therapy if responsiveness does not improve.

Anemia due to zidovudine in HIV-infected patients: Titrate dosage to use the minimum effective dose that will maintain a hemoglobin level sufficient to avoid red blood cell transfusions. Hemoglobin levels should not exceed 12 g/dL. Children 8 months to 17 years (based on limited data): IV, SubQ: Reported dosing range: 50 to 400 units/kg 2 to 3 times a week

Renal Impairment No dosage adjustment necessary.

Hepatic Impairment There are no dosage adjustments provided in the manufacturer's labeling.

Administration

SubQ is the preferred route of administration **except** in patients with CKD on hemodialysis. In patients with CKD on hemodialysis, the IV route is recommended.

Do not shake. Epoetin is usually administered undiluted, although preservative-free (single-dose vial) formulations may be diluted in a syringe prior to administration as a 1:1 dilution using bacteriostatic NS.

Monitoring Parameters Transferrin saturation and serum ferritin (prior to and during treatment); hemoglobin (weekly after initiation and following dose adjustments until stable and sufficient to minimize need for RBC transfusion, CKD patients should be also be monitored at least monthly following hemoglobin stability); blood pressure; monitor for signs of seizures (CKD patients following initiation for first few months, includes new-onset or change in seizure frequency or premonitory symptoms).

Cancer patients: Examinations recommended by the ASCO/ASH guidelines (Rizzo 2010) prior to treatment include: peripheral blood smear (in some situations a bone marrow exam may be necessary), assessment for iron, folate, or vitamin B_{12} deficiency, reticulocyte count, renal function status, and occult blood loss; during ESA treatment, assess baseline and periodic iron, total iron-binding capacity, and transferrin saturation or ferritin levels.

Medication Guide Available Yes

Dosage Forms Excipient information presented when available (limited, particularly for generics); consult specific product labeling.
Solution, Injection:
Epogen: 10,000 units/mL (2 mL); 20,000 units/mL (1 mL) [contains benzyl alcohol]
Procrit: 10,000 units/mL (2 mL); 20,000 units/mL (1 mL) [contains benzyl alcohol]
Solution, Injection [preservative free]:
Epogen: 2000 units/mL (1 mL); 3000 units/mL (1 mL); 4000 units/mL (1 mL); 10,000 units/mL (1 mL)
Procrit: 2000 units/mL (1 mL); 3000 units/mL (1 mL); 4000 units/mL (1 mL); 10,000 units/mL (1 mL); 40,000 units/mL (1 mL)

Dosage Forms: Canada Information with regard to form, strength, and availability of products uniquely available in Canada but currently not available in the US. Refer also to Dosage Forms.

Excipient information presented when available (limited, particularly for generics); consult specific product labeling.
Injection, solution [preservative free]:
Eprex: 1000 units/0.5 mL (0.5 mL), 2000 units/0.5 mL (0.5 mL), 3000 units/0.3 mL (0.3 mL), 4000 units/0.4 mL (0.4 mL), 5000 units/0.5 mL (0.5 mL), 6000 units/0.6 mL (0.6 mL), 8000 units/0.8 mL (0.8 mL), 10,000 units/mL (1 mL), 20,000 units/0.5 mL (0.5 mL), 30,000 units/0.75 mL (0.75 mL), 40,000 units/mL (1 mL) [contains polysorbate 80; prefilled syringe, free of human serum albumin]

EriBULin (er i BUE lin)

Related Information

Common Toxicity Criteria *on page 2242*

Management of Chemotherapy-Induced Nausea and Vomiting in Adults *on page 2253*

Safe Handling of Hazardous Drugs *on page 2379*

Brand Names: US Halaven

Brand Names: Canada Halaven

Index Terms B1939; E7389; ER-086526; Eribulin Mesylate; Halichondrin B Analog

Pharmacologic Category Antineoplastic Agent, Antimicrotubular

Use

Breast cancer, metastatic: Treatment of metastatic breast cancer in patients who have received at least 2 prior chemotherapy regimens for the treatment of metastatic disease (prior treatment should have included an anthracycline and a taxane in either the adjuvant or metastatic setting)

Liposarcoma, unresectable or metastatic: Treatment of unresectable or metastatic liposarcoma in patients who have received a prior anthracycline-containing regimen

Labeled Contraindications

There are no contraindications listed in the manufacturer's labeling.

Canadian labeling (not in the US labeling): Hypersensitivity to eribulin mesylate, halichondrin B, or its chemical derivatives.

Pregnancy Considerations Adverse effects were observed in animal reproduction studies. Based on its mechanism of action, eribulin would be expected to cause fetal harm if administered during pregnancy. Women of reproductive potential should use effective contraception to avoid pregnancy during eribulin treatment and for at least 2 weeks following the last eribulin dose; males with female partners of reproductive potential should use effective contraception during eribulin treatment and for 3.5 months following the last dose. The Canadian labeling recommends effective contraception during and for at least 3 months after treatment in women of reproductive potential.

Breastfeeding Considerations It is not known if eribulin is excreted in breast milk. Due to the potential for serious adverse reactions in the nursing infant, breastfeeding is not recommended by the manufacturer during eribulin treatment and for 2 weeks after the last dose.

Warnings/Precautions Hematologic toxicity, including severe neutropenia and neutropenic fever, has occurred. Neutropenic sepsis (fatal) has also been reported (case reports). May require treatment delay and dosage reduction. A higher incidence of grade 4 neutropenia and neutropenic fever occurred in patients with ALT or AST >3 x ULN or bilirubin >1.5 x ULN. Monitor complete blood counts prior to each dose; more frequently if severe cytopenias develop. Patients with baseline neutrophils <1,500/mm^3 were not included in clinical studies.

Peripheral neuropathy commonly occurs. Peripheral neuropathy may be prolonged (>1 year in 5% of metastatic breast cancer patients and >60 days in close to 60% of liposarcoma patients); over 60% of liposarcoma patients with peripheral neuropathy had not recovered within a median follow-up of ~6 months in one clinical trial. The median time to the first occurrence of peripheral neuropathy (any severity) in liposarcoma patients was 5 months (range: 3.5 to 9 months). Monitor for signs of peripheral motor or sensory neuropathy. May require treatment delay or discontinuation. Some patients may have preexisting neuropathy due to prior chemotherapy; monitor closely for worsening neuropathy.

QT prolongation was observed on day 8 of eribulin therapy (in an uncontrolled study); monitor ECG in patients with heart failure, bradyarrhythmia, with concomitant medication known to prolong the QT interval, or with electrolyte imbalance; correct hypokalemia and hypomagnesemia prior to treatment; monitor electrolytes periodically during treatment. Avoid use in patients with congenital long QT syndrome.

Dosage reduction required in patients with mild to moderate (Child-Pugh class A or B) hepatic impairment; use has not been studied in patients with severe hepatic impairment; transaminase or bilirubin elevations are associated with a higher incidence of grade 4 neutropenia and neutropenic fever. Dosage reduction required in patients with moderate or severe renal impairment (CrCl 15 to 49 mL/minute). Potentially significant drug-drug interactions may exist, requiring dose or frequency adjustment, additional monitoring, and/or selection of alternative therapy. Some products available internationally may have vial strength and dosing expressed as the base (instead of as the salt); refer to prescribing information for specific dosing information.

Adverse Reactions

>10%:

Cardiovascular: Peripheral edema (≥5% to 12%)

Central nervous system: Fatigue (≤62%), peripheral neuropathy (29% to 35%; grades 3/4: 3% to 8%), headache (18% to 19%)

Dermatologic: Alopecia (35% to 45%)

Endocrine & metabolic: Hypokalemia (≥5% to 30%), hypocalcemia (28%), weight loss (21%), hypophosphatemia (20%)

Gastrointestinal: Nausea (35% to 41%), constipation (25% to 32%), abdominal pain (≥5% to 29%), anorexia (20%), decreased appetite (19%), vomiting (18% to 19%), diarrhea (17% to 18%), stomatitis (≥5% to 14%)

Genitourinary: Urinary tract infection (10% to 11%)

Hematologic & oncologic: Neutropenia (63% to 82%; grade 4: 29% grades 3/4: 12% to 57%; nadir: 13 days; recovery: 8 days), anemia (58% to 70%; grades 3/4: 2% to 4%)

Hepatic: Increased serum ALT (18% to 43%), increased serum AST (36%)

Neuromuscular & skeletal: Weakness (≤62%), arthralgia (≤22%), myalgia (≤22%), back pain (16%), ostealgia (12%), limb pain (11%)

Respiratory: Cough (14% to 18%), dyspnea (16%)

Miscellaneous: Fever (21% to 28%)

1% to 10%:

Cardiovascular: Hypotension (≥5% to <10%)

Central nervous system: Anxiety (≥5% to <10%), depression (≥5% to <10%), dizziness (≥5% to <10%), insomnia (≥5% to <10%), myasthenia (≥5% to <10%)

Dermatologic: Skin rash (≥5% to <10%)

Endocrine & metabolic: Hyperglycemia (≥5% to <10%)

Gastrointestinal: Dysgeusia (≥5% to <10%), dyspepsia (≥5% to <10%), xerostomia (≥5% to <10%), mucosal inflammation (9%)

Hematologic & oncologic: Thrombocytopenia (≥5% to <10%; grades ≥3: 1%), febrile neutropenia (≤5%)

Neuromuscular & skeletal: Muscle spasm (≥5% to <10%), musculoskeletal pain (≥5% to <10%),

◄ Ophthalmic: Increased lacrimation (≥5% to <10%)

Respiratory: Oropharyngeal pain (≥5% to <10%), upper respiratory tract infection (≥5% to <10%)

<1%, postmarketing, and/or case reports: Dehydration, drug-induced hypersensitivity, hepatotoxicity, hypomagnesemia, interstitial pulmonary disease, lymphocytopenia, neutropenic sepsis, pancreatitis, pneumonia, prolonged Q-T interval on ECG, pruritus, sepsis, Stevens-Johnson syndrome, toxic epidermal necrolysis

Drug Interactions

Metabolism/Transport Effects Substrate of CYP3A4 (minor); **Note:** Assignment of Major/Minor substrate status based on clinically relevant drug interaction potential

Avoid Concomitant Use

Avoid concomitant use of EriBULin with any of the following: BCG (Intravesical); Deferiprone; Dipyrone

Increased Effect/Toxicity

EriBULin may increase the levels/effects of: CloZAPine; Deferiprone; Highest Risk QTc-Prolonging Agents; Moderate Risk QTc-Prolonging Agents

The levels/effects of EriBULin may be increased by: Dipyrone; MiFEPRIStone; Palifermin; Promazine

Decreased Effect

EriBULin may decrease the levels/effects of: BCG (Intravesical); Lenograstim

Hazardous Drugs Handling Considerations

Hazardous agent (NIOSH 2016 [group 1]).

Use appropriate precautions for receiving, handling, administration, and disposal. Gloves (single) should be worn during receiving, unpacking, and placing in storage.

NIOSH recommends double gloving, a protective gown, ventilated engineering controls (a class II biological safety cabinet or a compounding aseptic containment isolator), and closed system transfer devices (CSTDs) for preparation. Double gloving, a gown, and (if dosage form allows) CSTDs are required during administration (NIOSH 2016).

Storage/Stability Store intact vials at 25°C (77°F); excursions permitted between 15°C and 30°C (59°F and 86°F); do not freeze. Store in original carton. Undiluted solutions in a syringe and solutions diluted in normal saline for infusion are stable for up to 4 hours at room temperature or up to 24 hours refrigerated at 4°C (40°F).

Preparation for Administration No dilution required. May prepare by drawing into a syringe for administration or may dilute in 100 mL NS. Discard unused portion of vial.

Mechanism of Action Eribulin is a non-taxane microtubule inhibitor which is a halichondrin B analog. It inhibits the growth phase of the microtubule by inhibiting formation of mitotic spindles causing mitotic blockage and arresting the cell cycle at the G_2/M phase; suppresses microtubule polymerization yet does not affect depolymerization.

Pharmacodynamics/Kinetics

Distribution: V_d: 43 to 114 L/m^2

Protein binding: 49% to 65%

Metabolism: Negligible

Half-life, elimination: ~40 hours

Excretion: Feces (~82%, predominantly as unchanged drug); urine (9%, primarily as unchanged drug)

Dosing

Adult & Geriatric Note: *International Considerations:* Some products available internationally may have vial strength and dosing expressed as the base (instead of as the salt). Refer to prescribing information for specific dosing information.

Breast cancer, metastatic: IV: Eribulin mesylate: 1.4 mg/m^2 on days 1 and 8 of a 21-day treatment cycle

Liposarcoma, unresectable or metastatic: IV: Eribulin mesylate: 1.4 mg/m^2 on days 1 and 8 of a 21-day treatment cycle

Renal Impairment Note: *International Considerations:* Some products available internationally may have vial strength and dosing expressed as the base (instead of as the salt). Refer to prescribing information for specific dosing information.

CrCl ≥50 mL/minute: No dosage adjustment necessary.

CrCl 15 to 49 mL/minute: Reduce dose to eribulin mesylate 1.1 mg/m^2.

ESRD (*Canadian labeling*): Use is not recommended.

Hepatic Impairment Note: *International Considerations:* Some products available internationally may have vial strength and dosing expressed as the base (instead of as the salt). Refer to prescribing information for specific dosing information.

Mild hepatic impairment (Child-Pugh class A): Reduce dose to eribulin mesylate 1.1 mg/m^2.

Moderate hepatic impairment (Child-Pugh class B): Reduce dose to eribulin mesylate 0.7 mg/m^2.

Severe hepatic impairment (Child-Pugh class C): There are no dosage adjustments provided in the manufacturer's US labeling (has not been studied); use is not recommended in the Canadian labeling.

Obesity *ASCO Guidelines for appropriate chemotherapy dosing in obese adults with cancer:* Utilize patient's actual body weight (full weight) for calculation of body surface area- or weight-based dosing, particularly when the intent of therapy is curative; manage regimen-related toxicities in the same manner as for nonobese patients; if a dose reduction is utilized due to toxicity, consider resumption of full weight-based dosing with subsequent cycles, especially if cause of toxicity (eg, hepatic or renal impairment) is resolved (Griggs, 2012).

Adjustment for Toxicity Note: *International Considerations:* Some products available internationally may have vial strength and dosing expressed as the base (instead of as the salt). Refer to prescribing information for specific dosing information.

ANC <1,000/mm^3 or platelets <75,000/mm^3 or grade 3 or 4 nonhematologic toxicity on day 1 or 8: Withhold dose; may delay day 8 dose up to 1 week. If toxicity resolves to ≤ grade 2 by day 15 administer a reduced dose and wait at least 2 weeks before beginning the next cycle. Omit dose if not resolved to ≤ grade 2 by day 15. Do not re-escalate dose after reduction.

Permanently reduce dose from eribulin mesylate 1.4 mg/m^2 to 1.1 mg/m^2 for the following:

ANC <500/mm^3 for >7 days

ANC <1000/mm^3 with fever or infection

Platelets <25,000/mm^3

Platelets <50,000/mm^3 requiring transfusion

Nonhematologic toxicity of grade 3 or 4

Dose omission or delay due to toxicity on day 8 of prior cycle

Permanently reduce dose from eribulin mesylate 1.1 mg/m^2 to 0.7 mg/m^2 for occurrence of any of the above events; discontinue treatment if the above toxicities occur at the 0.7 mg/m^2 dose level.

Administration IV: Infuse over 2 to 5 minutes. May be administered undiluted or diluted. Do not administer other medications through the same IV line, or through a line containing dextrose.

Emetic Potential Low (10% to 30%)

Monitoring Parameters CBC with differential prior to each dose (increase frequency with grades 3/4 cytopenias); renal and liver function tests; serum electrolytes, including potassium and magnesium. Assess for peripheral neuropathy prior to each dose. Monitor ECG in patients with heart failure, bradyarrhythmia, with concomitant medication known to prolong the QT interval, and electrolyte abnormalities (eg, hypokalemia, hypomagnesemia).

Additional Information *International considerations:* Eribulin mesylate 1.4 mg is equivalent to eribulin (base) 1.23 mg.

Dosage Forms Excipient information presented when available (limited, particularly for generics); consult specific product labeling.

Solution, Intravenous, as mesylate:

Halaven: 1 mg/2 mL (2 mL) [contains alcohol, usp]

◆ **Eribulin Mesylate** *see* EriBULin *on page 712*

◆ **Erismodegib** *see* Sonidegib *on page 1682*

◆ **Erivedge** *see* Vismodegib *on page 1921*

Erlotinib (er LOE tye nib)

Related Information

Management of Chemotherapy-Induced Nausea and Vomiting in Adults *on page 2253*

Management of EGFR Inhibitor Toxicities: Dermatologic, Ocular, and Gastro-intestinal *on page 2291*

Prevention of Chemotherapy-Induced Nausea and Vomiting in Children *on page 2310*

Safe Handling of Hazardous Drugs *on page 2379*

Brand Names: US Tarceva

Brand Names: Canada Tarceva; Teva-Erlotinib

Index Terms CP358774; Erlotinib Hydrochloride; OSI-774

Pharmacologic Category Antineoplastic Agent, Epidermal Growth Factor Receptor (EGFR) Inhibitor; Antineoplastic Agent, Tyrosine Kinase Inhibitor

Use

Non-small cell lung cancer, metastatic: Treatment of metastatic non-small cell lung cancer (NSCLC) in tumors with epidermal growth factor receptor (EGFR) exon 19 deletions or exon 21 (L858R) substitution mutations as detected by an approved test either as first-line, maintenance, or as second or greater line treatment after progression following at least 1 prior chemo-therapy regimen.

Limitations of use: Use in combination with platinum-based chemotherapy is not recommended. Safety and efficacy of treatment for metastatic NSCLC with EGFR mutations other than exon 19 deletion or exon 21 (L858R) substitution have not been established.

Pancreatic cancer: First-line treatment of locally advanced, unresectable, or metastatic pancreatic cancer (in combination with gemcitabine)

Labeled Contraindications

There are no contraindications listed in the manufacturer's US labeling.

Canadian labeling: Hypersensitivity to erlotinib or any component of the formulation

Pregnancy Considerations Adverse events were observed in animal reproduction studies. Erlotinib crosses the placenta (Ji 2015; Jovelet 2015). Information related to the use of erlotinib in pregnancy is limited (Ji 2015; Rivas 2012; Zambelli 2008). Based on the mechanism of action, erlotinib may cause fetal harm if administered in pregnancy. Advise females of reproductive potential to use effective contraception during treatment and for at least 1 month after the last erlotinib dose.

Breastfeeding Considerations It is not known if erlotinib is excreted in breast milk. Due to the potential for serious adverse reactions in the nursing infant (including bullous and exfoliative skin disorders, diarrhea, hepatotoxicity, interstitial lung disease, microangiopathic hemolytic anemia with thrombocytopenia, and ocular disorders) lactating women should not breastfeed during treatment and for 2 weeks after the final erlotinib dose.

Warnings/Precautions Rare, sometimes fatal, interstitial lung disease (ILD) has occurred; symptoms include acute respiratory distress syndrome, interstitial pneumonia, obliterative bronchiolitis, pneumonitis (including radiation and hypersensitivity), pulmonary fibrosis, and pulmonary infiltrates. The onset of symptoms has been within 5 days to more than 9 months after treatment initiation (median: 39 days). Interrupt treatment for unexplained new or worsening pulmonary symptoms (dyspnea, cough, and fever); permanently discontinue for confirmed ILD.

Hepatic failure and hepatorenal syndrome have been reported, particularly in patients with baseline hepatic impairment (although have also been observed in patients with normal hepatic function). Monitor liver function (transaminases, bilirubin, and alkaline phosphatase); patients with any hepatic impairment (total bilirubin >ULN; Child-Pugh class A, B, or C) should be closely and more frequently monitored, including those with hepatic disease due to tumor burden. Dosage reduction, interruption, or discontinuation may be necessary for changes in hepatic function. Use with extreme caution in patients with total bilirubin >3 times ULN. Interrupt therapy if total bilirubin is >3 times ULN or transaminases are >5 times ULN in patients without preexisting hepatic impairment. In patients with baseline hepatic dysfunction or biliary obstruction, interrupt therapy if bilirubin doubles or transaminases triple from baseline values. Increased monitoring of liver function is required in patients with preexisting hepatic impairment or biliary obstruction. Acute renal failure, renal insufficiency, and hepatorenal syndrome have been reported, either secondary to hepatic impairment at baseline or due to severe dehydration; use with caution in patients with or at risk for renal impairment. Monitor closely for dehydration; monitor renal function and electrolytes in patients at risk for dehydration. If severe renal impairment develops, interrupt therapy until toxicity resolves. Gastrointestinal perforation has been reported; risk for perforation is increased with concurrent anti-angiogenic agents, corticosteroids, NSAIDs, and/or taxane based-chemotherapy, and patients with history of peptic ulcers or diverticular disease; permanently discontinue in patients who develop perforation.

Bullous, blistering, and/or exfoliating skin conditions, some suggestive of Stevens-Johnson or toxic epidermal necrolysis (TEN) have been reported. An acne-like rash commonly appears on the face, back, and upper chest.

Generalized or severe acneiform, erythematous or maculopapular rash may occur. Skin rash may correlate with treatment response and prolonged survival (Saif 2008); management of skin rashes that are not serious should include alcohol-free lotions, topical antibiotics, or topical corticosteroids, or if necessary, oral antibiotics and systemic corticosteroids; avoid sunlight. Reduce dose or temporarily interrupt treatment for severe skin reactions; discontinue treatment for bullous, blistering or exfoliative skin toxicity. Corneal perforation and ulceration have been reported; decreased tear production, abnormal eyelash growth, keratoconjunctivitis sicca, or keratitis have also been reported and are known risk factors for corneal ulceration/perforation. Interrupt or discontinue treatment in patients presenting with eye pain or other acute or worsening ocular symptoms. Consider a baseline ophthalmologic exam and reassess for ocular toxicities at 4 to 8 weeks after treatment initiation (Renouf 2012).

MI, CVA, and microangiopathic hemolytic anemia with thrombocytopenia have been reported (rarely) with erlotinib in combination with gemcitabine. Elevated INR and bleeding events (including fatal hemorrhage) have been reported; monitor prothrombin time and INR closely.

Some factors which correlate positively with response to EGFR-tyrosine kinase inhibitor (TKI) therapy in NSCLC include patients who have never smoked, EGFR mutation, and patients of Asian origin. EGFR mutations, specifically exon 19 deletions and exon 21 mutation (L858R), are associated with better response to erlotinib in patients with NSCLC (Riely 2006). Erlotinib treatment is not recommended in patients with NSCLC with K-ras mutations; they are not likely to benefit from erlotinib treatment (Eberhard 2005; Miller 2008). K-ras mutations correlated with poorer outcome with EGFR-TKI therapy in patients with NSCLC (Jackman 2009; Masarelli 2007; Shepherd 2005). The cobas EGFR mutation test has been approved to detect EGFR mutation for NSCLC treatment. Concurrent erlotinib plus platinum-based chemotherapy is not recommended for treatment of locally-advanced or metastatic NSCLC due to a lack of clinical benefit. Treatment in patients with metastatic NSCLC with EGFR mutations other than exon 19 deletion or exon 21 (L858R) substitution has not been evaluated. Select patients for metastatic NSCLC treatment based on EGFR exon 19 deletions and exon 21 mutation (L858R) in tumor or plasma specimens; if these mutations are not detected in plasma specimen, tumor tissue (if available) may be tested.

Erlotinib levels may be lower in patients who smoke; advise patients to stop smoking. Smokers treated with 300 mg/day exhibited steady-state erlotinib levels comparable to former- and never-smokers receiving 150 mg/day (Hughes 2009). Potentially significant drug-drug interactions may exist, requiring dose or frequency adjustment, additional monitoring, and/or selection of alternative therapy. Avoid concomitant use with proton pump inhibitors. If taken with an H_2-receptor antagonist (eg, ranitidine), administer erlotinib 10 hours after the H_2-receptor antagonist dose and at least 2 hours prior to the next H_2-receptor dose. If an antacid is necessary, separate dosing by several hours. In patients with NSCLC, EGFR mutations, specifically exon 19 deletions and exon 21 mutation (L858R), are associated with better response to erlotinib (Riely 2006); erlotinib treatment is not recommended in patients with K-ras mutations; they are not likely to benefit from erlotinib treatment (Eberhard 2005; Miller 2008). Concurrent erlotinib plus platinum-based chemotherapy is not recommended for first line treatment of locally advanced or metastatic NSCLC due to a lack of clinical benefit. The cobas EGFR mutation test has been approved to detect EGFR mutation for NSCLC treatment. Product may contain lactose; avoid use in patients with Lapp lactase deficiency, glucose-galactose malabsorption, or glucose intolerance.

Adverse Reactions

Adverse reactions reported with monotherapy:

>10%:

Cardiovascular: Chest pain (≤18%)

Central nervous system: Fatigue (9% to 52%)

Dermatologic: Skin rash (49% to 85%; grade 3: 5% to 13%; grade 4: <1%; median onset: 8 days), xeroderma (4% to 21%), pruritus (7% to 16%), paronychia (4% to 16%), alopecia (14% to 15%), acne vulgaris (6% to 12%)

Gastrointestinal: Diarrhea (20% to 62%; grade 3: 2% to 6%; grade 4: <1%; median onset: 12 days), anorexia (9% to 52%), nausea (23% to 33%), decreased appetite (≤28%), vomiting (13% to 23%), mucositis (≤18%), stomatitis (11% to 17%), abdominal pain (3% to 11%), constipation (≤8%)

Genitourinary: Urinary tract infection (≤4%)

Hematologic & oncologic: Anemia (≤11%; grade 4: 1%)

Infection: Increased susceptibility to infection (4% to 24%)

Neuromuscular & skeletal: Weakness (≤53%), back pain (19%), arthralgia (≤13%), musculoskeletal pain (11%)

Ophthalmic: Conjunctivitis (12% to 18%), keratoconjunctivitis sicca (12%)

Respiratory: Cough (33% to 48%), dyspnea (41% to 45%; grades 3/4: 8% to 28%)

Miscellaneous: Fever (≤11%)

1% to 10%:

Cardiovascular: Peripheral edema (≤5%)

Central nervous system: Pain (≤9%), headache (≤7%), anxiety (≤5%), dizziness (≤4%), insomnia (≤4%), neurotoxicity (≤4%), paresthesia (≤4%), voice disorder (≤4%)

Dermatologic: Folliculitis (≤8%), nail disease (≤7%), exfoliative dermatitis (5%), hypertrichosis (5%), skin fissure (5%), acneiform eruption (4% to 5%), erythema (≤5%), dermatitis (4%), erythematous rash (≤4%), palmar-plantar erythrodysesthesia (≤4%), bullous dermatitis

Endocrine & metabolic: Weight loss (4% to 5%)

Gastrointestinal: Dyspepsia (≤5%), xerostomia (≤3%), taste disorder (≤1%)

Hematologic & oncologic: Lymphocytopenia (≤4%; grade 3: 1%), leukopenia (≤3%), thrombocytopenia (≤1%)

Hepatic: Hyperbilirubinemia (7%; grade 3: ≤1%), increased serum ALT (grade 2: 2% to 4%; grade 3: 1% to 3%), increased gamma-glutamyl transferase (≤4%), hepatic failure (≤1%)

Neuromuscular & skeletal: Muscle spasm (≤4%), musculoskeletal chest pain (≤4%), ostealgia (≤4%)

Otic: Tinnitus (≤1%)

Renal: Increased serum creatinine (≤1%), renal failure (≤1%),

Respiratory: Nasopharyngitis (≤7%), epistaxis (≤4%), pulmonary embolism (≤4%), respiratory tract infection (≤4%), pneumonitis (3%), pulmonary fibrosis (3%)

<1%: Interstitial pulmonary disease

Adverse reactions reported with combination (erlotinib plus gemcitabine) therapy:

>10%:

Cardiovascular: Edema (37%), thrombosis (grades 3/4: 11%)

◄

Central nervous system: Fatigue (73% to 79%), depression (19%), dizziness (15%), headache (15%), anxiety (13%)

Dermatologic: Skin rash (70%), alopecia (14%)

Gastrointestinal: Nausea (60%), anorexia (52%), diarrhea (48%), abdominal pain (46%), vomiting (42%), weight loss (39%), stomatitis (22%), dyspepsia (17%), flatulence (13%)

Hepatic: Increased serum ALT (grade 2: 31%, grade 3: 13%, grade 4: <1%), increased serum AST (grade 2: 24%, grade 3: 10%, grade 4 <1%), hyperbilirubinemia (grade 2: 17%, grade 3: 10%, grade 4: <1%)

Infection: Increased susceptibility to infection (39%)

Neuromuscular & skeletal: Ostealgia (25%), myalgia (21%), neuropathy (13%), rigors (12%)

Respiratory: Dyspnea (24%), cough (16%)

Miscellaneous: Fever (36%)

1% to 10%:

Cardiovascular: Cardiac arrhythmia (<5%), syncope (<5%), deep vein thrombosis (4%), cerebrovascular accident (3%; including cerebral hemorrhage), myocardial infarction (2%)

Gastrointestinal: Intestinal obstruction (<5%), pancreatitis (<5%)

Hematologic & oncologic: Hemolytic anemia (<5%), microangiopathic hemolytic anemia with thrombocytopenia (1%)

Renal: Renal insufficiency (<5%), renal failure (1%)

Respiratory: Interstitial pulmonary disease (<3%)

<1%: Bullous dermatitis, exfoliative dermatitis, hepatic failure

Mono- or combination therapy: <1%, postmarketing, and/or case reports: Acute peptic ulcer with hemorrhage, bronchiolitis, corneal perforation, corneal ulcer, decreased lacrimation, episcleritis, gastritis, gastrointestinal hemorrhage, gastrointestinal perforation, hearing loss, hematemesis, hematochezia, hepatorenal syndrome, hepatotoxicity, hirsutism, hyperpigmentation, hypokalemia, increased eyelash thickness, increased growth in number of eyelashes, keratitis, melena, misdirected growth of eyelashes, myopathy (in combination with statin therapy), ocular inflammation, peptic ulcer, rhabdomyolysis (in combination with statin therapy), skin photosensitivity, skin rash (acneiform; sparing prior radiation field), Stevens-Johnson syndrome, toxic epidermal necrolysis, tympanic membrane perforation, uveitis

Drug Interactions

Metabolism/Transport Effects Substrate of CYP1A2 (minor), CYP3A4 (major); **Note:** Assignment of Major/Minor substrate status based on clinically relevant drug interaction potential; **Inhibits** UGT1A1

Avoid Concomitant Use

Avoid concomitant use of Erlotinib with any of the following: Conivaptan; Fosphenytoin-Phenytoin; Fusidic Acid (Systemic); Idelalisib; Irinotecan Products; Proton Pump Inhibitors

Increased Effect/Toxicity

Erlotinib may increase the levels/effects of: Fosphenytoin-Phenytoin; Irinotecan Products; Warfarin

The levels/effects of Erlotinib may be increased by: Aprepitant; Ciprofloxacin (Systemic); Conivaptan; CYP3A4 Inhibitors (Moderate); CYP3A4 Inhibitors (Strong); Dasatinib; FluvoxaMINE; Fosaprepitant; Fusidic Acid (Systemic); Grapefruit Juice; Idelalisib; MiFEPRIStone; Netupitant; Palbociclib; Simeprevir; Stiripentol

Decreased Effect

The levels/effects of Erlotinib may be decreased by: Antacids; Bosentan; CYP3A4 Inducers (Moderate); CYP3A4 Inducers (Strong); Dabrafenib; Deferasirox; Enzalutamide; Fosphenytoin-Phenytoin; H2-Antagonists; Leflunomide; Mitotane; Proton Pump Inhibitors; Sarilumab; Siltuximab; St John's Wort; Teriflunomide; Tocilizumab

Food Interactions Erlotinib bioavailability is increased with food. Grapefruit or grapefruit juice may decrease metabolism and increase erlotinib plasma concentrations. Management: Take on an empty stomach at least 1 hour before or 2 hours after the ingestion of food. Avoid grapefruit and grapefruit juice. Maintain adequate nutrition and hydration, unless instructed to restrict fluid intake.

Hazardous Drugs Handling Considerations

Hazardous agent (NIOSH 2016 [group 1]).

Use appropriate precautions for receiving, handling, administration, and disposal. Gloves (single) should be worn during receiving, unpacking, and placing in storage.

NIOSH recommends single gloving for administration of intact tablets or capsules. If manipulating tablets/capsules (eg, to prepare an oral suspension), NIOSH recommends double gloving, a protective gown, and preparation in a controlled device; if not prepared in a controlled device, respiratory and eye/face protection as well as ventilated engineering controls are recommended. NIOSH recommends double gloving, a protective gown, and (if there is a potential for vomit or spit up) eye/face protection for administration of an oral liquid/feeding tube administration (NIOSH 2016).

Storage/Stability

Store at 25°C (77°F); excursions are permitted between 15°C to 30°C (59°F to 86°F).

An oral suspension (10 mg/mL) prepared using erlotinib 150 mg tablets and Ora-Plus:Ora-Sweet (1:1 vehicle) is stable for at least 28 days at room temperature; do not refrigerate due to potential increased viscosity (Li 2016).

Mechanism of Action Reversibly inhibits overall epidermal growth factor receptor (HER1/EGFR) - tyrosine kinase activity. Intracellular phosphorylation is inhibited which prevents further downstream signaling, resulting in cell death. Erlotinib has higher binding affinity for EGFR exon 19 deletion or exon 21 L858R mutations than for the wild type receptor.

Pharmacodynamics/Kinetics

Absorption: Oral: ~60% on an empty stomach; food increases to ~100%

Distribution: 232 L

Protein binding: 93% to albumin and alpha$_1$-acid glycoprotein

Metabolism: Hepatic, via CYP3A4 (major), CYP1A1 (minor), CYP1A2 (minor), and CYP1C (minor)

Bioavailability: ~100% when given with food; ~60% without food

Half-life elimination: 36.2 hours

Time to peak, plasma: 4 hours

Excretion: Primarily as metabolites: Feces (83%; 1% as unchanged drug); urine (8%; <1% as unchanged drug)

◀ **Dosing**

Adult & Geriatric

Non-small cell lung cancer (NSCLC), metastatic, in patients with EGFR exon 19 deletions or exon 21 (L858R) substitution mutations: Oral: 150 mg once daily until disease progression or unacceptable toxicity (Capuzzo 2010; Rosell 2012; Shepherd 2005).

Pancreatic cancer: Oral: 100 mg once daily (in combination with gemcitabine); continue until disease progression or unacceptable toxicity (Moore 2007).

Dosage adjustment for concomitant CYP inhibitors/inducers:

CYP3A4 inhibitors (strong): Avoid concurrent use if possible; reduce erlotinib dose for severe adverse reactions if erlotinib is administered concomitantly with strong CYP3A4 inhibitors. Dose reduction should be done in decrements of 50 mg (after toxicity has resolved to baseline or ≤ grade 1).

Concomitant CYP3A4 and CYP1A2 inhibitor (eg, ciprofloxacin): Avoid concurrent use if possible; if concomitant use cannot be avoided, reduce dose in decrements of 50 mg if severe adverse reactions occur (after toxicity has resolved to baseline or ≤ grade 1).

CYP3A4 inducers: Avoid concurrent use if possible; if concomitant administration with CYP3A4 inducers cannot be avoided, increase erlotinib dose in 50 mg increments at 2-week intervals to a maximum of 450 mg; reduce erlotinib dose to recommended starting dose when CYP3A4 inducer is discontinued.

CYP1A2 inducers: Avoid concurrent moderate CYP1A2 inducers if possible. If unavoidable, increase dose at 2-week intervals in 50 mg increments to a maximum dose of 300 mg (with careful monitoring); immediately reduce erlotinib dose to recommended starting dose (based on indication) upon discontinuation of the moderate CYP1A2 inducer.

Dosage adjustment for concomitant smoking: Avoid tobacco smoking if possible. If unavoidable, increase dose at 2-week intervals in 50 mg increments to a maximum dose of 300 mg (with careful monitoring); immediately reduce erlotinib dose to recommended starting dose (based on indication) upon smoking cessation.

Renal Impairment

Renal impairment at treatment initiation: There are no dosage adjustments provided in the manufacturer's labeling (has not been studied), although <9% of a single dose is excreted in the urine.

Renal toxicity during treatment:

Grades 3/4 renal toxicity: Withhold treatment and consider discontinuing. If treatment is resumed, reinitiate with a 50 mg dose reduction after toxicity has resolved to baseline or ≤ grade 1.

Renal failure associated with hepatorenal syndrome or due to dehydration: Withhold treatment until renal toxicity is resolved. If treatment is resumed, reinitiate with a 50 mg dose reduction after toxicity has resolved.

Hepatic Impairment

Hepatic impairment at treatment initiation:

Total bilirubin > ULN or Child-Pugh classes A, B, and C: There are no dosage adjustments provided in the manufacturer's labeling; use with caution and monitor closely during treatment.

Total bilirubin >3 times ULN: Use extreme caution.

The following adjustments have also been studied: A reduced starting dose (75 mg once daily) has been recommended in patients with hepatic dysfunction (AST ≥3 times ULN or direct bilirubin 1 to 7 mg/dL), with individualized dosage escalation if tolerated (Miller 2007); another study determined that pharmacokinetic and safety profiles were similar between patients with normal hepatic function and moderate hepatic impairment (O'Bryant 2012).

Hepatotoxicity during treatment:

Patients with normal hepatic function at baseline: If total bilirubin >3 times ULN and/or transaminases >5 times ULN: Interrupt therapy and consider discontinuing. If treatment is resumed, reinitiate with a 50 mg dose reduction after bilirubin and transaminases return to baseline.

Patients with baseline hepatic impairment or biliary obstruction: If bilirubin doubles or transaminases triple over baseline: Interrupt therapy and consider discontinuing. If treatment is resumed, reinitiate with a 50 mg dose reduction after bilirubin and transaminases return to baseline.

Severe hepatotoxicity that does not significantly improve or resolve within 3 weeks: Discontinue treatment.

Adjustment for Toxicity

Dermatologic toxicity:

Bullous, blistering, or exfoliative skin toxicity (severe): Discontinue treatment.

Severe rash (unresponsive to medical management): Withhold treatment; may reinitiate with a 50 mg dose reduction after toxicity has resolved to baseline or ≤ grade 1.

Gastrointestinal toxicity:

Diarrhea: Manage with loperamide; in persistent, severe diarrhea (unresponsive to loperamide) or dehydration due to diarrhea, withhold treatment; may reinitiate with a 50 mg dose reduction after toxicity has resolved to baseline or ≤ grade 1.

Gastrointestinal perforation: Discontinue treatment.

Ocular toxicities:

Acute or worsening ocular toxicities (eg, eye pain): Interrupt and consider discontinuing treatment. If therapy is resumed, reinitiate with a 50 mg dose reduction after toxicity has resolved to baseline or ≤ grade 1.

Corneal perforation or severe ulceration: Discontinue treatment.

Keratitis (grade 3 or 4 or grade 2 persisting >2 weeks): Withhold treatment; may reinitiate with a 50 mg dose reduction after toxicity has resolved to baseline or ≤ grade 1.

Pulmonary symptoms: Acute onset (or worsening) of pulmonary symptoms (eg, dyspnea, cough, fever): Withhold treatment while evaluating for drug-induced interstitial lung disease; if resuming treatment, reinitiate with a 50 mg dose reduction after symptoms resolve to grade 1 or lower. Discontinue permanently with development of interstitial lung disease

Combination Regimens

Pancreatic cancer: Erlotinib-Gemcitabine (Pancreatic) on page 2108

Administration The manufacturer recommends administration on an empty stomach (at least 1 hour before or 2 hours after the ingestion of food). Avoid concomitant use with proton pump inhibitors (if possible). If taken with an H_2-receptor antagonist (eg, ranitidine), administer erlotinib 10 hours after the H_2-receptor antagonist dose and at least 2 hours prior to the next H_2- receptor dose. If an antacid is necessary, separate dosing by several hours.

For patients unable to swallow whole, tablets may be dissolved in 100 mL water and administered orally or via feeding tube (silicone-based); to ensure full dose is received, rinse container with 40 mL water, administer residue and repeat rinse; administer immediately after preparation (data on file, Genentech [contact product manufacturer to obtain current information]; Siu 2007; Soulieres 2004). If necessary, an oral suspension may be prepared (see Extemporaneous Preparations).

Emetic Potential Children and Adults: Minimal (<10%)

Extemporaneous Preparations A 10 mg/mL oral suspension may be prepared using erlotinib 150 mg tablets and Ora-Plus:Ora-Sweet (1:1 vehicle). Determine necessary quantity of erlotinib 150 mg tablets; crush the tablets in a glass mortar and triturate to a fine powder (estimated powder volume for each erlotinib 150 mg tablet is 0.25 mL). Measure the necessary volume of Ora-Plus and add to the powder by geometric dilution until a smooth suspension is created. Measure the necessary volume of Ora-Sweet and add to the suspension. Transfer to an amber plastic bottle and label "Shake Well Before Use", "Do Not Refrigerate" and "Use by (date)". Suspension is stable for at least 28 days at room temperature (do not refrigerate due to potential increased viscosity).

Li Q, Liu Z, Kolli S, et al. Stability of extemporaneous erlotinib, lapatinib, and imatinib oral suspension. *Am J Health Syst Pharm.* 2016;73(17):1331-1337.

Monitoring Parameters

Liver function tests (transaminases, bilirubin, and alkaline phosphatase [periodic], monitor more frequently with worsening liver function); renal function tests (periodic) and serum electrolytes (in patients at risk for dehydration; periodic); prothrombin time and INR (in patients on concomitant warfarin therapy); EGFR mutation status in patients with NSCLC adenocarcinoma (Keedy 2011); the cobas EGFR mutation test has been approved to detect EGFR mutation for first-line NSCLC treatment, smoking status.

Consider a baseline ophthalmologic exam and reassess for ocular toxicities at 4 to 8 weeks after treatment initiation (Renouf 2012). Monitor hydration status; monitor for signs/symptoms of pulmonary toxicity, dermatologic toxicity, and ocular toxicity.

Dietary Considerations Avoid grapefruit and grapefruit juice.

Dosage Forms Excipient information presented when available (limited, particularly for generics); consult specific product labeling.

Tablet, Oral:

Tarceva: 25 mg [contains fd&c yellow #6 (sunset yellow)]

Tarceva: 100 mg, 150 mg

◆ **Erlotinib Hydrochloride** see Erlotinib on page 716

◆ **Erwinase (Can)** see Asparaginase (*Erwinia*) on page 184

◆ **Erwinaze** see Asparaginase (*Erwinia*) on page 184

◆ *Erwinia chrysanthemi* see Asparaginase (*Erwinia*) on page 184

◆ **Erythropoiesis-Stimulating Agent (ESA)** see Darbepoetin Alfa on page 515

◆ **Erythropoiesis-Stimulating Agent (ESA)** see Epoetin Alfa on page 702

◆ **Erythropoiesis-Stimulating Protein** see Darbepoetin Alfa on page 515

◆ **Erythropoietin** see Epoetin Alfa on page 702

Estramustine (es tra MUS teen)

Related Information

Management of Chemotherapy-Induced Nausea and Vomiting in Adults on page 2253

Brand Names: US Emcyt

Brand Names: Canada Emcyt

Index Terms Estramustine Phosphate; Estramustine Phosphate Sodium

Pharmacologic Category Antineoplastic Agent, Alkylating Agent; Antineoplastic Agent, Antimicrotubular; Antineoplastic Agent, Hormone (Estrogen/Nitrogen Mustard)

Use

Prostate cancer: Treatment (palliative) of progressive or metastatic prostate cancer

Limitation of use: A clinical practice guideline from the American Society of Clinical Oncology (ASCO) and Cancer Care Ontario recommends that estramustine not be offered to men with metastatic castration-resistant prostate cancer due to a lack of benefit in survival or quality of life (Basch, 2014).

Labeled Contraindications Hypersensitivity to estramustine, estradiol, nitrogen mustard, or any component of the formulation; active thrombophlebitis or thromboembolic disorders (except where tumor mass is the cause of thromboembolic disorder and the benefit may outweigh the risk)

Canadian labeling: Additional contraindications (not in the U.S. labeling): Severe hepatic or cardiac disease

Pregnancy Considerations Estramustine is not indicated for use in women. Some men who were impotent on estrogen therapy have regained potency while taking estramustine; effective contraception should be used for male patients with partners of childbearing potential.

Breastfeeding Considerations Estramustine is not indicated for use in women.

Warnings/Precautions Glucose tolerance may be decreased; use with caution in patients with diabetes. Hypertension (monitor blood pressure periodically), peripheral edema (new-onset or exacerbation), or congestive heart disease may occur; use with caution in patients where fluid accumulation may be poorly tolerated, including cardiovascular disease (HF or hypertension), migraine, seizure disorder or renal dysfunction. Estrogen treatment for prostate cancer is associated with an increased risk of thrombosis and MI; (including fatalities); use caution with history of thrombophlebitis, thrombosis, or thromboembolic disease or history of cerebrovascular or coronary artery disease. Liver enzyme and bilirubin abnormalities may occur; monitor during and for 2 months after treatment. Use with caution in patients with hepatic impairment (may be metabolized poorly) or with metabolic bone diseases. Allergic reactions and angioedema, including airway involvement, have been reported with use. Patients with prostate cancer and osteoblastic metastases are at risk for hypocalcemia; monitor calcium. Estrogenic effects may decrease testosterone levels; may cause gynecomastia and/or impotence. Potentially significant drug-drug/drug-food interactions may exist, requiring dose or frequency adjustment, additional monitoring, and/or selection of alternative therapy. Avoid vaccination with live vaccines during treatment (risk of infection may be increased due to immunosuppression). Although the response to vaccines may be diminished, inactivated vaccines may be administered during treatment. Estramustine is associated with a moderate emetic potential; antiemetics are recommended to prevent nausea and vomiting. A clinical practice guideline from the American Society of Clinical Oncology (ASCO) and Cancer Care Ontario recommends that estramustine not be offered to men with metastatic castration-resistant prostate cancer due to a lack of benefit in survival or quality of life (Basch, 2014).

◀ **Adverse Reactions** Frequency not always defined.

>10%:

Cardiovascular: Edema (20%)

Endocrine & metabolic: Gynecomastia (75%), increased lactate dehydrogenase (2% to 33%), decreased libido

Gastrointestinal: Nausea (16%), diarrhea (13%), gastrointestinal irritation (12%)

Genitourinary: Breast tenderness (71%)

Hepatic: Increased serum AST (2% to 33%)

Respiratory: Dyspnea (12%)

1% to 10%:

Cardiovascular: Cardiac failure (3%), local thrombophlebitis (3%), myocardial infarction (3%), cerebrovascular accident (2%), pulmonary embolism (2%), chest pain (1%), flushing (1%)

Central nervous system: Lethargy (4%), insomnia (3%), emotional lability (2%), anxiety (1%), headache (1%)

Dermatologic: Pruritus (2%), xeroderma (2%), exfoliation of skin (1%), skin rash (1%), thinning hair (1%)

Endocrine & metabolic: Increased thirst (1%)

Gastrointestinal: Anorexia (4%), flatulence (2%), gastrointestinal hemorrhage (1%), sore throat (1%), vomiting (1%)

Hematologic & oncologic: Leukopenia (4%), bruise (3%), thrombocytopenia (1%)

Hepatic: Increased serum bilirubin (1% to 2%)

Neuromuscular & skeletal: Leg cramps (9%)

Ophthalmic: Lacrimation (1%)

Respiratory: Hoarseness (1%), rhinorrhea (1%)

<1%, postmarketing, and/or case reports: Anemia, angina pectoris, angioedema, cerebral ischemia, confusion, depression, decreased glucose tolerance, hypercalcemia, hypocalcemia, hypersensitivity reaction, hypertension, impotence, ischemic heart disease, myasthenia, venous thrombosis

Drug Interactions

Metabolism/Transport Effects None known.

Avoid Concomitant Use

Avoid concomitant use of Estramustine with any of the following: BCG (Intravesical); Natalizumab; Pimecrolimus; Tacrolimus (Topical); Vaccines (Live)

Increased Effect/Toxicity

Estramustine may increase the levels/effects of: Fingolimod; Leflunomide; Natalizumab; Tofacitinib; Vaccines (Live)

The levels/effects of Estramustine may be increased by: Clodronate; Denosumab; Ocrelizumab; Palifermin; Pimecrolimus; Roflumilast; Tacrolimus (Topical); Trastuzumab

Decreased Effect

Estramustine may decrease the levels/effects of: BCG (Intravesical); Coccidioides immitis Skin Test; Lenograstim; Nivolumab; Sipuleucel-T; Tertomotide; Vaccines (Inactivated); Vaccines (Live)

The levels/effects of Estramustine may be decreased by: Calcium Salts; Echinacea

Food Interactions Estramustine serum levels may be decreased if taken with milk or other dairy products, calcium supplements, and vitamins containing calcium. Management: Take on an empty stomach at least 1 hour before or 2 hours after eating.

Hazardous Drugs Handling Considerations
Hazardous agent (NIOSH 2016 [group 1]).

Use appropriate precautions for receiving, handling, administration, and disposal. Gloves (single) should be worn during receiving, unpacking, and placing in storage. NIOSH recommends single gloving for administration of intact tablets or capsules (NIOSH 2016).

Storage/Stability Store refrigerated at 2°C to 8°C (36°F to 46°F).

Mechanism of Action Estradiol and nornitrogen mustard carbamate-linked combination which has antiandrogen effects (due to estradiol) and antimicrotubule effects (due to nornitrogen mustard); causes a marked decrease in plasma testosterone and an increase in estrogen levels.

Pharmacodynamics/Kinetics

Absorption: Incomplete (Bergenheim, 1998)

Metabolism: Initially dephosphorylated in the GI tract, then hepatically oxidated and hydrolyzed to estramustine, estromustine (oxidized isomer of estramustine), estrone, and estradiol.

Bioavailability: Oral: 44% to 75% (Bergenheim, 1998)

Half-life elimination: Estromustine: 13.6 hours (range: 9-23 hours); Estrone: 16.5 hours (Bergenheim, 1998)

Time to peak: 2-3 hours (Bergenheim, 1998)

Excretion: Feces (primarily); urine (trace amounts) (Bergenheim, 1998)

Dosing

Adult & Geriatric Note: Estramustine is associated with a moderate emetic potential; antiemetics are recommended to prevent nausea and vomiting.

Prostate cancer, progressive or metastatic: Males: Oral: 14 mg/kg/day (range: 10-16 mg/kg/day) in 3 or 4 divided doses

Renal Impairment There are no dosage adjustments provided in the manufacturer's labeling; use with caution.

Hepatic Impairment There are no dosage adjustments provided in the manufacturer's labeling; use with caution (may be poorly metabolized).

Obesity *ASCO Guidelines for appropriate chemotherapy dosing in obese adults with cancer:* Utilize patient's actual body weight (full weight) for calculation of body surface area- or weight-based dosing, particularly when the intent of therapy is curative; manage regimen-related toxicities in the same manner as for nonobese patients; if a dose reduction is utilized due to toxicity, consider resumption of full weight-based dosing with subsequent cycles, especially if cause of toxicity (eg, hepatic or renal impairment) is resolved (Griggs, 2012).

Administration Estramustine is associated with a moderate emetic potential; antiemetics are recommended to prevent nausea and vomiting.

Administer on an empty stomach, at least 1 hour before or 2 hours after eating. Administer with water; do not administer with milk, milk-based products, or calcium products.

Emetic Potential Moderate (30% to 90%)

Monitoring Parameters Serum calcium, liver function tests (during and for 2 months following treatment); blood pressure

Dietary Considerations Should be taken at least 1 hour before or 2 hours after eating. Milk products and calcium-rich foods or supplements may impair the oral absorption of estramustine phosphate sodium.

Dosage Forms Excipient information presented when available (limited, particularly for generics); consult specific product labeling.

Capsule, Oral, as phosphate sodium:

Emcyt: 140 mg

◆ **Estramustine Phosphate** see Estramustine on page 724
◆ **Estramustine Phosphate Sodium** see Estramustine on page 724
◆ **ET-743** see Trabectedin on page 1803

Ethiodized Oil (eth EYE oh dyezd oyl)

Pharmacologic Category Diagnostic Agent, Radiologic Examination of GI Tract

Use

Hysterosalpingography: For hysterosalpingography in adults

Lymphography: For lymphography in adult and pediatric patients

Selective hepatic intra-arterial injection: For imaging tumors in adults with known hepatocellular carcinoma (HCC)

Pregnancy Risk Factor C

Dosing

Adult Use the smallest possible dose based on anatomical area to be visualized; dose varies with procedure. Refer to prescribing information for detailed dosing and administration information.

Hysterosalpingography: Inject in 2 mL increments into the endometrial cavity until tubal patency is observed; discontinue use if excessive discomfort develops. Reimage after 24 hours to determine if ethiodized oil has entered the peritoneal cavity.

Lymphography: Note: Inject into lymphatic vessel under radiological monitoring. Interrupt injection if patient experiences pain; discontinue injection if lymphatic blockage is present (to minimize entry into the venous circulation via lymphovenous channels) and/or as soon as ethiodized oil is radiographically evident in the thoracic duct (to minimize entry into the subclavian vein and pulmonary embolization). Obtain immediate postinjection images; reimage at 24 to 48 hours to evaluate nodal architecture.

Unilateral lymphography of upper extremities: 2 to 4 mL

Unilateral lymphography of lower extremities: 6 to 8 mL

Penile lymphography: 2 to 3 mL

Cervical lymphography: 1 to 2 mL

Selective hepatic intra-arterial injection: Note: Dose depends on tumor size, local blood flow in liver and tumor: Dosage range: 1.5 to 15 mL administered slowly under continuous radiologic monitoring; discontinue administration when stagnation or reflux is evident. Limit dose to the quantity required for adequate visualization; maximum total dose: 20 mL

Pediatric Use the smallest possible dose based on anatomical area to be visualized; dose varies with procedure. Refer to prescribing information for detailed dosing and administration information.

Lymphography: 1 to 6 mL according to area to be visualized; Maximum dose: 0.25 mL/kg.

Note: Inject into lymphatic vessel under radiological monitoring. Interrupt injection if patient experiences pain; discontinue injection if lymphatic blockage is present (to minimize entry into the venous circulation via lymphovenous channels) and/or as soon as ethiodized oil is radiographically evident in the thoracic duct (to minimize entry into the subclavian vein and pulmonary embolization). Obtain immediate postinjection images; reimage at 24 to 48 hours to evaluate nodal architecture.

Renal Impairment There are no dosage adjustments provided in the manufacturer's labeling.

Hepatic Impairment There are no dosage adjustments provided in the manufacturer's labeling.

Additional Information Complete prescribing information should be consulted for additional detail.

Dosage Forms Excipient information presented when available (limited, particularly for generics); consult specific product labeling.
Injection: Iodine 37% (10 mL)

♦ **Ethiofos** see Amifostine on page 104

♦ **Ethoxynaphthamido Penicillin Sodium** see Nafcillin on page 1296

♦ **Ethyol** see Amifostine on page 104

♦ **ETOP** see Etoposide Phosphate on page 740

♦ **Etopophos** see Etoposide Phosphate on page 740

Etoposide (e toe POE side)

Related Information

Hematopoietic Cell Transplantation on page 2365

Management of Chemotherapy-Induced Nausea and Vomiting in Adults on page 2253

Management of Drug Extravasations on page 2271

Palliative Care Medicine (Cancer) on page 2352

Prevention of Chemotherapy-Induced Nausea and Vomiting in Children on page 2310

Safe Handling of Hazardous Drugs on page 2379

Brand Names: US Toposar

Brand Names: Canada Etoposide Injection; Etoposide Injection USP; Vepesid

Index Terms EPEG; Epipodophyllotoxin; VePesid; VP-16; VP-16-213; VP16

Pharmacologic Category Antineoplastic Agent, Podophyllotoxin Derivative; Antineoplastic Agent, Topoisomerase II Inhibitor

Use

Small cell lung cancer (oral and IV): Treatment (first-line) of small cell lung cancer (SCLC)

Testicular cancer (IV): Treatment of refractory testicular tumors (injectable formulation)

Canadian labeling: Treatment of small cell lung cancer (SCLC; first- and second-line); treatment of non-small cell lung cancer (NSCLC); treatment of non-Hodgkin lymphomas (first-line); treatment of testicular cancer (first-line [injectable formulation] and refractory)

Labeled Contraindications Hypersensitivity to etoposide or any component of the formulation

Canadian labeling: Additional contraindications (not in US labeling): Severe leukopenia or thrombocytopenia; severe hepatic impairment; severe renal impairment

◀ **Pregnancy Considerations** Adverse events were observed in animal reproduction studies. Fetal growth restriction and newborn myelosuppression have been observed following maternal use of regimens containing etoposide during pregnancy (NTP 2013; Peccatori 2013). The European Society for Medical Oncology has published guidelines for diagnosis, treatment, and follow-up of cancer during pregnancy. The guidelines recommend referral to a facility with expertise in cancer during pregnancy and encourage a multi-disciplinary team (obstetrician, neonatologist, oncology team). In general, if chemotherapy is indicated, it should be avoided during in the first trimester, there should be a 3-week time period between the last chemotherapy dose and anticipated delivery, and chemotherapy should not be administered beyond week 33 of gestation. Guidelines for the treatment of SCLC are not provided (Peccatori 2013).

In women of reproductive potential, product labeling for etoposide phosphate notes that it may cause amenorrhea, infertility, or premature menopause; effective contraception should be used during therapy and for ≥6 months after the last dose. In males, azoospermia, oligospermia, or permanent loss of fertility may occur. In addition, spermatozoa and testicular tissue may be damaged. Males with female partners of reproductive potential should use condoms during therapy and for ≥4 months after the last dose.

Breastfeeding Considerations Etoposide is excreted in breast milk. Based on data from one case report, concentrations are below the limit of detection 24 hours after the last dose (Azuno 1995). Due to the potential for serious adverse reactions in the nursing infant, the manufacturer recommends a decision be made whether to discontinue nursing or to discontinue the drug, taking into account the importance of treatment to the mother.

Warnings/Precautions [US Boxed Warning]: Severe dose-limiting and dose-related myelosuppression with resulting infection or bleeding may occur. Treatment should be withheld for platelets <50,000/mm^3 or absolute neutrophil count (ANC) <500/mm^3. May cause anaphylactic-like reactions manifested by chills, fever, tachycardia, bronchospasm, dyspnea, and hypotension. In addition, facial/tongue swelling, coughing, chest tightness, cyanosis, laryngospasm, diaphoresis, hypertension, back pain, loss of consciousness, and flushing have also been reported less commonly. Incidence is primarily associated with intravenous administration (up to 2%) compared to oral administration (<1%). Infusion should be interrupted and medications for the treatment of anaphylaxis should be available for immediate use. High drug concentration and rate of infusion, as well as presence of benzyl alcohol in the etoposide intravenous formulation have been suggested as contributing factors to the development of hypersensitivity reactions. Etoposide intravenous formulations may contain benzyl alcohol, while etoposide phosphate (the water soluble prodrug of etoposide) intravenous formulation does not contain benzyl alcohol. Case reports have suggested that etoposide phosphate has been used successfully in patients with previous hypersensitivity reactions to etoposide (Collier 2008; Siderov 2002). The use of concentrations higher than recommended were associated with higher rates of anaphylactic-like reactions in children.

Secondary acute leukemias have been reported with etoposide, either as monotherapy or in combination with other chemotherapy agents. Must be diluted; do not give IV push, infuse over at least 30 to 60 minutes; hypotension is associated with rapid infusion. If hypotension occurs, interrupt infusion and administer IV hydration and supportive care; decrease infusion upon reinitiation. Etoposide is an irritant; tissue irritation and inflammation have occurred following extravasation. Do not administer IM or SubQ. Dosage should be adjusted in patients with hepatic or renal impairment (Canadian labeling contraindicates use in severe hepatic and/or renal impairment). Use with caution in patients with low serum albumin; may increase risk for toxicities. Use with caution in elderly patients; may be more likely to develop severe myelosuppression and/or GI effects (eg, nausea/vomiting). **[US Boxed Warning]: Should be administered under the supervision of an experienced cancer chemotherapy physician.**

Oral etoposide is associated with a low (adults) or moderate (children) emetic potential; antiemetics may be recommended to prevent nausea and vomiting (Dupuis 2011; Roila 2016). Potentially significant drug-drug interactions may exist, requiring dose or frequency adjustment, additional monitoring, and/or selection of alternative therapy.

Benzyl alcohol and derivatives: Some dosage forms may contain benzyl alcohol; large amounts of benzyl alcohol (≥99 mg/kg/day) have been associated with a potentially fatal toxicity ("gasping syndrome") in neonates; the "gasping syndrome" consists of metabolic acidosis, respiratory distress, gasping respirations, CNS dysfunction (including convulsions, intracranial hemorrhage), hypotension, and cardiovascular collapse (AAP ["Inactive" 1997]; CDC 1982); some data suggests that benzoate displaces bilirubin from protein binding sites (Ahlfors 2001); avoid or use dosage forms containing benzyl alcohol with caution in neonates. See manufacturer's labeling.

Injectable formulation contains alcohol (~33% v/v); may contribute to adverse reactions, especially with higher etoposide doses.

Polysorbate 80: Some dosage forms may contain polysorbate 80 (also known as Tweens). Hypersensitivity reactions, usually a delayed reaction, have been reported following exposure to pharmaceutical products containing polysorbate 80 in certain individuals (Isaksson 2002; Lucente 2000; Shelley 1995). Thrombocytopenia, ascites, pulmonary deterioration, and renal and hepatic failure have been reported in premature neonates after receiving parenteral products containing polysorbate 80 (Alade 1986; CDC 1984). See manufacturer's labeling.

Adverse Reactions The following may occur with higher doses used in stem cell transplantation: Alopecia, ethanol intoxication, hepatitis, hypotension (infusion-related), metabolic acidosis, mucositis, nausea and vomiting (severe), secondary malignancy, skin lesions (resembling Stevens-Johnson syndrome).

>10%:
  Dermatologic: Alopecia (8% to 66%)
  Gastrointestinal: Nausea and vomiting (31% to 43%), anorexia (10% to 13%), diarrhea (1% to 13%)
  Hematologic & oncologic: Leukopenia (60% to 91%; grade 4: 3% to 17%; nadir: 7 to 14 days; recovery: by day 20), thrombocytopenia (22% to 41%; grades 3/4: 1% to 20%; nadir: 9 to 16 days; recovery: by day 20), anemia (≤33%)
1% to 10%:
  Cardiovascular: Hypotension (1% to 2%; due to rapid infusion)
  Central nervous system: Peripheral neuropathy (1% to 2%)
  Gastrointestinal: Stomatitis (1% to 6%), abdominal pain (≤2%)
  Hepatic: Hepatotoxicity (≤3%)

Hypersensitivity: Anaphylactoid reaction (intravenous: 1% to 2%; oral capsules: <1%; including bronchospasm, chills, dyspnea, fever, tachycardia) <1%, postmarketing, and/or case reports: Amenorrhea, apnea (hypersensitivity-associated), back pain, constipation, cortical blindness (transient), cough, cyanosis, diaphoresis, drowsiness, dysphagia, erythema, esophagitis, extravasation (induration/necrosis), facial swelling, fatigue, fever, hyperpigmentation, hypersensitivity reaction, interstitial pneumonitis, ischemic heart disease, laryngospasm, maculopapular rash, malaise, metabolic acidosis, mucositis, myocardial infarction, optic neuritis, ovarian failure, pruritic erythematous rash, pruritus, pulmonary fibrosis, radiation-recall phenomenon (dermatitis), reversible posterior leukoencephalopathy syndrome (RPLS), seizure, skin rash, Stevens-Johnson syndrome, tongue edema, toxic epidermal necrolysis, toxic megacolon, urticaria, vasospasm, weakness

Drug Interactions

Metabolism/Transport Effects Substrate of CYP1A2 (minor), CYP2E1 (minor), CYP3A4 (major), P-glycoprotein; **Note:** Assignment of Major/Minor substrate status based on clinically relevant drug interaction potential; **Inhibits** CYP2C9 (weak)

Avoid Concomitant Use

Avoid concomitant use of Etoposide with any of the following: BCG (Intravesical); Conivaptan; Deferiprone; Dipyrone; Fusidic Acid (Systemic); Idelalisib; Natalizumab; Pimecrolimus; Tacrolimus (Topical); Vaccines (Live)

Increased Effect/Toxicity

Etoposide may increase the levels/effects of: CloZAPine; Deferiprone; Fingolimod; Leflunomide; Natalizumab; Tofacitinib; Vaccines (Live); Vitamin K Antagonists

The levels/effects of Etoposide may be increased by: Aprepitant; Atovaquone; Conivaptan; CycloSPORINE (Systemic); CYP3A4 Inhibitors (Moderate); CYP3A4 Inhibitors (Strong); Dasatinib; Denosumab; Dipyrone; Fosaprepitant; Fusidic Acid (Systemic); Idelalisib; MiFEPRIStone; Netupitant; Ocrelizumab; Palbociclib; Palifermin; P-glycoprotein/ABCB1 Inhibitors; Pimecrolimus; Promazine; Ranolazine; Roflumilast; Simeprevir; Stiripentol; Tacrolimus (Topical); Trastuzumab

Decreased Effect

Etoposide may decrease the levels/effects of: BCG (Intravesical); Coccidioides immitis Skin Test; Lenograstim; Nivolumab; Sipuleucel-T; Tertomotide; Vaccines (Inactivated); Vaccines (Live)

The levels/effects of Etoposide may be decreased by: Bosentan; CYP3A4 Inducers (Moderate); CYP3A4 Inducers (Strong); Dabrafenib; Deferasirox; Enzalutamide; Mitotane; Sarilumab; Siltuximab; St John's Wort; Tocilizumab

Hazardous Drugs Handling Considerations

Hazardous agent (NIOSH 2016 [group 1]).

Use appropriate precautions for receiving, handling, administration, and disposal. Gloves (single) should be worn during receiving, unpacking, and placing in storage.

NIOSH recommends single gloving for administration of intact tablets or capsules. If manipulating tablets/capsules (eg, to prepare an oral suspension), NIOSH recommends double gloving, a protective gown, and preparation in a controlled device; if not prepared in a controlled device, respiratory and eye/face protection as well as ventilated engineering controls are recommended.

NIOSH recommends double gloving, a protective gown, and (if there is a potential for vomit or spit up) eye/face protection for administration of an oral liquid/feeding tube administration. For IV preparation, NIOSH recommends double gloving, a protective gown, ventilated engineering controls (a class II biological safety cabinet or a compounding aseptic containment isolator), and closed system transfer devices (CSTDs). Double gloving, a gown, and (if dosage form allows) CSTDs are required during IV administration (NIOSH 2016).

Storage/Stability

Capsules: Store oral capsules at 2°C to 8°C (36°F to 46°F); do not freeze. Dispense in a light-resistant container.

Injection: Store intact vials of injection at 20°C to 25°C (68°F to 77°F; do not freeze. According to the manufacturer's labeling, stability for solutions diluted for infusion in D5W or NS (in glass or plastic containers) varies based on concentration; 0.2 mg/mL solutions are stable for 96 hours at room temperature and 0.4 mg/mL solutions are stable for 24 hours at room temperature (precipitation may occur at concentrations above 0.4 mg/mL).

Etoposide injection contains polysorbate 80 which may cause leaching of diethylhexyl phthalate (DEHP), a plasticizer contained in polyvinyl chloride (PVC) bags and tubing. Higher concentrations and longer storage time after preparation in PVC bags may increase DEHP leaching. Preparation in glass or polyolefin containers will minimize patient exposure to DEHP When undiluted etoposide injection is stored in acrylic or ABS (acrylonitrile, butadiene and styrene) plastic containers, the containers may crack and leak.

Preparation for Administration

Etoposide should be diluted to a concentration of 0.2 to 0.4 mg/mL in D5W or NS for administration. Diluted solutions have concentration-dependent stability: More concentrated solutions have shorter stability times. Precipitation may occur with concentrations >0.4 mg/mL.

Mechanism of Action

Etoposide has been shown to delay transit of cells through the S phase and arrest cells in late S or early G_2 phase. The drug may inhibit mitochondrial transport at the NADH dehydrogenase level or inhibit uptake of nucleosides into HeLa cells. It is a topoisomerase II inhibitor and appears to cause DNA strand breaks. Etoposide does not inhibit microtubular assembly.

Pharmacodynamics/Kinetics

Absorption: Oral: Significant inter- and intrapatient variation

Distribution: Average V_d: Children: 10 L/m^2; Adults: 7 to 17 L/m^2; poor penetration across the blood-brain barrier; CSF concentrations <5% of plasma concentrations

Protein binding: 94% to 98%

Metabolism: Hepatic, via CYP3A4 and 3A5, to various metabolites; in addition, conversion of etoposide to the O-demethylated metabolites (catechol and quinine) via prostaglandin synthases or myeloperoxidase occurs, as well as glutathione and glucuronide conjugation via GSTT1/GSTP1 and UGT1A1 (Yang, 2009)

Bioavailability: Oral: ~50% (range: 25% to 75%)

Half-life elimination: Terminal: IV: Normal renal/hepatic function: Children: 6 to 8 hours: Adults: 4 to 11 hours

◄ Excretion:
   Children: IV: Urine (~55% as unchanged drug) in 24 hours
   Adults: IV: Urine (56%; 45% as unchanged drug) within 120 hours; feces (44%) within 120 hours

Dosing

Adult & Geriatric

US labeling:

Small cell lung cancer (combination chemotherapy):
   IV: 35 mg/m^2/day for 4 days, up to 50 mg/m^2/day for 5 days every 3 to 4 weeks
   Oral: Due to poor bioavailability, oral doses should be twice the IV dose (and rounded to the nearest 50 mg)

Testicular cancer (combination chemotherapy): IV: 50 to 100 mg/m^2/day for days 1 to 5 **or** 100 mg/m^2/day on days 1, 3, and 5 repeated every 3 to 4 weeks

Canadian labeling: Non-Hodgkin lymphoma (in combination with other agents), non-small cell lung cancer (alone or in combination), small cell lung cancer (first-line in combination; second-line alone or in combination), testicular cancer (in combination; oral therapy for refractory disease):

   IV: 50 to 100 mg/m^2/day for 5 days
   Oral: 100 to 200 mg/m^2/day for 5 days; administer daily doses >200 mg in 2 divided doses.

Adult off-label uses and/or dosing:

Hematopoietic stem cell transplant conditioning regimen, lymphoid malignancies: IV: 60 mg/kg over 4 hours as a single dose 3 or 4 days prior to transplantation (Horning 1994; Snyder 1993; Weaver 1994)

Non-small cell lung cancer: IV: 100 mg/m^2 days 1, 2, and 3 every 3 weeks for 4 cycles or every 4 weeks for 3 to 4 cycles (in combination with cisplatin) (Arriagada 2004) **or** 50 mg/m^2 days 1 to 5 and days 29 to 33 (in combination with cisplatin and radiation therapy) (Albain 2009)

Ovarian cancer, refractory: Oral: 50 mg/m^2 once daily for 21 days every 4 weeks until disease progression or unacceptable toxicity (Rose 1998)

Small cell lung cancer, limited stage: IV: 120 mg/m^2 on days 1, 2, and 3 every 3 weeks (in combination with cisplatin) for 4 courses (Turrisi 1999) **or** 100 mg/m^2 on days 1, 2, and 3 for induction therapy (in combination with cisplatin), followed by consolidation chemotherapy (Saito 2006) **or** 100 mg/m^2 on days 1, 2, and 3 every 3 weeks (in combination with carboplatin) up to a maximum of 6 cycles (Skarlos 2001) **or** 100 mg/m^2 IV on day 1 (in combination with cisplatin), followed by 200 mg/m^2 **orally** on days 2 through 4 every 3 weeks for a maximum of 5 courses (Sundstrom 2002). According to American Society of Clinical Oncology (ASCO) guidelines, platinum-based therapy (cisplatin or carboplatin) in combination with either etoposide or irinotecan for 4 cycles is recommended over other regimens for limited stage disease (Rudin 2015).

Small cell lung cancer, extensive stage: 100 mg/m^2 IV on days 1, 2, and 3 every 3 weeks (in combination with cisplatin) for 4 cycles (Lara 2009) **or** 100 mg/m^2 IV on day 1 (in combination with cisplatin), followed by 200 mg/m^2 **orally** on days 2 through 4 every 3 weeks for a maximum of 5 courses (Sundstrom 2002) **or** IV: 80 mg/m^2 on days 1, 2, and 3 every 3 weeks (in combination with cisplatin) up to 8 cycles (Ihede 1994). According to ASCO guidelines, platinum-based therapy (cisplatin or carboplatin) in combination with either etoposide or irinotecan for 4 to 6 cycles is recommended over other regimens for extensive stage disease (Rudin 2015).

Testicular cancer (combination chemotherapy):

Nonseminoma: IV: 100 mg/m^2/day on days 1 through 5 every 21 days for 3 to 4 courses (Saxman 1998)

Nonseminoma, metastatic (high-dose regimens): IV: 750 mg/m^2/day administered 5, 4, and 3 days before peripheral blood stem cell infusion, repeat for a second cycle after recovery of granulocyte and platelet counts (Einhorn 2007) **or** 400 mg/m^2/day (beginning on cycle 3) on days 1, 2, and 3, with peripheral blood stem cell support, administered at 14- to 21-day intervals for 3 cycles (Kondagunta 2007)

Thymoma, locally advanced or metastatic: IV: 120 mg/m^2 days 1, 2, and 3 every 3 weeks (in combination with cisplatin) for up to 8 cycles (Giaccone 1996)

Unknown primary adenocarcinoma: Oral: 50 mg once daily on days 1, 3, 5, 7, and 9 alternating with 100 mg once daily on days 2, 4, 6, 8, and 10 every 3 weeks (in combination with paclitaxel and carboplatin) (Greco 2000; Hainsworth 2006)

Pediatric Note: Oral etoposide is associated with a moderate emetic potential; antiemetics may be recommended to prevent nausea and vomiting (Dupuis 2011).

Acute myeloid leukemia (AML) induction (off-label use; combination chemotherapy) (Woods 1996): IV:
<3 years: 3.3 mg/kg/day continuous infusion for 4 days
≥3 years: 100 mg/m^2/day continuous infusion for 4 days

Central nervous system tumors (off-label use; combination chemotherapy): IV:
<3 years: 6.5 mg/kg/dose days 3 and 4 of each 28-day "B" treatment cycle (Duffner 1993)
≥3 years: 100 mg/m^2/day on days 1, 2, and 3 of a 3-week treatment cycle (Taylor 2003)
≥6 years: 150 mg/m^2/day on days 3 and 4 of a 3-week treatment course (Kovnar 1990)

Hematopoietic stem cell transplantation conditioning regimen: IV: 60 mg/kg/dose over 4 hours as a single dose 3 or 4 days prior to transplantation (Horning 1994; Snyder 1993)

Hodgkin lymphoma (off-label use): IV: 200 mg/m^2/day on days 1, 2, and 3 every 3 weeks (Kelly 2002)

Neuroblastoma (off-label use): IV:
Induction: 100 mg/m^2/day on days 1 to 5 of each cycle (Kaneko 2002)
Hematopoietic stem cell transplantation conditioning regimen: 200 mg/m^2/day for 4 days beginning 8 or 9 days prior to transplantation (Kaneko 2002)

Sarcoma, refractory (off-label use): IV: 100 mg/m^2/day on days 1 to 5 of cycle; repeat cycle every 21 days (Van Winkle 2005)

Renal Impairment Oral, IV:
The manufacturer's US labeling recommends the following adjustments:
CrCl >50 mL/minute: No adjustment required.
CrCl 15 to 50 mL/minute: Administer 75% of dose
CrCl <15 mL minute: Data not available; consider further dose reductions

The following adjustments have also been recommended:
> Aronoff, 2007:
>> Adults:
>>> CrCl 10 to 50 mL/minute: Administer 75% of dose.
>>> CrCl <10 mL minute: Administer 50% of dose.
>>> Hemodialysis: Administer 50% of dose; supplemental posthemodialysis dose is not necessary.
>>> Peritoneal dialysis: Administer 50% of dose; supplemental dose is not necessary.
>>> Continuous renal replacement therapy (CRRT): Administer 75% of dose.
>> Children:
>>> CrCl 10 to 50 mL/minute/1.73 m^2: Administer 75% of dose.
>>> CrCl <10 mL minute/1.73 m^2: Administer 50% of dose.
>>> Hemodialysis: Administer 50% of dose.
>>> Peritoneal dialysis: Administer 50% of dose.
>>> Continuous renal replacement therapy (CRRT): Administer 75% of dose and reduce for hyperbilirubinemia.
> Janus, 2010: Hemodialysis: Reduce dose by 50%; not removed by hemodialysis so may be administered before or after dialysis
> Kintzel, 1995:
>> CrCl 46 to 60 mL/minute: Administer 85% of dose
>> CrCl 31 to 45 mL/minute: Administer 80% of dose
>> CrCl ≤30 mL/minute: Administer 75% of dose

Hepatic Impairment
US labeling: There are no dosage adjustments provided in the manufacturer's labeling.
Canadian labeling:
> Mild-to-moderate impairment: There are no dosage adjustments provided in the manufacturer's labeling.
> Severe impairment: Use is contraindicated.

The following adjustments have also been recommended:
> Donelli 1998: Liver dysfunction may reduce the metabolism and increase the toxicity of etoposide. Normal doses of IV etoposide should be given to patients with liver dysfunction (dose reductions may result in subtherapeutic concentrations); however, use caution with concomitant liver dysfunction (severe) and renal dysfunction as the decreased metabolic clearance cannot be compensated by increased renal clearance.
> Floyd 2006: Bilirubin 1.5 to 3 mg/dL or AST >3 times ULN: Administer 50% of dose
> King 2001; Koren, 1992: Bilirubin 1.5 to 3 mg/dL or AST >180 units/L: Administer 50% of dose

Obesity
*American Society of Clinical Oncology (ASCO) Guidelines for appropriate chemotherapy dosing in obese adults with cancer (**Note:** Excludes HSCT dosing):* Utilize patient's actual body weight (full weight) for calculation of body surface area- or weight-based dosing, particularly when the intent of therapy is curative; manage regimen-related toxicities in the same manner as for nonobese patients; if a dose reduction is utilized due to toxicity, consider resumption of full weight-based dosing with subsequent cycles, especially if cause of toxicity (eg, hepatic or renal impairment) is resolved (Griggs, 2012).

American Society for Blood and Marrow Transplantation (ASBMT) practice guideline committee position statement on chemotherapy dosing in obesity: Utilize actual body weight (full weight) for calculation of body surface area (BSA) for BSA-based dosing and utilize adjusted body weight 25% (ABW25) for mg/kg dosing for hematopoietic stem cell transplant conditioning regimens in adults (Bubalo, 2014).

ABW25: Adjusted wt (kg) = Ideal body weight (kg) + 0.25 [actual wt (kg) - ideal body weight (kg)]

Adjustment for Toxicity Oral, IV:

Infusion (hypersensitivity) reactions: Interrupt infusion.

ANC <500/mm^3 or platelets <50,000/mm^3: Withhold treatment until recovery.

Severe adverse reactions (nonhematologic): Reduce dose or discontinue treatment.

WBC 2000-3000/mm^3 or platelets 75,000-100,000/mm^3: Canadian labeling (not in US labeling): Reduce dose by 50%

Combination Regimens

Bone sarcoma (Ewing sarcoma):

Ifosfamide-Carboplatin-Etoposide (Ewing Sarcoma) on page 2154

Ifosfamide-Etoposide (Ewing Sarcoma) on page 2155

VAC Alternating With IE (Ewing Sarcoma) on page 2224

Bone sarcoma (osteosarcoma): Ifosfamide-Carboplatin-Etoposide (Osteosarcoma) on page 2154

Brain tumors:

CDDP/VP-16 on page 2028

COPE on page 2074

Gestational trophoblastic tumor:

EMA/CO (Gestational Trophoblastic Tumor) on page 2101

EMA/EP (Gestational Trophoblastic Tumor) on page 2101

EMA (Gestational Trophoblastic Tumor) on page 2102

Leukemia, acute lymphocytic:

Clofarabine-Cyclophosphamide-Etoposide (ALL) on page 2065

Hyper-CVAD (Leukemia, Acute Lymphocytic) on page 2146

Leukemia, acute myeloid:

5 + 2 + 5 (Cytarabine-Daunorubicin-Etoposide) (AML Consolidation) on page 1971

7 + 3 + 7 (Cytarabine-Daunorubicin-Etoposide) (AML Induction) on page 1973

Cytarabine (High Dose)-Daunorubicin-Etoposide (AML Induction) on page 2080

MEC-G (AML Induction) on page 2170

Mitoxantrone-Etoposide (AML Induction) on page 2175

Mitoxantrone-Etoposide-Cytarabine (AML) on page 2175

Lung cancer (non-small cell):

Cisplatin-Etoposide (NSCLC) on page 2041

EC (NSCLC) on page 2099

Lung cancer (small cell):

Carboplatin-Etoposide (Small Cell Lung Cancer) on page 2015

Cisplatin–Etoposide (Small Cell Lung Cancer) on page 2042

Lymphoma, Hodgkin:

BEACOPP-14 (Hodgkin) on page 1981

BEACOPP Escalated (Hodgkin) on page 1982

BEACOPP Escalated Plus Standard (Hodgkin) on page 1983

BEACOPP Standard (Hodgkin) on page 1984

Administration

Oral etoposide is associated with a low (adults) or moderate (children) emetic potential; antiemetics may be recommended to prevent nausea and vomiting (Dupuis 2011; Roila 2016).

Oral: Doses ≤200 mg/day as a single once daily dose; doses >200 mg should be given in 2 divided doses. If necessary, the injection may be used for oral administration (see Extemporaneous Preparations). Canadian labeling recommends administering capsule on an empty stomach.

IV: Administer standard doses over at least 30 to 60 minutes to minimize the risk of hypotension. Higher (off-label) doses used in transplantation may be infused over longer time periods depending on the protocol. Etoposide injection contains polysorbate 80 which may cause leaching of diethylhexyl phthalate (DEHP), a plasticizer contained in polyvinyl chloride (PVC) tubing. Administration through non-PVC (low sorbing) tubing will minimize patient exposure to DEHP. Etoposide is an irritant; tissue irritation and inflammation have occurred following extravasation; avoid extravasation.

Concentrations >0.4 mg/mL are very unstable and may precipitate within a few minutes. For large doses, where dilution to ≤0.4 mg/mL is not feasible, consideration should be given to slow infusion of the undiluted drug through a running normal saline, dextrose or saline/dextrose infusion; or use of etoposide phosphate. Due to the risk for precipitation, an inline filter may be used; etoposide solutions of 0.1 to 0.4 mg/mL may be filtered through a 0.22 micron filter without damage to the filter; etoposide solutions of 0.2 mg/mL may be filtered through a 0.22 micron filter without significant loss of drug.

Vesicant/Extravasation Risk May be an irritant

Emetic Potential

Children:

Oral: Moderate (30% to 90%)

IV: Low (10% to 30%)

Adults:

Oral: Low (10% to 30%)

IV: Low (10% to 30%)

Extemporaneous Preparations Etoposide 10 mg/mL oral solution: Dilute etoposide for injection 1:1 with normal saline to a concentration of 10 mg/mL. This solution is stable in plastic oral syringes for 22 days at room temperature (McLeod 1992). Prior to oral administration, further mix with fruit juice (orange or apple **NOT** grapefruit juice) or lemonade to a concentration of <0.4 mg/mL; once mixed with fruit juice, use within 3 hours (Lam 2011).

Lam MS. Extemporaneous compounding of oral liquid dosage formulations and alternative drug delivery methods for anticancer drugs. *Pharmacotherapy.* 2011;31(2):164-92.

McLeod HL and Relling MV, "Stability of Etoposide Solution for Oral Use," *Am J Hosp Pharm,* 1992, 49(11):2784-5.

Monitoring Parameters CBC with differential; liver function (bilirubin, ALT, AST), albumin, renal function tests; vital signs (blood pressure); signs of an infusion reaction

Dosage Forms Excipient information presented when available (limited, particularly for generics); consult specific product labeling.

Capsule, Oral:

Generic: 50 mg

Solution, Intravenous:

Toposar: 100 mg/5 mL (5 mL); 500 mg/25 mL (25 mL); 1 g/50 mL (50 mL) [contains alcohol, usp, polyethylene glycol 300, polysorbate 80]

Generic: 100 mg/5 mL (5 mL); 500 mg/25 mL (25 mL); 1 g/50 mL (50 mL)

Etoposide Phosphate (e toe POE side FOS fate)

Related Information
Common Toxicity Criteria *on page 2242*
Management of Drug Extravasations *on page 2271*
Safe Handling of Hazardous Drugs *on page 2379*

Brand Names: US Etopophos

Index Terms Epipodophyllotoxin; ETOP

Pharmacologic Category Antineoplastic Agent, Podophyllotoxin Derivative; Antineoplastic Agent, Topoisomerase II Inhibitor

Use
Small cell lung cancer: First-line treatment of small cell lung cancer (in combination with cisplatin)

Testicular cancer, refractory: Treatment of refractory testicular tumors (in combination with other chemotherapy agents)

Labeled Contraindications Hypersensitivity to etoposide products or any component of the formulation

Pregnancy Considerations Based on animal reproduction studies and the mechanism of action, etoposide phosphate may cause fetal harm if administered during pregnancy. Women of reproductive potential should avoid pregnancy during treatment. Fetal growth restriction and newborn myelosuppression have been observed following maternal use of regimens containing etoposide during pregnancy (NTP 2013; Peccatori 2013). The European Society for Medical Oncology has published guidelines for diagnosis, treatment, and follow-up of cancer during pregnancy. The guidelines recommend referral to a facility with expertise in cancer during pregnancy and encourage a multidisciplinary team (obstetrician, neonatologist, oncology team). In general, if chemotherapy is indicated, it should be avoided during in the first trimester, there should be a 3-week time period between the last chemotherapy dose and anticipated delivery, and chemotherapy should not be administered beyond week 33 of gestation. Guidelines for the treatment of SCLC are not provided (Peccatori 2013).

In women of reproductive potential, etoposide phosphate may cause amenorrhea, infertility, or premature menopause; effective contraception should be used during therapy and for at least 6 months after the last dose. In males, azoospermia, oligospermia, or permanent loss of fertility may occur. In addition, spermatozoa and testicular tissue may be damaged. Males with female partners of reproductive potential should use condoms during therapy and for 4 months after the last dose.

Breastfeeding Considerations Etoposide is excreted in breast milk (Azuno 1995). Due to the potential for serious adverse reactions in the nursing infant, the manufacturer recommends against breastfeeding during therapy.

Warnings/Precautions Etoposide phosphate is associated with hematologic toxicity, including neutropenia and thrombocytopenia. The nadir typically occurs at 10 to 14 days with recovery by day 21 (Perry 2012). Infections due to neutropenia and bleeding due to thrombocytopenia have occurred, some fatal. Monitor blood counts prior to each cycle of etoposide phosphate and more frequently if needed.

Etoposide phosphate may cause hypersensitivity reactions, including rash, pruritus, urticaria, and anaphylaxis. Interrupt therapy immediately and begin supportive management if hypersensitivity reactions occur. Discontinue permanently in patients with severe hypersensitivity reactions. Underlying mechanisms behind the development of hypersensitivity reactions is unknown, but have been attributed to high drug concentration and rate of infusion. Another possible mechanism may be due to the differences between available etoposide intravenous formulations. Etoposide intravenous formulation contains polysorbate 80 and benzyl alcohol, while etoposide phosphate (the water soluble prodrug of etoposide) intravenous formulation does not contain either vehicle. Case reports have suggested that etoposide phosphate has been used successfully in patients with previous hypersensitivity reactions to etoposide (Collier 2008; Siderov 2002).

Etoposide phosphate may result in infertility in male and female patients. Oligospermia, azoospermia, and permanent loss of fertility may occur in males; amenorrhea and premature menopause may also occur in women. Secondary malignancies (acute leukemias) have been reported with long term use of etoposide phosphate. Use with caution in patients with renal and/or hepatic impairment; may require dosage adjustment. Potentially significant drug-drug interactions may exist, requiring dose or frequency adjustment, additional monitoring, and/or selection of alternative therapy. Each 100 mg vial of etoposide phosphate is equivalent to 100 mg of etoposide; equivalent doses should be used when converting from etoposide to etoposide phosphate.

Adverse Reactions Also see adverse reactions for etoposide; etoposide phosphate is converted to etoposide, adverse reactions experienced with etoposide would also be expected with etoposide phosphate.

>10%:

Central nervous system: Malaise (≤39%), chills (≤24%)

Dermatologic: Alopecia (33% to 44%)

Gastrointestinal: Nausea and vomiting (37%), anorexia (16%), mucositis (11%)

Hematologic & oncologic: Leukopenia (91%; grade 4: 17%; nadir: day 15 to 22; recovery: usually by day 21), neutropenia (88%; grade 4: 37%; nadir: day 12 to 19; recovery: usually by day 21), anemia (72%; grades 3/4: 19%), thrombocytopenia (23%; grade 4: 9%; nadir: day 10 to 15; recovery: usually by day 21)

Neuromuscular & skeletal: Weakness (≤39%)

Miscellaneous: Fever (≤24%)

1% to 10%:

Cardiovascular: Hypotension (1% to 5%), localized phlebitis (≤5%; including cellulitis at injection site, local pain, local swelling, local tissue necrosis, tissue necrosis at injection site), hypertension (3%), facial flushing (2%)

Central nervous system: Dizziness (5%)

Dermatologic: Skin rash (3%)

Gastrointestinal: Constipation (8%), abdominal pain (7%), diarrhea (6%), dysgeusia (6%)

Hypersensitivity: Anaphylactoid reaction (3%; including bronchospasm, chills, diaphoresis, dyspnea, fever, pruritus, rigors, tachycardia)

Local: Extravasation (≤5%; including cellulitis at injection site, local pain, local swelling, local tissue necrosis, tissue necrosis at injection site)

<1%, postmarketing, and/or case reports: Acute leukemia (with/without pre-leukemia phase), apnea (hypersensitivity-associated), back pain, cortical blindness (transient), cough, cyanosis, diaphoresis, dysphagia, erythema, facial swelling, febrile neutropenia, hepatotoxicity, hyperpigmentation, infection, interstitial pneumonitis, laryngospasm, maculopapular rash, optic neuritis, pruritic erythematous rash, pulmonary fibrosis, radiation recall

phenomenon, seizure, Stevens-Johnson syndrome, swollen tongue, toxic epidermal necrolysis, urticaria

Drug Interactions

Metabolism/Transport Effects Substrate of CYP1A2 (minor), CYP2E1 (minor), CYP3A4 (major), P-glycoprotein; **Note:** Assignment of Major/Minor substrate status based on clinically relevant drug interaction potential; **Inhibits** CYP2C9 (weak)

Avoid Concomitant Use

Avoid concomitant use of Etoposide Phosphate with any of the following: BCG (Intravesical); Conivaptan; Deferiprone; Dipyrone; Fusidic Acid (Systemic); Idelalisib; Natalizumab; Pimecrolimus; Tacrolimus (Topical); Vaccines (Live)

Increased Effect/Toxicity

Etoposide Phosphate may increase the levels/effects of: CloZAPine; Deferiprone; Fingolimod; Leflunomide; Natalizumab; Tofacitinib; Vaccines (Live); Vitamin K Antagonists

The levels/effects of Etoposide Phosphate may be increased by: Aprepitant; Atovaquone; Conivaptan; CycloSPORINE (Systemic); CYP3A4 Inhibitors (Moderate); CYP3A4 Inhibitors (Strong); Dasatinib; Denosumab; Dipyrone; Fosaprepitant; Fusidic Acid (Systemic); Idelalisib; MiFEPRIStone; Netupitant; Ocrelizumab; Palbociclib; Palifermin; P-glycoprotein/ABCB1 Inhibitors; Pimecrolimus; Promazine; Ranolazine; Roflumilast; Simeprevir; Stiripentol; Tacrolimus (Topical); Trastuzumab

Decreased Effect

Etoposide Phosphate may decrease the levels/effects of: BCG (Intravesical); Coccidioides immitis Skin Test; Lenograstim; Nivolumab; Sipuleucel-T; Tertomotide; Vaccines (Inactivated); Vaccines (Live)

The levels/effects of Etoposide Phosphate may be decreased by: Bosentan; CYP3A4 Inducers (Moderate); CYP3A4 Inducers (Strong); Dabrafenib; Deferasirox; Enzalutamide; Mitotane; Sarilumab; Siltuximab; St John's Wort; Tocilizumab

Hazardous Drugs Handling Considerations

Hazardous agent (NIOSH 2016 [group 1]).

Use appropriate precautions for receiving, handling, administration, and disposal. Gloves (single) should be worn during receiving, unpacking, and placing in storage.

NIOSH recommends double gloving, a protective gown, ventilated engineering controls (a class II biological safety cabinet or a compounding aseptic containment isolator), and closed system transfer devices (CSTDs) for preparation. Double gloving, a gown, and (if dosage form allows) CSTDs are required during administration (NIOSH 2016).

Storage/Stability Store intact vials at 2°C to 8°C (36°F to 46°F). Retain in original package to protect from light. Reconstituted solution is stable for 7 days refrigerated at 2°C to 8°C (36°F to 46°F). Reconstituted solutions are stable at room temperature for 24 hours when reconstituted with SWFI, D5W, or NS, or for 48 hours when reconstituted with bacteriostatic water for injection with benzyl alcohol or bacteriostatic sodium chloride for injection with benzyl alcohol. Solutions diluted for infusion are stable for up to 24 hours at room temperature 20°C to 25°C (68°F to 77°F) or under refrigeration 2°C to 8°C (36°F to 46°F).

Preparation for Administration Reconstitute vials with 5 mL or 10 mL SWFI, D5W, NS, bacteriostatic water for injection with benzyl alcohol, or bacteriostatic sodium chloride for injection with benzyl alcohol to a concentration of 20 mg/mL or 10 mg/mL etoposide equivalent. These solutions may be administered without further dilution or may be diluted in D5W or NS to a concentration as low as 0.1 mg/mL.

Mechanism of Action Etoposide phosphate is converted *in vivo* to the active moiety, etoposide, by dephosphorylation. Etoposide inhibits mitotic activity; inhibits cells from entering prophase; inhibits DNA synthesis. Initially thought to be mitotic inhibitors similar to podophyllotoxin, but actually have no effect on microtubule assembly. However, later shown to induce DNA strand breakage and inhibition of topoisomerase II (an enzyme which breaks and repairs DNA); etoposide acts in late S or early G2 phases.

Pharmacodynamics/Kinetics

Distribution: V_d (mean): 18 to 29 L; poor penetration across blood-brain barrier

Protein binding: 97% (primarily to albumin)

Metabolism:

Etoposide phosphate: Rapidly and completely converted to etoposide in plasma

Etoposide: Hepatic, via CYP3A4 and 3A5 to various metabolites; in addition, conversion of etoposide to the O-demethylated metabolites (catechol and quinine) via prostaglandin synthases or myeloperoxidase occurs, as well as glutathione and glucuronide conjugation via GSTT1/GSTP1 and UGT1A1 (Yang 2009)

Half-life elimination: Terminal: 4 to 11 hours; Children: Normal renal/hepatic function: 6 to 8 hours

Excretion: Urine (56%; 45% as etoposide, <8% as metabolites) within 120 hours; feces (44%) within 120 hours

Dosing

Adult & Geriatric Note: Etoposide phosphate is a prodrug of etoposide; equivalent doses should be used when converting from etoposide to etoposide phosphate. Each 100 mg vial of etoposide phosphate is equivalent to 100 mg of etoposide.

Small cell lung cancer: IV: Etoposide 35 mg/m^2/day for 4 days or 50 mg/m^2/day for 5 days every 21 to 28 days (in combination with cisplatin). According to American Society of Clinical Oncology (ASCO) guidelines, platinum-based therapy (cisplatin or carboplatin) in combination with either etoposide or irinotecan for 4 to 6 cycles is recommended over other regimens for limited stage or extensive stage disease (4 cycles preferred for limited stage) (Rudin 2015).

Testicular cancer, refractory (in combination with other approved chemotherapeutic agents): IV: Etoposide 50 to 100 mg/m^2/day on days 1 to 5 every 21 to 28 days or 100 mg/m^2/day on days 1, 3, and 5 every 21 to 28 days.

Indication-specific off-label dosing: Refer to Etoposide monograph.

Renal Impairment

CrCl >50 mL/minute: No dosage adjustment necessary.

CrCl 15 to 50 mL/minute: Reduce dose to 75% of recommended dose.

CrCl <15 mL minute: There is no dosage adjustment provided in the manufacturer's labeling (has not been studied); consider further dose reductions.

Etoposide phosphate is rapidly and completely converted to etoposide in plasma, please refer to Etoposide monograph for additional renal dosing adjustments (for etoposide).

Hepatic Impairment There are no dosage adjustments provided in the manufacturer's labeling. Etoposide phosphate is rapidly and completely converted to etoposide in plasma; refer to Etoposide monograph for etoposide hepatic dosing adjustments.

Obesity *ASCO Guidelines for appropriate chemotherapy dosing in obese adults with cancer (Note: Excludes HSCT dosing):* Utilize patient's actual body weight (full weight) for calculation of body surface area- or weight-based dosing, particularly when the intent of therapy is curative; manage regimen-related toxicities in the same manner as for nonobese patients; if a dose reduction is utilized due to toxicity, consider resumption of full weight-based dosing with subsequent cycles, especially if cause of toxicity (eg, hepatic or renal impairment) is resolved (Griggs 2012).

Adjustment for Toxicity

Hematologic (ANC <500/mm^3 and/or platelets <50,000/mm^3): Interrupt treatment until blood counts have sufficiently recovered.

Severe adverse reactions: Reduce dose, interrupt treatment, or discontinue.

Combination Regimens

Retinoblastoma: Carboplatin-Etoposide-Vincristine (Retinoblastoma) on page 2016

Administration Small cell lung cancer, testicular cancer (refractory): Infuse over 5 minutes to 3.5 hours. Do not administer as an IV bolus over less than 5 minutes. Etoposide phosphate may be an irritant; monitor infusion site; avoid extravasation.

Vesicant/Extravasation Risk May be an irritant

Emetic Potential Low (10% to 30%)

Monitoring Parameters CBC with differential and platelets (prior to each cycle; more frequently if necessary), bilirubin, AST/ALT, renal function, vital signs (blood pressure)

Dosage Forms Excipient information presented when available (limited, particularly for generics); consult specific product labeling.

Solution Reconstituted, Intravenous [strength expressed as base]:
  Etopophos: 100 mg (1 ea)

◆ **Etoposide Injection (Can)** *see* Etoposide *on page 729*

◆ **Etoposide Injection USP (Can)** *see* Etoposide *on page 729*

◆ **Euflex (Can)** *see* Flutamide *on page 839*

◆ **Eulexin** *see* Flutamide *on page 839*

◆ *Euphorbia peplus* **Derivative** *see* Ingenol Mebutate *on page 1011*

◆ **Euro-Cyproheptadine (Can)** *see* Cyproheptadine *on page 467*

Everolimus (e ver OH li mus)

Related Information

Common Toxicity Criteria *on page 2242*

Management of Chemotherapy-Induced Nausea and Vomiting in Adults *on page 2253*

Prevention of Chemotherapy-Induced Nausea and Vomiting in Children *on page 2310*

Safe Handling of Hazardous Drugs *on page 2379*

Brand Names: US Afinitor; Afinitor Disperz; Zortress

Brand Names: Canada Afinitor; Afinitor Disperz

Index Terms RAD001

Pharmacologic Category Antineoplastic Agent, mTOR Kinase Inhibitor; Immunosuppressant Agent; mTOR Kinase Inhibitor

Use

Breast cancer, advanced (Afinitor only): Treatment of advanced hormone receptor-positive, HER2-negative breast cancer in postmenopausal women (in combination with exemestane and after letrozole or anastrozole failure)

Neuroendocrine tumors (Afinitor only): Treatment of locally advanced, metastatic or unresectable progressive pancreatic neuroendocrine tumors (PNET); treatment of progressive, well-differentiated, nonfunctional GI or lung neuroendocrine tumors in patients with unresectable, locally advanced or metastatic disease

Limitations of use: Not indicated for the treatment of functional carcinoid tumors.

Renal angiomyolipoma with tuberous sclerosis complex (Afinitor only): Treatment of renal angiomyolipoma with tuberous sclerosis complex (TSC) not requiring immediate surgery

Renal cell carcinoma, advanced (Afinitor only): Treatment of advanced renal cell cancer (RCC) after sunitinib or sorafenib failure

Subependymal giant cell astrocytoma (Afinitor or Afinitor Disperz only): Treatment of subependymal giant cell astrocytoma (SEGA) associated with TSC which requires intervention, but cannot be curatively resected

Liver transplantation (Zortress only): Prophylaxis of allograft rejection in liver transplantation (in combination with corticosteroids and reduced doses of tacrolimus, everolimus should not be administered earlier than 30 days post-transplant)

Renal transplantation (Zortress only): Prophylaxis of organ rejection in renal transplant patients at low to moderate immunologic risk (in combination with basiliximab induction and concurrent with corticosteroids and reduced doses of cyclosporine)

Labeled Contraindications Hypersensitivity to everolimus, sirolimus, other rapamycin derivatives, or any component of the formulation.

Pregnancy Considerations Adverse events were observed in animal reproduction studies with exposures lower than expected with human doses. Based on the mechanism of action, may cause fetal harm if administered during pregnancy. Women of reproductive potential should be advised to avoid pregnancy and use highly effective birth control during treatment and for up to 8 weeks after everolimus discontinuation.

Everolimus may cause infertility. In females, menstrual irregularities, secondary amenorrhea, and increases in luteinizing hormone and follicle-stimulating hormone have occurred. Azoospermia and oligospermia have been observed in males. Females of reproductive potential should consider family planning options prior to therapy.

The National Transplantation Pregnancy Registry (NTPR) is a registry which follows pregnancies which occur in maternal transplant recipients or those fathered by male transplant recipients. The NTPR encourages reporting of pregnancies following solid organ transplant by contacting them at 877-955-6877 or NTPR@giftoflifeinstitute.org.

Breastfeeding Considerations It is not known if everolimus is excreted in breast milk. Due to the potential for serious adverse reactions in the nursing infant, breastfeeding is not recommended by the manufacturer during therapy (Afinitor, Zortress) and for 2 weeks following the last dose (Afinitor).

Warnings/Precautions To avoid potential contact with everolimus, care-givers should wear gloves when preparing suspension from tablets for oral suspension. Noninfectious pneumonitis, interstitial lung disease (ILD), and/or noninfectious fibrosis have been observed with mTOR inhibitors including everolimus; some cases were fatal. Symptoms include dyspnea, cough, hypoxia and/or pleural effusion; promptly evaluate worsening respiratory symptoms. Cases of ILD have been reported with pulmonary hypertension (including pulmonary arterial hypertension) as a secondary event. Consider opportunistic infections such as *Pneumocystis jirovecii* pneumonia (PCP) when evaluating clinical symptoms. May require treatment interruption followed by dose reduction (pneumonitis has developed even with reduced doses) and/or corticosteroid therapy; discontinue for grade 4 pneumonitis. Consider discontinuation for recurrence of grade 3 toxicity after dosage reduction. In patients who require steroid therapy for symptom management, consider PCP prophylaxis. Imaging may overestimate the incidence of clinical pneumonitis. **[US Boxed Warning]: Everolimus has immunosuppressant properties which may result in infection;** the risk of developing bacterial (including mycobacterial), viral, fungal and protozoal infections and for local, opportunistic (including polyomavirus infection), and/or systemic infections is increased; may lead to sepsis, respiratory failure, hepatic failure, or fatality. Polyomavirus infection in transplant patients may be serious and/or fatal. Polyoma virus-associated nephropathy (due to BK virus), which may result in serious cases of deteriorating renal function and renal graft loss, has been observed with use. JC virus-associated progressive multiple leukoencephalopathy (PML) may also be associated with everolimus use in transplantation. Reduced immunosuppression (taking into account the risks of rejection) should be considered with evidence of polyoma virus infection or PML. Reactivation of hepatitis B has been observed in patients receiving everolimus. Resolve preexisting invasive fungal infections prior to treatment initiation. Cases (some fatal) of *Pneumocystis jirovecii* pneumonia (PCP) have been reported with everolimus use. Consider PCP prophylaxis in patients receiving concomitant corticosteroid or other immunosuppressant therapy. In addition, transplant recipient patients should receive prophylactic therapy for PCP and for cytomegalovirus (CMV). Monitor for signs and symptoms of infection during treatment. Discontinue if invasive systemic fungal infection is diagnosed (and manage with appropriate antifungal therapy).

[US Boxed Warning]: Immunosuppressant use may result in the development of malignancy, including lymphoma and skin cancer. The risk is associated with treatment intensity and the duration of therapy. To minimize the risk for skin cancer, limit exposure to sunlight and ultraviolet light; wear protective clothing and use effective sunscreen.

[US Boxed Warning]: Due to the increased risk for nephrotoxicity in renal transplantation, avoid standard doses of cyclosporine in combination with everolimus; reduced cyclosporine doses are recommended when everolimus is used in combination with cyclosporine. Therapeutic monitoring of cyclosporine and everolimus concentrations is recommended. Monitor for proteinuria; the risk of proteinuria is increased when everolimus is used in combination with cyclosporine, and with higher serum everolimus concentrations. Everolimus and cyclosporine combination therapy may increase the risk for thrombotic microangiopathy/thrombotic thrombocytopenic purpura/hemolytic uremic syndrome (TMA/TTP/HUS); monitor blood counts. In liver transplantation, the tacrolimus dose and target range should be reduced to minimize the risk of nephrotoxicity. Eliminating calcineurin inhibitors from the immunosuppressive regimen may result in acute rejection. Elevations in serum creatinine (generally mild), renal failure, and proteinuria have been also observed with everolimus use; monitor renal function (BUN, creatinine, and/or urinary protein). Risk of nephrotoxicity may be increased when administered with calcineurin inhibitors (eg, cyclosporine, tacrolimus); dosage adjustment of calcineurin inhibitor is necessary. An increased incidence of rash, infection and dose interruptions have been reported in patients with renal insufficiency (CrCl ≤60 mL/minute) who received mTOR inhibitors for the treatment of renal cell cancer (Gupta 2011); serum creatinine elevations and proteinuria have been reported. Monitor renal function (BUN, serum creatinine, urinary protein) at baseline and periodically, especially if risk factors for further impairment exist; pharmacokinetic studies have not been conducted; dosage adjustments are not required based on renal impairment. **[US Boxed Warning]: An increased risk of renal arterial and venous thrombosis has been reported with use in renal transplantation, generally within the first 30 days after transplant; may result in graft loss.** MTOR inhibitors are associated with an increase in hepatic artery thrombosis, most cases have been reported within 30 days after transplant and usually proceeded to graft loss or death; do not use everolimus prior to 30 days post liver transplant.

Potentially significant drug-drug/drug-food interactions may exist, requiring dose or frequency adjustment, additional monitoring, and/or selection of alternative therapy. In transplant patients, avoid the use of certain HMG-CoA reductase inhibitors (eg, simvastatin, lovastatin); may increase the risk for rhabdomyolysis due to the potential interaction with cyclosporine (which may be given in combination with everolimus for transplantation).

Use is associated with mouth ulcers, mucositis and stomatitis; manage with topical therapy; avoid the use of alcohol-, hydrogen peroxide-, iodine-, or thyme-based mouthwashes (due to the high potential for drug interactions, avoid the use of systemic antifungals unless fungal infection has been diagnosed). Everolimus is associated with the development of angioedema; concomitant use with other agents known to cause angioedema (eg, ACE inhibitors) may increase the risk. Everolimus use may delay wound healing and increase the occurrence of wound-related complications (eg, wound dehiscence, infection, incisional hernia, lymphocele, seroma); may require surgical intervention; use with caution in the peri-surgical period. Generalized edema, including peripheral edema and lymphedema, and local fluid accumulation (eg, pericardial effusion, pleural effusion, ascites) may also occur.

Everolimus exposure is increased in patients with hepatic impairment. For patients with breast cancer, neuroendocrine tumors, RCC, or renal angiomyolipoma with mild and moderate hepatic impairment, reduced doses are recommended; in patients with severe hepatic impairment, use is recommended (at reduced doses) if the potential benefit outweighs risks. Reduced doses are recommended in transplant patients with hepatic impairment; pharmacokinetic information does not exist for renal transplant patients with severe impairment (Child-Pugh class B or C); monitor whole blood trough levels closely for patients with SEGA, reduced doses may be needed for mild and moderate hepatic impairment (based on therapeutic drug monitoring), and are recommended in severe hepatic impairment; monitor whole blood trough levels.

[US Boxed Warning]: Increased mortality (usually associated with infections) within the first 3 months after transplant was noted in a study of patients with de novo heart transplant receiving immunosuppressive regimens containing everolimus (with or without induction therapy). Use in heart transplantation is not recommended. The boxed warning in the labeling (Zortress) is based on severe infectious complications, rather than efficacy (reduction in the incidence of cardiac allograft vasculopathy). Despite labeled warnings for this off-label indication, some centers continue to use everolimus (with reduced calcineurin inhibitor exposure). However, everolimus initiation in heart transplantation is delayed until 3 to 6 months post-transplantation due to impaired wound healing and pericardial effusions early on in the postoperative period (Andreassen 2014; Andreassen 2016; Costanza 2010; Hirt 2013; Hollis 2015). Hyperglycemia, hyperlipidemia, and hypertriglyceridemia have been reported. Higher serum everolimus concentrations are associated with an increased risk for hyperlipidemia. Use has not been studied in patients with baseline cholesterol >350 mg/dL. Monitor fasting glucose and lipid profile prior to treatment initiation and periodically thereafter; monitor more frequently in patients with concomitant medications affecting glucose. Manage with appropriate medical therapy (if possible, optimize glucose control and lipids prior to treatment initiation). Antihyperlipidemic therapy may not normalize levels. May alter insulin and/or oral hypoglycemic therapy requirements in patients with diabetes; the risk for new onset diabetes is increased with everolimus use after transplantation. Decreases in hemoglobin, neutrophils, platelets, and lymphocytes have been reported; monitor blood counts at baseline and periodically. Increases in serum glucose are common; may alter insulin and/or oral hypoglycemic therapy requirements in patients with diabetes; the risk for new-onset diabetes is increased with everolimus use after transplantation. Patients should not be immunized with live viral vaccines during or shortly after treatment and should avoid close contact with recently vaccinated (live vaccine) individuals; consider the timing of routine immunizations prior to the start of therapy in pediatric patients treated for SEGA. In pediatric patients treated for SEGA, complete recommended series of live virus childhood vaccinations prior to treatment (if immediate everolimus treatment is not indicated); an accelerated vaccination schedule may be appropriate. Continue treatment with everolimus for renal cell cancer as long as clinical benefit is demonstrated or until occurrence of unacceptable toxicity. Safety and efficacy have not been established for the use of everolimus in the treatment of carcinoid tumors.

Tablets (Afinitor, Zortress) and tablets for oral suspension (Afinitor Disperz) are not interchangeable; Afinitor Disperz is only indicated in conjunction with therapeutic monitoring for the treatment of SEGA. Do not combine formulations to achieve total desired dose. May cause infertility; in females, menstrual irregularities, secondary amenorrhea, and increases in luteinizing hormone and follicle-stimulating hormone have occurred; azoospermia and oligospermia have been observed in males. Avoid use in patients with hereditary galactose intolerance, Lapp lactase deficiency, or glucose-galactose malabsorption; may result in diarrhea and malabsorption. The safety and efficacy of everolimus in renal transplantation patients with high-immunologic risk or in solid organ transplant other than renal or liver have not been established. **[US**

Boxed Warning]: In transplantation, everolimus should only be used by physicians experienced in immunosuppressive therapy and management of transplant patients. Adequate laboratory and supportive medical resources must be readily available. For indications requiring whole blood trough concentrations to determine dosage adjustments, a consistent method should be used; concentration values from different assay methods may not be interchangeable.

Adverse Reactions

Transplantation:

Reactions occur in kidney and liver transplantation unless otherwise specified.

>10%:

Cardiovascular: Peripheral edema (kidney transplant: 45%; liver transplant: 18%), hypertension (kidney transplant: 30%; liver transplant: 17%)

Central nervous system: Headache (18% to 19%), insomnia (kidney transplant: 17%), procedural pain (kidney transplant: 15%)

Endocrine & metabolic: Diabetes mellitus (new onset: liver transplant: 32%; kidney transplant: 9%), hypercholesterolemia (15% to 24%), hyperkalemia (renal transplant: 18%), hypomagnesemia (kidney transplant: 14%), hypophosphatemia (kidney transplant: 13%), hyperglycemia (kidney transplant: 12%), hypokalemia (kidney transplant: 12%)

Gastrointestinal: Constipation (kidney transplant: 38%), nausea (kidney transplant: 29%; liver transplant: 14%), diarrhea (19%), vomiting (kidney transplant: 15%), abdominal pain (13%)

Genitourinary: Urinary tract infection (kidney transplant: 22%), hematuria (kidney transplant: 12%), dysuria (kidney transplant: 11%)

Hematologic & oncologic: Anemia (kidney transplant: 26%), leukopenia (3% to 12%)

Infection: Infection (kidney transplant: 62%; liver transplant: 50%), viral infection (liver transplant: 17%; kidney transplant: 10%), bacterial infection (liver transplant: 16%), hepatitis C (liver transplant: 11%)

Local: Incisional pain (kidney transplant: 16%)

Neuromuscular & skeletal: Limb pain (kidney transplant: 12%), back pain (kidney transplant: 11%)

Renal: Increased serum creatinine (kidney transplant: 18%)

Respiratory: Upper respiratory tract infection (kidney transplant: 16%)

Miscellaneous: Postoperative wound complication (kidney transplant: 35%; liver transplant: 11%; includes incisional hernia, lymphocele, seroma, wound dehiscence), fever (13% to 19%)

1% to 10%:

Cardiovascular: Hypertensive crisis (1%), angina pectoris, atrial fibrillation, chest discomfort, chest pain, congestive heart failure, deep vein thrombosis, edema, hypotension, palpitations, pulmonary embolism, renal artery thrombosis, syncope, tachycardia, venous thromboembolism

Central nervous system: Fatigue (9%), agitation, anxiety, chills, depression, dizziness, drowsiness, hallucination, hemiparesis, hypoesthesia, lethargy, malaise, migraine, myasthenia, neuralgia, pain, paresthesia

Dermatologic: Acneiform eruption, acne vulgaris, alopecia, cellulitis, diaphoresis, folliculitis, hypertrichosis, night sweats, onychomycosis, pruritus, skin rash, tinea pedis

Endocrine & metabolic: Acidosis, amenorrhea, cushingoid appearance, cyanocobalmin deficiency, dehydration, fluid retention, gout, hirsutism, hypercalcemia, hyperparathyroidism, hypertriglyceridemia, hyperuricemia, hypocalcemia, hypoglycemia, hyponatremia, iron deficiency, ovarian cyst

Gastrointestinal: Stomatitis (kidney transplant: 8%), dyspepsia (kidney transplant: 4%), upper abdominal pain (kidney transplant: 3%), abdominal distention, anorexia, decreased appetite, dysphagia, epigastric distress, flatulence, gastroenteritis, gastroesophageal reflux disease, gingival hyperplasia, hematemesis, hemorrhoids, intestinal obstruction, oral candidiasis, oral herpes, oral mucosa ulcer, peritoneal effusion, peritonitis

Genitourinary: Erectile dysfunction (kidney transplant: 5%), bladder spasm, perinephric abscess, perinephric hematoma, pollakiuria, proteinuria, pyuria, scrotal edema, urethritis, urinary retention, urinary urgency

Hematologic & oncologic: Neoplasm (3% to 4%), leukocytosis, lymphadenopathy, lymphorrhea, neutropenia, pancytopenia, thrombocythemia, thrombocytopenia

Hepatic: Abnormal hepatic function tests (liver transplant: 7%), ascites (liver transplant: 4%), hepatitis (noninfections), increased liver enzymes, increased serum alkaline phosphatase, increased serum bilirubin

Hypersensitivity: Angioedema (<1%)

Infection: BK virus (kidney transplant: 1%), bacteremia, candidiasis, herpes virus infection, influenza, sepsis, wound infection

Neuromuscular & skeletal: Tremor (8% to 9%), arthralgia, joint swelling, muscle spasm, musculoskeletal pain, myalgia, osteomyelitis, osteonecrosis, osteoporosis, spondylitis, weakness

Ophthalmic: Blurred vision, cataract, conjunctivitis

Renal: Hydronephrosis, increased blood urea nitrogen, interstitial nephritis, polyuria, pyelonephritis, renal failure (acute), renal insufficiency, renal tubular necrosis

Respiratory: Cough (kidney transplant: 7%), atelectasis, bronchitis, dyspnea, epistaxis, lower respiratory tract infection, nasal congestion, nasopharyngitis, oropharyngeal pain, pleural effusion, pneumonia, pulmonary edema, rhinorrhea, sinus congestion, sinusitis, wheezing

Antineoplastic:
Antineoplastic indications include advanced hormone receptor-positive, advanced nonfunctional NET of gastrointestinal or lung origin, HER2-negative breast cancer (advanced HR + BC), pancreatic neuroendocrine tumors (PNET), renal cell carcinoma (RCC), renal angiomyolipoma and tuberous sclerosis complex (TSC), and subependymal giant cell astrocytoma (SEGA) >10%:

Cardiovascular: Edema (PNET: ≤39%), peripheral edema (advanced nonfunctional NET of gastrointestinal or lung origin, PNET: ≤39%; advanced HR + BC, RCC, TSC: 13% to 25%), hypertension (PNET, RCC, SEGA: 4% to 13%)

Central nervous system: Malaise (PNET: ≤45%), fatigue (advanced HR + BC, advanced nonfunctional NET of gastrointestinal or lung origin, PNET, RCC: 31% to ≤45%; SEGA: 14%), headache (PNET: ≤30%; advanced HR + BC, RCC: 19% to 21%), migraine (PNET: ≤30%), behavioral problems (SEGA: 21%; includes abnormal behavior, aggressive behavior, agitation, anxiety, obsessive compulsive symptoms, panic attack), insomnia (advanced HR + BC, PNET, RCC, SEGA: 6% to 14%), dizziness (PNET, RCC: 7% to 12%)

Dermatologic: Skin rash (PNET: 59%; advanced HR + BC, advanced nonfunctional NET of gastrointestinal or lung origin, RCC, SEGA: 21% to 39%; may include allergic dermatitis, macular eruption, maculopapular rash, papular rash, urticaria), cellulitis (SEGA: 29%), acne vulgaris (TSC: 22%;

SEGA: 10%), nail disease (PNET: 22%; RCC: 5%), pruritus (advanced HR + BC, advanced nonfunctional NET of gastrointestinal or lung origin, PNET, RCC: 13% to 21%), xeroderma (PNET, RCC: 13%)

Endocrine & metabolic: Hypercholesterolemia (TSC, SEGA: 81% to 85%; advanced nonfunctional NET of gastrointestinal or lung origin: 71%), decreased serum bicarbonate (PNET: 56%), hyperglycemia (advanced nonfunctional NET of gastrointestinal or lung origin: 55%; SEGA: 25%; advanced HR + BC: 14%), hypertriglyceridemia (TSC: 52%; advanced nonfunctional NET of gastrointestinal or lung origin, SEGA: 27% to 30%), hypophosphatemia (advanced nonfunctional NET of gastrointestinal or lung origin, TSC: 43% to 49%; SEGA: 9%), decreased serum calcium (PNET: 37%), hypokalemia (advanced nonfunctional NET of gastrointestinal or lung origin: 27%), hypoalbuminemia (advanced nonfunctional NET of gastrointestinal or lung origin: 18%), amenorrhea (TSC, SEGA: 15% to 17%)

Gastrointestinal: Stomatitis (advanced HR + BC, advanced nonfunctional NET of gastrointestinal or lung origin, PNET, SEGA, TSC: 62% to 78%; advanced nonfunctional NET of gastrointestinal or lung origin grade 3: 9%; grades 3/4: ≤9%; RCC: 44%, grades 3/4: ≤4%), diarrhea (advanced nonfunctional NET of gastrointestinal or lung origin, PNET: 41% to 50%; advanced HR + BC, RCC: 30% to 33%; TSC, SEGA: 14% to 17%; may include bowel urgency, colitis, enteritis, enterocolitis, steatorrhea), abdominal pain (PNET: 36%; RCC, SEGA: 5% to 9%), decreased appetite (advanced HR + BC, advanced nonfunctional NET of gastrointestinal or lung origin, PNET: 22% to 30%; TSC: 6%), nausea (advanced HR + BC, advanced nonfunctional NET of gastrointestinal or lung origin, RCC: 26% to 29%; SEGA: 8%), vomiting (15% to 29%), weight loss (advanced HR + BC, advanced nonfunctional NET of gastrointestinal or lung origin, PNET: 22% to 28%; RCC: 9%; SEGA: 5%), anorexia (RCC: 25%), dysgeusia (advanced HR + BC, advanced nonfunctional NET of gastrointestinal or lung origin, PNET: 18% to 22%; RCC: 10%; TSC: 5%), mucositis (RCC: 19%; grades 3/4: ≤1%), constipation (advanced HR + BC, PNET, SEGA: 10% to 14%), xerostomia (advanced HR + BC, PNET, RCC: 8% to 11%)

Genitourinary: Urinary tract infection (PNET: 16%; advanced HR + BC, RCC: 5% to 10%), irregular menses (TSC, PNET: 10% to 11%)

Hematologic & oncologic: Increase in fasting plasma glucose (PNET: 75%, grades 3/4: 17%; TSC: 14%), prolonged partial thromboplastin time (SEGA: 72%), anemia (advanced nonfunctional NET of gastrointestinal or lung origin: 81%; TSC: 61%; SEGA: 41%; advanced nonfunctional NET of gastrointestinal or lung origin grade 3: 5%), lymphocytopenia (advanced nonfunctional NET of gastrointestinal or lung origin: 66%, grade 3:15%; grade 4: 2%; TSC: 20%, grade 3: 1%), thrombocytopenia (advanced nonfunctional NET of gastrointestinal or lung origin: 33%; RCC, TSC: 19%; advanced HR + BC, advanced nonfunctional NET of gastrointestinal or lung origin grade 3: 2%; advanced nonfunctional NET of gastrointestinal or lung origin grade 4: 1%), leukopenia (advanced nonfunctional NET of gastrointestinal or lung origin: 49%; TSC: 37%; advanced nonfunctional NET of gastrointestinal or lung origin grade 3: 2%), neutropenia (SEGA: 46%, grade 3: 9%; advanced nonfunctional NET of gastrointestinal or lung origin: 32%)

Hepatic: Increased serum alkaline phosphatase (PNET: 74%; TSC: 32%, grade 3: 1%), increased serum AST (advanced HR + BC: 69%; advanced nonfunctional NET of gastrointestinal or lung origin, PNET: 56% to 57%; RCC, TSC, SEGA: 23% to 33%; advanced HR + BC, advanced nonfunctional NET of gastrointestinal or lung origin, RCC, TSC grade 3: ≤4%;

advanced HR + BC, advanced nonfunctional NET of gastrointestinal or lung origin, RCC grade 4: ≤1%), increased serum ALT (advanced HR + BC, advanced nonfunctional NET of gastrointestinal or lung origin, PNET: 46% to 51%, RCC, TSC, SEGA: 18% to 21%; advanced nonfunctional NET of gastrointestinal or lung origin grade 3: 5%; RCC, TSC grade 3: 1%; advanced HR + BC, advanced nonfunctional NET of gastrointestinal or lung origin grade 4: ≤1%)

Infection: Infection (advanced HR + BC, advanced nonfunctional NET of gastrointestinal or lung origin: 50% to 58%; RCC: 37%; advanced HR + BC, advanced nonfunctional NET of gastrointestinal or lung origin, RCC grade 3: 4% to 8%; advanced HR + BC, advanced nonfunctional NET of gastrointestinal or lung origin, RCC grade 4: 1% to 3%)

Neuromuscular & skeletal: Weakness (RCC: 33%; advanced nonfunctional NET of gastrointestinal or lung origin: 23%; advanced HR + BC: 13%), arthralgia (advanced HR + BC, PNET, TSC: 13% to 20%), back pain (advanced HR + BC, PNET: 14% to 15%), limb pain (PNET, RCC, SEGA: 8% to 14%)

Renal: Increased serum creatinine (RCC: 50%; advanced HR + BC, PNET: 19% to 24%, advanced HR + BC, RCC grade 3: 1% to 2%, PNET grades 3/4: 2%)

Respiratory: Respiratory tract infection (SEGA: 31%, grade 3: 1%, grade 4: 1%; includes viral respiratory tract infection), cough (advanced HR + BC, advanced nonfunctional NET of gastrointestinal or lung origin, PNET, RCC, TSC: 20% to 30%; includes productive cough), nasopharyngitis (PNET: ≤25%; advanced HR + BC, RCC: 6% to 10%), rhinitis (PNET: ≤25%), upper respiratory tract infection (PNET: ≤25%; TSC: 11%; advanced HR + BC: 5%), dyspnea (advanced HR + BC, advanced nonfunctional NET of gastrointestinal or lung origin, PNET, RCC: 20% to 24%; includes dyspnea on exertion), epistaxis (advanced HR + BC, advanced nonfunctional NET of gastrointestinal or lung origin, PNET, RCC, TSC, SEGA: 5% to 22%), pneumonitis (advanced HR + BC, advanced nonfunctional NET of gastrointestinal or lung origin, PNET, RCC: 14% to 19%; TSC, SEGA: 1%; advanced HR + BC, advanced nonfunctional NET of gastrointestinal or lung origin, PNET, RCC grade 3: 2% to 4%; advanced HR + BC, PNET grade 4: <1%; may include interstitial pulmonary disease, pulmonary alveolar hemorrhage, pulmonary alveolitis, pulmonary fibrosis, pulmonary infiltrates, pulmonary toxicity, restrictive pulmonary disease), oropharyngeal pain (PNET: 11%)

Miscellaneous: Fever (advanced HR + BC, advanced nonfunctional NET of gastrointestinal or lung origin, PNET, RCC, SEGA: 15% to 31%)

1% to 10%:

Cardiovascular: Chest pain (RCC: 5%), tachycardia (RCC: 3%), congestive heart failure (RCC: 1%), deep vein thrombosis (RCC: <1%)

Central nervous system: Depression (TSC: 5%), paresthesia (RCC: 5%), chills (RCC: 4%)

Dermatologic: Alopecia (advanced HR + BC: 10%), palmar-plantar erythrodysesthesia (RCC: 5%), erythema (RCC: 4%), onychoclasis (RCC: 4%), skin lesion (RCC: 4%), acneiform eruption (RCC: 3%)

Endocrine & metabolic: Diabetes mellitus (PNET: 10%; RCC: exacerbation of diabetes mellitus: 2%, new onset: <1%), hypermenorrhea (TSC, SEGA: 6% to 10%), menstrual disease (TSC, SEGA: 6% to 10%), decreased serum fibrinogen (SEGA: 8%), increased luteinizing hormone (TSC, SEGA: 1% to 4%), increased follicle-stimulating hormone (TSC: 3%), ovarian cyst (TSC: 3%)

Gastrointestinal: Gastroenteritis (SEGA: 10%; includes viral gastroenteritis, gastrointestinal infection), hemorrhoids (RCC: 5%), dysphagia (RCC: 4%)

Genitourinary: Vaginal hemorrhage (TSC: 8%), dysmenorrhea (SEGA: 6%), uterine hemorrhage (SEGA: 6%), cystitis (advanced HR + BC: 3%)

Hematologic & oncologic: Hemorrhage (RCC: 3%)

Hepatic: Increased serum bilirubin (RCC: 3%; grade 3: <1%, grade 4: <1%)

Hypersensitivity: Hypersensitivity reaction (TSC, SEGA: 3%; includes anaphylaxis, chest pain, dyspnea, flushing), angioedema (RCC, TSC: ≤1%)

Infection: Candidiasis (advanced HR + BC, RCC: <1%), hepatitis C (advanced HR + BC: <1%), sepsis (advanced HR + BC, RCC: <1%)

Neuromuscular & skeletal: Muscle spasm (PNET: 10%), jaw pain (RCC: 3%)

Ophthalmic: Eyelid edema (RCC: 4%), conjunctivitis (RCC: 2%)

Otic: Otitis media (TSC: 6%)

Renal: Renal failure (RCC: 3%)

Respiratory: Streptococcal pharyngitis (SEGA: 10%), pleural effusion (RCC: 7%), pneumonia (advanced HR + BC, RCC, SEGA: 4% to 6%), bronchitis (advanced HR + BC, RCC: 4%), pharyngolaryngeal pain (RCC: 4%), rhinorrhea (RCC: 3%), sinusitis (advanced HR + BC, RCC: 3%)

Miscellaneous: Postoperative wound complication (RC: <1%; wound healing impairment)

<1%, postmarketing, and/or case reports: Arterial thrombosis, aspergillosis, azoospermia, cholecystitis, cholelithiasis, complex regional pain syndrome, decreased plasma testosterono, hemolytic uremic syndrome, hypersensitivity angiitis, male infertility, nephrotoxicity, oligospermia, pancreatitis (including acute pancreatitis), pericardial effusion, pneumonia (*Pneumocystis jirovecii*), polyoma virus infection, progressive multifocal leukoencephalopathy, reactivation of HBV, respiratory distress, thrombosis of vascular graft (kidney), thrombotic thrombocytopenic purpura

Drug Interactions

Metabolism/Transport Effects Substrate of CYP3A4 (major), P-glycoprotein; **Note:** Assignment of Major/Minor substrate status based on clinically relevant drug interaction potential; **Inhibits** CYP3A4 (weak)

Avoid Concomitant Use

Avoid concomitant use of Everolimus with any of the following: Antihepaciviral Combination Products; BCG (Intravesical); Conivaptan; CYP3A4 Inducers (Strong); CYP3A4 Inhibitors (Strong); Deferiprone; Dipyrone; Fusidic Acid (Systemic); Grapefruit Juice; Idelalisib; Natalizumab; Pimecrolimus; Pimozide; St John's Wort; Tacrolimus (Topical); Vaccines (Live); Voriconazole

Increased Effect/Toxicity

Everolimus may increase the levels/effects of: ACE Inhibitors; ARIPiprazole; CloZAPine; Deferiprone; Dofetilide; Fingolimod; HYDROcodone; Leflunomide; Lomitapide; Natalizumab; NiMODipine; Pimozide; Tofacitinib; Vaccines (Live)

The levels/effects of Everolimus may be increased by: Antihepaciviral Combination Products; Conivaptan; CycloSPORINE (Systemic); CYP3A4 Inhibitors (Moderate); CYP3A4 Inhibitors (Strong); Dasatinib; Denosumab; Dipyrone; Fosaprepitant; Fusidic Acid (Systemic); Grapefruit Juice; Idelalisib; Ocrelizumab; Palbociclib; P-glycoprotein/ABCB1 Inhibitors; Pimecrolimus; Promazine; Roflumilast; Stiripentol; Tacrolimus (Topical); Trastuzumab; Venetoclax; Voriconazole

◀ **Decreased Effect**

Everolimus may decrease the levels/effects of: Antidiabetic Agents; BCG (Intravesical); Coccidioides immitis Skin Test; Nivolumab; Sipuleucel-T; Tertomotide; Vaccines (Inactivated); Vaccines (Live)

The levels/effects of Everolimus may be decreased by: Bosentan; CYP3A4 Inducers (Moderate); CYP3A4 Inducers (Strong); Dabrafenib; Deferasirox; Echinacea; Efavirenz; Sarilumab; Siltuximab; St John's Wort; Tocilizumab

Food Interactions Grapefruit juice may increase levels of everolimus. Absorption with food may be variable. Management: Avoid grapefruit juice. Take with or without food, but be consistent with regard to food.

Hazardous Drugs Handling Considerations

Hazardous agent (NIOSH 2016 [group 1]).

Use appropriate precautions for receiving, handling, administration, and disposal. Gloves (single) should be worn during receiving, unpacking, and placing in storage.

NIOSH recommends single gloving for administration of intact tablets or capsules. If manipulating tablets/capsules (eg, to prepare an oral suspension), NIOSH recommends double gloving, a protective gown, and preparation in a controlled device; if not prepared in a controlled device, respiratory and eye/face protection as well as ventilated engineering controls are recommended. NIOSH recommends double gloving, a protective gown, and (if there is a potential for vomit or spit up) eye/face protection for administration of an oral liquid/feeding tube administration (NIOSH 2016).

Storage/Stability Tablets and tablets for suspension: Store at room temperature of 25°C (77°F); excursions permitted to 15°C to 30°C (59°F to 86°F). Protect from light; protect from moisture.

Mechanism of Action Everolimus is a macrolide immunosuppressant and a mechanistic target of rapamycin (mTOR) inhibitor which has antiproliferative and antiangiogenic properties, and also reduces lipoma volume in patients with angiomyolipoma. Reduces protein synthesis and cell proliferation by binding to the FK binding protein-12 (FKBP-12), an intracellular protein, to form a complex that inhibits activation of mTOR (mechanistic target of rapamycin) serine-threonine kinase activity. Also reduces angiogenesis by inhibiting vascular endothelial growth factor (VEGF) and hypoxia-inducible factor (HIF-1) expression. Angiomyolipomas may occur due to unregulated mTOR activity in TSC-associated renal angiomyolipoma (Budde 2012); everolimus reduces lipoma volume (Bissler 2012).

Pharmacodynamics/Kinetics

Absorption: Rapid (Kirchner 2004)

Distribution: Apparent V_d: 128 to 589 L (Zortress); volume of distribution in pediatric renal transplant patients (3 to 16 years) lower than adults (Van Damme-Lombaerts 2002)

Protein binding: ~74% (Afinitor and Zortress)

Metabolism: Extensively metabolized in the liver via CYP3A4; forms 6 weak metabolites (Afinitor and Zortress)

Bioavailability:

Tablets: ~30% (Tabernero 2008 [Afinitor]); Systemic exposure reduced by 22% with a high-fat meal and by 32% with a light-fat meal (Afinitor); Systemic exposure reduced 16% with a high-fat meal (Zortress)

Tablets for suspension (Afinitor): AUC equivalent to tablets although peak concentrations are 20% to 36% lower; steady state concentrations are similar; Systemic exposure reduced by 12% with a high-fat meal and by 30% with a low-fat meal

Half-life elimination: ~30 hours (Afinitor and Zortress); in pediatric renal transplant patients (3 to 16 years), half-life similar to adult data (Van Damme-Lombaerts 2002)

Time to peak, plasma: 1 to 2 hours (Afinitor and Zortress)

Excretion: Feces (80%, based on solid organ transplant studies); Urine (~5%, based on solid organ transplant studies); clearance in pediatric renal transplant patients lower than adults possibly due to distributive differences (Van Damme-Lombaerts 2002)

Dosing

Adult & Geriatric Note: Tablets (Afinitor, Zortress) and tablets for oral suspension (Afinitor Disperz) are not interchangeable; Afinitor Disperz is only indicated for the treatment of subependymal giant cell astrocytoma (SEGA), in conjunction with therapeutic monitoring. Do not combine formulations to achieve total desired dose.

Breast cancer, advanced, hormone receptor-positive, HER2-negative: Oral: 10 mg once daily (in combination with exemestane), continue treatment until disease progression or unacceptable toxicity

Neuroendocrine tumors (GI, lung, or pancreatic origin), advanced: Oral: 10 mg once daily, continue treatment until disease progression or unacceptable toxicity

Renal angiomyolipoma: Oral: 10 mg once daily, continue treatment until disease progression or unacceptable toxicity

Renal cell cancer, advanced (RCC): Oral: 10 mg once daily, continue treatment until disease progression or unacceptable toxicity

Renal cell carcinoma, advanced (off-label dose/combination): Oral: 5 mg once daily (in combination with lenvatinib), continue until disease progression or unacceptable toxicity (Motzer 2015)

Liver transplantation, rejection prophylaxis (begin at least 30 days posttransplant): Oral: Initial: 1 mg twice daily (in combination with tacrolimus [reduced dose required] and a corticosteroid; adjust maintenance dose if needed at a 4- to 5-day interval (from prior dose adjustment) based on serum concentrations, tolerability, and response.

If trough is <3 ng/mL: Double total daily dose (using available tablet strengths)

If trough >8 ng/mL on 2 consecutive measures: Decrease dose by 0.25 mg twice daily.

Renal transplantation, rejection prophylaxis: Oral: Initial: 0.75 mg twice daily (in combination with basiliximab induction, cyclosporine [reduced dose required] and a corticosteroid); adjust maintenance dose if needed at a 4- to 5-day interval (from prior dose adjustment) based on serum concentrations, tolerability, and response.

If trough is <3 ng/mL: Double total daily dose (using available tablet strengths)

If trough >8 ng/mL on 2 consecutive measures: Decrease dose by 0.25 mg twice daily.

Subependymal giant cell astrocytoma (SEGA; dosing based on body surface area [BSA]): Oral:

Initial: 4.5 mg/m^2 once daily; round to nearest tablet (tablet or tablet for oral suspension) size; continue until disease progression or unacceptable toxicity.

◀

If trough <5 ng/mL: Increase dose by 2.5 mg daily (tablets) or 2 mg daily (tablets for oral suspension).

If trough >15 ng/mL: Reduce dose by 2.5 mg daily (tablets) or 2 mg daily (tablets for oral suspension). If dose reduction necessary in patients receiving the lowest strength available, administer every other day.

Therapeutic drug monitoring: Assess trough concentration ~2 weeks after initiation or with dosage modifications, initiation or changes to concurrent CYP3A4/P-glycoprotein (P-gp) inhibitor/inducer therapy, changes in hepatic impairment, or when changing dosage forms between tablets and tablets for oral suspension; adjust maintenance dose if needed at 2-week intervals to achieve and maintain trough concentrations between 5 and 15 ng/mL; once stable dose is attained and if BSA is stable throughout treatment, monitor trough concentrations every 6 to 12 months (monitor every 3 to 6 months if BSA is changing).

Carcinoid tumors, advanced (off-label use): Oral: 10 mg once daily (in combination with octreotide LAR) until disease progression or toxicity (Pavel 2010)

Heart transplantation (≥3 months posttransplantation) (off-label use): Oral: Initial: 0.75 mg twice daily; adjust everolimus dose based on everolimus trough concentrations (Eisen 2003; Eisen 2013; Hollis 2015). **Note:** Mortality was increased with 3 mg/day when used in combination with rabbit antithymocyte globulin (Eisen 2013).

Lung transplantation (>1 month posttransplantation) (off-label use): Oral: Initial: 0.75 to 1.5 mg twice daily; adjust everolimus dose based on everolimus trough concentrations (Glanville 2015; Snell 2006; Strueber 2016)

Cystic fibrosis lung transplant recipients: Consider initiating with 1.25 to 2 mg twice daily since bioavailability and absorption is reduced; administer at least 30 minutes prior to a meal and with a lipase supplement (De Pablo 2013).

Waldenström macroglobulinemia, relapsed or refractory (off-label use): Oral: 10 mg once daily until disease progression or toxicity (Ghobrial 2010)

Dosage adjustment for concomitant CYP3A4 inhibitors/inducers and/or P-gp inhibitors:

Breast cancer, neuroendocrine tumors, RCC, renal angiomyolipoma:

CYP3A4/P-gp inducers: Strong inducers: Avoid coadministration with strong CYP3A4/P-gp inducers (eg, carbamazepine, phenobarbital, phenytoin, rifabutin, rifampin, rifapentine, St. John's wort); if concomitant use cannot be avoided, consider doubling the everolimus dose, using increments of 5 mg or less, with careful monitoring. If the strong CYP3A4/P-gp enzyme inducer is discontinued, consider allowing 3 to 5 days to elapse prior to reducing the everolimus to the dose used prior to initiation of the CYP3A4/P-gp inducer.

CYP3A4/P-gp inhibitors:

Strong inhibitors: Avoid concomitant administration with strong CYP3A4/P-gp inhibitors (eg, atazanavir, clarithromycin, indinavir, itraconazole, ketoconazole, nefazodone, nelfinavir, ritonavir, saquinavir, telithromycin, voriconazole).

Moderate CYP3A4/P-gp inhibitors (eg, amprenavir, aprepitant, diltiazem, erythromycin, fluconazole, fosamprenavir, verapamil): Reduce everolimus dose to 2.5 mg once daily; may consider increasing from 2.5 mg to 5 mg once daily based on patient tolerance. When the moderate inhibitor is discontinued, allow ~2 to 3 days to elapse prior to adjusting the everolimus upward to the recommended starting dose or to the dose used prior to initiation of the moderate inhibitor.

Renal transplantation: Dosage adjustments may be necessary based on everolimus serum concentrations

SEGA:

CYP3A4/P-gp inducers: Strong inducers: Avoid concomitant administration with strong CYP3A4/P-gp inducers (eg, carbamazepine, phenobarbital, phenytoin, rifabutin, rifampin, rifapentine, St John's wort); if concomitant use cannot be avoided, an initial starting everolimus dose of 9 mg/m^2 once daily is recommended, or, double the everolimus dose and assess tolerability; assess trough concentration after ~2 weeks; adjust dose as necessary based on therapeutic drug monitoring to maintain target trough concentrations of 5 to 15 ng/mL. If the strong CYP3A4 enzyme inducer is discontinued, reduce the everolimus dose by ~50% or to the dose used prior to initiation of the CYP3A4/P-gp inducer; reassess trough concentration after ~2 weeks.

CYP3A4/P-gp inhibitors:

Strong inhibitors: Avoid concomitant administration with strong CYP3A4/P-gp inhibitors (eg, atazanavir, clarithromycin, indinavir, itraconazole, ketoconazole, nefazodone, nelfinavir, ritonavir, saquinavir, telithromycin, voriconazole).

Moderate CYP3A4/P-gp inhibitors (eg, amprenavir, aprepitant, diltiazem, erythromycin, fluconazole, fosamprenavir, verapamil):

Currently taking a moderate CYP3A4/P-gp inhibitor and starting everolimus: 2.5 mg/m^2 once daily.

Currently taking everolimus and starting a moderate CYP3A4/P-gp inhibitor: Reduce everolimus dose by ~50%; if dose reduction is required for patients receiving the lowest strength available, administer every other day.

Discontinuing a moderate CYP3A4/P-gp inhibitor after concomitant use with everolimus: Discontinue moderate inhibitor and allow 2 to 3 days to elapse prior to resuming the everolimus dose used prior to initiation of the moderate inhibitor.

Therapeutic drug monitoring: Assess trough concentration ~2 weeks after everolimus initiation or dosage modifications, or initiation or changes to concurrent CYP3A4/P-gp inhibitor therapy; adjust maintenance dose if needed at 2-week intervals to achieve and maintain trough concentrations between 5 and 15 ng/mL.

Pediatric Note: Tablets (Afinitor, Zortress) and tablets for oral suspension (Afinitor Disperz) are not interchangeable. Do not combine formulations to achieve total desired dose.

Subependymal giant cell astrocytoma (SEGA): Children ≥1 year: Refer to adult dosing.

Renal Impairment No dosage adjustment is necessary.

Hepatic Impairment

Mild impairment (Child-Pugh class A):

Breast cancer, neuroendocrine tumors, RCC, renal angiomyolipoma: Reduce dose to 7.5 mg once daily; if not tolerated, may further reduce to 5 mg once daily.

Liver or renal transplantation: Reduce initial dose by ~33%; individualize subsequent dosing based on therapeutic drug monitoring (target trough concentration: 3 to 8 ng/mL).

SEGA: Adjustment to initial dose may not be necessary; subsequent dosing is based on therapeutic drug monitoring (monitor ~2 weeks after initiation, dosage modifications, or after any change in hepatic status; target trough concentration: 5 to 15 ng/mL).

Moderate impairment (Child-Pugh class B):

Breast cancer, neuroendocrine tumors, RCC, renal angiomyolipoma: Reduce dose to 5 mg once daily; if not tolerated, may further reduce to 2.5 mg once daily.

Liver or renal transplantation: Reduce initial dose by ~50%; individualize subsequent dosing based on therapeutic drug monitoring (target trough concentration: 3 to 8 ng/mL).

SEGA: Adjustment to initial dose may not be necessary; subsequent dosing is based on therapeutic drug monitoring (monitor ~2 weeks after initiation, dosage modifications, or after any change in hepatic status; target trough concentration: 5 to 15 ng/mL).

Severe impairment (Child-Pugh class C):

Breast cancer, neuroendocrine tumors, RCC, renal angiomyolipoma: If potential benefit outweighs risks, a maximum dose of 2.5 mg once daily may be used.

Liver or renal transplantation: Reduce initial dose by ~50%; individualize subsequent dosing based on therapeutic drug monitoring (target trough concentration: 3 to 8 ng/mL).

SEGA: Reduce initial dose to 2.5 mg/m^2 once daily (or current dose by ~50%); subsequent dosing is based on therapeutic drug monitoring (monitor ~2 weeks after initiation, dosage modifications, or after any change in hepatic status; target trough concentration: 5 to 15 ng/mL).

Adjustment for Toxicity

Breast cancer (adjustments apply to everolimus), neuroendocrine tumors, RCC, renal angiomyolipoma, SEGA: Toxicities may require temporary dose interruption (with or without a subsequent dose reduction) or discontinuation; reduce everolimus dose by ~50% if dosage adjustment is necessary:

Noninfectious pneumonitis:

Grade 1 (asymptomatic radiological changes suggestive of pneumonitis): No dosage adjustment is necessary; monitor appropriately.

Grade 2 (symptomatic but not interfering with activities of daily living [ADL]): Consider interrupting treatment, rule out infection, and consider corticosteroids until symptoms improve to ≤ grade 1; reinitiate at a lower dose. Discontinue if recovery does not occur within 4 weeks.

Grade 3 (symptomatic, interferes with ADL; oxygen indicated): Interrupt treatment until symptoms improve to ≤ grade 1; rule out infection and consider corticosteroid treatment; may reinitiate at a lower dose. If grade 3 toxicity recurs, consider discontinuing.

Grade 4 (life-threatening; ventilatory support indicated): Discontinue treatment; rule out infection; consider corticosteroid treatment.

Stomatitis (avoid the use of products containing alcohol, hydrogen peroxide, iodine, or thyme derivatives):

Grade 1 (minimal symptoms, normal diet): No dosage adjustment is necessary; manage with mouth wash (nonalcoholic or isotonic salt water) several times a day

Grade 2 (symptomatic but can eat and swallow modified diet): Interrupt treatment until symptoms improve to ≤ grade 1; reinitiate at same dose; if stomatitis recurs at grade 2, interrupt treatment until symptoms improve to ≤ grade 1 and then reinitiate at a lower dose. Also manage with topical (oral) analgesics (eg, benzocaine, butyl aminobenzoate, tetracaine, menthol, or phenol) ± topical (oral) corticosteroids (eg, triamcinolone).

Grade 3 (symptomatic and unable to orally aliment or hydrate adequately): Interrupt treatment until symptoms improve to ≤ grade 1; then reinitiate at a lower dose. Also manage with topical (oral) analgesics (eg, benzocaine, butyl aminobenzoate, tetracaine, menthol, or phenol) ± topical (oral) corticosteroids (eg, triamcinolone).

Grade 4 (life-threatening symptoms): Discontinue treatment; initiate appropriate medical intervention.

Metabolic toxicity (eg, hyperglycemia, dyslipidemia):

Grade 1: No dosage adjustment is necessary; initiate appropriate medical intervention and monitor.

Grade 2: No dosage adjustment is necessary; manage with appropriate medical intervention and monitor.

Grade 3: Temporarily interrupt treatment; reinitiate at a lower dose; manage with appropriate medical intervention and monitor.

Grade 4: Discontinue treatment; manage with appropriate medical intervention.

Nonhematologic toxicities (excluding pneumonitis, stomatitis, or metabolic toxicity):

Grade 1: If toxicity is tolerable, no dosage adjustment is necessary; initiate appropriate medical intervention and monitor.

Grade 2: If toxicity is tolerable, no dosage adjustment is necessary; initiate appropriate medical intervention and monitor. If toxicity becomes intolerable, temporarily interrupt treatment until improvement to ≤ grade 1 and reinitiate at the same dose; if toxicity recurs at grade 2, temporarily interrupt treatment until improvement to ≤ grade 1 and then reinitiate at a lower dose.

Grade 3: Temporarily interrupt treatment until improvement to ≤ grade 1; initiate appropriate medical intervention and monitor. May reinitiate at a lower dose; if toxicity recurs at grade 3, consider discontinuing.

Grade 4 (life-threatening symptoms): Discontinue treatment; initiate appropriate medical intervention.

Liver or renal transplantation:

Evidence of polyoma virus infection or PML: Consider reduced immunosuppression (taking into account the allograft risks associated with decreased immunosuppression)

Pneumonitis (grade 4 symptoms) or invasive systemic fungal infection: Discontinue

SEGA: *Severe/intolerable adverse reactions:* Temporarily interrupt or permanently discontinue treatment; if dose reduction is required upon reinitiation, reduce dose by ~50%; if dose reduction is required for patients receiving the lowest available strength, consider alternate-day dosing.

Combination Regimens

Breast cancer: Everolimus-Exemestane (Breast) on page 2111
Renal cell cancer: Everolimus-Lenvatinib (RCC) on page 2111

Administration May be taken with or without food; to reduce variability, take consistently with regard to food. Afinitor missed doses may be taken up to 6 hours after regularly scheduled time; if >6 hours, resume at next regularly scheduled time.

◄ Tablets: Swallow whole with a glass of water. Do not break, chew, or crush (do not administer tablets that are crushed or broken). Avoid contact with or exposure to crushed or broken tablets.

Tablets for oral suspension: Administer as a suspension only. Administer immediately after preparation; discard if not administered within 60 minutes after preparation. Prepare suspension in water only. Do not break or crush tablets.

Preparation in an oral syringe: Place dose into 10 mL oral syringe (maximum: 10 mg/syringe; use an additional syringe for doses >10 mg). Draw ~5 mL of water and ~4 mL of air into oral syringe; allow to sit (tip up) in a container until tablets are in suspension (3 minutes). Gently invert syringe 5 times immediately prior to administration; administer contents, then add ~5 mL water and ~4 mL of air to same syringe, swirl to suspend remaining particles and administer entire contents.

Preparation in a small glass: Place dose into a small glass (≤100 mL) containing ~25 mL water (maximum: 10 mg/glass; use and additional glass for doses >10 mg); allow to sit until tablets are in suspension (3 minutes). Stir gently with spoon immediately prior to administration; administer contents, then add ~25 mL water to same glass, swirl with same spoon to suspend remaining particles and administer entire contents.

Breast cancer, neuroendocrine tumors, renal cell cancer, renal angiolipoma, SEGA: Administer at the same time each day.

Solid organ transplantation: Administer consistently ~12 hours apart; administer at the same time as cyclosporine or tacrolimus.

Emetic Potential Children and Adults: Low (10% to 30%)

Extemporaneous Preparations

Tablets for oral suspension (Afinitor Disperz): Administer as a suspension only. Administer immediately after preparation; discard if not administered within 60 minutes after preparation. Prepare suspension in water only. Do not break or crush tablets.

Preparation in an oral syringe: Place dose into 10 mL oral syringe (maximum 10 mg/syringe; use an additional syringe for doses >10 mg). Draw ~5 mL of water and ~4 mL of air into oral syringe; allow to sit (tip up) in a container until tablets are in suspension (3 minutes). Gently invert syringe 5 times immediately prior to administration; administer contents, then add ~5 mL water and ~4 mL of air to same syringe, swirl to suspend remaining particles and administer entire contents.

Preparation in a small glass: Place dose into a small glass (≤100 mL) containing ~25 mL water (maximum 10 mg/glass; use an additional glass for doses >10 mg); allow to sit until tablets are in suspension (3 minutes). Stir gently with spoon immediately prior to administration; administer contents, then add ~25 mL water to same glass, swirl with same spoon to suspend remaining particles and administer entire contents.

Administer immediately after preparation; discard if not administered within 60 minutes after preparation.

Afinitor and Afinitor Disperz (everolimus) [prescribing information]. East Hanover, NJ: Novartis Pharmaceuticals Corporation; February 2016.

Tablets (Afinitor): Although the manufacturer recommends that the tablets be swallowed whole, an oral liquid may be prepared using tablets (for patients unable to swallow tablets whole). Disperse tablet in ~30 mL (1 oz) of water; gently stir. Administer and rinse container with additional 30 mL (1 oz) water and administer to ensure entire dose is administered. Administer immediately after preparation.

Afinitor (everolimus) [prescribing information]. East Hanover, NJ: Novartis Pharmaceuticals Corporation; July 2012.

Monitoring Parameters

CBC with differential (baseline and periodic); liver function (baseline and periodic); serum creatinine (baseline and periodic), urinary protein (baseline and periodic), and BUN (baseline and periodic); fasting serum glucose, HbA1c, and lipid profile (baseline and periodic); monitor for signs and symptoms of infection, noninfectious pneumonitis, or malignancy

Solid organ transplantation: Monitor everolimus whole blood trough concentrations (based on an LC/MS/MS assay method), especially in patients with hepatic impairment, with concomitant CYP3A4 inhibitors and inducers, and when cyclosporine or tacrolimus formulations or doses are changed; dosage adjustments should be made on trough concentrations obtained 4 to 5 days after a previous dosage adjustment; monitor cyclosporine or tacrolimus concentrations; monitor for proteinuria

SEGA: Monitor everolimus whole blood trough concentrations ~2 weeks after treatment initiation or with dosage modifications, initiation or changes to concurrent CYP3A4/P-glycoprotein (P-gp) inhibitor/inducer therapy, changes in hepatic function and when changing dosage forms between Afinitor tablets and Afinitor Disperz. Maintain trough concentrations between 5 and 15 ng/mL; once stable dose is attained and if BSA is stable throughout treatment, monitor trough concentrations every 6 to 12 months (monitor every 3 to 6 months if BSA is changing).

Dietary Considerations Avoid grapefruit juice.

Medication Guide Available Yes

Dosage Forms Excipient information presented when available (limited, particularly for generics); consult specific product labeling.

Tablet, Oral:
Afinitor: 2.5 mg, 5 mg, 7.5 mg, 10 mg
Zortress: 0.25 mg, 0.5 mg, 0.75 mg

Tablet Soluble, Oral:
Afinitor Disperz: 2 mg, 3 mg, 5 mg

◆ **Evista** see Raloxifene on page 1568

◆ **Evomela** see Melphalan on page 1182

Exemestane (ex e MES tane)

Related Information

Safe Handling of Hazardous Drugs on page 2379

Brand Names: US Aromasin

Brand Names: Canada Aromasin; CO Exemestane

Pharmacologic Category Antineoplastic Agent, Aromatase Inhibitor

Use Breast cancer: Treatment of advanced breast cancer in postmenopausal women whose disease has progressed following tamoxifen therapy; adjuvant treatment of postmenopausal women with estrogen receptor-positive early breast cancer following 2 to 3 years of tamoxifen (for a total of 5 consecutive years of adjuvant therapy).

Labeled Contraindications Known hypersensitivity to exemestane or any component of the formulation

Pregnancy Considerations Exemestane is not indicated for use in premenopausal women. Based on the mechanism of action and on animal data, exemestane is expected to cause fetal harm if administered to a pregnant woman. Women of reproductive potential should use effective contraception during treatment and for 1 month after the final dose. Pregnancy testing is recommended (for females of reproductive potential) within 7 days prior to therapy initiation.

Breastfeeding Considerations Exemestane is indicated for use only in postmenopausal women. Due to the potential for serious adverse reactions in the breastfeeding infant, breastfeeding is not recommended by the manufacturer during treatment and for 1 month after the final dose.

Warnings/Precautions Exemestane is not indicated for use in premenopausal women. Due to decreased circulating estrogen levels, exemestane is associated with a reduction in bone mineral density over time; decreases (from baseline) in lumbar spine and femoral neck density have been observed (when compared to tamoxifen or placebo in studies where concomitant use of bisphosphonates, calcium and vitamin D were not allowed); assess bone mineral density at baseline in patients with, or at risk for osteoporosis; monitor during exemestane therapy and initiate osteoporosis treatment if indicated. Due to high prevalence of vitamin D deficiency in women with breast cancer, assess 25-hydroxy vitamin D levels at baseline and supplement accordingly. Grade 3 or 4 lymphopenia has been observed with exemestane, although most patients had preexisting lower grade lymphopenia; some patients improved or recovered while continuing exemestane; lymphopenia did not result in a significant increase in viral infections, and no opportunistic infections were observed. Elevations of AST, ALT, alkaline phosphatase, and gamma glutamyl transferase >5 times ULN have been observed (rarely) in patients with advanced breast cancer; may be attributable to underlying liver and/or bone metastases. In patients with early breast cancer, elevations of bilirubin, alkaline phosphatase, and serum creatinine were more common with exemestane treatment than with tamoxifen or placebo. Potentially significant drug-drug interactions may exist, requiring dose or frequency adjustment, additional monitoring, and/or selection of alternative therapy. Exemestane should not be administered concurrently with estrogen-containing agents. Dose adjustment recommended with concomitant strong CYP3A4 inducers.

Adverse Reactions

Frequency not always defined. *Incidence not specifically defined, but reported in the range of 1% to 10%.

Cardiovascular: Hypertension (5% to 15%), edema (6% to 7%), ischemic heart disease (2%; angina pectoris, myocardial infarction), chest pain*

Central nervous system: Fatigue (8% to 22%), insomnia (11% to 14%), pain (13%), headache (7% to 13%), depression (6% to 13%), dizziness (8% to 10%), anxiety (4% to 10%), paresthesia (3%), carpal tunnel syndrome (2%), confusion,* hypoesthesia*

Dermatological: Hyperhidrosis (4% to 18%), alopecia (15%), dermatitis (8%), pruritus,* skin rash*

Endocrine & metabolic: Hot flash (13% to 33%), weight gain (8%), increased follicle-stimulating hormone, increased luteinizing hormone, increased sex hormone binding globulin (with daily doses of ≥2.5 mg; dose-dependent)

Gastrointestinal: Nausea (9% to 18%), abdominal pain (6% to 11%), diarrhea (4% to 10%), vomiting (7%), anorexia (6%), constipation (5%), increased appetite (3%), dyspepsia*

Genitourinary: Urinary tract infection (2% to 5%)

Hematologic & oncologic: Lymphedema*

Hepatic: Increased serum alkaline phosphatase (14% to 15%), increased serum bilirubin (5% to 7%)

Infection: Infection*

Neuromuscular & skeletal: Arthralgia (15% to 29%), back pain (9%), limb pain (9%), myalgia (6%), osteoarthritis (6%), weakness (6%), osteoporosis (5%), pathological fracture (4%), muscle cramps (2%)

Ophthalmic: Visual disturbance (5%)

Renal: Increased serum creatinine (6%)

Respiratory: Dyspnea (10%), cough (6%), flu-like symptoms (6%), bronchitis,* pharyngitis,* rhinitis,* sinusitis,* upper respiratory tract infection*

Miscellaneous: Fever (5%)

<1%, postmarketing, and/or case reports: Abnormal bone growth (osteochondrosis), acute generalized exanthematous pustulosis, cardiac failure, cholestatic hepatitis, endometrial hyperplasia, endometrial polyps, gastric ulcer, hepatitis, hypersensitivity reaction, increased gamma-glutamyl transferase, increased serum transaminases, neuropathy, tenosynovitis (fingers), thromboembolism, urticaria

Drug Interactions

Metabolism/Transport Effects Substrate of CYP3A4 (major); **Note:** Assignment of Major/Minor substrate status based on clinically relevant drug interaction potential

Avoid Concomitant Use

Avoid concomitant use of Exemestane with any of the following: Estrogen Derivatives

Increased Effect/Toxicity

Exemestane may increase the levels/effects of: Methadone

Decreased Effect

The levels/effects of Exemestane may be decreased by: Bosentan; CYP3A4 Inducers (Moderate); CYP3A4 Inducers (Strong); Dabrafenib; Deferasirox; Enzalutamide; Estrogen Derivatives; Mitotane; Sarilumab; Siltuximab; St John's Wort; Tocilizumab

Food Interactions AUC and C_{max} were increased by 59% and 39%, respectively, when exemestane was administered with a high-fat breakfast. Management: Administer after a meal.

Hazardous Drugs Handling Considerations

Hazardous agent (NIOSH 2016 [group 1]).

Use appropriate precautions for receiving, handling, administration, and disposal. Gloves (single) should be worn during receiving, unpacking, and placing in storage. NIOSH recommends single gloving for administration of intact tablets or capsules (NIOSH 2016).

Storage/Stability Store at 25°C (77°F); excursions permitted to 15°C to 30°C (59°F to 86°F).

Mechanism of Action Exemestane is an irreversible, steroidal aromatase inactivator. It is structurally related to androstenedione, and is converted to an intermediate that irreversibly blocks the active site of the aromatase enzyme, leading to inactivation ("suicide inhibition") and thus preventing conversion of androgens to estrogens in peripheral tissues. Significantly lowers circulating estrogens in postmenopausal breast cancers where growth is estrogen-dependent.

Pharmacodynamics/Kinetics

Absorption: Rapid and moderate (~42%) following oral administration; AUC and C_{max} increased by 59% and 39%, respectively, following a high-fat breakfast (compared to fasted state)

Distribution: Extensive into tissues

◄ Protein binding: 90%, primarily to albumin and α_1-acid glycoprotein

Metabolism: Extensively hepatic; oxidation (CYP3A4) of methylene group, reduction of 17-keto group with formation of many secondary metabolites; metabolites are inactive

Half-life elimination: ~24 hours

Time to peak: Women with breast cancer: 1.2 hours

Excretion: Urine (<1% as unchanged drug, 39% to 45% as metabolites); feces (36% to 48%)

Dosing

Adult & Geriatric

Breast cancer, advanced: Postmenopausal females: Oral: 25 mg once daily; continue until tumor progression

Breast cancer, early (adjuvant treatment): Postmenopausal females: Oral: 25 mg once daily (following 2 to 3 years of tamoxifen therapy) for a total duration of 5 years of endocrine therapy (in the absence of recurrence or contralateral breast cancer).

Duration of therapy: American Society of Clinical Oncology (ASCO) guidelines for Adjuvant Endocrine Therapy of Hormone Receptor-Positive Breast Cancer (Focused Update) recommend a maximum duration of 5 years of aromatase inhibitor (AI) therapy for postmenopausal women; AIs may be combined with tamoxifen for a total duration of up to 10 years of endocrine therapy. Refer to the guidelines for specific recommendations based on menopausal status and tolerability (Burstein 2014). In a phase III study with another AI (letrozole), treatment with an additional 5 years of AI therapy (for a total of 10 years of aromatase inhibitor therapy) demonstrated a significantly improved rate of disease-free survival and a decreased risk of disease recurrence and contralateral breast cancer (when compared to placebo), although overall survival was not significantly different between groups and bone-related adverse events occurred more frequently with letrozole versus placebo (Goss 2016).

Breast cancer, early (first-line adjuvant treatment; off-label use): Postmenopausal females: Oral: 25 mg once daily for 5 years (Burstein 2010; van de Velde 2011).

Duration of therapy: ASCO guidelines for Adjuvant Endocrine Therapy of Hormone Receptor-Positive Breast Cancer (Focused Update) recommend a maximum duration of 5 years of aromatase inhibitor (AI) therapy for postmenopausal women; AIs may be combined with tamoxifen for a total duration of up to 10 years of endocrine therapy. Refer to the guidelines for specific recommendations based on menopausal status and tolerability (Burstein 2014). In a phase III study with another AI (letrozole), treatment with an additional 5 years of AI therapy (for a total of 10 years of aromatase inhibitor therapy) demonstrated a significantly improved rate of disease-free survival and a decreased risk of disease recurrence and contralateral breast cancer (when compared to placebo), although overall survival was not significantly different between groups and bone-related adverse events occurred more frequently with letrozole versus placebo (Goss 2016).

Breast cancer, risk reduction (off-label use): Postmenopausal females ≥35 years: Oral: 25 mg once daily for 5 years (Goss 2011; Visvanathan 2013)

Dosage adjustment with strong CYP3A4 inducers: 50 mg once daily when used with potent inducers (eg, rifampin, phenytoin)

Renal Impairment No adjustment necessary (although the safety of chronic doses in patients with moderate-to-severe renal impairment has not been studied, dosage adjustment does not appear necessary).

Hepatic Impairment No adjustment necessary (although the safety of chronic doses in patients with moderate-to-severe hepatic impairment has not been studied, dosage adjustment does not appear necessary).

Combination Regimens

Breast cancer: Everolimus-Exemestane (Breast) on page 2111

Administration Administer after a meal.

Monitoring Parameters 25-hydroxy vitamin D levels (at baseline); bone mineral density

Dietary Considerations Patients on aromatase inhibitor therapy should receive vitamin D and calcium supplements.

Dosage Forms Excipient information presented when available (limited, particularly for generics); consult specific product labeling.

Tablet, Oral:

Aromasin: 25 mg

Generic: 25 mg

◆ **Exjade** *see* Deferasirox *on page* 552

◆ **3 Factor PCC** *see* Factor IX Complex (Human) [(Factors II, IX, X)] *on page* 767

Factor VIIa (Recombinant) (FAK ter SEV en aye ree KOM be nant)

Brand Names: US NovoSeven RT

Brand Names: Canada Niastase; Niastase RT

Index Terms Coagulation Factor VIIa; Eptacog Alfa (Activated); rFVIIa

Pharmacologic Category Antihemophilic Agent

Use Bleeding episodes and perioperative management: Treatment of bleeding episodes and perioperative management in adults and children with hemophilia A or B with inhibitors, congenital factor VII (FVII) deficiency, and Glanzmann's thrombasthenia with refractoriness to platelet transfusions, with or without antibodies to platelets; treatment of bleeding episodes and perioperative management in adults with acquired hemophilia.

Dosing

Adult & Geriatric IV:

Congenital hemophilia A or B with inhibitors:

Bleeding episodes: 90 mcg/kg/dose every 2 hours until hemostasis is achieved or until the treatment is judged ineffective. Doses between 35 and 90 mcg/kg/dose have been used successfully in clinical trials. The dose, interval, and duration of therapy may be adjusted based upon the severity of bleeding and the degree of hemostasis achieved. For patients experiencing severe bleeds, dosing should be continued at 3- to 6-hour intervals post-hemostasis. The duration of any post-hemostatic dosing should be minimized.

Perioperative management: 90 mcg/kg/dose immediately before surgery (additional bolus doses may be administered for major surgery if required); repeat at 2-hour intervals for the duration of surgery. For minor surgery, continue 90 mcg/kg/dose postoperatively every 2 hours for 48 hours, then every 2 to 6 hours until healed. For major surgery, continue 90 mcg/kg/dose postoperatively every 2 hours for 5 days, then every 4 hours until healed.

◀ **Congenital factor VII deficiency:**

Bleeding episodes: 15 to 30 mcg/kg/dose every 4 to 6 hours until hemostasis is achieved. Doses as low as 10 mcg/kg have been effective.

Perioperative management: 15 to 30 mcg/kg/dose immediately before surgery; repeat every 4 to 6 hours for the duration of surgery and until hemostasis achieved. Doses as low as 10 mcg/kg have been effective.

Acquired hemophilia:

Bleeding episodes: 70 to 90 mcg/kg/dose every 2 to 3 hours until hemostasis is achieved.

Perioperative management: 70 to 90 mcg/kg/dose immediately before surgery; repeat every 2 to 3 hours for the duration of surgery and until hemostasis achieved.

Glanzmann's thrombasthenia:

Bleeding episodes (severe, refractory to platelet transfusions): 90 mcg/kg/dose every 2 to 6 hours until hemostasis is achieved.

Perioperative management: 90 mcg/kg/dose immediately before surgery; repeat at 2-hour intervals for the duration of surgery. Continue 90 mcg/kg/dose every 2 to 6 hours to prevent postoperative bleeding. **Note:** Higher average infused doses (median 100 mcg/kg) were noted for surgical patients who had clinical refractoriness with or without platelet-specific antibodies compared to those with neither.

Intracranial hemorrhage associated with danaparoid (off-label use): IV: 90 mcg/kg once (NCS/SCCM [Frontera 2016]).

Refractory bleeding after cardiac surgery in nonhemophiliac patients (off-label use): Dosing not established; doses in the range of 35 to 70 mcg/kg/dose have been recommended based on low-quality evidence (case series, observational studies) (Chapman 2011; Ferraris 2011; Karkouti 2007); in patients with a left ventricular assist device, lower doses (ie, 10 to 20 mcg/kg) may be preferred to reduce thromboembolic events (Bruckner 2009).

Pediatric

Congenital factor VII deficiency: Children and Adolescents: Refer to adult dosing.

Glanzmann's thrombasthenia: Children and Adolescents: Refer to adult dosing.

Congenital hemophilia A or B with inhibitors: Children and Adolescents: Refer to adult dosing.

Renal Impairment There are no dosage adjustments provided the in manufacturer's labeling.

Hepatic Impairment There are no dosage adjustments provided in the manufacturer's labeling; use with caution.

Additional Information Complete prescribing information should be consulted for additional detail.

Dosage Forms Excipient information presented when available (limited, particularly for generics); consult specific product labeling.

Solution Reconstituted, Intravenous [preservative free]:

NovoSeven RT: 1 mg (1 ea); 2 mg (1 ea); 5 mg (1 ea); 8 mg (1 ea) [contains polysorbate 80]

◆ **Factor VIII (Human)** *see* Antihemophilic Factor (Human) *on page 140*

◆ **Factor VIII (Recombinant [Fc Fusion Protein])** *see* Antihemophilic Factor (Recombinant [Fc Fusion Protein]) *on page 147*

- ♦ **Factor VIII (Recombinant [Pegylated])** *see* Antihemophilic Factor (Recombinant [Pegylated]) *on page* 149

- ♦ **Factor VIII (Recombinant [Porcine Sequence])** *see* Antihemophilic Factor (Recombinant [Porcine Sequence]) *on page* 151

- ♦ **Factor VIII (Recombinant)** *see* Antihemophilic Factor (Recombinant) *on page* 143

Factor IX Complex (Human) [(Factors II, IX, X)]

(FAK ter nyne KOM pleks HYU man FAK ter too nyne ten)

Brand Names: US Bebulin; Profilnine; Profilnine SD

Index Terms 3 Factor PCC; 3-Factor PCC; PCC (Caution: Confusion-prone synonym); Prothrombin Complex Concentrate (Caution: Confusion-prone synonym); Three-Factor PCC

Pharmacologic Category Antihemophilic Agent; Blood Product Derivative; Prothrombin Complex Concentrate (PCC)

Use

Factor IX deficiency (hemophilia B [Christmas disease]): Prevention and control of bleeding in patients with factor IX deficiency (hemophilia B or Christmas disease)

Limitations of use: Not indicated for the treatment of other factor deficiencies (eg, factor II, VII, VIII, X), treatment of hemophilia A patients with inhibitors to factor VIII, or treatment of bleeding caused by low levels of liver-dependent coagulation factors.

Pregnancy Risk Factor C

Dosing

Adult & Geriatric Note: Factor IX complex (Human) [Factors II, IX, X] (Bebulin, Profilnine) contains low or nontherapeutic levels of factor VII component and should not be confused with Prothrombin Complex Concentrate (Human) [(Factors II, VII, IX, X), Protein C, Protein S] (Kcentra, Octaplex) which contains therapeutic levels of factor VII.

Control or prevention of bleeding in patients with factor IX deficiency (hemophilia B [Christmas disease]): Dosage is expressed in units of factor IX activity and must be individualized based on severity of factor IX deficiency, extent and location of bleeding, and clinical status of patient. Close laboratory monitoring of the factor IX level is required to determine proper dosage, particularly with severe hemorrhage and major surgery. Larger doses than those derived from the formula below may be required, especially if treatment is delayed. When multiple doses are required, administer at 24-hour intervals unless otherwise specified.

Formula for units required to raise blood level %:

Bebulin: In general, factor IX 1 unit/kg will increase the plasma factor IX level by 0.8%

Number of Factor IX units required = body weight (kg) x desired factor IX increase (as % of normal) x 1.2 units/kg

Profilnine: In general, factor IX 1 unit/kg will increase the plasma factor IX level by 1%:

Number of factor IX units required = bodyweight (kg) x desired factor IX increase (as % of normal) x 1 unit/kg

For example, to increase factor IX level to 25% of normal in a 70 kg patient: Number of factor IX units needed = 70 kg x 25 x 1 unit/kg = 1,750 units

As a general rule, the level of factor IX required for treatment of different conditions is listed below:

Hemorrhage: IV:

Minor bleeding (early hemarthrosis, minor epistaxis, gingival bleeding, mild hematuria):

Bebulin: Raise factor IX level to 20% of normal (typical initial dose: 25 to 35 units/kg); average duration of treatment is 1 day. A single dose is usually sufficient or a second dose may be given after 24 hours.

Profilnine: Raise factor IX level to 20% to 30% of normal (initial dose: 20 to 30 units/kg) every 16 to 24 hours for 1 to 2 days for minor hemorrhage or until hemorrhage stops and healing has been achieved.

Moderate bleeding (severe joint bleeding, early hematoma, major open bleeding, minor trauma, minor hemoptysis, hematemesis, melena, major hematuria):

Bebulin: Raise factor IX level to 40% of normal (typical initial dose: 50 to 65 units/kg); average duration of treatment is 2 days or until adequate wound healing.

Profilnine: Raise factor IX level to 20% to 30% of normal (initial dose: 20 to 30 units/kg) every 16 to 24 hours for 2 to 7 days for moderate hemorrhage or until hemorrhage stops and healing has been achieved.

Major bleeding (severe hematoma, major trauma, severe hemoptysis, hematemesis, melena):

Bebulin: Raise factor IX level to ≥60% of normal (typical initial dose: 75 to 90 units/kg); average duration of treatment is 2 to 3 days or until adequate wound healing.

Profilnine: Raise factor IX level to 30% to 50% of normal (initial dose: 30 to 50 units/kg) every 16 to 24 hours; following this treatment period, maintain factor IX levels at 20% of normal (maintenance dose: 20 units/kg) for 3 to 10 days or until healing has been achieved.

Surgical procedures: IV:

Dental surgery:

Bebulin: Raise factor IX level to 40% to 60% of normal on day of surgery (typical dose: 50 to 75 units/kg). One infusion, administered 1 hour prior to surgery, is generally sufficient for the extraction of one tooth; for the extraction of multiple teeth, replacement therapy may be required for up to 1 week (See dosing guidelines for *Minor Surgery*).

Profilnine: Raise factor IX level to 50% of normal immediately prior to procedure; maintain factor IX levels at 30% to 50% of normal (maintenance dose: 30 to 50 units/kg) every 16 to 24 hours for 7 to 10 days following surgery or until healing has been achieved.

Minor surgery:

Bebulin: Raise factor IX level to 40% to 60% of normal on day of surgery (typical initial dose: 50 to 75 units/kg). Decrease factor IX level from 40% to 60% of normal to 20% to 40% of normal during initial postoperative period (1 to 2 weeks or until adequate wound healing) [typical dose: 26 to 65 units/kg]. The preoperative dose should be given 1 hour prior to surgery. The average dosing interval may be every 12 hours initially, then every 24 hours later in the postoperative period.

Profilnine: Raise factor IX level to 30% to 50% of normal (initial dose: 30 to 50 units/kg) prior to surgery (**Note:** Surgery type not specified by the manufacturer); maintain factor IX levels at 30% to 50% of normal (maintenance dose: 30 to 50 units/kg) every 16 to 24 hours for 7 to 10 days following surgery or until healing is achieved.

Major surgery:

Bebulin: Raise factor IX level to ≥60% of normal on day of surgery (typical initial dose: 75 to 90 units/kg). Decrease factor IX level from ≥60% of normal to 20% to 60% of normal during initial postoperative period (1 to 2 weeks) [typical dose: 25 to 75 units/kg]; further decrease to maintain a factor IX level of 20% of normal during late postoperative period (≥3 weeks) and continuing until adequate wound healing is achieved [typical dose: 25 to 35 units/kg]. The preoperative dose should be given 1 hour prior to surgery. The average dosing interval may be every 12 hours initially, then every 24 hours later in the postoperative period.

Profilnine: Raise Factor IX level to 30% to 50% of normal (initial dose: 30 to 50 units/kg) prior to surgery (**Note:** Surgery type not specified by the manufacturer); maintain factor IX levels at 30% to 50% of normal (maintenance dose: 30 to 50 units/kg) every 16 to 24 hours for 7 to 10 days following surgery or until healing is achieved.

Life-threatening hemorrhage associated with warfarin (off-label use):
IV: **Note:** Products contain low or nontherapeutic levels of factor VII component; therefore, additional fresh frozen plasma (FFP) or factor VIIa may be considered (Masotti 2011). When immediate INR reversal is required, concomitant use of 1 to 2 units of FFP should be considered to ensure acute INR reversal (Baker 2004; Holland 2009). Coadminister vitamin K (phytonadione) 5 to 10 mg by slow IV infusion (ACCP [Guyatt 2012]); vitamin K may be repeated every 12 hours if INR is persistently elevated. Factor IX complex (human) dosing has not been established in this setting; the following regimens have been used with some success.

The following 2 methods have been suggested, but are not product specific:

Adjusted-dose regimen, weight based (Liumbruno 2009):

INR <2: 20 units/kg

INR 2 to 4: 30 units/kg

INR >4: 50 units/kg

Note: If after administration, INR remains >1.5 consider repeating dose appropriate for INR.

May also determine dose based on presenting INR and estimated functional prothrombin complex (PC) expressed as percentage of normal plasma levels (see table; Masotti 2011):

Units needed to be infused = (**target** % of functional PC to be reached – **current** estimated % of functional PC) x kg of body weight

Example:
Patient (weight: 70 kg) presents with INR of 4.5 which corresponds to an **estimated % functional PC** of 10% (see table). Target INR of 1.4 corresponds to an **estimated target % functional PC** of 40%.
Units needed to be infused = (40 - 10) x 70 kg = 2,100 units

Conversion of the INR to Estimated Functional Prothrombin Complex (PC)

INR Value	Estimated Functional PC
≥5	5%
4 to 4.9	10%
2.6 to 3.2	15%
2.2 to 2.5	20%
1.9 to 2.1	25%
1.7 to 1.8	30%
1.4 to 1.6	40%
1 to 1.3	100%

Intracranial hemorrhage associated with warfarin (off-label use): IV: **Note:** Factor IX complex (human) products contain low or nontherapeutic levels of factor VII component (ie, considered a 3-factor PCC). Four-factor PCC is preferred. Administer with vitamin K IV (NCS/SCCM [Frontera 2016]).

Fixed-dose regimen, weight based: INR ≥1.4: 50 units/kg; repeat INR within 15 to 60 minutes and serially every 6 to 8 hours for the next 24 to 48 hours. If INR remains ≥1.4 within the first 24 to 48 hours after initial dose, use FFP (alone) for further correction. For initial reversal, it is suggested to administer factor IX complex (PCC) alone rather than combined with FFP or recombinant factor VIIa (NCS/SCCM [Frontera 2016]).

Pediatric Control or prevention of bleeding in patients with factor IX deficiency (hemophilia B [Christmas disease]) (off-label use): IV: Refer to adult dosing.

Renal Impairment There are no dosage adjustments provided in the manufacturer's labeling.

Hepatic Impairment There are no dosage adjustments provided in the manufacturer's labeling; monitor factor IX levels. Use with caution due to the risk of thromboembolic complications.

Additional Information Complete prescribing information should be consulted for additional detail.

Dosage Forms Considerations Strengths expressed as an approximate value. Consult individual vial labels for exact potency within each vial.

Dosage Forms Excipient information presented when available (limited, particularly for generics); consult specific product labeling.
Solution Reconstituted, Intravenous:
Bebulin: 200-1200 units (1 ea)
Profilnine: 500 units (1 ea); 1000 units (1 ea); 1500 units (1 ea) [contains polysorbate 80]
Profilnine SD: 500 units (1 ea); 1000 units (1 ea); 1500 units (1 ea) [contains polysorbate 80]

◆ **Factor IX Concentrate** see Factor IX (Human) on page 771

◆ **Factor IX Concentrate** *see* Factor IX (Recombinant [Albumin Fusion Protein]) *on page* 777

◆ **Factor IX Concentrate** *see* Factor IX (Recombinant [Fc Fusion Protein]) *on page* 778

◆ **Factor IX Concentrate** *see* Factor IX (Recombinant) *on page* 773

Factor IX (Human) (FAK ter nyne HYU man)

Brand Names: US AlphaNine SD; Mononine

Brand Names: Canada Immunine VH

Index Terms Factor IX Concentrate

Pharmacologic Category Antihemophilic Agent; Blood Product Derivative

Use Prevention and control of bleeding in patients with hemophilia B (congenital factor IX deficiency or Christmas disease)

NOTE: Contains **nondetectable levels of factors II, VII, and X**. Therefore, **NOT INDICATED** for replacement therapy of any other clotting factor besides factor IX or for reversal of anticoagulation due to either vitamin K antagonists or other anticoagulants (eg, dabigatran), for hemophilia A patients with factor VIII inhibitors, or for patients in a hemorrhagic state caused by reduced production of liver-dependent coagulation factors (eg, hepatitis, cirrhosis).

Pregnancy Risk Factor C

Dosing

Adult & Geriatric NOTE: Contains **nondetectable levels of factors II, VII, and X**. Therefore, **NOT INDICATED** for replacement therapy of any other clotting factor besides factor IX or for reversal of anticoagulation due to either vitamin K antagonists or other anticoagulants (eg, dabigatran), for hemophilia A patients with factor VIII inhibitors, or for patients in a hemorrhagic state caused by reduced production of liver-dependent coagulation factors (eg, hepatitis, cirrhosis).

Control or prevention of bleeding in patients with factor IX deficiency (hemophilia B or Christmas disease): IV: *AlphaNine SD, Mononine:* Dosage is expressed in units of factor IX activity; dosing must be individualized based on severity of factor IX deficiency, extent and location of bleeding, and clinical status of patient. Refer to product information for specific manufacturer recommended dosing. Alternatively, the World Federation of Hemophilia (WFH) has recommended general dosing for factor IX products.

Formula to determine units required to obtain desired factor IX level:
Note: If patient has severe hemophilia (ie, baseline factor IX level is or presumed to be <1%), then may just use "desired factor IX level" instead of "desired factor IX level increase".

Number of factor IX units required = patient weight (in kg) x desired factor IX level increase (as % or units/dL) x 1 unit/kg

For example, to attain an 80% level in a 70 kg patient who has a baseline level of 20%: Number of factor IX units needed = 70 kg x 60% x 1 unit/kg = 4200 units

◄ **Alternative dosing (off-label): Note:** The following recommendations may vary from those found within prescribing information or practitioner preference.

Prophylaxis: 15 to 30 units/kg/dose twice weekly (Utrecht protocol; WFH [Srivastava 2013]) **or** 25 to 40 units/kg/dose twice weekly (Malmö protocol; WFH [Srivastava 2013]); optimum regimen has yet to be defined.

Treatment:

2013 World Federation of Hemophilia Treatment Recommendations (When No Significant Resource Constraint Exists):

Site of Hemorrhage/ Clinical Situation	Desired Factor IX Level to Maintain	Duration
Joint	40 to 60 units/dL	1 to 2 days, may be longer if response is inadequate
Superficial muscle/no neurovascular compromise	40 to 60 units/dL	2 to 3 days, sometimes longer if response is inadequate
Iliopsoas and deep muscle with neurovascular injury, or substantial blood loss	*Initial:* 60 to 80 units/dL *Maintenance:* 30 to 60 units/dL	*Initial:* 1 to 2 days *Maintenance:* 3 to 5 days, sometimes longer as secondary prophylaxis during physiotherapy
CNS/head	*Initial:* 60 to 80 units/dL *Maintenance:* 30 units/dL	*Initial:* 1 to 7 days *Maintenance:* 8 to 21 days
Throat and neck	*Initial:* 60 to 80 units/dL *Maintenance:* 30 units/dL	*Initial:* 1 to 7 days *Maintenance:* 8 to 14 days
Gastrointestinal	*Initial:* 60 to 80 units/dL *Maintenance:* 30 units/dL	*Initial:* 7 to 14 days *Maintenance:* Not specified
Renal	40 units/dL	3 to 5 days
Deep laceration	40 units/dL	5 to 7 days
Surgery (major)	*Preop:* 60 to 80 units/dL	
	Postop: 40 to 60 units/dL 30 to 50 units/dL 20 to 40 units/dL	*Postop:* 1 to 3 days 4 to 6 days 7 to 14 days
Surgery (minor)	*Preop:* 50 to 80 units/dL	
	Postop: 30 to 80 units/dL	*Postop:* 1 to 5 days depending on procedure type

Note: Factor IX level may either be expressed as units/dL or as %. Dosing frequency most commonly corresponds to the half-life of factor IX but should be determined based on an assessment of factor IX levels before the next dose.

Continuous infusion (for patients who require prolonged periods of treatment [eg, intracranial hemorrhage or surgery] to avoid peaks and troughs associated with intermittent infusions) (Batorova, 2002; Poon, 2012; Rickard, 1995; WFH [Srivastava 2013]): Following initial bolus to achieve the desired factor IX level: Initiate 4 to 6 units/kg/hour; adjust dose based on frequent factor assays and calculation of factor IX clearance at steady-state using the following equations:

Factor IX clearance (mL/kg/hour) = (current infusion rate in units/kg/hour) divided by (plasma level in units/**m**L)

New infusion rate (units/kg/hour) = (factor IX clearance in mL/kg/hour) x (desired plasma level in units/**m**L)

Pediatric NOTE: Contains **nondetectable levels of factors II, VII, and X**. Therefore, **NOT INDICATED** for replacement therapy of any other clotting factor besides factor IX or for reversal of anticoagulation due to either vitamin K antagonists or other anticoagulants (eg, dabigatran), for hemophilia A patients with factor VIII inhibitors, or for patients in a hemorrhagic state caused by reduced production of liver-dependent coagulation factors (eg, hepatitis, cirrhosis).

Control or prevention of bleeding in patients with factor IX deficiency (hemophilia B or Christmas disease): Infants, Children, and Adolescents: IV: *AlphaNine SD, Mononine:* Dosage is expressed in units of factor IX activity; dosing must be individualized based on severity of factor IX deficiency, extent and location of bleeding, and clinical status of patient. Refer to product information for specific manufacturer recommended dosing. Alternatively, the World Federation of Hemophilia (WFH) has recommended general dosing for factor IX products.

Formula to determine units required to obtain desired factor IX level:
Note: If patient has severe hemophilia (ie, baseline factor IX level is or presumed to be <1%), then may just use "desired factor IX level" instead of "desired factor IX level increase".

Number of factor IX units required = patient weight (in kg) x desired factor IX level increase (as % or units/dL) x 1 unit/kg

For example, to attain an 80% level in a 70 kg patient who has a baseline level of 20%: Number of factor IX units needed = 70 kg x 60% x 1 unit/kg = 4200 units

Alternative recommendations (off-label): Infants, Children, and Adolescents:
Prophylaxis, primary: Refer to adult dosing.
Treatment: Refer to adult dosing.

Additional Information Complete prescribing information should be consulted for additional detail.

Dosage Forms Considerations Strengths expressed with approximate values. Consult individual vial labels for exact potency within each vial.

Dosage Forms Excipient information presented when available (limited, particularly for generics); consult specific product labeling. [DSC] = Discontinued product

Solution Reconstituted, Intravenous [preservative free]:
AlphaNine SD: 500 units (1 ea); 1000 units (1 ea); 1500 units (1 ea) [contains polysorbate 80]
Mononine: 250 units (1 ea [DSC]); 500 units (1 ea [DSC]); 1000 units (1 ea) [contains polysorbate 80]

Factor IX (Recombinant) (FAK ter nyne ree KOM be nant)

Brand Names: US BeneFIX; Ixinity; Rixubis
Brand Names: Canada BeneFix
Index Terms Factor IX Concentrate; rFIX
Pharmacologic Category Antihemophilic Agent

◄ **Use**

Factor IX deficiency: Prevention and control of bleeding episodes in patients with factor IX deficiency (hemophilia B [Christmas disease]); perioperative management in patients with hemophilia B; routine prophylaxis to prevent or reduce the frequency of bleeding episodes in patients with hemophilia B (Rixubis).

Limitations of use: These products are not indicated for the treatment of other factor deficiencies (eg, factor II, VII, VIII, X), for the treatment of hemophilia A patients with inhibitors to factor VIII, the reversal of coumarin-induced anticoagulation, or for the treatment of bleeding because of low levels of liver-dependent coagulation factors. Ixinity and Rixubis are not indicated for induction of immune tolerance in patients with hemophilia B.

Pregnancy Risk Factor C
Dosing

Adult & Geriatric Note: Contains **only factor IX**. Therefore, **NOT INDICATED** for the treatment of other factors deficiencies (eg, factors II, VII, VIII, and X), hemophilia A patients with inhibitors to factor VIII, reversal of coumarin-induced anticoagulation, and bleeding due to low levels of liver-dependent clotting factors.

Control or prevention of bleeding in patients with factor IX deficiency (hemophilia B or Christmas disease): IV: Dosage is expressed in units of factor IX activity; dosing must be individualized based on severity of factor IX deficiency, extent and location of bleeding, clinical status of patient, and recovery of factor IX. **Refer to product information for specific manufacturer recommended dosing.** Alternatively, the World Federation of Hemophilia (WFH) has recommended general dosing for factor IX products.

Formula for units required to raise blood level %: **Note:** If patient has severe hemophilia (ie, baseline factor IX level is or presumed to be <1%), then may just use "desired factor IX level" instead of "desired factor IX level *increase*". On average, the observed recovery for BeneFix is 0.8 units/dL per units/kg in adults.

Number of factor IX units required = patient weight (in kg) x desired factor IX level increase (as % or units/dL) x reciprocal of observed recovery (as units/kg per units/dL)

Alternative dosing (off-label): Note: The following recommendations may vary from those found within prescribing information or practitioner preference.

Prophylaxis: 15 to 30 units/kg/dose twice weekly (Utrecht protocol; WFH [Srivastava 2013]) **or** 25 to 40 units/kg/dose twice weekly (Malmö protocol; WFH [Srivastava 2013]); optimum regimen has yet to be defined.

Treatment:

2013 World Federation of Hemophilia
Treatment Recommendations
(When No Significant Resource Constraint Exists):

Site of Hemorrhage/Clinical Situation	Desired Factor IX Level to Maintain	Duration
Joint	40-60 units/dL	1-2 days, may be longer if response is inadequate
Superficial muscle/no neurovascular compromise	40-60 units/dL	2-3 days, sometimes longer if response is inadequate
Iliopsoas and deep muscle with neurovascular injury, or substantial blood loss	*Initial:* 60-80 units/dL *Maintenance:* 30-60 units/dL	*Initial:* 1-2 days *Maintenance:* 3-5 days, sometimes longer as secondary prophylaxis during physiotherapy
CNS/head	*Initial:* 60-80 units/dL *Maintenance:* 30 units/dL	*Initial:* 1-7 days *Maintenance:* 8-21 days
Throat and neck	*Initial:* 60-80 units/dL *Maintenance:* 30 units/dL	*Initial:* 1-7 days *Maintenance:* 8-14 days
Gastrointestinal	*Initial:* 60-80 units/dL *Maintenance:* 30 units/dL	*Initial:* 7-14 days *Maintenance:* Not specified
Renal	40 units/dL	3-5 days
Deep laceration	40 units/dL	5-7 days
Surgery (major)	*Preop:* 60-80 units/dL	
	Postop: 40-60 units/dL 30-50 units/dL 20-40 units/dL	*Postop:* 1-3 days 4-6 days 7-14 days
Surgery (minor)	*Preop:* 50-80 units/dL	
	Postop: 30-80 units/dL	*Postop:* 1-5 days depending on procedure type

Note: Factor IX level may either be expressed as units/dL or as %. Dosing frequency most commonly corresponds to the half-life of factor IX but should be determined based on an assessment of factor IX levels before the next dose.

Continuous infusion (For patients who require prolonged periods of treatment [eg, intracranial hemorrhage or surgery] to avoid peaks and troughs associated with intermittent infusions) (Batorova 2002; Poon 2012; Rickard, 1995; WFH [Srivastava 2013]): **Note:** Evidence supporting the use of continuous infusion is primarily with BeneFix (Chowdary 2001); however manufacturer's labeling states that safety and efficacy of BeneFIX administration by continuous infusion has not been established: Following initial bolus to achieve the desired factor IX level, initiate 4 to 6 units/kg/hour; adjust dose based on frequent factor assays and calculation of factor IX clearance at steady-state using the following equations:

Factor IX clearance (mL/kg/hour) = (current infusion rate in units/kg/hour)/ (plasma level in units/mL)

New infusion rate (units/kg/hour) = (factor IX clearance in mL/kg/hour) x (desired plasma level in units/mL)

Routine prophylaxis to prevent bleeding episodes in patients with factor IX deficiency (hemophilia B or Christmas disease): IV: Rixubis: 40 to 60 units/kg twice weekly; may titrate dose depending upon age, bleeding pattern, and physical activity

◀ **Pediatric Note:** Contains **only factor IX**. Therefore, **NOT INDICATED** for the treatment of other factors deficiencies (eg, factors II, VII, VIII, and X), hemophilia A patients with inhibitors to factor VIII, reversal of coumarin-induced anticoagulation, and bleeding due to low levels of liver-dependent clotting factors.

Control or prevention of bleeding in patients with factor IX deficiency (hemophilia B or Christmas disease): IV: Dosage is expressed in units of factor IX activity; dosing must be individualized based on severity of factor IX deficiency, extent and location of bleeding, clinical status of patient, and recovery of factor IX. **Refer to product information for specific manufacturer recommended dosing.** Alternatively, the World Federation of Hemophilia (WFH) has recommended general dosing for factor IX products.

Formula for units required to raise blood level %: **Note:** If patient has severe hemophilia (ie, baseline factor IX level is or presumed to be <1%), then may just use "desired factor IX level" instead of "desired factor IX level *increase*". On average, the observed recovery for BeneFix is 0.7 units/dL per units/kg in children <15 years of age.

Infants, Children, and Adolescents: IV: Number of factor IX units required = patient weight (in kg) x desired factor IX level increase (as % or units/dL) x reciprocal of observed recovery (as units/kg per units/dL)

Alternative recommendations (off label): Infants, Children, and Adolescents:

Prophylaxis: Refer to adult dosing.

Treatment: Refer to adult dosing.

Routine prophylaxis to prevent bleeding episodes in patients with factor IX deficiency (hemophilia B or Christmas disease): IV: Rixubis: Children <12 years: 60 to 80 units/kg twice weekly; may titrate dose depending upon age, bleeding pattern, and physical activity.

Children ≥12 years and Adolescents: 40 to 60 units/kg twice weekly; may titrate dose depending upon age, bleeding pattern, and physical activity.

Renal Impairment There are no dosage adjustments provided in the manufacturer's labeling; monitor factor IX levels.

Hepatic Impairment There are no dosage adjustments provided in the manufacturer's labeling; monitor factor IX levels. Use with caution due to the risk of thromboembolic complications.

Additional Information Complete prescribing information should be consulted for additional detail.

Dosage Forms Considerations Strengths expressed with approximate values. Consult individual vial labels for exact potency within each vial.

Dosage Forms Excipient information presented when available (limited, particularly for generics); consult specific product labeling.

Kit, Intravenous [preservative free]:

BeneFIX: 250 units, 500 units, 1000 units, 2000 units, 3000 units [contains polysorbate 80]

Solution Reconstituted, Intravenous [preservative free]:

Ixinity: 250 units (1 ea); 500 units (1 ea); 1000 units (1 ea); 1500 units (1 ea); 2000 units (1 ea); 3000 units (1 ea) [contains mouse (murine) and/or hamster protein, polysorbate 80]

Rixubis: 250 units (1 ea); 500 units (1 ea); 1000 units (1 ea); 2000 units (1 ea); 3000 units (1 ea) [contains polysorbate 80]

Factor IX (Recombinant [Albumin Fusion Protein])

(FAK ter nyne ree KOM be nant al BYOO min FYOO zhuhn PROE teen)

Brand Names: US Idelvion

Brand Names: Canada Idelvion

Index Terms Factor IX Concentrate; rFIX-FP; rIX-FP

Pharmacologic Category Antihemophilic Agent

Use

Hemophilia B (congenital factor IX deficiency): Prevention and on-demand control of bleeding episodes in adults and children; perioperative management of bleeding in adults and children; routine prophylaxis to prevent or reduce the frequency of bleeding episodes in adults and children

Limitations of use: Not indicated for immune tolerance induction in patients with hemophilia B.

Dosing

Adult & Geriatric Note: Dose and duration of treatment depends on the severity of factor IX deficiency, the location and extent of bleeding, and the patient's clinical condition, age, and recovery of factor IX. Adjust dosing regimen based on individual response.

Hemophilia B (congenital factor IX deficiency): The calculation of the required dose is based on 1 unit/kg body weight is expected to increase the factor IX circulating level by 1.3 units/dL in adults. The required dose is determined by the following formula:

Number of factor IX units required = patient weight (in kg) x desired factor IX level increase (as % or units/dL) x reciprocal of recovery (as units/kg per units/dL)

On-demand control and prevention of bleeding episodes: IV:

Type of bleeding episode	Required circulating factor IX activity	Dosing frequency	Duration of therapy
Minor or moderate (uncomplicated hemarthrosis, muscle bleeding [except iliopsoas] or oral bleeding)	30 to 60 units/dL	48 to 72 hours	At least 1 day, until bleeding stops and healing is achieved. Single dose should be sufficient for majority of bleeds.
Major (life or limb threatening hemorrhage, deep muscle bleeding, including iliopsoas, intracranial, retropharyngeal)	60 to 100 units/dL	48 to 72 hours	7 to 14 days, or until bleeding stops and healing is achieved. Maintenance dose weekly.

◄

Perioperative management of bleeding: IV:

Type of bleeding surgery	Required circulating factor IX activity	Dosing frequency	Duration of therapy
Minor (including uncomplicated tooth extraction)	50 to 80 units/dL	48 to 72 hours	At least 1 day, until bleeding stops and healing is achieved. Single dose should be sufficient for majority of minor surgeries.
Major (including intracranial, pharyngeal, retropharyngeal, retroperitoneal)	60 to 100 units/dL	48 to 72 hours	7 to 14 days, or until bleeding stops and healing is achieved. Repeat dose every 48 to 72 hours for the first week or until healing is achieved. Maintenance dose 1 to 2 times per week

Routine prophylaxis: IV: 25 to 40 units/kg once every 7 days; if well controlled may switch to 50 to 75 units/kg once every 14 days.

Pediatric Note: Dose and duration of treatment depends on the severity of factor IX deficiency, the location and extent of bleeding, and the patient's clinical condition, age, and recovery of factor IX. Adjust dosing regimen based on individual response.

Hemophilia B (congenital factor IX deficiency): The calculation of the required dose is based on 1 unit/kg body weight is expected to increase the factor IX circulating level by 1 units/dL in infants and children <12 years and by 1.3 units/dL in Children ≥12 years and Adolescents. The required dose is determined by the following formula:

Number of factor IX units required = patient weight (in kg) x desired factor IX level increase (as % or units/dL) x reciprocal of recovery (as units/kg per units/dL)

On-demand control and prevention of bleeding episodes: Infants, Children, and Adolescents: IV: Refer to adult dosing.

Perioperative management of bleeding: Infants, Children, and Adolescents: IV: Refer to adult dosing.

Routine prophylaxis:

US labeling:

Infants and Children <12 years: IV: 40 to 55 units/kg once every 7 days

Children ≥12 years and Adolescents: IV: Refer to adult dosing.

Canadian labeling: Infants, Children ≥12 years, and Adolescents: IV: Refer to adult dosing.

Renal Impairment There are no dosage adjustments provided in the manufacturers labeling.

Hepatic Impairment There are no dosage adjustments provided in the manufacturers labeling; use with caution in patients with hepatic disease.

Additional Information Complete prescribing information should be consulted for additional detail.

Dosage Forms Excipient information presented when available (limited, particularly for generics); consult specific product labeling.

Solution Reconstituted, Intravenous:

Idelvix: 250 units (1 ea); 500 units (1 ea); 1000 units (1 ea); 2000 units (1 ea) [contains hamster protein, polysorbate 80]

Factor IX (Recombinant [Fc Fusion Protein])

(FAK tor nyne ree KOM be nant eff see FYOO zhun PRO teen)

Brand Names: US Alprolix

Brand Names: Canada Alprolix

Index Terms Factor IX Concentrate; rFIX

Pharmacologic Category Antihemophilic Agent

Use

Factor IX deficiency: Prevention and control of bleeding in patients with factor IX deficiency (hemophilia B [Christmas disease]); perioperative management of bleeding in patients with hemophilia B; routine prophylaxis to reduce the frequency of bleeding episodes in patients with hemophilia B.

Limitations of use: Not indicated for induction of immune tolerance in patients with hemophilia B.

Pregnancy Risk Factor C
Dosing

Adult & Geriatric Note: Contains **only factor IX**. Therefore, **NOT INDI-CATED** for the treatment of other factors deficiencies (eg, factors II, VII, VIII, and X), hemophilia A patients with inhibitors to factor VIII, reversal of coumarin-induced anticoagulation, and bleeding due to low levels of liver-dependent clotting factors.

Control or prevention of bleeding in patients with factor IX deficiency (hemophilia B or Christmas disease): IV: Dosage is expressed in units of factor IX activity; dosing must be individualized based on severity of factor IX deficiency, extent and location of bleeding, clinical status of patient, and recovery of factor IX. **Refer to product information for specific manufacturer recommended dosing.** Alternatively, the World Federation of Hemophilia (WFH) has recommended general dosing for factor IX products.

Formula for units required to raise blood level %: **Note:** If patient has severe hemophilia (ie, baseline factor IX level is or presumed to be <1%), then may just use "desired factor IX level" instead of "desired factor IX level *increase*".

Number of factor IX units required = patient weight (in kg) x desired factor IX level increase (as % or units/dL) x reciprocal of observed recovery (as units/kg per units/dL)

Alternative dosing (off-label): Note: The following recommendations may vary from those found within prescribing information or practitioner preference.

Prophylaxis: 15 to 30 units/kg/dose twice weekly (Utrecht protocol; WFH [Srivastava 2013]) **or** 25 to 40 units/kg/dose twice weekly (Malmö protocol; WFH [Srivastava 2013]) **or** 40 to 100 units/kg/dose 2 to 3 times weekly (National Hemophilia Foundation, MASAC recommendation 2007); optimum regimen has yet to be defined.

Treatment:

2013 World Federation of Hemophilia Treatment Recommendations (When No Significant Resource Constraint Exists)

Site of Hemorrhage/ Clinical Situation	Desired Factor IX Level to Maintain	Duration
Joint	40-60 units/dL	1-2 days, may be longer if response is inadequate
Superficial muscle/ no neurovascular compromise	40-60 units/dL	2-3 days, sometimes longer if response is inadequate
Iliopsoas and deep muscle with neurovascular injury, or substantial blood loss	*Initial:* 60-80 units/dL *Maintenance:* 30-60 units/dL	*Initial:* 1-2 days *Maintenance:* 3-5 days, sometimes longer as secondary prophylaxis during physiotherapy
CNS/head	*Initial:* 60-80 units/dL *Maintenance:* 30 units/dL	*Initial:* 1-7 days *Maintenance:* 8-21 days
Throat and neck	*Initial:* 60-80 units/dL *Maintenance:* 30 units/dL	*Initial:* 1-7 days *Maintenance:* 8-14 days
Gastrointestinal	*Initial:* 60-80 units/dL *Maintenance:* 30 units/dL	*Initial:* 7-14 days *Maintenance:* Not specified
Renal	40 units/dL	3-5 days
Deep laceration	40 units/dL	5-7 days
Surgery (major)	*Preop:* 60-80 units/dL	
	Postop: 40-60 units/dL 30-50 units/dL 20-40 units/dL	*Postop:* 1-3 days 4-6 days 7-14 days
Surgery (minor)	*Preop:* 50-80 units/dL	
	Postop: 30-80 units/dL	*Postop:* 1-5 days depending on procedure type

Note: Factor IX level may either be expressed as units/dL or as %. Dosing frequency most commonly corresponds to the half-life of factor IX but should be determined based on an assessment of factor IX levels before the next dose.

Pediatric Note: Contains **only factor IX**. Therefore, **NOT INDICATED** for the treatment of other factors deficiencies (eg, factors II, VII, VIII, and X), hemophilia A patients with inhibitors to factor VIII, reversal of coumarin-induced anticoagulation, and bleeding due to low levels of liver-dependent clotting factors.

Control or prevention of bleeding in patients with factor IX deficiency (hemophilia B or Christmas disease): IV: Dosage is expressed in units of factor IX activity; dosing must be individualized based on severity of factor IX deficiency, extent and location of bleeding, clinical status of patient, and recovery of factor IX. **Refer to product information for specific manufacturer recommended dosing.** Alternatively, the World Federation of Hemophilia (WFH) has recommended general dosing for factor IX products.

Formula for units required to raise blood level %: **Note:** If patient has severe hemophilia (ie, baseline factor IX level is or presumed to be <1%), then may just use "desired factor IX level" instead of "desired factor IX level *increase*".

Infants, Children, and Adolescents: IV: Number of factor IX units required = patient weight (in kg) x desired factor IX level increase (as

% or units/dL) x reciprocal of observed recovery (as units/kg per units/dL)

Alternative recommendations (off label): Infants, Children, and Adolescents:

Prophylaxis: Refer to adult dosing.

Treatment: Refer to adult dosing.

Routine prophylaxis to prevent bleeding episodes in patients with factor IX deficiency (hemophilia B or Christmas disease): IV: 50 units/kg once weekly or 100 units/kg once every 10 days; adjust dose based on individual response

Renal Impairment There are no dosage adjustments provided in the manufacturer's labeling; monitor factor IX levels.

Hepatic Impairment There are no dosage adjustments provided in the manufacturer's labeling; monitor factor IX levels. Use with caution due to the risk of thromboembolic complications.

Additional Information Complete prescribing information should be consulted for additional detail.

Dosage Forms Excipient information presented when available (limited, particularly for generics); consult specific product labeling.

Solution Reconstituted, Intravenous [preservative free]:

Alprolix. 250 units (1 ea); 500 units (1 ea); 1000 units (1 ea); 2000 units (1 ea); 3000 units (1 ea); 4000 units (1 ea)

◆ **Factor 13** *see* Factor XIII Concentrate (Human) *on page 782*

Factor XIII A-Subunit (Recombinant)
(FAK ter THIR teen aye SUB yoo nit ree KOM be nant)

Brand Names: US Tretten

Brand Names: Canada Tretten

Index Terms Catridecacog; Recombinant Factor XIII A-Subunit; rFXIII

Pharmacologic Category Antihemophilic Agent

Use Factor XIII A-subunit deficiency: Routine prophylaxis of bleeding in patients with congenital factor XIII A-subunit deficiency

Pregnancy Risk Factor C

Dosing

Adult & Geriatric Factor XIII A-subunit deficiency: IV: 35 units/kg once monthly to achieve a target trough level of factor XIII activity ≥10% using a validated assay; consider dose adjustment if adequate coverage is not achieved (higher doses may not increase the levels of tetrameric factor XIII).
Note: Treatment should be initiated under the supervision of a healthcare provider experienced in the treatment of rare bleeding disorders.

Pediatric Infants, Children, and Adolescents: Refer to adult dosing.

Renal Impairment No dosage adjustment provided in manufacturer's labeling.

Hepatic Impairment No dosage adjustment provided in manufacturer's labeling.

Additional Information Complete prescribing information should be consulted for additional detail.

◀ **Dosage Forms** Excipient information presented when available (limited, particularly for generics); consult specific product labeling.
Solution Reconstituted, Intravenous:
Tretten: 2000 - 3125 units (1 ea)

Factor XIII Concentrate (Human)
(FAK ter THIR teen KON cen trate HYU man)
Brand Names: US Corifact
Brand Names: Canada Corifact
Index Terms Activated Factor XIII; Corifact; Factor 13; FXIII
Pharmacologic Category Antihemophilic Agent; Blood Product Derivative
Use Prophylaxis against bleeding episodes and management of perioperative surgical bleeding in patients with congenital factor XIII deficiency
Pregnancy Risk Factor C
Dosing
Adult & Geriatric Congenital factor XIII deficiency: IV:
Prophylaxis:
Initial: 40 units/kg
Maintenance: Dose adjustment should be based on factor XIII activity trough levels (target level of 5% to 20% using Berichrom activity assay) and clinical response; repeat every 28 days
One trough level of <5%: Increase dosage by 5 units/kg
Trough level of 5% to 20%: No dosage change
Two trough levels of >20%: Decrease dosage by 5 units/kg
One trough level of >25%: Decrease dosage by 5 units/kg
Perioperative management of surgical bleeding: Individualize dosing based on factor XIII activity level, type of surgery, and clinical response; monitor factor XIII activity levels during and after surgery:
If time since last prophylactic dose ≤7 days: Additional dose may not be needed.
If time since last prophylactic dose 8 to 21 days: Additional partial or full dose may be necessary based on factor XIII activity level
If time since last prophylactic dose 21 to 28 days: Administer full prophylactic dose
Pediatric Infants, Children, and Adolescents: Refer to adult dosing.
Renal Impairment There are no dosage adjustments provided in the manufacturer's labeling.
Hepatic Impairment There are no dosage adjustments provided in the manufacturer's labeling.
Additional Information Complete prescribing information should be consulted for additional detail.
Dosage Forms Excipient information presented when available (limited, particularly for generics); consult specific product labeling.
Kit, Intravenous [preservative free]:
Corifact: 1000-1600 units
Dosage Forms: Canada Information with regard to form, strength, and availability of products uniquely available in Canada but currently not available in the US. Refer also to Dosage Forms.

Excipient information presented when available (limited, particularly for generics); consult specific product labeling.
Solution Reconstituted, Intravenous [preservative free]
Corifact: 200-320 units

Famciclovir (fam SYE kloe veer)

Brand Names: US Famvir [DSC]

Brand Names: Canada Apo-Famciclovir; Ava-Famciclovir; CO Famciclovir; Famvir; PMS-Famciclovir; Sandoz-Famciclovir

Pharmacologic Category Antiviral Agent

Use Treatment of acute herpes zoster (shingles) in immunocompetent patients; treatment and suppression of recurrent episodes of genital herpes in immunocompetent patients; treatment of herpes labialis (cold sores) in immunocompetent patients; treatment of recurrent orolabial/genital (mucocutaneous) herpes simplex in HIV-infected adult patients

Pregnancy Risk Factor B

Dosing

Adult & Geriatric

Genital herpes simplex virus (HSV) infection: Oral: **Note:** Initiate therapy as soon as possible after diagnosis and within 72 hours of rash onset

Immunocompetent patients:

Initial episode (off-label use): 250 mg 3 times daily for 7 to 10 days. **Note:** Treatment can be extended if healing is incomplete after 10 days of therapy (CDC [Workowski 2015])

Recurrence:

Manufacturer's labeling: 1,000 mg twice daily for 1 day (**Note:** Initiate therapy as soon as possible and within 6 hours of symptoms/lesions onset)

Alternate dosing: 125 mg twice daily for 5 days or 500 mg as a single dose, followed by 250 mg twice daily for 2 days (CDC [Workowski 2015]).

Suppressive therapy: 250 mg twice daily. **Note:** Duration not established, but efficacy/safety have been demonstrated for 1 year (CDC [Workowski 2015]).

HIV-infected patients:

Manufacturer's labeling: Recurrent episodes: 500 mg twice daily for 7 days

Alternate dosing:

Initial or recurrent episodes: 500 mg twice daily for 5 to 10 days (HHS [OI adult 2016])

Chronic suppressive therapy (off-label use): 500 mg twice daily; suppressive therapy can be continued indefinitely regardless of CD4 count in patients with severe recurrences of genital herpes or in patients who want to minimize frequency of recurrences, or to reduce the risk of genital ulcer disease in patients with CD4 cell counts <250 cells/mm^3 who are starting antiretroviral therapy. However, continuation of therapy should be reviewed annually, particularly if immune reconstitution has occurred (HHS [OI adult 2016]).

Herpes labialis/orolabial (cold sores): Oral: **Note:** Initiate therapy as soon as possible after diagnosis and within 72 hours of rash onset

Immunocompetent patients:

Recurrent episodes: 1,500 mg as a single dose; initiate therapy at first sign or symptom such as tingling, burning, or itching (initiated within 1 hour in clinical studies)

HIV patients:

Manufacturer's labeling: Recurrent episodes: 500 mg twice daily for 7 days

◄ Alternate dosing: Treatment: 500 mg twice daily for 5 to 10 days (HHS [OI adult 2016])

Herpes zoster (shingles): Oral: **Note:** Initiate therapy as soon as possible after diagnosis and within 1 week of rash onset or any time before full crusting of lesions

Immunocompetent patients: 500 mg every 8 hours for 7 days

HIV-infected patients with acute localized dermatomal lesion (off-label use): 500 mg 3 times daily for 7 to 10 days; consider longer duration if lesions heal slowly (HHS [OI adult 2016])

HIV-infected patients with extensive cutaneous lesion or visceral involvement (off-label use): Initial therapy with acyclovir IV may be switched to famciclovir 500 mg 3 times daily to complete a 10 to 14 day course, when formation of new lesions has ceased and signs and symptoms of visceral VZV infection are improving (HHS [OI adult 2016])

Varicella infection (chickenpox) in HIV-infected patients (uncomplicated cases) (off-label use): Oral: 500 mg 3 times daily for 5 to 7 days (HHS [OI adult 2016])

Pediatric

Genital herpes simplex virus (HSV) in HIV-infected patients: Adolescents (off-label population): Oral:

Initial or recurrent episodes: 500 mg twice daily for 5 to 10 days (HHS [OI adult 2016])

Chronic suppressive therapy (off-label use): 500 mg twice daily; suppressive therapy can be continued indefinitely regardless of CD4 count in patients with severe recurrences of genital herpes or in patients who want to minimize frequency of recurrences, or to reduce the risk of genital ulcer disease in patients with CD4 cell counts <250 cells/mm^3 who are starting antiretroviral therapy. However, continuation of therapy should be reviewed annually, particularly if immune reconstitution has occurred (HHS [OI adult 2016]).

Herpes labialis/orolabial (cold sores) in HIV-infected patients: Adolescents (off-label population): Oral: Treatment: 500 mg twice daily for 5 to 10 days (HHS [OI adult 2016])

Herpes zoster (shingles) in HIV-infected patients (off-label use) (HHS [OI adult 2016]): Adolescents: Oral:

Acute localized dermatomal lesion: 500 mg 3 times daily for 7 to 10 days; consider longer duration if lesions heal slowly

Extensive cutaneous lesion or visceral involvement (off-label use): Initial therapy with acyclovir IV may be switched to famciclovir 500 mg 3 times daily to complete a 10- to 14-day course, when formation of new lesions has ceased and signs and symptoms of visceral VZV infection are improving

Varicella infection (chickenpox) in HIV-infected patients (uncomplicated cases) (off-label use): Adolescents: Oral: 500 mg 3 times daily for 5 to 7 days (HHS [OI adult 2016])

Renal Impairment

Herpes zoster:

CrCl ≥60 mL/minute: No dosage adjustment necessary.

CrCl 40 to 59 mL/minute: Administer 500 mg every 12 hours

CrCl 20 to 39 mL/minute: Administer 500 mg every 24 hours

CrCl <20 mL/minute: Administer 250 mg every 24 hours

Hemodialysis: Administer 250 mg after each dialysis session.

Recurrent genital herpes: Treatment:
Single-day regimen:
CrCl ≥60 mL/minute: No dosage adjustment necessary.
CrCl 40 to 59 mL/minute: Administer 500 mg every 12 hours for 1 day
CrCl 20 to 39 mL/minute: Administer 500 mg as a single dose
CrCl <20 mL/minute: Administer 250 mg as a single dose
Hemodialysis: Administer 250 mg as a single dose after a dialysis session.
Alternatively the following recommendations have been made (Famvir Canadian product labeling 2016):
CrCl >20 mL/minute/1.73 m^2: Administer 125 mg every 12 hours
CrCl <20 mL/minute/1.73 m^2: Administer 125 mg every 24 hours
Hemodialysis: Administer 125 mg after each dialysis session.
Recurrent genital herpes: Suppression:
CrCl ≥40 mL/minute: No dosage adjustment necessary.
CrCl 20 to 39 mL/minute: Administer 125 mg every 12 hours
CrCl <20 mL/minute: Administer 125 mg every 24 hours
Hemodialysis: Administer 125 mg after each dialysis session.
Recurrent herpes labialis: Treatment (single-dose regimen):
CrCl ≥60 mL/minute: No dosage adjustment necessary.
CrCl 40 to 59 mL/minute: Administer 750 mg as a single dose
CrCl 20 to 39 mL/minute: Administer 500 mg as a single dose
CrCl <20 mL/minute: Administer 250 mg as a single dose
Hemodialysis: Administer 250 mg as a single dose after a dialysis session.
Recurrent orolabial/genital (mucocutaneous) herpes in HIV-infected patients:
CrCl ≥40 mL/minute: No dosage adjustment necessary.
CrCl 20 to 39 mL/minute: Administer 500 mg every 24 hours
CrCl <20 mL/minute: Administer 250 mg every 24 hours
Hemodialysis: Administer 250 mg after each dialysis session.
Hepatic Impairment
Mild-to-moderate impairment: No dosage adjustment is necessary
Severe impairment: No dosage adjustment provided in manufacturer's labeling; has not been studied. However, a 44% decrease in the C_{max} of penciclovir (active metabolite) was noted in patients with mild-to-moderate impairment; impaired conversion of famciclovir to penciclovir may affect efficacy.
Additional Information Complete prescribing information should be consulted for additional detail.
Dosage Forms Excipient information presented when available (limited, particularly for generics); consult specific product labeling. [DSC] = Discontinued product
Tablet, Oral:
Famvir: 125 mg [DSC], 250 mg [DSC], 500 mg [DSC]
Generic: 125 mg, 250 mg, 500 mg

◆ **Famvir [DSC]** *see* Famciclovir *on page 783*

◆ **Famvir (Can)** *see* Famciclovir *on page 783*

◆ **2F-ara-AMP** *see* Fludarabine *on page 817*

◆ **Fareston** *see* Toremifene *on page 1798*

◆ **Faridak** *see* Panobinostat *on page 1445*

◆ **Farydak** *see* Panobinostat *on page 1445*

Ferric Gluconate (FER ik GLOO koe nate)

Brand Names: US Ferrlecit
Brand Names: Canada Ferrlecit
Index Terms Sodium Ferric Gluconate; Sodium Ferric Gluconate Complex
Pharmacologic Category Iron Salt
Use Iron deficiency anemia: Treatment of iron-deficiency anemia in patients undergoing hemodialysis in conjunction with erythropoietin therapy
Labeled Contraindications Known hypersensitivity to ferric gluconate or any component of the formulation
Pregnancy Considerations Adverse events were not observed in animal reproduction studies. It is recommended that pregnant women meet the dietary requirements of iron with diet and/or supplements in order to prevent adverse events associated with iron deficiency anemia in pregnancy. Treatment of iron deficiency anemia in pregnant women is the same as in nonpregnant women and in most cases, oral iron preparations may be used. Except in severe cases of maternal anemia, the fetus achieves normal iron stores regardless of maternal concentrations.
Breastfeeding Considerations Iron is normally found in breast milk. Breast milk or iron fortified formulas generally provide enough iron to meet the recommended dietary requirements of infants. The amount of iron in breast milk is generally not influenced by maternal iron status.
Warnings/Precautions Serious hypersensitivity reactions, including anaphylactic-type reactions, have occurred (may be life-threatening). Monitor during administration and for ≥30 minutes after administration and until clinically stable after infusion. Avoid rapid administration. Equipment for resuscitation and trained personnel experienced in handling medical emergencies should always be immediately available. Clinically significant hypotension may occur; usually resolves within 1-2 hours. May augment hemodialysis-induced hypotension. Use with caution in elderly patients. Use only in patients with documented iron deficiency; caution with hemoglobinopathies or other refractory anemias.

Benzyl alcohol and derivatives: Some dosage forms may contain benzyl alcohol; large amounts of benzyl alcohol (≥99 mg/kg/day) have been associated with a potentially fatal toxicity ("gasping syndrome") in neonates; the "gasping syndrome" consists of metabolic acidosis, respiratory distress, gasping respirations, CNS dysfunction (including convulsions, intracranial hemorrhage), hypotension and cardiovascular collapse (AAP ["Inactive" 1997]; CDC, 1982); some data suggests that benzoate displaces bilirubin from protein binding sites (Ahlfors, 2001); avoid or use dosage forms containing benzyl alcohol with caution in neonates. See manufacturer's labeling.

Adverse Reactions Percentages reported in adults unless otherwise noted.
>10%:
Cardiovascular: Hypotension (children: 35%; adults: 29%), hypertension (children: 23%; adults: 13%), tachycardia (children: 17%; adults: 5%)
Central nervous system: Headache (children: 24%; adults: 7%), dizziness (13%)
Gastrointestinal: Vomiting (adults: ≤35%; children: 11%), nausea (adults: ≤35%; children: 9%), diarrhea (adults: ≤35%; children: 8%)
Hematologic & oncologic: Abnormal erythrocytes (11%; changes in color, morphology, or number)
Local: Injection site reaction (33%)
Neuromuscular & skeletal: Muscle cramps (25%)
Respiratory: Dyspnea (11%)
1% to 10%:
Cardiovascular: Chest pain (10%), syncope (6%), thrombosis (children: 6%), edema (5%), angina pectoris, bradycardia, myocardial infarction, peripheral edema (including leg edema), vasodilatation
Central nervous system: Pain (10%), fatigue (6%), paresthesia (6%), agitation, chills, drowsiness, impaired consciousness, malaise, rigors
Dermatologic: Pruritus (6%), diaphoresis, skin rash
Endocrine & metabolic: Hyperkalemia (6%), hypermenorrhea, hypervolemia, hypoglycemia, hypokalemia
Gastrointestinal: Abdominal pain (children: 9%; adults: 6%), anorexia, dyspepsia, eructation, flatulence, gastrointestinal disease, melena, rectal disease
Genitourinary: Urinary tract infection
Hematologic & oncologic: Anemia, carcinoma, leukocytosis, lymphadenopathy
Infection: Abscess, infection, sepsis
Neuromuscular & skeletal: Leg cramps (10%), weakness (7%), arm pain, arthralgia, back pain, myalgia
Ophthalmic: Conjunctivitis, corneal changes (arcus senilis), diplopia, eye redness, eyelid edema, nystagmus, watery eyes
Otic: Deafness
Respiratory: Pharyngitis (children: 9%), cough (6%), rhinitis (children: 6%), upper respiratory tract infection (6%), flu-like symptoms, pneumonia, pulmonary edema
Miscellaneous: Fever (children: 9%; adults: 5%)
<1%, postmarketing, and/or case reports: Anaphylaxis, convulsions, dysgeusia, facial flushing, hemorrhage, hypersensitivity reaction, hypertonia, hypoesthesia, loss of consciousness, nervousness, pallor, phlebitis, shock, skin discoloration, xerostomia

Drug Interactions
Metabolism/Transport Effects None known.
Avoid Concomitant Use
Avoid concomitant use of Ferric Gluconate with any of the following: Dimercaprol
Increased Effect/Toxicity
Ferric Gluconate may increase the levels/effects of: Amifostine; Antipsychotic Agents (Second Generation [Atypical]); DULoxetine; Hypotension-Associated Agents; Levodopa; Nitroprusside; Pholcodine

▶

The levels/effects of Ferric Gluconate may be increased by: ACE Inhibitors; Alfuzosin; Barbiturates; Benperidol; Blood Pressure Lowering Agents; Brimonidine (Topical); Diazoxide; Dimercaprol; Herbs (Hypotensive Properties); Lormetazepam; Molsidomine; Naftopidil; Nicergoline; Nicorandil; Obinutuzumab; Pentoxifylline; Phosphodiesterase 5 Inhibitors; Prostacyclin Analogues; Quinagolide

Decreased Effect

Ferric Gluconate may decrease the levels/effects of: Entacapone

Storage/Stability Store at 20°C to 25°C (68°F to 77°F); excursions permitted to 15°C to 30°C (59°F to 86°F). Do not freeze. Use immediately after dilution in NS.

Preparation for Administration For IV infusion, dilute ferric gluconate in NS (children: 25 mL NS, adults: 100 mL NS).

Mechanism of Action Supplies a source to elemental iron necessary to the function of hemoglobin, myoglobin and specific enzyme systems; allows transport of oxygen via hemoglobin

Pharmacodynamics/Kinetics Half-life elimination: Bound iron: 1 hour

Dosing

Adult & Geriatric

Iron-deficiency anemia, hemodialysis patients: IV: 125 mg elemental iron per dialysis session. Most patients will require a cumulative dose of 1 g elemental iron over approximately 8 sequential dialysis treatments to achieve a favorable response.

Note: A test dose of 2 mL diluted in NS 50 mL administered over 60 minutes was previously recommended (not in current manufacturer labeling). Doses >125 mg are associated with increased adverse events.

Chemotherapy-associated anemia (off-label use): IV infusion: 125 mg once every week for 6 doses (Pedrazzoli, 2008) or for 8 doses (Henry, 2007)

Pediatric Iron-deficiency anemia, hemodialysis patients: Children ≥6 years: IV: 1.5 mg/kg of elemental iron (maximum: 125 mg/dose) per dialysis session. Doses >1.5 mg/kg are associated with increased adverse events.

Renal Impairment No dosage adjustment necessary. The ferric gluconate iron complex is not dialyzable.

Hepatic Impairment No dosage adjustment necessary.

Administration IV:

Children: Administer diluted in 25 mL NS over 1 hour.

Adults: Administer diluted in 100 mL NS over 1 hour or administer undiluted, slowly at a rate of up to 12.5 mg/minute.

Monitoring Parameters Hemoglobin and hematocrit, serum ferritin, iron saturation; vital signs; signs and symptoms of hypersensitivity (monitor for ≥30 minutes following the end of administration and until clinically stable)

NKF K/DOQI guidelines recommend that iron status should be monitored monthly during initiation through the percent transferrin saturation (TSAT) and serum ferritin.

Chemotherapy-associated anemia (off-label use): Iron, total iron-binding capacity, transferrin saturation, or ferritin levels at baseline and periodically (Rizzo, 2011).

Test Interactions Serum or transferrin bound iron levels may be falsely elevated if assessed within 24 hours of ferric gluconate administration. Serum ferritin levels may be falsely elevated for 5 days after ferric gluconate administration.

Dosage Forms Considerations Strength of ferric gluconate injection is expressed as elemental iron.

Dosage Forms Excipient information presented when available (limited, particularly for generics); consult specific product labeling.

Solution, Intravenous:

Ferrlecit: 12.5 mg/mL (5 mL) [contains benzyl alcohol, sucrose]

Generic: 12.5 mg/mL (5 mL)

◆ **Ferriprox** see Deferiprone on page 555
◆ **Ferrlecit** see Ferric Gluconate on page 786

Ferumoxytol (fer ue MOX i tol)

Brand Names: US Feraheme

Pharmacologic Category Iron Salt

Use Iron-deficiency anemia in chronic kidney disease: Treatment of iron-deficiency anemia in adults with chronic kidney disease

Labeled Contraindications Hypersensitivity to ferumoxytol, other IV iron products, or any component of the formulation

Pregnancy Considerations Adverse events were observed in animal reproduction studies.

Breastfeeding Considerations It is not known if ferumoxytol is excreted into breast milk. Due to the potential for serious adverse reactions in the nursing infant, the manufacturer recommends a decision be made whether to discontinue nursing or to discontinue the drug, taking into account the importance of treatment to the mother.

Warnings/Precautions [US Boxed Warning]: Serious hypersensitivity reactions, including anaphylactic-type reactions (some fatal), may occur, presenting with cardiac/cardiorespiratory arrest, clinically significant hypotension, syncope, or unresponsiveness even in patients who previously tolerated ferumoxytol. Equipment for resuscitation and trained personnel experienced in handling emergencies should be immediately available during use. Monitor patients for signs/symptoms of hypersensitivity reactions, including blood pressure and pulse during and ≥30 minutes (until clinically stable) following administration. Other hypersensitivity reactions have also occurred (pruritus, rash, urticaria, wheezing). Patients with multiple drug allergies may have greater risk of anaphylaxis; elderly patients with multiple or serious comorbidities who develop hypersensitivity and/or hypotension after ferumoxytol may be at greater risk for serious adverse events.

Do not administer in the presence of tissue iron overload; periodic monitoring of hemoglobin, serum ferritin, serum iron, and transferrin saturation is recommended. Serum iron and transferrin-bound iron may be overestimated in laboratory assays if level is drawn during the first 24 hours following administration. Administration may alter magnetic resonance (MR) imaging; conduct anticipated MRI studies prior to use. MR imaging alterations may persist for ≤3 months following use, with peak alterations anticipated in the first 2 days following administration. If MR imaging is required within 3 months after administration, use T1- or proton density-weighted MR pulse sequences to decrease effect on imagining. Do not use T2-weighted sequence MR imaging prior to 4 weeks following ferumoxytol administration. Ferumoxytol does not interfere with X-ray, computed tomography (CT), positron emission tomography (PET), single photon emission computed tomography (SPECT), ultrasound or nuclear medicine imaging. Potentially significant drug-drug

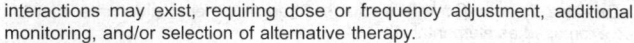

interactions may exist, requiring dose or frequency adjustment, additional monitoring, and/or selection of alternative therapy.

Adverse Reactions

1% to 10%:

Cardiovascular: Hypotension (≤3%), edema (2%), peripheral edema (2%), chest pain (1%), hypertension (1%)

Central nervous system: Dizziness (3%), headache (2%)

Dermatologic: Pruritus (1%), skin rash (1%)

Gastrointestinal: Diarrhea (4%), nausea (3%), constipation (2%), vomiting (2%), abdominal pain (1%)

Hypersensitivity: Hypersensitivity reactions (≤4%; serious hypersensitivity: <1%)

Neuromuscular & skeletal: Back pain (1%), muscle spasm (1%)

Respiratory: Cough (1%), dyspnea (1%)

Miscellaneous: Fever (1%)

<1%, postmarketing, and/or case reports: Anaphylactoid reaction, anaphylaxis, angioedema, cardiac arrhythmia, cardiac failure, cyanosis, fatigue, hypotension (clinically significant), infusion site reaction (including bruise, infusion site burning, infusion site erythema, infusion site irritation, infusion site swelling, infusion site warmth, local pain), ischemic heart disease, loss of consciousness, syncope, tachycardia, unresponsive to stimuli, urticaria, wheezing

Drug Interactions

Metabolism/Transport Effects None known.

Avoid Concomitant Use

Avoid concomitant use of Ferumoxytol with any of the following: Dimercaprol

Increased Effect/Toxicity

The levels/effects of Ferumoxytol may be increased by: Dimercaprol

Decreased Effect

Ferumoxytol may decrease the levels/effects of: Entacapone

Storage/Stability Store intact vials at 20°C to 25°C (68°F to 77°F); excursions are permitted between 15°C and 30°C (59°F and 86°F). Solutions diluted in NS or D5W at concentrations of 2 to 8 mg/mL elemental iron should be used immediately, but may be stored at 23°C to 27°C (73°F to 81°F) for up to 4 hours.

Preparation for Administration Must be diluted prior to administration. To prepare for intravenous infusion, dilute in 50 to 200 mL of NS or D5W.

Mechanism of Action Superparamagnetic iron oxide coated with a low molecular weight semisynthetic carbohydrate; iron-carbohydrate complex enters the reticuloendothelial system macrophages of the liver, spleen, and bone marrow where the iron is released from the complex. The released iron is either transported into storage pools or is transported via plasma transferrin for incorporation into hemoglobin.

Pharmacodynamics/Kinetics

Distribution: V_d: 3.16 L

Metabolism: Iron released from iron-carbohydrate complex after uptake in the reticuloendothelial system macrophages of the liver, spleen, and bone marrow

Half-life elimination: ~15 hours

Dialysis: Ferumoxytol is not removed by hemodialysis

Dosing

Adult & Geriatric

Doses expressed in mg of **elemental** iron. **Note:** Test dose: Product labeling does not indicate need for a test dose.

Iron-deficiency anemia in chronic kidney disease: IV: 510 mg as an IV infusion, followed by a second 510 mg IV infusion 3 to 8 days after initial dose. Assess response at least 30 days following the second dose. The recommended dose may be readministered in patients with persistent or recurrent iron-deficiency anemia.

Renal Impairment No dosage adjustment necessary.

Hemodialysis: Not removed by hemodialysis; however, administer dose after at least 1 hour of hemodialysis has been completed and once blood pressure has stabilized.

Hepatic Impairment There are no dosage adjustments provided in the manufacturer's labeling.

Administration

IV: Administer diluted as a slow IV infusion over at least 15 minutes. Patient should be in a reclined or semi-reclined position during the infusion; monitor for signs of hypersensitivity (including blood pressure and pulse) for at least 30 minutes after infusion. **Note:** Serious hypersensitivity reactions have been observed with rapid IV injection (<1 minute) (Macdougall, 2014; Vadhan-Raj, 2014). Wait ≥30 minutes between administration of ferumoxytol and other agents that may cause serious hypersensitivity reactions and/or hypotension (eg, chemotherapy, monoclonal antibodies).

Hemodialysis patients: Administer dose after at least 1 hour of hemodialysis has been completed and once blood pressure has stabilized.

Monitoring Parameters Hemoglobin, serum ferritin, serum iron, transferrin saturation (at least 1 month following second injection and periodically); signs/symptoms of hypersensitivity reactions, blood pressure, pulse (during and ≥30 minutes following administration)

Test Interactions May interfere with MR imaging; alterations may persist for ≤3 months following use, with peak alterations anticipated in the first 2 days following administration. If MR imaging is required within 3 months after administration, use T1- or proton density-weighted MR pulse sequences to decrease effect on imaging. Do not use T2-weighted sequence MR imaging prior to 4 weeks following administration.

Serum iron and transferrin-bound iron may be overestimated in laboratory assays if level is drawn during the first 24 hours following administration (due to contribution of iron in ferumoxytol).

Dosage Forms Considerations Strength of ferumoxytol is expressed as elemental iron

Dosage Forms Excipient information presented when available (limited, particularly for generics); consult specific product labeling.

Solution, Intravenous [preservative free]:

Feraheme: 510 mg/17 mL (17 mL)

Fibrinogen Concentrate (Human)

(fi BRIN o gin KON suhn trate HYU man)

Brand Names: US RiaSTAP

Brand Names: Canada RiaSTAP

Index Terms Coagulation Factor I; Fibryna

Pharmacologic Category Blood Product Derivative

◀ **Use Congenital fibrinogen deficiency:** Treatment of acute bleeding episodes in patients with congenital fibrinogen deficiency, including afibrinogenemia and hypofibrinogenemia.

Dosing

Adult & Geriatric Congenital fibrinogen deficiency: IV: **Note:** Maintain a target fibrinogen level of 100 mg/dL for minor bleeding and 150 mg/dL for major bleeding.

When baseline fibrinogen level is known:

Fibryna: Dose (mg/kg) = [Target level (mg/dL) - measured level (mg/dL)] **divided by** 1.8 (mg/dL per mg/kg body weight)

RiaSTAP: Dose (mg/kg) = [Target level (mg/dL) - measured level (mg/dL)] **divided by** 1.7 (mg/dL per mg/kg body weight)

When baseline fibrinogen level is not known: 70 mg/kg

Pediatric Congenital fibrinogen deficiency: IV:

Fibryna: Children ≥12 years and Adolescents: Refer to adult dosing.

RiaSTAP: Children ≥8 years and Adolescents: Refer to adult dosing.

Renal Impairment There are no dosage adjustments provided in the manufacturer's labeling.

Hepatic Impairment There are no dosage adjustments provided in the manufacturer's labeling.

Additional Information Complete prescribing information should be consulted for additional detail.

Product Availability Fibryna: FDA approved June 2017; anticipated availability is currently unknown.

Dosage Forms Excipient information presented when available (limited, particularly for generics); consult specific product labeling. [DSC] = Discontinued product

Injection, powder for reconstitution:

RiaSTAP: 900-1300 mg [contains albumin (human); exact potency labeled on vial]

◆ **Fibryna** *see* Fibrinogen Concentrate (Human) *on page 791*

Filgrastim (fil GRA stim)

Related Information

Hematopoietic Cell Transplantation *on page 2365*

Brand Names: US Granix; Neupogen; Zarxio

Brand Names: Canada Grastofil; Neupogen

Index Terms Filgrastim-sndz; G-CSF; Granulocyte Colony Stimulating Factor; Tbo-Filgrastim; Tevagrastim

Pharmacologic Category Colony Stimulating Factor; Hematopoietic Agent

Use

Myelosuppressive chemotherapy recipients with nonmyeloid malignancies:

Neupogen (filgrastim), Zarxio (filgrastim-sndz [biosimilar]), Grastofil [Canadian product]**:** To decrease the incidence of infection (neutropenic fever) in patients with nonmyeloid malignancies receiving myelosuppressive chemotherapy associated with a significant incidence of severe neutropenia with fever.

Granix (tbo-filgrastim): To decrease the duration of severe neutropenia in patients with nonmyeloid malignancies receiving myelosuppressive chemotherapy associated with a clinically significant incidence of neutropenic fever.

Acute myeloid leukemia (AML) following induction or consolidation chemotherapy (Neupogen, Zarxio, Grastofil [Canadian product]**):** To reduce the time to neutrophil recovery and the duration of fever following induction or consolidation chemotherapy in adults with AML.

Bone marrow transplantation (Neupogen, Zarxio, Grastofil [Canadian product]**):** To reduce the duration of neutropenia and neutropenia-related events (eg, neutropenic fever) in patients with nonmyeloid malignancies receiving myeloablative chemotherapy followed by marrow transplantation.

Hematopoietic radiation injury syndrome, acute (Neupogen): To increase survival in patients acutely exposed to myelosuppressive doses of radiation.

Peripheral blood progenitor cell collection and therapy (Neupogen, Zarxio, Grastofil [Canadian product]**):** Mobilization of autologous hematopoietic progenitor cells into the peripheral blood for apheresis collection.

Severe chronic neutropenia (Neupogen, Zarxio, Grastofil [Canadian product]**):** Long-term administration to reduce the incidence and duration of neutropenic complications (eg, fever, infections, oropharyngeal ulcers) in symptomatic patients with congenital, cyclic, or idiopathic neutropenia.

Labeled Contraindications

History of serious allergic reactions to human granulocyte colony-stimulating factors, such as filgrastim or pegfilgrastim, or any component of the formulation

Canadian labeling: Additional contraindications (not in the US labeling): Neupogen, Grastofil: Known hypersensitivity to *E. coli*-derived products

Pregnancy Considerations Adverse events were observed in animal reproduction studies. Filgrastim has been shown to cross the placenta in humans. Information related to the use of granulocyte colony stimulating factor (G-CSF) in pregnant patients with congenital, cyclic, or idiopathic neutropenia (Boxer 2015; Zeidler 2014) and G-CSF-induced allogeneic peripheral blood stem cells donation is limited (Leitner 2001; Shibata 2003). One review suggests avoiding use during the first trimester until additional outcome information is available (Pessach 2013). Data collected from the Severe Chronic Neutropenia International Registry (SCNIR) note dosing for chronic conditions may need adjusted in pregnant women; the lowest effective dose to maintain the absolute neutrophil count is recommended (Zeidler 2014).

Breastfeeding Considerations Endogenous G-CSF can be detected in breast milk, however, recombinant G-CSF, when administered orally to infants, was not found to be absorbed (Calhoun 2003). One review suggests waiting until 3 days after the last dose to resume breastfeeding until additional data is available (Pessach 2013).

The manufacturers recommend that caution be exercised when administering filgrastim products to breastfeeding women.

Warnings/Precautions Serious allergic reactions (including anaphylaxis) have been reported, usually with the initial exposure; may be managed symptomatically with administration of antihistamines, steroids, bronchodilators, and/or epinephrine. Allergic reactions may recur within days after the initial allergy management has been stopped. Do not administer filgrastim products to patients who experienced serious allergic reaction to filgrastim or pegfilgrastim. Permanently discontinue filgrastim products in patients with serious allergic reactions. Rare cases of splenic rupture have been reported (may be fatal); in patients with upper abdominal pain, left upper quadrant pain, or shoulder tip pain, withhold treatment and evaluate for enlarged spleen or splenic rupture. Moderate or severe cutaneous vasculitis has been reported, generally occurring in patients with severe chronic neutropenia on chronic therapy. Withhold treatment if cutaneous vasculitis occurs; may be restarted with a dose reduction once symptoms resolve and the absolute neutrophil count (ANC) has decreased. Capillary leak syndrome (CLS), characterized by hypotension, hypoalbuminemia, edema, and hemoconcentration, may occur in patients receiving human granulocyte colony-stimulating factors (G-CSF). CLS episode may vary in frequency and severity. If CLS develops, monitor closely and manage symptomatically (may require intensive care). CLS may be life-threatening if treatment is delayed.

White blood cell counts of ≥100,000/mm^3 have been reported with filgrastim doses >5 mcg/kg/day. When filgrastim products are used as an adjunct to myelosuppressive chemotherapy, discontinue when ANC exceeds 10,000/mm^3 after the ANC nadir has occurred (to avoid potential excessive leukocytosis). Doses that increase the ANC beyond 10,000/mm^3 may not result in additional clinical benefit. Monitor complete blood cell count (CBC) twice weekly during therapy. In patients receiving myelosuppressive chemotherapy, filgrastim discontinuation generally resulted in a 50% decrease in circulating neutrophils within 1 to 2 days, and a return to pretreatment levels in 1 to 7 days. When used for peripheral blood progenitor cell collection, discontinue filgrastim products if leukocytes >100,000/mm^3. Thrombocytopenia has also been reported with filgrastim products; monitor platelet counts. Filgrastim products should not be routinely used in the treatment of established neutropenic fever. Colony-stimulating factors may be considered in cancer patients with febrile neutropenia who are at high risk for infection-associated complications or who have prognostic factors indicative of a poor clinical outcome (eg, prolonged and severe neutropenia, age >65 years, hypotension, pneumonia, sepsis syndrome, presence of invasive fungal infection, uncontrolled primary disease, hospitalization at the time of fever development) (Freifeld 2011; Smith 2006). Colony-stimulating factors (CSF) should not be routinely used for patients with neutropenia who are afebrile. Dose-dense regimens that require colony-stimulating factors should only be used within the context of a clinical trial or if supported by convincing evidence (Smith 2015). Recommendations for the Use of WBC Growth Factors Clinical Practice Guideline Update recommend that prophylactic CSF be used in patients ≥65 years with diffuse aggressive lymphoma treated with curative chemotherapy (eg, rituximab, cyclophosphamide, doxorubicin, vincristine, prednisone), especially if patients have comorbid conditions (Smith 2015). CSF use in pediatric patients is typically directed by clinical pediatric protocols. The American Society of Clinical Oncology (ASCO) Recommendations for the Use of WBC Growth Factors Clinical Practice Guideline Update states that CSFs may be reasonable as primary prophylaxis in pediatric patients when chemotherapy regimens with a high likelihood of febrile neutropenia are employed. Likewise, secondary CSF prophylaxis should be limited to high-risk patients. In pediatric cancers in which dose-intense chemotherapy (with a survival benefit) is used, CSFs should be given to facilitate chemotherapy administration. CSFs should not be used in the pediatric population for nonrelapsed acute lymphoblastic or myeloid leukemia when no infection is present (Smith 2015). Do not use filgrastim products in the period 24 hours before to 24 hours after administration of cytotoxic chemotherapy because of the potential sensitivity of rapidly dividing myeloid cells to cytotoxic chemotherapy. Transient increase in neutrophil count is seen 1 to 2 days after filgrastim initiation; however, for sustained neutrophil response, continue until post-nadir ANC reaches 10,000/mm^3. Avoid simultaneous use of filgrastim products with chemotherapy and radiation therapy. Avoid concurrent radiation therapy with filgrastim; safety and efficacy have not been established with patients receiving radiation therapy. The G-CSF receptor through which filgrastim products act has been found on tumor cell lines. May potentially act as a growth factor for any tumor type (including myeloid malignancies and myelodysplasia). When used for stem cell mobilization, may release tumor cells from marrow, which could be collected in leukapheresis product; potential effect of tumor cell reinfusion is unknown.

May precipitate severe sickle cell crises, sometimes resulting in fatalities, in patients with sickle cell disorders (sickle cell trait or sickle cell disease); carefully evaluate potential risks and benefits. Discontinue in patients undergoing sickle cell crisis. Establish diagnosis of severe chronic neutropenia (SCN) prior to initiation; use prior to appropriate diagnosis of SCN may impair or delay proper evaluation and treatment for neutropenia due to conditions other than SCN. Based on findings of azotemia, hematuria (micro- and macroscopic), proteinuria, and renal biopsy, glomerulonephritis has occurred in patients receiving filgrastim. Glomerulonephritis usually resolved after filgrastim dose reduction or discontinuation. If glomerulonephritis is suspected, evaluate for cause; if likely due to filgrastim, consider dose reduction or treatment interruption. Myelodysplastic syndrome (MDS) and acute myeloid leukemia (AML) have been reported to occur in the natural history of congenital neutropenia (without cytokine therapy). Cytogenetic abnormalities and transformation to MDS and AML have been observed with filgrastim when used to manage SCN, although the risk for MDS and AML appears to be in patients with congenital neutropenia. Abnormal cytogenetics and MDS are associated with the development of AML. The effects of continuing filgrastim products in patients who have developed abnormal cytogenetics or MDS are unknown; consider risk versus benefits of continuing treatment. Acute respiratory distress syndrome (ARDS) has been reported. Evaluate patients who develop fever and lung infiltrates or respiratory distress for ARDS; discontinue in patients with ARDS. Reports of alveolar hemorrhage, manifested as pulmonary infiltrates and hemoptysis (requiring hospitalization), have occurred in healthy donors undergoing PBPC mobilization (off-label for use in healthy donors); hemoptysis resolved upon discontinuation. Increased bone marrow hematopoietic activity due to CSF use has been associated with transient bone-imaging changes; interpret results accordingly. Potentially significant drug-drug interactions may exist, requiring dose or frequency adjustment, additional monitoring, and/or selection of alternative therapy.

The packaging of some dosage forms may contain latex. Granix (tbo-filgrastim), including all components, is not made with natural rubber latex.

Some products available internationally may have vial strength and dosing expressed as units (instead of as micrograms). Refer to prescribing information for specific strength and dosing information.

Some dosage forms may contain polysorbate 80 (also known as Tweens). Hypersensitivity reactions, usually a delayed reaction, have been reported following exposure to pharmaceutical products containing polysorbate 80 in certain individuals (Isaksson 2002; Lucente 2000; Shelley 1995). Thrombocytopenia, ascites, pulmonary deterioration, and renal and hepatic failure have been reported in premature neonates after receiving parenteral products containing polysorbate 80 (Alade 1986; CDC 1984). See manufacturer's labeling.

Adverse Reactions

>10%:

Cardiovascular: Chest pain (5% to 13%)

Central nervous system: Fatigue (20%), dizziness (14%), pain (12%)

Dermatologic: Skin rash (2% to 14%)

Gastrointestinal: Nausea (10% to 43%)

Hematologic & oncologic: Thrombocytopenia (5% to 38%), splenomegaly (≥5%; severe chronic neutropenia: 30%), petechia (17%)

Hepatic: Increased serum alkaline phosphatase (6% to 11%)

Neuromuscular & skeletal: Ostealgia (5% to 33%; dose and cycle related), back pain (2% to 15%)

Respiratory: Epistaxis (2% to 15%), cough (14%), dyspnea (13%)

Miscellaneous: Fever (12% to 48%; dose and cycle related)

1% to 10%:

Cardiovascular: Peripheral edema (≥5%), hypertension (≥4%), cardiac arrhythmia (≤3%), myocardial infarction (≤3%)

Central nervous system: Headache (7% to 10%), hypoesthesia (≥5%), insomnia (≥5%), malaise (≥5%), mouth pain (≥5%)

Dermatologic: Alopecia (≥5%), erythema (≥2%), maculopapular rash (≥2%)

Endocrine & metabolic: Increased lactate dehydrogenase (6%)

Gastrointestinal: Vomiting (5% to 7%), decreased appetite (≥5%), constipation (≥2%), diarrhea (≥2%)

Genitourinary: Urinary tract infection (≥5%)

Hematologic & oncologic: Anemia (≥5%), leukocytosis (≤2%)

Hypersensitivity: Transfusion reaction (2% to 10%), hypersensitivity reaction (≥5%)

Immunologic: Antibody development (2% to 3%; no evidence of neutralizing response)

Infection: Sepsis (≥5%)

Neuromuscular & skeletal: Arthralgia (5% to 9%), limb pain (2% to 7%), muscle spasm (≥5%), musculoskeletal pain (≥5%) weakness (≥5%)

Respiratory: Bronchitis (≥5%), upper respiratory tract infection (≥5%)

<1%, postmarketing, and/or case reports: Anaphylaxis, capillary leak syndrome, cerebral hemorrhage, decreased bone mineral density, decreased hemoglobin, euthymia nodosum, exacerbation of psoriasis, facial edema, glomerulonephritis, hematuria, hemoptysis, hepatomegaly, hypersensitivity angiitis, hypotension, injection site reaction, osteoporosis, proteinuria, pulmonary alveolar hemorrhage, pulmonary infiltrates, renal insufficiency, respiratory distress syndrome, severe sickle cell crisis, splenic rupture, Sweet syndrome, tachycardia, urticaria, wheezing

Drug Interactions

Metabolism/Transport Effects None known.

Avoid Concomitant Use There are no known interactions where it is recommended to avoid concomitant use.

Increased Effect/Toxicity

Filgrastim may increase the levels/effects of: Belotecan; Bleomycin; Cyclophosphamide; Topotecan

Decreased Effect There are no known significant interactions involving a decrease in effect.

Storage/Stability

Neupogen: Store at 2°C to 8°C (36°F to 46°F). Store in the original carton. Protect from light. Protect from direct sunlight. Avoid freezing; if frozen, thaw in the refrigerator before administration. Discard if frozen more than once. Do not shake. Transport via a pneumatic tube has not been studied. Prior to injection, allow to reach room temperature for up to 30 minutes and a maximum of 24 hours. Discard any vial or prefilled syringe left at room temperature for more than 24 hours. Solutions diluted for infusion in D5W may be stored at room temperature for up to 24 hours (infusion must be completed within 24 hours of preparation).

Extended storage information may be available for undiluted filgrastim; contact product manufacturer to obtain current recommendations. Sterility has been assessed and maintained for up to 7 days when prepared under strict aseptic conditions (Jacobson 1996; Singh 1994). The manufacturer recommends using within 24 hours due to the potential for bacterial contamination.

Granix: Store prefilled syringes at 2°C to 8°C (36°F to 46°F). Protect from light. Do not shake. May be removed from 2°C to 8°C (36°F to 46°F) storage for a single period of up to 5 days between 23°C to 27°C (73°F to 81°F). If not used within 5 days, the product may be returned to 2°C to 8°C (36°F to 46°F) up to the expiration date. Dispose of syringes if stored at room temperature for more than 5 days. Exposure to -1°C to -5°C (23°F to 30°F) for up to 72 hours and temperatures as low as -15°C to -25°C (5°F to -13°F) for up to 24 hours do not adversely affect stability. Discard unused product.

Zarxio: Store at 2°C to 8°C (36°F to 46°F). Store in the original carton. Protect from light. Avoid freezing; if frozen, thaw in the refrigerator before administration. Discard if frozen more than once. Do not shake. Transport via a pneumatic tube has not been studied. Prior to injection, allow to reach room temperature for up to 30 minutes and a maximum of 24 hours. Discard any prefilled syringe left at room temperature for more than 24 hours. Solutions diluted for infusion may be stored at room temperature for up to 24 hours (infusion must be completed within 24 hours of preparation).

Grastofil [Canadian product]: Store at 2°C to 8°C (36°F to 46°F). Protect from light. Do not shake. Accidental one-time exposure to temperatures up to 30°C (86°F) or exposure to freezing temperatures <0°C (32°F) does not adversely affect stability. If exposure at >30°C or <0°C has been greater than 24 hours or frozen more than once, do not use. May be removed from the refrigerator and stored at room temperature (≤25°C) for a single period of up to 7 days. Do not return to refrigerator.

Preparation for Administration Visually inspect prior to use; discard if discolored or if particulates are present.

Neupogen: **Do not dilute with saline at any time; product may precipitate.** Filgrastim (vial only; do not use prefilled syringe for IV preparation) may be diluted with D5W to a concentration of 5 to 15 mcg/mL for IV infusion administration (minimum concentration: 5 mcg/mL). Concentrations of 5 to 15 mcg/mL require addition of albumin (final albumin concentration of 2 mg/mL) to prevent adsorption to plastics. Dilution to <5 mcg/mL is not recommended. Do not shake. May be prepared in glass bottles, polyvinyl chloride (PVC) or polyolefin bags, and polypropylene syringes. Discard unused portion of vial.

Granix: Remove needle shield and expel extra volume if needed (depending on dose). Prefilled syringe is for single use only; discard unused portion.

Grastofil [Canadian product]: **Do not dilute with saline at any time; product may precipitate.** May be diluted with D5W to a concentration of 5 to 15 mcg/mL for IV infusion administration. Concentrations of 5 to 15 mcg/mL require addition of albumin (final albumin concentration of 2 mg/mL) to prevent adsorption to plastics. Dilution to <5 mcg/mL is not recommended.

◀ Do not shake. May be prepared in glass if diluted with D5W or in PVC or polyolefin IV bags if diluted in D5W plus albumin. Discard unused portion of syringe.

Zarxio: **Do not dilute with saline at any time; product may precipitate.** Filgrastim-sndz may be diluted with D5W to a concentration of 5 to 15 mcg/mL for IV infusion administration. Concentrations of 5 to 15 mcg/mL require addition of albumin (final albumin concentration of 2 mg/mL) to prevent adsorption to plastics. Do not shake. May be prepared in glass, PVC, polyolefin, and polypropylene. Discard unused portion of syringe.

Mechanism of Action
Filgrastim, filgrastim-sndz, and tbo-filgrastim are granulocyte colony stimulating factors (G-CSF) produced by recombinant DNA technology. G-CSFs stimulate the production, maturation, and activation of neutrophils to increase both their migration and cytotoxicity.

Pharmacodynamics/Kinetics
Onset of action:
Filgrastim: 1 to 2 days
Tbo-filgrastim: Time to maximum ANC: 3 to 5 days
Duration:
Filgrastim: Neutrophil counts generally return to baseline within 4 days
Tbo-filgrastim: ANC returned to baseline by 21 days after completion of chemotherapy
Distribution: V_d: 150 mL/kg; Continuous infusion: No evidence of drug accumulation over a 11- to 20-day period
Metabolism: Systemically degraded
Bioavailability: Filgrastim: SubQ: 60% to 70%; Tbo-filgrastim: SubQ: 33%
Half-life elimination:
Neonates: 4.4 ± 0.4 hours (Gillan 1994)
Adults: Filgrastim: ~3.5 hours; Tbo-filgrastim: 3 to 4 hours
Time to peak, serum: SubQ: Filgrastim: 2 to 8 hours; Tbo-filgrastim: 4 to 6 hours

Dosing
Adult & Geriatric Note: Do not administer in the period 24 hours before to 24 hours after cytotoxic chemotherapy. May round the dose to the nearest vial size for convenience and cost minimization (Ozer 2000). **International considerations:** Dosages below expressed as micrograms; 1 mcg = 100,000 units (Hoglund 1998).

Myelosuppressive chemotherapy recipients with nonmyeloid malignancies (Neupogen [filgrastim], Zarxio [filgrastim-sndz; biosimilar], Grastofil [Canadian product]): SubQ, IV: 5 mcg/kg/day; doses may be increased by 5 mcg/kg (for each chemotherapy cycle) according to the duration and severity of the neutropenia; continue for up to 14 days until the absolute neutrophil count (ANC) reaches 10,000/mm³. Discontinue if the ANC surpasses 10,000/mm³ after the expected chemotherapy-induced neutrophil nadir.

Myelosuppressive chemotherapy recipients with nonmyeloid malignancies (Granix [tbo-filgrastim]): SubQ: 5 mcg/kg/day; continue until anticipated nadir has passed and neutrophil count has recovered to normal range.

Acute myeloid leukemia (AML) following induction or consolidation chemotherapy (Neupogen, Zarxio, Grastofil [Canadian product]): SubQ, IV: 5 mcg/kg/day; doses may be increased by 5 mcg/kg (for each chemotherapy cycle) according to the duration and severity of the neutropenia; continue for up to 14 days until the ANC reaches 10,000/mm³. Discontinue if the ANC surpasses 10,000/mm^3 after the expected chemotherapy-induced neutrophil nadir.

Bone marrow transplantation (Neupogen, Zarxio, Grastofil [Canadian product]): IV infusion: 10 mcg/kg/day (administer ≥24 hours after chemotherapy and ≥24 hours after bone marrow infusion); adjust the dose according to the duration and severity of neutropenia; recommended steps based on neutrophil response:

When ANC >1,000/mm^3 for 3 consecutive days: Reduce dose to 5 mcg/kg/day

If ANC remains >1,000/mm^3 for 3 more consecutive days: Discontinue

If ANC decreases to <1,000/mm^3: Resume at 5 mcg/kg/day.

If ANC decreases to <1,000/mm^3 during the 5 mcg/kg/day dose: Increase dose to 10 mcg/kg/day and follow the above steps.

Hematopoietic radiation injury syndrome, acute (Neupogen): SubQ: 10 mcg/kg once daily; begin as soon as possible after suspected or confirmed radiation doses >2 gray (Gy) and continue filgrastim until ANC remains >1,000/mm^3 for 3 consecutive CBCs or ANC exceeds 10,000/mm^3 after the radiation-induced nadir. ASCO guidelines recommend initiating within 24 hours of exposure of a dose ≥2 Gy and/or significant decrease in absolute lymphocyte count, or for anticipated neutropenia <500/mm^3 for ≥7 days (Smith 2015).

Peripheral blood progenitor (PBPC) cell collection and therapy (Neupogen, Zarxio, Grastofil [Canadian product]): SubQ: 10 mcg/kg daily, usually for 6 to 7 days (with apheresis occurring on days 5, 6, and 7). Begin at least 4 days before the first apheresis and continue until the last apheresis; discontinue for WBC >100,000/mm^3

Severe chronic neutropenia (Neupogen, Zarxio, Grastofil [Canadian product]): SubQ:

Congenital: Initial: 6 mcg/kg/day in 2 divided doses; adjust the dose based on ANC and clinical response; mean dose: 6 mcg/kg/day.

Idiopathic: Initial: 5 mcg/kg once daily; adjust the dose based on ANC and clinical response; total daily dose may be administered in 1 or 2 divided doses; mean dose: 1.2 mcg/kg/day

Cyclic: Initial: 5 mcg/kg once daily; adjust the dose based on ANC and clinical response; total daily dose may be administered in 1 or 2 divided doses; mean dose: 2.1 mcg/kg/day

Anemia in myelodysplastic syndrome (off-label use; in combination with epoetin): SubQ: 300 mcg weekly in 2 to 3 divided doses (Malcovati 2013) **or** 1 mcg/kg once daily (Greenberg 2009) **or** 75 mcg, 150 mcg, or 300 mcg per dose 3 times weekly (Hellstrom-Lindberg 2003)

Hematopoietic stem cell mobilization in autologous transplantation in patients with non-Hodgkin lymphoma or multiple myeloma (in combination with plerixafor; off-label combination): SubQ: 10 mcg/kg once daily; begin 4 days before initiation of plerixafor; continue G-CSF on each day prior to apheresis for up to 8 days (DiPersio 2009a; DiPersio 2009b)

Hepatitis C treatment-associated neutropenia (off-label use): SubQ: 150 mcg once weekly to 300 mcg 3 times weekly; titrate to maintain ANC between 750 and 10,000/mm^3 (Younossi 2008)

Neutropenia in advanced HIV infection (off-label use): SubQ: Initial: 1 mcg/kg once daily or 300 mcg one to three times per week; titrate to maintain ANC 2,000 to 10,000/mm^3; doses up to 10 mcg/kg/day or 600 mcg daily were studied (Kuritzkes 1998).

◄ **Pediatric Note:** Do not administer in the period 24 hours before to 24 hours after cytotoxic chemotherapy. **International considerations:** Dosages below expressed as micrograms; 1 mcg = 100,000 units (Hoglund 1998).

Myelosuppressive chemotherapy recipients with nonmyeloid malignancies (Neupogen [filgrastim], Zarxio [filgrastim-sndz; biosimilar], Gastrofil [Canadian product]): SubQ, IV: 5 mcg/kg/day; doses may be increased by 5 mcg/kg (for each chemotherapy cycle) according to the duration and severity of the neutropenia; continue for up to 14 days until the absolute neutrophil count (ANC) reaches 10,000/mm^3. Discontinue if the ANC surpasses 10,000/mm^3 after the expected chemotherapy-induced neutrophil nadir.

Bone marrow transplantation (Neupogen, Zarxio): IV infusion: 10 mcg/kg/day (administer ≥24 hours after chemotherapy and ≥24 hours after bone marrow infusion); adjust the dose according to the duration and severity of neutropenia; recommended steps based on neutrophil response:
When ANC >1,000/mm^3 for 3 consecutive days: Reduce dose to 5 mcg/kg/day
If ANC remains >1,000/mm^3 for 3 more consecutive days: Discontinue
If ANC decreases to <1,000/mm^3: Resume at 5 mcg/kg/day
If ANC decreases to <1,000/mm^3 during the 5 mcg/kg/day dose, increase dose to 10 mcg/kg/day and follow the above steps

Hematopoietic radiation injury syndrome, acute (Neupogen): SubQ: 10 mcg/kg once daily; begin as soon as possible after suspected or confirmed radiation doses >2 gray (Gy) and continue filgrastim until ANC remains >1,000/mm^3 for 3 consecutive CBCs or ANC exceeds 10,000/mm^3 after the radiation-induced nadir. ASCO guidelines recommend initiating within 24 hours of exposure of a dose ≥2 Gy and/or significant decrease in absolute lymphocyte count, or for anticipated neutropenia <500/mm^3 for ≥7 days (Smith 2015).

Peripheral blood progenitor cell collection and therapy (Neupogen, Zarxio): SubQ: 10 mcg/kg daily, usually for 6 to 7 days (with apheresis occurring on days 5, 6, and 7). Begin at least 4 days before the first apheresis and continue until the last apheresis; discontinue for WBC >100,000/mm^3

Severe chronic neutropenia (Neupogen, Zarxio, Grastofil [Canadian product]): Infants ≥1 month, Children, and Adolescents: SubQ:
Congenital: Initial: 6 mcg/kg/day in 2 divided doses; adjust the dose based on ANC and clinical response; mean dose: 6 mcg/kg/day.
Idiopathic: Initial: 5 mcg/kg once daily; adjust the dose based on ANC and clinical response; total daily dose may be administered in 1 or 2 divided doses; mean dose: 1.2 mcg/kg/day
Cyclic: Initial: 5 mcg/kg once daily; adjust the dose based on ANC and clinical response; total daily dose may be administered in 1 or 2 divided doses; mean dose: 2.1 mcg/kg/day

Neutropenia in advanced HIV infection (off-label use): Adolescents >13 years: SubQ: Refer to adult dosing.

Renal Impairment
Renal impairment at treatment initiation:
Neupogen, Zarxio: No dosage adjustment necessary.
Granix:
Mild impairment: No dosage adjustment necessary.
Moderate to severe impairment: There are no dosage adjustments provided in the manufacturer's labeling (has not been studied).

Renal toxicity during treatment: Glomerulonephritis due to filgrastim: Consider dose reduction or treatment interruption.

Hepatic Impairment

Neupogen, Zarxio: No dosage adjustment necessary.

Granix: There are no dosage adjustments provided in the manufacturer's labeling (has not been studied).

Combination Regimens

Lymphoma, non-Hodgkin (Burkitt):
Lymphoma, non-Hodgkin (DLBCL):
Lymphoma, non-Hodgkin (Mantle Cell):
Multiple myeloma:
Neuroblastoma:
Soft tissue sarcoma:
Soft tissue sarcoma (rhabdomyosarcoma):
Testicular cancer:
Unknown Primary (Adenocarcinoma):
Uterine sarcoma:
Wilms' tumor:

Administration Do not administer earlier than 24 hours after or in the 24 hours prior to cytotoxic chemotherapy.

IV (Neupogen, Zarxio, Grastofil [Canadian product]): May be administered IV as a short infusion over 15 to 30 minutes (chemotherapy-induced neutropenia) or by continuous infusion (chemotherapy-induced neutropenia) or as an infusion of no longer than 24 hours (bone marrow transplantation).

SubQ: May be administered SubQ (chemotherapy-induced neutropenia, peripheral blood progenitor cell collection, severe chronic neutropenia, hematopoietic radiation injury syndrome). Administer into the outer upper arm, abdomen (except within 2 inches of navel), front middle thigh, or the upper outer buttocks area. Rotate injection site; do not inject into areas that are tender, red, bruised, hardened, or scarred, or sites with stretch marks.

Some patients (or caregivers) may be appropriate candidates for SubQ self-administration with proper training; patients/caregivers should follow the manufacturer instructions for preparation and administration. Do not skip doses, change schedule, or discontinue without consulting with health care provider. Granix is available in prefilled syringes with and without a needle guard; the prefilled syringe without a safety needle guard is intended for patient/caregiver self-administration. If filgrastim comes in contact with the skin, wash area thoroughly with soap and water; if eye contact occurs, flush exposed eye(s) with water.

Monitoring Parameters

Chemotherapy-induced neutropenia: Complete blood cell count (CBC) with differential and platelets prior to chemotherapy and twice weekly during growth factor treatment.

Bone marrow transplantation: CBC with differential and platelets frequently.

Hematopoietic radiation injury syndrome (acute): CBC at baseline (do not delay filgrastim for baseline CBC) and approximately every 3 days until ANC remains >1,000/mm^3 for 3 consecutive CBCs. Estimate absorbed radiation dose (radiation exposure) based on information from public health authorities, biodosimetry (if available), or clinical findings (eg, onset of vomiting or lymphocyte depletion kinetics).

Peripheral progenitor cell collection: Neutrophil counts after 4 days of filgrastim treatment.

Severe chronic neutropenia: CBC with differential and platelets twice weekly during the first month of therapy and for 2 weeks following dose adjustments; once clinically stable, monthly for 1 year and quarterly thereafter. Monitor bone marrow and karyotype prior to treatment; and monitor marrow and cytogenetics annually throughout treatment.

Neutropenia in advanced HIV infection (off-label use): ANC 3 times weekly for 1st week then weekly thereafter (Kuritzkes 1999).

Test Interactions May interfere with bone imaging studies; increased hematopoietic activity of the bone marrow may appear as transient positive bone imaging changes

Dietary Considerations Some products may contain sodium.

Dosage Forms Considerations Filgrastim-sndz (Zarxio) is approved as a biosimilar to filgrastim (Neupogen).

Dosage Forms Excipient information presented when available (limited, particularly for generics); consult specific product labeling.

Solution, Injection:

Neupogen: filgrastim 300 mcg/mL (1 mL); filgrastim 480 mcg/1.6 mL (1.6 mL) [contains polysorbate 80]

Solution Prefilled Syringe, Injection [preservative free]:

Neupogen: filgrastim 300 mcg/0.5 mL (0.5 mL); filgrastim 480 mcg/0.8 mL (0.8 mL) [contains polysorbate 80]

Zarxio: filgrastim-sndz 300 mcg/0.5 mL (0.5 mL); filgrastim-sndz 480 mcg/ 0.8 mL (0.8 mL) [contains polysorbate 80]

Solution Prefilled Syringe, Subcutaneous [preservative free]:

Granix: tbo-filgrastim 300 mcg/0.5 mL (0.5 mL); tbo-filgrastim 480 mcg/0.8 mL (0.8 mL) [contains polysorbate 80]

Dosage Forms: Canada Information with regard to form, strength, and availability of products uniquely available in Canada but currently not available in the US. Refer also to Dosage Forms.

Excipient information presented when available (limited, particularly for generics); consult specific product labeling.

Solution Prefilled Syringe, Injection [preservative free]:

Gastrofil: 300 mcg/0.5 mL (0.5 mL); 480 mcg/0.8 mL [contains polysorbate 80]

- ◆ **Flagyl** *see* MetroNIDAZOLE (Systemic) *on page 1249*
- ◆ **Flagyl ER [DSC]** *see* MetroNIDAZOLE (Systemic) *on page 1249*
- ◆ **Flebogamma DIF** *see* Immune Globulin *on page 992*
- ◆ **Floxuridin** *see* Floxuridine *on page 804*

Floxuridine (floks YOOR i deen)

Related Information

Management of Chemotherapy-Induced Nausea and Vomiting in Adults *on page 2253*

Safe Handling of Hazardous Drugs *on page 2379*

Brand Names: Canada FUDR®

Index Terms 5-FUDR; FdUrD; Floxuridin; Fluorodeoxyuridine; FUDR

Pharmacologic Category Antineoplastic Agent, Antimetabolite; Antineoplastic Agent, Antimetabolite (Pyrimidine Analog)

Use Colorectal cancer, hepatic metastases: Palliative management of hepatic metastases of colorectal cancer (administered by continuous regional intra-arterial infusion) in select patients considered incurable by surgical resection or other means.

Labeled Contraindications Poor nutritional states; depressed bone marrow function; potentially serious infections

Pregnancy Considerations Teratogenic effects have been observed in animal reproduction studies. Medications that inhibit DNA synthesis are known to be teratogenic in humans. Women of childbearing potential should avoid pregnancy.

Breastfeeding Considerations It is not known if floxuridine is excreted in human milk; the manufacturer recommends against breastfeeding during floxuridine treatment.

Warnings/Precautions Use with extreme caution in patients with renal or hepatic impairment. Bleeding may occur; discontinue if hemorrhage (from any site) occurs. May cause severe hematologic toxicity (anemia, leukopenia, and thrombocytopenia). Discontinue if white blood count <3500/mm³ (or is falling rapidly) or if platelet count <100,000/mm³. May cause gastrointestinal toxicity. Discontinue at the first sign of stomatitis or esophagopharyngitis; discontinue for intractable vomiting, diarrhea, or gastrointestinal ulceration/bleeding. Myocardial ischemia has been reported; discontinue if occurs. Toxicities may occur; monitor closely. Severe toxicities are more likely to occur in high risk patients, patients with prior pelvic irradiation, or in those who have received prior alkylating agents.

[U.S. Boxed Warning]: Should be administered under the supervision of a physician experienced in cancer chemotherapy and in intra-arterial treatment. [U.S. Boxed Warning]: Due to the risk for severe toxic reactions, the manufacturer recommends that patients be hospitalized for initiation of the first treatment course. Not intended for use as an adjuvant to surgery or in patients with known disease extending beyond an area of single-artery infusion. Potentially significant drug-drug interactions may exist, requiring dose or frequency adjustment, additional monitoring, and/or selection of alternative therapy.

Adverse Reactions

>10%:

Gastrointestinal: Diarrhea (may be dose limiting), stomatitis

Hematologic & oncologic: Anemia, bone marrow depression (nadir: 7-10 days; may be dose limiting), leukopenia, thrombocytopenia

1% to 10%:

Dermatologic: Alopecia, dermatitis, localized erythema, skin hyperpigmentation, skin photosensitivity

Gastrointestinal: Anorexia, biliary sclerosis, cholecystitis

Hepatic: Jaundice

<1%, postmarketing, and/or case reports: Abdominal cramps, abdominal pain, BSP abnormality, change in prothrombin time, decreased erythrocyte sedimentation rate, decreased serum total protein, duodenal ulcer, duodenitis, enteritis, fever, gastritis, gastroenteritis, gastrointestinal hemorrhage, gastrointestinal ulcer, glossitis, hemorrhage, hepatic abscess, increased erythrocyte sedimentation rate, increased lactate dehydrogenase, increased serum alkaline phosphatase, increased serum bilirubin, increased serum total protein, increased serum transaminases, infusion related reaction (arterial aneurysm; arterial ischemia; arterial thrombosis; embolism; fibromyositis; thrombophlebitis; hepatic necrosis; abscesses; infection at catheter site; bleeding at catheter site; catheter blocked, displaced, or leaking), ischemic heart disease, lethargy, malaise, nausea, pharyngitis, skin rash, vomiting, weakness

Drug Interactions

Metabolism/Transport Effects Inhibits CYP2C9 (strong)

Avoid Concomitant Use

Avoid concomitant use of Floxuridine with any of the following: BCG (Intravesical); Deferiprone; Dipyrone; Gimeracil; Natalizumab; Pimecrolimus; Tacrolimus (Topical); Vaccines (Live)

Increased Effect/Toxicity

Floxuridine may increase the levels/effects of: Alitretinoin (Systemic); Bosentan; Cannabis; Carvedilol; CloZAPine; CYP2C9 Substrates; Deferiprone; Diclofenac (Systemic); Dronabinol; Fingolimod; Fosphenytoin; Lacosamide; Leflunomide; Natalizumab; Ospemifene; Parecoxib; Phenytoin; Ramelteon; Tetrahydrocannabinol; Tofacitinib; Vaccines (Live)

The levels/effects of Floxuridine may be increased by: Cimetidine; Denosumab; Dipyrone; Gimeracil; Ocrelizumab; Palifermin; Pimecrolimus; Promazine; Roflumilast; Tacrolimus (Topical); Trastuzumab

Decreased Effect

Floxuridine may decrease the levels/effects of: BCG (Intravesical); Coccidioides immitis Skin Test; Lenograstim; Nivolumab; Sipuleucel-T; Tertomotide; Vaccines (Inactivated); Vaccines (Live)

The levels/effects of Floxuridine may be decreased by: Echinacea

Hazardous Drugs Handling Considerations

Hazardous agent (NIOSH 2016 [group 1]).

Use appropriate precautions for receiving, handling, administration, and disposal. Gloves (single) should be worn during receiving, unpacking, and placing in storage.

NIOSH recommends double gloving, a protective gown, ventilated engineering controls (a class II biological safety cabinet or a compounding aseptic containment isolator), and closed system transfer devices (CSTDs) for preparation. Double gloving, a gown, and (if dosage form allows) CSTDs are required during administration (NIOSH 2016).

Storage/Stability Store intact vials at 20°C to 25°C (68°F to 77°F). Reconstituted vials are stable for up to 2 weeks under refrigeration at 2°C to 8°C (36°F to 46°F).

Preparation for Administration Reconstitute with 5 mL SWFI for a final concentration of 100 mg/mL. Further dilute in D5W or NS to a volume appropriate for intra-arterial administration.

Mechanism of Action Floxuridine is catabolized to fluorouracil after intra-arterial administration, resulting in activity similar to fluorouracil; inhibits thymidylate synthetase and disrupts DNA and RNA synthesis.

Pharmacodynamics/Kinetics

Metabolism: Hepatic; Active metabolites: Floxuridine monophosphate (FUDR-MP) and fluorouracil; Inactive metabolites: Urea, CO_2, α-fluoro-β-alanine, α-fluoro-β-guanidopropionic acid, α-fluoro-β-ureidopropionic acid, and dihydrofluorouracil

Excretion: Urine (as fluorouracil, urea, α-fluoro-β-alanine, α-fluoro-β-guanidopropionic acid, α-fluoro-β-ureidopropionic acid, and dihydrofluorouracil; Respiratory (as exhaled gases [CO_2])

Dosing

Adult Colorectal cancer, hepatic metastases: Intra-arterial: 0.1-0.6 mg/kg/day as a continuous infusion; continue until intolerable toxicity

Renal Impairment No dosage adjustment provided in the manufacturer's labeling; use with extreme caution.

Hepatic Impairment No dosage adjustment provided in the manufacturer's labeling; use with extreme caution. The following adjustments have been recommended (Floyd, 2006):

Serum bilirubin 1.2 times ULN or alkaline phosphatase 1.2 times ULN: Administer 80% of dose

Serum bilirubin 1.5 times ULN; transaminases 3 times baseline or alkaline phosphatase 1.5 times ULN: Administer 50% of dose

Serum bilirubin 2 times ULN; transaminases >3 times baseline or alkaline phosphatase 2 times ULN: No recommendation is available

Obesity *ASCO Guidelines for appropriate chemotherapy dosing in obese adults with cancer:* Utilize patient's actual body weight (full weight) for calculation of body surface area- or weight-based dosing, particularly when the intent of therapy is curative; manage regimen-related toxicities in the same manner as for nonobese patients; if a dose reduction is utilized due to toxicity, consider resumption of full weight-based dosing with subsequent cycles, especially if cause of toxicity (eg, hepatic or renal impairment) is resolved (Griggs, 2012).

Adjustment for Toxicity

Hematologic: Discontinue if white blood count <3500/mm³ (or is falling rapidly) or if platelet count <100,000/mm³.

Nonhematologic toxicity: Discontinue for myocardial ischemia, stomatitis/esophagopharyngitis, vomiting (intractable), diarrhea, gastrointestinal ulceration/bleeding, hemorrhage (from any site).

Administration Administer as a continuous intra-arterial infusion using an infusion pump.

Emetic Potential Low (10% to 30%)

Monitoring Parameters CBC with differential and platelet count; liver function; signs/symptoms of stomatitis/esophagopharyngitis, gastrointestinal ulceration/bleeding, hemorrhage, vomiting, and diarrhea

Dosage Forms Excipient information presented when available (limited, particularly for generics); consult specific product labeling.
Solution Reconstituted, Injection:
  Generic: 0.5 g (1 ea)

♦ **Fluciclovine 18F** *see* Fluciclovine F 18 *on page 807*
♦ **Fluciclovine F-18** *see* Fluciclovine F 18 *on page 807*

Fluciclovine F 18 (floo SYE kloe veen ef AYE teen)
Brand Names: US Axumin
Index Terms Axumin; Fluciclovine 18F; Fluciclovine F-18
Pharmacologic Category Radiopharmaceutical
Use Diagnostic imaging: Positron emission tomography (PET) in men with suspected prostate cancer recurrence based on elevated blood prostate specific antigen (PSA) levels following prior treatment
Dosing
Adult & Geriatric Diagnostic imaging: IV: 370 MBq (10 mCi); begin PET scanning 3 to 5 minutes after completion of fluciclovine F 18 administration.
Renal Impairment There are no dosage adjustments provided in the manufacturer's labeling.
Hepatic Impairment There are no dosage adjustments provided in the manufacturer's labeling.
Additional Information Complete prescribing information should be consulted for additional detail.
Dosage Forms Excipient information presented when available (limited, particularly for generics); consult specific product labeling.
Solution, Intravenous:
  Axumin: 335-8200 MBq/mL (9-221 mCi/mL)

♦ **Flucinom** *see* Flutamide *on page 839*

Fluconazole (floo KOE na zole)
Brand Names: US Diflucan
Brand Names: Canada ACT Fluconazole; Apo-Fluconazole; CanesOral; CO Fluconazole; Diflucan; Diflucan injection; Diflucan One; Diflucan PWS; Dom-Fluconazole; Fluconazole Injection; Fluconazole Injection SDZ; Fluconazole Omega; Monicure; Mylan-Fluconazole; Novo-Fluconazole; PHL-Fluconazole; PMS-Fluconazole; PRO-Fluconazole; Riva-Fluconazole; Taro-Fluconazole
Index Terms Diflucan
Pharmacologic Category Antifungal Agent, Oral; Antifungal Agent, Parenteral
Use Treatment of candidiasis (esophageal, oropharyngeal, peritoneal, urinary tract, vaginal); systemic candida infections (eg, candidemia, disseminated candidiasis, and pneumonia); cryptococcal meningitis; antifungal prophylaxis in allogeneic bone marrow transplant recipients
Pregnancy Risk Factor C (single dose for vaginal candidiasis)/D (all other indications)
Hazardous Drugs Handling Considerations
Hazardous agent (NIOSH 2016 [group 3]).

Use appropriate precautions for receiving, handling, administration, and disposal. Gloves (single) should be worn during receiving, unpacking, and placing in storage.

◀ NIOSH recommends single gloving for administration of intact tablets or capsules. NIOSH recommends double gloving, a protective gown, and (if there is a potential for vomit or spit up) eye/face protection for administration of an oral liquid/feeding tube administration. For IV preparation, double gloves, a protective gown, ventilated engineering controls (a class II biological safety cabinet or a compounding aseptic containment isolator), and closed system transfer devices (CSTDs) are recommended for compounding. Double gloving and a gown are required during IV administration (NIOSH 2016). Assess risk to determine appropriate containment strategy (USP-NF 2017).

Dosing

Adult & Geriatric The daily dose of fluconazole is the same for both oral and IV administration

Usual dosage range: Oral, IV: 150 mg once **or** Loading dose: 200 to 800 mg; maintenance: 200 to 800 mg once daily; duration and dosage depend on location and severity of infection

Indication-specific dosing:

Blastomycosis (off-label use): Oral: *CNS disease:* Consolidation: 800 mg daily for ≥12 months and until resolution of CSF abnormalities (Chapman 2008)

Candidiasis:

Candidemia (neutropenic and non-neutropenic patients) (off-label dose) (IDSA [Pappas 2016]): Oral, IV:

Initial therapy (ie, first-line): Loading dose: 800 mg (12 mg/kg) on day 1, then 400 mg daily (6 mg/kg/day) for 14 days after first negative blood culture and resolution of signs/symptoms. **Note:** Not recommended as first-line therapy in patients with previous azole exposure, critical illness, or if at high risk of *C. glabrata* infection (elderly, diabetic, malignancy)

Step down therapy (ie, after patient has responded to initial therapy): Oral:

Isolates other than *C. glabrata*: 400 mg daily

Isolates of *C. glabrata* (fluconazole-susceptible): 800 mg daily

Duration: Continue for 14 days after first negative blood culture and resolution of signs/symptoms; step-down therapy to fluconazole (usually after 5 to 7 days in non-neutropenic patients) is recommended only in clinically stable patients with negative repeat cultures and fluconazole-susceptible isolates

Chronic, disseminated (hepatosplenic) (fluconazole-susceptible isolates): Oral: 400 mg daily (6 mg/kg/day) following several weeks of initial therapy with an amphotericin B lipid formulation or an echinocandin. Continue fluconazole until lesion resolution (usually several months) (IDSA [Pappas 2016])

CNS candidiasis: Oral, IV: 400 to 800 mg daily (6 to 12 mg/kg/day) as step-down therapy following initial therapy with liposomal amphotericin B (with or without flucytosine); continue fluconazole until signs/symptoms and CSF/radiological abnormalities have resolved (IDSA [Pappas 2016])

Empiric therapy, suspected invasive candidiasis (non-neutropenic patients in the ICU) (alternative therapy) (off-label use): Oral, IV: Loading dose: 800 mg (12 mg/kg) on day 1, then 400 mg daily (6 mg/kg/day); treatment should continue for 14 days in patients with clinical improvement. Consider discontinuing after 4 to 5 days in patients with no clinical response. **Note:** Not recommended for patients with previous azole exposure or those colonized with azole-resistant *Candida* spp. (Pappas [IDSA 2016])

Endophthalmitis (with or without vitritis): Oral, IV: Loading dose: 800 mg (12 mg/kg) on day 1, then 400 to 800 mg daily (6 to 12 mg/kg/day) for at least 4 to 6 weeks until examination indicates resolution; for patients with vitritis or with macular involvement (with or without vitritis), an intravitreal injection with voriconazole or amphotericin B deoxycholate is also recommended (IDSA [Pappas 2016])

Esophageal: Oral, IV:

Manufacturer's labeling: Loading dose: 200 mg on day 1, then maintenance dose of 100 to 400 mg daily for 21 days and for at least 2 weeks following resolution of symptoms

Alternate recommendations: 200 to 400 mg daily for 14 to 21 days; chronic suppressive therapy of 100 to 200 mg 3 times weekly may be used for recurrent infections (IDSA [Pappas 2016])

Intertrigo (off-label use): Oral, IV: 50 mg daily or 150 mg once weekly (Coldiron 1991; Nozickova 1998; Stengel 1994)

Intra-abdominal infections: Oral, IV: Loading dose: 800 mg (12 mg/kg) on day 1, then 400 mg daily (6 mg/kg/day); duration of therapy determined by clinical response and source control (IDSA [Pappas 2016])

Intravascular infections (IDSA [Pappas 2016]): Oral, IV:

Endocarditis, native or prosthetic valve: 400 to 800 mg daily (6 to 12 mg/kg/day) for at least 6 weeks after valve replacement surgery (longer durations recommended in patients with perivalvular abscesses or other complications; fluconazole should only be used as step-down therapy in clinically stable, culture-negative patients following initial therapy with an amphotericin B lipid formulation (with or without flucytosine) or an echinocandin; long-term or chronic suppressive therapy with fluconazole in absence of valve replacement surgery or in patients with a prosthetic valve endocarditis: 400 to 800 mg daily

Implantable cardiac devices (eg, pacemaker, ICD, VAD) infection: 400 to 800 mg daily (6 to 12 mg/kg/day) for 4 to 6 weeks after device removal (4 weeks for infections limited to generator pockets and at least 6 weeks for infections involving the wires); fluconazole should only be used as step-down in clinically stable, culture-negative patients following initial therapy with an amphotericin B lipid formulation (with or without flucytosine) or an echinocandin; chronic suppressive therapy with fluconazole (following initial antifungal therapy) when VAD cannot be removed and as long as device remains in place: 400 to 800 mg daily

Thrombophlebitis, suppurative: 400 to 800 mg daily (6 to 12 mg/kg/day) for at least 2 weeks after candidemia has cleared; fluconazole may be used as initial therapy or as step-down therapy following initial therapy with an amphotericin B lipid formulation or an echinocandin in clinically stable patients with fluconazole-susceptible isolates.

Oropharyngeal: Oral, IV:

Manufacturer's labeling: Loading dose: 200 mg on day 1; maintenance dose 100 mg daily for ≥2 weeks. **Note:** Therapy with 100 mg daily is associated with resistance development (Rex 1995).

Alternate recommendations: 100 to 200 mg daily for 7 to 14 days for moderate-to-severe disease; in patients with recurrent infection, chronic therapy of 100 mg 3 times weekly is recommended, if required (IDSA [Pappas 2016])

Osteoarticular (osteomyelitis or septic arthritis): Oral, IV: 400 mg daily (6 mg/kg/day) for 6 to 12 months (osteomyelitis) or 6 weeks (septic arthritis); alternatively, fluconazole 400 mg daily for 6 to 12 months (osteomyelitis) or at least 4 weeks (septic arthritis) may also be used following 2 weeks of initial treatment with an echinocandin or an amphotericin B lipid formulation. In patients with fluconazole-susceptible isolates and septic arthritis involving a prosthetic device which cannot be removed, chronic suppressive therapy with fluconazole 400 mg daily is recommended (IDSA [Pappas 2016])

Peritonitis: Oral, IV: 50-200 mg/day. **Note:** Some clinicians do not recommend using <200 mg daily (Chen 2004).

Prophylaxis: Oral, IV:

Bone marrow transplant: 400 mg once daily. Patients anticipated to have severe granulocytopenia should start therapy several days prior to the anticipated onset of neutropenia and continue for 7 days after the neutrophil count is >1000 mm^3.

High-risk ICU patients in units with high incidence of invasive candidiasis (off-label use): Loading dose: 800 mg (12 mg/kg) on day 1, then 400 mg once daily (6 mg/kg/day) (IDSA [Pappas 2016])

Peritoneal dialysis associated infection (concurrently treated with antibiotics), prevention of secondary fungal infection: 200 mg every 48 hours (Restrepo 2010)

Solid organ transplant: 200 to 400 mg once daily for at least 7 to 14 days (Pappas 2009)

Surgical (perioperative) prophylaxis in high-risk patients undergoing liver, pancreas, kidney, or pancreas-kidney transplantation (off-label use): IV: 400 mg given in the perioperative period and continued in the postoperative period for ≤28 days. Time of initiation and duration varies with transplant type and operative protocol (Bratzler 2013).

Urinary tract infections:

Manufacturer's labeling: UTI: Oral, IV: 50 to 200 mg once daily

Alternate recommendations (IDSA [Pappas 2016]):

Candiduria (asymptomatic), patients undergoing a urologic procedure: Oral: 400 mg once daily (6 mg/kg/day) several days before and after the procedure.

Cystitis (symptomatic): Oral: 200 mg once daily (3 mg/kg/day) for 2 weeks

Fungus balls: Oral: 200 to 400 mg once daily (3 to 6 mg/kg/day); concomitant irrigation of amphotericin B deoxycholate via nephrostomy tubes, if present, is also recommended

Pyelonephritis: Oral: 200 to 400 mg once daily for 2 weeks

Vaginal/Vulvovaginal: Oral:

Uncomplicated: Manufacturer's labeling: 150 mg as a single dose

Complicated or severe: 150 mg every 72 hours for 2 or 3 doses (Pappas [IDSA 2016]) **or** 150 mg every 72 hours for 2 doses (CDC [Workowski 2015])

Recurrent: 150 mg once daily for 10 to 14 days, followed by 150 mg once weekly for 6 months (Pappas 2009) **or** fluconazole 100 mg, 150 mg, or 200 mg every 72 hours (day 1, 4, and 7) for a total of 3 doses, then 100 mg, 150 mg, or 200 mg once weekly for 6 months (CDC [Workowski 2015])

Coccidioidomycosis, treatment (off-label use):
HIV-infected (HHS [OI adult 2015]):
  Meningeal infections (consultation with specialist is advised): IV, Oral: 400 to 800 mg once daily; patients who complete initial therapy should be considered for lifelong suppressive therapy using fluconazole 400 mg once daily if CD4 counts remain <250 cells/mm^3.
  Mild infections (eg, focal pneumonia): Oral: 400 mg once daily; patients who complete initial therapy should be considered for lifelong suppressive therapy using fluconazole 400 mg once daily if CD4 counts remain <250 cells/mm^3.
Non-HIV infected:
  Extrapulmonary, bone and/or joint infection: Oral: A minimum dose of 800 mg once daily for 3 years to lifetime, depending on severity and host immunocompetence. **Note:** Amphotericin B may be used initially for severe disease and then switched to fluconazole (IDSA [Galgiani 2016])
  Extrapulmonary, soft tissue infection (not associated with bone infection): Oral: 400 mg once daily (some experts use up to 800 mg once daily) for a minimum of 6 to 12 months (IDSA [Galgiani 2016])
  HSCT (allogenic or autologous) or solid organ transplant clinically stable patients with active pulmonary infections (acute or chronic): Oral: 400 mg once daily, continued indefinitely or until discontinuation of antirejection therapy (IDSA [Galgiani 2016])
  Meningitis: Oral: Initial: 400 to 1200 mg once daily with a lifelong duration (IDSA [Galgiani 2016])
  Pneumonia, uncomplicated: Oral: 400 mg once daily (some experts use 800 mg once daily) for 3 to 6 months or longer, depending on response. **Note:** Antifungal treatment is recommended only for patients with severely debilitating illness or with extensive pulmonary involvement, concurrent diabetes, or frailty due to age or comorbidities (IDSA [Galgiani 2016])
  Pneumonia, symptomatic chronic cavitary: Oral: 400 mg once daily for 12 months (Galgiani 2000; IDSA [Galgiani 2016])
Coccidioidomycosis, prophylaxis (off-label use): Oral:
HIV-infected patients (HHS [OI adult 2015]):
  Primary prophylaxis in patients with a new positive IgM or IgG serologic test who live in disease-endemic areas and have CD4 counts <250 cells/mm^3: 400 mg once daily
  Chronic suppressive therapy (secondary prophylaxis): 400 mg once daily
Non-HIV-infected patients:
  Solid organ transplant patients: **Note:** The suggested regimens are for patients without active coccidioioimycosis who are undergoing organ transplantation in an endemic area.
    Seronegative patients: 200 mg once daily for 6 to 12 months (IDSA [Galgiani 2016]
    Seropositive patients: 400 mg once daily for 6 to 12 months (IDSA [Galgiani 2016]
Cryptococcosis:
Meningitis:
  Manufacturer's labeling: Oral, IV: 400 mg for 1 dose, then 200 to 400 mg once daily for 10 to 12 weeks following negative CSF culture

Alternate dosing: HIV-infected:

Induction (alternative to preferred therapy): Oral, IV: 800 to 1,200 mg once daily with concomitant flucytosine for 6 weeks (Perfect 2010) **or** 400 to 800 mg once daily with concomitant flucytosine for at least 2 weeks (HHS [OI adult 2015]) **or** 1,200 mg once daily as monotherapy for at least 2 weeks (HHS [OI adult 2015])

Consolidation (preferred therapy): Oral, IV: 400 mg once daily for at least 8 weeks (HHS [OI adult 2015])

Maintenance (suppression) (preferred therapy): Oral: 200 mg once daily for at least 12 months; maintenance therapy may be stopped if the following criteria are fulfilled: induction, consolidation, and at least 12 months of maintenance therapy has been completed, patient remains asymptomatic from cryptococcal infection, and CD4 count ≥100 cells/mm^3 for ≥3 months and HIV RNA suppressed in response to effective ART (HHS [OI adult 2015])

Pulmonary (immunocompetent) (off-label use): 400 mg once daily for 6 to 12 months (Perfect 2010)

Pediatric The daily dose of fluconazole is the same for oral and IV administration

Usual dosage range: Oral, IV: Loading dose: 6 to 12 mg/kg/dose; maintenance: 3 to 12 mg/kg/dose once daily; duration and dosage depend on location and severity of infection

Indication-specific dosing:

Candidiasis: Oral, IV:

Esophageal:

Manufacturer's recommendation: Loading dose: 6 mg/kg/dose; maintenance: 3-12 mg/kg/dose once daily for 21 days and for at least 2 weeks following resolution of symptoms (maximum: 600 mg/day)

HIV-exposed/-infected: Loading dose: 6 mg/kg/dose once on day 1; maintenance: 3 to 6 mg/kg/dose once daily for 4 to 21 days (maximum: 400 mg/day) (CDC 2009)

Relapse suppression (HIV-exposed/-infected): 3 to 6 mg/kg/dose once daily (maximum: 200 mg/day) (CDC 2009)

Invasive disease (alternative therapy): 5 to 6 mg/kg/dose every 12 hours for ≥28 days (maximum: 600 mg/day) (CDC 2009)

Oropharyngeal:

Manufacturer's recommendation: Loading dose: 6 mg/kg/dose; maintenance: 3 mg/kg/dose once daily for ≥2 weeks (maximum: 600 mg/day)

HIV-exposed/-infected: 3 to 6 mg/kg/dose once daily for 7 to 14 days (maximum: 400 mg/day) (CDC 2009)

Surgical (perioperative) prophylaxis in high-risk patients undergoing liver, pancreas, kidney, or pancreas-kidney transplantation (off-label use): IV: 6 mg/kg given in the perioperative period and continued in the postoperative period for ≤28 days (maximum dose 400 mg). Time of initiation and duration varies with transplant type and operative protocol (Bratzler 2013).

Coccidioidomycosis: Oral, IV:

Children: *Meningeal infection, or in a stable patient with diffuse pulmonary or disseminated disease (HIV-exposed/-infected):*

Treatment: 5 to 6 mg/kg/dose twice daily (maximum daily dose: 800 mg/**day**) (CDC 2009) followed by chronic suppressive therapy (see below)

Relapse suppression: 6 mg/kg/dose once daily (maximum daily dose: 400 mg/**day**) (CDC 2009)

Adolescents: Treatment, primary prophylaxis, or chronic suppressive therapy (secondary prophylaxis): Refer to adult dosing.

Cryptococcosis: Oral, IV:

Meningitis: Manufacturer's labeling: 12 mg/kg/dose for 1 dose, then 6 to 12 mg/kg/day for 10-12 weeks following negative CSF culture

HIV-exposed/-infected:

CNS disease (alternative therapy in patients intolerant of amphotericin B): Children:

Induction: 12 mg/kg/dose for 1 dose, then 6 to 12 mg/kg/day (maximum: 800 mg/day) for ≥2 weeks (in combination with flucytosine) (CDC 2009)

Consolidation: 10 to 12 mg/kg/day for 8 weeks (Perfect 2010) **or** 12 mg/kg/dose for 1 dose, then 6 to 12 mg/kg/day (maximum: 800 mg/day) for 8 weeks (CDC 2009)

Maintenance (suppression): 6 mg/kg/day (maximum: 200 mg/day) (CDC 2009; Perfect 2010)

Adolescents: Refer to adult dosing.

Non-CNS disease, disseminated (including severe pulmonary disease) (alternative therapy; off-label use): Induction: 12 mg/kg/dose for 1 dose, then 6 to 12 mg/kg/day (maximum: 600 mg/day) (CDC 2009)

Non-CNS disease, localized (including isolated pulmonary disease) (off-label use): 12 mg/kg/dose for 1 dose, then 6 to 12 mg/kg/day (maximum: 600 mg/day). **Note:** Duration depends upon infection site and severity (CDC 2009). For patients with pulmonary disease (not delineated by severity), the IDSA recommends a duration of 6 to 12 months (Perfect 2010).

Primary antifungal prophylaxis in pediatric oncology patients (guideline recommendations; Science 2014): Oral, IV:

Allogeneic hematopoietic stem cell transplant (HSCT): Infants ≥1 month, Children, and Adolescents <19 years: 6 to 12 mg/kg/day (maximum: 400 mg/day), begin at the start of conditioning; continue until engraftment

Allogeneic HSCT with grades 2 to 4 acute graft-versus-host-disease (GVHD) or chronic extensive GVHD: Begin with GVHD diagnosis, continue until GVHD resolves:

Infants ≥1 month and Children <13 years: 6 to 12 mg/kg/day (maximum: 400 mg/day)

Adolescents ≥13 years (where posaconazole is contraindicated): 6 to 12 mg/kg/day (maximum: 400 mg/day)

Autologous HSCT with neutropenia anticipated >7 days: Infants ≥1 month, Children, and Adolescents <19 years: 6 to 12 mg/kg/day (maximum: 400 mg/day), begin at the start of conditioning; continue until engraftment

Acute myeloid leukemia (AML) or myelodysplastic syndromes (MDS): Infants ≥1 month, Children, and Adolescents <19 years: 6 to 12 mg/kg/day (maximum: 400 mg/day) during chemotherapy associated neutropenia; alternative antifungals may be suggested for children ≥13 years in centers with a high local incidence of mold infections or if fluconazole is not available

Renal Impairment

Manufacturer's labeling: **Note:** Renal function estimated using the Cockcroft-Gault formula

No adjustment for vaginal candidiasis single-dose therapy

For multiple dosing in adults, administer loading dose of 50 to 400 mg, then adjust daily doses as follows (dosage reduction in children should parallel adult recommendations):

CrCl >50 mL/minute: No dosage adjustment necessary

CrCl ≤50 mL/minute (no dialysis): Reduce dose by 50%

End-stage renal disease on intermittent hemodialysis (IHD):

Manufacturer's labeling: 100% of daily dose (according to indication) after each dialysis session; on nondialysis days, patient should receive a reduced dose according to their CrCl.

Alternate recommendations: Doses of 200 to 400 mg every 48 to 72 hours **or** 100 to 200 mg every 24 hours have been recommended. **Note:** Dosing dependent on the assumption of 3 times/week, complete IHD sessions (Heintz 2009).

Continuous renal replacement therapy (CRRT) (Heintz 2009; Trotman 2005): Drug clearance is highly dependent on the method of renal replacement, filter type, and flow rate. Appropriate dosing requires close monitoring of pharmacologic response, signs of adverse reactions due to drug accumulation, as well as drug concentrations in relation to target trough (if appropriate). The following are general recommendations only (based on dialysate flow/ultrafiltration rates of 1 to 2 L/hour and minimal residual renal function) and should not supersede clinical judgment:

CVVH: Loading dose of 400 to 800 mg followed by 200 to 400 mg every 24 hours

CVVHD/CVVHDF: Loading dose of 400 to 800 mg followed by 400 to 800 mg every 24 hours (CVVHD or CVVHDF) **or** 800 mg every 24 hours (CVVHDF)

Note: Higher maintenance doses of 400 mg every 24 hours (CVVH), 800 mg every 24 hours (CVVHD), and 500 to 600 mg every 12 hours (CVVHDF) may be considered when treating resistant organisms and/or when employing combined ultrafiltration and dialysis flow rates of ≥2 L/hour for CVVHD/CVVHDF (Heintz 2009; Trotman 2005).

Hepatic Impairment There are no dosage adjustments provided in the manufacturer's labeling; use with caution.

Additional Information Complete prescribing information should be consulted for additional detail.

Dosage Forms Excipient information presented when available (limited, particularly for generics); consult specific product labeling.

Solution, Intravenous:

Generic: 100 mg (50 mL); 200 mg (100 mL); 400 mg (200 mL)

Solution, Intravenous [preservative free]:

Generic: 200 mg (100 mL); 400 mg (200 mL)

Suspension Reconstituted, Oral:

Diflucan: 10 mg/mL (35 mL); 40 mg/mL (35 mL) [orange flavor]

Generic: 10 mg/mL (35 mL); 40 mg/mL (35 mL)

Tablet, Oral:

Diflucan: 50 mg, 100 mg, 150 mg, 200 mg

Generic: 50 mg, 100 mg, 150 mg, 200 mg

◆ **Fluconazole Injection (Can)** *see* Fluconazole *on page 807*

◆ **Fluconazole Injection SDZ (Can)** *see* Fluconazole *on page 807*

◆ **Fluconazole Omega (Can)** *see* Fluconazole *on page 807*

Flucytosine (floo SYE toe seen)
Brand Names: US Ancobon
Index Terms 5-FC; 5-Fluorocytosine; 5-Flurocytosine
Pharmacologic Category Antifungal Agent, Oral
Use Candida/Cryptococcus infections: Adjunctive treatment of systemic fungal infections (eg, septicemia, endocarditis, UTI, meningitis, or pulmonary) caused by susceptible strains of *Candida* or *Cryptococcus*
Pregnancy Risk Factor C
Dosing
Adult & Geriatric Usual dosage ranges: Oral: 50 to 150 mg/kg/day in divided doses every 6 hours

Candidiasis (off-label dose) (IDSA [Pappas 2016]): Oral:

Central nervous system (eg, meningitis): 25 mg/kg/dose 4 times daily (with amphotericin B [liposomal]) until step-down therapy is clinically appropriate.

Cystitis, symptomatic: Fluconazole-resistant *C. glabrata*: 25 mg/kg/dose 4 times daily for 7 to 10 days as monotherapy.

Endocarditis (native or prosthetic valve) or infected implantable cardiac devices (eg, pacemaker, ICD, VAD): 25 mg/kg/dose 4 times daily (with an amphotericin B lipid formulation); for native or prosthetic valve endocarditis, therapy should continue for at least 6 weeks after valve replacement surgery (longer durations in patients with abscesses or other complications); for patients with implantable cardiac devices, therapy should continue for 4 to 6 weeks after surgery (4 weeks for infections limited to generator pockets and at least 6 weeks for infections involving the wires). **Note:** May transition to fluconazole if patient clinically stable with fluconazole-susceptible isolates in whom *Candida* has cleared from the bloodstream.

Endophthalmitis (with or without vitritis): Fluconazole- or voriconazole-resistant isolates: 25 mg/kg/dose 4 times daily (with amphotericin B [liposomal]) for at least 4 to 6 weeks until examination indicates resolution; for patients with vitritis or with macular involvement (with or without vitritis), an intravitreal injection with voriconazole or amphotericin B deoxycholate is also recommended.

Pyelonephritis, symptomatic: Fluconazole-resistant *C. glabrata*: 25 mg/kg/dose 4 times daily in combination with amphotericin B deoxycholate for 1 to 7 days or as monotherapy for 14 days.

Cryptococcal meningitis, treatment: Oral:

Non-HIV-infected, non-transplant: Induction: 25 mg/kg/dose (with amphotericin B) every 6 hours for at least 4 weeks; if clinical and microbiological improvement, may discontinue both amphotericin and flucytosine and follow with an extended course of fluconazole (IDSA [Perfect 2010]).

HIV-infected or solid organ transplant recipients: Induction: 25 mg/kg/dose (with amphotericin B) every 6 hours for at least 2 weeks; if clinical and microbiological improvement, may discontinue both amphotericin and flucytosine and follow with an extended course of fluconazole (HHS [OI adult 2017]; IDSA [Perfect 2010]).

Cerebral cryptococcomas: Induction: 25 mg/kg/dose (with amphotericin B and corticosteroids) every 6 hours for at least 6 weeks, followed with an extended course of fluconazole (IDSA [Perfect 2010])

◄ **Pediatric**

General dosing, susceptible infections: Infants, Children, and Adolescents (off-label population): Oral: 50 to 150 mg/kg/**day** in divided doses every 6 hours (*Red Book* [AAP 2015])

Cryptococcal meningitis, treatment:

Non-HIV-infected: Children (off-label population): Oral: Induction: 25 mg/kg/dose (with amphotericin B) every 6 hours for at least 4 weeks; if clinical improvement, may discontinue both amphotericin and flucytosine and follow with an extended course of fluconazole (Perfect 2010).

HIV-infected: Adolescents (off-label population): Refer to adult dosing.

Renal Impairment Adults: The manufacturer recommends dose reduction for elevated BUN or serum creatinine (or other signs of renal impairment); however, no specific dosage adjustments are provided. The following adjustments have been recommended (based on a usual dose of 25 mg/kg/dose every 6 hours):

CrCl >40 mL/minute: No dosage adjustment necessary (HHS [OI adult 2017]; IDSA [Perfect 2010])

CrCl 20 to 40 mL/minute: 25 mg/kg/dose every 12 hours (HHS [OI adult 2017])

CrCl 10 to 20 mL/minute: 25 mg/kg/dose every 24 hours (HHS [OI adult 2017])

CrCl <10 mL/minute: 25 mg/kg/dose every 48 hours (HHS [OI adult 2017])

ESRD on intermittent hemodialysis (IHD): 25 to 50 mg/kg/dose every 48 to 72 hours; administer dose after hemodialysis (Drew 1999; HHS [OI adult 2017])

Infants, Children, and Adolescents: The following adjustments have been recommended:

Aronoff 2007: Infants, Children, and non-HIV-exposed/positive Adolescents (based on a usual dose of 100 to 150 mg/kg/**day** divided every 6 hours):

GFR >50 mL/minute/1.73 m^2: No dosage adjustment necessary.

GFR 30 to 50 mL/minute/1.73 m^2: 25 to 37.5 mg/kg/dose every 8 hours

GFR 10 to 29 mL/minute/1.73 m^2: 25 to 37.5 mg/kg/dose every 12 hours

GFR <10 mL/minute/1.73 m^2: 25 to 37.5 mg/kg/dose every 24 hours

Hemodialysis: 25 to 37.5 mg/kg/dose every 24 hours

Peritoneal dialysis: 25 to 37.5 mg/kg/dose every 24 hours

Continuous renal replacement therapy: 25 to 37.5 mg/kg/dose every 8 hours (monitor serum concentrations)

HHS [OI pediatric] 2016: HIV-exposed/-positive: Children: Severe renal impairment: Avoid use.

HHS [OI adult] 2017: HIV-exposed/-positive: Adolescents (based on a usual dose of 25 mg/kg/dose every 6 hours):

CrCl >40 mL/minute: No dosage adjustment necessary.

CrCl 20 to 40 mL/minute: 25 mg/kg/dose every 12 hours

CrCl 10 to 20 mL/minute: 25 mg/kg/dose every 24 hours

CrCl <10 mL/minute: 25 mg/kg/dose every 48 hours

ESRD on hemodialysis: 25 to 50 mg/kg/dose every 48 to 72 hours; administer dose after hemodialysis

Hepatic Impairment There are no dosage adjustments provided in the manufacturer's labeling; use with caution.

Additional Information Complete prescribing information should be consulted for additional detail.

Dosage Forms Excipient information presented when available (limited, particularly for generics); consult specific product labeling.
Capsule, Oral:
Ancobon: 250 mg, 500 mg
Generic: 250 mg, 500 mg

◆ **Fludara** *see* Fludarabine *on page 817*

◆ **Fludara [DSC]** *see* Fludarabine *on page 817*

Fludarabine (floo DARE a been)

Related Information
Hematopoietic Cell Transplantation *on page 2365*
Management of Chemotherapy-Induced Nausea and Vomiting in Adults *on page 2253*
Prevention of Chemotherapy-Induced Nausea and Vomiting in Children *on page 2310*
Safe Handling of Hazardous Drugs *on page 2379*

Brand Names: US Fludara [DSC]

Brand Names: Canada Fludara; Fludarabine Phosphate for Injection; Fludarabine Phosphate for Injection, USP; Fludarabine Phosphate Injection, PPC STD.

Index Terms 2F-ara-AMP; Fludara; Fludarabine Monophosphate; Fludarabine Phosphate

Pharmacologic Category Antineoplastic Agent, Antimetabolite; Antineoplastic Agent, Antimetabolite (Purine Analog)

Use Chronic lymphocytic leukemia (refractory or progressive): Treatment of B-cell chronic lymphocytic leukemia (CLL) in adults who have not responded to or have progressed during treatment with at least one standard regimen containing an alkylating agent.

Labeled Contraindications
There are no contraindications listed in the manufacturer's US labeling.
Canadian labeling: Hypersensitivity to fludarabine or any component of the formulation; severe renal impairment (CrCl <30 mL/minute); decompensated hemolytic anemia; concurrent use with pentostatin

Pregnancy Considerations Adverse events were observed in animal reproduction studies. Based on the mechanism of action, fludarabine may cause fetal harm if administered during pregnancy. Effective contraception should be used to avoid pregnancy during and after treatment for women and men with female partners of reproductive potential.

Breastfeeding Considerations It is not known if fludarabine is present in breast milk. Due to the potential for serious adverse reactions in the breastfeeding infant, a decision should be made to discontinue breastfeeding or to discontinue fludarabine, taking into account the importance of treatment to the mother.

◄ **Warnings/Precautions [US Boxed Warning]: Life-threatening (and sometimes fatal) autoimmune effects, including hemolytic anemia, autoimmune thrombocytopenia/thrombocytopenic purpura (ITP), Evans syndrome, and acquired hemophilia have occurred; evaluate and monitor closely for hemolysis.** This has occurred in patients with and without a history of autoimmune hemolytic anemia or a positive Coombs test, and who may or may not be in remission from their disease. Corticosteroids may or may not effectively control the hemolytic episodes. Discontinue fludarabine if hemolysis occurs. The hemolytic effects recurred in most patients when rechallenged with fludarabine. Bone marrow suppression: **[US Boxed Warning]: Severe bone marrow suppression (anemia, thrombocytopenia, and neutropenia) may occur;** may be cumulative. The median time to nadir was 13 days (range: 3 to 25 days) for granulocytes and 16 days (range: 2 to 32 days) for platelets. Severe myelosuppression (trilineage bone marrow hypoplasia/aplasia) has been reported (rare) with a duration of significant cytopenias ranging from 2 months to 1 year. First-line combination therapy is associated with prolonged cytopenias, with anemia lasting up to 7 months, neutropenia up to 9 months, and thrombocytopenia up to 10 months; increased age is predictive for prolonged cytopenias (Gill 2010). Monitor patients with bone marrow impairment closely for excess toxicity; may require dosage reductions.

[US Boxed Warning]: Higher than recommended doses (up to 96 mg/m^2/day for 5 to 7 days) are associated with severe neurologic toxicity (delayed blindness, coma, death); similar neurotoxicity (agitation, coma, confusion, seizure) has been reported (rare) with standard CLL doses (25 mg/m^2/day for 5 days). Symptoms of neurotoxicity due to high doses appeared from 21 to 60 days following the last fludarabine dose, although neurotoxicity has been reported as early as 7 days and up to 225 days. Although administration of up to 15 courses of treatment have been used, the possible neurotoxic effects of chronic administration are unknown. Fatigue, weakness, visual disturbances, confusion, and seizures may occur; caution patients about performing tasks which require mental alertness (eg, operating machinery or driving).

Serious and sometimes fatal infections, including opportunistic infections and reactivations of latent viral infections such as VZV (herpes zoster) and Epstein-Barr virus have been reported with fludarabine. Prophylactic anti-infectives should be considered for patients with an increased risk for developing opportunistic infections. Use with caution in patients with documented infection, fever, immunodeficiency, or with a history of opportunistic infection. Progressive multifocal leukoencephalopathy (PML) (usually fatal) due to JC virus has been reported; most cases were in patients who had received prior and/or other concurrent chemotherapy. Onset may be a few weeks or may be delayed up to 1 year. Evaluate any neurological change promptly. May cause tumor lysis syndrome; risk is increased in patients with large tumor burden prior to treatment. Hydration and prophylactic antihyperuricemic therapy should be considered in patients at risk for tumor lysis syndrome. Graft-versus-host disease (GVHD) has been observed following transfusion of non-irradiated blood in patients treated with fludarabine; fatal outcome has been observed. Patients receiving fludarabine should only receive irradiated blood products due to the potential for transfusion-related GVHD.

[US Boxed Warning]: The use of fludarabine in combination with pentostatin (deoxycoformycin) for the treatment of refractory chronic lymphocytic leukemia has resulted in an unacceptably high incidence of fatal pulmonary toxicity. The use of fludarabine in combination with pentostatin is not recommended. Potentially significant drug-drug interactions may exist, requiring dose or frequency adjustment, additional monitoring, and/or selection of alternative therapy. Use with caution in patients with renal impairment; clearance of the primary metabolite 2-fluoro-ara-A is decreased in patients with renal impairment; dosage reductions are recommended (monitor closely for excessive toxicity) in patients with creatinine clearance between 30 and 79 mL/minute; use is not recommended if CrCl <30 mL/minute. Monitor the elderly closely for excessive toxicity; may require reduced doses. Avoid vaccination with live vaccines during and after fludarabine treatment. Fludarabine may damage testicular tissue and spermatozoa. **[US Boxed Warning]: Should be administered under the supervision of an experienced cancer chemotherapy physician.**

Adverse Reactions Frequency not always defined.

>10%:

Cardiovascular: Edema (8% to 19%)

Central nervous system: Fatigue (10% to 38%), neurological signs and symptoms (doses >96 mg/m^2 /day for 5 to 7 days: 36%; doses <125 mg/m^2/cycle: <1%; characterized by cortical blindness, coma, and paralysis; symptom onset may be delayed for 3 to 4 weeks), pain (20% to 22%), chills (11% to 19%), paresthesia (4% to 12%)

Dermatologic: Skin rash (15%), diaphoresis (1% to 13%)

Gastrointestinal: Nausea and vomiting (31% to 36%), anorexia (7% to 34%), diarrhea (13% to 15%), gastrointestinal hemorrhage (3% to 13%)

Genitourinary: Urinary tract infection (2% to 15%)

Hematologic & oncologic: Anemia (60%), neutropenia (grade 4: 59%; nadir: ~13 days), thrombocytopenia (55%; nadir: ~16 days), bone marrow depression (nadir: 10 to 14 days; recovery: 5 to 7 weeks; dose-limiting toxicity)

Infection: Infection (33% to 44%)

Neuromuscular & skeletal: Weakness (9% to 65%), myalgia (4% to 16%)

Ophthalmic: Visual disturbance (3% to 15%)

Respiratory: Cough (10% to 44%), pneumonia (16% to 22%), dyspnea (9% to 22%), upper respiratory tract infection (2% to 16%)

Miscellaneous: Fever (60% to 69%)

1% to 10%:

Cardiovascular: Angina pectoris (≤6%), cardiac arrhythmia (≤3%), cardiac failure (≤3%), cerebrovascular accident (≤3%), myocardial infarction (≤3%), supraventricular tachycardia (≤3%), deep vein thrombosis (1% to 3%), phlebitis (1% to 3%), aneurysm (≤1%), transient ischemic attacks (≤1%)

Central nervous system: Malaise (6% to 8%), headache (≤3%), sleep disorder (1% to 3%), cerebellar syndrome (≤1%), depression (≤1%), difficulty thinking (≤1%)

Dermatologic: Alopecia (≤3%), pruritus (1% to 3%), seborrhea (≤1%)

Endocrine & metabolic: Hyperglycemia (1% to 6%), dehydration (≤1%)

Gastrointestinal: Stomatitis (≤9%), cholelithiasis (≤3%), esophagitis (≤3%), constipation (1% to 3%), mucositis (≤2%), dysphagia (≤1%)

Genitourinary: Dysuria (3% to 4%), urinary hesitancy (≤3%), hematuria (2% to 3%), proteinuria (≤1%)

Hematologic & oncologic: Hemorrhage (≤1%), tumor lysis syndrome (≤1%)

Hepatic: Abnormal hepatic function tests (1% to 3%), hepatic failure (≤1%)

Hypersensitivity: Anaphylaxis (≤1%)

Neuromuscular & skeletal: Osteoporosis (≤2%), arthralgia (≤1%)

Otic: Hearing loss (2% to 6%)

Renal: Renal failure (≤1%), renal function test abnormality (≤1%)

Respiratory: Pharyngitis (≤9%), hypersensitivity pneumonitis (≤6%), hemoptysis (1% to 6%), sinusitis (≤5%), bronchitis (≤1%), epistaxis (≤1%), hypoxia (≤1%)

<1%, postmarketing, and/or case reports: Acquired blood coagulation disorder, acute myelocytic leukemia (usually associated with prior or concurrent treatment with other anticancer agents), adult respiratory distress syndrome, agitation, autoimmune hemolytic anemia, autoimmune thrombocytopenia, blindness, bone marrow aplasia (trilineage), bone marrow depression (trilineage), cerebral hemorrhage, coma, confusion, Epstein-Barr-associated lymphoproliferative disorder, erythema multiforme, Evans syndrome, flank pain, hemorrhagic cystitis, herpes zoster (reactivation), hyperkalemia, hyperphosphatemia, hyperuricemia, hypocalcemia, immune thrombocytopenia (autoimmune), increased liver enzymes, interstitial pneumonitis, malignant neoplasm of skin (new-onset or exacerbation), metabolic acidosis, myelodysplastic syndrome (usually associated with prior or concurrent treatment with other anticancer agents), myelofibrosis, opportunistic infection, optic neuritis, optic neuropathy, pancreatic disease (pancreatic enzymes abnormal), pancytopenia, pemphigus, pericardial effusion, peripheral neuropathy, pneumonitis, progressive multifocal leukoencephalopathy (PML), pulmonary fibrosis, pulmonary hemorrhage, reactivation of latent Epstein-Barr virus, respiratory distress, respiratory failure, seizure, Stevens-Johnson syndrome, toxic epidermal necrolysis, urate crystalluria, wrist-drop

Drug Interactions

Metabolism/Transport Effects None known.

Avoid Concomitant Use

Avoid concomitant use of Fludarabine with any of the following: BCG (Intravesical); Deferiprone; Dipyrone; Natalizumab; Pentostatin; Pimecrolimus; Tacrolimus (Topical); Vaccines (Live)

Increased Effect/Toxicity

Fludarabine may increase the levels/effects of: CloZAPine; Deferiprone; Fingolimod; Leflunomide; Natalizumab; Pentostatin; Tofacitinib; Vaccines (Live)

The levels/effects of Fludarabine may be increased by: Denosumab; Dipyrone; Ocrelizumab; Palifermin; Pentostatin; Pimecrolimus; Promazine; Roflumilast; Tacrolimus (Topical); Trastuzumab

Decreased Effect

Fludarabine may decrease the levels/effects of: BCG (Intravesical); Coccidioides immitis Skin Test; Lenograstim; Nivolumab; Sipuleucel-T; Tertomotide; Vaccines (Inactivated); Vaccines (Live)

The levels/effects of Fludarabine may be decreased by: Echinacea; Imatinib

Hazardous Drugs Handling Considerations

Hazardous agent (NIOSH 2016 [group 1]).

Use appropriate precautions for receiving, handling, administration, and disposal. Gloves (single) should be worn during receiving, unpacking, and placing in storage.

NIOSH recommends double gloving, a protective gown, ventilated engineering controls (a class II biological safety cabinet or a compounding aseptic containment isolator), and closed system transfer devices (CSTDs) for preparation. Double gloving, a gown, and (if dosage form allows) CSTDs are required during administration. In regions where an oral dosage form is available, NIOSH recommends single gloving for administration of intact tablets/capsules (NIOSH 2016).

Storage/Stability

IV: Store intact vials under refrigeration or at room temperature, as specified according to each manufacturer's labeling. Protect from light. Reconstituted solution or vials of the solution for injection that have been punctured (in use) should be used within 8 hours.

Tablet [Canadian product]: Store at 15°C to 30°C (59°F to 86°F); should be kept within packaging until use.

Preparation for Administration

Reconstitute lyophilized powder with 2 mL SWFI to a concentration of 25 mg/mL.

Dilute for infusion in 100 to 125 mL D5W or NS.

Mechanism of Action Fludarabine inhibits DNA synthesis by inhibition of DNA polymerase and ribonucleotide reductase; also inhibits DNA primase and DNA ligase I

Pharmacodynamics/Kinetics

Distribution: V_{ss}: 11 to 96 L/m^2 (Johnson 2000)

Protein binding: 2-fluoro-ara-A: ~19% to 29%

Metabolism: IV: Fludarabine phosphate is rapidly dephosphorylated in the plasma to 2-fluoro-ara-A (active metabolite), which subsequently enters tumor cells and is phosphorylated by deoxycytidine kinase to the active triphosphate derivative (2-fluoro-ara-ATP)

Bioavailability: Oral: 2-fluoro-ara-A: 50% to 65%

Half-life elimination: 2-fluoro-ara-A: Adults: ~20 hours

Time to peak, plasma: Oral: 1 to 2 hours

Excretion: Urine (primarily) (Johnson 2000)

Dosing

Adult & Geriatric

Chronic lymphocytic leukemia (CLL), refractory or progressive:

IV: 25 mg/m^2 once daily for 5 consecutive days every 28 days; continue for at least 3 additional cycles after maximal response is achieved

Oral (Canadian product; not available in US): 40 mg/m^2 once daily for 5 consecutive days every 28 days

CLL combination regimens (off-label dosing): IV:

FC regimen: 30 mg/m^2/day for 3 days every 28 days for 6 cycles (in combination with cyclophosphamide) (Eichhorst 2006) **or** 20 mg/m^2/day for 5 days every 28 days for 6 cycles (in combination with cyclophosphamide) (Flinn 2007)

FCR regimen: 25 mg/m^2/day for 3 days every 28 days for 6 cycles (in combination with cyclophosphamide and rituximab) (Keating 2005; Robak 2010; Wierda 2005)

FR regimen: 25 mg/m^2/day for 5 days every 28 days for 6 cycles (in combination with rituximab) (Byrd 2003)

OFAR regimen: 30 mg/m^2/day for 2 days every 28 days for 6 cycles (in combination with oxaliplatin, cytarabine, and rituximab) (Tsimberidou 2008)

Acute myeloid leukemia, newly diagnosed (off-label use): IV: 30 mg/m^2/day for 5 days (in combination with cytarabine ± G-CSF ± idarubicin (FA, FLAG, or FLAG-IDA regimens), followed by consolidation therapy (Borthakur 2008; Burnett 2013)

Acute myeloid leukemia, refractory or high/poor-risk patients (off-label use): IV: 30 mg/m^2/day for 5 days (in combination with cytarabine and filgrastim [FLAG regimen]), may repeat once for partial remission (Montillo 1998) **or** 30 mg/m^2/day for 5 days for 1 or 2 cycles (in combination with cytarabine, idarubicin, and filgrastim FLAG-IDA regimen]) (Virchis 2004)

Hematopoietic stem cell transplant (allogeneic) myeloablative conditioning regimen (off-label use): IV: 40 mg/m^2/day for 4 days (in combination with busulfan) beginning 6 days prior to transplantation (Rambaldi 2015).

Hematopoietic stem cell transplant (allogeneic) reduced-intensity conditioning regimen (off-label use): IV: 30 mg/m^2/day for 5 days (in combination with melphalan and alemtuzumab) prior to transplant (Tauro 2005) **or** 30 mg/m^2/day for 6 days beginning 10 days prior to transplant **or** 30 mg/m^2/day for 5 days beginning 6 days prior to transplant (in combination with busulfan with or without antithymocyte globulin) (Schetelig 2003)

Hematopoietic stem cell transplant (allogeneic) nonmyeloablative conditioning regimen (off-label use): IV: 30 mg/m^2/day for 3 doses beginning 5 days prior to transplant (in combination with cyclophosphamide and rituximab) (Khouri 2008) **or** 30 mg/m^2/day for 3 doses beginning 4 days prior to transplant (in combination with total body irradiation) (Hegenbart 2006; Rezvani 2008)

Non-Hodgkin lymphomas (off-label use): IV:

Follicular lymphoma, relapsed/refractory

FCR regimen: 25 mg/m^2/day for 3 days every 21 days for 4 cycles (in combination with cyclophosphamide and rituximab) (Sacchi 2007)

FCMR regimen: 25 mg/m^2/day for 3 days every 28 days for 4 cycles (in combination with cyclophosphamide, mitoxantrone, and rituximab) (Forstpointner 2004; Forstpointner 2006)

FNDR regimen: 25 mg/m^2/day for 3 days every 28 days for up to 8 cycles (in combination with mitoxantrone, dexamethasone, and rituximab) (McLaughlin 2000)

FR regimen: 25 mg/m^2/day for 5 days every 28 days for 6 cycles (in combination with rituximab) (Czuczman 2005)

Mantle cell lymphoma, relapsed or refractory:

FC regimen: 20 mg/m^2/day for 4 to 5 days or 25 mg/m^2/day for 3 to 5 days (in combination with cyclophosphamide) (Cohen 2001)

Waldenstrom macroglobulinemia (off-label use): IV: 25 mg/m^2/day for 5 days every 28 days (Foran 1999) **or** 25 mg/m^2 once daily for 5 days during weeks 5, 9, 13, 19, 23, and 27 (in combination with rituximab) (Treon 2009)

Pediatric

Acute lymphocytic leukemia, relapsed (off-label use): IV: 10.5 mg/m^2 bolus over 15 minutes followed by a continuous infusion of 30.5 mg/m^2/day for 48 hours in combination with cytarabine (Avramis 1998). Additional studies may be necessary to further define the role of fludarabine in the condition.

Acute myeloid leukemia, newly diagnosed (off-label use): IV: 10.5 mg/m^2 bolus infusion followed by a continuous infusion of 30.5 mg/m^2/day for 48 hours (in combination with cytarabine and idarubicin) during consolidation phase of treatment (Lange 2008)

Acute myeloid leukemia, relapsed (off-label use): IV: 10.5 mg/m^2 bolus over 15 minutes followed by a continuous infusion of 30.5 mg/m^2/day for 48 hours in combination with cytarabine (Avramis 1998). Additional studies may be necessary to further define the role of fludarabine in the condition.

Hematopoietic stem cell transplant (allogeneic), reduced-intensity conditioning regimen (off-label use): IV: 30 mg/m^2 once daily for 6 doses beginning 7 to 10 days prior to transplant (in combination with busulfan and antithymocyte globulin [rabbit]) (Pulsipher 2009)

Renal Impairment

Adults: CLL:

IV:

CrCl ≥80 mL/minute: No dosage adjustment necessary (administer the usual dose of 25 mg/m^2).

CrCl 50 to 79 mL/minute: Reduce dose to 20 mg/m^2.

CrCl 30 to 49 mL/minute: Reduce dose to 15 mg/m^2.

CrCl <30 mL/minute: Use is not recommended.

Oral (Canadian product; not available in US):

CrCl 30 to 70 mL/minute: Reduce dose by up to 50%.

CrCl <30 mL/minute: Use is contraindicated.

The following adjustments have also been used: Aronoff 2007: IV:

Adults:

CrCl 10 to 50 mL/minute: Reduce dose to 75% of usual dose.

CrCl <10 mL/minute: Reduce dose to 50% of usual dose.

Hemodialysis: Reduce dose to 50% of usual dose; administer after dialysis

Continuous ambulatory peritoneal dialysis (CAPD): Reduce dose to 50% of usual dose.

Continuous renal replacement therapy (CRRT): Reduce dose to 75% of usual dose.

Pediatrics:

CrCl 30 to 50 mL/minute: Reduce dose to 80% of usual dose.

CrCl <30 mL/minute: Use is not recommended.

Hemodialysis: Reduce dose to 25% of usual dose

Continuous ambulatory peritoneal dialysis (CAPD): Use is not recommended.

Continuous renal replacement therapy (CRRT): Reduce dose to 80% of usual dose.

Hepatic Impairment There are no dosage adjustments provided in the manufacturer's labeling.

Obesity

*American Society of Clinical Oncology (ASCO) Guidelines for appropriate chemotherapy dosing in obese adults with cancer (**Note:** Excludes leukemias and HSCT dosing):* Utilize patient's actual body weight (full weight) for calculation of body surface area- or weight-based dosing, particularly when the intent of therapy is curative; manage regimen-related toxicities in the same manner as for nonobese patients; if a dose reduction is utilized due to toxicity, consider resumption of full weight-based dosing with subsequent cycles, especially if cause of toxicity (eg, hepatic or renal impairment) is resolved (Griggs 2012).

American Society for Blood and Marrow Transplantation (ASBMT) practice guideline committee position statement on chemotherapy dosing in obesity: Utilize actual body weight (full weight) for calculation of body surface area

◀ in fludarabine dosing for hematopoietic stem cell transplant conditioning regimens in adults (Bubalo 2014).

Adjustment for Toxicity

Hematologic or nonhematologic toxicity (other than neurotoxicity): Consider treatment delay or dosage reduction.

Hemolysis: Discontinue treatment.

Neurotoxicity: Consider treatment delay or discontinuation.

Combination Regimens

Leukemia, acute myeloid:

FLAG (AML Induction) on page 2114

FLAG-IDA (AML Induction) on page 2115

Leukemia, chronic lymphocytic:

Fludarabine-Cyclophosphamide (CLL) on page 2116

Fludarabine-Cyclophosphamide-Ofatumumab (CLL) on page 2119

Fludarabine-Cyclophosphamide-Rituximab (CLL) on page 2119

Fludarabine-Rituximab (CLL) on page 2121

OFAR (CLL) on page 2181

Lymphoma, non-Hodgkin: Fludarabine-Mitoxantrone-Dexamethasone-Rituximab on page 2120

Lymphoma, non-Hodgkin (Follicular):

Fludarabine-Cyclophosphamide-Mitoxantrone-Rituximab (NHL-Follicular) on page 2117

Fludarabine-Cyclophosphamide-Rituximab (NHL-Follicular) on page 2120

Fludarabine-Rituximab (NHL-Follicular) on page 2122

Lymphoma, non-Hodgkin (Mantle Cell): Fludarabine-Cyclophosphamide (NHL-Mantle Cell) on page 2118

Administration

IV: The manufacturer recommends administering over ~30 minutes (for the treatment of CLL). Continuous infusions and IV bolus over 15 minutes have been used for some off-label protocols (refer to individual studies for infusion rate details).

Oral: Tablet [Canadian product] may be administered with or without food; should be swallowed whole with water; do not chew, break, or crush.

Emetic Potential Children and Adults:

Oral: Low (10% to 30%)

IV: Minimal (<10%)

Monitoring Parameters CBC with differential, platelet count, AST, ALT, serum creatinine, serum albumin, uric acid; monitor for signs of infection, neurotoxicity, and tumor lysis syndrome.

Dosage Forms Excipient information presented when available (limited, particularly for generics); consult specific product labeling. [DSC] = Discontinued product

Solution, Intravenous, as phosphate:

Generic: 50 mg/2 mL (2 mL)

Solution, Intravenous, as phosphate [preservative free]:

Generic: 50 mg/2 mL (2 mL)

Solution Reconstituted, Intravenous, as phosphate:

Fludara: 50 mg (1 ea [DSC])

Generic: 50 mg (1 ea)

Solution Reconstituted, Intravenous, as phosphate [preservative free]:

Generic: 50 mg (1 ea)

Dosage Forms: Canada Information with regard to form, strength, and availability of products uniquely available in Canada but currently not available in the US. Refer also to Dosage Forms.

Excipient information presented when available (limited, particularly for generics); consult specific product labeling.
Tablet, as phosphate:
  Fludara: 10 mg

◆ **Fludarabine Monophosphate** *see* Fludarabine *on page 817*

◆ **Fludarabine Phosphate** *see* Fludarabine *on page 817*

◆ **Fludarabine Phosphate for Injection (Can)** *see* Fludarabine *on page 817*

◆ **Fludarabine Phosphate for Injection, USP (Can)** *see* Fludarabine *on page 817*

◆ **Fludarabine Phosphate Injection, PPC STD. (Can)** *see* Fludarabine *on page 817*

◆ **Flugerel** *see* Flutamide *on page 839*

◆ **5-Fluorocytosine** *see* Flucytosine *on page 815*

◆ **Fluorodeoxyuridine** *see* Floxuridine *on page 804*

◆ **Fluoroplex** *see* Fluorouracil (Topical) *on page 835*

◆ **Fluoro Uracil** *see* Fluorouracil (Systemic) *on page 825*

◆ **5-Fluorouracil** *see* Fluorouracil (Systemic) *on page 825*

◆ **5-Fluorouracil** *see* Fluorouracil (Topical) *on page 835*

Fluorouracil (Systemic) (flure oh YOOR a sil)

Related Information
Management of Chemotherapy-Induced Nausea and Vomiting in Adults *on page 2253*
Management of Drug Extravasations *on page 2271*
Management of EGFR Inhibitor Toxicities: Dermatologic, Ocular, and Gastrointestinal *on page 2291*
Mucositis and Stomatitis *on page 2299*
Prevention of Chemotherapy-Induced Nausea and Vomiting in Children *on page 2310*
Safe Handling of Hazardous Drugs *on page 2379*

Brand Names: US Adrucil

Brand Names: Canada Fluorouracil Injection

Index Terms 5-Fluorouracil; 5-Fluracil; 5-FU; 5FU; Fluoro Uracil; Fluouracil; FU

Pharmacologic Category Antineoplastic Agent, Antimetabolite; Antineoplastic Agent, Antimetabolite (Pyrimidine Analog)

Use
Breast cancer: Management of breast cancer
Colon and rectal cancer: Management of colon and rectal cancer
Gastric cancer: Management of stomach (gastric) cancer
Pancreatic cancer: Management of pancreatic cancer

Labeled Contraindications There are no contraindications listed in the manufacturer's US labeling.

Canadian labeling: Known hypersensitivity to fluorouracil or any component of the formulation; debilitated patients; poor nutritional state; depressed bone marrow function following radiotherapy or therapy with other antineoplastic agents; potentially serious infections.

Pregnancy Considerations Adverse effects (increased resorptions, embryolethality, and teratogenicity) have been observed in animal reproduction studies. Based on the mechanism of action, fluorouracil may cause fetal harm if administered during pregnancy (according to the manufacturer's labeling). Females of reproductive potential and male patients with female partners of reproductive potential should use effective contraception during treatment and for 3 months following cessation of fluorouracil therapy.

Chemotherapy, if indicated, may be administered to pregnant women with breast cancer as part of a combination chemotherapy regimen (common regimens administered during pregnancy include doxorubicin [or epirubicin], cyclophosphamide, and fluorouracil); chemotherapy should not be administered during the first trimester, after 35 weeks' gestation, or within 3 weeks of planned delivery (Amant 2010; Loibl 2006). The European Society for Medical Oncology has published guidelines for diagnosis, treatment, and follow-up of cancer during pregnancy. The guidelines recommend referral to a facility with expertise in cancer during pregnancy and encourage a multidisciplinary team (obstetrician, neonatologist, oncology team). In general, if chemotherapy is indicated, it should be avoided during in the first trimester, there should be a 3-week time period between the last chemotherapy dose and anticipated delivery, and chemotherapy should not be administered beyond week 33 of gestation (Peccatori 2013).

Fertility (male and female) may be impaired during fluorouracil treatment.

Breastfeeding Considerations It is not known if fluorouracil is present in breast milk. Due to the potential for serious adverse reactions in the breastfed infant, the manufacturer recommends a decision be made to discontinue breastfeeding or to discontinue fluorouracil, taking into account the importance of treatment to the mother.

Warnings/Precautions Patients with select homozygous or compound heterozygous dihydropyrimidine dehydrogenase (DPD) gene mutations that result in complete or near complete absence of DPD activity are at increased risk for acute early-onset of toxicity and severe, life-threatening, or fatal adverse reactions (eg, mucositis, diarrhea, neutropenia, neurotoxicity) due to fluorouracil. Patients with partial DPD activity may also have increased risk of severe, life-threatening, or fatal adverse reactions when administered fluorouracil. Based on clinical assessment of toxicity onset, duration, and severity, withhold or permanently discontinue fluorouracil in patients with evidence of acute early-onset or unusually severe toxicity, which may indicate near complete or total absence of DPD activity. There is no fluorouracil dose that has been proven safe in patients with complete absence of DPD activity and data are insufficient to recommend a specific dose in patients with partial DPD activity as measured by any specific test.

Based on postmarketing reports, fluorouracil may cause cardiotoxicity (angina, MI/ischemia, arrhythmia, and heart failure). Risk factors for cardiotoxicity include continuous infusion administration (vs IV bolus) and coronary artery disease. Withhold fluorouracil for cardiotoxicity. The risks of resuming fluorouracil in patients with resolved cardiotoxicity have not been established. In a scientific statement from the AHA, fluorouracil has been determined to be an agent that may either cause reversible direct myocardial toxicity or exacerbate underlying myocardial dysfunction (magnitude: moderate/major) (AHA [Page 2016]). Fluorouracil may result in hyperammonemic encephalopathy in the absence of liver disease or other identifiable cause (postmarketing reports). The onset of hyperammonemic encephalopathy signs/symptoms (altered mental status, confusion, disorientation, coma, or ataxia in the presence of concomitant elevated serum ammonia level) was within 72 hours after fluorouracil infusion initiation. Withhold fluorouracil for hyperammonemic encephalopathy and initiate ammonia-lowering therapy. The risks of resuming fluorouracil in patients with resolved hyperammonemic encephalopathy have not been established. Fluorouracil may cause neurologic toxicity, including acute cerebellar syndrome and other neurologic events (postmarketing reports). Neurologic symptoms included confusion, disorientation, ataxia, or visual disturbances. Withhold fluorouracil for neurologic toxicity. There are insufficient data on the risks of resuming fluorouracil in patients with resolved neurologic toxicity.

Fluorouracil is associated with severe diarrhea. Withhold treatment for grade 3 or 4 diarrhea until resolved or to grade 1 or lower, then resume fluorouracil at a reduced dose. Administer fluids, electrolyte replacement, and/or antidiarrheal treatments as necessary. Mucositis, stomatitis, or esophagopharyngitis (which may lead to mucosal sloughing or ulceration) may occur with fluorouracil. The incidence of mucositis is reported to be higher with IV bolus fluorouracil administration (vs continuous infusion). Withhold fluorouracil grade 3 or 4 mucositis; resume at a reduced dose once mucositis has resolved to grade 1 or lower. Fluorouracil is associated with palmar-plantar erythrodysesthesia (hand-foot syndrome; HFS). Symptoms of HFS include a tingling sensation, pain, swelling, erythema with tenderness, and desquamation. HFS occurs more commonly when fluorouracil is administered as a continuous infusion (compared to IV bolus) and has been reported to occur more frequently in patients with prior chemotherapy exposure. The onset of HFS is usually after 8 to 9 weeks of fluorouracil, although may occur earlier. Initiate supportive care for symptomatic relief of HFS. Withhold fluorouracil for grade 2 or 3 HFS; resume at a reduced dose when HFS has resolved to grade 1 or lower. Fluorouracil can cause severe and fatal hematologic toxicity (neutropenia, thrombocytopenia, and anemia). The neutrophil nadir usually occurs between 9 to 14 days after administration. Monitor blood counts prior to each treatment cycle, weekly if administered on a weekly or similar schedule, and as clinically indicated. Withhold fluorouracil for grade 4 hematologic toxicity; when blood counts resolve to grade 1 or lower, resume at a reduced dose.

Serious errors have occurred when doses administered by continuous ambulatory infusion pumps have inadvertently been given over 1 to 4 hours instead of the intended extended continuous infusion duration. Depending on protocol, infusion duration may range from 46 hours to 7 days for fluorouracil continuous infusions. Ambulatory pumps utilized for continuous infusions should have safeguards to allow for detection of programming errors. If using an elastomeric device for ambulatory continuous infusion, carefully select the device and double check the flow rate. Appropriate prescribing (in single daily doses [not course doses] with instructions to infuse over a specific time period), appropriate training/certification/education of staff involved with dispensing and administration processes, and independent double checks should be utilized throughout dispensing and administration procedures (ISMP [Smetzer 2015]).

Uridine triacetate (formerly called vistonuridine), has been studied in cases of fluorouracil overdose. In a clinical study of 98 patients who received uridine triacetate for fluorouracil toxicity (due to overdose, accidental capecitabine ingestion, or possible DPD deficiency), 96 patients recovered fully (Bamat 2013). Of 17 patients receiving uridine triacetate beginning within 8 to 96 hours after fluorouracil overdose, all patients fully recovered (von Borstel 2009). Refer to Uridine Triacetate monograph. Potentially significant drug-drug interactions may exist, requiring dose or frequency adjustment, additional monitoring, and/or selection of alternative therapy. Clinically significant coagulation parameter elevations have been reported with concomitant use of warfarin and fluorouracil. Closely monitor INR and prothrombin time in patients receiving concomitant coumarin-derivative anticoagulants such as warfarin and adjust the anticoagulant dose accordingly.

Adverse Reactions Frequency not defined. Toxicity depends on duration of treatment and/or rate of administration.

Cardiovascular: Angina pectoris, cardiac arrhythmia, cardiac failure, cerebrovascular accident, ischemic heart disease, local thrombophlebitis, myocardial infarction, vasospasm, ventricular ectopy

Central nervous system: Cerebellar syndrome (acute), confusion, disorientation, euphoria, headache

Dermatologic: Alopecia, changes in nails (including nail loss), dermatitis, hyperpigmentation (supravenous), maculopapular rash (pruritic), palmar-plantar erythrodysesthesia, skin fissure, skin photosensitivity, Stevens-Johnson syndrome, toxic epidermal necrolysis, xeroderma

Gastrointestinal: Anorexia, diarrhea, esophagopharyngitis, gastrointestinal hemorrhage, gastrointestinal ulcer, mesenteric ischemia (acute), nausea, stomatitis, tissue sloughing (gastrointestinal), vomiting

Hematologic & oncologic: Agranulocytosis, anemia, leukopenia (nadir: days 9 to 14; recovery by day 30), pancytopenia, thrombocytopenia

Hypersensitivity: Anaphylaxis, hypersensitivity reaction (generalized)

Ophthalmic: Lacrimal stenosis, lacrimation, nystagmus, photophobia, visual disturbance

Respiratory: Epistaxis

<1%, postmarketing, and/or case reports: Dysgeusia (Syed 2016)

Drug Interactions

Metabolism/Transport Effects Inhibits CYP2C9 (strong)

Avoid Concomitant Use

Avoid concomitant use of Fluorouracil (Systemic) with any of the following: BCG (Intravesical); Deferiprone; Dipyrone; Gimeracil; Natalizumab; Pimecrolimus; Tacrolimus (Topical); Vaccines (Live)

Increased Effect/Toxicity

Fluorouracil (Systemic) may increase the levels/effects of: Alitretinoin (Systemic); Bosentan; Cannabis; Carvedilol; CloZAPine; CYP2C9 Substrates; Deferiprone; Diclofenac (Systemic); Dronabinol; Fingolimod; Fosphenytoin; Highest Risk QTc-Prolonging Agents; Lacosamide; Leflunomide; Moderate Risk QTc-Prolonging Agents; Natalizumab; Ospemifene; Parecoxib; Phenytoin; Ramelteon; Tetrahydrocannabinol; Tofacitinib; Vaccines (Live); Vitamin K Antagonists

The levels/effects of Fluorouracil (Systemic) may be increased by: Cimetidine; Denosumab; Dipyrone; Gemcitabine; Gimeracil; Leucovorin Calcium-Levoleucovorin; MetroNIDAZOLE (Systemic); MiFEPRIStone; Ocrelizumab; Palifermin; Pimecrolimus; Promazine; Roflumilast; SORAfenib; Tacrolimus (Topical); Trastuzumab

Decreased Effect

Fluorouracil (Systemic) may decrease the levels/effects of: BCG (Intra-vesical); Coccidioides immitis Skin Test; Lenograstim; Nivolumab; Sipuleucel-T; Tertomotide; Vaccines (Inactivated); Vaccines (Live)

The levels/effects of Fluorouracil (Systemic) may be decreased by: Echinacea; SORAfenib

Hazardous Drugs Handling Considerations

Hazardous agent (NIOSH 2016 [group 1]).

Use appropriate precautions for receiving, handling, administration, and disposal. Gloves (single) should be worn during receiving, unpacking, and placing in storage.

NIOSH recommends double gloving, a protective gown, ventilated engineering controls (a class II biological safety cabinet or a compounding aseptic containment isolator), and closed system transfer devices (CSTDs) for preparation. Double gloving, a gown, and (if dosage form allows) CSTDs are required during administration (NIOSH 2016).

Storage/Stability Store intact vials at 20°C to 25°C (68°F to 77°F). Do not freeze. Protect from light. Pharmacy bulk vials should be used within 4 hours of initial entry. Syringes and solutions diluted for infusion may be stored for up to 4 hours (at room temperature) prior to administration (according to the manufacturer). Fluorouracil 50 mg/mL in NS was stable in polypropylene infusion pump syringes for 7 days when stored at 30°C (86°F) (Stiles 1996). Stability of fluorouracil 1 mg/mL or 10 mg/mL in NS or D5W in PVC bags was demonstrated for up to 14 days at 4°C (39.2°F) and 21°C (69.8°F) (Martel 1996). Stability of undiluted fluorouracil (50 mg/mL) in ethylene-vinyl acetate ambulatory pump reservoirs was demonstrated for 3 days at 4°C (39.2°F) (precipitate formed after 3 days) and for 14 days at 33°C (91.4°F) (Martel 1996). Stability of undiluted fluorouracil (50 mg/mL) in PVC ambulatory pump reservoirs was demonstrated for 5 days at 4°C (39.2°F) (precipitate formed after 5 days) and for 14 days at 33°C (91.4°F) (Martel 1996). Follow USP 797 recommendations for beyond use dates based on the level of risk for preparation.

Preparation for Administration The 10 mL vial is a single-use vial; the bulk vial may be used to prepare multiple doses if a sterile transfer device is used. May dispense in a syringe or dilute for infusion.

Mechanism of Action A pyrimidine analog antimetabolite that interferes with DNA and RNA synthesis; after activation, F-UMP (an active metabolite) is incorporated into RNA to replace uracil and inhibit cell growth; the active metabolite F-dUMP, inhibits thymidylate synthetase, depleting thymidine triphosphate (a necessary component of DNA synthesis).

Pharmacodynamics/Kinetics

Distribution: Fluorouracil distributes throughout the body, including brain tissue, CSF, bone marrow, intestinal mucosa, and liver.

Metabolism: Hepatic; via a dehydrogenase enzyme; FU must be metabolized to form active metabolites, 5-fluoroxyuridine monophosphate (F-UMP) and 5-5-fluoro-2'-deoxyuridine-5'-O-monophosphate (F-dUMP)

Half-life elimination: Following bolus infusion: 8 to 20 minutes

Excretion: Urine (5% to 20% as unchanged drug within 6 hours; metabolites over 3 to 4 hours)

◀ **Dosing**

Adult & Geriatric

Breast cancer: IV:

CEF or FEC regimen: 500 mg/m² on days 1 and 8 every 28 days (in combination with cyclophosphamide and epirubicin) for 6 cycles (Levine 1998)

CMF regimen: 600 mg/m² on days 1 and 8 every 28 days (in combination with cyclophosphamide and methotrexate) for 6 cycles (Goldhirsch 1998; Levine 1998)

CAF or FAC regimen (off-label dosing): 500 mg/m² on days 1 and 8 every 21 to 28 days (in combination with cyclophosphamide and doxorubicin) for 6 cycles (Assikis 2003)

Colorectal cancer: IV: 400 mg/m² bolus on day 1, followed by 1,200 to 1,500 mg/m²/day continuous infusion for 2 days (over 46 hours) every 2 weeks (in combination with leucovorin ± either oxaliplatin or irinotecan) **or** *Roswell Park regimen:* 500 mg/m² (bolus) on days 1, 8, 15, 22, 29, and 36 (1 hour after leucovorin) every 8 weeks (in combination with leucovorin) for 4 cycles (Haller 2005)

FOLFOX6 and mFOLFOX6 regimen: 400 mg/m² bolus on day 1, followed by 1200 mg/m²/day continuous infusion for 2 days (over 46 hours) every 2 weeks (in combination with leucovorin and oxaliplatin) until disease progression or unacceptable toxicity (Cheeseman 2002)

FOLFIRI regimen: 400 mg/m² bolus on day 1, followed by 1200 mg/m²/day continuous infusion for 2 days (over 46 hours) every 2 weeks (in combination with leucovorin and irinotecan) until disease progression or unacceptable toxicity; after 2 cycles, may increase continuous infusion fluorouracil dose to 1500 mg/m²/day (over 46 hours) (Andre 1999)

FLOX regimen (off-label dosing): 500 mg/m² bolus on days 1, 8, 15, 22, 29, and 36 (1 hour after leucovorin) every 8 weeks (in combination with leucovorin and oxaliplatin) for 3 cycles (Kuebler 2007)

Gastric cancer: IV: 200 to 1,000 mg/m²/day as a continuous infusion over 24 hours (as part of a platinum-containing regimen); the duration and frequency of each cycle varies based on the dose and regimen.

CF regimen: 1,000 mg/m²/day continuous infusion days 1 to 4 and days 29 to 32 of a 35-day treatment cycle (preoperative chemoradiation; in combination with cisplatin) (Tepper 2008)

ECF regimen (resectable disease): 200 mg/m²/day continuous infusion days 1 to 21 every 3 weeks (in combination with epirubicin and cisplatin) for 6 cycles (3 cycles preoperatively and 3 cycles postoperatively) (Cunningham 2006)

ECF or EOF regimen (advanced disease): 200 mg/m²/day continuous infusion days 1 to 21 every 3 weeks (in combination with epirubicin and either cisplatin or oxaliplatin) for a planned duration of 24 weeks (Sumpter 2005)

TCF or DCF regimen: 750 mg/m²/day continuous infusion days 1 to 5 every 3 weeks or 1000 mg/m²/day continuous infusion days 1 to 5 every 4 weeks (in combination with docetaxel and cisplatin) until disease progression or unacceptable toxicity (Ajani 2007; Van Cutsem 2006)

ToGA regimen (HER2-positive): 800 mg/m²/day continuous infusion days 1 to 5 every 3 weeks (in combination with cisplatin and trastuzumab) until disease progression or unacceptable toxicity (Bang 2010)

Pancreatic cancer: IV:

FOLFIRINOX regimen: 400 mg/m^2 bolus on day 1, followed by 1,200 mg/m^2/day continuous infusion for 2 days (over 46 hours) every 14 days (in combination with leucovorin, irinotecan, and oxaliplatin) until disease progression or unacceptable toxicity for a recommended 12 cycles (Conroy 2011)

Chemoradiation therapy (off-label dosing): 250 mg/m^2/day continuous infusion for 3 weeks prior to and then throughout radiation therapy (Regine 2008)

Fluorouracil-Leucovorin (off-label dosing): 425 mg/m^2/day (bolus) days 1 to 5 every 28 days (in combination with leucovorin) for 6 cycles (Neoptolemos 2010)

Anal carcinoma (off-label use): IV: 1,000 mg/m^2/day continuous infusion days 1 to 4 and days 29 to 32 (in combination with mitomycin and radiation therapy) (Ajani 2008; Flam 1996)

Bladder cancer (off-label use): IV: 500 mg/m^2/day continuous infusion days 1 to 5 and days 16 to 20 (in combination with mitomycin and radiation therapy) (James 2012)

Cervical cancer (off-label use): IV: 1,000 mg/m^2/day continuous infusion days 1 to 4 (in combination with cisplatin and radiation therapy) every 3 weeks for 3 cycles (Eifel 2004; Morris 1999)

Esophageal cancer (off-label use): IV:

CF regimen: 1,000 mg/m^2/day continuous infusion days 1 to 4 and days 29 to 32 of a 35-day treatment cycle (preoperative chemoradiation; in combination with cisplatin) (Tepper 2008)

ECF regimen (resectable disease): 200 mg/m^2/day continuous infusion days 1 to 21 every 3 weeks (in combination with epirubicin and cisplatin) for 6 cycles (3 cycles preoperatively and 3 cycles postoperatively) (Cunningham 2006)

ECF or EOF regimen (advanced disease): 200 mg/m^2/day continuous infusion days 1 to 21 every 3 weeks (in combination with epirubicin and either cisplatin or oxaliplatin) for a planned duration of 24 weeks (Sumpter 2005)

MCF regimen: 300 mg/m^2/day continuous infusion for up to 6 months (in combination with mitomycin and cisplatin) (Ross 2002)

TCF or DCF regimen: 750 mg/m^2/day continuous infusion days 1 to 5 every 3 to 4 weeks (in combination with docetaxel and cisplatin) until disease progression or unacceptable toxicity (Ajani 2007; Van Cutsem 2006)

Head and neck cancer, squamous cell (off-label use): IV:

Platinum-Fluorouracil (CF) regimen: 1,000 mg/m^2/day continuous infusion days 1 to 4 every 3 weeks (in combination with cisplatin) for at least 6 cycles (Gibson 2005) **or** 1,000 mg/m^2/day continuous infusion days 1 to 4 every 4 weeks (in combination with carboplatin) for at least 6 cycles (Forastiere 1992) **or** 600 mg/m^2/day continuous infusion days 1 to 4, 22 to 25, and 43 to 46 (in combination with carboplatin and radiation) (Bourhis 2012; Denis 2004)

TPF regimen: 1,000 mg/m^2/day continuous infusion days 1 to 4 every 3 weeks (in combination with docetaxel and cisplatin) for 3 cycles, and followed by chemoradiotherapy (Posner 2007) **or** 750 mg/m^2/day continuous infusion days 1 to 5 every 3 weeks (in combination with docetaxel and cisplatin) for up to 4 cycles, followed by radiation in patients without progressive disease (Vermorken 2007)

831

Platinum, 5-FU, and cetuximab regimen: 1,000 mg/m²/day continuous infusion days 1 to 4 every 3 weeks (in combination with cetuximab and either cisplatin or carboplatin) for a total of up to 6 cycles (Vermorken 2008)

Hepatobiliary cancer (off-label use): IV: 600 mg/m² (bolus) on days 1, 8, and 15 every 4 weeks (in combination with gemcitabine and leucovorin) (Alberts 2005). Additional data may be needed to further define the role of fluorouracil in this condition.

Neuroendocrine tumors, pancreatic (off-label use): IV: 400 mg/m²/day (bolus) days 1 to 5 every 28 days (in combination with doxorubicin and streptozocin) for at least 4 cycles (Kouvaraki 2004). Additional data may be necessary to further define the role of fluorouracil in the management of this condition.

Penile cancer, advanced, squamous cell (off-label use): IV: 800 to 1,000 mg/m²/day continuous infusion for 4 days every 21 days (in combination with cisplatin) (Di Lorenzo 2012). Additional data may be needed to further define the role of fluorouracil in this condition.

Unknown primary cancer, squamous cell (off-label use): IV: 750 mg/m²/day continuous infusion for 5 days every 21 days (in combination with docetaxel and cisplatin) for 3 cycles (Pointreau 2009) **or** 500 mg/m²/day continuous infusion for 5 days every 21 days (in combination with paclitaxel and cisplatin) for 3 cycles (Hitt 2005) **or** 400 mg/m²/day (bolus) followed by 1,200 mg/m²/day continuous infusion for 2 days (over 46 hours) every 2 weeks (in combination with leucovorin and oxaliplatin) (Cheeseman 2002) **or** 700 mg/m²/day continuous infusion for 5 days (in combination with cisplatin) every 28 days until disease progression or unacceptable toxicity (Kusaba 2007). Additional data may be needed to further define the role of fluorouracil in this condition.

Vulvar cancer, advanced (off-label use): IV: 750 mg/m²/day continuous infusion days 1 to 5 every 14 days for 2 cycles (in combination with concomitant radiation and mitomycin) (Landoni 1996). Additional data may be needed to further define the role of fluorouracil in this condition.

Pediatric Nasopharyngeal carcinoma (off-label use): Children ≥8 years and Adolescents: IV: 1,000 mg/m²/day continuous infusion for 3 or 5 days every 3 or 4 weeks (in combination with cisplatin with or without either methotrexate or leucovorin, followed by radiation therapy [± interferon beta]) for 3 or 4 cycles (Buehrlen 2012; Casanova 2012; Mertens 2005; Rodriguez-Galindo 2005). Additional data may be needed to further define the role of fluorouracil in this condition.

Renal Impairment There are no dosage adjustments provided in the manufacturer's labeling; use with caution. The following adjustments have been suggested:

CrCl <50 mL/minute and continuous renal replacement therapy (CRRT): No dosage adjustment necessary (Aronoff 2007).

Hemodialysis:

Administer standard dose following hemodialysis on dialysis days (Janus 2010).

Administer 50% of standard dose following hemodialysis (Aronoff 2007).

Hepatic Impairment There are no dosage adjustments provided in the manufacturer's labeling; use with caution. The following adjustments have been suggested:

Bilirubin >5 mg/dL: Avoid use (Floyd 2006).

Hepatic impairment (degree not specified): Administer <50% of dose, then increase if toxicity does not occur (Koren 1992).

Obesity *ASCO Guidelines for appropriate chemotherapy dosing in obese adults with cancer:* Utilize patient's actual body weight (full weight) for calculation of body surface area- or weight-based dosing, particularly when the intent of therapy is curative; manage regimen-related toxicities in the same manner as for nonobese patients; if a dose reduction is utilized due to toxicity, consider resumption of full weight-based dosing with subsequent cycles, especially if cause of toxicity (eg, hepatic or renal impairment) is resolved (Griggs 2012).

Adjustment for Toxicity

Withhold treatment for the following (may resume at a reduced dose following resolution or improvement to grade 1):

Dermatologic toxicity: Grade 2 or 3 palmar-plantar erythrodysesthesia (hand-foot syndrome)

Gastrointestinal toxicity: Grade 3 or 4 diarrhea; grade 3 or 4 mucositis

Hematologic toxicity: Grade 4 myelosuppression

Withhold treatment for the following (there is no recommended dose for resumption):

Cardiovascular toxicity: Angina, MI/ischemia, arrhythmia, or heart failure in patients without a history of coronary artery disease or myocardial dysfunction

CNS toxicity: Acute cerebellar syndrome, confusion, disorientation, ataxia, or visual disturbances

Hyperammonemic encephalopathy

Combination Regimens

Anal cancer: Fluorouracil-Mitomycin (Anal Cancer) on page 2128

Bladder cancer: Cisplatin-Fluorouracil (Bladder Cancer) on page 2044

Breast cancer:

CAF IV (Breast) on page 2002

CAF Oral (Breast) on page 2003

CMF Oral (Breast) on page 2066

Docetaxel-Trastuzumab followed by FEC (Breast) on page 2095

FEC followed by Docetaxel Every 3 Weeks (Breast) on page 2112

FEC followed by Paclitaxel Weekly (Breast) on page 2112

FEC IV (Breast) on page 2112

FEC Oral (Breast) on page 2113

Cervical cancer: Cisplatin-Fluorouracil (Cervical Cancer) on page 2044

Colorectal cancer:

Bevacizumab-Fluorouracil-Leucovorin (Colorectal) on page 1992

Bevacizumab + FOLFIRI (Colorectal) on page 1992

Bevacizumab FOLFOX (Colorectal) on page 1993

Cetuximab + FOLFIRI (Colorectal) on page 2031

FLOX (Colorectal) on page 2116

Fluorouracil-Leucovorin Bolus (Colorectal) on page 2124

Fluorouracil-Leucovorin Infusional (Colorectal) on page 2125

Fluorouracil-Leucovorin-Irinotecan (Saltz Regimen) (Colorectal) on page 2126

FOLFIRI (Colorectal) on page 2128

FOLFOX1 (Colorectal) on page 2129

FOLFOX2 (Colorectal) on page 2130

FOLFOX3 (Colorectal) on page 2130

FOLFOX4 (Colorectal) on page 2130

◀

Administration IV administration rate varies by protocol; refer to specific reference for protocol. May be administered by IV push, IV bolus, or as a continuous infusion. Avoid extravasation (may be an irritant).

Vesicant/Extravasation Risk May be an irritant

Emetic Potential Children and Adults: Low (10% to 30%)

Monitoring Parameters CBC with differential and platelet count (prior to each treatment cycle, weekly if administered on a weekly or similar schedule, and as clinically indicated), renal function tests, LFTs, INR, and prothrombin time (in patients receiving concomitant coumarin-derivative anticoagulants); signs/symptoms of palmar-plantar erythrodysesthesia syndrome, cardiotoxicity, CNS toxicity, stomatitis, diarrhea, and hyperammonemic encephalopathy.

Dietary Considerations Increase dietary intake of thiamine.

Dosage Forms Excipient information presented when available (limited, particularly for generics); consult specific product labeling.
Solution, Intravenous:
Adrucil: 500 mg/10 mL (10 mL); 2.5 g/50 mL (50 mL); 5 g/100 mL (100 mL)
Generic: 500 mg/10 mL (10 mL); 1 g/20 mL (20 mL); 2.5 g/50 mL (50 mL); 5 g/100 mL (100 mL)
Solution, Intravenous [preservative free]:
Generic: 2.5 g/50 mL (50 mL); 5 g/100 mL (100 mL)

Fluorouracil (Topical) (flure oh YOOR a sil)

Related Information
Management of EGFR Inhibitor Toxicities: Dermatologic, Ocular, and Gastrointestinal *on page 2291*
Safe Handling of Hazardous Drugs *on page 2379*

Brand Names: US Carac; Efudex; Fluoroplex; Tolak

Brand Names: Canada Efudex; Fluoroplex

Index Terms 5-Fluorouracil; 5-FU; FU; Topical Fluorouracil

Pharmacologic Category Antineoplastic Agent, Antimetabolite; Antineoplastic Agent, Antimetabolite (Pyrimidine Analog); Topical Skin Product

Use
Actinic or solar keratosis: Management of multiple actinic or solar keratoses
Basal cell carcinoma (5%): Treatment of superficial basal cell carcinomas when conventional methods are impractical (eg, due to multiple lesions or difficult treatment sites)
Limitations of use: Establish diagnosis of superficial basal cell carcinoma prior to treatment (use has not been proven effective in other types of basal cell carcinomas); surgery is preferred with isolated, easily accessible basal cell carcinomas because success with such lesions is almost 100% and the success rate with fluorouracil cream and solution is ~93%.

Labeled Contraindications Hypersensitivity to fluorouracil or any component of the formulation; dihydropyrimidine dehydrogenase (DPD) enzyme deficiency; women who are or may become pregnant

Pregnancy Considerations Animal reproduction studies have not been conducted with topical fluorouracil, although teratogenic effects have been observed in animal studies with parenteral administration. Adverse effects have been reported following use of topical fluorouracil products in humans. Use is contraindicated during pregnancy. Women of reproductive potential should use effective contraception during and for one month after the final application of topical fluorouracil.

Breastfeeding Considerations It is not known if fluorouracil (topical) is excreted in breast milk. Due to the potential for serious adverse reactions in the nursing infant, a decision should be made to discontinue nursing or to discontinue the drug, taking into account the importance of treatment to the mother.

◄ **Warnings/Precautions** Individuals lacking dihydropyrimidine dehydrogenase (DPD) enzyme activity may exhibit severe toxicity with topical fluorouracil. Life-threatening systemic toxicity has been reported with the topical use of fluorouracil 5% in a patient with DPD enzyme deficiency; signs/symptoms included bloody diarrhea, stomatitis, esophagus, stomach, and small bowel inflammation, severe abdominal pain, vomiting, chills, fever, erythematous skin rash, neutropenia, and thrombocytopenia. It is unknown if patients with profound DPD enzyme deficiency would develop systemic toxicity with lower concentrations of topical fluorouracil. Discontinue if signs of DPD deficiency develop.

When applied to a lesion, erythema followed by vesiculation, desquamation, erosion and reepithelialization occurs. Local reactions and alterations in skin appearance may persist for several weeks after discontinuation. Bruising, burning, crusting, dryness, edema, irritation, pain, pruritus, scaling scarring, soreness, stinging, and ulceration may commonly result from topical therapy. Increased absorption through ulcerated or inflamed skin is possible. May be associated with delayed-type hypersensitivity reactions, including allergic contact dermatitis. Severe pruritus or eczema (at the application site or at a distant site) may be indicative of hypersensitivity; patch testing may not be useful in the evaluation of these reactions; discontinue immediately for signs of hypersensitivity. Topical fluorouracil is associated with photosensitivity, including severe sunburn. Avoid prolonged exposure to sunlight or UV irradiation during treatment; reaction intensity may be increased.

Appropriate use: Avoid topical application to mucous membranes due to potential for local inflammation and ulceration; cases of miscarriage and a birth defect (ventricular septal defect) have been reported when fluorouracil was applied to mucous membrane areas during pregnancy. The use of occlusive dressings with topical preparations may increase the severity of inflammation in nearby skin areas (a porous gauze dressing may be applied for cosmetic reasons without increase in reaction). Avoid eyelids, eyes, and periocular area when applying (corneal and conjunctival disorders have occurred with topical fluorouracil). Wash hands well following application; if ocular exposure occurs, flush with large amounts of water.

Benzyl alcohol and derivatives: Some dosage forms may contain benzyl alcohol; large amounts of benzyl alcohol (≥99 mg/kg/day) have been associated with a potentially fatal toxicity ("gasping syndrome") in neonates; the "gasping syndrome" consists of metabolic acidosis, respiratory distress, gasping respirations, CNS dysfunction (including convulsions, intracranial hemorrhage), hypotension and cardiovascular collapse (AAP ["Inactive"], 1997]; CDC, 1982); some data suggests that benzoate displaces bilirubin from protein binding sites (Ahlfors, 2001); avoid or use dosage forms containing benzyl alcohol with caution in neonates. See manufacturer's labeling. Some dosage forms contain peanut oil.

Adverse Reactions

>10%:

Dermatologic: Application site scaling (≤95%), application site dryness (70% to ≤95%), stinging of the skin (application site: ≤87%), skin erosion (application site: 25% to 68%)

Local: Application site erythema (90% to 99%), application site reaction (92% to 97%; crusting: 87%), application site burning (60% to ≤87%), application site pruritus (85%), application site edema (14% to 69%), application site pain (31% to 61%)

1% to 10%:
Central nervous system: Headache (4%)
Dermatologic: Skin irritation (1% to 2%)
Infection: Common cold (5%)
Ophthalmic: Eye irritation (3% to 7%; burning, watering, sensitivity, stinging, itching)
Respiratory: Sinusitis (5%)
<1%, postmarketing, and/or case reports: Allergic contact dermatitis, alopecia, anxiety, bullous pemphigoid, burning sensation of skin, conjunctival irritation, conjunctivitis, corneal disease, eosinophilia, eye irritation, herpes simplex infection, hyperpigmentation, ichthyosis, inflammation, insomnia, irritability, lacrimation, leukocytosis, lymphocytic leukemia, medicine-like taste, muscle tenderness, nasal discomfort, pain, pancytopenia, pruritus, scarring, skin blister, skin irritation, skin neoplasm (nonmelanoma), skin photosensitivity, skin rash, skin tenderness, stomatitis, suppuration, swelling, swelling of eye, telangiectasia, thrombocytopenia, toxic granulations, ulcer, urticaria

Drug Interactions
Metabolism/Transport Effects Inhibits CYP2C9 (weak)
Avoid Concomitant Use There are no known interactions where it is recommended to avoid concomitant use.
Increased Effect/Toxicity
Fluorouracil (Topical) may increase the levels/effects of: Fosphenytoin; Phenytoin; Vitamin K Antagonists

The levels/effects of Fluorouracil (Topical) may be increased by: Gemcitabine; Leucovorin Calcium-Levoleucovorin; SORAfenib
Decreased Effect
The levels/effects of Fluorouracil (Topical) may be decreased by: SORAfenib
Hazardous Drugs Handling Considerations
Hazardous agent (NIOSH 2016 [group 1]).

Use appropriate precautions for receiving, handling, administration, and disposal. Gloves (single) should be worn during receiving, unpacking, and placing in storage. NIOSH recommends double gloving, a protective gown, and (if liquid that could splash) eye/face protection for administration of a topical product; if there is potential for inhalation, respiratory protection is recommended (NIOSH 2016).
Storage/Stability Store at controlled room temperature of 15°C to 30°C (59°F to 86°F). Do not freeze.
Mechanism of Action A pyrimidine antimetabolite that interferes with DNA synthesis by blocking the methylation of deoxyuridylic acid to thymidylic acid; blocks DNA synthesis to prevent cell proliferation of fast growing cells and cause cell death.
Pharmacodynamics/Kinetics
Absorption: ~6% of a topical dose is absorbed systemically (5% cream)
Time to Peak: ~1 hour following application (4% cream)
Dosing
Adult & Geriatric
Actinic or solar keratosis: Topical:
Cream (0.5%): Apply thin film to lesions once daily for up to 4 weeks, as tolerated
Cream (1%): Apply to lesions twice daily for 2 to 6 weeks
Cream (4%): Apply to lesions once daily for 4 weeks as tolerated

Cream (5%) or solution (2% and 5%): Apply to lesions twice daily for 2 to 4 weeks; complete healing may not be evident for 1 to 2 months following treatment

Superficial basal cell carcinoma: Topical: Cream (5%) or solution (5%): Apply to affected lesions twice daily for 3 to 6 weeks; treatment may be continued for up to 10 to 12 weeks

Renal Impairment There are no dosage adjustments provided in the manufacturer's labeling.

Hepatic Impairment There are no dosage adjustments provided in the manufacturer's labeling.

Administration Topical: Apply 10 minutes after washing, rinsing, and drying the affected area. Apply a sufficient amount to cover lesions, preferably using a nonmetal applicator or suitable glove.

Cream (4%): Apply after washing, rinsing, and drying the affected area. Apply a sufficient amount to cover lesions of the face, ears, and/or scalp with a thin film, using fingertips to gently massage uniformly into skin.

If applied with fingertip, wash hands immediately after application. Do not cover area with an occlusive dressing. Topical preparations are for external use only; not for ophthalmic, oral, mucous membrane, or intravaginal use.

Dosage Forms Excipient information presented when available (limited, particularly for generics); consult specific product labeling.

Cream, External:

Carac: 0.5% (30 g) [contains methylparaben, polysorbate 80, propylene glycol, propylparaben, trolamine (triethanolamine)]

Efudex: 5% (40 g)

Fluoroplex: 1% (30 g) [contains benzyl alcohol]

Tolak: 4% (40 g) [contains cetyl alcohol, methylparaben, peanut oil, propylparaben]

Generic: 0.5% (30 g); 5% (40 g)

Solution, External:

Generic: 2% (10 mL); 5% (10 mL)

◆ **Fluorouracil Injection (Can)** see Fluorouracil (Systemic) on page 825

◆ **Fluouracil** see Fluorouracil (Systemic) on page 825

Fluoxymesterone (floo oks i MES te rone)

Brand Names: US Androxy

Index Terms Androxy; Halotestin

Pharmacologic Category Androgen

Use

Breast cancer, metastatic (females): Salvage treatment of inoperable metastatic breast cancer in postmenopausal females

Delayed puberty (males): Replacement therapy in the treatment of delayed male puberty

Hypogonadism (males): Treatment of male hypogonadism (primary or hypogonadotropic)

Pregnancy Risk Factor X

Hazardous Drugs Handling Considerations
Hazardous agent (NIOSH 2016 [group 2]).

Use appropriate precautions for receiving, handling, administration, and disposal. Gloves (single) should be worn during receiving, unpacking, and placing in storage. NIOSH recommends single gloving for administration of intact tablets or capsules (NIOSH 2016).

Dosing
Adult & Geriatric
Breast cancer, metastatic (females): Oral: Manufacturer labeling: 10 to 40 mg daily in divided doses for ≥3 months

Delayed puberty (males): Oral: 2.5 to 20 mg daily for 4 to 6 months

Hypogonadism, primary or hypogonadotropic (males): Oral: 5 to 20 mg daily

Renal Impairment There are no dosage adjustments provided in the manufacturer's labeling; use with caution.

Hepatic Impairment
Hepatic impairment prior to therapy: There are no dosage adjustments provided in the manufacturer's labeling; use with caution.

Hepatic impairment during therapy: Discontinue use if abnormal liver function tests or cholestatic hepatitis with jaundice occur.

Adjustment for Toxicity
Edema: If therapy is discontinued due to edema, may reinitiate (if indicated) at a reduced dosage

Hypercalcemia during therapy for metastatic breast cancer (females): Discontinue use

Hypogonadism (males) (off-label): Hematocrit (HCT) >50%: Use is not recommended; if HCT >54% during therapy, discontinue until HCT falls to a safe level, assess for hypoxia and sleep apnea; if reinitiating therapy, reduce the dose (Bhasin 2010)

Additional Information Complete prescribing information should be consulted for additional detail.

Dosage Forms Excipient information presented when available (limited, particularly for generics); consult specific product labeling.

Tablet, Oral:
Androxy: 10 mg [scored; contains fd&c blue #1 aluminum lake, fd&c yellow #10 aluminum lake, fd&c yellow #6 aluminum lake]

Controlled Substance C-III

♦ **5-Fluracil** see Fluorouracil (Systemic) on page 825
♦ **5-Flurocytosine** see Flucytosine on page 815

Flutamide (FLOO ta mide)
Related Information
Safe Handling of Hazardous Drugs on page 2379

Brand Names: Canada Apo-Flutamide; Euflex; PMS-Flutamide; Teva-Flutamide

Index Terms Eulexin; Flucinom; Flugerel; Niftolid; SCH 13521

Pharmacologic Category Antineoplastic Agent, Antiandrogen

Use Prostate cancer: Management of locally confined Stage B_2 to C and Stage D_2 metastatic prostate cancer (in combination with a luteinizing hormone-releasing hormone [LHRH] agonist). For Stage B_2 to C prostate cancer, flutamide treatment (and goserelin) should start 8 weeks prior to

◀ initiating radiation therapy and continue during radiation therapy. To achieve treatment benefit in Stage D_2 metastatic prostate cancer, initiate flutamide with the LHRH agonist and continue until disease progression.

Labeled Contraindications Hypersensitivity to flutamide or any component of the formulation; severe hepatic impairment (evaluate baseline hepatic enzymes prior to treatment).

Pregnancy Considerations Adverse events have been observed in animal reproduction studies. May cause fetal harm if administered in pregnancy. Flutamide is not indicated for use in women.

Breastfeeding Considerations According to the manufacturer, this product is not indicated for use in women. Information related to use in nursing women has not been located.

Warnings/Precautions [U.S. Boxed Warning]: Hospitalization and death (rare) due to liver failure have been reported in patients taking flutamide. Elevated serum transaminase levels, jaundice, hepatic encephalopathy, and acute hepatic failure have been reported. Hepatotoxicity was reversible after discontinuation in some cases. In about 50% of the cases, the onset of hepatotoxicity was within the first 3 months of treatment. Monitor serum transaminase levels at baseline, monthly for 4 months, and periodically thereafter. Also obtain liver function tests at the first symptoms suggestive of liver dysfunction (nausea, vomiting, abdominal pain, fatigue, anorexia, "flu-like" symptoms, hyperbilirubinuria, jaundice, or right upper quadrant tenderness). Use is not recommended in patients with ALT values greater than 2 times ULN; discontinue use immediately in patients with jaundice or if ALT rises above 2 times ULN. Use is contraindicated in patients with severe hepatic impairment. Androgen-deprivation therapy may increase the risk for cardiovascular disease (Levine, 2010). Not indicated for use in women and should not be used in women, particularly for nonserious or nonlife-threatening conditions.

Potentially significant drug-drug interactions may exist, requiring dose or frequency adjustment, additional monitoring, and/or selection of alternative therapy. Patients with glucose-6 phosphate dehydrogenase deficiency or hemoglobin M disease or smokers are at risk of toxicities associated with aniline exposure, including methemoglobinemia, hemolytic anemia, and cholestatic jaundice. Monitor methemoglobin levels. Gynecomastia may occur in patients receiving flutamide in combination with medical castration.

Adverse Reactions

>10%:

Endocrine & metabolic: Hot flash (46% to 61%), galactorrhea (9% to 42%), decreased libido (36%), increased lactate dehydrogenase (transient; mild)

Gastrointestinal: Diarrhea (12% to 40%), vomiting (11% to 12%)

Genitourinary: Impotence (33%), cystitis (16%), breast tenderness

Hematologic & oncologic: Rectal hemorrhage (14%), tumor flare

Hepatic: Increased serum AST (transient; mild)

1% to 10%:

Cardiovascular: Edema (4%), hypertension (1%)

Central nervous system: Anxiety, confusion, depression, dizziness, drowsiness, headache, insomnia, nervousness

Dermatologic: Skin rash (3% to 8%), ecchymoses, pruritus

Endocrine & metabolic: Gynecomastia (9%)

Gastrointestinal: Nausea (9%), proctitis (8%), gastric distress (4% to 6%), anorexia (4%), constipation, dyspepsia, increased appetite

Genitourinary: Hematuria (7%)

Hematologic & oncologic: Anemia (6%), leukopenia (3%), thrombocytopenia (1%)

Infection: Herpes zoster

Neuromuscular & skeletal: Weakness (1%)

<1%, postmarketing, and case reports: Cholestatic jaundice, hemolytic anemia, hepatic encephalopathy, hepatic failure, hepatic necrosis, hepatitis, hypersensitivity pneumonitis, increased blood urea nitrogen, increased gamma-glutamyl transferase, increased serum ALT, increased serum bilirubin, increased serum creatinine, jaundice, macrocytic anemia, malignant neoplasm of breast (male), methemoglobinemia, myocardial infarction, oligospermia, pulmonary embolism, skin photosensitivity, sulfhemoglobinemia, thrombophlebitis, urine discoloration (amber, yellow-green)

Drug Interactions

Metabolism/Transport Effects Substrate of CYP1A2 (major), CYP3A4 (minor); **Note:** Assignment of Major/Minor substrate status based on clinically relevant drug interaction potential

Avoid Concomitant Use

Avoid concomitant use of Flutamide with any of the following: Indium 111 Capromab Pendetide

Increased Effect/Toxicity

Flutamide may increase the levels/effects of: Prilocaine; Sodium Nitrite

The levels/effects of Flutamide may be increased by: Abiraterone Acetate; CYP1A2 Inhibitors (Moderate); CYP1A2 Inhibitors (Strong); Dapsone (Topical); Deferasirox; Nitric Oxide; Obeticholic Acid; Peginterferon Alfa-2b; Tetracaine (Topical); Vemurafenib

Decreased Effect

Flutamide may decrease the levels/effects of: Choline C 11; Indium 111 Capromab Pendetide

The levels/effects of Flutamide may be decreased by: Cannabis; CYP1A2 Inducers (Moderate); Cyproterone; Teriflunomide

Hazardous Drugs Handling Considerations

Hazardous agent (NIOSH 2016 [group 1]).

Use appropriate precautions for receiving, handling, administration, and disposal. Gloves (single) should be worn during receiving, unpacking, and placing in storage. NIOSH recommends single gloving for administration of intact tablets or capsules (NIOSH 2016).

Storage/Stability Store at 25°C (77°F); excursions permitted to 15°C to 30°C (59°F to 86°F). Dispense with a child-resistant closure in a tight, light-resistant container.

Mechanism of Action Nonsteroidal antiandrogen that inhibits androgen uptake and/or inhibits binding of androgen in target tissues.

Pharmacodynamics/Kinetics

Absorption: Oral: Rapid and complete

Protein binding: Parent drug: 94% to 96%; 2-hydroxyflutamide: 92% to 94%

Metabolism: Extensively hepatic to ≥6 metabolites, primarily 2-hydroxyflutamide (active)

Half-life elimination: ~6 hours (2-hydroxyflutamide)

Time to peak: ~2 hours (2-hydroxyflutamide)

Excretion: Primarily urine (as metabolites); feces (~4%)

◄ **Dosing**

Adult & Geriatric Prostate cancer, metastatic: Males: Oral: 250 mg 3
times daily (every 8 hours)

Renal Impairment No dosage adjustment is necessary in patients with
chronic renal insufficiency.

Hepatic Impairment

Mild to moderate impairment: There are no dosage adjustments provided in
the manufacturer's labeling.

Severe impairment: Use is contraindicated.

Administration May be administered with or without food. Administer orally in
3 divided doses (every 8 hours).

Monitoring Parameters Serum transaminases (at baseline, monthly for 4
months, and periodically thereafter); monitor liver function tests at the first sign
or symptom of liver dysfunction (eg, nausea, vomiting, abdominal pain,
fatigue, anorexia, flu-like symptoms, hyperbilirubinuria, jaundice, or right
upper quadrant tenderness); monitor prostate specific antigen (PSA)

Dosage Forms Excipient information presented when available (limited,
particularly for generics); consult specific product labeling.

Capsule, Oral:

Generic: 125 mg

Dosage Forms: Canada Information with regard to form, strength, and
availability of products uniquely available in Canada but currently not available
in the US. Refer also to Dosage Forms.

Excipient information presented when available (limited, particularly for
generics); consult specific product labeling.

Tablet, Oral: 250 mg

◆ **Folinate Calcium** *see* Leucovorin Calcium *on page 1124*

◆ **Folinic Acid (error prone synonym)** *see* Leucovorin Calcium *on page 1124*

◆ **Folotyn** *see* PRALAtrexate *on page 1540*

Fondaparinux (fon da PARE i nuks)

Brand Names: US Arixtra

Brand Names: Canada Arixtra

Index Terms Fondaparinux Sodium

Pharmacologic Category Anticoagulant; Anticoagulant, Factor Xa Inhibitor;
Pentasaccharide, Synthetic

Use

Acute deep vein thrombosis: Treatment of acute DVT in conjunction with
warfarin.

Acute pulmonary embolism: Treatment of acute PE in conjunction with
warfarin.

Deep vein thrombosis prophylaxis: Prophylaxis of DVT in patients undergoing surgery for hip replacement, knee replacement, hip fracture (including
extended prophylaxis following hip fracture surgery), or abdominal surgery
(in patients at risk for thromboembolic complications).

Pregnancy Risk Factor B

Dosing

Adult & Geriatric Note: PT and aPTT are insensitive measures of fondaparinux activity. If unexpected changes in coagulation parameters or major
bleeding occur, discontinue fondaparinux.

DVT prophylaxis: SubQ: Adults ≥50 kg: 2.5 mg once daily. **Note:** Prophylactic use contraindicated in patients <50 kg. Initiate dose after hemostasis has been established, no earlier than 6 to 8 hours postoperatively.

DVT prophylaxis with history of HIT (off-label use): SubQ: 2.5 mg once daily (Blackmer 2009; Harenberg 2004; Parody 2003)

Usual duration: 5 to 9 days (up to 10 days following abdominal surgery or up to 11 days following hip fracture, hip replacement, or knee replacement was administered in clinical trials). The American College of Chest Physicians recommends a minimum of 10 to 14 days for patients undergoing total hip arthroplasty, total knee arthroplasty, or hip fracture surgery; extended duration of up to 35 days suggested (Guyatt 2012).

Acute DVT/PE treatment: SubQ: **Note:** Start warfarin on the first or second treatment day and continue fondaparinux until INR is ≥2 for at least 24 hours (usually 5 to 7 days) (Guyatt 2012):

<50 kg: 5 mg once daily

50 to 100 kg: 7.5 mg once daily

>100 kg: 10 mg once daily

Usual duration: 5 to 9 days (administered up to 26 days in clinical trials)

Acute coronary syndrome (off-label use):

UA/NSTEMI: SubQ: 2.5 mg once daily; treat for the duration of hospitalization or until PCI performed (ACC/AHA [Amsterdam 2014])

STEMI: IV: 2.5 mg once; subsequent doses (starting the following day): SubQ: 2.5 mg once daily; treat for the duration of the hospitalization, up to 8 days, or until revascularization (ACCF/AHA [O'Gara 2013]; Yusuf 2006b)

Acute symptomatic superficial vein thrombosis (≥5 cm in length) of the legs (off-label use): SubQ: 2.5 mg once daily for 45 days (Decousus 2010; Guyatt 2012)

Acute thrombosis (unrelated to HIT) in patients with a past history of HIT (off-label use) (Guyatt 2012; Warkentin 2011): SubQ:

<50 kg: 5 mg once daily

50 to 100 kg: 7.5 mg once daily

>100 kg: 10 mg once daily

Renal Impairment

CrCl >50 mL/minute: There are no dosage adjustments provided in the manufacturer's labeling. Total clearance is reduced ~25% compared to patients with normal renal function.

CrCl 30 to 50 mL/minute: Use caution; total clearance ~40% lower compared to patients with normal renal function. When used for thromboprophylaxis, the American College of Chest Physicians suggests a 50% reduction in dose or use of low-dose heparin instead of fondaparinux (Garcia 2012).

CrCl <30 mL/minute: Use is contraindicated.

Hemodialysis: Dialyzable: Yes; clearance increased by 20% (NCS/SCCM [Frontera 2016])

Hepatic Impairment

Mild-to-moderate impairment (Child-Pugh class A and B): No dosage adjustment necessary; monitor for signs of bleeding.

Severe impairment (Child-Pugh class C): There are no dosage adjustment provided in the manufacturer's labeling (has not been studied). Use with caution; monitor closely for signs of bleeding.

Additional Information Complete prescribing information should be consulted for additional detail.

Dosage Forms Excipient information presented when available (limited, particularly for generics); consult specific product labeling.
Solution, Subcutaneous, as sodium:
Generic: 2.5 mg/0.5 mL (0.5 mL); 5 mg/0.4 mL (0.4 mL); 7.5 mg/0.6 mL (0.6 mL); 10 mg/0.8 mL (0.8 mL)
Solution, Subcutaneous, as sodium [preservative free]:
Arixtra: 2.5 mg/0.5 mL (0.5 mL); 5 mg/0.4 mL (0.4 mL); 7.5 mg/0.6 mL (0.6 mL); 10 mg/0.8 mL (0.8 mL)
Generic: 2.5 mg/0.5 mL (0.5 mL); 5 mg/0.4 mL (0.4 mL); 7.5 mg/0.6 mL (0.6 mL); 10 mg/0.8 mL (0.8 mL)

◆ **Fondaparinux Sodium** *see* Fondaparinux *on page 842*
◆ **5-Formyl Tetrahydrofolate** *see* Leucovorin Calcium *on page 1124*
◆ **Fortaz** *see* CefTAZidime *on page 360*
◆ **Fortaz in D5W** *see* CefTAZidime *on page 360*
◆ **Fortical [DSC]** *see* Calcitonin *on page 316*

Fosaprepitant (fos a PRE pi tant)

Related Information
Management of Chemotherapy-Induced Nausea and Vomiting in Adults *on page 2253*

Brand Names: US Emend
Brand Names: Canada Emend IV
Index Terms Aprepitant Injection; Fosaprepitant Dimeglumine; L-758,298; MK 0517
Pharmacologic Category Antiemetic; Substance P/Neurokinin 1 Receptor Antagonist

Use
Prevention of chemotherapy-induced nausea and vomiting:
Prevention of acute and delayed nausea and vomiting associated with highly emetogenic chemotherapy, including high-dose cisplatin (initial and repeat courses; in combination with other antiemetics)
Prevention of delayed nausea and vomiting associated with moderately emetogenic chemotherapy (initial and repeat courses; in combination with other antiemetics)
Limitations of use: Fosaprepitant has not been studied for the management of existing nausea and vomiting.

Labeled Contraindications
Hypersensitivity to fosaprepitant or any component of the formulation; concurrent use with pimozide
Canadian labeling: Additional contraindications (not in the US labeling): Concurrent use with astemizole, terfenadine, or cisapride

Pregnancy Considerations Adverse events were not observed in animal reproduction studies for aprepitant. Efficacy of hormonal contraceptive may be reduced; alternative or additional methods of contraception should be used both during treatment with fosaprepitant or aprepitant and for at least 1 month following the last fosaprepitant/aprepitant dose.

Breastfeeding Considerations It is not known if fosaprepitant is present in breast milk. According to the manufacturer, the decision to breastfeed during therapy should take into account the risk of exposure to the infant and the benefits of treatment to the mother.

Warnings/Precautions Fosaprepitant is rapidly converted to aprepitant, which has a high potential for drug interactions. Potentially significant drug-drug interactions may exist, requiring dose or frequency adjustment, additional monitoring, and/or selection of alternative therapy. Due to a drug interaction, a 50% reduction in the day 1 and 2 dexamethasone dose is recommended. Hypersensitivity reactions, including dyspnea, erythema, flushing, and anaphylaxis have been reported during infusions; if symptoms occur, stop infusion; do not reinitiate. Some dosage forms may contain polysorbate 80 (also known as Tweens). Hypersensitivity reactions, usually a delayed reaction, have been reported following exposure to pharmaceutical products containing polysorbate 80 in certain individuals (Isaksson 2002; Lucente 2000; Shelley 1995). Thrombocytopenia, ascites, pulmonary deterioration, and renal and hepatic failure have been reported in premature neonates after receiving parenteral products containing polysorbate 80 (Alade 1986; CDC 1984). See manufacturer's labeling. Use caution with hepatic impairment; has not been studied in patients with severe hepatic impairment (Child-Pugh class C). Not studied for treatment of existing nausea and vomiting. Chronic continuous administration of fosaprepitant is not recommended.

Adverse Reactions Adverse reactions reported with aprepitant and fosaprepitant (as part of a combination chemotherapy regimen) occurring at a higher frequency than standard antiemetic therapy:

>10%:

Central nervous system: Fatigue (1% to 15%)

Gastrointestinal: Diarrhea (13%)

1% to 10%:

Central nervous system: Peripheral neuropathy (3%), headache (2%)

Gastrointestinal: Hiccups (5%), anorexia (2%), constipation (2%), dyspepsia (2%), eructation (1%)

Genitourinary: Urinary tract infection (2%)

Hematologic & oncologic: Neutropenia (8%), anemia (3%), leukopenia (2%)

Hepatic: Increased serum ALT (1% to 3%), increased serum AST (1%)

Local: Infusion-site reaction (2%; includes induration at injection site, infusion-site pain, local pruritus, local thrombophlebitis, or localized erythema)

Neuromuscular & skeletal: Weakness (4%), limb pain (2%)

<1%, postmarketing, and/or case reports: Abdominal distention, abdominal pain, abnormal dreams, abnormal gait, acne vulgaris, anaphylaxis, anemia, angioedema, anxiety, bradycardia, candidiasis, cardiovascular signs and symptoms, chest discomfort, chills, cognitive dysfunction, colitis (neutropenic), conjunctivitis, cough, decreased visual acuity, diaphoresis, disorientation, dizziness, drowsiness, dysarthria, dysgeusia, dyspnea, dysuria, edema, epigastric distress, erythema, euphoria, febrile neutropenia, fecal impaction, flatulence, flushing, gastroesophageal reflux, gastroesophageal reflux disease, hallucination, hematuria (microscopic), hot flash, hyperglycemia, hypersensitivity reaction, hypertension, hypoesthesia, hyponatremia, impaired consciousness, increased serum alkaline phosphatase, insomnia, intestinal obstruction, lethargy, loss of consciousness, malaise, miosis, muscle cramps, myalgia, myasthenia, nausea, obstipation, oily skin, palpitations, paresthesia, perforated duodenal ulcer, pharyngitis, pollakiuria, polydipsia, polyuria, post nasal drip, pruritus, seizure, sensory disturbance, SIADH (syndrome of inappropriate antidiuretic hormone secretion), skin lesion, skin photosensitivity, skin rash, sneezing, staphylococcal infection, Stevens-Johnson syndrome, stomatitis, throat irritation, tinnitus, toxic ▶

epidermal necrolysis, urticaria, vomiting, weight changes (gain/loss), wheezing, xerostomia

Drug Interactions

Metabolism/Transport Effects Substrate of CYP1A2 (minor), CYP2C19 (minor), CYP3A4 (major); **Note:** Assignment of Major/Minor substrate status based on clinically relevant drug interaction potential; **Inhibits** CYP2C9 (weak), CYP3A4 (weak); **Induces** CYP2C9 (weak/moderate)

Avoid Concomitant Use

Avoid concomitant use of Fosaprepitant with any of the following: Astemizole; Cisapride; Conivaptan; Fusidic Acid (Systemic); Idelalisib; Pimozide; Terfenadine

Increased Effect/Toxicity

Fosaprepitant may increase the levels/effects of: ARIPiprazole; Astemizole; Cisapride; Corticosteroids (Systemic); CYP3A4 Substrates; DilTIAZem; Dofetilide; Flibanserin; HYDROcodone; Ifosfamide; Lomitapide; NiMODipine; Pimozide; Sirolimus; Terfenadine

The levels/effects of Fosaprepitant may be increased by: Aprepitant; Conivaptan; CYP3A4 Inhibitors (Moderate); CYP3A4 Inhibitors (Strong); Dasatinib; DilTIAZem; Fusidic Acid (Systemic); Idelalisib; MiFEPRIStone; Netupitant; Palbociclib; Simeprevir; Stiripentol

Decreased Effect

Fosaprepitant may decrease the levels/effects of: Contraceptives (Estrogens); Contraceptives (Progestins); PARoxetine; TOLBUTamide; Warfarin

The levels/effects of Fosaprepitant may be decreased by: Bosentan; CYP3A4 Inducers (Moderate); CYP3A4 Inducers (Strong); Dabrafenib; Deferasirox; Enzalutamide; Mitotane; PARoxetine; RifAMPin; Sarilumab; Siltuximab; St John's Wort; Tocilizumab

Food Interactions Aprepitant serum concentration may be increased when taken with grapefruit juice. Management: Avoid concurrent use.

Storage/Stability Store intact vials at 2°C to 8°C (36°F to 46°F). Solutions diluted to 1 mg/mL for infusion are stable for 24 hours at room temperature at ≤25°C (≤77°F). Solutions diluted in NS to a final volume of 250 mL (0.6 mg/mL) should be administered within 24 hours (data on file [Merck 2013]).

Preparation for Administration Reconstitute vial with 5 mL of NS, slowly directing diluent down side of vial to avoid foaming; swirl gently. Add reconstituted contents of the 150 mg vial to 145 mL NS (total volume of 150 mL), resulting in a final concentration of 1 mg/mL; gently invert bag 2 to 3 times to mix. Solutions may also be diluted to a final volume of 250 mL (0.6 mg/mL) (data on file [Merck 2013]).

Mechanism of Action Fosaprepitant is a prodrug of aprepitant, a substance P/neurokinin 1 (NK1) receptor antagonist. Fosaprepitant is rapidly converted to aprepitant, which prevents acute and delayed vomiting by inhibiting the substance P/neurokinin 1 (NK1) receptor; also augments the antiemetic activity of the 5-HT$_3$ receptor antagonist and corticosteroid activity and inhibits chemotherapy-induced emesis.

Pharmacodynamics/Kinetics

Distribution: Aprepitant: V_d: ~70 L; crosses the blood-brain barrier

Protein binding: Aprepitant: >95%

Metabolism:

Fosaprepitant: Hepatic and extrahepatic; rapidly (within 30 minutes after the end of infusion) converted to aprepitant (nearly complete conversion)

Aprepitant: Hepatic via CYP3A4 (major); CYP1A2 and CYP2C19 (minor); forms 7 weakly-active metabolites

Half-life elimination: Aprepitant: ~9 to 13 hours

Time to peak, plasma: Fosaprepitant is converted to aprepitant within 30 minutes after the end of infusion

Excretion: Urine (57%); feces (45%)

Dosing

Adult & Geriatric Prevention of chemotherapy-induced nausea/vomiting:

Highly emetogenic chemotherapy: IV: 150 mg ~30 minutes prior to chemotherapy on day 1 only (in combination with a 5-HT$_3$ antagonist on day 1 only and dexamethasone on days 1 to 4 [reduce dexamethasone dose by 50% on days 1 and 2])

Moderately emetogenic chemotherapy: IV: 150 mg ~30 minutes prior to chemotherapy on day 1 only (in combination with a 5-HT$_3$ antagonist and dexamethasone on day 1 [reduce dexamethasone dose by 50%])

Renal Impairment

There are no dosage adjustments provided in the manufacturer's labeling; however, due to modest decreases in protein binding of aprepitant, the AUC of pharmacologically active unbound drug is not significantly affected in patients with renal disease.

Hemodialysis: Aprepitant is not removed by hemodialysis.

Hepatic Impairment

Mild or moderate impairment (Child-Pugh class A or B): No dosage adjustment necessary.

Severe impairment (Child-Pugh class C): There is no dosage adjustment provided in the manufacturer's labeling (has not been studied); additional monitoring may be needed.

Administration
Infuse over 20 to 30 minutes ~30 minutes prior to chemotherapy

Monitoring Parameters
Monitor INR in patients on chronic warfarin therapy in the 2-week period (particularly at 7 to 10 days) following fosaprepitant administration; monitor for signs/symptoms of hypersensitivity reactions.

Dosage Forms
Excipient information presented when available (limited, particularly for generics); consult specific product labeling.

Solution Reconstituted, Intravenous:

Emend: 150 mg (1 ea) [contains disodium edta, polysorbate 80]

◆ **Fosaprepitant Dimeglumine** *see* Fosaprepitant *on page 844*

Foscarnet (fos KAR net)

Brand Names: US Foscavir

Brand Names: Canada Foscavir

Index Terms Foscavir; PFA; Phosphonoformate; Phosphonoformic Acid

Pharmacologic Category Antiviral Agent

Use

Cytomegalovirus retinitis: Treatment of cytomegalovirus (CMV) retinitis in persons with AIDS

Herpes simplex virus: Treatment of acyclovir-resistant mucocutaneous herpes simplex virus (HSV) infections in immunocompromised persons (eg, with advanced AIDS)

Pregnancy Risk Factor C

◄ **Dosing**

Adult & Geriatric

Cytomegalovirus (CMV) retinitis: IV:

Induction treatment: 60 mg/kg/dose every 8 hours for 14 to 21 days **or** 90 mg/kg every 12 hours for 14 to 21 days

Maintenance therapy: 90 to 120 mg/kg/day as a single daily infusion; due to lower toxicity, begin with 90 mg/kg once daily, may escalate to 120 mg/kg once daily if lower dose tolerated or for retinitis progression

CMV infection (preemptive therapy) after allogeneic stem cell transplantation (off-label use; second-line therapy): IV:

<100 days post-transplant: Induction: 60 mg/kg every 12 hours for 7 to 14 days, followed by maintenance therapy: 90 mg/kg once daily if CMV is still detectable and declining, continue until indicator test is negative. Minimum total duration (induction and maintenance) is 2 weeks (Tomblyn 2009)

>100 days post-transplant: 60 mg/kg every 12 hours for 14 days, continue treatment with 90 mg/kg once daily for 7 to 14 days or until indicator test is negative (Tomblyn 2009)

CMV infection (prophylaxis) after allogeneic stem cell transplantation (off-label use; second-line therapy): IV: 60 mg/kg every 12 hours for 7 days, followed by 90 to 120 mg/kg once daily until day 100 after transplant (Tomblyn 2009)

CMV esophagitis or colitis in HIV-infected patients (alternative to preferred therapy) (off-label use): IV: 60 mg/kg/dose every 8 hours or 90 mg/kg/dose every 12 hours for 21 to 42 days or until symptom resolution (HHS [OI adult 2015])

CMV neurological disease in HIV-infected patients (off-label use): IV: 60 mg/kg/dose every 8 hours or 90 mg/kg/dose every 12 hours plus ganciclovir until symptoms improve followed by chronic maintenance suppression (secondary prophylaxis) (HHS [OI adult 2015])

Herpes simplex infections (acyclovir-resistant): Induction: IV: 40 mg/kg/dose every 8 to 12 hours for 14 to 21 days

Pediatric

Cytomegalovirus (CMV) infection (preemptive therapy) after allogeneic stem cell transplantation (off-label use; second-line therapy): IV:

<100 days post-transplant: Induction: 60 mg/kg every 12 hours for 7 to 14 days, followed by maintenance therapy: 90 mg/kg once daily if CMV is still detectable and declining, continue until indicator test is negative. Minimum total duration (induction and maintenance) is 2 weeks (Tomblyn 2009)

>100 days post-transplant: 60 mg/kg every 12 hours for 14 days, continue treatment with 90 mg/kg once daily for 7 to 14 days or until indicator test is negative (Tomblyn 2009)

CMV infection (prophylaxis) after allogeneic stem cell transplantation (off-label use; second-line therapy): IV: 60 mg/kg every 12 hours for 7 days, followed by 90 to 120 mg/kg once daily until day 100 after transplant (Tomblyn 2009)

CMV esophagitis or colitis in HIV-infected patients (alternative to preferred therapy) (off-label use): Adolescents: Refer to adult dosing.

CMV neurological disease in HIV-infected patients (off-label use): Adolescents: Refer to adult dosing

Renal Impairment See tables.

Induction Dosing of Foscarnet in Patients With Abnormal Renal Function

CrCl (mL/min/kg)	HSV Equivalent to 40 mg/kg every 12 hours	HSV Equivalent to 40 mg/kg every 8 hours	CMV Equivalent to 60 mg/kg every 8 hours	CMV Equivalent to 90 mg/kg every 12 hours
<0.4	Not recommended	Not recommended	Not recommended	Not recommended
≥0.4-0.5	20 mg/kg every 24 hours	35 mg/kg every 24 hours	50 mg/kg every 24 hours	50 mg/kg every 24 hours
>0.5-0.6	25 mg/kg every 24 hours	40 mg/kg every 24 hours	60 mg/kg every 24 hours	60 mg/kg every 24 hours
>0.6-0.8	35 mg/kg every 24 hours	25 mg/kg every 12 hours	40 mg/kg every 12 hours	80 mg/kg every 12 hours
>0.8-1	20 mg/kg every 12 hours	35 mg/kg every 12 hours	50 mg/kg every 12 hours	50 mg/kg every 12 hours
>1-1.4	30 mg/kg every 12 hours	30 mg/kg every 8 hours	45 mg/kg every 8 hours	70 mg/kg every 12 hours
>1.4	40 mg/kg every 12 hours	40 mg/kg every 8 hours	60 mg/kg every 8 hours	90 mg/kg every 12 hours

Maintenance Dosing of Foscarnet in Patients With Abnormal Renal Function

CrCl (mL/min/kg)	CMV Equivalent to 90 mg/kg every 24 hours	CMV Equivalent to 120 mg/kg every 24 hours
<0.4	Not recommended	Not recommended
≥0.4-0.5	50 mg/kg every 48 hours	65 mg/kg every 48 hours
>0.5-0.6	60 mg/kg every 48 hours	80 mg/kg every 48 hours
>0.6-0.8	80 mg/kg every 48 hours	105 mg/kg every 48 hours
>0.8-1	50 mg/kg every 24 hours	65 mg/kg every 24 hours
>1-1.4	70 mg/kg every 24 hours	90 mg/kg every 24 hours
>1.4	90 mg/kg every 24 hours	120 mg/kg every 24 hours

Hemodialysis:
Foscarnet is highly removed by hemodialysis (up to ~38% in 2.5 hours HD with high-flux membrane) (Aweeka 1999)

Doses of 45 to 60 mg/kg/dose posthemodialysis (3 times/week) with the monitoring of weekly plasma concentrations to maintain peak plasma concentrations in the range of 500 to 800 micromolar for the treatment of CMV infection have been recommended (Aweeka 1999; Jayasekara 1999; MacGregor 1991)

Peritoneal dialysis: HSV infection (localized or disseminated): IV: 60 mg/kg/dose every 48 to 72 hours; higher doses may be necessary for herpes encephalitis or herpes zoster infection (Jayasekara 1999)

Hepatic Impairment There are no dosage adjustments provided in manufacturer's labeling.

Additional Information Complete prescribing information should be consulted for additional detail.

◀ **Dosage Forms** Excipient information presented when available (limited, particularly for generics); consult specific product labeling.
Solution, Intravenous, as sodium [preservative free]:
Foscavir: 24 mg/mL (250 mL)

Fulvestrant (fool VES trant)

Related Information

Common Toxicity Criteria *on page 2242*
Safe Handling of Hazardous Drugs *on page 2379*

Brand Names: US Faslodex
Brand Names: Canada Faslodex
Index Terms ICI-182,780; ZD9238
Pharmacologic Category Antineoplastic Agent, Estrogen Receptor Antagonist

Use

Breast cancer, metastatic: Treatment of hormone-receptor (HR)-positive metastatic breast cancer (as monotherapy) in postmenopausal women with disease progression following antiestrogen therapy

Breast cancer, advanced or metastatic (second-line endocrine-based combination therapy): Treatment of HR-positive, human epidermal growth factor receptor 2 (HER2)-negative advanced or metastatic breast cancer (in combination with palbociclib) in women with disease progression following endocrine therapy

Labeled Contraindications

Known hypersensitivity to fulvestrant or any component of the formulation
Canadian labeling: Additional contraindications (not in US labeling): Pregnant or lactating women

Pregnancy Considerations Adverse events were observed in animal reproduction studies. Based on the mechanism of action, fulvestrant may cause fetal harm if administered during pregnancy. For females of reproductive potential, pregnancy testing is recommended within 7 days prior to initiation of fulvestrant and effective contraception should be used during treatment and for 1 year after the last fulvestrant dose. Animal data suggest that fulvestrant may affect female and male fertility (although not approved for use in men).

Breastfeeding Considerations It is not known if fulvestrant is excreted into breast milk. Because of the potential for serious adverse reactions in the nursing infant, lactating women should not breast-feed during treatment and for 1 year after the final fulvestrant dose.

Warnings/Precautions Exposure is increased and dosage adjustment is recommended in patients with moderate hepatic impairment. Safety and efficacy have not been established in severe hepatic impairment. Use with caution in patients with a history of bleeding disorders (including thrombocytopenia) and/or patients on anticoagulant therapy; bleeding/hematoma may occur from IM administration. Events related to injection site, including sciatica, neuralgia, neuropathic pain, and peripheral neuropathy, have been reported with fulvestrant administration. Due to the proximity of underlying sciatic nerve, use caution if administering at the dorsogluteal site. Hypersensitivity reactions, including urticaria and angioedema, have been reported.

Benzyl alcohol and derivatives: Some dosage forms may contain benzyl alcohol; large amounts of benzyl alcohol (≥99 mg/kg/day) have been associated with a potentially fatal toxicity ("gasping syndrome") in neonates; the "gasping syndrome" consists of metabolic acidosis, respiratory distress, gasping respirations, CNS dysfunction (including convulsions, intracranial hemorrhage), hypotension and cardiovascular collapse (AAP ["Inactive" 1997]; CDC, 1982); some data suggests that benzoate displaces bilirubin from protein binding sites (Ahlfors 2001); avoid or use dosage forms containing benzyl alcohol with caution in neonates. See manufacturer's labeling.

Adverse Reactions Adverse reactions reported with 500 mg dose.
>10%:
Central nervous system: Fatique (8% to 29%), headache (8% to 20%)
Gastrointestinal: Nausea (10% to 28%), diarrhea (19%), constipation (5% to 16%), stomatitis (13%)
Hematologic & oncologic: Anemia (13% to 40%; grade 3: 2%)
Hepatic: Increased liver enzymes (>15%; grades 3/4: 1% to 2%)
Infection: Infection (31%; including nasopharyngitis, upper respiratory infection, urinary tract infection, influenza, bronchitis, rhinitis, conjunctivitis, pneumonia, sinusitis, cystitis, oral herpes, respiratory tract infection)
Local: Pain at injection site (12%; including neuralgia, peripheral neuropathy, sciatica)
1% to 10%:
Dermatologic: Alopecia (6%), skin rash (6%), xeroderma (1%)
Endocrine & metabolic: Hot flash (7%)
Gastrointestinal: Decreased appetite (8%), anorexia (6%), vomiting (6%), dysgeusia (3%)
Hematologic & oncologic: Decreased platelet count (10%), leukopenia (5%; grade 3: 1%; grade 4: 1%), neutropenia (4%; grade 3: 1%), febrile neutropenia (1%; grade 4: 1%)
Neuromuscular & skeletal: Ostealgia (9%), arthralgia (8%), back pain (8%), limb pain (7%), musculoskeletal pain (6%), weakness (5% to 6%)
Ophthalmic: Blurred vision (2%), dry eye syndrome (2%), increased lacrimation (1%)
Respiratory: Cough (5%), dyspnea (4%), epistaxis (2%)
<1%, postmarketing, and/or case reports (reported with 250 or 500 mg dose): Angioedema, hepatic failure, hepatitis, hypersensitivity reaction, increased gamma-glutamyl transferase, increased serum bilirubin, myalgia, thrombosis, urticaria, vaginal hemorrhage, vertigo

Drug Interactions
Metabolism/Transport Effects Substrate of CYP3A4 (minor); **Note:** Assignment of Major/Minor substrate status based on clinically relevant drug interaction potential

◀ **Avoid Concomitant Use** There are no known interactions where it is recommended to avoid concomitant use.

Increased Effect/Toxicity There are no known significant interactions involving an increase in effect.

Decreased Effect There are no known significant interactions involving a decrease in effect.

Hazardous Drugs Handling Considerations

Hazardous agent (NIOSH 2016 [group 1]).

Use appropriate precautions for receiving, handling, administration, and disposal. Gloves (single) should be worn during receiving, unpacking, and placing in storage.

NIOSH recommends double gloving, a protective gown, ventilated engineering controls (a class II biological safety cabinet or a compounding aseptic containment isolator), and closed system transfer devices (CSTDs) for preparation. Double gloving and a protective gown are recommended during administration (NIOSH 2016).

Storage/Stability Store in original carton at 2°C to 8°C (36°F to 46°F). Protect from light.

Mechanism of Action Estrogen receptor antagonist; competitively binds to estrogen receptors on tumors and other tissue targets, producing a nuclear complex that causes a dose-related down-regulation of estrogen receptors and inhibits tumor growth.

Pharmacodynamics/Kinetics

Duration: IM: Steady state concentrations reached within first month, when administered with additional dose given 2 weeks following the initial dose; plasma levels maintained for at least 1 month

Distribution: V_d: ~3 to 5 L/kg

Protein binding: 99%; to plasma proteins (VLDL, LDL and HDL lipoprotein fractions)

Metabolism: Hepatic via multiple biotransformation pathways (CYP3A4 substrate involved in oxidation pathway, although relative contribution to metabolism unknown); metabolites formed are either less active or have similar activity to parent compound

Half-life elimination:

Children 1 to 10 years: 70.4 ± 8.1 days (Sims 2012)

Adults 250 mg: ~40 days

Excretion: Feces (~90%); urine (<1%)

Clearance: Children 1 to 8 years (based on a 4 mg/kg dose): Decreased by 32% compared to adults

Dosing

Adult & Geriatric

Breast cancer, metastatic (postmenopausal women; HR positive): IM: Initial: 500 mg on days 1, 15, and 29; Maintenance: 500 mg once monthly. In studies, the 500 mg once monthly dose was administered at 28 days ± 3 days (Di Leo 2014).

Breast cancer, advanced or metastatic (second-line endocrine-based combination therapy): Adult females (HR positive, HER-2 negative): IM: Initial: 500 mg on days 1, 15, and 29; Maintenance: 500 mg once every 28 days. Administer in combination with palbociclib (and an LHRH agonist [eg, goserelin] if pre- or perimenopausal); continue until disease progression or unacceptable toxicity (Turner 2015). **Note:** Refer to Palbociclib monograph for dosing in combination with fulvestrant.

Renal Impairment There are no dosage adjustments provided in the manufacturer's labeling (has not been studied). However, renal elimination of fulvestrant is negligible.

Hepatic Impairment

Mild impairment (Child-Pugh class A): No dosage adjustment is necessary.

Moderate impairment (Child-Pugh class B): Reduce initial doses and maintenance dose to 250 mg.

Severe impairment (Child-Pugh class C): There are no dosage adjustments provided in the manufacturer's labeling (use has not been evaluated).

Combination Regimens

Breast cancer: Palbociclib-Fulvestrant (Breast) on page 2189

Administration For IM administration only. Administer 500 mg dose as two 5 mL IM injections (one in each buttocks [gluteal area]) slowly over 1 to 2 minutes per injection. If administering at the dorsogluteal site, use caution during injection due to the proximity of underlying sciatic nerve. Refer to facility policy for IM administration of large volumes. To prepare each syringe for administration, hold syringe upright; carefully tilt syringe cap back and forth (without twisting) until the cap disconnects for removal; pull cap off by pulling up without touching the syringe tip (to maintain sterility); attach safety needle to syringe tip and twist firmly to lock. Remove needle cap by pulling straight off to avoid damaging needle point, remove needle sheath and expel excess air from syringe prior to administration. Refer to product labeling for detailed instructions.

Monitoring Parameters Liver function tests; pregnancy testing is recommended within 7 days prior to fulvestrant initiation (for females of reproductive potential); monitor for signs/symptoms of bleeding

Test Interactions Due to a similarity in structures, fulvestrant may interfere with estradiol immunoassay, resulting in falsely elevated estradiol levels.

Dosage Forms Excipient information presented when available (limited, particularly for generics); consult specific product labeling.

Solution, Intramuscular:

Faslodex: 250 mg/5 mL (5 mL) [contains alcohol, usp, benzyl alcohol, benzyl benzoate]

♦ **Fungizone (Can)** *see* Amphotericin B (Conventional) *on page* 115

♦ **Fusilev** *see* LEVOleucovorin *on page* 1145

♦ **FXIII** *see* Factor XIII Concentrate (Human) *on page* 782

♦ **GA101** *see* Obinutuzumab *on page* 1341

♦ **⁶⁷Ga-Citrate** *see* Gallium Citrate Ga-67 *on page* 853

♦ **⁶⁷Ga-Gallium Citrate** *see* Gallium Citrate Ga-67 *on page* 853

♦ **Gallium Citrate Ga-67** *see* Gallium Citrate Ga-67 *on page* 853

Gallium Citrate Ga-67 (GAL ee um SIT rate jee aye SIX tee SEV en)

Index Terms ⁶⁷Ga-Citrate; ⁶⁷Ga-Gallium Citrate; Gallium Citrate Ga-67; Gallium Ga-67

Pharmacologic Category Radiopharmaceutical

Use Diagnostic imaging: Diagnostic imaging agent for use in identifying the presence and extent of Hodgkin disease, lymphoma, bronchogenic carcinoma, and acute inflammatory lesions

Pregnancy Risk Factor C

◀ **Dosing**
Adult Diagnostic imaging: IV:
Manufacturer's labeling: (based on 70 kg patient): 2 to 5 mCi (74 to 185 MBq).
Alternative dosing:
Scintigraphy for inflammation or infection: 4 to 6 mCi (150 to 220 MBq) (ACR/SPR 2014)
Tumor scintigraphy: 5 to 10 mCi (185 to 370 MBq) (ACR/SPR 2015)
Pediatric Diagnostic imaging: Scintigraphy for inflammation or infection (off-label use): IV: 0.07 mCi/kg (2.6 MBq/kg), with a minimum of 0.5 mCi (18.5 MBq) (ACR/SPR 2014) **or** alternatively for children >5 years: 0.04 to 0.07 mCi/kg (1.5 to 2.6 MBq/kg) (Palestro 2004)
Renal Impairment There are no dosage adjustments provided in the manufacturer's labeling.
Hepatic Impairment There are no dosage adjustments provided in the manufacturer's labeling.
Additional Information Complete prescribing information should be consulted for additional detail.

◆ **Gallium Ga-67** see Gallium Citrate Ga-67 on page 853
◆ **Gallium Ga-68** see Gallium Ga 68 Dotatate on page 854

Gallium Ga 68 Dotatate (GAL ee um jee aye SIX tee ATE doe tah TATE)

Brand Names: US Netspot
Index Terms Gallium Ga-68; Somakit-TATE
Pharmacologic Category Radiopharmaceutical
Use Diagnostic imaging: Use with positron emission tomography (PET) (after radiolabeling with Ga 68) for localization of somatostatin receptor-positive neuroendocrine tumors (NETs) in adult and pediatric patients.
Dosing
Adult Diagnostic imaging: IV: 2 MBq/kg (0.054 mCi/kg); maximum dose 200 MBq (5.4 mCi). Begin PET scanning 40 to 90 minutes after completion of gallium Ga 68 dotatate administration.
Pediatric Diagnostic imaging: IV: Refer to adult dosing.
Renal Impairment There are no dosage adjustments provided in the manufacturer's labeling.
Hepatic Impairment There are no dosage adjustments provided in the manufacturer's labeling.
Additional Information Complete prescribing information should be consulted for additional detail.
Dosage Forms Excipient information presented when available (limited, particularly for generics); consult specific product labeling.
Kit, Intravenous:
Netspot: Lyophilized dotatate mixture and reaction buffer solution [to be combined with Ga 68 (not included)]

◆ **GamaSTAN S/D** see Immune Globulin on page 992
◆ **Gamastan S/D (Can)** see Immune Globulin on page 992
◆ **Gammagard** see Immune Globulin on page 992
◆ **Gammagard Liquid (Can)** see Immune Globulin on page 992
◆ **Gammagard S/D [DSC]** see Immune Globulin on page 992

♦ **Gammagard S/D (Can)** *see* Immune Globulin *on page* 992

♦ **Gammagard S/D Less IgA** *see* Immune Globulin *on page* 992

♦ **Gamma Globulin** *see* Immune Globulin *on page* 992

♦ **Gammaked** *see* Immune Globulin *on page* 992

♦ **Gammaphos** *see* Amifostine *on page* 104

♦ **Gammaplex** *see* Immune Globulin *on page* 992

♦ **Gamunex (Can)** *see* Immune Globulin *on page* 992

♦ **Gamunex-C** *see* Immune Globulin *on page* 992

Ganciclovir (Systemic) (gan SYE kloe veer)

Brand Names: US Cytovene

Brand Names: Canada Cytovene; Ganciclovir for Injection

Index Terms DHPG Sodium; Ganciclovir Sodium; GCV Sodium; Nordeoxyguanosine

Pharmacologic Category Antiviral Agent

Use

Cytomegalovirus disease, prophylaxis (transplant patients): Prevention of cytomegalovirus (CMV) disease in adult transplant recipients at risk for CMV disease.

Cytomegalovirus retinitis (immunocompromised patients): Treatment of CMV retinitis in immunocompromised adult patients, including patients with AIDS.

Hazardous Drugs Handling Considerations

Hazardous agent (NIOSH 2016 [group 2]).

Use appropriate precautions for receiving, handling, administration, and disposal. Gloves (single) should be worn during receiving, unpacking, and placing in storage.

NIOSH recommends double gloving, a protective gown, ventilated engineering controls (a class II biological safety cabinet or a compounding aseptic containment isolator), and closed system transfer devices (CSTDs) for preparation. Double gloving, a gown, and (if dosage form allows) CSTDs are required during administration (NIOSH 2016).

Dosing

Adult & Geriatric

CMV retinitis (immunocompromised patients):

Manufacturer's labeling:

Induction therapy: IV: 5 mg/kg/dose every 12 hours for 14 to 21 days followed by maintenance therapy

Maintenance therapy: IV: 5 mg/kg/dose once daily for 7 days/week or 6 mg/kg/dose once daily for 5 days/week

Alternate dosing (HHS [OI adult 2017]):

Peripheral lesions (alternative agent): IV: Induction: 5 mg/kg/dose every 12 hours for 14 to 21 days followed by chronic maintenance (secondary prophylaxis)

Immediate sight-threatening lesions (adjacent to the optic nerve or fovea): Intravitreal injection (off-label route): Induction therapy: 2 mg of an extemporaneously prepared solution administered as intravitreal injections for 1 to 4 doses over a period of 7 to 10 days; administer with a concomitant systemically administered agent (oral valganciclovir preferred).

CMV disease prophylaxis in transplant patients: IV:

Manufacturer's labeling:

Induction therapy: 5 mg/kg/dose every 12 hours for 7 to 14 days

Maintenance therapy: 5 mg/kg/dose once daily for 7 days/week or 6 mg/kg/dose once daily for 5 days/week; duration is dependent on clinical condition and degree of immunosuppression

Alternate dosing:

Hematopoietic cell transplant recipients (allogeneic): 5 mg/kg/dose every 12 hours for 5 to 7 days, then 5 mg/kg/dose every 24 hours until day 100 post-transplant (Tomblyn 2009).

Solid organ transplant recipients: 5 mg/kg/dose every 24 hours; duration of prophylaxis is dependent on type of transplant, as well as donor and recipient CMV serostatus (Kotton 2013).

CMV disease, preemptive therapy (hematopoietic cell transplant recipients) (off-label use) (Tomblyn 2009): IV:

<100 days post-transplant: 5 mg/kg/dose every 12 hours for 7 days (autologous transplant) or 7 to 14 days (allogenic transplant), then 5 mg/kg/dose every 24 hours for 1 to 2 weeks or until the indicator test is negative (minimum total induction and maintenance treatment is 2 weeks when 14 days of twice daily is used and 3 weeks when a 7-day induction course is used).

>100 days post-transplant: 5 mg/kg/dose every 12 hours for 7 to 14 days, then 5 mg/kg/dose every 24 hours for 1 to 2 weeks or until the indicator test is negative.

CMV disease, treatment (solid organ transplant recipients) (off-label use): IV: 5 mg/kg/dose every 12 hours until 1 or 2 consecutive undetectable CMV viral load samples are obtained (minimum treatment course: 2 weeks) (Kotton 2013).

UL97 mutation for <5x ganciclovir EC50: 10 mg/kg/dose every 12 hours (Kotton 2013).

Ganciclovir-resistant strains: 5 mg/kg/dose every 24 hours in combination with daily foscarnet and monthly CMV hyperimmunoglobulin (Mylonakis 2002).

CMV esophagitis or colitis in HIV-infected patients (off-label use): IV: 5 mg/kg/dose every 12 hours, then change to oral valganciclovir therapy once oral therapy is tolerated; total duration of therapy: 21 to 42 days or until symptom resolution (HHS [OI adult 2017]).

CMV neurological disease in HIV-infected patients (off-label use): IV: 5 mg/kg/dose every 12 hours plus foscarnet until symptoms improve (HHS [OI adult 2017]).

CMV retinitis, chronic maintenance (secondary prophylaxis) in HIV-infected patients (off-label use; alternative agent): IV: 5 mg/kg/dose 5 to 7 times weekly; continue until sustained CD4 count >100 cells/mm^3 in response to ART for 3 to 6 months; discontinue only after consultation with an ophthalmologist) (HHS [OI adult 2017]).

Varicella-zoster: Acute retinal necrosis (ARN) in HIV-infected patients (off-label use): Intravitreal injection (off-label route): 2 mg of an extemporaneously prepared solution administered as an intravitreal injection twice weekly for 1 to 2 doses in combination with IV acyclovir for 10 to 14 days, followed by valacyclovir for 6 weeks (HHS [OI adult 2017]).

Varicella-zoster: Progressive outer retinal necrosis in HIV-infected patients (off-label use): IV: 5 mg/kg/dose every 12 hours (with or without IV foscarnet) **plus** intravitreal ganciclovir and/or intravitreal foscarnet (HHS [OI adult 2017]).

Pediatric

CMV disease, chronic maintenance (secondary prophylaxis) in HIV-exposed/-infected patients (off-label use):
Infants and Children: IV: 5 mg/kg/dose daily (CDC 2009)
Adolescents (alternative to preferred therapy): Refer to adult dosing.

CMV esophagitis or colitis in HIV-infected patients (off-label use):
Adolescents: Refer to adult dosing.

CMV neurological disease in HIV-exposed/-infected patients (off-label use): Infants, Children, and Adolescents: IV: Refer to adult dosing.

Varicella-zoster: Acute retinal necrosis (ARN) in HIV-infected patients (off-label use): Adolescents: Refer to adult dosing.

Varicella-zoster: Progressive outer retinal necrosis in HIV-exposed/-infected patients (off-label use):
Infants and Children: IV: 5 mg/kg/dose every 12 hours plus systemic foscarnet and intravitreal ganciclovir or intravitreal foscarnet (CDC 2009)
Adolescents: Refer to adult dosing.

Renal Impairment Note: Renally adjusted dose recommendations are based on an induction dose of 5 mg/kg/dose every 12 hours and a maintenance dose of 5 mg/kg/dose every 24 hours.

IV (Induction):
CrCl ≥70 mL/minute: No dosage adjustment necessary.
CrCl 50 to 69 mL/minute: Administer 2.5 mg/kg/dose every 12 hours
CrCl 25 to 49 mL/minute: Administer 2.5 mg/kg/dose every 24 hours
CrCl 10 to 24 mL/minute: Administer 1.25 mg/kg/dose every 24 hours
CrCl <10 mL/minute: Administer 1.25 mg/kg/dose 3 times/week following hemodialysis.

IV (Maintenance):
CrCl ≥70 mL/minute: No dosage adjustment necessary.
CrCl 50 to 69 mL/minute: Administer 2.5 mg/kg/dose every 24 hours
CrCl 25 to 49 mL/minute: Administer 1.25 mg/kg/dose every 24 hours
CrCl 10 to 24 mL/minute: Administer 0.625 mg/kg/dose every 24 hours
CrCl <10 mL/minute: Administer 0.625 mg/kg/dose 3 times/week following hemodialysis.

Intermittent hemodialysis (IHD) (administer after hemodialysis on dialysis days): Dialyzable (50%): CMV Infection: IV: Induction: 1.25 mg/kg every 48 to 72 hours; Maintenance: 0.625 mg/kg every 48 to 72 hours. **Note:** Dosing dependent on the assumption of 3 times/week, complete IHD sessions (Heintz 2009).

Peritoneal dialysis (PD): Dose as for CrCl <10 mL/minute (Aronoff 2007).

Continuous renal replacement therapy (CRRT) (Heintz 2009; Trotman 2005): Drug clearance is highly dependent on the method of renal replacement, filter type, and flow rate. Appropriate dosing requires close monitoring of pharmacologic response, signs of adverse reactions due to drug accumulation, as well as drug concentrations in relation to target trough (if appropriate). The following are general recommendations only (based on dialysate flow/ultrafiltration rates of 1 to 2 L/hour and minimal residual renal function) and should not supersede clinical judgment: CMV Infection:
CVVH: IV: Induction: 2.5 mg/kg every 24 hours; Maintenance: 1.25 mg/kg every 24 hours
CVVHD/CVVHDF: IV: Induction: 2.5 mg/kg every 12 hours; Maintenance: 2.5 mg/kg every 24 hours

Hepatic Impairment There are no dosage adjustments provided in the manufacturer's labeling (has not been studied).

◄ **Additional Information** Complete prescribing information should be consulted for additional detail.

Dosage Forms Excipient information presented when available (limited, particularly for generics); consult specific product labeling.

Solution Reconstituted, Intravenous:

Cytovene: 500 mg (1 ea)

Generic: 500 mg (1 ea)

Solution Reconstituted, Intravenous [preservative free]:

Generic: 500 mg (1 ea)

◆ **Ganciclovir for Injection (Can)** see Ganciclovir (Systemic) on page 855

◆ **Ganciclovir Sodium** see Ganciclovir (Systemic) on page 855

◆ **Gardasil 9** see Papillomavirus (9-Valent) Vaccine (Human, Recombinant) on page 1452

◆ **Gazyva** see Obinutuzumab on page 1341

◆ **G-CSF** see Filgrastim on page 792

◆ **G-CSF (PEG Conjugate)** see Pegfilgrastim on page 1467

◆ **GCV Sodium** see Ganciclovir (Systemic) on page 855

◆ **GDC-0199** see Venetoclax on page 1883

◆ **GDC-0449** see Vismodegib on page 1921

◆ **GDC-0973** see Cobimetinib on page 425

◆ **GD-Tranexamic Acid (Can)** see Tranexamic Acid on page 1816

Gefitinib (ge FI tye nib)

Related Information

Common Toxicity Criteria on page 2242

Management of Chemotherapy-Induced Nausea and Vomiting in Adults on page 2253

Management of EGFR Inhibitor Toxicities: Dermatologic, Ocular, and Gastrointestinal on page 2291

Prevention of Chemotherapy-Induced Nausea and Vomiting in Children on page 2310

Safe Handling of Hazardous Drugs on page 2379

Brand Names: US Iressa

Brand Names: Canada IRESSA

Index Terms ZD1839

Pharmacologic Category Antineoplastic Agent, Epidermal Growth Factor Receptor (EGFR) Inhibitor; Antineoplastic Agent, Tyrosine Kinase Inhibitor

Use

Non-small cell lung cancer:

US labeling: First-line treatment of metastatic non-small cell lung cancer (NSCLC) in tumors with epidermal growth factor receptor (EGFR) exon 19 deletions or exon 21 (L858R) substitution mutations as detected by an approved test.

Limitation of use: Safety and efficacy have not been established in patients with metastatic NSCLC whose tumors have EGFR mutations other than exon 19 deletions or exon 21 (L858R) substitution mutations

Canadian labeling: First-line treatment of locally advanced (nonresponsive to curative therapy) or metastatic NSCLC with activating mutations of the epidermal growth factor receptor tyrosine kinase (EGFR-TK).

Labeled Contraindications

There are no contraindications listed in the manufacturer's US labeling.

Canadian labeling: Hypersensitivity to gefitinib or any component of the formulation.

Pregnancy Considerations Adverse events have been observed in animal reproduction studies. Gefitinib may cause fetal harm when administered to a pregnant woman. Women of reproductive potential should use effective contraception during and for at least 2 weeks following gefitinib treatment.

Breastfeeding Considerations It is not known if gefitinib is excreted in breast milk. Due to the potential for serious adverse reactions in the nursing infant, breastfeeding is not recommended by the manufacturer.

Warnings/Precautions Interstitial lung disease (ILD) or ILD-like reactions (eg, acute respiratory distress syndrome, lung infiltration, pneumonitis, or pulmonary fibrosis) have occurred (rarely) with gefitinib; some cases were grade 3 or higher and some were fatal. Withhold gefitinib and promptly assess any patient with worsening respiratory symptoms (dyspnea, cough and fever); discontinue permanently if ILD is confirmed. Increased systemic gefitinib exposure is associated with an increased incidence of ILD. An increase in mortality was observed in patients with the following risk factors: Smoking, CT scan evidence of reduced normal lung (≤50%), preexisting ILD, increased age (≥65 years), and extensive areas adherent to pleura (≥50%).

Increases in ALT, AST, and bilirubin, including grade 3 or higher toxicity have been observed. Fatal hepatotoxicity has occurred rarely. Monitor liver functions tests periodically. Withhold gefitinib in patients with worsening liver function; discontinue for severe hepatic impairment. Gefitinib exposure is increased in patients with mild, moderate, and severe hepatic impairment due to cirrhosis. However, in a study of patients with liver metastases, patients with metastases and moderate impairment had similar systemic exposure as patients with metastases and normal hepatic function. Monitor for adverse reactions if administering to patients with moderate or severe hepatic impairment.

Gastrointestinal perforation has occurred (rarely); discontinue permanently if gastrointestinal perforation develops. Nausea, vomiting, decreased appetite, and stomatitis have also been reported. Diarrhea occurs in approximately one-third of patients; grade 3 or 4 diarrhea has been observed. Diarrhea symptoms should be managed as clinically indicated; avoid dehydration. Withhold gefitinib for severe or persistent (up to 14 days) diarrhea.

Ocular disorders, including keratitis, corneal erosion, abnormal eyelash growth, conjunctivitis, blepharitis, and dry eye have been reported; some events were grade 3. Recent corneal surgery and contact lens wearing may be risk factors for ocular toxicity. Advise patients to promptly report developing eye symptoms and promptly refer for ophthalmic evaluation if signs of keratitis (eg, acute or worsening of eye inflammation, lacrimation, blurred vision, pain, red eye, and/or light sensitivity). Interrupt gefitinib treatment or discontinue for severe or worsening ocular disorders. Skin reactions occurred in nearly one-half of patients taking gefitinib. Bullous skin disorders, including toxic epidermal necrolysis, Stevens Johnson syndrome, erythema multiforme, and dermatitis bullous have been reported. Interrupt gefitinib treatment or discontinue for development of severe bullous, blistering, or exfoliating dermatologic conditions.

Establish EGFR mutation status prior to treatment. Do not use in patients with EGFR mutation-negative tumors. Studies have demonstrated a subset of patients who are more likely to respond to gefitinib treatment. This subset includes patients of Asian origin, never-smokers, women, patients with bronchoalveolar adenocarcinoma, and patients with EGFR-mutated tumors. Deletion in exon 19 and mutation in exon 21 are the two most commonly found EGFR mutations; both mutations correlate with clinical response, resulting in increased response rates in patients with the mutation (Riely, 2006). Studies have compared gefitinib in treatment naïve patients to combination chemotherapy in the subsets of patients described above, resulting in a longer progression free survival in the gefitinib arm (Mok, 2009). ASCO guidelines state that the first-line use of gefitinib may be recommended in stage IV disease with activating EGFR mutations (Masters 2015). In patients with a KRAS mutation, however, EGFR-TKI therapy is not recommended.

Systemic exposure of gefitinib may be increased in CYP2D6 poor metabolizers; no dosage adjustment is recommended, although patients should be monitored closely for adverse reactions. Potentially significant drug-drug interactions may exist, requiring dose or frequency adjustment, additional monitoring, and/or selection of alternative therapy. Elevated gastric pH may reduce gefitinib plasma concentrations; if possible, avoid concomitant use with proton pump inhibitors. If proton pump inhibitor therapy is necessary, administer gefitinib 12 hours before or 12 hours after the proton pump inhibitor dose. May administer gefitinib 6 hours before or 6 hours after H_2-receptor antagonists or antacids. May contain lactose; consider intolerance risk in patients with galactose intolerance, Lapp lactase deficiency, or glucose-galactose malabsorption.

Adverse Reactions

>10%:

Central nervous system: Insomnia (15%), fatigue (14%)

Dermatologic: Dermatological reaction (47% to 58%), skin rash (52%), xeroderma (24%), pruritus (18%), paronychia (14%), acne vulgaris (11%), alopecia (5% to 11%)

Gastrointestinal: Diarrhea (29% to 47%; grades 3/4: 3%), anorexia (19% to 20%), nausea (17% to 18%), decreased appetite (17%), vomiting (13% to 14%), stomatitis (7% to 13%), constipation (12%)

Genitourinary: Proteinuria (8% to 35%)

Hepatic: Increased serum AST (8% to 40%; grades 3/4: 2% to 3%), increased serum ALT (11% to 38%; grades 3/4: 2% to 5%)

Neuromuscular & skeletal: Weakness (18%)

1% to 10%:

Central nervous system: Hypoesthesia (4%), peripheral sensory neuropathy (4%), peripheral neuropathy (2%)

Dermatologic: Nail disease (5% to 8%), acneiform eruption (6%)

Endocrine & metabolic: Dehydration (2%; secondary to diarrhea, nausea, vomiting, or anorexia)

Gastrointestinal: Xerostomia (2%)

Genitourinary: Cystitis (1%)

Hematologic & oncologic: Anemia (7%), pulmonary hemorrhage (4% to 5%), hemorrhage (4%; including epistaxis, hematuria), neutropenia (3%), leukopenia (2%), thrombocytopenia (1%)

Hepatic: Increased serum bilirubin (3%; grades 3/4: <1%)

Neuromuscular & skeletal: Myalgia (8%), arthralgia (6%)

Ophthalmic: Eye disease (6% to 7%; grades 3/4: <1%; including conjunctivitis, blepharitis, and dry eye)

Renal: Increased serum creatinine (2%)

Respiratory: Cough (9%), interstitial pulmonary disease (1%; grades 3/4: 3%)

Miscellaneous: Fever (9%)

<1%, postmarketing, and/or case reports: Angioedema, bullous skin disease, corneal erosion (reversible; may be associated with aberrant eyelash growth), decreased white blood cell count, erythema multiforme, fulminant hepatitis, gastrointestinal perforation, hemorrhagic cystitis, hepatic failure, hepatitis, hypersensitivity angiitis, hypersensitivity reaction, keratitis, keratoconjunctivitis sicca, pancreatitis, renal failure, skin fissure, Stevens-Johnson syndrome, toxic epidermal necrolysis, urticaria

Drug Interactions

Metabolism/Transport Effects Substrate of BCRP, CYP2D6 (major), CYP3A4 (major); **Note:** Assignment of Major/Minor substrate status based on clinically relevant drug interaction potential; **Inhibits** BCRP, CYP2D6 (weak)

Avoid Concomitant Use

Avoid concomitant use of Gefitinib with any of the following: Conivaptan; Fusidic Acid (Systemic); Idelalisib

Increased Effect/Toxicity

Gefitinib may increase the levels/effects of: ARIPiprazole; Perhexiline; Vinorelbine; Vitamin K Antagonists

The levels/effects of Gefitinib may be increased by: Abiraterone Acetate; Ajmaline; Aprepitant; Asunaprevir; Ceritinib; Cobicistat; Conivaptan; CYP2D6 Inhibitors (Moderate); CYP2D6 Inhibitors (Strong); CYP3A4 Inhibitors (Moderate); CYP3A4 Inhibitors (Strong); Darunavir; Dasatinib; Fosaprepitant; Fusidic Acid (Systemic); Idelalisib; Imatinib; Lumefantrine; MiFEPRIStone; Netupitant; Palbociclib; Panobinostat; Peginterferon Alfa-2b; Perhexiline; QuiNINE; Simeprevir; Stiripentol

Decreased Effect

The levels/effects of Gefitinib may be decreased by: Antacids; Bosentan; CYP3A4 Inducers (Moderate); CYP3A4 Inducers (Strong); Dabrafenib; Deferasirox; Enzalutamide; H2-Antagonists; Mitotane; Peginterferon Alfa-2b; Proton Pump Inhibitors; Sarilumab; Siltuximab; St John's Wort; Tocilizumab

Food Interactions Grapefruit juice may increase serum gefitinib concentrations. Management: Avoid concurrent use.

Hazardous Drugs Handling Considerations

Hazardous agent (meets NIOSH 2016 criteria). This medication is not on the NIOSH (2016) list; however, it meets the criteria for a hazardous drug. Drugs are classified as hazardous based on their properties; the properties of a hazardous drug include one or more of the following characteristics: carcinogenic, teratogenic (or other developmental toxicity), reproductive toxicity, organotoxic at low doses, genotoxic, and/or new agents with structural or toxicity profiles similar to existing hazardous agents.

Use appropriate precautions for receiving, handling, administration, and disposal. Gloves (single) should be worn during receiving, unpacking, and placing in storage.

◀ NIOSH recommends single gloving for administration of intact tablets or capsules. If manipulating tablets/capsules (eg, to prepare an oral suspension), NIOSH recommends double gloving, a protective gown, and preparation in a controlled device; if not prepared in a controlled device, respiratory and eye/face protection as well as ventilated engineering controls are recommended. NIOSH recommends double gloving, a protective gown, and (if there is a potential for vomit or spit up) eye/face protection for administration of an oral liquid/feeding tube administration (NIOSH 2016).

Storage/Stability Store at 20°C to 25°C (68°F to 77°F).

Mechanism of Action Gefitinib is a tyrosine kinase inhibitor (TKI) which reversibly inhibits kinase activity of wild-type and select activation mutations of epidermal growth factor receptor (EGFR). EGFR is expressed on cell surfaces of normal and cancer cells and has a role in cell growth and proliferation. Gefitinib prevents autophosphorylation of tyrosine residues associated with the EGFR receptor, which blocks downstream signaling and EGFR-dependent proliferation. Gefitinib has a higher binding affinity for EGFR exon 19 deletion and exon 21 (L858R) substitution mutation than for wild-type EGFR.

Pharmacodynamics/Kinetics

Absorption: Oral: Slow

Distribution: 1400 L

Protein binding: 90%, albumin and alpha$_1$-acid glycoprotein

Metabolism: Hepatic (extensive), primarily via CYP3A4, as well as CYP2D6; forms metabolites

Bioavailability: 60%

Half-life elimination: Oral: 41 hours

Time to peak, plasma: Oral: 3 to 7 hours

Excretion: Feces (86%); urine (<4%)

Dosing

Adult & Geriatric

Non-small cell lung cancer (NSCLC), metastatic, with EGFR exon 19 deletions or exon 21 (L858R) substitution mutations: Oral: 250 mg once daily until disease progression or unacceptable toxicity.

NSCLC, locally advanced or metastatic with EGFR mutations (Canadian labeling): Oral: 250 mg once daily.

Missed doses: Do not take a missed dose if it is within 12 hours of the next scheduled dose.

Dosage adjustment for concomitant therapy (US labeling): *Strong CYP3A4 inducers (eg, phenytoin, rifampin, or tricyclic antidepressants):* Increase gefitinib to 500 mg once daily (in the absence of severe adverse drug reactions); reduce gefitinib dose back to 250 mg once daily 7 days after discontinuing the strong CYP3A4 inducer.

Pediatric Non-small cell lung cancer (NSCLC), locally advanced or metastatic with EGFR mutations (Canadian labeling): Adolescents ≥17 years: Oral: Refer to Canadian adult dosing.

Renal Impairment

US labeling: There are no dosage adjustments provided in the manufacturer's labeling; however, due to minimal renal excretion (<4% of gefitinib and metabolites) the need for dosage adjustment is unlikely. Use has not been studied in patients with CrCl ≤20 mL/minute.

Canadian labeling: No dosage adjustment necessary. Use caution in severe impairment (CrCl ≤20 mL/minute).

Hepatic Impairment

Dosage adjustment for hepatic impairment at treatment initiation:

US labeling: There are no dosage adjustments provided in the manufacturer's labeling; systemic exposure is increased in hepatic impairment.

Canadian labeling: No dosage adjustment necessary. Use caution in moderate to severe impairment (Child-Pugh Class B or C) (systemic exposure may be increased); monitor closely.

Dosage adjustment for hepatotoxicity during treatment:

ALT and/or AST elevations (grade 2 or higher): Withhold treatment for up to 14 days; may resume treatment when fully resolved or improved to grade 1.

Severe hepatic impairment: Permanently discontinue.

Adjustment for Toxicity

Dermatologic toxicity:

Skin reactions (grade 3 or higher): Withhold treatment for up to 14 days; may resume treatment when fully resolved or improved to grade 1. *Canadian labeling:* Discontinue if unable to tolerate rechallenge following treatment interruption.

Severe bullous, blistering or exfoliating dermatologic conditions: Interrupt or discontinue treatment.

Gastrointestinal toxicity:

Diarrhea (grade 3 or higher): Withhold treatment for up to 14 days; may resume treatment when fully resolved or improved to grade 1. *Canadian labeling:* Discontinue if unable to tolerate rechallenge following treatment interruption.

Gastrointestinal perforation: Permanently discontinue.

Ocular toxicity:

Signs/symptoms of severe or worsening disorders, including keratitis: Withhold treatment for up to 14 days; may resume treatment when fully resolved or improved to grade 1. *Canadian labeling:* Discontinue if unable to tolerate rechallenge following treatment interruption.

Persistent ulcerative keratitis: Permanently discontinue.

Pulmonary toxicity:

Acute onset or worsening symptoms (dyspnea, cough, fever): Withhold treatment for up to 14 days; may resume treatment when fully resolved or improved to grade 1.

Interstitial lung disease (ILD), confirmed: Permanently discontinue.

Administration Oral: Administer with or without food.

For patients unable to swallow the tablet whole, place tablet in 120 to 240 mL water and stir for ~15 minutes; immediately drink the liquid or administer through a naso-gastric tube. Rinse the container with 120 to 240 mL water and immediately drink or administer through naso-gastric tube.

Emetic Potential Children and Adults: Minimal (<10%)

Extemporaneous Preparations For patients unable to swallow the tablet whole, place tablet in 120 to 240 ml water and stir for ~15 minutes; immediately drink the liquid or administer through a naso-gastric tube. Rinse the container with 120 to 240 mL water and immediately drink or administer through naso-gastric tube.

Iressa (gefitinib) [prescribing information]. Wilmington, DE: AstraZeneca; July 2015.

◄ **Monitoring Parameters** EGFR mutation status (prior to treatment initiation); liver function tests (ALT, AST, bilirubin at baseline and periodically thereafter); BUN, creatinine, and electrolytes (baseline and periodically thereafter); INR or prothrombin time (with concurrent warfarin treatment). Monitor for signs/symptoms of dermatologic toxicity, gastrointestinal perforation, ocular toxicity, and pulmonary toxicity; monitor closely for adverse reactions in CYP2D6 poor metabolizers and patients with hepatic impairment.

Dosage Forms Excipient information presented when available (limited, particularly for generics); consult specific product labeling.
Tablet, Oral:
  Iressa: 250 mg

Dosage Forms: Canada Information with regard to form, strength, and availability of products uniquely available in Canada but currently not available in the US. Refer also to Dosage Forms.

Excipient information presented when available (limited, particularly for generics); consult specific product labeling.
Tablet, oral:
  Iressa: 250 mg

◆ **Gelclair** *see* Mucosal Coating Agent *on page 1280*

Gemcitabine (jem SITE a been)

Related Information
  Common Toxicity Criteria *on page 2242*
  Management of Chemotherapy-Induced Nausea and Vomiting in Adults *on page 2253*
  Management of Drug Extravasations *on page 2271*
  Mucositis and Stomatitis *on page 2299*
  Prevention of Chemotherapy-Induced Nausea and Vomiting in Children *on page 2310*
  Safe Handling of Hazardous Drugs *on page 2379*

Brand Names: US Gemzar

Brand Names: Canada Gemcitabine For Injection; Gemcitabine For Injection Concentrate; Gemcitabine For Injection, USP; Gemcitabine Hydrochloride For Injection; Gemcitabine Injection; Gemcitabine Sun For Injection; Gemzar

Index Terms dFdC; dFdCyd; Difluorodeoxycytidine Hydrochlorothiazide; Gemcitabine HCl; Gemcitabine Hydrochloride; Gemzar, inj; LY-188011

Pharmacologic Category Antineoplastic Agent, Antimetabolite; Antineoplastic Agent, Antimetabolite (Pyrimidine Analog)

Use

Breast cancer: First-line treatment of metastatic breast cancer (in combination with paclitaxel) after failure of adjuvant chemotherapy which contained an anthracycline (unless contraindicated)

Non-small cell lung cancer (NSCLC): First-line treatment of inoperable, locally-advanced (stage IIIA or IIIB) or metastatic (stage IV) NSCLC (in combination with cisplatin)

Ovarian cancer: Treatment of advanced ovarian cancer (in combination with carboplatin) that has relapsed at least 6 months following completion of platinum-based chemotherapy

Pancreatic cancer (locally advanced or metastatic): First-line treatment of locally-advanced (nonresectable stage II or III) or metastatic (stage IV) pancreatic adenocarcinoma

Labeled Contraindications Hypersensitivity to gemcitabine or any component of the formulation

Pregnancy Considerations Adverse events were observed in animal reproduction studies. May cause fetal harm if administered during pregnancy; adverse effects in reproduction are anticipated based on the mechanism of action.

Breastfeeding Considerations It is not known if gemcitabine is excreted in breast milk. Due to the potential for serious adverse reactions in the nursing infant, the decision to discontinue gemcitabine or to discontinue breastfeeding should take into account the benefits of treatment to the mother.

Warnings/Precautions Gemcitabine may suppress bone marrow function (neutropenia, thrombocytopenia, and anemia); myelosuppression is usually the dose-limiting toxicity; toxicity is increased when used in combination with other chemotherapy; monitor blood counts; dosage adjustments are frequently required.

Hemolytic uremic syndrome (HUS) has been reported; may lead to renal failure and dialysis (including fatalities); monitor for evidence of anemia with microangiopathic hemolysis (elevation of bilirubin or LDH, reticulocytosis, severe thrombocytopenia, and/or renal failure) and monitor renal function at baseline and periodically during treatment. Permanently discontinue if HUS or severe renal impairment occurs; renal failure may not be reversible despite discontinuation. Serious hepatotoxicity (including liver failure and death) has been reported (when used alone or in combination with other hepatotoxic medications); use in patients with hepatic impairment (history of cirrhosis, hepatitis, or alcoholism) or in patients with hepatic metastases may lead to exacerbation of hepatic impairment. Monitor hepatic function at baseline and periodically during treatment; consider dose adjustments with elevated bilirubin; discontinue if severe liver injury develops. Capillary leak syndrome (CLS) with serious consequences has been reported, both with single-agent gemcitabine and with combination chemotherapy; discontinue if CLS develops.

Pulmonary toxicity, including adult respiratory distress syndrome, interstitial pneumonitis, pulmonary edema, and pulmonary fibrosis, has been observed; may lead to respiratory failure (some fatal) despite discontinuation. Onset of symptoms of pulmonary toxicity may be delayed up to 2 weeks beyond the last dose. Discontinue for unexplained dyspnea (with or without bronchospasm) or other evidence or pulmonary toxicity. Posterior reversible encephalopathy syndrome (PRES) has been reported, both with single-agent therapy and with combination chemotherapy. PRES may manifest with blindness, confusion, headache, hypertension, lethargy, seizure, and other visual and neurologic disturbances. If PRES diagnosis is confirmed (by MRI), discontinue therapy. Not indicated for use with concurrent radiation therapy; radiation toxicity, including tissue injury, severe mucositis, esophagitis, or pneumonitis, has been reported with concurrent and nonconcurrent administration; may have radiosensitizing activity when gemcitabine and radiation therapy are given ≤7 days apart; radiation recall may occur when gemcitabine and radiation therapy are given >7 days apart. Potentially significant drug-drug interactions may exist, requiring dose or frequency adjustment, additional monitoring, and/or selection of alternative therapy.

Prolongation of the infusion duration >60 minutes or more frequent than weekly dosing have been shown to alter the half-life and increase toxicity (hypotension, flu-like symptoms, myelosuppression, weakness); a fixed-dose rate (FDR) infusion rate of 10 mg/m^2/minute has been studied in adults in order to optimize the pharmacokinetics (off-label); prolonged infusion times increase the intracellular accumulation of the active metabolite, gemcitabine triphosphate (Ko 2006; Tempero 2003); patients who receive gemcitabine FDR experience more grade 3/4 hematologic toxicity (Ko 2006; Poplin 2009).

Adverse Reactions Frequency of adverse reactions reported for single-agent use of gemcitabine only; bone marrow depression is the dose-limiting toxicity.

>10%:

Cardiovascular: Peripheral edema (20%), edema (13%)

Central nervous system: Drowsiness (11%)

Dermatologic: Skin rash (30%), alopecia (15%)

Gastrointestinal: Nausea and vomiting (69%), diarrhea (19%), stomatitis (11%)

Genitourinary: Proteinuria (45%), hematuria (35%)

Hematologic & oncologic: Anemia (68%; grade 3: 7%; grade 4: 1%), neutropenia (63%; grade 3: 19%; grade 4: 6%), thrombocytopenia (24%; grade 3: 4%; grade 4: 1%), hemorrhage (17%; grade 3: <1%; grade 4: <1%)

Hepatic: Increased serum ALT (68%; grade 3: 8%, grade 4: 2%), increased serum AST (67%; grade 3: 6%; grade 4: 2%), increased serum alkaline phosphatase (55%; grade 3: 7%; grade 4: 2%), increased serum bilirubin (13%; grade 3: 2%, grade 4: <1%)

Infection: Infection (16%)

Renal: Increased blood urea nitrogen (16%)

Respiratory: Dyspnea (23%; grade 3: 3%; grade 4: <1%), flu-like symptoms (19%)

Miscellaneous: Fever (41%)

1% to 10%:

Central nervous system: Paresthesia (10%; grade 3: <1%)

Local: Injection site reaction (4%)

Renal: Increased serum creatinine (8%)

Respiratory: Bronchospasm (<2%)

<1%, postmarketing, and/or case reports (reported with single-agent use or with combination therapy): Adult respiratory distress syndrome, anaphylactoid reaction, anorexia, arthralgia, bullous skin disease, capillary leak syndrome, cardiac arrhythmia, cardiac failure, cellulitis, cerebrovascular accident (Kuenen 2002), constipation, desquamation, digital vasculitis, gangrene of skin or other tissue, hemolytic-uremic syndrome, hepatic failure, hepatic sinusoidal obstruction syndrome (formerly known as hepatic veno-occlusive disease), hepatotoxicity (rare), hyperglycemia, hypertension, hypocalcemia, hypotension, increased gamma-glutamyl transferase, interstitial pneumonitis, myocardial infarction, neuropathy, petechiae (Nishijima 2013; Zupancic 2007), pruritus (Curtis 2014), pulmonary edema, pulmonary fibrosis, radiation recall phenomenon, renal failure, respiratory failure, reversible posterior leukoencephalopathy syndrome, sepsis, supraventricular cardiac arrhythmia, thrombotic thrombocytopenic purpura (Nishijima 2013; Zupancic 2007)

Drug Interactions

Metabolism/Transport Effects None known.

Avoid Concomitant Use
Avoid concomitant use of Gemcitabine with any of the following: BCG (Intravesical); Deferiprone; Dipyrone; Natalizumab; Pimecrolimus; Tacrolimus (Topical); Vaccines (Live)

Increased Effect/Toxicity
Gemcitabine may increase the levels/effects of: Bleomycin; CloZAPine; Deferiprone; Fingolimod; Fluorouracil (Systemic); Fluorouracil (Topical); Leflunomide; Natalizumab; Tofacitinib; Vaccines (Live); Warfarin

The levels/effects of Gemcitabine may be increased by: Denosumab; Dipyrone; Ocrelizumab; Palifermin; Pimecrolimus; Promazine; Roflumilast; Tacrolimus (Topical); Trastuzumab

Decreased Effect
Gemcitabine may decrease the levels/effects of: BCG (Intravesical); Coccidioides immitis Skin Test; Lenograstim; Nivolumab; Sipuleucel-T; Vaccines (Inactivated); Vaccines (Live)

The levels/effects of Gemcitabine may be decreased by: Echinacea

Hazardous Drugs Handling Considerations
Hazardous agent (NIOSH 2016 [group 1]).

Use appropriate precautions for receiving, handling, administration, and disposal. Gloves (single) should be worn during receiving, unpacking, and placing in storage.

NIOSH recommends double gloving, a protective gown, ventilated engineering controls (a class II biological safety cabinet or a compounding aseptic containment isolator), and closed system transfer devices (CSTDs) for preparation. Double gloving, a gown, and (if dosage form allows) CSTDs are required during administration (NIOSH 2016).

Storage/Stability
Lyophilized powder: Store intact vials at room temperature of 20°C to 25°C (68°F to 77°F); excursions permitted to 15°C to 30°C (59°F to 86°F). Reconstituted vials are stable for 24 hours at room temperature. Do not refrigerate (may form crystals).
Solution for injection: Store intact vials refrigerated at 2°C to 8°C (36°F to 46°F); do not freeze.
Solutions diluted for infusion in NS are stable for 24 hours at room temperature. Do not refrigerate.

Preparation for Administration
Reconstitute lyophilized powder with preservative free NS; add 5 mL to the 200 mg vial, add 25 mL to the 1000 mg vial, or add 50 mL to the 2000 mg vial, resulting in a reconstituted concentration of 38 mg/mL (solutions must be reconstituted to ≤40 mg/mL to completely dissolve). Gemcitabine is also supplied as a concentrated solution for injection in different concentrations (40 mg/mL [Canada only] and 38 mg/mL); verify product concentration prior to preparation for administration.
Further dilute reconstituted lyophilized powder or concentrated solution for injection in NS for infusion; to concentrations as low as 0.1 mg/mL.

Mechanism of Action A pyrimidine antimetabolite that inhibits DNA synthesis by inhibition of DNA polymerase and ribonucleotide reductase, cell cycle-specific for the S-phase of the cycle (also blocks cellular progression at G1/S-phase). Gemcitabine is phosphorylated intracellularly by deoxycytidine kinase to gemcitabine monophosphate, which is further phosphorylated to active metabolites gemcitabine diphosphate and gemcitabine triphosphate.

Gemcitabine diphosphate inhibits DNA synthesis by inhibiting ribonucleotide reductase; gemcitabine triphosphate incorporates into DNA and inhibits DNA polymerase.

Pharmacodynamics/Kinetics

Distribution: Widely distributed into tissues; present in ascitic fluid; V_d: Infusions <70 minutes: 50 L/m^2; Long infusion times (70 to 285 minutes): 370 L/m^2

Protein binding: Negligible

Metabolism: Metabolized intracellularly by nucleoside kinases to the active diphosphate (dFdCDP) and triphosphate (dFdCTP) nucleoside metabolites

Half-life elimination:

Gemcitabine: Infusion time ≤70 minutes: 42 to 94 minutes; infusion time 3 to 4 hours: 4 to 10.5 hours (affected by age and gender)

Metabolite (gemcitabine triphosphate), terminal phase: 1.7 to 19.4 hours

Time to peak, plasma: 30 minutes after completion of infusion

Excretion: Urine (92% to 98%; primarily as inactive uracil metabolite); feces (<1%)

Dosing

Adult & Geriatric Note: Prolongation of the infusion duration >60 minutes and administration more frequently than once weekly have been shown to increase toxicity.

Breast cancer, metastatic: IV: 1250 mg/m^2 over 30 minutes days 1 and 8; repeat cycle every 21 days (in combination with paclitaxel) **or** (off-label dosing; as a single agent) 800 mg/m^2 over 30 minutes days 1, 8, and 15 of a 28-day treatment cycle (Carmichael 1995)

Non-small cell lung cancer, locally advanced or metastatic: IV: 1000 mg/m^2 over 30 minutes days 1, 8, and 15; repeat cycle every 28 days (in combination with cisplatin) **or** 1250 mg/m^2 over 30 minutes days 1 and 8; repeat cycle every 21 days (in combination with cisplatin) **or** (off-label dosing/combination) 1000 mg/m^2 over 30 minutes days 1 and 8; repeat cycle every 21 days (in combination with carboplatin) for up to 4 cycles (Grønberg 2009) **or** (off-label combination) 1000 mg/m^2 over 30 minutes days 1, 8, and 15; repeat cycle every 28 days (in combination with carboplatin) for up to 4 cycles (Danson 2003) **or** (off-label combination) 1000 mg/m^2 over 30 minutes days 1 and 8; repeat cycle every 21 days (in combination with docetaxel) for 8 cycles (Pujol 2005) **or** (off-label combination) 1000 mg/m^2 days 1, 8, and 15; repeat cycle every 28 days (in combination with vinorelbine) for 6 cycles (Greco 2007)

Ovarian cancer, advanced: IV: 1000 mg/m^2 over 30 minutes days 1 and 8; repeat cycle every 21 days (in combination with carboplatin) **or** (off-label dosing; as a single agent) 1000 mg/m^2 over 30 to 60 minutes days 1 and 8; repeat cycle every 21 days (Mutch 2007)

Pancreatic cancer (locally advanced or metastatic): IV: Initial: 1000 mg/m^2 over 30 minutes once weekly for 7 weeks followed by 1 week rest; then once weekly for 3 weeks out of every 4 weeks **or** (off-label combinations) 1000 mg/m^2 over 30 minutes weekly for up to 7 weeks followed by 1 week rest; then weekly for 3 weeks out of every 4 weeks (in combination with erlotinib) (Moore 2007) **or** 1000 mg/m^2 over 30 minutes days 1, 8, and 15 every 28 days (in combination with capecitabine) (Cunningham 2009) **or** 1000 mg/m^2 over 30 minutes days 1 and 15 every 28 days (in combination with cisplatin) (Heinemann 2006) **or** 1000 mg/m^2 infused at 10 mg/m^2/minute every 14 days (in combination with oxaliplatin)

(Louvet 2005) **or** 1000 mg/m^2 days 1, 8, and 15 every 28 days (in combination with paclitaxel [protein bound]) (Von Hoff 2013)

Pancreatic cancer (adjuvant therapy) (off-label use): IV: 1000 mg/m^2 on days 1, 8 and 15 every 28 days (in combination with capecitabine) for 6 cycles beginning within 12 weeks of resection (Neoptolemos 2017). American Society of Clinical Oncology guidelines recommend initiating within 8 weeks of resection (ASCO [Khorana 2017]).

Bladder cancer (off-label use):

Advanced or metastatic: IV: 1000 mg/m^2 over 30 to 60 minutes days 1, 8, and 15; repeat cycle every 28 days (in combination with cisplatin) (von der Maase 2000) **or** 1000 mg/m^2 over 30 minutes days 1 and 8; repeat cycle every 21 days (in combination with carboplatin) until disease progression or unacceptable toxicity (De Santis 2012)

Transitional cell carcinoma: Intravesicular instillation: 2000 mg (in 100 mL NS; retain for 1 hour) twice weekly for 3 weeks; repeat cycle every 4 weeks for at least 2 cycles (Dalbagni 2006)

Cervical cancer, recurrent or persistent (off-label use): IV: 1000 mg/m^2 days 1 and 8; repeat cycle every 21 days (in combination with cisplatin) (Monk 2009) **or** 1250 mg/m^2 over 30 minutes days 1 and 8; repeat cycle every 21 days (in combination with cisplatin) (Burnett 2000) **or** 800 mg/m^2 over 30 minutes days 1, 8, and 15; repeat cycle every 28 days (as a single-agent) (Schilder 2005) **or** 800 mg/m^2 days 1 and 8; repeat cycle every 28 days (in combination with cisplatin) (Brewer 2006)

Head and neck cancer, nasopharyngeal (off-label use): IV: 1000 mg/m^2 over 30 minutes days 1, 8, and 15 every 28 days (Zhang 2008) **or** 1000 mg/m^2 over 30 minutes days 1 and 8 every 21 days (in combination with vinorelbine) (Chen 2012)

Hepatobiliary cancer, advanced (off-label use): IV: 1000 mg/m^2 over 30 minutes days 1 and 8; repeat cycle every 21 days (in combination with cisplatin) (Valle 2010) **or** 1000 mg/m^2 over 30 minutes days 1 and 8; repeat cycle every 21 days (in combination with capecitabine) (Knox 2005) **or** 1000 mg/m^2 infused at 10 mg/m^2/minute every 2 weeks (in combination with oxaliplatin) (Andre 2004)

Hodgkin lymphoma, relapsed (off-label use): IV: 1000 mg/m^2 (800 mg/m^2 for post-transplant patients) over 30 minutes days 1 and 8; repeat cycle every 21 days (in combination with vinorelbine and doxorubicin liposomal) (Bartlett 2007) **or** 800 mg/m^2 days 1 and 4; repeat cycle every 21 days (in combination with ifosfamide, mesna, vinorelbine, and prednisolone) (Santoro 2007)

Malignant pleural mesothelioma (off-label use; in combination with cisplatin): IV: 1000 mg/m^2 over 30 minutes days 1, 8 and 15 every 28 days for up to 6 cycles (Nowak 2002) **or** 1250 mg/m^2 over 30 minutes days 1 and 8 every 21 days for up to 6 cycles (van Haarst 2002)

Non-Hodgkin lymphoma, refractory (off-label use): IV: 1000 mg/m^2 over 30 minutes days 1 and 8; repeat cycle every 21 days (in combination with cisplatin and dexamethasone) (Crump 2004) **or** 1000 mg/m^2 every 15 to 21 days (in combination with oxaliplatin and rituximab) (Lopez 2008)

Sarcoma (off-label uses): IV:

Ewing's sarcoma, refractory: 675 mg/m^2 over 90 minutes days 1 and 8; repeat cycle every 21 days (in combination with docetaxel) (Navid 2008)

Osteosarcoma, refractory: 675 mg/m^2 over 90 minutes days 1 and 8; repeat cycle every 21 days (in combination with docetaxel) (Navid 2008) **or** 1000 mg/m^2 weekly for 7 weeks followed by 1 week rest; then weekly for 3 weeks out of every 4 weeks (Merimsky 2000)

◄ *Soft tissue sarcoma, advanced:* 800 mg/m^2 over 90 minutes days 1 and 8; repeat cycle every 21 days (in combination with vinorelbine) (Dileo 2007) **or** 675 mg/m^2 over 90 minutes days 1 and 8; repeat cycle every 21 days (in combination with docetaxel) (Leu 2004) **or** 900 mg/m^2 over 90 minutes days 1 and 8; repeat cycle every 21 days (in combination with docetaxel) (Maki 2007)

Small cell lung cancer, refractory or relapsed (off-label use): IV: 1000 to 1250 mg/m^2 over 30 minutes days 1, 8, and 15 every 28 days (as a single agent) (Masters 2003)

Testicular cancer, refractory germ cell (off-label use): IV: 1000 to 1250 mg/m^2 over 30 minutes days 1 and 8 every 21 days (in combination with oxaliplatin) (DeGiorgi 2006; Kohllmannsberger 2004; Pectasides 2004) **or** 1000 mg/m^2 over 30 minutes days 1, 8, and 15 every 28 days for up to 6 cycles (in combination with paclitaxel) (Hinton 2002) **or** 800 mg/m^2 over 30 minutes days 1 and 8 every 21 days (in combination with oxaliplatin and paclitaxel) (Bokemeyer 2008)

Unknown-primary, adenocarcinoma (off-label use): IV: 1250 mg/m^2 days 1 and 8 every 21 days (in combination with cisplatin) (Culine 2003) **or** 1000 mg/m^2 over 30 minutes days 1 and 8 every 21 days for up to 6 cycles (in combination with docetaxel) (Pouessel 2004)

Uterine cancer (off-label use): IV: 900 mg/m^2 over 90 minutes days 1 and 8 every 21 days (in combination with docetaxel) (Hensley 2008) **or** 1000 mg/m^2 over 30 minutes days 1, 8, and 15 every 28 days (Look 2004)

Pediatric Note: Prolongation of the infusion duration >60 minutes and administration more frequently than once weekly have been shown to increase toxicity. Refer to specific references for ages of populations studied:

Germ cell tumor, refractory (off-label use): IV: 1000 mg/m^2 over 30 minutes days 1, 8, and 15 every 28 days (in combination with paclitaxel) for up to 6 cycles (Hinton 2002)

Hodgkin lymphoma, relapsed (off-label use): IV: 1000 mg/m^2 over 100 minutes days 1 and 8; repeat cycle every 21 days (in combination with vinorelbine) (Cole 2009) **or** 800 mg/m^2 days 1 and 4; repeat cycle every 21 days (in combination with ifosfamide, mesna, vinorelbine, and prednisolone) (Santoro 2007)

Sarcomas (off-label use): IV:

Ewing's sarcoma, refractory: 675 mg/m^2 over 90 minutes days 1 and 8; repeat cycle every 21 days (in combination with docetaxel) (Navid 2008)

Osteosarcoma, refractory: 675 mg/m^2 over 90 minutes days 1 and 8; repeat cycle every 21 days (in combination with docetaxel) (Navid 2008) **or** 1000 mg/m^2 weekly for 7 weeks followed by 1 week rest; then weekly for 3 weeks out of every 4 weeks (Merimsky 2000)

Renal Impairment There are no dosage adjustments provided in the manufacturer's labeling; use with caution in patients with preexisting renal dysfunction. Discontinue if severe renal toxicity or hemolytic uremic syndrome (HUS) occur during gemcitabine treatment.

Mild-to-severe renal impairment: No dosage adjustment necessary (Janus 2010; Li 2007).

ESRD (on hemodialysis): Hemodialysis should begin 6 to 12 hours after gemcitabine infusion (Janus 2010; Li 2007).

Hepatic Impairment There are no dosage adjustments provided in the manufacturer's labeling; use with caution. Discontinue if severe hepatotoxicity occurs during gemcitabine treatment. The following adjustments have been reported:

Transaminases elevated (with normal bilirubin): No dosage adjustment necessary (Venook 2000).

Serum bilirubin >1.6 mg/dL: Use initial dose of 800 mg/m^2; may escalate if tolerated (Ecklund 2005; Floyd 2006; Venook 2000).

Obesity *ASCO Guidelines for appropriate chemotherapy dosing in obese adults with cancer:* Utilize patient's actual body weight (full weight) for calculation of body surface area- or weight-based dosing, particularly when the intent of therapy is curative; manage regimen-related toxicities in the same manner as for nonobese patients; if a dose reduction is utilized due to toxicity, consider resumption of full weight-based dosing with subsequent cycles, especially if cause of toxicity (eg, hepatic or renal impairment) is resolved (Griggs 2012).

Adjustment for Toxicity

Nonhematologic toxicity (all indications):

Hold or decrease gemcitabine dose by 50% for the following: Severe (grade 3 or 4) nonhematologic toxicity until resolved (excludes nausea, vomiting, or alopecia [no dose modifications recommended])

Permanently discontinue gemcitabine for any of the following: Unexplained dyspnea (or other evidence of severe pulmonary toxicity), severe hepatotoxicity, hemolytic uremic syndrome (HUS), capillary leak syndrome (CLS), posterior reversible encephalopathy syndrome (PRES)

Hematologic toxicity:

Breast cancer:

Day 1:

Absolute granulocyte count (AGC) ≥1500/mm^3 and platelet count ≥100,000/mm^3: Administer 100% of full dose

AGC <1500/mm^3 or platelet count <100,000/mm^3: Hold dose

Day 8:

AGC ≥1200/mm^3 and platelet count >75,000/mm^3: Administer 100% of full dose

AGC 1000 to 1199/mm^3 or platelet count 50,000 to 75,000/mm^3: Administer 75% of full dose

AGC 700 to 999/mm^3 and platelet count ≥50,000/mm^3: Administer 50% of full dose

AGC <700/mm^3 or platelet count <50,000/mm^3: Hold dose

Non-small cell lung cancer (cisplatin dosage may also require adjustment):

AGC ≥1000/mm^3 and platelet count ≥100,000/mm^3: Administer 100% of full dose

AGC 500 to 999/mm^3 or platelet count 50,000 to 99,999/mm^3: Administer 75% of full dose

AGC <500/mm^3 or platelet count <50,000/mm^3: Hold dose

Ovarian cancer:

Day 1:

AGC ≥1500/mm^3 and platelet count ≥100,000/mm^3: Administer 100% of full dose

AGC <1500/mm^3 or platelet count <100,000/mm^3: Delay treatment cycle

Day 8:
AGC ≥1500/mm^3 and platelet count ≥100,000/mm^3: Administer 100% of full dose

AGC 1000 to 1499/mm^3 or platelet count 75,000 to 99,999/mm^3: Administer 50% of full dose

AGC <1000/mm^3 or platelet count <75,000/mm^3: Hold dose

Hematologic toxicity in previous cycle (dosing adjustment for subsequent cycles):

Initial occurrence: AGC <500/mm^3 for >5 days, AGC <100/mm^3 for >3 days, neutropenic fever, platelet count <25,000/mm^3, or cycle delay >1 week due to toxicity: Permanently reduce gemcitabine to 800 mg/m^2 on days 1 and 8.

Subsequent occurrence: AGC <500/mm^3 for >5 days, AGC <100/mm^3 for >3 days, neutropenic fever, platelet count <25,000/mm^3, or cycle delay >1 week due to toxicity: Permanently reduce gemcitabine to 800 mg/m^2 and administer on day 1 only.

Pancreatic cancer (locally advanced or metastatic):
AGC ≥1000/mm^3 and platelet count ≥100,000/mm^3: Administer 100% of full dose

AGC 500 to 999/mm^3 or platelet count 50,000 to 99,999/mm^3: Administer 75% of full dose

AGC <500/mm^3 or platelet count <50,000/mm^3: Hold dose

Combination Regimens

Biliary adenocarcinoma:
Gemcitabine-Capecitabine (Biliary Cancer) on page 2134
Gemcitabine-Cisplatin (Biliary Cancer) on page 2135
GEMOX (Biliary Cancer) on page 2141

Bladder cancer:
Carboplatin-Gemcitabine (Bladder) on page 2017
Cisplatin-Docetaxel-Gemcitabine (Bladder) on page 2038
Cisplatin-Gemcitabine (Bladder) on page 2051
Gemcitabine-Paclitaxel (Bladder) on page 2138
PCG (Bladder) on page 2191

Bone sarcoma (Ewing sarcoma): Docetaxel-Gemcitabine (Ewing Sarcoma) on page 2091

Bone sarcoma (osteosarcoma): Docetaxel-Gemcitabine (Osteosarcoma) on page 2091

Breast cancer: Gemcitabine-Paclitaxel (Breast) on page 2138

Cervical cancer: Cisplatin-Gemcitabine (Cervical) on page 2052

Head and neck cancer: Gemcitabine-Vinorelbine (Head and Neck) on page 2140

Lung cancer (non-small cell):
Bevacizumab-Cisplatin-Gemcitabine (NSCLC) on page 1991
Carboplatin-Gemcitabine (NSCLC) on page 2017
Cisplatin-Gemcitabine-Necitumumab (NSCLC) on page 2053
Cisplatin-Gemcitabine (NSCLC) on page 2054
Docetaxel-Gemcitabine (NSCLC) on page 2091
Gemcitabine-Vinorelbine (NSCLC) on page 2140

Lymphoma, Hodgkin:
GDP (Hodgkin) on page 2134
Gemcitabine-Dexamethasone-Carboplatin (Hodgkin) on page 2136
GVD (Hodgkin) on page 2143
IGEV (Hodgkin) on page 2155

Administration Infuse over 30 minutes; for off-label uses, infusion times may vary (refer to specific references). **Note:** Prolongation of the infusion time >60 minutes has been shown to increase toxicity. Gemcitabine has been administered at a fixed-dose rate (FDR) infusion rate of 10 mg/m^2/minute to optimize the pharmacokinetics (off-label); prolonged infusion times increase the intracellular accumulation of the active metabolite, gemcitabine triphosphate (Ko 2006; Tempero 2003). Patients who receive gemcitabine FDR experience more grade 3/4 hematologic toxicity (Ko 2006; Poplin 2009).

For intravesicular (bladder) instillation (off-label route), gemcitabine was diluted in 50 to 100 mL normal saline; patients were instructed to retain in the bladder for 1 hour (Addeo 2010; Dalbaghi 2006)

Vesicant/Extravasation Risk May be an irritant

Emetic Potential Children and Adults: Low (10% to 30%)

Monitoring Parameters CBC with differential and platelet count (prior to each dose); hepatic and renal function (prior to initiation of therapy and periodically, thereafter); monitor electrolytes, including potassium, magnesium, and calcium (when in combination therapy with cisplatin); monitor pulmonary function; signs/symptoms of capillary leak syndrome and posterior reversible encephalopathy syndrome

◀ **Dosage Forms** Excipient information presented when available (limited, particularly for generics); consult specific product labeling.
Solution, Intravenous:
Generic: 200 mg/5.26 mL (5.26 mL); 1 g/26.3 mL (26.3 mL); 2 g/52.6 mL (52.6 mL)
Solution, Intravenous [preservative free]:
Generic: 200 mg/5.26 mL (5.26 mL); 1 g/26.3 mL (26.3 mL); 2 g/52.6 mL (52.6 mL)
Solution Reconstituted, Intravenous:
Gemzar: 200 mg (1 ea); 1 g (1 ea)
Generic: 200 mg (1 ea); 1 g (1 ea); 2 g (1 ea)
Solution Reconstituted, Intravenous [preservative free]:
Generic: 200 mg (1 ea); 1 g (1 ea); 2 g (1 ea)

Dosage Forms: Canada Information with regard to form, strength, and availability of products uniquely available in Canada but currently not available in the US. Refer also to Dosage Forms.

Excipient information presented when available (limited, particularly for generics); consult specific product labeling.
Solution, Intravenous: 200 mg/5mL, 1 g/25 mL, 2 g/50 mL [40 mg/mL]
Solution, Intravenous: 200 mg/5.3 mL, 1 g/26.3 mL, 2 g/52.6 mL [38 mg/mL]
Solution Reconstituted, Intravenous: 200 mg, 1 g, 2 g

◆ **Gemcitabine For Injection (Can)** *see* Gemcitabine *on page 864*

◆ **Gemcitabine For Injection Concentrate (Can)** *see* Gemcitabine *on page 864*

◆ **Gemcitabine For Injection, USP (Can)** *see* Gemcitabine *on page 864*

◆ **Gemcitabine HCl** *see* Gemcitabine *on page 864*

◆ **Gemcitabine Hydrochloride** *see* Gemcitabine *on page 864*

◆ **Gemcitabine Hydrochloride For Injection (Can)** *see* Gemcitabine *on page 864*

◆ **Gemcitabine Injection (Can)** *see* Gemcitabine *on page 864*

◆ **Gemcitabine Sun For Injection (Can)** *see* Gemcitabine *on page 864*

Gemtuzumab Ozogamicin (gem TOO zoo mab oh zog a MY sin)

Related Information
Management of Chemotherapy-Induced Nausea and Vomiting in Adults *on page 2253*
Prevention of Chemotherapy-Induced Nausea and Vomiting in Children *on page 2310*
Safe Handling of Hazardous Drugs *on page 2379*

Index Terms CMA-676; Mylotarg

Pharmacologic Category Antineoplastic Agent, Anti-CD33; Antineoplastic Agent, Antibody Drug Conjugate; Antineoplastic Agent, Monoclonal Antibody

Use Acute myeloid leukemia: Gemtuzumab was withdrawn from the US commercial market in 2010. However, as of September 2017, Mylotarg has been approved for reintroduction into the US market. Information pertaining to this updated approval in the monograph is pending revision. Consult the prescribing information for additional information.

Labeled Contraindications Known hypersensitivity to gemtuzumab ozogamicin, calicheamicin derivatives, or any component of the formulation; patients with anti-CD33 antibody

Pregnancy Considerations Teratogenic effects have been observed in animal reproduction studies. May cause fetal harm when administered to a pregnant woman. Women of reproductive potential should avoid becoming pregnant while receiving treatment.

Breastfeeding Considerations It is not known if gemtuzumab ozogamicin is present in breast milk. Because human IgG is secreted in breast milk and the potential for serious adverse reactions in the breastfed infant exists, a decision should be made whether to discontinue breastfeeding or to discontinue the drug, taking into account the importance of treatment to the mother.

Warnings/Precautions Gemtuzumab has been associated with hepatotoxicity, including severe hepatic sinusoidal obstruction syndrome (SOS; formerly called veno-occlusive disease [VOD]). Symptoms of SOS include right upper quadrant pain, rapid weight gain, ascites, hepatomegaly, and bilirubin/transaminase elevations. Risk may be increased by combination chemotherapy, underlying hepatic disease, or hematopoietic stem cell transplant.

Severe hypersensitivity reactions (including anaphylaxis) and other infusion-related reactions may occur. Infusion-related events are common, generally reported to occur with the first dose after the end of the 2-hour intravenous infusion. These symptoms usually resolved after 2-4 hours with a supportive therapy of acetaminophen, diphenhydramine, and intravenous fluids. Other severe and potentially fatal infusion related pulmonary events (including dyspnea and hypoxia) have been reported infrequently. Symptomatic intrinsic lung disease or high peripheral blast counts may increase the risk of severe reactions. Fewer infusion-related events were observed after the second dose. Postinfusion reactions (may include fever, chills, hypotension, or dyspnea) may occur during the first 24 hours after administration. Consider discontinuation in patients who develop severe infusion-related reactions. In addition to infusion-related pulmonary events, gemtuzumab therapy is also associated with acute respiratory distress syndrome, pulmonary infiltrates, pleural effusion, noncardiogenic pulmonary edema, and pulmonary insufficiency.

Severe myelosuppression occurs in all patients at recommended dosages. Monitor blood counts. Tumor lysis syndrome (including renal failure) may occur as a consequence of leukemia treatment, adequate hydration and prophylactic antihyperuricemic medication must be instituted prior to use. Other methods to lower WBC <30,000 cells/mm^3 may be considered (hydroxyurea or leukapheresis) to minimize the risk of tumor lysis syndrome, and/or severe infusion reactions. An increased number of deaths have been reported in patients receiving gemtuzumab in combination with chemotherapy, compared to those receiving chemotherapy alone. Potentially significant drug-drug interactions may exist, requiring dose or frequency adjustment, additional monitoring, and/or selection of alternative therapy.

Adverse Reactions Frequency not defined.

Cardiovascular: hepatic sinusoidal obstruction syndrome (formerly known as hepatic veno-occlusive disease); higher frequency in patients with prior history of or subsequent hematopoietic stem cell transplant), hypertension, hypotension, peripheral edema, tachycardia

Central nervous system: Anxiety, cerebral hemorrhage, chills, depression, dizziness, headache, insomnia, intracranial hemorrhage, pain

Dermatologic: Pruritus, skin rash

◀ Endocrine & metabolic: Hyperglycemia, hypocalcemia, hypokalemia, hypomagnesemia, hypophosphatemia, increased lactate dehydrogenase

Gastrointestinal: Abdominal pain, anorexia, diarrhea, dyspepsia, gingival hemorrhage, melena, mucositis, nausea, stomatitis, vomiting

Genitourinary: Hematuria, vaginal hemorrhage

Hematologic & oncologic: Anemia, bruise, disseminated intravascular coagulation (DIC), febrile neutropenia, hemorrhage, leukopenia, lymphocytopenia, neutropenia (median recovery: 40 to 51 days), petechia, prolonged partial thromboplastin time, prolonged prothrombin time, thrombocytopenia (median recovery: 36 to 51 days)

Hepatic: Ascites, hyperbilirubinemia, increased serum alkaline phosphatase, increased serum ALT, increased serum AST

Infection: Herpes simplex infection, infection, sepsis

Local: Injection site reaction

Neuromuscular & skeletal: Arthralgia, back pain, myalgia, weakness

Renal: Increased serum creatinine

Respiratory: Cough, dyspnea, epistaxis, hypoxia, pharyngitis, pneumonia, rhinitis

Miscellaneous: Fever, infusion-related reaction

<1%, postmarketing, and/or case reports: Acute respiratory distress, anaphylaxis, bradycardia, Budd-Chiari syndrome, gastrointestinal hemorrhage, hepatic failure, hepatosplenomegaly, hypersitivity reaction, jaundice, neutropenic sepsis, non-cardiogenic pulmonary edema, portal vein thrombosis, pulmonary hemorrhage, renal insufficiency, renal failure (including renal failure secondary to tumor lysis syndrome)

Drug Interactions

Metabolism/Transport Effects None known.

Avoid Concomitant Use

Avoid concomitant use of Gemtuzumab Ozogamicin with any of the following: BCG (Intravesical); Belimumab; Deferiprone; Dipyrone; Natalizumab; Pimecrolimus; Tacrolimus (Topical); Vaccines (Live)

Increased Effect/Toxicity

Gemtuzumab Ozogamicin may increase the levels/effects of: Belimumab; CloZAPine; Deferiprone; Fingolimod; Leflunomide; Natalizumab; Tofacitinib; Vaccines (Live)

The levels/effects of Gemtuzumab Ozogamicin may be increased by: Denosumab; Dipyrone; Ocrelizumab; Pimecrolimus; Promazine; Roflumilast; Tacrolimus (Topical); Trastuzumab

Decreased Effect

Gemtuzumab Ozogamicin may decrease the levels/effects of: BCG (Intravesical); Coccidioides immitis Skin Test; Nivolumab; Sipuleucel-T; Tertomotide; Vaccines (Inactivated); Vaccines (Live)

The levels/effects of Gemtuzumab Ozogamicin may be decreased by: Echinacea

Hazardous Drugs Handling Considerations

Hazardous agent (NIOSH 2016 [group 1]).

Use appropriate precautions for receiving, handling, administration, and disposal. Gloves (single) should be worn during receiving, unpacking, and placing in storage.

NIOSH recommends double gloving, a protective gown, ventilated engineering controls (a class II biological safety cabinet or a compounding aseptic containment isolator), and closed system transfer devices (CSTDs) for preparation. Double gloving, a gown, and (if dosage form allows) CSTDs are required during administration (NIOSH 2016).

Storage/Stability

Light sensitive; protect from light (including direct and indirect sunlight, and unshielded fluorescent light). The infusion container should be placed in a UV protectant bag immediately after preparation.

Store intact vials at 2°C to 8°C (36°F to 46°F). Reconstituted solutions may be stored for up to 2 hours at room temperature or under refrigeration. Following dilution for infusion in NS, solutions are stable for up to 16 hours at room temperature. Administration requires 2 hours; therefore, the maximum elapsed time from initial reconstitution to completion of infusion should be 20 hours.

Preparation for Administration Protect from light during preparation (and administration). Prepare in biologic safety hood with shielded fluorescent light; (some institutions prepare in a darkened room with the lights in the biologic safety cabinet turned off). Allow to warm to room temperature prior to reconstitution. Reconstitute each 5 mg vial with sterile water for injection to a concentration of 1 mg/mL. Dilute in 100 mL of NS injection.

Mechanism of Action Gemtuzumab ozogamicin is an antibody to CD33 antigen, which is expressed on leukemic blasts in 80% of AML patients. Binds to the CD33 antigen, resulting in internalization of the antibody-antigen complex. Following internalization, the calicheamicin derivative is released inside the myeloid cell. The calicheamicin derivative binds to DNA resulting in double strand breaks and cell death. Pluripotent stem cells and nonhematopoietic cells are not affected.

Pharmacodynamics/Kinetics Half-life elimination: Based on a 9 mg/m^2 dose: Total calicheamicin: Initial dose: 41 hours, Repeat dose: 64 hours; Unconjugated: Initial dose: 143 hours

Dosing

Adult & Geriatric

Note: Gemtuzumab was withdrawn from the US commercial market in 2010. However, as of September 2017, Mylotarg has been approved for reintroduction into the US market. Information pertaining to this updated approval in the monograph is pending revision.

Note: Patients should receive diphenhydramine 50 mg orally and acetaminophen 650 to 1000 mg orally 1 hour prior to administration of each dose. Acetaminophen dosage should be repeated as needed every 4 hours for 2 additional doses. Pretreatment with methylprednisolone may ameliorate infusion-related symptoms.

Acute myeloid leukemia (off-label/investigational use): IV:

Favorable cytogenetics: Adults <60 years: 3 mg/m^2 on day 1 of course 1 (in combination with induction chemotherapy) and on day 1 of course 3 (in combination with chemotherapy) (Burnett 2011)

Newly diagnosed:

Adults 50 to 70 years: 3 mg/m^2 (maximum dose: 5 mg) on days 1, 4, and 7 of induction course 1 (in combination with cytarabine and daunorubicin), followed by 3 mg/m^2 (maximum dose: 5 mg) on day 1 of consolidation courses 1 and 2 (platelet dependent; in combination with cytarabine and daunorubicin) (Castaigne 2012; Castaigne 2014)

Adults ≥61 years: 6 mg/m^2 on day 1 and 3 mg/m^2 on day 8; for patients with complete or partial response or stable disease, follow with 2 mg/m^2 once a month for up to 8 monthly doses (Amidori 2016).

Acute promyelocytic leukemia (off-label/investigational use): IV:

Single-agent therapy (relapsed disease): 6 mg/m^2 infused over 2 hours on days 1 and 15; for patients testing PCR negative after 2 doses, a third dose was administered (LoCoco 2004). Additional data may be necessary to further define the role of gemtuzumab in this condition.

Combination therapy (high-risk patients with newly diagnosed disease) (Ravandi 2009):

Induction: 9 mg/m^2 as a single dose on day 1 (in combination with arsenic trioxide and tretinoin)

Post remission therapy (if arsenic trioxide or tretinoin discontinued due to toxicity): 9 mg/m^2 once every 4 to 5 weeks until 28 weeks after complete remission.

Renal Impairment There are no dosage adjustments provided in the manufacturer's labeling (has not been studied).

Hepatic Impairment There are no dosage adjustments provided in the manufacturer's labeling (has not been studied); use with caution.

Adjustment for Toxicity

Dyspnea or significant hypotension: Interrupt infusion; monitor

Anaphylaxis, pulmonary edema, acute respiratory distress syndrome: Strongly consider discontinuing treatment

Administration Administer via IV infusion, over 2 hours through a low protein-binding (0.2 to 1.2 micron) in-line filter. Protect from light during infusion. Do not administer as IV push or bolus. Premedicate with acetaminophen and diphenhydramine prior to each infusion. Monitor for infusion reactions.

Emetic Potential Children: Minimal (<10%)

Monitoring Parameters Monitor electrolytes, liver function (total bilirubin and transaminases), CBC with differential and platelets frequently. Monitor vital signs during the infusion and for 4 hours following the infusion. Monitor for signs/symptoms of postinfusion reaction. Monitor for signs and symptoms of hepatic sinusoidal obstruction syndrome (SOS; veno-occlusive disease; weight gain [rapid], right upper quadrant abdominal pain, hepatomegaly, ascites) and tumor lysis syndrome.

Product Availability Gemtuzumab was withdrawn from the US commercial market in 2010. However, as of September 2017, Mylotarg has been approved for reintroduction into the US market. Information pertaining to this updated approval in the monograph is pending revision. Consult the prescribing information for additional information. https://www.accessdata.fda.gov/drug-satfda_docs/label/2017/761060lbl.pdf.

Prescribing and Access Restrictions As of June 2010, gemtuzumab was withdrawn from the US market; however, as of September 2017, Mylotarg has been approved for reintroduction into the US market. Information pertaining to this updated approval in the monograph is pending revision. Consult the prescribing information for additional information.

In Canada, gemtuzumab is available through a special access program (access information is available from Health Canada).

◆ **Gemzar** see Gemcitabine on page 864

◆ **Gemzar, inj** see Gemcitabine on page 864

◆ **Gengraf** see CycloSPORINE (Systemic) on page 452

◆ **Gen-Medroxy (Can)** *see* MedroxyPROGESTERone *on page 1175*

Gentamicin (Systemic) (jen ta MYE sin)

Brand Names: Canada Gentamicin Injection, USP
Index Terms Gentamicin Sulfate
Pharmacologic Category Antibiotic, Aminoglycoside
Use Serious infections: Treatment of serious infections (eg, sepsis, meningitis, urinary tract infections, respiratory tract infections, peritonitis, bone infections, skin and soft tissue infections) caused by susceptible strains of the following microorganisms: *P. aeruginosa*, *Proteus* species (indole-positive and indole-negative), *Escherichia coli*, *Klebsiella* species, *Enterobacter* species, *Serratia* species, *Citrobacter* species, and *Staphylococcus* species (coagulase-positive and coagulase-negative); treatment of infective endocarditis caused by enterococci, in combination with other antibiotics.
Pregnancy Risk Factor D
Dosing
Adult & Geriatric In underweight and nonobese patients, use of total body weight (TBW) instead of ideal body weight for determining the initial mg/kg/dose is widely accepted (Nicolau 1995). Ideal body weight (IBW) also may be used to determine doses for patients who are neither underweight nor obese (Gilbert 2009).

Initial and periodic plasma drug levels (eg, peak and trough with conventional dosing, post dose level at a prespecified time with extended-interval dosing) should be determined, particularly in critically-ill patients with serious infections or in disease states known to significantly alter aminoglycoside pharmacokinetics (eg, cystic fibrosis, burns, or major surgery).

Usual dosage ranges:
Conventional: IM, IV: 3 to 5 mg/kg/day in divided doses every 8 hours
Once daily (extended-interval dosing [EID]): IV: 5 to 7 mg/kg/day once daily; not recommended in patients with ascites, burns covering >20% of the total body surface area, cystic fibrosis, end-stage renal disease (eg, requiring hemodialysis), endocarditis, infants, mycobacterial infections, or pregnancy (Bailey 1997; Nicolau 1995)

Indication-specific dosing: IM, IV:
Brucellosis (off-label use): 5 mg/kg once daily for 7 days (range: 5 to 14 days); administered in combination with 6 weeks of doxycycline (Ariza 2007). Additional data may be necessary to further define the role of gentamicin in this condition.
Cerebrospinal fluid (CSF) shunt infection (off-label route): Intraventricular (use a preservative-free preparation): 4 to 8 mg/day (IDSA [Tunkel 2004])
Gonococcal infection, uncomplicated (patients with severe cephalosporin allergy) (off-label use): IM: 240 mg as a single dose in combination with oral azithromycin (CDC [Workowski 2015])
Granuloma inguinale (donovanosis) (off-label use): 1 mg/kg/dose every 8 hours; gentamicin must be used in addition to the recommended antibiotic agent and only if improvement is not evident within the first days of therapy (CDC [Workowski 2015])

▶

◀ **Infective endocarditis, treatment** (AHA [Baddour 2015]):

Enterococcus (native or prosthetic valve) (off-label dose): IV, IM: 3 mg/kg/day in 2 or 3 divided doses in combination with a beta-lactam or vancomycin (choice of concomitant antibiotic and treatment duration are dependent on organism sensitivity testing and source of infection)

S. aureus (prosthetic valve; methicillin-susceptible or methicillin-resistant) (off-label dose): IV, IM: 3 mg/kg/day in 2 or 3 divided doses for 2 weeks; use in combination with other antibiotics (choice of concomitant antibiotic dependent on organism sensitivity testing)

Viridans group streptococcus (VGS) and *S. bovis* (native or prosthetic valve) (off-label use): IV, IM: 3 mg/kg/day once daily (preferred) or in 3 divided doses (alternative) in combination with other antibiotics (choice of concomitant antibiotic and treatment duration are dependent on organism sensitivity testing and source of infection)

Meningitis due to *Enterococcus* spp (off-label use), *Listeria monocytogenes* (off-label use), *Streptococcus agalactiae* (off-label use), or *Pseudomonas aeruginosa*: IV: 5 mg/kg/day in divided doses every 8 hours (administered with other antimicrobials [varies by causative organism and susceptibility]) (IDSA [Tunkel 2004])

Intra-abdominal infections (off-label dose): IV: 5 to 7 mg/kg once daily for 4 to 7 days (unless it is difficult to achieve source control) (IDSA [Solomkin 2010])

Pelvic inflammatory disease (off-label): Loading dose: 2 mg/kg IV or IM, then 1.5 mg/kg IV every 8 hours or 3 to 5 mg/kg IV once daily in combination with clindamycin IV. Transition from parenteral to oral therapy can usually be initiated within 24 to 48 hours of clinical improvement for a total treatment duration of 14 days (CDC [Workowski 2015])

Peritoneal dialysis-associated peritonitis (off-label use) (ISPD [Li 2016]): Intraperitoneal:

Intermittent dosing: 0.6 mg/kg per exchange once daily; allow to dwell ≥6 hours

Continuous dosing (all exchanges): Loading dose: 8 mg/**L**; maintenance dose: 4 mg/**L**

Plague (*Yersinia pestis*), treatment (off-label use): 5 mg/kg/dose once daily **or** 2 mg/kg loading dose, then 1.7 mg/kg/dose every 8 hours; duration of therapy is 10 to 14 days, or until 2 days after patient is afebrile (CDC 2015)

Pneumonia, hospital-acquired or ventilator-associated (off-label): IV: 5 to 7 mg/kg/day once daily for 7 days; may consider shorter or longer duration depending on rate of clinical improvement. When used as empiric therapy, use in combination with an agent active against *S. aureus* and an additional antipseudomonal agent. **Note:** Aminoglycosides are not recommended as monotherapy in patients with hospital-acquired or ventilator-associated pneumonia due to *P. aeruginosa* (Kalil 2016).

Sepsis/septic shock (empiric or targeted therapy) (off-label): IV: 5 to 7 mg/kg once daily; first dose administered as soon as possible and within 1 hour of identifying sepsis/septic shock. A duration of therapy of 7 to 10 days is generally adequate for serious infections; a variety of factors play a role in determining optimal duration of therapy; infectious diseases consultation may be necessary (SSC [Rhodes 2017]).

Surgical (preoperative) prophylaxis (off-label use): IV: 5 mg/kg within 60 minutes prior to surgical incision with or without other antibiotics (procedure dependent). **Note:** Dose is based on actual body weight unless >20% above ideal body weight, then dosage requirement may best be estimated using a dosing weight of IBW + 0.4 (TBW - IBW) (Bratzler 2013)

Synergy (for gram-positive infections): 3 mg/kg/day in 1-3 divided doses (with ampicillin)

Tularemia (off-label use): 5 mg/kg/dose once daily for 10 days (Dennis 2001) or 5 mg/kg/day in 2 divided doses for ≥10 days (WHO 2007)

Pediatric Note: Dosage should be based on an estimate of ideal body weight. In morbidly obese children and adolescents, dosage requirement may best be estimated using a dosing weight of IBW + 0.4 (TBW - IBW). Dosage should be individualized based upon serum concentration monitoring. Initial and periodic plasma drug concentrations (eg, peak and trough with conventional dosing, post dose level at a prespecified time with extended-interval dosing) should be determined, particularly in critically ill patients with serious infections or in disease states known to significantly alter aminoglycoside pharmacokinetics (eg, cystic fibrosis, burns, or major surgery). Some dosing based on gentamicin studies:

General dosing, susceptible infection:

Conventional dosing:

Manufacturer's labeling:

Infants: IM, IV: 2.5 mg/kg/dose every 8 hours

Children and Adolescents: IM, IV: 2 to 2.5 mg/kg/dose every 8 hours

Alternate dosing: Infants, Children, and Adolescents: IM, IV: 2 to 2.5 mg/kg/dose every 8 hours; some pediatric patients may require larger doses (ie, patients undergoing continuous hemofiltration, patients with major burns, febrile granulocytopenic patients); modify dose based on individual patient requirements as determined by renal function, serum drug concentrations, and patient-specific clinical parameters (*Red Book* [AAP 2015])

Extended-interval dosing: Limited data available:

Weight-directed: Infants, Children, and Adolescents: IV: 4.5 to 7.5 mg/kg/dose every 24 hours in patients with normal renal function (Contopoulos-Ioannidis 2004; *Red Book* (AAP 2015])

Age-directed: Based on data from 114 patients, the following has been suggested (McDade 2010):

Infants and Children ≥3 months to <2 years: IV: 9.5 mg/kg/dose every 24 hours

Children 2 to <8 years: IV: 8.5 mg/kg/dose every 24 hours

Children ≥8 years and Adolescents: IV: 7 mg/kg/dose every 24 hours

Surgical (preoperative) prophylaxis (off-label use): Infants, Children, and Adolescents: IV: 2 to 2.5 mg/kg as a single dose; in children and adolescents, a dose of 2.5 mg/kg is typically suggested; administer within 60 minutes prior to surgical incision with or without other antibiotics (procedure dependent) (Bratzler 2013; *Red Book* [AAP 2015]).

Renal Impairment

Adults:

Conventional dosing:

Manufacturer's labeling: Administer usual dosage for initial dose, then estimate reduced dose by dividing initial dose by patient's serum creatinine level (in mg/dL) and administer every 8 hours (eg, a 60 kg patient with serum creatinine of 2 mg/dL at a dose of 1 mg/kg would receive an initial dose of 60 mg, followed by 30 mg every 8 hours)

◄

Alternate dosing (Aronoff 2007): **Note:** Renally adjusted dose recommendations are based on doses of 1.7 mg/kg/dose every 8 hours or 5 to
7 mg/kg/dose once daily.

GFR >50 mL/minute: No dosage adjustment necessary.

GFR 10 to 50 mL/minute: Administer every 12 to 48 hours

GFR <10 mL/minute: Administer every 48 to 72 hours

Once daily (extended-interval dosing [EID]) (Bailey 1997; Nicolau 1995):
Note: Base initial dosing interval on the following; adjust interval based on
serum levels using institution-specific policies.

CrCl ≥60 mL/minute: Administer every 24 hours

CrCl 40 to 59 mL/minute: Administer every 36 hours

CrCl 20 to 39 mL/minute: Administer every 48 hours

CrCl <20 mL/minute: Monitor serum levels and redose when gentamicin
level is less than 1 mcg/mL or use conventional dosing.

Note: In patients with sepsis/septic shock and severe renal impairment,
the SSC guidelines do not recommend use of once-daily dosing.
Patients with mild renal impairment should still receive once-daily dosing
with an extended interval (ie, up to 3 days) (SSC [Rhodes 2017]).

Intermittent hemodialysis (IHD) (administer after hemodialysis on dialysis
days) (Heintz 2009): Dialyzable (~50%; variable; dependent on filter,
duration, and type of IHD):

Loading dose of 2 to 3 mg/kg loading dose followed by:

Mild UTI or synergy: 1 mg/kg/dose every 48 to 72 hours; consider
redosing for pre-HD or post-HD concentrations <1 mg/L

Moderate-to-severe UTI: 1 to 1.5 mg/kg/dose every 48 to 72 hours;
consider redosing for pre-HD concentrations <1.5 to 2 mg/L or post-
HD concentrations <1 mg/L

Systemic gram-negative rod infection: 1.5 to 2 mg/kg/dose every 48 to
72 hours; consider redosing for pre-HD concentrations <3 to 5 mg/L or
post-HD concentrations <2 mg/L

Note: Dosing dependent on the assumption of 3 times/week, complete
IHD sessions.

Continuous renal replacement therapy (CRRT) (Heintz 2009; Trotman
2005): Drug clearance is highly dependent on the method of renal
replacement, filter type, and flow rate. Appropriate dosing requires close
monitoring of pharmacologic response, signs of adverse reactions due to
drug accumulation, as well as target drug concentrations (if appropriate).
Note: The following are general recommendations only (based on dialysate flow/ultrafiltration rates of 1 to 2 L/hour and minimal residual renal
function) and should not supersede clinical judgment:

CVVH/CVVHD/CVVHDF:

Mild UTI or synergy: Loading dose of 2 to 3 mg/kg/dose followed by
1 mg/kg every 24 to 36 hours (redose when concentration <1 mg/L
[Heintz 2009])

Moderate to severe UTI: Loading dose of 2 to 3 mg/kg/dose followed by
1 to 1.5 mg/kg every 24 to 36 hours (redose when concentration <1.5
to 2 mg/L [Heintz 2009])

Systemic gram-negative infection: Loading dose of 2 to 3 mg/kg/dose
followed by 1.5 to 2.5 mg/kg every 24 to 48 hours (generally accepted
to redose when concentration <2 mg/L; one reference suggests redosing when <3 mg/L [Heintz 2009])

Infants, Children, and Adolescents:
Conventional dosing:
The following adjustments have been recommended (Aronoff 2007):
Note: Renally adjusted dose recommendations are based on doses of 2.5 mg/kg/dose every 8 hours:
GFR >50 mL/minute/1.73 m^2: No dosage adjustment necessary.
GFR 30 to 50 mL/minute/1.73 m^2: Administer every 12 to 18 hours
GFR 10 to 29 mL/minute/1.73 m^2: Administer every 18 to 24 hours
GFR <10 mL/minute/1.73 m^2: Administer every 48 to 72 hours
Intermittent hemodialysis (IHD): 2 mg/kg/dose; redose as indicated by serum concentration
Peritoneal dialysis (PD): 2 mg/kg/dose; redose as indicated by serum concentration
Continuous renal replacement therapy (CRRT): 2 to 2.5 mg/kg/dose every 12 to 24 hours, monitor serum concentrations.

Hepatic Impairment There are no dosage adjustments provided in the manufacturer's labeling; however dosage adjustment is not likely to be necessary (does not undergo hepatic metabolism).

Obesity In moderate obesity (TBW/IBW ≥1.25) or greater (eg, morbid obesity [TBW/IBW >2]), initial dosage requirement may be estimated using a dosing weight of IBW + 0.4 (TBW - IBW) (Traynor 1995).

Additional Information Complete prescribing information should be consulted for additional detail.

Dosage Forms Excipient information presented when available (limited, particularly for generics); consult specific product labeling. [DSC] = Discontinued product
Solution, Injection:
Generic: 10 mg/mL (2 mL); 40 mg/mL (2 mL, 20 mL)
Solution, Injection [preservative free]:
Generic: 10 mg/mL (2 mL)
Solution, Intravenous:
Generic: 60 mg (50 mL); 70 mg (50 mL); 80 mg (50 mL, 100 mL); 90 mg (100 mL); 100 mg (50 mL, 100 mL); 120 mg (100 mL); 10 mg/mL (6 mL, 8 mL [DSC], 10 mL)

◆ **Gentamicin Injection, USP (Can)** *see* Gentamicin (Systemic) *on page* 879

◆ **Gentamicin Sulfate** *see* Gentamicin (Systemic) *on page* 879

◆ **Gilotrif** *see* Afatinib *on page* 65

◆ **Giotrif (Can)** *see* Afatinib *on page* 65

◆ **Gleevec** *see* Imatinib *on page* 972

◆ **Gleostine** *see* Lomustine *on page* 1159

◆ **Gliadel Wafer** *see* Carmustine *on page* 346

◆ **Glivec** *see* Imatinib *on page* 972

◆ **Gln** *see* Glutamine *on page* 886

Glucarpidase (gloo KAR pid ase)

Brand Names: US Voraxaze
Index Terms Carboxypeptidase-G2; CPDG2; CPG2; Voraxaze
Pharmacologic Category Antidote; Enzyme

Use

Methotrexate toxicity: Treatment of toxic methotrexate plasma concentrations (>1 micromole/L) in patients with delayed clearance due to renal impairment.

Limitations of use: Due to the risk of subtherapeutic methotrexate exposure, glucarpidase is **NOT** indicated when methotrexate clearance is within the expected range (plasma methotrexate concentration within 2 standard deviations of mean methotrexate excretion curve specific for methotrexate dose administered) **or** in patients with normal renal function or mild renal impairment

Labeled Contraindications There are no contraindications listed in the manufacturer's labeling.

Pregnancy Considerations Animal reproduction studies have not been conducted. If administered to a pregnant woman, the risk to the fetus is unknown; use only if clearly needed. In general, medications used as antidotes should take into consideration the health and prognosis of the mother.

Breastfeeding Considerations It is not known if glucarpidase is present in breast milk. Caution should be used if administered to a breastfeeding woman.

Warnings/Precautions Serious allergic reactions have been reported.

Leucovorin calcium administration should be continued after glucarpidase; the same dose as was given prior to glucarpidase should be continued for the first 48 hours after glucarpidase; after 48 hours, leucovorin doses should be based on methotrexate concentrations. A single methotrexate concentration should not determine when leucovorin should be discontinued; continue leucovorin until the methotrexate concentration remains below the threshold for leucovorin treatment for ≥3 days. Leucovorin calcium is a substrate for glucarpidase and may compete with methotrexate for binding sites; **do not administer leucovorin calcium within 2 hours before or after glucarpidase.** In addition to leucovorin, glucarpidase use should be accompanied with adequate hydration and urinary alkalinization. During the first 48 hours following glucarpidase administration, the only reliable method of measuring methotrexate concentrations is the chromatographic method. DAMPA, an inactive methotrexate metabolite with a half-life of 9 hours, may interfere with immunoassay and result in the overestimation of the methotrexate concentration (when collected within 48 hours of glucarpidase administration). The utility of more than one glucarpidase dose in reducing plasma methotrexate levels was evaluated in a study of 100 patients with high-dose methotrexate-induced nephrotoxicity (Widemann 2010). Glucarpidase 50 units/kg IV was administered either as a single dose (n=65), 2 doses given 24 hours apart (n=28), or 3 doses given at 4 hour intervals (n=7). Six of the 65 patients randomized to a single dose also received a second delayed glucarpidase dose (>24 hours later) due to persistent methotrexate concentrations ≥1 micromole/L in spite of a ≥90% decrease in the plasma methotrexate concentration after the initial dose. The use of scheduled second and third glucarpidase doses did not result in additional methotrexate concentration decreases; and only 2 of the 6 patients who received a second delayed glucarpidase dose (>24 hours later) experienced a ≥50% methotrexate concentration reduction. Glucarpidase use for intrathecal methotrexate overdose (off-label route/use) should be used in conjunction with immediate lumbar drainage; concurrent dexamethasone (4 mg IV every 6 hours for 4 doses) may minimize methotrexate-induced chemical arachnoiditis;

leucovorin calcium (100 mg IV every 6 hours for 4 doses) may prevent systemic methotrexate toxicity (Widemann 2004).

Adverse Reactions
>10%: Immunologic: Antibody development (21%)
1% to 10%:
Cardiovascular: Flushing (2%), hypotension (1%)
Central nervous system: Headache (1%)
Gastrointestinal: Nausea/vomiting (2%)
Neuromuscular & skeletal: Paresthesia (2%)
<1%, postmarketing, and/or case reports: Blurred vision, diarrhea, hypersensitivity reaction, hypertension, localized warm feeling, skin rash, throat irritation, tremor

Drug Interactions
Metabolism/Transport Effects None known.
Avoid Concomitant Use There are no known interactions where it is recommended to avoid concomitant use.
Increased Effect/Toxicity There are no known significant interactions involving an increase in effect.
Decreased Effect
Glucarpidase may decrease the levels/effects of: Leucovorin Calcium-Levoleucovorin

Storage/Stability Store intact vials refrigerated at 2°C to 8°C (36°F to 46°F); do not freeze. Reconstituted solutions should be used immediately or may be stored for up to 4 hours under refrigeration.

Preparation for Administration
IV: Reconstitute each vial (1,000 units/vial) with 1 mL normal saline. Mix gently by rolling or tilting vial; do not shake. Upon reconstitution, solution should be clear, colorless and free of particulate matter.
Intrathecal (off-label route/use): Reconstitute 2,000 units with 12 mL preservative-free normal saline (Widemann 2004)

Mechanism of Action Glucarpidase is a recombinant enzyme which rapidly hydrolyzes the carboxyl-terminal glutamate residue from extracellular methotrexate into inactive metabolites (DAMPA and glutamate), resulting in a rapid reduction of methotrexate concentrations independent of renal function

Pharmacodynamics/Kinetics
Onset of action: Methotrexate toxicity: Reduces methotrexate concentrations by ≥97% within 15 minutes of IV administration
Duration: Methotrexate toxicity: Maintains a >95% reduction of methotrexate concentrations for up to 8 days
Distribution: V_d: IV: 3.6 L; distribution restricted to plasma volume
Half-life elimination: IV: Normal renal function: Serum glucarpidase activity levels: 5.6 hours; Serum total glucarpidase: ~9 hours. Impaired renal function (CrCl <30 mL/minute): 8 to 10 hours (Phillips 2008)

Dosing
Adult & Geriatric Note: Leucovorin calcium is a substrate for glucarpidase and may compete with methotrexate for binding sites; **do not administer leucovorin calcium within 2 hours before or after glucarpidase.**
Methotrexate toxicity: IV: 50 units/kg as a single dose (Buchen 2005; Widemann 1997; Widemann 2010); may require a second dose 24 hours later (Schwartz 2007; Widemann 1997)
Intrathecal methotrexate overdose (off-label route/use): Intrathecal: 2,000 units as soon as possible after accidental methotrexate overdose (Widemann 2004)

Pediatric Note: Leucovorin calcium is a substrate for glucarpidase and may compete with methotrexate for binding sites; **do not administer leucovorin calcium within 2 hours before or after glucarpidase.**

Methotrexate toxicity: IV: Refer to adult dosing.

Intrathecal methotrexate overdose (off-label route/use): Intrathecal: Refer to adult dosing.

Renal Impairment No dosage adjustment necessary.

Hepatic Impairment There are no dosage adjustments provided in the manufacturer's labeling (has not been studied).

Administration

IV: Infuse over 5 minutes; flush IV line before and after glucarpidase administration. Leucovorin calcium is a substrate for glucarpidase and may compete with methotrexate for binding sites; do not administer leucovorin calcium within 2 hours before or after glucarpidase.

Intrathecal (for intrathecal methotrexate overdose; off-label route/use): Glucarpidase was administered within 3 to 9 hours of accidental intrathecal methotrexate overdose in conjunction with lumbar drainage or ventriculolumbar perfusion (Widemann 2004). Administered over 5 minutes via lumbar route, ventriculostomy, Ommaya reservoir, or lumbar and ventriculostomy (O'Marcaigh 1996; Widemann 2004). In one case report, 1,000 units were administered through the ventricular catheter over 5 minutes and another 1,000 units were administered through the lumbar catheter (O'Marcaigh 1996).

Monitoring Parameters

Serum methotrexate levels: Use chromatographic method if <48 hours from glucarpidase administration (DAMPA interferes with immunoassay results until >48 hours)

CBC with differential, bilirubin, ALT, AST, serum creatinine; evaluate for signs/symptoms of methotrexate toxicity

Test Interactions Methotrexate levels: During the first 48 hours following glucarpidase administration, the only reliable method of measuring methotrexate concentrations is the chromatographic method. DAMPA, an inactive methotrexate metabolite with a half-life of 9 hours, may interfere with immunoassay and result in the overestimation of the methotrexate concentration (when collected within 48 hours of glucarpidase administration).

Prescribing and Access Restrictions Voraxaze is distributed through ASD Healthcare; procurement information is available (24 hours a day; 365 days a year) at 1-855-7-VORAXAZE (1-855-786-7292). Voraxaze is also commercially available in the U.S. through certain pharmacy wholesalers on a drop-ship basis; orders will only be processed during business hours for overnight delivery. For additional information, refer to http://www.btgplc.com/products/specialty-pharmaceuticals/voraxaze.

Dosage Forms Excipient information presented when available (limited, particularly for generics); consult specific product labeling.

Solution Reconstituted, Intravenous [preservative free]:

Voraxaze: 1000 units (1 ea)

◆ **GlutaMent [OTC]** see Glutamine on page 886

Glutamine (GLOO ta meen)

Brand Names: US GlutaMent [OTC]; Glutasolve [OTC]; GlutImmune [OTC]; NutreStore; Sympt-X [OTC]

Index Terms Endari; Gln; L-Glutamine

Pharmacologic Category Amino Acid; Gastrointestinal Agent, Miscellaneous

Use

Short bowel syndrome (NutreStore): For the treatment of short bowel syndrome in patients receiving specialized nutritional support when used in conjunction with a recombinant growth hormone that is approved for this indication.

Sickle cell disease (Endari): To reduce the acute complications of sickle cell disease in adult and pediatric patients 5 years and older.

Supplement (nutritional): Medical food used to promote GI tract healing and nutritional supplementation with GI disorders, HIV/AIDS, cancer, and other critical illnesses.

Note: A medical food is formulated to be administered enterally under the supervision of a physician and is intended for the specific dietary management of a disease or condition for which distinctive nutritional requirements are established by medical evaluation. Medical foods are not drugs and, therefore, are not subject to any FDA regulatory requirements that specifically apply to drugs (eg, requirement for written/oral prescription prior to dispensing, premarket review or approval, proof of safety and efficacy).

Pregnancy Risk Factor C

Dosing

Adult & Geriatric

Short bowel syndrome: NutreStore: Oral: 30 g/day administered as 5 g 6 times daily for up to 16 weeks; to be used in combination with growth hormone and nutritional support

Sickle cell disease: Endari: Oral:
<30 kg: 5 g (1 packet) twice daily (total dose 10 g/day)
30 to 65 kg: 10 g (2 packets) twice daily (total dose 20 g/day)
>65 kg: 15 g (3 packets) twice daily (total dose 30 g/day)

Supplement (nutritional):
GlutImmune, GlutaMent, GlutaSolve, Glutapak-10, Sympt-X: Oral: Average dose: 10 g 3 times/day; dosing range: 5 to 30 g/day
Glutamine (capsules): Oral: 500 mg daily

Pediatric

Sickle cell disease: Endari: Oral: Children ≥5 years and Adolescents:
<30 kg: 5 g (1 packet) twice daily (total dose 10 g/day)
30 to 65 kg: 10 g (2 packets) twice daily (total dose 20 g/day)
>65 kg: 15 g (3 packets) twice daily (total dose 30 g/day)

Supplement (nutritional): Sympt-X: Oral: 0.25 to 0.5 g/kg/day given in 3 divided doses

Renal Impairment There are no dosage adjustments provided in the manufacturer's labeling; use with caution.

Hepatic Impairment There are no dosage adjustments provided in the manufacturer's labeling; use with caution.

Additional Information Complete prescribing information should be consulted for additional detail.

Product Availability

Endari: FDA approved July 2017; anticipated availability is fourth quarter 2017. Information pertaining to this product within the monograph is pending revision. Consult the prescribing information for additional information.

Sympt-X is available in US in 300 g jars, 500 g jars and packets (10 g L-glutamine + 5 g maltodextrin)

◄ **Dosage Forms** Excipient information presented when available (limited, particularly for generics); consult specific product labeling. [DSC] = Discontinued product

Capsule, Oral:
  Generic: 500 mg
Packet, Oral:
  GlutaMent: 10 g (50 ea)
  Glutasolve: 15 g (56 ea)
  NutreStore: 5 g (84 ea)
  Sympt-X: 15 g (60s)
  Sympt-X G.I.: 10 g (60 ea [DSC])
Powder, Oral:
  GlutImmune: (454 g)
  Sympt-X: (300 g, 500 g)
Tablet, Oral:
  Generic: 500 mg

◆ **Glutasolve [OTC]** see Glutamine on page 886
◆ **GlutImmune [OTC]** see Glutamine on page 886
◆ **GM-CSF** see Sargramostim on page 1656
◆ **GM-CSF-Encoding Oncolytic Herpes Simplex Virus** see Talimogene Laherparepvec on page 1729
◆ **GnRH Agonist** see Histrelin on page 912

Goserelin (GOE se rel in)

Related Information
  Safe Handling of Hazardous Drugs on page 2379
Brand Names: US Zoladex
Brand Names: Canada Zoladex; Zoladex LA
Index Terms Goserelin Acetate; ICI-118630; ZDX
Pharmacologic Category Antineoplastic Agent, Gonadotropin-Releasing Hormone Agonist; Gonadotropin Releasing Hormone Agonist
Use

US labeling:

  Breast cancer, advanced (3.6 mg only): Palliative treatment of advanced breast cancer in pre- and perimenopausal women (estrogen and progesterone receptor values may help to predict if goserelin is likely to be beneficial).

  Endometrial thinning (3.6 mg only): Endometrial-thinning agent prior to endometrial ablation for dysfunctional uterine bleeding.

  Endometriosis (3.6 mg only): Management of endometriosis, including pain relief and reduction of endometriotic lesions for the duration of therapy (goserelin experience for endometriosis has been limited to women 18 years and older treated for 6 months).

  Prostate cancer, advanced (3.6 mg or 10.8 mg): Palliative treatment of advanced carcinoma of the prostate.

  Prostate cancer, stage B2 to C (3.6 mg or 10.8 mg):: Management of locally confined stage T2b to T4 (stage B2 to C) prostate cancer (in combination with an antiandrogen [eg, flutamide]); begin goserelin and antiandrogen therapy 8 weeks prior to initiating radiation therapy and continue during radiation therapy.

Canadian labeling:

Breast cancer, advanced (3.6 mg only): Palliative treatment of advanced breast cancer in pre- and perimenopausal women (with estrogen and/or progesterone receptor-positive tumors).

Breast cancer, early (3.6 mg only): Alternative to standard adjuvant chemotherapy in pre- and perimenopausal women with early breast cancer (with estrogen and/or progesterone receptor-positive tumors) who are unsuitable for, intolerant to, or decline chemotherapy.

Endometrial thinning (3.6 mg only): Endometrial-thinning agent prior to endometrial ablation.

Endometriosis (3.6 mg or 10.8 mg): Hormonal management of endometriosis, including pain relief and reduction of endometriotic lesions (goserelin experience for endometriosis has been limited to women 18 years and older treated for 6 months).

Prostate cancer, advanced (3.6 mg or 10.8 mg): Palliative treatment of hormone-dependent advanced carcinoma of the prostate (stage M1 or D2).

Prostate cancer, locally advanced (3.6 mg or 10.8 mg): Management of locally advanced (T3 or T4) or bulky stage T2b to T2c prostate cancer (in combination with a nonsteroidal antiandrogen and radiation therapy); begin goserelin and antiandrogen therapy 8 weeks prior to initiating radiation therapy and continue until completion of radiation therapy.

Prostate cancer, locally advanced (3.6 mg or 10.8 mg): Adjuvant hormone therapy to external beam irradiation in locally advanced prostate cancer (stage T3 to T4).

Labeled Contraindications

US labeling: Hypersensitivity to goserelin, GnRH, GnRH agonist analogues, or any component of the formulation; pregnancy (except if using for palliative treatment of advanced breast cancer)

Canadian labeling: Hypersensitivity to goserelin or any component of the formulation; undiagnosed vaginal bleeding

Pregnancy Considerations Adverse events were observed in animal reproduction studies. Goserelin induces hormonal changes which increase the risk for fetal loss and use is contraindicated in pregnancy unless being used for palliative treatment of advanced breast cancer.

Breast cancer: If used for the palliative treatment of breast cancer during pregnancy, the potential for increased fetal loss should be discussed with the patient.

Endometriosis, endometrial thinning: Use is contraindicated during pregnancy. Women of childbearing potential should not receive therapy until pregnancy has been excluded. Nonhormonal contraception is recommended for premenopausal women during therapy and for 12 weeks after therapy is discontinued. Although ovulation is usually inhibited and menstruation may stop, pregnancy prevention is not ensured during goserelin therapy. Changes in reproductive function may occur following chronic administration.

Breastfeeding Considerations It is not known if goserelin is excreted in breast milk, although goserelin is inactivated when used orally. Due to the potential for serious adverse reactions in the breastfeeding infant, a decision should be made to discontinue breastfeeding or to discontinue the drug, taking into account the importance of treatment to the mother.

Warnings/Precautions Transient increases in serum testosterone (in men with prostate cancer) and estrogen (in women with breast cancer) may result in a worsening of disease signs and symptoms (tumor flare) during the first few weeks of treatment. Some patients experienced a temporary worsening of ▶

bone pain, which may be managed symptomatically. Spinal cord compression and urinary tract obstruction have been reported when used for prostate cancer; closely observe patients for symptoms (eg, ureteral obstruction, weakness, paresthesias) in first few weeks of therapy. Manage with standard treatment; consider orchiectomy for extreme cases.

Androgen deprivation therapy may increase the risk for cardiovascular disease (Levine, 2010). An increased risk for MI, sudden cardiac death, and stroke has been observed. Monitor for signs/symptoms of cardiovascular disease; manage according to current clinical practice. Androgen deprivation therapy may cause prolongation of the QT/QTc interval; evaluate risk versus benefit in patients with congenital long QT syndrome, heart failure, frequent electrolyte abnormalities, and in patients taking medication known to prolong the QT interval. Correct electrolytes prior to initiation and consider periodic electrolyte and ECG monitoring. Hyperglycemia has been reported in males and may manifest as diabetes or worsening of preexisting diabetes (worsening glycemic control); monitor blood glucose and HbA_{1c} and manage diabetes appropriately.

Injection site and vascular injury, including pain, hematoma, hemorrhage and hemorrhagic shock (requiring blood transfusions or surgical intervention) have been reported with goserelin. Use extra caution when administering to patients with a low BMI and/or to patients receiving full dose anticoagulation (Canadian labeling does not recommend use of goserelin in these patients due to the risk of vascular injury/bleeding). Use caution while injecting goserelin into the anterior abdominal wall (due to the proximity of underlying inferior epigastric artery and its branches). Monitor for signs/symptoms of abdominal hemorrhage. Inform patient to immediately report abdominal pain, abdominal distention, dyspnea, dizziness, hypotension, and/or altered level of consciousness. Hypersensitivity reactions (including acute anaphylactic reactions) and antibody formation may occur; monitor. Hypercalcemia has been reported in prostate and breast cancer patients with bone metastases; initiate appropriate management if hypercalcemia occurs. Rare cases of pituitary apoplexy (frequently secondary to pituitary adenoma) have been observed with GnRH agonist administration (onset from 1 hour to usually <2 weeks); may present as sudden headache, vomiting, visual or mental status changes, and infrequently cardiovascular collapse; immediate medical attention required. A decreased AUC may be observed when using the 3-month implant in obese patients; monitor testosterone levels if desired clinical response is not observed. Use extra care when administering to patients with a low BMI. If implant removal is necessary, implant may be located by ultrasound.

Decreased bone density has been reported in women and may be irreversible; use caution if other risk factors are present; evaluate and institute preventive treatment if necessary. Cervical resistance may be increased; use caution when dilating the cervix for endometrial ablation. Women of childbearing potential should not receive therapy until pregnancy has been excluded. Nonhormonal contraception is recommended during therapy and for 12 weeks after therapy is discontinued. Chronic administration may result in effects on reproductive function due to antigonadotropic properties. Potentially significant drug-drug interactions may exist, requiring dose or frequency adjustment, additional monitoring, and/or selection of alternative therapy.

Adverse Reactions Some frequencies not defined. Percentages reported with the 1-month implant:

>10%:

Cardiovascular: Vasodilatation (females 57%), peripheral edema (females 21%)

Central nervous system: Headache (females 32% to 75%; males 1% to 5%), emotional lability (females 60%), depression (females 54%; males 1% to 5%), pain (8% to 17%), dyspareunia (females 14%), insomnia (5% to 11%)

Dermatologic: Diaphoresis (females 16% to 45%; males 6%), acne vulgaris (females 42%; usually within 1 month after starting treatment), seborrhea (females 26%)

Endocrine & metabolic: Hot flash (females 57% to 96%; males 64%), decreased libido (females 48% to 61%), increased libido (females 12%)

Gastrointestinal: Abdominal pain (females 7% to 11%), nausea (5% to 11%)

Genitourinary: Vaginitis (75%), breast atrophy (females 33%), sexual disorder (males 21%), breast hypertrophy (females 18%), decrease in erectile frequency (18%), pelvic symptoms (females 18%), genitourinary signs and symptoms (lower; males 13%)

Hematologic & oncologic: Tumor flare (females 23%; males: Incidence not reported)

Infection: Infection (females 13%; males: Incidence not reported)

Neuromuscular & skeletal: Decreased bone mineral density (females 23%; ~4% decrease from baseline in 6 months; male: Incidence not reported), weakness (females 11%)

1% to 10%:

Cardiovascular: Edema (females 5%; male 7%), hypertension (1% to 6%), cardiac failure (males 5%), cardiac arrhythmia (males >1% to <5%), cerebrovascular accident (males >1% to <5%), peripheral vascular disease (males >1% to <5%), varicose veins (males >1% to <5%), chest pain (1% to <5%), myocardial infarction (males <1% to <5%), palpitations, tachycardia (females)

Central nervous system: Lethargy (females ≤8%), migraine (females 1% to 7%), dizziness (females 6%; male 5%), malaise (females ≤5%), chills (males >1% to <5%), anxiety (1% to <5%), nervousness (females 3% to 5%), voice disorder (females 3%), abnormality in thinking, drowsiness, paresthesia

Dermatologic: Skin rash (males 6% to 8%; female frequency not reported), hair disease (females 4%), pruritus (females 2%), alopecia, skin discoloration, xeroderma

Endocrine & metabolic: Gynecomastia (males 8%), hirsutism (7%), gout (males >1% to <5%), hyperglycemia (males >1% to <5%), weight gain (>1% to <5%)

Gastrointestinal: Anorexia (1% to 5%), gastric ulcer (males >1% to <5%), constipation (1% to <5%), diarrhea (1% to <5%), vomiting (1% to <5%), increased appetite (females 2%), dyspepsia, flatulence, xerostomia

Genitourinary: Pelvic pain (females 9%; males 6%), mastalgia (>1% to 7%), uterine hemorrhage (6%), vulvovaginitis (5%), breast swelling (males >1% to <5%), urinary tract obstruction (males: >1% to <5%), urinary tract infection (1% to <5%), urinary frequency, vaginal hemorrhage

Hematologic & oncologic: Anemia (males >1% to <5%), bruise, hemorrhage

Hypersensitivity: Hypersensitivity reaction

Infection: Sepsis (males >1% to <5%)

Local: Application site reaction (females 6%)

◄ Neuromuscular & skeletal: Myalgia (females 3%, males frequency not reported), leg cramps (females 2%, males frequency not reported), hypertonia (females 1%; male frequency not reported), arthralgia, arthropathy

Ophthalmic: Amblyopia, dry eye syndrome

Renal: Renal insufficiency (<1% to >5%)

Respiratory: Upper respiratory tract infection (males 7%), chronic obstructive pulmonary disease (males 5%), flu-like symptoms (females 5%, male frequency not reported), pharyngitis (females 5%), sinusitis (females ≥1%; male frequency not reported), bronchitis, cough, epistaxis, rhinitis

Miscellaneous: Fever

<1%, postmarketing, and/or case reports (with monthly or 3-month implant): Anaphylaxis, bone fracture, convulsions, decreased glucose tolerance, decreased HDL cholesterol, deep vein thrombosis, diabetes mellitus, hypercalcemia, hypercholesterolemia, hyperlipidemia, hypotension, increased HDL cholesterol, increased LDL cholesterol, increased serum ALT, increased serum AST, increased serum triglycerides, injection site reaction (including vascular injury, pain, hematoma, hemorrhage, hemorrhagic shock), osteoporosis, ovarian cyst, ovarian hyperstimulation syndrome, pituitary apoplexy, pituitary neoplasm (including adenoma), pulmonary embolism, psychotic reaction, transient ischemic attacks

Drug Interactions

Metabolism/Transport Effects None known.

Avoid Concomitant Use

Avoid concomitant use of Goserelin with any of the following: Corifollitropin Alfa; Highest Risk QTc-Prolonging Agents; Hydroxychloroquine; Indium 111 Capromab Pendetide; MiFEPRIStone; Probucol; Promazine; Vinflunine

Increased Effect/Toxicity

Goserelin may increase the levels/effects of: Corifollitropin Alfa; Highest Risk QTc-Prolonging Agents; Moderate Risk QTc-Prolonging Agents

The levels/effects of Goserelin may be increased by: Hydroxychloroquine; MiFEPRIStone; Probucol; Promazine; QTc-Prolonging Agents (Indeterminate Risk and Risk Modifying); Vinflunine; Xipamide

Decreased Effect

Goserelin may decrease the levels/effects of: Antidiabetic Agents; Choline C 11; Indium 111 Capromab Pendetide

Hazardous Drugs Handling Considerations

Hazardous agent (NIOSH 2016 [group 1]).

Use appropriate precautions for receiving, handling, administration, and disposal. Gloves (single) should be worn during receiving, unpacking, and placing in storage.

NIOSH recommends double gloving, a protective gown, ventilated engineering controls (a class II biological safety cabinet or a compounding aseptic containment isolator), and closed system transfer devices (CSTDs) for preparation. Double gloves and a protective gown are required during administration (NIOSH 2016).

Storage/Stability Store at room temperature not to exceed 25°C (77°F). Keep in foil pouch until ready to use to protect from light and moisture.

Mechanism of Action Goserelin (a gonadotropin-releasing hormone [GnRH] analog) causes an initial increase in luteinizing hormone (LH) and follicle stimulating hormone (FSH), chronic administration of goserelin results in a sustained suppression of pituitary gonadotropins. Serum testosterone falls to levels comparable to surgical castration. The exact mechanism of this effect is unknown, but may be related to changes in the control of LH or down-regulation of LH receptors.

Pharmacodynamics/Kinetics

Onset:

Females: Estradiol suppression reaches postmenopausal levels within 3 weeks and FSH and LH are suppressed to follicular phase levels within 4 weeks of initiation

Males: Testosterone suppression reaches castrate levels within 2 to 4 weeks after initiation

Duration:

Females: Estradiol, LH and FSH generally return to baseline levels within 12 weeks following the last monthly implant.

Males: Testosterone levels maintained at castrate levels throughout the duration of therapy.

Absorption: SubQ: Rapid and can be detected in serum in 30 to 60 minutes; 3.6 mg: released slowly in first 8 days, then rapid and continuous release for 28 days

Distribution: V_d: Male: 44.1 L; Female: 20.3 L

Protein binding: ~27%

Metabolism: Hepatic hydrolysis of the C-terminal amino acids

Time to peak, serum: SubQ: Male: 12 to 15 days, Female: 8 to 22 days

Excretion: Urine (>90%; 20% as unchanged drug)

Dosing

Adult

US labeling:

Prostate cancer, advanced: Males: SubQ:

28-day implant: 3.6 mg every 28 days

12-week implant: 10.8 mg every 12 weeks

Prostate cancer, stage B2 to C (in combination with an antiandrogen and radiotherapy; begin 8 weeks prior to radiotherapy): Males: SubQ:
Combination 28-day/12-week implant: 3.6 mg implant, followed in 28 days by 10.8 mg implant

28-day implant (alternate dosing): 3.6 mg; repeated every 28 days for a total of 4 doses

Breast cancer, advanced: Females: SubQ: 3.6 mg every 28 days

Endometriosis: Females: SubQ: 3.6 mg every 28 days for 6 months

Endometrial thinning: Females: SubQ: 3.6 mg every 28 days for 1 or 2 doses

Canadian labeling:

Prostate cancer, advanced: Males: SubQ:

28-day implant: 3.6 mg every 28 days

3-month implant: 10.8 mg every 13 weeks

Prostate cancer, stage B2 to C (in combination with an antiandrogen and radiotherapy; begin 8 weeks prior to radiotherapy): Males: SubQ:
Combination 28-day/3-month implant: 3.6 mg implant, followed in 28 days by 10.8 mg implant

28-day implant (alternate dosing): 3.6 mg; repeated every 28 days for a total of 4 doses

Breast cancer, advanced: Females: SubQ: 3.6 mg every 28 days

Breast cancer, early: Females: SubQ: 3.6 mg every 28 days

Endometriosis: Females: SubQ:
  28-day implant: 3.6 mg every 28 days for 6 months
  3-month implant: 10.8 mg every 12 weeks for 6 months
Endometrial thinning: Females: SubQ: 3.6 mg every 28 days for 2 doses

Off-label dosing:
  Prevention of early menopause during chemotherapy for early stage hormone receptor negative breast cancer (off-label use): Adult females: SubQ: 3.6 mg every 28 days starting 1 week prior to the first chemotherapy dose; continue until within 2 weeks before or after the final chemotherapy dose (Moore, 2015).

Geriatric Males: Refer to adult dosing.

Renal Impairment No dosage adjustment necessary.

Hepatic Impairment No dosage adjustment necessary.

Administration SubQ: Administer implant by inserting needle at a 30 to 45 degree angle into the anterior abdominal wall below the navel line. Use caution while injecting goserelin into the anterior abdominal wall (due to the proximity of underlying inferior epigastric artery and its branches). Goserelin is an implant; therefore, do not attempt to eliminate air bubbles prior to injection (may displace implant). Do not attempt to aspirate prior to injection; if a large vessel is penetrated, blood will be visualized in the syringe chamber (if vessel is penetrated, withdraw needle and inject elsewhere with a new syringe). Do not penetrate into muscle or peritoneum. Implant may be detected by ultrasound if removal is required. Monitor for signs/symptoms of abdominal hemorrhage. Use extra care when administering goserelin to patients with a low BMI and/or to patients receiving full dose anticoagulation (Canadian labeling does not recommend use in these patients due to the risk of vascular injury/bleeding).

Monitoring Parameters Monitor blood glucose and HbA$_{1c}$ (periodically), bone mineral density, serum calcium, cholesterol/lipids; monitor for signs/symptoms of abdominal hemorrhage following injection.
  Prostate cancer: Consider periodic ECG and electrolyte monitoring. Monitor for weakness, paresthesias, tumor flare, urinary tract obstruction, and spinal cord compression in first few weeks of therapy.

Test Interactions Interferes with pituitary gonadotropic and gonadal function tests during and for up to 12 weeks after discontinued

Dosage Forms Excipient information presented when available (limited, particularly for generics); consult specific product labeling.
  Implant, Subcutaneous:
    Zoladex: 3.6 mg (1 ea); 10.8 mg (1 ea)

Dosage Forms: Canada Information with regard to form, strength, and availability of products uniquely available in Canada but currently not available in the US. Refer also to Dosage Forms.

  Excipient information presented when available (limited, particularly for generics); consult specific product labeling.
  Implant, Subcutaneous:
    Zoladex: 3.6 mg
    Zoladex LA: 10.8 mg

◆ **Goserelin Acetate** see Goserelin on page 888
◆ **GR38032R** see Ondansetron on page 1380

Granisetron (gra NI se tron)

Related Information

Management of Chemotherapy-Induced Nausea and Vomiting in Adults *on page 2253*

Prevention of Chemotherapy-Induced Nausea and Vomiting in Children *on page 2310*

Brand Names: US Granisol [DSC]; Sancuso; Sustol

Brand Names: Canada Granisetron Hydrochloride Injection; Granisetron Hydrochloride Injection SDZ; Nat-Granisetron

Index Terms BRL 43694; Granisetron HCl; Granisetron Hydrochloride; Granisol; Kytril

Pharmacologic Category Antiemetic; Selective 5-HT$_3$ Receptor Antagonist

Use

Chemotherapy-associated nausea and vomiting: Prevention of nausea and vomiting associated with initial and repeat courses of emetogenic chemotherapy, including high-dose cisplatin (injection and tablets); prevention of nausea and vomiting associated with anthracycline/cyclophosphamide chemotherapy regimens; prevention of nausea and vomiting associated with moderately and/or highly emetogenic chemotherapy regimens of up to 5 consecutive days of duration (transdermal).

Radiation-associated nausea and vomiting: Prevention of nausea and vomiting associated with radiation therapy, including total body radiation and fractionated abdominal radiation (tablets).

Labeled Contraindications

Hypersensitivity to granisetron or any component of the formulation or to other 5-HT3 receptor antagonists

Canadian labeling: Additional contraindications (not in US labeling): Concomitant use with apomorphine

Pregnancy Considerations Adverse events have not been observed in animal reproduction studies. In an ex vivo placental perfusion study, granisetron was shown to cross the placenta in a concentration (dose) dependent manner (Julius 2014). Initial studies note the pharmacokinetics of the transdermal system may be different in pregnant women. A relationship between granisetron plasma concentrations and relief of symptoms of nausea and vomiting of pregnancy was also observed (Cartis 2016). Some dosage forms (injection) may contain benzyl alcohol.

Breastfeeding Considerations It is not known if granisetron is excreted in breast milk. According to the manufacturer, the decision to continue or discontinue breastfeeding during therapy should take into account the risk of infant exposure, the benefits of breastfeeding to the infant, benefits of treatment to the mother, and the underlying maternal condition.

Warnings/Precautions Constipation may occur with all formulations, although a higher incidence is observed with tablets and the extended release subcutaneous injection. Hospitalization due to constipation or fecal impaction has been reported with the extended release subcutaneous injection. Progressive ileus and/or gastric distention may be masked by the extended release subcutaneous injection (assess risks/benefits in patients with recent abdominal surgery). Monitor for development of constipation and for decreased bowel activity, particularly in patients at risk for gastrointestinal obstruction. Granisetron does not stimulate gastric or intestinal peristalsis; do not use it in place of nasogastric suction.

Use with caution in patients with congenital long QT syndrome or other risk factors for QT prolongation (eg, medications known to prolong QT interval, electrolyte abnormalities, and cumulative high-dose anthracycline therapy). 5-HT$_3$ antagonists have been associated with a number of dose-dependent increases in ECG intervals (eg, PR, QRS duration, QT/QTc, JT), usually occurring 1 to 2 hours after IV administration. In general, these changes are not clinically relevant, however, when used in conjunction with other agents that prolong these intervals, arrhythmia may occur. When used with agents that prolong the QT interval (eg, Class I and III antiarrhythmics), clinically relevant QT interval prolongation may occur resulting in torsade de pointes. IV formulations of 5-HT$_3$ antagonists have more association with ECG interval changes, compared to oral formulations.

Antiemetics are most effective when used prophylactically (Roila 2016). If emesis occurs despite optimal antiemetic prophylaxis, re-evaluate emetic risk, disease, concurrent morbidities and medications to assure antiemetic regimen is optimized (Basch 2011).

Serotonin syndrome has been reported with 5-HT$_3$ receptor antagonists, predominantly when used in combination with other serotonergic agents (eg, SSRIs, SNRIs, MAOIs, mirtazapine, fentanyl, lithium, tramadol, and/or methylene blue). Some of the cases have been fatal. The majority of serotonin syndrome reports due to 5-HT$_3$ receptor antagonist have occurred in a postanesthesia setting or in an infusion center. Serotonin syndrome has also been reported following overdose of another 5-HT$_3$ receptor antagonist. Monitor patients for signs of serotonin syndrome, including mental status changes (eg, agitation, hallucinations, delirium, coma); autonomic instability (eg, tachycardia, labile blood pressure, diaphoresis, dizziness, flushing, hyperthermia); neuromuscular changes (eg, tremor, rigidity, myoclonus, hyperreflexia, incoordination); gastrointestinal symptoms (eg, nausea, vomiting, diarrhea); and/or seizures. If serotonin syndrome occurs, discontinue 5-HT$_3$ receptor antagonist treatment and begin supportive management. Potentially significant drug-drug interactions may exist, requiring dose or frequency adjustment, additional monitoring, and/or selection of alternative therapy.

Hypersensitivity reactions (including anaphylaxis) have been reported with granisetron in patients who have experienced hypersensitivity to other 5-HT$_3$ antagonists (cross-reactivity has been reported). Due to the extended release properties of the subcutaneous formulation, granisetron exposure may continue for 5 to 7 days following administration; hypersensitivity reactions may occur up to 7 days or longer following administration and may have an extended course. Monitor for signs/symptoms of hypersensitivity.

Extended-release (subcutaneous) injection: Injection site reactions are associated with the subcutaneous extended release formulation. Injection site infections have been reported (median onset: 9 days); infections were managed with antibiotics and completely resolved. Bruising and/or hematomas occur in over one-third of patients (median onset: 2 days); may be delayed (~5 days or later following administration). Severe bruising has also been reported. Patients receiving anticoagulant or antiplatelet medications are at higher risk for severe bruising/hematoma at the injection site (consider risk/benefit in these patients). Injection site bleeding has also been observed, occasionally lasting >5 days. Injection site pain/tenderness was commonly reported, usually lasting 5 to 7 days. Pain/tenderness interfered with activity or caused significant discomfort at rest (rare); some patients required pain medications. Injection site nodules occurred in less than one-fifth of patients, usually persisting for 15 to 21 days. Monitor for injection site reactions for at least 2 weeks after administration. If injection site reaction is not yet resolved prior to the next dose, rotate injection site with next administration.

Transdermal patch: Do not apply patch to red, irritated, or damaged skin. Application-site reactions have occurred with transdermal patch use; local reactions were generally mild and did not require discontinuation. If skin reaction is severe or generalized (allergic rash including erythematous, macular, or papular rash or pruritus), remove patch. Cover patch application site with clothing to protect from natural or artificial sunlight exposure while patch is applied and for 10 days following removal; granisetron may potentially be affected by natural or artificial sunlight. Do not apply heat (eg, heating pad) over or in area of the transdermal patch; avoid prolonged exposure to heat (may increase plasma concentrations).

Benzyl alcohol and derivatives: Some dosage forms may contain benzyl alcohol; large amounts of benzyl alcohol (≥99 mg/kg/day) have been associated with a potentially fatal toxicity ("gasping syndrome") in neonates; the "gasping syndrome" consists of metabolic acidosis, respiratory distress, gasping respirations, CNS dysfunction (including convulsions, intracranial hemorrhage), hypotension and cardiovascular collapse (AAP ["Inactive" 1997]; CDC 1982), some data suggests that benzoate displaces bilirubin from protein binding sites (Ahlfors 2001); avoid or use dosage forms containing benzyl alcohol with caution in neonates. See manufacturer's labeling.

Polysorbate 80: Some dosage forms may contain polysorbate 80 (also known as Tweens). Hypersensitivity reactions, usually a delayed reaction, have been reported following exposure to pharmaceutical products containing polysorbate 80 in certain individuals (Isaksson 2002; Lucente 2000; Shelley 1995). Thrombocytopenia, ascites, pulmonary deterioration, and renal and hepatic failure have been reported in premature neonates after receiving parenteral products containing polysorbate 80 (Alade 1986; CDC 1984). See manufacturer's labeling.

Adverse Reactions

>10%:

Central nervous system: Headache (oral and IV: 3% to 21%; transdermal: <1%)

Gastrointestinal: Nausea (20%), constipation (oral and IV: 3% to 18%; transdermal: 5%), vomiting (12%)

Neuromuscular & skeletal: Weakness (oral: 14% to 18%; IV: 5%)

1% to 10%:

Cardiovascular: Prolonged Q-T interval on ECG (1% to 3%; >450 milliseconds, not associated with any arrhythmias), hypertension (oral and IV: 1% to 2%)

Central nervous system: Dizziness (5%), insomnia (oral and IV: ≤5%), drowsiness (1% to 4%), anxiety (oral and IV: ≤2%), agitation (IV: <2%), central nervous system stimulation (IV: <2%)

Dermatologic: Alopecia (3%), skin rash (IV: 1%)

Gastrointestinal: Diarrhea (oral and IV: 4% to 9%), decreased appetite (6%), dyspepsia (oral: 6%), abdominal pain (4% to 6%), dysgeusia (IV: 2%)

Hematologic & oncologic: Leukopenia (9%), anemia (4%), thrombocytopenia (2%)

Hepatic: Increased serum ALT (>2 x ULN: 3% to 6%), increased serum AST (>2 x ULN: 3% to 5%)

Miscellaneous: Fever (3% to 9%)

<1%, postmarketing, and/or case reports (all routes): Angina pectoris, application site reaction (including allergic rash, burn, discoloration, erythema, erythematous rash, irritation, macular rash, pain, papular rash, pruritus, urticaria, vesicles), atrial fibrillation, atrioventricular block, bradycardia, cardiac arrhythmia, chest pain, ECG abnormality, extrapyramidal reaction, hypersensitivity reaction (includes anaphylaxis, dyspnea, hypotension, urticaria), hypotension, palpitations, serotonin syndrome, sick sinus syndrome, sinus bradycardia, syncope, ventricular ectopy (includes non-sustained tachycardia)

Drug Interactions

Metabolism/Transport Effects Substrate of CYP3A4 (minor); **Note:** Assignment of Major/Minor substrate status based on clinically relevant drug interaction potential

Avoid Concomitant Use

Avoid concomitant use of Granisetron with any of the following: Apomorphine; Highest Risk QTc-Prolonging Agents; Hydroxychloroquine; MiFEPRIStone; Probucol; Promazine; Vinflunine

Increased Effect/Toxicity

Granisetron may increase the levels/effects of: Apomorphine; Highest Risk QTc-Prolonging Agents; Moderate Risk QTc-Prolonging Agents; Panobinostat; Serotonin Modulators

The levels/effects of Granisetron may be increased by: Hydroxychloroquine; MiFEPRIStone; Probucol; Promazine; QTc-Prolonging Agents (Indeterminate Risk and Risk Modifying); Vinflunine; Xipamide

Decreased Effect

Granisetron may decrease the levels/effects of: Tapentadol; TraMADol

Storage/Stability

IV: Store at 15°C to 30°C (59°F to 86°F). Protect from light. Do not freeze vials. Stable when mixed in NS or D5W for at least 24 hours at room temperature.

Oral: Store tablet or oral solution at 15°C to 30°C (59°F to 86°F). Protect from light.

SubQ (extended-release injection): Store at 2°C to 8°C (36°F to 46°F); do not freeze. May be placed back in refrigerator after being kept at room temperature; may remain at room temperature for a maximum of 7 days. Protect from light.

Transdermal patch: Store at 20°C to 25°C (68°F to 77°F). Keep patch in original packaging until immediately prior to use.

Preparation for Administration

IV: May be given undiluted or may be further diluted in NS or D5W.

SubQ (extended-release injection): Remove extended-release injection kit from refrigeration at least 60 minutes prior to administration. Allow the syringe and all other contents to warm to room temperature. Activate 1 syringe warming pouch and wrap the syringe in the warming pouch for 5 to 6 minutes to allow to reach body temperature. Do not substitute non-kit components for any components of the administration kit.

Mechanism of Action Selective 5-HT$_3$-receptor antagonist, blocking serotonin, both peripherally on vagal nerve terminals and centrally in the chemoreceptor trigger zone

Pharmacodynamics/Kinetics

Onset of action: IV: 1 to 3 minutes

Duration: Oral, IV: Generally up to 24 hours; SubQ (extended-release): Remains detectable in the plasma for 7 days

Absorption: Oral: Tablets and oral solution are bioequivalent; Transdermal patch: ~66% over 7 days

Distribution: V_d: 2 to 4 L/kg; widely throughout body

Protein binding: ~65%

Metabolism: Hepatic via CYP1A1 and CYP3A4 N-demethylation, oxidation, and conjugation; some metabolites may have 5-HT$_3$ antagonist activity

Half-life elimination: Oral: 6 hours; IV: Mean range: 5 to 9 hours; SubQ (extended-release): ~24 hours

Time to peak, plasma: Transdermal patch: Maximum systemic concentrations: ~48 hours after application (range: 24 to 168 hours); SubQ (extended-release): ~24 hours

Excretion: Urine (11% to 12% as unchanged drug, 48% to 49% as metabolites); feces (34% to 38% as metabolites)

Dosing

Adult & Geriatric Note: Granisol oral solution has been discontinued in the US for more than 1 year.

Prevention of chemotherapy-associated nausea and vomiting:

Oral: 2 mg once daily up to 1 hour before chemotherapy or 1 mg twice daily; the first 1 mg dose should be given up to 1 hour before chemotherapy (with the second 1 mg dose 12 hours later). Administer only on the day(s) chemotherapy is given.

IV: 10 mcg/kg within 30 minutes prior to chemotherapy; only on the day(s) chemotherapy is given.

SubQ (extended-release injection): Moderately emetogenic chemotherapy or anthracycline/cyclophosphamide chemotherapy: 10 mg at least 30 minutes prior to chemotherapy on day 1 (in combination with IV dexamethasone on day 1 and [for anthracycline/cyclophosphamide chemotherapy] oral dexamethasone on days 2 to 4); do not administer more frequently than once every 7 days. May also be administered in combination with an NK$_1$ receptor antagonist antiemetic regimen.

Transdermal patch: Prophylaxis of chemotherapy-related emesis. Apply 1 patch at least 24 hours prior to chemotherapy; may be applied up to 48 hours before chemotherapy. Remove patch a minimum of 24 hours after chemotherapy completion. Maximum duration: Patch may be worn up to 7 days, depending on chemotherapy regimen duration.

Adult guideline recommendations:

American Society of Clinical Oncology (ASCO; Basch 2011). High emetic risk:

IV: 1 mg or 10 mcg/kg on the day(s) chemotherapy is administered (antiemetic regimen also includes dexamethasone and aprepitant or fosaprepitant)

Oral: 2 mg on the day(s) chemotherapy is administered (antiemetic regimen also includes dexamethasone and aprepitant or fosaprepitant)

Multinational Association of Supportive Care in Cancer (MASCC) and European Society of Medical Oncology (ESMO) (Roila 2016):

Highly emetic chemotherapy:

IV: 1 mg or 10 mcg/kg (antiemetic regimen includes dexamethasone and aprepitant/fosaprepitant) prior to chemotherapy on day 1

Oral: 1 mg or 2 mg (antiemetic regimen includes dexamethasone and aprepitant/fosaprepitant) prior to chemotherapy on day 1

Moderately emetic chemotherapy:

IV: 1 mg or 10 mcg/kg (antiemetic regimen includes dexamethasone [and aprepitant/fosaprepitant for AC chemotherapy regimen]) prior to chemotherapy on day 1

Oral: 1 mg or 2 mg (antiemetic regimen includes dexamethasone [and aprepitant/fosaprepitant for AC chemotherapy regimen]) prior to chemotherapy on day 1

Low emetic risk:

IV: 1 mg or 10 mcg/kg prior to chemotherapy on day 1

Oral: 1 mg or 2 mg prior to chemotherapy on day 1

Prophylaxis of radiation therapy-associated emesis: Oral: 2 mg once daily within 1 hour of radiation therapy.

Prevention of postoperative nausea and vomiting (off-label use): IV: 0.35 to 3 mg (5 to 20 **mcg**/kg) administered at the end of surgery (Gan 2014).

Pediatric Note: Granisol oral solution has been discontinued in the US for more than 1 year.

Prevention of chemotherapy-associated nausea and vomiting: Children ≥2 years and Adolescents: IV: 10 mcg/kg 30 minutes prior to chemotherapy; only on the day(s) chemotherapy is given.

Pediatric guideline recommendations:

Prevention of chemotherapy-induced nausea and vomiting (off-label dosing; Dupuis 2013):

Highly emetogenic chemotherapy: Infants ≥1 month and Children <12 years: IV: 40 mcg/kg as a single daily dose prior to chemotherapy. Antiemetic regimen also includes dexamethasone.

Highly emetogenic chemotherapy: Children ≥12 years and Adolescents: IV: 40 mcg/kg as a single daily dose prior to chemotherapy. Antiemetic regimen includes dexamethasone and (if no known or suspected drug interactions) aprepitant.

Moderately emetogenic chemotherapy: Infants ≥1 month, Children, and Adolescents:

IV: 40 mcg/kg as a single daily dose. Antiemetic regimen also includes dexamethasone

Oral: 40 mcg/kg every 12 hours. Antiemetic regimen also includes dexamethasone

Low emetogenic chemotherapy: Infants ≥1 month, Children, and Adolescents:

IV: 40 mcg/kg as a single daily dose.

Oral: 40 mcg/kg every 12 hours.

Renal Impairment

IV, Oral, Transdermal: No dosage adjustment necessary.

SubQ (extended-release injection):

CrCl ≥60 mL/minute: No dosage adjustment necessary.

CrCl 30 to 59 mL/minute: 10 mg on day 1 of chemotherapy; do not administer more frequently than once every 14 days.

CrCl <30 mL/minute: Avoid use.

Hepatic Impairment

Total clearance may be reduced by ~50% in patients with hepatic impairment. However, inter-subject variability limits interpretation of kinetic studies.

IV, Oral, Transdermal: No dose adjustment necessary (standard doses are well tolerated).

SubQ (extended-release injection): There is no dosage adjustment provided in the manufacturer's labeling.

Administration

Oral: Doses should be given up to 1 hour prior to initiation of chemotherapy/radiation

IV: Administer IV push over 30 seconds or as a 5-minute infusion

SubQ (extended-release injection): For subcutaneous administration only. Administer as a single injection at the back of the upper arm or in abdomen (at least one inch away from the umbilicus). Avoid using areas where the skin is burned, hardened, inflamed, swollen, or otherwise compromised. Inject slowly; may take up to 20 to 30 seconds (product is viscous, pressing the syringe plunger will not result in faster expulsion). A topical anesthetic may be applied at injection site prior to administration. Do not administer if particulate matter or discoloration is observed, if the tip cap is missing or has been tampered with, or the luer fitting is missing or dislodged. Remove from refrigerator at least 60 minutes prior to administration; remove from pack and activate 1 syringe warming pouch and wrap syringe with warming pouch for 5 to 6 minutes to allow warming to body temperature. Injection site reactions may occur; if injection site reaction is not yet resolved prior to the next dose, rotate injection site with next administration.

Transdermal (Sancuso): Apply patch to clean, dry, intact skin on upper outer arm. Do not use on red, irritated, or damaged skin. Remove patch from pouch immediately before application. Do not cut patch. Cover patch application site with clothing to protect from natural or artificial sunlight exposure while patch is applied and for 10 days following removal; granisetron may potentially be affected by natural or artificial sunlight. Do not apply heat (eg, heating pad) over or in area of the transdermal patch; avoid prolonged exposure to heat (may increase plasma concentrations).

Extemporaneous Preparations Note: Commercial oral solution is available (0.2 mg/mL)

A 0.2 mg/mL oral suspension may be made with tablets. Crush twelve 1 mg tablets in a mortar and reduce to a fine powder. Add 30 mL distilled water, mix well, and transfer to a bottle. Rinse the mortar with 10 mL cherry syrup and add to bottle. Add sufficient quantity of cherry syrup to make a final volume of 60 mL. Label "shake well". Stable 14 days at room temperature or refrigerated (Quercia 1997).

A 50 mcg/mL oral suspension may be made with tablets and one of three different vehicles (Ora-Sweet®, Ora-Plus®, or a mixture of methylcellulose 1% and Simple Syrup, N.F.). Crush one 1 mg tablet in a mortar and reduce to a fine powder. Add 20 mL of the chosen vehicle and mix to a uniform paste; transfer to a calibrated bottle. Label "shake well" and "refrigerate". Stable for 91 days refrigerated (Nahata 1998).

Nahata MC, Morosco RS, and Hipple TF, "Stability of Granisetron Hydrochloride in Two Oral Suspensions," *Am J Health Syst Pharm,* 1998, 55(23):2511-3.

Quercia RA, Zhang J, Fan C, et al, "Stability of Granisetron Hydrochloride in an Extemporaneously Prepared Oral Liquid," *Am J Health Syst Pharm,* 1997, 54(12):1404-6.

Monitoring Parameters

Monitor for constipation and for decreased bowel activity. Monitor for signs/symptoms of hypersensitivity. Monitor patients for signs of serotonin syndrome.

◀ Extended-release subcutaneous injection: Monitor for injection site reactions for at least 2 weeks after administration.

Product Availability Granisol oral solution has been discontinued in the US for more than 1 year.

Medication Guide Available Yes

Dosage Forms Excipient information presented when available (limited, particularly for generics); consult specific product labeling. [DSC] = Discontinued product

Patch, Transdermal:
Sancuso: 3.1 mg/24 hr (1 ea)
Prefilled Syringe, Subcutaneous:
Sustol: 10 mg/0.4 mL (0.4 mL) [contains polyethylene glycol]
Solution, Intravenous:
Generic: 0.1 mg/mL (1 mL [DSC]); 1 mg/mL (1 mL); 4 mg/4 mL (4 mL)
Solution, Intravenous [preservative free]:
Generic: 0.1 mg/mL (1 mL); 1 mg/mL (1 mL)
Solution, Oral:
Granisol: 2 mg/10 mL (30 mL [DSC]) [contains fd&c yellow #6 (sunset yellow), sodium benzoate; orange flavor]
Tablet, Oral:
Generic: 1 mg

Dosage Forms: Canada Information with regard to form, strength, and availability of products uniquely available in Canada but currently not available in the US. Refer also to Dosage Forms.

Excipient information presented when available (limited, particularly for generics); consult specific product labeling.

◆ **HAL** *see* Hexaminolevulinate *on page 911*

◆ **Halaven** *see* EriBULin *on page 712*

◆ **Haldol** *see* Haloperidol *on page 903*

◆ **Haldol Decanoate** *see* Haloperidol *on page 903*

◆ **Halichondrin B Analog** *see* EriBULin *on page 712*

Haloperidol (ha loe PER i dole)

Brand Names: US Haldol; Haldol Decanoate

Brand Names: Canada Apo-Haloperidol; Haloperidol Injection, USP; Haloperidol-LA; Haloperidol-LA Omega; Novo-Peridol; PMS-Haloperidol; PMS-Haloperidol LA

Index Terms Haloperidol Decanoate; Haloperidol Lactate

Pharmacologic Category First Generation (Typical) Antipsychotic

Use

Behavioral disorders (tablet, concentrate): Treatment of severe behavioral problems in children with combative, explosive hyperexcitability that cannot be accounted for by immediate provocation. Reserve for use in these children only after failure to respond to psychotherapy or medications other than antipsychotics.

Hyperactivity (tablet, concentrate): Short-term treatment of hyperactive children who show excessive motor activity with accompanying conduct disorders consisting of some or all of the following symptoms: impulsivity, difficulty sustaining attention, aggression, mood lability, or poor frustration tolerance. Reserve for use in these children only after failure to respond to psychotherapy or medications other than antipsychotics.

Psychotic disorders (tablet, concentrate): Management of manifestations of psychotic disorders.

Schizophrenia:

IM, lactate: Treatment of schizophrenia.

IM, decanoate: Treatment of patients with schizophrenia who require prolonged parenteral antipsychotic therapy.

Tourette disorder (tablet, concentrate, IM lactate): Control of tics and vocal utterances in Tourette syndrome in adults and children.

Pregnancy Risk Factor C

Dosing

Adult

Psychosis:

Manufacturer's labeling: Oral: 0.5 to 5 mg 2 to 3 times daily; adjust dose based on response and tolerability. According to the manufacturer, daily dosages up to 100 mg may be necessary in some cases to achieve an optimal response; infrequently, doses >100 mg have been used in severely treatment resistant patients. Recommended dose range for schizophrenia: 5 to 20 mg/day (APA [Lehman 2004)].

Schizophrenia:

IM (as lactate): 2 to 5 mg; subsequent doses may be administered as often as every 60 minutes, although 4- to 8-hour intervals may be satisfactory.

IM (as decanoate): **Note:** Establish tolerance to oral haloperidol prior to changing to IM decanoate injection.

Initial: 10 to 20 times the daily oral dose. The initial dose should not exceed 100 mg regardless of previous antipsychotic requirements. If the initial dose conversion requires >100 mg, administer the dose in 2 injections (maximum of 100 mg for first injection) separated by 3 to 7 days.

Oral haloperidol ≤10 mg/day, elderly, or debilitated: Initiate dose at 10 to 15 times the daily oral dose

Oral haloperidol >10 mg/day or high risk of relapse: Initiate dose at 20 times the daily oral dose

Maintenance dose: 10 to 15 times the previous daily oral dose or 50 to 200 mg administer doses at 4-week intervals (Buchanan 2009; Hasan 2013).

Oral overlap: Following initial dose, taper the oral dose and discontinue following the subsequent 2 or 3 injections (ie, 60 to 90 days) (McEvoy 2006). Alter rate of taper based on clinical response and presence of adverse events.

Alternative dosing regimen:

Loading dose regimen: Initial: 20 times the previous daily oral dose, divide total dose and give every 3 to 7 days, do not exceed 250 mg per injection; discontinue oral haloperidol prior to first injection. Reduce the dose by 25% each month, depending on clinical response, in months 2 to 4, and establish the maintenance dose.

Usual maintenance dose: 200 mg per month (Ereshefsky 1993)

Tourette syndrome: Oral: 0.5 to 5 mg 2 to 3 times daily; adjust dose based on response and tolerability. Tourette Canada Guidelines recommend a dosing range of 0.5 to 3 mg/day (Pringsheim 2012) and European Society for the Study of Tourette Syndrome recommend a dosing range of 0.25 to 15 mg/day (Roessner 2011). According to the manufacturer, daily dosages up to 100 mg may be necessary in some cases to achieve an optimal response; infrequently doses >100 mg have been used in severely treatment resistant patients.

Chemotherapy-induced nausea and vomiting (off-label use): Breakthrough nausea/vomiting: Oral, IV (off-label route): 0.5 to 1 mg every 6 hours as needed (Lohr 2008)

Chorea of Huntington disease (off-label use): Oral: Initial: 0.5 to 2 mg/day; adjust dose based on response and tolerability up to a maximum dose of 10 mg/day (Reilmann 2013). Additional data may be necessary to further define the role of haloperidol in this condition.

Delirium in the intensive care unit, treatment (off-label use): Note: The optimal dose and regimen of haloperidol for the treatment of severe agitation and/or delirium has not been established. Currently, there are no studies evaluating the role of haloperidol on duration or severity of delirium. Haloperidol has been used for symptomatic treatment (severe agitation) of delirious patients. Current guidelines do not advocate use of haloperidol for the treatment or prevention of delirium due to insufficient evidence (Barr 2013).

IV (off-label route): Initial: 0.5 to 10 mg depending on degree of agitation; if inadequate response, may repeat bolus dose (with sequential doubling of initial bolus dose) every 15 to 30 minutes until calm achieved, then administer 25% of the last bolus dose every 6 hours; monitor ECG and QTc interval. After the patient is controlled, haloperidol therapy should be tapered over several days. This strategy is based upon expert opinion; efficacy and safety have not been formally evaluated (Tesar 1988).

Note: Continuous infusions have also been used with doses in the range of 0.5 to 2 mg/hour with an optional loading dose of 2.5 mg (Reade 2009).

Delirium in the intensive care unit (patients at high risk of delirium), prevention (off-label use): Note: The optimal dose and regimen of haloperidol for prevention of ICU delirium has not been established. Current guidelines do not advocate use of haloperidol for the treatment or prevention of delirium due to insufficient evidence (Barr 2013). Haloperidol may decrease the incidence of delirium (Van den Boogaard 2013; Wang 2012).

IV (off-label route): 0.5 mg followed by a continuous infusion of 0.1 mg/hour for 12 hours (Wang 2012) **or** 0.5 to 1 mg every 8 hours (Van den Boogaard 2013)

Nausea and vomiting in advanced or terminal illness (palliative care; off-label use): Oral, SubQ (off-label route): Initial: 1.5 to 3 mg/day; titrate daily based on response and tolerability up to a maximum of 6 mg per 24 hours (Hardy 2010, Mercadante 1995). Additional data may be necessary to further define the role of haloperidol in this condition.

Nausea and vomiting in advanced cancer (Glare 2008):

Oral: 1.5 to 2.5 mg once or twice daily

SubQ: 1 to 2 mg 2 to 3 times a day **or** as a continuous subcutaneous infusion at 1 to 5 mg per 24 hours

Obsessive-compulsive disorder (off-label use): Oral: Initial: 2 mg/day; adjust dose based on response and tolerability by 2 mg every 3 days up to a maximum dose of 10 mg/day. Average dose in clinical trial was 6 mg/day (McDougle 1994). Additional data may be necessary to further define the role of haloperidol in this condition.

Postoperative nausea and vomiting (PONV), prevention (off-label use): IM, IV (off-label route): 0.5 to 2 mg (Gan 2014)

Rapid tranquilization (agitation/aggression/violent behavior) (off-label use): IM (as lactate): 2.5 to 10 mg (Clinton 1987; MacDonald 2012; Powney 2012; Wilson 2012)

Discontinuation of therapy: The manufacturer and the American Psychiatric Association (APA), Canadian Psychiatric Association (CPA), and World Federation of Societies of Biological Psychiatry (WFSBP) guidelines recommend gradually tapering antipsychotics to avoid withdrawal symptoms and minimize the risk of relapse (APA [Lehman 2004], Cerovecki 2013; CPA [Addington 2005]; WFSBP [Hasan 2012]); risk for withdrawal symptoms may be highest with highly anti-cholinergic or dopaminergic antipsychotics (Cerovecki 2013). When stopping antipsychotic therapy in patients with schizophrenia, the CPA guidelines recommend a gradual taper over 6 to 24 months, and the APA guidelines recommend reducing the dose by 10% each month (APA [Lehman 2004]; CPA [Addington 2005]). Continuing anti-parkinsonism agents for a brief period after discontinuation may prevent withdrawal symptoms (Cerovecki 2013). When switching antipsychotics, 3 strategies have been suggested: cross-titration (gradually discontinuing the first antipsychotic while gradually increasing the new antipsychotic), overlap and taper (maintaining the dose of the first antipsychotic while gradually increasing the new antipsychotic, then tapering the first antipsychotic), and abrupt change (abruptly discontinuing the first antipsychotic and either increasing the new antipsychotic gradually or starting it at a treatment dose). Evidence supporting ideal switch strategies and taper rates is limited, and results are conflicting (Cerovecki 2013; Remington 2005).

◀ **Geriatric**

Psychosis: Oral: 0.5 to 2 mg 2 to 3 times daily; adjust dose based on response and tolerability. Maximum dosage per manufacturer's labeling: 100 mg/day. Recommended dose range for schizophrenia: 5 to 20 mg/day (APA [Lehman 2004]).

Psychosis/agitation associated with dementia (off-label use): Oral: Initial: 0.25 to 2 mg daily; slowly increase dose based on response and tolerability every 4 to 7 days in increments of 0.25 to 1 mg (De Deyn 1999; Devanand 1998); doses up to 6 mg/day in 1 to 2 divided doses were evaluated in clinical trials (Lonergan 2002). APA guidelines recommend against the first-line use of haloperidol for non-emergent situations (ie, longer-term treatment). If used, in patients without a clinically significant response after 4 weeks, taper and withdraw therapy. In patients with an adequate response, attempt to taper and withdraw therapy within 4 months, unless symptoms recurred with a previous taper attempt. Assess symptoms at least monthly during taper and for at least 4 months after withdrawal of therapy (APA [Reus 2016]).

Pediatric

Behavior disorders, nonpsychotic:

Children 3 to 12 years weighing 15 to 40 kg: Oral: Initial: 0.5 mg/day in 2 to 3 divided doses; may increase by 0.5 mg every 5 to 7 days to usual maintenance range of 0.05 to 0.075 mg/kg/day in 2 to 3 divided doses; maximum dose not established; children with severe, nonpsychotic disturbance may require higher doses; however, no improvement has been shown with doses >6 mg/day.

Children >40 kg and Adolescents (off-label dose): Oral: 0.5 to 15 mg/day in 2 to 3 divided doses; begin at lower end of the range and may increase as needed (no more frequently than every 5 to 7 days); maximum daily dose: 15 mg/day. **Note:** Higher doses may be necessary in severe or refractory cases (Kliegman 2011).

Psychosis:

Children 3 to 12 years weighing 15 to 40 kg: Oral: Initial: 0.5 mg/day in 2 to 3 divided doses; increase by 0.5 mg every 5 to 7 days to usual maintenance range of 0.05 to 0.15 mg/kg/day in 2 to 3 divided doses; higher doses may be necessary in severe or refractory cases; maximum dose not established; in adolescents, the maximum daily dose is 15 mg/day (Kliegman 2011)

Children >40 kg and Adolescents (off-label dose): Oral: 0.5 to 15 mg/day in 2 to 3 divided doses; begin at lower end of the range and may increase as needed (no more frequently than every 5 to 7 days); maximum daily dose: 15 mg/day (Kliegman 2011; Willner 1969). **Note:** Higher doses may be necessary in severe or refractory cases (Kliegman 2011).

Tourette syndrome:

Children 3 to 12 years weighing 15 to 40 kg: Oral:

Manufacturer's labeling: Initial: 0.5 mg/day in 2 to 3 divided doses; increase by 0.5 mg every 5 to 7 days to usual maintenance of 0.05 to 0.075 mg/kg/day in 2 to 3 divided doses; maximum dose not established; however, no improvement has been shown with doses >6 mg/day in patients with nonpsychotic disturbances

Alternate dosing: Initial: 0.25 to 0.5 mg/day in 2 to 3 divided doses titrated to a usual daily dose range of 1 to 4 mg/day (Roessner 2011; Scahill 2006)

Children >40 kg and Adolescents (off-label dose): Oral: 0.25 to 15 mg/day in 2 to 3 divided doses; begin at lower end of the range and may increase as needed (no more frequently than every 5 to 7 days) (Kleigman 2011; Roessner 2011); usual dose range: 1 to 4 mg/day (Roessner 2011; Scahill 2006); maximum dose not established; however, no improvement has been shown with doses >6 mg/day in patients with nonpsychotic disturbances

Renal Impairment There are no dosage adjustments provided in the manufacturer's labeling.

Hepatic Impairment There are no dosage adjustments provided in the manufacturer's labeling.

Additional Information Complete prescribing information should be consulted for additional detail.

Dosage Forms Excipient information presented when available (limited, particularly for generics); consult specific product labeling.

Concentrate, Oral, as lactate [strength expressed as base]:
Generic: 2 mg/mL (5 mL, 15 mL, 120 mL)

Solution, Intramuscular, as decanoate [strength expressed as base]:
Haldol Decanoate: 50 mg/mL (1 mL); 100 mg/mL (1 mL) [contains benzyl alcohol, sesame oil]
Generic: 50 mg/mL (1 mL, 5 mL); 100 mg/mL (1 mL, 5 mL)

Solution, Injection, as lactate [strength expressed as base]:
Haldol: 5 mg/mL (1 mL)
Generic: 5 mg/mL (1 mL, 10 mL)

Solution, Injection, as lactate [strength expressed as base, preservative free]:
Generic: 5 mg/mL (1 mL)

Tablet, Oral:
Generic: 0.5 mg, 1 mg, 2 mg, 5 mg, 10 mg, 20 mg

Heparin (HEP a rin)

Brand Names: US Hep Flush-10 [DSC]

Brand Names: Canada Heparin Leo; Heparin Lock Flush; Heparin Sodium Injection, USP

Index Terms Heparin Calcium; Heparin Lock Flush; Heparin Sod/Sod Chloride; Heparin Sodium; Heparinized Saline

Pharmacologic Category Anticoagulant; Anticoagulant, Heparin

Use

Anticoagulation: Prophylaxis and treatment of thromboembolic disorders (eg, venous thromboembolism, pulmonary embolism) and thromboembolic complications associated with atrial fibrillation; prevention of clotting in ▶

arterial and cardiac surgery; as an anticoagulant for extracorporeal circulation and dialysis procedures

Note: Heparin lock flush solution is intended only to maintain patency of IV devices and is **not** to be used for systemic anticoagulant therapy.

Pregnancy Risk Factor C

Dosing

Adult Note: Many concentrations of heparin are available ranging from 1 unit/mL to 20,000 units/mL. Carefully examine each prefilled syringe or vial prior to use ensuring that the correct concentration is chosen. Heparin lock flush solution is intended only to maintain patency of IV devices and is not to be used for anticoagulant therapy.

Acute coronary syndromes (off-label use): IV infusion (weight-based dosing per institutional nomogram recommended):

STEMI: Adjunct to fibrinolysis (full-dose alteplase, reteplase, or tenecteplase): Initial bolus of 60 units/kg (maximum: 4,000 units), then 12 units/kg/hour (maximum: 1,000 units/hour) as continuous infusion. Adjust to target aPTT of 1.5 to 2 times control (approximately 50 to 70 seconds). Continue for a minimum of 48 hours, and preferably for the duration of hospitalization (up to 8 days) or until revascularization (if performed) (ACCF/AHA [O'Gara 2013]).

NSTE-ACS: Initial bolus of 60 units/kg (maximum: 4,000 units), followed by an initial infusion of 12 units/kg/hour (maximum: 1,000 units/hour). Adjust to target aPTT of 1.5 to 2 times control (approximately 50 to 70 seconds). Recommended duration is 48 hours or until percutaneous coronary intervention (PCI) is performed.

Note: If PCI is performed while patient on fondaparinux, 85 units/kg of heparin (60 units/kg if a GP IIb/IIIa inhibitor [eg, abciximab, eptifibatide, tirofiban] is used concomitantly) should be given immediately before PCI with subsequent heparin dosing based on the target activated clotting time (AHA/ACC [Amsterdam 2014]).

Anticoagulation (Intermittent administration): IV: Initial: 10,000 units, then 50 to 70 units/kg (5,000 to 10,000 units) every 4 to 6 hours

Atrial fibrillation (off-label use): Guidelines pertaining to peri-cardioversion use (ACCP [You 2012]):

Patients with atrial fibrillation (for more than 48 hours or unknown duration) undergoing cardioversion: IV heparin to maintain an aPTT prolongation that corresponds to plasma heparin levels of 0.3 to 0.7 units/mL anti-Xa activity started at the time of transesophageal echocardiography (TEE) is recommended with cardioversion performed within 24 hours of the TEE if no thrombus is seen.

Patients with atrial fibrillation (for 48 hours or less) undergoing cardioversion: Cardioversion may be performed without prolonged anticoagulation. However, anticoagulation with IV heparin to maintain an aPTT prolongation that corresponds to plasma heparin levels of 0.3 to 0.7 units/mL anti-Xa activity should be started at presentation in patients with no contraindications to anticoagulation.

Emergency cardioversion in hemodynamically unstable patient: Cardioversion may be performed without prolonged anticoagulation. Anticoagulation with IV heparin to maintain an aPTT prolongation that corresponds to plasma heparin levels of 0.3 to 0.7 units/mL anti-Xa activity should be started prior to cardioversion in patients with no contraindications to anticoagulation.

Cardiothoracic surgery (cardiopulmonary bypass): IV: Initial: 300 to 400 units/kg prior to arterial or venous cannulation; titrate to ACT. Cardiopulmonary bypass may be initiated once ACT is at least 400 seconds; measure ACT every 30 minutes and administer additional heparin as necessary (Kincaid 2014).

Interstitial cystitis (bladder pain syndrome) (off-label use): Intravesical: **Note:** Various dosage regimens of heparin (20,000 to 50,000 units) alone or with alkalinized lidocaine (1% to 4%) have been used. When lidocaine and heparin are mixed, there is a risk of precipitation if proper alkalinization does not occur. Lidocaine stability and pH should be determined after the components have been mixed, prior to administration.

Single-dose regimen: Instill the combination of 50,000 units of heparin, lidocaine 200 mg, and sodium bicarbonate 420 mg in 15 mL of sterile water into the bladder via catheter and allow to dwell for 30 minutes before draining (Parsons 2012).

Once-weekly dosing regimen: Instill the combination of 20,000 units of heparin, lidocaine 4% (5 mL), and sodium bicarbonate 7% (25 mL) into an empty bladder via catheter once weekly for 12 weeks and allow to dwell for 30 minutes before draining (Nomiya 2013).

Twice-weekly dosing regimen: Instill 25,000 units of heparin (diluted with 5 mL of sterile water) into bladder via catheter twice weekly for 3 months (Kuo 2001).

Maintenance of catheter patency (continuous infusion): Using heparin 2 unit/mL large volume IV solutions, may administer at an infusion rate of 3 mL/hour (equivalent to 6 units/hour); however, rate of infusion dependent upon age, weight, clinical condition of patient, and procedure being employed. Do not use as a "catheter lock flush".

Maintenance of line patency (line flushing): When using daily flushes of heparin to maintain patency of single and double lumen central catheters, 10 units/mL is commonly used for younger infants (eg, <10 kg) while 100 units/mL is used for older infants, children, and adults. Capped PVC catheters and peripheral heparin locks require flushing more frequently (eg, every 6 to 8 hours). Volume of heparin flush is usually similar to volume of catheter (or slightly greater). Additional flushes should be given when stagnant blood is observed in catheter, after catheter is used for drug or blood administration, and after blood withdrawal from catheter.

Parenteral nutrition: Addition of heparin (0.5 to 3 unit/mL) to peripheral and central parenteral nutrition has not been shown to decrease catheter-related thrombosis. The final concentration of heparin used for TPN solutions may need to be decreased to 0.5 units/mL in small infants receiving larger amounts of volume in order to avoid approaching therapeutic amounts. Arterial lines are heparinized with a final concentration of 1 unit/mL.

Percutaneous coronary intervention (off-label use; Levine 2011): IV:

No prior anticoagulant therapy:

If no GPIIb/IIIa inhibitor use planned: Initial bolus of 70 to 100 units/kg (target ACT 250 to 300 seconds for HemoTec®, 300 to 350 seconds for Hemochron®)

or

If planning GPIIb/IIIa inhibitor use: Initial bolus of 50 to 70 units/kg (target ACT 200 to 250 seconds regardless of device)

Prior anticoagulant therapy:

If no GPIIb/IIIa inhibitor use planned: Additional heparin as needed (eg, 2,000 to 5,000 units) (target ACT 250 to 300 seconds for HemoTec®, 300 to 350 seconds for Hemochron®)

or

If planning GPIIb/IIIa inhibitor use: Additional heparin as needed (eg, 2,000 to 5,000 units) (target ACT 200 to 250 seconds regardless of device)

Thromboprophylaxis (low-dose heparin): SubQ: 5,000 units every 8 to 12 hours. **Note:** The American College of Chest Physicians recommends a minimum of 10 to 14 days for patients undergoing total hip arthroplasty, total knee arthroplasty, or hip fracture surgery (Guyatt 2012).

Venous thromboembolism (treatment): Note: Start warfarin on the first or second treatment day and continue heparin until INR is ≥2 for at least 24 hours (usually 5 to 7 days) (Guyatt, 2012).

DVT/PE (off-label dosing): IV: 80 units/kg (or alternatively 5,000 units) IV push followed by an initial continuous infusion of 18 units/kg/hour (or alternatively 1,000 units/hour) (Guyatt 2012)

or

DVT/PE (off-label dosing): SubQ: *Unmonitored dosing regimen:* Initial: 333 units/kg then 250 units/kg every 12 hours (Guyatt 2012; Kearon 2006)

Geriatric Patients >60 years of age may have higher serum levels and clinical response (longer aPTTs) as compared to younger patients receiving similar dosages. Lower dosages may be required.

Pediatric Note: Many concentrations of heparin are available ranging from 1 unit/mL to 20,000 units/mL. Carefully examine each prefilled syringe or vial prior to use ensuring that the correct concentration is chosen. Heparin lock flush solution is intended only to maintain patency of IV devices and is not to be used for anticoagulant therapy.

Thrombosis, treatment: *Systemic heparinization:*

Infants: IV: Initial loading dose: 75 units/kg over 10 minutes; then initial continuous maintenance infusion at: 28 units/kg/hour; adjust dose to maintain an anti-Xa activity of 0.35 to 0.7 units/mL or an aPTT range that correlates to this anti-Xa range or a protamine titration range of 0.2 to 0.4 units/mL (ACCP [Monagle 2012])

Children and Adolescents: IV: Initial loading dose: 75 units/kg over 10 minutes, then initial continuous maintenance infusion at: 20 units/kg/hour; adjust dose to maintain an anti-Xa activity of 0.35 to 0.7 units/mL or an aPTT range that correlates to this anti-Xa range or a protamine titration range of 0.2 to 0.4 units/mL (ACCP [Monagle 2012])

Note: Because of variation among hospitals with reagents (lot numbers) and corresponding control of aPTT values, individual institutions should establish unique, institution-specific nomograms. Due to extensive variability within reagents and anti-Xa levels with corresponding aPTTs, a specific nomogram has not been provided; refer to guidelines for a specific nomogram (ACCP [Monagle 2012]).

Renal Impairment

No dosage adjustment required; adjust therapeutic heparin according to aPTT or anti-Xa activity.

Hemodialysis: Not dialyzable (NCS/SCCM [Frontera 2016])

Hepatic Impairment No dosage adjustment required; adjust therapeutic heparin according to aPTT or anti-Xa activity.

Additional Information Complete prescribing information should be consulted for additional detail.

Dosage Forms Excipient information presented when available (limited, particularly for generics); consult specific product labeling. [DSC] = Discontinued product

Solution, Injection, as sodium:
  Generic: 1000 units (500 mL); 2000 units (1000 mL); 12,500 units (250 mL); 25,000 units (250 mL, 500 mL); 1000 units/mL (1 mL, 10 mL, 30 mL); 2500 units/mL (10 mL [DSC]); 5000 units/mL (1 mL, 10 mL); 10,000 units/mL (1 mL, 4 mL, 5 mL); 20,000 units/mL (1 mL)

Solution, Injection, as sodium [preservative free]:
  Generic: 1000 units/mL (2 mL); 5000 units/0.5 mL (0.5 mL)

Solution, Intravenous, as sodium:
  Hep Flush-10: 10 units/mL (10 mL [DSC])
  Generic: 10,000 units (250 mL); 12,500 units (250 mL); 20,000 units (500 mL); 25,000 units (250 mL, 500 mL); 1 units/mL (1 mL, 2 mL, 2.5 mL, 3 mL, 5 mL, 10 mL); 2 units/mL (3 mL [DSC]); 10 units/mL (1 mL, 2 mL, 2.5 mL, 3 mL, 5 mL, 10 mL, 30 mL [DSC]); 100 units/mL (1 mL, 2 mL, 2.5 mL, 3 mL, 5 mL, 10 mL, 30 mL [DSC], 100 mL [DSC], 250 mL); 2000 units/mL (5 mL [DSC]); 1000 units/L in NaCl 0.9% (1000 mL); 15,000 units/500 mL in NaCl 0.9% (500 mL); 2000 units/500 mL in NaCl 0.9% (500 mL); 250 units/250 mL in NaCl 0.45% (250 mL)

Solution, Intravenous, as sodium [preservative free]:
  Generic: 1 units/mL (3 mL [DSC]); 10 units/mL (1 mL, 3 mL, 5 mL); 100 units/mL (1 mL, 3 mL, 5 mL)

Hexaminolevulinate (hex a mee noe LEV ue lin ate)

Brand Names: US Cysview

Index Terms HAL; Hexaminolevulinate HCl; Hexaminolevulinate Hydrochloride

Pharmacologic Category Contrast Agent

Use

Detection of bladder cancer: Imaging agent for cystoscopic detection of non-muscle-invasive papillary cancer of the bladder in patients with suspected or known lesion(s) based on a prior cystoscopy. Hexaminolevulinate is used with the Karl Storz D-Light C Photodynamic Diagnostic (PDD) system to perform cystoscopy with the blue light setting (mode 2) as an adjunct to the white light setting (mode 1).

◀ Limitations of use: Not a replacement for random bladder biopsies or other procedures used to detect bladder cancer. Not for repeat use (risks associated with repeat exposures have not been evaluated).

Pregnancy Risk Factor C

Dosing

Adult Detection of bladder cancer: Intravesical instillation: 100 mg (50 mL) instilled into empty bladder via urinary catheter

Renal Impairment There are no dosage adjustments provided in the manufacturer's labeling.

Hepatic Impairment There are no dosage adjustments provided in the manufacturer's labeling.

Additional Information Complete prescribing information should be consulted for additional detail.

Dosage Forms Excipient information presented when available (limited, particularly for generics); consult specific product labeling.

Solution Reconstituted, Intravesical, as hydrochloride:

Cysview: 100 mg (1 ea)

♦ **Hexaminolevulinate HCl** see Hexaminolevulinate on page 911

♦ **Hexaminolevulinate Hydrochloride** see Hexaminolevulinate on page 911

♦ **HHT** see Omacetaxine on page 1375

♦ **High-Molecular-Weight Iron Dextran (DexFerrum)** see Iron Dextran Complex on page 1053

Histrelin (his TREL in)

Related Information

Safe Handling of Hazardous Drugs on page 2379

Brand Names: US Supprelin LA; Vantas

Brand Names: Canada Vantas

Index Terms GnRH Agonist; Histrelin Acetate; LH-RH Agonist

Pharmacologic Category Antineoplastic Agent, Gonadotropin-Releasing Hormone Agonist; Gonadotropin Releasing Hormone Agonist

Use

Central precocious puberty (Supprelin LA): Treatment of children with central precocious puberty

Prostate cancer, advanced (Vantas): Palliative treatment of advanced prostate cancer

Labeled Contraindications Hypersensitivity to histrelin acetate, gonadotropin-releasing hormone (GnRH), GnRH-agonist analogs, or any component of the formulation; females who are or may become pregnant

Pregnancy Considerations Histrelin is contraindicated for use during pregnancy or in women who may become pregnant. Adverse events were observed in animal reproduction studies. May cause fetal harm or spontaneous abortion if administered during pregnancy.

Breastfeeding Considerations It is not known if histrelin is present in breast milk. The products are not indicated for use in postpubertal women.

Warnings/Precautions Proper surgical insertion technique is essential to avoid complications. Patients should keep arm dry for 24 hours and avoid heavy lifting/strenuous exertion of insertion arm for 7 days after implantation. Potentially significant drug-drug interactions may exist, requiring dose or frequency adjustment, additional monitoring, and/or selection of alternative therapy.

CPP: Transient increases in estradiol serum levels (female) or testosterone levels (female and male) may occur during the first week of use. Worsening symptoms may occur, however, manifestations of puberty should decrease within 4 weeks. If the implant breaks during removal, the remaining pieces should be removed; confirm the removal of the entire implant (refer to manufacturer's instructions for removal procedure). Psychiatric events have been described with GnRH agonists, including histrelin; symptoms of emotional lability, irritability, impatience, anger, and aggression have been reported in postmarketing accounts. Monitor for development or worsening of psychiatric symptoms. Seizures have been reported in patients receiving GnRH agonists, including histrelin. Reports have occurred in patients with a history of seizures, epilepsy, cerebrovascular disorders, CNS anomalies, or tumors, and patients on concomitant medications associated with seizures (eg, bupropion, SSRIs). Seizures have also been reported in patients without underlying conditions.

Prostate cancer: Transient increases in testosterone serum levels occur during the first week of use (initial tumor flare), which may result in a worsening of disease signs and symptoms such as bone pain, hematuria, neuropathy, ureteral or bladder outlet obstruction, and spinal cord compression. Spinal cord compression may contribute to paralysis; close attention should be given during the first few weeks of therapy to both patients having metastatic vertebral lesions and/or urinary tract obstructions, and to any patients reporting weakness, paresthesias, or poor urine output. Androgen-deprivation therapy (ADT) may increase the risk for cardiovascular disease (Levine 2010); an increased risk of MI, sudden cardiac death, and stroke has been reported with GnRH agonist use in men; monitor for symptoms associated with cardiovascular disease. ADT may prolong the QT/QTc interval; consider the benefits of ADT versus the risk for QT prolongation in patients with a history of QTc prolongation, congenital long QT syndrome, heart failure, frequent electrolyte abnormalities, and in patients with medications known to prolong the QT interval, or with preexisting cardiac disease. Consider periodic monitoring of electrocardiograms and electrolytes in at-risk patients. Hyperglycemia has been reported with androgen deprivation therapy (in prostate cancer) and may manifest as diabetes or worsening of preexisting diabetes; monitor blood glucose and/or HbA$_{1c}$. Rare cases of pituitary apoplexy (frequently secondary to pituitary adenoma) have been observed with GnRH agonist administration (onset from 1 hour to usually <2 weeks); may present as sudden headache, vomiting, visual or mental status changes, and infrequently, cardiovascular collapse; immediate medical attention required. In studies, the implant was not recovered in a small number of patients. Serum testosterone rose above castrate level and the implant was not palpable or visualized (via ultrasound); it was believed to have been extruded. Some patients had continued testosterone levels below castration level even though the implant was not palpable.

Adverse Reactions

CPP:

>10%: Dermatologic: Dermatological reaction (51%; insertion site reaction includes bruise, discomfort, pain, protrusion of implant area, pruritus, soreness, swelling, tingling)

>2% to 10%:

Dermatologic: Scarring (6%)

Genitourinary: Uterine hemorrhage (4%)

Local: Application site pain (4%)

Neuromuscular & skeletal: Keloid-like scar (6%)

Miscellaneous: Procedural complications (6%; suture-related), postoperative pain (4%)

≤2%, postmarketing, and/or case reports: Amblyopia, breast tenderness, dysmenorrhea, emotional lability, epistaxis, erythema, flu-like symptoms, gynecomastia, headache, hypermenorrhea, localized infection (implant site), migraine, pituitary apoplexy, pituitary neoplasm, precocious puberty (progression of central precocious puberty), pruritus, seizure, sensation of cold, weight gain

Prostate cancer:

>10%:

Dermatologic: Dermatological reaction (66%; implant site reaction includes bruise, erythema, pain, soreness, swelling, tenderness)

Endocrine & metabolic: Hot flash (66%)

2% to 10%:

Central nervous system: Fatigue (10%), headache (3%), insomnia (3%)

Endocrine & metabolic: Gynecomastia (4%), decreased libido (2%), weight gain (2%)

Gastrointestinal: Constipation (4%)

Genitourinary: Testicular atrophy (5%; expected pharmacological consequence of testosterone suppression), sexual disorder (4%)

Renal: Renal insufficiency (5%)

<2%, postmarketing, and/or case reports: Abdominal distress, alopecia, anemia, arthralgia, back pain, breast tenderness, bruise, decreased bone mineral density, depression, diaphoresis, dizziness, dyspnea on exertion, dysuria, fluid retention, flushing, food craving, genital pruritus, hematoma, hematuria, hepatic disease, hepatic injury (severe), hypercalcemia, hypercholesterolemia, hyperglycemia, increased appetite, increased lactate dehydrogenase, increased prostatic acid phosphatase, increased serum AST, increased serum creatinine, increased testosterone level, irritability, lethargy, limb pain, malaise, mastalgia, muscle twitching, myalgia, nausea, neck pain, nephrolithiasis, night sweats, ostealgia, pain, palpitations, peripheral edema, pruritus, pituitary apoplexy, renal failure, sensation of cold, stent occlusion, tremor, urinary frequency, urinary retention, ventricular premature contractions, weakness, weight loss

Drug Interactions

Metabolism/Transport Effects None known.

Avoid Concomitant Use

Avoid concomitant use of Histrelin with any of the following: Corifollitropin Alfa; Indium 111 Capromab Pendetide

Increased Effect/Toxicity

Histrelin may increase the levels/effects of: Corifollitropin Alfa; Highest Risk QTc-Prolonging Agents; Moderate Risk QTc-Prolonging Agents

The levels/effects of Histrelin may be increased by: MiFEPRIStone

Decreased Effect

Histrelin may decrease the levels/effects of: Antidiabetic Agents; Choline C 11; Indium 111 Capromab Pendetide

Hazardous Drugs Handling Considerations

Hazardous agent (NIOSH 2016 [group 1]).

Use appropriate precautions for receiving, handling, administration, and disposal. Gloves (single) should be worn during receiving, unpacking, and placing in storage.

NIOSH recommends double gloving, a protective gown, ventilated engineering controls (a class II biological safety cabinet or a compounding aseptic containment isolator), and (when dosage form allows) closed system transfer devices (CSTDs) for compounding. Double gloving and a protective gown are recommended during administration (NIOSH 2016).

Storage/Stability Upon delivery, separate contents of implant carton. Store implant (small carton containing amber plastic pouch and glass vial) under refrigeration at 2°C to 8°C (36°F to 46°F) until the day of insertion; excursions permitted to 25°C (77°F) for 7 days (if unused within 7 days, may return to proper refrigeration until product expiration date). Keep implant wrapped in the amber pouch for protection from light; do not freeze. Do not open implant vial until just before the time of insertion. The implantation insertion kit should be stored at room temperature (do not refrigerate insertion kit).

Preparation for Administration The implant may be slightly curved and/or partially flattened when removed from refrigerator; may roll implant (in sterile-gloved hands) a few times between fingers and thumb. If resistance is felt when inserting implant into insertion tool cannula, remove and manually manipulate or roll as needed and reinsert into cannula.

Mechanism of Action Potent inhibitor of gonadotropin secretion; continuous administration results in, after an initiation phase, the suppression of luteinizing hormone (LH), follicle-stimulating hormone (FSH), and a subsequent decrease in testosterone and dihydrotestosterone (males) and estrone and estradiol (premonopausal females). Testosterone levels are reduced to castrate levels in males (treated for prostate cancer) within 2 to 4 weeks. Additionally, in patients with CPP, linear growth velocity is slowed (improves chance of attaining predicted adult height).

Pharmacodynamics/Kinetics

Onset of action: Prostate cancer: Chemical castration: Within 2 to 4 weeks; CPP: Progression of sexual development stops and growth is decreased within 1 month

Duration: 12 months (plus a few additional weeks of histrelin release)

Distribution: Adults: V_d: ~58.4 L ± 7.86 L

Protein binding: Adults: ~70% ± 9%

Metabolism: Hepatic via C-terminal dealkylation and hydrolysis

Bioavailability: Adults: SubQ: 92%

Half-life elimination: Adults: Terminal: ~4 hours

Time to peak, serum: Adults: 12 hours

Dosing

Adult & Geriatric Prostate cancer, advanced (Vantas): SubQ: 50 mg implant surgically inserted every 12 months

Pediatric Central precocious puberty (Supprelin LA): Children ≥2 years: SubQ: 50 mg implant surgically inserted every 12 months. Discontinue at the appropriate time for the onset of puberty.

Renal Impairment

Vantas: CrCl ≥15 mL/minute: No dosage adjustment necessary.

Supprelin LA: There are no dosage adjustments provided in the manufacturer's labeling.

Hepatic Impairment There are no dosage adjustments provided in the manufacturer's labeling (has not been studied).

Administration SubQ: Surgical implantation (using a sterile field) into the inner portion of the upper arm requires the use of the implantation device provided. Do not bend or pinch the implant. Use the patient's nondominant arm for placement; implant should be placed halfway between the shoulder and the elbow at the crease between the tricep and the bicep. Implant removal should occur after ~12 months; a replacement implant may be inserted if therapy is to be continued. Palpate area of incision to locate implant for removal. If not readily palpated, ultrasound, CT, or MRI may be used to locate implant; plain films are not recommended because the implant is not radio-paque. Refer to manufacturer's labeling for full insertion and removal details.

Monitoring Parameters

Central precocious puberty (CPP): Luteinizing hormone, follicle-stimulating hormone, estradiol, or testosterone (after 1 month then every 6 months); height, bone age (every 6 to 12 months); Tanner staging; monitor for clinical evidence of suppression of CPP manifestations; monitor for development or worsening of psychiatric symptoms, including depression.

Prostate cancer: Serum testosterone levels, prostate specific antigen (PSA); bone mineral density; weakness, paresthesias, and urinary tract obstruction (especially during first few weeks of therapy); screen for diabetes; monitor for symptoms associated with cardiovascular disease. Consider periodic mon-itoring of electrocardiograms and electrolytes.

Test Interactions Results of diagnostic test of pituitary gonadotropic and gonadal functions may be affected during and after therapy

Medication Guide Available Yes

Dosage Forms Excipient information presented when available (limited, particularly for generics); consult specific product labeling.

Kit, Subcutaneous:
Supprelin LA: 50 mg
Vantas: 50 mg

Hyaluronidase (hye al yoor ON i dase)

Related Information

Management of Drug Extravasations *on page 2271*

Brand Names: US Amphadase; Hylenex; Vitrase

Index Terms Wydase

Pharmacologic Category Antidote, Extravasation; Enzyme

Use

Absorption and dispersion of injected drugs: As an adjuvant to increase the absorption and dispersion of other injected drugs.

Subcutaneous fluid administration: As an adjuvant in subcutaneous fluid administration (hypodermoclysis) for achieving hydration.

Subcutaneous urography: As an adjunct in subcutaneous urography for improving resorption of radiopaque agents.

Labeled Contraindications Hypersensitivity to hyaluronidase or any component of the formulation

Pregnancy Considerations Adverse events have not been observed in animal reproduction studies (not conducted with all products). Administration during labor did not cause any increase in blood loss or differences in cervical trauma. It is not known whether it affects the fetus if used during labor. Hyaluronidase has been evaluated for use prior to intracytoplasmic sperm injection (ICSI) to increase male fertility (DeVos, 2008; Evison, 2009).

Breastfeeding Considerations It is not known if hyaluronidase is excreted in breast milk. The manufacturer recommends that caution be exercised when administering hyaluronidase to nursing women.

Warnings/Precautions For labeled indications, do not administer intravenously (enzyme is rapidly inactivated and desired effects will not be produced); do not inject in or around infected or inflamed areas; may spread localized infection. Do not apply directly to the cornea; not for topical use. Hyaluronidase is ineffective for extravasation management of vasoconstrictors (eg, dopamine, epinephrine, norepinephrine, phenylephrine, vasopressin) or to reduce swelling of bites or stings; do not use in these settings. Use with caution in patients with reported history of bee sting allergy; hyaluronidase is an active component in bee venom. Discontinue if sensitization occurs (a skin test may be performed to determine hypersensitivity). Some products may contain albumin; albumin carries an extremely remote risk for transmission of viral diseases, Creutzfeldt-Jakob disease (CJD) and variant CJD (vCJD). No cases of transmission of viral diseases, CJD, or vCJD have been identified for licensed albumin or albumin contained in other licensed products. Potentially significant interactions may exist, requiring dose or frequency adjustment, additional monitoring, and/or selection of alternative therapy.

Adverse Reactions Frequency not defined.

Cardiovascular: Edema

Local: Injection site reaction

<1%, postmarketing, and/or case reports: Anaphylactic-like reactions (retrobulbar block or IV injections), anaphylaxis, angioedema, hypersensitivity reaction, urticaria

Drug Interactions

Metabolism/Transport Effects None known.

Avoid Concomitant Use

Avoid concomitant use of Hyaluronidase with any of the following: Phenylephrine (Systemic)

◀ **Increased Effect/Toxicity**

Hyaluronidase may increase the levels/effects of: Alpha-/Beta-Agonists; DOPamine; Local Anesthetics; Phenylephrine (Systemic)

Decreased Effect

The levels/effects of Hyaluronidase may be decreased by: Antihistamines; Corticosteroids; Estrogen Derivatives; Salicylates

Storage/Stability

Amphadase, Hylenex: Store intact vials in refrigerator at 2°C to 8°C (36°F to 46°F); do not freeze.

Vitrase: Store intact vials in refrigerator at 2°C to 8°C (36°F to 46°F); do not freeze. Protect from light. If adding to other injectable solutions, store admixture at 15°C to 25°C (59°F to 77°F) and use within 6 hours.

Preparation for Administration Extravasation management (off-label use): To make a 15 units/mL concentration, mix 0.1 mL (of 150 units/mL) with 0.9 mL NS.

Mechanism of Action Enzymatically modifies the permeability of connective tissue through hydrolysis of hyaluronic acid, one of the chief components of tissue cement which offers resistance to diffusion of liquids through tissues; hyaluronidase increases the distribution/dispersion and absorption of locally injected or extravasated substances.

Pharmacodynamics/Kinetics

Onset of action: SubQ: Immediate; when used for extravasation, there is usually a reduction in swelling within 15-30 minutes after administration (Zenk, 1981b)

Duration: 24-48 hours (variable)

Dosing

Adult & Geriatric

Skin test: Intradermal: 0.02 mL (Amphadase 3 units, Hylenex 3 units, or Vitrase 4 units) of a 150 units/mL (Amphadase, Hylenex) or 200 units/mL (Vitrase) solution. Positive reaction consists of a wheal with pseudopods appearing within 5 minutes and persisting for 20-30 minutes with localized itching (transient erythema is not considered a positive reaction). Skin testing is not necessary prior to use for extravasation management.

Dehydration: *Hypodermoclysis:* SubQ: 150 or 200 units followed by subcutaneous isotonic fluid administration ≥1000 mL **or** may be added to small volumes (≤200 mL) of subcutaneous replacement fluid. Rate and volume of a single clysis should not exceed those used for infusion of IV fluids.

Dispersion/absorption enhancement of injected drugs: SubQ: 50-300 units (usual dose: 150 units) either injected prior to drug administration or added to injection solution (consult compatibility reference prior to mixing)

Extravasation management (off-label use): Note: Administer as soon as extravasation is recognized. Do not use for extravasation of vasoconstrictors (eg, dopamine, norepinephrine [manage with phentolamine]). For extravasation management, skin testing is not necessary prior to use. The concentration of doses used to manage extravasation ranges from **15 units/mL to 150 units/mL**; refer to specific vesicant (below) for a description of doses/concentrations used in published case reports and/or reviews:

Aminophylline, calcium solutions, dextrose 10%, nafcillin, parenteral nutrition, potassium solutions, and radiocontrast media extravasation: Intradermal or SubQ: Inject a total of 1 mL (15 units/mL) as five separate 0.2 mL injections (using a 25-gauge needle) into area of extravasation at the leading edge in a clockwise manner (MacCara, 1983; Zenk, 1981b)

Contrast media extravasation: The injection of a total of 5 mL (150 units/mL) as five separate 1 mL injections around the extravasation site has been also used successfully (Rowlett, 2012).

Dextrose 50% extravasation: Injection of a total of 1 mL (150 units/mL) as five separate 0.2 mL injections administered along the leading edge of erythema has also been used successfully for dextrose 50% extravasation (Wiegand, 2009).

Mannitol: SubQ: Administer multiple injections of 0.5-1 mL (15 units/mL) around the periphery of the extravasation (Kumar, 2003)

Paclitaxel: IV: Administer 1-6 mL (150 units/mL) into existing IV line, and/or, if needle/cannula has been removed, inject subcutaneously in a clockwise manner around area of extravasation; usual dose is 1 mL hyaluronidase for each 1 mL of extravasated drug; may repeat several times over the next 3-4 hours (Ener, 2004)

Sodium bicarbonate: SubQ: Administer 4-5 separate 0.2 mL injections (15 units/mL) around area of extravasation (Hurst, 2004)

Vinca alkaloid (vinblastine, vincristine, vindesine, vinorelbine) extravasation:

If needle/cannula still in place: IV: After gently aspirating to remove extravasated vesicant, administer 1-6 mL hyaluronidase (150 units/mL) into existing IV line; the usual dose is 1 mL hyaluronidase for each 1 ml of extravasated drug (Perez Fidalgo, 2012; Schulmeister, 2011).

If needle/cannula has been removed: SubQ: Inject 1-6 mL (150 units/mL) in a clock wise manner using 1 mL for every 1 mL of drug extravasated (Schulmeister, 2011) **or** administer 1 mL (150 units/mL) as 5 separate 0.2 mL injections (using a 25-gauge needle) into the extravasation site (Polovich, 2009).

Retrobulbar/peribulbar block (adjuvant in bupivacaine-lidocaine mixture) (off-label use): 3.75 units (150 units/mL concentration) or 7.5 units (150 units/mL concentration) for every 1 mL of a 1:1 mixture of bupivacaine 0.75% and lidocaine 2%; administer a total of 6-8 mL of mixture divided evenly between retrobulbar and peribulbar injections (Kallio, 2000).

Pediatric

Skin test: Children and Adolescents: Intradermal: 0.02 mL (Amphadase 3 units, Hylenex 3 units, or Vitrase 4 units) of a 150 units/mL (Amphadase, Hylenex) or 200 units/mL (Vitrase) solution. Positive reaction consists of a wheal with pseudopods appearing within 5 minutes and persisting for 20-30 minutes with localized itching (transient erythema is not considered a positive reaction). Skin testing is not necessary prior to use for extravasation management.

Dehydration: Hypodermoclysis: SubQ: 150 or 200 units followed by subcutaneous isotonic fluid administration ≥1000 mL **or** may be added to small volumes (≤200 mL) of subcutaneous replacement fluid

Premature Infants: Volume of a single clysis/day should not exceed 25 mL/kg and the rate of administration should not exceed 2 mL/minute

Children <3 years: Volume of a single clysis should not exceed 200 mL

Children ≥3 years and Adolescents: Rate and volume of a single clysis should not exceed those used for infusion of IV fluids

Dispersion/absorption enhancement of injected drugs: Children and Adolescents: SubQ: 50-300 units (usual dose: 150 units) either injected prior to drug administration or added to injection solution (consult compatibility reference prior to mixing)

◄

Subcutaneous urography: Infants and Children: SubQ: 75 units over each scapula followed by injection of contrast medium at the same site; patient should be in the prone position during drug administration

Renal Impairment There are no dosage adjustments provided in the manufacturer's labeling.

Hepatic Impairment There are no dosage adjustments provided in the manufacturer's labeling.

Administration Do **not** administer IV for labeled uses (enzyme is rapidly inactivated and desired effects will not be produced).

Extravasation management (off-label use): Stop vesicant infusion immediately and disconnect IV line (leave needle/cannula in place); gently aspirate extravasated solution from the IV line (do **NOT** flush the line). Keep needle/cannula in place for vinca alkaloid extravasation, if appropriate, remove needle/cannula for other vesicants; elevate extremity.

Hyaluronidase administration:

Local administration (intradermal or subQ): Using a 150 units/mL concentration, mix 0.1 mL (of 150 units/mL) with 0.9 mL NS in 1 mL syringe to make final concentration of 15 units/mL; administer 5 x 0.2 mL (15 units/mL) intradermally and/or subcutaneously into area of extravasation (Mac-Cara, 1983).

Vinca alkaloids: If needle/cannula still in place, administer 1-6 mL hyaluronidase (150 units/mL) into the existing IV line; the usual dose is 1 mL hyaluronidase for each 1 mL of extravasated drug (Perez Fidalgo, 2012; Schulmeister, 2011). If needle/cannula has been removed, inject 1-6 mL (150 units/mL) subcutaneously in a clockwise manner using 1 mL for 1 mL of drug extravasated (Schulmeister, 2011) **or** administer 1 mL (150 units/mL) as 5 separate 0.2 mL injections (25-gauge needle) subcutaneously into the extravasation site (Polovich, 2009).

Retrobulbar/peribulbar administration (off-label use): After combining hyaluronidase with a 1:1 mixture of bupivacaine 0.75% and lidocaine 2%, administer according to standard anesthetic technique (Kallio, 2000).

Monitoring Parameters Extravasation management (off-label use): Document and monitor extravasation site.

Additional Information

Amphadase: pH: 6.8 (solution in vial)
Hylenex: pH: 7 (solution in vial)
Vitrase: pH: 6.4-7.2 (solution in vial)

Dosage Forms Excipient information presented when available (limited, particularly for generics); consult specific product labeling. [DSC] = Discontinued product

Solution, Injection:
Amphadase: 150 units/mL (1 mL) [contains edetate disodium, thimerosal]
Solution, Injection [preservative free]:
Hylenex: 150 units/mL (1 mL [DSC]) [contains albumin human, edetate disodium]
Hylenex: 150 units/mL (1 mL) [contains albumin human, polysorbate 80]
Vitrase: 200 units/mL (1.2 mL)
Generic: 150 units/mL (1 mL)

◆ **Hyaluronidase and Rituximab** *see* Rituximab and Hyaluronidase *on page 1623*

◆ **Hycamptamine** *see* Topotecan *on page 1790*

♦ **Hycamtin** see Topotecan on page 1790
♦ **Hydrea** see Hydroxyurea on page 925

Hydrocortisone (Systemic) (hye droe KOR ti sone)
Brand Names: US A-Hydrocort [DSC]; Cortef; Solu-CORTEF
Brand Names: Canada Cortef; Solu-Cortef
Index Terms A-hydroCort; Compound F; Cortisol; Hydrocortisone Sodium Succinate
Pharmacologic Category Corticosteroid, Systemic
Use

Allergic states: Control of severe or incapacitating allergic conditions intractable to adequate trials of conventional treatment in drug hypersensitivity reactions, perennial or seasonal allergic rhinitis, serum sickness, transfusion reactions, or acute noninfectious laryngeal edema (epinephrine is the drug of first choice).

Dermatologic diseases: Atopic dermatitis; bullous dermatitis herpetiformis; contact dermatitis; exfoliative dermatitis; exfoliative erythroderma; pemphigus; severe erythema multiforme (Stevens-Johnson syndrome); severe psoriasis; severe seborrheic dermatitis; mycosis fungoides.

Edematous states: To induce diuresis or remission of proteinuria in the nephrotic syndrome, without uremia, of the idiopathic type or that due to lupus erythematosus.

Endocrine disorders: Acute adrenocortical insufficiency; congenital adrenal hyperplasia; hypercalcemia associated with cancer; nonsuppurative thyroiditis; primary or secondary adrenocortical insufficiency; preoperatively and in the event of serious trauma or illness, in patients with known adrenal insufficiency or when adrenocortical reserve is doubtful; shock unresponsive to conventional therapy if adrenocortical insufficiency exists or is suspected.

GI diseases: To tide the patient over a critical period of the disease in ulcerative colitis and regional enteritis.

Hematologic disorders: Acquired (autoimmune) hemolytic anemia; congenital (erythroid) hypoplastic anemia (Diamond Blackfan anemia); erythroblastopenia (RBC anemia); immune thrombocytopenia (formerly known as idiopathic thrombocytopenic purpura) in adults; pure red cell aplasia; select cases of secondary thrombocytopenia.

Neoplastic diseases: Palliative management of leukemias and lymphomas (adults); acute leukemia of childhood.

Nervous system: Acute exacerbations of multiple sclerosis; cerebral edema associated with primary or metastatic brain tumor, or craniotomy. **Note**: Treatment guidelines recommend the use of high-dose IV or oral methylprednisolone for acute exacerbations of multiple sclerosis (AAN [Scott 2011]; NICE 2014).

Ophthalmic diseases: Severe acute and chronic allergic and inflammatory processes involving the eye, such as allergic conjunctivitis; allergic corneal marginal ulcers; anterior segment inflammation; chorioretinitis; diffuse posterior uveitis and choroiditis; herpes zoster ophthalmicus; iritis and iridocyclitis; keratitis; optic neuritis; sympathetic ophthalmia; other ocular inflammatory conditions unresponsive to topical corticosteroids.

Respiratory diseases: Aspiration pneumonitis; bronchial asthma; berylliosis; fulminating or disseminated pulmonary tuberculosis when used concurrently with appropriate antituberculous chemotherapy; idiopathic eosinophilic pneumonias; Loeffler syndrome (not manageable by other means); symptomatic sarcoidosis.

◄ **Rheumatic disorders:** As adjunctive therapy for short-term administration in acute and subacute bursitis, acute gouty arthritis, acute nonspecific tenosynovitis, ankylosing spondylitis, epicondylitis, posttraumatic osteoarthritis, psoriatic arthritis, rheumatoid arthritis, including juvenile rheumatoid arthritis, synovitis of osteoarthritis; during an exacerbation or as maintenance therapy in acute rheumatic carditis, dermatomyositis (polymyositis), temporal arteritis, and systemic lupus erythematosus.

Miscellaneous: Trichinosis with neurologic or myocardial involvement; tuberculous meningitis with subarachnoid block or impending block when used concurrently with appropriate antituberculous chemotherapy.

Pregnancy Risk Factor C

Dosing

Adult & Geriatric Note: Adjust dose depending upon condition being treated and response of patient. The lowest possible dose should be used to control the condition; when dose reduction is possible, the dose should be reduced gradually. In life-threatening situations, parenteral doses larger than the oral dose may be needed.

Anti-inflammatory or immunosuppressive:
IM, IV: Initial: 100 to 500 mg/dose at intervals of 2, 4, or 6 hours.
Oral: Initial: 20 to 240 mg/day.

Multiple sclerosis, acute exacerbations:
Note: Treatment guidelines recommend the use of high-dose IV or oral methylprednisolone for acute exacerbations of multiple sclerosis (AAN [Scott 2011]; NICE 2014).
IM, IV: 800 mg/day for 1 week, followed by 320 mg every other day for 1 month.
Oral: 200 mg/day for 1 week, followed by 80 mg every other day for 1 month.

Adrenal insufficiency:
Acute adrenal insufficiency (adrenal crisis) (off-label dose): 100 mg IV bolus, immediately followed by 200 mg over 24 hours as a continuous IV infusion or in divided doses (IM or IV) every 6 hours, then 100 mg over 24 hours the following day (Allolio 2015; ES [Bornstein 2016]). Alternatively, may administer 100 mg IV bolus, then 50 to 75 mg IV every 6 hours for 24 hours, followed by a slow taper over the next 72 hours (administering doses every 4 to 6 hours during taper) (Gardner 2011). **Note:** Appropriate fluid resuscitation is also required (ES [Bornstein 2016]; Gardner 2011).

Chronic primary adrenal insufficiency (physiologic replacement) (off-label dose): Oral: 15 to 25 mg daily in 2 to 3 divided doses. Administer the largest dose in the morning upon awakening, followed by next dose 2 hours after lunch (two-dose regimen) or next dose at lunch, followed by smallest dose in the afternoon no later than 4 to 6 hours before bedtime (three-dose regimen) (ES [Bornstein 2016]).

Temporary adrenal insufficiency (temporary), physiologic replacement following resection of an ACTH-producing tumor or unilateral adrenalectomy (off-label dose): Oral: 10 to 12 mg/m2/day in 2 to 3 divided doses, with the first dose taken as soon as possible after waking; continue hydrocortisone until HPA axis recovers, generally 6 to 12 months following resection of ACTH-producing tumors or 18 months following unilateral adrenalectomy (ES [Neiman 2015]).

Congenital adrenal hyperplasia (off-label dose): Oral: 15 to 25 mg/day in 2 to 3 divided doses (Speiser 2010).

Stress dosing in patients known to be adrenally-suppressed (ie, prevention of adrenal crisis in glucocorticoid-treated patients) (off-label dose):

Sickness:

Illness with fever: Oral: Double the routine oral hydrocortisone dose until recovery for fever >38°C [100.4°F] or triple the routine oral hydrocortisone dose until recovery for fever >39°C [102.2°F]); return to standard dose within 1 to 2 days (Allolio 2015)

Gastroenteritis with vomiting and/or diarrhea: IM, SubQ: 100 mg dose given early in course of illness; repeat after 6 to 12 hours (Allolio 2015)

Severe infection (eg, pneumonia/with altered cognition): IM, SubQ: 100 mg dose given early in course of illness; repeat after 6 to 12 hours until recovery (Allolio 2015)

Surgery:

Minor stress (ie, inguinal herniorrhaphy): IV: 25 mg/day for 1 day (Coursin 2002; Salem 1994)

Moderate stress (ie, joint replacement, cholecystectomy): IV: 50 to 75 mg/day (25 mg every 8 to 12 hours) for 1 to 2 days (Coursin 2002; Salem 1994)

Major stress (pancreatoduodenectomy, esophagogastrectomy, cardiac surgery): IV: 100 to 150 mg/day (50 mg every 8 to 12 hours) for 2 to 3 days (Coursin 2002; Salem 1994)

Septic shock (off-label use): IV: 200 mg/day as a continuous infusion (Rhodes 2017; Weber-Carstens 2007) **or** 50 mg IV bolus every 6 hours (Annane 2002; Sprung 2008). Taper slowly (over several days) when vasopressors are no longer required; do not stop abruptly. **Note:** Low-dose hydrocortisone in septic shock patients may cause a significant increase in hyperglycemia and hypernatremia. A small study demonstrated that repetitive bolus doses of hydrocortisone caused significant hyperglycemia that was not seen during continuous infusion (Weber-Carstens 2007); practice guidelines recommend strategies for avoidance and/or detection of these side effects (eg, the use of continuous infusion) (Rhodes 2017).

Thyroid storm (off-label use): IV: 300 mg loading dose, followed by 100 mg every 8 hours (ATA [Ross 2016])

Pediatric Note: Adjust dose depending upon condition being treated and response of patient. The lowest possible dose should be used to control the condition; when dose reduction is possible, the dose should be reduced gradually. In life-threatening situations, parenteral doses larger than the oral dose may be needed.

Anti-inflammatory or immunosuppressive:

Infants and Children:

Oral: 2.5 to 10 mg/kg/day **or** 75 to 300 mg/m^2/day in divided doses every 6 to 8 hours (Kliegman 2007).

IM, IV:

Manufacturer labeling: Initial: 0.56 to 8 mg/kg/day or 20 to 240 mg/m^2/day in 3 or 4 divided doses.

Alternate dosing: 1 to 5 mg/kg/day **or** 30 to 150 mg/m^2/day divided every 12 to 24 hours (Kliegman 2007).

Adolescents: Oral, IM, IV, SubQ: 15 to 240 mg every 12 hours (Kliegman 2007).

Congenital adrenal hyperplasia (off-label dose): Oral: (tablets): Infants, Children, and Adolescents: **Note:** Administer morning dose as early as possible. Tablets may result in more reliable serum concentrations than oral liquid formulation; use of oral suspension is not recommended. Doses must be individualized by monitoring growth, bone age, and hormonal levels; mineralocorticoid (eg, fludrocortisone) and sodium supplement may be required in salt losers (AAP 2000; AAP 2010; Endocrine Society [Speiser 2010]).

Initial: 10 to 15 mg/m^2/day in 3 divided doses; higher initial doses (20 mg/m^2/day) may be required to achieve initial target hormone serum concentrations (AAP 2010; Endocrine Society [Speiser 2010]).

Maintenance dose: Usual requirement:

Infants: 2.5 to 5 mg/**dose** 3 times daily.

Children: 5 to 10 mg/**dose** 3 times daily.

Adolescents: Refer to adult dosing.

Physiologic replacement (off-label dose): Infants and Children: Oral: 8 to 10 mg/m^2/day divided every 8 hours; up to 12 mg/m^2/day in some patients; to replicate diurnal variation, the highest doses are typically administered in the morning and mid-day dose with the lower dose in the evening (Ahmet 2011; Elder 2015; Gupta 2008; Maguire 2007; Shulman 2007).

Septic shock (off-label use): Infants, Children, and Adolescents: IV: 50 to 100 mg/m^2/day (Marx 2014; Shulman 2007); in some cases, doses may be titrated up to 50 mg/**kg**/day for shock reversal; however, efficacy data variable with the higher doses (Brierley 2009; Menon 2012). **Note:** Use recommended only in fluid refractory, catecholamine-resistant shock, and suspected or proven absolute (classic) adrenal insufficiency.

Renal Impairment There are no dosage adjustments provided in the manufacturer's labeling; use with caution.

Hepatic Impairment There are no dosage adjustments provided in the manufacturer's labeling; use with caution.

Additional Information Complete prescribing information should be consulted for additional detail.

Dosage Forms Excipient information presented when available (limited, particularly for generics); consult specific product labeling. [DSC] = Discontinued product

Solution Reconstituted, Injection, as sodium succinate [strength expressed as base]:

A-Hydrocort: 100 mg (1 ea [DSC])

Solution Reconstituted, Injection, as sodium succinate [strength expressed as base, preservative free]:

Solu-CORTEF: 100 mg (1 ea); 250 mg (1 ea); 500 mg (1 ea); 1000 mg (1 ea)

Tablet, Oral, as base:

Cortef: 5 mg, 10 mg, 20 mg [scored]

Generic: 5 mg, 10 mg, 20 mg

◆ **Hydrocortisone Sodium Succinate** see Hydrocortisone (Systemic) on page 921

◆ **Hydroxycarbamide** see Hydroxyurea on page 925

◆ **Hydroxydaunomycin Hydrochloride** see DOXOrubicin (Conventional) on page 624

◆ **Hydroxyldaunorubicin Hydrochloride** see DOXOrubicin (Conventional) on page 624

Hydroxyurea (hye droks ee yoor EE a)

Related Information

Management of Chemotherapy-Induced Nausea and Vomiting in Adults *on page 2253*

Prevention of Chemotherapy-Induced Nausea and Vomiting in Children *on page 2310*

Safe Handling of Hazardous Drugs *on page 2379*

Brand Names: US Droxia; Hydrea

Brand Names: Canada Apo-Hydroxyurea; Hydrea; Mylan-Hydroxyurea

Index Terms HU; Hydroxycarbamide; Hydurea

Pharmacologic Category Antineoplastic Agent, Miscellaneous

Use

Chronic myeloid leukemia (Hydrea): Treatment of refractory chronic myeloid leukemia (CML)

Head and neck cancer (Hydrea): Management (with concomitant radiation therapy) of locally advanced squamous cell head and neck cancer (excluding lip cancer)

Sickle cell anemia (Droxia): Management of sickle cell anemia (to reduce the frequency of painful crises and to reduce the need for blood transfusions in patients with recurrent moderate to severe painful crises)

Labeled Contraindications

US labeling: Hypersensitivity to hydroxyurea or any component of the formulation

Canadian labeling: Additional contraindications (not in the US labeling): Severe bone marrow depression (eg, leukopenia [<2,500/mm^3], thrombocytopenia [<100,000/mm^3], or severe anemia)

Pregnancy Considerations Adverse effects have been observed in animal reproduction studies. Based on its mechanism of action, hydroxyurea may cause fetal harm if administered during pregnancy. Women of reproductive potential should be advised to avoid becoming pregnant during treatment (verify pregnancy status prior to starting hydroxyurea therapy) and should use effective contraception during and for at least 6 months after completion of therapy. Hydroxyurea use may damage spermatozoa and testicular tissue; males with female partners of reproductive potential should use effective contraception during and for at least 1 year after therapy. Azoospermia or oligospermia (sometimes reversible) has been observed in male patients; counsel males of reproductive potential about sperm banking prior to therapy initiation.

Breastfeeding Considerations Hydroxyurea is excreted in breast milk. Due to the potential for serious adverse reactions in the nursing infant, breastfeeding is not recommended by the manufacturer.

Warnings/Precautions To decrease risk of exposure, wear gloves when handling and wash hands before and after contact. **[US Boxed Warning]: Hydroxyurea may cause severe myelosuppression. Monitor blood counts at baseline and throughout treatment. Interrupt treatment and reduce dose as necessary.** Leukopenia and neutropenia commonly occur (thrombocytopenia and anemia are less common); leukopenia/neutropenia occur first. Severe or life-threatening myelosuppression may occur at the recommended dose. Hematologic toxicity reversible (rapid) with treatment interruption. Correct severe anemia prior to initiating treatment. Do not initiate therapy if bone marrow function is markedly reduced. Hydroxyurea should not be used in sickle cell anemia with severe bone marrow suppression (neutrophils <2,000/mm^3, platelets <80,000/mm^3, hemoglobin <4.5 g/dL, or reticulocytes <80,000/mm^3 when hemoglobin <9 g/dL per manufacturer's labeling). Use with caution in patients with a history of prior chemotherapy or radiation therapy; myelosuppression is more common. Patients with a history of radiation therapy are also at risk for exacerbation of post irradiation erythema. Self-limiting macrocytosis/megaloblastic erythropoiesis may be seen early in treatment (may resemble pernicious anemia, but is unrelated to vitamin B$_{12}$ or folic acid deficiency). Prophylactic folic acid supplementation is recommended. Plasma iron clearance may be delayed and iron utilization rate (by erythrocytes) may be reduced. Potentially significant drug-drug interactions may exist, requiring dose or frequency adjustment, additional monitoring, and/or selection of alternative therapy. When treated concurrently with hydroxyurea and antiretroviral agents (including didanosine and stavudine), HIV-infected patients are at higher risk for potentially fatal pancreatitis, hepatotoxicity, hepatic failure, and severe peripheral neuropathy; discontinue immediately if signs of these toxicities develop. Hyperuricemia may occur with antineoplastic treatment; adequate hydration and initiation or dosage adjustment of uricosuric agents (eg, allopurinol) may be necessary.

In patients with sickle cell anemia, Droxia is not recommended if neutrophils <2,000/mm^3, platelets <80,000/mm^3, hemoglobin <4.5 g/dL, or reticulocytes <80,000/mm^3 when hemoglobin <9 g/dL per manufacturer's labeling. May cause macrocytosis, which can mask folic acid deficiency; prophylactic folic acid supplementation is recommended. **[US Boxed Warning]: Hydroxyurea is carcinogenic. Advise sun protection and monitor patients for malignancies.** Treatment of myeloproliferative disorders (eg, polycythemia vera, thrombocythemia) with long-term hydroxyurea is associated with secondary leukemia; it is unknown if this is drug-related or disease-related. Skin cancer has been reported with long-term hydroxyurea use. Monitor for signs/symptoms of secondary malignancies. Cutaneous vasculitic toxicities (vasculitic ulceration and gangrene) have been reported with hydroxyurea treatment, most often in patients with a history of or receiving concurrent interferon therapy; discontinue hydroxyurea and consider alternate cytoreductive therapy if cutaneous vasculitic toxicity develops. Use caution with renal dysfunction; may require dose reductions. Elderly patients may be more sensitive to the effects of hydroxyurea; may require lower doses. Avoid use of live vaccines during hydroxyurea therapy. Concomitant use may potentiate viral replication and may possibly increase vaccine adverse reactions due to suppression of normal defense mechanisms by hydroxyurea; the antibody response to vaccines may be decreased. Immunization with live vaccines may result in severe infection. Consider consultation with a specialist if immunization with a live vaccine is necessary.

Adverse Reactions Frequency not always defined.

Cardiovascular: Edema, hypersensitivity angiitis

Central nervous system: Chills, disorientation, dizziness, drowsiness (dose-related), hallucination, headache, malaise, peripheral neuropathy (HIV-infected patients), seizure, vasculitic ulcerations

Dermatologic: Eczema (infants and children 9 to 18 months: 13% [Thornburg 2012]), leg ulcer (7% [Hernández-Boluda 2011]), dermal ulcer (3% [Antonioli 2012]), nail discoloration (2% [Randi 2005]), alopecia (infrequent, [Hernández-Boluda 2011]), changes in nails (infrequent, [Hernández-Boluda 2011]), hyperpigmentation (infrequent, [Hernández-Boluda 2011]), atrophy of nail, dermatomyositis-like skin changes, desquamation, erythema (peripheral), facial erythema, gangrene of skin or other tissue, maculopapular rash, papule (violet), skin atrophy, skin carcinoma

Endocrine & metabolic: Increased uric acid

Gastrointestinal: Acute mucocutaneous toxicity (5% [Hernández-Boluda 2011]), diarrhea (infrequent, [Antonioli 2012]), gastric distress (infrequent, [Antonioli 2012]), nausea (infrequent, [Antonioli 2012]), oral mucosa ulcer (infrequent, [Hernández-Boluda 2011]), anorexia, BSP abnormality (retention), constipation, gastrointestinal irritation (potentiated with radiation therapy), mucositis (potentiated with radiation therapy), pancreatitis (HIV-infected patients), stomatitis, vomiting

Genitourinary: Dysuria

Hematologic & oncologic: Leukemia (4% [Hernández-Boluda 2011]; secondary; long-term use), leukopenia (2% [Hernández-Boluda 2011]), bone marrow depression (neutropenia [common], thrombocytopenia; hematologic recovery: within 2 weeks); abnormal erythropoiesis (megaloblastic; self-limiting), macrocytosis (MCV >97: 42% [Randi 2005]), reticulocytopenia (infants and children 9 to 18 months [Wang 2011])

Hepatic: Hepatic failure (HIV-infected patients), hepatotoxicity, increased liver enzymes

Neuromuscular & skeletal: Panniculitis (Antonioli 2012), weakness

Renal: Increased blood urea nitrogen, increased serum creatinine, renal tubular disease

Respiratory: Asthma (infants and children 9 to 18 months: 9% [Thornburg 2012]), dyspnea, pulmonary fibrosis (rare), pulmonary infiltrates (diffuse, rare)

<1%, postmarketing, and/or case reports: Actinic keratosis (Antonioli 2012), azoospermia, basal cell carcinoma (Antonioli 2012), cholestasis, hepatitis, hyperkeratosis (Antonioli 2012), lesion (dyschromic [Antonioli 2012]), malignant neoplasm (Wong 2014), mucous membrane lesion (Antonioli 2012), oligospermia, pneumonitis (Antonioli 2012), squamous cell carcinoma (Antonioli 2012), tumor lysis syndrome

Drug Interactions

Metabolism/Transport Effects None known.

Avoid Concomitant Use

Avoid concomitant use of Hydroxyurea with any of the following: BCG (Intravesical); Deferiprone; Didanosine; Dipyrone; Natalizumab; Pimecrolimus; Stavudine; Tacrolimus (Topical); Vaccines (Live)

Increased Effect/Toxicity

Hydroxyurea may increase the levels/effects of: CloZAPine; Deferiprone; Didanosine; Fingolimod; Leflunomide; Natalizumab; Stavudine; Tofacitinib; Vaccines (Live)

The levels/effects of Hydroxyurea may be increased by: Denosumab; Didanosine; Dipyrone; Ocrelizumab; Palifermin; Pimecrolimus; Promazine; Roflumilast; Stavudine; Tacrolimus (Topical); Trastuzumab

Decreased Effect

Hydroxyurea may decrease the levels/effects of: BCG (Intravesical); Coccidioides immitis Skin Test; Lenograstim; Nivolumab; Sipuleucel-T; Tertomotide; Vaccines (Inactivated); Vaccines (Live)

The levels/effects of Hydroxyurea may be decreased by: Echinacea

◄ **Hazardous Drugs Handling Considerations**
Hazardous agent (NIOSH 2016 [group 1]).

Use appropriate precautions for receiving, handling, administration, and disposal. Gloves (single) should be worn during receiving, unpacking, and placing in storage.

NIOSH recommends single gloving for administration of intact tablets or capsules. If manipulating tablets/capsules (eg, to prepare an oral suspension), NIOSH recommends double gloving, a protective gown, and preparation in a controlled device; if not prepared in a controlled device, respiratory and eye/face protection as well as ventilated engineering controls are recommended. NIOSH recommends double gloving, a protective gown, and (if there is a potential for vomit or spit up) eye/face protection for administration of an oral liquid/feeding tube administration (NIOSH 2016).

Storage/Stability Store at 25°C (77°F); excursions permitted between 15°C and 30°C (59°F and 86°F). Keep bottle tightly closed.

Mechanism of Action Antimetabolite which selectively inhibits ribonucleoside diphosphate reductase, preventing the conversion of ribonucleotides to deoxyribonucleotides, halting the cell cycle at the G1/S phase and therefore has radiation sensitizing activity by maintaining cells in the G_1 phase and interfering with DNA repair. In sickle cell anemia, hydroxyurea increases red blood cell (RBC) hemoglobin F levels, RBC water content, deformability of sickled cells, and alters adhesion of RBCs to endothelium.

Pharmacodynamics/Kinetics Note: In pediatric patients, large interpatient variability and phenotypic differences have been reported (Ware 2011).

Onset: Sickle cell anemia: Fetal hemoglobin increase: 4 to 12 weeks

Absorption: Readily absorbed (≥80%); relatively rapid (Rodriguez 1998)

Distribution: Distributes widely into tissues (including into the brain); estimated volume of distribution approximates total body water (Gwilt 1998); concentrates in leukocytes and erythrocytes

V_d: Children: ~12 L (range: 2.5 to 52) (Ware 2011); Adults: ~20 L/m² (Rodriguez 1998)

Metabolism: Up to 60% via hepatic metabolism and urease found in intestinal bacteria

Bioavailability: ~100% (Rodriguez 1998)

Protein binding: 75% to 80% bound to serum proteins (Gwilt 1998)

Half-life elimination: 1.9 to 3.9 hours (Gwilt 1998); Children: Sickle cell anemia: 1.7 hours (range: 0.7 to 3 hours) (Ware 2011)

Time to peak: Children: "Fast" phenotype: 15 to 30 minutes; "Slow" phenotype: 60 to 120 minutes (Ware 2011); Adults: 1 to 4 hours

Excretion: Urine (sickle cell anemia: ~40% of administered dose)

Clearance: Children: ~7 L/hour (range: 1.6 to 22) (Ware 2011); Adults: ~7.5 L/hour (Rodriguez 1998)

Dosing

Adult Note: Doses should be based on ideal or actual body weight, whichever is less (per manufacturer). Prophylactic administration of folic acid is recommended.

US labeling:

Chronic myeloid leukemia (CML), head and neck cancer: Oral: Initial: 15 mg/kg/day; individualize treatment based on tumor type, disease state, response to treatment, patient risk factors, and current clinical practice standards. May be used alone or in combination with other agents or radiation.

Sickle cell anemia: Oral:

Manufacturer's labeling: Initial: 15 mg/kg/day as a single dose; if blood counts are in an acceptable range, may increase by 5 mg/kg/day every 12 weeks until the maximum tolerated dose of 35 mg/kg/day is achieved or the dose that does not produce toxic effects over 24 consecutive weeks (do not increase dose if blood counts are between acceptable and toxic ranges). Monitor for toxicity every 2 weeks; if toxicity occurs, withhold treatment until the bone marrow recovers, then restart with a dose reduction of 2.5 mg/kg/day; if no toxicity occurs over the next 12 weeks, then the subsequent dose may be increased by 2.5 mg/kg/day every 12 weeks to a maximum tolerated dose (dose which does not produce hematologic toxicity for 24 consecutive weeks). If hematologic toxicity recurs a second time at a specific dose, discontinue treatment.

Acceptable hematologic ranges: Neutrophils ≥2,500/mm³; platelets ≥95,000/mm³; hemoglobin >5.3 g/dL, and reticulocytes ≥95,000/mm³ if the hemoglobin concentration is <9 g/dL

Toxic hematologic ranges: Neutrophils <2,000/mm³; platelets <80,000/mm³; hemoglobin <4.5 g/dL; and reticulocytes <80,000/mm³ if the hemoglobin concentration is <9 g/dL

Alternate recommendations (off-label dose): Initial: 15 mg/kg/day; if dosage escalation is warranted based on clinical/laboratory findings, may increase by 5 mg/kg/day increments every 8 weeks. Monitor for toxicity at least every 4 weeks when adjusting dose; aim for a target absolute neutrophils ≥2,000/mm³ (younger patients with lower baseline counts may safely tolerate absolute neutrophils down to 1,250/mm³; maintain platelet count ≥80,000/mm³. Give until mild myelosuppression is achieved (absolute neutrophils: 2,000/mm³ to 4,000/mm³), up to a maximum dose of 35 mg/kg/day. If toxicity occurs (neutropenia or thrombocytopenia), withhold treatment until the bone marrow recovers (monitor weekly), then restart at a dose 5mg/kg/day lower than the dose given prior to onset of cytopenias (NHLBI 2014). **Note:** A clinical response to treatment may take 3 to 6 months; a 6 month trial on the maximum tolerated dose is recommended prior to considering discontinuation due to treatment failure; effectiveness of hydroxyurea depends upon daily dosing adherence. For patients who have a clinical response, long-term hydroxyurea therapy is indicated (NHLBI 2014)

Canadian labeling:

Note: Titrate dose to patient response; if WBC count falls to <2,500/mm³, or the platelet count to <100,000/mm³, therapy should be interrupted for at least 3 days and resumed when values rise toward normal.

Chronic myeloid leukemia (resistant): Continuous therapy: Oral: 20 to 30 mg/kg once daily

Solid tumors (eg, head and neck cancer): Oral:

Intermittent therapy: 80 mg/kg as a single dose every third day

Concomitant therapy with irradiation (head and neck cancer): 80 mg/kg as a single dose every third day starting at least 7 days before initiation of irradiation

Acute myeloid leukemia (AML), cytoreduction (off-label use): Oral: 50 to 100 mg/kg/day until WBC <100,000/mm³ (Grund 1977) **or** 50 to 60 mg/kg/day until WBC <10,000 to 20,000/mm³ (Dohner 2010)

Essential thrombocythemia, high-risk (off-label use): Oral: 500 to 1000 mg daily; adjust dose to maintain platelets <400,000/mm³ (Harrison 2005)

◄ **Head and neck cancer (off-label dosing; with concurrent radiation therapy and fluorouracil):** Oral: 1000 mg every 12 hours for 11 doses per cycle (Garden 2004)

Hypereosinophilic syndrome (off-label use): Oral: 1,000 to 3,000 mg/day (Klion 2006)

Meningioma (off-label use): Oral: 20 mg/kg once daily (Newton 2000; Rosenthal 2002)

Polycythemia vera, high-risk (off-label use): Oral: 15 to 20 mg/kg/day (Finazzi 2007)

Geriatric Refer to adult dosing. May require lower doses.

Pediatric Note: Doses should be based on ideal or actual body weight, whichever is less (per manufacturer). Prophylactic administration of folic acid is recommended.

Sickle cell anemia (off-label use): Infants ≥6 months, Children, and Adolescents: Oral: 20 mg/kg/dose once daily; increase by 5 mg/kg/**day** every 8 weeks until mild myelosuppression (target ANC 2,000 to 4,000/mm^3 [a lower ANC limit of 1,500/mm^3 has been used in some studies]) is achieved; maximum dose: 35 mg/kg/**day** (Hankins 2005; NHLBI 2014; Strouse 2012; Thornburg 2009; Wang 2001; Wang 2011); initial starting dose of 15 mg/kg/dose once daily has also been studied (Kinney 1999; Zimmerman 2004).

If myelosuppression occurs (platelets <80,000/mm^3, neutrophils <2,000/mm^3; younger patients with lower baseline counts may safely tolerate ANC down to 1,250/mm^3), hold therapy until counts recover (monitor weekly); reinitiate at a dose 5 mg/kg/**day** lower than the dose given prior to onset of cytopenias (NHLBI 2014); some have recommended reinitiating at a dose 2.5 mg/kg/**day** lower (Hankins 2005; Heeney 2008; Wang 2001; Wang 2011; Zimmerman 2004). **Note:** A clinical response to treatment may take 3 to 6 months; a 6-month trial of the maximum tolerated dose is recommended prior to considering discontinuation due to treatment failure; effectiveness of hydroxyurea depends upon daily dosing adherence. For patients who have a clinical response, long-term hydroxyurea therapy is indicated (NHLBI 2014).

Renal Impairment

US labeling: The manufacturer's labeling recommends the following adjustments:

CML, head and neck cancer:

    CrCl ≥60 mL/minute: No dosage adjustment (of initial dose) necessary.

    CrCl <60 mL/minute: Reduce initial dose by 50% to 7.5 mg/kg/day; titrate to response/avoidance of toxicity

    End-stage renal disease (ESRD): Reduce initial dose by 50% to 7.5 mg/kg/dose (administer after dialysis on dialysis days); titrate to response/avoidance of toxicity

Sickle cell anemia:

    CrCl ≥60 mL/minute: No dosage adjustment (of initial dose) necessary.

    CrCl <60 mL/minute: Reduce initial dose by 50% to 7.5 mg/kg/day (Yan 2005); titrate to response/avoidance of toxicity (refer to usual dosing).

    ESRD: Reduce initial dose by 50% to 7.5 mg/kg/dose (administer after dialysis on dialysis days); titrate to response/avoidance of toxicity.

The following adjustments have also been reported:

Aronoff 2007: Adults:

    CrCl >50 mL/minute: No dosage adjustment necessary

    CrCl 10 to 50 mL/minute: Administer 50% of dose.

CrCl <10 mL/minute: Administer 20% of dose.

Hemodialysis: Administer dose after dialysis on dialysis days.

Continuous renal replacement therapy (CRRT): Administer 50% of dose.

NHLBI 2014: Sickle cell anemia: Adults: Chronic kidney disease: Initial 5 to 10 mg/kg/day

Kintzel 1995:

CrCl 46 to 60 mL/minute: Administer 85% of dose.

CrCl 31 to 45 mL/minute: Administer 80% of dose.

CrCl <30 mL/minute: Administer 75% of dose.

Canadian labeling: There are no specific dosage adjustments provided in the manufacturer's labeling; however, a dose reduction should be considered. Closely monitor for bone marrow toxicity.

Hepatic Impairment There are no dosage adjustments provided in the manufacturer's labeling; closely monitor for bone marrow toxicity.

Obesity *ASCO Guidelines for appropriate chemotherapy dosing in obese adults with cancer (solid tumors):* Utilize patient's actual body weight (full weight) for calculation of body surface area- or weight-based dosing, particularly when the intent of therapy is curative; manage regimen-related toxicities in the same manner as for nonobese patients; if a dose reduction is utilized due to toxicity, consider resumption of full weight-based dosing with subsequent cycles, especially if cause of toxicity (eg, hepatic or renal impairment) is resolved (Griggs 2012). **Note:** The manufacturer recommends dosing based on ideal or actual body weight, whichever is less.

Adjustment for Toxicity

Cutaneous vasculitic ulcerations: Discontinue

Gastrointestinal toxicity (severe nausea, vomiting, severe mucositis, anorexia) (*Canadian labeling*): Temporarily interrupt treatment

Hepatitis and cholestasis (*Canadian labeling*): Discontinue

Pancreatitis: Discontinue permanently

Hematologic toxicity: CML, head and neck cancer:

US labeling: Do not initiate therapy if bone marrow function is markedly reduced. Monitor blood counts prior to and during treatment; modify dose or discontinue hydroxyurea as needed.

Canadian labeling: WBC <2,500/mm^3 or platelets <100,000/mm^3: Interrupt treatment (for at least 3 days), may resume when values rise toward normal. Do not initiate therapy if bone marrow function is markedly reduced. Monitor blood counts prior to and during treatment; modify dose or discontinue hydroxyurea as needed.

Sickle cell anemia:

Manufacturer's labeling: Neutrophils <2,000/mm^3, platelets <80,000/mm^3, hemoglobin <4.5 g/dL, or reticulocytes <80,000/mm^3 with hemoglobin <9 g/dL: Interrupt treatment; following recovery, may resume with a dose reduction of 2.5 mg/kg/day. Hydroxyurea may then be titrated up or down every 12 weeks in 2.5 mg/kg/day increments until the patient is at a stable dosage that does not result in hematologic toxicity for 24 weeks. If hematologic toxicity recurs a second time at a specific dose, discontinue treatment.

Alternate recommendations (off-label dose): Absolute neutrophils <2,000/mm^3 (younger patients with lower baseline counts may safely tolerate absolute neutrophils down to 1,250/mm^3), platelets <80,000/mm^3: Interrupt treatment; following recovery, may restart at a dose 5mg/kg/day lower than the dose given prior to onset of cytopenias (NHLBI 2014).

◀ **Combination Regimens**
Head and neck cancer: Fluorouracil-Hydroxyurea (Head and Neck Cancer) on page 2124

Administration Administer at the same time each day.

Impervious gloves should be worn when handling bottles containing hydroxyurea or when handling/administering intact capsules (single gloves are recommended for administration of intact capsules). Wash hands with soap and water before and after contact with the bottle or capsules when handling. Avoid exposure to crushed or open capsules. If skin contact with crushed or opened capsules occurs, immediately wash the affected area thoroughly with soap and water. If eye(s) contact with crushed or opened capsules occurs, the affected area should be flushed thoroughly with water or isotonic eyewash designated for that purpose for at least 15 minutes. If the powder from the capsule is spilled, immediately wipe it up with a damp disposable towel and discard (along with the empty capsules) in a closed container, such as a plastic bag. The spill areas should then be cleaned 3 times using a detergent solution followed by clean water.

Emetic Potential Children and Adults: Minimal (<10%)

Extemporaneous Preparations A 40 mg/mL oral suspension may be prepared with capsules and either a 1:1 mixture of Ora-Sweet® and Ora-Plus® or a 1:1 mixture of methylcellulose 1% and simple syrup NF. Empty the contents of eight 500 mg capsules into a mortar. Add small portions of chosen vehicle and mix to a uniform paste; mix while incrementally adding the vehicle to almost 100 mL; transfer to a calibrated bottle, rinse mortar with vehicle, and add sufficient quantity of vehicle to make 100 mL. Label "shake well" and "refrigerate". Store in plastic prescription bottles. Stable for 14 days at room temperature or refrigerated (preferred) (Nahata 2003).

A 100 mg/mL oral solution may be prepared with capsules. Mix the contents of twenty 500 mg capsules with enough room temperature sterile water (~50 mL) to initially result in a 200 mg/mL concentration. Stir vigorously using a magnetic stirrer for several hours, then filter to remove insoluble contents. Add 50 mL Syrpalta® (flavored syrup, HUMCO) to filtered solution, resulting in 100 mL of a 100 mg/mL hydroxyurea solution. Stable for 1 month at room temperature in amber plastic bottle (Heeney 2004).

Heeney MM, Whorton MR, Howard TA, et al, "Chemical and Functional Analysis of Hydroxyurea Oral Solutions," *J Pediatr Hematol Oncol* 2004, 26(3):179-84.

Nahata MC, Morosco RS, Boster EA, et al, "Stability of Hydroxyurea in Two Extemporaneously Prepared Oral Suspensions Stored at Two Temperatures," 2003, 38:P-161(E) [abstract from 2003 ASHP Midyear Clinical Meeting].

Monitoring Parameters CBC with differential and platelets (once weekly for antineoplastic indications; every 2 weeks initially for sickle cell anemia), renal function and liver function tests, serum uric acid; hemoglobin F levels (sickle cell disease); pregnancy status prior to therapy initiation in women of reproductive potential; monitor for cutaneous toxicities

Sickle cell disease: Monitor for toxicity every 2 weeks during dose escalation (neutrophils, platelets, hemoglobin, reticulocytes) (manufacturer's labeling) or at least every 4 weeks when adjusting the dose (CBC with WBC differential, reticulocytes) [NHLBI 2014]). Once on a stable dose, may monitor CBC with differential, reticulocyte count and platelets every 2 to 3 months (NHLBI 2014). Monitor RBC, MCV (mean corpuscular volume) and HbF (fetal hemoglobin) levels for evidence of consistent or progressive laboratory response (NHLBI 2014).

Test Interactions False-negative triglyceride measurement by a glycerol oxidase method. An analytical interference between hydroxyurea and enzymes (lactate dehydrogenase, urease, and uricase) may result in false elevations of lactic acid, urea, and uric acid.

Dietary Considerations Supplemental administration of folic acid is recommended; hydroxyurea may mask development of folic acid deficiency.

Dosage Forms Excipient information presented when available (limited, particularly for generics); consult specific product labeling.

Capsule, Oral:

Droxia: 200 mg, 300 mg [contains brilliant blue fcf (fd&c blue #1)]

Droxia: 400 mg [contains fd&c yellow #10 (quinoline yellow)]

Hydrea: 500 mg

Generic: 500 mg

◆ **Hydurea** see Hydroxyurea on page 925

◆ **Hylenex** see Hyaluronidase on page 917

◆ **HyperRHO S/D** see $Rh_o(D)$ Immune Globulin on page 1591

◆ **Hyqvia** see Immune Globulin on page 992

◆ **I^{123} Iobenguane** see Iobenguane I 123 on page 1029

◆ **I-123 MIBG** see Iobenguane I 123 on page 1029

Ibandronate (oye BAN droh nate)

Related Information

Hypercalcemia of Malignancy on page 2341

Brand Names: US Boniva

Index Terms Bondronate; Ibandronate Sodium; Ibandronic Acid

Pharmacologic Category Bisphosphonate Derivative

Use

Postmenopausal osteoporosis: Treatment and prevention of osteoporosis in postmenopausal females.

Limitations of use: The optimal duration has not been determined. Safety and efficacy for osteoporosis treatment are based on clinical data of 3-years duration (oral) and 1-year duration (IV). All patients on bisphosphonate therapy should be re-evaluated periodically for the need to continue therapy. Consider discontinuing after 3 to 5 years in patients at low-risk for fracture. Re-evaluate fracture risk periodically in patients who discontinue therapy.

Labeled Contraindications

Known hypersensitivity to ibandronate or any component of the formulation; hypocalcemia; oral tablets are also contraindicated in patients unable to stand or sit upright for at least 60 minutes and in patients with abnormalities of the esophagus which delay esophageal emptying, such as stricture or achalasia.

Documentation of allergenic cross-reactivity for bisphosphonates is limited. However, because of similarities in chemical structure and/or pharmacologic actions, the possibility of cross-sensitivity cannot be ruled out with certainty.

Pregnancy Considerations Adverse effects were observed in animal reproduction studies. It is not known if bisphosphonates cross the placenta, but fetal exposure is expected (Djokanovic, 2008; Stathopoulos, 2011). Bisphosphonates are incorporated into the bone matrix and gradually released over time. The amount available in the systemic circulation varies by dose and duration of therapy. Theoretically, there may be a risk of fetal harm when pregnancy follows the completion of therapy; however, available data have not shown that exposure to bisphosphonates during pregnancy significantly increases the risk of adverse fetal events (Djokanovic, 2008; Levy, 2009; Stathopoulos, 2011). Until additional data is available, most sources recommend discontinuing bisphosphonate therapy in women of reproductive potential as early as possible prior to a planned pregnancy; use in premenopausal women should be reserved for special circumstances when rapid bone loss is occurring (Bhalla, 2010; Pereira, 2012; Stathopoulos, 2011). Because hypocalcemia has been described following in utero bisphosphonate exposure, exposed infants should be monitored for hypocalcemia after birth (Djokanovic, 2008; Stathopoulos, 2011).

Breastfeeding Considerations It is not known if ibandronate is excreted into breast milk.

Warnings/Precautions Hypocalcemia must be corrected before therapy initiation. Ensure adequate calcium and vitamin D intake.

Atypical femur fractures have been reported in patients receiving bisphosphonates for treatment/prevention of osteoporosis. The fractures include subtrochanteric femur (bone just below the hip joint) and diaphyseal femur (long segment of the thigh bone). Some patients experience prodromal pain weeks or months before the fracture occurs. It is unclear if bisphosphonate therapy is the cause for these fractures, although the majority of cases have been reported in patients taking bisphosphonates. Patients receiving long-term (>3-5 years) therapy may be at an increased risk. Discontinue bisphosphonate therapy in patients who develop a femoral shaft fracture.

Infrequently, severe (and occasionally debilitating) bone, joint, and/or muscle pain have been reported during bisphosphonate treatment. The onset of pain ranged from a single day to several months. Discontinue intravenous ibandronate therapy in patients who experience severe symptoms; symptoms usually resolve upon discontinuation. Some patients experienced recurrence when rechallenged with same drug or another bisphosphonate; avoid use in patients with a history of these symptoms in association with bisphosphonate therapy.

Oral bisphosphonates may cause dysphagia, esophagitis, esophageal or gastric ulcer; risk may increase in patients unable to comply with dosing instructions; discontinue use if new or worsening symptoms develop. Intravenous bisphosphonates may cause transient decreases in serum calcium and have also been associated with renal toxicity.

Osteonecrosis of the jaw (ONJ), also referred to as medication-related osteonecrosis of the jaw (MRONJ), has been reported in patients receiving bisphosphonates. Known risk factors for MRONJ include invasive dental procedures (eg, tooth extraction, dental implants, boney surgery), cancer diagnosis, concomitant therapy (eg, chemotherapy, corticosteroids, angiogenesis inhibitors), poor oral hygiene, ill-fitting dentures, and comorbid disorders (anemia, coagulopathy, infection, preexisting dental or periodontal disease). Risk may increase with increased duration of bisphosphonate use. According to a position paper by the American Association of Maxillofacial Surgeons (AAOMS), MRONJ has been associated with bisphosphonates and other antiresorptive agents (denosumab), and antiangiogenic agents (eg, bevacizumab, sunitinib) used for the treatment of osteoporosis or malignancy; risk is significantly higher in cancer patients receiving antiresorptive therapy compared to patients receiving osteoporosis treatment (regardless of medication used or dosing schedule). MRONJ risk is also increased with monthly

IV antiresorptive therapy compared to the minimal risk associated with oral bisphosphonate use, although risk appears to increase with oral bisphosphonates when duration of therapy exceeds 4 years (AAOMS [Ruggiero 2014]). The manufacturer's labeling states that discontinuing bisphosphonates in patients requiring invasive dental procedures may reduce the risk of ONJ and clinical judgment by physician and/or oral surgeon should be used. However, the AAOMS suggests there is currently no evidence that interrupting oral bisphosphonate therapy alters the risk of ONJ following tooth extraction, and that no alternations or delay in any procedure common to oral/maxillofacial surgeons, periodontists, and other dental providers is necessary in patients receiving oral bisphosphonates for <4 years who have no clinical risk factors (special considerations apply to patients receiving dental implants). Conversely, in patients receiving oral bisphosphonates for >4 years **or** in patients receiving oral bisphosphonates for <4 years who have also taken corticosteroids or antiangiogenic medications concomitantly, the AAOMS recommends considering a 2-month drug free period prior to invasive dental procedures based on a theoretical benefit. Patients developing ONJ during therapy should receive care by an oral surgeon (AAOMS [Ruggiero 2014]). According to the manufacturer, discontinuation of oral bisphosphonate therapy should be considered (based on risk/benefit evaluation) in patients who develop ONJ.

Allergic reactions, including anaphylactic reaction/shock (some fatal), angioedema, bronchospasm, exacerbation of asthma, rash, Stevens-Johnson syndrome, erythema multiforme, and dermatitis bullous have been reported; discontinue immediately if anaphylactic or other severe hypersensitivity/allergic reactions occur. Use not recommended with severe renal impairment (CrCl <30 mL/minute). In the management of osteoporosis, re-evaluate the need for continued therapy periodically; the optimal duration of treatment has not yet been determined. Consider discontinuing after 3-5 years of use in patients at low-risk for fracture; following discontinuation, re-evaluate fracture risk periodically. Potentially significant drug-drug interactions may exist, requiring dose or frequency adjustment, additional monitoring, and/or selection of alternative therapy.

Adverse Reactions Percentages vary based on frequency of administration (daily vs monthly). Unless specified, percentages are reported with oral use.
>10%:
  Gastrointestinal: Dyspepsia (4% to 12%)
  Neuromuscular & skeletal: Back pain (4% to 14%)
  Respiratory: Upper respiratory tract infection (2% to 34%)
1% to 10%:
  Cardiovascular: Hypertension (6% to 7%)
  Central nervous system: Headache (3% to 7%), dizziness (1% to 4%), fatigue (3%), insomnia (1% to 2%), depression (2%)
  Dermatologic: Skin rash (1% to 2%)
  Gastrointestinal: Abdominal pain (5% to 8%), diarrhea (2% to 7%), nausea (4% to 5%), dental disease (4%), constipation (3% to 4%), vomiting (3%), gastritis (2%), gastroenteritis (3%)
  Genitourinary: Urinary tract infection (2% to 6%), cystitis (3%)
  Hypersensitivity: Acute phase reaction-like symptoms (IV: 10%; oral: 3% to 9%), hypersensitivity reaction (3%)
  Infection: Influenza (4% to 8%)
  Local: Injection site reaction (<2%)

Neuromuscular & skeletal: Limb pain (1% to 8%), arthralgia (4% to 9%), myalgia (1% to 6%), arthropathy (4%), weakness (4%), localized osteoarthritis (1% to 3%), muscle cramps (2%)

Respiratory: Bronchitis (3% to 10%), pneumonia (6%), nasopharyngitis (3% to 4%), flu-like symptoms (1% to 3%), pharyngitis (3%)

Postmarketing and/or case reports: Acute renal failure, anaphylactic shock, anaphylaxis, angioedema, bronchospasm, bullous dermatitis, erythema multiforme, exacerbation of asthma, femur fracture (diaphyseal or subtrochanteric), hypocalcemia, iritis, musculoskeletal pain (bone, joint, or muscle; incapacitating), ophthalmic inflammation, osteonecrosis (oro-facial sites including the external auditory canal), osteonecrosis of the jaw, prolonged Q-T interval on ECG (Bonilla 2014), scleritis, Stevens-Johnson syndrome, uveitis

Drug Interactions

Metabolism/Transport Effects None known.

Avoid Concomitant Use There are no known interactions where it is recommended to avoid concomitant use.

Increased Effect/Toxicity

Ibandronate may increase the levels/effects of: Deferasirox; Highest Risk QTc-Prolonging Agents; Moderate Risk QTc-Prolonging Agents

The levels/effects of Ibandronate may be increased by: Aminoglycosides; MiFEPRIStone; Nonsteroidal Anti-Inflammatory Agents; Systemic Angiogenesis Inhibitors

Decreased Effect

The levels/effects of Ibandronate may be decreased by: Antacids; Calcium Salts; Iron Salts; Magnesium Salts; Multivitamins/Minerals (with ADEK, Folate, Iron); Multivitamins/Minerals (with AE, No Iron); Proton Pump Inhibitors

Food Interactions Food may reduce absorption; mean oral bioavailability is decreased up to 90% when given with food. Management: Take with a full glass (6-8 oz) of plain water, at least 60 minutes prior to any food, beverages, or medications. Mineral water with a high calcium content should be avoided. Wait at least 60 minutes after taking ibandronate before taking anything else.

Storage/Stability Store at 25°C (77°F); excursions permitted to 15°C to 30°C (59°F to 86°F).

Mechanism of Action A bisphosphonate which inhibits bone resorption via actions on osteoclasts or on osteoclast precursors; decreases the rate of bone resorption, leading to an indirect increase in bone mineral density.

Pharmacodynamics/Kinetics

Distribution: Terminal V_d: 90 L; 40% to 50% of circulating ibandronate binds to bone

Protein binding: 85.7% to 99.5%

Metabolism: Not metabolized

Bioavailability: Oral: Minimal; reduced ~90% following standard breakfast

Half-life elimination:

Oral: 150 mg dose: Terminal: 37 to 157 hours

IV: Terminal: ~5 to 25 hours

Time to peak, plasma: Oral: 0.5 to 2 hours

Excretion: Urine (50% to 60% of absorbed dose, excreted as unchanged drug); feces (unabsorbed drug)

Dosing
Adult & Geriatric
Postmenopausal osteoporosis (treatment): Note: Consider discontinuing after 3 to 5 years of use for osteoporosis in patients at low-risk for fracture. Patients should receive supplemental calcium and vitamin D if dietary intake is inadequate.

Oral: 150 mg once monthly

IV: 3 mg every 3 months

Postmenopausal osteoporosis (prevention): Oral: 150 mg once monthly. **Note:** Patients should receive supplemental calcium and vitamin D if dietary intake is inadequate.

Hypercalcemia of malignancy (off-label use): IV: 2 to 6 mg over 1-2 hours (Pecherstorfer 2003; Ralston 1997)

Metastatic bone disease due to breast cancer (off-label use): IV: 6 mg every 3 to 4 weeks (Diel 2004)

Missed doses:

Oral: If once-monthly oral dose is missed, it should be given the next morning after remembered if the next month's scheduled dose is >7 days away. If the next month's scheduled dose is within 7 days, wait until the next month's scheduled dose. May then return to the original monthly schedule (original scheduled day of the month). Do not give >150 mg within 7 days.

IV: If an IV dose is missed, it should be administered as soon as it can be rescheduled. Thereafter, it should be given every 3 months from the date of the last injection.

Renal Impairment
Osteoporosis: Oral, IV:

CrCl ≥30 mL/minute: No dosage adjustment necessary.

CrCl <30 mL/minute: Use not recommended.

Oncologic uses (off-label): IV: CrCl <30 mL/minute: 2 mg every 3 to 4 weeks (von Moos 2005)

Hepatic Impairment There are no dosage adjustments provided in the manufacturer's labeling (has not been studied); however, ibandronate does not undergo hepatic metabolism.

Administration
Oral: Administer 60 minutes before the first food or drink of the day (other than water) and prior to taking any oral medications or supplements (eg, calcium, antacids, vitamins). Ibandronate should be taken in an upright position with a full glass (6-8 oz) of plain water and the patient should avoid lying down for 60 minutes to minimize the possibility of GI side effects. Mineral water with a high calcium content should be avoided. The tablet should be swallowed whole; do not chew or suck. Do not eat or drink anything (except water) for 60 minutes following administration of ibandronate.

IV: Administer as a 15-30 second bolus intravenously; avoid paravenous or intraarterial administration (may cause tissue damage). Do not mix with calcium-containing solutions or other drugs. For osteoporosis, do not administer more frequently than every 3 months. Infuse over 1 hour for metastatic bone disease due to breast cancer (Diel, 2004) and over 1-2 hours for hypercalcemia of malignancy (Pecherstorfer, 2003; Ralston, 1997).

Monitoring Parameters
Osteoporosis: Bone mineral density (BMD) should be evaluated 1 to 2 years after initiating therapy and every 2 years thereafter (NOF [Cosman 2014]); annual measurements of height and weight, assessment of chronic back

pain; serum calcium and 25(OH)D; may consider measuring biochemical markers of bone turnover

Serum creatinine prior to each IV dose

Test Interactions Bisphosphonates may interfere with diagnostic imaging agents such as technetium-99m-diphosphonate in bone scans.

Dietary Considerations

Ensure adequate calcium and vitamin D intake; if dietary intake is inadequate, dietary supplementation is recommended. Women and men should consume:

Calcium: 1,000 mg/day (men: 50 to 70 years) **or** 1,200 mg/day (women ≥51 years and men ≥71 years) (IOM 2011; NOF [Cosman 2014])

Vitamin D: 800 to 1,000 int. units daily (men and women ≥50 years) (NOF [Cosman 2014]). Recommended Dietary Allowance (RDA): 600 int. units daily (men and women ≤70 years) **or** 800 int. units daily (men and women ≥71 years) (IOM 2011).

Ibandronate tablet should be taken with a full glass (6 to 8 oz) of plain water, at least 60 minutes prior to any food, beverages, or medications. Mineral water with a high calcium content should be avoided.

Medication Guide Available Yes

Dosage Forms Excipient information presented when available (limited, particularly for generics); consult specific product labeling.

Solution, Intravenous:

Boniva: 3 mg/3 mL (3 mL)

Generic: 3 mg/3 mL (3 mL)

Solution, Intravenous [preservative free]:

Generic: 3 mg/3 mL (3 mL)

Tablet, Oral:

Boniva: 150 mg

Generic: 150 mg

◆ **Ibandronate Sodium** *see* Ibandronate *on page 933*

◆ **Ibandronic Acid** *see* Ibandronate *on page 933*

◆ **Ibenzmethyzin** *see* Procarbazine *on page 1557*

◆ **Ibrance** *see* Palbociclib *on page 1421*

Ibritumomab (ib ri TYOO mo mab)

Related Information

Management of Drug Extravasations *on page 2271*

Brand Names: US Zevalin Y-90

Brand Names: Canada Zevalin

Index Terms Ibritumomab Tiuxetan; IDEC-Y2B8; Y-90 Ibritumomab; Y-90 Zevalin

Pharmacologic Category Antineoplastic Agent, Anti-CD20; Antineoplastic Agent, Monoclonal Antibody; Radiopharmaceutical

Use Non-Hodgkin lymphoma: Treatment of relapsed or refractory, low-grade or follicular B-cell non-Hodgkin lymphoma (NHL); treatment of previously untreated follicular NHL in patients who achieve a partial or complete response to first-line chemotherapy

Labeled Contraindications There are no contraindications listed within the manufacturer's labeling.

Pregnancy Considerations Animal reproduction studies have not been conducted. Based on the radioactivity, Y-90 ibritumomab may cause fetal harm if administered during pregnancy. IgG molecules are known to cross the placenta. Women of reproductive potential should avoid becoming pregnant during treatment with ibritumomab. Females of reproductive potential and males with female partners of reproductive potential should use effective contraception for at least 12 months following treatment. The effect on future fertility is unknown.

Breastfeeding Considerations It is not known whether ibritumomab is present in breast milk. Because many immunoglobulins are excreted in milk and due to the potential for serious adverse reactions in the breastfeeding infant, a decision should be made to either discontinue breastfeeding or to not administer ibritumomab, taking into account the importance of treatment to the mother.

Warnings/Precautions Radiopharmaceutical; use appropriate precautions for handling, disposal, and minimizing exposure to patients and healthcare personnel. Use only under supervision of individuals with experience/training in the handling of radioactive materials approved by the applicable regulatory authority. **[US Boxed Warning]: Severe cutaneous and mucocutaneous skin reactions have been reported (with fatalities). Discontinue all components of the therapeutic regimen in patients experiencing severe cutaneous or mucocutaneous skin reactions,** including erythema multiforme, Stevens-Johnson syndrome, toxic epidermal necrolysis, bullous dermatitis, and exfoliative dermatitis. Onset may occur within days to 4 months following infusion.

To be used as part of the Zevalin therapeutic regimen (in combination with rituximab). **[US Boxed Warning]: Do not exceed the Y-90 ibritumomab maximum allowable dose of 32 mCi (1184 MBq).** Use should be reserved to physicians and other professionals qualified and experienced in the safe handling of radiopharmaceuticals, and in monitoring and emergency treatment of infusion reactions. The contents of the kit are not radioactive until radiolabeling occurs. During and after radiolabeling, adequate shielding should be used with this product, minimize radiation exposure (to patient and healthcare professionals) in accordance with institutional radiation safety practices.

[US Boxed Warning]: Serious fatal infusion reactions may occur with the rituximab component of the therapeutic regimen. Immediately stop infusion and discontinue all components of the therapeutic regimen in patients who develop severe infusion reactions. Fatalities due to rituximab infusion were associated with acute respiratory distress syndrome, hypoxia, pulmonary infiltrates, cardiogenic shock, MI, or ventricular fibrillation; 80% of fatalities occurred with the first rituximab infusion. Administer in a facility with immediate access to resuscitative measures. Infusion reactions typically occur with the first rituximab infusion (onset within 30 to 120 minutes). Reactions may also include hypotension, angioedema, bronchospasm, and urticaria. Less severe reactions may be managed by slowing or interrupting infusion.

[US Boxed Warning]: Delayed, prolonged, and severe cytopenias (thrombocytopenia and neutropenia) are common. Do not administer to patients with ≥25% lymphoma marrow involvement, patients with impaired bone marrow reserve (eg, prior myeloablative treatment, platelet count <100,000/mm³, neutrophil count <1,500/mm³, hypocellular marrow), or to patients with prior stem cell collection failure. In studies, the median platelet, ANC, and hemoglobin nadir was 49 to 53 days, 61 to 62 days, and 68 to 69 days, respectively. Cytopenias may persist beyond 12 weeks. The median ▶

duration of thrombocytopenia and neutropenia was 24 to 35 days and 22 to 29 days respectively, and the median time to platelet and ANC recovery was 13 to 14 days and 12 to 15 days, respectively. Patients with mild baseline thrombocytopenia may experience higher incidences of severe neutropenia and thrombocytopenia. Hemorrhage may occur due to thrombocytopenia; avoid concomitant use of medications interfering with coagulation or platelet function. Monitor CBC and platelets weekly until recovery or as clinically indicated. Closely monitor patients for complications of cytopenias (eg, febrile neutropenia, hemorrhage) for up to 3 months after administration.

American Society of Clinical Oncology (ASCO) provisional clinical opinion update on hepatitis B virus screening recommendations (Hwang 2015): Patients receiving anti-CD20 antibodies are at high risk for hepatitis B virus (HBV) reactivation. Screen for HBV infection with hepatitis B surface antigen (HBsAg) and hepatitis B core antibody (anti-HBc) tests prior to treatment initiation; either a total anti-HBc (with both IgG and IgM) or anti-HBc IgG test should be used to screen for chronic or resolved HBV infection (do not use anti-HBc IgM as it may only confirm acute HBV infection). In addition, patients who have risk factors for HBV infection (eg, birthplace in a country with ≥2% HBV prevalence, household or sexual contact with HBV infected patients, high-risk behaviors [eg, IV drug use], and HIV infection) should also be screened prior to beginning therapy. Initiate prophylactic antiviral therapy (utilizing antivirals with low rates of viral resistance) for HBsAg positive/anti-HBc positive patients (without delaying cancer therapy) and continue the antivirals during and for ~6 to 12 months after completing treatment. HBsAg negative/anti-HBc positive patients should be monitored for HBV reactivation with HBV DNA and ALT testing approximately every 3 months during treatment; antiviral therapy may be initiated prophylactically or begun promptly at the first sign of HBV reactivation. Malignancies due to the radiation dose from therapeutic exposure may occur. Secondary malignancies (acute myelogenous leukemia and/or myelodysplastic syndrome) have been reported following use; the median time to diagnosis (secondary malignancy) following ibritumomab treatment was 1.9 years with a range of 0.4 to 6.3 years (Czuczman 2007). Product contains albumin, which confers a theoretical risk of transmission of viral disease or Creutzfeldt-Jakob disease. The safety of immunization with live vaccines following ibritumomab therapy has not been studied; do not administer live viral vaccines to patients who have recently received ibritumomab treatment; the ability to generate a response to any vaccine after receiving treatment has not been studied. Potentially significant drug-drug interactions may exist, requiring dose or frequency adjustment, additional monitoring, and/or selection of alternative therapy. Infusion site erythema and ulceration have been reported following extravasation; monitor infusion site; promptly terminate infusion with symptoms/signs of extravasation (restart in another limb). There is a case report of (delayed) erythema and ulceration, which is described as radiation necrosis following yttrium-90-ibritumomab extravasation (Williams 2006). Delayed (up to 1 month) radiation injury has occurred in or near areas of lymphomatous involvement. In a postmarketing registry of biodistribution images, biodistribution was altered in a limited number of patients.

Adverse Reactions

>10%:

Central nervous system: Fatigue (33%)

Gastrointestinal: Nausea (18%), abdominal pain (17%), diarrhea (11%)

Hematologic & oncologic: Thrombocytopenia (62% to 95%; grades 3/4: 51% to 63%; nadir: 49-53 days; median duration: 24 days; median time to recovery: 13 days), neutropenia (45% to 77%; grades 3/4: 41% to 60%; nadir: 61-62 days; median duration: 22 days; median time to recovery: 12 days), anemia (22% to 61%; grades 3/4: 5% to 17%; nadir: 68-69 days), leukopenia (43%; grades 3/4: 36%), lymphocytopenia (26%; grades 3/4: 18%), metastases (1% to 13%; includes acute myelogenous leukemia and myelodysplastic syndrome)

Infection: Infection (within first 3 months: 29%; serious: 1% to 3%; 3 months to 4 years after treatment: 6%)

Neuromuscular & skeletal: Weakness (15%)

Respiratory: Nasopharyngitis (19%), cough (11%)

1% to 10%:

Cardiovascular: Hypertension (7%)

Central nervous system: Dizziness (7%)

Dermatologic: Night sweats (8%), pruritus (7%), skin rash (7%)

Gastrointestinal: Anorexia (8%)

Genitourinary: Urinary tract infection (7%)

Hematologic & oncologic: Petechia (8%), bruise (7%), severe cytopenia (prolonged: 5%)

Immunologic: Antibody development (HAMA/HACA: 1% to 3%)

Neuromuscular & skeletal: Myalgia (9%)

Respiratory: Bronchitis (8%), flu-like symptoms (8%), rhinitis (8%), pharyngolaryngeal pain (7%), sinusitis (7%), epistaxis (5%)

Miscellaneous: Fever (10%), biodistribution altered (1%)

<1%, postmarketing, and/or case reports: Adult respiratory distress syndrome, angioedema, bullous dermatitis, cardiogenic shock, chills, dyspnea, erythema multiforme, exfoliative dermatitis, febrile neutropenia, headache, hypoxia, infusion-related reaction, injection site reaction (erythema/ulceration following extravasation), myocardial infarction, pain, pulmonary infiltrates, radiation injury (delayed [~1 month]; in tissues in or near areas of lymphomatous involvement), sepsis, Stevens-Johnson syndrome, tissue necrosis (following Yttrium-90-ibritumomab extravasation), toxic epidermal necrolysis, ventricular fibrillation, vomiting

Drug Interactions

Metabolism/Transport Effects None known.

Avoid Concomitant Use

Avoid concomitant use of Ibritumomab with any of the following: BCG (Intravesical); Belimumab; Deferiprone; Dipyrone; Natalizumab; Pimecrolimus; Tacrolimus (Topical); Vaccines (Live)

Increased Effect/Toxicity

Ibritumomab may increase the levels/effects of: Belimumab; CloZAPine; Deferiprone; Fingolimod; Leflunomide; Natalizumab; Tofacitinib; Vaccines (Live)

The levels/effects of Ibritumomab may be increased by: Agents with Antiplatelet Properties; Anticoagulants; Denosumab; Dipyrone; Ocrelizumab; Pimecrolimus; Promazine; Roflumilast; Tacrolimus (Topical); Trastuzumab

Decreased Effect

Ibritumomab may decrease the levels/effects of: BCG (Intravesical); Coccidioides immitis Skin Test; Nivolumab; Sipuleucel-T; Tertomotide; Vaccines (Inactivated); Vaccines (Live)

The levels/effects of Ibritumomab may be decreased by: Echinacea

◀ **Storage/Stability** Store kits at 2°C to 8°C (36°F to 46°F). Do not freeze. Administer Y-90 ibritumomab tiuxetan within 8 hours of radiolabeling.

Preparation for Administration Radiopharmaceutical; use appropriate precautions for handling and disposal. To prepare radiolabeled injection and determine radiochemical purity, follow detailed preparation guidelines provided by manufacturer. Use appropriate shielding during and after radiolabeling.

Mechanism of Action Ibritumomab is a monoclonal antibody directed against the CD20 antigen found on pre-B and mature B lymphocytes (normal and malignant). Ibritumomab binding induces apoptosis in B lymphocytes *in vitro*. It is combined with the chelator tiuxetan, which acts as a specific chelation site for Yttrium-90 (Y-90). The monoclonal antibody acts as a delivery system to direct the radioactive isotope to the targeted cells, however, binding has been observed in lymphoid cells throughout the body and in lymphoid nodules in organs such as the large and small intestines. Beta-emission induces cellular damage through the formation of free radicals (in both target cells and surrounding cells).

Pharmacodynamics/Kinetics

Duration: B cell recovery begins in ~12 weeks; generally in normal range within 9 months

Distribution: To lymphoid cells throughout the body and in lymphoid nodules in organs such as the large and small intestines, spleen, testes, and liver

Metabolism: Has not been characterized; the product of yttrium-90 radioactive decay is zirconium-90 (nonradioactive)

Half-life elimination: Y-90 ibritumomab: 30 hours; Yttrium-90 decays with a physical half-life of 64 hours

Excretion: A median of 7.2% of the radiolabeled activity was excreted in urine over 7 days

Dosing

Adult & Geriatric Note: Premedicate with oral acetaminophen 650 mg and oral diphenhydramine 50 mg prior to **each** rituximab infusion. Allow at least 6 weeks, but no more than 12 weeks following first-line chemotherapy before treatment initiation; platelets should recover to ≥150,000/mm^3 prior to initiation of treatment regimen.

Non-Hodgkin lymphoma: Ibritumomab is administered **only** as part of the Zevalin therapeutic regimen (a combined treatment regimen with rituximab). The regimen consists of two steps:

Day 1:
Rituximab: IV: 250 mg/m^2 at an initial rate of 50 mg/hour. If hypersensitivity or infusion-related events do not occur, increase infusion in increments of 50 mg/hour every 30 minutes, to a maximum of 400 mg/hour. Stop rituximab and discontinue regimen for severe infusion reaction. For less severe infusion reactions, temporarily slow or interrupt; the infusion may be resumed at one-half the previous rate upon improvement of symptoms.

Day 7, 8, or 9 of treatment:
Rituximab: IV: 250 mg/m^2 at an initial rate of 100 mg/hour (50 mg/hour if infusion-related events occurred with the day 1 infusion). If hypersensitivity or infusion-related events do not occur, increase infusion in increments of 100 mg/hour every 30 minutes, to a maximum of 400 mg/hour, as tolerated (increase in 50 mg/hour increments every 30 minutes if initial infusion rate was 50 mg/hour).

Y-90 ibritumomab (within 4 hours after completion of the rituximab infusion): IV:

Platelet count ≥150,000 cells/mm^3: 0.4 mCi/kg (14.8 MBq/kg) actual body weight over 10 minutes; maximum dose: 32 mCi (1184 MBq)

Platelet count between 100,000 to 149,000 cells/mm^3 (in relapsed or refractory patients): 0.3 mCi/kg (11.1 MBq/kg) actual body weight over 10 minutes; maximum dose: 32 mCi (1184 MBq)

Platelet count <100,000 cells/mm^3: Do **not** administer

Maximum dose: The prescribed, measured, and administered dose of Y-90 ibritumomab must not exceed 32 mCi (1184 MBq), regardless of the patient's body weight

Renal Impairment There are no dosage adjustments provided in the manufacturer's labeling.

Hepatic Impairment There are no dosage adjustments provided in the manufacturer's labeling.

Administration

Rituximab: Administer the first infusion of rituximab at an initial rate of 50 mg/hour. If hypersensitivity or infusion-related events do not occur, escalate the infusion rate in 50 mg/hour increments every 30 minutes, to a maximum of 400 mg/hour. Immediately stop infusion for severe infusion reaction (discontinue ibritumomab regimen); less severe reactions may be managed by slowing or interrupting infusion. For less severe reactions, infusion may continue at one-half the previous rate upon improvement of patient symptoms. If infusion reaction did not occur in initial rituximab infusion, subsequent rituximab infusion can be administered at an initial rate of 100 mg/hour and increased in 100 mg/hour increments at 30-minute intervals, to a maximum of 400 mg/hour as tolerated. If infusion reaction occurred with initial rituximab infusion, initiate at 50 mg/hour with increases of 50 mg/hour increments every 30 minutes.

Y-90 ibritumomab: Begin within 4 hours of completion of rituximab infusion. Inject slowly, over 10 minutes through a 0.22 micron low protein binding in-line filter (filter placed between syringe and infusion port) into a free-flowing IV line. After injection, flush line with at least 10 mL normal saline. Avoid extravasation; closely monitor infusion site; if signs or symptoms of extravasation occur, stop infusion and restart in another limb.

Radiopharmaceutical; use appropriate precautions for handling and disposal.

Vesicant/Extravasation Risk May be an irritant; there is an isolated case report of (delayed) erythema and ulceration, which is described as radiation necrosis following yttrium-90-ibritumomab extravasation (Williams 2006).

Monitoring Parameters

CBC with differential and platelet counts weekly until recovery, or as clinically indicated. Platelet count must be obtained prior to day 7, 8, or 9; monitor for cytopenias (and related complications) for up to 3 months after use.

Hepatitis B virus screening recommendations (ASCO provisional clinical opinion update [Hwang 2015]): Screen for hepatitis B virus (HBV) infection with hepatitis B surface antigen (HBsAg) and hepatitis B core antibody (anti-HBc) tests prior to treatment initiation; either a total anti-HBc (with both IgG and IgM) or anti-HBc IgG test should be used to screen for chronic or resolved HBV infection (do not use anti-HBc IgM as it may only confirm acute HBV infection). HBsAg negative/anti-HBc positive patients should be monitored for HBV reactivation with HBV DNA and ALT testing approximately every 3 months during treatment.

◀ Monitor for signs of active hepatitis B infection (during and for up to 12 months after therapy completion). Monitor for infusion-related allergic reactions (typically within 30 to 120 minutes of administration), for extravasation during ibritumomab infusion; and for severe cutaneous and mucocutaneous reactions.

Additional Information Ibritumomab tiuxetan is produced in Chinese hamster ovary cell cultures. Kit is not radioactive. Radiolabeling of ibritumomab with Yttrium-90 must be performed by appropriate personnel in a specialized facility.

Dosage Forms Excipient information presented when available (limited, particularly for generics); consult specific product labeling.

Kit, Intravenous [preservative free]:

Zevalin Y-90: 3.2 mg/2 mL [pyrogen free; contains albumin human]

◆ **Ibritumomab Tiuxetan** *see* Ibritumomab *on page 938*

Ibrutinib (eye BROO ti nib)

Related Information
Hematopoietic Cell Transplantation *on page 2365*
Safe Handling of Hazardous Drugs *on page 2379*

Brand Names: US Imbruvica
Brand Names: Canada Imbruvica
Index Terms BTK Inhibitor PCI-32765; CRA-032765; PCI-32765
Pharmacologic Category Antineoplastic Agent; Antineoplastic Agent, Bruton Tyrosine Kinase Inhibitor; Antineoplastic Agent, Tyrosine Kinase Inhibitor

Use

Chronic graft-versus-host disease (refractory): Treatment of chronic graft-versus-host disease (cGVHD) after failure of one or more lines of systemic therapy.

Chronic lymphocytic leukemia/small lymphocytic lymphoma: Treatment of chronic lymphocytic leukemia/small lymphocytic lymphoma (CLL/SLL); treatment of CLL/SLL in patients with 17p deletion.

Mantle cell lymphoma, previously treated: Treatment of mantle cell lymphoma (MCL) in patients who have received at least 1 prior therapy

Marginal zone lymphoma, relapsed/refractory: Treatment of marginal zone lymphoma (MZL) in patients who require systemic therapy and have received at least one prior anti-CD20-based therapy.

Waldenström macroglobulinemia: Treatment of Waldenström macroglobulinemia

Labeled Contraindications
There are no contraindications listed in the manufacturer's US labeling.
Canadian labeling: Known hypersensitivity to ibrutinib or any component of the formulation.

Pregnancy Considerations Based on animal reproduction studies, ibrutinib may cause fetal harm if administered during pregnancy. For women of reproductive potential, verify pregnancy status prior to treatment initiation. Women of reproductive potential should avoid pregnancy during therapy and for up to 1 month after treatment cessation; males should avoid fathering a child during treatment and for 1 month after the last dose.

Breastfeeding Considerations It is not known if ibrutinib is present in breast milk. According to the manufacturer, the decision to breastfeed during therapy should take into account the risk of exposure to the breastfeeding infant and the benefits of treatment to the mother.

Warnings/Precautions Grade 3 and 4 neutropenia, thrombocytopenia, and anemia occurred commonly during clinical studies in patients who received single-agent ibrutinib for B-cell malignancies. Monitor blood counts monthly or as clinically necessary. Lymphocytosis (≥50% increase from baseline) may occur upon therapy initiation, generally within the first few weeks of therapy. The increase in lymphocytes is temporary, and resolves by a median of 8 weeks (mantle cell lymphoma) or 14 weeks (chronic lymphocytic leukemia). Some patients who developed lymphocytosis (lymphocytes >400,000/mcL) have developed intracranial hemorrhage, lethargy, headache, and gait instability (some cases may have been associated with disease progression). Monitor for leukostasis, particularly in patients experiencing a rapid increase in lymphocytes to >400,000/mcL. Grade 3 or higher bleeding events (intracranial hemorrhage [including subdural hematoma], gastrointestinal bleeding, hematuria, and post-procedural bleeding) have occurred; some events were fatal. Bleeding events of any grade, including bruising and petechiae, have occurred in approximately half of patients receiving ibrutinib. Monitor for signs of bleeding. Patients receiving concurrent antiplatelet or anticoagulant treatment may have an increased risk for bleeding. Evaluate the risk-benefit of withholding ibrutinib for 3 to 7 days prior to and after surgery, depending on the procedure type and risk of bleeding. Serious infections (some fatal) have been observed, including bacterial, viral, and fungal infections. Cases of *Pneumocystis jirovecii* pneumonia (PCP) have also been reported (Ahn 2016). Monitor and evaluate for fever and other signs/symptoms of infection and manage appropriately. Consider prophylaxis (according to standard of care) for patients at increased risk for opportunistic infections. Evaluate promptly. Progressive multifocal oncephalopathy (PML) has been observed; evaluate for symptoms and manage appropriately. Patients treated with ibrutinib have developed second primary malignancies, including skin cancers and other carcinomas. Evaluate for sign/symptoms of malignancy during treatment.

Atrial fibrillation and atrial flutter have occurred, particularly in patients with cardiac risk factors, hypertension, infections (acute), or with a history of atrial fibrillation. Monitor periodically for clinical symptoms of atrial fibrillation (eg, palpitations, light-headedness); an ECG should be performed if symptoms or new-onset dyspnea develop. Manage atrial fibrillation appropriately; for persistent atrial fibrillation, evaluate the risk-benefit of ibrutinib treatment and dose modification. Hypertension has been reported with ibrutinib therapy. The median onset of hypertension was 4.6 months (range: 0.03 to 22 months). Monitor for new onset hypertension or hypertension that is not adequately controlled after treatment initiation. May require antihypertensive therapy or adjustment of existing antihypertensive regimen. Hyperviscosity may require plasmapheresis prior to or during ibrutinib treatment in patients with Waldenström macroglobulinemia; adjustment of ibrutinib dose due to plasmapheresis is not necessary. Use with caution in patients with preexisting renal impairment; has not been studied in those with severe impairment or in patients on dialysis. Renal failure has been reported with use; some cases were fatal. Clinical trials report serum creatinine increases of up to 3 times ULN; monitor renal function periodically and maintain hydration. Tumor lysis syndrome has been reported (rare); increased uric acid levels have been observed, including grade 4 elevations. Assess risk for tumor lysis syndrome (eg, high tumor burden); monitor closely in patients at risk and manage appropriately. A retrospective analysis of a phase 3 efficacy trial in previously treated patients with chronic lymphocytic leukemia/small lymphocytic lymphoma evaluated the effect of dose intensity on progression-free survival (PFS) and overall response rate (ORR). A higher dose intensity was associated with longer median PFS and a higher ORR; optimal outcomes were achieved in patients with sustained adherence to a 420 mg/day dosing schedule (Barr 2017). Ibrutinib is hepatically metabolized, and exposure is increased in patients with hepatic dysfunction. Dosage adjustment is recommended in patients with mild (Child-Pugh class A) impairment; avoid use in patients with moderate or severe (Child-Pugh class B or C) impairment. Monitor closely for toxicity. May cause dizziness, fatigue, and/or weakness, which may impair physical or mental abilities; patients must be cautioned about performing tasks that require mental alertness (eg, operating machinery, driving). Potentially significant drug-drug/drug-food interactions may exist, requiring dose or frequency adjustment, additional monitoring, and/or selection of alternative therapy.

Adverse Reactions

>10%:

Cardiovascular: Peripheral edema (19% to 35%), hypertension (6% to 17%)

Central nervous system: Fatigue (21% to 44%), dizziness (11% to 20%), headache (12% to 18%), anxiety (16%), chills (12%)

Dermatologic: Skin rash (21% to 29%), skin infection (14% to 16%), pruritus (11% to 14%)

Endocrine & metabolic: Hyperuricemia (15% to 16%), hypoalbuminemia (14%), hypokalemia (13%), dehydration (12%)

Gastrointestinal: Diarrhea (37% to 59%), nausea (20% to 31%), constipation (14% to 25%), abdominal pain (14% to 24%), vomiting (11% to 23%), decreased appetite (16% to 21%), stomatitis (14% to 20%), dyspepsia (11% to 19%), gastroesophageal reflux disease (13%), upper abdominal pain (13%)

Genitourinary: Urinary tract infection (10% to 14%)

Hematologic & oncologic: Thrombocytopenia (43% to 69%; grades 3/4: 5% to 17%), neutropenia (22% to 53%; grades 3/4: 13% to 29%), bruise (12% to 51%; grades 3/4: ≤2%), decreased hemoglobin (13% to 43%; grades 3/4: ≤13%), hemorrhage (30%; grades ≥3: ≤6%; ≥ grade 3 bleeding events include gastrointestinal bleeding, hematuria, postprocedural hemorrhage, intracranial hemorrhage, subdural hematoma), petechia (11% to 16%), malignant neoplasm (secondary; 3% to 16%; non-melanoma skin cancer was most frequently reported; also includes carcinoma and one case of histiocytic sarcoma)

Infection: Infection

Neuromuscular & skeletal: Musculoskeletal pain (25% to 40%), arthralgia (11% to 24%), muscle spasm (11% to 21%), weakness (14%), arthropathy (13%)

Ophthalmic: Dry eye syndrome (17%), increased lacrimation (13%), blurred vision (10% to 13%), decreased visual acuity (11%)

Respiratory: Upper respiratory tract infection (16% to 47%), dyspnea (12% to 27%), cough (13% to 22%), sinusitis (11% to 22%), epistaxis (11% to 19%), pneumonia (11% to 15%), oropharyngeal pain (14%), bronchitis (11%)

Miscellaneous: Fever (17% to 25%)

1% to 10%:

Cardiovascular: Atrial fibrillation (≤9%), atrial flutter (≤9%)

Renal: Increased serum creatinine (1.5 to 3 x ULN: 9)

<1%, postmarketing, and/or case reports: Abnormal platelet aggregation (Kamel 2015), hepatic failure, hypersensitivity (includes anaphylactic shock, angioedema, urticaria), interstitial pulmonary disease, onychoclasis,

pneumonia due to *Pneumocystis carinii*, pneumonitis (Mato 2016), progressive multifocal leukoencephalopathy, renal failure, Stevens-Johnson syndrome, tumor lysis syndrome

Drug Interactions

Metabolism/Transport Effects Substrate of CYP2D6 (minor), CYP3A4 (major); **Note:** Assignment of Major/Minor substrate status based on clinically relevant drug interaction potential

Avoid Concomitant Use

Avoid concomitant use of Ibrutinib with any of the following: BCG (Intravesical); Bitter Orange; Conivaptan; CYP3A4 Inducers (Strong); CYP3A4 Inhibitors (Strong); Deferiprone; DilTIAZem; Dipyrone; Fusidic Acid (Systemic); Grapefruit Juice; Idelalisib; Natalizumab; Pimecrolimus; St John's Wort; Tacrolimus (Topical); Vaccines (Live)

Increased Effect/Toxicity

Ibrutinib may increase the levels/effects of: Agents with Antiplatelet Properties; Anticoagulants; CloZAPine; Deferiprone; Digoxin; Fingolimod; Leflunomide; Methotrexate; Natalizumab; Tofacitinib; Vaccines (Live)

The levels/effects of Ibrutinib may be increased by: Bitter Orange; Cimetidine; Ciprofloxacin (Systemic); Clotrimazole (Oral); Conivaptan; CycloSPORINE (Systemic); CYP3A4 Inhibitors (Moderate); CYP3A4 Inhibitors (Strong); Dasatinib; Denosumab; DilTIAZem; Dipyrone; Flaxseed Oil; FluvoxaMINE; Fosaprepitant; Fusidic Acid (Systemic); Grapefruit Juice; Idelalisib; Ocrelizumab; Omega-3 Fatty Acids; Palbociclib; Pimecrolimus; Posaconazole; Promazine; Roflumilast; Simeprevir; Stiripentol; Tacrolimus (Topical); Tofisopam; Trastuzumab; Vitamin E (Systemic); Voriconazole

Decreased Effect

Ibrutinib may decrease the levels/effects of: BCG (Intravesical); Coccidioides immitis Skin Test; Nivolumab; Sipuleucel-T; Tertomotide; Vaccines (Inactivated); Vaccines (Live)

The levels/effects of Ibrutinib may be decreased by: Bosentan; CYP3A4 Inducers (Moderate); CYP3A4 Inducers (Strong); Dabrafenib; Deferasirox; Echinacea; Sarilumab; Siltuximab; St John's Wort; Tocilizumab

Food Interactions Grapefruit and Seville oranges inhibit CYP3A (moderately or strongly) and may increase ibrutinib exposure. Management: Avoid grapefruit and Seville oranges during therapy.

Hazardous Drugs Handling Considerations

This medication is not on the NIOSH (2016) list; however, it may meet the criteria for a hazardous drug. Drugs are classified as hazardous based on their properties; the properties of a hazardous drug include one or more of the following characteristics: carcinogenic, teratogenic (or other developmental toxicity), reproductive toxicity, organotoxic at low doses, genotoxic, and/or new agents with structural or toxicity profiles similar to existing hazardous agents. Assess risk to determine appropriate containment strategy (USP-NF 2017).

Use appropriate precautions for receiving, handling, administration, and disposal. Gloves (single) should be worn during receiving, unpacking, and placing in storage. NIOSH recommends single gloving for administration of intact tablets or capsules. If manipulating tablets/capsules (eg, if unable to swallow whole), NIOSH recommends double gloving, a protective gown, and preparation in a controlled device; if not prepared in a controlled device, respiratory and eye/face protection as well as ventilated engineering controls are recommended. NIOSH recommends double gloving, a protective gown, and (if there is a potential for vomit or spit up) eye/face protection for administration of an oral liquid/feeding tube administration (NIOSH 2016).

Storage/Stability Store at 20°C to 25°C (68°F to 77°F); excursions are permitted between 15°C and 30°C (59°F and 86°F). Keep in original container until dispensing.

Mechanism of Action Ibrutinib is a potent and irreversible inhibitor of Bruton's tyrosine kinase (BTK), an integral component of the B-cell receptor (BCR) and cytokine receptor pathways. Constitutive activation of B-cell receptor signaling is important for survival of malignant B-cells; BTK inhibition results in decreased malignant B-cell proliferation and survival.

Pharmacodynamics/Kinetics

Distribution: ~10,000 L (Marostica 2015)

Bioavailability: Absolute bioavailability in fasted condition was 2.9% and doubled when combined with a meal. Administration with food increased the C_{max} by ~2- to 4-fold and the AUC 2-fold (compared with overnight fasting). Administration under fasting conditions resulted in exposure of ~60% compared to when administered either 30 minutes before or after a meal, or 2 hours after a high-fat meal (de Jong 2015).

Protein binding: ~97%

Metabolism: Hepatic via CYP3A (major) and CYP2D6 (minor) to active metabolite PCI-45227

Half-life elimination: 4 to 6 hours

Time to peak: 1 to 2 hours (4 hours under fed conditions [de Jong 2015])

Excretion: Feces (80%; 1% as unchanged drug); urine (<10%, as metabolites)

Dosing

Adult & Geriatric

Chronic graft-versus-host disease (cGVHD; refractory): Oral: 420 mg once daily; continue until cGVHD disease progression, recurrence of underlying malignancy, or unacceptable toxicity (Miklos 2016). When cGVHD treatment is no longer required, discontinue ibrutinib based on medical assessment of patient.

Chronic lymphocytic leukemia/small lymphocytic lymphoma (CLL/SLL): Oral: 420 mg once daily (either as monotherapy or in combination with bendamustine and rituximab); continue until disease progression or unacceptable toxicity (Byrd 2014; Chanan-Khan 2016).

CLL/SLL with 17p deletion: Oral: 420 mg once daily; continue until disease progression or unacceptable toxicity (Byrd 2014).

Mantle cell lymphoma (MCL), previously treated: Oral: 560 mg once daily; continue until disease progression or unacceptable toxicity (Wang 2013; Wang 2015).

Marginal zone lymphoma (MZL), relapsed/refractory: Oral: 560 mg once daily; continue until disease progression or unacceptable toxicity (Noy 2017).

Waldenström macroglobulinemia (WM): Oral: 420 mg once daily; continue until disease progression or unacceptable toxicity (Treon 2015).

Missed doses: Administer as soon as the missed dose is remembered on the same day; return to normal scheduling the following day. Do not take extra capsules to make up for the missed dose.

Dosage adjustment for concomitant therapy:
B-cell malignancies:

Moderate CYP3A inhibitors, posaconazole at doses ≤200 mg twice daily, and voriconazole (any dose): Reduce ibrutinib dose to 140 mg once daily. Monitor closely and interrupt ibrutinib treatment as recommended for toxicities.

Other strong CYP3A inhibitors and posaconazole at doses >200 mg twice daily: Avoid concurrent use. If these inhibitors will be used short-term (eg, anti-infectives for ≤7 days), interrupt ibrutinib treatment.

cGVHD:

Moderate CYP3A inhibitors: Administer ibrutinib at 420 mg once daily. Monitor closely and interrupt ibrutinib treatment as recommended for toxicities.

Posaconazole immediate release 200 mg twice daily or delayed release 300 mg once daily or voriconazole (any dose): Reduce ibrutinib dose to 280 mg once daily. Monitor closely and interrupt ibrutinib treatment as recommended for toxicities.

Other strong CYP3A inhibitors and posaconazole at doses >200 mg immediate release twice daily or >300 mg delayed release once daily: Avoid concurrent use. If these inhibitors will be used short-term (eg, anti-infectives for ≤7 days), interrupt ibrutinib treatment.

Renal Impairment

CrCl ≥25 mL/minute: There are no dosage adjustments provided in the manufacturer's labeling; however, renal excretion is minimal and drug exposure is not altered in patients with mild to moderate impairment.

CrCl <25 mL/minute: There are no dosage adjustments provided in the manufacturer's labeling (has not been studied).

End-stage renal disease (ESRD) requiring dialysis: There are no dosage adjustments provided in the manufacturer's labeling (has not been studied).

Hepatic Impairment

Mild impairment (Child-Pugh class A): Reduce dose to 140 mg once daily. Monitor for toxicities; may require treatment interruption.

Moderate and severe impairment (Child-Pugh classes B and C): Avoid use.

Adjustment for Toxicity

Hematologic toxicity: ≥ Grade 3 neutropenia with infection or fever, or grade 4 toxicity: Interrupt therapy; upon improvement to grade 1 toxicity or baseline, resume dosing at the starting dose. If toxicity recurs, reduce daily dose by 140 mg. If toxicity recurs after first dose reduction, reduce daily dose by an additional 140 mg. If toxicity persists following 2 dose reductions, discontinue therapy.

Nonhematologic toxicity: ≥ Grade 3 toxicity: Interrupt therapy; upon improvement to grade 1 toxicity or baseline, resume dosing at the starting dose. If toxicity recurs, reduce daily dose by 140 mg. If toxicity recurs after first dose reduction, reduce daily dose by an additional 140 mg. If toxicity persists following 2 dose reductions, discontinue therapy.

Recommend dose reductions for toxicity (following recovery):

Chronic lymphocytic leukemia/small lymphocytic lymphoma, chronic graft-versus-host disease, **and** *Waldenström macroglobulinemia:*
First occurrence: Restart at 420 mg once daily
Second occurrence: Restart at 280 mg once daily
Third occurrence: Restart at 140 mg once daily
Fourth occurrence: Discontinue

Mantle cell lymphoma **and** *marginal zone lymphoma:*
  First occurrence: Restart at 560 mg once daily
  Second occurrence: Restart at 420 mg once daily
  Third occurrence: Restart at 280 mg once daily
  Fourth occurrence: Discontinue

Combination Regimens

Leukemia, chronic lymphocytic: Ibrutinib-Bendamustine-Rituximab (CLL) on page 2152

Administration

Administer orally with water at approximately the same time every day. Swallow capsules whole; do not open, break, or chew the capsules. Maintain adequate hydration during treatment.

Based on an analysis of 3 pharmacokinetic studies, it is suggested that ibrutinib may be administered without regard to food (de Jong 2015).

Ibrutinib was administered via nasogastric (NG) and percutaneous endoscopic gastrostomy (PEG) tube (single case report) by opening the capsule contents and flushing the contents down the tube(s) with water (Maddox 2016).

Emetic Potential Low (10% to 30%)

Monitoring Parameters Monitor blood counts monthly or as clinically necessary; renal and hepatic function; uric acid levels as clinically necessary; verify pregnancy status prior to treatment initiation (in women of reproductive potential); sign/symptoms of bleeding, infections, progressive multifocal encephalopathy, tumor lysis syndrome, and second primary malignancies; signs/symptoms of atrial fibrillation; ECG prior to initiation (patients with cardiac risk factors or history of atrial fibrillation) and during therapy if clinically indicated. Monitor adherence.

Dietary Considerations Avoid grapefruit, grapefruit juice, and Seville oranges during therapy.

Dosage Forms Excipient information presented when available (limited, particularly for generics); consult specific product labeling.
  Capsule, Oral:
    Imbruvica: 140 mg

IDArubicin (eye da ROO bi sin)

Related Information

Management of Chemotherapy-Induced Nausea and Vomiting in Adults *on page 2253*

Management of Drug Extravasations *on page 2271*

Prevention of Chemotherapy-Induced Nausea and Vomiting in Children *on page 2310*

Safe Handling of Hazardous Drugs *on page 2379*

Brand Names: US Idamycin PFS

Brand Names: Canada Idamycin PFS; Idarubicin Hydrochloride Injection

Index Terms 4-Demethoxydaunorubicin; 4-DMDR; Idarubicin Hydrochloride; IDR; IMI 30; SC 33428

Pharmacologic Category Antineoplastic Agent, Anthracycline; Antineoplastic Agent, Topoisomerase II Inhibitor

Use Acute myeloid leukemia: Treatment of acute myeloid leukemia (AML) in adults (in combination with other approved chemotherapy agents).

Labeled Contraindications Bilirubin >5 mg/dL

Documentation of allergenic cross-reactivity for drugs in this class is limited. However, because of similarities in chemical structure and/or pharmacologic actions, the possibility of cross-sensitivity cannot be ruled out with certainty.

Pregnancy Considerations Adverse events were observed in animal reproduction studies. Fetal fatality was noted in a case report following second trimester exposure in a pregnant woman. The manufacturer recommends that women of childbearing potential avoid pregnancy.

Breastfeeding Considerations It is not known if idarubicin is excreted in breast milk. Due to the potential for serious adverse reactions in the nursing infant, breastfeeding is not recommended by the manufacturer.

Warnings/Precautions [US Boxed Warning]: May cause myocardial toxicity; may lead to heart failure. Cardiotoxicity is more common in patients who have previously received anthracyclines or have preexisting cardiac disease. The risk of myocardial toxicity is also increased in patients with concomitant or prior mediastinal/pericardial irradiation, patients with anemia, bone marrow depression, infections, leukemic pericarditis or myocarditis. Patients with active or dormant cardiovascular disease, concurrent administration of cardiotoxic drugs, prior therapy with other anthracyclines or anthracenediones are also at increased risk for cardiotoxicity. Potentially fatal heart failure, acute arrhythmias (may be life-threatening) or other cardiomyopathies may also occur. Regular monitoring of LVEF and discontinuation at the first sign of impairment is recommended, especially in patients with cardiac risk factors or impaired cardiac function. The half-life of other cardiotoxic agents (eg, trastuzumab) must be considered. Avoid the use of anthracycline-based therapy for at least 5 half-lives after discontinuation of the cardiotoxic agent. Monitor cardiac function during treatment. Patients >60 years who were undergoing induction therapy experienced heart failure, serious arrhythmias, chest pain, MI, and asymptomatic declines in LVEF more frequently than younger patients.

[US Boxed Warning]: Vesicant; may cause severe local tissue damage and necrosis if extravasation occurs. For IV administration only. NOT for IM or SubQ administration. Administer through a rapidly flowing IV line. Ensure proper needle or catheter placement prior to and during infusion. Avoid extravasation.

◄ **[US Boxed Warning]: May cause severe myelosuppression when used at therapeutic doses.** Patients are at risk of developing infection and bleeding (may be fatal) due to neutropenia and thrombocytopenia, respectively. Monitor blood counts frequently. Do not use in patients with preexisting bone marrow suppression unless the benefit outweighs the risk. **[US Boxed Warning]: Dosage reductions are recommended in patients with renal or hepatic impairment.** Do not use if bilirubin >5 mg/dL. Rapid lysis of leukemic cells may lead to hyperuricemia. Ensure adequate hydration and consider use of antihyperuricemic prophylaxis. Systemic infections should be controlled prior to initiation of treatment. **[US Boxed Warning]: Should be administered under the supervision of an experienced cancer chemotherapy physician.** Use in facilities with laboratory and supportive resources adequate to monitor drug tolerance and protect and maintain a patient compromised by drug toxicity. The physician and institution must be capable of responding rapidly and completely to severe hemorrhagic conditions and/or overwhelming infection. Idarubicin is associated with a moderate emetic potential; antiemetics are recommended to prevent nausea and vomiting (Basch, 2011; Dupuis, 2011; Roila, 2010). Abdominal pain, diarrhea, and mucositis may commonly occur. Potentially significant drug-drug interactions may exist, requiring dose or frequency adjustment, additional monitoring, and/or selection of alternative therapy.

Adverse Reactions The relative cardiotoxicity of idarubicin compared to doxorubicin is unclear. Some investigators report no increase in cardiac toxicity for adults at cumulative oral idarubicin doses up to 540 mg/m^2; other reports suggest a maximum cumulative intravenous dose of 150 mg/m^2.

>10%:

Cardiovascular: Cardiac failure (dose-related), ECG abnormalities (transient; includes atrial premature contractions, S-T wave changes, supraventricular tachycardia, ventricular premature contractions; generally asymptomatic and self-limiting)

Central nervous system: Headache

Dermatologic: Alopecia (25% to 30%), skin rash (11%), urticaria

Gastrointestinal: Vomiting (30% to 60%), gastrointestinal hemorrhage (30%), diarrhea (9% to 22%), stomatitis (11%), nausea

Genitourinary: Urine discoloration (darker yellow)

Hematologic & oncologic: Anemia (effects are generally less severe with oral dosing), bone marrow suppression (nadir: 10 to 15 days; recovery: 21 to 28 days; primarily leukopenia; effects are generally less severe with oral dosing), thrombocytopenia (effects are generally less severe with oral dosing)

Hepatic: Increased serum bilirubin (≤44%), increased serum transaminases (≤44%)

Miscellaneous: Radiation recall phenomenon

1% to 10%:

Central nervous system: Peripheral neuropathy, seizure

<1%, postmarketing, and/or case reports: Cardiomyopathy, hyperuricemia, myocarditis, typhlitis (neutropenic)

Drug Interactions

Metabolism/Transport Effects Substrate of P-glycoprotein

Avoid Concomitant Use

Avoid concomitant use of IDArubicin with any of the following: BCG (Intravesical); Deferiprone; Dipyrone; Natalizumab; Pimecrolimus; Tacrolimus (Topical); Vaccines (Live)

Increased Effect/Toxicity

IDArubicin may increase the levels/effects of: CloZAPine; Deferiprone; Fingolimod; Leflunomide; Natalizumab; Tofacitinib; Vaccines (Live)

The levels/effects of IDArubicin may be increased by: Ado-Trastuzumab Emtansine; Bevacizumab; Cyclophosphamide; Denosumab; Dipyrone; Lumacaftor; Ocrelizumab; Palifermin; P-glycoprotein/ABCB1 Inhibitors; Pimecrolimus; Promazine; Ranolazine; Roflumilast; Tacrolimus (Topical); Taxane Derivatives; Trastuzumab

Decreased Effect

IDArubicin may decrease the levels/effects of: BCG (Intravesical); Cardiac Glycosides; Coccidioides immitis Skin Test; Lenograstim; Nivolumab; Sipuleucel-T; Tertomotide; Vaccines (Inactivated); Vaccines (Live)

The levels/effects of IDArubicin may be decreased by: Cardiac Glycosides; Echinacea; Lumacaftor; P-glycoprotein/ABCB1 Inducers

Hazardous Drugs Handling Considerations

Hazardous agent (NIOSH 2016 [group 1]).

Use appropriate precautions for receiving, handling, administration, and disposal. Gloves (single) should be worn during receiving, unpacking, and placing in storage.

NIOSH recommends double gloving, a protective gown, ventilated engineering controls (a class II biological safety cabinet or a compounding aseptic containment isolator), and closed system transfer devices (CSTDs) for preparation. Double gloving, a gown, and (if dosage form allows) CSTDs are required during administration (NIOSH 2016).

Storage/Stability Store intact vials of solution refrigerated at 2°C to 8°C (36°F to 46°F). Protect from light.

Preparation for Administration May draw up 1 mg/mL solution into a syringe (for administration) or further dilute in NS or D5W.

Mechanism of Action Similar to daunorubicin, idarubicin inhibits DNA and RNA synthesis by intercalation between DNA base pairs and by steric obstruction. Although the exact mechanism is unclear, it appears that direct binding to DNA (intercalation) and inhibition of DNA repair (topoisomerase II inhibition) result in blockade of DNA and RNA synthesis and fragmentation of DNA.

Pharmacodynamics/Kinetics

Distribution: V_{dss}: 1,500 L/m^2 (Robert, 1993); extensive tissue binding; CSF

Protein binding: 94% (idarubicinol) to 97% (idarubicin)

Metabolism: Hepatic to idarubicinol (active metabolite)

Half-life elimination:

Children: Children ≥1 year and adolescents: 17.6 ± 6.8 hours (range: 8.3 to 29.6 hours) (Reid 1990)

Adults: Adults: 22 hours (range: 4 to 48 hours); >45 hours (idarubicinol)

Excretion: Primarily biliary; urine (8 to 10% as idarubicinol, ~2% to 5% as unchanged drug [Robert 1993])

Dosing

Adult & Geriatric Idarubicin is associated with a moderate emetic potential; antiemetics are recommended to prevent nausea and vomiting (Basch, 2011; Roila, 2010).

Acute myeloid leukemia (AML): IV:

Manufacturer labeling: Induction: 12 mg/m²/day for 3 days (in combination with cytarabine); a second induction cycle may be administered if necessary.

Indication-specific dosing:

AML, relapsed/refractory: FLAG-IDA regimen: 10 mg/m²/day for 3 days (in combination with fludarabine, cytarabine, and filgrastim); a second course was given for consolidation upon hematologic recovery (Parker, 1997)

Acute promyelocytic leukemia (APL):

LPA 2005 (high-risk patients; Sanz, 2010):

Induction (all patients): 12 mg/m²/day on days 2, 4, 6, and 8 (day 8 dose was omitted in patients >70 years) in combination with ATRA (tretinoin) (Sanz, 2010)

Consolidation (patients ≤60 years): 5 mg/m²/day for 4 days in consolidation cycle 1 and 12 mg/m²/day for 1 day in consolidation cycle 3 (in combination with ATRA [tretinoin] and cytarabine) (Sanz, 2010)

APML4 protocol (Iland, 2012): Induction (age-adjusted dosing):

Age <60 years: 12 mg/m²/day on days 2, 4, 6, and 8 (in combination with ATRA [tretinoin] and arsenic trioxide)

Age 61 to 70 years: 9 mg/m²/day on days 2, 4, 6, and 8 (in combination with ATRA [tretinoin] and arsenic trioxide)

Age >70 years: 6 mg/m²/day on days 2, 4, 6, and 8 (in combination with ATRA [tretinoin] and arsenic trioxide)

Pediatric Note: Idarubicin is associated with a moderate emetic potential; antiemetics are recommended to prevent nausea and vomiting (Dupuis, 2011).

Acute myeloid leukemia (AML) (off-label use): IV:

Newly diagnosed (CCG-2961) (Lange, 2008):

Induction: IdaDCTER: Idarubicin 5 mg/m²/dose daily for 4 days on days 0 to 3 in combination with cytarabine, etoposide, thioguanine, and dexamethasone

Consolidation:

IdaDCTER: Idarubicin 5 mg/m²/dose daily for 4 days on days 0 to 3 in combination with cytarabine, etoposide, thioguanine, and dexamethasone

or

Idarubicin 12 mg/m²/dose daily for 3 days on days 0 to 2 in combination with fludarabine and cytarabine

Relapsed/refractory: 12 mg/m² once daily for 3 days on days 0 to 2 in combination with fludarabine and cytarabine (Dinndorf, 1997; Leahey, 1997)

Renal Impairment There are no dosage adjustments provided in the manufacturer's labeling; however, it does recommend that dosage reductions be made. Patients with S_{cr} ≥2 mg/dL did not receive treatment in many clinical trials. The following adjustments have been recommended (Aronoff, 2007):

Adults:

CrCl >50 mL/minute: No dosage adjustment is necessary.

CrCl 10 to 50 mL/minute: Administer 75% of dose.

CrCl <10 mL/minute: Administer 50% of dose.

Hemodialysis: Supplemental dose not needed.

Continuous ambulatory peritoneal dialysis (CAPD): Supplemental dose not needed.

Infants, Children, and Adolescents:
GFR >50 mL/minute/1.73 m^2: No dosage adjustment is necessary.
GFR ≤50 mL/minute/1.73 m^2: Administer 75% of dose
Intermittent hemodialysis: Administer 75% of dose
Peritoneal dialysis (PD): Administer 75% of dose
Continuous renal replacement therapy (CRRT): Administer 75% of dose

Hepatic Impairment
Bilirubin 2.6 to 5 mg/dL: Administer 50% of dose (Perry, 2012)
Bilirubin >5 mg/dL: Avoid use

Adjustment for Toxicity Manufacturer labeling: If patients experience severe mucositis during the first induction cycle, delay administration of the second cycle until mucositis has resolved; consider reducing the dose by 25%.

Combination Regimens
Leukemia, acute myeloid:
5 + 2 (Cytarabine-Idarubicin) (AML Consolidation) on page 1970
7 + 3 (Cytarabine-Idarubicin) (AML Induction) on page 1972
FLAG-IDA (AML Induction) on page 2115
Leukemia, acute promyelocytic: Tretinoin-Idarubicin (APL) on page 2221

Administration Idarubicin is associated with a moderate emetic potential; antiemetics are recommended to prevent nausea and vomiting (Basch, 2011; Dupuis, 2011; Roila, 2010).

For IV administration only. Do not administer IM or SubQ; administer as slow injection over 10 to 15 minutes into a free-flowing IV solution of NS or D5W. In some pediatric protocols (off label use), idarubicin was infused over 15 minutes or over at least 30 minutes (Lange, 2008; Leahy, 1997); refer to individual protocols for infusion rate details.

Vesicant; ensure proper needle or catheter placement prior to and during infusion; avoid extravasation.

Extravasation management: If extravasation occurs, stop infusion immediately and disconnect (leave cannula/needle in place); gently aspirate extravasated solution (do **NOT** flush the line); remove needle/cannula; elevate extremity. Initiate antidote (dexrazoxane or dimethyl sulfate [DMSO]). Apply dry cold compresses for 20 minutes 4 times daily for 1 to 2 days (Perez Fidalgo, 2012); withhold cooling beginning 15 minutes before dexrazoxane infusion; continue withholding cooling until 15 minutes after infusion is completed. Topical DMSO should not be administered in combination with dexrazoxane; may lessen dexrazoxane efficacy.
Dexrazoxane: Adults: 1000 mg/m^2 (maximum dose: 2000 mg) IV (administer in a large vein remote from site of extravasation) over 1 to 2 hours days 1 and 2, then 500 mg/m^2 (maximum dose: 1000 mg) IV over 1 to 2 hours day 3; begin within 6 hours of extravasation. Day 2 and day 3 doses should be administered at approximately the same time (± 3 hours) as the dose on day 1 (Mouridsen, 2007; Perez Fidalgo, 2012). **Note:** Reduce dexrazoxane dose by 50% in patients with moderate to severe renal impairment (CrCl <40 mL/minute).
DMSO: Children and Adults: Apply topically to a region covering twice the affected area every 8 hours for 7 days; begin within 10 minutes of extravasation; do not cover with a dressing (Perez Fidalgo, 2012).

Vesicant/Extravasation Risk Vesicant
Emetic Potential Children and Adults: Moderate (30% to 90%)

Monitoring Parameters CBC with differential and platelet count (frequently), cardiac function (LVEF; prior and during treatment), serum electrolytes, renal function (serum creatinine; prior to and during treatment), uric acid, liver function (ALT, AST, bilirubin; prior to and during treatment); monitor infusion site for signs of extravasation; monitor for gastrointestinal toxicity and infection

Dosage Forms Excipient information presented when available (limited, particularly for generics); consult specific product labeling.

Solution, Intravenous, as hydrochloride [preservative free]:

Idamycin PFS: 5 mg/5 mL (5 mL); 10 mg/10 mL (10 mL); 20 mg/20 mL (20 mL)

Generic: 5 mg/5 mL (5 mL); 10 mg/10 mL (10 mL); 20 mg/20 mL (20 mL)

♦ **Idarubicin Hydrochloride** *see* IDArubicin *on page 951*

♦ **Idarubicin Hydrochloride Injection (Can)** *see* IDArubicin *on page 951*

♦ **IDEC-C2B8** *see* RiTUXimab *on page 1610*

♦ **IDEC-Y2B8** *see* Ibritumomab *on page 938*

Idelalisib (eye del a LIS ib)

Related Information

Common Toxicity Criteria *on page 2242*

Safe Handling of Hazardous Drugs *on page 2379*

Brand Names: US Zydelig

Brand Names: Canada Zydelig

Index Terms CAL-101; GS-1101; PI_3K Delta Inhibitor CAL-101

Pharmacologic Category Antineoplastic Agent, Phosphatidylinositol 3-Kinase Inhibitor

Use

Chronic lymphocytic leukemia: Treatment of relapsed chronic lymphocytic leukemia (CLL) (in combination with rituximab) when rituximab alone is appropriate therapy due to other comorbidities

Follicular B-cell non-Hodgkin lymphoma: Treatment of relapsed follicular B-cell non-Hodgkin lymphoma after at least 2 prior systemic therapies

Small lymphocytic lymphoma: Treatment of relapsed small lymphocytic lymphoma (SLL) after at least 2 prior systemic therapies

Limitations of use: Idelalisib is not indicated or recommended for first-line treatment of CLL, follicular B-cell non-Hodgkin lymphoma, or SLL.

Labeled Contraindications

Serious hypersensitivity reactions (including anaphylaxis and toxic epidermal necrolysis) to idelalisib or any component of the formulation

Canadian labeling: Additional contraindications (not in US labeling): Use in first-line chronic lymphocytic leukemia and early-line indolent non-Hodgkin lymphoma outside of a clinical trial

Pregnancy Considerations Adverse events were observed in animal reproduction studies. Women of reproductive potential should use effective contraception during therapy and for at least 1 month after treatment discontinuation.

Breastfeeding Considerations It is not known if idelalisib is excreted in breast milk. Because of the potential for serious adverse reactions in the nursing infant, the manufacturer recommends a decision be made to discontinue nursing or the drug, taking into account the importance of treatment to the mother.

Warnings/Precautions [US Boxed Warning]: Serious hepatotoxicity (some fatal) has been observed. Monitor hepatic function at baseline and during therapy. May require treatment interruption and/or dosage reduction. ALT/AST elevations >5 times ULN have occurred, and were generally observed during the first 12 weeks of therapy; transaminase elevations were reversible upon therapy interruption. Hepatotoxicity may recur upon rechallenge, even at a reduced dose; discontinue for recurrent hepatotoxicity. Avoid concomitant use with other hepatotoxic agents. Monitor ALT/AST at baseline and every 2 weeks for the first 6 months, every 4 weeks for the next 3 months, then every 1 to 3 months thereafter, or as clinically necessary. Increase monitoring to weekly if ALT or AST >3 times ULN until resolved. Interrupt therapy if ALT/AST >5 times ULN; monitor LFTs weekly until resolved. **[US Boxed Warning]: Serious and/or fatal diarrhea and colitis have been reported. Monitor closely; may require treatment interruption, dosage reduction, and/or discontinuation.** Grade 3 or higher diarrhea or colitis have been reported in clinical trials. Diarrhea may occur at any time during therapy and responds poorly to antidiarrheal (antimotility) medications. The median time to resolution of diarrhea was 1 week to 1 month (following therapy interruption); corticosteroids were used in some cases to manage toxicity. Avoid concomitant use with other promotility agents. **[US Boxed Warning]: Serious and/or fatal intestinal perforation may occur; discontinue permanently if perforation develops.** In some patients, perforation was preceded by moderate to severe diarrhea. Monitor closely for new or worsening abdominal pain, chills, fever, nausea, or vomiting.

[US Boxed Warning]: Fatal and/or serious infection has occurred in Idelalisib-treated patients. Monitor for signs and symptoms of infection. Interrupt idelalisib if infection is suspected. Commonly reported infections include pneumonia, sepsis, and febrile neutropenia. Serious cases (some fatal) of *Pneumocystis jirovecii* pneumonia (PCP) and cytomegalovirus (CMV) have been reported, rarely. Consider PCP prophylaxis throughout idelalisib treatment (and after discontinuation if infection risk persists); interrupt treatment if PCP infection of any grade is suspected; permanently discontinue if PCP infection is confirmed. Interrupt idelalisib for positive CMV PCR or antigen test until the infection has resolved. If idelalisib is reinitiated, monitor for CMV reactivation by PCR or antigen test at least monthly.

[US Boxed Warning]: Serious and/or fatal pneumonitis may occur. Monitor for pulmonary symptoms and bilateral interstitial infiltrates. May require therapy interruption or discontinuation. Symptoms such as cough, dyspnea, hypoxia, interstitial infiltrates, or an oxygen saturation decrease of more than 5% should be promptly evaluated. Time to onset of symptoms ranged from less than 1 month to 15 months after therapy initiation. Interrupt therapy for suspected pneumonitis; if diagnosis is confirmed, discontinue idelalisib and administer corticosteroids as appropriate. Serious allergic/hypersensitivity reactions, including anaphylaxis, have been reported. Discontinue permanently for serious reactions and manage appropriately.

Cases of Stevens Johnson syndrome (SJS) and toxic epidermal necrolysis (TEN) have been reported (some fatal). Severe and/or life-threatening cutaneous/mucocutaneous reactions (grade 3 or higher), including exfoliative dermatitis, rash (generalized, erythematous, maculopapular, papular, pruritic, exfoliative), and skin disorder, have been observed. Monitor closely for dermatologic toxicity and discontinue for severe reactions. Grade 3 or 4 neutropenia occurred in close to one-third of patients in clinical trials;

◄ thrombocytopenia and anemia (any grade) have also been reported. Monitor blood counts at least every 2 weeks for the first 3 months, and at least weekly in patients with neutropenia (ANC <1,000/mm^3). May require treatment interruption and dosage reduction. Potentially significant interactions may exist, requiring dose or frequency adjustment, additional monitoring, and/or selection of alternative therapy. Consult drug interactions database for more detailed information.

Adverse Reactions As reported with monotherapy.

>10%:

Central nervous system: Fatigue (30%), insomnia (12%), headache (11%)

Dermatologic: Skin rash (21%), night sweats (12%)

Gastrointestinal: Diarrhea (47%), nausea (29%), abdominal pain (26%), decreased appetite (16%), vomiting (15%)

Hematologic & oncologic: Decreased neutrophils (53%; grade 3: 14%; grade 4: 11%), decreased hemoglobin (28%; grade 3: 2%), decreased platelet count (26%; grade 3: 3%; grade 4: 3%)

Hepatic: Increased serum ALT (50%), increased serum AST (41%), severe hepatotoxicity (18%)

Infection: Severe infection (21%; including sepsis, febrile neutropenia)

Neuromuscular & skeletal: Weakness (12%)

Respiratory: Cough (29%), pneumonia (15% to 25%), dyspnea (17%), upper respiratory tract infection (12%)

Miscellaneous: Fever (28%)

1% to 10%:

Cardiovascular: Peripheral edema (10%)

Respiratory: Pneumonitis (4%)

<1%, postmarketing, and/or case reports: Anaphylaxis, cytomegalovirus disease, erythematous rash, exfoliative dermatitis, hypersensitivity reaction, intestinal perforation, macular eruption, maculopapular rash, papular rash, pneumonia due to pneumocystis carinii, pruritic rash, Stevens-Johnson syndrome, toxic epidermal necrolysis

Drug Interactions

Metabolism/Transport Effects Substrate of CYP3A4 (major), P-glycoprotein, UGT1A4; **Note:** Assignment of Major/Minor substrate status based on clinically relevant drug interaction potential; **Inhibits** CYP2C8 (weak), CYP3A4 (strong), UGT1A1

Avoid Concomitant Use

Avoid concomitant use of Idelalisib with any of the following: Ado-Trastuzumab Emtansine; Alfuzosin; Amodiaquine; Aprepitant; Astemizole; Asunaprevir; Avanafil; Axitinib; Barnidipine; BCG (Intravesical); Blonanserin; Bosutinib; Bromocriptine; Budesonide (Systemic); Ceritinib; Cobimetinib; Conivaptan; Crizotinib; CYP3A4 Inducers (Strong); CYP3A4 Substrates; Dabrafenib; Dapoxetine; Domperidone; Dronedarone; Eletriptan; Eplerenone; Everolimus; Flibanserin; Fluticasone (Nasal); Halofantrine; Ibrutinib; Isavuconazonium Sulfate; Ivabradine; Lapatinib; Lercanidipine; Lomitapide; Lovastatin; Lurasidone; Macitentan; Naloxegol; Natalizumab; Neratinib; Nilotinib; NiMODipine; Nisoldipine; Olaparib; Palbociclib; Pimecrolimus; Pimozide; Radotinib; Ranolazine; Red Yeast Rice; Regorafenib; Rupatadine; Salmeterol; Silodosin; Simeprevir; Simvastatin; Sonidegib; St John's Wort; Suvorexant; Tacrolimus (Topical); Tamsulosin; Terfenadine; Ticagrelor; Tolvaptan; Toremifene; Trabectedin; Udenafil; Ulipristal; Vaccines (Live); Vemurafenib; VinCRIStine (Liposomal); Vinflunine; Vorapaxar

Increased Effect/Toxicity

Idelalisib may increase the levels/effects of: Ado-Trastuzumab Emtansine; Alfuzosin; Almotriptan; Alosetron; Amodiaquine; Apixaban; Aprepitant; Astemizole; Asunaprevir; Avanafil; Axitinib; Barnidipine; Bedaquiline; Benperidol; Blonanserin; Bortezomib; Bosentan; Bosutinib; Brentuximab Vedotin; Brinzolamide; Bromocriptine; Budesonide (Nasal); Budesonide (Oral Inhalation); Budesonide (Systemic); Budesonide (Topical); Calcifediol; Cannabidiol; Cannabis; Ceritinib; CloZAPine; Cobimetinib; Conivaptan; Corticosteroids (Orally Inhaled); Corticosteroids (Systemic); Crizotinib; CYP3A4 Substrates; Dabrafenib; Dapoxetine; Delamanid; Dexamethasone (Ophthalmic); Dienogest; Dofetilide; Domperidone; Dronabinol; Dronedarone; Drospirenone; Dutasteride; Eletriptan; Eplerenone; Estazolam; Everolimus; Evogliptin; Fingolimod; Flibanserin; Fluticasone (Nasal); Halofantrine; HydrOXYzine; Ibrutinib; Iloperidone; Imatinib; Imidafenacin; Isavuconazonium Sulfate; Ivabradine; Lacosamide; Lapatinib; Leflunomide; Lercanidipine; Levobupivacaine; Lomitapide; Lovastatin; Lumefantrine; Lurasidone; Macitentan; MedroxyPROGESTERone; MethylPREDNISolone; Naldemedine; Naloxegol; Natalizumab; Neratinib; Nilotinib; NiMODipine; Nisoldipine; Olaparib; Ospemifene; Oxybutynin; Palbociclib; Parecoxib; Paricalcitol; Pimozide; PONATinib; Pranlukast; PrednisoLONE (Systemic); PredniSONE; Propafenone; Radotinib; Ramelteon; Ranolazine; Red Yeast Rice; Regorafenib; Repaglinide; Retapamulin; Rilpivirine; RomiDEPsin; Rupatadine; Salmeterol; Silodosin; Simeprevir; Simvastatin; Sonidegib; SORAfenib; Suvorexant; Tamsulosin; TasImelteon; Terfenadine; Tetrahydrocannabinol; Ticagrelor; Tolvaptan; Toremifene; Trabectedin; TraMADol; Udenafil; Ulipristal; Vaccines (Live); Vemurafenib; Vilazodone; VinCRIStine (Liposomal); Vindesine; Vinflunine; Vorapaxar; Zolpidem; Zuclopenthixol

The levels/effects of Idelalisib may be increased by: CYP3A4 Inhibitors (Strong); Denosumab; Ocrelizumab; Pimecrolimus; Roflumilast; Tacrolimus (Topical); Trastuzumab

Decreased Effect

Idelalisib may decrease the levels/effects of: BCG (Intravesical); Coccidioides immitis Skin Test; Doxercalciferol; Ifosfamide; Nivolumab; Prasugrel; Sipuleucel-T; Tertomotide; Ticagrelor; Vaccines (Inactivated); Vaccines (Live)

The levels/effects of Idelalisib may be decreased by: Bosentan; CYP3A4 Inducers (Moderate); CYP3A4 Inducers (Strong); Deferasirox; Echinacea; Sarilumab; Siltuximab; St John's Wort; Tocilizumab

Hazardous Drugs Handling Considerations

Hazardous agent (meets NIOSH 2016 criteria). This medication is not on the NIOSH (2016) list; however, it meets the criteria for a hazardous drug. Drugs are classified as hazardous based on their properties; the properties of a hazardous drug include one or more of the following characteristics: carcinogenic, teratogenic (or other developmental toxicity), reproductive toxicity, organotoxic at low doses, genotoxic, and/or new agents with structural or toxicity profiles similar to existing hazardous agents.

Use appropriate precautions for receiving, handling, administration, and disposal. Gloves (single) should be worn during receiving, unpacking, and placing in storage. NIOSH recommends single gloving for administration of intact tablets or capsules (NIOSH 2016).

Storage/Stability Store at 20°C to 30°C (68°F to 86°F); excursions are permitted between 15°C and 30°C (59°F and 86°F). Dispense in the original container.

◀ **Mechanism of Action** Potent small molecule inhibitor of the delta isoform of phosphatidylinositol 3-kinase (PI3Kδ), which is highly expressed in malignant lymphoid B-cells. PI3Kδ inhibition results in apoptosis of malignant tumor cells. In addition, idelalisib inhibits several signaling pathways, including B-cell receptor, CXCR4 and CXCR5 signaling which may play important roles in CLL pathophysiology (Furman, 2014).

Pharmacodynamics/Kinetics

Distribution: 23 L

Protein binding: >84%

Metabolism: Hepatic; primarily via aldehyde oxidase and CYP3A (to major metabolite GS-563117); minor metabolism via UGT1A4

Half-life elimination: ~8 hours

Time to peak: Median: 1.5 hours

Excretion: Feces (78%; 44% as GS-563117); urine (14%; 49% as GS-563117)

Dosing

Adult & Geriatric Note: The maximum recommended starting dose is 150 mg twice daily. Optimal duration and safety of therapy beyond several months is currently unknown.

Chronic lymphocytic leukemia, relapsed: Oral: 150 mg twice daily (in combination with rituximab); continue until disease progression or unacceptable toxicity (Furman 2014)

Follicular B-cell non-Hodgkin lymphoma, relapsed: Oral: 150 mg twice daily; continue until disease progression or unacceptable toxicity (Gopal 2014)

Small lymphocytic lymphoma, relapsed: Oral: 150 mg twice daily; continue until disease progression or unacceptable toxicity (Gopal 2014)

Renal Impairment

CrCl ≥15 mL/minute: No dosage adjustment necessary (Jin 2015b).

CrCl <15 mL/minute: There are no dosage adjustments provided in the manufacturer's labeling (has not been studied).

Hepatic Impairment

Preexisting hepatic impairment: Exposure is increased in patients with ALT/AST or bilirubin >ULN as compared to patients with normal hepatic function; patients with ALT/AST >2.5 times ULN or bilirubin >1.5 times ULN were excluded from some studies. Based on a pharmacokinetic study in patients with moderate and severe hepatic impairment (Child Pugh classes B and C) compared to healthy subjects, single oral doses of 150 mg were well tolerated; idelalisib and GS-563117 exposure differences were observed but not considered clinically relevant (Jin 2015a). Monitor closely for toxicity.

Hepatotoxicity during treatment:

ALT/AST >3 to 5 times ULN or bilirubin >1.5 to 3 times ULN: Continue current dose; monitor LFTs at least weekly until ALT/AST and/or bilirubin ≤1 times ULN.

ALT/AST >5 to 20 times ULN or bilirubin >3 to 10 times ULN: Temporarily interrupt therapy. Monitor LFTs at least weekly until ALT/AST and/or bilirubin ≤1 times ULN, then may reinitiate therapy at 100 mg twice daily.

ALT/AST >20 times ULN or bilirubin >10 times ULN: Discontinue permanently.

Recurrent hepatotoxicity: Discontinue.

Adjustment for Toxicity

Anaphylaxis or other serious allergic reactions: Permanently discontinue.

Dermatologic toxicity:

Severe cutaneous reactions: Discontinue.

Suspected Stevens-Johnson syndrome (SJS) or toxic epidermal necrolysis (TEN): Interrupt therapy; discontinue permanently if SJS or TEN are confirmed.

Hematologic toxicity:

Neutropenia:

ANC 1,000 to <1,500 cells/mm^3: Continue current dose.

ANC 500 to <1,000 cells/mm^3: Continue current dose; monitor blood counts at least weekly.

ANC <500 cells/mm^3: Temporarily interrupt therapy; monitor blood counts at least weekly until ANC ≥500 cells/mm^3, then may reinitiate therapy at 100 mg twice daily.

Thrombocytopenia:

Platelets 50,000 to <75,000 cells/mm^3: Continue current dose.

Platelets 25,000 to <50,000 cells/mm^3: Continue current dose; monitor platelet counts at least weekly.

Platelets <25,000 cells/mm^3: Temporarily interrupt therapy; monitor platelet counts at least weekly, may reinitiate therapy at 100 mg twice daily when platelets recover to ≥25,000 cells/mm^3.

Gastrointestinal toxicity:

Moderate diarrhea (increase of 4 to 6 stools/day over baseline): Continue current dose; monitor at least weekly until resolved.

Severe diarrhea (increase of ≥7 stools/day over baseline) or hospitalization: Temporarily interrupt therapy; monitor at least weekly until resolved, then may reinitiate therapy at 100 mg twice daily.

Life-threatening diarrhea: Discontinue permanently.

Infection:

Sepsis, pneumonia, or other infection (grade 3 or higher): Interrupt therapy until infection has resolved.

Cytomegalovirus (CMV) infection or viremia: Interrupt therapy for evidence of CMV infection of any grade or viremia (positive PCR or antigen test) until infection has resolved. If idelalisib is reinitiated, monitor for CMV reactivation by PCR or antigen test at least monthly.

Pneumocystis jirovecii pneumonia (PCP) infection: Interrupt therapy for suspected PCP infection of any grade; permanently discontinue if PCP infection is confirmed.

Pulmonary toxicity: If pneumonitis is suspected, interrupt therapy and evaluate; discontinue for symptomatic pneumonitis of any severity thought to be associated with therapy (may also require corticosteroids).

Other toxicity (not listed above): If severe or life-threatening toxicities occur, interrupt therapy until toxicity is resolved. If the decision is made to resume therapy, reduce the dose to 100 mg twice daily. Discontinue permanently if severe or life-threatening toxicities recur upon rechallenge.

Combination Regimens

Leukemia, chronic lymphocytic: Idelalisib-Rituximab (CLL) on page 2154

Administration Administer orally twice daily with or without food. Swallow tablets whole.

Missed doses: May administer a missed dose if within 6 hours of usual dosing time. If >6 hours, skip the missed dose and resume therapy with the next scheduled dose.

Emetic Potential Low (10% to 30%)

Monitoring Parameters Complete blood counts with differential at least every 2 weeks for the first 6 months, and at least weekly in patients with neutropenia (ANC <1,000/mm^3), or as clinically necessary; liver function tests at baseline and every 2 weeks for the first 3 months, every 4 weeks for the next 3 months, then every 1 to 3 months thereafter, or as clinically necessary; monitor for infections (including sepsis, pneumonia, PCP, and CMV); monitor for signs/symptoms of diarrhea/colitis, intestinal perforation, pneumonitis, dermatologic toxicity, and hypersensitivity reactions

Prescribing and Access Restrictions Available through specialty pharmacies. Further information may be obtained at http://www.zydeligaccess-connect.com/.

Medication Guide Available Yes

Dosage Forms Excipient information presented when available (limited, particularly for generics); consult specific product labeling.
Tablet, Oral:
Zydelig: 100 mg, 150 mg

♦ **Idelvion** *see* Factor IX (Recombinant [Albumin Fusion Protein]) *on page* 777

♦ **IDH2 inhibitor** *see* Enasidenib *on page* 676

♦ **Idhifa** *see* Enasidenib *on page* 676

♦ **IDHIFA** *see* Enasidenib *on page* 676

♦ **IDR** *see* IDArubicin *on page* 951

♦ **Ifex** *see* Ifosfamide *on page* 962

Ifosfamide (eye FOSS fa mide)

Related Information

Management of Chemotherapy-Induced Nausea and Vomiting in Adults *on page* 2253

Management of Drug Extravasations *on page* 2271

Prevention of Chemotherapy-Induced Nausea and Vomiting in Children *on page* 2310

Safe Handling of Hazardous Drugs *on page* 2379

Brand Names: US Ifex

Brand Names: Canada Ifex; Ifosfamide for Injection

Index Terms Isophosphamide; Z4942

Pharmacologic Category Antineoplastic Agent, Alkylating Agent; Antineoplastic Agent, Alkylating Agent (Nitrogen Mustard)

Use Testicular cancer: Treatment (third-line) of germ cell testicular cancer (in combination with other chemotherapy drugs and with concurrent mesna for prophylaxis of hemorrhagic cystitis)

Labeled Contraindications

Known hypersensitivity to ifosfamide or any component of the formulation; urinary outflow obstruction

Canadian labeling: Additional contraindications (not in US labeling): Severe leukopenia/thrombocytopenia; severe renal and/or hepatic impairment; cystitis; active infection; advanced cerebral arteriosclerosis

Pregnancy Considerations Adverse effects have been observed in animal reproduction studies. Fetal growth retardation and neonatal anemia have been reported with exposure to ifosfamide-containing regimens during human pregnancy. Male and female fertility may be affected (dose and duration dependent). Ifosfamide interferes with oogenesis and spermatogenesis; amenorrhea, azoospermia, and sterility have been reported and may be irreversible. Avoid pregnancy during treatment; male patients should not father a child during and for at least 6 months after completion of therapy.

Breastfeeding Considerations Ifosfamide is excreted in breast milk. Breastfeeding is not recommended during ifosfamide treatment; due to the potential for serious adverse reactions in the breastfeeding infant, the manufacturer recommends a decision be made to discontinue ifosfamide or to discontinue breastfeeding, taking into account the benefits of treatment to the mother.

Warnings/Precautions [US Boxed Warning]: Hemorrhagic cystitis may occur (may be severe); concomitant mesna reduces the risk of hemorrhagic cystitis. Hydration (at least 2 L/day in adults), dose fractionation, and/or mesna administration will reduce the incidence of hematuria and protect against hemorrhagic cystitis. Obtain urinalysis prior to each dose; if microscopic hematuria is detected, withhold until complete resolution. Exclude or correct urinary tract obstructions prior to treatment. Use with caution (if at all) in patients with active urinary tract infection. Hemorrhagic cystitis is dose-dependent and is increased with high single doses (compared with fractionated doses); past or concomitant bladder radiation or busulfan treatment may increase the risk for hemorrhagic cystitis. **[US Boxed Warning]: May cause severe nephrotoxicity, resulting in renal failure.** Nephrotoxicity may be fatal. Acute and chronic renal failure as well as renal parenchymal and tubular necrosis (including acute) have been reported; tubular damage may be delayed (months to years) and may persist. Renal manifestations include decreased glomerular rate, increased creatinine, proteinuria, enzymuria, cylindruria, tubular acidosis, aminoaciduria, phosphaturia, and glycosuria. Syndrome of inappropriate antidiuretic hormone (SIADH), renal rickets, and Fanconi syndrome have been reported. Evaluate renal function prior to and during treatment; monitor urine for erythrocytes and signs of urotoxicity.

[US Boxed Warning]: May cause CNS toxicity which may be severe, resulting in encephalopathy and death; monitor for CNS toxicity; discontinue for encephalopathy. Symptoms of CNS toxicity (somnolence, confusion, dizziness, disorientation, hallucinations, cranial nerve dysfunction, psychotic behavior, extrapyramidal symptoms, seizures, coma, peripheral neuropathy, blurred vision, and/or urinary incontinence) have been observed within a few hours to a few days after initial dose and generally resolve within 2 to 3 days of treatment discontinuation (although symptoms may persist longer); maintain supportive care until complete resolution. Recurrence of CNS toxicity (after several cycles with no CNS incidents) has been reported. Risk factors may include hypoalbuminemia, renal dysfunction, and high-dose antiemetic therapy. Concomitant centrally-acting medications may result in additive CNS effects. Peripheral neuropathy has been reported.

[US Boxed Warning]: Bone marrow suppression may occur (may be severe and lead to fatal infections); monitor blood counts before and after each cycle. Leukopenia, neutropenia, thrombocytopenia and anemia are associated with ifosfamide. Myelosuppression is dose dependent, increased with single high doses (compared to fractionated doses) and ▶

increased with decreased renal function. Severe myelosuppression may occur when administered in combination with other chemotherapy agents or radiation therapy. Use with caution in patients with compromised bone marrow reserve. Unless clinically necessary, avoid administering to patients with WBC <2,000/mm^3 and platelets <50,000/mm^3. Bleeding events due to thrombocytopenia may occur. Antimicrobial prophylaxis may be necessary in some neutropenic patients; administer antibiotics and/or antifungal agents for neutropenic fever. May cause significant suppression of the immune responses; may lead to serious infection, sepsis or septic shock; reported infections have included bacterial, viral, fungal, and parasitic; latent viral infections may be reactivated; use with caution with other immunosuppressants or in patients with infection.

Ifosfamide-induced cardiotoxicity has been reported; may be fatal. Arrhythmias (eg, atrial/supraventricular tachycardia, atrial fibrillation, pulseless ventricular tachycardia), ST-segment or T-wave changes, cardiomyopathy, pericardial effusion, pericarditis, and epicardial fibrosis have been observed; the risk for cardiotoxicity is dose-dependent; concomitant cardiotoxic agents (eg, anthracyclines), irradiation of the cardiac region, and renal impairment may also increase the risk; use with caution in patients with cardiac risk factors or preexisting cardiac disease. In a scientific statement from the American Heart Association, ifosfamide has been determined to be an agent that may either cause reversible direct myocardial toxicity or exacerbate underlying myocardial dysfunction (magnitude: moderate/major) (AHA [Page 2016]). Interstitial pneumonitis, pulmonary fibrosis, and pulmonary toxicity leading to respiratory failure (may be fatal) have been reported; monitor for signs and symptoms of pulmonary toxicity.

Anaphylactic/anaphylactoid reactions have been associated with ifosfamide; cross sensitivity with similar agents may occur. Hepatic sinusoidal obstruction syndrome (SOS), formerly called veno-occlusive disease (VOD), has been reported with ifosfamide-containing regimens. Secondary malignancies may occur (onset may be delayed); the risk for myelodysplastic syndrome (which may progress to acute leukemia) is increased with treatment. May interfere with wound healing. Potentially significant drug-drug interactions may exist, requiring dose or frequency adjustment, additional monitoring, and/or selection of alternative therapy. Use with caution in patients with prior radiation therapy. Ifosfamide is associated with a moderate emetic potential; antiemetics are recommended to prevent nausea and vomiting (Basch 2011; Dupuis 2011; Roila 2010).

Adverse Reactions

>10%:

Central nervous system: Brain disease (≤15%), central nervous system toxicity (≤15%)

Dermatologic: Alopecia (83% to 90%; combination therapy: 100%)

Endocrine & metabolic: Metabolic acidosis (31%)

Gastrointestinal: Nausea (≤58%), vomiting (≤58%)

Hematologic & oncologic: Leukopenia (≤100%; grade 4: ≤50%; nadir: 8 to 14 days), anemia (38%), thrombocytopenia (20%; grades 3/4: ≤8%)

Renal: Hematuria (6% to 92%, reduced with mesna; grade 2 [gross hematuria]: 8% to 12%)

1% to 10%:

Cardiovascular: Localized phlebitis (2% to 3%)

Gastrointestinal: Anorexia (1%)

Hematologic & oncologic: Febrile neutropenia (1%)

Hepatic: Hepatic insufficiency (2% to 3%), increased serum bilirubin (2% to 3%), increased serum transaminases (2% to 3%)

Infection: Infection (8% to 10%)

Renal: Renal insufficiency (6%)

Miscellaneous: Fever (1%)

<1%, postmarketing, and/or case reports: Abdominal pain, abnormal gait, acute renal failure, agranulocytosis, altered hormone level (increased gonadotropin), amenorrhea, amnesia, anaphylaxis, angina pectoris, angioedema, anovulation, anuria, arthralgia, asterixis, atrial premature contractions, atrial fibrillation, atrial flutter, atrial premature contractions, azoospermia, blood coagulation disorder, blurred vision, bone marrow failure, bradycardia, bradyphrenia, bronchospasm, bundle branch block, capillary leak syndrome, cardiac arrhythmia, cardiac failure, cardiogenic shock, cardiomyopathy, cardiotoxicity, casts in urine, catatonia, chest pain, chills, cholestasis, chronic renal failure, colitis, conjunctivitis, constipation, cough, increased serum creatinine, decreased creatinine clearance, decreased plasma estrogen concentration, deep vein thrombosis, delirium, delusions, dermatitis, diarrhea, disseminated intravascular coagulation, dysarthria, dysesthesia, dyspnea, dysuria, ECG abnormality (QRS complex abnormal), edema, enterocolitis, erythema, extrapyramidal reaction, facial swelling, Fanconi's syndrome, fatigue, fecal incontinence, flushing, fulminant hepatitis, gastrointestinal hemorrhage, glycosuria, granulocytopenia, growth suppression (children), hearing loss, hemolytic anemia, hemolytic-uremic syndrome, hemorrhage (including myocardial), hemorrhagic cystitis, hepatic failure, hepatic sinusoidal obstruction syndrome (formerly known as hepatic veno-occlusive disease), hepatitis (cytolytic), hepatorenal syndrome, herpes zoster, hyperglycemia, hyperhidrosis, hypertension, hyperpigmentation, hypersensitivity pneumonitis, hypersensitivity reaction, hypocalcemia, hypoesthesia, hypokalemia, hyponatremia, hypophosphatemia, hypotension, hypoxia, intestinal obstruction, immunosuppression, increased blood urea nitrogen, increased creatinine clearance, increased gamma-glutamyl transferase, increased lactate dehydrogenase, increased serum alkaline phosphatase, infertility, infusion site reaction (erythema, inflammation, pain, pruritus, swelling, tenderness), inhibition of spermatogenesis, interstitial nephritis, interstitial pneumonitis, interstitial pulmonary disease, inversion T wave on ECG, irritable bladder, jaundice, left ventricular dysfunction (failure), leukoencephalopathy, limb pain, lymphocytopenia, malaise, mania, menopause (premature), mental status changes, metastases (including ALL, AML, APL, lymphoma, MDS, RCC, sarcomas, thyroid cancer), methemoglobinemia, mucosal inflammation, mucous membrane ulceration, multi-organ failure, muscle twitching, mutism, myalgia, myocardial infarction, myocarditis, nail disease, nephrogenic diabetes insipidus, neuralgia, neutropenia, oligospermia, oliguria, osteomalacia (adults), ovarian failure, pain, palmar-plantar erythrodysesthesia, pancreatitis, pancytopenia, panic attack, paranoia, parenchymal damage (renal), paresthesia, pericardial effusion, pericarditis, peripheral neuropathy, petechia, phosphaturia, physical health deterioration, pleural effusion, pneumonia (including *Pneumocystis jirovecii*), pneumonitis, pollakiuria, polydipsia, polyneuropathy, polyuria, portal vein thrombosis, progressive multifocal leukoencephalopathy, proteinuria, pruritus, pulmonary edema, pulmonary embolism, pulmonary fibrosis, pulmonary hypertension, reduced ejection fraction, renal tubular acidosis, renal tubular necrosis, respiratory distress syndrome (acute), respiratory failure, reversible posterior leukoencephalopathy syndrome, rhabdomyolysis, rickets, salivation,

seizure, sepsis, septic shock, SIADH, skin abnormalities related to radiation recall, skin necrosis, skin rash (including macular and papular), status epilepticus, sterility, Stevens-Johnson syndrome, stomatitis, ST segment changes on ECG, supraventricular extrasystole, tachycardia, talkativeness (logorrhea), tinnitus, toxic epidermal necrolysis, tumor lysis syndrome, typhlitis, uremia, urinary incontinence, urine abnormality (aminoaciduria and enzymuria), urticaria, vasculitis, ventricular fibrillation, ventricular premature contractions, ventricular tachycardia, vertigo, viral hepatitis, visual impairment, wound healing impairment

Drug Interactions

Metabolism/Transport Effects Substrate of CYP2B6 (major), CYP2C19 (minor), CYP2C8 (minor), CYP2C9 (minor), CYP3A4 (minor); **Note:** Assignment of Major/Minor substrate status based on clinically relevant drug interaction potential; **Induces** CYP2C9 (weak/moderate)

Avoid Concomitant Use

Avoid concomitant use of Ifosfamide with any of the following: BCG (Intravesical); Deferiprone; Dipyrone; Natalizumab; Pimecrolimus; Tacrolimus (Topical); Vaccines (Live)

Increased Effect/Toxicity

Ifosfamide may increase the levels/effects of: CloZAPine; Deferiprone; Fingolimod; Leflunomide; Natalizumab; Tofacitinib; Vaccines (Live); Vitamin K Antagonists

The levels/effects of Ifosfamide may be increased by: Aprepitant; Busulfan; CYP3A4 Inducers (Moderate); CYP3A4 Inducers (Strong); Denosumab; Dipyrone; Fosaprepitant; MiFEPRIStone; Ocrelizumab; Palifermin; Pimecrolimus; Promazine; Roflumilast; Tacrolimus (Topical); Thiotepa; Trastuzumab

Decreased Effect

Ifosfamide may decrease the levels/effects of: BCG (Intravesical); Coccidioides immitis Skin Test; Lenograstim; Nivolumab; Sipuleucel-T; Tertomotide; Vaccines (Inactivated); Vaccines (Live)

The levels/effects of Ifosfamide may be decreased by: CYP2B6 Inducers (Moderate); CYP3A4 Inducers (Moderate); CYP3A4 Inducers (Strong); CYP3A4 Inhibitors (Moderate); CYP3A4 Inhibitors (Strong); Dabrafenib; Echinacea; Lumacaftor; Nilotinib

Hazardous Drugs Handling Considerations

Hazardous agent (NIOSH 2016 [group 1]).

Use appropriate precautions for receiving, handling, administration, and disposal. Gloves (single) should be worn during receiving, unpacking, and placing in storage.

NIOSH recommends double gloving, a protective gown, ventilated engineering controls (a class II biological safety cabinet or a compounding aseptic containment isolator), and closed system transfer devices (CSTDs) for preparation. Double gloving, a gown, and (if dosage form allows) CSTDs are required during administration (NIOSH 2016).

Storage/Stability Store intact vials of powder for injection at room temperature of 20°C to 25°C (68°F to 77°F); avoid temperatures >30°C (86°F). Store intact vials of solution at 2°C to 8°C (36°F to 46°F). Reconstituted solutions and solutions diluted in D5W, NS, or LR for administration are stable for 24 hours refrigerated.

Preparation for Administration Reconstitute powder with SWFI or bacteriostatic SWFI (1 g in 20 mL or 3 g in 60 mL) to a concentration of 50 mg/mL.

Further dilution in 50 to 1,000 mL D5W, NS, or lactated Ringer's (to a final concentration of 0.6 to 20 mg/mL) is recommended for IV infusion (may also dilute in D2.5W, $\frac{1}{2}$NS, or D5NS).

Mechanism of Action Causes cross-linking of strands of DNA by binding with nucleic acids and other intracellular structures, resulting in cell death; inhibits protein synthesis and DNA synthesis

Pharmacodynamics/Kinetics Pharmacokinetics are dose dependent

Distribution: V_d: Approximates total body water; penetrates CNS, but not in therapeutic levels

Protein binding: Negligible

Metabolism: Hepatic to active metabolites isofosforamide mustard, 4-hydroxy-ifosfamide, acrolein, and inactive dichloroethylated and carboxy metabolites; acrolein is the agent implicated in development of hemorrhagic cystitis

Half-life elimination (increased in the elderly):

High dose (3,800 to 5,000 mg/m^2): ~15 hours

Lower dose (1,600 to 2,400 mg/m^2): ~7 hours

Excretion:

High dose (5,000 mg/m^2): Urine (70% to 86%; 61% as unchanged drug)

Lower dose (1,600 to 2,400 mg/m^2): Urine (12% to 18% as unchanged drug)

Dosing

Adult & Geriatric Note: To prevent bladder toxicity, ifosfamide should be given with mesna and hydration (at least 2 L of oral or IV fluid per day). Ifosfamide is associated with a moderate emetic potential; antiemetics are recommended to prevent nausea and vomiting (Basch 2011; Roila 2010).

Testicular cancer: IV:

Manufacturer's labeling; as part of combination chemotherapy and with mesna: 1,200 mg/m^2/day for 5 days every 3 weeks or after hematologic recovery

VIP regimen: 1,200 mg/m^2/day for 5 days every 3 weeks for 4 cycles (in combination with etoposide, mesna, and cisplatin) (Nichols 1998)

VeIP regimen: 1,200 mg/m^2/day for 5 days every 3 weeks for 4 cycles (in combination with vinblastine, mesna, and cisplatin) (Loehrer 1998)

Off-label dosing/combinations:

TIP regimen (off-label dosing): 1,500 mg/m^2/day for 4 days (days 2 to 5) every 3 weeks for 4 cycles (in combination with paclitaxel, mesna, and cisplatin) (Kondagunta 2005)

TICE regimen (off-label dosing): 2,000 mg/m^2/day for 3 days (days 2 to 4) over 4 hours every 2 weeks for 2 cycles (in combination with paclitaxel and mesna; followed by carboplatin and etoposide) (Kondagunta 2007)

Bladder cancer, advanced (off-label use): IV: 1,500 mg/m^2/day for 5 days every 3 weeks (with mesna) until disease progression (Witte 1997)

Cervical cancer, recurrent or metastatic (off-label use): IV: 1,500 mg/m^2/day for 5 days every 3 weeks (with mesna) (Coleman 1986; Sutton 1993)

Ewing sarcoma (off-label use): IV:

VAC/IE regimen: Adults ≤30 years: IE: 1,800 mg/m^2/day for 5 days (in combination with mesna and etoposide) alternate with VAC (vincristine, doxorubicin, and cyclophosphamide) every 3 weeks for a total of 17 courses (Grier 2003)

VAIA regimen: 3,000 mg/m^2 day on days 1, 2, 22, 23, 43, and 44 for 4 courses (in combination with vincristine, doxorubicin, dactinomycin, and mesna) (Paulussen 2001) **or** Adults ≤35 years: 2,000 mg/m^2/day for 3 days every 3 weeks for 14 courses (in combination with vincristine, doxorubicin, dactinomycin, and mesna) (Paulussen 2008)

VIDE regimen: Adults ≤50 years: 3,000 mg/m²/day over 1 to 3 hours for 3 days every 3 weeks for 6 courses (in combination with vincristine, doxorubicin, etoposide, and mesna) (Juergens 2006)

IE regimen: 1,800 mg/m²/day over 1 hour for 5 days every 3 weeks for 12 cycles (in combination with etoposide and mesna) (Miser 1987)

ICE regimen: Adults ≤22 years: 1,800 mg/m²/day for 5 days every 3 weeks for up to 12 cycles (in combination with carboplatin and etoposide [and mesna]) (van Winkle 2005)

Hodgkin lymphoma, relapsed or refractory (off-label use): IV:

ICE regimen: 5,000 mg/m² (over 24 hours) beginning on day 2 every 2 weeks for 2 cycles (in combination with mesna, carboplatin, and etoposide) (Moskowitz 2001)

IGEV regimen: 2,000 mg/m²/day for 4 days every 3 weeks for 4 cycles (in combination with mesna, gemcitabine, vinorelbine, and prednisolone) (Santoro 2007)

Non-Hodgkin lymphomas (off-label use): IV:

Burkitt lymphoma (CODOX-M/IVAC regimen):

Adults ≤65 years: Cycles 2 and 4 (IVAC): 1,500 mg/m²/day for 5 days (IVAC is combination with cytarabine, mesna, and etoposide; IVAC alternates with CODOX-M) (Mead 2008)

Adults >65 years: Cycles 2 and 4 (IVAC): 1,000 mg/m²/day for 5 days (IVAC is combination with cytarabine, mesna, and etoposide; IVAC alternates with CODOX-M) (Mead 2008)

Diffuse large B-cell lymphoma (RICE regimen): 5,000 mg/m² (over 24 hours) beginning on day 4 every 2 weeks for 3 cycles (in combination with mesna, carboplatin, etoposide, and rituximab) (Kewalramani 2004)

Osteosarcoma (off-label use): IV:

Ifosfamide/cisplatin/doxorubicin/HDMT regimen: Adults <40 years: 3,000 mg/m²/day continuous infusion for 5 days during weeks 4 and 10 (preop) and during weeks 16, 25, and 34 (postop) (in combination with cisplatin, doxorubicin, methotrexate [high-dose], and mesna) (Bacci 2003)

Ifosfamide/cisplatin/epirubicin regimen: 2,000 mg/m²/day over 4 hours for 3 days (days 2, 3, and 4) every 3 weeks for 3 cycles (preop) and every 4 weeks for 3 cycles (postop) (in combination with cisplatin, epirubicin, and mesna) (Basaran 2007)

ICE regimen (adults ≤22 years): 1,800 mg/m²/day for 5 days every 3 weeks for up to 12 cycles (in combination with carboplatin and etoposide [and mesna]) (van Winkle 2005)

Ovarian cancer, advanced (platinum-resistant): IV: 1,000 to 1,200 mg/m²/day for 5 days (with mesna) every 28 days for up to 6 cycles (Markman 1992). Additional trials may be necessary to further define the role of ifosfamide in this condition.

Soft tissue sarcoma (off-label use): IV:

Single-agent ifosfamide: 3,000 mg/m²/day over 4 hours for 3 days every 3 weeks for at least 2 cycles or until disease progression (van Oosterom 2002)

EIA regimen: 1,500 mg/m²/day for 4 days every 3 weeks until disease progression or unacceptable toxicity (in combination with etoposide, doxorubicin, and regional hyperthermia) (Issels 2010)

MAID regimen: 2,000 mg/m²/day continuous infusion for 3 days every 3 weeks (in combination with mesna, doxorubicin, and dacarbazine) (Antman 1993; Antman 1998) **or** 2,500 mg/m²/day continuous infusion for 3 days every 3 weeks (in combination with mesna, doxorubicin, and dacarbazine); reduce ifosfamide to 1,500 mg/m^2/day if prior pelvic irradiation (Elias 1989)

Ifosfamide/epirubicin: 1,800 mg/m^2/day over 1 hour for 5 days every 3 weeks for 5 cycles (in combination with mesna and epirubicin) (Frustaci 2001)

AIM regimens: 1,500 mg/m^2/day over 2 hours for 4 days every 3 weeks for 4 to 6 cycles (in combination with mesna and doxorubicin) (Worden 2005) **or** 2,000 to 3,000 mg/m^2/day over 3 hours for 3 days (in combination with mesna and doxorubicin) (Grobmyer 2004)

Thymomas and thymic cancers, advanced (off-label use): IV: 1,200 mg/m^2/day for 4 days every 3 weeks for 4 cycles (in combination with mesna, cisplatin, and etoposide); colony-stimulating growth factor support was administered on days 5 to 15 (or until WBC ≥10,000/mm^3) (Loehrer 2001) **or** 1,500 mg/m^2/day for 5 days (with mesna) every 3 weeks for up to 9 cycles (Highley 1999). Additional trials may be necessary to further define the role of ifosfamide in this condition.

Pediatric Note: To prevent bladder toxicity, ifosfamide should be given with mesna and hydration (at least 2 L of oral or IV fluid per day). Ifosfamide is associated with a moderate emetic potential; antiemetics are recommended to prevent nausea and vomiting (Dupuis 2011).

Ewing sarcoma (off-label use): IV:

VAC/IE regimen: IE: 1,800 mg/m^2/day for 5 days (in combination with mesna and etoposide) alternate with VAC (vincristine, doxorubicin, and cyclophosphamide) every 3 weeks for a total of 17 courses (Grier 2003)

ICE CAV regimen: ICE: 1,800 mg/m^2/day for 5 days every 3 to 4 weeks for 2 courses (in combination with carboplatin and etoposide [and mesna]), followed by CAV (cyclophosphamide, doxorubicin, and vincristine) (Milano 2006)

VAIA regimen: 3,000 mg/m^2/day on days 1, 2, 22, 23, 43, and 44 for 4 courses (in combination with vincristine, doxorubicin, dactinomycin, and mesna) (Paulussen 2001) **or** 2,000 mg/m^2/day for 3 days every 3 weeks for 14 courses (in combination with vincristine, doxorubicin, dactinomycin, and mesna) (Paulussen 2008)

VIDE regimen: 3,000 mg/m^2/day over 1 to 3 hours for 3 days every 3 weeks for 6 courses (In combination with vincristine, doxorubicin, etoposide, and mesna) (Juergens 2006)

IE regimen: 1,800 mg/m^2/day over 1 hour for 5 days every 3 weeks for 12 cycles (in combination with etoposide and mesna) (Miser 1987)

ICE regimen: 1,800 mg/m^2/day for 5 days every 3 weeks for up to 12 cycles (in combination with carboplatin and etoposide [and mesna]) (van Winkle 2005)

Osteosarcoma (off-label use): IV:

Ifosfamide/cisplatin/doxorubicin/HDMT regimen: 3,000 mg/m^2/day continuous infusion for 5 days during weeks 4 and 10 (preop) and during weeks 16, 25, and 34 (postop) (in combination with cisplatin, doxorubicin, methotrexate [high-dose], and mesna) (Bacci 2003)

Ifosfamide/cisplatin/epirubicin regimen: Children ≥15 years: 2,000 mg/m^2/day over 4 hours for 3 days (days 2, 3, and 4) every 3 weeks for 3 cycles (preop) and every 4 weeks for 3 cycles (postop) (in combination with cisplatin, epirubicin, and mesna) (Basaran 2007)

IE regimen: 3,000 mg/m^2/day over 3 hours for 4 days every 3 to 4 weeks (in combination with etoposide and mesna) (Gentet 1997)

ICE regimen: Children ≥1 year: 1,800 mg/m^2/day for 5 days every 3 weeks for up to 12 cycles (in combination with carboplatin and etoposide [and mesna]) (van Winkle 2005)

Ifosfamide/HDMT/etoposide regimen: 3,000 mg/m^2/day over 3 hours for 4 days during weeks 4 and 9 (3 additional postop courses were administered in good responders) (in combination with methotrexate [high-dose], etoposide, and mesna) (Le Deley 2007)

Renal Impairment

Consider dosage reduction in patients with renal impairment; however, there are no dosage adjustments provided in the manufacturer's labeling; ifosfamide (and metabolites) are excreted renally and may accumulate in patients with renal dysfunction. Ifosfamide and metabolites are dialyzable. The following adjustments have also been recommended:

Aronoff 2007:

CrCl ≥10 mL/minute: Children and Adults: No dosage adjustment necessary.

CrCl <10 mL/minute: Children and Adults: Administer 75% of dose.

Hemodialysis (supplement for dialysis):

Children: 1 g/m^2 followed by hemodialysis 6 to 8 hours later

Adults: No supplemental dose needed

Kintzel 1995:

CrCl 46 to 60 mL/minute: Administer 80% of dose

CrCl 31 to 45 mL/minute: Administer 75% of dose

CrCl <30 mL/minute: Administer 70% of dose

Hepatic Impairment There are no dosage adjustments provided in the manufacturer's labeling; however, ifosfamide is extensively hepatically metabolized to both active and inactive metabolites; use with caution. The following adjustments have been recommended:

Floyd 2006: Bilirubin >3 mg/dL: Administer 25% of dose.

Obesity *ASCO Guidelines for appropriate chemotherapy dosing in obese adults with cancer:* Utilize patient's actual body weight (full weight) for calculation of body surface area- or weight-based dosing, particularly when the intent of therapy is curative; manage regimen-related toxicities in the same manner as for nonobese patients; if a dose reduction is utilized due to toxicity, consider resumption of full weight-based dosing with subsequent cycles, especially if cause of toxicity (eg, hepatic or renal impairment) is resolved (Griggs 2012).

Adjustment for Toxicity

WBC <2,000/mm^3 and/or platelets <50,000/mm^3: Avoid administering treatment (unless clinically necessary)

Encephalopathy: Discontinue treatment

Combination Regimens

Bone sarcoma (Ewing sarcoma):

Bone sarcoma (osteosarcoma):

Administration Ifosfamide is associated with a moderate emetic potential; antiemetics are recommended to prevent nausea and vomiting (Basch 2011; Dupuis 2011; Roila 2010).

Administer IV over at least 30 minutes (infusion times may vary by protocol; refer to specific protocol for infusion duration). To prevent bladder toxicity, ifosfamide should be given with mesna and hydration.

Vesicant/Extravasation Risk May be an irritant

Emetic Potential Children and Adults: Moderate (30% to 90%)

Monitoring Parameters CBC with differential (prior to each cycle and as clinically appropriate), urine output, urinalysis (prior to each dose), liver function, and renal function tests; signs and symptoms of neurotoxicity, pulmonary toxicity, and/or hemorrhagic cystitis

Dosage Forms Excipient information presented when available (limited, particularly for generics); consult specific product labeling

Solution, Intravenous:
  Generic: 1 g/20 mL (20 mL); 3 g/60 mL (60 mL)
Solution, Intravenous [preservative free]:
  Generic: 1 g/20 mL (20 mL); 3 g/60 mL (60 mL)
Solution Reconstituted, Intravenous:
  Ifex: 1 g (1 ea); 3 g (1 ea)
  Generic: 1 g (1 ea); 3 g (1 ea)

Imatinib (eye MAT eh nib)

Related Information

Common Toxicity Criteria *on page 2242*

Hematopoietic Cell Transplantation *on page 2365*

Management of Chemotherapy-Induced Nausea and Vomiting in Adults *on page 2253*

Prevention of Chemotherapy-Induced Nausea and Vomiting in Children *on page 2310*

Safe Handling of Hazardous Drugs *on page 2379*

Brand Names: US Gleevec

Brand Names: Canada ACT-Imatinib; Apo-Imatinib; Gleevec; Teva-Imatinib

Index Terms CGP-57148B; Glivec; Imatinib Mesylate; STI-571

Pharmacologic Category Antineoplastic Agent, BCR-ABL Tyrosine Kinase Inhibitor; Antineoplastic Agent, Tyrosine Kinase Inhibitor

Use

Acute lymphoblastic leukemia: Treatment of relapsed or refractory Philadelphia chromosome-positive (Ph+) acute lymphoblastic leukemia (ALL) in adults

Treatment of newly diagnosed Ph+ ALL in children (in combination with chemotherapy)

Aggressive systemic mastocytosis: Treatment of aggressive systemic mastocytosis without D816V c-Kit mutation as determined by an approved test (or c-Kit mutational status unknown) in adults

Chronic myeloid leukemia: Treatment of Ph+ chronic myeloid leukemia (CML) in chronic phase (newly diagnosed) in adults and children

Treatment of Ph+ CML in blast crisis, accelerated phase, or chronic phase after failure of interferon-alfa therapy

Dermatofibrosarcoma protuberans: Treatment of unresectable, recurrent, and/or metastatic dermatofibrosarcoma protuberans (DFSP) in adults

Gastrointestinal stromal tumors: Treatment of Kit (CD117)-positive unresectable and/or metastatic malignant gastrointestinal stromal tumors (GIST)

Adjuvant treatment of Kit (CD117)-positive GIST following complete gross resection

Hypereosinophilic syndrome and/or chronic eosinophilic leukemia: Treatment of hypereosinophilic syndrome (HES) and/or chronic eosinophilic leukemia (CEL) in adult patients who have the FIP1L1-platelet-derived growth factor (PDGF) receptor alpha fusion kinase (mutational analysis or fluorescent in situ hybridization [FISH] demonstration of CHIC2 allele deletion) and for patients with HES and/or CEL who are FIP1L1-PDGF receptor alpha fusion kinase negative or unknown

Myelodysplastic/Myeloproliferative diseases: Treatment of myelodysplastic syndrome/myeloproliferative diseases (MDS/MPD) associated with PDGF receptor gene rearrangements as determined by an approved test in adults

Labeled Contraindications

There are no contraindications listed in the manufacturer's US labeling.

Canadian labeling: Hypersensitivity to imatinib or any component of the formulation

Pregnancy Considerations Adverse events have been observed in animal reproduction studies. Women of childbearing potential are advised not to become pregnant (female patients and female partners of male patients); highly effective contraception should be used during treatment and for 2 weeks after the last imatinib dose. Case reports of pregnancies while on therapy (both males and females) include reports of spontaneous abortion, minor abnormalities (hypospadias, pyloric stenosis, and small intestine rotation) at or shortly after birth, and other congenital abnormalities including skeletal malformations, hypoplastic lungs, exomphalos, kidney abnormalities, hydrocephalus, cerebellar hypoplasia, and cardiac defects.

Retrospective case reports of women with CML in complete hematologic response (CHR) with cytogenic response (partial or complete) who interrupted imatinib therapy due to pregnancy, demonstrated a loss of response in some patients while off treatment. At 18 months after treatment reinitiation following delivery, CHR was again achieved in all patients and cytogenic response was achieved in some patients. Cytogenetic response rates may not be at as high as compared to patients with 18 months of uninterrupted therapy (Ault 2006; Pye 2008).

Breastfeeding Considerations Imatinib and its active metabolite are found in human breast milk; the milk/plasma ratio is 0.5 for imatinib and 0.9 for the active metabolite. Based on body weight, up to 10% of a therapeutic maternal dose could potentially be received by a breast-fed infant. Due to the potential for serious adverse reactions in the breastfeeding infant, breastfeeding is not recommended by the manufacturer during treatment and for 1 month after the last imatinib dose.

Warnings/Precautions Imatinib is commonly associated with fluid retention, weight gain, and edema (risk increases with higher doses and age >65 years); may be occasionally serious and lead to significant complications, including pleural effusion, pericardial effusion, pulmonary edema, and ascites. Monitor regularly for rapid weight gain or other signs/symptoms of fluid retention; rapid unexpected weight gain should be evaluated and managed appropriately. Use with caution in patients where fluid accumulation may be poorly tolerated, such as in cardiovascular disease (heart failure [HF] or hypertension) and pulmonary disease. Severe HF and left ventricular dysfunction (LVD) have been reported occasionally. Cardiac adverse events usually occur in patients with advanced age or comorbidities; carefully monitor patients with preexisting cardiac disease or risk factors for HF or history of renal failure. With initiation of imatinib treatment, cardiogenic shock and/or LVD have been reported in patients with hypereosinophilic syndrome (HES) and cardiac involvement (reversible with systemic steroids, circulatory support and temporary cessation of imatinib). Echocardiogram and serum troponin monitoring may be considered in patients with HES/chronic eosinophilic leukemia (CEL) and in patients with myelodysplastic/myeloproliferative (MDS/MPD) disease or aggressive systemic mastocytosis associated with high eosinophil levels. Patients with high eosinophil levels and an abnormal echocardiogram or abnormal serum troponin level may benefit from prophylactic systemic steroids (for 1 to 2 weeks) with the initiation of imatinib. In a scientific statement from the American Heart Association, imatinib has been determined to be an agent that may either cause direct myocardial toxicity (rare) or exacerbate underlying myocardial dysfunction (magnitude: moderate) (AHA [Page 2016]).

Severe bullous dermatologic reactions (including erythema multiforme and Stevens-Johnson syndrome) have been reported; recurrence has been described with rechallenge. Case reports of successful resumption at a lower dose (with corticosteroids and/or antihistamine) have been described; however, some patients may experience recurrent reactions. Drug reaction with eosinophilia and systemic symptoms (DRESS) has been reported; if DRESS occurs, interrupt therapy and consider permanent discontinuation.

Hepatotoxicity may occur (may be severe); fatal hepatic failure and severe hepatic injury requiring liver transplantation have been reported with both short- and long-term use; monitor liver function (transaminases, bilirubin, and alkaline phosphatase) prior to initiation and monthly or as needed thereafter; therapy interruption or dose reduction may be necessary. Transaminase and bilirubin elevations, and acute liver failure have been observed with imatinib in combination with chemotherapy. Use with caution in patients with preexisting hepatic impairment; dosage adjustment recommended in patients with severe impairment. Use with caution in renal impairment; dosage adjustment recommended for moderate and severe impairment (CrCl <40 mL/minute). Imatinib is associated with acute kidney injury and a decline in renal function (may be associated with duration of therapy); monitor renal function periodically during treatment (Marcolino 2011). Tumor lysis syndrome (TLS), including fatalities, has been reported in patients with acute lymphoblastic leukemia (ALL), chronic myeloid leukemia (CML) eosinophilic leukemias, and gastrointestinal stromal tumors (GIST); risk for TLS is higher in patients with a high tumor burden or high proliferation rate; monitor closely; correct clinically significant dehydration and treat high uric acid levels prior to initiation of imatinib.

Imatinib is associated with a moderate emetic potential; antiemetics may be recommended to prevent nausea and vomiting (Dupuis, 2011; Roila, 2010). May cause GI irritation; take with food and water to minimize irritation. There have been rare reports (including fatalities) of GI perforation. Severe hemorrhage (grades 3 and 4) have been reported with use, including GI hemorrhage and/or tumor hemorrhage. The incidence of hemorrhage is higher in patients with GIST (GI tumors may have been hemorrhage source); gastric antral vascular ectasia has also been reported (Alshehry 2014; Saad Aldin 2012). May cause hematologic toxicity (anemia, neutropenia, and thrombocytopenia; usually occurring within the first several months of treatment). Monitor blood counts weekly for the first month, biweekly for the second month, and as clinically necessary thereafter; median duration of neutropenia is 2 to 3 weeks; median duration of thrombocytopenia is 2 to 4 weeks. In CML, cytopenias are more common in accelerated or blast phase than in chronic phase. Hypothyroidism has been reported in patients who were receiving thyroid hormone replacement therapy prior to the initiation of imatinib; monitor thyroid function; the average onset for imatinib-induced hypothyroidism is 2 weeks; consider doubling levothyroxine doses upon initiation of imatinib (Hamnvik 2011). Potentially significant drug-drug interactions may exist, requiring dose or frequency adjustment, additional monitoring, and/or selection of alternative therapy. Imatinib exposure may be reduced in patients who have had gastric surgery (eg, bypass, major gastrectomy, or resection); monitor imatinib trough concentrations (Liu 2011; Pavlovsky 2009; Yoo 2010). Growth retardation has been reported in children receiving imatinib for the treatment of CML; generally where treatment was initiated in prepubertal children; growth velocity was usually restored as pubertal age was reached (Shima 2011); monitor growth closely. The incidence of edema was increased with age older than 65 years in CML and GIST studies. Reports of accidents have been received but it is unclear if imatinib has been the direct cause in any case; advise patients regarding side effects such as dizziness, blurred vision, or somnolence; use caution when driving/operating motor vehicles and heavy machinery. Determine PDGFRb gene rearrangements status (for MDS/MPD), D816V c-Kit mutation status (for aggressive systemic mastocytosis [ASM]), Philadelphia chromosome status for acute lymphoblastic leukemia and chronic myeloid leukemia, Kit (CD117)-positivity for GIST, and FIP1L1–platelet-derived growth factor (PDGF) receptor status for HES or CEL prior to initiating treatment.

Adverse Reactions Adverse reactions listed as a composite of data across many trials, except where noted for a specific indication.

>10%:

Cardiovascular: Edema (11% to 86%; includes aggravated edema, anasarca, ascites, pericardial effusion, pulmonary edema, and superficial edema), peripheral edema (20% to 41%), facial edema (≤17%), chest pain (7% to 11%), hypotension (Ph+ ALL; children, adolescents, adults)

Central nervous system: Fatigue (20% to 75%), pain (≤47%), headache (8% to 37%), dizziness (5% to 19%), insomnia (9% to 15%), depression (3% to 15%), taste disorder (≤13%), rigors (10% to 12%), anxiety (8% to 12%), paresthesia (≤12%), chills (≤11%)

Dermatologic: Skin rash (9% to 50%), dermatitis (GIST: ≤39%), pruritus (7% to 26%), night sweats (CML: 13% to 17%), alopecia (7% to 15%), diaphoresis (GIST: ≤13%)

Endocrine & metabolic: Increased lactate dehydrogenase (≤60%), weight gain (5% to 32%), decreased serum albumin (≤21%), hypokalemia (6% to 13%)

Gastrointestinal: Nausea (41% to 73%), diarrhea (25% to 59%), vomiting (11% to 58%), abdominal pain (3% to 57%), anorexia (≤36%), dyspepsia (11% to 27%), flatulence (≤25%), abdominal distension (≤19%), constipation (8% to 16%), stomatitis (≤16%), upper abdominal pain (14%)

Hematologic & oncologic: Hemorrhage (3% to 53%; grades 3/4: ≤19%), leukopenia (GIST: 5% to 47%; grades 3/4: 2%), hypoproteinemia (≤32%), anemia, neutropenia, thrombocytopenia

Hepatic: Increased serum AST (≤38%), increased serum ALT (≤34%), increased alkaline phosphatase (≤17%), increased serum bilirubin (≤13%), increased serum transaminases

Infection: Influenza (Ph+ CML: ≤14%), infection (Ph+ ALL; children, adolescents, adults

Neuromuscular & skeletal: Muscle cramps (16% to 62%), musculoskeletal pain (adults: 38% to 49%; children: 21%), arthralgia (11% to 40%), myalgia (9% to 32%), weakness (≤21%), back pain (≤17%), limb pain (≤16%), ostealgia (≤11%)

Ophthalmic: Periorbital edema (15% to 74%), increased lacrimation (DFSP: 25%; GIST: ≤18%), eyelid edema (Ph+ CML: 19%), blurred vision (≤11%)

Renal: Increased serum creatinine (≤44%)

Respiratory: Nasopharyngitis (1% to 31%), cough (11% to 27%), upper respiratory tract infection (3% to 21%), dyspnea (≤21%), pharyngolaryngeal pain (≤18%), rhinitis (DFSP: 17%), pharyngitis (CML: 10% to 15%), flu-like symptoms (1% to 14%), pneumonia (CML: 4% to 13%), sinusitis (4% to 11%)

Miscellaneous: Fever (6% to 41%)

1% to 10%:

Cardiovascular: Palpitations (≤5%), hypertension (≤4%), cardiac failure (Ph+ CML: 1%), flushing

Central nervous system: Cerebral hemorrhage (≤9%), hypoesthesia, peripheral neuropathy

Dermatologic: Skin photosensitivity (4% to 7%), xeroderma (≤7%), erythema, nail disease

◀

Endocrine & metabolic: Hypophosphatemia (10%), hyperglycemia (≤10%), weight loss (≤10%), hypocalcemia (GIST: ≤6%), fluid retention (Ph+ CML: 3%; pleural effusion, pericardial effusion, ascites, or pulmonary edema: 2%), hyperkalemia (1%)

Gastrointestinal: Decreased appetite (10%), gastroenteritis (≤10%), gastrointestinal hemorrhage (1% to 8%), gastritis, gastroesophageal reflux, increased serum lipase, xerostomia

Hematologic & oncologic: Lymphocytopenia (≤10%; grades 3/4: 1% to 2%), eosinophilia, febrile neutropenia, pancytopenia, purpura

Neuromuscular & skeletal: Joint swelling

Ophthalmic: Conjunctivitis (5% to 8%), conjunctival hemorrhage, dry eyes

Respiratory: Hypoxia (9%), oropharyngeal pain (Ph+ CML: ≤6%), epistaxis, pleural effusion, pneumonitis (Ph+ ALL; children, adolescents, adults)

<1%, postmarketing, and/or case reports: Actinic keratosis, acute generalized exanthematous pustulosis, anaphylactic shock, angina pectoris, angioedema, aplastic anemia, arthritis, ascites, atrial fibrillation, avascular necrosis of bones, blepharitis, bullous rash, cardiac arrhythmia, cardiac tamponade, cardiogenic shock, cataract, cellulitis, cerebral edema, cheilitis, cold extremities, colitis, confusion, decreased libido, decreased linear skeletal growth rate (children), dehydration, diverticulitis, DRESS syndrome, drowsiness, dyschromia, dysphagia, embolism, eructation, erythema multiforme, esophagitis, exfoliative dermatitis, folliculitis, fungal infection, gastric ulcer, gastrointestinal obstruction, gastrointestinal perforation, glaucoma, gout, gynecomastia, hearing loss, hematemesis, hematoma, hematuria, hemolytic anemia, hepatic failure, hepatic necrosis, hepatitis, hepatotoxicity, herpes simplex infection, herpes zoster, hypercalcemia, hypermenorrhea, hypersensitivity angiitis, hyperuricemia, hypomagnesemia, hyponatremia, hypothyroidism, IgA vasculitis, increased creatine phosphokinase, increased intracranial pressure, inflammatory bowel disease, interstitial pneumonitis, interstitial pulmonary disease, intestinal obstruction, jaundice, left ventricular dysfunction, lichen planus, lower respiratory tract infection, lymphadenopathy, macular edema, melena, memory impairment, menstrual disease, migraine, myocardial infarction, myopathy, onychoclasis, optic neuritis, oral mucosa ulcer, osteonecrosis (hip), ovarian cyst (hemorrhagic), palmar-plantar erythrodysesthesia, pancreatitis, papilledema, pericarditis, petechia, pleuritic chest pain, polyuria, psoriasis, pulmonary fibrosis, pulmonary hemorrhage, pulmonary hypertension, Raynaud phenomenon, reactivation of HBV, renal failure, respiratory failure, restless leg syndrome, retinal hemorrhage, rhabdomyolysis, ruptured corpus luteal cyst, sciatica, scrotal edema, seizure, sepsis, sexual disorder, Stevens-Johnson syndrome, subconjunctival hemorrhage, subdural hematoma, Sweet syndrome, syncope, tachycardia, telangiectasia (gastric antral), thrombocythemia, thrombosis, tinnitus, toxic epidermal necrolysis, tremor, tumor hemorrhage (GIST), tumor lysis syndrome, urinary tract infection, urticaria, vertigo, vesicular eruption, vitreous hemorrhage

Drug Interactions

Metabolism/Transport Effects Substrate of CYP1A2 (minor), CYP2C19 (minor), CYP2C8 (minor), CYP2C9 (minor), CYP2D6 (minor), CYP3A4 (major), P-glycoprotein; **Note:** Assignment of Major/Minor substrate status based on clinically relevant drug interaction potential; **Inhibits** BCRP, CYP2C9 (weak), CYP3A4 (moderate)

Avoid Concomitant Use

Avoid concomitant use of Imatinib with any of the following: Aprepitant; Asunaprevir; BCG (Intravesical); Bosutinib; Budesonide (Systemic); Cobimetinib; Deferiprone; Dipyrone; Domperidone; Flibanserin; Grapefruit Juice; Ivabradine; Lomitapide; Naloxegol; Natalizumab; Neratinib; Olaparib; Pimecrolimus; Pimozide; Simeprevir; Tacrolimus (Topical); Tolvaptan; Trabectedin; Ulipristal; Vaccines (Live)

Increased Effect/Toxicity

Imatinib may increase the levels/effects of: AmLODIPine; Apixaban; Aprepitant; ARIPiprazole; Asunaprevir; Avanafil; Blonanserin; Bosentan; Bosutinib; Brexpiprazole; Bromocriptine; Budesonide (Systemic); Budesonide (Topical); Cannabis; Cilostazol; CloZAPine; Cobimetinib; Colchicine; Cyclo-SPORINE (Systemic); CYP2D6 Substrates; CYP3A4 Substrates; Dapoxetine; Deferiprone; Deflazacort; Dofetilide; Domperidone; DOXOrubicin (Conventional); Dronabinol; Eletriptan; Eliglustat; Eplerenone; Everolimus; FentaNYL; Fingolimod; Flibanserin; GuanFACINE; Halofantrine; HYDROcodone; HydrOXYzine; Ibrutinib; Ivabradine; Ivacaftor; Leflunomide; Lomitapide; Lurasidone; Manidipine; Mirodenafil; Naldemedine; Naloxegol; Natalizumab; Neratinib; NiMODipine; Olaparib; OxyCODONE; Pimozide; Propafenone; Ranolazine; Rupatadine; Salmeterol; SAXagliptin; Sildenafil; Simeprevir; Simvastatin; Sonidegib; Suvorexant; Telithromycin; Tetrahydrocannabinol; Ticagrelor; Tofacitinib; Tolvaptan; Trabectedin; Udenafil; Ulipristal; Vaccines (Live); Venetoclax; Vilazodone; Vindesine; Warfarin; Zopiclone; Zuclopenthixol

The levels/effects of Imatinib may be increased by: Acetaminophen; CYP3A4 Inhibitors (Moderate); CYP3A4 Inhibitors (Strong); Denosumab; Dipyrone; Grapefruit Juice; Lansoprazole; Ocrelizumab; P-glycoprotein/ABCB1 Inhibitors; Pimecrolimus; Promazine; Propacetamol; Roflumilast; Tacrolimus (Topical); Trastuzumab

Decreased Effect

Imatinib may decrease the levels/effects of: BCG (Intravesical); Coccidioides immitis Skin Test; Fludarabine; Ifosfamide; Nivolumab; Sipuleucel-T, Terlumotide; Vaccines (Inactivated); Vaccines (Live)

The levels/effects of Imatinib may be decreased by: Bosentan; CYP3A4 Inducers (Moderate); CYP3A4 Inducers (Strong); Dabrafenib; Deferasirox; Dexamethasone (Systemic); Echinacea; Enzalutamide; Gemfibrozil; Ibuprofen; Mitotane; Rifamycin Derivatives; Sarilumab; Siltuximab; St John's Wort; Tocilizumab

Food Interactions Food may reduce GI irritation. Grapefruit juice may increase imatinib plasma concentration. Management: Take with a meal and a large glass of water. Avoid grapefruit juice. Maintain adequate hydration, unless instructed to restrict fluid intake.

Hazardous Drugs Handling Considerations

Hazardous agent (NIOSH 2016 [group 1]).

Use appropriate precautions for receiving, handling, administration, and disposal. Gloves (single) should be worn during receiving, unpacking, and placing in storage.

◀ NIOSH recommends single gloving for administration of intact tablets or capsules. If manipulating tablets/capsules (eg, to prepare an oral suspension), NIOSH recommends double gloving, a protective gown, and preparation in a controlled device; if not prepared in a controlled device, respiratory and eye/ face protection as well as ventilated engineering controls are recommended. NIOSH recommends double gloving, a protective gown, and (if there is a potential for vomit or spit up) eye/face protection for administration of an oral liquid/feeding tube administration (NIOSH 2016).

Storage/Stability
Store at 25°C (77°F); excursions permitted between 15°C to 30°C (59°F to 86°F). Protect from moisture.

An oral suspension (40 mg/mL) prepared using imatinib 400 mg tablets and Ora-Sweet is stable for up to 14 days at both room temperature and 4°C (39.2°F) (Li 2016).

Mechanism of Action
Inhibits Bcr-Abl tyrosine kinase, the constitutive abnormal gene product of the Philadelphia chromosome in chronic myeloid leukemia (CML). Inhibition of this enzyme blocks proliferation and induces apoptosis in Bcr-Abl positive cell lines as well as in fresh leukemic cells in Philadelphia chromosome positive CML. Also inhibits tyrosine kinase for platelet-derived growth factor (PDGF), stem cell factor (SCF), c-Kit, and cellular events mediated by PDGF and SCF.

Pharmacodynamics/Kinetics
Absorption: Rapid

Protein binding: Parent drug and metabolite: ~95% to albumin and alpha$_1$-acid glycoprotein

Metabolism: Hepatic via CYP3A4 (minor metabolism via CYP1A2, CYP2D6, CYP2C9, CYP2C19); primary metabolite (active): N-demethylated piperazine derivative (CGP74588); severe hepatic impairment (bilirubin >3 to 10 times ULN) increases AUC by 45% to 55% for imatinib and its active metabolite, respectively

Bioavailability: 98%; may be decreased in patients who have had gastric surgery (eg, bypass, total or partial resection) (Liu 2011; Pavlovsky 2009; Yoo 2010)

Half-life elimination: Adults: Parent drug: ~18 hours; N-desmethyl metabolite: ~40 hours; Children: Parent drug: ~15 hours

Time to peak: 2 to 4 hours

Excretion: Feces (68% primarily as metabolites, 20% as unchanged drug); urine (13% primarily as metabolites, 5% as unchanged drug)

Dosing
Adult & Geriatric Note: Treatment may be continued until disease progression or unacceptable toxicity. The optimal duration of therapy for chronic myeloid leukemia (CML) in complete remission is not yet determined. Discontinuing CML treatment is not recommended unless part of a clinical trial (Baccarani 2009). Imatinib is associated with a moderate emetic potential; antiemetics may be recommended to prevent nausea and vomiting (Roila 2010).

Philadelphia chromosome-positive (Ph+) chronic myeloid leukemia (CML): Oral:
Chronic phase: 400 mg once daily; may be increased to 600 mg daily, if tolerated, for disease progression, lack of hematologic response after 3 months, lack of cytogenetic response after 6 to 12 months, or loss of previous hematologic or cytogenetic response. An increase to 800 mg daily has been used (Cortes, 2010; Hehlmann, 2014).

Accelerated phase or blast crisis: 600 mg once daily; may be increased to 800 mg daily (400 mg twice daily), if tolerated, for disease progression, lack of hematologic response after 3 months, lack of cytogenetic response after 6 to 12 months, or loss of previous hematologic or cytogenetic response

Ph+ acute lymphoblastic leukemia (ALL) (relapsed or refractory): Oral: 600 mg once daily

Gastrointestinal stromal tumors (GIST) (adjuvant treatment following complete resection): Oral: 400 mg once daily; recommended treatment duration: 3 years

GIST (unresectable and/or metastatic malignant): Oral: 400 mg once daily; may be increased up to 800 mg daily (400 mg twice daily), if tolerated, for disease progression. **Note:** Significant improvement (progression-free survival, objective response rate) was demonstrated in patients with KIT exon 9 mutation with 800 mg (versus 400 mg), although overall survival (OS) was not impacted. The higher dose did not demonstrate a difference in time to progression or OS patients with Kit exon 11 mutation or wild-type status (Debiec-Rychter, 2006; Heinrich, 2009).

Aggressive systemic mastocytosis (ASM) with eosinophilia: Oral: Initiate at 100 mg once daily; titrate up to a maximum of 400 mg once daily (if tolerated) for insufficient response to lower dose

ASM without D816V c-Kit mutation or c-Kit mutation status unknown: Oral: 400 mg once daily

Dermatofibrosarcoma protuberans (DFSP): Oral: 400 mg twice daily

Hypereosinophilic syndrome (HES) and/or chronic eosinophilic leukemia (CEL): Oral: 400 mg once daily

HES/CEL with FIP1L1-PDGFRα fusion kinase: Oral: Initiate at 100 mg once daily; titrate up to a maximum of 400 mg once daily (if tolerated) if insufficient response to lower dose

Myelodysplastic/myeloproliferative disease (MDS/MPD) with PDGF receptor gene rearrangements: Oral: 400 mg once daily

Chordoma, progressive, advanced, or metastatic expressing PDGFRB and/or PDGFB (off-label use): Oral: 400 mg twice daily (Stacchiotti 2012)

Desmoid tumors, unresectable and/or progressive (off-label use): Oral: 300 mg twice daily (BSA ≥1.5 m^2), 200 mg twice daily (BSA 1 to 1.49 m^2), 100 mg twice daily (BSA <1 m^2) (Chugh 2010) **or** 400 mg once daily; may increase to 400 mg twice daily if progressive disease on 400 mg daily (Penel 2011)

Melanoma, advanced or metastatic with C-KIT mutation (off-label use): Oral: 400 mg twice daily (Carvajal 2011)

Stem cell transplant (SCT, off-label use) for CML (in patients who have not failed imatinib therapy prior to transplant): Oral:

Prophylactic use to prevent relapse post SCT: 400 mg daily starting after engraftment for 1 year post transplant (Carpenter 2007) **or** 300 mg daily starting on day +35 post SCT (increased to 400 mg within 4 weeks) and continued until 12 months post transplant (Olavarria 2007)

Relapse post SCT: Initial: 400 mg daily; if inferior response after 3 months, dose may be increased to 600 to 800 mg daily (Hess 2005) **or** 400 to 600 mg daily (chronic phase) **or** 600 mg daily (blast or accelerated phase) (DeAngelo 2004)

Dosage adjustment with concomitant strong CYP3A4 inducers: Avoid concomitant use of strong CYP3A4 inducers (eg, dexamethasone, carbamazepine, phenobarbital, phenytoin, rifabutin, rifampin); if concomitant use cannot be avoided, increase imatinib dose by at least 50% with careful monitoring.

Pediatric Note: Treatment may be continued until disease progression or unacceptable toxicity. The optimal duration of therapy for CML in complete remission is not yet determined. Imatinib is associated with a moderate emetic potential; antiemetics may be recommended to prevent nausea and vomiting (Dupuis, 2011).

Philadelphia chromosome-positive (Ph+) acute lymphoblastic leukemia (ALL) (newly diagnosed): Children ≥1 year and Adolescents: Oral: 340 mg/m²/day (in combination with chemotherapy); maximum: 600 mg daily

Ph+ chronic myeloid leukemia (CML), chronic phase, newly diagnosed: Children ≥1 year and Adolescents: Oral: 340 mg/m²/day; maximum: 600 mg daily

Dosage adjustment with concomitant strong CYP3A4 inducers: Avoid concomitant use of strong CYP3A4 inducers (eg, dexamethasone, carbamazepine, phenobarbital, phenytoin, rifabutin, rifampin); if concomitant use cannot be avoided, increase imatinib dose by at least 50% with careful monitoring.

Dosage adjustment for hepatotoxicity: Refer to Dosing: Hepatic Impairment.

Dosage adjustment for hematologic adverse reactions: Refer to Dosing: Adjustment for Toxicity.

Dosage adjustment for nonhematologic adverse reactions: Refer to Dosing: Adjustment for Toxicity.

Renal Impairment

CrCl 40 to 59 mL/minute: Maximum recommended dose: 600 mg.

CrCl 20 to 39 mL/minute: Decrease recommended starting dose by 50%; dose may be increased as tolerated; maximum recommended dose: 400 mg.

CrCl <20 mL/minute: Use caution; a dose of 100 mg daily has been tolerated in a limited number of patients with severe impairment (Gibbons 2008).

Hepatic Impairment

Mild-to-moderate impairment: No dosage adjustment necessary.

Severe impairment: Reduce dose by 25%.

Dosage adjustment for hepatotoxicity (during therapy): If elevations of bilirubin >3 times ULN or transaminases >5 times ULN occur, withhold treatment until bilirubin <1.5 times ULN and transaminases <2.5 times ULN. Resume treatment at a reduced dose as follows (**Note:** The decision to resume treatment should take into consideration the initial severity of hepatotoxicity):

Adults:

If current dose 400 mg daily, reduce dose to 300 mg daily

If current dose 600 mg daily, reduce dose to 400 mg daily

If current dose 800 mg daily, reduce dose to 600 mg daily

Children ≥1 year and Adolescents: If current dose 340 mg/m²/day, reduce dose to 260 mg/m²/day

Adjustment for Toxicity

Hematologic toxicity:

Chronic phase CML (initial dose 400 mg daily in adults or 340 mg/m^2/day in children); ASM, MDS/MPD, and HES/CEL (initial dose 400 mg daily); or GIST (initial dose 400 mg daily): If ANC <1 x 10^9/L and/or platelets <50 x 10^9/L: Withhold until ANC ≥1.5 x 10^9/L and platelets ≥75 x 10^9/L; resume treatment at original starting dose. For recurrent neutropenia and/or thrombocytopenia, withhold until recovery, and reinstitute treatment at a reduced dose as follows:

Children ≥1 year and Adolescents: If initial dose 340 mg/m^2/day, reduce dose to 260 mg/m^2/day.

Adults: If initial dose 400 mg daily, reduce dose to 300 mg daily.

CML (accelerated phase or blast crisis): Adults (initial dose 600 mg daily): If ANC <0.5 x 10^9/L and/or platelets <10 x 10^9/L, establish whether cytopenia is related to leukemia (bone marrow aspirate or biopsy). If unrelated to leukemia, reduce dose to 400 mg daily. If cytopenia persists for an additional 2 weeks, further reduce dose to 300 mg daily. If cytopenia persists for 4 weeks and is still unrelated to leukemia, withhold treatment until ANC ≥1 x 10^9/L and platelets ≥20 x 10^9/L, then resume treatment at 300 mg daily.

ASM associated with eosinophilia and HES/CEL with FIP1L1-PDGFRα fusion kinase: Adults (starting dose 100 mg daily): If ANC <1 x 10^9/L and/or platelets <50 x 10^9/L: Withhold until ANC ≥1.5 x 10^9/L and platelets ≥75 x 10^9/L; resume treatment at previous dose.

DFSP: Adults (initial dose 800 mg daily): If ANC <1 x 10^9/L and/or platelets <50 x 10^9/L, withhold until ANC ≥1.5 x 10^9/L and platelets ≥75 x 10^9/L; resume treatment at reduced dose of 600 mg daily. For recurrent neutropenia and/or thrombocytopenia, withhold until recovery, and reinstitute treatment with a further dose reduction to 400 mg daily.

Ph+ ALL:

Pediatrics (Schultz 2009): Hematologic toxicity requiring dosage adjustments was not observed in the study. No major toxicities were observed with imatinib at 340 mg/m^2/day in combination with intensive chemotherapy.

Adults (initial dose 600 mg daily): If ANC <0.5 x 10^9/L and/or platelets <10 x 10^9/L, establish whether cytopenia is related to leukemia (bone marrow aspirate or biopsy). If unrelated to leukemia, reduce dose to 400 mg daily. If cytopenia persists for an additional 2 weeks, further reduce dose to 300 mg daily. If cytopenia persists for 4 weeks and is still unrelated to leukemia, withhold treatment until ANC ≥1 x 10^9/L and platelets ≥20 x 10^9/L, then resume treatment at 300 mg daily.

Nonhematologic toxicity (eg, severe edema):
Withhold treatment until toxicity resolves; may resume if appropriate (depending on initial severity of adverse event).

Combination Regimens

Leukemia, acute lymphocytic: Hyper-CVAD + Imatinib on page 2145

Administration

Imatinib is associated with a moderate emetic potential; antiemetics may be recommended to prevent nausea and vomiting (Dupuis 2011; Roila 2010).

Should be administered with a meal and a large glass of water. For daily dosing ≥800 mg, the 400 mg tablets should be used in order to reduce iron exposure. Do not crush tablets. Tablets may be dispersed in water or apple juice (using ~50 mL for 100 mg tablet, ~200 mL for 400 mg tablet); stir until dissolved and administer immediately. If necessary, an oral suspension may ▶

be prepared (see Extemporaneous Preparations). Avoid skin or mucous membrane contact with crushed tablets; if contact occurs, wash thoroughly. Avoid exposure to crushed tablets.

Adults: Doses ≤600 mg may be given once daily; 800 mg dose should be administered as 400 mg twice daily.

Children: Dosing may be once or twice daily for chronic myeloid leukemia (CML) and once daily for Philadelphia chromosome-positive (Ph+) acute lymphoblastic leukemia (ALL).

Emetic Potential Children and Adults: Moderate (30% to 60%)

Extemporaneous Preparations An oral suspension may be prepared by placing tablets (whole, do not crush) in a glass of water or apple juice. Use ~50 mL for 100 mg tablet, or ~200 mL for 400 mg tablet. Stir until tablets are disintegrated, then administer immediately. To ensure the full dose is administered, rinse the glass and administer residue.

Gleevec (imatinib) [prescribing information]. East Hanover, NJ: Novartis Pharmaceuticals; August 2016.

A 40 mg/mL oral suspension may be prepared using imatinib 400 mg tablets and Ora-Sweet. Determine necessary quantity of imatinib 400 mg tablets; crush the tablets in a glass mortar and triturate to a fine powder (estimated powder volume for each imatinib 400 mg tablet is 0.4 mL). Measure the necessary volume of Ora-Sweet (to make a 40 mg/mL suspension) and add to the powder by geometric dilution until a smooth suspension is created. Transfer to an amber plastic bottle and label "Shake Well Before Use" and "Use by (date)". Suspension is stable for up to 14 days at both room temperature and 4°C (39.2°F).

Li Q, Liu Z, Kolli S, et al. Stability of extemporaneous erlotinib, lapatinib, and imatinib oral suspension. Am J Health Syst Pharm. 2016;73(17):1331-1337.

Monitoring Parameters CBC (weekly for first month, biweekly for second month, then periodically thereafter), liver function tests (at baseline and monthly or as clinically indicated; more frequently [at least weekly] in patients with moderate-to-severe hepatic impairment [Ramanathan 2008]), renal function (at baseline and periodically thereafter), serum electrolytes (including calcium, phosphorus, potassium and sodium levels); bone marrow cytogenetics (in CML; at 6-, 12-, and 18 months), pregnancy test; fatigue, weight, and edema/fluid status; consider echocardiogram and serum troponin levels in patients with HES/CEL, and in patients with MDS/MPD or ASM with high eosinophil levels; in pediatric patients, also monitor serum glucose, albumin, and growth

Gastric surgery (eg, bypass, major gastrectomy, or resection) patients: Monitor imatinib trough concentrations (Liu 2011; Pavlovsky 2009; Yoo 2010)

Thyroid function testing (Hamnvik 2011):
   Preexisting levothyroxine therapy: Obtain baseline TSH levels, then monitor every 4 weeks until levels and levothyroxine dose are stable, then monitor every 2 months
   Without preexisting thyroid hormone replacement: TSH at baseline, then every 4 weeks for 4 months, then every 2 to 3 months

Monitor for signs/symptoms of CHF in patients with at risk for cardiac failure or patients with preexisting cardiac disease. Monitor for signs/symptoms of gastrointestinal irritation or perforation and dermatologic toxicities.

Dietary Considerations Avoid grapefruit juice.

Dosage Forms Excipient information presented when available (limited, particularly for generics); consult specific product labeling.
Tablet, Oral:
Gleevec: 100 mg, 400 mg [scored]
Generic: 100 mg, 400 mg

Imipenem and Cilastatin (i mi PEN em & sye la STAT in)

Brand Names: US Primaxin I.V.
Brand Names: Canada Imipenem and Cilastatin for Injection; Imipenem and Cilastatin for Injection, USP; Primaxin; RAN-Imipenem-Cilastatin
Index Terms Cilastatin and Imipenem; Imipemide; Imipenem/Cilastatin; Primaxin I.M. [DSC]
Pharmacologic Category Antibiotic, Carbapenem
Use

Bacterial septicemia: Treatment of septicemia caused by *Enterococcus faecalis*, *Staphylococcus aureus* (penicillinase-producing), *Escherichia coli*, *Klebsiella* species, *Pseudomonas aeruginosa*, *Serratia* species, *Enterobacter* species, *Bacteroides* species (including *Bacteroides fragilis*).

Bone and joint infections: Treatment of bone and joint infections caused by *E. faecalis*, *S. aureus* (penicillinase-producing), *Staphylococcus epidermidis*, *Enterobacter* species, *P. aeruginosa*.

Endocarditis: Treatment of endocarditis caused by *S. aureus* (penicillinase-producing).

Gynecologic infections: Treatment of gynecologic infections caused by *E. faecalis*; *S. aureus* (penicillinase-producing), *S. epidermidis*, *Streptococcus agalactiae* (group B streptococci), *E. coli*, *Klebsiella* species, *Proteus* species, *Enterobacter* species, *Bifidobacterium* species, *Bacteroides* species (including *B. fragilis*), *Gardnerella vaginalis*; *Peptococcus* species, *Peptostreptococcus* species, *Cutibacterium* species.

Intra-abdominal infections: Treatment of intra-abdominal infections caused by *E. faecalis*, *S. aureus* (penicillinase-producing), *S. epidermidis*, *E. coli*, *Klebsiella* species, *Enterobacter* species, *Proteus* species, *Morganella morganii*, *P. aeruginosa*, *Citrobacter* species, *Clostridium* species, *Bacteroides* ▶

species (including *B. fragilis*), *Fusobacterium* species, *Peptococcus* species, *Peptostreptococcus* species, *Eubacterium* species, *Cutibacterium* species, *Bifidobacterium* species.

Lower respiratory tract infections: Treatment of lower respiratory tract infections caused by *S. aureus* (penicillinase-producing), *E. coli*, *Klebsiella* species, *Enterobacter* species, *Haemophilus influenzae*, *Haemophilus para-influenzae*, *Acinetobacter* species, *Serratia marcescens*.

Skin and skin structure infections: Treatment of skin and skin structure infections caused by *E. faecalis*, *S. aureus* (penicillinase-producing), *S. epidermidis*, *E. coli*, *Klebsiella* species, *Enterobacter species*, *Proteus vulgaris*, *Providencia rettgeri*, *M. morganii*, *P. aeruginosa*, *Serratia* species, *Citrobacter* species, *Acinetobacter* species, *Bacteroides* species (including *B. fragilis*), *Fusobacterium* species, *Peptococcus* species, *Peptostreptococcus* species.

Urinary tract infections (complicated and uncomplicated): Treatment of uncomplicated and complicated urinary tract infections caused by *E. faecalis*, *S. aureus* (penicillinase-producing), *E. coli*, *Klebsiella* species, *Enterobacter* species, *P. vulgaris*, *Providencia rettgeri*, *M. morganii*, *P. aeruginosa*.

Limitations of use: Not indicated in patients with meningitis because safety and efficacy have not been established; not recommend in pediatric patients with CNS infections because of the risk of seizures.

Pregnancy Risk Factor C

Dosing

Adult & Geriatric Doses based on **imipenem** content.

  Usual dosage range: IV:

    Susceptible bacterial species: 500 mg every 6 hours or 1,000 mg every 8 hours (maximum dose: 4,000 mg/day)

    Intermediate susceptibility bacterial species: 1,000 mg every 6 hours (maximum dose: 4,000 mg/day)

  Indication-specific dosing:

    ***Burkholderia pseudomallei* (melioidosis) (off-label use):** IV: Initial: 20 mg/kg every 8 hours for at least 10 days (White 2003) **or** 25 mg/kg (up to 1 g) every 6 hours for at least 10 days (Currie 2003); continue parenteral therapy until clinical improvement then switch to oral therapy if tolerated and/or appropriate. Additional data may be necessary to further define the role of imipenem/cilastatin in this condition.

    Intra-abdominal infections, complicated: IV: 500 mg every 6 hours **or** 1 g every 8 hours for 4 to 7 days (provided source controlled). **Note:** Not recommended for mild to moderate, community-acquired intra-abdominal infections due to risk of toxicity and the development of resistant organisms (Solomkin 2010).

    Neutropenic fever (off-label use): IV: 500 mg every 6 hours (Paul 2006)

    Nontuberculous mycobacterial disease (off-label use): IV: *M. abscessus* skin, soft tissue, or bone infections: 500 mg every 6 to 12 hours; use in combination with other antibacterial agents (ATS/IDSA [Griffith 2007]).

    Pneumonia, hospital acquired or ventilator-associated (off-label dose): IV: 500 mg every 6 hours for 7 days; may consider shorter or longer duration depending on rate of clinical improvement. When used as empiric therapy, use in combination with an agent active against MRSA (unless coverage of MSSA only is appropriate) with or without an additional antipseudomonal agent (dependent on patient and institution-specific risk factors). **Note:** May need to decrease dose in patients weighing less than 70 kg to prevent seizures (Kalil 2016).

Skin and soft tissue necrotizing infections (off-label use): IV: 1 g every 6 to 8 hours in combination with an agent effective against MRSA (eg, vancomycin, linezolid, daptomycin) for empiric therapy of polymicrobial [mixed] infections. Continue until further debridement is not necessary, patient has clinically improved, and patient is afebrile for 48 to 72 hours (IDSA [Stevens 2014]).

Surgical-site infection (intestinal or genitourinary tract surgery) (off-label use): IV: 500 mg every 6 hours (IDSA [Stevens 2014]).

Pediatric Dosage based on **imipenem** content:

Non-CNS infections: IV: Infants ≥3 months, Children, and Adolescents: 15 to 25 mg/kg every 6 hours
Maximum dosage: 4,000 mg/day

***Burkholderia pseudomallei* (melioidosis) (off-label use):** IV: Initial: 20 mg/kg every 8 hours for at least 10 days (White 2003) **or** 25 mg/kg (up to 1 g) every 6 hours for at least 10 days (Currie 2003); continue parenteral therapy until clinical improvement, then switch to oral therapy if tolerated and/or appropriate. Additional data may be necessary to further define the role of imipenem/cilastatin in this condition.

Cystic fibrosis exacerbations: IV: Infants, Children, and Adolescents: Up to 100 mg/kg/**day** divided every 6 hours (Strandvik 1988; Zobell 2012); maximum dose: 4 g daily has been used (Zobell 2012). **Note:** Efficacy in exacerbations may be limited due to rapid development of resistance (Zobell 2012).

Renal Impairment *Adults:*

US labeling (estimation of renal function for the purpose of dosing adjustment should be done using the Cockcroft-Gault formula):

Usual dosing regimen of 500 mg every 6 hours:
CrCl ≥90 mL/minute: No dosage adjustment necessary.
CrCl ≥60 to <90 mL/minute: 400 mg every 6 hours
CrCl ≥30 to <60 mL/minute: 300 mg every 6 hours
CrCl ≥15 to <30 mL/minute: 200 mg every 6 hours
CrCl <15 mL/minute: Do not administer imipenem and cilastatin unless hemodialysis is instituted within 48 hours.

Usual dosing regimen of 1,000 mg every 8 hours:
CrCl ≥90 mL/minute: No dosage adjustment necessary.
CrCl ≥60 to <90 mL/minute: 500 mg every 6 hours
CrCl ≥30 to <60 mL/minute: 500 mg every 8 hours
CrCl ≥15 to <30 mL/minute: 500 mg every 12 hours
CrCl <15 mL/minute: Do not administer imipenem and cilastatin unless hemodialysis is instituted within 48 hours.

Usual dosing regimen of 1,000 mg every 6 hours:
CrCl ≥90 mL/minute: No dosage adjustment necessary.
CrCl ≥60 to <90 mL/minute: 750 mg every 8 hours
CrCl ≥30 to <60 mL/minute: 500 mg every 6 hours
CrCl ≥15 to <30 mL/minute: 500 mg every 12 hours
CrCl <15 mL/minute: Do not administer imipenem and cilastatin unless hemodialysis is instituted within 48 hours.

◄ **Canadian labeling:** Reduced IV dosage regimen based on creatinine clearance (mL/minute/1.73 m^2) and body weight ≥70 kg (**Note:** The manufacturer labeling recommends further proportionate dose reductions for patients <70 kg, but does not provide specific dosing recommendations):

Mild renal impairment (CrCl 31 to 70 mL/minute/1.73 m^2):

Fully susceptible organisms: Maximum dosage: 500 mg every 8 hours

Less susceptible organisms (primarily some *Pseudomonas* strains): Maximum dosage: 500 mg every 6 hours

Moderate renal impairment (CrCl 21 to 30 mL/minute/1.73 m^2):

Fully susceptible organisms: Maximum dosage: 500 mg every 12 hours

Less susceptible organisms (primarily some *Pseudomonas* strains): Maximum dosage: 500 mg every 8 hours

Severe renal impairment (CrCl 0 to 20 mL/minute/1.73 m^2):

Fully susceptible organisms: Maximum dosage: 250 mg every 12 hours

Less susceptible organisms (primarily some *Pseudomonas* strains): Maximum dosage: 500 mg every 12 hours

Note: Patients with CrCl 6 to 20 mL/minute/1.73 m^2 should receive 250 mg every 12 hours or 3.5 mg/kg (whichever is lower) every 12 hours for most pathogens; seizure risk may increase with higher dosing.

End-stage renal disease (ESRD) on intermittent hemodialysis (IHD): Use the dosing recommendation (for US labeling) for patients with a CrCl ≥15 to <30 mL/minute; administer dose after dialysis session and at intervals timed from the end of that dialysis session **or** 250 to 500 mg every 12 hours (Heintz 2009). **Note:** Dosing dependent on the assumption of 3 times/week, complete IHD sessions.

Continuous renal replacement therapy (CRRT) (Heintz 2009; Trotman 2005): Drug clearance is highly dependent on the method of renal replacement, filter type, and flow rate. Appropriate dosing requires close monitoring of pharmacologic response, signs of adverse reactions due to drug accumulation, as well as drug concentrations in relation to target trough (if appropriate). The following are general recommendations only (based on dialysate flow/ultrafiltration rates of 1 to 2 L/hour and minimal residual renal function) and should not supersede clinical judgment:

CVVH: Loading dose of 1 g followed by either 250 mg every 6 hours **or** 500 mg every 8 hours

CVVHD: Loading dose of 1 g followed by either 250 mg every 6 hours **or** 500 mg every 6 to 8 hours

CVVHDF: Loading dose of 1 g followed by either 250 mg every 6 hours **or** 500 mg every 6 hours

Note: Data suggest that 500 mg every 8 to 12 hours may provide sufficient time above MIC to cover organisms with MIC values ≤2 mg/L; however, a higher dose of 500 mg every 6 hours is recommended for resistant organisms (particularly *Pseudomonas* spp) with MIC ≥4 mg/L or deep-seated infections (Fish 2005).

Hepatic Impairment There are no dosage adjustments provided in the manufacturer's labeling.

Additional Information Complete prescribing information should be consulted for additional detail.

Dosage Forms Excipient information presented when available (limited, particularly for generics); consult specific product labeling.

Injection, powder for reconstitution: Imipenem 250 mg and cilastatin 250 mg; imipenem 500 mg and cilastatin 500 mg

Primaxin® I.V.: Imipenem 250 mg and cilastatin 250 mg [contains sodium 18.8 mg (0.8 mEq)]; imipenem 500 mg and cilastatin 500 mg [contains sodium 37.5 mg (1.6 mEq)]

◆ **Imipenem and Cilastatin for Injection (Can)** *see* Imipenem and Cilastatin *on page* 983

◆ **Imipenem and Cilastatin for Injection, USP (Can)** *see* Imipenem and Cilastatin *on page* 983

◆ **Imipenem/Cilastatin** *see* Imipenem and Cilastatin *on page* 983

Imiquimod (i mi KWI mod)

Brand Names: US Aldara; Zyclara; Zyclara Pump
Brand Names: Canada Aldara P; Apo-Imiquimod; Vyloma; Zyclara
Pharmacologic Category Skin and Mucous Membrane Agent; Topical Skin Product

Use

Actinic keratosis (2.5%, 3.75% and 5% cream): Topical treatment of clinically typical, nonhyperkeratotic, nonhypertrophic, visible or palpable actinic keratoses on the full face or scalp in immunocompetent adults.

Genital and perianal warts (3.75% and 5% cream): Treatment of external genital and perianal warts (condyloma acuminata) in patients 12 years and older.

Superficial basal cell carcinoma (Aldara 5% cream): Topical treatment of biopsy-confirmed, primary superficial basal cell carcinoma in immunocompetent adults with a maximum tumor diameter of 2 cm located on the trunk (excluding anogenital skin), neck, or extremities (excluding hands and feet), only when surgical methods are medically less appropriate and patient follow-up can be reasonably assured.

Limitations of use: Safety and efficacy has not been established in immunosuppressed patients and in patients with basal cell nevus syndrome or xeroderma pigmentosum, or for prevention or transmission of HPV. Imiquimod should be used with caution in patients with preexisting autoimmune conditions. Imiquimod has been evaluated in pediatrics ages 2 to 12 with molluscum, contagiosum, however, studies failed to demonstrate efficacy.

Labeled Contraindications

There are no contraindications listed in the manufacturer's US labeling.

Canadian labeling: Hypersensitivity to imiquimod or any component of the formulation

Pregnancy Considerations Adverse events were observed in some animal reproduction studies following oral administration. Imiquimod may weaken condoms and vaginal diaphragms. Imiquimod appears to pose a low risk, but use in pregnant women should be avoided until additional data are available (CDC [Workowski 2015]).

Breastfeeding Considerations It is not known if imiquimod is present in breast milk. The manufacturer recommends that caution be exercised when administering imiquimod to breastfeeding women.

Warnings/Precautions Intense local inflammatory reactions (including skin weeping or erosion) may occur after a few applications; may require treatment interruption and may be accompanied by systemic symptoms (fever, malaise, myalgia); reactions may extend beyond the application site. Imiquimod has the potential to exacerbate inflammatory conditions of the skin (including chronic graft-versus-host disease). Due to the potential for increased sensitivity to sunlight, avoid or minimize sunlight exposure (including sunlamps or other artificial sunlight exposure) during treatment. Advise patients to wear protective clothing (eg, a hat) during treatment. Patients with sunburn should not to use imiquimod until full recovery form sunburn. Patients with a potential for considerable sun exposure (eg, due to their occupations) or inherent sensitivity to sunlight should use caution during imiquimod treatment. Flu-like symptoms (arthralgias, chills, fatigue, fever, malaise, myalgias, nausea, rigors) may accompany or precede local inflammatory reactions; may require treatment interruption. Severe local inflammation of female external genitalia following topical application may lead to severe vulvar swelling and urinary retention; interrupt or discontinue treatment for severe symptoms.

Safety and efficacy have not been established in the treatment of actinic keratosis with repeat use (more than 1 treatment course) in the same area. Safety of imiquimod 5% applied to areas of skin larger than 25 cm^2 has not been established. Lymphadenopathy has occurred in patients being treated for actinic keratosis; lymphadenopathy resolved within 4 weeks after completion of treatment. Safety and efficacy in immunosuppressed patients have not been established. Use with caution in patients with preexisting autoimmune disorders (onset or exacerbation of disease has been reported). Use in basal cell carcinoma (BCC) should be limited to superficial carcinomas with a maximum diameter of 2 cm. Safety and efficacy in treatment of other types of BCC lesions of the face, head, and anogenital area, or other subtypes of BCC (including nodular and morpheaform), have not been established. Patients with superficial BCC treated with imiquimod should have regular follow up of the treatment site. Imiquimod has not been evaluated for the treatment of urethral, intravaginal, cervical, rectal, or intra-anal human papilloma viral disease and is not recommended for these conditions.

Not intended for oral, nasal, intravaginal, or ophthalmic use. Administration is not recommended until tissue is healed from any previous drug or surgical treatment. Treatment should not be prolonged beyond recommended period due to missed doses or rest periods. Safety and efficacy have not been established for basal cell nevus syndrome, in immunocompromised patients, or for xeroderma pigmentosum. Safety and efficacy of the 2.5% cream in the treatment of external genital warts have not been established. Potentially significant drug-drug interactions may exist, requiring dose or frequency adjustment, additional monitoring, and/or selection of alternative therapy. Some dosage forms may contain benzyl alcohol; large amounts of benzyl alcohol (≥99 mg/kg/day) have been associated with a potentially fatal toxicity ("gasping syndrome") in neonates; the "gasping syndrome" consists of metabolic acidosis, respiratory distress, gasping respirations, CNS dysfunction (including convulsions, intracranial hemorrhage), hypotension and cardiovascular collapse (AAP 1997; CDC 1982); some data suggests that benzoate displaces bilirubin from protein binding sites (Ahlfors 2001); avoid or use dosage forms containing benzyl alcohol with caution in neonates See manufacturer's labeling.

Adverse Reactions Note: Frequency of reactions vary and are related to the degree of inflammation associated with the treated disease, number of weekly applications, product formulation, and individual sensitivity.

>10%:
  Dermatologic: Localized erythema (58% to 100%; remote: 2%), xeroderma (local; including flaking, scaling; 18% to 93%; remote: 1%), crusted skin (local; 4% to 93%), skin sclerosis (local; 5% to 84%), dermal ulcer (local; 4% to 62%; remote: 2%), localized vesiculation (2% to 31%), excoriation (local; remote: 1%)
  Infection: Fungal infection (2% to 11%)
  Local: Localized edema (12% to 78%; remote: 1%), application site discharge (22% to 51%), local pruritus (3% to 32%), localized burning (9% to 26%)
  Respiratory: Upper respiratory tract infection (15% to 33%)
1% to 10%:
  Cardiovascular: Chest pain, localized blanching
  Central nervous system: Headache (2% to 6%), fatigue (1% to 4%), dizziness (<1% to 3%), local discomfort (soreness; ≤3%), rigors (1%), anxiety, pain, tingling of skin (local)
  Dermatologic: Skin pain (local; 1% to 8%), skin hypertrophy (local; 3%), skin infection (local; 1% to 3%), eczema (2%), cheilitis (≤2%), alopecia (1%), dermal hemorrhage (local), localized rash, papule (local), seborrhoeic keratosis, skin tenderness (local), stinging of the skin (local), tinea (cruris)
  Endocrine & metabolic: Increased serum glucose
  Gastrointestinal: Nausea (1% to 4%), diarrhea (1% to 3%), anorexia (≤3%), vomiting (1%), dyspepsia
  Genitourinary: Bacterial vaginosis (3%), urinary tract infection (1%)
  Hematologic & oncologic: Squamous cell carcinoma (4%), lymphadenopathy (2% to 3%)
  Infection: Herpes simplex (≤3%)
  Local: Local irritation (3% to 6%)
  Neuromuscular & skeletal: Arthralgia (1% to 3%), myalgia (≥1%), back pain
  Respiratory: Sinusitis (7%), flu-like symptoms (<1% to 4%), cough, pharyngitis, rhinitis
  Miscellaneous: Fever (≤3%)
Postmarketing and/or case reports: Abdominal pain, acute exacerbations of multiple sclerosis, agitation, anemia, angioedema, atrial fibrillation, capillary leak syndrome, cardiac failure, cardiomyopathy, cellulitis (local), cerebrovascular accident, chills, depression, dermatitis, dyspnea, dysuria, erythema multiforme, erythema (scrotal), exacerbation of psoriasis, exacerbation of ulcerative colitis, exfoliative dermatitis, febrile seizures, Henoch-Schönlein purpura (IgA vasculitis), hepatic insufficiency, herpes zoster, hyperpigmentation, immune thrombocytopenia (ITP), insomnia, ischemia, lethargy, leukopenia, malignant lymphoma, myocardial infarction, pain (scrotal), palpitations, pancytopenia, paresis, proteinuria, psoriasis, pulmonary edema, scrotal edema, seizure, squamous cell carcinoma, supraventricular tachycardia, syncope, tachycardia, thrombocytopenia, thyroiditis, ulcerative colitis, ulcer (scrotal), urinary retention, urticaria, vertebral disk disease (spondylitis onset or exacerbated)

Drug Interactions

Metabolism/Transport Effects Substrate of CYP1A2 (minor), CYP3A4 (minor); **Note:** Assignment of Major/Minor substrate status based on clinically relevant drug interaction potential

Avoid Concomitant Use

Avoid concomitant use of Imiquimod with any of the following: BCG (Intravesical); Natalizumab; Pimecrolimus; Tacrolimus (Topical); Vaccines (Live)

◄ **Increased Effect/Toxicity**

Imiquimod may increase the levels/effects of: Fingolimod; Leflunomide; Natalizumab; Tofacitinib; Vaccines (Live)

The levels/effects of Imiquimod may be increased by: Denosumab; Ocrelizumab; Pimecrolimus; Roflumilast; Tacrolimus (Topical); Trastuzumab

Decreased Effect

Imiquimod may decrease the levels/effects of: BCG (Intravesical); Coccidioides immitis Skin Test; Nivolumab; Sipuleucel-T; Tertomotide; Vaccines (Inactivated); Vaccines (Live)

The levels/effects of Imiquimod may be decreased by: Echinacea

Storage/Stability

2.5% and 3.75% cream: Store at 25°C (77°F); excursions permitted to 15°C to 30°C (59°F to 86°F); do not freeze. Store pump upright. Discard pump after a full course of therapy has been completed. Discard partially used packets; do not reuse.

5% cream: Store at 4°C to 25°C (39°F to 77°F); do not freeze. Discard partially used packets; do not reuse.

Vyloma (Canadian product; not available in the US): Store at 15°C to 25°C (59°F to 77°F); do not freeze.

Mechanism of Action Imiquimod, an immune response modifier, is a Toll-like receptor 7 agonist that activates immune cells. Topical application to the skin is associated with increases in markers for cytokines and immune cells.

Pharmacodynamics/Kinetics

Absorption: Minimal; systemic absorption more dependent upon surface area of application as opposed to dose

Time to peak: 9 to 12 hours

Excretion: Urine (<3% of applied dose as imiquimod and metabolites)

Dosing

Adult & Geriatric

Actinic keratosis: Topical:

2.5% and 3.75% cream: Apply thin film (using up to 2 packets or 2 full pump actuations) once daily before bedtime for 2 weeks to the skin of the affected area (either the entire face or balding scalp, but not both concurrently); leave on for ~8 hours, then remove with mild soap and water. After a 2-week period of no treatment, repeat with a second 2-week treatment (do not extend treatment cycles because of missed doses or rest periods). Maximum to be prescribed: 56 packets or 2 x 7.5 g pumps per 2 cycles of treatment. Treatment should continue for the full treatment course even if all actinic keratoses appear to be gone (do not extend the treatment period because of missed doses or rest periods).

5% cream: Apply 2 times per week (using up to 1 packet per application), prior to normal sleeping hours, to a defined treatment area(s) on the face or scalp (but not both concurrently; treatment should be limited to areas ≤25 cm²); leave on for ~8 hours, then remove with mild soap and water. Maximum to be prescribed: 36 packets per 16-week treatment period. Treatment should continue for 16 weeks (do not extend the treatment period beyond 16 weeks because of missed doses or rest periods).

Genital and perianal warts: Topical:

3.75% cream: Apply a thin layer once daily (using up to 1 packet or 1 full actuation of pump) prior to bedtime; leave on skin for ~8 hours, then remove with mild soap and water. Continue treatment until there is total clearance of the warts or for a maximum duration of therapy of 8 weeks.

Maximum to be prescribed: 56 packets or 2 x 7.5 g pumps per course of treatment.

5% cream: Apply a thin layer 3 times per week (on alternate days) prior to bedtime; leave on skin for 6 to 10 hours, then remove with mild soap and water. Continue until there is total clearance of the genital/perianal warts or for a maximum duration of therapy of 16 weeks.

Superficial basal cell carcinoma (Aldara 5% cream): Topical: Apply once daily 5 days per week, prior to normal sleeping hours, for 6 weeks; leave on skin for ~8 hours, then remove with mild soap and water. Apply enough cream to cover the treatment area, including 1 cm of skin surrounding the tumor. Tumor treatment area should not exceed 3 cm (maximum of 2 cm tumor diameter plus a 1 cm margin of skin around the tumor). The diameter of cream droplet applied should range from 4 mm to 7 mm for tumor areas of 0.5 cm to 2 cm, respectively. Maximum to be prescribed: 36 packets during the 6-week treatment period. Safety/efficacy of repeated use in a previously treated area have not been established.

Cutaneous flat warts (off-label use): Topical (5% cream): Apply once daily at bedtime until warts completely disappear up to a maximum of 12 weeks (Kim 2006). Additional data may be necessary to further define the role of imiquimod in this condition.

Herpes simplex virus (HSV) infection, acyclovir-resistant (off-label use): Topical: Apply to lesions once daily for 5 consecutive days (CDC [Workowski 2015])

Pediatric Genital and perianal warts (3.75% and 5% cream): Children ≥12 years and Adolescents: Topical: Refer to adult dosing.

Renal Impairment There are no dosage adjustments provided in the manufacturer's labeling.

Hepatic Impairment There are no dosage adjustments provided in the manufacturer's labeling.

Adjustment for Toxicity

Local skin reactions (eg, erythema, edema, skin erosion/weeping, scabbing): Temporarily interrupt treatment for up to several days for severe or intolerable reactions; may consider resuming therapy once reaction subsides.

Systemic/flu-like reactions (eg, malaise, fever, rigors): Consider temporary interruption of therapy.

Vulvar swelling: Interrupt or discontinue therapy for severe vulvar swelling.

Administration Topical: Wash hands prior to and following application. For topical use only; not for ophthalmic, oral, intra-anal, or intravaginal use. Avoid use in or on the lips and nostrils; do not use in or near the eyes. Do not occlude the application site. Pump (Zyclara) should be primed prior to first use only by pressing top of pump completely down repeatedly until cream appears; discard cream obtained during priming; no further priming is required throughout therapy.

Actinic keratosis: The treatment area should be washed with mild soap and thoroughly dried (~10 minutes) prior to application. Apply 5% cream over a single contiguous area (~25 cm^2) on the face or scalp or 2.5% and 3.75% cream over an area on the face or scalp. Both face and scalp should not be treated concurrently. Apply a thin layer to the affected area and rub in until the cream is no longer visible. A transient increase in actinic keratosis lesion counts may be observed during treatment.

◄ *Genital/perianal warts:* Apply a thin layer to external or perianal wart area and rub in until the cream is no longer visible. Avoid use of excessive amounts of cream. Nonocclusive dressings (such as cotton gauze or cotton underwear) may be used in the management of skin reactions.

Superficial basal cell carcinoma (Aldara): Treatment area should have a maximum diameter no more than 2 cm on the trunk, neck, or extremities (excluding the hands, feet, and anogenital skin). Treatment area should include a 1 cm margin around the tumor. Wash and thoroughly dry treatment area prior to application; apply a thin layer to the affected area (and margin) and rub in until the cream is no longer visible.

Monitoring Parameters Assess response to therapy periodically (reduction in lesion size is indicative of a therapeutic response); monitor for local skin reactions and for signs and symptoms of hypersensitivity to imiquimod.

Dosage Forms Excipient information presented when available (limited, particularly for generics); consult specific product labeling.

Cream, External:

Aldara: 5% (12 ea) [contains benzyl alcohol, cetyl alcohol, methylparaben, propylparaben, sorbitan monostearate(sorbitan stearate)]

Zyclara: 3.75% (28 ea) [contains benzyl alcohol, cetyl alcohol, methylparaben, propylparaben]

Zyclara Pump: 2.5% (7.5 g); 3.75% (7.5 g) [contains benzyl alcohol, cetyl alcohol, methylparaben, propylparaben]

Generic: 5% (1 ea, 12 ea, 24 ea)

Dosage Forms: Canada Information with regard to form, strength, and availability of products uniquely available in Canada but currently not available in the US. Refer also to Dosage Forms.

Excipient information presented when available (limited, particularly for generics); consult specific product labeling.

Cream, topical:

Vyloma: 3.75% (28s) [contains benzyl alcohol; 0.25 g/packet]

♦ **Imlygic** *see* Talimogene Laherparepvec *on page 1729*

♦ **ImmuCyst (Can)** *see* BCG (Intravesical) *on page 219*

Immune Globulin (i MYUN GLOB yoo lin)

Brand Names: US Bivigam; Carimune NF; Cuvitru; Flebogamma DIF; GamaSTAN S/D; Gammagard; Gammagard S/D Less IgA; Gammagard S/D [DSC]; Gammaked; Gammaplex; Gamunex-C; Hizentra; Hyqvia; Octagam; Privigen

Brand Names: Canada Cuvitru; Gamastan S/D; Gammagard Liquid; Gammagard S/D; Gamunex; Hizentra; IGIVnex; Octagam 10%; Panzyga; Privigen

Index Terms Gamma Globulin; Human Normal Immunoglobulin; IG; IGIM; IGIV; IGSC; IMIG; Immune Globulin IV; Immune Globulin Subcutaneous (Human); Immune Serum Globulin; ISG; IV Immune Globulin; IVIG; Normal Immunoglobulin; Panglobulin; Polygam; Sandoglobulin; SCIG

Pharmacologic Category Blood Product Derivative; Immune Globulin

Use

Chronic inflammatory demyelinating polyneuropathy: Treatment of chronic inflammatory demyelinating polyneuropathy (CIDP) (Gammaked, Gamunex-C)

Chronic lymphocytic leukemia: Prevention of bacterial infection in patients with hypogammaglobulinemia and/or recurrent bacterial infections with B-cell chronic lymphocytic leukemia (CLL) (Gammagard S/D)

Immune thrombocytopenia:
Treatment of acute immune thrombocytopenia (ITP) (Carimune NF, Gammagard S/D, Gammaked, Gamunex-C).
Treatment of chronic ITP (Carimune NF, Flebogamma DIF 10%, Gammagard S/D, Gammaked, Gammaplex, Gamunex-C, Octagam 10%, Panzyga [Canadian product], Privigen)

Immunodeficiency syndromes: Treatment of primary humoral immunodeficiency syndromes (congenital agammaglobulinemia, severe combined immunodeficiency syndromes [SCIDS], common variable immunodeficiency, X-linked agammaglobulinemia, Wiskott-Aldrich syndrome) (Bivigam, Carimune NF, Cuvitru, Flebogamma DIF, HyQvia, Gammagard Liquid, Gammagard S/D, Gammaked, Gammaplex, Gamunex-C, Hizentra, Octagam 5%, Panzyga [Canadian product], Privigen); Treatment of secondary immunodeficiency (Panzyga [Canadian product])

Kawasaki syndrome: Prevention of coronary artery aneurysms associated with Kawasaki syndrome (in combination with aspirin) (Gammagard S/D)

Multifocal motor neuropathy: Treatment of multifocal motor neuropathy (MMN) (Gammagard Liquid)

Passive immunity: Provision of passive immunity in the following susceptible individuals (GamaSTAN S/D):
Hepatitis A: Pre-exposure prophylaxis; postexposure: within 14 days and/or prior to manifestation of disease
Measles: For use within 6 days of exposure in an unvaccinated person, who has not previously had measles
Rubella: Postexposure prophylaxis to reduce the risk of infection and fetal damage in exposed pregnant women who will not consider therapeutic abortion
Varicella: For immunosuppressed patients when varicella zoster immune globulin is not available

Pregnancy Risk Factor C

Dosing

Adult Note: Some clinicians may administer IGIV formulations FDA approved only for intravenous administration as a subcutaneous infusion based on clinical judgment and patient tolerability.

B-cell chronic lymphocytic leukemia (CLL) with hypogammaglobulinemia, prevention of bacterial infections (Gammagard S/D): IV: 400 mg/kg every 3 to 4 weeks

Chronic inflammatory demyelinating polyneuropathy (CIDP) (Gammaked, Gamunex-C): IV: Loading dose: 2,000 mg/kg (in divided doses over 2 to 4 consecutive days); Maintenance: 1,000 mg/kg administered over 1 day every 3 weeks. Alternatively, administer 500 mg/kg/day for 2 consecutive days every 3 weeks.

Hepatitis A (GamaSTAN S/D): IM:
Preexposure prophylaxis upon travel into endemic areas (hepatitis A vaccine preferred):
0.02 **mL**/kg for anticipated risk of exposure <3 months
0.06 **mL**/kg for anticipated risk of exposure ≥3 months; repeat every 4 to 6 months.
Postexposure prophylaxis: 0.02 **mL**/kg given within 14 days of exposure and/or prior to manifestation of disease; not needed if at least 1 dose of hepatitis A vaccine was given at ≥1 month before exposure (CDC 2006)

◀ **Immune thrombocytopenia (ITP):**

Carimune NF: IV: Initial: 400 mg/kg/day for 2 to 5 consecutive days (6% solution recommended); Maintenance: 400 mg/kg (no more frequent than daily) as needed to maintain platelet count ≥30,000/mm^3 and/or to control significant bleeding; may increase dose if needed (range: 800 to 1,000 mg/kg).

Flebogamma DIF 10%: IV: 1,000 mg/kg once daily for 2 consecutive days

Gammagard S/D: IV: 1,000 mg/kg; up to 3 total doses may be given on alternate days based on patient response and/or platelet count.

Gammaked, Gamunex-C: IV: 1,000 mg/kg/day for 2 consecutive days (second dose may be withheld if adequate platelet response in 24 hours) **or** 400 mg/kg once daily for 5 consecutive days

Gammaplex, Octagam 10%, Privigen: IV: 1,000 mg/kg/day for 2 consecutive days

Panzyga [Canadian product]: IV: 1,000 mg/kg/day for 2 consecutive days; may repeat treatment in patients who relapse

American College of Obstetricians and Gynecologists Guidelines: IV: Initial: 1,000 mg/kg as a one-time dose for pregnant women with ITP refractory to corticosteroids, when significant side effects occur with corticosteroids, or a more rapid platelet increase is necessary; may repeat if necessary (ACOG 2016).

American Society of Hematology Guidelines: Newly diagnosed ITP with platelets <30,000/mm^3: First line treatment: IV: 1,000 mg/kg as a single dose, may repeat if necessary (Neunert 2011)

Measles:

GamaSTAN S/D: IM:

Immunocompetent: 0.25 **mL**/kg given within 6 days of exposure

Immunocompromised children: 0.5 **mL**/kg (maximum dose: 15 **mL**) immediately following exposure

Postexposure prophylaxis, any nonimmune person (off-label population): Patients ≤30 kg: 0.5 **mL**/kg (maximum dose: 15 **mL**) within 6 days of exposure. If patient >30 kg, patient will have lower titers than what is recommended due to the maximum volume that can be administered (CDC 2013)

Gammaked, Gamunex-C, Octagam 5%: IV:

Preexposure prophylaxis in patients with primary humoral immunodeficiency (**ONLY** if routine dose is <400 mg/kg): ≥400 mg/kg immediately before expected exposure followed by resumption of prior dosing in 3 to 4 weeks.

Postexposure prophylaxis in patients with primary humoral immunodeficiency: 400 mg/kg administered as soon as possible after exposure followed by resumption of prior dosing in 3 to 4 weeks.

Postexposure prophylaxis, any nonimmune person (off-label population): 400 mg/kg within 6 days of exposure (CDC 2013)

Hizentra: SubQ infusion:

Preexposure prophylaxis in patients with primary humoral immunodeficiency at risk of measles exposure (eg, during an outbreak; travel to endemic area):

Patients receiving weekly or more frequent dosing: Ensure total weekly dose of ≥200 mg/kg for 2 consecutive weeks followed by resumption of prior dosing schedule

Patients receiving biweekly dosing: Administer ≥400 mg/kg once followed by resumption of prior dosing schedule.

Postexposure prophylaxis in patients with primary humoral immunodeficiency regardless of prior dosing schedule (daily, weekly, or biweekly): 400 mg/kg administered as soon as possible after exposure followed by resumption of prior dosing schedule.

ACIP recommendations: The Advisory Committee on Immunization Practices (ACIP) recommends postexposure prophylaxis with immune globulin (IG) to any nonimmune person exposed to measles. The following patient groups are at risk for severe measles complications and should receive IG therapy: Infants <12 months of age, pregnant women without evidence of immunity; severely compromised persons (eg, persons with severe primary immunodeficiency; some bone marrow transplant patients; some ALL patients; and some patients with AIDS or HIV infection [refer to guidelines for additional details]). IGIM is recommended for infants <12 months of age. IGIV is recommended for pregnant women and immunocompromised persons. Although prophylaxis may be given to any nonimmune person, priority should be given to those at greatest risk for measles complications and also to persons exposed in settings with intense, prolonged, close contact (eg, households, daycare centers, classrooms). Following IG administration, any nonimmune person should then receive the measles mumps and rubella (MMR) vaccine if the person is ≥12 months of age at the time of vaccine administration and the vaccine is not otherwise contraindicated. MMR should not be given until 6 months following IGIM or 8 months following IGIV administration. If a person is already receiving IGIV therapy, a dose of 400 mg/kg IV within 3 weeks prior to exposure (or 200 mg/kg SubQ for 2 consecutive weeks prior to exposure if previously on SubQ therapy) should be sufficient to prevent measles infection. IG therapy is not indicated for any person who already received one dose of a measles-containing vaccine at ≥12 months of age unless they are severely immunocompromised (CDC 2013).

Multifocal motor neuropathy (MMN) (Gammagard Liquid): IV: 500 to 2400 mg/kg/**month** based upon response

Primary humoral immunodeficiency disorders:

IV infusion dosing:

Bivigam, Gammaplex: IV: 300 to 800 mg/kg every 3 to 4 weeks; dose adjusted based on monitored trough serum IgG concentrations and clinical response

Carimune NF: IV: 400 to 800 mg/kg every 3 to 4 weeks. **Note:** In previously untreated agammaglobulinemic or hypogammaglobulinemic patients use a 3% solution; may administer subsequent infusions with a higher concentration if patient tolerates lower concentration.

Flebogamma DIF 5%, Flebogamma DIF 10%, Gammagard Liquid, Gammagard S/D, Gammaked, Gamunex-C, Octagam 5%: IV: 300 to 600 mg/kg every 3 to 4 weeks; dose adjusted based on monitored trough serum IgG concentrations and clinical response

Privigen, Panzyga [Canadian product]: IV: 200 to 800 mg/kg every 3 to 4 weeks; dose adjusted based on monitored trough serum IgG concentrations and clinical response

Switching to weekly subcutaneous infusion dosing:

Gammagard Liquid, Gammaked, Gamunex-C: SubQ infusion: Begin 1 week after last IV dose. Use the following equation to calculate initial dose:

Initial weekly dose (grams) = [1.37 x IGIV dose (grams)] divided by [IV dose interval (weeks)]

Note: For subsequent dose adjustments, refer to product labeling.

◀

Hizentra: SubQ infusion: For weekly or frequent (up to daily) dosing, begin 1 week after last IV infusion or SubQ infusion. For biweekly (every 2 week) dosing, begin 1 or 2 weeks after last IV infusion or 1 week after the last SubQ weekly infusion. **Note:** Patient should have received an IV immune globulin routinely for at least 3 months before switching to SubQ. Use the following equation to calculate initial weekly dose:

Initial weekly dose (grams) = [Previous IGIV dose (grams)] divided by [IV dose interval (eg, 3 or 4 weeks)] then multiply by 1.37. For patients switching to Hizentra from a different SubQ formulation, the previous weekly SubQ dose should be used initially. To convert the dose (in grams) to mL, multiply the calculated dose (in g) by 5.

Note: Provided the total weekly dose is maintained, any dosing interval from daily up to biweekly (every 2 weeks) may be used. For patients switching to Hizentra from a different SubQ formulation, the previous weekly SubQ dose should be used initially. Use the following calculations to calculate frequent or biweekly dosing:

Biweekly dosing (grams) = multiply the calculated or previous weekly dose by 2.

Frequent (2 to 7 times per week) dosing (grams) = divide the calculated or previous weekly dose by the desired number of times per week (eg, for 3 times per week dosing, divide weekly dose by 3)

Note: For subsequent dose adjustments, refer to product labeling.

SubQ infusion dosing:

Cuvitru: SubQ:

Patients switching from another IG SubQ product: SubQ infusion:

Weekly dosing (grams): Weekly dose is the same as the prior immune globulin subcutaneous weekly dose

Biweekly dosing (grams): Multiply the calculated weekly dose by 2

Frequent (2 to 7 times per week) dosing (grams): Divide the calculated weekly dose by the desired number of administration times per week

Note: For subsequent dose adjustments, refer to product labeling.

Patients switching from IGIV therapy or Hyqvia: SubQ infusion: Begin treatment one week after patient's last immune globulin IV or Hyqvia infusion

Initial weekly dosing (grams): Divide the previous immune globulin IV or Hyqvia dose (grams) by the number of weeks between IV doses, then multiply this dose by 1.3 (dose adjustment factor)

Biweekly dosing (grams): Multiply the calculated weekly dose by 2

Frequent (2 to 7 times per week) dosing (grams): Divide the calculated weekly dose by the desired number of times per week

Note: For subsequent dose adjustments, refer to product labeling.

HyQvia: SubQ: See manufacturer's labeling for initial ramp-up schedule (initiating treatment with a full monthly dose has not been evaluated); dose adjusted based on monitored trough serum IgG concentrations and clinical response after initial ramp-up. **Note:** For patients previously on another IgG treatment, administer the first dose ~1 week after the last infusion of previous treatment.

Patients naive to IgG therapy or switching from IG SubQ therapy: SubQ infusion: 300 to 600 mg/kg every 3 to 4 weeks, after the initial dose ramp-up

Patients switching from IGIV therapy: SubQ infusion: Administer the same dose and frequency as the previous IGIV therapy after the initial dose ramp-up. For subsequent dose adjustments, refer to product labeling.

Rubella (GamaSTAN S/D): IM: Postexposure prophylaxis during pregnancy: 0.55 **mL**/kg

Secondary immunodeficiency: Panzyga [Canadian product]: IV: 200 to 800 mg/kg every 3 to 4 weeks; dose adjusted based on monitored trough serum IgG concentrations and clinical response

Varicella (GamaSTAN S/D): IM: Prophylaxis: 0.6 to 1.2 **mL**/kg (varicella zoster immune globulin preferred) within 72 hours of exposure (Gershon 1978). **Note:** For patients at risk of thrombosis, administer at the lower end of the recommended dosage range.

Off-label uses: IV:

Acquired hypogammaglobulinemia secondary to malignancy (off-label use): 400 mg/kg/dose every 3 weeks; reevaluate every 4 to 6 months (Anderson 2007)

Antibody-mediated rejection in cardiac transplantation, treatment (off-label use): Dose/frequency/duration of treatment varies greatly: 100 to 2,000 mg/kg (dose may be divided into 2 or 4 doses) 1 to 3 times per week, often given after each plasmapheresis; may be re-dosed monthly, if re-dose necessary and based on response (AHA [Colvin 2015]; ISHLT [Costanzo 2010]).

Dermatomyositis/polymyositis (refractory) (use in combination with other agents in patients with dermatomyositis) (off-label use): 2,000 mg/kg per treatment course administered in divided doses over 2 to 5 consecutive days (eg, 400 mg/kg/day for 5 days); maximum (per treatment course): 2,000 mg/kg (Feasby 2007).

Guillain-Barré syndrome (off-label use): A total dose of 2 g/kg per treatment course, given in divided doses over 2 to 5 consecutive days (eg, 400 mg/kg/day for 5 days) (Feasby 2007; Hughes 2014). European Federation of Neurological Societies (EFNS) guidelines recommend the 5-day treatment regimen (Elovaara, 2008).

Hematopoietic cell transplantation (HCT) with hypogammaglobulinemia (IgG <400 mg/dL), prevention of bacterial infection (off-label use): **Note:** Increase dose or frequency to maintain IgG concentration >400 mg/dL.

≤100 days post-HCT: 500 mg/kg/dose once weekly (Tomblyn 2009)

>100 days post-HCT: 500 mg/kg/dose every 3 to 4 weeks (Tomblyn 2009)

HIV-associated thrombocytopenia (off-label use): 1,000 mg/kg/day for 2 days (Anderson 2007)

Lambert-Eaton myasthenic syndrome (LEMS) (off-label use): 1,000 mg/kg/day for 2 days (Bain 1996; Patwa 2012)

Myasthenia gravis (acute exacerbation) (off-label use): Adjunctive therapy: 2 g/kg per treatment course, administered in divided doses over 2 to 5 consecutive days (eg, 400 mg/kg/day for 5 days) (Barth 2011; Feasby 2007; Zinman 2007). **Note:** A single dose of 1 g/kg may have similar efficacy to 1 g/kg given on 2 consecutive days (Gajdos 2005)

Relapsing-remitting multiple sclerosis (off-label use): 1,000 mg/kg per month, with or without an induction of 400 mg/kg/day for 5 days (Feasby 2007). Optimal dosing has not been established.

Geriatric Refer to adult dosing. Use with caution; administer the minimum dose and infusion rate practicable.

Pediatric Note: HyQvia and Octagam 10% are **not** FDA-approved for use in children.

Children and Adolescents:

Hepatitis A: Refer to adult dosing.

Immune thrombocytopenia (ITP):

Carimune NF: IV: Initial: 400 mg/kg/day for 2 to 5 consecutive days (6% solution recommended); Maintenance: 400 mg/kg (no more frequent than daily) as needed to maintain platelet count ≥30,000/mm^3 and/or to control significant bleeding; may increase dose if needed (range: 800 to 1,000 mg/kg). For acute ITP, may discontinue after day 2 if platelet response is adequate (30,000 to 50,000/mm^3) after the first 2 doses.

Flebogamma DIF 10%: Children ≥2 years and Adolescents: IV: 1,000 mg/kg once daily for 2 consecutive days

Gammaked, Gamunex-C: IV: 1,000 mg/kg/day for 2 consecutive days (second dose may be withheld if adequate platelet response in 24 hours) or 400 mg/kg once daily for 5 consecutive days.

Privigen: IV: 1,000 mg/kg/day for 2 consecutive days (not approved for use in pediatric patients <15 years of age).

American Society of Hematology Guidelines: Newly diagnosed ITP: Initial pharmacologic management: Children and Adolescents: IV: 800 to 1,000 mg/kg as a single dose (Neunert 2011).

Kawasaki syndrome: IV:

Gammagard S/D: 1,000 mg/kg as a single dose or 400 mg/kg/day for 4 consecutive days. Begin within 7 days of onset of fever.

AHA guidelines (2004): 2,000 mg/kg as a single dose within 10 days of disease onset

Note: Must be used in combination with aspirin: 80 to 100 mg/kg/day orally, divided every 6 hours for up to 14 days (until fever resolves for at least 48 hours); then decrease dose to 3 to 5 mg/kg/day once daily. In patients without coronary artery abnormalities, give lower dose for 6 to 8 weeks. In patients with coronary artery abnormalities, low-dose aspirin should be continued indefinitely.

Measles: Refer to adult dosing.

Primary humoral immunodeficiency disorders:

IV infusion dosing:

Bivigam: IV: Children ≥6 years and Adolescents: 300 to 800 mg/kg every 3 to 4 weeks; dose adjusted based on monitored trough serum IgG concentrations and clinical response

Carimune NF: IV: Children and Adolescents: 400 to 800 mg/kg every 3 to 4 weeks. **Note:** In previously untreated agammaglobulinemic or hypogammaglobulinemic patients use a 3% solution; may administer subsequent infusions with a higher concentration if patient tolerates lower concentration.

Flebogamma DIF 5%: IV: Children ≥2 years, and Adolescents: 300 to 600 mg/kg every 3 to 4 weeks; dose adjusted based on monitored trough serum IgG concentrations and clinical response

Gammagard Liquid, Gammagard S/D: IV: Children ≥2 years and Adolescents: 300 to 600 mg/kg every 3 to 4 weeks; dose adjusted based on monitored trough serum IgG concentrations and clinical response.

Gammaked, Gamunex-C: IV: Children ≥2 years and Adolescents: 300 to 600 mg/kg every 3 to 4 weeks; dose adjusted based on monitored trough serum IgG concentrations and clinical response.

Gammaplex: IV: Children ≥2 years, and Adolescents: 300 to 800 mg/kg every 3 to 4 weeks; dose adjusted based on monitored trough serum IgG concentrations and clinical response.

Octagam 5%: IV: Children and Adolescents: 300 to 600 mg/kg every 3 to 4 weeks; dose adjusted based on monitored trough serum IgG concentrations and clinical response.

Panzyga [Canadian product]: IV: Children ≥2 years and Adolescents: 200 to 800 mg/kg every 3 to 4 weeks; dose adjusted based on monitored trough serum IgG concentrations and clinical response.

Privigen: IV: Children ≥3 years and Adolescents: 200 to 800 mg/kg every 3 to 4 weeks; dose adjusted based on monitored trough serum IgG concentrations and clinical response

Switching to weekly subcutaneous infusion dosing:

Gammagard Liquid, Gammaked, Gamunex-C: Children ≥2 years and Adolescents:

SubQ infusion: Begin 1 week after last IV dose. Use the following equation to calculate initial dose:

Initial weekly dose (grams) = [1.37 x IGIV dose (grams)] divided by [IV dose interval (weeks)]

Note: For subsequent dose adjustments, refer to product labeling.

Hizentra: SubQ infusion: Children ≥2 years and Adolescents: For weekly or frequent (up to daily) dosing, begin 1 week after last IV infusion or SubQ infusion. For biweekly (every 2 week) dosing, begin 1 or 2 weeks after last IV infusion or 1 week after the last SubQ weekly infusion. **Note:** Patient should have received an IV immune globulin routinely for at least 3 months before switching to SubQ. Use the following equation to calculate initial weekly dose:

Initial weekly dose (grams) = [Previous IGIV dose (grams)] divided by [IV dose interval (eg, 3 or 4 weeks)] then multiply by 1.37. If switching from a different SubQ formulation to Hizentra, maintain previous weekly SubQ dose initially. To convert the dose (in grams) to mL, multiply the calculated dose (in grams) by 5.

Note: Provided the total weekly dose is maintained, any dosing interval from daily up to biweekly (every 2 weeks) may be used. Use the following calculations to calculate frequent or biweekly dosing:

Biweekly dosing (grams) = multiply the calculated or previous weekly dose by 2.

Frequent (2 to 7 times per week) dosing (grams) = divide the calculated or previous weekly dose by the desired number of times per week (eg, for 3 times per week dosing, divide weekly dose by 3).

Note: For subsequent dose adjustments, refer to product labeling.

SubQ infusion dosing:

Cuvitru: SubQ infusion: Children ≥2 years and Adolescents: Refer to adult dosing.

Secondary immunodeficiency: Panzyga [Canadian product]: IV: Children ≥2 years and Adolescents: 200 to 800 mg/kg every 3 to 4 weeks; dose adjusted based on monitored trough serum IgG concentrations and clinical response.

Varicella: Refer to adult dosing.

Dermatomyositis/polymyositis (refractory) (use in combination with other agents in patients with dermatomyositis) (off-label use): IV: 2,000 mg/kg per treatment course administered in divided doses over 2 consecutive days (eg, 1,000 mg/kg/day for 2 days); maximum (per treatment course): 2,000 mg/kg (Feasby 2007)

Guillain-Barré syndrome (off-label use): Children and Adolescents: IV: 1,000 mg/kg/day for 2 days (Feasby 2007; Korinthenberg 2005) **or** 400 mg/kg/day for 5 days (El-Bayoumi 2011; Korinthenberg 2005).Two-day regimens have been associated with a higher incidence of early relapse (Korinthenberg 2005). American Academy of Neurology guidelines state optimal dosing has not been established (Patwa 2012).

◀ **Hematopoietic cell transplantation (HCT) with hypogammaglobuline-mia (IgG <400 mg/dL), prevention of bacterial infection (off-label use) (Tomblyn 2009):** IV: *Note*: Increase dose or frequency to maintain IgG concentration >400 mg/dL.

≤100 days post-HCT:

Infants and Children (Allogeneic HCT recipients): IV: 400 mg/kg/dose once monthly

Adolescents: IV: 500 mg/kg/dose once weekly

>100 days post-HCT: Infants, Children, and Adolescents: IV: 500 mg/kg/dose every 3 to 4 weeks

HIV infection [prophylaxis of bacterial infection in patients with hypogammaglobulinemia (IgG <400 mg/dL)] (off-label use): Infants and Children: IV:

Primary prophylaxis for serious bacterial infections: 400 mg/kg/dose every 2 to 4 weeks (DHHS [pediatric] 2013)

Secondary prophylaxis for invasive bacterial infections: Should only be used if subsequent infections are frequent severe infections (>2 infections during a 1-year period): 400 mg/kg/dose every 2 to 4 weeks (DHHS [pediatric] 2013)

Myasthenia gravis (acute exacerbation) (off-label use): Adolescents: Refer to adult dosing.

Renal Impairment

IV: Use with caution due to risk of immune globulin-induced renal dysfunction; the rate of infusion and concentration of solution should be minimized. Discontinue if renal function deteriorates during treatment.

IM: There are no dosage adjustments provided in the manufacturer's labeling.

SubQ infusion: There are no dosage adjustments provided in the manufacturer's labeling; consider lower, more frequent dosing.

Hepatic Impairment IM, IV, SubQ infusion: There are no dosage adjustments provided in the manufacturer's labeling.

Obesity Some clinicians dose IGIV on ideal body weight or an adjusted ideal body weight in morbidly obese patients (Siegel 2010).

Additional Information Complete prescribing information should be consulted for additional detail.

Dosage Forms Considerations

Carimune NF may contain a significant amount of sodium and also contains sucrose.

Gammagard S/D may contain a significant amount of sodium and also contains glucose.

Octagam contains maltose.

Hyqvia Kit is supplied with a Hyaluronidase (Human Recombinant) component intended for injection prior to Immune Globulin administration to improve dispersion and absorption of the Immune Globulin.

Dosage Forms Excipient information presented when available (limited, particularly for generics); consult specific product labeling. [DSC] = Discontinued product

Injectable, Intramuscular [preservative free]:

GamaSTAN S/D: 15% to 18% [150 to 180 mg/mL] (2 mL, 10 mL)

Kit, Subcutaneous:

Hyqvia: 2.5 g/25 mL, 5 g/50 mL, 10 g/100 mL, 20 g/200 mL, 30 g/300 mL [contains albumin human, edetate disodium dihydrate, mouse (murine) and/or hamster protein]

Solution, Injection [preservative free]:
  Gammagard: 1 g/10 mL (10 mL); 2.5 g/25 mL (25 mL); 5 g/50 mL (50 mL); 10 g/100 mL (100 mL); 20 g/200 mL (200 mL); 30 g/300 mL (300 mL) [latex free]
  Gammaked: 1 g/10 mL (10 mL); 2.5 g/25 mL (25 mL); 5 g/50 mL (50 mL); 10 g/100 mL (100 mL); 20 g/200 mL (200 mL) [latex free]
  Gamunex-C: 1 g/10 mL (10 mL); 2.5 g/25 mL (25 mL); 5 g/50 mL (50 mL); 10 g/100 mL (100 mL); 20 g/200 mL (200 mL); 40 g/400 mL (400 mL) [latex free]
Solution, Intravenous [preservative free]:
  Bivigam: 5 g/50 mL (50 mL); 10 g/100 mL (100 mL) [sugar free; contains polysorbate 80]
  Flebogamma DIF: 0.5 g/10 mL (10 mL); 5 g/50 mL (50 mL); 5 g/100 mL (100 mL); 10 g/100 mL (100 mL); 20 g/200 mL (200 mL); 20 g/400 mL (400 mL); 10 g/200 mL (200 mL); 2.5 g/50 mL (50 mL) [contains polyethylene glycol]
  Gammaplex: 5 g/50 mL (50 mL); 5 g/100 mL (100 mL) [contains polysorbate 80]
  Gammaplex: 10 g/100 mL (100 mL)
  Gammaplex: 20 g/200 mL (200 mL); 20 g/400 mL (400 mL); 10 g/200 mL (200 mL); 2.5 g/50 mL (50 mL [DSC]) [contains polysorbate 80]
  Octagam: 1 g/20 mL (20 mL); 2 g/20 mL (20 mL); 5 g/50 mL (50 mL); 5 g/100 mL (100 mL); 10 g/100 mL (100 mL); 20 g/200 mL (200 mL); 25 g/500 mL (500 mL); 10 g/200 mL (200 mL); 2.5 g/50 mL (50 mL) [sucrose free]
  Privigen: 5 g/50 mL (50 mL); 10 g/100 mL (100 mL); 20 g/200 mL (200 mL); 40 g/400 mL (400 mL)
Solution, Subcutaneous [preservative free]:
  Cuvitru: 1 g/5 mL (5 mL); 2 g/10 mL (10 mL); 4 g/20 mL (20 mL); 8 g/40 mL (40 mL)
  Hizentra: 1 g/5 mL (5 mL); 2 g/10 mL (10 mL); 4 g/20 mL (20 mL); 10 g/50 mL (50 mL) [contains polysorbate 80]
Solution Reconstituted, Intravenous [preservative free]:
  Carimune NF: 3 g (1 ea [DSC]); 6 g (1 ea); 12 g (1 ea)
  Gammagard S/D: 5 g (1 ea [DSC]); 10 g (1 ea [DSC])
  Gammagard S/D Less IgA: 5 g (1 ea); 10 g (1 ea)
Dosage Forms: Canada Information with regard to form, strength, and availability of products uniquely available in Canada but currently not available in the US. Refer also to Dosage Forms.
  Excipient information presented when available (limited, particularly for generics); consult specific product labeling.
  Solution, Intravenous [preservative free]:
    Panzyga: 1 g/10 mL (10 mL), 2.5 g/25 mL (25 mL), 5 g/50 mL (50 mL), 10 g/100 mL (100 mL), 20 g/200 mL (200 mL), 30 g/300 mL (30 mL)

◆ **Immune Globulin IV** see Immune Globulin on page 992

◆ **Immune Globulin Subcutaneous (Human)** see Immune Globulin on page 992

◆ **Immune Serum Globulin** see Immune Globulin on page 992

◆ **Immunine VH (Can)** see Factor IX (Human) on page 771

◆ **INCB424** see Ruxolitinib on page 1645

◆ **INCB 18424** see Ruxolitinib on page 1645

◆ **Indium In-111 Pentetreotide Kit** see Indium In-111 Pentetreotide on page 1002

Indium In-111 Pentetreotide
(IN dee um eye en won e LEV en pen te TREE oh tide)
Brand Names: US OctreoScan®
Index Terms ¹¹¹In-Pentetreotide; Indium In-111 Pentetreotide Kit; Octreo-Scan® (Prep Kit)
Pharmacologic Category Radiopharmaceutical
Use Scintigraphic localization of primary and metastatic neuroendocrine tumors with somatostatin receptors
Pregnancy Risk Factor C
Dosing
Adult
Planar imaging: IV: 3 mCi (111 MBq)
Single photon emission computed tomograph (SPECT) imaging: IV: 6 mCi (222 MBq)
Pediatric IV: 0.14 mCi/kg (5 MBq/kg)
Renal Impairment No dosage adjustment provided in manufacturer's labeling; use with caution.
Hepatic Impairment No dosage adjustment provided in manufacturer's labeling.
Additional Information Complete prescribing information should be consulted for additional detail.
Dosage Forms Excipient information presented when available (limited, particularly for generics); consult specific product labeling.
Kit, [preservative free]:
OctreoScan®:
Injection, powder for reconstitution: Pentetreotide 10 mcg
Injection, solution: Indium In-111 chloride 111 MBq (3.0 mCi) per 1 mL (1.1 mL)

◆ **INF-alpha 2** see Interferon Alfa-2b on page 1018
◆ **Infed** see Iron Dextran Complex on page 1053
◆ **Inflectra** see InFLIXimab on page 1002

InFLIXimab (in FLIKS e mab)
Related Information
Hematopoietic Cell Transplantation on page 2365
Brand Names: US Inflectra; Remicade; Renflexis
Brand Names: Canada Inflectra; Remicade; Remsima
Index Terms Avakine; Infliximab, Recombinant; Infliximab-abda; Infliximab-dyyb
Pharmacologic Category Antirheumatic, Disease Modifying; Gastrointestinal Agent, Miscellaneous; Immunosuppressant Agent; Monoclonal Antibody; Tumor Necrosis Factor (TNF) Blocking Agent
Use
Ankylosing spondylitis: Treatment of adults with active ankylosing spondylitis (to reduce signs/symptoms)
Crohn disease: Treatment of adults and pediatric patients ≥6 years with moderately to severely active Crohn disease who have had inadequate responses to conventional therapy (to reduce signs/symptoms and induce and maintain clinical remission) or to reduce the number of draining enterocutaneous and rectovaginal fistulas and maintain fistula closure in adults

Plaque psoriasis: Treatment of adults with chronic, severe (extensive and/or disabling) plaque psoriasis as an alternative to other systemic therapy

Psoriatic arthritis: Treatment of adults with psoriatic arthritis (to reduce signs/symptoms of active arthritis and inhibit progression of structural damage and improve physical function)

Rheumatoid arthritis: Treatment of adults with moderately to severely active rheumatoid arthritis (with methotrexate) (to reduce signs/symptoms of active arthritis and inhibit progression of structural damage and improve physical function)

Ulcerative colitis: Treatment of adults and pediatric patients ≥6 years (Remicade only) with moderately to severely active ulcerative colitis with inadequate response to conventional therapy (to reduce signs/symptoms and induce and maintain clinical remission and mucosal healing and eliminate corticosteroid use)

Note: Renflexis, Inflectra, and Remsima [Canadian product] are approved as biosimilar to Remicade; approved uses may vary (see product labeling).

Labeled Contraindications

Hypersensitivity to infliximab, murine proteins, or any component of the formulation; doses >5 mg/kg in patients with moderate or severe heart failure (NYHA Class III/IV)

Canadian labeling: Additional contraindications (not in US labeling): Severe infections (eg, sepsis, abscesses, tuberculosis, and opportunistic infections); use in patients with moderate or severe heart failure (NYHA Class III/IV)

Pregnancy Considerations Animal reproduction studies have not been conducted. Infliximab crosses the placenta and can be detected in the serum of infants for up to 6 months following in utero exposure. A fatal outcome has been reported in an infant who received a live vaccine (BCG) after in utero exposure to infliximab; it is recommended to wait ≥6 months following birth before administering any live vaccine to infants exposed to infliximab in utero. If a biologic agent such as infliximab is needed to treat inflammatory bowel disease during pregnancy, it is recommended to hold therapy after 30 weeks gestation (Habal 2012).

Health care providers are also encouraged to enroll women exposed to infliximab during pregnancy in the MotherToBaby Autoimmune Diseases Study by contacting the Organization of Teratology Information Specialists (OTIS) (877-311-8972).

Breastfeeding Considerations Small amounts of infliximab are present in breast milk. Information is available from three postpartum women who were administered infliximab 5 mg/kg 1 to 24 weeks after delivery. Infliximab was detected within 12 hours and the highest milk concentrations (0.09 to 0.105 mcg/mL) were seen 2 to 3 days after the dose. Corresponding maternal serum concentrations were 18 to 64 mcg/mL (Ben-Horin 2011). Due to the potential for serious adverse reactions in the breastfeeding infant, the manufacturer recommends a decision be made whether to discontinue breastfeeding or the drug, taking into account the importance of treatment to the mother.

Warnings/Precautions [US Boxed Warning]: Patients receiving infliximab are at increased risk for serious infections which may result in hospitalization and/or fatality; infections usually developed in patients receiving concomitant immunosuppressive agents (eg, methotrexate or corticosteroids) and may present as disseminated (rather than local) disease. Active tuberculosis (or reactivation of latent tuberculosis), invasive fungal (including aspergillosis, blastomycosis, candidiasis,

coccidioidomycosis, histoplasmosis, and pneumocystosis) and bacterial, viral or other opportunistic infections (including legionellosis and listeriosis) have been reported. Monitor closely for signs/symptoms of infection. Discontinue for serious infection or sepsis. Consider risks versus benefits prior to use in patients with a history of chronic or recurrent infection. Consider empiric antifungal therapy in patients who are at risk for invasive fungal infection and develop severe systemic illness. Caution should be exercised when considering use the elderly or in patients with conditions that predispose them to infections (eg, diabetes) or residence/travel from areas of endemic mycoses (blastomycosis, coccidioidomycosis, histoplasmosis), or with latent or localized infections. Do not initiate infliximab therapy in patients with an active infection, including clinically important localized infection. Patients who develop a new infection while undergoing treatment should be monitored closely. Potentially significant drug interactions may exist, requiring dose or frequency adjustment, additional monitoring, and/or selection of alternative therapy.

[US Boxed Warning]: Infliximab treatment has been associated with active tuberculosis (may be disseminated or extrapulmonary) or reactivation of latent infections; evaluate patients for tuberculosis risk factors and latent tuberculosis infection (with a tuberculin skin test) prior to and during therapy; treatment of latent tuberculosis should be initiated before use. Patients with initial negative tuberculin skin tests should receive continued monitoring for tuberculosis throughout treatment. Most cases of reactivation have been reported within the first couple months of treatment. Caution should be exercised when considering the use of infliximab in patients who have been exposed to tuberculosis.

Patients should be brought up to date with all immunizations before initiating therapy. Live vaccines should not be given concurrently; there is no data available concerning secondary transmission of live vaccines in patients receiving therapy. A fatal outcome has been reported in an infant who received a live vaccine (BCG) after in utero exposure to infliximab; infliximab crosses the placenta and has been detected in infants' serum for up to 6 months. It is recommended to wait ≥6 months following birth before administering any live vaccine to infants exposed to infliximab in utero. Reactivation of hepatitis B virus (HBV) has occurred in chronic virus carriers (may be fatal); use with caution; evaluate prior to initiation and during treatment.

[US Boxed Warning]: Lymphoma and other malignancies (may be fatal) have been reported in children and adolescent patients receiving TNF-blocking agents including infliximab. Half the cases are lymphomas (Hodgkin's and non-Hodgkin's). **[US Boxed Warning]: Postmarketing cases of hepatosplenic T-cell lymphoma have been reported in patients treated with infliximab. Almost all patients had received and concurrent or prior treatment with azathioprine or mercaptopurine at or prior to diagnosis and the majority of reported cases occurred in adolescent and young adult males with Crohn disease or ulcerative colitis.** Malignancies occurred after a median of 30 months (range: 1 to 84 months) after the first dose of TNF blocker therapy; most patients were receiving concomitant immunosuppressants. The impact of infliximab on the development and course of malignancies is not fully defined. As compared to the general population, an increased risk of lymphoma has been noted in clinical trials; however, rheumatoid arthritis alone has been previously associated with an increased rate of lymphoma. Use caution in patients with a history of COPD, higher rates of malignancy were reported in COPD patients treated with infliximab. Psoriasis patients with a history of phototherapy had a higher incidence of nonmelanoma skin cancers. Melanoma and Merkel cell carcinoma have been reported in patients receiving TNF-blocking agents including infliximab. Perform periodic skin examinations in all patients during therapy, particularly those at increased risk for skin cancer.

Severe hepatic reactions (including hepatitis, jaundice, acute hepatic failure, and cholestasis) have been reported during treatment; reactions occurred between 2 weeks to >1 year after initiation of therapy and some cases were fatal or necessitated liver transplantation; discontinue with jaundice and/or marked increase in liver enzymes (≥5 times ULN). Use caution with heart failure; if a decision is made to use with heart failure, monitor closely and discontinue if exacerbated or new symptoms occur. Doses >5 mg/kg should not be administered in patients with moderate to severe heart failure (HF) (NYHA Class III/IV). In a scientific statement from the American Heart Association, TNF blockers have been determined to be agents that may either cause direct myocardial toxicity or exacerbate underlying myocardial dysfunction (magnitude: major) (AHA [Page 2016]). Use caution with history of hematologic abnormalities; hematologic toxicities (eg, leukopenia, neutropenia, thrombocytopenia, pancytopenia) have been reported (may be fatal); discontinue if significant abnormalities occur. Positive antinuclear antibody titers have been detected in patients (with negative baselines). Rare cases of autoimmune disorder, including lupus-like syndrome, have been reported; monitor and discontinue if symptoms develop. Rare cases of optic neuritis and demyelinating disease (including multiple sclerosis, systemic vasculitis, and Guillain-Barré syndrome) have been reported; use with caution in patients with preexisting or recent onset CNS demyelinating disorders, or seizures; discontinue if significant CNS adverse reactions develop.

Acute infusion reactions may occur. Hypersensitivity reaction may occur within 2 hours of infusion. Medication and equipment for management of hypersensitivity reaction should be available for immediate use. Interruptions and/or reinstitution at a slower rate may be required (consult protocols). Pretreatment may be considered, and may be warranted in all patients with prior infusion reactions. Serum sickness-like reactions have occurred; may be associated with a decreased response to treatment. The development of antibodies to infliximab may increase the risk of hypersensitivity and/or infusion reactions; concomitant use of immunosuppressants may lessen the development of anti-infliximab antibodies. The risk of infusion reactions may be increased with retreatment after an interruption or discontinuation of prior maintenance therapy. Retreatment in psoriasis patients should be resumed as a scheduled maintenance regimen without any induction doses; use of an induction regimen should be used cautiously for retreatment of all other patients.

Some dosage forms may contain polysorbate 80 (also known as Tweens). Hypersensitivity reactions, usually a delayed reaction, have been reported following exposure to pharmaceutical products containing polysorbate 80 in certain individuals (Isaksson 2002; Lucente 2000; Shelley 1995). Thrombocytopenia, ascites, pulmonary deterioration, and renal and hepatic failure have been reported in premature neonates after receiving parenteral products containing polysorbate 80 (Alade 1986; CDC 1984). See manufacturer's labeling.

Efficacy was not established in a study to evaluate infliximab use in juvenile idiopathic arthritis (JIA).

Adverse Reactions

>10%:

Central nervous system: Headache (18%)

Gastrointestinal: Abdominal pain (Crohn disease: 26%; other indications: 12%), nausea (21%)

Hepatic: Increased serum ALT (<3x ULN: 17% to 51%; ≥3x ULN: 2% to 10%; ≥5x ULN: 1% to 4%)

Immunologic: Increased ANA titer (~50%), antibody development (double-stranded DNA, 20%), antibody development (anti-infliximab; variable; ~10% to 15% [range: 6% to 61%]; Mayer 2006)

Infection: Infection (Crohn disease: 50% to 59%; other indications: 27% to 36%), abscess (Crohn disease patients with fistulizing disease: 6% to 15%)

Respiratory: Upper respiratory tract infection (32%), sinusitis (14%), cough (12%), pharyngitis (12%)

Miscellaneous: Infusion related reaction (18%; severe: <1%)

1% to 10%:

Cardiovascular: Flushing (Crohn disease: 9%), hypertension (7%), chest pain (1%), bradycardia (≥0.2%), edema (≥0.2%), hypotension (≥0.2%), thrombophlebitis (deep) (≥0.2%)

Central nervous system: Fatigue (9%), pain (8%), chills (≤3%), dizziness (≥0.2%)

Dermatologic: Skin rash (1% to 10%), pruritus (≤7%), cellulitis (≥0.2%), diaphoresis (≥0.2%)

Endocrine & metabolic: Dehydration (≥0.2%)

Gastrointestinal: Dyspepsia (10%), GI moniliasis (5%), constipation (≥0.2%), intestinal obstruction (≥0.2%)

Genitourinary: Urinary tract infection (8%)

Hematologic & oncologic: Anemia (children with Crohn disease: 11%; adults: ≥0.2%), hemolytic anemia (≥0.2%), leukopenia (Crohn disease: 9%; other indications: ≥0.2%), lymphadenopathy (≥0.2%), malignant lymphoma (≥0.2%), neutropenia (Crohn disease: 7%), pancytopenia (≥0.2%), sarcoidosis (≥0.2%), thrombocytopenia (≥0.2%)

Hepatic: Hepatitis (≥0.2%)

Hypersensitivity: Hypersensitivity reaction (Crohn disease: 6%; other indications: ≥0.2%), delayed hypersensitivity (plaque psoriasis: 1%), serum sickness (≥0.2%)

Infection: Viral infection (Crohn disease: 8%), bacterial infection (Crohn disease: 6%), serious infection (1% to 5%; other indications: 12%), sepsis (≥0.2%)

Neuromuscular & skeletal: Arthralgia (1% to 8%), bone fracture (Crohn disease: 7%), myalgia (1%)

Respiratory: Bronchitis (10%), dyspnea (≤1%), lower respiratory tract infection (≥0.2%), pleurisy (≥0.2%), pulmonary edema (≥0.2%)

Miscellaneous: Fever (≤3% to 7%)

<1%, postmarketing, and/or case reports: Acute hepatic failure, agranulocytosis, anaphylactic shock, anaphylaxis, angina pectoris, antibody development, autoimmune hepatitis, bronchospasm, cardiac failure (worsening), cholecystitis, cholestasis, chronic inflammatory demyelinating polyneuropathy, confusion, convulsions, demyelinating disease of the central nervous system (eg, multiple sclerosis, optic neuritis), demyelinating disease (peripheral; eg, Guillain-Barré syndrome, chronic inflammatory demyelinating

polyneuropathy, multifocal motor neuropathy), dysgeusia, erythema multiforme, erythematous rash, exacerbation of psoriasis, gastrointestinal hemorrhage, hepatic carcinoma, hepatic failure, hepatic injury, hepatitis B (reactivation), hepatotoxicity (idiosyncratic) (Chalasani 2014), hepatosplenic T-cell lymphomas (mainly young adult or adolescent males), Hodgkin lymphoma, immune thrombocytopenia, interstitial fibrosis, interstitial pneumonitis, intestinal stenosis, jaundice, laryngeal edema, leukemia, liver function tests increased (transient), lupus-like syndrome (drug-induced), malignant melanoma, malignant neoplasm (leiomyosarcoma), meningitis, Merkel cell carcinoma, myocardial infarction, nephrolithiasis, neuritis, neuropathy, numbness, opportunistic infection, pancreatitis, pericardial effusion, peripheral neuropathy, pharyngeal edema, pleural effusion, pneumonia, psoriasis (including new onset, palmoplantar, pustular, or exacerbation), pulmonary disease, pulmonary fibrosis, reactivated tuberculosis, renal cell carcinoma, renal failure, seizure, Stevens-Johnson syndrome, syncope, tachycardia, tendon disease, thrombotic thrombocytopenia purpura, tingling sensation, toxic epidermal necrolysis, transverse myelitis, tuberculosis, ulcer, urticaria, vasculitis (systemic and cutaneous), vision loss (transient)

Drug Interactions

Metabolism/Transport Effects None known.

Avoid Concomitant Use

Avoid concomitant use of InFLIXimab with any of the following: Abatacept; Adalimumab; Anakinra; BCG (Intravesical); Belimumab; Canakinumab; Certolizumab Pegol; Etanercept; Golimumab; Natalizumab; Pimecrolimus; Rilonacept; Tacrolimus (Topical); Tocilizumab; Tofacitinib; Ustekinumab; Vaccines (Live); Vedolizumab

Increased Effect/Toxicity

InFLIXimab may Increase the levels/effects of: Abatacept; Anakinra; Belimumab; Canakinumab; Certolizumab Pegol; Fingolimod; Leflunomide; Natalizumab; Rilonacept; Tofacitinib; Vaccines (Live); Vedolizumab

The levels/effects of InFLIXimab may be increased by: Adalimumab; Denosumab; Etanercept; Golimumab; Ocrelizumab; Pimecrolimus; Roflumilast; Tacrolimus (Topical); Tocilizumab; Trastuzumab; Ustekinumab

Decreased Effect

InFLIXimab may decrease the levels/effects of: BCG (Intravesical); Coccidioides immitis Skin Test; Nivolumab; Sipuleucel-T; Tertomotide; Vaccines (Inactivated); Vaccines (Live)

The levels/effects of InFLIXimab may be decreased by: Echinacea

Storage/Stability Store intact vials at 2°C to 8°C (36°F to 46°F). The manufacturer recommends that solutions diluted in NS for infusion should be used within 3 hours of preparation. However, a stability study of infliximab 0.4 mg/mL prepared in NS in polyvinyl chloride (PVC) bags found no loss of biological activity when stored refrigerated at 4°C for up to 14 days (Ikeda 2012).

Preparation for Administration Reconstitute vials with 10 mL sterile water for injection (SWFI) with a 21-gauge or smaller needle, directing the SWFI towards the wall of the vial. Swirl vial gently to dissolve powder; do not shake. Allow solution to stand for 5 minutes. Total dose of reconstituted product should be further diluted to 250 mL of NS injection (add reconstituted infliximab slowly) to a final concentration of 0.4 to 4 mg/mL. Do not dilute reconstituted infliximab solution with any other diluent. Infusion should begin within 3 hours of preparation (see Storage/Stability for additional information). ▶

◀ **Mechanism of Action** Infliximab is a chimeric monoclonal antibody that binds to human tumor necrosis factor alpha (TNFα), thereby interfering with endogenous TNFα activity. Elevated TNFα levels have been found in involved tissues/fluids of patients with rheumatoid arthritis, ankylosing spondylitis, psoriatic arthritis, plaque psoriasis, Crohn disease and ulcerative colitis. Biological activities of TNFα include the induction of proinflammatory cytokines (interleukins), enhancement of leukocyte migration, activation of neutrophils and eosinophils, and the induction of acute phase reactants and tissue degrading enzymes. Animal models have shown TNFα expression causes polyarthritis, and infliximab can prevent disease as well as allow diseased joints to heal.

Pharmacodynamics/Kinetics Note: Pharmacokinetic data in pediatric patients (6 to 17 years) reported to be similar to adult values.

Onset of action: Crohn disease: 1 to 2 weeks; Rheumatoid arthritis: 3 to 7 days

Duration of action: Crohn disease: 8 to 48 weeks; Rheumatoid arthritis: 6 to 12 weeks

Distribution: Within the vascular compartment; V_d: 3 to 6 L (Klotz 2007)

Half-life elimination: 7 to 12 days (Klotz 2007)

Dosing

Adult & Geriatric Note: Premedication with antihistamines (H_1-antagonist +/- H_2-antagonist), acetaminophen, and/or corticosteroids may be considered to prevent and/or manage infusion-related reactions. Renflexis, Inflectra, and Remsima [Canadian product] are approved as biosimilar to Remicade. Approved uses for biosimilar agents may vary (consult product labeling).

Ankylosing spondylitis: IV: 5 mg/kg at 0, 2, and 6 weeks, followed by 5 mg/kg every 6 weeks thereafter

Crohn disease: IV: 5 mg/kg at 0, 2, and 6 weeks, followed by 5 mg/kg every 8 weeks thereafter; dose may be increased to 10 mg/kg in patients who respond but then lose their response. If no response by week 14, consider discontinuing therapy.

Plaque psoriasis: IV: 5 mg/kg at 0, 2, and 6 weeks, followed by 5 mg/kg every 8 weeks thereafter.

Psoriatic arthritis (with or without methotrexate): IV: 5 mg/kg at 0, 2, and 6 weeks, followed by 5 mg/kg every 8 weeks thereafter.

Rheumatoid arthritis (in combination with methotrexate therapy): IV 3 mg/kg at 0, 2, and 6 weeks, followed by 3 mg/kg every 8 weeks thereafter; Remicade doses have ranged from 3 to 10 mg/kg repeated at 4- to 8-week intervals

Ulcerative colitis: IV: 5 mg/kg at 0, 2, and 6 weeks, followed by 5 mg/kg every 8 weeks thereafter. Doses up to 10 mg/kg were studied in clinical trials with similar efficacy observed with both doses (Rutgeerts 2005).

Pustular psoriasis (off-label use): IV: 5 mg/kg at week 0, 2, and 6, followed by 5 mg/kg every 8 weeks for up to 46 weeks (Suguira 2014; Torii 2011)

Dosage adjustment with heart failure (HF): Weigh risk versus benefits for individual patient:

Mild HF (NYHA Class I/II): No dosage adjustment necessary; use with caution and monitor closely for worsening of HF

Moderate to severe (NYHA Class III or IV): ≤5 mg/kg

Pediatric Note: Premedication with antihistamines (H_1-antagonist +/- H_2-antagonist), acetaminophen, and/or corticosteroids may be considered to prevent and/or manage infusion-related reactions. Renflexis, Inflectra, and Remsima [Canadian product] are approved as biosimilar to Remicade. Approved uses for biosimilar agents may vary (consult product labeling).

Crohn disease: Children ≥6 years and Adolescents: IV: 5 mg/kg at 0, 2, and 6 weeks, followed by 5 mg/kg every 8 weeks thereafter; in adult patients with Crohn disease, it has been observed that patients who do not respond by week 14 are unlikely to respond with continued dosing; consider discontinuing therapy.

Ulcerative colitis: Children ≥6 years and Adolescents: IV (Remicade only): 5 mg/kg at 0, 2, and 6 weeks, followed by 5 mg/kg every 8 weeks thereafter

Juvenile idiopathic arthritis (off-label use): Children ≥4 years and Adolescents: IV: Initial: 3 mg/kg at 0, 2, and 6 weeks; then 3 to 6 mg/kg/dose every 8 weeks thereafter, in combination with methotrexate during induction and maintenance (Ruperto 2010). Alternatively, some studies used 6 mg/kg starting at week 14 of a methotrexate induction regimen (weeks 0 to 13); repeat dose (6 mg/kg) at week 16 and 20, then every 8 weeks thereafter (Ruperto 2007; Visvanathan 2012).

Renal Impairment There are no dosage adjustments provided in the manufacturer's labeling.

Hepatic Impairment There are no dosage adjustments provided in the manufacturer's labeling.

Administration The infusion should begin within 3 hours of reconstitution and dilution. Infuse over at least 2 hours; do not infuse with other agents; use in-line low protein binding filter (≤1.2 micron). Temporarily discontinue or decrease infusion rate with infusion-related reactions. Antihistamines (H_1-antagonist +/- H_2-antagonist), acetaminophen and/or corticosteroids may be used to manage reactions. Infusion may be reinitiated at a lower rate upon resolution of mild to moderate symptoms.

Guidelines for the treatment and prophylaxis of infusion reactions: (**Note:** Limited to adult patients and dosages used in Crohn disease; prospective data for other populations [pediatrics, other indications/dosing] are not available).

A protocol for the treatment of infusion reactions, as well as prophylactic therapy for repeat infusions, has been published (Mayer, 2006).

Treatment of infusion reactions: Medications for the treatment of hypersensitivity reactions should be available for immediate use. For mild reactions, the rate of infusion should be decreased to 10 mL/hour. Initiate a normal saline infusion (500 to 1,000 mL/hour) and appropriate symptomatic treatment (eg, acetaminophen and diphenhydramine); monitor vital signs every 10 minutes until normal. After 20 minutes, the infusion may be increased at 15-minute intervals, as tolerated, to completion (initial increase to 20 mL/hour, then 40 mL/hour, then 80 mL/hour, etc [maximum of 125 mL/hour]). For moderate reactions, the infusion should be stopped or slowed. Initiate a normal saline infusion (500 to 1,000 mL/hour) and appropriate symptomatic treatment. Monitor vital signs every 5 minutes until normal. After 20 minutes, the infusion may be reinstituted at 10 mL/hour; then increased at 15-minute intervals, as tolerated, to completion (initial increase 20 mL/hour, then 40 mL/hour, then 80 mL/hour, etc [maximum of 125 mL/hour]). For severe reactions, the infusion should be stopped with administration of appropriate symptomatic treatment (eg, hydrocortisone/methylprednisolone, diphenhydramine and epinephrine) and frequent monitoring of vitals (consult institutional policies, if available). Re-treatment after a severe reaction should only be done if the benefits outweigh the risks and with appropriate prophylaxis. Delayed infusion reactions typically occur 1 to 7 days after an infusion. Treatment should consist of appropriate symptomatic treatment (eg, acetaminophen, antihistamine, methylprednisolone).

Prophylaxis of infusion reactions: Premedication with acetaminophen and diphenhydramine 90 minutes prior to infusion may be considered in all patients with prior infusion reactions, and in patients with severe reactions corticosteroid administration is recommended. Steroid dosing may be oral (prednisone 50 mg orally every 12 hours for 3 doses prior to infusion) or intravenous (a single dose of hydrocortisone 100 mg or methylprednisolone 20 to 40 mg administered 20 minutes prior to the infusion). On initiation of the infusion, begin with a test dose at 10 mL/hour for 15 minutes. Thereafter, the infusion may be increased at 15-minute intervals, as tolerated, to completion (initial increase 20 mL/hour, then 40 mL/hour, then 80 mL/hour, etc). A maximum rate of 125 mL/hour is recommended in patients who experienced prior mild to moderate reactions and 100 mL/hour is recommended in patients who experienced prior severe reactions. In patients with cutaneous flushing, aspirin may be considered (Becker, 2004). For delayed infusion reactions, premedicate with acetaminophen and diphenhydramine 90 minutes prior to infusion. On initiation of the infusion, begin with a test dose at 10 mL/hour for 15 minutes. Thereafter, the infusion may be increased to infuse over 3 hours. Postinfusion therapy with acetaminophen for 3 days and an antihistamine for 7 days is recommended.

Monitoring Parameters Monitor improvement of symptoms and physical function assessments. During infusion, if reaction is noted, monitor vital signs every 2 to 10 minutes, depending on reaction severity, until normal. Active and latent TB screening prior to initiating and during therapy; signs/symptoms of infection (prior to, during, and following therapy); CBC with differential; signs/symptoms/worsening of heart failure; HBV screening prior to initiating (all patients), HBV carriers (during and for several months following therapy); signs and symptoms of hypersensitivity reaction; symptoms of lupus-like syndrome; LFTs (discontinue if >5 times ULN); signs and symptoms of malignancy (eg, splenomegaly, hepatomegaly, abdominal pain, persistent fever, night sweats, weight loss).

Psoriasis patients with history of phototherapy should be monitored for nonmelanoma skin cancer.

Medication Guide Available Yes

Dosage Forms Considerations Remicade contains sucrose 500 mg per vial

Dosage Forms Excipient information presented when available (limited, particularly for generics); consult specific product labeling.

Solution Reconstituted, Intravenous:

Inflectra: 100 mg (1 ea) [contains polysorbate 80]

Solution Reconstituted, Intravenous [preservative free]:

Remicade: 100 mg (1 ea) [contains polysorbate 80]

Renflexis: 100 mg (1 ea) [contains polysorbate 80]

Dosage Forms: Canada Information with regard to form, strength, and availability of products uniquely available in Canada but currently not available in the US. Refer also to Dosage Forms.

Excipient information presented when available (limited, particularly for generics); consult specific product labeling.
Solution Reconstituted, Intravenous (preservative free):
  Remicade: 100 mg (contains polysorbate 80, sucrose 500 mg)
  Inflectra: 100 mg (contains polysorbate 80, sucrose 500 mg; biosimilar agent)
  Remsima 100 mg (contains polysorbate 80, sucrose 500 mg; biosimilar agent)

◆ **Infliximab-abda** *see* InFLIXimab *on page* 1002
◆ **Infliximab-dyyb** *see* InFLIXimab *on page* 1002
◆ **Infliximab, Recombinant** *see* InFLIXimab *on page* 1002
◆ **Infufer (Can)** *see* Iron Dextran Complex *on page* 1053

Ingenol Mebutate (IN je nol MEB u tate)
Brand Names: US Picato
Brand Names: Canada Picato
Index Terms *Euphorbia peplus* Derivative; PEP005
Pharmacologic Category Topical Skin Product
Use Actinic keratosis: Topical treatment of actinic keratosis
Pregnancy Risk Factor C
Dosing
Adult & Geriatric Actinic keratosis: Topical:
  Face or scalp: Apply 0.015% gel once daily to affected area for 3 consecutive days; patients not achieving clearance or that experience recurrence after achieving clearance ≥8 weeks after initial treatment may benefit from a second treatment course.
  Trunk or extremities: Apply 0.05% gel once daily to affected area for 2 consecutive days
Renal Impairment There are no dosage adjustments provided in the manufacturer's labeling. However, dosage adjustment unlikely due to low systemic absorption.
Hepatic Impairment There are no dosage adjustments provided in the manufacturer's labeling. However, dosage adjustment unlikely due to low systemic absorption.
Additional Information Complete prescribing information should be consulted for additional detail.
Dosage Forms Excipient information presented when available (limited, particularly for generics); consult specific product labeling.
Gel, External:
  Picato: 0.015% (3 ea); 0.05% (2 ea) [contains benzyl alcohol, isopropyl alcohol]

◆ **Inlyta** *see* Axitinib *on page* 201

Inotuzumab Ozogamicin (in oh TOOZ ue mab oh zoe ga MYE sin)
Related Information
  Safe Handling of Hazardous Drugs *on page* 2379
Brand Names: US Besponsa

▶

◀ **Index Terms** CMC-544; Way 207294; WAY-207294

Pharmacologic Category Antineoplastic Agent, Anti-CD22; Antineoplastic Agent, Antibody Drug Conjugate; Antineoplastic Agent, Monoclonal Antibody

Use Acute lymphoblastic leukemia (relapsed/refractory): Treatment of relapsed or refractory B-cell precursor acute lymphoblastic leukemia (ALL) in adults.

Labeled Contraindications There are no contraindications listed in the manufacturer's labeling.

Pregnancy Considerations Based on the mechanism of action and information from animal reproduction studies, inotuzumab ozogamicin may be expected to cause adverse events if used during pregnancy. Pregnancy status should be evaluated prior to therapy. Women of reproductive potential should use effective contraception during therapy and for at least 8 months after the last dose. Effective contraception should also be used for at least 5 months after the last dose when treating males who have female partners of reproductive potential.

Inotuzumab ozogamicin may impair fertility in males and females of reproductive potential.

Breastfeeding Considerations It is not known if inotuzumab ozogamicin is present in breast milk. Due to the potential for serious adverse reactions in the nursing infant, breastfeeding is not recommended by the manufacturer during therapy and for at least 2 months after the last dose.

Warnings/Precautions [US Boxed Warning]: Hepatotoxicity, including severe, life-threatening, and sometimes fatal sinusoidal obstructions syndrome (formerly called veno-occlusive disease [VOD]) has occurred in patients with relapsed or refractory acute lymphoblastic leukemia (ALL) who received inotuzumab ozogamicin. The risk of VOD was greater in patients who received a hematopoietic stem cell transplant (HSCT) following inotuzumab ozogamicin treatment. The use of HSCT conditioning regimens containing 2 alkylating agents (eg, busulfan in combination with other alkylating agents) and a total bilirubin level ≥ upper limit of normal (ULN) before HSCT were significantly associated with increasing the risk of VOD. Other risk factors for VOD associated with inotuzumab ozogamicin included ongoing or prior liver disease, prior HSCT, increased age, later salvage lines, and a higher number of inotuzumab ozogamicin treatment cycles. Liver function test elevations may require treatment interruption, dose reduction, or permanent discontinuation; discontinue permanently if VOD occurs. Patients with a history of VOD or who have serious ongoing hepatic liver disease (eg, cirrhosis, nodular regenerative hyperplasia, active hepatitis) are at an increased risk for worsening of liver disease, including developing VOD, following inotuzumab ozogamicin therapy. VOD was reported up to 56 days after the last dose during treatment or during follow-up without an intervening HSCT. For patients receiving HSCT after inotuzumab ozogamicin, the median time to onset of VOD was 15 days (range: 3 to 57 days). Due to the VOD risk, the recommended treatment duration with inotuzumab ozogamicin is 2 cycles in patients proceeding to HSCT; an additional cycle may be considered for patients not in CR or CRi and MRD negativity after 2 cycles. For patients not proceeding to HSCT, the recommended maximum is 6 cycles. Monitor closely for signs and symptoms of VOD (eg, total bilirubin elevations, hepatomegaly [may be painful], rapid weight gain, and ascites). For patients who proceed to HSCT, monitor liver tests closely during the first month post-HSCT. Utilize standard medical management for severe VOD. Other hepatotoxicity events have been reported, including grades 3 and 4 AST, ALT, and total bilirubin elevations. Monitor liver function tests (ALT, AST, total bilirubin, and alkaline phosphatase) prior to and following each inotuzumab ozogamicin dose in all patients. Elevations of liver function tests may require dosing interruption, dose reduction, or permanent discontinuation of inotuzumab ozogamicin.

[US Boxed Warning]: A higher post-HSCT non-relapse mortality rate was observed in patients who received inotuzumab ozogamicin, resulting in a higher Day 100 post-HSCT mortality rate. The most common causes of post-HSCT non-relapse mortality included VOD and/or infection. Among patients with ongoing VOD, multiorgan failure or infection resulting in fatality occurred. Monitor closely for toxicities post-HSCT, including signs/symptoms of infection and VOD.

Hematologic toxicity, including thrombocytopenia and neutropenia commonly occur (including grades 3 and 4). Neutropenic fever occurred in over one-fourth of patients; may be life-threatening. For patients who were in complete remission (CR) or CR with incomplete hematologic recovery (CRi) at the end of treatment, the time to platelet recovery (to >50,000/mm^3) was >45 days after the last dose in some patients. Complications associated with myelo-suppression (including infections and bleeding/hemorrhagic events) have been observed. Monitor complete blood counts prior to each dose and monitor for signs and symptoms of effects of myelosuppression during treatment; may require treatment interruption, dose reduction, or permanent discontinuation. Infections, including serious infections (some life-threatening or fatal), were reported in nearly half of patients treated with inotuzumab ozogamicin. Fatal infections, including pneumonia, neutropenic sepsis, sepsis, septic shock, and pseudomonal sepsis, have been reported; bacterial, viral, and fungal infections occurred. Monitor for signs and symptoms of infection during treatment. Administer prophylactic anti-infectives and employ surveillance testing during and after treatment. Severe infection may require treatment interruption, dose reduction, or permanent discontinuation. Hemorrhagic events associated with thrombocytopenia have been reported, including grades 3 or 4 hemorrhagic events and one grade 5 (fatal) intra-abdominal hemorrhage. The most common hemorrhagic event was epistaxis. Monitor for signs and symptoms of bleeding/hemorrhage during treatment; may require treatment interruption, dose reduction, or permanent discontinuation.

Grade 2 infusion related reactions were reported with inotuzumab ozogamicin administration in a small percentage of patients. Infusion reactions (eg, fever, chills, rash, dyspnea) usually occurred in cycle 1 shortly after the end of the infusion and resolved spontaneously or with medical management. Premedicate with a corticosteroid, antipyretic, and antihistamine prior to dosing. Monitor closely during the infusion and for at least 1 hour after the end of the infusion for potential reactions. If an infusion reaction occurs, interrupt infusion and manage appropriately. Depending on the severity, consider discontinuing the infusion or administering corticosteroids and antihistamines. Permanently discontinue if a severe or life-threatening infusion reaction occurs. Hypersensitivity reactions have been reported. Increases in the corrected QT interval of ≥60 msec from baseline were observed in a small number of patients (including grade 2 prolongation in some patients), although none had QTcF values greater than 500 msec. There were no grade 3 or higher QT prolongations or cases of torsades de pointes reported. Use inotuzumab ozogamicin with caution in patients with a history of (or predisposition for) QTc prolongation, patients taking drugs known to prolong the QT interval, and/or in patients with electrolyte abnormalities. Obtain ECG and electrolytes prior to treatment initiation, after initiation of any drug known to prolong QTc, and periodically as clinically indicated during treatment. Potentially significant drug-drug interactions may exist, requiring dose or frequency adjustment, additional monitoring, and/or selection of alternative therapy.

Adverse Reactions

>10%:

Cardiovascular: Hepatic veno-occlusive disease (≤23%)

Central nervous system: Fatigue (35%), headache (28%), chills (11%)

Endocrine & metabolic: Increased gamma-glutamyl transferase (21% to 67%), hyperuricemia (4% to 16%)

Gastrointestinal: Increased serum lipase (9% to 32%), nausea (31%), abdominal pain (23%), diarrhea (17%), constipation (16%), vomiting (15%), increased serum amylase (5% to 15%), stomatitis (13%), decreased appetite (12%)

Hematologic & oncologic: Thrombocytopenia (51%; grade 3: 14%; grade 4: 28%), neutropenia (49%; grade 3: 20% to 49%; grade 4: 27%), anemia (36%; grade ≥3%: 24%), leukopenia (35%; grade ≥3: 33%), hemorrhage (grade ≥3: 5% to 33%), febrile neutropenia (26%; grade ≥3: 26%), lymphocytopenia (18%; grade ≥3: 16%)

Hepatic: Increased serum AST (71%), increased serum alkaline phosphatase (13% to 57%), increased serum ALT (49%), increased serum transaminases (26%), hyperbilirubinemia (21%), hepatotoxicity (14%)

Infection: Infection (48%)

Respiratory: Epistaxis (15%)

Miscellaneous: Fever (32%)

1% to 10%:

Cardiovascular: Prolonged Q-T interval on ECG (1%)

Gastrointestinal: Abdominal distention (6%)

Hematologic & oncologic: Bone marrow failure (2%; includes bone marrow failure, febrile bone marrow aplasia), tumor lysis syndrome (2%)

Hepatic: Ascites (4%)

Immunologic: Antibody development (anti-inotuzumab antibodies: 3%)

Miscellaneous: Infusion related reaction (2%; grade 2: 2%; includes hypersensitivity)

Frequency not defined: Infection: Bacterial infection, fungal infection, viral infection

Drug Interactions

Metabolism/Transport Effects None known.

Avoid Concomitant Use

Avoid concomitant use of Inotuzumab Ozogamicin with any of the following: BCG (Intravesical); Deferiprone; Dipyrone; Highest Risk QTc-Prolonging Agents; Hydroxychloroquine; MiFEPRIStone; Natalizumab; Pimecrolimus; Probucol; Promazine; Tacrolimus (Topical); Vaccines (Live); Vinflunine

Increased Effect/Toxicity

Inotuzumab Ozogamicin may increase the levels/effects of: Deferiprone; Fingolimod; Highest Risk QTc-Prolonging Agents; Leflunomide; Moderate Risk QTc-Prolonging Agents; Natalizumab; Tofacitinib; Vaccines (Live)

The levels/effects of Inotuzumab Ozogamicin may be increased by: Denosumab; Dipyrone; Hydroxychloroquine; MiFEPRIStone; Ocrelizumab; Pimecrolimus; Probucol; Promazine; QTc-Prolonging Agents (Indeterminate Risk and Risk Modifying); Roflumilast; Tacrolimus (Topical); Trastuzumab; Vinflunine; Xipamide

Decreased Effect

Inotuzumab Ozogamicin may decrease the levels/effects of: BCG (Intravesical); Coccidioides immitis Skin Test; Nivolumab; Sipuleucel-T; Tertomotide; Vaccines (Inactivated); Vaccines (Live)

The levels/effects of Inotuzumab Ozogamicin may be decreased by: Echinacea

Hazardous Drugs Handling Considerations

Hazardous agent. This medication is not on the NIOSH (2016) list; however, it meets the criteria for a hazardous drug.

Use appropriate precautions for receiving, handling, administration, and disposal. Gloves (single) should be worn during receiving, unpacking, and placing in storage. NIOSH recommends double gloving, a protective gown, ventilated engineering controls (a class II biological safety cabinet or a compounding aseptic containment isolator), and closed system transfer devices (CSTDs) for preparation. Double gloving, a gown, and (if dosage form allows) CSTDs are required during administration (NIOSH 2016).

Storage/Stability Store intact vials at 2°C to 8°C (36°F to 46°F); do not freeze. Store vials in original carton to protect from light. Protect from light following reconstitution and dilution for infusion and do not freeze. Reconstituted solutions may be used immediately or after being refrigerated for up to 4 hours. Solutions diluted for infusion may be used immediately, after storage at room temperature for up to 4 hours, or after being refrigerated for up to 3 hours. The maximum time from reconstitution to the end of the infusion should be ≤8 hours, with ≤4 hours between reconstitution and dilution. If refrigerated, allow solutions diluted for infusion to reach room temperature for ~1 hour prior to administration.

Preparation for Administration Reconstitute each vial with 4 mL of SWFI to a concentration of 0.25 mg/mL; gently swirl to dissolve. Do not shake. Inspect reconstituted solution for particulates or discoloration; reconstituted solution should be clear to opalescent, colorless to slightly yellow, and free of visible foreign matter. Each vial delivers 3.6 mL (0.9 mg). Calculate required volume and add reconstituted solution to an infusion container with NS to a total volume of 50 mL. Infusion containers made of polyvinyl chloride (PVC; DEHP-or non-DEHP-containing), polyolefin (polypropylene and/or polyethylene), or ethylene vinyl acetate (EVA) are recommended. Gently invert to mix (do not shake).

Mechanism of Action Inotuzumab ozogamicin is a humanized CD22-directed monoclonal antibody-drug conjugate which is composed of the IgG4 kappa antibody inotuzumab (which is specific for human CD22), a calicheamicin component (a cytotoxic agent that causes double-stranded DNA breaks), and an acid-cleavable linker that covalently binds the calicheamicin to inotuzumab. After the antibody-drug conjugate binds to CD22, the CD22-conjugate complex is internalized, and releases calicheamicin. Calicheamicin binds to the minor groove of DNA to induce double strand cleavage and subsequent cell cycle arrest and apoptosis (Kantarjian 2016).

Pharmacodynamics/Kinetics Note: Body surface area was found to significantly affect distribution.

Distribution: ~12 L

Protein binding: Calicheamicin: ~97% bound to human plasma proteins

Metabolism: Calicheamicin: Primarily via nonenzymatic reduction

Half-life, elimination: 12.3 days

Excretion: Clearance (steady state): 0.0333 L/hour.

◄ **Dosing**

Adult & Geriatric

Acute lymphoblastic leukemia, B-cell precursor (relapsed/refractory):
IV: Premedication is recommended prior to dosing. Prior to the first dose, cytoreduction to a peripheral blast count of ≤10,000/mm^3 with a combination of hydroxyurea, steroids, and/or vincristine is recommended for patients with circulating lymphoblasts.

Cycle 1: 0.8 mg/m2 on day 1 and 0.5 mg/m^2 on days 8 and 15 of a 21-day treatment cycle (total dose/cycle 1: 1.8 mg/m^2); treatment cycle may be extended to 4 weeks if complete remission (CR) is achieved, or CR with incomplete hematologic recovery (CRi) and/or to allow for recovery from toxicity.

Subsequent cycles:
Patients who achieve CR or CRi: 0.5 mg/m^2 on days 1, 8 and 15 of a 28-day treatment cycle (total dose/cycle: 1.5 mg/m^2)

Patients who do NOT achieve CR or CRi: 0.8 mg/m^2 on day 1 and 0.5 mg/m^2 on days 8 and 15 of a 28-day treatment cycle (total dose/cycle: 1.8 mg/m^2); if CR or CRi is not achieved within 3 cycles, discontinue treatment.

Treatment duration: The recommended duration of treatment is 2 cycles for patients proceeding to hematopoietic stem cell transplant (HSCT); may consider a third cycle in patients who do not achieve CR or CRi and minimal residual disease (MRD) negativity after 2 cycles. For patients not proceeding to HSCT, may continue treatment for a maximum of up to 6 cycles.

Premedication: A corticosteroid, an antipyretic, and an antihistamine are recommended prior to dosing (observe for symptoms of infusion reaction during and for at least 1 hour after the end of the infusion).

Note: Doses on days 8 and 15 may be varied by ±2 days (maintain a minimum of 6 days between doses). CR is defined as <5% blasts in bone marrow and the absence of peripheral blood leukemic blasts, full recovery of peripheral blood counts (platelets ≥100,000/mm^3 and ANC ≥1,000/mm^3) and resolution of any extramedullary disease. CRi is defined as <5% blasts in bone marrow and the absence of peripheral blood leukemic blasts, incomplete recovery of peripheral blood counts (platelets <100,000/mm^3 and/or ANC <1,000/mm^3) and resolution of any extramedullary disease.

Renal Impairment

CrCl 15 to 89 mL/minute: There are no dosage adjustments provided in the manufacturer's labeling; however pharmacokinetics in this patient population are similar to those in patients with normal renal function.

End-stage renal disease (ESRD) with or without hemodialysis: There are no dosage adjustments provided in the manufacturer's labeling (has not been studied).

Hepatic Impairment

Hepatic impairment prior to treatment initiation:
Total bilirubin ≤1.5 times ULN and AST/ALT ≤2.5 times ULN: No initial dosage adjustment necessary.

Total bilirubin >1.5 times ULN and/or AST/ALT >2.5 times ULN: There are no dosage adjustments provided in the manufacturer's labeling.

Hepatotoxicity during treatment:
Sinusoidal obstruction syndrome (also known as veno-occlusive disease) or other severe liver toxicity: Discontinue permanently.

Total bilirubin >1.5 times ULN and AST/ALT >2.5 times ULN: Interrupt treatment until recovery of total bilirubin to ≤1.5 times ULN and AST/ALT to ≤2.5 times ULN prior to each dose unless due to Gilbert syndrome or hemolysis. Permanently discontinue treatment if total bilirubin does not recover to ≤1.5 times ULN or AST/ALT does not recover to ≤2.5 times ULN. Refer to Dosing: Adjustment for Toxicity for dose modifications depending on duration of treatment interruption.

Adjustment for Toxicity Modify the inotuzumab ozogamicin dose for toxicities; doses within a treatment cycle (eg, day 8 and/or day 15 doses) do not need to be interrupted due to neutropenia or thrombocytopenia; however, dosing interruptions within a cycle are recommended for non-hematologic toxicities. If a dose is reduced due to toxicity, do not re-escalate the dose.

Hematologic toxicity:

If ANC decreases, and the ANC prior to inotuzumab ozogamicin treatment was ≥1,000/mm³, interrupt the next cycle of treatment until ANC recovers to ≥1,000/mm³. Discontinue inotuzumab ozogamicin if low ANC persists for >28 days and is suspected to be related to inotuzumab ozogamicin.

If platelet count decreases, and the platelet count prior to inotuzumab ozogamicin treatment was ≥50,000/mm³, interrupt the next cycle of treatment until platelets recover to ≥50,000/mm³. Discontinue inotuzumab ozogamicin if low platelets persist for >28 days and is suspected to be related to inotuzumab ozogamicin.

If ANC or platelet counts decrease and ANC <1,000/mm³ and/or platelet count was <50,000/mm³ prior to inotuzumab ozogamicin treatment, then interrupt the next cycle of treatment until at least one of the following occurs:

- ANC and platelet counts recover to at least baseline levels for the prior cycle **or**
- ANC recovers to ≥1,000/mm³ and platelet count recovers to ≥50,000/mm³ **or**
- Based on most recent bone marrow assessment, disease is stable or improved and the ANC and platelet count decrease is considered to be due to underlying disease (not considered to be an inotuzumab ozogamicin-related toxicity).

Nonhematologic toxicity:

Dose modifications depending on duration of treatment interruption due to nonhematologic toxicity:

If interruption is <7 days (within a cycle): Interrupt the next dose (maintain a minimum of 6 days between doses).

If interruption is ≥7 days: Omit the next dose within the cycle.

If interruption is ≥14 days: Once recovery is adequate, decrease the total inotuzumab ozogamicin dose by 25% for the subsequent cycle. If further dose modification is necessary, then reduce the number of doses to 2 per cycle for subsequent cycles. If a 25% decrease in the total dose followed by a decrease to 2 doses per cycle is not tolerated, then permanently discontinue treatment.

If interruption is >28 days: Consider permanently discontinuing.

Hepatotoxicity: Refer to Dosing: Hepatic Impairment.

Infusion reaction: Interrupt infusion and institute appropriate medical management; depending on the severity of the reaction, consider discontinuing the infusion or administer steroids and antihistamines. For severe or life-threatening infusion reactions, discontinue permanently.

◀ **Other nonhematologic toxicity ≥ grade 2:** Interrupt treatment until recovery to grade 1 or pretreatment grade levels prior to each dose.

Administration Infuse over 1 hour (at a rate of 50 mL/hour). If refrigerated, allow to reach room temperature for ~1 hour prior to administration. Infuse at room temperature and protect from light during infusion. Infusion sets made of PVC (DEHP-or non-DEHP-containing), polyolefin (polypropylene and/or polyethylene), or polybutadiene are recommended for administration. An inline filter is not required during administration; however, if the diluted solution is filtered, polyethersulfone (PES)-, polyvinylidene fluoride (PVDF)-, or hydrophilic polysulfone (HPS)-based filters are recommended (do not use filters made of nylon or mixed cellulose ester). Do not mix or administer with other medications.

Monitoring Parameters

Complete blood counts (prior to each dose), liver function tests including ALT, AST, total bilirubin, and alkaline phosphatase (prior to and following each dose); for patients who proceed to HSCT, monitor liver function tests closely during the first month post-HSCT, then less frequently thereafter, according to standard medical practice; electrolytes (prior to treatment initiation, after initiation of any drug known to prolong QTc, and periodically as clinically indicated during treatment); pregnancy status (prior to treatment in females of reproductive potential). Obtain ECG (prior to treatment initiation, after initiation of any drug known to prolong QTc, and periodically as clinically indicated during treatment).

Monitor closely for signs and symptoms of VOD (eg, hepatomegaly with or without pain, rapid weight gain, ascites); monitor for signs/symptoms of effects of myelosuppression (bleeding, hemorrhage, infection) during treatment; monitor closely during the infusion and for at least 1 hour after the end of the infusion for the potential infusion reactions.

Dosage Forms Excipient information presented when available (limited, particularly for generics); consult specific product labeling.

Solution Reconstituted, Intravenous [preservative free]:

Besponsa: 0.9 mg (1 ea) [contains polysorbate 80]

◆ **¹¹¹In-Pentetreotide** see Indium In-111 Pentetreotide on page 1002

◆ **Interferon Alfa-2b (PEG Conjugate)** see Peginterferon Alfa-2b on page 1473

Interferon Alfa-2b (in ter FEER on AL fa too bee)

Related Information

Malignant Pleural Effusions on page 2346

Management of Chemotherapy-Induced Nausea and Vomiting in Adults on page 2253

Prevention of Chemotherapy-Induced Nausea and Vomiting in Children on page 2310

Brand Names: US Intron A

Brand Names: Canada Intron A

Index Terms INF-alpha 2; Interferon Alpha-2b; rLFN-α2; α-2-interferon

Pharmacologic Category Antineoplastic Agent, Biological Response Modulator; Biological Response Modulator; Immunomodulator, Systemic; Interferon

Use

AIDS-related Kaposi sarcoma: Treatment of patients 18 years and older with AIDS-related Kaposi sarcoma

Chronic hepatitis B: Treatment of chronic hepatitis B in patients 1 year and older with compensated liver disease

Chronic hepatitis C: Treatment of chronic hepatitis C in patients 18 years and older with compensated liver disease who have a history of blood or blood-product exposure and/or are hepatitis C virus (HCV) antibody-positive; in combination with ribavirin for treatment of chronic hepatitis C in patients 3 years and older with compensated liver disease previously untreated with alpha interferon therapy and in patients 18 years and older who have relapsed following alpha interferon therapy

Condylomata acuminata: Treatment of patients 18 years and older with condylomata acuminata involving external surfaces of the genital and perianal areas

Follicular lymphoma: Initial treatment of clinically aggressive follicular non-Hodgkin lymphoma in conjunction with anthracycline-containing combination chemotherapy in patients 18 years and older

Hairy cell leukemia: Treatment of patients 18 years and older with hairy cell leukemia

Melanoma (malignant): Adjuvant to surgical treatment in patients 18 years and older with malignant melanoma who are free of disease but at high risk for systemic recurrence, within 56 days of surgery

Labeled Contraindications

Hypersensitivity to interferon alfa or any component of the formulation; decompensated liver disease; autoimmune hepatitis

Combination therapy with interferon alfa-2b and ribavirin is also contraindicated in women who are pregnant, in males with pregnant partners; in patients with hemoglobinopathies (eg, thalassemia major, sickle-cell anemia); creatinine clearance <50 mL/minute; or hypersensitivity to ribavirin or any component of the formulation

Documentation of allergenic cross-reactivity for interferons is limited. However, because of similarities in chemical structure and/or pharmacologic actions, the possibility of cross-sensitivity cannot be ruled out with certainty.

Pregnancy Considerations Animal reproduction studies have demonstrated abortifacient effects. Disruption of the normal menstrual cycle was also observed in animal studies; therefore, the manufacturer recommends that reliable contraception is used in women of childbearing potential. Alfa interferon is endogenous to normal amniotic fluid. In vitro administration studies have reported that when administered to the mother, it does not cross the placenta. Case reports of use in pregnant women are limited. The Perinatal HIV Guidelines Working Group does not recommend that interferon-alfa be used during pregnancy. Interferon alfa-2b monotherapy should only be used in pregnancy when the potential benefit to the mother justifies the possible risk to the fetus. Combination therapy with ribavirin is contraindicated in pregnancy; two forms of contraception should be used during combination therapy and patients should have monthly pregnancy tests. A pregnancy registry has been established for women inadvertently exposed to ribavirin while pregnant (800-593-2214).

Breastfeeding Considerations Breast milk samples obtained from a lactating mother prior to and after administration of interferon alfa-2b showed that interferon alfa is present in breast milk and administration of the medication did not significantly affect endogenous levels. Breastfeeding is not linked to the spread of hepatitis C virus; however, if nipples are cracked or bleeding, breastfeeding is not recommended. Mothers coinfected with HIV are discouraged from breastfeeding to decrease potential transmission of HIV.

Warnings/Precautions [US Boxed Warning]: May cause or aggravate fatal or life-threatening autoimmune disorders, neuropsychiatric symptoms (including depression and/or suicidal thoughts/behaviors), ischemic, and/or infectious disorders; monitor closely with clinical and laboratory evaluations (periodic); discontinue treatment for severe persistent or worsening symptoms; some cases may resolve with discontinuation.

Neuropsychiatric disorders: May cause neuropsychiatric events, including depression, psychosis, mania, suicidal behavior/ideation, attempts and completed suicides and homicidal ideation; may occur in patients with or without previous psychiatric symptoms. Effects are usually rapidly reversible upon therapy discontinuation, but have persisted up to three weeks. If psychiatric symptoms persist or worsen, or suicidal or homicidal ideation or aggressive behavior towards others is identified, discontinue treatment, and follow the patient closely. Careful neuropsychiatric monitoring is recommended during and for 6 months after treatment in patients who develop psychiatric disorders (including clinical depression). New or exacerbated neuropsychiatric or substance abuse disorders are best managed with early intervention. Use with caution in patients with a history of psychiatric disorders. Drug screening and periodic health evaluation (including monitoring of psychiatric symptoms) is recommended if initiating treatment in patients with coexisting psychiatric condition or substance abuse disorders. Suicidal ideation or attempts may occur more frequently in pediatric patients (eg, adolescents) when compared to adults. Higher doses, usually in elderly patients, may result in increased CNS toxicity (eg, obtundation and coma).

Hepatic disease: May cause hepatotoxicity; monitor closely if abnormal liver function tests develop. A transient increase in ALT (≥ 2 times baseline) may occur in patients treated with interferon alfa-2b for chronic hepatitis B. Therapy generally may continue; monitor. Worsening and potentially fatal liver disease, including jaundice, hepatic encephalopathy, and hepatic failure have been reported in patients receiving interferon alfa for chronic hepatitis B and C with decompensated liver disease, autoimmune hepatitis, history of autoimmune disease, and immunosuppressed transplant recipients; avoid use in these patients; use is contraindicated in decompensated liver disease. Patients with cirrhosis are at increased risk of hepatic decompensation. Therapy should be discontinued for any patient developing signs and symptoms of liver failure. Permanently discontinue for severe (grade 3) hepatic injury or hepatic decompensation (Child-Pugh class B and C [score >6]). Chronic hepatitis B or C patients with a history of autoimmune disease or who are immunosuppressed transplant recipients should not receive interferon alfa-2b.

Bone marrow suppression: Causes bone marrow suppression, including potentially severe cytopenias, and very rarely, aplastic anemia. Discontinue treatment for severe neutropenia (ANC <500/mm^3) or thrombocytopenia (platelets <25,000/mm^3). Hemolytic anemia (hemoglobin <10 g/dL) was observed when combined with ribavirin; anemia occurred within 1 to 2 weeks of initiation of therapy. Use caution in patients with preexisting myelosuppression and in patients with concomitant medications which cause myelosuppression.

Autoimmune disorders: Avoid use in patients with history of autoimmune disorders; development of autoimmune disorders (thrombocytopenia, vasculitis, Raynaud's disease, rheumatoid arthritis, lupus erythematosus and rhabdomyolysis) has been associated with use. Monitor closely; consider discontinuing. Worsening of psoriasis and sarcoidosis (and the development of new sarcoidosis) have been reported; use extreme caution.

Cardiovascular disease/coagulation disorders: Use caution and monitor closely in patients with cardiovascular disease (ischemic or thromboembolic), arrhythmias, hypertension, and in patients with a history of MI or prior therapy with cardiotoxic drugs. Patients with preexisting cardiac disease and/or advanced cancer should have baseline and periodic ECGs. May cause hypotension (during administration or delayed up to 2 days), arrhythmia, tachycardia (≥150 bpm), cardiomyopathy (~2% in AIDS-related Kaposi Sarcoma patients), and/or MI. Some experiencing cardiovascular adverse effects had no prior history of cardiac disease. Supraventricular arrhythmias occur rarely, and are associated with preexisting cardiac disease or prior therapy with cardiotoxic agents. Dose modification, discontinuation, and/or additional therapies may be necessary. In a scientific statement from the American Heart Association, interferon has been determined to be an agent that may either cause reversible direct myocardial toxicity or exacerbate underlying myocardial dysfunction (magnitude: moderate/major) (AHA [Page 2016]). Hemorrhagic cerebrovascular events have been observed with therapy. Use caution in patients with coagulation disorders.

Endocrine disorders: Thyroid disorders (possibly reversible) have been reported; use caution in patients with preexisting thyroid disease. TSH levels should be within normal limits prior to initiating interferon. Treatment should not be initiated in patients with preexisting thyroid disease who cannot be maintained in normal ranges by medication. Discontinue interferon use in patients who develop thyroid abnormalities during treatment and in patients with thyroid disease who subsequently cannot maintain normal ranges with thyroid medication. Discontinuation of interferon therapy may or may not reverse thyroid dysfunction. Diabetes mellitus has been reported; discontinue if cannot effectively manage with medication. Use with caution in patients with a history of diabetes mellitus, particularly if prone to DKA. Hypertriglyceridemia has been reported; discontinue if persistent and severe, and/or combined with symptoms of pancreatitis.

Pulmonary disease: Dyspnea, pulmonary infiltrates, pulmonary hypertension, interstitial pneumonitis, pneumonia, bronchiolitis obliterans, and sarcoidosis may be induced or aggravated by treatment, sometimes resulting in respiratory failure or fatality. Has been reported more in patients being treated for chronic hepatitis C, although has also occurred with use for oncology indications. Patients with fever, cough, dyspnea or other respiratory symptoms should be evaluated with a chest x-ray; monitor closely and consider discontinuing treatment with evidence of impaired pulmonary function. Use with caution in patients with a history of pulmonary disease.

Ophthalmic disorders: Decreased or loss of vision, macular edema, optic neuritis, retinal hemorrhages, cotton wool spots, papilledema, retinal detachment (serous), and retinal artery or vein thrombosis have occurred (or been aggravated) in patients receiving alpha interferons. Use caution in patients with preexisting eye disorders; monitor closely; a complete eye exam should be done promptly in patients who develop ocular symptoms; discontinue with new or worsening ophthalmic disorders.

Dental and periodontic disorders: In patients receiving combination interferon and ribavirin therapy, dental and periodontal disorders have been reported; additionally, dry mouth can damage teeth and mouth mucous membranes during chronic therapy.

Commonly associated with fever and flu-like symptoms; rule out other causes/ infection with persistent fever; use with caution in patients with debilitating conditions. Acute hypersensitivity reactions (eg, urticaria, angioedema, bronchoconstriction, anaphylaxis) have been reported (rarely) with alfa interferons. If an acute reaction develops, discontinue therapy immediately; transient rashes have occurred in some patients following injection, but have not necessitated treatment interruption. Do not treat patients with visceral AIDS-related Kaposi sarcoma associated with rapidly-progressing or life-threatening disease. Some formulations contain albumin, which may carry a remote risk of viral transmission. Due to differences in dosage, patients should not change brands of interferons without the concurrence of their healthcare provider. Combination therapy with ribavirin is associated with birth defects and/or fetal mortality and hemolytic anemia. Do not use combination therapy with ribavirin in patients with CrCl <50 mL/minute. Interferon alfa-2b at doses ≥10 million units/m^2 is associated with a moderate emetic potential; antiemetics may be recommended to prevent nausea and vomiting. Potentially significant drug-drug interactions may exist, requiring dose or frequency adjustment, additional monitoring, and/or selection of alternative therapy.

Some dosage forms may contain polysorbate 80 (also known as Tweens). Hypersensitivity reactions, usually a delayed reaction, have been reported following exposure to pharmaceutical products containing polysorbate 80 in certain individuals (Isaksson 2002; Lucente 2000; Shelley 1995). Thrombocytopenia, ascites, pulmonary deterioration, and renal and hepatic failure have been reported in premature neonates after receiving parenteral products containing polysorbate 80 (Alade 1986; CDC 1984). See manufacturer's labeling.

Adverse Reactions Note: In a majority of patients, a flu-like symptom (fever, chills, tachycardia, malaise, myalgia, headache), occurs within 1-2 hours of administration; may last up to 24 hours and may be dose limiting.

>10%:
  Cardiovascular: Chest pain (≤28%)
  Central nervous system: Fatigue (8% to 96%), headache (21% to 62%), chills (≤54%), rigors (≤42%), depression (3% to 40%; grades 3/4: 2%), drowsiness (≤33%), dizziness (≤24%), irritability (≤22%), paresthesia (1% to 21%), pain (≤18%), right upper quadrant pain (≤15%), amnesia (≤14%), lack of concentration (≤14%), malaise (≤14%), confusion (≤12%), insomnia (≤12%)
  Dermatologic: Alopecia (≤38%), skin rash (≤25%), diaphoresis (1% to 21%), pruritus (≤11%)
  Endocrine & metabolic: Weight loss (<1% to 13%), amenorrhea (≤12%)
  Gastrointestinal: Anorexia (1% to 69%), nausea, (17% to 66%), diarrhea (2% to 45%), vomiting (children 27%; adults 2% to 32%), xerostomia (≤28%), dysgeusia (≤24%), abdominal pain (1% to 23%), constipation (≤14%), gingivitis (≤14%)

Hematologic & oncologic: Neutropenia (≤92%; grade 4: 1% to 4%), leukopenia (≤68%), anemia (≤32%), thrombocytopenia (≤15%)

Hepatic: Increased serum AST (≤63%; grades 3/4: 14%), increased serum ALT (≤15%), increased serum alkaline phosphatase (≤13%)

Infection: Candidiasis (≤17%)

Local: Injection site reaction (≤20%)

Neuromuscular & skeletal: Myalgia (28% to 75%), weakness (≤63%), skeletal pain (≤21%), arthralgia (≤19%), back pain (≤19%)

Renal: Increased blood urea nitrogen (≤12%)

Respiratory: Flu-like symptoms (≤79%), dyspnea (≤34%), cough (≤31%), pharyngitis (≤31%), sinusitis (≤21%)

Miscellaneous: Fever (34% to 94%; more common in children)

5% to 10%:

Cardiovascular: Edema (≤10%), hypertension (≤9%)

Central nervous system: Hypoesthesia (≤10%), anxiety (≤9%), vertigo (≤8%), agitation (≤7%)

Dermatologic: Xeroderma (≤10%), dermatitis (≤8%)

Endocrine & metabolic: Decreased libido (≤5%)

Gastrointestinal: Loose stools (≤10%), dyspepsia (≤8%)

Genitourinary: Urinary tract infection (≤5%)

Hematologic & oncologic: Purpura (≤5%)

Infection: Infection (≤7%), herpes virus infection (≤5%)

Renal: Polyuria (≤10%), increased serum creatinine (≤6%)

Respiratory: Bronchitis (≤10%), nasal congestion (<10%), epistaxis (≤7%)

<5%, postmarketing, and/or case reports:

Cardiovascular: Angina pectoris, arteritis, atrial fibrillation, bradycardia, cardiac arrhythmia, cardiac failure, cardiomegaly, cardiomyopathy, cerebrovascular accident, coronary artery disease, extrasystoles, flushing, heart valve disease, hypotension, myocardial infarction, palpitations, peripheral ischemia, periarteritis nodosa, pulmonary embolism, Raynaud's phenomenon, reduced ejection fraction, retinal vein occlusion, syncope, tachycardia, thrombosis, vasculitis

Central nervous system: Nervousness (≤3%), aggressive behavior, aphasia, ataxia, Bell's palsy, carpal tunnel syndrome, coma, dysphasia, extrapyramidal reaction, hallucination, homicidal ideation, hyporeflexia, hypothermia, mania, migraine, neuralgia, neuropathy, paranoia, peripheral neuropathy, psychoneurosis, psychosis, suicidal ideation, seizure

Dermatologic: Cellulitis, eczema, epidermal cyst, erythema, erythema multiforme, erythematous rash, exacerbation of psoriasis, folliculitis, lichenoid dermatitis, lipoma, maculopapular rash, psoriasis, skin photosensitivity, Stevens-Johnson syndrome, toxic epidermal necrolysis, urticaria

Endocrine & metabolic: Increased lactate dehydrogenase (≤1%), albuminuria, dehydration, diabetes mellitus, goiter, hirsutism, hot flash, hypercalcemia, hyperglycemia, hyperthyroidism, hypertriglyceridemia, hypothyroidism, pituitary insufficiency, menorrhagia

Gastrointestinal: Aphthous stomatitis, biliary colic, colitis, esophagitis, gastritis, gastrointestinal hemorrhage, mucositis, pancreatitis, stomatitis

Genitourinary: Cystitis, dysuria, hematuria, impotence, leukorrhea, mastitis, nephrotic syndrome, nocturia, pelvic pain, proteinuria, sexual disorder, urinary incontinence, uterine hemorrhage

◄

Hematologic & oncologic: Aplastic anemia (rarely), exacerbation of sarcoidosis, granulocytopenia, hemolytic anemia, hypochromic anemia, immune thrombocytopenia, lipoma, lymphadenitis, lymphadenopathy, lymphocytopenia, lymphocytosis, pancytopenia, pure red cell aplasia, rectal hemorrhage, sarcoidosis, thrombotic thrombocytopenic purpura

Hepatic: Abnormal hepatic function tests, ascites, hepatic encephalopathy, hepatic failure, hepatitis, hepatotoxicity, hyperbilirubinemia, jaundice

Hypersensitivity: Anaphylaxis, angioedema, hypersensitivity reaction (acute)

Infection: Abscess, fungal infection, sepsis

Local: Tissue necrosis at injection site

Neuromuscular & skeletal: Amyotrophy, arthritis, leg cramps, myositis, rhabdomyolysis, rheumatoid arthritis, spondylitis, systemic lupus erythematosus, tendonitis, tremor

Ophthalmic: Blurred vision, conjunctivitis, macular edema, nystagmus, optic neuritis, papilledema, photophobia, retinal cotton-wool spot, retinal detachment (serous), retinal thrombosis, Vogt-Koyanagi-Harada syndrome

Otic: Auditory impairment, hearing loss

Renal: Renal failure, renal insufficiency

Respiratory: Asthma, bronchiolitis obliterans, bronchoconstriction, bronchospasm, cyanosis, hemoptysis, hypoventilation, interstitial pneumonitis, pleural effusion, pneumonia, pneumothorax, pulmonary fibrosis, pulmonary hypertension, pulmonary infiltrates, respiratory insufficiency, upper respiratory tract infection, wheezing

Miscellaneous: Abscess, alcohol intolerance

Drug Interactions

Metabolism/Transport Effects Inhibits CYP1A2 (weak)

Avoid Concomitant Use

Avoid concomitant use of Interferon Alfa-2b with any of the following: BCG (Intravesical); Deferiprone; Dipyrone; Telbivudine

Increased Effect/Toxicity

Interferon Alfa-2b may increase the levels/effects of: Aldesleukin; CloZAPine; Deferiprone; Methadone; Ribavirin (Oral Inhalation); Ribavirin (Systemic); Telbivudine; Theophylline Derivatives; TiZANidine; Zidovudine

The levels/effects of Interferon Alfa-2b may be increased by: Dipyrone; Promazine

Decreased Effect

Interferon Alfa-2b may decrease the levels/effects of: BCG (Intravesical)

Storage/Stability Store intact vials under refrigeration at 2°C to 8°C (36°F to 46°F); do not freeze. After reconstitution of powder for injection, product should be used immediately, but may be stored under refrigeration for ≤24 hours.

Preparation for Administration Powder for injection: The manufacturer recommends reconstituting vial with the diluent provided (SWFI). When reconstituted with SWFI 1 mL, the 10 million unit vial concentration is 10 million units/mL, the 18 million unit vial concentration is 18 million units/mL, and the 50 million unit vial concentration is 50 million units/mL. Swirl gently. To prepare solution for infusion, further dilute appropriate dose in NS 100 mL. Final concentration should be ≥10 million units/100 mL.

Mechanism of Action Binds to a specific receptor on the cell wall to initiate intracellular activity; multiple effects can be detected including induction of gene transcription. Inhibits cellular growth, alters the state of cellular differentiation, interferes with oncogene expression, alters cell surface antigen expression, increases phagocytic activity of macrophages, and augments cytotoxicity of lymphocytes for target cells

Pharmacodynamics/Kinetics

Distribution: V_d: 31 L; but has been noted to be much greater (370 to 720 L) in leukemia patients receiving continuous infusion IFN; IFN does not penetrate the CSF

Metabolism: Primarily renal, filtered and absorbed at the renal tubule

Bioavailability: IM: 83%; SubQ: 90%

Half-life elimination: IV: ~2 hours; IM, SubQ: ~2 to 3 hours

Time to peak, serum: IM, SubQ: ~3 to 12 hours; IV: By the end of a 30-minute infusion

Dosing

Adult & Geriatric Consider premedication with acetaminophen prior to administration to reduce the incidence of some adverse reactions. Not all dosage forms and strengths are appropriate for all indications; refer to product labeling for details. Interferon alfa-2b at doses ≥10 million units/m^2 is associated with a moderate emetic potential; antiemetics may be recommended to prevent nausea and vomiting.

Hairy cell leukemia: IM, SubQ: 2 million units/m^2 3 times weekly for up to 6 months (may continue treatment with sustained treatment response); discontinue for disease progression or failure to respond after 6 months

Lymphoma (follicular): SubQ: 5 million units 3 times weekly for up to 18 months

Malignant melanoma: Induction: 20 million units/m^2 IV for 5 consecutive days per week for 4 weeks, followed by maintenance dosing of 10 million units/m^2 SubQ 3 times weekly for 48 weeks

AIDS-related Kaposi sarcoma: IM, SubQ: 30 million units/m^2 3 times weekly; continue until disease progression or until maximal response has been achieved after 16 weeks

Chronic hepatitis B: IM, SubQ: 5 million units daily or 10 million units 3 times weekly for 16 weeks

Chronic hepatitis C: IM, SubQ: 3 million units 3 times weekly. In patients with normalization of ALT at 16 weeks, continue treatment (if tolerated) for 18-24 months; consider discontinuation if normalization does not occur at 16 weeks. **Note:** May be used in combination therapy with ribavirin in previously untreated patients or in patients who relapse following alpha interferon therapy.

Condyloma acuminata: Intralesionally: 1 million units/lesion (maximum: 5 lesions per treatment) 3 times weekly (on alternate days) for 3 weeks. May administer a second course at 12-16 weeks.

Pediatric Consider premedication with acetaminophen prior to administration to reduce the incidence of some adverse reactions. Not all dosage forms and strengths are appropriate for all indications; refer to product labeling for details.

Note: The following dosing may also be used in **infants** in the setting of HIV-exposure/-infection (CDC 2009).

Chronic hepatitis B (including HIV coinfection): SubQ: Children and Adolescents 1 to 17 years: 3 million units/m^2 3 times weekly for 1 week, followed by 6 million units/m^2 3 times weekly (maximum: 10 million units per dose); total duration of therapy 16 to 24 weeks (treat for 24 weeks in HIV-exposure/-infection)

Chronic hepatitis C with HIV coinfection: IM, SubQ: Children and Adolescents 1 to 17 years: 3 to 5 million units/m^2 3 times weekly (maximum: 3 million units per dose) with ribavirin for 48 weeks, regardless of HCV genotype (CDC 2009)

Renal Impairment

Renal impairment at treatment initiation: Combination therapy with ribavirin (hepatitis C) is contraindicated in patients with CrCl <50 mL/minute; use combination therapy with ribavirin (hepatitis C) with caution in patients with impaired renal function and CrCl ≥50 mL/minute.

Renal toxicity during treatment: *Indication-specific adjustments:* Lymphoma (follicular): Serum creatinine >2 mg/dL: Permanently discontinue.

Hepatic Impairment

Hepatic impairment at treatment initiation: There are no dosage adjustments provided in the manufacturer's labeling. Contraindicated in patients with decompensated liver disease or autoimmune hepatitis.

Hepatotoxicity during treatment: Permanently discontinue for severe (grade 3) hepatic injury or hepatic decompensation (Child-Pugh class B and C [score >6]).

Indication-specific adjustments:

Lymphoma (follicular): AST >5 times ULN: Permanently discontinue.

Malignant melanoma (induction and maintenance):

ALT/AST >5 to 10 times ULN: Temporarily withhold; resume with a 50% dose reduction when adverse reaction abates

ALT/AST >10 times ULN: Permanently discontinue.

Adjustment for Toxicity

Hematologic toxicity (also refer to indication specified adjustments below): ANC <500/mm^3 or platelets <25,000/mm^3: Discontinue treatment.

Hypersensitivity reaction (acute, serious), ophthalmic disorders (new or worsening), thyroid abnormality development (which cannot be normalized with medication), signs or symptoms of liver failure: Discontinue treatment.

Liver function abnormality, pulmonary infiltrate development, evidence of pulmonary function impairment, or autoimmune disorder development, triglycerides >1,000 mg/dL: Monitor closely and discontinue if appropriate. Permanently discontinue for severe (grade 3) hepatic injury or hepatic decompensation (Child-Pugh class B and C [score >6]).

Neuropsychiatric disorders (during treatment):

Clinical depression or other psychiatric problem: Monitor closely during and for 6 months after treatment.

Severe depression or other psychiatric disorder: Discontinue treatment.

Persistent or worsening psychiatric symptoms, suicidal ideation, aggression towards others: Discontinue treatment and follow with appropriate psychiatric intervention.

Manufacturer-recommended adjustments, listed according to indication:

Lymphoma (follicular):

Neutrophils >1000/mm^3 to <1,500/mm^3: Reduce dose by 50%; may re-escalate to starting dose when neutrophils return to >1,500/mm^3

Severe toxicity (neutrophils <1000/mm^3 or platelets <50,000/mm^3): Temporarily withhold.

AST >5 times ULN or serum creatinine >2 mg/dL: Permanently discontinue.

Hairy cell leukemia:

Platelet count <50,000/mm^3: Do not administer intramuscularly (administer SubQ instead).

Severe toxicity: Reduce dose by 50% or temporarily withhold and resume with 50% dose reduction; permanently discontinue if persistent or recurrent severe toxicity is noted.

Chronic hepatitis B:
WBC <1,500/mm^3, granulocytes <750/mm^3, or platelet count <50,000/mm^3, or other laboratory abnormality or severe adverse reaction: Reduce dose by 50%; may re-escalate to starting dose upon resolution of hematologic toxicity. Discontinue for persistent intolerance.
WBC <1,000/mm^3, granulocytes <500/mm^3, or platelet count <25,000/mm^3: Permanently discontinue

Chronic hepatitis C: Severe toxicity: Reduce dose by 50% or temporarily withhold until subsides; permanently discontinue for persistent toxicities after dosage reduction.

AIDS-related Kaposi sarcoma: Severe toxicity: Reduce dose by 50% or temporarily withhold; may resume at reduced dose with toxicity resolution; permanently discontinue for persistent/recurrent toxicities.

Malignant melanoma (induction and maintenance):
Severe toxicity including neutrophils >250/mm^3 to <500/mm^3 or ALT/AST >5 to 10 times ULN: Temporarily withhold; resume with a 50% dose reduction when adverse reaction abates.
Neutrophils <250/mm^3, ALT/AST >10 times ULN, or severe/persistent adverse reactions: Permanently discontinue.

Combination Regimens
Leukemia, acute lymphocytic: Hyper-CVAD (Leukemia, Acute Lymphocytic) on page 2146
Lymphoma, non-Hodgkin: Fludarabine-Mitoxantrone-Dexamethasone-Rituximab on page 2120
Melanoma: CVD-Interleukin-Interferon (Melanoma) on page 2075
Multiple myeloma: Melphalan-Prednisone (Multiple Myeloma) on page 2171
Renal cell cancer:
Bevacizumab-Interferon Alfa (RCC) on page 1994
Interleukin 2-Interferon Alfa-2 (RCC) on page 2156

Administration Administer dose in the evening (if possible) to enhance tolerability. Not all dosage forms are recommended for all administration routes; refer to manufacturer's labeling. Interferon alfa-2b at doses ≥10 million units/m^2 is associated with a moderate emetic potential; antiemetics may be recommended to prevent nausea and vomiting.

IM: Rotate injection sites; preferred sites for injection are anterior thigh, deltoid, and superolateral buttock. Some patients may be appropriate for self-administration with appropriate training. Allow to reach room temperature prior to injection. In hairy cell leukemia treatment, if platelets are <50,000/mm^3, do not administer intramuscularly (administer SubQ instead).

IV: Infuse over ~20 minutes

SubQ: Suggested for those who are at risk for bleeding or are thrombocytopenic. Rotate SubQ injection site; preferred sites for injection are abdomen (except around the navel), anterior thigh, and outer upper arm. Patient should be well hydrated. Some patients may be appropriate for self-administration with appropriate training. Allow to reach room temperature prior to injection.

Intralesional: Inject at an angle nearly parallel to the plane of the skin, directing the needle to center of the base of the wart to infiltrate the lesion core and cause a small wheal. Only infiltrate the keratinized layer; avoid administration which is too deep or shallow. Allow to reach room temperature prior to injection.

Emetic Potential

Children: Minimal (<10%)

Adults:

$\geq$10 million units/m^2: Moderate (30% to 90%)

>5 to <10 million units/m^2: Low (10% to 30%)

$\leq$5 million units/m^2: Minimal (<10%)

Monitoring Parameters

General monitoring parameters for *all indications*:

At baseline (repeat during therapy if clinically indicated): Chest x-ray, serum creatinine, albumin, prothrombin time, triglycerides.

At baseline and periodically thereafter: CBC with differential, platelets and hemoglobin, liver function tests, electrolytes and TSH; ophthalmic exam (or with new ocular symptoms); ECG (in patients with preexisting cardiac abnormalities or in advanced stages of cancer). Monitor serum bilirubin, ALT, AST, alkaline phosphatase and LDH at 2, 8 and 12 weeks following initiation, then every 6 months during treatment. Permanently discontinue for severe (grade 3) hepatic injury or hepatic decompensation (Child-Pugh class B and C [score >6]).

During therapy: Weight; neuropsychiatric changes during and for 6 months after therapy.

Additional *indication-specific* monitoring parameters:

Chronic hepatitis B: CBC with differential and platelets and liver function tests: Baseline, weeks 1, 2, 4, 8, 12, and 16, at the end of treatment, and then 3 and 6 months post treatment

Chronic hepatitis C:

CBC with differential and platelets: Baseline, weeks 1 and 2, then monthly

Liver function: Every 3 months

TSH: Baseline and periodically during treatment; in patients with preexisting thyroid disorders also repeat at 3 months and 6 months

Condyloma acuminate (intralesional administration): Monitor CBC with differential, liver function tests (elevations have been reported).

Malignant melanoma: CBC with differential and platelets and liver function tests: Weekly during induction phase, then monthly during maintenance

Oncology patients: Thyroid function monitoring (Hamnvik 2011): TSH and anti-TPO antibodies at baseline; if TPO antibody positive, monitor TSH every 2 months; if TPO antibody negative, monitor TSH every 6 months

Medication Guide Available Yes

Dosage Forms Excipient information presented when available (limited, particularly for generics); consult specific product labeling.

Solution, Injection:

Intron A: 6,000,000 units/mL (3.8 mL); 10,000,000 units/mL (3.2 mL) [contains edetate disodium, metacresol, polysorbate 80]

Solution Reconstituted, Injection [preservative free]:

Intron A: 10,000,000 units (1 ea); 18,000,000 units (1 ea); 50,000,000 units (1 ea) [contains albumin human]

Dosage Forms: Canada Information with regard to form, strength, and availability of products uniquely available in Canada but currently not available in the US. Refer also to Dosage Forms.

Excipient information presented when available (limited, particularly for generics); consult specific product labeling.

Solution, Injection:
Intron A: 10,000,000 units/mL (1 mL, 2.5 mL) [contains edetate disodium, metacresol, polysorbate 80]
Solution, Injection (prefilled pen):
Intron A: 6,000,000 units/mL (3 mL); 15,000,000 units/mL (1.2 mL); 25,000,000 units/mL (1.2 mL); 50,000,000 units/mL (1.2 mL) [contains edetate disodium, metacresol, polysorbate 80]

◆ **Interferon Alpha-2b** *see* Interferon Alfa-2b *on page 1018*

◆ **Interleukin 2** *see* Aldesleukin *on page 71*

◆ **Intrapleural Talc** *see* Talc (Sterile) *on page 1728*

◆ **Intron A** *see* Interferon Alfa-2b *on page 1018*

Iobenguane I 123 (eye oh BEN gwane eye one TWEN tee three)

Brand Names: US AdreView™

Index Terms 123 Meta-Iodobenzlyguanidine Sulfate; 123I-Metaiodobenzyl-guanidine (MIBG); I-123 MIBG; I^{123} Iobenguane; Iobenguane Sulfate I 123; Iobenguane Sulfate I-123

Pharmacologic Category Radiopharmaceutical

Use As an adjunct to other diagnostic tests, in the detection of primary or metastatic pheochromocytoma or neuroblastoma; scintigraphic assessment of sympathetic myocardium innervation (by measurement of heart to mediastinum [H/M] ratio of radioactivity uptake) in patients with New York Heart Association class II or class III heart failure and LVEF ≤35% (may help identify lower 1 and 2 year mortality risks, indicated by H/M ratio ≥1.6)

Pregnancy Risk Factor C

Dosing

Adult & Geriatric Note: Thyroid protective agents (SSKI, Lugol's solution or potassium iodide), should be given at least 1 hour prior to administration (in patients at risk for accumulation in thyroid).

Radioimaging: IV: 10 mCi (370 MBq)

Heart failure: Adults: Begin anterior planar chest imaging 4 hours (± 10 minutes) following administration; single photon emission computed tomography (SPECT) may then be performed. Low-energy high-resolution is the recommended imaging collimator; the recommended matrix for planar images is 128x128; position camera to include entire heart and as much of upper chest as possible within field. Follow details within manufacturer's labeling to determine heart to mediastinum (H/M) ratio.

Pheochromocytoma and neuroblastoma: Perform whole body planar scintigraphy imaging 18-30 hours after iobenguane I 123 administration; SPECT may be performed following planar scintigraphy (as appropriate).

Pediatric Note: Thyroid protective agents (SSKI, Lugol's solution or potassium iodide), should be given at least 1 hour prior to administration (in patients at risk for accumulation in thyroid).

Radioimaging: *Pheochromocytoma and neuroblastoma:* Perform whole body planar scintigraphy imaging 18-30 hours after iobenguane I 123 administration; single photon emission computed tomography (SPECT) may be performed following planar scintigraphy (as appropriate). IV:
Children 1 month to 16 years and <70 kg: Dose according to body weight; see table on next page.
Children <16 years and ≥70 kg: 10 mCi (370 MBq)
Children ≥16 years: Refer to adult dosing

Iobenguane I 123 Pediatric Dosing by Body Weight

(Children 1 Month to 16 Years and <70 kg)

Weight (kg)	mCi Dose	MBq Dose
3	1	37
4	1.4	52
6	1.9	70
8	2.3	85.1
10	2.7	99.9
12	3.2	118.4
14	3.6	133.2
16	4	148
18	4.4	162.8
20	4.6	170.2
22	5	185
24	5.3	196.1
26	5.6	207.2
28	5.8	214.6
30	6.2	229.4
32	6.5	240.5
34	6.8	251.6
36	7.1	262.7
38	7.3	270.1
40	7.6	281.2
42	7.8	288.6
44	8	296
46	8.2	303.4
48	8.5	314.5
50	8.8	325.6
52-54	9	333
56-58	9.2	340.4
60-62	9.6	355.2
64-66	9.8	362.6
68	9.9	366.3

Renal Impairment No dosage adjustment provided in manufacturer's labeling (has not been studied). However, radiation exposure may be increased in patients with severe renal impairment, use with caution.

Hepatic Impairment No dosage adjustment provided in manufacturer's labeling.

Additional Information Complete prescribing information should be consulted for additional detail.

Dosage Forms Excipient information presented when available (limited, particularly for generics); consult specific product labeling.
Injection, solution:
AdreView™: Iobenguane sulfate 0.08 mg and I 123 74 MBq (2 mCi) per mL (5 mL) [contains benzyl alcohol]

♦ **Iobenguane Sulfate I 123** *see* Iobenguane I 123 *on page 1029*

♦ **Iodine I 131 Tositumomab and Tositumomab** *see* Tositumomab and Iodine I 131 Tositumomab *on page 1801*

♦ **IPG-Ondansetron (Can)** *see* Ondansetron *on page 1380*

Ipilimumab (ip i LIM u mab)

Related Information
Common Toxicity Criteria *on page 2242*

Management of Chemotherapy-Induced Nausea and Vomiting in Adults *on page 2253*

Brand Names: US Yervoy

Brand Names: Canada Yervoy

Index Terms Ipilimumab, inj; MDX-010; MDX-CTLA-4; MOAB-CTLA-4

Pharmacologic Category Antineoplastic Agent, Monoclonal Antibody

Use
Melanoma, unresectable or metastatic: Treatment of unresectable or metastatic melanoma in adult and pediatric patients 12 years and older

Melanoma, adjuvant treatment: Adjuvant treatment of cutaneous melanoma in patients with pathologic involvement of regional lymph nodes of more than 1 mm who have undergone complete resection, including total lymphadenectomy

Labeled Contraindications
There are no contraindications listed in the manufacturer's US labeling.

Canadian labeling: Hypersensitivity to ipilimumab or any component of the formulation; active life-threatening autoimmune disease, or with organ transplantation graft where further immune activation is potentially imminently life-threatening

Pregnancy Considerations
Adverse effects were observed in animal reproduction studies. Ipilimumab is an IgG1 immunoglobulin and human IgG1 is known to cross the placenta, therefore, ipilimumab may be expected to reach the fetus. Ipilimumab may cause fetal harm if administered during pregnancy (based on the mechanism of action). Women of reproductive potential should use effective contraception during treatment and for 3 months following the last ipilimumab dose.

A pregnancy registry has been established to collect information about women exposed to ipilimumab during pregnancy. Advise pregnant women to enroll in the Pregnancy Safety Surveillance Study by calling 1-844-593-7869.

Breastfeeding Considerations
It is not known if ipilimumab is present in breast milk. The manufacturer recommends to discontinue breastfeeding during treatment and for 3 months following the final dose.

Warnings/Precautions
[US Boxed Warning]: Severe and fatal immune-mediated adverse effects may occur. While any organ system may be involved, common severe effects include dermatitis (including toxic epidermal necrolysis), endocrinopathy, enterocolitis, hepatitis, and neuropathy. Reactions generally occur during treatment, although some reactions have occurred weeks to months after treatment discontinuation. Discontinue treatment (permanently) and initiate high-dose systemic corticosteroid treatment for severe immune mediated reactions. Evaluate liver function, adrenocorticotropic hormone (ACTH) level, and thyroid function tests at baseline and prior to each dose. Assess for signs and symptoms of enterocolitis, dermatitis, neuropathy, and endocrinopathy at baseline and prior to each dose. Initiate systemic

corticosteroids (prednisone 1 to 2 mg/kg/day or equivalent) for severe reactions. Uncommon immune-mediated adverse effects reported include eosinophilia, hemolytic anemia, iritis, meningitis, myocarditis (fatal), nephritis, pancreatitis, pericarditis, pneumonitis, sarcoidosis, and uveitis. Other rare immune-mediated reactions reported in clinical trials include angiopathy, arthritis, autoimmune central neuropathy (encephalitis), autoimmune thyroiditis, blepharitis, conjunctivitis, episcleritis, erythema multiforme, leukocytoclastic vasculitis, myositis, neurosensory hypoacusis, ocular myositis, polymyalgia rheumatica, polymyositis, psoriasis, scleritis, temporal arteritis, and vasculitis. Administer corticosteroid ophthalmic drops in patients who develop episcleritis, iritis, or uveitis; permanently discontinue ipilimumab if unresponsive to topical ophthalmic immunosuppressive treatments. For severe immune-mediated episcleritis or uveitis, initiate systemic corticosteroids (prednisone 1 to 2 mg/kg/day or equivalent); taper over at least 1 month (Weber 2012).

Immune-mediated enterocolitis (including fatal cases) may occur. The median time to onset of grade 3 to 5 enterocolitis was 1.1 to 1.7 months. Monitor for signs and symptoms of enterocolitis (abdominal pain, blood in stool, diarrhea, or mucous in stool; with or without fever) and intestinal perforation (peritoneal signs, ileus). If enterocolitis develops, infectious causes should be ruled out; consider endoscopy for persistent or severe symptoms. Withhold ipilimumab treatment and administer antidiarrheals for moderate enterocolitis (diarrhea with ≤6 stools over baseline abdominal pain, mucous or blood in stool); if persists for >1 week, initiate systemic corticosteroids (prednisone at 0.5 mg/kg/day or equivalent). If severe enterocolitis (diarrhea ≥7 stools above baseline, fever, ileus, peritoneal signs) develops, permanently discontinue ipilimumab and initiate systemic corticosteroids (prednisone 1 to 2 mg/kg/day or equivalent); when resolved to ≤ grade 1, taper corticosteroids slowly over ≥1 month (rapid tapering may cause recurrence or worsen symptoms). May consider adding anti-tumor necrosis factor (TNF) or other immunosuppressive therapy for management of immune-mediated enterocolitis unresponsive to 3 to 5 days of systemic corticosteroids or recurring after symptomatic improvement.

Severe, life-threatening or fatal hepatotoxicity and immune-mediated hepatitis have been observed. The median time to onset for grade 3 or 4 immune-mediated hepatitis in patients receiving ipilimumab for adjuvant treatment of melanoma was 2 months. Monitor liver function tests (LFTs) and evaluate for signs of hepatotoxicity prior to each dose; if hepatotoxicity develops, infectious or malignant causes should be ruled out and liver function should be monitored more frequently until resolves. Withhold treatment for grade 2 hepatotoxicity (ALT or AST 2.5 to 5 times ULN or total bilirubin 1.5 to 3 times ULN). If severe or grade 3 or 4 hepatotoxicity develops (ALT or AST >5 times ULN or total bilirubin >3 times ULN), permanently discontinue ipilimumab and initiate systemic corticosteroids (prednisone 1 to 2 mg/kg/day or equivalent). If transaminases do not decrease within 48 hours of steroid initiation, consider adding mycophenolate mofetil (Weber 2012). May begin tapering corticosteroid (over 1 month) when LFTs show sustained improvement or return to baseline

Severe, life-threatening, or fatal immune-mediated dermatitis has been reported. The median time to onset for dermatologic toxicity is 2 to 3 weeks. Monitor for signs/symptoms of dermatitis, including rash and pruritus; dermatitis should be considered immune-mediated unless identified otherwise. Mild-to-moderate dermatitis (localized rash and pruritus) should be treated symptomatically; topical or systemic corticosteroids should be administered if not resolved within 1 week. Withhold treatment for moderate to severe dermatologic symptoms. Permanently discontinue ipilimumab and initiate systemic corticosteroid (prednisone 1 to 2 mg/kg/day or equivalent) for Stevens-Johnson syndrome, toxic epidermal necrolysis, or rash complicated by dermal ulceration (full thickness) or necrotic, bullous, or hemorrhagic manifestations; when dermatitis is controlled, taper corticosteroid over at least 1 month.

Severe or life-threatening endocrine disorders (hypophysitis, adrenal insufficiency [including adrenal crisis], hyperthyroidism and hypothyroidism) have been reported; may require hospitalization. Endocrine disorders of moderate severity (including hypothyroidism, adrenal insufficiency, hypopituitarism, and less commonly hyperthyroidism and Cushing's syndrome) which have required hormone replacement therapy or medical intervention have also been reported. The median onset for moderate-to-severe endocrine disorders was 2.2 to 2.5 months; long-term hormone replacement therapy has been required in many cases. Monitor thyroid function tests, adrenocorticotropic hormone (ACTH) level, and serum chemistries prior to each dose and as clinically necessary; also monitor for signs of hypophysitis, adrenal insufficiency and thyroid disorders (eg, abdominal pain, fatigue, headache, hypotension, mental status changes, unusual bowel habits); rule out other potential causes such as underlying disease or brain metastases. Endocrine disorders should be considered immune-mediated unless identified otherwise; consider endocrinology referral for further evaluation. If symptomatic, withhold ipilimumab treatment and initiate systemic corticosteroids (prednisone 1 to 2 mg/kg/day or equivalent) and appropriate hormone replacement therapy.

Immune-mediated neuropathies (some fatal) may occur. Severe peripheral motor neuropathy and fatal Guillain-Barré syndrome have been reported (rare). The median time to onset of grade 2 to 5 immune-mediated neuropathy in patients receiving ipilimumab for adjuvant treatment of melanoma was 1.4 to 27.4 months. Monitor for signs of motor or sensory neuropathy (unilateral or bilateral weakness, sensory changes or paresthesia). Withhold treatment in patients with neuropathy that does not interfere with daily activities (moderate neuropathy). Permanently discontinue for severe neuropathy (interferes with daily activities, including symptoms similar to Guillain-Barré syndrome) and treat accordingly. Consider initiating systemic corticosteroids (prednisone 1 to 2 mg/kg/day or equivalent) for severe neuropathies.

Adverse Reactions

>10%:

Central nervous system: Fatigue (41% to 46%), headache (15% to 33% [Hodi 2010])

Dermatologic: Pruritus (24% to 45% [Hodi 2010]), skin rash (19% to 50% [Hodi 2010]), dermatitis (grade 2: 12% to 21%; grades 3/4: 2% to 4% [includes Stevens-Johnson syndrome, toxic epidermal necrolysis, dermal ulceration, necrotic, bullous or hemorrhagic dermatitis])

Endocrine & metabolic: Weight loss (32%), pituitary insufficiency (4%; grade 2: ≤2% to 16%; grades 3/4: 2% to 7%)

Gastrointestinal: Diarrhea (32% to 49%), nausea (25% to 35% [Hodi 2010]), decreased appetite (14% to 27% [Hodi 2010]), increased serum lipase (26%), vomiting (13% to 24% [Hodi 2010]), constipation (21% [Hodi 2010]), colitis (8% to 16%), enterocolitis (grade 2: 5% to 14%; grades 3 to 5: 7% to 16%), increased serum amylase (17%), abdominal pain (15% [Hodi 2010])

Hematologic & oncologic: Decreased hemoglobin (25%), anemia (12% [Hodi 2010])

Hepatic: Increased serum ALT (≤2% to 46% [Hodi 2010]), increased serum AST (≤38% [Hodi 2010]), increased serum alkaline phosphatase (17%), increased serum bilirubin (11%), hepatitis (grade 2: 5%; grades 3/4: 11%)

Respiratory: Cough (16% [Hodi 2010]), dyspnea (15% [Hodi 2010])

Miscellaneous: Fever (12% to 18% [Hodi 2010])

1% to 10%:

Central nervous system: Insomnia (10%), neuropathy (grade 2: <1%; grades 3 to 5: 2%)

Dermatologic: Urticaria (2%), vitiligo (2% [Hodi 2010])

Endocrine & metabolic: Hypophysitis (2% [Hodi 2010]), adrenal insufficiency (≤2% [Hodi 2010]), hypothyroidism (≤2% [Hodi 2010])

Gastrointestinal: Intestinal perforation (1% to 2%), pancreatitis (1%)

Hematologic & oncologic: Eosinophilia (1% to 2%)

Hepatic: Hepatotoxicity (grade 2: 3%)

Immunologic: Antibody development (1%)

Renal: Increased serum creatinine (10%), nephritis (≤1%)

<1%, postmarketing, and/or case reports: Acute respiratory distress, adrenocortical insufficiency (Hodi 2010), arthritis, blepharitis, bronchiolitis obliterans organizing pneumonia (Barjaktarevic 2013), capillary leak syndrome (Hodi 2010), conjunctivitis, Cushing syndrome, DRESS syndrome, encephalitis, episcleritis, erythema multiforme, esophagitis, gastrointestinal ulcer, giant-cell arteritis, Graves' ophthalmopathy, Guillain-Barré syndrome, hemolytic anemia, hepatic failure, hepatitis (immune-mediated), hypersensitivity angiitis, hyperthyroidism, hypoacusis (neurosensory), hypogonadism, increased thyroid stimulating hormone level, infusion related reaction, iritis, meningitis, myasthenia gravis, myelofibrosis, myocarditis, myositis, myositis (ocular), pericarditis, peripheral motor neuropathy, peritonitis, pneumonitis, polymyalgia rheumatica, polymyositis, psoriasis, renal failure, sarcoidosis, scleritis, sepsis, thyroiditis (autoimmune), uveitis, vascular disease, vasculitis

Drug Interactions

Metabolism/Transport Effects None known.

Avoid Concomitant Use There are no known interactions where it is recommended to avoid concomitant use.

Increased Effect/Toxicity

Ipilimumab may increase the levels/effects of: Vemurafenib

Decreased Effect There are no known significant interactions involving a decrease in effect.

Storage/Stability Store intact vials refrigerated at 2°C to 8°C (36°F to 46°F); do not freeze. Protect from light. Prior to preparation, allow vials to sit at room temperature for ~5 minutes. Solutions diluted for infusion in NS or D5W are stable for up to 24 hours refrigerated or at room temperature.

Preparation for Administration Prior to preparation, allow vials to sit at room temperature for ~5 minutes. Inspect vial prior to use; solution may have a pale yellow color or may contain translucent or white amorphous ipilimumab particles; discard if cloudy or discolored. Withdraw appropriate ipilimumab volume and transfer to IV bag, dilute with NS or D5W to a final concentration between 1 to 2 mg/mL. Mix by gently inverting, do not shake.

Mechanism of Action Ipilimumab is a recombinant human IgG1 immunoglobulin monoclonal antibody which binds to the cytotoxic T-lymphocyte associated antigen 4 (CTLA-4). CTLA-4 is a down-regulator of T-cell activation pathways. Blocking CTLA-4 allows for enhanced T-cell activation and proliferation. In melanoma, ipilimumab may indirectly mediate T-cell immune responses against tumors.

Pharmacodynamics/Kinetics Half-life elimination: Terminal: 15.4 days

Dosing

Adult

Melanoma, unresectable or metastatic: IV: 3 mg/kg every 3 weeks for a maximum of 4 doses (Hodi 2010); doses may be delayed due to toxicity, but all doses must be administered within 16 weeks of the initial dose.

Melanoma, adjuvant treatment: IV: 10 mg/kg every 3 weeks for 4 doses, followed by 10 mg/kg every 12 weeks for up to 3 years unless disease progression or unacceptable toxicity occur (Eggermont 2016); if toxicity occurs, doses are omitted (not delayed).

Melanoma, unresectable or metastatic, first-line combination therapy (off-label use): IV: 3 mg/kg every 3 weeks for 4 doses (in combination with nivolumab; with nivolumab continued until disease progression or unacceptable toxicity) (Larkin 2015).

Small cell lung cancer, progressive (off-label use): IV: 3 mg/kg every 3 weeks (in combination with nivolumab) for 4 doses, followed by nivolumab monotherapy (Antonia 2016).

Pediatric Melanoma, unresectable or metastatic: Children ≥12 years and Adolescents: IV: 3 mg/kg every 3 weeks for a maximum of 4 doses; doses may be delayed due to toxicity, but all doses must be administered within 16 weeks of the initial dose.

Renal Impairment No dosage adjustment necessary.

Hepatic Impairment

Impairment at baseline:

Mild impairment (total bilirubin >1 to 1.5 x ULN **or** AST >ULN): No dosage adjustment necessary.

Moderate or severe impairment (total bilirubin >1.5 x ULN and any AST): There are no dosage adjustments provided in the manufacturer's labeling (has not been studied).

Impairment during treatment:

AST or ALT >2.5 to ≤5 x ULN or bilirubin >1.5 to ≤3 x ULN: Temporarily withhold treatment.

ALT or AST >5 times ULN, or total bilirubin >3 times ULN: Permanently discontinue; also administer systemic corticosteroids (prednisone 1 to 2 mg/kg/day or equivalent). May begin tapering corticosteroid (over 1 month) when LFTs show sustained improvement or return to baseline.

Adjustment for Toxicity

Dermatologic toxicity: Treat symptomatically for mild to moderate dermatitis (eg, localized rash and pruritus); topical or systemic corticosteroids should be administered if not resolved within 1 week. Withhold ipilimumab for moderate to severe dermatologic symptoms. Permanently discontinue for ▶

◄

Stevens-Johnson syndrome, toxic epidermal necrolysis, or rash complicated by dermal ulceration (full thickness) or necrotic, bullous, or hemorrhagic manifestations; also initiate systemic corticosteroids (prednisone 1 to 2 mg/kg/day or equivalent). When dermatitis is controlled, taper corticosteroid over at least 1 month.

Endocrinopathy: Temporarily withhold ipilimumab for symptomatic endocrinopathy; initiate systemic corticosteroids (prednisone at 1 to 2 mg/kg/day or equivalent), and begin appropriate hormone replacement therapy. Resume treatment in patients with complete or partial resolution of toxicity (≤ grade 1) and who are receiving prednisone <7.5 mg daily (or equivalent). Permanently discontinue ipilimumab for symptomatic endocrinopathy lasting 6 weeks or longer, or if unable to reduce corticosteroid dose to prednisone ≤7.5 mg daily (or equivalent).

Gastrointestinal toxicity:

Moderate enterocolitis: Withhold ipilimumab and administer antidiarrheal treatment; if moderate enterocolitis persists for >1 week, initiate systemic corticosteroids (prednisone at 0.5 mg/kg/day or equivalent). May resume treatment in patients with complete or partial resolution of toxicity (≤ grade 1) and who are receiving prednisone <7.5 mg daily (or equivalent).

Severe enterocolitis: Permanently discontinue. Initiate systemic corticosteroids (prednisone 1 to 2 mg/kg/day or equivalent). Upon improvement to ≤ grade 1, taper corticosteroids slowly over ≥1 month (rapid tapering may cause recurrence or worsen symptoms). May consider adding anti-tumor necrosis factor (TNF) or other immunosuppressive therapy for management of immune-mediated enterocolitis unresponsive to 3 to 5 days of systemic corticosteroids or recurring after symptomatic improvement.

Neuropathy: Withhold therapy for moderate neuropathy (not interfering with daily activities). Permanently discontinue for severe neuropathy which interferes with daily activities, such as Guillain-Barré-like syndromes. Consider initiating systemic corticosteroids (prednisone 1 to 2 mg/kg/day or equivalent) for severe neuropathies.

Ophthalmologic toxicity: Administer corticosteroid eye drops for uveitis, iritis, or episcleritis. Permanently discontinue for grade 2 through 4 immune-mediated reactions which do not improve to ≤ grade 1 within 2 weeks while receiving topical therapy or which require systemic treatment.

Pancreatitis, immune-mediated: Permanent discontinuation is recommended for grades 3 or 4 amylase or lipase increases (Weber 2012)

Other toxicity: Temporarily withhold ipilimumab for grade 2 adverse reactions. May resume treatment in patients (with grade 2 toxicity) with complete or partial resolution of toxicity (≤ grade 1) and who are receiving prednisone <7.5 mg daily (or equivalent). Initiate systemic corticosteroids (prednisone 1 to 2 mg/kg/day or equivalent) for severe immune-mediated adverse reactions. Permanently discontinue for clinically significant or severe immune-mediated adverse reactions, grade 2 reactions lasting 6 weeks or longer, grade 3 or 4 toxicity, or if unable to reduce corticosteroid dose to prednisone ≤7.5 mg daily (or equivalent).

Combination Regimens

Melanoma: Ipilimumab-Nivolumab (Melanoma) on page 2157

Administration IV: Infuse over 90 minutes through a non-pyrogenic, low protein-binding in-line filter. Do not administer with other medications. Flush with NS or D5W at the end of infusion

Emetic Potential Low (10% to 30%)

Monitoring Parameters Monitor liver function and evaluate for signs of hepatotoxicity prior to each dose; if hepatotoxicity develops, liver function should be monitored more frequently until resolves. If liver functions tests are >8 times ULN, monitor every other day until begin to fall, then weekly until normal (Weber 2012). Monitor serum chemistries and adrenocorticotropic hormone (ACTH) prior to each dose. Monitor for signs of hypophysitis, adrenal insufficiency and thyroid disorders (eg, abdominal pain, fatigue, headache, hypotension, mental status changes, unusual bowel habits). Monitor TSH, free T_4 and cortisol levels (morning) at baseline, prior to dose, and as clinically indicated. Monitor for signs and symptoms of enterocolitis (abdominal pain, blood or mucus in stool or diarrhea, and intestinal perforation (peritoneal signs, ileus). Monitor for rash, pruritus, and other signs of dermatologic toxicity. Monitor for signs of motor or sensory neuropathy (unilateral or bilateral weakness, sensory changes or paresthesia). Monitor for ocular toxicity at baseline, then at 4 to 8 weeks with further evaluations as clinically indicated (Renouf 2012).

Medication Guide Available Yes

Dosage Forms Excipient information presented when available (limited, particularly for generics); consult specific product labeling.

Solution, Intravenous [preservative free]:

Yervoy: 50 mg/10 mL (10 mL); 200 mg/40 mL (40 mL) [contains polysorbate 80]

♦ **Ipilimumab, inj** *see* Ipilimumab *on page* 1031

♦ **Iressa** *see* Gefitinib *on page* 858

♦ **IRESSA (Can)** *see* Gefitinib *on page* 858

Irinotecan (Conventional) (eye rye no TEE kan con VEN sha nal)

Related Information

Management of Chemotherapy-Induced Nausea and Vomiting in Adults *on page* 2253

Management of Drug Extravasations *on page* 2271

Management of EGFR Inhibitor Toxicities: Dermatologic, Ocular, and Gastrointestinal *on page* 2291

Mucositis and Stomatitis *on page* 2299

Prevention of Chemotherapy-Induced Nausea and Vomiting in Children *on page* 2310

Safe Handling of Hazardous Drugs *on page* 2379

Brand Names: US Camptosar

Brand Names: Canada Camptosar; Irinotecan For Injection; Irinotecan Hydrochloride Injection; Irinotecan Hydrochloride Trihydrate For Injection; Irinotecan Hydrochloride Trihydrate Injection

Index Terms Camptothecin-11; Conventional Irinotecan; CPT-11; Irinotecan HCl; Irinotecan Hydrochloride

Pharmacologic Category Antineoplastic Agent, Camptothecin; Antineoplastic Agent, Topoisomerase I Inhibitor

Use Colorectal cancer, metastatic: Treatment of metastatic carcinoma of the colon or rectum

Labeled Contraindications Hypersensitivity to irinotecan or any component of the formulation

◀ **Pregnancy Considerations** Adverse events were observed in animal reproduction studies. Information related to the use of irinotecan (conventional) during pregnancy is limited (Cirillo 2012; Taylor 2009). May cause fetal harm if administered during pregnancy. Women of childbearing potential should avoid becoming pregnant while receiving treatment.

Breastfeeding Considerations It is not known if irinotecan is excreted in breast milk. Due to the potential for serious adverse reactions in the nursing infant, the manufacturer recommends a decision be made to discontinue nursing or to discontinue the drug, taking into account the importance of treatment to the mother.

Warnings/Precautions Severe hypersensitivity reactions (including anaphylaxis) have occurred. Monitor closely; discontinue therapy if hypersensitivity occurs. Irinotecan is an irritant; avoid extravasation. If extravasation occurs, the manufacturer recommends flushing the external site with sterile water and applying ice.

[US Boxed Warning]: Severe diarrhea may be dose-limiting and potentially fatal; early-onset and late-onset diarrhea may occur. Early diarrhea occurs during or within 24 hours of receiving irinotecan and is characterized by cholinergic symptoms; may be prevented or treated with atropine. Late diarrhea may be life-threatening and should be promptly treated with loperamide. Antibiotics may be necessary if patient develops ileus, fever, or severe neutropenia. Interrupt treatment and reduce subsequent doses for severe diarrhea. Early diarrhea is generally transient and rarely severe; cholinergic symptoms may include increased salivation, rhinitis, miosis, diaphoresis, flushing, abdominal cramping, and lacrimation; bradycardia may also occur. Cholinergic symptoms may occur more frequently with higher irinotecan doses. Late diarrhea occurs more than 24 hours after treatment, which may lead to dehydration, electrolyte imbalance, or sepsis. Late diarrhea may be complicated by colitis, ulceration, bleeding, ileus, obstruction, or infection; cases of megacolon and intestinal perforation have been reported. The median time to onset for late diarrhea is 5 days with every-3-week irinotecan dosing and 11 days with weekly dosing. Advise patients to have loperamide readily available for the treatment of late diarrhea. Patients with diarrhea should be carefully monitored and treated promptly; may require fluid and electrolyte therapy. Bowel function should be returned to baseline for at least 24 hours prior to resumption of weekly irinotecan dosing. Avoid diuretics and laxatives in patients experiencing diarrhea. Patients >65 years of age are at greater risk for early and late diarrhea. A dose reduction is recommended for patients ≥70 years of age receiving the every-3-week regimen. Irinotecan is associated with a moderate emetic potential; antiemetics are recommended to prevent nausea and vomiting (Basch 2011; Dupuis 2011; Roila 2016).

[US Boxed Warning]: May cause severe myelosuppression. Deaths due to sepsis following severe neutropenia have been reported. Complications due to neutropenia should be promptly managed with antibiotics. Therapy should be temporarily withheld if neutropenic fever occurs or if the absolute neutrophil count is <1,000/mm^3; reduce the dose upon recovery to an absolute neutrophil count ≥1,000/mm^3. Patients who have previously received pelvic/abdominal radiation therapy have an increased risk of severe bone marrow suppression; the incidence of grade 3 or 4 neutropenia was higher in patients receiving weekly irinotecan who have previously received pelvic/ abdominal radiation therapy. Concurrent radiation therapy is not recommended with irinotecan (based on limited data). Fatal cases of interstitial pulmonary disease (IPD)-like events have been reported with single-agent and combination therapy. Risk factors for pulmonary toxicity include preexisting lung disease, use of pulmonary toxic medications, radiation therapy, and colony-stimulating factors. Patients with risk factors should be monitored for respiratory symptoms before and during irinotecan treatment. Promptly evaluate progressive changes in baseline pulmonary symptoms or any new-onset pulmonary symptoms (eg, dyspnea, cough, fever). Discontinue all chemotherapy if IPD is diagnosed.

Patients with even modest elevations in total serum bilirubin levels (1 to 2 mg/dL) have a significantly greater likelihood of experiencing first-course grade 3 or 4 neutropenia than those with bilirubin levels that were <1 mg/dL. Patients with abnormal glucuronidation of bilirubin, such as those with Gilbert's syndrome, may also be at greater risk of myelosuppression when receiving therapy with irinotecan. Use caution when treating patients with known hepatic dysfunction or hyperbilirubinemia exposure to the active metabolite (SN-38) is increased; toxicities may be increased. Dosage adjustments should be considered.

Patients homozygous for the UGT1A1*28 allele are at increased risk of neutropenia; initial one-level dose reduction should be considered for both single-agent and combination regimens. Heterozygous carriers of the UGT1A1*28 allele may also be at increased neutropenic risk; however, most patients have tolerated normal starting doses. A test is available for clinical determination of UGT phenotype, although a dose reduction is already recommended in patients who have experienced toxicity.

Renal impairment and acute renal failure have been reported, possibly due to dehydration secondary to diarrhea. Use with caution in patients with renal impairment; not recommended in patients on dialysis. Patients with bowel obstruction should not be treated with irinotecan until resolution of obstruction. Contains sorbitol; do not use in patients with hereditary fructose intolerance. Thromboembolic events have been reported. Higher rates of hospitalization, neutropenic fever, thromboembolism, first-cycle discontinuation, and early mortality were observed in patients with a performance status of 2 than in patients with a performance status of 0 or 1. Except as part of a clinical trial, use in combination with fluorouracil and leucovorin administered for 4 or 5 consecutive days ("Mayo Clinic" regimen) is not recommended due to increased toxicity. Potentially significant interactions may exist, requiring dose or frequency adjustment, additional monitoring, and/or selection of alternative therapy. CYP3A4 enzyme inducers may decrease exposure to irinotecan and SN-38 (active metabolite); enzyme inhibitors may increase exposure; for use in patients with CNS tumors (off-label use), selection of antiseizure medications that are not enzyme inducers is preferred. Irinotecan (conventional) and irinotecan (liposomal) are **NOT** interchangeable. Dosing differs between formulations; verify intended product and dose prior to preparation and administration.

Adverse Reactions Frequency of adverse reactions reported for single-agent use of irinotecan only. In limited pediatric experience, dehydration (often associated with severe hypokalemia and hyponatremia) was among the most significant grade 3/4 adverse events, with a frequency up to 29%. In addition, grade 3/4 infection was reported in 24%.

>10%:

Cardiovascular: Vasodilatation (9% to 11%)

Central nervous system: Cholinergic syndrome (47%; includes diaphoresis, flushing, increased peristalsis, lacrimation, miosis, rhinitis, sialorrhea), pain (23% to 24%), dizziness (15% to 21%), insomnia (19%), headache (17%), chills (14%)

Dermatologic: Alopecia (46% to 72%), diaphoresis (16%), skin rash (13% to 14%)

Endocrine & metabolic: Weight loss (30%), dehydration (15%)

Gastrointestinal: Diarrhea (late: 83% to 88%, grades 3/4: 14% to 31%; early: 43% to 51%, grades 3/4: 7% to 22%), nausea (70% to 86%), abdominal pain (57% to 68%), vomiting (62% to 67%), abdominal cramps (57%), anorexia (44% to 55%), constipation (30% to 32%), mucositis (30%), flatulence (12%), stomatitis (12%)

Hematologic & oncologic: Anemia (60% to 97%; grades 3/4: 5% to 7%), leukopenia (63% to 96%, grades 3/4: 14% to 28%), thrombocytopenia (96%, grades 3/4: 1% to 4%), neutropenia (30% to 96%; grades 3/4: 14% to 31%)

Hepatic: Increased serum bilirubin (84%), increased serum alkaline phosphatase (13%)

Infection: Infection (14%)

Neuromuscular & skeletal: Weakness (69% to 76%), back pain (14%)

Respiratory: Dyspnea (22%), cough (17% to 20%), rhinitis (16%)

Miscellaneous: Fever (44% to 45%)

1% to 10%:

Cardiovascular: Edema (10%), hypotension (6%), thromboembolism (5%)

Central nervous system: Drowsiness (9%), confusion (3%)

Gastrointestinal: Abdominal distention (10%), dyspepsia (10%)

Hematologic & oncologic: Febrile neutropenia (grades 3/4: 2% to 6%), hemorrhage (grades 3/4: 1% to 5%), neutropenic infection (grades 3/4: 1% to 2%)

Hepatic: Increased serum AST (10%), ascites (grades 3/4: ≤9%), jaundice (grades 3/4: ≤9%)

Respiratory: Pneumonia (4%)

<1%, postmarketing, and/or case reports: Acute renal failure, anaphylactoid reaction, anaphylaxis, angina pectoris, arterial thrombosis, bradycardia, cardiac arrhythmia, cerebral infarction, cerebrovascular accident, circulatory shock, colitis, deep vein thrombophlebitis, dysarthria, embolism, gastrointestinal hemorrhage, gastrointestinal obstruction, hepatomegaly, hiccups, hyperglycemia, hypersensitivity reaction, hyponatremia, immune thrombocytopenia, increased serum amylase, increased serum ALT, increased serum lipase, interstitial pulmonary disease, intestinal obstruction, intestinal perforation, ischemic colitis, ischemic heart disease, lymphocytopenia, megacolon, muscle cramps, myocardial infarction, pancreatitis, paresthesia, peripheral vascular disease, pulmonary embolism; pulmonary toxicity (includes dyspnea, fever, reticulonodular infiltrates on chest x-ray), renal insufficiency, syncope, thrombophlebitis, thrombosis, typhlitis (including neutropenic typhlitis), ulcer, ulcerative colitis, vertigo

Drug Interactions

Metabolism/Transport Effects Substrate of BCRP, CYP3A4 (major), P-glycoprotein, SLCO1B1, UGT1A1; **Note:** Assignment of Major/Minor substrate status based on clinically relevant drug interaction potential

Avoid Concomitant Use

Avoid concomitant use of Irinotecan (Conventional) with any of the following: BCG (Intravesical); Conivaptan; CYP3A4 Inducers (Strong); CYP3A4

Inhibitors (Strong); Deferiprone; Dipyrone; Fusidic Acid (Systemic); Idelalisib; Natalizumab; Pimecrolimus; St John's Wort; Tacrolimus (Topical); UGT1A1 Inhibitors; Vaccines (Live)

Increased Effect/Toxicity

Irinotecan (Conventional) may increase the levels/effects of: CloZAPine; Deferiprone; Fingolimod; Leflunomide; Natalizumab; Tofacitinib; Vaccines (Live)

The levels/effects of Irinotecan (Conventional) may be increased by: Aprepitant; Conivaptan; CYP3A4 Inhibitors (Moderate); CYP3A4 Inhibitors (Strong); Dasatinib; Denosumab; Dipyrone; Fosaprepitant; Fusidic Acid (Systemic); Idelalisib; Netupitant; Ocrelizumab; Palbociclib; Palifermin; P-glycoprotein/ABCB1 Inhibitors; Pimecrolimus; Promazine; Ranolazine; Roflumilast; Simeprevir; SORAfenib; Stiripentol; Tacrolimus (Topical); Teriflunomide; Trastuzumab; UGT1A1 Inhibitors

Decreased Effect

Irinotecan (Conventional) may decrease the levels/effects of: BCG (Intravesical); Coccidioides immitis Skin Test; Lenograstim; Nivolumab; Sipuleucel-T; Tertomotide; Vaccines (Inactivated); Vaccines (Live)

The levels/effects of Irinotecan (Conventional) may be decreased by: Bosentan; CYP3A4 Inducers (Moderate); CYP3A4 Inducers (Strong); Dabrafenib; Deferasirox; Echinacea; Sarilumab; Siltuximab; St John's Wort; Tocilizumab

Hazardous Drugs Handling Considerations

Hazardous agent (NIOSH 2016 [group 1]).

Use appropriate precautions for receiving, handling, administration, and disposal. Gloves (single) should be worn during receiving, unpacking, and placing in storage.

NIOSH recommends double gloving, a protective gown, ventilated engineering controls (a class II biological safety cabinet or a compounding aseptic containment isolator), and closed system transfer devices (CSTDs) for preparation. Double gloving, a gown, and (if dosage form allows) CSTDs are required during administration (NIOSH 2016).

Storage/Stability Store intact vials at 15°C to 30°C (59°F to 86°F). Protect from light; retain vials in original carton until use. Solutions diluted in NS may precipitate if refrigerated. Solutions diluted in D5W are stable for 24 hours at room temperature or 48 hours under refrigeration at 2°C to 8°C (36°F to 46°F), although the manufacturer recommends use within 24 hours if refrigerated, or within 4 to 12 hours (manufacturer dependent; refer to specific prescribing information) at room temperature (including infusion time) only if prepared under strict aseptic conditions (eg, laminar flow hood). Do not freeze. Undiluted commercially available injectable solution prepared in oral syringes is stable for 21 days under refrigeration (Wagner 2010).

Preparation for Administration Dilute in D5W (preferred) or NS to a final concentration of 0.12 to 2.8 mg/mL.

Mechanism of Action Irinotecan and its active metabolite (SN-38) bind reversibly to topoisomerase I-DNA complex preventing religation of the cleaved DNA strand. This results in the accumulation of cleavable complexes and double-strand DNA breaks. As mammalian cells cannot efficiently repair these breaks, cell death consistent with S-phase cell cycle specificity occurs, leading to termination of cellular replication.

◄ **Pharmacodynamics/Kinetics**

Distribution:

Children and Adolescents: ~37 L/m^2 (range: 15.2-77 L/m^2) (Ma, 2000); distributes to pleural fluid, sweat, and saliva

Adults: 33-150 L/m^2

Protein binding, plasma: Predominantly albumin; Irinotecan: 30% to 68%, SN-38 (active metabolite): ~95%

Metabolism: Primarily hepatic to SN-38 (active metabolite) by carboxylesterase enzymes; may also undergo CYP3A4-mediated metabolism to inactive metabolites (one of which may be hydrolyzed to release SN-38). SN-38 undergoes conjugation by UDP-glucuronosyl transferase 1A1 (UGT1A1) to form a glucuronide metabolite. SN-38 is increased by UGT1A1*28 polymorphism (10% of North Americans are homozygous for UGT1A1*28 allele).

Bioavailability: Median: 9%; increased in presence of gefitinib (median: 42%) (Furman 2009)

Half-life elimination:

Children and Adolescents (Ma 2000): Irinotecan: 2.66 hours (range: 1.82-4.47 hours); SN-38 (active metabolite): 1.58 hours (range: 0.29-8.28 hours)

Adults: Irinotecan: 6 to 12 hours; SN-38: ~10 to 20 hours

Time to peak:

Irinotecan: Oral: Children and Adolescents: 3 hours (Wagner 2010a)

SN-38: Following 90-minute infusion: ~1 hour

Excretion: Urine: Irinotecan (11% to 20%), metabolites (SN-38 <1%, SN-38 glucuronide, 3%)

Dosing

Adult Note: A reduction in the starting dose by one dose level should be considered for prior pelvic/abdominal radiotherapy, performance status of 2, or known homozygosity for UGT1A1*28 allele (subsequent dosing/adjustments should be based on individual tolerance). Irinotecan (conventional) and irinotecan (liposomal) are **NOT** interchangeable. Dosing differs between formulations; verify intended product and dose prior to preparation and administration.

Premedications: Consider premedication of atropine 0.25 to 1 mg IV or SubQ in patients with cholinergic symptoms (eg, increased salivation, rhinitis, miosis, diaphoresis, abdominal cramping) or early-onset diarrhea. Irinotecan is associated with a moderate emetic potential; antiemetics are recommended to prevent nausea and vomiting (Basch 2011; Dupuis 2011; Roila 2016).

Colorectal cancer, metastatic (single-agent therapy): IV:

Weekly regimen: 125 mg/m^2 over 90 minutes on days 1, 8, 15, and 22 of a 6-week treatment cycle (may adjust upward to 150 mg/m^2 if tolerated)

Adjusted dose level -1: 100 mg/m^2

Adjusted dose level -2: 75 mg/m^2

Further adjust to 50 mg/m^2 (in decrements of 25 to 50 mg/m^2) if needed

Once-every-3-week regimen: 350 mg/m^2 over 90 minutes, once every 3 weeks

Adjusted dose level -1: 300 mg/m^2

Adjusted dose level -2: 250 mg/m^2

Further adjust to 200 mg/m^2 (in decrements of 25 to 50 mg/m^2) if needed

Colorectal cancer, metastatic (in combination with fluorouracil and leucovorin): IV: Six-week (42-day) cycle:

Regimen 1: 125 mg/m^2 over 90 minutes on days 1, 8, 15, and 22; to be given in combination with bolus leucovorin and fluorouracil (leucovorin administered immediately following irinotecan; fluorouracil immediately following leucovorin)

Adjusted dose level -1: 100 mg/m^2

Adjusted dose level -2: 75 mg/m^2

Further adjust if needed in decrements of ~20%

Regimen 2: 180 mg/m^2 over 90 minutes on days 1, 15, and 29; to be given in combination with infusional leucovorin and bolus/infusion fluorouracil (leucovorin administered immediately following irinotecan; fluorouracil immediately following leucovorin)

Adjusted dose level -1: 150 mg/m^2

Adjusted dose level -2: 120 mg/m^2

Further adjust if needed in decrements of ~20%

Colorectal cancer, metastatic (off-label dosing): IV: FOLFOXIRI regimen: 165 mg/m^2 over 1 hour once every 2 weeks (in combination with oxaliplatin, leucovorin, and fluorouracil) (Falcone 2007)

Cervical cancer, recurrent or metastatic (off-label use): IV: 125 mg/m^2 over 90 minutes once weekly for 4 consecutive weeks followed by a 2-week rest during each 6 week treatment cycle (Verschraegen 1997)

CNS tumor, recurrent glioblastoma (off-label use): IV: 125 mg/m^2 over 90 minutes once every 2 weeks (in combination with bevacizumab). **NOTE:** In patients taking concurrent antiepileptic enzyme-inducing medications irinotecan dose was increased to 340 mg/m^2 (Friedman 2009; Vredenburgh 2007).

Esophageal cancer, metastatic or locally advanced (off-label use): IV: 65 mg/m^2 over 90 minutes days 1, 8, 15, and 22 of a 6-week treatment cycle (in combination with cisplatin) (Ajani 2002; Ilson 1999) **or** 180 mg/m^2 over 90 minutes every 2 weeks (in combination with leucovorin and fluorouracil) (Guimbaud 2014) **or** 250 mg/m^2 every 3 weeks (in combination with capecitabine) (Leary 2009; Moehler 2010)

Ewing sarcoma, recurrent or progressive (off-label use): IV: 20 mg/m^2 days 1 to 5 and days 8 to 12 every 3 weeks (in combination with temozolomide) (Casey 2009)

Gastric cancer, metastatic or locally advanced (off-label use): IV: 150 mg/m^2 (as a single agent) on days 1 and 15 of a 4-week treatment cycle (Hironaka 2013) **or** 65 mg/m^2 over 90 minutes days 1, 8, 15, and 22 of a 6-week treatment cycle (in combination with cisplatin) (Ajani 2002) **or** 70 mg/m^2 over 90 minutes on days 1 and 15 of a 4-week treatment cycle (in combination with cisplatin) for up to 6 cycles (Park 2005) **or** 180 mg/m^2 over 90 minutes every 2 weeks (in combination with leucovorin and fluorouracil) (Bouche 2004; Guimbaud 2014) **or** 250 mg/m^2 every 3 weeks (in combination with capecitabine) (Moehler 2010)

Non-small cell lung cancer, advanced (off-label use): IV: 60 mg/m^2 days 1, 8, and 15 every 4 weeks (in combination with cisplatin) (Ohe 2007)

Ovarian cancer, recurrent, platinum- and taxane-resistant (off-label use): IV: 100 mg/m^2 days 1, 8, and 15 every 4 weeks (as a single-agent) for up to 6 cycles (Matsumoto 2006)

◄

Pancreatic cancer, advanced (off-label use): IV: FOLFIRINOX regimen: 180 mg/m^2 over 90 minutes every 2 weeks (in combination with oxaliplatin, leucovorin, and fluorouracil) (Conroy 2005; Conroy 2011)

Small cell lung cancer, extensive stage (off-label use): IV: 60 mg/m^2 days 1, 8, and 15 every 4 weeks (in combination with cisplatin) (Noda 2002) **or** 65 mg/m^2 days 1 and 8 every 3 weeks (in combination with cisplatin) (Hanna 2006) **or** 175 mg/m^2 day 1 every 3 weeks (in combination with carboplatin) (Hermes 2008) **or** 50 mg/m^2 days 1, 8 and 15 every 4 weeks (in combination with carboplatin) (Schmittel 2006). According to American Society of Clinical Oncology (ASCO) guidelines, platinum-based therapy (cisplatin or carboplatin) in combination with either etoposide or irinotecan for 4 to 6 cycles is recommended over other regimens for extensive stage disease (Rudin 2015).

Geriatric

Weekly dosing schedule: No dosing adjustment is recommended

Every 3-week dosing colorectal cancer schedule: Recommended initial dose is 300 mg/m^2/dose for patients ≥70 years

Pediatric See "Note" in adult dosing.

Ewing sarcoma, recurrent or progressive (off-label use): IV: Refer to adult dosing.

Rhabdomyosarcoma, relapsed/refractory (off-label use; Vassal 2007): IV:

Children <10 kg: 20 mg/kg once every 3 weeks

Children ≥10 kg and Adolescents: 600 mg/m^2 once every 3 weeks

Renal Impairment

Renal impairment: There are no dosage adjustments provided in the manufacturer's labeling (has not been studied); use with caution.

Dialysis: Use in patients with dialysis is not recommended by the manufacturer; however, literature suggests reducing weekly dose from 125 mg/m^2 to 50 mg/m^2 and administer after hemodialysis or on nondialysis days (Janus 2010).

Hepatic Impairment

Manufacturer's labeling:

Liver metastases with normal hepatic function: No dosage adjustment necessary.

Bilirubin >ULN to ≤2 mg/dL: Consider reducing initial dose by one dose level

Bilirubin >2 mg/dL: Use is not recommended

Alternate recommendations: The following adjustments have also been recommended:

Bilirubin 1.5 to 3 mg/dL: Administer 75% of dose (Floyd 2006)

Bilirubin 1.51 to 3 times ULN: Reduce dose from 350 mg/m^2 every 3 weeks to 200 mg/m^2 every 3 weeks (Raymond 2002)

Obesity *ASCO Guidelines for appropriate chemotherapy dosing in obese adults with cancer:* Utilize patient's actual body weight (full weight) for calculation of body surface area- or weight-based dosing, particularly when the intent of therapy is curative; manage regimen-related toxicities in the same manner as for nonobese patients; if a dose reduction is utilized due to toxicity, consider resumption of full weight-based dosing with subsequent cycles, especially if cause of toxicity (eg, hepatic or renal impairment) is resolved (Griggs 2012).

Adjustment for Toxicity It is recommended that new courses begin only after the granulocyte count recovers to ≥1,500/mm^3, the platelet counts recover to ≥100,000/mm^3, and treatment-related diarrhea has fully resolved. Depending on the patient's ability to tolerate therapy, doses should be adjusted in increments of 25 to 50 mg/m^2. Treatment should be delayed 1 to 2 weeks to allow for recovery from treatment-related toxicities. If the patient has not recovered after a 2-week delay, consider discontinuing irinotecan. See tables below and on following pages.

Colorectal Cancer: Single-Agent Schedule: Recommended Dosage Modifications[1]

Toxicity NCI Grade[2] (Value)	During a Cycle of Therapy	At Start of Subsequent Cycles of Therapy (After Adequate Recovery), Compared to Starting Dose in Previous Cycle[1]	
	Weekly	Weekly	Once Every 3 Weeks
No toxicity	Maintain dose level	↑ 25 mg/m^2 up to a maximum dose of 150 mg/m^2	Maintain dose level
Neutropenia			
Grade 1 (1,500 to 1,999/mm^3)	Maintain dose level	Maintain dose level	Maintain dose level
Grade 2 (1,000 to 1,499/mm^3)	↓ 25 mg/m^2	Maintain dose level	Maintain dose level
Grade 3 (500 to 999/mm^3)	Omit dose until resolved to ≤ grade 2, then ↓ 25 mg/m^2	↓ 25 mg/m^2	↓ 50 mg/m^2
Grade 4 (<500/mm^3)	Omit dose until resolved to ≤ grade 2, then ↓ 50 mg/m^2	↓ 50 mg/m^2	↓ 50 mg/m^2
Neutropenic Fever (grade 4 neutropenia and ≥ grade 2 fever)	Omit dose until resolved, then ↓ 50 mg/m^2	↓ 50 mg/m^2	↓ 50 mg/m^2
Other Hematologic Toxicities	Dose modifications for leukopenia, thrombocytopenia, and anemia during a course of therapy and at the start of subsequent courses of therapy are also based on NCI toxicity criteria and are the same as recommended for neutropenia above.		
Diarrhea			
Grade 1 (2 to 3 stools/day > pretreatment)	Maintain dose level	Maintain dose level	Maintain dose level
Grade 2 (4 to 6 stools/day > pretreatment)	↓ 25 mg/m^2	Maintain dose level	Maintain dose level
Grade 3 (7 to 9 stools/day > pretreatment)	Omit dose until resolved to ≤ grade 2, then ↓ 25 mg/m^2	↓ 25 mg/m^2	↓ 50 mg/m^2
Grade 4 (≥10 stools/day > pretreatment)	Omit dose until resolved to ≤ grade 2, then ↓ 50 mg/m^2	↓ 50 mg/m^2	↓ 50 mg/m^2

(continued)

Colorectal Cancer: Single-Agent Schedule: Recommended Dosage Modifications[1] (continued)

Toxicity NCI Grade[2] (Value)	During a Cycle of Therapy	At Start of Subsequent Cycles of Therapy (After Adequate Recovery), Compared to Starting Dose in Previous Cycle[1]	
	Weekly	Weekly	Once Every 3 Weeks
Other Nonhematologic Toxicities[3]			
Grade 1	Maintain dose level	Maintain dose level	Maintain dose level
Grade 2	$\downarrow$ 25 mg/m^2	$\downarrow$ 25 mg/m^2	$\downarrow$ 50 mg/m^2
Grade 3	Omit dose until resolved to $\leq$ grade 2, then $\downarrow$ 25 mg/m^2	$\downarrow$ 25 mg/m^2	$\downarrow$ 50 mg/m^2
Grade 4	Omit dose until resolved to $\leq$ grade 2, then $\downarrow$ 50 mg/m^2	$\downarrow$ 50 mg/m^2	$\downarrow$ 50 mg/m^2

[1] All dose modifications should be based on the worst preceding toxicity.

[2] National Cancer Institute Common Toxicity Criteria (version 1.0).

[3] Excludes alopecia, anorexia, asthenia.

Colorectal Cancer: Combination Schedules: Recommended Dosage Modifications[1]

Toxicity NCI[2] Grade (Value)	During a Cycle of Therapy	At the Start of Subsequent Cycles of Therapy (After Adequate Recovery), Compared to the Starting Dose in the Previous Cycle[1]
No toxicity	Maintain dose level	Maintain dose level
Neutropenia		
Grade 1 (1,500 to 1,999/mm^3)	Maintain dose level	Maintain dose level
Grade 2 (1,000 to 1,499/mm^3)	$\downarrow$ 1 dose level	Maintain dose level
Grade 3 (500 to 999/mm^3)	Omit dose until resolved to $\leq$ grade 2, then $\downarrow$ 1 dose level	$\downarrow$ 1 dose level
Grade 4 (<500/mm^3)	Omit dose until resolved to $\leq$ grade 2, then $\downarrow$ 2 dose levels	$\downarrow$ 2 dose levels
Neutropenic Fever (grade 4 neutropenia and $\geq$ grade 2 fever)	Omit dose until resolved, then $\downarrow$ 2 dose levels	
Other Hematologic Toxicities	Dose modifications for leukopenia or thrombocytopenia during a course of therapy and at the start of subsequent courses of therapy are also based on NCI toxicity criteria and are the same as recommended for neutropenia above.	
Diarrhea		
Grade 1 (2 to 3 stools/day > pretreatment)	Delay dose until resolved to baseline, then give same dose	Maintain dose level
Grade 2 (4 to 6 stools/day > pretreatment)	Omit dose until resolved to baseline, then $\downarrow$ 1 dose level	Maintain dose level
Grade 3 (7 to 9 stools/day > pretreatment)	Omit dose until resolved to baseline, then $\downarrow$ by 1 dose level	$\downarrow$ 1 dose level
Grade 4 ($\geq$10 stools/day > pretreatment)	Omit dose until resolved, then $\downarrow$ 2 dose levels	$\downarrow$ 2 dose levels

(continued)

Colorectal Cancer: Combination Schedules: Recommended Dosage Modifications[1] (continued)

Toxicity NCI[2] Grade (Value)	During a Cycle of Therapy	At the Start of Subsequent Cycles of Therapy (After Adequate Recovery), Compared to the Starting Dose in the Previous Cycle[1]
Other Nonhematologic Toxicities[3]		
Grade 1	Maintain dose level	Maintain dose level
Grade 2	Omit dose until resolved to ≤ grade 1, then ↓ 1 dose level	Maintain dose level
Grade 3	Omit dose until resolved to ≤ grade 2, then ↓ 1 dose level	↓ 1 dose level
Grade 4	Omit dose until resolved to ≤ grade 2, then ↓ 2 dose levels	↓ 2 dose levels
Mucositis and/or stomatitis	Decrease only 5-FU, not irinotecan	Decrease only 5-FU, not irinotecan

[1]All dose modifications should be based on the worst preceding toxicity.

[2]National Cancer Institute Common Toxicity Criteria (version 1.0).

[3]Excludes alopecia, anorexia, asthenia.

Combination Regimens

Bone sarcoma (Ewing sarcoma): Irinotecan-Temozolomide (Ewing Sarcoma) on page 2161

Brain tumors: Bevacizumab-Irinotecan (Glioblastoma) on page 1994

Colorectal cancer:

Bevacizumab + FOLFIRI (Colorectal) on page 1992

Cetuximab (Biweekly)-Irinotecan (Colorectal) on page 2029

Cetuximab + FOLFIRI (Colorectal) on page 2031

Cetuximab-Irinotecan (Colorectal) on page 2032

Fluorouracil-Leucovorin-Irinotecan (Saltz Regimen) (Colorectal) on page 2126

FOLFIRI (Colorectal) on page 2128

FOLFOXIRI (Colorectal) on page 2132

Panitumumab + FOLFIRI (Colorectal) on page 2189

Ramucirumab-FOLFIRI (Colorectal) on page 2200

Ziv-Aflibercept + FOLFIRI (Colorectal) on page 2234

Esophageal cancer:

Irinotecan-Capecitabine (Esophageal Cancer) on page 2157

Irinotecan-Cisplatin (Esophageal Cancer) on page 2159

Irinotecan-Fluorouracil-Leucovorin (Esophageal Cancer) on page 2160

Gastric cancer:

Cisplatin-Irinotecan (Gastric) on page 2056

Irinotecan-Capecitabine (Gastric Cancer) on page 2158

Irinotecan-Leucovorin-Fluorouracil (Gastric Cancer) on page 2160

Lung cancer (non-small cell): Cisplatin-Irinotecan (NSCLC) on page 2056

Lung cancer (small cell):

Carboplatin-Irinotecan (Small Cell Lung Cancer) on page 2018

Cisplatin-Irinotecan (Small Cell Lung Cancer) on page 2057

Pancreatic cancer: FOLFIRINOX (Pancreatic) on page 2129

Administration Administer by IV infusion, usually over 90 minutes. Irinotecan is associated with a moderate emetic potential (Basch 2011; Dupuis 2011; Roila 2016); premedication with dexamethasone and a 5-HT$_3$ blocker is recommended 30 minutes prior to administration; prochlorperazine may be considered for subsequent use (if needed). Consider atropine 0.25 to 1 mg IV or SubQ as premedication for or treatment of cholinergic symptoms (eg, increased salivation, rhinitis, miosis, diaphoresis, abdominal cramping) or early onset diarrhea.

The recommended regimen to manage late diarrhea is loperamide 4 mg orally at onset of late diarrhea, followed by 2 mg every 2 hours (or 4 mg every 4 hours at night) until 12 hours have passed without a bowel movement. If diarrhea recurs, then repeat administration. Loperamide should not be used for more than 48 consecutive hours.

Vesicant/Extravasation Risk May be an irritant

Emetic Potential Children and Adults: Moderate (30% to 90%)

Monitoring Parameters CBC with differential, platelet count, and hemoglobin with each dose; bilirubin, electrolytes (with severe diarrhea); bowel movements and hydration status; signs/symptoms of pulmonary toxicity or hypersensitivity reactions; monitor infusion site for signs of inflammation and avoid extravasation

A test is available for genotyping of UGT1A1; however, use of the test is not widely accepted and a dose reduction is already recommended in patients who have experienced toxicity.

Dietary Considerations Contains sorbitol; do not use in patients with hereditary fructose intolerance.

Dosage Forms Excipient information presented when available (limited, particularly for generics); consult specific product labeling.
Solution, Intravenous, as hydrochloride:
  Camptosar: 40 mg/2 mL (2 mL); 100 mg/5 mL (5 mL); 300 mg/15 mL (15 mL)
  Generic: 40 mg/2 mL (2 mL); 100 mg/5 mL (5 mL); 500 mg/25 mL (25 mL)
Solution, Intravenous, as hydrochloride [preservative free]:
  Generic: 40 mg/2 mL (2 mL); 100 mg/5 mL (5 mL)

Irinotecan (Liposomal) (eye rye no TEE kan lye po SO mal)

Related Information

Common Toxicity Criteria *on page 2242*

Management of Chemotherapy-Induced Nausea and Vomiting in Adults *on page 2253*

Safe Handling of Hazardous Drugs *on page 2379*

Brand Names: US Onivyde

Index Terms Irinotecan Liposome; Liposomal Irinotecan; Liposome-Encapsulated Irinotecan Hydrochloride PEP02; MM-398; Onivyde

Pharmacologic Category Antineoplastic Agent, Camptothecin; Antineoplastic Agent, Topoisomerase I Inhibitor

Use

Pancreatic adenocarcinoma, metastatic: Treatment of metastatic adenocarcinoma of the pancreas (in combination with fluorouracil and leucovorin) disease progression following gemcitabine-based therapy.

Limitations of use: Irinotecan (liposomal) is not indicated as a single agent for the treatment of metastatic adenocarcinoma of the pancreas.

Labeled Contraindications Severe hypersensitivity to irinotecan (liposomal), irinotecan hydrochloride, or any component of the formulation

Pregnancy Considerations Animal reproduction studies have not been conducted with the liposomal formulation. Based on the mechanism of action as well as animal data using irinotecan (conventional), irinotecan (liposomal) may cause fetal harm if administered during pregnancy. Women of child-bearing potential should use effective contraception while receiving treatment and avoid pregnancy for one month following the last dose. Males with female partners of reproductive potential should use condoms during therapy and for four months following the last dose.

Breastfeeding Considerations It is not known if irinotecan (liposomal) is excreted in breast milk. Due to the potential for serious adverse reactions in the nursing infant, the manufacturer does not recommend breastfeeding during therapy or for one month following the last dose.

Warnings/Precautions [US Boxed Warning]: Fatal neutropenic sepsis occurred in nearly 1% of patients receiving irinotecan (liposomal). Severe or life-threatening neutropenic fever or sepsis occurred in 3% and severe or life-threatening neutropenia occurred in 20% of patients receiving irinotecan (liposomal) in combination with fluorouracil and leucovorin. Withhold irinotecan (liposomal) for absolute neutrophil count below 1,500/mm³ or neutropenic fever. Monitor blood cell counts periodically during treatment (days 1 and 8 of each cycle and more frequently if clinically necessary). May require therapy interruption, dose reduction, and/or discontinuation. Anemia, lymphopenia, and thrombocytopenia also commonly occur. The incidence of neutropenia was higher in Asian patients (compared to white patients).

[US Boxed Warning]: Severe diarrhea (may be life-threatening) occurred in 13% of patients receiving irinotecan (liposomal) in combination with fluorouracil and leucovorin. Do not administer irinotecan (liposomal) to patients with bowel obstruction. Withhold irinotecan (liposomal) for diarrhea of grade 2 to 4 severity. Administer loperamide for late diarrhea of any severity. Administer atropine, if not contraindicated, for early diarrhea of any severity. Early onset diarrhea occurs within 24 hours of chemotherapy, and may cause other symptoms of cholinergic reaction. Late onset diarrhea occurs more than 24 hours following chemotherapy. Diarrhea may require therapy interruption, dosage reduction, and/or discontinuation. Nausea, vomiting and stomatitis commonly occur. The pharmacokinetics of irinotecan (liposomal) have not been studied in patients with hepatic impairment. However, exposure to the active metabolite (SN-38) is increased in patients with hepatic impairment receiving irinotecan (conventional); toxicities may be increased.

Irinotecan (conventional) may cause severe and fatal interstitial lung disease (ILD). Withhold irinotecan (liposomal) during diagnostic evaluation if new or progressive dyspnea, cough, or fever occurs during use. Discontinue therapy if ILD diagnosis is confirmed. Severe hypersensitivity reactions (including anaphylaxis) have occurred with irinotecan (conventional). Monitor closely; permanently discontinue irinotecan (liposomal) therapy if severe hypersensitivity occurs. Irinotecan (liposomal) and irinotecan (conventional) are NOT interchangeable. Dosing differs between formulations; verify intended product and dose prior to preparation and administration. Potentially significant interactions may exist, requiring dose or frequency adjustment, additional monitoring, and/or selection of alternative therapy. CYP3A4 enzyme inducers may decrease exposure to irinotecan and SN-38 (active metabolite); avoid concomitant use (substitute non-enzyme inducing therapies at least 2 weeks prior to irinotecan [liposomal] initiation). Enzyme inhibitors may increase exposure; avoid concomitant use (discontinue strong CYP3A4 inhibitors at least 1 week prior to irinotecan [liposomal] initiation).

Adverse Reactions Frequency not always defined. Percentages reported as part of combination chemotherapy regimens.

Cardiovascular: Septic shock (≥2%)

Central nervous system: Fatigue (≤56%)

Dermatologic: Alopecia (14%)

Endocrine & metabolic: Hypoalbuminemia (43%), hypomagnesemia (35%), hypocalcemia (32%), hypokalemia (32%), hypophosphatemia (29%), hyponatremia (27%), weight loss (17%), dehydration (8%)

Gastrointestinal: Diarrhea (59%, grade 3/4: 13%; early onset 30%, grade 3/4: 3%; late onset 43%, grade 3/4: 9%), vomiting (52%), nausea (51%), decreased appetite (44%), stomatitis (32%), gastroenteritis (3%)

Hematologic & oncologic: Anemia (97%, grades 3/4: 6%), lymphocytopenia (81%, grades 3/4: 27%), neutropenia (52%, grades 3/4: 20%; incidence of neutropenia was higher among Asian patients), thrombocytopenia (41%, grades 3/4: 2%), febrile neutropenia (≤3%, grades 3/4: ≤3%)

Hepatic: Increased serum ALT (51%)

Hypersensitivity: Severe hypersensitivity

Infection: Sepsis (4%, grades 3/4: 3%), neutropenic sepsis (≤3%, grades 3/4: ≤3%)

Local: Catheter infection (3%)

Neuromuscular & skeletal: Weakness (≤56%)

Renal: Increased creatinine clearance (18%), acute renal failure (≥2%)

Respiratory: Pneumonia (≥2%), interstitial pulmonary disease

Miscellaneous: Fever (23%)

Drug Interactions

Metabolism/Transport Effects Substrate of BCRP, CYP3A4 (major), P-glycoprotein, SLCO1B1, UGT1A1; **Note:** Assignment of Major/Minor substrate status based on clinically relevant drug interaction potential

Avoid Concomitant Use

Avoid concomitant use of Irinotecan (Liposomal) with any of the following: BCG (Intravesical); Conivaptan; CYP3A4 Inducers (Strong); CYP3A4 Inhibitors (Strong); Deferiprone; Dipyrone; Fusidic Acid (Systemic); Idelalisib; Natalizumab; Pimecrolimus; St John's Wort; Tacrolimus (Topical); UGT1A1 Inhibitors; Vaccines (Live)

Increased Effect/Toxicity

Irinotecan (Liposomal) may increase the levels/effects of: CloZAPine; Deferiprone; Fingolimod; Leflunomide; Natalizumab; Tofacitinib; Vaccines (Live)

The levels/effects of Irinotecan (Liposomal) may be increased by: Aprepitant; Conivaptan; CYP3A4 Inhibitors (Moderate); CYP3A4 Inhibitors (Strong); Dasatinib; Denosumab; Dipyrone; Fosaprepitant; Fusidic Acid (Systemic); Idelalisib; Netupitant; Ocrelizumab; Palbociclib; Palifermin; P-glycoprotein/ABCB1 Inhibitors; Pimecrolimus; Promazine; Ranolazine; Roflumilast; Simeprevir; SORAfenib; Stiripentol; Tacrolimus (Topical); Teriflunomide; Trastuzumab; UGT1A1 Inhibitors

Decreased Effect

Irinotecan (Liposomal) may decrease the levels/effects of: BCG (Intravesical); Coccidioides immitis Skin Test; Lenograstim; Nivolumab; Sipuleucel-T; Tertomotide; Vaccines (Inactivated); Vaccines (Live)

The levels/effects of Irinotecan (Liposomal) may be decreased by: Bosentan; CYP3A4 Inducers (Moderate); CYP3A4 Inducers (Strong); Dabrafenib; Deferasirox; Echinacea; Sarilumab; Siltuximab; St John's Wort; Tocilizumab

Food Interactions Irinotecan serum concentrations may be increased when taken with grapefruit juice. Management: Avoid ingestion of large quantities and/or concentrated grapefruit juice

Hazardous Drugs Handling Considerations

Hazardous agent (NIOSH 2016 [group 1]).

Use appropriate precautions for receiving, handling, administration, and disposal. Gloves (single) should be worn during receiving, unpacking, and placing in storage.

NIOSH recommends double gloving, a protective gown, ventilated engineering controls (a class II biological safety cabinet or a compounding aseptic containment isolator), and closed system transfer devices (CSTDs) for preparation. Double gloving, a gown, and (if dosage form allows) CSTDs are required during administration (NIOSH 2016).

Storage/Stability Store intact vials at 2°C to 8°C (36°F to 46°F); do not freeze. Protect from light. Solution diluted for administration in D5W or NS is stable for up to 4 hours when stored at room temperature, or up to 24 hours when refrigerated (administration should be completed within these time frames). Allow diluted solution to come to room temperature prior to administration.

Preparation for Administration Withdraw appropriate dose from the vial and dilute in 500 mL D5W or NS. Mix by gentle inversion; protect diluted solution from light.

Mechanism of Action Irinotecan (liposomal) is a topoisomerase 1 inhibitor encapsulated in a lipid bilayer (liposome). Irinotecan and its active metabolite (SN-38) bind reversibly to topoisomerase I-DNA complex preventing re-ligation of the cleaved DNA strand. This results in the accumulation of cleavable complexes and double-strand DNA breaks. As mammalian cells cannot efficiently repair these breaks, cell death consistent with S-phase cell cycle specificity occurs, leading to termination of cellular replication.

Pharmacodynamics/Kinetics

Distribution: 4.1 L; 95% of irinotecan remains liposome-encapsulated

Protein binding: <1%

Metabolism: Irinotecan hydrochloride: Primarily hepatic to SN-38 (active metabolite) by carboxylesterase enzymes; may also undergo CYP3A4-mediated metabolism to inactive metabolites (one of which may be hydrolyzed to release SN-38). SN-38 undergoes conjugation by UDP-glucuronosyl transferase 1A1 (UGT1A1) to form a glucuronide metabolite. SN-38 is increased by UGT1A1*28 polymorphism (10% of North Americans are homozygous for UGT1A1*28 allele).

Half-life elimination: Total irinotecan: ~26 hours; SN-38: ~68 hours

Excretion: Urine: Irinotecan hydrochloride (11% to 20%), metabolites (SN-38 <1%, SN-38 glucuronide, 3%)

Dosing

Adult & Geriatric Note: Premedicate with a corticosteroid and an antiemetic 30 minutes prior to infusion. Irinotecan (liposomal) and irinotecan (conventional) are NOT interchangeable. Dosing differs between formulations; verify intended product and dose prior to preparation and administration.

◀ **Pancreatic adenocarcinoma, metastatic:** IV: 70 mg/m^2 once every 2 weeks (in combination with fluorouracil and leucovorin). **Note:** Reduce initial starting dose to 50 mg/m^2 in patients known to be homozygous for the UGT1A1*28 allele; the dose may be increased to 70 mg/m^2 as tolerated in subsequent cycles.

Renal Impairment

CrCl 30 to 89 mL/minute: There are no dosage adjustments provided in the manufacturer's labeling; however, a population pharmacokinetic analysis showed no effect on total SN-38 exposure in patients with mild to moderate renal impairment.

CrCl <30 mL/minute: There are no dosage adjustments provided in the manufacturer's labeling (insufficient data).

Hepatic Impairment Bilirubin >ULN: There are no dosage adjustments provided in the manufacturer's labeling.

Adjustment for Toxicity **Note:** Fluorouracil and leucovorin may also require dosage adjustment.

Hematologic toxicity: ANC <1,500/mm^3 or neutropenic fever: Withhold treatment. Resume therapy when ANC ≥1,500/mm^3 with a reduced dose for grade 3 or 4 neutropenia or neutropenic fever in subsequent cycles:

First occurrence: Reduce dose to 50 mg/m^2 (in patients receiving 70 mg/m^2); reduce dose to 43 mg/m^2 in patients homozygous for UGT1A1*28 without previous increase to 70 mg/m^2

Second occurrence: Reduce dose to 43 mg/m^2 (in patients receiving 50 mg/m^2); reduce dose to 35 mg/m^2 in patients homozygous for UGT1A1*28 previously receiving 43 mg/m^2

Third occurrence: Discontinue

Nonhematologic toxicity:

Anaphylactic reaction: Discontinue permanently

Diarrhea: Withhold therapy for grade 2 to 4 diarrhea. Administer IV or SubQ atropine 0.25 to 1 mg (unless clinically contraindicated) for early-onset diarrhea of any severity. Administer loperamide for late-onset diarrhea of any severity. Following recovery to ≤ grade 1 diarrhea, resume treatment at a reduced dose:

First occurrence: Reduce dose to 50 mg/m^2 (in patients receiving 70 mg/m^2); reduce dose to 43 mg/m^2 in patients homozygous for UGT1A1*28 without previous increase to 70 mg/m^2

Second occurrence: Reduce dose to 43 mg/m^2 (in patients receiving 50 mg/m^2); reduce dose to 35 mg/m^2 in patients homozygous for UGT1A1*28 previously receiving 43 mg/m^2

Third occurrence: Discontinue

Interstitial lung disease (ILD): Discontinue

Other grade 3 or 4 adverse reactions: Withhold therapy. Upon recovery to ≤ grade 1 toxicity, resume treatment at a reduced dose:

First occurrence: Reduce dose to 50 mg/m^2 (in patients receiving 70 mg/m^2); reduce dose to 43 mg/m^2 in patients homozygous for UGT1A1*28 without previous increase to 70 mg/m^2

Second occurrence: Reduce dose to 43 mg/m^2 (in patients receiving 50 mg/m^2); reduce dose to 35 mg/m^2 in patients homozygous for UGT1A1*28 previously receiving 43 mg/m^2

Third occurrence: Discontinue

Combination Regimens

Pancreatic cancer: Fluorouracil-Leucovorin-Irinotecan (Liposomal) (Pancreatic) on page 2126

Administration

Administer by IV infusion over 90 minutes. Premedicate with a corticosteroid and an antiemetic 30 minutes prior to infusion. Administer irinotecan (liposomal) prior to fluorouracil and leucovorin. Do not use in-line filters for administration.

Administer IV or SubQ atropine 0.25 to 1 mg (unless clinically contraindicated) for early onset diarrhea of any severity; initiate loperamide for late-onset diarrhea of any severity.

Emetic Potential Low (10% to 30%)

Monitoring Parameters Complete blood counts on days 1 and 8 of each cycle and as clinically indicated; bilirubin, electrolytes (with severe diarrhea); bowel movements (diarrhea episodes) and hydration status; signs/symptoms of pulmonary toxicity or hypersensitivity reactions

Dosage Forms Excipient information presented when available (limited, particularly for generics); consult specific product labeling.

Injectable, Intravenous:

Onivyde: 43 mg/10 mL (10 mL) [contains mpeg-2000-dspe (methoxy-terminated peg)]

◆ **Irinotecan For Injection (Can)** *see* Irinotecan (Conventional) *on page* 1037

◆ **Irinotecan HCl** *see* Irinotecan (Conventional) *on page* 1037

◆ **Irinotecan Hydrochloride** *see* Irinotecan (Conventional) *on page* 1037

◆ **Irinotecan Hydrochloride Injection (Can)** *see* Irinotecan (Conventional) *on page* 1037

◆ **Irinotecan Hydrochloride Trihydrate For Injection (Can)** *see* Irinotecan (Conventional) *on page* 1037

◆ **Irinotecan Hydrochloride Trihydrate Injection (Can)** *see* Irinotecan (Conventional) *on page* 1037

◆ **Irinotecan Liposome** *see* Irinotecan (Liposomal) *on page* 1048

◆ **Iron (III) Hydroxide Sucrose Complex** *see* Iron Sucrose *on page* 1057

◆ **Iron Dextran** *see* Iron Dextran Complex *on page* 1053

Iron Dextran Complex (EYE ern DEKS tran KOM pleks)

Brand Names: US Dexferrum [DSC]; Infed

Brand Names: Canada Dexiron; Infufer

Index Terms High-Molecular-Weight Iron Dextran (DexFerrum); Imferon; Iron Dextran; Low-Molecular-Weight Iron Dextran (INFeD)

Pharmacologic Category Iron Salt

Use Iron deficiency: Treatment of iron deficiency in patients in whom oral administration is unsatisfactory or infeasible

Labeled Contraindications Hypersensitivity to iron dextran or any component of the formulation; any anemia not associated with iron deficiency

Pregnancy Considerations Adverse events have been observed in animal reproduction studies. It is not known if iron dextran (as iron dextran) crosses the placenta. It is recommended that pregnant women meet the dietary requirements of iron with diet and/or supplements in order to prevent adverse events associated with iron deficiency anemia in pregnancy. Treatment of iron deficiency anemia in pregnant women is the same as in nonpregnant women and in most cases, oral iron preparations may be used. Except in severe cases of maternal anemia, the fetus achieves normal iron stores regardless of maternal concentrations.

◄ **Breastfeeding Considerations** Trace amounts of iron dextran (as iron dextran) are found in human milk. Iron is normally found in breast milk. Breast milk or iron fortified formulas generally provide enough iron to meet the recommended dietary requirements of infants. The amount of iron in breast milk is generally not influenced by maternal status.

Warnings/Precautions [U.S. Boxed Warning]: Deaths associated with parenteral administration following anaphylactic-type reactions have been reported (use only where resuscitation equipment and personnel are available). A test dose should be administered to all patients prior to the first therapeutic dose. Fatal reactions have occurred even in patients who tolerated the test dose. Monitor patients for signs/symptoms of anaphylactic reactions during any iron dextran administration; fatalities have occurred with the test dose. A history of drug allergy (including multiple drug allergies) and/or the concomitant use of an ACE inhibitor may increase the risk of anaphylactic-type reactions. Adverse events (including life-threatening) associated with iron dextran usually occur with the high-molecular-weight formulation (Dexferrum), compared to low-molecular-weight (INFeD) (Chertow, 2006). Delayed (1-2 days) infusion reaction (including arthralgia, back pain, chills, dizziness, and fever) may occur with large doses (eg, total dose infusion) of IV iron dextran; usually subsides within 3-4 days. Delayed reaction may also occur (less commonly) with IM administration; subsiding within 3-7 days. Use with caution in patients with a history of significant allergies, asthma, serious hepatic impairment, preexisting cardiac disease (may exacerbate cardiovascular complications), and rheumatoid arthritis (may exacerbate joint pain and swelling). Avoid use during acute kidney infection.

In patients with chronic kidney disease (CKD) requiring iron supplementation, the IV route is preferred for hemodialysis patients; either oral iron or IV iron may be used for nondialysis and peritoneal dialysis CKD patients. In patients with cancer-related anemia (either due to cancer or chemotherapy-induced) requiring iron supplementation, the IV route is superior to oral therapy; IM administration is not recommended for parenteral iron supplementation.

[U.S. Boxed Warning]: Use only in patients where the iron deficient state is not amenable to oral iron therapy. Discontinue oral iron prior to initiating parenteral iron therapy. Exogenous hemosiderosis may result from excess iron stores; patients with refractory anemias and/or hemoglobinopathies may be prone to iron overload with unwarranted iron supplementation. Anemia in the elderly is often caused by "anemia of chronic disease" or associated with inflammation rather than blood loss. Iron stores are usually normal or increased, with a serum ferritin >50 ng/mL and a decreased total iron binding capacity. IV administration of iron dextran is often preferred over IM in the elderly secondary to a decreased muscle mass and the need for daily injections. Intramuscular injections of iron-carbohydrate complexes may have a risk of delayed injection site tumor development. Iron dextran products differ in chemical characteristics. The high-molecular-weight formulation (Dexferrum) and the low-molecular-weight formulation (INFeD) are not clinically interchangeable. Intramuscular iron dextran use in neonates may be associated with an increased incidence of gram-negative sepsis.

Adverse Reactions Frequency not defined. Adverse event risk is reported to be higher with the high-molecular-weight iron dextran formulation.

Cardiovascular: Bradycardia, cardiac arrhythmia, chest pain, chest tightness, flushing, hypertension, hypotension, shock, syncope, tachycardia

Central nervous system: Chills, disorientation, dizziness, headache, loss of consciousness, malaise, paresthesia, seizure, unresponsive to stimuli

Dermatologic: Diaphoresis, pruritus, skin rash, urticaria

Gastrointestinal: Abdominal pain, diarrhea, dysgeusia, nausea, vomiting

Genitourinary: Hematuria, urine discoloration

Hematologic & oncologic: Leukocytosis, lymphadenopathy, purpura

Hypersensitivity: Anaphylaxis (includes acute respiratory distress, circulatory shock)

Infection: Sterile abscess

Local: Injection site reaction (includes injection site cellulitis, inflammation at injection site, injection site phlebitis, local soreness/soreness at injection site, pain at injection site, swelling at injection site), local discoloration (at the site of intramuscular injection)

Neuromuscular & skeletal: Amyotrophy (with intramuscular injection), arthralgia, arthritis, back pain, exacerbation of arthritis, myalgia, weakness

Respiratory: Bronchospasm, cyanosis, dyspnea, wheezing

Miscellaneous: Fever, fibrosis (with intramuscular injection)

<1%, postmarketing, and/or case reports: Angioedema, neoplasm (at former injection site)

Drug Interactions

Metabolism/Transport Effects None known.

Avoid Concomitant Use

Avoid concomitant use of Iron Dextran Complex with any of the following: Dimercaprol

Increased Effect/Toxicity

The levels/effects of Iron Dextran Complex may be increased by: ACE Inhibitors; Dimercaprol

Decreased Effect

Iron Dextran Complex may decrease the levels/effects of: Entacapone

Storage/Stability Store at 20°C to 25°C (68°F to 77°F); excursions permitted to 15°C to 30°C (59°F to 86°F).

Preparation for Administration Solutions for infusion should be diluted in 250-1000 mL NS.

Mechanism of Action The released iron, from the plasma, eventually replenishes the depleted iron stores in the bone marrow where it is incorporated into hemoglobin

Pharmacodynamics/Kinetics

Onset of action: Hematologic response to either oral or parenteral iron salts is essentially the same; red blood cell form and color changes within 3 to 10 days

Maximum effect: Peak reticulocytosis occurs in 5 to 10 days, and hemoglobin values increase within 2 to 4 weeks; serum ferritin peak: 7 to 9 days after IV dose

Absorption:

IM: 60% absorbed after 3 days; 90% after 1 to 3 weeks, the balance is slowly absorbed over months

IV: Uptake of iron by the reticuloendothelial system appears to be constant at about 10 to 20 mg/hour

Half-life elimination: 48 hours

Excretion: Urine and feces via reticuloendothelial system

Dosing

Adult & Geriatric Note: Dexferrum has been discontinued in the US for more than 1 year.

Note: A 0.5 mL test dose should be given prior to starting iron dextran therapy.

Iron-deficiency anemia: IM (INFeD), IV (Dexferrum, INFeD):

Dose (mL) = 0.0442 (desired hemoglobin - observed hemoglobin) x LBW + (0.26 x LBW)

Desired hemoglobin: Usually 14.8 g/dL

LBW = Lean body weight in kg

Iron replacement therapy for blood loss: (INFeD), IV (Dexferrum, INFeD):

Replacement iron (mg) = blood loss (mL) x Hct

Maximum daily dosage: Manufacturer's labeling: **Note:** Replacement of larger estimated iron deficits may be achieved by serial administration of smaller incremental dosages. Daily dosages should be limited to 100 mg iron (2 mL)

Cancer-/chemotherapy-associated anemia: IV: **Note:** Use the iron-deficiency anemia equation for determining a calculated dose, when applicable.

Weekly administration (off-label dosing; INFed):

Weeks 1-3: Test dose of 25 mg (over 1-2 minutes), followed by 75 mg (bolus) once weekly

Weeks 4 and after: 100 mg over 5 minutes once weekly until the calculated dose is reached (Auerbach, 2004)

or

Week 1: Test dose of 25 mg (slow IV push), followed 1 hour later by 75 mg over 5 minutes

Weeks 2-10: 100 mg over 5 minutes once weekly for a total cumulative dose of 1000 mg (NCCN anemia guidelines v.2.2014)

Total dose infusion (off-label dosing; INFeD):

Test dose of 25 mg (over 1-2 minutes), followed 1 hour later by the balance of the calculated total dose mixed in 500 mL NS and infused at 175 mL/hour (Auerbach, 2004)

or

Test dose of 25 mg (slow IV push) followed 1 hour later by the balance of the total dose as a single infusion over several hours; if calculated dose exceeds 1000 mg, administer remaining dose in excess of 1000 mg after 4 weeks if inadequate hemoglobin response (NCCN anemia guidelines v.2.2014)

Pediatric Note: Dexferrum has been discontinued in the US for more than 1 year.

Note: A 0.5 mL test dose (0.25 mL in infants) should be given prior to starting iron dextran therapy.

Iron-deficiency anemia: IM (INFeD), IV (Dexferrum, INFeD):

Children 5-15 kg: Should not normally be given in the first 4 months of life: Dose (mL) = 0.0442 (desired hemoglobin - observed hemoglobin) x W + (0.26 x W)

Desired hemoglobin: Usually 12 g/dL

W = Total body weight in kg

Children >15 kg: Refer to adult dosing.

Iron replacement therapy for blood loss: Refer to adult dosing.

Maximum daily dose:

Children <5 kg: 25 mg iron (0.5 mL)

Children 5-10 kg: 50 mg iron (1 mL)

Children ≥10 kg: Refer to adult dosing.

Renal Impairment Hemodialysis: Nondialyzable. No dosage adjustment provided in manufacturer's labeling.

Hepatic Impairment No dosage adjustment provided in manufacturer's labeling.

Administration Note: A test dose should be given on the first day of therapy; patient should be observed for 1 hour for hypersensitivity reaction, then the remainder of the day's dose (dose minus test dose) should be given. Resuscitation equipment, medication, and trained personnel should be available. An uneventful test dose does not ensure an anaphylactic-type reaction will not occur during administration of the therapeutic dose.

IM (INFeD): Use Z-track technique (displacement of the skin laterally prior to injection); injection should be deep into the upper outer quadrant of buttock; alternate buttocks with subsequent injections. Administer test dose at same recommended site using the same technique.

IV: Test dose should be given gradually over at least 30 seconds (INFeD) or 5 minutes (Dexferrum), or over 1-2 minutes (INFeD) for cancer-/chemotherapy-associated anemia (Auerbach, 2004). Subsequent dose(s) may be administered by IV bolus undiluted at a rate not to exceed 50 mg/minute (maximum 100 mg). For total dose infusion in patients with cancer-/chemotherapy-associated anemia (off-label dose): 1 hour after the test dose, administer the balance of the dose diluted in 500 mL NS and infuse at 175 mL/hour (Auerbach, 2004) or administer over several hours (NCCN Anemia guidelines v.2.2104). Avoid dilutions with dextrose (increased incidence of local pain and phlebitis).

Monitoring Parameters Hemoglobin, hematocrit, reticulocyte count, serum ferritin, serum iron, TIBC; monitor for anaphylaxis/hypersensitivity reaction (during test dose and therapeutic dose)

Test Interactions May cause falsely elevated values of serum bilirubin and falsely decreased values of serum calcium. Residual iron dextran may remain in reticuloendothelial cells; may affect accuracy of examination of bone marrow iron stores. Bone scans with 99m Tc-labeled bone seeking agents may show reduced bony uptake, marked renal activity, and excess blood pooling and soft tissue accumulation following IV iron dextran infusion or with high serum ferritin levels. Following IM iron dextran, bone scans with 99m Tc-diphosphonate may show dense activity in the buttocks.

Product Availability Note: Dexferrum has been discontinued in the US for more than 1 year.

Dosage Forms Considerations Strength of iron dextran complex is expressed as elemental iron.

Dosage Forms Excipient information presented when available (limited, particularly for generics); consult specific product labeling. [DSC] = Discontinued product

Solution, Injection:

Dexferrum: 50 mg/mL (1 mL [DSC], 2 mL [DSC])

Infed: 50 mg/mL (2 mL)

Iron Sucrose (EYE ern SOO krose)

Brand Names: US Venofer

Brand Names: Canada Venofer

Index Terms Iron (III) Hydroxide Sucrose Complex; Iron sucrose complex, inj

Pharmacologic Category Iron Salt

Use Iron deficiency anemia: Treatment of iron-deficiency anemia in chronic kidney disease (CKD)

Labeled Contraindications Known hypersensitivity to iron sucrose or any component of the formulation

Pregnancy Considerations Teratogenic effects were not observed in animal studies. There are no adequate and well-controlled studies in pregnant women. Based on limited data, iron sucrose may be effective for the treatment of iron-deficiency anemia in pregnancy. It is recommended that pregnant women meet the dietary requirements of iron with diet and/or supplements in order to prevent adverse events associated with iron deficiency anemia in pregnancy. Treatment of iron deficiency anemia in pregnant women is the same as in nonpregnant women and in most cases, oral iron preparations may be used. Except in severe cases of maternal anemia, the fetus achieves normal iron stores regardless of maternal concentrations.

Breastfeeding Considerations Iron is normally found in breast milk. Breast milk or iron fortified formulas generally provide enough iron to meet the recommended dietary requirements of infants. The amount of iron in breast milk is generally not influenced by maternal iron status.

Warnings/Precautions Hypersensitivity reactions, including rare postmarketing anaphylactic and anaphylactoid reactions (some fatal), have been reported; monitor patients during and for ≥30 minutes postadministration; discontinue immediately for signs/symptoms of a hypersensitivity reaction (shock, hypotension, loss of consciousness). Equipment for resuscitation and trained personnel experienced in handling medical emergencies should always be immediately available. Significant hypotension has been reported frequently in hemodialysis-dependent patients. Hypotension has also been reported in peritoneal dialysis and nondialysis patients. Hypotension may be related to total dose or rate of administration (avoid rapid IV injection), follow recommended guidelines. Withhold iron in the presence of tissue iron overload; periodic monitoring of hemoglobin, hematocrit, serum ferritin, and transferrin saturation is recommended.

Adverse Reactions Events and incidences are associated with use in adults unless otherwise specified.

>10%:
- Cardiovascular: Hypotension (2% to 3%; children: 2%; hemodialysis patients: 39%; may be related to total dose or rate of administration)
- Central nervous system: Headache (3% to 13%; children: 6%)
- Gastrointestinal: Nausea (5% to 15%; children: 3%)
- Neuromuscular & skeletal: Muscle cramps (1% to 3%; hemodialysis patients: 29%)
- Respiratory: Nasopharyngitis (2% to 16%), pharyngitis (2% to 16%), sinusitis (2% to 16%), upper respiratory tract infection (2% to 16%; children: 4%)

1% to 10%:
- Cardiovascular: Hypertension (7% to 8%; children: 2%), peripheral edema (3% to 7%), chest pain (1% to 6%), thrombosis (children: 2%; arteriovenous fistula), cardiac failure (>1%)
- Central nervous system: Dizziness (1% to 7%; children: 4%)
- Dermatologic: Pruritus (2% to 4%)
- Endocrine & metabolic: Hypoglycemia (≤4%), hypervolemia (1% to 3%), gout (≤3%), hyperglycemia (≤3%)
- Gastrointestinal: Vomiting (5% to 9%; children: 4%), diarrhea (5% to 8%), dysgeusia (≤8%), peritonitis (children: 4%), abdominal pain (1% to 4%)
- Immunologic: Graft complications (≤10%)
- Infection: Sepsis (>1%)
- Local: Injection site reaction (≤6%)

Neuromuscular & skeletal: Limb pain (3% to 6%), arthralgia (1% to 4%), myalgia (≤4%), weakness (1% to 3%), back pain (1% to 2%)

Ophthalmic: Conjunctivitis (≤3%)

Otic: Otalgia (≤2%)

Respiratory: Dyspnea (1% to 6%), cough (1% to 3%; children: 4%), nasal congestion (≤1%)

Miscellaneous: Fever (1% to 3%; children: 4%)

<1%, postmarketing, and/or case reports: Anaphylactic shock, anaphylactoid reaction, angioedema, bradycardia, bronchospasm, circulatory shock, confusion, facial rash, hyperhidrosis, hypersensitivity reaction (including wheezing), hypoesthesia, joint swelling, local discoloration (at injection site following extravasation), loss of consciousness, necrotizing enterocolitis (reported in premature infants; no causal relationship established), paresthesia, seizure, shock, urine discoloration, urticaria

Drug Interactions

Metabolism/Transport Effects None known.

Avoid Concomitant Use

Avoid concomitant use of Iron Sucrose with any of the following: Dimercaprol

Increased Effect/Toxicity

Iron Sucrose may increase the levels/effects of: Amifostine; Antipsychotic Agents (Second Generation [Atypical]); DULoxetine; Hypotension-Associated Agents; Levodopa; Nitroprusside; Pholcodine

The levels/effects of Iron Sucrose may be increased by: Alfuzosin; Barbiturates; Benperidol; Blood Pressure Lowering Agents; Brimonidine (Topical); Diazoxide; Dimercaprol; Herbs (Hypotensive Properties); Lormetazepam; Molsidomine; Naftopidil; Nicergoline; Nicorandil; Obinutuzumab; Pentoxifylline; Phosphodiesterase 5 Inhibitors; Prostacyclin Analogues; Quinagolide

Decreased Effect

Iron Sucrose may decrease the levels/effects of: Entacapone

Storage/Stability Store intact vials at controlled room temperature of 20°C to 25°C (68°F to 77°F); excursions permitted to 15°C to 30°C (59°F to 86°F); do not freeze. Iron sucrose is stable for 7 days at room temperature (23°C to 27°C [73°F to 81°F]) or under refrigeration (2°C to 6°C [36°F to 43°F]) when undiluted in a plastic syringe or following dilution in normal saline in a plastic syringe (concentration 2-10 mg/mL) or for 7 days at room temperature (23°C to 27°C [73°F to 81°F]) following dilution in normal saline in an IV bag (concentration 1-2 mg/mL).

Preparation for Administration

Children: May administer undiluted or diluted in 25 mL of NS. Do not dilute to concentrations <1 mg/mL.

Adults: Doses ≤200 mg may be administered undiluted or diluted in a maximum of 100 mL NS. Doses >200 mg should be diluted in a maximum of 250 mL NS. Do not dilute to concentrations <1 mg/mL.

Mechanism of Action Iron sucrose is dissociated by the reticuloendothelial system into iron and sucrose. The released iron increases serum iron concentrations and is incorporated into hemoglobin.

Pharmacodynamics/Kinetics

Onset of action: Hematologic response to either oral or parenteral iron salts is essentially the same; red blood cell form and color changes within 3-10 days

Maximum effect: Peak reticulocytosis occurs in 5-10 days, and hemoglobin values increase within 2-4 weeks

Distribution: V_{dss}: Healthy adults: 7.9 L

◀ Metabolism: Dissociated into iron and sucrose by the reticuloendothelial system

Half-life elimination: Healthy adults: 6 hours; Nondialysis-dependent adolescents: 8 hours

Excretion: Healthy adults: Urine (5%) within 24 hours

Dosing

Adult & Geriatric Doses expressed in mg of **elemental** iron. **Note:** Test dose: Product labeling does not indicate need for a test dose in product-naive patients.

Iron-deficiency anemia in chronic kidney disease (CKD): IV:

Hemodialysis-dependent patient: 100 mg administered during consecutive dialysis sessions to a cumulative total dose of 1000 mg (10 doses); may repeat treatment if clinically indicated.

Peritoneal dialysis-dependent patient: Two infusions of 300 mg administered 14 days apart, followed by a single 400 mg infusion 14 days later (total cumulative dose of 1000 mg in 3 divided doses); may repeat treatment if clinically indicated.

Nondialysis-dependent patient: 200 mg administered on 5 different occasions within a 14-day period (total cumulative dose: 1000 mg in 14-day period); may repeat treatment if clinically indicated. **Note:** Dosage has also been administered as 2 infusions of 500 mg on day 1 and day 14 (limited experience).

Chemotherapy-associated anemia (off-label use): IV: 200 mg once every 3 weeks for 5 doses (Bastit, 2008) or 100 mg once weekly during weeks 0 to 6, followed by 100 mg every other week from weeks 8 to 14 (Hedenus, 2007)

Pediatric Doses expressed in mg of **elemental** iron. **Note:** Test dose: Product labeling does not indicate need for a test dose in product-naive patients.

Iron-deficiency anemia in chronic kidney disease (CKD): Children ≥2 years and Adolescents: IV: **Note:** Not indicated for iron replacement treatment in children and adolescents.

Hemodialysis-dependent patient: Maintenance therapy: 0.5 mg/kg/dose (maximum: 100 mg) every 2 weeks for 6 doses; may repeat if clinically indicated.

Nondialysis-dependent patient: Maintenance therapy: 0.5 mg/kg/dose (maximum: 100 mg) every 4 weeks for 3 doses; may repeat if clinically indicated

Peritoneal dialysis-dependent patient: Maintenance therapy: 0.5 mg/kg/dose (maximum: 100 mg) every 4 weeks for 3 doses; may repeat if clinically indicated

Renal Impairment

No dosage adjustment provided in manufacturer's labeling.

Hemodialysis: Not dialyzable

Hepatic Impairment No dosage adjustment provided in manufacturer's labeling.

Administration Administer intravenously as a slow IV injection (**not** for rapid IV injection) or as an IV infusion. Can be administered through dialysis line.

Children and Adolescents:

Slow IV injection: Administer undiluted over 5 minutes

Infusion: Infuse diluted solution over 5-60 minutes

Adults:

Slow IV injection: May administer doses ≤200 mg undiluted by slow IV injection over 2-5 minutes. When administering to hemodialysis-dependent patients, give iron sucrose early during the dialysis session.

Infusion: Infuse diluted doses ≤200 mg over at least 15 minutes; infuse diluted 300 mg dose over 1.5 hours; infuse diluted 400 mg dose over 2.5 hours; infuse diluted 500 mg dose over 3.5-4 hours (limited experience). When administering to hemodialysis-dependent patients, give iron sucrose early during the dialysis session.

Monitoring Parameters

CKD patients: Hematocrit, hemoglobin, serum ferritin, serum iron, transferrin, percent transferrin saturation (TSAT), TIBC (takes ~4 weeks of treatment to see increased serum iron and ferritin, and decreased TIBC); iron status should be assessed ≥48 hours after last dose (due to rapid increase in values following administration); signs/symptoms of hypersensitivity reactions (during and ≥30 minutes following infusion); hypotension (during and following infusion)

Chemotherapy-associated anemia (off-label use): Iron, total iron-binding capacity, transferrin saturation, or ferritin levels at baseline and periodically (Rizzo, 2011)

Dosage Forms Considerations Strength of iron sucrose is expressed as elemental iron.

Dosage Forms Excipient information presented when available (limited, particularly for generics); consult specific product labeling.

Solution, Intravenous [preservative free]:

Venofer: 20 mg/mL (2.5 mL, 5 mL, 10 mL)

♦ **Iron sucrose complex, inj** see Iron Sucrose on page 1057

♦ **Isavuconazole** see Isavuconazonium Sulfate on page 1061

Isavuconazonium Sulfate (eye sa vue koe na ZOE nee um sul FATE)

Brand Names: US Cresemba

Index Terms BAL8557; Isavuconazole

Pharmacologic Category Antifungal Agent, Azole Derivative; Antifungal Agent, Oral; Antifungal Agent, Parenteral

Use

Aspergillosis: Treatment of invasive aspergillosis in adults

Mucormycosis: Treatment of invasive mucormycosis in adults

Pregnancy Risk Factor C

Dosing

Adult & Geriatric Note: Dosage expressed as milligrams of isavuconazonium sulfate; switching between the intravenous (IV) and oral formulations of isavuconazonium sulfate is acceptable; for maintenance dosing, it is not necessary to restart dosing with the initial dose regimen when switching between formulations.

Aspergillosis, invasive:

IV: Initial: 372 mg (isavuconazole 200 mg) every 8 hours for 6 doses; Maintenance: 372 mg (isavuconazole 200 mg) once daily. Start maintenance dose 12 to 24 hours after the last loading dose.

Oral: Initial: 372 mg (isavuconazole 200 mg) every 8 hours for 6 doses; Maintenance: 372 mg (isavuconazole 200 mg) once daily. Start maintenance dose 12 to 24 hours after the last loading dose.

Duration of therapy: Minimum of 6 to 12 weeks, although duration is highly dependent on degree/duration of immunosuppression, disease site, and evidence of disease improvement (IDSA [Patterson 2016])

Mucormycosis, invasive:

IV: Initial: 372 mg (isavuconazole 200 mg) every 8 hours for 6 doses; Maintenance: 372 mg (isavuconazole 200 mg) once daily. Start maintenance dose 12 to 24 hours after the last loading dose.

Oral: Initial: 372 mg (isavuconazole 200 mg) every 8 hours for 6 doses; Maintenance: 372 mg (isavuconazole 200 mg) once daily. Start maintenance dose 12 to 24 hours after the last loading dose.

Renal Impairment No dosage adjustment necessary.

Hepatic Impairment

Mild or moderate impairment (Child-Pugh class A or B): No dosage adjustment necessary.

Severe impairment (Child-Pugh class C): There are no dosage adjustments provided in the manufacturer's labeling (has not been studied); use with caution.

Additional Information Complete prescribing information should be consulted for additional detail.

Dosage Forms Excipient information presented when available (limited, particularly for generics); consult specific product labeling.

Capsule, Oral:

Cresemba: 186 mg [contains disodium edta]

Solution Reconstituted, Intravenous:

Cresemba: 372 mg (1 ea)

◆ **ISG** *see* Immune Globulin *on page 992*

◆ **Isophosphamide** *see* Ifosfamide *on page 962*

Isosulfan Blue (eye soe SUL fan bloo)

Index Terms Lymphazurin

Pharmacologic Category Contrast Agent

Use Lymphatic vessel delineation: Adjunct to lymphography to delineate lymphatic vessels in primary and secondary lymphedema of the extremities; chyluria, chylous ascites or chylothorax; lymph node involvement by primary or secondary neoplasm; and lymph node response to therapeutic modalities for visualization of the lymphatic system draining the region of injection.

Pregnancy Risk Factor C

Dosing

Adult Lymphatic vessel delineation: SubQ: Inject 0.5 mL into 3 interdigital spaces of each extremity per study; maximum dose: 3 mL (30 mg)

Renal Impairment There are no dosage adjustments provided in the manufacturer's labeling.

Hepatic Impairment There are no dosage adjustments provided in the manufacturer's labeling.

Additional Information Complete prescribing information should be consulted for additional detail.

Dosage Forms Excipient information presented when available (limited, particularly for generics); consult specific product labeling.

Solution, Subcutaneous:

Generic: 1% (5 mL)

Solution, Subcutaneous [preservative free]:

Generic: 1% (5 mL)

ISOtretinoin (eye soe TRET i noyn)

Related Information

Management of EGFR Inhibitor Toxicities: Dermatologic, Ocular, and Gastro-intestinal *on page 2291*

Safe Handling of Hazardous Drugs *on page 2379*

Brand Names: US Absorica; Amnesteem; Claravis; Myorisan; Zenatane

Brand Names: Canada Accutane; Clarus; Epuris

Index Terms 13-*cis*-Retinoic Acid; 13-*cis*-Vitamin A Acid; 13-CRA; *Cis*-Retinoic Acid; Accutane; Isotretinoinum

Pharmacologic Category Acne Products; Antineoplastic Agent, Retinoic Acid Derivative; Retinoic Acid Derivative

Use Acne, severe recalcitrant nodular: Treatment of severe recalcitrant nodular acne unresponsive to conventional therapy (including systemic antibiotics)

Labeled Contraindications

Hypersensitivity to isotretinoin or any component of the formulation; sensitivity to parabens (Zenatane only) or vitamin A; pregnant women or those who may become pregnant

Canadian labeling: Additional contraindications not in the US labeling: Breast-feeding, hepatic or renal insufficiency, hypervitaminosis A, excessive hyperlipidemia, concurrent tetracycline therapy.

Documentation of allergenic cross-reactivity for retinoids is limited. However, because of similarities in chemical structure and/or pharmacologic actions, the possibility of cross-sensitivity cannot be ruled out with certainty.

Pregnancy Considerations Isotretinoin and its metabolites can be detected in fetal tissue following maternal use during pregnancy (Benifla 1995; Kraft 1989). **[US Boxed Warnings]: Use of isotretinoin is contraindicated in females who are or may become pregnant. Birth defects (facial, eye, ear, skull, central nervous system, cardiovascular, thymus and parathyroid gland abnormalities) have been noted following isotretinoin exposure during pregnancy and the risk for severe birth defects is high, with any dose or even with short treatment duration. Low IQ scores have also been reported. The risk for spontaneous abortion and premature births is increased. Because of the high likelihood of teratogenic effects, all patients (male and female), prescribers, wholesalers, and dispensing pharmacists must register and be active in the iPLEDGE™ risk evaluation and mitigation strategy (REMS) program; do not prescribe isotretinoin for women who are or who are likely to become pregnant while using the drug. If pregnancy occurs during therapy, isotretinoin should be discontinued immediately and the patient referred to an obstetrician-gynecologist specializing in reproductive toxicity.** This medication is contraindicated in females of childbearing potential unless they are able to comply with the guidelines of the iPLEDGE™ pregnancy prevention program. Females of childbearing potential must have two negative pregnancy tests with a sensitivity of at least 25 milliunits/mL prior to beginning therapy and testing should continue monthly during therapy. Females of childbearing potential should not become pregnant during therapy or for 1 month following discontinuation of isotretinoin. Upon discontinuation of treatment, females of childbearing potential should have a pregnancy test after their last dose and again one month after their last dose. Two forms of contraception should be continued during this time. Any pregnancies should be reported to the

◄ iPLEDGE™ program (www.ipledgeprogram.com or 866-495-0654) and the FDA through MedWatch (800-FDA-1088).

Breastfeeding Considerations It is not known if isotretinoin is present in breast milk. A case report describes a green discharge from the breast of a nonbreastfeeding woman that was determined to be iatrogenic galactorrhea due to isotretinoin (Larsen 1985). Due to the potential for serious adverse reactions in the breastfed infant, breastfeeding is not recommended by the manufacturer.

Warnings/Precautions This medication should only be prescribed by prescribers competent in treating severe recalcitrant nodular acne and experienced with the use of systemic retinoids. Anaphylaxis and other types of allergic reactions, including cutaneous reactions and serious cases of allergic vasculitis, often with purpura of the extremities and extracutaneous involvement (including renal) have been reported. Discontinue therapy if a serious allergic reaction occurs and institute appropriate medical management. **[US Boxed Warnings]: Birth defects (facial, eye, ear, skull, central nervous system, cardiovascular, thymus and parathyroid gland abnormalities) have been noted following isotretinoin exposure during pregnancy and the risk for severe birth defects is high, with any dose or even with short treatment duration. Low IQ scores have also been reported. The risk for spontaneous abortion and premature births is increased. Because of the high likelihood of teratogenic effects, all patients (male and female), prescribers, wholesalers, and dispensing pharmacists must register and be active in the iPLEDGE risk evaluation and mitigation strategy (REMS) program; do not prescribe isotretinoin for women who are or who are likely to become pregnant while using the drug. If pregnancy occurs during therapy, isotretinoin should be discontinued immediately and the patient referred to an obstetrician-gynecologist specializing in reproductive toxicity.** Women of childbearing potential must be capable of complying with effective contraceptive measures. Patients must select and commit to two forms of contraception. Therapy is begun after two negative pregnancy tests; effective contraception must be used for at least 1 month before beginning therapy, during therapy, and for 1 month after discontinuation of therapy. Prescriptions should be written for no more than a 30-day supply, and pregnancy testing and counseling should be repeated monthly.

May cause depression, psychosis, mood disturbance, and rarely, suicidal ideation, suicide attempts, suicide, and aggressive and/or violent behaviors. All patients should be observed closely for symptoms of depression or suicidal thoughts. Discontinue therapy if depression, mood disturbance, psychosis, or aggression develops. Discontinuation of treatment alone may not be sufficient, further evaluation may be necessary. Use with extreme caution in patients with a history of psychiatric disorder. Retinoids have been associated with pseudotumor cerebri (benign intracranial hypertension), especially in children. Concurrent use of other drugs associated with this effect (eg, tetracyclines) may increase risk. Early signs and symptoms include papilledema, headache, nausea, vomiting, and visual disturbances; discontinue immediately and refer patient to a neurologist if papilledema occurs. Hearing impairment, which can continue after therapy is discontinued, may occur. Clinical hepatitis, elevated liver enzymes, inflammatory bowel disease, skeletal hyperostosis, premature epiphyseal closure, vision impairment, corneal opacities, decreased tolerance to contact lenses (due to dry eyes), and decreased night vision have also been reported with the use of isotretinoin. Postmarketing reports of erythema multiforme and severe skin reactions (eg, Stevens-Johnson syndrome, toxic epidermal necrolysis), including fatalities, have been reported; monitor for severe skin reactions; discontinue use if severe skin reaction occurs.

Use with caution in patients with diabetes mellitus; impaired glucose control has been reported. Acute pancreatitis may occur in patients with normal or elevated triglyceride levels; fatal hemorrhagic pancreatitis (rare) has been reported; discontinue therapy if hypertriglyceridemia cannot be controlled at an acceptable level or symptoms of pancreatitis occur. Marked elevations of serum triglycerides have been reported; use with caution in patients with hypertriglyceridemia or those who may be at high risk (eg, patients with diabetes, obesity, increased alcohol intake, family history of or those with lipid metabolism disorder). The effects on triglycerides, HDL, and cholesterol have been reversible upon discontinuation of therapy. Instruct patients to avoid or limit ethanol; may increase triglyceride levels if taken in excess.

May decrease bone mineral density; osteoporosis, osteopenia, bone fractures, and delayed healing of bone fractures have been reported. Use caution in patients with a genetic predisposition for bone loss (eg, age-related osteoporosis, history of childhood osteoporosis conditions, osteomalacia or other disorders of bone metabolism; including patients diagnosed with anorexia nervosa and those on concomitant medications that may cause drug-induced osteoporosis/osteomalacia and/or affect vitamin D metabolism (eg, systemic corticosteroids, anticonvulsants). Patients may be at increased risk when participating in activities with repetitive impact (such as sports) where the risk of spondylolisthesis with and without pars fractures and hip growth plate injuries in early and late adolescence are known. Patients should be instructed not to donate blood during therapy and for 1 month following discontinuation of therapy due to risk of donated blood being given to a pregnant female. Safety of long-term use is not established and is not recommended; the effect on bone loss is unknown. Some products may contain tartrazine (FD&C yellow no. 5), which may cause allergic reactions, including bronchial asthma, in certain individuals. Allergy is frequently seen in patients who also have an aspirin hypersensitivity.

Absorica: Absorption is ~83% greater than Accutane when administered under fasting conditions; they are bioequivalent when taken with a high-fat meal. Absorica is **not** interchangeable with other generic isotretinoin products. Isotretinoin and tretinoin (which is also known as all-*trans* retinoic acid, or ATRA) may be confused, while both products may be used in cancer treatment, they are **not** interchangeable; verify product prior to dispensing and administration to prevent medication errors.

Musculoskeletal symptoms (including arthralgia) have been reported; generally symptoms were mild to moderate, but occasionally required discontinuation of therapy. Transient pain in the chest has occurred; symptoms generally cleared after discontinuation of therapy, but in some cases persisted. Rhabdomyolysis, some associated with strenuous physical activity, has been reported (rarely).

Acute pancreatitis may occur in patients with normal or elevated triglyceride levels; fatal hemorrhagic pancreatitis (rare) has been reported; discontinue therapy if hypertriglyceridemia cannot be controlled at an acceptable level or symptoms of pancreatitis occurs. Neutropenia and rare cases of agranulocytosis have been reported; discontinue if clinically significant decreases in white cell counts occur. Avoid prolonged exposure to UV rays or sunlight. Avoid skin resurfacing procedures (eg, dermabrasion, laser) and wax epilation during therapy and for at least 6 months after discontinuation of isotretinoin due to the risk of scarring. Potentially significant interactions may exist, requiring dose or frequency adjustment, additional monitoring, and/or selection of alternative therapy.

Adverse Reactions

>10%:

Endocrine & metabolic: Increased serum triglycerides (25%)

Neuromuscular & skeletal: Back pain (children: 29%)

1% to 10%:

Ophthalmic: Conjunctivitis (4%), blepharitis (1%), chalazion (1%), hordeolum (1%)

Frequency not defined:

Cardiovascular: Cerebrovascular accident, chest pain, edema, flushing, palpitations, syncope, tachycardia, thrombosis

Central nervous system: Aggressive behavior, attempted suicide, depression, dizziness, drowsiness, emotional lability, fatigue, headache, insomnia, lethargy, malaise, nervousness, paresthesia, pseudotumor cerebri, psychosis, seizure, suicidal ideation, vasculitis (renal), violent behavior

Dermatologic: Acne fulminans, allergic skin reaction, alopecia, cheilitis, diaphoresis, eczema, eruptive xanthoma, facial erythema, hair disease, hirsutism, hyperpigmentation, hypopigmentation, nail disease, paronychia, pruritus, pyogenic granuloma, scaling of skin of feet, skin atrophy, skin photosensitivity, skin rash, sunburn (increased susceptibility), superficial peeling of palms, xeroderma

Endocrine & metabolic: Decreased HDL cholesterol, increased gammaglutamyl transferase, increased lactate dehydrogenase, increased serum cholesterol, increased serum glucose, hyperuricemia, menstrual disease, weight loss

Gastrointestinal: Colitis, esophagitis, esophageal ulcer, gastrointestinal symptoms (nonspecific), gingival hemorrhage, gingivitis, inflammatory bowel disease, nausea, pancreatitis, xerostomia

Genitourinary: Genitourinary disease (nonspecific findings), hematuria, proteinuria, pyuria

Hematologic & oncologic: Anemia, bruise, lymphadenopathy, neutropenia, purpura, thrombocytopenia

Hepatic: Increased serum alkaline phosphatase, increased serum ALT, increased serum AST, hepatitis

Hypersensitivity: Anaphylaxis, hypersensitivity reaction

Infection: Herpes simplex infection (disseminated), infection

Neuromuscular & skeletal: Arthralgia, arthritis, bone disease, calcification of ligament, calcification of tendon, decreased bone mineral density, increased creatine phosphokinase, myalgia, premature epiphyseal closure, skeletal hyperostosis, tendonitis, weakness

Ophthalmic: Cataract, corneal opacity, keratitis, nocturnal amblyopia, optic neuritis, photophobia, vision color changes, visual disturbance

Otic: Auditory impairment, tinnitus

Renal: Glomerulonephritis

Respiratory: Bronchospasm, dry nose, epistaxis, respiratory tract infection, voice disorder, Wegener's granulomatosis

Miscellaneous: Wound healing impairment

<1%, postmarketing, and/or case reports: Agranulocytosis, contact lens intolerance, decreased visual acuity, dry eye syndrome, erythema multiforme, eye pain, eyelid disease (meibomian gland dysfunction/atrophy; Neudorfer 2012), myopia, rhabdomyolysis, Stevens-Johnson syndrome, toxic epidermal necrolysis

Drug Interactions

Metabolism/Transport Effects None known.

Avoid Concomitant Use

Avoid concomitant use of ISOtretinoin with any of the following: Aminolevulinic Acid (Systemic); Multivitamins/Fluoride (with ADE); Multivitamins/Minerals (with ADEK, Folate, Iron); Multivitamins/Minerals (with AE, No Iron); Tetracycline Derivatives; Vitamin A

Increased Effect/Toxicity

ISOtretinoin may increase the levels/effects of: Aminolevulinic Acid (Systemic); Aminolevulinic Acid (Topical); Mipomersen; Porfimer; Verteporfin

The levels/effects of ISOtretinoin may be increased by: Alcohol (Ethyl); Multivitamins/Fluoride (with ADE); Multivitamins/Minerals (with ADEK, Folate, Iron); Multivitamins/Minerals (with AE, No Iron); Tetracycline Derivatives; Vitamin A

Decreased Effect

ISOtretinoin may decrease the levels/effects of: Contraceptives (Estrogens); Contraceptives (Progestins)

Food Interactions Isotretinoin bioavailability increased if taken with food or milk. Management: Administer orally with a meal (except Absorica which may be taken without regard to meals).

Hazardous Drugs Handling Considerations

Hazardous agent (meets NIOSH 2016 criteria). This medication is not on the NIOSH (2016) list; however, it meets the criteria for a hazardous drug. Drugs are classified as hazardous based on their properties; the properties of a hazardous drug include one or more of the following characteristics: carcinogenic, teratogenic (or other developmental toxicity), reproductive toxicity, organotoxic at low doses, genotoxic, and/or new agents with structural or toxicity profiles similar to existing hazardous agents.

Use appropriate precautions for receiving, handling, administration, and disposal. Gloves (single) should be worn during receiving, unpacking, and placing in storage.

NIOSH recommends single gloving for administration of intact tablets or capsules. If manipulating tablets/capsules (eg, to prepare an oral suspension), NIOSH recommends double gloving, a protective gown, and preparation in a controlled device; if not prepared in a controlled device, respiratory and eye/face protection as well as ventilated engineering controls are recommended. NIOSH recommends double gloving, a protective gown, and (if there is a potential for vomit or spit up) eye/face protection for administration of an oral liquid/feeding tube administration (NIOSH 2016).

Storage/Stability Store at 20°C to 25°C (68°F to 77°F); excursions permitted between 15°C to 30°C (59°F to 86°F). Protect from light.

Mechanism of Action Reduces sebaceous gland size and reduces sebum production in acne treatment; in neuroblastoma, decreases cell proliferation and induces differentiation

Pharmacodynamics/Kinetics Note: Pharmacokinetic parameters in adolescents (12 to 15 years) are similar to adults.

◀ Absorption: Enhanced with a high-fat meal; Absorica absorption is ~83% greater than Accutane when administered under fasting conditions; they are bioequivalent when taken with a high-fat meal.

Protein binding: 99% to 100%; primarily albumin

Metabolism: Hepatic via CYP2B6, 2C8, 2C9, 2D6, 3A4; forms metabolites; major metabolite: 4-oxo-isotretinoin (active)

Half-life elimination: Terminal: Parent drug: 21 hours; Metabolite: 21 to 24 hours

Time to peak, serum: 3 to 5 hours

Excretion: Urine and feces (equal amounts)

Dosing

Adult & Geriatric

Acne (severe recalcitrant nodular):

Manufacturer's labeling: 0.5 to 1 mg/kg/day in 2 divided doses for 15 to 20 weeks; may discontinue earlier if the total cyst count decreases by >70%. Adults with very severe disease/scarring or primarily involves the trunk may require dosage adjustment up to 2 mg/kg/day, as tolerated. Adjust dose according to the appearance of clinical side effects and/or response of the disease.

Alternate dosing: 0.5 mg/kg/day in 2 divided doses for 1 month, then increase to 1 mg/kg/day in 2 divided doses as tolerated until a cumulative dose of 120 to 150 mg/kg is reached (AAD [Zaenglein 2016]).

Acne (moderate) (off-label use): Oral: Low-dose regimens: 20 mg/day (~0.3 to 0.4 mg/kg/day) for 6 months (Amichai 2006) **or** 0.25 to 0.4 mg/kg daily for 24 weeks (Lee 2011)

Cutaneous T-cell lymphomas (off-label use): Oral: Induction: 1 mg/kg/day (in 2 divided doses and in combination with interferon alfa-2b) for 3 to 4 months (Duvic 2003; Knobler 1991). If response occurs, may continue therapy for an additional 3 months; if response continues after 6 months of therapy, may administer isotretinoin and interferon alfa-2b at a 50% reduced dose for an additional 3 months, followed by interferon alfa-2b maintenance therapy (Knobler 1991). Additional trials may be necessary to further define the role of isotretinoin in the management of this condition.

Squamous cell skin cancer, prevention in high-risk patients (off-label use): Oral: Initial: 0.25 mg/kg every other day for 1 month, then 0.25 mg/kg daily for one month, then 0.5 mg/kg daily. Adjust dose as needed based on tolerance; higher doses may be more effective for severe skin cancer (Otley 2006). Additional data may be necessary to further define the role of isotretinoin in this setting.

Pediatric

Acne (severe recalcitrant nodular): Children ≥12 years to Adolescents ≤17 years: Oral:

Manufacturer's labeling: 0.5 to 1 mg/kg/day in 2 divided doses for 1 to 20 weeks; may discontinue earlier if the total cyst count decreases by >70%. Adjust dose according to the appearance of clinical side effects and/or response of the disease.

Alternate dosing: 0.5 mg/kg/day in 2 divided doses for 1 month, then increase to 1 mg/kg/day in 2 divided doses as tolerated until a cumulative dose of 120 to 150 mg/kg is reached (AAD [Zaenglein 2016]).

Acne (moderate) (off-label use): Children ≥12 years to Adolescents ≤17 years: Oral: 20 mg/day (~0.3 to 0.4 mg/kg/day) for 6 months (Amichai 2006) **or** 0.3 to 0.5 mg/kg/day for 15 to 20 weeks (AAD [Zaenglein 2016])

Neuroblastoma, high-risk (off-label use): Children and Adolescents: Oral: 160 mg/m^2/day (in 2 divided doses) days 15 through 28 of a 28-day treatment cycle for 6 cycles (regimen also includes dinutuximab, sargramostim, and aldesleukin) (Yu 2010) **or** 160 mg/m^2/day (in 2 divided doses) days 1 through 14 every 28 days for 6 cycles, beginning after continuation chemotherapy or transplantation (Matthay 1999)

Renal Impairment There are no dosage adjustments provided in the manufacturer's labeling.

Hepatic Impairment

Hepatic impairment prior to treatment: There are no dosage adjustments provided in the manufacturer's labeling.

Hepatotoxicity during treatment: Liver enzymes may normalize with dosage reduction or with continued treatment; discontinue if normalization does not readily occur or if hepatitis is suspected.

Administration

Oral: Administer with a meal (except Absorica, which may be taken without regard to meals). According to the manufacturer's labeling, capsules should be swallowed whole with a full glass of liquid; do not chew or suck on the capsule. For patients unable to swallow capsule whole, an oral liquid may be prepared (see Extemporaneous Preparations); may irritate esophagus if contents are removed from the capsule. Safety of once-daily dosing of isotretinoin has not been established and is not recommended.

Neuroblastoma (off-label use): In a pharmacokinetic study, the end of the capsule was punctured/cut and capsule contents extruded into ice cream or yogurt if patients were unable to swallow capsules whole; if capsule is opened, contents must be consumed immediately to avoid degradation (Veal 2007). Refer to Extemporaneous Preparations for additional information.

Extemporaneous Preparations

For patients unable to swallow the capsules whole, an oral liquid may be prepared with softgel capsules (not recommended by the manufacturers) by one of the following methods:

Place capsules (softgel formulations only) in small container and add warm (~37°C [97°F]) water or milk to cover capsule(s); wait 2 to 3 minutes until capsule is softened and then drink the milk or water with the softened capsule, or swallow softened capsule.

Puncture capsule (softgel formulations only) with needle or cut with scissors; squeeze capsule contents into 5 to 10 mL of milk or tube feed formula; draw mixture up into oral syringe and administer via feeding tube; flush feeding tube with ≥30 mL additional milk or tube feeding formula.

Puncture capsule (softgel formulations only) with needle or cut with scissors and draw contents into oral syringe; add 1 to 5 mL of medium chain triglyceride, soybean, or safflower oil to the oral syringe; mix gently and administer via feeding tube; flush feeding tube with ≥30 mL milk or tube feeding formula.

Lam MS. Extemporaneous compounding of oral liquid dosage formulations and alternative drug delivery methods for anticancer drugs. *Pharmacotherapy.* 2011;31(2):164-192.

Monitoring Parameters CBC with differential and platelet count, baseline sedimentation rate, glucose, CPK; signs of depression, mood alteration, psychosis, aggression, severe skin reactions; changes in vision

Pregnancy test (for all female patients of childbearing potential): Two negative tests with a sensitivity of at least 25 milliunits/mL prior to beginning therapy (the second performed at least 19 days after the first test and performed during the first 5 days of the menstrual period immediately preceding the start

◀ of therapy); monthly tests to rule out pregnancy prior to refilling prescription and one month after discontinuation (Absorica).

Lipids: Prior to treatment and at weekly or biweekly intervals until response to treatment is established. Test should not be performed <36 hours after consumption of ethanol.

Liver function tests: Prior to treatment and at weekly or biweekly intervals until response to treatment is established.

When used for oncology indications, monitor adherence.

Dietary Considerations Should be taken with food, except Absorica which may be taken without regard to meals. Limit intake of vitamin A; avoid use of other vitamin A products. Some formulations may contain soybean oil.

Additional Information All patients (male and female), must be registered in the iPLEDGE™ risk management program. Females of childbearing potential must receive oral and written information reviewing the hazards of therapy and the effects that isotretinoin can have on a fetus. Therapy should not begin without two negative pregnancy tests at least 19 days apart. Two forms of contraception (a primary and secondary form as described in the iPLEDGE™ program materials) must be used simultaneously beginning 1 month prior to treatment, during treatment, and for 1 month after therapy is discontinued; limitations to their use must be explained. Micro-dosed progesterone products that do not contain an estrogen ("mini-pills") are not an acceptable form of contraception during isotretinoin treatment. Prescriptions should be written for no more than a 30-day supply, and pregnancy testing and counseling should be repeated monthly. During therapy, pregnancy tests must be conducted by a CLIA-certified laboratory. Prescriptions must be filled and picked up from the pharmacy within 7 days of specimen collection for pregnancy test for women of childbearing potential. Prescriptions for males and females of nonchildbearing potential must be filled and picked up within 30 days of prescribing.

Any cases of accidental pregnancy should be reported to the iPLEDGE™ program or FDA MedWatch. All patients (male and female) must read and sign the informed consent material provided in the pregnancy prevention program.

Medication Guide Available Yes

Dosage Forms Excipient information presented when available (limited, particularly for generics); consult specific product labeling.

Capsule, Oral:

Absorica: 10 mg, 20 mg [contains soybean oil]

Absorica: 25 mg [contains brilliant blue fcf (fd&c blue #1), fd&c yellow #6 (sunset yellow), soybean oil, tartrazine (fd&c yellow #5)]

Absorica: 30 mg [contains soybean oil]

Absorica: 35 mg [contains fd&c blue #2 (indigotine), soybean oil]

Absorica: 40 mg [contains soybean oil]

Amnesteem: 10 mg, 20 mg, 40 mg [contains soybean oil]

Claravis: 10 mg [contains fd&c yellow #6 (sunset yellow), soybean oil]

Claravis: 20 mg [contains soybean oil]

Claravis: 30 mg

Claravis: 40 mg [contains fd&c yellow #6 (sunset yellow), soybean oil]

Myorisan: 10 mg, 20 mg [contains soybean oil]

Myorisan: 30 mg

Myorisan: 40 mg [contains fd&c yellow #6 (sunset yellow), soybean oil]

Zenatane: 10 mg [contains brilliant blue fcf (fd&c blue #1), edetate disodium, fd&c yellow #10 (quinoline yellow), methylparaben, propylparaben, soybean oil]

Zenatane: 20 mg [contains edetate disodium, methylparaben, propylparaben, soybean oil]

Zenatane: 30 mg [contains edetate disodium, fd&c blue #2 aluminum lake, fd&c yellow #10 (quinoline yellow), methylparaben, propylparaben, soybean oil]

Zenatane: 40 mg [contains brilliant blue fcf (fd&c blue #1), edetate disodium, fd&c blue #2 (indigotine), fd&c yellow #10 (quinoline yellow), methylparaben, propylparaben, soybean oil]

Dosage Forms: Canada Information with regard to form, strength, and availability of products uniquely available in Canada but currently not available in the US.

Excipient information presented when available (limited, particularly for generics); consult specific product labeling.

Capsule, Oral:

Accutane: 10 mg, 40 mg

Clarus 10 mg, 40 mg

Epuris 10 mg, 20 mg, 30 mg, 40 mg

◆ **Isotretinoinum** see ISOtretinoin on page 1063

◆ **Istodax [DSC]** see RomiDEPsin on page 1634

◆ **Istodax (Can)** see RomiDEPsin on page 1634

◆ **Istodax (Overfill)** see RomiDEPsin on page 1634

Itraconazole (i tra KOE na zole)

Brand Names: US Onmel; Sporanox; Sporanox Pulsepak

Brand Names: Canada Sporanox

Pharmacologic Category Antifungal Agent, Oral

Use

Aspergillosis (capsules): Treatment of pulmonary and extrapulmonary aspergillosis in immunocompromised and nonimmunocompromised patients who are intolerant of or refractory to amphotericin B therapy. **Note:** IDSA Aspergillosis guidelines recommend amphotericin B formulations for invasive aspergillosis (initial or salvage) only when voriconazole is contraindicated or not tolerated (IDSA [Patterson 2016]).

Blastomycosis (capsules): Treatment of pulmonary and extrapulmonary blastomycosis in immunocompromised and nonimmunocompromised patients.

Histoplasmosis (capsules): Treatment of histoplasmosis, including chronic cavitary pulmonary disease and disseminated, nonmeningeal histoplasmosis in immunocompromised and nonimmunocompromised patients.

Onychomycosis:

Capsules: Treatment of onychomycosis of the toenail, with or without fingernail involvement, and onychomycosis of the fingernail caused by dermatophytes (tinea unguium) in nonimmunocompromised patients

Tablets: Treatment of onychomycosis of the toenail caused by *Trichophyton rubrum* or *Trichophyton mentagrophytes* in nonimmunocompromised patients

Oropharyngeal/Esophageal candidiasis (oral solution): Treatment of oropharyngeal and esophageal candidiasis

◀ *Canadian labeling:* **Oral capsules: Additional indications (not in US labeling):**

Candidiasis, oral and/or esophageal: Treatment of oral and/or esophageal candidiasis in immunocompromised and immunocompetent patients

Chromomycosis: Treatment of chromomycosis in immunocompromised and immunocompetent patients

Dermatomycoses: Treatment of dermatomycoses due to tinea pedis, tinea cruris, tinea corporis, and of pityriasis versicolor in patients for whom oral therapy is appropriate

Onychomycosis: Treatment of onychomycosis in immunocompromised and immunocompetent patients

Paracoccidioidomycosis: Treatment of paracoccidioidomycosis in immunocompromised and immunocompetent patients

Sporotrichosis: Treatment of cutaneous and lymphatic sporotrichosis in immunocompromised and immunocompetent patients

Pregnancy Risk Factor C

Dosing

Adult & Geriatric Note: Capsule and oral solution formulations are not bioequivalent (oral solution has higher bioavailability) and thus are not interchangeable. Generally, oral solution is the preferred formulation because of improved absorption (IDSA [Kauffman 2007]; HHS [OI adult 2016]).

Aspergillosis, invasive (salvage therapy):

Manufacturer's labeling: Oral capsule: 200 to 400 mg daily. For life-threatening infections, administer a loading dose of 200 mg 3 times daily (total: 600 mg daily) for the first 3 days of therapy. Continue treatment for at least 3 months and until clinical and laboratory evidence suggest that infection has resolved.

Alternate recommendations: Oral solution: 200 mg twice daily; duration of therapy is a minimum of 6 to 12 weeks, although duration is highly dependent on degree/duration of immunosuppression, disease site, and evidence of disease improvement (IDSA [Patterson 2016])

Blastomycosis: *Manufacturer labeling:* Oral capsule: Initial: 200 mg once daily; if no clinical improvement or evidence of progressive infection, may increase dose in increments of 100 mg up to maximum of 400 mg daily. Doses >200 mg daily should be administered in 2 divided doses. **Note:** For life-threatening infections, the US labeling recommends administering a loading dose of 200 mg 3 times daily (total: 600 mg daily) for the first 3 days of therapy. Continue treatment for at least 3 months and until clinical and laboratory evidence suggest that infection has resolved.

Alternative dosing: 200 mg 3 times daily for 3 days, then 200 mg twice daily for 6 to 12 months; in moderately severe to severe infection, therapy should be initiated with ~2 weeks of amphotericin B (Chapman 2008).

Candidiasis: Oral:

Esophageal:

US labeling: Oral solution: 100 to 200 mg once daily for a minimum of 3 weeks; continue dosing for 2 weeks after resolution of symptoms

Alternate dosing: Oral solution: Fluconazole-refractory disease: 200 mg once daily for 14 to 21 days (IDSA [Pappas 2016])

Canadian labeling:

Oral solution: 100 to 200 mg once daily for a minimum of 3 weeks; continue dosing for 2 weeks after resolution of symptoms

Oral capsules: 100 mg once daily for 4 weeks; increase dose to 200 mg once daily in patients with AIDS and neutropenic patients

Alternate dosing: HIV-infected patients: Oral solution: 200 mg once daily for 14 to 21 days (HHS [OI adult 2016])

Oropharyngeal:

US labeling: Oral solution: 200 mg once daily for 1 to 2 weeks; in patients unresponsive or refractory to fluconazole: 100 mg twice daily (clinical response expected in 2 to 4 weeks)

Alternate dosing: Oral solution: Fluconazole-refractory disease: 200 mg once daily for up to 28 days (IDSA [Pappas 2016])

Canadian labeling:

Oral solution: 200 mg once daily or in divided doses daily for 1 to 2 weeks

Oral capsules: 100 mg once daily for 2 weeks; increase dose to 200 mg once daily in patients with AIDS and neutropenic patients

Alternate dosing: HIV-infected patients (alternative to preferred therapy): Oral solution: 200 mg once daily for 7 to 14 days (HHS [OI adult 2016])

Vulvo-vaginal (uncomplicated) in HIV-infected patients (alternative to preferred therapy) (off-label use): Oral solution: 200 mg once daily for 3 to 7 days (HHS [OI adult 2016])

Chromomycosis: Canadian labeling (not in US labeling): Oral: 200 mg once daily for 6 months (when due to *Fonsecaea pedrosoi*) or 100 mg once daily for 3 months (when due to *Cladosporium carrioni*)

Coccidioidomycosis, extrapulmonary (non-HIV infected) (off-label use): Oral:

Soft tissue infection (not associated with bone infection): 200 mg twice daily for at least 6 to 12 months (IDSA [Galgiani 2016])

Bone and/or joint infection: 200 mg twice daily for 3 years to lifetime, depending on severity and host immunocompetence. **Note:** Amphotericin B may be used initially in severe cases and then switched to itraconazole (IDSA [Galgiani 2016])

Coccidioidal pneumonia (off-label use): Oral:

Non-HIV infected (symptomatic, chronic cavitary): Oral: 200 mg twice daily for at least 12 months (IDSA [Galgiani 2016])

HIV-infected patients (focal pneumonia): 200 mg twice daily (HHS [OI adult 2016])

Coccidioidal meningitis (off-label use):

Non-HIV infected: Oral: 200 mg 2 to 4 times daily; close monitoring required to assure adequate absorption (IDSA [Galgiani 2016])

HIV-infected patients (HHS [OI adult 2015]) (alternative to preferred therapy): Oral:

Treatment: 200 mg 3 times daily for 3 days, then 200 mg twice daily, followed by chronic suppressive therapy

Chronic suppressive therapy: 200 mg twice daily continued indefinitely, even with increase in CD4 count on ART

Cryptococcosis in HIV-infected patients (off-label use) (alternative to preferred therapy): Oral: *Treatment, consolidation therapy:* 200 mg twice daily for ≥8 weeks (HHS [OI adult 2016])

Histoplasmosis:

Treatment:

Manufacturer's labeling: Oral capsule: Initial: 200 mg once daily; if no clinical improvement or evidence of progressive infection, may increase dose in increments of 100 mg up to maximum of 400 mg daily. Doses

>200 mg daily should be administered in 2 divided doses. **Note:** For life-threatening infections, the US labeling recommends administering a loading dose of 200 mg 3 times daily (total: 600 mg daily) for the first 3 days of therapy. Continue treatment for at least 3 months and until clinical and laboratory evidence suggest that infection has resolved.

Alternate dosing: 200 mg 3 times daily for 3 days, then 200 mg twice daily (or once daily in mild-moderate disease) for 6 to 12 weeks in mild-moderate disease or ≥12 months in progressive disseminated or chronic cavitary pulmonary histoplasmosis; in moderately-severe to severe infection, therapy should be initiated with ~2 weeks of a lipid formation of amphotericin B (Wheat, 2007). Duration of twice daily maintenance therapy should be at least 12 months in HIV-infected patients (HHS [OI adult 2016])

Prophylaxis (off-label use):

Primary prophylaxis in HIV-infected patients: 200 mg once daily; primary prophylaxis is indicated when CD4 count <150 cells/mm^3 and at increased risk of exposure (HHS [OI adult 2016])

Long-term suppression therapy (secondary prophylaxis) in HIV-infected patients: 200 mg once daily; long-term suppressive therapy is indicated in patients who relapse despite appropriate therapy or in patients with CNS or severe disseminated infection (HHS [OI adult 2016])

Microsporidiosis, disseminated (caused by *Trachipleistophora* or *Anncaliia*) in HIV-infected patients (off-label use): Oral: 400 mg once daily in combination with albendazole (HHS [OI adult 2016])

Onychomycosis (fingernail involvement only): Oral capsule: 200 mg twice daily for 1 week; repeat 1-week course after 3-week off-time

Onychomycosis (toenails due to *Trichophyton rubrum* or *T. mentagrophytes*): Oral tablet: 200 mg once daily for 12 consecutive weeks.

Onychomycosis (toenails with or without fingernail involvement): Oral capsule: 200 mg once daily for 12 consecutive weeks

Canadian labeling (not in US labeling): "Pulse-dosing": 200 mg twice daily for 1 week; repeat 1-week course twice with 3-week off-time between each course

Paracoccidioidomycosis: Canadian labeling (not in US labeling): Oral capsule: 100 mg once daily for 6 months

Penicilliosis in HIV-infected patients (off-label use) (HHS [OI adult 2016]): Oral:

Primary prophylaxis: 200 mg once daily for patients with a CD4 count <100 cells/mm^3 who spend extensive time in northern Thailand, Vietnam, and Southern China, especially rural areas

Treatment: 200 mg twice daily for 8 weeks (mild disease) or 10 weeks (severe infections), then continue with maintenance therapy. In severely-ill patients, initiate therapy with 2 weeks of liposomal amphotericin B.

Chronic maintenance (secondary prophylaxis): 200 mg once daily until CD4 count >100 cells/mm^3 for ≥6 months in response to ART

Pityriasis versicolor: Canadian labeling (not in US labeling): Oral: 200 mg once daily for 7 days

Sporotrichosis: Oral:

Lymphocutaneous: 200 mg daily for 3 to 6 months (Kauffman, 2007)

 Canadian labeling (not in US labeling): 100 mg once daily for 3 months

Osteoarticular and pulmonary: 200 mg twice daily for ≥1 years (may use amphotericin B initially for stabilization) (Kauffman, 2007)

Tinea corporis or tinea cruris: Canadian labeling (not in US labeling): Oral capsule: 100 mg once daily for 14 consecutive days or 200 mg once daily for 7 consecutive days. **Note:** Equivalency between regimens not established.

Tinea pedis: Canadian labeling (not in US labeling): Oral capsule: 100 mg once daily for 28 consecutive days or 200 mg twice daily for 7 consecutive days. **Note:** Equivalency between regimens not established. Patients with chronic resistant infection may benefit from lower dose and extended treatment time (100 mg once daily for 28 days).

Pediatric Note: Capsule and oral solution formulations are not bioequivalent (oral solution has higher bioavailability) and thus are not interchangeable. Generally, oral solution is the preferred formulation because of improved absorption (HHS [OI pediatric 2013]).

Usual dosage range: Limited data available: Infants, Children, and Adolescents: Oral capsule or solution: 2.5 to 5 mg/kg/dose every 12 hours for treatment; for relapse prevention, once daily dose may be considered; usual maximum daily dose: 200 mg/day (Bradley 2015; *Red Book* [AAP 2015]); some infections may require up to 400 mg/day.

Indication-specific dosing:

Blastomycosis (off-label population) (Chapman 2008; *Red Book* [AAP 2015]): Limited data available: Infants, Children, and Adolescents: Oral capsule or solution:

Mild to moderate pulmonary and extrapulmonary disease: 5 mg/kg/dose twice daily for 6 to 12 months; maximum dose: 200 mg/dose.

Severe or CNS infection (step down therapy after amphotericin B response): 5 mg/kg/dose twice daily; total therapy duration: At least 12 months; maximum dose: 200 mg/dose.

Candidiasis (HIV-exposed/-positive) (HHS [OI adult 2016]; HHS [OI pediatric 2013]): Oral solution: Limited data available:

Oropharyngeal, treatment (off-label population):

Infants and Children: If fluconazole-refractory: 2.5 mg/kg/dose twice daily for 7 to 14 days; maximum dose range: 200 to 400 mg/**day**

Adolescents: 200 mg once daily for 7 to 14 days

Esophageal, treatment (off-label population):

Infants and Children: 2.5 mg/kg/dose twice daily for at least 21 days and at least 2 weeks following resolution of symptoms

Adolescents: 200 mg once daily for 14 to 21 days

Vulvovaginal, uncomplicated (off-label use): Adolescents: 200 mg once daily for 3 to 7 days

Secondary prophylaxis (off-label use):

Infants and Children: 2.5 mg/kg/dose twice daily, maximum daily dose: 200 mg/**day**

Adolescents: Oropharyngeal candidiasis (suppressive): 200 mg once daily

Candidiasis, invasive (off-label use): Oral solution: Limited data available:

Primary prophylaxis (ESCMID [Hope 2012]): Children ≥2 years and Adolescents:

AML and recurrent leukemia: 2.5 mg/kg every 12 hours after last dose of chemotherapy; continue until neutrophil recovery.

HSCT, allogeneic: 2.5 mg/kg every 12 hours after completion of the conditioning regimen; continue until at least day +100.

HSCT, autologous: 2.5 mg/kg every 12 hours after last dose of chemotherapy; continue until neutrophil recovery.

Coccidioidomycosis, (HIV-exposed/-positive) (off-label use) (HHS [OI adult 2016]; HHS [OI pediatric 2013]):

Treatment:

Mild to moderate infection, non-CNS (eg, focal pneumonitis):

Infants and Children: Oral solution: 2 to 5 mg/kg/dose 3 times daily for 3 days followed by 2 to 5 mg/kg/dose twice daily; maximum dose: 200 mg/dose. Duration of treatment determined by rate of clinical response. For skeletal infection, 5 mg/kg/dose twice daily for 12 months (Bradley 2015).

Adolescents: Oral: 200 mg twice daily.

Severe infection, non-CNS (with amphotericin B or as step down therapy after amphotericin B response):

Infants and Children: Oral: 5 mg/kg/dose twice daily; total therapy duration: at least 12 months; maximum dose: 200 mg/dose. Product formulation not specified.

Adolescents: Oral: 200 mg twice daily.

CNS disease/meningitis:

Infants and Children: Not recommended; drug of choice for this age group is fluconazole.

Adolescents: Oral: 200 mg 3 times daily for 3 days, then 200 mg twice daily; product formulation not specified.

Relapse prevention:

Infants and Children: Oral: 2 to 5 mg/kg/dose twice daily; maximum dose: 200 mg/dose

Adolescents: Oral: 200 mg twice daily

Cryptococcus (HIV-exposed/-positive) (off-label use) (HHS [OI pediatric 2013]): Infants and Children: Oral solution: Limited data available:

Treatment, consolidation therapy: Oral solution (preferred): Initial: 2.5 to 5 mg/kg/dose 3 times daily (maximum daily dose: 600 mg daily) for 3 days (9 doses) followed by 5 to 10 mg/kg/day divided once or twice daily (maximum daily dose: 400 mg daily) for a minimum of 8 weeks

Relapse prevention: 5 mg/kg/dose once daily (maximum daily dose: 200 mg/day).

Histoplasmosis (off-label population) (HHS [OI adult 2016]; HHS [OI pediatric 2013]; IDSA [Wheat 2007]; *Red Book* [AAP 2015]): Oral solution (preferred): Limited data available:

Primary prophylaxis in HIV-infected patients: Adolescents: Refer to adult dosing.

Treatment, acute primary pulmonary disease: Infants and Children: 2 to 5 mg/kg/dose 3 times daily for 3 days (9 doses) followed by 2 to 5 mg/kg/dose twice daily; maximum dose: 200 mg/dose. Duration of therapy for HIV-exposed/-positive patients is 12 months or for HIV-exposed/-positive children with functional cellular immunity (CD4 percentage >20% or >300 cells/mm^3 if age ≥6 years) 12 weeks of treatment may be adequate if clinically improved and urine antigen concentrations decreased. For non-HIV-exposed/-positive patients, a duration of 6 to 12 weeks is recommended depending on severity.

Treatment, mild disseminated disease:

Infants and Children: 2 to 5 mg/kg/dose 3 times daily for 3 days (9 doses) followed by 2 to 5 mg/kg/dose twice daily; maximum dose: 200 mg/dose. Duration for HIV-exposed/-positive patients: At least 12 months. Duration for non-HIV-exposed/-positive: 3 months.

Adolescents: 200 mg 3 times daily for 3 days, then 200 mg twice daily. Duration for HIV-exposed/-positive patients: At least 12 months. Duration for non-HIV-exposed/-positive: 3 months.

Consolidation treatment for moderate-severe to severe disseminated disease, including CNS infection (following appropriate induction therapy):

Infants and Children: 2 to 5 mg/kg/dose 3 times daily for 3 days (9 doses) followed by 2 to 5 mg/kg/dose twice daily; maximum dose: 200 mg/dose. Duration for HIV-exposed/-positive patients: 12 months for non-CNS disseminated disease or for ≥12 months for CNS infection as determined by clinical response. Duration for non-HIV-exposed/-positive: At least 3 months.

Adolescents: 200 mg 3 times daily for 3 days (disseminated disease) or until resolution of abnormal CSF findings (CNS infection), then 200 mg twice daily. Duration for HIV-exposed/-positive patients: 12 months for non-CNS disseminated disease or for ≥12 months for CNS infection as determined by clinical response. Duration for non-HIV-exposed/-positive: At least 3 months.

Long-term suppression therapy (secondary prophylaxis):

Infants and Children: 5 to 10 mg/kg/dose once daily; maximum dose: 200 mg/dose

Adolescents: Refer to adult dosing.

Microsporidiosis, disseminated (caused by *Trachipleistophora* or *Anncaliia*) in HIV-infected patients (off-label use): Adolescents: Refer to adult dosing.

Penicilliosis in HIV-infected patients (off-label use): Adolescents: Refer to adult dosing.

Sporotrichosis (off-label population) (Kauffman 2007; *Red Book* [AAP 2015]): Limited data available: Infants, Children, and Adolescents: Oral solution (preferred):

Lymphocutaneous or localized cutaneous: 3 to 5 mg/kg/dose twice daily; continue until 2 to 4 weeks after all lesions have resolved, usual total duration: 3 to 6 months; maximum dose: 200 mg/dose.

Visceral or disseminated (step down therapy after amphotericin B response): 3 to 5 mg/kg/dose twice daily; continue until total therapy duration: at least 12 months; maximum dose: 200 mg/dose.

Renal Impairment

The manufacturer's labeling states to use with caution in patients with renal impairment; dosage adjustment may be needed. Limited data suggest that no dosage adjustments are required in renal impairment; wide variations observed in plasma concentrations versus time profiles in patients with uremia, or receiving hemodialysis or continuous ambulatory peritoneal dialysis (Boelaert, 1988).

Hemodialysis: Nondialyzable

Hepatic Impairment There are no dosage adjustments provided in the manufacturer's labeling; however, use caution and monitor closely for signs/symptoms of toxicity.

Additional Information Complete prescribing information should be consulted for additional detail.

Dosage Forms Excipient information presented when available (limited, particularly for generics); consult specific product labeling.

Capsule, Oral:

Sporanox: 100 mg [contains brilliant blue fcf (fd&c blue #1), d&c red #22 (eosine), fd&c blue #2 (indigotine)]

Sporanox Pulsepak: 100 mg [contains brilliant blue fcf (fd&c blue #1), d&c red #22 (eosine), fd&c blue #2 (indigotine)]

Generic: 100 mg

Solution, Oral:

Sporanox: 10 mg/mL (150 mL) [contains propylene glycol, saccharin sodium, sorbitol]

Tablet, Oral:

Onmel: 200 mg

♦ **IVIG** see Immune Globulin on page 992

♦ **IV Immune Globulin** see Immune Globulin on page 992

Ixabepilone (ix ab EP i lone)

Related Information

Chemotherapy-Induced Peripheral Neuropathy on page 2236

Common Toxicity Criteria on page 2242

Management of Chemotherapy-Induced Nausea and Vomiting in Adults on page 2253

Management of Drug Extravasations on page 2271

Prevention of Chemotherapy-Induced Nausea and Vomiting in Children on page 2310

Safe Handling of Hazardous Drugs on page 2379

Brand Names: US Ixempra Kit

Index Terms Azaepothilone B; BMS-247550; Epothilone B Lactam

Pharmacologic Category Antineoplastic Agent, Antimicrotubular; Antineoplastic Agent, Epothilone B Analog

Use Breast cancer: Treatment of metastatic or locally-advanced breast cancer resistant to treatment with an anthracycline and a taxane, or if taxane-resistant and further anthracycline therapy is contraindicated (in combination with capecitabine) or as monotherapy in tumors are resistant or refractory to anthracyclines, taxanes, and capecitabine.

Anthracycline resistance is defined as progression during treatment or within 3 months in the metastatic setting (within 6 months in the adjuvant setting). Taxane resistance is defined as progression during treatment within 4 months in the metastatic setting (within 12 months in the adjuvant setting).

Labeled Contraindications History of severe (grade 3 or 4) hypersensitivity to polyoxyethylated castor oil (Cremophor EL) or its derivatives; neutrophil count <1,500/mm^3 or platelet count <100,000/mm^3; combination therapy with ixabepilone and capecitabine in patients with AST or ALT >2.5 times ULN or bilirubin >1 times ULN

Pregnancy Considerations Adverse events were observed in animal reproduction studies. Women of childbearing potential should be advised to use effective contraception during treatment.

Breastfeeding Considerations It is not known if ixabepilone is excreted in breast milk. Due to the potential for serious adverse reactions in the nursing infant, a decision should be made to discontinue breastfeeding or to discontinue the drug, taking into account the importance of treatment to the mother.

Warnings/Precautions [U.S. Boxed Warning]: Due to increased risk of toxicity and neutropenia-related mortality, combination therapy with capecitabine is contraindicated in patients with AST or ALT >2.5 times ULN or bilirubin >1 times ULN. Use (as monotherapy) is not recommended if AST or ALT >10 times ULN or bilirubin >3 times ULN; use caution in patients with AST or ALT >5 times ULN. Toxicities and serious adverse reactions are increased (in mono- and combination therapy) with hepatic dysfunction; dosage reductions are necessary. Diluent contains polyoxyethylated castor oil (Cremophor EL), which is associated with hypersensitivity reactions; use is contraindicated in patients with a history of severe hypersensitivity to polyoxyethylated castor oil (Cremophor EL) or its derivatives. Medications for the treatment of reaction should be available for immediate use; reactions may also be managed with a reduction of infusion rate. Premedicate with an H_1- and H_2-antagonist 1 hour prior to infusion; patients who experience hypersensitivity (eg, bronchospasm, dyspnea, flushing, rash) should also be premedicated with a corticosteroid for all subsequent cycles if treatment is continued.

Dose-dependent myelosuppression, particularly neutropenia, may occur with mono- or combination therapy. Neutropenic fever and infection have been reported with use. The risk for neutropenia is increased with hepatic dysfunction, especially when used in combination with capecitabine. Severe neutropenia and/or thrombocytopenia may require dosage adjustment and/or treatment delay. Peripheral (sensory and motor) neuropathy occurs commonly; may require dose reductions, treatment delays or discontinuation. Usually occurs during the first 3 cycles. Use with caution in patients with preexisting neuropathy. Patients with diabetes may have an increased risk for severe peripheral neuropathy. Use with caution in patients with a history of cardiovascular disease; the incidence of MI, ventricular dysfunction, and supraventricular arrhythmias is higher when ixabepilone is used in combination with capecitabine (as compared to capecitabine alone). Consider discontinuing ixabepilone in patients who develop cardiac ischemia or impaired cardiac function.

Potentially significant drug-drug interactions may exist, requiring dose or frequency adjustment, additional monitoring, and/or selection of alternative therapy. Due to the ethanol content in the diluent, may cause cognitive impairment; patients must be cautioned about performing tasks which require mental alertness (eg, operating machinery or driving). Toxicities or serious adverse events with combination therapy may be increased in the elderly.

Adverse Reactions Percentages reported with monotherapy.
>10%:
  Central nervous system: Peripheral neuropathy (63%; grades 3/4: 14%; grade 3/4 median onset: cycle 4), peripheral sensory neuropathy (62%; grades 3/4: 14%), headache (11%)
  Dermatologic: Alopecia (48%)

Gastrointestinal: Nausea (42%), vomiting (29%), mucositis (≤29%), stomatitis (≤29%), diarrhea (22%), anorexia (19%), constipation (16%), abdominal pain (13%)

Hematologic & oncologic: Leukopenia (grade 3: 36%; grade 4: 13%), neutropenia (grade 3: 31%; grade 4: 23%)

Neuromuscular & skeletal: Weakness (56%), arthralgia (≤49%), myalgia (≤49%), musculoskeletal pain (20%)

1% to 10%:

Cardiovascular: Edema (9%), chest pain (5%)

Central nervous system: Peripheral motor neuropathy (10%; grade 3: 1%), pain (8%), dizziness (7%), insomnia (5%)

Dermatologic: Nail disease (9%), skin rash (9%), palmar-plantar erythrodysesthesia (8%), pruritus (6%), desquamation (2%), hyperpigmentation (2%)

Endocrine & metabolic: Hot flash (6%), weight loss (6%), dehydration (2%)

Gastrointestinal: Dysgeusia (6%), gastroesophageal reflux (6%)

Hematologic & oncologic: Anemia (grade 3: 6%; grade 4: 2%), febrile neutropenia (3%; grade 3: 3%), thrombocytopenia (grade 3: 5%; grade 4: 2%)

Hypersensitivity: Hypersensitivity (5%; grade 3: 1%)

Infection: Infection (5%)

Ophthalmic: Increased lacrimation (4%)

Respiratory: Dyspnea (9%), upper respiratory tract infection (6%), cough (2%)

Miscellaneous: Fever (8%)

Mono- and combination therapy: <1%, postmarketing, and/or case reports: Acute hepatic failure, acute pulmonary edema, angina pectoris, atrial flutter, autonomic neuropathy, blood coagulation disorder, cardiomyopathy, cerebral hemorrhage, colitis, delayed gastric emptying, dysphagia, embolism, enterocolitis, erythema multiforme, gastrointestinal hemorrhage, hemorrhage, hypokalemia, hyponatremia, hypotension, hypovolemia, hypovolemic shock, hypoxia, increased gamma-glutamyl transferase, increased serum alkaline phosphatase, increased serum transaminases, interstitial pneumonitis, intestinal obstruction, jaundice, left ventricular dysfunction, metabolic acidosis, myocardial infarction, nephrolithiasis, neutropenic infection, orthostatic hypotension, pneumonia, pneumonitis, radiation recall phenomenon, renal failure, respiratory failure, sepsis, septic shock, supraventricular cardiac arrhythmia, syncope, thrombosis, trismus, urinary tract infection, vasculitis, voice disorder

Drug Interactions

Metabolism/Transport Effects Substrate of CYP3A4 (major); **Note:** Assignment of Major/Minor substrate status based on clinically relevant drug interaction potential

Avoid Concomitant Use

Avoid concomitant use of Ixabepilone with any of the following: BCG (Intravesical); Conivaptan; Deferiprone; Dipyrone; Fusidic Acid (Systemic); Idelalisib; St John's Wort

Increased Effect/Toxicity

Ixabepilone may increase the levels/effects of: CloZAPine; Deferiprone

The levels/effects of Ixabepilone may be increased by: Aprepitant; Conivaptan; CYP3A4 Inhibitors (Moderate); CYP3A4 Inhibitors (Strong); Dasatinib; Dipyrone; Fosaprepitant; Fusidic Acid (Systemic); Idelalisib; MiFEPRIStone; Netupitant; Palbociclib; Palifermin; Promazine; Simeprevir; Stiripentol

Decreased Effect

Ixabepilone may decrease the levels/effects of: BCG (Intravesical); Lenograstim

The levels/effects of Ixabepilone may be decreased by: Bosentan; CYP3A4 Inducers (Moderate); CYP3A4 Inducers (Strong); Dabrafenib; Deferasirox; Dexamethasone (Systemic); Enzalutamide; Mitotane; Sarilumab; Siltuximab; St John's Wort; Tocilizumab

Food Interactions Grapefruit juice may increase plasma concentrations of ixabepilone. Management: Avoid grapefruit juice.

Hazardous Drugs Handling Considerations

Hazardous agent (NIOSH 2016 [group 1]).

Use appropriate precautions for receiving, handling, administration, and disposal. Gloves (single) should be worn during receiving, unpacking, and placing in storage.

NIOSH recommends double gloving, a protective gown, ventilated engineering controls (a class II biological safety cabinet or a compounding aseptic containment isolator), and closed system transfer devices (CSTDs) for preparation. Double gloving, a gown, and (if dosage form allows) CSTDs are required during administration (NIOSH 2016).

Storage/Stability Store intact vials under refrigeration at 2°C to 8°C (36°F to 46°F); protect from light. Reconstituted solution (in the vial) is stable for up to 1 hour at room temperature; infusion solution diluted in appropriate solution for infusion is stable for 6 hours at room temperature if a pH range of 6 to 9 is maintained (infusion must be completed within 6 hours).

Preparation for Administration Allow to reach room temperature for ~30 minutes prior to reconstitution. Diluent vial may contain a white precipitate which should dissolve upon reaching room temperature. **Reconstitute only with the provided diluent.** Dilute the 15 mg vial with 8 mL and the 45 mg vial with 23.5 mL (using provided diluent) to a concentration of 2 mg/mL (contains overfill). Gently swirl and invert vial until dissolved completely. Prior to administration, further dilute using a non-DEHP container (eg, glass, polypropylene or polyolefin), to a final concentration of 0.2 to 0.6 mg/mL in ~250 mL lactated Ringer's, adjusted sodium chloride 0.9% (pH adjusted prior to ixabepilone addition with 2 mEq sodium bicarbonate per 250 to 500 mL sodium chloride) or PLASMA-LYTE A Injection pH 7.4. Mix thoroughly.

Mechanism of Action Epothilone B analog; binds to the beta-tubulin subunit of the microtubule, stabilizing microtubular promoting tubulin polymerization and stabilizing microtubular function, thus arresting the cell cycle (at the G2/M phase) and inducing apoptosis. Activity in taxane-resistant cells has been demonstrated.

Pharmacodynamics/Kinetics

Distribution: >1,000 L

Protein binding: 67% to 77%

Metabolism: Extensively hepatic, via CYP3A4; >30 metabolites (inactive) formed

Half-life elimination: ~52 hours

Time to peak, plasma: At the end of infusion (3 hours)

Excretion: Feces (65%; 2% of the total dose as unchanged drug); urine (21%; 6% of the total dose as unchanged drug)

Dosing

Adult & Geriatric Note: Premedicate with an H_1-antagonist (eg, oral diphenhydramine 50 mg) and H_2-antagonist (eg, oral ranitidine 150 to 300 mg) ~1 hour prior to infusion. Patients with a history of hypersensitivity should also be premedicated with corticosteroids (dexamethasone 20 mg orally 1 hour before or IV 30 minutes before infusion). For dose calculation, body surface area (BSA) is capped at a maximum of 2.2 m^2.

Breast cancer (metastatic or locally advanced): IV: 40 mg/m^2/dose over 3 hours every 3 weeks (maximum dose: 88 mg) either as monotherapy or in combination with capecitabine

Dosage adjustment with concomitant strong CYP3A4 inhibitors/inducers:

CYP3A4 inhibitors: Avoid concomitant administration with strong CYP3A4 inhibitors (eg, itraconazole, ketoconazole, voriconazole, clarithromycin, telithromycin, nefazodone, atazanavir, delavirdine, indinavir, nelfinavir, ritonavir, saquinavir); if concomitant administration with a strong CYP3A4 inhibitor cannot be avoided, consider a dose reduction to 20 mg/m^2. When a strong CYP3A4 inhibitor is discontinued, allow ~1 week to elapse prior to adjusting ixabepilone dose upward to the indicated dose.

CYP3A4 inducers: Avoid concomitant administration with strong CYP3A4 inducers (eg, dexamethasone, phenytoin, carbamazepine, rifampin, phenobarbital); if concomitant administration with a strong CYP3A4 inducer cannot be avoided and after maintenance on the strong CYP3A4 inducer is established, consider adjusting the ixabepilone dose gradually up to 60 mg/m^2 (as a 4-hour infusion), with careful monitoring. If the strong CYP3A4 enzyme inducer is discontinued, reduce ixabepilone dose to the dose used prior to initiation of the CYP3A4 inducer.

Renal Impairment There are no dosage adjustments provided in the manufacturer's labeling, however, renal excretion is minimal. Pharmacokinetics (monotherapy) are not affected in patients with mild-to-moderate renal insufficiency (CrCl >30 mL/minute); monotherapy has not been studied in patients with serum creatinine >1.5 times ULN. Combination therapy with capecitabine has not been studied in patients with CrCl <50 mL/minute.

Hepatic Impairment

Ixabepilone monotherapy (initial cycle; adjust doses for subsequent cycles based on toxicity):

AST and ALT ≤2.5 times ULN and bilirubin ≤1 times ULN: No dosage adjustment necessary

AST and ALT >2.5 to ≤10 times ULN and bilirubin >1 to ≤1.5 times ULN: Reduce dose to 32 mg/m^2

AST and ALT ≤10 times ULN and bilirubin >1.5 to ≤3 times ULN: Reduce dose to 20 to 30 mg/m^2 (initiate treatment at 20 mg/m^2, may escalate up to a maximum of 30 mg/m^2 in subsequent cycles if tolerated)

AST or ALT >10 times ULN or bilirubin >3 times ULN: Use is not recommended

Combination therapy of ixabepilone with capecitabine:

AST and ALT ≤2.5 times ULN and bilirubin ≤1 times ULN: No dosage adjustment necessary

AST or ALT >2.5 times ULN or bilirubin >1 times ULN: Use is contraindicated

Obesity *ASCO Guidelines for appropriate chemotherapy dosing in obese adults with cancer:* In general, utilize patient's actual body weight (full weight) for calculation of body surface area- or weight-based dosing, particularly when the intent of therapy is curative; manage regimen-related toxicities in the same manner as for nonobese patients; if a dose reduction is utilized due to toxicity, consider resumption of full weight-based dosing with subsequent cycles, especially if cause of toxicity (eg, hepatic or renal impairment) is resolved (Griggs, 2012). **Note:** According to the manufacturer, patients with a body surface area (BSA) >2.2 m^2 should be dosed based upon a maximum BSA of 2.2 m^2

Adjustment for Toxicity

Hematologic:

Neutrophils <500/mm^3 for ≥7 days: Reduce ixabepilone dose by 20%

Neutropenic fever: Reduce ixabepilone dose by 20%

Platelets <25,000/mm^3 (or <50,000/mm^3 with bleeding): Reduce ixabepilone dose by 20%

Nonhematologic:

Neuropathy:

Grade 2 (moderate) for ≥7 days: Reduce ixabepilone dose by 20%

Grade 3 (severe) for <7 days: Reduce ixabepilone dose by 20%

Grade 3 (severe or disabling) for ≥7 days: Discontinue ixabepilone treatment

Grade 3 toxicity (severe; other than neuropathy): Reduce ixabepilone dose by 20%

Grade 3 arthralgia/myalgia or fatigue (transient): Continue ixabepilone at current dose

Grade 3 hand-foot syndrome: Continue ixabepilone at current dose

Grade 4 toxicity (disabling): Discontinue ixabepilone treatment

Note: Adjust dosage at the start of a cycle are based on toxicities (hematologic and nonhematologic) from the previous cycle; delay new cycles until neutrophils have recovered to ≥1,500/mm^3, platelets have recovered to ≥100,000/mm^3 and nonhematologic toxicities have resolved or improved to at least grade 1. If toxicities persist despite initial dose reduction, reduce dose an additional 20%.

Capecitabine dosage adjustments for combination therapy with ixabepilone: Refer to Capecitabine monograph.

Combination Regimens

Breast cancer: Capecitabine-Ixabepilone (Breast) on page 2008

Administration IV: Infuse over 3 hours. Use non-DEHP administration set (eg, polyethylene); filter with a 0.2 to 1.2 micron inline filter. Administration should be completed within 6 hours of preparation. If the dose is increased (above 40 mg/m^2) due to concomitant CYP3A4 inducer use, infuse over 4 hours.

Vesicant/Extravasation Risk Irritant

Emetic Potential Children and Adults: Low (10% to 30%)

Monitoring Parameters CBC with differential; hepatic function (ALT, AST, bilirubin); monitor for hypersensitivity, signs/symptoms of neuropathy

Dietary Considerations Avoid grapefruit juice (may increase plasma concentrations of ixabepilone).

Dosage Forms Considerations Diluent supplied in Ixempra Kit contains polyoxyethylated castor oil (Cremophor EL)

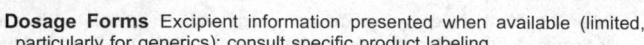

Dosage Forms Excipient information presented when available (limited, particularly for generics); consult specific product labeling.

Solution Reconstituted, Intravenous:

Ixempra Kit: 15 mg (1 ea); 45 mg (1 ea) [contains alcohol, usp, cremophor el]

Ixazomib (ix AZ oh mib)

Related Information

Common Toxicity Criteria *on page* 2242

Management of Chemotherapy-Induced Nausea and Vomiting in Adults *on page* 2253

Safe Handling of Hazardous Drugs *on page* 2379

Brand Names: US Ninlaro

Index Terms Ixazomib Citrate; MLN9708; Proteasome Inhibitor MLN9708

Pharmacologic Category Antineoplastic Agent, Proteasome Inhibitor

Use Multiple myeloma: Treatment of multiple myeloma (in combination with lenalidomide and dexamethasone) in patients who have received at least one prior therapy

Labeled Contraindications There are no contraindications listed In the manufacturer's labeling.

Pregnancy Considerations Based on animal data and the mechanism of action, ixazomib is expected to cause fetal harm if used during pregnancy. Males and females of reproductive potential should use effective contraception during therapy and for 90 days after the last dose.

When used for the treatment of multiple myeloma, ixazomib is indicated to be used with lenalidomide and dexamethasone. Lenalidomide is contraindicated for use during pregnancy (refer to Lenalidomide monograph for details). Dexamethasone is a weak to moderate CYP3A4 inducer, and may decrease the efficacy of hormonal contraceptives. Women using hormonal contraception should also use a barrier method.

Breastfeeding Considerations It is not known if ixazomib is excreted into breast milk. Due to the potential for serious adverse events in a nursing infant, the manufacturer recommends that breastfeeding be discontinued during therapy and for 90 days after the last ixazomib dose.

Warnings/Precautions Neutropenia and thrombocytopenia were reported commonly in clinical trials; grade 3 and 4 toxicity was also observed. Platelet nadirs generally occurred between days 14 to 21 of each cycle with a recovery to baseline by the start of the subsequent cycle. Monitor platelet counts at least monthly during treatment, and consider more frequent monitoring during the initial 3 cycles. May require therapy interruption, dosage reduction and/or platelet transfusions. Monitor complete blood counts (with differential) for neutropenia; therapy interruption or dosage modification may be necessary. Diarrhea, constipation, nausea, and vomiting have been reported. Antidiarrheals, antiemetics, and supportive care may be required to manage toxicity. Dosage adjustment is recommended for grade 3 or 4 symptoms.

Peripheral neuropathy (mostly grade 1 or 2) was observed. Peripheral sensory neuropathy was the most commonly reported symptom, while peripheral motor neuropathy was rarely seen. Monitor closely for signs/symptoms of neuropathy; may require dosage adjustment (of ixazomib and/or lenalidomide) or treatment discontinuation. Peripheral edema was reported in one-quarter of patients receiving ixazomib (generally grade 1 or 2 reactions). If peripheral edema occurs, evaluate for potential underlying causes and provide supportive care. If necessary, grade 3 or 4 symptoms may require dosage adjustment of dexamethasone and/or ixazomib. Rash was reported with ixazomib use; the majority of cases were grade 1 or 2 (grade 3 rash was observed in a small number of patients). Maculopapular and macular rashes were the most commonly reported cutaneous reactions. Monitor for dermatologic toxicity and manage with supportive care or with dosage modification of ixazomib and/or lenalidomide (for grade 2 or higher toxicity).

Drug-induced livery injury, hepatocellular injury, hepatic steatosis, hepatitis cholestatic and hepatotoxicity were reported rarely in clinical trials. Monitor liver enzymes regularly; may require dosage adjustment for grade 3 or 4 toxicity. Reduced initial doses are recommended for patients with moderate and severe hepatic impairment (exposure is increased). In patients with CrCl less than 30 mL/minute or end stage renal disease requiring dialysis, reduced initial doses are recommended (exposure is increased). Concomitant lenalidomide may also require dose reduction. Herpes zoster infection has been reported; patients receiving antiviral prophylaxis had a lower incidence of infection. Consider antiviral prophylaxis during ixazomib treatment to decrease the risk of herpes zoster reactivation. Potentially significant drug-drug interactions may exist, requiring dose or frequency adjustment, additional monitoring, and/or selection of alternative therapy.

Adverse Reactions Adverse reaction percentages reported as part of a combination regimen with lenalidomide and dexamethasone.
>10%
Cardiovascular: Peripheral edema (25%)
Central nervous system: Peripheral neuropathy (28%; grade 3: 2%), peripheral sensory neuropathy (19%)
Dermatologic: Skin rash (19%)
Gastrointestinal: Diarrhea (42%), constipation (34%), nausea (26%), vomiting (22%)
Hematologic & oncologic: Thrombocytopenia (78%; grades 3/4: 26%), neutropenia (67%; grades 3/4: 26%)
Neuromuscular & skeletal: Back pain (21%)
Ophthalmic: Eye disease (26%)
Respiratory: Upper respiratory tract infection (19%)
1% to 10%:
Hepatic: Hepatic insufficiency (6%)
Infection: Herpes zoster (4%; <1% with antiviral prophylaxis)
Ophthalmic: Blurred vision (6%), conjunctivitis (6%), xerophthalmia (5%)
<1%, postmarketing, and/or case reports: Cholestatic hepatitis, hepatocellular hepatitis, hepatotoxicity, liver steatosis, peripheral motor neuropathy, reversible posterior leukoencephalopathy syndrome, Stevens-Johnson syndrome, Sweet's syndrome, thrombotic thrombocytopenic purpura, transverse myelitis, tumor lysis syndrome

Drug Interactions
Metabolism/Transport Effects Substrate of CYP3A4 (major), P-glycoprotein; **Note:** Assignment of Major/Minor substrate status based on clinically relevant drug interaction potential

Avoid Concomitant Use
Avoid concomitant use of Ixazomib with any of the following: BCG (Intravesical); Contraceptives (Progestins); CYP3A4 Inducers (Strong); Deferiprone; Dipyrone; St John's Wort

◀ **Increased Effect/Toxicity**

Ixazomib may increase the levels/effects of: CloZAPine; Deferiprone

The levels/effects of Ixazomib may be increased by: Dipyrone; Promazine

Decreased Effect

Ixazomib may decrease the levels/effects of: BCG (Intravesical); Contraceptives (Estrogens); Contraceptives (Progestins)

The levels/effects of Ixazomib may be decreased by: Bosentan; CYP3A4 Inducers (Moderate); CYP3A4 Inducers (Strong); Dabrafenib; Deferasirox; Sarilumab; Siltuximab; St John's Wort; Tocilizumab

Hazardous Drugs Handling Considerations

Hazardous agent (NIOSH 2016 [group 1]).

Use appropriate precautions for receiving, handling, administration, and disposal. Gloves (single) should be worn during receiving, unpacking, and placing in storage. NIOSH recommends single gloving for administration of intact tablets or capsules (NIOSH 2016).

Storage/Stability Store at ≤30°C (86°F). Do not freeze. Store in original packaging until immediately prior to use.

Mechanism of Action Ixazomib reversibly inhibits proteasomes, enzyme complexes which regulate protein homeostasis within the cell. Specifically, it reversibly inhibits chymotrypsin-like activity of the beta 5 subunit of the 20S proteasome, leading to activation of signaling cascades, cell-cycle arrest, and apoptosis.

Pharmacodynamics/Kinetics

Absorption: High-fat meals decreased AUC by 28% and C_{max} by 69%

Distribution: 543 L

Protein binding: 99% to plasma proteins

Metabolism: Likely hepatic via multiple CYP enzymes and non-CYP proteins. At clinically relevant concentrations, no specific CYP isoform contributes predominantly to metabolism; possible CYP isoforms involved in metabolism include CYP3A4, 1A2, 2B6, 2C8, 2D6, 2C19, and 2C9.

Bioavailability: 58%

Half-life elimination: Terminal: 9.5 days

Time to peak: Median: 1 hour

Excretion: Urine (62%; <3.5% as unchanged drug); Feces (22%)

Dosing

Adult Note: ANC should be ≥1,000/mm³, platelets should be ≥75,000/mm³, and nonhematologic toxicities should be at baseline or ≤ grade 1 (per prescriber discretion) prior to initiating a new cycle of therapy. Consider antiviral prophylaxis to decrease the risk of herpes zoster reactivation.

Multiple myeloma: Oral: 4 mg once weekly on days 1, 8, and 15 of a 28-day treatment cycle (in combination with lenalidomide and dexamethasone); continue until disease progression or unacceptable toxicity (Moreau 2016).

Missed doses: If a dose is delayed or missed, administer only if the next scheduled dose is ≥72 hours away. Do not take a missed dose within 3 days of the next scheduled dose; do not double up on doses to make up for the missed dose. If vomiting occurs, do not repeat the dose; resume dosing at the next scheduled dose.

Renal Impairment The International Myeloma Working Group (IMWG) recommends the use of the Chronic Kidney Disease Epidemiology Collaboration (CKD-EPI) equation (preferred) or the Modification of Diet in Renal

Disease (MDRD) formula to evaluate renal function estimation in multiple myeloma patients with a stable serum creatinine (Dimopoulos 2016).

Preexisting renal impairment:

CrCl ≥30 mL/minute: The IMWG suggest that ixazomib (in combination with lenalidomide and dexamethasone) may be safely administered to patients with a CrCl ≥30 mL/minute (Dimopoulos 2016).

CrCl <30 mL/minute: Reduce initial dose to 3 mg once weekly on days 1, 8, and 15 of a 28-day treatment cycle

ESRD requiring dialysis: Reduce initial dose to 3 mg once weekly on days 1, 8, and 15 of a 28-day treatment cycle; ixazomib is not dialyzable and may be administered without regarding to dialysis timing.

Renal toxicity during treatment: Grade 3 or 4 toxicity: Withhold ixazomib until recovery to baseline or improvement to ≤ grade 1 (at prescriber's discretion). If attributable to ixazomib, resume ixazomib at the next lower dose.

Hepatic Impairment

Preexisting hepatic impairment:

Mild impairment (total bilirubin ≤ ULN and AST > ULN or total bilirubin >1 to 1.5 times ULN and any AST): No dosage adjustment is necessary.

Moderate (total bilirubin >1.5 to 3 times ULN) or severe (total bilirubin >3 times ULN) impairment: Reduce initial dose to 3 mg once weekly on days 1, 8, and 15 of a 28-day treatment cycle

Hepatotoxicity during treatment: Grade 3 or 4 toxicity: Withhold ixazomib until recovery to baseline or improvement to ≤ grade 1 (at prescriber's discretion). If attributable to ixazomib, resume ixazomib at the next lower dose.

Adjustment for Toxicity
Also refer to Lenalidomide monograph for dosage modification recommendations.

Recommended ixazomib dosage reductions for toxicity:

Initial starting dose: 4 mg

First dose reduction: 3 mg

Second dose reduction: 2.3 mg

If unable to tolerate 2.3 mg, discontinue ixazomib

Hematologic toxicity:

Neutropenia: ANC <500/mm^3: Withhold ixazomib and lenalidomide until ANC is ≥500/mm^3. Consider adding growth-colony stimulating factor (G-CSF). Upon recovery, resume lenalidomide at the next lower dose and resume ixazomib at the dose used prior to therapy interruption. If neutropenia to ≤500/mm^3 recurs, interrupt ixazomib and lenalidomide until ANC is ≥500/mm^3. Following recovery, resume ixazomib at the next lower dose and resume lenalidomide at the dose used prior to therapy interruption. For additional occurrences, alternate dose modification of lenalidomide and ixazomib.

Thrombocytopenia: Platelet count <30,000/mm^3: Withhold ixazomib and lenalidomide until platelet count is ≥30,000/mm^3. Upon recovery, resume lenalidomide at the next lower dose and resume ixazomib at the dose used prior to therapy interruption. If thrombocytopenia to ≤30,000/mm^3 recurs, interrupt ixazomib and lenalidomide until platelets are ≥30,000/mm^3. Following recovery, resume ixazomib at the next lower dose and resume lenalidomide at the dose used prior to therapy interruption. For additional occurrences, alternate dose modification of lenalidomide and ixazomib.

◀

Nonhematologic toxicity:
  Dermatologic toxicity:
    Grade 2 or 3 rash: Withhold lenalidomide until rash recovers to ≤ grade 1. Upon recovery, resume lenalidomide at the next lower dose and resume ixazomib at the dose used prior to therapy interruption. If grade 2 or 3 rash recurs, interrupt ixazomib and lenalidomide until rash recovers to ≤ grade 1. Following recovery, resume ixazomib at the next lower dose and resume lenalidomide at the dose used prior to therapy interruption. For additional occurrences, alternate dose modification of lenalidomide and ixazomib.
    Grade 4 rash: Discontinue treatment regimen.
  Peripheral neuropathy:
    Grade 1 (with pain) or grade 2: Interrupt ixazomib until peripheral neuropathy recovers to ≤ grade 1 without pain or to baseline. Upon recovery, resume ixazomib at the dose used prior to therapy interruption.
    Grade 2 (with pain) or grade 3: Withhold ixazomib until recovery to baseline or improvement to ≤ grade 1 (at prescriber's discretion). Following recovery, resume ixazomib at the next lower dose.
    Grade 4: Discontinue treatment regimen.
  Other toxicities (nonhematologic): Grade 3 or 4 toxicity: Withhold ixazomib until recovery to baseline or improvement to ≤ grade 1 (at prescriber's discretion). If attributable to ixazomib, resume ixazomib at the next lower dose.

Combination Regimens
  Multiple myeloma: Ixazomib-Lenalidomide-Dexamethasone (Multiple Myeloma) on page 2162

Administration Oral: Administer on the same day of the week and at approximately the same time on that day; take at least 1 hour before or at least 2 hours after eating. Swallow capsule whole; do not crush, chew, or open the capsule. Avoid skin or eye exposure to capsule contents. If skin contact occurs, wash thoroughly with soap and water; if eye contact occurs, flush thoroughly with water.

Emetic Potential Low (10% to 30%)

Monitoring Parameters Platelet counts at least monthly during treatment (consider more frequent monitoring during the first 3 cycles), complete blood count (with differential) as clinically necessary, renal and liver function tests; signs/symptoms of gastrointestinal and dermatologic toxicity; signs/symptoms of peripheral neuropathy and peripheral edema.

Prescribing and Access Restrictions Available through specialty pharmacies and distributors. Further information may be obtained from the manufacturer, Takeda Oncology, at 1-800-390-5663 or at http://www.ninlarohcp.com.

Dosage Forms Excipient information presented when available (limited, particularly for generics); consult specific product labeling.
  Capsule, Oral:
    Ninlaro: 2.3 mg, 3 mg, 4 mg

- ◆ **Jadenu Sprinkle** *see* Deferasirox *on page* 552
- ◆ **Jakafi** *see* Ruxolitinib *on page* 1645
- ◆ **Jakavi (Can)** *see* Ruxolitinib *on page* 1645
- ◆ **JAMP-Allopurinol (Can)** *see* Allopurinol *on page* 94
- ◆ **JAMP-Anastrozole (Can)** *see* Anastrozole *on page* 135
- ◆ **JAMP-Bicalutamide (Can)** *see* Bicalutamide *on page* 252
- ◆ **JAMP-Ciprofloxacin (Can)** *see* Ciprofloxacin (Systemic) *on page* 393
- ◆ **JAMP-Letrozole (Can)** *see* Letrozole *on page* 1119
- ◆ **JAMP-Methotrexate (Can)** *see* Methotrexate *on page* 1205
- ◆ **JAMP-Mycophenolate (Can)** *see* Mycophenolate *on page* 1283
- ◆ **JAMP Olanzapine FC (Can)** *see* OLANZapine *on page* 1364
- ◆ **JAMP-Olanzapine ODT (Can)** *see* OLANZapine *on page* 1364
- ◆ **JAMP-Ondansetron (Can)** *see* Ondansetron *on page* 1380
- ◆ **JAMP-Tobramycin (Can)** *see* Tobramycin (Systemic) *on page* 1787
- ◆ **JAMP-Valacyclovir (Can)** *see* ValACYclovir *on page* 1852
- ◆ **JAMP-Vancomycin (Can)** *see* Vancomycin *on page* 1861
- ◆ **Jevtana** *see* Cabazitaxel *on page* 305
- ◆ **JNJ-54767414** *see* Daratumumab *on page* 509
- ◆ **Kadcyla** *see* Ado-Trastuzumab Emtansine *on page* 57
- ◆ **Kemsol (Can)** *see* Dimethyl Sulfoxide *on page* 598
- ◆ **Keoxifene Hydrochloride** *see* Raloxifene *on page* 1568
- ◆ **Kepivance** *see* Palifermin *on page* 1425
- ◆ **Keratinocyte Growth Factor, Recombinant Human** *see* Palifermin *on page* 1425

Ketoconazole (Systemic) (kee toe KOE na zole)

Brand Names: Canada Apo-Ketoconazole; Teva-Ketoconazole

Index Terms Nizoral

Pharmacologic Category Antifungal Agent, Imidazole Derivative; Antifungal Agent, Oral

Use Fungal infections (systemic):

US labeling: Treatment of susceptible systemic fungal infections, including blastomycosis, histoplasmosis, paracoccidioidomycosis, coccidioidomycosis, and chromomycosis in patients who have failed or who are intolerant to other antifungal therapies

Limitations of use: Ketoconazole should only be used when other effective antifungal therapy is not available or tolerated **and** the potential benefits outweigh the potential risks.

Canadian labeling: Treatment of serious or life-threatening systemic fungal infections (eg, systemic candidiasis, chronic mucocutaneous candidiasis, coccidioidomycosis, paracoccidioidomycosis, histoplasmosis, and chromomycosis) where alternate therapy is inappropriate or ineffective; may be considered for severe dermatophytoses unresponsive to other therapy

Pregnancy Risk Factor C

◀ **Dosing**
  Adult & Geriatric
    Fungal infections (systemic): Oral: 200 mg once daily; may increase to 400 mg once daily if response is insufficient. Continue until active fungal infection is resolved; some infections may require a treatment duration of up to 6 months.
    Prostate cancer, advanced (off-label use): Oral: 400 mg 3 times daily (in combination with oral hydrocortisone) until disease progression (Ryan 2007; Small 2004)
    Cushing syndrome (off-label use): Oral: Initial: 400 to 600 mg daily in 2 or 3 divided doses; may increase dose by 200 mg daily every 7 to 28 days up to a maximum of 1,200 mg daily in 2 or 3 divided doses; dosage range: 200 to 1,200 mg daily; mean effective dose in most studies: 600 to 800 mg daily in 2 divided doses (Castinetti 2014; ES [Nieman 2015]; Miller 1993)
  Pediatric Fungal infections (systemic): Children >2 years: Oral: 3.3 to 6.6 mg/kg once daily. Continue until active fungal infection is resolved; some infections may require a treatment duration of up to 6 months.
  Renal Impairment There are no dosage adjustments provided in the manufacturer's labeling. However, some resources suggest that no dosage adjustment is necessary in mild-to-severe impairment (Aronoff 2007).
    End-stage renal disease (ESRD) on intermittent hemodialysis: Supplemental dose is not necessary (Aronoff 2007). Not dialyzable.
  Hepatic Impairment Use is contraindicated in acute or chronic liver disease.
    Hepatotoxicity during treatment:
      US labeling: If ALT >ULN or 30% above baseline (or if patient is symptomatic), interrupt therapy and obtain full hepatic function panel. Upon normalization of liver function, may consider resuming therapy if benefit outweighs risk (hepatotoxicity has been reported on rechallenge).
      Canadian labeling: Discontinue therapy for liver function tests >3 times ULN or if abnormalities persist, worsen, or are associated with hepatotoxicity symptoms.
  Additional Information Complete prescribing information should be consulted for additional detail.
  Medication Guide Available Yes
  Dosage Forms Excipient information presented when available (limited, particularly for generics); consult specific product labeling.
    Tablet, Oral:
      Generic: 200 mg

- **Kogenate FS Bio-Set** *see* Antihemophilic Factor (Recombinant) *on page 143*
- **Kovaltry** *see* Antihemophilic Factor (Recombinant) *on page 143*
- **KU-0059436** *see* Olaparib *on page 1368*
- **Kymriah** *see* Tisagenlecleucel *on page 1787*
- **Kyprolis** *see* Carfilzomib *on page 337*
- **Kytril** *see* Granisetron *on page 895*
- **L-758,298** *see* Fosaprepitant *on page 844*
- **L 754030** *see* Aprepitant *on page 165*
- **Ladakamycin** *see* AzaCITIDine *on page 206*
- **L-AmB** *see* Amphotericin B (Liposomal) *on page 123*
- **Lambrolizumab** *see* Pembrolizumab *on page 1486*

Lanreotide (lan REE oh tide)

Brand Names: US Somatuline Depot
Brand Names: Canada Somatuline Autogel
Index Terms Lanreotide (Long-Acting Aqueous); Lanreotide Acetate; Lanreotide Autogel
Pharmacologic Category Somatostatin Analog
Use

US labeling:

Acromegaly: Long-term treatment of acromegalic patients who have had an inadequate response to surgery and/or radiotherapy, or for whom surgery and/or radiotherapy is not an option.

Gastroenteropancreatic neuroendocrine tumors: Treatment (to improve progression-free survival) of unresectable, well- or moderately-differentiated, locally advanced or metastatic gastroenteropancreatic neuroendocrine tumors (GEP-NETs).

Canadian labeling:

Acromegaly: Long-term treatment of patients with acromegaly due to pituitary tumors who have had an inadequate response to surgery and/or radiotherapy, or for whom surgery and/or radiotherapy is not an option; relief of symptoms associated with acromegaly.

Enteropancreatic neuroendocrine tumors: Treatment (to delay progression) of enteropancreatic neuroendocrine tumors in patients with grade 1 or a subset of grade 2 (equivalent to Ki67 <10%) unresectable, locally advanced, or metastatic disease.

Labeled Contraindications

Hypersensitivity to lanreotide or any component of the formulation

Canadian labeling: Additional contraindications (not in the US labeling): Hypersensitivity to somatostatin or related peptides; complicated, untreated bile duct lithiasis

Pregnancy Considerations Adverse events were observed in animal reproduction studies. Information related to the use of lanreotide in pregnancy is limited (deMenis, 1999) and it is recommended to discontinue therapy during pregnancy (Chandraharan 2003; Melmed 2012).

Breastfeeding Considerations It is not known if lanreotide is excreted in breast milk. Due to the potential for serious adverse reactions in the breastfeeding infant, the manufacturer recommends a decision should be made to discontinue breastfeeding or to discontinue the drug, taking into account the importance of treatment to the mother.

Warnings/Precautions Inhibition of insulin and glucagon secretion may affect glucose regulation, leading to hyper-/hypoglycemia, especially in patients with diabetes. Monitor serum glucose levels with the initiation of therapy and with dosage changes; dose adjustments in antidiabetic medications may be necessary. May reduce gall bladder motility, leading to cholelithiasis (may be dose- or duration-related); may require periodic monitoring (consider ultrasonography at baseline and periodically thereafter). Slight decreases in thyroid function have been observed during therapy; may require monitoring of thyroid function tests.

Bradycardia, sinus bradycardia, and hypertension have been observed with therapy; use with caution in patients with preexisting cardiac disease; monitor heart rate. Patients without preexisting cardiac disease may experience a decrease in heart rate though not to the level of bradycardia. Appropriate medical therapy should be initiated if patients develop symptomatic bradycardia. Use with caution in patients with moderate to severe renal and hepatic impairment; lower initial doses may be recommended. Diarrhea and loose stools may occur (may affect intestinal absorption of concurrently-administered medication); abdominal pain may also occur. Potentially significant drug-drug interactions may exist, requiring dose or frequency adjustment, additional monitoring, and/or selection of alternative therapy. Allergic reactions, including angioedema and anaphylaxis, have been reported.

Adverse Reactions
>10%:
  Cardiovascular: Bradycardia (3% to 18%), hypertension (5% to 14%)
  Central nervous system: Headache (5% to 16%)
  Endocrine & metabolic: Weight loss (5% to 11%)
  Gastrointestinal: Diarrhea (26% to 65%; dose related), abdominal pain (7% to 34%; dose related), vomiting (5% to 19%), flatulence (≤14%; dose related), nausea (9% to 11%)
  Hematologic & oncologic: Anemia (3% to 14%)
  Hepatic: Cholelithiasis (2% to 27%), gallbladder sludge (20%)
  Local: Injection site reaction (6% to 22%; induration 5%; pain 4%; mass 2%)
  Neuromuscular & skeletal: Musculoskeletal pain (19%)
1% to 10%:
  Cardiovascular: Sinus bradycardia (3% to 7%)
  Central nervous system: Dizziness (9%), depression (7%)
  Endocrine & metabolic: Hyperglycemia (≤7%)
  Gastrointestinal: Loose stools (6% to 9%), constipation (5% to 8%)
  Immunologic: Antibody development (<1% to 4%)
  Neuromuscular & skeletal: Arthralgia (7% to 10%)
<1%, postmarketing, and/or case reports: Anaphylaxis, angioedema, aortic insufficiency, cholecystitis, decreased heart rate, dysautonomia, hypersensitivity, hypothyroidism, induration at injection site (persistent), injection site pruritus, malaise, mitral valve insufficiency, pancreatitis, steatorrhea

Drug Interactions
  Metabolism/Transport Effects None known.
  Avoid Concomitant Use
    Avoid concomitant use of Lanreotide with any of the following: Ceritinib

Increased Effect/Toxicity

Lanreotide may increase the levels/effects of: Bradycardia-Causing Agents; Bromocriptine; Ceritinib; Codeine; Hypoglycemia-Associated Agents; Ivabradine; Lacosamide; Pegvisomant

The levels/effects of Lanreotide may be increased by: Androgens; Antidiabetic Agents; Bretylium; Herbs (Hypoglycemic Properties); MAO Inhibitors; Pegvisomant; Prothionamide; Quinolone Antibiotics; Ruxolitinib; Salicylates; Selective Serotonin Reuptake Inhibitors; Tofacitinib

Decreased Effect

Lanreotide may decrease the levels/effects of: Antidiabetic Agents; Cyclo-SPORINE (Systemic); Gallium Ga 68 Dotatate

The levels/effects of Lanreotide may be decreased by: Quinolone Antibiotics

Storage/Stability Store at 2°C to 8°C (36°F to 46°F). Protect from light; store in the original package.

Preparation for Administration Allow to reach room temperature by removing sealed pouch from refrigerator 30 minutes prior to administration; keep in sealed pouch until just prior to administration.

Mechanism of Action Synthetic octapeptide analogue of somatostatin which is a peptide inhibitor of multiple endocrine, neuroendocrine, and exocrine mechanisms. Displays a greater affinity for somatostatin type 2 (SSTR2) and type 5 (SSTR5) receptors found in pituitary gland, pancreas, and growth hormone (GH) secreting neoplasms of pituitary gland and a lesser affinity for somatostatin receptors 1, 3, and 4. Reduces GH secretion and also reduces the levels of insulin-like growth factor 1.

Pharmacodynamics/Kinetics

Distribution: V_{ss}: ~0.2 L/kg (Somatuline Canadian labeling 2015)

Protein binding: 79% to 83% (Somatuline Canadian labeling 2015)

Metabolism: Extensively within GI tract after biliary excretion (Somatuline Canadian labeling 2015)

Bioavailability: 69% to ~78%

Half-life, elimination: *Depot*: 23 to 30 days

Time to peak, plasma: Mean: 7 to 12 hours (Somatuline Canadian labeling 2015)

Excretion: Urine (~5% as unchanged drug); feces (<0.5% as unchanged drug)

Dosing

Adult & Geriatric

US labeling:

Acromegaly: SubQ: Initial dose: 90 mg once every 4 weeks for 3 months; after initial 90 days of therapy, adjust dose based on clinical response of patient, growth hormone (GH) levels, and/or insulin-like growth factor 1 (IGF-1) levels as follows:

GH ≤1 ng/mL, IGF-1 normal, symptoms stable: 60 mg once every 4 weeks; once stabilized on 60 mg once every 4 weeks, may consider regimen of 120 mg once every 6 or 8 weeks (extended-interval dosing)

GH >1 to 2.5 ng/mL, IGF-1 normal, symptoms stable: 90 mg once every 4 weeks; once stabilized on 90 mg once every 4 weeks, may consider regimen of 120 mg once every 6 or 8 weeks (extended-interval dosing)

GH >2.5 ng/mL, IGF-1 elevated and/or uncontrolled symptoms: 120 mg once every 4 weeks

Gastroenteropancreatic neuroendocrine tumors (GEP-NETs): SubQ: 120 mg once every 4 weeks until disease progression or unacceptable toxicity

Canadian labeling:

Acromegaly: SubQ: Initial dose: 90 mg once every 4 weeks for 3 months; after initial 90 days of therapy, adjust dose based on clinical response of patient, growth hormone (GH) levels, and/or insulin-like growth factor 1 (IGF-1) levels as follows:

GH ≤1 ng/mL, IGF-1 normal, symptoms stable: 60 mg once every 4 weeks; once stabilized on 60 mg once every 4 weeks, may consider regimen of 120 mg once every 6 or 8 weeks (extended-interval dosing)

GH >1 to 2.5 ng/mL, IGF-1 normal, symptoms stable: 90 mg once every 4 weeks; once stabilized on 90 mg once every 4 weeks, may consider regimen of 120 mg once every 6 or 8 weeks (extended-interval dosing)

GH >2.5 ng/mL, IGF-1 elevated and/or uncontrolled symptoms: 120 mg once every 4 weeks

Enteropancreatic neuroendocrine tumors (NETs): SubQ: 120 mg once every 4 weeks, continue until disease progression

Pediatric Acromegaly: Adolescents ≥16 years (*Canadian labeling*): Refer to adult dosing.

Renal Impairment

Acromegaly:

CrCl 60 to 89 mL/minute: No dosage adjustment necessary.

CrCl ≤59 mL/minute: Initial dose: 60 mg once every 4 weeks for 3 months; adjust dose based on clinical response of patient, GH levels, and/or IGF-1 levels; use of an extended-interval dose of 120 mg once every 6 or 8 weeks should be done with caution.

Gastroenteropancreatic or enteropancreatic neuroendocrine tumors (GEP-NETs):

CrCl ≥30 mL/minute: No dosage adjustment necessary.

CrCl <30 mL/minute: There are no dosage adjustments provided in the manufacturer's labeling (has not been studied).

Hepatic Impairment

Acromegaly:

Mild impairment: No dosage adjustment necessary.

Moderate to severe impairment: Initial dose: 60 mg once every 4 weeks for 3 months; adjust dose based on clinical response of patient, GH levels, and/or IGF-1 levels; use of an extended-interval dose of 120 mg once every 6 or 8 weeks should be done with caution.

Gastroenteropancreatic or enteropancreatic neuroendocrine tumors (GEP-NETs): There are no dosage adjustments provided in the manufacturer's labeling (has not been studied).

Administration Administer by deep subcutaneous injection into superior outer quadrant of buttocks. Alternate injection sites between the right and left sides from one injection to the next. Remove sealed pouch from refrigerator 30 minutes prior to administration.

Monitoring Parameters Serum GH and IGF-1 at 3 months and as clinically indicated in acromegaly patients (obtain levels 6 weeks after dose adjustment when switching to extended-interval dosing), glucose levels, thyroid function (where clinically indicated); heart rate, consider gall bladder ultrasonography (baseline and periodically during therapy)

Dosage Forms Excipient information presented when available (limited, particularly for generics); consult specific product labeling.

Solution, Subcutaneous:

Somatuline Depot: 120 mg/0.5 mL (0.5 mL); 60 mg/0.2 mL (0.2 mL); 90 mg/0.3 mL (0.3 mL)

Dosage Forms: Canada Information with regard to form, strength, and availability of products uniquely available in Canada but currently not available in the US. Refer also to Dosage Forms.

Excipient information presented when available (limited, particularly for generics); consult specific product labeling.

Solution, Subcutaneous:
Somatuline Autogel: 60 mg/0.5 mL (0.5 mL); 90 mg/0.5 mL (0.5 mL); 120 mg/0.5 mL (0.5 mL)

◆ **Lanreotide Acetate** *see* Lanreotide *on page 1091*

◆ **Lanreotide Autogel** *see* Lanreotide *on page 1091*

◆ **Lanreotide (Long-Acting Aqueous)** *see* Lanreotide *on page 1091*

◆ **Lanvis (Can)** *see* Thioguanine *on page 1774*

Lapatinib (la PA ti nib)

Related Information
Common Toxicity Criteria *on page 2242*
Management of Chemotherapy-Induced Nausea and Vomiting in Adults *on page 2253*
Management of EGFR Inhibitor Toxicities: Dermatologic, Ocular, and Gastrointestinal *on page 2291*
Prevention of Chemotherapy-Induced Nausea and Vomiting in Children *on page 2310*
Safe Handling of Hazardous Drugs *on page 2379*
Brand Names: US Tykerb
Brand Names: Canada Tykerb
Index Terms GW572016; Lapatinib Ditosylate
Pharmacologic Category Antineoplastic Agent, Anti-HER2; Antineoplastic Agent, Epidermal Growth Factor Receptor (EGFR) Inhibitor; Antineoplastic Agent, Tyrosine Kinase Inhibitor
Use
Breast cancer: Treatment of human epidermal growth receptor type 2 (HER2) overexpressing advanced or metastatic breast cancer (in combination with capecitabine) in patients who have received prior therapy (with an anthracycline, a taxane, and trastuzumab); HER2 overexpressing hormone receptor-positive metastatic breast cancer in postmenopausal women where hormone therapy is indicated (in combination with letrozole)
Limitations of use: Patients should have disease progression on trastuzumab prior to initiation of treatment with lapatinib in combination with capecitabine.
Labeled Contraindications Known severe hypersensitivity to lapatinib or any component of the formulation
Pregnancy Considerations Adverse events were demonstrated in animal reproduction studies. Lapatinib may cause fetal harm if administered during pregnancy. Women of childbearing potential should be advised to avoid pregnancy during treatment.

European Society for Medical Oncology (ESMO) guidelines for cancer during pregnancy recommend delaying treatment with HER-2 targeted agents until after delivery in pregnant patients with HER-2 positive disease (Peccatori 2013).

◀ **Breastfeeding Considerations** It is not known if lapatinib is excreted in breast milk. Due to the potential for serious adverse reactions in the nursing infant, the decision to discontinue lapatinib or discontinue breastfeeding during treatment should take in account the benefits of treatment to the mother.

Warnings/Precautions Decreases in left ventricular ejection fraction (LVEF) have been reported (usually within the first 3 months of treatment); baseline and periodic LVEF evaluations are recommended; interrupt treatment with decreased LVEF ≥ grade 2 or LVEF < LLN; may reinitiate with a reduced dose after a minimum of 2 weeks if the LVEF recovers and the patient is asymptomatic. In a scientific statement from the American Heart Association, lapatinib has been determined to be an agent that may either cause reversible direct myocardial toxicity or exacerbate underlying myocardial dysfunction (magnitude: moderate/major) (AHA [Page 2016]). QTC prolongation has been observed; use caution in patients with a history of QTC prolongation or with medications known to prolong the QT interval; a baseline and periodic 12-lead ECG should be considered; correct electrolyte (potassium, calcium and magnesium) abnormalities prior to and during treatment. Use with caution in conditions which may impair left ventricular function and in patients with a history of or predisposed to (prior treatment with anthracyclines, chest wall irradiation) left ventricular dysfunction. Interstitial lung disease (ILD) and pneumonitis have been reported (with lapatinib monotherapy and with combination chemotherapy); monitor for pulmonary symptoms which may indicate ILD or pneumonitis; discontinue treatment for grade 3 (or higher) pulmonary symptoms indicative of ILD or pneumonitis (eg, dyspnea, dry cough).

[US Boxed Warning]: Hepatotoxicity (ALT or AST >3 times ULN and total bilirubin >2 times ULN) has been reported with lapatinib; may be severe and/or fatal. Onset of hepatotoxicity may occur within days to several months after treatment initiation. Monitor (at baseline and every 4 to 6 weeks during treatment, and as clinically indicated); discontinue with severe changes in liver function; do not reinitiate. Use caution in patients with hepatic dysfunction; dose reductions should be considered in patients with preexisting severe (Child-Pugh class C) hepatic impairment. Potentially significant drug-drug interactions may exist, requiring dose or frequency adjustment, additional monitoring, and/or selection of alternative therapy. Patients who carry the HLA alleles DQA1*02:01 and DRB1*07:01 may experience a greater incidence of severe liver injury than patients who are noncarriers. These alleles are present in ~15% to 25% of Caucasian, Asian, African, and Hispanic patient populations and 1% in Japanese populations. May cause diarrhea (onset is generally within 6 days and duration is 4 to 5 days); may be severe and/or fatal; instruct patients to immediately report any bowel pattern changes. After first unformed stool, administer antidiarrheal agents; severe diarrhea may require hydration, electrolytes, antibiotics (if duration >24 hours, fever, or grade 3/4 neutropenia), and/or treatment interruption, dose reduction, or discontinuation. Severe cutaneous reactions have been reported with use. Discontinue therapy if life-threatening dermatologic reactions (eg, progressive skin rash with blisters or mucosal lesions) such as erythema multiforme, Stevens-Johnson syndrome, or toxic epidermal necrolysis occur.

Adverse Reactions Percentages reported for combination therapy.
>10%:
  Central nervous system: Fatigue (≤20%), headache (14%)
  Dermatologic: Palmar-plantar erythrodysesthesia (with capecitabine: 53%), skin rash (28% to 44%), alopecia (13%), xeroderma (10% to 13%), pruritus (12%), nail disease (11%)
  Gastrointestinal: Diarrhea (64% to 65%), nausea (31% to 44%), vomiting (17% to 26%), mucositis (15%), stomatitis (14%), anorexia (11%), dyspepsia (11%)
  Hematologic & oncologic: Decreased hemoglobin (with capecitabine: 56%; grade 3: <1%), decreased neutrophils (with capecitabine: 22%; grade 3: 3%; grade 4: <1%), decreased platelet count (with capecitabine: 18%; grade 3: <1%)
  Hepatic: Increased serum AST (49% to 53%), increased serum ALT (37% to 46%), increased serum bilirubin (22% to 45%)
  Neuromuscular & skeletal: Limb pain (12%), weakness (12%), back pain (11%)
  Respiratory: Dyspnea (12%), epistaxis (11%)
1% to 10%:
  Cardiovascular: Decreased left ventricular ejection fraction (with letrozole: 5%; with capecitabine: grade 2: 2%; grade 3: <1%)
  Central nervous system: Insomnia (10%)
<1%, postmarketing, and/or case reports: Anaphylaxis, hepatotoxicity, hypersensitivity, interstitial pulmonary disease, paronychia, pneumonitis, prolonged Q-T interval on ECG, severe dermatological reaction, Stevens-Johnson syndrome, torsades de pointes, toxic epidermal necrolysis, ventricular arrhythmia

Drug Interactions
  Metabolism/Transport Effects Substrate of CYP3A4 (major), P-glycoprotein; **Note:** Assignment of Major/Minor substrate status based on clinically relevant drug interaction potential; **Inhibits** BCRP, CYP2C8 (moderate), CYP3A4 (weak), P-glycoprotein

Avoid Concomitant Use
  Avoid concomitant use of Lapatinib with any of the following: Amodiaquine; Conivaptan; CYP3A4 Inducers (Strong); CYP3A4 Inhibitors (Strong); Dexamethasone (Systemic); Fusidic Acid (Systemic); Grapefruit Juice; Idelalisib; PAZOPanib; Pimozide; Silodosin; St John's Wort; Topotecan; VinCRIStine (Liposomal)

Increased Effect/Toxicity
  Lapatinib may increase the levels/effects of: Afatinib; Amodiaquine; ARIPiprazole; Betrixaban; Bilastine; Brentuximab Vedotin; Celiprolol; Colchicine; CYP2C8 Substrates; Dabigatran Etexilate; DOXOrubicin (Conventional); Edoxaban; Everolimus; Flibanserin; Highest Risk QTc-Prolonging Agents; HYDROcodone; Lomitapide; Moderate Risk QTc-Prolonging Agents; Naldemedine; Naloxegol; NiMODipine; PAZOPanib; P-glycoprotein/ABCB1 Substrates; Pimozide; Prucalopride; Ranolazine; RifAXIMin; Selexipag; Silodosin; Topotecan; Venetoclax; VinCRIStine (Liposomal)

  The levels/effects of Lapatinib may be increased by: Aprepitant; Conivaptan; CYP3A4 Inhibitors (Moderate); CYP3A4 Inhibitors (Strong); Dasatinib; Fosaprepitant; Fusidic Acid (Systemic); Grapefruit Juice; Idelalisib; Netupitant; Palbociclib; P-glycoprotein/ABCB1 Inhibitors; Ranolazine; Simeprevir; Stiripentol

▶

◀ **Decreased Effect**
The levels/effects of Lapatinib may be decreased by: Bosentan; CYP3A4 Inducers (Moderate); CYP3A4 Inducers (Strong); Dabrafenib; Deferasirox; Dexamethasone (Systemic); Sarilumab; Siltuximab; St John's Wort; Tocilizumab

Food Interactions Systemic exposure of lapatinib is increased when administered with food (AUC three- to fourfold higher). Grapefruit juice may increase the levels/effects of lapatinib. Management: Administer once daily on an empty stomach, 1 hour before or 1 hour after a meal at the same time each day. Avoid grapefruit juice. Maintain adequate hydration, unless instructed to restrict fluid intake.

Hazardous Drugs Handling Considerations

Hazardous agent (meets NIOSH 2016 criteria). This medication is not on the NIOSH (2016) list; however, it meets the criteria for a hazardous drug. Drugs are classified as hazardous based on their properties; the properties of a hazardous drug include one or more of the following characteristics: carcinogenic, teratogenic (or other developmental toxicity), reproductive toxicity, organotoxic at low doses, genotoxic, and/or new agents with structural or toxicity profiles similar to existing hazardous agents.

Use appropriate precautions for receiving, handling, administration, and disposal. Gloves (single) should be worn during receiving, unpacking, and placing in storage.

NIOSH recommends single gloving for administration of intact tablets or capsules. If manipulating tablets/capsules (eg, to prepare an oral suspension), NIOSH recommends double gloving, a protective gown, and preparation in a controlled device; if not prepared in a controlled device, respiratory and eye/face protection as well as ventilated engineering controls are recommended. NIOSH recommends double gloving, a protective gown, and (if there is a potential for vomit or spit up) eye/face protection for administration of an oral liquid/feeding tube administration (NIOSH 2016).

Storage/Stability

Store at room temperature of 25°C (77°F); excursions permitted between 15°C to 30°C (59°F to 86°F).

An oral suspension (50 mg/mL) prepared using lapatinib 250 mg tablets and Ora-Plus:Ora-Sweet (1:1 vehicle) is stable for at least 28 days at room temperature; do not refrigerate due to potential increased viscosity (Li 2016).

Mechanism of Action Tyrosine kinase (dual kinase) inhibitor; inhibits EGFR (ErbB1) and HER2 (ErbB2) by reversibly binding to tyrosine kinase, blocking phosphorylation and activation of downstream second messengers (Erk1/2 and Akt), regulating cellular proliferation and survival in ErbB- and ErbB2-expressing tumors. Combination therapy with lapatinib and endocrine therapy may overcome endocrine resistance occurring in HER2+ and hormone receptor positive disease.

Pharmacodynamics/Kinetics

Absorption: Incomplete and variable

Protein binding: >99% to albumin and alpha$_1$-acid glycoprotein

Metabolism: Hepatic; extensive via CYP3A4 and 3A5, and to a lesser extent via CYP2C19 and 2C8 to oxidized metabolites

Half-life elimination: ~24 hours

Time to peak, plasma: ~4 hours (Burris 2009)

Excretion: Feces (27% as unchanged drug; range 3% to 67%); urine (<2%)

Dosing

Adult & Geriatric

Breast cancer, metastatic, HER2+ (with prior anthracycline, taxane, and trastuzumab therapy): Oral: 1,250 mg once daily (in combination with capecitabine) until disease progression or unacceptable toxicity (Geyer 2006)

Breast cancer, metastatic, HER2+, hormonal therapy indicated: Oral: 1,500 mg once daily (in combination with letrozole) until disease progression (Johnston 2009)

Breast cancer, metastatic, HER2+ with brain metastases, first-line therapy (off-label use): Oral: 1,250 mg once daily (in combination with capecitabine) until disease progression or unacceptable toxicity (Bachelot 2013)

Breast cancer, metastatic, HER2+, with progression on prior trastuzumab therapy (off-label use): Oral: 1,000 mg once daily (in combination with trastuzumab) (Blackwell 2010; Blackwell 2012)

Missed doses: If a dose is missed, resume with the next scheduled daily dose; do not double the dose the next day.

Dosage adjustment for concomitant CYP3A4 inhibitors/inducers:

CYP3A4 inhibitors: Avoid the use of concomitant strong CYP3A4 inhibitors. If concomitant use cannot be avoided, consider reducing lapatinib to 500 mg once daily with careful monitoring. When a strong CYP3A4 inhibitor is discontinued, allow ~1 week to elapse prior to adjusting the lapatinib dose upward.

CYP3A4 inducers: Avoid the use of concomitant strong CYP3A4 inducers. If concomitant use cannot be avoided, consider gradually titrating lapatinib from 1,250 mg once daily up to 4,500 mg daily (in combination with capecitabine) **or** from 1,500 mg once daily up to 5,500 mg daily (in combination with letrozole), based on tolerability and with careful monitoring. If the strong CYP3A4 enzyme inducer is discontinued, reduce the lapatinib dose to the indicated dose.

Renal Impairment There are no dosage adjustments provided in the manufacturer's labeling (has not been studied); however, due to the minimal renal elimination (<2%), dosage adjustments may not be necessary.

Hepatic Impairment

Mild or moderate preexisting impairment (Child-Pugh class A or B): There are no dosage adjustments provided in the manufacturer's labeling.

Severe preexisting impairment (Child-Pugh class C): The following adjustments should be considered (and are predicted to normalize the AUC), however, there are no clinical data associated with the adjustments.

In combination with capecitabine: Reduce dose from 1,250 mg once daily to 750 mg once daily.

In combination with letrozole: Reduce dose from 1,500 mg once daily to 1,000 mg once daily.

Severe hepatotoxicity during treatment: Discontinue permanently (do not rechallenge).

Adjustment for Toxicity

Cardiac toxicity: Discontinue treatment for at least 2 weeks for LVEF < LLN or decreased LVEF ≥ grade 2; may be restarted at 1,000 mg once daily (in combination with capecitabine) **or** 1,250 mg once daily (in combination with letrozole) if LVEF recovers to normal and patient is asymptomatic.

Dermatologic toxicity: Discontinue treatment for suspected erythema multiforme, Stevens-Johnson syndrome, or toxic epidermal necrolysis.

Diarrhea:
Grade 3 diarrhea or grade 1 or 2 diarrhea with complicating features (moderate-to-severe abdominal cramping, grade 2 or higher nausea/vomiting, decreased performance status, fever, sepsis, neutropenia, frank bleeding, or dehydration): Interrupt treatment; may restart at a reduced dose (from 1,500 mg once daily to 1,250 mg once daily or from 1,250 mg once daily to 1,000 mg once daily) when diarrhea resolves to ≤ grade 1. Grade 4 diarrhea: Permanently discontinue.

Pulmonary toxicity: Discontinue treatment with pulmonary symptoms indicative of interstitial lung disease or pneumonitis which are ≥ grade 3

Other toxicities: Withhold for any toxicity (other than cardiac) ≥ grade 2 until toxicity resolves to ≤ grade 1 and reinitiate at the standard dose of 1,250 or 1,500 mg once daily; for persistent toxicity, reduce dosage to 1,000 mg once daily (in combination with capecitabine) **or** 1,250 mg once daily (in combination with letrozole)

Combination Regimens
Breast cancer:
Capecitabine + Lapatinib (Breast) on page 2008
Lapatinib-Letrozole (Breast) on page 2162
Lapatinib-Trastuzumab (Breast) on page 2162

Administration Administer once daily, on an empty stomach, 1 hour before or 1 hour after a meal. Take full dose at the same time each day; dividing dose throughout the day is not recommended.

Note: For combination treatment with capecitabine, capecitabine should be administered in 2 doses (approximately 12 hours apart) and taken with food or within 30 minutes after a meal.

Emetic Potential
Children: Minimal (<10%)
Adults: Low (10% to 30%)

Extemporaneous Preparations A 50 mg/mL oral suspension may be prepared using lapatinib 250 mg tablets and Ora-Plus:Ora-Sweet (1:1 vehicle). Determine necessary quantity of lapatinib 250 mg tablets; crush the tablets in a glass mortar and triturate to a fine powder (estimated powder volume for each lapatinib 250 mg tablet is 0.6 mL). Measure the necessary volume of Ora-Plus and add to the powder by geometric dilution until a smooth suspension is created. Measure the necessary volume of Ora-Sweet and add to the suspension. Transfer to an amber plastic bottle and label "Shake Well Before Use", "Do Not Refrigerate" and "Use by (date)". Suspension is stable for at least 28 days at room temperature; do not refrigerate due to potential for increased viscosity.

Li Q, Liu Z, Kolli S, et al. Stability of extemporaneous erlotinib, lapatinib, and imatinib oral suspension. *Am J Health Syst Pharm.* 2016;73(17):1331-1337.

Monitoring Parameters LVEF (baseline and periodic), CBC with differential, liver function tests, including transaminases, bilirubin, and alkaline phosphatase (baseline and every 4-6 weeks during treatment); electrolytes including calcium, potassium, magnesium; monitor for fluid retention; ECG monitoring if at risk for QTc prolongation; symptoms of ILD or pneumonitis; monitor for diarrhea and dermatologic toxicity

Dietary Considerations Avoid grapefruit juice.

Prescribing and Access Restrictions Lapatinib is available through specialty pharmacies only. Information is available at www.gskcta.com or 1-866-265-6491.

Dosage Forms Excipient information presented when available (limited, particularly for generics); consult specific product labeling.

Tablet, Oral:

Tykerb: 250 mg [contains fd&c yellow #6 (sunset yellow), fd&c yellow #6 aluminum lake]

♦ **Lapatinib Ditosylate** *see* Lapatinib *on page 1095*

♦ **Lartruvo** *see* Olaratumab *on page 1372*

♦ **L-ASP** *see* Asparaginase (*E. coli*) *on page 178*

♦ **L-asparaginase (*E. coli*)** *see* Asparaginase (*E. coli*) *on page 178*

♦ **L-asparaginase (*Erwinia*)** *see* Asparaginase (*Erwinia*) *on page 184*

♦ **L-asparaginase with Polyethylene Glycol** *see* Pegaspargase *on page 1462*

♦ **LBH589** *see* Panobinostat *on page 1445*

♦ **LDE225** *see* Sonidegib *on page 1682*

♦ **LDK378** *see* Ceritinib *on page 371*

♦ **LDP-341** *see* Bortezomib *on page 271*

♦ **Lederle Leucovorin (Can)** *see* Leucovorin Calcium *on page 1124*

♦ **LEE-011** *see* Ribociclib *on page 1602*

♦ **Lemtrada** *see* Alemtuzumab *on page 82*

Lenalidomide (le na LID oh mide)

Related Information

Common Toxicity Criteria *on page 2242*

Management of Chemotherapy-Induced Nausea and Vomiting in Adults *on page 2253*

Prevention of Chemotherapy-Induced Nausea and Vomiting in Children *on page 2310*

Safe Handling of Hazardous Drugs *on page 2379*

Brand Names: US Revlimid

Brand Names: Canada Revlimid

Index Terms CC-5013; IMid-1

Pharmacologic Category Angiogenesis Inhibitor; Antineoplastic Agent; Immunomodulator, Systemic

Use

Mantle cell lymphoma: Treatment of patients with mantle cell lymphoma that has relapsed or progressed after 2 prior therapies (one of which included bortezomib).

Multiple myeloma: Treatment of multiple myeloma (in combination with dexamethasone) and as maintenance therapy following autologous hematopoietic stem cell transplantation.

Myelodysplastic syndromes: Treatment of patients with transfusion-dependent anemia due to low- or intermediate-1-risk myelodysplastic syndromes (MDS) associated with a deletion 5q (del 5q) cytogenetic abnormality with or without additional cytogenetic abnormalities

Limitations of use: Lenalidomide is not indicated and is not recommended for the treatment of chronic lymphocytic leukemia (CLL) outside of controlled clinical trials.

◄ **Labeled Contraindications**

Hypersensitivity (eg, angioedema, Stevens-Johnson syndrome, toxic epidermal necrolysis) to lenalidomide or any component of the formulation; pregnancy

Canadian labeling: Additional contraindications (not in the US labeling): Platelet count <50,000/mm³ (in MDS patients); hypersensitivity to thalidomide or pomalidomide; women capable of becoming pregnant; breastfeeding women; male patients unable to follow or comply with required contraceptive measures

Pregnancy Considerations [US Boxed Warning]: Do not use lenalidomide in pregnant women. Lenalidomide is an analogue of thalidomide (a human teratogen) and could potentially cause severe birth defects or embryo-fetal death; use is contraindicated during pregnancy and pregnancy must be avoided while taking lenalidomide. Obtain 2 negative pregnancy tests prior to initiation of treatment; 2 forms of contraception (or abstain from heterosexual intercourse) must be used at least 4 weeks prior to, during, and for 4 weeks after lenalidomide treatment (and during treatment interruptions). In order to decrease the risk of embryo-fetal exposure, lenalidomide is available only through a restricted distribution program (Revlimid REMS).

Women of childbearing potential should be treated only if they are able to comply with the conditions of the Revlimid REMS program. Women of reproductive potential must avoid pregnancy beginning 4 weeks prior to therapy, during therapy, during therapy interruptions, and for ≥4 weeks after therapy is discontinued. Two forms of effective/reliable contraception (eg, tubal ligation, IUD, hormonal birth control methods, male latex or synthetic condom, diaphragm, or cervical cap) or total abstinence from heterosexual intercourse must be used by females who are not infertile or who have not had a hysterectomy. A negative pregnancy test (sensitivity of at least 50 milliunits/mL) 10 to 14 days prior to therapy, within 24 hours prior to beginning therapy, weekly during the first 4 weeks, and every 4 weeks (every 2 weeks for women with irregular menstrual cycles) thereafter is required for women of childbearing potential. Lenalidomide must be immediately discontinued for a missed period, abnormal pregnancy test or abnormal menstrual bleeding; refer patient to a reproductive toxicity specialist if pregnancy occurs during treatment.

Lenalidomide is also present in the semen of males. Males (including those vasectomized) should use a latex or synthetic condom during any sexual contact with women of childbearing age during treatment, during treatment interruptions, and for 4 weeks after discontinuation. Male patients should not donate sperm during, and for 4 weeks after treatment, and during therapy interruptions.

A pregnancy exposure registry has been created to monitor outcomes in females exposed to lenalidomide during pregnancy and female partners of male patients and to understand the root cause for the pregnancy. The pregnancy exposure registry may be contacted at 1-888-423-5436. The parent or legal guardian for patients between 12 and 18 years of age must agree to ensure compliance with the required guidelines. Any suspected fetal exposure should be reported to the FDA via the MedWatch program (1-800-FDA-1088) and to Celgene Corporation (1-888-423-5436).

Breastfeeding Considerations It is not known if lenalidomide is present in breast milk. Due to the potential for serious adverse reactions in the infant, breastfeeding is not recommended by the manufacturer.

Warnings/Precautions [US Boxed Warning]: Hematologic toxicity (neutropenia and thrombocytopenia) occurs in a majority of patients (grade 3/4: 80% in patients with del 5q myelodysplastic syndrome) and may require dose reductions and/or delays; the use of blood product support and/or growth factors may be needed. CBC should be monitored weekly for the first 8 weeks and at least monthly thereafter in patients being treated for del 5q myelodysplastic syndromes. In patients being treated for multiple myeloma, monitor CBC weekly for the first 2 cycles, every 2 weeks during cycle 3, and monthly thereafter. In patients receiving lenalidomide for mantle cell lymphoma (MCL), monitor CBC weekly for the first cycle, every 2 weeks during cycles 2 to 4, and monthly thereafter. Monitor for signs of infection, bleeding, or bruising; may require dosage adjustment. Lenalidomide use (≥4 cycles) may decrease the number of CD34+ cells collected for autologous stem cell transplant. Transplant eligible patients receiving lenalidomide should be referred to an appropriate transplant center in order to optimize the timing of stem cell collection. Cyclophosphamide in combination with G-CSF or G-CSF in combination with a CXC chemokine receptor 4 inhibitor (eg, plerixafor) may be considered when CD34+ cell collection is impaired. **[US Boxed Warning]: Lenalidomide has been associated with a significant increase in risk for arterial and venous thromboembolic events in multiple myeloma patients treated with lenalidomide and dexamethasone combination therapy. Deep vein thrombosis (DVT), pulmonary embolism (PE), myocardial infarction, and stroke have occurred; monitor for signs and symptoms of thromboembolism (shortness of breath, chest pain, or arm or leg swelling) and seek prompt medical attention with development of these symptoms. Thromboprophylaxis is recommended; the choice of regimen should be based on assessment of the patient's underlying risk factors.** Erythropoietin-stimulating agents (ESAs) and estrogens may contribute to thromboembolic risk; use with caution. Patients with a prior history of arterial thromboembolic events may be at greater risk; minimize modifiable factors such as hyperlipidemia, hypertension, and smoking. Anticoagulant prophylaxis should be individualized and selected based on the thromboembolism risk of the combination treatment regimen, using the safest and easiest to administer (Palumbo 2008).

In a scientific statement from the American Heart Association, lenalidomide has been determined to be an agent that may either cause direct myocardial toxicity or exacerbate underlying myocardial dysfunction (magnitude: major) (AHA [Page 2016]).

In a clinical trial comparing lenalidomide versus chlorambucil single agent therapy in patients >65 years of age with chronic lymphocytic leukemia patients (not an FDA-approved indication), increased mortality was observed in the lenalidomide treatment arm. Atrial fibrillation, cardiac failure, and MI were observed more frequently in lenalidomide-treated patients; lenalidomide (alone or in combination) is not currently recommended for first-line treatment of CLL. Second primary malignancies (SPMs), including hematologic (primarily AML and MDS) and solid tumor malignancies, and non-melanoma skin cancers, have been reported with lenalidomide when used for the treatment of MDS and multiple myeloma; the incidence may be higher when lenalidomide is used in combination with an alkylating agent. Monitor for development of secondary malignancies. Both hypothyroidism and hyperthyroidism have been reported with lenalidomide use; monitor thyroid function prior to therapy initiation and periodically throughout treatment.

Angioedema, Stevens-Johnson syndrome (SJS), and toxic epidermal necrolysis (TEN) have been reported; may be fatal. Consider interrupting or discontinuing treatment with grade 2 or 3 skin rash; discontinue and do not reinitiate treatment with grade 4 rash, exfoliative or bullous rash, or for suspected SJS or TEN. Patients with a history of grade 4 rash with thalidomide should not receive lenalidomide. Discontinue treatment with angioedema. Use caution in renal impairment; may experience an increased rate of toxicities (due to reduced clearance and increased half-life); initial dosage adjustments are recommended for moderate-to-severe and dialysis-dependent renal impairment. Tumor lysis syndrome (with fatalities) has been reported with lenalidomide; patients with a high tumor burden may be at risk for tumor lysis syndrome; monitor closely; institute appropriate management for hyperuricemia. Tumor flare reaction has been observed in studies of lenalidomide for the treatment of chronic lymphocytic leukemia (CLL) and lymphoma; clinical presentation includes low grade fever, pain, rash, and tender lymph node swelling. In patients with MCL, tumor flare may mimic disease progression; monitor closely. In clinical trials, the majority of tumor flare events occurred in the first cycle of therapy. Treatment with corticosteroids, nonsteroidal anti-inflammatory drugs (NSAIDs), and/or analgesics may be considered; therapy interruption may be necessary as well. Hepatic failure, including fatalities, has occurred in patients treated with combination lenalidomide and dexamethasone therapy; may have hepatocellular, cholestatic, or mixed characteristics. Risk factors may include preexisting viral liver disease, elevated liver enzymes at baseline, and concomitant medications. Monitor closely; interrupt therapy in patients with abnormal hepatic function tests. May consider resuming treatment at a lower dose upon return to baseline. Certain adverse reactions (DVT, pulmonary embolism, atrial fibrillation, renal failure) are more likely in elderly patients. Monitor renal function closely, and select dose accordingly.

[US Boxed Warning]: Do not use lenalidomide in pregnant women. Lenalidomide is an analogue of thalidomide (a human teratogen) and could potentially cause severe birth defects or embryo-fetal death; use is contraindicated during pregnancy and pregnancy must be avoided while taking lenalidomide. Obtain 2 negative pregnancy testes prior to initiation of treatment; 2 forms of contraception (or abstain from heterosexual intercourse) must be used at least 4 weeks prior to, during and for 4 weeks after lenalidomide treatment (and during treatment interruptions). Distribution is restricted; physicians, pharmacies, and patients must be registered with the Revlimid REMS program. In order to decrease the risk of embryo-fetal exposure, lenalidomide is available only through a restricted distribution program (Revlimid REMS). Prescribers and pharmacies must be certified with the program to prescribe or dispense lenalidomide. Males taking lenalidomide (even those vasectomized) must use a latex or synthetic condom during any sexual contact with women of childbearing potential and for up to 28 days following discontinuation of therapy. Males taking lenalidomide must not donate sperm. Patients should be advised not to donate blood during therapy and for 1 month following completion of therapy. May cause dizziness or fatigue; caution patients about performing tasks which require mental alertness (eg, operating machinery or driving). Potentially significant drug-drug interactions may exist, requiring dose or frequency adjustment, additional monitoring, and/or selection of alternative therapy. Formulation contains lactose; avoid use in patients with Lapp lactase deficiency, glucose-galactose malabsorption, or glucose intolerance. Lenalidomide should only be prescribed to patients (male and female) who can understand and comply with the conditions of the Revlimid REMS program. If used in patients between 12 to 18 years of age, the parent or legal guardian must agree to ensure compliance with the Revlimid REMS program.

Adverse Reactions Frequency not always defined; may vary based on indication and/or concomitant therapy.

Cardiovascular: Peripheral edema (8% to 26%), edema (10%), deep vein thrombosis (4% to 10%; grades 3/4: ≤8%), hypotension (7% to 10%), hypertension (6% to 8%), chest pain (5% to 8%), atrial fibrillation (3% to 7%; grades 3/4: ≤4%), palpitations (5%), myocardial infarction (1% to <5%), pulmonary embolism (2% to 4%; grades 3/4: 1% to 4%), syncope (grades 3/4: 1% to 3%), tachycardia (grades 3/4: 2%), cerebrovascular accident (≤2%), angina pectoris (≥1%), bradycardia (≥1%), cerebral ischemia (≥1%), cardiac failure (1%), cardiac arrest, cardiogenic shock, cardiomyopathy, cardiorespiratory arrest, cerebral infarction, increased cardiac enzymes (troponin I), ischemia, ischemic heart disease, septic shock, subarachnoid hemorrhage, supraventricular cardiac arrhythmia, tachyarrhythmia, thrombophlebitis, thrombosis, transient ischemic attacks, ventricular dysfunction

Central nervous system: Fatigue (29% to 44%), insomnia (10% to 28%), dizziness (20% to 23%), headache (10% to 20%), depression (5% to 11%), chills (5% to 10%), falling (5% to 8%), hypoesthesia (7%), lethargy (7%), pain (7%), neuropathy (including peripheral, 5% to 7%), rigors (6%), noncardiac chest pain (3% to 6%), emotional lability (≥1%), glossalgia (≥1%), hallucination (≥1%), malaise (≥1%), abnormal gait, aphasia, cerebellar infarction, confusion, dysarthria, impaired consciousness, migraine, spinal cord compression, vertigo

Dermatologic: Pruritus (4% to 42%), skin rash (19% to 36%), xeroderma (9% to 14%), diaphoresis (7% to 10%), night sweats (8%), ecchymoses (5%), erythema (5%), cellulitis (≤5%), hyperpigmentation (≥1%), Sweet's syndrome

Endocrine & metabolic: Weight loss (9% to 20%), hypokalemia (7% to 17%), hyperglycemia (4% to 12%), hypocalcemia (3% to 11%), hypothyroidism (7%), hypomagnesemia (6% to 7%), dehydration (3% to 7%), diabetes mellitus (<5%), gout (<5%), hypophosphatemia (<5%, grades 3/4: ≤3%), hyponatremia (2% to <5%), hirsutism (≥1%), loss of libido (≥1%), Graves' disease, hypernatremia, hypoglycemia

Gastrointestinal: Diarrhea (17% to 49%), constipation (16% to 41%), nausea (24% to 30%), decreased appetite (7% to 23%), abdominal pain (8% to 21%), anorexia (10% to 16%), dysgeusia (4% to 15%), vomiting (10% to 12%), dyspepsia (5% to 11%), xerostomia (7%), loose stools (6%), gastroenteritis (2% to 6%), gastrointestinal hemorrhage (≥1%), biliary obstruction, cholecystitis, colonic polyps, diverticulitis, dysphagia, gastritis, gastroesophageal reflux disease, infection of mouth, inguinal hernia (obstructive), intestinal obstruction, intestinal perforation, irritable bowel syndrome, ischemic colitis, melena

Genitourinary: Urinary tract infection (4% to 14%), dysuria (7%), erectile dysfunction (≥1%), azotemia, hematuria, pelvic pain, perirectal obsess, urolithiasis, urosepsis

Hematologic & oncologic: Thrombocytopenia (19% to 62%; grades 3/4: 8% to 50%; MDS: Onset: 28 days [range: 8 to 290 days]; recovery: 22 days [range: 5 to 224 days]), neutropenia (33% to 61%; grades 3/4: 27% to 53%; MDS: Onset: 42 days [range: 14 to 411 days]; recovery: 17 days [range: 2 to 170 days]), anemia (12% to 44%; grades 3/4: 6% to 19%), leukopenia (8% to 15%; grades 3/4: 4% to 7%), tumor flare (10%), lymphocytopenia (5% to 7%; grades 3/4: 3% to 4%), bruise (3% to 6%), febrile neutropenia (1% to 6%; grades 3/4: 1% to 6%), second primary malignant neoplasms (≤5%, including AML, lymphomas, solid tumors), squamous cell carcinoma of skin (3% to <5%; grades 3/4: ≤3%), pancytopenia (<5%; grades 3/4: ≤2%), basal cell carcinoma (<5%; grades 3/4: <1%), granulocytopenia (grades 3/4: 2%), autoimmune hemolytic anemia (≥1%), acute leukemia, blood coagulation disorder, bone marrow depression, bronchogenic carcinoma, decreased hemoglobin, hemolysis, hemolytic anemia (including warm type), lung carcinoma, malignant lymphoma, myelocytic leukemia, neutropenic infection, pancreatitis, postoperative hemorrhage, prostate carcinoma, rectal hemorrhage, splenic infarction

Hepatic: Increased serum ALT (8%), abnormal hepatic function tests (≥1%), hepatic failure, hyperbilirubinemia

Hypersensitivity: Hypersensitivity reaction, transfusion reaction

Infection: Influenza (3% to 6%), sepsis (including *Enterobacter*, 3% to 6%; grades 3/4: 2% to 5%), bacteremia (1%), bacterial infection, clostridium infection, fungal infection, herpes virus infection, kidney infection, Klebsiella infection, localized infection, pseudomonas infection, staphylococcal infection

Local: Catheter infection

Neuromuscular & skeletal: Muscle cramps (18% to 33%), back pain (13% to 32%), weakness (14% to 28%), arthralgia (8% to 22%), tremor (21%), muscle spasm (11% to 21%), ostealgia (1% to 16%), limb pain (5% to 15%), musculoskeletal pain (7% to 13%), musculoskeletal chest pain (7% to 11%), myalgia (9%), myasthenia (5% to 8%), neck pain (2% to 8%), arthritis, bone fracture (femur, femoral neck, pelvis, hip, rib, spinal compression), calcium pyrophosphate deposition disease

Ophthalmic: Blurred vision (17%), cataract (≤14%; grades 3/4: ≤6%), subcapsular posterior cataract (<5%), blindness (≥1%), ocular hypertension (≥1%)

Otic: Otic infection

Renal: Renal failure (4% to 10%), increased serum creatinine

Respiratory: Cough (13% to 28%), upper respiratory tract infection (6% to 25%), dyspnea (17% to 24%), nasopharyngitis (6% to 23%), pneumonia (9% to 18%), bronchitis (6% to 17%), pharyngitis (14% to 16%), epistaxis (3% to 15%), oropharyngeal pain (3% to 10%), sinusitis (7% to 8%), pleural effusion (7%; grades 3/4: 1%), dyspnea on exertion (≤7%), respiratory tract infection (4% to 7%), rhinitis (3% to 7%), lower respiratory tract infection (2% to 6%), hypoxia (2%; grades 3/4: 1%), hoarseness (≥1%), pneumonitis (grades 3/4: 1%), pulmonary hypertension (grades 3/4: 1%), respiratory distress (1%; grades 3/4: 1% to 2%), chronic obstructive pulmonary disease, interstitial pulmonary disease, pulmonary edema, pulmonary infiltrates, respiratory failure, wheezing

Miscellaneous: Fever (14% to 28%), physical health deterioration (2%), multiorgan failure (grades 3/4: 1%), mass (renal), nodule

<1%, postmarketing, and/or case reports: Angioedema, atrial flutter, catheter infection, circulatory shock, desquamation, drug overdose, erythema multiforme, Fanconi's syndrome, hematologic disease (impaired stem cell

mobilization), hemorrhage, hemorrhagic diathesis, hepatitis, intracranial hemorrhage, leukoencephalopathy, myopathy, nephrolithiasis, orthostatic hypotension, peripheral ischemia, pseudomembranous colitis, pseudomonas infection, pulmonary edema, pulmonary infiltrates, rectal hemorrhage, renal tubular necrosis, Stevens-Johnson syndrome, stomatitis, toxic epidermal necrolysis, tumor lysis syndrome, urinary retention, urticaria, viral infection

Drug Interactions

Metabolism/Transport Effects Substrate of P-glycoprotein

Avoid Concomitant Use

Avoid concomitant use of Lenalidomide with any of the following: Abatacept; Anakinra; BCG (Intravesical); Canakinumab; Certolizumab Pegol; Deferiprone; Dipyrone; Natalizumab; Pimecrolimus; Rilonacept; Tacrolimus (Topical); Tocilizumab; Tofacitinib; Vaccines (Live); Vedolizumab

Increased Effect/Toxicity

Lenalidomide may increase the levels/effects of: Abatacept; Anakinra; Bisphosphonate Derivatives; Canakinumab; Certolizumab Pegol; CloZAPine; Deferiprone; Digoxin; Fingolimod; Leflunomide; Natalizumab; Rilonacept; Tofacitinib; Vaccines (Live); Vedolizumab

The levels/effects of Lenalidomide may be increased by: Denosumab; Dexamethasone (Systemic); Dipyrone; Erythropoiesis-Stimulating Agents; Estrogen Derivatives; Ocrelizumab; Pimecrolimus; Promazine; Roflumilast; Tacrolimus (Topical); Tocilizumab; Trastuzumab

Decreased Effect

Lenalidomide may decrease the levels/effects of: BCG (Intravesical); Coccidioides immitis Skin Test; Nivolumab; Sipuleucel-T; Tertomotide; Vaccines (Inactivated); Vaccines (Live)

The levels/effects of Lenalidomide may be decreased by: Echinacea

Hazardous Drugs Handling Considerations

Hazardous agent (NIOSH 2016 [group 2]).

Use appropriate precautions for receiving, handling, administration, and disposal. Gloves (single) should be worn during receiving, unpacking, and placing in storage. NIOSH recommends single gloving for administration of intact tablets or capsules (NIOSH 2016).

Storage/Stability Store at 20°C to 25°C (68°F to 77°F); excursions permitted to 15°C and 30°C (59°F and 86°F).

Mechanism of Action Lenalidomide has immunomodulatory, antiangiogenic, and antineoplastic characteristics via multiple mechanisms. It selectively inhibits secretion of proinflammatory cytokines (potent inhibitor of tumor necrosis factor-alpha secretion); enhances cell-mediated immunity by stimulating proliferation of anti-CD3 stimulated T cells (resulting in increased IL-2 and interferon gamma secretion); inhibits trophic signals to angiogenic factors in cells. Inhibits the growth of myeloma cells by inducing cell cycle arrest and cell death.

Pharmacodynamics/Kinetics

Absorption: Rapid

Protein binding: ~30%

Half-life elimination: 3 to 5 hours

Time, to peak, plasma: MDS or myeloma patients: 0.5 to 6 hours

Excretion: Urine (~82%; as unchanged drug)

Hemodialysis effect: ~30% of the drug in body is removed in a 4-hour hemodialysis session; Hemodialysis patients: 80% decrease in drug clearance compared with healthy subjects.

Dosing

Adult

Mantle cell lymphoma (MCL): Oral: 25 mg once daily for 21 days of a 28-day treatment cycle; continue until disease progression or unacceptable toxicity

Multiple myeloma: Oral: 25 mg once daily for 21 days of a 28-day treatment cycle (in combination with dexamethasone). In patients not eligible for autologous stem cell transplantation, continue until disease progression or unacceptable toxicity; in transplant eligible patients, hematopoietic stem cell mobilization should occur within 4 cycles of a lenalidomide-containing therapy.

Multiple myeloma, maintenance (following autologous stem cell transplant): Oral: 10 mg once daily (begin after adequate hematologic recovery); continue until disease progression or unacceptable toxicity. If tolerated, may increase dose to 15 mg once daily after 3 cycles (each cycle is 28 days).
Off-label dosing: 10 mg once daily for 21 days of a 28-day treatment cycle until relapse (Palumbo 2010)

Myelodysplastic syndrome (MDS) with deletion 5q: Oral: 10 mg once daily

Chronic lymphocytic leukemia (CLL), relapsed/refractory (off-label use): Oral: 10 mg once daily beginning on day 9 of cycle 1; administer continuously in combination with cyclic rituximab (Badoux 2013)

Diffuse large B-cell lymphoma, relapsed/refractory (off-label use): Oral: 25 mg once daily for 21 days of a 28-day treatment cycle for up to 1 year (Wiernik 2008)

Multiple myeloma, newly diagnosed (off-label combination): Oral: 25 mg once daily for 14 days of a 21-day cycle (in combination with bortezomib and dexamethasone) for 8 cycles (Kumar 2012; Richardson 2010) **or** 25 mg once daily for 21 days of a 28-day cycle (in combination with carfilzomib and dexamethasone) for up to 8 cycles (Jakubowiak 2012)

Multiple myeloma, relapsed (off-label combinations): Adults: Oral: 25 mg once daily for 21 days of 28-day cycle (in combination with carfilzomib and dexamethasone) until disease progression or unacceptable toxicity (Stewart 2015) **or** 25 mg once daily for 21 days of a 28-day cycle (in combination with daratumumab and dexamethasone) until disease progression or unacceptable toxicity; refer to the IMWG recommendations for Dosing in Renal Impairment (Dimopoulos 2016a; Dimopoulos 2016b).

Myelodysplastic syndrome (MDS), lower risk, without deletion 5q (off-label use): Oral: 10 mg once daily (Raza 2008)

Systemic light chain amyloidosis (off-label use): Oral: 15 mg once daily for 21 days of a 28-day cycle (in combination with dexamethasone) (Nair 2012; Sanchorawala 2007)

Geriatric Refer to adult dosing. Due to the potential for decreased renal function in the elderly, select dose carefully and closely monitor renal function.

Renal Impairment Note: *Maintain appropriate number of treatment days per cycle based on indication and/or protocol.* Further individualize (increase or decrease dose) based on tolerance.

Recommended initial dose adjustment in the manufacturer's labeling:
  MCL and multiple myeloma (combination therapy with dexamethasone):
    CrCl >60 mL/minute: No dosage adjustment necessary.
    CrCl 30 to 60 mL/minute: 10 mg once daily (for multiple myeloma, may increase to 15 mg once daily after 2 cycles if nonresponsive but tolerating treatment)
    CrCl <30 mL/minute (nondialysis dependent): 15 mg every 48 hours
    ESRD: CrCl <30 mL/minute and dialysis dependent: 5 mg once daily (administer after dialysis on dialysis days)
  MDS and multiple myeloma (maintenance treatment after autologous stem cell transplant):
    CrCl >60 mL/minute: No dosage adjustment necessary.
    CrCl 30 to 60 mL/minute: 5 mg once daily
    CrCl <30 mL/minute (nondialysis dependent): 2.5 mg once daily
    ESRD: CrCl <30 mL/minute and dialysis dependent: 2.5 mg once daily (administer after dialysis on dialysis days)
  Dialysis removal: Approximately 30% removed during a 4-hour hemodialysis session
  The International Myeloma Working Group (IMWG) recommendations (Dimopoulos 2016b):
    The IMWG recommends use of the Chronic Kidney Disease Epidemiology Collaboration (CKD-EPI) equation (preferred) or the Modification of Diet in Renal Disease (MDRD) formula to evaluate renal function estimation in multiple myeloma patients with a stable serum creatinine.
    Combination therapy with dexamethasone:
      CrCl ≥60 mL/minute: 25 mg once daily (no dosage adjustment necessary).
      CrCl 30 to 59 mL/minute: 10 mg once daily (may increase to 15 mg once daily in the absence of toxicity).
      CrCl 15 to 29 mL/minute: 15 mg once every other day; may adjust to 10 mg once daily.
      CrCl <15 mL/minute: 5 mg once daily
      ESRD on dialysis: 5 mg once daily.
Hepatic Impairment There are no dosage adjustments provided in the manufacturer's labeling (has not been studied). However, lenalidomide undergoes minimal hepatic metabolism.
Adjustment for Toxicity
NONHEMATOLOGIC toxicities:
Dermatologic toxicities:
  Skin rash, grade 2 or 3: Consider interrupting or discontinuing treatment
  Angioedema, grade 4 rash, exfoliative or bullous rash, or suspected Stevens-Johnson syndrome or toxic epidermal necrolysis: Discontinue treatment; do not rechallenge
Tumor flare reaction:
  Grade 1 or 2: Continue therapy at physician's discretion; may consider symptom management with corticosteroids, nonsteroidal anti-inflammatory drugs (NSAIDs) and/or analgesic therapy.
  Grade 3 or 4: Interrupt therapy until resolved to ≤ grade 1; consider symptom management with corticosteroids, nonsteroidal anti-inflammatory drugs (NSAIDs) and/or analgesic therapy.
Other toxicities: For additional treatment-related grade 3/4 toxicities, hold treatment and restart (if appropriate) at next lower dose level when toxicity has resolved to ≤ grade 2.

◄ **HEMATOLOGIC toxicities:**
Adjustment for thrombocytopenia in MCL:
Platelets <50,000/mm^3: Hold treatment, check CBC weekly
When platelets return to ≥50,000/mm^3: Resume treatment at 5 mg below previous dose; do not dose below 5 mg daily

Adjustment for neutropenia in MCL:
ANC <1,000/mm^3 for at least 7 days or associated with fever (≥38.5°C [101°F]): Hold treatment, check CBC weekly
ANC <500/mm^3: Hold treatment, check CBC weekly
When ANC returns to ≥1,000/mm^3: Resume treatment at 5 mg below previous dose; do not dose below 5 mg daily

Adjustment for thrombocytopenia in MDS:
*Thrombocytopenia developing **within** 4 weeks of beginning treatment at 10 mg daily:*
Baseline platelets ≥100,000/mm^3:
 If platelets <50,000/mm^3: Hold treatment
 When platelets return to ≥50,000/mm^3: Resume treatment at 5 mg daily
Baseline platelets <100,000/mm^3:
 If platelets fall to 50% of baseline: Hold treatment
 If baseline ≥60,000/mm^3 and platelet level returns to ≥50,000/mm^3: Resume at 5 mg daily
 If baseline <60,000/mm^3 and platelet level returns to ≥30,000/mm^3: Resume at 5 mg daily
*Thrombocytopenia developing **after** 4 weeks of beginning treatment at 10 mg daily:*
Platelets <30,000/mm^3 **or** <50,000/mm^3 with platelet transfusions: Hold treatment
When platelets return to ≥30,000/mm^3 (without hemostatic failure): Resume at 5 mg daily
Thrombocytopenia developing during treatment at 5 mg daily:
Platelets <30,000/mm^3 **or** <50,000/mm^3 with platelet transfusions: Hold treatment
When platelets return to ≥30,000/mm^3 (without hemostatic failure): Resume at 2.5 mg once daily

Adjustment for neutropenia in MDS:
*Neutropenia developing **within** 4 weeks of beginning treatment at 10 mg daily:*
For baseline absolute neutrophil count (ANC) ≥1,000/mm^3:
 ANC <750/mm^3: Hold treatment
 When ANC returns to ≥1,000/mm^3: Resume at 5 mg daily
For baseline absolute neutrophil count (ANC) <1,000/mm^3:
 ANC <500/mm^3: Hold treatment
 When ANC returns to ≥500/mm^3: Resume at 5 mg daily
*Neutropenia developing **after** 4 weeks of beginning treatment at 10 mg daily:*
ANC <500/mm^3 for ≥7 days or associated with fever (≥38.5°C [101°F]): Hold treatment
When ANC returns to ≥500/mm^3: Resume at 5 mg daily
Neutropenia developing during treatment at 5 mg daily:
ANC <500/mm^3 for ≥7 days or associated with fever (≥38.5°C [101°F]): Hold treatment
When ANC returns to ≥500/mm^3: Resume at 2.5 mg once daily

Adjustment for thrombocytopenia in multiple myeloma:

Combination therapy with dexamethasone:

Platelets <30,000/mm^3: Hold treatment, check CBC weekly

When platelets return to ≥30,000/mm^3: Resume at next lower dose; do not dose below 2.5 mg daily

Additional occurrence of platelets <30,000/mm^3: Hold treatment

When platelets return to ≥30,000/mm^3: Resume treatment at next lower dose; do not dose below 2.5 mg daily

Maintenance following autologous stem cell transplant:

Platelets <30,000/mm^3: Hold treatment, check CBC weekly

When platelets return to ≥30,000/mm^3: Resume at next lower dose; maintain continuous daily dosing

Additional occurrence of platelets <30,000/mm^3 (and current dose is 5 mg once daily): Hold treatment

When platelets return to ≥30,000/mm^3 (and current dose is 5 mg once daily): Resume treatment at 5 mg daily on days 1 to 21 of a 28-day cycle; do not dose below 5 mg daily on days 1 to 21 of a 28-day cycle.

Adjustment for neutropenia in multiple myeloma:

Combination therapy with dexamethasone:

ANC <1,000/mm^3: Hold treatment, check CBC weekly

When ANC returns to ≥1,000/mm^3 (with neutropenia as only toxicity): Resume at 25 mg daily or initial starting dose

When ANC returns to ≥1,000/mm^3 (with additional toxicities): Resume at next lower dose; do not dose below 2.5 mg daily

Additional occurrence of ANC <1,000/mm^3: Hold treatment

When ANC returns to ≥1,000/mm^3: Resume treatment at next lower dose; do not dose below 2.5 mg daily

Maintenance following autologous stem cell transplant:

ANC <500/mm^3: Hold treatment, check CBC weekly

When ANC returns to ≥500/mm^3: Resume at next lower dose; maintain continuous daily dosing

Additional occurrence of ANC <500/mm^3 (and current dose is 5 mg daily): Hold treatment

When ANC returns to ≥500/mm^3: Resume treatment at 5 mg daily on days 1 to 21 of a 28-day cycle; do not dose below 5 mg daily on days 1 to 21 of a 28-day cycle.

Combination Regimens

◀ **Administration** Administer at about the same time each day with water; administer with or without food. Swallow capsule whole; do not break, open, or chew.

Missed doses: May administer a missed dose if within 12 hours of usual dosing time. If greater than 12 hours, patient should skip dose for that day and resume usual dosing the following day. Patient should **not** take 2 doses to make up for a missed dose.

Emetic Potential
Children: Minimal (<10%)
Adults: Low (10% to 30%)

Monitoring Parameters
CBC with differential (MCL - weekly for the first cycle, every 2 weeks during cycles 2 to 4; MDS - weekly for first 8 weeks; Multiple myeloma - weekly for the first 2 cycles, every 2 weeks during the third cycle), then monthly thereafter; serum creatinine, liver function tests, thyroid function tests (TSH at baseline then every 2 to 3 months during lenalidomide treatment [Hamnvik 2011]); ECG when clinically indicated; monitor for signs and symptoms of infection (if neutropenic), secondary malignancies, thromboembolism, tumor lysis syndrome, or tumor flare reaction

Women of childbearing potential: Pregnancy test 10 to 14 days **and** 24 hours prior to initiating therapy, weekly during the first 4 weeks of treatment, then every 2 to 4 weeks through 4 weeks after therapy discontinued

Prescribing and Access Restrictions In Canada, distribution is restricted through RevAid (www.RevAid.ca or 1-888-738-2431).

Medication Guide Available Yes

Dosage Forms Excipient information presented when available (limited, particularly for generics); consult specific product labeling.
Capsule, Oral:
Revlimid: 2.5 mg [contains fd&c blue #2 (indigotine)]
Revlimid: 5 mg
Revlimid: 10 mg, 15 mg, 20 mg [contains fd&c blue #2 (indigotine)]
Revlimid: 25 mg

Lenvatinib (len VA ti nib)

Related Information
Common Toxicity Criteria *on page 2242*
Management of Chemotherapy-Induced Nausea and Vomiting in Adults *on page 2253*
Safe Handling of Hazardous Drugs *on page 2379*

Brand Names: US Lenvima 10 MG Daily Dose; Lenvima 14 MG Daily Dose; Lenvima 18 MG Daily Dose; Lenvima 20 MG Daily Dose; Lenvima 24 MG Daily Dose; Lenvima 8 MG Daily Dose

Brand Names: Canada Lenvima

Index Terms E7080; Lenvatinib Mesylate; Lenvima

Pharmacologic Category Antineoplastic Agent, Tyrosine Kinase Inhibitor; Antineoplastic Agent, Vascular Endothelial Growth Factor (VEGF) Inhibitor

Use
Renal cell carcinoma, advanced: Treatment of advanced renal cell carcinoma (in combination with everolimus) following one prior anti-angiogenic therapy.

Thyroid cancer, differentiated: Treatment of locally recurrent or metastatic, progressive, radioactive iodine-refractory differentiated thyroid cancer (DTC)

Labeled Contraindications There are no contraindications listed in the manufacturer's US labeling.

Canadian labeling: Hypersensitivity to lenvatinib or any component of the formulation.

Pregnancy Considerations Adverse events were observed in animal reproduction studies. Based on the mechanism of action, lenvatinib may cause fetal harm if administered in pregnancy. Females of reproductive potential should use effective contraception during lenvatinib treatment and for at least 2 weeks after completion of therapy.

Breastfeeding Considerations It is not known if lenvatinib is excreted into breast milk. The manufacturer recommends that breastfeeding be discontinued during therapy.

Warnings/Precautions Hypertension, including grade 3 and 4 toxicity, occurred in clinical trials; the median time to onset of new or worsening hypertension was 16 to 35 days. Blood pressure should be controlled prior to initiating therapy; monitor frequently throughout treatment. Other cardiac events such as decreased left or right ventricular function, decreased ejection fraction, cardiac failure, or pulmonary edema were also reported, including grades 2, 3, and 4 events. In patients with thyroid cancer, decreased ejection fraction (EF) was the most commonly reported of these events; some patients experienced greater than 20% EF reduction. Monitor for signs/symptoms of cardiac decompensation. QT/QTc prolongation was also observed in lenvatinib treated patients, including prolongation >500 msec and increases >60 msec from baseline. Monitor and correct electrolyte abnormalities in all patients; obtain electrocardiograms in patients with congenital long QT syndrome, heart failure, bradyarrhythmias, or in those on concomitant medications known to prolong the QT interval. Cardiac effects may require therapy interruption, dosage reduction, or discontinuation. An increased incidence of hypocalcemia (including grade 3 events) was observed in lenvatinib-treated patients compared to the control group in clinical trials. Calcium replacement therapy and dosage interruption or reduction generally corrected hypocalcemia. Monitor serum calcium levels at least monthly; replace calcium as necessary. May require therapy interruption or dosage reduction. Arterial thromboembolic events, including grade 3 or higher events, have been reported. Discontinue treatment if arterial thrombosis occurs; the safety of resuming therapy after such an event has not been established. Lenvatinib has not been studied in patients who have had an arterial thromboembolic event within the preceding 6 months. Hemorrhagic events (most frequently epistaxis) occurred in over one-third of lenvatinib-treated patients. Serious tumor-related bleeding events (including cases of fatal hemorrhage) have been observed in clinical trials and postmarketing surveillance. Serious and fatal carotid artery hemorrhages were reported more frequently in patients with anaplastic thyroid carcinoma (ATC) than with other tumor types. Safety and efficacy of lenvatinib have not been established in the treatment of ATC. Consider the risk of hemorrhage associated with tumor infiltration/invasion into major blood vessels. Monitor for bleeding; may require therapy interruption, dosage reduction, or discontinuation.

Lenvatinib impairs exogenous thyroid suppression. In patients with differentiated thyroid cancer and a normal thyroid stimulating hormone (TSH) level at baseline, TSH elevations were observed in over half of lenvatinib-treated patients. Grades 1 and 2 hypothyroidism occurred in renal cell cancer patients receiving lenvatinib and everolimus; TSH elevations occurred in over half of in patients with a normal or low TSH at baseline. Monitor TSH levels at baseline and at least monthly; adjust thyroid hormone therapy or manage hypothyroidism as clinically necessary. Gastrointestinal perforation, fistula formation, or abscess were reported in a small percentage of patients in a clinical trial. Discontinue use in patients who develop perforation or life-threatening fistula. Lenvatinib is associated with a moderate emetic potential; antiemetics are recommended to prevent nausea and vomiting. Nausea, vomiting, and diarrhea were commonly observed. Initiate appropriate management prior to therapy interruption or dosage reduction; initiate active management of diarrhea and other gastrointestinal symptoms for grade 1 or higher events. Monitor closely for dehydration; dehydration or hypovolemia due to diarrhea and vomiting are risk factors for renal toxicity. Diarrhea may require treatment interruption, dose reduction, and or discontinuation. The incidence of diarrhea is higher in when lenvatinib is used in combination with everolimus; recurrent diarrhea occurred despite dose reduction. Diarrhea was the most common reason for dose reduction or treatment interruption in patients with renal cell cancer. Reversible posterior leukoencephalopathy syndrome (RPLS) has occurred (rarely). If RPLS diagnosis is confirmed through MRI, interrupt treatment until fully resolved. Therapy may resume at a reduced dose or be discontinued, depending on the severity and persistence of neurologic symptoms. Palmar-plantar erythrodysesthesia (usually grades 1 to 2) was observed in nearly one-third of patients receiving lenvatinib.

Elevations in transaminases (including grade 3 or greater events) were observed. There have been case reports of hepatic failure (some fatal) and acute hepatitis with single-agent lenvatinib. Monitor liver function tests at baseline and throughout therapy. May require therapy interruption, dosage reduction, or discontinuation. If hepatic failure occurs, discontinue treatment. Proteinuria (including grade 3 toxicity) was commonly observed. Monitor for proteinuria at baseline and periodically throughout therapy. If urine dipstick for proteinuria is 2+, obtain a 24-hour urine protein. Withhold treatment for proteinuria ≥2 g/24 hours; resume at a reduced dose when proteinuria is <2 g/24 hours. Discontinue for nephrotic syndrome. Renal impairment may also occur (may be grade 3 or higher); a primary risk factor for severe renal impairment is dehydration or hypovolemia due to diarrhea and vomiting. Monitor renal function throughout treatment; may require therapy interruption, dosage reduction, or discontinuation. Potentially significant drug-drug interactions may exist, requiring dose or frequency adjustment, additional monitoring, and/or selection of alternative therapy.

Adverse Reactions

>10%:

Cardiovascular: Hypertension (73%), peripheral edema (21%)

Central nervous system: Fatigue (67%), headache (38%), voice disorder (31%), mouth pain (25%), dizziness (15%), insomnia (12%)

Dermatologic: Palmar-plantar erythrodysesthesia (32%), skin rash (21%), alopecia (12%)

Endocrine & metabolic: Increased thyroid stimulating hormone level (57%), weight loss (51%)

Gastrointestinal: Diarrhea (67%), decreased appetite (54%), nausea (47%), stomatitis (41%), vomiting (36%), abdominal pain (31%), constipation (29%), dysgeusia (18%), xerostomia (17%), dyspepsia (13%)

Genitourinary: Proteinuria (34%), urinary tract infection (11%)

Hematologic & oncologic: Hemorrhage (35%; grades ≥3: 2%)

Neuromuscular & skeletal: Arthralgia (≤62%), myalgia (≤62%)

Renal: Renal insufficiency (14%)

Respiratory: Cough (24%), epistaxis (12%)

1% to 10%:

Cardiovascular: Hypotension (9%), prolonged Q-T interval on ECG (9%), thromboembolic complications (5%), pulmonary embolism (3%), reduced ejection fraction (2%; ejection fraction reduced by >20%)

Dermatologic: Hyperkeratosis (7%)

Endocrine & metabolic: Dehydration (9%), hypocalcemia (grades 3/4: 9%), hypokalemia (grades 3/4: 6%), hypercalcemia (>5%), hypercholesterolemia (>5%), hyperkalemia (>5%), hypoalbuminemia (>5%), hypoglycemia (>5%), hypomagnesemia (>5%)

Gastrointestinal: Infection of mouth (10%), increased serum amylase (>5%), increased serum lipase (grades 3/4: 4%), gastrointestinal fistula (2%)

Hematologic & oncologic: Decreased platelet count (grades 3/4: 2%)

Hepatic: Hyperbilirubinemia (>5%), increased serum alkaline phosphatase (>5%), increased serum AST (grades 3 or higher: 5%), increased serum ALT (grades 3 or higher: 4%)

Renal: Increased serum creatinine (grades 3/4: 3%)

Respiratory: Pulmonary edema (7%)

<1%, postmarketing, and/or case reports: Pancreatitis, reversible posterior leukoencephalopathy syndrome, tumor hemorrhage

Drug Interactions

Metabolism/Transport Effects Substrate of BCRP, CYP3A4 (minor), P-glycoprotein; **Note:** Assignment of Major/Minor substrate status based on clinically relevant drug interaction potential; **Inhibits** BSEP, OAT1, OAT3, OCT1, OCT2, SLCO1B1, UGT1A1, UGT1A4

Avoid Concomitant Use

Avoid concomitant use of Lenvatinib with any of the following: Highest Risk QTc-Prolonging Agents; Hydroxychloroquine; Irinotecan Products; MiFEPRIStone; Probucol; Promazine; Vinflunine

Increased Effect/Toxicity

Lenvatinib may increase the levels/effects of: Highest Risk QTc-Prolonging Agents; Irinotecan Products; Moderate Risk QTc-Prolonging Agents

The levels/effects of Lenvatinib may be increased by: Hydroxychloroquine; MiFEPRIStone; Probucol; Promazine; QTc-Prolonging Agents (Indeterminate Risk and Risk Modifying); Vinflunine; Xipamide

Decreased Effect There are no known significant interactions involving a decrease in effect.

Hazardous Drugs Handling Considerations

Hazardous agent (meets NIOSH 2016 criteria). This medication is not on the NIOSH (2016) list; however, it meets the criteria for a hazardous drug. Drugs are classified as hazardous based on their properties; the properties of a hazardous drug include one or more of the following characteristics: carcinogenic, teratogenic (or other developmental toxicity), reproductive toxicity, organotoxic at low doses, genotoxic, and/or new agents with structural or toxicity profiles similar to existing hazardous agents.

Use appropriate precautions for receiving, handling, administration, and disposal. Gloves (single) should be worn during receiving, unpacking, and placing in storage.

NIOSH recommends single gloving for administration of intact tablets or capsules. If manipulating tablets/capsules (eg, to prepare an oral suspension), NIOSH recommends double gloving, a protective gown, and preparation in a controlled device; if not prepared in a controlled device, respiratory and eye/face protection as well as ventilated engineering controls are recommended. NIOSH recommends double gloving, a protective gown, and (if there is a potential for vomit or spit up) eye/face protection for administration of an oral liquid/feeding tube administration (NIOSH 2016).

Storage/Stability Store at 25°C (77°F); excursions are permitted between 15°C and 30°C (59°F and 86°F).

Mechanism of Action Lenvatinib is a multitargeted tyrosine kinase inhibitor of vascular endothelial growth factor (VEGF) receptors VEGFR1 (FLT1), VEGFR2 (KDR), VEGFR3 (FLT4), fibroblast growth factor (FGF) receptors FGFR1, 2, 3, and 4, platelet derived growth factor receptor alpha (PDGFRα), KIT, and RET. Inhibition of these receptor tyrosine kinases leads to decreased tumor growth and slowing of cancer progression. Combining lenvatinib with everolimus has demonstrated increased antiangiogenic and antitumor activity by decreasing human endothelial cell proliferation, tube formation, and VEGF signaling (in vitro) compared to either drug alone.

Pharmacodynamics/Kinetics

Protein binding: 98% to 99%

Metabolism: Primarily enzymatic through CYP3A and aldehyde oxidase; nonenzymatic metabolism also occurs

Half-life elimination: ~28 hours

Time to peak: 1 to 4 hours

Excretion: Feces (~64%); urine (~25%)

Dosing

Adult & Geriatric Note: Lenvatinib is associated with a moderate emetic potential; antiemetics are recommended to prevent nausea and vomiting.

Renal cell carcinoma, advanced: Oral: 18 mg once daily (in combination with everolimus), continue until disease progression or unacceptable toxicity (Motzer 2015)

Thyroid cancer, differentiated: Oral: 24 mg once daily until disease progression or unacceptable toxicity (Schlumberger 2015)

Missed doses: Do not take a missed dose within 12 hours of the next dose (if within 12 hours, skip the missed dose and return to regular administration time).

Renal Impairment

Preexisting renal impairment:

CrCl ≥30 mL/minute: No dosage adjustment necessary.

CrCl <30 mL/minute:

Renal cell cancer, advanced: 10 mg once daily

Thyroid cancer, differentiated: 14 mg once daily

End-stage renal disease (ESRD): There are no dosage adjustments provided in the manufacturer's labeling (has not been studied).

Hemodialysis: Lenvatinib is not expected to be dialyzable (due to high protein binding).

Renal toxicity during treatment: Interrupt therapy or discontinue if grade 3 or 4 renal failure or impairment develops. Consider resuming at a reduced dose if resolves to ≤ grade 1 or baseline (depending on severity and persistence of toxicity).

Hepatic Impairment

Preexisting hepatic impairment:

Mild or moderate impairment (Child-Pugh class A or B): No dosage adjustment necessary.

Severe impairment (Child-Pugh class C):

    Renal cell cancer, advanced: 10 mg once daily

    Thyroid cancer, differentiated: 14 mg once daily

Hepatotoxicity during treatment: Interrupt therapy if grade 3 or 4 hepatotoxicity develops. When improved to ≤ grade 1 or baseline, may either resume at a reduced dose or discontinue, depending on severity and persistence of toxicity. Discontinue for hepatic failure; do not resume.

Adjustment for Toxicity

Recommended dose modifications for persistent and intolerable grade 2 or grade 3 adverse reactions or grade 4 laboratory abnormalities:

Renal cell cancer, advanced:

    First occurrence: Interrupt therapy until resolved to ≤ grade 1 or baseline, then resume dosing at 14 mg once daily

    Second occurrence (same or different toxicity): Interrupt therapy until resolved to ≤ grade 1 or baseline, then resume dosing at 10 mg once daily.

    Third occurrence (same or different toxicity): Interrupt therapy until resolved to ≤ grade 1 or baseline, then resume dosing at 8 mg once daily.

    Note: For toxicities related only to everolimus, reduce frequency to every other day or interrupt or discontinue everolimus (refer to Everolimus monograph for dosage adjustment for toxicity). For toxicities related to both lenvatinib and everolimus, first reduce lenvatinib, and then everolimus.

Thyroid cancer, differentiated:

    First occurrence: Interrupt therapy until resolved to ≤ grade 1 or baseline, then resume dosing at 20 mg once daily

    Second occurrence (same or different toxicity): Interrupt therapy until resolved to ≤ grade 1 or baseline, then resume dosing at 14 mg once daily

    Third occurrence (same or different toxicity): Interrupt therapy until resolved to ≤ grade 1 or baseline, then resume dosing at 10 mg once daily

    Note: There are currently no recommendations for resuming therapy in patients who experience grade 4 clinical adverse reactions that resolve.

Arterial thrombotic event: Discontinue therapy; do not resume.

Cardiac:

    Cardiac dysfunction: Temporarily interrupt therapy for a grade 3 event until improved to ≤ grade 1 or baseline; depending on severity and persistence of toxicity, may either resume therapy at a reduced dose or discontinue treatment. Discontinue for a grade 4 event; do not resume.

    Hypertension: Monitor blood pressure prior to and throughout therapy; initiate or adjust antihypertensive medication to control blood pressure. Temporarily interrupt therapy for grade 3 hypertension that persists despite optimal medical management. When hypertension is ≤ grade 2, resume therapy at a reduced dose. Discontinue therapy for life-threatening hypertension; do not resume.

    QT prolongation: Temporarily interrupt therapy for ≥ grade 3 QT prolongation (>500 msec). When improved to ≤ grade 1 (<480 msec) or baseline, resume therapy at a reduced dose

◀

Gastrointestinal toxicity:

Nausea, vomiting, or diarrhea:

Grade 3: Initiate prompt medical management prior to interrupting therapy (or reducing dose) until resolves to ≤ grade 1 or baseline; then resume (may require dose reduction).

Grade 4 vomiting or diarrhea despite optimal medical management: Discontinue therapy; do not resume.

Perforation (any grade) or fistula formation (grade 3 or 4; life-threatening): Discontinue therapy; do not resume.

Hemorrhage: Temporarily interrupt therapy for a grade 3 event until improved to ≤ grade 1 or baseline; depending on severity and persistence of toxicity, may either resume therapy at a reduced dose or discontinue treatment. Discontinue for a grade 4 event; do not resume.

Hypocalcemia: Administer calcium replacement therapy as necessary; may require treatment interruption or dose reduction depending on the severity, presence of ECG changes, and persistence of hypocalcemia.

Nephrotic syndrome: Discontinue therapy; do not resume.

Proteinuria: Temporarily interrupt therapy for ≥2 g proteinuria/24 hours; resume therapy at a reduced dose when improved to <2 g proteinuria/24 hours.

Reversible posterior leukoencephalopathy syndrome (RPLS): Interrupt or discontinue therapy until fully resolved; consider resuming at a reduced dose if resolves to ≤ grade 1, depending on severity and persistence of neurologic symptoms.

Combination Regimens

Renal cell cancer: Everolimus-Lenvatinib (RCC) on page 2111

Administration

Lenvatinib is associated with a moderate emetic potential; antiemetics are recommended to prevent nausea and vomiting.

Oral: Administer orally at the same time each day (administer lenvatinib and everolimus at the same time each day when used for the treatment of renal cell cancer). May be administered without regards to meals.

Capsules should be swallowed whole, however, if unable to swallow whole, the capsules may be dissolved in a small glass of liquid. Measure 15 mL of water or apple juice into a glass; add whole capsule and leave in liquid for at least 10 minutes, then stir for at least 3 minutes. Administer liquid, then add 15 mL of additional water or apple juice to glass, swirl a few times and then swallow additional liquid.

Emetic Potential Moderate (30% to 90%)

Extemporaneous Preparations An oral solution may be prepared in a glass. Measure 15 mL of water or apple juice into a glass; add whole capsule and leave in liquid for at least 10 minutes, then stir for at least 3 minutes. Administer liquid, then add 15 mL of additional water or apple juice to glass, swirl a few times and then swallow additional liquid.

Lenvima (lenvatinib) [prescribing information]. Woodcliff Lake, NJ: Eisai Inc.; May 2016.

Monitoring Parameters Liver function tests (at baseline, every 2 weeks for 2 months, and at least monthly thereafter); renal function; electrolytes; serum calcium at least monthly; TSH levels at baseline and monthly or as clinically indicated; monitor for proteinuria at baseline and periodically during treatment (urine dipstick; if 2+ then 24-hour urine protein); monitor blood pressure after 1 week, then every 2 weeks for 2 months, and at least monthly thereafter; electrocardiogram in select patients; monitor for signs/symptoms of cardiac

decompensation, arterial thrombosis, reversible posterior leukoencephalopathy syndrome, signs/symptoms of gastrointestinal perforation/fistula, and hemorrhagic events

Prescribing and Access Restrictions Lenvatinib is available only through specialty pharmacies. For further information on patient assistance, product availability, and prescribing instructions, please refer to the following website: http://www.lenvima.com/hcp/pharmacy-financial-options

Dosage Forms Considerations Each Lenvima Therapy Pack contains a 30 day supply of dosage units

Dosage Forms Excipient information presented when available (limited, particularly for generics); consult specific product labeling.

Capsule Therapy Pack, Oral:
Lenvima 10 MG Daily Dose: 10 mg (30 ea)
Lenvima 14 MG Daily Dose: 10 mg & 4 mg (60 ea)
Lenvima 18 MG Daily Dose: 10 mg & 2x4 mg (15 ea, 90 ea)
Lenvima 20 MG Daily Dose: 2x10 mg (60 ea)
Lenvima 24 MG Daily Dose: 2x10 mg & 4 mg (90 ea)
Lenvima 8 MG Daily Dose: 2x4 mg (10 ea, 60 ea)

◆ **Lenvatinib Mesylate** see Lenvatinib on page 1112

◆ **Lenvima** see Lenvatinib on page 1112

◆ **Lenvima 8 MG Daily Dose** see Lenvatinib on page 1112

◆ **Lenvima 10 MG Daily Dose** see Lenvatinib on page 1112

◆ **Lenvima 14 MG Daily Dose** see Lenvatinib on page 1112

◆ **Lenvima 18 MG Daily Dose** see Lenvatinib on page 1112

◆ **Lenvima 20 MG Daily Dose** see Lenvatinib on page 1112

◆ **Lenvima 24 MG Daily Dose** see Lenvatinib on page 1112

Letrozole (LET roe zole)

Related Information
Safe Handling of Hazardous Drugs on page 2379

Brand Names: US Femara

Brand Names: Canada ACH-Letrozole; Apo-Letrozole; Auro-Letrozole; Bio-Letrozole; Femara; JAMP-Letrozole; Mar-Letrozole; MED-Letrozole; Nat-Letrozole; PMS-Letrozole; RAN-Letrozole; Riva-Letrozole; Sandoz-Letrozole; Teva-Letrozole; Van-Letrozole; Zinda-Letrozole

Index Terms CGS-20267

Pharmacologic Category Antineoplastic Agent, Aromatase Inhibitor

Use Breast cancer in postmenopausal women: Adjuvant treatment of hormone receptor-positive early breast cancer, extended adjuvant treatment of early breast cancer after 5 years of tamoxifen; treatment of advanced breast cancer with disease progression following antiestrogen therapy; first-line treatment of hormone receptor-positive or hormone receptor-unknown, locally-advanced, or metastatic breast cancer

Labeled Contraindications
Hypersensitivity to letrozole or any component of the formulation; pregnancy
Canadian labeling: Additional contraindications (not in the US labeling): Hypersensitivity to other aromatase inhibitors; use in patients <18 years of age; premenopausal endocrine status; breastfeeding

◄ **Pregnancy Considerations** Use is contraindicated in women with an established pregnancy.

Breast cancer: Letrozole is approved for the treatment of breast cancer in postmenopausal women. Based on the mechanism of action and data from animal reproduction studies, letrozole may cause fetal harm if used during pregnancy. A pregnancy test is recommended prior to therapy in women of reproductive potential and effective contraception should be used during therapy and for at least 3 weeks following the last dose.

Infertility associated with polycystic ovarian syndrome (PCOS): Letrozole is used off-label to induce ovulation in infertile anovulatory women with PCOS (Balen 2016; Franik 2014; Legro 2013; Legro 2014; Misso 2012). Baseline testing is done prior to letrozole therapy to rule out unexpected ovulation which prevents exposure in early pregnancy (Legro 2016).

Breastfeeding Considerations It is not known if letrozole is present in breast milk. Due to the potential for serious adverse reactions in the breastfed infant, breastfeeding is not recommended by the manufacturer during therapy and for at least 3 weeks after the last dose.

Warnings/Precautions Use caution with hepatic impairment; dose adjustment recommended in patients with cirrhosis or severe hepatic dysfunction. May cause dizziness, fatigue, and somnolence; patients should be cautioned before performing tasks which require mental alertness (eg, operating machinery or driving). May increase total serum cholesterol; in patients treated with adjuvant therapy and cholesterol levels within normal limits, an increase of ≥1.5 x ULN in total cholesterol (non-fasting) has been demonstrated in 8.2% of letrozole-treated patients (25% requiring lipid-lowering medications) vs 3.2% of tamoxifen-treated patients (16% requiring medications); monitor cholesterol panel; may require antihyperlipidemics. May cause decreases in bone mineral density (BMD). In one study, a decrease in hip BMD by 3.8% from baseline in letrozole-treated patients vs 2% in placebo at 2 years was demonstrated, however, while lumbar spine BMD was decreased, the difference was not statistically. Results of a safety study did demonstrate a decrease in lumbar spine BMD with letrozole (compared to tamoxifen). Osteoporosis and bone fractures have occurred at higher rates when compared to tamoxifen or to placebo; monitor BMD. Potentially significant drug-drug interactions may exist, requiring dose or frequency adjustment, additional monitoring, and/or selection of alternative therapy.

Adverse Reactions

>10%:

Cardiovascular: Edema (7% to 18%)

Central nervous system: Headache (4% to 20%), dizziness (3% to 14%), fatigue (8% to 13%)

Dermatologic: Diaphoresis (≤24%), night sweats (15%)

Endocrine & metabolic: Hypercholesterolemia (3% to 52%), hot flash (6% to 50%), weight gain (2% to 13%)

Gastrointestinal: Nausea (9% to 17%), constipation (2% to 11%)

Neuromuscular & skeletal: Weakness (4% to 34%), arthralgia (8% to 25%), arthritis (7% to 25%), ostealgia (5% to 22%), back pain (5% to 18%), decreased bone mineral density (≤5% to 15%), osteoporosis (≤5% to 15%), bone fracture (10% to 14%)

Respiratory: Dyspnea (6% to 18%), cough (6% to 13%)

1% to 10%:

Cardiovascular: Chest pain (6% to 8%), hypertension (5% to 8%), chest wall pain (6%), peripheral edema (5%), cerebrovascular accident (2% to 3%; including hemorrhagic stroke, thrombotic stroke), thromboembolism (2% to 3%; including portal vein thrombosis, pulmonary embolism, thrombophlebitis, venous thrombosis), angina pectoris (1% to 2%), myocardial infarction (1% to 2%), transient ischemic attacks

Central nervous system: Insomnia (6% to 7%), pain (5%), anxiety (<5%), depression (<5%), vertigo (<5%), drowsiness (3%)

Dermatologic: Skin rash (5%), alopecia (3% to 5%), pruritus (1%)

Endocrine & metabolic: Weight loss (6% to 7%), hypercalcemia (<5%)

Gastrointestinal: Diarrhea (5% to 8%), vomiting (3% to 7%), abdominal pain (6%), anorexia (1% to 5%), dyspepsia (3%)

Genitourinary: Mastalgia (2% to 7%), urinary tract infection (6%), vaginal dryness (5%), vaginal hemorrhage (5%), vaginal irritation (5%)

Hematologic & oncologic: Metastases (2% to 4%)

Infection: Infection (7%), influenza (6%), viral infection (6%)

Neuromuscular & skeletal: Limb pain (4% to 10%), myalgia (7% to 9%)

Ophthalmic: Cataract (2%)

Renal: Renal disease (5%)

Respiratory: Pleural effusion (<5%)

<1%, postmarketing, and/or case reports: Anaphylaxis, angioedema, arterial thrombosis, blurred vision, cardiac failure, carpal tunnel syndrome, dysesthesia, dysgeusia, endometrial carcinoma, endometrial hyperplasia, erythema multiforme, eye irritation, fever, hepatitis, hypoesthesia, increased appetite, increased liver enzymes, increased thirst, irritability, leukopenia, memory Impairment, nervousness, palpitations, paresthesia, stomatitis, tachycardia, tenosynovitis (trigger finger), thrombocytopenia, toxic epidermal necrolysis, urinary frequency, urticaria, vaginal discharge, xeroderma, xerostomia

Drug Interactions

Metabolism/Transport Effects Substrate of CYP2A6 (minor), CYP3A4 (minor); **Note:** Assignment of Major/Minor substrate status based on clinically relevant drug interaction potential; **Inhibits** CYP2A6 (strong)

Avoid Concomitant Use

Avoid concomitant use of Letrozole with any of the following: Artesunate; Tegafur

Increased Effect/Toxicity

Letrozole may increase the levels/effects of: Artesunate; CYP2A6 Substrates; Methadone

Decreased Effect

Letrozole may decrease the levels/effects of: Artesunate; Tegafur

The levels/effects of Letrozole may be decreased by: Tamoxifen

Hazardous Drugs Handling Considerations

Hazardous agent (NIOSH 2016 [group 1]).

Use appropriate precautions for receiving, handling, administration, and disposal. Gloves (single) should be worn during receiving, unpacking, and placing in storage. NIOSH recommends single gloving for administration of intact tablets or capsules (NIOSH 2016).

Storage/Stability Store at room temperature of 25°C (77°F); excursions permitted to 15°C to 30°C (59°F to 86°F).

◄ **Mechanism of Action** Letrozole is a nonsteroidal competitive inhibitor of the aromatase enzyme system which binds to the heme group of aromatase, a cytochrome P450 enzyme which catalyzes conversion of androgens to estrogens (specifically, androstenedione to estrone and testosterone to estradiol). This leads to inhibition of the enzyme and a significant reduction in plasma estrogen (estrone, estradiol and estrone sulfate) levels. Letrozole does not appear to affect synthesis of adrenal or thyroid hormones, aldosterone, or androgens.

Pharmacodynamics/Kinetics

Absorption: Rapid and well absorbed; not affected by food

Distribution: V_d: ~1.9 L/kg

Protein binding, plasma: Weak

Metabolism: Hepatic via CYP3A4 and 2A6 to an inactive carbinol metabolite

Half-life elimination: Terminal: ~2 days

Time to steady state, plasma: 2 to 6 weeks; steady state serum concentrations are 1.5 to 2 times higher than single-dose values. In girls 3 to 9 years, steady state concentrations were 25% to 67% that of the mean adult values (Feuillan 2007)

Excretion: Urine (~90%; 6% as unchanged drug, 75% as glucuronide carbinol metabolite, 9% as unidentified metabolites)

Dosing

Adult & Geriatric

Breast cancer, advanced (first- or second-line treatment): Females: Postmenopausal: Oral: 2.5 mg once daily; continue until tumor progression

Breast cancer, early (adjuvant treatment): Females: Postmenopausal: Oral: 2.5 mg once daily for a planned duration of 5 years; discontinue at relapse.

Duration of therapy: American Society of Clinical Oncology (ASCO) guidelines for Adjuvant Endocrine Therapy of Hormone Receptor-Positive Breast Cancer (Focused Update) recommend a maximum duration of 5 years of aromatase inhibitor therapy for postmenopausal women; aromatase inhibitors may be combined with tamoxifen for a total duration of up to 10 years of endocrine therapy. Refer to the guidelines for specific recommendations based on menopausal status and tolerability (Burstein 2014). Treatment with an additional 5 years of therapy (for a total of 10 years of aromatase inhibitor therapy) has demonstrated a significantly improved rate of disease-free survival and a decreased risk of disease recurrence and contralateral breast cancer (when compared to placebo), although overall survival was not significantly different between groups and bone-related adverse events occurred more frequently with letrozole versus placebo (Goss 2016).

Breast cancer, early (extended adjuvant treatment): Females: Postmenopausal: Oral: 2.5 mg once daily for a planned duration of 5 years (after 5 years of tamoxifen); discontinue at relapse. In clinical trials, letrozole was initiated within 3 months of discontinuing tamoxifen (Goss 2003; Jin 2012).

Duration of therapy: ASCO guidelines for Adjuvant Endocrine Therapy of Hormone Receptor-Positive Breast Cancer (Focused Update) recommend a maximum duration of 5 years of aromatase inhibitor therapy for postmenopausal women; aromatase inhibitors may be combined with tamoxifen for a total duration of up to 10 years of endocrine therapy. Refer to the guidelines for specific recommendations based on menopausal status and tolerability (Burstein 2014). Treatment with an additional 5 years of therapy (for a total of 10 years of aromatase inhibitor therapy) has demonstrated a significantly improved rate of disease-free survival and a decreased risk of disease recurrence and contralateral breast cancer (when compared to placebo), although overall survival was not significantly different between groups and bone-related adverse events occurred more frequently with letrozole versus placebo (Goss 2016).

Off-label combinations:

Breast cancer, advanced, estrogen receptor-positive, HER2-negative: Females: Oral: 2.5 mg once daily (in combination with palbociclib) until disease progression or unacceptable toxicity (Finn 2015) **or** 2.5 mg once daily (in combination with ribociclib) until disease progression or unacceptable toxicity (Hortobagyi 2016)

Breast cancer, metastatic, hormone receptor-positive, HER2-positive: Females: Oral: 2.5 mg once daily (in combination with lapatinib) until disease progression or unacceptable toxicity (Johnston 2009)

Infertility/ovulation stimulation in anovulatory women with polycystic ovarian syndrome (PCOS; off-label use): Oral: 2.5 to 7.5 mg daily on cycle days 3 to 7 (Franik 2014; Legro 2013; Legro 2014; Misso 2012). Up to 5 treatment cycles may be administered with the dose increased in subsequent cycles for nonresponse or poor ovulatory response as determined by progesterone levels; maximum dose 7.5 mg daily (Legro 2014). Additional trials may be necessary to further define the routine use of letrozole in infertile women with PCOS.

Ovarian (epithelial) cancer, recurrent (off-label use): Oral: 2.5 mg once daily; continue until disease progression or unacceptable toxicity (Ramirez 2008)

Renal Impairment
CrCl ≥10 mL/minute: No dosage adjustment necessary.
CrCl <10 mL/minute: There are no dosage adjustments provided in the manufacturer's labeling.

Hepatic Impairment
Mild to moderate impairment (Child-Pugh class A or B): No dosage adjustment necessary.
Severe impairment (Child-Pugh class C) and cirrhosis: 2.5 mg every other day
Noncirrhotic patients with elevated bilirubin: There are no dosage adjustments provided in the manufacturer's labeling (effect has not been determined).

Combination Regimens
Breast cancer:
Lapatinib-Letrozole (Breast) on page 2162
Letrozole-Ribociclib (Breast Cancer Regimen) on page 2167
Palbociclib-Letrozole (Breast) on page 2189

Administration Administer orally without regard to meals.

Monitoring Parameters
Cholesterol, hepatic function tests; bone density; pregnancy test (prior to treatment in females of reproductive potential).
For infertility/ovarian stimulation (off-label use), a pregnancy test is recommended prior to initiation. Midluteal progestin concentrations (in a clinical study, nonresponse to treatment was defined as a progesterone concentration <3 ng/mL during the midluteal phase; poor ovulatory response was defined as progesterone concentrations indicating ovulation but just above the cutoff point) (Legro 2014).

Dietary Considerations Calcium and vitamin D supplementation are recommended.

Dosage Forms Excipient information presented when available (limited, particularly for generics); consult specific product labeling.
Tablet, Oral:
Femara: 2.5 mg
Generic: 2.5 mg

◆ **Letrozole and Ribociclib** see Ribociclib and Letrozole on page 1608

◆ **Leucovorin** see Leucovorin Calcium on page 1124

Leucovorin Calcium (loo koe VOR in KAL see um)

Related Information

Mucositis and Stomatitis on page 2299

Brand Names: Canada Lederle Leucovorin; Leucovorin Calcium Injection; Leucovorin Calcium Injection USP

Index Terms 5-Formyl Tetrahydrofolate; Calcium Folinate; Calcium Leucovorin; Citrovorum Factor; Folinate Calcium; Folinic Acid (error prone synonym); Leucovorin

Pharmacologic Category Antidote; Chemotherapy Modulating Agent; Rescue Agent (Chemotherapy); Vitamin, Water Soluble

Use

Colorectal cancer, advanced: Injection: Palliative treatment of advanced colorectal cancer to prolong survival (in combination with 5-fluorouracil).

Methotrexate toxicity:
Injection: Rescue agent after high-dose methotrexate treatment in osteosarcoma and to diminish the toxicity and counteract the effects of impaired methotrexate elimination and of inadvertent overdosage of folic acid antagonists.
Oral: Rescue agent to diminish toxicity and counteract effects of impaired methotrexate elimination and inadvertent overdoses of folic acid antagonists.

Megaloblastic anemia: Injection: Treatment of megaloblastic anemias due to folic acid deficiency (when oral therapy is not feasible).

Labeled Contraindications Pernicious anemia and other megaloblastic anemias secondary to vitamin B_{12}-deficiency

Pregnancy Considerations Animal reproduction studies have not been conducted. Leucovorin is a biologically active form of folic acid. Adequate amounts of folic acid are recommended during pregnancy.

Breastfeeding Considerations Leucovorin is a biologically active form of folic acid. Adequate amounts of folic acid are recommended in breastfeeding women.

Warnings/Precautions When used for the treatment of accidental folic acid antagonist overdose, administer as soon as possible. When used for the treatment of a methotrexate overdose, administer IV leucovorin as soon as possible. Monitoring of the serum methotrexate concentration is essential to determine the optimal dose/duration of leucovorin; however, do not wait for the results of a methotrexate level before initiating therapy. It is important to adjust the leucovorin dose once a methotrexate level is known. When used for methotrexate rescue therapy, methotrexate serum concentrations should be monitored to determine dose and duration of leucovorin therapy. The dose may need to be increased or administration prolonged in situations where methotrexate excretion may be delayed (eg, ascites, pleural effusion, renal insufficiency, inadequate hydration); **never administer leucovorin intrathecally**. Parenteral administration may be preferred to oral if vomiting or malabsorption is likely. Potentially significant drug-drug interactions may exist, requiring dose or frequency adjustment, additional monitoring, and/or selection of alternative therapy. Combination of leucovorin and sulfamethoxazole-trimethoprim for the acute treatment of PCP in patients with HIV infection has been reported to cause increased rates of treatment failure. Leucovorin may increase the toxicity of 5-fluorouracil; deaths from severe enterocolitis, diarrhea, and dehydration have been reported (in elderly patients); granulocytopenia and fever have also been reported.

Hypersensitivity, including allergic reactions, anaphylactoid reactions, and urticaria have been reported with leucovorin. Because leucovorin is typically administered in combination with other chemotherapy agents, it may be difficult to determine the causative agent for hypersensitivity reactions. In a series of 44 patients with hypersensitivity to leucovorin-containing regimens, hypersensitivity/infusion reaction to leucovorin was confirmed in 5 patients; reactions also occurred with subsequent rechallenge with LEVOleucovorin (Ureña-Tavera, 2015).

Leucovorin is inappropriate treatment for pernicious anemia and other megaloblastic anemias secondary to a lack of vitamin B_{12}; a hematologic remission may occur while neurologic manifestations progress. Leucovorin is excreted renally; the risk for toxicities may be increased in patients with renal impairment.

Benzyl alcohol and derivatives: When doses >10 mg/m^2 are required using the powder for injection, reconstitute using sterile water for injection, not a solution containing benzyl alcohol; large amounts of benzyl alcohol (≥99 mg/kg/day) have been associated with a potentially fatal toxicity ("gasping syndrome") in neonates; the "gasping syndrome" consists of metabolic acidosis, respiratory distress, gasping respirations, CNS dysfunction (including convulsions, intracranial hemorrhage), hypotension, and cardiovascular collapse (AAP ["Inactive" 1997]; CDC, 1982); some data suggests that benzoate displaces bilirubin from protein binding sites (Ahlfors, 2001); avoid or use dosage forms containing benzyl alcohol with caution in neonates. See manufacturer's labeling.

Injection: Due to calcium content, do not administer IV solutions at a rate >160 mg/minute. Not intended for intrathecal use.

Adverse Reactions Frequency not defined. Toxicities (especially gastrointestinal toxicity) of fluorouracil are enhanced when used in combination with leucovorin.

Dermatologic: Erythema, pruritus, skin rash, urticaria

Hematologic & oncologic: Thrombocythemia

Hypersensitivity: Anaphylactoid reaction, hypersensitivity reaction

Respiratory: Wheezing

Drug Interactions

Metabolism/Transport Effects None known.

Avoid Concomitant Use

Avoid concomitant use of Leucovorin Calcium with any of the following: Raltitrexed; Trimethoprim

Increased Effect/Toxicity

Leucovorin Calcium may increase the levels/effects of: Capecitabine; Fluorouracil (Systemic); Fluorouracil (Topical); Tegafur

◀

Decreased Effect

Leucovorin Calcium may decrease the levels/effects of: Fosphenytoin; PHENobarbital; Phenytoin; Primidone; Raltitrexed; Trimethoprim

The levels/effects of Leucovorin Calcium may be decreased by: Glucarpidase

Storage/Stability

Powder for injection: Powder for injection: Store intact vials and reconstituted solution at 25°C (77°F); excursions permitted between 15°C and 30°C (59°F and 86°F). Protect from light. Solutions reconstituted with bacteriostatic water for injection U.S.P., must be used within 7 days. Solutions reconstituted with SWFI must be used immediately.

Solution for injection: Prior to dilution, store vials under refrigeration at 2°C to 8°C (36°F to 46°F). Protect from light.

Tablet: Store at room temperature of 15°C to 30°C (59°F to 86°F).

Preparation for Administration

Powder for injection: Reconstitute with SWFI or BWFI; dilute in D5W or NS for infusion. When doses >10 mg/m^2 are required, reconstitute using sterile water for injection, not a solution containing benzyl alcohol.

For methanol toxicity, dilute in D5W (Barceloux, 2002).

Mechanism of Action A reduced form of folic acid, leucovorin supplies the necessary cofactor blocked by methotrexate. Leucovorin actively competes with methotrexate for transport sites, displaces methotrexate from intracellular binding sites, and restores active folate stores required for DNA/RNA synthesis. Stabilizes the binding of 5-dUMP and thymidylate synthetase, enhancing the activity of fluorouracil. When administered with pyrimethamine for the treatment of opportunistic infections, leucovorin reduces the risk for hematologic toxicity (HHS [OI adult 2015]).

Methanol toxicity treatment: Formic acid (methanol's toxic metabolite) is normally metabolized to carbon dioxide and water by 10-formyltetrahydrofolate dehydrogenase after being bound to tetrahydrofolate. Administering a source of tetrahydrofolate may aid the body in eliminating formic acid (Barceloux, 2002).

Pharmacodynamics/Kinetics

Absorption: Oral, IM: Well absorbed

Metabolism: Intestinal mucosa and hepatically to 5-methyl-tetrahydrofolate (5MTHF; active)

Bioavailability: Saturable at oral doses >25 mg; 25 mg (97%), 50 mg (75%), 100 mg (37%)

Half-life elimination: ~4 to 8 hours

Time to peak: Oral: ~2 hours; IV: Total folates: 10 minutes; 5MTHF: ~1 hour; IM: Total folates: 52 minutes; 5MTHF: 2.8 hours

Excretion: Urine (primarily); feces

Dosing

Adult & Geriatric

Colorectal cancer, advanced: IV: 200 mg/m^2/day over at least 3 minutes for 5 days every 4 weeks for 2 cycles, then every 4 to 5 weeks (in combination with fluorouracil) **or** 20 mg/m^2/day for 5 days every 4 weeks for 2 cycles, then every 4 to 5 weeks (in combination with fluorouracil). **Note:** Multiple leucovorin-containing regimens are available for the treatment of colorectal cancer. Refer to appropriate literature/guidelines for additional details.

Folic acid antagonist (eg, trimethoprim, pyrimethamine) overdose: Oral: 5 to 15 mg once daily

Folate-deficient megaloblastic anemia: IM, IV: ≤1 mg once daily

High-dose methotrexate-rescue: Initial: Oral, IM, IV: 15 mg (~10 mg/m^2); start 24 hours after beginning methotrexate infusion; continue every 6 hours for 10 doses, until methotrexate level is <0.05 micromolar. Adjust dose as follows:

Normal methotrexate elimination (serum methotrexate level ~10 micromolar at 24 hours after administration, 1 micromolar at 48 hours, and <0.2 micromolar at 72 hours): Oral, IM, IV: 15 mg every 6 hours for 60 hours (10 doses) beginning 24 hours after the start of methotrexate infusion

Delayed late methotrexate elimination (serum methotrexate level remaining >0.2 micromolar at 72 hours and >0.05 micromolar at 96 hours after administration): Continue leucovorin calcium 15 mg (oral, IM or IV) every 6 hours until methotrexate level is <0.05 micromolar

Delayed early methotrexate elimination and/or acute renal injury (serum methotrexate level ≥50 micromolar at 24 hours, or ≥5 micromolar at 48 hours, or a doubling of serum creatinine level at 24 hours after methotrexate administration): IV: 150 mg every 3 hours until methotrexate level is <1 micromolar, then 15 mg every 3 hours until methotrexate level is <0.05 micromolar

High-dose methotrexate overexposure: Leucovorin nomogram dosing for high-dose methotrexate overexposure (off-label dosing; generalized dosing derived from reference nomogram figures, refer to each reference [Bleyer, 1978; Bleyer, 1981; Widemann, 2006] or institution-specific nomogram for details):

At 24 hours:
For methotrexate levels of ≥100 micromolar at ~24 hours, leucovorin is initially dosed at 1,000 mg/m^2 every 6 hours
For methotrexate levels of ≥10 to <100 micromolar at 24 hours, leucovorin is initially dosed at 100 mg/m^2 every 3 or 6 hours
For methotrexate levels of ~1 to 10 micromolar at 24 hours, leucovorin is initially dosed at 10 mg/m^2 every 3 or 6 hours

At 48 hours:
For methotrexate levels of ≥100 micromolar at 48 hours, leucovorin is dosed at 1,000 mg/m^2 every 6 hours
For methotrexate levels of ≥10 to <100 micromolar at 48 hours, leucovorin is dosed at 100 mg/m^2 every 3 hours
For methotrexate levels of ~1 to 10 micromolar at 48 hours, leucovorin is dosed at 100 mg/m^2 every 6 hours **or** 10 to 100 mg/m^2 every 3 hours

At 72 hours:
For methotrexate levels of ≥10 micromolar at 72 hours, leucovorin is dosed at 100 to 1,000 mg/m^2 every 3 to 6 hours
For methotrexate levels of ~1 to 10 micromolar at 72 hours, leucovorin is dosed at 10 to 100 mg/m^2 every 3 hours
For methotrexate levels of ~0.1 to 1 micromolar at 72 hours, leucovorin is dosed at 10 mg/m^2 every 3 to 6 hours

If serum creatinine is increased more than 50% above baseline, increase the standard leucovorin dose to 100 mg/m^2 every 3 hours, then adjust according to methotrexate levels above.

Follow methotrexate levels daily, leucovorin may be discontinued when methotrexate level is <0.1 micromolar

◀

Methotrexate overdose (inadvertent) (begin as soon as possible after overdose): Oral, IM, IV: 10 mg/m² every 6 hours until the methotrexate level is <0.01 micromolar. If serum creatinine is increased more than 50% above baseline 24 hours after methotrexate administration, if 24 hour methotrexate level is >5 micromolar, or if 48 hour methotrexate level is >0.9 micromolar, increase leucovorin dose to 100 mg/m² IV every 3 hours until the methotrexate level is <0.01 micromolar.

Do not administer leucovorin intrathecally; the use of intrathecal leucovorin is not advised (Jardine, 1996; Smith, 2008).

Bladder cancer, neoadjuvant treatment (off-label use): IV, Oral: 15 mg every 6 hours for 4 doses on days 2 and 9, starting 24 hours after each methotrexate dose (in combination with methotrexate, vinblastine, and cisplatin) (Griffiths, 2011).

Cofactor therapy in methanol toxicity (off-label use): IV: 1 mg/kg (maximum dose: 50 mg) over 30 to 60 minutes every 4 to 6 hours. Therapy should continue until methanol and formic acid have been completely eliminated (Barceloux, 2002).

Esophageal cancer, advanced or metastatic (off-label use): IV: 400 mg/m² over 2 hours once every 2 weeks (in combination with fluorouracil and irinotecan [FOLFIRI]) until disease progression or unacceptable toxicity (Guimbaud, 2014) **or** 200 mg/m² over 2 hours once every 2 weeks (in combination with fluorouracil and oxaliplatin) until disease progression or unacceptable toxicity (Al-Batran, 2008).

Gastric cancer, advanced or metastatic (off-label use): IV: 400 mg/m² over 2 hours once every 2 weeks (in combination with fluorouracil and irinotecan [FOLFIRI]) until disease progression or unacceptable toxicity (Guimbaud, 2014) **or** 200 mg/m² over 2 hours once every 2 weeks (in combination with fluorouracil and oxaliplatin) until disease progression or unacceptable toxicity (Al-Batran, 2008).

Pancreatic cancer, metastatic (off-label use): IV: 400 mg/m² over 2 hours once every 2 weeks (in combination with fluorouracil, oxaliplatin, and irinotecan [FOLFIRINOX]) for at least 6 months (Conroy, 2011).

Pemetrexed toxicity (off-label dose): IV: 100 mg/m² once, followed by 50 mg/m² every 6 hours for 8 days (used in clinical trial for CTC grade 4 leukopenia ≥3 days; CTC grade 4 neutropenia ≥3 days; immediately for CTC grade 4 thrombocytopenia, bleeding associated with grade 3 thrombocytopenia, or grade 3 or 4 mucositis) (Alimta [prescribing information], 2013).

Prevention of pyrimethamine hematologic toxicity in HIV-infected patients (off-label use; HHS [OI adult 2015]): Oral:

Isosporiasis (*Isospora belli*):
  Treatment: 10 to 25 mg once daily (in combination with pyrimethamine)
  Chronic maintenance (secondary prophylaxis): 5 to 10 mg once daily (in combination with pyrimethamine)

Pneumocystis pneumonia (PCP): Prophylaxis (primary and secondary): 25 mg once weekly (in combination with pyrimethamine [with dapsone]) **or** 10 mg once daily (in combination with pyrimethamine [with atovaquone])

Toxoplasma gondii encephalitis:
  Primary prophylaxis: 25 mg once weekly (in combination with pyrimethamine [with dapsone]) **or** 10 mg once daily (in combination with pyrimethamine [with atovaquone])
  Treatment: 10 to 25 mg once daily (in combination with pyrimethamine [with either sulfadiazine, clindamycin, atovaquone, or azithromycin]).

Note: May increase leucovorin to 50 to 100 mg/day in divided doses in cases of pyrimethamine toxicity (rash, nausea, bone marrow suppression).

Chronic maintenance (secondary prophylaxis): 10 to 25 mg once daily (in combination with pyrimethamine [with either sulfadiazine or clindamycin]) **or** 10 mg once daily (in combination with pyrimethamine [with atovaquone])

Pediatric

Folic acid antagonist (eg, trimethoprim, pyrimethamine) overdose: Refer to adult dosing.

Folate-deficient megaloblastic anemia: Refer to adult dosing.

High-dose methotrexate-rescue: Refer to adult dosing.

Cofactor therapy in methanol toxicity (off-label use): Refer to adult dosing.

Prevention of pyrimethamine hematologic toxicity in HIV-exposed/-positive patients (off-label uses; CDC, 2009):

Infants and Children >1 month of age: **Note:** Leucovorin should continue for 1 week after pyrimethamine is discontinued.

Toxoplasmosis (*Toxoplasma gondii*):

Primary prophylaxis: Oral: 5 mg once every 3 days (in combination with pyrimethamine [with either dapsone or atovaquone])

Secondary prophylaxis: Oral: 5 mg once every 3 days (in combination with pyrimethamine [with either sulfadiazine, atovaquone, or clindamycin])

Treatment (congenital): Oral or IM: 10 mg with every pyrimethamine dose (in combination with either sulfadiazine or clindamycin); treatment duration: 12 months

Treatment (acquired): Oral: Acute induction: 10-25 mg once daily (in combination with pyrimethamine [with either sulfadiazine, clindamycin, or atovaquone]) for ≥6 weeks

Adolescents: Refer to adult dosing

Renal Impairment There are no dosage adjustments provided in the manufacturer's labeling.

Hepatic Impairment There are no dosage adjustments provided in the manufacturer's labeling.

Combination Regimens

Bladder cancer: CMV (Bladder) on page 2068

Bone sarcoma (osteosarcoma):

HDMTX on page 2144

MAP (Osteosarcoma) on page 2170

Colorectal cancer:

Bevacizumab-Fluorouracil-Leucovorin (Colorectal) on page 1992

Bevacizumab + FOLFIRI (Colorectal) on page 1992

Bevacizumab FOLFOX (Colorectal) on page 1993

Cetuximab + FOLFIRI (Colorectal) on page 2031

FLOX (Colorectal) on page 2116

Fluorouracil-Leucovorin Bolus (Colorectal) on page 2124

Fluorouracil-Leucovorin Infusional (Colorectal) on page 2125

Fluorouracil-Leucovorin-Irinotecan (Saltz Regimen) (Colorectal) on page 2126

FOLFIRI (Colorectal) on page 2128

FOLFOX1 (Colorectal) on page 2129

FOLFOX2 (Colorectal) on page 2130

Administration Due to calcium content, do not administer IV solutions at a rate >160 mg/minute; not intended for intrathecal use.

Refer to individual protocols. Should be administered IM, IV push, or IV infusion (15 minutes to 2 hours). Leucovorin should not be administered concurrently with methotrexate. It is commonly initiated 24 hours after the start of methotrexate. Toxicity to normal tissues may be irreversible if leucovorin is not initiated by ~40 hours after the start of methotrexate.

As a rescue after folate antagonists: Administer by IV bolus, IM, or orally.

Do not administer orally in the presence of nausea or vomiting. Doses >25 mg should not be administered orally (should be converted to parenteral therapy).

Combination therapy with fluorouracil: Fluorouracil is usually given after, or at the midpoint, of the leucovorin infusion. Leucovorin is usually administered by IV bolus injection or short (10 to 120 minutes) IV infusion. Other administration schedules have been used; refer to individual protocols.

For the treatment of methanol toxicity, infuse over 30 to 60 minutes (Barceloux, 2002)

Extemporaneous Preparations A 5 mg/mL oral suspension may be prepared with tablets, Cologel, and a 2:1 mixture of simple syrup and wild cherry syrup. Crush twenty-four 25 mg tablets in a glass mortar and reduce to a fine powder; transfer powder to amber bottle. Add 30 mL Cologel and shake mixture thoroughly. Add a quantity of syrup mixture sufficient to make 120 mL. Label "shake well" and "refrigerate". Stable for 28 days refrigerated.

Lam MS. Extemporaneous Compounding of Oral Liquid Dosage Formulations and Alternative Drug Delivery Methods for Anticancer Drugs. *Pharmacotherapy.* 2011;31(2):164-192.

Monitoring Parameters

High-dose methotrexate therapy: Plasma methotrexate concentration; leucovorin is continued until the plasma methotrexate level <0.05 micromolar. With 4- to 6-hour high-dose methotrexate infusions, plasma drug values in excess of 50 and 1 micromolar at 24 and 48 hours after starting the infusion, respectively, are often predictive of delayed methotrexate clearance.

Fluorouracil therapy: CBC with differential and platelets, liver function tests, electrolytes

Dietary Considerations Solutions for injection contain calcium 0.004 mEq per leucovorin 1 mg

Dosage Forms Excipient information presented when available (limited, particularly for generics); consult specific product labeling. [DSC] = Discontinued product

Solution, Injection [strength expressed as base]:
Generic: 300 mg/30 mL (30 mL [DSC])

Solution Reconstituted, Injection [strength expressed as base]:
Generic: 100 mg (1 ea); 200 mg (1 ea); 350 mg (1 ea); 500 mg (1 ea)

Solution Reconstituted, Injection [strength expressed as base, preservative free]:
Generic: 50 mg (1 ea); 100 mg (1 ea); 200 mg (1 ea); 350 mg (1 ea)

Tablet, Oral [strength expressed as base]:
Generic: 5 mg, 10 mg, 15 mg, 25 mg

◆ **Leucovorin Calcium Injection (Can)** *see* Leucovorin Calcium *on page 1124*

◆ **Leucovorin Calcium Injection USP (Can)** *see* Leucovorin Calcium *on page 1124*

◆ **Leukeran** *see* Chlorambucil *on page 383*

◆ **Leukine** *see* Sargramostim *on page 1656*

Leuprolide (loo PROE lide)

Related Information
Safe Handling of Hazardous Drugs *on page 2379*

Brand Names: US Eligard; Lupron Depot (1-Month); Lupron Depot (3-Month); Lupron Depot (4-Month); Lupron Depot (6-Month); Lupron Depot-Ped (1-Month); Lupron Depot-Ped (3-Month)

Brand Names: Canada Eligard; Lupron; Lupron Depot

Index Terms Abbott-43818; Leuprolide Acetate; Leuprorelin Acetate; TAP-144

Pharmacologic Category Antineoplastic Agent; Gonadotropin-Releasing Hormone Agonist; Gonadotropin Releasing Hormone Agonist

Use

Central precocious puberty: Treatment of children with central precocious puberty (CPP). CPP is defined as early onset of secondary sexual characteristics (usually <8 years of age in girls and <9 years of age in boys) associated with pubertal pituitary gonadotropin activation; may have a significantly advanced bone age resulting in diminished adult height.

Limitations of use: Prior to treatment initiation, confirm clinical diagnosis of CPP with blood concentrations of luteinizing hormone (LH) (basal or stimulated with a gonadotropin-releasing hormone [GnRH] analog), sex steroids, and bone age assessment (versus chronological age). Baseline evaluations should include height and weight measurements, diagnostic brain imaging (to rule out intracranial tumor), pelvic/testicular/adrenal ultrasound (to rule out steroid-secreting tumors), human chorionic gonadotropin levels (to rule out a chorionic gonadotropin-secreting tumor), and adrenal steroid measurements (to exclude congenital adrenal hyperplasia).

Endometriosis: Management of endometriosis, including pain relief and reduction of endometriotic lesions. Initial management of endometriosis and symptom recurrence (in combination with norethindrone acetate).

Limitations of use: Experience with leuprolide depot in females has been limited to women ≥18 years; treatment should be limited to 6 months.

Prostate cancer, advanced: Palliative treatment of advanced prostate cancer

Uterine leiomyomata (fibroids): Treatment (preoperative) of anemia caused by uterine leiomyomata (fibroids).

Limitations of use: Experience with leuprolide depot in females has been limited to women ≥18 years.

Labeled Contraindications

Hypersensitivity to leuprolide, GnRH, GnRH-agonist analogs, or any component of the formulation; women who are or may become pregnant; breast-feeding (Lupron Depot 3.75 mg [monthly] and Lupron Depot 11.25 mg [3-month]); undiagnosed abnormal vaginal bleeding (Lupron Depot 3.75 mg [monthly] and Lupron Depot 11.25 mg [3-month]).

Lupron Depot 22.5 mg, 30 mg, and 45 mg and Eligard (all strengths) are also not indicated for use in women

Pregnancy Considerations Use is contraindicated in pregnant women.

Adverse events were observed in animal reproduction studies. Pregnancy must be excluded prior to the start of treatment. Although leuprolide usually inhibits ovulation and stops menstruation, contraception is not ensured and a nonhormonal contraceptive should be used.

Breastfeeding Considerations It is not known if leuprolide is present in breast milk; use is contraindicated in breastfeeding women.

Warnings/Precautions Guidelines from the American Society of Clinical Oncology (ASCO) for hormonal management of advanced prostate cancer which is androgen-sensitive (Loblaw 2007) recommend either orchiectomy or luteinizing hormone-releasing hormone (LHRH) agonists as initial treatment for androgen deprivation. Transient increases in testosterone serum levels (~50% above baseline) occur at the start of treatment. Androgen-deprivation therapy (ADT) may increase the risk for cardiovascular disease (Levine 2010); sudden cardiac death and stroke have been reported in men receiving GnRH agonists; ADT may prolong the QT/QTc interval; consider the benefits of ADT versus the risk for QT prolongation in patients with a history of QTc prolongation, congenital long QT syndrome, heart failure, frequent electrolyte abnormalities, and in patients with medications known to prolong the QT interval, or with preexisting cardiac disease. Consider periodic monitoring of electrocardiograms and electrolytes in at-risk patients. Tumor flare, bone pain, neuropathy, urinary tract obstruction, and spinal cord compression have been reported when used for prostate cancer; closely observe patients for weakness, paresthesias, hematuria, and urinary tract obstruction in first few weeks of therapy. Observe patients with metastatic vertebral lesions or urinary obstruction closely. Exacerbation of endometriosis or uterine leiomyomata may occur initially. Decreased bone density has been reported when used for ≥6 months; use caution in patients with additional risk factors for bone loss (eg, chronic alcohol use, corticosteroid therapy). In patients with prostate cancer, androgen deprivation therapy may increase the risk for cardiovascular disease, diabetes, insulin resistance, obesity, alterations in lipids, and fractures; monitor as clinically necessary. Psychiatric events have been described with GnRH agonists, including leuprolide; symptoms of emotional lability, irritability, impatience, anger, and aggression have been reported in post-marketing accounts. Monitor for development or worsening of psychiatric symptoms. Use with caution in patients with a history of psychiatric illness. Rare cases of pituitary apoplexy (frequently secondary to pituitary adenoma) have been observed with GnRH agonist administration (onset from 1 hour to usually <2 weeks); may present as sudden headache, vomiting, visual or mental status changes, and infrequently cardiovascular collapse; immediate medical attention required. Convulsions have been observed in postmarketing reports in patients receiving GnRH agonists, including leuprolide; patients affected included both those with and without a history of cerebrovascular disorders, central nervous system anomalies or tumors, epilepsy, seizures, and those on concomitant medications which may lower the seizure threshold (eg, bupropion, SSRIs). If seizures occur, manage accordingly. Females treated for precocious puberty may experience menses or spotting during the first 2 months of treatment; notify healthcare provider if bleeding continues after the second month.

The American Society of Clinical Oncology (ASCO) Guideline Update on Ovarian Suppression for Adjuvant Endocrine Therapy for Women With Hormone Receptor-Positive Breast Cancer (Burstein 2016) recommends that premenopausal women with higher-risk disease receive ovarian suppression (in addition to adjuvant endocrine therapy), although lower-risk patients should not; premenopausal women with stage II or stage III breast cancers who would ordinarily be advised to receive adjuvant chemotherapy should also receive ovarian suppression (in addition to endocrine therapy). Additionally, women with stage I or II breast cancers at higher risk of recurrence who might consider chemotherapy may be offered ovarian suppression (in addition to endocrine therapy). Women with stage 1 disease which does not require chemotherapy should receive endocrine therapy, but not ovarian suppression. Likewise, women with node-negative cancers 1 cm or less (T1a, T1b) should receive endocrine therapy, but not ovarian suppression. Guidelines from ASCO for Endocrine Therapy in Hormone Receptor-Positive Metastatic Breast Cancer (Rugo 2016) recommend that premenopausal women with ER-positive metastatic breast cancer start ovarian suppression, preferably in combination with hormonal therapy. While premenopausal patients without prior hormone therapy exposure can be treated with tamoxifen, or ovarian suppression, or ablation alone, combination therapy is preferred. In metastatic breast cancer, ovarian suppression with GnRH agonists or ablation with oophorectomy appear to achieve similar results.

Benzyl alcohol and derivatives: Some dosage forms may contain benzyl alcohol; large amounts of benzyl alcohol (≥99 mg/kg/day) have been associated with a potentially fatal toxicity ("gasping syndrome") in neonates; the "gasping syndrome" consists of metabolic acidosis, respiratory distress, gasping respirations, CNS dysfunction (including convulsions, intracranial hemorrhage), hypotension, and cardiovascular collapse (AAP ["Inactive" 1997]; CDC 1982); some data suggests that benzoate displaces bilirubin from protein binding sites (Ahlfors 2001); avoid or use dosage forms containing benzyl alcohol with caution in neonates.

Some dosage forms may contain polysorbate 80 (also known as Tweens). Hypersensitivity reactions, usually a delayed reaction, have been reported following exposure to pharmaceutical products containing polysorbate 80 in certain individuals (Isaksson 2002; Lucente 2000; Shelley 1995). Thrombocytopenia, ascites, pulmonary deterioration, and renal and hepatic failure have been reported in premature neonates after receiving parenteral products containing polysorbate 80 (Alade 1986; CDC 1984). See manufacturer's labeling.

The Atrigel delivery system is a nongelatin-based, biodegradable, polymer matrix. Vehicle used in depot injectable formulations (polylactide-co-glycolide microspheres) has rarely been associated with retinal artery occlusion in patients with abnormal arteriovenous anastomosis. Due to different release properties, combinations of dosage forms or fractions of dosage forms should not be interchanged. Potentially significant interactions may exist, requiring dose or frequency adjustment, additional monitoring, and/or selection of alternative therapy.

Adverse Reactions

Children (percentages based on 1-month and 3-month pediatric formulations combined):

>10%: Local: Pain at injection site (≤20%)

2% to 10%:

Cardiovascular: Vasodilatation (2%)

Central nervous system: Emotional lability (5%), mood changes (5%), headache (3% to 5%), pain (3%)

Dermatologic: Acne vulgaris (3%), seborrhea (3%), skin rash (3% including erythema multiforme)

Endocrine & metabolic: Weight gain (≤7%)

Genitourinary: Vaginal discharge (3%), vaginal hemorrhage (3%), vaginitis (3%)

Local: Injection site reaction (≤9%)

<2%: Abnormal gait, alopecia, arthralgia, asthma, body odor, bradycardia, cervix disease, constipation, cough, decreased appetite, decreased visual acuity, depression, dizziness, drowsiness, dysmenorrhea, dyspepsia, dysphagia, epistaxis, excessive crying, feminization, fever, flu-like symptoms, gingivitis, goiter, growth suppression, gynecomastia, hirsutism, hyperhidrosis, hyperkinesia, hypersensitivity reaction, hypertension, increased appetite, infection, lacrimation, leukoderma, limb pain, musculoskeletal pain, myalgia, myopathy, nausea, nervousness, obesity, pallor, peripheral edema, personality disorder, pharyngitis, precocious puberty, purpura, rhinitis, sinusitis, skin striae, syncope, urinary incontinence, vomiting, weakness

Adults: Note: For prostate cancer treatment, an initial rise in serum testosterone concentrations may cause "tumor flare" or worsening of symptoms, including bone pain, neuropathy, hematuria, or ureteral or bladder outlet obstruction during the first 2 weeks. Similarly, an initial increase in estradiol levels, with a temporary worsening of symptoms, may occur in women treated with leuprolide.

Delayed release formulations:

>10%:

Cardiovascular: Edema (≤14%)

Central nervous system: Headache (≤65%), pain (<2% to 33%), depression (≤31%), insomnia (≤31%), fatigue (≤17%), dizziness (≤16%)

Dermatologic: Allergic skin reaction (≤12%)

Endocrine & metabolic: Hot flash (25% to 98%), weight changes (≤13%), hyperlipidemia (≤12%), decreased libido (≤11%)

Gastrointestinal: Nausea and vomiting (≤25%), gastrointestinal disease (14%), change in bowel habits (≤14%)

Genitourinary: Vaginitis (11% to 28%), testicular atrophy (≤20%), genitourinary complaint (13% to 15%)

Local: Burning sensation at injection site burning (transient: ≤35%)

Neuromuscular & skeletal: Weakness (≤18%), arthropathy (≤12%)

Respiratory: Flu-like symptoms (≤12%), respiratory tract disease (11%)

1% to 10% (limited to important or life-threatening):

Cardiovascular: Angina pectoris (<5%), atrial fibrillation (<5%), bradycardia (<5%), cardiac arrhythmia (<5%), cardiac failure (<5%), deep thrombophlebitis (<5%), hyper-/hypotension (<5%), palpitations (<5%), syncope (<5%), tachycardia (<5%)

Central nervous system: Nervousness (≤8%), paresthesia (≤8%), anxiety (≤6%), agitation (<5%), confusion (<5%), delusions (<5%), dementia (<5%), neuropathy (<5%), paralysis (<5%), seizure (<5%), ostealgia (<2%)

Dermatologic: Acne vulgaris (≤10%), alopecia (≤5%), diaphoresis (≤5%), cellulitis (<5%), hair disease (<5%), pruritus (≤3%), skin rash (≤2%)

Endocrine & metabolic: Dehydration (≤8%), gynecomastia (≤7%), decreased serum bicarbonate (≥5%), hypercholesterolemia (≥5%), hyperglycemia (≥5%), hyperphosphatemia (≥5%), hyperuricemia (≥5%), hypoalbuminemia (≥5%), hypocholesterolemia (≥5%), hypoproteinemia (≥5%), increased lactate dehydrogenase (≥5%), increased prostatic acid phosphatase (≥5%), menstrual disorder (≤2%), hirsutism (<2%)

Gastrointestinal: Anorexia (<5%), dysphagia (<5%), eructation (<5%), gastric ulcer (<5%), gastrointestinal hemorrhage (<5%), intestinal obstruction (<5%), peptic ulcer (<5%), constipation (≤3%), gastroenteritis (≤3%), diarrhea (≤2%)

Genitourinary: Mastalgia (≤6%), impotence (≤5%), balanitis (<5%), breast hypertrophy (<5%), lactation (<5%), penile disease (<5%), testicular disease (<5%), urinary incontinence (<5%), urinary tract infection (<5%), nocturia (≤4%), testicular pain (≤4%), dysuria (≤2%), bladder spasm (<2%), erectile dysfunction (<2%), hematuria (<2%), urinary retention (<2%), urinary urgency (<2%)

Hematologic & oncologic: Change in platelet count (increased; ≥5%), decreased prostatic acid phosphatase (≥5%), eosinophilia (≥5%), leukopenia (≥5%), bruise (≤5%), ecchymoses (<5%), lymphadenopathy (<5%), neoplasm (<5%), anemia, decreased hematocrit, decreased hemoglobin

Hepatic: Abnormal hepatic function tests (≥5%), increased serum AST (≥5%), prolonged partial thromboplastin time (≥5%), prolonged prothrombin time (≥5%), hepatomegaly (<5%)

◀

Hypersensitivity: Hypersensitivity reaction (<5%)

Infection: Infection (5%)

Local: Pain at injection site (2% to 5%), injection site reaction (<5%), erythema at injection site (1% to 3%)

Neuromuscular & skeletal: Myalgia (≤8%), neuromuscular disease (<5%), pathological fracture (<5%), arthralgia (≤1%)

Renal: Decreased urine specific gravity (≥5%), increased blood urea nitrogen (≥5%), increased serum creatinine (≥5%), increased urine specific gravity (≥5%), polyuria (2% to 4%)

Respiratory: Emphysema (<5%), epistaxis (<5%), hemoptysis (<5%), increased bronchial secretions (<5%), pleural effusion (<5%), pulmonary edema (<5%), dyspnea (≤2%), cough (≤1%)

Miscellaneous: Fever (<5%)

Immediate release formulation:

>10%:

Cardiovascular: ECG changes (19%), peripheral edema (12%)

Central nervous system: Pain (13%)

Endocrine & metabolic: Hot flash (55%)

1% to 10% (limited to important or life-threatening):

Cardiovascular: Hypertension (8%), heart murmur (3%), thrombophlebitis (2%), cardiac failure (1%), angina pectoris, cardiac arrhythmia, myocardial infarction, pulmonary embolism, syncope

Central nervous system: Headache (7%), insomnia (7%), dizziness (5%), ostealgia (5%), anxiety, depression, fatigue, fever, nervousness, peripheral neuropathy

Dermatologic: Dermatitis (5%), alopecia, hyperpigmentation, pruritus, skin lesion

Endocrine & metabolic: Decreased libido, diabetes mellitus, goiter, gynecomastia, hypercalcemia, hypoglycemia

Gastrointestinal: Constipation (7%), anorexia (6%), nausea and vomiting (5%), diarrhea, dysphagia, gastrointestinal hemorrhage, peptic ulcer, rectal polyps

Genitourinary: Decreased testicular size (7%), hematuria (6%), urinary frequency (6%), impotence (4%), urinary tract infection (3%), bladder spasm, dysuria, incontinence, mastalgia, testicular pain, urinary tract obstruction

Hematologic & oncologic: Anemia (5%), bruise

Infection: Infection

Local: Injection site reaction

Neuromuscular & skeletal: Weakness (10%)

Ophthalmic: Blurred vision

Renal: Increased blood urea nitrogen, increased serum creatinine

Respiratory: Dyspnea (2%), cough, pneumonia, pulmonary fibrosis

Miscellaneous: Fever, inflammation

Children and Adults: *Any formulations:* Postmarketing and/or case reports: Abdominal pain, abscess at injection site, anaphylaxis, anaphylactoid reaction, asthma, bone fracture (spine), cerebrovascular accident, convulsions, coronary artery disease, decreased white blood cell count, diabetes mellitus, fibromyalgia syndrome (arthralgia/myalgia), headaches, GI distress), flushing, hemoptysis, hepatic injury, hepatic insufficiency, hepatotoxicity, hyperuricemia, hypokalemia, hypoproteinemia, induration at injection site, interstitial pulmonary disease, leukocytosis, myocardial infarction, osteopenia, paralysis, penile swelling, peripheral neuropathy, pituitary apoplexy (cardiovascular collapse, mental status altered, ophthalmoplegia, sudden headache, visual changes, vomiting), prolonged QT interval on ECG, prostate pain, pulmonary embolism, pulmonary infiltrates, retroperitoneal fibrosis (pelvic), seizure, skin photosensitivity, suicidal ideation (rare), tenosynovitis (symptoms), thrombocytopenia, transient ischemic attacks, urticaria

Drug Interactions

Metabolism/Transport Effects None known.

Avoid Concomitant Use

Avoid concomitant use of Leuprolide with any of the following: Corifollitropin Alfa; Highest Risk QTc-Prolonging Agents; Hydroxychloroquine; Indium 111 Capromab Pendetide; MiFEPRIStone; Probucol; Promazine; Vinflunine

Increased Effect/Toxicity

Leuprolide may increase the levels/effects of: Corifollitropin Alfa; Highest Risk QTc-Prolonging Agents; Moderate Risk QTc-Prolonging Agents

The levels/effects of Leuprolide may be increased by: Hydroxychloroquine; MiFEPRIStone; Probucol; Promazine; QTc-Prolonging Agents (Indeterminate Risk and Risk Modifying); Vinflunine; Xipamide

Decreased Effect

Leuprolide may decrease the levels/effects of: Antidiabetic Agents; Choline C 11; Indium 111 Capromab Pendetide

Hazardous Drugs Handling Considerations

Hazardous agent (NIOSH 2016 [group 1]).

Use appropriate precautions for receiving, handling, administration, and disposal. Gloves (single) should be worn during receiving, unpacking, and placing in storage.

NIOSH recommends double gloving, a protective gown, ventilated engineering controls (a class II biological safety cabinet or a compounding aseptic containment isolator), and (when dosage form allows) closed system transfer devices (CSTDs) for compounding. Double gloving and a gown are required during administration (NIOSH 2016).

Storage/Stability

Eligard: Store at 2°C to 8°C (36°F to 46°F). Allow to reach room temperature prior to using. Once outside the refrigerator, the kit may be stored (in its original packaging) at 15°C to 30°C (59°F to 86 °F) for up to 8 weeks prior to mixing and administration. Once mixed, must be administered within 30 minutes (discard if not used within 30 minutes).

Lupron Depot, Lupron Depot-Ped: Store at room temperature of 25°C (77°F); excursions permitted to 15°C to 30°C (59°F to 86°F). Upon reconstitution, the suspension does not contain a preservative and should be used immediately; discard if not used within 2 hours.

Leuprolide acetate 5 mg/mL solution: Store at 20°C to 25°C (68°F to 77°F); excursions permitted to 15°C to 30°C (59°F to 86°F). Protect from light and store vial in carton until use. Do not freeze.

Preparation for Administration

Eligard: Packaged in two syringes; one contains the Atrigel polymer system and the second contains leuprolide acetate powder; follow package instructions for mixing

Lupron Depot, Lupron Depot-Ped: Reconstitute only with diluent provided

◄ **Mechanism of Action** Leuprolide, is an agonist of gonadotropin releasing hormone (GnRH) receptors. Acting as a potent inhibitor of gonadotropin secretion, leuprolide produces an initial increase in luteinizing hormone (LH) and follicle stimulating hormone (FSH), which leads to a transient increase (5 to 12 days [Cook 2000]) in testosterone and dihydrotestosterone (in males) and estrone and estradiol (in premenopausal females). Continuous leuprolide administration then results in suppression of ovarian and testicular steroidogenesis due to decreased levels of LH and FSH with subsequent decrease in testosterone (male) and estrogen (female) levels. In males, testosterone levels are reduced to below castrate levels. Leuprolide may also have a direct inhibitory effect on the testes, and act by a different mechanism not directly related to reduction in serum testosterone.

Pharmacodynamics/Kinetics

Onset of action: Following transient increase, testosterone suppression occurs in ~2 to 4 weeks of continued therapy

Onset of therapeutic suppression for precocious puberty: Leuprolide: 2 to 4 weeks; Leuprolide depot: 1 month

Distribution: Males: V_d: 27 L

Protein binding: 43% to 49%

Metabolism: Major metabolite, pentapeptide (M-1)

Bioavailability: SubQ: 94%

Half-life elimination: ~3 hours

Excretion: Urine (<5% as parent and major metabolite)

Dosing

Adult & Geriatric

Prostate cancer, advanced: Note: Treatment is usually continued after development of metastatic (castration-resistant) disease.

IM:

Lupron Depot 7.5 mg (monthly): 7.5 mg every month **or**

Lupron Depot 22.5 mg (3 month): 22.5 mg every 12 weeks **or**

Lupron Depot 30 mg (4 month): 30 mg every 16 weeks **or**

Lupron Depot 45 mg (6 month): 45 mg every 24 weeks

SubQ:

Eligard: 7.5 mg monthly **or** 22.5 mg every 3 months **or** 30 mg every 4 months **or** 45 mg every 6 months

Leuprolide acetate 5 mg/mL solution: 1 mg daily

Endometriosis: IM: Initial therapy may be with leuprolide alone or in combination with norethindrone; if re-treatment for an additional 6 months is necessary, concomitant norethindrone should be used. Re-treatment is not recommended for longer than one additional 6-month course.

Lupron Depot: 3.75 mg every month for up to 6 months **or**

Lupron Depot-3 month: 11.25 mg every 3 months for up to 2 doses (6 months total duration of treatment)

Uterine leiomyomata (fibroids): IM (in combination with iron):

Lupron Depot: 3.75 mg every month for up to 3 months **or**

Lupron Depot-3 month: 11.25 mg as a single injection

Breast cancer, premenopausal ovarian supression (off-label use): IM:

Lupron Depot: 3.75 mg every 28 days for up to 24 months (Boccardo 1999) **or**

Lupron Depot-3 month: 11.25 mg every 3 months for up to 24 months (Boccardo 1999; Schmid 2007)

Treatment of paraphilia/hypersexuality (off-label use; Guay 2009; Reilly 2000): Males: IM:

Note: Additional trials may be necessary to further define the role of leuprolide in this condition. May cause an initial increase in androgen concentrations which may be treated with an antiandrogen (eg, flutamide, cyproterone) for 1 to 2 months (Guay 2009). Avoid use in patients with osteoporosis or active pituitary pathology.

SubQ: Test dose: 1 mg (observe for hypersensitivity)

Depot IM: 3.75 to 7.5 mg monthly

Pediatric

Precocious puberty (consider discontinuing by age 11 for females and by age 12 for males):

IM:

Lupron Depot-Ped (monthly):

≤25 kg: 7.5 mg every month

>25 to 37.5 kg: 11.25 mg every month

>37.5 kg: 15 mg every month

Titrate dose upward in increments of 3.75 mg every 4 weeks if down-regulation is not achieved.

Lupron Depot-Ped (3 month): 11.25 mg or 30 mg every 12 weeks

SubQ (leuprolide acetate 5 mg/mL solution): Initial: 50 mcg/kg/day; titrate dose upward by 10 mcg/kg/day if down-regulation is not achieved. **Note:** Higher mg/kg doses may be required in younger children.

Renal Impairment There are no dosage adjustments provided in the manufacturer's labeling (has not been studied).

Hepatic Impairment There are no dosage adjustments provided in the manufacturer's labeling (has not been studied).

Administration

Do not use concurrently a fractional dose of the 3-, 4-, or 6-month depot formulation, or a combination of doses of the monthly depot formulation or any depot formulation due to different release characteristics. Do not use a combination of syringes to achieve a particular dose.

IM: Lupron Depot, Lupron Depot-Ped: Administer as a single injection into the gluteal area, anterior thigh, or deltoid. Vary injection site periodically.

SubQ:

Eligard: Vary/rotate injection site; choose site with adequate subcutaneous tissue (eg, upper or mid-abdomen, upper buttocks) that does not have excessive pigment, nodules, lesions, or hair. Avoid areas with brawny or fibrous tissues or areas that may be compressed or rubbed (eg, belt or waistband). Administer within 30 minutes of preparation.

Leuprolide acetate 5 mg/mL solution: Vary injection site; if an alternate syringe from the syringe provided is required, insulin syringes should be used

Monitoring Parameters Bone mineral density; monitor for development or worsening of psychiatric symptoms

Precocious puberty: GnRH testing (blood LH and FSH levels), measurement of height and bone age every 6 to 12 months, testosterone in males and estradiol in females (IM [monthly] and SubQ formulations: 1 to 2 months after initiation of therapy or with dosage change; IM [3 month] formulation: 2 to 3 months after initiation of therapy, month 6, and as clinically indicated there-after); Tanner staging

◀ Prostatic cancer: LH and FSH levels, serum testosterone (~4 weeks after initiation of therapy), PSA; weakness, paresthesias, and urinary tract obstruction in first few weeks of therapy. Screen for diabetes (blood glucose and HbA_{1c}) and cardiovascular risk prior to initiating and periodically during treatment. Consider periodic monitoring of electrocardiograms and electrolytes.

Treatment of paraphilia/hypersexuality (off-label use; Reilly 2000): CBC (baseline, monthly for 4 months then every 6 months); serum testosterone (baseline, monthly for 4 months then every 6 months); serum LH (baseline and every 6 months), FSH (baseline), serum BUN and creatinine (baseline and every 6 months); bone density (baseline and yearly); ECG (baseline)

Test Interactions Interferes with pituitary gonadotropic and gonadal function tests during and up to 3 months after monthly administration of leuprolide therapy.

Medication Guide Available Yes

Dosage Forms Excipient information presented when available (limited, particularly for generics); consult specific product labeling.

Kit, Injection, as acetate:
Generic: 1 mg/0.2 mL
Kit, Intramuscular, as acetate:
Lupron Depot (1-Month): 7.5 mg [latex free; contains polysorbate 80]
Lupron Depot (6-Month): 45 mg [latex free; contains polysorbate 80]
Kit, Intramuscular, as acetate [preservative free]:
Lupron Depot (1-Month): 3.75 mg [latex free; contains polysorbate 80]
Lupron Depot (3-Month): 11.25 mg, 22.5 mg [latex free; contains polysorbate 80]
Lupron Depot (4-Month): 30 mg [latex free; contains polysorbate 80]
Lupron Depot-Ped (1-Month): 7.5 mg, 11.25 mg, 15 mg [latex free; contains polysorbate 80]
Lupron Depot-Ped (3-Month): 30 mg (Ped), 11.25 mg (Ped) [latex free; contains polysorbate 80]
Kit, Subcutaneous, as acetate:
Eligard: 7.5 mg, 22.5 mg, 30 mg, 45 mg

◆ **Leuprolide Acetate** *see* Leuprolide *on page* 1131

◆ **Leuprorelin Acetate** *see* Leuprolide *on page* 1131

◆ **Leurocristine Sulfate** *see* VinCRIStine *on page* 1895

◆ **Leustatin** *see* Cladribine *on page* 411

◆ **Levaquin** *see* LevoFLOXacin (Systemic) *on page* 1140

◆ **Levaquin in 5% Dextrose Injection (Can)** *see* LevoFLOXacin (Systemic) *on page* 1140

◆ **Leva Set** *see* Lidocaine and Prilocaine *on page* 1150

LevoFLOXacin (Systemic) (lee voe FLOKS a sin)

Brand Names: US Levaquin

Brand Names: Canada ACT Levofloxacin; APO-Levofloxacin; Levaquin; Levaquin in 5% Dextrose Injection; Mylan-Levofloxacin; PMS-Levofloxacin; Sandoz-Levofloxacin; Teva-Levofloxacin

Pharmacologic Category Antibiotic, Fluoroquinolone; Antibiotic, Respiratory Fluoroquinolone

Use

Treatment of community-acquired pneumonia, including multidrug resistant strains of *S. pneumoniae* (MDRSP); nosocomial pneumonia; acute bacterial exacerbation of chronic bronchitis; acute bacterial rhinosinusitis (ABRS); prostatitis (chronic bacterial); urinary tract infection (uncomplicated or complicated); acute pyelonephritis; skin or skin structure infections (uncomplicated or complicated); reduce incidence or disease progression of inhalational anthrax (postexposure); prophylaxis and treatment of plague (pneumonic and septicemic) due to *Y. pestis*

Limitations of use: Because fluoroquinolones have been associated with disabling and potentially irreversible serious adverse reactions (eg, tendinitis and tendon rupture, peripheral neuropathy, CNS effects), reserve levofloxacin for use in patients who have no alternative treatment options for acute exacerbation of chronic bronchitis, acute bacterial sinusitis, and uncomplicated urinary tract infections.

Pregnancy Risk Factor C

Dosing

Adult & Geriatric Note: Sequential therapy (intravenous to oral) may be instituted based on prescriber's discretion.

Acute bacterial rhinosinusitis: Oral, IV:

Manufacturer's labeling: 750 mg every 24 hours for 5 days or 500 mg every 24 hours for 10 to 14 days

Alternate recommendations: 500 mg every 24 hours for 5 to 7 days (Chow 2012)

Anthrax (inhalational): Oral, IV: 500 mg every 24 hours for 60 days, beginning as soon as possible after exposure

Bite wounds (animal/human) (off-label use): Oral, IV: **Note:** Recommended as an alternative therapy for human bite wound in patients hypersensitive to beta-lactams: 750 mg once daily; in combination with metronidazole or clindamycin (IDSA [Stevens 2014])

***Chlamydia trachomatis* urogenital infection (alternative to preferred therapy) (off-label use):** Oral: 500 mg once daily for 7 days (CDC [Workowski 2015])

Chronic bronchitis (acute bacterial exacerbation): Oral: 500 mg every 24 hours for 7 days; Canadian labeling (not in US labeling) also includes a dosage regimen of 750 mg every 24 hours for 5 days

Diabetic foot infections, moderate to severe (off-label use): Oral, IV: **Note:** Initial treatment should begin with an IV regimen for severe infections; moderate infections may initially be treated with IV or oral regimen (IDSA [Lipsky 2012]): 750 mg once daily (Graham 2002); use in combination with clindamycin (limited evidence supporting clindamycin for severe *S. aureus* infections) (IDSA [Lipsky 2012])

Diverticulitis, peritonitis (off-label use) (Solomkin, [IDSA] 2010): Oral, IV: 750 mg every 24 hours for 7 to 10 days; use adjunctive metronidazole therapy

Epididymitis (off-label use; CDC [Workowski 2015]): Oral:

Likely caused by enteric organisms: 500 mg once daily for 10 days

Likely caused by sexually-transmitted chlamydia and gonorrhea and enteric organisms in men who practice insertive anal sex: 500 mg once daily for 10 days in combination with ceftriaxone

Intra-abdominal infection, complicated, community-acquired (in combination with metronidazole) (off-label use) (Solomkin, [IDSA] 2010): IV: 750 mg once daily for 4 to 7 days (provided source controlled). **Note:** Avoid using in settings where *E. coli* susceptibility to fluoroquinolones is <90%.

Neutropenia (chemotherapy-induced), antibacterial prophylaxis (off-label use): Oral: 500 mg once daily (Bucaneve 2005; Cullen 2005)

Pelvic inflammatory disease (in patients allergic to cephalosporins; off-label use): Oral: 500 mg once daily for 14 days with concomitant metronidazole; **Note:** The CDC recommends use as an alternative therapy only if standard parenteral cephalosporin therapy is not feasible, community prevalence, and individual risk of quinolone-resistant gonococcal organisms is low. Culture sensitivity must be confirmed (CDC [Workowski 2015]).

Plague (prophylaxis and treatment): Oral, IV: 500 mg every 24 hours for 10 to 14 days, beginning as soon as possible after exposure. **Note:** Dose of 750 mg once daily may be considered if clinically warranted.

Pneumonia:

Community-acquired (CAP): Oral, IV: 500 mg every 24 hours for 7 to 14 days or 750 mg every 24 hours for 5 days; **Note:** CAP guidelines recommend the 750 mg dose (IDSA/ATS [Mandell 2007])

Hospital-acquired or ventilator- associated pneumonia: IV: 750 mg every 24 hours for 7 days; may consider shorter or longer duration depending on rate of clinical improvement. When used as empiric therapy, use in combination with an agent active against MRSA (unless coverage of MSSA only is appropriate) with or without an additional antipseudomonal agent (dependent on patient and institution-specific risk factors) (Kalil 2016).

Prostatitis (chronic bacterial): Oral, IV: 500 mg every 24 hours for 28 days

Skin and skin structure infections: Oral, IV:

Uncomplicated: 500 mg every 24 hours for 7 to 10 days

Complicated: 750 mg every 24 hours for 7 to 14 days

Surgical (preoperative) prophylaxis (off-label use): IV: 500 mg within 120 minutes prior to surgical incision (Bratzler 2013)

Surgical site infections (intestinal or genitourinary tract; perineum or axilla) (off-label use): IV: 750 mg every 24 hours, in combination with metronidazole (IDSA [Stevens 2014])

Traveler's diarrhea (off-label use): Oral: 500 mg once daily for 1 to 3 days (IDSA [Hill 2006])

Tuberculosis, drug-resistant tuberculosis, or intolerance to first-line agents (off-label use): Oral: 500 to 1,000 mg every 24 hours (CDC 2003)

Urethritis, nongonococcal (off-label use): Oral: 500 mg every 24 hours for 7 days (CDC [Workowski 2015])

Urinary tract infections: Oral, IV:

Uncomplicated: 250 mg once daily for 3 days

Complicated, including pyelonephritis: 250 mg once daily for 10 days **or** 750 mg once daily for 5 days

Pediatric

Acute bacterial rhinosinusitis (off-label use): Oral, IV: 10 to 20 mg/kg/day divided every 12 to 24 hours for 10 to 14 days (maximum: 500 mg daily). **Note:** Recommended in patients with a type I penicillin allergy, after failure of initial therapy or in patients at risk for antibiotic resistance (eg, daycare attendance, age <2 years, recent hospitalization, antibiotic use within the past month) (Chow 2012).

Anthrax (inhalational, postexposure): Oral, IV:

Infants ≥6 months and Children ≤50 kg: 8 mg/kg every 12 hours for 60 days (do not exceed 250 mg/dose), beginning as soon as possible after exposure

Children >50 kg: 500 mg every 24 hours for 60 days, beginning as soon as possible after exposure

Chlamydia trachomatis **urogenital infection (alternative to preferred therapy) (off-label use):** Adolescents: Refer to adult dosing.

Community-acquired pneumonia (CAP) (IDSA/PIDS 2011): Note: May consider addition of vancomycin or clindamycin to empiric therapy if community-acquired MRSA suspected; alternative to ceftriaxone or cefotaxime in patients not fully immunized for *H. influenzae* type b and *S. pneumoniae*, or significant local resistance to penicillin in invasive pneumococcal strains.

Infants ≥6 months and Children ≤4 years:

S. pneumoniae (MICs to penicillin ≤2.0 mcg/mL), mild infection or step-down therapy (alternative to amoxicillin): Oral: 8 to 10 mg/kg/dose every 12 hours (maximum: 750 mg daily)

S. pneumoniae (MICs to penicillin ≥4.0 mcg/mL):

Moderate-to-severe infection (alternative to ceftriaxone): IV: 8 to 10 mg/kg/dose every 12 hours (maximum: 750 mg daily)

Mild infection, step-down therapy (preferred): Oral: 8 to 10 mg/kg/dose every 12 hours (maximum: 750 mg daily)

H. influenzae, moderate-to-severe infection (alternative to ampicillin, ceftriaxone, or cefotaxime): IV: 8 to 10 mg/kg/dose every 12 hours (maximum: 750 mg daily)

Atypical pathogens, moderate-to-severe infection (alternative to azithromycin) or empiric treatment (alternative to azithromycin +/- beta-lactam; should be limited to macrolide allergic/intolerant patients): Oral, IV: 8 to 10 mg/kg/dose every 12 hours (maximum: 750 mg daily)

Children 5 to 16 years:

S. pneumoniae (MICs to penicillin ≤2.0 mcg/mL), mild infection or step-down therapy (alternative to amoxicillin): Oral: 8 to 10 mg/kg/dose once daily (maximum: 750 mg daily)

S. pneumoniae (MICs to penicillin ≥4.0 mcg/mL):

Moderate-to-severe infection (alternative to ceftriaxone): IV: 8 to 10 mg/kg/dose once daily (maximum: 750 mg daily)

Mild infection, step-down therapy (preferred): Oral: 8 to 10 mg/kg/dose once daily (maximum: 750 mg daily)

H. influenzae, moderate-to-severe infection (alternative to ampicillin, ceftriaxone, or cefotaxime): IV: 8 to 10 mg/kg/dose once daily (maximum: 750 mg daily)

Atypical pathogens:

Moderate-to-severe infection (alternative to azithromycin): Oral, IV: 8 to 10 mg/kg/dose once daily (maximum: 750 mg daily)

Mild infection, step-down therapy (alternative to azithromycin in adolescents with skeletal maturity): Oral: 500 mg once daily

Plague (prophylaxis and treatment): Infants ≥6 months and Children: Oral, IV:

≤50 kg: 8 mg/kg every 12 hours for 10 to 14 days (do not exceed 250 mg/dose), beginning as soon as possible after exposure

>50 kg: 500 mg every 24 hours for 10 to 14 days, beginning as soon as possible after exposure. **Note:** Dose of 750 mg once daily may be considered if clinically warranted.

Surgical (preoperative) prophylaxis (off-label use): Children ≥1 year: IV: 10 mg/kg within 120 minutes prior to surgical incision (maximum: 500 mg) (Bratzler 2013)

Renal Impairment IV, Oral:

Normal renal function dosing of 250 mg daily:

CrCl 20 to 49 mL/minute: No dosage adjustment required.

CrCl 10 to 19 mL/minute: Administer 250 mg every 48 hours (except in uncomplicated UTI, where no dosage adjustment is required).

Hemodialysis/chronic ambulatory peritoneal dialysis (CAPD): No information available.

Normal renal function dosing of 500 mg daily:

CrCl 20 to 49 mL/minute: Administer 500 mg initial dose, followed by 250 mg every 24 hours.

CrCl 10 to 19 mL/minute: Administer 500 mg initial dose, followed by 250 mg every 48 hours.

Hemodialysis/chronic ambulatory peritoneal dialysis (CAPD): Administer 500 mg initial dose, followed by 250 mg every 48 hours; supplemental doses are not required following either hemodialysis or CAPD

Normal renal function dosing of 750 mg daily:

CrCl 20 to 49 mL/minute: Administer 750 mg every 48 hours.

CrCl 10 to 19 mL/minute: Administer 750 mg initial dose, followed by 500 mg every 48 hours.

Hemodialysis/chronic ambulatory peritoneal dialysis (CAPD): Administer 750 mg initial dose, followed by 500 mg every 48 hours; supplemental doses are not required following either hemodialysis or CAPD.

Normal renal function dosing of 750 or 1,000 mg daily (treatment of tuberculosis **only**) (CDC 2003): CrCl <30 mL/minute: Administer 750 or 1,000 mg 3 times per week (in hemodialysis patients administer after dialysis on dialysis days).

Continuous renal replacement therapy (CRRT) (Heintz 2009; Trotman 2005): Drug clearance is highly dependent on the method of renal replacement, filter type, and flow rate. Appropriate dosing requires close monitoring of pharmacologic response, signs of adverse reactions due to drug accumulation, as well as drug concentrations in relation to target trough (if appropriate). The following are general recommendations only (based on dialysate flow/ultrafiltration rates of 1 to 2 L/hour and minimal residual renal function) and should not supersede clinical judgment:

CVVH: Loading dose of 500 to 750 mg followed by 250 mg every 24 hours.

CVVHD: Loading dose of 500 to 750 mg followed by 250 to 500 mg every 24 hours.

CVVHDF: Loading dose of 500 to 750 mg followed by 250 to 750 mg every 24 hours.

Hepatic Impairment IV, Oral: No dosage adjustment provided in manufacturer's labeling (has not been studied). However, dosage adjustment unlikely due to limited hepatic metabolism.

Additional Information Complete prescribing information should be consulted for additional detail.

Medication Guide Available Yes

Dosage Forms Excipient information presented when available (limited, particularly for generics); consult specific product labeling. [DSC] = Discontinued product

Solution, Intravenous:
  Generic: 250 mg/50 mL (50 mL); 500 mg/100 mL (100 mL); 750 mg/150 mL (150 mL)
Solution, Intravenous [preservative free]:
  Levaquin: 250 mg/50 mL (50 mL [DSC]); 500 mg/100 mL (100 mL [DSC]); 750 mg/150 mL (150 mL [DSC])
  Generic: 250 mg/50 mL (50 mL); 500 mg/100 mL (100 mL); 750 mg/150 mL (150 mL); 25 mg/mL (20 mL, 30 mL)
Solution, Oral:
  Levaquin: 25 mg/mL (480 mL [DSC]) [contains propylene glycol]
  Generic: 25 mg/mL (10 mL, 20 mL, 100 mL, 200 mL, 480 mL)
Tablet, Oral:
  Levaquin: 250 mg, 500 mg, 750 mg
  Generic: 250 mg, 500 mg, 750 mg

◆ **Levo-folinic Acid** see LEVOleucovorin on page 1145

LEVOleucovorin (lee voe loo koe VOR in)

Brand Names: US Fusilev
Index Terms 6S-leucovorin; Calcium Levoleucovorin; L-leucovorin; Levo-folinic Acid; Levo-leucovorin; Levoleucovorin Calcium Pentahydrate; S-leucovorin
Pharmacologic Category Antidote; Chemotherapy Modulating Agent; Rescue Agent (Chemotherapy)
Use
  Colorectal cancer, metastatic: Palliative treatment of advanced, metastatic colorectal cancer (In combination with fluorouracil).
  Folic acid antagonist overdose: Antidote to diminish toxicity in inadvertent overdosage of folic acid antagonists.
  High-dose methotrexate rescue: Rescue agent after high-dose methotrexate therapy in osteosarcoma treatment.
  Impaired methotrexate elimination: Antidote to diminish toxicity and counteract effects of impaired methotrexate elimination.
  Limitations of use: Levoleucovorin is not indicated for the treatment of pernicious anemia or megaloblastic anemias secondary to the lack of vitamin B_{12} (improper use may result in hematologic remission with progressive neurologic manifestations).
Labeled Contraindications Severe hypersensitivity or previous allergic reaction to leucovorin products, folinic acid, folic acid, or any component of the formulation.
Pregnancy Considerations Animal reproduction studies have not been conducted. Levoleucovorin is the levo isomeric form of racemic leucovorin, a biologically active form of folic acid. Adequate amounts of folic acid are recommended during pregnancy.
Breastfeeding Considerations It is not known if levoleucovorin is present in breast milk. Due to the potential for serious adverse reactions in the breastfed infant, a decision should be made to discontinue breastfeeding or to discontinue levoleucovorin, taking into account the importance of treatment to the mother. Levoleucovorin is the levo isomeric form of racemic leucovorin, a

biologically active form of folic acid. Adequate amounts of folic acid are recommended in breastfeeding women.

Warnings/Precautions For IV administration only; do not administer intrathecally. Due to calcium content, do not administer IV solutions at a rate >160 mg levoleucovorin/minute. Methotrexate serum concentrations should be monitored to determine dose and duration of levoleucovorin therapy; dose may need to be increased or administration prolonged in situations where methotrexate excretion may be delayed (eg, ascites, pleural effusion, renal insufficiency, inadequate hydration, concurrent interacting medications). Although levoleucovorin may lessen hematologic toxicity due to methotrexate, it has no effect on other toxicities associated with methotrexate (eg, nephrotoxicity). When used for the treatment of accidental folic acid antagonist overdose, administer as soon as possible.

Levoleucovorin and leucovorin calcium enhance the toxicity of fluorouracil. Deaths due to severe enterocolitis, diarrhea, and dehydration have been reported in elderly patients receiving weekly leucovorin calcium in combination with fluorouracil. Levoleucovorin is indicated in combination with fluorouracil for the palliative treatment of colorectal cancer; when administered together, the fluorouracil dose is reduced (compared to fluorouracil dosing without levoleucovorin). The typical fluorouracil gastrointestinal toxicities (eg, diarrhea, stomatitis) may be of greater severity or longer duration with fluorouracil and levoleucovorin combination therapy. Symptoms of gastrointestinal toxicity should be completely resolved prior to treatment. Elderly and/or debilitated patients are at higher risk for severe gastrointestinal toxicity. Concomitant use of leucovorin calcium and sulfamethoxazole-trimethoprim for the acute treatment of PCP in patients with HIV infection has been associated with increased rates of treatment failure and morbidity; may also occur with levoleucovorin. Seizures and/or syncope have been reported with leucovorin calcium; generally in patients with CNS metastases or other underlying risk factors. Potentially significant drug-drug interactions may exist, requiring dose or frequency adjustment, additional monitoring, and/or selection of alternative therapy.

Adverse Reactions Adverse reactions reported with levoleucovorin either as a part of combination chemotherapy or following chemotherapy.
>10%:
  Central nervous system: Fatigue (≤29%), malaise (≤29%)
  Dermatologic: Dermatitis (6% to 29%), alopecia (≤26%)
  Gastrointestinal: Stomatitis (38% to 72%; grades 3/4: 6% to 12%), diarrhea (6% to 70%; grades 3/4: ≤19%), nausea (19% to 62%), vomiting (38% to 40%), anorexia (≤24%), decreased appetite (≤24%), abdominal pain (≤14%)
  Neuromuscular & skeletal: Weakness (≤29%)
1% to 10%:
  Central nervous system: Confusion (6%), neuropathy (6%)
  Gastrointestinal: Dysgeusia (6%), dyspepsia (6%), typhlitis (6%)
  Renal: Renal insufficiency (6%)
  Respiratory: Dyspnea (6%)
<1%, postmarketing, and/or case reports: Disruption of body temperature regulation, hypersensitivity reaction, pruritus, rigors, skin rash

Drug Interactions
  Metabolism/Transport Effects None known.

Avoid Concomitant Use

Avoid concomitant use of LEVOleucovorin with any of the following: Raltitrexed; Trimethoprim

Increased Effect/Toxicity

LEVOleucovorin may increase the levels/effects of: Capecitabine; Fluorouracil (Systemic); Fluorouracil (Topical); Tegafur

Decreased Effect

LEVOleucovorin may decrease the levels/effects of: Fosphenytoin; PHENobarbital; Phenytoin; Primidone; Raltitrexed; Trimethoprim

The levels/effects of LEVOleucovorin may be decreased by: Glucarpidase

Storage/Stability

Lyophilized powder: Prior to reconstitution, store intact vials at 25°C (77°F); excursions permitted from 15°C to 30°C (59°F to 86°F). Protect from light. Initial reconstituted solution in the vial may be stored for 12 hours (50 mg vial) or 24 hours (175 mg vial) at room temperature. Solutions further diluted for infusion in NS are stable for 12 hours (50 mg vial) or 24 hours (175 mg vial) at room temperature. Storage times may vary based on manufacturer and/or product; refer to manufacturer's labeling. Solutions further diluted for infusion in D5W are stable for 4 hours at room temperature.

Injection solution: Store intact vials between 2°C and 8°C (36°F and 46°F). Protect from light. Store in carton until contents are used. Solutions further diluted for infusion in NS or D5W are stable for up to 4 hours at room temperature.

Preparation for Administration

Lyophilized powder: Reconstitute the 50 mg vial with 5.3 mL NS (preservative free) to a concentration of 10 mg/mL. Reconstitute 175 mg vial with 17.7 mL NS (preservative free) to a concentration of 10 mg/mL. Do not use if solution appears cloudy or contains a precipitate. May further dilute for infusion in NS or D5W to a final concentration of 0.5 to 5 mg/mL.

Injection solution: May further dilute for infusion in NS or D5W to a concentration of 0.5 mg/mL.

Do not prepare with other products in the same admixture; may cause precipitation.

Mechanism of Action

Levoleucovorin counteracts the toxic (and therapeutic) effects of folic acid antagonists (eg, methotrexate) which act by inhibiting dihydrofolate reductase. Levoleucovorin is the levo isomeric and pharmacologic active form of leucovorin (levoleucovorin does not require reduction by dihydrofolate reductase). A reduced derivative of folic acid, leucovorin supplies the necessary cofactor blocked by methotrexate.

Leucovorin enhances the activity (and toxicity) of fluorouracil by stabilizing the binding of 5-fluoro-2'-deoxyuridine-5'-monophosphate (FdUMP; a fluorouracil metabolite) to thymidylate synthetase resulting in inhibition of this enzyme.

Pharmacodynamics/Kinetics

Metabolism: Converted to the active reduced form of folate, 5-methyl-tetrahydrofolate (5-methyl-THF; active)

Half-life elimination: Total-tetrahydrofolate: 5.1 hours; (6S)-5-methyl-5,6,7,8-tetrahydrofolate: 6.8 hours

Time to peak, serum: IV (healthy volunteers; 15 mg dose): 0.9 hours

Dosing

Adult & Geriatric Note: Levoleucovorin, when substituted in place of leucovorin calcium (the racemic form), is dosed at **one-half** the usual dose of leucovorin calcium:

Colorectal cancer, metastatic: IV: The following regimens have been used (in combination with fluorouracil; fluorouracil doses may need to be adjusted for toxicity; no adjustment is required for the levoleucovorin dose): 100 mg/m^2/day over at least 3 minutes (followed by fluorouracil 370 mg/m^2/day) for 5 days every 4 weeks for 2 cycles, then every 4 to 5 weeks depending on recovery from toxicities, **or**

10 mg/m^2/day (followed by fluorouracil 425 mg/m^2/day) for 5 days every 4 weeks for 2 cycles, then every 4 to 5 weeks depending on recovery from toxicities, **or**

Substitution dosing: Levoleucovorin, when substituted in place of leucovorin calcium within a chemotherapy regimen, is dosed at **one-half** the usual dose of leucovorin calcium (Goldberg 1997; Kovoor 2009)

High-dose methotrexate rescue: IV: Usual dose: 7.5 mg (~5 mg/m^2) every 6 hours for 10 doses, beginning 24 hours after the start of the methotrexate infusion (based on a methotrexate dose of 12 g/m^2 IV over 4 hours). Levoleucovorin (and hydration and urinary alkalinization to pH ≥7) should be continued and/or adjusted until the methotrexate level is <0.05 micromolar (5 x 10^{-8} M) as follows:

Normal methotrexate elimination (serum methotrexate levels ~10 micromolar at 24 hours post administration, 1 micromolar at 48 hours and <0.2 micromolar at 72 hours post infusion): 7.5 mg IV every 6 hours for 10 doses

Delayed late methotrexate elimination (serum methotrexate levels >0.2 micromolar at 72 hours and >0.05 micromolar at 96 hours post methotrexate infusion): Continue 7.5 mg IV every 6 hours until methotrexate level is <0.05 micromolar

Delayed early methotrexate elimination and/or evidence of acute renal injury (serum methotrexate level ≥50 micromolar at 24 hours, ≥5 micromolar at 48 hours or a doubling or more of the serum creatinine level at 24 hours post methotrexate infusion [likely to develop reversible renal failure]): 75 mg IV every 3 hours until methotrexate level is <1 micromolar, followed by 7.5 mg IV every 3 hours until methotrexate level is <0.05 micromolar

Significant clinical toxicity in the presence of impaired methotrexate elimination or renal impairment (as described above): Extend levoleucovorin treatment for an additional 24 hours (total of 14 doses) in subsequent treatment cycles.

Delayed methotrexate elimination due to third space fluid accumulation, renal insufficiency, or inadequate hydration: May require higher levoleucovorin doses or prolonged administration.

Folic acid antagonist overdose: IV: 7.5 mg (~5 mg/m^2) every 6 hours; continue until the methotrexate level is <0.01 micromolar (10^{-8} M). Initiate treatment as soon as possible after methotrexate overdose. Increase the levoleucovorin dose to 50 mg/m^2 IV every 3 hours if the 24-hour serum creatinine has increased 50% over baseline, or if the 24 hour methotrexate level is >5 micromolar (5 x 10^{-6} M), or if the 48-hour methotrexate level is >0.9 micromolar (9 x 10^{-7} M); continue levoleucovorin until the methotrexate level is <0.01 micromolar (10^{-8} M). Hydration (aggressive) and urinary alkalinization (urinary pH ≥7 with sodium bicarbonate) should also be maintained.

Impaired methotrexate elimination: IV: 7.5 mg (~5 mg/m²) every 6 hours; continue until the methotrexate level is <0.01 micromolar (10^{-8} M). Initiate treatment within 24 hours of methotrexate administration if elimination is impaired. Increase the levoleucovorin dose to 50 mg/m² IV every 3 hours if the 24-hour serum creatinine has increased 50% over baseline, or if the 24-hour methotrexate level is >5 micromolar (5×10^{-6} M), or if the 48-hour methotrexate level is >0.9 micromolar (9×10^{-7} M); continue levoleucovorin until the methotrexate level is <0.01 micromolar (10^{-8} M). Hydration (aggressive) and urinary alkalinization (urinary pH ≥7 with sodium bicarbonate) should also be maintained.

Pediatric Note: Levoleucovorin, when substituted in place of leucovorin calcium (the racemic form), is dosed at **one-half** the usual dose of leucovorin calcium:

High-dose methotrexate rescue: Children and Adolescents: Refer to adult dosing.

Folic acid antagonist overdose: Children and Adolescents: Refer to adult dosing.

Impaired methotrexate elimination: Children and Adolescents: Refer to adult dosing.

Renal Impairment There are no initial dosage adjustments provided in the manufacturer's labeling; in patients with impaired methotrexate elimination, adjust levoleucovorin dose based on methotrexate levels.

Hepatic Impairment There are no dosage adjustments provided in the manufacturer's labeling.

Administration For IV administration only; do not administer intrathecally. Administer by slow IV push or infusion over at least 3 minutes, not to exceed 160 mg/minute (due to calcium content).

For colorectal cancer: Levoleucovorin has also been administered (off-label administration rate) as IV infusion over 2 hours (Comella 2000; Tournigand 2006).

Monitoring Parameters High-dose methotrexate therapy, impaired methotrexate elimination, or methotrexate overdose (inadvertent): Serum methotrexate and creatinine levels at least once daily. Monitor urine pH. Monitor fluid and electrolyte status in patients with delayed methotrexate elimination (likely to experience renal toxicity). For colorectal cancer, monitor for diarrhea and stomatitis.

Dosage Forms Excipient information presented when available (limited, particularly for generics); consult specific product labeling.

Solution, Intravenous:
  Generic: 175 mg/17.5 mL (17.5 mL)
Solution, Intravenous [preservative free]:
  Generic: 175 mg/17.5 mL (17.5 mL); 250 mg/25 mL (25 mL)
Solution Reconstituted, Intravenous:
  Fusilev: 50 mg (1 ea)
  Generic: 50 mg (1 ea)
Solution Reconstituted, Intravenous [preservative free]:
  Generic: 175 mg (1 ea)

◆ **Levo-leucovorin** see LEVOleucovorin on page 1145
◆ **Levoleucovorin Calcium Pentahydrate** see LEVOleucovorin on page 1145
◆ **Levulan Kerastick** see Aminolevulinic Acid (Topical) on page 114

- ◆ **L-Glutamine** *see* Glutamine *on page 886*
- ◆ **LH-RH Agonist** *see* Histrelin *on page 912*
- ◆ **Lido BDK** *see* Lidocaine and Prilocaine *on page 1150*

Lidocaine and Prilocaine (LYE doe kane & PRIL oh kane)

Brand Names: US AgonEaze; Anodyne LPT; DermacinRx Empricaine; DermacinRx Prizopak; Dolotranz; EMLA [DSC]; Leva Set; Lido BDK; Lidopril; Lidopril XR; LiProZonePak; Livixil Pak; LP Lite Pak; Medolor Pak; Oraqix; Prilolid; Priloxx LP; Relador Pak; Venipuncture CPI

Brand Names: Canada EMLA; Oraqix

Index Terms Lidocaine/Prilocaine; Prilocaine and Lidocaine

Pharmacologic Category Local Anesthetic

Use

US labeling:

Cream: Topical anesthetic for use on normal intact skin to provide local analgesia; for use on genital mucous membranes for superficial minor surgery; and as pretreatment for infiltration anesthesia.

Periodontal gel: Topical anesthetic for use in periodontal pockets during scaling and/or root planing procedures

Canadian labeling:

Cream: Topical anesthetic for use on intact skin in connection with: IV cannulation or venipuncture; superficial surgical procedures (eg, split skin grafting, electrolysis, removal of molluscum contagiosum); laser treatment for superficial skin surgery (eg, telangiectasia, port wine stains, warts, moles, skin nodules, scar tissue); surgical procedures of genital mucosa (≤10 minutes) on small superficial localized lesions (eg, removal of condylomata by laser or cautery, biopsies); local infiltration anesthesia in genital mucous membranes; mechanical cleansing/debridement of leg ulcers; vaccination with measles-mumps-rubella (MMR), diphtheria-pertussis-tetanus-poliovirus (DPTP), *Haemophilus influenzae* b, and hepatitis B.

Patch: Topical anesthetic for use on intact skin in connection with IV cannulation or venipuncture; vaccination with measles-mumps-rubella (MMR), diphtheria-pertussis-tetanus-poliovirus (DPTP), *Haemophilus influenzae* b, and hepatitis B.

Periodontal gel: Topical anesthetic for use in periodontal pockets during scaling and/or root planing procedures

Pregnancy Risk Factor B

Dosing

Adult Anesthetic: Topical:

Cream (intact skin): **Note:** Apply a thick layer to intact skin and cover with an occlusive dressing. Dermal analgesia can be expected to increase for up to 3 hours under occlusive dressing and persist for 1 to 2 hours after removal of the cream.

US labeling:

Minor dermal procedures (eg, IV cannulation or venipuncture): Apply 2.5 g (1/2 of the 5 g tube) over 20 to 25 cm^2 of skin surface area) for at least 1 hour

Major dermal procedures (eg, more painful dermatological procedures involving a larger skin area such as split thickness skin graft harvesting): Apply 2 g per 10 cm^2 of skin and allow to remain in contact with the skin for at least 2 hours.

Adult male genital skin (eg, pretreatment prior to local anesthetic infiltration): Apply 1 g per 10 cm^2 to the skin surface for 15 minutes. Local anesthetic infiltration should be performed immediately after removal of cream.

Adult female genital mucous membranes: Minor procedures (eg, removal of condylomata acuminata, pretreatment for local anesthetic infiltration): Apply 5 to 10 g for 5 to 10 minutes. The local anesthetic infiltration or procedure should be performed immediately after removal of cream.

Canadian labeling:

Minor dermal procedures (eg, IV cannulation, venipuncture, surgical or laser treatment): Apply 2 g (~1/2 of the 5 g tube) over ~13.5 cm^2 for at least 1 hour but no longer than 5 hours

Major dermal procedures (eg, split-skin grafting): 1.5 to 2 g per 10 cm^2 (maximum: 60 g per 400 cm^2) for at least 2 hours but no longer than 5 hours

Genital mucosa (eg, surgical procedures ≤10 minutes such as localized wart removal, and prior to local anesthetic infiltration): Apply 2 g (~1/2 of 5 g tube) per lesion (maximum: 10 g) for 5 to 10 minutes. Initiate procedure immediately after removing cream.

Leg ulcers (eg, mechanical cleansing/surgical debridement): Apply ~1 to 2 g per 10 cm^2 (maximum: 10 g) for at least 30 minutes and up to 60 minutes for necrotic tissue that is more difficult to penetrate. Initiate procedure immediately after removing cream.

Periodontal gel (Oraqix): Apply on gingival margin around selected teeth using the blunt-tipped applicator included in package. Wait 30 seconds, then fill the periodontal pockets using the blunt-tipped applicator until gel becomes visible at the gingival margin. Wait another 30 seconds before starting treatment. May reapply; maximum recommended dose: One treatment session: 5 cartridges (8.5 g)

Transdermal patch [Canadian product]: Minor procedures (eg, needle insertion): Apply 1 or more patches to intact skin surface area <10 cm^2 for at least 1 hour (maximum application time: 5 hours)

Geriatric Smaller areas of treatment may be necessary depending on status of patient (eg, debilitated, impaired hepatic function). Refer to adult dosing.

Pediatric Although the incidence of systemic adverse effects is very low, caution should be exercised, particularly when applying over large areas and leaving on for >2 hours

Local anesthetic (procedures): Infants and Children (intact skin): Topical:
Note: If a patient >3 months of age does not meet the minimum weight requirement, the maximum total dose should be restricted to the corresponding maximum based on patient weight.

Cream: Should **not** be used in neonates with a gestation age <37 weeks nor in infants <12 months of age who are receiving treatment with methemoglobin-inducing agents

Dosing is based on child's age and weight:

Age 0 to 3 months or <5 kg: Apply a maximum of 1 g over no more than 10 cm^2 of skin; leave on for no longer than 1 hour

Age 3 months to 12 months and >5 kg: Apply no more than a maximum 2 g total over no more than 20 cm^2 of skin; leave on for no longer than 4 hours

◀

Age 1 to 6 years and >10 kg: Apply no more than a maximum of 10 g total over no more than 100 cm^2 of skin. US labeling recommends leaving on for no longer than 4 hours. Canadian labeling recommends leaving on for no longer than 5 hours.

Age 7 to 12 years and >20 kg: Apply no more than a maximum 20 g total over no more than 200 cm^2 of skin. US labeling recommends leaving on for no longer than 4 hours. Canadian labeling recommends leaving on for no longer than 5 hours.

Transdermal patch [Canadian product]: **Note:** Should not be used in neonates with a gestation age <37 weeks nor in infants <12 months of age who are receiving treatment with methemoglobin-inducing agents *Dosing is based on child's age and weight: Apply patch(es) to skin area(s) <10 cm^2:*

Age 0 to 3 months or <5 kg: Apply 1 patch and leave on for ~1 hour (do not exceed 1-hour application time); do not apply more than 1 patch at same time; safety of repeated dosing not established

Age 3 months to 12 months and >5 kg: Apply 1 to 2 patches for ~1 hour (maximum application time: 4 hours); do not apply more than 2 patches at the same time

Age 1 to 6 years and >10 kg: Apply 1 or more patches for minimum of 1 hour (maximum application time: 5 hours); maximum dose: 10 patches

Age 7 to 12 years and >20 kg: Apply 1 or more patches for a minimum of 1 hour (maximum application time: 5 hours); maximum dose: 20 patches

Renal Impairment There are no dosage adjustments provided in the manufacturer labeling. Lidocaine and prilocaine primarily undergo hepatic metabolism and their pharmacokinetics are not expected to be changed significantly in renal impairment.

Hepatic Impairment Smaller areas of treatment are recommended for patients with severe hepatic impairment.

Additional Information Complete prescribing information should be consulted for additional detail.

Dosage Forms Excipient information presented when available (limited, particularly for generics); consult specific product labeling. [DSC] = Discontinued product

Cream, topical:

AgonEaze: Lidocaine 2.5% and prilocaine 2.5% (2 x 30 g) [packaged with occlusive dressing]

Anodyne LPT: Lidocaine 2.5% and prilocaine 2.5% (3 x 30 g) [packaged with occlusive dressing]

DermacinRx Empricaine: Lidocaine 2.5% and prilocaine 2.5% (1 x 30 g) [packaged with occlusive dressing]

DermacinRx Prizopak: Lidocaine 2.5% and prilocaine 2.5% (3 x 30 g) [packaged with occlusive dressing]

Dolotranz: Lidocaine 2.5% and prilocaine 2.5% (3 x 30 g) [packaged with lidocaine gel 4%]

EMLA: Lidocaine 2.5% and prilocaine 2.5% (5 g [DSC], 30 g [DSC])

Leva Set: Lidocaine 2.5% and prilocaine 2.5% (3 x 30 g) [packaged with occlusive dressing]

Lido BDK: Lidocaine 2.5% and prilocaine 2.5% (5 g)

Lidopril: Lidocaine 2.5% and prilocaine 2.5% (3 x 30 g) [packaged with occlusive dressing]

Lidopril XR: Lidocaine 2.5% and prilocaine 2.5% (2 x 30 g) [packaged with occlusive dressing]

LiProZonePak: Lidocaine 2.5% and prilocaine 2.5% (3 x 30 g) [packaged with occlusive dressing]

Livixil Pak: Lidocaine 2.5% and prilocaine 2.5% (3 x 30 g) [packaged with occlusive dressing]

LP Lite Pak: Lidocaine 2.5% and prilocaine 2.5% (2 x 30 g) [packaged with occlusive dressing]

Medolor Pak: Lidocaine 2.5% and prilocaine 2.5% (3 x 30 g) [packaged with occlusive dressing]

Prilolid: Lidocaine 2.5% and prilocaine 2.5% (1 x 30 g) [packaged with occlusive dressing]

Priloxx LP: Lidocaine 2.5% and prilocaine 2.5%

Relador Pak: Lidocaine 2.5% and prilocaine 2.5% (3 x 30 g) [packaged with occlusive dressing]

Venipuncture CPI: Lidocaine 2.5% and prilocaine 2.5% (5 g)

Generic: Lidocaine 2.5% and prilocaine 2.5% (5 g, 30 g, 5800 g, 18,000 g)

Gel, periodontal:

Oraqix: Lidocaine 2.5% and prilocaine 2.5% (1.7 g)

Dosage Forms: Canada Information with regard to form, strength, and availability of products uniquely available in Canada but currently not available in the US. Refer also to Dosage Forms.

Excipient information presented when available (limited, particularly for generics); consult specific product labeling.

Patch, transdermal:

EMLA Patch: Lidocaine 2.5% and prilocaine 2.5% per patch (2s, 20s) [active contact surface area of each 1 g patch: 10 cm^2; surface area of entire patch: 40 cm^2]

♦ **Lidocaine/Prilocaine** *see* Lidocaine and Prilocaine *on page 1150*

♦ **Lidopril** *see* Lidocaine and Prilocaine *on page 1150*

♦ **Lidopril XR** *see* Lidocaine and Prilocaine *on page 1150*

♦ **Lilly CT-3231** *see* Vindesine *on page 1910*

Linezolid (li NE zoh lid)

Brand Names: US Zyvox

Brand Names: Canada Apo-Linezolid; Linezolid Injection; Sandoz-Linezolid; Zyvoxam

Pharmacologic Category Antibiotic, Oxazolidinone

Use

Enterococcal infections (vancomycin-resistant): Treatment of vancomycin-resistant (VRE) *Enterococcus faecium* infections, including cases with concurrent bacteremia. **Note:** Not a preferred agent in resistant *E. faecalis* infections which are usually susceptible to beta-lactams (O'Driscoll 2015).

Pneumonia:

Community-acquired: Treatment of community-acquired pneumonia (CAP) caused by *Streptococcus pneumoniae*, including cases with concurrent bacteremia, or *Staphylococcus aureus* (methicillin-susceptible isolates only). **Note:** Not a preferred agent for CAP; may be used as an alternate choice in multi-drug resistant *S. pneumoniae* and MRSA pneumonia. For methicillin-susceptible *S. aureus,* the use of beta-lactams is preferred (IDSA/ATS [Mandell 2007]).

◄ *Hospital-acquired or healthcare-associated:* Treatment of hospital-acquired or healthcare-associated pneumonia caused by *S. aureus* (methicillin-susceptible and -resistant isolates), or *S. pneumoniae*. **Note:** For methicillin-susceptible *S. aureus*, the use of beta-lactams is preferred (IDSA/ATS [Kalil 2016]).

Skin and skin structure infections:

Complicated: Treatment of complicated skin and skin structure infections, including diabetic foot infections, without concomitant osteomyelitis, caused by *S. aureus* (methicillin-susceptible and -resistant isolates), *Streptococcus pyogenes*, or *Streptococcus agalactiae*.

Uncomplicated: Treatment of uncomplicated skin and skin structure infections caused by *S. aureus* (methicillin-susceptible isolates) or *S. pyogenes*. **Note:** Generally reserved as alternate for skin and skin structure infections due to MRSA (IDSA [Liu 2011]; IDSA [Stevens 2014]).

Limitations of use: Linezolid has not been studied in the treatment of decubitus ulcers. Linezolid is not indicated for treatment of gram-negative infections; if a concomitant gram-negative pathogen is documented or suspected, initiate specific therapy immediately.

Pregnancy Risk Factor C

Dosing

Adult & Geriatric Note: Linezolid is not a preferred agent in treatment of infections requiring prolonged therapy (ie, >2 weeks) due to the risk of serious hematologic and neurologic toxicity. Use of linezolid is generally reserved for treatment of infections due to drug-resistant organisms (eg, MRSA, VRE).

Enterococcal infections (vancomycin-resistant [VRE]), including concurrent bacteremia: Oral, IV: 600 mg every 12 hours

Pneumonia:

Community-acquired (CAP) due to multi-drug resistant *S. pneumoniae*: Oral, IV: 600 mg every 12 hours; duration dependent upon severity of illness and clinical response

CAP due to MRSA: Oral, IV: 600 mg every 12 hours for 7 to 21 days (IDSA [Liu 2011])

Hospital-acquired (HAP) or ventilator-associated (VAP) due to MRSA, MSSA, and *S. pneumoniae* (generally reserved for MRSA): Oral, IV: 600 mg every 12 hours for 7 days; may consider a shorter or longer duration depending on rate of clinical improvement. When used as empiric therapy, use in combination with an antipseudomonal agent (one or two antipseudomonal agents depending on patient and institution specific risk factors) (IDSA/ATS [Kalil 2016])

Skin and skin structure infections (SSI), complicated: Oral, IV: 600 mg every 12 hours for 10 to 14 days. **Note:** Generally reserved as an alternative for MRSA infections. For diabetic foot infections, may extend treatment duration up to 4 weeks if slow to resolve (IDSA [Lipsky 2012]).

Skin and skin structure infections (SSI), uncomplicated: Oral: 400 mg every 12 hours for 10 to 14 days. **Note:** Generally reserved as an alternative for MRSA infections. The dose most commonly employed clinically is 600 mg every 12 hours; a 5- to 10-day treatment course may be sufficient (IDSA [Liu 2011]; IDSA [Stevens 2014]).

CNS infection due to MRSA (off-label use): Oral, IV: 600 mg every 12 hours; duration may vary depending on type and severity of infection, as well as clinical response (IDSA [Liu 2011])

Infective endocarditis (treatment), native or prosthetic valve (off-label use): IV, Oral: *Enterococcus (resistant to penicillin, aminoglycosides, and vancomycin):* 600 mg every 12 hours for a minimum of 6 weeks (AHA [Baddour 2015])

Intravascular catheter-associated bloodstream infection due to MRSA, methicillin-resistant coagulase negative staphylococci, or ampicillin- or vancomycin-resistant enterococcus (off-label use): Oral, IV: 600 mg every 12 hours (IDSA [Mermel 2009])

Osteomyelitis due to MRSA (off-label use): Oral, IV: 600 mg every 12 hours for a minimum of 8 weeks (for MRSA, some experts combine with rifampin, unless patient has concurrent bacteremia; in this case, clearance of bacteremia should occur first) (Birmingham 2003; IDSA [Liu 2011]; Rao 2004).

Osteomyelitis, native vertebral (off-label use): Staphylococci (oxacillin-susceptible or -resistant) or *Enterococcus* spp (penicillin-susceptible or – resistant): Oral, IV: 600 mg every 12 hours for 6 weeks (IDSA [Berbari 2015])

Prosthetic joint infection (off-label use):
Enterococcus spp (penicillin-susceptible or -resistant) (alternative treatment): Oral, IV: 600 mg every 12 hours for 4 to 6 weeks (consider adding an aminoglycoside) followed by an oral antibiotic suppressive regimen (IDSA [Osmon 2013]). **Note:** Generally reserved for VRE.
Staphylococci (oxacillin-sensitive or -resistant) (alternative treatment): Oral, IV: 600 mg every 12 hours for 2 to 6 weeks used in combination with rifampin followed by oral antibiotic treatment and suppressive regimens (IDSA [Osmon 2013]). **Note:** Generally reserved for VRE.

Septic arthritis due to MRSA (off-label use): Oral, IV: 600 mg every 12 hours for 3 to 4 weeks (IDSA [Liu 2011])

Tuberculosis, extensively drug-resistant (off-label use): Oral, IV: 600 mg once daily in addition to existing regimen; continue this dose until negative sputum smears for 2 consecutive weeks or until completion of 4 months of therapy then reduce dose to 300 mg once daily and continue for at least an additional 18 months; some patients may require continued therapy with 600 mg once daily instead if there is concern for resistance due to low exposure. Patient must be monitored closely for hematologic and neurologic toxicities (Lee 2012).

Pediatric

Usual dosage: Oral, IV:
Children ≤11 years: 10 mg/kg (maximum: 600 mg/dose) every 8 hours
Children ≥12 years and Adolescents: Refer to adult dosing.

Indication-specific dosing:

Enterococcal infections, vancomycin-resistant, including concurrent bacteremia: Oral, IV:
Infants and Children ≤11 years: 10 mg/kg every 8 hours for 14 to 28 days
Children ≥12 years and Adolescents: Refer to adult dosing.

Pneumonia:
Community-acquired (CAP):
Manufacturer's labeling (includes concurrent bacteremia): Oral, IV:
Infants and Children ≤11 years: 10 mg/kg/dose every 8 hours for 10 to 14 days
Children ≥12 years and Adolescents: Refer to adult dosing.

◄

Alternate dosing:

Infants >3 months and Children ≤11 years (IDSA/PIDS 2011):

S. pneumoniae (MICs to penicillin ≤2.0 mcg/mL), mild infection or step-down therapy (alternative to amoxicillin): Oral: 10 mg/kg/dose every 8 hours

S. pneumoniae (MICs to penicillin ≥4.0 mcg/mL):

Severe infection (alternative to ceftriaxone): IV: 10 mg/kg/dose every 8 hours

Mild infection, step-down therapy (preferred): Oral: 10 mg/kg/dose every 8 hours

S. aureus (methicillin-resistant/clindamycin-susceptible):

Severe infection (alternative to vancomycin or clindamycin): IV: 10 mg/kg/dose every 8 hours

Mild infection, step-down therapy (alternative to clindamycin): Oral: 10 mg/kg/dose every 8 hours

S. aureus (methicillin- and clindamycin-resistant):

Severe infection (alternative to vancomycin): IV: 10 mg/kg/dose every 8 hours

Mild infection, step-down therapy (preferred): Oral: 10 mg/kg/dose every 8 hours

Children ≤11 years (Liu 2011): Oral, IV: *S. aureus* (methicillin-resistant): 10 mg/kg/dose every 8 hours for 7 to 21 days (maximum: 600 mg/dose)

Children ≥12 years and Adolescents (IDSA/PIDS 2011):

S. pneumoniae (MICs to penicillin ≤2.0 mcg/mL), mild infection or step-down therapy (alternative to amoxicillin): Oral: 10 mg/kg/dose every 12 hours

S. pneumoniae (MICs to penicillin ≥4.0 mcg/mL)

Severe infection (alternative to ceftriaxone): IV: 10 mg/kg/dose every 12 hours

Mild infection, step-down therapy (preferred): Oral: 10 mg/kg/dose every 12 hours

S. aureus (methicillin-resistant/clindamycin-susceptible):

Severe infection (alternative to vancomycin/clindamycin): IV: 10 mg/kg/dose every 12 hours

Mild infection, step-down therapy (alternative to clindamycin): Oral: 10 mg/kg/dose every 12 hours

S. aureus (methicillin- and clindamycin-resistant):

Severe infection (alternative to vancomycin): IV: 10 mg/kg/dose every 12 hours

Mild infection, step-down therapy (preferred): Oral: 10 mg/kg/dose every 12 hours

Children ≥12 years and Adolescents (Liu 2011): *S. aureus* (methicillin-resistant): Refer to adult dosing.

Hospital-acquired or healthcare-associated: Oral, IV:

Manufacturer's labeling:

Infants and Children ≤11 years: 10 mg/kg every 8 hours for 10 to 14 days

Children ≥12 years and Adolescents: Refer to adult dosing.

Alternate dosing (Liu 2011): *S. aureus* (methicillin-resistant):

Infants and Children ≤11 years: 10 mg/kg/dose every 8 hours for 7 to 21 days (maximum: 600 mg/dose)

Children ≥12 years and Adolescents: Refer to adult dosing.

Skin and skin structure infections, complicated: Oral, IV:

Infants and Children ≤11 years: 10 mg/kg every 8 hours for 10 to 14 days

Children ≥12 years and Adolescents: Refer to adult dosing.

Skin and skin structure infections, uncomplicated: Oral:

Infants and Children <5 years: 10 mg/kg every 8 hours for 10 to 14 days

Children 5 to 11 years: 10 mg/kg every 12 hours for 10 to 14 days

Children ≥12 years and Adolescents: 600 mg every 12 hours for 10 to 14 days

Brain abscess, subdural empyema, spinal epidural abscess (*S. aureus* [methicillin-resistant]) (off-label use) (Liu 2011): Oral, IV: **Note:** The manufacturer does not recommend the use of linezolid for empiric treatment of pediatric CNS infections since therapeutic linezolid concentrations are not consistently achieved or maintained in the CSF of patients with ventriculoperitoneal shunts.

Children ≤11 years: 10 mg/kg every 8 hours for 4 to 6 weeks (maximum: 600 mg/dose)

Children ≥12 years and Adolescents: Refer to adult dosing.

Meningitis (*S. aureus* [methicillin-resistant]) (off-label use) (Liu 2011): Oral, IV:

Infants and Children ≤11 years: 10 mg/kg every 8 hours for 2 weeks (maximum: 600 mg/dose)

Children ≥12 years and Adolescents: Refer to adult dosing.

Osteomyelitis (*S. aureus* [methicillin-resistant]) (off-label use) (Liu 2011): Oral, IV:

Infants and Children ≤11 years: 10 mg/kg every 8 hours for a minimum of 4 to 6 weeks (maximum: 600 mg/dose)

Children ≥12 years and Adolescents: Refer to adult dosing.

Septic arthritis (*S. aureus* [methicillin-resistant]) (off-label use) (Liu 2011): Oral, IV:

Infants and Children ≤11 years: 10 mg/kg every 8 hours for 3 to 4 weeks (maximum: 600 mg/dose)

Children ≥12 years and Adolescents: Refer to adult dosing.

Septic thrombosis of cavernous or dural venous sinus (*S. aureus* [methicillin-resistant]) (off-label use) (Liu 2011): Oral, IV:

Children ≤11 years: 10 mg/kg every 8 hours for 4 to 6 weeks (maximum: 600 mg/dose)

Children >12 years and Adolescents: Refer to adult dosing.

Renal Impairment

Mild to severe impairment: No dosage adjustment necessary. The two primary metabolites may accumulate in patients with renal impairment but the clinical significance is unknown; use with caution.

End-stage renal disease (ESRD) on intermittent hemodialysis (IHD):

Manufacturer's labeling: Dialyzable (~30% removed during 3-hour dialysis session): No dosage adjustment necessary; administer after hemodialysis on dialysis days. The two primary metabolites may accumulate in patients with renal impairment but the clinical significance is unknown; use with caution.

Alternate dosing: If administration time is not immediately after dialysis session, may consider administration of a supplemental dose especially early in the treatment course to maintain levels above the MIC (Brier 2003). However, others have recommended no supplemental dose or dosage adjustment for patients on IHD (Heintz 2009; Trotman 2005)

Peritoneal dialysis: No supplemental dose or dosage adjustment needed (Heintz 2009; Trotman 2005)

Continuous renal replacement therapy (CVVH, CVVHD, CVVHDF): Some have suggested no supplemental dose or dosage adjustment needed (Heintz 2009; Trotman 2005). Others have postulated that achievement of MIC 2 mg/L may be suboptimal in ~30% of patients undergoing CVVHD or CVVHDF given 600 mg every 12 hours; however, no alternative dosing recommendations suggested (Roger 2016).

Hepatic Impairment

Mild to moderate impairment (Child-Pugh class A or B): No dosage adjustment necessary.

Severe impairment (Child-Pugh class C): There are no dosage adjustments provided in the manufacturer's labeling (has not been studied).

Obesity According to one study, the use of the standard dose of 600 mg every 12 hours for patients who are ≤150 kg will provide AUC values similar to that seen in non-obese adult patients; patients >150 kg were not included in the study. Use standard dosing for patients with weights ≤150 kg (Bhalodi 2013).

Additional Information Complete prescribing information should be consulted for additional detail.

Dosage Forms Excipient information presented when available (limited, particularly for generics); consult specific product labeling.

Solution, Intravenous:

Zyvox: 200 mg/100 mL (100 mL); 600 mg/300 mL (300 mL)

Generic: 600 mg/300 mL (300 mL)

Suspension Reconstituted, Oral:

Zyvox: 100 mg/5 mL (150 mL) [orange flavor]

Generic: 100 mg/5 mL (150 mL)

Tablet, Oral:

Zyvox: 600 mg

Generic: 600 mg

Lomustine (loe MUS teen)

Related Information

Management of Chemotherapy-Induced Nausea and Vomiting in Adults *on page* 2253

Prevention of Chemotherapy-Induced Nausea and Vomiting in Children *on page* 2310

Safe Handling of Hazardous Drugs *on page* 2379

Brand Names: US Gleostine

Brand Names: Canada CeeNU

Index Terms CCNU; CeeNU; Lomustinum

Pharmacologic Category Antineoplastic Agent, Alkylating Agent; Antineoplastic Agent, Alkylating Agent (Nitrosourea)

Use

Brain tumors: Treatment of primary and metastatic brain tumors (after appropriate surgical and/or radiotherapeutic procedures).

Hodgkin lymphoma: Treatment (in combination with other chemotherapy agents) of Hodgkin lymphoma which has progressed following initial chemotherapy; however, the use of lomustine in the management of Hodgkin lymphoma is limited due to efficacy of other chemotherapy agents/regimens.

Labeled Contraindications

US labeling: There are no contraindications listed in the manufacturer's labeling.

Canadian labeling: Hypersensitivity to lomustine or any component of the formulation; severe leukopenia and/or thrombocytopenia.

Pregnancy Considerations Adverse effects have been observed in animal reproduction studies. Based on the mechanism of action, lomustine may cause fetal harm when administered to a pregnant woman. Women of reproductive potential should use effective contraception during treatment and for 2 weeks after the final lomustine dose. Males with female partners of reproductive potential should use effective contraception during treatment and for 3.5 months (US labeling) or 6 months (Canadian labeling) after the final lomustine dose.

Breastfeeding Considerations It is not known if lomustine is excreted in breast milk. Due to the potential for serious adverse reactions in the nursing infant, the manufacturer recommends that women not breast-feed during treatment and for 2 weeks after the final lomustine dose.

Warnings/Precautions Wear gloves when handling the bottle/capsules; if contact with skin occurs, immediately wash area (thoroughly).

◀ **[US Boxed Warnings]:** Lomustine causes bone marrow suppression, including fatal myelosuppression. Hematologic toxicity is dose-related, cumulative, and delayed (occurring 4 to 6 weeks after drug administration and persisting for 1 to 2 weeks). Thrombocytopenia is generally more severe than leukopenia. Cumulative myelosuppression from lomustine is manifested by greater severity and longer duration of cytopenias. Monitor blood counts for at least 6 weeks after each dose. Do not administer lomustine more frequently than once every 6 weeks. Dose adjustments should be based on nadir counts from prior dose. The Canadian labeling contraindicates use in patients with severe leukopenia and/or thrombocytopenia.

[US Boxed Warning]: Lomustine should only be prescribed and dispensed as a single dose once every 6 weeks. Serious and fatal adverse events have occurred with overdosage (when lomustine was inadvertently administered daily). Health care providers, including pharmacists, should emphasize to the patient that only one dose of lomustine is taken every 6 weeks. The Institute for Safe Medication Practices (ISMP) recommends that prescribers only prescribe one dose at a time and pharmacies dispense only enough capsules for a single dose; in addition, patients should receive both verbal counseling and written instructions regarding proper dose and administration (ISMP 2014).

May cause pulmonary toxicity (infiltrates and/or fibrosis). Pulmonary toxicity is usually related to cumulative doses >1,100 mg/m^2. May be delayed 6 months or longer after treatment initiation. Patients with baseline below 70% of predicted forced vital capacity or carbon monoxide diffusing capacity are at increased risk. Patients treated at a younger age may also be at increased risk for pulmonary toxicity. Monitor pulmonary function tests at baseline and frequently during treatment. Discontinue lomustine permanently in patients diagnosed with pulmonary fibrosis. Lomustine is associated with a moderate emetic potential; antiemetics are recommended to prevent nausea and vomiting (Dupuis 2011). Stomatitis has also been reported. Hepatotoxicity (transaminase, alkaline phosphatase and bilirubin elevations) has been reported; monitor liver function. Progressive renal failure with a decrease in kidney size has been reported. Use with caution in patients with renal impairment; may require dosage adjustment. Monitor renal function. Long-term use of nitrosoureas is associated with the development of secondary malignancies, including acute leukemia and myelodysplasia. Avoid immunization with live viral vaccines; may result in severe infection or lack of vaccine response. Potentially significant drug-drug interactions may exist, requiring dose or frequency adjustment, additional monitoring, and/or selection of alternative therapy.

Adverse Reactions

>10%:

Gastrointestinal: Nausea and vomiting, (onset: 3 to 6 hours after oral administration; duration: <24 hours)

Hematologic & oncologic: Leukopenia (65%; nadir: 5 to 6 weeks; recovery 6 to 8 weeks), bone marrow depression (dose-limiting, delayed, cumulative), thrombocytopenia (nadir: 4 weeks; recovery 5 to 6 weeks)

Frequency not defined:

Central nervous system: Ataxia, disorientation, dysarthria, lethargy

Dermatologic: Alopecia

Gastrointestinal: Stomatitis

Genitourinary: Azotemia (progressive), nephron atrophy, nephrotoxicity

Hematologic & oncologic: Acute leukemia, anemia, bone marrow dysplasia

Hepatic: Hepatotoxicity, increased serum alkaline phosphatase, increased serum bilirubin, increased serum transaminases

Ophthalmic: Blindness, optic atrophy, visual disturbance

Renal: Renal failure

Respiratory: Pulmonary fibrosis, pulmonary infiltrates

Drug Interactions

Metabolism/Transport Effects Substrate of CYP2D6 (minor); **Note:** Assignment of Major/Minor substrate status based on clinically relevant drug interaction potential

Avoid Concomitant Use

Avoid concomitant use of Lomustine with any of the following: BCG (Intravesical); Deferiprone; Dipyrone; Natalizumab; Pimecrolimus; Tacrolimus (Topical); Vaccines (Live)

Increased Effect/Toxicity

Lomustine may increase the levels/effects of: CloZAPine; Deferiprone; Fingolimod; Leflunomide; Natalizumab; Tofacitinib; Vaccines (Live)

The levels/effects of Lomustine may be increased by: Denosumab; Dipyrone; Ocrelizumab; Palifermin; Pimecrolimus; Promazine; Roflumilast; Tacrolimus (Topical); Trastuzumab

Decreased Effect

Lomustine may decrease the levels/effects of: BCG (Intravesical); Coccidioides immitis Skin Test; Lenograstim; Nivolumab; Sipuleucel-T; Tertomotide; Vaccines (Inactivated); Vaccines (Live)

The levels/effects of Lomustine may be decreased by: Echinacea

Hazardous Drugs Handling Considerations

Hazardous agent (NIOSH 2016 [group 1]).

Use appropriate precautions for receiving, handling, administration, and disposal. Gloves (single) should be worn during receiving, unpacking, and placing in storage. NIOSH recommends single gloving for administration of intact tablets or capsules (NIOSH 2016).

Storage/Stability Store at 25°C (77°F); excursions permitted between 15°C and 30°C (59°F and 86°F). Avoid temperatures over 40°C (104°F).

Mechanism of Action Inhibits DNA, RNA, and protein synthesis via alkylation and carbamylation of DNA and RNA; lomustine is cell cycle non-specific (Perry 2012)

Pharmacodynamics/Kinetics

Distribution: Crosses blood-brain barrier; CNS concentrations are high (Perry 2012)

Metabolism: Hepatic to active metabolites (Perry 2012)

Half-life elimination: Metabolites: 16 to 48 hours

Time to peak, serum: ~3 hours (Perry 2012)

Excretion: Urine (~50%, as metabolites)

Dosing

Adult & Geriatric Note: Dispense only enough capsules for a single dose; do not dispense more than one dose at a time (ISMP 2014). Repeat courses should only be administered after adequate recovery of leukocytes to >4,000/mm^3 and platelets to >100,000/mm^3. Doses should be rounded to the nearest 5 mg. Lomustine is associated with a moderate emetic potential; antiemetics are recommended to prevent nausea and vomiting.

Brain tumors: *Manufacturer's labeling:* Oral: 130 mg/m² as a single dose once every 6 weeks; reduce dose to 100 mg/m² as a single dose once every 6 weeks in patients with compromised bone marrow function (dosage reductions may be recommended for combination chemotherapy regimens).

Anaplastic oligodendroglioma: PCV regimen (off-label combination): Oral: 130 mg/m² on day 1 every 6 weeks for up to 4 cycles prior to radiation therapy (in combination with procarbazine and vincristine) (Cairncross 2013; Cairncross 2006).

Astrocytoma, high grade: POC regimen (off-label dosing): Adults ≤21 years: Oral: 100 mg/m² on day 1 every 6 weeks for 8 cycles (in combination with vincristine and prednisone) (Finlay 1995).

Glioblastoma, recurrent:

PCV regimen (off-label dosing): Oral: 110 mg/m² on day 1 every 6 weeks for 7 cycles (in combination with procarbazine and vincristine) (Levin 2000).

Single-agent therapy: Oral: 100 to 130 mg/m² every 6 weeks until disease progression or unacceptable toxicity (Wick 2010).

Medulloblastoma (off-label dosing): Adults ≤21 years: Oral: 75 mg/m² once every 6 weeks for 8 cycles (in combination with cisplatin and vincristine) (Packer 2006; Packer 1999).

Hodgkin lymphoma: *Manufacturer's labeling:* Oral: 130 mg/m² as a single dose once every 6 weeks; reduce dose to 100 mg/m² as a single dose once every 6 weeks in patients with compromised bone marrow function (dosage reductions may be recommended for combination chemotherapy regimens). **Note:** The use of lomustine in the management of Hodgkin lymphoma is limited due to efficacy of other chemotherapy agents/regimens.

Pediatric Note: Dispense only enough capsules for a single dose; do not dispense more than one dose at a time (ISMP 2014). Repeat courses should only be administered after adequate recovery of leukocytes to >4,000/mm³ and platelets to >100,000/mm³. Doses should be rounded to the nearest 5 mg. Lomustine is associated with a moderate emetic potential; antiemetics are recommended to prevent nausea and vomiting (Dupuis 2011).

Brain tumors: *Manufacturer's labeling:* Oral: 130 mg/m² as a single dose once every 6 weeks; reduce dose to 100 mg/m² as a single dose once every 6 weeks in patients with compromised bone marrow function (dosage reductions may be recommended for combination chemotherapy regimens)

Astrocytoma, high grade: POC regimen (off-label dosing): Children ≥18 months and Adolescents: Oral: 100 mg/m² on day 1 every 6 weeks for 8 cycles (in combination with vincristine and prednisone) (Finlay 1995)

Medulloblastoma (off-label dosing): Children ≥3 years and Adolescents: Oral: 75 mg/m² once every 6 weeks for 8 cycles (in combination with cisplatin and vincristine) (Packer 2006; Packer 1999)

Hodgkin lymphoma: *Manufacturer's labeling:* Oral: 130 mg/m² as a single dose once every 6 weeks; reduce dose to 100 mg/m² as a single dose once every 6 weeks in patients with compromised bone marrow function (dosage reductions may be recommended for combination chemotherapy regimens). **Note:** The use of lomustine in the management of Hodgkin lymphoma is limited due to efficacy of other chemotherapy agents/regimens.

Renal Impairment There are no dosage adjustments provided in the manufacturer's labeling. The following adjustments have been recommended:

Aronoff 2007: Adults:
  CrCl 10 to 50 mL/minute: Reduce dose to 75% of normal dose
  CrCl <10 mL/minute: Reduce dose to 25% to 50% of normal dose
  Continuous ambulatory peritoneal dialysis (CAPD): Reduce dose to 25% to 50% of normal dose

Kintzel 1995:
  CrCl 46 to 60 mL/minute: Reduce dose to 75% of normal dose
  CrCl 31 to 45 mL/minute: Reduce dose to 70% of normal dose
  CrCl ≤30 mL/minute: Avoid use

Hemodialysis: Due to its lipophilic nature, lomustine is not dialyzable (Canadian labeling). Supplemental dose is not necessary (Aronoff 2007).

Hepatic Impairment There are no dosage adjustments provided in the manufacturer's labeling. However, lomustine is hepatically metabolized and caution should be used in patients with hepatic dysfunction.

Obesity *ASCO Guidelines for appropriate chemotherapy dosing in obese adults with cancer:* Utilize patient's actual body weight (full weight) for calculation of body surface area- or weight-based dosing, particularly when the intent of therapy is curative; manage regimen-related toxicities in the same manner as for nonobese patients; if a dose reduction is utilized due to toxicity, consider resumption of full weight-based dosing with subsequent cycles, especially if cause of toxicity (eg, hepatic or renal impairment) is resolved (Griggs 2012).

Adjustment for Toxicity

Hematologic toxicity: Dosing adjustment (based on nadir) for subsequent cycles:
  Leukocytes ≥3,000/mm^3, platelets ≥75,000/mm^3: No dosage adjustment required
  Leukocytes 2,000 to 2,999/mm^3, platelets 25,000 to 74,999/mm^3: Reduce dose to 70% of prior dose
  Leukocytes <2,000/mm^3, platelets <25,000/mm^3: Reduce dose to 50% of prior dose

Nonhematologic toxicity: Pulmonary fibrosis: Discontinue permanently.

Combination Regimens

Brain tumors:
  PCV (Brain Tumor Regimen) on page 2191
  POC on page 2196

Administration

Lomustine is associated with a moderate emetic potential; antiemetics are recommended to prevent nausea and vomiting (Dupuis 2011).

Oral: Administering on an empty stomach may reduce the incidence of nausea and vomiting.

Varying strengths of capsules may be required to obtain necessary dose. Dispense only enough capsules for a single dose; do not dispense more than one dose at a time (ISMP 2014). Do not break capsules. If contact with skin occurs, immediately wash area (thoroughly). Avoid exposure to broken capsules.

Emetic Potential Children and Adults: Moderate (30% to 90%)

Monitoring Parameters CBC with differential and platelet count (weekly for at least 6 weeks after a dose), hepatic and renal function tests (periodic), pulmonary function tests (baseline and periodic)

◄ **Dosage Forms** Excipient information presented when available (limited, particularly for generics); consult specific product labeling. [DSC] = Discontinued product

Capsule, Oral:

Gleostine: 5 mg, 10 mg, 40 mg, 100 mg

Generic: 10 mg [DSC], 40 mg [DSC], 100 mg [DSC]

Dosage Forms: Canada Information with regard to form, strength, and availability of products uniquely available in Canada but currently not available in the US.

Excipient information presented when available (limited, particularly for generics); consult specific product labeling.

Capsule, Oral:

CeeNu: 10 mg, 40 mg, 100 mg

♦ **Lomustinum** see Lomustine on page 1159

♦ **Longastatin** see Octreotide on page 1348

♦ **Lonsurf** see Trifluridine and Tipiracil on page 1837

LORazepam (lor A ze pam)

Brand Names: US Ativan; LORazepam Intensol

Brand Names: Canada Apo-Lorazepam; Ativan; Dom-Lorazepam; Lorazepam Injection, USP; PHL-Lorazepam; PMS-Lorazepam; PRO-Lorazepam; Teva-Lorazepam

Pharmacologic Category Anticonvulsant, Benzodiazepine; Benzodiazepine

Use

Anxiety (oral): Management of anxiety disorders, short-term (≤4 months) relief of anxiety symptoms, or anxiety associated with depressive symptoms, or anxiety/stress-associated insomnia.

Anesthesia premedication (parenteral): Anesthesia premedication in adults to relieve anxiety or to produce amnesia (diminish recall) or sedation.

Anesthesia premedication (sublingual) [Canadian product]: Anesthesia premedication to relieve anxiety prior to surgical procedures.

Status epilepticus (parenteral): Treatment of status epilepticus.

Dosing

Adult

Anxiety disorder: Oral: Initial: 2 to 3 mg daily in 2 to 3 divided doses; usual dose: 2 to 6 mg daily in divided doses; however, daily dose may vary from 1 to 10 mg/day

Insomnia due to anxiety or stress: Oral:

<65 years: 0.5 to 2 mg at bedtime (Winkelman 2015)

≥65 years: 0.5 to 1 mg at bedtime (Winkelman 2015)

Note: The manufacturer recommends higher dosing (ie, 2 to 4 mg at bedtime); however, generally, it is a safer approach to employ the above recommended doses.

Premedication for anesthesia:

IM: 0.05 mg/kg administered 2 hours before surgery (maximum dose: 4 mg)

IV: 0.044 mg/kg administered 15 to 20 minutes before surgery (usual dose: 2 mg; maximum dose: 4 mg). **Note:** Doses >2 mg should generally not be exceeded in patients >50 years.

Sublingual tablet [Canadian product]: 0.05 mg/kg 1 to 2 hours before surgery (maximum dose: 4 mg)

Status epilepticus: IV:

American Epilepsy Society and Neurocritical Care Society recommendations: 0.1 mg/kg (maximum dose: 4 mg) given at a maximum rate of 2 mg/minute; may repeat in 5 to 10 minutes (AES [Glauser 2016]; NCS [Brophy 2012]). **Note:** Dilute dose 1:1 with saline.

Manufacturer's labeling: 4 mg given slowly (2 mg/minute); may repeat in 10 to 15 minutes. May be given IM, but IV preferred.

Agitation in the ICU patient (off-label use): IV: Loading dose: 0.02 to 0.04 mg/kg (maximum single dose: 2 mg); Maintenance: 0.02 to 0.06 mg/kg every 2 to 6 hours as needed **or** 0.01 to 0.1 mg/kg/hour; maximum dose: ≤10 mg/hour (Barr 2013)

Alcohol withdrawal delirium (off-label use) (Mayo-Smith 2004):

IV: 1 to 4 mg every 5 to 15 minutes until calm, then every hour as needed to maintain light somnolence

IM: 1 to 4 mg every 30 to 60 minutes until calm, then every hour as needed to maintain light somnolence

Alcohol withdrawal syndrome (off-label use) (Mayo-Smith, 1997):

Oral, IM, IV (fixed-dose regimen): 2 mg every 6 hours for 4 doses, then 1 mg every 6 hours for 8 additional doses

Oral, IM, IV (symptom-triggered regimen): 2 to 4 mg every 1 hour as needed; dose determined by a validated severity assessment scale

Chemotherapy-associated nausea and vomiting (off-label use): Breakthrough nausea/vomiting or as adjunct to standard antiemetics: Oral, IV, Sublingual (off-label route): 0.5 to 2 mg every 6 hours as needed (Lohr 2008)

Partial complex seizures, refractory (off-label use): Oral: 1 mg twice daily; increase biweekly in increments of 1 mg twice daily until seizures stop or side effects occur (Walker, 1984); however, additional data may be necessary to further define the role of lorazepam in this condition

Psychogenic catatonia (off-label use):

IM, Sublingual (off-label route): 1 to 2 mg; repeat dose in 3 hours then again in another 3 hours if initial and subsequent doses, respectively, are ineffective (Rosebush, 1990; Rosebush 2010); however, additional data may be necessary to further define the role of lorazepam in this condition

or

Oral, IM, IV: Initial: 1 mg; may repeat in 5 minutes if necessary. If initial challenge is unsuccessful, may increase dose up to 4 to 8 mg per day; may continue treatment for up to 5 days (Bush, 1996); however, additional data may be necessary to further define the role of lorazepam in this condition

Rapid tranquilization of the agitated patient (off-label use): Oral, IM, IV: 1 to 3 mg administered every 30 to 60 minutes; may be administered with an antipsychotic (eg, haloperidol) (Allen 2005; Battaglia 2005; De Fruyt 2004; Wilson 2012). **Note:** When administering IM, may consider a lower initial dose (eg, 0.5 mg) (Allen 2005).

Dosage adjustment for lorazepam with concomitant medications: *Probenecid or valproic acid:* Reduce lorazepam dose by 50%

Geriatric Refer also to adult dosing. Dose selection should generally be on the low end of the dosage range (initial dose not to exceed 2 mg).

Anxiety disorder: Oral: Initial: 1 to 2 mg daily in divided doses

◀ **Pediatric**

Chemotherapy-associated nausea and vomiting (off-label use):

Anticipatory nausea/vomiting (prevention and treatment): Infants ≥1 month, Children, and Adolescents: Oral: 0.04 to 0.08 mg/kg/dose (maximum dose: 2 mg) once at bedtime the evening prior to chemotherapy and once the next day before chemotherapy (Dupuis 2014)

Breakthrough nausea/vomiting: Children ≥2 years and Adolescents: IV: 0.025 to 0.05 mg/kg/dose (maximum dose: 2 mg) every 6 hours as needed (Dupuis 2003); however, additional data may be necessary to further define the role of lorazepam in children for chemotherapy-associated nausea and vomiting

Status epilepticus: Infants, Children, and Adolescents (off-label use):

American Epilepsy Society and Neurocritical Care Society recommendations: IV: 0.1 mg/kg (maximum dose: 4 mg) given at a maximum rate of 2 mg/minute; may repeat in 5 to 10 minutes (AES [Glauser 2016]; NCS [Brophy 2012]). **Note:** Dilute dose 1:1 with saline.

American Academy of Pediatrics recommendation: IV, IM: 0.05 to 0.1 mg/kg (maximum dose: 4 mg); may repeat dose every 10 to 15 minutes if seizure continues (AAP [Hegenbarth 2008])

Dosage adjustment for lorazepam with concomitant medications: *Probenecid or valproic acid:* Reduce lorazepam dose by 50%

Renal Impairment

Oral: No dosage adjustment necessary (Aronoff 2007).

Parenteral:

Mild-to-moderate impairment: No dosage adjustment necessary for acute doses; use repeated doses with caution; may increase the risk of propylene glycol toxicity. Monitor closely if using for prolonged periods of time or at high doses.

Severe impairment or failure: Use is not recommended.

Hepatic Impairment

Oral:

Mild-to-moderate impairment: No dosage adjustment necessary.

Severe impairment and/or encephalopathy: Use with caution; may require lower doses.

Parenteral:

Mild-to-moderate impairment: No dosage adjustment necessary; use with caution.

Severe impairment or failure: Use is not recommended.

Additional Information Complete prescribing information should be consulted for additional detail.

Dosage Forms Excipient information presented when available (limited, particularly for generics); consult specific product labeling. [DSC] = Discontinued product

Concentrate, Oral:

LORazepam Intensol: 2 mg/mL (30 mL) [alcohol free, dye free, sugar free; unflavored flavor]

Generic: 2 mg/mL (30 mL)

Solution, Injection:

Ativan: 2 mg/mL (1 mL, 10 mL); 4 mg/mL (1 mL, 10 mL) [contains benzyl alcohol, polyethylene glycol, propylene glycol]

Generic: 2 mg/mL (1 mL, 10 mL); 4 mg/mL (1 mL, 10 mL)

Solution, Intravenous:
Generic: 100 mg/100 mL in NaCl 0.9% (100 mL); 60 mg/60 mL in NaCl 0.9% (60 mL [DSC])
Tablet, Oral:
Ativan: 0.5 mg, 1 mg [DSC]
Ativan: 1 mg [scored]
Ativan: 2 mg [DSC]
Ativan: 2 mg [scored]
Generic: 0.5 mg, 1 mg, 2 mg
Dosage Forms: Canada Information with regard to form, strength, and availability of products uniquely available in Canada but currently not available in the US. Refer also to Dosage Forms.

Excipient information presented when available (limited, particularly for generics); consult specific product labeling.
Tablet, Sublingual: 0.5 mg, 1 mg, 2 mg
Controlled Substance C-IV

◆ **Lorazepam Injection, USP (Can)** see LORazepam on page 1164
◆ **LORazepam Intensol** see LORazepam on page 1164
◆ **Lovenox** see Enoxaparin on page 680
◆ **Lovenox HP (Can)** see Enoxaparin on page 680
◆ **Lovenox With Preservative (Can)** see Enoxaparin on page 680
◆ **Low-Molecular-Weight Iron Dextran (INFeD)** see Iron Dextran Complex on page 1053
◆ **L-PAM** see Melphalan on page 1182
◆ **L-Phenylalanine Mustard** see Melphalan on page 1182
◆ **LP Lite Pak** see Lidocaine and Prilocaine on page 1150
◆ **L-Sarcolysin** see Melphalan on page 1182
◆ **Lupron (Can)** see Leuprolide on page 1131
◆ **Lupron Depot (Can)** see Leuprolide on page 1131
◆ **Lupron Depot (1-Month)** see Leuprolide on page 1131
◆ **Lupron Depot (3-Month)** see Leuprolide on page 1131
◆ **Lupron Depot (4-Month)** see Leuprolide on page 1131
◆ **Lupron Depot (6-Month)** see Leuprolide on page 1131
◆ **Lupron Depot-Ped (1-Month)** see Leuprolide on page 1131
◆ **Lupron Depot-Ped (3-Month)** see Leuprolide on page 1131
◆ **LX1032** see Telotristat Ethyl on page 1744
◆ **LX1606** see Telotristat Ethyl on page 1744
◆ **LY170053** see OLANZapine on page 1364
◆ **LY-188011** see Gemcitabine on page 864
◆ **LY231514** see PEMEtrexed on page 1494
◆ **LY303366** see Anidulafungin on page 139
◆ **LY3012207** see Olaratumab on page 1372
◆ **Lymphazurin** see Isosulfan Blue on page 1062
◆ **Lymphocyte Immune Globulin** see Antithymocyte Globulin (Equine) on page 154

Mechlorethamine (Systemic) (me klor ETH a meen)

Related Information

Management of Chemotherapy-Induced Nausea and Vomiting in Adults *on page 2253*

Management of Drug Extravasations *on page 2271*

Prevention of Chemotherapy-Induced Nausea and Vomiting in Children *on page 2310*

Safe Handling of Hazardous Drugs *on page 2379*

Brand Names: US Mustargen

Index Terms Chlorethazine; Chlorethazine Mustard; HN_2; Mechlorethamine Hydrochloride; Mustine; Nitrogen Mustard

Pharmacologic Category Antineoplastic Agent, Alkylating Agent; Antineoplastic Agent, Alkylating Agent (Nitrogen Mustard)

Use

Hodgkin lymphoma: Palliative treatment of Hodgkin lymphoma

Malignant effusion: Palliative treatment of effusions from metastatic carcinomas

Additional approved uses (manufacturer labeling): Treatment of lymphosarcoma, chronic myelocytic or chronic lymphocytic leukemia, polycythemia vera, mycosis fungoides, and bronchogenic carcinoma

Labeled Contraindications Hypersensitivity to mechlorethamine or any component of the formulation; presence of known infection

Pregnancy Considerations Adverse events have been observed in animal reproduction studies. Women of childbearing potential are advised not to become pregnant during treatment. **[U.S. Boxed Warning]: Avoid exposure during pregnancy.**

Breastfeeding Considerations It is not known if mechlorethamine is excreted in human breast milk. Due to the potential for serious adverse reactions in the nursing infant, the decision to discontinue mechlorethamine or to discontinue breastfeeding should take into account the importance of treatment to the mother.

Warnings/Precautions [U.S. Boxed Warning]: Mechlorethamine is a highly toxic nitrogen mustard; avoid inhalation of vapors or dust; review and follow special handling procedures. Avoid dust or vapor contact with skin or eyes. If accidental skin exposure occurs, wash/irrigate thoroughly with water for at least 15 minutes, followed by 2% sodium thiosulfate solution; remove and destroy any contaminated clothing. If exposure to eye(s) occurs, promptly irrigate for at least 15 minutes with copious amounts of water, normal saline, or balanced salt ophthalmic irrigating solution; obtain ophthalmology consultation. The manufacturer recommends neutralizing remaining unused mechlorethamine, empty or partial vials, gloves, tubing, glassware, etc., after mechlorethamine administration; soak in an aqueous solution containing equal volumes of sodium thiosulfate (5%) and sodium bicarbonate (5%) for 45 minutes; rinse with water; dispose of properly.

[U.S. Boxed Warning]: Mechlorethamine is a potent vesicant; extravasation results in painful inflammation with induration and sloughing. If extravasation occurs, promptly manage by infiltrating area with 1/6 molar sodium thiosulfate solution, followed by dry cold compresses for 6-12 hours. Ensure proper needle or catheter placement prior to and during infusion. Avoid extravasation.

Bone marrow suppression: May cause lymphopenia, leukopenia, granulocytopenia, thrombocytopenia and anemia. Agranulocytopenia may occur (rare); persistent pancytopenia has been reported. Monitor blood counts. Bleeding due to thrombocytopenia may occur. Use with caution in patients where neoplasm has bone marrow involvement or in those who have received prior myelosuppressive chemotherapy; marrow function may be further compromised (possibly fatal). Bone marrow function should recover after mechlorethamine administration prior to initiating radiation therapy or other chemotherapy regimens.

Hyperuricemia may occur, especially with lymphomas; ensure adequate hydration; consider antihyperuricemic therapy if appropriate. Mechlorethamine is associated with a high emetic potential (Basch, 2011; Dupuis, 2011; Roila, 2010); antiemetics are recommended to prevent nausea and vomiting. Hypersensitivity reactions, including anaphylaxis, have been reported. Mechlorethamine has immunosuppressant properties; may predispose patients to infections (bacterial, viral, or fungal). Alkylating agents, including mechlorethamine, are associated with in increased incidence of secondary malignancies; concurrent radiation therapy or combination chemotherapy may increase the risk. Potentially significant drug-drug interactions may exist, requiring dose or frequency adjustment, additional monitoring, and/or selection of alternative therapy.

◄ **[U.S. Boxed Warning]: Avoid exposure during pregnancy.** Impaired spermatogenesis, azoospermia, and total germinal aplasia may occur in male patients treated with mechlorethamine, particularly when used in combination with other chemotherapy agents. Delayed menses, oligomenorrhea, or temporary or permanent amenorrhea may be observed in female patients treated with mechlorethamine.

Bone marrow failure and other toxicities are more common in chronic lymphocytic leukemia (CLL); in general, mechlorethamine is no longer used in the treatment of CLL. Bone and nervous system tumors typically respond poorly to treatment with mechlorethamine. The routine use of mechlorethamine in widely disseminated tumors is discouraged. **[U.S. Boxed Warning]: Should be administered under the supervision of an experienced cancer chemotherapy physician.**

Adverse Reactions Frequency not defined.

Cardiovascular: Local thrombophlebitis

Central nervous system: Brain disease (high dose), drowsiness, headache, lethargy, metallic taste, sedation, vertigo

Dermatologic: Alopecia, diaphoresis, erythema multiforme, maculopapular rash, skin rash

Endocrine & metabolic: Amenorrhea, hyperuricemia, oligomenorrhea

Gastrointestinal: Anorexia, diarrhea, mucositis, nausea, vomiting

Genitourinary: Inhibition of spermatogenesis

Hematologic & oncologic: Agranulocytosis, granulocytopenia (onset: 6 to 8 days; recovery: 10 to 21 days), hemolytic anemia, leukopenia, lymphocytopenia, pancytopenia, petechia, thrombocytopenia

Hepatic: Jaundice

Hypersensitivity: Anaphylaxis, hypersensitivity reaction

Infection: Herpes zoster

Neuromuscular & skeletal: Weakness

Ophthalmic: Lacrimation

Otic: Deafness, tinnitus

Miscellaneous: Fever, tissue necrosis (extravasation)

Drug Interactions

Metabolism/Transport Effects None known.

Avoid Concomitant Use

Avoid concomitant use of Mechlorethamine (Systemic) with any of the following: BCG (Intravesical); Deferiprone; Dipyrone; Natalizumab; Pimecrolimus; Tacrolimus (Topical); Vaccines (Live)

Increased Effect/Toxicity

Mechlorethamine (Systemic) may increase the levels/effects of: CloZAPine; Deferiprone; Fingolimod; Leflunomide; Natalizumab; Tofacitinib; Vaccines (Live)

The levels/effects of Mechlorethamine (Systemic) may be increased by: Denosumab; Dipyrone; Ocrelizumab; Palifermin; Pimecrolimus; Promazine; Roflumilast; Tacrolimus (Topical); Trastuzumab

Decreased Effect

Mechlorethamine (Systemic) may decrease the levels/effects of: BCG (Intravesical); Coccidioides immitis Skin Test; Lenograstim; Nivolumab; Sipuleucel-T; Tertomotide; Vaccines (Inactivated); Vaccines (Live)

The levels/effects of Mechlorethamine (Systemic) may be decreased by: Echinacea

Hazardous Drugs Handling Considerations
Hazardous agent (NIOSH 2016 [group 1]).

Use appropriate precautions for receiving, handling, administration, and disposal. Gloves (single) should be worn during receiving, unpacking, and placing in storage.

NIOSH recommends double gloving, a protective gown, ventilated engineering controls (a class II biological safety cabinet or a compounding aseptic containment isolator), and closed system transfer devices (CSTDs) for preparation. Double gloving, a gown, and (if dosage form allows) CSTDs are required during administration (NIOSH 2016).

Storage/Stability Store intact vials at room temperature of 15°C to 30°C (59°F to 86°F). Protect from light. Protect from humidity. **Must be prepared immediately before use;** degradation begins shortly after dilution.

Preparation for Administration Must be prepared immediately before use; degradation begins shortly after dilution. Dilute powder with 10 mL SWFI or NS to a final concentration of 1 mg/mL. May be further diluted in 50-100 mL NS for intracavitary administration.

Mechanism of Action Bifunctional alkylating agent that inhibits DNA and RNA synthesis via formation of carbonium ions; produces interstrand and intrastrand cross-links in DNA resulting in miscoding, breakage, and failure of replication. Although not cell phase-specific *per se,* mechlorethamine effect is most pronounced in the S phase, and cell proliferation is arrested in the G_2 phase.

Pharmacodynamics/Kinetics
Metabolism: Rapid hydrolysis in the plasma to active metabolites (Perry, 2012)

Half-life elimination: 15-20 minutes (Perry, 2012)

Dosing
Adult & Geriatric Dosage should be based on ideal dry weight (evaluate the presence of edema or ascites so that dosage is based on actual weight unaugmented by edema/ascites). Mechlorethamine is associated with a high emetic potential (Basch, 2011; Roila, 2010); antiemetics are recommended to prevent nausea and vomiting

Hodgkin lymphoma (off-label dosing): IV:

MOPP regimen: 6 mg/m^2 on days 1 and 8 of a 28-day treatment cycle for 6 to 8 cycles (Canelos, 1992; DeVita, 1970)

Stanford V regimen: 6 mg/m^2 as a single dose on day 1 in weeks 1, 5, and 9 (Horning, 2000; Horning, 2002)

Malignant effusion: Intracavitary: 0.4 mg/kg as a single dose; although 0.2 mg/kg (10-20 mg) as a single dose has been used by the *intrapericardial* route

Renal Impairment No dosage adjustment provided in manufacturer's labeling.

Hepatic Impairment No dosage adjustment provided in manufacturer's labeling.

The following have also been reported:

Mild-to-moderate impairment: No dosage adjustment necessary (Ecklund, 2005).

Severe liver impairment: No dosage adjustment necessary; concomitant chemotherapy may require alteration until improvement in hepatic function (Ecklund, 2005)

◀

Obesity *ASCO Guidelines for appropriate chemotherapy dosing in obese adults with cancer:* In general, utilize patient's actual body weight (full weight) for calculation of body surface area- or weight-based dosing, particularly when the intent of therapy is curative; manage regimen-related toxicities in the same manner as for nonobese patients; if a dose reduction is utilized due to toxicity, consider resumption of full weight-based dosing with subsequent cycles, especially if cause of toxicity (eg, hepatic or renal impairment) is resolved (Griggs, 2012). **Note:** The manufacturer recommends dosing be based on ideal dry body weight and the presence of edema or ascites should be considered so the dose will be based on unaugmented weight.

Combination Regimens

Lymphoma, Hodgkin:

MOPP/ABVD (Hodgkin) on page 2176

MOPP/ABV Hybrid (Hodgkin) on page 2177

MOPP (Hodgkin) on page 2178

Stanford V (Hodgkin) on page 2209

Administration

IV: Administer as a slow IV push over a few minutes into a free-flowing IV solution. Mechlorethamine is associated with a high emetic potential (Basch, 2011; Dupuis, 2011; Roila, 2010); antiemetics are recommended to prevent nausea and vomiting.

Intracavitary: May further dilute in 50-100 mL of normal saline prior to instillation; rotate patient position every 5-10 minutes for 1 hour after instillation to obtain uniform distribution.

Prepare immediately prior to administration.

Vesicant; ensure proper needle or catheter placement prior to and during infusion; avoid extravasation.

Extravasation management: If extravasation occurs, stop infusion immediately and disconnect (leave cannula/needle in place); gently aspirate extravasated solution (do **NOT** flush the line); remove needle/cannula; elevate extremity.

Sodium thiosulfate 1/6 M solution: Inject subcutaneously into extravasation area using 2 mL for each mg of mechlorethamine suspected to have extravasated (Perez Fidalgo, 2012; Polovich, 2009). Apply ice for 6-12 hours after sodium thiosulfate administration (Mustargen prescribing information, 2013; Polovich, 2009) **or** may apply dry cold compresses for 20 minutes 4 times daily for 1-2 days (Perez Fidalgo, 2012).

Vesicant/Extravasation Risk Vesicant

Emetic Potential Children and Adults: High (>90%)

Monitoring Parameters CBC with differential and platelet count; renal and hepatic function; signs/symptoms of hypersensitivity reactions, infection, and extravasation

Additional Information A topical gel is commercially approved for topical treatment of cutaneous T-cell lymphoma (mycosis fungoides type), please refer to Mechlorethamine (Topical) monograph.

Product Availability Mustargen: Mustargen was acquired by Recordati Rare Diseases in 2013; availability information is currently unknown.

Dosage Forms Excipient information presented when available (limited, particularly for generics); consult specific product labeling.

Solution Reconstituted, Injection, as hydrochloride:

Mustargen: 10 mg (1 ea)

Mechlorethamine (Topical) (me klor ETH a meen)

Brand Names: US Valchlor

Index Terms Mechlorethamine HCl (Topical); Mechlorethamine Topical Gel

Pharmacologic Category Antineoplastic Agent, Alkylating Agent; Antineoplastic Agent, Alkylating Agent (Nitrogen Mustard)

Use Cutaneous T-cell lymphoma: Topical treatment of stage IA and IB mycosis fungoides-type cutaneous T-cell lymphoma in patients who have received prior skin-directed therapy

Labeled Contraindications Known severe hypersensitivity to mechlorethamine or any component of the formulation

Pregnancy Considerations Adverse events have been observed in animal reproduction studies. There have been case reports of teratogenic events following systemic use in humans. Pregnancy should be avoided if therapy is needed.

Breastfeeding Considerations It is not known if mechlorethamine is excreted into breast milk following topical application. Due to the potential for serious adverse reactions in the nursing infant following topical or systemic exposure from the mother's skin, the manufacturer recommends a decision be made whether to discontinue nursing or to discontinue the drug, taking into account the importance of treatment to the mother.

Warnings/Precautions Caregivers should wear nitrile gloves when applying to patients. Wash hands thoroughly with soap and water after handling/application. If accidental skin exposure occurs, wash thoroughly for at least 15 minutes with soap and water; remove any contaminated clothing. Eye exposure may result in pain, burning, inflammation, photophobia, and blurred vision. Blindness and severe anterior eye injury (irreversible) may occur. If exposure to eye(s) occurs, promptly irrigate for at least 15 minutes with copious amounts of water, normal saline, or balanced salt ophthalmic irrigating solution; obtain ophthalmology consultation. Exposure to mucous membranes may cause pain, redness, and ulceration; may be severe. If mucosal contact occurs, irrigate promptly for at least 15 minutes with copious amounts of water and obtain medical consultation.

Dermatitis commonly occurs; may be moderately severe or severe. Monitor for redness, swelling, itching, blistering, ulceration, and secondary skin infections. Facial, genitalia, anus and intertriginous skin areas are at increased risk for dermatitis. Dermatitis may require dosage reduction. Avoid direct contact with mechlorethamine (other than intended treatment areas for the patient). Secondary exposure risks include dermatitis, mucosal injury, and secondary malignancies. To prevent secondary exposure, follow recommended application procedures. In a clinical study, non-melanoma skin cancers developed during or within 1 year following treatment. Some instances occurred in patients who had received previous treatments that were associated with non-melanoma skin cancer. Monitor for non-melanoma skin cancers during and following treatment; may occur anywhere on the skin, including untreated areas.

Mechlorethamine gel contains alcohol and is flammable; follow recommended application procedures and avoid fire, flame, and smoking until mechlorethamine has dried.

Adverse Reactions

>10%:

Dermatologic: Dermatitis (56%; moderately severe or severe: 23%), pruritus (20%), bacterial skin infection (11%)

Hematologic & oncologic: Hematologic abnormality (decreased hemoglobin, neutrophils, or platelets; 13%)

1% to 10%:

Dermatologic: Dermal ulcer (6%), skin hyperpigmentation (5%)

Hematologic & oncologic: Malignant neoplasm (nonmelanoma skin cancer; 2%)

Postmarketing and/or case reports: Anaphylaxis, hypersensitivity reaction

Drug Interactions

Metabolism/Transport Effects None known.

Avoid Concomitant Use There are no known interactions where it is recommended to avoid concomitant use.

Increased Effect/Toxicity There are no known significant interactions involving an increase in effect.

Decreased Effect There are no known significant interactions involving a decrease in effect.

Hazardous Drugs Handling Considerations

Hazardous agent (NIOSH 2016 [group 1]).

Use appropriate precautions for receiving, handling, administration, and disposal. Gloves (single) should be worn during receiving, unpacking, and placing in storage. NIOSH recommends double gloving, a protective gown, and (if liquid that could splash) eye/face protection for administration of a topical product; if there is potential for inhalation, respiratory protection is recommended (NIOSH 2016).

Storage/Stability Prior to dispensing, store in freezer at -25°C to -15°C (-13°F to 5°F). After dispensing, refrigerate at 2°C to 8°C (36°F to 46°F); apply immediately (or within 30 minutes) after removal from refrigerator; return to refrigerator promptly after each use. Discard unused product 60 days after opening.

Mechanism of Action Mechlorethamine is a nitrogen mustard alkylating agent which forms inter- and intra-strand DNA cross-links, resulting in inhibition of DNA synthesis. Topical application allows for skin-directed treatment while minimizing systemic nitrogen mustard exposure (Lessin, 2013).

Pharmacodynamics/Kinetics

Absorption: Topical: None detected (Lessin, 2013)

Distribution: Topical: No detectable systemic exposure in a clinical study (Lessin, 2013)

Dosing

Adult & Geriatric

Cutaneous T-cell lymphoma (mycosis fungoides-type): Topical: Apply a thin film once daily to affected areas of skin

Note: Concurrent use of topical or systemic corticosteroids was not allowed in the clinical study (Lessin, 2013).

Renal Impairment No dosage adjustment provided in the manufacturer's labeling; however, based on the lack of systemic exposure, dosage adjustment is likely not necessary.

Hepatic Impairment No dosage adjustment provided in the manufacturer's labeling; however, based on the lack of systemic exposure, dosage adjustment is likely not necessary.

Adjustment for Toxicity Skin ulceration (any grade), blistering, or dermatitis (moderately severe-to-severe): Withhold treatment; upon improvement, may reinitiate treatment with a reduced frequency of once every 3 days; if every 3-day application is tolerated for at least 1 week, may increase to every other day for at least 1 week, then (if tolerated) may increase to once daily.

Administration Apply a thin film topically to affected area. Apply immediately (or within 30 minutes) after removal from refrigerator; return to refrigerator promptly after each use. Apply to completely dry skin at least 4 hours before or 30 minutes after showering/washing. Allow treated area(s) to dry for 5-10 minutes after application before covering with clothing. May apply emollients (moisturizers) to treated area 2 hours before or 2 hours after mechlorethamine application. Do not use occlusive dressings over treatment areas. Avoid fire, flame, and smoking until mechlorethamine has dried.

Caregivers should wear nitrile gloves when applying to patients. Wash hands thoroughly with soap and water after handling/application. If accidental skin exposure occurs, wash thoroughly for at least 15 minutes with soap and water; remove any contaminated clothing.

Monitoring Parameters Monitor for dermatologic toxicity (skin ulcers, blistering, dermatitis, secondary skin infections) and signs/symptoms of non-melanoma skin cancer.

Prescribing and Access Restrictions Valchlor is only available through a specialty pharmacy; information regarding prescribing and access may be found at www.valchlor.com.

Medication Guide Available Yes

Dosage Forms Considerations Valchlor 0.016% is equivalent to 0.02% mechlorethamine hydrochloride

Dosage Forms Excipient information presented when available (limited, particularly for generics); consult specific product labeling.

Gel, External:
Valchlor: 0.016% (60 g) [contains edetate disodium, isopropyl alcohol, menthol, propylene glycol]

◆ **Mechlorethamine HCl (Topical)** *see* Mechlorethamine (Topical) *on page* 1173

◆ **Mechlorethamine Hydrochloride** *see* Mechlorethamine (Systemic) *on page* 1168

◆ **Mechlorethamine Topical Gel** *see* Mechlorethamine (Topical) *on page* 1173

◆ **Med-Anastrozole (Can)** *see* Anastrozole *on page* 135

◆ **Med-Cyproterone (Can)** *see* Cyproterone *on page* 468

◆ **MEDI4736** *see* Durvalumab *on page* 652

◆ **MED-Letrozole (Can)** *see* Letrozole *on page* 1119

◆ **Medolor Pak** *see* Lidocaine and Prilocaine *on page* 1150

◆ **Medrol** *see* MethylPREDNISolone *on page* 1227

◆ **Medrol Dose Pack** *see* MethylPREDNISolone *on page* 1227

◆ **Medroxy (Can)** *see* MedroxyPROGESTERone *on page* 1175

MedroxyPROGESTERone (me DROKS ee proe JES te rone)

Brand Names: US Depo-Provera; Depo-SubQ Provera 104; Provera

◄ **Brand Names: Canada** Alti-MPA; Apo-Medroxy; Depo-Prevera; Depo-Provera; Dom-Medroxyprogesterone; Gen-Medroxy; Medroxy; Medroxyprogesterone Acetate Injectable Suspension USP; Novo-Medrone; PMS-Medroxyprogesterone; Provera; Provera-Pak; Teva-Medroxyprogesterone

Index Terms Acetoxymethylprogesterone; Medroxyprogesterone Acetate; Methylacetoxyprogesterone; MPA

Pharmacologic Category Contraceptive; Progestin

Use

Abnormal uterine bleeding (tablet): Treatment of abnormal uterine bleeding due to hormonal imbalance in the absence of organic pathology, such as fibroids or uterine cancer.

Amenorrhea, secondary (tablet): Treatment of secondary amenorrhea due to hormonal imbalance in the absence of organic pathology, such as fibroids or uterine cancer.

Contraception (104 mg/0.65 mL and 150 mg/mL injection): Prevention of pregnancy in women of childbearing potential.

Endometrial hyperplasia (tablet): Prevention of endometrial hyperplasia in nonhysterectomized postmenopausal women receiving daily oral conjugated estrogens 0.625 mg.

Endometrial carcinoma (400 mg/mL injection) (100 mg tablet [Canadian product]): Adjunctive therapy and/or palliative treatment of inoperable, recurrent, and/or metastatic endometrial carcinoma.

Endometriosis (104 mg/0.65 mL injection): Management of endometriosis-associated pain.

Pregnancy Risk Factor X (tablet)

Hazardous Drugs Handling Considerations

Hazardous agent (NIOSH 2016 [group 2]).

Use appropriate precautions for receiving, handling, administration, and disposal. Gloves (single) should be worn during receiving, unpacking, and placing in storage. NIOSH recommends single gloving for administration of intact tablets or capsules. For injectable products, NIOSH recommends double gloving, a protective gown, and ventilated engineering controls (a class II biological safety cabinet or a compounding aseptic containment isolator) for preparation. Double gloving and a protective gown are required during IM or subcutaneous administration (NIOSH 2016).

Dosing

Adult & Geriatric

Abnormal uterine bleeding: Oral: 5 or 10 mg daily for 5 to 10 days starting on day 16 or 21 of menstrual cycle. Secretory transformation of the endometrium will occur when adequately primed with endogenous or exogenous estrogen. Withdrawal bleeding may be expected within 3 to 7 days after discontinuing medroxyprogesterone.

Amenorrhea, secondary: Oral: 5 or 10 mg daily for 5 to 10 days. Therapy may be started at any time. Secretory transformation of the endometrium will occur when adequately primed with endogenous or exogenous estrogen. Withdrawal bleeding may be expected within 3 to 7 days after discontinuing medroxyprogesterone.

Contraception:

Depo-Provera Contraceptive: IM: 150 mg every 3 months (every 13 weeks)

Depo-subQ Provera 104: SubQ: 104 mg every 3 months (every 12 to 14 weeks)

Endometrial carcinoma, recurrent or metastatic (adjunctive/palliative treatment):
IM (Depo-Provera): Initial: 400 to 1,000 mg/week
Oral (100 mg tablet [Canadian product]): Manufacturer's labeling: Usual dose: 200 to 400 mg daily. Doses >200 mg daily may not confer additional benefit (Thigpen 1999). If improvement or disease stabilization occurs, 200 mg daily may be sufficient for maintenance. Discontinue use if no improvement within 2 to 3 months.

Endometrial hyperplasia reduction: Oral: 5 or 10 mg daily for 12 to 14 consecutive days each month, starting on day 1 or day 16 of the cycle. When treating postmenopausal women, use for the shortest duration possible at the lowest effective dose consistent with treatment goals. Reevaluate patients as clinically appropriate to determine if treatment is still necessary. Consider use of an estrogen with a progestin in postmenopausal women with a uterus. Women who have had a hysterectomy generally do not need a progestin. Adjust dose based on patient response. Attempt to taper or discontinue at 3- to 6-month intervals.

Endometriosis (Depo-subQ Provera 104): SubQ: 104 mg every 3 months (every 12 to 14 weeks)

Hot flashes (off-label use): IM: 400 mg as single dose (Loprinzi 2006)

Paraphilia/hypersexuality (off-label use) (Reilly 2000): Males (**Note:** Avoid use if active pituitary pathology, hepatic failure, or thrombocmbolic disease):
IM (Depo-Provera): 100 to 600 mg weekly
Oral: 100 to 500 mg daily

Pediatric Adolescents:
Abnormal uterine bleeding: Refer to adult dosing.
Amenorrhea, secondary: Refer to adult dosing.
Contraception: Refer to adult dosing.
Endometriosis: Refer to adult dosing.

Renal Impairment There are no dosage adjustments provided in the manufacturer's labeling (has not been studied).

Hepatic Impairment Medroxyprogesterone is extensively metabolized in the liver. Most products are contraindicated in patients with hepatic impairment. If needed for the palliative treatment metastatic endometrial carcinoma, monitor closely; withhold or discontinue treatment if liver dysfunction develops and do not resume until hepatic function has returned to normal.

Additional Information Complete prescribing information should be consulted for additional detail.

Dosage Forms Excipient information presented when available (limited, particularly for generics); consult specific product labeling.
Suspension, Intramuscular, as acetate:
Depo-Provera: 150 mg/mL (1 mL); 400 mg/mL (2.5 mL)
Generic: 150 mg/mL (1 mL)
Suspension Prefilled Syringe, Intramuscular, as acetate:
Depo-Provera: 150 mg/mL (1 mL) [contains methylparaben, polyethylene glycol, polysorbate 80, propylparaben]
Generic: 150 mg/mL (1 mL)
Suspension Prefilled Syringe, Subcutaneous, as acetate:
Depo-SubQ Provera 104: 104 mg/0.65 mL (0.65 mL) [contains methylparaben, propylparaben]

Tablet, Oral, as acetate:
Provera: 2.5 mg, 5 mg, 10 mg [scored]
Generic: 2.5 mg, 5 mg, 10 mg
Dosage Forms: Canada Information with regard to form, strength, and availability of products uniquely available in Canada but currently not available in the US. Refer also to Dosage Forms.

Excipient information presented when available (limited, particularly for generics); consult specific product labeling.
Tablet, Oral, as acetate: 100 mg

♦ **Medroxyprogesterone Acetate** *see* MedroxyPROGESTERone *on page 1175*

♦ **Medroxyprogesterone Acetate Injectable Suspension USP (Can)** *see* MedroxyPROGESTERone *on page 1175*

♦ **Megace ES** *see* Megestrol *on page 1178*

♦ **Megace Oral [DSC]** *see* Megestrol *on page 1178*

♦ **Megace OS (Can)** *see* Megestrol *on page 1178*

Megestrol (me JES trole)
Related Information
Palliative Care Medicine (Cancer) *on page 2352*
Safe Handling of Hazardous Drugs *on page 2379*
Brand Names: US Megace ES; Megace Oral [DSC]
Brand Names: Canada Megace OS; Megestrol
Index Terms 5071-1DL(6); Megestrol Acetate
Pharmacologic Category Antineoplastic Agent, Hormone; Appetite Stimulant; Progestin
Use
Anorexia or cachexia: *Suspension:* Treatment of anorexia, cachexia, or unexplained significant weight loss in patients with AIDS
Limitations of use: Treatment of AIDS-related weight loss should only be initiated after addressing the treatable causes (eg, malignancy, infection, malabsorption, endocrine disease, renal disease, psychiatric disorder) for weight loss. Megestrol is not intended to prevent weight loss.
Breast cancer: *Tablet:* Treatment (palliative) of advanced breast cancer
Endometrial cancer: *Tablet:* Treatment (palliative) of advanced endometrial carcinoma
Labeled Contraindications
Hypersensitivity to megestrol or any component of the formulation; known or suspected pregnancy (suspension).
Documentation of allergenic cross-reactivity for progestins is limited. However, because of similarities in chemical structure and/or pharmacologic actions, the possibility of cross-sensitivity cannot be ruled out with certainty.
Pregnancy Considerations Adverse events were demonstrated in animal reproduction studies. May cause fetal harm if administered to a pregnant woman. Use during pregnancy is contraindicated (suspension) and appropriate contraception is recommended in women who may become pregnant. In clinical studies, megestrol was shown to cause breakthrough vaginal bleeding in women.

Breastfeeding Considerations Megestrol is present in breast milk. Information is available from five breastfeeding women, ~8 weeks postpartum, who were administered megestrol 4 mg in combination with ethinyl estradiol 50 mcg daily for contraception. Maternal serum and milk samples were obtained over 5 days, beginning 10 days after therapy began. The highest concentrations of megestrol were found at the samples taken 3 hours after the maternal dose. Mean concentrations of megestrol were 6.5 ng/mL (maternal serum; range: 3.7 to 10.8 ng/mL), 4.6 ng/mL (foremilk; range: 1.1 to 12.7 ng/mL), and 5.6 ng/mL (hindmilk; range: 1.2 to 18.5 ng/mL) (Nilsson 1977). Due to the potential for adverse reaction in the breastfed newborn, the manufacturer recommends discontinuing breastfeeding while receiving megestrol.

Warnings/Precautions May suppress hypothalamic-pituitary-adrenal (HPA) axis during chronic administration; consider the possibility of adrenal suppression in any patient receiving or being withdrawn from chronic therapy when signs/symptoms suggestive of hypoadrenalism are noted (during stress or in unstressed state). Laboratory evaluation and replacement/stress doses of rapid-acting glucocorticoid should be considered. Cushing syndrome has been reported with long-term use. New-onset diabetes and exacerbation of preexisting diabetes have been reported with long-term use. Use with caution in patients with a history of thromboembolic disease. Vaginal bleeding or discharge may occur in females. The effects on HIV viral replications are unknown in patients with AIDS related cachexia. Potentially significant drug-drug interactions may exist, requiring dose or frequency adjustment, additional monitoring, and/or selection of alternative therapy.

Megace ES suspension is not equivalent to other formulations on a mg per mg basis; Megace ES suspension 625 mg/5 mL is equivalent to megestrol acetate suspension 800 mg/20 mL.

Benzyl alcohol and derivatives: Some dosage forms may contain sodium benzoate/benzoic acid; benzoic acid (benzoate) is a metabolite of benzyl alcohol; large amounts of benzyl alcohol (≥99 mg/kg/day) have been associated with a potentially fatal toxicity ("gasping syndrome") in neonates; the "gasping syndrome" consists of metabolic acidosis, respiratory distress, gasping respirations, CNS dysfunction (including convulsions, intracranial hemorrhage), hypotension, and cardiovascular collapse (AAP ["Inactive" 1997]; CDC 1982); some data suggests that benzoate displaces bilirubin from protein binding sites (Ahlfors 2001); avoid or use dosage forms containing benzyl alcohol derivative with caution in neonates. See manufacturer's labeling.

Adverse Reactions Frequency not always defined.

Cardiovascular: Hypertension (4% to 8%), cardiomyopathy (1% to 3%), chest pain (1% to 3%), edema (1% to 3%), palpitations (1% to 3%), peripheral edema (1% to 3%), cardiac failure

Central nervous system: Headache (3% to 10%), pain (4% to 6%, similar to placebo), insomnia (1% to 6%), abnormality in thinking (1% to 3%), confusion (1% to 3%), convulsions (1% to 3%), depression (1% to 3%), hypoesthesia (1% to 3%), neuropathy (1% to 3%), paresthesia (1% to 3%), carpal tunnel syndrome, lethargy, malaise, mood changes

Dermatologic: Skin rash (6% to 12%), alopecia (1% to 3%), dermatological disease (1% to 3%), diaphoresis (1% to 3%), pruritus (1% to 3%), vesiculobullous dermatitis (1% to 3%)

Endocrine & metabolic: Hyperglycemia (6%), decreased libido (1% to 5%), albuminuria (1% to 3%), gynecomastia (1% to 3%), increased lactate dehydrogenase (1% to 3%), adrenocortical insufficiency, amenorrhea, Cushing's syndrome, diabetes mellitus, hot flash, HPA-axis suppression, hypercalcemia, weight gain (not attributed to edema or fluid retention)

Gastrointestinal: Diarrhea (10%, similar to placebo), flatulence (6% to 10%), vomiting (4% to 6%), nausea (4% to 5%), dyspepsia (2% to 3%), abdominal pain (1% to 3%), constipation (1% to 3%), oral moniliasis (1% to 3%), sialorrhea (1% to 3%), xerostomia (1% to 3%)

Genitourinary: Impotence (4% to 14%), urinary incontinence (1% to 3%), urinary tract infection (1% to 3%), urinary frequency (1% to 2%), break-through bleeding

Hematologic & oncologic: Leukopenia (1% to 3%), sarcoma (1% to 3%), tumor flare

Hepatic: Hepatomegaly (1% to 3%)

Infection: Candidiasis (1% to 3%), herpes virus infection (1% to 3%), infection (1% to 3%)

Neuromuscular & skeletal: Weakness (5% to 6%)

Ophthalmic: Amblyopia (1% to 3%)

Respiratory: Cough (1% to 3%), dyspnea (1% to 3%), pharyngitis (1% to 3%), pulmonary disorder (1% to 3%), pneumonia (1%), hyperventilation

Miscellaneous: Fever (1% to 6%)

Postmarketing and/or case reports: Decreased glucose tolerance, thromboembolic phenomena (including deep vein thrombosis, pulmonary embolism, thrombophlebitis)

Drug Interactions

Metabolism/Transport Effects None known.

Avoid Concomitant Use

Avoid concomitant use of Megestrol with any of the following: Dofetilide; Indium 111 Capromab Pendetide; Ulipristal

Increased Effect/Toxicity

Megestrol may increase the levels/effects of: C1 inhibitors; Dofetilide; Pomalidomide

The levels/effects of Megestrol may be increased by: Herbs (Progestogenic Properties)

Decreased Effect

Megestrol may decrease the levels/effects of: Anticoagulants; Antidiabetic Agents; Choline C 11; Indium 111 Capromab Pendetide; Ulipristal

The levels/effects of Megestrol may be decreased by: Ulipristal

Hazardous Drugs Handling Considerations

Hazardous agent (NIOSH 2016 [group 1]).

Use appropriate precautions for receiving, handling, administration, and disposal. Gloves (single) should be worn during receiving, unpacking, and placing in storage. NIOSH recommends single gloving for administration of intact tablets or capsules. NIOSH recommends double gloving, a protective gown, and (if there is a potential for vomit or spit up) eye/face protection for administration of an oral liquid/feeding tube administration (NIOSH 2016).

Storage/Stability

Suspension: Store at 15°C to 25°C (59°F to 77°F); protect from heat. Store/dispense in a tight container.

Tablet: Store at 15°C to 30°C (59°F to 86°F); protect from light. Protect from temperatures above 40°C (104°F).

Mechanism of Action A synthetic progestin with antiestrogenic properties which disrupt the estrogen receptor cycle. Megestrol interferes with the normal estrogen cycle and results in a lower LH titer. May also have a direct effect on the endometrium. Megestrol is an antineoplastic progestin thought to act through an antileutenizing effect mediated via the pituitary. May stimulate appetite by antagonizing the metabolic effects of catabolic cytokines.

Pharmacodynamics/Kinetics

Onset of action: Breast or endometrial cancer: At least 2 months of continuous therapy; Weight gain: 2 to 4 weeks

Absorption: Well absorbed

Metabolism: Hepatic (to free steroids and glucuronide conjugates)

Half-life elimination: Suspension: 20 to 50 hours; Tablet: Mean: 34.2 hours (range: 13 to 105 hours)

Time to peak, serum: Suspension: 5 hours; Tablet: 2.2 hours (range: 1 to 3 hours)

Excretion: Urine (57% to 78%; 5% to 8% as metabolites); feces (8% to 30%) within 10 days

Dosing

Adult Note: Megace ES suspension is not equivalent to other formulations on a mg-per-mg basis.

Anorexia or cachexia associated with AIDS: Oral: Suspension: Initial: 625 mg daily (of the 125 mg/mL suspension) or 800 mg daily (of the 40 mg/mL suspension); daily doses of 400 mg to 800 mg have been found to be effective

Breast cancer, advanced: Oral: Tablet: 160 mg per day in divided doses of 40 mg 4 times daily for at least 2 months

Endometrial cancer, advanced: Oral: Tablet: 40 to 320 mg daily in divided doses for at least 2 months

Cancer-related cachexia (off-label use): Oral: Doses ranging from 160 to 800 mg per day were effective in achieving weight gain, higher doses (>160 mg) were associated with more weight gain (Beller 1997; Loprinzi 1990; Loprinzi 1993; Vadell 1998); based on a meta-analysis, an optimal dose has not been determined (Ruiz Garcia 2013)

Geriatric Use with caution; refer to adult dosing.

Renal Impairment There are no dosage adjustments provided in the manufacturer's labeling; however, the urinary excretion of megestrol acetate is substantial, use with caution.

Hepatic Impairment There are no dosage adjustments provided in the manufacturer's labeling.

Administration

Oral: Shake suspension well before use.

The 625 mg/5 mL suspension may be administered without regard to meals.

Monitoring Parameters Observe for signs of thromboembolic events; blood pressure, weight; serum glucose

Dosage Forms Excipient information presented when available (limited, particularly for generics); consult specific product labeling. [DSC] = Discontinued product

Suspension, Oral, as acetate:

Megace ES: 625 mg/5 mL (150 mL) [contains alcohol, usp, sodium benzoate; lemon-lime flavor]

Megace Oral: 40 mg/mL (240 mL [DSC]) [lemon-lime flavor]

Generic: 40 mg/mL (10 mL, 240 mL, 480 mL); 400 mg/10 mL (10 mL); 625 mg/5 mL (150 mL)
Tablet, Oral, as acetate:
Generic: 20 mg, 40 mg
Dosage Forms: Canada Information with regard to form, strength, and availability of products uniquely available in Canada but currently not available in the US. Refer also to Dosage Forms.

Excipient information presented when available (limited, particularly for generics); consult specific product labeling.
Tablet, Oral, as acetate: 160 mg

◆ **Megestrol Acetate** see Megestrol on page 1178
◆ **Mekinist** see Trametinib on page 1809

Melphalan (MEL fa lan)
Related Information
Hematopoietic Cell Transplantation on page 2365
Management of Chemotherapy-Induced Nausea and Vomiting in Adults on page 2253
Management of Drug Extravasations on page 2271
Mucositis and Stomatitis on page 2299
Prevention of Chemotherapy-Induced Nausea and Vomiting in Children on page 2310
Safe Handling of Hazardous Drugs on page 2379
Brand Names: US Alkeran; Evomela
Brand Names: Canada Alkeran
Index Terms L-PAM; L-Phenylalanine Mustard; L-Sarcolysin; Melphalan HCl; Melphalan Hydrochloride; Phenylalanine Mustard
Pharmacologic Category Antineoplastic Agent, Alkylating Agent; Antineoplastic Agent, Alkylating Agent (Nitrogen Mustard)
Use
Multiple myeloma: Palliative treatment of multiple myeloma (injection [Alkeran and Evomela] and tablets); high-dose conditioning treatment prior to hematopoietic stem cell transplantation (HSCT) (Evomela only).
Ovarian cancer: Palliative treatment of nonresectable epithelial ovarian carcinoma (tablets)
Labeled Contraindications Hypersensitivity to melphalan or any component of the formulation; patients whose disease was resistant to prior melphalan therapy (Alkeran only).
Pregnancy Considerations Adverse effects have been observed in animal reproduction studies. May cause fetal harm if administered during pregnancy. Women of reproductive potential should be advised to avoid pregnancy while on and after melphalan therapy. Males with female partners of reproductive potential should use effective contraception during and after melphalan treatment. Therapy may suppress ovarian function leading to amenorrhea. Reversible and irreversible testicular suppression has been reported in male patients after melphalan administration.
Breastfeeding Considerations It is not known if melphalan is excreted in breast milk. Due to the potential for serious adverse reactions in the nursing infant, breastfeeding is not recommended by the manufacturer.

Warnings/Precautions [US Boxed Warning]: Bone marrow suppression is common; may be severe and result in infection or bleeding; has been demonstrated more with the IV formulation (compared to oral). Myelosuppression is dose-related; myeloablation is expected when used in high doses for conditioning regimens prior to stem cell transplantation. Do not administer melphalan-containing conditioning regimen unless the stem cell product is available for rescue. Monitor blood counts; supportive care for infections, anemia, and thrombocytopenia may be necessary. When used for palliative treatment, may require treatment delay or dose modification for thrombocytopenia or neutropenia. Use with caution in patients with prior bone marrow suppression, impaired renal function (consider dose reduction), or who have received prior (or concurrent) chemotherapy or irradiation. Myelotoxicity is generally reversible, although irreversible bone marrow failure has been reported. In patients who are candidates for autologous transplantation, avoid melphalan-containing induction regimens if future transplant may be necessary (due to the effects on stem cell reserve).

[US Boxed Warning]: Hypersensitivity reactions (including anaphylaxis) have occurred in ~2% of patients receiving IV melphalan, usually after multiple treatment cycles. Symptoms may include urticaria, pruritus, edema, skin rashes, tachycardia, bronchospasm, dyspnea, and hypotension. Discontinue infusion and treat symptomatically. Hypersensitivity may also occur (rarely) with oral melphalan. Do not readminister (oral or IV) in patients who experience hypersensitivity to melphalan.

Gastrointestinal toxicities, including nausea, vomiting, diarrhea and mucositis, are common, particularly when used in high doses for conditioning regimens (the incidence of grade 3 or 4 mucositis was 13% in clinical trials). When administering high-dose melphalan in autologous transplantation, cryotherapy is recommended to prevent oral mucositis (Lalla 2014). Melphalan is associated with a moderate emetic potential (depending on dose and/or administration route); antiemetics may be recommended to prevent nausea and vomiting (Dupuis 2011). Nutritional support and/or analgesics may be necessary in patients with severe mucositis. Abnormal liver function tests may occur; hepatitis and jaundice have also been reported; hepatic sinusoidal obstruction syndrome (SOS; formerly called veno-occlusive disease) has been reported with IV melphalan. Monitor liver function tests. Pulmonary fibrosis (some fatal) and interstitial pneumonitis have been observed with treatment. Dosage reduction is recommended with IV melphalan in patients with renal impairment (when used for palliative treatment); reduced initial doses may also be recommended with oral melphalan. Closely monitor patients with azotemia. High-dose melphalan with autologous stem cell transplant is feasible in patients with multiple myeloma and renal impairment (Dimopoulos 2016). Prolonged mucositis has occurred when standard melphalan doses were administered to patients with chronic kidney disease (Bodge 2014).

[US Boxed Warning]: Produces chromosomal changes in vitro and in vivo. Melphalan should be considered potentially leukemogenic in humans. Secondary malignancies (including acute myeloid leukemia, myeloproliferative disease, and carcinoma) have been reported (some patients were receiving combination chemotherapy or radiation therapy); the risk is increased with increased treatment duration and cumulative doses. Suppresses ovarian function and produces amenorrhea; may also cause reversible or irreversible testicular suppression.

Intravenous melphalan is available in different formulations. Evomela (melphalan for injection) is a lyophilized powder which is reconstituted with normal saline to a 5 mg/mL concentration. Alkeran (melphalan hydrochloride for injection) and generic melphalan hydrochloride are also powder formulations which are reconstituted with the supplied diluent (which contains propylene glycol and ethanol) to a 5 mg/mL concentration. Indications for use, product preparation, storage, and dosing differ between formulations. Use caution when selecting melphalan formulations for preparation and administration. Do not mix or combine the formulations.

Melphalan is an irritant; local reactions may occur (Perez Fidalgo 2012). Extravasation may cause local tissue damage; administration by slow injection into a fast running IV solution into an injection port or via a central line is recommended; do not administer directly into a peripheral vein. Some dosage forms may contain propylene glycol; large amounts are potentially toxic and have been associated hyperosmolality, lactic acidosis, seizures and respiratory depression; use caution (AAP 1997; Zar 2007). **[US Boxed Warning]: Should be administered under the supervision of an experienced cancer chemotherapy physician.** Avoid vaccination with live vaccines during treatment if immunocompromised. Toxicity may be increased in elderly; start with lowest recommended adult doses. Potentially significant drug-drug interactions may exist, requiring dose or frequency adjustment, additional monitoring, and/or selection of alternative therapy.

Adverse Reactions

>10%:

Cardiovascular: Peripheral edema (conditioning: 33%)

Central nervous system: Fatigue (≥50%; conditioning: 77%), dizziness (conditioning: 38%)

Endocrine & metabolic: Hypokalemia (≥50% conditioning: 74%), hypophosphatemia (conditioning: 49%)

Gastrointestinal: Diarrhea (≥50%; conditioning: 93%), nausea (≥50%; conditioning: 90%), vomiting (≥50%; conditioning: 64%), decreased appetite (conditioning: 49%), constipation (conditioning: 48%), mucositis (conditioning: 38%), abdominal pain (conditioning: 28%), dysgeusia (conditioning: 28%), stomatitis (conditioning: 28%), dyspepsia (conditioning: 26%)

Hematologic & oncologic: Anemia (≥50%), decreased absolute lymphocyte count (≥50%), decreased neutrophils (≥50%), decreased platelet count (≥50%; nadir: 14 to 21 days; recovery: 28 to 35 days), decreased white blood cell count (≥50%; nadir: 14 to 21 days; recovery: 28 to 35 days), febrile neutropenia (conditioning: 41%; grades 3/4: 28%)

Miscellaneous: Fever (conditioning: 48%)

1% to 10%:

Gastrointestinal: Hematochezia

Genitourinary: Amenorrhea (9%)

Hypersensitivity: Hypersensitivity reaction (IV: 2%; less common in oral formula; includes bronchospasm, dyspnea, edema, hypotension, pruritus, skin rash, tachycardia, urticaria), anaphylaxis (≤2%)

Renal: Renal failure

Frequency not defined:

Cardiovascular: hepatic sinusoidal obstruction syndrome (formerly known as hepatic veno-occlusive disease), vasculitis

Central nervous system: Flushing sensation, tingling sensation

Endocrine & metabolic: SIADH (dose related; Greenbaum-Lefkoe 1985)

Genitourinary: Infertility, inhibition of testicular function

Hematologic & oncologic: Bone marrow depression

Hepatic: Hepatitis, increased serum transaminases, jaundice

Renal: Increased blood urea nitrogen

Miscellaneous: Chromosomal abnormality

<1%, postmarketing, and/or case reports: Alopecia, bone marrow failure (irreversible), hemolytic anemia, interstitial pneumonitis, maculopapular rash, pulmonary fibrosis, skin ulceration at injection site, tissue necrosis at injection site (rarely requiring skin grafting)

Drug Interactions

Metabolism/Transport Effects None known.

Avoid Concomitant Use

Avoid concomitant use of Melphalan with any of the following: BCG (Intravesical); Deferiprone; Dipyrone; Natalizumab; Pimecrolimus; Tacrolimus (Topical); Vaccines (Live)

Increased Effect/Toxicity

Melphalan may increase the levels/effects of: Carmustine; CloZAPine; CycloSPORINE (Systemic); Deferiprone; Fingolimod; Leflunomide; Natalizumab; Tofacitinib; Vaccines (Live)

The levels/effects of Melphalan may be increased by: Denosumab; Dipyrone; Nalidixic Acid; Ocrelizumab; Palifermin; Pimecrolimus; Promazine; Roflumilast; Tacrolimus (Topical); Trastuzumab

Decreased Effect

Melphalan may decrease the levels/effects of: BCG (Intravesical); Coccidioides immitis Skin Test; Lenograstim; Nivolumab; Sipuleucel-T; Tertomotide; Vaccines (Inactivated); Vaccines (Live)

The levels/effects of Melphalan may be decreased by: Echinacea

Food Interactions Food interferes with oral absorption. Management: Administer on an empty stomach.

Hazardous Drugs Handling Considerations

Hazardous agent (NIOSH 2016 [group 1]).

Use appropriate precautions for receiving, handling, administration, and disposal. Gloves (single) should be worn during receiving, unpacking, and placing in storage. NIOSH recommends single gloving for administration of intact tablets or capsules. For IV preparation, NIOSH recommends double gloving, a protective gown, ventilated engineering controls (a class II biological safety cabinet or a compounding aseptic containment isolator), and closed system transfer devices (CSTDs). Double gloving, a gown, and (if dosage form allows) CSTDs are required during IV administration (NIOSH 2016).

Storage/Stability

Alkeran injection: Store intact vials at 15°C to 30°C (59°F to 86°F). Protect from light. The manufacturer recommends administration be completed within 60 minutes of reconstitution; **immediately** dilute dose in NS. Do not refrigerate reconstituted solution; precipitation occurs.

Evomela injection: Store intact vials at 25°C (77°F); excursions are permitted between 15°C to 30°C (59°F to 86°F). Protect from light (store in original container). The reconstituted solution is stable for 1 hour at room temperature or for 24 hours at 5°C (41°F). Solutions diluted in NS for infusion are stable for 4 hours at room temperature (in addition to the 1 hour at room temperature following reconstitution).

Tablet: Store at 2°C to 8°C (36°F to 46°F). Protect from light.

◄ **Preparation for Administration Note:** Intravenous melphalan is available in different formulations. Indications for use, product preparation, storage, and dosing differ between formulations. Use caution when selecting melphalan formulations for preparation and administration. Do not mix or combine the formulations.

Alkeran injection: Stability is limited; must be prepared fresh. **The time between reconstitution/dilution and administration of parenteral melphalan (Alkeran) must be kept to a minimum (manufacturer recommends <60 minutes) because reconstituted and diluted solutions are unstable.** Dissolve powder initially with 10 mL of supplied diluent to a concentration of 5 mg/mL; shake immediately and vigorously to dissolve. **Immediately** dilute dose in NS to a concentration of ≤0.45 mg/mL (manufacturer recommended concentration). Do not refrigerate solution; precipitation occurs if stored at 5°C. The manufacturer recommends administration within 60 minutes of reconstitution.

Evomela injection: Reconstitute each vial with 8.6 mL of NS to a 5 mg/mL concentration. The NS should appear to be "pulled" into the vial by negative pressure due to a partial vacuum present in the vial. If no vacuum is present, discard the vial. Further dilute the appropriate dose in NS to a concentration of 0.45 mg/mL.

Mechanism of Action Alkylating agent which is a derivative of mechlorethamine that inhibits DNA and RNA synthesis via formation of carbonium ions; cross-links strands of DNA; acts on both resting and rapidly dividing tumor cells.

Pharmacodynamics/Kinetics

Absorption: Oral: Variable and incomplete

Distribution: V_d: 0.5 L/kg; Evomela: Penetrates CSF; Alkeran: Low penetration into CSF

Protein binding: ~50% to 92%; primarily to albumin (~40% to 60%), ~20% to alpha$_1$-acid glycoprotein

Metabolism: Hepatic; chemical hydrolysis to monohydroxymelphalan and dihydroxymelphalan

Bioavailability: Oral: Variable; 56% to 93%; exposure is reduced by 36% to 54% with a high-fat meal

Half-life elimination: Terminal: IV: ~75 minutes; Oral: 1.5 ± 0.83 hours

Time to peak, serum: Oral: ~1 to 2 hours

Excretion: Oral: Feces (20% to 50%); urine (~10% as unchanged drug)

Dosing

Adult Note: Intravenous melphalan is available in different formulations. Indications for use, product preparation, storage, and dosing differ between formulations. Use caution when selecting melphalan formulations for preparation and administration. Do not mix or combine the formulations. Melphalan is associated with a moderate emetic potential (depending on dose and/or administration route); antiemetics may be recommended to prevent nausea and vomiting. Adjust dose based on patient response and weekly blood counts.

Multiple myeloma (conditioning regimen prior to hematopoietic stem cell transplantation): IV (Evomela only): 100 mg/m^2 daily for 2 days on day -3 and day -2 prior to autologous stem cell transplantation on day 0 (Hari 2015). **Note:** Per the manufacturer, if patients weigh more than 130% of their ideal body weight, body surface area should be calculated using adjusted ideal body weight.

Multiple myeloma conditioning regimen for autologous hematopoietic stem cell transplantation (off-label doses): IV:

200 mg/m^2 alone 2 days prior to transplantation (Fermand 2005; Moreau 2002) **or**

140 mg/m^2 2 days prior to transplantation (combined with busulfan) (Fermand 2005) **or**

140 mg/m^2 2 days prior to transplantation (combined with total body irradiation [TBI]) (Moreau 2002) **or**

140 mg/m^2 5 days prior to transplantation (combined with TBI) (Barlogie 2006)

Multiple myeloma (palliative treatment): Note: Response is gradual; may require repeated courses to realize benefit:

Oral: Usual dose (as described in the manufacturer's labeling):

6 mg once daily for 2 to 3 weeks initially, followed by up to 4 weeks rest, then a maintenance dose of 2 mg daily as hematologic recovery begins **or**

10 mg daily for 7 to 10 days; institute 2 mg daily maintenance dose after WBC >4,000 cells/mm^3 and platelets >100,000 cells/mm^3 (~4 to 8 weeks); titrate maintenance dose to hematologic response **or**

0.15 mg/kg/day for 7 days, with a 2 to 6 week rest, followed by a maintenance dose of ≤0.05 mg/kg/day as hematologic recovery begins **or**

0.25 mg/kg/day for 4 days (or 0.2 mg/kg/day for 5 days); repeat at 4- to 6-week intervals as ANC and platelet counts return to normal

Other dosing regimens in **combination therapy** *(off-label doses):*

4 mg/m^2/day for 7 days every 4 weeks (in combination with prednisone **or** with prednisone and thalidomide) (Palumbo 2006; Palumbo 2008) **or**

6 mg/m^2/day for 7 days every 4 weeks (in combination with prednisone) (Palumbo 2004) **or**

0.25 mg/kg/day for 4 days every 6 weeks (in combination with prednisone [Facon 2006; Facon 2007] **or** with prednisone and thalidomide [Facon 2007]) **or**

9 mg/m^2/day for 4 days every 6 weeks (in combination with prednisone **or** with prednisone and bortezomib) (Dimopoulos 2009; San Miguel 2008) **or**

IV (Alkeran and Evomela): 16 mg/m^2 administered at 2-week intervals for 4 doses, then administer at 4-week intervals after adequate hematologic recovery.

Ovarian cancer: Oral: 0.2 mg/kg/day for 5 days, repeat every 4 to 5 weeks **or**

Off-label dosing: 7 mg/m^2/day in 2 divided doses for 5 days, repeat every 28 days (Wadler 1996)

Amyloidosis, light chain (off-label use): Oral: 0.22 mg/kg/day for 4 days every 28 days (in combination with oral dexamethasone) (Palladini 2004) **or** 10 mg/m^2/day for 4 days every month (in combination with oral dexamethasone) for 12 to 18 treatment cycles (Jaccard 2007)

Hodgkin lymphoma, relapsed/refractory (off-label use): IV: 30 mg/m^2 over 15 minutes on day 6 (in combination with carmustine, etoposide, and cytarabine [mini-BEAM regimen]); repeat cycle every 4 to 6 weeks (Colwill 1995; Martin 2001)

Geriatric Refer to adult dosing. Use caution and begin at the lower end of dosing range.

◀ **Pediatric Note:** Intravenous melphalan is available in different formulations. Indications for use, product preparation, storage, and dosing differ between formulations. Use caution when selecting melphalan formulations for preparation and administration. Do not mix or combine the formulations. Melphalan is associated with a moderate emetic potential (depending on dose and/or administration route); antiemetics may be recommended to prevent nausea and vomiting (Dupuis 2011).

Conditioning regimen for autologous hematopoietic stem cell transplantation (off-label use): IV:

140 mg/m^2 2 days prior to transplantation (combined with busulfan) (Canete 2009) **or**

180 mg/m^2 (with pre- and posthydration) 12 to 30 hours prior to transplantation (Pritchard 2005) **or**

45 mg/m^2/day for 4 days starting 8 days prior to transplantation (combined with busulfan or etoposide and carboplatin) (Berthold 2005)

Renal Impairment

The manufacturer's labeling contains the following adjustment recommendations (for approved dosing levels) based on route of administration:

Oral: Moderate to severe renal impairment: Consider a reduced dose initially.

IV:

Conditioning regimen for multiple myeloma: No dosage adjustment is necessary.

Palliative treatment of multiple myeloma: BUN ≥30 mg/dL: Reduce dose by up to 50%.

Hemodialysis: Melphalan is not removed (to any significant degree) by hemodialysis.

The following adjustments have also been recommended:

Aronoff 2007: Adults: Oral (based on a 6 mg once-daily dose):

CrCl 10 to 50 mL/minute: Reduce dose to 75% of normal dose.

CrCl <10 mL/minute: Reduce dose to 50% of normal dose.

Hemodialysis: Administer dose after hemodialysis.

Continuous ambulatory peritoneal dialysis (CAPD): Reduce dose to 50% of normal dose.

Continuous renal replacement therapy (CRRT): Reduce dose to 75% of normal dose.

Carlson 2005: Oral (for melphalan-prednisone combination therapy; based on a study evaluating toxicity with melphalan dosed at 0.25 mg/kg/day for 4 days/cycle):

CrCl >10 to <30 mL/minute: Reduce dose to 75% of normal dose

CrCl ≤10 mL/minute: Data is insufficient for a recommendation

Kintzel 1995:

Oral: Adjust dose in the presence of hematologic toxicity

IV:

CrCl 46 to 60 mL/minute: Reduce dose to 85% of normal dose.

CrCl 31 to 45 mL/minute: Reduce dose to 75% of normal dose.

CrCl <30 mL/minute: Reduce dose to 70% of normal dose.

Badros 2001: IV: Autologous stem cell transplant (single-agent conditioning regimen; no busulfan or irradiation): Serum creatinine >2 mg/dL: Reduce dose from 200 mg/m^2 over 2 days (as 100 mg/m^2/day for 2 days) to 140 mg/m^2 given as a single-dose infusion

International Myeloma Working Group (IMWG) Recommendations (Dimo-poulos 2016):

The IMWG recommends the use of the Chronic Kidney Disease Epidemi-ology Collaboration (CKD-EPI) equation (preferred) or the Modification of Diet in Renal Disease (MDRD) formula to evaluate renal function estimation in multiple myeloma patients with a stable serum creatinine.

Oral:

CrCl >60 mL/minute: Usual dose: 0.15 to 0.25 mg/kg/day for 4 to 7 days

CrCl 15 to 59 mL/minute: Reduce dose to 75% of usual dose

CrCl <15 mL/minute: Reduce dose to 50% of usual dose

Hemodialysis: Reduce dose to 50% of usual dose

IV (high-dose melphalan for autologous stem cell transplant conditioning regimen):

CrCl >60 mL/minute: Usual dose: 200 mg/m^2 per treatment course

CrCl <15 to 59 mL/minute: Reduce dose to 140 mg/m^2 per treatment course; 100 mg/m^2 (per treatment course) may be appropriate in some patients

Hemodialysis: Reduce dose to 100 to 140 mg/m^2 per treatment course

Hepatic Impairment Melphalan is hepatically metabolized; however, dos-age adjustment does not appear to be necessary (King, 2001).

Obesity

*American Society of Clinical Oncology (ASCO) Guidelines for appropriate chemotherapy dosing in obese adults with cancer (**Note:** Excludes HSCT dosing):* Utilize patient's actual body weight (full weight) for calculation of body surface area- or weight-based dosing, particularly when the intent of therapy is curative; manage regimen-related toxicities in the same manner as for nonobese patients; if a dose reduction is utilized due to toxicity, consider resumption of full weight-based dosing with subsequent cycles, especially if cause of toxicity (eg, hepatic or renal impairment) is resolved (Griggs 2012).

American Society for Blood and Marrow Transplantation (ASBMT) practice guideline committee position statement on chemotherapy dosing in obesity: Utilize actual body weight (full weight) for calculation of body surface area in melphalan dosing for hematopoietic stem cell transplant conditioning regimens in adults (Bubalo 2014). **Note:** The manufacturer of Evomela recommends that if patients weigh more than 130% of their ideal body weight, body surface area should be calculated using adjusted ideal body weight.

Adjustment for Toxicity

Oral:

WBC <3000/mm^3: Withhold treatment until recovery

Platelets <100,000/mm^3: Withhold treatment until recovery

IV: Palliative treatment of multiple myeloma: Adjust dose based on blood cell count at the nadir and day of treatment

Combination Regimens

Lymphoma, Hodgkin:

Dexa-BEAM (Hodgkin) on page 2086

mini-BEAM (Hodgkin) on page 2174

Multiple myeloma:

Melphalan-Prednisone (Multiple Myeloma) on page 2171

Melphalan-Prednisone-Thalidomide (Multiple Myeloma) on page 2172

VBMCP (Multiple Myeloma) on page 2227

Administration Melphalan is associated with a moderate emetic potential (depending on dose and/or administration route); antiemetics may be recommended to prevent nausea and vomiting (Dupuis 2011).

Intravenous melphalan is available in different formulations. Indications for use, product preparation, storage, and dosing differ between formulations. Use caution when selecting melphalan formulations for preparation and administration. Do not mix or combine the formulations.

Oral: Administer on an empty stomach (Schmidt 2002)
IV:
 Alkeran: Due to limited stability, complete administration of IV dose should occur within 60 minutes of reconstitution. Infuse over 15 to 20 minutes.
 Evomela: Infuse over 15 to 20 minutes (palliative treatment for multiple myeloma) or 30 minutes (conditioning regimen for autologous stem cell transplantation).
 Melphalan (IV) is an irritant; local reactions may occur (Perez Fidalgo 2012). Extravasation may cause local tissue damage; administration by slow injection into a fast running IV solution into an injection port or via a central line is recommended; do not administer by direct injection into a peripheral vein.

Vesicant/Extravasation Risk May be an irritant

Emetic Potential
 Children:
  IV: >50 mg/m^2: Moderate (30% to 90%)
  IV (lower dose): Minimal (<10%)
  Oral: Minimal (<10%)
 Adults:
  IV: Moderate (30% to 90%)
  Oral: Minimal (<10%)

Monitoring Parameters CBC with differential and platelet count, serum electrolytes, renal/liver function tests, serum uric acid; signs/symptoms of hypersensitivity reaction, pulmonary toxicity, and gastrointestinal toxicity; monitor infusion site.

Test Interactions False-positive Coombs' test [direct]

Dosage Forms Considerations Different formulations of intravenous melphalan are available. Alkeran (melphalan hydrochloride for injection) and generic melphalan hydrochloride are reconstituted with the supplied diluent (which contains propylene glycol and ethanol). Evomela (melphalan for injection) is reconstituted with normal saline. Use caution when selecting melphalan formulations for preparation and administration. Do not mix or combine the formulations.

Dosage Forms Excipient information presented when available (limited, particularly for generics); consult specific product labeling.
Solution Reconstituted, Intravenous:
 Alkeran: 50 mg (1 ea) [contains alcohol, usp, propylene glycol]
 Evomela: 50 mg (1 ea)
 Generic: 50 mg (1 ea)
Solution Reconstituted, Intravenous [preservative free]:
 Generic: 50 mg (1 ea)
Tablet, Oral:
 Alkeran: 2 mg
 Generic: 2 mg

♦ **Melphalan HCl** see Melphalan on page 1182

♦ **Melphalan Hydrochloride** see Melphalan on page 1182

♦ **Mercaptoethane Sulfonate** see Mesna on page 1199

Mercaptopurine (mer kap toe PURE een)

Related Information

Management of Chemotherapy-Induced Nausea and Vomiting in Adults on page 2253

Prevention of Chemotherapy-Induced Nausea and Vomiting in Children on page 2310

Safe Handling of Hazardous Drugs on page 2379

Brand Names: US Purinethol [DSC]; Purixan

Brand Names: Canada Purinethol

Index Terms 6-Mercaptopurine (error-prone abbreviation); 6-MP (error-prone abbreviation); Purinethol

Pharmacologic Category Antineoplastic Agent, Antimetabolite; Antineoplastic Agent, Antimetabolite (Purine Analog); Immunosuppressant Agent

Use Acute lymphoblastic leukemia: Treatment of acute lymphoblastic leukemia (ALL), as part of a combination chemotherapy regimen

Labeled Contraindications Hypersensitivity to mercaptopurine or any component of the formulation; patients whose disease showed prior resistance to mercaptopurine

Pregnancy Considerations May cause fetal harm if administered during pregnancy. Case reports of fetal loss have been noted with mercaptopurine administration during the first trimester; adverse effects have also been noted with second and third trimester use. Women of child bearing potential should avoid becoming pregnant during treatment.

Breastfeeding Considerations Mercaptopurine is the active metabolite of azathioprine. Following administration of azathioprine, mercaptopurine can be detected in breast milk (Gardiner 2006). It is not known if/how much mercaptopurine is found in breast milk following oral administration. According to the manufacturer, the decision to discontinue mercaptopurine or discontinue breastfeeding during therapy should take into account the benefits of treatment to the mother.

Warnings/Precautions Hepatotoxicity has been reported, including jaundice, ascites, hepatic necrosis (may be fatal), intrahepatic cholestasis, parenchymal cell necrosis, and/or hepatic encephalopathy; may be due to direct hepatic cell damage or hypersensitivity. While hepatotoxicity or hepatic injury may occur at any dose, dosages exceeding the recommended dose are associated with a higher incidence. Signs of jaundice generally appear early in treatment, after ~1 to 2 months (range: 1 week to 8 years) and may resolve following discontinuation; recurrence with rechallenge has been noted. Monitor liver function tests, including transaminases, alkaline phosphatase, and bilirubin weekly with treatment initiation, then monthly thereafter (monitor more frequently if used in combination with other hepatotoxic drugs or in patients with preexisting hepatic impairment). Consider a reduced dose in patients with baseline hepatic impairment; monitor closely for toxicity. Withhold treatment for clinical signs of jaundice (hepatomegaly, anorexia, tenderness), deterioration in liver function tests, toxic hepatitis, or biliary stasis until hepatotoxicity is ruled out.

Dose-related leukopenia, thrombocytopenia, and anemia are common; however, may be indicative of disease progression. Hematologic toxicity may be delayed. Bone marrow may appear hypoplastic (could also appear normal). Monitor blood counts; dose may require adjusting for severe neutropenia or thrombocytopenia. Monitor for bleeding (due to thrombocytopenia) or infection (due to neutropenia). Profound severe or repeated hematologic toxicity may be indicative of TPMT deficiency. Patients with homozygous genetic defect of thiopurine methyltransferase (TPMT) are more sensitive to myelosuppressive effects; generally associated with rapid myelosuppression. Significant mercaptopurine dose reductions will be necessary (possibly with continued concomitant chemotherapy at normal doses). Patients who are heterozygous for TPMT defects will have intermediate activity; may have increased toxicity (primarily myelosuppression) although will generally tolerate normal mercaptopurine doses. Consider TPMT testing for severe toxicities/excessive myelosuppression. A germline variant in nucleoside diphophate-linked moiety X-type motif 15 (NUDT15) is strongly correlated with mercaptopurine intolerance in children receiving treatment for acute lymphoblastic leukemia (ALL). A genome-wide association study was performed in two prospective clinical childhood ALL trials, and showed that patients homozygous for the TT genotype were extremely sensitive to mercaptopurine, and achieved an average dose intensity of only 8.3%. The NUDT15 genetic variant is most common in East Asian and Hispanic patients. In patients homozygous for either TPMT or NUDT15 (or heterozygous for both), mercaptopurine dose reductions of ≥50% were required in 100% of patients (Yang 2015). Potentially significant drug-drug interactions may exist, requiring dose or frequency adjustment, additional monitoring, and/or selection of alternative therapy. Because azathioprine is metabolized to mercaptopurine, concomitant use with azathioprine may result in a significant increase in hematologic toxicity and profound myelosuppression; avoid concurrent use. Hematologic toxicity may be exacerbated by other medications which inhibit TPMT (eg, mesalamine, olsalazine, sulfasalazine) or by other myelosuppressive drugs. Minimize sun exposure due to possible photosensitivity. Cases of symptomatic hypoglycemia have been reported in children receiving mercaptopurine for the treatment of ALL; cases were reported in children less than 6 years of age or with a low body mass index.

Immunosuppressive agents, including mercaptopurine, are associated with the development of lymphoproliferative disorders and other malignancies. In an analysis of T-cell lymphomas associated with TNF blockers (with or without thiopurines) for the treatment of rheumatoid arthritis, Crohn disease, ulcerative colitis, or ankylosing spondylitis (off-label uses for thiopurines), an increase in the incidence of T-cell lymphomas, most commonly mycosis fungoides/Sézary syndrome and hepatosplenic T-cell lymphoma (HSTCL) was reported (Deepak 2013). HSTCL is a rare white blood cell cancer that is usually fatal. Most HSTCL cases occurred in patients treated with a combination of TNF blockers and thiopurines, although cases of HSTCL also occurred in patients receiving azathioprine or mercaptopurine monotherapy. Skin cancers (melanoma and non-melanoma), Kaposi and non-Kaposi sarcomas, and uterine cervical cancer in situ have been reported in patients receiving immunosuppressive treatment (including mercaptopurine); risk of development may be related to the degree and duration of immunosuppression. Partial regression of lymphoproliferative disorders may occur upon therapy discontinuation. Regimens containing multiple immunosuppressants increase the risk of Epstein-Barr virus (EBV)-associated lymphoproliferative disorders; use with caution.

Mercaptopurine is immunosuppressive; immune responses to infections may be impaired and the risk for infection is increased; common signs of infection, such as fever and leukocytosis may not occur; lethargy and confusion may be more prominent signs of infection. Immune response to vaccines may be diminished; live virus vaccines impose a risk for infection. Consider adjusting dosage in patients with renal impairment. Some renal adverse effects may be minimized with hydration and prophylactic antihyperuricemic therapy. To avoid potentially serious dosage errors, the terms "6-mercaptopurine" or "6-MP" should be avoided; use of these terms has been associated with six-fold overdosages.

Macrophage activation syndrome (MAS), also known as hemophagocytic lymphohistiocytosis, is a life-threatening disorder which may develop in patients with autoimmune disorders (particularly inflammatory bowel disease); mercaptopurine use for the treatment of autoimmune conditions (off-label use) may cause increased susceptibility to MAS. Discontinue mercaptopurine if MAS develops or is suspected. Monitor; promptly treat infections such as Epstein-Barr virus and cytomegalovirus (which are known triggers for MAS).

Adverse Reactions Frequency not always defined.

Central nervous system: Malaise (5% to 20%), drug fever

Dermatologic: Skin rash (5% to 20%), hyperpigmentation (<5%), urticaria (<5%), alopecia

Endocrine & metabolic: Hyperuricemia (<5%)

Gastrointestinal: Anorexia (5% to 20%), diarrhea (5% to 20%), nausea (5% to 20%; minimal), vomiting (5% to 20%; minimal), oral lesion (<5%), pancreatitis (<5%), cholestasis, mucositis, sprue-like symptoms, stomach pain, ulcerative bowel lesion

Genitourinary: Oligospermia, renal toxicity, uricosuria

Hematologic & oncologic: Bone marrow depression (>20%; onset 7 to 10 days; nadir 14 days; recovery: 21 days), anemia, granulocytopenia, hemorrhage, hepatosplenic T-cell lymphomas, leukopenia, lymphocytopenia, metastases, neutropenia, thrombocytopenia

Hepatic: Hyperbilirubinemia (<5%), increased serum transaminases (<5%), ascites, hepatic encephalopathy, hepatic fibrosis, hepatic injury, hepatic necrosis, hepatomegaly, hepatotoxicity, intrahepatic cholestasis, jaundice, toxic hepatitis

Immunologic: Immunosuppression

Infection: Infection

Respiratory: Pulmonary fibrosis

<1%, postmarketing, and/or case reports: Hypoglycemia, portal hypertension, skin photosensitivity

Drug Interactions

Metabolism/Transport Effects None known.

Avoid Concomitant Use

Avoid concomitant use of Mercaptopurine with any of the following: Aza-THIOprine; BCG (Intravesical); Deferiprone; Dipyrone; Febuxostat; Natalizumab; Pimecrolimus; Tacrolimus (Topical)

◀ **Increased Effect/Toxicity**

Mercaptopurine may increase the levels/effects of: CloZAPine; Deferiprone; Fingolimod; Leflunomide; Natalizumab; Tofacitinib; Vaccines (Live)

The levels/effects of Mercaptopurine may be increased by: 5-ASA Derivatives; Allopurinol; AzaTHIOprine; Denosumab; Dipyrone; DOXOrubicin (Conventional); Febuxostat; Ocrelizumab; Palifermin; Pimecrolimus; Promazine; Roflumilast; Sulfamethoxazole; Tacrolimus (Topical); Trastuzumab; Trimethoprim

Decreased Effect

Mercaptopurine may decrease the levels/effects of: BCG (Intravesical); Coccidioides immitis Skin Test; Lenograstim; Nivolumab; Sipuleucel-T; Tertomotide; Vaccines (Inactivated); Vaccines (Live); Vitamin K Antagonists

The levels/effects of Mercaptopurine may be decreased by: Echinacea

Food Interactions Absorption is variable with food. Management: Preferably, take on an empty stomach at the same time each day 1 hour before or 2 hours after a meal. Maintain adequate hydration, unless instructed to restrict fluid intake.

Hazardous Drugs Handling Considerations

Hazardous agent (NIOSH 2016 [group 1]).

Use appropriate precautions for receiving, handling, administration, and disposal. Gloves (single) should be worn during receiving, unpacking, and placing in storage.

NIOSH recommends single gloving for administration of intact tablets or capsules. If manipulating tablets/capsules (eg, to prepare an oral suspension), NIOSH recommends double gloving, a protective gown, and preparation in a controlled device; if not prepared in a controlled device, respiratory and eye/face protection as well as ventilated engineering controls are recommended. NIOSH recommends double gloving, a protective gown, and (if there is a potential for vomit or spit up) eye/face protection for administration of an oral liquid/feeding tube administration (NIOSH 2016).

Storage/Stability

Tablets: Store at 15°C to 25°C (59°F to 77°F). Store in a dry place.

Suspension: Store at 15°C to 25°C (59°F to 77°F). Do not store above 25°C (77°F). Store in a dry place. Use within 8 weeks after opening.

Preparation for Administration Suspension: Wear disposable gloves when handling. Shake bottle vigorously for at least 30 seconds prior to administration. Attach the bottle adaptor into the neck of the bottle (do not remove after insertion). Measure dose with an oral dosing syringe to assure proper dose is administered. Oral syringe provided by the manufacturer is intended to be reused, wash with warm soapy water and rinse well (hold syringe under water and move plunger several times to ensure inside of syringe is clean); allow to dry completely.

Mechanism of Action Mercaptopurine is a purine antagonist which inhibits DNA and RNA synthesis; acts as false metabolite and is incorporated into DNA and RNA, eventually inhibiting their synthesis; specific for the S phase of the cell cycle

Pharmacodynamics/Kinetics

Absorption: Variable and incomplete (~50% of a dose is absorbed); C_{max} of suspension is 34% higher than the tablet

Distribution: V_d: > total body water; CNS penetration is poor

Protein binding: ~19%

Metabolism: Hepatic and in GI mucosa; hepatically via xanthine oxidase and methylation via thiopurine methyltransferase to sulfate conjugates, 6-thiouric acid, and other inactive compounds; first-pass effect

Half-life elimination: Tablets: Children: 21 minutes; Adults: 47 minutes; Suspension: ~2 hours

Time to peak, serum: Within 2 hours

Excretion: Urine (46% as mercaptopurine and metabolites)

Dosing

Adult Note: Patients with minimal or no thiopurine S-methyltransferase (TPMT) activity are at increased risk for severe toxicity at conventional mercaptopurine doses and generally require dose reduction; consider TPMT gene polymorphism testing in patients who experience severe bone marrow suppression (homozygous deficient patients may require up to a 90% dosage reduction; heterozygous patients usually tolerate recommended doses, although some may require dosage reduction).

Acute lymphoblastic leukemia (ALL): Maintenance: Oral: 1.5 to 2.5 mg/kg once daily (50 to 75 mg/m² once daily); continue based on blood counts **or**

Off-label ALL dosing (combination chemotherapy; refer to specific reference for combinations):

Early intensification (two 4-week courses): 60 mg/m²/day days 1 to 14 (Larson 1995; Larson 1998)

Interim maintenance (12-week course): 60 mg/m²/day days 1 to 70 (Larson 1995; Larson 1998)

Maintenance (prolonged): 50 mg 3 times/day for 2 years (Kantarjian 2000) **or** 60 mg/m²/day for 2 years from diagnosis (Larson 1995; Larson 1998)

Larsen 2016: Patients ≤30 years:

Consolidation: Oral: 60 mg/m² once daily on days 1 to 14 and 29 to 42 of a 56-day cycle (in combination with cyclophosphamide, cytarabine, vincristine, pegaspargase, and intrathecal methotrexate)

Interim Maintenance 1 and 2: Oral: 25 mg/m² once daily on days 1 to 56 (in combination with vincristine, high-dose methotrexate, and intrathecal methotrexate)

Maintenance phase: Oral: 75 mg/m² once daily on days 1 to 84 of an 84-day cycle (in combination with vincristine, steroid, oral methotrexate, and intrathecal methotrexate). Maintenance cycles are repeated for a total duration of 2 years (females) and 3 years (males) from the start of Interim Maintenance I. During Maintenance, the mercaptopurine (and oral methotrexate) dose may be titrated to target absolute neutrophil count (ANC) and platelet count goals.

Acute promyelocytic leukemia, maintenance (off-label use): 60 mg/m²/day for 1 year (in combination with tretinoin and methotrexate) (Powell 2010)

Crohn disease, remission maintenance or reduction of steroid use (off-label use): Oral: 1 to 1.5 mg/kg/day (Lichtenstein 2009)

Lymphoblastic lymphoma (off-label use): Maintenance (prolonged): 50 mg 3 times daily for 2 years (Kantarjian 2000; Thomas 2004)

Ulcerative colitis (off-label use): Oral:

Initial: 50 mg once daily; titrate dose up if clinical remission not achieved or down if leukopenia occurs (Lobel 2004) **or**

Initial: 50 mg (25 mg if heterozygous for TPMT activity) once daily; titrate up to goal of 1.5 mg/kg (0.75 mg/kg if heterozygous for TPMT activity) if WBC >4,000/mm^3 (and at least 50% of baseline) and LFTs and amylase are stable (Siegel 2005) **or**

Maintenance: 1 to 1.5 mg/kg/day (Carter 2004) **or**

Remission maintenance: 1.5 mg/kg/day (Danese 2011)

Dosage adjustment with concurrent allopurinol: Avoid concomitant use. If administered concurrently, reduce mercaptopurine dosage to 25% to 33% of the usual dose.

Geriatric Due to renal decline with age, initiate treatment at the low end of recommended dose range.

Pediatric Note: Patients with minimal or no thiopurine S-methyltransferase (TPMT) activity are at increased risk for severe toxicity at conventional mercaptopurine doses and generally require dose reduction; consider TPMT gene polymorphism testing in patients who experience severe bone marrow suppression (homozygous deficient patients may require up to a 90% dosage reduction; heterozygous patients usually tolerate recommended doses, although some may require dosage reduction).

Acute lymphoblastic leukemia (ALL): Maintenance: Oral: 1.5 to 2.5 mg/kg once daily (50 to 75 mg/m^2 once daily); continue based on blood counts **or**

Risk-stratified ALL dosing *(combination chemotherapy; refer to specific reference for combinations):*

Standard Risk (Bostrom 2003; Stork 2010): Children 1 to <10 years: *Consolidation, Interim Maintenance I and Maintenance:* Oral: 50 to 75 mg/m^2/day; cycle duration and frequency are dependent on protocol phase (in combination with vincristine, steroid, methotrexate [oral and/or intrathecal]); refer to specific protocol for details. Maintenance cycles are repeated for a total duration of 2 years (females) and 3 years (males) from the start of Interim Maintenance I. During Maintenance, mercapto-purine (and oral methotrexate) doses are adjusted to maintain a target absolute neutrophil count (ANC) goal (generally 1,000 to 2,000/mm^3) and platelet goal (≥100,000/mm^3), varies based on protocol)

High risk (Larsen 2016): Children and Adolescents:

Consolidation: Oral: 60 mg/m^2 once daily on days 1 to 14 and 29 to 42 of a 56-day cycle (in combination with cyclophosphamide, cytarabine, vincristine, pegaspargase, and intrathecal methotrexate)

Interim Maintenance1 and 2: Oral: 25 mg/m^2 once daily on days 1 to 56 (in combination with vincristine, high-dose methotrexate, and intra-thecal methotrexate)

Maintenance phase: Oral: 75 mg/m^2 once daily on days 1 to 84 of an 84-day cycle (in combination with vincristine, steroid, oral methotrexate, and intrathecal methotrexate). Maintenance cycles are repeated for a total duration of 2 years (females) and 3 years (males) from the start of Interim Maintenance I. During Maintenance, the mercaptopurine (and oral methotrexate) dose may be titrated to target ANC and platelet count goals.

Acute promyelocytic leukemia, maintenance (off-label use):
Children and Adolescents ≤17 years: Oral: 50 mg/m^2/day for 2 years (in combination with methotrexate and tretinoin). Doses of mercaptopurine (and methotrexate) were decreased by 50% if the WBC count was <3,500/mm^3 and discontinued for WBC <2,500/mm^3 (Ortega 2005) **or**
Adolescents ≥15 years: Oral: 60 mg/m^2/day for 1 year (in combination with tretinoin and methotrexate) (Powell 2010) **or**
Children and Adolescents <14 years: Oral: 100 mg/m^2/day for 14 days of a 28-day cycle (in combination with tretinoin and methotrexate) for 2 years (Zhang 2011)

Autoimmune hepatitis (off-label use): Oral: 1.5 mg/kg/day (in combination with prednisone) (Manns 2010)

Crohn disease, remission maintenance (off-label use): Doses range from 1 to 1.5 mg/kg/day (Grossman 2008; Markowitz 2000); children ≤6 years may require higher doses to achieve clinical improvement (Grossman 2008).

Lymphoblastic lymphoma (off-label use): Adolescents ≥15 years: Maintenance (prolonged): 50 mg 3 times daily for 2 years (Kantarjian 2000; Thomas 2004) **or** 60 mg/m^2/day for 2 years from diagnosis (Stock 2008) **or** 75 mg/m^2/day for 2 years (girls) or 3 years (boys) from first interim maintenance (Stock 2008)

Ulcerative colitis, remission maintenance (off-label use): Doses range from 1 to 1.5 mg/kg/day (Grossman 2008; Sandhu 2010); children ≤6 years may require higher doses to achieve clinical improvement (Grossman 2008); additional trials may be necessary to further define the role of mercaptopurine in pediatric patients with this condition.

Dosage adjustment with concurrent allopurinol: Avoid concomitant use. If administered concurrently, reduce mercaptopurine dosage to 25% to 33% of the usual dose.

Renal Impairment The manufacturer's labeling recommends starting with reduced doses (starting at the low end of the dosing range) or increasing the dosing interval to every 36 to 48 hours to avoid accumulation in patients with renal impairment; however, no specific dosage adjustment is provided. The following adjustments have also been recommended (Aronoff 2007): Children:
CrCl ≤50 mL/minute/1.73 m^2: Administer every 48 hours
Hemodialysis: Administer every 48 hours
Continuous ambulatory peritoneal dialysis (CAPD): Administer every 48 hours
Continuous renal replacement therapy (CRRT): Administer every 48 hours

Hepatic Impairment The manufacturer's labeling recommends considering a reduced dose (starting at the low end of the dosing range) with close monitoring for toxicity dose in patients with baseline hepatic impairment; however, no specific dosage adjustment is provided.

Adjustment for Toxicity Adjust dosage for excessive hematologic toxicity.

Combination Regimens
Leukemia, acute lymphocytic:
CALGB 8811 Regimen (ALL) on page 2003
CALGB 9111 Regimen (ALL) on page 2004
Hyper-CVAD (Leukemia, Acute Lymphocytic) on page 2146
MTX/6-MP/VP (Maintenance) on page 2178
POMP on page 2197
PVA (POG 8602) on page 2197

Leukemia, acute promyelocytic:
Tretinoin-Daunorubicin-Cytarabine Induction, Consolidation, Maintenance (APL) on page 2218
Tretinoin-Idarubicin (APL) on page 2221

Administration Administer preferably on an empty stomach (Burton 1986; Kantarjian 2000); avoid concomitant milk products if possible (de Lemos 2007). Administer at the same time(s) each day.

Acute lymphoblastic leukemia (ALL) treatment in children (Schmiegelow 1997): Administration in the evening has demonstrated superior outcome; administration with food did not significantly affect outcome.

If adherence is limited by administering on an empty stomach in the evening or by avoiding concomitant milk products, simplification of administration (eg, take with food/dairy without regard to time of day) should be considered. In adherent patients (taking mercaptopurine regularly), no association was seen between risk of ALL relapse and mercaptopurine ingestion habits; there was also no association noted with red cell thioguanine nucleotide (TGN) levels and administration with food, dairy, or time of day (Landier 2017).

Suspension: Shake well for at least 30 seconds to ensure suspension is mixed thoroughly (suspension is viscous). Measure dose with an oral dosing syringe (a 1 mL and a 5 mL oral dosing syringe are supplied by the manufacturer) to assure proper dose is administered. Patients and caregivers should be trained on appropriate measuring and administration, handling, storage, disposal, cleanup of accidental spills, and proper cleaning of oral dosing syringe. Use within 8 weeks after opening.

Emetic Potential Children and Adults: Minimal (<10%)

Extemporaneous Preparations A 50 mg/mL oral suspension may be prepared in a vertical flow hood with tablets and a mixture of sterile water for injection (SWFI), simple syrup, and cherry syrup. Crush thirty 50 mg tablets in a mortar and reduce to a fine powder. Add ~5 mL SWFI and mix to a uniform paste; then add ~10 mL simple syrup; mix while continuing to add cherry syrup to make a final volume of 30 mL; transfer to a calibrated bottle. Label "shake well" and "caution chemotherapy". Stable for 35 days at room temperature.

Aliabadi HM, Romanick M, Desai, S, et al, "Effect of Buffer and Antioxidant on Stability of a Mercaptopurine Suspension," *Am J Health Syst Pharm* 2008, 65(5):441-7.

Monitoring Parameters CBC with differential (weekly initially, although clinical status may require increased frequency), bone marrow exam (to evaluate marrow status), liver function tests (transaminases, alkaline phosphatase, and bilirubin; weekly initially, then monthly; monitor more frequently if on concomitant hepatotoxic agents or in patients with preexisting hepatic impairment), renal function, urinalysis; consider thiopurine methyltransferase (TPMT) genotyping to identify TPMT defect (if severe hematologic toxicity occurs); signs/symptoms of macrophage activating syndrome; photosensitivity reactions. Monitor adherence.

For use as immunomodulatory therapy in CD or UC, monitor CBC with differential weekly for 1 month, then biweekly for 1 month, followed by monitoring every 1 to 2 months throughout the course of therapy. LFTs should be assessed every 3 months. Monitor for signs/symptoms of malignancy (eg, splenomegaly, hepatomegaly, abdominal pain, persistent fever, night sweats, weight loss).

Test Interactions TPMT testing: Recent transfusions may result in a misinterpretation of the actual TPMT activity. Concomitant drugs may influence TPMT activity in the blood.

Prescribing and Access Restrictions For specialty or local pharmacy distribution and availability contact AnovoRx at http://www.purixan-us.com/find-purixan/ or call 888-470-0904.

Dosage Forms Excipient information presented when available (limited, particularly for generics); consult specific product labeling. [DSC] = Discontinued product

Suspension, Oral:
  Purixan: 2000 mg/100 mL (100 mL) [contains aspartame, methylparaben, propylparaben]
Tablet, Oral:
  Purinethol: 50 mg [DSC] [scored]
  Generic: 50 mg

◆ **6-Mercaptopurine (error-prone abbreviation)** *see* Mercaptopurine *on page 1191*

Mesna (MES na)

Brand Names: US Mesnex
Brand Names: Canada Mesna for injection; Uromitexan
Index Terms Mercaptoethane Sulfonate; Sodium 2-Mercaptoethane Sulfonate
Pharmacologic Category Antidote; Chemoprotective Agent
Use

Prevention of ifosfamide-induced hemorrhagic cystitis: Preventive agent to reduce the incidence of ifosfamide-induced hemorrhagic cystitis

Limitations of use: Mesna is not indicated to reduce the risk of hematuria due to other conditions such as thrombocytopenia

Labeled Contraindications Hypersensitivity to mesna or any component of the formulation

Pregnancy Considerations Adverse effects were not observed in animal reproduction studies. Use during pregnancy only if clearly needed.

Breastfeeding Considerations It is not known if mesna is excreted in breast milk. Benzyl alcohol, a component in some formulations, does enter breast milk and may be absorbed by a nursing infant. Due to the potential for adverse reactions in the nursing infant, a decision should be made to discontinue breastfeeding or to discontinue mesna, taking into account the importance of treatment to the mother.

Warnings/Precautions Monitor urine for hematuria. Severe hematuria despite utilization of mesna may require ifosfamide dose reduction or discontinuation. Examine morning urine specimen for hematuria prior to ifosfamide or cyclophosphamide treatment; if hematuria (>50 RBC/HPF) develops, reduce the ifosfamide/cyclophosphamide dose or discontinue the drug; will not prevent hemorrhagic cystitis in all patients. Mesna will not reduce the risk of hematuria related to thrombocytopenia. Patients should receive adequate hydration during treatment. Mesna is intended for the prevention of hemorrhagic cystitis and will not prevent or alleviate other toxicities associated with ifosfamide or cyclophosphamide.

Hypersensitivity reactions have been reported; symptoms ranged from mild hypersensitivity to systemic anaphylactic reactions and may include fever, hypotension, tachycardia, acute renal impairment, hypoxia, respiratory distress, urticaria, angioedema, signs of disseminated intravascular coagulation, hematologic abnormalities, increased liver enzymes, nausea, vomiting, arthralgia, and myalgia. Reactions may occur with the first exposure, or after several months of treatment. Monitor for signs/symptoms of reactions. May require discontinuation. Patients with autoimmune disorders receiving cyclophosphamide and mesna may be at increased risk. Mesna is a thiol compound; it is unknown if the risk for reaction is increased in patients who have had a reaction to other thiol compounds (eg, amifostine). Drug rash with eosinophilia and systemic symptoms and bullous/ulcerative skin and mucosal reactions consistent with Stevens-Johnson syndrome (SJS) or toxic epidermal necrolysis (TEN) have been reported. The skin and mucosal reactions may be characterized by rash, pruritus, urticaria, erythema, burning sensation, angioedema, periorbital edema, flushing, and stomatitis. Reactions may occur with the first exposure, or after several months of treatment. May require discontinuation.

Benzyl alcohol and derivatives: Some dosage forms may contain benzyl alcohol; large amounts of benzyl alcohol (≥99 mg/kg/day) have been associated with a potentially fatal toxicity ("gasping syndrome") in neonates; the "gasping syndrome" consists of metabolic acidosis, respiratory distress, gasping respirations, CNS dysfunction (including convulsions, intracranial hemorrhage), hypotension, and cardiovascular collapse (AAP ["Inactive" 1997]; CDC, 1982); some data suggests that benzoate displaces bilirubin from protein binding sites (Ahlfors, 2001); avoid or use dosage forms containing benzyl alcohol with caution in neonates. See manufacturer's labeling.

Adverse Reactions Mesna alone (frequency not defined):

Cardiovascular: Flushing

Central nervous system: Dizziness, drowsiness, headache, hyperesthesia, rigors

Dermatologic: Skin rash

Gastrointestinal: Anorexia, constipation, diarrhea, dysgeusia (with oral administration), flatulence, nausea, unpleasant taste (with oral administration), vomiting

Local: Injection site reaction

Neuromuscular & skeletal: Arthralgia, back pain

Ophthalmic: Conjunctivitis

Respiratory: Cough, flu-like symptoms, pharyngitis, rhinitis

Miscellaneous: Fever

<1%, postmarketing and/or case reports (mesna alone or in combination): Anaphylaxis, erythema at injection site, hypersensitivity reaction, hypertension, hypotension, increased serum transaminases, increased ST segment on ECG, limb pain, malaise, myalgia, pain at injection site, tachycardia, tachypnea, thrombocytopenia

Drug Interactions

Metabolism/Transport Effects None known.

Avoid Concomitant Use There are no known interactions where it is recommended to avoid concomitant use.

Increased Effect/Toxicity There are no known significant interactions involving an increase in effect.

Decreased Effect There are no known significant interactions involving a decrease in effect.

Storage/Stability Store intact vials and tablets at room temperature of 20°C to 25°C (68°F to 77°F); excursions are permitted between 15°C and 30°C (59°F and 86°F). Opened multidose vials may be stored and used for use up to 8 days after initial puncture. Solutions diluted for infusion in D5W, NS, D5^{1}/$_4$NS, D5^{1}/$_3$NS, D5^{1}/$_2$NS, or lactated Ringer's and stored at room temperature should be used within 24 hours. According to the manufacturer, mesna and ifosfamide may be mixed in the same bag if the final ifosfamide concentration is ≤50 mg/mL. Solutions of mesna and ifosfamide (1:1) in NS at a concentration of up to 20 mg/mL are stable for 14 days in PVC bags (Zhang, 2014). Solutions of mesna (0.5 to 3.2 mg/mL) and cyclophosphamide (1.8 to 10.8 mg/mL) in D5W are stable for 48 hours refrigerated or 6 hours at room temperature (Menard, 2003). Mesna injection prepared for oral administration is stable for at least 9 days undiluted in polypropylene syringes and stored at 5°C, 24°C, 35°C; for 7 days when diluted 1:2 or 1:5 with syrups and stored at 24°C in capped tubes; or for 24 hours at 5°C when diluted to 1:2, 1:10, and 1:100 in orange or apple juice, milk, or carbonated beverages (Goren, 1991).

Preparation for Administration IV: Dilute in D5W, NS, D5^{1}/$_4$NS, D5^{1}/$_3$NS, D5^{1}/$_2$NS, or lactated Ringer's to a final concentration of 20 mg/mL.

Mechanism of Action In blood, mesna is oxidized to dimesna which in turn is reduced in the kidney back to mesna, supplying a free thiol group which binds to and inactivates acrolein, the urotoxic metabolite of ifosfamide and cyclophosphamide

Pharmacodynamics/Kinetics

Distribution: 0.65 ± 0.24 L/kg; distributed to total body water

Protein binding: 69% to 75%

Metabolism: Rapidly oxidized to mesna disulfide (dimesna) in the intravascular compartment. Mesna and dimesna do not undergo hepatic metabolism.

Bioavailability: Oral: Free mesna: 58% (range: 45% to 71%); not affected by food

Half-life elimination: Mesna: ~22 minutes; Dimesna: ~70 minutes

Time to peak, plasma: Oral: Free mesna: 1.5 to 4 hours

Excretion: Urine (32% as mesna; 33% as dimesna), majority of IV dose excreted within 4 hours

Dosing

Adult & Geriatric Note: Mesna dosing schedule should be repeated each day ifosfamide is received. If ifosfamide dose is adjusted (decreased or increased), the mesna dose should also be modified to maintain the mesna-to-ifosfamide ratio.

Prevention of ifosfamide-induced hemorrhagic cystitis:

Standard-dose ifosfamide (manufacturer's labeling): IV: Mesna dose is equal to 20% of the ifosfamide dose given for 3 doses: With the ifosfamide dose, hour 4, and at hour 8 after the ifosfamide dose (total daily mesna dose is 60% of the ifosfamide dose)

Oral mesna (following IV mesna; for ifosfamide doses ≤2 g/m^2/day): Mesna dose (IV) is equal to 20% of the ifosfamide dose at hour 0, followed by mesna dose (orally) equal to 40% of the ifosfamide dose given 2 and 6 hours after the ifosfamide dose (total daily mesna dose is 100% of the ifosfamide dose). **Note:** If the oral mesna dose is vomited within 2 hours of administration, repeat the dose or administer IV mesna.

◄ Short infusion standard-dose ifosfamide (<2.5 g/m²/day): ASCO guidelines: IV: Total mesna dose is equal to 60% of the ifosfamide dose, in 3 divided doses (each mesna dose as 20% of ifosfamide dose), given 15 minutes before the ifosfamide dose, and 4 and 8 hours after each dose of ifosfamide (Hensley, 2009)

Continuous infusion standard-dose ifosfamide (<2.5 g/m²/day): ASCO guidelines: IV: Mesna dose (as a bolus) is equal to 20% of the ifosfamide dose, followed by a continuous infusion of mesna at 40% of the ifosfamide dose; continue mesna infusion for 12-24 hours after completion of ifosfamide infusion (Hensley, 2009)

High-dose ifosfamide (>2.5 g/m²/day): ASCO guidelines: Evidence for use is inadequate; more frequent and prolonged mesna administration regimens may be required (Hensley, 2009)

Other dosing strategies used in combination with ifosfamide (off-label dosing):

Mesna continuous infusion: IV: 1.8 g/m²/day to 5 g/m²/day as a continuous infusion (100% of the ifosfamide dose), repeated each day ifosfamide is received; see protocols for specific details (Bacci, 2003; Kolb, 2003; Moskowitz, 2011)

Mesna bolus followed by continuous infusion: IV: 1000 mg/m² 1 hour prior to ifosfamide on day 1, followed by 3000 mg/m²/day continuous infusion (continuous infusion is 100% of the ifosfamide dose) on days 1, 2, and 3 (with sufficient hydration) every 3 weeks for 6 courses (Juergens, 2006)

Prevention of cyclophosphamide-induced hemorrhagic cystitis (off-label use):

HDCAV/IE regimen for Ewing sarcoma: Children ≥4 years and Adults <40 years: IV: 2100 mg/m²/day continuous infusion (mesna dose is equivalent to the cyclophosphamide dose) for 2 days with cyclophosphamide infusion during cycles 1, 2, 3, and 6 (Kolb, 2003)

Hyper-CVAD regimen for ALL: Adults: IV: 600 mg/m²/day continuous infusion (mesna continuous infusion is same total dose as cyclophosphamide) on days 1, 2, and 3, beginning with cyclophosphamide and ending 6 hours after the last cyclophosphamide dose during odd-numbered cycles (cycles 1, 3, 5, 7) of an 8-cycle phase (Kantarjian, 2000)

Pediatric

Prevention of ifosfamide-induced hemorrhagic cystitis (off-label use):

Short infusion standard-dose ifosfamide (<2.5 g/m²/day): ASCO guidelines: Refer to adult dosing.

Continuous infusion standard-dose ifosfamide (<2.5 g/m²/day): ASCO guidelines: Refer to adult dosing.

Other dosing strategies used in combination with ifosfamide (off-label dosing):

Mesna continuous infusion: IV: 1.8 g/m²/day to 5 g/m²/day as a continuous infusion (100% of the ifosfamide dose), repeated each day ifosfamide is received; see protocols for specific details (Bacci, 2003; Kolb, 2003; Moskowitz, 2011)

Mesna bolus followed by continuous infusion: IV: 1000 mg/m² 1 hour prior to ifosfamide on day 1, followed by 3000 mg/m²/day continuous infusion (continuous infusion is 100% of the ifosfamide dose) on days 1, 2, and 3 (with sufficient hydration) every 3 weeks for 6 courses (Juergens, 2006)

Mesna (20% higher than ifosfamide) continuous infusion: IV: 3600 mg/m^2/
day continuous infusion for 4 days (mesna dose is 20% higher than
ifosfamide), with hydration, during weeks 4 and 9 (3 additional postop
courses were administered in good responders) (Le Deley, 2007)

**Prevention of cyclophosphamide-induced hemorrhagic cystitis (off-
label use):** HDCAV/IE regimen for Ewing sarcoma: Children ≥4 years
and Adults <40 years: IV: 2100 mg/m^2/day continuous infusion (mesna
dose is equivalent to the cyclophosphamide dose) for 2 days with cyclophosphamide infusion during cycles 1, 2, 3, and 6 (Kolb, 2003)

Renal Impairment There are no dosage adjustments provided in the
manufacturer's labeling (has not been studied)

Hepatic Impairment There are no dosage adjustments provided in the
manufacturer's labeling (has not been studied)

Combination Regimens

Bone sarcoma (osteosarcoma): Ifosfamide-Cisplatin-Epirubicin (Osteosarcoma) on page 2155

Leukemia, acute lymphocytic:
Hyper-CVAD + Imatinib on page 2145
Hyper-CVAD (Leukemia, Acute Lymphocytic) on page 2146

Lymphoma, Hodgkin:
ICE (Hodgkin) on page 2153
IGEV (Hodgkin) on page 2155
MINE-ESHAP (Hodgkin) on page 2174
VIM-D (Hodgkin) on page 2231

Lymphoma, non-Hodgkin (Burkitt):
CODOX-M/IVAC (NHL-Burkitt) on page 2068
Hyper-CVAD Alternating With High-Dose Methotrexate-Cytarabine + Ritux-
imab + CNS Prophylaxis (NHL-Burkitt) on page 2144

Lymphoma, non-Hodgkin (DLBCL): R-ICE (NHL-DLBCL) on page 2205

Lymphoma, non-Hodgkin (Mantle cell): Rituximab-Hyper-CVAD (NHL-Mantle
Cell) on page 2208

Multiple myeloma: Hyper-CVAD (Multiple Myeloma) on page 2152

Penile cancer: Paclitaxel-Ifosfamide-Cisplatin (Penile) on page 2186

Soft tissue sarcoma: Epirubicin-Ifosfamide (Soft Tissue Sarcoma) on
page 2103

Testicular cancer:
TIP (Testicular) on page 2214
VeIP (Testicular) on page 2231
VIP (Testicular) on page 2233

Wilms' tumor: Regimen I (Wilms' Tumor) on page 2203

Administration Maintain adequate hydration and urinary output during
ifosfamide treatment

IV: Administer as an IV bolus (per manufacturer); may also be administered by
short infusion or continuous infusion (maintain continuous infusion for 12-24
hours after completion of ifosfamide infusion) (Hensley, 2009); refer to
specific protocol for administration rate/details

Oral: Administer orally in tablet formulation; patients who vomit within 2 hours
after taking oral mesna should repeat the dose or receive IV mesna. A
solution may be prepared from solution for injection by dilution in syrup, juice,
carbonate beverages, or milk (Goren, 1991); see Extemporaneous Preparations section.

◀ **Extemporaneous Preparations** An oral solution may be prepared from mesna solution for injection. Dilute solution for injection to 20 mg/mL or 50 mg/mL with orange or grape syrup. Prior to administration, syrup-diluted solutions may be diluted to a final concentration of 1, 10, or 50 mg/mL with any of the following: Carbonated beverages, apple juice, orange juice, or milk. Mesna injection prepared for oral administration is stable for at least 9 days undiluted in polypropylene syringes and stored at 5°C, 24°C, 35°C; for 7 days when diluted 1:2 or 1:5 with syrups and stored at 24°C in capped tubes; or for 24 hours at 5°C when diluted to 1:2, 1:10, and 1:100 in orange or apple juice, milk, or carbonated beverages. Dilution of mesna with diet or sugar-free preparations has not been evaluated.

Goren MP, Lyman BA, Li JT. The stability of mesna in beverages and syrup for oral administration. *Cancer Chemother Pharmacol*. 1991;28(4):298-301.

Monitoring Parameters Monitor urine for hematuria; urine output and hydration status; monitor for signs/symptoms of hypersensitivity or dermatologic toxicity

Test Interactions

Urinary ketones: False-positive tests for urinary ketones may occur in patients receiving mesna with the use of nitroprusside-based urine tests, including dipstick tests.

CPK activity: Mesna may interfere with enzymatic creatine kinase (CPK) activity tests which use a thiol compound (eg, N-acetylcysteine) for CPK reactivation; may result in a falsely low CPK level.

Ascorbic acid: Mesna may result in false-positive reactions in Tillman's reagent-based urine screening tests for ascorbic acid.

Additional Information Oncology Comment: Guidelines from the American Society of Clinical Oncology (ASCO) for the use of chemotherapy and radiotherapy protectants (Hensley, 2009 [update]; Schuchter, 2002) recommend mesna to decrease the incidence of ifosfamide-induced urotoxicity associated with short infusion and continuous infusion standard-dose ifosfamide (<2.5 g/m^2/day). Although evidence is inadequate regarding mesna's uroprotective effects in high-dose ifosfamide (>2.5 g/m^2/day), the guidelines suggest more frequent and prolonged mesna administration times may be required. For prevention of high-dose cyclophosphamide-induced urotoxicity (associated with stem cell transplantation), the guidelines recommend mesna in conjunction with saline diuresis (or forced saline diuresis alone).

Dosage Forms Excipient information presented when available (limited, particularly for generics); consult specific product labeling.

Solution, Intravenous:

Mesnex: 100 mg/mL (10 mL) [contains benzyl alcohol, edetate disodium]

Generic: 100 mg/mL (10 mL)

Tablet, Oral:

Mesnex: 400 mg [scored]

Dosage Forms: Canada Information with regard to form, strength, and availability of products uniquely available in Canada but currently not available in the US. Refer also to Dosage Forms.

Excipient information presented when available (limited, particularly for generics); consult specific product labeling.
Solution, Intravenous:
  Mesna for injection: 100 mg/mL (10 mL) [contains benzyl alcohol, edetate disodium]
  Uromitexan: 100 mg/mL (4 mL, 10 mL) [contains edetate disodium]
  Uromitexan: 100 mg/mL (10 mL, 50 mL) [contains benzyl alcohol, edetate disodium]

◆ **Mesna for injection (Can)** *see* Mesna *on page 1199*

◆ **Mesnex** *see* Mesna *on page 1199*

◆ **123 Meta-Iodobenzlyguanidine Sulfate** *see* Iobenguane I 123 *on page 1029*

◆ **Metastron** *see* Strontium-89 *on page 1697*

Methotrexate (meth oh TREKS ate)
Related Information
  Common Toxicity Criteria *on page 2242*
  Hematopoietic Cell Transplantation *on page 2365*
  Management of Chemotherapy-Induced Nausea and Vomiting in Adults *on page 2253*
  Mucositis and Stomatitis *on page 2299*
  Prevention of Chemotherapy-Induced Nausea and Vomiting in Children *on page 2310*
  Safe Handling of Hazardous Drugs *on page 2379*
Brand Names: US Otrexup; Rasuvo; Rheumatrex [DSC]; Trexall; Xatmep
Brand Names: Canada Apo-Methotrexate; JAMP Methotrexate; Methotrexate Injection USP; Methotrexate Injection, BP; Methotrexate Sodium Injection; Metoject; ratio-Methotrexate Sodium
Index Terms Amethopterin; Methotrexate Sodium; Methotrexalum; MTX (error-prone abbreviation)
Pharmacologic Category Antineoplastic Agent, Antimetabolite (Antifolate); Antirheumatic, Disease Modifying; Immunosuppressant Agent
Use
  Oncology uses: Acute lymphoblastic leukemia (ALL) maintenance treatment, ALL meningeal leukemia (preservative-free only; prophylaxis and treatment); treatment of trophoblastic neoplasms (gestational choriocarcinoma, chorioadenoma destruens and hydatidiform mole), breast cancer, head and neck cancer (epidermoid), cutaneous T-Cell lymphoma (advanced mycosis fungoides), lung cancer (squamous cell and small cell), advanced non-Hodgkin lymphomas (NHL), osteosarcoma (preservative-free only).
  Nononcology uses: Treatment of psoriasis (severe, recalcitrant, disabling) that is unresponsive to other therapies; severe, active rheumatoid arthritis (RA) that is unresponsive to or intolerant of first-line therapy including full dose nonsteroidal anti-inflammatory agents (NSAIDs); active polyarticular-course juvenile idiopathic arthritis (pJIA) that is unresponsive to or intolerant of first-line therapy including full dose nonsteroidal anti-inflammatory agents (NSAIDs).

◄ Limitations of use: Otrexup and Rasuvo are not indicated for the treatment of neoplastic diseases.

Guideline recommendations: Rheumatoid arthritis: Treatment initiation with a disease-modifying antirheumatic drug (DMARD) is recommended in DMARD-naïve patients with either early rheumatoid arthritis (RA) (disease duration <6 months) or established RA (disease duration ≥6 months). Methotrexate is the preferred initial DMARD for most early or established RA patients (Singh [ACR 2016]).

Labeled Contraindications

Known hypersensitivity to methotrexate or any component of the formulation; breastfeeding

Additional contraindications for patients with psoriasis, rheumatoid arthritis or polyarticular-course juvenile idiopathic arthritis: Pregnancy, alcoholism, alcoholic liver disease or other chronic liver disease, immunodeficiency syndromes (overt or laboratory evidence); preexisting blood dyscrasias (eg, bone marrow hypoplasia, leukopenia, thrombocytopenia, significant anemia)

Pregnancy Considerations [US Boxed Warning]: Some products are contraindicated in pregnant women. Methotrexate has been reported to cause fetal death and/or congenital abnormalities. Methotrexate is not recommended for women of childbearing potential unless there is clear medical evidence that the benefits can be expected to outweigh the considered risks. Pregnant women with psoriasis or rheumatoid arthritis should not receive methotrexate. Studies in animals and pregnant women have shown evidence of fetal abnormalities; therefore, the manufacturer classifies methotrexate as pregnancy category X (for psoriasis or RA). A pattern of congenital malformations associated with maternal methotrexate use is referred to as the aminopterin/methotrexate syndrome. Features of the syndrome include CNS, skeletal, and cardiac abnormalities. Low birth weight and developmental delay have also been reported. The use of methotrexate may impair fertility and cause menstrual irregularities or oligospermia during treatment and following therapy. It is not known if fertility impairment is reversible. Methotrexate is approved for the treatment of trophoblastic neoplasms (gestational choriocarcinoma, chorioadenoma destruens, and hydatidiform mole) and has been used for the medical management of ectopic pregnancy and the medical management of abortion. Pregnancy should be excluded prior to therapy in women of childbearing potential. Use for the treatment of neoplastic diseases only when the potential benefit to the mother outweighs the possible risk to the fetus. Pregnancy should be avoided for ≥3 months following treatment in male patients and at least 6 months and ≥1 ovulatory cycle in female patients. A registry is available for pregnant women exposed to autoimmune medications including methotrexate. For additional information contact the Organization of Teratology Information Specialists, OTIS Autoimmune Diseases Study, at 877-311-8972.

Breastfeeding Considerations Low amounts of methotrexate are present in breast milk. Due to the potential for serious adverse reactions in a breastfed infant, use is contraindicated in breastfeeding mothers.

Warnings/Precautions [US Boxed Warning]: Methotrexate causes hepatotoxicity, fibrosis, and cirrhosis, but generally only after prolonged use. Acutely, liver enzyme elevations are frequently seen. These are usually transient and asymptomatic, and also do not appear predictive of subsequent hepatic disease. Liver biopsy after sustained use often shows histologic changes, and fibrosis and cirrhosis have been reported; these latter lesions often are not preceded by symptoms or

abnormal liver function tests in the psoriasis population. For this reason, periodic liver biopsies are usually recommended for psoriatic patients who are under long-term treatment. Persistent abnormalities in liver function tests may precede appearance of fibrosis or cirrhosis in the rheumatoid arthritis population. Risk is related to cumulative dose (≥1.5 g) and prolonged exposure. Monitor closely (with liver function tests, including serum albumin) for liver toxicities. Liver enzyme elevations may be noted, but may not be predictive of hepatic disease in long term treatment for psoriasis (but generally is predictive in rheumatoid arthritis [RA] treatment). Discontinue methotrexate with moderate to severe change in liver biopsy. Risk factors for hepatotoxicity include history of above moderate ethanol consumption, persistent abnormal liver chemistries, history of chronic liver disease (including hepatitis B or C), family history of inheritable liver disease, diabetes, obesity, hyperlipidemia, lack of folate supplementation during methotrexate therapy, cumulative methotrexate dose exceeding 1.5 g, continuous daily methotrexate dosing, history of significant exposure to hepatotoxic drugs, and advanced age. Use caution with preexisting liver impairment; may require dosage reduction. Use caution when used with other hepatotoxic agents (azathioprine, retinoids, sulfasalazine). **[US Boxed Warning]: Methotrexate elimination is reduced in patients with ascites and pleural effusions;** resulting in prolonged half-life and toxicity; may require dose reduction or discontinuation. Monitor closely for toxicity.

May cause renal damage leading to acute renal failure, especially with high-dose methotrexate; monitor renal function and methotrexate levels closely, maintain adequate hydration and urinary alkalinization. Use caution in osteosarcoma patients treated with high-dose methotrexate in combination with nephrotoxic chemotherapy (eg, cisplatin). **[US Boxed Warning]: Methotrexate elimination is reduced in patients with renal impairment; monitor closely for toxicity; may require dose reduction or, in some cases, discontinuation of methotrexate administration. [US Boxed Warning]: Tumor lysis syndrome may occur in patients with high tumor burden; appropriate supportive and pharmacologic measures may prevent or alleviate tumor lysis syndrome.**

[US Boxed Warning]: Methotrexate-induced lung disease, including acute or chronic interstitial pneumonitis, is a potentially dangerous lesion, which may occur acutely at any time during therapy and has been reported at low doses. It is not always fully reversible and fatalities have been reported. Pulmonary symptoms (especially a dry, nonproductive cough) may require interruption of treatment and careful investigation. Pulmonary symptoms may occur at any time during therapy and at any dosage; monitor closely for pulmonary symptoms, particularly dry, nonproductive cough. Other potential symptoms include fever, dyspnea, hypoxemia, or pulmonary infiltrate. **[US Boxed Warning]: Methotrexate elimination is reduced in patients with pleural effusions;** may require dose reduction or discontinuation. Monitor closely for toxicity.

[US Boxed Warning]: Unexpectedly severe (sometimes fatal) bone marrow suppression and aplastic anemia have been reported with concomitant administration of methotrexate (usually in high dosage) along with some nonsteroidal anti-inflammatory drugs (NSAIDs); anemia, pancytopenia, leukopenia, neutropenia, and/or thrombocytopenia may occur. Monitor blood counts. Use caution in patients with preexisting bone marrow suppression. Discontinue treatment (immediately) in RA or psoriasis if a significant decrease in hematologic components is noted. **[US Boxed Warning]: Malignant lymphomas, which may regress following withdrawal of methotrexate, may occur in patients receiving low-dose methotrexate and, thus, may not require cytotoxic treatment. Discontinue methotrexate first and, if the lymphoma does not regress, appropriate treatment should be instituted.** Other secondary tumors have been reported.

[US Boxed Warning]: Gastrointestinal toxicity may occur (may be unexpectedly severe, usually occurs with high doses along with concomitant use of some NSAIDs); diarrhea and ulcerative stomatitis may require treatment interruption; otherwise hemorrhagic enteritis and death from intestinal perforation may occur. Diarrhea or stomatitis may also require discontinuation. Use with caution in patients with peptic ulcer disease or ulcerative colitis; the risk of gastrointestinal adverse effects may be increased. In children, doses ≥12 g/m^2 (IV) are associated with a high emetic potential; doses ≥250 mg/m^2 (IV) in adults and children are associated with moderate emetic potential (Dupuis 2011). Antiemetics may be recommended to prevent nausea and vomiting.

May cause neurotoxicity. Leukoencephalopathy has been reported (case reports), usually in patients who have received cranial irradiation and IV methotrexate. Chronic leukoencephalopathy has been reported with high-dose methotrexate (with leucovorin rescue and even without cranial irradiation) and with intrathecal methotrexate; discontinuing methotrexate does not always result in complete recovery; may be progressive and fatal. Serious neurotoxicity, including generalized and focal seizures has occurred (usually in pediatric ALL patients receiving intermediate-dose (1 g/m^2 IV methotrexate); leukoencephalopathy and/or microangiopathic calcifications were noted on diagnostic imaging studies in symptomatic patients. A transient acute stroke-like encephalopathy has been observed, usually with high-dose regimens; manifestations may include confusion, hemiparesis, transient blindness, seizure, and coma. Chemical arachnoiditis (headache, back pain, nuchal rigidity, fever) and myelopathy may result from intrathecal administration. May cause dizziness and fatigue; may affect the ability to drive or operate heavy machinery.

[US Boxed Warning]: Severe, occasionally fatal skin reactions have been reported following single or multiple doses of methotrexate. Reactions have occurred within days of oral, intramuscular, intravenous, or intrathecal methotrexate administration. Recovery has been reported with discontinuation of therapy. Severe dermatologic reactions have included toxic epidermal necrolysis, Stevens-Johnson syndrome, exfoliative dermatitis, skin necrosis, and erythema multiforme; discontinue methotrexate if severe reactions occur. Radiation recall dermatitis and sunburn may be precipitated by methotrexate administration. Psoriatic lesions may be worsened by concomitant exposure to ultraviolet radiation.

Anaphylaxis may occur; if anaphylaxis or other serious hypersensitivity reaction occurs, discontinue methotrexate immediately and institute appropriate management. Potentially significant drug-drug interactions may exist, requiring dose or frequency adjustment, additional monitoring, and/or selection of alternative therapy. Do not administer NSAIDs prior to or during high-dose methotrexate therapy; may increase and prolong serum methotrexate levels. Doses used for psoriasis may still lead to unexpected toxicities; use caution when administering NSAIDs or salicylates with lower doses of methotrexate for RA. Methotrexate may increase the levels and effects of mercaptopurine; may require dosage adjustments. Vitamins containing folate may decrease response to systemic methotrexate; folate deficiency may increase methotrexate toxicity. Concomitant use of proton pump inhibitors with methotrexate (primarily high-dose methotrexate) may elevate and prolong serum methotrexate and metabolite (hydroxymethotrexate) levels; may lead to toxicities; use with caution. Immunization may be ineffective during methotrexate treatment. Immunization with live vaccines is not recommended; cases of disseminated vaccinia infections due to live vaccines have been reported. **[US Boxed Warning]: Concomitant methotrexate administration with radiotherapy may increase the risk of soft tissue necrosis and osteonecrosis.**

[US Boxed Warnings]: Because of the possibility of serious toxic reactions (which can be fatal), methotrexate should be used only in life threatening neoplastic diseases or in patients with psoriasis or rheumatoid arthritis with severe, recalcitrant, disabling disease which is not adequately responsive to other forms of therapy. Deaths have been reported with the use of methotrexate in the treatment of malignancy, psoriasis, and rheumatoid arthritis. Patients should be closely monitored for bone marrow, liver, lung, skin, and kidney toxicities. Patients should be informed by their physician of the risks involved and be under a physician's care throughout therapy. The use of methotrexate high-dose regimens recommended for osteosarcoma requires meticulous care. High-dose regimens of methotrexate injection for other neoplastic diseases are investigational, and a therapeutic advantage has not been established. Should be administered under the supervision of a physician experienced in the use of antimetabolite therapy. Immune suppression may lead to potentially fatal opportunistic infections, including *Pneumocystis jirovecii* pneumonia (PCP). Methotrexate use increases the risk for developing life-threatening or fatal bacterial, fungal, or viral infections, including invasive fungal infections, hepatitis B reactivation, tuberculosis (primary infection or reactivation), disseminated herpes zoster infection and/or cytomegalovirus infection. Use methotrexate with extreme caution in patients with an active infection (contraindicated in patients with immunodeficiency syndrome). Monitor for signs/symptoms of infection during and after treatment; manage promptly if infections occurs. Dose reduction or discontinuation may be necessary for serious infection. **[US Boxed Warnings]: Use only preservative-free methotrexate formulations and diluents for intrathecal and high-dose therapy. Do NOT use formulations or diluents containing preservatives for intrathecal and high-dose therapy because they contain benzyl alcohol. Methotrexate has been reported to cause fetal death and/or congenital abnormalities. Methotrexate is not recommended for women of childbearing potential unless there is clear medical evidence that the benefits can be expected to outweigh the considered risks. Pregnant women with psoriasis or rheumatoid arthritis should not receive methotrexate. Some products are contraindicated in pregnant women.** May cause impairment of fertility, oligospermia, and menstrual dysfunction; it is not known if fertility impairment is reversible. Toxicity from methotrexate or any immunosuppressive is increased in the elderly. Methotrexate injection may contain benzyl alcohol and should not be used in neonates. Errors have occurred (some resulting in death) when methotrexate was administered as a "daily" dose instead of a "weekly" dose intended for some indications. The ISMP Targeted Medication Safety Best Practices for Hospitals recommends hospitals use a weekly dosage regimen default for oral methotrexate orders, with a hard stop override requiring verification of appropriate oncology indication; manual systems should require verification of an oncology indication prior to dispensing oral methotrexate for daily administration. Pharmacists should provide patient education for patients discharged on weekly oral methotrexate; education should include written leaflets that contain clear instructions about the weekly dosing schedule and explain the danger of taking extra doses (ISMP 2014).

When used for intrathecal administration, should not be prepared during the preparation of any other agents; after preparation, store intrathecal medications in an isolated location or container clearly marked with a label identifying as "intrathecal" use only; delivery of intrathecal medications to the patient should only be with other medications intended for administration into the central nervous system (Jacobson 2009).

Benzyl alcohol and derivatives: Some dosage forms may contain benzyl alcohol; large amounts of benzyl alcohol ($\geq$99 mg/kg/day) have been associated with a potentially fatal toxicity ("gasping syndrome") in neonates; the "gasping syndrome" consists of metabolic acidosis, respiratory distress, gasping respirations, CNS dysfunction (including convulsions, intracranial hemorrhage), hypotension, and cardiovascular collapse (AAP ["Inactive" 1997]; CDC 1982); some data suggests that benzoate displaces bilirubin from protein binding sites (Ahlfors 2001); avoid or use dosage forms containing benzyl alcohol with caution in neonates. See manufacturer's labeling.

Glucarpidase is an enzyme that rapidly hydrolyzes extracellular methotrexate into inactive metabolites, allowing for a rapid reduction of methotrexate concentrations. Glucarpidase may be used for methotrexate overexposure; it is approved for the treatment of toxic plasma methotrexate concentrations (>1 micromole/L) in patients with delayed clearance due to renal impairment.

Adverse Reactions Note: Adverse reactions vary by route and dosage. Frequency not always defined.

Cardiovascular: Arterial thrombosis, cerebral thrombosis, chest pain, deep vein thrombosis, hypotension, pericardial effusion, pericarditis, plaque erosion (psoriasis), pulmonary embolism, retinal thrombosis, thrombophlebitis, vasculitis

Central nervous system: Dizziness ($\leq$3%), headache (pJIA 1%), abnormal cranial sensation, brain disease, chemical arachnoiditis (intrathecal; acute), chills, cognitive dysfunction (has been reported at low dosage), drowsiness, fatigue, leukoencephalopathy (intravenous administration after craniospinal irradiation or repeated high-dose therapy; may be chronic), malaise, mood changes (has been reported at low dosage), neurological signs and symptoms (at high dosages; including confusion, hemiparesis, transient blindness, seizures, and coma), severe neurotoxicity (reported with unexpectedly increased frequency among pediatric patients with acute lymphoblastic leukemia who were treated with intermediate-dose intravenous methotrexate), speech disturbance

Dermatologic: Alopecia (≤10%), burning sensation of skin (psoriasis 3% to 10%), skin photosensitivity (3% to 10%), skin rash (≤3%), dermatitis (rheumatoid arthritis 1% to 3%), pruritus (rheumatoid arthritis 1% to 3%), acne vulgaris, dermal ulcer, diaphoresis, ecchymoses, erythema multiforme, erythematous rash, exfoliative dermatitis, furunculosis, hyperpigmentation, hypopigmentation, skin abnormalities related to radiation recall, skin necrosis, Stevens-Johnson syndrome, telangiectasia, toxic epidermal necrolysis, urticaria

Endocrine & metabolic: Decreased libido, decreased serum albumin, diabetes mellitus, gynecomastia, menstrual disease

Gastrointestinal: Diarrhea (≤11%), nausea and vomiting (≤11%), stomatitis (2% to 10%), abdominal distress, anorexia, aphthous stomatitis, enteritis, gastrointestinal hemorrhage, gingivitis, hematemesis, intestinal perforation, melena

Genitourinary: Azotemia, cystitis, defective oogenesis, defective spermatogenesis, dysuria, hematuria, impotence, infertility, oligospermia, pancreatitis, proteinuria, severe renal disease, vaginal discharge

Hematologic & oncologic: Thrombocytopenia (rheumatoid arthritis 3% to 10%; platelet count <100,000/mm^3), leukopenia (1% to 3%; WBC <3000/mm^3), pancytopenia (rheumatoid arthritis 1% to 3%), agranulocytosis, anemia, aplastic anemia, bone marrow depression (nadir: 7-10 days), decreased hematocrit, eosinophilia, gastric ulcer, hypogammaglobulinemia, lymphadenopathy, lymphoma, lymphoproliferative disorder, neutropenia, non-Hodgkin's lymphoma (in patients receiving low-dose oral methotrexate), tumor lysis syndrome

Hepatic: Increased liver enzymes (14% to 15%), cirrhosis (chronic therapy), hepatic failure, hepatic fibrosis (chronic therapy), hepatitis (acute), hepatotoxicity

Hypersensitivity: Anaphylactoid reaction

Infection: Cryptococcosis, cytomegalovirus disease (including cytomegaloviral pneumonia, sepsis, nocardiosis), herpes simplex infection, herpes zoster, histoplasmosis, infection, vaccinia (disseminated; following smallpox immunization)

Neuromuscular & skeletal: Arthralgia, myalgia, myelopathy (subacute), osteonecrosis (with radiotherapy), osteoporosis

Ophthalmic: Blurred vision, conjunctivitis, eye pain, visual disturbance

Otic: Tinnitus

Renal: Renal failure

Respiratory: Interstitial pneumonitis (rheumatoid arthritis 1%), chronic obstructive pulmonary disease, cough, epistaxis, pharyngitis, pneumonia (including *Pneumocystis jirovecii*), pulmonary alveolitis, pulmonary disease, pulmonary fibrosis, respiratory failure, upper respiratory tract infection

Miscellaneous: Fever, nodule, tissue necrosis

<1%, postmarketing, and/or case reports: Acute respiratory distress (Morgan 2011), bone fracture (stress), cerebrovascular accident (Morgan 2011), mesenteric ischemia (acute; Morgan 2011)

Drug Interactions

Metabolism/Transport Effects Substrate of BCRP, OAT3, P-glycoprotein, SLCO1B1

Avoid Concomitant Use

Avoid concomitant use of Methotrexate with any of the following: Acitretin; BCG (Intravesical); Deferiprone; Dipyrone; Foscarnet; Natalizumab; Pimecrolimus; Tacrolimus (Topical)

Increased Effect/Toxicity

Methotrexate may increase the levels/effects of: CloZAPine; CycloSPORINE (Systemic); Deferiprone; Dipyrone; Fingolimod; Leflunomide; Loop Diuretics; Natalizumab; Tegafur; Theophylline Derivatives; Tofacitinib; Vaccines (Live)

The levels/effects of Methotrexate may be increased by: Acitretin; Alitretinoin (Systemic); Ciprofloxacin (Systemic); CycloSPORINE (Systemic); Denosumab; Dexketoprofen; Diethylamine Salicylate; Dipyrone; Eltrombopag; Foscarnet; Fosphenytoin-Phenytoin; Gemfibrozil; Ibrutinib; LevETIRAcetam; Loop Diuretics; Lumacaftor; Mipomersen; Nonsteroidal Anti-Inflammatory Agents; Ocrelizumab; Palifermin; Penicillins; P-glycoprotein/ABCB1 Inhibitors; Pimecrolimus; Probenecid; Promazine; Proton Pump Inhibitors; Ranolazine; Roflumilast; Salicylates; SulfaSALAzine; Sulfonamide Derivatives; Tacrolimus (Topical); Teriflunomide; Trastuzumab; Trimethoprim

Decreased Effect

Methotrexate may decrease the levels/effects of: BCG (Intravesical); Coccidioides immitis Skin Test; Fosphenytoin-Phenytoin; Lenograstim; Loop Diuretics; Nivolumab; Sapropterin; Sipuleucel-T; Tertomotide; Vaccines (Inactivated); Vaccines (Live)

The levels/effects of Methotrexate may be decreased by: Bile Acid Sequestrants; Cephalothin; Echinacea; Lumacaftor; P-glycoprotein/ABCB1 Inducers

Food Interactions Methotrexate peak serum levels may be decreased if taken with food. Milk-rich foods may decrease methotrexate absorption. Management: Administer without regard to food.

Hazardous Drugs Handling Considerations

Hazardous agent (NIOSH 2016 [group 1]).

Use appropriate precautions for receiving, handling, administration, and disposal. Gloves (single) should be worn during receiving, unpacking, and placing in storage. NIOSH recommends single gloving for administration of intact tablets or capsules. Double gloving, a protective gown, and (if there is a potential for vomit or spit up) eye/face protection are recommended for administration of an oral liquid/feeding tube administration. For injection preparation, NIOSH recommends double gloving, a protective gown, ventilated engineering controls (a class II biological safety cabinet or a compounding aseptic containment isolator), and closed system transfer devices (CSTDs). Double gloving, a gown, and (if dosage form allows) CSTDs are required during injection administration (NIOSH 2016).

Storage/Stability

Tablets: Store between 20°C and 25°C (68°F and 77°F). Protect from light.

Injection: Store intact vials and autoinjectors between 20°C and 25°C (68°F and 77°F); excursions may be permitted between 15°C and 30°C (59°F and 86°F). Protect from light.

IV: Solution diluted in D5W or NS is stable for 24 hours at room temperature (21°C to 25°C).

Intrathecal: Intrathecal dilutions are preservative free and should be used as soon as possible after preparation. After preparation, store intrathecal medications (until use) in an isolated location or container clearly marked with a label identifying as "intrathecal" use only.

Oral solution: Prior to dispensing, store at 2°C to 8°C (36°F to 46°F). Avoid freezing and excessive heat. After dispensing, patients may store methotrexate oral solution at room temperature (20°C to 25°C [68°F to 77°F]) for up to 60 days; excursions permitted to 15°C to 30°C (59°F to 86°F).

Preparation for Administration Use preservative-free preparations for intrathecal or high-dose methotrexate administration.

IV: Dilute powder with D5W or NS to a concentration of ≤25 mg/mL (20 mg and 50 mg vials) and 50 mg/mL (1 g vial). May further dilute in D5W or NS.

Intrathecal: Prepare intrathecal solutions with preservative-free NS, lactated Ringer's, or Elliot's B solution to a final volume of up to 12 mL (volume generally based on institution or practitioner preference). Intrathecal methotrexate concentrations may be institution specific or based on practitioner preference, generally ranging from a final concentration of 1 mg/mL (per prescribing information; Grossman 1993; Lin 2008) up to ~2 to 4 mg/mL (de Lemos 2009; Glantz 1999). For triple intrathecal therapy (methotrexate 12 mg/hydrocortisone 24 mg/cytarabine 36 mg), preparation to final volume of 12 mL is reported (Lin 2008). Intrathecal medications should **NOT** be prepared during the preparation of any other agents.

Mechanism of Action Methotrexate is a folate antimetabolite that inhibits DNA synthesis, repair, and cellular replication. Methotrexate irreversibly binds to and inhibits dihydrofolate reductase, inhibiting the formation of reduced folates, and thymidylate synthetase, resulting in inhibition of purine and thymidylic acid synthesis, thus interfering with DNA synthesis, repair, and cellular replication. Methotrexate is cell cycle specific for the S phase of the cycle. Actively proliferative tissues are more susceptible to the effects of methotrexate.

The MOA in the treatment of rheumatoid arthritis and polyarticular-course juvenile idiopathic arthritis is unknown, but may affect immune function. In psoriasis, methotrexate is thought to target rapidly proliferating epithelial cells in the skin.

In Crohn disease, it may have immune modulator and anti-inflammatory activity.

Pharmacodynamics/Kinetics

Onset of action: Antirheumatic: 3 to 6 weeks; additional improvement may continue longer than 12 weeks

Absorption:

Oral: Highly variable; dose dependent; decreased absorption at higher doses (pediatric patients: >40 mg/m^2; adult patients: >80 mg/m^2); possibly due to saturation effect

IM injection: Complete

Distribution: Penetrates slowly into third space fluids (eg, pleural effusions, ascites), exits slowly from these compartments (slower than from plasma); sustained concentrations retained in kidney and liver

V_d: IV: 0.18 L/kg (initial); 0.4 to 0.8 L/kg (steady state)

Protein binding: ~50%

Metabolism: Partially metabolized by intestinal flora (after oral administration) to DAMPA by carboxypeptidase; hepatic aldehyde oxidase converts methotrexate to 7-hydroxy methotrexate; polyglutamates are produced intracellularly and are just as potent as methotrexate; their production is dose- and duration-dependent and they are slowly eliminated by the cell once formed. Polyglutamated forms can be converted back to methotrexate.

Bioavailability: Oral: Children: Highly variable: 23% to 95%; Adults: Low doses (≤30 mg/m^2): ~60%; in general, bioavailability is dose dependent and decreases as the dose increases (especially at doses >80 mg/m^2 [>40 mg/m^2 in pediatric patients])

◄ Half-life elimination:
  Children: ALL: 0.7 to 5.8 hours (dose range: 6.3 to 30 mg/m^2); pJIA: 0.9 to 2.3 hours (dose range: 3.75 to 26.2 mg/m^2)
  Adults: Low dose: 3 to 10 hours; High dose: 8 to 15 hours
Time to peak, serum: Oral: Children: 0.7 to 4 hours (reported for a 15 mg/m^2 dose); Adults: 1 to 2 hours; IM: Children and Adults: 30 to 60 minutes
Excretion: Dose and route dependent; IV: Urine (80% to 90% as unchanged drug; 5% to 7% as 7-hydroxy methotrexate); feces (<10%)

Dosing

Adult Note: Methotrexate doses between 100 to 500 mg/m^2 **may require** leucovorin calcium rescue. Doses >500 mg/m^2 **require** leucovorin calcium rescue (refer to Dosing: Adjustment for Toxicity for leucovorin calcium dosing). Doses ≥250 mg/m^2 (IV) are associated with moderate emetic potential. Antiemetics may be recommended to prevent nausea and vomiting.

Acute lymphoblastic leukemia (ALL):
  Meningeal leukemia prophylaxis or treatment: Intrathecal: Manufacturer's labeling: 12 mg (maximum 15 mg/dose) every 2 to 7 days; continue for 1 dose beyond CSF cell count normalization. **Note:** Optimal intrathecal chemotherapy dosing should be based on age rather than on body surface area (BSA); CSF volume correlates with age and not to BSA (Bleyer 1983; Kerr 2001).
  CALGB 8811 regimen (Larson 1995; combination therapy):
    Early intensification: Intrathecal: 15 mg day 1 of early intensification phase, repeat in 4 weeks
    CNS prophylaxis/interim maintenance phase:
    Intrathecal: 15 mg day 1, 8, 15, 22, and 29
    Oral: 20 mg/m^2 days 36, 43, 50, 57, and 64
    Prolonged maintenance: Oral: 20 mg/m^2 days 1, 8, 15, and 22 every 4 weeks for 24 months from diagnosis
  Dose-intensive regimen (Kantarjian 2000; combination therapy):
    IV: 200 mg/m^2 over 2 hours, followed by 800 mg/m^2 over 24 hours beginning day 1, (followed by leucovorin rescue) of even numbered cycles (in combination with cytarabine; alternates with Hyper-CVAD)
    CNS prophylaxis: Intrathecal: 12 mg on day 2 of each cycle; duration depends on risk
    Maintenance: IV: 10 mg/m^2/day for 5 days every month for 2 years (in combination with prednisone, vincristine, and mercaptopurine)
  Breast cancer: IV: CMF regimen: 40 mg/m^2 days 1 and 8 every 4 weeks (in combination with cyclophosphamide and fluorouracil) for 6 to 12 cycles (Bonadonna 1995; Levine 1998)
  Choriocarcinoma, chorioadenoma, gestational trophoblastic diseases: 15 to 30 mg oral or IM daily for a 5 day course; may repeat for 3 to 5 courses (manufacturer's labeling) **or** 100 mg/m^2 IV over 30 minutes followed by 200 mg/m^2 IV over 12 hours (with leucovorin 24 hours after the start of methotrexate), administer a second course if hCG levels plateau for 3 consecutive weeks (Garrett 2002) **or** 100 mg/m^2 IV push followed by 200 mg/m^2 IV over 12 hours on day 1 (with leucovorin 24 hours after the start of methotrexate; in combination with dactinomycin, etoposide, vincristine, and cyclophosphamide) every 14 days and continuing for at least 2 cycles after hCG level is normal (Escobar 2003; Lurain 2006)

Head and neck cancer, advanced: IV: 40 mg/m^2 once weekly until disease progression or unacceptable toxicity (Forastiere 1992; Guardiola 2004; Stewart 2009)

Lymphoma, non-Hodgkin: IV:

  CODOX-M/IVAC regimen (Mead 2008): Cycles 1 and 3 of CODOX-M (CODOX-M alternates with IVAC)

  Adults ≤65 years: IV: 300 mg/m^2 over 1 hour (on day 10) followed by 2,700 mg/m^2 over 23 hours (with leucovorin rescue)

  Adults >65 years: IV: 100 mg/m^2 over 1 hour (on day 10) followed by 900 mg/m^2 over 23 hours (with leucovorin rescue)

  Hyper-CVAD alternating with high-dose methotrexate/cytarabine regimen: IV: 1,000 mg/m^2 over 24 hours on day 1 during even courses (2, 4, 6, and 8) of 21-day treatment cycles (Thomas 2006) **or** 200 mg/m^2 bolus day 1 followed by 800 mg/m^2 over 24 hours during even courses (2, 4, 6, and 8) of 21-day treatment cycles (Khouri 1998) with leucovorin rescue

Mycosis fungoides (cutaneous T-cell lymphoma): 5 to 50 mg once weekly or 15 to 37.5 mg twice weekly orally or IM for early stages (manufacturer's labeling) **or** 25 mg orally once weekly, may increase to 50 mg once weekly (Zackheim 2003)

Osteosarcoma: Adults ≤30 years: IV: MAP regimen: 12 g/m^2 (maximum: 20 g/dose) over 4 hours (followed by leucovorin rescue) for 4 doses during induction (before surgery) at weeks 4, 5, 9, and 10, and for 8 doses during maintenance (after surgery) at weeks 15, 16, 20, 21, 24, 25, 28, and 29 (in combination with doxorubicin and cisplatin) (Bielack 2015; Whelan 2015); other combinations, intervals, age ranges, and doses (8 to 14 g/m^2/dose) have been described (with leucovorin rescue), refer to specific reference for details (Bacci 2000; Bacci 2003; Goorin 2003; Le Deley 2007; Meyers 1992; Meyers 2005; Weiner 1986; Winkler 1988)

Psoriasis: Note: Some experts recommend concomitant folic acid 1 to 5 mg daily (except the day of methotrexate) to reduce hematologic, gastrointestinal, and hepatic adverse events related to methotrexate.

  Oral: Initial: 2.5 to 5 mg/dose every 12 hours for 3 doses per week **or**

  Oral, IM, IV, SubQ: Initial: 10 to 25 mg given once weekly; adjust dose gradually to optimal response (doses above 20 mg once weekly are associated with an increased incidence of toxicity); doses >30 mg per week should not be exceeded.

  Note: An initial test dose of 2.5 to 5 mg is recommended in patients with risk factors for hematologic toxicity or renal impairment. (Kalb 2009).

Rheumatoid arthritis: Note: Some experts recommend concomitant folic acid at a dose of at least 5 mg per week (except the day of methotrexate) to reduce hematologic, gastrointestinal, and hepatic adverse events related to methotrexate.

  Oral (manufacturer labeling): Initial: 7.5 mg once weekly or 2.5 mg every 12 hours for 3 doses per week; adjust dose gradually to optimal response (dosage exceeding 20 mg once weekly are associated with an increased incidence of toxicity; *alternatively*, 10 to 15 mg once weekly, increased by 5 mg every 2 to 4 weeks to a maximum of 20 to 30 mg once weekly has been recommended by some experts. Consider parenteral therapy with inadequate response or intolerance to oral therapy (Visser 2009).

  SubQ: Initial: 7.5 mg once weekly; adjust dose gradually to optimal response (doses above 20 mg once weekly are associated with an increased incidence of toxicity)

◄ IM: 7.5 mg once weekly; adjust dose gradually to optimal response (doses above 20 mg once weekly are associated with an increased incidence of toxicity)

Off-label uses:

Acute promyelocytic leukemia (APL) maintenance phase:
Oral: 15 mg/m^2 once weekly for 2 years (Ades 2008) or 20 mg/m^2 once weekly for 1 year (Powell 2010)
IM: 15 mg/m^2 once weekly for 2 years (Sanz 2004)

Bladder cancer (off-label use):
Dose-dense MVAC regimen: 30 mg/m^2 day 1 every 2 weeks (in combination with vinblastine, doxorubicin, and cisplatin) (Sternberg 2001)
CMV regimen: 30 mg/m^2 days 1 and 8 every 3 weeks for 3 cycles (in combination with cisplatin, vinblastine and leucovorin rescue) (Griffiths 2011)

CNS lymphoma (off-label use): IV: 8,000 mg/m^2 over 4 hours (followed by leucovorin rescue) every 14 days until complete response or a maximum of 8 cycles; if complete response, follow with 2 consolidation cycles at the same dose every 14 days (with leucovorin rescue), followed by 11 maintenance cycles of 8,000 mg/m^2 every 28 days with leucovorin rescue (Batchelor 2003) **or** 2,500 mg/m^2 over 2 to 3 hours every 14 days for 5 doses (in combination with vincristine, procarbazine, intrathecal methotrexate, leucovorin, dexamethasone, and cytarabine) (De Angelis 2002) **or** 3,500 mg/m^2 over 2 hours on day 2 every 2 weeks (in combination with rituximab, vincristine, procarbazine, and leucovorin [with intra-omaya methotrexate 12 mg between days 5 and 12 of each cycle if positive CSF cytology]) for 5 to 7 induction cycles (Shah 2007)

Crohn disease, moderate/severe, corticosteroid-dependent or refractory (off-label use):
Remission induction or reduction of steroid use: IM, SubQ: 25 mg once weekly (Lichtenstein 2009)
Remission maintenance: IM: 15 mg once weekly (Feagan 2000; Lichtenstein 2009)

Dermatomyositis/polymyositis (off-label uses):
Oral: Initial: 7.5 to 15 mg per week, often adjunctively with high-dose corticosteroid therapy; may increase in weekly 2.5 mg increments to target dose of 10 to 25 mg per week (**Note:** Administration of folate 5 to 7 mg per week has been used to reduce side effects) (Briemberg 2003; Newman 1995; Wiendl 2008).
IV, IM: Doses of 20 to 60 mg/week have been employed if failure with oral therapy (doses >50 mg/week may require leucovorin calcium rescue) (Briemberg 2003)

Ectopic pregnancy (off-label use): IM:
Single-dose regimen: Methotrexate 50 mg/m^2 on day 1; Measure serum hCG levels on days 4 and 7; if needed, repeat dose on day 7 (ACOG 2008; ASRM 2006; Barnhart 2009)
Two-dose regimen: Methotrexate 50 mg/m^2 on day 1; Measure serum hCG levels on day 4 and administer a second dose of methotrexate 50 mg/m^2; Measure serum hCG levels on day 7 and if needed, administer a third dose of 50 mg/m^2 (ACOG 2008; Barnhart 2009)

Multidose regimen: Methotrexate 1 mg/kg on day 1; leucovorin calcium 0.1 mg/kg IM on day 2; measure serum hCG on day 2; methotrexate 1 mg/kg on day 3; leucovorin calcium 0.1 mg/kg on day 4; measure serum hCG on day 4; continue up to a total of 4 courses based on hCG concentrations (ACOG 2008; ASRM 2006; Barnhart 2009)

Graft-versus-host disease, acute (aGVHD), prophylaxis: IV: 15 mg/m^2/dose on day 1 and 10 mg/m^2/dose on days 3 and 6 after allogeneic transplant (in combination with cyclosporine and prednisone) (Chao 1993; Chao 2000; Ross 1999) **or** 15 mg/m^2/dose on day 1 and 10 mg/m^2/dose on days 3, 6, and 11 after allogeneic transplant (in combination with cyclosporine) (Chao 2000) **or** 15 mg/m^2/dose on day 1 and 10 mg/m^2/dose on days 3, 6, and 11 after allogeneic transplant (in combination with cyclosporine, followed by leucovorin); may omit day 11 methotrexate for grade 2 or higher toxicity (Ruutu 2013)

Multiple sclerosis (off-label use): Oral: 7.5 or 20 mg once weekly either alone or as add-on therapy to interferon beta-1a (Calabresi 2002; Goodkin 1996; Lugaresi 2001)

Nonleukemic meningeal cancer (off-label uses): Intrathecal: 12 mg/dose twice weekly for 4 weeks, then weekly for 4 doses, then monthly for 4 doses (Glantz 1998) **or** 10 mg twice weekly for 4 weeks, then weekly for 1 month, then every 2 weeks for 2 months (Glantz 1999) **or** 10 to 15 mg twice weekly for 4 weeks, then once weekly for 4 weeks, then a maintenance regimen of once a month (Chamberlain 2010)

Soft tissue sarcoma (desmoid tumors, aggressive fibromatosis), advanced (off-label use): IV: 30 mg/m^2 every 7 to 10 days (dose usually rounded to 50 mg) in combination with vinblastine for 1 year (Azzarelli 2001)

Systemic lupus erythematosus, moderate-to-severe (off-label use): Oral: Initial: 7.5 mg once weekly; may increase by 2.5 mg increments weekly (maximum: 20 mg once weekly), in combination with prednisone (Fortin 2008)

Takayasu arteritis, refractory or relapsing disease (off-label use): Oral: Initial dose: 0.3 mg/kg/week (maximum: 15 mg per week), titrated by 2.5 mg increments every 1 to 2 weeks until reaching a maximum tolerated weekly dose of 25 mg (use in combination with a corticosteroid; Hoffman 1994)

Uveitis (off-label use): Oral: 7.5 to 20 mg once weekly either alone or in conjunction with other corticosteroids/immunosuppressants (Diaz-Llopis 2009; Galor 2008; Kaplan-Messas 2003; Munoz-Fernandez 2009)

Geriatric Refer to adult dosing; adjust for renal impairment.

Breast cancer: Patients >60 years: IV: CMF regimen: 30 mg/m^2 days 1 and 8 every 4 weeks (in combination with cyclophosphamide and fluorouracil) for up to 12 cycles (Bonadonna 1995)

Meningeal leukemia: Intrathecal: Consider a dose reduction (CSF volume and turnover may decrease with age)

Non-Hodgkin lymphoma: CODOX-M/IVAC regimen (Mead 2008): Cycles 1 and 3 of CODOX-M (CODOX-M alternates with IVAC): IV: 100 mg over 1 hour (on day 10) followed by 900 mg over 23 hours (with leucovorin rescue)

Rheumatoid arthritis/psoriasis: Oral: Initial: 5 to 7.5 mg per week, not to exceed 20 mg per week

◄ **Pediatric Note:** Methotrexate doses between 100 to 500 mg/m^2 **may require** leucovorin calcium rescue. Doses >500 mg/m^2 **require** leucovorin calcium rescue (refer to Dosing: Adjustment for Toxicity for leucovorin calcium dosing). In children, doses ≥12 g/m^2 (IV) are associated with a high emetic potential; doses ≥250 mg/m^2 (IV) are associated with moderate emetic potential (Dupuis 2011). Antiemetics may be recommended to prevent nausea and vomiting.

Polyarticular juvenile idiopathic arthritis (pJIA): Oral, IM, SubQ: Initial: 10 mg/m^2 once weekly, adjust gradually to optimum response; doses up to 20 to 30 mg/m^2 once weekly (0.65 to 1 mg/kg/week) have been used (doses above 20 mg/m^2 once weekly may be associated with an increased risk of toxicity)

Acute lymphoblastic leukemia (ALL; intrathecal therapy is also administered [refer to specific reference]):
Consolidation/intensification phases (as part of a combination regimen): 1,000 mg/m^2 IV over 24 hours in week 1 of intensification and 20 mg/m^2 IM (use 50% dose reduction if on same day as intrathecal methotrexate) on day 1 of week 2 of intensification phase; Intensification repeats every 2 weeks for a total of 12 courses (Mahoney 2000) **or** 5000 mg/m^2 IV over 24 hours days 8, 22, 36, and 50 of consolidation phase (Schrappe 2000) with leucovorin rescue

Interim maintenance (as part of a combination regimen): 15 mg/m^2 orally days 0, 7, 14, 21, 28, and 35 of interim maintenance phase (Seibel 2008) **or** 100 mg/m^2 (escalate dose by 50 mg/m^2 each dose) IV days 0, 10, 20, 30, and 40 of increased intensity interim maintenance phase (Seibel 2008)

Maintenance (as part of a combination regimen; adjust dose for excessive hematologic toxicity): 20 mg/m^2 IM once weekly on day 1 of weeks 25 to 130 (Mahoney 2000) **or** 20 mg/m^2 orally days 7, 14, 21, 28, 35, 42, 49, 56, 63, 70, and 77 (Seibel 2008)

T-cell acute lymphoblastic leukemia (Asselin 2011; triple intrathecal therapy is also administered [refer to specific reference]):
Induction (weeks 1 to 6; as part of a combination regimen): IV:
Low dose: 40 mg/m^2 day 2
High dose: 500 mg/m^2 over 30 minutes followed by 4500 mg/m^2 over 23.5 hours (with leucovorin rescue) day 22
Consolidation (weeks 7 to 33; combination chemotherapy): IV: High dose: 500 mg/m^2 over 30 minutes followed by 4500 mg/m^2 over 23.5 hours (with leucovorin rescue) in weeks 7, 10, and 13 with leucovorin rescue
Continuation (weeks 34 to 108; combination chemotherapy): IV, IM: 30 mg/m^2 weekly until 2 years after documented complete remission

ALL, CNS prophylaxis triple intrathecal therapy (off-label dosing): Intrathecal: Age-based dosing (in combination with cytarabine and hydrocortisone): Days of administration vary based on risk status and protocol; refer to institutional protocols or reference for details (Matloub 2006):
<2 years: 8 mg
2 to <3 years: 10 mg
3 to ≤8 years: 12 mg
>8 years: 15 mg

Meningeal leukemia, prophylaxis or treatment: Intrathecal: 6 to 12 mg/dose (based on age) every 2 to 7 days; continue for 1 dose beyond CSF cell count normalization. **Note:** Optimal intrathecal chemotherapy dosing should be based on age rather than on body surface area (BSA); CSF volume correlates with age and not to BSA (Bleyer 1983; Kerr 2001):

<1 year: 6 mg/dose
1 year: 8 mg/dose
2 years: 10 mg/dose
≥3 years: 12 mg/dose

Osteosarcoma: IV: MAP regimen: 12 g/m^2 (maximum: 20 g/dose) over 4 hours (followed by leucovorin rescue) for 4 doses during induction (before surgery) at weeks 4, 5, 9, and 10, and for 8 doses during maintenance (after surgery) at weeks 15, 16, 20, 21, 24, 25, 28, and 29 (in combination with doxorubicin and cisplatin) (Bielack 2015; Whelan 2015); other combinations, intervals, and doses (8 to 14 g/m^2/dose) have been described (with leucovorin rescue), refer to specific reference for details (Bacci 2000; Bacci 2003; Goorin 2003; Le Deley 2007; Meyers 1992; Meyers 2005; Weiner 1986; Winkler 1988)

Crohn disease, induction and maintenance (off-label use): SubQ: 15 mg/m^2 once weekly; maximum dose: 25 mg (Rufo 2012)

Dermatomyositis (off-label use): Oral, SubQ (preferred): The lesser of 15 mg/m^2 or 1 mg/kg once weekly (maximum dose: 40 mg/week) in combination with corticosteroids (Huber 2010) **or** 15 mg/m^2 once weekly (range: 10 to 20 mg/m^2 once weekly; maximum dose: 25 mg/week) in combination with prednisone (Ramanan 2005)

Graft-versus-host disease, acute (aGVHD) prophylaxis (off-label use): IV: Refer to adult dosing.

Renal Impairment There are no dosage adjustments provided in the manufacturer's labeling. The following adjustments have been recommended:

Aronoff 2007:
Adults:
CrCl 10 to 50 mL/minute: Administer 50% of dose
CrCl <10 mL/minute: Avoid use
Intermittent hemodialysis: Administer 50% of dose (post dialysis)
Continuous renal replacement therapy (CRRT): Administer 50% of dose
Children:
CrCl 10 to 50 mL/minute/1.73 m^2: Administer 50% of dose
CrCl <10 mL/minute/1.73 m^2: Administer 30% of dose
Intermittent hemodialysis: Administer 30% of dose (post dialysis)
Continuous ambulatory peritoneal dialysis (CAPD): Administer 30% of dose
Continuous renal replacement therapy (CRRT): Administer 50% of dose

Kintzel 1995:
CrCl 46 to 60 mL/minute: Administer 65% of normal dose
CrCl 31 to 45 mL/minute: Administer 50% of normal dose
CrCl <30 mL/minute: Avoid use

Hemodialysis patients with cancer (Janus 2010): Administer 25% of dose after hemodialysis; monitor closely for toxicity

High-dose methotrexate, dose-intensive regimen for ALL (200 mg/m^2 over 2 hours, followed by 800 mg/m^2 over 24 hours with leucovorin rescue [Kantarjian 2000]):
Serum creatinine <1.5 mg/dL: No dosage adjustment necessary

◄

Serum creatinine 1.5 to 2 mg/dL: Administer 75% of dose
Serum creatinine >2 mg/dL: Administer 50% of dose

Hepatic Impairment There are no dosage adjustments provided in the manufacturer's labeling; use with caution in patients with impaired hepatic function or preexisting hepatic damage. The following adjustments have been recommended (Floyd 2006):

Bilirubin 3.1 to 5 mg/dL **or** transaminases >3 times ULN: Administer 75% of dose

Bilirubin >5 mg/dL: Avoid use

Obesity *ASCO Guidelines for appropriate chemotherapy dosing in obese adults with cancer (excludes leukemias):* Utilize patient's actual body weight (full weight) for calculation of body surface area- or weight-based dosing, particularly when the intent of therapy is curative; manage regimen-related toxicities in the same manner as for nonobese patients; if a dose reduction is utilized due to toxicity, consider resumption of full weight-based dosing with subsequent cycles, especially if cause of toxicity (eg, hepatic or renal impairment) is resolved (Griggs 2012).

Adjustment for Toxicity

Methotrexate toxicities:
Nonhematologic toxicity: Diarrhea, stomatitis, or vomiting which may lead to dehydration: Discontinue until recovery
Hematologic toxicity:
Psoriasis, rheumatoid arthritis: Significant blood count decrease: Discontinue immediately
Oncologic uses: Profound granulocytopenia and fever: Evaluate immediately; consider broad-spectrum parenteral antimicrobial coverage

Leucovorin calcium dosing (from methotrexate injection prescribing information; other leucovorin dosing/schedules may be specific to chemotherapy protocols):
Normal methotrexate elimination (serum methotrexate level ~10 micromolar at 24 hours after administration, 1 micromolar at 48 hours, and <0.2 micromolar at 72 hours): Leucovorin calcium 15 mg (oral, IM, or IV) every 6 hours for 60 hours (10 doses) beginning 24 hours after the start of methotrexate infusion
Delayed late methotrexate elimination (serum methotrexate level remaining >0.2 micromolar at 72 hours and >0.05 micromolar at 96 hours after administration): Continue leucovorin calcium 15 mg (oral, IM or IV) every 6 hours until methotrexate level is <0.05 micromolar
Delayed early methotrexate elimination and/or acute renal injury (serum methotrexate level ≥50 micromolar at 24 hours, or ≥5 micromolar at 48 hours, or a doubling of serum creatinine level at 24 hours after methotrexate administration): Leucovorin calcium 150 mg IV every 3 hours until methotrexate level is <1 micromolar, then 15 mg IV every 3 hours until methotrexate level <0.05 micromolar

Leucovorin nomogram dosing for high-dose methotrexate overexposure (**generalized dosing** derived from reference nomogram figures, refer to each reference [Bleyer 1978; Bleyer 1981; Widemann 2006] or institution-specific nomogram for details):

At 24 hours:
For methotrexate levels of ≥100 micromolar at ~24 hours, leucovorin is initially dosed at 1000 mg/m^2 every 6 hours
For methotrexate levels of ≥10 to <100 micromolar at 24 hours, leucovorin is initially dosed at 100 mg/m^2 every 3 or 6 hours

For methotrexate levels of ~1 to 10 micromolar at 24 hours, leucovorin is initially dosed at 10 mg/m² every 3 or 6 hours

At 48 hours:

For methotrexate levels of ≥100 micromolar at 48 hours, leucovorin is dosed at 1000 mg/m² every 6 hours

For methotrexate levels of ≥10 to <100 micromolar at 48 hours, leucovorin is dosed at 100 mg/m² every 3 hours

For methotrexate levels of ~1 to 10 micromolar at 48 hours, leucovorin is dosed at 100 mg/m² every 6 hours **or** 10 to 100 mg/m² every 3 hours

At 72 hours:

For methotrexate levels of ≥10 micromolar at 72 hours, leucovorin is dosed at 100 to 1000 mg/m² every 3 to 6 hours

For methotrexate levels of ~1 to 10 micromolar at 72 hours, leucovorin is dosed at 10 to 100 mg/m² every 3 hours

For methotrexate levels of ~0.1 to 1 micromolar at 72 hours, leucovorin is dosed at 10 mg/m² every 3 to 6 hours

If serum creatinine is increased more than 50% above baseline, increase the standard leucovorin dose to 100 mg/m² every 3 hours, then adjust according to methotrexate levels above.

Follow methotrexate levels daily, leucovorin may be discontinued when methotrexate level is <0.1 micromolar

Combination Regimens

Bladder cancer:

Bone sarcoma (osteosarcoma):

Breast cancer:

Gestational trophoblastic tumor:

Leukemia, acute lymphocytic:

Leukemia, acute promyelocytic:

Lymphoma, Hodgkin:

◀

Administration In children, doses ≥ 12 g/m^2 are associated with a high emetic potential; doses ≥ 250 mg/m^2 (IV) in adults and children are associated with moderate emetic potential (Dupuis 2011). Antiemetics may be recommended to prevent nausea and vomiting.

Methotrexate may be administered orally, IM, IV, intrathecally, or SubQ; IV administration may be as slow push (10 mg/minute), bolus infusion, or 24-hour continuous infusion (route and rate of administration depend on indication and/or protocol; refer to specific references). Must use preservative-free formulation for intrathecal or high-dose methotrexate administration.

Specific dosing schemes vary, but high doses should be followed by leucovorin calcium rescue to prevent toxicity.

Oral solution: Ensure accuracy when dispensing and administering to prevent dosing errors. A calibrated oral syringe/dosing cup that can measure and deliver the prescribed dose accurately should be used; do not use a household teaspoon or tablespoon to measure dose.

Otrexup and Rasuvo are autoinjectors for once weekly subcutaneous use in the abdomen or thigh; patient may self-administer after appropriate training. All schedules should be continually tailored to the individual patient. An initial test dose may be given prior to the regular dosing schedule to detect any extreme sensitivity to adverse effects.

Emetic Potential
Children:
IV:
≥ 12 g/m^2: High (>90%)
≥ 250 mg/m^2 to <12 g/m^2: Moderate (30% to 90%)
>50 mg/m^2 to <250 mg/m^2: Low (10% to 30%)
≤ 50 mg/m^2: Minimal (<10%)
Oral: Minimal (<10%)
Adults:
IV:
≥ 250 mg/m^2: Moderate (30% to 90%)
>50 to <250 mg/m^2: Low (10% to 30%)
≤ 50 mg/m^2: Minimal (<10%)
Oral: Minimal (<10%)

Monitoring Parameters
Oncologic uses: Baseline and frequently during treatment: CBC with differential and platelets, serum creatinine, BUN, liver function tests (LFTs); methotrexate levels and urine pH (with high-dose methotrexate); closely monitor fluid and electrolyte status in patients with impaired methotrexate elimination; chest x-ray (baseline); pulmonary function test (if methotrexate-induced lung disease suspected); monitor carefully for toxicities (due to

impaired elimination) in patients with ascites, pleural effusion, decreased folate stores, renal impairment, and/or hepatic impairment

Psoriasis (Kalb 2009; Menter 2009):

CBC with differential and platelets (baseline, 7 to 14 days after initiating therapy or dosage increase, every 2 to 4 weeks for first few months, then every 1 to 3 months depending on leukocyte count and stability of patient) monitor more closely in patients with risk factors for hematologic toxicity (eg, renal insufficiency, advanced age, hypoalbuminemia); BUN and serum creatinine (baseline and every 2 to 3 months) calculate glomerular filtration rate if at risk for renal dysfunction; consider PPD for latent TB screening (baseline); LFTs (baseline, monthly for first 6 months, then every 1 to 2 months; more frequently if at risk for hepatotoxicity or if clinically indicated; liver function tests should be performed at least 5 days after the last dose); pregnancy test (if female of reproductive potential); chest x-ray (baseline if underlying lung disease); pulmonary function test (if methotrexate-induced lung disease suspected)

Liver biopsy for patients **with** risk factors for hepatotoxicity: Baseline or after 2 to 6 months of therapy and with each 1 to 1.5 g cumulative dose interval

Liver biopsy for patients **without** risk factors for hepatotoxicity: If persistent elevations in 5 of 9 AST levels during a 12-month period, or decline of serum albumin below the normal range with normal nutritional status. Consider biopsy after cumulative dose of 3.5 to 4 g and after each additional 1.5 g.

Rheumatoid arthritis:

CBC with differential and platelets, serum creatinine, and LFTs: Baseline and every 2 to 4 weeks for 3 months after initiation or following dose increases, then every 8 to 12 weeks during 3 to 6 months of treatment, followed by every 12 weeks beyond 6 months of treatment; monitor more frequently if clinically indicated (Singh [ACR 2016]).

Chest x-ray (within 1 year prior to initiation), Hepatitis B and C serology (if at high risk); tuberculosis testing annually for patients who live, travel or work in areas with likely TB exposure (Kremer 1994).

Liver biopsy: Baseline (consider only for patients with persistent abnormal baseline LFTs, history of alcoholism, or chronic hepatitis B or C) or during treatment if persistent LFT elevations (6 of 12 tests abnormal over 1 year or 5 of 9 results when LFTs performed at 6-week intervals) (Kremer 1994).

Polyarticular-course juvenile idiopathic arthritis: Complete blood counts (at least monthly), renal function (every 1 to 2 months), liver function (every 1 to 2 months). Increase monitoring frequency during initial dosing, dose changes, or during periods of increased risk of elevated methotrexate blood levels (eg, dehydration). Pregnancy test (prior to initiation) in females of reproductive potential. Monitor pulmonary function tests if methotrexate-induced lung disease is suspected, especially if baseline values are available.

Crohn disease (off-label use; Lichtenstein 2009): CBC with differential and platelets (baseline and periodic) and liver function tests (baseline and every 1 to 2 months); baseline liver biopsy (in patients with abnormal baseline LFTs or with chronic liver disease); liver biopsy at 1 year if (over a 1-year span) AST consistently elevated or serum albumin consistently decreased; chest x-ray (baseline)

Ectopic pregnancy (off-label use; Barnhart 2009): Prior to therapy, measure serum hCG, CBC with differential and platelets, liver function tests, serum creatinine. Serum hCG concentrations should decrease between treatment days 4 and 7. If hCG decreases by >15%, additional courses are not needed however, continue to measure hCG weekly until no longer detectable. If <15% decrease is observed, repeat dose per regimen.

Dietary Considerations Some products may contain sodium.

Product Availability Xatmep (methotrexate 2.5 mg/mL oral solution): FDA approved April 2017; availability anticipated in June 2017. Consult the prescribing information for additional information.

Dosage Forms Excipient information presented when available (limited, particularly for generics); consult specific product labeling. [DSC] = Discontinued product

Solution, Injection:
Generic: 250 mg/10 mL (10 mL); 50 mg/2 mL (2 mL)

Solution, Injection [preservative free]:
Generic: 1 g/40 mL (40 mL); 100 mg/4 mL (4 mL); 200 mg/8 mL (8 mL); 250 mg/10 mL (10 mL); 50 mg/2 mL (2 mL)

Solution, Oral:
Xatmep: 2.5 mg/mL (120 mL) [contains methylparaben sodium, propylparaben sodium]

Solution Auto-injector, Subcutaneous [preservative free]:
Otrexup: 7.5 mg/0.4 mL (0.4 mL [DSC]); 10 mg/0.4 mL (0.4 mL); 12.5 mg/0.4 mL (0.4 mL); 15 mg/0.4 mL (0.4 mL); 17.5 mg/0.4 mL (0.4 mL); 20 mg/0.4 mL (0.4 mL); 22.5 mg/0.4 mL (0.4 mL); 25 mg/0.4mL (0.4 mL)
Rasuvo: 7.5 mg/0.15 mL (0.15 mL); 10 mg/0.2 mL (0.2 mL); 12.5 mg/0.25 mL (0.25 mL); 15 mg/0.3 mL (0.3 mL); 17.5 mg/0.35 mL (0.35 mL); 20 mg/0.4 mL (0.4 mL); 22.5 mg/0.45 mL (0.45 mL); 25 mg/0.5 mL (0.5 mL); 27.5 mg/0.55 mL (0.55 mL [DSC]); 30 mg/0.6 mL (0.6 mL)

Solution Reconstituted, Injection [preservative free]:
Generic: 1 g (1 ea)

Tablet, Oral:
Rheumatrex: 2.5 mg [DSC] [scored]
Trexall: 5 mg, 7.5 mg, 10 mg, 15 mg [scored]
Generic: 2.5 mg

Methylene Blue (METH i leen bloo)

Brand Names: US ProvayBlue

Index Terms Methylthionine Chloride; Methylthioninium Chloride

Pharmacologic Category Antidote; Phenothiazine Derivative

Use

Methemoglobinemia (acquired) (Provayblue only): Treatment of pediatric and adult patients with acquired methemoglobinemia

Methemoglobinemia (drug induced) (generic only): Treatment of drug-induced methemoglobinemia

Pregnancy Risk Factor X

Dosing

Adult & Geriatric

Methemoglobinemia (acquired): IV: 1 mg/kg over 5 to 30 minutes, may repeat dose 1 hour later if methemoglobin level remains above 30% or symptoms persist; consider alternative therapy if resolution does not occur after 2 doses

Methemoglobinemia (drug induced): IV: 1 to 2 mg/kg or 25 to 50 mg/m^2 over several minutes; may be repeated in 1 hour if necessary

Chromoendoscopy (off label use): Topical: 0.1% to 1% solution sprayed via catheter or directly applied onto gastrointestinal mucosa during procedure (Areia 2008; Ichimasa 2014; Kaminski 2014; Ngamruengphong 2009)

Ifosfamide-induced encephalopathy (off-label use): Oral, IV: **Note:** Treatment may not be necessary; encephalopathy may improve spontaneously (Patel 2006):

Prevention: 50 mg every 6 to 8 hours (Turner 2003). Additional data may be necessary to further define the role of methylene blue in this condition.

Treatment: 50 mg as a single dose or every 4 to 8 hours until symptoms resolve (Patel 2006; Turner 2003). Additional data may be necessary to further define the role of methylene blue in this condition.

Onychomycosis (toenail; off-label use): Topical: 2% solution applied to affected area(s) at 15 day intervals for 6 months; used in conjunction with photodynamic therapy (Figueiredo Souza 2014). Additional data may be necessary to further define the role of methylene blue in this condition.

Sentinel node mapping in breast cancer surgery (off label use): Intraparenchymal: 5 mg of a 1% solution administered once during procedure (Simmons 2001; Simmons 2003; Thevarajah 2005). Additional data may be necessary to further define the role of methylene blue in this condition.

Vasoplegia syndrome associated with cardiac surgery (off-label use): IV: 1.5 to 2 mg/kg over 20 to 60 minutes administered once (Levin 2004; Leyh 2003). **Note:** Improvement of vasoplegia (eg, increased systemic vascular resistance, reduced vasopressor dosage) has been observed within 1 to 2 hours following methylene blue administration. Some have employed the use of continuous infusion (0.5 to 1 mg/kg/hour) after administration of the bolus dose; however, prospective clinical trials are necessary to validate this dosing schema (Grayling 2003; Omar 2014; Weiner 2013).

Pediatric

Methemoglobinemia (acquired): Neonates, Infants, Children, and Adolescents: IV: Refer to adult dosing.

Methemoglobinemia (drug induced): Children and Adolescents: IV: Refer to adult dosing.

Renal Impairment There are no dosage adjustments provided in the manufacturer's labeling. However, use with caution in severe renal impairment.

Hepatic Impairment There are no dosage adjustments provided in the manufacturer's labeling.

Additional Information Complete prescribing information should be consulted for additional detail.

◄ **Dosage Forms** Excipient information presented when available (limited, particularly for generics); consult specific product labeling.
Solution, Injection:
Generic: 1% (1 mL, 10 mL)
Solution, Intravenous:
ProvayBlue: 50 mg/10 mL (10 mL)

Methylnaltrexone (meth il nal TREKS one)

Brand Names: US Relistor
Brand Names: Canada Relistor
Index Terms Methylnaltrexone Bromide; N-methylnaltrexone Bromide
Pharmacologic Category Gastrointestinal Agent, Miscellaneous; Opioid Antagonist, Peripherally-Acting

Use

Opioid-induced constipation with advanced illness (injection only): Treatment of opioid-induced constipation in adults with advanced illness or pain caused by active cancer who require opioid dosage escalation for palliative care.

Opioid-induced constipation with chronic non-cancer pain (tablets and injection): Treatment of opioid-induced constipation in adults with chronic non-cancer pain, including patients with chronic pain related to prior cancer or its treatment who do not require frequent (eg, weekly) opioid dosage escalation.

Dosing

Adult & Geriatric

Opioid-induced constipation with advanced illness: SubQ: Dosing is according to body weight: Administer 1 dose every other day as needed; maximum: 1 dose/24 hours
<38 kg: 0.15 mg/kg (round dose up to nearest 0.1 mL of volume)
38 to <62 kg: 8 mg
62 to 114 kg: 12 mg
>114 kg: 0.15 mg/kg (round dose up to nearest 0.1 mL of volume)

Opioid-induced constipation with chronic non-cancer pain: Note: Discontinue all maintenance laxatives prior to initiation of therapy; if response is not optimal after 3 days, laxative therapy may be reinitiated.
Oral: 450 mg once daily
SubQ: 12 mg once daily

Renal Impairment

CrCl ≥60 mL/minute: No dosage adjustment necessary.
CrCl <60 mL/minute:
Opioid-induced constipation with advanced illness: SubQ:
<38 kg: 0.075 mg/kg every other day (round dose up to nearest 0.1 mL of volume)
38 to <62 kg: 4 mg every other day
62 to 114 kg: 6 mg every other day
>114 kg: 0.075 mg/kg every other day (round dose up to nearest 0.1 mL of volume)
Opioid-induced constipation with chronic non-cancer pain:
Oral: 150 mg once daily
SubQ: 6 mg once daily
End-stage renal impairment (dialysis-dependent): There are no dosage adjustments provided in the manufacturer's labeling (has not been studied).

Hepatic Impairment

Opioid-induced constipation with advanced illness: There are no dosage adjustments provided in the manufacturer's labeling. For the injection, consider following the subcutaneous dosing recommendations for opioid-induced constipation with chronic non-cancer pain in patients with severe impairment (Child-Pugh class C).

Opioid-induced constipation with chronic non-cancer pain:

Oral:

Mild impairment (Child-Pugh class A): No dosage adjustment necessary.

Moderate or severe impairment (Child-Pugh class B and C): 150 mg once daily

SubQ:

Mild or moderate impairment (Child-Pugh class A or B): No dosage adjustment necessary.

Severe impairment (Child Pugh class C):

<38 kg: 0.075 mg/kg once daily (round dose up to nearest 0.1 mL of volume)

38 to <62 kg: 4 mg once daily

62 to 114 kg: 6 mg once daily

>114 kg: 0.075 mg/kg once daily (round dose up to nearest 0.1 mL of volume)

Additional Information Complete prescribing information should be consulted for additional detail.

Medication Guide Available Yes

Dosage Forms Excipient information presented when available (limited, particularly for generics); consult specific product labeling.

Kit, Subcutaneous:

Relistor: 12 mg/0.6 mL [contains edetate calcium disodium]

Solution, Subcutaneous:

Relistor: 8 mg/0.4 mL (0.4 mL); 12 mg/0.6 mL (0.6 mL) [contains edetate calcium disodium]

Tablet, Oral, as bromide:

Relistor: 150 mg [contains edetate calcium disodium]

◆ **Methylnaltrexone Bromide** *see* Methylnaltrexone *on page 1226*

MethylPREDNISolone (meth il pred NIS oh lone)

Related Information

Corticosteroids Systemic Equivalencies *on page 2417*

Hematopoietic Cell Transplantation *on page 2365*

Management of Chemotherapy-Induced Nausea and Vomiting in Adults *on page 2253*

Palliative Care Medicine (Cancer) *on page 2352*

Brand Names: US A-Methapred [DSC]; DEPO-Medrol; Medrol; P-Care D40; P-Care D80; ReadySharp Methylprednisolone; SOLU-medrol

Brand Names: Canada Depo-Medrol; Medrol; Methylprednisolone Acetate; Methylprednisolone Sodium Succinate For Injection; Methylprednisolone Sodium Succinate For Injection USP; Solu-Medrol

Index Terms 6-α-Methylprednisolone; A-Methapred; Medrol Dose Pack; Methylprednisolone Acetate; Methylprednisolone Sodium Succinate; Solumedrol

Pharmacologic Category Corticosteroid, Systemic

Use
Oral, IM, and IV administration:
Allergic: Control of severe or incapacitating allergic conditions intractable to adequate trials of conventional treatment in atopic dermatitis, drug hypersensitivity reactions, seasonal or perennial allergic rhinitis, serum sickness, and/or transfusion reactions.

Dermatologic: Bullous dermatitis herpetiformis; contact dermatitis; exfoliative dermatitis; exfoliative erythroderma; mycosis fungoides; pemphigus; erythema multiforme (Stevens-Johnson syndrome); severe psoriasis; severe seborrheic dermatitis.

Endocrine: Congenital adrenal hyperplasia; hypercalcemia associated with cancer; nonsuppurative thyroiditis; primary or secondary adrenocortical insufficiency (hydrocortisone or cortisone is the first choice; synthetic analogs may be used in conjunction with mineralocorticoids where applicable).

GI: To tide the patient over a critical period of the disease in Crohn disease or ulcerative colitis.

Hematologic: Acquired (autoimmune) hemolytic anemia; congenital (erythroid) hypoplastic anemia (Diamond Blackfan anemia); erythroblastopenia (RBC anemia; oral only); immune thrombocytopenia (formerly known as idiopathic thrombocytopenic purpura) (adults; oral and IV only); pure red cell aplasia (excluding oral); secondary thrombocytopenia.

Neoplastic: Palliative management of leukemias and lymphomas.

Nervous system: Acute exacerbations of multiple sclerosis; cerebral edema associated with primary or metastatic brain tumor, craniotomy, or head injury (excluding oral).

Ophthalmic:

Oral: Severe acute and chronic allergic and inflammatory processes involving the eye and its adnexa such as allergic conjunctivitis; allergic corneal marginal ulcers; anterior segment inflammation; chorioretinitis; diffuse posterior uveitis and choroiditis; herpes zoster ophthalmicus; iritis and iridocyclitis; keratitis; optic neuritis; sympathetic ophthalmia; uveitis.

Injection: Sympathetic ophthalmia; temporal arteritis, uveitis and other ocular inflammatory conditions unresponsive to topical corticosteroids.

Renal: To induce diuresis or remission of proteinuria in nephrotic syndrome, with or without uremia, of the idiopathic type or that due to lupus erythematosus.

Respiratory: Aspiration pneumonitis (oral only); asthma; berylliosis; fulminating or disseminated pulmonary tuberculosis when used concurrently with appropriate antituberculous chemotherapy; idiopathic eosinophilic pneumonias; symptomatic sarcoidosis.

Rheumatic: As adjunctive therapy for short-term administration in acute rheumatic carditis, acute gouty arthritis, ankylosing spondylitis, dermatomyositis, polymyositis, psoriatic arthritis, rheumatoid arthritis (including juvenile rheumatoid arthritis), systemic lupus erythematosus; as adjunctive therapy for short-term administration in acute and subacute bursitis, acute nonspecific tenosynovitis, epicondylitis, posttraumatic osteoarthritis, relapsing polychondritis, synovitis of osteoarthritis (oral only).

Miscellaneous: Trichinosis with neurologic or myocardial involvement; tuberculous meningitis with subarachnoid block or impending block when used concurrently with appropriate antituberculous chemotherapy.

Intra-articular or soft tissue administration (methylprednisolone acetate only): As adjunctive therapy for short-term administration in acute gouty arthritis, acute and subacute bursitis, acute nonspecific tenosynovitis, epicondylitis, rheumatoid arthritis, and/or synovitis of osteoarthritis.

Intralesional administration (methylprednisolone acetate only): Alopecia areata; discoid lupus erythematosus; keloids; localized hypertrophic; infiltrated, inflammatory lesions of granuloma annulare; lichen planus; lichen simplex chronicus (neurodermatitis); psoriatic plaques; necrobiosis lipoidica diabeticorum. May be useful in cystic tumor of an aponeurosis or tendon (ganglia).

Labeled Contraindications

Hypersensitivity to methylprednisolone or any component of the formulation; systemic fungal infection (except intra-articular injection for localized joint conditions); intrathecal administration; live or attenuated virus vaccines (with immunosuppressive doses of corticosteroids); use in premature infants (formulations containing benzyl alcohol preservative only); immune thrombocytopenia (formerly known as idiopathic thrombocytopenic purpura) (IM administration only)

Canadian labeling: Additional contraindications (not in US labeling):

Methylprednisolone tablets: Herpes simplex of the eye, vaccinia and varicella (except for short-term or emergency therapy)

Methylprednisolone acetate injection: Epidural or intravascular administration; intra-articular injections in unstable joints; herpes simplex of the eye, vaccinia and varicella (except for short-term or emergency therapy)

Methylprednisolone sodium succinate: Hypersensitivity to cow's milk or its components or other dairy products which may contain trace amounts of milk ingredients; epidural administration; herpes simplex of the eye, vaccinia and varicella, arrested tuberculosis, acute psychoses, Cushing syndrome, peptic ulcer, markedly elevated serum creatinine (except for short-term or emergency therapy)

Documentation of allergenic cross-reactivity for corticosteroids is limited. However, because of similarities in chemical structure and/or pharmacologic actions, the possibility of cross-sensitivity cannot be ruled out with certainty.

Pregnancy Considerations Adverse events have been observed with corticosteroids in animal reproduction studies. Methylprednisolone crosses the placenta (Anderson 1981). Some studies have shown an association between first trimester systemic corticosteroid use and oral clefts or decreased birth weight; however, information is conflicting and may be influenced by maternal dose/indication for use (Lunghi 2010; Park-Wyllie 2000; Pradat 2003). Hypoadrenalism may occur in newborns following maternal use of corticosteroids in pregnancy; monitor.

When systemic corticosteroids are needed in pregnancy for rheumatic disorders, it is generally recommended to use the lowest effective dose for the shortest duration of time, avoiding high doses during the first trimester (Götestam Skorpen 2016; Makol 2011; Østensen 2009).

For dermatologic disorders in pregnant women, systemic corticosteroids are generally not preferred for initial therapy; should be avoided during the first trimester; and used during the second or third trimester at the lowest effective dose (Bae 2012; Leachman 2006).

Pregnant women with poorly controlled asthma or asthma exacerbations may have a greater fetal/maternal risk than what is associated with appropriately used medications. Uncontrolled asthma is associated with an increased risk of perinatal mortality, preeclampsia, preterm birth, and low birth weight infants. Inhaled corticosteroids are recommended for the treatment of asthma during pregnancy; however, systemic corticosteroids should be used to control acute exacerbations or treat severe persistent asthma (ACOG 2008; GINA 2016; Namazy 2016).

The National Transplantation Pregnancy Registry (NTPR) is a registry which follows pregnancies which occur in maternal transplant recipients or those fathered by male transplant recipients. The NTPR encourages reporting of pregnancies following solid organ transplant by contacting them at 877-955-6877 or NTPR@giftoflifeinstitute.org.

Breastfeeding Considerations Methylprednisolone is present in breast milk (Cooper 2015; Strijbos 2015).

The relative infant dose (RID) of methylprednisolone is 2.8% to 5.6% when calculated using the highest breast milk concentration located and compared to a weight-adjusted infant dose of 15 to 30 mg/kg/day. In general, breastfeeding is considered acceptable when the RID is <10%; when an RID is >25% breastfeeding should generally be avoided (Anderson 2016; Ito 2000). Using the highest milk concentration (5.55 mcg/mL), the estimated daily infant dose via breast milk is 0.8325 mg/kg/day. This milk concentration was obtained following maternal administration of methylprednisolone 1,000 mg IV infused over 2 hours. The maximum milk concentration occurred 1 hour after the maternal dose and methylprednisolone was below the limits of quantification 12 hours after the dose (Cooper 2015).

The manufacturer notes that when used systemically, maternal use of corticosteroids have the potential to cause adverse events in a breastfeeding infant (eg, growth suppression, interfere with endogenous corticosteroid production) and therefore recommends a decision be made whether to discontinue breastfeeding or to discontinue the drug, taking into account the importance of treatment to the mother.

Corticosteroids are generally considered acceptable in breastfeeding women when used in usual doses (Götestam Skorpen 2016; WHO 2002); however, monitoring of the nursing infant is recommended (WHO 2002). If there is concern about exposure to the infant, some guidelines recommend waiting 4 hours after the maternal dose of an oral systemic corticosteroid before breastfeeding in order to decrease potential exposure to the breastfeeding infant (based on a study using prednisolone) (Bae 2012; Butler 2014; Götestam Skorpen 2016; Leachman 2006; Makol 2011; Ost 1985).

Warnings/Precautions Corticosteroids are not approved for epidural injection. Serious neurologic events (eg, spinal cord infarction, paraplegia, quadriplegia, cortical blindness, stroke), some resulting in death, have been reported with epidural injection of corticosteroids, with and without use of fluoroscopy.

High doses of methylprednisolone IV (usually doses of 1 g/day) may induce a toxic form of acute hepatitis (rare); serious hepatic injury may occur, resulting in acute liver failure and death. Time to onset can be several weeks or longer; resolution has been observed after discontinuation of therapy. Discontinue methylprednisolone if toxic hepatitis occurs. Avoid use of high doses in patients with a history of methylprednisone-induced toxic hepatitis.

Use with caution in patients with thyroid disease, hepatic impairment, renal impairment, cardiovascular disease, diabetes, glaucoma, cataracts, myasthenia gravis, osteoporosis, seizures, or GI diseases (diverticulitis, fresh intestinal anastomoses, active or latent peptic ulcer, ulcerative colitis, abscess or other pyogenic infection) due to perforation risk. Not recommended for the treatment of optic neuritis; may increase frequency of new episodes. Use with caution in patients with a history of ocular herpes simplex; corneal perforation has occurred; do not use in active ocular herpes simplex. Use caution following acute MI (corticosteroids have been associated with myocardial rupture).

Use with caution in the elderly with the smallest possible effective dose for the shortest duration. May affect growth velocity; growth should be routinely monitored in pediatric patients. Withdraw therapy with gradual tapering of dose. Patients may require higher doses when subject to stress (ie, trauma, surgery, severe infection).

May cause hypercortisolism or suppression of hypothalamic-pituitary-adrenal (HPA) axis, particularly in younger children or in patients receiving high doses for prolonged periods. HPA axis suppression may lead to adrenal crisis. Withdrawal and discontinuation of a corticosteroid should be done slowly and carefully. Particular care is required when patients are transferred from systemic corticosteroids to inhaled products due to possible adrenal insufficiency or withdrawal from steroids, including an increase in allergic symptoms. Patients receiving >20 mg per day of prednisone (or equivalent) may be most susceptible. Fatalities have occurred due to adrenal insufficiency in asthmatic patients during and after transfer from systemic corticosteroids to aerosol steroids; aerosol steroids do not provide the systemic steroid needed to treat patients having trauma, surgery, or infections. Use in septic shock or sepsis syndrome may increase mortality in some populations (eg, patients with elevated serum creatinine, patients who develop secondary infections after use).

Acute myopathy has been reported with high dose corticosteroids, usually in patients with neuromuscular transmission disorders; may involve ocular and/or respiratory muscles; monitor creatine kinase; recovery may be delayed. Corticosteroid use may cause psychiatric disturbances, including euphoria, insomnia, mood swings, personality changes, severe depression, or psychotic manifestations. Preexisting psychiatric conditions may be exacerbated by corticosteroid use. Prolonged use of corticosteroids may increase the incidence of secondary infection, cause activation of latent infections, mask acute infection (including fungal infections), prolong or exacerbate viral or parasitic infections, or limit response to killed or inactivated vaccines. Exposure to chickenpox or measles should be avoided; corticosteroids should not be used to treat ocular herpes simplex. Corticosteroids should not be used for cerebral malaria, fungal infections, or viral hepatitis. Close observation is required in patients with latent tuberculosis and/or TB reactivity; restrict use in active TB (only fulminating or disseminated TB in conjunction with antituberculosis treatment). Amebiasis should be ruled out in any patient with recent travel to tropic climates or unexplained diarrhea prior to initiation of corticosteroids. Use with extreme caution in patients with *Strongyloides* infections; hyperinfection, dissemination and fatalities have occurred. Prolonged treatment with corticosteroids has been associated with the development of Kaposi sarcoma (case reports); discontinuation may result in clinical improvement (Goedert 2002).

High-dose corticosteroids should not be used to manage acute head injury. Rare cases of anaphylactoid reactions have been observed in patients receiving corticosteroids. Avoid injection or leakage into the dermis; dermal and/or subdermal skin depression may occur at the site of injection. Avoid deltoid muscle injection; subcutaneous atrophy may occur. Septic arthritis may occur as a complication to parenteral therapy; institute appropriate antimicrobial therapy as required. Potentially significant drug-drug interactions may exist, requiring dose or frequency adjustment, additional monitoring, and/or selection of alternative therapy.

Methylprednisolone **acetate** IM injection (multiple-dose vial) and the diluent for methylprednisolone **sodium succinate** injection may contain benzyl alcohol; large amounts of benzyl alcohol ($\geq$99 mg/kg/day) have been associated with a potentially fatal toxicity ("gasping syndrome") in neonates; the "gasping syndrome" consists of metabolic acidosis, respiratory distress, gasping respirations, CNS dysfunction (including convulsions, intracranial hemorrhage), hypotension, and cardiovascular collapse (AAP ["Inactive" 1997]; CDC 1982); some data suggests that benzoate displaces bilirubin from protein binding sites (Ahlfors 2001); avoid or use dosage forms containing benzyl alcohol with caution in neonates.

Some dosage forms may contain polysorbate 80 (also known as Tweens). Hypersensitivity reactions, usually a delayed reaction, have been reported following exposure to pharmaceutical products containing polysorbate 80 in certain individuals (Isaksson 2002; Lucente 2000; Shelley 1995). Thrombocytopenia, ascites, pulmonary deterioration, and renal and hepatic failure have been reported in premature neonates after receiving parenteral products containing polysorbate 80 (Alade 1986; CDC 1984). See manufacturer's labeling.

Adverse Reactions

Frequency not defined:

Cardiovascular: Bradycardia, cardiac arrest, cardiac arrhythmia, cardiac failure, cardiomegaly, circulatory shock, congestive heart failure, edema, embolism (fat), hypertension, hypertrophic cardiomyopathy (in neonates), myocardial rupture (post MI), syncope, tachycardia, thromboembolism, thrombophlebitis, vasculitis

Central nervous system: Arachnoiditis, depression, emotionallability, euphoria, headache, increased intracranial pressure, insomnia, malaise, meningitis, myasthenia, neuritis, neuropathy, paraplegia, paresthesia, personality changes, psychic disorders, pseudotumor cerebri (usually following discontinuation), seizure, sensory disturbance, vertigo

Dermatologic: Acne vulgaris, allergic dermatitis, alopecia, atrophic striae, diaphoresis, ecchymoses, epidermal thinning, erythema, exfoliation of skin, facial erythema, hyperpigmentation, hypertrichosis, hypopigmentation, skin atrophy, skin rash, suppression of skin test reaction, thinning hair, urticaria, xeroderma

Endocrine & metabolic: Adrenal suppression, calcinosis, cushingoid state, Cushing syndrome, decreased glucose tolerance, diabetes mellitus, fluid retention, glycosuria, growth suppression (children), hirsutism, HPA-axis suppression, hyperglycemia, hyperlipidemia, hypokalemia, hypokalemic alkalosis, insulin resistance (increased requirements for insulin or oral hypoglycemic agents in diabetes), menstrual disease, moon face, negative nitrogen balance, protein catabolism, sodium retention, weight gain

Gastrointestinal: Abdominal distention, bladder dysfunction (after intrathecal administration, including bowel dysfunction), carbohydrate intolerance (increased), gastrointestinal hemorrhage, gastrointestinal perforation, hiccups, increased appetite, intestinal perforation (of both of the small and large intestines; especially in patients with inflammatory bowel disease), nausea, pancreatitis, peptic ulcer, spermatozoa disorder (decreased motility and number of spermatozoa), ulcerative esophagitis

Hematologic: Leukocytosis (transient), malignant neoplasm (secondary), petechia

Hepatic: Hepatomegaly, increased liver enzymes, increased serum transaminases

Hypersensitivity: Anaphylactoid reaction, anaphylaxis, angioedema, hypersensitivity reaction

Infection: Increased susceptibility to infection, infection (ophthalmic), sterile abscess

Local: Injection site infection

Neuromuscular & skeletal: Amyotrophy, arthropathy, aseptic necrosis of femoral head, aseptic necrosis of humoral head, bone fracture, Charcotlike arthropathy, lipotrophy, osteoporosis, rupture of tendon, steroid myopathy, vertebral compression fracture

Ophthalmic: Blindness, exophthalmoses, glaucoma, increased intraocular pressure, ophthalmic inflammation (ophthalmic), subcapsular posterior cataract, visual impairment

Respiratory: Pulmonary edema, rhinitis

Miscellaneous: Anaphylactoid reaction, anaphylaxis, angioedema, hypersensitivity reactions, tissue sloughing (residue or slough at injection site), wound healing Impairment

<1%, postmarketing, and/or case reports: Venous thrombosis (Johannesdottir 2013)

Drug Interactions

Metabolism/Transport Effects Substrate of CYP3A4 (minor); **Note:** Assignment of Major/Minor substrate status based on clinically relevant drug interaction potential; **Inhibits** CYP2C8 (weak)

Avoid Concomitant Use

Avoid concomitant use of MethylPREDNISolone with any of the following: Aldesleukin; Amodiaquine; BCG (Intravesical); Desmopressin; Indium 111 Capromab Pendetide; MiFEPRIStone; Natalizumab; Pimecrolimus; Tacrolimus (Topical)

Increased Effect/Toxicity

MethylPREDNISolone may increase the levels/effects of: Acetylcholinesterase Inhibitors; Amodiaquine; Amphotericin B; Androgens; CycloSPORINE (Systemic); Deferasirox; Desirudin; Desmopressin; Fingolimod; Leflunomide; Loop Diuretics; Natalizumab; Nicorandil; NSAID (COX-2 Inhibitor); NSAID (Nonselective); Quinolone Antibiotics; Thiazide and Thiazide-Like Diuretics; Tofacitinib; Vaccines (Live); Warfarin

The levels/effects of MethylPREDNISolone may be increased by: Aprepitant; CycloSPORINE (Systemic); CYP3A4 Inhibitors (Strong); Denosumab; DilTIAZem; Estrogen Derivatives; Fosaprepitant; Indacaterol; MiFEPRIStone; Neuromuscular-Blocking Agents (Nondepolarizing); Ocrelizumab; Pimecrolimus; Roflumilast; Salicylates; Tacrolimus (Topical); Telaprevir; Trastuzumab

◄ **Decreased Effect**

MethylPREDNISolone may decrease the levels/effects of: Aldesleukin; Antidiabetic Agents; BCG (Intravesical); Calcitriol (Systemic); Coccidioides immitis Skin Test; Corticorelin; CycloSPORINE (Systemic); Hyaluronidase; Indium 111 Capromab Pendetide; Isoniazid; Nivolumab; Salicylates; Sipuleucel-T; Telaprevir; Tertomotide; Urea Cycle Disorder Agents; Vaccines (Inactivated); Vaccines (Live)

The levels/effects of MethylPREDNISolone may be decreased by: Antacids; Bile Acid Sequestrants; CYP3A4 Inducers (Strong); Echinacea; MiFEPRIStone; Mitotane

Storage/Stability

Methylprednisolone acetate injection and tablets: Store at 20°C to 25°C (68°F to 77°F). Do not autoclave vials.

Methylprednisolone sodium succinate injection: Store intact vials at 20°C to 25°C (68°F to 77°F). Protect from light. Do not autoclave. Store reconstituted solutions at 20°C to 25°C (68°F to 77°F) and use within 48 hours.

Preparation for Administration Methylprednisolone sodium succinate injection: Reconstitute vials only with provided diluent or bacteriostatic water with benzyl alcohol (see manufacturer's labeling for details). For IV infusion, dilute reconstituted dose in D5W, NS, or D5NS. Formulations containing benzyl alcohol should not be used in neonates. Neonates should only receive doses reconstituted with preservative free SWFI.

Mechanism of Action In a tissue-specific manner, corticosteroids regulate gene expression subsequent to binding specific intracellular receptors and translocation into the nucleus. Corticosteroids exert a wide array of physiologic effects including modulation of carbohydrate, protein, and lipid metabolism and maintenance of fluid and electrolyte homeostasis. Moreover cardiovascular, immunologic, musculoskeletal, endocrine, and neurologic physiology are influenced by corticosteroids. Decreases inflammation by suppression of migration of polymorphonuclear leukocytes and reversal of increased capillary permeability.

Pharmacodynamics/Kinetics

Onset of action: IV (succinate): Within 1 hour; Intra-articular (IV acetate): 1 week

Duration: Intra-articular (IV acetate): 1 to 5 weeks

Absorption: Oral: Well absorbed (Czock 2005)

Bioavailability: Oral: 88% ± 23% (Czock 2005)

Distribution: V_d: IV (succinate): 24 L ± 6 L (Czock 2005)

Metabolism: Hepatic to metabolites (Czock 2005)

Half-life elimination:

Adolescents: IV: 1.9 ± 0.7 hours (age range: 12 to 20 years; Rouster-Stevens 2008)

Adults: Oral: 2.5 ± 1.2 hours (Czock 2005); IV (succinate): 0.25 ± 0.1 hour (Czock 2005)

Time to peak, plasma:

Oral: 2.1 ± 0.7 hours (Czock 2005)

IV (succinate): 0.8 hours (Czock 2005)

Excretion: Urine (1.3% [oral], 9.2% [IV succinate] as unchanged drug) (Czock 2005)

Dosing

Adult & Geriatric The lowest possible dose should be used to control the condition; when dose reduction is possible, the dose should be reduced gradually. **Only sodium succinate salt may be given IV.**

Allergic conditions: Oral: Tapered-dosage schedule (eg, dose-pack containing 21 x 4 mg tablets):

Day 1: 24 mg on day 1 administered as 8 mg (2 tablets) before breakfast, 4 mg (1 tablet) after lunch, 4 mg (1 tablet) after supper, and 8 mg (2 tablets) at bedtime **OR** 24 mg (6 tablets) as a single dose or divided into 2 or 3 doses upon initiation (regardless of time of day)

Day 2: 20 mg on day 2 administered as 4 mg (1 tablet) before breakfast, 4 mg (1 tablet) after lunch, 4 mg (1 tablet) after supper, and 8 mg (2 tablets) at bedtime

Day 3: 16 mg on day 3 administered as 4 mg (1 tablet) before breakfast, 4 mg (1 tablet) after lunch, 4 mg (1 tablet) after supper, and 4 mg (1 tablet) at bedtime

Day 4: 12 mg on day 4 administered as 4 mg (1 tablet) before breakfast, 4 mg (1 tablet) after lunch, and 4 mg (1 tablet) at bedtime

Day 5: 8 mg on day 5 administered as 4 mg (1 tablet) before breakfast and 4 mg (1 tablet) at bedtime

Day 6: 4 mg on day 6 administered as 4 mg (1 tablet) before breakfast

Anti-inflammatory or immunosuppressive: Note: Initial dosage depends upon condition being treated; adjust subsequent doses based on patient response.

Oral: 4 to 48 mg/day in 1 to 4 divided doses initially, followed by gradual reduction in dosage to the lowest possible level consistent with maintaining an adequate clinical response.

IM (succinate): 10 to 40 mg/day initially

IM (acetate): 4 to 120 mg single dose; repeated injections may be necessary for recurrent or chronic conditions.

IV (succinate): 10 to 40 mg over a period of several minutes and repeated IV or IM at intervals depending on clinical response; when high dosages are needed, administer 30 mg/kg over a period ≥30 minutes and may be repeated every 4 to 6 hours for 48 hours.

Intralesional (acetate): 20 to 60 mg; for large lesions, it may be necessary to distribute doses ranging from 20 to 40 mg by repeated local injections; 1 to 4 injections are usually employed with intervals between injections varying with the type of lesion being treated and clinical response.

Soft tissue (acetate): 4 to 30 mg; repeated injections may be necessary for recurrent or chronic conditions.

Arthritis: Intra-articular (acetate): Administer every 1 to 5 weeks.

Large joints (eg, knee, ankle, shoulder): 20 to 80 mg

Medium joints (eg, elbow, wrist): 10 to 40 mg

Small joints (eg, metacarpophalangeal, interphalangeal, sternoclavicular, acromioclavicular): 4 to 10 mg

Asthma, exacerbations:

Acute, short-course "burst" (NAEPP 2007):

Oral: 40 to 60 mg/day in divided doses once or twice daily for 3 to 10 days; **Note:** Burst should be continued until symptoms resolve and peak expiratory flow is at least 80% of personal best; usually requires 3 to 10 days of treatment; longer treatment may be required.

IM (**acetate**): 240 mg as a one-time dose; **Note:** This may be given in place of short-course "burst" of oral steroids in patients who are vomiting or if compliance is a problem.

Hospital/emergency medical care doses: Oral, IV: 40 to 80 mg/day in divided doses once or twice daily until peak expiratory flow is 70% of predicted or personal best.

Asthma, long-term (maintenance) (NAEPP 2007): Oral: 7.5 to 60 mg once daily in the morning or every other day as needed for asthma control

Multiple sclerosis, acute exacerbation:

Note: Treatment guidelines recommend high-dose IV methylprednisolone succinate or oral methylprednisolone for acute exacerbations of multiple sclerosis (AAN [Scott 2011]); NICE 2014).

Manufacturer's labeling: Oral, IV (succinate only), IM (acetate or succinate): 160 mg daily for 1 week, followed by 64 mg every other day for 1 month.

Off-label dosing:

Oral: 500 mg daily for 5 days (NICE 2014).

IV (succinate only): 1,000 mg daily for 3 to 7 days (AAN [Scott 2011]; NICE 2014).

Bronchiolitis obliterans syndrome, prevention (off-label use): IV (sodium succinate): 1000 mg daily for 3 days. **Note:** Many centers use 10 to 15 mg/kg/day for smaller patients (Meyer 2014).

Cadaveric organ recovery (hormonal resuscitation) (off-label use): IV (sodium succinate): 15 mg/kg **or** 2,000 mg bolus administered to the brain-dead donor who is hemodynamically unstable requiring significant vasopressor support; give concomitantly with vasopressin, levothyroxine or liothyronine (preferred), dextrose (if bolus dose insulin used), and regular insulin (bolus dose or continuous infusion). If continuous infusion insulin is employed, maintain blood glucose 120 to 180 mg/dL (Rosendale 2003a; Rosendale 2003b; Rosengard 2002; Salim 2007; Zaroff 2002).

Cardiac transplant: Acute cellular rejection (treatment) or antibody-mediated rejection (treatment) (off-label use): IV (sodium succinate): 250 to 1,000 mg daily for 3 days (AHA [Colvin 2015]; ISHLT [Costanzo 2010]).

COPD exacerbation (off-label use): Note: Dose, frequency, and duration of therapy not established. GOLD guidelines recommend the use of oral prednisone; however, methylprednisolone may be used as an alternative (GOLD [Decramer 2014]). No comparative studies exist to examine safety and efficacy between low-, medium-, or high-dose regimens. While several clinical trials have examined the use of methylprednisolone in this setting, these trials included low numbers of patients, employed vastly different regimens, and/or examined different clinical outcomes (Albert 1980; Alía 2011; Niewoehner 1999; Sayiner 2001; Shortall 2002; Vrondracek 2006; Willaert 2002). Current dosing strategies are empiric and have not been established by clinical trials. Based on expert opinion, commonly used regimens ranging from 60 to 125 mg IV administered 1 to 4 times daily followed by oral therapy (eg, prednisone 40 mg once daily) for a total of 5 to 14 days of therapy may be employed; the shorter duration (ie, 5 days) may be preferred (Leuppi 2013); however, comparative prospective data does not exist. IV administration with a higher dose (eg, ≥60 mg) may be preferred for those patients with impending or actual acute respiratory failure; outcome trials not available for this approach.

Dermatomyositis/polymyositis (off-label dosing): IV (succinate): 1,000 mg daily for 3 to 5 days for severe muscle weakness, followed by conversion to oral prednisone (Drake 1996)

Gout, acute (off-label dosing): IV (succinate), IM: Initial: 0.5 to 2 mg/kg; may be repeated as clinically indicated (ACR guidelines [Khanna 2012])

Lupus nephritis (off-label dosing): High-dose "pulse" therapy: IV (succinate): 0.5 to 1 g/day for 3 days (Ponticelli 2010)

Pneumocystis **pneumonia in AIDS patients (off-label use):** IV (succinate): 30 mg twice daily on days 1 to 5, then 30 mg once daily on days 6 to 10, then 15 mg once daily on days 11 to 21 (CDC 2009a).

Spinal cord injury, acute (off-label use): IV (succinate): 30 mg/kg over 15 minutes followed in 45 minutes by a continuous infusion of 5.4 mg/kg/hour for 23 hours; **Note:** Due to insufficient evidence of clinical efficacy (ie, preserving or improving spinal cord function), the routine use of methylprednisolone in the treatment of acute spinal cord injury is no longer recommended. If used in this setting, methylprednisolone should not be initiated >8 hours after the injury; not effective in penetrating trauma (eg, gunshot) (Consortium for Spinal Cord Medicine 2008).

Pediatric The lowest possible dose should be used to control the condition; when dose reduction is possible, the dose should be reduced gradually. **Only sodium succinate salt may be given IV.**

Anti-inflammatory or immunosuppressive: Note: Initial dosage depends upon condition being treated; adjust subsequent doses based on patient response.

Infants, Children, and Adolescents: Oral, IM (acetate or succinate), IV (succinate): Initial: 0.11 to 1.6 mg/kg/day or 3.2 to 48 mg/m^2/day in 3 to 4 divided doses; usual range: 0.5 to 1.7 mg/kg/day (Kliegman 2015); for oral, IM (succinate), and IV (succinate) may also administer in divided doses every 6 to 12 hours (Kliegman 2015); for IM (acetate) administer as a single daily dose

"Pulse" therapy: IV (succinate): 30 mg/kg/dose once daily for 1 to 5 days; maximum: 1,000 mg/day (Kliegman 2015)

Long-acting: IM (acetate): 4 to 80 mg every 1 to 2 weeks

Asthma, exacerbations:

Acute, short-course "burst" (NAEPP 2007):

Infants and Children <12 years:

Oral: 1 to 2 mg/kg/day in divided doses once or twice daily for 3 to 10 days; maximum daily dose: 60 mg/**day**; **Note:** Burst should be continued until symptoms resolve or patient achieves peak expiratory flow 80% of personal best; usually requires 3 to 10 days of treatment (~5 days on average); longer treatment may be required

IM (**acetate**): **Note:** This may be given in place of short-course "burst" of oral steroids in patients who are vomiting or if compliance is a problem. Children ≤4 years: 7.5 mg/kg as a one-time dose; maximum dose: 240 mg

Children 5 to 11 years: 240 mg as a one-time dose

Children ≥12 years and Adolescents: Oral, IM (acetate): Refer to adult dosing.

Hospital/emergency medical care doses:

Infants and Children <12 years: Oral, IV: 1 to 2 mg/kg/day in 2 divided doses; maximum daily dose: 60 mg/day; continue until peak expiratory flow is 70% of predicted or personal best

Children ≥12 years and Adolescents: Oral, IV: Refer to adult dosing

◀ *Status asthmaticus* (previous NAEPP guidelines; still used by some clinicians): Children: IV: Loading dose: 2 mg/kg/dose, then 0.5 to 1 mg/kg/dose every 6 hours; **Note:** See NAEPP 2007 guidelines for asthma exacerbations (emergency medical care or hospital doses) listed above

Asthma, long-term treatment (maintenance) (NAEPP, 2007):
Infants and Children <12 years: Oral: 0.25 to 2 mg/kg/day once daily in the morning or every other day as needed for asthma control; maximum daily dose: 60 mg/day

Children ≥12 years and Adolescents: Oral: Refer to adult dosing

Lupus nephritis (off-label dosing): Children and Adolescents: IV (succinate): High-dose "pulse" therapy: 30 mg/kg/dose or 600 to 1,000 mg/m^2/dose once daily for 3 days; maximum dose: 1,000 mg/day (Adams 2006; Marks 2010)

***Pneumocystis* pneumonia; moderate or severe infection (off-label use):**
Note: Initiate therapy within 72 hours of diagnosis, if possible.
Infants and Children: IV (succinate): 1 mg/kg/dose every 6 hours on days 1 to 7, then 1 mg/kg/dose twice daily on days 8 and 9, then 0.5 mg/kg/dose twice daily on days 10 and 11, and then 1 mg/kg/dose once daily on days 12 to 16 (CDC 2009)

Adolescents: IV (succinate): Refer to adult dosing

Spinal cord injury, acute (off-label use): IV (succinate): 30 mg/kg over 15 minutes, followed in 45 minutes by a continuous infusion of 5.4 mg/kg/hour for 23 hours. **Note:** Due to insufficient evidence of clinical efficacy (ie, preserving or improving spinal cord function), the routine use of methylprednisolone in the treatment of acute spinal cord injury is no longer recommended. If used in this setting, methylprednisolone should not be initiated >8 hours after the injury; not effective in penetrating trauma (eg, gunshot) (Consortium for Spinal Cord Medicine 2008).

Renal Impairment There are no dosage adjustments provided in the manufacturer's labeling; use with caution.

Hepatic Impairment There are no dosage adjustments provided in the manufacturer's labeling; use with caution.

Combination Regimens
Leukemia, acute lymphocytic: Hyper-CVAD (Leukemia, Acute Lymphocytic) on page 2146
Lymphoma, Hodgkin:
ESHAP (Hodgkin) on page 2110
MINE-ESHAP (Hodgkin) on page 2174
Lymphoma, non-Hodgkin: ESHAP on page 2109
Lymphoma, non-Hodgkin (DLBCL): R-ESHAP (NHL-DLBCL) on page 2204

Administration
Oral: Administer tablets after meals or with food or milk to decrease GI upset. If prescribed once daily, administer in the morning.

IM (acetate, succinate): Avoid injection into the deltoid muscle due to a high incidence of subcutaneous atrophy. Avoid injection or leakage into the dermis. Do not inject into areas that have evidence of acute local infection.

IV (succinate): Rate dependent upon dose; typically, intermittent infusion is administered over 15 to 60 minutes. Do not administer moderate- or high-dose IV push; severe adverse effects, including hypotension, cardiac arrhythmia, and sudden death, have been reported in patients receiving high-dose methylprednisolone IV push over <20 minutes (Barron 1982,

Ditzian-Kadanoff 1987, Garin 1986, Liebling 1981, Lucas 1993). **Do not give acetate form IV.**

Low dose (eg, ≤1.8 mg/kg or ≤125 mg/dose): IV push over 3 to 15 minutes; maximum concentration: 125 mg/mL

Moderate dose (eg, ≥2 mg/kg or 250 mg/dose): Administer over 15 to 30 minutes

High dose (eg, ≥15 mg/kg or ≥500 mg/dose): Administer over 30 to 60 minutes; doses ≥1,000 mg: Administer over 60 minutes. **Note:** In some of the adult spinal cord injury trials, bolus doses (30 mg/kg) have been administered over 15 minutes.

Intra-articular or soft tissue (acetate): See manufacturer's labeling for details.

Intralesional: Inject directly into the lesion. For large lesions, administer multiple small injections (20 to 40 mg) into the area of the lesion. Avoid injection of sufficient material to cause blanching because this may be followed by a small slough.

Monitoring Parameters Blood pressure, blood glucose, electrolytes; weight; intraocular pressure (use >6 weeks); bone mineral density; growth and development in children; HPA axis suppression

Test Interactions Decreased response to skin tests

Dietary Considerations Take tablets with meals to decrease GI upset; need diet rich in pyridoxine, vitamin C, vitamin D, folate, calcium, phosphorus, and protein.

Additional Information Sodium content of 1 g sodium succinate injection: 2.01 mEq; 53 mg of sodium succinate salt is equivalent to 40 mg of methylprednisolone base

Methylprednisolone acetate: Depo-Medrol

Methylprednisolone sodium succinate: Solu-Medrol

Dosage Forms Excipient information presented when available (limited, particularly for generics); consult specific product labeling. [DSC] = Discontinued product

Kit, Injection, as acetate:

P-Care D40: 40 mg/mL [contains polyethylene glycol]

P-Care D80: 40 mg/mL [contains polyethylene glycol]

ReadySharp Methylprednisolone: 80 mg/mL [contains polyethylene glycol]

Solution Reconstituted, Injection, as sodium succinate [strength expressed as base]:

A-Methapred: 40 mg (1 ea [DSC]); 125 mg (1 ea [DSC]) [contains benzyl alcohol]

SOLU-medrol: 500 mg (1 ea); 1000 mg (1 ea)

SOLU-medrol: 2 g (1 ea) [contains benzyl alcohol]

Generic: 40 mg (1 ea); 125 mg (1 ea); 1000 mg (1 ea)

Solution Reconstituted, Injection, as sodium succinate [strength expressed as base, preservative free]:

SOLU-medrol: 40 mg (1 ea); 125 mg (1 ea); 500 mg (1 ea); 1000 mg (1 ea)

Suspension, Injection, as acetate:

DEPO-Medrol: 20 mg/mL (5 mL); 40 mg/mL (5 mL, 10 mL) [contains benzyl alcohol, polyethylene glycol, polysorbate 80]

DEPO-Medrol: 40 mg/mL (1 mL) [contains polyethylene glycol]

DEPO-Medrol: 80 mg/mL (1 mL)

DEPO-Medrol: 80 mg/mL (5 mL) [contains benzyl alcohol, polyethylene glycol, polysorbate 80]

DEPO-Medrol: 80 mg/mL (1 mL) [contains polyethylene glycol]

◀ Generic: 40 mg/mL (1 mL, 5 mL [DSC], 10 mL); 80 mg/mL (1 mL, 5 mL)
Suspension, Injection, as acetate [preservative free]:
  Generic: 80 mg/mL (1 mL [DSC])
Tablet, Oral:
  Medrol: 2 mg [DSC]
  Medrol: 2 mg, 8 mg, 16 mg, 32 mg, 4 mg [scored]
  Generic: 8 mg, 16 mg, 32 mg, 4 mg
Tablet Therapy Pack, Oral:
  Medrol: 4 mg (21 ea) [scored]
  Generic: 4 mg (21 ea)

♦ **6-α-Methylprednisolone** see MethylPREDNISolone on page 1227

♦ **Methylprednisolone Acetate** see MethylPREDNISolone on page 1227

♦ **Methylprednisolone Sodium Succinate** see MethylPREDNISolone on page 1227

♦ **Methylprednisolone Sodium Succinate For Injection (Can)** see Methyl-PREDNISolone on page 1227

♦ **Methylprednisolone Sodium Succinate For Injection USP (Can)** see MethylPREDNISolone on page 1227

♦ **Methylthionine Chloride** see Methylene Blue on page 1224

♦ **Methylthioninium Chloride** see Methylene Blue on page 1224

♦ **3-methyl TTNEB** see Bexarotene (Systemic) on page 246

Metoclopramide (met oh KLOE pra mide)

Related Information

Management of Chemotherapy-Induced Nausea and Vomiting in Adults on page 2253

Palliative Care Medicine (Cancer) on page 2352

Brand Names: US Metozolv ODT [DSC]; Reglan

Brand Names: Canada Apo-Metoclop; Metoclopramide Hydrochloride Injection; Metoclopramide Omega; Metonia

Index Terms Metoclopramide HCl; Reglan

Pharmacologic Category Antiemetic; Gastrointestinal Agent, Prokinetic

Use

Injection:

Diabetic gastroparesis (diabetic gastric stasis): Relief of symptoms associated with acute and recurrent diabetic gastric stasis.

Prevention of nausea and vomiting associated with emetogenic cancer chemotherapy: Prophylaxis of vomiting associated with emetogenic cancer chemotherapy.

Prevention of postoperative nausea and vomiting: Prophylaxis of postoperative nausea and vomiting in circumstances where nasogastric suction is undesirable.

Radiological examination: To stimulate gastric emptying and intestinal transit of barium when delayed emptying interferes with radiological examination of the stomach and/or small intestine.

Small bowel intubation: To facilitate small bowel intubation in adults and pediatrics in whom the tube does not pass the pylorus with conventional maneuvers.

Oral:

Diabetic gastroparesis (diabetic gastric stasis): Relief of symptoms associated with acute and recurrent diabetic gastroparesis (gastric stasis) in adults.

Gastroesophageal reflux: Short-term (4 to 12 weeks) therapy for adults with documented symptomatic GERD who fail to respond to conventional therapy.

Limitations of use: Oral metoclopramide is indicated for adults only. Treatment should not exceed 12-week duration.

Labeled Contraindications

Known sensitivity or intolerance to metoclopramide or any component of the formulation; situations where stimulation of gastrointestinal (GI) motility may be dangerous, including mechanical GI obstruction, perforation, or hemorrhage (except when used prior to endoscopy for evaluation of acute upper GI bleeding [Barkun 2010]); pheochromocytoma; history of seizure disorder (eg, epilepsy), concomitant use with other agents likely to increase extrapyramidal reactions. **Note:** Use of metoclopramide in patients with paragangliomas or other catecholamine-secreting tumors (ie, conditions similar to pheochromocytoma) should likely be avoided due to the risk of hypertensive crisis.

Canadian labeling: Additional contraindications (not in the US labeling): Infants <1 year of age.

Pregnancy Considerations Adverse events were not observed in animal reproduction studies. Metoclopramide crosses the placenta and can be detected in cord blood and amniotic fluid (Arvela 1983; Bylsma-Howell 1983). Available evidence suggests safe use during pregnancy (ACOG 2015; Berkovitch 2002; Matok 2009; Sørensen 2000). Evidence related to the efficacy for the treatment of nausea and vomiting of pregnancy is limited (ACOG 2015; Arsenault 2002); metoclopramide may be used for prophylaxis of nausea and vomiting associated with cesarean delivery (ASA 2016; Smith 2011).

Breastfeeding Considerations Metoclopramide is present in breast milk.

The relative infant dose (RID) of metoclopramide is ~5% when calculated using the highest breast milk concentration located and compared to an infant therapeutic dose of 0.5 mg/kg/day. In general, breastfeeding is considered acceptable when the RID is <10%; when an RID is >25% breastfeeding should generally be avoided (Anderson 2016; Ito 2000). Using the highest milk concentration (0.1565 mcg/mL), the estimated daily infant dose via breast milk is 0.024 mg/kg/day. This milk concentration was obtained following maternal administration of oral metoclopramide 10 mg three times daily. Peak milk concentrations appeared approximately the same time as peak maternal serum concentrations, 2 to 3 hours after the dose. Metoclopramide was also detected in the serum of a breastfeeding infant (Kauppila 1983).

Although not commonly reported, transient intestinal discomfort has been noted in two breastfed infants following exposure via breast milk (Zuppa 2010).

Metoclopramide may increase prolactin concentrations and cause galactorrhea and gynecomastia, but studies which evaluated its use to increase milk production for women who want to breastfeed have had mixed results. In addition, due to the potential for adverse events, nonpharmacologic measure should be considered prior to the use of medications as galactagogues (ABM 2011).

The manufacturer recommends that caution be used if administered to a breastfeeding woman. When treatment for nausea and vomiting is needed, the WHO recommends metoclopramide be avoided due to insufficient data on long-term side effects to the infant (WHO 2002).

Warnings/Precautions [US Boxed Warning]: May cause tardive dyskinesia, a serious movement disorder which is often irreversible; the risk of developing tardive dyskinesia increases with duration of treatment and total cumulative dose. Discontinue metoclopramide in patients who develop signs/symptoms of tardive dyskinesia. There is no known treatment for tardive dyskinesia. In some patients, symptoms lessen or resolve after metoclopramide treatment is stopped. Avoid metoclopramide treatment longer than 12 weeks in all but rare cases in which therapeutic benefit is thought to outweigh the risk of developing tardive dyskinesia. Tardive dyskinesia is characterized by involuntary movements of the face, tongue, or extremities and may be disfiguring. An analysis of utilization patterns showed that ~20% of patients who used metoclopramide took it for longer than 12 weeks. Metoclopramide may mask underlying tardive disease by suppressing or partially suppressing tardive dyskinesia signs (metoclopramide should not be used to control tardive dyskinesia symptoms as the long-term course is unknown). The risk for tardive dyskinesia appears to be increased in the elderly, women, and diabetics, although it is not possible to predict which patients will develop tardive dyskinesia. There is no known effective treatment for established cases of tardive dyskinesia, although in some patients, tardive dyskinesia may remit (partially or completely) within several weeks to months after metoclopramide is withdrawn.

May cause extrapyramidal symptoms (EPS), generally manifested as acute dystonic reactions within the initial 24 to 48 hours of use at the usual adult dose (30 to 40 mg/day). Risk of these reactions is increased at higher doses, and in pediatric patients and adults <30 years of age. Symptoms may include involuntary limb movements, facial grimacing, torticollis, oculogyric crisis, rhythmic tongue protrusion, bulbar type speech, trismus, or dystonic reactions resembling tetanus. May also rarely present as stridor and dyspnea (may be due to laryngospasm). Dystonic symptoms may be managed with IM diphenhydramine or benztropine. Pseudoparkinsonism (eg, bradykinesia, tremor, rigidity, mask-like facies) may also occur (usually within first 6 months of therapy) and is generally reversible within 2 to 3 months following discontinuation. Symptoms of Parkinson disease may be exacerbated by metoclopramide; use with extreme caution (or avoid use) in patients with Parkinson disease.

Metoclopramide has been known to cause sinus arrest (usually with rapid IV administration or higher doses) (Bentsen, 2002; Malkoff 1995). The torsadogenic potential for metoclopramide is considered to be low (Claassen, 2005). Based on case reports, however, metoclopramide may cause QT prolongation and torsades de pointes in certain individuals (eg, heart failure patients with renal impairment); use with caution in these patients (Siddiquie, 2009). There is data in healthy male volunteers to show that metoclopramide actually shortens the QT interval while at the same time increasing QT variance (Ellidokuz, 2003). No human data other than case reports; however, has demonstrated a consistent QT prolonging effect with metoclopramide nor is there any substantiated evidence to show a direct association with the development of torsades de pointes.

Metoclopramide use may be associated (rarely) with neuroleptic malignant syndrome (NMS); may be fatal. Monitor for manifestations of NMS, which include hyperthermia, muscle rigidity, altered consciousness, and autonomic instability (irregular pulse or blood pressure, tachycardia, diaphoresis, and cardiac arrhythmias). Discontinue immediately if signs/symptoms of NMS appear and begin intensive symptomatic management and monitoring. Bromocriptine and dantrolene have been used to manage NMS, although effectiveness have not been established.

Mental depression has occurred (in patients with and without a history of depression), and symptoms range from mild to severe (suicidal ideation and suicide); use in patients with a history of depression only if anticipated benefits outweigh potential risks.

In a study in hypertensive patients, IV metoclopramide was associated with catecholamine release. Use with caution in patients with hypertension. There are reports of hypertensive crises in some patients with undiagnosed pheochromocytoma. Immediately discontinue with any rapid rise in blood pressure that is associated with metoclopramide. Hypertensive crises may be managed with phentolamine. Use with caution in patients who are at risk of fluid overload (HF, cirrhosis); metoclopramide causes a transient increase in serum aldosterone and increases the risk for fluid retention/overload; discontinue if adverse events or signs/symptoms appear.

Patients with NADH-cytochrome b5 reductase deficiency are at increased risk of methemoglobinemia and/or sulfhemoglobinemia. Use with caution in patients with renal impairment; dosage adjustment may be needed. Use with caution following surgical anastomosis/closure; promotility agents may theoretically increase pressure in suture lines.

For patients with diabetic gastroparesis, the usual manifestations of delayed gastric emptying (eg, nausea, vomiting, heartburn, persistent fullness after meals, anorexia) appear to respond to metoclopramide within different time intervals. Significant relief of nausea occurs early and continues to improve over a 3-week period; relief of vomiting and anorexia may precede the relief of abdominal fullness by a week or more. If gastroesophageal reflux symptoms are confined to particular situations, such as following the evening meal, consider use of metoclopramide as a single dose prior to the provocative situation, rather than using the drug throughout the day. Symptoms of postprandial and daytime heartburn respond better to metoclopramide, with less observed effect on nocturnal symptoms. Because there is no documented correlation between symptoms and healing of esophageal lesions, patients with documented lesions should be monitored endoscopically. Healing of esophageal ulcers and erosions has been endoscopically demonstrated at the end of a 12-week trial using a dosage of 15 mg 4 times daily.

EPS are increased in pediatric patients. In neonates, prolonged clearance of metoclopramide may lead to increased serum concentrations. Neonates may also have decreased levels of NADH-cytochrome b5 reductase which increases the risk of methemoglobinemia. Potentially significant drug-drug interactions may exist, requiring dose or frequency adjustment, additional monitoring, and/or selection of alternative therapy. CNS effects may be potentiated when used with other sedative drugs or ethanol. Abrupt discontinuation may (rarely) result in withdrawal symptoms (dizziness, headache, nervousness).

◄ Benzyl alcohol and derivatives: Some dosage forms may contain sodium benzoate/benzoic acid; benzoic acid (benzoate) is a metabolite of benzyl alcohol; large amounts of benzyl alcohol (≥99 mg/kg/day) have been associated with a potentially fatal toxicity ("gasping syndrome") in neonates; the "gasping syndrome" consists of metabolic acidosis, respiratory distress, gasping respirations, CNS dysfunction (including convulsions, intracranial hemorrhage), hypotension, and cardiovascular collapse (AAP ["Inactive" 1997]; CDC, 1982); some data suggest that benzoate displaces bilirubin from protein binding sites (Ahlfors, 2001); avoid or use dosage forms containing benzyl alcohol derivative with caution in neonates. See manufacturer's labeling.

Adverse Reactions Frequency not always defined.

Cardiovascular: Atrioventricular block, bradycardia, congestive heart failure, flushing (following high IV doses), hypertension, hypotension, supraventricular tachycardia

Central nervous system: Drowsiness (~10% to 70%; dose related), dystonic reaction (<1% to 25%; dose and age related), lassitude (~10%), restlessness (~10%), fatigue (2% to 10%), headache (4% to 5%), dizziness (1% to 4%), somnolence (2% to 3%), akathisia, confusion, depression, drug-induced Parkinson's disease, hallucination (rare), insomnia, neuroleptic malignant syndrome (rare), seizure, suicidal ideation, tardive dyskinesia

Dermatologic: Skin rash, urticaria

Endocrine & metabolic: Amenorrhea, fluid retention, galactorrhea, gynecomastia, hyperprolactinemia, porphyria

Gastrointestinal: Nausea (4% to 6%), vomiting (1% to 2%), diarrhea

Genitourinary: Impotence, urinary frequency, urinary incontinence

Hematologic & oncologic: Agranulocytosis, leukopenia, methemoglobinemia, neutropenia, sulfhemoglobinemia

Hepatic: Hepatotoxicity (rare)

Hypersensitivity: Angioedema (rare), hypersensitivity reaction

Neuromuscular & skeletal: Laryngospasm (rare)

Ophthalmic: Visual disturbance

Respiratory: Bronchospasm, laryngeal edema (rare)

Drug Interactions

Metabolism/Transport Effects Substrate of CYP1A2 (minor), CYP2D6 (minor); **Note:** Assignment of Major/Minor substrate status based on clinically relevant drug interaction potential

Avoid Concomitant Use

Avoid concomitant use of Metoclopramide with any of the following: Antipsychotic Agents; Droperidol; Promethazine; Rivastigmine; Tetrabenazine; Trimetazidine

Increased Effect/Toxicity

Metoclopramide may increase the levels/effects of: Antipsychotic Agents; CycloSPORINE (Systemic); Highest Risk QTc-Prolonging Agents; Levosulpiride; Moderate Risk QTc-Prolonging Agents; Prilocaine; Promethazine; Selective Serotonin Reuptake Inhibitors; Serotonin/Norepinephrine Reuptake Inhibitors; Sodium Nitrite; Tetrabenazine; Thiopental; Tricyclic Antidepressants; Trimetazidine

The levels/effects of Metoclopramide may be increased by: Dapsone (Topical); Deutetrabenazine; Droperidol; MetyroSINE; MiFEPRIStone; Nitric Oxide; Rivastigmine; Serotonin Modulators; Tetracaine (Topical)

Decreased Effect

Metoclopramide may decrease the levels/effects of: Anti-Parkinson Agents (Dopamine Agonist); Atovaquone; Posaconazole; Quinagolide

The levels/effects of Metoclopramide may be decreased by: Analgesics (Opioid); Anticholinergic Agents

Storage/Stability

Injection: Store intact vials at 20°C to 25°C (68°F to 77°F); injection is photosensitive and should be protected from light during storage; parenteral admixtures in D5W, D5½NS, NS, LR, or Ringer's injection are stable for up to 24 hours after preparation at normal light conditions or up to 48 hours if protected from light. When mixed with NS, can be stored frozen for up to 4 weeks; metoclopramide is degraded when admixed and frozen with D5W.

Oral solution: Store at 20°C to 25°C (68°F to 77°F). Do not freeze. Dispense in tight, light-resistant container.

Tablet: Store at 20°C to 25°C (68°F to 77°F). Dispense in tight, light-resistant container.

Tablet, orally disintegrating: Store at 20°C to 25°C (68°F to 77°F). Keep in original packaging until just prior to use.

Preparation for Administration Injection: Lower doses (≤10 mg): No dilution required; Higher doses (>10 mg): Dilute in 50 mL of compatible solution (preferably NS).

Mechanism of Action Blocks dopamine receptors and (when given in higher doses) also blocks serotonin receptors in chemoreceptor trigger zone of the CNS; enhances the response to acetylcholine of tissue in upper GI tract causing enhanced motility and accelerated gastric emptying without stimulating gastric, biliary, or pancreatic secretions; increases lower esophageal sphincter tone

Pharmacodynamics/Kinetics

Onset of action: Oral: 30 to 60 minutes; IV: 1 to 3 minutes; IM: 10 to 15 minutes

Duration: Therapeutic: 1 to 2 hours, regardless of route

Absorption: Oral: Rapid, well absorbed

Distribution: V_d: Neonates, PMA 31 to 40 weeks: 6.94 L/kg (Kearns 1998); Infants: 4.4 L/kg; Children: 3 L/kg; Adults: ~3.5 L/kg

Protein binding: ~30%

Bioavailability: Oral: 80 ± 15.5%

Half-life elimination: Normal renal function: Neonates, PMA 31 to 40 weeks: 5.4 hours (Kearns, 1998); Infants: 4.15 hours (range: 2.23 to 10.3 hours) (Kearns 1988); Children: ~4 hours (range: 2 to 12.5 hours); half-life and clearance may be dose-dependent; Adults: 5 to 6 hours (may be dose dependent)

Time to peak, serum: Neonates, PMA 31 to 40 weeks: 2.45 hours (Kearns, 1998); Infants: 2.2 hours; Adults: 1 to 2 hours

Excretion: Urine (~85%); feces

Dosing

Adult

Diabetic gastroparesis: Note: American Diabetes Association guidelines state that use should be reserved for severe cases that are unresponsive to other therapies; when used, duration should be ≤5 days (ADA 2017).

Oral (early manifestations): 10 mg up to 4 times daily 30 minutes before meals or food and at bedtime for 2 to 8 weeks. Treatment >12 weeks is not recommended per product labeling.

IM, IV (for severe symptoms): 10 mg over 1 to 2 minutes; 10 days of IV therapy may be necessary before symptoms are controlled to allow transition to oral administration.

Gastroparesis management, regardless of etiology (off-label use): American College of Gastroenterology Guidelines: Oral: Initial: 5 mg 3 times daily before meals. Dosage range: 5 to 10 mg 2 to 3 times daily before meals (maximum: 40 mg daily). Liquid formulation is preferred (to increase absorption) and the use of drug holidays or dose reductions (eg, 5 mg before the two main meals of the day) is also recommended when clinically possible (Camilleri 2013).

Gastroesophageal reflux: Oral: 10 to 15 mg up to 4 times daily 30 minutes before meals and at bedtime; alternatively, single doses of up to 20 mg (rather than continuous treatment) may be administered prior to provoking situation if symptoms are intermittent. Treatment >12 weeks is not recommended.

Prevention of nausea and vomiting associated with emetogenic chemotherapy: IV: **Note:** Pretreatment with diphenhydramine will decrease risk of extrapyramidal reactions.

Highly emetogenic: Initial dose: 2 mg/kg over 15 minutes 30 minutes before chemotherapy; repeat every 2 hours for 2 doses, then every 3 hours for 3 doses.

Less emetogenic: Initial dose: 1 mg/kg over 15 minutes 30 minutes before chemotherapy; repeat every 2 hours for 2 doses, then every 3 hours for 3 doses.

Delayed-emesis prophylaxis (off-label): Oral: 20 to 40 mg (or 0.5 mg/kg/dose) 2 to 4 times daily for 3 to 4 days in combination with dexamethasone (ASCO guidelines (Kris 2006]).

Refractory or intolerant to antiemetics with a higher therapeutic index (off-label; Hesketh 2008):

IV: 1 to 2 mg/kg/dose before chemotherapy and repeat 2 hours after chemotherapy.

Oral: 0.5 mg/kg every 6 hours on days 2 to 4.

Prevention of postoperative nausea and vomiting:

IM, IV (off-label route): Usual dose: 10 mg near end of surgery; some patients may require 20 mg. **Note:** Guidelines discourage use of 10 mg metoclopramide due to lack of effectiveness (Gan 2007); comparative study indicates higher dose (20 mg) may be efficacious (Quaynor 2002).

Oral (off-label route): 20 mg orally 2 hours prior to anesthesia has been recommended (Metonia Canadian product labeling).

Radiological exam:

IV: 10 mg as a single dose

Oral (off-label route): 20 mg as a single dose 5 to 10 minutes prior to exam (Metonia Canadian product labeling 2014).

Small bowel intubation (postpyloric feeding tube placement): IV: 10 mg as a single dose.

Gastric bezoars (off-label use): Oral, IV: 5 to 10 mg 3 to 4 times daily until resolution (Gaya 2002; Winkler 1983). To prevent further bezoar formation, metoclopramide was continued for up to 16 months in one study (Winkler 1983). Additional data may be necessary to further define the role of metoclopramide in the treatment of this condition.

Continuous infusion: IV: 40 mg administered over 24 hours for 3 days; may repeat if bezoar is not cleared (Delpre 1984).

Hiccups (off-label use): Note: Additional data may be necessary to further define the role of metoclopramide in the prevention and treatment of this condition.

Prevention:

IV: 0.17 mg/kg as a single dose starting the day of or 1 day before anticipated hiccup-precipitating event (Stav 1992).

Oral: 10 mg every 6 to 8 hours starting the day of or 1 day before anticipated hiccup-precipitating event (Baethge 1986; Cersosimo 1998).

Treatment:

IV, IM: 5 to 10 mg every 8 hours (Madanagopolan 1975; Middleton 1973). Therapy may begin with parenteral dosing and transition to oral dosing (10 mg orally every 6 to 8 hours) when hiccups are controlled. Treatment usually continues until metoclopramide can be withdrawn without provoking a recurrence (Friedman 1996).

Oral: 10 mg every 6 to 8 hours (Madanagopolan 1975; Middleton 1973).

Migraine (acute) (off-label use): Note: The IV route is preferred by the American Headache Society (AHS [Orr 2016]).

Oral: 10 to 20 mg as a single dose (EFNS [Evers 2009]).

IM, SubQ: 10 mg as a single dose (EFNS [Evers 2009]).

IV: 10 to 20 mg as a single dose (AHS [Orr 2016]; EFNS [Evers 2009]).

Prevention of radiation therapy-induced nausea and vomiting (minimal emetic risk) (off-label use): Oral: 20 mg as rescue therapy; if rescue therapy is used, then administer prior to each fraction until the end of radiation therapy (Basch 2011).

Treatment of nausea and vomiting in advanced cancer (off-label use): Oral, IV, IM, SubQ (off-label route): 5 mg four times a day (30 minutes prior to meals and at bedtime) (Protus 2015).

Geriatric Initial: Dose at the lower end of the recommended range (may require only 5 mg/dose) and use the lowest effective dose. Refer to adult dosing.

Pediatric

Small bowel intubation (postpyloric feeding tube placement): Children and Adolescents: IV:

<6 years: 0.1 mg/kg as a single dose

6 to 14 years: 2.5 to 5 mg as a single dose

>14 years: Refer to adult dosing.

Prevention of chemotherapy-associated nausea and vomiting (off-label use): Children and Adolescents: Moderately emetogenic chemotherapy (patients who cannot receive corticosteroids): IV: 1 mg/kg prior to chemotherapy, followed by Oral: 0.0375 mg/kg every 6 hours; regimen also includes ondansetron or granisetron; coadministration of diphenhydramine or benztropine is recommended to prevent metoclopramide-induced adverse effects (Dupuis 2013).

Renal Impairment

CrCl <40 mL/minute: Administer 50% of normal dose.

Not dialyzable (0% to 5%); supplemental dose is not necessary (Aronoff, 2007).

Hepatic Impairment There are no dosage adjustments provided in the manufacturer's labeling. However, metoclopramide has been used safely in patients with advanced liver disease with normal renal function.

◀ **Administration**

Injection: May be given IM, direct IV push, short infusion (at least 15 minutes), or continuous infusion; lower doses (≤10 mg) of metoclopramide can be given IV push undiluted over 1 to 2 minutes; higher doses (>10 mg) to be diluted in 50 mL of compatible solution (preferably NS) and given IVPB over at least 15 minutes. **Note:** Rapid IV administration may be associated with a transient (but intense) feeling of anxiety and restlessness, followed by drowsiness.

Tablets: When used for gastroparesis/reflux, administer 30 minutes prior to meals and at bedtime.

Orally disintegrating tablets: When used for gastroparesis/reflux, administer on an empty stomach at least 30 minutes prior to food and at bedtime (do not repeat if inadvertently taken with food). Do not remove from packaging until time of administration. If tablet breaks or crumbles while handling, discard and remove new tablet. Using dry hands, place tablet on tongue and allow to dissolve (disintegrates within ~1 minute [range: 10 seconds to 14 minutes]). Swallow with saliva (formulation is designed to be taken without liquids).

Oral solution: When used for gastroparesis/reflux, administer 30 minutes prior to meals and at bedtime.

Subcutaneous administration (off-label route) has been reported, either as an intermittent bolus injection or as continuous infusion (Bruera 1996; McCallum 1991).

Monitoring Parameters Signs of tardive dyskinesias, extrapyramidal symptoms; signs/symptoms of neuroleptic malignant syndrome

Medication Guide Available Yes

Dosage Forms Excipient information presented when available (limited, particularly for generics); consult specific product labeling. [DSC] = Discontinued product

Solution, Injection:
  Generic: 5 mg/mL (2 mL)
Solution, Injection [preservative free]:
  Generic: 5 mg/mL (2 mL)
Solution, Oral:
  Generic: 5 mg/5 mL (10 mL, 473 mL); 10 mg/10 mL (10 mL)
Tablet, Oral:
  Reglan: 5 mg [contains fd&c blue #1 aluminum lake, fd&c yellow #10 aluminum lake]
  Reglan: 10 mg [dye free]
  Generic: 5 mg, 10 mg
Tablet Disintegrating, Oral:
  Metozolv ODT: 5 mg [DSC]
  Generic: 5 mg, 10 mg

♦ **Metoclopramide HCl** see Metoclopramide on page 1240

♦ **Metoclopramide Hydrochloride Injection (Can)** see Metoclopramide on page 1240

♦ **Metoclopramide Omega (Can)** see Metoclopramide on page 1240

♦ **Metoject (Can)** see Methotrexate on page 1205

♦ **Metonia (Can)** see Metoclopramide on page 1240

♦ **Metozolv ODT [DSC]** see Metoclopramide on page 1240

♦ **Metro** see MetroNIDAZOLE (Systemic) on page 1249

MetroNIDAZOLE (Systemic) (met roe NYE da zole)

Brand Names: US First-Metronidazole 100; First-Metronidazole 50; Flagyl; Flagyl ER [DSC]; Metro; MetroNIDAZOLE Benzo+SyrSpend

Brand Names: Canada Flagyl; Metronidazole Injection USP; Novo-Nidazol; PMS-Metronidazole

Index Terms Benzoyl Metronidazole; Flagyl; Metronidazole Benzoate; Metronidazole Hydrochloride

Pharmacologic Category Amebicide; Antibiotic, Miscellaneous; Antiprotozoal, Nitroimidazole

Use

Amebiasis: Oral immediate-release tablet and capsule: Treatment of acute intestinal amebiasis (amebic dysentery) and amebic liver abscess

Limitations of use (oral immediate-release tablet, capsule and injection): When used for amebic liver abscess, may be used concurrently with percutaneous needle aspiration when it is clinically indicated.

Anaerobic bacterial infections (caused by _Bacteroides_ spp., including the _B. fragilis_ group): Oral immediate-release tablet, capsule, and injection:

Bacterial septicemia: Treatment of bacterial septicemia (also caused by _Clostridium_ spp.)

Bone and joint infections: Treatment (adjunctive therapy) of bone and joint infections

CNS Infections: Treatment of CNS infections, including meningitis and brain abscess

Endocarditis: Treatment of endocarditis

Gynecologic infections: Treatment of gynecologic infections including endometritis, endomyometritis, tubo-ovarian abscess, or postsurgical vaginal cuff infection (also caused by _Clostridium_ spp., _Peptococcus_ spp., _Peptostreptococcus_ spp., and _Fusobacterium_ spp.)

Intra-abdominal infections: Treatment of intra-abdominal infections, including peritonitis, intra-abdominal abscess and liver abscess (also caused by _Clostridium_ spp., _Eubacterium_ spp., _Peptococcus_ spp., and _Peptostreptococcus_ spp.)

Lower respiratory tract infections: Treatment of lower respiratory tract infections, including pneumonia, empyema and lung abscess

Skin and skin structure infections: Treatment of skin and skin structure infections (also caused by _Clostridium_ spp., _Peptococcus_ spp., _Peptostreptococcus_ spp., and _Fusobacterium_ spp.)

Bacterial vaginosis: Oral extended-release tablet: Treatment of bacterial vaginosis in nonpregnant women

Surgical prophylaxis (colorectal surgery): Injection: Preoperative, intraoperative, and postoperative prophylaxis to reduce the incidence of postoperative infection in patients undergoing elective colorectal surgery classified as contaminated or potentially contaminated

Trichomoniasis: Oral immediate-release tablet, capsule, and injection: Treatment of infections caused by _Trichomonas vaginalis_, including treatment of asymptomatic sexual partners

Pregnancy Risk Factor B

Dosing

Adult & Geriatric

Amebiasis (acute dysentery): Oral: Immediate-release tablets and capsules: 750 mg every 8 hours for 5 to 10 days

Amebic liver abscess: Oral:

Immediate-release tablets: 500 to 750 mg every 8 hours for 5 to 10 days

◄ Capsules: 750 mg every 8 hours for 5 to 10 days

Bacterial vaginosis or vaginitis due to _Gardnerella, Mobiluncus:_ Oral:
Tablet:

Immediate release (off-label use): 500 mg twice daily for 7 days (CDC [Workowski 2015])

Extended release: 750 mg once daily for 7 days

Intra-abdominal infection:

Manufacturer's labeling: Oral (immediate release), IV: 500 mg every 6 hours (maximum: 4 g/day); **Note:** Initial: 1 g IV loading dose may be administered

Alternate dosing:

Acute diverticulitis, outpatient treatment: Oral (immediate release): 500 mg every 6 to 8 hours; use in combination with a fluoroquinolone (eg, ciprofloxacin) or sulfamethoxazole and trimethoprim (Jacobs 2007)

Complicated, community-acquired, mild to moderate (in combination with cephalosporin or fluoroquinolone): IV: 500 mg every 8 to 12 hours **or** 1.5 g every 24 hours for 4 to 7 days (provided source controlled) (Solomkin 2010)

Pelvic inflammatory disease (off-label dose): Oral (immediate release):

Mild to moderately severe: 500 mg twice daily for 14 days (may be added to a combination of a third-generation parenteral cephalosporin and doxycycline) (CDC [Workowski 2015])

With tubo-ovarian abscess: 500 mg twice daily to complete at least 14 days of therapy (in combination with doxycycline following a parenteral therapy regimen)

Trichomoniasis (index case and sex partner): Oral:

Immediate-release tablets:

Manufacturer's labeling: 250 mg every 8 hours for 7 days **or** 1 g twice daily for 2 doses (on same day) **or** 2 g as a single dose

Alternate dosing: 2 g as a single dose (preferred regimen) **or** 500 mg twice daily for 7 days (off-label dose) (CDC [Workowski 2015])

Capsules: 375 mg twice daily for 7 days

Trichomoniasis in HIV-infected women (off-label dose): Oral (immediate release): 500 mg twice daily for 7 days (CDC [Workowski 2015])

Trichomoniasis, persistent or recurrent (ie, treatment failure of nitro-imidazole [eg metronidazole] single-dose therapy) (index case; treatment of sex partner; off-label dose): Oral (immediate release): 500 mg twice daily for 7 days. If this regimen also fails, consider 2 g once daily for 7 days (CDC [Workowski 2015])

Balantidiasis (off-label use): IV, Oral (immediate release): 750 mg 3 times daily for ≥5 days (Anagyrou 2003; Schuster 2008)

Bite wounds (animal/human) (off-label use) (IDSA [Stevens 2014]):
Note: Use in combination with a second- or third-generation cephalosporin, levofloxacin, or sulfamethoxazole/trimethoprim for animal bites, or in combination with ciprofloxacin or levofloxacin for human bites.

Oral: 250 to 500 mg 3 times daily

IV: 500 mg every 8 hours

Clostridium difficile-**associated diarrhea (CDAD) (off-label use): Note:** Recent guideline recommends converting to oral vancomycin therapy if the patient does not show a clear clinical response after 5 to 7 days of metronidazole therapy (Surawicz 2013)

Mild to moderate infection: Oral (immediate release): 500 mg 3 times daily for 10 to 14 days (Cohen 2010; Surawicz 2013)

Severe complicated infection (no abdominal distention): IV: 500 mg 3 times daily with oral vancomycin for 10 to 14 days (Surawicz 2013)

Severe complicated infection (with ileus, toxic colitis, and/or abdominal distention): IV: 500 mg 3 times daily with oral and rectal vancomycin for 10 to 14 days (Surawicz 2013)

Crohn disease, mild to moderate (off-label use): Oral (immediate release): 10 to 20 mg/kg/day (Lichtenstein 2009) or 500 mg twice daily (in combination with ciprofloxacin) (Steinhart 2002).

Dientamoeba fragilis **infections (off-label use):** Oral (immediate release): 500 to 750 mg 3 times daily for 10 days (CDC 2012)

Giardiasis (off-label use): Oral (immediate release): 250 to 500 mg 3 times daily for 5 to 10 days (Granados 2012)

Helicobacter pylori **eradication (off-label use):** Oral (immediate release):

Triple therapy: Metronidazole 500 mg twice daily for 10 to 14 days, in combination with clarithromycin and a proton pump inhibitor (Chey 2007)

Quadruple therapy: Metronidazole 250 mg 4 times daily for 10 to 14 days, in combination with bismuth subsalicylate, a tetracycline, and either ranitidine or a proton pump inhibitor (Chey 2007)

Periodontitis (associated with aggressive disease; off-label use): Oral (immediate release): 250 mg every 8 hours in combination with amoxicillin for 10 days; used in addition to scaling, root planing and pocket irrigation (Silva-Senem 2013)

Pouchitis (post ileal pouch-anal anastomosis, acute treatment; off-label use): Oral (immediate release): 400 to 500 mg three times daily for 7 days (Holubar 2010; Wall 2011)

Prophylaxis against sexually-transmitted diseases following sexual assault (off-label use): Oral (immediate release): 2 g as a single dose in combination with ceftriaxone and azithromycin (CDC [Workowski 2015])

Skin and soft tissue necrotizing infections (off-label use): IV: 500 mg every 6 hours, in combination with cefotaxime or ceftriaxone for empiric therapy of polymicrobial infections. Continue until further debridement is not necessary, patient has clinically improved, and patient is afebrile for 48 to 72 hours (IDSA [Stevens 2014]).

Surgical prophylaxis:

Manufacturer's labeling: IV: 15 mg/kg 1 hour prior to surgical incision; followed by 7.5 mg/kg 6 and 12 hours after initial dose

Alternate dosing:

IV: 500 mg within 60 minutes prior to surgical incision in combination with other antibiotics (Bratzler 2013). **Note:** Considered a recommended agent for select procedures other than colorectal surgery (off-label use) (Bratzler 2013).

Oral (for colorectal surgical prophylaxis only; immediate release; off-label use): 1 g every 3 to 4 hours for 3 doses, starting after mechanical bowel preparation the afternoon and evening before the procedure with or without additional oral antibiotics and with an appropriate IV antibiotic prophylaxis regimen (Bratzler 2013).

Surgical site infections (intestinal or GU tract; axilla or perineum) (off-label use): IV: 500 mg every 8 hours; in combination with ceftriaxone, ciprofloxacin, or levofloxacin (IDSA [Stevens 2014]).

Tetanus (*Clostridium tetani*** infection; off-label use):** Oral (immediate release): 500 mg every 6 hours for 7 to 10 days in combination with supportive therapy (Ahmadsyah, 1985)

Urethritis, nongonococcal (recurrent or persistent urethritis in men who have sex with women and who live in regions where *T. vaginalis* is prevalent; off-label use): Oral (immediate release): 2 g as a single dose. **Note:** Compliance with initial regimen and lack of re-exposure to an untreated sex partner should be excluded prior to use (CDC [Workowski 2015])

Pediatric

Infants, Children, and Adolescents:

Amebiasis: Oral: 35 to 50 mg/kg/day in divided doses every 8 hours for 7 to 10 days (*Red Book* [AAP 2012])

Trichomoniasis: Oral: 15 mg/kg/day in divided doses every 8 hours for 7 days (*Red Book* [AAP 2012])

Anaerobic infections (off-label dosing):

Oral: 30 to 50 mg/kg/day in divided doses every 8 hours (maximum: 2,250 mg/day) (*Red Book* [AAP 2012])

IV: 22.5 to 40 mg/kg/day in divided doses every 8 hours (maximum: 1,500 mg/day) (*Red Book* [AAP 2012])

Balantidiasis (off-label use): Oral: 35 to 50 mg/kg/day in 3 divided doses for 5 days (*Red Book* [AAP 2012]; Schuster 2008)

***Clostridium difficile*-associated diarrhea (CDAD; off-label use):** Oral: 30 mg/kg/day divided every 6 hours for ≥10 days (maximum: 2 g/day) (*Red Book* [AAP 2012]; Schutze 2013). **Note:** Recommended agent for the initial treatment of mild to moderate disease and for first relapse (*Red Book* [AAP 2012]; Schutze 2013).

Giardiasis (off-label use): Oral: 15 mg/kg/day in divided doses every 8 hours for 5 to 10 days (Granados 2012; *Red Book* [AAP 2012])

***Helicobacter pylori* eradication (off-label use):** Oral: 20 mg/kg/day in 2 divided doses for 10 to 14 days in combination therapy with amoxicillin and either a proton pump inhibitor or bismuth subsalicylate daily or 20 mg/kg/day in 2 divided doses on days 6 through 10 in combination therapy with a proton pump inhibitor and clarithromycin (after treatment with amoxicillin and a proton pump inhibitor for days 1 through 5) (maximum: 1 g/day) (Koletzko 2011)

Skin and soft tissue necrotizing infections (off-label use): IV: 7.5 mg/kg every 6 hours, in combination with cefotaxime for empiric therapy of polymicrobial infections. Continue until further debridement is not necessary, patient has clinically improved, and patient is afebrile for 48 to 72 hours (IDSA [Stevens 2014]).

Surgical (preoperative) prophylaxis (off-label use):

Infants <1,200 g: IV: 7.5 mg/kg within 60 minutes prior to surgical incision in combination with other antibiotics (Bratzler 2013).

Infants ≥1,200 g and Children ≥1 year:

IV: 15 mg/kg within 60 minutes prior to surgical incision in combination with other antibiotics (maximum: 500 mg per dose) (Bratzler 2013).

Oral (for colorectal surgical prophylaxis only): 15 mg/kg (maximum: 1,000 mg) every 3 to 4 hours for 3 doses, starting after mechanical bowel preparation the afternoon and evening before the procedure, with or without additional oral antibiotics and with an appropriate IV antibiotic prophylaxis regimen (Bratzler 2013).

Tetanus (*Clostridium tetani* infection, off-label use): Oral, IV: 30 mg/kg per day in divided doses every 6 hours for 10 to 14 days in combination with tetanus immune globulin and supportive therapy (maximum: 4 g/day) (*Red Book* [AAP 2012])

Adolescents: Oral:

Pelvic inflammatory disease (off-label dosing): Refer to adult dosing

Prophylaxis against sexually-transmitted diseases following sexual assault (off-label use): Refer to adult dosing.

Vaginal infections:

Vaginitis (*Trichomonas vaginalis*; off-label use): 2 g as a single dose (*Red Book* [AAP 2012])

Vaginosis (bacterial; off-label use): 500 mg twice daily for 7 days (*Red Book* [AAP 2012])

Renal Impairment

Manufacturer's labeling:

Mild, moderate, or severe impairment: There are no dosage adjustments provided in the manufacturer's labeling; however, decreased renal function does not alter the single-dose pharmacokinetics

End-stage renal disease (ESRD) requiring dialysis: Metronidazole metabolites may accumulate; monitor for adverse events. Accumulated metabolites may be rapidly removed by dialysis:

Intermittent hemodialysis (IHD): If administration cannot be separated from hemodialysis, consider supplemental dose following hemodialysis.

Peritoneal dialysis (PD): No dosage adjustment necessary.

Alternate dosing:

Intermittent hemodialysis (IHD) (administer after hemodialysis on dialysis days): Dialyzable (50% to 100%): 500 mg every 8 to 12 hours. **Note:** Dosing regimen highly dependent on clinical indication (trichomoniasis vs *C. difficile* colitis) (Heintz 2009). **Note:** Dosing dependent on the assumption of thrice weekly, complete IHD sessions.

Continuous renal replacement therapy (CRRT) (Heintz 2009; Trotman 2005): Drug clearance is highly dependent on the method of renal replacement, filter type, and flow rate. Appropriate dosing requires close monitoring of pharmacologic response, signs of adverse reactions due to drug accumulation, as well as drug concentrations in relation to target trough (if appropriate). The following are general recommendations only (based on dialysate flow/ultrafiltration rates of 1 to 2 L/hour and minimal residual renal function) and should not supersede clinical judgment:

CVVH/CVVHD/CVVHDF: 500 mg every 6 to 12 hours (or per clinical indication; dosage reduction generally not necessary)

Hepatic Impairment

Manufacturer's labeling:

Mild or moderate impairment (Child-Pugh class A or B): No dosage adjustment necessary; use with caution and monitor for adverse events

Severe impairment (Child-Pugh class C):

Extended-release tablets: Use is not recommended.

Immediate-release capsules:

Amebiasis: 375 mg 3 times daily

Trichomoniasis: 375 mg once daily

Immediate-release tablets, injection: Reduce dose by 50%

◄ *Alternate dosing:* The pharmacokinetics of a single oral 500 mg dose were not altered in patients with cirrhosis; initial dose reduction is therefore not necessary (Daneshmend, 1982). In one study of IV metronidazole, patients with alcoholic liver disease (with or without cirrhosis), demonstrated a prolonged elimination half-life (eg, ~18 hours). The authors recommended the dose be reduced accordingly (clearance was reduced by ~62%) and the frequency may be prolonged (eg, every 12 hours instead of every 6 hours) (Lau, 1987). In another single IV dose study using metronidazole metabolism to predict hepatic function, patients classified as Child-Pugh class C demonstrated a half-life of ~21.5 hours (Muscara, 1995).

Additional Information Complete prescribing information should be consulted for additional detail.

Dosage Forms Considerations

Parenteral solution contains 28 mEq of sodium/gram of metronidazole.

First-Metronidazole and MetroNIDAZOLE Benzo+SyrSpend oral suspensions are a compounding kits. Refer to manufacturer's labeling for compounding instructions.

Dosage Forms Excipient information presented when available (limited, particularly for generics); consult specific product labeling. [DSC] = Discontinued product

Capsule, Oral:
  Flagyl: 375 mg
  Generic: 375 mg
Solution, Intravenous:
  Metro: 500 mg (100 mL)
  Generic: 500 mg (100 mL)
Solution, Intravenous [preservative free]:
  Generic: 500 mg (100 mL [DSC])
Suspension Reconstituted, Oral:
  First-Metronidazole 50: 50 mg/mL (150 mL) [contains saccharin sodium, sodium benzoate]
  First-Metronidazole 100: 100 mg/mL (150 mL) [contains saccharin sodium, sodium benzoate]
  MetroNIDAZOLE Benzo+SyrSpend: 50 mg/mL (120 mL)
Tablet, Oral:
  Flagyl: 250 mg, 500 mg
  Generic: 250 mg, 500 mg
Tablet Extended Release 24 Hour, Oral:
  Flagyl ER: 750 mg [DSC]

Dosage Forms: Canada Information with regard to form, strength, and availability of products uniquely available in Canada but currently not available in the United States. Refer also to Dosage Forms.

Excipient information presented when available (limited, particularly for generics); consult specific product labeling.
  Capsule, Oral:
    Flagyl: 500 mg

♦ **Metronidazole Benzoate** *see* MetroNIDAZOLE (Systemic) *on page 1249*

♦ **MetroNIDAZOLE Benzo+SyrSpend** *see* MetroNIDAZOLE (Systemic) *on page 1249*

♦ **Metronidazole Hydrochloride** *see* MetroNIDAZOLE (Systemic) *on page 1249*

◆ **Metronidazole Injection USP (Can)** *see* MetroNIDAZOLE (Systemic) *on page 1249*

◆ **MET Tyrosine Kinase Inhibitor PF-02341066** *see* Crizotinib *on page 432*

◆ **Miacalcin** *see* Calcitonin *on page 316*

Micafungin (mi ka FUN gin)

Brand Names: US Mycamine
Brand Names: Canada Mycamine
Index Terms Micafungin Sodium
Pharmacologic Category Antifungal Agent, Parenteral; Echinocandin
Use

Candidemia, acute disseminated candidiasis, *Candida* peritonitis and abscesses: Treatment of candidemia, acute disseminated candidiasis, *Candida* peritonitis and abscesses

Esophageal candidiasis: Treatment of esophageal candidiasis

Prophylaxis of *Candida* infections: Prophylaxis of *Candida* infections in patients undergoing hematopoietic stem cell transplantation (HSCT)

Pregnancy Risk Factor C

Dosing

Adult & Geriatric

Aspergillosis, invasive (salvage therapy) (off-label use): IV: 100 to 150 mg once daily. Minimum duration of therapy is 6 to 12 weeks, although duration is highly dependent on degree/duration of immunosuppression, disease site, and evidence of disease improvement (IDSA [Patterson 2016])

Candidemia, acute disseminated candidiasis, and *Candida* peritonitis and abscesses: IV: 100 mg once daily; mean duration of therapy (from clinical trials) was 15 days (range: 10 to 47 days). **Note:** For treatment of candidemia, IDSA Candidiasis guidelines recommend a total duration of antifungal therapy of at least 2 weeks *after* the documented clearance of *Candida* from the bloodstream and resolution of candidemia-associated symptoms in patients without metastatic complications; may transition to fluconazole (eg, after 5 to 7 days in non-neutropenic patients) in clinically stable patients, with fluconazole-susceptible isolates and negative repeat cultures (IDSA [Pappas 2016]).

Candidiasis, chronic disseminated (hepatosplenic) (off-label use): IV: 100 mg daily for several weeks, followed by oral fluconazole therapy (IDSA [Pappas 2016])

Candidiasis, empiric therapy (suspected invasive candidiasis in non-neutropenic ICU patients) (off-label use): IV: 100 mg daily; treatment should continue for 14 days in patients showing clinical improvement. Consider discontinuing after 4 to 5 days in patients with no clinical response (IDSA [Pappas 2016]).

Candidiasis, intravascular infections (native or prosthetic valve endocarditis, infection of implantable cardiac devices, suppurative thrombophlebitis) (off-label use): IV: 150 mg daily. For native or prosthetic valve endocarditis, therapy should continue for at least 6 weeks after valve replacement surgery (longer durations in patients with abscesses or other complications); for patients with implantable cardiac devices, therapy should continue for 4 to 6 weeks after surgery (4 weeks for infections limited to generator pockets and at least 6 weeks for infections involving the wires); for suppurative thrombophlebitis, after catheter removal, continue ▶

for at least 2 weeks after candidemia has cleared. **Note:** Step-down to fluconazole therapy is recommended in clinically stable patients and fluconazole-susceptible isolates with negative repeat cultures (IDSA [Pappas 2016]).

Candidiasis, osteoarticular infections (osteomyelitis or septic arthritis) (alternative therapy) (off-label use): IV: 100 mg daily for at least 14 days, followed by fluconazole therapy (IDSA [Pappas 2016])

Candidiasis, oropharyngeal (refractory disease) (alternative therapy) (off-label use): IV: 100 mg once daily (IDSA [Pappas 2016])

Empiric antifungal therapy (neutropenic fever) (off-label use): IV: 100 mg once daily (IDSA [Patterson 2016])

Esophageal candidiasis: IV: 150 mg once daily; mean duration of therapy (from clinical trials) was 15 days (range: 10 to 30 days). **Note:** IDSA Candidiasis guidelines suggest considering a transition to oral fluconazole therapy once oral intake tolerable. In patients with fluconazole-refractory disease, continue micafungin for 14 to 21 days (IDSA [Pappas 2016]).

Prophylaxis of *Candida* infections: IV:
In hematopoietic stem cell transplantation: 50 mg once daily; mean duration of therapy (from clinical trials) was 19 days (range: 6 to 51 days)
In high-risk ICU patients in units with high incidence of invasive candidiasis (alternative therapy; off-label use): 100 mg daily (Pappas [IDSA 2016])

Pediatric

Candidemia, acute disseminated candidiasis, and *Candida* peritonitis and abscesses: Infants ≥4 months, Children, and Adolescents: IV: 2 mg/kg once daily; maximum: 100 mg once daily

Esophageal candidiasis: Infants ≥4 months, Children, and Adolescents: IV:
≤30 kg: 3 mg/kg once daily
>30 kg: 2.5 mg/kg once daily; maximum: 150 mg once daily

Prophylaxis of *Candida* infection in hematopoietic stem cell transplantation: Infants ≥4 months, Children, and Adolescents: IV: 1 mg/kg once daily; maximum: 50 mg once daily

Primary antifungal prophylaxis in allogeneic HSCT (when fluconazole is contraindicated; off-label dosing/population; guideline recommendation): Infants ≥1 month, Children, and Adolescents <19 years: IV: 1 mg/kg once daily; maximum: 50 mg once daily (Science, 2014)

Renal Impairment
No dosage adjustment necessary.
Poorly dialyzed; no supplemental dose or dosage adjustment necessary, including patients on intermittent hemodialysis.

Hepatic Impairment No dosage adjustment necessary.

Additional Information Complete prescribing information should be consulted for additional detail.

Dosage Forms Excipient information presented when available (limited, particularly for generics); consult specific product labeling.
Solution Reconstituted, Intravenous, as sodium:
Mycamine: 50 mg (1 ea); 100 mg (1 ea)
Solution Reconstituted, Intravenous, as sodium [preservative free]:
Mycamine: 50 mg (1 ea); 100 mg (1 ea)

◆ **Micafungin Sodium** see Micafungin on page 1255

◆ **MICRhoGAM Ultra-Filtered Plus** see Rh₀(D) Immune Globulin on page 1591

Midostaurin (mye doe STAW rin)

Related Information

Common Toxicity Criteria *on page* 2242

Safe Handling of Hazardous Drugs *on page* 2379

Brand Names: US Rydapt

Brand Names: Canada Rydapt

Index Terms CGP 41251; N-benzoyl-staurosporine; PKC 412

Pharmacologic Category Antineoplastic Agent, FLT3 Inhibitor; Antineoplastic Agent, Tyrosine Kinase Inhibitor

Use

Acute myeloid leukemia, FLT3-positive: Treatment of adult patients with newly diagnosed FLT3 mutation-positive (as detected by an approved test) acute myeloid leukemia (AML), in combination with standard cytarabine and daunorubicin induction and cytarabine consolidation chemotherapy

Limitations of use: Not indicated as single-agent induction therapy for the treatment of patients with AML.

Mast cell leukemia: Treatment of adult patients with mast cell leukemia (MCL)

Systemic mastocytosis: Treatment of adult patients with aggressive systemic mastocytosis (ASM) or systemic mastocytosis with associated hematological neoplasm (SM-AHN)

Labeled Contraindications Hypersensitivity to midostaurin or any component of the formulation

Pregnancy Considerations Adverse events were observed in animal reproduction studies with doses providing less than the human exposure at the recommended dose based on AUC. Based on the mechanism of action, midostaurin may cause fetal harm if used in pregnant women.

Pregnancy status should be verified within 7 days prior to therapy initiation. Females of reproductive potential and males with female partners of reproductive potential should use effective contraception during therapy and for at least 4 months after the last dose. Based on animal data, treatment with midostaurin may impair fertility in males and females.

Breastfeeding Considerations It is not known if midostaurin is present in breast milk. Due to the potential for adverse reactions in the breastfed infant, breastfeeding is not recommended by the manufacturer during therapy and for at least 4 months after the last dose.

Warnings/Precautions Lymphopenia, leukopenia, neutropenia, thrombocytopenia and anemia have been commonly observed in patients with systemic mastocytosis. Although the incidence of hematologic toxicity in acute myeloid leukemia (AML) may be confounded by concomitant chemotherapy, febrile neutropenia was reported at a slightly higher incidence in patients with AML receiving chemotherapy plus midostaurin (compared to chemotherapy plus placebo). Monitor blood counts. Nausea and vomiting commonly occur; premedicate with antiemetics prior to administration. Diarrhea, abdominal pain, and constipation also occur frequently. Mucositis has also been reported.

Hypersensitivity reactions, including anaphylactic shock, angioedema, dyspnea, chest pain and flushing have been observed. Interstitial lung disease and pneumonitis have been reported with midostaurin (either as monotherapy or in combination with other chemotherapy), some cases have been fatal. Monitor for pulmonary symptoms; discontinue in patients who develop signs/symptoms of interstitial lung disease or pneumonitis (without an infectious etiology).

◄ Potentially significant interactions may exist, requiring dose or frequency adjustment, additional monitoring, and/or selection of alternative therapy.

Adverse Reactions

>10%:

Cardiovascular: Edema (40%), prolonged Q-T interval on ECG (11%)

Central nervous system: Headache (26% to 46%), fatigue (34%), dizziness (13%), insomnia (11% to 12%)

Dermatologic: Hyperhidrosis (14%), skin rash (14%)

Endocrine & metabolic: Hyperglycemia (20% to 80%), hypocalcemia (39% to 74%), hyperuricemia (8% to 37%), increased gamma-glutamyl transferase (35%), hyponatremia (34%), hypoalbuminemia (27%), hypokalemia (25%), hyperkalemia (23%), hypophosphatemia (22%), hypernatremia (21%), hypomagnesemia (20%)

Gastrointestinal: Nausea (47% to 83%), vomiting (19% to 68%), mucositis (66%), diarrhea (54%), increased serum lipase (37%), abdominal pain (34%), constipation (29%), increased serum amylase (20%), hemorrhoids (15%), gastrointestinal hemorrhage (14%)

Genitourinary: Urinary tract infection (16%)

Hematologic & oncologic: Febrile neutropenia (8% to 83%; grades ≥3: 84%), lymphocytopenia (66%; grades ≥3: 42%), leukopenia (61%; grades ≥3: 19%), anemia (60%; grades ≥3: 38%), thrombocytopenia (50%; grades ≥3: 27%), neutropenia (49%; grades ≥3: 22%), petechia (36%), prolonged partial thromboplastin time (13%; grades ≥3: 3%)

Hepatic: Increased serum ALT (31% to 71%), increased serum alkaline phosphatase (39%), increased serum AST (32%), hyperbilirubinemia (29%)

Infection: Localized infection (24%; device related)

Neuromuscular & skeletal: Musculoskeletal pain (33% to 35%), arthralgia (14% to 19%)

Renal: Increased serum creatinine (25%), renal insufficiency (11% to 12%)

Respiratory: Upper respiratory tract infection (20% to 30%), epistaxis (12% to 28%), dyspnea (23%), cough (18%), pleural effusion (6% to 13%)

Miscellaneous: Fever (27%)

1% to 10%:

Cardiovascular: Hypotension (9%), hypertension (8%), cardiac failure (6%), thrombosis (5%), pericardial effusion (4%), ischemia (≤4%), myocardial infarction (≤4%)

Central nervous system: Disturbance in attention (7%), chills (5%), vertigo (5%), mental status changes (4%)

Dermatologic: Xeroderma (7%), cellulitis (≤7%), erysipelas (≤5%)

Endocrine & metabolic: Weight gain (6% to 7%), hypercalcemia (3%)

Gastrointestinal: Dyspepsia (6%), gastritis (3%)

Hematologic & oncologic: Bruise (6%), hematoma (6%)

Hypersensitivity: Hypersensitivity (4%)

Infection: Herpes virus infection (10%), sepsis (9%), fungal infection (7%)

Neuromuscular & skeletal: Tremor (4% to 6%)

Ophthalmic: Eyelid edema (3%)

Respiratory: Pneumonia (10%), bronchitis (6%), oropharyngeal pain (4%), pulmonary edema (3%), interstitial pulmonary disease (≤2%), pneumonitis (≤2%)

Drug Interactions

Metabolism/Transport Effects Substrate of CYP3A4 (major); **Note:** Assignment of Major/Minor substrate status based on clinically relevant drug interaction potential; **Inhibits** SLCO1A1; **Induces** MRP2

Avoid Concomitant Use

Avoid concomitant use of Midostaurin with any of the following: BCG (Intravesical); CYP3A4 Inducers (Strong); Deferiprone; Dipyrone; Fusidic Acid (Systemic); Highest Risk QTc-Prolonging Agents; Hydroxychloroquine; Idelalisib; MiFEPRIStone; Probucol; Promazine; St John's Wort; Vinflunine

Increased Effect/Toxicity

Midostaurin may increase the levels/effects of: Deferiprone; Highest Risk QTc-Prolonging Agents; Moderate Risk QTc-Prolonging Agents

The levels/effects of Midostaurin may be increased by: Aprepitant; Conivaptan; CYP3A4 Inhibitors (Moderate); CYP3A4 Inhibitors (Strong); Dasatinib; DilTIAZem; Dipyrone; Fosaprepitant; Fusidic Acid (Systemic); Grapefruit Juice; Hydroxychloroquine; Idelalisib; MiFEPRIStone; Netupitant; Palbociclib; Probucol; Promazine; QTc-Prolonging Agents (Indeterminate Risk and Risk Modifying); Simeprevir; Stiripentol; Vinflunine; Xipamide

Decreased Effect

Midostaurin may decrease the levels/effects of: Antidiabetic Agents; BCG (Intravesical)

The levels/effects of Midostaurin may be decreased by: Bosentan; CYP3A4 Inducers (Moderate); CYP3A4 Inducers (Strong); Dabrafenib; Deferasirox; Sarilumab; Siltuximab; St John's Wort; Tocilizumab

Food Interactions Grapefruit juice may increase midostaurin plasma concentration. Management: Avoid grapefruit juice.

Hazardous Drugs Handling Considerations Hazardous agent (meets NIOSH 2016 criteria). This medication is not on the NIOSH (2016) list; however, it meets the criteria for a hazardous drug. Drugs are classified as hazardous based on their properties; the properties of a hazardous drug include one or more of the following characteristics: carcinogenic, teratogenic (or other developmental toxicity), reproductive toxicity, organotoxic at low doses, genotoxic, and/or new agents with structural or toxicity profiles similar to existing hazardous agents.

Use appropriate precautions for receiving, handling, administration, and disposal. Gloves (single) should be worn during receiving, unpacking, and placing in storage. NIOSH recommends single gloving for administration of intact tablets or capsules (NIOSH 2016).

Storage/Stability Store at 25°C (77°F); excursions permitted to 15°C to 30°C (59°F to 86°F). Store in the original package to protect from moisture.

Mechanism of Action

Midostaurin is a tyrosine kinase inhibitor which inhibits multiple receptors, such as wild type FLT3, FLT3 mutant kinases ITD and TKD, KIT (wild type and D816V mutant), PDGFRα/β, VEGFR2, and members of the serine/threonine protein kinase C (PKC) family.

Midostaurin inhibits FLT3 receptor signaling and cell proliferation, and induces apoptosis in ITD- and TKD- mutant expressing leukemic cells, as well as in cells overexpressing wild type FLT3 and PDGFR. It also may inhibit KIT signaling, cell proliferation, and histamine release (and induces apoptosis) in mast cells.

◄ **Pharmacodynamics/Kinetics**

Absorption: Exposure was increased 1.2- or 1.6-fold when administered with a standard or high-fat meal, respectively, compared to the fasted state. Midostaurin C_{max} was reduced 20% and 27%, respectively, when administered with a standard or high-fat meal compared to a fasted state.

Distribution: 95.2 L

Protein binding: >99.8% bound to plasma proteins (parent drug, CGP62221, and CGP52421); midostaurin is mainly bound to α1-acid glycoprotein

Metabolism: Primarily hepatic via CYP3A4 to active metabolites CGP62221 and CGP52421

Half-life elimination: 21 hours (midostaurin); 32 hours (CGP62221); 482 hours (CGP52421)

Time to peak: 1 to 3 hours (fasted state); 2.5 to 3 hours (with standard or high-fat meal)

Excretion: Feces (95%; 91% as metabolites and 4% as unchanged drug); urine (5%)

Dosing

Adult & Geriatric Note: Administer prophylactic antiemetics prior to midostaurin therapy.

Acute myeloid leukemia (AML), FLT3-positive: Oral: 50 mg twice daily on days 8 to 21 of each induction cycle (in combination with daunorubicin and cytarabine) and on days 8 to 21 of each consolidation cycle (in combination with high-dose cytarabine)

Mast cell leukemia: Oral: 100 mg twice daily until disease progression or unacceptable toxicity (Gotlib 2016)

Systemic mastocytosis (aggressive systemic mastocytosis or systemic mastocytosis with associated hematological neoplasm): Oral: 100 mg twice daily until disease progression or unacceptable toxicity (Gotlib 2016)

Missed doses: If a dose is missed or vomited, do not make up the dose; take the next dose at the usually scheduled time.

Renal Impairment

CrCl ≥30 mL/minute: There are no dosage adjustments provided in the manufacturer's labeling; however, the pharmacokinetics of midostaurin and active metabolites were not significantly altered.

CrCl 15 to 29 mL/minute: There are no dosage adjustments provided in the manufacturer's labeling (has not been studied).

Hepatic Impairment

Mild (total bilirubin >1 to 1.5 times ULN or AST > ULN) or moderate (total bilirubin 1.5 to 3 times ULN and any AST) impairment: There are no dosage adjustments provided in the manufacturer's labeling; however, the pharmacokinetics of midostaurin and active metabolites were not significantly altered.

Severe impairment (total bilirubin >3 times ULN and any AST): There are no dosage adjustments provided in the manufacturer's labeling (has not been studied).

Adjustment for Toxicity

Systemic mastocytosis (aggressive systemic mastocytosis, systemic mastocytosis with associated hematological neoplasm, or mast cell leukemia):

Hematologic toxicity (attributed to midostaurin):

ANC <1,000/mm^3 (in patients *without* mast cell leukemia) or ANC <500/mm^3 (in patients with baseline ANC of 500 to 1,500/mm^3): Interrupt midostaurin; when ANC has improved to ≥1,000/mm³, resume therapy at a reduced dose of 50 mg twice daily and if tolerated, may increase dose to 100 mg twice daily.

Persistently low ANC for >21 days (associated with midostaurin): Discontinue midostaurin

Platelets <50,000/mm³ (in patients *without* mast cell leukemia) or platelets <25,000/mm³ (in patients with baseline platelet count of 25,000 to 75,000/mm³): Interrupt midostaurin; when platelets have improved to ≥50,000/mm³, resume therapy at a reduced dose of 50 mg twice daily and if tolerated, may increase dose to 100 mg twice daily.

Persistently low platelet count for >21 days (associated with midostaurin): Discontinue midostaurin

Hemoglobin <8 g/L (in patients *without* mast cell leukemia) or life-threatening anemia in patients with baseline hemoglobin of 8 to 10 g/L: Interrupt midostaurin; when hemoglobin has improved to ≥8 g/L, resume therapy at a reduced dose of 50 mg twice daily and if tolerated, may increase dose to 100 mg twice daily.

Persistently low hemoglobin for >21 days (associated with midostaurin): Discontinue midostaurin

Nonhematologic toxicity:

Nausea/vomiting, grade 3 or 4 (despite optimal antiemetic prophylaxis): Interrupt midostaurin for 3 days (6 doses), then resume therapy at a reduced dose of 50 mg twice daily. If tolerated, increase dose to 100 mg twice daily.

Other grade 3 or 4 toxicities: Interrupt midostaurin until improvement to ≤ grade 2, then resume therapy at a reduced dose of 50 mg twice daily. If tolerated, increase dose to 100 mg twice daily.

All indications: Pulmonary toxicity: Signs/symptoms of interstitial lung disease or pneumonitis without infectious etiology): Discontinue midostaurin.

Administration Administer with food at approximately 12-hour intervals. Do not open or crush the capsules. Administer prophylactic antiemetics prior to midostaurin therapy.

Monitoring Parameters FLT3 mutation status (in AML); CBC with differential (in patients with systemic mastocytosis, at least weekly for the first 4 weeks, every other week for the next 8 weeks, and monthly thereafter or as clinically indicated); pregnancy status within 7 days of therapy initiation in women of reproductive potential; signs/symptoms of pulmonary toxicity (interstitial lung disease and pneumonitis); consider ECG for QT interval assessment in patients on concurrent medications that may prolong the QT interval.

Dosage Forms Excipient information presented when available (limited, particularly for generics); consult specific product labeling.

Capsule, Oral:

Rydapt: 25 mg [contains cremophor rh40]

- ◆ **MITC** *see* MitoMYcin (Systemic) *on page 1262*
- ◆ **MITO** *see* MitoMYcin (Systemic) *on page 1262*
- ◆ **MITO-C** *see* MitoMYcin (Systemic) *on page 1262*
- ◆ **Mitomycin-X** *see* MitoMYcin (Systemic) *on page 1262*
- ◆ **Mitomycin-C** *see* MitoMYcin (Ophthalmic) *on page 1266*
- ◆ **Mitomycin-C** *see* MitoMYcin (Systemic) *on page 1262*

MitoMYcin (Systemic) (mye toe MYE sin)

Related Information

Management of Chemotherapy-Induced Nausea and Vomiting in Adults *on page 2253*

Management of Drug Extravasations *on page 2271*

Mucositis and Stomatitis *on page 2299*

Prevention of Chemotherapy-Induced Nausea and Vomiting in Children *on page 2310*

Safe Handling of Hazardous Drugs *on page 2379*

Brand Names: Canada Mitomycin For Injection; Mitomycin For Injection USP; Mutamycin

Index Terms MITC; MITO; MITO-C; Mitomycin-C; Mitomycin-X; MMC; MTC; Mutamycin

Pharmacologic Category Antineoplastic Agent, Antibiotic

Use

Gastric cancer: Treatment of disseminated adenocarcinoma of the stomach (in combination with other chemotherapy agents) and as palliative treatment when other modalities have failed.

Pancreatic cancer: Treatment of disseminated adenocarcinoma of the pancreas (in combination with other chemotherapy agents) and as palliative treatment when other modalities have failed.

Limitations of use: Not recommended for single-agent primary therapy or to replace appropriate surgery and/or radiotherapy in the treatment of these conditions.

Labeled Contraindications Hypersensitivity to mitomycin or any component of the formulation; thrombocytopenia; coagulation disorders, or other increased bleeding tendency

Pregnancy Considerations Adverse events have been observed in animal reproduction studies.

Breastfeeding Considerations It is not known if mitomycin is present in breast milk. Due to the potential for serious adverse reactions in the breastfed infant, breastfeeding is not recommended by the manufacturer.

Warnings/Precautions [US Boxed Warning]: Bone marrow suppression (thrombocytopenia and leukopenia) is common and may be severe and/or contribute to infections. WBC and platelet nadir usually occurs at 4 weeks, although may occur at up to 8 weeks; recovery occurs within 10 weeks. Fatalities due to sepsis have been reported; monitor for infections. Myelosuppression is dose-limiting, delayed in onset, and cumulative; therefore, monitor blood counts closely during and for at least 8 weeks following treatment; treatment delay or dosage adjustment may be required for significant thrombocytopenia (platelets <100,000/mm^3) or leukopenia (WBC<4,000/mm^3) or a progressive decline in either value. Monitor for renal toxicity; do not administer if serum creatinine is >1.7 mg/dL. **[US Boxed Warning]: Hemolytic-uremic syndrome (HUS) has been reported**

(incidence not defined); condition usually involves microangiopathic hemolytic anemia (hematocrit ≤25%), thrombocytopenia (≤100,000/mm³), and irreversible renal failure (serum creatinine ≥1.6 mg/dL). HUS may occur at any time (either with single agent or combination therapy), is generally associated with single doses ≥60 mg, and HUS symptoms may be exacerbated by blood transfusion. Other less common effects may include pulmonary edema, neurologic abnormalities, and hypertension. A high mortality from HUS has been reported. Bladder fibrosis/contraction has been reported with intravesical administration (unlabeled administration route). Mitomycin is a potent vesicant; ensure proper needle or catheter placement prior to and during infusion. Avoid extravasation. May cause necrosis and tissue sloughing; delayed erythema and/or ulceration have been reported.

In a scientific statement from the American Heart Association, mitomycin has been determined to be an agent that may either cause reversible direct myocardial toxicity or exacerbate underlying myocardial dysfunction (magnitude: moderate) (AHA [Page 2016]). Cases of acute respiratory distress syndrome (ARDS) have been reported in patients receiving mitomycin in combination with other chemotherapy who were maintained at FIO_2 concentrations >50% perioperatively; use caution to provide only enough oxygen to maintain adequate arterial saturation and avoid overhydration. Pulmonary toxicity has also been reported as dyspnea with nonproductive cough and appearance of pulmonary infiltrates on radiograph; discontinue therapy if pulmonary toxicity occurs and other potential etiologies have been ruled out. Shortness of breath and bronchospasm have been reported in patients receiving vinca alkaloids in combination with mitomycin or who received mitomycin previously; this acute respiratory distress has occurred within minutes to hours following the vinca alkaloid; may be managed with bronchodilators, steroids and/or oxygen. Potentially significant interactions may exist, requiring dose or frequency adjustment, additional monitoring, and/or selection of alternative therapy. **[US Boxed Warning]: Should be administered under the supervision of an experienced cancer chemotherapy physician.**

Adverse Reactions

>10%:
  Gastrointestinal: Anorexia (14%), nausea (14%), vomiting (14%)
  Hematologic & oncologic: Bone marrow depression (64%; onset: 4 weeks; recovery: 8 to 10 weeks), hemolytic-uremic syndrome (HUS; ≤15%), thrombotic thrombocytopenic purpura (TTP; ≤15%)
  Miscellaneous: Fever (14%)
1% to 10%:
  Dermatologic: Alopecia (4%)
  Gastrointestinal: Mucous membrane disease (toxicity: 4%), stomatitis (4%)
  Renal: Increased serum creatinine (2%)
<1%, postmarketing, and/or case reports: Adult respiratory distress syndrome (ARDS), bladder spasm (intravesical administration), cardiac failure, dyspnea, extravasation reactions, fibrosis (bladder; intravesical administration), hepatic sinusoidal obstruction syndrome (formerly known as hepatic veno-occlusive disease), interstitial fibrosis, malaise, nonproductive cough, pulmonary infiltrates, renal failure (irreversible), skin rash, weakness

Drug Interactions

Metabolism/Transport Effects Substrate of P-glycoprotein

Avoid Concomitant Use

Avoid concomitant use of MitoMYcin (Systemic) with any of the following: BCG (Intravesical); Deferiprone; Dipyrone; Natalizumab; Pimecrolimus; Tacrolimus (Topical); Vaccines (Live)

Increased Effect/Toxicity

MitoMYcin (Systemic) may increase the levels/effects of: CloZAPine; Deferiprone; Fingolimod; Leflunomide; Natalizumab; Tofacitinib; Vaccines (Live)

The levels/effects of MitoMYcin (Systemic) may be increased by: Antineoplastic Agents (Vinca Alkaloids); Denosumab; Dipyrone; Lumacaftor; Ocrelizumab; Palifermin; P-glycoprotein/ABCB1 Inhibitors; Pimecrolimus; Promazine; Ranolazine; Roflumilast; Tacrolimus (Topical); Trastuzumab

Decreased Effect

MitoMYcin (Systemic) may decrease the levels/effects of: BCG (Intravesical); Coccidioides immitis Skin Test; Lenograstim; Nivolumab; Sipuleucel-T; Tertomotide; Vaccines (Inactivated); Vaccines (Live)

The levels/effects of MitoMYcin (Systemic) may be decreased by: Echinacea; Lumacaftor; P-glycoprotein/ABCB1 Inducers

Hazardous Drugs Handling Considerations

Hazardous agent (NIOSH 2016 [group 1]).

Use appropriate precautions for receiving, handling, administration, and disposal. Gloves (single) should be worn during receiving, unpacking, and placing in storage.

NIOSH recommends double gloving, a protective gown, ventilated engineering controls (a class II biological safety cabinet or a compounding aseptic containment isolator), and closed system transfer devices (CSTDs) for preparation. Double gloving, a gown, and (if dosage form allows) CSTDs are required during administration (NIOSH 2016).

Storage/Stability
Store intact vials at 25°C (77°F); avoid exposure to temperatures >40°C (104°F). Reconstituted solution is stable for 7 days at room temperature and 14 days when refrigerated. Protect reconstituted solution from light. Solutions further diluted for infusion (concentration 20 to 40 mcg/mL) are stable for 12 hours at room temperature when diluted in NS and 24 hours at room temperature when diluted in sodium lactate.

Preparation for Administration
Reconstitute powder with SWFI to a concentration of 0.5 mg/mL; shake to dissolve. If powder does not dissolve immediately, allow to stand at room temperature until dispersion. May further dilute in NS or sodium lactate to 20 to 40 mcg/mL.

Intravesicular preparation (off-label route): For bladder instillation, mix 20 to 40 mg mitomycin in 20 to 40 mL of normal saline or sterile water for injection (final concentration 1 to 2 mg/mL) (Au 2001; Hall 2007; O'Brien 2013).

Mechanism of Action
Mitomycin alkylates DNA to produce DNA cross-linking (primarily with guanine and cytosine pairs) and inhibits DNA and RNA synthesis. Mitomycin is not cell cycle specific but has its maximum effect against cells in late G and early S phases (Perry 2012).

Pharmacodynamics/Kinetics

Metabolism: Primarily hepatic

Half-life elimination: 17 minutes (30 mg dose)

Excretion: Feces (primarily [Perry 2012]); Urine

Dosing

Adult & Geriatric

Gastric cancer: IV: 20 mg/m^2 once every 6 to 8 weeks

Off-label dosing: IV: 7 mg/m^2 (maximum dose: 14 mg) once every 6 weeks for 4 cycles (in combination with cisplatin and fluorouracil) (Ross 2002)

Pancreatic cancer: IV: 20 mg/m^2 once every 6 to 8 weeks

Anal carcinoma (off-label use): IV: 10 mg/m^2 as an IV bolus on days 1 and 29 (maximum: 20 mg/dose) in combination with fluorouracil and radiation therapy (Ajani 2008; Flam 1996) **or** 10 mg/m^2 on day 1 (maximum dose: 15 mg) in combination with capecitabine and radiation therapy (Meulendijks 2014) **or** 12 mg/m^2 on day 1 (maximum dose: 20 mg) in combination with capecitabine and radiation therapy (Thind 2014)

Bladder cancer (off-label use):

Muscle invasive: IV: 12 mg/m^2 on day 1 (in combination with fluorouracil and radiation) (James 2012)

Nonmuscle invasive (off-label route): Intravesicular instillation:

Low risk of recurrence (uncomplicated): 40 mg as a single dose postoperatively; retain in bladder for 1 to 2 hours (Hall 2007; O'Brien 2013)

Increased risk of recurrence: 20 mg weekly for 6 weeks, followed by 20 mg monthly for 3 years; retain in bladder for 1 to 2 hours (Friedrich 2007) **or** 40 mg weekly for 6 weeks (with urine alkalinization and decreased urine volume to increase drug concentration); retain in bladder for 2 hours (Au 2001)

Cervical cancer, recurrent or metastatic (off-label use): IV: 6 mg/m^2 on day 1 once every 4 weeks (in combination with cisplatin) for a minimum of 2 cycles (preferably 9 cycles) (Wagenaar 2001)

Esophageal cancer, advanced (off-label use): IV: 7 mg/m^2 (maximum dose: 14 mg) once every 6 weeks for 4 cycles (in combination with cisplatin and fluorouracil) (Ross 2002)

Vulvar cancer, advanced (off-label use): IV: 15 mg/m^2 on day 1 every 14 days for 2 cycles (in combination with concomitant radiation and fluorouracil) (Landoni 1996)

Renal Impairment The manufacturer's labeling states to avoid use in patients with serum creatinine >1.7 mg/dL, although no other dosage modifications are provided. The following adjustments have been recommended (Aronoff 2007): Adults:

CrCl <10 mL/minute: Reduce dose to 75% of usual dose.

Continuous ambulatory peritoneal dialysis (CAPD): Reduce dose to 75% of usual dose.

Hepatic Impairment There are no dosage adjustments provided in the manufacturer's labeling (has not been studied).

Obesity *ASCO Guidelines for appropriate chemotherapy dosing in obese adults with cancer:* Utilize patient's actual body weight (full weight) for calculation of body surface area- or weight-based dosing, particularly when the intent of therapy is curative; manage regimen-related toxicities in the same manner as for nonobese patients; if a dose reduction is utilized due to toxicity, consider resumption of full weight-based dosing with subsequent cycles, especially if cause of toxicity (eg, hepatic or renal impairment) is resolved (Griggs, 2012).

Adjustment for Toxicity

Leukocytes 2,000 to <3,000/mm^3: Hold therapy until leukocyte count ≥4,000/mm^3; reduce to 70% of prior dose in subsequent cycles

Leukocytes <2,000/mm^3: Hold therapy until leukocyte count ≥4,000/mm^3; reduce to 50% of prior dose in subsequent cycles

Platelets 25,000 to <75,000/mm^3: Hold therapy until platelets ≥100,000/mm^3; reduce to 70% of prior dose in subsequent cycles

Platelets <25,000/mm^3: Hold therapy until platelets ≥100,000 mm^3; reduce to 50% of prior dose in subsequent cycles

Combination Regimens

Anal cancer: Fluorouracil-Mitomycin (Anal Cancer) on page 2128

Administration

IV: Administer by slow IV push/bolus via a freely-running saline infusion. Consider using a central venous catheter.

Vesicant; ensure proper needle or catheter placement prior to and during infusion; avoid extravasation.

Extravasation management: If extravasation occurs, stop infusion immediately and disconnect (leave cannula/needle in place); gently aspirate extravasated solution (do **NOT** flush the line); remove needle/cannula; elevate extremity. Initiate dimethyl sulfate (DMSO) antidote. Apply dry cold compress for 20 minutes 4 times/day for 1 to 2 days (Pérez Fidalgo 2012).

DMSO: Apply topically to a region covering twice the affected area every 8 hours for 7 days; begin within 10 minutes of extravasation; do not cover with a dressing (Perez Fidalgo 2012).

Intravesicular (off-label route): Instill into bladder and retain for 1 to 2 hours (Au 2001; Friedrich 2007; Hall 2007; O'Brien 2013); rotate patient every 15 to 30 minutes

Vesicant/Extravasation Risk Vesicant

Emetic Potential Children and Adults: Low (10% to 30%)

Monitoring Parameters Monitor CBC with differential (repeatedly during therapy and for ≥8 weeks following therapy); serum creatinine; pulmonary function tests; monitor for signs/symptoms of HUS; monitor infusion site.

Dosage Forms Excipient information presented when available (limited, particularly for generics); consult specific product labeling.

Solution Reconstituted, Intravenous:

Generic: 5 mg (1 ea); 20 mg (1 ea); 40 mg (1 ea)

MitoMYcin (Ophthalmic) (mye toe MYE sin)

Brand Names: US Mitosol

Index Terms Mitomycin-C; MMC

Pharmacologic Category Antineoplastic Agent, Antibiotic; Ophthalmic Agent, Miscellaneous

Use Glaucoma surgery: Adjunct to ab externo glaucoma surgery

Pregnancy Risk Factor X

Hazardous Drugs Handling Considerations

Hazardous agent (NIOSH 2016 [group 1]).

Use appropriate precautions for receiving, handling, administration, and disposal. Gloves (single) should be worn during receiving, unpacking, and placing in storage.

NIOSH recommends double gloving, a protective gown, and preparation in a controlled device or use of ventilated engineering controls (a class II biological safety cabinet or a compounding aseptic containment isolator) for preparation; if not prepared in a controlled device, respiratory and eye/face protection as well as ventilated engineering controls are recommended. NIOSH recommends double gloving, a protective gown, and (if liquid that could splash) eye/face protection for topical administration (NIOSH 2016).

Dosing

Adult & Geriatric Glaucoma surgery (adjunctive therapy): Topical ophthalmic: 0.2 mg solution is aseptically applied via saturated sponges to surgical site of glaucoma filtration surgery for 2 minutes

Renal Impairment There are no dosage adjustments provided in the manufacturer's labeling.

Hepatic Impairment There are no dosage adjustments provided in the manufacturer's labeling.

Additional Information Complete prescribing information should be consulted for additional detail.

Dosage Forms Excipient information presented when available (limited, particularly for generics); consult specific product labeling.

Kit, Ophthalmic:

Mitosol: 0.2 mg

◆ **Mitomycin For Injection (Can)** see MitoMYcin (Systemic) on page 1262

◆ **Mitomycin For Injection USP (Can)** see MitoMYcin (Systemic) on page 1262

◆ **Mitosol** see MitoMYcin (Ophthalmic) on page 1266

Mitotane (MYE toe tane)

Related Information

Management of Chemotherapy-Induced Nausea and Vomiting In Adults on page 2253

Prevention of Chemotherapy-Induced Nausea and Vomiting in Children on page 2310

Safe Handling of Hazardous Drugs on page 2379

Brand Names: US Lysodren

Brand Names: Canada Lysodren

Index Terms Chloditan; Chlodithane; Khloditan; Mytotan; o,p'-DDD; Ortho, para-DDD

Pharmacologic Category Antineoplastic Agent, Miscellaneous

Use Adrenocortical carcinoma: Treatment of inoperable (functional or nonfunctional) adrenocortical carcinoma

Labeled Contraindications

There are no contraindications listed in the manufacturer's US labeling.

Canadian labeling: Hypersensitivity to mitotane or any component of the formulation

Pregnancy Considerations Mitotane crosses the placenta (Gerl 1992) and may cause fetal harm if administered during pregnancy. Although use in pregnancy is limited, preterm birth and early pregnancy loss have been reported (Baszko-Błaszyk 2011; Kojori 2011; Tripto-Shkolnik 2013).

Mitotane has a long elimination half-life. Women of reproductive potential should use effective contraception during treatment and after treatment until plasma levels are no longer detected. When used to treat Cushing disease, available guidelines recommend avoiding pregnancy for years after stopping mitotane therapy (Nieman 2015).

Breastfeeding Considerations Mitotane is present in breast milk. Because of the potential for serious adverse reactions in the breastfed infant, the manufacturer recommends discontinuing breastfeeding until after mitotane is discontinued and until plasma levels are no longer detected.

Warnings/Precautions [US Boxed Warning]: Adrenal crisis occurs in the setting of shock or severe trauma and response to shock is impaired in patients taking mitotane. Administer hydrocortisone, monitor for escalating signs of shock and discontinue mitotane until recovery occurs. Patients treated with mitotane may develop adrenal insufficiency; steroid replacement therapy may be required. Monitor free cortisol and corticotropin (ACTH) levels to achieve optimal steroid replacement. CNS adverse effects, including lethargy, sedation, and vertigo may occur; mitotane plasma concentrations above 20 mcg/mL are associated with higher incidence of toxicity. Patients must be cautioned about performing tasks which require mental alertness (eg, operating machinery or driving). Ovarian macrocysts (often bilateral and multiple) have been reported in premenopausal females receiving mitotane. Complications due to the cysts have been reported (including adnexal torsion and hemorrhagic cyst rupture). Improvement following discontinuation of mitotane has occurred in some cases. Female patients should obtain medical care if they experience vaginal bleeding and/or pelvic pain. Although uncommon, prolonged bleeding time may occur; consider bleeding possibility prior to any surgical intervention. If currently on anticoagulant therapy, monitor coagulation parameters and adjust anticoagulant dose as needed.

Use with caution in patients with hepatic impairment; hepatic impairment may interfere with mitotane metabolism and may result in accumulation. Potentially significant drug-drug interactions may exist, requiring dose or frequency adjustment, additional monitoring, and/or selection of alternative therapy. Mitotane is associated with a moderate emetic potential; antiemetics may be needed to prevent nausea and vomiting.

Adverse Reactions

>10%:

Central nervous system: Depression (≤40%), dizziness (≤40%), vertigo (≤40%)

Dermatologic: Skin rash (15%)

Gastrointestinal: Anorexia (≤80%), diarrhea (≤80%), nausea (≤80%), vomiting (≤80%)

Frequency not defined:

Cardiovascular: Flushing, hypertension, orthostatic hypotension

Central nervous system: Ataxia, central nervous system toxicity (including sedation, lethargy), confusion, dysarthria, generalized ache, headache, mental deficiency

Endocrine & metabolic: Adrenocortical insufficiency, albuminuria, altered hormone level (decreased serum androstenedione), decreased plasma testosterone (males and females), growth suppression, gynecomastia, hypercholesterolemia, hypertriglyceridemia, hypothyroidism, increased sex hormone binding globulin, ovarian cyst (including bilateral, multiple)

Genitourinary: Hematuria, hemorrhagic cystitis

Hematologic & oncologic: Neutropenia, prolonged bleeding time

Hepatic: Hepatitis, increased liver enzymes

Neuromuscular & skeletal: Weakness

Ophthalmic: Blurred vision, cataract, diplopia, maculopathy, retinopathy

Miscellaneous: Fever

Drug Interactions
Metabolism/Transport Effects Induces CYP3A4 (strong)
Avoid Concomitant Use
Avoid concomitant use of Mitotane with any of the following: Abiraterone Acetate; Antihepaciviral Combination Products; Apixaban; Apremilast; Aprepitant; Artemether; Asunaprevir; Axitinib; Bedaquiline; Boceprevir; Bortezomib; Bosutinib; Brigatinib; Cariprazine; Ceritinib; CloZAPine; Cobimetinib; Crizotinib; Daclatasvir; Dasabuvir; Deflazacort; Delamanid; Dienogest; Dronedarone; Eliglustat; Enzalutamide; Everolimus; Flibanserin; Gemigliptin; Grazoprevir; Ibrutinib; Idelalisib; Irinotecan Products; Isavuconazonium Sulfate; Itraconazole; Ivabradine; Ivacaftor; Ixazomib; Lapatinib; Lumefantrine; Lurasidone; Macitentan; Midostaurin; MiFEPRIStone; Naldemedine; Naloxegol; Neratinib; Netupitant; NIFEdipine; Nilotinib; NiMODipine; Nisoldipine; Olaparib; Palbociclib; Panobinostat; PAZOPanib; PONATinib; Praziquantel; Ranolazine; Regorafenib; Ribociclib; Rivaroxaban; Roflumilast; RomiDEPsin; Simeprevir; Sonidegib; SORAfenib; Suvorexant; Tasimelteon; Telaprevir; Ticagrelor; Tofacitinib; Tolvaptan; Toremifene; Trabectedin; Ulipristal; Valbenazine; Vandetanib; Velpatasvir; Venetoclax; VinCRIStine (Liposomal); Vinflunine; Vorapaxar; Voxilaprevir

Increased Effect/Toxicity
Mitotane may increase the levels/effects of: Clarithromycin; Doxercalciferol; Ifosfamide

The levels/effects of Mitotane may be increased by: Clarithromycin
Decreased Effect
Mitotane may decrease the levels/effects of: Abiraterone Acetate; Antihepaciviral Combination Products; Apixaban; Apremilast; Aprepitant; ARIPiprazole; ARIPiprazole Lauroxil; Artemether; Asunaprevir; Axitinib; Bedaquiline; Benperidol; Boceprevir; Bortezomib; Bosutinib; Brentuximab Vedotin; Brexpiprazole; Brigatinib; Cabozantinib; Calcifediol; Cannabidiol; Cannabis; Cariprazine; Ceritinib; Clarithromycin; Clindamycin (Systemic); CloZAPine; Cobimetinib; Corticosteroids (Systemic); Crizotinib; CYP3A4 Substrates; Dabrafenib; Daclatasvir; Dasabuvir; Dasatinib; Deflazacort; Delamanid; Dexamethasone (Systemic); Dienogest; Diethylstilbestrol; DOXOrubicin (Conventional); Dronabinol; Dronedarone; Eliglustat; Enzalutamide; Erlotinib; Estriol (Systemic); Estriol (Topical); Etoposide; Etoposide Phosphate; Everolimus; Evogliptin; Exemestane; FentaNYL; Flibanserin; Gefitinib; Gemigliptin; Glecaprevir and Pibrentasvir; Grazoprevir; GuanFACINE; Ibrutinib; Idelalisib; Ifosfamide; Imatinib; Irinotecan Products; Isavuconazonium Sulfate; Itraconazole; Ivabradine; Ivacaftor; Ixabepilone; Ixazomib; Lapatinib; Linagliptin; Lumefantrine; Lurasidone; Macitentan; Manidipine; Maraviroc; MethylPREDNISolone; Midostaurin; MiFEPRIStone; Mirodenafil; Naldemedine; Naloxegol; Neratinib; Netupitant; NIFEdipine; Nilotinib; NiMODipine; Nisoldipine; Olaparib; Osimertinib; Palbociclib; Panobinostat; PAZOPanib; Perampanel; Pimavanserin; PONATinib; Praziquantel; Propafenone; QUEtiapine; Radotinib; Ramelteon; Ranolazine; Reboxetine; Regorafenib; Ribociclib; Rivaroxaban; Roflumilast; Rolapitant; RomiDEPsin; SAXagliptin; Sertraline; Simeprevir; Sirolimus; Sonidegib; SORAfenib; SUFentanil; SUNItinib; Suvorexant; Tadalafil; Tasimelteon; Telaprevir; Temsirolimus; Tetrahydrocannabinol; TiaGABine; Ticagrelor; Tofacitinib; Tolvaptan; Toremifene; Trabectedin; Tropisetron; Udenafil; Ulipristal; Valbenazine; Vandetanib; Velpatasvir; Vemurafenib; Venetoclax; Vilazodone; VinCRIStine (Liposomal); Vinflunine; Vorapaxar; Vortioxetine; Voxilaprevir; Zaleplon; Zuclopenthixol

The levels/effects of Mitotane may be decreased by: Spironolactone

Hazardous Drugs Handling Considerations

Hazardous agent (NIOSH 2016 [group 1]).

Use appropriate precautions for receiving, handling, administration, and disposal. Gloves (single) should be worn during receiving, unpacking, and placing in storage. NIOSH recommends single gloving for administration of intact tablets or capsules (NIOSH 2016).

Storage/Stability Store at 25°C (77°F); excursions are permitted between 15°C and 30°C (59°F and 86°F).

Mechanism of Action Mitotane is an adrenolytic agent that suppresses (directly) the adrenal cortex and alters the peripheral metabolism of steroids

Pharmacodynamics/Kinetics

Onset of action: Antitumor response: Achieved at serum concentrations ≥14 mcg/mL; Pediatric patients: In experience with treatment of adenocarcinoma reported 1.5 to 12.5 months to reach 10 mcg/mL with subsequent rapid escalation of serum concentration, clinical response may be observed earlier (Rodriguez-Galindo 2005; Zancanella 2006).

Duration: Measurable serum levels may persist for months after discontinuation (Veytsman 2009).

Absorption: Oral: ~40%

Distribution: Stored primarily in fat tissue but is found in all body tissues

Metabolism: Hepatic and other tissues; converted to a water soluble metabolite

Half-life elimination: 18 to 159 days (median: 53 days)

Excretion: Urine (~10%, as metabolites); feces (1% to 17%, as metabolites)

Dosing

Adult & Geriatric Note: Mitotane is associated with a moderate emetic potential; antiemetics may be needed to prevent nausea and vomiting.

Adrenocortical carcinoma: Oral: Initial: 2 to 6 g per day in 3 to 4 divided doses, then increase incrementally to achieve a blood concentration of 14 to 20 mcg/mL or as tolerated.

Off-label dosing: Initial 1 to 2 g per day; increase by 1 to 2 g per day at 1- to 2-week intervals as tolerated; usual dose 4 to 6 g per day; maximum of 6 to 10 g per day (Veytsman 2009)

Cushing syndrome (off-label use): Oral: Initial: 500 mg 3 times daily (Biller 2008); may increase dose rapidly during the first 4 to 6 weeks up to a maximum of 4,000 mg to 8,000 mg per day in 3 divided doses, with the largest dose given in the evening to minimize discomfort (Baudry 2012; ES [Neiman 2015]; Schteingart 1980); after achieving control of cortisol secretion, gradually taper to the minimal dose required to maintain remission (Baudry 2012)

Pediatric Adrenocortical carcinoma (stage III or IV) (off-label use): Based on limited data (efficacy results are variable; optimal dose not fully established): Children and Adolescents: Oral: Initial: 0.5 to 1 g/day divided 3 times a day, increase weekly to a target dose of 4 g/m^2/day (divided 3 times a day) in combination with 8 cycles of the CED regimen (cisplatin, etoposide, and doxorubicin); titrate dose to achieve a target serum concentration of 14 to 20 mcg/mL (Zancanella 2006). Additional data may be necessary to further define the role of mitotane in the treatment of adrenocortical carcinoma in pediatric patients.

Renal Impairment There are no dosage adjustments provided in the manufacturer's labeling.

Hepatic Impairment There are no dosage adjustments provided in the manufacturer's labeling. However, accumulation may occur in patients with hepatic impairment; use with caution.

Adjustment for Toxicity

Adrenal crisis in the setting of shock or severe trauma: Discontinue mitotane until recovery occurs.

CNS toxicity: Discontinue mitotane until symptoms resolve; 7 to 10 days after symptoms resolve, restart at a lower dose (eg, decrease dose by 500 to 1,000 mg).

Significant neuropsychiatric adverse effects: Withhold treatment for at least 1 week and restart at a lower dose (Allolio 2006).

Administration Note: Mitotane is associated with a moderate emetic potential; antiemetics may be needed to prevent nausea and vomiting.

Administer in 3 to 4 divided doses/day.

Emetic Potential Moderate (30% to 90%)

Monitoring Parameters

Monitor for therapeutic mitotane levels; monitor free cortisol and corticotropin levels; monitor adrenal function; signs/symptoms of CNS toxicity, signs/symptoms of ovarian macrocysts (eg, vaginal bleeding and/or pelvic pain). Monitor adherence.

Mitotane level monitoring (gas chromatography-flame ionization assay): Adults: Every 4 to 8 weeks until target levels are attained, then monitor every 3 months; urinary free cortisol levels; TSH and free thyroxine every few months (Veytsman 2009).

Pediatrics (adrenocortical carcinoma): Monitor mitotane serum concentrations initially every 2 to 4 weeks until serum concentration of 10 mcg/mL is achieved, then monitor every 1 to 2 weeks (even after target concentration of 14 to 20 mcg/mL is reached) and use conservative dose adjustments due to drug accumulation and narrow therapeutic window (Zancanella 2006).

Dosage Forms Excipient information presented when available (limited, particularly for generics); consult specific product labeling.

Tablet, Oral:

Lysodren: 500 mg [scored]

MitoXANTRONE (mye toe ZAN trone)

Related Information

Hematopoietic Cell Transplantation *on page 2365*

Management of Chemotherapy-Induced Nausea and Vomiting in Adults *on page 2253*

Management of Drug Extravasations *on page 2271*

Prevention of Chemotherapy-Induced Nausea and Vomiting in Children *on page 2310*

Safe Handling of Hazardous Drugs *on page 2379*

Brand Names: Canada Mitoxantrone Injection; Mitoxantrone Injection USP

Index Terms CL-232315; DHAD; DHAQ; Dihydroxyanthracenedione; Dihydroxyanthracenedione Dihydrochloride; Mitoxantrone Dihydrochloride; Mitoxantrone HCl; Mitoxantrone Hydrochloride; Mitozantrone; Novantrone

Pharmacologic Category Antineoplastic Agent, Anthracenedione; Antineoplastic Agent, Topoisomerase II Inhibitor

Use Initial treatment of acute nonlymphocytic leukemias (ANLL [includes myelogenous, promyelocytic, monocytic and erythroid leukemias]); treatment of advanced hormone-refractory prostate cancer; secondary progressive or relapsing-remitting multiple sclerosis (MS)

Canadian labeling: Additional uses (not in U.S. labeling): Treatment of metastatic breast cancer, relapsed leukemia (adults), lymphoma, and hepatocellular carcinoma

Labeled Contraindications Hypersensitivity to mitoxantrone or any component of the formulation

Canadian labeling: Additional contraindications (not in U.S. labeling): Prior hypersensitivity to anthracyclines; prior substantial anthracycline exposure and abnormal cardiac function prior to initiation of mitoxantrone therapy; presence of severe myelosuppression due to prior chemo- and/or radiotherapy; severe hepatic impairment; intrathecal administration

Pregnancy Considerations Adverse events have been observed in animal reproduction studies. Based on the mechanism of action, mitoxantrone may cause fetal harm if administered during pregnancy. Use of effective contraception during therapy is recommended. Information related to pregnancy outcomes following maternal use of mitoxantrone in pregnancy is limited (Amato 2015; Houtchens 2013; NTP 2013).

Infertility and amenorrhea have been reported in women with MS using mitoxantrone (Amato 2015; Houtchens 2013). Women with multiple sclerosis who are of reproductive potential should have a pregnancy test prior to each dose. Women who wish to become pregnant should discontinue therapy at least 2 to 3 months prior to conception (Houtchens 2013).

The European Society for Medical Oncology has published guidelines for diagnosis, treatment, and follow-up of cancer during pregnancy. The guidelines recommend referral to a facility with expertise in cancer during pregnancy and encourage a multidisciplinary team (obstetrician, neonatologist, oncology team). In general, if chemotherapy is indicated, it should be avoided in the first trimester, there should be a 3-week time period between the last chemotherapy dose and anticipated delivery, and chemotherapy should not be administered beyond week 33 of gestation (Peccatori 2013).

Breastfeeding Considerations Mitoxantrone is excreted in human milk and significant concentrations (18 ng/mL) have been reported for 28 days after the last administration. Due to the potential for serious adverse reactions in the nursing infant, the manufacturer recommends that breastfeeding be discontinued before starting treatment.

Warnings/Precautions [U.S. Boxed Warning]: Usually should not be administered if baseline neutrophil count <1500 cells/mm³ (except for treatment of ANLL). Monitor blood counts and monitor for infection due to neutropenia. Treatment may lead to severe myelosuppression; unless the expected benefit outweighs the risk, use is generally not recommended in patients with preexisting myelosuppression from prior chemotherapy.

[U.S. Boxed Warning]: May cause myocardial toxicity and potentially-fatal heart failure (HF); risk increases with cumulative dosing. Effects may occur during therapy or may be delayed (months or years after completion of therapy). Predisposing factors for mitoxantrone-induced cardiotoxicity include prior anthracycline or anthracenedione therapy, prior cardiovascular disease, concomitant use of cardiotoxic drugs, and mediastinal/pericardial irradiation, although may also occur in patients without risk factors. Prior to therapy initiation, evaluate all patients for

cardiac-related signs/symptoms, including history, physical exam, and ECG; and evaluate baseline left ventricular ejection fraction (LVEF) with echocardiogram or multigated radionuclide angiography (MUGA) or MRI. Not recommended for use in MS patients when LVEF <50%, or baseline LVEF below the lower limit of normal (LLN). Evaluate for cardiac signs/symptoms (by history, physical exam, and ECG) and evaluate LVEF (using same method as baseline LVEF) in MS patients prior to each dose and if signs/symptoms of HF develop. Use in MS should be limited to a cumulative dose of ≤140 mg/m^2, and discontinued if LVEF falls below LLN or a significant decrease in LVEF is observed; decreases in LVEF and HF have been observed in patients with MS who have received cumulative doses <100 mg/m^2. Patients with MS should undergo annual LVEF evaluation following discontinuation of therapy to monitor for delayed cardiotoxicity.

[U.S. Boxed Warning]: For IV administration only, into a free-flowing IV; may cause severe local tissue damage if extravasation occurs; do not administer subcutaneously, intramuscularly, or intra-arterially. Do not administer intrathecally; may cause serious and permanent neurologic damage. Irritant with vesicant-like properties; extravasation resulting in burning, erythema, pain, swelling and skin discoloration (blue) has been reported; may result in tissue necrosis and require debridement for skin graft. Ensure proper needle or catheter placement prior to and during infusion. Avoid extravasation. May cause urine, saliva, tears, and sweat to turn blue-green for 24 hours postinfusion. Whites of eyes may have blue-green tinge. **[U.S. Boxed Warning]:** Treatment with mitoxantrone increases the risk of developing secondary acute myelogenous leukemia (AML) in patients with cancer and in patients with MS; acute promyelocytic leukemia (APL) has also been observed. Symptoms of acute leukemia include excessive bruising, bleeding and recurrent infections. The risk for secondary leukemia is increased in patients who are heavily pretreated, with higher doses, and with combination chemotherapy.

[U.S. Boxed Warning]: Should be administered under the supervision of a physician experienced in cancer chemotherapy agents. Dosage should be reduced in patients with impaired hepatobiliary function (clearance is reduced). Canadian labeling contraindicates use in severe hepatic impairment. Not for treatment of multiple sclerosis in patients with concurrent hepatic impairment. Not for treatment of primary progressive multiple sclerosis. Rapid lysis of tumor cells may lead to hyperuricemia.

Adverse Reactions Includes events reported with any indication; incidence varies based on treatment, dose, and/or concomitant medications.

>10%:

  Cardiovascular: Edema (10% to 30%), cardiac disease (≤18%), cardiac arrhythmia (3% to 18%), ECG changes (≤11%)

  Central nervous system: Pain (8% to 41%), fatigue (≤39%), headache (6% to 13%)

  Dermatologic: Alopecia (20% to 61%), nail bed changes (≤11%)

  Endocrine & metabolic: Menstrual disease (26% to 61%), amenorrhea (28% to 53%), hyperglycemia (10% to 31%), weight gain (≤17%), weight loss (≤17%), increased gamma-glutamyl transferase (3% to 15%)

Gastrointestinal: Nausea (26% to 76%), vomiting (6% to 72%), diarrhea (14% to 47%), mucositis (10% to 29%; onset: ≤1 week), stomatitis (8% to 29%; onset: ≤1 week), anorexia (22% to 25%), constipation (10% to 16%), gastrointestinal hemorrhage (2% to 16%), abdominal pain (9% to 15%), dyspepsia (5% to 14%)

Genitourinary: Urinary tract infection (7% to 32%), hematuria (≤11%), urine abnormality (5% to 11%)

Hematologic & oncologic: Neutropenia (79% to 100%; onset: ≤3 weeks; grade 4: 23% to 54%), leukopenia (9% to 100%), lymphocytopenia (72% to 95%), anemia (≤75%), decreased hemoglobin (≤75%), thrombocytopenia (33% to 39%; grades 3/4: 3% to 4%), bruise (≤11%), febrile neutropenia (≤11%), petechia (≤11%)

Hepatic: Increased serum alkaline phosphatase (≤37%), increased serum transaminases (5% to 20%)

Infection: Infection (4% to 60%), sepsis (≤34%), fungal infection (9% to 15%)

Neuromuscular & skeletal: Weakness (≤24%)

Renal: Increased blood urea nitrogen (≤22%), increased serum creatinine (≤13%)

Respiratory: Upper respiratory tract infection (7% to 53%), pharyngitis (≤19%), dyspnea (6% to 18%), cough (5% to 13%)

Miscellaneous: Fever (6% to 78%)

1% to 10%:

Cardiovascular: Cardiac failure (≤5%), ischemia (≤5%), decreased left ventricular ejection fraction (≤5%), hypertension (≤4%)

Central nervous system: Chills (≤5%), anxiety (5%), depression (5%), seizure (2% to 4%)

Dermatologic: Diaphoresis (≤9%), skin infection (≤5%)

Endocrine & metabolic: Hypocalcemia (10%), hypokalemia (7% to 10%), hyponatremia (9%), hypermenorrhea (7%)

Gastrointestinal: Aphthous stomatitis (≤10%)

Genitourinary: Impotence (≤7%), proteinuria (≤6%), sterility (≤5%)

Hematologic & oncologic: Granulocytopenia (6%), hemorrhage (5% to 6%), acute leukemia (≤3%; secondary; includes AML, APL)

Hepatic: Jaundice (3% to 7%)

Infection: Fungal infection (cutaneous: ≤10%)

Neuromuscular & skeletal: Back pain (6% to 8%), arthralgia (≤5%), myalgia (≤5%)

Ophthalmic: Conjunctivitis (≤5%), blurred vision (≤3%)

Renal: Renal failure (≤8%)

Respiratory: Rhinitis (10%), pneumonia (≤9%), sinusitis (≤6%)

<1%, postmarketing, and/or case reports: Anaphylactoid reaction, anaphylaxis, chest pain, dehydration, hypersensitivity reaction, interstitial pneumonitis (with combination chemotherapy), hyperuricemia, hypotension, ocular discoloration (blue discoloration of sclera), phlebitis (at infusion site), skin rash, tachycardia, urine discoloration (blue-green), urticaria

Drug Interactions

Metabolism/Transport Effects Substrate of BCRP

Avoid Concomitant Use

Avoid concomitant use of MitoXANTRONE with any of the following: BCG (Intravesical); Deferiprone; Dipyrone; Natalizumab; Pimecrolimus; Tacrolimus (Topical); Vaccines (Live)

Increased Effect/Toxicity

MitoXANTRONE may increase the levels/effects of: CloZAPine; Deferiprone; Fingolimod; Leflunomide; Natalizumab; Tofacitinib; Vaccines (Live)

The levels/effects of MitoXANTRONE may be increased by: CycloSPORINE (Systemic); Denosumab; Dipyrone; Ocrelizumab; Palifermin; Pimecrolimus; Promazine; Roflumilast; Tacrolimus (Topical); Trastuzumab

Decreased Effect

MitoXANTRONE may decrease the levels/effects of: BCG (Intravesical); Coccidioides immitis Skin Test; Lenograstim; Nivolumab; Sipuleucel-T; Tertomotide; Vaccines (Inactivated); Vaccines (Live)

The levels/effects of MitoXANTRONE may be decreased by: Echinacea

Hazardous Drugs Handling Considerations

Hazardous agent (NIOSH 2016 [group 1]).

Use appropriate precautions for receiving, handling, administration, and disposal. Gloves (single) should be worn during receiving, unpacking, and placing in storage.

NIOSH recommends double gloving, a protective gown, ventilated engineering controls (a class II biological safety cabinet or a compounding aseptic containment isolator), and closed system transfer devices (CSTDs) for preparation. Double gloving, a gown, and (if dosage form allows) CSTDs are required during administration (NIOSH 2016).

Storage/Stability Store intact vials at 15°C to 25°C (59°F to 77°F); do not freeze. Opened vials may be stored at room temperature for 7 days or under refrigeration for up to 14 days. Solutions diluted in D5W or NS for administration are stable for 7 days at room temperature or under refrigeration, although the manufacturer recommends immediate use.

Preparation for Administration Dilute in at least 50 mL of NS or D5W. May further dilute in D5W, NS or D5NS, use immediately after preparation.

Mechanism of Action Related to the anthracyclines, mitoxantrone intercalates into DNA resulting in cross-links and strand breaks; binds to nucleic acids and inhibits DNA and RNA synthesis by template disordering and steric obstruction; replication is decreased by binding to DNA topoisomerase II and seems to inhibit the incorporation of uridine into RNA and thymidine into DNA; active throughout entire cell cycle (cell-cycle nonspecific)

Pharmacodynamics/Kinetics

Absorption: Oral: Poor

Distribution: V_d: 14 L/kg; V_{dss}: >1,000 L/m^2; distributes extensively into pleural fluid, kidney, thyroid, liver, heart, pancreas, spleen, bone marrow, and red blood cells; prolonged retention in tissues

Protein binding: 78%

Metabolism: Hepatic; pathway not determined

Half-life elimination: Terminal: 23 to 215 hours (median: ~75 hours); may be prolonged with hepatic impairment

Excretion: Feces (25%); urine (6% to 11%; 65% as unchanged drug)

Dosing

Adult & Geriatric Details concerning dosing in combination regimens should also be consulted.

US labeling:

Acute nonlymphocytic leukemias (ANLL): IV:

Acute myeloid leukemia (AML) induction: 12 mg/m^2 once daily for 3 days (in combination with cytarabine); for incomplete response, may repeat

(7-10 days later) at 12 mg/m^2 once daily for 2 days (in combination with cytarabine) (Arlin 1990)

AML consolidation (beginning ~6 weeks after initiation of the final induction course): 12 mg/m^2 once daily for 2 days (in combination with cytarabine), repeat in 4 weeks (Arlin 1990)

Multiple sclerosis: IV: 12 mg/m^2 every 3 months (maximum lifetime cumulative dose: 140 mg/m^2; discontinue use with LVEF <50% or clinically significant reduction in LVEF)

Prostate cancer (advanced, hormone-refractory): IV: 12 to 14 mg/m^2 every 3 weeks (in combination with corticosteroids)

Canadian labeling:

Acute nonlymphocytic leukemias (ANLL): IV:

AML induction: 10 to 12 mg/m^2 once daily for 3 days (in combination with cytarabine); for incomplete response, may repeat at 10 to 12 mg/m^2 once daily for 2 days (in combination with cytarabine)

AML consolidation (beginning ~6 weeks after initiation of the final induction course): 12 mg/m^2 once daily for 2 days (in combination with cytarabine), repeat in 4 weeks

Acute leukemias (relapsed): IV: Induction: 12 mg/m^2 once daily for 5 consecutive days; may repeat once if needed (at the same dose and duration)

Breast cancer (metastatic), lymphoma: IV: Initial: Single agent: 14 mg/m^2 every 21 days; reduce initial dose to ≤12 mg/m^2 for myelosuppression due to previous treatment or for poor general health. When used in combination with other agents, reduce initial dose to 10 to 12 mg/m^2.

Hepatocellular cancer: IV: Initial: Single agent: 14 mg/m^2 every 21 days; reduce initial dose to ≤12 mg/m^2 for myelosuppression due to previous treatment or for poor general health

Adult off-label uses and/or dosing:

AML, refractory: IV:

CLAG-M regimen: 10 mg/m^2 once daily for 3 days (in combination with cladribine, cytarabine, and filgrastim), may repeat once if needed (Wierzbowska 2008)

MEC or EMA regimen: 6 mg/m^2 once daily for 6 days (in combination with cytarabine and etoposide) (Amadori 1991)

Mitoxantrone/Etoposide: 10 mg/m^2 once daily for 5 days (in combination with etoposide) (Ho 1988)

APL consolidation phase (second course): IV: 10 mg/m^2 once daily for 5 days (Sanz 2004)

Hodgkin lymphoma, refractory: IV:

MINE-ESHAP regimen: 10 mg/m^2 on day 1 every 28 days for up to 2 cycles (MINE is combination with mesna, ifosfamide, mitoxantrone, and etoposide; MINE alternates with ESHAP for up to 2 cycles of each) (Fernandez 2010)

VIM-D regimen: 10 mg/m^2 on day 1 every 28 days (in combination with etoposide, ifosfamide, mesna, and dexamethasone) (Phillips 1990)

Non-Hodgkin lymphoma (as part of combination chemotherapy regimens): IV:

CNOP regimen: 10 mg/m^2 every 21 days (Bessell 2003)

FCMR regimen: 8 mg/m^2 every 28 days (Forstpointner 2004)

FMR regimen: 10 mg/m^2 every 21 days (Zinzani 2004)

FND regimen: 10 mg/m^2 every 28 days (Tsimberidou 2002)

MINE-ESHAP regimen: 8 mg/m² every 21 days for 6 cycles (MINE is combination with mesna, ifosfamide, mitoxantrone, and etoposide; followed by ESHAP) (Rodriguez 1995)

Stem cell transplantation, autologous: IV: 60 mg/m² administered 4 to 5 days prior to autografting (as 3 divided doses over 1 hour each at 1-2 hour intervals on the same day; in combination with other chemotherapeutic agent[s]) (Oyan 2006; Tarella 2001)

Pediatric Details concerning dosing in combination regimens should also be consulted.

Acute nonlymphocytic leukemias: IV:

Acute myeloid leukemia (AML) consolidation phase (second course; off-label use): 10 mg/m² once daily for 5 days (in combination with cytarabine) (Stevens, 1998)

Acute promyelocytic leukemia (APL) consolidation phase (second course; off-label use): 10 mg/m² once daily for 5 days (Ortega, 2005; Sanz, 2004)

Renal Impairment No dosage adjustment provided in manufacturer's labeling (has not been studied).

Hemodialysis: Supplemental dose is not necessary

Peritoneal dialysis: Supplemental dose is not necessary

Elderly: Clearance is decreased in elderly patients; use with caution

Hepatic Impairment

U.S. labeling: No dosage adjustment provided in the manufacturer's labeling; however, clearance is reduced in hepatic dysfunction. Patients with severe hepatic dysfunction (bilirubin >3.4 mg/dL) have an AUC of 3 times greater than patients with normal hepatic function; consider dose adjustments. **Note:** MS patients with hepatic impairment should not receive mitoxantrone.

Canadian labeling:

Mild-to-moderate impairment: No specific dosage adjustment provided; consider dose adjustments and monitor closely.

Severe impairment: Use is contraindicated.

Obesity *ASCO Guidelines for appropriate chemotherapy dosing in obese adults with cancer:* Utilize patient's actual body weight (full weight) for calculation of body surface area- or weight-based dosing, particularly when the intent of therapy is curative, manage regimen-related toxicities in the same manner as for nonobese patients; if a dose reduction is utilized due to toxicity, consider resumption of full weight-based dosing with subsequent cycles, especially if cause of toxicity (eg, hepatic or renal impairment) is resolved (Griggs, 2012).

Adjustment for Toxicity

ANLL patients: Severe or life-threatening nonhematologic toxicity: Withhold treatment until toxicity resolves

MS patients:

Neutrophils <1500/mm³: Use is not recommended.

Signs/symptoms of HF: Evaluate for cardiac signs/symptoms and LVEF.

LVEF <50% or baseline LVEF below the lower limit of normal (LLN): Use is not recommended.

***Canadian labeling (not in U.S. labeling):* Hepatocellular cancer, lymphoma, or breast cancer (metastatic):**

WBC nadir >1500/mm³ **and** platelet nadir >50,000/mm³ and recovery ≤21 days: Repeat previous dose or increase dose by 2 mg/m² if myelosuppression is inadequate.

WBC nadir >1500/mm^3 **and** platelet nadir >50,000/mm^3 and recovery >21 days: Withhold treatment until recovery then resume at previous dose.

WBC nadir <1500/mm^3 **or** platelet nadir <50,000/mm^3 (regardless of recovery time): Withhold treatment until recovery then decrease previous dose by 2 mg/m^2.

WBC nadir <1000/mm^3 **or** platelet nadir <25,000/mm^3 (regardless of recovery time): Withhold treatment until recovery then decrease previous dose by 4 mg/m^2.

Combination Regimens

Leukemia, acute myeloid:

5 + 2 (Cytarabine-Mitoxantrone) (AML Consolidation) on page 1970

7 + 3 (Cytarabine-Mitoxantrone) (AML Induction) on page 1972

CLAG-M (AML Induction) on page 2065

MEC-G (AML Induction) on page 2170

Mitoxantrone-Etoposide (AML Induction) on page 2175

Mitoxantrone-Etoposide-Cytarabine (AML) on page 2175

Leukemia, acute promyelocytic: Tretinoin-Idarubicin (APL) on page 2221

Lymphoma, Hodgkin:

MINE-ESHAP (Hodgkin) on page 2174

VIM-D (Hodgkin) on page 2231

Lymphoma, non-Hodgkin: Fludarabine-Mitoxantrone-Dexamethasone-Rituximab on page 2120

Lymphoma, non-Hodgkin (Follicular): Fludarabine-Cyclophosphamide-Mitoxantrone-Rituximab (NHL-Follicular) on page 2117

Prostate cancer: Mitoxantrone-Prednisone (Prostate) on page 2175

Administration For IV administration only; do not administer intrathecally, subcutaneously, intramuscularly or intra-arterially. Must be diluted prior to use. Usually administered as a short IV infusion over 5-15 minutes; do not infuse over <3-5 minutes.

High doses for bone marrow transplant (off-label use) are usually given as 3 divided doses over 1 hour each at 1-2 hour intervals on the same day (Oyan, 2006; Tarella, 2001).

Irritant with vesicant-like properties; ensure proper needle or catheter placement prior to and during infusion; avoid extravasation.

Extravasation management: If extravasation occurs, stop infusion immediately and disconnect (leave cannula/needle in place); gently aspirate extravasated solution (do **NOT** flush the line); remove needle/cannula; elevate extremity. Initiate antidote (dexrazoxane or dimethyl sulfate [DMSO]). Apply dry cold compresses for 20 minutes 4 times daily for 1-2 days (Perez Fidalgo, 2012); withhold cooling beginning 15 minutes before dexrazoxane infusion; continue withholding cooling until 15 minutes after infusion is completed. Topical DMSO should not be administered in combination with dexrazoxane; may lessen dexrazoxane efficacy.

Dexrazoxane: Adults: 1000 mg/m^2 (maximum dose: 2000 mg) IV (administer in a large vein remote from site of extravasation) over 1-2 hours days 1 and 2, then 500 mg/m^2 (maximum dose: 1000 mg) IV over 1-2 hours day 3; begin within 6 hours of extravasation. Day 2 and day 3 doses should be administered at approximately the same time (± 3 hours) as the dose on day 1 (Mouridsen, 2007; Perez Fidalgo, 2012). **Note:** Reduce dexrazoxane dose by 50% in patients with moderate to severe renal impairment (CrCl <40 mL/minute).

DMSO: Children and Adults: Apply topically to a region covering twice the affected area every 8 hours for 7 days; begin within 10 minutes of extravasation; do not cover with a dressing (Perez Fidalgo, 2012).

Vesicant/Extravasation Risk Vesicant; see Management of Drug Extravasations on page 2271.

Emetic Potential Children and Adults: Low (10% to 30%)

Monitoring Parameters CBC with differential, serum uric acid (for leukemia treatment), liver function tests; for the treatment of multiple sclerosis, obtain pregnancy test; monitor injection site for extravasation

Cardiac monitoring: Prior to initiation, evaluate all patients for cardiac-related signs/symptoms, including history, physical exam, and ECG; evaluate baseline and periodic left ventricular ejection fraction (LVEF) with echocardiogram or multigated radionuclide angiography (MUGA) or MRI. In patients with MS, evaluate for cardiac signs/symptoms (by history, physical exam, and ECG) and evaluate LVEF (using same method as baseline LVEF) prior to each dose and if signs/symptoms of HF develop. Patients with MS should undergo annual LVEF evaluation following discontinuation of therapy to monitor for delayed cardiotoxicity.

Medication Guide Available Yes

Dosage Forms Excipient information presented when available (limited, particularly for generics); consult specific product labeling.

Concentrate, Intravenous:
Generic: 20 mg/10 mL (10 mL); 25 mg/12.5 mL (12.5 mL); 30 mg/15 mL (15 mL)

◆ **Mitoxantrone Dihydrochloride** *see* MitoXANTRONE *on page 1271*

◆ **Mitoxantrone HCl** *see* MitoXANTRONE *on page 1271*

◆ **Mitoxantrone Hydrochloride** *see* MitoXANTRONE *on page 1271*

◆ **Mitoxantrone Injection (Can)** *see* MitoXANTRONE *on page 1271*

◆ **Mitoxantrone Injection USP (Can)** *see* MitoXANTRONE *on page 1271*

◆ **Mitozantrone** *see* MitoXANTRONE *on page 1271*

◆ **MK 0517** *see* Fosaprepitant *on page 844*

◆ **MK 869** *see* Aprepitant *on page 165*

◆ **MK-3475** *see* Pembrolizumab *on page 1486*

◆ **MK4827** *see* Niraparib *on page 1324*

◆ **MLN341** *see* Bortezomib *on page 271*

◆ **MLN9708** *see* Ixazomib *on page 1084*

◆ **MM-398** *see* Irinotecan (Liposomal) *on page 1048*

◆ **MMC** *see* MitoMYcin (Ophthalmic) *on page 1266*

◆ **MMC** *see* MitoMYcin (Systemic) *on page 1262*

◆ **MMF** *see* Mycophenolate *on page 1283*

◆ **MOAB 2C4** *see* Pertuzumab *on page 1506*

◆ **MOAB ABX-EGF** *see* Panitumumab *on page 1440*

◆ **MOAB C225** *see* Cetuximab *on page 377*

◆ **MoAb CD52** *see* Alemtuzumab *on page 82*

◆ **MOAB Ch14.18** *see* Dinutuximab *on page 600*

◆ **MOAB-CTLA-4** *see* Ipilimumab *on page 1031*

Mucosal Coating Agent (myoo KOH sul KOH ting AY gent)

Brand Names: US Episil; Gelclair; Mucotrol; MuGard; Orafate; ProThelial

Index Terms Mucosal Adherent Agent; Mucosal Barrier Agent; Mucosal Barrier Gel; Mucosal Bioadherent Agent; Mucosal Protective Agent; Oral Wound Care Products; Sucralfate Paste (Orafate, ProThelial)

Pharmacologic Category Gastrointestinal Agent, Miscellaneous

Use Mucosal protection: Management of oral mucosal pain and protection from further irritation caused by oral mucositis/stomatitis (resulting from chemotherapy or radiation therapy); irritation; lesions, periodontal and gingival inflammation, tooth extractions, and wounds/lesions due to oral surgery; chafing; minor lesions; traumatic ulcers, and abrasions caused by braces/ill-fitting dentures or disease; diffuse aphthous ulcers (canker sores).

Labeled Contraindications

Hypersensitivity to any ingredient or component of the formulation

Additional product-specific contraindications: Episil: Hypersensitivity to peanuts, soya, or peppermint oil

Warnings/Precautions

May decrease absorption of sublingually administered medications. Episil contains alcohol (may cause irritation when applied), propylene glycol (may cause skin irritation), soy, and peppermint oil (may cause allergic reaction). Avoid eating or drinking for at least 1 hour (Mucotrol, MuGard, Orafate, ProThelial) or 30 to 60 minutes (Gelclair) following use. Consult a health care provider if no improvement is seen after 7 days of use. Orafate and ProThelial are safe if swallowed; however, evaluate swallowing capability prior to use to minimize incidental ingestion. Orafate and ProThelial may cause constipation if swallowed.

Adverse Reactions

<1%, postmarketing, and/or case reports: Burning sensation of mouth, mild stinging sensation (oral cavity), oral inflammation (mild)

Drug Interactions

Metabolism/Transport Effects None known.

Avoid Concomitant Use There are no known interactions where it is recommended to avoid concomitant use.

Increased Effect/Toxicity There are no known significant interactions involving an increase in effect.

Decreased Effect There are no known significant interactions involving a decrease in effect.

Storage/Stability

Store at room temperature. Protect from direct sunlight.

Episil: Store bottle in outer carton; use within 1 month of first use.

Gelclair: Use immediately after mixing with water.

Mucotrol: Do not refrigerate. Protect from moisture.

MuGard: Tightly seal bottle after use.

Preparation for Administration

Episil, Orafate, ProThelial: Does not require reconstitution.

Gelclair: Pour 15 mL (the contents of a single-use packet) into a glass and mix with water (refer to product information for details). Stir well and use immediately.

MuGard: Dilution prior to use is not recommended.

Mechanism of Action

Adheres to the mucosal surface of mouth forming a protective film or coating over the irritated areas and lesions, protecting the lesion from further irritation and pain.

Dosing

Adult & Geriatric Mucosal protection: Oral:

Episil: Apply 1 to 3 pumps to the oral cavity 2 to 3 times daily, or as needed; maximum duration for continuous use: 30 days

Gelclair: Rinse, gargle, and spit 15 mL (1 single-use packet) mixed in water 3 times daily, or as needed.

Mucotrol: Slowly dissolve 1 wafer by swishing around in the mouth, 3 times daily, or as needed

MuGard: Rinse with 5 mL 4 to 6 times daily (for oral mucositis/stomatitis) or 4 to 6 times daily or as needed (for other ulcerative conditions); may use up to 10 mL if needed to fully coat inside of mouth

Orafate:

Oral inflammation: Brush 1.25 to 2.5 mL across the front and back of gingiva 2 times daily for the first day then once daily at bedtime until healed (maximum: 10 mL per 24 hours)

Following dental cleaning (scaling/root planing): Brush 1.25 to 2.5 mL into gingival area daily for 4 weeks as directed (maximum: 10 mL per 24 hours)

Following tooth extraction or gingival (gum) surgery: Place 1.25 to 2.5 mL into wound 3 times daily the first day, then twice daily or as instructed until healed (maximum: 10 mL per 24 hours)

Following tonsillectomy or other oral soft tissue surgery: Place 2.5 to 5 mL into wound 3 times daily on the first day then twice daily or as directed (maximum: 10 mL per 24 hours)

ProThelial: Usual dosage: 2.5 to 5 mL every 8 hours on the first day; 2.5 to 5 mL every 12 hours thereafter (maximum: 40 mL daily)

Prevention of chemo-radiation mucositis (beginning the first day of cancer treatment):

Grade 1 or 2: 2.5 to 5 mL 3 times a day for 1 day, followed by 2.5 to 5 mL twice daily until 1 week after completion of chemo-radiation therapy

Grade 3 or 4: 10 mL 3 times a day, continue until 1 week after completion of chemo-radiation therapy

Treatment of chemo-radiation mucositis:

Grade 1 or 2: 2.5 to 5 mL 3 times a day for 1 day, followed by 2.5 to 5 mL twice daily until 1 week after completion of chemo-radiation therapy

Grade 3 or 4: 10 mL 3 times a day for 2 days, followed by 5 to 10 mL twice daily until 1 week after completion of chemo-radiation therapy

Pediatric Mucosal protection: Children ≥12 years and Adolescents: Oral: Orafate: Refer to adult Orafate dosing.

Administration

Episil: Remove protective cap from pump and prime pump by pumping into a paper cloth until an even liquid stream develops; firmly press pump (1 to 3 times) to apply liquid stream to oral cavity, distribute to affected areas of mouth and wait for gel and protective film to form. Do not swallow. Wait 5 minutes after use before eating and drinking.

Gelclair: Use before meals or as directed. Add 15 mL (1 single use packet) to water and stir (refer to product information for details); rinse around the mouth for a minimum of 1 minute (as long as possible) to coat the tongue, palate, throat, inside of cheeks, and all oral tissue thoroughly. Mixture should be gargled and spit out. Avoid eating or drinking for at least 30 to 60 minutes following treatment. If water is not available, may use undiluted. If unable to rinse and gargle, apply directly to mouth using a sponge or swab. No adverse effects are anticipated is accidently swallowed.

Mucotrol: Wafer should be swished around the mouth and allowed to slowly dissolve. Avoid eating or drinking for at least 1 hour following treatment.

MuGard: Gently pour 5 mL into mouth and rinse entire oral cavity for at least 1 minute (if rinsing is painful, spread throughout mouth by gently rotating head). Ensure all parts of the oral cavity are coated; may use up to 10 mL to coat entire oral cavity if needed. May spit or swallow excess rinse. Avoid eating or drinking for at least 1 hour following treatment.

Orafate: Apply in any of the following ways: either brushed alone or with toothpaste over affected tooth-gum line area for 2 minutes with an up and down motion; mix with equal portions of dentifrice (tooth paste, powder, gel) and layer over areas of soft tissue adjacent to teeth cleaned by the dental clinician; dab directly on to affected gum margin (allow to sit 2 minutes, then gargle and spit); layer onto affected oral area (allow to sit 2 minutes, then remove manually or spit); or place in mouth and suck back and forth through spaces between teeth. Safe if swallowed. Avoid eating or drinking for at least 1 hour following use.

ProThelial: Scoop paste from jar and place in mouth for 30 seconds. Use tongue or cotton-tipped swab to apply paste throughout oral mucosa. Can be swished and then expectorated or swallowed. May be mixed (1:1) with yogurt, pudding, apple sauce, tapioca, or ice cream to improve taste. Avoid eating or drinking for at least 1 hour following use.

Monitoring Parameters Monitor mucositis/stomatitis symptoms/severity

Dosage Forms Considerations Orafate and ProThelial each contain sucralfate (as a 10% paste).

Dosage Forms Excipient information presented when available (limited, particularly for generics); consult specific product labeling. [DSC] = Discontinued product

Gel, Mouth/Throat:
Gelclair: 15 mL/packet (15 mL)
Liquid, Mouth/Throat:
Episil: (10 mL)
MuGard: (5 mL, 240 mL) [contains benzyl alcohol]
Paste, Mouth/Throat:
Orafate: 10% (30 mL) [contains methylparaben, propylparaben, saccharin sodium; strawberry flavor]
ProThelial: 10% (125 mL, 250 mL, 500 mL) [contains methylparaben, propylparaben, saccharin sodium]
Wafer, Mouth/Throat:
Mucotrol: (21 ea, 45 ea) [sugar free; mild licorice flavor]

◆ **Mucosal Protective Agent** see Mucosal Coating Agent on page 1280

◆ **Mucotrol** see Mucosal Coating Agent on page 1280

◆ **MuGard** see Mucosal Coating Agent on page 1280

◆ **Mustargen** see Mechlorethamine (Systemic) on page 1168

◆ **Mustine** see Mechlorethamine (Systemic) on page 1168

◆ **Mutamycin** see MitoMYcin (Systemic) on page 1262

◆ **Mycamine** see Micafungin on page 1255

◆ **Mycelex** see Clotrimazole (Oral) on page 424

Mycophenolate (mye koe FEN oh late)

Related Information
Hematopoietic Cell Transplantation on page 2365
Safe Handling of Hazardous Drugs on page 2379

Brand Names: US CellCept; CellCept Intravenous; Myfortic

Brand Names: Canada Ach-Mycophenolate; Apo-Mycophenolate; CellCept; CellCept I.V.; CO Mycophenolate; JAMP-Mycophenolate; Myfortic; Mylan-Mycophenolate; Novo-Mycophenolate; Sandoz-Mycophenolate Mofetil; Vanc-Mycophenolate

Index Terms MMF; MPA; Mycophenolate Mofetil; Mycophenolate Sodium; Mycophenolic Acid

Pharmacologic Category Immunosuppressant Agent

Use Organ transplantation: Prophylaxis of organ rejection concomitantly with cyclosporine and corticosteroids in patients receiving allogeneic renal (CellCept, Myfortic), cardiac (CellCept), or hepatic (CellCept) transplants

◄ **Labeled Contraindications**

Hypersensitivity to mycophenolate mofetil, mycophenolic acid, mycophenolate sodium, or any component of the formulation

Cellcept: Intravenous formulation is also contraindicated in patients who are allergic to polysorbate 80

Canadian labeling: Additional contraindications (not in US labeling): Cellcept: Pregnancy; women of childbearing potential and not using highly effective contraceptive methods; women of childbearing potential not providing a pregnancy test result; breastfeeding

Pregnancy Considerations [US Boxed Warning]: Mycophenolate is associated with an increased risk of congenital malformations and first trimester pregnancy loss when used by pregnant women. Females of reproductive potential must be counseled about pregnancy prevention and planning. Alternative agents with less potential for embryofetal toxicity should be considered for women planning a pregnancy. The following congenital malformations have been reported following exposure during pregnancy: External ear abnormalities, cleft lip and palate, anomalies of the distal limbs, heart, esophagus, kidney, and nervous system. The combination of ear, eye, and lip/palate abnormalities has been identified as mycophenolate embryopathy (Perez-Aytes 2017). Spontaneous abortions have also been noted.

Females of reproductive potential (girls who have entered puberty and women with a uterus who have not passed through clinically confirmed menopause) should have a negative pregnancy test with a sensitivity of ≥25 milliunits/mL immediately before mycophenolate therapy and the test should be repeated 8 to 10 days later. Pregnancy tests should then be repeated during routine follow-up visits. Acceptable forms of contraception should be used during treatment and for 6 weeks after therapy is discontinued. The effectiveness of hormonal contraceptive agents may be affected by mycophenolate.

Current guidelines recommend that pregnancy be delayed following a kidney transplant until 1 year has passed without an acute rejection; this time period may be adjusted as clinically appropriate. Women planning a pregnancy and who are already taking mycophenolate following a kidney transplant should be switched to a different medication and mycophenolate should be discontinued for at least 6 weeks before pregnancy is attempted (KDIGO 2009). Mycophenolate is not recommended for the treatment of psoriasis in pregnant women (Menter 2009). Mycophenolate should not be used during pregnancy in women with lupus nephritis; women who become pregnant during mycophenolate therapy should be switched to a different medication (KDIGO 2012). For women with lupus nephritis taking mycophenolate and who are planning a pregnancy, mycophenolate should be discontinued at least 6 weeks prior to trying to conceive (Hahn 2012).

Health care providers should report female exposures to mycophenolate during pregnancy or within 6 weeks of discontinuing therapy to the Mycophenolate Pregnancy Registry (800-617-8191).

The National Transplantation Pregnancy Registry (NTPR) is a registry which follows pregnancies which occur in maternal transplant recipients or those fathered by male transplant recipients. The NTPR encourages reporting of pregnancies following solid organ transplant by contacting them at 877-955-6877 or NTPR@giftoflifeinstitute.org.

Breastfeeding Considerations It is not known if mycophenolate is present in human milk. Due to the potential for serious adverse reactions in the breastfed infant, the manufacturer recommends a decision be made whether to discontinue breastfeeding or to discontinue the drug (during therapy or within 6 weeks after treatment is complete), taking into account the importance of treatment to the mother.

Warnings/Precautions [US Boxed Warning]: Risk for bacterial, viral, fungal, and protozoal infections, including opportunistic infections, is increased with immunosuppressant therapy; infections may be serious and potentially fatal. Due to the risk of oversuppression of the immune system, which may increase susceptibility to infection, combination immunosuppressant therapy should be used with caution. Polyomavirus associated nephropathy (PVAN), JC virus-associated progressive multifocal leukoencephalopathy (PML), cytomegalovirus (CMV) infections, reactivation of hepatitis B (HBV) or hepatitis C (HCV), have been reported with use. A reduction in immunosuppression should be considered for patients with new or reactivated viral infections; however, in transplant recipients, the risk that reduced immunosuppression presents to the functioning graft should also be considered. PVAN, primarily from activation of BK virus, may lead to the deterioration of renal function and/or renal graft loss. PML, a potentially fatal condition, commonly presents with apathy, ataxia, cognitive deficiencies, confusion, and hemiparesis. Risk factors for development of PML include treatment with immunosuppressants and immune function impairment; consultation with a neurologist should be considered in any patient with neurological symptoms receiving immunosuppressants. Risk of CMV viremia or disease is increased in transplant recipients CMV seronegative at the time of transplant who receive a graft from a CMV seropositive donor. In patients infected with HBV or HCV, viral reactivation may occur; these patients should be monitored for signs of active HBV or HCV. **[US Boxed Warning]: Risk of development of lymphoma and skin malignancy is increased.** The risk for malignancies is related to intensity/duration of therapy. Patients should be monitored appropriately, instructed to limit exposure to sunlight/UV light to decrease the risk of skin cancer, and given supportive treatment should these conditions occur. Post-transplant lymphoproliferative disorder related to EBV infection has been reported in immunosuppressed organ transplant patients; risk is highest in EBV seronegative patients (including many young children). Neutropenia (including severe neutropenia) may occur, requiring dose reduction or interruption of treatment (risk greater from day 31-180 post-transplant). Use may rarely be associated with gastric or duodenal ulcers, GI bleeding and/or perforation. Use caution in patients with active serious digestive system disease; patients with active peptic ulcers were not included in clinical studies. Use caution in renal impairment as toxicity may be increased; may require dosage adjustment in severe impairment.

[US Boxed Warning]: Mycophenolate is associated with an increased risk of congenital malformations and first trimester pregnancy loss when used by pregnant women. Females of reproductive potential must be counseled about pregnancy prevention and planning. Alternative agents should be considered for women planning a pregnancy. Females of reproductive potential should have a negative pregnancy test with a sensitivity of ≥25 milliunits/mL immediately before therapy and the test should be repeated 8-10 days later. Pregnancy tests should be repeated during routine follow-up visits. Acceptable forms of contraception should be used during treatment and for 6 weeks after therapy is discontinued. Females of childbearing potential should have a negative pregnancy test within 1 week prior to beginning therapy. Two reliable forms of contraception should be used beginning 4 weeks prior to, during, and for 6 weeks after therapy. Because mycophenolate mofetil has demonstrated teratogenic effects in rats and rabbits, tablets should not be crushed, and capsules should not be opened or crushed. Avoid inhalation or direct contact with skin or mucous membranes of the powder contained in the capsules and the powder for oral suspension. Caution should be exercised in the handling and preparation of solutions of intravenous mycophenolate. Avoid skin contact with the intravenous solution and reconstituted suspension. If such contact occurs, wash thoroughly with soap and water, rinse eyes with plain water.

Theoretically, use should be avoided in patients with the rare hereditary deficiency of hypoxanthine-guanine phosphoribosyltransferase (such as Lesch-Nyhan or Kelley-Seegmiller syndrome). Intravenous solutions should be given over at least 2 hours; never administer intravenous solution by rapid or bolus injection. Live attenuated vaccines should be avoided during use; vaccinations may be less effective during therapy. **[US Boxed Warning]: Should be administered under the supervision of a physician experienced in immunosuppressive therapy.**

Mycophenolate sodium and mycophenolate mofetil should not be used interchangeably without health care provider supervision because the rate of absorption following the administration of these two products is not equivalent. Single dose pharmacokinetic studies in adult renal transplant patients suggest that bioavailability is similar between oral mycophenolate mofetil (1,000 mg) and delayed release mycophenolic acid (720 mg) (Arns, 2005). In clinical trials, comparative efficacy and safety profiles have been observed in adult renal transplant patients randomized to either oral mycophenolate mofetil (1,000 mg twice daily) or delayed release mycophenolic acid (720 mg twice daily) (Budde, 2004; Salvadori, 2003).

Some dosage forms may contain phenylalanine. Some dosage forms may contain polysorbate 80 (also known as Tweens). Hypersensitivity reactions, usually a delayed reaction, have been reported following exposure to pharmaceutical products containing polysorbate 80 in certain individuals (Isaksson, 2002; Lucente 2000; Shelley, 1995). Thrombocytopenia, ascites, pulmonary deterioration, and renal and hepatic failure have been reported in premature neonates after receiving parenteral products containing polysorbate 80 (Alade, 1986; CDC, 1984). See manufacturer's labeling.

Adverse Reactions Data for incidence >20% as reported in adults following oral dosing of CellCept alone in renal, cardiac, and hepatic allograft rejection studies. Profile in 3% to <20% range reflects use in combination with cyclosporine and corticosteroids. In general, lower doses used in renal rejection patients had less adverse effects than higher doses. Rates of adverse effects were similar for each indication, except for those unique to the specific organ involved. The type of adverse effects observed in pediatric patients was similar to those seen in adults, with the exception of abdominal pain, anemia, diarrhea, fever, hypertension, infection, pharyngitis, respiratory tract infection, sepsis, and vomiting, which were more frequent in pediatric patients; lymphoproliferative disorder was the only type of malignancy observed. Percentages of adverse reactions were similar in studies comparing CellCept to Myfortic in patients following renal transplant.

>20%:

Cardiovascular: Hypertension (28% to 78%), hypotension (33%), peripheral edema (27% to 64%), edema (27% to 28%), chest pain (26%), tachycardia (20% to 22%)

Central nervous system: Pain (31% to 76%), headache (16% to 54%), insomnia (41% to 52%), dizziness (29%), anxiety (28%), paresthesia (21%)

Dermatologic: Skin rash (22%)

Endocrine & metabolic: Hyperglycemia (44% to 47%), hypercholesterolemia (41%), hypomagnesemia (39%), hypokalemia (32% to 37%), hypocalcemia (30%), increased lactate dehydrogenase (23%), hyperkalemia (22%)

Gastrointestinal: Abdominal pain (25% to 63%), nausea (20% to 55%), diarrhea (31% to 51%), constipation (19% to 41%), vomiting (33% to 34%), anorexia (25%), dyspepsia (22%)

Genitourinary: Urinary tract infection (37%)

Hematologic & oncologic: Leukopenia (23% to 46%), anemia (26% to 43%), leukocytosis (22% to 41%), thrombocytopenia (24% to 38%), hypochromic anemia (25%)

Hepatic: Abnormal hepatic function tests (25%), ascites (24%)

Infection: Sepsis (27%), infection (18% to 27%), candidiasis (17% to 22%), herpes simplex infection (10% to 21%)

Neuromuscular & skeletal: Back pain (35% to 47%), weakness (35% to 43%), tremor (24% to 34%)

Renal: Increased serum creatinine (39%), increased blood urea nitrogen (35%), renal function abnormality (22% to 26%)

Respiratory: Dyspnea (31% to 37%), respiratory tract infection (22% to 37%), pleural effusion (34%), cough (31%), pulmonary disease (22% to 30%), sinusitis (26%)

Miscellaneous: Fever (21% to 52%)

3% to <20%:

Cardiovascular: Angina pectoris, arterial thrombosis, atrial fibrillation, atrial flutter, bradycardia, cardiac arrhythmia, cardiac failure, extrasystoles, facial edema, increased venous pressure, orthostatic hypotension, palpitations, pericardial effusion, peripheral vascular disorder, supraventricular extrasystole, supraventricular tachycardia, syncope, thrombosis, vasodilatation, vasospasm, ventricular premature contractions, ventricular tachycardia

Central nervous system: Abnormality in thinking, agitation, confusion, delirium, depression, drowsiness, emotional lability, hallucination, hypertonia, hypoesthesia, malaise, myasthenia, nervousness, neuropathy, psychosis, seizure, vertigo, voice disorder

Dermatologic: Acne vulgaris, alopecia, cellulitis, dermal ulcer, diaphoresis, fungal dermatitis, pallor, pruritus, skin hypertrophy, vesiculobullous dermatitis

Endocrine & metabolic: Acidosis, albuminuria, alkalosis, Cushing's syndrome, dehydration, diabetes mellitus, gout, hirsutism, hypercalcemia, hyperphosphatemia, hyperlipidemia, hypervolemia, hypochloremia, hypoglycemia, hyponatremia, hypophosphatemia, hypoproteinemia, hypothyroidism, hypovolemia, increased gamma-glutamyl transferase, increased thirst, parathyroid disease, weight gain, weight loss

Gastrointestinal: Mucocutaneous candidiasis (16% to 18%), cholangitis, dysphagia, enlargement of abdomen, esophagitis, flatulence, gastric disease, gastric ulcer, gastritis, gastroenteritis, gastrointestinal hemorrhage, GI moniliasis, gingival hyperplasia, gingivitis, hernia, hiccups, intestinal obstruction, melena, oral candidiasis, oral mucosa ulcer, peritonitis, stomatitis, xerostomia

◀

Genitourinary: Dysuria, hematuria, impotence, nocturia, oliguria, pelvic pain, prostatic disease, scrotal edema, urinary frequency, urinary incontinence, urinary retention, urinary tract abnormality

Hematologic & oncologic: Blood coagulation disorder, bruise, hemophthalmos, hemorrhage, neoplasm, neutropenia, pancytopenia, petechia, polycythemia, prolonged prothrombin time, prolonged partial thromboplastin time, skin carcinoma

Hepatic: Cholestatic jaundice, hepatic insuffiency, hepatitis, hyperbilirubinemia, increased serum alkaline phosphatase, increased serum transaminases, jaundice

Infection: Cytomegalovirus disease (viremia/syndrome: 12% to 14%; tissue invasive disease: 6% to 12%), herpes zoster (cutaneous disease: 4% to 10%), abscess (local), infection (of ileus)

Neuromuscular & skeletal: Arthralgia, arthropathy, leg cramps, myalgia, neck pain, osteoporosis

Ophthalmic: Abnormal lacrimation, amblyopia, cataract, conjunctivitis, visual disturbance

Otic: Deafness, ear disease, otalgia, tinnitus

Renal: Hydronephrosis, increased serum creatinine, pyelonephritis, renal failure, renal tubular necrosis

Respiratory: Apnea, asthma, atelectasis, bronchitis, epistaxis, flu-like symptoms, hemoptysis, hyperventilation, hypoxia, increased bronchial secretions, pharyngitis, pneumonia, pneumothorax, pulmonary edema, pulmonary hypertension, respiratory acidosis, respiratory tract infection (moniliasis), rhinitis

Miscellaneous: Abnormal healing, cyst, fever and chills

<1%, postmarketing and/or case reports: Atypical mycobacterial infection, bronchiectasis (Boddana 2011, Rook 2006), colitis, endocarditis (infectious), gastrointestinal perforation, hypogammaglobulinemia (Boddana 2011; Keven 2003; Robertson 2009), interstitial pulmonary disease, lymphoproliferative disorder, malabsorption (intestinal villous atrophy), malignant lymphoma, malignant neoplasm, meningitis, pancreatitis, progressive multifocal leukoencephalopathy, pulmonary fibrosis, pure red cell aplasia, renal disease (BK virus-associated), tuberculosis

Drug Interactions

Metabolism/Transport Effects Substrate of OAT3, SLCO1B1, SLCO1B3, UGT1A10, UGT1A8, UGT1A9, UGT2B7

Avoid Concomitant Use

Avoid concomitant use of Mycophenolate with any of the following: BCG (Intravesical); Bile Acid Sequestrants; Cholestyramine Resin; Natalizumab; Pimecrolimus; Rifamycin Derivatives; Tacrolimus (Topical); Vaccines (Live)

Increased Effect/Toxicity

Mycophenolate may increase the levels/effects of: Acyclovir-Valacyclovir; Fingolimod; Ganciclovir-Valganciclovir; Leflunomide; Natalizumab; Tofacitinib; Vaccines (Live)

The levels/effects of Mycophenolate may be increased by: Acyclovir-Valacyclovir; Denosumab; Ganciclovir-Valganciclovir; Isavuconazonium Sulfate; Ocrelizumab; Pimecrolimus; Probenecid; Roflumilast; Tacrolimus (Topical); Teriflunomide; Trastuzumab

Decreased Effect

Mycophenolate may decrease the levels/effects of: BCG (Intravesical); Coccidioides immitis Skin Test; Contraceptives (Estrogens); Contraceptives (Progestins); Nivolumab; Sipuleucel-T; Tertomotide; Vaccines (Inactivated); Vaccines (Live)

The levels/effects of Mycophenolate may be decreased by: Antacids; Bile Acid Sequestrants; Cholestyramine Resin; CycloSPORINE (Systemic); Echinacea; Magnesium Salts; MetroNIDAZOLE (Systemic); Penicillins; Proton Pump Inhibitors; Quinolone Antibiotics; Rifamycin Derivatives; Sevelamer

Food Interactions Food decreases C_{max} of MPA by 40% following CellCept administration and 33% following Myfortic use; the extent of absorption is not changed. Management: Take CellCept or Myfortic on an empty stomach to decrease variability; however, Cellcept may be taken with food if necessary in stable renal transplant patients.

Hazardous Drugs Handling Considerations

Hazardous agent (NIOSH 2016 [group 2]).

Use appropriate precautions for receiving, handling, administration, and disposal. Gloves (single) should be worn during receiving, unpacking, and placing in storage.

NIOSH recommends single gloving for administration of intact tablets or capsules. If manipulating tablets/capsules (eg, to prepare an oral suspension), NIOSH recommends double gloving, a protective gown, and preparation in a controlled device; If not prepared in a controlled device, respiratory and eye/face protection as well as ventilated engineering controls are recommended. NIOSH recommends double gloving, a protective gown, and (if there is a potential for vomit or spit up) eye/face protection for administration of an oral liquid/feeding tube administration. For IV preparation, NIOSH recommends double gloving, a protective gown, ventilated engineering controls (a class II biological safety cabinet or a compounding aseptic containment isolator), and closed system transfer devices (CSTDs). Double gloving, a gown, and (if dosage form allows) CSTDs are required during IV administration (NIOSH 2016).

Storage/Stability

Capsules: Store at 25°C (77°F); excursions permitted to 15°C to 30°C (59°F to 86°F).

Tablets: Store at 25°C (77°F); excursions permitted to 15°C to 30°C (59°F to 86°F). Protect from moisture and light.

Oral suspension: Store powder for oral suspension at 25°C (77°F); excursions permitted to 15°C to 30°C (59°F to 86°F). Once reconstituted, the oral solution may be stored at room temperature or under refrigeration. Do not freeze. The mixed suspension is stable for 60 days.

Injection: Store intact vials and solutions diluted in D5W at 25°C (77°F); excursions permitted to 15°C to 30°C (59°F to 86°F). Begin infusion within 4 hours of reconstitution.

Preparation for Administration

Oral suspension: Should be constituted prior to dispensing to the patient and **not** mixed with any other medication. Add 47 mL of water to the bottle and shake well for ~1 minute. Add another 47 mL of water to the bottle and shake well for an additional minute. Final concentration is 200 mg/mL of mycophenolate mofetil.

◄ IV: Reconstitute the contents of each vial with 14 mL of 5% dextrose injection; dilute the contents of a vial with 5% dextrose in water to a final concentration of 6 mg mycophenolate mofetil per mL. **Note:** Vial is vacuum-sealed; if a lack of vacuum is noted during preparation, the vial should not be used.

Mechanism of Action MPA exhibits a cytostatic effect on T and B lymphocytes. It is an inhibitor of inosine monophosphate dehydrogenase (IMPDH) which inhibits *de novo* guanosine nucleotide synthesis. T and B lymphocytes are dependent on this pathway for proliferation.

Pharmacodynamics/Kinetics

Onset of action: Peak effect: Correlation of toxicity or efficacy is still being developed, however, one study indicated that 12-hour AUCs >40 mcg/mL/ hour were correlated with efficacy and decreased episodes of rejection

Absorption: Rapid and extensive; early post-transplant period mycophenolic acid (MPA) AUC values are lower (~45% to 53%) than later post-transplant period (>3 months) MPA AUC values in both pediatric patients and adults
Oral: Myfortic: 93%

Distribution:
CellCept: MPA: Oral: 4 L/kg; IV: 3.6 L/kg
Myfortic: MPA: Oral: 54 L (at steady state); 112 L (elimination phase)

Protein binding: MPA: >97%, MPAG 82%

Metabolism: Hepatic and via GI tract; CellCept is completely hydrolyzed in the liver to mycophenolic acid (MPA; active metabolite); enterohepatic recirculation of MPA may occur; MPA is glucuronidated to MPAG (inactive metabolite)

Bioavailability: Oral: CellCept: 80.7% to 94%; enterohepatic recirculation contributes to MPA concentration (Staatz 2007); two 500 mg tablets have been shown to be bioequivalent to four 250 mg capsules or 1,000 mg of oral suspension; Myfortic: 72%

Half-life elimination:
CellCept: MPA: Oral: 18 hours; IV: 17 hours
Myfortic: MPA: Oral: 8 to 16 hours; MPAG: 13 to 17 hours

Time to peak, plasma: Oral: MPA:
CellCept: 1 to 1.5 hours
Myfortic: 1.5 to 2.75 hours

Excretion:
CellCept: MPA: Urine (<1%), feces (6%); MPAG: Urine (87%)
Myfortic: MPA: Urine (3%), feces; MPAG: Urine (>60%)

Dosing

Adult Note: May be used IV for up to 14 days; transition to oral therapy as soon as tolerated.

Renal transplant:
CellCept:
Oral: 1 g twice daily. Doses >2 g daily are not recommended.
IV: 1 g twice daily
Myfortic: Oral: 720 mg twice daily (total daily dose: 1440 mg)

Cardiac transplantation: *CellCept:*
Oral: 1.5 g twice daily
IV: 1.5 g twice daily

Hepatic transplantation: *CellCept:*
Oral: 1.5 g twice daily
IV: 1 g twice daily

Autoimmune hepatitis, refractory (off-label use): *CellCept:* Oral: 2 g daily (Manns, 2010)

Lupus nephritis (off-label use): CellCept: Oral:

Induction: 1 g twice daily for 6 months in combination with a glucocorticoid (Ong, 2005) **or** 2-3 g daily for 6 months in combination with glucocorticoids (Hahn, 2012)

Maintenance: 0.5-3 g daily (Contreras, 2004) **or** 1 g twice daily (Dooley, 2011) **or** 1-2 g daily (Hahn, 2012)

Myasthenia gravis (off-label use): *CellCept:* Oral: 1 g twice daily (range: 1-3 g daily) (Cahoon, 2006; Ciafaloni, 2001; Merriggioli, 2003)

Psoriasis, moderate-to-severe (off-label use): *CellCept:* Oral: 2-3 g daily (Menter, 2009)

Geriatric Dosage is the same as younger patients, however, dosing should be cautious due to possibility of increased hepatic, renal, or cardiac dysfunction. Elderly patients may be at an increased risk of certain infections, gastrointestinal hemorrhage, and pulmonary edema, as compared to younger patients.

Pediatric

Renal transplant: Oral:

CellCept: Infants ≥3 months, Children, and Adolescents: *Cellcept suspension:* 600 mg/m^2/dose twice daily; maximum dose: 1 g twice daily

Alternatively, may use Cellcept solid dosage forms according to BSA as follows:

BSA 1.25 to 1.5 m^2: 750 mg capsule twice daily

BSA >1.5 m^2: 1 g capsule or tablet twice daily

Myfortic: Children ≥5 years and Adolescents: Usual dosage: 400 mg/m^2/dose twice daily; maximum dose: 720 mg twice daily

BSA <1.19 m^2: Use of this formulation is not recommended

BSA 1.19 to 1.58 m^2: 540 mg twice daily (maximum: 1080 mg daily)

BSA >1.58 m^2: 720 mg twice daily (maximum: 1440 mg daily)

Renal Impairment

Renal transplant: GFR <25 mL/minute/1.73 m^2 in patients outside the immediate post-transplant period:

CellCept: Doses of >1 g administered twice daily should be avoided; patients should also be carefully observed; no dose adjustments are needed in renal transplant patients experiencing delayed graft function postoperatively

Myfortic: No dose adjustments are needed in renal transplant patients experiencing delayed graft function postoperatively; however, monitor carefully for potential concentration dependent adverse events

Cardiac or liver transplant: No data available; mycophenolate may be used in cardiac or hepatic transplant patients with severe chronic renal impairment if the potential benefit outweighs the potential risk.

Autoimmune disease (off-label use): There have been no specific dosage adjustments identified, although use of lower doses may be required. MPA exposure appears to be inversely related to renal function (Abd Rahman, 2013); monitor closely for efficacy and adverse effects, especially in patients with end-stage renal disease (Haubitz, 2002; MacPhee, 2000).

Hemodialysis: Not removed; supplemental dose is not necessary.

Peritoneal dialysis: Supplemental dose is not necessary.

Hepatic Impairment No dosage adjustment is recommended for renal patients with severe hepatic parenchymal disease; however, it is not currently known whether dosage adjustments are necessary for hepatic disease with other etiologics.

◄ **Adjustment for Toxicity** Neutropenia (ANC <1.3 x 10³/μL): Dosing should be interrupted or the dose reduced, appropriate diagnostic tests performed and patients managed appropriately

Administration

Oral dosage formulations (tablet, capsule, suspension) should be administered on an empty stomach (1 hour before or 2 hours after meals) to avoid variability in MPA absorption. The oral solution may be administered via a nasogastric tube (minimum 8 French, 1.7 mm interior diameter); oral suspension should not be mixed with other medications. Delayed release tablets should not be crushed, cut, or chewed. Cellcept may be administered with food in stable renal transplant patients when necessary. If a dose is missed, administer as soon as it is remembered. If it is close to the next scheduled dose, skip the missed dose and resume at next regularly scheduled time; do not double a dose to make up for a missed dose.

Intravenous solutions should be administered over at least 2 hours (either peripheral or central vein); do **not** administer intravenous solution by rapid or bolus injection.

Extemporaneous Preparations A 50 mg/mL oral suspension may be made with mycophenolate mofetil capsules, Ora-Plus, and cherry syrup. In a vertical flow hood, empty six 250 mg capsules into a mortar; add 7.5 mL Ora-Plus and mix to a uniform paste. Mix while adding 15 mL of cherry syrup in incremental proportions; transfer to a calibrated bottle, rinse mortar with cherry syrup, and add sufficient quantity of cherry syrup to make 30 mL. Label "shake well". Stable for 210 days at 5°C, for 28 days at 25°C to 37°C, and for 11 days at 45°C.

Venkataramanan R, McCombs JR, Zuckerman S, et al, "Stability of Mycophenolate Mofetil as an Extemporaneous Suspension," *Ann Pharmacother*, 1998, 32(7-8):755-7.

Monitoring Parameters Complete blood count (weekly for first month, twice monthly during months 2 and 3, then monthly thereafter through the first year); renal and liver function; signs and symptoms of organ rejection; signs and symptoms of bacterial, fungal, protozoal, new or reactivated viral, or opportunistic infections; neurological symptoms (eg, hemiparesis, confusion, cognitive deficiencies, ataxia) suggestive of PML, pregnancy test (immediately prior to initiation and 8-10 days later in females of childbearing potential, followed by repeat tests during therapy); monitor skin (for lesions suspicious of skin cancer); monitor for signs of lymphoma

Dietary Considerations Some products may contain phenylalanine.

Additional Information Females of reproductive potential are required to have contraceptive counseling and use acceptable birth control unless heterosexual intercourse is completely avoided. Use of an intrauterine device (IUD), tubal sterilization, or vasectomy of the female patient's partner are acceptable contraceptive methods that can be used alone. If a hormonal contraceptive is used (eg, combination oral contraceptive pills, transdermal patches, vaginal rings, or progestin only products), then one barrier method must also be used (eg, diaphragm or cervical cap with spermicide, contraceptive sponge, male or female condom). Alternatively, the use of two barrier methods is also acceptable (eg, diaphragm or cervical cap with spermicide, or contraceptive sponge **PLUS** male or female condom). Refer to manufacturer's labeling for full details.

Medication Guide Available Yes

Dosage Forms Excipient information presented when available (limited, particularly for generics); consult specific product labeling.

Capsule, Oral, as mofetil:
  CellCept: 250 mg [contains fd&c blue #2 (indigotine)]
  Generic: 250 mg

Solution Reconstituted, Intravenous, as mofetil hydrochloride:
  CellCept Intravenous: 500 mg (1 ea) [contains polysorbate 80]
  Generic: 500 mg (1 ea)

Suspension Reconstituted, Oral, as mofetil:
  CellCept: 200 mg/mL (160 mL) [contains aspartame, methylparaben, sorbitol, soybean lecithin; mixed fruit flavor]
  Generic: 200 mg/mL (160 mL)

Tablet, Oral, as mofetil:
  CellCept: 500 mg [contains fd&c blue #2 aluminum lake]
  Generic: 500 mg

Tablet Delayed Release, Oral, as mycophenolic acid:
  Myfortic: 180 mg [contains fd&c blue #2 (indigotine)]
  Myfortic: 360 mg
  Generic: 180 mg, 360 mg

Nabilone (NA bi lone)

Related Information

Management of Chemotherapy-Induced Nausea and Vomiting in Adults on page 2253

Brand Names: US Cesamet

◄ **Brand Names: Canada** ACT Nabilone; Cesamet; PMS-Nabilone; RAN™-Nabilone; Teva-Nabilone

Pharmacologic Category Antiemetic

Use Treatment of refractory nausea and vomiting associated with cancer chemotherapy

Labeled Contraindications Hypersensitivity to nabilone, other cannabinoids, or any component of the formulation

Pregnancy Considerations Adverse events have been observed in animal reproduction studies.

Breastfeeding Considerations Because some cannabinoids are excreted in breast milk, use in breastfeeding is not recommended.

Warnings/Precautions May cause tachycardia and orthostatic hypotension; use caution with cardiovascular disease. May affect CNS function (dizziness, drowsiness, ataxia, depression, hallucinations, and psychosis have been reported); use with caution in the elderly and those with preexisting CNS depression. May cause additive CNS effects with sedatives, hypnotics, or other psychoactive agents; patients must be cautioned about performing tasks which require mental alertness (eg, operating machinery or driving). Use caution in patients with mania, depression, or schizophrenia; cannabinoid use may reveal symptoms of psychiatric disorders. Careful psychiatric monitoring is recommended; psychiatric adverse reactions may persist for up to 3 days after discontinuing treatment. Has potential for abuse and or dependence, use caution in patients with substance abuse history or potential.

Adverse Reactions

>10%:

Central nervous system: Drowsiness (52% to 66%), dizziness (59%), vertigo (52% to 59%), euphoria (11% to 38%), ataxia (13% to 14%), depression (14%), lack of concentration (12%), sleep disorder (11%)

Gastrointestinal: Xerostomia (22% to 36%)

Ophthalmic: Visual disturbance (13%)

1% to 10%:

Cardiovascular: Hypotension (8%)

Central nervous system: Dysphoria (9%), headache (6% to 7%), sedation (3%), depersonalization (2%), disorientation (2%)

Gastrointestinal: Anorexia (8%), nausea (4%), increased appetite (2%)

Neuromuscular & skeletal: Weakness (8%)

Frequency not defined:

Cardiovascular: Cardiac arrhythmia, cerebrovascular accident, chest pain, flushing, hypertension, orthostatic hypotension, palpitations, syncope, tachycardia

Central nervous system: Abnormal dreams, akathisia, anxiety, apathy, chills, confusion, difficulty thinking, dystonia, emotional disturbance, emotional lability, equilibrium disturbance, fatigue, hallucination, hyperactivity, illusion, insomnia, malaise, memory impairment, nervousness, numbness, pain, psychoneurosis (phobic), panic disorder, paranoia, paresthesia, psychological disorder (withdrawal), psychosis (including toxic), seizure, speech disturbance, stupor, voice disorder

Dermatologic: Anhidrosis, diaphoresis, skin photosensitivity, pruritus, skin rash

Endocrine & metabolic: Hot flash, increased thirst

Gastrointestinal: Abdominal pain, aphthous stomatitis, constipation, diarrhea, dysgeusia, dyspepsia, gastritis, mouth irritation, vomiting

Genitourinary: Altered micturition (decreased/increased), urinary retention

Hematologic & oncologic: Anemia, leukopenia

Hypersensitivity: Hypersensitivity reaction

Infection: Infection

Neuromuscular & skeletal: Arthralgia, back pain, myalgia, neck pain, tremor

Ophthalmic: Amblyopia, eye irritation, mydriasis, photophobia, visual field defect, xerophthalmia

Otic: Tinnitus

Renal: Polyuria

Respiratory: Cough, dyspnea, epistaxis, nasal congestion, pharyngitis, sinus headache, wheezing

Miscellaneous: Fever

Drug Interactions

Metabolism/Transport Effects None known.

Avoid Concomitant Use There are no known interactions where it is recommended to avoid concomitant use.

Increased Effect/Toxicity

Nabilone may increase the levels/effects of: Alcohol (Ethyl); Amifostine; CNS Depressants; DULoxetine; Hypotension-Associated Agents; Levodopa; Nitroprusside; Pholcodine; Sympathomimetics

The levels/effects of Nabilone may be increased by: Alfuzosin; Anticholinergic Agents; Benperidol; Blood Pressure Lowering Agents; Brimonidine (Topical); Cocaine; Diazoxide; Herbs (Hypotensive Properties); Lormetazepam; Molsidomine; Naftopidil; Nicergoline; Nicorandil; Obinutuzumab; Pentoxifylline; Phosphodiesterase 5 Inhibitors; Prostacyclin Analogues; Quinagolide

Decreased Effect There are no known significant interactions involving a decrease in effect.

Storage/Stability Store at 25°C (77°F); excursion permitted to 15°C and 30°C (59°F and 86°F).

Mechanism of Action Antiemetic activity may be due to effect on cannabinoid receptors (CB1) within the central nervous system.

Pharmacodynamics/Kinetics

Absorption: Rapid and complete

Distribution: ~12.5 L/kg

Metabolism: Extensively metabolized to several active metabolites by oxidation and stereospecific enzyme reduction; CYP450 enzymes may also be involved

Half-life elimination: Parent compound: ~2 hours; Metabolites: ~35 hours

Time to peak, serum: Within 2 hours

Excretion: Feces (~60%); renal (~24%)

Dosing

Adult Nausea and vomiting associated with cancer chemotherapy: Oral: 1-2 mg twice daily (maximum: 6 mg divided in 3 doses daily); begin with the lower dose in the range and increase if needed. May administer 2 or 3 times per day during the entire chemotherapy course; continue for up to 48 hours after the last chemotherapy dose. A dose of 1-2 mg the night before chemotherapy may also be of benefit.

Geriatric Refer to adult dosing. Use the lower end of the dosing range (to minimize adverse events).

◀ **Pediatric Nausea and vomiting associated with cancer chemotherapy (off-label use; Dupuis, 2003):** Oral: Children >4 years:
<18 kg: 0.5 mg every 12 hours
18-30 kg: 1 mg every 12 hours
>30 kg: 1 mg every 8-12 hours

Renal Impairment No dosage adjustment provided in manufacturer's labeling (has not been studied).

Hepatic Impairment No dosage adjustment provided in manufacturer's labeling (has not been studied).

Administration Initial dose should be given 1-3 hours before chemotherapy.

Monitoring Parameters Blood pressure, heart rate; signs and symptoms of excessive use, abuse, or misuse

Dosage Forms Excipient information presented when available (limited, particularly for generics); consult specific product labeling.
Capsule, Oral:
Cesamet: 1 mg [contains fd&c blue #2 (indigotine)]

Controlled Substance C-II

◆ **nab-Paclitaxel** *see* PACLitaxel (Protein Bound) *on page 1411*

Nafcillin (naf SIL in)

Index Terms Ethoxynaphthamido Penicillin Sodium; Nafcillin Sodium; Nallpen; Sodium Nafcillin

Pharmacologic Category Antibiotic, Penicillin

Use Staphylococcal infections: Treatment of infections caused by susceptible penicillinase-producing staphylococci

Pregnancy Risk Factor B

Dosing

Adult & Geriatric

Catheter-related bloodstream infections (off-label use): IV: 2 g every 4 hours (IDSA [Mermel 2009])

Endocarditis: Methicillin-susceptible *Staphylococcus aureus* (MSSA) (off-label dose): IV:

Native valve: 12 g/day in 4 or 6 divided doses (ie, 2 g every 4 hours or 3 g every 6 hours) for 6 weeks. **Note:** Duration intended for *complicated* right-sided infective endocarditis (IE) or left-sided IE. For *uncomplicated* right-sided IE, 2 weeks of therapy may be adequate (AHA [Baddour 2015]).

Prosthetic valve: 12 g/day in 6 divided doses (ie, 2 g every 4 hours) for ≥6 weeks (use with rifampin for entire course and gentamicin for first 2 weeks) (AHA [Baddour 2015])

Osteomyelitis: Methicillin-susceptible *S. aureus* (MSSA) (off-label dose): IV: 1.5 to 2 g every 4 to 6 hours or via continuous infusion (IDSA [Berbari 2015])

Prosthetic joint infections: Methicillin-susceptible *S. aureus* (MSSA) (off-label dose): 1.5 to 2 g every 4 to 6 hours (IDSA [Osmon 2013])

Skin and soft tissue infections (IDSA [Stevens 2014]):

Due to methicillin-susceptible Staphylococcus aureus (MSSA) (off-label dose): IV: 1 to 2 g every 4 hours for 7 to 14 days

Necrotizing infection due to MSSA (off-label use): IV: 1 to 2 g every 4 hours; continue until further debridement is not necessary, patient has clinically improved, and patient is afebrile for 48 to 72 hours

Streptococcal skin infections (off-label use): IV: 1 to 2 g every 4 to 6 hours (IDSA [Stevens 2014])

Surgical site infections (trunk or extremity [away from axilla or perineum]) (off-label use): IV: 2 g every 6 hours (IDSA [Stevens 2014])

Pediatric

Mild-to-moderate infections: IM, IV: 100 to 150 mg/kg/day in divided doses every 6 hours (maximum dose: 4,000 mg daily) (*Red Book* [AAP 2015])

Severe infections: IM, IV: 150 to 200 mg/kg/day in divided doses every 4 to 6 hours (*Red Book* [AAP 2015]); for life-threatening infection (eg, meningitis), 200 mg/kg/day in divided doses every 6 hours (maximum dose: 12 g daily) (Tunkel 2004)

Skin and soft tissue infections (IDSA [Stevens 2014]):

Due to methicillin-susceptible Staphylococcus aureus (MSSA): IV: 100 to 150 mg/kg/day in divided doses every 6 hours for 7 to 14 days

Necrotizing infection due to MSSA (off-label use): IV: 200 mg/kg/day in divided doses every 6 hours; continue until further debridement is not necessary, patient has clinically improved, and patient is afebrile for 48 to 72 hours

Streptococcal skin infections (off-label use): IV: 200 mg/kg/day in divided doses every 6 hours (IDSA [Stevens 2014])

Renal Impairment No dosage adjustment necessary; use with caution in patients with concomitant hepatic impairment.

Poorly dialyzed. No supplemental dose or dosage adjustment necessary, including patients on intermittent hemodialysis, peritoneal dialysis, or continuous renal replacement therapy (eg, CVVHD) (Aronoff 2007; Heintz 2009).

Hepatic Impairment There are no dosage adjustments provided in the manufacturer's labeling. Nafcillin primarily undergoes hepatic metabolism; dosage adjustment may be necessary, particularly in the setting of concomitant renal impairment.

Additional Information Complete prescribing information should be consulted for additional detail.

Dosage Forms Considerations

Nafcillin lyophilized powder contains sodium approximately 66 mg [2.9 mEq] per gram of nafcillin.

Nafcillin in Dextrose (iso-osmotic) contains sodium 76.6 mg [3.33 mEq] per gram of nafcillin.

Dosage Forms Excipient information presented when available (limited, particularly for generics); consult specific product labeling.

Solution, Intravenous:

Generic: 1 g/50 mL (50 mL); 2 g/100 mL (100 mL)

Solution Reconstituted, Injection:

Generic: 1 g (1 ea); 2 g (1 ea); 10 g (1 ea)

Solution Reconstituted, Injection [preservative free]:

Generic: 1 g (1 ea); 2 g (1 ea); 10 g (1 ea)

Solution Reconstituted, Intravenous:

Generic: 1 g (1 ea); 2 g (1 ea)

◆ **Nafcillin Sodium** *see* Nafcillin *on page 1296*

Naldemedine (nal DEM e deen)

Index Terms Naldemedine Tosylate; Symproic

◀ **Pharmacologic Category** Gastrointestinal Agent, Miscellaneous; Opioid Antagonist, Peripherally-Acting

Use Opioid-induced constipation: Treatment of opioid-induced constipation (OIC) in adults with chronic noncancer pain, including patients with chronic pain related to prior cancer or its treatment who do not require frequent (eg, weekly) opioid dosage escalation.

Dosing

Adult & Geriatric Opioid-induced constipation: Oral: 0.2 mg once daily. Discontinue treatment if opioid pain medication is discontinued.

Renal Impairment No dosage adjustment necessary.

Hepatic Impairment

Mild to moderate impairment (Child-Pugh classes A and B): No dosage adjustment necessary.

Severe impairment (Child-Pugh class C): Avoid use (has not been studied).

Additional Information Complete prescribing information should be consulted for additional detail.

Medication Guide Available Yes

Controlled Substance C-II

Necitumumab (ne si TOOM oo mab)

Related Information

Management of EGFR Inhibitor Toxicities: Dermatologic, Ocular, and Gastrointestinal on page 2291

Brand Names: US Portrazza

Index Terms Anti-EGFR Monoclonal Antibody IMC-11F8; IMC-11F8; Portrazza

Pharmacologic Category Antineoplastic Agent, Epidermal Growth Factor Receptor (EGFR) Inhibitor; Antineoplastic Agent, Monoclonal Antibody

Use

Non-small cell lung cancer (squamous), metastatic: First-line treatment of metastatic squamous non-small cell lung cancer (NSCLC) in combination with gemcitabine and cisplatin

Limitations of use: Not indicated for treatment of non-squamous non-small cell lung cancer.

Labeled Contraindications There are no contraindications listed in the manufacturer's labeling.

Pregnancy Considerations Necitumumab is expected to cross the placenta. Based on animal data and the mechanism of action, necitumumab is expected to cause fetal harm if administered during pregnancy. Women of reproductive potential should use effective contraception during therapy and for 3 months after the last dose.

Breastfeeding Considerations It is not known if necitumumab is excreted into breast milk; however, human IgG antibodies can be detected in breast milk. Due to the potential for serious adverse reactions in the nursing infant, breastfeeding is not recommended by the manufacturer during therapy or for 3 months after the last dose.

Warnings/Precautions [US Boxed Warning]: Cardiopulmonary arrest and/or sudden death occurred in a small percentage of patients treated with necitumumab in combination with gemcitabine and cisplatin. Monitor serum electrolytes closely, including serum magnesium, potassium, and calcium, with aggressive replacement when warranted during and after necitumumab administration. Continue electrolyte monitoring for at least 8 weeks after the last dose. Some cardiopulmonary events were fatal; many of those patients had comorbid conditions (including a history of coronary artery disease, hypomagnesemia, COPD, and/or hypertension). Patients with significant coronary artery disease, MI within 6 months, uncontrolled hypertension or uncontrolled heart failure were excluded from the squamous cell non-small cell lung cancer study. **[US Boxed Warning]: Hypomagnesemia occurred in a majority of patients receiving necitumumab in combination with gemcitabine and cisplatin; hypomagnesemia was severe in one-fifth of patients. Monitor for hypomagnesemia, hypocalcemia, and hypokalemia prior to each dose of necitumumab during treatment and for at least 8 weeks following completion of necitumumab. Withhold necitumumab for Grade 3 or 4 electrolyte abnormalities. Replete electrolytes as appropriate.** May resume treatment when hypomagnesemia and related electrolyte abnormalities are improved to grade 2 or lower. The median time to development of hypomagnesemia was 6 weeks after treatment initiation.

Dermatologic toxicity, including rash, dermatitis anceiform, acne, dry skin, pruritus, generalized rash, skin fissures, maculo-papular rash, and/or erythema occurs commonly; may be severe. Skin toxicity usually developed within the first 2 weeks of treatment and resolved within 17 weeks after onset. May require treatment interruption, dose reduction, or discontinuation. Patients should minimize exposure to the sun. Infusion-related reactions have been reported with necitumumab, usually after the first or second infusion. Premedication was not routinely administered prior to the first dose in the squamous cell NSCLC study. Monitor for signs/symptoms of infusion reaction. Discontinue for serious or life-threatening reactions. Venous and arterial thromboembolic events (VTE and ATE) were observed with necitumumab, including grades 3 and 4 events and some fatalities. The most common VTEs were deep vein thrombosis and pulmonary embolism and the most common ATEs were cerebral stroke and ischemia and MI. Discontinue necitumumab for serious or life-threatening VTE or ATE. The incidence of VTE may be higher in patients ≥70 years of age (compared to patients under age 70).

Necitumumab is not indicated for use in patients with non-squamous NSCLC. In a study of necitumumab in combination with pemetrexed and cisplatin for the treatment of metastatic non-squamous NSCLC, patients experienced increased serious and fatal toxicities and cardiopulmonary arrest/sudden death within 30 days of the last dose of necitumumab (compared to peme-trexed and cisplatin without necitumumab).

Adverse Reactions Adverse reaction percentages reported as part of a combination regimen with gemcitabine and cisplatin.

>10%:

Central nervous system: Headache (11%)

Dermatologic: Skin toxicity (79%; grades 3/4: 8%), skin rash (44%; grades 3/4: 4%), acneiform eruption (15%; grades 3/4: 1%)

Endocrine & metabolic: Hypomagnesemia (43% to 83%; grades 3/4: 20%), hypocalcemia (45%; grades 3/4: 6%; with albumin corrected: 36%; grades 3/4: 4%), hypophosphatemia (31%; grades 3/4: 8%), hypokalemia (28%; grades 3/4: 5%), weight loss (13%)

Gastrointestinal: Vomiting (29%), diarrhea (16%), stomatitis (11%)

1% to 10%:

Cardiovascular: Venous thromboembolism (9%; grades 3/4: 5%), arterial thromboembolism (5%; grades 3/4: 4%), pulmonary embolism (5%; cardiorespiratory arrest (3%), deep vein thrombosis (2%), cerebrovascular accident (≤2%), ischemia (≤2%), myocardial infarction (1%)

Dermatologic: Acne vulgaris (9%), paronychia (7%), pruritus (7%), xeroderma (7%), skin fissure (5%)

Immunologic: Antibody development (4%; neutralizing: 1%)

Ophthalmic: Conjunctivitis (7%)

Respiratory: Hemoptysis (10%)

Miscellaneous: Infusion related reaction (2%; grade 3: <1%)

Drug Interactions

Metabolism/Transport Effects None known.

Avoid Concomitant Use There are no known interactions where it is recommended to avoid concomitant use.

Increased Effect/Toxicity There are no known significant interactions involving an increase in effect.

Decreased Effect There are no known significant interactions involving a decrease in effect.

Storage/Stability Store intact vials at 2°C to 8°C (36°F to 46°F). Do not freeze. Store in original carton to protect from light. Do not shake. Solutions diluted for infusion in NS are stable for up to 4 hours at room temperature or 24 hours at 2°C to 8°C (36°F to 46°F); do not freeze or shake.

Preparation for Administration Dilute for infusion in NS to a total volume of 250 mL (do not use solutions containing dextrose). Gently invert to mix; do not shake.

Mechanism of Action Necitumumab is a recombinant human IgG1 EGFR monoclonal antibody which binds (with a high affinity) to the ligand binding site of the EGFR receptor to prevent receptor activation and downstream signaling (Thatcher 2015).

Pharmacodynamics/Kinetics

Distribution: V_{dss}: 7 L

Half-life elimination: ~14 days

Dosing

Adult & Geriatric Note: For patients with a prior grade 1 or 2 infusion reaction, premedicate (prior to all subsequent necitumumab infusions) with diphenhydramine (or equivalent). For patients with a recurrent grade 1 or 2 infusion reaction, premedicate (prior to all subsequent necitumumab infusions) with diphenhydramine (or equivalent), acetaminophen, and dexamethasone (or equivalent).

Non-small cell lung cancer (squamous), metastatic: IV: 800 mg on days 1 and 8 of each 3-week treatment cycle (in combination with gemcitabine and cisplatin); continue until disease progression or unacceptable toxicity (Thatcher 2015).

In the study, gemcitabine and cisplatin were administered for a maximum of 6 cycles, while patients without disease progression continued necitumumab as single agent therapy (Thatcher 2015).

Renal Impairment There are no dosage adjustments provided in the manufacturer's labeling; however, based on pharmacokinetics, dosage adjustment is not likely necessary.

Hepatic Impairment

Mild to moderate impairment: There are no dosage adjustments provided in the manufacturer's labeling; however, based on pharmacokinetics, dosage adjustment is not likely necessary.

Severe impairment: There is no dosage adjustment provided in the manufacturer's labeling (has not been studied).

Adjustment for Toxicity

Dermatologic toxicity:

Grade 3 rash or acneiform rash: Withhold treatment until symptoms resolve to grade 2 or lower, then resume necitumumab with the dose reduced to 400 mg for at least 1 treatment cycle. If symptoms do not worsen, may increase the dose to 600 mg and then 800 mg in subsequent cycles.

Grade 3 rash or acneiform rash that does not resolve to grade 2 or lower within 6 weeks: Permanently discontinue.

Grade 3 rash or acneiform rash that worsens or is intolerable at the 400 mg dose: Permanently discontinue.

Grade 3 skin induration/fibrosis: Permanently discontinue.

Grade 4 dermatologic toxicity: Permanently discontinue.

Electrolyte abnormality: Grade 3 or 4 electrolyte abnormality: Withhold treatment; may resume when electrolyte abnormality has improved to grade 2 or lower (replete electrolytes as appropriate).

Infusion-related reactions:

Grade 1: Reduce infusion rate by 50%.

Grade 2: Interrupt infusion until signs/symptoms have resolved to grade 1 or 0, then resume with the rate reduced by 50% for all subsequent infusions.

Grade 3 or 4: Permanently discontinue.

Thromboembolic events: Serious or life-threatening VTE or ATE: Discontinue treatment.

Combination Regimens

Lung cancer (non-small cell): Cisplatin-Gemcitabine-Necitumumab (NSCLC) on page 2053

Administration

IV: Infuse over 60 minutes using an infusion pump. Infuse through a separate line. Flush with sodium chloride 0.9% at the end of infusion. Do not infuse with other medications or with electrolytes. Monitor for infusion reactions; reduce infusion rate by 50% for grade 1 infusion reaction; interrupt infusion for grade 2 infusion reaction.

Necitumumab should be administered prior to gemcitabine and cisplatin (Thatcher 2015).

Emetic Potential Low (10% to 30%)

Monitoring Parameters Serum electrolytes, including magnesium, potassium, and calcium (prior to each dose during treatment and for at least 8 weeks following completion). Signs/symptoms of infusion-related reactions, dermatologic toxicity, and thromboembolism.

Dosage Forms Considerations Portrazza is produced in genetically engineered mammalian NS0 cells.

Dosage Forms Excipient information presented when available (limited, particularly for generics); consult specific product labeling.

Solution, Intravenous [preservative free]:

Portrazza: 800 mg/50 mL (50 mL) [contains polysorbate 80]

Nelarabine (nel AY re been)

Related Information

Common Toxicity Criteria *on page 2242*

Management of Chemotherapy-Induced Nausea and Vomiting in Adults *on page 2253*

Prevention of Chemotherapy-Induced Nausea and Vomiting in Children *on page 2310*

Safe Handling of Hazardous Drugs *on page 2379*

Brand Names: US Arranon

Brand Names: Canada Atriance

Index Terms 2-Amino-6-Methoxypurine Arabinoside; 506U78; GW506U78

Pharmacologic Category Antineoplastic Agent, Antimetabolite; Antineoplastic Agent, Antimetabolite (Purine Analog)

Use T-cell acute lymphoblastic leukemia/lymphoma: Treatment of relapsed or refractory T-cell acute lymphoblastic leukemia/lymphoma following at least 2 chemotherapy regimens.

Labeled Contraindications

There are no contraindications listed in the US labeling.

Canadian labeling: Hypersensitivity to nelarabine or any component of the formulation.

Pregnancy Considerations Adverse effects were observed in animal reproduction studies and nelarabine may cause fetal harm if administered during pregnancy. Women of childbearing potential should be advised to use effective contraception and avoid becoming pregnant during therapy.

The European Society for Medical Oncology has published guidelines for diagnosis, treatment, and follow-up of cancer during pregnancy. The guidelines recommend referral to a facility with expertise in cancer during pregnancy and encourage a multidisciplinary team (obstetrician, neonatologist, oncology team). In general, if chemotherapy is indicated, it should be avoided during the first trimester, there should be a 3-week time period between the last chemotherapy dose and anticipated delivery, and chemotherapy should not be administered beyond week 33 of gestation. Specific use of nelarabine is not discussed (Peccatori 2013).

Breastfeeding Considerations It is not known if nelarabine or ara-G are excreted in breast milk. Due to the potential for serious adverse reactions in the nursing infant, the manufacturer recommends a decision be made whether to discontinue nursing or to discontinue the drug taking into account the importance of treatment to the mother.

Warnings/Precautions **[US Boxed Warning]: Severe neurotoxicities, including mental status changes, severe somnolence, seizures, and peripheral neuropathy (ranging from numbness and paresthesias to**

motor weakness and paralysis), have been reported. Observe closely for signs and symptoms of neurotoxicity; discontinue if ≥ grade 2. Adverse reactions associated with demyelination and ascending peripheral neuropathies similar to Guillain-Barré syndrome have also been reported. Neurologic toxicities may not fully return to baseline after treatment cessation. Neurologic toxicity is dose-limiting. Risk of neurotoxicity may increase in patients with concurrent or previous intrathecal chemotherapy or history of craniospinal irradiation. Fatal neurological outcomes have been reported following concurrent use of nelarabine with intrathecal chemotherapy. The Canadian labeling does not recommend concurrent use with intrathecal therapy and/or craniospinal radiation. Tumor lysis syndrome (TLS) may occur as a consequence of leukemia treatment. May lead to life threatening acute renal failure; adequate hydration and prophylactic allopurinol should be instituted prior to treatment to prevent hyperuricemia and TLS; monitor closely. Bone marrow suppression, including leukopenia, thrombocytopenia, anemia, neutropenia and febrile neutropenia are associated with treatment; monitor blood counts regularly. Use caution in patients with renal impairment; ara-G clearance may be reduced with renal dysfunction. Use caution with severe hepatic impairment; risk of adverse reactions may be higher with severe hepatic dysfunction. Avoid administration of live vaccines. Potentially significant drug-drug interactions may exist, requiring dose or frequency adjustment, additional monitoring, and/or selection of alternative therapy.

Adverse Reactions Pediatric adverse reactions fell within a range similar to adults except where noted.

>10%:

Cardiovascular: Peripheral edema (15%), edema (11%)

Central nervous system: Fatigue (50%), drowsiness (7% to 23%), dizziness (21%), peripheral neuropathy (12% to 21%; grades 2/3: 11% to 14%; may be similar to Guillain-Barré syndrome), headache (15% to 17%), hypoesthesia (6% to 17%), paresthesia (4% to 15%), pain (1% to 11%; includes neuropathic pain)

Endocrine & metabolic: Hypokalemia (11%)

Gastrointestinal: Nausea (41%), diarrhea (22%), vomiting (10% to 22%), constipation (21%)

Hematologic & oncologic: Anemia (95% to 99%, grade 4: 10% to 14%), neutropenia (81% to 94%; grade 4: children 62%, adults 49%), thrombocytopenia (86% to 88%; grade 4: 22% to 32%), leukopenia (38%; grade 4: 7%), febrile neutropenia (12%; grade 4: 1%), petechia (12%)

Hepatic: Increased serum transaminases (12%)

Neuromuscular & skeletal: Weakness (6% to 17%), myalgia (13%)

Respiratory: Cough (25%), dyspnea (7% to 20%)

Miscellaneous: Fever (23%)

1% to 10%:

Cardiovascular: Hypotension (8%), sinus tachycardia (8%), chest pain (5%)

Central nervous system: Ataxia (1% to 9%), confusion (8%), myasthenia (8%), rigors (8%), insomnia (7%), abnormal gait (6%), depression (6%), impaired consciousness (6%), noncardiac chest pain (5%), motor dysfunction (4%), amnesia (3%), equilibrium disturbance (2%), sensory disturbance (1% to 2%), disturbance in attention (1%), dysarthria (1%), hydrocephalus (1%), hypertonia (1%), hyporeflexia (1%), lethargy (1%), mental status changes (1%), nerve palsy (1%), paralysis (1%; including nerve paralysis), sciatica (1%), speech disturbance (1%), aphasia, brain disease, cerebral hemorrhage, coma, hemiparesis, intracranial hemorrhage, leukoencephalopathy, loss of consciousness, seizure

Endocrine & metabolic: Decreased serum albumin (10%), hypocalcemia (8%), dehydration (7%), hyperglycemia (6%), hypoglycemia (6%), hypomagnesemia (6%)

Gastrointestinal: Abdominal pain (9%), anorexia (9%), stomatitis (8%), abdominal distention (6%), dysgeusia (3%)

Hepatic: Increased serum bilirubin (10%), increased serum AST (6%)

Infection: Infection (5% to 9%)

Neuromuscular & skeletal: Arthralgia (9%), back pain (8%), limb pain (7%), tremor (4% to 5%)

Ophthalmic: Blurred vision (4%), nystagmus (1%)

Renal: Increased serum creatinine (6%)

Respiratory: Pleural effusion (10%), epistaxis (8%), pneumonia (8%), sinusitis (7%), wheezing (5%), sinus headache (1%)

<1%, postmarketing, and/or case reports: Demyelinating disease (craniospinal demyelination), increased creatine phosphokinase, opportunistic infection, pneumothorax, progressive multifocal leukoencephalopathy, rhabdomyolysis, tumor lysis syndrome

Drug Interactions

Metabolism/Transport Effects None known.

Avoid Concomitant Use

Avoid concomitant use of Nelarabine with any of the following: BCG (Intravesical); Deferiprone; Dipyrone; Natalizumab; Pentostatin; Pimecrolimus; Tacrolimus (Topical); Vaccines (Live)

Increased Effect/Toxicity

Nelarabine may increase the levels/effects of: CloZAPine; Deferiprone; Fingolimod; Leflunomide; Natalizumab; Tofacitinib; Vaccines (Live)

The levels/effects of Nelarabine may be increased by: Denosumab; Dipyrone; Ocrelizumab; Palifermin; Pimecrolimus; Promazine; Roflumilast; Tacrolimus (Topical); Trastuzumab

Decreased Effect

Nelarabine may decrease the levels/effects of: BCG (Intravesical); Coccidioides immitis Skin Test; Lenograstim; Nivolumab; Sipuleucel-T; Tertomotide; Vaccines (Inactivated); Vaccines (Live)

The levels/effects of Nelarabine may be decreased by: Echinacea; Pentostatin

Hazardous Drugs Handling Considerations

Hazardous agent (NIOSH 2016 [group 1]).

Use appropriate precautions for receiving, handling, administration, and disposal. Gloves (single) should be worn during receiving, unpacking, and placing in storage.

NIOSH recommends double gloving, a protective gown, ventilated engineering controls (a class II biological safety cabinet or a compounding aseptic containment isolator), and closed system transfer devices (CSTDs) for preparation. Double gloving, a gown, and (if dosage form allows) CSTDs are required during administration (NIOSH 2016).

Storage/Stability Store unopened vials at 25°C (77°F); excursions permitted to 15°C to 30°C (59°F to 86°F). Stable in plastic (PVC) or glass containers for up to 8 hours at room temperature.

Preparation for Administration Reconstitution is not required; do not dilute; the appropriate dose should be added to empty plastic (PVC) bag or glass container.

Mechanism of Action Nelarabine, a prodrug of ara-G, is demethylated by adenosine deaminase to ara-G and then converted to ara-GTP. Ara-GTP is incorporated into the DNA of the leukemic blasts, leading to inhibition of DNA synthesis and inducing apoptosis. Ara-GTP appears to accumulate at higher levels in T-cells, which correlates to clinical response.

Pharmacodynamics/Kinetics

Distribution: V_{ss}:

Nelarabine: Pediatric patients: 213 ± 358 L/m^2; Adults: 197 ± 216 L/m^2

Ara-G: Pediatric patients: 33 ± 9.3 L/m^2; Adults: 50 ± 24 L/m^2

Protein binding: Nelarabine and Ara-G: <25%

Metabolism: Hepatic; demethylated by adenosine deaminase to form ara-G (active); also hydrolyzed to form methylguanine. Both ara-G and methyl-guanine metabolized to guanine. Guanine is deaminated into xanthine, which is further oxidized to form uric acid, which is then oxidized to form allantoin.

Half-life elimination: Pediatric patients: Nelarabine: 13 minutes, Ara-G: 2 hours; Adults: Nelarabine: 18 minutes, Ara-G: 3 hours

Time to peak: Ara-G: Adults: 3 to 25 hours (of day 1)

Excretion: Urine (nelarabine 5% to 10%, Ara-G 20% to 30%)

Clearance: Nelarabine clearance is ~30% higher in pediatric patients (259 ± 409 L/hour/m^2) than in adults (197 ± 189 L/hour/m^2); Ara-G clearance in pediatric patients (11.3 ± 4.2 L/hour/m^2) is similar to adults (10.5 ± 4.5 L/hour/m^2)

Dosing

Adult & Geriatric T-cell acute lymphoblastic leukemia/lymphoma: IV: 1,500 mg/m^2/dose on days 1, 3, and 5; repeat every 21 days until a transplant candidate, disease progression, or unacceptable toxicity.

Pediatric T-cell acute lymphoblastic leukemia/lymphoma: IV: 650 mg/m^2/dose on days 1 through 5; repeat every 21 days until a transplant candidate, disease progression, or unacceptable toxicity.

Renal Impairment

CrCl ≥50 mL/minute: No dosage adjustment necessary.

CrCl <50 mL/minute: There are no dosage adjustments provided in the manufacturer's labeling, (although ARA-G clearance is decreased as renal function declines, data is insufficient for a dosing recommendation); monitor closely.

Hepatic Impairment There are no dosage adjustments provided in the manufacturer's labeling (has not been studied); closely monitor with severe impairment (total bilirubin >3 times ULN).

Adjustment for Toxicity

Neurologic toxicity ≥ grade 2: Discontinue treatment.

Hematologic or other (non-neurologic) toxicity: Consider treatment delay.

Administration Adequate IV hydration recommended to prevent tumor lysis syndrome; allopurinol may be used if hyperuricemia is anticipated.

IV:

Children: Infuse over 1 hour daily for 5 consecutive days

Adults: Infuse over 2 hours on days 1, 3, and 5

Emetic Potential Children and Adults: Minimal (<10%)

◄ **Monitoring Parameters** CBC with differential, liver and kidney function; monitor closely for neurologic toxicity (severe somnolence, seizure, peripheral neuropathy, confusion, ataxia, paresthesia, hypoesthesia, coma, or craniospinal demyelination); signs and symptoms of tumor lysis syndrome; hydration status

Dosage Forms Excipient information presented when available (limited, particularly for generics); consult specific product labeling.
Solution, Intravenous:
  Arranon: 5 mg/mL (50 mL)

Dosage Forms: Canada Information with regard to form, strength, and availability of products uniquely available in Canada but currently not available in the US. Refer also to Dosage Forms.

Excipient information presented when available (limited, particularly for generics); consult specific product labeling.
Injection, solution:
  Atriance: 5 mg/mL (50 mL)

◆ **Neoral** see CycloSPORINE (Systemic) on page 452
◆ **Neosar** see Cyclophosphamide on page 438
◆ **NEPA** see Netupitant and Palonosetron on page 1311

Neratinib (ne RA ti nib)

Related Information

Common Toxicity Criteria on page 2242
Management of EGFR Inhibitor Toxicities: Dermatologic, Ocular, and Gastrointestinal on page 2291
Safe Handling of Hazardous Drugs on page 2379

Brand Names: US Nerlynx

Index Terms HKI-272

Pharmacologic Category Antineoplastic Agent, Anti-HER2; Antineoplastic Agent, Epidermal Growth Factor Receptor (EGFR) Inhibitor; Antineoplastic Agent, Tyrosine Kinase Inhibitor

Use Breast cancer: Extended adjuvant treatment of early stage human epidermal growth receptor type 2 (HER2) overexpressed/amplified breast cancer (following adjuvant trastuzumab-based therapy).

Labeled Contraindications There are no contraindications listed in the manufacturer's labeling.

Pregnancy Considerations Based on the mechanism of action and data from animal reproduction studies, use of neratinib in pregnancy may cause fetal harm. Women of reproductive potential should have a pregnancy test prior to treatment; effective contraception should be used during therapy and for at least 1 month after the last dose. Male patients with female partners of reproductive potential should also use effective contraception during therapy and for at least 3 months after the last dose.

Breastfeeding Considerations It is not known if neratinib is present in breast milk. According to the manufacturer, breastfeeding is not recommended during therapy or for at least 1 month after the last dose.

Warnings/Precautions Severe diarrhea, which may result in dehydration, hypotension, and renal failure has been observed commonly with neratinib treatment. Almost all patients receiving neratinib in a clinical trial experienced diarrhea; the majority developed diarrhea during the first month of treatment.

The median time to onset of grade 3 or higher diarrhea was 8 days (range: 1 day to 350 days); the median cumulative duration of toxicity was 5 days (range: 1 day to 139 days). Antidiarrheal prophylaxis with loperamide has been shown to lower the incidence and severity of diarrhea and is recommended during the first 2 cycles of therapy (begin with the first dose of neratinib). Monitor closely for diarrhea and subsequent complications; additional antidiarrheals may be necessary. Administer fluid and electrolytes as needed; stool cultures may be needed to exclude infectious etiologies for diarrhea. Diarrhea may require therapy interruption and dosage reductions and/or discontinuation. Nausea, vomiting, abdominal pain, and stomatitis have also been reported.

Hepatotoxicity characterized by elevated liver enzymes has been reported with neratinib therapy. ALT and AST elevations have been observed, and have led to treatment discontinuation is some patients. Monitor liver function tests (ALT, AST, total bilirubin, and alkaline phosphatase) prior to treatment initiation, monthly for the first 3 months, then every 3 months thereafter and as clinically indicated. Assess liver function tests in patients with grade 3 or higher diarrhea or in those with signs/symptoms of hepatotoxicity (worsening fatigue, nausea, vomiting, right upper quadrant tenderness, fever, rash, or eosinophilia). May require therapy interruption, dose reduction, or permanent discontinuation. Use with caution in patients with hepatic impairment; neratinib clearance may be reduced in patients with severe hepatic dysfunction. Dose reduction is required in patients with preexisting severe (Child-Pugh class C) hepatic impairment.

Potentially significant interactions may exist, requiring dose or frequency adjustment, additional monitoring, and/or selection of alternative therapy. Concomitant use of neratinib with drugs that affect gastric pH may result in decreased neratinib exposure and reduced efficacy; avoid concomitant use with proton pump inhibitors and H_2-receptor antagonists. If antacid administration is necessary, administer neratinib 3 hours after the antacid. The incidence of serious adverse reactions and treatment discontinuation was higher in patients 65 years and older (compared to patients younger than 65 years) in a clinical trial. The most commonly reported serious adverse reactions in elderly patients included vomiting, diarrhea, renal failure, and dehydration.

Adverse Reactions

>10%:
  Central nervous system: Fatigue (27%)
  Dermatologic: Skin rash (18%)
  Gastrointestinal: Diarrhea (95%), nausea (43%), abdominal pain (36%), vomiting (26%), stomatitis (14%), decreased appetite (12%)
  Neuromuscular & skeletal: Muscle spasm (11%)
1% to 10%:
  Dermatologic: Nail disease (8%), xeroderma (6%), skin fissure (2%)
  Endocrine & metabolic: Weight loss (5%), dehydration (4%)
  Gastrointestinal: Dyspepsia (10%), abdominal distension (5%), xerostomia (3%)
  Genitourinary: Urinary tract infection (5%)
  Hepatic: Increased serum ALT (9% to 10%), increased serum AST (5% to 7%)
  Respiratory: Epistaxis (5%)

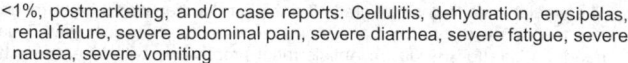

<1%, postmarketing, and/or case reports: Cellulitis, dehydration, erysipelas, renal failure, severe abdominal pain, severe diarrhea, severe fatigue, severe nausea, severe vomiting

Drug Interactions

    Metabolism/Transport Effects Substrate of CYP3A4 (major); **Note:** Assignment of Major/Minor substrate status based on clinically relevant drug interaction potential; **Inhibits** P-glycoprotein

    Avoid Concomitant Use

    Avoid concomitant use of Neratinib with any of the following: Cimetidine; Conivaptan; CYP3A4 Inducers (Moderate); CYP3A4 Inducers (Strong); CYP3A4 Inhibitors (Moderate); CYP3A4 Inhibitors (Strong); Fusidic Acid (Systemic); H2-Antagonists; Idelalisib; PAZOPanib; Proton Pump Inhibitors; Silodosin; Topotecan; VinCRIStine (Liposomal)

    Increased Effect/Toxicity

    Neratinib may increase the levels/effects of: Afatinib; Betrixaban; Bilastine; Brentuximab Vedotin; Celiprolol; Colchicine; Dabigatran Etexilate; Digoxin; DOXOrubicin (Conventional); Edoxaban; Everolimus; Naldemedine; Naloxegol; PAZOPanib; P-glycoprotein/ABCB1 Substrates; Prucalopride; Ranolazine; RifAXIMin; Silodosin; Topotecan; Venetoclax; VinCRIStine (Liposomal)

    The levels/effects of Neratinib may be increased by: Cimetidine; Ciprofloxacin (Systemic); Clotrimazole (Oral); Conivaptan; CycloSPORINE (Systemic); CYP3A4 Inhibitors (Moderate); CYP3A4 Inhibitors (Strong); Dasatinib; FluvoxaMINE; Fosaprepitant; Fusidic Acid (Systemic); Idelalisib; Palbociclib; Simeprevir; Stiripentol; Tofisopam

    Decreased Effect

    The levels/effects of Neratinib may be decreased by: Antacids; Cimetidine; CYP3A4 Inducers (Moderate); CYP3A4 Inducers (Strong); Deferasirox; H2-Antagonists; Proton Pump Inhibitors; Sarilumab; Siltuximab; Tocilizumab

Food Interactions

    Grapefruit juice may increase neratinib exposure. Management: Avoid grapefruit juice.

    Maintain adequate hydration.

Hazardous Drugs Handling Considerations

    Hazardous agent (meets NIOSH 2016 criteria). This medication is not on the NIOSH (2016) list; however, it meets the criteria for a hazardous drug. Drugs are classified as hazardous based on their properties; the properties of a hazardous drug include one or more of the following characteristics: carcinogenic, teratogenic (or other developmental toxicity), reproductive toxicity, organotoxic at low doses, genotoxic, and/or new agents with structural or toxicity profiles similar to existing hazardous agents.

    Use appropriate precautions for receiving, handling, administration, and disposal. Gloves (single) should be worn during receiving, unpacking, and placing in storage. NIOSH recommends single gloving for administration of intact tablets or capsules (NIOSH 2016).

Storage/Stability Store at 20°C to 25°C (68°F to 77°F); excursions permitted between 15°C and 30°C (59°F and 86°F).

Mechanism of Action Neratinib is an irreversible tyrosine kinase inhibitor of human growth factor receptor 1, 2, and 4 (HER1, HER2, and HER 4) (Chan 2016), as well as epidermal growth factor receptor (EGFR). Neratinib reduces EGFR and HER2 autophosphorylation and downstream MAPK and AKT signaling pathways and demonstrates antitumor activity in EGFR and/or HER2 expressing cancer cell lines.

Pharmacodynamics/Kinetics

Absorption: A high-fat meal increases neratinib C_{max} and AUC_{inf} by 1.7- and 2.2-fold, respectively. A standard breakfast increased neratinib C_{max} by 1.2-fold and AUC_{inf} by 1.1-fold.

Distribution: V_{ss}/F: 6,433 L

Protein binding: >99% to serum albumin and alpha-1 acid glycoprotein

Metabolism: Primarily hepatic via CYP3A4 (major) and flavin-containing monooxygenase (minor) to active metabolites M3, M6, M7, and M1

Half-life elimination: 7 to 17 hours

Time to peak: 2 to 8 hours (parent drug and active metabolites M3, M6, and M7)

Excretion: Feces (~97%); urine (~1%)

Dosing

Adult & Geriatric Note: Antidiarrheal prophylaxis is recommended during the first 2 cycles of therapy; initiate with the first neratinib dose (see Premedications below)

Breast cancer (HER2-positive), extended adjuvant therapy: Oral: 240 mg once daily for 1 year (Chan 2016)

Missed dose: If a dose is missed, resume therapy with the next scheduled daily dose; do not replace the missed dose.

Premedication: Antidiarrheal prophylaxis is recommended during the first 2 cycles of therapy; initiate with the first neratinib dose. Titrate to 1 to 2 bowel movements/day. Additional antidiarrheal medication may be required for loperamide-refractory diarrhea.

Days 1 to 14: Loperamide 4 mg orally 3 times daily

Days 15 to 56: Loperamide 4 mg orally twice daily

Days 57 to 365: Loperamide 4 mg as needed (maximum: 16 mg/day)

Renal Impairment There are no dosage adjustments provided in the manufacturer's labeling; however, renal function does not have a clinically significant effect on neratinib pharmacokinetics.

Hepatic Impairment

Preexisting hepatic impairment:

Mild to moderate (Child-Pugh class A or B) impairment: No dosage adjustment is necessary.

Severe (Child-Pugh class C) impairment: Reduce initial dose to 80 mg once daily.

Hepatotoxicity during treatment:

ALT >5 to 20 times ULN (grade 3) or bilirubin >3 to 10 times ULN (grade 3): Interrupt neratinib until recovery to ≤ grade 1 (evaluate for alternative hepatotoxic causes); resume therapy at the next lower dose level (see Dosing: Adjustment for Toxicity) if recovery to ≤ grade 1 occurs within 3 weeks.

Recurrent grade 3 ALT or bilirubin elevation despite one dose reduction: Discontinue permanently.

ALT >20 times ULN (grade 4) or bilirubin >10 times ULN (grade 4): Permanently discontinue and evaluate for alternative hepatotoxic causes.

Adjustment for Toxicity Discontinue neratinib if toxicity does not recover to ≤ grade 1, for toxicities that result in a treatment delay of more than 3 weeks, or in patients unable to tolerate the 120 mg once daily dose.

Recommended neratinib dose reductions for toxicity:

First dose reduction: 200 mg once daily

Second dose reduction: 160 mg once daily

Third dose reduction: 120 mg once daily

Diarrhea:

Grade 1: Increase of <4 stools/day over baseline

Grade 2: Increase of 4 to 6 stools/day over baseline

Grade 3: Increase of ≥7 stools/day over baseline; incontinence; hospitalization indicated; limiting self-care activities of daily living

Grade 4: Life-threatening consequences; urgent intervention necessary

Grade 1, grade 2 (lasting <5 days), or grade 3 diarrhea (lasting <2 days): Adjust antidiarrheal medication and diet; maintain fluid intake of ~2 L. When diarrhea has improved to ≤ grade 1 or baseline, initiate loperamide 4 mg with each subsequent neratinib dose.

Grade 2 diarrhea lasting ≥5 days or grade 3 diarrhea lasting longer than 2 days (despite optimal antidiarrheal management), or any grade diarrhea with complicating features (eg, dehydration, fever, hypotension, renal failure, or grade 3/4 neutropenia): Interrupt treatment. Modify diet; maintain fluid intake of ~2 L. If diarrhea improves to ≤ grade 1 in 1 week or less, resume neratinib at the same dose. If diarrhea improves to ≤ grade 1 in more than 1 week, resume neratinib at the next lower dose. When diarrhea has improved to ≤ grade 1 or baseline, initiate loperamide 4 mg with each subsequent neratinib dose.

Recurrent ≥ grade 2 diarrhea (occurring at 120 mg once daily dose): Permanently discontinue neratinib.

Grade 4 diarrhea (life-threatening consequences; urgent intervention necessary): Permanently discontinue neratinib.

Other toxicities:

Grade 3: Interrupt treatment until toxicity improves to ≤ grade 1 or baseline within 3 weeks of stopping neratinib. Upon recovery, resume neratinib at the next lower dose.

Grade 4: Permanently discontinue neratinib.

Administration Administer orally once daily with food at approximately the same time each day. Swallow tablets whole; do not crush, chew or split tablets. Antidiarrheal prophylaxis is recommended during the first 2 cycles (see Dosing). Avoid concomitant use with proton pump inhibitors and H_2-receptor antagonists; if antacids are necessary, administer neratinib 3 hours after antacids.

Monitoring Parameters Liver function tests (ALT, AST, bilirubin, and alkaline phosphatase) prior to treatment initiation, monthly for the first 3 months, then every 3 months thereafter or as clinically indicated; fractionated bilirubin and prothrombin time if clinically necessary; pregnancy test prior to therapy initiation in women of reproductive potential; monitor for diarrhea and signs/symptoms of dehydration and hepatotoxicity (eg, worsening fatigue, nausea, vomiting, right upper quadrant pain, fever, rash, or eosinophilia). Monitor adherence.

Product Availability Nerlynx: FDA approved July 2017; anticipated availability is September 2017

Prescribing and Access Restrictions Neratinib is available through select specialty pharmacies. Refer to http://www.nerlynx.com for further information.

Dosage Forms Excipient information presented when available (limited, particularly for generics); consult specific product labeling.

Tablet, Oral:

Nerlynx: 40 mg

◆ **Nerlynx** *see* Neratinib *on page 1306*

◆ **NESP** *see* Darbepoetin Alfa *on page 515*

◆ **Netspot** *see* Gallium Ga 68 Dotatate *on page 854*

Netupitant and Palonosetron (net UE pi tant & pal oh NOE se tron)

Related Information

Management of Chemotherapy-Induced Nausea and Vomiting in Adults *on page 2253*

Brand Names: US Akynzeo

Index Terms NEPA; Netupitant/Palonosetron HCl; Palonosetron and Netupitant; Palonosetron Hydrochloride and Netupitant

Pharmacologic Category Antiemetic; Selective 5-HT$_3$ Receptor Antagonist; Substance P/Neurokinin 1 Receptor Antagonist

Use Chemotherapy-induced nausea and vomiting: Prevention of acute and delayed nausea and vomiting associated with initial and repeat courses of cancer chemotherapy, including, but not limited to, highly emetogenic chemotherapy.

Labeled Contraindications There are no contraindications listed in the manufacturer's labeling.

Pregnancy Considerations Adverse events were observed in some animal reproduction studies using the components of this combination product.

Breastfeeding Considerations It is not known if netupitant or palonosetron are excreted in breast milk. Due to the potential for serious adverse reactions in the nursing infant, the manufacturer recommends a decision be made whether to discontinue nursing or to discontinue the drug, taking into account the importance of treatment to the mother.

Warnings/Precautions Serotonin syndrome has been reported with 5-HT$_3$ receptor antagonists, predominantly when used in combination with other serotonergic agents (eg, SSRIs, SNRIs, MAOIs, mirtazapine, fentanyl, lithium, tramadol, and methylene blue). Some of the cases have been fatal. The majority of serotonin syndrome reports with 5-HT$_3$ receptor antagonists occurred in a postanesthesia setting or in an infusion center. Serotonin syndrome has also been reported following overdose of another 5-HT$_3$ receptor antagonist. Monitor patients for signs of serotonin syndrome, including mental status changes (eg, agitation, hallucinations, delirium, coma); autonomic instability (eg, tachycardia, labile blood pressure, diaphoresis, dizziness, flushing, hyperthermia); neuromuscular changes (eg, tremor, rigidity, myoclonus, hyperreflexia, incoordination); gastrointestinal symptoms (eg, nausea, vomiting, diarrhea); and/or seizures. If serotonin syndrome occurs, discontinue 5-HT$_3$ receptor antagonist treatment and begin supportive management.

Hypersensitivity (including anaphylaxis) has been reported with or without known hypersensitivity to other 5-HT$_3$ receptor antagonists. Avoid use in severe hepatic impairment; dosage adjustment not necessary in mild or moderate impairment. Avoid use in severe renal impairment or end stage renal disease; dosage adjustment not necessary in mild or moderate impairment. Potentially significant drug-drug interactions may exist, requiring dose or frequency adjustment, additional monitoring, and/or selection of alternative therapy. Use caution when dosing elderly patients due to a higher frequency of decreased hepatic, renal, cardiac function, and concomitant disease or drug therapy.

Adverse Reactions

1% to 10%:

Central nervous system: Headache (9%), fatigue (4% to 7%)

Dermatologic: Erythema (3%)

Gastrointestinal: Dyspepsia (4%), constipation (3%)

Neuromuscular & skeletal: Weakness (8%)

Drug Interactions

Metabolism/Transport Effects Refer to individual components.

Avoid Concomitant Use

Avoid concomitant use of Netupitant and Palonosetron with any of the following: Apomorphine; Aprepitant; Asunaprevir; Bosutinib; Budesonide (Systemic); Cobimetinib; CYP3A4 Inducers (Strong); Domperidone; Flibanserin; Ivabradine; Lomitapide; Naloxegol; Neratinib; Olaparib; Pimozide; Simeprevir; Tolvaptan; Trabectedin; Ulipristal

Increased Effect/Toxicity

Netupitant and Palonosetron may increase the levels/effects of: AmLODIPine; Apixaban; Apomorphine; Aprepitant; ARIPiprazole; Asunaprevir; Avanafil; Blonanserin; Bosentan; Bosutinib; Brexpiprazole; Bromocriptine; Budesonide (Systemic); Budesonide (Topical); Cannabis; Cilostazol; Cobimetinib; Colchicine; CYP3A4 Substrates; Dapoxetine; Deflazacort; Dexamethasone (Systemic); Dofetilide; Domperidone; DOXOrubicin (Conventional); Dronabinol; Eletriptan; Eliglustat; Eplerenone; Everolimus; FentaNYL; Flibanserin; GuanFACINE; Halofantrine; HYDROcodone; HydrOXYzine; Ibrutinib; Imatinib; Ivabradine; Ivacaftor; Lomitapide; Lurasidone; Manidipine; Mirodenafil; Naldemedine; Naloxegol; Neratinib; NiMODipine; Olaparib; OxyCODONE; Pimecrolimus; Pimozide; Propafenone; Ranolazine; Rupatadine; Salmeterol; SAXagliptin; Serotonin Modulators; Sildenafil; Simeprevir; Sonidegib; Suvorexant; Telithromycin; Tetrahydrocannabinol; Ticagrelor; Tolvaptan; Trabectedin; Udenafil; Ulipristal; Venetoclax; Vilazodone; Vindesine; Zopiclone; Zuclopenthixol

Decreased Effect

Netupitant and Palonosetron may decrease the levels/effects of: Ifosfamide; Tapentadol; TraMADol

The levels/effects of Netupitant and Palonosetron may be decreased by: Bosentan; CYP3A4 Inducers (Moderate); CYP3A4 Inducers (Strong); Dabrafenib; Deferasirox; Sarilumab; Siltuximab; St John's Wort; Tocilizumab

Storage/Stability Store at 20°C to 25°C (68°F to 77°F); excursions are permitted between 15°C and 30°C (59°F and 86°F)

Mechanism of Action Netupitant is a selective substance P/neurokinin (NK_1) receptor antagonist, which augments the antiemetic activity of $5-HT_3$ receptor antagonists and corticosteroids to inhibit acute and delayed chemotherapy-induced emesis. Palonosetron is a selective $5-HT_3$ receptor antagonist, which blocks serotonin, both on vagal nerve terminals in the periphery and centrally in the chemoreceptor trigger zone. Palonosetron inhibits the cross-talk between the $5-HT_3$ and NK_1 receptors. The combination of palonosetron and netupitant works synergistically to inhibit substance P response to a greater extent than either agent alone (Aapro, 2014).

Pharmacodynamics/Kinetics

Netupitant:

Absorption: Within 15 minutes to 3 hours

Distribution: V_d: 1,982 ± 906 L

Protein binding: >99.5% for netupitant; >97% for major metabolites

Metabolism: Extensively hepatic via CYP3A4 (major), CYP2C9 (minor) and CYP2D6 (minor); forms active metabolites M1, M2, and M3

Half-life elimination: 80 ± 29 hours

Time to peak: ~5 hours

Excretion: Feces (~71%); urine (~4%)

Palonosetron:

Absorption: Well absorbed

Distribution: V_d: 8.3 ± 2.5 L/kg

Protein binding: ~62%

Metabolism: ~50% metabolized to relatively inactive metabolites (N-oxide-palonosetron and 6-S-hydroxy-palonosetron); CYP2D6, 3A4, and 1A2 contribute to metabolism

Half-life elimination: 48 ± 19 hours

Time to peak: ~5 hours

Excretion: Feces (5% to 8%); urine (85% to 93%; 40% as unchanged drug)

Dosing

Adult

Highly-emetogenic chemotherapy (including cisplatin-based): Oral: One capsule ~1 hour prior to initiation of chemotherapy on day 1 (Gralla 2014). **Note:** Antiemetic regimen also includes dexamethasone 12 mg orally ~30 minutes prior to initiation of chemotherapy on day 1, and 8 mg orally once daily on days 2 to 4.

Anthracycline and cyclophosphamide-based chemotherapy and chemotherapy not considered highly emetogenic: Oral: One capsule ~1 hour prior to initiation of chemotherapy on day 1 (Gralla 2014). **Note:** Antiemetic regimen also includes dexamethasone 12 mg orally ~30 minutes prior to chemotherapy on day 1.

Geriatric No dosage adjustment necessary. Refer to adult dosing.

Renal Impairment

Mild or moderate impairment: No dosage adjustment is necessary.

Severe impairment or ESRD: Avoid use.

Hepatic Impairment

Mild or moderate impairment (Child-Pugh score 5 to 8): No dosage adjustment is necessary.

Severe impairment (Child-Pugh score >9): Avoid use.

Administration Oral: May administer with or without food.

Dosage Forms Excipient information presented when available (limited, particularly for generics); consult specific product labeling.

Capsule, Oral:

Akynzeo: Netupitant 300 mg and palonosetron 0.5 mg

- ◆ **Netupitant/Palonosetron HCl** *see* Netupitant and Palonosetron *on page 1311*
- ◆ **Neulasta** *see* Pegfilgrastim *on page 1467*
- ◆ **Neulasta Onpro** *see* Pegfilgrastim *on page 1467*
- ◆ **Neulasta Onpro kit** *see* Pegfilgrastim *on page 1467*
- ◆ **Neupogen** *see* Filgrastim *on page 792*
- ◆ **NeutraSal** *see* Saliva Substitute *on page 1653*
- ◆ **NexAVAR** *see* SORAfenib *on page 1685*
- ◆ **Nexavar (Can)** *see* SORAfenib *on page 1685*
- ◆ **Niastase (Can)** *see* Factor VIIa (Recombinant) *on page 765*
- ◆ **Niastase RT (Can)** *see* Factor VIIa (Recombinant) *on page 765*
- ◆ **Niftolid** *see* Flutamide *on page 839*
- ◆ **Nilandron** *see* Nilutamide *on page 1321*

Nilotinib (nye LOE ti nib)

Related Information

Common Toxicity Criteria *on page 2242*

Management of Chemotherapy-Induced Nausea and Vomiting in Adults *on page 2253*

Safe Handling of Hazardous Drugs *on page 2379*

Brand Names: US Tasigna

Brand Names: Canada Tasigna

Index Terms AMN107; Nilotinib HCl; Nilotinib Hydrochloride Monohydrate

Pharmacologic Category Antineoplastic Agent, BCR-ABL Tyrosine Kinase Inhibitor; Antineoplastic Agent, Tyrosine Kinase Inhibitor

Use Chronic myelogenous leukemia:

Treatment of adults with newly diagnosed Philadelphia chromosome-positive chronic myelogenous leukemia (CML) in chronic phase.

Treatment of chronic- and accelerated-phase Philadelphia chromosome-positive CML in adults resistant or intolerant to prior therapy that included imatinib.

Labeled Contraindications

Hypokalemia, hypomagnesemia, or long QT syndrome

Canadian labeling: Additional contraindication (not in US labeling): Hypersensitivity to nilotinib or any component of the formulation; persistent QTc >480 msec

Pregnancy Considerations Adverse effects were observed in animal reproduction studies. May cause fetal harm if administered during pregnancy. Women of childbearing potential should be advised to use effective contraception during treatment.

Breastfeeding Considerations It is not known if nilotinib is excreted in breast milk. Due to the potential for serious adverse reactions in the nursing infant, the decision to discontinue breastfeeding during therapy or to discontinue nilotinib should take into account the benefits of treatment to the mother.

Warnings/Precautions [US Boxed Warnings]: May prolong the QT interval; sudden deaths have been reported. Use in patients with hypokalemia, hypomagnesemia, or long QT syndrome is contraindicated. Correct hypomagnesemia and hypokalemia prior to initiating therapy; monitor electrolytes periodically. Monitor ECG and QTc (baseline, at 7 days, with dose change, and periodically). Avoid the use of QT-prolonging agents. Avoid concurrent use with antiarrhythmics and other drugs which may prolong QT interval; may increase the risk of potentially-fatal arrhythmias. Sudden deaths appear to be related to dose-dependent ventricular repolarization abnormalities. Prolonged QT interval may result in torsade de pointes, which may cause syncope, seizure, and/or death. Patients with uncontrolled or significant cardiovascular disease were excluded from studies. **[US Boxed Warning]: Administer on an empty stomach, at least 1 hour before and 2 hours after food;** administration with food may prolong the QT$_c$. Nilotinib solubility is decreased at higher pH; concurrent use with proton pump inhibitors is not recommended. If necessary, H$_2$-receptor blockers may be administered ~10 hours before and 2 hours after a nilotinib dose. Antacids (eg, aluminum hydroxide, magnesium hydroxide, simethicone) may be administered ~2 hours before or 2 hours after nilotinib. Potentially significant drug-drug/drug-food interactions may exist, requiring dose or frequency adjustment, additional monitoring, and/or selection of alternative therapy. **[US Boxed Warning]: Avoid concurrent use with strong CYP3A4 inhibitors.**

Cardiovascular events such as ischemic heart disease-related events, arterial vascular occlusive events, peripheral arterial occlusive disease, and ischemic cerebrovascular accident have been reported. Use caution in patients with preexisting risk factors, and monitor for new or worsening symptoms suggestive of cardiovascular events. Fluid retention, including pleural and pericardial effusions, ascites, and pulmonary edema were reported; may be severe. Monitor closely for signs/symptoms of fluid retention (eg, rapid weight gain or swelling) and for symptoms of respiratory or cardiac distress (eg, shortness of breath). Evaluate promptly and manage as appropriate. In a clinical study comparing nilotinib and imatinib in the treatment of newly diagnosed Ph+ chronic phase CML, hemorrhagic events (eg, gastrointestinal hemorrhage, including grade 3 or 4 events) occurred more frequently in the nilotinib arm.

Dosage reduction is recommended in patients with hepatic impairment, along with close monitoring of the QT interval. Nilotinib metabolism is primarily hepatic (exposure is increased in patients with hepatic impairment). May cause hepatotoxicity, including dose-limiting elevations in bilirubin, transaminases, and alkaline phosphatase; monitor liver function. UGT1A1 polymorphisms may be a risk factor for increased toxicity (eg, hyperbilirubinemia) (Shibata, 2013).

Reversible myelosuppression, including grades 3 and 4 thrombocytopenia, neutropenia, and anemia may occur; may require dose reductions and/or treatment delay; monitor blood counts. Use with caution in patients with a history of pancreatitis; may cause dose-limiting elevations of serum lipase and amylase; monitor. In patients with abdominal symptoms in conjunction with lipase increases, withhold treatment and consider diagnostics to exclude pancreatitis. Tumor lysis syndrome (TLS) has been reported in patients with resistant or intolerant CML; the majority of cases had malignant disease progression, high WBC counts, and/or dehydration; maintain adequate hydration and treat high uric acid levels prior to nilotinib. Consider alternative therapy or a dosage increase (with more frequent monitoring) in patients with total gastrectomy (nilotinib exposure is reduced). Capsules contain lactose; do not use with galactose intolerance, severe lactase deficiency, or glucose-galactose malabsorption syndromes.

Adverse Reactions

>10%:

Cardiovascular: Peripheral edema (≤15%), hypertension (10% to 11%)

Central nervous system: Headache (20% to 35%), fatigue (21% to 32%), insomnia (7% to 12%), dizziness (≤12%)

Dermatologic: Skin rash (≤38%), pruritus (20% to 32%), night sweats (12% to 27%), alopecia (11% to 13%), xeroderma (>5% to 12%)

Endocrine & metabolic: Increased serum glucose (50%), hyperglycemia (≤50%), increased serum cholesterol (28%), hypophosphatemia (≥10%)

Gastrointestinal: Nausea (22% to 37%), vomiting (13% to 29%), diarrhea (19% to 28%), increased serum lipase (28%), constipation (19% to 26%), upper abdominal pain (12% to 18%), abdominal pain (15% to 16%), decreased appetite (including anorexia; 15% to 17%)

Hematologic & oncologic: Neutropenia (1% to 15%; grades 3/4: 12% to 42%; median duration: 15 days), thrombocytopenia (18%; grades 3/4: 10% to 42%; median duration: 22 days), anemia (8%; grades 3/4: 4% to 27%)

Hepatic: Hepatic: Increased serum ALT (10% to 72%), increased serum AST (10% to 47%), hyperbilirubinemia (≥10%)

Infection: Influenza (≤13%)

◄

Neuromuscular & skeletal: Arthralgia (16% to 26%), limb pain (15% to 20%), back pain (15% to 19%), myalgia (16% to 19%), weakness (14% to 16%), ostealgia (14% to 15%), muscle spasm (12% to 15%), musculoskeletal pain (11% to 12%)

Respiratory: Cough (17% to 27%), nasopharyngitis (≤27%), upper respiratory tract infection (≤17%), dyspnea (9% to 15%; exertional), oropharyngeal pain (≤12%), flu-like symptoms (11%)

Miscellaneous: Fever (14% to 28%)

1% to 10%:

Cardiovascular: Ischemic heart disease (5% to 9%), peripheral arterial disease (3% to 4%), cerebral ischemia (1% to 3%), pericardial effusion (≤2%), angina pectoris, cardiac arrhythmia (including AV block, atrial fibrillation, bradycardia, cardiac flutter, extrasystoles, and tachycardia), chest discomfort, chest pain (including noncardiac), flushing, palpitations, prolonged Q-T interval on ECG

Central nervous system: Anxiety, depression, flank pain, hypoesthesia, malaise, myasthenia, pain, paresthesia, peripheral neuropathy, vertigo, voice disorder

Dermatologic: Acne vulgaris, dermatitis (including allergic and acneiform), eczema, erythema, folliculitis, hyperhidrosis, urticaria

Endocrine & metabolic: Decreased serum albumin, diabetes mellitus, fluid retention, hypercalcemia, hypercholesterolemia, hyperkalemia, hyperlipidemia, hyperphosphatemia, hypertriglyceridemia, hypocalcemia, hypokalemia, hypomagnesemia, hyponatremia, increased gamma-glutamyl transferase, increased HDL cholesterol, increased VLDL, weight gain, weight loss

Gastrointestinal: Dyspepsia (4% to 10%), gastrointestinal hemorrhage (≤5%), abdominal distension, abdominal distress, dysgeusia, flatulence, increased serum amylase, pancreatitis

Genitourinary: Pollakiuria

Hematologic & oncologic: Bruise, cutaneous papilloma, decreased hemoglobin, eosinophilia, febrile neutropenia, hemophthalmos, hemorrhage, leukopenia, lymphocytopenia, pancytopenia

Hepatic: Ascites (≤2%), hepatic insufficiency, increased serum alkaline phosphatase

Immunologic: Change in serum protein (decreased globulins)

Neuromuscular & skeletal: Increased creatine phosphokinase, neck pain

Ophthalmic: Eyelid edema (1%), conjunctivitis, eye pruritus, periorbital edema, xerophthalmia

Respiratory: Pleural effusion (≤2%), pulmonary edema (≤2%), epistaxis

Frequency not defined:

Cardiovascular: Hypotension, occlusive arterial disease (basilar, peripheral), pericarditis, reduced ejection fraction, shock (hemorrhagic), thrombosis, ventricular dysfunction

Central nervous system: Amnesia, breast induration, cerebral edema, confusion, disorientation, dysesthesia, dysphoria, lethargy, restless leg syndrome

Dermatologic: Dermal ulcer, erythema multiforme, erythema nodosum, exfoliative dermatitis, furuncle, hyperkeratosis, palmar-plantar erythrodysesthesia, psoriasis, skin atrophy, skin blister, skin discoloration, skin hyperpigmentation, skin hypertrophy, skin photosensitivity, tinea pedis

Endocrine & metabolic: Altered hormone level (insulin C-peptide decreased), hypermenorrhea, hyperparathyroidism (secondary), hyperuricemia, hypoglycemia, thyroiditis

Gastrointestinal: Cholestasis, enterocolitis, gastric ulcer (perforation possible), gingivitis, hematemesis, hemorrhoids, hiatal hernia, intestinal obstruction, oral lesion (papilloma), rectal hemorrhage, ulcerative esophagitis

Genitourinary: Hematuria, urinary incontinence, urine discoloration

Hematologic & oncologic: Increased parathyroid hormone, leukocytosis, paraproteinemia, petechiae, retroperitoneal hemorrhage, thrombocythemia

Hepatic: Hepatomegaly

Hypersensitivity: Hypersensitivity

Infection: Abscess, reactivation of HBV, sepsis

Local: Local swelling (nipple), localized edema

Neuromuscular & Skeletal: Arthritis

Ophthalmic: Blepharitis, diplopia, eye pain, optic neuritis, papilledema, photophobia, retinopathy (central serous chorioretinopathy), swelling of eye

Otic: Auditory impairment, otalgia, tinnitus

Renal: Renal failure

Respiratory: Pulmonary hypertension, wheezing

Miscellaneous: Benign nodule (sebaceous hyperplasia), cyst (dermal), troponin increased

<1%, postmarketing, and/or case reports: Allergic skin reaction, arteriosclerosis, ascorbic acid deficiency (Oak 2016), blurred vision, bronchitis, candidiasis, cardiac failure, cardiomegaly, cerebral infarction, chills, conjunctival hemorrhage, coronary artery disease, cyanosis, decreased visual acuity, dehydration, dysuria, ecchymoses, erectile dysfunction, esophageal pain, exfoliation of skin, eye irritation, facial edema, gastritis, gastroenteritis, gastroesophageal reflux disease, gout, gynecomastia, heart murmur, hematoma, hepatitis, hepatotoxicity, herpes simplex infection, hyperemia (scleral, conjunctival, ocular), hyperesthesia, hypertensive crisis, hyperthyroidism, hypothyroidism, increased appetite, increased blood urea nitrogen, increased lactate dehydrogenase, increased serum creatinine, intermittent claudication, interstitial pulmonary disease, intracranial hemorrhage, jaundice, joint swelling, lack of concentration, local alterations in temperature sensations, local discomfort (sensitive teeth), loss of consciousness, mastalgia, melena, mesenteric artery occlusion, migraine, myocardial infarction, nocturia, nonhemorrhagic stroke, occlusive arterial disease (coronary), oral mucosa ulcer, pharyngolaryngeal pain, photopsia, pleurisy, pleuritic chest pain, pneumonia, sinusitis, skin pain, stiffness, stomatitis, syncope, throat irritation, transient ischemic attacks, tremor, tumor lysis syndrome, urinary tract infection, urinary urgency, xerostomia

Drug Interactions

Metabolism/Transport Effects Substrate of CYP3A4 (major), P-glycoprotein; **Note:** Assignment of Major/Minor substrate status based on clinically relevant drug interaction potential; **Inhibits** CYP2C8 (moderate), CYP2C9 (weak), CYP3A4 (moderate), UGT1A1; **Induces** CYP2C8 (weak/moderate), CYP2C9 (weak/moderate)

Avoid Concomitant Use

Avoid concomitant use of Nilotinib with any of the following: Amifampridine; Amodiaquine; Aprepitant; Asunaprevir; BCG (Intravesical); Bosutinib; Budesonide (Systemic); Cobimetinib; Conivaptan; CYP3A4 Inducers (Strong); CYP3A4 Inhibitors (Strong); Deferiprone; Dexamethasone (Systemic); Dipyrone; Domperidone; Flibanserin; Fusidic Acid (Systemic); Highest Risk QTc-Prolonging Agents; Hydroxychloroquine; Idelalisib; Irinotecan Products; Ivabradine; MiFEPRIStone; Mizolastine; Moderate Risk QTc-Prolonging Agents; Naloxegol; Natalizumab; Neratinib; Olaparib; Pimecrolimus;

▶

Pimozide; Probucol; Promazine; Simeprevir; St John's Wort; Tacrolimus (Topical); Tolvaptan; Trabectedin; Uliprisral; Vaccines (Live); Vinflunine

Increased Effect/Toxicity

Nilotinib may increase the levels/effects of: AmLODIPine; Amodiaquine; Apixaban; Aprepitant; Asunaprevir; Avanafil; Blonanserin; Bosentan; Bosutinib; Brexpiprazole; Bromocriptine; Budesonide (Systemic); Budesonide (Topical); Cannabis; Cilostazol; Cobimetinib; Colchicine; CYP2C8 Substrates; CYP3A4 Substrates; Dapoxetine; Deferiprone; Deflazacort; Domperidone; DOXOrubicin (Conventional); Dronabinol; Eletriptan; Eplerenone; Everolimus; FentaNYL; Fingolimod; Flibanserin; GuanFACINE; Highest Risk QTc-Prolonging Agents; HYDROcodone; HydrOXYzine; Ibrutinib; Imatinib; Irinotecan Products; Ivabradine; Ivacaftor; Leflunomide; Lomitapide; Lurasidone; Manidipine; Mirodenafil; Naldemedine; Naloxegol; Natalizumab; Neratinib; NiMODipine; Olaparib; OxyCODONE; Pimozide; Ranolazine; Rupatadine; SAXagliptin; Selexipag; Sildenafil; Simeprevir; Sonidegib; Suvorexant; Tetrahydrocannabinol; Ticagrelor; Tofacitinib; Tolvaptan; Trabectedin; Udenafil; Uliprisral; Vaccines (Live); Venetoclax; Vilazodone; Vindesine; Zopiclone

The levels/effects of Nilotinib may be increased by: Amifampridine; Bilastine; Buprenorphine; Conivaptan; CYP3A4 Inhibitors (Moderate); CYP3A4 Inhibitors (Strong); Denosumab; Dipyrone; Fosaprepitant; Fusidic Acid (Systemic); Hydroxychloroquine; Idelalisib; Indapamide; MiFEPRIStone; Mizolastine; Moderate Risk QTc-Prolonging Agents; Netupitant; Ocrelizumab; Palbociclib; Pimecrolimus; Probucol; Promazine; QTc-Prolonging Agents (Indeterminate Risk and Risk Modifying); Roflumilast; Stiripentol; Tacrolimus (Topical); Teneligliptin; Trastuzumab; Vinflunine; Xipamide

Decreased Effect

Nilotinib may decrease the levels/effects of: Antidiabetic Agents; BCG (Intravesical); Coccidioides immitis Skin Test; CYP2B6 Substrates; Ifosfamide; Nivolumab; Sipuleucel-T; Tertomotide; Vaccines (Inactivated); Vaccines (Live)

The levels/effects of Nilotinib may be decreased by: Antacids; Bosentan; CYP3A4 Inducers (Moderate); CYP3A4 Inducers (Strong); Dabrafenib; Deferasirox; Dexamethasone (Systemic); Echinacea; H2-Antagonists; Proton Pump Inhibitors; Sarilumab; Siltuximab; St John's Wort; Tocilizumab

Food Interactions Grapefruit juice may result in increased concentrations of nilotinib and potentiate QT prolongation. Management: Avoid grapefruit juice.

Hazardous Drugs Handling Considerations

Hazardous agent (NIOSH 2016 [group 1]).

Use appropriate precautions for receiving, handling, administration, and disposal. Gloves (single) should be worn during receiving, unpacking, and placing in storage. NIOSH recommends single gloving for administration of intact tablets or capsules (NIOSH 2016).

Storage/Stability Store at 25°C (77°F); excursions are permitted between 15°C and 30°C (59°F and 86°F).

Mechanism of Action Selective tyrosine kinase inhibitor that targets BCR-ABL kinase, c-KIT and platelet derived growth factor receptor (PDGFR); does not have activity against the SRC family. Inhibits BCR-ABL mediated proliferation of leukemic cell lines by binding to the ATP-binding site of BCR-ABL and inhibiting tyrosine kinase activity. Nilotinib has activity in imatinib-resistant BCR-ABL kinase mutations.

Pharmacodynamics/Kinetics

Protein binding: ~98%

Metabolism: Hepatic; oxidation and hydroxylation, via CYP3A4 to primarily inactive metabolites

Bioavailability: Capsule: ~50% (when compared to oral solution with pH of 1.2 to 1.3); two 200 mg capsules sprinkled on applesauce was determined to be bioequivalent to two 200 mg intact capsules; bioavailability is increased 82% when administered 30 minutes after a high-fat meal

Half-life elimination: ~15 to 17 hours

Time to peak: 3 hours

Excretion: Feces (93%; 69% as parent drug)

Dosing

Adult & Geriatric Note: If clinically indicated, may be administered in combination with hematopoietic growth factors (eg, erythropoietin, filgrastim) and with hydroxyurea or anagrelide.

Chronic myeloid leukemia (CML), Ph+, newly-diagnosed in chronic phase: Oral: 300 mg twice daily

CML, Ph+, resistant or intolerant in chronic or accelerated phase: Oral: 400 mg twice daily

Gastrointestinal stromal tumor (GIST), refractory (off-label use): Oral: 400 mg twice daily until disease progression or unacceptable toxicity (Reichardt, 2012)

Missed doses: If a dose is missed, do not make up, resume with next scheduled dose.

Dosage adjustment for concomitant CYP3A4 inhibitors/inducers:

CYP3A4 inhibitors: Avoid the concomitant use of a strong CYP3A4 inhibitor with nilotinib. If a strong CYP3A4 inhibitor is required, interruption of nilotinib treatment is recommended.

If therapy cannot be interrupted and concurrent use with a strong CYP3A4 inhibitor cannot be avoided, consider reducing the nilotinib dose to 300 mg once daily in patients with resistant or intolerant Ph+ CML (chronic or accelerated phase) or to 200 mg once daily in newly diagnosed chronic phase Ph+ CML, with careful monitoring, especially of the QT interval. When a strong CYP3A4 inhibitor is discontinued, allow a washout period prior to adjusting nilotinib dose upward.

CYP3A4 inducers: Avoid the concomitant use of a strong CYP3A4 inducer with nilotinib (based on pharmacokinetic parameters, an increased nilotinib dose is not likely to compensate for decreased exposure).

Renal Impairment There are no dosage adjustments provided in the manufacturer's labeling (has not been studied in patients with serum creatinine >1.5 times ULN); however, nilotinib and its metabolites have minimal renal excretion; dosage adjustments for renal dysfunction may not be necessary.

Hepatic Impairment

For hepatic impairment at treatment initiation: Note: Consider alternative therapies first if possible; recommendations vary by indication

Newly diagnosed Ph+ CML in chronic phase: Mild to severe impairment (Child-Pugh class A, B, or C): Initial: 200 mg twice daily; may increase to 300 mg twice daily based on patient tolerability

◀

Resistant or intolerant Ph+ CML in chronic or accelerated phase:
Mild to moderate impairment (Child-Pugh class A or B): Initial: 300 mg twice daily; may increase to 400 mg twice daily based on patient tolerability
Severe impairment (Child-Pugh class C): Initial: 200 mg twice daily; may increase to 300 mg twice daily and then further increase to 400 mg twice daily based on patient tolerability

For hepatotoxicity during treatment:
If bilirubin >3 times ULN (≥ grade 3): Withhold treatment, monitor bilirubin, resume treatment at 400 mg once daily when bilirubin returns to ≤1.5 times ULN (≤ grade 1)
If ALT or AST >5 times ULN (≥ grade 3): Withhold treatment, monitor transaminases, resume treatment at 400 mg once daily when ALT or AST returns to ≤2.5 times ULN (≤ grade 1)

Adjustment for Toxicity
Dosage adjustment for hematologic toxicity unrelated to underlying leukemia:
ANC <1000/mm^3 and/or platelets <50,000/mm^3: Withhold treatment, monitor blood counts
If ANC >1000/mm^3 and platelets >50,000/mm^3 within 2 weeks: Resume at prior dose
If ANC <1000/mm^3 and/or platelets <50,000/mm^3 for >2 weeks: Reduce dose to 400 mg once daily

Dosage adjustment for nonhematologic toxicity:
Amylase or lipase >2 times ULN (≥ grade 3): Withhold treatment, monitor serum amylase or lipase, resume treatment at 400 mg once daily when lipase or amylase returns to ≤1.5 times ULN (≤ grade 1)
Lipase increases in conjunction with abdominal symptoms: Withhold treatment and consider diagnostics to exclude pancreatitis.
Clinically-significant moderate or severe nonhematologic toxicity: Withhold treatment, upon resolution of toxicity, resume at 400 mg once daily; may escalate back to initial dose (300 mg twice daily or 400 mg twice daily depending on indication) if clinically appropriate.

Dosage adjustment for QT prolongation: Note: Repeat ECG ~7 days after any dosage adjustment.
QT$_c$ >480 msec: Withhold treatment, monitor and correct potassium and magnesium levels; review concurrent medications.
If QT$_c$F returns to <450 msec and to within 20 msec of baseline within 2 weeks: Resume at prior dose.
If QT$_c$F returns to 450 to 480 msec after 2 weeks: Reduce dose to 400 mg once daily.
If QT$_c$F >480 msec after dosage reduction to 400 mg once daily: Discontinue treatment.

Administration Administer twice daily with doses ~12 hours apart. Administer on an empty stomach, at least 1 hour before or 2 hours after food. Capsules should be swallowed whole with water. If unable to swallow whole, may empty contents into 5 mL applesauce and administer within 15 minutes (do not save for later use).

Emetic Potential Children and Adults: Low (10% to 30%)

Monitoring Parameters CBC with differential (every 2 weeks for first 2 months, then monthly); electrolytes (including potassium, calcium, and magnesium; baseline and periodic); lipid profile and glucose (baseline and periodically during the first year, then at least yearly), hepatic function (ALT/AST, bilirubin, alkaline phosphatase; baseline and monthly or as clinically indicated); serum lipase/amylase (baseline and monthly or as clinically indicated), uric acid (baseline); bone marrow assessments; ECG and QTc (baseline, 7 days after treatment initiation or dosage adjustments, and periodically thereafter); signs/symptoms of cardiovascular events, hemorrhage, or fluid retention.

Thyroid function testing (Hamnvik, 2011):
Preexisting levothyroxine therapy: Obtain baseline TSH levels, then monitor every 4 weeks until levels and levothyroxine dose are stable, then monitor every 2 months
Without preexisting thyroid hormone replacement: TSH at baseline, then monthly for 4 months, then every 2 to 3 months

Dietary Considerations The bioavailability of nilotinib is increased with food. Take on an empty stomach, at least 1 hour before or 2 hours after food. Avoid grapefruit juice.

Medication Guide Available Yes

Dosage Forms Excipient information presented when available (limited, particularly for generics); consult specific product labeling.
Capsule, Oral:
Tasigna: 150 mg, 200 mg

◆ **Nilotinib HCl** *see* Nilotinib *on page 1314*

◆ **Nilotinib Hydrochloride Monohydrate** *see* Nilotinib *on page 1314*

Nilutamide (ni LOO ta mide)

Related Information
Safe Handling of Hazardous Drugs *on page 2379*

Brand Names: US Nilandron

Brand Names: Canada Anandron

Index Terms RU-23908

Pharmacologic Category Antineoplastic Agent, Antiandrogen

Use Prostate cancer, metastatic: Treatment of metastatic prostate cancer (in combination with surgical castration)

Labeled Contraindications
Hypersensitivity to nilutamide or any component of the formulation; severe hepatic impairment; severe respiratory insufficiency
Canadian labeling: Additional contraindications (not in US labeling): Use in women and children

Pregnancy Considerations Animal reproduction studies have not been conducted. Nilutamide is not indicated for use in women.

Breastfeeding Considerations Nilutamide is not indicated for use in women.

Warnings/Precautions [US Boxed Warning]: Interstitial pneumonitis has been reported in 2% of patients exposed to nilutamide in controlled studies. An increased incidence has been observed in one small study of Japanese patients. Symptoms typically include exertional dyspnea, cough, chest pain and fever; interstitial changes (including pulmonary fibrosis) leading to hospitalization and fatalities have been reported (rarely). Most cases occurred within the first 3 months of treatment and most reversed after discontinuation. X-rays showed interstitial or alveolo-interstitial changes; pulmonary function tests revealed a restrictive pattern with decreased DL_{co}. Perform chest x-ray prior to treatment

◀ **initiation and consider baseline pulmonary function testing. Instruct patients to report new or worsening dyspnea. Discontinue nilutamide immediately if signs and/or symptoms of interstitial pneumonitis are observed until a causal effect can be ruled out.**

Androgen-deprivation therapy may increase the risk for cardiovascular disease (Levine, 2010). Androgen deprivation therapy with other antiandrogen agents has resulted in prolongation of the QT/QTc interval (Garnick, 2004). Correct electrolytes prior to initiation and consider periodic electrolyte and ECG monitoring in patients at risk for QT prolongation.

Hepatitis or marked increases in liver enzymes leading to drug discontinuation occurred in 1% of patients receiving nilutamide in controlled studies. Rare cases of hospitalization or deaths due to severe liver injury have been reported, with the onset of hepatotoxicity usually occurring within first 3 to 4 months of therapy. Monitor transaminases. Signs/symptoms of hepatic dysfunction (nausea/vomiting, abdominal pain, anorexia, fatigue, flu-like symptoms, dark urine, jaundice, and/or right upper quadrant pain) should prompt liver function testing. Discontinue treatment immediately for jaundice or ALT >2 times the upper limit of normal (ULN). Approximately 5% of patients experience intolerance (facial flushing, hypotension, malaise) when ethanol is combined with nilutamide. Instruct patients to avoid ethanol. Hyperglycemia has been observed; use with caution in diabetic patients and monitor for loss of glucose control. Prolonged use of antiandrogen therapy is associated with decreased bone mineral density and an increased risk of osteoporosis and fracture (Smith, 2003). Anemia may occur with testosterone suppression.

A delay in adaptation to dark has been reported; in clinical studies, this was reported by 13% to 57% of patients; the delay ranged from seconds to a few minutes after passing from a light to a dark area (this may not abate with continued treatment although may be alleviated by wearing tinted sunglasses); caution patients who experience adaptation delay about driving at night or through tunnels. Not indicated for use in women and pediatric patients. Patients with disease progression while receiving antiandrogen therapy may experience clinical improvement with discontinuation of the antiandrogen. Potentially significant drug-drug interactions may exist, requiring dose or frequency adjustment, additional monitoring, and/or selection of alternative therapy.

Adverse Reactions Reactions reported from monotherapy and combination therapy.

>10%:

Endocrine & metabolic: Hot flash (28%)

Ophthalmic: Nocturnal amblyopia (13% to 57%)

1% to 10%:

Cardiovascular: Hypertension (5%), cardiac failure (3%), angina pectoris (2%), edema (2%), syncope (2%)

Central nervous system: Dizziness (7%), paresthesia (3%), malaise (2%), nervousness (2%)

Dermatologic: Pruritus (2%)

Endocrine & metabolic: Hyperglycemia (4%), increased haptoglobin (2%), weight loss (2%)

Gastrointestinal: Nausea (10%), constipation (7%), diarrhea (2%), gastrointestinal hemorrhage (2%), melena (2%), xerostomia (2%)

Hematologic & oncologic: Leukopenia (3%)

Hepatic: Increased serum ALT (8%), increased serum AST (8%), increased serum alkaline phosphatase (3%)

Neuromuscular & skeletal: Arthritis (2%)

Ophthalmic: Visual disturbance (7%), cataract (2%), photophobia (2%)

Renal: Increased blood urea nitrogen (2%), increased serum creatinine (2%)

Respiratory: Dyspnea (6%), cough (2%), interstitial pneumonitis (2%), rhinitis (2%)

Miscellaneous: Alcohol intolerance (5%)

<1%, postmarketing, and/or case reports: Anxiety, aplastic anemia, cold extremities, gynecomastia, headache, hepatic injury, hepatitis, maculopapular rash, palpitations, prolonged Q-T interval on ECG, urticaria, vomiting, weight gain

Drug Interactions

Metabolism/Transport Effects Substrate of CYP2C19 (major); Note: Assignment of Major/Minor substrate status based on clinically relevant drug interaction potential

Avoid Concomitant Use

Avoid concomitant use of Nilutamide with any of the following: Alcohol (Ethyl); Indium 111 Capromab Pendetide

Increased Effect/Toxicity

Nilutamide may increase the levels/effects of: Alcohol (Ethyl)

The levels/effects of Nilutamide may be increased by: CYP2C19 Inhibitors (Moderate); CYP2C19 Inhibitors (Strong)

Decreased Effect

Nilutamide may decrease the levels/effects of: Choline C 11; Indium 111 Capromab Pendetide

The levels/effects of Nilutamide may be decreased by: CYP2C19 Inducers (Strong); Dabrafenib; Enzalutamide; Lumacaftor

Hazardous Drugs Handling Considerations

Hazardous agent (meets NIOSH 2016 criteria). This medication is not on the NIOSH (2016) list; however, it meets the criteria for a hazardous drug. Drugs are classified as hazardous based on their properties; the properties of a hazardous drug include one or more of the following characteristics: carcinogenic, teratogenic (or other developmental toxicity), reproductive toxicity, organotoxic at low doses, genotoxic, and/or new agents with structural or toxicity profiles similar to existing hazardous agents.

Use appropriate precautions for receiving, handling, administration, and disposal. Gloves (single) should be worn during receiving, unpacking, and placing in storage. NIOSH recommends single gloving for administration of intact tablets or capsules (NIOSH 2016).

Storage/Stability Store at 25°C (77°F); excursions permitted between 15°C to 30°C (59°F to 86°F). Protect from light.

Mechanism of Action Nilutamide is a nonsteroidal antiandrogen which blocks testosterone effects at the androgen receptor level, preventing androgen response.

Pharmacodynamics/Kinetics

Absorption: Rapid and complete

Metabolism: Hepatic (extensive), forms active metabolites

Half-life elimination: Terminal: 38 to 59 hours; Metabolites: 59 to 126 hours

Excretion: Urine (62%; <2% as unchanged drug); feces (1% to 7%)

◀ **Dosing**

Adult & Geriatric Prostate cancer, metastatic: Oral: 300 mg once daily (starting the same day or day after surgical castration) for 30 days, followed by 150 mg once daily. Consider therapy discontinuation in patients with evidence of disease progression.

Renal Impairment There are no dosage adjustments provided in the manufacturer's labeling.

Hepatic Impairment

Hepatic impairment at treatment initiation:

Mild or moderate impairment: There are no dosage adjustments provided in the manufacturer's labeling.

Severe impairment: Use is contraindicated.

Hepatotoxicity during treatment: ALT >2 times ULN or jaundice: Discontinue treatment.

Administration Administer without regard to meals.

Monitoring Parameters CBC (periodic), liver function tests (transaminases; at baseline, regularly during the first 4 months of treatment, and then periodically thereafter; more frequently if clinically indicated), electrolytes, serum testosterone, PSA, blood glucose and/or glycosylated hemoglobin (HbA1c) in patients with diabetes; chest x-ray (baseline); consider pulmonary function testing (baseline); bone-mineral density (as clinically indicated in patients at risk of osteoporosis); ECG; signs and symptoms of liver dysfunction; vision changes. If initiating nilutamide in patients who are on warfarin, closely monitor prothrombin time.

Dosage Forms Excipient information presented when available (limited, particularly for generics); consult specific product labeling. [DSC] = Discontinued product

Tablet, Oral:

Nilandron: 150 mg [DSC]

Nilandron: 150 mg [contains corn starch]

Generic: 150 mg

Dosage Forms: Canada Information with regard to form, strength, and availability of products uniquely available in Canada but currently not available in the US. Refer also to Dosage Forms.

Excipient information presented when available (limited, particularly for generics); consult specific product labeling.

Tablet, Oral:

Anandron: 50 mg

♦ **Ninlaro** see Ixazomib on page 1084

♦ **Nipent** see Pentostatin on page 1501

Niraparib (nye RAP a rib)

Related Information

Common Toxicity Criteria on page 2242

Safe Handling of Hazardous Drugs on page 2379

Brand Names: US Zejula

Index Terms MK4827; Niraparib Tosylate; Zejula

Pharmacologic Category Antineoplastic Agent, PARP Inhibitor

Use Ovarian, fallopian tube, or primary peritoneal cancer: Maintenance treatment of recurrent epithelial ovarian, fallopian tube, or primary peritoneal cancer in patients who are in a complete or partial response to platinum-based chemotherapy.

Labeled Contraindications There are no contraindications listed in the manufacturer's labeling.

Pregnancy Considerations Animal reproduction studies have not been conducted, however based on the mechanism of action, niraparib may cause fetal harm if used during pregnancy. Pregnancy testing should be conducted prior to treatment and effective contraception should be used during therapy and for at least 6 months after the last dose in women of reproductive potential. Fertility may be impaired if administered to males.

Breastfeeding Considerations It is not known if niraparib is present in breast milk. Due to the potential for adverse events, breastfeeding is not recommended during therapy and for 1 month after the last dose.

Warnings/Precautions Myelodysplastic syndrome/acute myeloid leukemia (MDS/AML) have been reported (rare), including fatal cases. The duration of niraparib treatment prior to the development of MDS/AML varied from <1 month to 2 years. All patients had received prior chemotherapy, including platinum-based regimens. Discontinue niraparib if MDS/AML is confirmed. Thrombocytopenia, anemia and neutropenia commonly occur, including grade 3 and 4 events (which rarely required discontinuation). Monitor blood counts weekly for the first month, then monthly for 11 months, then periodically thereafter. Do not initiate niraparib until hematologic toxicity due to previous chemotherapy has resolved to grade 1 or lower. Hematologic toxicity may require treatment interruption, dose reduction, or discontinuation. If hemato-logic toxicities do not resolve within 28 days following interruption, discontinue niraparib and obtain consult with hematology for further assessment, including marrow and cytogenetic analysis.

Hypertension and hypertensive crisis have been reported, including grade 3 and 4 hypertension (hypertension required discontinuation in rare cases). Monitor blood pressure and heart rate monthly during the first year and periodically thereafter. Patients with cardiac disorders (especially coronary insufficiency, arrhythmias and hypertension) should be monitored closely. If necessary, hypertension should be managed with antihypertensives and niraparib dose adjustment. Nausea, vomiting, constipation and mucositis/stomatitis have been reported. Consider administering niraparib at bedtime to diminish the potential for nausea and vomiting. Potentially drug-drug significant interactions may exist, requiring dose or frequency adjustment, additional monitoring, and/or selection of alternative therapy.

Adverse Reactions

>10%:

Cardiovascular: Hypertension (20%)

Central nervous system: Fatigue (≤57%), insomnia (27%), headache (26%), dizziness (18%), anxiety (11%)

Dermatologic: Skin rash (21%)

Gastrointestinal: Nausea (74%), constipation (40%), vomiting (34%), decreased appetite (25%), mucositis (≤20%), stomatitis (≤20%), dyspepsia (18%)

Genitourinary: Urinary tract infection (13%)

Hematologic & oncologic: Thrombocytopenia (61%; grades 3/4: 29%), anemia (50%; grades 3/4: 25%), neutropenia (30%; grades 3/4: 20%), leukopenia (17%; grades 3/4: 5%)

◄ Hepatic: Increased serum AST (≤10% to 36%), increased serum ALT (≤10% to 28%)

Neuromuscular & skeletal: Weakness (≤57%), back pain (18%)

Respiratory: Nasopharyngitis (23%), dyspnea (20%), cough (16%)

1% to 10%:

Cardiovascular: Palpitations (10%), peripheral edema, tachycardia

Central nervous system: Depression

Endocrine & metabolic: Hypokalemia, increased gamma-glutamyl transferase, weight loss

Gastrointestinal: Dysgeusia (10%), xerostomia (10%)

Hepatic: Increased serum alkaline phosphatase

Ophthalmic: Conjunctivitis

Renal: Increased serum creatinine

Respiratory: Bronchitis, epistaxis

<1%, postmarketing, and/or case reports: Acute myelocytic leukemia, hypertensive crisis, myelodysplastic syndrome

Drug Interactions

Metabolism/Transport Effects Substrate of BCRP, P-glycoprotein; **Inhibits** BCRP

Avoid Concomitant Use

Avoid concomitant use of Niraparib with any of the following: BCG (Intravesical); Deferiprone; Dipyrone

Increased Effect/Toxicity

Niraparib may increase the levels/effects of: CloZAPine; Deferiprone

The levels/effects of Niraparib may be increased by: Dipyrone; Promazine

Decreased Effect

Niraparib may decrease the levels/effects of: BCG (Intravesical)

Hazardous Drugs Handling Considerations

Hazardous agent (meets NIOSH 2016 criteria). This medication is not on the NIOSH (2016) list; however, it meets the criteria for a hazardous drug. Drugs are classified as hazardous based on their properties; the properties of a hazardous drug include one or more of the following characteristics: carcinogenic, teratogenic (or other developmental toxicity), reproductive toxicity, organotoxic at low doses, genotoxic, and/or new agents with structural or toxicity profiles similar to existing hazardous agents.

Use appropriate precautions for receiving, handling, administration, and disposal. Gloves (single) should be worn during receiving, unpacking, and placing in storage. NIOSH recommends single gloving for administration of intact tablets or capsules (NIOSH 2016).

Storage/Stability Store at 20°C to 25°C (68°F to 77°F); excursions permitted from 15°C to 30°C (59°F to 86°F).

Mechanism of Action Niraparib is a poly (ADP-ribose) polymerase (PARP) enzyme inhibitor, which is highly selective for PARP-1 and PARP-2. PARP-1 and PARP-2 are involved in detecting DNA damage and promote repair (Mirza 2016). Inhibiting PARP enzymatic activity results in DNA damage, apoptosis and cell death. Niraparib induces cytotoxicity in tumor cell lines with and without BRCA1/2 deficiencies.

Pharmacodynamics/Kinetics

Distribution: $V_{d/F}$: 1,074 L

Protein binding: 83%

Metabolism: Metabolized by carboxylesterases to an inactive metabolite, which subsequently undergoes glucuronidation.

Bioavailability: ~73%

Half-life elimination: 36 hours

Time to peak: Within 3 hours

Excretion: Urine (~48% [at 21 days]; 11% [pooled samples collected over 6 days] as unchanged drug); Feces (~39% [at 21 days]; 19% [pooled samples collected over 6 days] as unchanged drug)

Dosing

Adult & Geriatric Ovarian, fallopian tube, or primary peritoneal cancer, recurrent (maintenance treatment): Oral: 300 mg once daily, continue until disease progression or unacceptable toxicity (Mirza 2016). Begin treatment no later than 8 weeks following the most recent platinum-containing regimen.

Missed/vomited doses: If a dose is missed or vomited, an additional dose should not be taken that day. Resume dosing with the next scheduled daily dose.

Renal Impairment Renal function estimated using the Cockcroft-Gault formula.

CrCl 30 to <90 mL/minute: No dosage adjustment necessary.

CrCl <30 mL/minute: There are no dosage adjustments provided in the manufacturer's labeling (has not been studied).

End stage renal disease (ESRD): There are no dosage adjustments provided in the manufacturer's labeling (has not been studied).

Hepatic Impairment Hepatic function estimated using the National Cancer Institute Organ Dysfunction Working Group Criteria.

Mild impairment: No dosage adjustment necessary.

Moderate to severe impairment: There are no dosage adjustments provided in the manufacturer's labeling (has not been studied).

Adjustment for Toxicity Adverse reactions may be managed with treatment interruption, dose reduction, or discontinuation.

Recommended niraparib dosage adjustment levels:

Starting dose: 300 mg/day

First dose reduction: Reduce to 200 mg/day.

Second dose reduction: Reduce to 100 mg/day.

If further dose reduction below 100 mg/day is needed, discontinue niraparib.

Hematologic toxicity:

Platelets <100,000/mm^3:

First occurrence: Withhold treatment for a maximum of 28 days and monitor blood counts weekly. When platelets are ≥100,000/mm^3, resume niraparib at the same or at a reduced dose. If platelet count was <75,000/mm^3, resume at a reduced dose.

Second occurrence: Withhold treatment for a maximum of 28 days and monitor blood counts weekly. When platelets are ≥100,000/mm^3, resume niraparib at a reduced dose. Discontinue if platelet count has not returned to acceptable levels within 28 days of interrupting dose, or if dose has already been reduced to 100 mg/day.

Neutrophils <1,000/mm^3 or hemoglobin <8 g/dL: Withhold treatment for a maximum of 28 days and monitor blood counts weekly. When neutrophils are ≥1,500/mm^3 or hemoglobin is ≥9 g/dL, resume niraparib at a reduced dose. Discontinue if neutrophils and/or hemoglobin have not returned to acceptable levels within 28 days of interrupting dose, or if dose has already been reduced to 100 mg/day.

◀

Hematologic toxicity requiring transfusion: Withhold niraparib. Consider platelet transfusion for platelets ≤10,000/mm^3. If other risk factors (eg, concurrent anticoagulation or antiplatelet therapy), consider interrupting the anticoagulant/antiplatelet and/or transfusing to a higher platelet count. Resume niraparib at a reduced dose.

Secondary myelodysplastic syndrome (MDS) or acute myeloid leukemia (AML): Discontinue niraparib with confirmed diagnosis of MDS or AML.

Nonhematologic toxicity:

Grade 3 or higher adverse reaction (where prophylactic management is not feasible or persistent despite management): Withhold niraparib for up to 28 days or until resolution; may resume with the dose reduced (up to two dose reductions are permitted).

Grade 3 or higher adverse reaction lasting more than 28 days at a dose of 100 mg/day: Discontinue treatment.

Administration Administer at approximately the same time each day, either with or without food. Swallow capsules whole. Consider administering at bedtime to diminish the potential for nausea and vomiting.

Monitoring Parameters CBC with differential (weekly for the first month, then monthly for 11 months, then periodically); pregnancy test (prior to treatment; in females of reproductive potential). Monitor blood pressure and heart rate monthly during the first year and periodically thereafter.

Dosage Forms Excipient information presented when available (limited, particularly for generics); consult specific product labeling.

Capsule, Oral, as tosylate:

Zejula: 100 mg [contains fd&c blue #1 aluminum lake, fd&c yellow #5 aluminum lake]

◆ **Niraparib Tosylate** see Niraparib on page 1324

◆ **Nitrogen Mustard** see Mechlorethamine (Systemic) on page 1168

Nivolumab (nye VOL ue mab)

Related Information

Common Toxicity Criteria on page 2242

Management of Chemotherapy-Induced Nausea and Vomiting in Adults on page 2253

Brand Names: US Opdivo

Brand Names: Canada Opdivo

Index Terms Anti-PD-1 Human Monoclonal Antibody MDX-1106; BMS-936558; MDX-1106; Nivolumab, inj; ONO-4538

Pharmacologic Category Antineoplastic Agent, Anti-PD-1 Monoclonal Antibody; Antineoplastic Agent, Immune Checkpoint Inhibitor; Antineoplastic Agent, Monoclonal Antibody

Use

Colorectal cancer, metastatic (microsatellite instability-high or mismatch repair deficient): Treatment of microsatellite instability-high (MSI-H) or mismatch repair deficient (dMMR) metastatic colorectal cancer (CRC) in adults and pediatric patients 12 years and older that has progressed following treatment with a fluoropyrimidine, oxaliplatin, and irinotecan.

Head and neck cancer, squamous cell (recurrent or metastatic): Treatment of recurrent or metastatic squamous cell carcinoma of the head and neck in patients with disease progression on or after platinum-based therapy.

Hodgkin lymphoma, classical: Treatment of classical Hodgkin lymphoma (cHL) in adult patients that have relapsed or progressed following autologous hematopoietic stem cell transplant (HSCT) and brentuximab vedotin, or 3 or more lines of systemic therapy that includes autologous HSCT.

Melanoma, unresectable or metastatic: Treatment (as a single agent) of BRAF V600 wild-type or BRAF V600 mutation-positive unresectable or metastatic melanoma; treatment of unresectable or metastatic melanoma (in combination with ipilimumab)

Non-small cell lung cancer, metastatic, progressive: Treatment of metastatic non-small cell lung cancer (NSCLC) that has progressed on or after platinum-based chemotherapy. Patients with EGFR or ALK genomic tumor aberrations should have disease progression (on approved EGFR- or ALK-directed therapy) prior to receiving nivolumab.

Renal cell cancer, advanced: Treatment of advanced renal cell cancer in patients who have received prior anti-angiogenic therapy.

Urothelial carcinoma, locally advanced or metastatic: Treatment of locally advanced or metastatic urothelial carcinoma in patients with disease progression during or following a platinum-containing therapy or disease progression within 12 months of neoadjuvant or adjuvant treatment with a platinum-containing therapy.

Labeled Contraindications There are no contraindications listed in the manufacturer's US labeling.

Canadian labeling: Hypersensitivity to nivolumab or any component of the formulation.

Pregnancy Considerations Adverse events were observed in animal reproduction studies. Nivolumab may be expected to cross the placenta; effects to the fetus may be greater in the second and third trimesters. Based on its mechanism of action, nivolumab is expected to cause fetal harm if used during pregnancy. Women of reproductive potential should use highly effective contraception during therapy and for at least 5 months after the last nivolumab dose.

Breastfeeding Considerations It is not known if nivolumab is present in breast milk. Due to the potential for serious adverse reactions in the breastfed infant, the manufacturer recommends to discontinue breastfeeding during treatment.

Warnings/Precautions Nivolumab may cause immune-mediated pneumonitis (severe pneumonitis or interstitial lung disease); fatal cases have been reported. Immune-mediated pneumonitis is defined as no other clear etiology and requiring corticosteroid use. The median time to onset was 1.6 to 3.5 months (range: 1 day to 22.3 months) across several clinical trials. Some cases developed after nivolumab was discontinued for other reasons. High-dose systemic corticosteroids (followed by a corticosteroid taper) were administered for a median duration of 26 to 30 days (range 1 day to 11.8 months). Most patients improved to grade 0 or 1; some patients with grade 2 or 3 pneumonitis had complete resolution (after completing corticosteroid therapy) and nivolumab was reinitiated without recurrence in some patients. Monitor for signs (with radiographic imaging) and symptoms of pneumonitis. May require treatment interruption, corticosteroid therapy, and/or permanent discontinuation. Grades 2, 3, or 4 pneumonitis should be managed with corticosteroids (prednisone 1 to 2 mg/kg daily or equivalent) followed by a corticosteroid taper. Withhold treatment until resolution for moderate (grade 2) immune-mediated pneumonitis; permanently discontinue for severe (grade 3) or life-threatening (grade 4) immune-mediated pneumonitis.

◀

Diarrhea or colitis occurred commonly in patients receiving nivolumab (some cases were fatal). Immune-mediated colitis (defined as no other clear etiology and requiring corticosteroid use), including cases of grades 2 and 3 colitis, occurred in some patients. The median time to onset of colitis was 1.6 to 5.3 months (range: 2 days to 21 months) from nivolumab initiation; some cases developed after nivolumab was discontinued for other reasons. In studies, the median duration of high-dose systemic corticosteroid therapy was 23 days to 1.1 months (range: 1 day to 12 months). Most patients with grade 2 or 3 immune-related colitis had complete resolution (improvement to grade 0); after resolution, nivolumab was reinitiated in some patients without recurrence, although was permanently discontinued in other patients. Monitor for signs and symptoms of colitis. May require treatment interruption, corticosteroid therapy, and/or permanent discontinuation. Severe colitis (grade 3) or life threatening colitis (grade 4) should be managed with corticosteroids (prednisone 1 to 2 mg/kg daily or equivalent) followed by a corticosteroid taper. Moderate colitis (grade 2) of >5 days duration should be managed with corticosteroids (prednisone 0.5 to 1 mg/kg daily or equivalent) followed by a corticosteroid taper; may increase to prednisone 1 to 2 mg/kg daily (or equivalent) if colitis worsens or does not improve despite corticosteroid therapy. Some cases required the addition of infliximab to corticosteroid therapy. Permanently discontinue nivolumab for grade 4 colitis or diarrhea, or colitis that recurs upon reinitiation (single-agent therapy) or for severe or life-threatening colitis (grade 3 or 4) or for colitis that recurs upon reinitiation (in combination with ipilimumab).

ALT, AST, alkaline phosphatase, and total bilirubin elevations have occurred in nivolumab-treated patients. Immune-mediated hepatitis (defined as no other clear etiology and requiring corticosteroid use) occurred in patients receiving nivolumab; most cases included grade 2 and grade 3 hepatitis, although grade 4 toxicity also occurred. The median time to onset was 2.1 to 3.3 months (range: 6 days to 11 months) after nivolumab initiation. Immune-mediated hepatitis was managed with high-dose systemic corticosteroids; in some cases, mycophenolate was added to corticosteroid therapy. In studies, the median duration of high-dose systemic corticosteroid therapy was 23 days to 1.1 months (range: 1 day to 13.2 months). Immune-mediated hepatitis resolved and did not recur with continued corticosteroid use in some patients, although some patients experienced recurrence and permanently discontinued treatment. When used in combination with ipilimumab, a majority of patients had complete resolution of hepatitis after completion of steroid therapy, and some patients had recurrence or worsening hepatitis when nivolumab and ipilimumab were restarted. Monitor liver function at baseline and periodically for changes. Initiate corticosteroids (prednisone 0.5 to 1 mg/kg daily or equivalent for grade 2 or prednisone 1 to 2 mg/kg daily or equivalent followed by a corticosteroid taper for grade 3 or 4) transaminase elevations (with or without total bilirubin elevations). Withhold treatment for moderate (grade 2) immune-mediated hepatitis; permanently discontinue for severe (grade 3) or life-threatening (grade 4) immune-mediated hepatitis.

Renal dysfunction has occurred with nivolumab therapy. Immune-mediated nephritis (defined as renal dysfunction or ≥ grade 2 creatinine elevations with no other clear etiology and requiring corticosteroid use) or autoimmune nephritis may occur with nivolumab treatment. The median time to onset was 2.7 to 4.6 months (range: 9 days to 12.3 months). For single-agent nivolumab, all patients received high-dose systemic corticosteroids (at least

40 mg prednisone or equivalent per day) for a median duration of 3 weeks (range: 1 day to 15.4 months); complete resolution occurred in about one-half of patients, with no recurrence upon rechallenge. When used in combination with ipilimumab, two-thirds of patients received high-dose systemic corticosteroids (at least 40 mg prednisone or equivalent per day) for a median duration of 2 weeks (range: 1 day to 1.1 months); complete resolution occurred in all patients, some patients resumed combination therapy with no recurrence. Monitor serum creatinine at baseline and periodically during treatment. Initiate corticosteroids (prednisone 1 to 2 mg/kg daily or equivalent) followed by a corticosteroid taper for life-threatening (grade 4) serum creatinine elevation and permanently discontinue nivolumab. Withhold treatment for moderate (grade 2) and severe (grade 3) creatinine elevations and administer corticosteroids (prednisone 0.5 to 1 mg/kg daily or equivalent) followed by a corticosteroid taper; if toxicity worsens or does not improve, increase to prednisone 1 to 2 mg/kg daily (or equivalent).

Immune-mediated rash, including Stevens-Johnson syndrome (SJS) and toxic epidermal necrolysis (TEN) have been observed in patients receiving nivolumab; some cases have been fatal. The median time to onset of immune-mediated rash was 18 days to 2.8 months (range: 1 day to 25.8 months) after nivolumab initiation. Withhold treatment for signs or symptoms of SJS or TEN and refer to specialist for assessment and treatment; discontinue permanently if confirmed. Withhold treatment for grade 3 rash and permanently discontinue for life-threatening (grade 4) rash and administer corticosteroids (prednisone 1 to 2 mg/kg/day or equivalent followed by a taper) for severe (grade 3) or life-threatening (grade 4) immune-mediated rash. High-dose systemic corticosteroids (followed by a corticosteroid taper) were administered to some patients for a median duration of 12 to 14 days (range: 1 day to 9 months); topical corticosteroids were also used to manage dermatologic toxicity. Complete resolution occurred in nearly half of patients; some patient experienced recurrence with rechallenge.

Type 1 diabetes mellitus may occur, including cases of diabetic ketoacidosis. The median time to onset was 2.5 to 4.4 months (range: 15 days to 22 months). Monitor for hyperglycemia. Withhold nivolumab for severe (grade 3) hyperglycemia until blood sugar has been appropriately controlled. Permanently discontinue for life-threatening (grade 4) hyperglycemia.

Immune-mediated encephalitis (without clear etiology) may occur. Withhold nivolumab for new-onset moderate to severe neurologic signs/symptoms; evaluate to rule out other neurologic causes or infection. Evaluate with neurology consultation, brain MRI, and lumbar puncture. For confirmed immune-mediated encephalitis felt to be caused by nivolumab (if other etiologies are ruled out), administer corticosteroids (prednisone 1 to 2 mg/kg/day or equivalent), followed by a corticosteroid taper. Permanently discontinue nivolumab if immune-mediated encephalitis occurs.

Hypophysitis may occur; some patients developed grades 1, 2, or 3 toxicity. Most patients received corticosteroids; combination therapy was restarted for the majority of the patients without worsening hypophysitis (several patients continued on corticosteroid therapy). The median time to onset was 2.7 to 4.9 months (range: from 27 days to 11 months). Monitor for signs/symptoms of hypophysitis. Administer hormone replacement therapy as clinically indicated and corticosteroids (prednisone 1 mg/kg/day or equivalent followed by a taper) for grade 2 or higher toxicity. In studies, the median duration of high-dose systemic corticosteroid therapy was 14 to 19 days (range: 1 day to 2 months). Withhold nivolumab for moderate (grade 2) or severe (grade 3) and permanently discontinue treatment for life-threatening (grade 4) hypophysitis. Adrenal insufficiency may occur; may require hormone replacement therapy and/or corticosteroid therapy. The median time to onset across several clinical trials was 3 to 4.3 months (range: 15 days to 21 months). In studies, the median duration of high-dose systemic corticosteroid therapy was 9 to 11 days (range: 1 day to 2.7 months). Monitor for signs/symptoms of adrenal insufficiency both during and after treatment. Administer corticosteroids (prednisone 1 to 2 mg/kg/day or equivalent followed by a taper) for severe (grade 3) or life-threatening (grade 4) adrenal insufficiency. Withhold nivolumab for moderate (grade 2) and permanently discontinue for severe (grade 3) or life-threatening (grade 4) toxicity.

Immune-mediated hyperthyroidism and hypothyroidism/thyroiditis have occurred, mostly grades 1 and 2 hyper-/hypothyroidism (one patient receiving nivolumab in combination with ipilimumab experienced grade 3 autoimmune thyroiditis). The median onset for hyperthyroidism was 23 days to 1.5 months (range: 1 day to 14.2 months); most cases resolved (may require medical management, including corticosteroids and methimazole). Hypothyroidism occurred with a median onset of 2 to 3 months (range: 1 day to 16.6 months). Most patients received subsequent nivolumab (with or without ipilimumab) treatment while continuing thyroid replacement therapy. Monitor thyroid function at baseline and for changes periodically during treatment (in one study patients were evaluated at baseline, treatment day 1, and every 6 weeks). Isolated hypothyroidism may be managed with hormone replacement therapy; initiate medical management (eg, methimazole) to control hyperthyroidism.

Other clinically relevant immune-mediated disorders may occur; may develop after discontinuation of nivolumab. Immune-mediated adverse reactions observed included facial/abducens nerve paresis, autoimmune neuropathy, demyelination, duodenitis, gastritis, Guillain-Barré syndrome, histiocytic necrotizing lymphadenitis (Kikuchi lymphadenitis), hypopituitarism, motor dysfunction, myasthenic syndrome, myocarditis, myositis, pancreatitis, polymyalgia rheumatica, rhabdomyolysis, sarcoidosis, systemic inflammatory response syndrome, uveitis, iritis, and vasculitis. If an immune-mediated adverse event is suspected, evaluate to exclude other causes. Based on symptom severity, withhold or permanently discontinue nivolumab, administer high-dose corticosteroids, and if appropriate, initiate hormone replacement therapy. Upon improvement to grade 0 or 1, begin corticosteroid taper (over at least 1 month). After corticosteroid taper is completed and based on the severity of the reaction, may consider reinitiating nivolumab. Infusion-related reactions have occurred with both single-agent nivolumab and when used in combination with ipilimumab; severe reactions, although rare, were observed when given as a single agent. Monitor closely; discontinue for severe or life-threatening reactions. Mild or moderate reactions may be managed by interrupting or decreasing the infusion rate. Patients who received allogeneic hematopoietic stem cell transplant (HSCT) following discontinuation of nivolumab therapy experienced complications (some fatal), including severe or refractory acute graft-versus-host disease (some cases occurring within 14 days after stem cell infusion), non-infectious febrile syndrome (requiring corticosteroids), lymphocytic encephalitis, viral encephalitis, and sinusoidal obstructive syndrome (SOS; formerly called veno-occlusive disease). These complications may occur despite intervening therapy between nivolumab and HSCT. Monitor closely for early signs/symptoms of transplant-related complications and manage promptly. Potentially significant drug-drug interactions may exist, requiring dose or frequency adjustment, additional monitoring, and/or selection of alternative therapy.

Adverse Reactions

>10%:

Cardiovascular: Edema (≤13%), peripheral edema (≤13%)

Central nervous system: Fatigue (≤53%), malaise (≤46%), headache (17%), peripheral neuropathy (new onset and exacerbations: ≤14%)

Dermatologic: Skin rash (1% to 40%; immune-mediated: 9%), pruritus (10% to 23%), vitiligo (≤11%)

Endocrine & metabolic: Hyperglycemia (≤42%), hyponatremia (20% to 41%), increased serum triglycerides (32%), hyperkalemia (15% to 30%), hypocalcemia (13% to 26%), increased serum cholesterol (21%), hypercalcemia (2% to 19%), hypokalemia (16%), hypomagnesemia (14% to 16%), hypothyroidism (≤12%; including immune-mediated events), thyroiditis (≤12%; including immune-mediated events)

Gastrointestinal: Diarrhea (2% to 33%), increased serum lipase (20% to 29%), decreased appetite (22% to 28%), nausea (20% to 28%), constipation (14% to 23%), vomiting (12% to 19%), increased serum amylase (10% to 18%), abdominal pain (13% to 16%)

Genitourinary: Urinary tract infection (17%)

Hematologic & oncologic: Lymphocytopenia (32% to 42%; grade 3/4: 4% to 11%), anemia (26% to 40%; grade 3/4: 3% to 8%), leukopenia (11% to 38%, grades 3/4: ≤5%), neutropenia (37%; grade 3/4: 5%), thrombocytopenia (15% to 37%; grade 3/4: 2% to 3%)

Hepatic: Increased serum AST (24% to 33%), increased serum alkaline phosphatase (10% to 33%), increased serum ALT (16% to 31%), increased serum bilirubin (11% to 13%)

Immunologic: Graft versus host disease (>10%; within 14 days of stem cell infusion: 20%), antibody development (11%; neutralizing: <1%; no evidence of altered pharmacokinetic profile)

Neuromuscular & skeletal: Weakness (≤56%), musculoskeletal pain (19% to 33%), back pain (21%), arthralgia (10% to 20%)

Renal: Increased serum creatinine (16% to 42%)

Respiratory: Upper respiratory tract infection (11% to 44%), cough (17% to 36%; includes productive cough), dyspnea (2% to 27%; includes exertional dyspnea), bronchopneumonia (≤13%), pneumonia (≤13%), nasal congestion (11%)

Miscellaneous: Febrile reaction (35%; events without an infectious cause that required steroids), fever (≤29%; may include tumor-associated fever), infusion related reaction (≤14%)

1% to 10%:

Cardiovascular: Pulmonary embolism (2% to 3%)

Central nervous system: Neuritis (<10%), peripheral nerve palsy (peroneal: <10%)

Dermatologic: Erythema (10%)

Endocrine & metabolic: Hyperthyroidism (3%; including immune-mediated events), adrenocortical insufficiency (1%; including immune-mediated events), increased gamma-glutamyl transferase

Gastrointestinal: Intestinal perforation (<10%), stomatitis (<10%), colitis (including immune-mediated events: 2% to 3%)

Hepatic: Hepatitis (immune-mediated: 2%)

Immunologic: Sjogren syndrome (<10%)

Neuromuscular & skeletal: Myopathy (<10%), rheumatic disease (spondyloarthropathy: <10%)

Renal: Acute renal failure (≥2%), nephritis (≤1%; immune-mediated), renal insufficiency (≤1%; immune-mediated)

Respiratory: Interstitial pulmonary disease (6%), pleural effusion (1% to 5%), pneumonitis (≤5%; including immune-mediated events), respiratory failure (≥2%)

Frequency not defined:

Central nervous system: Migraine

Dermatologic: Palmar-plantar erythrodysesthesia

Endocrine & metabolic: Weight loss

Gastrointestinal: Abdominal distress

Neuromuscular & skeletal: Limb pain

<1%, postmarketing, and/or case reports: Demyelinating disease (immune-mediated), diabetic ketoacidosis, duodenitis (immune-mediated), encephalitis (limbic/lymphocytic/viral; may be immune-mediated), facial paralysis (immune-mediated), gastritis (immune-mediated), Guillain-Barré syndrome (immune-mediated), hepatic sinusoidal obstruction syndrome (formerly known as hepatic veno-occlusive disease), hypophysitis (including immune-mediated events), iritis (immune-mediated), lymphadenitis (immune-mediated; histiocytic necrotizing lymphadenitis [Kikuchi lymphadenitis]), motor dysfunction (immune-mediated), myasthenia (myasthenic syndrome; immune-mediated), myocarditis (immune-mediated), myositis (immune-mediated), neuropathy (autoimmune; immune-mediated), pancreatitis (immune-mediated), pituitary insufficiency (immune-mediated), pneumonia due to *Pneumocystis carinii*, polymyalgia rheumatica (immune-mediated), rhabdomyolysis (immune-mediated), sarcoidosis (immune-mediated), sepsis (systemic inflammatory response), sixth nerve palsy (abducens nerve palsy; immune-mediated), type I diabetes mellitus (immune-mediated event), uveitis (immune-mediated), vasculitis

Drug Interactions

Metabolism/Transport Effects None known.

Avoid Concomitant Use

Avoid concomitant use of Nivolumab with any of the following: Belimumab

Increased Effect/Toxicity

Nivolumab may increase the levels/effects of: Belimumab

Decreased Effect

The levels/effects of Nivolumab may be decreased by: Immunosuppressants

Storage/Stability Store intact vials at 2°C to 8°C (36°F to 46°F); do not freeze. Protect from light. Do not shake. After preparation in NS or D5W, store the infusion solution at room temperature for no more than 8 hours (including infusion time) or refrigerated at 2°C to 8°C (36°F to 46°F) for up to 24 hours (including infusion time). Infusion must be completed within 24 hours of preparation. Do not freeze solutions prepared for infusion.

Preparation for Administration Withdraw the required volume and transfer into an IV container. Dilute with either NS or D5W to a final concentration of 1 to 10 mg/mL. Mix by gentle inversion; do not shake.

Mechanism of Action

Nivolumab is a fully human immunoglobulin G4 (IgG4) monoclonal antibody that selectively inhibits programmed cell death-1 (PD-1) activity by binding to the PD-1 receptor to block the ligands PD-L1 and PD-L2 from binding. The negative PD-1 receptor signaling that regulates T-cell activation and proliferation is therefore disrupted (Robert 2015). This releases PD-1 pathway-mediated inhibition of the immune response, including the antitumor immune response.

Combining nivolumab (anti-PD-1) with ipilimumab (anti-CTLA-4) results in enhanced T-cell function that is greater than that of either antibody alone, resulting in improved anti-tumor responses in metastatic melanoma.

Pharmacodynamics/Kinetics

Distribution: V_{dss}: 6.8 L (single-agent); ~8 L (combination therapy with ipilimumab)

Half-life elimination: ~25 days (single-agent and combination therapy with ipilimumab)

Dosing

Adult & Geriatric

Colorectal cancer, metastatic (microsatellite instability-high or mismatch repair deficient): IV: 240 mg (flat dose) once every 2 weeks until disease progression or unacceptable toxicity

Off-label dosing: 3 **mg/kg** once every 2 weeks until disease progression or unacceptable toxicity (Overman 2017)

Head and neck cancer, squamous cell, recurrent or metastatic: IV: 3 mg/kg once every 2 weeks until disease progression or unacceptable toxicity (Ferris 2016).

Hodgkin lymphoma, classical: IV: 3 **mg/kg** once every 2 weeks until disease progression or unacceptable toxicity (Ansell 2015; Younes 2016).

Melanoma, unresectable or metastatic: IV: 240 **mg** (flat dose) once every 2 weeks (as a single agent) until disease progression or unacceptable toxicity

Off-label dosing: 3 **mg/kg** once every 2 weeks (as a single agent) until disease progression or unacceptable toxicity (Robert 2015; Weber 2015).

Melanoma, unresectable or metastatic, first-line combination therapy: IV: 1 **mg/kg** once every 3 weeks (in combination with ipilimumab) for 4 doses, followed by 240 **mg** (flat dose) once every 2 weeks (nivolumab monotherapy) until disease progression or unacceptable toxicity. **Note:** If nivolumab therapy is withheld, ipilimumab should also be withheld.

Off-label dosing: 1 **mg/kg** once every 3 weeks (in combination with ipilimumab) for 4 doses, followed by 3 **mg/kg** once every 2 weeks (nivolumab monotherapy) until disease progression or unacceptable toxicity (Larkin 2015).

Non-small cell lung cancer, metastatic, progressive: IV: 240 **mg** (flat dose) once every 2 weeks until disease progression or unacceptable toxicity.

Off-label dosing: 3 **mg/kg** once every 2 weeks until disease progression or unacceptable toxicity (Borghaei 2015; Brahmer 2015).

Renal cell cancer, advanced: IV: 240 **mg** (flat dose) once every 2 weeks until disease progression or unacceptable toxicity.

Off-label dosing: 3 **mg/kg** once every 2 weeks until disease progression or unacceptable toxicity (Motzer 2015).

◀ **Urothelial carcinoma (locally advanced or metastatic):** IV: 240 **mg** (flat dose) once every 2 weeks until disease progression or unacceptable toxicity.

Off-label dosing: 3 **mg/kg** once every 2 weeks until disease progression or unacceptable toxicity (Sharma 2017).

Small cell lung cancer, progressive (off-label use):

Single agent: IV: 3 **mg/kg** once every 2 weeks until disease progression or unacceptable toxicity (Antonia 2016).

Combination therapy: IV: 1 **mg/kg** once every 3 weeks (in combination with ipilimumab) for 4 doses, followed by 3 **mg/kg** once every 2 weeks (nivolumab monotherapy) until disease progression or unacceptable toxicity (Antonia 2016).

Pediatric Colorectal cancer, metastatic (microsatellite instability-high or mismatch repair deficient): Children ≥12 years and Adolescents: IV: 240 mg (flat dose) once every 2 weeks until disease progression or unacceptable toxicity

Renal Impairment

*Renal impairment **prior to** treatment initiation:* No dosage adjustment necessary.

*Renal toxicity **during** treatment:*

Creatinine >1.5 to 6 times ULN: Withhold treatment; administer corticosteroids (prednisone 0.5 to 1 mg/kg daily or equivalent) followed by a corticosteroid taper; may resume therapy upon recovery to grade 0 or 1 toxicity. If toxicity worsens or does not improve, increase corticosteroid dose to prednisone 1 to 2 mg/kg daily (or equivalent).

Creatinine >6 times ULN or life-threatening: Permanently discontinue; initiate high-dose systemic corticosteroids (prednisone 1 to 2 mg/kg daily or equivalent) followed by a corticosteroid taper.

Hepatic Impairment

*Hepatic impairment **prior to** treatment initiation:*

Mild impairment (total bilirubin ≤ ULN and AST > ULN or total bilirubin <1 to 1.5 times ULN and any AST): No dosage adjustment necessary.

Moderate (total bilirubin >1.5 to 3 times ULN and any AST) to severe (total bilirubin >3 times ULN and any AST) impairment: There are no dosage adjustments provided in the manufacturer's labeling (has not been studied).

*Hepatotoxicity **during** treatment:*

AST or ALT >3 to 5 times ULN or total bilirubin >1.5 to 3 times ULN: Withhold treatment; may resume therapy upon recovery to grade 0 or 1 toxicity.

AST or ALT >5 times ULN or total bilirubin >3 times ULN: Permanently discontinue.

Immune-mediated hepatitis:

Grade 2 transaminase elevations (with or without total bilirubin elevations): Withhold treatment and initiate high-dose systemic corticosteroids (prednisone 0.5 to 1 mg/kg daily or equivalent)

Severe (grade 3) or life-threatening (grade 4) transaminase elevations (with or without bilirubin elevations): Permanently discontinue treatment and initiate high-dose systemic corticosteroids (prednisone 1 to 2 mg/kg daily or equivalent)

Adjustment for Toxicity

Withhold treatment for any of the following (may resume upon recovery to grade 0 or 1 toxicity):

Note: If receiving combination therapy with ipilimumab, when nivolumab is withheld, ipilimumab should also be withheld.

Adrenal insufficiency (grade 2)

Colitis:

Grade 2 colitis or diarrhea; for grade 2 colitis with a duration >5 days; also administer systemic corticosteroids (prednisone 0.5 to 1 mg/kg daily or equivalent) followed by a corticosteroid taper; may increase to prednisone 1 to 2 mg/kg daily (or equivalent) if colitis worsens or does not improve despite corticosteroid use

Grade 3 colitis or diarrhea (single-agent nivolumab); also administer systemic corticosteroids (prednisone 1 to 2 mg/kg daily or equivalent) followed by a corticosteroid taper

Diabetes mellitus, type 1 (grade 3 hyperglycemia)

Encephalitis (new onset moderate or severe neurologic toxicity)

Hypophysitis (grade 2 or 3); also administer high-dose systemic corticosteroids (prednisone 1 mg/kg daily or equivalent)

Pneumonitis (grade 2); also administer high-dose systemic corticosteroids (prednisone 1 to 2 mg/kg daily or equivalent) followed by a corticosteroid taper

Rash (grade 3), suspected Stevens-Johnson syndrome or toxic epidermal necrolysis; also administer high-dose systemic corticosteroids (prednisone 1 to 2 mg/kg daily or equivalent)

Other immune mediated toxicities; also administer high-dose systemic corticosteroids followed by a corticosteroid taper (over 1 month)

Other treatment-related toxicity (severe or grade 3, first occurrence)

Permanently discontinue for:

Adrenal insufficiency (grade 3 or 4); also administer high-dose systemic corticosteroids (prednisone 1 to 2 mg/kg daily or equivalent)

Colitis or diarrhea (grade 3, if in combination with ipilimumab) or colitis or diarrhea (grade 4); also administer high-dose systemic corticosteroids (prednisone 1 to 2 mg/kg daily or equivalent) followed by a corticosteroid taper

Colitis (recurrent)

Diabetes mellitus, type 1 (grade 4 hyperglycemia)

Encephalitis (immune mediated); also administer high-dose systemic corticosteroids (prednisone 1 to 2 mg/kg daily or equivalent) followed by a corticosteroid taper

Hypophysitis (grade 4); also administer high-dose systemic corticosteroids (prednisone 1 mg/kg daily or equivalent)

Pneumonitis (grade 3 or 4); also administer high-dose systemic corticosteroids (prednisone 1 to 2 mg/kg daily or equivalent) followed by a corticosteroid taper

Rash (grade 4), or confirmed Stevens-Johnson syndrome or toxic epidermal necrolysis; also administer high-dose systemic corticosteroids (prednisone 1 to 2 mg/kg daily or equivalent)

Any toxicity requiring corticosteroid dose of prednisone ≥10 mg/day (or equivalent) for longer than 12 weeks.

Other adverse reactions that are life-threatening or grade 4, severe or grade 3 adverse reactions that recur, or persistent grade 2 or 3 treatment-related toxicity lasts beyond 12 weeks.

Infusion-related reaction:
Mild or moderate reaction: Interrupt or slow the infusion rate
Severe or life-threatening reaction: Discontinue

Thyroid disorder (hyperthyroidism or hypothyroidism):
There are no recommended dosage modifications. Initiate antithyroid therapy for hyperthyroidism; administer thyroid hormone replacement therapy for hypothyroidism.

Combination Regimens
Melanoma: Ipilimumab-Nivolumab (Melanoma) on page 2157

Administration
Administer as an IV infusion over 60 minutes through a line with a sterile, nonpyrogenic, low protein binding 0.2 to 1.2 micrometer in-line filter. Do not administer other medications through the same IV line. Flush IV line at the end of the infusion.

Combination therapy with ipilimumab: When administered in combination with ipilimumab, infuse nivolumab first followed by ipilimumab on the same day. Use separate infusion bags and filters for each infusion. If nivolumab therapy is withheld, ipilimumab should also be withheld.

Emetic Potential Minimal (<10%)

Monitoring Parameters Hepatic and renal function tests (baseline and periodic), thyroid function (baseline and periodically [eg, at treatment day 1 and every 6 weeks]); blood glucose. Monitor for signs/symptoms of adrenal insufficiency, hypophysitis, thyroid disorders, immune-mediated colitis, pneumonitis, rash/dermatologic toxicity, encephalitis (changes in neurologic function); monitor for infusion reactions.

Medication Guide Available Yes

Dosage Forms Excipient information presented when available (limited, particularly for generics); consult specific product labeling.
Solution, Intravenous [preservative free]:
Opdivo: 40 mg/4 mL (4 mL); 100 mg/10 mL (10 mL) [contains polysorbate 80]

◆ **Novo-Nidazol (Can)** *see* MetroNIDAZOLE (Systemic) *on page 1249*

◆ **Novo-Peridol (Can)** *see* Haloperidol *on page 903*

◆ **Novo-Purol (Can)** *see* Allopurinol *on page 94*

◆ **NovoSeven RT** *see* Factor VIIa (Recombinant) *on page 765*

◆ **Noxafil** *see* Posaconazole *on page 1536*

◆ **Nplate** *see* RomiPLOStim *on page 1638*

◆ **N-trifluoroacetyladriamycin-14-valerate** *see* Valrubicin *on page 1858*

◆ **Numoisyn** *see* Saliva Substitute *on page 1653*

◆ **Nu-Ondansetron (Can)** *see* Ondansetron *on page 1380*

◆ **Nu-Prochlor (Can)** *see* Prochlorperazine *on page 1563*

◆ **NutreStore** *see* Glutamine *on page 886*

◆ **Nuwiq** *see* Antihemophilic Factor (Recombinant) *on page 143*

◆ **NVP-LDE225** *see* Sonidegib *on page 1682*

◆ **Nyaderm (Can)** *see* Nystatin (Topical) *on page 1340*

◆ **Nyamyc** *see* Nystatin (Topical) *on page 1340*

◆ **Nyata** *see* Nystatin (Topical) *on page 1340*

Nystatin (Oral) (nye STAT in)

Brand Names: US Bio-Statin

Brand Names: Canada PMS-Nystatin

Pharmacologic Category Antifungal Agent, Oral Nonabsorbed/Partially Absorbed

Use Treatment of susceptible cutaneous, mucocutaneous, and oral cavity fungal infections normally caused by the *Candida* species

Pregnancy Risk Factor C

Dosing

Adult & Geriatric

Oral candidiasis: Suspension (swish and swallow): 400,000-600,000 units 4 times/day; swish in the mouth and retain for as long as possible (several minutes) before swallowing

Intestinal infections: Oral tablets: 500,000-1,000,000 units every 8 hours

Note: Powder for compounding: ⅛ teaspoon (500,000 units) to equal approximately ½ cup of water; give 4 times/day

Pediatric Oral candidiasis:

Suspension:

Premature infants: 100,000 units 4 times/day; paint suspension into recesses of the mouth

Infants: 200,000 units 4 times/day or 100,000 units to each side of mouth 4 times/day; paint suspension into recesses of the mouth

Children and Adolescents: 400,000 to 600,000 units 4 times/day; swish in the mouth and retain for as long as possible (several minutes) before swallowing

Powder for compounding: Children and Adolescents: Refer to adult dosing.

Renal Impairment There are no dosage adjustments provided in the manufacturer's labeling.

Hepatic Impairment There are no dosage adjustments provided in the manufacturer's labeling.

Additional Information Complete prescribing information should be consulted for additional detail.

◄ **Dosage Forms** Excipient information presented when available (limited, particularly for generics); consult specific product labeling. [DSC] = Discontinued product

Capsule, Oral [preservative free]:
  Bio-Statin: 500,000 units, 1,000,000 units [dye free]
Powder, Oral:
  Bio-Statin: (1 ea)
  Generic: (1 ea [DSC])
Suspension, Mouth/Throat:
  Generic: 100,000 units/mL (5 mL, 60 mL, 473 mL, 480 mL)
Tablet, Oral:
  Generic: 500,000 units

Nystatin (Topical) (nye STAT in)

Brand Names: US Nyamyc; Nyata; Nystop; Pedi-Dri [DSC]; Pediaderm AF Complete [DSC]

Brand Names: Canada Nyaderm; Ratio-Nystatin

Pharmacologic Category Antifungal Agent, Topical

Use Fungal infections (cutaneous and mucocutaneous): Treatment of cutaneous and mucocutaneous fungal infections caused by *Candida albicans* and other susceptible *Candida* species.

Pregnancy Risk Factor C

Dosing

Adult & Geriatric Fungal infections (cutaneous and mucocutaneous): Topical: **Note:** Cream is usually preferred to ointment for intertriginous areas; very moist lesions are best treated with topical powder

Cream, ointment: Apply to the affected areas twice daily or as indicated until healing is complete

Powder: Apply to the affected areas 2 to 3 times daily until healing is complete

Pediatric Fungal infections (cutaneous and mucocutaneous): Infants, Children, and Adolescents: Topical: Refer to adult dosing.

Renal Impairment There are no dosage adjustments provided in the manufacturer's labeling. However, dosage adjustment unlikely due to low systemic absorption

Hepatic Impairment There are no dosage adjustments provided in the manufacturer's labeling. However, dosage adjustment unlikely due to low systemic absorption

Additional Information Complete prescribing information should be consulted for additional detail.

Dosage Forms Considerations

Nyata Kit contains nystatin powder and Curatin exfoliating serum.

Pediaderm AF Complete Kit contains nystatin cream and Pediaderm Diaper Defense cream.

Dosage Forms Excipient information presented when available (limited, particularly for generics); consult specific product labeling. [DSC] = Discontinued product

Cream, External:
  Generic: 100,000 units/g (15 g, 30 g)
Kit, External:
  Nyata: 100,000 units/g [DSC]
  Pediaderm AF Complete: 100,000 units/g [DSC] [contains methylparaben, propylene glycol, propylparaben]

Ointment, External:
  Generic: 100,000 units/g (15 g, 30 g)
Powder, External:
  Nyamyc: 100,000 units/g (15 g, 30 g, 60 g)
  Nyata: 100,000 units/g (45 g)
  Nystop: 100,000 units/g (15 g, 30 g, 60 g)
  Pedi-Dri: 100,000 units/g (56.7 g [DSC])
  Generic: 100,000 units/g (15 g, 30 g, 60 g)

◆ **Nystop** see Nystatin (Topical) on page 1340
◆ **Oasis** see Saliva Substitute on page 1653

Obinutuzumab (oh bi nue TOOZ ue mab)

Related Information
  Management of Chemotherapy-Induced Nausea and Vomiting in Adults on page 2253
Brand Names: US Gazyva
Brand Names: Canada Gazyva
Index Terms GA101; R05072759; R7159
Pharmacologic Category Antineoplastic Agent, Anti-CD20; Antineoplastic Agent, Monoclonal Antibody
Use
Chronic lymphocytic leukemia: Treatment of patients with previously untreated chronic lymphocytic leukemia (CLL) in combination with chlorambucil
Follicular lymphoma: Treatment of follicular lymphoma (in combination with bendamustine followed by obinutuzumab monotherapy) in patients who relapsed after, or are refractory to, a rituximab-containing regimen.
Labeled Contraindications
  There are no contraindications listed in the manufacturer's US labeling.
  Canadian labeling: Known hypersensitivity (IgE mediated) to obinutuzumab or any component of the formulation.
Pregnancy Considerations Adverse effects were observed in animal reproduction studies. Monoclonal antibodies are known to cross the placenta. Based on the mechanism of action and on animal data, if exposure occurs during pregnancy, B-cell counts may be depleted and immunologic function may be affected in the neonate after birth. Administration of live vaccines to neonates and infants exposed in utero should be avoided until after B-cell recovery. It has been recommended that women of childbearing potential use effective contraception during therapy and for 18 months after the last treatment (Gazyva Canadian product labeling 2016).
Breastfeeding Considerations It is not known if obinutuzumab is present in breast milk. However, endogenous human immunoglobulin can be detected in milk. Although antibodies in breast milk may not enter the breastfed infant's circulations in substantial amounts, the manufacturer recommends the decision to breastfeed during therapy should take into account the risk of exposure to the infant and the benefits of treatment to the mother. Alternatively, it has been recommended to discontinue breastfeeding during therapy and for 18 months after the last treatment (Gazyva Canadian product labeling 2016).
Warnings/Precautions [US Boxed Warning]: Hepatitis B virus (HBV) reactivation may occur with use of CD20-directed cytolytic antibodies (including obinutuzumab) and may result in fulminant hepatitis, hepatic failure, and death. Screen all patients for HBV infection by measuring

◀ **hepatitis B surface antigen (HBsAg) and hepatitis B core antibody (anti-HBc) prior to therapy initiation; monitor patients for clinical and laboratory signs of hepatitis or HBV during and for several months after treatment. Discontinue obinutuzumab (and concomitant chemotherapy) if viral hepatitis develops** and initiate appropriate antiviral therapy. Reactivation has occurred in patients who are HBsAg positive as well as in those who are HBsAg negative but are anti-HBc positive; HBV reactivation has also been observed in patients who had previously resolved HBV infection. HBV reactivation has been reported for other CD20-directed antibodies after therapy discontinuation. Reactivation of HBV replication is often followed by hepatitis. Use cautiously in patients who show evidence of prior HBV infection (eg, HBsAg positive [regardless of antibody status] or HBsAG negative but anti-HBc positive); consult with appropriate clinicians regarding monitoring and consideration of antiviral therapy before and/or during obinutuzumab treatment. The safety of resuming obinutuzumab treatment following HBV reactivation is not known; discuss reinitiation of therapy in patients with resolved HBV reactivation with physicians experienced in HBV management. American Society of Clinical Oncology (ASCO) provisional clinical opinion update on HBV screening recommendations (Hwang 2015): Patients receiving anti-CD20 antibodies are at high risk for HBV reactivation. Screen for HBV infection with HBsAG and anti-HBc tests prior to treatment initiation; either a total anti-HBc (with both immunoglobulin [IgG] and immunoglobulin [IgM]) or anti-HBc IgG test should be used to screen for chronic or resolved HBV infection (do not use anti-HBc IgM as it may only confirm acute HBV infection). In addition, patients who have risk factors for HBV infection (eg, birthplace in a country with ≥2% HBV prevalence, household or sexual contact with HBV-infected patients, high-risk behaviors [eg, intravenous drug use], and HIV infection) should also be screened prior to beginning therapy. Initiate prophylactic antiviral therapy (utilizing antivirals with low rates of viral resistance) for HBsAg-positive/anti-HBc-positive patients (without delaying cancer therapy) and continue the antivirals during and for ~6 to 12 months after completing treatment. HBsAg-negative/anti-HBc-positive patients should be monitored for HBV reactivation with HBV DNA and ALT testing approximately every 3 months during treatment; antiviral therapy may be initiated prophylactically or begun promptly at the first sign of HBV reactivation.

[US Boxed Warning]: Progressive multifocal leukoencephalopathy (PML) resulting in death may occur with treatment. PML is due to JC virus infection. Consider PML in any patient with new onset or worsening neurological symptoms and if PML is suspected, discontinue obinutuzumab (consider discontinuation or dose reduction of any concomitant chemotherapy or immunosuppressive therapy) and evaluate promptly.

May cause severe and life-threatening infusion reactions; reactions may include bronchospasm, dyspnea, tachycardia, larynx and throat irritation, wheezing, laryngeal edema, flushing, hypertension, hypotension, fever, dizziness, nausea, vomiting, diarrhea, headache, fatigue, and/or chills. Infusion reactions occur more frequently with the first 1,000 mg infused. Delayed reactions (up to 24 hours later) and reactions with subsequent infusions have occurred. Premedicate with acetaminophen, an antihistamine, and an IV glucocorticoid (dexamethasone or methylprednisolone) prior to infusion. Hydrocortisone has not been effective in reducing the rate of infusion reactions and is not recommended). Infusion reactions may require rate reduction, interruption of therapy, or treatment discontinuation. Monitor during the entire infusion; monitor patients with preexisting cardiac or pulmonary conditions closely. Due to the risk for hypotension, consider temporarily withholding antihypertensive therapies for 12 hours prior to, during, and for 1 hour after administration. Administer in a facility with immediate access to resuscitative measures (eg, glucocorticoids, epinephrine, bronchodilators, and/or oxygen).

Severe and life-threatening (grade 3 and 4) neutropenia (including neutropenic fever) have been observed in clinical trials. Neutropenia may have a late onset (>28 days after therapy completion) and/or be prolonged (duration >28 days). Consider administration of granulocyte colony-stimulating factors in patients who develop grade 3 or 4 neutropenia. Monitor for signs/symptoms of infection; antimicrobial prophylaxis is recommended in neutropenic patients with severe neutropenia that lasts more than 1 week (continue prophylaxis until neutropenia improves to ≤ grade 2). Antiviral and/or antifungal prophylaxis should also be considered. Severe and life-threatening thrombocytopenia has also been reported when used in combination with chlorambucil or bendamustine. In a small percentage of patients, thrombocytopenia occurred acutely (within 24 hours) after obinutuzumab administration; platelet transfusions may be necessary. Fatal hemorrhagic events during the first cycle of therapy for CLL have been reported; monitor frequently for thrombocytopenia and bleeding episodes, particularly during the initial cycle. Thrombocytopenia may require dose delays of obinutuzumab and chemotherapy and/or dose reductions of chemotherapy. Consider withholding platelet inhibitors, anticoagulants, or other medications which may increase bleeding risk (especially during the first cycle). Leukopenia, lymphopenia, and anemia commonly occur. Monitor blood counts frequently throughout therapy. Bacterial, fungal, and new or reactivated viral infections may occur during and/or following therapy; fatal infections have been reported. Do not administer to patients with an active infection. Patients with a history of recurrent or chronic infections may be at increased risk. Tumor lysis syndrome (TLS) has been reported with obinutuzumab (some cases fatal). Acute renal failure, hyperkalemia, hypocalcemia, hyperuricemia, and/or hyperphosphatemia may occur. Administer prophylaxis (antihyperuricemic therapy [eg, allopurinol or rasburicase] and hydration) in patients at high risk (high circulating lymphocyte counts [>25,000/mm^3], high tumor burden, or renal impairment) prior to initiating obinutuzumab therapy (administer prior to each subsequent cycle if needed). Monitor lab parameters during initial treatment days in patients at risk for TLS. Correct electrolyte abnormalities; monitor renal function and hydration status, and administer supportive care, including dialysis as indicated. Administration of live virus vaccines during treatment (and until B-cell recovery) is not recommended; the safety and efficacy of immunization with live or attenuated viral vaccines during or after obinutuzumab therapy has not been determined. If obinutuzumab exposure occurs during pregnancy, the safety and timing of live virus vaccinations for the infant should be evaluated. Potentially significant drug-drug interactions may exist, requiring dose or frequency adjustment, additional monitoring, and/or selection of alternative therapy.

Adverse Reactions Adverse reactions reported in combination with chlorambucil or bendamustine in addition to reaction incidence during the monotherapy phase.

>10%:

Endocrine & metabolic: Hypophosphatemia (25% to 41%), hypocalcemia (37% to 38%;), hyperkalemia (33%), hyponatremia (26%), hypoalbumine-mia (23%), hypokalemia (14%)

Gastrointestinal: Constipation (8% to 19%), vomiting

Hematologic & oncologic: Lymphocytopenia (80% to 99%; grades 3/4: 39% to 93%), leukopenia (6% to 86%; grades 3/4: 4% to 47%), neutropenia (11% to 76%; grades 3/4: 10% to 52%; onset ≥28 days after completion of treatment: 16%; lasting ≥28 days: 3%), decreased hemoglobin (50%), thrombocytopenia (11% to 48%; grades 3/4: 1% to 13% onset within 24 hours of infusion: 4%), anemia (12% to 39%; grades 3/4: 1% to 10%), hemorrhage (11%; grades 3/4: 5%)

Hepatic: Increased serum AST (24% to 27%), increased serum ALT (21% to 35%), increased serum alkaline phosphatase (18%)

Infection: Infection (38% to 66%)

Neuromuscular & skeletal: Musculoskeletal signs and symptoms (18% to 41%; including pain), back pain (5%), arthralgia (7% to 12%), weakness (11%)

Renal: Decreased creatinine clearance (43% to 58%), increased serum creatinine (30%)

Respiratory: Cough (10% to 26%), upper respiratory tract infection (12% to 13%), sinusitis (10% to 12%)

1% to 10%:

Central nervous system: Fatigue (8%)

Dermatologic: Pruritus (9%)

Gastrointestinal: Diarrhea (8% to 10%), nausea (8%), dyspepsia (5%)

Genitourinary: Urinary tract infection (5% to 10%)

Hematologic & oncologic: Tumor lysis syndrome, febrile neutropenia

Hepatic: Increased liver enzymes (4%; may be secondary or exacerbated by premedications)

Immunologic: Antibody development (1% to 7%)

Infection: Sepsis

Neuromuscular & skeletal: Limb pain (9%), back pain (5%)

Respiratory: Nasopharyngitis (6% to 9%), bronchitis (7%), nasal congestion (7%)

Miscellaneous: Infusion related reaction (initial infusion: 53% to 69%; grades 3/4: 9% to 20%; second infusion: 3% to 25%; subsequent infusions: ≤8%), fever (6% to 18%)

Frequency Not Defined:

Cardiovascular: Exacerbation of cardiac disease

Central nervous system: Progressive multifocal leukoencephalopathy

Infection: JCV (John Cunningham virus) infection, reactivation of HBV, viral infection (new or reactivation)

Drug Interactions

Metabolism/Transport Effects None known.

Avoid Concomitant Use

Avoid concomitant use of Obinutuzumab with any of the following: BCG (Intravesical); Belimumab; Deferiprone; Dipyrone; Natalizumab; Pimecrolimus; Tacrolimus (Topical); Vaccines (Live)

Increased Effect/Toxicity

Obinutuzumab may increase the levels/effects of: Amifostine; Antipsychotic Agents (Second Generation [Atypical]); Belimumab; Blood Pressure

Lowering Agents; Deferiprone; DULoxetine; Fingolimod; Leflunomide; Natalizumab; Pholcodine; Tofacitinib; Vaccines (Live)

The levels/effects of Obinutuzumab may be increased by: Agents with Antiplatelet Properties; Alfuzosin; Anticoagulants; Barbiturates; Benperidol; Brimonidine (Topical); Denosumab; Diazoxide; Dipyrone; Herbs (Hypotensive Properties); Lormetazepam; Molsidomine; Naftopidil; Nicergoline; Nicorandil; Ocrelizumab; Pentoxifylline; Phosphodiesterase 5 Inhibitors; Pimecrolimus; Prostacyclin Analogues; Quinagolide; Roflumilast; Tacrolimus (Topical); Trastuzumab

Decreased Effect

Obinutuzumab may decrease the levels/effects of: BCG (Intravesical); Coccidioides immitis Skin Test; Nivolumab; Sipuleucel-T; Tertomotide; Vaccines (Inactivated); Vaccines (Live)

The levels/effects of Obinutuzumab may be decreased by: Echinacea

Storage/Stability Store intact vials at 2°C to 8°C (36°F to 46°F); do not freeze or shake. Protect from light. Solutions diluted in NS for infusion should be used immediately. If not used immediately, the diluted solutions may be stored up to 24 hours at 2°C to 8°C (36°F to 46°F) followed by 48 hours (including infusion time) at room temperature of ≤30°C (≤86°F).

Preparation for Administration

Chronic lymphocytic leukemia:

Cycle 1, day 1 and 2 doses (100 mg and 900 mg, respectively): Withdraw 40 mL of obinutuzumab solution from vial. Dilute 4 mL into a 100 mL infusion bag of NS (100 mg dose; use immediately). Dilute remaining 36 mL into a 250 mL NS infusion bag (900 mg dose, for use on day 2); store at 2°C to 8°C (36°F to 46°F) for up to 24 hours; use immediately after reaching room temperature. Gently invert to mix; do not shake or freeze.

Cycle 1 (day 8 and 15 doses) and cycles 2 through 6 (1,000 mg): Withdraw 40 mL of obinutuzumab solution from vial. Dilute into a 250 mL NS infusion bag. Gently invert to mix; do not shake or freeze.

Do not use other diluents (eg, dextrose) to prepare the infusion. Final concentration for administration should be 0.4 to 4 mg/mL. May use PVC or non-PVC infusion bags.

Follicular lymphoma (1,000 mg): Withdraw 40 mL of obinutuzumab solution from vial. Dilute into a 250 mL NS infusion bag. Gently invert to mix; do not shake or freeze.

Do not use other diluents (eg, dextrose) to prepare the infusion. Final concentration for administration should be 0.4 to 4 mg/mL. May use PVC or non-PVC infusion bags.

Mechanism of Action Obinutuzumab is a glycoengineered type II anti-CD20 monoclonal antibody. The CD20 antigen is expressed on the surface of pre B- and mature B-lymphocytes; upon binding to CD20, obinutuzumab activates complement-dependent cytotoxicity, antibody-dependent cellular cytotoxicity and antibody-dependent cellular phagocytosis, resulting in cell death (Sehn 2012).

Pharmacodynamics/Kinetics

Distribution: V_d: ~4.1 to 4.3 L

Half-life elimination: ~26.4 to 36.8 days

Dosing

Adult & Geriatric Note: Premedication with acetaminophen, an antihistamine, and a glucocorticoid (dexamethasone or methylprednisolone) 30 to 60 minutes prior to treatment may be necessary (see Administration).

Antihyperuricemic prophylaxis and adequate hydration are recommended for patients at high risk for tumor lysis syndrome. Antimicrobial, antiviral, and antifungal prophylaxis may be considered in certain patients.

Chronic lymphocytic leukemia (CLL): IV:

Cycle 1: 100 mg on day 1, followed by 900 mg on day 2, followed by 1,000 mg weekly for 2 doses (days 8 and 15)

Cycles 2 through 6: 1,000 mg on day 1 every 28 days for 5 doses

Missed doses: Administer the missed dose as soon as possible; adjust dosing schedule accordingly. In some cases, patients who do not complete the day 1 cycle 1 dose may proceed to the day 2 cycle 1 treatment (if appropriate).

Follicular lymphoma: IV: **Note:** Patients with stable disease, complete response, or partial response after 6 cycles of combination therapy with obinutuzumab and bendamustine should continue on obinutuzumab monotherapy for 2 years.

Cycle 1 (in combination with bendamustine): 1,000 mg weekly for 3 doses on day 1, day 8, and day 15

Cycles 2 through 6 (in combination with bendamustine): 1,000 mg on day 1 every 28 days for 5 doses

Obinutuzumab monotherapy: 1,000 mg once every 2 months for 2 years

Missed doses: Administer the missed dose as soon as possible; adjust dosing schedule accordingly. During obinutuzumab monotherapy, maintain the original dosing schedule for subsequent doses.

Renal Impairment

CrCl ≥30 mL/minute: There are no dosage adjustments provided in the manufacturer's labeling; however, dosage adjustment is not likely necessary as pharmacokinetics are not affected.

CrCl <30 mL/minute: There are no dosage adjustments provided in the manufacturer's labeling (has not been studied)

Hepatic Impairment There are no dosage adjustments provided in the manufacturer's labeling (has not been studied)

Adjustment for Toxicity

Hematologic:

Grade 3 or 4 neutropenia: Consider treatment interruption and use of granulocyte colony-stimulating factors. In patients with severe and long-lasting (>1 week) neutropenia, antimicrobial prophylaxis is recommended until neutropenia improves to grade 1 or 2.

Grade 3 or 4 thrombocytopenia: Consider treatment interruption.

Infusion reactions:

Mild to moderate (Grades 1 and 2): Reduce infusion rate or interrupt infusion and manage symptoms as appropriate. Upon symptom resolution, continue or resume infusion. If no further infusion reaction symptoms occur, may resume infusion rate escalation as appropriate for the treatment cycle dose. For CLL only, day 1 (cycle 1) infusion rate may be increased back up to a maximum of 25 mg/hour after 1 hour.

Severe (Grade 3): Interrupt therapy; manage symptoms as appropriate. Upon symptom resolution, may reinitiate infusion at no more than 50% of the rate at which the reaction occurred. If no further infusion reaction symptoms occur, may resume infusion rate escalation as appropriate for the treatment cycle dose. For CLL only, day 1 (cycle 1) infusion rate may be increased back up to a maximum of 25 mg/hour after 1 hour. Permanently discontinue if ≥ grade 3 infusion-related symptoms occur upon rechallenge.

Life-threatening (Grade 4): Discontinue infusion immediately; permanently discontinue therapy.

Infection: Consider treatment interruption.

Other toxicity: Consider treatment interruption for ≥ grade 2 nonhematologic toxicity.

Combination Regimens

Leukemia, chronic lymphocytic: Chlorambucil-Obinutuzumab (CLL) on page 2034

Lymphoma, non-Hodgkin (Follicular): Bendamustine-Obinutuzumab (NHL-Follicular) on page 1986

Administration For IV infusion only. Do not administer IV push or as a bolus. Administer through a dedicated IV line; do not mix with or infuse with other medications. May use PVC or non-PVC administration sets. Premedication with acetaminophen, an antihistamine, and a glucocorticoid (dexamethasone or methylprednisolone) may be required to prevent infusion reactions (see below). In patients with severe (grade 3 or 4) neutropenia lasting more than 1 week, antimicrobial prophylaxis is strongly recommended (continue until neutropenia resolves to grade 1 or 2); antiviral and antifungal prophylaxis should be considered.

Premedication to prevent infusion reactions:

Chronic lymphocytic leukemia (CLL) (cycle 1 [days 1 and 2]) and follicular lymphoma (FL) (day 1): All patients should receive acetaminophen (650 to 1,000 mg) and an antihistamine (eg, diphenhydramine 50 mg) at least 30 minutes prior to infusion. In addition, an IV glucocorticoid (dexamethasone 20 mg or methylprednisolone 80 mg) should be administered at least 1 hour prior to infusion.

All subsequent infusions: All patients should receive acetaminophen 650 to 1,000 mg at least 30 minutes prior to infusion.

If patients experienced grade 1 or 2 infusion-related reaction with previous infusion: Administer an antihistamine (eg, diphenhydramine 50 mg) in addition to acetaminophen at least 30 minutes prior to infusion.

If patients experienced a grade 3 infusion-related reaction with previous infusion **or** have a lymphocyte count >25,000 cells/mm^3 prior to next treatment: Administer an IV glucocorticoid (dexamethasone 20 mg or methylprednisolone 80 mg) at least 1 hour prior to infusion, in addition to acetaminophen and an antihistamine at least 30 minutes prior to infusion.

Infusion rate:

CLL:

Cycle 1 (day 1): Infuse at 25 mg/hour over 4 hours; do not increase the infusion rate

Cycle 1 (day 2): If no reaction to previous infusion, initiate infusion at 50 mg/hour for 30 minutes; if tolerated, may escalate rate in increments of 50 mg/hour every 30 minutes to a maximum rate of 400 mg/hour.

Cycle 1 (days 8 and 15), and cycles 2 through 6: If no reaction to previous infusion and the final infusion rate was 100 mg/hour or faster, initiate infusion at 100 mg/hour for 30 minutes; if tolerated, may escalate infusion rate in increments of 100 mg/hour every 30 minutes to a maximum rate of 400 mg/hour.

FL:

Cycle 1 (day 1): Initiate infusion at 50 mg/hour; if tolerated, may escalate rate in increments of 50 mg/hour every 30 minutes to a maximum rate of 400 mg/hour.

◄ *All subsequent infusions:* If no reaction to previous infusion and the final infusion rate was 100 mg/hour or faster, initiate infusion at 100 mg/hour for 30 minutes; if tolerated, may escalate rate in increments of 100 mg/hour every 30 minutes to a maximum rate of 400 mg/hour.

Emetic Potential Minimal (<10%)

Monitoring Parameters

CBC with differential (at regular intervals), renal function, electrolytes, uric acid (if at risk for tumor lysis syndrome); hepatitis B screening in all patients (HBsAG and anti-HBc measurements) prior to therapy initiation. Hepatitis B virus (HBV) screening recommendations (American Society of Clinical Oncology provisional clinical opinion update [Hwang 2015]): Screen for HBV infection with hepatitis B surface antigen (HBsAG) and hepatitis B core antibody (anti-HBc) tests prior to treatment initiation; either a total anti-HBc (with both immunoglobulin G [IgG] and immunoglobulin M [IgM]) or anti-HBc IgG test should be used to screen for chronic or resolved HBV infection (do not use anti-HBc IgM as it may only confirm acute HBV infection). HBsAg-negative/anti-HBc–positive patients should be monitored for HBV reactivation with HBV DNA and ALT testing approximately every 3 months during treatment.

Monitor for signs of active hepatitis B infection (during and for up to 12 months after therapy completion). Monitor for signs or symptoms of infusion reaction; signs of infection; fluid status; signs/symptoms of progressive multifocal leukoencephalopathy (PML; focal neurologic deficits, which may present as hemiparesis, visual field deficits, cognitive impairment, aphasia, ataxia, and/or cranial nerve deficits); evaluate for PML with brain MRI, lumbar puncture, and neurologist consultation.

Dosage Forms Excipient information presented when available (limited, particularly for generics); consult specific product labeling.

Solution, Intravenous [preservative free]:

Gazyva: 1000 mg/40 mL (40 mL)

◆ **Obizur** *see* Antihemophilic Factor (Recombinant [Porcine Sequence]) *on page 151*

◆ **Ocphyl (Can)** *see* Octreotide *on page 1348*

◆ **Octacog Alfa** *see* Antihemophilic Factor (Recombinant) *on page 143*

◆ **Octagam** *see* Immune Globulin *on page 992*

◆ **Octagam 10% (Can)** *see* Immune Globulin *on page 992*

◆ **Octostim (Can)** *see* Desmopressin *on page 573*

◆ **OctreoScan®** *see* Indium In-111 Pentetreotide *on page 1002*

◆ **OctreoScan® (Prep Kit)** *see* Indium In-111 Pentetreotide *on page 1002*

Octreotide (ok TREE oh tide)

Related Information

Management of EGFR Inhibitor Toxicities: Dermatologic, Ocular, and Gastrointestinal *on page 2291*

Brand Names: US SandoSTATIN; SandoSTATIN LAR Depot

Brand Names: Canada Ocphyl; Octreotide Acetate Omega; Octreotide Injection; Sandostatin; Sandostatin LAR

Index Terms Longastatin; Octreotide Acetate

Pharmacologic Category Antidiarrheal; Antidote; Somatostatin Analog

Use
Acromegaly:

Injection solution: To reduce blood levels of growth hormone (GH) and insulin-like growth factor 1 (IGF-1) in patients with inadequate response to or who cannot be treated with surgical resection, pituitary irradiation, and bromocriptine mesylate at maximally tolerated doses; goal of therapy is to achieve normalization of GH and IGF-1 levels.

LAR depot suspension: Long-term maintenance treatment of acromegaly in patients with an inadequate response to surgery and/or radiotherapy (or for whom surgery/radiotherapy are not options) with a goal of therapy to reduce GH and IGF-1 levels to normal.

Carcinoid tumors:

Injection solution: Management of symptoms (diarrhea and flushing) in patients with metastatic carcinoid tumors.

LAR depot suspension: Long-term treatment of severe diarrhea and flushing episodes associated with metastatic carcinoid tumors.

Vasoactive intestinal peptide-secreting tumors:

Injection solution: Treatment of profuse watery diarrhea associated with vasoactive intestinal peptide-secreting tumors (VIPomas).

LAR depot suspension: Long-term treatment of profuse watery diarrhea associated with VIPomas.

Limitations of use: The effects of octreotide (injection solution and LAR depot suspension) on tumor size, rate of growth, and development of metastases in patients with carcinoid syndrome and VIPomas have not been determined.

Labeled Contraindications Hypersensitivity to octreotide or any component of the formulation

Pregnancy Considerations Adverse events have not been observed in animal reproduction studies. Octreotide crosses the placenta and can be detected in the newborn at delivery (Caron 1995; Fassnacht 2001; Maffei 2010); data concerning use in pregnancy is limited. In case reports of acromegalic women who received normal doses of octreotide during pregnancy, no congenital malformations were reported. Because normalization of IGF-1 and GH may restore fertility in women with acromegaly, women of childbearing potential should use adequate contraception during treatment. Long-acting formulations should be discontinued ~2 months prior to a planned pregnancy, use short acting octreotide as needed until conception. Octreotide therapy may be considered in pregnant women with worsening symptoms if needed. Monitoring of IGF-1 and/or GH is not recommended during pregnancy (Katznelson 2014).

Breastfeeding Considerations Octreotide is excreted in breast milk. In a case report, a woman was taking octreotide SubQ in doses up to 2400 mcg/day prior to and throughout pregnancy. Octreotide was measurable in the colostrum in concentrations similar to those in the maternal serum (Maffei 2010); however, oral absorption of octreotide is considered to be poor (Battershill, 1989). The manufacturer recommends that caution be exercised when administering octreotide to nursing women.

Warnings/Precautions May impair gallbladder function; monitor patients for cholelithiasis. The incidence of gallbladder stone or biliary sludge increases with a duration of therapy of ≥12 months. Prophylactic cholecystectomy is recommended in patients with gastrointestinal or pancreatic neuroendocrine tumors undergoing abdominal surgery if octreotide treatment is planned (Oberg 2004). Use with caution in patients with renal and/or hepatic impairment; dosage adjustment may be required in patients receiving dialysis and in patients with established cirrhosis. Somatostatin analogs may affect glucose regulation. In type I diabetes, severe hypoglycemia may occur; in type II diabetes or patients without diabetes, hyperglycemia may occur. Insulin and other hypoglycemic medication requirements may change. Octreotide may worsen hypoglycemia in patients with insulinomas; use with caution. Do not use depot formulation for the treatment of sulfonylurea-induced hypoglycemia (Dougherty 2010). Bradycardia, conduction abnormalities, and arrhythmia have been observed in acromegalic and carcinoid syndrome patients; use caution with CHF or concomitant medications that alter heart rate or rhythm. Cardiovascular medication requirements may change. Octreotide may enhance the adverse/toxic effects of other QTc-prolonging agents. May alter absorption of dietary fats; monitor for pancreatitis. May reduce excessive fluid loss in patients with conditions that cause such loss; monitor for elevations in zinc levels in such patients that are maintained on total parenteral nutrition (TPN). Chronic treatment has been associated with abnormal Schillings test; monitor vitamin B_{12} levels. Suppresses secretion of TSH; monitor for hypothyroidism.

Postmarketing cases of serious and fatal events, including hypoxia and necrotizing enterocolitis, have been reported with octreotide use in children (usually with serious underlying conditions), particularly in children <2 years of age. In studies with octreotide depot, the incidence of cholelithiasis in children is higher than the reported incidences for adults and efficacy was not demonstrated. Therapy may restore fertility; females of childbearing potential should use adequate contraception. Dosage adjustment may be necessary in the elderly; significant increases in elimination half-life have been observed in older adults. Mild to moderate injection-site pain (usually lasting 1 hour) may occur with the depot formulation. Vehicle used in depot injection (polylactide-co-glycolide microspheres) has rarely been associated with retinal artery occlusion in patients with abnormal arteriovenous anastomosis. Therapy with immediate release octreotide (solution) should be withheld 24 hours prior to administration of radiolabeled somatostatin analogs; the IM (depot) formulation should be withheld at least 2 months before administration of radiolabeled somatostatin analogs (Oberg 2004). Potentially significant drug-drug interactions may exist, requiring dose or frequency adjustment, additional monitoring, and/or selection of alternative therapy.

Adverse Reactions Adverse reactions vary by route of administration and dosage form. Frequency of cardiac, endocrine, and gastrointestinal adverse reactions was generally higher in patients with acromegaly.

>10%:

Cardiovascular: Sinus bradycardia (19% to 25%), chest pain (≤20%; non-depot formulations), palpitations (5% to 15%), peripheral edema (5% to 15%), hypertension (≤13%)

Central nervous system: Fatigue (1% to 32%), headache (6% to 30%), malaise (16% to 20%), dizziness (5% to 20%), anxiety (5% to 15%), confusion (5% to 15%), hypoesthesia (5% to 15%), insomnia (5% to 15%), paresthesia (5% to 15%), rigors (5% to 15%), pain (4% to 15%)

Dermatologic: Pruritus (≤18%), skin rash (15%; depot formulation), diaphoresis (5% to 15%), alopecia (≤13%)

Endocrine & metabolic: Hyperglycemia (2% to 27%), hypothyroidism (≤12%; non-depot formulations)

Gastrointestinal: Diarrhea (34% to 61%), abdominal pain (5% to 61%), loose stools (5% to 61%), nausea (5% to 61%), flatulence (≤38%), cholelithiasis (13% to 38%; length of therapy-dependent), gallbladder sludge (24%; length of therapy-dependent), constipation (9% to 21%), vomiting (4% to 21%), biliary obstruction (duct dilatation: 12%), anorexia (5% to 15%), abdominal cramps (5% to 15%)

Hematologic & oncologic: Anemia (≤15%; non-depot formulations: <1%)

Hypersensitivity: Hypersensitivity reaction (5% to 15%)

Immunologic: Antibody development (≤25%; to octreotide; no efficacy change)

Local: Pain at injection site (2% to 50%; formulation-related)

Neuromuscular & skeletal: Back pain (1% to 27%), arthropathy (8% to 19%), myalgia (≤18%), arthralgia (1% to 15%), weakness (5% to 15%)

Otic: Otalgia (5% to 15%)

Renal: Nephrolithiasis (5% to 15%)

Respiratory: Upper respiratory tract infection (10% to 23%), dyspnea (≤20%; non-depot formulations), flu-like symptoms (1% to 20%), cough (5% to 15%), pharyngitis (5% to 15%), rhinitis (5% to 15%), sinusitis (5% to 15%)

Miscellaneous: Fever (16% to 20%)

1% to 10%:

Cardiovascular: Cardiac conduction disturbance (9% to 10%), cardiac arrhythmia (3% to 9%), angina pectoris (1% to 4%), cardiac failure (1% to 4%), edema (1% to 4%), flushing (1% to 4%), phlebitis (1% to 4%)

Central nervous system: Abnormal gait (1% to 4%), amnesia (1% to 4%), depression (1% to 4%), drowsiness (1% to 4%), hallucination (1% to 4%), hypertonia (1% to 4%), nervousness (1% to 4%), neuralgia (1% to 4%), neuropathy (1% to 4%), vertigo (1% to 4%), voice disorder (1% to 4%)

Dermatologic: Acne vulgaris (1% to 4%), cellulitis (1% to 4%)

Endocrine & metabolic: Goiter (≤8%; non-depot formulations), hypoglycemia (2% to 4%), albuminuria (1% to 4%), hypokalemia (1% to 4%), gout (1% to 4%), cachexia (1% to 4%)

Gastrointestinal: Dyspepsia (4% to 6%), fecal discoloration (4% to 6%), steatorrhea (4% to 6%), tenesmus (4% to 6%), colitis (1% to 4%), diverticulitis (1% to 4%), dysgeusia (1% to 4%), dysphagia (1% to 4%), gastritis (1% to 4%), gastroenteritis (1% to 4%), gingivitis (1% to 4%), glossitis (1% to 4%), malabsorption (fat: 1% to 4%), melena (1% to 4%), stomatitis (1% to 4%), xerostomia (1% to 4%)

Genitourinary: Impotence (1% to 4%), mastalgia (1% to 4%), pollakiuria (1% to 4%; non-depot formulations), urinary incontinence (1% to 4%), urinary tract infection (1% to 4%)

Hematologic & oncologic: Bruise (1% to 4%), hematoma (1% to 4%), hypoproteinemia (1% to 4%)

Infection: Abscess (renal: 1% to 4%), bacterial infection (1% to 4%), candidiasis (1% to 4%), cold symptoms (1% to 4%)

Local: Hematoma at injection site (1% to 4%)

Neuromuscular & skeletal: Hyperkinesia (1% to 4%), tremor (1% to 4%)

Ophthalmic: Blurred vision (1% to 4%), visual disturbance (1% to 4%)

Otic: Tinnitus (1% to 4%)

Respiratory: Bronchitis (1% to 4%), epistaxis (1% to 4%)

<1%, postmarketing, and/or case reports: Adrenocortical insufficiency, amenorrhea, anaphylactic shock, anaphylactoid reaction, aneurysm, aphasia, appendicitis, arthritis, ascites, atrial fibrillation, basal cell carcinoma, Bell's palsy, biliary obstruction, breast carcinoma, cardiac failure, cerebrovascular disease, cholangitis (ascending), cholecystitis, cholestatic hepatitis,

cyanocobalamin deficiency, deafness, decreased libido, diabetes insipidus, diabetes mellitus, erythema (with wheal), facial edema, galactorrhea, gastrointestinal hemorrhage, gastrointestinal ulcer, glaucoma, gynecomastia, hematuria, hemiparesis, hemorrhoids, hepatitis, hyperesthesia, hypoxia (children), increased creatine phosphokinase, increased intraocular pressure, increased liver enzymes, increased serum creatinine, intestinal obstruction, intracranial hemorrhage, iron deficiency, ischemia, jaundice, joint effusion, liver steatosis, malignant hyperthermia, menstrual disease (polymenorrhea), migraine, myocardial infarction, necrotizing enterocolitis (neonates), nephrolithiasis, neuritis, nodule (pulmonary), oligomenorrhea, orthostatic hypotension, pancreatitis, pancytopenia, paranoia, paresis, petechia, pituitary apoplexy, pleural effusion, pneumonia, pneumothorax, polyp (gallbladder), prolonged Q-T interval on ECG, pulmonary embolism, pulmonary hypertension, Raynaud's phenomenon, rectal hemorrhage, renal failure, renal insufficiency, scotoma, seizure, status asthmaticus, syncope, tachycardia, thrombocytopenia, thrombophlebitis, thrombosis (including retinal vein), urticaria, vaginitis, visual field defect, weight loss

Drug Interactions

Metabolism/Transport Effects None known.

Avoid Concomitant Use

Avoid concomitant use of Octreotide with any of the following: Ceritinib

Increased Effect/Toxicity

Octreotide may increase the levels/effects of: Bradycardia-Causing Agents; Bromocriptine; Ceritinib; Codeine; Highest Risk QTc-Prolonging Agents; Hypoglycemia-Associated Agents; Ivabradine; Lacosamide; Moderate Risk QTc-Prolonging Agents; Pegvisomant

The levels/effects of Octreotide may be increased by: Androgens; Antidiabetic Agents; Bretylium; Herbs (Hypoglycemic Properties); MAO Inhibitors; MiFEPRIStone; Pegvisomant; Prothionamide; Quinolone Antibiotics; Ruxolitinib; Salicylates; Selective Serotonin Reuptake Inhibitors; Tofacitinib

Decreased Effect

Octreotide may decrease the levels/effects of: Antidiabetic Agents; CycloSPORINE (Systemic); Gallium Ga 68 Dotatate; Telotristat Ethyl

The levels/effects of Octreotide may be decreased by: Quinolone Antibiotics

Food Interactions Octreotide may alter absorption of dietary fats. Management: Administer injections between meals to decrease GI effects.

Storage/Stability

Injection solution: Octreotide is a clear solution and should be stored at refrigerated temperatures between 2°C and 8°C (36°F and 46°F). Protect from light. May be stored at room temperature of 20°C to 30°C (68°F and 86°F) for up to 14 days when protected from light. Stable as a parenteral admixture in NS or D5W for 24 hours. Discard multidose vials within 14 days after initial entry.

LAR depot suspension: Prior to dilution, store at refrigerated temperatures between 2°C and 8°C (36°F and 46°F). Protect from light. Additionally, the manufacturer reports that octreotide suspension may be stored at room temperature of 20°C to 25°C (68°F and 77°F) for up to 10 days when protected from light (data on file [Novartis 2011]). Depot drug product kit may be at room temperature for 30 to 60 minutes prior to use. Use suspension immediately after preparation.

Preparation for Administration

IV infusion: Dilute injection solution in 50 to 200 mL NS or D5W

IM depot: Allow vial and provided diluent-filled syringe to reach room temperature slowly (approximately 30 to 60 minutes). Reconstitute with provided diluent; refer to product labeling for detailed mixing instructions.

Mechanism of Action

Mimics natural somatostatin by inhibiting serotonin release, and the secretion of gastrin, VIP, insulin, glucagon, secretin, motilin, and pancreatic polypeptide. Decreases growth hormone and IGF-1 in acromegaly. Octreotide provides more potent inhibition of growth hormone, glucagon, and insulin as compared to endogenous somatostatin. Also suppresses LH response to GnRH, secretion of thyroid-stimulating hormone and decreases splanchnic blood flow.

Pharmacodynamics/Kinetics

Duration: SubQ: 6 to 12 hours; when using Sandostatin LAR Depot formulation, steady-state levels are achieved after 3 injections (3 months of therapy)

Absorption: SubQ: Rapid and complete; IM (depot formulation): Released slowly (via microsphere degradation in the muscle)

Distribution: V_d: 14 L (21.6 ± 8.5 L in acromegaly)

Protein binding: 65%, primarily to lipoprotein (41% in acromegaly)

Metabolism: Extensively hepatic

Bioavailability: SubQ: 100%; IM: 60% to 63% of SubQ dose

Half-life elimination: 1.7 to 1.9 hours; Increased in elderly patients; Cirrhosis: Up to 3.7 hours; Fatty liver disease: Up to 3.4 hours; Renal impairment: Up to 3.1 hours

Time to peak, plasma: SubQ: 0.4 hours (0.7 hours acromegaly); IM: 1 hour

Excretion: Urine (32% as unchanged drug)

Clearance: Adults: 10 L/hour; Adults with acromegaly: 18 L/hour

Dosing

Adult

Acromegaly:

SubQ, IV: Initial: 50 mcg 3 times/day; titrate to achieve growth hormone levels <5 ng/mL or IGF-I (somatomedin C) levels <1.9 units/mL in males and <2.2 units/mL in females. Usual effective dose: 100 mcg 3 times/day; range: 300 to 1,500 mcg/day. Doses above 300 mcg/day rarely result in additional benefit; if increased dose fails to provide additional benefit, the dose should be reduced. **Note:** Should be withdrawn yearly for a 4-week interval (8 weeks for depot injection) in patients who have received irradiation. Resume if levels increase and signs/symptoms recur.

IM depot injection: Patients must be stabilized on subcutaneous octreotide for at least 2 weeks before switching to the long-acting depot. Upon switch: 20 mg IM intragluteally every 4 weeks for 3 months, then the dose may be modified based upon response.

Dosage adjustment for acromegaly: After 3 months of depot injections, the dosage may be continued or modified as follows:

GH ≤1 ng/mL, IGF-1 normal, and symptoms controlled: Reduce octreotide depot to 10 mg IM every 4 weeks

GH ≤2.5 ng/mL, IGF-1 normal, and symptoms controlled: Maintain octreotide depot at 20 mg IM every 4 weeks

GH >2.5 ng/mL, IGF-1 elevated, and/or symptoms uncontrolled: Increase octreotide depot to 30 mg IM every 4 weeks

Note: Patients not adequately controlled at a dose of 30 mg may increase dose to 40 mg every 4 weeks. Dosages >40 mg are not recommended.

Carcinoid tumors:

SubQ, IV: Initial 2 weeks: 100 to 600 mcg/day in 2 to 4 divided doses; usual range: 50 to 750 mcg/day (some patients may require up to 1,500 mcg/day); experience with doses above 750 mcg/day is limited.

IM depot injection: Patients must be stabilized on subcutaneous octreotide for at least 2 weeks before switching to the long-acting depot. Upon switch: 20 mg IM intragluteally every 4 weeks for 2 months, then the dose may be modified based upon response.

Note: Patients should continue to receive their SubQ injections for the first 2 weeks at the same dose in order to maintain therapeutic levels (some patients may require 3 to 4 weeks of continued SubQ injections). Patients who experience periodic exacerbations of symptoms may require temporary SubQ injections in addition to depot injections (at their previous SubQ dosing regimen) until symptoms have resolved.

Dosage adjustment for carcinoid tumors: After 2 months of depot injections, the dosage may be continued or modified as follows:

Increase to 30 mg IM every 4 weeks if symptoms are inadequately controlled

Decrease to 10 mg IM every 4 weeks, for a trial period, if initially responsive to 20 mg dose

Dosage >30 mg is not recommended

Vasoactive intestinal peptide tumors (VIPomas):

SubQ, IV: Initial 2 weeks: 200 to 300 mcg/day in 2 to 4 divided doses; titrate dose based on response/tolerance. Range: 150 to 750 mcg/day (doses >450 mcg/day are rarely required)

IM depot injection: Patients must be stabilized on subcutaneous octreotide for at least 2 weeks before switching to the long-acting depot. Upon switch: 20 mg IM intragluteally every 4 weeks for 2 months, then the dose may be modified based upon response.

Note: Patients receiving depot injection should continue to receive their SubQ injections for the first 2 weeks at the same dose in order to maintain therapeutic levels (some patients may require 3 to 4 weeks of continued SubQ injections). Patients who experience periodic exacerbations of symptoms may require temporary SubQ injections in addition to depot injections (at their previous SubQ dosing regimen) until symptoms have resolved.

Dosage adjustment for VIPomas: After 2 months of depot injections, the dosage may be continued or modified as follows:

Increase to 30 mg IM every 4 weeks if symptoms are inadequately controlled

Decrease to 10 mg IM every 4 weeks, for a trial period, if initially responsive to 20 mg dose

Dosage >30 mg is not recommended

Carcinoid crisis, prevention (off-label use): Immediate release octreotide solution (Oberg 2004):

Patients controlled with octreotide IM (depot) 20 to 30 mg: SubQ: 250 to 500 mcg within 1 to 2 hours prior to procedure.

Emergency surgery in somatostatin analog-naïve patients with functional neuroendocrine tumors:

IV bolus: 500 to 1000 mcg 1 to 2 hours prior to procedure **or**

SubQ: 500 mcg 1 to 2 hours prior to procedure

Intraoperative use for carcinoid crisis with hypotension: IV: 500 to 1,000 mcg bolus, repeat at 5 minute intervals until symptoms are controlled or IV: 500 to 1,000 mcg bolus followed by 50 to 200 mcg/hour continuous infusion during the procedure.

Postoperative dose (if supplemental doses required during procedure): IV: 50 to 200 mcg/hour continuous infusion for 24 hours, followed by resumption of the preoperative treatment schedule.

Diarrhea (off-label use): IV: Initial: 50 to 100 mcg every 8 hours; increase by 100 mcg/dose at 48-hour intervals; maximum dose: 500 mcg every 8 hours

Diarrhea (refractory) associated with chemotherapy (off-label use):

Low grade or uncomplicated: SubQ: 100 to 150 mcg every 8 hours (Benson 2004; Kornblau 2000)

Severe: Initial: SubQ: 100 to 150 mcg every 8 hours; may increase to 500 to 1500 mcg IV or SubQ every 8 hours (Kornblau 2000)

Complicated: IV, SubQ: Initial: 100 to 150 mcg 3 times/day or IV Infusion: 25 to 50 mcg/hour; may escalate to 500 mcg 3 times/day until controlled (Benson 2004)

Diarrhea associated with acute graft-versus-host disease (GVHD) (off-label use): IV: 500 mcg every 8 hours; discontinue within 24 hours of diarrhea resolution to avoid ileus; Maximum duration of therapy if diarrhea is not resolved: 7 days (Kornblau 2000)

Esophageal varices bleeding (off-label use): IV bolus: 25 to 100 mcg (usual bolus dose: 50 mcg) followed by continuous IV infusion of 25 to 50 mcg/hour for 2 to 5 days; may repeat bolus in first hour if hemorrhage not controlled (Corley 2001; Erstad 2001; Garcia-Tsao 2010)

Gastroenteropancreatic neuroendocrine tumors (off-label use):

IM (depot): 30 mg every 4 weeks until tumor progression or death (Rinke 2009) **or**

SubQ: Initial: 100 to 500 mcg 2 to 4 times daily (usually 150 mcg 3 times daily), may increase to response (symptom control) by doubling the dose every 3 to 4 days or a continuous subQ infusion of 1,000 to 2,000 mcg/day (Oberg 2004) **or**

IM (depot): Assure tolerability by initiating with the SubQ formulation for 3 to 7 days (and continue with SubQ for the first ~14 days after the initial IM depot dose). Then initiate IM (depot): 20 to 30 mg every 28 days (SubQ doses of 200 to 600 mcg/day should receive 20 mg IM and SubQ doses of 750 to 1,500 mcg/day should receive 30 mg IM); IM (depot) range: 20 to 60 mg every 28 days (Oberg 2004).

Hepatorenal syndrome (off-label use): SubQ: Initial: 100 mcg 3 times daily; may increase to 200 mcg 3 times daily (with a goal to increase mean arterial pressure [MAP] by at least 15 mm Hg from baseline) (Angeli 1999; Esrailian 2007; Garcia-Tsao 2009; AASLD [Runyon 2012])

Malignant bowel obstruction (off-label use): SubQ: 200 to 900 mcg/day in 2 to 3 divided doses (Mercadante 2007; Mercadante 2012) or 300 mcg/day by continuous SubQ infusion (Mercadante 2000)

Sulfonylurea-induced hypoglycemia (off-label use): Note: Although octreotide use has been advocated as a first line therapy, indications and dosing for octreotide are not firmly established (Glatstein 2012). Octreotide may reduce the incidence of recurrent hypoglycemia seen with dextrose-alone therapy (Fasano 2008). In addition, although subcutaneous administration is the preferred route, administration via intravenous bolus and intravenous infusion have also been described in the literature (Barkin 2013; Braatvedt 1997; Carr 2002; Crawford 2004; Dougherty 2010;

Dougherty 2013; Fasano 2008; Graudins 1997; Green 2003; Hung 1997; McLaughlin 2000; Mordel 1998). Optimal care decisions should be made based upon patient-specific details. Repeat dosing, dose escalation, or initiation of a continuous infusion may be required in patients who experience recurrent hypoglycemia. Duration of treatment may exceed 24 hours.
SubQ: 50 to 75 mcg; repeat every 6 hours as needed based upon blood glucose concentrations (Fasano 2008; Howland 2011)
IV: Doses up to 125 mcg/hour have been used successfully (McLaughlin 2000)

Thymoma/thymic malignancies, advanced (off-label use): SubQ: 500 mcg 3 times daily; evaluate after 2 months, patients with remission (complete or partial) continued octreotide for up to a maximum of 12 months; patients with stable disease continued octreotide and also received prednisone for up to 12 months or until disease progression or unacceptable toxicity (Loehrer 2004).

Geriatric Refer to adult dosing. Elimination half-life is increased by 46% and clearance is decreased by 26%; dose adjustment may be required. Dosing should generally begin at the lower end of dosing range.

Pediatric Infants and Children:

Congenital hyperinsulinism (off-label use): SubQ: Initial: 2 to 10 mcg/kg/day; up to 40 mcg/kg/day have been used (Stanley 1997).

Secretory diarrhea (off-label use): IV, SubQ: Doses of 1 to 10 mcg/kg every 12 hours have been used in children beginning at the low end of the range and increasing by 0.3 mcg/kg/dose at 3-day intervals. Suppression of growth hormone (animal data) is of concern when used as long-term therapy.

Sulfonylurea-induced hypoglycemia (off-label use): Note: Although octreotide use has been advocated as a first line therapy, indications and dosing for octreotide are not firmly established (Glatstein 2012). Octreotide may reduce the incidence of recurrent hypoglycemia seen with dextrose-alone therapy (Fasano 2008). In addition, although subcutaneous administration is the preferred route, administration via intravenous bolus and intravenous infusion have also been described in the literature (Barkin 2013; Braatvedt 1997; Carr 2002; Crawford 2004; Dougherty 2010; Dougherty 2013; Fasano 2008; Graudins 1997; Green 2003; Hung 1997; McLaughlin 2000; Mordel 1998). Optimal care decisions should be made based upon patient-specific details. Repeat dosing, dose escalation, or initiation of a continuous infusion may be required in patients who experience recurrent hypoglycemia. Duration of treatment may exceed 24 hours. SubQ: 1 to 1.25 mcg/kg; repeat in 6 hours as needed based upon blood glucose concentrations (Howland 2011). Children generally need only a single dose (Dougherty 2013).

Renal Impairment

Regular injection (solution):
Mild to severe impairment: There are no dosage adjustments provided in the manufacturer's labeling.
Severe impairment requiring dialysis: There are no specific dosage adjustments provided in the manufacturer's labeling; however, a dosage adjustment may be needed since clearance is reduced by ~50%.

Depot injection:
Mild to severe impairment: No initial dosage adjustment necessary.
Severe impairment requiring dialysis: Initial dose: 10 mg IM every 4 weeks; titrate based upon response (clearance is reduced by ~50%)

Hepatic Impairment

Regular injection (solution): There are no dosage adjustments provided in the manufacturer's labeling. Half-life is prolonged and total body clearance is decreased in patients with cirrhosis and fatty liver disease.

Depot injection: Patients with established cirrhosis of the liver: Initial dose: 10 mg IM every 4 weeks; titrate based upon response.

Usual Infusion Concentrations: Adult IV infusion: 500 mcg in 250 mL (concentration: 2 **mcg**/mL) of D5W or NS

Administration

Regular injection formulation: Administer SubQ or IV; IV administration may be IV push (undiluted over 3 minutes), intermittent IV infusion (over 15 to 30 minutes), or continuous IV infusion (off-label route). In emergency situations (eg, carcinoid crisis), octreotide may be given as a rapid IV bolus.

SubQ: Use the concentration with smallest volume to deliver dose to reduce injection site pain. Rotate injection site; may bring to room temperature prior to injection.

Depot formulation: Administer IM intragluteal (avoid deltoid administration); alternate gluteal injection sites to avoid irritation. For IM administration only; **do not** administer depot formulation (Sandostatin LAR) intravenously or subcutaneously; must be administered immediately after mixing.

Monitoring Parameters

Acromegaly: Growth hormone, somatomedin C (IGF-1)

Carcinoid: 5-HIAA, plasma serotonin and plasma substance P

VIPomas: Vasoactive intestinal peptide

Chronic therapy: Thyroid function (baseline and periodic), vitamin B_{12} level, blood glucose, glycemic control and antidiabetic regimen (patients with diabetes mellitus); cardiac function (heart rate, ECG), zinc level (patients with excessive fluid loss maintained on TPN)

Dietary Considerations Schedule injections between meals to decrease GI effects. May alter absorption of dietary fats.

Dosage Forms Excipient information presented when available (limited, particularly for generics); consult specific product labeling.

Kit, Intramuscular:

SandoSTATIN LAR Depot: 10 mg, 20 mg, 30 mg

Solution, Injection:

SandoSTATIN: 50 mcg/mL (1 mL); 100 mcg/mL (1 mL)

SandoSTATIN: 200 mcg/mL (5 mL) [contains phenol]

SandoSTATIN: 500 mcg/mL (1 mL)

SandoSTATIN: 1000 mcg/mL (5 mL) [contains phenol]

Generic: 50 mcg/mL (1 mL); 100 mcg/mL (1 mL); 200 mcg/mL (5 mL); 1000 mcg/5 mL (5 mL); 500 mcg/mL (1 mL); 1000 mcg/mL (5 mL)

Solution, Injection [preservative free]:

Generic: 100 mcg/mL (1 mL); 500 mcg/mL (1 mL)

◆ **Octreotide Acetate** *see* Octreotide *on page 1348*

◆ **Octreotide Acetate Omega (Can)** *see* Octreotide *on page 1348*

◆ **Octreotide Injection (Can)** *see* Octreotide *on page 1348*

◆ **Odomzo** *see* Sonidegib *on page 1682*

Ofatumumab (oh fa TOOM yoo mab)

Related Information

Management of Chemotherapy-Induced Nausea and Vomiting in Adults *on page 2253*

Brand Names: US Arzerra

Brand Names: Canada Arzerra

Index Terms HuMax-CD20

Pharmacologic Category Antineoplastic Agent, Anti-CD20; Antineoplastic Agent, Monoclonal Antibody

Use

Chronic lymphocytic leukemia, previously untreated: Treatment of previously untreated chronic lymphocytic leukemia (CLL) (in combination with chlorambucil) when fludarabine-based therapy is considered inappropriate

Chronic lymphocytic leukemia, relapsed: Treatment of relapsed CLL (in combination with fludarabine and cyclophosphamide).

Chronic lymphocytic leukemia, refractory: Treatment of CLL refractory to fludarabine and alemtuzumab

Chronic lymphocytic leukemia, extended treatment: Extended treatment of patients who are in complete or partial response after at least two lines of therapy for recurrent or progressive CLL

Labeled Contraindications

There are no contraindications listed in the manufacturer's US labeling.

Canadian labeling: Hypersensitivity to ofatumumab or any component of the formulation; presence or history of progressive multifocal leukoencephalopathy.

Pregnancy Considerations Adverse events were observed in some animal reproduction studies. Based on animal data, prolonged depletion of circulating B cells may occur; avoid administering live vaccines to newborns exposed to ofatumumab in utero until B cell recovery occurs.

Breastfeeding Considerations It is not known if ofatumumab is present in human milk. However, human IgG is excreted in breast milk, and therefore, ofatumumab may also be excreted in milk. Available data suggest antibodies present in breast milk do not significantly enter the neonatal and infant circulation. According to the manufacturer, the decision to breastfeed during therapy should take into account the risk of exposure to the infant and the benefits of treatment to the mother.

Warnings/Precautions [US Boxed Warning]: Hepatitis B virus (HBV) reactivation may occur in patients receiving CD20-directed antibody treatment, including ofatumumab; may result in fulminant hepatitis, hepatic failure, and death. Fatal cases of HBV have also occurred in patients not previously infected with HBV. Prior to initiating therapy, obtain hepatitis B surface antigen (HBsAg) and hepatitis B core antibody (anti-HBc) measurements in all patients; monitor for clinical and laboratory signs of hepatitis or HBV during and for several months after treatment. HBV reactivation has been reported up to 12 months after therapy discontinuation. Discontinue ofatumumab (and concomitant medications) if viral hepatitis develops and initiate appropriate antiviral therapy. Reactivation has occurred in patients who are HBsAg positive as well as in those who are HBsAg negative but are anti-HBc positive; HBV reactivation has also been observed in patients who had previously resolved HBV infection. Use cautiously in patients who show evidence of prior HBV infection (eg, HBsAg positive [regardless of antibody status] or HBsAg negative but anti-HBc positive); consult with appropriate clinicians regarding monitoring and consideration of antiviral therapy before and/or during ofatumumab treatment. The safety of resuming ofatumumab treatment following HBV reactivation is not known; discuss reinitiation of therapy in patients with resolved HBV reactivation with physicians experienced in HBV management. Bacterial, fungal, and other new or reactivated viral infections may occur during and/or following therapy; monitor closely for signs/symptoms of infection.

American Society of Clinical Oncology (ASCO) provisional clinical opinion update on hepatitis B virus screening [Hwang 2015]) recommendations: Patients receiving anti-CD20 antibodies are at high risk for hepatitis B virus (HBV) reactivation. Screen for HBV infection with hepatitis B surface antigen (HBsAg) and hepatitis B core antibody (anti-HBc) tests prior to treatment initiation; either a total anti-HBc (with both IgG and IgM) or anti-HBc IgG test should be used to screen for chronic or resolved HBV infection (do not use anti-HBc IgM as it may only confirm acute HBV infection). In addition, patients who have risk factors for HBV infection (eg, birthplace in a country with ≥2% HBV prevalence, household or sexual contact with HBV infected patients, high-risk behaviors [eg, intravenous drug use], and HIV infection) should also be screened prior to beginning therapy. Initiate prophylactic antiviral therapy (utilizing antivirals with low rates of viral resistance) for HBsAg positive/anti-HBc positive patients (without delaying cancer therapy) and continue the antivirals during and for ~6 to 12 months after completing treatment. HBsAg negative/anti-HBc positive patients should be monitored for HBV reactivation with HBV DNA and ALT testing approximately every 3 months during treatment; antiviral therapy may be initiated prophylactically or begun promptly at the first sign of HBV reactivation.

May cause serious infusion reaction (some fatal); reactions may include bronchospasm, dyspnea, laryngeal edema, pulmonary edema, flushing, hypertension, hypotension, syncope, cardiac ischemia/infarction, acute coronary syndrome, arrhythmia, bradycardia, back pain, abdominal pain, fever, rash, urticaria, angioedema, cytokine release syndrome, and/or anaphylactoid/anaphylactic reactions. Infusion reactions occur more frequently with the first 2 infusions and may occur despite premedication. Premedicate prior to infusion with acetaminophen, an antihistamine, and a corticosteroid. Interrupt infusion for reaction of any severity and institute appropriate treatment; may require subsequent rate modification. Discontinue immediately and permanently if anaphylactic reaction occurs.

[US Boxed Warning]: Progressive multifocal leukoencephalopathy (PML) resulting in death may occur with CD20-directed antibody treatment, including ofatumumab. Consider PML in any patient with new onset or worsening neurological symptoms, and if suspected, discontinue ofatumumab and evaluate promptly. Severe and prolonged (≥1 week) cytopenias (neutropenia, thrombocytopenia, and anemia) may occur. Grade 3 or 4 late-onset neutropenia (onset ≥42 days after last treatment dose) and/or prolonged neutropenia (not resolved 24 to 42 days after last dose) has been reported. Pancytopenia, agranulocytosis, and fatal neutropenic sepsis have occurred when used in combination with chlorambucil. Monitor blood counts regularly during and after treatment; more frequently if grade 3 or 4 cytopenias develop. Tumor lysis syndrome (TLS) has occurred in patients receiving ofatumumab; patients with a high tumor burden and/or high circulating lymphocyte counts (>25,000/mm^3) are at increased risk for TLS. Administer prophylactic antihyperuricemic therapy and aggressive hydration beginning 12 to 24 hours

◀ prior to ofatumumab treatment. Correct electrolyte abnormalities; monitor renal function and hydration status.

Potentially significant drug-drug interactions may exist, requiring dose or frequency adjustment, additional monitoring, and/or selection of alternative therapy. Live vaccines should not be given to patients who have recently received ofatumumab; there is no data concerning secondary transmission; the ability to generate an immune response to any vaccine following treatment is unknown. Patients ≥65 years experienced a higher incidence of adverse reactions (compared with younger patients).

Adverse Reactions

>10%:

Central nervous system: Fatigue (15%)

Dermatologic: Skin rash (14%)

Gastrointestinal: Diarrhea (18%), nausea (11%)

Hematologic & oncologic: Neutropenia (24%; ≥ grade 3: ≥22%; may be prolonged >2 weeks), anemia (16%; grades 3/4: 5%)

Infection: Infection (65% to 70%; includes bacterial, fungal, or viral), serious infection (20%)

Respiratory: Pneumonia (8% to 23%), cough (19%), upper respiratory tract infection (11% to 19%), dyspnea (14%), bronchitis (9% to 11%)

Miscellaneous: Infusion related reaction (46%; day 1 reactions: 25% to 44%; subsequent infusions: 2% to 29%), fever (20%)

1% to 10%:

Cardiovascular: Peripheral edema (9%), hypertension (5%), hypotension (5%), tachycardia (5%)

Central nervous system: Chills (8%), insomnia (5% to 7%), headache (6%)

Dermatologic: Urticaria (8%), hyperhidrosis (5%)

Hematologic & oncologic: Hypogammaglobulinemia (5%; grades 3/4: <1%)

Infection: Sepsis (8%), influenza (6%), herpes zoster (5% to 6%)

Neuromuscular & skeletal: Back pain (5% to 8%), muscle spasm (5%)

Respiratory: Nasopharyngitis (8%), sinusitis (5%)

<1%, postmarketing, and/or case reports: Antibody development, hepatitis B (new-onset or reactivation), porphyria cutanea tarda, progressive multifocal leukoencephalopathy, Stevens Johnson syndrome, tumor lysis syndrome

Drug Interactions

Metabolism/Transport Effects None known.

Avoid Concomitant Use

Avoid concomitant use of Ofatumumab with any of the following: BCG (Intravesical); Belimumab; Natalizumab; Pimecrolimus; Tacrolimus (Topical); Vaccines (Live)

Increased Effect/Toxicity

Ofatumumab may increase the levels/effects of: Belimumab; Fingolimod; Leflunomide; Natalizumab; Tofacitinib; Vaccines (Live)

The levels/effects of Ofatumumab may be increased by: Denosumab; Ocrelizumab; Pimecrolimus; Roflumilast; Tacrolimus (Topical); Trastuzumab

Decreased Effect

Ofatumumab may decrease the levels/effects of: BCG (Intravesical); Coccidioides immitis Skin Test; Nivolumab; Sipuleucel-T; Tertomotide; Vaccines (Inactivated); Vaccines (Live)

The levels/effects of Ofatumumab may be decreased by: Echinacea

Storage/Stability Store intact vials at 2°C to 8°C (36°F to 46°F); do not freeze. Protect from light. Solutions diluted in NS for infusion must be started within 12 hours of preparation (may store at 2°C to 8°C [36°F to 46°F] if not used immediately); discard any remaining solution 24 hours after preparation.

Preparation for Administration Prepare all doses in 1,000 mL NS. Begin infusion within 12 hours of preparation.

300 mg dose: Withdraw 15 mL from a 1,000 mL NS bag. Add contents of 3 ofatumumab 100 mg vials to NS bag. Gently invert to mix; do not shake.

1,000 mg dose: Withdraw 50 mL from a 1,000 mL NS bag. Add contents of 1 ofatumumab 1,000 mg vial. Gently invert to mix; do not shake.

2,000 mg dose: Withdraw 100 mL from a 1,000 mL NS bag. Add contents of 2 ofatumumab 1,000 mg vials to NS bag. Gently invert to mix; do not shake.

Mechanism of Action Ofatumumab is a monoclonal antibody which binds specifically the extracellular (large and small) loops of the CD20 molecule (which is expressed on normal B lymphocytes and in B-cell CLL) resulting in potent complement-dependent cell lysis and antibody-dependent cell-mediated toxicity in cells that overexpress CD20.

Pharmacodynamics/Kinetics

Distribution: V_{dss}: 6.1 L (following repeated infusions)

Half-life elimination: 17.6 days (following repeated infusions)

Dosing

Adult & Geriatric Note: Premedicate with acetaminophen, an antihistamine, and a corticosteroid 30 to 120 minutes prior to treatment (see Premedication below).

Chronic lymphocytic leukemia (CLL), previously untreated: IV: Cycle 1 (cycle is 28 days): 300 mg on day 1, followed by 1,000 mg on day 8; Subsequent cycles: 1,000 mg on day 1 every 28 days; continue for at least 3 cycles until best response or a maximum of 12 cycles (in combination with chlorambucil) (Hillmen 2015)

Premedication: Premedicate with oral acetaminophen (1,000 mg) or equivalent, an oral or IV antihistamine (eg, diphenhydramine 50 mg or cetirizine 10 mg orally or equivalent), and an IV corticosteroid (prednisolone 50 mg or equivalent). Full dose corticosteroid is recommended for the first 2 infusions; in the absence of infusion reaction ≥ grade 3, may reduce or omit corticosteroid dose for subsequent infusions.

CLL, relapsed: IV: Cycle 1 (cycle is 28 days): 300 mg on day 1, followed by 1,000 mg on day 8; Subsequent cycles: 1,000 mg on day 1 every 28 days; continue for a maximum of 6 cycles (in combination with fludarabine and cyclophosphamide) (Robak 2017)

Premedication: Premedicate with oral acetaminophen (1,000 mg) or equivalent, an oral or IV antihistamine (eg, diphenhydramine 50 mg or cetirizine 10 mg orally or equivalent), and an IV corticosteroid (prednisolone 50 mg or equivalent). Full dose corticosteroid is recommended for the first 2 infusions; in the absence of infusion reaction ≥ grade 3, may reduce or omit corticosteroid dose for subsequent infusions.

CLL, refractory: IV: Initial dose: 300 mg on day 1, followed 1 week later by 2,000 mg once weekly for 7 doses (doses 2 to 8), followed 4 weeks later by 2,000 mg once every 4 weeks for 4 doses (doses 9 to 12; for a total of 12 doses) (Wierda 2010)

Premedication: Premedicate with oral acetaminophen (1,000 mg) or equivalent, an oral or IV antihistamine (eg, diphenhydramine 50 mg or cetirizine 10 mg orally or equivalent), and an IV corticosteroid (prednisolone 100 mg or equivalent). Full dose corticosteroid is recommended for doses 1, 2, and 9; in the absence of infusion reaction ≥ grade 3, may reduce or omit corticosteroid dose for doses 3 to 8; may administer reduced corticosteroid dose (ranging from half to full dose) with doses 10 to 12 if ≥ grade 3 reaction did not occur with dose 9.

CLL, extended treatment: IV: 300 mg on day 1, followed by 1,000 mg on day 8, followed by 1,000 mg 7 weeks later and then every 8 weeks for up to a maximum of 2 years (van Oers 2015)

Premedication: Premedicate with oral acetaminophen (1,000 mg) or equivalent, an oral or IV antihistamine (eg, diphenhydramine 50 mg or cetirizine 10 mg orally or equivalent), and an IV corticosteroid (prednisolone 50 mg or equivalent). Full dose corticosteroid is recommended for the first 2 infusions; in the absence of infusion reaction ≥ grade 3, may reduce or omit corticosteroid dose for subsequent infusions.

Renal Impairment

CrCl ≥30 mL/minute: There are no dosage adjustments provided in the US manufacturer's labeling; however, there were no clinically relevant pharmacokinetic effects observed in patients with baseline CrCl ≥30 mL/minute.

CrCl <30 mL/minute: There are no dosage adjustments provided in the manufacturer's labeling (has not been studied).

Hepatic Impairment
There are no dosage adjustments provided in the manufacturer's labeling (has not been studied).

Adjustment for Toxicity
Infusion reaction: Interrupt infusion for infusion reaction (any severity). If the reaction resolves or remains at ≤ grade 2, resume with the following modifications (based on the grade of the initial reaction):

Grade 1 or 2 infusion reaction:
Resume at one-half of the previous rate; may increase (see Administration) based on patient tolerance.

Grade 3 or 4 infusion reaction: Resume infusion at 12 mL/hour; may increase (see Administration) based on patient tolerance.

If reaction severity does not resolve to ≤ grade 2 despite management: Consider permanent discontinuation

Anaphylactic reaction: Discontinue permanently

Combination Regimens

Leukemia, chronic lymphocytic:
Chlorambucil-Ofatumumab (CLL) on page 2034
Fludarabine-Cyclophosphamide-Ofatumumab (CLL) on page 2119

Administration
Do not administer IV push, IV bolus, or as a subcutaneous injection. Premedicate with acetaminophen, an antihistamine, and a corticosteroid 30 to 120 minutes prior to administration (see Dosing). Infuse in an environment equipped to monitor for and manage infusion reactions. Administer with infusion pump and administration set. Do not exceed infusion rates below. Do not mix with or infuse with other medications. Flush line before and after infusion with NS. Begin infusion within 12 hours of preparation. Interrupt infusion for any severity of infusion reaction; if the reaction resolves or remains at ≤ grade 2, may resume infusion (see Dosing: Adjustment for Toxicity).

Previously untreated chronic lymphocytic leukemia (CLL), relapsed CLL, and extended treatment of CLL:

Initial 300 mg dose: Initiate infusion at 12 mL/hour for 30 minutes, if tolerated (no infusion reaction) increase to 25 mL/hour for 30 minutes, if tolerated, increase to 50 mL/hour for 30 minutes, if tolerated, increase to 100 mL/hour for 30 minutes, if tolerated, increase to 200 mL/hour for 30 minutes, if tolerated increase to 300 mL/hour for 30 minutes, if tolerated, increase to 400 mL/hour for remainder of infusion. Median duration of infusion: 4.8 to 5.2 hours.

Subsequent 1,000 mg infusions (if no reaction to previous infusion): Initiate infusion at 25 mL/hour for 30 minutes, if tolerated (no infusion reaction) increase to 50 mL/hour for 30 minutes, if tolerated, increase to 100 mL/hour for 30 minutes, if tolerated, increase to 200 mL/hour for 30 minutes, if tolerated, increase to 400 mL/hour for remainder of infusion. Median duration of infusion: 4.2 to 4.4 hours.

Refractory CLL:

Doses 1 and 2: Initiate infusion at 12 mL/hour for 30 minutes, if tolerated (no infusion reaction) increase to 25 mL/hour for 30 minutes, if tolerated, increase to 50 mL/hour for 30 minutes, if tolerated, increase to 100 mL/hour for 30 minutes, if tolerated, increase to 200 mL/hour for remainder of infusion. Median duration of infusion: 6.8 hours.

Doses 3 to 12: Initiate infusion at 25 mL/hour for 30 minutes, if tolerated (no infusion reaction) increase to 50 mL/hour for 30 minutes, if tolerated, increase to 100 mL/hour for 30 minutes, if tolerated, increase to 200 mL/hour for 30 minutes, if tolerated, increase to 400 mL/hour for remainder of infusion. Median duration of infusion: 4.2 to 4.4 hours.

Emetic Potential Minimal (<10%)

Monitoring Parameters CBC with differential (at regular intervals during and after therapy; more frequently if grades 3 or 4 cytopenias develop), renal function, electrolytes

Hepatitis B virus screening recommendations (ASCO provisional clinical opinion update [Hwang 2015]): Screen for hepatitis B virus (HBV) infection with hepatitis B surface antigen (HBsAg) and hepatitis B core antibody (anti-HBc) tests prior to treatment initiation; either a total anti-HBc (with both IgG and IgM) or anti-HBc IgG test should be used to screen for chronic or resolved HBV infection (do not use anti-HBc IgM as it may only confirm acute HBV infection). HBsAg negative/anti-HBc positive patients should be monitored for HBV reactivation with HBV DNA and ALT testing approximately every 3 months during treatment.

Signs of active hepatitis B infection (during and for up to 12 months after therapy completion); signs/symptoms of hepatitis; signs or symptoms of infusion reaction; signs of infection; fluid status; signs/symptoms of intestinal obstruction (eg, abdominal pain, repeated vomiting); signs/symptoms of progressive multifocal leukoencephalopathy (focal neurologic deficits, which may present as hemiparesis, visual field deficits, cognitive impairment, aphasia, ataxia, and/or cranial nerve deficits).

Dosage Forms Excipient information presented when available (limited, particularly for generics); consult specific product labeling.

Concentrate, Intravenous [preservative free]:

Arzerra: 100 mg/5 mL (5 mL); 1000 mg/50 mL (50 mL) [contains edetate disodium, mouse (murine) and/or hamster protein, polysorbate 80]

OLANZapine (oh LAN za peen)

Brand Names: US ZyPREXA; ZyPREXA Relprevv; ZyPREXA Zydis

Brand Names: Canada ACT Olanzapine; ACT Olanzapine ODT; Apo-Olanzapine; Apo-Olanzapine ODT; Auro-Olanzapine ODT; JAMP Olanzapine FC; JAMP-Olanzapine ODT; Mar-Olanzapine; Mar-Olanzapine ODT; Mint-Olanzapine ODT; Mylan-Olanzapine; Mylan-Olanzapine ODT; Olanzapine for injection; Olanzapine ODT; PHL-Olanzapine; PHL-Olanzapine ODT; PMS-Olanzapine; PMS-Olanzapine ODT; RAN-Olanzapine; RAN-Olanzapine ODT; Riva-Olanzapine; Riva-Olanzapine ODT; Sandoz-Olanzapine; Sandoz-Olanzapine ODT; Teva-Olanzapine; Teva-Olanzapine ODT; Van-Olanzapine; Zyprexa; Zyprexa Intramuscular; Zyprexa Zydis

Index Terms LY170053; Olanzapine Pamoate; Zyprexa Zydis

Pharmacologic Category Antimanic Agent; Second Generation (Atypical) Antipsychotic

Use

Oral: Treatment of the manifestations of schizophrenia; treatment of acute or mixed mania episodes associated with bipolar I disorder (as monotherapy or in combination with lithium or valproate); maintenance treatment of bipolar I disorder; in combination with fluoxetine for treatment-resistant or bipolar I depression

IM, extended-release (Zyprexa Relprevv): Treatment of schizophrenia

IM, short-acting (Zyprexa IntraMuscular): Treatment of acute agitation associated with schizophrenia and bipolar I mania

Pregnancy Risk Factor C

Dosing

Adult & Geriatric

Schizophrenia:

Oral: Initial: 5 to 10 mg once daily (increase to 10 mg once daily within 5 to 7 days); thereafter, adjust by 5 mg daily at 1-week intervals, up to a recommended maximum of 20 mg/day. Maintenance: 10 to 20 mg once daily. Doses up to 60 mg daily have been used in treatment-resistant schizophrenia; however, supporting evidence is limited (APA [Lehman 2004]).

Special risk patients: Initial: 5 mg once daily is recommended in patients who are debilitated, who have a predisposition to hypotensive reactions, who exhibit a combination of factors that may result in slower metabolism of olanzapine (eg, nonsmoking female patients ≥65 years), or who may be more pharmacodynamically sensitive to olanzapine; increase dose with caution as clinically indicated.

Extended-release injection: IM: **Note:** Establish tolerance to oral olanzapine prior to changing to extended-release injection. Maximum dose: 300 mg every 2 weeks or 405 mg every 4 weeks

Patients established on oral olanzapine 10 mg daily: Initial dose: 210 mg every 2 weeks for 4 doses or 405 mg every 4 weeks for 2 doses; Maintenance dose: 150 mg every 2 weeks or 300 mg every 4 weeks

Patients established on oral olanzapine 15 mg daily: Initial dose: 300 mg every 2 weeks for 4 doses; Maintenance dose: 210 mg every 2 weeks or 405 mg every 4 weeks

Patients established on oral olanzapine 20 mg daily: Initial and maintenance dose: 300 mg every 2 weeks

Special risk patients: Initial: 150 mg every 4 weeks is recommended in patients who are debilitated, who have a predisposition to hypotensive reactions, who exhibit a combination of factors that may result in slower metabolism of olanzapine (eg, nonsmoking female patients ≥65 years), or who may be more pharmacodynamically sensitive to olanzapine; increase dose with caution as clinically indicated.

Bipolar I (acute mixed or manic episodes: Oral:

Monotherapy: Initial: 10 to 15 mg once daily; increase by 5 mg daily at intervals of not less than 24 hours. Maintenance: 5 to 20 mg daily; recommended maximum dose: 20 mg/day.

Combination therapy (with lithium or valproate): Initial: 10 mg once daily; dosing range: 5 to 20 mg daily

Agitation (acute, associated with bipolar disorder or schizophrenia):

Short-acting injection: IM: Initial dose: 10 mg (a lower dose of 5 to 7.5 mg may be considered when clinical factors warrant); additional doses (up to 10 mg) may be considered; however, 2 hours after the initial dose and 4 hours after the second dose should be allowed between doses to evaluate response (maximum total dose: 30 mg/day)

Special risk patients: Consider a lower dose of 2.5 mg in patients who are debilitated, who have a predisposition to hypotensive reactions, or who may be more pharmacodynamically sensitive to olanzapine.

Short-acting injection: IV (off-label route): **Note**: The IV route has only been studied in emergency departments, where patients can be closely monitored for respiratory depression (Chan 2013; Cole 2017; Martel 2015; Taylor 2017). The World Federation of Societies of Biological Psychiatry (WFSBP) expert consensus panel recommends against the use of intravenous medications in the management of agitation except in cases where there is no alternative (WFSBP [Garriga 2016]).

Monotherapy: IV: Initial: 10 mg; may provide two additional 5 mg doses in 5-minute intervals if needed; maximum: 20 mg (Taylor 2017). **Note:** Lower doses of 5 mg as a single dose have been studied concomitantly with midazolam (Chan 2013), however, concomitant use of parenteral olanzapine and benzodiazepines is not recommended due to potential for excessive sedation and cardiorespiratory depression.

Depression:

Depression associated with bipolar disorder (in combination with fluoxetine): Oral: Initial: 5 mg in the evening; adjust as tolerated to usual range of 5 to 12.5 mg daily. See **"Note"**

Treatment-resistant depression (in combination with fluoxetine): Oral: Initial: 5 mg in the evening; adjust as tolerated to range of 5 to 20 mg daily. See **"Note"**

Note (olanzapine/fluoxetine combination [Symbyax]): When using individual components of fluoxetine with olanzapine rather than fixed dose combination product (Symbyax), approximate dosage correspondence is as follows:

Olanzapine 2.5 mg + fluoxetine 20 mg = Symbyax 3/25
Olanzapine 5 mg + fluoxetine 20 mg = Symbyax 6/25
Olanzapine 12.5 mg + fluoxetine 20 mg = Symbyax 12/25
Olanzapine 5 mg + fluoxetine 50 mg = Symbyax 6/50
Olanzapine 12.5 mg + fluoxetine 50 mg = Symbyax 12/50

Special risk patients: Initial: 2.5 to 5 mg once daily is recommended in patients who have a predisposition to hypotensive reactions, who have hepatic impairment, who exhibit a combination of factors that may result in slower metabolism of olanzapine (eg, female, elderly, nonsmoking status), or who may be more pharmacodynamically sensitive to olanzapine; increase dose with caution as clinically indicated.

◀ **Chemotherapy-associated acute and delayed nausea or vomiting, prevention (off-label use):** Oral: 10 mg on the day of chemotherapy (day 1) followed by 10 mg once daily days 2 to 4 (in combination with dexamethasone and palonosetron on day 1 only) (Navari 2007; Navari 2011).

Chemotherapy-associated breakthrough nausea or vomiting (off-label use): Oral: 10 mg once daily for 3 days (Navari 2013).

Delirium (off-label use): Oral: 5 mg once daily for up to 5 days (NICE 2010).

Delusional parasitosis (off-label use): Oral: Initial: 2.5 mg once daily; increase gradually based on response and tolerability up to 5 to 10 mg/day. Maximum: 20 mg/day (Freudenmann 2008; Heller 2013). Additional data may be necessary to further define the role of olanzapine in this condition.

Post-traumatic stress disorder (off-label use): Oral: Initial: 5 to 10 mg daily; adjust dose based on response and tolerability every 1 to 2 weeks, up to 20 mg daily (Carey 2012; Stein 2002).

Tourette syndrome (off-label use): Initial: 2.5 to 5 mg daily; increase gradually based on response and tolerability to a usual dosage range of 2.5 to 20 mg daily (Pringsheim 2012; Roessner 2011). After initial dosage, increments of 2.5 to 5 mg weekly or biweekly were commonly used for dosage adjustments in clinical trials up to a maximum dosage of 20 mg/day (Budman 2001; Onofrj 2000; Stamenkovic 2000).

Discontinuation of therapy: American Psychiatric Association (APA), Canadian Psychiatric Association (CPA), and World Federation of Societies of Biological Psychiatry (WFSBP) guidelines recommend gradually tapering antipsychotics to avoid withdrawal symptoms and minimize the risk of relapse (APA [Lehman 2004]; Cerovecki 2013; CPA [Addington 2005]; WFSBP [Hasan 2012]); risk for withdrawal symptoms may be highest with highly anti-cholinergic or dopaminergic antipsychotics (Cerovecki 2013). When stopping antipsychotic therapy in patients with schizophrenia, the CPA guidelines recommend a gradual taper over 6 to 24 months, and the APA guidelines recommend reducing the dose by 10% each month (APA [Lehman 2004]; CPA [Addington 2005]). Continuing anti-parkinsonism agents for a brief period after discontinuation may prevent withdrawal symptoms (Cerovecki 2013). When switching antipsychotics, 3 strategies have been suggested: cross-titration (gradually discontinuing the first antipsychotic while gradually increasing the new antipsychotic), overlap and taper (maintaining the dose of the first antipsychotic while gradually increasing the new antipsychotic, then tapering the first antipsychotic), and abrupt change (abruptly discontinuing the first antipsychotic and either increasing the new antipsychotic gradually or starting it at a treatment dose). Evidence supporting ideal switch strategies and taper rates is limited, and results are conflicting (Cerovecki 2013; Remington 2005).

Pediatric

Bipolar I (acute mixed or manic episodes): Adolescents ≥13 years: Oral: Initial: 2.5 to 5 mg once daily; adjust by 2.5 to 5 mg daily to target dose of 10 mg daily; dosing range: 2.5 to 20 mg daily

Depression associated with bipolar I disorder (in combination with fluoxetine): Children and Adolescents 10 to 17 years: Oral: Initial: 2.5 mg once daily in the evening (in combination with fluoxetine); adjust dose, if needed, as tolerated; safety of doses >12 mg of olanzapine in combination with fluoxetine doses >50 mg has not been studied in pediatrics.

Schizophrenia: Adolescents ≥13 years: Oral: Initial: 2.5 to 5 mg once daily; adjust by 2.5 to 5 mg daily to target dose of 10 mg daily; dosing range: 2.5 to 20 mg daily

Chemotherapy-associated breakthrough or refractory nausea or vomiting (off-label use): Infants, Children, and Adolescents: Oral: 0.1 mg/kg/dose once daily (maximum: 10 mg/dose); if necessary, may increase to 0.14 mg/kg/dose once daily (maximum: 10 mg/dose) (Flank 2016).

Tourette syndrome (off-label use): Children and Adolescents: Initial: 2.5 to 5 mg once daily; increase gradually based on response and tolerability to a usual dosage of 2.5 to 12.5 mg once daily (AACAP [Murphy 2013]; Pringsheim 2012). After initial dosage, increments of 2.5 to 5 mg weekly or biweekly were used for dosage adjustments in clinical trials up to a maximum dosage of 20 mg/day (McCracken 2008; Stephens 2004)

Renal Impairment No dosage adjustment necessary. Not removed by dialysis.

Hepatic Impairment There are no dosage adjustments provided in the manufacturer's labeling except when used in combination with fluoxetine (as separate components) the initial olanzapine dose should be limited to 2.5 to 5 mg daily. Use with caution (cases of hepatitis and liver injury have been reported with olanzapine use).

Additional Information Complete prescribing information should be consulted for additional detail.

Medication Guide Available Yes

Dosage Forms Excipient information presented when available (limited, particularly for generics); consult specific product labeling.

Solution Reconstituted, Intramuscular:
ZyPREXA: 10 mg (1 ea) [contains tartaric acid]
Generic: 10 mg (1 ea)

Suspension Reconstituted, Intramuscular:
ZyPREXA Relprevv: 210 mg (1 ea); 300 mg (1 ea); 405 mg (1 ea) [contains polysorbate 80]

Tablet, Oral:
ZyPREXA: 2.5 mg, 5 mg, 7.5 mg, 10 mg
ZyPREXA: 15 mg [contains fd&c blue #2 aluminum lake]
ZyPREXA: 20 mg
Generic: 2.5 mg, 5 mg, 7.5 mg, 10 mg, 15 mg, 20 mg

Tablet Disintegrating, Oral:
ZyPREXA Zydis: 5 mg, 10 mg, 15 mg, 20 mg [contains aspartame, methylparaben sodium, propylparaben sodium]
Generic: 5 mg, 10 mg, 15 mg, 20 mg

Dosage Forms: Canada Information with regard to form, strength, and availability of products uniquely available in Canada but currently not available in the US. Refer also to Dosage Forms.

Excipient information presented when available (limited, particularly for generics); consult specific product labeling.

◆ **Olanzapine for injection (Can)** see OLANZapine on page 1364

◆ **Olanzapine ODT (Can)** see OLANZapine on page 1364

◆ **Olanzapine Pamoate** see OLANZapine on page 1364

Olaparib (oh LAP a rib)

Related Information

Common Toxicity Criteria *on page 2242*

Management of Chemotherapy-Induced Nausea and Vomiting in Adults *on page 2253*

Safe Handling of Hazardous Drugs *on page 2379*

Brand Names: US Lynparza

Brand Names: Canada Lynparza

Index Terms AZD2281; KU-0059436; PARP Inhibitor AZD2281

Pharmacologic Category Antineoplastic Agent, PARP Inhibitor

Use

Ovarian cancer, advanced (BRCA-mutated): Capsules, tablets: Treatment of deleterious or suspected deleterious germline BRCA-mutated (as detected by an approved test) advanced ovarian cancer in patients who have been treated with 3 or more prior lines of chemotherapy

Ovarian cancer, recurrent (maintenance): Tablets: Maintenance treatment of recurrent epithelial ovarian, fallopian tube, or primary peritoneal cancer in patients who are in a complete or partial response to platinum-based chemotherapy.

Labeled Contraindications

There are no contraindications listed in the manufacturer's US labeling.

Canadian labeling: Hypersensitivity to olaparib or any component of the formulation.

Pregnancy Considerations Adverse events were observed in animal reproduction studies at doses less than human exposure. Based on animal reproduction studies and the mechanism of action, olaparib may be expected to cause adverse events to the fetus. Women of reproductive potential should use highly effective contraception during therapy and for at least 6 months after the last olaparib dose. In women of reproductive potential, pregnancy testing is recommended prior to treatment initiation.

Breastfeeding Considerations It is not known if olaparib is present in breast milk. Due to the potential for serious adverse reactions in the breastfed infant, the manufacturer recommends that lactating women should not breast-feed during treatment and for 1 month after the last olaparib dose.

Warnings/Precautions Anemia, neutropenia, thrombocytopenia and lymphopenia have been reported. Monitor complete blood counts at baseline and monthly thereafter; do not initiate olaparib until any hematologic toxicity caused by previous chemotherapy has resolved to ≤ grade 1. Myelodysplastic syndrome/acute myeloid leukemia (MDS/AML) has been reported (rarely) in clinical trials and long-term follow up, mostly in patients with documented BRCA mutation. Most MDS/AML cases were fatal. Additional cases of MDS/AML have been reported in patients treated with olaparib in combination studies. The duration of olaparib therapy prior to development of the secondary cancers ranged from less than 6 months to greater than 2 years; all patients had received prior chemotherapy with platinum agents and/or other DNA-damaging medications, including radiation; some of these patients had a prior history of cancer or bone marrow dysplasia. If prolonged hematologic toxicity occurs during therapy, interrupt treatment and monitor blood counts weekly until recovered; if counts do not recover to ≤ grade 1 after 4 weeks, further evaluation (including bone marrow and cytogenetic analyses) is necessary. If MDS/AML is confirmed, discontinue therapy.

Pneumonitis (including some fatalities) has occurred rarely. Interrupt treatment for new or worsening respiratory symptoms such as cough, dyspnea, fever, wheezing, or radiologic abnormalities; evaluate promptly. Discontinue treatment if pneumonitis is confirmed. Monitor closely for toxicity in patients with mild or moderate renal impairment; dosage adjustment is recommended for moderate impairment. Nausea and vomiting (usually mild to moderate) may commonly occur. Hypersensitivity reactions, including rash and dermatitis, have been reported. Olaparib is associated with a moderate emetic potential; antiemetics are recommended to prevent nausea and vomiting. Potentially significant drug-drug interactions may exIst, requiring dose or frequency adjustment, additional monitoring, and/or selection of alternative therapy. Olaparib is available as 100 mg and 150 mg tablets and as 50 mg capsules. Do not substitute the 50 mg capsules for the 100 mg or 150 mg tablets on a mg-per-mg basis due to differences in dosing and bioavailability.

Adverse Reactions

≥10%:
  Cardiovascular: Peripheral edema (10% to <20%)
  Central nervous system: Fatigue (including weakness; 66% to 68%), headache (10% to 25%), dizziness (10% to <20%)
  Dermatologic: Skin rash (10% to 25%)
  Gastrointestinal: Nausea (64% to 75%), abdominal pain (43%), vomiting (32% to 43%), diarrhea (28% to 31%), dyspepsia (25%), decreased appetite (22% to 25%), dysgeusia (10% to 21%), constipation (10% to <20%)
  Genitourinary: Urinary tract infection (10% to <20%)
  Hematologic & oncologic: Decreased hemoglobin (85% to 90%; grades 3/4: 8% to 15%), increased MCV (57% to 85%), decreased absolute lymphocyte count (56%; grades 3/4: 17%), anemia (25% to 34%; grades 3/4: 4% to 18%), decreased neutrophils (25% to 32%; grades 3/4: 7% to 8%), decreased platelet count (26% to 30%; grades 3/4: 3% to 6%)
  Neuromuscular & skeletal: Musculoskeletal pain (21% to 32%), myalgia (22% to 25%), back pain (10% to 25%)
  Renal: Increased serum creatinine (26% to 30%)
  Respiratory: Upper respiratory tract infection (26% to 43%), cough (10% to 21%), dyspnea (10% to <20%)
1% to ≤10%:
  Cardiovascular: Hypertension, venous thrombosis (including pulmonary embolism)
  Central nervous system: Anxiety, depression, insomnia, peripheral neuropathy
  Dermatologic: Pruritus, xeroderma (including eczema)
  Endocrine & metabolic: Hot flash, hyperglycemia, hypomagnesemia
  Gastrointestinal: Stomatitis
  Genitourinary: Dysuria, urinary incontinence, vulvovaginal disease
  Hematologic & oncologic: Myelodysplastic syndrome (acute myeloid leukemia; 2%), leukopenia
  Miscellaneous: Fever
<1%, postmarketing, and/or case reports: Pneumonitis

Drug Interactions

Metabolism/Transport Effects Substrate of CYP3A4 (major), P-glycoprotein; **Note:** Assignment of Major/Minor substrate status based on clinically relevant drug interaction potential

◀ **Avoid Concomitant Use**

Avoid concomitant use of Olaparib with any of the following: BCG (Intravesical); Bitter Orange; Conivaptan; CYP3A4 Inducers (Moderate); CYP3A4 Inducers (Strong); CYP3A4 Inhibitors (Moderate); CYP3A4 Inhibitors (Strong); Deferiprone; Dipyrone; Fusidic Acid (Systemic); Idelalisib

Increased Effect/Toxicity

Olaparib may increase the levels/effects of: CloZAPine; Deferiprone

The levels/effects of Olaparib may be increased by: Bitter Orange; Conivaptan; CYP3A4 Inhibitors (Moderate); CYP3A4 Inhibitors (Strong); Dasatinib; Dipyrone; Fosaprepitant; Fusidic Acid (Systemic); Idelalisib; Palbociclib; Promazine; Simeprevir; Stiripentol

Decreased Effect

Olaparib may decrease the levels/effects of: BCG (Intravesical)

The levels/effects of Olaparib may be decreased by: CYP3A4 Inducers (Moderate); CYP3A4 Inducers (Strong); Deferasirox; Sarilumab; Siltuximab; Tocilizumab

Food Interactions Coadministration with grapefruit or Seville oranges may increase olaparib plasma concentrations. Management: Avoid concomitant administration with grapefruit, grapefruit juice, Seville oranges, or Seville orange juice.

Hazardous Drugs Handling Considerations

This medication is not on the NIOSH (2016) list; however, it may meet the criteria for a hazardous drug. Drugs are classified as hazardous based on their properties; the properties of a hazardous drug include one or more of the following characteristics: carcinogenic, teratogenic (or other developmental toxicity), reproductive toxicity, organotoxic at low doses, genotoxic, and/or new agents with structural or toxicity profiles similar to existing hazardous agents. Assess risk to determine appropriate containment strategy (USP-NF 2017).

Use appropriate precautions for receiving, handling, administration, and disposal. Gloves (single) should be worn during receiving, unpacking, and placing in storage. NIOSH recommends single gloving for administration of intact tablets or capsules (NIOSH 2016).

Storage/Stability

Capsules: Store at 25°C (77°F); excursions permitted to 15°C to 30°C (59°F to 86°F). Do not expose capsules to temperatures >40°C (104°F).

Tablets: Store at 20°C to 25°C (68°F to 77°F); excursions permitted to 15°C to 30°C (59°F to 86°F). Protect from moisture.

Mechanism of Action Olaparib is a poly (ADP-ribose) polymerase (PARP) enzyme inhibitor, including PARP1, PARP2, and PARP3. PARP enzymes are involved in DNA transcription, cell cycle regulation, and DNA repair. Olaparib is a potent oral PARP inhibitor which induces synthetic lethality in BRCA1/2 deficient tumor cells through the formation of double-stranded DNA breaks which cannot be accurately repaired, which leads to disruption of cellular homeostasis and cell death (Ledermann 2012).

Pharmacodynamics/Kinetics

Absorption: Rapid; delayed with a high-fat meal (extent of absorption not significantly altered)

Distribution: Capsule: 167 ± 196 L; Tablet: 158 ± 136 L

Protein binding: ~82%

Metabolism: Primarily hepatic via CYP3A4; the majority of metabolism is through oxidation with some metabolites undergoing subsequent glucuronide or sulfate conjugation

Bioavailability: Tablet formulation has higher bioavailability than the capsule formulation.

Half-life elimination, terminal: Capsule: 11.9 ± 4.8 hours; Tablet: 14.9 ± 8.2 hours

Time to peak: Capsule: 1 to 3 hours; Tablet: 1.5 hours

Excretion: Urine (44%, mostly metabolites); feces (42%, mostly metabolites)

Dosing

Adult & Geriatric Note: Olaparib is available as 100 mg and 150 mg tablets and as 50 mg capsules. Do not substitute the 50 mg capsules for the 100 mg or 150 mg tablets on a mg-per-mg basis due to differences in dosing and bioavailability.

Ovarian cancer, advanced (BRCA-mutated): Oral:

Capsules: 400 mg twice daily (12 hours apart) until disease progression or unacceptable toxicity (Domchek 2016)

Tablets: 300 mg twice daily (12 hours apart) until disease progression or unacceptable toxicity

Ovarian cancer, recurrent (maintenance): Oral: *Tablets:* 300 mg twice daily (12 hours apart) until disease progression or unacceptable toxicity

Breast cancer, metastatic, HER2-negative, BRCA-mutated (off-label use): Oral: *Tablets:* 300 mg twice daily until disease progression or unacceptable toxicity (Robson 2017)

Missed doses: If a dose is missed, administer the next dose at its scheduled time.

Dosage adjustment for concomitant therapy with CYP3A inhibitors: Avoid concomitant use with moderate or strong CYP3A inhibitors (consider alternative agents with less CYP3A inhibition). If coadministration with a **moderate** CYP3A inhibitor cannot be avoided, reduce dose to 200 mg twice daily (capsules) or 150 mg twice daily (tablets). If coadministration with a **strong** CYP3A inhibitor cannot be avoided, reduce dose to 150 mg twice daily (capsules) or 100 mg twice daily (tablets).

Renal Impairment

CrCl 51 to 80 mL/minute: No dosage adjustment necessary; monitor closely for toxicity, as an increase in mean AUC has been observed in patients with mild impairment.

CrCl 31 to 50 mL/minute:

Capsules: Reduce dose to 300 mg twice daily.

Tablets: Reduce dose to 200 mg twice daily.

CrCl ≤30 mL/minute: There are no dosage adjustments provided in the manufacturer's labeling (has not been studied).

ESRD: There are no dosage adjustments provided in the manufacturer's labeling (has not been studied).

Hepatic Impairment

Mild impairment (Child-Pugh class A): No dosage adjustment necessary.

Moderate-to-severe impairment (Child-Pugh classes B and C): There are no dosage adjustments provided in the manufacturer's labeling (has not been studied).

Adjustment for Toxicity

Consider therapy interruption or dose reduction if adverse reactions occur.

Capsules: The recommended dose reduction is to 200 mg twice daily; if further reduction is required, reduce dose to 100 mg twice daily.

Tablets: The recommended dose reduction is to 250 mg twice daily; if further reduction is required, reduce dose to 200 mg twice daily.
Pneumonitis: Discontinue
Secondary AML/MDS: Discontinue

Administration

Administer with or without food. Swallow capsules whole; do not chew, dissolve, or open capsule. Do not administer if capsules appear deformed or show evidence of leakage. Swallow tablets whole; do not chew, crush, dissolve, or divide tablet.

Based on a pharmacokinetic study, the rate of absorption was slower and the peak exposure was decreased when administered with a high-fat meal; however, the extent of absorption was not affected; nausea and vomiting were reported more frequently when olaparib was administered in a fasted state (Plummer 2015).

Olaparib is available as 100 mg and 150 mg tablets and as 50 mg capsules. Due to differences in dosing and bioavailability, do **not** substitute the 50 mg capsules for the 100 mg or 150 mg tablets on a mg-per-mg basis.

Emetic Potential Low (10% to 30%)

Monitoring Parameters Complete blood count at baseline and monthly thereafter, or as clinically indicated (weekly until recovery for prolonged hematologic toxicity), renal function, pregnancy test (prior to treatment initiation in women of reproductive potential); monitor for signs/symptoms of AML/MDS and pneumonitis. Monitor adherence.

Dietary Considerations Avoid grapefruit, grapefruit juice, Seville oranges, or Seville orange juice.

Prescribing and Access Restrictions Olaparib is available only through the designated specialty pharmacy Biologics, Inc. For further information on patient assistance, product availability, and prescribing instructions, please refer to the following website: http://myaccess360.com/hcp/reimbursement/Oncology.aspx?product=lynparza or call 1-844-275-2360.

Medication Guide Available Yes

Dosage Forms Excipient information presented when available (limited, particularly for generics); consult specific product labeling.
Capsule, Oral:
  Lynparza: 50 mg
Tablet, Oral:
  Lynparza: 100 mg, 150 mg

Olaratumab (oh lar AT ue mab)

Related Information

Safe Handling of Hazardous Drugs *on page 2379*

Brand Names: US Lartruvo

Index Terms Anti-PDGFR Alpha Monoclonal Antibody IMC-3G3; IMC-3G3; LY3012207

Pharmacologic Category Antineoplastic Agent, Monoclonal Antibody; Antineoplastic Agent, PDGFR-alpha Blocker

Use Soft tissue sarcoma: Treatment (in combination with doxorubicin) of adults with soft tissue sarcoma (STS) with a histologic subtype for which an anthracycline-containing regimen is appropriate and which is not amenable to curative treatment with radiotherapy or surgery.

Labeled Contraindications There are no contraindications listed in the manufacturer's labeling.

Pregnancy Considerations Based on its mechanism of action, olaratumab would be expected to cause fetal harm if administered to a pregnant woman. Animal reproduction studies have not been conducted. Adequate contraception during therapy and for 3 months following the last dose is recommended in women of reproductive potential.

Breastfeeding Considerations It is not known if olaratumab is excreted in breast milk. Due to the potential for serious adverse reactions in a nursing infant, breastfeeding is not recommended by the manufacturer during therapy and for 3 months following the last dose.

Warnings/Precautions Olaratumab is associated with infusion reactions; most infusion reactions occurred with the first or second cycle. Grade 3 or higher reactions have occurred, including a fatal case. Symptoms of infusion reactions have included flushing, dyspnea, bronchospasm, and/or fever/chills; severe cases included hypotension, anaphylactic shock, or cardiac arrest. Premedication with diphenhydramine and dexamethasone is recommended. Monitor for signs/symptoms of infusion reactions during and after infusion (resuscitation equipment should be readily available). May require treatment interruption (followed by rate reduction) or permanent discontinuation.

Nausea, vomiting, diarrhea, mucositis, and abdominal pain have been reported, with a higher incidence in patients treated with olaratumab and doxorubicin, compared to doxorubicin alone. A higher incidence of grade 3 and 4 lymphopenia and neutropenia have been reported in patients treated with olaratumab and doxorubicin, compared to doxorubicin alone. Thrombocytopenia (all grades) also had a higher incidence in the combination arm. Potentially significant drug-drug interactions may exist, requiring dose or frequency adjustment, additional monitoring, and/or selection of alternative therapy.

Adverse Reactions

>10%:

Central nervous system: Fatigue (69%), neuropathy (22%), headache (20%), anxiety (11%)

Dermatologic: Alopecia (52%)

Endocrine & metabolic: Hyperglycemia (52%), hypokalemia (21%), hypophosphatemia (21%), hypomagnesemia (16%)

Gastrointestinal: Nausea (73%), mucositis (53%), vomiting (45%), diarrhea (34%), decreased appetite (31%), abdominal pain (23%)

Hematologic & oncologic: Lymphocytopenia (77%, grades 3/4: 44%), neutropenia (65%, grades 3/4: 48%), thrombocytopenia (63%, grades 3/4: 6%), prolonged partial thromboplastin time (33%, grades 3/4: 5%)

Hepatic: Increased serum alkaline phosphatase (16%)

Neuromuscular & skeletal: Musculoskeletal pain (64%)

Ophthalmic: Xerophthalmia (11%)

Miscellaneous: Infusion related reaction (13% to 14%)

1% to 10%: Immunologic: Development of IgG antibodies (4%; all patients had neutralizing antibodies; however, therapeutic effects of antibodies could not be assessed)

Drug Interactions

Metabolism/Transport Effects None known.

Avoid Concomitant Use

Avoid concomitant use of Olaratumab with any of the following: BCG (Intravesical); Deferiprone; Dipyrone

◀ **Increased Effect/Toxicity**
  Olaratumab may increase the levels/effects of: CloZAPine; Deferiprone

  The levels/effects of Olaratumab may be increased by: Dipyrone; Promazine
Decreased Effect
  Olaratumab may decrease the levels/effects of: BCG (Intravesical)
Hazardous Drugs Handling Considerations
Hazardous agent (meets NIOSH 2016 criteria). This medication is not on the NIOSH (2016) list; however, it meets the criteria for a hazardous drug. Drugs are classified as hazardous based on their properties; the properties of a hazardous drug include one or more of the following characteristics: carcinogenic, teratogenic (or other developmental toxicity), reproductive toxicity, organotoxic at low doses, genotoxic, and/or new agents with structural or toxicity profiles similar to existing hazardous agents.

Use appropriate precautions for receiving, handling, administration, and disposal. Gloves (single) should be worn during receiving, unpacking, and placing in storage. NIOSH recommends double gloving, a protective gown, ventilated engineering controls (a class II biological safety cabinet or a compounding aseptic containment isolator), and closed system transfer devices (CSTDs) for preparation. Double gloving, a gown, and CSTDs are required during administration (NIOSH 2016).

Storage/Stability Store intact vials at 2°C to 8°C (36°F to 46°F); do not freeze. Keep in original carton to protect from light. Do not shake. Solutions diluted for infusion may be stored for up to 24 hours refrigerated and for an additional 4 hours at room temperature (infusion must be completed within this time frame). If refrigerated, allow infusion solution to reach room temperature prior to administration.

Preparation for Administration Withdraw calculated dose volume and dilute in NS to a total volume of 250 mL. Gently invert to mix (do not shake). Do not freeze the diluted solution. Dilute with NS only; do not use dextrose-containing or other solutions.

Mechanism of Action Olaratumab is a human (recombinant) IgG1 antibody which expressly binds to platelet-derived growth receptor alpha (PDGFR-α) to prevent binding of PDGF-AA, PDGF-BB, and PDGF-CC and block receptor activation and disrupt PDGF receptor signaling. The PDGF-alpha receptor has a role in cell differentiation, growth, and angiogenesis and has demonstrated antitumor activity in sarcomas (Tap 2016).
Pharmacodynamics/Kinetics
Distribution: V_{ss}: 7.7 L
Half-life, elimination: ~11 days (range: 6 to 24 days)
Dosing
Adult
Soft tissue sarcoma: IV: 15 mg/kg on days 1 and 8 every 3 weeks (in combination with doxorubicin) for 8 cycles; after 8 cycles are completed, continue olaratumab (as a single agent) until disease progression or unacceptable toxicity (Tap 2016).
  Premedications: On day 1 of cycle 1, premedicate with diphenhydramine (25 to 50 mg IV) and dexamethasone (10 to 20 mg IV) prior to olaratumab.
Note: Dexrazoxane was allowed on day 1 of cycles 5 to 8 to reduce the potential for doxorubicin-related cardiotoxicity (Tap 2016).

Renal Impairment

CrCl 30 to 89 mL/minute: There are no dosage adjustments provided in the manufacturer's labeling; however, mild to moderate impairment has no clinically relevant impact on olaratumab pharmacokinetics.

CrCl <30 mL/minute: There are no dosage adjustments provided in the manufacturer's labeling (has not been studied).

Hepatic Impairment

Mild (total bilirubin within normal limits and AST greater than the upper limit of normal [ULN] or total bilirubin >1 up to 1.5 times ULN and any AST) to moderate (total bilirubin >1.5 up to 3 times ULN and any AST) impairment: There are no dosage adjustments provided in the manufacturer's labeling; however, mild to moderate impairment has no clinically relevant impact on olaratumab pharmacokinetics.

Severe impairment (total bilirubin >3 times ULN and any AST): There are no dosage adjustments provided in the manufacturer's labeling (has not been studied).

Adjustment for Toxicity

Hematologic toxicity: Neutropenic fever/infection or grade 4 neutropenia lasting longer than 1 week: Withhold olaratumab until the absolute neutrophil count (ANC) is ≥1,000/mm^3 and then resume with the dose permanently reduced to 12 mg/kg.

Infusion reaction:

Grade 1 or 2: Interrupt infusion; after resolution resume with the rate reduced by 50%.

Grade 3 or 4: Discontinue permanently.

Note: Doxorubicin may also require dosage modification.

Combination Regimens

Soft tissue sarcoma: Olaratumab-Doxorubicin (Soft Tissue Sarcoma) on page 2181

Administration

Infuse over 60 minutes. Do not infuse as an IV push or bolus. Flush the IV line with normal saline at the end of infusion. Do not coadminister electrolytes or other medications through the same IV line.

If refrigerated, allow infusion solution to reach room temperature prior to administration. Infusion must be completed within 28 hours of dilution (when stored appropriately; see Storage/Stability).

Monitoring Parameters CBC with differential. Monitor for signs/symptoms of infusion reactions.

Dosage Forms Excipient information presented when available (limited, particularly for generics); consult specific product labeling.

Solution, Intravenous [preservative free]:

Lartruvo: 190 mg/19 mL (19 mL); 500 mg/50 mL (50 mL)

Omacetaxine (oh ma se TAX een)

Related Information

Safe Handling of Hazardous Drugs *on page* 2379

Brand Names: US Synribo

Index Terms CGX-625; HHT; Homoharringtonine; Omacetaxine Mepesuccinate

Pharmacologic Category Antineoplastic Agent, Cephalotaxine; Antineoplastic Agent, Protein Synthesis Inhibitor

◄ **Use Chronic myeloid leukemia:** Treatment of chronic or accelerated phase chronic myeloid leukemia (CML) in adult patients resistant and/or intolerant to 2 or more tyrosine kinase inhibitors

Labeled Contraindications There are no contraindications listed in the manufacturer's labeling.

Pregnancy Considerations Adverse events were observed in animal reproduction studies at doses less than the equivalent human dose (based on BSA). Based on the mechanism of action, omacetaxine may cause fetal harm if administered during pregnancy. Women of reproductive potential should avoid pregnancy during therapy. Omacetaxine may impair fertility in males.

Breastfeeding Considerations It is not known if omacetaxine is present in breast milk. Due to the potential for serious adverse reactions in the breastfed infant, the decision to discontinue omacetaxine or to discontinue breastfeeding should take into account the importance of treatment to the mother.

Warnings/Precautions Grade 3/4 neutropenia, thrombocytopenia, and anemia commonly occur; generally reversible, although may require treatment delay and/or a reduction in the number of treatment days with future cycles. Myelosuppression may rarely be fatal. Monitor blood counts (in induction and maintenance cycles). Neutropenia may increase the risk for infection. Thrombocytopenia may increase the risk of bleeding; cerebrovascular hemorrhages have been reported (some fatal); gastrointestinal hemorrhages have occurred. Due to the increased risk of bleeding, avoid the use of anticoagulants, aspirin, and NSAIDs when the platelet count is <50,000/mm^3. Patients ≥65 years of age are more likely to experience toxicity, especially hematologic toxicity. Omacetaxine may induce glucose intolerance; hyperglycemia (including grade 3 and 4 events) has been observed; hyperosmolar nonketotic hyperglycemia has been reported (case report). Monitor blood glucose frequently, especially in patients with diabetes or with risk factors for diabetes. Avoid use in patients with poorly controlled diabetes; may initiate after glycemic control has been established. Potentially significant interactions may exist, requiring dose or frequency adjustment, additional monitoring, and/or selection of alternative therapy.

Adverse Reactions

>10%:

Cardiovascular: Peripheral edema (16%)

Central nervous system: Fatigue (29% to 31%), headache (13% to 20%), chills (13%), insomnia (12%)

Dermatologic: Alopecia (15%), skin rash (11%)

Endocrine & metabolic: Increased uric acid (grades 3/4: 56% to 57%), hyperglycemia (grades 3/4: 10% to 15%; hyperosmolar nonketotic hyperglycemia <1%)

Gastrointestinal: Diarrhea (35% to 41%), nausea (29% to 35%), abdominal pain (16% to 23%), vomiting (12% to 15%), constipation (14%), anorexia (10% to 13%)

Hematologic & oncologic: Thrombocytopenia (58% to 76%; grades 3/4: 49% to 88%), neutropenia (20% to 53%; grades 3/4: 18% to 81%), anemia (51% to 61%; grades 3/4: 36% to 80%), leukocyte disorder (decreased: grades 3/4: 61% to 72%), febrile neutropenia (10% to 20%; grades 3/4: 10% to 16%), lymphocytopenia (17%; grades 3/4: 16%)

Infection: Infection (46% to 56%; grades 3/4: 11% to 20%)

Local: Injection site reaction (22% to 35%; includes edema, erythema, hematoma, hemorrhage, hypersensitivity, induration, inflammation, infusion related reaction, irritation, mass, pruritus, rash)

Neuromuscular & skeletal: Weakness (23% to 24%), arthralgia (19%), limb pain (11% to 13%), back pain (12%), myalgia (11%)

Renal: Increased serum creatinine (grades 3/4: 9% to 16%)

Respiratory: Epistaxis (11% to 17%), cough (≤16%), dyspnea (11%)

Miscellaneous: Fever (25% to 29%)

1% to 10%:

Cardiovascular: Acute coronary syndrome, angina pectoris, bradycardia, cardiac arrhythmia, chest pain, edema, hypertension, hypotension, palpitations, tachycardia, ventricular premature contractions

Central nervous system: Agitation, anxiety, cerebral hemorrhage, confusion, depression, dizziness, hyperthermia, hypoesthesia, lethargy, malaise, mental status changes, mouth pain, myasthenia, pain, paresthesia, sciatica, seizure, voice disorder

Dermatologic: Burning sensation of skin, dermal ulcer, desquamation, erythema, hyperhidrosis, hyperpigmentation, night sweats, pruritus, skin lesion, xeroderma

Endocrine & metabolic: Decreased serum glucose (grades 3/4: 6% to 8%), dehydration, diabetes mellitus, gout, hot flash

Gastrointestinal: Abdominal distention, anal fissure, aphthous stomatitis, decreased appetite, dysgeusia, dyspepsia, dysphagia, gastritis, gastroesophageal reflux disease, gastrointestinal hemorrhage, gingival hemorrhage, gingival pain, gingivitis, hemorrhoids, melena, mucosal inflammation, oral mucosa ulcer, stomatitis, xerostomia

Genitourinary: Dysuria

Hematologic & oncologic: Bone marrow failure (10%; grades 3/4: 10%), bruise, hematoma, hemorrhage (ear), oral hemorrhage, petechia, purpura

Hepatic: Increased serum bilirubin (grades 3/4: 6% to 9%), increased serum ALT (grades 3/4: 2% to 6%)

Hypersensitivity: Hypersensitivity reaction, transfusion reaction

Neuromuscular & skeletal: Muscle spasm, musculoskeletal chest pain, musculoskeletal pain (or discomfort), ostealgia, stiffness, tremor

Ophthalmic: Blurred vision, cataract, conjunctival hemorrhage, conjunctivitis, diplopia, eyelid edema, eye pain, increased lacrimation, xerophthalmia

Otic: Otalgia, tinnitus

Respiratory: Flu-like symptoms, hemoptysis, nasal congestion, pharyngolaryngeal pain, rales, rhinorrhea, sinus congestion

Drug Interactions

Metabolism/Transport Effects Substrate of P-glycoprotein

Avoid Concomitant Use

Avoid concomitant use of Omacetaxine with any of the following: Anticoagulants; Aspirin; BCG (Intravesical); Natalizumab; Nonsteroidal Anti-Inflammatory Agents; Pimecrolimus; Tacrolimus (Topical); Vaccines (Live)

Increased Effect/Toxicity

Omacetaxine may increase the levels/effects of: Fingolimod; Leflunomide; Natalizumab; Tofacitinib; Vaccines (Live)

The levels/effects of Omacetaxine may be increased by: Anticoagulants; Aspirin; Denosumab; Nonsteroidal Anti-Inflammatory Agents; Ocrelizumab; Pimecrolimus; Roflumilast; Tacrolimus (Topical); Trastuzumab

◀ **Decreased Effect**

Omacetaxine may decrease the levels/effects of: Antidiabetic Agents; BCG (Intravesical); Coccidioides immitis Skin Test; Nivolumab; Sipuleucel-T; Tertomotide; Vaccines (Inactivated); Vaccines (Live)

The levels/effects of Omacetaxine may be decreased by: Echinacea

Hazardous Drugs Handling Considerations

Hazardous agent (NIOSH 2016 [group 1]).

Use appropriate precautions for receiving, handling, administration, and disposal. Gloves (single) should be worn during receiving, unpacking, and placing in storage.

NIOSH recommends double gloving, a protective gown, ventilated engineering controls (a class II biological safety cabinet or a compounding aseptic containment isolator), and closed system transfer devices (CSTDs) for preparation. Double gloving, a gown, and (if dosage form allows) CSTDs are required during administration (NIOSH 2016).

Storage/Stability Store intact vials at 20°C to 25°C (68°F to 77°F); excursions are permitted between 15°C and 30°C (59°F and 86°F). Protect from light (intact vial and reconstituted solutions). Reconstituted solution should be used within 12 hours if stored at room temperature or within 6 days (144 hours) if refrigerated at 2°C to 8°C (36°F to 46°F).

Preparation for Administration Avoid skin and eye contact; wear protective eyewear and gloves during handling and administration. Reconstitute each 3.5 mg vial with sodium chloride 0.9% (NS) 1 mL, resulting in a concentration of 3.5 mg/mL. Gently swirl until solution is clear (lyophilized powder dissolves completely in <1 minute).

Mechanism of Action Omacetaxine is a reversible protein synthesis inhibitor which binds to the A-site cleft of the ribosomal subunit to interfere with chain elongation and inhibit protein synthesis. It acts independently of BCR-ABL1 kinase-binding activity, and has demonstrated activity against tyrosine kinase inhibitor-resistant BCR-ABL mutations.

Pharmacodynamics/Kinetics

Onset:

Chronic phase CML: Mean time to major cytogenetic response: 3.5 months

Accelerated phase CML: Mean time to response: 2.3 months

Duration:

Chronic phase CML: Median duration of major cytogenetic response: 12.5 months

Accelerated phase CML: Median duration of major hematologic response: 4.7 months

Absorption: SubQ: Rapid (Nemunaitis 2013)

Distribution: V_{dss}: 141 ± 93.4 L

Protein binding: ≤50%

Metabolism: Hydrolyzed by plasma esterases to 4'-DMHHT; minimal hepatic metabolism

Half-life elimination: 14.6 hours

Time to peak: SubQ: ~30 minutes

Excretion: Urine (~37); feces (~44%)

Dosing

Adult & Geriatric Chronic myeloid leukemia (CML), chronic or accelerated phase: SubQ:

Induction: 1.25 mg/m^2 twice daily for 14 consecutive days of a 28-day treatment cycle; continue until hematologic response is achieved

Maintenance: 1.25 mg/m^2 twice daily for 7 consecutive days of a 28-day treatment cycle; continue until no longer achieving clinical treatment benefit

Missed doses: If a dose is missed, skip that dose and resume with the next regularly scheduled dose. Do not administer 2 doses at the same time to make up for a missed dose.

Renal Impairment There are no dosage adjustments provided in the manufacturer's labeling (has not been studied). Based on the minimal amount of unchanged drug excreted in the urine, dosage adjustment is not likely necessary (Nemunaitis 2013).

Hepatic Impairment There are no dosage adjustments provided in the manufacturer's labeling (has not been studied).

Adjustment for Toxicity

Hematologic toxicity: May delay treatment cycles and/or reduce the number of treatment days during a cycle for hematologic toxicities.

Neutropenia grade 4 (ANC <500/mm^3) or thrombocytopenia ≥ grade 3 (platelets <50,000/mm^3) during a cycle: Delay the start of the next cycle until ANC ≥1000/mm^3 and platelets ≥50,000/mm^3 **AND** reduce the number of treatment days by 2 days (eg, reduce from 14 days to 12 days or reduce from 7 days to 5 days)

Nonhematologic toxicity: Manage symptomatically; interrupt and/or delay treatment until toxicity resolves.

Administration Administer subcutaneously at approximately 12 hour intervals. If home administration is to occur, advise patient on proper handling, storage conditions, administration, disposal, and clean-up of accidental spillage; ensure that the patient or patient's caregiver is an appropriate candidate for home administration. Avoid skin and eye contact; wear protective eyewear and gloves during handling and administration.

Emetic Potential Low (10% to 30%)

Monitoring Parameters CBC with differential and platelets (weekly during induction and initial maintenance cycles, then every 2 weeks or as clinically indicated after initial maintenance cycles); blood glucose (frequently); signs/symptoms of infection; signs of bleeding

Medication Guide Available Yes

Dosage Forms Excipient information presented when available (limited, particularly for generics); consult specific product labeling.

Solution Reconstituted, Subcutaneous, as mepesuccinate [preservative free]:
Synribo: 3.5 mg (1 ea)

Ondansetron (on DAN se tron)

Related Information

Management of Chemotherapy-Induced Nausea and Vomiting in Adults on page 2253

Prevention of Chemotherapy-Induced Nausea and Vomiting in Children on page 2310

Brand Names: US Zofran; Zofran ODT; Zuplenz

Brand Names: Canada ACT Ondansetron; AG-Ondansetron; Apo-Ondansetron; Bio-Ondansetron; Dom-Ondansetron; IPG-Ondansetron; JAMP-Ondansetron; Mar-Ondansetron; Mint-Ondansetron; Mylan-Ondansetron; NAT-Ondansetron; Nu-Ondansetron; Ondansetron Hydrochloride Dihydrate Injection; Ondansetron Injection; Ondansetron Injection USP; Ondansetron-Omega; Ondissolve ODF; PHL-Ondansetron; PMS-Ondansetron; Priva-Ondansetron; RAN-Ondansetron; ratio-Ondansetron; Sandoz-Ondansetron; Sandoz-Ondansetron ODT; Septa-Ondansetron; Teva-Ondansetron; Vanc-Ondansetron; Zofran ODT

Index Terms GR38032R; Ondansetron HCl; Ondansetron Hydrochloride

Pharmacologic Category Antiemetic; Selective 5-HT$_3$ Receptor Antagonist

Use

Cancer chemotherapy-induced nausea and vomiting:

IV: Prevention of nausea and vomiting associated with initial and repeat courses of emetogenic cancer chemotherapy (including high-dose cisplatin)

Oral:

Prevention of nausea and vomiting associated with highly emetogenic cancer chemotherapy (including cisplatin ≥50 mg/m^2).

Prevention of nausea and vomiting associated with initial and repeat courses of moderately emetogenic cancer chemotherapy.

Radiotherapy-associated nausea and vomiting: Oral: Prevention of nausea and vomiting associated with radiotherapy in patients receiving either total body irradiation, single high-dose fraction to the abdomen, or daily fractions to the abdomen.

Postoperative nausea and/or vomiting: IV and Oral: Prevention of postoperative nausea and/or vomiting (PONV). If nausea/vomiting occur in a patient who had not received prophylactic ondansetron, IV ondansetron may be administered to prevent further episodes.

Limitations of use: Routine prophylaxis for PONV in patients with minimal expectation of nausea and/or vomiting is not recommended, although use is recommended in patients when nausea and vomiting must be avoided in the postoperative period, even if the incidence of PONV is low.

Labeled Contraindications Hypersensitivity to ondansetron or any component of the formulation; concomitant use with apomorphine

Pregnancy Considerations Adverse events were not observed in animal reproduction studies. Ondansetron readily crosses the human placenta in the first trimester of pregnancy and can be detected in fetal tissue (Siu 2006). Due to pregnancy-induced physiologic changes, clearance of ondansetron may increase as pregnancy progresses (Lemon 2016).

Although ondansetron has been evaluated for the treatment of nausea and vomiting of pregnancy, current guidelines note data related to fetal safety is conflicting (ACOG 2015); ondansetron is generally reserved for use when other agents have failed (Arsenault 2002). Because a dose-dependent QT-interval prolongation occurs with use, the manufacturer recommends ECG monitoring in patients with electrolyte abnormalities (which can be associated with some cases of NVP; Koren 2012). An international consensus panel recommends that 5-HT$_3$ antagonists (including ondansetron) should not be withheld in pregnant patients receiving chemotherapy for the treatment of gynecologic cancers, when chemotherapy is given according to general recommendations for chemotherapy use during pregnancy (Amant 2010).

Breastfeeding Considerations It is not known if ondansetron is excreted into breast milk. According to the manufacturer, the decision to continue or discontinue breastfeeding during therapy should take into account the risk of infant exposure, the benefits of breastfeeding to the infant, and benefits of treatment to the mother.

Warnings/Precautions Antiemetics are most effective when used prophylactically (Roila 2016). If emesis occurs despite optimal antiemetic prophylaxis, reevaluate emetic risk, disease, concurrent morbidities and medications to assure antiemetic regimen is optimized (Basch 2011). Ondansetron does not stimulate gastric or intestinal peristalsis (do not use in place of nasogastric suction). Ondansetron may mask progressive ileus and/or gastric distension; monitor for decreased bowel activity. Hypersensitivity reactions (including anaphylaxis and bronchospasm) have been reported; discontinue if hypersensitivity occurs. Use with caution in patients allergic to other 5-HT$_3$ receptor antagonists; cross-reactivity has been reported.

ECG changes, including dose-dependent QT interval prolongation have been observed with ondansetron. Cases of torsade de pointes have also been reported. Selective 5-HT$_3$ antagonists, including ondansetron, have been associated with a number of dose-dependent increases in ECG intervals (eg, PR, QRS duration, QT/QTc, JT), usually occurring 1 to 2 hours after IV administration. Single doses >16 mg ondansetron IV are no longer recommended due to the potential for an increased risk of QT prolongation. In most patients, these changes are not clinically relevant; however, when used in conjunction with other agents that prolong these intervals or in those at risk for QT prolongation, arrhythmia may occur. When used with agents that prolong the QT interval (eg, Class I and III antiarrhythmics) or in patients with cardiovascular disease, clinically relevant QT interval prolongation may occur resulting in torsade de pointes. Avoid ondansetron use in patients with congenital long QT syndrome. Use caution and monitor ECG in patients with other risk factors for QT prolongation (eg, medications known to prolong QT interval, electrolyte abnormalities [hypokalemia or hypomagnesemia], heart failure, bradyarrhythmias, and cumulative high-dose anthracycline therapy). IV formulations of 5-HT$_3$ antagonists have more association with ECG interval changes, compared to oral formulations. Dose limitations are recommended for patients with severe hepatic impairment (Child-Pugh class C); use with caution in mild-moderate hepatic impairment; clearance is decreased and half-life increased in hepatic impairment.

Serotonin syndrome has been reported with 5-HT$_3$ receptor antagonists, predominantly when used in combination with other serotonergic agents (eg, SSRIs, SNRIs, MAOIs, mirtazapine, fentanyl, lithium, tramadol, and/or methylene blue). Some of the cases have been fatal. The majority of serotonin syndrome reports due to 5-HT$_3$ receptor antagonist have occurred in a postanesthesia setting or in an infusion center. Serotonin syndrome has also been reported following overdose of ondansetron. Monitor patients for signs of serotonin syndrome, including mental status changes (eg, agitation, hallucinations, delirium, coma); autonomic instability (eg, tachycardia, labile blood pressure, diaphoresis, dizziness, flushing, hyperthermia); neuromuscular changes (eg, tremor, rigidity, myoclonus, hyperreflexia, incoordination); gastrointestinal symptoms (eg, nausea, vomiting, diarrhea); and/or seizures. If serotonin syndrome occurs, discontinue 5-HT$_3$ receptor antagonist treatment and begin supportive management. Potentially significant drug-drug interactions may exist, requiring dose or frequency adjustment, additional monitoring, and/or selection of alternative therapy. Orally disintegrating tablets contain phenylalanine.

Benzyl alcohol and derivatives: Some dosage forms may contain sodium benzoate/benzoic acid; benzoic acid (benzoate) is a metabolite of benzyl alcohol; large amounts of benzyl alcohol (≥99 mg/kg/day) have been associated with a potentially fatal toxicity ("gasping syndrome") in neonates; the "gasping syndrome" consists of metabolic acidosis, respiratory distress, gasping respirations, CNS dysfunction (including convulsions, intracranial hemorrhage), hypotension, and cardiovascular collapse (AAP ["Inactive" 1997]; CDC 1982); some data suggests that benzoate displaces bilirubin from protein binding sites (Ahlfors 2001); avoid or use dosage forms containing benzyl alcohol derivative with caution in neonates. See manufacturer's labeling.

Adverse Reactions Note: Percentages reported in adult patients unless otherwise specified.
>10%:
  Central nervous system: Headache (oral: 9% to 27%; IV: 17%), fatigue (oral: ≤9% to 13%), malaise (oral: ≤9% to 13%)
  Gastrointestinal: Constipation (6% to 11%)
1% to 10%:
  Central nervous system: Drowsiness (IV: ≤8%), sedation (IV: ≤8%), (dizziness (7%), agitation (oral: ≤6%), anxiety (oral: ≤6%), paresthesia (IV: 2%), sensation of cold (IV: 2%)
  Dermatologic: Pruritus (2% to 5%), skin rash (1%)
  Gastrointestinal: Diarrhea (oral: 6% to 7%; IV: Children 1 to 24 months of age: 2%)
  Genitourinary: Gynecologic disease (oral: 7%), urinary retention (oral: 5%)
  Hepatic: Increased serum ALT (>2 times ULN: 1% to 5%; transient), increased serum AST (>2 times ULN: 1% to 5%; transient)
  Local: Injection site reaction (IV: 4%; includes burning sensation at injection site, erythema at injection site, injection site pain)
  Respiratory: Hypoxia (oral: 9%)
  Miscellaneous: Fever (2% to 8%)
<1%, postmarketing, and/or case reports: Abdominal pain, accommodation disturbance, anaphylactoid reaction, anaphylaxis, angina pectoris, angioedema, atrial fibrillation, bradycardia, bronchospasm, bullous skin disease, cardiac arrhythmia, cardiorespiratory arrest (IV), chest pain, chills, depression of ST segment on ECG, dyspnea, dystonic reaction, ECG changes, extrapyramidal reaction (IV), flushing, hepatic failure (when used with other hepatotoxic medications), hiccups, hypersensitivity reaction, hypokalemia, hypotension, ischemic heart disease, laryngeal edema, laryngospasm (IV), liver enzyme disorder, mucosal tissue reaction, myocardial infarction, neuroleptic malignant syndrome, oculogyric crisis, palpitations, positive lymphocyte transformation test, prolonged Q-T interval on ECG (dose dependent), second-degree atrioventricular block, serotonin syndrome, shock (IV), Stevens-Johnson syndrome, stridor, supraventricular tachycardia, syncope, tachycardia, tonic-clonic seizures, torsades de pointes, toxic epidermal

necrolysis, transient blindness (lasted ≤48 hours), transient blurred vision (following infusion), urticaria, vascular occlusive events, ventricular premature contractions, ventricular tachycardia, weakness, xerostomia

Drug Interactions

Metabolism/Transport Effects Substrate of CYP1A2 (minor), CYP2C9 (minor), CYP2D6 (minor), CYP2E1 (minor), CYP3A4 (major), P-glycoprotein; **Note:** Assignment of Major/Minor substrate status based on clinically relevant drug interaction potential; **Inhibits** CYP2C9 (weak)

Avoid Concomitant Use

Avoid concomitant use of Ondansetron with any of the following: Apomorphine; Highest Risk QTc-Prolonging Agents; Hydroxychloroquine; MiFEPRIStone; Probucol; Promazine; Vinflunine

Increased Effect/Toxicity

Ondansetron may increase the levels/effects of: Apomorphine; Highest Risk QTc-Prolonging Agents; MetFORMIN; Moderate Risk QTc-Prolonging Agents; Panobinostat; Serotonin Modulators

The levels/effects of Ondansetron may be increased by: Hydroxychloroquine; MiFEPRIStone; P-glycoprotein/ABCB1 Inhibitors; Probucol; Promazine; QTc-Prolonging Agents (Indeterminate Risk and Risk Modifying); Ranolazine; Vinflunine; Xipamide

Decreased Effect

Ondansetron may decrease the levels/effects of: Tapentadol; TraMADol

The levels/effects of Ondansetron may be decreased by: Bosentan; CYP3A4 Inducers (Moderate); CYP3A4 Inducers (Strong); Dabrafenib; Deferasirox; Enzalutamide; Mitotane; Sarilumab; Siltuximab; St John's Wort; Tocilizumab

Food Interactions Tablet: Food slightly increases the extent of absorption. Management: Administer without regard to meals.

Storage/Stability

Oral soluble film: Store between 20°C and 25°C (68°F and 77°F). Store pouches in cartons; keep film in individual pouch until ready to use.

Oral solution: Store between 15°C and 30°C (59°F and 86°F). Protect from light.

Tablet: Store between 2°C and 30°C (36°F and 86°F).

Vial: Store between 2°C and 30°C (36°F and 86°F). Protect from light. Chemically and physically stable when mixed in D5W or NS for 48 hours at room temperature; however, diluents generally do not contain a preservative and sterile precautions should be observed. After dilution, do not use beyond 24 hours.

Premixed bag in D5W: Store at 20°C to 25°C (68°F to 77°F), excursions permitted from 15°C to 30°C (59°F to 86°F); may refrigerate; avoid freezing and excessive heat; protect from light.

Preparation for Administration Vial:

Prevention of chemotherapy-induced nausea and vomiting: Dilution is required prior to IV infusion. Dilute in 50 mL D5W or NS. In pediatric patients between 6 months and 1 year of age and/or ≤10 kg, may dilute in 10 to 50 mL D5W or NS, depending on fluid needs of the patient. Use diluted solutions within 24 hours of preparation.

Prevention of postoperative nausea and vomiting: No dilution is required.

Mechanism of Action Selective 5-HT$_3$-receptor antagonist, blocking serotonin, both peripherally on vagal nerve terminals and centrally in the chemoreceptor trigger zone

Pharmacodynamics/Kinetics

Onset of action: ~30 minutes

Absorption: Oral: 100%; nonlinear absorption occurs with increasing oral doses; Zofran ODT tablets are bioequivalent to Zofran tablets; absorption does not occur via oral mucosa

Distribution: V_d:

Infants and Children: Surgical patients:
  1 to 4 months: 3.5 L/kg
  5 to 24 months: 2.3 L/kg
  3 to 12 years: 1.65 L/kg

Children and Adolescents: Cancer patients: 4 to 18 years: 1.9 L/kg

Adults: 1.9 L/kg

Protein binding, plasma: 70% to 76%

Metabolism: Extensively hepatic via hydroxylation, followed by glucuronide or sulfate conjugation; CYP1A2, CYP2D6, and CYP3A4 substrate; some demethylation occurs

Bioavailability: Oral: 50% to 70% due to some first-pass metabolism; in cancer patients (adults) 85% to 87% bioavailability possibly related to changes in metabolism

Half-life elimination:

Children: Cancer patients: Children and Adolescents: 4 to 18 years: 2.8 hours; Surgical patients: Infants 1 to 4 months: 6.7 hours; Infants and Children 5 months to 12 years: 2.9 hours

Adults: 3 to 6 hours; Mild-to-moderate hepatic impairment (Child-Pugh classes A and B): 12 hours; Severe hepatic impairment (Child-Pugh class C): 20 hours

Time to peak: Oral: ~2 hours; Oral soluble film: ~1 hour

Excretion: Urine (44% to 60% as metabolites, ~5% as unchanged drug); feces (~25%)

Clearance:

Cancer patients: Children and Adolescents 4 to 18 years: 0.599 L/kg/hour

Surgical patients: Infants and Children: 1 to 4 months: 0.401 L/kg/hour; 5 to 24 months: 0.581 L/kg/hour; 3 to 12 years: 0.439 L/kg/hour

Adult (normal): 19 to 40 years: 0.381 L/kg/hour; 61 to 74 years: 0.319 L/kg/hour; >75 years: 0.262 L/kg/hour

Dosing

Adult

Prevention of chemotherapy-induced nausea and vomiting:

Prevention of nausea and vomiting associated with emetogenic chemotherapy: IV: 0.15 mg/kg/dose (maximum: 16 mg/dose) administered over 15 minutes for 3 doses, beginning 30 minutes prior to chemotherapy, followed by subsequent doses 4 and 8 hours after the first dose

Prevention of nausea and vomiting associated with highly emetogenic chemotherapy: Oral: 24 mg 30 minutes prior to the start of single-day chemotherapy

Prevention of nausea and vomiting associated with moderately emetogenic chemotherapy: Oral: 8 mg beginning 30 minutes before chemotherapy; repeat dose 8 hours after initial dose, then 8 mg every 12 hours for 1 to 2 days after chemotherapy completed

Guideline recommendations: **Prevention of chemotherapy-induced nausea and vomiting:**

American Society of Clinical Oncology (ASCO; Basch 2011):

High emetic risk: Day(s) chemotherapy is administered (antiemetic regimen also includes dexamethasone and aprepitant or fosaprepitant):

IV: 8 mg or 0.15 mg/kg. **Note:** Single IV doses >16 mg are no longer recommended by the manufacturer due to the potential for QT prolongation.

Oral: 8 mg twice daily

Multinational Association of Supportive Care in Cancer (MASCC) and European Society of Medical Oncology (ESMO) (Roila 2016):

Highly emetic chemotherapy (antiemetic regimen includes dexamethasone and aprepitant/fosaprepitant):

IV: 8 mg or 0.15 mg/kg as a single dose prior to chemotherapy. **Note:** Single IV doses >16 mg are no longer recommended by the manufacturer due to the potential for QT prolongation

Oral: 16 mg as a single dose prior to chemotherapy (8 mg twice daily has also been used)

Moderately emetic chemotherapy (antiemetic regimen includes dexamethasone [and aprepitant/fosaprepitant for AC chemotherapy regimen]):

IV: 8 mg or 0.15 mg/kg as a single dose prior to chemotherapy. **Note:** Single IV doses >16 mg are no longer recommended by the manufacturer due to the potential for QT prolongation.

Oral: 16 mg (as 8 mg twice daily)

Low emetic risk: Ondansetron (dose not specified) prior to chemotherapy on day 1

Prevention of radiation therapy-induced nausea and vomiting:

Total body irradiation: Oral: 8 mg administered 1 to 2 hours before each daily fraction of radiotherapy

Single high-dose fraction radiotherapy to abdomen: Oral: 8 mg administered 1 to 2 hours before irradiation, then 8 mg every 8 hours after first dose for 1 to 2 days after completion of radiotherapy

Daily fractionated radiotherapy to abdomen: Oral: 8 mg administered 1 to 2 hours before irradiation, then 8 mg every 8 hours after first dose for each day of radiotherapy

American Society of Clinical Oncology Antiemetic Guideline recommendations (Basch 2011): Give before each fraction throughout radiation therapy for high emetic risk (continue for at least 24 hours after completion) and for moderate emetic risk. For low emetic risk, may give either as prevention or rescue; for minimal emetic risk, give as rescue (if rescue used for either low or minimal emetic risk, then prophylaxis should be given until the end of radiation therapy).

IV (off-label route/dosing): 8 mg or 0.15 mg/kg. **Note:** Single IV doses >16 mg are no longer recommended by the manufacturer due to the potential for QT prolongation.

Prevention of postoperative nausea and vomiting (PONV):

IM, IV: 4 mg as a single dose (over 2 to 5 minutes if giving IV) administered ~30 minutes before the end of anesthesia (see **Note** below).

Note: The manufacturer recommends administration immediately before induction of anesthesia; however, this has been shown not to be as effective as administration at the end of surgery (Sun, 1997). Repeat doses given in response to inadequate control of nausea/vomiting from preoperative doses are generally ineffective.

Oral: 16 mg administered 1 hour prior to induction of anesthesia

Treatment of postoperative nausea and vomiting (off-label): IV: 4 mg as a single dose for failure when an agent from a different class was utilized as prophylaxis **or** 1 mg may be effective when a prophylactic agent was not utilized (Gan 2007)

Nausea and vomiting of pregnancy (severe or refractory) (off-label use):

IV: 8 mg administered over 15 minutes every 12 hours (Arsenault 2002)

Oral: 8 mg every 12 hours (Arsenault 2002)

Geriatric Oral, IV: No dosing adjustment required; refer to adult dosing.

Pediatric

Prevention of chemotherapy-induced nausea and vomiting:

Prevention of nausea and vomiting associated with emetogenic chemotherapy: Infants ≥6 months, Children, and Adolescents: IV: 0.15 mg/kg/dose (maximum: 16 mg/dose) over 15 minutes for 3 doses, beginning 30 minutes prior to chemotherapy, followed by subsequent doses administered 4 and 8 hours after the first dose

Prevention of nausea and vomiting associated with moderately emetogenic chemotherapy: Oral:

Children 4 to 11 years: 4 mg 30 minutes before chemotherapy; repeat 4 and 8 hours after initial dose, then 4 mg every 8 hours for 1 to 2 days after chemotherapy completed

Children ≥12 years:

Tablet: 8 mg 30 minutes before chemotherapy; repeat 4 and 8 hours after initial dose, then 8 mg every 8 hours for 1 to 2 days after chemotherapy completed.

Soluble film: 8 mg orally twice a day. The first dose should be administered 30 minutes before the start of emetogenic chemotherapy, with a subsequent dose 8 hours after the first dose, then 8 mg twice a day (every 12 hours) for 1 to 2 days after completion of chemotherapy.

Pediatric guideline recommendations:

Prevention of chemotherapy-induced nausea and vomiting (off-label dosing; Dupuis 2013):

Highly emetogenic chemotherapy: Infants ≥1 month and Children <12 years: IV, Oral: 0.15 mg/kg/dose (5 mg/m^2/dose) prior to chemotherapy and then every 8 hours; maximum recommended IV dose: 16 mg. Antiemetic regimen also includes dexamethasone

Highly emetogenic chemotherapy: Children ≥12 years and Adolescents: IV, Oral: 0.15 mg/kg/dose (5 mg/m^2/dose) prior to chemotherapy and then every 8 hours; maximum recommended IV dose: 16 mg. Antiemetic regimen includes dexamethasone and if no known or suspected drug interactions, aprepitant.

Moderately emetogenic chemotherapy: Infants ≥1 month, Children, and Adolescents: IV, Oral: 0.15 mg/kg/dose (5 mg/m^2/dose; maximum: 8 mg dose); prior to chemotherapy and then every 12 hours. Antiemetic regimen also includes dexamethasone.

Low emetogenicity chemotherapy: Infants ≥1 month, Children, and Adolescents: IV, Oral: 0.3 mg/kg/dose (10 mg/m^2/dose; maximum IV dose: 16 mg) prior to chemotherapy

Prevention of postoperative nausea and vomiting (PONV): *US labeling:*
Infants ≥1 month and Children ≤12 years: IV:
   ≤40 kg: 0.1 mg/kg as a single dose over 2 to 5 minutes
   >40 kg: 4 mg as a single dose over 2 to 5 minutes
Adolescents >12 years: IV, IM: Refer to adult dosing.

Renal Impairment
IV: No dosage adjustment is necessary.
Oral: No dosage adjustment necessary; however, according to the manufacturer, there is no experience for oral ondansetron in renal impairment beyond first-day administration (has not been studied beyond day 1).

Hepatic Impairment
Mild to moderate impairment: No dosage adjustment necessary.
Severe impairment (Child-Pugh class C):
   IV: Day 1: Maximum daily dose: 8 mg; however, according to the manufacturer, (there is no experience beyond first-day administration (has not been studied beyond day 1)
   Oral: Maximum daily dose: 8 mg

Administration
Oral: Oral dosage forms should be administered 30 minutes prior to chemotherapy; 1 to 2 hours before radiotherapy; 1 hour prior to the induction of anesthesia
Orally disintegrating tablets: Do not remove from blister until needed. Peel backing off the blister, do not attempt to push tablet through the foil. Using dry hands, place tablet on tongue and allow to dissolve. Swallow with saliva (no need to administer with liquids).
Oral soluble film: Do not remove from pouch until immediately before use. Using dry hands, place film on top of tongue and allow to dissolve (4 to 20 seconds). Swallow with or without liquid. If using more than one film, each film should be allowed to dissolve completely before administering the next film.
IM: Should be administered undiluted.
IV:
   IVPB: Infuse diluted solution over 15 minutes; 24-hour continuous infusions have been reported, but are rarely used.
   Chemotherapy-induced nausea and vomiting: Give first dose 30 minutes prior to beginning chemotherapy.
   IV push: Prevention of postoperative nausea and vomiting: Single doses may be administered IV injection as undiluted solution over at least 30 seconds but preferably over 2 to 5 minutes

Extemporaneous Preparations Note: Commercial oral solution is available (0.8 mg/mL)

If commercial oral solution is unavailable, a 0.8 mg/mL syrup may be made with ondansetron tablets, Ora-Plus® (Paddock), and any of the the following syrups: Cherry syrup USP, Syrpalta® (HUMCO), Ora-Sweet® (Paddock), or Ora-Sweet® Sugar-Free (Paddock). Crush ten 8 mg tablets in a mortar and reduce to a fine powder (flaking of the tablet coating occurs). Add 50 mL Ora-Plus® in 5 mL increments, mixing thoroughly; mix while adding the chosen syrup in incremental proportions to **almost** 100 mL; transfer to a calibrated bottle, rinse mortar with syrup, and add sufficient quantity of syrup to make 100 mL. Label "shake well" and "refrigerate". Stable for 42 days refrigerated (Trissel, 1996).

Rectal suppositories: Calibrate a suppository mold for the base being used. Determine the displacement factor (DF) for ondansetron for the base being used (Fattibase® = 1.1; Polybase® = 0.6). Weigh the ondansetron tablet(s). Divide the tablet weight by the DF; this result is the weight of base displaced by the drug. Subtract the weight of base displaced from the calculated weight of base required for each suppository. Grind the ondansetron tablets in a mortar and reduce to a fine powder. Weigh out the appropriate weight of suppository base. Melt the base over a water bath (<55°C). Add the ondansetron powder to the suppository base and mix well. Pour the mixture into the suppository mold and cool. Stable for at least 30 days refrigerated (Tenjarla, 1998).

Tenjarla SN, Ward ES, and Fox JL, "Ondansetron Suppositories: Extemporaneous Preparation, Drug Release, Stability and Flux Through Rabbit Rectal Membrane," *Int J Pharm Compound*, 1998, 2(1):83-8.

Trissel LA, *Trissel's Stability of Compounded Formulations*, Washington, DC: American Pharmaceutical Association, 1996.

Monitoring Parameters ECG (if applicable in high-risk or elderly patients); potassium, magnesium. Monitor for signs of serotonin syndrome; monitor for decreased bowel activity.

Dietary Considerations Some products may contain phenylalanine.

Dosage Forms Excipient information presented when available (limited, particularly for generics); consult specific product labeling. [DSC] = Discontinued product

Film, Oral:
Zuplenz: 4 mg (1 ea, 10 ea, 30 ea); 8 mg (1 ea, 10 ea, 30 ea)

Solution, Injection, as hydrochloride [strength expressed as base]:
Zofran: 40 mg/20 mL (20 mL [DSC]) [contains methylparaben, propylparaben]
Generic: 4 mg/2 mL (2 mL); 40 mg/20 mL (20 mL)

Solution, Injection, as hydrochloride [strength expressed as base, preservative free]:
Generic: 4 mg/2 mL (2 mL)

Solution, Oral, as hydrochloride [strength expressed as base]:
Zofran: 4 mg/5 mL (50 mL) [strawberry flavor]
Generic: 4 mg/5 mL (50 mL)

Tablet, Oral:
Generic: 24 mg

Tablet, Oral, as hydrochloride [strength expressed as base]:
Zofran: 4 mg, 8 mg
Generic: 4 mg, 8 mg

Tablet Disintegrating, Oral:
Zofran ODT: 4 mg, 8 mg [contains aspartame, methylparaben sodium, propylparaben sodium; strawberry flavor]
Generic: 4 mg, 8 mg

Dosage Forms: Canada Information with regard to form, strength, and availability of products uniquely available in Canada but currently not available in the US. Refer also to Dosage Forms.

Excipient information presented when available (limited, particularly for generics); consult specific product labeling.

◆ **Ondansetron HCl** *see* Ondansetron *on page 1380*

◆ **Ondansetron Hydrochloride** *see* Ondansetron *on page 1380*

Osimertinib (oh si mer ti nib)

Related Information

Common Toxicity Criteria *on page 2242*

Management of Chemotherapy-Induced Nausea and Vomiting in Adults *on page 2253*

Management of EGFR Inhibitor Toxicities: Dermatologic, Ocular, and Gastrointestinal *on page 2291*

Safe Handling of Hazardous Drugs *on page 2379*

Brand Names: US Tagrisso

Brand Names: Canada Tagrisso

Index Terms AZD9291; Tagrisso

Pharmacologic Category Antineoplastic Agent, Epidermal Growth Factor Receptor (EGFR) Inhibitor; Antineoplastic Agent, Tyrosine Kinase Inhibitor

Use Non-small cell lung cancer, metastatic: Treatment of metastatic epidermal growth factor receptor (EGFR) T790M mutation-positive non-small cell lung cancer (NSCLC), as detected by an approved test, in patients who have progressed on or after EGFR tyrosine kinase inhibitor (TKI) therapy

Labeled Contraindications

There are no contraindications listed in the manufacturer's US labeling.

Canadian labeling: Additional contraindications (not in US labeling): Hypersensitivity to osimertinib or any component of the formulation.

Pregnancy Considerations Based on data from animal reproduction studies and the mechanism of action, use during pregnancy is expected to cause fetal harm. Women of reproductive potential should use effective contraception during therapy and for 6 weeks after the last dose. Males with female partners of reproductive potential should also use effective contraception during therapy and for 4 months after the last dose.

Breastfeeding Considerations It is not known if osimertinib is present in breast milk. Because of the potential for serious adverse reactions in the breastfed infant, breastfeeding is not recommended by the manufacturer during therapy and for 2 weeks after the last dose.

◀ **Warnings/Precautions** Interstitial lung disease (ILD) and pneumonitis was observed in clinical studies; some events were fatal. Withhold treatment with worsening respiratory symptoms (dyspnea, cough, fever) which may be indicative of ILD; permanently discontinue if ILD is confirmed.

Cardiomyopathy (cardiac failure, congestive heart failure, pulmonary edema, decreased ejection fraction, or stress cardiomyopathy) has been observed; some events were fatal. In patients who had baseline and at least one follow up assessment, a left ventricular ejection fraction (LVEF) decline of ≥10% and a drop to below 50% was noted. Assess LVEF prior to treatment, while on treatment in patients with cardiac risk factors, and in patients who develop cardiac signs/symptoms during treatment. Permanently discontinue for symptomatic heart failure or persistent, asymptomatic left ventricular dysfunction that does not resolve within 4 weeks. Prolongation of the QTc interval may occur; QTc >500 msec and an increase from baseline of >60 msec have been reported, although no QTc-related arrhythmias have been reported. Patients with a baseline QTc of ≥470 were excluded from clinical trials. Monitor ECG and electrolytes periodically in patients with a history of congenital long QTc syndrome, heart failure, electrolyte abnormalities, and/or those taking concurrent medications known to prolong the QTc interval. Permanently discontinue in patients who develop QTc interval prolongation with signs/symptoms of life-threatening arrhythmia.

Lymphopenia, thrombocytopenia, neutropenia, and anemia may occur (usually grades 1 and 2) with osimertinib. Diarrhea (usually grades 1 and 2) was observed in almost half the patients receiving osimertinib. Skin reactions, including rash, dry skin, and itching may occur. Nail toxicity may also occur. Keratitis has been reported (rarely) in clinical trials. Promptly refer patients for ophthalmologic evaluation if signs/symptoms of keratitis (eye inflammation, lacrimation, light sensitivity, blurred vision, eye pain and/or red eye) develop. Osimertinib may impair fertility; effects may be reversible in females. Potentially significant drug-drug interactions may exist, requiring dose or frequency adjustment, additional monitoring, and/or selection of alternative therapy. Confirm the presence of a T790M epidermal growth factor receptor (EGFR) mutation in tumor sample or plasma specimen prior to treatment initiation. Mutation status should be determined from tumor sample; if tumor was not biopsied, a plasma sample may be used. Circulating tumor cells from plasma sample may be used as a surrogate marker for detection of T790M in tumor tissue (Remon 2017). If mutation is not detected in plasma sample, re-evaluate the feasibility of tumor biopsy for tissue testing. Information on diagnostic tests approved for detection of T790M mutations may be found at www.fda.gov/companiondiagnostics.

Adverse Reactions

>10%:

Central nervous system: Fatigue (22%)

Dermatologic: Skin rash (34%), xeroderma (23%), nail disease (22%), pruritus (13%)

Gastrointestinal: Diarrhea (41%), decreased appetite (18%), nausea (16%), stomatitis (15%), constipation (14%), vomiting (11%)

Hematologic & oncologic: Lymphocytopenia (63%, grades 3/4: 8%), leukopenia (61%; grades 3/4: 1%), thrombocytopenia (46%, grades 3/4: <1%), neutropenia (27%, grades 3/4: 2%)

Respiratory: Cough (17%)

1% to 10%:

Cardiovascular: Decreased left ventricular ejection fraction (4%), prolonged Q-T interval on ECG (≤3%; prolonged from baseline), cardiomyopathy (2%)

Neuromuscular & skeletal: Back pain (10%)

Respiratory: Interstitial pneumonitis (4%)

<1%, postmarketing, and/or case reports: Keratitis

Drug Interactions

Metabolism/Transport Effects Substrate of BCRP, CYP3A4 (major), P-glycoprotein; **Note:** Assignment of Major/Minor substrate status based on clinically relevant drug interaction potential; **Inhibits BCRP**

Avoid Concomitant Use

Avoid concomitant use of Osimertinib with any of the following: BCG (Intravesical); Deferiprone; Dipyrone; Highest Risk QTc-Prolonging Agents; Hydroxychloroquine; MiFEPRIStone; Natalizumab; PAZOPanib; Pimecrolimus; Probucol; Promazine; St John's Wort; Tacrolimus (Topical); Vaccines (Live); Vinflunine

Increased Effect/Toxicity

Osimertinib may increase the levels/effects of: BCRP/ABCG2 Substrates; Deferiprone; Fingolimod; Highest Risk QTc-Prolonging Agents; Leflunomide; Moderate Risk QTc-Prolonging Agents; Natalizumab; PAZOPanib; Tofacitinib; Topotecan; Vaccines (Live)

The levels/effects of Osimertinib may be increased by: Denosumab; Dipyrone; Hydroxychloroquine; MiFEPRIStone; Ocrelizumab; Pimecrolimus; Probucol; Promazine; QTc-Prolonging Agents (Indeterminate Risk and Risk Modifying); Roflumilast; Tacrolimus (Topical); Trastuzumab; Vinflunine; Xipamide

Decreased Effect

Osimertinib may decrease the levels/effects of: BCG (Intravesical); Coccidioides immitis Skin Test; Nivolumab; Sipuleucel-T; Tertomotide; Vaccines (Inactivated); Vaccines (Live)

The levels/effects of Osimertinib may be decreased by: Bosentan; CYP3A4 Inducers (Moderate); CYP3A4 Inducers (Strong); Dabrafenib; Deferasirox; Echinacea; Enzalutamide; Mitotane; Sarilumab; Siltuximab; St John's Wort; Tocilizumab

Hazardous Drugs Handling Considerations

Hazardous agent (meets NIOSH 2016 criteria). This medication is not on the NIOSH (2016) list; however, it meets the criteria for a hazardous drug. Drugs are classified as hazardous based on their properties; the properties of a hazardous drug include one or more of the following characteristics: carcinogenic, teratogenic (or other developmental toxicity), reproductive toxicity, organotoxic at low doses, genotoxic, and/or new agents with structural or toxicity profiles similar to existing hazardous agents.

Use appropriate precautions for receiving, handling, administration, and disposal. Gloves (single) should be worn during receiving, unpacking, and placing in storage. NIOSH recommends single gloving for administration of intact tablets or capsules (NIOSH 2016). If manipulating tablets/capsules (eg, to prepare an oral suspension), NIOSH recommends double gloving, a protective gown, and preparation in a controlled device; if not prepared in a controlled device, respiratory and eye/face protection as well as ventilated engineering controls are recommended. NIOSH recommends double-gloving, a protective gown, and (if there is a potential for vomit or spit up) eye/face ▶

protection for administration of an oral liquid/feeding tube administration (NIOSH 2016).

Storage/Stability

Store at 25°C (77°F); excursions are permitted between 15°C and 30°C (59°F and 86°F).

Preparation for Administration For patients who have difficulty swallowing tablets, disperse tablet in 60 mL of noncarbonated water (only), stir until tablet is dispersed into small pieces (will not dissolve completely) and use immediately; rinse container with 120 to 240 mL water and drink or administer immediately. For nasogastric administration, disperse the tablet in 15 mL of noncarbonated water; use an additional 15 mL of water to transfer residue to the syringe. Administer the 30 mL of liquid via the nasogastric tube and flush appropriately (with ~30 mL of water). Do not crush, heat, or ultrasonicate during preparation.

Mechanism of Action Osimertinib is an irreversible epidermal growth factor receptor (EGFR) tyrosine kinase inhibitor which binds to select mutant forms of EGFR, including T790M, L858R, and exon 19 deletion at lower concentrations than wild-type. Osimertinib exhibits less activity against wild-type EGFR (as compared to other EGFR inhibitors) and is selective for sensitizing mutations and the T790M resistance mutation, which is the most common mechanism of resistance to EGFR tyrosine kinase inhibitors (Janne 2015).

Pharmacodynamics/Kinetics

Distribution: V_{ss}/F: 997 L

Protein binding: Binding is likely high

Metabolism: Hepatic; predominantly oxidation (via CYP3A) and dealkylation to 2 active metabolites (AZ7550 and AZ5104)

Bioavailability: AUC is increased by 19% with a high-fat, high-calorie meal

Half-life, elimination: Mean (estimated): 48 hours

Time to peak: Median: 6 hours (range: 3 to 24 hours)

Excretion: Feces (68%; ~2% as unchanged drug); Urine (14%; ~2% as unchanged drug)

Dosing

Adult & Geriatric Note: Confirm tumor T790M EGFR mutation status prior to treatment initiation (in the absence of tumor biopsy, a plasma specimen may be utilized).

Non-small cell lung cancer, metastatic (T790M EGFR mutation-positive): Oral: 80 mg once daily until disease progression or unacceptable toxicity (Janne 2015; Mok 2017)

Missed doses: If a dose is missed, do not make up the missed dose, take the next dose as scheduled.

Dosage adjustment for concomitant strong CYP3A4 inducers: Avoid concomitant use. If coadministration with a strong CYP3A4 inducer cannot be avoided, increase osimertinib dose to 160 mg once daily. Reduce osimertinib dose to 80 mg once daily 3 weeks after discontinuation of the strong CYP3A4 inducer.

Renal Impairment Note: Renal function may be estimated using the Cockcroft Gault formula.

CrCl 15 to 89 mL/minute: No dosage adjustment necessary.

End-stage renal disease (ESRD): There are no dosage adjustments provided in the manufacturer's labeling (has not been studied).

Hepatic Impairment

Mild (total bilirubin ≤ULN and AST >ULN **or** total bilirubin 1 to 1.5 times ULN and any AST) or moderate (total bilirubin 1.5 to 3 times ULN and any AST) impairment: No dosage adjustment necessary.

Severe impairment (total bilirubin 3 to 10 times ULN and any AST): There are no dosage adjustments provided in the manufacturer's labeling (has not been studied).

Adjustment for Toxicity

Cardiotoxicity:

QTc interval >500 msec on at least 2 separate ECGs: Withhold treatment until QTc interval is <481 msec or recovers to baseline (if baseline QTc ≥481 msec) and then resume at a dose of 40 mg once daily.

QTc interval prolongation with signs/symptoms of life-threatening arrhythmia: Permanently discontinue.

Symptomatic heart failure or asymptomatic left ventricular dysfunction that persists for 4 weeks or longer: Permanently discontinue.

Pulmonary toxicity: Interstitial lung disease/pneumonitis: Permanently discontinue.

Other toxicities: Grade 3 or higher adverse reaction: Withhold treatment for up to 3 weeks. If improves to grade 2 or lower within 3 weeks, resume at either 80 mg once daily or 40 mg once daily. If not improved within 3 weeks, permanently discontinue.

Administration Oral: May be administered with or without food.

For patients who have difficulty swallowing tablets, disperse tablet in 60 mL of noncarbonated water (only), stir until tablet is dispersed into small pieces (will not dissolve completely) and immediately swallow. Rinse container with 120 to 240 mL of water and immediately drink. For nasogastric administration, disperse the tablet in 15 mL of noncarbonated water; use an additional 15 mL of water to transfer residue to the syringe. Administer the 30 mL of liquid via the nasogastric tube and flush appropriately (with ~30 mL of water). Do not crush, heat, or ultrasonicate during preparation.

Emetic Potential Minimal (<10%)

Monitoring Parameters T790M epidermal growth factor receptor (EGFR) mutation status (prior to treatment). Monitor ECG and electrolytes periodically (in patients with a history of congenital long QTc syndrome, heart failure, electrolyte abnormalities, and/or those taking concurrent medications known to prolong the QTc interval). Assess LVEF prior to treatment, and while on treatment in patients with cardiac risk factors, and assess in patients who develop cardiac signs/symptoms. Monitor for signs/symptoms of interstitial lung disease or pneumonitis, dermatologic, and gastrointestinal toxicity.

Prescribing and Access Restrictions Available through specialty pharmacies and distributors. Further information may be obtained from the manufacturer, Astra Zeneca, at 1-844-275-2360 or at https://www.tagrisso.com.

Dosage Forms Excipient information presented when available (limited, particularly for generics); consult specific product labeling.

Tablet, Oral:

Tagrisso: 40 mg, 80 mg

◆ **Otrexup** *see* Methotrexate *on page 1205*

◆ **Oxalatoplatin** *see* Oxaliplatin *on page 1394*

◆ **Oxalatoplatinum** *see* Oxaliplatin *on page 1394*

Oxaliplatin (ox AL i pla tin)

Related Information
Chemotherapy-Induced Peripheral Neuropathy *on page 2236*
Common Toxicity Criteria *on page 2242*
Management of Chemotherapy-Induced Nausea and Vomiting in Adults *on page 2253*
Management of Drug Extravasations *on page 2271*
Mucositis and Stomatitis *on page 2299*
Prevention of Chemotherapy-Induced Nausea and Vomiting in Children *on page 2310*
Safe Handling of Hazardous Drugs *on page 2379*

Brand Names: US Eloxatin [DSC]

Brand Names: Canada Eloxatin; Oxaliplatin Injection; PMS-Oxaliplatin

Index Terms Diaminocyclohexane Oxalatoplatinum; Eloxatin; L-OHP; Oxalatoplatin; Oxalatoplatinum

Pharmacologic Category Antineoplastic Agent, Alkylating Agent; Antineoplastic Agent, Platinum Analog

Use

Colon cancer, stage III (adjuvant therapy): Adjuvant treatment of stage III colon cancer (in combination with infusional fluorouracil and leucovorin) after complete resection of primary tumor.

Colorectal cancer, advanced: Treatment of advanced colorectal cancer (in combination with infusional fluorouracil and leucovorin).

Labeled Contraindications

Hypersensitivity to oxaliplatin, other platinum-containing compounds, or any component of the formulation

Canadian labeling: Additional contraindications (not in the US labeling): Pregnancy, breastfeeding; severe renal impairment (CrCl <30 mL/minute)

Pregnancy Considerations Adverse events were observed in animal reproduction studies at one-tenth the equivalent human dose. Women of childbearing potential should be advised to avoid pregnancy and use effective contraception during treatment. Males and females of reproductive potential desiring children should consider fertility preservation prior to therapy (Levi 2015; O'Neil 2011).

Breastfeeding Considerations It is not known if oxaliplatin is present in breast milk. Due to the potential for serious adverse reactions in the breastfed infant, a decision should be made to discontinue breastfeeding or to discontinue oxaliplatin taking into account the importance of treatment to the mother.

Warnings/Precautions [US Boxed Warning]: Anaphylactic reactions have been reported with oxaliplatin (may occur within minutes of administration); symptoms may be managed with epinephrine, corticosteroids, antihistamines, and discontinuation; oxygen and bronchodilators have also been used (Kim 2009). Grade 3 or 4 hypersensitivity has been observed. Allergic reactions are similar to reactions reported with other platinum analogs, and may occur with any cycle. Reactions typically occur after multiple cycles; in retrospective reviews, reaction occurred at a median of 7 to 9 cycles, with an onset of 5 to 70 minutes (Kim 2009; Polyzos 2009). Symptoms may include bronchospasm (rare), erythema, hypotension (rare), pruritus, rash, and/or urticaria; previously-untreated patients have also experienced flushing, diaphoresis, diarrhea, shortness of breath, chest pain, hypotension, syncope, and disorientation. According to the manufacturer, rechallenge is contraindicated (deaths due to anaphylaxis have been associated with platinum derivatives). In patients rechallenged after mild hypersensitivity, reaction recurred at a higher level of severity; for patients with severe hypersensitivity, rechallenge (with 2 to 3 days of antihistamine and corticosteroid premedication, and prolongation of infusion time) allowed for 2 to 4 additional oxaliplatin cycles; however, rechallenge was not feasible in nearly two-thirds of patients due to the severity of the initial reaction (Polyzos 2009).

Two different types of peripheral sensory neuropathy may occur: The first type of neuropathy is an acute presentation (within hours to 1 to 2 days), reversible (resolves within 14 days), with primarily peripheral symptoms that are often exacerbated by cold (may include pharyngolaryngeal dysesthesia); commonly recur with subsequent doses; avoid mucositis prophylaxis with ice chips, exposure to cold temperatures, or consumption of cold food/beverages during or within hours after oxaliplatin infusion. Cold-triggered neuropathy may last up to 7 days after oxaliplatin administration (Grothey 2011). The second type of neuropathy is a more persistent (>14 days) presentation that often interferes with daily activities (eg, writing, buttoning, swallowing), these symptoms may improve in some patients upon discontinuing treatment. In a retrospective evaluation of patients treated with oxaliplatin for colorectal cancer, the incidence of peripheral sensory neuropathy was similar between diabetic and nondiabetic patients (Ramanathan 2010). Several retrospective studies (as well as a small, underpowered randomized trial) have suggested calcium and magnesium infusions before and after oxaliplatin administration may reduce incidence of cumulative sensory neuropathy; however, a recent abstract of an ongoing randomized, placebo-controlled, double-blind study in patients with colorectal cancer suggests there is no benefit of calcium and magnesium in preventing sensory neuropathy or in decreasing oxaliplatin discontinuation rates (Loprinzi 2013).

Grade 3 and 4 neutropenia occurs commonly with oxaliplatin in combination with fluorouracil and leucovorin; sepsis, neutropenic sepsis, and septic shock have been reported with oxaliplatin (some fatal). Delay oxaliplatin treatment until neutrophils are ≥1500/mm^3; withhold treatment for sepsis or septic shock. Reduce the dose after recovery from grade 4 neutropenia or neutropenic fever. QT prolongation and ventricular arrhythmias, including fatal torsades de pointes have been reported in postmarketing surveillance. ECG monitoring is recommend in patients with heart failure, bradyarrhythmias, concomitant medications known to cause QT prolongation (including class Ia and III antiarrhythmics), and electrolyte abnormalities. Avoid use in patients with congenital long QT syndrome. Monitor potassium and magnesium prior to and periodically during treatment; correct hypokalemia and hypomagnesemia prior to treatment initiation.

Oxaliplatin is associated with a moderate emetic potential; antiemetics are recommended to prevent nausea and vomiting (Basch 2011; Dupuis 2011; Roila 2016). Fluorouracil and leucovorin are associated with GI adverse events; the incidence of GI toxicity is increased when oxaliplatin is administered with fluorouracil and leucovorin. Mucositis, stomatitis, GI bleeding, and GI obstruction have been reported. Cases of reversible posterior leukoencephalopathy syndrome (RPLS) have been reported. Signs/symptoms include headache, mental status changes, seizure, blurred vision, blindness and/or other vision changes; may be associated with hypertension; diagnosis is confirmed with brain imaging. May cause pulmonary fibrosis (may be fatal);

withhold treatment for unexplained pulmonary symptoms (eg, crackles, dyspnea, nonproductive cough, pulmonary infiltrates) until interstitial lung disease or pulmonary fibrosis are excluded. Hepatotoxicity (including rare cases of hepatitis and hepatic failure) has been reported. Liver biopsy has revealed peliosis, idiopathic noncirrhotic portal hypertension (including nodular regenerative hyperplasia), sinusoidal alterations, perisinusoidal fibrosis, and veno-occlusive lesions; the presence of hepatic vascular disorders (including veno-occlusive disease) should be considered, especially in individuals developing portal hypertension or who present with increased liver function tests. Rhabdomyolysis (including fatal cases) has been reported with oxaliplatin; discontinue if signs/symptoms of rhabdomyolysis occur. Use caution with renal dysfunction; increased toxicity may occur; reduce initial dose in severe impairment. Potentially significant drug-drug interactions may exist, requiring dose or frequency adjustment, additional monitoring, and/or selection of alternative therapy. Elderly patients are more sensitive to some adverse events including diarrhea, dehydration, hypokalemia, leukopenia, fatigue and syncope. Oxaliplatin is for IV administration. Administration via the intraperitoneal route (not an approved administration route) is associated with peritoneal hemorrhage and hemorrhagic complications (Charrier 2016). Oxaliplatin is an irritant with vesicant-like properties; ensure proper needle or catheter placement prior to and during infusion; avoid extravasation.

Adverse Reactions Percentages reported with monotherapy.

>10%:

Central nervous system: Peripheral neuropathy (may be dose limiting; 76% to 92%; acute 65%; grades 3/4: 5%; persistent 43%; grades 3/4: 3%), fatigue (61%), pain (14%), headache (13%), insomnia (11%)

Gastrointestinal: Nausea (64%), diarrhea (46%), vomiting (37%), abdominal pain (31%), constipation (31%), anorexia (20%), stomatitis (14%)

Hematologic & oncologic: Anemia (64%; grades 3/4: 1%), thrombocytopenia (30%; grades 3/4: 3%), leukopenia (13%)

Hepatic: Increased serum AST (54%; grades 3/4: 4%), increased serum ALT (36%; grades 3/4: 1%), increased serum bilirubin (13%; grades 3/4: 5%)

Neuromuscular & skeletal: Back pain (11%)

Respiratory: Dyspnea (13%), cough (11%)

Miscellaneous: Fever (25%)

1% to 10%:

Cardiovascular: Edema (10%), chest pain (5%), peripheral edema (5%), flushing (3%), thromboembolism (2%)

Central nervous system: Rigors (9%), dizziness (7%)

Dermatologic: Skin rash (5%), alopecia (3%), palmar-plantar erythrodysesthesia (1%)

Endocrine & metabolic: Dehydration (5%), hypokalemia (3%)

Gastrointestinal: Dyspepsia (7%), dysgeusia (5%), flatulence (3%), hiccups (2%), mucositis (2%), dysphagia (acute 1% to 2%), gastroesophageal reflux disease (1%)

Genitourinary: Dysuria (1%)

Hematologic & oncologic: Neutropenia (7%)

Hypersensitivity: Hypersensitivity reaction (3%; includes urticaria, pruritus, facial flushing, shortness of breath, bronchospasm, diaphoresis, hypotension, syncope: grades 3/4: 2% to 3%)

Local: Injection site reaction (9%; redness, swelling, pain)

Neuromuscular & skeletal: Arthralgia (7%)

Ocular: Abnormal lacrimation (1%)

Renal: Increased serum creatinine (5% to 10%)

Respiratory: Upper respiratory tract infection (7%), rhinitis (6%), epistaxis (2%), pharyngitis (2%), pharyngolaryngeal dysesthesia (grades 3/4: 1% to 2%)

<1%, postmarketing, and/or case reports (reported with mono- and combination therapy): Abnormal gait, acute renal failure, anaphylaxis, anaphylactic shock, anaphylactoid reaction, angioedema, aphonia, ataxia, blepharoptosis, cerebral hemorrhage, colitis, cranial nerve palsy, decreased deep tendon reflex, deafness, decreased visual acuity, diplopia, dysarthria, eosinophilic pneumonitis, fasciculations, febrile neutropenia, hematuria, hemolysis, hemolytic anemia (immuno-allergic), hemolytic-uremic syndrome, hemorrhage, hepatic failure, hepatic fibrosis (perisinusoidal), hepatic sinusoidal obstruction syndrome (SOS; veno-occlusive disease), hepatitis, hepatotoxicity, hypertension, hypomagnesemia, hypoxia, idiopathic noncirrhotic portal hypertension (nodular regenerative hyperplasia), increased INR, increased serum alkaline phosphatase, infusion related reaction (extravasation [including necrosis]), interstitial nephritis (acute), interstitial pulmonary disease, intestinal obstruction, laryngospasm, Lhermittes' sign, metabolic acidosis, muscle spasm, myoclonus, neutropenic enterocolitis, neutropenic infection (sepsis), optic neuritis, pancreatitis, prolonged Q-T interval on ECG, prolonged prothrombin time, pulmonary fibrosis, purpura, rectal hemorrhage, renal tubular necrosis, reversible posterior leukoencephalopathy syndrome (RPLS), rhabdomyolysis, seizure, sepsis, septic shock, temporary vision loss, thrombocytopenia (immuno-allergic), torsades de pointes, trigeminal neuralgia, ventricular arrhythmia, visual field loss, voice disorder

Drug Interactions

Metabolism/Transport Effects Substrate of OCT2

Avoid Concomitant Use

Avoid concomitant use of Oxaliplatin with any of the following: BCG (Intravesical); Deferiprone; Dipyrone; Natalizumab; Pimecrolimus; Tacrolimus (Topical); Vaccines (Live)

Increased Effect/Toxicity

Oxaliplatin may increase the levels/effects of: CloZAPine; Deferiprone; Fingolimod; Highest Risk QTc-Prolonging Agents; Leflunomide; Moderate Risk QTc-Prolonging Agents; Natalizumab; Taxane Derivatives; Tofacitinib; Topotecan; Vaccines (Live)

The levels/effects of Oxaliplatin may be increased by: BuPROPion; Denosumab; Dipyrone; MiFEPRIStone; Ocrelizumab; Palifermin; Pimecrolimus; Promazine; Roflumilast; Tacrolimus (Topical); Trastuzumab

Decreased Effect

Oxaliplatin may decrease the levels/effects of: BCG (Intravesical); Coccidioides immitis Skin Test; Fosphenytoin-Phenytoin; Lenograstim; Nivolumab; Sipuleucel-T; Tertomotide; Vaccines (Inactivated); Vaccines (Live)

The levels/effects of Oxaliplatin may be decreased by: Echinacea

Hazardous Drugs Handling Considerations

Hazardous agent (NIOSH 2016 [group 1]).

Use appropriate precautions for receiving, handling, administration, and disposal. Gloves (single) should be worn during receiving, unpacking, and placing in storage.

◀ NIOSH recommends double gloving, a protective gown, ventilated engineering controls (a class II biological safety cabinet or a compounding aseptic containment isolator), and closed system transfer devices (CSTDs) for preparation. Double gloving, a gown, and (if dosage form allows) CSTDs are required during administration (NIOSH 2016).

Storage/Stability Store intact vials at 25°C (77°F); excursions permitted to 15°C to 30°C (59°F to 86°F); do not freeze. Protect concentrated solution from light (store in original outer carton). According to the manufacturer, solutions diluted in D5W for infusion are stable up to 6 hours at room temperature of 20°C to 25°C (68°F to 77°F) or up to 24 hours under refrigeration at 2°C to 8°C (36°F to 46°F). Oxaliplatin solution diluted with D5W to a final concentration of 0.7 mg/mL (polyolefin container) has been shown to retain >90% of the original concentration for up to 30 days when stored at room temperature or refrigerated; artificial light did not affect the concentration (Andre 2007). As this study did not examine sterility, refrigeration would be preferred to limit microbial growth. Solutions diluted for infusion do not require protection from light.

Preparation for Administration Do not prepare using a chloride-containing solution such as NaCl due to rapid conversion to monochloroplatinum, dichloroplatinum, and diaquoplatinum; all highly reactive in sodium chloride (Takimoto 2007). Do not use needles or administration sets containing aluminum during preparation.

Aqueous solution: Dilution with D5W (250 or 500 mL) is required prior to administration.

Lyophilized powder: Use only SWFI or D5W to reconstitute powder. To obtain final concentration of 5 mg/mL add 10 mL of diluent to 50 mg vial or 20 mL diluent to 100 mg vial. Gently swirl vial to dissolve powder. Dilution with D5W (250 or 500 mL) is required prior to administration. Discard unused portion of vial.

Mechanism of Action Oxaliplatin, a platinum derivative, is an alkylating agent. Following intracellular hydrolysis, the platinum compound binds to DNA forming cross-links which inhibit DNA replication and transcription, resulting in cell death. Cytotoxicity is cell-cycle nonspecific.

Pharmacodynamics/Kinetics

Distribution: V_d: 440 L

Protein binding: >90% primarily albumin and gamma globulin (irreversible binding to platinum)

Metabolism: Nonenzymatic (rapid and extensive), forms active and inactive derivatives

Half-life elimination:

Children: Oxaliplatin ultrafilterable platinum (terminal): Median: 293 hours; range: 187 to 662 hours (Beaty 2010)

Adults: Oxaliplatin ultrafilterable platinum: Distribution: Alpha phase: 0.4 hours; Beta phase: 16.8 hours; Terminal: 391 hours

Excretion: Urine (~54%); feces (~2%)

Dosing

Adult Note: Oxaliplatin is associated with a moderate emetic potential; antiemetics are recommended to prevent nausea and vomiting (Basch 2011; Dupuis 2011; Roila 2016).

Colorectal cancer (advanced): IV: 85 mg/m² every 2 weeks until disease progression or unacceptable toxicity (in combination with infusional fluorouracil/leucovorin)

Colon cancer, stage III (adjuvant therapy): IV: 85 mg/m^2 every 2 weeks for 6 months (12 cycles; in combination with infusional fluorouracil/leucovorin)

Colon/colorectal cancer (off-label doses or combinations): IV: 85 mg/m^2/dose on days 1, 15, and 29 of an 8-week treatment cycle in combination with fluorouracil/leucovorin (Kuebler 2007) **or** 85 mg/m^2 every 2 weeks in combination with fluorouracil/leucovorin/irinotecan (Falcone 2007) **or** 130 mg/m^2 every 3 weeks in combination with capecitabine (Cassidy 2008; Haller 2011)

Biliary adenocarcinoma, advanced (off-label use): IV:

GEMOX regimen: 100 mg/m^2 on day 2 every 2 weeks (in combination with gemcitabine) until disease progression or unacceptable toxicity (Andre 2004) **or**

CAPOX regimen: 130 mg/m^2 on day 1 every 3 weeks (in combination with capecitabine) until disease progression or unacceptable toxicity (Nehls 2008)

Chronic lymphocytic leukemia, fludarabine-refractory (off-label use): IV: OFAR regimen: 25 mg/m^2/day for 4 days every 4 weeks (in combination with fludarabine, cytarabine, and rituximab) for up to 6 cycles (Tsimberidou 2008)

Esophageal/gastric cancers (off-label use): IV: 130 mg/m^2 on day 1 every 3 weeks (in combination with epirubicin and either capecitabine or fluorouracil) for up to 8 cycles (Cunningham 2008) **or** 85 mg/m^2 on day 1 every 2 weeks (in combination with docetaxel, leucovorin, and fluorouracil) for up to 8 cycles (Al-Batran 2008) **or** 85 mg/m^2 on day 1 every 2 weeks (in combination with leucovorin and fluorouracil; FOLFOX4) for 6 cycles (Conroy 2010) **or**

Gastric cancer: IV: 130 mg/m^2 on day 1 every 3 weeks (in combination with capecitabine) for 8 cycles (Bang 2012)

Neuroendocrine tumors (carcinoid), refractory (off-label use): IV: 130 mg/m^2 on day 1 every 3 weeks (in combination with capecitabine) for up to 6 cycles (Bajetta 2007)

Non-Hodgkin lymphoma, relapsed/refractory (off-label use): IV: 100 mg/m^2 on day 1 every 3 weeks (in combination with gemcitabine and rituximab) (Lopez 2008; Rodriguez 2007)

Ovarian cancer, advanced (off-label use): IV: 130 mg/m^2 once every 3 weeks until disease progression or unacceptable toxicity (Dieras 2002; Piccart 2000)

Pancreatic cancer, advanced (off-label use): IV: 85 mg/m^2 every 2 weeks (in combination with fluorouracil, leucovorin, and irinotecan; FOLFIRINOX regimen) for up to 6 months (Conroy 2011) **or** 110 to 130 mg/m^2 on day 1 every 3 weeks (in combination with capecitabine) until disease progression or unacceptable toxicity (Xiong 2008)

Testicular cancer, refractory (off-label use): IV: 130 mg/m^2 every 3 weeks in combination with gemcitabine (De Georgi 2006; Kollmannsberger 2004; Pectasides 2004) **or** 130 mg/m^2 on day 1 every 3 weeks (in combination with gemcitabine and paclitaxel) for up to 8 cycles (Bokemeyer 2008)

Unknown primary cancer, recurrent or refractory (off-label use): IV: 130 mg/m^2 on day 1 of a 21-day cycle (in combination with capecitabine) for 6 cycles or may continue until clinical benefit no longer realized (Hainsworth 2010)

Geriatric No dosage adjustment necessary. Refer to adult dosing.

◄ **Renal Impairment**
Manufacturer's US labeling:
CrCl ≥30 mL/minute: No dosage adjustment necessary.
CrCl <30 mL/minute: Reduce dose from 85 mg/m² to 65 mg/m².
Alternate recommendations: CrCl ≥20 mL/minute: In a study with a limited number of patients with mild to moderate impairment, defined by the authors as CrCl 20 to 59 mL/minute (determined using 24-hour urine collection), oxaliplatin was well tolerated, suggesting a dose reduction may not be necessary in patients with CrCl ≥20 mL/minute receiving every-3-week dosing (dose range: 80 to 130 mg/m² every 3 weeks) (Takimoto 2003).

Hepatic Impairment Mild, moderate, or severe impairment: No dosage adjustment necessary (Doroshow 2003; Synold 2007).

Obesity *ASCO Guidelines for appropriate chemotherapy dosing in obese adults with cancer:* Utilize patient's actual body weight (full weight) for calculation of body surface area- or weight-based dosing, particularly when the intent of therapy is curative; manage regimen-related toxicities in the same manner as for nonobese patients; if a dose reduction is utilized due to toxicity, consider resumption of full weight-based dosing with subsequent cycles, especially if cause of toxicity (eg, hepatic or renal impairment) is resolved (Griggs 2012).

Adjustment for Toxicity
Acute toxicities: Longer infusion time (6 hours) may mitigate acute toxicities (eg, pharyngolaryngeal dysesthesia).
Neurosensory events:
Persistent (>7 days) grade 2 neurosensory events:
Adjuvant treatment of stage III colon cancer: Reduce dose to 75 mg/m²
Advanced colorectal cancer: Reduce dose to 65 mg/m²
Consider withholding oxaliplatin for grade 2 neuropathy lasting >7 days despite dose reduction.
Persistent (>7 days) grade 3 neurosensory events: Consider discontinuing oxaliplatin.
Gastrointestinal toxicity (grade 3/4) occurring despite prophylactic treatment:
Adjuvant treatment of stage III colon cancer: Delay next dose until recovery from toxicity, then reduce dose to 75 mg/m².
Advanced colorectal cancer: Delay next dose until recovery from toxicity, then reduce dose to 65 mg/m².
Hematologic toxicity (grade 4 neutropenia [Canadian labeling: grade 3 or 4 neutropenia], febrile neutropenia, or grade 3/4 thrombocytopenia):
Adjuvant treatment of stage III colon cancer: Delay next dose until neutrophils recover to ≥1500/mm³ and platelets recover to ≥75,000/mm³, then reduce dose to 75 mg/m².
Advanced colorectal cancer: Delay next dose until neutrophils recover to ≥1500/mm³ and platelets recover to ≥75,000/mm³, then reduce dose to 65 mg/m².
Pulmonary toxicity (unexplained respiratory symptoms including non-productive cough, dyspnea, crackles, pulmonary infiltrates): Discontinue until interstitial lung disease or pulmonary fibrosis have been excluded.
Rhabdomyolysis: Discontinue for signs/symptoms of rhabdomyolysis.
Sepsis or septic shock: Withhold treatment.

Combination Regimens

Biliary adenocarcinoma: GEMOX (Biliary Cancer) on page 2141

Colorectal cancer:

Esophageal cancer:

Gastric cancer:

Gastrointestinal cancer: CAPOX (Biliary Cancer) on page 2010

Leukemia, chronic lymphocytic: OFAR (CLL) on page 2181

Lymphoma, non-Hodgkin (DLBCL): GEMOX-R (NHL-DLBCL) on page 2141

Lymphoma, non-Hodgkin (Mantle Cell): GEMOX-R (NHL-Mantle Cell) on page 2141

Pancreatic cancer:

Testicular cancer:

Unknown primary, adenocarcinoma: Capecitabine-Oxaliplatin (Unknown Primary, Adenocarcinoma) on page 2009

Administration Administer as IV infusion over 2 hours; extend infusion time to 6 hours for acute toxicities. Flush infusion line with D5W prior to administration of any concomitant medication. Avoid mucositis prophylaxis with ice chips, exposure to cold temperatures, or consumption of cold food/beverages during or within hours after oxaliplatin infusion (may exacerbate acute neurological symptoms). Do not use needles or administration sets containing aluminum. When used in combination with a fluoropyrimidine (eg, 5-FU), infuse oxaliplatin first.

Oxaliplatin is associated with a moderate emetic potential; antiemetics are recommended to prevent nausea and vomiting (Basch 2011; Dupuis 2011; Roila 2016).

Irritant with vesicant-like properties; ensure proper needle or catheter placement prior to and during infusion. Avoid extravasation; monitor IV site for redness, swelling, or pain.

Extravasation management: If extravasation occurs, stop infusion immediately and disconnect (leave cannula/needle in place); gently aspirate extravasated solution (do **NOT** flush the line); remove needle/cannula; elevate extremity. Information conflicts regarding use of warm or cold compresses. Cold compresses could potentially precipitate or exacerbate peripheral neuropathy (de Lemos 2005).

Vesicant/Extravasation Risk Irritant with vesicant-like properties

Cold compress may cause local vasoconstriction and reduce cellular injury; however, may cause or exacerbate peripheral neuropathy; warm compresses may increase local drug removal, although may also increase cellular uptake and injury (de Lemos 2005).

Emetic Potential Children and Adults: Moderate (30% to 90%)

Monitoring Parameters CBC with differential, blood chemistries, including serum creatinine, ALT, AST, and bilirubin (prior to each cycle), electrolytes, including potassium and magnesium (prior to and periodically during treatment); INR and prothrombin time (in patients on oral anticoagulant therapy); neurologic evaluation prior to each dose and periodically thereafter; hypersensitivity; respiratory effects; RPLS

Dosage Forms Excipient information presented when available (limited, particularly for generics); consult specific product labeling. [DSC] = Discontinued product

Solution, Intravenous [preservative free]:
  Eloxatin: 50 mg/10 mL (10 mL [DSC]); 100 mg/20 mL (20 mL [DSC])
  Generic: 50 mg/10 mL (10 mL); 100 mg/20 mL (20 mL)
Solution Reconstituted, Intravenous [preservative free]:
  Generic: 50 mg (1 ea); 100 mg (1 ea)

◆ **Oxaliplatin Injection (Can)** see Oxaliplatin on page 1394

PACLitaxel (Conventional) (pac li TAKS el con VEN sha nal)

Related Information

Chemotherapy-Induced Peripheral Neuropathy on page 2236
Chronic Pain Management (Cancer) on page 2327
Management of Chemotherapy-Induced Nausea and Vomiting in Adults on page 2253
Management of Drug Extravasations on page 2271
Mucositis and Stomatitis on page 2299
Prevention of Chemotherapy-Induced Nausea and Vomiting in Children on page 2310
Safe Handling of Hazardous Drugs on page 2379

Brand Names: Canada Apo-Paclitaxel; Paclitaxel for Injection; Paclitaxel Injection USP

Index Terms Conventional Paclitaxel; Onxol; Taxol

Pharmacologic Category Antineoplastic Agent, Antimicrotubular; Antineoplastic Agent, Taxane Derivative

Use

Breast cancer: Adjuvant treatment of node-positive breast cancer; treatment of metastatic breast cancer after failure of combination chemotherapy or relapse within 6 months of adjuvant chemotherapy (prior therapy should have included an anthracycline)

Kaposi sarcoma (AIDS-related): Second-line treatment of AIDS-related Kaposi sarcoma

Non-small cell lung cancer: First-line treatment of non-small cell lung cancer (in combination with cisplatin) in patients who are not candidates for potentially curative surgery and/or radiation therapy

Ovarian cancer: Subsequent therapy for treatment of advanced ovarian cancer; first-line therapy of ovarian cancer (in combination with cisplatin)

Labeled Contraindications Hypersensitivity to paclitaxel, polyoxyl 35/polyoxyethylated castor oil (Cremophor EL), or any component of the formulation; treatment of solid tumors in patients with baseline neutrophil counts <1,500/mm^3; treatment of Kaposi sarcoma in patients with baseline neutrophil counts <1,000/mm^3.

Pregnancy Considerations Adverse events (embryotoxicity, fetal toxicity, and maternal toxicity) have been observed in animal reproduction studies at doses less than the recommended human dose. An *ex vivo* human placenta perfusion model illustrated that paclitaxel crossed the placenta at term. Placental transfer was low and affected by the presence of albumin; higher albumin concentrations resulted in lower paclitaxel placental transfer (Berveiller, 2012). Some pharmacokinetic properties of paclitaxel may be altered in pregnant women (van Hasselt, 2014). Women of childbearing potential should be advised to avoid becoming pregnant. A pregnancy registry is available for all cancers diagnosed during pregnancy at Cooper Health (877-635-4499).

Breastfeeding Considerations Paclitaxel is excreted in breast milk (case report). The mother (3 months postpartum) was treated with paclitaxel 30 mg/m^2 (56.1 mg) and carboplatin once weekly for papillary thyroid cancer. Milk samples were obtained 4-316 hours after the infusion given at the sixth and final week of therapy. The average paclitaxel milk concentration over the testing interval was 0.78 mg/L. Although maternal serum concentrations were not noted in the report, the relative infant dose to a nursing infant was calculated to be ~17% of the maternal dose. Paclitaxel continued to be detected in breast milk when sampled at 172 hours after the dose and was below the limit of detection when sampled at 316 hours after the infusion (Griffin, 2012). Due to the potential for serious adverse reactions in a nursing infant, breastfeeding is not recommended.

Warnings/Precautions [US Boxed Warning]: Anaphylaxis and severe hypersensitivity reactions (dyspnea requiring bronchodilators, hypotension requiring treatment, angioedema, and/or generalized urticaria) have occurred in 2% to 4% of patients in clinical studies; premedicate with corticosteroids, diphenhydramine, and H$_2$ antagonists prior to infusion. Some reactions have been fatal despite premedication. If severe hypersensitivity occurs, stop infusion and do not rechallenge. Minor hypersensitivity reactions (flushing, skin reactions, dyspnea, hypotension, or tachycardia) do not require interruption of treatment. Infusion-related hypotension, bradycardia, and/or hypertension may occur; frequent monitoring of vital signs is recommended, especially during the first hour of the infusion. Conventional paclitaxel formulations contain polyoxyl 35/polyoxyethylated castor oil (Cremophor EL) which is associated with hypersensitivity reactions.

Formulations also contain dehydrated alcohol which may cause adverse CNS effects.

[US Boxed Warning]: Bone marrow suppression (primarily neutropenia; may be severe or result in infection) may occur. Monitor blood counts frequently. Do not administer if baseline neutrophil count is <1,500/mm^3 (for solid tumors) or <1,000/mm^3 (for patients with AIDS-related Kaposi sarcoma). Bone marrow suppression (usually neutropenia) is dose-dependent and is the dose-limiting toxicity; neutrophil nadir is usually at a median of 11 days. Subsequent cycles should not be administered until neutrophils are >1,500/mm^3 (for solid tumors) and 1,000/mm^3 (for Kaposi sarcoma); platelets should recover to 100,000/mm^3. Reduce future doses by 20% for severe neutropenia (<500/mm^3 for 7 days or more) and consider the use of supportive therapy, including growth factor treatment.

Use extreme caution with hepatic dysfunction (myelotoxicity may be worsened in patients with total bilirubin >2 times ULN); dose reductions are recommended. Peripheral neuropathy may commonly occur; patients with preexisting neuropathies from prior chemotherapy or coexisting conditions (eg, diabetes mellitus) may be at a higher risk; reduce dose by 20% for severe neuropathy. Rare but severe conduction abnormalities have been reported; conduct continuous cardiac monitoring during subsequent infusions for these patients. In a scientific statement from the American Heart Association, conventional paclitaxel has been determined to be an agent that may either cause direct myocardial toxicity or exacerbate underlying myocardial dysfunction (magnitude: moderate) (AHA [Page 2016]). Elderly patients have an increased risk of toxicity (neutropenia, neuropathy, and cardiovascular events); use with caution. Intraperitoneal administration of paclitaxel is associated with a higher incidence of chemotherapy-related toxicity (Armstrong 2006).

Paclitaxel is an irritant with vesicant-like properties; ensure proper needle or catheter placement prior to and during infusion; avoid extravasation. Injection site reactions are generally mild (skin discoloration, tenderness, erythema, or swelling) and occur more commonly with an extended infusion duration (eg, 24 hours); injection site reactions may be delayed (7 to 10 days). More severe reactions (phlebitis, cellulitis, skin exfoliation, necrosis, fibrosis, and induration) have also been reported. Recall skin reactions may occur despite administering through a different IV site. **[US Boxed Warning]: Should be administered under the supervision of an experienced cancer chemotherapy physician; administer in a facility sufficient to appropriately diagnose and manage complications.** Potentially significant drug-drug interactions may exist, requiring dose or frequency adjustment, additional monitoring, and/or selection of alternative therapy.

Adverse Reactions Percentages reported with single-agent therapy.

>10%:

Cardiovascular: Flushing (28%), ECG abnormality (14% to 23%), edema (21%), hypotension (4% to 12%)

Central nervous system: Peripheral neuropathy (42% to 70%; grades 3/4: ≤7%)

Dermatologic: Alopecia (87%), skin rash (12%)

Gastrointestinal: Nausea (≤52%), vomiting (≤52%), diarrhea (38%), mucositis (17% to 35%), stomatitis (15%; most common at doses >390 mg/m^2), abdominal pain (with intraperitoneal administration)

Hematologic & oncologic: Neutropenia (78% to 98%; grade 4: 14% to 75%; onset: 8 to 10 days; median nadir: 11 days; recovery: 15 to 21 days), leukopenia (90%; grade 4: 17%), anemia (47% to 90%; grades 3/4: 2% to 16%), thrombocytopenia (4% to 20%; grades 3/4: 1% to 7%), hemorrhage (14%)

Hepatic: Increased serum alkaline phosphatase (22%), increased serum AST (19%)

Hypersensitivity: Hypersensitivity reaction (31% to 45%; grades 3/4: ≤2%)

Infection: Infection (15% to 30%)

Local: Injection site reaction (erythema at injection site, skin discoloration at injection site, swelling at injection site, tenderness at injection site: 13%)

Neuromuscular & skeletal: Arthralgia (≤60%), myalgia (≤60%), weakness (17%)

Renal: Increased serum creatinine (observed in Kaposi sarcoma patients only: 18% to 34%, severe: 5% to 7%)

1% to 10%:

Cardiovascular: Bradycardia (3%), tachycardia (2%), hypertension (1%), cardiac arrhythmia (1%), syncope (1%), venous thrombosis (1%)

Dermatologic: Changes in nails (2%)

Hematologic & oncologic: Febrile neutropenia (2%)

Hepatic: Increased serum bilirubin (7%)

Respiratory: Dyspnea (2%)

<1%, postmarketing, and/or case reports: Anaphylaxis, ataxia, atrial fibrillation, atrioventricular block, back pain, brain disease (neurological), cardiac conduction disturbance, cardiac failure, cellulitis, chills, conjunctivitis, dehydration, desquamation, enterocolitis, exacerbation of scleroderma, fibrosis at injection site, hepatic encephalopathy, hepatic necrosis, increased lacrimation, induration at injection site, intestinal obstruction, intestinal perforation, interstitial pneumonitis, ischemic colitis, ischemic heart disease, maculopapular rash, malaise, myocardial infarction, neutropenic enterocolitis, ototoxicity (tinnitus and hearing loss), pancreatitis, paralytic ileus, phlebitis, pneumonitis, pruritus, pulmonary embolism, pulmonary fibrosis, radiation recall phenomenon, radiation pneumonitis, renal insufficiency, seizure, skin edema (diffuse), skin necrosis, skin sclerosis, Stevens-Johnson syndrome, supraventricular tachycardia, thickening of skin, toxic epidermal necrolysis, typhlitis (neutropenic), ventricular tachycardia (asymptomatic), visual disturbance (scintillating scotomata)

Drug Interactions

Metabolism/Transport Effects Substrate of CYP2C8 (major), CYP3A4 (major), P-glycoprotein; **Note:** Assignment of Major/Minor substrate status based on clinically relevant drug interaction potential

Avoid Concomitant Use

Avoid concomitant use of PACLitaxel (Conventional) with any of the following: Atazanavir; BCG (Intravesical); Conivaptan; Deferiprone; Dipyrone; Fusidic Acid (Systemic); Idelalisib; Natalizumab; Pimecrolimus; SORAfenib; Tacrolimus (Topical); Vaccines (Live)

Increased Effect/Toxicity

PACLitaxel (Conventional) may increase the levels/effects of: Amifostine; Antineoplastic Agents (Anthracycline, Systemic); Antipsychotic Agents (Second Generation [Atypical]); Bexarotene (Systemic); CloZAPine; Deferiprone; DOXOrubicin (Conventional); DULoxetine; Fingolimod; Hypotension-Associated Agents; Leflunomide; Levodopa; Natalizumab; Nitroprusside; Pholcodine; Tofacitinib; Trastuzumab; Vaccines (Live); Vinorelbine

◀

The levels/effects of PACLitaxel (Conventional) may be increased by: Abiraterone Acetate; Alfuzosin; Aprepitant; Atazanavir; Barbiturates; Benperidol; Blood Pressure Lowering Agents; Brimonidine (Topical); Clopidogrel; Conivaptan; CYP2C8 Inhibitors (Moderate); CYP2C8 Inhibitors (Strong); CYP3A4 Inhibitors (Moderate); CYP3A4 Inhibitors (Strong); Dasatinib; Deferasirox; Denosumab; Diazoxide; Dipyrone; Fosaprepitant; Fusidic Acid (Systemic); Herbs (Hypotensive Properties); Idelalisib; Lormetazepam; MiFEPRIStone; Molsidomine; Naftopidil; Netupitant; Nicergoline; Nicorandil; Obinutuzumab; Ocrelizumab; Palbociclib; Palifermin; Pentoxifylline; P-glycoprotein/ABCB1 Inhibitors; Phosphodiesterase 5 Inhibitors; Pimecrolimus; Platinum Derivatives; Promazine; Prostacyclin Analogues; Quinagolide; Ranolazine; Roflumilast; Simeprevir; SORAfenib; Stiripentol; Tacrolimus (Topical)

Decreased Effect

PACLitaxel (Conventional) may decrease the levels/effects of: BCG (Intravesical); Coccidioides immitis Skin Test; Lenograstim; Nivolumab; Sipuleucel-T; Tertomotide; Vaccines (Inactivated); Vaccines (Live)

The levels/effects of PACLitaxel (Conventional) may be decreased by: Bexarotene (Systemic); Bosentan; CYP2C8 Inducers (Strong); CYP3A4 Inducers (Moderate); CYP3A4 Inducers (Strong); Dabrafenib; Deferasirox; Echinacea; Enzalutamide; Mitotane; Sarilumab; Siltuximab; St John's Wort; Tocilizumab; Trastuzumab

Hazardous Drugs Handling Considerations

Hazardous agent (NIOSH 2016 [group 1]).

Use appropriate precautions for receiving, handling, administration, and disposal. Gloves (single) should be worn during receiving, unpacking, and placing in storage.

NIOSH recommends double gloving, a protective gown, ventilated engineering controls (a class II biological safety cabinet or a compounding aseptic containment isolator), and (if compatible) closed system transfer devices (CSTDs) for preparation. Double gloving, a gown, and (if dosage form allows) CSTDs are required during administration (NIOSH 2016).

Storage/Stability Store intact vials at room temperature of 20°C to 25°C (68°F to 77°F). Protect from light. Solutions diluted for infusion in D5W and NS are stable for up to 27 hours at ambient temperature (~25°C).

Paclitaxel should be dispensed in either glass or non-PVC containers (eg, Excel/PAB). Use **nonpolyvinyl** (non-PVC) tubing (eg, polyethylene) to minimize leaching. Formulated in a vehicle known as polyoxyl 35/polyoxyethylated castor oil (Cremophor EL), which has been found to leach the plasticizer DEHP from polyvinyl chloride infusion bags or administration sets. Contact of the undiluted concentrate with plasticized polyvinyl chloride (PVC) equipment or devices is not recommended.

Preparation for Administration Dilute for infusion in 250 to 1,000 mL D5W, D$_5$LR, D$_5$NS, or NS to a concentration of 0.3 to 1.2 mg/mL, use a non-PVC container (glass or polyethylene). Chemotherapy dispensing devices (eg, Chemo Dispensing Pin) should not be used to withdraw paclitaxel from the vial; closed system transfer devices may not be compatible with undiluted paclitaxel.

Mechanism of Action Paclitaxel promotes microtubule assembly by enhancing the action of tubulin dimers, stabilizing existing microtubules, and inhibiting their disassembly, interfering with the late G$_2$ mitotic phase, and inhibiting cell replication. In addition, the drug can distort mitotic spindles, resulting in the breakage of chromosomes. Paclitaxel may also suppress cell proliferation and modulate immune response.

Pharmacodynamics/Kinetics

V_{dss}: 24-hour infusion: 227 to 688 L/m^2; biphasic with initial rapid distribution to the peripheral compartment; later phase is a slow efflux of paclitaxel from the peripheral compartment; widely distributed into body fluids and tissues; affected by dose and duration of infusion

Protein binding: 89% to 98%

Metabolism: Hepatic via CYP2C8 and 3A4; forms metabolites (primarily 6α-hydroxypaclitaxel)

Half-life elimination:

Children: 4.6 to 17 hours (varies with dose and infusion duration)

Adults:

3-hour infusion: Mean (terminal): ~13 to 20 hours

24-hour infusion: Mean (terminal): ~16 to 53 hours

Excretion: Feces (~71%; ~5% as unchanged drug); urine (~14%)

Dosing

Adult & Geriatric Note: Premedication with dexamethasone (20 mg orally at 12 and 6 hours prior to the dose [reduce dexamethasone dose to 10 mg orally with advanced HIV disease]), diphenhydramine (50 mg IV 30 to 60 minutes prior to the dose), and cimetidine, famotidine, or ranitidine (IV 30 to 60 minutes prior to the dose) is recommended.

Breast cancer, adjuvant treatment: IV: 175 mg/m^2 over 3 hours every 3 weeks for 4 cycles (administer sequentially following an anthracycline-containing regimen)

Breast cancer, metastatic or relapsed: IV: 175 mg/m^2 over 3 hours every 3 weeks

Non-small cell lung cancer: IV: 135 mg/m^2 over 24 hours every 3 weeks (in combination with cisplatin)

Ovarian cancer, advanced:

Previously treated: IV: 135 or 175 mg/m^2 over 3 hours every 3 weeks

Previously untreated: IV: 175 mg/m^2 over 3 hours every 3 weeks (in combination with cisplatin) or 135 mg/m^2 over 24 hours administered every 3 weeks (in combination with cisplatin)

Intraperitoneal (off-label route): 60 mg/m^2 on day 8 of a 21-day treatment cycle for 6 cycles, in combination with IV paclitaxel (135 mg/m^2 over 24 hours on day 1) and intraperitoneal cisplatin (Armstrong, 2006). **Note:** Administration of intraperitoneal paclitaxel should include the standard paclitaxel premedication regimen.

Previously untreated (off-label combination): IV: 175 mg/m^2 over 3 hours every 3 weeks (in combination with carboplatin) for 6 cycles, or 60 mg/m^2 over 1 hour weekly (in combination with carboplatin) for 18 weeks (Pignata, 2014)

Kaposi sarcoma, AIDS related: IV: 135 mg/m^2 over 3 hours every 3 weeks **or** 100 mg/m^2 over 3 hours every 2 weeks (due to dose-related toxicity, the 100 mg/m^2 dose should be used for patients with a lower performance status). **Note:** Reduce the dexamethasone premedication dose to 10 mg.

Bladder cancer, advanced or metastatic (off-label use): IV: 150 mg/m^2 every 2 weeks (in combination with gemcitabine) (Sternberg, 2001) **or** 200 mg/m^2 over 1 hour every 3 weeks (in combination with gemcitabine) for 6 cycles (Meluch, 2001)

◀ **Cervical cancer, advanced (off-label use):** IV: 135 or 175 mg/m^2 every 3 weeks (in combination with bevacizumab and cisplatin) until disease progression or unacceptable toxicity (Tewari, 2014) **or** 175 mg/m^2 every 3 weeks (in combination with bevacizumab and topotecan) until disease progression or unacceptable toxicity (Tewari, 2014) **or** 135 mg/m^2 over 24 hours every 3 weeks (in combination with cisplatin) for 6 cycles (Monk, 2009; Moore, 2004).

Esophageal/gastric cancer, preoperative chemoradiation (off-label use): IV: 50 mg/m^2 on days 1, 8, 15, 22, and 29 (in combination with carboplatin and radiation therapy) followed by surgery within 4 to 6 weeks (van Hagen, 2012)

Head and neck cancers, advanced (off-label use): IV: 175 mg/m^2 over 3 hours every 3 weeks (in combination with cisplatin) for at least 6 cycles (Gibson, 2005)

Penile cancer, metastatic (off-label use): IV: 175 mg/m^2 over 3 hours every 3 to 4 weeks (in combination with ifosfamide and cisplatin) for 4 cycles (Pagliaro, 2010)

Small cell lung cancer, relapsed/refractory (off-label use): IV: 175 mg/m^2 over 3 hours every 3 weeks (as a single agent) for up to 5 cycles (Smit, 1998) **or** 80 mg/m^2 over 1 hour weekly for 6 weeks of an 8-week treatment cycle (as a single agent) until disease progression or unacceptable toxicity (Yamamoto, 2006)

Soft tissue sarcoma (angiosarcoma), advanced/unresectable (off-label use): IV: 80 mg/m^2 over 1 hour on days 1, 8, and 15 of a 4-week treatment cycle (as a single agent) for up to 6 cycles (Penel, 2008) **or** 135 to 175 mg/m^2 over 3 hours every 3 weeks (as a single agent) (Schlemmer, 2008) **or** 75 to 100 mg/m^2 once weekly (as a single agent) (Schlemmer, 2008)

Testicular germ cell tumors, relapsed/refractory (off-label use): IV: 80 mg/m^2 over 1 hour on days 1 and 8 of a 3-week treatment cycle (in combination with gemcitabine and oxaliplatin) for 2 cycles beyond best response and up to a maximum of 8 cycles (Bokemeyer, 2008) **or** 250 mg/m^2 over 24 hours on day 1 of a 3-week treatment cycle (in combination with ifosfamide, mesna, cisplatin, and filgrastim) for 4 cycles (Kondagunta, 2005) **or** 100 mg/m^2 over 1 hour on days 1, 8, and 15 of a 4-week treatment cycle (in combination with gemcitabine) for up to 6 cycles (Einhorn, 2007)

Thymoma/thymic carcinoma, advanced (off-label use): IV: 225 mg/m^2 over 3 hours every 3 weeks (in combination with carboplatin) for up to 6 cycles (Lemma, 2011)

Unknown primary adenocarcinoma (off-label use): IV: 200 mg/m^2 over 3 hours every 3 weeks (in combination with carboplatin) for 6 to 8 cycles (Briasoulis, 2000) **or** 200 mg/m^2 over 1 hour every 3 weeks (in combination with carboplatin and etoposide) for 4 to 8 cycles (Greco, 2000)

Renal Impairment There are no dosage adjustments provided in the manufacturer's labeling. The following have been recommended:

CrCl <50 mL/minute: Adults: No dosage adjustment is necessary (Aron-off 2007).

Hemodialysis: Paclitaxel may be used in cancer patients on hemodialysis and because paclitaxel is not dialyzable, it may be used either before or after hemodialysis (Janus 2010).

Hepatic Impairment Note: The manufacturer's labeling recommendations are based upon the patient's first course of therapy where the usual dose would be 135 mg/m² dose over 24 hours or the 175 mg/m² dose over 3 hours in patients with normal hepatic function. Dosage in subsequent courses should be based upon individual tolerance. Adjustments for other regimens are not available.

24-hour infusion:

Transaminases <2 times upper limit of normal (ULN) and bilirubin level ≤1.5 mg/dL: 135 mg/m²

Transaminases 2 to <10 times ULN and bilirubin level ≤1.5 mg/dL: 100 mg/m²

Transaminases <10 times ULN and bilirubin level 1.6 to 7.5 mg/dL: 50 mg/m²

Transaminases ≥10 times ULN or bilirubin level >7.5 mg/dL: Avoid use

3-hour infusion:

Transaminases <10 times ULN and bilirubin level ≤1.25 times ULN: 175 mg/m²

Transaminases <10 times ULN and bilirubin level 1.26 to 2 times ULN: 135 mg/m²

Transaminases <10 times ULN and bilirubin level 2.01 to 5 times ULN: 90 mg/m²

Transaminases ≥10 times ULN or bilirubin level >5 times ULN: Avoid use

Obesity *ASCO Guidelines for appropriate chemotherapy dosing in obese adults with cancer:* Utilize patient's actual body weight (full weight) for calculation of body surface area- or weight-based dosing, particularly when the intent of therapy is curative; manage regimen-related toxicities in the same manner as for nonobese patients; if a dose reduction is utilized due to toxicity, consider resumption of full weight-based dosing with subsequent cycles, especially if cause of toxicity (eg, hepatic or renal impairment) is resolved (Griggs, 2012).

Adjustment for Toxicity

Dosage modification for toxicity (solid tumors, including ovary, breast, and lung carcinoma): Courses of paclitaxel should not be repeated until the neutrophil count is ≥1,500/mm³ and the platelet count is ≥100,000/mm³; reduce dosage by 20% for patients experiencing severe peripheral neuropathy or severe neutropenia (neutrophil <500/mm³ for a week or longer)

Dosage modification for immunosuppression in advanced HIV disease: Paclitaxel should not be given to patients with HIV if the baseline or subsequent neutrophil count is <1000 cells/mm³. Additional modifications include: Reduce dosage of dexamethasone in premedication to 10 mg orally; reduce dosage by 20% in patients experiencing severe peripheral neuropathy or severe neutropenia (neutrophil <500/mm³ for a week or longer); initiate concurrent hematopoietic growth factor (G-CSF) as clinically indicated

Combination Regimens

Bladder cancer:

Gemcitabine-Paclitaxel (Bladder) on page 2138

PCG (Bladder) on page 2191

Breast cancer:

AC (Dose-Dense) followed by Paclitaxel (Dose-Dense) (Breast) on page 1976

AC (Dose-Dense) followed by Paclitaxel (Dose-Dense)-Trastuzumab (Breast) on page 1977

Administration

IV: Infuse over 3 or 24 hours (depending on indication/protocol); some off-label protocols use a 1-hour infusion. Infuse through a 0.22-micron in-line filter and polyethylene-lined (non-PVC) administration set. When administered as a part of a combination chemotherapy regimen, sequence of administration may vary by regimen; refer to specific protocol for sequence recommendation.

Premedication with dexamethasone (20 mg orally or IV at 12 and 6 hours before the dose; reduce to 10 mg with advanced HIV disease), diphenhydramine (50 mg IV 30 to 60 minutes prior to the dose), and cimetidine 300 mg, famotidine 20 mg, or ranitidine 50 mg (IV 30 to 60 minutes prior to the dose) is recommended.

Irritant with vesicant-like properties; avoid extravasation. Ensure proper needle or catheter position prior to administration.

Extravasation management: If extravasation occurs, stop infusion immediately and disconnect (leave cannula/needle in place); gently aspirate extravasated solution (do **NOT** flush the line); remove needle/cannula; initiate antidote (hyaluronidase); remove needle/cannula; elevate extremity. Information conflicts regarding the use of warm or cold compresses (Perez Fidalgo, 2012; Polovich, 2009).

Hyaluronidase: If needle/cannula still in place: Administer 1 to 6 mL (150 units/mL) into existing IV line; usual dose is 1 mL for each 1 mL of extravasated drug; if needle/cannula has been removed, inject subcutaneously in a clockwise manner around area of extravasation; may repeat several times over the next 3 to 4 hours (Ener, 2004).

Intraperitoneal (off-label route): Solution was prepared in warmed saline and infused as rapidly as possible through an implantable intraperitoneal catheter (Armstrong, 2006).

Vesicant/Extravasation Risk Irritant with vesicant-like properties

Emetic Potential Children and Adults: Low (10% to 30%)

Monitoring Parameters CBC with differential and platelet count, liver and kidney function; monitor for hypersensitivity reactions, vital signs (frequently during the first hour of infusion), continuous cardiac monitoring (patients with conduction abnormalities); monitor infusion site during infusion.

Dosage Forms Considerations Paclitaxel injection contains polyoxyl 35/ olyoxyethylated castor oil (Cremophor EL)

Dosage Forms Excipient information presented when available (limited, particularly for generics); consult specific product labeling.

Concentrate, Intravenous:

Generic: 100 mg/16.7 mL (16.7 mL); 30 mg/5 mL (5 mL); 150 mg/25 mL (25 mL); 300 mg/50 mL (50 mL)

Concentrate, Intravenous [preservative free]:

Generic: 100 mg/16.7 mL (16.7 mL); 30 mg/5 mL (5 mL); 300 mg/50 mL (50 mL)

PACLitaxel (Protein Bound) (pac li TAKS el PROE teen bownd)

Related Information

Management of Drug Extravasations *on page 2271*

Prevention of Chemotherapy-Induced Nausea and Vomiting in Children *on page 2310*

Safe Handling of Hazardous Drugs *on page 2379*

Brand Names: US Abraxane

Brand Names: Canada Abraxane for Injectable Suspension

Index Terms ABI-007; Albumin-Bound Paclitaxel; Albumin-Stabilized Nanoparticle Paclitaxel; nab-Paclitaxel; Nanoparticle Albumin-Bound Paclitaxel; Paclitaxel (Nanoparticle Albumin Bound); Paclitaxel, Albumin-Bound; Protein-Bound Paclitaxel

◀ **Pharmacologic Category** Antineoplastic Agent, Antimicrotubular; Antineoplastic Agent, Taxane Derivative

Use

US labeling:

Breast cancer, metastatic: Treatment of refractory (metastatic) or relapsed (within 6 months of adjuvant therapy) breast cancer after failure of combination chemotherapy (including anthracycline-based therapy unless clinically contraindicated)

Non-small cell lung cancer (NSCLC): First-line treatment of locally advanced or metastatic NSCLC (in combination with carboplatin) in patients ineligible for curative surgery or radiation therapy

Pancreatic adenocarcinoma: First-line treatment of metastatic adenocarcinoma of the pancreas (in combination with gemcitabine)

Canadian labeling:

Breast cancer, metastatic: Treatment of metastatic breast cancer

Pancreatic adenocarcinoma: First-line treatment of metastatic adenocarcinoma of the pancreas (in combination with gemcitabine)

Labeled Contraindications Baseline neutrophil count of <1500/mm^3; severe hypersensitivity reaction to paclitaxel (protein bound) or any component of the formulation

Pregnancy Considerations Adverse events were observed in animal reproduction studies. An *ex vivo* human placenta perfusion model illustrated that paclitaxel (non-protein bound preparation) crossed the placenta at term. Placental transfer was low and affected by the presence of albumin; higher albumin concentrations resulted in lower paclitaxel placental transfer (Berveiller 2012). Women of childbearing potential should be advised to avoid becoming pregnant during therapy; may cause fetal harm if administered during pregnancy. Additionally, testicular atrophy/degeneration was observed in animal studies; males should be advised to not father a child during therapy. A pregnancy registry is available for all cancers diagnosed during pregnancy at Cooper Health (877-635-4499).

Breastfeeding Considerations Paclitaxel (non-protein bound) is excreted in breast milk (case report). The mother (3 months postpartum) was treated with paclitaxel 30 mg/m^2 (56.1 mg) and carboplatin once weekly for papillary thyroid cancer. Milk samples were obtained 4-316 hours after the infusion given at the sixth and final week of therapy. The average paclitaxel milk concentration over the testing interval was 0.78 mg/L. Although maternal serum concentrations were not noted in the report, the relative infant dose to a nursing infant was calculated to be ~17% of the maternal dose. Paclitaxel continued to be detected in breast milk when sampled at 172 hours after the dose and was below the limit of detection when sampled at 316 hours after the infusion (Griffin 2012).

Due to the potential for serious adverse reactions in the nursing infant, the decision to discontinue the drug or to discontinue breastfeeding should take into consideration the benefit of treatment to the mother.

Warnings/Precautions [US Boxed Warning]: Paclitaxel (protein-bound) is not interchangeable with other forms of paclitaxel, including Cremophor-based or unbound paclitaxel.

[US Boxed Warning]: Bone marrow suppression, primarily neutropenia, may occur; monitor peripheral blood counts frequently. Baseline neutrophils should be ≥1,500/mm^3 for administration on day 1 of each cycle; platelets should recover to >100,000/mm^3 prior to day 1 of the next treatment cycle. Hematologic toxicity is dose-dependent and dose-limiting. For severe neutropenia, dose reductions may be recommended for subsequent cycles. Dose- and schedule-related cumulative sensory neuropathy is common; severe sensory neuropathy may occur. If ≥ grade 3 sensory neuropathy occurs, withhold therapy until resolution to grade 1 or 2 (breast cancer) or ≤ grade 1 (non-small cell lung cancer [NSCLC] and pancreatic cancer). Upon recovery, subsequent cycles should be dose reduced. Prior therapy with neurotoxic agents may influence the frequency and severity of neurologic toxicity. Severe hypersensitivity (including anaphylaxis) have been reported; do not rechallenge after severe hypersensitivity reaction. Premedication is not generally necessary prior to paclitaxel (protein bound), but may be needed in patients with prior mild-to-moderate hypersensitivity reactions. Use has not been studied in patients with a prior hypersensitivity reaction to conventional paclitaxel or to albumin.

In a scientific statement from the American Heart Association, conventional paclitaxel has been determined to be an agent that may either cause direct myocardial toxicity or exacerbate underlying myocardial dysfunction (magnitude: moderate) (AHA [Page 2016]). Pneumonitis (including fatal cases) was observed in clinical trials when used in combination with gemcitabine. Monitor for signs/symptoms of pneumonitis; interrupt therapy during diagnostic process. If pneumonitis is confirmed, permanently discontinue. Sepsis was observed in both neutropenic and non-neutropenic patients treated with paclitaxel (protein bound) in combination with gemcitabine for pancreatic cancer; biliary obstruction or the presence of a biliary stent may be risk factors for severe and/or fatal sepsis. Treat promptly with broad spectrum antibiotics if fever occurs (regardless of neutrophil count). May require therapy interruption and/or dosage reduction. Exposure may be increased in patients with hepatic impairment; monitor closely; the risk of toxicities (particularly myelosuppression) is increased. Reduced initial dosages are recommended for breast cancer and NSCLC patients with moderate and severe hepatic impairment; use is not recommended in pancreatic patients with moderate or severe impairment (bilirubin >1.5 times ULN and AST ≤10 times ULN). Use is not recommended in patients with AST >10 times ULN or total bilirubin >5 times ULN.

Vision disturbances, including decreased visual acuity associated with cystoid macular edema (CME), have been observed; resolution observed in most cases following therapy discontinuation. Consider prompt/complete ophthalmologic evaluation in patients with vision changes/decreased acuity; the Canadian labeling recommends discontinuing therapy if CME is confirmed. Certain adverse events (myelosuppression, peripheral neuropathy, arthralgia, diarrhea, decreased appetite, dehydration, fatigue, and epistaxis) occurred more frequently in older adults ≥65 years compared to younger adults. Product contains albumin, which confers a remote risk of viral disease transmission and a theoretical risk of transmission of Creutzfeldt-Jakob disease. Potentially significant drug-drug interactions may exist, requiring dose or frequency adjustment, additional monitoring, and/or selection of alternative therapy.

Adverse Reactions Frequency may vary based on indication and/or concomitant therapy.
>10%:
  Cardiovascular: ECG abnormality (60%; 35% in patients with a normal baseline), peripheral edema (10% to 46%)

◄ Central nervous system: Peripheral sensory neuropathy (71%; grades 3/4: 10%; dose dependent; cumulative), fatigue (25% to 59%), peripheral neuropathy (48% to 54%; grade 3: 3% to 17%), headache (14%), depression (12%)

Dermatologic: Alopecia (50% to 90%), skin rash (10% to 30%)

Endocrine & metabolic: Dehydration (21%), increased gamma-glutamyl transferase (grades 3/4: 14%), hypokalemia (12%)

Gastrointestinal: Nausea (27% to 54%; grades 3/4: 3% to 6%), diarrhea (15% to 44%; grades 3/4: ≤6%), decreased appetite (17% to 36%), vomiting (12% to 36%; grades 3/4: 4% to 6%), constipation (16%), dysgeusia (16%)

Genitourinary: Urinary tract infection (11%)

Hematologic & oncologic: Anemia (33% to 98%; grades 3/4: 1% to 28%), neutropenia (73% to 85%; grades 3/4: 34% to 47%), thrombocytopenia (2% to 74%; grades 3/4: <1% to 18%), bone marrow depression (dose-related)

Hepatic: Increased serum AST (39%), increased serum alkaline phosphatase (36%)

Infection: Infection (24%; primarily included oral candidiasis, respiratory tract infection, and pneumonia)

Neuromuscular & skeletal: Weakness (16% to 47%; severe: 8%), musculoskeletal pain (10% to 44%; myalgia/arthralgia), limb pain (11%)

Ophthalmic: Visual disturbance (13%; severe [keratitis, blurred vision]: 1%)

Renal: Increased serum creatinine (11%; severe 1%)

Respiratory: Cough (7% to 17%), epistaxis (7% to 15%), dyspnea (12%)

Miscellaneous: Fever (41%)

1% to 10%:

Cardiovascular: Edema (10%), cardiac failure (<10%), hypotension (5%), significant cardiovascular event (grades 3/4: 3%; included chest pain, cardiac arrest, supraventricular tachycardia, thrombosis, pulmonary thromboembolism, pulmonary emboli, and hypertension)

Gastrointestinal: Mucositis (7% to 10%; grades 3/4: ≤1%)

Hematologic & oncologic: Hemorrhage (2%), febrile neutropenia (2%)

Hepatic: Increased serum bilirubin (7%)

Hypersensitivity: Hypersensitivity reaction (4%, includes anaphylactic reactions, chest pain, dyspnea, flushing, hypotension; severe: <1%)

Infection: Sepsis (5%)

Ophthalmic: Cystoid macular edema (<10%)

Respiratory: Pneumonitis (4%)

<1%, postmarketing, and/or case reports: Atrioventricular block, autonomic neuropathy, bradycardia, cardiac arrhythmia, cerebrovascular accident, cranial nerve palsy, decreased visual acuity, embolism, erythema, hepatic encephalopathy, hepatic necrosis, injection site reaction (mild), intestinal obstruction, intestinal perforation, ischemic colitis, ischemic heart disease, left ventricular dysfunction, maculopapular rash, myocardial infarction, nail discoloration, neutropenic sepsis, optic nerve damage (rare), palmar-plantar erythrodysesthesia (in patients previously exposed to capecitabine), pancreatitis, pancytopenia, paralytic ileus, peripheral motor neuropathy, pneumonia, pneumothorax, pruritus, pulmonary embolism, radiation pneumonitis (with concurrent radiation therapy), radiation recall phenomenon, skin photosensitivity, Stevens-Johnson syndrome, thrombosis, toxic epidermal necrolysis, transient ischemic attacks, ventricular dysfunction, vocal cord paralysis

Drug Interactions

Metabolism/Transport Effects Substrate of CYP2C8 (major), CYP3A4 (major), P-glycoprotein; **Note:** Assignment of Major/Minor substrate status based on clinically relevant drug interaction potential

Avoid Concomitant Use

Avoid concomitant use of PACLitaxel (Protein Bound) with any of the following: BCG (Intravesical); Conivaptan; Deferiprone; Dipyrone; Fusidic Acid (Systemic); Idelalisib; Natalizumab; Pimecrolimus; Tacrolimus (Topical); Vaccines (Live)

Increased Effect/Toxicity

PACLitaxel (Protein Bound) may increase the levels/effects of: Antineoplastic Agents (Anthracycline, Systemic); CloZAPine; Deferiprone; DOXOrubicin (Conventional); Fingolimod; Leflunomide; Natalizumab; Tofacitinib; Vaccines (Live); Vinorelbine

The levels/effects of PACLitaxel (Protein Bound) may be increased by: Abiraterone Acetate; Aprepitant; Clopidogrel; Conivaptan; CYP2C8 Inhibitors (Moderate); CYP2C8 Inhibitors (Strong); CYP3A4 Inhibitors (Moderate); CYP3A4 Inhibitors (Strong); Dasatinib; Deferasirox; Denosumab; Dipyrone; Fosaprepitant; Fusidic Acid (Systemic); Idelalisib; MiFEPRIStone; Netupitant; Ocrelizumab; Palbociclib; Palifermin; P-glycoprotein/ABCB1 Inhibitors; Pimecrolimus; Platinum Derivatives; Promazine; Ranolazine; Roflumilast; Simeprevir; Stiripentol; Tacrolimus (Topical); Trastuzumab

Decreased Effect

PACLitaxel (Protein Bound) may decrease the levels/effects of: BCG (Intravesical); Coccidioides immitis Skin Test; Lenograstim; Nivolumab; Sipuleucel-T; Tertomotide; Vaccines (Inactivated); Vaccines (Live)

The levels/effects of PACLitaxel (Protein Bound) may be decreased by: Bosentan; CYP2C8 Inducers (Strong); CYP3A4 Inducers (Moderate); CYP3A4 Inducers (Strong); Dabrafenib; Deferasirox; Echinacea; Enzalutamide; Mitotane; Sarilumab; Siltuximab; St John's Wort; Tocilizumab

Food Interactions Paclitaxel (protein bound) serum concentrations may be increased when taken with grapefruit or grapefruit juice. Management: Avoid concurrent use.

Hazardous Drugs Handling Considerations

Hazardous agent (NIOSH 2016 [group 1]).

Use appropriate precautions for receiving, handling, administration, and disposal. Gloves (single) should be worn during receiving, unpacking, and placing in storage.

NIOSH recommends double gloving, a protective gown, ventilated engineering controls (a class II biological safety cabinet or a compounding aseptic containment isolator), and closed system transfer devices (CSTDs) for preparation. Double gloving, a gown, and (if dosage form allows) CSTDs are required during administration (NIOSH 2016).

Storage/Stability

US labeling: Store intact vials at 20°C to 25°C (68°F to 77°F) and protect from bright light. Freezing or refrigerating do not adversely affect the stability of intact vials. Reconstituted solution in the vial as well as solution in infusion container for administration may be stored under refrigeration at 2°C to 8°C (36°F to 46°F) for up to 24 hours, although the manufacturer recommends immediate use. Protect solution from light. The total combined refrigerated storage time of both reconstituted solution in the vial and administration bag

◀ is 24 hours; solution may then be stored at room temperature (~25°C [77°F]) and ambient light for up to 4 hours.

Canadian labeling: Store intact vials at 20°C to 25°C (68°F to 77°F) and protect from bright light. Freezing or refrigerating do not adversely affect the stability of intact vials. Reconstituted solution in the vial may be stored under refrigeration at 2°C to 8°C (36°F to 46°F) for up to 8 hours, although the manufacturer recommends immediate use. Protect solution from light. Once transferred from vial to infusion bag for administration, use immediately or, if necessary, may store at 20°C to 25°C (68°F to 77°F) and ambient light for up to 8 hours.

Preparation for Administration

Reconstitute vial with 20 mL NS to a concentration of 5 mg/mL. Add NS slowly (over a minimum of 1 minute), directing it along inside vial wall; allow vial to sit for 5 minutes, then gently swirl for 2 minutes; avoid foaming. If foaming or clumping occurs, allow solution to stand for at least 15 minutes until foaming subsides. Reconstituted solution will appear milky and homogenous without visible particulates; if particulates or settling are visible, gently invert vial to re-suspend. Discard reconstituted suspension if precipitates are observed. Draw calculated dose slowly into syringe, then place without further dilution into an empty sterile container. **Note:** Use of DEHP-free containers or administration sets is not necessary.

The use of syringes or IV bags containing silicone oil as a lubricant; may result in formation of proteinaceous strands. **Note:** The Canadian labeling recommends administering the infusion solution through a 15-micron filter if syringes/IV bags containing silicone oil are used and proteinaceous strands are observed; discard the solution if a filter is not available. Do not use a filter with a pore size <15 microns.

Mechanism of Action Albumin-bound paclitaxel nanoparticle formulation; paclitaxel promotes microtubule assembly by enhancing the action of tubulin dimers, stabilizing existing microtubules, and inhibiting their disassembly, interfering with the late G_2 mitotic phase, and inhibiting cell replication. May also distort mitotic spindles, resulting in the breakage of chromosomes. Paclitaxel may also suppress cell proliferation and modulate immune response.

Pharmacodynamics/Kinetics

Distribution: V_d: 1741 L (extensive extravascular distribution and/or tissue binding)

Protein binding: 94%

Metabolism: Hepatic primarily via CYP2C8 to 6-alpha-hydroxypaclitaxel; also to minor metabolites via CYP3A4

Half-life elimination: Terminal: 13 to 27 hours

Excretion: Feces (~20%); urine (4% as unchanged drug, <1% as metabolites)

Dosing

Adult & Geriatric Note: When administered as part of a combination chemotherapy regimen, sequence of administration may vary by regimen; refer to specific protocol for sequence of administration. Premedication is not generally necessary prior to paclitaxel (protein bound), but may be needed in patients with prior mild-to-moderate hypersensitivity reactions.

Breast cancer, metastatic: IV: 260 mg/m² every 3 weeks (Gradishar 2005)

Off-label dosing: IV: 100 to 150 mg/m² on days 1, 8, and 15 of a 28-day cycle (Gradishar 2009)

Non-small cell lung cancer (NSCLC), locally advanced or metastatic: IV: 100 mg/m² on days 1, 8, and 15 of each 21-day cycle (in combination with carboplatin) (Socinski 2012)

Pancreatic adenocarcinoma, metastatic: IV: 125 mg/m² on days 1, 8, and 15 of a 28-day cycle (in combination with gemcitabine) (Von Hoff 2013)

Melanoma, metastatic (off-label use): IV:

Previously treated patients: 100 mg/m² on days 1, 8, and 15 of a 28-day cycle; if tolerated, may increase dose by 25 mg/m² in cycle 2 and beyond (Hersh 2010)

Previously untreated patients: 150 mg/m² on days 1, 8, and 15 of a 28-day cycle (Hersh 2010)

Ovarian, fallopian tube, or primary peritoneal cancer, recurrent (off-label use): IV: 260 mg/m² on day 1 of a 21-day cycle for 6 to 8 cycles (Teneriello 2009) **or** 100 mg/m² on days 1, 8, and 15 of a 28-day cycle until disease progression or unacceptable toxicity (Coleman 2011)

Renal Impairment

CrCl ≥30 mL/minute: No dosage adjustment necessary

CrCl <30 mL/minute: There are no dosage adjustments provided in the manufacturer's labeling (has not been studied)

End-stage renal disease (ESRD): There are no dosage adjustments provided in the manufacturer's labeling (has not been studied)

Hepatic Impairment Dosage adjustment for hepatic impairment at treatment initiation:

Breast cancer (every 3 week regimen):

Mild impairment (AST ≤10 times ULN and bilirubin >1 to <1.5 times ULN): No dosage adjustment necessary.

Moderate impairment (AST ≤10 times ULN and bilirubin >1.5 to ≤3 times ULN): Reduce dose to 200 mg/m²; may increase up to 260 mg/m² if the reduced dose is tolerated for 2 cycles

Severe impairment:

AST ≤10 times ULN and bilirubin >3 to ≤5 times ULN: Reduce dose to 200 mg/m²; may increase up to 260 mg/m² in subsequent cycles if the reduced dose is tolerated for 2 cycles

AST >10 times ULN or bilirubin >5 times ULN: Use is not recommended (has not been studied)

Non-small cell lung cancer (NSCLC) regimen:

Mild impairment (AST ≤10 times ULN and bilirubin >1 to ≤1.5 times ULN): No dosage adjustment necessary.

Moderate impairment (AST ≤10 times ULN and bilirubin >1.5 to ≤3 times ULN): Reduce dose to 80 mg/m²; may increase up to 100 mg/m² in subsequent cycles if the reduced dose is tolerated for 2 cycles

Severe impairment:

AST ≤10 times ULN and bilirubin >3 to ≤5 times ULN: Reduce dose to 80 mg/m²; may increase up to 100 mg/m² in subsequent cycles if the reduced dose is tolerated for 2 cycles

AST >10 times ULN or bilirubin >5 times ULN: Use is not recommended (has not been studied).

Pancreatic adenocarcinoma:

Mild impairment (AST ≤10 times ULN and bilirubin >1 to ≤1.5 times ULN): No dosage adjustment necessary.

Moderate impairment (AST ≤10 times ULN and bilirubin >1.5 to ≤3 times ULN): Use is not recommended.

Severe impairment:

AST ≤10 times ULN and bilirubin >3 to ≤5 times ULN: Use is not recommended.

AST >10 times ULN or bilirubin >5 times ULN: Use is not recommended.

Dosage adjustment for hepatic impairment during treatment: AST >10 times ULN or bilirubin >5 times ULN: Withhold treatment

Obesity *ASCO Guidelines for appropriate chemotherapy dosing in obese adults with cancer:* Utilize patient's actual body weight (full weight) for calculation of body surface area- or weight-based dosing, particularly when the intent of therapy is curative; manage regimen-related toxicities in the same manner as for nonobese patients; if a dose reduction is utilized due to toxicity, consider resumption of full weight-based dosing with subsequent cycles, especially if cause of toxicity (eg, hepatic or renal impairment) is resolved (Griggs 2012).

Adjustment for Toxicity

Breast cancer (every 3 week regimen):

Severe neutropenia (<500 cells/mm^3) ≥1 week: Reduce dose to 220 mg/m^2 for subsequent courses

Recurrent severe neutropenia: Reduce dose to 180 mg/m^2 for subsequent courses

Sensory neuropathy

Grade 1 or 2: Dosage adjustment generally not required

Grade 3: Hold treatment until resolved to grade 1 or 2, then resume with reduced dose for all subsequent cycles

Severe sensory neuropathy: Reduce dose to 220 mg/m^2 for subsequent courses

Recurrent severe sensory neuropathy: Reduce dose to 180 mg/m^2 for subsequent courses

Non-small cell lung cancer (NSCLC):

Neutropenia: ANC <1,500 cells/mm^3: Withhold therapy until ANC is ≥1,500 cells/mm^3 on day 1 or ≥500 cells/mm^3 on days 8 or 15. Reduce dose upon therapy reinitiation if:

Neutropenic fever (ANC <500 cells/mm^3 with fever >38°C) **or** delay of next cycle by >7 days due to ANC <1,500 cells/mm^3 **or** ANC <500 cells/mm^3 for >7 days:

First occurrence: Permanently reduce dose to 75 mg/m^2

Second occurrence: Permanently reduce dose to 50 mg/m^2

Third occurrence: Discontinue therapy.

Thrombocytopenia: Platelet count <100,000 cells/mm^3: Withhold therapy until platelet count is ≥100,000 cells/mm^3 on day 1 or ≥50,000 cells/mm^3 on days 8 or 15. Reduce dose upon therapy reinitiation if:

Platelet count <50,000 cells/mm^3:

First occurrence: Permanently reduce dose to 75 mg/m^2

Second occurrence: Discontinue therapy.

Sensory neuropathy: Withhold therapy for grade 3 or 4 peripheral neuropathy. Resume therapy at reduced doses when neuropathy resolves completely or improves to grade 1:

First occurrence: Permanently reduce dose to 75 mg/m^2

Second occurrence: Permanently reduce dose to 50 mg/m^2

Third occurrence: Discontinue therapy.

Pancreatic adenocarcinoma:

Note: Dose level reductions for toxicity:

Full dose: 125 mg/m^2

First dose reduction: 100 mg/m^2

Second dose reduction: 75 mg/m^2

If additional dose reduction is necessary: Discontinue.

Hematologic toxicity (neutropenia and/or thrombocytopenia):

Day 1: If ANC is <1,500 cells/mm^3 or platelet count is <100,000 cells/mm^3: Withhold therapy until ANC is ≥1,500 cells/mm^3 and platelet count is ≥100,000 cells/mm^3

Day 8:

If ANC is 500 to <1,000 cells/mm^3 **or** platelet count is 50,000 to <75,000 cells/mm^3: Reduce 1 dose level

If ANC is <500 cells/mm^3 **or** platelet count is <50,000 cells/mm^3: Withhold day 8 dose

Day 15:

US labeling:

If day 8 doses were reduced or given without modification:

If ANC is 500 to <1,000 cells/mm^3 **or** platelet count is 50,000 to <75,000 cells/mm^3: Reduce 1 dose level from day 8

If ANC is <500 cells/mm^3 **or** platelet count is <50,000 cells/mm^3: Withhold day 15 dose

If day 8 doses were withheld:

If ANC is ≥1000 cells/mm^3 **or** platelet count is ≥75,000 cells/mm^3: Reduce 1 dose level from day 1

If ANC is 500 to <1,000 cells/mm^3 **or** platelet count is 50,000 to <75,000 cells/mm^3: Reduce 2 dose levels from day 1

If ANC is <500 cells/mm^3 **or** platelet count is <50,000 cells/mm^3: Withhold day 15 dose

Canadian labeling:

If day 8 doses were given without modification:

If ANC is 500 to <1,000 cells/mm^3 or platelet count is 50,000 to <75,000 cells/mm^3: Treat at current dose and follow with WBC growth factors or reduce 1 dose level from day 8 if growth factors are not available

If ANC is <500 cells/mm^3 or platelet count is <50,000 cells/mm^3: Withhold day 15 dose

If day 8 doses were reduced:

If ANC is ≥1,000 cells/mm^3 and platelet count is ≥75,000 cells/mm^3: Treat with day 1 dose and follow with WBC growth factors or reduce 1 dose level from day 1 if growth factors are not available

If ANC is 500 to <1,000 cells/mm^3 or platelet count is 50,000 to <75,000 cells/mm^3: Treat with day 8 dose and follow with WBC growth factors or reduce 1 dose level from day 8 if growth factors are not available

If ANC is <500 cells/mm^3 or platelet count is <50,000 cells/mm^3: Withhold day 15 dose

If day 8 doses were withheld:

If ANC is ≥1,000 cells/mm^3 and platelet count is ≥75,000 cells/mm^3: Treat with day 1 dose and follow with WBC growth factors or reduce 1 dose level from day 1 if growth factors are not available

If ANC is 500 to <1,000 cells/mm^3 or platelet count is 50,000 to <75,000 cells/mm^3: Reduce 1 dose level from day 1 and follow with WBC growth factors or reduce 2 dose levels from day 1 if growth factors are not available

If ANC is <500 cells/mm^3 or platelet count is <50,000 cells/mm^3: Withhold day 15 dose

Neutropenic fever: Withhold therapy for grade 3 or 4 fever. Resume therapy at next lower dose level when fever resolves and ANC is ≥1500 cells/mm^3.

Peripheral neuropathy: Withhold therapy for grade 3 or 4 peripheral neuropathy. Resume therapy at next lower dose level when neuropathy improves to ≤ grade 1.

Dermatologic toxicity: For grade 2 or 3 toxicity, reduce dose to next lower dose level; if toxicity persists, discontinue.

Gastrointestinal toxicity: Withhold therapy for grade 3 mucositis or diarrhea. Resume therapy at next lower dose level when improves to ≤ grade 1.

Combination Regimens

Lung cancer (non-small cell): Carboplatin-Paclitaxel (Protein Bound) (NSCLC) on page 2022

Pancreatic cancer: Gemcitabine-Paclitaxel (Protein Bound) (Pancreatic) on page 2139

Administration IV: Administer over 30 minutes (breast cancer and NSCLC) or over 30 to 40 minutes (pancreatic cancer); limiting the infusion rate to 30 minutes reduces the risk for infusion-related reaction. Monitor infusion site; avoid extravasation. When given on a weekly (off-label) schedule, infusions were administered over ~30 minutes (Gradishar 2009; Hersh 2010; Rizvi 2008). When administered as part of a combination chemotherapy regimen, sequence of administration may vary by regimen; refer to specific protocol for sequence of administration. According to the manufacturer, paclitaxel (protein bound should be given first, followed immediately by carboplatin (NSCLC) or gemcitabine (pancreatic cancer).

Vesicant/Extravasation Risk May be an irritant

Emetic Potential Children and Adults: Low (10% to 30%)

Monitoring Parameters CBC with differential (prior to day 1 of cycle for metastatic breast cancer and prior to days 1, 8, and 15 for NSCLC); hepatic function; monitor infusion site; monitor for neuropathy and signs/symptoms of pneumonitis and sepsis

Dosage Forms Excipient information presented when available (limited, particularly for generics); consult specific product labeling.

Suspension Reconstituted, Intravenous:

Abraxane: 100 mg (1 ea)

◆ **Paclitaxel, Albumin-Bound** *see* PACLitaxel (Protein Bound) *on page* 1411

◆ **Paclitaxel for Injection (Can)** *see* PACLitaxel (Conventional) *on page* 1402

◆ **Paclitaxel Injection USP (Can)** *see* PACLitaxel (Conventional) *on page* 1402

◆ **Paclitaxel (Nanoparticle Albumin Bound)** *see* PACLitaxel (Protein Bound) *on page* 1411

Palbociclib (pal boe SYE klib)

Related Information

Common Toxicity Criteria *on page 2242*
Safe Handling of Hazardous Drugs *on page 2379*

Brand Names: US Ibrance

Brand Names: Canada Ibrance

Index Terms Palbociclib Isethionate; PD 0332991; PD-0332991; PD-332991

Pharmacologic Category Antineoplastic Agent, Cyclin-Dependent Kinase Inhibitor

Use

Breast cancer, advanced (initial endocrine-based therapy): Treatment of hormone receptor (HR)-positive, human epidermal growth factor receptor 2 (HER2)-negative advanced or metastatic breast cancer (in combination with an aromatase inhibitor) in postmenopausal women as initial endocrine-based therapy

Breast cancer, advanced (with disease progression following endocrine therapy): Treatment of HR-positive, HER2-negative advanced or metastatic breast cancer (in combination with fulvestrant) in women with disease progression following endocrine therapy

Labeled Contraindications

There are no contraindications listed in the US manufacturer's labeling.
Canadian labeling: Hypersensitivity to palbociclib or any component of the formulation

Pregnancy Considerations Adverse events were observed in animal reproduction studies. Based on the mechanism of action, palbociclib may be expected to cause fetal harm if used during pregnancy. In women of reproductive potential, a pregnancy test is recommended prior to treatment initiation. Women of reproductive potential should use effective contraception during treatment and for at least 3 weeks after the last dose. Males with female partners of reproductive potential should use effective contraception during treatment and for 3 months after the last dose. Although not approved for use in men, animal data suggests that palbociclib may affect male fertility.

Breastfeeding Considerations It is not known if palbociclib is present in breast milk. Due to the potential for serious adverse reactions in the breastfed infant, breastfeeding is not recommended by the manufacturer during treatment and for at least 3 weeks after the last dose.

Warnings/Precautions Neutropenia was commonly observed in clinical studies, including grades 3 and 4 neutropenia. The median time to the first neutropenia episode (any grade) was 15 days; the median duration of grade 3 or higher neutropenia was 7 days. Leukopenia, anemia, lymphocytopenia, thrombocytopenia, neutropenic fever, and neutropenic sepsis have also been reported. Monitor blood counts prior to initiating therapy and at the beginning of each cycle (as well as on day 15 of the first 2 cycles), and as clinically necessary; if neutropenia is limited to grades 1 or 2 in the first 6 cycles, monitor every 3 months (prior to the beginning of a cycle) and as clinically indicated for subsequent cycles. Treatment interruption, delay, or dose reduction is recommended for grade 3 or 4 neutropenia.

Infections (including grades 3 and 4) were reported more frequently in patients receiving palbociclib and an antiestrogen compared with those receiving an antiestrogen only. Monitor for signs/symptoms of infection and manage appropriately. Nausea, vomiting, diarrhea, and stomatitis (generally grade 1 or 2) were reported from clinical studies. Potentially significant drug-drug ▶

interactions may exist, requiring dose or frequency adjustment, additional monitoring, and/or selection of alternative therapy.

Adverse Reactions Percentages reported as part of combination therapy.

>10%:

Central nervous system: Fatigue (41%), headache (26%), peripheral neuropathy (13%)

Dermatologic: Alopecia (18% to 22%), skin rash (17%)

Gastrointestinal: Nausea (25% to 34%), stomatitis (25% to 28%), diarrhea (21% to 24%), constipation (20%), vomiting (15% to 19%), decreased appetite (16%)

Hematologic & oncologic: Neutropenia (75% to 83%; grade 3: 48% to 55%; grade 4: 6% to 11%), decreased absolute lymphocyte count (81%; grade 3: 17%; grade 4: 1%), anemia (30% to 78%; grade 3: 3% to 5%; grade 4: ≤1%), leukopenia (43% to 53%; grade 3: 19% to 30%; grade 4: ≤1%), thrombocytopenia (17% to 23%; grade 3: 2%; grade 4: ≤1%)

Infection: Infection (47% to 55%)

Neuromuscular & skeletal: Weakness (8% to 13%)

Respiratory: Upper respiratory tract infection (31%), epistaxis (7% to 11%)

Miscellaneous: Fever (13%)

1% to 10%:

Cardiovascular: Pulmonary embolism (1% to 5%)

Dermatologic: Xeroderma (6%)

Gastrointestinal: Dysgeusia (7%)

Hematologic & oncologic: Febrile neutropenia (1%; grade 3: 1%)

Ophthalmic: Blurred vision (6%), increased lacrimation (6%), dry eye syndrome (4%)

Drug Interactions

Metabolism/Transport Effects Substrate of CYP3A4 (major); **Note:** Assignment of Major/Minor substrate status based on clinically relevant drug interaction potential; **Inhibits** CYP3A4 (weak)

Avoid Concomitant Use

Avoid concomitant use of Palbociclib with any of the following: BCG (Intravesical); Conivaptan; CYP3A4 Inducers (Strong); CYP3A4 Inhibitors (Strong); Deferiprone; Dipyrone; Fusidic Acid (Systemic); Grapefruit Juice; Idelalisib; Natalizumab; Pimecrolimus; Pimozide; St John's Wort; Tacrolimus (Topical); Vaccines (Live)

Increased Effect/Toxicity

Palbociclib may increase the levels/effects of: ARIPiprazole; CloZAPine; CYP3A4 Substrates; Deferiprone; Dofetilide; Fingolimod; Flibanserin; HYDROcodone; Leflunomide; Lomitapide; Natalizumab; NiMODipine; Pimozide; Tofacitinib; Vaccines (Live)

The levels/effects of Palbociclib may be increased by: Aprepitant; Conivaptan; CYP3A4 Inhibitors (Moderate); CYP3A4 Inhibitors (Strong); Dasatinib; Denosumab; Dipyrone; Fosaprepitant; Fusidic Acid (Systemic); Grapefruit Juice; Idelalisib; Netupitant; Ocrelizumab; Pimecrolimus; Promazine; Roflumilast; Simeprevir; Stiripentol; Tacrolimus (Topical); Trastuzumab

Decreased Effect

Palbociclib may decrease the levels/effects of: BCG (Intravesical); Coccidioides immitis Skin Test; Nivolumab; Sipuleucel-T; Tertomotide; Vaccines (Inactivated); Vaccines (Live)

The levels/effects of Palbociclib may be decreased by: CYP3A4 Inducers (Moderate); CYP3A4 Inducers (Strong); Dabrafenib; Deferasirox; Echinacea; Sarilumab; Siltuximab; St John's Wort; Tocilizumab

Food Interactions Coadministration with grapefruit may increase palbociclib plasma concentrations. Management: Avoid concomitant administration with grapefruit.

Hazardous Drugs Handling Considerations

Hazardous agent (meets NIOSH 2016 criteria). This medication is not on the NIOSH (2016) list; however, it meets the criteria for a hazardous drug. Drugs are classified as hazardous based on their properties; the properties of a hazardous drug include one or more of the following characteristics: carcinogenic, teratogenic (or other developmental toxicity), reproductive toxicity, organotoxic at low doses, genotoxic, and/or new agents with structural or toxicity profiles similar to existing hazardous agents.

Use appropriate precautions for receiving, handling, administration, and disposal. Gloves (single) should be worn during receiving, unpacking, and placing in storage. NIOSH recommends single gloving for administration of intact tablets or capsules (NIOSH 2016).

Storage/Stability Store at 20°C to 25°C (68°F to 77°F); excursions are permitted between 15°C and 30°C (59°F and 86°F).

Mechanism of Action Palbociclib is a reversible small molecule cyclin-dependent kinase (CDK) inhibitor which is selective for CDK 4 and 6. CDKs have a role in regulating progression through the cell cycle at the G1/S phase by blocking retinoblastoma (Rb) hyperphosphorylation (Finn 2015). Palbociclib reduces proliferation of breast cancer cell lines by preventing progression from the G1 to the S cell cycle phase. The combination of palbociclib with an antiestrogen provides for increased inhibition of Rb phosphorylation, downstream signaling, and tumor growth compared with each agent alone.

Pharmacodynamics/Kinetics

Absorption: Increased with high-fat, high-calorie food

Distribution: V_d (mean): 2,583 L

Protein binding: ~85%

Metabolism: Extensively hepatic; Major pathways: Oxidation and sulfonation, primarily by CYP3A and sulfotransferase (SULT) enzyme SULT2A1; Minor pathways: Acylation and glucuronidation

Bioavailability: Mean absolute bioavailability: 46%

Half-life elimination: 29 ± 5 hours

Time to peak: 6 to 12 hours

Excretion: Feces (~74%, primarily as metabolites); Urine (~18%; primarily as metabolites)

Dosing

Adult & Geriatric Note: Refer to aromatase inhibitor or fulvestrant monographs for respective dosing in combination with palbociclib.

Breast cancer, advanced, initial endocrine-based therapy: Females (HER-2 negative): Oral: 125 mg once daily for 21 days, followed by 7 days off, repeat every 28 days (in combination with continuous aromatase inhibitor therapy); continue until disease progression or unacceptable toxicity (Finn 2015).

Breast cancer, advanced (with disease progression following endocrine therapy): Females (HER-2 negative): Oral: 125 mg once daily for 21 days, followed by 7 days off, repeat every 28 days (in combination with fulvestrant [and an LHRH agonist (eg, goserelin) if pre- or perimenopausal]); continue until disease progression or unacceptable toxicity (Turner 2015).

Missed/vomited doses: If a dose is vomited or missed, an additional dose should not be taken that day. Resume dosing with the next scheduled daily dose.

Dosage adjustment for concomitant therapy:

Strong CYP3A inhibitors: Avoid concomitant use with strong CYP3A inhibitors (eg, azole antifungals, clarithromycin, nefazodone, protease inhibitors, telithromycin, verapamil, grapefruit or grapefruit juice) and consider alternatives with no or minimal CYP3A inhibition. If coadministration with a strong CYP3A inhibitor cannot be avoided, reduce palbociclib dose to 75 mg once daily. If the strong inhibitor is discontinued, increase palbociclib dose (after 3 to 5 inhibitor half-lives have elapsed) to the dose used prior to initiating the strong CYP3A inhibitor.

CYP3A inducers: Avoid concomitant use with strong CYP3A inducers.

Renal Impairment

CrCl 30 to <90 mL/minute: There are no dosage adjustments provided in the manufacturer's labeling, however, since palbociclib exposure is not increased, dosage adjustments are not likely necessary.

CrCl <30 mL/minute: There are no dosage adjustments provided in the manufacturer's labeling (has not been studied).

Hepatic Impairment

Mild impairment (total bilirubin ≤ ULN and AST > ULN or total bilirubin >1 to 1.5 times ULN and any AST): There are no dosage adjustments provided in the manufacturer's labeling, however, since palbociclib exposure is not increased, dosage adjustments are not likely necessary.

Moderate to severe impairment (total bilirubin >1.5 times ULN and any AST): There are no dosage adjustments provided in the manufacturer's labeling (has not been studied).

Adjustment for Toxicity May require treatment interruption/delay, dose reduction, or discontinuation for some adverse reactions. The recommended first dose reduction is to 100 mg daily; if a second reduction is required, reduce dose to 75 mg daily. If dose reduction below 75 mg daily is required, discontinue treatment.

Hematologic toxicity (except lymphopenia unless associated with clinical events [eg, opportunistic infection]), according to Common Toxicity Criteria for Adverse Events Version 4:

Grade 1 or 2: No dosage adjustment required.

Grade 3:

Day 1 of cycle: Withhold palbociclib therapy and repeat CBC with differential within 1 week. When improved to ≤ grade 2, initiate the next cycle at the same dose.

Day 15 of first 2 cycles: If at grade 3, continue palbociclib therapy at current dose to complete the cycle. Repeat CBC with differential on day 22. If at grade 4 on day 22, withhold palbociclib treatment until resolved to ≤ grade 2. After resolution, resume at next lower dose. Consider dose reduction in future cycles if recovery from grade 3 neutropenia is prolonged (>1 week) or for recurrent grade 3 neutropenia on day 1 of subsequent cycles.

Grade 3 (ANC 500/mm^3 to <1,000/mm^3) plus fever ≥38.5°C and/or infection at any time: Withhold palbociclib treatment until resolved to ≤ grade 2. Resume at next lower dose upon restarting.

Grade 4 at any time: Withhold palbociclib treatment until resolved to ≤ grade 2. After resolution, resume at next lower dose.

Nonhematologic toxicity (according to Common Toxicity Criteria for Adverse Events Version 4):

Grade 1 or 2: No dosage adjustment required.

Grade 3 or higher (if persistent despite optimal medical management): Withhold palbociclib until symptoms resolve to ≤ grade 1 or ≤ grade 2 (if toxicity is not a safety risk); after resolution, resume at the next lower dose.

Combination Regimens

Breast cancer:

Palbociclib-Fulvestrant (Breast) on page 2189

Palbociclib-Letrozole (Breast) on page 2189

Administration Oral: Administer with food. Take at approximately the same time each day. Swallow whole, do not crush, chew, or open capsules prior to swallowing (do not ingest if capsules are broken, cracked, or not fully intact).

Emetic Potential Low (10% to 30%)

Monitoring Parameters CBC with differential (prior to treatment initiation, every 2 weeks for first 2 cycles, then prior to each cycle, and as clinically indicated; if neutropenia is limited to grades 1 or 2 in the first 6 cycles, monitor every 3 months [prior to the beginning of a cycle] and as clinically indicated for subsequent cycles); pregnancy test prior to treatment initiation (in women of reproductive potential); monitor for signs/symptoms of infection.

Dietary Considerations Avoid grapefruit.

Prescribing and Access Restrictions Palbociclib is available through specialty pharmacies. For more information, refer to http://www.ibrance.com/getting-ibrance

Dosage Forms Excipient information presented when available (limited, particularly for generics); consult specific product labeling.

Capsule, Oral:

Ibrance: 75 mg, 100 mg, 125 mg

◆ **Palbociclib Isethionate** *see* Palbociclib *on page* 1421

Palifermin (pal ee FER min)

Related Information

Hematopoietic Cell Transplantation *on page* 2365

Mucositis and Stomatitis *on page* 2299

Safe Handling of Hazardous Drugs *on page* 2379

Brand Names: US Kepivance

Index Terms AMJ 9701; Keratinocyte Growth Factor, Recombinant Human; rhKGF; rhu Keratinocyte Growth Factor; rHu-KGF

Pharmacologic Category Chemoprotective Agent; Keratinocyte Growth Factor

Use

Oral mucositis: To decrease the incidence and duration of severe oral mucositis associated with hematologic malignancies in patients receiving myelotoxic therapy in the setting of autologous hematopoietic stem cell support (when the preparative regimen is expected to result in mucositis ≥ grade 3 in most patients).

◄ Limitations of use: Use (safety and efficacy) is not established for non-hematologic malignancies; use is not recommended with conditioning regimens containing melphalan 200 mg/m^2. Palifermin was not effective in decreasing the incidence of severe mucositis in patients with hematologic malignancies receiving myelotoxic therapy in the setting of allogeneic hematopoietic stem cell support.

Labeled Contraindications There are no contraindications listed in the manufacturer's labeling.

Pregnancy Considerations Adverse events were observed in animal reproduction studies.

Breastfeeding Considerations It is not known if palifermin is excreted in breast milk. Because of the potential for serious adverse reactions in the nursing infant, the manufacturer recommends a decision be made to discontinue nursing or the drug, taking into account the importance of treatment to the mother.

Warnings/Precautions Edema, erythema, pruritus, rash, oral/perioral dysesthesia, taste alteration, tongue discoloration, and tongue thickening may occur (median onset of cutaneous toxicities following initial dose is 6 days; median duration is 5 days); instruct patients to report mucocutaneous effects. Safety and efficacy have not been established with nonhematologic malignancies; effect on the growth of keratinocyte growth factor (KGF) receptor expressing, nonhematopoietic human tumors is not known. Palifermin has been shown to enhance epithelial tumor cell lines *in vitro*. Do not administer within 24 hours before, during, or after myelotoxic chemotherapy. If administered during or within 24 hours of (before or after) chemotherapy, palifermin may increase the severity and duration of mucositis due to the increased sensitivity of rapidly dividing epithelial cells.

The Multinational Association of Supportive Care in Cancer and the International Society for Oral Oncology (MASCC/ISOO) guidelines for the prevention and treatment of mucositis recommend palifermin (at the FDA-approved dose) for the prevention of oral mucositis in patients with hematologic malignancies who are receiving high-dose chemotherapy and total body irradiation with autologous stem cell transplantation (Lalla 2014). Guidelines from the American Society of Clinical Oncology (ASCO) for the use of chemotherapy and radiotherapy protectants (Hensley 2008) recommend the use of palifermin to decrease the incidence of severe mucositis in patients undergoing autologous stem-cell transplantation with a total body irradiation (TBI) conditioning regimen. According to the ASCO guidelines, data are insufficient to recommend palifermin when the conditioning regimen is chemotherapy only. Palifermin may be considered in patients undergoing myeloablative allogeneic stem-cell transplantation with a TBI conditioning regimen, however data are again insufficient to recommend palifermin when the conditioning regimen is chemotherapy only. Due to a lack of appropriate data, the guidelines also do not recommend palifermin use in non-stem-cell transplantation treatment regimens or for use when treating solid tumors.

Adverse Reactions

>10%:

Cardiovascular: Edema (28%)

Central nervous system: Pain (16%), dysesthesia (12%; includes hypoesthesia, oral hyperesthesia, paresthesia)

Dermatologic: Skin rash (62%; grade 3: 3%), pruritus (35%), erythema (32%)

Gastrointestinal: Increased serum amylase (62%, grades 3/4: 38%), increased serum lipase (28%, grades 3/4: 11%), mouth discoloration (≤17%), swelling of mouth (≤17%), tongue discoloration (≤17%), tongue edema (≤17%), dysgeusia (16%)

Miscellaneous: Fever (39%)

1% to 10%:

Immunologic: Antibody development (2%)

Neuromuscular & skeletal: Arthralgia (10%)

<1%, postmarketing, and/or case reports: Cataract, cough, genital edema (vaginal), hyperpigmentation (flexural), palmar-plantar erythrodysesthesia (hand-foot syndrome), perineal pain, rhinitis, vaginal disease (erythema)

Drug Interactions

Metabolism/Transport Effects None known.

Avoid Concomitant Use There are no known interactions where it is recommended to avoid concomitant use.

Increased Effect/Toxicity

Palifermin may increase the levels/effects of: Antineoplastic Agents

The levels/effects of Palifermin may be increased by: Heparin; Heparin (Low Molecular Weight)

Decreased Effect There are no known significant interactions involving a decrease in effect.

Hazardous Drugs Handling Considerations

Hazardous agent (NIOSH 2016 [group 2]).

Use appropriate precautions for receiving, handling, administration, and disposal. Gloves (single) should be worn during receiving, unpacking, and placing in storage.

NIOSH recommends double gloving, a protective gown, ventilated engineering controls (a class II biological safety cabinet or a compounding aseptic containment isolator), and closed system transfer devices (CSTDs) for preparation. Double gloving, a gown, and (if dosage form allows) CSTDs are required during administration (NIOSH 2016).

Storage/Stability Store intact vials at 2°C to 8°C (36°F to 46°F). Protect from light. Although the manufacturer recommends immediate use, reconstituted vials are stable for up to 24 hours refrigerated. Bring to room temperature for up to 1 hour prior to administration; however, do not use if left at room temperature >1 hour. Protect reconstituted solution from light. Do not freeze reconstituted product.

Preparation for Administration To reconstitute, slowly add 1.2 mL SWFI, to a final concentration of 5 mg/mL. Swirl gently; do not shake or vigorously agitate. May take up to 3 minutes to dissolve; reconstituted solution should be clear and colorless. Do not filter during preparation or administration.

Mechanism of Action Palifermin is a recombinant keratinocyte growth factor (KGF) produced in *E. coli*. Endogenous KGF is produced by mesenchymal cells in response to epithelial tissue injury. KGF binds to the KGF receptor resulting in proliferation, differentiation and migration of epithelial cells in multiple tissues, including (but not limited to) the tongue, buccal mucosa, esophagus, and salivary gland.

Pharmacodynamics/Kinetics

Onset of action: Epithelial cell proliferation (dose-dependent): 48 hours

Half-life elimination: 4.5 hours (range: 3.3 to 5.7 hours)

◀ **Dosing**

Adult & Geriatric Oral mucositis associated with autologous hematopoietic stem cell transplant (HSCT) conditioning regimens: IV: 60 mcg/kg/day for 3 consecutive days before and 3 consecutive days after myelotoxic therapy; total of 6 doses (Spielberger, 2004)

> **Note:** Administer first 3 doses prior to myelotoxic therapy, with the third dose given 24 to 48 hours before beginning the myelotoxic conditioning regimen. Administer the last 3 doses after completion of the myelotoxic conditioning regimen, with the first of these doses after (but on the same day) as HSCT infusion and at least 7 days after the most recent dose of palifermin.

Renal Impairment There are no dosage adjustments provided in the manufacturer's labeling; however, based on a pharmacokinetic study, renal impairment has minimal to no impact on palifermin pharmacokinetics.

Hepatic Impairment There are no dosage adjustments provided in the manufacturer's labeling (has not been studied).

Administration Administer by IV bolus. If heparin is used to maintain the patency of the IV line, flush line with saline prior to and after palifermin administration. Do not administer palifermin during or within 24 hours before or after chemotherapy. Allow solution to reach room temperature prior to administration; do not use if at room temperature >1 hour. Do not filter.

Monitoring Parameters Monitor for oral mucositis

Dosage Forms Excipient information presented when available (limited, particularly for generics); consult specific product labeling.

Solution Reconstituted, Intravenous [preservative free]:
  Kepivance: 6.25 mg (1 ea)

Palonosetron (pal oh NOE se tron)

Related Information

Management of Chemotherapy-Induced Nausea and Vomiting in Adults *on page 2253*

Prevention of Chemotherapy-Induced Nausea and Vomiting in Children *on page 2310*

Brand Names: US Aloxi

Brand Names: Canada Aloxi

Index Terms Palonosetron Hydrochloride; Palonosetron, inj; RS-25259; RS-25259-197

Pharmacologic Category Antiemetic; Selective 5-HT$_3$ Receptor Antagonist

Use

Chemotherapy-induced nausea and vomiting: Prevention of acute and delayed nausea and vomiting associated with initial and repeat courses in patients treated with moderately emetogenic cancer chemotherapy in adults; prevention of acute nausea and vomiting associated with initial and repeat courses in patients treated with highly emetogenic cancer chemotherapy in adults; prevention of acute nausea and vomiting associated with initial and repeat courses of emetogenic cancer chemotherapy (including highly emetogenic chemotherapy) in pediatric patients 1 month to <17 years.

Capsules [Canadian product]: Prevention of acute nausea and vomiting associated with moderately emetogenic cancer chemotherapy in adults.

Postoperative nausea and vomiting: Prevention of postoperative nausea and vomiting (PONV) for up to 24 hours following surgery in adults.

Limitations of use: Routine prophylaxis for PONV in patients with minimal expectation of nausea and/or vomiting is not recommended, although use is recommended in patients when nausea and vomiting must be avoided in the postoperative period, even if the incidence of PONV is low.

Labeled Contraindications Known hypersensitivity to palonosetron or any component of the formulation

Pregnancy Considerations Adverse events have not been observed in animal reproduction studies. Use during pregnancy only if clearly needed.

Breastfeeding Considerations It is not known if palonosetron is present in breast milk. Due to the potential for adverse reactions in the breastfed infant, the manufacturer recommends a decision be made whether to discontinue breastfeeding or to discontinue palonosetron, taking into account the importance of treatment to the mother.

Warnings/Precautions Hypersensitivity (including anaphylaxis) has been reported in patients with or without known hypersensitivity to other 5-HT$_3$ receptor antagonists. Serotonin syndrome has been reported with 5-HT$_3$ receptor antagonists, predominantly when used in combination with other serotonergic agents (eg, SSRIs, SNRIs, MAOIs, mirtazapine, fentanyl, lithium, tramadol, and/or methylene blue). Some of the cases have been fatal. The majority of serotonin syndrome reports due to 5-HT$_3$ receptor antagonists have occurred in a post-anesthesia setting or in an infusion center. Serotonin syndrome has also been reported following overdose of another 5-HT$_3$ receptor antagonist. Monitor patients for signs of serotonin syndrome, including mental status changes (eg, agitation, hallucinations, delirium, coma); autonomic instability (eg, tachycardia, labile blood pressure, diaphoresis, dizziness, flushing, hyperthermia); neuromuscular changes (eg, tremor, rigidity, myoclonus, hyperreflexia, incoordination); gastrointestinal symptoms (eg, nausea, vomiting, diarrhea); and/or seizures. If serotonin syndrome occurs, discontinue 5-HT$_3$ receptor antagonist treatment and begin supportive management.

Selective 5-HT$_3$ receptor antagonists have been associated with dose-dependent increases in ECG intervals (eg, PR, QRS duration, QT/QTc, JT). A thorough QT/QTc study evaluating the effect of palonosetron on QT/QTc demonstrated a magnitude of effect less than the threshold for regulatory concern (Morganroth 2016). Reduction in heart rate may occur with the 5-HT$_3$ antagonists, including palonosetron (Gonullu 2012). Antiemetics are most effective when used prophylactically (Roila 2016). Potentially significant drug-drug interactions may exist, requiring dose or frequency adjustment, additional monitoring, and/or selection of alternative therapy. If emesis occurs despite optimal antiemetic prophylaxis, re-evaluate emetic risk, disease, concurrent morbidities and medications to assure antiemetic regimen is optimized (Basch 2011). For postoperative nausea and vomiting (PONV), may use for low expectation of PONV if it is essential to avoid nausea and vomiting in the postoperative period; use is not recommended if there is little expectation of nausea and vomiting.

Adverse Reactions Frequencies reported for both indications (chemotherapy-associated nausea and vomiting and postoperative nausea and vomiting) and in adults unless otherwise noted.

1% to 10%:

Cardiovascular: Prolonged Q-T interval on ECG (PONV 1% to 5%; chemotherapy-associated <1%), bradycardia (chemotherapy-associated 1%), sinus bradycardia (PONV: 1%), tachycardia (may be nonsustained; 1%), hypotension (≤1%)

Central nervous system: Headache (chemotherapy-associated: Adults 9%; infants, children, and adolescents <1%), anxiety (chemotherapy-associated: 1%), dizziness (infants, children, and adults ≤1%)

Dermatologic: Pruritus (PONV: 1%)

Endocrine & metabolic: Hyperkalemia (chemotherapy-associated: 1%)

Gastrointestinal: Constipation (chemotherapy-associated: 5%), diarrhea (≤1%), flatulence (≤1%)

Genitourinary: Urinary retention (≤1%)

Hepatic: Increased serum ALT (≤1%; may be transient), increased serum AST (≤1%; may be transient)

Neuromuscular & skeletal: Weakness (chemotherapy-associated: 1%)

<1%, postmarketing, and/or case reports: Abdominal pain, allergic dermatitis, amblyopia, anaphylactic shock (very rare), anaphylaxis (very rare), anasarca, anemia, anorexia, arthralgia, cardiac arrhythmia, chills, decreased appetite, decreased blood pressure, decreased gastrointestinal motility, decreased platelet count, dermatological disease (infants, children, and adolescents), distended vein, drowsiness, dyskinesia (infants, children, and adolescents), dyspepsia, electrolyte disturbance, epistaxis, erythema, euphoria, extrasystoles, eye irritation, fatigue, fever, flattened T wave on ECG, flu-like symptoms, glycosuria, hiccups, hot flash, hyperglycemia, hypersensitivity (very rare), hypersomnia, hypertension, hypokalemia, hypoventilation, increased bilirubin (transient), increased liver enzymes, infusion site pain (infants, children, and adolescents), injection site reaction (very rare; includes burning sensation at injection site, discomfort at injection site, induration at injection site, pain at injection site), insomnia, ischemic heart disease, laryngospasm, limb pain, metabolic acidosis, motion sickness, paresthesia, serotonin syndrome, sialorrhea, sinus arrhythmia, sinus tachycardia, skin rash, supraventricular extrasystole, tinnitus, vein discoloration, ventricular premature contractions, xerostomia

Drug Interactions

Metabolism/Transport Effects Substrate of CYP1A2 (minor), CYP2D6 (minor), CYP3A4 (minor); **Note:** Assignment of Major/Minor substrate status based on clinically relevant drug interaction potential

Avoid Concomitant Use

Avoid concomitant use of Palonosetron with any of the following: Apomorphine

Increased Effect/Toxicity

Palonosetron may increase the levels/effects of: Apomorphine; Serotonin Modulators

Decreased Effect

Palonosetron may decrease the levels/effects of: Tapentadol; TraMADol

Storage/Stability

Store intact vials at 20°C to 25°C (68°F to 77°F); excursions permitted to 15°C to 30°C (59°F to 86°F). Do not freeze. Protect from light. Solutions of 5 mcg/mL and 30 mcg/mL in NS, D5W, D5½NS, and D5LR injection are stable for 48 hours at room temperature and 14 days under refrigeration (Trissel 2004).

Capsules [Canadian product]: Store at 20°C to 25°C (68°F to 77°F); excursions permitted to 15°C to 30°C (59°F to 86°F).

Mechanism of Action Palonosetron is a selective 5-HT$_3$ receptor antagonist, blocking serotonin, both on vagal nerve terminals in the periphery and centrally in the chemoreceptor trigger zone

Pharmacodynamics/Kinetics

Absorption: Capsules [Canadian product]: Well absorbed

Distribution: V_d:

Children 1 month to 17 years: Mean range: 5.3 to 6.3 L/kg

Adults: 8.3 ± 2.5 L/kg

Protein binding: ~62%

Metabolism: ~50% metabolized via CYP enzymes (and likely other pathways) to relatively inactive metabolites (N-oxide-palonosetron and 6-S-hydroxy-palonosetron); CYP1A2, 2D6, and 3A4 contribute to its metabolism

Bioavailability: Capsules [Canadian product]: 97%

Half-life elimination: IV: Children 1 month to 17 years: Median: 29.5 hours (range: 20 to 30 hours); Adults: ~40 hours

Time to peak (plasma): Capsules [Canadian product]: 5.1 ± 5.9 hours

Excretion: Urine (80%; 40% as unchanged drug)

Clearance:

Infants and children <2 years: 0.31 L/hour/kg

Children 2 to <12 years: Mean range: 0.19 to 0.23 L/hour/kg

Children ≥12 years, Adolescents, and Adults: 0.160 L/hour/kg

Dosing

Adult

Prevention of chemotherapy-induced nausea and vomiting (moderately and highly emetogenic chemotherapy): IV: 0.25 mg beginning ~30 minutes prior to the start of chemotherapy

Capsule [Canadian product]: Moderately emetogenic chemotherapy: Oral: 0.5 mg ~1 hour prior to the start of chemotherapy.

Prevention of postoperative nausea and vomiting: IV: 0.075 mg immediately prior to anesthesia induction

Geriatric No dosage adjustment necessary. Refer to adult dosing.

Pediatric

Prevention of chemotherapy-induced nausea and vomiting (highly emetogenic chemotherapy): Infants ≥1 month, Children, and Adolescents <17 years: IV: 20 **mcg**/kg (maximum dose: 1.5 **mg**) beginning ~30 minutes prior to the start of chemotherapy

Pediatric guideline recommendations:

Prevention of chemotherapy-induced nausea and vomiting for highly emetogenic chemotherapy (Patel 2017):

Infants ≥1 month to 6 months: IV: 20 **mcg**/kg once prior to chemotherapy (maximum: 1.5 **mg**/dose). Antiemetic regimen also includes dexamethasone (if no contraindications to corticosteroids).

Infants ≥6 months, Children and Adolescents <17 years: IV: 20 **mcg**/kg once prior to chemotherapy (maximum: 1.5 **mg**/dose). Antiemetic regimen also includes aprepitant (if **no** potential drug interactions) and dexamethasone (if no contraindications to corticosteroids).

Adolescents ≥17 years:

IV: 0.25 mg once prior to chemotherapy. Antiemetic regimen also includes aprepitant (if **no** potential drug interactions) and dexamethasone (if no contraindications to corticosteroids).

Oral [Canadian product]: 0.5 mg once prior to chemotherapy. Antiemetic regimen also includes aprepitant (if **no** potential drug interactions) and dexamethasone (if no contraindications to corticosteroids).

Prevention of chemotherapy-induced nausea and vomiting for moderately emetogenic chemotherapy (off-label; Patel 2017):

Infants ≥1 month to 6 months: IV: 20 **mcg**/kg once prior to chemotherapy (maximum: 1.5 **mg**/dose. Antiemetic regimen also includes dexamethasone (if no contraindications to corticosteroids).

Infants ≥6 months, Children and Adolescents <17 years: IV: 20 **mcg**/kg once prior to chemotherapy (maximum: 1.5 **mg**/dose). Antiemetic regimen also includes dexamethasone; if patient cannot receive corticosteroids, antiemetic regimen may include aprepitant (if **no** potential drug interactions).

Adolescents ≥17 years:

IV: 0.25 mg once prior to chemotherapy. Antiemetic regimen also includes dexamethasone; if patient cannot receive corticosteroids, antiemetic regimen may include aprepitant (if **no** potential drug interactions).

Oral [Canadian product]: 0.5 mg once prior to chemotherapy. Antiemetic regimen also includes dexamethasone; if patient cannot receive corticosteroids, antiemetic regimen may include aprepitant (if **no** potential drug interactions).

Renal Impairment No dosage adjustment is necessary.

Hepatic Impairment No dosage adjustment is necessary.

Administration Flush IV line with NS prior to and following administration.

Prevention of chemotherapy-induced nausea and vomiting:

Children: Infuse over 15 minutes, beginning ~30 minutes prior to the start of chemotherapy

Adults: Infuse over 30 seconds, beginning ~30 minutes prior to the start of chemotherapy

Capsule [Canadian product]: May be administered with or without food.

Prevention of postoperative nausea and vomiting: Infuse over 10 seconds immediately prior to anesthesia induction

Dosage Forms Excipient information presented when available (limited, particularly for generics); consult specific product labeling.

Solution, Intravenous:

Aloxi: 0.25 mg/5 mL (5 mL) [contains edetate disodium]

Dosage Forms: Canada Information with regard to form, strength, and availability of products uniquely available in Canada but currently not available in the US. Refer also to Dosage Forms.

Excipient information presented when available (limited, particularly for generics); consult specific product labeling.

Capsule, Oral:

Aloxi: 0.5 mg

◆ **Palonosetron and Netupitant** *see* Netupitant and Palonosetron *on page 1311*

◆ **Palonosetron Hydrochloride** *see* Palonosetron *on page 1428*

◆ **Palonosetron Hydrochloride and Netupitant** *see* Netupitant and Palonosetron *on page 1311*

◆ **Palonosetron, inj** *see* Palonosetron *on page 1428*

Pamidronate (pa mi DROE nate)

Related Information

Chronic Pain Management (Cancer) *on page* 2327
Hypercalcemia of Malignancy *on page* 2341
Safe Handling of Hazardous Drugs *on page* 2379

Brand Names: Canada Aredia; Pamidronate Disodium; Pamidronate Disodium Omega; PMS-Pamidronate

Index Terms Pamidronate Disodium

Pharmacologic Category Bisphosphonate Derivative

Use

Hypercalcemia of malignancy: Treatment of moderate or severe hypercalcemia associated with malignancy, with or without bone metastases, in conjunction with adequate hydration.

Osteolytic bone metastases of breast cancer and osteolytic lesions of multiple myeloma: Treatment of osteolytic bone metastases of breast cancer and osteolytic lesions of multiple myeloma in conjunction with standard antineoplastic therapy.

Paget disease: Treatment of patients with moderate to severe Paget disease of bone.

Labeled Contraindications Hypersensitivity to pamidronate, other bisphosphonates, or any component of the formulation

Pregnancy Considerations Adverse events were observed in animal reproduction studies. It is not known if bisphosphonates cross the placenta, but fetal exposure is expected (Djokanovic, 2008; Stathopoulos, 2011). Bisphosphonates are incorporated into the bone matrix and gradually released over time. The amount available in the systemic circulation varies by dose and duration of therapy. Theoretically, there may be a risk of fetal harm when pregnancy follows the completion of therapy; however, available data have not shown that exposure to bisphosphonates during pregnancy significantly increases the risk of adverse fetal events (Djokanovic, 2008; Levy, 2009; Stathopoulos, 2011). Until additional data is available, most sources recommend discontinuing bisphosphonate therapy in women of reproductive potential as early as possible prior to a planned pregnancy; use in premenopausal women should be reserved for special circumstances when rapid bone loss is occurring (Bhalla, 2010; Pereira, 2012; Stathopoulos, 2011). Because hypocalcemia has been described following *in utero* bisphosphonate exposure, exposed infants should be monitored for hypocalcemia after birth (Djokanovic, 2008; Stathopoulos, 2011).

Breastfeeding Considerations It is not known if pamidronate is present in breast milk. Pamidronate was not detected in the milk of a breastfeeding woman receiving pamidronate 30 mg IV monthly (therapy started ~6 months postpartum). Following the first infusion, milk was pumped and collected for 0 to 24 hours and 25 to 48 hours and each day pooled for analysis. Pamidronate readings were below the limit of quantification (<0.4 micromole/L). During therapy, breast milk was pumped and discarded for the first 48 hours following each infusion prior to resuming breastfeeding. The infant was breastfed >80% of the time; adverse events were not observed in the breastfed infant (Simonoski, 2000). Monitoring the serum calcium concentrations of breastfed infants is recommended (Stathopoulos 2011). Due to the potential for serious adverse reactions in the breastfed infant, the manufacturer recommends a decision be made whether to discontinue breastfeeding or to discontinue the drug, taking into account the importance of treatment to the mother.

Warnings/Precautions Atypical femur fractures (after minimal or no trauma) have been reported. The fractures include subtrochanteric femur (bone just below the hip joint) and diaphyseal femur (long segment of the thigh bone). Some patients experience prodromal pain weeks or months before the fracture occurs. It is unclear if bisphosphonate therapy is the cause for these fractures. Patients receiving long-term (>3 to 5 years) bisphosphonate therapy may be at an increased risk. Consider discontinuing pamidronate in patients with a suspected femoral shaft fracture. Patients who present with thigh or groin pain in the absence of trauma should be evaluated. Infrequently, severe (and occasionally debilitating) musculoskeletal (bone, joint, and/or muscle) pain have been reported during bisphosphonate treatment. The onset of pain ranged from a single day to several months. Consider discontinuing therapy in patients who experience severe symptoms; symptoms usually resolve upon discontinuation. Some patients experienced recurrence when rechallenged with same drug or another bisphosphonate; avoid use in patients with a history of these symptoms in association with bisphosphonate therapy.

Initial or single doses have been associated with renal deterioration, progressing to renal failure and dialysis. Withhold pamidronate treatment (until renal function returns to baseline) in patients with evidence of renal deterioration. Glomerulosclerosis (focal segmental) with or without nephrotic syndrome has also been reported. Longer infusion times (>2 hours) may reduce the risk for renal toxicity, especially in patients with preexisting renal insufficiency. Single pamidronate doses should not exceed 90 mg. Patients with serum creatinine >3 mg/dL were not studied in clinical trials; limited data are available in patients with CrCl <30 mL/minute. Evaluate serum creatinine prior to each treatment. For the treatment of bone metastases, use is not recommended in patients with severe renal impairment; for renal impairment in indications other than bone metastases, use clinical judgment to determine if benefits outweigh potential risks.

Use has been associated with asymptomatic electrolyte abnormalities (including hypophosphatemia, hypokalemia, hypomagnesemia, and hypocalcemia). Rare cases of symptomatic hypocalcemia, including tetany have been reported. Patients with a history of thyroid surgery may have relative hypoparathyroidism; predisposing them to pamidronate-related hypocalcemia. Patients with preexisting anemia, leukopenia, or thrombocytopenia should be closely monitored during the first 2 weeks of treatment.

Osteonecrosis of the jaw (ONJ), also referred to as medication-related osteonecrosis of the jaw (MRONJ), has been reported in patients receiving bisphosphonates. Known risk factors for MRONJ include invasive dental procedures (eg, tooth extraction, dental implants, boney surgery), cancer diagnosis, concomitant therapy (eg, chemotherapy, corticosteroids, angiogenesis inhibitors), poor oral hygiene, ill-fitting dentures, and comorbid disorders (anemia, coagulopathy, infection, preexisting dental or periodontal disease). Risk may increase with increased duration of bisphosphonate use and/or may be reported at a greater frequency based on tumor type (eg, advanced breast cancer, multiple myeloma). According to a position paper by the American Association of Maxillofacial Surgeons (AAOMS), MRONJ has been associated with bisphosphonates and other antiresorptive agents (denosumab), and antiangiogenic agents (eg, bevacizumab, sunitinib) used for the treatment of osteoporosis or malignancy; risk is significantly higher in cancer patients receiving antiresorptive therapy compared to patients receiving osteoporosis treatment (regardless of medication used or dosing schedule).

MRONJ risk is also increased with monthly IV antiresorptive therapy compared to the minimal risk associated with oral bisphosphonate use, although risk appears to increase with oral bisphosphonates when duration of therapy exceeds 4 years. The AAOMS suggests that if medically permissible, initiation of IV bisphosphonates for cancer therapy should be delayed until optimal dental health is attained (if extractions are required, antiresorptive therapy should delayed until the extraction site has mucosalized or until after adequate osseous healing). Once IV bisphosphonate therapy is initiated for oncologic disease, procedures that involve direct osseous injury and placement of dental implants should be avoided. Patients developing ONJ during therapy should receive care by an oral surgeon (AAOMS [Ruggiero 2014]).

Hypercalcemia of malignancy (HCM): Adequate hydration is required during treatment (urine output ~2 L/day); avoid overhydration, especially in patients with heart failure.

Multiple myeloma: Patients with Bence-Jones proteinuria and dehydration should be adequately hydrated prior to therapy. The American Society of Clinical Oncology (ASCO) has also published guidelines on bisphosphonates use for prevention and treatment of bone disease in multiple myeloma (Kyle, 2007). Bisphosphonate (pamidronate or zoledronic acid) use is recommended in multiple myeloma patients with lytic bone destruction or compression spine fracture from osteopenia. Bisphosphonates may also be considered in patients with pain secondary to osteolytic disease, adjunct therapy to stabilize fractures or impending fractures, and for multiple myeloma patients with osteopenia but no radiographic evidence of lytic bone disease. Bisphosphonates are not recommended in patients with solitary plasmacytoma, smoldering (asymptomatic) or indolent myeloma, or monoclonal gammopathy of undetermined significance. The guidelines recommend monthly treatment for a period of 2 years. At that time, consider discontinuing in responsive and stable patients, and reinitiate if a new-onset skeletal-related event occurs. The ASCO guidelines are in alignment with the prescribing information for dosing, renal dose adjustments, infusion times, prevention and management of osteonecrosis of the jaw, and monitoring of laboratory parameter recommendations. According to the guidelines, in patients with extensive bone disease with existing severe renal disease (a serum creatinine >3 mg/dL or CrCl <30 mL/minute) pamidronate at a dose of 90 mg over 4 to 6 hours should be used (unless preexisting renal disease in which case a reduced initial dose should be considered). Monitor for albuminuria every 3 to 6 months; in patients with unexplained albuminuria >500 mg/24 hours, withhold the dose until level returns to baseline, then recheck every 3 to 4 weeks. Pamidronate may be reinitiated at a dose not to exceed 90 mg every 4 weeks with a longer infusion time of at least 4 hours.

Breast cancer (metastatic): The American Society of Clinical Oncology (ASCO) updated guidelines on the role of bone-modifying agents (BMAs) in the prevention and treatment of skeletal-related events for metastatic breast cancer patients (Van Poznak, 2011). The guidelines recommend initiating a BMA (denosumab, pamidronate, zoledronic acid) in patients with metastatic breast cancer to the bone. There is currently no literature indicating the superiority of one particular BMA. Optimal duration is not yet defined; however, the guidelines recommend continuing therapy until substantial decline in patient's performance status. The ASCO guidelines are in alignment with prescribing information for dosing, renal dose adjustments, infusion times, prevention and management of osteonecrosis of the jaw, and monitoring of laboratory parameter recommendations. BMAs are not the first-line therapy for pain. BMAs are to be used as adjunctive therapy for cancer-related bone pain associated with bone metastasis, demonstrating a modest pain control benefit. BMAs should be used in conjunction with agents such as NSAIDS, opioid and nonopioid analgesics, corticosteroids, radiation/surgery, and interventional procedures.

Adverse Reactions Note: Actual percentages may vary by indication and duration of infusion; treatment for multiple myeloma is associated with higher percentage.

>10%:

Central nervous system: Fatigue (≤37%), headache (≤26%), insomnia (≤22%)

Endocrine & metabolic: Hypophosphatemia (≤18%), hypokalemia (4% to 18%), hypocalcemia (≤3% to 17%), hypomagnesemia (10% to 12%)

Gastrointestinal: Nausea (≤54%), vomiting (≤36%), anorexia (≤26%), abdominal pain (≤23%), dyspepsia (≤23%)

Genitourinary: Urinary tract infection (≤19%)

Hematologic & oncologic: Anemia (≤43%), metastases (21% to 31%), granulocytopenia (≤20%)

Local: Infusion site reaction (≤18%; includes induration, pain, redness, and swelling)

Neuromuscular & skeletal: Myalgia (≤26%), weakness (≤22%), arthralgia (≤14%), osteonecrosis of the jaw (cancer patients: 1% to 11%)

Renal: Increased serum creatinine (≤19%)

Respiratory: Dyspnea (≤30%), cough (≤26%), upper respiratory tract infection (≤24%), sinusitis (≤16%), pleural effusion (≤11%)

Miscellaneous: Fever (18% to 39%; transient)

1% to 10%:

Cardiovascular: Atrial fibrillation (≤6%), hypertension (≤6%), syncope (≤6%), tachycardia (≤6%), atrial flutter (≤1%), cardiac failure (≤1%), edema (≤1%)

Central nervous system: Drowsiness (≤6%), psychosis (≤4%), seizure (≤2%)

Endocrine & metabolic: Hypothyroidism (≤6%)

Gastrointestinal: Constipation (≤6%), gastrointestinal hemorrhage (≤6%), diarrhea (≤1%), stomatitis (≤1%)

Genitourinary: Uremia (≤4%)

Hematologic & oncologic: Leukopenia (≤4%), neutropenia (≤1%), thrombocytopenia (≤1%)

Infection: Candidiasis (≤6%)

Neuromuscular & skeletal: Back pain, ostealgia

Respiratory: Rales (≤6%), rhinitis (≤6%)

<1%, postmarketing, and/or case reports: Acute renal failure, anaphylactic shock, angioedema, bronchospasm, cardiac failure, confusion, conjunctivitis, electrolyte disturbance, episcleritis, flu-like symptoms, focal segmental glomerulosclerosis (including collapsing variant), hallucination (visual), hematuria, herpes virus infection (reactivation), hyperkalemia, hypernatremia, hypersensitivity reaction, hypervolemia, hypotension, inflammation at injection site, injection site phlebitis, iridocyclitis, iritis, left heart failure, lymphocytopenia, malaise, mineral abnormalities, nephrotic syndrome, osteonecrosis (other than jaw), paresthesia, pruritus, renal failure, renal insufficiency, scleritis, skin rash, tetany, uveitis, xanthopsia

Drug Interactions

Metabolism/Transport Effects None known.

Avoid Concomitant Use There are no known interactions where it is recommended to avoid concomitant use.

Increased Effect/Toxicity

Pamidronate may increase the levels/effects of: Deferasirox

The levels/effects of Pamidronate may be increased by: Aminoglycosides; Nonsteroidal Anti-Inflammatory Agents; Systemic Angiogenesis Inhibitors; Thalidomide

Decreased Effect

The levels/effects of Pamidronate may be decreased by: Proton Pump Inhibitors

Hazardous Drugs Handling Considerations

Hazardous agent (NIOSH 2016 [group 3]).

Use appropriate precautions for receiving, handling, administration, and disposal. Gloves (single) should be worn during receiving, unpacking, and placing in storage.

NIOSH recommends double gloving, a protective gown, ventilated engineering controls (a class II biological safety cabinet or a compounding aseptic containment isolator), and closed-system transfer devices (CSTDs) when compounding. Double gloving and a gown are required during administration (NIOSH 2016). Assess risk to determine appropriate containment strategy (USP-NF 2017).

Storage/Stability

Powder for reconstitution: Store at 20°C to 25°C (68°F to 77°F). The reconstituted solution is stable for 24 hours stored under refrigeration at 2°C to 8°C (36°F to 46°F). The diluted solution for infusion is stable in D5W or NS at room temperature for up to 24 hours.

Solution for injection: Store at 20°C to 25°C (68°F to 77°F). The diluted solution for infusion is stable in D5W or NS at room temperature for up to 24 hours.

Preparation for Administration

Powder for injection: Reconstitute by adding 10 mL of SWFI to each vial of lyophilized powder, the resulting solution will be 30 mg/10 mL or 90 mg/10 mL.

Pamidronate may be further diluted in 250 to 1000 mL of 1/2NS or NS or D5W. (The manufacturers recommend dilution in 1000 mL for hypercalcemia of malignancy, 500 mL for Paget's disease and bone metastases of myeloma, and 250 mL for bone metastases of breast cancer.)

Mechanism of Action Nitrogen-containing bisphosphonate; inhibits bone resorption and decreases mineralization by disrupting osteoclast activity (Gralow 2009; Rogers 2011)

Pharmacodynamics/Kinetics

Onset of action:

Hypercalcemia of malignancy (HCM): Reduction of albumin-corrected serum calcium: Children: ~48 hours (Kerdudo 2005); Adults: ≤24 hours for decrease in albumin-corrected serum calcium, maximum effect: ≤7 days

Paget disease: ~1 month for ≥50% decrease in serum alkaline phosphatase

Maximum effect: Hypercalcemia of malignancy: ≤7 days

Duration: HCM: 7 to 14 days; Paget disease: 1 to 372 days

Absorption: Poorly from the GI tract

◄ Distribution: 38% to 70% over 120 hours

Metabolism: Not metabolized

Half-life elimination: 28 ± 7 hours

Excretion: Biphasic; urine (30% to 62% as unchanged drug; lower in patients with renal dysfunction) within 120 hours

Dosing

Adult Note: Single doses should not exceed 90 mg.

Hypercalcemia of malignancy: IV:

Moderate cancer-related hypercalcemia (corrected serum calcium: 12 to 13.5 mg/dL): 60 to 90 mg, as a single dose over 2 to 24 hours

Severe cancer-related hypercalcemia (corrected serum calcium: >13.5 mg/dL): 90 mg, as a single dose over 2 to 24 hours

Re-treatment in patients who show an initial complete or partial response (allow at least 7 days to elapse prior to re-treatment): May re-treat at the same dose if serum calcium does not return to normal or does not remain normal after initial treatment.

Multiple myeloma, osteolytic bone lesions: IV: 90 mg over 4 hours once monthly:

Lytic disease: American Society of Clinical Oncology (ASCO) guidelines: 90 mg over at least 2 hours once every 3 to 4 weeks for 2 years; discontinue after 2 years in patients with responsive and/or stable disease; resume therapy with new-onset skeletal-related events (Kyle 2007)

Newly-diagnosed, symptomatic (off-label dose): 30 mg over 2.5 hours once monthly for at least 3 years (Gimsing 2010)

Breast cancer, osteolytic bone metastases: IV: 90 mg over 2 hours once every 3 to 4 weeks

Paget's disease (moderate-to-severe): IV: 30 mg over 4 hours once daily for 3 consecutive days (total dose = 90 mg); may re-treat at initial dose if clinically indicated

Hyperparathyroidism (off-label use): IV: 15 to 90 mg as a single dose (Ammann 2003; Jansson 2004; Lu 2003); may be repeated every 1 to 2 months or when hypercalcemia recurs (Jansson 1991; Torregrosa 2003). The treatment period in clinical trials was up to 1 year (Torregrosa 2003).

Prevention of androgen deprivation-induced osteoporosis (off-label use): Males: IV: 60 mg over 2 hours once every 3 months (Smith 2001)

Geriatric Refer to adult dosing. Begin at lower end of adult dosing range.

Renal Impairment Patients with serum creatinine >3 mg/dL were excluded from clinical trials; there are only limited pharmacokinetic data in patients with CrCl <30 mL/minute.

Manufacturer recommends the following guidelines:

Treatment of bone metastases: Use is not recommended in patients with severe renal impairment.

Renal impairment in indications other than bone metastases: Use clinical judgment to determine if benefits outweigh potential risks.

Multiple myeloma: American Society of Clinical Oncology (ASCO) guidelines (Kyle 2007):

Severe renal impairment (serum creatinine >3 mg/dL **or** CrCl <30 mL/minute) and extensive bone disease: 90 mg over 4 to 6 hours. However, a reduced initial dose should be considered if renal impairment was preexisting.

Albuminuria >500 mg/24 hours (unexplained): Withhold dose until returns to baseline, then recheck every 3 to 4 weeks; consider reinitiating at a dose not to exceed 90 mg every 4 weeks and with a longer infusion time of at least 4 hours

Dosing adjustment in renal toxicity: In patients with bone metastases, treatment should be withheld for deterioration in renal function (increase of serum creatinine ≥0.5 mg/dL in patients with normal baseline [serum creatinine <1.4 mg/dL] or ≥1 mg/dL in patients with abnormal baseline [serum creatinine ≥1.4 mg/dL]). Resumption of therapy may be considered when serum creatinine returns to within 10% of baseline.

Hepatic Impairment

Mild to moderate impairment: No dosage adjustment necessary.

Severe impairment: There are no dosage adjustments provided in the manufacturer's labeling (has not been studied).

Administration IV: Infusion rate varies by indication. Longer infusion times (>2 hours) may reduce the risk for renal toxicity, especially in patients with preexisting renal insufficiency. The manufacturer recommends infusing over 2 to 24 hours for hypercalcemia of malignancy; over 2 hours for osteolytic bone lesions with metastatic breast cancer; and over 4 hours for Paget's disease and for osteolytic bone lesions with multiple myeloma. The ASCO guidelines for bisphosphonate use in multiple myeloma recommend infusing pamidronate over at least 2 hours; if therapy is withheld due to renal toxicity, infuse over at least 4 hours upon reintroduction of treatment after renal recovery (Kyle 2007).

Monitoring Parameters Serum creatinine (prior to each treatment); serum electrolytes, including calcium, phosphate, magnesium, and potassium; CBC with differential; monitor for hypocalcemia for at least 2 weeks after therapy; dental exam and preventive dentistry prior to therapy for patients at risk of osteonecrosis, including all cancer patients; patients with preexisting anemia, leukopenia, or thrombocytopenia should be closely monitored during the first 2 weeks of treatment; in addition, monitor urine albumin every 3 to 6 months in multiple myeloma patients

Test Interactions Bisphosphonates may interfere with diagnostic imaging agents such as technetium-99m-diphosphonate in bone scans.

Dietary Considerations Multiple myeloma or metastatic bone lesions from solid tumors or Paget's disease: Take adequate daily calcium and vitamin D supplement (if patient is not hypercalcemic).

Dosage Forms Excipient information presented when available (limited, particularly for generics); consult specific product labeling. [DSC] = Discontinued product

Solution, Intravenous, as disodium:

Generic: 30 mg/10 mL (10 mL); 90 mg/10 mL (10 mL)

Solution, Intravenous, as disodium [preservative free]:

Generic: 30 mg/10 mL (10 mL [DSC]); 6 mg/mL (10 mL); 90 mg/10 mL (10 mL [DSC])

Solution Reconstituted, Intravenous, as disodium:

Generic: 30 mg (1 ea); 90 mg (1 ea)

◆ **Pamidronate Disodium** see Pamidronate on page 1433

◆ **Pamidronate Disodium Omega (Can)** see Pamidronate on page 1433

◆ **Panglobulin** see Immune Globulin on page 992

Panitumumab (pan i TOOM yoo mab)

Related Information

Management of Chemotherapy-Induced Nausea and Vomiting in Adults *on page 2253*

Management of EGFR Inhibitor Toxicities: Dermatologic, Ocular, and Gastro-intestinal *on page 2291*

Prevention of Chemotherapy-Induced Nausea and Vomiting in Children *on page 2310*

Brand Names: US Vectibix

Brand Names: Canada Vectibix

Index Terms ABX-EGF; MOAB ABX-EGF; Monoclonal Antibody ABX-EGF; rHuMAb-EGFr

Pharmacologic Category Antineoplastic Agent, Epidermal Growth Factor Receptor (EGFR) Inhibitor; Antineoplastic Agent, Monoclonal Antibody

Use

Colorectal cancer (metastatic): Treatment of patients with wild-type *RAS* (defined as wild-type in both *KRAS* and *NRAS* as determined by an approved test) metastatic colorectal cancer (mCRC), either as first-line therapy in combination with FOLFOX (fluorouracil, leucovorin, and oxaliplatin) or as a single agent following disease progression after prior treatment with fluoropyrimidine-, oxaliplatin-, and irinotecan-containing chemotherapy

Limitations of use: Panitumumab is not indicated for the treatment of patients with *RAS*-mutant mCRC or for whom *RAS* mutation status is unknown.

Labeled Contraindications

There are no contraindications listed in the manufacturer's US labeling.

Canadian labeling: History of severe or life-threatening hypersensitivity reactions to panitumumab or any component of the formulation.

Pregnancy Considerations Based on animal reproduction studies and on the mechanism of action, panitumumab may cause fetal harm if administered during pregnancy. Panitumumab is a human IgG monoclonal antibody and may be transferred across the placenta. Because panitumumab inhibits epidermal growth factor (EGF), a component of fetal development, adverse effects on pregnancy would be expected. Females of reproductive potential should use effective contraception during treatment and for at least 2 months after the last dose. Panitumumab may reduce fertility in females of reproductive potential (based on animal data).

In the US and Canada, women who become pregnant during panitumumab treatment are encouraged to enroll in Amgen's Pregnancy Surveillance Program (US: 1-800-772-6436; Canada: 1-866-512-6436).

Breastfeeding Considerations

It is not known if panitumumab is present in breast milk. Panitumumab is an IgG monoclonal antibody and maternal IgG immunoglobulins are excreted in breast milk; however, breast milk antibodies are not expected to enter neonatal and infant circulation in substantial amounts. Due to the potential for serious adverse reactions in the breastfeeding infant, the manufacturer recommends women not breastfeed during therapy and for 2 months after the final panitumumab dose.

In the US and Canada, women who breastfeed during panitumumab treatment are encouraged to enroll in Amgen's Lactation Surveillance Program (US: 1-800-772-6436; Canada: 1-866-512-6436).

Warnings/Precautions [US Boxed Warning]: Dermatologic toxicities have been reported in 90% of patients receiving single agent panitumumab and were severe (grade 3 or higher) in 15% of patients); may include dermatitis acneiform, pruritus, erythema, rash, skin exfoliation, paronychia, dry skin, and skin fissures. Severe skin toxicities may be complicated by infection, sepsis, necrotizing fasciitis, or abscesses. The median time to development of skin (or ocular) toxicity was 2 weeks, with resolution ~12 weeks after discontinuation. Monitor all dermatologic toxicities for development of inflammation or infection. Rare cases of Stevens-Johnson syndrome and toxic epidermal necrolysis have been reported; bullous mucocutaneous disease (life-threatening/fatal) have been observed. Withhold treatment for severe or life-threatening dermatologic or soft tissue toxicities associated with severe/life-threatening inflammatory or infectious complications; dermatologic toxicity may require dose reduction or permanent discontinuation. The severity of dermatologic toxicity is predictive for response; grades 2 to 4 skin toxicity correlates with improved progression free survival and overall survival, compared to grade 1 skin toxicity (Peeters 2009; Van Cutsem 2007). Patients should minimize sunlight exposure and wear sunscreen and protective clothing/hat; sunlight may exacerbate skin reactions. Keratitis and ulcerative keratitis (known risk factors for corneal perforation) have occurred. Monitor for evidence of ocular toxicity; interrupt or discontinue treatment for acute or worsening keratitis. Gastric mucosal and nail toxicities have also been reported.

Severe infusion reactions (bronchospasm, dyspnea, fever, chills, and hypotension) have been reported in ~1% of patients; fatal infusion reactions have been reported with postmarketing surveillance. Discontinue infusion for severe reactions; permanently discontinue in patients with persistent severe infusion reactions. Appropriate medical support for the management of infusion reactions should be readily available. Mild to moderate infusion reactions are managed by slowing the infusion rate.

Pulmonary fibrosis and interstitial lung disease have been observed (rarely) in clinical trials; fatalities have been reported. Interrupt treatment for acute onset or worsening of pulmonary symptoms; permanently discontinue treatment if interstitial lung disease is confirmed. Patients with a history of or evidence of interstitial pneumonitis or pulmonary fibrosis were excluded from most clinical trials; consider the benefits of therapy versus the risk of pulmonary complications in such patients. May cause diarrhea; the incidence and severity of chemotherapy-induced diarrhea and other toxicities (rash, electrolyte abnormalities, stomatitis) is increased with combination chemotherapy; severe diarrhea and dehydration (which may lead to acute renal failure) has been observed with panitumumab in combination with chemotherapy. In a study of bevacizumab with combination chemotherapy ± panitumumab, the use of panitumumab resulted in decreased progression-free and overall survival and significantly increased toxicity compared to regimens without panitumumab (Hecht 2009). Toxicities included rash/acneiform dermatitis, diarrhea/dehydration, electrolyte disturbances, mucositis/stomatitis, and an increased incidence of pulmonary embolism. Magnesium and/or calcium depletion may occur during treatment (may be delayed; hypomagnesemia occurred ≥8 weeks after completion of panitumumab) and after treatment is discontinued; electrolyte repletion may be necessary; monitor for hypomagnesemia and hypocalcemia during treatment and for at least 8 weeks after completion. Hypokalemia has also been reported. Patients >65 years of age receiving panitumumab plus FOLFOX experienced a higher incidence of serious adverse events including severe diarrhea.

Confirm absence of *RAS* mutation prior to treatment; patients with colorectal cancer with tumors with codons 12 and 13 (exon 2), codons 59 and 61 (exon 3), or codons 117 and 146 (exon 4) *RAS* (*KRAS* or *NRAS*) mutations are unlikely to benefit from EGFR inhibitor therapy. Panitumumab is not indicated patients with *RAS* mutation-positive metastatic colorectal cancer or patients in whom *RAS* mutation status is unknown. Utilizing an anti-EGFR-directed antibody in patients whose tumors contain *RAS* mutations resulted in increased toxicity without clinical benefit. In a study of FOLFOX4 (fluorouracil, leucovorin, and oxaliplatin) ± panitumumab, patients with a *KRAS* mutation who received panitumumab with FOLFOX4 experienced a significantly shortened progression-free survival (Douillard 2010). In addition, a subset analysis of patients with wild-type *KRAS* identified additional *RAS* (*KRAS* [exons 3 and 4] or *NRAS* [exons 2, 3, 4]) mutations; progression-free survival and overall survival were significantly shortened in patients with *RAS* mutations who received FOLFOX4 in combination with panitumumab (Douillard 2013). The American Society of Clinical Oncology (ASCO) provisional clinical opinion update recommends that all patients with metastatic colorectal cancer who are candidates for anti-EGFR therapy should be tested (in a certified lab) for mutations in both *KRAS* and *NRAS* exon 2 (codons 12 and 13), exon 3 (codons 59 and 61), and exon 4 (codons 117 and 146); anti-EGFR monoclonal antibody therapy should only be considered in patients whose tumors lack mutations after extended *RAS* testing (Allegra 2016). Information on tests approved for detection of RAS mutation is available at www.fda.gov/CompanionDiagnostics. Panitumumab is also reported to be ineffective in patients with BRAF V600E mutation (Di Nicolantonio 2008). Potentially significant drug-drug interactions may exist, requiring dose or frequency adjustment, additional monitoring, and/or selection of alternative therapy.

Adverse Reactions
Monotherapy:
>10%:
  Central nervous system: Fatigue (26%)
  Dermatologic: Skin toxicity (90%; grades 3/4: 15%), erythema (66%; grades 3/4: 6%), pruritus (58%; grades 3/4: 3%), acneiform eruption (57%; grades 3/4: 7%), paronychia (25%; grades 3/4: 2%), rash (22%; grades 3/4: 1%), skin fissure (20%; grades 3/4: 1%), exfoliative dermatitis (18%; grades 3/4: 2%), acne vulgaris (14%; grades 3/4: 1%)
  Endocrine & metabolic: Hypomagnesemia (grades 3/4: 7%)
  Gastrointestinal: Nausea (23%), diarrhea (21%; grades 3/4: 2%), vomiting (19%)
  Ophthalmic: Ocular toxicity (16%)
  Respiratory: Dyspnea (18%), cough (15%)
  Miscellaneous: Fever (17%)
1% to 10%:
  Cardiovascular: Pulmonary embolism (1%)
  Central nervous system: Chills (3%)
  Dermatologic: Nail toxicity (10%), xeroderma (10%), desquamation (9%; grades 3/4: <1%), dermal ulcer (6%; grades 3/4: <1%), pustular rash (4%), papular rash (2%)
  Endocrine & metabolic: Dehydration (3%)
  Gastrointestinal: Mucositis (7%), stomatitis (7%), xerostomia (5%)
  Immunologic: Antibody formation (≤5%)

Ophthalmic: Abnormal eyelash growth (6%), conjunctivitis (5%)

Respiratory: Epistaxis (4%), interstitial pulmonary disease (1%)

Miscellaneous: Infusion related reaction (3%; grades 3/4: <1%)

<1%: Hypersensitivity reaction, pulmonary fibrosis

Combination therapy with FOLFOX:

>10%:

Dermatologic: Skin rash (56%; grades 3/4: 17% to 26%), acneiform eruption (32%; grades 3/4: 10%), pruritus (23%; grades 3/4: <1%), paronychia (21%; grades 3/4: 3%), xeroderma (21%; grades 3/4: 2%), erythema (16%; grades 3/4: 2%), skin fissure (16%; grades 3/4: <1%), alopecia (15%), acne vulgaris (14%; grades 3/4: 3%)

Endocrine & metabolic: Hypomagnesemia (30%), hypokalemia (21%), weight loss (18%)

Gastrointestinal: Diarrhea (62%), anorexia (36%), abdominal pain (28%), stomatitis (27%), mucosal inflammation (25%)

Neuromuscular & skeletal: Weakness (25%)

Ophthalmic: Conjunctivitis (18%)

Respiratory: Epistaxis (14%)

1% to 10%:

Cardiovascular: Deep vein thrombosis (5%)

Central nervous system: Fatigue (≥1%), paresthesia (≥1%)

Dermatologic: Nail disorder (10%; grades 3/4: 1%), palmar-plantar erythrodysesthesia (9%; grades 3/4: 1%), cellulitis (3%)

Endocrine & metabolic: Dehydration (8%), hypocalcemia (6%)

Hypersensitivity: Hypersensitivity (≥1%)

Local: Localized infection (4%)

<1%: Antibody development

Postmarketing and/or case reports (mono- and combination therapy): Abscess, angioedema, bullous skin disease (mucocutaneous), corneal ulcer, keratitis, necrotizing fasciitis, sepsis, skin necrosis, Stevens-Johnson syndrome, toxic epidermal necrolysis

Drug Interactions

Metabolism/Transport Effects None known.

Avoid Concomitant Use

Avoid concomitant use of Panitumumab with any of the following: Amino levulinic Acid (Systemic)

Increased Effect/Toxicity

Panitumumab may increase the levels/effects of: Aminolevulinic Acid (Systemic); Aminolevulinic Acid (Topical); Porfimer; Verteporfin

Decreased Effect There are no known significant interactions involving a decrease in effect.

Storage/Stability Store intact vials in the original carton at 2°C to 8°C (36°F to 46°F) until the time of use. Do not freeze; do not shake. Protect from direct sunlight. Solutions diluted in NS for infusion should be used within 6 hours of preparation if stored at room temperature or within 24 hours of dilution if stored at 2°C to 8°C (36°F to 46°F); do not freeze.

Preparation for Administration Inspect vial prior to use; solution is colorless but may contain a small amount of translucent to white amorphous panitumumab protein particles. Do not shake vial. Use a 21-gauge (or larger gauge/smaller bore) needle to withdraw appropriate volume from vial; do not use needle-free devices or vial adapters to withdraw vial contents. The manufacturer recommends diluting to a total volume of 100 mL (for doses ≤1,000 mg) or 150 mL (doses >1,000 mg) of NS. The final concentration should not exceed 10 mg/mL. Gently invert to mix; do not shake. Discard any unused portion remaining in the vial.

Mechanism of Action Panitumumab is a recombinant human IgG2 mono-clonal antibody which binds specifically to the epidermal growth factor receptor (EGFR, HER1, c-ErbB-1) and competitively inhibits the binding of epidermal growth factor (EGF) and other ligands. Binding to the EGFR blocks phosphorylation and activation of intracellular tyrosine kinases, resulting in inhibition of cell survival, growth, proliferation, and transformation. EGFR signal transduction may result in *KRAS* and *NRAS* wild-type activation; cells with *RAS* mutations appear to be unaffected by EGFR inhibition.

Pharmacodynamics/Kinetics Half-life elimination: ~7.5 days (range: 4 to 11 days)

Dosing

Adult & Geriatric Note: Establish *RAS* mutation status (to confirm *RAS* wild-type) prior to treatment initiation.

Colorectal cancer, metastatic, *RAS* wild-type: IV: 6 mg/kg every 14 days as a single agent (Van Cutsem 2007) or in combination with FOLFOX (fluorouracil, leucovorin, and oxaliplatin) (Douillard 2010; Douillard 2013); continue until disease progression or unacceptable toxicity (Douillard 2010; Van Cutsem 2007)

Colorectal cancer, metastatic, *RAS* wild-type in combination with FOLFIRI (fluorouracil, leucovorin, and irinotecan; off-label combination): IV: 6 mg/kg every 14 days; continue until disease progression or unacceptable toxicity (Peeters 2010)

Renal Impairment There are no dosage adjustments provided in the manufacturer's labeling (has not been studied).

Hepatic Impairment There are no dosage adjustments provided in the manufacturer's labeling (has not been studied).

Adjustment for Toxicity

Infusion reactions, mild-to-moderate (grade 1 or 2): Reduce the infusion rate by 50% for the duration of infusion.

Infusion reactions, severe (grade 3 or 4): Stop infusion; consider permanent discontinuation (depending on severity or persistence of reaction).

Dermatologic toxicity:

Grade 3 toxicity (first occurrence): Withhold 1 to 2 doses; if reaction improves to <grade 3, resume therapy at initial dose.

Grade 3 toxicity (second occurrence): Withhold 1 to 2 doses; if reaction improves to <grade 3, resume therapy at 80% of initial dose.

Grade 3 toxicity (third occurrence): Withhold 1 to 2 doses; if reaction improves to <grade 3, resume therapy at 60% of initial dose.

Grade 3 toxicity (fourth occurrence), grade 3 toxicity that does not recover to <grade 3 after withholding 1 or 2 doses, or grade 4 toxicity: Permanently discontinue.

Ocular toxicity (acute or worsening keratitis): Interrupt or discontinue treatment.

Pulmonary toxicity:

Acute onset or worsening pulmonary symptoms: Interrupt treatment.

Interstitial lung disease: Permanently discontinue treatment.

Combination Regimens

Colorectal cancer:

Panitumumab + FOLFIRI (Colorectal) on page 2189

Panitumumab + FOLFOX4 (Colorectal) on page 2190

Administration IV: For IV infusion only; do not administer IV push or as a bolus. Administer via infusion pump through a low protein-binding 0.2 or 0.22 micrometer in-line filter. Doses ≤1,000 mg, infuse over 1 hour; if first infusion is tolerated, subsequent doses may be administered over 30 to 60 minutes. Doses >1,000 mg, infuse over 90 minutes. Flush line with NS before and after infusion; do not mix or administer with other medications. Reduce infusion rate by 50% for mild to moderate infusion reactions (grades 1 and 2); stop infusion for severe infusion reactions (grades 3 and 4) and consider permanent discontinuation. Appropriate medical support for the management of infusion reactions should be readily available.

Emetic Potential
Children: Minimal (<10%)
Adults: Low (10% to 30%)

Monitoring Parameters *RAS* genotyping of tumor tissue to establish *RAS* mutation status and confirm *RAS* wild-type (prior to treatment initiation). Monitor serum electrolytes, including magnesium and calcium (periodically during and for at least 8 weeks after therapy), and potassium. Monitor vital signs and temperature before, during, and after infusion. Monitor for skin toxicity, for evidence of ocular toxicity, and for acute onset or worsening pulmonary symptoms.

Dosage Forms Excipient information presented when available (limited, particularly for generics); consult specific product labeling.
Solution, Intravenous [preservative free]:
Vectibix: 100 mg/5 mL (5 mL); 400 mg/20 mL (20 mL)

Panobinostat (pan oh BIN oh stat)

Related Information
Common Toxicity Criteria *on page 2242*
Management of Chemotherapy-Induced Nausea and Vomiting in Adults *on page 2253*
Safe Handling of Hazardous Drugs *on page 2379*

Brand Names: US Farydak

Index Terms Faridak; LBH589; Panobinostat Lactate

Pharmacologic Category Antineoplastic Agent, Histone Deacetylase (HDAC) Inhibitor

Use Multiple myeloma: Treatment of multiple myeloma (in combination with bortezomib and dexamethasone) in patients who have received at least 2 prior regimens, including bortezomib and an immunomodulatory agent.

Labeled Contraindications There are no contraindications listed in the manufacturer's labeling.

Pregnancy Considerations Adverse events were observed in animal reproduction studies. Pregnancy should be ruled out prior to treatment. Women of reproductive potential should avoid pregnancy and use an effective contraceptive during therapy and for at least 3 months after the last panobinostat dose. Males should use condoms during therapy and for at least 6 months after the last dose of panobinostat.

Breastfeeding Considerations It is not known if panobinostat is excreted into breast milk. Due to the potential for serious adverse reactions in the nursing infant, the manufacturer recommends a decision be made to discontinue nursing or to discontinue the drug, taking into account the importance of treatment to the mother.

Warnings/Precautions [US Boxed Warning]: Severe diarrhea occurred in one-fourth of panobinostat treated patients. Monitor for symptoms, institute antidiarrheal treatment, interrupt panobinostat, and then reduce dose or discontinue panobinostat. Any grade diarrhea was reported in over two-thirds of patients, and may occur at any time. Monitor hydration status and serum electrolytes (including magnesium, potassium, and phosphate). Patients should have antidiarrheal medications available for use; begin antidiarrheal medications at the first sign of diarrhea, loose stools, or abdominal cramping. Interrupt panobinostat treatment for moderate diarrhea (4 to 6 stools per day). Panobinostat is associated with nausea and vomiting (moderate emetic potential); consider antiemetics to prevent nausea and vomiting. Some antiemetics known to prolong the QT interval (eg, dolasetron or ondansetron) may be used with frequent ECG monitoring.

[US Boxed Warning]: Severe and fatal cardiac ischemic events, severe arrhythmias, and ECG changes have occurred in patients receiving panobinostat. Arrhythmias may be exacerbated by electrolyte abnormalities. Obtain ECG and electrolytes at baseline and periodically during treatment as clinically indicated. ECG abnormalities including ST-segment depression and T-wave abnormalities have been observed. Monitor and correct electrolyte abnormalities as needed. Panobinostat may prolong the QT interval. Do not initiate treatment in patients with a QTcF >450 msec or with clinically significant baseline ST-segment or T-wave abnormalities. Interrupt treatment if QTcF increases to ≥480 msec; correct electrolyte abnormalities; if QT prolongation does not resolve, permanently discontinue panobinostat. Concomitant use with medications known to prolong the QT interval is not recommended. Do not initiate panobinostat treatment in patients with a history of recent MI or unstable angina.

Severe thrombocytopenia, neutropenia and anemia have occurred; may require treatment interruption, dosage modification, discontinuation, transfusion or granulocyte colony-stimulating factor support. Monitor CBC with differential at baseline and during treatment; patients >65 years may require more frequent monitoring. Serious and fatal hemorrhage has occurred, including grade 3 and 4 hemorrhage. All patients with hemorrhage also experienced thrombocytopenia at the time of hemorrhage. Localized and systemic infections (including pneumonia, bacterial infections, invasive fungal infections, and viral infections) have been observed; infections may be severe (or fatal). Do not initiate treatment in patients with active infections. Monitor for sings/symptoms of infections during treatment. If infection occurs, begin appropriate management and consider interrupting or discontinuing panobinostat.

Hepatic dysfunction (transaminase and total bilirubin elevations) has been reported. Monitor liver function prior to and during treatment. If liver function tests are abnormal, consider dosage adjustments and monitor until liver function returns to normal or baseline. Initial dose should be reduced in patients with mild-to-moderate hepatic impairment; avoid use in patients with severe impairment. Potentially significant drug-drug/drug-food interactions may exist, requiring dose or frequency adjustment, additional monitoring, and/or selection of alternative therapy.

Adverse Reactions Frequency not always defined.

>10%:

Cardiovascular: Abnormal T waves on ECG (40%), peripheral edema (29%; grades 3/4: 2%), depression of ST segment on ECG (22%), cardiac arrhythmia (12%; grades 3/4: 3%)

Central nervous system: Fatigue (≤60%, grades 3/4: ≤25%), lethargy (≤60%; grades 3/4: ≤25%), malaise (≤60%; grades 3/4: ≤25%)

Endocrine & metabolic: Hypocalcemia (67%; grades 3/4: 5%), hypoalbuminemia (63%; grades 3/4: 2%), hypophosphatemia (63%; grades 3/4: 20%), hypokalemia (52%; grades 3/4: 18%), hyponatremia (49%; grades 3/4: 13%), hyperphosphatemia (29%; grades 3/4: 2%), hypermagnesemia (27%; grades 3/4: 5%), weight loss (12%; grades 3/4: 2%)

Gastrointestinal: Diarrhea (68%; grades 3/4: 25%), nausea (36%; grades 3/4: 6%), decreased appetite (28%; grades 3/4: 3%), vomiting (26%; grades 3/4: 7%)

Hematologic & oncologic: Thrombocytopenia (97%; grades 3/4: 67%), lymphocytopenia (82%; grades 3/4: 53%), leukopenia (81%; grades 3/4: 23%), neutropenia (75%; grades 3/4: 34%), anemia (62%; grades 3/4: 18%)

Hepatic: Hyperbilirubinemia (21%, grades 3/4: 1%)

Infection: Severe infection (31%; includes bacterial, fungal, and viral infections)

Neuromuscular & skeletal: Weakness (≤60%; grades ≥3: ≤25%)

Renal: Increased serum creatinine (41%; grades 3/4: 1%)

Miscellaneous: Fever (26%)

1% to 10%:

Cardiovascular: Hypertension (>2% to <10%), hypotension (>2% to <10%), orthostatic hypotension (>2% to <10%), palpitations (>2% to <10%), syncope (>2% to <10%), ischemic heart disease (4%), ECG changes, prolonged Q-T interval on ECG

Central nervous system: Chills (>2% to <10%), dizziness (>2% to <10%), headache (>2% to <10%), insomnia (>2% to <10%)

Dermatologic: Cheilitis (>2% to <10%), erythema (>2% to <10%), skin lesion (>2% to <10%), skin rash (>2% to <10%)

Endocrine & metabolic: Dehydration (>2% to <10%), fluid retention (>2% to <10%), hyperglycemia (>2% to <10%), hyperuricemia (>2% to <10%), hypomagnesemia (>2% to <10%), hypothyroidism (>2% to <10%)

Gastrointestinal: Abdominal distention (>2% to <10%), abdominal pain (>2% to <10%), colitis (>2% to <10%), dysgeusia (>2% to <10%), dyspepsia (>2% to <10%), flatulence (>2% to <10%), gastritis (>2% to <10%), gastrointestinal pain (>2% to <10%), xerostomia (>2% to <10%), gastrointestinal toxicity

Genitourinary: Urinary incontinence (>2% to <10%)

Hematologic & oncologic: Hemorrhage (grades 3/4: 4%)

Hepatic: Hepatitis B (>2% to <10%), increased serum alkaline phosphatase (>2% to <10%), increased serum transaminases, increased serum bilirubin

Infection: Sepsis (6%)

Neuromuscular & skeletal: Joint swelling (>2% to <10%), tremor (>2% to <10%)

Renal: Increased blood urea nitrogen (>2% to <10%), mean glomerular filtration rate decreased (>2% to <10%), renal failure (>2% to <10%)

Respiratory: Cough (>2% to <10%), dyspnea (>2% to <10%), rales (>2% to <10%), respiratory failure (>2% to <10%), wheezing (>2% to <10%)

Drug Interactions

Metabolism/Transport Effects Substrate of CYP2C19 (minor), CYP2D6 (minor), CYP3A4 (major), P-glycoprotein; **Note:** Assignment of Major/Minor substrate status based on clinically relevant drug interaction potential; **Inhibits** CYP2D6 (weak)

Avoid Concomitant Use

Avoid concomitant use of Panobinostat with any of the following: BCG (Intravesical); Conivaptan; CYP3A4 Inducers (Strong); Fusidic Acid (Systemic); Grapefruit Juice; Highest Risk QTc-Prolonging Agents; Hydroxychloroquine; Idelalisib; MiFEPRIStone; Natalizumab; Pimecrolimus; Pomegranate; Probucol; Promazine; Star Fruit; Tacrolimus (Topical); Vaccines (Live); Vinflunine

Increased Effect/Toxicity

Panobinostat may increase the levels/effects of: CYP2D6 Substrates; Fingolimod; Highest Risk QTc-Prolonging Agents; Leflunomide; Moderate Risk QTc-Prolonging Agents; Natalizumab; Tofacitinib; Vaccines (Live)

The levels/effects of Panobinostat may be increased by: Aprepitant; Conivaptan; CYP3A4 Inhibitors (Moderate); CYP3A4 Inhibitors (Strong); Dasatinib; Denosumab; Dolasetron; Fosaprepitant; Fusidic Acid (Systemic); Granisetron; Grapefruit Juice; Hydroxychloroquine; Idelalisib; MiFEPRIStone; Netupitant; Ocrelizumab; Ondansetron; Palbociclib; Pimecrolimus; Pomegranate; Probucol; Promazine; QTc-Prolonging Agents (Indeterminate Risk and Risk Modifying); Roflumilast; Simeprevir; Star Fruit; Stiripentol; Tacrolimus (Topical); Trastuzumab; Vinflunine; Xipamide

Decreased Effect

Panobinostat may decrease the levels/effects of: BCG (Intravesical); Coccidioides immitis Skin Test; Nivolumab; Sipuleucel-T; Tertomotide; Vaccines (Inactivated); Vaccines (Live)

The levels/effects of Panobinostat may be decreased by: Bosentan; CYP3A4 Inducers (Moderate); CYP3A4 Inducers (Strong); Dabrafenib; Deferasirox; Echinacea; Sarilumab; Siltuximab; St John's Wort; Tocilizumab

Food Interactions Star fruit, pomegranate or pomegranate juice, grapefruit or grapefruit juice may interfere with panobinostat metabolism. Management: Avoid star fruit, pomegranate or pomegranate juice, and grapefruit or grapefruit juice.

Hazardous Drugs Handling Considerations

Hazardous agent (NIOSH 2016 [group 1]).

Use appropriate precautions for receiving, handling, administration, and disposal. Gloves (single) should be worn during receiving, unpacking, and placing in storage. NIOSH recommends single gloving for administration of intact tablets or capsules (NIOSH 2016).

Storage/Stability Store at 20°C to 25°C (68°F to 77°F); excursions are permitted between 15°C and 30°C (59°F and 86°F). Store blister pack in original carton. Protect from light.

Mechanism of Action Panobinostat is a histone deacetylase (HDAC) inhibitor; inhibits enzymatic activity of HDACs resulting in increased acetylation of histone proteins. Accumulation of acetylated histones and other proteins induces cell cycle arrest and/or apoptosis of some transformed cells. Panobinostat has minimal activity in multiple myeloma as a single-agent; however, synergistic activity is demonstrated when combined with bortezomib and dexamethasone (San-Miguel 2014).

Pharmacodynamics/Kinetics

Protein binding: ~90% to plasma proteins

Metabolism: Extensive via reduction, hydrolysis, oxidation, and glucuronidation; CYP3A accounts for ~40% of elimination, CYP2D6 and CYP2C19 are minor pathways.

Bioavailability: ~21%; AUC is 16% lower (compared with fasting) when administered with a high-fat meal.

Half-life elimination: ~37 hours

Time to peak: Within 2 hours

Excretion: Feces (44% to 77%; <4% as unchanged drug); Urine (29% to 51%; <3% as unchanged drug)

Dosing

Adult & Geriatric Determine QTcF prior to the start of therapy and verify that QTcF <450 msec prior to panobinostat initiation. Baseline ANC should be at least 1,500/mm^3 and platelets at least 100,000/mm^3 prior to treatment. Panobinostat is associated with a moderate emetic potential; consider antiemetics to prevent nausea and vomiting.

Multiple myeloma: Adults: Oral: 20 mg once every other day for 3 doses each week during weeks 1 and 2 of a 21-day treatment cycle (eg, Monday, Wednesday, and Friday of weeks 1 and 2 only, rest during week 3) for up to 8 cycles (in combination with bortezomib and dexamethasone); treatment may continue (the same schedule for panobinostat; bortezomib and dexamethasone schedules are modified) for an additional 8 cycles in patients experiencing clinical benefit and acceptable toxicity (San-Miguel 2014). The total duration of therapy may be up to 16 cycles (48 weeks).

Missed doses: Missed doses may be taken up to 12 hours after the scheduled time. Do not repeat the dose if vomiting occurs; patients should take the next usual scheduled dose.

Dosage adjustment for concomitant therapy:

CYP2D6 substrates: Avoid coadministration with sensitive CYP2D6 substrates (eg, atomoxetine, desipramine, dextromethorphan, metoprolol, nebivolol, perphenazine, tolterodine, venlafaxine) or CYP2D6 substrates that have a narrow therapeutic index (eg, thioridazine, pimozide).

Strong CYP3A inducers: Avoid concomitant use with strong CYP3A inducers.

Strong CYP3A inhibitors: Reduce the starting panobinostat dose to 10 mg with strong CYP3A inhibitors (eg, boceprevir, clarithromycin, conivaptin, indinavir, itraconazole, ketoconazole, lopinavir/ritonavir, nefazodone, nelfinavir, posaconazole, ritonavir, saquinavir, telaprevir, telithromycin, voriconazole).

Renal Impairment

CrCl <80 mL/minute: There are no dosage adjustments provided in the manufacturer's labeling. However, based on a pharmacokinetic study of a single 30 mg dose, renal impairment does not appear to impact panobinostat exposure in patients with mild, moderate, and severe renal impairment (excluding dialysis patients), and initial dosage adjustment is not necessary (Sharma 2015).

End-stage renal disease (ESRD) and ESRD on dialysis: There are no dosage adjustments provided in the manufacturer's labeling (has not been studied). The dialyzability of panobinostat is unknown.

◀ **Hepatic Impairment**

Hepatic impairment *prior to* treatment:

Mild impairment (bilirubin ≤1 times ULN and AST >1 times ULN or bilirubin >1 to 1.5 times ULN and any AST): Reduce initial dose to 15 mg; monitor frequently for adverse events and adjust dose as needed for toxicity.

Moderate impairment (bilirubin >1.5 to 3 times ULN and any AST): Reduce initial dose to 10 mg; monitor frequently for adverse events and adjust dose as needed for toxicity.

Severe impairment: Avoid use.

Hepatic impairment *during* treatment: If liver function tests are abnormal, consider dosage adjustments and monitor until liver function returns to normal or baseline.

Adjustment for Toxicity If dose reductions are necessary, keep the same treatment schedule and reduce panobinostat dose in increments of 5 mg (from 20 mg to 15 mg, from 15 mg to 10 mg); if dose reduction below 10 mg 3 times a week is necessary, discontinue treatment.

Hematologic toxicity:

Thrombocytopenia:

Grade 3 (platelets <50,000/mm^3): No dosage adjustments are necessary; monitor platelets weekly.

Grade 3 (platelets <50,000/mm^3) with bleeding: Interrupt panobinostat treatment, monitor platelets weekly until platelets ≥50,000/mm^3 and then restart panobinostat at a reduced dose. (Interrupt bortezomib until platelets ≥50,000/mm^3; if only 1 dose omitted, restart bortezomib at the same dose; if ≥2 consecutive doses or doses within the same cycle are omitted, then restart bortezomib at a reduced dose.)

Grade 4 (platelets <25,000/mm^3): Interrupt panobinostat treatment, monitor platelets weekly until platelets ≥50,000/mm^3 and then restart panobinostat at a reduced dose. (Interrupt bortezomib until platelets ≥50,000/mm^3; if only 1 dose omitted, restart bortezomib at the same dose; if ≥2 consecutive doses or doses within the same cycle are omitted, then restart bortezomib at a reduced dose.)

Severe thrombocytopenia: Consider platelet transfusions. Discontinue panobinostat if thrombocytopenia does not improve despite treatment modifications or if repeated platelet transfusions are required.

Neutropenia:

Grade 3 (ANC 750 to 1,000/mm^3): No dosage adjustments are necessary.

Grade 3 (ANC 500 to 750/mm^3 [2 or more occurrences]): Interrupt panobinostat treatment until ANC ≥1,000/mm^3 and then restart at the same dose. (Bortezomib dosage adjustment is not necessary.)

Grade 3 (ANC <1,000/mm^3) with neutropenic fever: Interrupt panobinostat treatment until neutropenic fever resolves and ANC ≥1,000/mm^3 and then restart at a reduced dose. (Interrupt bortezomib until neutropenic fever resolves and ANC ≥1,000/mm^3; if only 1 dose omitted, restart bortezomib at the same dose; if ≥2 consecutive doses or doses within the same cycle are omitted, then restart bortezomib at a reduced dose.)

Grade 4 (ANC <500/mm^3): Interrupt panobinostat treatment until ANC ≥1,000/mm^3 and then restart at a reduced dose. (Interrupt bortezomib until ANC ≥1,000/mm^3; if only 1 dose omitted, restart bortezomib at the same dose; if ≥2 consecutive doses or doses within the same cycle are omitted, then restart bortezomib at a reduced dose.)

Neutropenia, grade 3 or 4: Consider growth factor support or dose modification; if neutropenia does not improve or if severe infection occurs despite dose modification or growth factor support, discontinue panobinostat.

Anemia: Grade 3 (hemoglobin <8 g/dL): Interrupt panobinostat until hemoglobin ≥10 g/dL and then restart at a reduced dose.

Nonhematologic toxicity:

Cardiovascular: QTcF increase to ≥480 msec: Interrupt panobinostat treatment; correct electrolyte abnormalities. If QT prolongation does not resolve then permanently discontinue panobinostat.

Diarrhea:

First sign of abdominal cramping, loose stools, or onset of diarrhea: Begin antidiarrheal medication (eg, loperamide).

Grade 2 (moderate diarrhea; 4 to 6 stools per day): Interrupt panobinostat until resolved and then restart at the same dose. (Consider interruption of bortezomib until resolved and then restart at the same dose.)

Grade 3 (severe diarrhea; ≥7 stools per day, IV fluids or hospitalization required): Interrupt panobinostat treatment until resolved and then restart at a reduced dose. (Interrupt bortezomib until resolved and then restart at a reduced dose.)

Grade 4 (life-threatening): Permanently discontinue panobinostat. (Permanently discontinue bortezomib.)

Infection: Consider interrupting or discontinuing panobinostat.

Nausea or vomiting (panobinostat is associated with nausea and vomiting; consider prophylactic antiemetics):

Severe nausea (grades 3/4): Interrupt panobinostat treatment until resolved and then restart at a reduced dose.

Severe/life-threatening vomiting (grades 3/4): Interrupt panobinostat treatment until resolved and then restart at a reduced dose.

Other toxicities:

Grade 3 or 4 toxicity or recurrent grade 2 toxicity: Withhold panobinostat treatment until recovery to grade 1 or less and then restart at a reduced dose.

Recurrent grade 3 or 4 toxicity: Withhold panobinostat treatment until recovery to grade 1 or less and then restart at a reduced dose.

Combination Regimens

Multiple myeloma: Panobinostat-Bortezomib-Dexamethasone (Multiple Myeloma) on page 2190

Administration Panobinostat is associated with a moderate emetic potential; consider antiemetics to prevent nausea and vomiting. Administer orally at approximately the same time on scheduled days. May administer with or without food. Swallow capsule whole with a cup of water. Do not open, crush, or chew the capsules. Avoid exposure to crushed and/or broken capsules. Avoid direct skin or mucous membrane contact with powder inside the capsules; if contact occurs, wash thoroughly.

Emetic Potential Moderate (30% to 90%)

Monitoring Parameters CBC with differential and platelets (prior to treatment initiation then weekly or more often if clinically indicated during treatment); serum electrolytes, including potassium and magnesium prior to treatment and during treatment (in the clinical trial, electrolytes were monitored prior to the start of each cycle, after the fifth panobinostat dose in week 2 through cycle 8 and then at the beginning of cycles 9 to 16); liver function tests at baseline and regularly during treatment; pregnancy test (in women of reproductive potential, rule out pregnancy prior to and intermittently during treatment); ECG (prior to treatment initiation and periodically as clinically indicated during treatment); hydration status; monitor for gastrointestinal toxicity (eg, diarrhea, nausea, vomiting), signs/symptoms of hemorrhage and/or infection.

Dietary Considerations Avoid star fruit, pomegranate or pomegranate juice, and grapefruit or grapefruit juice.

Medication Guide Available Yes

Dosage Forms Excipient information presented when available (limited, particularly for generics); consult specific product labeling.

Capsule, Oral:

Farydak: 10 mg [contains brilliant blue fcf (fd&c blue #1)]

Farydak: 15 mg, 20 mg

♦ **Panobinostat Lactate** see Panobinostat on page 1445

♦ **Panretin** see Alitretinoin (Topical) on page 93

♦ **Panzyga (Can)** see Immune Globulin on page 992

Papillomavirus (9-Valent) Vaccine (Human, Recombinant)

(pap ih LO ma VYE rus nine VAY lent vak SEEN YU man ree KOM be nant)

Brand Names: US Gardasil 9

Brand Names: Canada Gardasil 9

Index Terms 9-Valent HPV; 9vHPV; HPV Vaccine (9-valent); HPV9; Human Papillomavirus Vaccine (9-valent)

Pharmacologic Category Vaccine; Vaccine, Inactivated (Viral)

Use Prevention of human papillomavirus infection:

Females 9 to 26 years of age:

For the prevention of the following diseases:

Cervical, vulvar, vaginal, and anal cancer caused by human papillomavirus (HPV) types 16, 18, 31, 33, 45, 52, and 58

Genital warts (condyloma acuminata) caused by HPV types 6 and 11

For the prevention of the following precancerous or dysplastic lesions caused by HPV types 6, 11, 16, 18, 31, 33, 45, 52, and 58:

Cervical intraepithelial neoplasia (CIN) grades 1, 2, and 3

Cervical adenocarcinoma in situ (AIS)

Vulvar intraepithelial neoplasia (VIN) grades 2 and 3

Vaginal intraepithelial neoplasia (VaIN) grades 2 and 3

Anal intraepithelial neoplasia (AIN) grades 1, 2, and 3

Males 9 through 26 years of age:

For the prevention of the following diseases:

Anal cancer caused by HPV types 16, 18, 31, 33, 45, 52, and 58

Genital warts (condyloma acuminata) caused by HPV types 6 and 11

For the prevention of the following precancerous or dysplastic lesions caused by HPV types 6, 11, 16, 18, 31, 33, 45, 52, and 58:

Anal intraepithelial neoplasia (AIN) grades 1, 2, and 3

The Advisory Committee on Immunization Practices (ACIP) recommends routine vaccination for females and males 11 to 12 years; for patients with any history of sexual abuse or assault, vaccination should be started at 9 years. Catch-up vaccination is recommended for females and transgender persons 13 to 26 years and males 13 to 21 years. Vaccination for males 22 through 26 years is recommended if immunocompromised (including HIV) and for men who have sex with men and may be considered for any other male in this age group (CDC/ACIP [Meites 2016]).

Dosing

Adult Immunization: IM:

Manufacturer's labeling: Adults ≤26 years: 3-dose series: 0.5 mL at 0, 2, and 6 months

CDC/ACIP recommended immunization schedule: Adults ≤26 years: Vaccination recommended in females and transgender persons ≤26 years or males ≤21 years if not previously vaccinated or completed the 3-dose series (typically administer first dose at age 11 to 12 years). Vaccination for males 22 through 26 years is recommended if immunocompromised (including HIV) and for men who have sex with men and may be considered for any other male in this age group. Second and third doses may be given after age 26 years to complete a previously initiated series (CDC/ACIP [Markowitz 2014]; CDC/ACIP [Meites 2016]).

Have not received any doses: 3-dose series: IM: 0.5 mL at 0, 1 to 2, and 6 months. There should be a 4-week minimum interval between the first and second dose; a 12-week minimum interval between the second and third dose; a 5-month minimum interval between the first and third dose.

Partially vaccinated, first dose before 15 years of age:
If 2 doses administered at least 5 months apart: no more doses needed
If only a single dose or if doses <5 months apart: IM: Administer one additional 0.5 mL dose

Partially vaccinated, first dose at 15 years of age or later: Complete 3-dose series: IM: There should be a 4-week minimum interval between the first and second dose; a 12-week minimum interval between the second and third dose; a 5-month minimum interval between the first and third dose.

Pediatric Immunization:

Manufacturer's labeling:

Children ≥9 years and Adolescents <15 years:
2-dose series: IM: 0.5 mL at 0, and 6 to 12 months. If the second dose is inadvertently administered earlier than 5 months after the first dose, then patient should be converted to a 3-dose series.
3-dose series: IM: 0.5 mL at 0, 2, and 6 months

Adolescents ≥15 years: 3-dose series: IM: 0.5 mL at 0, 2, and 6 months

CDC/ACIP recommended immunization schedule: Routine vaccination at 11 to 12 years of age; may start as early as 9 years of age. In a 2-dose schedule, minimum interval between first and second doses is 5 months. In a 3-dose schedule, minimum interval between first and second doses is 4 weeks; the minimum interval between the second and third dose is 12 weeks; the minimum interval between first and third doses is 5 months. (CDC/ACIP [Meites 2016]).

Non-immunocompromised patients and certain medical conditions: Asplenia, asthma, chronic granulomatous disease, chronic liver disease, chronic lung disease, chronic renal disease, CNS anatomic barrier defects (eg, cochlear implant), complement deficiency, diabetes, heart disease, or sickle cell disease:
Children ≥9 years and Adolescents <15 years: 2-dose series: IM: 0.5 mL at 0, and 6 to 12 months. Administer first dose at age 11 to 12 years. For patients with any history of sexual abuse or assault, vaccination should be started at 9 years.
Adolescents ≥15 years: 3-dose series: IM: 0.5 mL at 0, 1 to 2, and 6 months

◀ Immunocompromised patients: Children ≥9 years and Adolescents: 3-dose series: IM: 0.5 mL at 0, 1 to 2, and 6 months. **Note**: Includes immuno-compromising conditions that might reduce cell-mediated or humoral immunity (eg, lymphocyte antibody deficiencies, T lymphocyte complete or partial defects, HIV infection, malignant neoplasms, transplantation, autoimmune disease, immunosuppressive therapy).

Renal Impairment There are no dosage adjustments provided in the manufacturer's labeling.

Hepatic Impairment There are no dosage adjustments provided in the manufacturer's labeling.

Additional Information Complete prescribing information should be consulted for additional detail.

Medication Guide Available Yes

Dosage Forms Excipient information presented when available (limited, particularly for generics); consult specific product labeling.

Suspension, Intramuscular [preservative free]:

  Gardasil 9: (0.5 mL) [contains polysorbate 80, yeast extract]

Suspension Prefilled Syringe, Intramuscular [preservative free]:

  Gardasil 9: (0.5 mL) [contains polysorbate 80, yeast extract]

◆ **Paraplatin** see CARBOplatin on page 327

◆ **PARP Inhibitor AZD2281** see Olaparib on page 1368

PAZOPanib (paz OH pa nib)

Related Information

Management of Chemotherapy-Induced Nausea and Vomiting in Adults on page 2253

Safe Handling of Hazardous Drugs on page 2379

Brand Names: US Votrient

Brand Names: Canada Votrient

Index Terms GW786034; Pazopanib HCl; Pazopanib Hydrochloride

Pharmacologic Category Antineoplastic Agent, Tyrosine Kinase Inhibitor; Antineoplastic Agent, Vascular Endothelial Growth Factor (VEGF) Inhibitor

Use

Renal cell carcinoma, advanced: Treatment of advanced renal cell carcinoma

Soft tissue sarcoma, advanced: Treatment of advanced soft tissue sarcoma (in patients who have received prior chemotherapy)

Limitations of use: The efficacy of pazopanib for the treatment of adipocytic soft tissue sarcoma or gastrointestinal stromal tumors (GIST) has not been demonstrated.

Labeled Contraindications

There are no contraindications listed in the manufacturer's US labeling.

Canadian labeling: Hypersensitivity to pazopanib or any component of the formulation; use in pediatric patients <2 years of age (due to the antiangiogenic effects)

Pregnancy Considerations Adverse effects were observed in animal reproduction studies. Based on its mechanism of action, pazopanib would be expected to cause fetal harm if administered to a pregnant woman. Verify pregnancy status in women of reproductive potential prior to initiating treatment. Women of reproductive potential should avoid becoming pregnant during treatment and use effective contraception during therapy and for at least 2 weeks after the last pazopanib dose. Male patients (including vasectomized patients) with pregnant partners or with female partners of reproductive potential should use condoms during treatment and for at least 2 weeks after the last pazopanib dose. Pazopanib may impair fertility in both men and women of reproductive potential.

Breastfeeding Considerations It is not known if pazopanib is present in breast milk. Due to the potential for serious adverse reactions in the breastfed infant, the manufacturer recommends discontinuing breastfeeding during treatment and for 2 weeks after the last pazopanib dose.

Warnings/Precautions [US Boxed Warning]: Severe and fatal hepatotoxicity (transaminase and bilirubin elevations) has been observed in studies. Monitor hepatic function and interrupt treatment, reduce dose, or discontinue as recommended. Liver function tests (ALT, AST, and bilirubin) should be monitored at baseline; at weeks 3, 5, 7, and 9; at months 3 and 4; and as clinically necessary, then periodically (after month 4). Transaminase elevations usually occur early in the treatment course. Use is not recommended in patients with preexisting severe hepatic impairment (bilirubin >3 times ULN with any ALT level); dosage reductions is recommended for preexisting moderate hepatic impairment (bilirubin >1.5 to 3 times ULN). Mild indirect (unconjugated) hyperbilirubinemia may occur in patients with Gilbert's syndrome; for patients with known Gilbert syndrome (only a mild indirect bilirubin elevation) and ALT >3 times ULN, follow isolated ALT elevation dosage modification recommendations. A pooled analysis of TA repeat polymorphism of UGT1A1 showed a statistically significant increase of hyperbilirubinemia in patients with the (TA)7/TA7 genotype (UGT1A1*28/*28), relative to the (TA)6/(TA)6 and (TA6/(TA)7 genotypes. In a large pooled analysis, grade 2 and 3 ALT elevations (ALT >3 to <20 x ULN) were observed more frequently in patients carrying the HLA-B*57:01 allele versus noncarriers. Monitor liver function in all patients receiving pazopanib.

Venous and arterial thromboembolism have been reported. DVT, pulmonary embolism, angina, transient ischemic attack, MI, and ischemic stroke were observed more frequently in the pazopanib group (versus placebo) in clinical trials. Fatalities were observed. Monitor for signs/symptoms of venous thrombotic events and pulmonary embolism. Use with caution in patients with a history of or an increased risk for these events. Use in patients with recent arteriothrombotic event (within 6 months) has not been studied and is not recommended. Thrombotic microangiopathy (TMA), including thrombotic thrombocytopenic purpura (TTP) and hemolytic uremic syndrome (HUS), has been observed in clinical studies. TMA has occurred with pazopanib monotherapy or when used in combination with bevacizumab or topotecan (off-label use); it typically occurs within 90 days of treatment initiation. Monitor for signs/symptoms and permanently discontinue in patients who develop TMA. Hemorrhagic events (including fatal events) have been reported. In clinical studies, the most common events in renal cell carcinoma patients were hematuria, epistaxis, hemoptysis, and rectal hemorrhage. Epistaxis, mouth hemorrhage, and anal hemorrhage were most common in soft tissue sarcoma patients. Use is not recommended in patients with a history of hemoptysis, cerebral hemorrhage or clinically significant gastrointestinal hemorrhage within 6 months (these populations were excluded from clinical trials).

May cause and/or worsen hypertension (hypertensive crisis has been observed); monitor frequently; blood pressure should be controlled prior to treatment initiation; antihypertensive therapy should be used if needed. Hypertension usually occurs early in the treatment course. Dosage reduction may be necessary for hypertension that is persistent despite management with antihypertensive therapy; discontinue for hypertensive crisis, or for severe and persistent hypertension which is refractory to dose reduction and antihypertensive therapy. May cause new-onset or worsening of existing heart failure; baseline and periodic LVEF monitoring is recommended in patients at increased risk of heart failure (eg, prior anthracycline treatment). Concurrent hypertension may increase the risk for cardiac dysfunction. Monitor for signs/symptoms of heart failure. QTc prolongation, including torsade de pointes, has been observed; use caution in patients with a history of QTc prolongation, with medications known to prolong the QT interval, or with preexisting cardiac disease. Obtain baseline and periodic ECGs; correct electrolyte (potassium, calcium, and magnesium) abnormalities prior to and during treatment.

Gastrointestinal perforation and fistula (including fatal events) have been reported; monitor for symptoms of gastrointestinal perforation and fistula. Proteinuria has been reported with use. Obtain baseline and periodic urinalysis and 24-hour urine protein when clinically indicated. Dosage reduction may be necessary for significant proteinuria (≥3 g/24 hours); discontinue for recurrent proteinuria. Interstitial lung disease (ILD)/pneumonitis has been reported with pazopanib; may be fatal. Monitor for pulmonary symptoms which could indicate ILD/pneumonitis; discontinue if ILD or pneumonitis develop. Hypothyroidism has been reported with use; monitor thyroid function tests. Vascular endothelial growth factor (VEGF) receptor inhibitors are associated with impaired wound healing. Discontinue treatment at least 7 days prior to scheduled surgery; treatment reinitiation should be guided by clinical judgment. Discontinue if wound dehiscence occurs.

Patients with mild-to-moderate renal impairment (CrCl ≥30 mL/minute) were included in trials. There are no pharmacokinetic data in patients with severe renal impairment undergoing dialysis (peritoneal and hemodialysis); however, renal impairment is not expected to significantly influence pazopanib pharmacokinetics or exposure. Potentially significant drug-drug interactions may exist, requiring dose or frequency adjustment, additional monitoring, and/or selection of alternative therapy. Increased toxicity and mortality has been observed in trials evaluating concurrent use of pazopanib with other chemotherapeutic agents (pemetrexed, lapatinib). Pazopanib is not approved for use in combination with other chemotherapy.

Hand-foot skin reaction (HFSR) observed with tyrosine kinase inhibitors (TKIs) is distinct from hand-foot syndrome (palmar-plantar erythrodysesthesia) associated with traditional chemotherapy agents. HFSR due to TKIs is localized with defined hyperkeratotic lesions; symptoms include burning, dysesthesia, paresthesia, or tingling of the palms/soles, and generally occur within the first 2 to 4 weeks of treatment. Pressure and flexor areas may develop blisters (callus-like), dry/cracked skin, edema, erythema, desquamation, or hyperkeratosis. The incidence of HFSR is lower with pazopanib (compared to other tyrosine kinase inhibitors). Examine skin at baseline (remove calluses with pedicure prior to treatment) and with each visit; apply an emollient based moisturizer twice daily during treatment. If HFSR develops, consider changing moisturizer to a urea-based product; topical steroids may be utilized for the anti-inflammatory effect; avoid excessive friction or pressure to affected areas and avoid restrictive footwear. Temporary dose reduction or treatment interruption may be necessary (Appleby 2011).

Reversible posterior leukoencephalopathy syndrome (RPLS) has been reported (rarely); may be fatal. Monitor for neurological changes or symptoms (blindness, confusion, headache, lethargy, seizure, visual or neurologic disturbances); permanently discontinue pazopanib in patients who develop RPLS. Serious, including fatal, infections have been reported; monitor for signs and symptoms of infection. Temporarily or permanently discontinue therapy for serious infections as clinically indicated. Cases of retinal detachment or tear have been reported. In an analysis of pooled clinical trials, grade 3 and 4 neutropenia, thrombocytopenia, and palmar-plantar erythrodysesthesia syndrome (hand-foot syndrome) were more frequently observed in patients of East Asian descent than in non-East Asian patients. Patients >65 years of age may be at greater risk for transaminase elevations (ALT >3 time ULN). Patients ≥65 years of age experienced increased incidences of grade 3 or 4 fatigue, hypertension, decreased appetite, and transaminase elevations and are at increased risk for hepatotoxicity. Pazopanib is not approved for use in pediatric patients. Based on its mechanism of action, organ growth and maturation during early postnatal development may be affected. May potentially cause serious adverse effects on organ development, particularly in children <2 years of age.

Adverse Reactions

>10%:

Cardiovascular: Hypertension (40% to 42%; grade 3: 4% to 7%, early in treatment), bradycardia (2% to 19%), peripheral edema (STS: 14%), cardiac insufficiency (11% to 13%)

Central nervous system: Fatigue (19%, grade 3: 2%; STS: 65%, grades 3/4: 1% to 13%), tumor pain (STS: 29%, grade 3: 8%), headache (10%; STS: 23%, grade 3: 1%), dizziness (11%)

Dermatologic: Hair discoloration (38% to 39%, grade 3: <1%), exfoliative dermatitis (STS: 18%, grade 3: <1%), alopecia (8% to 12%), dermatological disease (STS: 11%, grade 3: 2%), hypopigmentation (STS, skin: 11%), palmar-plantar erythrodysesthesia (6% to 11%)

Endocrine & metabolic: Weight loss (9%, STS: 48%, grade 3: 4%), increased serum glucose (41% to 45%, grade 3: <1%), increased thyroid-stimulating hormone (TSH), decreased serum albumin (STS: 34%, grade 3: 1%), decreased serum phosphate (34%, grade 3: 4%), decreased serum sodium (31%, grade 3: 1% to 4%), decreased serum magnesium (26%, grades 3/4: ≤1%), decreased serum glucose (17%, grade 4: <1%), increased serum potassium (STS: 16%, grade 3: 1%)

Gastrointestinal: Diarrhea (52% to 59%; grades 3/4: ≤5%), nausea (26%, grade 3: <1%; STS: 56%, grade 3: 3%), decreased appetite (STS: 40%, grade 3: 6%), anorexia (22%, grade 3: 2%), vomiting (21%, grades 3/4: ≤2%; STS: 33%, grade 3: 3%), dysgeusia (8%, STS: 28%), increased serum lipase (27%, grades 3/4: 4%), gastrointestinal pain (STS: 23%, grade 3: 3%), abdominal pain (11%, grade 3: 2%), mucositis (STS: 12%, grade 3: 2%), stomatitis (STS: 11%, grade 3: <1%)

Hematologic & oncologic: Leukopenia (37% to 44%; STS, grade 3: 1%), lymphocytopenia (31%, grades 3/4: ≤4%; STS: 43%, grade 3: 10%), thrombocytopenia (32% to 36%; grades 3/4: ≤6%; grade 4: ≤1%), neutropenia (33% to 34%; grades 3/4 [in patients of East Asian descent]: 12%; grades 3/4 [in patients of non-East Asian descent]: ≤4%), hemorrhage (13% to 22%, including pulmonary, gastrointestinal, and genitourinary, grade 4: 1%, including intracranial, subarachnoid, and peritoneal)

◄ Hepatic: Increased serum AST (51% to 53%; grades 3/4: ≤7%), increased serum ALT (4% to 53%; grades 3/4: 2% to 10%), increased serum bilirubin (29% to 36%; grades 3/4: ≤3%), increased serum alkaline phosphatase (STS: 32%, grade 3: 3%)

Neuromuscular & skeletal: Musculoskeletal pain (STS: 23%, grade 3: 2%), myalgia (STS: 23%, grade 3: 2%), weakness (14%, grade 3: 3%)

Respiratory: Dyspnea (STS: 20%, grades 3/4: ≤5%), cough (STS: 17%)

Miscellaneous: Tumor pain (29%)

1% to 10%:

Cardiovascular: Chest pain (5% to 10%; STS, grade 3: 2%), left ventricular systolic dysfunction (STS: 8%), venous thrombosis (STS: 5%), ischemia (≤2%), myocardial infarction (≤2%), prolonged Q-T interval on ECG (2%), facial edema (RCC: 1%), transient ischemic attacks (RCC: 1%)

Central nervous system: Insomnia (STS: 9%), voice disorder (4% to 8%), chills (STS: 5%)

Dermatologic: Skin rash (RCC: 8%), skin depigmentation (RCC: 3%), xeroderma (STS: 6%), nail disease (STS: 5%)

Endocrine & metabolic: Hypothyroidism (4% to 8%)

Gastrointestinal: Dyspepsia (5% to 7%), anal hemorrhage (STS: 2%), gastrointestinal fistula (≤1%), gastrointestinal perforation (≤1%)

Genitourinary: Proteinuria (1% to 9%), hematuria (RCC: 4%)

Hematologic & oncologic: Oral hemorrhage (STS: 3%), rectal hemorrhage (RCC: 1%)

Ophthalmic: Blurred vision (STS: 5%)

Respiratory: Epistaxis (2% to 8%), pneumothorax (≤3%), hemoptysis (RCC: 2%)

Frequency not defined:

Cardiovascular: Decreased left ventricular ejection fraction, hypertensive crisis

Central nervous system: Reversible posterior leukoencephalopathy syndrome

Hematologic & oncologic: Hemolytic-uremic syndrome, neutropenic infection, thrombotic thrombocytopenic purpura

Hepatic: Hepatotoxicity, severe hepatotoxicity

Infection: Serious infection

Neuromuscular & skeletal: Arthralgia (RCC), muscle spasm (RCC)

<1%, postmarketing, and/or case reports: Cardiac disease, cerebral hemorrhage, cerebrovascular accident, congestive heart failure, interstitial pneumonitis, nephrotic syndrome, pancreatitis, retinal changes (tear), retinal detachment, torsades de pointes

Drug Interactions

Metabolism/Transport Effects Substrate of BCRP, CYP1A2 (minor), CYP2C8 (minor), CYP3A4 (major), P-glycoprotein; **Note:** Assignment of Major/Minor substrate status based on clinically relevant drug interaction potential; **Inhibits** CYP2C8 (weak), CYP3A4 (weak), SLCO1B1, UGT1A1

Avoid Concomitant Use

Avoid concomitant use of PAZOPanib with any of the following: Amodiaquine; AtorvaSTATin; BCG (Intravesical); BCRP/ABCG2 Inhibitors; Conivaptan; CYP3A4 Inducers (Strong); Fusidic Acid (Systemic); Grapefruit Juice; H2-Antagonists; Highest Risk QTc-Prolonging Agents; Hydroxychloroquine; Idelalisib; Irinotecan Products; Lapatinib; MiFEPRIStone; Natalizumab; P-glycoprotein/ABCB1 Inhibitors; Pimecrolimus; Pimozide; Probucol;

Promazine; Proton Pump Inhibitors; Tacrolimus (Topical); Vaccines (Live); Voxilaprevir

Increased Effect/Toxicity

PAZOPanib may increase the levels/effects of: Amodiaquine; ARIPiprazole; Bisphosphonate Derivatives; Fingolimod; Highest Risk QTc-Prolonging Agents; HYDROcodone; Irinotecan Products; Leflunomide; Lomitapide; Moderate Risk QTc-Prolonging Agents; Natalizumab; NiMODipine; Pimozide; Tofacitinib; Vaccines (Live); Vinflunine

The levels/effects of PAZOPanib may be increased by: Aprepitant; AtorvaSTATin; BCRP/ABCG2 Inhibitors; Conivaptan; CYP3A4 Inhibitors (Moderate); CYP3A4 Inhibitors (Strong); Dasatinib; Denosumab; Fosaprepitant; Fusidic Acid (Systemic); Grapefruit Juice; HMG-CoA Reductase Inhibitors; Hydroxychloroquine; Idelalisib; Lapatinib; MiFEPRIStone; Netupitant; Ocrelizumab; Palbociclib; P-glycoprotein/ABCB1 Inhibitors; Pimecrolimus; Probucol; Promazine; QTc-Prolonging Agents (Indeterminate Risk and Risk Modifying); Roflumilast; Stiripentol; Tacrolimus (Topical); Trastuzumab; Voxilaprevir; Xipamide

Decreased Effect

PAZOPanib may decrease the levels/effects of: BCG (Intravesical); Coccidioides immitis Skin Test; Nivolumab; Sipuleucel-T; Tertomotide; Vaccines (Inactivated); Vaccines (Live)

The levels/effects of PAZOPanib may be decreased by: Antacids; Bosentan; CYP3A4 Inducers (Moderate); CYP3A4 Inducers (Strong); Dabrafenib; Deferasirox; Echinacea; H2-Antagonists; Proton Pump Inhibitors; Sarilumab; Siltuximab; St John's Wort; Tocilizumab

Food Interactions Systemic exposure of pazopanib is increased when administered with food (AUC twofold higher with a meal). Grapefruit juice may increase the levels/effects of pazopanib. Management: Take on an empty stomach 1 hour before or 2 hours after a meal. Maintain adequate nutrition and hydration, unless instructed to restrict fluid intake. Avoid grapefruit/grapefruit juice.

Hazardous Drugs Handling Considerations

Hazardous agent (NIOSH 2016 [group 1]).

Use appropriate precautions for receiving, handling, administration, and disposal. Gloves (single) should be worn during receiving, unpacking, and placing in storage. NIOSH recommends single gloving for administration of intact tablets or capsules (NIOSH 2016).

Storage/Stability Store at 20°C to 25°C (68°F to 77°F); excursions are permitted between 15°C and 30°C (59°F and 86°F).

Mechanism of Action Tyrosine kinase (multikinase) inhibitor; limits tumor growth via inhibition of angiogenesis by inhibiting cell surface vascular endothelial growth factor receptors (VEGFR-1, VEGFR-2, VEGFR-3), platelet-derived growth factor receptors (PDGFR-alpha and -beta), fibroblast growth factor receptor (FGFR-1 and -3), cytokine receptor (cKIT), interleukin-2 receptor inducible T-cell kinase, lymphocyte-specific protein tyrosine kinase (Lck), and transmembrane glycoprotein receptor tyrosine kinase (c-Fms)

Pharmacodynamics/Kinetics

Protein binding: >99%

Metabolism: Hepatic; primarily via CYP3A4, minor metabolism via CYP1A2 and CYP2C8

Bioavailability: Rate and extent of bioavailability are increased with food and increased if tablets are crushed (do not crush tablets)

Half-life elimination: ~31 hours

Time to peak, plasma: 2 to 4 hours

Excretion: Feces (primarily); urine (<4%)

Dosing

Adult & Geriatric

Renal cell carcinoma (RCC), advanced: Oral: 800 mg once daily (Sternberg 2010)

Soft tissue sarcoma (STS), advanced: Oral: 800 mg once daily (Van Der Graaf 2012)

Thyroid cancer, advanced differentiated (off-label use): Oral: 800 mg once daily until disease progression or unacceptable toxicity (Bible 2010; Bible 2014)

Missed doses: If a dose is missed, do not take if <12 hours until the next dose.

Concomitant CYP3A4 inhibitors/inducers:

CYP3A4 inhibitors: Avoid concomitant strong CYP3A4 inhibitors (may increase pazopanib concentrations). If pazopanib must be administered concomitantly with a potent enzyme inhibitor, reduce pazopanib to 400 mg once daily with careful monitoring; further dosage reductions may be needed if adverse events occur.

CYP3A4 inducers: Avoid concomitant strong CYP3A4 inducers (may decrease pazopanib concentrations); use of pazopanib is not recommended in situations where the chronic use of a strong CYP3A4 inducer is required.

Renal Impairment

CrCl ≥30 mL/minute: No dosage adjustment necessary (renal impairment is not expected to influence pazopanib exposure).

CrCl <30 mL/minute: There are no dosage adjustments provided in the manufacturer's labeling (has not been studied); however, renal impairment is not expected to influence pazopanib exposure.

Hepatic Impairment

Preexisting impairment:

Mild (bilirubin ≤1.5 times ULN or ALT >ULN): No dosage adjustment required (Shibata 2013).

Moderate (bilirubin >1.5 to 3 times ULN): Consider alternative therapy or reduce to 200 mg once daily (maximum tolerated dose in patients with moderate hepatic impairment) (Shibata 2013).

Severe (bilirubin >3 times ULN with any ALT level): Use is not recommended.

During treatment:

Isolated ALT elevations 3 to 8 times ULN: Continue treatment, monitor liver function weekly until ALT returns to grade 1 or baseline.

Isolated ALT elevations >8 times ULN: Interrupt treatment until ALT returns to grade 1 or baseline. If therapy benefit is greater than the risk of hepatotoxicity, may reinitiate treatment at ≤400 mg once daily (with liver function monitored weekly for 8 weeks); permanently discontinue if ALT >3 times ULN occurs with reinitiation.

ALT >3 times ULN concurrently with bilirubin >2 times ULN: Permanently discontinue; monitor until resolution.

Gilbert syndrome with mild indirect bilirubin elevation and ALT >3 times ULN: Refer to isolated ALT elevations dosage recommendations above.

Adjustment for Toxicity
  Initial dosage reduction: Note: Prior to dose reduction, temporarily discontinue therapy if 24-hour urine protein ≥3 g or for other toxicities when clinically indicated.
  RCC: Reduce to 400 mg once daily
  STS: Reduce to 600 mg once daily
  Further modification: *RCC, STS:* Adjust dose in 200 mg increments or decrements based on individual tolerance; maximum dose: 800 mg
  Hypertension: Manage as appropriate with antihypertensive therapy and interrupt treatment or reduce dose as clinically warranted.
  Hypertension (severe, persistent, and refractory to antihypertensives and dose reduction) or evidence of hypertensive crisis: Discontinue treatment.
  Infection, serious: Consider treatment interruption or discontinuation.
  Proteinuria (24-hour urine protein ≥3 g): Interrupt treatment and reduce the dose.
  Proteinuria (recurrent 24-hour urine protein ≥3 g refractory to dose reduction): Discontinue treatment.
  Pulmonary toxicity: Interstitial lung disease (ILD) or pneumonitis: Discontinue treatment.
  Reversible posterior leukoencephalopathy syndrome (RPLS): Permanently discontinue.
  Thrombotic microangiopathy (TMA): Permanently discontinue.
  Wound dehiscence: Discontinue treatment.
Administration Administer on an empty stomach, 1 hour before or 2 hours after a meal. Do not crush tablet (rate of absorption may be increased; may affect systemic exposure).
Emetic Potential Low (10% to 30%)
Monitoring Parameters Monitor liver function tests (ALT, AST, bilirubin) at baseline; at weeks 3, 5, 7, and 9; at months 3 and 4; and as clinically necessary, then periodically after month 4 (monitor more frequently if clinically indicated); serum electrolytes (eg, calcium, magnesium, potassium); urinalysis (for proteinuria; baseline and periodic), 24-hour urine protein (if clinically indicated); thyroid function (TSH and T_4 at baseline and TSH every 6 to 8 weeks during treatment [Appleby 2011]); verify pregnancy status (in women of reproductive potential) prior to therapy initiation; blood pressure; ECG (baseline and periodic); LVEF (if at risk for cardiac dysfunction; baseline and periodic); signs/symptoms of GI perforation or fistula, venous/arterial thrombotic events, pulmonary embolism, interstitial lung disease/pneumonitis, infection, heart failure, or neurological changes. Monitor adherence.
Dietary Considerations Avoid grapefruit juice.
Medication Guide Available Yes
Dosage Forms Excipient information presented when available (limited, particularly for generics); consult specific product labeling.
  Tablet, Oral:
  Votrient: 200 mg

◆ **Pazopanib HCl** *see* PAZOPanib *on page 1454*
◆ **Pazopanib Hydrochloride** *see* PAZOPanib *on page 1454*
◆ **P-Care D40** *see* MethylPREDNISolone *on page 1227*
◆ **P-Care D80** *see* MethylPREDNISolone *on page 1227*
◆ **PCB** *see* Procarbazine *on page 1557*

- ◆ **PCC (Caution: Confusion-prone synonym)** *see* Factor IX Complex (Human) [(Factors II, IX, X)] *on page* 767
- ◆ **PCI-32765** *see* Ibrutinib *on page* 944
- ◆ **PCZ** *see* Procarbazine *on page* 1557
- ◆ **PD 0332991** *see* Palbociclib *on page* 1421
- ◆ **PDL-063** *see* Elotuzumab *on page* 663
- ◆ **PDX** *see* PRALAtrexate *on page* 1540
- ◆ **Pediaderm AF Complete [DSC]** *see* Nystatin (Topical) *on page* 1340
- ◆ **Pedi-Dri [DSC]** *see* Nystatin (Topical) *on page* 1340
- ◆ **PEG-L-asparaginase** *see* Pegaspargase *on page* 1462
- ◆ **PEG-ASP** *see* Pegaspargase *on page* 1462
- ◆ **PEG-asparaginase** *see* Pegaspargase *on page* 1462

Pegaspargase (peg AS par jase)

Related Information

Management of Chemotherapy-Induced Nausea and Vomiting in Adults *on page* 2253

Prevention of Chemotherapy-Induced Nausea and Vomiting in Children *on page* 2310

Brand Names: US Oncaspar

Index Terms L-asparaginase with Polyethylene Glycol; PEG-ASP; PEG-asparaginase; PEG-L-asparaginase; PEGLA; Polyethylene Glycol-L-asparaginase

Pharmacologic Category Antineoplastic Agent, Enzyme; Antineoplastic Agent, Miscellaneous

Use

Acute lymphoblastic leukemia and hypersensitivity to asparaginase: Treatment of acute lymphoblastic leukemia (ALL) in patients with hypersensitivity to native forms of L-asparaginase (as a component of a multiagent chemotherapy regimen)

Acute lymphoblastic leukemia, first-line: First-line treatment of ALL (as a component of a multiagent chemotherapy regimen)

Labeled Contraindications

History of serious allergic reactions to pegaspargase or any component of the formulation; history of any of the following with prior L-asparaginase treatment: serious thrombosis, pancreatitis, and/or serious hemorrhagic events

Canadian labeling: Additional contraindications (not in the US labeling): Severe hepatic impairment (bilirubin >3 times upper limit of normal [ULN]; transaminases >10 times ULN).

Pregnancy Considerations Animal reproduction studies have not been conducted with pegaspargase.

Breastfeeding Considerations It is not known if pegaspargase is excreted in breast milk. Due to the potential for serious adverse reactions in the nursing infant, the manufacturer recommends a decision be made to discontinue nursing or to discontinue the drug, taking into account the importance of treatment to the mother.

Warnings/Precautions Anaphylaxis and serious allergic reactions (eg, bronchospasm, hypotension, laryngeal edema, local erythema or swelling, systemic rash, urticaria) may occur; discontinue in patients with serious allergic reaction. The risk of serious allergic reactions is increased in patients with a history of hypersensitivity reactions to other L-asparaginase products. Observe patients for 1 hour after administration; equipment and immediate treatment for hypersensitivity reactions should be available during administration.

Serious thrombotic events, including sagittal sinus thrombosis may occur; discontinue with serious thrombotic event. Anticoagulation prophylaxis during therapy may be considered in some patients (Farge 2013). Pancreatitis may occur; promptly evaluate patients with abdominal pain. The manufacturer recommends discontinuing pegaspargase if pancreatitis occurs during treatment. May consider continuing therapy for asymptomatic chemical pancreatitis (amylase or lipase >3 times ULN) or only radiologic abnormalities; monitor closely for rising amylase and/or lipase levels (Stock 2011). Discontinue permanently for clinical pancreatitis (eg, vomiting, severe abdominal pain) with amylase/lipase elevation >3 times ULN for >3 days and/or development of a pancreatic pseudocyst. Avoid alcohol use (Stock 2011). May cause glucose intolerance; irreversible in some cases; use with caution in patients with hyperglycemia, or diabetes. Monitor serum glucose. Increased prothrombin time, increased partial thromboplastin time, and hypofibrinogenemia may occur. Severe or symptomatic coagulopathy may require treatment with fresh-frozen plasma; use with caution in patients with underlying coagulopathy or previous hematologic complications from asparaginase. Monitor coagulation parameters at baseline and periodically during and after therapy. Altered liver function tests (eg, increased AST, ALT, alkaline phosphatase, bilirubin [direct and indirect], and decreased serum albumin, plasma fibrinogen) may occur with therapy. Use with caution in patients with preexisting hepatic impairment. Monitor liver function tests at baseline and periodically during treatment.

In a study comparing IV pegaspargase to IM native *E. coli* asparaginase for post-induction treatment in children with ALL, 5-year disease-free survival did not differ and the overall frequency of asparaginase-related toxicities (including allergy, pancreatitis, and thrombotic or bleeding complications) did not differ between the IV pegaspargase and IM native *E. coli* apsaraginase groups. The median nadir serum asparaginase activity was significantly higher in the IV pegaspargase group. Reported treatment-related anxiety was significantly lower (for both patients and guardians) in the group that received IV pegaspargase (Place 2015).

Potentially significant drug-drug interactions may exist, requiring dose or frequency adjustment, additional monitoring, and/or selection of alternative therapy. Do not interchange pegaspargase for asparaginase (*E. coli*) or asparaginase (*Erwinia*); ensure the proper asparaginase formulation, route of administration, and dose prior to administration.

Adverse Reactions

>10%:

Hepatic: Increased serum transaminases (ALT, AST; grades 3/4: 3% to 11%)

Hypersensitivity: Hypersensitivity reaction (grades 3/4: 1%, includes anaphylaxis, bronchospasm, erythema, hives, hypotension, laryngeal edema, skin rash, swelling, urticaria; relapsed acute lymphoblastic leukemia [ALL] with no prior asparaginase hypersensitivity: 10%; relapsed ALL with prior asparaginase hypersensitivity: 32%)

1% to 10%:

Cardiovascular: Thrombosis (4%)

Central nervous system: Cerebral thrombosis (or hemorrhage of the brain: 2%; grades 3/4: 3%)

◄ Endocrine & metabolic: Hyperglycemia (3% [some patients required insulin therapy]; grades 3/4: 5%)

Gastrointestinal: Pancreatitis (1%; grades 3/4: 2% [includes 3 deaths])

Hematologic: Blood coagulation disorder (grades 3/4: 2% to 7%; includes prolonged prothrombin time or partial thromboplastin time or decreased serum fibrogen)

Hepatic: Abnormal hepatic function tests (grades 3/4: 5%), hyperbilirubine-mia (grades 3/4: 1% to 2%)

Immunologic: Hypersensitivity to L-asparaginase (grades 3/4: 2%)

<1%, postmarketing, case reports, and/or frequency not defined: Abdominal pain, anemia, anorexia, antithrombin III deficiency, arthralgia, ascites, bac-teremia, bronchospasm, bruise, chest pain, chills, coagulation time increased, colitis, confusion, constipation, cough, deep vein thrombosis, disseminated intravascular coagulation, dizziness, dyspnea, edema, emo-tional lability, endocarditis, epistaxis, facial edema, fatigue, fever, gastro-intestinal pain, headache, hematuria, hemolytic anemia, hemorrhagic cystitis, hepatic failure, hepatomegaly, hyperammonemia, hypertension, hyperuricemia, hypoalbuminemia, hypoglycemia, hyponatremia, increased blood urea nitrogen, increased serum amylase, increased serum creatinine, increased serum lipase, increased thirst, injection site pain, jaundice, leukopenia, lip edema, liver steatosis, malaise, metabolic acidosis, myalgia, nausea, night sweats, ostealgia, pancytopenia, paresthesia, petechial rash, prolonged prothrombin time, proteinuria, purpura, renal failure, renal function abnormality, sagittal sinus thrombosis, seizure, sepsis, septic shock, sub-acute bacterial endocarditis, superficial venous thrombosis, tachycardia, thrombocytopenia, uric acid nephropathy, urticaria, vomiting

Drug Interactions

Metabolism/Transport Effects None known.

Avoid Concomitant Use

Avoid concomitant use of Pegaspargase with any of the following: BCG (Intravesical); Natalizumab; Pimecrolimus; Tacrolimus (Topical); Vaccines (Live)

Increased Effect/Toxicity

Pegaspargase may increase the levels/effects of: Fingolimod; Leflunomide; Natalizumab; Tofacitinib; Vaccines (Live)

The levels/effects of Pegaspargase may be increased by: Denosumab; Ocrelizumab; Pimecrolimus; Roflumilast; Tacrolimus (Topical); Trastuzumab

Decreased Effect

Pegaspargase may decrease the levels/effects of: BCG (Intravesical); Coccidioides immitis Skin Test; Nivolumab; Sipuleucel-T; Tertomotide; Vac-cines (Inactivated); Vaccines (Live)

The levels/effects of Pegaspargase may be decreased by: Echinacea; Pegloticase

Storage/Stability Store intact vials at 2°C to 8°C (36°F to 46°F); do not freeze. Do not shake; protect from light. Discard vial if previously frozen, stored at room temperature for >48 hours, excessively shaken/agitated, or if cloudy, discolored, or if precipitate is present. If not used immediately, solutions diluted for infusion in NS or D5W should be protected from light, refrigerated at 2°C to 8°C (36°F to 46°F) and used within 48 hours (including administration time).

Preparation for Administration IV: Dilute in 100 mL NS or D5W.

Mechanism of Action Pegaspargase is a modified version of L-asparaginase, conjugated with polyethylene glycol. In leukemic cells, asparaginase hydrolyzes L-asparagine to ammonia and L-aspartic acid, leading to depletion of asparagine. Leukemia cells, especially lymphoblasts, require exogenous asparagine; normal cells can synthesize asparagine. Asparagine depletion in leukemic cells leads to inhibition of protein synthesis and apoptosis. Asparaginase is cycle-specific for the G_1 phase of the cell cycle.

Pharmacodynamics/Kinetics

Onset: Asparagine depletion: IM: Within 4 days

Duration: Asparagine depletion: IV (in asparaginase naive adults): 2 to 4 weeks (Douer 2007); IM: ~21 days

Absorption: Not absorbed from the GI tract; therefore, requires parenteral administration; IM: Slow

Distribution: Apparent V_d: Plasma volume: IM: Children: 1.5 L/m²; IV: Adults (asparaginase naive): 2.4 L/m² (Douer 2007)

Metabolism: Systemically degraded

Half-life elimination:

IM: Children: 5.8 days; Adults: 5.5-6 days; 3.2 ± 1.8 days in patients who previously had a hypersensitivity reaction to native L-asparaginase

IV: Adults (asparaginase naive): 7 days (Douer 2007)

Time to peak: IM: 3 to 4 days

Excretion: Clearance is unaffected by age, renal function, or hepatic function; not detected in urine

Dosing

Adult & Geriatric Acute lymphoblastic leukemia (ALL): IM, IV: 2500 units/m² (as part of a combination chemotherapy regimen), do not administer more frequently than every 14 days

Pediatric Acute lymphoblastic leukemia (ALL): IM, IV: Refer to adult dosing.

Renal Impairment There are no dosage adjustments provided in the manufacturer's labeling.

Hepatic Impairment There are no initial dosage adjustments provided in the manufacturer's labeling. The following adjustments have been recommended (Stock 2011):

ALT/AST >3 to 5 times ULN: Continue therapy.

ALT/AST >5 to 20 times ULN: Delay next dose until transaminases <3 times ULN.

ALT/AST >20 times ULN: Discontinue therapy if it takes longer than 1 week for transaminases to return to <3 times ULN.

Direct bilirubin <3 mg/dL: Continue therapy.

Direct bilirubin 3.1 to 5 mg/dL: Hold pegaspargase and resume when direct bilirubin <2 mg/dL; consider switching to alternate asparaginase product.

Direct bilirubin >5 mg/dL: Discontinue pegaspargase; do not substitute other asparaginase products; do not make up for missed doses.

Adjustment for Toxicity The following adjustments have been recommended (Stock 2011):

Hyperammonemia-related fatigue: Continue therapy for grade 2 toxicity. If grade 3 toxicity occurs, reduce dose by 25%; resume full dose when toxicity ≤ grade 2 (make up for missed doses). If grade 4 toxicity occurs, reduce dose by 50%; resume full dose when toxicity ≤ grade 2 (make up for missed doses).

◄ *Hyperglycemia:* Continue therapy for uncomplicated hyperglycemia. If hyperglycemia requires insulin therapy, hold pegaspargase (and any concomitant corticosteroids) until blood glucose controlled; resume dosing at prior dose level. For life-threatening hyperglycemia or toxicity requiring urgent intervention, hold pegaspargase (and corticosteroids) until blood glucose is controlled with insulin; resume pegaspargase and do not make up for missed doses.

Hypersensitivity reactions: May continue dosing for urticaria without bronchospasm, hypotension, edema, or need for parenteral intervention. If wheezing or other symptomatic bronchospasm with or without urticaria, angioedema, hypotension, and/or life-threatening hypersensitivity reactions occur, discontinue pegaspargase. Replace pegaspargase with asparaginase (Erwinia).

Hypertriglyceridemia: If serum triglyceride level <1,000 mg/dL, continue pegaspargase but monitor closely for pancreatitis. If triglyceride level >1,000 mg/dL, hold pegaspargase and monitor; resume therapy at prior dose level after triglyceride level returns to baseline.

Pancreatitis:

Asymptomatic amylase or lipase >3 times ULN (chemical pancreatitis) or radiologic abnormalities only: Continue pegaspargase and monitor levels closely.

Clinical pancreatitis (abdominal pain with amylase or lipase >3 times ULN for >3 days and/or development of pancreatic pseudocyst): Permanently discontinue pegaspargase.

Thrombosis and bleeding, CNS:

Thrombosis: Continue therapy for abnormal laboratory findings without a clinical correlate. If grade 3 toxicity occurs, discontinue therapy; if CNS signs/symptoms are fully resolved and further pegaspargase doses are required, may resume therapy at a lower dose and/or longer intervals between doses. Discontinue therapy for grade 4 toxicity.

Hemorrhage: Discontinue therapy; do not withhold therapy for abnormal laboratory findings without a clinical correlate. If grade 3 toxicity occurs, discontinue therapy; if CNS signs/symptoms are fully resolved and further pegaspargase doses are required, may resume therapy at a lower dose and/or longer intervals between doses. Discontinue therapy for grade 4 toxicity.

Thrombosis and bleeding, non-CNS:

Thrombosis: Continue therapy for abnormal laboratory findings without a clinical correlate. If grade 3 or 4 toxicity occurs, withhold therapy until acute toxicity and clinical signs resolve and anticoagulant therapy is stable or completed. Do not withhold therapy for abnormal laboratory findings without clinical correlate.

Hemorrhage: If grade 2 bleeding in conjunction with hypofibrinogenemia occurs, withhold therapy until bleeding ≤ grade 1. Do not withhold therapy for abnormal laboratory findings without clinical correlate. For grade 3 or 4 bleeding, withhold therapy until bleeding ≤ grade 1 and until acute toxicity and clinical signs resolve and coagulant replacement therapy is stable or completed.

Combination Regimens

Leukemia (acute lymphocytic): Hyper-CVAD (Leukemia, Acute Lymphocytic) on page 2146

Administration Have available appropriate agents for maintenance of an adequate airway and treatment of a hypersensitivity reaction (antihistamine, epinephrine, oxygen, IV corticosteroids). Be prepared to treat anaphylaxis at each administration.

IM: Must only be administered as a deep intramuscular injection into a large muscle. Do not exceed 2 mL per injection site; use multiple injection sites for IM injection volume >2 mL.

IV: Administer over 1 to 2 hours through a running IV infusion line; **do not administer IV push.**

Emetic Potential Children and Adults: Minimal (<10%)

Monitoring Parameters CBC with differential, platelets, amylase/lipase, liver function tests (baseline and periodically during treatment), fibrinogen, PT, PTT (coagulation parameters [baseline and periodically during and after treatment]), renal function tests; urine glucose, blood glucose; triglycerides; uric acid; vital signs during administration; monitor for onset of abdominal pain; observe for allergic reaction (for 1 hour after administration); signs/symptoms of thrombosis or bleeding

Dosage Forms Excipient information presented when available (limited, particularly for generics); consult specific product labeling.

Solution, Injection [preservative free]:

Oncaspar: 750 units/mL (5 mL)

Pegfilgrastim (peg fil GRA stim)

Brand Names: US Neulasta; Neulasta Onpro

Brand Names: Canada Neulasta

Index Terms G-CSF (PEG Conjugate); Granulocyte Colony Stimulating Factor (PEG Conjugate); Neulasta Onpro kit; Pegylated G-CSF; SD/01

Pharmacologic Category Colony Stimulating Factor; Hematopoietic Agent

Use

US labeling:

Prevention of chemotherapy-induced neutropenia: To decrease the incidence of infection (as manifested by febrile neutropenia), in patients with nonmyeloid malignancies receiving myelosuppressive cancer chemotherapy associated with a clinically significant incidence of febrile neutropenia.

Limitation of use: Pegfilgrastim is not indicated for mobilization of peripheral blood progenitor cells for hematopoietic stem cell transplant.

Hematopoietic radiation injury syndrome (acute): To increase survival in patients acutely exposed to myelosuppressive doses of radiation.

Canadian labeling:

Prevention of chemotherapy-induced neutropenia: To decrease the incidence of infection (as manifested by febrile neutropenia), in adult patients with nonmyeloid malignancies receiving myelosuppressive cancer chemotherapy.

Labeled Contraindications

Hypersensitivity (serious allergic reaction) to pegfilgrastim, filgrastim, or any component of the formulation

Canadian labeling: Additional contraindications (not in US labeling): Hypersensitivity to *E. coli*-derived proteins.

Pregnancy Considerations Adverse events were observed in some animal reproduction studies.

◄ Women who are exposed to Neulasta during pregnancy are encouraged to enroll in the Amgen Pregnancy Surveillance Program (800-772-6436).

Breastfeeding Considerations It is not known if pegfilgrastim is excreted in breast milk. The manufacturer recommends that caution be exercised when administering pegfilgrastim to nursing women.

Warnings/Precautions Do not use pegfilgrastim in the period 14 days before to 24 hours after administration of cytotoxic chemotherapy because of the potential sensitivity of rapidly dividing myeloid cells to cytotoxic chemotherapy. Safety and efficacy have not been established with dose-dense chemotherapy regimens (Smith 2006). Not indicated for peripheral blood progenitor cell (PBPC) mobilization for hematopoietic stem cell transplantation.

Serious allergic reactions (including anaphylaxis) may occur, usually with the initial dose; may recur within days after discontinuation of initial antiallergic treatment. Permanently discontinue for severe reactions. Do not administer in patients with a history of serious allergic reaction to pegfilgrastim or filgrastim. Acute respiratory distress syndrome (ARDS) has been reported with use; evaluate patients with pulmonary symptoms such as fever, pulmonary infiltrates, or respiratory distress for ARDS. Discontinue pegfilgrastim if ARDS occurs. Rare cases of splenic rupture have been reported (some fatal); patients must be instructed to report left upper abdominal pain or shoulder pain. May precipitate sickle cell crises in patients with sickle cell disorders (severe and sometimes fatal sickle cell crises have occurred with filgrastim). The granulocyte-colony stimulating factor (G-CSF) receptor through which pegfilgrastim (and filgrastim) work has been located on tumor cell lines. May potentially act as a growth factor for any tumor type, including myeloid malignancies and myelodysplasia (pegfilgrastim is not approved for myeloid malignancies). Capillary leak syndrome (CLS), characterized by hypotension, hypoalbuminemia, edema, and hemoconcentration, may occur in patients receiving human granulocyte colony-stimulating factors (G-CSF), including pegfilgrastim. CLS episodes vary in frequency and severity. If CLS develops, monitor closely and manage symptomatically (may require intensive care). CLS may be life-threatening if treatment is delayed.

Leukocytosis (WBC $\geq 100,000/mm^3$) has been reported in patients receiving pegfilgrastim. Monitor complete blood counts during therapy. Glomerulonephritis has occurred, and generally resolved after pegfilgrastim dose reduction or discontinuation. Diagnosis was made by the presence of azotemia, microscopic and macroscopic hematuria, proteinuria, and renal biopsy. Evaluate if glomerulonephritis is suspected; if felt due to pegfilgrastim, consider dose reduction or therapy interruption.

The On-body injector is not recommended for use in patients with acute hematopoietic radiation injury syndrome. The On-body injector contains an acrylic adhesive; may result in a significant reaction in patients who react to acrylic adhesives. A health care provider must fill the On-body injector prior to applying to the patient's skin. The On-body delivery system may be applied on the same day as chemotherapy administration as long as pegfilgrastim is delivered no less than 24 hours after chemotherapy is administered. The prefilled syringe provided in the On-body kit contains overfill to compensate for loss during delivery; do not use for manual subcutaneous injection (will result in higher than recommended dose). Do not use prefilled syringe intended for manual injection to fill the On-body injector; may result in lower than intended dose. The On-body injector is only for use with pegfilgrastim; do not use to deliver other medications. Do not expose the On-body injector to oxygen-rich environments (eg, hyperbaric chambers), MRI, x-ray (including airport x-ray), CT scan, or ultrasound (may damage injector system). Keep the On-body injector at least 4 inches away from electrical equipment, including cell phones, cordless phones, microwaves, and other common appliances (injector may not work properly).

Colony-stimulating factors may be considered in cancer patients with febrile neutropenia who are at high risk for infection-associated complications or who have prognostic factors indicative of a poor clinical outcome (eg, prolonged and severe neutropenia, age >65 years, hypotension, pneumonia, sepsis syndrome, presence of invasive fungal infection, uncontrolled primary disease, hospitalization at the time of fever development) (Freifeld 2011; Smith 2006). Colony-stimulating factors should not be routinely used for patients with neutropenia who are afebrile. Dose-dense regimens that require colony-stimulating factors should only be used within the context of a clinical trial or if supported by convincing evidence. The safety/efficacy of pegfilgrastim in the setting of dose-dense therapy has not been fully established (Smith 2015).

ASCO guidelines recommend that prophylactic colony-stimulating factors be used in patients ≥65 years with diffuse aggressive lymphoma treated with curative chemotherapy (eg, rituximab, cyclophosphamide, doxorubicin, vincristine, prednisone), especially if patients have comorbid conditions (Smith 2015). The 6 mg fixed dose should not be used in infants, children, and adolescents weighing <45 kg. CSF use in pediatric patients is typically directed by clinical pediatric protocols. ASCO Recommendations for the Use of WBC Growth Factors Clinical Practice Guideline Update states that CSFs may be reasonable as primary prophylaxis in pediatric patients when chemotherapy regimens with a high likelihood of febrile neutropenia are employed. Likewise, secondary CSF prophylaxis should be limited to high-risk patients. In pediatric cancers in which dose-intense chemotherapy (with a survival benefit) is used, CSFs should be given to facilitate chemotherapy administration. CSFs should not be used in the pediatric population for non-relapsed acute lymphoblastic or myeloid leukemia when no infection is present (Smith 2015). The On-body injector has not been studied for use in pediatrics. The packaging (needle cover) contains latex.

Adverse Reactions

Neuromuscular & skeletal: Ostealgia (31%), limb pain (9%)

<1%, postmarketing, and/or case reports: Acute respiratory distress syndrome (ARDS), alopecia, anaphylaxis, antibody development, arthralgia, back pain, bruising at injection site, capillary leak syndrome, chest pain, constipation, diarrhea, erythema, fatigue, fever, flushing, glomerulonephritis, headache, hypersensitivity angiitis, hypertonia, increased serum alkaline phosphatase, increased uric acid, influenza, injection site reaction, leukocytosis, musculoskeletal pain, myalgia, neck pain, pain, pain at injection site, periorbital edema, peripheral edema, polyarthralgia, polymyalgia rheumatica, rhinitis, severe sickle cell crisis, skeletal pain, splenic rupture, splenomegaly, Sweet syndrome, urticaria, vomiting, weakness

Drug Interactions

Metabolism/Transport Effects None known.

Avoid Concomitant Use There are no known interactions where it is recommended to avoid concomitant use.

Increased Effect/Toxicity

Pegfilgrastim may increase the levels/effects of: Belotecan; Topotecan

◀ **Decreased Effect**
The levels/effects of Pegfilgrastim may be decreased by: Pegloticase

Storage/Stability Store under refrigeration at 2°C to 8°C (36°F to 46°F); do not freeze. If syringe for manual injection is inadvertently frozen, allow to thaw in refrigerator; discard if frozen more than one time. Protect from light. Do not shake. Allow prefilled syringe to reach room temperature for at least 30 minutes prior to injection; discard if kept at room temperature for longer than 48 hours. The On-body injector kit should not be held at room temperature for longer than 12 hours prior to use (discard if stored at room temperature for >12 hours).

Preparation for Administration

Subcutaneous administration from the prefilled syringe: For doses of 6 mg, the prefilled syringe may be used. **Direct** administration of doses <6 mg using the prefilled syringe is not recommended by the manufacturer (it does not have graduation marks necessary for accurate measurement of doses other than 6 mg).

On-body injector: A health care provider must fill the On-body injector prior to applying to the patient's skin. The On-body delivery system may be applied on the same day as chemotherapy administration as long as pegfilgrastim is delivered no less than 24 hours after chemotherapy is administered.

The prefilled syringe provided in the On-body kit contains overfill to compensate for loss during delivery; do not use for manual subcutaneous injection (will result in higher than recommended dose). Do not use prefilled syringe intended for manual injection to fill the On-body injector; may result in lower than intended dose. The On-body injector has not been studied for use in pediatrics.

Mechanism of Action Stimulates the production, maturation, and activation of neutrophils, pegfilgrastim activates neutrophils to increase both their migration and cytotoxicity. Pegfilgrastim has a prolonged duration of effect relative to filgrastim and a reduced renal clearance.

Pharmacodynamics/Kinetics

Half-life elimination: SubQ: Pediatrics (100 mcg/kg dose): 0 to 5 years: 30.1 ± 38.2 hours; 6 to 11 years: 20.2 ± 11.3 hours; 12 years and older: 21.2 ± 16 hours; Adults: 15 to 80 hours. Pharmacokinetics (in adults) were comparable between manual subcutaneous injection and the On-body injector system.

Excretion: Primarily through binding to neutrophils

Dosing

Adult & Geriatric

Prevention of chemotherapy-induced neutropenia: SubQ: 6 mg once per chemotherapy cycle, beginning at least 24 hours after completion of chemotherapy; **Note:** Do not administer in the period between 14 days before and 24 hours after administration of cytotoxic chemotherapy.

Hematopoietic radiation injury syndrome (acute): SubQ: 6 mg once weekly for 2 doses. Obtain a baseline CBC prior to administration, but do not delay pegfilgrastim use if a CBC is not readily obtainable. Administer the first dose as soon as possible after suspected or confirmed radiation exposure greater than 2 gray (Gy). Administer the second dose 1 week after the first dose.

Pediatric

Prevention of chemotherapy-induced neutropenia: Note: Do not administer in the period between 14 days before and 24 hours after administration of cytotoxic chemotherapy.

Children and Adolescents <45 kg: SubQ: Administer once per chemotherapy cycle, beginning at least 24 hours after completion of chemotherapy (dose and volume are based on patient weight). Maximum dose: 6 mg (Andre 2007; Borinstein 2009). **Note:** The prefilled syringe is not designed to allow for direct administration of doses less than 6 mg (0.6 mL). Due to the potential for dosing errors, the manufacturer does not recommend direct administration of doses less than 6 mg (0.6 mL); use caution to avoid dosing errors.

Patients <10 kg: 0.1 **mg/kg** (0.01 **mL/kg** volume)

Patients 10 to 20 kg: 1.5 **mg** (0.15 **mL** volume)

Patients 21 to 30 kg: 2.5 **mg** (0.25 **mL** volume)

Patients 31 to 44 kg: 4 **mg** (0.4 **mL** volume)

Children and Adolescents ≥45 kg: SubQ: 6 mg once per chemotherapy cycle, beginning at least 24 hours after completion of chemotherapy

Hematopoietic radiation injury syndrome (acute): Obtain a baseline CBC prior to administration, but do not delay pegfilgrastim use if a CBC is not readily obtainable. Administer the first dose as soon as possible after suspected or confirmed radiation exposure greater than 2 gray (Gy). Administer the second dose 1 week after the first dose.

Children and Adolescents <45 kg: SubQ: Administer 2 doses of pegfilgrastim one week apart (dose and volume are based on patient weight).

Patients <10 kg: 0.1 **mg/kg** (0.01 **mL/kg** volume)

Patients 10 to 20 kg: 1.5 **mg** (0.15 **mL** volume)

Patients 21 to 30 kg: 2.5 **mg** (0.25 **mL** volume)

Patients 31 to 44 kg: 4 **mg** (0.4 **mL** volume)

Children and Adolescents ≥45 kg: SubQ: 6 mg once weekly for 2 doses (the second dose should be administered 1 week after the first dose).

Renal Impairment No dosage adjustment necessary.

Hepatic Impairment There are no dosage adjustments provided in the manufacturer's labeling (has not been studied).

Combination Regimens

Bone sarcoma (Ewing sarcoma): Docetaxel-Gemcitabine (Ewing Sarcoma) on page 2091

Bone sarcoma (osteosarcoma): Docetaxel-Gemcitabine (Osteosarcoma) on page 2091

Breast cancer: AC (Dose-Dense) followed by Paclitaxel (Dose-Dense)-Trastuzumab (Breast) on page 1977

Endometrial cancer: Cisplatin-Doxorubin-Paclitaxel (Endometrial) on page 2041

Lymphoma, non-Hodgkin (AIDS-Related): EPOCH Dose-Adjusted-Rituximab (NHL-AIDS-Related) on page 2107

Lymphoma, non-Hodgkin (Mantle Cell): Cladribine-Rituximab (NHL-Mantle Cell) on page 2064

Soft tissue sarcoma: Docetaxel-Gemcitabine (Soft Tissue Sarcoma) on page 2092

Uterine sarcoma: Docetaxel-Gemcitabine (Uterine Leiomyosarcoma) on page 2093

Administration Administer subcutaneously. Do not use 6 mg fixed dose in infants, children, or adolescents <45 kg (Smith 2006). Pegfilgrastim is available in prefilled syringes for manual subcutaneous administration or as a kit for use with the On-body injector. **Direct** administration of doses <6 mg using the prefilled syringe is not recommended by the manufacturer (it does not have graduation marks necessary for accurate measurement of doses other than 6 mg); use caution to avoid dosing errors.

Manual subcutaneous administration: Administer to outer upper arms, abdomen (except within 2 inches of navel), front middle thigh, or upper outer buttocks. Allow prefilled syringe to reach room temperature for at least 30 minutes prior to injection. Engage/activate needle guard following use to prevent accidental needlesticks

On-body injector: A health care provider must fill the On-body injector prior to applying to the patient's skin. Apply to intact, nonirritated skin on the back of the arm or abdomen (only use the back of the arm if caregiver is available to monitor On-body injection status). The On-body injector system will deliver pegfilgrastim over ~45 minutes approximately 27 hours after application. The On-body delivery system may be applied on the same day as chemotherapy administration as long as pegfilgrastim is delivered at least 24 hours after chemotherapy is administered. Keep the On-body injector dry for ~3 hours before dose delivery. A missed dose may occur if the On-body injector fails or leaks; if a dose is missed, administer a new dose by manual subcutaneous injection as soon as possible after discovery of missed dose. Do not expose the On-body injector to oxygen-rich environments (eg, hyperbaric chambers), MRI, x-ray (including airport x-ray), CT-scan, or ultrasound (may damage injector system). Keep the On-body injector at least 4 inches away from electrical equipment, including cell phones, cordless phones, microwaves, and other common appliances (injector may not work properly). The On-body injector is not recommended for use in patients with acute hematopoietic radiation injury syndrome. The On-body injector has not been studied in pediatric patients. Refer to prescribing information for further details.

The prefilled syringe provided in the On-body kit contains overfill to compensate for loss during delivery; do not use for manual subcutaneous injection (will result in higher than recommended dose). Do not use prefilled syringe intended for manual injection to fill the On-body injector; may result in lower than intended dose. The On-body injector is only for use with pegfilgrastim; do not use to deliver other medications.

Monitoring Parameters

Chemotherapy-induced neutropenia: Complete blood count (with differential) and platelet count should be obtained prior to chemotherapy and as clinically necessary.

Hematopoietic radiation injury syndrome: CBC at baseline (do not delay administration if CBC not readily available); estimate absorbed radiation dose.

Evaluate fever, pulmonary infiltrates, and respiratory distress; evaluate for left upper abdominal pain, shoulder tip pain, or splenomegaly. Monitor for signs/symptoms of glomerulonephritis (azotemia, hematuria, proteinuria) and capillary leak syndrome (hypotension, hypoalbuminemia, edema and hemoconcentration). Monitor for sickle cell crisis (in patients with sickle cell anemia).

Test Interactions May interfere with bone imaging studies; increased hematopoietic activity of the bone marrow may appear as transient positive bone imaging changes

Dosage Forms Excipient information presented when available (limited, particularly for generics); consult specific product labeling.
Prefilled Syringe Kit, Subcutaneous [preservative free]:
 Neulasta Onpro: 6 mg/0.6 mL (0.6 mL)
Solution, Subcutaneous [preservative free]:
 Neulasta: 6 mg/0.6 mL (0.6 mL)
Dosage Forms: Canada Information with regard to form, strength, and availability of products uniquely available in Canada but currently not available in the US. Refer also to Dosage Forms.

Excipient information presented when available (limited, particularly for generics); consult specific product labeling.

◆ **PEG-IFN Alfa-2b** *see* Peginterferon Alfa-2b *on page 1473*

Peginterferon Alfa-2b (peg in ter FEER on AL fa too bee)
Related Information
 Common Toxicity Criteria *on page 2242*
 Management of Chemotherapy-Induced Nausea and Vomiting in Adults *on page 2253*
 Prevention of Chemotherapy-Induced Nausea and Vomiting in Children *on page 2310*
Brand Names: US Peg-Intron Redipen Pak 4 [DSC]; Peg-Intron Redipen [DSC]; PegIntron; Sylatron
Brand Names: Canada PegIntron
Index Terms Interferon Alfa-2b (PEG Conjugate); PEG-IFN Alfa-2b; Pegylated Interferon Alfa-2b; Polyethylene Glycol Interferon Alfa-2b
Pharmacologic Category Antineoplastic Agent, Biological Response Modulator; Biological Response Modulator; Immunomodulator, Systemic; Interferon
Use
Chronic hepatitis C (CHC): Peg-Intron: Treatment of chronic hepatitis C (CHC) in compensated liver disease.
 Combination therapy with ribavirin and an approved hepatitis C virus [HCV] NS3/4A protease inhibitor in adult patients with HCV genotype 1 infection. **Note:** Regimen is **not** recommended for hepatitis C virus (HCV) genotype 1 in HCV treatment guidelines (treatment-naive or treatment-experienced) (AASLD/IDSA 2015).
 Combination therapy with ribavirin in adult patients with HCV genotypes other than 1, in pediatric patients (3 to 17 years), or in patients with HCV genotype 1 with contraindications or intolerance to HCV NS3/4A protease inhibitor use. **Note:** Combination therapy with peginterferon (**without** the addition of another preferred HCV antiviral agent) is **not** recommended for HCV genotypes other than 1 (ie, genotypes 2, 3, 4, 5, or 6) in HCV adult treatment guidelines (treatment-naive or treatment-experienced) (AASLD/IDSA 2015).
 Monotherapy in adult patients with contraindications or significant intolerance to ribavirin if previously untreated. **Note:** Monotherapy with peginterferon is **not** recommended in HCV treatment guidelines (treatment-naive or treatment-experienced) (AASLD/IDSA 2015).
 Limitations of use: *Manufacturer's labeling:* Combination therapy with ribavirin provides substantially better response rates than monotherapy.

◀ ***Guideline recommendations:*** Current AASLD/IDSA recommendations do not specify a particular peginterferon (eg, 2a or 2b); however, guideline recommendations are based on clinical trials that used peginterferon alfa-2a (AASLD/IDSA 2015). Hepatitis C treatment guidelines are constantly changing with the advent of new treatment therapies and information; consult current clinical practice guidelines for the most recent treatment recommendations.

Melanoma: Sylatron: Adjuvant treatment of melanoma (with microscopic or gross nodal involvement within 84 days of definitive surgical resection, including complete lymphadenectomy)

Labeled Contraindications

Hypersensitivity (including urticaria, angioedema, bronchoconstriction, anaphylaxis, Stevens Johnson syndrome, and toxic epidermal necrolysis) to peginterferon alfa-2b, interferon alfa-2b, other alfa interferons, or any component of the formulation; autoimmune hepatitis; decompensated liver disease (Child-Pugh score >6, classes B and C)

Documentation of allergenic cross-reactivity for interferons is limited. However, because of similarities in chemical structure and/or pharmacologic actions, the possibility of cross-sensitivity cannot be ruled out with certainty

Combination therapy with peginterferon alfa-2b and ribavirin is also contraindicated in pregnancy, women who may become pregnant, males with pregnant partners; hemoglobinopathies (eg, thalassemia major, sickle-cell anemia); renal dysfunction (CrCl <50 mL/minute)

Pregnancy Considerations Use with ribavirin is contraindicated in pregnant women and males whose female partners are pregnant.

[US Boxed Warning]: Combination therapy with ribavirin may cause birth defects and/or fetal mortality; avoid pregnancy in females and female partners of male patients. Two forms of contraception should be used along with monthly pregnancy tests during combination therapy and for 6 months after therapy has been discontinued. If used in combination with ribavirin, all warnings related to the use of ribavirin and pregnancy and/or contraception should be followed.

Reproduction studies with pegylated interferon alfa have not been conducted. Animal reproduction studies with nonpegylated interferon alfa-2b have demonstrated abortifacient effects. Disruption of the normal menstrual cycle was also observed in animal studies; therefore, the manufacturer recommends that reliable contraception is used in women of childbearing potential. Alfa interferon is endogenous to normal amniotic fluid (Lebon 1982). In vitro administration studies have reported that when administered to the mother, it does not cross the placenta (Waysbort 1993). Case reports of use in pregnant women are limited.

The HHS Perinatal HIV Guidelines do not recommend that peginterferon alfa be used during pregnancy (HHS [perinatal] 2016). Mother-to-child transmission of HCV does not occur if the woman is not viremic, therefore, HCV-infected women of childbearing potential should postpone pregnancy until therapy is complete. Treatment of HCV is not recommended for women who are already pregnant (AASLD/IDSA 2015).

A pregnancy registry has been established for women inadvertently exposed to ribavirin while pregnant (800-593-2214).

Breastfeeding Considerations Breast milk samples obtained from a lactating mother prior to and after administration of interferon alfa-2b showed that interferon alfa is present in breast milk and administration of the medication did not significantly affect endogenous levels (Kumar, 2000). Breastfeeding is not linked to the spread of hepatitis C virus (ACOG 2007); however, if nipples are cracked or bleeding, breastfeeding is not recommended (CDC [Workowski] 2015). Mothers coinfected with HIV are discouraged from breastfeeding to decrease potential transmission of HIV (HHS [perinatal] 2015).

Warnings/Precautions [US Boxed Warnings]: May cause or aggravate severe depression or other neuropsychiatric adverse events (including suicide and suicidal ideation) in patients with and without a history of psychiatric disorder; monitor closely with clinical evaluations (periodic); discontinue treatment with worsening or persistently severe signs/ symptoms of neuropsychiatric disorders (eg, depression, encephalopathy, psychosis). Many cases resolve upon discontinuation, although some cases may persist. May cause or aggravate fatal or life-threatening autoimmune disorders, infectious disorders, ischemic disorders; monitor closely with clinical evaluations (periodic); discontinue treatment in patients with worsening or persistently severe signs/symptoms of infectious disorders; may resolve with discontinuation. May also cause hemorrhagic cerebrovascular events.

Neuropsychiatric disorders: Neuropsychiatric effects may occur in patients with and without a history of psychiatric disorder; addiction relapse, aggression, depression, homicidal ideation and suicidal behavior/ideation have been observed with peginterferon alfa-2b; bipolar disorder, encephalopathy, hallucinations, mania, and psychosis have been observed with other alfa interferons. Onset may be delayed (up to 6 months after discontinuation). Higher doses may be associated with the development of encephalopathy (higher risk in elderly patients). Use with caution in patients with a history of psychiatric disorders, including depression or substance abuse history. New or exacerbated neuropsychiatric or substance abuse disorders are best managed with early intervention. Drug screening and periodic health evaluation (including monitoring of psychiatric symptoms) is recommended if initiating treatment in patients with coexisting psychiatric condition or substance abuse disorders. Monitor all patients for evidence of depression and other psychiatric symptoms; patients being treated for melanoma should be monitored for depression and psychiatric symptoms every 3 weeks during the first 8 weeks of treatment and every 6 months thereafter; permanently discontinue treatment if psychiatric symptoms persist, worsen or if suicidal behavior develops. Patients should continue to be monitored for 6 months after completion of therapy.

Bone marrow suppression: Causes bone marrow suppression, including potentially severe cytopenias; alfa interferons may (rarely) cause aplastic anemia. Use with caution in patients who are chronically immunosuppressed, with low peripheral blood counts or myelosuppression, including concurrent use of myelosuppressive therapy. Dosage modification may be necessary for hematologic toxicity. Combination therapy with ribavirin may potentiate the neutropenic effects of alfa interferons. When used in combination with ribavirin, an increased incidence of anemia was observed when using ribavirin weight-based dosing, as compared to flat-dose ribavirin.

Hepatic disease: Use is contraindicated in patients with hepatic decompensation or autoimmune hepatitis. Discontinue treatment immediately with hepatic decompensation (Child Pugh score >6) or evidence of severe hepatic injury. Patients with chronic hepatitis C (CHC) with cirrhosis receiving peginterferon alfa-2b are at risk for hepatic decompensation. CHC patients coinfected with human immunodeficiency virus (HIV) are at increased risk for hepatic decompensation when receiving antiretroviral therapy; monitor closely. A transient increase in ALT (2 to 5 times above baseline) which is not associated with deterioration of liver function may occur with peginterferon alfa-2b use (for the treatment of chronic hepatitis C); therapy generally may continue with monitoring. Instruct patients to avoid alcohol; may increase hepatic effects.

Gastrointestinal disorders: Pancreatitis (including fatal cases) has been observed with alfa interferon therapy; discontinue therapy if known or suspected pancreatitis develops. Ulcerative or hemorrhagic/ischemic colitis has been observed with alfa interferons (within 12 weeks of initiation); withhold treatment for suspected pancreatitis; discontinue therapy for known pancreatitis. Ulcerative or hemorrhagic/ischemic colitis has been observed with alfa interferons; discontinue therapy if signs of colitis (abdominal pain, bloody diarrhea, fever) develop; symptoms typically resolve within 1 to 3 weeks.

Autoimmune disorders: Thyroiditis, thrombotic microangiopathy, immune thrombocytopenia, rheumatoid arthritis, interstitial nephritis, systemic lupus erythematosus, and psoriasis have been reported with therapy; use with caution in patients with autoimmune disorders.

Cardiovascular disease: Use with caution in patients with cardiovascular disease or a history of cardiovascular disease; hypotension, arrhythmia, bundle branch block, tachycardia, cardiomyopathy, angina pectoris and MI have been observed with treatment. Patients with preexisting cardiac abnormalities should have baseline ECGs prior to combination treatment with ribavirin; closely monitor patients with a history of MI or arrhythmia. Patients with a history of significant or unstable cardiac disease should not receive combination treatment with ribavirin. Discontinue treatment (permanently) for new-onset ventricular arrhythmia or cardiovascular decompensation.

Endocrine disorders: Diabetes mellitus (including new-onset type I diabetes), hyperglycemia, and thyroid disorders have been reported; discontinue peginterferon alfa-2b if cannot be effectively managed with medication. Use caution in patients with a history of diabetes mellitus, particularly if prone to DKA. Use with caution in patients with thyroid disorders; may cause or aggravate hyper- or hypothyroidism.

Pulmonary disease: May cause or aggravate dyspnea, pulmonary infiltrates, pneumonia, bronchiolitis obliterans, interstitial pneumonitis, pulmonary hypertension, and sarcoidosis which may result in respiratory failure; may recur upon rechallenge with treatment; monitor closely. Use with caution in patients with existing pulmonary disease (eg, chronic obstructive pulmonary disease). Withhold combination therapy with ribavirin for development of pulmonary infiltrate or pulmonary function impairment.

Ophthalmic disorders: Ophthalmologic disorders (including decreased visual acuity, blindness, macular edema, retinal hemorrhages, optic neuritis, papilledema, cotton wool spots, retinal detachment [serous], and retinal artery or vein thrombosis) have occurred with peginterferon alfa-2b and/or with other alfa interferons. Prior to start of therapy, ophthalmic exams are recommended for all patients; patients with diabetic or hypertensive retinopathy should have periodic ophthalmic exams during treatment; a complete eye exam should be done promptly in patients who develop ocular symptoms. Permanently discontinue treatment with new or worsening ophthalmic disorder.

[US Boxed Warning]: Combination treatment with ribavirin may cause birth defects and/or fetal mortality (avoid pregnancy in females and female partners of male patients); hemolytic anemia (which may worsen cardiac disease), genotoxicity, mutagenicity, and may possibly be carcinogenic. Potentially significant drug-drug interactions may exist, requiring dose or frequency adjustment, additional monitoring, and/or selection of alternative therapy. Peripheral neuropathy has been reported with alpha interferons when used in combination with telbivudine. Interferon therapy is commonly associated with flu-like symptoms, including fever; rule out other causes/infection with persistent or high fever. Acute hypersensitivity reactions (eg, urticaria, angioedema, bronchoconstriction, anaphylaxis) and cutaneous reactions (eg, Stevens-Johnson syndrome, toxic epidermal necrolysis) have been reported (rarely) with alfa interferons; prompt discontinuation is recommended; transient rashes do not require interruption of therapy. Hypertriglyceridemia has been reported (may result in pancreatitis); periodically monitor and manage with appropriate treatment; consider discontinuing peginterferon if persistent and severe (triglycerides >1000 mg/dL), particularly if combined with symptoms of pancreatitis. Interferons are commonly associated with flu-like symptoms. Use with caution in patients with debilitating conditions. Use with caution in patients with renal impairment (CrCl <50 mL/minute); monitor closely for signs of interferon toxicity. For the treatment of chronic hepatitis C, dosage adjustments are recommended with monotherapy in patients with moderate-to-severe impairment; do not use combination therapy with ribavirin in adult patients renal dysfunction (CrCl <50 mL/minute); discontinue if serum creatinine >2 mg/dL in children. Dosage adjustment is also recommended when used for the treatment of melanoma. Serum creatinine increases have been reported in patients with renal insufficiency. Use with caution in the elderly; the potential adverse effects (eg, neuropsychiatric events, cardiac events, systemic effects) may be more pronounced. Encephalopathy has also been observed in primarily elderly patients treated with higher doses of peginterferon alfa-2b. For the treatment of hepatitis, elderly patients generally do not respond to interferon treatment as well as younger patients. When used in combination with ribavirin, closely monitor adults >50 years of age for the development of anemia. Dental/periodontal disorders have been reported with combination therapy; dry mouth may affect teeth and mucous membranes; instruct patients to brush teeth twice daily; encourage regular dental exams; rinse mouth thoroughly after vomiting.

Combination therapy with ribavirin or monotherapy for the treatment of chronic hepatitis C is not a recommended treatment regimen (AASLD/IDSA 2015). Safety and efficacy have not been established in patients who have received organ transplants or are coinfected with HIV or hepatitis B. Patients with significant bridging fibrosis or cirrhosis, genotype 1 infection or who have not responded to prior therapy, including previous pegylated interferon treatment are less likely to benefit from combination therapy with peginterferon alfa-2b and ribavirin. Growth velocity (height and weight) was decreased in children on combination treatment with ribavirin during the length of treatment. Severely inhibited growth velocity has been noted. Long-term follow-up data indicate that combination therapy may inhibit growth, resulting in reduced adult height in some patients. Growth should be closely monitored in pediatric patients during therapy and posttreatment. **[US Boxed Warning]: Combination therapy with ribavirin is contraindicated in pregnancy.** Due to differences in dosage, patients should not change brands of interferon. Some dosage forms may contain polysorbate 80 (also known as Tweens). Hypersensitivity reactions, usually a delayed reaction, have been reported following exposure to pharmaceutical products containing polysorbate 80 in certain individuals (Isaksson, 2002; Lucente 2000; Shelley, 1995). Thrombocytopenia, ascites, pulmonary deterioration, and renal and hepatic failure have been reported in premature neonates after receiving parenteral products containing polysorbate 80 (Alade, 1986; CDC, 1984). See manufacturer's labeling.

Adverse Reactions

Antiviral:

>10%:

Central nervous system: Headache (56%), fatigue (including asthenia; ≤52%), depression (29%), anxiety (≤28%), emotional lability (≤28%), irritability (≤28%), insomnia (23%), rigors (23%), dizziness (12%)

Dermatologic: Alopecia (22%), pruritus (12%)

Endocrine & metabolic: Weight Loss (11%)

Gastrointestinal: Nausea (26%), anorexia (20%), diarrhea (18%), abdominal pain (15%)

Infection: Viral infection (11%)

Local: Inflammation at injection site (47%), injection site reaction (47%)

Neuromuscular & skeletal: Myalgia (54%), weakness (52%), musculoskeletal pain (28%), arthralgia (23%)

Miscellaneous: Fever (22%)

1% to 10%:

Cardiovascular: Chest pain (6%), flushing (6%)

Central nervous system: Lack of concentration (10%), right upper quadrant pain (8%), malaise (7%), nervousness (4%), agitation (2%), suicidal ideation (≤2%)

Dermatologic: Diaphoresis (6%), skin rash (6%)

Endocrine & metabolic: Hypothyroidism (5%), menstrual disease (4%), hyperthyroidism (3%)

Gastrointestinal: Vomiting (7%), dyspepsia (6%), xerostomia (6%), constipation (1%)

Hematologic & oncologic: Thrombocytopenia (7%), neutropenia (6%)

Hepatic: Increased serum ALT (10%), hepatomegaly (6%)

Immunologic: Antibody development (neutralizing: 2%)

Local: Pain at injection site (2% to 3%)

Ophthalmic: Conjunctivitis (4%), blurred vision (2%)

Respiratory: Pharyngitis (10%), cough (8%), sinusitis (7%), dyspnea (4%), rhinitis (2%)

Antineoplastic:

>10%:

Central nervous system: Fatigue (94%), headache (70%), chills (63%), depression (59%, grades 3/4: 7%), dizziness (35%), neuropathy (olfactory) (23%), paresthesia (21%)

Dermatologic: Exfoliative rash (36%), alopecia (34%)

Endocrine & metabolic: Weight loss (11%)

Gastrointestinal: Anorexia (69%), nausea (64%), dysgeusia (38%), diarrhea (37%), vomiting (26%)

Hepatic: Increased serum ALT (≤77%, grades 3/4: ≤11%), increased serum AST (≤77%, grades 3/4: ≤11%), increased serum alkaline phosphatase (23%)

Immunologic: Antibody development (binding antibodies: 35%)

Local: Injection site reaction (62%)

Neuromuscular & skeletal: Myalgia (68%), arthralgia (51%)

Miscellaneous: Fever (75%)

1% to 10%:

Cardiovascular: Bundle branch block (≤4%), myocardial infarction (≤4%), supraventricular cardiac arrhythmia (≤4%), ventricular tachycardia (≤4%)

Endocrine & metabolic: Increased gamma-glutamyl transferase (8%, grades 3/4: 4%)

Genitourinary: Proteinuria (7%)

Hematologic & oncologic: Anemia (6%)

Respiratory: Dyspnea (6%), cough (5%)

<1%, postmarketing, and/or case reports: Aggressive behavior, amnesia, anaphylaxis, angina pectoris, angioedema, aphthous stomatitis, aplastic anemia, auditory impairment, bacterial infection, bipolar mood disorder, brain disease (including exacerbations), bronchiolitis obliterans, bronchoconstriction, cardiac arrest, cardiac arrhythmia, cardiomyopathy, cerebrovascular accident, colitis, cytopenia, dehydration, diabetes mellitus, diabetic ketoacidosis, drug dependence (including relapse), drug overdose, dysgeusia, erythema multiforme, exacerbation of autoimmune disease, fungal infection, hallucination, hearing loss, hemorrhagic colitis, homicidal ideation, hyperglycemia, hypersensitivity reaction, hypertension, hypertriglyceridemia, hypotension, immune thrombocytopenia, interstitial nephritis, interstitial pneumonitis, ischemic colitis, leukopenia, lupus-like syndrome, macular edema, mania, migraine, myositis, optic neuritis, palpitations, pancreatitis, papilledema, paresthesia, peripheral neuropathy, pneumonia, psoriasis, pulmonary fibrosis, pulmonary hypertension, pulmonary infiltrates, pure red cell aplasia, renal failure, renal insufficiency (includes increases in serum creatinine), retinal cotton-wool spot, retinal detachment, retinal hemorrhage, retinal thrombosis, retinopathy, rhabdomyolysis, rheumatoid arthritis, sarcoidosis, seizure, sepsis, Stevens-Johnson syndrome, systemic lupus erythematosus, tachycardia, thrombotic thrombocytopenic purpura, thyroiditis, toxic epidermal necrolysis, ulcerative colitis, urticaria, vertigo, vision loss, visual disturbance, Vogt-Koyanagi-Harada syndrome

Drug Interactions

Metabolism/Transport Effects Inhibits CYP1A2 (weak)

Avoid Concomitant Use

Avoid concomitant use of Peginterferon Alfa-2b with any of the following: BCG (Intravesical); Deferiprone; Dipyrone; Telbivudine

Increased Effect/Toxicity

Peginterferon Alfa-2b may increase the levels/effects of: Aldesleukin; CloZAPine; CYP1A2 Substrates; CYP2D6 Substrates; Deferiprone; Methadone; Ribavirin (Oral Inhalation); Ribavirin (Systemic); Telbivudine; TiZANidine; Zidovudine

The levels/effects of Peginterferon Alfa-2b may be increased by: Dipyrone; Promazine

Decreased Effect

Peginterferon Alfa-2b may decrease the levels/effects of: BCG (Intravesical); CYP2D6 Substrates; FLUoxetine

The levels/effects of Peginterferon Alfa-2b may be decreased by: Pegloticase

Storage/Stability Prior to reconstitution, store Redipen at 2°C to 8°C (36°F to 46°F). Store intact vials at 25°C (77°F); excursions permitted to 15°C to 30°C (59°F to 86°F). Do not freeze. Once reconstituted each product should be used immediately or may be stored for ≤24 hours at 2°C to 8°C (36°F to 46°F); do not freeze. Do not shake. Keep away from heat. Products do not contain preservative (single use; do not reuse).

Preparation for Administration

Redipen: Hold cartridge upright and press the two halves together until there is a "click". Gently invert to mix; do not shake; do not reuse (single use).

Peg-Intron (vial): Add 0.7 mL sterile water for injection, USP (supplied single-use diluent; discard unused portion) to the vial. Gently swirl. Do not re-enter vial after dose removed.

Sylatron (vial): Add 0.7 mL sterile water for injection and swirl gently (do not shake), resulting in the following concentrations (do not withdraw more than 0.5 mL from each vial):

296 mcg vial: 40 mcg/0.1 mL

444 mcg vial: 60 mcg/0.1 mL

888 mcg vial: 120 mcg/0.1 mL

Mechanism of Action Alpha interferons are a family of proteins, produced by nucleated cells, that have antiviral, antiproliferative, and immune-regulating activity. There are 16 known subtypes of alpha interferons. Interferons interact with cells through high affinity cell surface receptors. Following activation, multiple effects can be detected including induction of gene transcription. Inhibits cellular growth, alters the state of cellular differentiation, interferes with oncogene expression, alters cell surface antigen expression, increases phagocytic activity of macrophages, and augments cytotoxicity of lymphocytes for target cells.

Pharmacodynamics/Kinetics

Bioavailability: Increases with chronic dosing

Half-life elimination: CHC: ~40 hours (range: 22 to 60 hours); Melanoma: ~43 to 51 hours

Time to peak: CHC: 15 to 44 hours

Excretion: Urine (~30%); clearance reduced in renal impairment by 17% in moderate dysfunction, 44% in severe dysfunction

Dosing

Adult & Geriatric

Melanoma: SubQ: Initial: 6 mcg/kg/week for 8 doses; Maintenance: 3 mcg/kg/week for up to 5 years. **Note:** Premedicate with acetaminophen (500-1000 mg orally) 30 minutes prior to the first dose and as needed for subsequent doses thereafter.

Chronic hepatitis C (CHC): SubQ:

Manufacturer's labeling: **Note:** Discontinue after 12 weeks in patients with HCV (genotype 1) if HCV RNA does not decrease by at least 2 log (compared to pretreatment) or if detectable HCV RNA present at 24. Discontinuation is also recommended in patients who previously failed therapy (regardless of genotype) if detectable HCV RNA present at 12 or 24 weeks.

Combination therapy with ribavirin: **Note:** Combination therapy with ribavirin (without the addition of another preferred HCV antiviral agent) is **not** recommended in HCV treatment guidelines (treatment-naive or treatment-experienced patients) (AASLD/IDSA 2015). Current AASLD/IDSA recommendations do not specify a particular peginterferon (eg, 2a or 2b); however, guideline recommendations are based on clinical trials that used peginterferon alfa-2a.

Initial dose (based on an average weekly dose of 1.5 mcg/kg):
  <40 kg: 50 mcg once weekly (with ribavirin 800 mg/day)
  40 to 50 kg: 64 mcg once weekly (with ribavirin 800 mg/day)
  51 to 60 kg: 80 mcg once weekly (with ribavirin 800 mg/day)
  61 to 65 kg: 96 mcg once weekly (with ribavirin 800 mg/day)
  66 to 75 kg: 96 mcg once weekly (with ribavirin 1,000 mg/day)
  76 to 80 kg: 120 mcg once weekly (with ribavirin 1,000 mg/day)
  81 to 85 kg: 120 mcg once weekly (with ribavirin 1200 mg/day)
  86 to 105 kg: 150 mcg once weekly (with ribavirin 1,200 mg/day)
  >105 kg: 1.5 mcg/kg once weekly (with ribavirin 1,400 mg/day)

Treatment duration: 48 weeks for genotype 1, 24 weeks for genotypes 2 and 3, or 48 weeks for patients who previously failed therapy (regardless of genotype)

Monotherapy: **Note:** Monotherapy is **not** recommended in HCV treatment guidelines (treatment-naive or treatment-experienced patients) (AASLD/IDSA 2015). Current AASLD/IDSA recommendations do not specify a particular peginterferon (eg, 2a or 2b); however, guideline recommendations are based on clinical trials that used peginterferon alfa-2a. It is not known whether peginterferon alfa 2b could be used interchangeably. Please refer to AASLD/IDSA clinical practice guidelines for further guidance.

Initial dose (based on average weekly dose of 1 mcg/kg):
  ≤45 kg: 40 mcg once weekly
  46 to 56 kg: 50 mcg once weekly
  57 to 72 kg: 64 mcg once weekly
  73 to 88 kg: 80 mcg once weekly
  89 to 106 kg: 96 mcg once weekly
  107 to 136 kg: 120 mcg once weekly
  137 to 160 kg: 150 mcg once weekly

Treatment duration: 1 year

Pediatric Chronic hepatitis C (CHC):

Manufacturer labeling: Children 3 to 17 years: SubQ: Combination therapy with ribavirin: 60 mcg/m^2 once weekly; **Note:** Children who reach their 18th birthday during treatment should remain on the pediatric regimen. Treatment duration is 48 weeks for genotype 1, 24 weeks for genotypes 2 and 3. Discontinue combination therapy in patients with HCV (genotype 1) at 12 weeks if HCV-RNA does not decrease by at least 2 log (compared to pretreatment) or if detectable HCV-RNA present at 24 weeks.

Renal Impairment Chronic hepatitis C:

Peginterferon alfa-2b combination with ribavirin:
  Adults: CrCl <50 mL/minute: Combination therapy with ribavirin is not recommended.
  Children: Serum creatinine >2 mg/dL: Discontinue treatment.

Peginterferon alfa-2b monotherapy:
  CrCl 30 to 50 mL/minute: Reduce dose by 25%
  CrCl 10 to 29 mL/minute: Reduce dose by 50%

◄   Hemodialysis: Reduce dose by 50%

Discontinue use if renal function declines during treatment.

Melanoma:

CrCl >50 mL/minute/1.73 m^2: No dosage adjustment is necessary.

CrCl 30 to 50 mL/minute/1.73 m^2: Reduce initial dose to 4.5 mcg/kg/week; reduce maintenance dose to 2.25 mcg/kg/week

CrCl <30 mL/minute/1.73 m^2 and ESRD on dialysis: Reduce initial dose to 3 mcg/kg/week; reduce maintenance dose to 1.5 mcg/kg/week

Hemodialysis: Following a single 1 mcg/kg/ dose, no clinically meaningful amount of peginterferon alfa-2b was removed during hemodialysis.

Hepatic Impairment

Decompensated liver disease or autoimmune hepatitis: Use is contraindicated.

Hepatic decompensation or severe hepatic injury during treatment (Child-Pugh score >6 [class B or C]): Discontinue immediately.

Adjustment for Toxicity

Melanoma:

Discontinue for any of the following: Persistent or worsening severe neuropsychiatric disorders (depression, psychosis, encephalopathy), grade 4 nonhematologic toxicity, new or worsening retinopathy, new-onset ventricular arrhythmia or cardiovascular decompensation, evidence of hepatic injury (severe) or hepatic decompensation (Child-Pugh score >6 [Class B or C]), development of hyper- or hypothyroidism or diabetes that cannot be effectively managed with medication, or inability to tolerate a dose of 1 mcg/kg/week

Temporarily withhold for any of the following: ANC <500/mm^3, platelets <50,000/mm^3, ECOG performance status (PS) ≥2, nonhematologic toxicity ≥ grade 3

May reinitiate at a reduced dose once ANC ≥500/mm^3, platelets ≥50,000/mm^3, ECOG PS at 0 to 1, and nonhematologic toxicity completely resolved or improved to grade 1.

Reduced dose schedule, Weeks 1 to 8:

First dose reduction (if prior dose 6 mcg/kg/week): 3 mcg/kg/week

Second dose reduction (if prior dose 3 mcg/kg/week): 2 mcg/kg/week

Third dose reduction (if prior dose 2 mcg/kg/week): 1 mcg/kg/week

Discontinue permanently if unable to tolerate 1 mcg/kg/week

Reduced dose schedule, Weeks 9 to 260:

First dose reduction (if prior dose 3 mcg/kg/week): 2 mcg/kg/week

Second dose reduction (if prior dose 2 mcg/kg/week): 1 mcg/kg/week

Discontinue permanently if unable to tolerate 1 mcg/kg/week

Chronic hepatitis C: Dosage adjustment for depression (severity based upon DSM-IV criteria):

Mild depression: No dosage adjustment required; evaluate once weekly by visit/phone call. If depression remains stable, continue weekly visits. If depression improves, resume normal visit schedule. For worsening depression, see "Moderate depression" or "Severe depression".

Moderate depression: **Note:** Evaluate once weekly (visit or phone) with an office visit at least every other week. If depression remains stable, consider psychiatric evaluation and continue with reduced dosing. If symptoms improve and remain stable for 4 weeks, resume normal visit schedule; continue reduced dosing or return to normal dose. For worsening depression, see "Severe depression".

Children: Decrease peginterferon alfa-2b dose to 40 mcg/m^2/week, may further decrease to 20 mcg/m^2/week if needed

Adults:

Peginterferon alfa-2b combination therapy: Refer to adult weight-based dosage reduction with combination therapy for depression below

Peginterferon alfa-2b monotherapy: Refer to adult weight-based dosage reduction with monotherapy for depression below

Severe depression: Discontinue peginterferon alfa-2b and ribavirin permanently. Obtain immediate psychiatric consultation. Utilize followup psychiatric therapy as needed.

Chronic hepatitis C: Dosage adjustment in hematologic toxicity:

Children:

Hemoglobin decrease ≥2 g/dL in any 4-week period and stable cardiac disease: Decrease peginterferon alfa-2b dose by 50%; decrease ribavirin dose by 200 mg daily (regardless of the patient's initial dose); monitor and evaluate weekly. If hemoglobin <8.5 g/dL any time after dose reduction or <12 g/dL after 4 weeks of dose reduction, permanently discontinue both peginterferon alfa-2b and ribavirin.

Hemoglobin 8.5 to <10 g/dL and no history of cardiac disease: Decrease ribavirin dose to 12 mg/kg/day; may further reduce to 8 mg/kg/day; no dosage adjustment necessary for peginterferon alfa-2b.

WBC 1000 to <1500/mm^3, neutrophils 500 to <750/mm^3, or platelets 50,000 to <70,000/mm^3: Reduce peginterferon alfa-2b dose to 40 mcg/m^2/week; may further reduce to 20 mcg/m^2/week

Hemoglobin <8.5 g/dL, WBC <1000/mm^3, neutrophils <500/mm^3, or platelets <50,000/mm^3: Permanently discontinue peginterferon alfa-2b and ribavirin

Adults:

Hemoglobin decrease ≥2 g/dL in any 4-week period and stable cardiac disease: Decrease peginterferon alfa-2b dose by 50%; decrease ribavirin dose by 200 mg daily. If hemoglobin <8.5 g/dL any time after dose reduction or <12 g/dL after 4 weeks of dose reduction, permanently discontinue both peginterferon alfa-2b and ribavirin.

Hemoglobin 8.5 to <10 g/dL and no history of cardiac disease: Decrease ribavirin dose by 200 mg daily (patients receiving 1400 mg daily should decrease dose by 400 mg daily [ie, first dose reduction to 1000 mg daily]); may further reduce ribavirin dose by additional 200 mg daily if needed. No dosage adjustment necessary for peginterferon alfa-2b.

WBC 1000 to <1500/mm^3, neutrophils 500 to <750/mm^3, or platelets 25,000 to <50,000/mm^3:

Peginterferon alfa-2b combination therapy: Refer to adult weight-based dosage reduction with combination therapy for hematologic toxicity below.

Peginterferon alfa-2b monotherapy: Refer to adult weight-based dosage reduction monotherapy for hematologic toxicity below.

Hemoglobin <8.5 g/dL, WBC <1000/mm^3, neutrophils <500/mm^3, or platelets <25,000/mm^3: Permanently discontinue peginterferon alfa-2b and ribavirin.

◄

Chronic hepatitis C: **Adult weight-based dosage reduction for depression or hematologic toxicity:**

Peginterferon alfa-2b combination therapy: Initially reduce to average weekly dose of 1 mcg/kg; may further reduce to average weekly dose of 0.5 mcg/kg if needed as follows:

<40 kg: 35 mcg once weekly; may further reduce to 20 mcg once weekly if needed

40 to 50 kg: 45 mcg once weekly; may further reduce to 25 mcg once weekly if needed

51 to 60 kg: 50 mcg once weekly; may further reduce to 30 mcg once weekly if needed

61 to 75 kg: 64 mcg once weekly; may further reduce to 35 mcg once weekly if needed

76 to 85 kg: 80 mcg once weekly; may further reduce to 45 mcg once weekly if needed

86 to 104 kg: 96 mcg once weekly; may further reduce to 50 mcg once weekly if needed

105 to 125 kg: 108 mcg once weekly; may further reduce to 64 mcg once weekly if needed

>125 kg: 135 mcg once weekly; may further reduce to 72 mcg once weekly if needed

Peginterferon alfa-2b monotherapy: Reduce to average weekly dose of 0.5 mcg/kg as follows:

≤45 kg: 20 mcg once weekly

46 to 56 kg: 25 mcg once weekly

57 to 72 kg: 30 mcg once weekly

73 to 88 kg: 40 mcg once weekly

89 to 106 kg: 50 mcg once weekly

107 to 136 kg: 64 mcg once weekly

≥137 kg: 80 mcg once weekly

Administration For SubQ administration; rotate injection site; thigh, outer surface of upper arm, and abdomen are preferred injection sites; do not inject near navel or waistline; patients who are thin should only use thigh or upper arm. Do not inject into bruised, infected, irritated, red, or scarred skin. The weekly dose may be administered at bedtime to reduce flu-like symptoms. For the treatment of CHC, the administration volume depends on the patient's weight and the peginterferon concentration used.

Emetic Potential Children and Adults: Minimal (<10%)

Monitoring Parameters

Manufacturer's labeling:

Baseline and periodic TSH (for patients being treated for melanoma, obtain baseline within 4 weeks prior to treatment initiation, and then at 3 and 6 months, and every 6 months thereafter during treatment); CBC with differential and platelets; serum chemistries, liver function tests (for patients with melanoma, monitor serum bilirubin, ALT, AST, alkaline phosphatase, and LDH at 2 and 8 weeks, and 2 and 3 months following initiation, then every 6 months during therapy), renal function, triglycerides; serum glucose or HbA_{1c} (for patients with diabetes mellitus). Clinical studies (for combination therapy) tested as follows: CBC (including hemoglobin, WBC, and platelets) and chemistries (including liver function tests and uric acid) measured at weeks 2, 4, 8, and 12, and then every 6 weeks; TSH measured every 12 weeks during treatment. ECG at baseline for patients with preexisting cardiac abnormalities (for combination therapy with ribavirin).

Evaluate for depression and other psychiatric symptoms before and after initiation of therapy; patients being treated for melanoma should be monitored for depression and psychiatric symptoms every 3 weeks during the first eight weeks of treatment and every 6 months thereafter, and continued monitoring for 6 months after the last dose; baseline ophthalmic eye examination; periodic ophthalmic exam in patients with diabetic or hypertensive retinopathy; baseline ECG in patients with cardiac disease; serum glucose or HbA$_{1c}$ (for patients with diabetes mellitus). In combination therapy with ribavirin, pregnancy tests (for women of childbearing age who are receiving treatment or who have male partners who are receiving treatment), continue monthly up to 6 months after discontinuation of therapy. In pediatric patients, growth velocity and weight should also be monitored during and periodically after treatment discontinuation.

Hepatitic C: Serum HCV RNA levels (pretreatment, 12 and 24 weeks after therapy initiation, 24 weeks after completion of therapy).

Alternate recommendations (AASLD/IDSA 2015): Chronic Hepatitis C:

Baseline (within 12 weeks prior to starting antiviral therapy): CBC, INR, hepatic function panel (albumin, total and direct bilirubin, ALT, AST, and alkaline phosphatase), calculated GFR.

Baseline (at any time prior to starting antiviral therapy): HCV genotype and subtype, quantitative HCV viral load.

During therapy: CBC, serum creatinine, calculated GFR, hepatic function panel (after 4 weeks of therapy and as clinically indicated); quantitative HCV viral load testing (after 4 weeks of therapy and at 12 weeks after completion of therapy). If quantitative HCV viral load is detectable at treatment week 4, repeat testing is recommended after 2 additional weeks of treatment (treatment week 6).

Medication Guide Available Yes

Dosage Forms Excipient information presented when available (limited, particularly for generics); consult specific product labeling. [DSC] = Discontinued product

Kit, Subcutaneous:

Sylatron: 4 x 200 mcg, 4 x 300 mcg [contains polysorbate 80]

Kit, Subcutaneous [preservative free]:

Peg-Intron Redipen: 50 mcg/0.5 mL [DSC], 80 mcg/0.5 mL [DSC], 120 mcg/0.5 mL [DSC], 150 mcg/0.5 mL [DSC]

Peg-Intron Redipen Pak 4: 50 mcg/0.5 mL [DSC], 80 mcg/0.5 mL [DSC], 120 mcg/0.5 mL [DSC], 150 mcg/0.5 mL [DSC]

PegIntron: 50 mcg/0.5 mL, 80 mcg/0.5 mL, 120 mcg/0.5 mL, 150 mcg/0.5 mL [contains polysorbate 80]

Sylatron: 200 mcg, 300 mcg, 600 mcg [contains polysorbate 80]

◆ **PegIntron** *see* Peginterferon Alfa-2b *on page* 1473

◆ **Peg-Intron Redipen [DSC]** *see* Peginterferon Alfa-2b *on page* 1473

◆ **Peg-Intron Redipen Pak 4 [DSC]** *see* Peginterferon Alfa-2b *on page* 1473

◆ **PEGLA** *see* Pegaspargase *on page* 1462

◆ **Pegylated DOXOrubicin Liposomal** *see* DOXOrubicin (Liposomal) *on page* 636

◆ **Pegylated G-CSF** *see* Pegfilgrastim *on page* 1467

◆ **Pegylated Interferon Alfa-2b** *see* Peginterferon Alfa-2b *on page* 1473

◆ **Pegylated Liposomal DOXOrubicin** *see* DOXOrubicin (Liposomal) *on page* 636

◆ **Pegylated Liposomal DOXOrubicin Hydrochloride (Doxil, Caelyx)** *see* DOXOrubicin (Liposomal) *on page 636*

Pembrolizumab (pem broe LIZ ue mab)

Brand Names: US Keytruda

Brand Names: Canada Keytruda

Index Terms Anti-PD-1 Monoclonal Antibody MK-3475; Lambrolizumab; MK-3475; SCH 90045

Pharmacologic Category Antineoplastic Agent, Anti-PD-1 Monoclonal Antibody; Antineoplastic Agent, Monoclonal Antibody

Use

Head and neck cancer, squamous cell (recurrent or metastatic): Treatment of recurrent or metastatic squamous cell carcinoma of the head and neck in patients with disease progression on or after platinum-containing chemotherapy.

Hodgkin lymphoma, classical (relapsed or refractory): Treatment of adult and pediatric patients with refractory classical Hodgkin lymphoma or patients who have relapsed after 3 or more prior lines of therapy.

Melanoma (unresectable or metastatic): Treatment of unresectable or metastatic melanoma.

Microsatellite instability-high cancer (unresectable or metastatic):

Solid tumors: Treatment of unresectable or metastatic, microsatellite instability-high (MSI-H) or mismatch repair deficient solid tumors in adult and pediatric patients that have progressed following prior treatment and have no satisfactory alternate treatment options.

Limitation of use: Safety and efficacy in pediatric patients with MSI-H central nervous system cancers have not been established.

Colorectal cancer: Treatment of unresectable or metastatic, MSI-H or mismatch repair deficient colorectal cancer in patients that have progressed following treatment with a fluoropyrimidine, oxaliplatin, and irinotecan.

Non-small cell lung cancer (metastatic):

First-line, single-agent treatment of metastatic non-small cell lung cancer (NSCLC) in patients with tumors with high PD-L1 expression (tumor proportion score [TPS] ≥50%), as determined by an approved test, and with no EGFR or ALK genomic tumor aberrations.

First-line treatment (in combination with pemetrexed and carboplatin) of metastatic nonsquamous NSCLC

Single-agent treatment of metastatic NSCLC in patients with tumors with PD-L1 expression (TPS ≥1%), as determined by an approved test, and with disease progression on or following platinum-containing chemotherapy. Patients with EGFR or ALK genomic tumor aberrations should have disease progression (on approved EGFR- or ALK-directed therapy) prior to receiving pembrolizumab.

Urothelial carcinoma (locally advanced or metastatic):

Treatment of locally advanced or metastatic urothelial cancer in patients who are not eligible for cisplatin-containing treatment.

Treatment of locally advanced or metastatic urothelial cancer in patients with disease progression during or after platinum-containing chemotherapy or within 12 months of neoadjuvant or adjuvant platinum-containing chemotherapy.

Labeled Contraindications There are no contraindications listed in the manufacturer's US labeling.

Canadian labeling: Hypersensitivity to pembrolizumab or any component of the formulation.

Pregnancy Considerations Animal reproduction studies have not been conducted. Immunoglobulins are known to cross the placenta; therefore fetal exposure to pembrolizumab is expected. Based on the mechanism of action, pembrolizumab may cause fetal harm if administered during pregnancy; an alteration in the immune response or immune mediated disorders may develop following in utero exposure. Women of reproductive potential should use highly effective contraception during therapy and for at least 4 months after treatment is complete.

Breastfeeding Considerations It is not known if pembrolizumab is present in breast milk. The manufacturer recommends that breastfeeding be discontinued during therapy and for 4 months following the final dose. Immunoglobulins are excreted in breast milk; therefore pembrolizumab may be expected to appear in breast milk.

Warnings/Precautions Immune-mediated pneumonitis has been observed, including fatal cases. The median time to development was 3.3 months (range: 2 days to ~19 months) and the median duration was 1.5 months (range: 1 day to over 17 months). Many patients required initial management with high-dose systemic corticosteroids, the median duration of initial corticosteroid therapy was 8 days (range: 1 day to ~10 months) followed by a corticosteroid taper. Pneumonitis resolved in half of the affected patients. May require treatment interruption, corticosteroid therapy (prednisone 1 to 2 mg/kg /day [or equivalent] followed by a taper, for grade 2 or higher pneumonitis), and/or permanent discontinuation. Monitor for signs and symptoms of pneumonitis; if pneumonitis is suspected, evaluate with radiographic imaging and administer systemic corticosteroids for grade 2 or higher pneumonitis. Pneumonitis occurred more frequently in patients with a history of prior thoracic radiation.

Immune-mediated colitis has occurred, including cases of grade 2 to 4 colitis. The median time to onset of colitis was 3.5 months (range: 10 days to 16.2 months) and the median duration was 1.3 months (range: 1 day to over 8 months). In many patients, colitis was managed with high-dose systemic corticosteroids for a median duration of 7 days (range: 1 day to 5.3 months), followed by a corticosteroid taper. Most patients with colitis experienced resolution. May require treatment interruption, systemic corticosteroid therapy, and/or permanent discontinuation. Monitor for signs and symptoms of colitis; administer systemic corticosteroids for grade 2 or higher colitis.

Immune-mediated hepatitis occurred (grades 2 to 4 hepatitis). The median onset for hepatitis was 1.3 months (range: 8 days to 21.4 months); the median duration was 1.8 months (range: 8 days to over 20 months). Hepatitis resolved in most patients. Administer corticosteroids (prednisone 0.5 to 1 mg/kg/day [or equivalent] for grade 2 hepatitis, and prednisone 1 to 2 mg/kg/day [or equivalent] for grade 3 or higher, each followed by a taper), and withhold or discontinue therapy based on the severity of liver enzyme elevations. Systemic corticosteroids were used to manage immune-mediated hepatitis in many patients; the median duration of high-dose corticosteroid therapy was 5 days (range: 1 to 26 days), followed by a taper. Monitor for liver function changes. May require treatment interruption, systemic corticosteroids (for grade 2 or higher toxicity), and/or permanent discontinuation.

Immune-mediated hypophysitis occurred (grades 2, 3, and 4). The median time to onset was 3.7 months (range: 1 days to 12 months) and the median duration was 4.7 months (range: 8 days to over 12 months). Most cases were managed with systemic corticosteroids. Nearly half of patients with hypophysitis experienced resolution. Monitor for signs/symptoms of hypophysitis (eg, hypopituitarism, adrenal insufficiency). May require treatment interruption, systemic corticosteroids, hormone replacement (as clinically indicated), and/or permanent discontinuation.

Immune-mediated nephritis has occurred. The onset for autoimmune nephritis was 5.1 months (range: 12 days to 12.8 months) and the median duration was 3.3 months (range: 12 days to over 9 months). Grade 2 or higher nephritis should be managed with systemic corticosteroids (prednisone initial dose of 1 to 2 mg/kg/day [or equivalent], followed by a taper). Most patients required systemic corticosteroids. The median duration of corticosteroid use was 15 days (range: 3 days to 4 months), followed by a taper. Nephritis resolved in over half of affected patients. Monitor for renal function changes. May require treatment interruption, systemic corticosteroids (for grade 2 or higher toxicity), and/or permanent discontinuation.

Immune-mediated hyperthyroidism, hypothyroidism, and thyroiditis have occurred. The median onset for hyperthyroidism was 1.4 months (range: 1 day to ~22 months) and the median duration was 2.1 months (range: 1 day to over 15 months). Hyperthyroidism resolved in nearly three-fourths of affected patients. Hypothyroidism occurred with a median onset of 3.5 months (range: 1 day to 19 months) and median duration was not reached (range: 2 days to over 27 months). Hypothyroidism resolved in one-fifth of affected patients. The incidence of new or worsening hypothyroidism was higher in patients with squamous cell cancer of the head and neck. Monitor for changes in thyroid function (at baseline, periodically during treatment, and as clinically indicated) and for signs/symptoms of thyroid disorders. Administer thionamides and beta-blockers for hyperthyroidism as appropriate; may require treatment interruption and/or permanent discontinuation. Isolated hypothyroidism may be managed with replacement therapy. Thyroiditis occurred with a median onset of 1.2 months (range: 0.5 to 3.5 months). Type 1 diabetes mellitus has occurred (including diabetic ketoacidosis). Insulin therapy may be required; if severe hyperglycemia is observed, administer antihyperglycemics and withhold pembrolizumab treatment until glucose control has been accomplished.

Immune-mediated rashes, including Stevens-Johnson syndrome (SJS), toxic epidermal necrolysis (TEN, some fatal), exfoliative dermatitis, and bullous pemphigoid may occur with pembrolizumab. Monitor for suspected severe skin reactions and exclude other causes. Based on the severity of the dermatologic toxicity, withhold or permanently discontinue pembrolizumab and administer corticosteroids. Withhold pembrolizumab for signs/symptoms of SJS or TEN and refer for specialized care for assessment and management. Permanently discontinue pembrolizumab if SJS or TEN is confirmed. Other clinically relevant immune-mediated disorders have been observed (may involve any organ system), including rash, exfoliative dermatitis, bullous pemphigoid, uveitis, arthritis, vasculitis, myositis, Guillain-Barré syndrome, pancreatitis, hemolytic anemia, serum sickness, myasthenia gravis, myelitis, myocarditis, and partial seizures (in a patient with inflammatory foci in brain parenchyma). If an immune-mediated adverse event is suspected, evaluate appropriately to confirm or exclude other causes; withhold treatment and administer systemic corticosteroids based on severity of reaction. Upon resolution to grade 0 or 1, initiate corticosteroid taper (continue tapering over at least 1 month). When reaction remains at grade 1 or less during taper may reinitiate pembrolizumab. Immune-mediated adverse reactions that do not resolve with systemic corticosteroids may be managed with other systemic immunosuppressants (based on limited data). Discontinue permanently for severe or grade 3 immune-mediated adverse event that is recurrent or life-threatening. Infusion-related reactions (including severe and life-threatening cases) have occurred. Interrupt infusion for severe (grade 3) or life-threatening (grade 4) reactions; and permanently discontinue for severe (grade 3) or life-threatening (grade 4) infusion-related reactions. Hypersensitivity and anaphylaxis have been observed (rare).

Patients who received allogeneic hematopoietic stem cell transplant (HSCT) following discontinuation of pembrolizumab therapy experienced immune-mediated complications (some fatal) including graft versus host disease (GVHD) and severe sinusoidal obstructive syndrome (SOS; formerly called veno-occlusive disease) following reduced-intensity conditioning. Fatal hyperacute GVHD post HSCT has also been reported in lymphoma patients who received an anti PD-1 antibody prior to transplant. These complications may occur despite intervening therapy between pembrolizumab and HSCT. Monitor closely for early signs/symptoms of transplant-related complications (eg, hyperacute GVHD, severe [grade 3 to 4] acute GVHD, steroid-requiring febrile syndrome, SOS, and other immune-mediated adverse reactions) and manage promptly. Solid organ transplant rejection has been reported in postmarketing surveillance. Pembrolizumab may increase the risk of rejection; consider benefit versus risk of pembrolizumab treatment in solid organ transplant patients.

Adverse Reactions Incidence of adverse reactions include unapproved dosing regimens.

>10%:
  Cardiovascular: Peripheral edema (14%)
  Central nervous system: Fatigue (26% to 43%), headache (11%)
  Dermatologic: Pruritus (11% to 28%), skin rash (20% to 24%; immune-mediated: 1%)
  Endocrine & metabolic: Hyperglycemia (49%), hypoalbuminemia (37%), hyponatremia (10% to 37%), hypertriglyceridemia (33%), decreased serum phosphate (29%), increased serum potassium (28%), decreased serum bicarbonate (22%), hypocalcemia (21%), hypothyroidism (immune-mediated; 9% to 14%)
  Gastrointestinal: Decreased appetite (20% to 22%), constipation (19% to 22%), nausea (13% to 22%), diarrhea (18% to 20%), abdominal pain (13% to 18%), vomiting (12% to 15%)
  Genitourinary: Urinary tract infection (15% to 19%), hematuria (12% to 13%)
  Hematologic & oncologic: Anemia (17% to 44%; grades 3/4: 6% to 10%), lymphocytopenia (40%; grades 3/4: 9%), thrombocytopenia (27%; grades 3/4: 4%), neutropenia (24%; grades 3/4: 7%)
  Hepatic: Increased serum alkaline phosphatase (17% to 37%), increased serum AST (24% to 28%), increased serum ALT (21%)
  Neuromuscular & skeletal: Musculoskeletal pain (21% to 32%), arthralgia (10% to 14%)
  Renal: Increased serum creatinine (11% to 35%)
  Respiratory: Cough (14% to 24%), upper respiratory tract infection (13%), dyspnea (11% to 14%)
  Miscellaneous: Fever (11% to 24%)

◀ 1% to 10%:
   Cardiovascular: Facial edema (10%)
   Central nervous system: Peripheral neuropathy (2% to 10%), confu-
      sion (≥2%)
   Endocrine & metabolic: Weight loss (10%), hyperthyroidism (immune-medi-
      ated; 3%)
   Gastrointestinal: Colitis (immune-mediated; 2%)
   Genitourinary: Urosepsis (≥2%)
   Hepatic: Hyperbilirubinemia (10%)
   Immunologic: Antibody development (2%)
   Infection: Herpes zoster (≥1%)
   Neuromuscular & skeletal: Weakness (10%), arthritis (immune-mediated;
      2%), myositis (immune-mediated; ≤1%)
   Ophthalmic: Uveitis (immune-mediated; ≤1%)
   Renal: Acute renal failure (≥2%)
   Respiratory: Pneumonitis (3%), pleural effusion (≥2%), respiratory failure
      (≥2%), pneumonia (≥1%)
   Miscellaneous: Infusion-related reaction (≤9%; including anaphylaxis, hyper-
      sensitivity reaction)
<1%, postmarketing, and/or case reports: Adrenocortical insufficiency
   (immune-mediated), bullous pemphigoid (immune-mediated), chronic
   inflammatory demyelinating polyradiculoneuropathy (Maleissye 2016), diabetic ketoacidosis, exfoliative dermatitis (immune-mediated), Guillain-Barré
   syndrome (immune-mediated), hemolytic anemia (immune-mediated), hepatitis (including autoimmune hepatitis), hypophysitis, interstitial nephritis
   (with renal failure), myasthenia gravis (immune-mediated), myelitis
   (immune-mediated), myocarditis (immune-mediated), nephritis (autoimmune), organ transplant rejection (solid; immune-mediated), pancreatitis
   (immune-mediated), partial epilepsy (immune-mediated; in a patient with
   inflammatory foci in brain parenchyma), septic shock, thyroiditis, type 1
   diabetes mellitus, vasculitis (immune-mediated)

Drug Interactions
Metabolism/Transport Effects None known.
Avoid Concomitant Use There are no known interactions where it is
   recommended to avoid concomitant use.
Increased Effect/Toxicity There are no known significant interactions
   involving an increase in effect.
Decreased Effect There are no known significant interactions involving a
   decrease in effect.

Storage/Stability Lyophilized powder (50 mg vial) and injection solution
   (100 mg/4 mL vial): Store intact vials refrigerated at 2°C to 8°C (36°F to
   46°F); protect injection solution vials from light and do not shake or freeze.
   Reconstituted solutions and solutions diluted for infusion in NS or D5W may
   be stored at room temperature for up to 6 hours (infusion must be completed
   within 6 hours of reconstitution) or refrigerated at 2°C to 8°C (36°F to 46°F) for
   no more than 24 hours from the time of reconstitution. Do not freeze. If
   refrigerated, allow to reach room temperature prior to administration.

Preparation for Administration
   Injection solution (100 mg/4 mL vial): Withdraw appropriate volume from vial
   and transfer to IV bag containing NS or D5W; final concentration should be
   between 1 to 10 mg/mL. Mix by gently inverting bag. Discard unused portion
   of the vial.

Lyophilized powder (50 mg vial): Reconstitute by adding 2.3 mL SWFI along the vial wall (do not add directly to lyophilized powder); resulting vial concentration is 25 mg/mL. Slowly swirl vial; do not shake. Allow up to 5 minutes for bubbles to dissipate. Reconstituted solution is a clear to slightly opalescent and colorless to slightly yellow solution; discard if visible particles present. Withdraw appropriate volume from vial and transfer to IV bag containing NS or D5W; final concentration should be between 1 to 10 mg/mL. Mix by gently inverting bag. Discard unused portion of the vial.

Mechanism of Action Highly selective anti-PD-1 humanized monoclonal antibody which inhibits programmed cell death-1 (PD-1) activity by binding to the PD-1 receptor on T-cells to block PD-1 ligands (PD-L1 and PD-L2) from binding. Blocking the PD-1 pathway inhibits the negative immune regulation caused by PD-1 receptor signaling (Hamid 2013). Anti-PD-1 antibodies (including pembrolizumab) reverse T-cell suppression and induce antitumor responses (Robert 2014).

Pharmacodynamics/Kinetics Note: Clearance is ~21% lower at steady state than with the first dose. With weight-based dosing (2 mg/kg), pembrolizumab concentrations in pediatric patients are comparable to those of adults (at the same dose).

Distribution: V_{dss}: 6 L

Half-life elimination: 22 days

Dosing

Adult & Geriatric

Head and neck cancer, squamous cell, (recurrent or metastatic): IV: 200 **mg** once every 3 weeks until disease progression, unacceptable toxicity, or (in patients without disease progression) for up to 24 months.

Hodgkin lymphoma, classical (relapsed or refractory): IV: 200 **mg** once every 3 weeks until disease progression, unacceptable toxicity, or (in patients without disease progression) up to 24 months.

Melanoma (unresectable or metastatic): IV: 200 **mg** once every 3 weeks until disease progression or unacceptable toxicity.

Off-label dosing: 2 mg/kg once every 3 weeks until disease progression or unacceptable toxicity (Ribas 2015).

Microsatellite Instability-high cancer (unresectable or metastatic): IV: 200 **mg** once every 3 weeks until disease progression, unacceptable toxicity, or (in patients without disease progression) for up to 24 months.

Non-small cell lung cancer (metastatic), single-agent therapy: IV: 200 **mg** once every 3 weeks until disease progression, unacceptable toxicity, or (in patients without disease progression) up to 24 months.

Off-label dosing (in patients with disease progression following platinum-containing chemotherapy): 2 mg/kg once every 3 weeks for 24 months or until disease progression or unacceptable toxicity (Herbst 2016).

Non-small cell lung cancer (metastatic, nonsquamous), combination therapy: IV: 200 **mg** once every 3 weeks (in combination with pemetrexed and carboplatin) for 4 cycles, followed by pembrolizumab monotherapy of 200 **mg** once every 3 weeks (with or without optional indefinite pemetrexed maintenance therapy) until disease progression, unacceptable toxicity, or (in patients without disease progression) up to 24 months (Langer 2016).

Urothelial carcinoma (locally advanced or metastatic): IV: 200 **mg** once every 3 weeks until disease progression, unacceptable toxicity, or (in patients without disease progression) for up to 24 months (Belmunt 2017).

◄

Merkel cell carcinoma, advanced (off-label use): IV: 2 **mg/kg** once every 3 weeks for up to 2 years or until complete response, or until disease progression or unacceptable toxicity (Nghiem 2016).

Pediatric

Hodgkin lymphoma, classical (relapsed or refractory): Children ≥2 years and Adolescents: IV: 2 **mg/kg** (maximum: 200 mg) once every 3 weeks until disease progression, unacceptable toxicity, or (in patients without disease progression) up to 24 months.

Microsatellite instability-high cancer (unresectable or metastatic): Children ≥2 years and Adolescents: IV: 2 **mg/kg** (maximum: 200 mg) once every 3 weeks until disease progression, unacceptable toxicity, or (in patients without disease progression) up to 24 months.

Renal Impairment No dosage adjustment necessary. In a pharmacokinetic study, no difference in clearance was noted for patients with eGFR ≥15 mL/minute/1.73 m².

Hepatic Impairment

*Hepatic impairment **prior** to treatment initiation:*

Mild impairment (total bilirubin ≤ ULN and AST > ULN or total bilirubin >1 to 1.5 times ULN and any AST): No dosage adjustment necessary.

Moderate (total bilirubin >1.5 to 3 times ULN and any AST) to severe (total bilirubin >3 times ULN and any AST) impairment: There are no dosage adjustments provided in the manufacturer's labeling (has not been studied).

*Hepatotoxicity **during** treatment:* **Note:** For patients with baseline grade 2 ALT or AST abnormalities due to liver metastases, permanently discontinue if AST or ALT increases by ≥50% (relative to baseline) and persists at least 1 week.

AST or ALT >3 to 5 times ULN or total bilirubin >1.5 to 3 times ULN: Withhold treatment; may resume therapy upon recovery to grade 0 or 1 toxicity. Also administer corticosteroids (prednisone 0.5 to 1 mg/kg/day [or equivalent] followed by a taper).

AST or ALT >5 times ULN or total bilirubin >3 times ULN: Permanently discontinue. Also administer corticosteroids (prednisone 1 to 2 mg/kg/day [or equivalent] followed by a taper).

Adjustment for Toxicity

Withhold treatment for any of the following (may resume upon recovery to grade 0 or 1 toxicity):

Colitis, moderate (grade 2) or severe (grade 3); also administer corticosteroids (prednisone 1 to 2 mg/kg/day [or equivalent] followed by a taper).

Dermatologic toxicity: Grade 3 severe skin reactions or suspected Stevens-Johnson syndrome (SJS) or toxic epidermal necrolysis (TEN).

Endocrinopathies:

Hyperglycemia, severe; also administer antihyperglycemics.

Hyperthyroidism, severe (grade 3) or life threatening (grade 4); manage with thionamides and beta-blockers as appropriate.

Hypophysitis, grade 2 (symptomatic); also administer corticosteroids (followed by a taper) and hormone replacement therapy if appropriate.

Hematologic toxicity, grade 4 (in patients with classical Hodgkin lymphoma)

Nephritis, grade 2; also administer corticosteroids (prednisone 1 to 2 mg/kg/day [or equivalent] followed by a taper).

Pneumonitis, moderate (grade 2); also administer corticosteroids (prednisone 1 to 2 mg/kg/day [or equivalent] followed by a taper).

Other treatment-related toxicity, severe or grade 3; may require corticosteroids (based on severity). Upon improvement to grade 0 or 1, initiate corticosteroid taper and continue to taper over at least 1 month. Restart pembrolizumab if the adverse reaction remains at grade 0 or 1 following corticosteroid taper. May consider other systemic immunosuppressants if not controlled by corticosteroids (based on limited data).

Withhold (may resume upon recovery to grade 0 or 1 toxicity) or discontinue for:

Hyperthyroidism, severe (grade 3) or life-threatening (grade 4); manage with thionamides and beta-blockers as appropriate.

Hypophysitis, severe (grade 3) or life-threatening (grade 4); also administer corticosteroids and hormone replacement as appropriate.

Permanently discontinue for:

Adverse reactions that are life-threatening (excluding endocrinopathies controlled with hormone replacement therapy, or hematologic toxicity [in patients with classical Hodgkin lymphoma]), persistent grade 2 or 3 adverse reaction (excluding endocrinopathies controlled with hormone replacement therapy) that does not recover to grade 0 or 1 within 12 weeks after the last pembrolizumab dose, or any recurrent severe or grade 3 treatment-related adverse reaction. Also administer corticosteroids (may consider other systemic immunosuppressants if not controlled by corticosteroids [based on limited data]).

Colitis, life-threatening (grade 4); also administer corticosteroids (prednisone 1 to 2 mg/kg/day [or equivalent] followed by a taper).

Dermatologic toxicity: Grade 4 severe skin reactions or confirmed SJS or TEN.

Immune mediated adverse reactions: Discontinue permanently if unable to reduce corticosteroid dose to prednisone ≤10 mg/day (or equivalent) within 12 weeks.

Infusion-related reaction, grade 3 or 4.

Nephritis, severe (grade 3) or life-threatening (grade 4); also administer corticosteroids (prednisone 1 to 2 mg/kg/day [or equivalent] followed by a taper).

Pneumonitis, severe (grade 3), life-threatening (grade 4), or moderate (grade 2) that recurs; also administer corticosteroids (prednisone 1 to 2 mg/kg/day [or equivalent] followed by a taper).

Combination Regimens

Lung cancer (non-small cell): Carboplatin-Pemetrexed-Pembrolizumab (NSCLC) on page 2024

Administration IV: Infuse over 30 minutes through a 0.2 to 5 micron sterile, nonpyrogenic, low-protein binding inline or add-on filter. Do not infuse other medications through the same infusion line.

Non-small cell lung cancer (metastatic): When administered in combination with chemotherapy (pemetrexed and carboplatin), pembrolizumab should be administered prior to chemotherapy if scheduled to be administered on the same day.

Emetic Potential Minimal (<10%)

Monitoring Parameters PD-L1 expression status in patients with NSCLC (when used as single-agent therapy); liver function tests (AST, ALT, and total bilirubin); renal function; thyroid function (at baseline, periodically during treatment and as clinically indicated); glucose; CBC with differential (in patients with Hodgkin lymphoma); signs/symptoms of colitis, dermatologic toxicity, hypophysitis, thyroid disorders, pneumonitis, infusion reactions.

◀ **Medication Guide Available** Yes

Dosage Forms Excipient information presented when available (limited, particularly for generics); consult specific product labeling.

Solution, Intravenous [preservative free]:

Keytruda: 100 mg/4 mL (4 mL) [contains polysorbate 80]

Solution Reconstituted, Intravenous [preservative free]:

Keytruda: 50 mg (1 ea) [contains polysorbate 80]

PEMEtrexed (pem e TREKS ed)

Related Information

Common Toxicity Criteria on page 2242

Management of Chemotherapy-Induced Nausea and Vomiting in Adults on page 2253

Prevention of Chemotherapy-Induced Nausea and Vomiting in Children on page 2310

Safe Handling of Hazardous Drugs on page 2379

Brand Names: US Alimta

Brand Names: Canada Alimta

Index Terms LY231514; Pemetrexed Disodium

Pharmacologic Category Antineoplastic Agent, Antimetabolite; Antineoplastic Agent, Antimetabolite (Antifolate)

Use

Mesothelioma: Treatment of unresectable malignant pleural mesothelioma (in combination with cisplatin)

Non-small cell lung cancer (NSCLC), nonsquamous: Treatment of locally advanced or metastatic NSCLC (as initial treatment in combination with cisplatin; as maintenance treatment after 4 cycles of initial platinum-based first-line therapy; as single-agent treatment after prior chemotherapy)

Limitation of use: Not indicated for the treatment of **squamous** cell NSCLC

Labeled Contraindications

Severe hypersensitivity to pemetrexed or any component of the formulation

Canadian labeling: Additional contraindications; not in US labeling: Concomitant yellow fever vaccine

Pregnancy Considerations Adverse effects were observed in animal reproduction studies. Based on the mechanism of action, pemetrexed may cause fetal harm if administered to a pregnant woman. Women of childbearing potential should use effective contraceptive measures to avoid becoming pregnant during treatment. A negative serum pregnancy test prior to treatment is recommended in the Canadian labeling. The Canadian labeling also recommends that males receiving therapy use effective contraceptive measures and not father a child during, and for up to 6 months after, therapy. Additionally, the Canadian labeling recommends counseling on sperm storage prior to treatment, as irreversible infertility has been reported in males.

Breastfeeding Considerations According to the manufacturer, due to the potential for serious adverse reactions in the nursing infant, a decision should be made to discontinue pemetrexed or to discontinue breastfeeding during therapy, taking into account the benefits of treatment to the mother. The Canadian labeling recommends discontinuing nursing.

Warnings/Precautions Hypersensitivity (including anaphylaxis) has been reported with use. May cause bone marrow suppression (anemia, neutropenia, thrombocytopenia and/or pancytopenia); frequent laboratory monitoring is necessary (myelosuppression is often dose-limiting). Dose reductions in subsequent cycles may be required. Prophylactic folic acid and vitamin B_{12} supplements are necessary to reduce hematologic and gastrointestinal toxicity and infection; initiate supplementation 1 week before the first dose of pemetrexed. Pretreatment with dexamethasone is necessary to reduce the incidence and severity of cutaneous reactions. Rarely, Stevens-Johnson syndrome and toxic epidermal necrolysis have been reported. Although the effect of third space fluid is not fully defined, studies have determined pemetrexed concentrations in patients with mild-to-moderate ascites/pleural effusions were similar to concentrations in trials of patients without third space fluid accumulation. Drainage of fluid from ascites/effusions may be considered, but is not likely necessary. Use caution with hepatic dysfunction not due to metastases; may require dose adjustment. Interstitial pneumonitis with respiratory insufficiency has been observed with use; interrupt therapy and evaluate promptly with progressive dyspnea and cough.

The manufacturer does not recommend use in patients with CrCl <45 mL/ minute. Decreased renal function results in increased toxicity. Potentially significant drug-drug interactions may exist, requiring dose or frequency adjustment, additional monitoring, and/or selection of alternative therapy. Use caution in patients receiving concurrent nephrotoxins; may result in delayed pemetrexed clearance. NSAIDs may reduce the clearance of pemetroxed. In patients with CrCl 45 to 79 mL/minute, interruption of NSAID therapy may be necessary prior to, during, and immediately after pemetrexed therapy. Not indicated for use in patients with squamous cell NSCLC.

Adverse Reactions

>10%:
 Central nervous system: Fatigue (18% to 34%; dose-limiting)
 Dermatologic: Desquamation (≤14%), skin rash (≤14%)
 Gastrointestinal: Nausea (12% to 31%), anorexia (19% to 22%), vomiting (6% to 16%), stomatitis (5% to 15%), diarrhea (5% to 13%)
 Hematologic & oncologic: Anemia (15% to 19%; grades 3/4: 3% to 5%), leukopenia (6% to 12%; grades 3/4: 2% to 4%), neutropenia (6% to 11%; grades 3/4: 3% to 5%; dose-limiting; nadir: 8 to 10 days; recovery: 4 to 8 days after nadir)
 Respiratory: Pharyngitis (15%)
1% to 10%:
 Cardiovascular: Edema (1% to 5%)
 Central nervous system: Neuropathy (sensory: ≤9%; motor: ≤5%)
 Dermatologic: Pruritus (1% to 7%), alopecia (1% to 6%), erythema multiforme (≤5%)
 Endocrine & metabolic: Weight loss (1%)
 Gastrointestinal: Constipation (1% to 6%), abdominal pain (≤5%)
 Hematologic & oncologic: Thrombocytopenia (1% to 8%; grades 3/4: 2%; dose-limiting), febrile neutropenia (grades 3/4: 2%)
 Hepatic: Increased serum ALT (8% to 10%; grades 3/4: ≤2%), increased serum AST (7% to 8%; grades 3/4: ≤1%)
 Hypersensitivity: Hypersensitivity reaction (≤5%)
 Infection: Infection (≤5%), sepsis (1%)
 Ophthalmic: Conjunctivitis (≤5%), increased lacrimation (≤5%)
 Renal: Decreased creatinine clearance (≤5%), increased serum creatinine (≤5%)
 Miscellaneous: Fever (1% to 8%)

<1%, postmarketing, and/or case reports: Cardiac arrhythmia, chest pain, colitis, dehydration, depression, esophagitis, gastrointestinal obstruction, hemolytic anemia, hepatobiliary disease (failure), hypertension, increased gamma-glutamyl transferase, interstitial pneumonitis, pain, pancreatitis, pancytopenia, peripheral ischemia, pulmonary embolism, radiation recall phenomenon (median onset: 6 days; range: 1 to 35 days), renal failure, Stevens-Johnson syndrome, supraventricular cardiac arrhythmia, syncope, thromboembolism, toxic epidermal necrolysis, ventricular tachycardia

Drug Interactions

Metabolism/Transport Effects None known.

Avoid Concomitant Use

Avoid concomitant use of PEMEtrexed with any of the following: BCG (Intravesical); Deferiprone; Dipyrone; Natalizumab; Pimecrolimus; Tacrolimus (Topical); Vaccines (Live)

Increased Effect/Toxicity

PEMEtrexed may increase the levels/effects of: CloZAPine; Deferiprone; Fingolimod; Leflunomide; Natalizumab; Tofacitinib; Vaccines (Live)

The levels/effects of PEMEtrexed may be increased by: Denosumab; Dipyrone; NSAID (Nonselective); Ocrelizumab; Palifermin; Pimecrolimus; Promazine; Roflumilast; Tacrolimus (Topical); Trastuzumab

Decreased Effect

PEMEtrexed may decrease the levels/effects of: BCG (Intravesical); Coccidioides immitis Skin Test; Lenograstim; Nivolumab; Sipuleucel-T; Tertomotide; Vaccines (Inactivated); Vaccines (Live)

The levels/effects of PEMEtrexed may be decreased by: Echinacea

Hazardous Drugs Handling Considerations

Hazardous agent (NIOSH 2016 [group 1]).

Use appropriate precautions for receiving, handling, administration, and disposal. Gloves (single) should be worn during receiving, unpacking, and placing in storage.

NIOSH recommends double gloving, a protective gown, ventilated engineering controls (a class II biological safety cabinet or a compounding aseptic containment isolator), and closed system transfer devices (CSTDs) for preparation. Double gloving, a gown, and (if dosage form allows) CSTDs are required during administration (NIOSH 2016).

Storage/Stability Store intact vials at room temperature of 25°C (77°F); excursions permitted to 15°C to 30°C (59°F to 86°F). Reconstituted solution and infusion solution are stable for 24 hours when refrigerated at 2°C to 8°C (36°F to 46°F).

Preparation for Administration Reconstitute with NS (preservative free); add 4.2 mL to the 100 mg vial and 20 mL to the 500 mg vial, resulting in a 25 mg/mL concentration. Gently swirl. Solution may be colorless to green-yellow. Further dilute in 100 mL NS prior to infusion (the manufacturer recommends a total volume of 100 mL).

Mechanism of Action Antifolate; disrupts folate-dependent metabolic processes essential for cell replication. Inhibits thymidylate synthase (TS), dihydrofolate reductase (DHFR), glycinamide ribonucleotide formyltransferase (GARFT), and aminoimidazole carboxamide ribonucleotide formyltransferase (AICARFT), the enzymes involved in folate metabolism and DNA synthesis, resulting in inhibition of purine and thymidine nucleotide and protein synthesis.

Pharmacodynamics/Kinetics

Distribution: V_{dss}: 16.1 L

Protein binding: ~81%

Metabolism: Minimal

Half-life elimination: Normal renal function: 3.5 hours

Excretion: Urine (70% to 90% as unchanged drug)

Dosing

Adult & Geriatric Note: Start vitamin supplements 1 week before initial pemetrexed dose: Folic acid 400 to 1000 mcg daily orally (begin 7 days prior to treatment initiation; continue daily during treatment and for 21 days after last pemetrexed dose) and vitamin B_{12} 1000 mcg IM 7 days prior to treatment initiation and then every 3 cycles. Give dexamethasone 4 mg orally twice daily for 3 days, beginning the day before treatment to minimize cutaneous reactions. New treatment cycles should not begin unless ANC ≥1500/mm^3, platelets ≥100,000/mm^3, and CrCl ≥45 mL/minute.

Malignant pleural mesothelioma: IV: 500 mg/m^2 on day 1 of each 21-day cycle (in combination with cisplatin) **or** (off-label) in combination with carboplatin (Castagneto 2008; Ceresoli 2006) **or** (off-label) as single-agent therapy (Taylor 2008)

Non-small cell lung cancer, nonsquamous: IV:

Initial treatment: 500 mg/m^2 on day 1 of each 21-day cycle (in combination with cisplatin)

Maintenance or second-line treatment: 500 mg/m^2 on day 1 of each 21-day cycle (as a single-agent)

Bladder cancer, metastatic (off-label use): IV: 500 mg/m^2 on day 1 of each 21-day cycle until disease progression or unacceptable toxicity (Sweeney 2006)

Cervical cancer, persistent or recurrent (off-label use): IV: 500 mg/m^2 on day 1 of each 21-day cycle until disease progression or unacceptable toxicity occurs (Lorusso 2010) **or** 900 mg/m^2 on day 1 of each 21-day cycle (Miller 2008)

Ovarian cancer, platinum-resistant (off-label use): IV: 500 mg/m^2 on day 1 of each 21-day cycle (Vergote 2009)

Thymic malignancies, metastatic (off-label use): IV: 500 mg/m^2 on day 1 of each 21-day cycle for 6 cycles or until disease progression or unacceptable toxicity occurs (Loehrer 2006)

Renal Impairment

Renal function may be estimated using the Cockcroft-Gault formula (using actual body weight) or glomerular filtration rate (GFR) measured by Tc99m-DPTA serum clearance.

CrCl ≥45 mL/minute: No dosage adjustment necessary.

CrCl <45 mL/minute: Use is not recommended by the manufacturer (an insufficient number of patients have been studied for dosage recommendations).

According to a phase I study in advanced cancer patients with renal impairment, pemetrexed doses up to 500 mg/m^2 (with vitamin supplementation) were well tolerated in patients with glomerular filtration rate (GFR) 40 to 79 mL/minute; however, accrual was halted in patients with GFR <29 mL/minute (due to toxicity) and accrual did not occur in patients with GFR 30 to 39 mL/minute. Patients with GFR ≥80 mL/minute tolerated doses of 600 mg/m^2 (Mita 2006).

◄ *Concomitant NSAID use with renal dysfunction:*
CrCl ≥80 mL/minute: No dosage adjustment necessary.
CrCl 45 to 79 mL/minute and NSAIDs with short half-lives (eg, ibuprofen, indomethacin, ketoprofen, ketorolac): Avoid NSAID for 2 days before, the day of, and for 2 days following a dose of pemetrexed.
Any creatinine clearance and NSAIDs with long half-lives (eg, nabumetone, naproxen, oxaprozin, piroxicam): Avoid NSAID for 5 days before, the day of, and 2 days following a dose of pemetrexed.

Hepatic Impairment Grade 3 (5.1 to 20 times ULN) **or** 4 (>20 times ULN) transaminase elevation during treatment: Reduce pemetrexed dose to 75% of previous dose (and cisplatin).

Obesity *ASCO Guidelines for appropriate chemotherapy dosing in obese adults with cancer:* Utilize patient's actual body weight (full weight) for calculation of body surface area- or weight-based dosing, particularly when the intent of therapy is curative; manage regimen-related toxicities in the same manner as for nonobese patients; if a dose reduction is utilized due to toxicity, consider resumption of full weight-based dosing with subsequent cycles, especially if cause of toxicity (eg, hepatic or renal impairment) is resolved (Griggs, 2012).

Adjustment for Toxicity
Toxicity: Discontinue if patient develops grade 3 or 4 toxicity after two dose reductions or immediately if grade 3 or 4 neurotoxicity develops
Hematologic toxicity: Upon recovery, reinitiate therapy
Nadir ANC <500/mm^3 and nadir platelets ≥50,000/mm^3: Reduce dose to 75% of previous dose of pemetrexed (and cisplatin)
Nadir platelets <50,000/mm^3 **without bleeding** (regardless of nadir ANC): Reduce dose to 75% of previous dose of pemetrexed (and cisplatin)
Nadir platelets <50,000/mm^3 **with bleeding** (regardless of nadir ANC): Reduce dose to 50% of previous dose of pemetrexed (and cisplatin)
Nonhematologic toxicity ≥ grade 3 (excluding neurotoxicity): Withhold treatment until recovery to baseline; upon recovery, reinitiate therapy as follows:
Grade 3 or 4 toxicity (excluding mucositis): Reduce dose to 75% of previous dose of pemetrexed (and cisplatin)
Grade 3 or 4 diarrhea or any diarrhea requiring hospitalization: Reduce dose to 75% of previous dose of pemetrexed (and cisplatin)
Grade 3 or 4 mucositis: Reduce pemetrexed dose to 50% of previous dose (continue cisplatin at 100% of previous dose)
Neurotoxicity:
Grade 0 to 1: Continue pemetrexed at 100% of previous dose (and cisplatin)
Grade 2: Continue pemetrexed at 100% of previous dose; reduce cisplatin dose to 50% of previous dose

Combination Regimens
Lung cancer (non-small cell):
Bevacizumab-Carboplatin-Pemetrexed (NSCLC) on page 1990
Carboplatin-Pemetrexed (NSCLC) on page 2024
Carboplatin-Pemetrexed-Pembrolizumab (NSCLC) on page 2024
Cisplatin-Pemetrexed (NSCLC) on page 2059
Malignant pleural mesothelioma:
Carboplatin-Pemetrexed (Mesothelioma) on page 2024
Cisplatin-Pemetrexed (Mesothelioma) on page 2059

Administration IV: Infuse over 10 minutes.

Emetic Potential Children and Adults: Low (10% to 30%)

Monitoring Parameters CBC with differential and platelets (before each cycle and as needed; monitor for nadir and recovery); renal function tests (serum creatinine, creatinine clearance, BUN; prior to each cycle and as needed) total bilirubin, ALT, AST (periodic); signs/symptoms of mucositis and diarrhea

Dietary Considerations Initiate folic acid supplementation 1 week before first dose of pemetrexed, continue for full course of therapy, and for 21 days after last dose. Institute vitamin B_{12} 1 week before the first dose; administer every 9 weeks thereafter.

Dosage Forms Excipient information presented when available (limited, particularly for generics); consult specific product labeling.
Solution Reconstituted, Intravenous:
Alimta: 100 mg (1 ea); 500 mg (1 ea)

◆ **Pemetrexed Disodium** *see* PEMEtrexed *on page 1494*

◆ **Pentahydrate** *see* Sodium Thiosulfate *on page 1678*

◆ **Pentam** *see* Pentamidine (Systemic) *on page 1499*

Pentamidine (Systemic) (pen TAM i deen)

Brand Names: US Pentam
Brand Names: Canada Pentamidine Isetionate for Injection BP
Index Terms Pentamidine Diisetionate; Pentamidine Isethionate; Pentamidine Isetionate
Pharmacologic Category Antifungal Agent; Antiprotozoal
Use Treatment of pneumonia caused by *Pneumocystis jirovecii* pneumonia (PCP)
Pregnancy Risk Factor C
Dosing
  Adult & Geriatric
    Pneumocystis jirovecii **pneumonia (PCP), treatment:**
      Manufacturer labeling: IM, IV: 4 mg/kg once daily for 14 to 21 days
      HIV-infected patients (alternative to preferred therapy): IV: 4 mg/kg/dose once daily for 21 days; may reduce to 3 mg/kg/dose once daily if toxicity occurs (HHS [OI adult 2015])
    Trypanosomiasis (off-label use): IM, IV: 4 mg/kg once daily for 7 to 10 days (CDC 2013)
  Pediatric
    Pneumocystis jirovecii **pneumonia (PCP), prophylaxis (primary and secondary) in oncology patients (including HSCT recipients) (off-label use): Note:** For patients intolerant to sulfamethoxazole and trimethoprim: Children ≥2 years and Adolescents: IV: 4 mg/kg/dose once a month (Kim 2008; Prasad 2007); in HSCT recipient, doses have been administered every 2 to 4 weeks (Tomblyn [CDC/IDSA 2009])
    Pneumocystis jirovecii **pneumonia (PCP), treatment (moderate-severe disease): Note:** For patients who cannot tolerate or who fail to respond to 5 to 7 days of sulfamethoxazole and trimethoprim.
      Manufacturer's labeling: Infants ≥5 months, Children, and Adolescents: IM, IV: 4 mg/kg/dose once daily for 14 to 21 days
      HIV-exposed/-positive:
        Infants and Children: IV: 4 mg/kg/dose once daily; if clinical improvement after 7 to 10 days of therapy, may change to an oral regimen to complete a 21-day course (HHS [OI pediatric 2013])
        Adolescents: IV: Refer to adult dosing.

Non-HIV-exposed/-positive: Infants, Children, and Adolescents: IV: 3 to 4 mg/kg/dose once daily for 21 days (Bradley 2015)

Trypanosomiasis, treatment (non-CNS disease) (off-label use): Infants, Children, Adolescents, and Adults: IM, IV: 4 mg/kg/dose once daily for 7 to 10 days (Bradley 2015; CDC 2013; *Red Book* [AAP 2015])

Renal Impairment IV: The FDA-approved labeling recommends that caution should be used in patients with renal impairment; however, no specific dosage adjustment guidelines are available. The following guidelines have been used by some clinicians (Aronoff 2007):

Adults:

CrCl ≥10 mL/minute: No dosage adjustment necessary.

CrCl <10 mL/minute: Administer 4 mg/kg every 24 to 36 hours.

Children:

CrCl >30 mL/minute: No dosage adjustment necessary.

CrCl 10 to 30 mL/minute: Administer 4 mg/kg every 36 hours.

CrCl <10 mL/minute and peritoneal dialysis: Administer 4 mg/kg every 48 hours.

Hemodialysis: Administer 4 mg/kg every 48 hours, after dialysis on dialysis days.

Hepatic Impairment There are no dosage adjustments provided in the manufacturer's labeling (has not been studied). Use with caution.

Additional Information Complete prescribing information should be consulted for additional detail.

Dosage Forms Excipient information presented when available (limited, particularly for generics); consult specific product labeling.

Solution Reconstituted, Injection, as isethionate:

Pentam: 300 mg (1 ea)

Pentamidine (Oral Inhalation) (pen TAM i deen)

Brand Names: US Nebupent

Index Terms Pentamidine Diisetionate; Pentamidine Isethionate; Pentamidine Isetionate

Pharmacologic Category Antifungal Agent; Antiprotozoal

Use Prevention of *Pneumocystis jirovecii* pneumonia (PCP) in high-risk, HIV-infected patients either with a history of PCP or with a CD4+ count ≤200/mm^3

Pregnancy Risk Factor C

Dosing

Adult & Geriatric *Pneumocystis jirovecii* pneumonia (PCP), prevention: Primary or secondary prophylaxis (alternative to preferred therapy): Inhalation: 300 mg once every 4 weeks via Respirgard II nebulizer (HHS [OI adult 2015])

Pediatric

***Pneumocystis jirovecii* pneumonia (PCP), prevention:**

Children ≥5 years (off-label population): Inhalation: 300 mg once every 4 weeks via Respirgard II nebulizer (HHS [OI pediatric 2013]; *Redbook* [AAP 2015]; Tomblyn 2009)

Adolescents (off-label population): Refer to adult dosing.

Renal Impairment There are no dosage adjustments provided in manufacturer's labeling (has not been studied). Use with caution.

Hepatic Impairment There are no dosage adjustments provided in manufacturer's labeling (has not been studied). Use with caution.

Additional Information Complete prescribing information should be consulted for additional detail.

Dosage Forms Excipient information presented when available (limited, particularly for generics); consult specific product labeling.
Solution Reconstituted, Inhalation, as isethionate:
  Nebupent: 300 mg (1 ea)

♦ **Pentamidine Diisetionate** *see* Pentamidine (Oral Inhalation) *on page 1500*

♦ **Pentamidine Diisetionate** *see* Pentamidine (Systemic) *on page 1499*

♦ **Pentamidine Isethionate** *see* Pentamidine (Oral Inhalation) *on page 1500*

♦ **Pentamidine Isethionate** *see* Pentamidine (Systemic) *on page 1499*

♦ **Pentamidine Isetionate** *see* Pentamidine (Oral Inhalation) *on page 1500*

♦ **Pentamidine Isetionate** *see* Pentamidine (Systemic) *on page 1499*

♦ **Pentamidine Isetionate for Injection BP (Can)** *see* Pentamidine (Systemic) *on page 1499*

Pentostatin (pen toe STAT in)

Related Information

Hematopoietic Cell Transplantation *on page 2365*

Management of Chemotherapy-Induced Nausea and Vomiting in Adults *on page 2253*

Prevention of Chemotherapy-Induced Nausea and Vomiting in Children *on page 2310*

Safe Handling of Hazardous Drugs *on page 2379*

Brand Names: US Nipent

Brand Names: Canada Nipent

Index Terms 2'-Deoxycoformycin; Co-Vidarabine; dCF; Deoxycoformycin

Pharmacologic Category Antineoplastic Agent, Antimetabolite; Antineoplastic Agent, Antimetabolite (Purine Analog)

Use Hairy cell leukemia: Treatment (as a single-agent) of untreated and interferon-refractory hairy cell leukemia in patients with active disease (clinically significant anemia, neutropenia, thrombocytopenia, or disease-related symptoms)

Labeled Contraindications Hypersensitivity to pentostatin or any component of the formulation

Pregnancy Considerations Adverse events were observed in animal reproduction studies. Women of childbearing potential should be advised to avoid becoming pregnant during treatment.

Breastfeeding Considerations It is not known if pentostatin is excreted in breast milk. Due to the potential for serious adverse reactions in nursing the infant, a decision should be made to discontinue pentostatin or to discontinue breast feeding, taking into account the importance of treatment to the mother.

Warnings/Precautions [U.S. Boxed Warnings]: Severe renal, liver, pulmonary, and CNS toxicities have occurred with doses higher than recommended; do not exceed the recommended dose. May cause elevations (usually reversible) in liver function tests. Withhold treatment or discontinue for CNS toxicity. Serum creatinine elevations occurring at recommended doses are usually minor and reversible. Withhold treatment for elevated serum creatinine and determine creatinine clearance. May require dosage adjustment or therapy discontinuation. Use with caution in patients with renal dysfunction (CrCl <60 mL/minute); the terminal half-life is prolonged; may require dosage adjustment.

Myelosuppression may occur, primarily early in treatment (first few courses). Neutropenia may worsen during initial courses for the treatment of hairy cell leukemia. If severe neutropenia persists beyond early cycles, evaluate for disease status. Monitor blood counts during treatment (more frequently in the initial cycles). In patients who present with infections prior to treatment, infections should be resolved, if possible, prior to initiation of treatment; preexisting infections may worsen with pentostatin treatment. Treatment should be temporarily withheld for active infections during therapy. Use in patients with infections only if the potential benefit justifies the potential risk.

Severe rashes may occur and worsen with therapy continuation; may require treatment interruption or discontinuation. Potentially significant drug-drug interactions may exist, requiring dose or frequency adjustment, additional monitoring, and/or selection of alternative therapy. **[U.S. Boxed Warnings]: Do not administer concurrently with fludarabine; concomitant use has resulted in serious or fatal pulmonary toxicity.** Fatal pulmonary edema and hypotension have been reported in patients treated with pentostatin in combination with carmustine, etoposide, or high-dose cyclophosphamide as part of a myeloablative regimen for bone marrow transplant. **[U.S. Boxed Warning]: Should be administered under the supervision of an experienced cancer chemotherapy physician.**

Adverse Reactions

>10%:

Central nervous system: Fatigue (29% to 42%), pain (8% to 20%), chills (11% to 19%), headache (13% to 17%), central nervous system toxicity (1% to 11%)

Dermatologic: Skin rash (26% to 43%), pruritus (10% to 21%), skin changes (4% to 17%)

Gastrointestinal: Nausea (≤63%), vomiting (≤63%), diarrhea (15% to 17%), anorexia (13% to 16%), abdominal pain (4% to 16%), stomatitis (5% to 12%)

Hematologic & oncologic: Leukopenia (22% to 60%), anemia (8% to 35%), thrombocytopenia (6% to 32%), bone marrow depression (nadir: 7 days; recovery: 10 to 14 days)

Hepatic: Increased serum transaminases (2% to 19%)

Hypersensitivity: Hypersensitivity reaction (2% to 11%)

Infection: Infection (7% to 36%)

Neuromuscular & skeletal: Myalgia (11% to 19%), weakness (10% to 12%)

Respiratory: Cough (17% to 20%), upper respiratory tract infection (13% to 16%), rhinitis (10% to 11%), dyspnea (8% to 11%)

Miscellaneous: Fever (42% to 46%)

1% to 10%:

Cardiovascular: Chest pain (3% to 10%), facial edema (3% to 10%), hypotension (3% to 10%), peripheral edema (3% to 10%), angina pectoris (<3%), atrioventricular block (<3%), bradycardia (<3%), cardiac arrhythmia (<3%), cardiac failure (<3%), deep vein thrombophlebitis (<3%), hypertension (<3%), localized phlebitis (<3%), pericardial effusion (<3%), sinoatrial arrest (<3%), syncope (<3%), tachycardia (<3%), vasculitis (<3%), ventricular premature contractions (<3%)

Central nervous system: Anxiety (3% to 10%), confusion (3% to 10%), depression (3% to 10%), dizziness (3% to 10%), drowsiness (3% to 10%), insomnia (3% to 10%), nervousness (3% to 10%), paresthesia (3% to 10%), abnormal dreams (<3%), abnormality in thinking (<3%), amnesia (<3%), ataxia (<3%), dysarthria (<3%), emotional lability (<3%), encephalitis (<3%), hallucination (<3%), hostility (<3%), meningism (<3%), neuralgia (<3%), neuritis (<3%), neuropathy (<3%), paralysis (<3%), psychoneurosis (<3%), seizure (<3%), twitching (<3%), vertigo (<3%)

Dermatologic: Diaphoresis (8% to 10%), cellulitis (6%), furunculosis (4%), xeroderma (3% to 10%), urticaria (3% to 10%), acne vulgaris (<3%), alopecia (<3%), eczema (<3%), skin photosensitivity (<3%)

Endocrine & metabolic: Amenorrhea (<3%), decreased libido (<3%), hypercalcemia (<3%), hyponatremia (<3%), gout (<3%), loss of libido (<3%)

Gastrointestinal: Dyspepsia (3% to 10%), flatulence (3% to 10%), gingivitis (3% to 10%), constipation (<3%), dysgeusia (<3%), dysphagia (<3%), glossitis (<3%), intestinal obstruction (<3%), oral candidiasis (2%)

Genitourinary: Urinary tract infection (3%), impotence (<3%)

Hematologic & oncologic: Agranulocytosis (3% to 10%), hemorrhage (3% to 10%), acute leukemia (<3%), aplastic anemia (<3%), hemolytic anemia (<3%), petechia (<3%)

Infection: Herpes zoster (8%), viral infection (≤8%), bacterial infection (5%), herpes simplex infection (4%), sepsis (3%), abscess (2%)

Neuromuscular & skeletal: Arthralgia (3% to 10%), arthritis (<3%), hyperkinesia (<3%), osteomyelitis (1%)

Ophthalmic: Conjunctivitis (4%), amblyopia (<3%), lacrimal dysfunction (<3%), nonreactive pupils (<3%), photophobia (<3%), retinopathy (<3%), visual disturbance (<3%), watery eyes (<3%), xerophthalmia (<3%)

Otic: Deafness (<3%), labyrinthitis (<3%), otalgia (<3%), tinnitus (<3%)

Renal: Increased serum creatinine (3% to 10%), nephrolithiasis (<3%), renal disease (<3%), renal failure (<3%), renal function abnormality (<3%), renal insufficiency (<3%)

Respiratory: Pharyngitis (8% to 10%), sinusitis (6%), pneumonia (5%), asthma (3% to 10%), bronchitis (3%), bronchospasm (<3%), flu-like symptoms (<3%), laryngeal edema (<3%), pulmonary embolism (<3%)

<1%, postmarketing, and/or case reports: Dysuria, fungal skin infection, hematuria, lethargy, pulmonary edema, pulmonary toxicity (in combination with fludarabine), uveitis, vision loss

Drug Interactions

Metabolism/Transport Effects None known.

Avoid Concomitant Use

Avoid concomitant use of Pentostatin with any of the following: BCG (Intravesical); Deferiprone; Dipyrone; Fludarabine; Natalizumab; Nelarabine; Pegademase Bovine; Pimecrolimus; Tacrolimus (Topical); Vaccines (Live)

Increased Effect/Toxicity

Pentostatin may increase the levels/effects of: CloZAPine; Cyclophosphamide; Deferiprone; Fingolimod; Fludarabine; Leflunomide; Natalizumab; Tofacitinib; Vaccines (Live)

The levels/effects of Pentostatin may be increased by: Denosumab; Dipyrone; Fludarabine; Ocrelizumab; Palifermin; Pimecrolimus; Promazine; Roflumilast; Tacrolimus (Topical); Trastuzumab

Decreased Effect

Pentostatin may decrease the levels/effects of: BCG (Intravesical); Coccidioides immitis Skin Test; Lenograstim; Nelarabine; Nivolumab; Pegademase Bovine; Sipuleucel-T; Tertomotide; Vaccines (Inactivated); Vaccines (Live)

The levels/effects of Pentostatin may be decreased by: Echinacea; Pegademase Bovine

◄ **Hazardous Drugs Handling Considerations**
Hazardous agent (NIOSH 2016 [group 1]).

Use appropriate precautions for receiving, handling, administration, and disposal. Gloves (single) should be worn during receiving, unpacking, and placing in storage.

NIOSH recommends double gloving, a protective gown, ventilated engineering controls (a class II biological safety cabinet or a compounding aseptic containment isolator), and closed system transfer devices (CSTDs) for preparation. Double gloving, a gown, and (if dosage form allows) CSTDs are required during administration (NIOSH 2016).

Storage/Stability Store intact vials under refrigeration at 2°C to 8°C (36°F to 46°F). Reconstituted vials and solutions diluted for infusion (in D5W or NS) may be stored at room temperature for 8 hours.

Preparation for Administration Reconstitute with 5 mL SWFI to a concentration of 2 mg/mL. The solution may be further diluted in 25 to 50 mL NS or D5W for infusion. When diluted for infusion in D5W or NS at concentrations of 0.18 to 0.33 mg/mL, pentostatin is compatible with PVC containing infusion bags and infusion sets.

Mechanism of Action Pentostatin is a purine antimetabolite that inhibits adenosine deaminase, preventing the deamination of adenosine to inosine. Accumulation of deoxyadenosine (dAdo) and deoxyadenosine 5'-triphosphate (dATP) results in a reduction of purine metabolism which blocks DNA synthesis and leads to cell death.

Pharmacodynamics/Kinetics
Distribution: V_d: IV: 20 L/m^2 (Lathia, 2002)
Protein binding: ~4%
Half-life elimination: Terminal: ~6 hours; Renal impairment (CrCl <50 mL/minute): 18 hours (range: 11 to 23 hours [Lathia, 2002])
Excretion: Urine (~50% to 96%) within 24 hours (30% to 90% as unchanged drug)
Clearance: Adults: 68 mL/minute/m^2 (mean)

Dosing
Adult & Geriatric

Hairy cell leukemia: IV: 4 mg/m^2 every 2 weeks. **Note:** The optimal duration has not been determined; in the absence of unacceptable toxicity, may continue until complete response is achieved or until 2 doses after complete response. Discontinue after 6 months if partial or complete response is not achieved.

Acute graft-versus-host disease (GVHD), steroid-refractory (off-label use): IV:
Initial therapy: 1.5 mg/m^2 days 1 to 3 and days 15 to 17 (in combination with corticosteroids) (Alousi, 2009)
Steroid-refractory disease: 1.5 mg/m^2 daily for 3 days; may repeat after 2 weeks if needed (Bolanos-Meade, 2005)

Chronic graft-versus-host disease (GVHD), steroid-refractory (off-label use): IV: 4 mg/m^2 once every 2 weeks; discontinue after 6 months for sustained objective response, or continue every 2 to 4 weeks for up to 12 months if still improving (Jacobsohn, 2007; Jacobsohn, 2009) **or** 4 mg/m^2 once every 2 weeks for 3 months (Wolff, 2011)

Chronic lymphocytic leukemia (CLL; off-label use): IV:
Previously treated: 4 mg/m^2 once every 3 weeks (in combination with cyclophosphamide and rituximab) for 6 cycles (Lamanna, 2006)

Previously untreated: 2 mg/m² once every 3 weeks (in combination with cyclophosphamide and rituximab) for 6 cycles (Kay, 2007)

Cutaneous T-cell lymphoma, mycosis fungoides/Sezary syndrome (off-label use): IV: 4 mg/m² once weekly for 3 weeks, then every 2 weeks for 6 weeks, then once monthly for a maximum of 6 months (Ho, 1999)

T-cell prolymphocytic leukemia, refractory (off-label use): IV: 4 mg/m² once weekly for 4 weeks then every 2 weeks until optimum response is achieved (Mercieca, 1994) **or** 4 mg/m² once weekly for 4 weeks then every 2 weeks (in combination with alemtuzumab) until complete or best response or up to a total of 14 doses (Ravandi, 2009)

Pediatric Chronic graft-versus-host disease (GVHD), steroid-refractory: IV: 4 mg/m² once every 2 weeks; discontinue after 6 months for sustained objective response, or continue every 2 to 4 weeks for up to 12 months if still improving (Jacobsohn, 2007; Jacobsohn, 2009) **or** 4 mg/m² once every 2 weeks for 3 months (Wolff, 2011)

Renal Impairment There are no dosage adjustments provided in the manufacturer's labeling; although not adequately studied, two patients with CrCl 50 to 60 mL/minute achieved responses when treated with 2 mg/m²/dose. For renal toxicity *during* treatment, withhold for elevated serum creatinine and determine creatinine clearance. The following adjustments have also been recommended:

Kintzel, 1995:

CrCl 46 to 60 mL/minute: Administer 70% of dose
CrCl 31 to 45 mL/minute: Administer 60% of dose
CrCl <30 mL/minute: Consider use of alternative drug

Lathia, 2002:

CrCl ≥60 mL/minute: Administer 4 mg/m²/dose
CrCl 40 to 59 mL/minute: Administer 3 mg/m²/dose
CrCl 20 to 39 mL/minute: Administer 2 mg/m²/dose

Alousi, 2009; Jacobsohn, 2009; Poi, 2013 (for GVHD treatment):

CrCl 30 to 50 mL/minute/1.73 m²: Reduce dose by 50%
CrCl <30 mL/minute/1.73 m²: Withhold dose

Lamanna, 2006 (for previously treated CLL): Serum creatinine >2 mg/dL or 20% above patient's baseline: Withhold treatment until serum creatinine ≤2 mg/dL or returns to baseline, or until CrCl ≥50 mL/minute

Hepatic Impairment There are no dosage adjustments provided in the manufacturer's labeling.

Obesity

American Society of Clinical Oncology (ASCO) Guidelines for appropriate chemotherapy dosing in obese adults with cancer: Utilize patient's actual body weight (full weight) for calculation of body surface area- or weight-based dosing, particularly when the intent of therapy is curative; manage regimen-related toxicities in the same manner as for nonobese patients; if a dose reduction is utilized due to toxicity, consider resumption of full weight-based dosing with subsequent cycles, especially if cause of toxicity (eg, hepatic or renal impairment) is resolved (Griggs, 2012).

American Society for Blood and Marrow Transplantation (ASBMT) practice guideline committee position statement on chemotherapy dosing in obesity: Utilize actual body weight (full weight) for calculation of body surface area in pentostatin dosing for hematopoietic stem cell transplant conditioning regimens in adults (Bubalo, 2014).

◀ **Adjustment for Toxicity**
ANC <200/mm^3 (with baseline ANC >500/mm^3): Temporarily interrupt treatment until ANC returns to pre-dose levels.
CNS toxicity: Withhold treatment or discontinue.
Infection, active: Interrupt treatment until infection is controlled.
Rash: Severe rashes may require treatment interruption or discontinuation.
Other severe adverse reactions: Withhold treatment or discontinue.

Combination Regimens
Leukemia, chronic lymphocytic: Pentostatin-Cyclophosphamide-Rituximab (CLL) on page 2193

Administration Administer IV over 20 to 30 minutes or as a bolus infusion. Hydrate with 500 to 1,000 mL fluid prior to infusion and 500 mL after infusion.

Emetic Potential
Children: Minimal (<10%)
Adults: Low (10% to 30%)

Monitoring Parameters CBC with differential and platelet count (prior to each dose; more frequently during initial cycles), peripheral blood smears (periodically for hairy cells and to assess treatment response), liver function, serum uric acid, renal function (serum creatinine and/or creatinine clearance at baseline, and serum creatinine prior to each dose), bone marrow evaluation, signs/symptoms of pulmonary and CNS toxicity

Dosage Forms Excipient information presented when available (limited, particularly for generics); consult specific product labeling.
Solution Reconstituted, Intravenous:
Nipent: 10 mg (1 ea)

♦ **PEP005** see Ingenol Mebutate on page 1011
♦ **Periactin** see Cyproheptadine on page 467
♦ **Perjeta** see Pertuzumab on page 1506

Pertuzumab (per TU zoo mab)

Related Information
Management of Chemotherapy-Induced Nausea and Vomiting in Adults on page 2253
Safe Handling of Hazardous Drugs on page 2379

Brand Names: US Perjeta

Brand Names: Canada Perjeta

Index Terms 2C4 Antibody; MOAB 2C4; Monoclonal Antibody 2C4; Omnitarg; rhuMAb-2C4

Pharmacologic Category Antineoplastic Agent, Anti-HER2; Antineoplastic Agent, Monoclonal Antibody

Use
Breast cancer, metastatic: Treatment of human epidermal growth factor receptor 2 (HER2)-positive metastatic breast cancer (in combination with trastuzumab and docetaxel) in patients who have not received prior anti-HER2 therapy or chemotherapy to treat metastatic disease.

Breast cancer, neoadjuvant treatment: Neoadjuvant treatment of locally advanced, inflammatory, or early stage HER2-positive, breast cancer (either greater than 2 cm in diameter or node positive) in combination with trastuzumab and docetaxel (as part of a complete treatment regimen for early breast cancer).

Limitations of use: The safety of pertuzumab as part of a doxorubicin-containing regimen has not been established; the safety of pertuzumab administered for more than 6 cycles for early breast cancer has not been established.

Labeled Contraindications Known hypersensitivity to pertuzumab or any component of the formulation

Pregnancy Considerations [US Boxed Warning]: Pertuzumab exposure during pregnancy may result in embryo-fetal mortality and birth defects. Advise patients of the risks and the need for effective contraception. Verify pregnancy status prior to treatment initiation (in women of reproductive potential). Based on the mechanism of action of pertuzumab and data from similar agents, oligohydramnios or oligohydramnios sequence may occur resulting in pulmonary hypoplasia, skeletal anomalies, and neonatal death. Monitor for oligohydramnios if exposure occurs during pregnancy or within 7 months prior to conception; conduct appropriate fetal testing if oligohydramnios occurs. Effective contraception should be used during therapy and for 7 months after the last dose (of pertuzumab in combination with trastuzumab) for women of childbearing potential. Advise patients to immediately report to healthcare provider if pregnancy is suspected during treatment. If pertuzumab exposure occurs during pregnancy or exposure to pertuzumab in combination with trastuzumab occurs within 7 months prior to conception, healthcare providers should report the exposure to the Genentech Adverse Event Line (888-835-2555).

Women exposed to pertuzumab during pregnancy or exposed to pertuzumab in combination with trastuzumab within 7 months prior to conception are encouraged to enroll in MotHER Pregnancy Registry (1-800-690-6720 or www.motherpregnancyregistry.com).

European Society for Medical Oncology (ESMO) guidelines for cancer during pregnancy recommend delaying treatment with HER2-targeted agents until after delivery in pregnant patients with HER2-positive disease (Peccatori 2013).

Breastfeeding Considerations It is not known if pertuzumab is excreted in human milk. Because many immunoglobulins are excreted in human milk, and the potential for serious adverse reactions in the breastfeeding infant exists, the decision to discontinue breastfeeding or to discontinue pertuzumab should take into account the benefits of treatment to the mother. The extended half-life of pertuzumab and the 7-month wash out period for trastuzumab should be considered for decisions regarding breastfeeding after treatment is completed.

Warnings/Precautions [US Boxed Warning]: May result in cardiac failure (clinical and subclinical) manifesting as decreased left ventricular ejection fraction (LVEF) and heart failure (HF). Assess cardiac function at baseline and during treatment. Discontinue for confirmed clinically significant decline in left ventricular function. Decreases in LVEF are associated with HER-2 inhibitors, including pertuzumab. Patients who received prior anthracycline therapy or chest irradiation may be at an increased risk for cardiotoxicity. In studies of pertuzumab (versus placebo) in combination with trastuzumab and docetaxel for the treatment of metastatic breast cancer, the rate of cardiotoxicity (LVEF decline or symptomatic LV systolic dysfunction) was not increased in the pertuzumab group when compared to placebo. In the neoadjuvant setting, the incidence of LV dysfunction was higher in patients treated with pertuzumab. In a study of pertuzumab, trastuzumab and docetaxel, compared with trastuzumab and docetaxel, the incidence of LVEF decline (of >10% decrease from baseline or to <50%) was 8.4% and 1.9%, respectively; LVEF recovered to ≥50% in all patients. In another neoadjuvant study, LVEF declines (of >10% decrease from baseline or to <50%) were noted in 6.9% to 16% of patients receiving various combinations and sequences of pertuzumab plus trastuzumab with FEC (fluorouracil, epirubicin, and cyclophosphamide), docetaxel, and/or carboplatin; LVEF recovered to ≥50% in most patients. Of note, patients with pretreatment LVEF ≤50%, CHF, LVEF decreases to <50% during prior trastuzumab treatment, or conditions which could impair LV function (eg, uncontrolled hypertension, recent MI, serious arrhythmia requiring treatment, or cumulative lifetime anthracycline exposure >360 mg/m^2 doxorubicin or its equivalent) were excluded from studies. Assess LVEF at baseline, every 3 months during treatment (metastatic patients) or every 6 weeks during treatment (neoadjuvant setting), and every 6 months after therapy discontinuation up to 24 months after the last dose of pertuzumab and/or trastuzumab. Withhold pertuzumab and trastuzumab if LVEF <45% **or** 45% to 49% with a ≥10% absolute decline from baseline; repeat LVEF assessment in ~3 weeks; discontinue if LVEF has not improved or has declined further (unless potential benefits outweigh risks).

Infusion reactions (either during or on the day of infusion) have been associated with pertuzumab; commonly described as fever, chills, fatigue, headache, weakness, myalgia, hypersensitivity, abnormal taste or vomiting. The incidence of hypersensitivity/anaphylaxis was slightly higher in the group receiving pertuzumab (compared to placebo) in combination with trastuzumab and docetaxel. Monitor for 1 hour after the first infusion and for 30 minutes after subsequent infusions. For significant infusion reactions, interrupt or slow infusion rate; for severe infusion reactions, consider permanently discontinuing. Medications and equipment for the treatment of hypersensitivity should be available for immediate use during infusion. Diarrhea occurred more frequently in patients receiving pertuzumab in combination with trastuzumab and docetaxel, compared to patients receiving only trastuzumab and docetaxel.

[US Boxed Warning]: Pertuzumab exposure during pregnancy may result in embryo-fetal mortality and birth defects. Advise patients of the risks and the need for effective contraception. Verify pregnancy status prior to treatment initiation. Effective contraception should be used by all patients receiving pertuzumab during therapy and for 7 months after the last dose (of pertuzumab in combination with trastuzumab) in women of child-bearing potential.

Establish HER2 status prior to treatment; has only been studied in patients with evidence of HER2 overexpression, either as 3+ IHC (Dako Herceptest) or FISH amplification ratio ≥2 (Dako *HER*2 FISH pharmDx test). Safety of combination or sequential therapy with doxorubicin-containing regimens has not been established. For early breast cancer, the safety of treatment beyond 6 cycles has not been determined. Potentially significant drug-drug interactions may exist, requiring dose or frequency adjustment, additional monitoring, and/or selection of alternative therapy.

Adverse Reactions Note: Reactions reported in combination therapy with trastuzumab and docetaxel unless otherwise noted.

>10%:

Central nervous system: Fatigue (26% to 38%), headache (11% to 21%), decreased left ventricular ejection fraction (8% to 16%), insomnia (8% to 13%), dizziness (3% to 13%)

Dermatologic: Alopecia (52% to 65%), skin rash (11% to 34%; grades 3/4: <1%), pruritus (4% to 14%), palmar-plantar erythrodysesthesia (11%), xeroderma (9% to 11%)

Gastrointestinal: Diarrhea (46% to 67%; grades 3/4: 5% to 8%), nausea (39% to 53%; monotherapy 24%), vomiting (13% to 36%; monotherapy 15%), decreased appetite (11% to 29%), constipation (23%), mucositis (20% to 28%), stomatitis (17% to 19%), dysgeusia (13% to 18%), abdominal pain (monotherapy 12%)

Hematologic & oncologic: Neutropenia (47% to 53%; grades 3/4: 43% to 49%), anemia (3% to 23%; grades 3/4: 3% to 4%), leukopenia (9% to 16%; grades 3/4: 5% to 12%), febrile neutropenia (8% to 14%; grades 3/4: 9% to 13%)

Hypersensitivity: Hypersensitivity (1% to 11%; grades 3/4: 2%)

Neuromuscular & skeletal: Weakness (15% to 26%), myalgia (11% to 23%), arthralgia (10% to 12%)

Respiratory: Upper respiratory tract infection (4% to 17%; grades 3/4: <1%), epistaxis (11%)

Miscellaneous: Fever (9% to 19%; grades 3/4: 1%), infusion reactions (13%; grades 3/4: <1%)

1% to 10%:

Cardiovascular: Left ventricular dysfunction (3% to 4%), peripheral edema (3% to 4%)

Central nervous system: Peripheral sensory neuropathy (8%; grades 3/4: 1%), peripheral neuropathy (1%)

Dermatologic: Nail disease (7%), paronychia (1% to 7%)

Gastrointestinal: Dyspepsia (8%), anorexia (monotherapy 5%)

Hematologic & oncologic: Thrombocytopenia (1%)

Hepatic: Increased serum ALT (3%)

Ophthalmic: Increased lacrimation (4% to 5%)

Respiratory: Dyspnea (5% to 8%), nasopharyngitis (7%), oropharyngeal pain (7%), cough (5%)

<1%, postmarketing, and/or case reports with combination therapy: Heart failure, pleural effusion, sepsis

Drug Interactions

Metabolism/Transport Effects None known.

Avoid Concomitant Use

Avoid concomitant use of Pertuzumab with any of the following: Belimumab

Increased Effect/Toxicity

Pertuzumab may increase the levels/effects of: Belimumab

Decreased Effect There are no known significant interactions involving a decrease in effect.

Hazardous Drugs Handling Considerations

Hazardous agent (NIOSH 2016 [group 1]).

Use appropriate precautions for receiving, handling, administration, and disposal. Gloves (single) should be worn during receiving, unpacking, and placing in storage.

NIOSH recommends double gloving, a protective gown, ventilated engineering controls (a class II biological safety cabinet or a compounding aseptic containment isolator), and closed system transfer devices (CSTDs) for preparation. Double gloving, a gown, and (if dosage form allows) CSTDs are required during administration (NIOSH 2016).

Storage/Stability Store intact vials at 2°C to 8°C (36°F to 46°F) until time of use. Protect from light. Do not freeze. Do not shake. Solutions diluted for infusion in NS should be used immediately; if not used immediately, maybe stored at 2°C to 8°C (36°F to 46°F) for up to 24 hours.

Preparation for Administration Dilute in 250 mL NS only (do not use dextrose 5% solutions) in PVC or non-PVC (polyolefin) bags. Gently invert to mix (avoid foaming); do not shake. Do not mix with other medications.

Mechanism of Action Pertuzumab is a recombinant humanized monoclonal antibody which targets the extracellular human epidermal growth factor receptor 2 protein (HER2) dimerization domain. Inhibits HER2 dimerization and blocks HER downstream signaling halting cell growth and initiating apoptosis. Pertuzumab binds to a different HER2 epitope than trastuzumab so that when pertuzumab is combined with trastuzumab, a more complete inhibition of HER2 signaling occurs (Baselga, 2012).

Pharmacodynamics/Kinetics

Distribution: V_d: 5.12 L (Gianni, 2010)

Half-life elimination: Terminal: 18 days

Dosing

Adult & Geriatric Note: For pertuzumab, trastuzumab, and docetaxel combination regimens, pertuzumab and trastuzumab may be administered in any order; however, docetaxel should be given after pertuzumab and trastuzumab. Observe patients for 30 to 60 minutes after each pertuzumab infusion and before subsequent infusions of trastuzumab or docetaxel.

Breast cancer, metastatic HER2+: IV: 840 mg over 60 minutes followed by a maintenance dose of 420 mg over 30 to 60 minutes every 3 weeks until disease progression or unacceptable toxicity (in combination with trastuzumab and docetaxel) (Baselga, 2012; Swain, 2015).

Breast cancer, neoadjuvant treatment HER2+: Adults: IV: 840 mg over 60 minutes followed by a maintenance dose of 420 mg over 30 to 60 minutes every 3 weeks for 3 to 6 cycles; may be administered as one of the regimens below. Postoperatively, continue trastuzumab to complete 1 year of treatment.

Four preoperative cycles of pertuzumab, trastuzumab, and docetaxel, followed by 3 postoperative cycles of fluorouracil, epirubicin, and cyclophosphamide (FEC) (Gianni, 2012) **or**

Three preoperative cycles of FEC (alone) followed by 3 preoperative cycles of pertuzumab, trastuzumab, and docetaxel (Schneeweiss, 2013) **or**

Six preoperative cycles of pertuzumab, trastuzumab, docetaxel, and carboplatin (Schneeweiss, 2013)

Missed doses or delays: If <6 weeks has elapsed, administer the 420 mg maintenance dose; do not wait until the next planned dose. If ≥6 weeks has elapsed, readminister the 840 mg initial dose (over 60 minutes), and then follow with a maintenance dose of 420 mg (over 30 to 60 minutes) every 3 weeks.

Renal Impairment
CrCl ≥30 mL/minute: No dosage adjustment necessary.

CrCl <30 mL/minute: There are no dosage adjustments provided in the manufacturer's labeling (has not been studied).

Hepatic Impairment
There are no dosage adjustments provided in the manufacturer's labeling (has not been studied).

Adjustment for Toxicity Note: Dose reductions are not recommended for pertuzumab; if trastuzumab is withheld, pertuzumab should also be withheld; if trastuzumab is discontinued, pertuzumab should be discontinued; pertuzumab and trastuzumab may be continued if docetaxel is discontinued.

Infusion-related reaction: Slow or interrupt the infusion

Serious hypersensitivity: Discontinue immediately

Cardiotoxicity: Left ventricular ejection fraction (LVEF) declines to <45% **or** LVEF 45% to 49% with ≥10% absolute decrease below pretreatment values: Withhold treatment (pertuzumab and trastuzumab) for at least 3 weeks; may resume if LVEF returns to >49% **or** to 45% to 49% with <10% absolute decrease below pretreatment values. If after a repeat assessment within ~3 weeks, LVEF has not improved (or has declined further), discontinue pertuzumab and trastuzumab (unless the benefit of treatment outweighs risks).

Combination Regimens
Breast cancer:

Paclitaxel-Pertuzumab-Trastuzumab (Breast) on page 2186

Pertuzumab-Trastuzumab-Docetaxel (Metastatic Breast) on page 2195

Pertuzumab-Trastuzumab-Docetaxel (Neoadjuvant Breast) on page 2195

Administration For IV infusion only, as a short infusion; infuse initial dose (840 mg) over 60 minutes; infuse maintenance dose (420 mg) over 30 to 60 minutes. Do not administer IV push or as a rapid bolus. Do not mix with other medications. For pertuzumab, trastuzumab, and docetaxel combination regimens, pertuzumab and trastuzumab may be administered in any order; however, docetaxel should be given after pertuzumab and trastuzumab. Observe patients for 30 to 60 minutes after each pertuzumab infusion and before subsequent infusions of trastuzumab or docetaxel.

Emetic Potential Low (<10% to 30%)

Monitoring Parameters HER2 expression (either as 3+ IHC [Dako Herceptest™] or FISH amplification ratio ≥2 [Dako *HER2* FISH pharmDx™ test]); pregnancy test; assess LVEF at baseline, every 3 months during treatment (more frequently for declines) in metastatic treatment and every 6 weeks for neoadjuvant treatment, and every 6 months following discontinuation for up to 24 months from the last dose of pertuzumab and/or trastuzumab); monitor for infusion reaction and hypersensitivity

Dosage Forms Excipient information presented when available (limited, particularly for generics); consult specific product labeling.

Solution, Intravenous [preservative free]:

Perjeta: 420 mg/14 mL (14 mL) [contains mouse (murine) and/or hamster protein]

◆ **PF-01367338** *see* Rucaparib *on page 1641*

◆ **PF-01367338 BW** *see* Rucaparib *on page 1641*

◆ **PF-02341066** *see* Crizotinib *on page 432*

◆ **PFA** *see* Foscarnet *on page 847*

Pilocarpine (Systemic) (pye loe KAR peen)

Brand Names: US Salagen
Brand Names: Canada Salagen
Index Terms Pilocarpine HCl; Pilocarpine Hydrochloride
Pharmacologic Category Cholinergic Agonist
Use Xerostomia: Treatment of symptoms of dry mouth from salivary gland hypofunction caused by radiotherapy for cancer of the head and neck; treatment of symptoms of dry mouth in patients with Sjögren syndrome.
Pregnancy Risk Factor C
Dosing
  Adult & Geriatric
    Xerostomia: Oral:
      Associated with head and neck cancer: Initial: 5 mg 3 times daily; may titrate dose based on response and tolerability; usual dosage range: 15 to 30 mg/day; maximum: 10 mg/dose
      Sjögren syndrome: 5 mg 4 times daily
  Renal Impairment There are no dosage adjustments provided in the manufacturer's labeling.
  Hepatic Impairment
    Mild impairment (Child-Pugh score 5 to 6): No dosage adjustment necessary.
    Moderate impairment (Child-Pugh score 7 to 9): Initial: 5 mg twice daily; adjust dose based on response and tolerability.
    Severe impairment (Child-Pugh score 10 to 15): Use is not recommended.
Additional Information Complete prescribing information should be consulted for additional detail.

Dosage Forms Excipient information presented when available (limited, particularly for generics); consult specific product labeling.
Tablet, Oral, as hydrochloride:
 Salagen: 5 mg
 Salagen: 7.5 mg [contains fd&c blue #2 aluminum lake]
 Generic: 5 mg, 7.5 mg

◆ **Pilocarpine HCl** *see* Pilocarpine (Systemic) *on page 1512*

◆ **Pilocarpine Hydrochloride** *see* Pilocarpine (Systemic) *on page 1512*

Piperacillin and Tazobactam (pi PER a sil in & ta zoe BAK tam)

Brand Names: US Zosyn
Brand Names: Canada AJ-PIP/TAZ; Piperacillin and Tazobactam for Injection; Tazocin
Index Terms Piperacillin and Tazobactam Sodium; Piperacillin Sodium and Tazobactam Sodium; Piperacillin Sodium/Tazobactam; Piperacillin/Tazobactam Sod; Tazobactam and Piperacillin
Pharmacologic Category Antibiotic, Penicillin
Use
 Intra-abdominal infections: Treatment of appendicitis complicated by rupture or abscess and peritonitis caused by beta-lactamase-producing strains of *Escherichia coli*, *Bacteroides fragilis*, *Bacteroides ovatus*, *Bacteroides thetaiotaomicron*, or *Bacteroides vulgatus*.
 Pelvic infections: Treatment of postpartum endometriosis or pelvic inflammatory disease caused by beta-lactamase-producing strains of *E. coli*.
 Pneumonia, community-acquired: Treatment of moderate severity community-acquired pneumonia (CAP) caused by beta-lactamase-producing strains of *Haemophilus influenzae*. Infectious Diseases Society of America/ American Thoracic Society (IDSA/ATS) guidelines only recommend piperacillin/tazobactam for CAP caused by *P. aeruginosa* or due to aspiration (Mandell 2007).
 Pneumonia, hospital-acquired (nosocomial): Treatment of moderate to severe hospital-acquired (nosocomial) pneumonia caused by beta-lactamase-producing strains of *Staphylococcus aureus* and by piperacillin/tazobactam-susceptible *Acinetobacter baumanii*, *H. influenzae*, *Klebsiella pneumoniae*, and *Pseudomonas aeruginosa*.
 Skin and skin structure infections: Treatment of skin and skin structure infections, including cellulitis, cutaneous abscesses, and ischemic/diabetic foot infections caused by beta-lactamase–producing strains of *S. aureus*.
Dosing
 Adult & Geriatric Note: Dosing presented is based on traditional infusion method (IV infusion over 30 minutes) unless otherwise specified as the extended infusion method (IV infusion over 4 hours [off-label method]).
  Usual dosage range: IV: 3.375 g every 6 hours or 4.5 g every 6 to 8 hours; maximum: 18 g daily
   Extended infusion method (off-label dosing): 3.375 to 4.5 g IV over 4 hours every 8 hours (Kim 2007; Shea 2009); an alternative regimen of 4.5 g IV over 3 hours every 6 hours has also been described (Kim 2007)

  Indication-specific dosing:
   Appendicitis, diverticulitis, intra-abdominal abscess, peritonitis: IV: 3.375 g every 6 hours for 7 to 10 days

Pneumonia:

Community-acquired pneumonia (CAP): IV: 3.375 g every 6 hours for 7 to 10 days. **Note:** IDSA/ATS guidelines only recommend piperacillin/tazobactam for CAP caused by *P. aeruginosa* or due to aspiration (Mandell 2007).

Hospital-acquired or ventilator-associated: IV: 4.5 g every 6 hours for 7 days; may consider shorter or longer duration depending on rate of clinical improvement. Administration as an extended infusion may be considered. When used as empiric therapy, use in combination with an agent active against MRSA (unless coverage of MSSA only is appropriate) with or without an additional antipseudomonal agent (dependent on patient and institution-specific risk factors) (Kalil 2016).

Skin and soft tissue infection: IV: 3.375 g every 6 hours for 7 to 10 days. **Note:** For severe diabetic foot infections, recommended treatment duration is up to 4 weeks depending on severity of infection and response to therapy (Lipsky 2012).

Necrotizing infections (off-label use): IV:3.375 g every 6 to 8 hours (in combination with vancomycin for empiric therapy); continue until further debridement is not necessary, patient has clinically improved, and patient is afebrile for 48 to 72 hours (IDSA [Stevens 2014]).

Bite wound infection (animal) (off-label use): IV: 3.375 g every 6 to 8 hours (IDSA [Stevens 2014])

Intra-abdominal infection, complicated (off-label use): IV: 3.375 g every 6 hours for 4 to 7 days (provided source controlled). **Note:** Increase to 3.375 g every 4 hours or 4.5 g every 6 hours if *P. aeruginosa* is suspected. Not recommended for mild-to-moderate, community-acquired intra-abdominal infections due to risk of toxicity and the development of resistant organisms (Solomkin 2010).

Surgical (perioperative) prophylaxis (off-label use): IV: 3.375 g within 60 minutes prior to surgery. Doses may be repeated in 2 hours if procedure is lengthy or if there is excessive blood loss (Bratzler 2013).

Surgical site infections (intestinal or genitourinary tract) (off-label use): IV: 3.375 g every 6 hours or 4.5 g every 8 hours (IDSA [Stevens 2014])

Pediatric Note: Piperacillin and tazobactam is a combination product; each 3.375 g vial contains 3 g piperacillin sodium and 0.375 g tazobactam sodium in an 8:1 ratio. Dosage recommendations in **pediatric** patients are based on the **piperacillin** component. Dosing presented is based on traditional infusion method (IV infusion over 30 minutes) unless otherwise specified as the extended infusion method (IV infusion over 4 hours [off-label method]).

Usual dosage range: IV:

Infants 2 to 9 months: 80 mg piperacillin/kg/dose every 8 hours (Red Book [AAP] 2012):

Infants >9 months, Children, and Adolescents: 100 mg piperacillin/kg/dose every 8 hours (maximum dose: 16 g piperacillin/day) (Red Book [AAP] 2012):

Children and Adolescents: Extended-infusion method: Limited data available: 100 mg piperacillin/kg/dose infused over 4 hours 3 times daily. Dosing based on a prospective, observational study (n=332) in a single children's hospital comparing the extended interval method to traditional dosing (Nichols 2012).

Indication-specific dosing: Infants, Children, and Adolescents: **Note:** In pediatric patients, dosage recommendations are based on the **piperacillin** component. Dosing is presented in mg/kg/**dose** and mg/kg/**day**; use caution.

Appendicitis, peritonitis:
Infants 2 to 9 months: IV: 80 mg piperacillin/kg/dose every 8 hours
Infants >9 months, Children, and Adolescents ≤40 kg: IV: 100 mg piper-acillin/kg/dose every 8 hours (maximum: 3,000 mg piperacillin/dose)
Children and Adolescents >40 kg: Refer to adult dosing.

Cystic fibrosis, pseudomonal lung infections (off-label use):
Standard dosing: IV: 240 to 400 mg piperacillin/kg/**day** divided every 8 hours (Kliegman, 2011); others have used 350 to 400 mg/kg/**day** divided every 4 hours in early piperacillin trials (Zobell, 2013)
High-dose: Limited data available: IV: 450 mg piperacillin/kg/**day** divided every 4 to 6 hours or 600 mg piperacillin/kg/**day** divided every 4 hours has been described from early studies of piperacillin alone; usual maximum daily dose: 18 to 24 g piperacillin/**day**. **Note:** Piperacillin doses >600 mg/kg/day or an extended duration of therapy (>14 days) have been associated with dose-related adverse effects including serum sickness, immune-mediated hemolytic anemia and bone marrow sup-pression (Zobell 2013).

Intra-abdominal infection, complicated (off-label use): IV: 200 to 300 mg piperacillin/kg/day divided every 6 to 8 hours (maximum dose: 12 g piperacillin/day) (Solomkin, 2010).

Skin and soft tissue necrotizing infections (off-label use): IV: 60 to 75 mg piperacillin/kg every 6 hours (in combination with vancomycin for empiric therapy); continue until further debridement is not necessary, patient has clinically improved, and patient is afebrile for 48 to 72 hours. (IDSA [Stevens 2014])

Surgical (perioperative) prophylaxis (off-label use): Note: Doses may be repeated in 2 hours if procedure is lengthy or if there is excessive blood loss (Bratzler 2013): IV:
Infants 2 to 9 months: 80 mg piperacillin/kg within 60 minutes prior to surgical incision (maximum: 3,000 mg piperacillin/dose)
Infants >9 months, Children, and Adolescents ≤40 kg: 100 mg piperacillin/kg within 60 minutes prior to surgical incision (maximum: 3,000 mg piperacillin/dose).
Children and Adolescents >40 kg: Refer to adult dosing.

Renal Impairment
Adults:
Traditional infusion method (ie, IV infusion over 30 minutes): Manufac-turer's labeling:
CrCl >40 mL/minute: No dosage adjustment necessary.
CrCl 20 to 40 mL/minute: Administer 2.25 g every 6 hours (3.375 g every 6 hours for hospital-acquired or ventilator-associated pneumonia)
CrCl <20 mL/minute: Administer 2.25 g every 8 hours (2.25 g every 6 hours for hospital-acquired or ventilator-associated pneumonia)
Note: Some clinicians suggest adjusting the dose at CrCl ≤20 mL/minute (rather than CrCl <40 mL/minute) in patients receiving either traditional or extended-infusion methods, particularly if treating serious gram-negative infections (empirically or definitively) (Patel 2010).
Extended infusion method (off-label dosing): CrCl ≤20 mL/minute: 3.375 g IV over 4 hours every 12 hours (Patel 2010)

◄

End-stage renal disease (ESRD):

Intermittent hemodialysis (IHD): 2.25 g every 12 hours (2.25 g every 8 hours for hospital-acquired or ventilator-associated pneumonia); Hemodialysis removes 30% to 40% of a piperacillin/tazobactam dose. **Note:** Dosing dependent on the assumption of 3 times/week, complete IHD sessions. Administer scheduled doses after hemodialysis on dialysis days; if next regularly scheduled dose is not due right after dialysis session, administer an additional dose of 0.75 g after the dialysis session.

Peritoneal dialysis (PD): 2.25 g every 12 hours (2.25 g every 8 hours for hospital-acquired or ventilator-associated pneumonia); peritoneal dialysis removes 6% of piperacillin and 21% of tazobactam.

Continuous renal replacement therapy (CRRT) (Heintz 2009; Trotman 2005): Drug clearance is highly dependent on the method of renal replacement, filter type, and flow rate. Appropriate dosing requires close monitoring of pharmacologic response, signs of adverse reactions due to drug accumulation, as well as drug concentrations in relation to target trough (if appropriate). The following are general recommendations only (based on dialysate flow/ultrafiltration rates of 1 to 2 L/hour and minimal residual renal function) and should not supersede clinical judgment (Trotman 2005):

CVVH: 2.25 to 3.375 g every 6 to 8 hours

CVVHD: 2.25 to 3.375 g every 6 hours

CVVHDF: 3.375 g every 6 hours

Note: Higher dose of 3.375 g should be considered when treating resistant pathogens (especially *Pseudomonas* spp); alternative recommendations suggest dosing of 4.5 g every 8 hours (Valtonen 2001); regardless of regimen, there is some concern of tazobactam (TAZ) accumulation, given its lower clearance relative to piperacillin (PIP). Some clinicians advocate dosing with PIP to alternate with PIP/TAZ, particularly in CVVH-dependent patients, to lessen this concern.

Infants, Children, and Adolescents: There are no dosage adjustments provided in the manufacturer's labeling; however, the following adjustments have been recommended (Aronoff, 2007): Dosing based on a usual dose of 200 to 300 mg piperacillin/kg/day in divided doses every 6 hours.

GFR >50 mL/minute/1.73 m^2: No dosage adjustment necessary.

GFR 30 to 50 mL/minute/1.73 m^2: 35 to 50 mg piperacillin/kg/dose every 6 hours

GFR <30 mL/minute/1.73 m^2: 35 to 50 mg piperacillin/kg/dose every 8 hours

End-stage renal disease (ESRD) on intermittent hemodialysis (IHD): Hemodialysis removes 30% to 40% of a piperacillin/tazobactam dose: 50 to 75 mg piperacillin/kg/dose every 12 hours

Peritoneal dialysis (PD): Peritoneal dialysis removes 21% of tazobactam and 6% of piperacillin: 50 to 75 mg piperacillin/kg/dose every 12 hours

Continuous renal replacement therapy (CRRT): 35 to 50 mg piperacillin/kg/dose every 8 hours

Hepatic Impairment No dosage adjustment necessary.

Additional Information Complete prescribing information should be consulted for additional detail.

Dosage Forms Excipient information presented when available (limited, particularly for generics); consult specific product labeling.

Note: 8:1 ratio of piperacillin sodium/tazobactam sodium

Infusion [premixed iso-osmotic solution]:

Zosyn: 2.25 g: Piperacillin 2 g and tazobactam 0.25 g (50 mL) [contains edetate disodium, sodium 128 mg (5.58 mEq)]

Zosyn: 3.375 g: Piperacillin 3 g and tazobactam 0.375 g (50 mL) [contains edetate disodium, sodium 192 mg (8.38 mEq)]

Zosyn: 4.5 g: Piperacillin 4 g and tazobactam 0.5 g (100 mL) [contains edetate disodium, sodium 256 mg (11.17 mEq)]

Injection, powder for reconstitution: 2.25 g: Piperacillin 2 g and tazobactam 0.25 g; 3.375 g: Piperacillin 3 g and tazobactam 0.375 g; 4.5 g: Piperacillin 4 g and tazobactam 0.5 g; 40.5 g: Piperacillin 36 g and tazobactam 4.5 g

Zosyn: 2.25 g: Piperacillin 2 g and tazobactam 0.25 g [contains edetate disodium, sodium 130 mg (5.68 mEq)]

Zosyn: 3.375 g: Piperacillin 3 g and tazobactam 0.375 g [contains edetate disodium, sodium 195 mg (8.52 mEq)]

Zosyn: 4.5 g: Piperacillin 4 g and tazobactam 0.5 g [contains edetate disodium, sodium 260 mg (11.36 mEq)]

Zosyn: 40.5 g: Piperacillin 36 g and tazobactam 4.5 g [contains edetate disodium, sodium 2304 mg (100.4 mEq); bulk pharmacy vial]

◆ **Piperacillin and Tazobactam for Injection (Can)** *see* Piperacillin and Tazobactam *on page* 1513

◆ **Piperacillin and Tazobactam Sodium** *see* Piperacillin and Tazobactam *on page* 1513

◆ **Piperacillin Sodium and Tazobactam Sodium** *see* Piperacillin and Tazobactam *on page* 1513

◆ **Piperacillin Sodium/Tazobactam** *see* Piperacillin and Tazobactam *on page* 1513

◆ **Piperacillin/Tazobactam Sod** *see* Piperacillin and Tazobactam *on page* 1513

◆ **PKC 412** *see* Midostaurin *on page* 1257

◆ **Platinol** *see* CISplatin *on page* 400

◆ **Platinol-AQ** *see* CISplatin *on page* 400

Plerixafor (pler IX a fore)

Related Information

Hematopoietic Cell Transplantation *on page* 2365

Safe Handling of Hazardous Drugs *on page* 2379

Brand Names: US Mozobil

Brand Names: Canada Mozobil

Index Terms AMD3100; LM3100

Pharmacologic Category Hematopoietic Agent; Hematopoietic Stem Cell Mobilizer

Use Peripheral stem cell mobilization: Mobilization of hematopoietic stem cells (HSC) for collection and subsequent autologous transplantation (in combination with filgrastim) in patients with non-Hodgkin lymphoma (NHL) and multiple myeloma (MM)

Labeled Contraindications History of hypersensitivity to plerixafor or any component of the formulation (anaphylactic shock has occurred).

Pregnancy Considerations Adverse effects have been observed in animal reproduction studies. May cause fetal harm if administered to pregnant women. Women of childbearing potential should use effective contraceptive measures to avoid becoming pregnant during treatment.

Breastfeeding Considerations It is not known if plerixafor is excreted in breast milk. Due to the potential for serious adverse reactions in the nursing infant, a decision should be made to discontinue plerixafor or to discontinue breastfeeding, taking into account the importance of treatment to the mother.

Warnings/Precautions Serious hypersensitivity reactions, including anaphylactic-type reactions (may be life-threatening with serious hypotension and shock) have been reported. Observe patients for hypersensitivity symptoms during, for 30 minutes after administration, and until clinically stable. Medication, personnel, and equipment for hypersensitivity management should be available. Mild-to-moderate allergic reactions may also occur, usually within 30 minutes of administration. Increases circulating leukocytes when used in conjunction with filgrastim; monitor WBC counts. Thrombocytopenia has been observed; monitor platelet counts. Not intended for mobilization in patients with leukemia; may contaminate apheresis product by mobilizing leukemic cells. When used in combination with filgrastim, tumor cells released from marrow could be collected in leukapheresis product; potential effect of tumor cell reinfusion is unknown. Splenomegaly and splenic rupture have been reported (rarely) with filgrastim use; instruct patients to report left upper quadrant pain or scapular/shoulder tip pain; promptly evaluate in any patient who report these symptoms.

Primary route of elimination is renal; dosage reduction is recommended in patients with moderate-to-severe renal impairment (CrCl ≤50 mL/minute). Medications that may reduce renal function or compete for active tubular secretion may increase serum concentrations of plerixafor. Use has not been studied in patients weighing >175% of ideal body weight.

Adverse Reactions Adverse reactions reported with filgrastim combination therapy.

>10%:
Central nervous system: Fatigue (27%), headache (22%), dizziness (11%)
Gastrointestinal: Diarrhea (37%), nausea (34%)
Local: Injection site reaction (34%, including edema, erythema, hematoma, hemorrhage, induration, inflammation, irritation, pain, paresthesia, pruritus, skin rash, urticaria)
Neuromuscular & skeletal: Arthralgia (13%)

1% to 10%:
Central nervous system: Insomnia (7%), malaise (<5%)
Dermatologic: Erythema (<5%), hyperhidrosis (<5%)
Gastrointestinal: Vomiting (10%), flatulence (7%), abdominal distension (<5%), abdominal distress (<5%), abdominal pain (<5%), constipation (<5%), dyspepsia (<5%), oral hypoesthesia (<5%), xerostomia (<5%)
Hematologic & oncologic: Hyperleukocytosis (7%)
Neuromuscular & skeletal: Musculoskeletal pain (<5%)

<1%, postmarketing, and/or case reports: Abnormal dreams, anaphylaxis, diaphoresis, dyspnea, hypersensitivity reaction, hypoxia, leukocytosis, nightmares, orthostatic hypotension, periorbital swelling, syncope, thrombocytopenia

Drug Interactions

Metabolism/Transport Effects None known.

Avoid Concomitant Use There are no known interactions where it is recommended to avoid concomitant use.

Increased Effect/Toxicity There are no known significant interactions involving an increase in effect.

Decreased Effect There are no known significant interactions involving a decrease in effect.

Hazardous Drugs Handling Considerations

Hazardous agent (NIOSH 2016 [group 3]).

Use appropriate precautions for receiving, handling, administration, and disposal. Gloves (single) should be worn during receiving, unpacking, and placing in storage.

NIOSH recommends double gloving, a protective gown, ventilated engineering controls (a class II biological safety cabinet or a compounding aseptic containment isolator), and closed system transfer devices (CSTDs) for preparation. Double gloving and a protective gown are required during administration (NIOSH 2016).

Storage/Stability Store at 25°C (77°F); excursions permitted to 15°C to 30°C (59°F to 86°F).

Mechanism of Action Reversibly inhibits binding of stromal cell-derived factor-1-alpha (SDF-1α), expressed on bone marrow stromal cells, to the CXC chemokine receptor 4 (CXCR4), resulting in mobilization of hematopoietic stem and progenitor cells from bone marrow into peripheral blood. Plerixafor used in combination with filgrastim results in synergistic increase in CD34+ cell mobilization. Mobilized CD34+ cells are capable of engrafting with extended repopulating capacity.

Pharmacodynamics/Kinetics

Onset of action: Peak CD34+ mobilization (healthy volunteers): Plerixafor monotherapy: 6 to 9 hours after administration; Plerixafor + filgrastim: 10 to 14 hours

Duration: Sustained elevation in CD34+ cells (healthy volunteers): 4 to 18 hours after administration

Absorption: SubQ: Rapid; exposure using the mg/kg dosing increases with increasing body weight; the fixed dosing (20 mg) results in higher exposure than the mg/kg dose, but the median time to reach the target cell count is the same for both dosing regimens

Distribution: 0.3 L/kg; primarily to extravascular fluid space

Protein binding: ≤58%

Metabolism: Not metabolized

Half-life elimination: Terminal: 3 to 5 hours

Time to peak, plasma: SubQ: 30 to 60 minutes

Excretion: Urine (~70%; as parent drug)

Dosing

Adult & Geriatric Note: Dosing is based on actual body weight. Begin plerixafor after patient has received filgrastim (10 mcg/kg once daily) for 4 days; plerixafor, filgrastim, and apheresis should be continued daily until sufficient cell collection up to a maximum of 4 days.

Hematopoietic stem cell mobilization (in non-Hodgkin lymphoma and multiple myeloma): SubQ: Administer ~11 hours prior to apheresis

◀ **Pregnancy Considerations [US Boxed Warning]:** Pomalidomide is an analogue of thalidomide (a known human teratogen) and may cause severe birth defects or embryo-fetal death if taken during pregnancy. Pomalidomide cannot be used in women who are pregnant or may become pregnant during therapy. Obtain 2 negative pregnancy tests prior to initiation of treatment; 2 forms of contraception (or abstain from heterosexual intercourse) must be used at least 4 weeks prior to, during, and for ≥4 weeks after pomalidomide treatment (and during treatment interruptions) in females of reproductive potential. In order to decrease the risk of embryo-fetal exposure, pomalidomide is available only through a restricted distribution program (Pomalyst REMS).

Studies in animals have shown evidence of fetal abnormalities and use is contraindicated in women who are or may become pregnant. Women of childbearing potential should be treated only if they are able to comply with the conditions of the Pomalyst REMS Program. Reliable contraception is required even with a history of infertility (unless due to hysterectomy or if ≥24 consecutive months postmenopausal (natural). Reliable methods of birth control include one highly effective method (eg, tubal ligation, IUD, hormonal [birth control pills, injections, hormonal patches, vaginal rings, or implants], or partner's vasectomy) and one additional effective method (eg, male latex or synthetic condom, diaphragm, or cervical cap). Pregnancy tests should be performed 10 to 14 days and 24 hours prior to beginning therapy; weekly for the first 4 weeks and then every 4 weeks (every 2 weeks if menstrual cycle irregular) thereafter and during therapy interruptions for at least 4 weeks after discontinuation. Pomalidomide must be immediately discontinued for a missed period, abnormal pregnancy test or abnormal menstrual bleeding; refer patient to a reproductive toxicity specialist if pregnancy occurs during treatment. Pomalidomide is present in the semen of males taking this medication. Males (including those vasectomized) should use a latex or synthetic condom during any sexual contact with women of childbearing age during treatment, during treatment interruptions, and for 28 days after discontinuation. Male patients should not donate sperm. Any suspected fetal exposure should be reported to the FDA via the MedWatch program (1-800-332-1088) and to Celgene Corporation (1-888-423-5436).

Breastfeeding Considerations It is not known if pomalidomide is excreted into breast milk. Due to the potential for serious adverse reactions in the nursing infant, a decision should be made to discontinue nursing or to discontinue treatment with pomalidomide, taking into account the importance of treatment to the mother.

Warnings/Precautions Due to the embryo-fetal risk, pomalidomide is only available through a restricted distribution program under the Pomalyst REMS program. Pomalidomide should only be prescribed to patients who can understand and comply with the conditions of the Pomalyst REMS program. Prescribers and pharmacies must be certified with the REMS program.

[US Boxed Warning]: Pomalidomide is a thalidomide (human teratogen) analog and may cause severe life-threatening birth defects or embryo-fetal deaths; use is contraindicated in pregnancy. Pregnancy must be excluded prior to therapy initiation with 2 negative pregnancy tests; prevent pregnancy during therapy with 2 reliable forms of contraception (or abstain from heterosexual intercourse) beginning 4 weeks prior to, during and for 4 weeks after pomalidomide therapy (and during treatment interruptions) in females of reproductive potential. In order to

decrease the risk of embryo-fetal exposure, pomalidomide is available only through a restricted distribution program (Pomalyst REMS). Reliable methods of birth control include one highly effective method (eg, tubal ligation, IUD, hormonal [birth control pills, injections, hormonal patches, vaginal rings, or implants], or partner's vasectomy) and one additional effective method (eg, male latex or synthetic condom, diaphragm, or cervical cap). Males taking pomalidomide must use a latex or synthetic condom during any sexual contact with a woman of childbearing potential during therapy and for up to 28 days after treatment discontinuation, even if successfully vasectomized. Patients should not donate blood during pomalidomide treatment and for 1 month after therapy discontinuation; male patients receiving pomalidomide must not donate sperm.

Neutropenia, anemia, and thrombocytopenia were frequently reported in clinical trials; neutropenia was the most frequently reported grade 3/4 adverse event, followed by anemia and thrombocytopenia. Neutropenic fever has also been reported. Monitor complete blood counts weekly for the first 8 weeks of therapy and monthly or as clinically indicated thereafter; may require therapy interruption, reduction and/or discontinuation. Acute myelogenous leukemia (AML) as a secondary malignancy has been reported in patients receiving pomalidomide in the investigational treatment of condition(s) other than multiple myeloma. **[US Boxed Warning]: Venous and arterial thromboembolic events such as deep vein thrombosis (DVT), pulmonary embolism (PE), MI, and stroke have occurred during pomalidomide therapy. Clinical trials utilized antithrombotic prophylaxis. Thromboprophylaxis is recommended; and should be based on assessment of the patient's underlying risk factors.** Arterial thrombotic events also included cerebrovascular ischemia and ischemic heart disease. Monitor for signs/symptoms of thromboembolism (shortness of breath, chest pain, or arm or leg swelling) and advise patients to promptly seek medical attention should symptoms occur. May cause dizziness and/or confusion; caution patients to avoid tasks that require mental alertness (eg, operating machinery or driving). Avoid concomitant medications which may exacerbate dizziness and confusion. Angioedema and severe dermatologic reactions have been reported. Discontinue (permanently) for angioedema, skin exfoliation, bullae, or any other severe dermatologic toxicity. Use with caution in patients with a prior history of serious hypersensitivity reactions to thalidomide or lenalidomide; such patients were excluded from pomalidomide clinical trials and may therefore be at risk for hypersensitivity reactions when administered pomalidomide. Peripheral and sensory neuropathy occurred in clinical trials, including some cases of grade 3 neuropathy, although no cases of grade 4 neuropathy were observed. Monitor closely for signs/symptoms of neuropathy; may require therapy interruption, dose modification and/or discontinuation.

Interstitial lung disease (ILD) and related events (eg, pneumonitis) have been reported. Use with caution in hepatic impairment; initial dosage adjustment is recommended. Hepatic failure (with fatalities) has been reported; elevated bilirubin and ALT have also been observed. Monitor liver function tests. Interrupt treatment for elevated liver enzymes; consider dose reduction after enzymes return to baseline. Use with caution in patients receiving hemodialysis; initial dosage adjustment is recommended. Patients with a high tumor burden may be at risk for tumor lysis syndrome; monitor closely; institute appropriate management for hyperuricemia. Potentially significant drug-drug interactions may exist, requiring dose or frequency adjustment, additional ▶

◀ monitoring, and/or selection of alternative therapy. Cigarette smoking may induce CYP1A2 mediated metabolism of pomalidomide, potentially reducing its systemic exposure and efficacy.

Adverse Reactions Frequency not always defined.

Cardiovascular: Peripheral edema (25%), angina pectoris, congestive cardiac failure, hypotension, myocardial infarction, septic shock, syncope

Central nervous system: Fatigue (≤58%), dizziness (22%; grades 3/4: <5%), peripheral neuropathy (22%), neuropathy (18%; grades 3/4: 2%), headache (15%), anxiety (13%), confusion (12%; grades 3/4: 6%), chills (10%), insomnia (7%), pain (6%), altered mental status, depression, falling, noncardiac chest pain

Dermatologic: Skin rash (21%), pruritus (15%), xeroderma (9%), hyperhidrosis (8%), cellulitis

Endocrine & metabolic: Hypercalcemia (22%; grades 3/4: 10%), hypokalemia (12%; grades 3/4: <5%), hyperglycemia (11%; grades 3/4: <5%), hyponatremia (11%; grades 3/4: <5%), dehydration (<10%; grade 3/4: 5%), hypocalcemia (6%), weight gain (≤5%)

Gastrointestinal: Constipation (36%), nausea (36%), diarrhea (35%), decreased appetite (23%), weight loss (15%), vomiting (14%), abdominal pain, *Clostridium difficile*

Genitourinary: Urinary tract infection (10%, grades 3/4: 2%), urosepsis

Hematologic & oncologic: Neutropenia (53%; grades 3/4: 48%), anemia (38%; grades 3/4: 23%), thrombocytopenia (26%; grades 3/4: 22%), leukopenia (13%; grades 3/4: 7%), febrile neutropenia (<10%), lymphocytopenia (4%; grades 3/4: 2%), decreased hemoglobin

Hepatic: Increased serum ALT

Infection: Sepsis (<10%), bacteremia, pneumonia due to *Streptococcal* species, viral infection

Neuromuscular & skeletal: Weakness (≤58%), back pain (35%), musculoskeletal chest pain (23%), muscle spasm (22%), arthralgia (17%), myasthenia (14%), musculoskeletal pain (12%), ostealgia (12%), tremor (10%), limb pain (8%), fracture, vertebral compression fracture

Renal: Increased serum creatinine (19%), renal failure (15%)

Respiratory: Upper respiratory tract infection (37%), dyspnea (36%), pneumonia (28%; includes streptococcal pneumonia), cough (17%), epistaxis (17%), productive cough (9%), oropharyngeal pain (6%), bronchospasm, lobar pneumonia, pulmonary infection

Miscellaneous: Fever (23%), night sweats (5%), failure to thrive, multiorgan failure, physical health deterioration

<1%, postmarketing, and/or case reports: Acute cytolytic hepatitis, acute hepatoxicity, acute myelocytic leukemia, atrial fibrillation, hepatic failure, hepatitis (includes cytolytic hepatitis), hyperbilirubinemia, hyperkalemia, hypersensitivity reaction, increased liver enzymes, interstitial pulmonary disease, liver steatosis, neutropenic sepsis, pancytopenia, pelvic pain, pneumonia (*Pneumocystis jirovecii*), pneumonitis, prolonged prothrombin time, pulmonary fibrosis, respiratory syncytial virus infection, thrombosis, tumor lysis syndrome, urinary retention, vertigo, weight gain

Drug Interactions

Metabolism/Transport Effects Substrate of CYP1A2 (major), CYP2C19 (minor), CYP2D6 (minor), CYP3A4 (minor), P-glycoprotein; **Note:** Assignment of Major/Minor substrate status based on clinically relevant drug interaction potential

Avoid Concomitant Use

Avoid concomitant use of Pomalidomide with any of the following: Abatacept; Anakinra; Azelastine (Nasal); BCG (Intravesical); Canakinumab; Certolizumab Pegol; Deferiprone; Dipyrone; Natalizumab; Orphenadrine; Oxomemazine; Paraldehyde; Pimecrolimus; Rilonacept; Tacrolimus (Topical); Thalidomide; Tocilizumab; Tofacitinib; Vaccines (Live); Vedolizumab

Increased Effect/Toxicity

Pomalidomide may increase the levels/effects of: Abatacept; Alcohol (Ethyl); Anakinra; Analgesics (Opioid); Azelastine (Nasal); Bisphosphonate Derivatives; Blonanserin; Buprenorphine; Canakinumab; Certolizumab Pegol; CloZAPine; CNS Depressants; Deferiprone; Estrogen Derivatives; Fingolimod; Flunitrazepam; HYDROcodone; Leflunomide; Methotrimeprazine; MetyroSINE; Mirtazapine; Natalizumab; Orphenadrine; OxyCODONE; Paraldehyde; Piribedil; Pramipexole; Rilonacept; ROPINIRole; Rotigotine; Selective Serotonin Reuptake Inhibitors; Suvorexant; Thalidomide; Tofacitinib; Vaccines (Live); Vedolizumab; Zolpidem

The levels/effects of Pomalidomide may be increased by: Abiraterone Acetate; Brimonidine (Topical); Cannabis; Chlormethiazole; Chlorphenesin Carbamate; Ciprofloxacin (Systemic); CYP1A2 Inhibitors (Moderate); CYP1A2 Inhibitors (Strong); Deferasirox; Denosumab; Dimethindene (Topical); Dipyrone; Doxylamine; Dronabinol; Droperidol; Erythropoiesis-Stimulating Agents; HydrOXYzine; Kava Kava; Lofexidine; Magnesium Sulfate; Methotrimeprazine; Minocycline; Nabilone; Obeticholic Acid; Ocrelizumab; Oxomemazine; Peginterferon Alfa-2b; Perampanel; Pimecrolimus; Progestins; Promazine; Roflumilast; Rufinamide; Sodium Oxybate; Tacrolimus (Topical); Tapentadol; Tetrahydrocannabinol; Tocilizumab; Trastuzumab; Trimeprazine; Vemurafenib

Decreased Effect

Pomalidomide may decrease the levels/effects of: BCG (Intravesical); Coccidioides immitis Skin Test; Nivolumab; Sipuleucel-T; Tertomotide; Vaccines (Inactivated); Vaccines (Live)

The levels/effects of Pomalidomide may be decreased by: Echinacea

Hazardous Drugs Handling Considerations

Hazardous agent (NIOSH 2016 [group 1]).

Use appropriate precautions for receiving, handling, administration, and disposal. Gloves (single) should be worn during receiving, unpacking, and placing in storage. NIOSH recommends single gloving for administration of intact tablets or capsules (NIOSH 2016).

Storage/Stability Store at 20°C to 25°C (68°F to 77°F); excursions permitted to 15°C to 30°C (59°F to 86°F).

Mechanism of Action Induces cell cycle arrest and apoptosis directly in multiple myeloma cells; enhances T cell- and natural killer (NK) cell-mediated cytotoxicity; inhibits production of proinflammatory cytokines tumor necrosis factor-α (TNF-α), IL-1, IL-6, and IL-12; inhibits angiogenesis (Zhu 2013)

Pharmacodynamics/Kinetics

Absorption: Rapid; slowed by food.

Distribution: V_{dss}: 62 to 138 L; semen distribution is ~67% of plasma levels

Protein binding: 12% to 44%

Metabolism: Hepatic via CYP1A2 and CYP3A4; CYP2C19 and CYP2D6 (minor)

◄ Half-life elimination: ~9.5 hours (healthy subjects); ~7.5 hours (multiple myeloma patients)

Time to peak: 2 to 3 hours

Excretion: Urine (73%; 2% as unchanged drug); feces (15%; 8% as unchanged drug)

Dosing

Adult & Geriatric Note: ANC should be ≥500 cells/mm^3 and platelets ≥50,000 cells/mm^3 prior to initiating new cycles of therapy.

Multiple myeloma, relapsed/refractory: Oral: 4 mg once daily on days 1 to 21 of 28-day cycles (in combination with dexamethasone); continue until disease progression or unacceptable toxicity (Richardson 2014; San Miguel 2013).

Dosage adjustment for concomitant therapy with strong CYP1A2 inhibitors: Avoid concomitant use of strong CYP1A2 inhibitors. If concomitant use of strong CYP1A2 inhibitors cannot be avoided, reduce the pomalidomide dose by 50%.

Renal Impairment

CrCl ≥15 to <60 mL/minute: There are no dosage adjustments provided in the manufacturer's labeling. Compared to patients with normal renal function, pomalidomide pharmacokinetics were not significantly altered in patients with CrCl between 15 to 60 mL/minute.

Hemodialysis: Initial: 3 mg once daily. Administer after hemodialysis on dialysis days. Hemodialysis can remove pomalidomide from circulation.

The International Myeloma Working Group (IMWG) recommendations (Dimopoulos 2016): The IMWG recommends use of the Chronic Kidney Disease Epidemiology Collaboration (CKD-EPI) equation (preferred) or the Modification of Diet in Renal Disease (MDRD) formula to evaluate renal function estimation in multiple myeloma patients with a stable serum creatinine.

CrCl ≥45 mL/minute: No dosage adjustment required.

CrCl <45 mL/minute: Data is insufficient at this time to make a determination.

ESRD on dialysis: Data is insufficient at this time to make a determination.

Hepatic Impairment

*Hepatic impairment **prior** to treatment:*

Mild or moderate impairment (Child-Pugh class A or B): Initial: 3 mg once daily

Severe impairment (Child-Pugh class C): Initial: 2 mg once daily

*Hepatic impairment **during** treatment:* If liver enzymes are elevated, stop pomalidomide and evaluate; after liver enzymes return to baseline, may consider restarting at a lower dose

Adjustment for Toxicity

Hematologic:

If ANC <500 cells/mm^3 (or ANC <1,000 cells/mm^3 with fever ≥38.5°C) and/or platelets <25,000 cells/mm^3: Interrupt therapy and follow weekly CBCs. When ANC ≥500 cells/mm^3 and/or platelets ≥50,000 cells/mm^3: Resume dosing at 3 mg once daily.

For each subsequent drop of ANC <500 cells/mm^3 and/or platelets <25,000 cells/mm^3: Interrupt therapy. When ANC ≥500 cells/mm^3 and/or platelets ≥50,000 cells/mm^3: Resume dosing at 1 mg less than the previous dose. If toxicities occur at 1 mg daily dose, discontinue treatment.

Nonhematologic: If grade 3 or 4 toxicity occurs, interrupt therapy until resolved to ≤ grade 2; if appropriate, may restart therapy at 1 mg less than the previous dose. If toxicities occur at 1 mg daily dose, discontinue treatment.

Dermatologic toxicity:

Angioedema, skin exfoliation, bullae, or any other severe dermatologic toxicity: Permanently discontinue.

Combination Regimens

Multiple myeloma:

Daratumumab-Pomalidomide-Dexamethasone (Multiple Myeloma) on page 2085

Pomalidomide-Dexamethasone (Multiple Myeloma) on page 2196

Administration Administer without regard to meals. Swallow whole with water; do not break, chew, or open the capsules.

Missed doses: May administer a missed dose if within 12 hours of usual dosing time. If >12 hours, skip the dose for that day and resume usual dosing the following day. Do not take 2 doses to make up for a skipped dose.

Emetic Potential Minimal (<10%)

Monitoring Parameters CBC with differential and platelets weekly for the first 8 weeks and monthly or as clinically necessary thereafter; renal function (ie, serum creatinine, creatinine clearance); liver function tests (monthly); monitor for signs/symptoms of thromboembolism, neuropathy, tumor lysis syndrome (in patients at risk), and interstitial lung disease. Consider thyroid function tests (TSH recommended at baseline and every 2 to 3 months during treatment for structurally similar medications [Hamnvik 2011]).

Women of childbearing potential: Pregnancy test 10 to 14 days **and** 24 hours prior to initiating therapy, weekly during the first month, then monthly thereafter in women with regular menstrual cycles or every 2 weeks in women with irregular menstrual cycles. Pregnancy tests should be continued for at least 4 weeks after discontinuation.

Prescribing and Access Restrictions In Canada, pomalidomide is only available through a restricted distribution program called RevAid. Only physicians and pharmacists registered with the program are authorized to prescribe or dispense pomalidomide. Patients must also be registered and meet all conditions of the program. Two negative pregnancy tests with a sensitivity of at least 25 milliunits/mL are required prior to initiating therapy in women of childbearing potential. Further information is available at 1-888-738-2431 or www.RevAid.ca.

Medication Guide Available Yes

Dosage Forms Excipient information presented when available (limited, particularly for generics); consult specific product labeling.

Capsule, Oral:

Pomalyst: 1 mg, 2 mg, 3 mg [contains fd&c blue #2 (indigotine)]

Pomalyst: 4 mg [contains brilliant blue fcf (fd&c blue #1), fd&c blue #2 (indigotine)]

♦ **Pomalyst** *see* Pomalidomide *on page* 1521

PONATinib (poe NA ti nib)

Related Information

Safe Handling of Hazardous Drugs *on page* 2379

Brand Names: US Iclusig

◄ **Brand Names: Canada** Iclusig

Index Terms AP24534; Ponatinib HCl; Ponatinib Hydrochloride

Pharmacologic Category Antineoplastic Agent, BCR-ABL Tyrosine Kinase Inhibitor; Antineoplastic Agent, Tyrosine Kinase Inhibitor

Use

Acute lymphoblastic leukemia: Treatment of Philadelphia chromosome-positive acute lymphoblastic leukemia (Ph+ ALL) in patients for whom no other tyrosine kinase inhibitor therapy is indicated or who are T315I-positive.

Chronic myeloid leukemia: Treatment of chronic myeloid leukemia (CML) in chronic, accelerated, or blast phase in patients for whom no other tyrosine kinase inhibitor therapy is indicated or who are T315I-positive.

Limitations of use: Ponatinib is not indicated and not recommended for treatment of newly diagnosed chronic phase CML.

Labeled Contraindications

There are no contraindications listed in the manufacturer's US labeling.

Canadian labeling: Hypersensitivity to ponatinib or any component of the formulation; unmanaged cardiovascular risk factors, including uncontrolled hypertension; patients not adequately hydrated and with uncorrected hyperuricemia

Pregnancy Considerations Based on animal data and its mechanism of action, ponatinib is expected to cause fetal harm if used during pregnancy. Verify pregnancy status prior to initiating ponatinib treatment. Women of childbearing potential should use effective contraception during treatment and for 3 weeks after the last dose.

Breastfeeding Considerations It is not known if ponatinib is excreted in breast milk. Due to the potential for serious adverse reactions in the nursing infant, the manufacturer recommends that breastfeeding be discontinued during therapy and for 6 days after the last dose.

Warnings/Precautions **[US Boxed Warning]: Arterial occlusions have occurred in at least 35% of ponatinib-treated patients. Some patients experienced more than 1 type of event. Events included fatal myocardial infarction (MI), stroke, stenosis of large arterial vessels of the brain, severe peripheral vascular disease, and the need for urgent revascularization procedures; incidents were observed in patients with and without cardiovascular risk factors (including patients ≤50 years of age). Monitor closely for arterial occlusion; interrupt or discontinue therapy immediately for arterial occlusion. Consider risk:benefit ratio when deciding to restart therapy.** Fatal and life-threatening arterial occlusion may occur within 2 weeks of therapy initiation and is not dose dependent (events have occurred at doses as low as 15 mg daily), and may cause recurrent or multisite occlusion. The most common risk factors for developing arterial occlusive events were hypertension, hyperlipidemia, and history of cardiac disease. Increasing age and a prior history of ischemia, hypertension, diabetes, or hyperlipidemia are also risk factors for development of ponatinib-associated vascular occlusion. Patients have required a revascularization procedure (cerebrovascular, coronary, and peripheral arterial) due to serious arterial thrombosis/occlusion. MI and coronary artery occlusion may result in heart failure due to myocardial ischemia. Cerebrovascular occlusion (including fatal stroke) has occurred; may cause stenosis over multiple segments in major arterial vessels that supply the brain. Peripheral arterial occlusive events, including fatal mesenteric artery occlusion and life-threatening peripheral arterial disease, have occurred. Some patients have required amputation due to digital or distal extremity necrosis. Renal artery stenosis (associated with worsening or refractory hypertension) has been reported. **[US Boxed Warning]: Venous occlusive events have occurred in 6% of ponatinib-treated patients. Monitor for evidence of venous thromboembolism. Consider dose modification or discontinuation of ponatinib in patients who develop serious venous thromboembolism.** Venous thromboembolism, including deep vein thrombosis, pulmonary embolism, superficial thrombophlebitis, and retinal vein thrombosis have been reported.

[US Boxed Warning]: Serious heart failure (HF) or left ventricular dysfunction, including fatalities, were reported in clinical trials. Monitor for signs/symptoms of HF; interrupt or discontinue ponatinib therapy for new or worsening HF. The most commonly reported heart failure events were congestive heart failure and decreased ejection fraction. Treat as clinically warranted if HF develops. Consider ponatinib discontinuation in the event of serious HF. Cardiac arrhythmias (bradyarrhythmias and tachyarrhythmias) have also been reported. The most commonly reported arrhythmia was atrial fibrillation; ~50% of events were grade 3 or 4. Other grade 3 or 4 rhythm disorders have occurred (case reports). Some events required hospitalization; symptomatic bradyarrhythmia which required pacemaker implantation occurred in a few cases. Monitor for sign/symptoms of bradycardia (fainting, dizziness, chest pain) and tachycardia (palpitations, dizziness). May require therapy interruption and further evaluation. Treatment-emergent blood pressure elevations (systolic or diastolic) developed in over two-thirds of ponatinib-treated patients; symptomatic hypertension or hypertensive crisis were reported in several patients, requiring urgent intervention. Blood pressure may worsen in patients with preexisting hypertension. Monitor blood pressure closely, and manage elevated pressures as clinically indicated. May require therapy interruption, dosage reduction, or discontinuation if hypertension is resistant to medical management. Renal artery stenosis (associated with worsening, labile, or treatment-resistant hypertension) has occurred in some patients receiving ponatinib. Evaluate for renal artery stenosis for hypertension that significantly worsens, is labile, or treatment-resistant.

[US Boxed Warning]: Liver failure and death resulting from ponatinib-induced hepatotoxicity were observed; monitor liver function prior to and at least monthly (or as clinically indicated) during treatment. The median time to onset was 3 months (range: less than 1 month to 47 months). Hepatotoxicity may require treatment interruption (followed by dose reduction) or discontinuation. One case of fulminant hepatic failure leading to death occurred within 1 week of therapy initiation; acute liver failure has also occurred. Treatment may result in ALT and/or AST, bilirubin, and alkaline phosphatase elevations. ALT/AST elevations may be irreversible. A single-dose (30 mg) pharmacokinetic study found that ponatinib exposure was not increased in patients with hepatic impairment (Child-Pugh class A, B, or C) as compared to patients with normal hepatic function. While generally well tolerated, patients with hepatic impairment did have an increased overall incidence of adverse reactions (eg, gastrointestinal disorders, pancreatitis). Monitor closely when administering to patients with impaired hepatic function. The starting dose should be reduced in patients with hepatic impairment.

Severe myelosuppression (grade 3 or 4) is commonly observed with ponatinib, and the incidence was greater in patients with accelerated or blast phase CML and Ph+ ALL. The median onset to severe myelosuppression was 1 month (range: up to 40 months). Monitor blood counts closely; may require therapy interruption and/or dosage reduction. Hemorrhagic events occurred in ponatinib-treated patients, including serious events such as cerebral (subdural hematoma) and gastrointestinal hemorrhages; fatalities were reported. Serious bleeding episodes occurred more frequently in patients with accelerated or blast phase CML, and Ph+ ALL; most patients had grade 4 thrombocytopenia. Monitor platelet levels closely and for signs/symptoms of bleeding, and interrupt therapy if necessary.

Treatment-related lipase elevations and clinical pancreatitis occurred in clinical studies, including grade 3 and 4 events. The median time to onset was 14 days (range: 3 days to ~48 months); the majority of cases resolved within 2 weeks of therapy interruption or dose reduction. Monitor serum lipase every 2 weeks for the first 2 months and monthly thereafter or as clinically indicated; more frequent monitoring may be considered in patients with a history of pancreatitis or alcohol abuse. Monitor for clinical signs of pancreatitis, such as abdominal symptoms; interrupt therapy if necessary. Do not reinitiate treatment until complete resolution of symptoms and lipase level is <1.5 times ULN. Serious gastrointestinal perforation (fistula) occurred very rarely; monitor for signs/symptoms of perforation and/or fistula. Serious fluid retention events, including fatality due to brain edema (case report), were observed in ponatinib-treated patients. Peripheral edema, pleural effusions, pericardial effusions, and peripheral swelling were commonly seen. Monitor patients for fluid retention; may require therapy interruption, dosage reduction, or discontinuation.

Peripheral and cranial neuropathy have been reported. Peripheral neuropathy, paresthesia, hypoesthesia, hyperesthesia, dysguesia, and muscular weakness occurred most frequently; cranial neuropathy occurred rarely. In one-quarter of patients who experienced symptoms, neuropathy developed during the first month of therapy. Monitor for signs/symptoms of neuropathy; consider interrupting treatment if neuropathy develops. Reversible posterior leukoencephalopathy syndrome (RPLS) has been reported in postmarketing surveillance. Signs/symptoms include seizure, headache, decreased awareness, altered mental status, vision loss, and other visual and/or neurological disturbances. Hypertension is common; RPLS is diagnosed through MRI of the brain. Discontinue ponatinib for RPLS diagnosis; resume only if RPLS resolves and the benefit of treatment outweighs the risk.

Serious ocular events such as blindness and blurred vision have occurred with ponatinib use. Macular edema, retinal vein occlusion, and retinal hemorrhage have been reported in a small percentage of patients; conjunctival irritation, corneal erosion or abrasion, dry eye, conjunctivitis, conjunctival hemorrhage, hyperaemia and edema, or eye pain occurred more frequently. Other toxicities include cataracts, periorbital edema, blepharitis, glaucoma, eyelid edema, ocular hyperaemia, iritis, iridocyclitis, and ulcerative keratitis. Perform comprehensive ophthalmic exams prior to therapy initiation and periodically during treatment.

In a randomized study of first-line treatment of newly diagnosed chronic phase CML, a 2-fold increased risk of serious adverse reaction was demonstrated for ponatinib as compared to imatinib; the study was stopped due to safety concerns. Arterial and venous thrombosis and occlusion events occurred at least twice as frequently in the ponatinib arm of the study (compared to the imatinib arm); a higher incidence of hematologic toxicity, pancreatitis, hepatotoxicity, heart failure, hypertension, and dermatologic/subcutaneous tissue disorders was also observed in patients receiving ponatinib. Ponatinib is not indicated and not recommended for treatment of newly diagnosed chronic phase CML.

Hyperuricemia and serious tumor lysis syndrome (rare) were reported. Patients should receive adequate hydration and be monitored for elevated uric acid levels and/or the development of tumor lysis syndrome. Manage elevated uric acid levels prior to initiating therapy. As ponatinib inhibits VEGF activity, therapy may impair wound healing. Hold therapy for at least 1 week prior to major surgery; resume therapy post procedure based on clinical judgment of appropriate wound healing. Potentially significant drug-drug interactions may exist, requiring dose or frequency adjustment, additional monitoring, and/or selection of alternative therapy. Patients ≥65 years of age may be more likely to experience weakness, decreased appetite, dyspnea, increased lipase, muscle spasms, peripheral edema, and thrombocytopenia; monitor closely. Cautious dose selection is recommended based on greater frequency of decreased hepatic, renal, or cardiac function, and of concomitant disease or other drug therapy.

Adverse Reactions

>10%:

Cardiovascular: Hypertension (53% to 71%), peripheral edema (13% to 22%; grades 3/4: ≤1%), arterial ischemia (3% to 20%; grades 3/4: ≤11%; including cardiac, cerebrovascular, and peripheral-vascular ischemia), cardiac failure (6% to 15%; including congestive heart failure, reduced ejection fraction, pulmonary edema, cardiogenic shock, cardiorespiratory arrest, right ventricular failure), myocardial infarction (12%)

Central nervous system: Fatigue or weakness (31% to 39%), headache (25% to 39%), pain (6% to 16%), chills (7% to 13%), insomnia (7% to 12%), dizziness (3% to 11%)

Dermatologic: Skin rash (34% to 54%), xeroderma (24% to 39%), cellulitis (≤11%)

Endocrine & metabolic: Increased serum glucose (58%), decreased serum phosphate (57%), decreased serum calcium (52%), decreased serum sodium (29%), decreased serum glucose (24%), decreased serum potassium (16%), increased serum potassium (15%), decreased serum bicarbonate (11%)

Gastrointestinal: Abdominal pain (34% to 49%), constipation (24% to 47%), increased serum lipase (41%; grades 3/4: 15%), nausea (22% to 32%), decreased appetite (8% to 31%), diarrhea (13% to 26%), vomiting (13% to 24%), stomatitis (9% to 23%), weight loss (5% to 13%), gastrointestinal hemorrhage (2% to 11%; grades 3/4: ≤6%)

Genitourinary: Urinary tract infection (≤12%)

Hematologic & oncologic: Neutropenia (grades 3/4: 24% to 63%), leukopenia (grades 3/4: 14% to 63%), thrombocytopenia (grades 3/4: 36% to 57%), anemia (grades 3/4: 9% to 55%), bone marrow depression (severe grade 3 or 4: 48%), lymphocytopenia (grades 3/4: 10% to 37%), febrile neutropenia (1% to 25%), hemorrhage (24%; including cerebral hemorrhage and gastrointestinal hemorrhage)

Hepatic: Increased serum ALT (53%; grades 3/4: 8%), increased serum AST (41%; grades 3/4: 4%), increased serum alkaline phosphatase (37%), decreased serum albumin (28%), increased serum bilirubin (19%)

Infection: Sepsis (1% to 22%)

Miscellaneous: Fever (23% to 32%)

◀ Neuromuscular & skeletal: Arthralgia (13% to 31%), myalgia (6% to 22%), limb pain (9% to 17%), back pain (11% to 16%), peripheral neuropathy (6% to 16%; including burning sensation), muscle spasm (5% to 13%), ostealgia (9% to 12%)

Respiratory: Dyspnea (6% to 21%), pleural effusion (3% to 19%; grades 3/4: ≤3%), cough (6% to 18%), pneumonia (3% to 13%), nasopharyngitis (3% to 12%), upper respiratory tract infection (≤11%)

1% to 10%:

Cardiovascular: Peripheral ischemia (8%), supraventricular tachycardia (5%), venous thromboembolism (5%); atrial fibrillation (4%), pericardial effusion (1% to 3%), cerebral hemorrhage (2%), bradycardia (1%; symptomatic)

Endocrine & metabolic: Increased serum sodium (10%), hyperuricemia (7%), increased serum calcium (5%), increased serum triglycerides (3%)

Gastrointestinal: Pancreatitis (6%; grade 3: 5%), increased serum amylase (3%)

Ophthalmic: Blurred vision (6%), retinal toxicity (3%, including macular edema, retinal vein occlusion, retinal hemorrhage)

Renal: Increased serum creatinine (7%)

Frequency not defined:

Cardiovascular: Cerebrovascular accident

Gastrointestinal: Mouth pain, oral mucosa ulcer, oropharyngeal pain, throat ulcer, tongue ulcer

Ophthalmic: Cataract, conjunctival irritation, corneal ulcer, dry eye syndrome, eye pain, glaucoma, iridocyclitis, iritis, keratitis

<1%, postmarketing, and/or case reports: Acute hepatic failure, ascites, atrial flutter, atrial tachycardia, cerebral edema, complete atrioventricular block, gastrointestinal fistula, gastrointestinal perforation, mesenteric artery occlusion, pulmonary embolism, retinal vein thrombosis, sick sinus syndrome, tumor lysis syndrome (serious)

Drug Interactions

Metabolism/Transport Effects Substrate of BCRP, CYP2C8 (minor), CYP2D6 (minor), CYP3A4 (minor), P-glycoprotein; **Note:** Assignment of Major/Minor substrate status based on clinically relevant drug interaction potential; **Inhibits** BCRP, BSEP

Avoid Concomitant Use

Avoid concomitant use of PONATinib with any of the following: BCG (Intravesical); CYP3A4 Inducers (Strong); Deferiprone; Dipyrone; St John's Wort

Increased Effect/Toxicity

PONATinib may increase the levels/effects of: CloZAPine; Deferiprone

The levels/effects of PONATinib may be increased by: CYP3A4 Inhibitors (Strong); Dipyrone; Grapefruit Juice; Promazine

Decreased Effect

PONATinib may decrease the levels/effects of: BCG (Intravesical)

The levels/effects of PONATinib may be decreased by: CYP3A4 Inducers (Strong); St John's Wort

Food Interactions Ponatinib serum concentrations may be increased when taken with grapefruit or grapefruit juice. Management: Reduce initial dose.

Hazardous Drugs Handling Considerations

Hazardous agent (NIOSH 2016 [group 1]).

Use appropriate precautions for receiving, handling, administration, and disposal. Gloves (single) should be worn during receiving, unpacking, and placing in storage. NIOSH recommends single gloving for administration of intact tablets or capsules (NIOSH 2016).

Storage/Stability Store at 20°C to 25°C (68°F to 77°F); excursions permitted between 15°C to 30°C (59°F to 86°F).

Mechanism of Action Ponatinib is a pan-BCR-ABL tyrosine kinase inhibitor with *in vitro* activity against cells expressing native or mutant BCR-ABL (including T315I); it also inhibits VEGFR, FGFR, PDGFR, EPH, and SRC kinases, as well as KIT, RET, TIE2, and FLT3.

Pharmacodynamics/Kinetics

Absorption: Plasma concentrations not affected by food

Distribution: V_d: 1223 L

Protein binding: >99% to plasma proteins

Metabolism: Primarily hepatic through CYP3A4; CYP2C8, CYP2D6, and CYP3A5 are also involved in metabolism. Phase II metabolism occurs via esterases and/or amidases.

Half-life elimination: ~24 hours (range: 12 to 66 hours)

Time to peak: ≤6 hours

Excretion: Feces (~87%); urine (~5%)

Dosing

Adult & Geriatric Note: The optimal ponatinib dose has not been identified. Consider discontinuing therapy if no response has occurred by 3 months (90 days) of therapy.

Acute lymphoblastic leukemia (ALL), Philadelphia chromosome-positive (Ph+), T315I-positive or in patients for whom no other tyrosine kinase inhibitor therapy is indicated: Oral: Initial: 45 mg once daily

Chronic myeloid leukemia (CML; chronic, accelerated, or blast phase), T315I-positive or in patients for whom no other tyrosine kinase inhibitor therapy is indicated: Oral: Initial: 45 mg once daily; consider reducing the dose for patients in chronic or accelerated phase who have achieved a major cytogenetic response

Note: Ponatinib is not recommended for treatment of **newly diagnosed** chronic phase CML.

Dosage adjustment for strong CYP3A inhibitors: Reduce ponatinib dose to 30 mg once daily when administered with concomitant strong CYP3A inhibitors (eg, boceprevir, clarithromycin, conivaptan, grapefruit juice, indinavir, itraconazole, ketoconazole, lopinavir/ritonavir, nefazodone, nelfinavir, posaconazole, ritonavir, saquinavir, telaprevir, telithromycin, voriconazole).

Renal Impairment There are no dosage adjustments provided in the manufacturer's labeling (has not been studied); although renal excretion is not a major excretion route for ponatinib.

Hepatic Impairment

Hepatic impairment prior to treatment initiation: Mild-to-severe impairment (Child-Pugh class A, B, or C): Initial: 30 mg once daily; monitor closely for toxicity.

Hepatotoxicity during treatment:

AST or ALT >3 times ULN (≥ Grade 2): If toxicity occurs at a dose of 45 mg daily, interrupt therapy; upon recovery to ≤ grade 1 (<3 times ULN), resume therapy at 30 mg daily. If toxicity occurs at a dose of 30 mg daily, interrupt therapy; upon recovery to ≤ grade 1, resume therapy at 15 mg daily. If toxicity occurs at a dose of 15 mg daily, discontinue therapy.

ALT or AST ≥3 times ULN with bilirubin >2 times ULN and alkaline phosphatase <2 times ULN: Discontinue therapy.

Adjustment for Toxicity

Hematologic: ANC <1000/mm^3 or platelets <50,000/mm^3:

First occurrence: Interrupt therapy; upon recovery of ANC to ≥1500/mm^3 and platelets to ≥75,000/mm^3, resume therapy at 45 mg daily.

Second occurrence: Interrupt therapy; upon recovery of ANC to ≥1500/mm^3 and platelets to ≥75,000/mm^3, resume therapy at a reduced dose of 30 mg daily.

Third occurrence: Interrupt therapy; upon recovery of ANC to ≥1500/mm^3 and platelets to ≥75,000/mm^3, resume therapy at a reduced dose of 15 mg daily.

Nonhematologic toxicity:

Arterial or venous occlusive reactions: Interrupt therapy; do not resume ponatinib in the event of serious occlusive events unless the potential benefit of therapy outweighs the risk of recurrent occlusions and other treatment options are not available.

Pancreatitis and lipase elevations:

Asymptomatic grade 1 or 2 serum lipase elevation: Consider interrupting therapy or dose reduction.

Asymptomatic grade 3 or 4 serum lipase elevation (>2 times ULN) or asymptomatic radiologic pancreatitis (grade 2): If toxicity occurs at a dose of 45 mg daily, interrupt therapy; upon recovery to ≤ grade 1 (<1.5 times ULN), resume therapy at a reduced dose of 30 mg daily. If toxicity occurs at a dose of 30 mg daily, interrupt therapy; upon recovery to ≤ grade 1, resume therapy at a reduced dose of 15 mg daily. If toxicity occurs at a dose of 15 mg daily, discontinue therapy.

Symptomatic grade 3 pancreatitis: If toxicity occurs at a dose of 45 mg daily, interrupt therapy; upon recovery of serum lipase elevation to ≤ grade 1 and complete symptom resolution, resume therapy at a reduced dose of 30 mg daily. If toxicity occurs at a dose of 30 mg daily, interrupt therapy; upon recovery of serum lipase elevation to ≤ grade 1 and complete symptom resolution, resume therapy at a reduced dose of 15 mg daily. If toxicity occurs at a dose of 15 mg daily, discontinue therapy.

Grade 4 pancreatitis: Discontinue therapy.

Reversible posterior leukoencephalopathy syndrome (RPLS): Interrupt therapy for RPLS diagnosis; resume only if RPLS resolves and if the benefit outweighs the risk.

Other nonhematologic toxicities: For serious reactions (other than arterial or venous occlusion), modify the dose or interrupt treatment; do not restart therapy until symptom resolution or unless the benefit of therapy outweighs the risk of recurrent toxicity.

Administration Administer with or without food. Swallow tablets whole (do not crush or dissolve).

Emetic Potential Low (10% to 30%)

Monitoring Parameters CBC with differential and platelets every 2 weeks for the first 3 months, then monthly or as clinically needed; liver function tests at baseline and at least monthly thereafter or more frequently if clinically warranted; serum lipase every 2 weeks for the first 2 months and monthly thereafter (more frequently in patients with a history of pancreatitis or alcohol abuse); serum electrolytes and uric acid; monitor cardiac function and blood pressure. Monitor for signs/symptoms of arterial/venous occlusion or thromboembolism, hemorrhage, fluid retention, pancreatitis (clinical signs), gastrointestinal perforation/fistula, hepatotoxicity (jaundice, anorexia, bleeding, bruising), reversible posterior leukoencephalopathy syndrome; comprehensive ocular exam at baseline and periodically; signs/symptoms of neuropathy

Dietary Considerations Avoid grapefruit juice.

Prescribing and Access Restrictions Patient access and support is available through the ARIAD PASS program. Information regarding program enrollment may be found at http://www.ariadpass.com or by calling 1-855-447-PASS (7277). In Canada, ponatinib is available through the Iclusig Controlled Distribution Program; information about the program may be found at www.iclusigcdp.ca or by calling 1-888-867-7426.

Medication Guide Available Yes

Dosage Forms Excipient information presented when available (limited, particularly for generics); consult specific product labeling.

Tablet, Oral:
Iclusig: 15 mg, 45 mg

◆ **Ponatinib HCl** see PONATinib on page 1527

◆ **Ponatinib Hydrochloride** see PONATinib on page 1527

Porfimer (POR ti mer)

Brand Names: US Photofrin

Brand Names: Canada Photofrin

Index Terms CL-184116; Dihematoporphyrin Ether; Porfimer Sodium

Pharmacologic Category Antineoplastic Agent, Miscellaneous

Use

Barrett esophagus dysplasia (photodynamic therapy): Ablation of high-grade dysplasia in Barrett esophagus (in patients who do not undergo esophagectomy)

Endobronchial cancer (photodynamic therapy): Treatment of microinvasive endobronchial non-small cell lung cancer (NSCLC) in patients for whom surgery and radiation therapy are not indicated; reduction of obstruction and symptom palliation in patients with obstructing (partial or complete) endobronchial NSCLC

Esophageal cancer (photodynamic therapy): Palliation of completely obstructing esophageal cancer, or partially obstructing esophageal cancer in patients who cannot be treated satisfactorily with Nd:YAG laser therapy.

Pregnancy Risk Factor C

Dosing

Adult & Geriatric

Esophageal cancer or endobronchial non-small cell lung cancer (photodynamic therapy): IV: 2 mg/kg, followed by endoscopic exposure to the appropriate laser light and debridement; repeat courses must be separated by at least 30 days (delay subsequent treatment for insufficient healing) for a maximum of 3 courses

Barrett esophagus dysplasia (photodynamic therapy): IV: 2 mg/kg, followed by endoscopic exposure to the appropriate laser light; repeat courses must be separated by at least 90 days (delay subsequent treatment for insufficient healing) for a maximum of 3 courses

◀

Renal Impairment There are no dosage adjustments provided in the manufacturer's labeling (has not been studied); use caution as porfimer elimination may be prolonged.

Hepatic Impairment There are no dosage adjustments provided in the manufacturer's labeling (has not been studied); use caution as porfimer elimination may be prolonged.

Additional Information Complete prescribing information should be consulted for additional detail.

Dosage Forms Excipient information presented when available (limited, particularly for generics); consult specific product labeling.

Solution Reconstituted, Intravenous, as sodium [preservative free]:
Photofrin: 75 mg (1 ea)

Dosage Forms: Canada Information with regard to form, strength, and availability of products uniquely available in Canada but currently not available in the US. Refer also to Dosage Forms.

Excipient information presented when available (limited, particularly for generics); consult specific product labeling.

Solution Reconstituted, Intravenous, as sodium [preservative free]:
Photofrin: 15 mg, 75 mg

◆ **Porfimer Sodium** see Porfimer on page 1535
◆ **Portrazza** see Necitumumab on page 1298

Posaconazole (poe sa KON a zole)

Brand Names: US Noxafil
Brand Names: Canada Posanol
Index Terms SCH 56592
Pharmacologic Category Antifungal Agent, Oral
Use

Prophylaxis of invasive Aspergillus and Candida infections: Suspension and delayed-release tablets (13 years and older) and injection (18 years and older): Prophylaxis of invasive Aspergillus and Candida infections in patients who are at high risk of developing these infections due to being severely immunocompromised (eg, hematopoietic stem cell transplant [HSCT] recipients with graft-versus-host disease [GVHD] or those with prolonged neutropenia secondary to chemotherapy for hematologic malignancies).

Oropharyngeal candidiasis: Suspension (13 years and older): Treatment of oropharyngeal candidiasis (including patients refractory to itraconazole and/or fluconazole)

Dosing

Adult & Geriatric Note: The delayed-release tablet and oral suspension are not to be used interchangeably due to dosing differences for each formulation. Since the delayed-release tablet is easier to administer, better tolerated, and more reliably absorbed, the use of delayed-release tablets are preferred. The bioavailability of a once daily 300 mg dose given as the delayed-release tablet appears to be similar or greater than the bioavailability of 200 mg given 3 to 4 times daily, based upon available pharmacokinetic studies (Cumpston 2015; Durani 2015).

Aspergillosis, invasive:
Prophylaxis (immunocompromised host):
Oral:
Suspension: 200 mg 3 times daily; duration of therapy is based on recovery from neutropenia or immunosuppression. In patients with acute myelogenous leukemia (AML) or myelodysplastic syndromes (MDS), posaconazole was initiated at the time of chemotherapy initiation (or if receiving anthracyclines, 24 hours after the last anthracycline dose) and was continued until recovery from neutropenia, until complete remission, or for up to 12 weeks, whichever occurred first (Cornely 2007). In patients with graft-versus-host disease (GVHD) receiving immunosuppressive therapy, posaconazole was continued for 112 days (Ullmann 2007), although the optimal duration in GVHD has not been fully defined (Tomblyn 2009). It is recommended to continue throughout the duration of immunosuppression (ie, corticosteroid equivalent of >1 mg/kg/day of prednisone for >2 weeks and/or the use of other anti-GVHD therapies) (IDSA [Patterson 2016]).
Tablets (delayed release): Initial: 300 mg twice daily on day 1 followed by 300 mg once daily on day 2 and thereafter. Duration is based on recovery from neutropenia or immunosuppression.
Missed doses: Take as soon as remembered. If it is <12 hours until the next dose, skip the missed does and return to the regular schedule. Do not double doses.
IV: Loading dose: 300 mg twice a day on day 1 followed by 300 mg once daily on day 2 and thereafter. Duration is based on recovery from neutropenia or immunosuppression.
Treatment (refractory to or intolerant of conventional therapy) (off-label use):
Oral:
Suspension: 200 mg 3 times daily (IDSA [Patterson 2016])
Tablets (delayed release): Initial dose: 300 mg twice daily on day 1; Maintenance dose: 300 mg once daily (IDSA [Patterson 2016])
IV: Loading dose: 300 mg twice daily on day 1; Maintenance dose: 300 mg once daily (IDSA [Patterson 2016])
Duration of therapy: Minimum of 6 to 12 weeks, although duration is highly dependent on degree/duration of immunosuppression, disease site, and evidence of disease improvement (IDSA [Patterson 2016])
Alternative dosing recommendations (Posanol Canadian product labeling 2016):
Oral:
Suspension: 400 mg twice daily; in patients unable to tolerate food or nutritional supplement, administer 200 mg 4 times daily; duration of therapy is based on severity of underlying disease, recovery from immunosuppression, and clinical response.
Tablets (delayed release): Initial: 300 mg twice daily on day 1; Maintenance dose: 300 mg once daily; duration of therapy is based on disease severity, recovery from immunosuppression, and clinical response.
IV: Loading dose: 300 mg twice daily on day 1; Maintenance dose: 300 mg once daily on day 2 and thereafter. Duration of therapy is based on disease severity, recovery from immunosuppression, and clinical response.

◀

Candidal infections:
  Prophylaxis (disseminated candidiasis, immunocompromised host):
  Oral:
    Suspension: 200 mg 3 times daily; duration of therapy is based on recovery from neutropenia or immunosuppression
    Tablets (delayed release): Oral: Initial: 300 mg twice daily on day 1; Maintenance dose: 300 mg once daily on day 2 and thereafter; duration of therapy is based on recovery from neutropenia or immunosuppression
      Missed doses: Take as soon as remembered. If it is <12 hours until the next dose, skip the missed does and return to the regular schedule. Do not double doses.
  IV: Initial: 300 mg twice daily on day 1; Maintenance dose: 300 mg once daily on day 2 and thereafter; duration of therapy is based on recovery from neutropenia or immunosuppression.
  Treatment:
  Oral:
    Oropharyngeal infection: Suspension: Initial: 100 mg twice daily on day 1; Maintenance: 100 mg once daily on day 2 and thereafter for 13 days
    Oropharyngeal infection (refractory to fluconazole):
      Manufacturer's labeling: Suspension: 400 mg twice daily; duration of therapy is based on underlying disease and clinical response
      Alternate dosing: Suspension: 400 mg twice daily for 3 days, then 400 mg once daily for up to 28 days (IDSA [Pappas 2016])
        HIV-infected patients (alternative to fluconazole or azole refractory): Suspension: 400 mg twice daily on day 1, then 400 mg once daily for 7 to 14 days for initial episodes (continue for 28 days in azole refractory patients) (HHS [OI adult 2015])
    Esophageal infections (off-label use):
      Fluconazole-refractory (alternate therapy):
      Tablets, delayed-release: 300 mg once daily (IDSA [Pappas 2016])
      Suspension: 400 mg twice daily (IDSA [Pappas 2016])
      HIV-infected patients (azole refractory): Suspension: 400 mg twice daily for 28 days. **Note:** If patient has frequent or severe recurrences, may continue for suppressive therapy; consider discontinuing when CD4 >200/mm^3 (HHS [OI adult 2015])

Coccidioidomycosis in HIV-infected patients (alternative to preferred therapy) (off-label use) (HHS [OI adult 2015]; Anstead 2005; Schein 2011; Stevens 2007):
  Mild infections (eg, focal pneumonia): Oral: Suspension: 200 to 400 mg twice daily; patients who complete initial therapy should be considered for lifelong suppressive therapy.
  Chronic suppressive therapy: Oral: Suspension: 200 mg twice daily

Mucormycosis, salvage and step-down therapy (off-label use): Oral:
  Suspension: 800 mg daily in 2 or 4 divided doses; duration of therapy is based on response and risk of relapse due to immunosuppression (Danion 2015; ECIL [Skiada 2013]; ESCMID/ECMM [Cornely 2014]; Greenberg 2006)
  Tablets (delayed release): 300 mg once daily (Danion 2015)

Cryptococcal infections:
Pulmonary, nonimmunosuppressed (off-label use): Oral: Suspension: 400 mg twice daily. **Note:** Fluconazole is considered first-line treatment (Perfect 2010; Raad 2006).

Salvage treatment of relapsed infection (off-label use): Oral: Suspension: 400 mg twice daily (or 200 mg 4 times daily) for 10 to 12 weeks. **Note:** Salvage treatment should only be started after an appropriate course of an induction regimen (Perfect 2010; Pitisuttitihum 2005).

Pediatric Note: The delayed-release tablet and oral suspension are not to be used interchangeably due to dosing differences for each formulation.

Candidal infections: Oral: Adolescents ≥13 years: Refer to adult dosing.

Coccidioidomycosis in HIV-infected patients (alternative to preferred therapy) (off-label use): Adolescents: Oral: Refer to adult dosing.

Primary antifungal prophylaxis in allogeneic HSCT with grades 2 to 4 acute graft-versus-host-disease (GVHD) or chronic extensive GVHD (guideline recommendation): Adolescents ≥13 years: Oral: Suspension: 200 mg 3 times daily beginning with GVHD diagnosis, continue until GVHD resolves (Science 2014)

Primary antifungal prophylaxis in AML or MDS in centers with a high local incidence of mold infections (alternative to fluconazole; guideline recommendation): Adolescents ≥13 years: Oral: Suspension: 200 mg 3 times daily during chemotherapy-associated neutropenia (Science 2014)

Renal Impairment
Delayed-release tablets and oral suspension:
eGFR 20 to 80 mL/minute/1.73 m^2: No dosage adjustment necessary.
eGFR <20 mL/minute/1.73 m^2: No dosage adjustment necessary; however, monitor for breakthrough fungal infections due to variability in posaconazole exposure.

Intravenous infusion:
eGFR ≥50 mL/minute/1.73 m^2: No dosage adjustment recommended
eGFR <50 mL/minute/1.73 m^2: Avoid use unless risk/benefit has been assessed; the intravenous vehicle (cyclodextrin) may accumulate. Monitor serum creatinine levels; if increases occur, consider oral therapy.

Continuous venovenous hemofiltration (CVVH): In a critically ill patient undergoing CVVH, IV posaconazole administered at standard dosing demonstrated no evidence of SBECD accumulation; however, no specific dosing recommendations can be made (Morris 2015).

Hepatic Impairment
Preexisting mild-to-severe impairment (Child-Pugh class A, B, or C): No dosage adjustment necessary.
Hepatotoxicity during treatment: There are no dosage adjustments provided in the manufacturer's labeling; consider discontinuing therapy.

Additional Information Complete prescribing information should be consulted for additional detail.

Dosage Forms Excipient information presented when available (limited, particularly for generics); consult specific product labeling.
Solution, Intravenous:
Noxafil: 300 mg/16.7 mL (16.7 mL) [contains edetate disodium]
Suspension, Oral:
Noxafil: 40 mg/mL (105 mL) [contains polysorbate 80, sodium benzoate; cherry flavor]
Tablet Delayed Release, Oral:
Noxafil: 100 mg

- **Posanol (Can)** *see* Posaconazole *on page 1536*
- **PR-171** *see* Carfilzomib *on page 337*

PRALAtrexate (pral a TREX ate)

Related Information

Management of Chemotherapy-Induced Nausea and Vomiting in Adults *on page 2253*

Safe Handling of Hazardous Drugs *on page 2379*

Brand Names: US Folotyn

Index Terms PDX

Pharmacologic Category Antineoplastic Agent, Antimetabolite; Antineoplastic Agent, Antimetabolite (Antifolate)

Use Peripheral T-cell lymphoma: Treatment of relapsed or refractory peripheral T-cell lymphoma (PTCL)

Labeled Contraindications There are no contraindications listed in the manufacturer's labeling.

Pregnancy Considerations Adverse effects were observed in animal reproduction studies. May cause fetal harm if administered to a pregnant woman.

Breastfeeding Considerations It is not known if pralatrexate is excreted in breast milk. Due to the potential for serious adverse reactions in the nursing infant, a decision should be made to discontinue breastfeeding or to discontinue pralatrexate, taking into account the benefits of treatment to the mother.

Warnings/Precautions May cause bone marrow suppression (thrombocytopenia, neutropenia and anemia); may require dosage modification; monitor blood counts. Mucositis, including stomatitis or mucosal inflammation of gastrointestinal and genitourinary tracts, may occur; monitor weekly; may require dosage modification. Prophylactic folic acid and vitamin B_{12} supplements are necessary to reduce hematologic toxicity and treatment-related mucositis. Severe and potentially fatal dermatologic reactions, including skin exfoliation, ulceration, and toxic epidermal necrolysis (TEN) have been reported. Skin reaction may be progressive; severity may increase with continued treatment; may also involve skin and subcutaneous tissues which are affected by lymphoma; monitor all dermatologic reactions closely; withhold or discontinue treatment for severe dermatologic reaction.

Pralatrexate may cause tumor lysis syndrome (TLS); monitor closely, if TLS develops, treat for associated complications. Use with caution in patients with moderate to severe renal impairment (has not been studied in patients with renal impairment); monitor renal function and for systemic toxicity due to increased exposure. Concurrent use with drugs with substantial renal clearance (eg, NSAIDs, sulfamethoxazole/trimethoprim) may result in delayed pralatrexate clearance. Liver function test abnormalities have been observed with use; monitor liver function; persistent abnormalities may indicate hepatotoxicity and may require dosage modification or discontinuation.

Patients with moderate-to-severe renal impairment are at higher risk for increased exposure and toxicity. Monitor renal function and for systemic toxicity due to increased exposure. Dosage adjustment is recommended in patients with severe renal impairment (eGFR 15 to <30 mL/minute/1.73 m^2). Unless the potential benefits outweigh potential risks, avoid use in patients with end-stage renal disease (ESRD), including patients undergoing dialysis.

Serious adverse reactions, including toxic epidermal necrolysis and mucositis were reported in patients with ESRD undergoing dialysis. Potentially significant drug-drug interactions may exist, requiring dose or frequency adjustment, additional monitoring, and/or selection of alternative therapy.

Adverse Reactions

>10%:

Cardiovascular: Edema (30%)

Central nervous system: Fatigue (36%)

Dermatologic: Skin rash (15%), pruritus (14%; grade 3: 2%), night sweats (11%)

Endocrine & metabolic: Hypokalemia (15%)

Gastrointestinal: Mucositis (70%; grade 3: 17%; grade 4: 4%), nausea (40%), constipation (33%), vomiting (25%), diarrhea (21%), anorexia (15%), abdominal pain (12%)

Hematologic & oncologic: Thrombocytopenia (41%; grade 3: 14%; grade 4: 19%), anemia (34%; grade 3: 15%; grade 4: 2%), neutropenia (24%; grade 3: 13%; grade 4: 7%), leukopenia (11%; grade 3: 3%; grade 4: 4%)

Hepatic: Increased serum transaminases (13%; grade 3: 5%)

Infection: Infection

Neuromuscular & skeletal: Limb pain (12%), back pain (11%)

Respiratory: Cough (28%), epistaxis (26%), dyspnea (19%), pharyngolaryngeal pain (14%)

Miscellaneous: Fever (32%)

1% to 10%:

Cardiovascular: Tachycardia (10%)

Endocrine & metabolic: Severe dehydration (>3%)

Hematologic & oncologic: Febrile neutropenia (serious: >3%)

Infection: Sepsis (serious: >3%)

Neuromuscular & skeletal: Weakness (10%)

Respiratory: Upper respiratory tract infection (10%)

<1%, postmarketing, and/or case reports: Dermal ulcer, desquamation, intestinal obstruction, lymphocytopenia, odynophagia, pancytopenia, toxic epidermal necrolysis, tumor lysis syndrome

Drug Interactions

Metabolism/Transport Effects Substrate of BCRP

Avoid Concomitant Use

Avoid concomitant use of PRALAtrexate with any of the following: BCG (Intravesical); Natalizumab; Pimecrolimus; Tacrolimus (Topical); Vaccines (Live)

Increased Effect/Toxicity

PRALAtrexate may increase the levels/effects of: Fingolimod; Leflunomide; Natalizumab; Tofacitinib; Vaccines (Live)

The levels/effects of PRALAtrexate may be increased by: Denosumab; Nonsteroidal Anti-Inflammatory Agents; Ocrelizumab; Palifermin; Pimecrolimus; Probenecid; Roflumilast; Salicylates; Sulfamethoxazole; Tacrolimus (Topical); Trastuzumab; Trimethoprim

Decreased Effect

PRALAtrexate may decrease the levels/effects of: BCG (Intravesical); Coccidioides immitis Skin Test; Lenograstim; Nivolumab; Sapropterin; Sipuleucel-T; Tertomotide; Vaccines (Inactivated); Vaccines (Live)

The levels/effects of PRALAtrexate may be decreased by: Echinacea

Hazardous Drugs Handling Considerations
Hazardous agent (NIOSH 2016 [group 1]).

Use appropriate precautions for receiving, handling, administration, and disposal. Gloves (single) should be worn during receiving, unpacking, and placing in storage.

NIOSH recommends double gloving, a protective gown, ventilated engineering controls (a class II biological safety cabinet or a compounding aseptic containment isolator), and closed system transfer devices (CSTDs) for preparation. Double gloving, a gown, and (if dosage form allows) CSTDs are required during administration (NIOSH 2016).

Storage/Stability Store intact vials refrigerated at 2°C to 8°C (36°F to 46°F). Store in original carton to protect from light until use. Unopened vials (stored in the original carton) are stable for up to 72 hours at room temperature (discard after 72 hours).

Preparation for Administration Withdraw into syringe for administration; do not dilute (manufacturer recommends immediate use after placing in syringe). Discard unused portion in the vial.

Mechanism of Action Antifolate analog; inhibits DNA, RNA, and protein synthesis by selectively entering cells expressing reduced folate carrier (RFC-1), is polyglutamylated by folylpolyglutamate synthetase (FPGS) and then competes for the DHFR-folate binding site to inhibit dihydrofolate reductase (DHFR)

Pharmacodynamics/Kinetics
Distribution: *S*-diastereomer: 105 L; *R*-diastereomer: 37 L

Protein binding: ~67%

Metabolism: Not significantly metabolized by phase I hepatic isoenzymes or phase II glucuronidases.

Half-life elimination: 12 to 18 hours

Excretion: Urine (~34% as unchanged drug; parent drug [racemic pralatrexate]: ~39%); Feces (34%); Respiratory (10% [exhaled])

Dosing

Adult & Geriatric Note: Initiate vitamin supplements before initial pralatrexate dose: Folic acid 1 to 1.25 mg/day orally beginning 10 days prior to initial pralatrexate dose; continue during treatment and for 30 days after last pralatrexate dose; vitamin B_{12} 1,000 mcg IM within 10 weeks prior to initial pralatrexate dose and every 8 to 10 weeks thereafter (after first dose, subsequent B_{12} doses may be administered on the same day as pralatrexate).

Prior to administering any dose, mucositis should be ≤ grade 1 and absolute neutrophil count (ANC) should be ≥1,000/mm³; platelets should be ≥100,000/mm³ for the first dose and ≥50,000/mm³ for subsequent doses

Peripheral T-cell lymphoma (PTCL), relapsed or refractory: IV: 30 mg/m² once weekly for 6 weeks of a 7-week treatment cycle; continue until disease progression or unacceptable toxicity (O'Connor 2011)

Cutaneous T-cell lymphoma, relapsed or refractory (off-label use): IV: 15 mg/m² once weekly for 3 weeks of a 4-week treatment cycle (Horwitz 2012)

Renal Impairment Peripheral T-cell lymphoma (PTCL), relapsed or refractory:

Estimated glomerular filtration rate (eGFR) ≥30 mL/minute/1.73 m²: No dosage adjustment necessary.

eGFR 15 to <30 mL/minute/1.73 m^2: Initial: Reduce dose to 15 mg/m^2; if dose reductions for toxicity are necessary, reduce each dose to 10 mg/m^2. End-stage renal disease (ESRD), including dialysis: Avoid use (unless the potential benefit outweighs risks).

Hepatic Impairment Patients with total bilirubin >1.5 mg/dL, AST or ALT >2.5 times the upper limit of normal (ULN), or ALT or AST >5 times ULN if documented hepatic lymphoma involvement were excluded from clinical trials. Persistent abnormalities may indicate hepatotoxicity requiring dosage modification:

Grade 3 (AST or ALT >5 to 20 times ULN or bilirubin >3 to 10 times ULN): Omit dose; decrease to 20 mg/m^2 when recovers to ≤ grade 2

Grade 4 (AST or ALT >20 times ULN or bilirubin >10 times ULN): Discontinue treatment.

Obesity *ASCO Guidelines for appropriate chemotherapy dosing in obese adults with cancer:* Utilize patient's actual body weight (full weight) for calculation of body surface area- or weight-based dosing, particularly when the intent of therapy is curative; manage regimen-related toxicities in the same manner as for nonobese patients; if a dose reduction is utilized due to toxicity, consider resumption of full weight-based dosing with subsequent cycles, especially if cause of toxicity (eg, hepatic or renal impairment) is resolved (Griggs, 2012).

Adjustment for Toxicity Severe or intolerable adverse events may require dose omission, reduction or interruption. Do not make up omitted doses at the end of a cycle; do not re-escalate dose after a reduction due to toxicity.

Hematologic toxicity:

Platelets:

<50,000/mm^3 (for 1-week duration): Omit dose; continue at previous dose if platelets recover within 1 week

<50,000/mm^3 (for 2-week duration): Omit dose; decrease to 20 mg/m^2 (10 mg/m^2 in patients with eGFR 15 to <30 mL/minute/1.73 m^2) if platelets recover within 2 weeks

<50,000/mm^3 (for 3-week duration): Discontinue treatment.

ANC:

500 to 1,000/mm^3 without fever (for 1-week duration): Omit dose; continue at previous dose if ANC recovers within 1 week

500 to 1,000/mm^3 with fever **or** ANC <500/mm^3 (for 1-week duration): Omit dose, give filgrastim or sargramostim support; continue at previous dose (with growth factor support) if ANC recovers within 1 week

500 to 1,000/mm^3 with fever **or** ANC <500/mm^3 (recurrent or for 2-week duration): Omit dose and give filgrastim or sargramostim support; decrease to 20 mg/m^2 (10 mg/m^2 in patients with eGFR 15 to <30 mL/minute/1.73 m^2) with growth factor support if ANC recovers within 2 weeks

500 to 1,000/mm^3 with fever **or** ANC <500/mm^3 (second recurrence or for 3 week duration): Discontinue treatment.

Nonhematologic toxicity: Mucositis (on day of treatment):

Grade 2: Omit dose; continue at previous dose when recovers to ≤ grade 1

Grade 3 or recurrent grade 2: Omit dose and decrease to 20 mg/m^2 (10 mg/m^2 in patients with eGFR 15 to <30 mL/minute/1.73 m^2) when recovers to ≤ grade 1

Grade 4: Discontinue treatment.

◄ **Nonhematologic toxicity (other than mucositis):**
Grade 3: Omit dose; decrease to 20 mg/m^2 (10 mg/m^2 in patients with eGFR 15 to <30 mL/minute/1.73 m^2) when recovers to ≤ grade 2
Grade 4: Discontinue treatment.

Administration Administer IV push (undiluted) over 3 to 5 minutes into the line of a free-flowing normal saline IV

Emetic Potential Minimal (<10%)

Monitoring Parameters CBC with differential (baseline and weekly), serum chemistries, including renal and liver function tests (prior to the first and fourth doses in each cycle); mucositis severity (baseline and weekly); monitor for signs of tumor lysis syndrome and for dermatologic reactions

Dosage Forms Excipient information presented when available (limited, particularly for generics); consult specific product labeling.
Solution, Intravenous [preservative free]:
Folotyn: 20 mg/mL (1 mL); 40 mg/2 mL (2 mL)

◆ **Pred Forte** see PrednisoLONE (Ophthalmic) on page 1544
◆ **Pred Mild** see PrednisoLONE (Ophthalmic) on page 1544

PrednisoLONE (Ophthalmic) (pred NISS oh lone)

Brand Names: US Omnipred; Pred Forte; Pred Mild

Brand Names: Canada Minims Prednisolone Sodium Phosphate; PMS-Prednisolone Sodium Phosphate Forte; Pred Forte; Pred Mild; Ratio-Prednisolone; Sandoz Prednisolone

Index Terms Econopred; Prednisolone Acetate, Ophthalmic; Prednisolone Sod Phosphate; Prednisolone Sodium Phosphate, Ophthalmic

Pharmacologic Category Corticosteroid, Ophthalmic

Use

Corneal injury: Treatment of corneal injury from chemical or thermal burns (excluding Pred Forte) or radiation burns or penetration of foreign bodies (Omnipred only).

Ophthalmic inflammatory conditions:
0.12%: Treatment of mild to moderate noninfectious allergic and inflammatory disorders of the lid, conjunctiva, cornea, and sclera.
1%: Treatment of steroid-responsive inflammatory conditions of the palpebral and bulbar conjunctiva, cornea, and anterior segment of the globe such as acne rosacea, allergic conjunctivitis, cyclitis, herpes zoster keratitis, iritis, superficial punctate keratitis, and selected infective conjunctivitis.

Pregnancy Risk Factor C

Dosing

Adult & Geriatric

Ophthalmic inflammatory conditions/corneal injury: Ophthalmic:
Prednisolone acetate: Instill 1 to 2 drops in the affected eye(s) 2 to 4 times daily. During the initial 24 to 48 hours, the dosing frequency may be increased if necessary. If signs and symptoms fail to improve after 2 days, re-evaluate. Do not discontinue therapy prematurely; withdraw therapy with gradual tapering of dose in chronic conditions.
Prednisolone sodium phosphate: Instill 1 to 2 drops into conjunctival sac every hour during the day and every 2 hours at night until satisfactory response is obtained, then use 1 drop every 4 hours; subsequent reduction to 1 drop 3 to 4 times daily may be adequate. Do not discontinue therapy prematurely; withdraw therapy with gradual tapering of dose in chronic conditions.

Pediatric Ophthalmic inflammation, treatment: Children and Adolescents (off-label use): Ophthalmic: Prednisolone acetate 1%: Limited data available: Instill 1 to 2 drops into conjunctival sac 3 to 6 times daily. If signs and symptoms fail to improve after 2 days, re-evaluate. Initiate with more frequent dosing, and decrease as clinically indicated. If signs and symptoms fail to improve after 2 days, re-evaluate (Wilson 2009).

Renal Impairment There are no dosage adjustments provided in the manufacturer's labeling.

Hepatic Impairment There are no dosage adjustments provided in the manufacturer's labeling.

Additional Information Complete prescribing information should be consulted for additional detail.

Dosage Forms Excipient information presented when available (limited, particularly for generics); consult specific product labeling.

Solution, Ophthalmic, as sodium phosphate:
Generic: 1% (10 mL)
Suspension, Ophthalmic, as acetate:
Omnipred: 1% (5 mL, 10 mL) [contains benzalkonium chloride, edetate disodium, polysorbate 80]
Pred Forte: 1% (1 mL, 5 mL, 10 mL, 15 mL) [contains benzalkonium chloride, edetate disodium, polysorbate 80, sodium bisulfite]
Pred Mild: 0.12% (5 mL, 10 mL)
Generic: 1% (5 mL, 10 mL, 15 mL)

◆ **Prednisolone Acetate, Ophthalmic** *see* PrednisoLONE (Ophthalmic) *on page 1544*

◆ **Prednisolone Sodium Phosphate, Ophthalmic** *see* PrednisoLONE (Ophthalmic) *on page 1544*

◆ **Prednisolone Sod Phosphate** *see* PrednisoLONE (Ophthalmic) *on page 1544*

PredniSONE (PRED ni sone)

Related Information
Corticosteroids Systemic Equivalencies *on page 2417*
Palliative Care Medicine (Cancer) *on page 2352*

Brand Names: US Deltasone; PredniSONE Intensol; Rayos

Brand Names: Canada Apo-Prednisone; JAA-Prednisone; Teva-Prednisone; Winpred

Index Terms Deltacortisone; Deltadehydrocortisone; Deltasone

Pharmacologic Category Corticosteroid, Systemic

Use

Allergic states: Control of severe or incapacitating allergic conditions intractable to adequate trials of conventional treatment in drug hypersensitivity reactions, seasonal or perennial allergic rhinitis; serum sickness.

Dermatologic diseases: Atopic dermatitis; bullous dermatitis herpetiformis; contact dermatitis; exfoliative dermatitis/erythroderma; mycosis fungoides; pemphigus; severe erythema multiforme (Stevens-Johnson syndrome). *Immediate-release only:* Severe psoriasis, severe seborrheic dermatitis.

Endocrine disorders: Congenital adrenal hyperplasia; hypercalcemia of malignancy; nonsuppurative thyroiditis; primary or secondary adrenocortical insufficiency (hydrocortisone or cortisone is the first choice; synthetic analogues may be used in conjunction with mineralocorticoids where applicable.

GI diseases: During acute episodes in regional enteritis (Crohn disease) and ulcerative colitis.

Hematologic disorders: Acquired (autoimmune) hemolytic anemia; congenital (erythroid) hypoplastic anemia/Diamond-Blackfan anemia; immune thrombocytopenia (formerly known as idiopathic thrombocytopenic purpura) in adults; secondary thrombocytopenia in adults.

Delayed-release only: Pure red cell aplasia.

Immediate-release only: Erythroblastopenia (red blood cell anemia).

Neoplastic diseases:

Delayed-release only: Treatment of acute leukemia and aggressive lymphomas.

Immediate-release only: Palliative management of leukemias and lymphomas in adults; acute leukemia of childhood.

Nervous system (delayed-release only): Acute exacerbations of multiple sclerosis; cerebral edema associated with primary or metastatic brain tumor, craniotomy, or head injury. **Note:** Treatment guidelines recommend the use of high dose IV or oral methylprednisolone for acute exacerbations of multiple sclerosis (Scott 2011; NICE 2014).

Ophthalmic diseases:

Delayed-release only: Severe acute and chronic allergic and inflammatory processes involving the eye and its adnexa, such as sympathetic ophthalmia; uveitis and ocular inflammatory conditions unresponsive to topical steroids.

Immediate-release only: Severe acute and chronic allergic and inflammatory processes involving the eye and its adnexa, such as allergic conjunctivitis, allergic corneal marginal ulcers, anterior segment inflammation, chorioretinitis, diffuse posterior uveitis and choroiditis, herpes zoster ophthalmicus, iridocyclitis, iritis, keratitis, optic neuritis, sympathetic ophthalmia.

Renal diseases: To induce a diuresis or remission of proteinuria in the nephrotic syndrome, without uremia, of the idiopathic type or that is caused by lupus erythematosus.

Respiratory diseases: Aspiration pneumonitis; asthma; fulminating or disseminated pulmonary tuberculosis when used concurrently with appropriate chemotherapy; symptomatic sarcoidosis.

Delayed-release only: Acute exacerbations of chronic obstructive pulmonary disease (COPD); allergic bronchopulmonary aspergillosis; hypersensitivity pneumonitis; idiopathic bronchiolitis obliterans with organizing pneumonia; idiopathic eosinophilic pneumonias; idiopathic pulmonary fibrosis; *Pneumocystis carinii* pneumonia (PCP) associated with hypoxemia occurring in an HIV-positive individual who is also under treatment with appropriate anti-PCP antibiotics.

Immediate-release only: Berylliosis; Loeffler syndrome not manageable by other means.

Rheumatic disorders:

Maintenance therapy:

Delayed-release only: During an exacerbation or as maintenance therapy in selected cases of ankylosing spondylitis, dermatomyositis/polymyositis, polymyalgia rheumatica, psoriatic arthritis, relapsing polychondritis, rheumatoid arthritis including juvenile rheumatoid arthritis, Sjögren syndrome, systemic lupus erythematosus, vasculitis.

Immediate-release only: During an exacerbation or as maintenance therapy in selected cases of acute rheumatic carditis, systemic dermatomyositis (polymyositis), systemic lupus erythematosus.

Short-term therapy:

Delayed release only: As adjunctive therapy for short-term administration in acute gouty arthritis.

Immediate-release only: As adjunctive therapy for short-term administration in acute and subacute bursitis; acute gouty arthritis; acute nonspecific tenosynovitis; ankylosing spondylitis; epicondylitis; posttraumatic osteoarthritis; psoriatic arthritis; rheumatoid arthritis including juvenile rheumatoid arthritis; synovitis of osteoarthritis.

Miscellaneous: Trichinosis with neurologic or myocardial involvement; tuberculous meningitis with subarachnoid block or impending block when used concurrently with appropriate antituberculous chemotherapy.

Delayed-release only: Acute or chronic solid organ rejection.

Labeled Contraindications Hypersensitivity to prednisone or any component of the formulation; administration of live or live attenuated vaccines with immunosuppressive doses of prednisone; systemic fungal infections

Documentation of allergenic cross-reactivity for corticosteroids is limited. However, because of similarities in chemical structure and/or pharmacologic actions, the possibility of cross-sensitivity cannot be ruled out with certainty.

Pregnancy Considerations Adverse events have been observed with corticosteroids in animal reproduction studies. Prednisone and its metabolite, prednisolone, cross the human placenta. In the mother, prednisone is converted to the active metabolite prednisolone by the liver. Prior to reaching the fetus, prednisolone is converted by placental enzymes back to prednisone. As a result, the level of prednisone remaining in the maternal serum and reaching the fetus are similar; however, the amount of prednisolone reaching the fetus is ~8 to 10 times lower than the maternal serum concentration (healthy women at term) (Beitins 1972).

Some studies have shown an association between first trimester systemic corticosteroid use and oral clefts or decreased birth weight; however, information is conflicting and may be influenced by maternal dose/indication for use (Lunghi 2010; Park Wyllic 2000; Pradat 2003). Hypoadrenalism may occur in newborns following maternal use of corticosteroids in pregnancy; monitor.

When systemic corticosteroids are needed in pregnancy for rheumatic disorders, it is generally recommended to use the lowest effective dose for the shortest duration of time, avoiding high doses during the first trimester (Götestam Skorpen 2016; Makol 2011; Østensen 2009).

For dermatologic disorders in pregnant women, systemic corticosteroids are generally not preferred for initial therapy; should be avoided during the first trimester; and used during the second or third trimester at the lowest effective dose (Bae 2012; Leachman 2006). Prednisone is preferred by some guidelines when an oral corticosteroid is needed because placental enzymes limit passage to the embryo (Murase 2014).

Pregnant women with poorly controlled asthma or asthma exacerbations may have a greater fetal/maternal risk than what is associated with appropriately used medications. Uncontrolled asthma is associated with an increased risk of perinatal mortality, preeclampsia, preterm birth, and low birth weight infants. Inhaled corticosteroids are recommended for the treatment of asthma during pregnancy; however, systemic corticosteroids, including prednisone, should be used to control acute exacerbations or treat severe persistent asthma (ACOG 2008; GINA 2016; Namazy 2016).

◀ Prednisone may be used to treat lupus nephritis in pregnant women who have active nephritis or substantial extrarenal disease activity (Hahn 2012). Prednisone is recommended for use in fetal-neonatal alloimmune thrombocytopenia and pregnancy-associated immune thrombocytopenia (ACOG 2016). Prednisone may be used (alternative agent) to treat primary adrenal insufficiency (PAI) in pregnant women. Pregnant women with PAI should be monitored at least once each trimester (Bornstein 2016).

The National Transplantation Pregnancy Registry (NTPR) is a registry which follows pregnancies which occur in maternal transplant recipients or those fathered by male transplant recipients. The NTPR encourages reporting of pregnancies following solid organ transplant by contacting them at 877-955-6877 or NTPR@giftoflifeinstitute.org.

Breastfeeding Considerations

Prednisone and its metabolite, prednisolone, are present in breast milk. Actual concentrations are dependent upon maternal dose (Berlin 1979; Katz 1975; Sagraves 1981). Peak concentrations of prednisone and prednisolone in breast milk occur ~2 hours after an oral maternal dose (Berlin 1979; Sagraves 1981); the half-life in breast milk is 1.9 hours (prednisone) and 4.2 hours (prednisolone) (Sagraves 1981).

In a study which included six mother-infant pairs, adverse events were not observed in nursing infants (maternal prednisone dose not provided) (Ito 1993).

The manufacturer notes that when used systemically, maternal use of corticosteroids have the potential to cause adverse events in a breastfeeding infant (eg, growth suppression, interfere with endogenous corticosteroid production) and therefore, a decision should be made whether to discontinue nursing or to discontinue the drug, taking into account the importance of treatment to the mother. Corticosteroids are generally considered acceptable in breastfeeding women when used in usual doses (Götestam Skorpen 2016; WHO 2002); however, monitoring of the breastfeeding infant is recommended (WHO 2002). Prednisone is one of the oral corticosteroids preferred for use in breastfeeding women (Butler 2014). If there is concern about exposure to the infant, some guidelines recommend waiting 4 hours after the maternal dose of an oral systemic corticosteroid before breastfeeding in order to decrease potential exposure to the breastfeeding infant (based on a study using prednisolone) (Bae 2012; Butler 2014; Götestam Skorpen 2016; Leachman 2006; Makol 2011; Ost 1985).

Warnings/Precautions May cause hypercortisolism or suppression of hypothalamic-pituitary-adrenal (HPA) axis, particularly in younger children or in patients receiving high doses for prolonged periods. HPA axis suppression may lead to adrenal crisis. Withdrawal and discontinuation of a corticosteroid should be done slowly and carefully. Particular care is required when patients are transferred from systemic corticosteroids to inhaled products due to possible adrenal insufficiency or withdrawal from steroids, including an increase in allergic symptoms. Patients receiving >20 mg per day of prednisone (or equivalent) may be most susceptible. Fatalities have occurred due to adrenal insufficiency in asthmatic patients during and after transfer from systemic corticosteroids to aerosol steroids; aerosol steroids do **not** provide the systemic steroid needed to treat patients having trauma, surgery, or infections.

Acute myopathy has been reported with high dose corticosteroids, usually in patients with neuromuscular transmission disorders; may involve ocular and/ or respiratory muscles; monitor creatine kinase; recovery may be delayed. Prolonged use of corticosteroids may increase the incidence of secondary infection, mask acute infection (including fungal infections), prolong or exacerbate viral infections, or limit response to killed or inactivated vaccines. Exposure to chickenpox or measles should be avoided. Corticosteroids should not be used to treat viral hepatitis or cerebral malaria. Close observation is required in patients with latent tuberculosis and/or TB reactivity; restrict use in active TB (only fulminating or disseminated TB in conjunction with antituberculosis treatment). Latent or active amebiasis should be ruled out in any patient with recent travel to tropic climates or unexplained diarrhea prior to corticosteroid initiation. Use with extreme caution in patients with Strongyloides infections; hyperinfection, dissemination and fatalities have occurred. Prolonged treatment with corticosteroids has been associated with the development of Kaposi sarcoma (case reports); if noted, discontinuation of therapy should be considered (Goedert 2002). Use with caution in patients with cataracts and/or glaucoma; increased intraocular pressure, open-angle glaucoma, and cataracts have occurred with prolonged use. Use with caution in patients with a history of ocular herpes simplex; corneal perforation has occurred; do not use in active ocular herpes simplex. Consider routine eye exams in chronic users. Corticosteroid use may cause psychiatric disturbances, including euphoria, insomnia, mood swings, personality changes, severe depression or frank psychotic manifestations. Preexisting psychiatric conditions may be exacerbated by corticosteroid use. Rare cases of anaphylactoid reactions have been observed in patients receiving corticosteroids.

Use with caution in patients with HF, hypertension, diabetes, GI diseases (diverticulitis, fresh intestinal anastomoses, active or latent peptic ulcer, ulcerative colitis [nonspecific]), hepatic impairment, myasthenia gravis, MI, patients with or who are at risk for osteoporosis, renal impairment, seizure disorders or thyroid disease. May affect growth velocity; growth and development should be routinely monitored in pediatric patients. Use with caution in the elderly in the smallest possible effective dose for the shortest duration.

Withdraw therapy with gradual tapering of dose. Increased mortality was observed in patients receiving high-dose IV methylprednisolone; high-dose corticosteroids should not be used for the management of head injury. Patients may require higher doses when subject to stress (ie, trauma, surgery, severe infection). Potentially significant drug-drug interactions may exist, requiring dose or frequency adjustment, additional monitoring, and/or selection of alternative therapy.

Some dosage forms may contain sodium benzoate/benzoic acid; benzoic acid (benzoate) is a metabolite of benzyl alcohol; large amounts of benzyl alcohol (≥99 mg/kg/day) have been associated with a potentially fatal toxicity ("gasping syndrome") in neonates; the "gasping syndrome" consists of metabolic acidosis, respiratory distress, gasping respirations, CNS dysfunction (including convulsions, intracranial hemorrhage), hypotension, and cardiovascular collapse (AAP ["Inactive" 1997]; CDC 1982); some data suggests that benzoate displaces bilirubin from protein binding sites (Ahlfors 2001); avoid or use dosage forms containing benzyl alcohol derivative with caution in neonates. See manufacturer's labeling.

◀ Some dosage forms may contain propylene glycol; large amounts are potentially toxic and have been associated hyperosmolality, lactic acidosis, seizures, and respiratory depression; use caution (AAP ["Inactive" 1997]; Zar 2007).

Adverse Reactions Frequency not defined.

Cardiovascular: Cardiac failure (in susceptible patients), hypertension

Central nervous system: Emotional lability, headache, increased intracranial pressure (with papilledema), myasthenia, psychiatric disturbance (including euphoria, insomnia, mood swings, personality changes, severe depression), seizure, vertigo

Dermatologic: Diaphoresis, facial erythema, skin atrophy, urticaria

Endocrine & metabolic: Cushing's syndrome, decreased serum potassium, diabetes mellitus, fluid retention, growth suppression (children), hypokalemic alkalosis, hypothyroidism (enhanced), menstrual disease, negative nitrogen balance (due to protein catabolism), sodium retention

Gastrointestinal: Abdominal distention, carbohydrate intolerance, pancreatitis, peptic ulcer (with possible perforation and hemorrhage), ulcerative esophagitis

Hematologic & oncologic: Bruise, Kaposi's sarcoma, petechia

Hepatic: Increased serum alkaline phosphatase, increased serum ALT, increased serum AST

Hypersensitivity: Anaphylaxis, hypersensitivity reaction

Infection: Infection

Neuromuscular & skeletal: Amyotrophy, aseptic necrosis of bones (femoral and humeral heads), osteoporosis, pathological fracture (long bones), rupture of tendon (particularly Achilles tendon), steroid myopathy, vertebral compression fracture

Ophthalmic: Exophthalmos, glaucoma, increased intraocular pressure, subcapsular posterior cataract

Miscellaneous: Wound healing impairment

<1%, postmarketing, and/or case reports: Venous thrombosis (Johannesdottir 2013)

Drug Interactions

Metabolism/Transport Effects Substrate of CYP3A4 (minor); **Note:** Assignment of Major/Minor substrate status based on clinically relevant drug interaction potential

Avoid Concomitant Use

Avoid concomitant use of PredniSONE with any of the following: Aldesleukin; BCG (Intravesical); Desmopressin; Indium 111 Capromab Pendetide; MiFEPRIStone; Natalizumab; Pimecrolimus; Tacrolimus (Topical)

Increased Effect/Toxicity

PredniSONE may increase the levels/effects of: Acetylcholinesterase Inhibitors; Amphotericin B; Androgens; Ceritinib; CycloSPORINE (Systemic); Deferasirox; Desirudin; Desmopressin; Fingolimod; Leflunomide; Loop Diuretics; Natalizumab; Nicorandil; NSAID (COX-2 Inhibitor); NSAID (Nonselective); Quinolone Antibiotics; Thiazide and Thiazide-Like Diuretics; Tofacitinib; Vaccines (Live); Warfarin

The levels/effects of PredniSONE may be increased by: Aprepitant; Boceprevir; CycloSPORINE (Systemic); CYP3A4 Inhibitors (Strong); Denosumab; DilTIAZem; Estrogen Derivatives; Fluconazole; Fosaprepitant; Indacaterol; MiFEPRIStone; Neuromuscular-Blocking Agents (Nondepolarizing); Ocrelizumab; Pimecrolimus; Ritonavir; Roflumilast; Salicylates; Tacrolimus (Topical); Telaprevir; Trastuzumab

Decreased Effect

PredniSONE may decrease the levels/effects of: Aldesleukin; Antidiabetic Agents; BCG (Intravesical); Calcitriol (Systemic); Coccidioides immitis Skin Test; Corticorelin; CycloSPORINE (Systemic); Hyaluronidase; Indium 111 Capromab Pendetide; Isoniazid; Nivolumab; Salicylates; Sipuleucel-T; Telaprevir; Tertomotide; Urea Cycle Disorder Agents; Vaccines (Inactivated); Vaccines (Live)

The levels/effects of PredniSONE may be decreased by: Antacids; Bile Acid Sequestrants; CYP3A4 Inducers (Strong); Echinacea; MiFEPRIStone; Mitotane; Somatropin; Tesamorelin

Storage/Stability

Store at 25°C (77°F); excursions permitted to 15°C to 30°C (59°F to 86°F). Protect from light and moisture.

Oral solution, concentrate: Discard opened bottle after 90 days.

Mechanism of Action Decreases inflammation by suppression of migration of polymorphonuclear leukocytes and reversal of increased capillary permeability; suppresses the immune system by reducing activity and volume of the lymphatic system; suppresses adrenal function at high doses. Antitumor effects may be related to inhibition of glucose transport, phosphorylation, or induction of cell death in immature lymphocytes. Antiemetic effects are thought to occur due to blockade of cerebral innervation of the emetic center via inhibition of prostaglandin synthesis.

Pharmacodynamics/Kinetics

Absorption: 50% to 90% (may be altered in hepatic failure, chronic renal failure, inflammatory bowel disease, hyperthyroidism, and in the elderly) (Frey 1990)

Protein binding (concentration dependent): <50% (Frey 1990)

Metabolism: Hepatic to metabolite prednisolone (active)

Half-life elimination: 2 to 3 hours

Time to peak: Oral: Immediate-release tablet: 2 hours; Delayed-release tablet: 6 to 6.5 hours

Excretion: Urine (as conjugates)

Dosing

Adult General dosing; anti-inflammatory/immunosuppressive/endocrine disorders: Oral: Initial: 5 to 60 mg daily:

Note: Dose depends upon condition being treated and response of patient. Consider alternate day therapy for long-term therapy. Discontinuation of long-term therapy requires gradual withdrawal by tapering the dose.

Prednisone taper (other regimens also available):

Day 1: 30 mg divided as 10 mg before breakfast, 5 mg at lunch, 5 mg at dinner, 10 mg at bedtime

Day 2: 5 mg at breakfast, 5 mg at lunch, 5 mg at dinner, 10 mg at bedtime

Day 3: 5 mg 4 times daily (with meals and at bedtime)

Day 4: 5 mg 3 times daily (breakfast, lunch, bedtime)

Day 5: 5 mg 2 times daily (breakfast, bedtime)

Day 6: 5 mg before breakfast

Indication-specific dosing:

Acute asthma (off-label dose): Oral: 40 to 60 mg/day for 3 to 10 days; administer as single or 2 divided doses (NAEPP 2007).

Acute exacerbations of chronic obstructive pulmonary disease (COPD) (off-label use for immediate release products; off-label dose): Oral: 40 mg once daily for 5 days (GOLD 2014).

◀

Acute gout (off-label dose): Oral: Initial: ≥0.5 mg/kg for 5 to 10 days (ACR guidelines [Khanna 2012])

Anaphylaxis, adjunctive treatment (off-label dose): Oral: 0.5 mg/kg (Lieberman 2005)

Antineoplastic: Oral: Usual range: 10 mg daily to 100 mg/m²/day (depending on indication). Refer to specific protocol for dosing and administration details.

Autoimmune hepatitis (off-label use): Oral: Initial: 60 mg daily for 1 week, *followed by* 40 mg daily for 1 week, *then* 30 mg daily for 2 weeks, *then* 20 mg daily. Half this dose should be given when used in combination with azathioprine (AASLD [Manns 2010]).

Bell palsy (off-label use): Oral: 60 mg daily for 5 days, followed by a 5-day taper. Treatment should begin within 72 hours of onset of symptoms (OHNS [Baugh 2013]).

Crohn disease, moderate/severe (off-label dose): Oral: 40 to 60 mg daily until resolution of symptoms and resumption of weight gain (usual duration: 7 to 28 days) (Lichtenstein 2009).

Dermatomyositis/polymyositis (off-label dose): Oral: 1 mg/kg daily (range: 0.5 to 1.5 mg/kg/day), often in conjunction with steroid-sparing therapies; depending on response/tolerance, consider slow tapering after 2 to 8 weeks depending on response; taper regimens vary widely, but often involve 5 to 10 mg decrements per week and may require 6 to 12 months to reach a low once-daily or every-other-day dose to prevent disease flare (Briemberg 2003; Hengstman 2009; Iorizzo 2008; Wiendl 2008).

Duchenne muscular dystrophy (off-label use): Oral: 0.75 mg/kg/day or 10 mg/kg/weekend, divided over 2 days. When used daily, the dose may be decreased to 0.3 mg/kg/day in patients who experience adverse reactions. Doses as high as 1.5 mg/kg/day have been studied, but there is no evidence that doses above 0.75 mg/kg/day provide greater efficacy (AAN [Gloss 2016]; Escolar 2011; Matthews 2016).

Giant cell arteritis (off-label use): Oral: Initial: 40 to 60 mg daily; typically requires 1 to 2 years of treatment, but may begin to taper after 2 to 3 months; alternative dosing of 30 to 40 mg daily has demonstrated similar efficacy (Hiratzka 2010).

Glucocorticoid remediable aldosteronism, treatment (off-label use): Oral: Initial: 2.5 to 5 mg once daily preferably at bedtime to suppress early morning ACTH surge (Funder 2016)

Graves orbitopathy (off-label use): Oral: 0.4 to 0.5 mg/kg/day, starting 1 to 3 days after radioactive iodine treatment, and continued for 1 month, then gradually taper over 2 months (Ross 2016).

Herpes zoster (off-label use): Oral: 60 mg daily for 7 days, *followed by* 30 mg daily for 7 days, *then* 15 mg daily for 7 days (Dworkin 2007).

Immune thrombocytopenia (off-label dose): Oral: 1 to 2 mg/kg/day (American Society of Hematology 1997).

Immune thrombocytopenia in pregnancy: Initial: 10 to 20 mg/day (ACOG 2016). Adjust to the minimum effective dose to achieve response; generally continue for at least 21 days, then taper to the minimum effective dose required to maintain platelet count (ACOG 2016; Neunert 2011).

Lupus nephritis, induction (off-label dose): Oral:
Class III-IV lupus nephritis: 0.5 to 1 mg/kg/day (after glucocorticoid pulse) tapered after a few weeks to lowest effective dose, in combination with an immunosuppressive agent (Hahn 2012).

Class V lupus nephritis: 0.5 mg/kg/day for 6 months in combination mycophenolate mofetil; if not improved after 6 months, use 0.5 to 1 mg/kg/day (after a glucocorticoid pulse) for an additional 6 months in combination with cyclophosphamide (Hahn 2012).

Multiple sclerosis, acute exacerbations:

Note: Treatment guidelines recommend the use of high dose IV or oral methylprednisolone for acute exacerbations of multiple sclerosis (AAN [Scott 2011]; NICE 2014).

Oral: 200 mg daily for 1 week, followed by 80 mg every other day for 1 month.

Pericarditis (off-label use):

Recurrent pericarditis: Oral: 1 to 1.5 mg/kg once daily for at least 1 month; taper dose over a 3-month period (Maisch 2004)

Tuberculosis pericarditis: Oral: 1 to 2 mg/kg once daily for 5 to 7 days followed by 6 to 8 weeks of tapering (Maisch 2004) **or** 60 mg once daily for 4 weeks, followed by 30 mg once daily for 4 weeks, 15 mg once daily for 2 weeks, and 5 mg once daily for 1 week (Reuter 2006).

***Pneumocystis* pneumonia (adjunctive therapy) in HIV-infected patients (off-label dose):** Oral: 40 mg twice daily for 5 days beginning as early as possible and within 72 hours of PCP therapy, followed by 40 mg once daily on days 6 through 10, followed by 20 mg once daily on days 11 through 21 (DHHS [adult] 2015).

Polymyalgia rheumatica (off-label dose): Oral: Evidence to support an optimal dose and duration are lacking; recommendations provided are general guidelines only. Individualize therapy using the minimum effective dose and duration (Dejaco [EULAR/ACR 2015]):

Initial: Dosage range: 12.5 to 25 mg daily; consider higher doses within this range for patients at high risk of relapse and low risk of adverse events; consider lower doses within this range for patients with high risk factors for side effects (eg, diabetes, osteoporosis, glaucoma). Single daily doses are preferred over divided daily doses. Avoid initial doses ≤7.5 mg/day or >30 mg/day.

Tapering: For initial dosing, taper to a dose of 10 mg/day within 4 to 8 weeks. If relapse occurs, increase dosing to the prerelapse dose and gradually taper back to the dose which relapse occurred within 4 to 8 weeks. Once remission is achieved (initial or relapse therapy), taper daily dose by 1 mg every 4 weeks (or by 1.25 mg decrements if using schedules such as 10 mg and 7.5 mg on alternate days) until discontinuation.

Prostate cancer, metastatic (off-label use): Oral: 5 mg twice daily (in combination with abiraterone) until disease progression or unacceptable toxicity (de Bono 2011; Ryan 2015) **or** 10 mg once daily (in combination with cabazitaxel) for up to 10 cycles (de Bono 2010) **or** 5 mg twice daily (in combination with docetaxel) for up to 10 cycles (Berthold 2008; Tannock 2004).

Rheumatoid arthritis (off-label dose): Oral: ≤10 mg daily (American College of Rheumatology 2002).

Subacute thyroiditis (off-label use): Oral: Initial: 40 mg/day for 1 to 2 weeks; gradually taper over 2 to 4 weeks or longer depending on clinical response (Ross 2016).

Takayasu arteritis (off-label use): Oral: Initial: 40 to 60 mg daily; taper to lowest effective dose when ESR and CRP levels are normal; usual duration: 1 to 2 years (Hiratzka 2010).

◀ **Thyrotoxicosis, type 2 amiodarone-induced (off-label use):** Oral: 40 mg once daily for 14 to 28 days; gradually taper over 2 to 3 months depending on clinical response. **Note:** Use in combination with an antithyroid agent if etiology of thyrotoxicosis (eg, type 1 or type 2) cannot be unequivocally determined or if patient is too clinically unstable to allow a trial of monotherapy (Ross 2016).

Tuberculosis, severe, paradoxical reactions (off-label dose): Oral: 1 mg/kg/day, gradually reduce after 1 to 2 weeks (AIDS*info* guidelines 2008).

Geriatric Refer to adult dosing; use the lowest effective dose.

Pediatric

General dosing; anti-inflammatory/immunosuppressive/endocrine disorders: Children and Adolescents: Oral: Refer to adult dosing.

Note: Dose depends upon condition being treated and response of patient; dosage for infants and children should be based on severity of the disease and response of the patient rather than on strict adherence to dosage indicated by age, weight, or body surface area. Consider alternate day therapy for long-term therapy. Discontinuation of long-term therapy requires gradual withdrawal by tapering the dose.

Indication-specific dosing:

Acute asthma (off-label dose): Oral:

Infants and Children <12 years: 1 to 2 mg/kg/day for 3 to 10 days (maximum: 60 mg/day) (NAEPP 2007).

Children ≥12 years and Adolescents: Refer to adult dosing.

Antineoplastic: Children and Adolescents: Oral: Refer to adult dosing or to specific protocol.

Autoimmune hepatitis (monotherapy or in combination with azathioprine) (off-label use): Infants, Children, and Adolescents: Oral: Initial: 1 to 2 mg/kg/day for 2 weeks (maximum: 60 mg/day), followed by a taper over 6 to 8 weeks to a dose of 0.1 to 0.2 mg/kg/day or 2.5 to 5 mg daily (AASLD [Manns 2010]; Della Corte 2012).

Bell palsy (off-label use):

Infants, Children, and Adolescents <16 years: Oral: 1 mg/kg/day for 1 week, then taper over 1 week; ideally start within the 72 hours of onset of symptoms; maximum daily dose: 60 mg/day

Adolescents ≥16 years: Oral: Refer to adult dosing.

Duchenne muscular dystrophy (off-label use): Children ≥4 years and Adolescents: Oral: 0.75 mg/kg/day or 10 mg/kg/weekend, divided over 2 days. The dose may be decreased to 0.3 mg/kg/day in patients who experience adverse reactions. Doses as high as 1.5 mg/kg/day have been studied, but there is no evidence that doses above 0.75 mg/kg/day provide greater efficacy (AAN [Gloss 2016]; Escolar 2011; Matthews 2016).

Nephrotic syndrome; steroid sensitive (SSNS) (off-label dose): Children and Adolescents: Oral:

Initial episode: 2 mg/kg/day or 60 mg/m^2/day once daily, maximum daily dose: 60 mg/day for 4 to 6 weeks; then adjust to an alternate-day schedule of 1.5 mg/kg/dose or 40 mg/m^2/dose on alternate days as a single dose, maximum dose: 40 mg/dose (Gipson 2009; KDIGO 2012; KDOQI 2013); duration of therapy based on patient response.

Relapse: 2 mg/kg/day or 60 mg/m^2/day once daily, maximum daily dose: 60 mg/day, continue until complete remission for at least 3 days; then adjust to an alternate-day schedule of 1.5 mg/kg/dose or 40 mg/m^2/dose on alternate days as a single dose, maximum dose: 40 mg/dose, recommended duration of alternate day dosing is variable: may continue for at least 4 weeks then taper. Longer duration of treatment may be necessary in patients who relapse frequently, some patients may require up to 3 months of treatment (Gipson 2009; KDIGO 2012; KDOQI 2013).

Maintenance therapy for frequently relapsing SSNS: Taper previous dose down to lowest effective dose which maintains remission using an alternate day schedule; usual effective range: 0.1 to 0.5 mg/kg/day on alternating days; other patients may require doses up to 0.7 mg/kg/dose every other day (KDIGO 2012; KDOQI 2013).

Pneumocystis pneumonia (adjunctive therapy) in HIV-infected patients (off-label dose): Oral:

Infants and Children: 1 mg/kg twice daily on days 1 to 5, *followed by* 0.5 to 1 mg/kg twice daily on days 6 to 10, *followed by* 0.5 mg/kg once daily on days 11 through 21 (DHHS [pediatric] 2013).

Adolescents: Refer to adult dosing.

Renal Impairment There are no dosage adjustments provided in the manufacturer's labeling.

Hemodialysis: Supplemental dose is not necessary.

Hepatic Impairment There are no dosage adjustments provided in the manufacturer's labeling.

Combination Regimens Note: In the US, prednisone is the preferred corticosteroid. However, in the British literature, prednisolone is often used. The oral doses of these two agents are equivalent (ie, 1 mg prednisone = 1 mg prednisolone). Also, early clinical trials gave prednisone only with the first and fourth cycles. Some clinicians give prednisone with every cycle.

Lymphoma, non-Hodgkin:
Lymphoma, non-Hodgkin (AIDS-Related):
Lymphoma, non-Hodgkin (DLBCL):
Lymphoma, non-Hodgkin (Follicular):
Lymphoma, non-Hodgkin (Mantle Cell):
Multiple myeloma:
Prostate cancer:

Administration

Administer after meals or with food or milk to decrease GI upset. May administer antacids between meals to help prevent peptic ulcers.

Delayed-release tablets: Swallow whole; do not break, divide, crush, or chew.

Oral solution, concentrate: Administer only with provided calibrated dropper.

Monitoring Parameters Blood pressure; weight; serum glucose; electrolytes; growth in pediatric patients; presence of infection, bone mineral density; assess HPA axis suppression (eg, ACTH stimulation test, morning plasma cortisol test, urinary free cortisol test); Hgb, occult blood loss; chest x-ray (at regular intervals during prolonged therapy); IOP with therapy >6 weeks.

Test Interactions Decreased response to skin tests

Dietary Considerations May require increased dietary intake of pyridoxine, vitamin C, vitamin D, folate, calcium, and phosphorus; may require decreased dietary intake of sodium and potassium supplementation

Additional Information Tapering of corticosteroids after a short course of therapy (<7-10 days) is generally not required unless the disease/inflammatory process is slow to respond. Tapering after prolonged exposure is dependent upon the individual patient, duration of corticosteroid treatments, and size of steroid dose. Recovery of the HPA axis may require several months. Subtle but important HPA axis suppression may be present for as long as several months after a course of as few as 10-14 days duration. Testing of HPA axis (cosyntropin) may be required, and signs/symptoms of adrenal insufficiency should be monitored in patients with a history of use.

Dosage Forms Excipient information presented when available (limited, particularly for generics); consult specific product labeling. [DSC] = Discontinued product

Concentrate, Oral:
PredniSONE Intensol: 5 mg/mL (30 mL) [contains alcohol, usp; unflavored flavor]

Solution, Oral:
Generic: 5 mg/5 mL (5 mL [DSC], 120 mL, 500 mL)

Tablet, Oral:
Deltasone: 20 mg [scored; contains fd&c yellow #10 aluminum lake, fd&c yellow #6 aluminum lake]
Generic: 1 mg, 2.5 mg, 5 mg, 10 mg, 20 mg, 50 mg, 10 mg, 5 mg

Tablet Delayed Release, Oral:
Rayos: 1 mg, 2 mg, 5 mg

Tablet Therapy Pack, Oral:
Generic: 10 mg (21 ea, 48 ea); 5 mg (21 ea, 48 ea)

◆ **PredniSONE Intensol** see PredniSONE on page 1545
◆ **Prilocaine and Lidocaine** see Lidocaine and Prilocaine on page 1150
◆ **Prilolid** see Lidocaine and Prilocaine on page 1150
◆ **Priloxx LP** see Lidocaine and Prilocaine on page 1150
◆ **Primaxin (Can)** see Imipenem and Cilastatin on page 983
◆ **Primaxin I.M. [DSC]** see Imipenem and Cilastatin on page 983
◆ **Primaxin I.V.** see Imipenem and Cilastatin on page 983
◆ **Priva-Ondansetron (Can)** see Ondansetron on page 1380
◆ **Priva-Valacyclovir (Can)** see ValACYclovir on page 1852
◆ **Privigen** see Immune Globulin on page 992
◆ **PRO-Bicalutamide (Can)** see Bicalutamide on page 252

Procarbazine (proe KAR ba zeen)

Related Information

Management of Chemotherapy-Induced Nausea and Vomiting in Adults on page 2253

Prevention of Chemotherapy-Induced Nausea and Vomiting in Children on page 2310

Safe Handling of Hazardous Drugs on page 2379

Brand Names: US Matulane

Brand Names: Canada Matulane; Natulan

Index Terms Benzmethyzin; Ibenzmethyzin; N-Methylhydrazine; PCB; PCZ; Procarbazine HCl; Procarbazine Hydrochloride

Pharmacologic Category Antineoplastic Agent, Alkylating Agent

Use Treatment of Hodgkin lymphoma

Labeled Contraindications Hypersensitivity to procarbazine or any component of the formulation; inadequate bone marrow reserve

Pregnancy Considerations Adverse events were observed in animal reproduction studies. There are case reports of fetal malformations in the offspring of pregnant women exposed to procarbazine as part of a combination chemotherapy regimen. Women of reproductive potential should avoid becoming pregnant during treatment.

◀ **Breastfeeding Considerations** It is not known if procarbazine is excreted in breast milk. Due to the potential for serious adverse reactions in the nursing infant, nursing is not recommended during treatment with procarbazine.

Warnings/Precautions Hematologic toxicity (leukopenia and thrombocytopenia) may occur 2-8 weeks after treatment initiation. Allow ≥1 month interval between radiation therapy or myelosuppressive chemotherapy and initiation of procarbazine treatment. Withhold treatment for leukopenia (WBC <4000/mm^3) or thrombocytopenia (platelets <100,000/mm^3). Monitor for infections due to neutropenia. May cause hemolysis and/or presence of Heinz inclusion bodies in erythrocytes. Procarbazine is associated with a high emetic potential; antiemetics are recommended to prevent nausea and vomiting (Dupuis, 2011; Roila, 2010). May cause diarrhea and stomatitis; withhold treatment for diarrhea or stomatitis. Withhold treatment for CNS toxicity, hemorrhage, or hypersensitivity. Azoospermia and infertility have been reported with procarbazine when used in combination with other chemotherapy agents. Possibly carcinogenic; acute myeloid leukemia and lung cancer have been reported following use.

Use with caution in patients with hepatic or renal impairment. Potentially significant drug-drug interactions may exist, requiring dose or frequency adjustment, additional monitoring, and/or selection of alternative therapy. Possesses MAO inhibitor activity and has potential for severe drug and food interactions; follow MAOI diet (avoid tyramine-containing foods). Avoid ethanol consumption, may cause disulfiram-like reaction. **[U.S. Boxed Warning]: Should be administered under the supervision of an experienced cancer chemotherapy physician.**

Adverse Reactions Frequency not always defined.

Cardiovascular: Edema, flushing, hypotension, syncope, tachycardia

Central nervous system: Apprehension, ataxia, chills, coma, confusion, depression, dizziness, drowsiness, falling, fatigue, hallucination, headache, hyporeflexia, insomnia, lethargy, nervousness, neuropathy, nightmares, pain, paresthesia, seizure, slurred speech, unsteadiness

Dermatologic: Alopecia, dermatitis, diaphoresis, hyperpigmentation, pruritus, skin rash, urticaria

Endocrine & metabolic: Gynecomastia (in prepubertal and early pubertal males)

Gastrointestinal: Nausea and vomiting (60% to 90%; increasing the dose in a stepwise fashion over several days may minimize), abdominal pain, anorexia, constipation, diarrhea, dysphagia, hematemesis, melena, stomatitis, xerostomia

Genitourinary: Reduced fertility (>10%), azoospermia (reported with combination chemotherapy), hematuria, nocturia

Hematologic & oncologic: Malignant neoplasm (2% to 15%; secondary; nonlymphoid; reported with combination therapy), anemia, bone marrow depression, eosinophilia, hemolysis (in patients with G6PD deficiency), hemolytic anemia, pancytosis, petechia, purpura, thrombocytopenia

Hepatic: Hepatic insufficiency, jaundice

Hypersensitivity: Hypersensitivity reaction

Infection: Herpes virus infection, increased susceptibility to infection

Neuromuscular & skeletal: Arthralgia, foot-drop, myalgia, tremor, weakness

Ophthalmic: Accommodation disturbance, diplopia, nystagmus, papilledema, photophobia, retinal hemorrhage

Otic: Hearing loss

Renal: Polyuria

Respiratory: Cough, epistaxis, hemoptysis, hoarseness, pleural effusion, pneumonitis, pulmonary toxicity (<1%)

Miscellaneous: Fever

Drug Interactions

Metabolism/Transport Effects Inhibits Monoamine Oxidase

Avoid Concomitant Use

Avoid concomitant use of Procarbazine with any of the following: Alpha-/Beta-Agonists (Indirect-Acting); Alpha1-Agonists; Amphetamines; Antidepressants (Serotonin Reuptake Inhibitor/Antagonist); Apraclonidine; AtoMOXetine; Atropine (Ophthalmic); BCG (Intravesical); Bezafibrate; Buprenorphine; BuPROPion; BusPIRone; CarBAMazepine; Cyclobenzaprine; Cyproheptadine; Dapoxetine; Deferiprone; Deutetrabenazine; Dexmethylphenidate; Dextromethorphan; Diethylpropion; Dipyrone; Droxidopa; EPINEPHrine (Oral Inhalation); FentaNYL; Guanethidine; Heroin; HYDROmorphone; Indoramin; Isometheptene; Levonordefrin; Linezolid; MAO Inhibitors; Maprotiline; Meperidine; Meptazinol; Mequitazine; Methyldopa; Methylene Blue; Methylphenidate; Mianserin; Mirtazapine; Moclobemide; Morphine (Liposomal); Morphine (Systemic); Natalizumab; Nefopam; OxyMORphone; Pheniramine; Pholcodine; Pimecrolimus; Pizotifen; Reboxetine; Selective Serotonin Reuptake Inhibitors; Serotonin 5-HT1D Receptor Agonists; Serotonin/Norepinephrine Reuptake Inhibitors; SUFentanil; Tacrolimus (Topical); Tapentadol; Tetrabenazine; Tetrahydrozoline (Nasal); Tianeptine; Tricyclic Antidepressants; Tryptophan; Vaccines (Live); Valbenazine

Increased Effect/Toxicity

Procarbazine may increase the levels/effects of: Alpha-/Beta-Agonists (Indirect-Acting); Alpha1-Agonists; Amphetamines; Antidepressants (Serotonin Reuptake Inhibitor/Antagonist); Antipsychotic Agents; Apraclonidine; AtoMOXetine; Atropine (Ophthalmic); Beta2-Agonists; Betahistine; Bezafibrate; Blood Glucose Lowering Agents; Brimonidine (Ophthalmic); Brimonidine (Topical); BuPROPion; Carbocisteine; CloZAPine; Codeine; Cyproheptadine; Deferiprone; Deutetrabenazine; Dexmethylphenidate; Dextromethorphan; Diethylpropion; Domperidone; DOPamine; Doxapram; Droxidopa; EPINEPHrine (Nasal); EPINEPHrine (Oral Inhalation); Epinephrine (Racemic); EPINEPHrine (Systemic); Fingolimod; Heroin; HYDROcodone; HYDROmorphone; Indoramin; Iohexol; Iomeprol; Iopamidol; Isometheptene; Leflunomide; Levonordefrin; Levosulpiride; Linezolid; Lithium; MAO Inhibitors; Meperidine; Meptazinol; Mequitazine; Metaraminol; Methyldopa; Methylene Blue; Methylphenidate; Metoclopramide; Mianserin; Mirtazapine; Moclobemide; Morphine (Liposomal); Morphine (Systemic); Natalizumab; Nefopam; Norepinephrine; Pindolol; Pizotifen; Reboxetine; Reserpine; Selective Serotonin Reuptake Inhibitors; Serotonin 5-HT1D Receptor Agonists; Serotonin Modulators; Serotonin/Norepinephrine Reuptake Inhibitors; Tetrahydrozoline (Nasal); Tofacitinib; TraMADol; Tricyclic Antidepressants; Vaccines (Live)

The levels/effects of Procarbazine may be increased by: Altretamine; Analgesics (Opioid); Antiemetics (5HT3 Antagonists); Antipsychotic Agents; Buprenorphine; BusPIRone; CarBAMazepine; Cerebrolysin; Chlorphenesin Carbamate; COMT Inhibitors; Cyclobenzaprine; Dapoxetine; Denosumab; Dihydrocodeine; Dipyrone; FentaNYL; Guanethidine; Levodopa; Maprotiline; Metaxalone; Methadone; Methylene Blue; Ocrelizumab; OxyCODONE; OxyMORphone; Palifermin; Pheniramine; Pholcodine; Pimecrolimus; Promazine; Roflumilast; SUFentanil; Tacrolimus (Topical); Tapentadol; ▶

◀ **Hepatic Impairment** No dosage adjustment provided in manufacturer's labeling; use with caution; may result in increased toxicity. The following adjustments have been reported in literature:

Floyd, 2006:

Transaminases 1.6-6 times ULN: Administer 75% of dose

Transaminases >6 times ULN: Use clinical judgment

Serum bilirubin >5 mg/dL or transaminases >3 times ULN: Avoid use

King, 2001: Serum bilirubin >5 mg/dL or transaminases >180 units/L: Avoid use

Obesity *ASCO Guidelines for appropriate chemotherapy dosing in obese adults with cancer:* Utilize patient's actual body weight (full weight) for calculation of body surface area- or weight-based dosing, particularly when the intent of therapy is curative; manage regimen-related toxicities in the same manner as for nonobese patients; if a dose reduction is utilized due to toxicity, consider resumption of full weight-based dosing with subsequent cycles, especially if cause of toxicity (eg, hepatic or renal impairment) is resolved (Griggs, 2012). **Note:** The manufacturer suggests that an estimated lean body mass be used in obese patients and patients with rapid weight gain due to edema, ascites, or abnormal fluid retention.

Adjustment for Toxicity Withhold treatment (promptly) for any of the following: CNS toxicity (eg, paresthesia, confusion, neuropathy), hematologic toxicity (WBC <4000/mm^3 or platelets <100,000/mm^3), hypersensitivity, gastrointestinal toxicities (stomatisis, diarrhea), and hemorrhage or bleeding.

Combination Regimens

Brain tumors: PCV (Brain Tumor Regimen) on page 2191

Lymphoma, Hodgkin:

BEACOPP-14 (Hodgkin) on page 1981

BEACOPP Escalated (Hodgkin) on page 1982

BEACOPP Escalated Plus Standard (Hodgkin) on page 1983

BEACOPP Standard (Hodgkin) on page 1984

ChIVPP (Hodgkin) on page 2033

C-MOPP/ABV Hybrid (Hodgkin) on page 2067

MOPP/ABVD (Hodgkin) on page 2176

MOPP/ABV Hybrid (Hodgkin) on page 2177

MOPP (Hodgkin) on page 2178

Lymphoma, non-Hodgkin (DLBCL): CEPP (NHL-DLBCL) on page 2029

Lymphoma, non-Hodgkin (NHL): PEP-C (NHL) on page 2194

Lymphoma, non-Hodgkin (Mantle cell): PEP-C (NHL-Mantle Cell) on page 2194

Administration Oral: May be given as a single daily dose or in 2 to 3 divided doses. Procarbazine is associated with a high emetic potential; antiemetics are recommended to prevent nausea and vomiting (Dupuis, 2011; Roila, 2010).

Emetic Potential Children and Adults: High (>90%)

Extemporaneous Preparations A 10 mg/mL oral suspension may be prepared using capsules, glycerin, and strawberry syrup. Empty the contents of ten 50 mg capsules into a mortar. Add 2 mL glycerin and mix to a thick uniform paste. Add 10 mL strawberry syrup in incremental proportions; mix until uniform. Transfer the mixture to an amber glass bottle and rinse mortar with small amounts of strawberry syrup; add rinses to the bottle in sufficient quantity to make 50 mL. Label "shake well" and "protect from light". Stable for 7 days at room temperature.

Matulane® data on file, Sigma Tau Pharmaceuticals, Inc.

Monitoring Parameters CBC with differential, platelet and reticulocyte count, urinalysis, liver function test, renal function test. Monitor for infections, CNS toxicity, and gastrointestinal toxicities.

Dietary Considerations Avoid tyramine-containing foods/beverages. Some examples include aged or matured cheese, air-dried or cured meats (including sausages and salamis), fava or broad bean pods, tap/draft beers, Marmite concentrate, sauerkraut, soy sauce and other soybean condiments.

Dosage Forms Excipient information presented when available (limited, particularly for generics); consult specific product labeling.

Capsule, Oral, as hydrochloride:
Matulane: 50 mg

♦ **Procarbazine HCl** see Procarbazine on page 1557

♦ **Procarbazine Hydrochloride** see Procarbazine on page 1557

Prochlorperazine (proe klor PER a zeen)

Brand Names: US Compazine [DSC]; Compro

Brand Names: Canada Apo-Prochlorperazine; Nu-Prochlor; PMS-Prochlorperazine; Sandoz-Prochlorperazine

Index Terms Chlormeprazine; Compazine; Prochlorperazine Edisylate; Prochlorperazine Maleate; Prochlorperazine Mesylate

Pharmacologic Category Antiemetic; First Generation (Typical) Antipsychotic; Phenothiazine Derivative

Use Nausea/vomiting: Management of severe nausea and vomiting

Dosing

Adult Note: Injection solution mesylate formulation is a Canadian product (not available in the US).

Nausea/vomiting:

Oral (tablet): 5 to 10 mg 3 to 4 times/day; usual maximum: 40 mg/day; larger doses may rarely be required for resistant nausea/vomiting

IM (as edisylate): 5 to 10 mg every 3 to 4 hours; maximum dose: 40 mg/day

IM (as mesylate): 5 to 10 mg 2 to 3 times/day; usual maximum: 40 mg/day

IV (as edisylate): 2.5 to 10 mg; maximum: 10 mg/dose or 40 mg/day; may repeat dose every 3 to 4 hours as needed

Rectal: 25 mg twice daily

Canadian product (10 mg suppository): 5 to 10 mg 3 to 4 times/day

Breakthrough chemotherapy-induced nausea and vomiting: IM, IV, Oral: 5 to 10 mg every 4 to 6 hours as needed (Lohr 2008)

Nausea and vomiting due to low emetogenic chemotherapy: 5 to 10 mg IV or orally prior to chemotherapy followed by 5 to 10 mg orally every 6 hours if needed following chemotherapy (Hesketh 2008)

Nausea and vomiting due to minimally emetogenic radiation therapy: IV, Oral: 10 mg (Basch 2011)

Surgical nausea/vomiting: Note: Should not exceed 40 mg/day

IM (as edisylate): 5 to 10 mg 1 to 2 hours before anesthesia induction or to control symptoms during or after surgery; may repeat once in 30 minutes if necessary

IM (as mesylate): 5 to 10 mg 1 to 2 hours before anesthesia induction; may repeat once if needed during surgery; postoperatively: 5 to 10 mg every 3 to 4 hours as needed up to maximum of 40 mg daily

▶

◀ *IV (as edisylate):* 5 to 10 mg 15 to 30 minutes before anesthesia induction or to control symptoms during or after surgery; may repeat once if necessary

IV (as mesylate): 20 mg/L of IV solution during surgery or postoperatively; usual maximum: 30 mg daily

Rectal: 25 mg (Golembiewski 2005)

Geriatric Initiate at lower end of dosage range; increase dose slowly and cautiously. Refer to adult dosing.

Pediatric Note: Injection solution mesylate formulation is a Canadian product (not available in US).

Use is contraindicated in children <9 kg or <2 years.

Nausea/vomiting:

Oral (therapy >1 day usually not required):

9 to 13 kg: 2.5 mg 1 to 2 times/day as needed (maximum: 7.5 mg/day)

>13 to 18 kg: 2.5 mg 2 to 3 times/day as needed (maximum: 10 mg/day)

>18 to 39 kg: 2.5 mg 3 times/day or 5 mg 2 times/day as needed (maximum: 15 mg/day)

IM (as edisylate): 0.13 mg/kg/dose; convert to oral therapy as soon as possible

IM (as mesylate): 0.14 mg/kg/dose; convert to oral therapy at equivalent or greater dose (if necessary) as soon as possible

Breakthrough chemotherapy-induced nausea and vomiting, refractory (off-label dosing; Dupuis 2003):

IV: 0.1 to 0.15 mg/kg/dose every 3 to 4 hours as needed (maximum: 10 mg/dose and 40 mg/day)

Oral: 0.1 mg/kg/dose every 6 hours as needed (maximum: 10 mg/dose and 40 mg/day)

Renal Impairment There are no dosage adjustments provided in the manufacturer's labeling.

Hepatic Impairment There are no dosage adjustments provided in the manufacturer's labeling; systemic exposure may be increased as drug undergoes hepatic metabolism.

Additional Information Complete prescribing information should be consulted for additional detail.

Dosage Forms Excipient information presented when available (limited, particularly for generics); consult specific product labeling. [DSC] = Discontinued product

Solution, Injection, as edisylate [strength expressed as base]:

Generic: 5 mg/mL (2 mL, 10 mL [DSC])

Suppository, Rectal:

Compazine: 25 mg (12 ea [DSC])

Compro: 25 mg (12 ea)

Generic: 25 mg (1 ea, 12 ea, 1000 ea)

Tablet, Oral, as maleate [strength expressed as base]:

Compazine: 5 mg [DSC], 10 mg [DSC]

Generic: 5 mg, 10 mg

Dosage Forms: Canada Information with regard to form, strength, and availability of products uniquely available in Canada but currently not available in the US. Refer also to Dosage Forms.

Excipient information presented when available (limited, particularly for generics); consult specific product labeling.

Injection, solution, as mesylate [strength expressed as base]: 5 mg/mL (2 mL)

Suppository, rectal: 10 mg (10s)

♦ **Radium-223 Dichloride** *see* Radium Ra 223 Dichloride *on page 1566*

Radium Ra 223 Dichloride

(RAY dee um R A two twenty-three dye KLOR ide)

Brand Names: US Xofigo

Index Terms 223Ra; Alpharadin; BAY88-8223; Radium-223 Chloride; Radium-223 Dichloride

Pharmacologic Category Radiopharmaceutical

Use Prostate cancer: Treatment of castration-resistant prostate cancer in patients with symptomatic bone metastases and no known visceral metastatic disease.

Labeled Contraindications Use in women who are or may become pregnant

Pregnancy Considerations Contraindicated in pregnancy; use is contraindicated in women who are or may become pregnant.

Based on the mechanism of action, radium Ra 223 dichloride has the potential to cause fetal harm if administered during pregnancy. Not indicated for use in women. Men who are sexually active should use condoms during and for 6 months after completing treatment; their female partners of reproductive potential should use a highly effective contraceptive method during and for 6 months after treatment is completed.

Breastfeeding Considerations It is not known if radium Ra 223 dichloride is excreted in breast milk. Not indicated for use in women.

Warnings/Precautions Radiopharmaceutical; use appropriate precautions for handling, disposal, and minimizing exposure to patients and healthcare personnel. Use only under supervision of individuals with experience/training in the handling of radioactive materials approved by the applicable regulatory authority.

Hematologic toxicity, including anemia, lymphocytopenia, thrombocytopenia, leukopenia, and neutropenia commonly occur; monitor blood counts at baseline and prior to each dose. Bone marrow failure occurred in 2% of patients receiving radium Ra 223 dichloride in clinical studies (did not occur in patients who received placebo). Bone marrow failure may be prolonged and fatal (rare); may require blood transfusion support. Vascular hemorrhage due to thrombocytopenia has been reported. Infection may occur due to neutropenia. Prior to initial dose, ANC should be ≥1,500/mm^3, platelets ≥100,000/mm^3, and hemoglobin ≥10 g/dL; prior to subsequent doses, ANC should be ≥1,000/mm^3 and platelets ≥50,000/mm^3. Neutrophils and platelet nadirs typically occurred 2 to 3 weeks after administration; recovery generally occurred ~6 to 8 weeks after administration. If recovery does not occur within 6 to 8 weeks from the last dose (despite supportive care), treatment should be discontinued. Closely monitor patients with compromised bone marrow reserve; discontinue if life-threatening complications occur despite supportive care.

The safety and efficacy of concurrent chemotherapy have not been established. Due to the potential for additive bone marrow toxicity, concurrent use with chemotherapy is not recommended outside of a clinical trial. If chemotherapy, other systemic radioisotopes, or external radiotherapy are required, radium Ra 223 dichloride should be discontinued. Potentially significant drug-drug interactions may exist, requiring dose or frequency adjustment, additional monitoring, and/or selection of alternative therapy. Although fewer malignancies were reported for radium Ra 223 dichloride than for placebo (from clinical studies), long-term cumulative radiation exposure may increase the risk for malignancies (onset may be delayed). Dehydration may occur due to gastrointestinal adverse events (diarrhea, nausea, vomiting); monitor oral intake, hydration status, and urine output. Patients and caregivers should use the following precautions to minimize exposure: When handling bodily fluids, wear gloves and wash hands after handling; wash any clothing soiled with radium Ra 223 dichloride promptly and separately from other clothing; where a normal toilet is available, use in preference to a urinal; flush toilet several times after use; wash hands thoroughly after urination.

Adverse Reactions

>10%:
  Cardiovascular: Peripheral edema (13%)
  Gastrointestinal: Nausea (36%), diarrhea (25%), vomiting (19%)
  Hematologic & oncologic: Anemia (93%; grades 3/4: 6%), lymphocytopenia (72%; grades 3/4: 20%), leukopenia (35%; grades 3/4: 3%), thrombocytopenia (31%; grades 3/4: 1% to 6%), neutropenia (18%; grades 3/4: 1% to 3%)

1% to 10%:
  Endocrine & metabolic: Dehydration (3%)
  Hematologic & oncologic: Pancytopenia (2%; grades 3/4: 1%)
  Local: Injection site reactions (erythema, pain, swelling: 1%)
  Renal: Renal failure/insufficiency (3%)

<1%: Aplastic anemia

Drug Interactions

Metabolism/Transport Effects None known.

Avoid Concomitant Use
  Avoid concomitant use of Radium Ra 223 Dichloride with any of the following: BCG (Intravesical); Deferiprone; Dipyrone

Increased Effect/Toxicity
  Radium Ra 223 Dichloride may increase the levels/effects of: CloZAPine; Deferiprone

  The levels/effects of Radium Ra 223 Dichloride may be increased by: Dipyrone; Promazine

Decreased Effect
  Radium Ra 223 Dichloride may decrease the levels/effects of: BCG (Intravesical)

Storage/Stability Store at room temperature <40°C (104°F). Keep in original container or equivalent radiation shielding.

Preparation for Administration Do not dilute or mix with any solutions. Radiopharmaceutical; use appropriate precautions for handling and disposal. Wear gloves and use adequate shielding for handling and administration.

Mechanism of Action Alpha particle-emitting isotope; emits high energy, short-range alpha particles which target bone metastases; mimics calcium to form complexes with bone mineral in areas with increased bone turnover. Alpha emission induces double strand DNA breaks in adjacent cells, which results in an antitumor effect on the bone metastases.

Pharmacodynamics/Kinetics

Onset: A significant response in pain index was seen at week 2 (Nilsson 2012).

Duration: Mean duration of pain relief: 44 days (Nilsson 2012)

Distribution: Primarily to the bone or excreted in to intestine

Metabolism: Decays (is not metabolized)

Half-life elimination: 11.4 days (Nilsson 2007)

Excretion: Feces (13%); urine (2%)

Dosing

Adult & Geriatric Note: Calculate administration volume using patient weight, radioactivity content (at the reference date), and decay correction factor; determine net patient dose immediately before and after administration with an appropriate radioisotope dose calibrator; refer to product labeling for further details. Prior to initial dose, ANC should be ≥1,500/mm^3, platelets ≥100,000/mm^3, and hemoglobin ≥10 g/dL.

Prostate cancer, castration-resistant with symptomatic bone metastases: Males: IV: 55 kBq/kg (1.49 microcurie/kg) every 4 weeks for 6 doses.

Renal Impairment

CrCl 30 to 89 mL/minute: No dosage adjustment necessary.

CrCl <30 mL/minute: There are no dosage adjustments provided in the manufacturer's labeling, (has not been studied).

Hepatic Impairment

Mild impairment: No dosage adjustment necessary.

Moderate to severe impairment: There are no dosage adjustments provided in the manufacturer's labeling (has not been studied); however, dosage adjustment is not likely needed because not metabolized hepatically or eliminated in bile.

Adjustment for Toxicity

ANC <1,000/mm^3 or platelets <50,000/mm^3 (prior to subsequent doses): Withhold treatment until hematologic recovery; if recovery does not occur within 6 to 8 weeks from the last dose (despite supportive care), discontinue treatment.

Compromised bone marrow reserve: Closely monitor; discontinue if life-threatening complications occur despite supportive care

Administration Administer as a slow IV injection over 1 minute. Flush IV line or cannula before and after administration with saline. Radiopharmaceutical; use appropriate precautions for handling and disposal.

Monitoring Parameters CBC with differential at baseline and prior to each dose. Monitor fluid intake, hydration status, and urine output.

Dosage Forms Excipient information presented when available (limited, particularly for generics); consult specific product labeling.

Solution, Intravenous:

Xofigo: 1100 kBq/mL (30 microcurie/mL) (6 mL)

◆ **rAHF** see Antihemophilic Factor (Recombinant [Porcine Sequence]) on page 151

◆ **rAHF** see Antihemophilic Factor (Recombinant) on page 143

◆ **rAHF (Fc Fusion Protein)** see Antihemophilic Factor (Recombinant [Fc Fusion Protein]) on page 147

Raloxifene (ral OKS i feen)

Related Information

Safe Handling of Hazardous Drugs on page 2379

Brand Names: US Evista

Brand Names: Canada ACT Raloxifene; Apo-Raloxifene; Evista; PMS-Raloxifene; Teva-Raloxifene

Index Terms Keoxifene Hydrochloride; Raloxifene HCl; Raloxifene Hydrochloride

Pharmacologic Category Selective Estrogen Receptor Modulator (SERM)

Use

Osteoporosis: Treatment and prevention of osteoporosis in postmenopausal women

Risk reduction for invasive breast cancer: Risk reduction of invasive breast cancer in postmenopausal women with osteoporosis; risk reduction of invasive breast cancer in postmenopausal women with high risk for invasive breast cancer (high risk is defined as at least 1 breast biopsy showing lobular carcinoma in situ or atypical hyperplasia, one or more first-degree relatives with breast cancer, or a 5-year predicted risk of breast cancer 1.66% or more [based on the modified Gail model]; factors included in the modified Gail model include current age, number of first-degree relatives with breast cancer, number of breast biopsies, age at menarche, nulliparity, or age of first live birth).

Limitations of use: Raloxifene does not eliminate the risk of breast cancer; patients should have a breast exam and mammogram prior to initiating raloxifene and continue regular breast exams and mammograms as per current guideline recommendations. Raloxifene is not indicated for the treatment of invasive breast cancer or reduction of the risk of recurrence. Raloxifene is not indicated for the reduction of the risk of noninvasive breast cancer. There are no data available regarding the effect of raloxifene on invasive breast cancer incidence in women with inherited mutations BRCA1, BRCA2 to be able to make specific recommendations on the effectiveness of raloxifene.

Labeled Contraindications History of or current venous thromboembolic disorders (including deep vein thrombosis [DVT], pulmonary embolism [PE], and retinal vein thrombosis); pregnancy or women who could become pregnant; breastfeeding

Pregnancy Considerations Adverse events were observed in in animal reproduction studies. Raloxifene is contraindicated for use in women who are or may become pregnant.

Breastfeeding Considerations It is not known if raloxifene is excreted into breast milk. Breastfeeding is contraindicated by the manufacturer.

Warnings/Precautions [US Boxed Warning]: Raloxifene may increase the risk for DVT and PE; use is contraindicated in patients with history of or current venous thromboembolic disorders (including DVT, PE, or retinal vein thrombosis). Consider risks versus benefits in women at risk for thromboembolism (HF, superficial thrombophlebitis, active malignancy). The risk for DVT and PE are higher during the first 4 months of treatment. Superficial thrombophlebitis has also been reported. Discontinue raloxifene at least 72 hours prior to and during prolonged immobilization (postoperative recovery or prolonged bed rest); restart only once patient fully ambulatory. Advise patients to move periodically during prolonged travel.

[US Boxed Warning]: The risk of death due to stroke is increased in postmenopausal women with coronary heart disease or at increased risk for major coronary events; consider risks versus benefits in women at risk for stroke. Do not use for primary or secondary prevention of cardiovascular disease. Assess risks versus benefits in women at risk for stroke (eg, prior stroke, TIA, atrial fibrillation, hypertension, or smokers). Women with a history of marked elevated triglycerides (>5.6 mmol/L or >500 mg/dL) in response to treatment with oral estrogens (or estrogen/progestin) may also

◄ develop elevated triglycerides when treated with raloxifene; monitor triglycerides.

The use of raloxifene has not been adequately studied in women with a prior history of breast cancer. Safety has not been established in premenopausal women; use in premenopausal women is not indicated and not recommended. Raloxifene does not eliminate the risk of breast cancer; investigate unexplained breast abnormality that occurs during treatment. Raloxifene is not indicated for treatment of invasive breast cancer, to reduce the risk of recurrence of invasive breast cancer, or to reduce the risk of noninvasive breast cancer. The efficacy (for breast cancer risk reduction) in women with inherited BRCA1 and BRCA1 mutations has not been established. The American Society of Clinical Oncology (ASCO) guidelines for breast cancer risk reduction (Visvanathan 2013) recommend raloxifene (for 5 years) as an option to reduce the risk of ER-positive invasive breast cancer in postmenopausal women with a 5-year projected risk (based on NCI trial model) of ≥1.66%, or with lobular carcinoma in situ. Raloxifene should not be used in premenopausal women. Women with osteoporosis may use raloxifene beyond 5 years of treatment. Investigate unexplained uterine bleeding.

Use with caution in patients with hepatic or renal impairment; safety and efficacy have not been established. Safety and efficacy have not been established in men; raloxifene is not indicated for use in men. Potentially significant drug-drug interactions may exist, requiring dose or frequency adjustment, additional monitoring, and/or selection of alternative therapy. Concurrent use with systemic estrogen therapy is not recommended; safety has not been established.

Adverse Reactions

>10%:

Cardiovascular: Peripheral edema (3% to 14%)

Endocrine & metabolic: Hot flash (8% to 29%)

Infection: Infection (11%)

Neuromuscular & skeletal: Arthralgia (11% to 16%), leg cramps (≤12%), muscle spasm (≤12%)

Respiratory: Flu-like symptoms (14% to 15%)

1% to 10%:

Cardiovascular: Chest pain (3%), syncope (<2%), venous thromboembolism (1% to 2%; includes deep vein thrombosis, pulmonary embolism, retinal vein thrombosis)

Central nervous system: Insomnia (6%), hypoesthesia (<2%), neuralgia (<2%)

Dermatologic: Skin rash (6%), diaphoresis (3%)

Endocrine & metabolic: Weight gain (9%)

Gastrointestinal: Abdominal pain (7%), vomiting (5%), gastrointestinal disease (3%), flatulence (2% to 3%), gastroenteritis (≤3%)

Genitourinary: Vaginal hemorrhage (3% to 6%), mastalgia (4%), leukorrhea (3%), urinary tract abnormality (3%), uterine disease (3%), endometrium disease (≤3%)

Neuromuscular & skeletal: Myalgia (8%), tendon disease (4%)

Respiratory: Bronchitis (10%), sinusitis (10%), pharyngitis (8%), pneumonia (3%), laryngitis (≤2%)

<1%, postmarketing, and/or case reports: Cerebrovascular accident, decreased LDL cholesterol (Delmas 1997; Walsh 1998), decreased serum cholesterol (Delmas 1997; Walsh 1998), decreased serum fibrinogen (Walsh 1998), hypertriglyceridemia (in women with a history of increased triglycerides in response to oral estrogens), retinal vein occlusion, superficial thrombophlebitis

Drug Interactions

Metabolism/Transport Effects None known.

Avoid Concomitant Use

Avoid concomitant use of Raloxifene with any of the following: Ospemifene

Increased Effect/Toxicity

Raloxifene may increase the levels/effects of: Ospemifene

Decreased Effect

Raloxifene may decrease the levels/effects of: Levothyroxine; Ospemifene

The levels/effects of Raloxifene may be decreased by: Bile Acid Sequestrants

Hazardous Drugs Handling Considerations

Hazardous agent (NIOSH 2016 [group 2]).

Use appropriate precautions for receiving, handling, administration, and disposal. Gloves (single) should be worn during receiving, unpacking, and placing in storage. NIOSH recommends single gloving for administration of intact tablets or capsules (NIOSH 2016).

Storage/Stability Store at 20°C to 25°C (68°F to 77°F); excursions permitted to 15°C to 30°C (59°F to 86°F).

Mechanism of Action Raloxifene is an estrogen agonist/antagonist (a selective estrogen receptor modulator [SERM]); selective binding activates estrogenic pathways in some tissues and antagonizes estrogenic pathways in other tissues. Raloxifene acts like an estrogen agonist in the bone to prevent bone loss and has estrogen antagonist activity to block some estrogen effects in the breast and uterine tissues. Raloxifene decreases bone resorption, increasing bone mineral density and decreasing fracture incidence.

Pharmacodynamics/Kinetics

Absorption: Rapid; ~60%

Distribution: 2,348 L/kg

Protein binding: Highly protein bound (95% to albumin and α-glycoprotein); does not bind to sex-hormone-binding globulin

Metabolism: Hepatic, extensive first-pass metabolism; metabolized to glucuronide conjugates

Bioavailability: ~2%

Half-life elimination: 27.7 hours (following a single dose); 32.5 hours (following multiple doses)

Excretion: Feces (primarily); urine (<0.2% as unchanged drug; <6% as glucuronide conjugates)

Dosing

Adult & Geriatric

Osteoporosis: Females: Oral: 60 mg once daily

Risk reduction for invasive breast cancer: Females (postmenopausal): Oral: 60 mg once daily.

Duration of therapy for breast cancer risk reduction: 5 years; may be used longer than 5 years in women with osteoporosis where breast cancer risk reduction is a secondary benefit (Visvanathan 2013).

Renal Impairment CrCl ≤50 mL/minute: There are no dosage adjustments provided in the manufacturer's labeling; use with caution.

Hepatic Impairment There are no dosage adjustments provided in the manufacturer's labeling (has not been studied); use with caution.

Administration May be administered at any time of day without regard to meals.

Monitoring Parameters Lipid profile (in women at risk for hypertriglyceridemia); mammogram and breast exam (prior to and regularly during treatment)

Osteoporosis: Bone mineral density (BMD) should be evaluated 1 to 2 years after initiating therapy and every 2 years thereafter (NOF [Cosman 2014]); annual measurements of height and weight; serum calcium and 25(OH)D; may consider monitoring biochemical markers of bone turnover

Dietary Considerations Osteoporosis prevention or treatment: Ensure adequate calcium and vitamin D intake; if dietary intake is inadequate, dietary supplementation is recommended. Women and men should consume:

Calcium: 1,000 mg/day (men: 50 to 70 years) **or** 1,200 mg/day (women ≥51 years and men ≥71 years) (IOM 2011; NOF [Cosman 2014])

Vitamin D: 800 to 1,000 int. units daily (men and women ≥50 years) (NOF [Cosman 2014]). Recommended Dietary Allowance (RDA): 600 int. units daily (men and women ≤70 years) **or** 800 int. units daily (men and women ≥71 years) (IOM 2011).

Medication Guide Available Yes

Dosage Forms Excipient information presented when available (limited, particularly for generics); consult specific product labeling.

Tablet, Oral, as hydrochloride:

Evista: 60 mg [contains fd&c blue #2 aluminum lake]

Generic: 60 mg

◆ **Raloxifene HCl** *see* Raloxifene *on page* 1568

◆ **Raloxifene Hydrochloride** *see* Raloxifene *on page* 1568

Raltitrexed (ral ti TREX ed)

Related Information

Common Toxicity Criteria *on page* 2242

Safe Handling of Hazardous Drugs *on page* 2379

Brand Names: Canada Tomudex

Index Terms D1694; ICI-D1694; Raltitrexed Disodium; TDX; ZD1694

Pharmacologic Category Antineoplastic Agent, Antimetabolite; Antineoplastic Agent, Antimetabolite (Antifolate)

Use Note: Not approved in the US.

Colorectal cancer, advanced: Treatment of advanced colorectal cancer

Labeled Contraindications Hypersensitivity to raltitrexed or any component of the formulation; severe renal and/or hepatic impairment; pregnancy or breastfeeding; use in women who may become pregnant; use in children.

Pregnancy Considerations

Use is contraindicated in women who are or may become pregnant during treatment.

Adverse events were observed in animal reproduction studies. Pregnancy should be excluded prior to treatment, and should be avoided during treatment and for at least 6 months following treatment (including women with male partners receiving treatment). Pregnant women should not handle this medication.

Breastfeeding Considerations Use in nursing women is contraindicated by the manufacturer.

Warnings/Precautions Neutropenia, leukopenia, anemia, and thrombocytopenia may occur; neutropenia and thrombocytopenia may be severe. Bone marrow suppression is typically mild to moderate and generally occurs 7 to 14 days after treatment; recovery usually occurs by day 21. Use with caution in patients with preexisting bone marrow suppression. Nausea, vomiting, and diarrhea are common; mucositis and stomatitis may also occur. Severe diarrhea with concomitant hematologic toxicity (neutropenia) may be life-threatening and may require discontinuation or subsequent dose reduction. Nausea and vomiting are usually responsive to antiemetics.

Use caution in elderly patients; monitor closely, especially for GI toxicity such as diarrhea or mucositis. Use with caution in patients with mild to moderate hepatic impairment. Use is contraindicated in severe impairment and is not recommended in clinical jaundice or decompensated liver disease. Therapy interruption is required in patients with hepatotoxicity; may reinitiate therapy when hepatic enzymes return to grade 2 or lower. Asymptomatic and self-limiting reversible ALT and AST elevations may also occur. Use with caution in patients with mild to moderate renal impairment (clearance is reduced ~50%). Use is contraindicated in severe impairment. Use with caution in patients who have received prior radiation therapy.

Potentially significant interactions may exist, requiring dose or frequency adjustment, additional monitoring, and/or selection of alternative therapy. May cause malaise/weakness (caution patients concerning operation of machinery/driving).

Adverse Reactions

>10%:

Dermatologic: Skin rash (14%)

Gastrointestinal: Nausea (57% to 58%; grades 3/4: ≤12%), diarrhea (37% to 38%; grades 3/4: 11%), vomiting (37% to 38%; grades 3/4: ≤12%), anorexia (26% to 28%), abdominal pain (17% to 18%), constipation (13% to 15%), mucositis (12%; grades 3/4: ≤2%), stomatitis (11%; grades 3/4: ≤2%)

Hematologic & oncologic: Leukopenia (20% to 22%; grade 3/4: 12% to 13%; nadir within 7 to 14 days, recovery by 21 days), anemia (15% to 18%; grades 3/4: 7% to 8%)

Hepatic: Increased serum AST (16% to 18%), increased serum ALT (14% to 15%)

Neuromuscular & skeletal: Weakness (46% to 49%)

Miscellaneous: Fever (2% to 23%)

1% to 10%:

Cardiovascular: Peripheral edema (10%), cardiac arrhythmia (3%; including sinus tachycardia, supraventricular tachycardia, atrial fibrillation), cardiac abnormality (2%; including congestive heart failure)

Central nervous system: Headache (6%), dizziness (4% to 5%), chills (4%), malaise (4%), pain (4%), insomnia (3% to 4%), depression (3%), paresthesia (2% to 3%), hypertonia (<2%)

Dermatologic: Alopecia (6%), diaphoresis (3% to 4%), cellulitis (3%), pruritus (3%)

Endocrine & metabolic: Dehydration (6% to 7%), weight loss (6%), hypokalemia (2%)

Gastrointestinal: Dysgeusia (6%), dyspepsia (6%), flatulence (2% to 3%), xerostomia (2% to 3%)

Genitourinary: Urinary tract infection (3%)

Hematologic & oncologic: Thrombocytopenia (5% to 6%; grades 3/4: 4%)

Hepatic: Hyperbilirubinemia (2% to 3%; grades 3/4: 2%), increased serum alkaline phosphatase (2% to 3%)

Infection: Infection (3%), sepsis (2% to 3%)

Neuromuscular & skeletal: Myalgia (3%), arthralgia (<2%)

Ophthalmic: Conjunctivitis (2% to 3%)

Renal: Increased serum creatinine (2% to 3%)

Respiratory: Flu-like symptoms (6% to 8%), cough (5%), dyspnea (4% to 5%), pharyngitis (4% to 5%)

<1%, postmarketing, and/or case reports: Desquamation

Drug Interactions

Metabolism/Transport Effects None known.

Avoid Concomitant Use

Avoid concomitant use of Raltitrexed with any of the following: BCG (Intravesical); Deferiprone; Dipyrone; Folic Acid; Leucovorin Calcium-Levoleucovorin; Levomefolate; Methylfolate; Multivitamins/Minerals (with ADEK, Folate, Iron)

Increased Effect/Toxicity

Raltitrexed may increase the levels/effects of: CloZAPine; Deferiprone

The levels/effects of Raltitrexed may be increased by: Dipyrone; Palifermin; Promazine

Decreased Effect

Raltitrexed may decrease the levels/effects of: BCG (Intravesical); Lenograstim

The levels/effects of Raltitrexed may be decreased by: Folic Acid; Leucovorin Calcium-Levoleucovorin; Levomefolate; Methylfolate; Multivitamins/Minerals (with ADEK, Folate, Iron)

Hazardous Drugs Handling Considerations

Hazardous agent (meets NIOSH 2016 criteria). This medication is not on the NIOSH (2016) list; however, it meets the criteria for a hazardous drug. Drugs are classified as hazardous based on their properties; the properties of a hazardous drug include one or more of the following characteristics: carcinogenic, teratogenic (or other developmental toxicity), reproductive toxicity, organotoxic at low doses, genotoxic, and/or new agents with structural or toxicity profiles similar to existing hazardous agents.

Use appropriate precautions for receiving, handling, administration, and disposal. Gloves (single) should be worn during receiving, unpacking, and placing in storage.

NIOSH recommends double gloving, a protective gown, ventilated engineering controls (a class II biological safety cabinet or a compounding aseptic containment isolator), and closed system transfer devices (CSTDs) for preparation. Double gloving, a gown, and (if dosage form allows) CSTDs are required during administration (NIOSH 2016).

Storage/Stability Store intact vials at 2°C to 25°C (36°F to 77°F). Protect from light. Reconstituted solutions and solutions diluted for IV infusion are stable for up to 24 hours at 2°C to 8°C (36°F to 46°F), although the manufacturer recommends use as soon as possible after preparation. Discard after 24 hours; infusion must be completed within 24 hours of reconstitution.

Preparation for Administration Reconstitute each 2 mg vial with 4 mL SWFI resulting in a concentration of 0.5 mg/mL; further dilute for infusion by adding to 50 to 250 mL NS or D5W.

Mechanism of Action Raltitrexed is a folate analogue that selectively inhibits thymidylate synthase, blocking purine synthesis. This results in an overall inhibition of DNA synthesis.

Pharmacodynamics/Kinetics

Distribution: V_{ss}: 548 L

Protein binding: 93%

Metabolism: Undergoes extensive intracellular metabolism to active polyglutamate forms; appears to be little or no systemic metabolism of the drug

Half-life elimination: Triphasic; Beta: ~2 hours; Terminal: 198 hours

Excretion: Urine (~50% as unchanged drug); feces (~15%)

Dosing

Adult Note: Treatment should be administered only if WBC >4,000/mm^3, ANC >2,000/mm^3, and platelets >100,000/mm^3

Colorectal cancer, advanced: IV: 3 mg/m^2 once every 3 weeks in the absence of toxicity

Malignant pleural mesothelioma (off-label use): IV: 3 mg/m^2 once every 3 weeks (in combination with cisplatin) until disease progression or unacceptable toxicity occurs (van Meerbeeck 2005)

Geriatric Refer to adult dosing; use with caution.

Renal Impairment

CrCl >65 mL/minute: No dosage adjustment necessary.

CrCl 55 to 65 mL/minute: Reduce dose to 75% of usual dose once every 4 weeks.

CrCl 25 to 54 mL/minute: Reduce dose to percentage of dose equivalent to CrCl once every 4 weeks (eg, reduce dose to 25% of usual dose for CrCl of 25 mL/minute)

CrCl <25 mL/minute: Do not administer (use is contraindicated in severe renal impairment)

Hepatic Impairment

Preexisting impairment: Use is not recommended in clinical jaundice or decompensated liver disease.

Mild to moderate impairment: No dosage adjustment necessary; use with caution.

Severe impairment: Use is contraindicated.

Hepatotoxicity during treatment: Interrupt therapy until toxicity returns to grade 2 or lower.

Obesity *ASCO Guidelines for appropriate chemotherapy dosing in obese adults with cancer:* Utilize patient's actual body weight (full weight) for calculation of body surface area- or weight-based dosing, particularly when the intent of therapy is curative; manage regimen-related toxicities in the same manner as for nonobese patients (Griggs 2012).

Adjustment for Toxicity Delay dose in subsequent cycles until recovery from toxicity. May consider administering leucovorin if appropriate. Once a dose reduction has been made, do not escalate dose in subsequent cycles. Grade 4 gastrointestinal toxicity (diarrhea or mucositis) or grade 3 gastrointestinal toxicity in combination with grade 4 hematologic toxicity: Discontinue therapy and manage with supportive measures (consider administering leucovorin).

◀ Grade 3 hematologic toxicity (neutropenia or thrombocytopenia) or grade 2 gastrointestinal toxicity (diarrhea or mucositis): Reduce dose by 25%.

Grade 4 hematologic toxicity (neutropenia or thrombocytopenia) or grade 3 gastrointestinal toxicity (diarrhea or mucositis): Reduce dose by 50%.

Combination Regimens

Malignant pleural mesothelioma: Cisplatin-Raltitrexed (Mesothelioma) on page 2060

Administration

IV: Administer as an infusion over 15 minutes.

When used in combination with cisplatin for malignant pleural mesothelioma (off-label use), administer raltitrexed first, followed by cisplatin (van Meerbeeck 2005).

Monitoring Parameters CBC with differential (at baseline, prior to each treatment, or weekly if gastrointestinal toxicity observed); hepatic function tests and serum creatinine (at baseline and prior to each treatment); signs of gastrointestinal toxicity

Dietary Considerations Avoid folic acid, folinic acid (leucovorin calcium), and multivitamins with folic acid close to and during administration.

Product Availability Not available in the US

Dosage Forms: Canada Information with regard to form, strength, and availability of products uniquely available in Canada but currently not available in the US.

Excipient information presented when available (limited, particularly for generics); consult specific product labeling.

Injection, powder for reconstitution, as disodium:
Tomudex: 2 mg

◆ **Raltitrexed Disodium** *see* Raltitrexed *on page 1572*

Ramucirumab (ra mue SIR ue mab)

Related Information

Common Toxicity Criteria *on page 2242*

Brand Names: US Cyramza

Brand Names: Canada Cyramza

Index Terms IMC-1121B

Pharmacologic Category Antineoplastic Agent, Monoclonal Antibody; Antineoplastic Agent, Vascular Endothelial Growth Factor (VEGF) Inhibitor; Antineoplastic Agent, Vascular Endothelial Growth Factor Receptor 2 (VEGFR2) Inhibitor

Use

Colorectal cancer, metastatic: Treatment (in combination with FOLFIRI [irinotecan, leucovorin, and fluorouracil]) of metastatic colorectal cancer (mCRC) in patients with disease progression on or after prior therapy with bevacizumab, oxaliplatin, and a fluoropyrimidine.

Gastric cancer, advanced or metastatic: Treatment (single-agent or in combination with paclitaxel) of advanced or metastatic gastric or gastroesophageal junction adenocarcinoma in patients with disease progression on or following fluoropyrimidine- or platinum-containing chemotherapy

Non-small cell lung cancer, metastatic: Treatment (in combination with docetaxel) of metastatic non-small cell lung cancer (NSCLC) in patients with disease progression on or after platinum-based chemotherapy. Patients with EGFR or ALK genomic tumor aberrations should have disease progression on FDA-approved therapy for these aberrations prior to receiving ramucirumab.

Labeled Contraindications

There are no contraindications listed in the manufacturer's US labeling.

Canadian labeling: Hypersensitivity to ramucirumab or any component of the formulation.

Pregnancy Considerations Ramucirumab inhibits angiogenesis, which is of critical importance to human fetal development. Based on the mechanism of action, ramucirumab may cause fetal harm if administered during pregnancy. Women of reproductive potential should use effective contraception during and for at least 3 months after the last ramucirumab dose. Ramucirumab may impair fertility in women.

Breastfeeding Considerations It is not known if ramucirumab is excreted in breast milk. Immunoglobulins are excreted in breast milk, and it is assumed that ramucirumab may appear in breast milk. Due to the potential for serious adverse reactions in the nursing infant, breastfeeding is not recommended by the manufacturer.

Warnings/Precautions [US Boxed Warning]: **Ramucirumab is associated with an increased risk of hemorrhage and gastrointestinal hemorrhage, which may be severe or sometimes fatal. Discontinue ramucirumab permanently in patients who experience serious bleeding.** Patients receiving NSAIDs were excluded from some clinical trials; the risk of gastric hemorrhage in patients with gastric tumors receiving NSAIDs is not known. In addition, NSCLC patients receiving therapeutic anticoagulation or chronic NSAID or other antiplatelet therapy (other than aspirin), or with radiograph evidence of major airway or blood vessel involvement or intra-tumor cavitation were also excluded from the clinical study; the risk of pulmonary hemorrhage in such patients is not known. Serious and fatal arterial thrombotic events, including MI, cardiac arrest, cerebrovascular accident, and cerebral ischemia, have occurred with ramucirumab. Discontinue permanently in patients who experience serious arterial thrombotic events.

Ramucirumab is associated with infusion-related reactions (may be severe), generally occurring with the first or second dose. Symptoms of infusion reactions have included chills, flushing, hypotension, bronchospasm, dyspnea, hypoxia, wheezing, chest pain/tightness, supraventricular tachycardia, back pain/spasms, rigors/tremors, and/or paresthesia. Monitor for infusion reaction symptoms during infusion; discontinue immediately and permanently for grade 3 or 4 reactions. Administer in a facility equipped to manage infusion reactions. May cause and/or worsen hypertension; the incidence of severe hypertension is increased with ramucirumab. Blood pressure (BP) should be controlled prior to treatment initiation. Monitor BP every 2 weeks (more frequently if indicated) during treatment. If severe hypertension occurs, temporarily withhold until medically controlled. Discontinue permanently if medically significant hypertension cannot be controlled with antihypertensive therapy or in patients with hypertensive crisis or hypertensive encephalopathy. Ramucirumab is associated with proteinuria (may be severe). Monitor proteinuria during treatment by urine dipstick and/or urinary protein creatinine ratio for the development of and/or worsening of proteinuria. Withhold treatment for urine protein levels ≥2 g/24 hours. Discontinue permanently for urine protein >3 g/24 hours or for nephrotic syndrome.

◄ **[US Boxed Warning]: Ramucirumab may increase the risk of gastro-intestinal perforation, a potentially fatal event. Discontinue permanently in patients who experience a gastrointestinal perforation.** Cases of reversible posterior leukoencephalopathy syndrome (RPLS) have been reported (may be fatal). Symptoms of RPLS include headache, seizure, confusion, lethargy, blindness and/or other vision, or neurologic disturbances. Confirm diagnosis of RPLS with MRI; discontinue ramucirumab with confirmed RPLS diagnosis. Resolution of symptoms may occur within days after dis-continuation, although neurologic sequelae may remain in some patients. **[US Boxed Warning]: Impaired wound healing can occur with antibodies inhibiting the VEGF pathway. Discontinue ramucirumab in patients with impaired wound healing. Withhold ramucirumab prior to surgery and discontinue in patients who develop wound healing complications.** Following surgery, use clinical judgment to resume based on adequate wound healing. If wound healing complications develop during treatment, withhold ramucirumab until wound is fully healed. Ramucirumab was not studied in patients with serious or nonhealing wounds. Clinical deterioration, including new onset or worsening encephalopathy, ascites, or hepatorenal syndrome has been reported in patients with Child-Pugh class B or C cirrhosis receiving ramucirumab. Use in patients with Child-Pugh class B or C cirrhosis only if the potential benefits outweigh the potential risks. Hypothyroidism has been observed; monitor thyroid function during treatment.

A higher incidence of neutropenia and thrombocytopenia were observed when ramucirumab was used in combination with paclitaxel (compared to paclitaxel with placebo); monitor CBC with differential when used in combination with paclitaxel. Antiangiogenic medications may increase the risk for heart failure (HF); events consistent with HF have been reported with ramucirumab. Use with caution in patients with known (or at risk of) coronary artery disease. Ramucirumab may enhance the cardiotoxicity of other chemotherapy with cardiotoxic potential (Cyramza Canadian labeling 2015).

Adverse Reactions As reported with monotherapy. Frequency not always defined.

Cardiovascular: Hypertension (16%; grades 3/4: 8%), arterial thrombosis (including myocardial infarction, cardiac arrest, cerebrovascular accident, and cerebral ischemia; 2%)

Central nervous system: Headache (9%)

Dermatologic: Skin rash (4%)

Endocrine & metabolic: Hyponatremia (6%)

Gastrointestinal: Diarrhea (14%), intestinal obstruction (2%)

Genitourinary: Proteinuria (8% to 17%; grade ≥3: 1%)

Hematologic & oncologic: Decreased red blood cells (requiring transfusion; 11%), neutropenia (5%), anemia (4%), hemorrhage (2% to 4%)

Immunologic: Antibody development (3%; neutralizing: 1%)

Respiratory: Epistaxis (5%)

Miscellaneous: Infusion related reaction (≤16%; reactions minimized with premedications)

<1% and frequency not defined: Gastrointestinal perforation, reversible posterior leukoencephalopathy syndrome

Drug Interactions

Metabolism/Transport Effects None known.

Avoid Concomitant Use

Avoid concomitant use of Ramucirumab with any of the following: Belimumab

Increased Effect/Toxicity

Ramucirumab may increase the levels/effects of: Belimumab; Bisphosphonate Derivatives

Decreased Effect There are no known significant interactions involving a decrease in effect.

Storage/Stability Store intact vials at 2°C to 8°C (36°F to 46°F); do not freeze. Retain in original carton to protect from light. Do not shake. Solutions diluted in NS for infusion may be stored at 2°C to 8°C (36°F to 46°F) for no longer than 24 hours (do not freeze) or may be stored for 4 hours at room temperature (below 25°C [77°F]); do not shake diluted product.

Preparation for Administration Dilute total dose in NS 250 mL prior to administration (the manufacturer recommends a final volume of 250 mL). Do not use dextrose containing solutions. Invert gently to mix thoroughly; do not shake. Discard unused portion of the vial.

Mechanism of Action Ramucirumab is a recombinant monoclonal antibody which inhibits vascular endothelial growth factor receptor 2 (VEGFR2). Ramucirumab has a high affinity for VEGFR2 (Spratlin, 2010), binding to it and blocking binding of VEGFR ligands, VEGF-A, VEGF-C, and VEGF-D to inhibit activation of VEGFR2, thereby inhibiting ligand-induced proliferation and migration of endothelial cells. VEGFR2 inhibition results in reduced tumor vascularity and growth (Fuchs, 2014).

Pharmacodynamics/Kinetics Half-life elimination: 14 days

Dosing

Adult & Geriatric Note: Premedicate prior to infusion with an IV H_1 antagonist (for patients who experienced a grade 1 or 2 infusion reaction with a prior infusion, also premedicate with dexamethasone or equivalent and acetaminophen).

Colorectal cancer, metastatic: IV: 8 mg/kg every 2 weeks in combination with FOLFIRI (irinotecan, leucovorin, and fluorouracil); continue until disease progression or unacceptable toxicity.

Gastric cancer, advanced or metastatic: IV: 8 mg/kg every 2 weeks as a single agent or in combination with paclitaxel; continue until disease progression or unacceptable toxicity.

Non-small cell lung cancer, metastatic: IV: 10 mg/kg on day 1 every 21 days in combination with docetaxel; continue until disease progression or unacceptable toxicity

Renal Impairment No dosage adjustment necessary.

Hepatic Impairment

Mild impairment (normal bilirubin with AST > ULN **or** total bilirubin >1 to 1.5 times ULN and any AST): No dosage adjustment necessary.

Moderate impairment (total bilirubin >1.5 to 3 times ULN and any AST): No dosage adjustment necessary.

Severe impairment (total bilirubin >3 times ULN and any AST): There are no dosage adjustments provided in the manufacturer's labeling (has not been studied). Use in patients with Child-Pugh class B or C cirrhosis only if the potential benefits outweigh the potential risks.

Adjustment for Toxicity

Infusion-related reaction:

Grade 1 or 2: Reduce infusion rate by 50%

Grade 3 or 4: Permanently discontinue

Hypertension:
Severe hypertension: Interrupt infusion until controlled with medical management

Severe hypertension, uncontrolled: Permanently discontinue

Proteinuria:
Urine protein ≥2 g/24 hours (first dose reduction): Withhold treatment; when urine protein returns to <2 g/24 hours, reinitiate at a reduced dose of 6 mg/kg (if initial dose was 8 mg/kg) or 8 mg/kg (if initial dose was 10 mg/kg)

Recurrent urine protein ≥2 g/24 hours (second dose reduction): Withhold treatment; when urine protein returns to <2 g/24 hours, reinitiate at a reduced dose of 5 mg/kg (if first dose reduction was to 6 mg/kg) or 6 mg/kg (if first dose reduction was to 8 mg/kg)

Urine protein >3 g/24 hours: Discontinue permanently

Nephrotic syndrome: Discontinue permanently

Arterial thrombotic events: Discontinue permanently

Bleeding, grade 3 or 4: Discontinue permanently

Gastrointestinal perforation: Discontinue permanently

Reversible posterior leukoencephalopathy syndrome (RPLS): Discontinue permanently for confirmed diagnosis

Wound healing complications: Withhold treatment prior to surgery; do not reinitiate until the surgical wound is fully healed. If wound healing complications develop during treatment, withhold ramucirumab until the wound is fully healed.

Combination Regimens

Colorectal cancer: Ramucirumab-FOLFIRI (Colorectal) on page 2200

Gastric cancer: Paclitaxel-Ramucirumab (Gastric) on page 2187

Lung cancer (non-small cell): Docetaxel-Ramucirumab (NSCLC) on page 2094

Administration Premedicate prior to infusion with an IV H$_1$ antagonist; for patients who experienced a grade 1 or 2 infusion reaction with a prior infusion, also premedicate with dexamethasone (or equivalent) and acetaminophen.

Infuse over 60 minutes through a separate infusion line using an infusion pump; the use of a 0.22 micron protein sparing filter is recommended. Do not administer as an IV push or bolus. Flush the line with NS after infusion is complete. Do not infuse in the same IV line with electrolytes or other medications. Administer ramucirumab prior to docetaxel, paclitaxel, or FOLFIRI if administering in combination. Monitor for infusion reaction; reduce infusion rate (by 50%) for grade 1 or 2 infusion reaction; discontinue permanently for grade 3 or 4 infusion reaction.

Emetic Potential Minimal (<10%)

Monitoring Parameters Liver function tests; urine protein (by urine dipstick and/or urinary protein creatinine ratio); thyroid function; CBC with differential (when used as a part of combination chemotherapy); blood pressure (every 2 weeks; more frequently if indicated); signs/symptoms of infusion-related reactions (during infusion); signs/symptoms of arterial thromboembolic events, bleeding/hemorrhage, gastrointestinal perforation, wound healing impairment, and reversible posterior leukoencephalopathy syndrome

Dosage Forms Excipient information presented when available (limited, particularly for generics); consult specific product labeling.

Solution, Intravenous [preservative free]:

Cyramza: 100 mg/10 mL (10 mL); 500 mg/50 mL (50 mL) [contains polysorbate 80]

Rasburicase (ras BYOOR i kayse)

Brand Names: US Elitek

Brand Names: Canada Fasturtec

Index Terms Recombinant Urate Oxidase; Urate Oxidase

Pharmacologic Category Enzyme; Enzyme, Urate-Oxidase (Recombinant)

Use

Hyperuricemia associated with malignancy: Initial management of uric acid levels in pediatric and adult patients with leukemia, lymphoma, and solid tumor malignancies receiving chemotherapy expected to result in tumor lysis and elevation of plasma uric acid

Limitations of use: Indicated only for a single course of treatment

Labeled Contraindications History of anaphylaxis or severe hypersensitivity to rasburicase or any component of the formulation; history of hemolytic reaction or methemoglobinemia associated with rasburicase; glucose-6-phosphatase dehydrogenase (G6PD) deficiency

Pregnancy Considerations Adverse effects were observed in animal reproduction studies. Use during pregnancy only if the benefit to the mother outweighs the potential risk to the fetus.

Breastfeeding Considerations It is not known if rasburicase is present in breast milk. Due to the potential for serious adverse reactions in the breastfed infant, a decision should be made to discontinue breastfeeding or to discontinue the drug, taking into account the importance of treatment to the mother.

Warnings/Precautions [US Boxed Warning]: Serious and fatal hypersensitivity reactions (including anaphylaxis) have been reported; immediately and permanently discontinue in patients developing serious hypersensitivity reaction; reactions may occur at any time during treatment, including the initial dose. Signs and symptoms of hypersensitivity may include bronchospasm, chest pain/tightness, dyspnea, hypotension, hypoxia, shock, or urticaria. The safety and efficacy of more than one course of administration has not been established. **[US Boxed Warning]: Due to the risk for hemolysis (<1%), rasburicase is contraindicated in patients with G6PD deficiency; discontinue immediately and permanently in any patient developing hemolysis. Patients at higher risk for G6PD deficiency (eg, African or Mediterranean descent) should be screened prior to therapy;** severe hemolytic reactions occurred within 2 to 4 days of rasburicase initiation. **[US Boxed Warning]: Methemoglobinemia has been reported (<1%). Discontinue immediately and permanently in any patient**

developing methemoglobinemia; initiate appropriate treatment (eg, transfusion, methylene blue) if methemoglobinemia occurs.

[US Boxed Warning]: Enzymatic degradation of uric acid in blood samples will occur if left at room temperature, which may interfere with serum uric acid measurements; specific guidelines for the collection of plasma uric acid samples must be followed, including collection in prechilled tubes with heparin anticoagulant, immediate ice water bath immersion and assay within 4 hours (sample should remain on ice until analyzed). Patients at risk for tumor lysis syndrome should receive appropriate IV hydration as part of uric acid management; however, alkalinization (with sodium bicarbonate) concurrently with rasburicase is not recommended (Coiffier 2008). Rasburicase is immunogenic and can elicit an antibody response; efficacy may be reduced with subsequent courses of therapy.

Adverse Reactions

>10%:

Cardiovascular: Peripheral edema (50%)

Central nervous system: Headache (26%), anxiety (24%)

Dermatologic: Rash (13%; serious: <1%)

Endocrine & metabolic: Hypophosphatemia (17%), hypervolemia (12%)

Gastrointestinal: Nausea (27% to 58%), vomiting (38% to 50%), abdominal pain (20% to 22%), constipation (20%), diarrhea (20%), mucositis (15%)

Hepatic: Hyperbilirubinemia (16%), increased serum ALT (11%)

Immunologic: Antibody development (children: 11%; IgE: 6%), development of IgG antibodies (18%; neutralizing 8%)

Infection: Sepsis (12%; serious: 5%)

Respiratory: Pharyngolaryngeal pain (14%)

Miscellaneous: Fever (46%)

1% to 10%:

Cardiovascular: Ischemic heart disease (≥2%), supraventricular arrhythmia (≥2%)

Endocrine & metabolic: Hyperphosphatemia (10%)

Gastrointestinal: Gastrointestinal infection (≥2%)

Hematologic & oncologic: Pulmonary hemorrhage (≥2%)

Hypersensitivity: Hypersensitivity (4%)

Infection: Infection (abdominal, ≥2%)

Respiratory: Respiratory failure (≥2%)

<1%, postmarketing, and/or case reports: Anaphylaxis, hemolysis, methemoglobinemia, muscle spasm, seizure

Drug Interactions

Metabolism/Transport Effects None known.

Avoid Concomitant Use There are no known interactions where it is recommended to avoid concomitant use.

Increased Effect/Toxicity There are no known significant interactions involving an increase in effect.

Decreased Effect There are no known significant interactions involving a decrease in effect.

Storage/Stability The lyophilized drug product and the diluent for reconstitution should be stored at 2°C to 8°C (36°F to 46°F); do not freeze. Protect from light. Reconstituted solution and solution diluted for infusion may be stored for up to 24 hours at 2°C to 8°C (36°F to 46°F). Discard unused product.

Preparation for Administration Reconstitute with provided diluent (use 1 mL diluent for the 1.5 mg vial and 5 mL diluent for the 7.5 mg vial). Mix by gently swirling; do **not** shake or vortex. Discard if discolored or containing particulate matter. Total dose should be further diluted in NS to a final volume of 50 mL. The manufacturer's labeling states that filters should not be used during reconstitution or administration. However, because the provided diluent is in a glass ampule, it should be filtered **prior** to reconstitution (ISMP [Smetzer 2017]).

Mechanism of Action Rasburicase is a recombinant urate-oxidase enzyme, which converts uric acid to allantoin (an inactive and soluble metabolite of uric acid); it does not inhibit the formation of uric acid.

Pharmacodynamics/Kinetics

Onset: Uric acid levels decrease within 4 hours of initial administration
Distribution: Children: 110 to 127 mL/kg; Adults: 76 to 138 mL/kg
Half-life elimination: ~16 to 23 hours

Dosing

Adult & Geriatric Hyperuricemia associated with malignancy: IV: 0.2 mg/kg once daily for up to 5 days (use beyond 5 days or administration of more than 1 course is not recommended) **or**

Alternate dosing (off-label; Coiffier 2008): 0.05 to 0.2 mg/kg once daily for 1 to 7 days (average of 2 to 3 days) with the duration of treatment dependent on plasma uric acid levels and clinical judgment (patients with significant tumor burden may require an increase to twice daily); the following dose levels are recommended based on risk of tumor lysis syndrome (TLS):

High risk: 0.2 mg/kg once daily (duration is based on plasma uric acid levels)

Intermediate risk: 0.15 mg/kg once daily (duration is based on plasma uric acid levels)

Low risk: 0.1 mg/kg once daily (duration is based on clinical judgment); a dose of 0.05 mg/kg was used effectively in one trial

Single-dose rasburicase (off-label dosing; based on limited data): 0.15 mg/kg (Campara 2009; Liu 2005) **or** 3 to 7.5 mg as a single dose (Hutcherson 2006; McBride 2013; McDonnell 2006; Reeves 2008; Trifilio 2006); repeat doses (1.5 to 6 mg) may be needed based on serum uric acid levels

Prevention in high-risk patients with hematologic malignancies (off-label dosing): 3 mg as a single dose (Jones 2015)

Pediatric Hyperuricemia associated with malignancy: IV: 0.2 mg/kg once daily for up to 5 days (use beyond 5 days or administration of more than 1 course is not recommended) **or**

Alternate dosing (off-label; Coiffier 2008): 0.05 to 0.2 mg/kg once daily for 1 to 7 days (average of 2 to 3 days) with the duration of treatment dependent on plasma uric acid levels and clinical judgment (patients with significant tumor burden may require an increase to twice daily); the following dose levels are recommended based on risk of tumor lysis syndrome (TLS):

High risk: 0.2 mg/kg once daily (duration is based on plasma uric acid levels)

Intermediate risk: 0.15 mg/kg once daily (duration is based on plasma uric acid levels); may consider managing initially with a single dose

Low risk: 0.1 mg/kg once daily (duration is based on clinical judgment); a dose of 0.05 mg/kg was used effectively in one trial

Single-dose rasburicase (off-label dosing; based on limited data): 0.15 mg/kg; additional doses may be needed based on serum uric acid levels (Liu 2005)

Prevention in high-risk patients with hematologic malignancies (off-label dosing): 0.2 mg/kg as a single dose (Jones 2015)

Renal Impairment There are no dosage adjustments provided in the manufacturer's labeling.

Hepatic Impairment There are no dosage adjustments provided in the manufacturer's labeling.

Administration

IV infusion over 30 minutes; do **not** administer as a bolus infusion. Do **not** filter during infusion. If not possible to administer through a separate line, IV line should be flushed with at least 15 mL saline prior to and following rasburicase infusion.

The optimal timing of rasburicase administration (with respect to chemotherapy administration) is not specified in the US labeling. In some studies, chemotherapy was administered 4 to 24 hours after the first rasburicase dose (Cortes 2010; Kikuchi 2009; Vadhan-Raj 2012); however, rasburicase generally may be administered irrespective of chemotherapy timing.

Monitoring Parameters Plasma uric acid levels (4 hours after rasburicase administration, then every 6 to 8 hours until TLS resolution), CBC, G6PD deficiency screening (in patients at high risk for deficiency); monitor for hypersensitivity reactions

Test Interactions Specific handling procedures must be followed to prevent the degradation of uric acid in plasma samples. Blood must be collected in prechilled tubes containing heparin anticoagulant. Samples must then be **immediately** immersed and maintained in an ice water bath. Prepare samples by centrifugation in a precooled centrifuge (4°C). Samples must be analyzed within 4 hours of collection.

Dosage Forms Excipient information presented when available (limited, particularly for generics); consult specific product labeling.

Solution Reconstituted, Intravenous:

Elitek: 1.5 mg (1 ea); 7.5 mg (1 ea)

Regorafenib (re goe RAF e nib)

Related Information

Common Toxicity Criteria *on page 2242*

Management of Chemotherapy-Induced Nausea and Vomiting in Adults *on page 2253*

Safe Handling of Hazardous Drugs *on page 2379*

Brand Names: US Stivarga

Brand Names: Canada Stivarga

Index Terms BAY 73-4506

Pharmacologic Category Antineoplastic Agent, Tyrosine Kinase Inhibitor; Antineoplastic Agent, Vascular Endothelial Growth Factor (VEGF) Inhibitor

Use

Colorectal cancer, metastatic: Treatment of metastatic colorectal cancer in patients previously treated with fluoropyrimidine-, oxaliplatin-, and irinotecan-based chemotherapy, anti-VEGF therapy, and anti-EGFR therapy (if *RAS* wild type)

Gastrointestinal stromal tumors: Treatment of locally-advanced, unresectable, or metastatic gastrointestinal stromal tumor (GIST) in patients previously treated with imatinib and sunitinib

Hepatocellular carcinoma: Treatment of hepatocellular carcinoma in patients previously treated with sorafenib

Labeled Contraindications There are no contraindications listed in the manufacturer's US labeling.

Canadian labeling: Hypersensitivity to regorafenib, any component of the formulation, or sorafenib.

Pregnancy Considerations In animal reproduction studies, teratogenic effects were observed with doses less than the equivalent human dose. Based on animal reproduction studies and on the mechanism of action, regorafenib may cause fetal harm if administered during pregnancy. Patients (male and female) should use effective contraception during therapy and for at least 2 months following treatment.

Breastfeeding Considerations It is not known if regorafenib is present in breast milk. Due to the potential for serious adverse reactions in the breastfed infant, breastfeeding is not recommended by the manufacturer during treatment and for 2 weeks after the last dose.

Warnings/Precautions Myocardial ischemia and infarction were observed at a higher incidence than placebo in a clinical trial. Interrupt therapy in patients who develop new or acute onset ischemia or infarction; resume only if the benefit of therapy outweighs the cardiovascular risk. Skin reactions occurred commonly, including hand-foot skin reaction (HFSR), also known as palmar-plantar erythrodysesthesia syndrome (PPES), and severe rash requiring dose reduction. Grade 3 or 4 HFSR was observed more frequently in regorafenib-treated patients (compared to placebo), and although rare, erythema multiforme and Stevens Johnson syndrome were also observed more frequently in regorafenib-treated patients. Toxic epidermal necrolysis has also been reported (rare). Onset of HFSR typically occurs in the first cycle of treatment. Therapy interruptions, dosage reductions, and/or discontinuation may be necessary depending on the severity and persistence. Supportive treatment may be of benefit for symptomatic relief. Pooled data from several clinical trials showed a higher incidence of HFSR in Asian patients compared to Caucasians. In addition to recommended dosage modifications, the following treatments may be used for management of HFSR (McLellan 2015): A manicure/pedicure to remove hyperkeratotic areas/calluses which may predispose to HFSR and mechanical support/correction for abnormal weight bearing prior to treatment are recommended. During treatment, patients should use alcohol-free moisturizers liberally, reduce exposure to hot water (may exacerbate hand-foot symptoms), avoid constrictive footwear and excessive skin friction, and avoid vigorous exercise/activities that may stress hands or feet. Patients should wear thick cotton gloves/socks and wear shoes with padded insoles. Grade 1 HFSR may be relieved with moisturizing creams, cotton gloves and socks (at night) and/or keratolytic creams such as urea (10% to 40%) or salicylic acid (6%) along with a topical analgesic (eg, lidocaine gel) to relieve pain. Apply topical steroid (eg, clobetasol ointment or foam) twice daily to erythematous areas of grade 2 HFSR (in addition to continuing grade 1 management); topical analgesics and then systemic analgesics (if appropriate) may be used for pain control; dose reduction may be necessary. Grade 3 HFSR should be managed by continuing grades 1 and 2 symptomatic management and interrupting treatment for at least 7 days until resolved to grade 1 or lower.

Gastrointestinal perforation or fistula has occurred in a small number of patients treated with regorafenib; some cases were fatal. Monitor for signs/symptoms of perforation (fever, abdominal pain with constipation, and/or nausea/vomiting); permanently discontinue therapy if perforation or fistula develop. The incidence of hemorrhage was increased with regorafenib. Hemorrhage of the respiratory, gastrointestinal, or genitourinary tracts was observed in trials; some cases were fatal. Permanently discontinue in patients who experience severe or life-threatening bleeding. In patients receiving concomitant warfarin, monitor INR frequently.

[US Boxed Warning]: Severe and sometimes fatal hepatotoxicity has been observed in clinical trials. Monitor hepatic function at baseline and during treatment. Interrupt therapy for hepatotoxicity; dose reductions or discontinuation are necessary depending on the severity and persistence. Hepatic dysfunction, characterized by a hepatocellular injury pattern, typically occurred with the first 2 months of treatment in clinical trials. Closely monitor for adverse effects in patients with mild or moderate impairment; use is not recommended in severe hepatic impairment. A higher incidence of hepatotoxicity has been observed in Asian patients (particularly Japanese), compared to Caucasians (Li 2015). A higher incidence of hepatotoxicity and hand-foot skin reactions were observed in Asian patients, particularly in Japanese patients, compared to non-Asian patients (Li 2015).

Elevated blood pressure was observed in clinical trials (onset typically in the first cycle of therapy); ensure blood pressure is adequately controlled prior to initiation. Monitor blood pressure weekly for the first 6 weeks and monthly thereafter or as clinically indicated; if hypertension develops, interrupt therapy or permanently discontinue for severe or uncontrolled hypertension. Hypertensive crisis has occurred in some patients. Patients 65 years and older had an increased incidence of grade 3 or higher hypertension (compared to younger patients).

Reversible posterior leukoencephalopathy syndrome (RPLS) occurred very rarely in regorafenib-treated patients; evaluate promptly if symptoms (eg, seizures, severe headache, visual disturbances, confusion, or altered mental function) occur. Discontinue if diagnosis is confirmed. An increased rate of infection (including fatal events) was observed in regorafenib-treated patients in clinical trials. The most commonly reported infections were urinary tract infections, nasopharyngitis, mucocutaneous and systemic fungal infections, and pneumonia. Respiratory infections were the most commonly reported fatal infections. Interrupt therapy for grade 3 or 4 infections (or worsening infection of any grade). Regorafenib inhibits vascular endothelial growth factor, which may lead to impaired wound healing. Discontinue regorafenib at least 2 weeks prior to scheduled surgery; resume regorafenib postsurgery based on clinical judgment of wound healing; discontinue therapy if wound dehiscence occurs. Hypersensitivity reactions have been observed with regorafenib.

Potentially significant drug-drug or drug-food interactions may exist, requiring dose or frequency adjustment, additional monitoring, and/or selection of alternative therapy.

Adverse Reactions

>10%:

Cardiovascular: Hypertension (30% to 59%; grade ≥3: 8% to 28%)

Central nervous system: Fatigue (52% to 64%), voice disorder (30% to 39%), pain (29%), headache (10% to 16%)

Dermatologic: Palmar-plantar erythrodysesthesia (45% to 67%; grade ≥3: 17% to 22%), skin rash (26% to 30%; grade ≥3: 6% to 7%), alopecia (24%)

Endocrine & metabolic: Hypocalcemia (17% to 59%), hypophosphatemia (55% to 57%), weight loss (14% to 32%), hyponatremia (30%), increased amylase (26%), hypokalemia (21% to 26%), hypothyroidism (18%)

Gastrointestinal: Diarrhea (43% to 47%), decreased appetite (31% to 47%), increased serum lipase (14% to 46%), mucositis (33% to 40%), nausea (20%), vomiting (17%)

Hematologic & oncologic: Anemia (79%; grade 3: 5%; grade 4: 1%), lymphocytopenia (30% to 54%; grade 3: 8% to 9%), thrombocytopenia (13% to 41%; grade 3: 1% to 2%; grade 4: <1%), increased INR (24%), hemorrhage (11% to 21%; grade ≥3: 2% to 4%), neutropenia (3% to 16%; grade 3: 1%)

Hepatic: Increased serum AST (58% to 65%; grade 3: 5%; grade 4: 1%), increased serum ALT (45%; grade 3: 4% to 5%; grade 4: 1%), hyperbilirubinemia (33% to 45%)

Infection: Infection (31% to 32%; grade ≥3: 5% to 9%)

Neuromuscular & skeletal: Stiffness (14%)

Renal: Proteinuria (33% to 60%)

Miscellaneous: Fever (21% to 28%)

1% to 10%:

Cardiovascular: Ischemic heart disease (≤1%), myocardial infarction (≤1%)

Gastrointestinal: Gastrointestinal fistula (≤2%), gastrointestinal perforation (≤2%)

Hepatic: Hepatic failure (≤2%)

<1%, postmarketing, and/or case reports: Erythema multiforme, hepatic injury (severe), hypersensitivity reaction, hypertensive crisis, keratoacanthoma, reversible posterior leukoencephalopathy syndrome (RPLS), squamous cell carcinoma of skin, Stevens-Johnson syndrome, toxic epidermal necrolysis

Drug Interactions

Metabolism/Transport Effects Substrate of CYP3A4 (major), UGT1A9; **Note:** Assignment of Major/Minor substrate status based on clinically relevant drug interaction potential; **Inhibits** BCRP, UGT1A1, UGT1A9

Avoid Concomitant Use

Avoid concomitant use of Regorafenib with any of the following: Conivaptan; CYP3A4 Inducers (Strong); CYP3A4 Inhibitors (Strong); Fusidic Acid (Systemic); Grapefruit Juice; Idelalisib; Irinotecan Products; PAZOPanib; St John's Wort

Increased Effect/Toxicity

Regorafenib may increase the levels/effects of: BCRP/ABCG2 Substrates; Beta-Blockers; Bisphosphonate Derivatives; Calcium Channel Blockers (Nondihydropyridine); Digoxin; Irinotecan Products; Ivabradine; PAZOPanib; Topotecan

The levels/effects of Regorafenib may be increased by: Aprepitant; Conivaptan; CYP3A4 Inhibitors (Moderate); CYP3A4 Inhibitors (Strong); Dasatinib; Fosaprepitant; Fusidic Acid (Systemic); Grapefruit Juice; Idelalisib; Netupitant; Palbociclib; Simeprevir; Stiripentol; Warfarin

Decreased Effect

The levels/effects of Regorafenib may be decreased by: Bosentan; CYP3A4 Inducers (Moderate); CYP3A4 Inducers (Strong); Dabrafenib; Deferasirox; Neomycin; Sarilumab; Siltuximab; St John's Wort; Tocilizumab

Food Interactions Regorafenib serum concentrations may be altered when taken with grapefruit or grapefruit juice. Management: Avoid concurrent use.

Hazardous Drugs Handling Considerations

Hazardous agent (NIOSH 2016 [group 1]).

Use appropriate precautions for receiving, handling, administration, and disposal. Gloves (single) should be worn during receiving, unpacking, and placing in storage. NIOSH recommends single gloving for administration of intact tablets or capsules (NIOSH 2016).

Storage/Stability Store at 25°C (77°F); excursions permitted to 15°C to 30°C (59°F to 86°F). Store tablets in the original bottle and protect from moisture (do not remove the desiccant); keep container tightly closed. Discard any unused tablets 7 weeks after opening the bottle.

Mechanism of Action Regorafenib is a multikinase inhibitor; it targets kinases involved with tumor angiogenesis, oncogenesis, and maintenance of the tumor microenvironment which results in inhibition of tumor growth. Specifically, it inhibits VEGF receptors 1-3, KIT, PDGFR-alpha, PDGFR-beta, RET, FGFR1 and 2, TIE2, DDR2, TrkA, Eph2A, RAF-1, BRAF, BRAF^{V600E}, SAPK2, PTK5, and Abl.

Pharmacodynamics/Kinetics

Absorption: A high-fat meal increased the mean AUC of the parent drug by 48% compared to the fasted state and decreased the mean AUC of the M-2 (N-oxide) and M-5 (N-oxide and N-desmethyl) active metabolites by 20% and 51%, respectively. A low-fat meal increased the mean AUC of regorafenib, M-2, and M-5 by 36%, 40% and 23%, respectively (as compared to the fasted state).

Protein binding: 99.5% (active metabolites M-2 and M-5 are also highly protein bound)

Metabolism: Hepatic via CYP3A4 and UGT1A9, primarily to active metabolites M-2 (N-oxide) and M-5 (N-oxide and N-desmethyl)

Bioavailability: Tablets: 69%; Oral solution: 83%

Half-life elimination: Regorafenib: 28 hours (range: 14 to 58 hours); M-2 metabolite: 25 hours (range: 14 to 32 hours); M-5 metabolite: 51 hours (range: 32 to 70 hours)

Time to peak: 4 hours

Excretion: Feces (71%; 47% as parent compound; 24% as metabolites); Urine (19%)

Dosing

Adult & Geriatric

Colorectal cancer, metastatic: Oral: 160 mg once daily for the first 21 days of each 28-day cycle; continue until disease progression or unacceptable toxicity (Grothey 2013)

Gastrointestinal stromal tumor (GIST), locally-advanced, unresectable, or metastatic: Oral: 160 mg once daily for the first 21 days of each 28-day cycle; continue until disease progression or unacceptable toxicity (Demetri 2013)

Hepatocellular carcinoma: Oral: 160 mg once daily for the first 21 days of a 28-day cycle; continue until disease progression or unacceptable toxicity (Bruix 2017)

Missed doses: Do not administer 2 doses on the same day to make up for a missed dose from the previous day.

Renal Impairment

CrCl ≥15 mL/minute: No dosage adjustment necessary

ESRD on dialysis: There are no dosage adjustments provided in the manufacturer's labeling (has not been studied).

Hepatic Impairment

Preexisting mild (total bilirubin ≤ ULN and AST > ULN or total bilirubin > ULN to ≤1.5 times ULN) or moderate (total bilirubin >1.5 times to ≤3 times ULN and any AST) impairment: No dosage adjustment necessary; closely monitor for adverse effects.

Preexisting severe impairment (total bilirubin >3 times ULN): Use is not recommended (has not been studied).

Hepatotoxicity during treatment:

Grade 3 AST and/or ALT elevation: Withhold dose until recovery. If benefit of treatment outweighs toxicity risk, resume therapy at a reduced dose of 120 mg once daily.

AST or ALT >20 times ULN: Discontinue permanently.

AST or ALT >3 times ULN **and** bilirubin >2 times ULN: Discontinue permanently.

Recurrence of AST or ALT >5 times ULN despite dose reduction to 120 mg: Discontinue permanently.

◄ **Adjustment for Toxicity** If dose reduction is necessary, reduce in 40 mg increments; the lowest recommended dose is 80 mg/day.

Dermatologic:

Grade 2 hand-foot skin reaction (HFSR; palmar-plantar erythrodysesthesia syndrome [PPES]) of any duration: Reduce dose to 120 mg once daily for first occurrence. If grade 2 HFSR recurs at this dose, further reduce the dose to 80 mg once daily. Interrupt therapy for grade 2 HFSR that is recurrent or fails to improve within 7 days in spite of dosage reduction.

Grade 3 HFSR: Interrupt therapy for a minimum of 7 days. Upon recovery, reduce dose to 120 mg once daily. If grade 2 to 3 toxicity recurs at this dose, further reduce dose to 80 mg once daily upon recovery. Interrupt therapy for grade 2 to 3 HFSR that is recurrent or fails to improve within 7 days in spite of dosage reduction.

Recurrent or persistent HFSR at 80 mg once daily: Discontinue treatment.

Other dermatologic toxicity: Withhold treatment, reduce dose or permanently discontinue treatment depending on the severity and persistence of the dermatologic toxicity. Symptomatic relief may be managed with supportive measures.

Hypertension: Grade 2 (symptomatic): Interrupt therapy.

Infection: Grade 3 or 4 (or worsening infection of any grade): Interrupt therapy; resume regorafenib at the same dose following infection resolution.

Other toxicity: Any grade 3 or 4 adverse reaction (other than hepatotoxicity or infection): Interrupt therapy; upon recovery, reduce dose to 120 mg once daily (except infection). If any grade 3 or 4 adverse reaction occurs (other than hepatotoxicity or infection) while on this reduced dose, may further reduce dose to 80 mg once daily upon recovery. For any grade 4 adverse reaction, only resume therapy if the benefit outweighs the risk. Permanently discontinue therapy if unable to tolerate 80 mg once daily.

Gastrointestinal perforation/fistula: Discontinue permanently.

Hemorrhage (severe or life-threatening): Discontinue permanently.

Reversible posterior leukoencephalopathy syndrome (RPLS): Discontinue.

Wound dehiscence: Discontinue.

Administration Oral: Take at the same time each day. Swallow tablet whole with water after a low-fat meal (containing <600 calories and <30% fat).

Emetic Potential Low (10% to 30%)

Monitoring Parameters Obtain liver function tests at baseline, every 2 weeks during the first 2 months of treatment, then monthly or more frequently if clinically necessary (weekly until improvement if liver function tests are elevated). CBC with differential and platelets and serum electrolytes (baseline and periodic). Monitor INR more frequently if receiving warfarin. Monitor blood pressure weekly for the first 6 weeks of therapy and with every subsequent cycle, or more frequently if indicated. Monitor for hand-foot skin reaction (HFSR)/palmar-plantar erythrodysesthesia syndrome (PPES); it is recommended to monitor for signs of HFSR during the first weeks of treatment, then every 1 to 2 weeks for 2 cycles, then every 4 to 6 weeks thereafter (McLellan 2015). Monitor for signs/symptoms of cardiac ischemia or infarction, bleeding, GI perforation or fistula, infection, and reversible posterior leukoencephalopathy syndrome (severe headaches, seizure, confusion, or change in vision). Monitor for impaired wound healing.

Dietary Considerations Avoid grapefruit juice.

Prescribing and Access Restrictions Regorafenib is available only through the REACH support program. Information regarding program enrollment may be found at http://www.stivarga-us.com/hcp/mcrc/support.html or by calling 1-866-639-2827.

Dosage Forms Excipient information presented when available (limited, particularly for generics); consult specific product labeling.
Tablet, Oral:
  Stivarga: 40 mg [contains soybean lecithin]

Rh$_o$(D) Immune Globulin (ar aych oh (dee) i MYUN GLOB yoo lin)

Brand Names: US HyperRHO S/D; MICRhoGAM Ultra-Filtered Plus; RhoGAM Ultra-Filtered Plus; Rhophylac; WinRho SDF

Brand Names: Canada WinRho SDF

Index Terms Anti-D Immunoglobulin; RhIG; Rho(D) Immune Globulin (Human); RhoIGIV; RhoIVIM

Pharmacologic Category Blood Product Derivative; Immune Globulin

Use

Immune thrombocytopenia (ITP):

Rhophylac: To increase platelet counts in Rh$_o$(D) positive nonsplenectomized adults with chronic ITP.

WinRho SDF: To increase platelet counts in Rh$_o$(D) positive nonsplenectomized patients with the following conditions: acute ITP (children), chronic ITP (adults and children), or ITP secondary to HIV infection (adults and children).

◄ **Pregnancy and other obstetric conditions:**

Prevention of rhesus (Rh) isoimmunization in an Rh-incompatible pregnancy. All products are for use in Rh$_o$(D) negative mothers who are not already sensitized to the Rh$_o$(D) factor. An Rh-incompatible pregnancy is assumed if the fetus/baby is either Rh$_o$(D) positive or Rh$_o$(D) unknown or if the father is either Rh$_o$(D) positive or Rh$_o$(D) unknown. Use is not needed if the father or baby is conclusively Rh$_o$(D) negative. Product specific indications are as follows based on the above criteria:

HyperRHO S/D Full Dose: For antepartum prophylaxis at ~28 weeks gestation; for administration within 72 hours of birth for the prevention of hemolytic disease of the newborn; for administration within 72 hours of spontaneous or induced abortion, ruptured tubal pregnancy, amniocentesis or abdominal trauma.

HyperRHO S/D Mini Dose: For administration within 3 hours (or as soon as possible) of spontaneous or induced abortion up to 12 weeks' gestation.

MICRhoGAM Ultra-Filtered Plus: For administration within 72 hours of actual or threatened termination of pregnancy (spontaneous or induced) up to and including 12 weeks' gestation.

RhoGAM Ultra-Filtered Plus: For antepartum prophylaxis at 26 to 28 weeks' gestation; for administration within 72 hours of birth for prevention of hemolytic disease of the newborn; for administration within 72 hours of amniocentesis, chorionic villus sampling (CVS), percutaneous umbilical blood sampling (PUBS), abdominal trauma or obstetrical manipulation, ectopic pregnancy, threatened pregnancy loss after 12 weeks' gestation (with continuation of pregnancy), pregnancy termination (spontaneous or induced) after 12 weeks' gestation.

Rhophylac: For antepartum prophylaxis at 28 to 30 weeks' gestation; for administration within 72 hours of birth for the prevention of hemolytic disease of the newborn; for administration within 72 hours of obstetric complications including miscarriage, abortion, threatened abortion, ectopic pregnancy or hydatiform mole, transplacental hemorrhage resulting from antepartum hemorrhage; for administration within 72 hours of invasive procedures during pregnancy including amniocentesis, chorionic biopsy, or obstetric manipulative procedures such as external version or abdominal trauma.

WinRho SDF: For antepartum prophylaxis at 28 weeks' gestation; for administration within 72 hours of birth for the prevention of hemolytic disease of the newborn; for administration following obstetric complications including miscarriage, abortion, threatened abortion, ectopic pregnancy or hydatiform mole, transplacental hemorrhage resulting from antepartum hemorrhage; for administration following invasive procedures during pregnancy including amniocentesis, chorionic biopsy, or obstetric manipulative procedures such as external version or abdominal trauma.

Transfusion:

HyperRHO S/D Full Dose, MICRhoGAM Ultra-Filtered Plus, RhoGAM Ultra-Filtered Plus, Rhophylac, and WinRho SDF: To prevent isoimmunization in Rh$_o$(D) negative individuals who have been transfused with Rh$_o$(D) positive red blood cells or blood components containing red blood cells.

Labeled Contraindications

HyperRHO S/D Full Dose, HyperRHO S/D Mini Dose: There are no contraindications listed in the manufacturer's labeling.

MICRhoGAM Ultra-Filtered Plus, RhoGAM Ultra-Filtered Plus: Use in Rh-positive individuals.

Rhophylac: Anaphylactic or severe systemic reaction to a previous dose of human immune globulin; use in IgA-deficient patients with antibodies to IgA and a history of hypersensitivity; administration to the neonate of a mother who received Rhophylac postpartum.

WinRho SDF: Anaphylactic or severe systemic reaction to a previous dose of human immune globulin; use in IgA-deficient patients with antibodies to IgA and a history of hypersensitivity; autoimmune hemolytic anemia; preexisting hemolysis or at high risk for hemolysis; suppression of Rh$_O$(D) isoimmunization in infants.

WinRho SDF Canadian labeling: Additional contraindications (not in US labeling): All uses: Use in IgA-deficient patients; hypersensitivity to Rh$_O$(D) immune globulin or any component of the formulation.

Rh Immunization prophylaxis: Use in Rh$_O$(D)-positive women; Rh$_O$(D) negative women who are Rh immunized.

Immune thrombocytopenia (ITP): Rh$_O$(D)-negative patients; splenectomized patients; ITP secondary to other conditions including leukemia, lymphoma, or active viral infections with EBV or HCV; elderly patients with underlying cardiac, renal, or hepatic comorbidities that would predispose them to acute hemolytic reactions (AHR) complications; autoimmune hemolytic anemia (Evan syndrome); systemic lupus erythematosus (SLE); antiphospholipid antibody syndrome.

Documentation of allergenic cross-reactivity for immune globulins is limited. However, because of similarities in chemical structure and/or pharmacologic actions, the possibility of cross-sensitivity cannot be ruled out with certainty.

Pregnancy Considerations Animal reproduction studies have not been conducted.

Rh$_O$(D) immune globulin (RhIG) is administered to pregnant women to prevent alloimmunization of Rh$_O$(D) negative mothers who may potentially have a fetus who is Rh$_O$(D) positive. Administration of the immune globulin prevents the mother from developing antibodies to the D antigen and the development of hemolytic anemia in the newborn. Current guidelines recommend administration of RhIG to pregnant women who are Rh$_O$(D) negative and who are not already Rh$_O$(D) alloimmunized at ~28 weeks gestation (unless the father is known to be Rh$_O$(D) negative), within 72 hours of delivery of an Rh$_O$(D) positive infant, after a first trimester pregnancy loss, or after invasive procedures such as amniocentesis, chorionic villus sampling (CVS), or fetal blood sampling (ACOG 1999). Available evidence suggests that Rh$_O$(D) immune globulin administration during pregnancy does not harm the fetus or affect future pregnancies.

In pregnant women who require treatment for ITP, other agents are preferred. RhIG for this indication in pregnancy is limited to case reports and small studies (Neunert 2011).

Breastfeeding Considerations Adverse events in the nursing infant have not been observed when administered to women for the suppression of Rh isoimmunization. The manufacturer recommends that caution be used if administered to nursing women. The purified immune globulin in these products is obtained from human donors; the Rh$_O$(D) antibodies are endogenous to human plasma.

Warnings/Precautions Rhophylac, WinRho SDF: **[US Boxed Warning]: May cause fatal intravascular hemolysis (IVH) in Rh$_O$(D)-positive patients treated with intravenous (IV) Rh$_O$(D) immune globulin for immune thrombocytopenia (ITP). IVH may result in clinically compromising anemia and**

multiorgan system failure including acute respiratory distress syndrome. Acute renal insufficiency, renal failure, severe anemia, and disseminated intravascular coagulation (DIC) have also been reported. Patients should be closely monitored for at least 8 hours after administration. Alert patients to, and monitor them for back pain, shaking chills, fever, and discolored urine or hematuria. Absence of these signs and/or symptoms within 8 hours does not indicate IVH cannot occur subsequently. If signs and/or symptoms of intravascular hemolysis are present or suspected, perform post-treatment laboratory tests, including plasma hemoglobin, haptoglobin, LDH, and plasma bilirubin (direct and indirect). Previous administration of IV Rh₀(D) immune globulin does not preclude the possibility of IVH. Transfuse patients with hemolysis and clinically compromising anemia after receiving Rh₀(D) immune globulin; use Rh₀(D)-negative packed red blood cells.

Severe hypersensitivity reactions may occur. Immediate treatment (including epinephrine 1 mg/mL) for anaphylactoid and/or hypersensitivity reactions should be available during use. Some products are specifically contraindicated in patients with a previous anaphylactic or severe systemic reaction to an immune globulin. If symptoms of allergic or early signs of hypersensitivity reactions occur, discontinue immediately and institute appropriate treatment. Use with caution in patients with IgA deficiency, may contain trace amounts of IgA; patients with known antibodies to IgA have a greater risk of developing potentially anaphylactic reactions. Some products are specifically contraindicated in patients with antibodies against IgA.

Acute renal dysfunction/failure, osmotic nephropathy, and death may occur with IGIV products. Use with caution and administer at the minimum infusion rate possible in patients at risk for renal disease (eg, diabetes mellitus, >65 years of age, volume depletion, sepsis, paraproteinemia, concomitant use of nephrotoxic medications); ensure adequate hydration prior to administration in these patients. Thrombotic events have been reported with administration of intravenous immune globulins (IVIG); use with caution in patients with a history of atherosclerosis or cardiovascular and/or thrombotic risk factors or patients with known/suspected hyperviscosity. Consider a baseline assessment of blood viscosity in patients at risk for hyperviscosity. Administer at the minimum practical infusion rate. Monitor for adverse pulmonary events including transfusion-related acute lung injury (TRALI); noncardiogenic pulmonary edema has been reported with IVIG use. TRALI is characterized by severe respiratory distress, pulmonary edema, hypoxemia, and fever in the presence of normal left ventricular function and usually occurs within 1 to 6 hours after infusion; may be managed with oxygen and respiratory support.

Use with caution in patients with thrombocytopenia or coagulation disorders; bleeding/hematoma may occur from IM administration. Use with caution in patients with renal impairment or those at risk for renal disease (eg, diabetes mellitus, advanced age [>65 years], volume depletion, sepsis, paraproteinemia, concomitant use of nephrotoxic medications). In patients at risk of renal dysfunction, ensure adequate hydration prior to administration; administer at the minimum practical infusion rate. Product of human plasma; may potentially contain infectious agents which could transmit disease. Screening of donors, as well as testing and/or inactivation or removal of certain viruses, reduces the risk. Infections thought to be transmitted by this product should be reported to the manufacturer.

Some products may contain maltose, which may result in falsely elevated blood glucose readings. Some dosage forms may contain polysorbate 80 (also known as Tweens). Hypersensitivity reactions, usually a delayed reaction, have been reported following exposure to pharmaceutical products containing polysorbate 80 in certain individuals (Isaksson 2002; Lucente 2000; Shelley 1995). Thrombocytopenia, ascites, pulmonary deterioration, and renal and hepatic failure have been reported in premature neonates after receiving parenteral products containing polysorbate 80 (Alade 1986; CDC 1984). See manufacturer's labeling.

Immune globulin deficiency syndromes: Not for replacement therapy in immune globulin deficiency syndromes.

ITP: Appropriate use: Safety and efficacy of WinRho not established in $Rh_0(D)$ negative, non-ITP thrombocytopenia, or splenectomized patients; safety and efficacy of Rhophylac not established in patients with preexisting anemia (may increase the severity of preexisting anemia). Dose adjustment may be required with decreased hemoglobin. Do not administer IM or SubQ; administer dose IV only. Although $Rh_0(D)$ immune globulin is not the preferred pharmacologic agent for the management of ITP, a single dose may be used in nonsplenectomized children who are $Rh_0(D)$ positive and require treatment, or in adults when corticosteroids are contraindicated (Neunert 2011).

$Rh_0(D)$ suppression: For use in the mother; do not administer to the neonate. If $Rh_0(D)$ antibodies are already present in the mother, use of the $Rh_0(D)$ immune globulin is not beneficial. In addition, if the father is known to be $Rh_0(D)$ negative, administration of the immune globulin is not needed. When treatment is indicated, administration should be within the time frame recommended. However, there may still be benefit if therapy is given as late as 28 days postpartum. The longer treatment is delayed, the less protection will be provided (ACOG 1999).

Adverse Reactions Frequency not defined.

Cardiovascular: Hypertension, hypotension, vasodilatation

Central nervous system: Chills, dizziness, drowsiness, headache, malaise, shivering

Dermatologic: Diaphoresis, pallor, pruritus, skin rash, skin sclerosis (at injection site)

Endocrine & metabolic: Decreased haptoglobins, increased lactate dehydrogenase

Gastrointestinal: Abdominal pain, diarrhea, nausea, vomiting

Hematologic & oncologic: Acute intravascular hemolysis (patients with ITP), decreased hemoglobin (patients with ITP)

Hepatic: Increased serum bilirubin

Hypersensitivity: Anaphylaxis

Immunologic: Antibody development (positive anti-C antibody test)

Local: Injection site reaction: Discomfort at injection site, erythema at injection site, pain at injection site (mild), swelling at injection site

Neuromuscular & skeletal: Arthralgia, back pain, hyperkinesia, myalgia, weakness

Renal: Renal insufficiency (can be acute)

Miscellaneous: Fever, infusion related reaction

<1%, postmarketing, and/or case reports: Adult respiratory distress syndrome, anemia (clinically compromising), anuria, cardiac failure, chest pain, disseminated intravascular coagulation, edema, erythema, fatigue, hematuria, hemoglobinemia, hemoglobinuria (transient in patients with ITP),

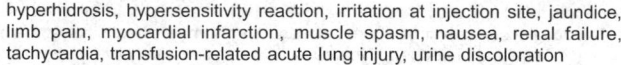

hyperhidrosis, hypersensitivity reaction, irritation at injection site, jaundice, limb pain, myocardial infarction, muscle spasm, nausea, renal failure, tachycardia, transfusion-related acute lung injury, urine discoloration

Drug Interactions

Metabolism/Transport Effects None known.

Avoid Concomitant Use There are no known interactions where it is recommended to avoid concomitant use.

Increased Effect/Toxicity There are no known significant interactions involving an increase in effect.

Decreased Effect

Rho(D) Immune Globulin may decrease the levels/effects of: Measles, Mumps, and Rubella Virus Vaccine; Measles, Mumps, Rubella, and Varicella Virus Vaccine; Vaccines (Live); Varicella Virus Vaccine

Storage/Stability

Store at 2°C to 8°C (35°F to 46°F); do not freeze.

Rhophylac: Store at 2°C to 8°C (35°F to 46°F); do not freeze. Protect from light.

Preparation for Administration

Rhophylac: Bring prefilled syringe to room temperature before use.

WinRho SDF: ITP: May dilute in NS prior to IV administration if needed; do not dilute with D5W.

Mechanism of Action

Rh suppression: Not completely characterized; prevents isoimmunization by suppressing the immune response and antibody formation by Rh_o(D)-negative individuals to Rh_o(D)-positive red blood cells. When administered within 72 hours of a full term delivery, the incidence of Rh isoimmunization decreases from 12% to 13% to 1% to 2%. The rate further decreases to <1% with administration at both 28 weeks' gestation and postpartum.

ITP: Not completely characterized; Rh_o(D) immune globulin is thought to form anti-D-coated red blood cell complexes which bind to macrophage Fc receptors within the reticuloendothelial system (RES); blocks or saturates the RES ability to clear antibody-coated cells, including platelets. Thus, platelets are spared from destruction.

Pharmacodynamics/Kinetics

Onset of platelet increase: ITP: WinRho: Platelets should rise within 1 to 2 days

Peak effect: WinRho: In 7 to 14 days

Duration: Suppression of Rh isoimmunization: Rhophylac 300 mcg dose: Rh_o(D) immune globulin titers detected up to and at least 9 weeks; WinRho SDF 120 mcg dose: ≤6 weeks; Treatment of ITP: 30 days (variable)

Distribution: V_d: IM: RhoGAM Ultra Filtered Plus: 7.3 ± 1.5 L

Bioavailability: IM: Rhophylac: 69%

Half-life elimination: RhoGAM Ultra Filtered Plus: 30.9 ± 13.8 days (IM); Rhophylac: 16 ± 4 days (IV), 18 ± 5 days (IM); WinRho SDF ~24 days (IV), ~30 days (IM)

Time to peak, plasma: RhoGAM Ultra Filtered Plus: 4 days (IM); Rhophylac: 2 to 7 days (IM); WinRho SDF: ≤2 hours (IV), 5 to 10 days (IM)

Dosing

Adult Note: Rh_o(D) immune globulin 300 mcg has traditionally been referred to as a "full dose". Potency and dosing recommendations may also be expressed in international units by comparison to the WHO anti-Rh_o(D) standard where 1 mcg = 5 international units

Immune thrombocytopenia (ITP):
Rhophylac: IV: 50 mcg/kg
WinRho SDF: IV:
Initial: 50 mcg/kg as a single injection, or can be given as a divided dose on separate days. If hemoglobin is <10 g/dL: Dose should be reduced to 25 to 40 mcg/kg.
Subsequent dosing: 25 to 60 mcg/kg can be used if required to increase platelet count; frequency of dosing is dependent upon clinical response
Maintenance dosing if patient **did respond** to initial dosing: 25 to 60 mcg/kg based on platelet count and hemoglobin concentration
Maintenance dosing if patient **did not respond** to initial dosing:
Hemoglobin <8 g/dL: Alternative treatment should be used
Hemoglobin 8 to 10 g/dL: Redose between 25 to 40 mcg/kg
Hemoglobin >10 g/dL: Redose between 50 to 60 mcg/kg

Rh$_o$(D) suppression: Note: In general, a 300 mcg dose will suppress the immune response to a fetal-maternal hemorrhage with ≤15 mL of Rh-positive RBC. If exposure to >15 mL of Rh-positive RBC is suspected, an appropriate dose should be calculated. If the first dose is administered early in pregnancy, additional doses may be needed to ensure adequate levels of passively acquired anti-D at delivery (ACOG 1999). If delivery occurs within 3 weeks after the last antepartum dose, a postpartum dose may be withheld, but testing for fetal-maternal hemorrhage of >15 mL should be performed (ACOG 1999).

Pregnancy prophylaxis: Note: if antepartum prophylaxis is indicated, the mother may also need a postpartum dose if the infant is Rh-positive.
Antepartum prophylaxis:
HyperRHO S/D Full Dose: IM: 300 mcg at ~28 weeks' gestation.
RhoGAM: IM: 300 mcg at 26 to 28 weeks' gestation; If delivery does not occur within 12 weeks after the dose, a second 300 mcg dose is recommended. If the first dose is prior to 26 weeks' gestation, administer every 12 weeks to ensure adequate levels of passively acquired anti-D. If delivery occurs within 3 weeks after the last antepartum dose, a postpartum dose may be withheld, but testing for fetal-maternal hemorrhage of >15 mL should be performed.
Rhophylac: IM, IV: 300 mcg at 28 to 30 weeks' gestation.
WinRho SDF: IM, IV: 300 mcg at 28 weeks' gestation. If the first dose is administered early in pregnancy, administer every 12 weeks to ensure adequate levels of passively acquired anti-D.
Postpartum prophylaxis:
HyperRHO S/D Full Dose: IM: 300 mcg provides sufficient antibody if volume of Rh-positive RBC exposure is ≤15 mL. If exposure to >15 mL of Rh-positive RBC is suspected, an appropriate dose should be calculated (see dosing for excessive fetomaternal hemorrhage). The dose should be administered within 72 hours of delivery, but may provide some benefit if given later.
RhoGAM: IM: 300 mcg provides sufficient antibody if volume of Rh-positive RBC exposure is ≤15 mL. If exposure to >15 mL of Rh-positive RBC is suspected, an appropriate dose should be calculated. The dose should be administered within 72 hours of delivery.

Rhophylac: IM, IV: 300 mcg provides sufficient antibody if volume of Rh-positive RBC exposure is ≤15 mL. If exposure to >15 mL of Rh-positive RBC is suspected, an appropriate dose should be calculated (see dosing for excessive fetomaternal hemorrhage). The dose should be administered within 72 hours of delivery.

WinRho SDF: IM, IV: 120 mcg. The dose should be administered within 72 hours of delivery but may be given up to 28 days after delivery.

Other pregnancy/obstetric conditions:

Abdominal trauma:

HyperRHO S/D Full Dose: IM: 300 mcg following abdominal trauma in the second or third trimester. If exposure to >15 mL of Rh-positive RBC is suspected, an appropriate dose should be calculated (see dosing for excessive fetomaternal hemorrhage).

RhoGam: IM: 300 mcg within 72 hours following abdominal trauma or obstetrical manipulation occurring at ≥13 weeks' gestation. If exposure to >15 mL of Rh-positive RBC is suspected, an appropriate dose should be calculated.

Rhophylac: IV, IM: 300 mcg within 72 hours of complication. If exposure to >15 mL of Rh-positive RBC is suspected, an appropriate dose should be calculated (see dosing for excessive fetomaternal hemorrhage).

Amniocentesis:

HyperRHO S/D Full Dose: IM: 300 mcg at 15 to 18 weeks' gestation or during the third trimester. If exposure to >15 mL of Rh-positive RBC is suspected, an appropriate dose should be calculated (see dosing for excessive fetomaternal hemorrhage).

RhoGam: IM: 300 mcg within 72 hours of a procedure occurring at ≥13 weeks' gestation. If exposure to >15 mL of Rh-positive RBC is suspected, an appropriate dose should be calculated.

Rhophylac: IV, IM: 300 mcg within 72 hours of procedure. If exposure to >15 mL of Rh-positive RBC is suspected, an appropriate dose should be calculated (see dosing for excessive fetomaternal hemorrhage).

WinRho SDF: IV, IM: 300 mcg immediately after amniocentesis occurring before 34 weeks' gestation; repeat dose every 12 weeks during pregnancy. Administer 120 mcg within 72 hours of amniocentesis occurring after 34 weeks' gestation.

Ectopic pregnancy:

HyperRHO S/D Full Dose: IM: 300 mcg for complications occurring at ≥13 weeks' gestation. If exposure to >15 mL of Rh-positive RBC is suspected, an appropriate dose should be calculated (see dosing for excessive fetomaternal hemorrhage).

RhoGam: IM: 300 mcg within 72 hours of complications occurring at ≥13 weeks' gestation. If exposure to >15 mL of Rh-positive RBC is suspected, an appropriate dose should be calculated.

Rhophylac: IV, IM: 300 mcg within 72 hours of complication. If exposure to >15 mL of Rh-positive RBC is suspected, an appropriate dose should be calculated (see dosing for excessive fetomaternal hemorrhage).

Termination of pregnancy (spontaneous or induced):

HyperRHO S/D Mini Dose: IM: 50 mcg within 3 hours or as soon as possible following spontaneous or induced abortion occurring <13 weeks' gestation; administer within 72 hours of termination if prompt administration is not possible.

HyperRHO S/D Full Dose: IM: 300 mcg following miscarriage or abortion occurring ≥13 weeks' gestation. If exposure to >15 mL of Rh-positive RBC is suspected, an appropriate dose should be calculated (see dosing for excessive fetomaternal hemorrhage).

MICRhoGAM: IM: 50 mcg within 72 hours of actual or threatened termination occurring <13 weeks' gestation. **Note:** RhoGAM may be administered if MICRhoGAM is not available.

RhoGAM: IM: 300 mcg within 72 hours following spontaneous or induced termination occurring ≥13 weeks' gestation. If exposure to >15 mL of Rh-positive RBC is suspected, an appropriate dose should be calculated.

Rhophylac: IV, IM: 300 mcg within 72 hours of miscarriage or abortion. If exposure to >15 mL of Rh-positive RBC is suspected, an appropriate dose should be calculated (see dosing for excessive fetomaternal hemorrhage).

WinRho SDF: IV, IM: 120 mcg within 72 hours of abortion occurring after 34 weeks' gestation.

Threatened pregnancy loss with continuation of pregnancy:

HyperRHO S/D Full Dose: IM: 300 mcg following threatened loss at any time during pregnancy; administer as soon as possible. If exposure to >15 mL of Rh-positive RBC is suspected, an appropriate dose should be calculated (see dosing for excessive fetomaternal hemorrhage).

MICRhoGAM: IM: 50 mcg within 72 hours of threatened termination occurring <13 weeks' gestation. **Note:** RhoGAM may be administered if MICRhoGAM is not available.

RhoGAM: IM: 300 mcg within 72 hours following threatened loss ≥13 weeks' gestation. If exposure to >15 mL of Rh-positive RBC is suspected, an appropriate dose should be calculated.

Rhophylac: IV, IM: 300 mcg within 72 hours of threatened abortion. If exposure to >15 mL of Rh-positive RBC is suspected, an appropriate dose should be calculated (see dosing for excessive fetomaternal hemorrhage).

WinRho SDF: IV, IM: 300 mcg immediately following a threatened abortion occurring at any time during pregnancy

Additional invasive/manipulative procedures or obstetric complications:

RhoGam: IM: 300 mcg within 72 hours of chorionic villus sampling or percutaneous umbilical blood sampling ≥13 weeks' gestation. If exposure to >15 mL of Rh-positive RBC is suspected, an appropriate dose should be calculated.

Rhophylac: IV, IM: 300 mcg within 72 hours of procedures such as chorionic biopsy or external version, or within 72 hours of complications such as hydatidiform mole, or transplacental hemorrhage resulting from antepartum hemorrhage. If exposure to >15 mL of Rh-positive RBC is suspected, an appropriate dose should be calculated (see dosing for excessive fetomaternal hemorrhage).

WinRho SDF: IV, IM: 300 mcg immediately after chorionic villus sampling before 34 weeks' gestation; repeat dose every 12 weeks during pregnancy. Administer 120 mcg within 72 hours of manipulation occurring after 34 weeks' gestation.

Dosing for excessive fetomaternal hemorrhage:

HyperRHO S/D Full Dose: IM: When exposure to >15 mL Rh-positive RBC or >30 mL whole blood is suspected, a fetal red cell count should be calculated. The fetal RBC volume is then divided by 15 mL, providing the number of 300 mcg doses (vials/syringes) to administer. If the dose calculated results in a fraction, round up to the next higher whole 300 mcg dose (vial/syringe).

Rhophylac: IV, IM: When exposure to >15 mL Rh-positive RBC, administer 300 mcg; in addition, administer 20 mcg per mL fetal RBC in excess of 15 mL if bleeding can be quantified or an additional 300 mcg if excess bleeding cannot be quantified. Total dose should be administered within 72 hours of complication.

Transfusion: Note: Actual dose is based upon volume of blood/blood product exposure.

WinRho SDF: Administer within 72 hours after exposure of incompatible blood transfusion.

IV: Calculate dose as follows; administer 600 mcg every 8 hours until the total dose is administered:

Exposure to Rh$_o$(D) positive whole blood: 9 mcg/mL blood

Exposure to Rh$_o$(D) positive red blood cells: 18 mcg/mL cells

IM: Calculate dose as follows; administer 1,200 mcg every 12 hours until the total dose is administered:

Exposure to Rh$_o$(D) positive whole blood: 12 mcg/mL blood

Exposure to Rh$_o$(D) positive red blood cells: 24 mcg/mL cells

HyperRHO S/D Full Dose: IM: Multiply the volume of Rh-positive whole blood administered by the hematocrit of the donor unit to equal the volume of RBCs transfused. The volume of RBCs is then divided by 15 mL, providing the number of 300 mcg doses (vials/syringes) to administer. If the dose calculated results in a fraction, round up to the next higher whole 300 mcg dose (vial/syringe). Administer as soon as possible and within 72 hours after an incompatible transfusion.

MICRhoGAM: IM: <2.5 mL of Rh-positive red blood cell exposure: 50 mcg. Administer within 72 hours after an incompatible transfusion.

RhoGAM: IM:

2.5 to 15 mL Rh-positive red blood cell exposure: 300 mcg. Administer within 72 hours after an incompatible transfusion.

>15 mL Rh-positive red blood cell exposure: 20 mcg per mL of Rh-positive red blood cell exposure. Multiple doses may be given at the same time or spaced at intervals; total dose must be given within 72 hours of exposure.

Rhophylac: IM, IV: 20 mcg per 2 mL transfused blood or 20 mcg per mL erythrocyte concentrate. Administer within 72 hours after an incompatible transfusion.

Geriatric Refer to adult dosing. Patients >65 years of age with a concurrent comorbid condition may be at increased risk of developing acute hemolytic reactions. Fatal outcomes associated with IVH have occurred most frequently in those >65 years. Use with caution; consider starting at lower doses.

Pediatric Immune thrombocytopenia (ITP): Children and Adolescents: WinRho SDF: Refer to adult dosing.

Renal Impairment There are no dosage adjustments provided in the manufacturer's labeling.

Hepatic Impairment There are no dosage adjustments provided in the manufacturer's labeling.

Administration

When used for the prevention of rhesus (Rh) isoimmunization in an Rh-incompatible pregnancy, the dose is administered to the mother, not the neonate.

HyperRHO S/D Full Dose, HyperRHO S/D Mini Dose, MICRhoGAM Ultra-Filtered Plus and RhoGAM Ultra-Filtered Plus are for IM administration only. Rhophylac and WinRho SDF may be administered IM or IV (based on indication). Do not administer Rhophylac subcutaneously into the fatty tissue. There have been reports of lack of effect in patients with a BMI ≥ 30 kg/m^2 when Rhophylac was administered IM.

IM: Administer into the deltoid muscle of the upper arm or anterolateral aspect of the upper thigh; avoid gluteal region due to risk of sciatic nerve injury. If large doses (>5 mL) are needed, administration in divided doses at different sites is recommended. HyperRHO S/D, MICRhoGAM Ultra-Filtered Plus and RhoGAM Ultra-Filtered Plus should not be administered intravenously.

IV:

Rhophylac: ITP: Infuse at 2 mL per 15 to 60 seconds

WinRho SDF: Infuse at 2 mL per 5 to 15 seconds when used for the prevention of rhesus (Rh) isoimmunization or over 3 to 5 minutes when used for the treatment of ITP.

Monitoring Parameters

Immune thrombocytopenia (ITP): Signs and symptoms of intravascular hemolysis (IVH), including anemia, renal insufficiency, back pain, shaking, chills, discolored urine, or hematuria; observe patient for 8 hours following administration. In addition, CBC (prior to therapy and 1 to 3 days after first infusion); differential and peripheral blood smear (prior to therapy), direct antiglobulin test and antibody screen (prior to therapy); reticulocyte count (prior to therapy); urinalysis (prior to therapy and 1 to 2 hours after treatment [product labeling specifies dipstick urinalysis at baseline and 2, and 4 hours prior to the end of the monitoring period]); serum creatinine and BUN (prior to therapy; monitor after therapy if post treatment hemoglobin decreases by >1 g/dL) (Despotovic 2012). For patients with suspected IVH, monitor plasma hemoglobin, haptoglobin, LDH, and plasma bilirubin (direct and indirect).

Pregnancy/obstetric conditions: Monitor for systemic reactions for 20 minutes after administration

Transfusion: Signs and symptoms of hemolytic reaction

Test Interactions Rh_o(D) immune globulin may affect the results of blood typing, the antibody screening test, and the direct antiglobulin (Coombs') test in the mother and neonate. Fetal-maternal hemorrhage may cause false blood-typing result in the mother; when there is any doubt to the patients' Rh type, Rh_o(D) immune globulin should be administered. WinRho SDF liquid contains maltose; may result in falsely elevated blood glucose levels with dehydrogenase pyrroloquinolinequinone or glucose-dye-oxidoreductase testing methods. WinRho SDF also contains trace amounts of anti-A, B, C and E; may alter Coombs' tests. Rhophylac can contain antibodies to other Rh antigens (eg, anti-C antibodies), which might be detected by sensitive serological tests.

Dosage Forms Excipient information presented when available (limited, particularly for generics); consult specific product labeling. [DSC] = Discontinued product

Solution, Injection:

WinRho SDF: 2500 units/2.2 mL (2.2 mL); 5000 units/4.4 mL (4.4 mL); 1500 units/1.3 mL (1.3 mL); 15,000 units/13 mL (13 mL)

◀

Solution, Injection [preservative free]:
  WinRho SDF: 2500 units/2.2 mL (2.2 mL); 5000 units/4.4 mL (4.4 mL); 1500
    units/1.3 mL (1.3 mL); 15,000 units/13 mL (13 mL) [contains polysor-
    bate 80]
Solution Prefilled Syringe, Injection [preservative free]:
  Rhophylac: 1500 units/2 mL (2 mL)
Solution Prefilled Syringe, Intramuscular:
  HyperRHO S/D: 250 units (1 ea [DSC])
Solution Prefilled Syringe, Intramuscular [preservative free]:
  HyperRHO S/D: 250 units (1 ea); 1500 units (1 ea) [latex free]
  MICRhoGAM Ultra-Filtered Plus: 250 units (1 ea) [latex free, thimerosal free;
    contains polysorbate 80]
  RhoGAM Ultra-Filtered Plus: 1500 units (1 ea) [latex free, thimerosal free;
    contains polysorbate 80]

- ◆ **RhoGAM Ultra-Filtered Plus** see Rh_o(D) Immune Globulin on page 1591
- ◆ **RhoIGIV** see Rh_o(D) Immune Globulin on page 1591
- ◆ **RhoIVIM** see Rh_o(D) Immune Globulin on page 1591
- ◆ **Rhophylac** see Rh_o(D) Immune Globulin on page 1591
- ◆ **Rh-TSH** see Thyrotropin Alfa on page 1784
- ◆ **rHuEPO** see Epoetin Alfa on page 702
- ◆ **rhuGM-CSF** see Sargramostim on page 1656
- ◆ **rhu Keratinocyte Growth Factor** see Palifermin on page 1425
- ◆ **rHu-KGF** see Palifermin on page 1425
- ◆ **rhuMAb-2C4** see Pertuzumab on page 1506
- ◆ **rHuMAb-EGFr** see Panitumumab on page 1440
- ◆ **rhuMAb HER2** see Trastuzumab on page 1822
- ◆ **rhuMAb-VEGF** see Bevacizumab on page 237
- ◆ **RiaSTAP** see Fibrinogen Concentrate (Human) on page 791

Ribociclib (rye boe SYE klib)

Related Information

Common Toxicity Criteria on page 2242
Safe Handling of Hazardous Drugs on page 2379

Brand Names: US Kisqali 200 Dose; Kisqali 400 Dose; Kisqali 600 Dose

Index Terms LEE-011; LEE011

Pharmacologic Category Antineoplastic Agent, Cyclin-Dependent Kinase
Inhibitor

Use Breast cancer, advanced or metastatic: Treatment of hormone receptor
(HR)-positive, human epidermal growth factor receptor 2 (HER2)-negative
advanced or metastatic breast cancer (in combination with an aromatase
inhibitor) in postmenopausal women as initial endocrine-based therapy.

Labeled Contraindications There are no contraindications listed in the
manufacturer's labeling.

Pregnancy Considerations Adverse events were observed in animal
reproduction studies. Based on the mechanism of action, ribociclib may be
expected to cause fetal harm if used during pregnancy. Women of reproductive potential should have a pregnancy test prior to treatment and use effective
contraception during treatment and for at least 3 weeks after the last dose.

Although not approved for use in men, animal data suggests that ribociclib may affect male fertility.

Breastfeeding Considerations It is not known if ribociclib is present in breast milk. Due to the potential for adverse events in the breastfed infant, the manufacturer does not recommend breastfeeding during therapy or for at least 3 weeks after the last dose.

Warnings/Precautions Ribociclib is associated with concentration-dependent QT prolongation, with an estimated mean increase in the QT interval exceeding 20 msec at the mean steady-state C_{max} of a 600 mg once daily dose. QTcF interval prolongation >500 msec has been observed, as well as QTcF prolongations >60 msec from baseline. QT interval changes occurred within the initial 4 weeks of ribociclib therapy and were reversible with treatment interruption. Torsades de pointes has not been reported, although syncope occurred in a small percentage of patients. One sudden death was reported in a patient with grade 3 hypokalemia and grade 2 QT prolongation who was receiving ribociclib in combination with letrozole. Evaluate ECG prior to treatment initiation. Initiate treatment only in patients with QTcF <450 msec. Repeat ECG on day 14 of cycle 1, at the beginning of cycle 2, and as clinically indicated. Monitor serum electrolytes (including potassium, magnesium, calcium, and phosphorous) prior to treatment, at the beginning of the first 6 cycles, and as clinically indicated. Correct electrolyte abnormality prior to treatment. QT prolongation may require treatment interruption, dose reduction and/or discontinuation. Avoid ribociclib use in patients who have or are at risk for developing QTc prolongation, including patients with long QT syndrome, uncontrolled or significant cardiac disease (eg, recent MI, HF, unstable angina, bradyarrhythmias), or electrolyte abnormalities. Also avoid using ribociclib with medications known to prolong the QTc interval and/or strong CYP3A inhibitors (may prolong the QTcF interval).

ALT and/or AST elevations have been observed, including grade 3 or 4 events. The median time to onset for grade 3 or higher transaminase elevations was 57 days; the median time for grade 3 or higher elevations to resolve to grade 2 or lower was 24 days. Concurrent elevation of ALT or AST >3 times ULN and total bilirubin >2 times ULN (with normal alkaline phosphatase and in the absence of cholestasis) occurred (rare); all cases resolved following ribociclib discontinuation. Monitor liver function tests (baseline, every 2 weeks for the first 2 cycles, at the beginning of each subsequent 4 cycles and as clinically necessary). Depending on the severity, hepatobiliary toxicity may require treatment interruption, dose reduction and/or discontinuation. Reduced initial doses are recommended for moderate to severe hepatic impairment. Neutropenia commonly occurs, including grades 3 and 4 neutropenia. The median time to onset for grade 2 or higher neutropenia was 16 days. The median recovery for grade 3 or higher neutropenia was 15 days (resolution to normal levels or to less than grade 3 toxicity). Neutropenic fever has been observed. Monitor blood counts (baseline, every 2 weeks for the first 2 cycles, at the beginning of each subsequent 4 cycles and as clinically necessary). Neutropenia may require treatment interruption, dose reduction and/or discontinuation (depending on the severity). Anemia, thrombocytopenia, and lymphopenia have also been observed. Potentially significant drug-drug interactions may exist, requiring dose or frequency adjustment, additional monitoring, and/or selection of alternative therapy.

Adverse Reactions

>10%:

Cardiovascular: Peripheral edema (12%)

Central nervous system: Fatigue (37%), headache (22%), insomnia (12%)

Dermatologic: Alopecia (33%), skin rash (17%), pruritus (14%)

Endocrine & metabolic: Decreased serum potassium (11%)

Gastrointestinal: Nausea (52%), diarrhea (35%), vomiting (29%), constipation (25%), decreased appetite (19%), stomatitis (12%), abdominal pain (11%)

Genitourinary: Urinary tract infection (11%)

Hematologic & oncologic: Neutropenia (75%; grade 3: 50%; grade 4: 10%), leukopenia (33%; grade 3: 20%; grade 4: 1%), decreased platelet count (29%; grade 3: 1%), anemia (18%; grade 4: <1%), abnormal phosphorus levels (decreased; 13%; grade 3: 5%; grade 4: 1%), lymphocytopenia (11%; grade 3: 6%; grade 4: 1%)

Hepatic: Increased serum ALT (≤46%), increased serum AST (≤44%), increased serum bilirubin (≤18%)

Neuromuscular & skeletal: Back pain (20%)

Renal: Increased serum creatinine (20%)

Respiratory: Dyspnea (12%)

Miscellaneous: Fever (13%)

1% to 10%:

Cardiovascular: Prolonged Q-T interval on ECG (3%), syncope (3%)

Hematologic & oncologic: Febrile neutropenia (2%)

Hepatic: Decreased serum bilirubin (≤1%)

Drug Interactions

Metabolism/Transport Effects Substrate of CYP3A4 (major); **Note:** Assignment of Major/Minor substrate status based on clinically relevant drug interaction potential; **Inhibits** CYP3A4 (moderate)

Avoid Concomitant Use

Avoid concomitant use of Ribociclib with any of the following: Amifampridine; Aprepitant; Asunaprevir; BCG (Intravesical); Bosutinib; Budesonide (Systemic); Cobimetinib; Conivaptan; CYP3A4 Inducers (Strong); Deferiprone; Dipyrone; Domperidone; Flibanserin; Fusidic Acid (Systemic); Grapefruit Juice; Highest Risk QTc-Prolonging Agents; Hydroxychloroquine; Idelalisib; Ivabradine; Lomitapide; MiFEPRIStone; Mizolastine; Moderate Risk QTc-Prolonging Agents; Naloxegol; Natalizumab; Neratinib; Olaparib; Pimecrolimus; Pimozide; Pomegranate; Probucol; Promazine; Simeprevir; St John's Wort; Tacrolimus (Topical); Tolvaptan; Trabectedin; Ulipristal; Vaccines (Live); Vinflunine

Increased Effect/Toxicity

Ribociclib may increase the levels/effects of: AmLODIPine; Apixaban; Aprepitant; Asunaprevir; Avanafil; Blonanserin; Bosentan; Bosutinib; Brexpiprazole; Bromocriptine; Budesonide (Systemic); Budesonide (Topical); Cannabis; Cilostazol; Cobimetinib; Colchicine; CYP3A4 Substrates; Dapoxetine; Deferiprone; Deflazacort; Domperidone; DOXOrubicin (Conventional); Dronabinol; Eletriptan; Eplerenone; Everolimus; FentaNYL; Fingolimod; Flibanserin; GuanFACINE; Highest Risk QTc-Prolonging Agents; HYDROcodone; HydrOXYzine; Ibrutinib; Imatinib; Ivabradine; Ivacaftor; Leflunomide; Lomitapide; Lurasidone; Manidipine; Mirodenafil; Naldemedine; Naloxegol; Natalizumab; Neratinib; NiMODipine; Olaparib; OxyCODONE; Pimozide; Ranolazine; Rupatadine; SAXagliptin; Sildenafil; Simeprevir; Sonidegib; Suvorexant; Tetrahydrocannabinol; Ticagrelor; Tofacitinib; Tolvaptan; Trabectedin; Udenafil; Ulipristal; Vaccines (Live); Venetoclax; Vilazodone; Vindesine; Zopiclone

The levels/effects of Ribociclib may be increased by: Amifampridine; Bilastine; Buprenorphine; Conivaptan; CYP3A4 Inhibitors (Moderate); CYP3A4 Inhibitors (Strong); Denosumab; Dipyrone; Fosaprepitant; Fusidic Acid (Systemic); Grapefruit Juice; Hydroxychloroquine; Idelalisib; Indapamide; MiFEPRIStone; Mizolastine; Moderate Risk QTc-Prolonging Agents; Netupitant; Ocrelizumab; Palbociclib; Pimecrolimus; Pomegranate; Probucol; Promazine; QTc-Prolonging Agents (Indeterminate Risk and Risk Modifying); Roflumilast; Stiripentol; Tacrolimus (Topical); Teneligliptin; Trastuzumab; Vinflunine; Xipamide

Decreased Effect

Ribociclib may decrease the levels/effects of: BCG (Intravesical); Coccidioides immitis Skin Test; Ifosfamide; Nivolumab; Sipuleucel-T; Tertomotide; Vaccines (Inactivated); Vaccines (Live)

The levels/effects of Ribociclib may be decreased by: Bosentan; CYP3A4 Inducers (Moderate); CYP3A4 Inducers (Strong); Dabrafenib; Deferasirox; Echinacea; Sarilumab; Siltuximab; St John's Wort; Tocilizumab

Food Interactions

Food: A high-fat, high-calorie meal does not affect the rate or extent of ribociclib absorption.

Pomegranates, pomegranate juice, and grapefruits may inhibit the metabolism of ribociclib and increase its systemic exposure. Management: Avoid pomegranate, pomegranate juice, and grapefruits during therapy.

Hazardous Drugs Handling Considerations

Hazardous agent (meets NIOSH 2016 criteria). This medication is not on the NIOSH (2016) list; however, it meets the criteria for a hazardous drug. Drugs are classified as hazardous based on their properties; the properties of a hazardous drug include one or more of the following characteristics: carcinogenic, teratogenic (or other developmental toxicity), reproductive toxicity, organotoxic at low doses, genotoxic, and/or new agents with structural or toxicity profiles similar to existing hazardous agents.

Use appropriate precautions for receiving, handling, administration, and disposal. Gloves (single) should be worn during receiving, unpacking, and placing in storage. NIOSH recommends single gloving for administration of intact tablets or capsules (NIOSH 2016).

Storage/Stability Store at 20°C to 25°C (68°F to 77°F). Store in the original package.

Mechanism of Action Ribociclib is a small molecule cyclin-dependent kinase (CDK) inhibitor which is selective for CDK 4 and 6; it blocks retinoblastoma protein phosphorylation and prevents progression through the cell cycle, resulting in arrest at the G1 phase (Hortobagyi 2016). The combination of ribociclib and an aromatase inhibitor causes increased inhibition of tumor growth compared with each agent alone.

Pharmacodynamics/Kinetics

Distribution: V_{ss}/F: 1,090 L

Protein binding: ~70%

Metabolism: Extensively hepatic, predominantly via CYP3A4; undergoes oxidation to circulating metabolites M13, M4, and M1, although clinical activity is primarily due to the parent drug.

Half-life elimination; Terminal: ~30 to 55 hours

Time to peak: 1 to 4 hours

◀ Excretion: Feces (69%; 17% as parent drug, 14% as metabolite M1, ≤3% as other metabolites); Urine (23%; 12% as parent drug, 4% as M1, ≤3% as other metabolites)

Dosing

Adult & Geriatric

Breast cancer, advanced or metastatic: Females (HR-positive, HER-2 negative): Oral: 600 mg once daily for 21 days, followed by a 7-day rest period to complete a 28-day treatment cycle (in combination with continuous letrozole); continue until disease progression or unacceptable toxicity (Hortobagyi 2016). May also be administered in combination with other aromatase inhibitors.

Missed doses: If a dose is missed or vomited, do not administer an additional dose that day. Resume ribociclib dosing with the next usual dose.

Dosage adjustment for concomitant strong CYP3A inhibitors: Avoid concomitant use with strong CYP3A inhibitors and consider alternatives with less potential for CYP3A inhibition. If coadministration with a strong CYP3A inhibitor cannot be avoided, reduce ribociclib dose to 400 mg once daily. If the strong inhibitor is discontinued, increase ribociclib dose (after at least 5 inhibitor half-lives have elapsed) to the dose used prior to initiating the strong CYP3A inhibitor.

Renal Impairment

CrCl 30 to <90 mL/minute: There are no dosage adjustments provided in the manufacturer's labeling; however, based on a pharmacokinetic analysis, exposure was not affected.

CrCl <30 mL/minute: There are no dosage adjustments provided in the manufacturer's labeling (has not been studied).

Hepatic Impairment

Hepatic impairment at baseline:

Mild impairment (Child-Pugh class A): No dosage adjustment necessary.

Moderate or severe impairment (Child-Pugh class B or C): Reduce initial dose to 400 mg/day.

Hepatobiliary toxicity *during* treatment (see Dosing: Adjustment for Toxicity for dose adjustment levels):

Elevations from baseline **without** total bilirubin increase >2 times the upper limit of normal (ULN):

Grade 1 (ALT and/or AST elevated >1 to 3 times ULN): No dosage adjustment necessary.

Grade 2 (ALT and/or AST elevated >3 to 5 times ULN): If baseline was below grade 2, interrupt treatment until recovery to baseline or lower and then resume ribociclib at the same dose level. For recurrent grade 2 elevations, interrupt treatment until recovery and then resume ribociclib at the next lower dose level. If baseline was at grade 2, no dosage adjustment necessary.

Grade 3 (ALT and/or AST elevated >5 to 20 times ULN): Interrupt treatment until recovery to baseline or lower and then resume ribociclib at the next lower dose level. For recurrent grade 3 elevations, discontinue ribociclib.

Grade 4 (ALT and/or AST elevated >20 times ULN): Discontinue ribociclib.

Combined ALT and/or AST elevations >3 times ULN **with** total bilirubin increase >2 times ULN (in the absence of cholestasis), regardless of baseline grade: Discontinue ribociclib.

Adjustment for Toxicity

Recommended ribociclib dosage adjustment levels:

Starting dose: 600 mg/day.

First dose reduction: Reduce to 400 mg/day.

Second dose reduction: Reduce to 200 mg/day.

If further dose reduction below 200 mg/day is needed, discontinue ribociclib.

Note: For dosage adjustment of concomitant aromatase inhibitor therapy refer to monograph and/or prescribing information.

Hematologic toxicity:

Grade 1 or 2 neutropenia (ANC 1,000/mm^3 to below the lower limit of normal): No dosage adjustment necessary.

Grade 3 neutropenia (ANC 500 to <1,000/mm^3): Interrupt treatment until recovery to grade 2 or lower and then resume ribociclib at the same dose. For recurrent grade 3 neutropenia, interrupt treatment until recovery and then resume ribociclib at the next lower dose level.

Grade 3 neutropenia with neutropenic fever (a single episode of fever >38.3°C or fever above 38°C for more than 1 hour and/or concurrent infection): Interrupt treatment until recovery to grade 2 or lower and then resume ribociclib at the next lower dose level.

Grade 4 neutropenia (ANC <500/mm^3): Interrupt treatment until recovery to grade 2 or lower and then resume ribociclib at the next lower dose level.

Nonhematologic toxicity:

Cardiovascular: QT prolongation:

QTcF >480 msec: Interrupt treatment; when QTcF resolves to <481 msec, may resume ribociclib at the same dose level. If QTcF ≥481 msec recurs, interrupt treatment until QTcF resolves to <481 msec and resume ribociclib at the next lower dose level.

QTcF >500 msec: Interrupt treatment for QTcF >500 msec on at least 2 separate ECGs (within the same visit); if QTcF resolves to <481 msec, may resume ribociclib at the next lower dose level. If QTcF interval prolongation is **either** >500 msec **or** >60 msec increase from baseline **AND** associated with torsades de pointes, polymorphic ventricular tachycardia, unexplained syncope, or signs/symptoms of serious arrhythmia, permanently discontinue ribociclib.

Other nonhematologic toxicities (based on Common Toxicity Criteria for Adverse Events Version 4):

Grade 1 or 2: No dosage adjustment necessary. Initiate appropriate medical management and monitoring as indicated.

Grade 3: Interrupt treatment until recovery to grade 1 or lower and then resume ribociclib at the same dose level. If grade 3 toxicity recurs, interrupt treatment until recovery to grade 1 or lower and then resume ribociclib at the next lower dose level.

Grade 4: Discontinue ribociclib.

Combination Regimens

Breast cancer: Letrozole-Ribociclib (Breast Cancer Regimen) on page 2167

Administration Oral: May be administered with or without food. Administer at approximately the same time each day (and at the same time as letrozole [or other aromatase inhibitor]), preferably in the morning. Swallow tablets whole; do not crush, chew, or split tablets (do not ingest broken or cracked tablets). ▶

◀ **Monitoring Parameters** Complete blood count (baseline, every 2 weeks for the first 2 cycles, at the beginning of each subsequent 4 cycles and as clinically necessary); liver function tests (baseline, every 2 weeks for the first 2 cycles, at the beginning of each subsequent 4 cycles and as clinically necessary); serum electrolytes (including potassium, magnesium, calcium, and phosphorous) prior to treatment, at the beginning of the first 6 cycles, and as clinically indicated; pregnancy test prior to treatment (in females of reproductive potential). ECG (prior to treatment initiation; repeat on day 14 of cycle 1, at the beginning of cycle 2, and as clinically indicated).

Dietary Considerations Avoid pomegranate, pomegranate juice, and grape-fruits.

Dosage Forms Excipient information presented when available (limited, particularly for generics); consult specific product labeling.

Tablet, Oral:

Kisqali 200 Dose: 200 mg (21s) [contains soybean lecithin]
Kisqali 400 Dose: 200 mg (42s) [contains soybean lecithin]
Kisqali 600 Dose: 200 mg (63s) [contains soybean lecithin]

Ribociclib and Letrozole (rye boe SYE klib & LET roe zole)

Brand Names: US Kisqali Femara Co-Pack

Index Terms Letrozole and Ribociclib; Ribociclib Succinate and Letrozole

Use Breast cancer, advanced or metastatic: Ribociclib and letrozole (Kisqali Femara Co-Pack) is packaged as a 28-day treatment pack and is indicated as initial endocrine-based therapy for the treatment of postmenopausal women with hormone receptor (HR)-positive, human epidermal growth factor receptor 2 (HER2)-negative advanced or metastatic breast cancer. Refer to the individual Ribociclib and Letrozole Lexicomp monographs and/or the prescribing information for complete information.

Adverse Reactions Also see individual agents.

>10%:

Cardiovascular: Peripheral edema (12%)

Central nervous system: Fatigue (37%), headache (22%), insomnia (12%)

Dermatologic: Alopecia (33%), skin rash (17%), pruritus (14%)

Endocrine & metabolic: Increased serum ALT (46%), increased serum AST (44%), decreased serum potassium (11%)

Gastrointestinal: Nausea (52%), diarrhea (35%), vomiting (29%), constipation (25%), decreased appetite (19%), stomatitis (12%), abdominal pain (11%)

Genitourinary: Urinary tract infection (11%)

Hematologic & oncologic: Neutropenia (75%; grade 3: 50%; grade 4: 10%), leukopenia (33%; grade 3: 20%; grade 4: 1%), decreased platelet count (29%; grade 3: 1%), anemia (18%; grade 4: <1%), abnormal phosphorus levels (13%; grade 3: 5%; grade 4: 1%; decreased), lymphocytopenia (11%; grade 3: 6%; grade 4: 1%)

Hepatic: Abnormal hepatic function tests (18%)

Neuromuscular & skeletal: Back pain (20%)

Renal: Increased serum creatinine (20%)

Respiratory: Dyspnea (12%)

Miscellaneous: Fever (13%)

1% to 10%:

Cardiovascular: Syncope (3%), prolonged Q-T interval on ECG (≤3%)

Hepatic: Increased serum bilirubin (1%)

Drug Interactions

Metabolism/Transport Effects Refer to individual components.

Avoid Concomitant Use

Avoid concomitant use of Ribociclib and Letrozole with any of the following: Amifampridine; Aprepitant; Artesunate; Asunaprevir; BCG (Intravesical); Bosutinib; Budesonide (Systemic); Cobimetinib; Conivaptan; CYP3A4 Inducers (Strong); Deferiprone; Dipyrone; Domperidone; Flibanserin; Fusidic Acid (Systemic); Grapefruit Juice; Highest Risk QTc-Prolonging Agents; Hydroxychloroquine; Idelalisib; Ivabradine; Lomitapide; MiFEPRIStone; Mizolastine; Moderate Risk QTc-Prolonging Agents; Naloxegol; Natalizumab; Neratinib; Olaparib; Pimecrolimus; Pimozide; Pomegranate; Probucol; Promazine; Simeprevir; St John's Wort; Tacrolimus (Topical); Tegafur; Tolvaptan; Trabectedin; Ulipristal; Vaccines (Live); Vinflunine

Increased Effect/Toxicity

Ribociclib and Letrozole may increase the levels/effects of: AmLODIPine; Apixaban; Aprepitant; Artesunate; Asunaprevir; Avanafil; Blonanserin; Bosentan; Bosutinib; Brexpiprazole; Bromocriptine; Budesonide (Systemic); Budesonide (Topical); Cannabis; Cilostazol; Cobimetinib; Colchicine; CYP2A6 Substrates; CYP3A4 Substrates; Dapoxetine; Deferiprone; Deflazacort; Domperidone; DOXOrubicin (Conventional); Dronabinol; Eletriptan; Eplerenone; Everolimus; FentaNYL; Fingolimod; Flibanserin; GuanFACINE; Highest Risk QTc-Prolonging Agents; HYDROcodone; HydrOXYzine; Ibrutinib; Imatinib; Ivabradine; Ivacaftor; Leflunomide; Lomitapide; Lurasidone; Manidipine; Mirodenafil; Naldemedine; Naloxegol; Natalizumab; Neratinib; NiMODipine; Olaparib; OxyCODONE; Pimozide; Ranolazine; Rupatadine; SAXagliptin; Sildenafil; Simeprevir; Sonidegib; Suvorexant; Tetrahydrocannabinol; Ticagrelor; Tofacitinib; Tolvaptan; Trabectedin; Udenafil; Ulipristal; Vaccines (Live); Venetoclax; Vilazodone; Vindesine; Zopiclone

The levels/effects of Ribociclib and Letrozole may be increased by: Amifampridine; Bilastine; Buprenorphine; Conivaptan; CYP3A4 Inhibitors (Moderate); CYP3A4 Inhibitors (Strong); Denosumab; Dipyrone; Fosaprepitant; Fusidic Acid (Systemic); Grapefruit Juice; Hydroxychloroquine; Idelalisib; Indapamide; MiFEPRIStone; Mizolastine; Moderate Risk QTc-Prolonging Agents; Netupitant; Ocrelizumab; Palbociclib; Pimecrolimus; Pomegranate; Probucol; Promazine; QTc-Prolonging Agents (Indeterminate Risk and Risk Modifying); Roflumilast; Stiripentol; Tacrolimus (Topical); Teneligliptin; Trastuzumab; Vinflunine; Xipamide

Decreased Effect

Ribociclib and Letrozole may decrease the levels/effects of: Artesunate; BCG (Intravesical); Coccidioides immitis Skin Test; Ifosfamide; Nivolumab; Sipuleucel-T; Tegafur; Tertomotide; Vaccines (Inactivated); Vaccines (Live)

The levels/effects of Ribociclib and Letrozole may be decreased by: Bosentan; CYP3A4 Inducers (Moderate); CYP3A4 Inducers (Strong); Dabrafenib; Deferasirox; Echinacea; Sarilumab; Siltuximab; St John's Wort; Tocilizumab

Combination Regimens

Breast cancer: Letrozole-Ribociclib (Breast Cancer Regimen) on page 2167

Dosage Forms Considerations Kisqali Femara Co-Pack consists of two drugs (a 21-day supply of ribociclib 200 mg tablets provided as weekly blister dose cards and a separate bottle containing 28 letrozole 2.5 mg tablets) co-packaged together and dispensed in a single carton for a single 28-day cycle.

Dosage Forms Excipient information presented when available (limited, particularly for generics); consult specific product labeling.
Tablet Therapy Pack, Oral:
  Kisqali Femara Co-Pack:
    200 mg daily dose: Kisqali (ribociclib) 200 mg (21s), and Femara (letrozole) 2.5 mg (28s)
    400 mg daily dose: Kisqali (ribociclib) 200 mg (42s), and Femara (letrozole) 2.5 mg (28s)
    600 mg daily dose: Kisqali (ribociclib) 200 mg (63s), and Femara (letrozole) 2.5 mg (28s)

- ◆ **Ribociclib Succinate and Letrozole** see Ribociclib and Letrozole on page 1608
- ◆ **Rimso-50** see Dimethyl Sulfoxide on page 598
- ◆ **Rituxan** see RiTUXimab on page 1610
- ◆ **Rituxan Hycela** see Rituximab and Hyaluronidase on page 1623

RiTUXimab (ri TUK si mab)

Related Information
  Common Toxicity Criteria on page 2242
  Hematopoietic Cell Transplantation on page 2365
  Management of Chemotherapy-Induced Nausea and Vomiting in Adults on page 2253
  Prevention of Chemotherapy-Induced Nausea and Vomiting in Children on page 2310

Brand Names: US Rituxan
Brand Names: Canada Rituxan
Index Terms Anti-CD20 Monoclonal Antibody; C2B8 Monoclonal Antibody; IDEC-C2B8; Rituximab Conventional; Rituximab Intravenous; Rituximab, IV
Pharmacologic Category Antineoplastic Agent, Anti-CD20; Antineoplastic Agent, Monoclonal Antibody; Antirheumatic Miscellaneous; Immunosuppressant Agent; Monoclonal Antibody

Use
Chronic lymphocytic leukemia: Treatment of previously untreated or previously treated CD20-positive chronic lymphocytic leukemia (CLL) (in combination with fludarabine and cyclophosphamide).
Granulomatosis with polyangiitis: Treatment of granulomatosis with polyangiitis (GPA; Wegener granulomatosis) (in combination with glucocorticoids).
Microscopic polyangiitis: Treatment of microscopic polyangiitis (MPA) (in combination with glucocorticoids).
Non-Hodgkin lymphomas: Treatment of CD20-positive non-Hodgkin lymphomas (NHL):
  Relapsed or refractory, low-grade or follicular B-cell NHL (as a single agent)
  Follicular B-cell NHL, previously untreated (in combination with first-line chemotherapy, and as single-agent maintenance therapy if complete or partial response to first-line rituximab with chemotherapy)
  Nonprogressing (including stable disease), low-grade B-cell NHL (as a single agent after first-line CVP treatment)
  Diffuse large B-cell NHL, previously untreated (in combination with CHOP chemotherapy [or other anthracycline-based regimen])

Rheumatoid arthritis: Treatment of moderately to severely active rheumatoid arthritis (in combination with methotrexate) in adult patients with inadequate response to one or more TNF antagonist therapies.

Limitations of use: Rituximab is not recommended for use in patients with severe, active infections.

Labeled Contraindications

There are no contraindications listed in the manufacturer's US labeling.

Canadian labeling: Known type 1 hypersensitivity or anaphylactic reaction to murine proteins, Chinese Hamster Ovary (CHO) cell proteins, or any component of the formulation; patients who have or have had progressive multifocal leukoencephalopathy (PML); patients with severe, active infections

Pregnancy Considerations Animal reproduction studies have demonstrated adverse effects including decreased (reversible) B-cells and immunosuppression. Rituximab crosses the placenta and can be detected in the newborn. In one infant born at 41 weeks' gestation, in utero exposure occurred from week 16 to 37; rituximab concentrations were higher in the neonate at birth (32,095 ng/mL) than the mother (9,750 ng/mL) and still measurable at 18 weeks of age (700 ng/mL infant; 500 ng/mL mother) (Friedrichs 2006).

B-cell lymphocytopenia lasting <6 months may occur in exposed infants. Retrospective case reports of inadvertent pregnancy during rituximab treatment collected by the manufacturer (often combined with concomitant teratogenic therapies) describe premature births and infant hematologic abnormalities and infections; no specific pattern of birth defects has been observed (limited data) (Chakravarty 2010).

Effective contraception should be used in women of reproductive potential during and for 12 months following treatment with rituximab.

The European Society for Medical Oncology has published guidelines for diagnosis, treatment, and follow-up of cancer during pregnancy. The guidelines recommend referral to a facility with expertise in cancer during pregnancy and encourage a multidisciplinary team (obstetrician, neonatologist, oncology team). Based on limited data, if pregnancy occurs during rituximab treatment, the pregnancy may continue provided rituximab treatment is withheld. In general, although the risk of B-cell depletion in the newborn is increased, if postponing rituximab treatment would significantly compromise maternal outcome in patients diagnosed with B-cell lymphoma during pregnancy, rituximab use is not discouraged during the pregnancy (Peccatori 2013). An international consensus panel has published guidelines for hematologic malignancies during pregnancy. In patients with aggressive lymphomas, rituximab (as a component of the R-CHOP chemotherapy regimen) may be administered in the second and third trimesters, however, the cytotoxic portion of the regimen should not be administered within 3 weeks prior to anticipated delivery (Lishner 2016).

Other agents are preferred for treating lupus nephritis in pregnant women (Hahn 2012). When treating rheumatoid arthritis, it is recommended to discontinue use and switch to a safer medication prior to conception unless no other pregnancy compatible medication is able to control maternal disease (Götestam Skorpen 2016).

◄ Data collection to monitor pregnancy and infant outcomes following exposure to rituximab is ongoing. A pregnancy registry is available for all cancers diagnosed during pregnancy at Cooper Health (877-635-4499).

Breastfeeding Considerations It is not known if rituximab is present in human milk. However, human IgG is excreted in breast milk, and therefore, rituximab may also be excreted in milk. Although rituximab would not be expected to enter the circulation of a breastfed infant in significant amounts, the unknown risks to the breastfed infant from oral rituximab ingestion should be weighed against the known benefits of breastfeeding. When treating rheumatoid arthritis, it is recommended to avoid breastfeeding during therapy unless no other compatible medication is able to control maternal disease. Breastfeeding should not be discouraged if no other agent is available (Götestam Skorpen 2016).

Warnings/Precautions [US Boxed Warning]: Serious (including fatal) infusion-related reactions have been reported, usually with the first infusion; fatalities have been reported within 24 hours of infusion; monitor closely during infusion; discontinue for severe reactions and provide medical intervention for grades 3 or 4 infusion reactions. Reactions usually occur within 30 to 120 minutes and may include hypotension, angioedema, bronchospasm, hypoxia, urticaria, and in more severe cases pulmonary infiltrates, acute respiratory distress syndrome, myocardial infarction, ventricular fibrillation, cardiogenic shock, and/or anaphylactoid events. Closely monitor patients with a history of prior cardiopulmonary reactions or with preexisting cardiac or pulmonary conditions and patients with high numbers of circulating malignant cells (>25,000/mm^3). Prior to infusion, premedicate patients with acetaminophen and an antihistamine (and methylprednisolone for patients with RA). Medications for the treatment of hypersensitivity reactions (eg, bronchodilators, epinephrine, corticosteroids, oxygen) should be available for immediate use; treatment is symptomatic. If infusion reaction occurs, temporarily or permanently discontinue infusion (depending on the severity of the reaction and required interventions). After symptoms resolve, infusion may be resumed with at least a 50% infusion rate reduction. Discontinue infusion for serious or life-threatening cardiac arrhythmias. Perform cardiac monitoring during and after the infusion in patients who develop clinically significant arrhythmias or who have a history of arrhythmia or angina.

[US Boxed Warning]: Hepatitis B virus (HBV) reactivation may occur with rituximab and in some cases may result in fulminant hepatitis, hepatic failure, and death. Screen all patients for HBV infection prior to treatment initiation, and monitor patients during and after treatment with rituximab. Discontinue rituximab and concomitant medications in the event of HBV reactivation. Screening should include hepatitis B surface antigen (HBsAg) and hepatitis B core antibody (anti-HBc); monitor patients for clinical and laboratory signs of hepatitis or HBV reactivation during and for several months after treatment. If viral hepatitis develops, initiate appropriate antiviral therapy. Reactivation has occurred in patients who are HBsAg positive as well as in those who are HBsAg negative but are anti-HBc positive; HBV reactivation has also been observed in patients who had previously resolved HBV infection. HBV reactivation has been reported up to 24 months after discontinuation. Use cautiously in patients who show evidence of prior HBV infection (eg, HBsAg positive [regardless of antibody status] or HBsAg negative but anti-HBc positive); consult with appropriate clinicians regarding monitoring and consideration of antiviral therapy before and/or during rituximab treatment. The safety of resuming rituximab treatment following HBV reactivation is not known; discuss reinitiation of therapy in patients with resolved HBV reactivation with physicians experienced in HBV management. American Society of Clinical Oncology (ASCO) provisional clinical opinion update on hepatitis B virus screening recommendations (Hwang 2015): Patients receiving anti-CD20 antibodies are at high risk for hepatitis B virus (HBV) reactivation. Screen for HBV infection with HBsAg and anti-HBc tests prior to treatment initiation; either a total anti-HBc (with both IgG and IgM) or anti-HBc IgG test should be used to screen for chronic or resolved HBV infection (do not use anti-HBc IgM as it may only confirm acute HBV infection). In addition, patients who have risk factors for HBV infection (eg, birthplace in a country with ≥2% HBV prevalence, household or sexual contact with HBV infected patients, high-risk behaviors [eg, intravenous drug use], and HIV infection) should also be screened prior to beginning therapy. Initiate prophylactic antiviral therapy (utilizing antivirals with low rates of viral resistance) for HBsAg positive/anti-HBc positive patients (without delaying cancer therapy) and continue the antivirals during and for ~6 to 12 months after completing treatment. HBsAg negative/anti-HBc positive patients should be monitored for HBV reactivation with HBV DNA and ALT testing approximately every 3 months during treatment; antiviral therapy may be initiated prophylactically or begun promptly at the first sign of HBV reactivation.

[US Boxed Warning]: Progressive multifocal leukoencephalopathy (PML) due to JC virus infection has been reported with rituximab; may be fatal. Cases were reported in patients with hematologic malignancies receiving rituximab either with combination chemotherapy, or with hematopoietic stem cell transplant. Cases were also reported in patients receiving rituximab for autoimmune diseases who had received concurrent or prior immunosuppressant therapy. Onset may be delayed, although most cases were diagnosed within 12 months of the last rituximab dose. A retrospective analysis of patients (n=57) diagnosed with PML following rituximab therapy, found a median of 16 months (following rituximab initiation), 5.5 months (following last rituximab dose), and 6 rituximab doses preceded PML diagnosis. Clinical findings included confusion/disorientation, motor weakness/hemiparesis, altered vision/speech, and poor motor coordination with symptoms progressing over weeks to months (Carson 2009). Promptly evaluate any patient presenting with neurological changes; consider neurology consultation, brain MRI and lumbar puncture for suspected PML. Discontinue rituximab in patients who develop PML; consider reduction/discontinuation of concurrent chemotherapy or immunosuppressants. Use is not recommended in patients with severe active infection. Serious and potentially fatal bacterial, fungal, and either new or reactivated viral infections may occur during treatment and after completing rituximab. Infections have been observed in patients with prolonged hypogammaglobulinemia, defined as hypogammaglobulinemia >11 months after rituximab exposure. Associated new or reactivated viral infections have included cytomegalovirus, herpes simplex virus, parvovirus B19, varicella zoster virus, West Nile virus, and hepatitis B and C. Discontinue rituximab (and concomitant chemotherapy) in patients who develop viral hepatitis and initiate antiviral therapy. Discontinue rituximab in patients who develop other serious infections and initiate appropriate anti-infective treatment.

Tumor lysis syndrome leading to acute renal failure requiring dialysis (some fatal) may occur within 12 to 24 hours following the first dose when used as a single agent in the treatment of NHL. Hyperkalemia, hypocalcemia, hyperuricemia, and/or hyperphosphatemia may occur. Administer prophylaxis (antihyperuricemic therapy, aggressive hydration) in patients at high risk (high numbers of circulating malignant cells ≥25,000/mm^3 or high tumor burden). Correct electrolyte abnormalities; monitor renal function and hydration status, and administer supportive care as indicated. May cause fatal renal toxicity in patients with NHL. Patients who received combination therapy with cisplatin and rituximab for NHL experienced renal toxicity during clinical trials; this combination is not an approved treatment regimen. Renal toxicity also occurred due to tumor lysis syndrome. Monitor for signs of renal failure; discontinue rituximab with increasing serum creatinine or oliguria.

[US Boxed Warning]: Severe and sometimes fatal mucocutaneous reactions (lichenoid dermatitis, paraneoplastic pemphigus, Stevens-Johnson syndrome, toxic epidermal necrolysis and vesiculobullous dermatitis) have been reported; onset has been variable but has occurred as early as the first day of exposure. Discontinue in patients experiencing severe mucocutaneous skin reactions; the safety of re-exposure following mucocutaneous reactions has not been evaluated. Abdominal pain, bowel obstruction, and perforation have been reported (rarely fatal), with an average onset of symptoms of ~6 days (range: 1 to 77 days); evaluate abdominal pain or repeated vomiting. Rituximab is associated with lymphopenia, leukopenia, neutropenia, thrombocytopenia, and anemia; the duration of cytopenias may be prolonged and may extend months beyond treatment. Monitor blood counts. Live vaccines should not be given concurrently with rituximab; there is no data available concerning secondary transmission of live vaccines with or following rituximab treatment. Rheumatoid arthritis patients should be brought up to date with nonlive immunizations (following current guidelines) at least 4 weeks before initiating therapy; response to some immunizations may be lower in some patients receiving rituximab. Potentially significant drug-drug interactions may exist, requiring dose or frequency adjustment, additional monitoring, and/or selection of alternative therapy.

Use with caution in the elderly. There is a higher risk of cardiac (supraventricular arrhythmia) and pulmonary adverse events (pneumonia, pneumonitis) and the incidence of serious infections and/or grade 3 or 4 adverse reactions are higher in elderly patients. The safety of concomitant immunosuppressants other than corticosteroids has not been evaluated in patients with granulomatosis with polyangiitis (GPA; Wegener granulomatosis) or microscopic polyangiitis (MPA) after rituximab-induced B-cell depletion. There are only limited data on subsequent courses of rituximab for GPA or MPA; safety and efficacy of re-treatment have not been established. There is limited data on the safety of other biologics or disease-modifying antirheumatic drugs (DMARDs) other than methotrexate in patients with rheumatoid arthritis with B-cell depletion following rituximab treatment. Monitor patients closely for infection if biologic agents or DMARDS are used concomitantly. The use of rituximab is not recommended in RA patients who have not had prior inadequate response to one or more TNF antagonists.

Some dosage forms may contain polysorbate 80 (also known as Tweens). Hypersensitivity reactions, usually a delayed reaction, have been reported following exposure to pharmaceutical products containing polysorbate 80 in certain individuals (Isaksson 2002; Lucente 2000; Shelley 1995).

Thrombocytopenia, ascites, pulmonary deterioration, and renal and hepatic failure have been reported in premature neonates after receiving parenteral products containing polysorbate 80 (Alade 1986; CDC 1984). See manufacturer's labeling.

Adverse Reactions Patients treated with rituximab for rheumatoid arthritis (RA) may experience fewer adverse reactions.

>10%:

Cardiovascular: Peripheral edema (8% to 16%), hypertension (6% to 12%)

Central nervous system: Fatigue (13% to 39%), chills (3% to 33%), neuropathy (≤30%), headache (17% to 19%), insomnia (≤14%), pain (12%)

Dermatologic: Skin rash (10% to 17%), pruritus (5% to 17%), night sweats (15%)

Endocrine & metabolic: Weight gain (11%)

Gastrointestinal: Nausea (8% to 23%), diarrhea (10% to 17%), abdominal pain (2% to 14%)

Hematologic & oncologic: Lymphocytopenia (48%; grades 3/4: 40%; median duration: 14 days), anemia (8% to 35%; grades 3/4: 3%), leukopenia (NHL: 14%, grades 3/4: 4%; CLL: grades 3/4: 23%; GPA/MPA: 10%), neutropenia (NHL: 14%, grades 3/4: 4% to 6%, median duration: 13 days; CLL: grades 3/4: 30% to 49%; late-onset: <1%, occurs >40 days after last dose), thrombocytopenia (12%; grades 3/4: 2% to 11%), cytopenia (may be prolonged), febrile neutropenia (CLL)

Hepatic: Increased serum ALT (≤13%)

Hypersensitivity: Angioedema (11%)

Immunologic: Antibody development (human antichimeric antibody [HACA] positive: 1% to 23%)

Infection: Infection (19% to 62%), bacterial infection (19%)

Neuromuscular & skeletal: Weakness (2% to 26%), muscle spasm (≤17%), arthralgia (6% to 13%)

Respiratory: Cough (13%), rhinitis (3% to 12%), epistaxis (≤11%)

Miscellaneous: Infusion related reaction (lymphoma: first dose: 77%, decreases with subsequent infusions and may include rigors; CLL: 59%, grades 3/4: 7% to 9%; RA: first infusion: 32%; GPA/MPA: 12%), fever (5% to 53%)

1% to 10%:

Cardiovascular: Hypotension (10%), flushing (5%)

Central nervous system: Dizziness (10%), anxiety (2% to 5%), migraine (RA: 2%), paresthesia (2%)

Dermatologic: Urticaria (2% to 8%)

Endocrine & metabolic: Hyperglycemia (9%), increased lactate dehydrogenase (7%)

Gastrointestinal: Vomiting (10%), dyspepsia (RA: 3%)

Infection: Viral infection (10%), fungal infection (1%)

Neuromuscular & skeletal: Back pain (10%), myalgia (10%)

Respiratory: Dyspnea (≤10%), throat irritation (2% to 9%), bronchospasm (8%), upper respiratory tract infection (RA: 7%), sinusitis (6%)

<1%, postmarketing and/or case reports: Acute mucocutaneous toxicity, acute renal failure, acute respiratory distress, anaphylactoid reaction, anaphylaxis, angina pectoris, aplastic anemia, arthritis (polyarticular), bone marrow depression, bronchiolitis obliterans, cardiac arrhythmia, cardiac failure, cardiogenic shock, encephalitis, fulminant hepatitis, gastrointestinal perforation, hemolytic anemia, hepatic failure, hepatitis, hypogammaglobulinemia (prolonged), hypoxia, increased serum immunoglobulins (hyperviscosity

syndrome in Waldenstrom's macroglobulinemia), interstitial pneumonitis, intestinal obstruction, intestinal perforation, Kaposi's sarcoma (progression), laryngeal edema, lichenoid dermatitis, lupus-like syndrome, mucositis, myelitis, myocardial infarction, nephrotoxicity, optic neuritis, pancytopenia (prolonged), pemphigus (paraneoplastic; uncommon), pleurisy, pneumonia, pneumonitis, polymyositis, progressive multifocal leukoencephalopathy, pure red cell aplasia, reactivated tuberculosis, reactivation of HBV, reversible posterior leukoencephalopathy syndrome, serum sickness, Stevens-Johnson syndrome, supraventricular cardiac arrhythmia, toxic epidermal necrolysis, tumor lysis syndrome, uveitis, vasculitic rash, vasculitis (systemic), ventricular fibrillation, ventricular tachycardia, vesiculobullous dermatitis, viral infection (reactivation; includes JC virus infection, cytomegalovirus, herpes simplex virus, parvovirus B19, varicella-zoster virus, West Nile disease, and hepatitis C), wheezing

Drug Interactions

Metabolism/Transport Effects None known.

Avoid Concomitant Use

Avoid concomitant use of RiTUXimab with any of the following: Abatacept; BCG (Intravesical); Belimumab; Certolizumab Pegol; Deferiprone; Dipyrone; Natalizumab; Pimecrolimus; Tacrolimus (Topical); Tofacitinib; Vaccines (Live)

Increased Effect/Toxicity

RiTUXimab may increase the levels/effects of: Abatacept; Belimumab; Certolizumab Pegol; CloZAPine; Deferiprone; Fingolimod; Leflunomide; Natalizumab; Tofacitinib; Vaccines (Live)

The levels/effects of RiTUXimab may be increased by: Denosumab; Dipyrone; Ocrelizumab; Pimecrolimus; Promazine; Roflumilast; Tacrolimus (Topical); Trastuzumab

Decreased Effect

RiTUXimab may decrease the levels/effects of: BCG (Intravesical); Coccidioides immitis Skin Test; Nivolumab; Sipuleucel-T; Tertomotide; Vaccines (Inactivated); Vaccines (Live)

The levels/effects of RiTUXimab may be decreased by: Echinacea

Storage/Stability Store intact vials at 2°C to 8°C (36°F to 46°F); do not freeze. Do not shake. Protect vials from direct sunlight. Solutions for infusion in NS or D5W are stable at 2°C to 8°C (36°F to 46°F) for 24 hours and at room temperature for an additional 24 hours (although because there is no preservative, the manufacturer recommends storing refrigerated).

Preparation for Administration IV: Withdraw necessary amount of rituximab and dilute to a final concentration of 1 to 4 mg/mL with NS or D5W. Gently invert the bag to mix the solution. Do not shake. Do not mix or dilute with other medications. Compatible in polyvinyl chloride (PVC) and polyethylene bags.

Mechanism of Action Rituximab is a monoclonal antibody directed against the CD20 antigen on the surface of B-lymphocytes. CD20 regulates cell cycle initiation; and, possibly, functions as a calcium channel. Rituximab binds to the antigen on the cell surface, activating complement-dependent B-cell cytotoxicity; and to human Fc receptors, mediating cell killing through an antibody-dependent cellular toxicity. B-cells are believed to play a role in the development and progression of rheumatoid arthritis. Signs and symptoms of RA are reduced by targeting B-cells and the progression of structural damage is delayed.

Pharmacodynamics/Kinetics

Onset:

Immune thrombocytopenia: Initial response: 7 to 56 days; Peak response: 14 to 180 days (Neunert 2011).

NHL: B-cell depletion: Within 3 weeks.

Rheumatoid arthritis (RA): B-cell depletion: Within 2 weeks.

Duration:

NHL: Detectable in serum 3 to 6 months after completion of treatment; B-cell depletion is sustained for up to 6 to 9 months and B-cell recovery begins ~6 months following completion of treatment; median B-cell levels return to normal by 12 months following completion of treatment

RA: B-cell depletion persists for at least 6 months.

Distribution: RA: 3.1 L; GPA/MPA: 4.5 L

Half-life elimination:

CLL: Median terminal half-life: 32 days (range: 14 to 62 days)

NHL: Median terminal half-life: 22 days (range: 6 to 52 days)

RA: Mean terminal half-life: 18 days (range: 5 to 78 days)

GPA/MPA: 23 days (range: 9 to 49 days)

Dosing

Adult & Geriatric Note: Pretreatment with acetaminophen and an antihistamine is recommended for all indications. For oncology uses, antihyperuricemic therapy and aggressive hydration are recommended for patients at risk for tumor lysis syndrome (high tumor burden or lymphocytes >25,000/mm^3). In patients with chronic lymphocytic leukemia (CLL), *Pneumocystis jirovecii* pneumonia (PCP) and antiherpetic viral prophylaxis is recommended during treatment (and for up to 12 months following treatment). In patients with granulomatosis with polyangiitis (GPA) and microscopic polyangiitis (MPA), PCP prophylaxis is recommended during and for 6 months after rituximab treatment. For patients with rheumatoid arthritis (RA), premedication with methylprednisolone 100 mg IV (or equivalent) is recommended 30 minutes prior to each dose.

Chronic lymphocytic leukemia: IV: 375 mg/m^2 on the day prior to fludarabine/cyclophosphamide in cycle 1, then 500 mg/m^2 on day 1 (every 28 days) of cycles 2 to 6 (in combination with fludarabine and cyclophosphamide)

Chronic lymphocytic leukemia (off-label combinations): IV: 375 mg/m^2 on the day prior to bendamustine in cycle 1, then 500 mg/m^2 on day 1 (every 28 days) of cycles 2 to 6 (in combination with bendamustine) (Eichorst 2016) **or** 375 mg/m^2 on day 1, followed by 500 mg/m^2 every 14 days for 4 doses and then 500 mg/m^2 every 28 days for 3 doses (in combination with idelalisib) (Furman 2014)

Granulomatosis with polyangiitis (GPA; Wegener granulomatosis): IV: 375 mg/m^2 once weekly for 4 doses (in combination with methylprednisolone IV for 1 to 3 days followed by daily prednisone)

Microscopic polyangiitis (MPA): IV: 375 mg/m^2 once weekly for 4 doses (in combination with methylprednisolone IV for 1 to 3 days followed by daily prednisone)

Non-Hodgkin lymphoma (NHL; relapsed/refractory, low-grade or follicular CD20-positive, B-cell): IV: 375 mg/m^2 once weekly for 4 or 8 doses (as a single agent)

Re-treatment following disease progression: 375 mg/m^2 once weekly for 4 doses

◀ *For maintenance therapy (as a single agent, in patients with response to induction therapy), the following recommendations have been made:* IV: 375 mg/m^2 every 3 months until disease progression or maximum duration of 2 years (Rituxan IV Canadian product labeling 2016)

NHL (diffuse large B-cell): IV: 375 mg/m^2 given on day 1 of each chemotherapy cycle for up to 8 doses (in combination with CHOP chemotherapy [or other anthracycline-based regimen])

NHL (follicular, CD20-positive, B-cell, previously untreated): IV: 375 mg/m^2 given on day 1 of each chemotherapy cycle for up to 8 doses (in combination with first-line chemotherapy)

Maintenance therapy (as a single agent, in patients with partial or complete response to rituximab plus chemotherapy; begin 8 weeks after completion of rituximab in combination with chemotherapy): IV: 375 mg/m^2 once every 8 weeks for 12 doses

NHL (nonprogressing, low-grade, CD20-positive, B-cell, after 6 to 8 cycles of first line CVP are completed): IV: 375 mg/m^2 once weekly for 4 doses every 6 months for a maximum of 16 doses (as a single agent)

NHL: Combination therapy with ibritumomab: IV: 250 mg/m^2 IV day 1; repeat in 7 to 9 days with ibritumomab (also see Ibritumomab monograph)

Rheumatoid arthritis: IV: 1,000 mg on days 1 and 15 (in combination with methotrexate); subsequent courses may be administered every 24 weeks (based on clinical evaluation), if necessary may be repeated no sooner than every 16 weeks

Antibody-mediated rejection in cardiac transplantation, treatment (off-label use): IV: 375 mg/m^2 once weekly for 1 to 4 doses (AHA [Colvin 2015]; ISHLT [Costanzo 2010]) **or** 1,000 **mg** on days 7 and 21 or on days 7 and 22 (AHA [Colvin 2015])

Autoimmune hemolytic anemia, refractory (off-label use): IV: 375 mg/m^2 once weekly for 4 doses (may continue systemic corticosteroids); a second course may be administered for relapse (Gobert 2011; Reynaud 2015; Roumier 2014)

Burkitt lymphoma (off-label use): IV: 375 mg/m^2 on day 1 and 11 of cycles 1 and 3 and days 2 and 8 of cycles 2 and 4 (Thomas 2006) **or** 375 mg/m^2 at the start of each chemotherapy cycle, followed by 2 additional doses 3 and 6 weeks after the completion of chemotherapy (Hoelzer 2014) **or** 50 mg/m^2 on day 8 and 375 mg/m^2 on days 10 and 12 of cycle 2 followed by 375 mg/m^2 on day 8 of cycles 3 to 7 (Rizzieri 2014).

CNS lymphoma (off-label use): IV:

Newly diagnosed: 375 mg/m^2 on day 3 every 14 days (in combination with high-dose methotrexate) until disease progression or unacceptable toxicity, or for 2 doses beyond a complete response followed by monthly treatments for up to a total of 1 year (Holdhoff 2014) **or** 500 mg/m^2 on day 1 of each cycle for 5 to 7 induction cycles (in combination with high-dose methotrexate, vincristine, and procarbazine, followed by whole-brain radiotherapy and cytarabine consolidation) (Shah 2007)

Refractory disease: 375 mg/m^2 on day 1 every 28 days (in combination with temozolomide) for 4 cycles, then followed by temozolomide monotherapy (Wong 2004)

Graft-versus-host disease (GVHD), chronic, refractory (off-label use): IV: 375 mg/m^2 once weekly for 4 doses; a second course of 4 weekly doses may be administered 8 weeks after initial therapy for lack of or incomplete response (Cutler 2006) **or** 375 mg/m^2 once weekly for 4 to 8 doses (Wolff 2011)

Hodgkin lymphoma, nodular lymphocyte-predominate, advanced (off-label use): IV: 375 mg/m^2 once weekly for 4 weeks (Ekstrand 2003; Schulz 2008) **or** 375 mg/m^2 once weekly for 4 weeks followed by maintenance dosing of 375 mg/m^2 once weekly for 4 weeks every 6 months for 2 years (Advani 2014). May be administered as a single agent or in combination with cyclophosphamide, doxorubicin, vincristine, and prednisone [R-CHOP], or for relapsed disease, in combination with ifosfamide, carboplatin and etoposide [RICE]) (Advani 2013).

Idiopathic membranous nephropathy, resistant (off-label use): IV: 375 mg/m^2 once weekly for 4 doses; repeat cycle at 6 months (Fervenza 2010) **or** 1,000 mg (flat dose) on days 1 and 15; may repeat cycle at 6 months (Fervenza 2008) **or** 375 mg/m^2 once weekly for 2 doses (Dahan 2016) **or** 375 mg/m^2 once weekly for 4 doses (Ruggenenti 2012; Ruggenenti 2015) **or** 375 mg/m^2 as a single dose and repeated at least 1 week later only if circulating B-cells >5/mm^3 were detected (Ruggenenti 2012; Ruggenenti 2015)

Immune thrombocytopenia, refractory (off-label use): IV: 375 mg/m^2 once weekly for 4 doses (Arnold 2007; Godeau 2008; Provan 2010) **or** some patients may have a response with a dose of 100 mg (flat dose) once weekly for 4 weeks (Zaja 2010).

Lupus nephritis, refractory (off-label use): IV: 375 mg/m^2 once weekly for 4 doses (Diaz-Largares 2012; Melander 2009) **or** 1,000 mg (flat dose) on days 0 and 15 (Diaz-Largares 2012) **or** 500 to 1,000 mg (flat dose) on days 1 and 15 (Vigna-Perez 2006)

Mucosa-associated lymphoid tissue lymphoma (gastric), advanced (off-label use): IV: 375 mg/m^2 once weekly for 4 doses (Martinelli 2005)

Myasthenia gravis, severe, refractory (off-label use): IV: 375 mg/m^2 once weekly for 4 weeks, then once a month for 2 months; repeat if symptomatic (Diaz-Manera 2012) **or** 375 mg/m^2 once weekly for 4 weeks; may repeat if clinically indicated (Tandan 2017). Additional data may be necessary to further define the role of rituximab in the management of refractory myasthenia gravis.

Neuromyelitis optica, relapse prevention (off-label use): IV: 1,000 mg once every 2 weeks for 2 doses, repeat every 6 months or when monthly CD19 cells counts are >0.1% of total lymphocytes (Damato 2016; Mealy 2014; Trebst 2014) **or** 375 mg/m^2 once weekly for 4 weeks, repeat every 6 months (Damato 2016; Trebst 2014). Additional data may be necessary to further define the role of rituximab in the prevention of neuromyelitis optica relapse.

Pemphigus vulgaris, newly diagnosed (off-label use): IV: 1,000 mg once every 2 weeks for 2 doses (in combination with prednisone), followed by 500 mg at months 12 and 18 (Joly 2017). Additional data may be necessary to further define the role of rituximab as initial therapy for newly diagnosed pemphigus vulgaris.

Pemphigus vulgaris, refractory (off-label use): IV: 375 mg/m^2 once weekly for 4 doses (some patients also continued immunosuppressant therapy); may repeat a second time (based on response) if needed (Cholera 2016; El Tal 2006; Kasperkiewicz 2008) **or** 375 mg/m^2 once weekly of weeks 1, 2, and 3 of a 4-week cycle, repeat for 1 additional cycle, then 1 dose per month for 4 months (total of 10 doses in 6 months), in combination with IV immune globulin (Ahmed 2006) **or** 1,000 mg once every 2 weeks for 2 doses (some patients also continued immunosuppressant therapy) (Cholera 2016; Kasperkiewicz 2008)

◄

Posttransplant lymphoproliferative disorder (off-label use): IV: 375 mg/m^2 once weekly for 4 doses (Choquet 2006) **or** 375 mg/m^2 once weekly for 4 doses, followed 4 weeks later with 4 cycles of CHOP (cyclophosphamide, doxorubicin, vincristine, prednisone) chemotherapy (Trappe 2012)

Splenic marginal zone lymphoma (off-label use): IV: 375 mg/m^2 once weekly for 6 weeks followed by 375 mg/m^2 once every 2 months for 1 to 2 years (Kalpadakis 2013) **or** 375 mg/m^2 once weekly for 4 weeks as monotherapy or 375 mg/m^2 on day 1 of each chemotherapy cycle for up to 6 cycles; 1 to 2 additional cycles of rituximab monotherapy may be administered for consolidation or to improve response (Else 2012). Additional data may be necessary to further define the role of rituximab in this condition.

Thrombotic thrombocytopenic purpura (acquired) (off-label use): IV: 375 mg/m^2 once weekly for 4 doses (in combination with plasma exchange); up to 4 additional doses may be administered for ADAMTS13 levels remaining below normal or for persistently detectable anti-ADAMTS13 IgG antibodies (Scully 2007; Scully 2011). Rituximab should be timed to be administered immediately following plasma exchange; allow 24 hours after rituximab before the next plasma exchange (McDonald 2010; Sayani 2015).

Waldenström macroglobulinemia (off-label use): IV:

Single-agent rituximab: 375 mg/m^2 once weekly for 4 weeks as a single agent; may repeat cycle one time after 12 weeks (Dimopoulos 2002).

In combination with cyclophosphamide and dexamethasone: 375 mg/m^2 on day 1 every 21 days for 6 cycles (Dimopoulos 2007).

In combination with bortezomib: 375 mg/m^2 on days 1, 8, 15, and 22 every 28 days during cycles 1 and 4; treatment is continued for 6 cycles, with a total of 8 rituximab doses (Ghobrial 2010).

In combination with bortezomib and dexamethasone: 375 mg/m^2 on days 1, 8, 15, and 22 every 35 days during cycles 2 and 5; treatment is administered for 6 cycles, with a total of 8 rituximab doses (Dimopoulos 2013) **or** 375 mg/m^2 on day 11 every 21 days for 4 cycles (induction); after a 12-week break, 4 additional maintenance cycles (spaced 12 weeks apart) were administered (Treon 2009).

In combination with bendamustine: 375 mg/m^2 on day 1 every 28 days for 4 cycles; single rituximab doses were also administered 1 week prior to the first cycle and 4 weeks after the last cycles (for a total of 6 rituximab doses) (Rummel 2005).

In combination with carfilzomib and dexamethasone: 375 mg/m^2 on days 2 and 9 every 21 days for 6 induction cycles, followed by 375 mg/m^2 on day 2 every 8 weeks for 8 maintenance cycles (Treon 2014).

Pediatric Note: Pretreatment with acetaminophen and an antihistamine is recommended.

Autoimmune hemolytic anemia, refractory (off-label use): IV: 375 mg/m^2 once weekly for 2 to 4 doses (may continue systemic corticosteroids); a second course may be administered for relapse (Rao 2008; Zecca 2003).

Immune thrombocytopenia, refractory (off-label use): IV: 375 mg/m^2 once weekly for 4 doses (Parodi 2009; Provan 2010; Wang 2005)

Nephrotic syndrome, severe, refractory (off-label use): IV: 375 mg/m^2 once weekly for 2 to 4 doses **or** 375 mg/m^2 (maximum dose: 500 mg) as a single dose (Dello Strologo 2009; Fujinaga 2010; Guigonis 2008; Prytula 2010). Additional data may be necessary to further define the role of rituximab in this condition.

Renal Impairment There are no dosage adjustments provided in the manufacturer's labeling (has not been studied).

Hepatic Impairment There are no dosage adjustments provided in the manufacturer's labeling (has not been studied).

Adjustment for Toxicity Dosage adjustments for rituximab are not recommended; however, adjustments for concomitant chemotherapy may be necessary.

Combination Regimens

Rituximab-Hyper-CVAD (NHL-Mantle Cell) on page 2208
VcR-CAP (NHL-Mantle Cell) on page 2228
Primary CNS Lymphoma: Temozolomide-Rituximab (CNS Lymphoma) on page 2212
Waldenstrom Macroglobulinemia:
Bendamustine-Rituximab (Waldenstrom Macroglobulinemia) on page 1988
Bortezomib-Dexamethasone-Rituximab (Waldenstrom Macroglobulinemia) on page 1998
Bortezomib-Rituximab (Waldenstrom Macroglobulinemia) on page 2000
Cladribine-Rituximab (Waldenstrom Macroglobulinemia) on page 2064
R-CHOP (Waldenstrom Macroglobulinemia) on page 2201

Administration Note: Some pediatric protocols utilize an alternate rituximab administration rate. Refer to specific protocol for administration rate guidelines.

For IV administration only. Do **not** administer IV push or bolus. If an infusion reaction occurs, slow or stop the infusion. If the reaction abates, restart infusion at 50% of the previous rate. Discontinue infusion in the event of serious or life-threatening cardiac arrhythmias.

IV: Initial infusion: Start infusion at a rate of 50 mg/hour; if there is no infusion reaction, increase the rate by 50 mg/hour increments every 30 minutes, to a maximum rate of 400 mg/hour.

Subsequent infusions:

Standard infusion rate: If patient tolerated initial infusion, start at 100 mg/hour; if there is no infusion reaction, increase the rate by 100 mg/hour increments every 30 minutes, to a maximum rate of 400 mg/hour.

Accelerated infusion rate (90 minutes): For patients with previously untreated follicular NHL and diffuse large B-cell NHL who are receiving a corticosteroid as part of their combination chemotherapy regimen, have a circulating lymphocyte count <5,000/mm^3, or have no significant cardiovascular disease. After tolerance has been established (no grade 3 or 4 infusion-related event) at the recommended infusion rate in cycle 1, a rapid infusion rate may be used beginning with cycle 2. The daily corticosteroid, acetaminophen, and diphenhydramine are administered prior to treatment, then the rituximab dose is administered over 90 minutes, with 20% of the dose administered over the first 30 minutes and the remaining 80% is given over 60 minutes (Sehn 2007). If the 90-minute infusion in cycle 2 is tolerated, the same rate may be used for the remainder of the treatment regimen (through cycles 6 or 8).

Emetic Potential Children and Adults: Minimal (<10%)

Monitoring Parameters CBC with differential and platelets (obtain prior to treatment and at weekly to monthly intervals and more frequently in patients with lymphoid malignancies, or at 2- to 4-month intervals in rheumatoid arthritis patients, GPA and MPA), electrolytes (in patients at risk for TLS), renal function (in patients at risk for TLS), fluid/hydration status balance; blood pressure, vital signs.

Screen all patients for HBV infection prior to therapy initiation (eg, HBsAG and anti-HBc measurements). In addition, carriers and patients with evidence of current infection or recovery from prior hepatitis B infection should be monitored closely for clinical and laboratory signs of HBV reactivation and/or infection during therapy and for up to 2 years following completion of treatment. Hepatitis B virus (HBV) screening recommendations (ASCO provisional clinical opinion update [Hwang 2015]): Screen for HBV infection with hepatitis B surface antigen (HBsAG) and hepatitis B core antibody (anti-HBc) tests prior to treatment initiation; either a total anti-HBc (with both IgG and IgM) or anti-HBc IgG test should be used to screen for chronic or resolved HBV infection (do not use anti-HBc IgM as it may only confirm acute HBV infection). HBsAg negative/anti-HBc positive patients should be monitored for HBV reactivation with HBV DNA and ALT testing approximately every 3 months during treatment.

Monitor for infusion reactions; signs of active hepatitis B infection (during and for up to 12 months after therapy completion); cardiac monitoring during and after infusion (in rheumatoid arthritis patients and in patients with preexisting cardiac disease or if arrhythmias develop during or after subsequent infusions); monitor for signs/symptoms of bowel obstruction/perforation (abdominal pain, vomiting); signs or symptoms of progressive multifocal leukoencephalopathy (focal neurologic deficits, which may present as hemiparesis, visual field deficits, cognitive impairment, aphasia, ataxia, and/or cranial nerve deficits); if PML is suspected, obtain brain MRI scan and lumbar puncture; signs/symptoms of TLS and/or mucocutaneous skin reactions.

Medication Guide Available Yes

Dosage Forms Excipient information presented when available (limited, particularly for generics); consult specific product labeling.

Solution, Intravenous [preservative free]:

Rituxan: 10 mg/mL (10 mL, 50 mL) [contains polysorbate 80]

♦ **Rituximab, IV** see RiTUXimab on page 1610

Rituximab and Hyaluronidase (ri TUK si mab & hye al yoor ON i dase)

Related Information

Common Toxicity Criteria on page 2242

Management of EGFR Inhibitor Toxicities: Dermatologic, Ocular, and Gastrointestinal on page 2291

Brand Names: US Rituxan Hycela

Index Terms Anti-CD20 Monoclonal Antibody; Hyaluronidase and Rituximab; Rituximab Subcutaneous

Pharmacologic Category Antineoplastic Agent, Anti-CD20; Antineoplastic Agent, Monoclonal Antibody

Use

Chronic lymphocytic leukemia: Treatment of adult patients with previously untreated and previously treated chronic lymphocytic leukemia (CLL) (in combination with fludarabine and cyclophosphamide)

Diffuse large B-cell lymphoma: Treatment of adult patients with previously untreated diffuse large B-cell lymphoma (DLBCL) in combination with cyclophosphamide, doxorubicin, vincristine, prednisone (CHOP) or other anthracycline-based chemotherapy regimens

Follicular lymphoma: Treatment of adult patients with:

Relapsed or refractory follicular lymphoma (FL) as a single agent;

Previously untreated FL (in combination with first-line chemotherapy) and, in patients achieving a complete or partial response to rituximab in combination with chemotherapy (as single-agent maintenance therapy);

Non-progressing (including stable disease) FL as a single agent after first-line cyclophosphamide, vincristine, and prednisone (CVP) chemotherapy

Limitations of use: Initiate treatment with rituximab/hyaluronidase only after patients have received at least 1 full dose of a rituximab product by intravenous infusion; rituximab/hyaluronidase is not indicated for the treatment of non-malignant conditions.

Labeled Contraindications

There are no contraindications listed in the manufacturer's labeling.

Canadian labeling: Known type 1 hypersensitivity or anaphylactic reaction to murine proteins, Chinese Hamster Ovary (CHO) cell proteins, or any component of the formulation; patients who have or have had progressive multifocal leukoencephalopathy (PML); patients with severe, active infections

Pregnancy Considerations Rituximab crosses the placenta; B-cell lymphocytopenia lasting <6 months may occur in exposed infants. Effective contraception should be used in women of reproductive potential during therapy and for 12 months following treatment. Refer to individual monographs for additional information.

Breastfeeding Considerations It is not known if rituximab or hyaluronidase are present in breast milk. However, human IgG is excreted in breast milk; therefore, rituximab may be present. According to the manufacturer, lactating women should not breastfeed during therapy or for at least 6 months after treatment is complete. Refer to individual monographs for additional information.

Warnings/Precautions [US Boxed Warning]: Hepatitis B virus (HBV) reactivation may occur with rituximab-containing products, including rituximab/hyaluronidase, in some cases resulting in fulminant hepatitis, hepatic failure, and death. Screen all patients for HBV infection before treatment initiation, and monitor patients during and after treatment with rituximab/hyaluronidase. Discontinue rituximab/hyaluronidase and concomitant medications in the event of HBV reactivation. Screening should include hepatitis B surface antigen (HBsAg) and hepatitis B core antibody (anti-HBc); monitor patients for clinical and laboratory signs of hepatitis or HBV reactivation during and for several months after treatment. If viral hepatitis develops, initiate appropriate antiviral therapy. Reactivation has occurred in patients who are HBsAg positive as well as in those who are HBsAg negative but are anti-HBc positive; HBV reactivation has also been observed in patients who had previously resolved HBV infection. HBV reactivation has been reported up to 24 months after rituximab discontinuation. Use cautiously in patients who show evidence of prior HBV infection (eg, HBsAg positive [regardless of antibody status] or HBsAG negative but anti-HBc positive); consult with appropriate clinicians regarding monitoring and consideration of antiviral therapy before and/or during rituximab treatment. The safety of resuming rituximab-containing treatment following HBV reactivation is not known; discuss reinitiation of therapy in patients with resolved HBV reactivation with physicians experienced in HBV management. American Society of Clinical Oncology (ASCO) provisional clinical opinion update on hepatitis B virus screening recommendations (Hwang 2015): Patients receiving anti-CD20 antibodies are at high risk for hepatitis B virus (HBV) reactivation. Screen for HBV infection with HBsAG and anti-HBc tests prior to treatment initiation; either a total anti-HBc (with both IgG and IgM) or anti-HBc IgG test should be used to screen for chronic or resolved HBV infection (do not use anti-HBc IgM as it may only confirm acute HBV infection). In addition, patients who have risk factors for HBV infection (eg, birthplace in a country with ≥2% HBV prevalence, household or sexual contact with HBV infected patients, high-risk behaviors [eg, intravenous drug use], and HIV infection) should also be screened prior to beginning therapy. Initiate prophylactic antiviral therapy (utilizing antivirals with low rates of viral resistance) for HBsAg positive/anti-HBc positive patients (without delaying cancer therapy) and continue the antivirals during and for ~6 to 12 months after completing treatment. HBsAg negative/anti-HBc positive patients should be monitored for HBV reactivation with HBV DNA and ALT testing approximately every 3 months during treatment; antiviral therapy may be initiated prophylactically or begun promptly at the first sign of HBV reactivation.

[US Boxed Warning]: Severe, including fatal, mucocutaneous reactions may occur in patients receiving rituximab-containing products, including rituximab/hyaluronidase. Paraneoplastic pemphigus, Stevens-Johnson syndrome, lichenoid dermatitis, vesiculobullous dermatitis, and toxic epidermal necrolysis have been reported. Discontinue in patients experiencing severe mucocutaneous skin reactions; the safety of reexposure following mucocutaneous reactions has not been evaluated. Subcutaneous rituximab has been associated with localized cutaneous (and injection site) reactions (eg, pain, erythema, swelling, induration, rash, pruritus, hemorrhage); may occur >24 hours after administration. Reactions have been mostly mild to moderate and have resolved without intervention. Local reactions were most common during the first rituximab/hyaluronidase cycle (incidence decreases with subsequent injections).

[US Boxed Warning]: Progressive multifocal leukoencephalopathy (PML) (including fatalities) may occur in patients receiving rituximab-containing products, including rituximab/hyaluronidase. Promptly evaluate any patient presenting with neurological changes; consider neurology consultation, brain MRI and lumbar puncture for suspected PML. Discontinue rituximab/hyaluronidase in patients who develop PML; consider reduction/discontinuation of concurrent chemotherapy or immunosuppressants. Rituximab-containing products are associated with hypersensitivity reactions (may be related to cytokine release and/or other chemical mediators). Due to the higher risk of hypersensitivity and other acute reactions, patients must receive at least one full dose of intravenous rituximab prior to receiving subcutaneous rituximab/hyaluronidase. Infusion-related reactions (with the use of intravenous rituximab formulations) usually occur within 30 to 120 minutes and may include hypotension, angioedema, bronchospasm, hypoxia, urticaria, and in more severe cases pulmonary infiltrates, acute respiratory distress syndrome, myocardial infarction, ventricular fibrillation, cardiogenic shock, and/or anaphylactoid events. Anaphylactic and other hypersensitivity reactions may occur (typically occur within minutes of infusion initiation); severe cytokine release syndrome may occur within 1 to 2 hours of starting infusion. Patients with a history of pulmonary insufficiency or with pulmonary tumor infiltration may have a poorer outcome. Closely monitor patients with a history of prior cardiopulmonary reactions or with preexisting cardiac or pulmonary conditions and patients with high numbers of circulating malignant cells (>25,000/mm³). Prior to administration, premedicate patients with acetaminophen and an antihistamine (and consider glucocorticoids). Observe patients for at least 15 minutes following subcutaneous administration; increase observation time in patients at higher risk of hypersensitivity reactions. Interrupt rituximab/hyaluronidase administration immediately for signs of a severe reaction; initiate aggressive symtpmatic treatment. Medications for the treatment of hypersensitivity reactions (eg, bronchodilators, epinephrine, antihistamines, corticosteroids) should be available for immediate use.

Serious and potentially fatal bacterial, fungal, and either new or reactivated viral infections may occur during treatment and after completing therapy with rituximab-containing products. Infections have been observed in patients with prolonged hypogammaglobulinemia, defined as hypogammaglobulinemia >11 months after rituximab exposure. Associated new or reactivated viral infections have included cytomegalovirus, herpes simplex virus, parvovirus B19, varicella zoster virus, West Nile virus, and hepatitis B and C. Discontinue rituximab/hyaluronidase in patients who develop serious infections and initiate appropriate anti-infective treatment.

Rituximab-containing products may cause severe or fatal renal toxicity. Patients who received combination therapy with cisplatin and rituximab for NHL experienced renal toxicity (associated with tumor lysis syndrome) during clinical trials; this combination is not an approved treatment regimen. Renal toxicity also occurred due to tumor lysis syndrome. Monitor for signs of renal failure; discontinue rituximab-containing products with increasing serum creatinine or oliguria. Tumor lysis syndrome may occur within 12 to 24 hours after administration of a rituximab-containing product. Hyperkalemia, hypocalcemia, hyperuricemia, and/or hyperphosphatemia may occur. Administer prophylaxis (antihyperuricemic therapy, hydration) in patients at high risk (high numbers of circulating malignant cells ≥25,000/mm^3 or high tumor burden). Correct electrolyte abnormalities; monitor renal function and hydration status, and administer supportive care as indicated.

Cardiac events (eg, ventricular fibrillation, myocardial infarction, and cardiogenic shock) may occur with rituximab-containing products. Discontinue rituximab/hyaluronidase for serious or life-threatening cardiac arrhythmias. Perform cardiac monitoring during and after administration in patients who develop clinically significant arrhythmias or who have a history of arrhythmia or angina. Abdominal pain, bowel obstruction, and perforation have been reported (rarely fatal) in patients receiving rituximab-containing products, with an average onset of symptoms of ~6 days (range: 1 to 77 days); evaluate abdominal pain or repeated vomiting. Rituximab is associated with lymphopenia, leukopenia, neutropenia, thrombocytopenia, and anemia; the duration of cytopenias may be prolonged and may extend months beyond treatment. Monitor blood counts.

Potentially significant interactions may exist, requiring dose or frequency adjustment, additional monitoring, and/or selection of alternative therapy. Live vaccines should not be given concurrently with rituximab; there is no data available concerning secondary transmission of live vaccines with or following rituximab-containing treatment. Some dosage forms may contain polysorbate 80 (also known as Tweens). Hypersensitivity reactions, usually a delayed reaction, have been reported following exposure to pharmaceutical products containing polysorbate 80 in certain individuals (Isaksson 2002; Lucente 2000; Shelley 1995). Thrombocytopenia, ascites, pulmonary deterioration, and renal and hepatic failure have been reported in premature neonates after receiving parenteral products containing polysorbate 80 (Alade 1986; CDC 1984). See manufacturer's labeling.

Adverse Reactions Also see individual agents. All incidences are from combination therapy regimens.

>10%:

Central nervous system: Fatigue (11% to 20%), paresthesia (9% to 16%), headache (6% to 13%), peripheral neuropathy (12%; grades 3/4: ≤2%)

Dermatologic: Alopecia (14% to 24%), allergic skin reaction (16%; pain, swelling, induration, hemorrhage, erythema, pruritus, and rash, as well as injection site reactions), erythema (9% to 15%), skin rash (10% to 12%; including severe mucocutaneous reactions)

Gastrointestinal: Nausea (22% to 38%), constipation (8% to 25%), vomiting (11% to 21%), diarrhea (14% to 18%), abdominal pain (7% to 14%)

Hematologic & oncologic: Neutropenia (31% to 65%; grades 3/4: 25% to 56%), anemia (15% to 23%; grades 3/4: 5%), leukopenia (6% to 19%; grades 3/4: 3% to 4%), febrile neutropenia (8% to 14%; grades 3/4: 7% to 14%)

Immunologic: Antibody development (anti-hyaluronidase antibodies: 11% to 13%; anti-rituximab antibodies: 2%)

Infection: Serious infection (46% to 56%; including reactivation of viral infections)

Local: Erythema at injection site (13% to 26%)

Neuromuscular & skeletal: Weakness (8% to 17%), arthralgia (9% to 13%)

Respiratory: Cough (11% to 23%), upper respiratory tract infection (13% to 15%), dyspnea (4% to 11%), pneumonia (2% to 11%)

Miscellaneous: Fever (13% to 32%)

1% to 10%:

Cardiovascular: Peripheral edema (5% to 8%), chest pain (6%), hypertension (6%), hypotension (1%)

Central nervous system: Chills (8% to 13%), insomnia (1% to 9%), dizziness (7%)

Dermatologic: Pruritus (8% to 10%)

Endocrine & metabolic: Weight loss (8%)

Gastrointestinal: Decreased appetite (8%), dyspepsia (5% to 8%), mucosal inflammation (5% to 8%), stomatitis (6%), upper abdominal pain (5%)

Genitourinary: Urinary tract infection (2% to 8%)

Hematologic & oncologic: Lymphocytopenia (5%; grades 3/4: 1%)

Infection: Influenza (4%)

Local: Pain at injection site (8% to 16%)

Neuromuscular & skeletal: Limb pain (7% to 10%), ostealgia (6% to 10%), back pain (9%), muscle spasm (8%), myalgia (8%)

Ophthalmic: Conjunctivitis (5%)

Respiratory: Nasopharyngitis (10%), oropharyngeal pain (6% to 9%), bronchitis (7% to 8%), sinusitis (7%), flu-like symptoms (3%)

Frequency not defined:

Hypersensitivity: Hypersensitivity reaction

Infection: JC virus infection

Local: Infusion site reaction (≤7% monotherapy in maintenance setting; higher with combination therapy and initial infusions)

<1%, postmarketing, and/or case reports: Bone marrow depression, bronchiolitis obliterans, hypogammaglobulinemia (prolonged), interstitial pulmonary disease, intestinal obstruction, intestinal perforation, Kaposi sarcoma (disease progression), lupus-like syndrome, optic neuritis, pancytopenia (prolonged), pleurisy, polyarthritis, progressive multifocal leukoencephalopathy, serum sickness, uveitis, vasculitis (systemic; with rash), viral infection

◄ **Drug Interactions**

Metabolism/Transport Effects None known.

Avoid Concomitant Use

Avoid concomitant use of Rituximab and Hyaluronidase with any of the following: Abatacept; BCG (Intravesical); Belimumab; Certolizumab Pegol; Deferiprone; Dipyrone; Natalizumab; Phenylephrine (Systemic); Pimecrolimus; Tacrolimus (Topical); Tofacitinib; Vaccines (Live)

Increased Effect/Toxicity

Rituximab and Hyaluronidase may increase the levels/effects of: Abatacept; Alpha-/Beta-Agonists; Belimumab; Certolizumab Pegol; CloZAPine; Deferiprone; DOPamine; Fingolimod; Leflunomide; Local Anesthetics; Natalizumab; Phenylephrine (Systemic); Tofacitinib; Vaccines (Live)

The levels/effects of Rituximab and Hyaluronidase may be increased by: Denosumab; Dipyrone; Ocrelizumab; Pimecrolimus; Promazine; Roflumilast; Tacrolimus (Topical); Trastuzumab

Decreased Effect

Rituximab and Hyaluronidase may decrease the levels/effects of: BCG (Intravesical); Coccidioides immitis Skin Test; Nivolumab; Sipuleucel-T; Tertomotide; Vaccines (Inactivated); Vaccines (Live)

The levels/effects of Rituximab and Hyaluronidase may be decreased by: Antihistamines; Corticosteroids; Echinacea; Estrogen Derivatives; Salicylates

Storage/Stability Store intact vials at 2°C to 8°C (36°F to 46°F); do not freeze. Store in original packaging to protect from light. Following transfer from vial to syringe, the manufacturer recommends immediate use. If not used immediately, syringes may be stored for 48 hours at 2°C to 8°C (36°F to 46°F) and subsequently for 8 hours at 30°C (86°F) in diffused daylight.

Preparation for Administration Withdraw dose from the vial and transfer to a syringe; label with the peel-off sticker. To avoid clogging the needle, attach the injection needle to the syringe immediately prior to administration; rituximab/hyaluronidase is compatible with polypropylene and polycarbonate syringes and stainless steel transfer and injection needles.

Mechanism of Action

Rituximab is a monoclonal antibody directed against the CD20 antigen on the surface of pre-B and mature B-lymphocytes. CD20 regulates cell cycle initiation; and, possibly, functions as a calcium channel. Rituximab binds to the antigen on the cell surface, activating complement-dependent B-cell cytotoxicity; and to human Fc receptors, mediating cell killing through an antibody-dependent cellular toxicity.

Hyaluronidase increases the absorption rate of rituximab-containing products by increasing permeability of subcutaneous tissue through temporary depolymerization of hyaluronan; at the recommended doses, hyaluronidase acts locally and the effects are reversible. Permeability of the subcutaneous tissue is restored within 24 to 48 hours.

Pharmacodynamics/Kinetics

Onset of action:

CLL: B-cells begin to deplete following the first cycle of rituximab, with 28% of patients B-cell depleted prior to the dose in cycle 2; by cycle 6, 96% of patients were B-cell depleted.

FL: Peripheral B-cell counts decrease to levels below normal following the first cycle of rituximab and are maintained during treatment with rituximab/hyaluronidase.

Duration of action:
  CLL: Patients remained B-cell depleted until month 9, where signs of repletion were seen.
  FL: After discontinuing rituximab/hyaluronidase, B-cell repletion begins after 6 months (may be longer in some patients)
Distribution: V_{dss}: SubQ: 8.52 L (CLL); 8.09 L (FL)
Bioavailability (compared to IV rituximab): SubQ: 63.4% (CLL); 64.6% (FL)
Half-life elimination (terminal): 32 days (CLL); 34.1 days (FL)

Dosing

Adult & Geriatric Note: All patients must receive at least one full dose of intravenous rituximab (without experiencing severe adverse reactions) prior to initiating treatment with subcutaneous rituximab/hyaluronidase; patients who do not tolerate a full IV dose should continue to receive IV rituximab in subsequent cycles. May switch to SubQ rituximab/hyaluronidase when a full IV dose is successfully administered.

Premedicate with acetaminophen and an antihistamine prior to each dose (consider glucocorticoid premedication if necessary). Antihyperuricemic therapy and aggressive hydration are recommended for patients at risk for tumor lysis syndrome (high tumor burden or lymphocytes >25,000/mm³). In patients with chronic lymphocytic leukemia (CLL), *Pneumocystis jirovecii* pneumonia (PCP) and antiherpetic viral prophylaxis is recommended during treatment (and for up to 12 months following treatment).

Chronic lymphocytic leukemia: SubQ: Rituximab 1,600 mg/hyaluronidase 26,800 units (fixed dose) on day 1 of a 28-day cycle in cycles 2 through 6 (in combination with fludarabine and cyclophosphamide) (Assouline 2016) (IV rituximab should be administered in cycle 1).

Diffuse large B-cell lymphoma: SubQ: Rituximab 1,400 mg/hyaluronidase 23,400 units (fixed dose) on day 1 of cycles 2 through 8 in combination with cyclophosphamide, doxorubicin, vincristine, and prednisone (CHOP) (IV rituximab should be administered in cycle 1).

Follicular lymphoma:

Previously untreated: SubQ: Induction: Rituximab 1,400 mg/hyaluronidase 23,400 units (fixed dose) on day 1 of a 21-day cycle in cycles 2 through 8 (in combination with chemotherapy) (Davies 2017); IV rituximab should be administered in cycle 1. In patients with complete or partial response following combination chemotherapy, initiate maintenance treatment (see below).

Maintenance: SubQ: In patients with complete or partial response, initiate rituximab 1,400 mg/hyaluronidase 23,400 units (fixed dose) once every 8 weeks for 12 doses (Davies 2017). Maintenance treatment should be initiated 8 weeks following completion of initial combination chemotherapy treatment.

Non-progressing disease following 6 to 8 cycles of first-line CVP chemotherapy: SubQ: Rituximab 1,400 mg/hyaluronidase 23,400 units (fixed dose) once weekly for 3 weeks (IV rituximab should be administered in week 1 for a total of 4 weeks of therapy) at 6-month intervals to a maximum of 16 doses.

Relapsed or refractory: SubQ: Rituximab 1,400 mg/hyaluronidase 23,400 units (fixed dose) once weekly for 3 or 7 weeks (IV rituximab should be administered in week 1) for a total of 4 or 8 weeks of therapy

◀ **Use Chemotherapy-induced nausea and vomiting (CINV), prevention:** Prevention of delayed nausea and vomiting associated with initial and repeat courses of emetogenic cancer chemotherapy, including, but not limited to, highly-emetogenic chemotherapy in adults (in combination with other antiemetic agents).

Labeled Contraindications Concurrent use of thioridazine (a CYP2D6 substrate)

Pregnancy Considerations Adverse events were observed in some animal reproduction studies.

Breastfeeding Considerations It is not known if rolapitant is excreted into breast milk. According to the manufacturer, the decision to breast-feed during therapy should take into account the risk of exposure to the infant and the benefits of treatment to the mother.

Warnings/Precautions Avoid use in patients with severe hepatic impairment; if use cannot be avoided, monitor for adverse reactions related to rolapitant. Potentially significant drug-drug interactions may exist, requiring dose or frequency adjustment, additional monitoring, and/or selection of alternative therapy. Rolapitant's inhibitory effect on CYP2D6 may persist for at least 7 days (or longer); increased plasma concentrations of certain CYP2D6 substrates may result in QT prolongation and torsades de pointes. Monitor for adverse reactions if concomitant use with CYP2D6 substrates with a narrow therapeutic index cannot be avoided. Avoid concurrent use with pimozide; concurrent use with thioridazine is contraindicated.

Adverse Reactions Clinical trials were conducted in patients receiving combination therapy with a 5-HT3 receptor antagonist and dexamethasone. It is not possible to correlate frequency of adverse events with rolaprepitant alone.

1% to 10%:

Central nervous system: Dizziness (6%)

Gastrointestinal: Decreased appetite (9%), hiccups (5%), dyspepsia (4%), stomatitis (4%), abdominal pain (3%)

Genitourinary: Urinary tract infection (4%)

Hematologic & oncologic: Neutropenia (7% to 9%), anemia (3%)

Drug Interactions

Metabolism/Transport Effects Substrate of CYP3A4 (major); **Note:** Assignment of Major/Minor substrate status based on clinically relevant drug interaction potential; **Inhibits** BCRP, CYP2B6 (weak), CYP2C8 (weak), CYP2D6 (moderate), P-glycoprotein

Avoid Concomitant Use

Avoid concomitant use of Rolapitant with any of the following: Amodiaquine; PAZOPanib; Pimozide; Silodosin; Thioridazine; Topotecan; VinCRIStine (Liposomal)

Increased Effect/Toxicity

Rolapitant may increase the levels/effects of: Afatinib; Ajmaline; Amodiaquine; ARIPiprazole; BCRP/ABCG2 Substrates; Betrixaban; Bilastine; Brentuximab Vedotin; Brexpiprazole; BuPROPion; Celiprolol; CloZAPine; Colchicine; CYP2D6 Substrates; Dabigatran Etexilate; DOXOrubicin (Conventional); Edoxaban; Eliglustat; Everolimus; Fesoterodine; Indoramin; Metoprolol; Naldemedine; Naloxegol; Nebivolol; PAZOPanib; Perhexiline; P-glycoprotein/ABCB1 Substrates; Pimozide; Propafenone; Prucalopride; Ranolazine; RifAXIMin; Silodosin; Thioridazine; Topotecan; Venetoclax; VinCRIStine (Liposomal)

Decreased Effect

Rolapitant may decrease the levels/effects of: Codeine; Tamoxifen; TraMADol

The levels/effects of Rolapitant may be decreased by: Bosentan; CYP3A4 Inducers (Moderate); CYP3A4 Inducers (Strong); Dabrafenib; Deferasirox; Enzalutamide; Mitotane; Sarilumab; Siltuximab; St John's Wort; Tocilizumab

Storage/Stability Store at 20°C to 25°C (68°F to 77°F); excursions are permitted between 15°C and 30°C (59°F and 86°F)

Mechanism of Action Rolapitant prevents delayed nausea and vomiting associated with emetogenic chemotherapy by selectively and competitively inhibiting the substance P/neurokinin 1 (NK$_1$) receptor.

Pharmacodynamics/Kinetics

Distribution: V$_d$/F: 387 L

Protein binding: 99.8%

Metabolism: Hepatic; primarily by CYP3A4 to form active metabolite M19 (major)

Half-life elimination: ~7 days (range: 169 to 183 hours)

Time to peak: ~4 hours

Excretion: Feces (73%); urine (~14%; primarily as metabolites)

Dosing

Adult & Geriatric

Chemotherapy-induced nausea and vomiting (prevention): Oral: **Note:** Do not administer rolapitant at less than 2-week intervals. No dosage adjustment for concomitant dexamethasone is required.

Highly emetogenic chemotherapy (cisplatin-based): 180 mg administered ~1 to 2 hours prior to chemotherapy on day 1 only (in combination with dexamethasone given on days 1, 2, 3, and 4 and a 5-HT$_3$ receptor antagonist given on day 1)

Moderately emetogenic chemotherapy and anthracycline/cyclophosphamide combinations: 180 mg administered ~1 to 2 hours prior to chemotherapy on day 1 only (in combination with dexamethasone given on day 1 and a 5-HT$_3$ receptor antagonist given as appropriate based the agent selected)

Renal Impairment

CrCl 30 to 90 mL/minute: There are no dosage adjustments provided in the manufacturer's labeling; however, based on pharmacokinetics, dosage adjustment is not likely necessary.

CrCl <30 ml/minute and end-stage renal disease (ESRD): There are no dosage adjustments provided in the manufacturer's labeling (has not been studied).

Hepatic Impairment

Child-Pugh classes A and B: No dosage adjustment is necessary.

Child-Pugh class C: Avoid use if possible (has not been studied); if use cannot be avoided, monitor closely for adverse reactions related to rolapitant.

Administration Administer orally ~1 to 2 hours prior to each chemotherapy cycle (on day 1 only). May be administered without regard to meals.

Monitoring Parameters If concomitant use with CYP2D6 substrates with a narrow therapeutic index cannot be avoided, monitor for adverse reactions.

Dosage Forms Excipient information presented when available (limited, particularly for generics); consult specific product labeling.
Tablet, Oral:
Varubi: 90 mg [contains fd&c blue #2 aluminum lake]

◆ **Rolapitant Hydrochloride** see Rolapitant on page 1631
◆ **Rolapitant Monohydrate Hydrochloride** see Rolapitant on page 1631

RomiDEPsin (roe mi DEP sin)

Related Information
Common Toxicity Criteria on page 2242
Management of Chemotherapy-Induced Nausea and Vomiting in Adults on page 2253
Safe Handling of Hazardous Drugs on page 2379

Brand Names: US Istodax (Overfill); Istodax [DSC]
Brand Names: Canada Istodax
Index Terms Depsipeptide; FK228; FR901228
Pharmacologic Category Antineoplastic Agent, Histone Deacetylase (HDAC) Inhibitor

Use
Cutaneous T-cell lymphoma: Treatment of cutaneous T-cell lymphoma (CTCL) in patients who have received at least one prior systemic therapy
Peripheral T-cell lymphoma: Treatment of peripheral T-cell lymphoma (PTCL) in patients who have received at least one prior therapy

Labeled Contraindications
There are no contraindications listed in the manufacturer's US labeling.
Canadian labeling: Hypersensitivity to romidepsin or any component of the formulation.

Pregnancy Considerations Adverse events were observed in animal reproduction studies. Based on the mechanism of action, romidepsin may cause fetal harm if administered during pregnancy.

Breastfeeding Considerations It is not known if romidepsin is excreted in breast milk. Due to the potential for serious adverse reactions in the nursing infant, the manufacturer recommends a decision be made to discontinue nursing or to discontinue the drug, taking into account the importance of treatment to the mother.

Warnings/Precautions Anemia, leukopenia, neutropenia, lymphopenia and thrombocytopenia may occur; may require dosage modification; monitor blood counts during treatment. Serious infections (occasionally fatal), including pneumonia, sepsis, and viral reactivation (eg, Epstein Barr and hepatitis B) have occurred during or within 30 days of treatment. Monitor patients with a history of hepatitis B infections closely for viral reactivation; consider antiviral prophylaxis. Epstein Barr reactivation leading to liver failure has also been reported, with ganciclovir antiviral prophylaxis failure in one case. The risk of life-threatening infection may be increased in patients who have received prior with antilymphocytic monoclonal antibodies or who have disease involvement in the bone marrow. QTc prolongation has been observed; use caution in patients with a history of QTc prolongation, congenital long QT syndrome, with medications known to prolong the QT interval, or with preexisting cardiac disease. Obtain baseline and periodic ECG (12-lead); monitor and correct electrolyte (potassium, magnesium, and calcium) abnormalities prior to and during treatment. T-wave and ST-segment changes have also been reported. Use with caution in patients with moderate-to-severe hepatic impairment or end-stage renal disease. Tumor lysis syndrome (TLS) has been observed; closely monitor patients with advanced disease and/or with a high tumor burden (risk of TLS is higher); if TLS occurs, initiate appropriate treatment. Potentially significant drug-drug interactions may exist, requiring dose or frequency adjustment, additional monitoring, and/or selection of alternative therapy. Romidepsin is associated with a moderate emetic potential; antiemetics are recommended to prevent nausea and vomiting (MASCC 2016).

Adverse Reactions

>10%:

Cardiovascular: ECG changes (ST-T wave changes: 2% to 63%), hypotension (7% to 23%)

Central nervous system: Fatigue (53% to 77%), headache (15% to 34%), chills (11% to 17%)

Dermatologic: Pruritus (7% to 31%), dermatitis (≤27%), exfoliative dermatitis (≤27%)

Endocrine & metabolic: Hypocalcemia (4% to 52%), hyperglycemia (2% to 51%), hypoalbuminemia (3% to 48%), hyperuricemia (≤33%), hypomagnesemia (22% to 28%), hypermagnesemia (≤27%), hypophosphatemia (≤27%), hyponatremia (≤20%), hypokalemia (6% to 20%), weight loss (10% to 15%)

Gastrointestinal: Nausea (56% to 86%), anorexia (23% to 54%), vomiting (34% to 52%), dysgeusia (15% to 40%), constipation (12% to 40%), diarrhea (20% to 36%), abdominal pain (13% to 14%)

Hematologic & oncologic: Anemia (19% to 72%; grades 3/4: 3% to 28%), thrombocytopenia (17% to 72%; grades 3/4: ≤36%), neutropenia (11% to 66%; grades 3/4: 4% to 47%), lymphocytopenia (4% to 57%; grades 3/4: ≤37%), leukopenia (4% to 55%; grades 3/4: ≤45%)

Hepatic: Increased serum AST (3% to 28%), increased serum ALT (3% to 22%)

Infection: Infection (46% to 54%; including infection of central line)

Neuromuscular & skeletal: Weakness (53% to 77%)

Respiratory: Cough (18% to 21%), dyspnea (13% to 21%)

Miscellaneous: Fever (20% to 47%)

1% to 10%:

Cardiovascular: Tachycardia (≤10%), peripheral edema (6% to 10%), chest pain, deep vein thrombosis, edema, prolonged Q-T interval on ECG, pulmonary embolism, supraventricular cardiac arrhythmia, syncope, ventricular arrhythmia

Dermatologic: Cellulitis

Endocrine & metabolic: Dehydration

Gastrointestinal: Stomatitis (6% to 10%)

Hematologic & oncologic: Tumor lysis syndrome (1% to 2%), febrile neutropenia

Hepatic: Hyperbilirubinemia

Hypersensitivity: Hypersensitivity reaction

Infection: Sepsis

Respiratory: Hypoxia, pneumonia, pneumonitis

<1%, postmarketing, and/or case reports: Acute renal failure, acute respiratory distress, atrial fibrillation, bacteremia, candidiasis, cardiac failure, cardiogenic shock, ischemic heart disease, multi-organ failure, reactivation of latent Epstein-Barr virus, respiratory failure, septic shock

◄ **Drug Interactions**

Metabolism/Transport Effects Substrate of CYP3A4 (major), P-glyco-protein; **Note:** Assignment of Major/Minor substrate status based on clin-ically relevant drug interaction potential; **Inhibits** BSEP

Avoid Concomitant Use

Avoid concomitant use of RomiDEPsin with any of the following: BCG (Intravesical); CYP3A4 Inducers (Strong); Deferiprone; Dexamethasone (Systemic); Dipyrone; Natalizumab; Pimecrolimus; RifAMPin; St John's Wort; Tacrolimus (Topical); Vaccines (Live)

Increased Effect/Toxicity

RomiDEPsin may increase the levels/effects of: CloZAPine; Deferiprone; Fingolimod; Highest Risk QTc-Prolonging Agents; Leflunomide; Moderate Risk QTc-Prolonging Agents; Natalizumab; Tofacitinib; Vaccines (Live); Warfarin

The levels/effects of RomiDEPsin may be increased by: CYP3A4 Inhibitors (Strong); Denosumab; Dipyrone; MiFEPRIStone; Ocrelizumab; P-glycopro-tein/ABCB1 Inhibitors; Pimecrolimus; Promazine; Ranolazine; RifAMPin; Roflumilast; Tacrolimus (Topical); Trastuzumab

Decreased Effect

RomiDEPsin may decrease the levels/effects of: BCG (Intravesical); Cocci-dioides immitis Skin Test; Nivolumab; Sipuleucel-T; Tertomotide; Vaccines (Inactivated); Vaccines (Live)

The levels/effects of RomiDEPsin may be decreased by: Bosentan; CYP3A4 Inducers (Moderate); CYP3A4 Inducers (Strong); Dabrafenib; Deferasirox; Dexamethasone (Systemic); Echinacea; Sarilumab; Siltuximab; St John's Wort; Tocilizumab

Food Interactions Grapefruit juice may increase the levels/effects of romi-depsin. Management: Avoid grapefruit juice.

Hazardous Drugs Handling Considerations

Hazardous agent (NIOSH 2016 [group 1]).

Use appropriate precautions for receiving, handling, administration, and disposal. Gloves (single) should be worn during receiving, unpacking, and placing in storage.

NIOSH recommends double gloving, a protective gown, ventilated engineer-ing controls (a class II biological safety cabinet or a compounding aseptic containment isolator), and closed system transfer devices (CSTDs) for prep-aration. Double gloving, a gown, and (if dosage form allows) CSTDs are required during administration (NIOSH 2016).

Storage/Stability Store intact vials at room temperature of 20°C to 25°C (68°F to 77°F); excursions are permitted between 15°C and 30°C (59°F and 86°F). The reconstituted solution is stable for 8 hours at room temperature. Solutions diluted for infusion in NS are stable for 24 hours at room temper-ature; however, the manufacturer recommends use as soon as possible after dilution.

Preparation for Administration Reconstitute each vial of romidepsin with 2.2 mL of supplied diluent to a reconstituted concentration of 5 mg/mL (both the drug and diluent vials contain overfill to ensure the appropriate volume can be withdrawn); swirl until dissolved. The reconstituted vial will contain a deliverable volume of 2 mL of product. Further dilute in 500 mL normal saline; compatible with polyvinyl chloride (PVC), ethylene vinyl acetate (EVA), poly-ethylene (PE) and glass infusion containers.

Mechanism of Action Histone deacetylase inhibitor; catalyzes acetyl group removal from protein lysine residues (including histone and transcription factors). Inhibition of histone deacetylase results in accumulation of acetyl groups, leading to alterations in chromatin structure and transcription factor activation causing termination of cell growth (induces arrest in cell cycle at G_1 and G_2/M phases) leading to cell death.

Pharmacodynamics/Kinetics

Protein binding: 92% to 94%; primarily to α_1-acid glycoprotein

Metabolism: Hepatic, primarily via CYP3A4, minor metabolism from CYP3A5, 1A1, 2B6, and 2C19

Half-life elimination: ~3 hours

Dosing

Adult & Geriatric Note: Romidepsin is associated with a moderate emetic potential; antiemetics are recommended to prevent nausea and vomiting (MASCC 2016).

Cutaneous T-cell lymphoma: IV: 14 mg/m² days 1, 8, and 15 of a 28-day treatment cycle; repeat cycle as long as benefit continues and treatment is tolerated.

Peripheral T-cell lymphoma: IV: 14 mg/m² days 1, 8, and 15 of a 28-day treatment cycle; repeat cycle as long as benefit continues and treatment is tolerated.

Renal Impairment There are no dosage adjustments provided in the manufacturer's labeling (has not been studied). However, dosage adjustment is not likely necessary since pharmacokinetics are unaffected by renal impairment. Use with caution in patients with end-stage renal disease (has not been studied).

Hepatic Impairment

Mild impairment: There are no dosage adjustments provided in the manufacturer's labeling. However, mild hepatic impairment does not significantly influence the pharmacokinetics of romidepsin.

Moderate or severe impairment: There are no dosage adjustments provided in the manufacturer's labeling. Use with caution.

Obesity *American Society of Clinical Oncology (ASCO) Guidelines for appropriate chemotherapy dosing in obese adults with cancer:* Utilize patient's actual body weight (full weight) for calculation of body surface area- or weight-based dosing, particularly when the intent of therapy is curative; manage regimen-related toxicities in the same manner as for nonobese patients; if a dose reduction is utilized due to toxicity, consider resumption of full weight-based dosing with subsequent cycles, especially if cause of toxicity (eg, hepatic or renal impairment) is resolved (Griggs, 2012).

Adjustment for Toxicity

Nonhematologic toxicity (excluding alopecia):

Grade 2 or 3: Delay treatment until toxicity returns to ≤ grade 1 or baseline, may restart at 14 mg/m²

Grade 4 or recurrent grade 3 toxicity: Delay treatment until toxicity returns to ≤ grade 1 or baseline, permanently reduce dose to 10 mg/m²

Recurrent grade 3 or 4 toxicity despite dosage reduction: Discontinue treatment

Hematologic toxicity:

Grade 3 or 4 neutropenia or thrombocytopenia: Delay treatment until ANC ≥1500/mm³ and/or platelets ≥75,000/mm³ or baseline, may restart at 14 mg/m²

◀

Immunologic: Antibody formation (≤4%; no correlation between antibody development and drug safety or efficacy has been established)

Neuromuscular & skeletal: Shoulder pain (8%)

Frequency not defined:

Hematologic & oncologic: Myelofibrosis (bone marrow reticulin formation/deposition)

<1%, postmarketing, and/or case reports: Angioedema, erythromelalgia, hypersensitivity reaction, myelofibrosis (marrow fibrosis with collagen), thromboembolism, thrombosis

Drug Interactions

Metabolism/Transport Effects None known.

Avoid Concomitant Use There are no known interactions where it is recommended to avoid concomitant use.

Increased Effect/Toxicity There are no known significant interactions involving an increase in effect.

Decreased Effect There are no known significant interactions involving a decrease in effect.

Storage/Stability Store intact vials refrigerated at 2°C to 8°C (36°F to 46°F); do not freeze. Protect from light. Store in original carton until use. Reconstituted solution may be stored at room temperature of 25°C (77°F) or refrigerated at 2°C to 8°C (36°F to 46°F) for up to 24 hours prior to administration. Protect reconstituted solution from light; discard any unused portion.

Preparation for Administration Reconstitute with only preservative free SWFI (add 0.72 mL to 250 mcg vial or 1.2 mL to 500 mcg vial). Do not use bacteriostatic water for injection. Gently invert vial and swirl; do not shake. Usually dissolves within 2 minutes.

Mechanism of Action Thrombopoietin (TPO) peptide mimetic which increases platelet counts in ITP by binding to and activating the human TPO receptor.

Pharmacodynamics/Kinetics

Onset of action: Platelet count increase: SubQ: 4 to 9 days (Wang, 2004); Peak platelet count increase: Days 12 to 16 (Wang, 2004)

Duration: Platelet counts return to baseline by day 28 (Wang, 2004)

Absorption: SubQ: Slow (Wang, 2004)

Half-life elimination: Median: 3.5 days (range: 1 to 34 days)

Time to peak, plasma: SubQ: Median: 14 hours (range: 7 to 50 hours)

Dosing

Adult & Geriatric Note: Initial dose is based on actual body weight. Use the lowest dose sufficient to maintain platelet count ≥50,000/mm^3 as necessary to reduce the risk of bleeding. Adjust dose based on platelet count response; discontinue if platelet count does not respond to a level that avoids clinically important bleeding after 4 weeks at the maximum recommended dose. Do not use to normalize platelet counts.

Chronic immune thrombocytopenia (ITP): SubQ: Initial: 1 mcg/kg once weekly; adjust dose by 1 mcg/kg/week increments to achieve platelet count ≥50,000/mm^3 and to reduce the risk of bleeding; Maximum dose: 10 mcg/kg/week (median dose needed to achieve response in clinical trials: 2 mcg/kg)

Dosage adjustment recommendations:

Platelet count <50,000/mm^3: Increase weekly dose by 1 mcg/kg

Platelet count >200,000/mm^3 for 2 consecutive weeks: Reduce weekly dose by 1 mcg/kg

Platelet count >400,000/mm^3: Withhold dose; assess platelet count weekly; when platelet count <200,000/mm^3, resume with the weekly dose reduced by 1 mcg/kg

Renal Impairment There are no dosage adjustments provided in the manufacturer's labeling (has not been studied).

Hepatic Impairment There are no dosage adjustments provided in the manufacturer's labeling (has not been studied).

Administration Administer SubQ. Administration volume may be small; use appropriate syringe (with graduations to 0.01 mL) for administration. Verify calculations, final concentration, and volume drawn up for administration.

Monitoring Parameters CBC with differential and platelets (baseline, during treatment [weekly until platelet response stable for at least 4 weeks then monthly] and weekly for at least 2 weeks following discontinuation or completion of treatment)

Evaluate for neutralizing antibodies in patients with inadequate response (blood samples may be submitted to the manufacturer for assay [1-800-772-6436]).

Dietary Considerations Some products may contain sucrose.

Additional Information Restricted access to Nplate was previously a REMS requirement via the Nplate NEXUS (Network of Experts Understanding and Supporting Nplate and Patients) program. Patients, prescribers, and pharmacies were required to be enrolled in this program. However, the FDA eliminated this REMS requirement in December 2011. There is currently no restricted access to obtaining Nplate.

Medication Guide Available Yes

Dosage Forms Excipient information presented when available (limited, particularly for generics); consult specific product labeling.
Solution Reconstituted, Subcutaneous [preservative free]:
Nplate: 250 mcg (1 ea); 500 mcg (1 ea)

◆ **RP-6976** *see* DOCEtaxel *on page 606*

◆ **rpFVIII** *see* Antihemophilic Factor (Recombinant [Porcine Sequence]) *on page 151*

◆ **RPR-116258A** *see* Cabazitaxel *on page 305*

◆ **RS-25259** *see* Palonosetron *on page 1428*

◆ **RS-25259-197** *see* Palonosetron *on page 1428*

◆ **RU-23908** *see* Nilutamide *on page 1321*

◆ **Rubidomycin Hydrochloride** *see* DAUNOrubicin (Conventional) *on page 530*

◆ **Rubraca** *see* Rucaparib *on page 1641*

Rucaparib (roo KAP a rib)

Related Information
Common Toxicity Criteria *on page 2242*
Management of Chemotherapy-Induced Nausea and Vomiting in Adults *on page 2253*
Safe Handling of Hazardous Drugs *on page 2379*

Brand Names: US Rubraca

Index Terms AG014699; CO-338; PF-01367338; PF-01367338 BW; Rubraca; Rucaparib Camsylate

◀ **Pharmacologic Category** Antineoplastic Agent, PARP Inhibitor

Use Ovarian cancer, advanced: Treatment (monotherapy) of deleterious germline and/or somatic BRCA mutation associated (as detected by an approved test) advanced ovarian cancer in patients who have been treated with 2 or more prior lines of chemotherapy.

Labeled Contraindications There are no contraindications listed in the manufacturer's labeling.

Pregnancy Considerations Based on animal reproduction studies and its mechanism of action, rucaparib may be expected to cause adverse events to the fetus. Women of reproductive potential should use effective contraception during therapy and for 6 months after the last dose. Pregnancy testing is recommended prior to therapy initiation.

Breastfeeding Considerations It is not known if rucaparib is excreted in breast milk. Due to the potential for serious adverse reactions in the nursing infant, breastfeeding is not recommended by the manufacturer during treatment and for 2 weeks after the last dose.

Warnings/Precautions Anemia, neutropenia, lymphocytopenia, and thrombocytopenia were commonly observed in clinical trials. Monitor blood counts as clinically necessary. Do not initiate treatment until after hematologic recovery (to grade 1 or lower) from prior chemotherapy. Prolonged hematologic toxicity may require therapy interruption. Myelodysplastic syndrome/acute myeloid leukemia (MDS/AML) and AML have been reported (rarely) in a clinical trial of patients with ovarian cancer receiving rucaparib monotherapy. The duration of therapy prior to development of MDS/AML and AML ranged from 57 days to ~1.5 years and 107 days to 427 days, respectively; all patients had received prior chemotherapy with platinum agents and/or other DNA-damaging medications. Monitor blood counts at baseline and then monthly and as clinically indicated. If prolonged hematologic toxicity occurs and blood counts do not recover to ≤ grade 1 after 4 weeks, further evaluation (including bone marrow and cytogenetic analyses) is necessary. If MDS/AML is confirmed, discontinue therapy. Rucaparib is associated with a moderate emetic potential; antiemetics may be necessary to prevent nausea and vomiting.

Adverse Reactions

>10%:

Central nervous system: Fatigue (≤77%), dizziness (17%)

Dermatologic: Skin rash (13%)

Endocrine & metabolic: Increased serum cholesterol (40%)

Gastrointestinal: Nausea (77%), vomiting (46%), constipation (40%), decreased appetite (39%), dysgeusia (39%), diarrhea (34%), abdominal pain (32%)

Hematologic & oncologic: Decreased hemoglobin (67%, grades 3 to 4: 23%), decreased absolute lymphocyte count (45%, grades 3 to 4: 7%), anemia (44%, grades 3 to 4: 25%), thrombocytopenia (21%, grades 3 to 4: 5%), neutropenia (15%)

Hepatic: Increased serum ALT (74%), increased serum AST (73%)

Neuromuscular & skeletal: Weakness (≤77%)

Renal: Increased serum creatinine (92%)

Respiratory: Dyspnea (21%)

Miscellaneous: Fever (11%)

1% to 10%:

Dermatologic: Skin photosensitivity (10%), pruritus (9%), palmar-plantar erythrodysesthesia (2%)

Hematologic & oncologic: Febrile neutropenia (1%)

<1%, postmarketing, and/or case reports: Acute myelocytic leukemia, myelo-dysplastic syndrome

Drug Interactions

Metabolism/Transport Effects Substrate of BCRP, CYP1A2 (minor), CYP2D6 (minor), CYP3A4 (minor), P-glycoprotein; **Note:** Assignment of Major/Minor substrate status based on clinically relevant drug interaction potential

Avoid Concomitant Use

Avoid concomitant use of Rucaparib with any of the following: BCG (Intra-vesical); Deferiprone; Dipyrone

Increased Effect/Toxicity

Rucaparib may increase the levels/effects of: CloZAPine; Deferiprone

The levels/effects of Rucaparib may be increased by: Dipyrone; Promazine

Decreased Effect

Rucaparib may decrease the levels/effects of: BCG (Intravesical)

Hazardous Drugs Handling Considerations

Hazardous agent (meets NIOSH 2016 criteria). This medication is not on the NIOSH (2016) list; however, it meets the criteria for a hazardous drug. Drugs are classified as hazardous based on their properties; the properties of a hazardous drug include one or more of the following characteristics: carcino-genic, teratogenic (or other developmental toxicity), reproductive toxicity, organotoxic at low doses, genotoxic, and/or new agents with structural or toxicity profiles similar to existing hazardous agents.

Use appropriate precautions for receiving, handling, administration, and disposal. Gloves (single) should be worn during receiving, unpacking, and placing in storage. NIOSH recommends single gloving for administration of intact tablets or capsules (NIOSH 2016).

Storage/Stability Store at 20°C to 25°C (68°F to 77°F); excursions permitted to 15°C to 30°C (59°F to 86°F).

Mechanism of Action Rucaparib is a poly (ADP-ribose) polymerase (PARP) enzyme inhibitor, including PARP1, PARP2, and PARP3. PARP enzymes are involved in DNA transcription, cell cycle regulation, and DNA repair. By inhibiting PARP, rucaparib may cause increased formation of PARP-DNA complexes, resulting in DNA damage, apoptosis, and cell death. Increased cytotoxicity due to rucaparib was observed in tumor cell lines deficient in BRCA1/2 and other DNA repair genes.

Pharmacodynamics/Kinetics

Absorption: C_{max} is increased by 20%, AUC is increased by 38%, and T_{max} is delayed by 2.5 hours following a high-fat meal (as compared to the fasting state)

Distribution: 113 to 262 L (following a single IV dose of 12 to 40 mg)

Protein binding: 70%

Metabolism: Primarily hepatic via CYP2D6; minor pathways include CYP1A2 and CYP3A4

Bioavailability: 36% (range: 30% to 45%)

Half-life elimination: Terminal: 17 to 19 hours (following a single oral 600 mg dose)

Time to peak: 1.9 hours

Dosing

Adult & Geriatric Note: Administer only to patients with deleterious germ-line and/or somatic BRCA mutation, as detected by an approved test.

Rucaparib is associated with a moderate emetic potential; antiemetics may be necessary to prevent nausea and vomiting.

Ovarian cancer, advanced: Oral: 600 mg twice daily until disease progression or unacceptable toxicity.

Missed doses: If a dose is missed, administer the next dose at its scheduled time. Do not repeat a vomited dose.

Renal Impairment

CrCl ≥30 mL/minute: No dosage adjustment is necessary

CrCl <30 mL/minute: There are no dosage adjustments provided in the manufacturer's labeling (has not been studied).

Hemodialysis: There are no dosage adjustments provided in the manufacturer's labeling (has not been studied).

Hepatic Impairment

Mild impairment (total bilirubin ≤ ULN and AST > ULN **or** total bilirubin 1 to 1.5 times ULN and any AST): No dosage adjustment is necessary.

Moderate to severe impairment (total bilirubin >1.5 times ULN): There are no dosage adjustments provided in the manufacturer's labeling (has not been studied).

Adjustment for Toxicity Consider therapy interruption or dose reduction if adverse events occur.

Recommended rucaparib dose reductions:

Starting dose: 600 mg twice daily

1st dose reduction: 500 mg twice daily

2nd dose reduction: 400 mg twice daily

3rd dose reduction: 300 mg twice daily

Secondary myelodysplastic syndrome/acute myeloid leukemia (MDS/AML): Discontinue

Administration

Rucaparib is associated with a moderate emetic potential; antiemetics may be necessary to prevent nausea and vomiting.

Administer orally twice daily (~12 hours apart) with or without food. Do not repeat a vomited dose.

Emetic Potential Moderate (30% to 90%)

Monitoring Parameters Complete blood count at baseline and monthly thereafter, or as clinically indicated (weekly until recovery for prolonged hematologic toxicity); monitor for signs/symptoms of MDS/AML. Monitor adherence.

Product Availability Rubraca: FDA approved December 2016; anticipated availability is currently undetermined.

Dosage Forms Excipient information presented when available (limited, particularly for generics); consult specific product labeling.

Tablet, Oral:

Rubraca: 200 mg [contains fd&c blue #1 aluminum lake, fd&c blue #2 aluminum lake]

Rubraca: 250 mg, 300 mg

◆ **Rucaparib Camsylate** *see* Rucaparib *on page 1641*

Ruxolitinib (rux oh LI ti nib)

Related Information

Hematopoietic Cell Transplantation *on page 2365*

Management of Chemotherapy-Induced Nausea and Vomiting in Adults *on page 2253*

Safe Handling of Hazardous Drugs *on page 2379*

Brand Names: US Jakafi

Brand Names: Canada Jakavi

Index Terms INCB 18424; INCB018424; INCB424; Ruxolitinib Phosphate

Pharmacologic Category Antineoplastic Agent, Janus Associated Kinase Inhibitor; Antineoplastic Agent, Tyrosine Kinase Inhibitor; Janus Associated Kinase Inhibitor

Use

Myelofibrosis: Treatment of intermediate or high-risk myelofibrosis, including primary myelofibrosis, post-polycythemia vera myelofibrosis and post-essential thrombocythemia myelofibrosis

Polycythemia vera: Treatment of polycythemia vera with an inadequate response to or intolerance to hydroxyurea

Labeled Contraindications

There are no contraindications listed in the manufacturer's US labeling.

Canadian labeling: Hypersensitivity to ruxolitinib or any component of the formulation or container; history of or current progressive multifocal leukoencephalopathy

Pregnancy Considerations Increased resorptions (late) and reduced fetal weights were observed in animal reproduction studies.

Breastfeeding Considerations It is not known if ruxolitinib is excreted in breast milk. According to the manufacturer, due to the potential for serious adverse reactions in the nursing infant, a decision should be made to discontinue ruxolitinib or to discontinue breastfeeding during therapy, taking into account the benefits of treatment to the mother.

Warnings/Precautions Hematologic toxicity, including thrombocytopenia, anemia and neutropenia may occur; may require dosage modification; monitor complete blood counts at baseline, every 2 to 4 weeks during dose stabilization, and then as clinically necessary. Thrombocytopenia is generally reversible with treatment interruption or dose reduction; platelet transfusions may be administered during treatment if clinically indicated. Anemia may require blood transfusion; may consider dose modification. Neutropenia (ANC <500/mm^3) is generally reversible and managed by treatment interruption.

Serious bacterial, mycobacterial (including tuberculosis), fungal, or viral infections have occurred. Active serious infections should be resolved prior to treatment initiation. Monitor for infections (including signs/symptoms of active tuberculosis and herpes zoster) during treatment. Prompt treatment is recommended if symptoms of active tuberculosis and/or herpes zoster infection develop. Evaluate for tuberculosis risk factors prior to treatment initiation; patients at higher risk for tuberculosis (prior residence/travel to countries with a high tuberculosis prevalence, close contacts with active tuberculosis, or history of latent or active tuberculosis where adequate treatment course cannot be confirmed) should be tested for latent infection. For patients with evidence of tuberculosis (active or latent), decide risk-benefit of continuing treatment. Progressive multifocal leukoencephalopathy (PML) has been reported; discontinue and evaluate if suspected. Hepatitis B viral load (HBV-DNA titer) increases (with and without associated ALT or AST elevations) have been reported with ruxolitinib in patients with chronic hepatitis B infection, although the effect of ruxolitinib is unknown; monitor and manage appropriately.

May require initial dosage reduction for hepatic impairment; in patients with myelofibrosis, avoid use if platelets <50,000/mm^3 and with hepatic impairment (any degree). May require initial dosage reduction for renal impairment. Avoid use in patients with ESRD not requiring dialysis; in patients with myelofibrosis, avoid use if platelets <50,000/mm^3 and with moderate to severe renal impairment. Ruxolitinib is not removed by dialysis, however, some active metabolites may be removed. On dialysis days, patients are advised to take their dose following dialysis sessions. Potentially significant drug-drug interactions may exist, requiring dose or frequency adjustment, additional monitoring, and/or selection of alternative therapy. Ruxolitinib has been associated with increases in lipid parameters (eg, total cholesterol, LDL cholesterol, and triglycerides). Assess lipid parameters 8 to 12 weeks after ruxolitinib initiation; monitor and manage hyperlipidemia accordingly.

Discontinue treatment in myelofibrosis patients after 6 months if no reduction in spleen size or no improvement in symptoms. Consider gradually tapering off if discontinuing for reasons other than thrombocytopenia. Within ~1 week after discontinuation, symptoms of myelofibrosis generally return to pretreatment levels. Acute relapse of myelofibrosis symptoms (eg, fever, respiratory distress, hypotension, DIC, multiorgan failure), splenomegaly, worsening cytopenias, hemodynamic compensation, and septic shock-like syndrome have been reported with treatment tapering or discontinuation (Tefferi 2011). Symptoms generally return over approximately 1 week. Evaluate and treat any intercurrent illness and consider restarting or increasing dose. Consider gradually tapering off if discontinuing for reasons other than thrombocytopenia or neutropenia. Patients should not interrupt/discontinue treatment without consulting healthcare provider.

Non-melanoma skin cancers (basal cell, squamous cell, and Merkel cell carcinoma) have been reported in patients who have received ruxolitinib; periodic skin examinations should be performed.

Adverse Reactions

>10%:

Central nervous system: Dizziness (15% to 18%), headache (15% to 16%), fatigue (15%), insomnia (12%) (Verstovsek 2012)

Dermatologic: Bruise (23%), pruritus (14%)

Endocrine & metabolic: Increased serum cholesterol (17% to 35%), hypertriglyceridemia (15%)

Gastrointestinal: Diarrhea (15%), abdominal pain (15%)

Hematologic & oncologic: Anemia (72% to 96%; grade 3: ≤34%; grade 4: ≤11%), thrombocytopenia (27% to 70%; grade 3: 5% to 9%; grade 4: ≤4%), neutropenia (3% to 19%; grade 3: 5%; grade 4: ≤2%)

Hepatic: Increased serum ALT (25%; grade 3: <1%), increased serum AST (17% to 23%)

Neuromuscular & skeletal: Muscle spasm (12%)

Respiratory: Dyspnea (13%)

1% to 10%:

Cardiovascular: Edema (8%), hypertension (<6%)

Endocrine & metabolic: Weight gain (≤7%)

Gastrointestinal: Constipation (8%), nausea (6%), flatulence (5%), vomiting

Genitourinary: Urinary tract infection (≤9%)

Infection: Herpes zoster (2% to 6%)

Neuromuscular & skeletal: Weakness (7%)

Respiratory: Nasopharyngitis (9%), cough (8%), epistaxis (6%)

<1%, postmarketing, and/or case reports: Bradycardia, disseminated intravascular coagulation, fever, hemorrhagic diathesis, hypotension, multi-organ failure, myelofibrosis (symptom exacerbation), progressive multifocal leukoencephalopathy, prolonged Q-T interval on ECG, respiratory distress, systolic hypertension, tuberculosis, withdrawal syndrome

Drug Interactions

Metabolism/Transport Effects Substrate of CYP3A4 (major); **Note:** Assignment of Major/Minor substrate status based on clinically relevant drug interaction potential

Avoid Concomitant Use

Avoid concomitant use of Ruxolitinib with any of the following: BCG (Intravesical); Conivaptan; Deferiprone; Dipyrone; Fusidic Acid (Systemic); Idelalisib; Natalizumab; Pimecrolimus; Tacrolimus (Topical); Vaccines (Live)

Increased Effect/Toxicity

Ruxolitinib may increase the levels/effects of: Bradycardia-Causing Agents; CloZAPine; Deferiprone; Fingolimod; Leflunomide; Natalizumab; Tofacitinib; Vaccines (Live)

The levels/effects of Ruxolitinib may be increased by: Aprepitant; Conivaptan; CYP3A4 Inhibitors (Moderate); CYP3A4 Inhibitors (Strong); Dasatinib; Denosumab; Dipyrone; Fluconazole; Fosaprepitant; Fusidic Acid (Systemic); Grapefruit Juice; Idelalisib; MiFEPRIStone; Netupitant; Ocrelizumab; Palbociclib; Pimecrolimus; Promazine; Roflumilast; Simeprevir; Stiripentol; Tacrolimus (Topical); Trastuzumab

Decreased Effect

Ruxolitinib may decrease the levels/effects of: BCG (Intravesical); Coccidioides immitis Skin Test; Nivolumab; Sipuleucel-T; Tertomotide; Vaccines (Inactivated); Vaccines (Live)

The levels/effects of Ruxolitinib may be decreased by: Bosentan; CYP3A4 Inducers (Moderate); CYP3A4 Inducers (Strong); Dabrafenib; Deferasirox; Echinacea; Enzalutamide; Mitotane; Sarilumab; Siltuximab; St John's Wort; Tocilizumab

Food Interactions Grapefruit juice may increase the effects of ruxolitinib. Management: Avoid grapefruit juice.

Hazardous Drugs Handling Considerations

Hazardous agent (meets NIOSH 2016 criteria). This medication is not on the NIOSH (2016) list; however, it meets the criteria for a hazardous drug. Drugs are classified as hazardous based on their properties; the properties of a hazardous drug include one or more of the following characteristics: carcinogenic, teratogenic (or other developmental toxicity), reproductive toxicity, organotoxic at low doses, genotoxic, and/or new agents with structural or toxicity profiles similar to existing hazardous agents.

Use appropriate precautions for receiving, handling, administration, and disposal. Gloves (single) should be worn during receiving, unpacking, and placing in storage.

◄ NIOSH recommends single gloving for administration of intact tablets or capsules. If manipulating tablets/capsules (eg, to prepare an oral suspension), NIOSH recommends double gloving, a protective gown, and preparation in a controlled device; if not prepared in a controlled device, respiratory and eye/face protection as well as ventilated engineering controls are recommended. NIOSH recommends double gloving, a protective gown, and (if there is a potential for vomit or spit up) eye/face protection for administration of an oral liquid/feeding tube administration (NIOSH 2016).

Storage/Stability Store at 20°C to 25°C (68°F to 77°F); excursions are permitted between 15°C and 30°C (59°F and 86°F).

Mechanism of Action Kinase inhibitor which selectively inhibits Janus Associated Kinases (JAKs), JAK1 and JAK2. JAK1 and JAK2 mediate signaling of cytokine and growth factors responsible for hematopoiesis and immune function; JAK mediated signaling involves recruitment of STATs (signal transducers and activators of transcription) to cytokine receptors which leads to modulation of gene expression. In myelofibrosis and polycythemia vera, JAK1/2 activity is dysregulated; ruxolitinib modulates the affected JAK1/2 activity.

Pharmacodynamics/Kinetics

Absorption: Rapid

Distribution: V_d: Myelofibrosis: 72 L; Polycythemia vera: 75 L

Protein binding: ~97%; primarily to albumin

Metabolism: Hepatic, primarily via CYP3A4 (and minimally CYP2C9); forms active metabolites responsible for 20% to 50% of activity

Half-life elimination: Ruxolitinib: ~3 hours (hepatic impairment: 4.1 to 5 hours); Ruxolitinib + metabolites: ~5.8 hours

Time to peak: Within 1 to 2 hours

Excretion: Urine (74%, <1% as unchanged drug); feces (22%, <1% as unchanged drug)

Dosing

Adult Note: Consider gradually tapering off (by 5 mg twice daily each week) if discontinuing for reasons other than thrombocytopenia.

Myelofibrosis: Oral: Initial dose (based on platelet count, titrate dose thereafter based on efficacy and safety):

Platelets >200,000/mm³: 20 mg twice daily

Platelets 100,000 to 200,000/mm³: 15 mg twice daily

Platelets 50,000 to <100,000/mm³: 5 mg twice daily

Dosage modification based on response in patients with baseline platelet count ≥100,000/mm³ prior to initial treatment with ruxolitinib: For insufficient response (with adequate platelet and neutrophil counts), may increase the dose in 5 mg twice daily increments to a maximum dose of 25 mg twice daily. Do not increase during initial 4 weeks and no more frequently than every 2 weeks. Discontinue treatment after 6 months if no reduction in spleen size or no improvement in symptoms. When discontinuing for reasons other than thrombocytopenia, consider gradually tapering by ~5 mg twice daily per week.

Dose increases may be considered if meet all of the following situations:
- Failure to achieve either a 50% reduction (from baseline) in palpable spleen length or a 35% reduction (from baseline) in spleen volume (measured by CT or MRI)
- Platelet count >125,000/mm³ at 4 weeks (and never <100,000/mm³)
- Absolute neutrophil count (ANC) >750/mm³

Dosage modification for bleeding requiring intervention (regardless of platelet count): Interrupt treatment until bleeding resolved; may consider resuming at the prior dose if the underlying cause of bleeding has resolved or at a reduced dose if the underlying cause of bleeding persists.

Dosage modification based on response in patients with baseline platelet 50,000 to <100,000/mm^3 prior to initial treatment with ruxolitinib: US labeling: For insufficient response (with adequate platelet and neutrophil counts), may increase the dose in 5 mg daily increments to a maximum dose of 10 mg twice daily. Do not increase during initial 4 weeks and no more frequently than every 2 weeks. Discontinue treatment after 6 months if no reduction in spleen size or no improvement in symptoms.

Dose increases may be considered if meet all of the following situations:
- Platelet count remains ≥40,000/mm^3 and did not decrease more than 20% in prior 4 weeks
- Absolute neutrophil count (ANC) >1,000/mm^3
- No adverse event or hematological toxicity resulting in dose reduction or interruption occurred in prior 4 weeks

Polycythemia vera: Oral: Initial dose: 10 mg twice daily (titrate dose based on efficacy and safety)

Dose modification due to insufficient response: If response is insufficient and platelet, hemoglobin, and neutrophil counts are adequate, the dose may be increased in 5 mg twice daily increments to a maximum of 25 mg twice daily. Do not increase dose in the first 4 weeks of treatment and not more frequently than every 2 weeks. Consider dose increases in patients who meet all of the following conditions:
- Inadequate efficacy demonstrated by one or more of the following: Continued need for phlebotomy, WBC >ULN of normal range, platelet count >ULN of normal range, or palpable spleen that is reduced by <25% from baseline.
- Platelet count ≥140,000/mm^3
- Hemoglobin ≥12 g/dL
- ANC ≥1,500/mm^3

Dosage adjustment with concomitant strong CYP3A4 inhibitors (eg, azole antifungals, clarithromycin, conivaptin, grapefruit juice, mibefradil, nefazodone, protease inhibitors, telithromycin) and fluconazole (≤200 mg):
Note: Avoid concomitant use with fluconazole doses >200 mg daily.
Myelofibrosis: Initial dose:
Platelets ≥100,000/mm^3: 10 mg twice daily.
Platelets 50,000/mm^3 to <100,000/mm^3: 5 mg once daily.
Polycythemia vera: Initial dose: 5 mg twice daily
Patients stabilized on ruxolitinib ≥10 mg twice daily: Reduce dose by 50% (rounded up to the closest available tablet strength).
Patients stabilized on ruxolitinib 5 mg twice daily: Reduce dose to 5 mg once daily.
Patients stabilized on ruxolitinib 5 mg once daily: Avoid strong CYP3A4 inhibitors or fluconazole or interrupt treatment for the duration of strong CYP3A4 inhibitor or fluconazole use.
Monitor closely and further adjust dose based on safety and efficacy.

◀ **Renal Impairment**

Myelofibrosis:

CrCl 15 to 59 mL/minute and platelets >150,000/mm³: No dosage adjustment is necessary.

CrCl 15 to 59 mL/minute and platelets 100,000 to 150,000/mm³: Initial dose: 10 mg twice daily; additional dose adjustments should be made with careful monitoring.

CrCl 15 to 59 mL/minute and platelets 50,000 to <100,000/mm³: Initial dose: 5 mg once daily; additional dose adjustments should be made with careful monitoring.

CrCl 15 to 59 mL/minute and platelets <50,000/mm³: Avoid use.

End-stage renal disease (ESRD) on dialysis and platelets 100,000 to 200,000/mm³: Initial dose: 15 mg once after dialysis; administer subsequent doses after dialysis on dialysis days. Additional dose adjustments should be made with frequent monitoring.

ESRD on dialysis and platelets >200,000/mm³: Initial dose: 20 mg once after dialysis; administer subsequent doses after dialysis on dialysis days. Additional dose adjustments should be made with frequent monitoring

ESRD not requiring dialysis: Avoid use.

Polycythemia vera:

CrCl 15 to 59 mL/minute and any platelet count: Initial: 5 mg twice daily. Additional dose adjustments should be made with frequent monitoring.

End-stage renal disease (ESRD) on dialysis: Initial dose: 10 mg once after dialysis; additional dose adjustments should be made with careful monitoring

ESRD not requiring dialysis: Avoid use.

Hemodialysis is not expected to enhance the elimination of ruxolitinib.

Hepatic Impairment

Myelofibrosis:

Mild to severe impairment (Child-Pugh class A, B, or C) and platelets >150,000/mm³: No dosage adjustment is necessary.

Mild to severe impairment (Child-Pugh class A, B, or C) and platelets 100,000 to 150,000/mm³: Initial dose: 10 mg twice daily; additional dose adjustments should be made with careful monitoring.

Mild to severe impairment (Child-Pugh class A, B, or C) and platelets 50,000 to <100,000/mm³: Initial dose: 5 mg once daily; additional dose adjustments should be made with careful monitoring.

Mild to severe impairment (Child-Pugh class A, B, or C) and platelets <50,000/mm³: Avoid use.

Polycythemia vera: Mild to severe impairment (Child-Pugh class A, B, or C) and any platelet count: Initial dose: 5 mg twice daily; additional dose adjustments should be made with careful monitoring.

Adjustment for Toxicity

Myelofibrosis:

Dosage modification for treatment interruption:

If baseline platelet count ≥100,000/mm³ prior to initial treatment with ruxolitinib and:

Platelets <50,000/mm³ and ANC <500/mm³: Interrupt treatment; upon platelet recovery (to ≥50,000/mm³) or ANC recovery (to ≥750/mm³), dosing may be restarted or increased based on the following platelet or ANC levels

Platelets ≥125,000/mm^3: Dose should be at least 5 mg twice daily below the dose at treatment interruption, up to a maximum of 20 mg twice daily

Platelets 100,000 to <125,000/mm^3: Dose should be at least 5 mg twice daily below the dose at treatment interruption, up to a maximum of 15 mg twice daily

Platelets 75,000 to <100,000/mm^3: Dose should be at least 5 mg twice daily below the dose at treatment interruption, up to a maximum of 10 mg twice daily for at least 2 weeks; may increase to 15 mg twice daily if stable

Platelets 50,000 to <75,000/mm^3: 5 mg twice daily for at least 2 weeks; may increase to 10 mg twice daily if stable

Platelets <50,000/mm^3: Continue to withhold treatment

ANC ≥750/mm^3: Resume at 5 mg once daily or 5 mg twice daily below the largest dose in the week prior to treatment interruption, whichever is greater

Note: Long-term maintenance at 5 mg twice daily has not demonstrated responses; limit use of the dose level to patients where the benefits outweigh risks

If baseline platelet count 50,000 to <100,000/mm^3 prior to initial treatment with ruxolitinib and:

Platelets <25,000/mm^3 and ANC <500/mm^3: Interrupt treatment; upon platelet recovery (to ≥35,000/mm^3) or ANC recovery (to ≥750/mm^3), resume at 5 mg once daily or 5 mg twice daily below the largest dose in the week prior to treatment interruption, whichever is greater

Note: Long-term maintenance at 5 mg twice daily has not demonstrated responses; limit use of the dose level to patients where the benefits outweigh risks

Dosage reduction for thrombocytopenia in patients with baseline platelet count ≥100,000/mm^3 prior to initial treatment with ruxolitinib:

Platelet Count	Dose at Time of Thrombocytopenia				
	25 mg twice/day	20 mg twice/day	15 mg twice/day	10 mg twice/day	5 mg twice/day
	New Dose	New Dose	New Dose	New Dose	New Dose
100,000 to <125,000/mm^3	20 mg twice/day	15 mg twice/day	No change	No change	No change
75,000 to <100,000/mm^3	10 mg twice/day	10 mg twice/day	10 mg twice/day	No change	No change
50,000 to <75,000/mm^3	5 mg twice/day	5 mg twice/day	5 mg twice/day	5 mg twice/day	No change
<50,000/mm^3	Hold dose	Hold dose	Hold dose	Hold dose	Hold dose

Note: Long-term maintenance at 5 mg twice daily has not demonstrated responses; limit use of the dose level to patients where the benefits outweigh risks

Dosage reduction for thrombocytopenia in patients with baseline platelet count 50,000 to <100,000/mm^3 prior to initial treatment with ruxolitinib:

Platelets 25,000 to <35,000/mm^3 **and** platelet count decreased <20% during prior 4 weeks:

If current daily dose >5 mg: Reduce dose by 5 mg once daily

If current dose 5 mg once daily: Continue 5 mg once daily

Platelets 25,000 to <35,000/mm^3 **and** platelet count decreased ≥20% during prior four weeks:

If current daily dose >10 mg: Reduce dose by 5 mg twice daily

If current dose 5 mg twice daily: Reduce dose to 5 mg once daily

◀

If current dose 5 mg once daily: Continue 5 mg once daily

Platelets <25,000 mm^3: Continue to withhold treatment

Note: Long-term maintenance at 5 mg twice daily has not demonstrated responses; limit use of the dose level to patients where the benefits outweigh risks

Polycythemia vera:

Hematologic toxicity:

Hemoglobin ≥12 g/dL AND platelets ≥100,000/mm^3: No dosage adjustment necessary.

Hemoglobin 10 to <12 g/dL AND platelets 75,000 to <100,000/mm^3: Consider dosage adjustment to avoid dose interruptions due to anemia and thrombocytopenia.

Hemoglobin 8 to <10 g/dL OR platelets 50,000 to <75,000/mm^3: Reduce dose by 5 mg twice daily; for patients currently receiving 5 mg twice daily, reduce dose to 5 mg once daily.

Hemoglobin <8 g/dL OR platelets <50,000/mm^3 OR ANC <1,000/mm^3: Interrupt dosing.

Dosage reduction following treatment interruption (use the most severe category of hemoglobin, platelets or ANC to determine reinitiation dose):

Hemoglobin <8 g/dL OR platelets <50,000/mm^3 OR ANC <1,000/mm^3: Continue to hold.

Hemoglobin 8 to <10 g/dL OR platelets 50,000 to <75,000/mm^3 OR ANC 1,000 to <1,500/mm^3: Restart at a maximum of 5 mg twice daily (continue treatment for at least 2 weeks, if stable, then may increase dose by 5 mg twice daily) or no more than 5 mg twice daily less than the dose that resulted in dose interruption

Hemoglobin 10 to <12 g/dL OR platelets 75,000 to <100,000/mm^3 OR ANC 1,500 to <2,000/mm^3: Restart at a maximum of 10 mg twice daily (continue treatment for at least 2 weeks, if stable, then may increase dose by 5 mg twice daily) or no more than 5 mg twice daily less than the dose that resulted in dose interruption

Hemoglobin ≥12 g/dL OR platelets ≥100,000/mm^3 OR ANC ≥2,000/mm^3: Restart at a maximum of 15 mg twice daily (continue treatment for at least 2 weeks, if stable, then may increase dose by 5 mg twice daily) or no more than 5 mg twice daily less than the dose that resulted in dose interruption

Note: If dose interruption was required while receiving 5 mg twice daily, may restart at 5 mg twice daily or 5 mg once daily (but not higher) once hemoglobin is ≥10 g/dL, platelets are ≥75,000/mm^3, and ANC is ≥1,500/mm^3

Dose management after restarting treatment: After restarting following a dose interruption, the dose may be titrated, although the maximum total daily dose should not exceed 5 mg less than the dose resulting in the interruption (unless dose interruption following phlebotomy-associated anemia, in which case the maximum total daily dose is not limited).

Administration Oral: May be administered orally with or without food. If a dose is missed, return to the usual dosing schedule and do **not** administer an additional dose.

If unable to ingest tablets, may administer through a nasogastric (NG) tube (≥8 Fr): Suspend 1 tablet in ~40 mL water and stir for ~10 minutes and administer (within 6 hours after dispersion) with appropriate syringe; rinse NG tube with ~75 mL water (effect of enteral tube feeding on ruxolitinib exposure has not been evaluated)

Emetic Potential Minimal (<10%)

Extemporaneous Preparations A suspension for nasogastric administration may be prepared with tablets. Place one tablet into ~40 mL water; stir for approximately 10 minutes. Administer within 6 hour after preparation.

Jakafi (ruxolitinib) [prescribing information]. Wilmington, DE: Incyte Corporation; December 2014.

Monitoring Parameters CBC (baseline, every 2 to 4 weeks until dose stabilized, then as clinically indicated), lipid parameters (8 to 12 weeks after ruxolitinib initiation and as appropriate thereafter), renal function, hepatic function. Monitor hepatitis B viral load (HBV-DNA titer) in patients with chronic hepatitis B infection. Perform periodic skin examinations monitor for signs/symptoms of infection; Tuberculin skin test (prior to initiation).

Dietary Considerations Avoid grapefruit juice (may increase the effects of ruxolitinib).

Prescribing and Access Restrictions Available through specialty/network pharmacies. Further information may be obtained from the manufacturer, Incyte, at 1-855-452-5234 or at www.Jakafi.com.

Dosage Forms Excipient information presented when available (limited, particularly for generics); consult specific product labeling.

Tablet, Oral:
Jakafi: 5 mg, 10 mg, 15 mg, 20 mg, 25 mg

Saliva Substitute (sa LYE va SUB stee tute)

Brand Names: US Aquoral; Biotene Moisturizing Mouth Spray [OTC]; Biotene Oral Balance [OTC]; BocaSal; Caphosol; Entertainer's Secret [OTC]; Moi-Stir [OTC]; Mouth Kote [OTC]; NeutraSal; Numoisyn; Oasis; SalivaMAX; SalivaSure [OTC]; Salivate Rx

Index Terms Artificial Saliva

Pharmacologic Category Gastrointestinal Agent, Miscellaneous

Use

Mucositis (due to high-dose chemotherapy or radiation therapy): Adjunct to standard oral care in relief of symptoms associated with chemotherapy or radiation therapy-induced mucositis

Xerostomia: Relief of dry mouth and throat in xerostomia or hyposalivation

Dosing

Adult & Geriatric

Mucositis (due to high-dose chemotherapy or radiation therapy): Oral: Caphosol, NeutraSal: Swish and spit 4 to 10 doses daily (use for the duration of chemo- or radiation therapy).
SalivateRx: Swish and spit 2 to 10 doses daily.

◀ **Xerostomia:** Oral: Use as needed, or product-specific dosing:

Aquoral: 2 sprays 3 to 4 times daily.

Biotene Oral Balance gel: Apply one-half inch length onto tongue and spread evenly; repeat as often as needed.

Caphosol, NeutraSal, SalivateRx: Swish and spit 2 to 10 doses daily.

Entertainer's Secret: Spray as often as needed.

Mouth Kote spray: Spray 3 to 5 times, swish for 8 to 10 seconds, then spit or swallow; use as often as needed.

Numoisyn liquid: Use 2 mL as needed.

Numoisyn lozenges: Dissolve 1 lozenge slowly; maximum 16 lozenges/day.

Oasis mouthwash: Rinse mouth with ~30 mL twice daily or as needed; do not swallow.

Oasis spray: 1 to 2 sprays as needed; maximum 60 sprays/day.

SalivaSure: Dissolve 1 lozenge slowly as needed; for severe symptoms, 1 lozenge per hour is recommended.

Renal Impairment There are no dosage adjustments provided in the manufacturer's labeling.

Hepatic Impairment There are no dosage adjustments provided in the manufacturer's labeling.

Additional Information Complete prescribing information should be consulted for additional detail.

Dosage Forms Excipient information presented when available (limited, particularly for generics); consult specific product labeling. [DSC] = Discontinued product

Liquid, oral:

Biotene Oral Balance: Water, starch, sunflower oil, propylene glycol, xylitol, glycerine, purified milk extract (45 mL) [sugar-free]

Numoisyn: Water, sorbitol, linseed extract, *Chondrus crispus*, methylparaben, sodium benzoate, potassium sorbate, dipotassium phosphate, propylparaben (300 mL)

Lozenge, oral:

Numoisyn: Sorbitol 0.3 g/lozenge, polyethylene glycol, malic acid, sodium citrate, calcium phosphate dibasic, hydrogenated cottonseed oil, citric acid, magnesium stearate, silicon dioxide (100s)

SalivaSure: Xylitol, citric acid, apple acid, sodium citrate dihydrate, sodium carboxymethylcellulose, dibasic calcium phosphate, silica colloidal, magnesium stearate, stearic acid (90s)

Powder, for reconstitution, oral:

BocaSal: Calcium chloride, sodium bicarbonate, sodium chloride, and sodium phosphates (30s)

NeutraSal: Calcium chloride, sodium bicarbonate, sodium chloride, and sodium phosphates (30s, 120s)

SalivaMAX: Calcium chloride, sodium bicarbonate, sodium chloride, and sodium phosphates (30s, 120s)

Salivate Rx: Calcium chloride, sodium bicarbonate, sodium chloride, and sodium phosphates (30s)

Solution, oral:

Caphosol: Dibasic sodium phosphate 0.032%, monobasic sodium phosphate 0.009%, calcium chloride 0.052%, sodium chloride 0.569%, purified water (30 mL) [packaged in two 15 mL ampuls when mixed together provide one 30 mL dose]

Entertainer's Secret: Sodium carboxymethylcellulose, aloe vera gel, glycerin (60 mL) [ethanol free; honey-apple flavor]

Solution, oral [mouthwash/gargle]:
  Oasis: Water, glycerin, sorbitol, poloxamer 338, PEG-60, hydrogenated castor oil, copovidone, sodium benzoate, carboxymethylcellulose (473 mL) [ethanol free, sugar free; mild mint flavor]
Solution, oral [spray]:
  Aquoral: Oxidized glycerol triesters and silicon dioxide (5.6 mL, 40 mL [DSC]) [contains aspartame; citrus flavor]
  Biotene Moisturizing Mouth Spray: Water, polyglycitol, propylene glycol, sunflower oil, xylitol, milk protein extract, potassium sorbate, acesulfame K, potassium thiocyanate, lysozyme, lactoferrin, lactoperoxidase (45 mL)
  Moi-Stir: Water, sorbitol, sodium carboxymethylcellulose, methylparaben, propylparaben, potassium chloride, dibasic sodium phosphate, calcium chloride, magnesium chloride, sodium chloride (120 mL)
  Mouth Kote: Water, xylitol, sorbitol, yerba santa, citric acid, ascorbic acid, sodium saccharin, sodium benzoate (5 mL, 60 mL, 240 mL) [ethanol free, sugar free; lemon-lime flavor]
  Oasis: Glycerin, cetylpyridinium, copovidone (30 mL) [ethanol free, sugar free; contains sodium benzoate; delivers ~150 sprays, mild mint flavor]

◆ **SalivaSure [OTC]** see Saliva Substitute on page 1653
◆ **Salivate Rx** see Saliva Substitute on page 1653
◆ **Samarium-153 Lexidronam** see Samarium Sm 153 Lexidronam on page 1655

Samarium Sm 153 Lexidronam

(sa MAR ee um es em won fif tee three lex ID roe nam)

Brand Names: US Quadramet

Index Terms [153]Sm-Lexidronam; Samarium-153 Lexidronam

Pharmacologic Category Radiopharmaceutical

Use Osteoblastic metastatic bone lesion pain: Relief of pain associated with confirmed osteoblastic metastatic bone lesions that enhance on radionuclide bone scan.

Pregnancy Risk Factor D

Dosing

Adult Note: Dose adjustments for extremes of weight have not been studied; use caution when determining dose for very thin or obese patients.

  Osteoblastic metastatic bone lesion pain: IV: 1 mCi/kg (37 MBq/kg)

Renal Impairment There are no dosage adjustments provided in the manufacturer's labeling (has not been studied); use with caution, patients with renal insufficiency may not tolerate the recommended hydration.

Hepatic Impairment There are no dosage adjustments provided in the manufacturer's labeling. However, a need for dosage adjustment is unlikely since studies have not revealed hepatic excretion.

Additional Information Complete prescribing information should be consulted for additional detail.

Dosage Forms Excipient information presented when available (limited, particularly for generics); consult specific product labeling. [DSC] = Discontinued product
Solution, Intravenous:
  Quadramet: 1850 MBq/mL (1 ea, 3 mL [DSC])

◆ **Sancuso** see Granisetron on page 895
◆ **SandIMMUNE** see CycloSPORINE (Systemic) on page 452

Sargramostim (sar GRAM oh stim)

Related Information

Hematopoietic Cell Transplantation *on page 2365*
Mucositis and Stomatitis *on page 2299*

Brand Names: US Leukine

Brand Names: Canada Leukine

Index Terms GM-CSF; GMCSF; Granulocyte-Macrophage Colony Stimulating Factor; Prokine; Recombinant Granulocyte-Macrophage Colony Stimulating Factor; rhuGM-CSF

Pharmacologic Category Colony Stimulating Factor; Hematopoietic Agent

Use

Acute myeloid leukemia (AML; following induction chemotherapy): To shorten time to neutrophil recovery and to reduce the incidence of severe and life-threatening infections and infections resulting in death following induction chemotherapy in older adults (≥55 years of age)

Bone marrow transplant (allogeneic or autologous) failure or engraftment delay: For graft failure or engraftment delay in patients who have undergone allogeneic or autologous bone marrow transplantation (in the presence or absence of infection), to prolong survival (survival benefit may be greater in patients with autologous bone marrow transplant failure or engraftment delay, no previous total body irradiation, malignancy other than leukemia, or multiple organ failure score ≤2)

Myeloid reconstitution after allogeneic bone marrow transplantation: To accelerate myeloid recovery in patients undergoing allogeneic bone marrow transplant from HLA-matched related donors (safe and effective in accelerating myeloid engraftment, reducing the incidence of bacteremia and other culture-positive infections, and shortening the median hospitalization duration)

Myeloid reconstitution after autologous bone marrow transplantation: To accelerate myeloid recovery following transplantation in non-Hodgkin lymphoma (NHL), acute lymphoblastic leukemia (ALL), Hodgkin lymphoma patients undergoing autologous bone marrow transplant (safe and effective in accelerating myeloid engraftment, reducing the median duration of antibiotic administration, reducing the median duration of infectious episodes, and shortening the median hospitalization duration)

Peripheral stem cell transplantation (autologous), mobilization and post-transplant: Mobilization of hematopoietic progenitor cells for collection by leukapheresis (increases the number of progenitor cells capable of engraftment and may lead to more rapid engraftment); to accelerate myeloid reconstitution following peripheral blood progenitor cell transplantation

Labeled Contraindications Hypersensitivity to sargramostim, yeast-derived products, or any component of the formulation; concomitant use with cytotoxic chemotherapy and radiation therapy or within 24 hours preceding/following chemotherapy or radiation therapy; patients with excessive (≥10%) leukemic myeloid blasts in bone marrow or peripheral blood

Pregnancy Considerations Animal reproduction studies have not been conducted.

Breastfeeding Considerations It is not known if sargramostim is present in breast milk. Breastfeeding is not recommended by the manufacturer.

Warnings/Precautions Simultaneous administration or administration 24 hours preceding/following cytotoxic chemotherapy or radiotherapy is contraindicated due to the sensitivity of rapidly dividing hematopoietic progenitor cells. If there is a rapid increase in blood counts (ANC >20,000/mm³ or platelets >500,000/mm³), decrease the dose by 50% or discontinue therapy. Excessive blood counts should fall to normal within 3 to 7 days after the discontinuation of therapy. Monitor CBC with differential twice weekly during treatment. Limited response to sargramostim may be seen in patients who have received bone marrow purged by chemical agents which do not preserve an adequate number of responsive hematopoietic progenitors (eg, <1.2 x 10⁴/kg progenitors). In patients receiving autologous bone marrow transplant, response to sargramostim may be limited if extensive radiotherapy to the abdomen or chest or multiple myelotoxic agents were administered prior to transplantation. Limited in vitro data suggest that when using sargramostim to mobilize peripheral blood progenitor cells, tumor cells may be released and reinfused into patients in the leukapheresis product; the effect of tumor cell reinfusion has not been well studied. May potentially act as a growth factor for any tumor type, particularly myeloid malignancies; caution should be exercised when using in any malignancy with myeloid characteristics. Discontinue use if disease progression occurs during treatment.

Serious allergic and anaphylactic reactions have been reported; discontinue immediately and initiate appropriate therapy if a serious allergic or anaphylactic reaction occurs. A "first-dose effect", characterized by respiratory distress, hypoxia, flushing, hypotension, syncope, and/or tachycardia, may occur (rarely) with the first dose of a cycle and resolve with appropriate symptomatic treatment; symptoms do not usually occur with subsequent doses within that cycle. Sequestration of granulocytes in pulmonary circulation and dyspnea have been reported; monitor respiratory symptoms during and following IV infusion. Decrease infusion rate by 50% if dyspnea occurs; discontinue the infusion if dyspnea persists despite reduction in the rate of administration. Subsequent doses may be administered at the standard rate with careful monitoring. Use with caution in patients with hypoxia or preexisting pulmonary disease. Edema, capillary leak syndrome, pleural and/or pericardial effusion have been reported; fluid retention has been shown to be reversible with dosage reduction or discontinuation of sargramostim with or without concomitant use of diuretics. Use with caution in patients with preexisting fluid retention, pulmonary infiltrates, or congestive heart failure; may exacerbate fluid retention.

Use with caution in patients with preexisting cardiac disease. Reversible transient supraventricular arrhythmias have been reported, especially in patients with a history of arrhythmias. Use with caution in patients with hepatic impairment (hyperbilirubinemia and elevated transaminases have been observed) or renal impairment (serum creatinine elevations have been observed). Monitor hepatic and renal function at least every other week in patients with history of impairment. Treatment with sargramostim may induce neutralizing anti-drug antibodies. Antibody formation may be related to duration of sargramostim exposure; use sargramostim for the shortest duration necessary.

According to clinical practice guidelines, colony-stimulating factors (CSFs) should not be routinely used in the treatment of established neutropenic fever. Colony-stimulating factors may be considered in cancer patients with febrile neutropenia who are at high risk for infection-associated complications or who have prognostic factors indicative of a poor clinical outcome (eg, prolonged and severe neutropenia, age >65 years, hypotension, pneumonia, sepsis syndrome, presence of invasive fungal infection, uncontrolled primary disease, hospitalization at the time of fever development) (Freifeld 2011; Smith 2006). CSFs should not be routinely used for patients with neutropenia who are afebrile. Dose-dense regimens that require CSFs should only be used within the context of a clinical trial or if supported by convincing evidence (Smith 2015). The American Society of Clinical Oncology (ASCO) Recommendations for the Use of WBC Growth Factors Clinical Practice Guideline Update recommend that prophylactic colony-stimulating factors be used in patients ≥65 years with diffuse aggressive lymphoma treated with curative chemotherapy (eg, rituximab, cyclophosphamide, doxorubicin, vincristine, prednisone), especially if patients have comorbid conditions (Smith 2015). CSF use in pediatric patients is typically directed by clinical pediatric protocols. The ASCO Recommendations for the Use of WBC Growth Factors Clinical Practice Guideline Update states that CSFs may be reasonable as primary prophylaxis in pediatric patients when chemotherapy regimens with a high likelihood of febrile neutropenia are employed. Likewise, secondary CSF prophylaxis should be limited to high-risk patients. In pediatric cancers in which dose-intense chemotherapy (with a survival benefit) is used, CSFs should be given to facilitate chemotherapy administration. CSFs should not be used in the pediatric population for non-relapsed acute lymphoblastic or myeloid leukemia when no infection is present (Smith 2015).

Benzyl alcohol and derivatives: Some dosage forms may contain benzyl alcohol; large amounts of benzyl alcohol (≥99 mg/kg/day) have been associated with a potentially fatal toxicity ("gasping syndrome") in neonates; the "gasping syndrome" consists of metabolic acidosis, respiratory distress, gasping respirations, CNS dysfunction (including convulsions, intracranial hemorrhage), hypotension, and cardiovascular collapse (AAP ["Inactive" 1997]; CDC 1982); some data suggests that benzoate displaces bilirubin from protein binding sites (Ahlfors 2001); avoid or use dosage forms containing benzyl alcohol with caution in neonates. See manufacturer's labeling.

Adverse Reactions

>10%:

Cardiovascular: Hypertension (34%), edema (13% to 25%), pericardial effusion (4% to 25%), chest pain (15%), peripheral edema (11%), tachycardia (11%)

Central nervous system: Malaise (57%), headache (26%), chills (25%), anxiety (11%), insomnia (11%)

Dermatologic: Skin rash (44% to 77%), pruritus (23%)

Endocrine & metabolic: Weight loss (37%), hyperglycemia (25%), hypercholesterolemia (17%), hypomagnesemia (15%)

Gastrointestinal: Diarrhea (81% to 89%), nausea (58% to 70%), vomiting (46% to 70%), abdominal pain (38%), anorexia (13%), hematemesis (13%), dysphagia (11%), gastrointestinal hemorrhage (11%)

Genitourinary: Urinary tract infection (14%)

Hepatic: Hyperbilirubinemia (30%)

Neuromuscular & skeletal: Weakness (66%), ostealgia (21%), arthralgia (11% to 21%), myalgia (18%)

Ophthalmic: Retinal hemorrhage (11%)

Renal: Increased blood urea nitrogen (23%), increased serum creatinine (15%)

Respiratory: Pharyngitis (23%), epistaxis (17%), dyspnea (15%)

Miscellaneous: Fever (81%)

1% to 10%:

Immunologic: Antibody development (2%)

Respiratory: Pleural effusion (1%)

<1%, postmarketing, and/or case reports: Anaphylaxis, capillary leak syndrome, cardiac arrhythmia, dizziness, eosinophilia, flushing, hypotension, hypoxia, injection site reaction, leukocytosis, liver function impairment (transient), pain, prolonged prothrombin time, respiratory distress, supraventricular cardiac arrhythmia, syncope, thrombocythemia, thrombosis

Drug Interactions

Metabolism/Transport Effects None known.

Avoid Concomitant Use There are no known interactions where it is recommended to avoid concomitant use.

Increased Effect/Toxicity

Sargramostim may increase the levels/effects of: Bleomycin

The levels/effects of Sargramostim may be increased by: Cyclophosphamide

Decreased Effect There are no known significant interactions involving a decrease in effect.

◄ **Storage/Stability**

Store intact vials at 2°C to 8°C (36°F to 46°F); do not freeze. Do not shake.

Solution for injection: May be stored for up to 20 days at 2°C to 8°C (36°F to 46°F) once the vial has been entered. Discard remaining solution after 20 days.

Powder for injection: Preparations made with SWFI should be administered as soon as possible, and discarded within 6 hours of reconstitution. Solutions reconstituted with bacteriostatic water may be stored for up to 20 days at 2°C to 8°C (36°F to 46°F); do not freeze. When combining previously reconstituted solutions with freshly reconstituted solutions, administer within 6 hours following preparation; the contents of vials reconstituted with different diluents should not be mixed together.

Preparation for Administration

Powder for injection: May be reconstituted with 1 mL of preservative free SWFI or bacteriostatic water for injection. Direct the diluent toward the side of the vial and gently swirl to reconstitute; do not shake. Do not mix the contents of vials which have been reconstituted with different diluents.

SubQ: Administer without further dilution.

IV: Further dilution with NS is required. If the final sargramostim concentration is <10 mcg/mL, 1 mg of human albumin per 1 mL of NS should be added (eg, add 1 mL of 5% human albumin per 50 mL of NS).

Mechanism of Action Sargramostim stimulates proliferation, differentiation, and functional activity of neutrophils, eosinophils, monocytes, and macrophages.

Pharmacodynamics/Kinetics

Onset of action: Increase in WBC in 7 to 14 days

Duration: WBCs return to baseline within 1 to 2 weeks of discontinuing drug

Half-life elimination:

Children 6 months to 15 years: IV: Median: 1.6 hours; range: 0.9 to 2.5 hours; SubQ: Median: 2.3 hours (0.3 to 3.8 hours) (Stute 1995)

Adults: IV: ~60 minutes; SubQ: ~2.7 hours

Time to peak, serum: SubQ: 1 to 3 hours

Dosing

Adult & Geriatric Note: May round the dose to the nearest vial size (Ozer 2000).

Acute myeloid leukemia (following induction chemotherapy): Adults ≥55 years: IV: 250 mcg/m^2/day (infused over 4 hours) starting approximately on day 11 or 4 days following the completion of induction chemotherapy (if day 10 bone marrow is hypoplastic with <5% blasts), continue until ANC >1,500/mm^3 for 3 consecutive days or a maximum of 42 days. If ANC >20,000/mm^3, interrupt treatment or reduce the dose by 50%.

If a second cycle of chemotherapy is necessary, administer ~4 days after the completion of chemotherapy if the bone marrow is hypoplastic with <5% blasts

Discontinue sargramostim immediately if leukemic regrowth occurs. If a severe adverse reaction occurs, reduce the dose by 50% or temporarily discontinue the dose until the reaction abates.

Bone marrow transplantation (allogeneic or autologous) failure or engraftment delay: IV: 250 mcg/m^2/day (infused over 2 hours) for 14 days; If engraftment has not occurred after 7 days off sargramostim, may repeat. If engraftment still has not occurred after 7 days off sargramostim, a third course of 500 mcg/m^2/day for 14 days may be attempted. If there is still no improvement, it is unlikely that further dose escalation will be of benefit.

If a severe adverse reaction occurs, reduce the dose by 50% or temporarily discontinue the dose until the reaction abates

If blast cells appear or disease progression occurs, discontinue treatment

If ANC >20,000 cells/mm^3, interrupt treatment or reduce the dose by 50%.

Myeloid reconstitution after allogeneic or autologous bone marrow transplantation: IV: 250 mcg/m^2/day (infused over 2 hours), begin 2 to 4 hours after the marrow infusion and ≥24 hours after chemotherapy or radiotherapy, when the post marrow infusion ANC is <500/mm^3, and continue until ANC >1,500/mm^3 for 3 consecutive days. If ANC >20,000/mm^3, interrupt treatment or reduce the dose by 50%.

If a severe adverse reaction occurs, reduce dose by 50% or temporarily discontinue the dose until the reaction abates

If blast cells appear or progression of the underlying disease occurs, discontinue treatment

Peripheral stem cell transplantation (autologous), mobilization: IV, SubQ: 250 mcg/m^2/day IV (infused over 24 hours) or SubQ once daily; continue the same dose throughout peripheral blood progenitor cell collection. If WBC >50,000/mm^3, reduce the dose by 50%.

Note: The optimal schedule for peripheral blood progenitor cell collection has not been established (usually begun by day 5 and performed daily until protocol specified targets are achieved). If adequate numbers of progenitor cells are not collected, consider other mobilization therapy.

Peripheral stem cell transplantation (autologous), post-transplant: IV, SubQ: 250 mcg/m^2/day IV (infused over 24 hours) or SubQ once daily beginning immediately following infusion of progenitor cells; continue until ANC is >1,500/mm^3 for 3 consecutive days.

Hematopoietic radiation injury syndrome, acute (off-label use): SubQ: 250 mcg/m^2/day; continue until ANC >1,000/mm^3 (Waselenko 2004). ASCO guidelines recommend initiating within 24 hours of exposure of a dose ≥2 gray (Gy) and/or significant decrease in absolute lymphocyte count, or for anticipated neutropenia <500/mm^3 for ≥7 days (Smith 2015).

Primary prophylaxis of neutropenia in patients receiving chemotherapy (outside transplant and AML) or who are at high risk for neutropenic fever (off-label use): SubQ: 250 mcg/m^2/day (may round to the nearest vial size [Ozer 2000]) beginning at least 24 hours after chemotherapy administration; continue until ANC >1,500/mm^3 for 3 consecutive days (Smith 2015).

Pediatric

Hematopoietic radiation injury syndrome, acute (off-label use): Children and Adolescents: SubQ: 250 mcg/m^2/day; continue until ANC >1,000/mm^3 (Waselenko 2004). ASCO guidelines recommend initiating within 24 hours of exposure of a dose ≥2 gray (Gy) and/or significant decrease in absolute lymphocyte count, or for anticipated neutropenia <500/mm^3 for ≥7 days (Smith 2015).

Neuroblastoma, high-risk (off-label use): Children and Adolescents: SubQ or IV: 250 mcg/m^2 once daily for 14 days, beginning 3 days prior to administration of dinutuximab (each cycle is 28 days); sargramostim is administered during cycles 1, 3, and 5 (regimen also includes dinutuximab, isotretinoin, and aldesleukin) (Yu 2010).

Renal Impairment There are no dosage adjustments provided in the manufacturer's labeling.

Hepatic Impairment There are no dosage adjustments provided in the manufacturer's labeling.

Combination Regimens

Leukemia, acute myeloid: MEC-G (AML Induction) on page 2170

Lymphoma, non-Hodgkin (Burkitt): CODOX-M/IVAC (NHL-Burkitt) on page 2068

Administration Sargramostim is administered as a subcutaneous injection or intravenous infusion.

IV: Infuse over 2 hours, 4 hours or 24 hours (indication specific). An in-line membrane filter should **NOT** be used for intravenous administration.

SubQ: Administer subcutaneously into the thigh, abdomen (avoiding navel/waistline), or outer upper arm; rotate injection sites. Do not inject into areas that are tender, bruised, red, or hard. Allow to reach room temperature 30 minutes prior to injection. Administer without further dilution.

Monitoring Parameters CBC with differential (twice weekly during treatment), renal/liver function tests (at least every 2 weeks in patients displaying renal or hepatic dysfunction prior to treatment initiation); pulmonary function; vital signs; hydration status; weight

Test Interactions May interfere with bone imaging studies; increased hematopoietic activity of the bone marrow may appear as transient positive bone imaging changes

Dosage Forms Excipient information presented when available (limited, particularly for generics); consult specific product labeling. [DSC] = Discontinued product

Solution, Injection:

Leukine: 500 mcg/mL (1 mL [DSC]) [contains benzyl alcohol]

Solution Reconstituted, Intravenous [preservative free]:

Leukine: 250 mcg (1 ea)

Siltuximab (sil TUX i mab)

Brand Names: US Sylvant

Brand Names: Canada Sylvant

Index Terms CNTO 328

Pharmacologic Category Antineoplastic Agent, Monoclonal Antibody; Interleukin-6 Receptor Antagonist

Use Castleman disease: Treatment of multicentric Castleman disease (MCD) in patients who are human immunodeficiency virus (HIV) negative and human herpesvirus-8 (HHV-8) negative

Limitations of use: Has not been studied in patients with MCD who are HIV positive or HHV-8 positive because in a nonclinical study, siltuximab did not bind to virally produced IL-6

Labeled Contraindications Severe hypersensitivity to siltuximab or any component of the formulation

Pregnancy Considerations Adverse events were not observed in animal reproduction studies. However, decreased globulin levels were detected in the pregnant animals and their offspring. Infants born to pregnant women treated with siltuximab may be at increased risk for infection. Use during pregnancy only if the potential benefit outweighs the possible risk to the fetus. Women of childbearing potential should use effective contraception during and for 3 months following treatment discontinuation.

Breastfeeding Considerations It is not known if siltuximab is excreted in breast milk. Because many immunoglobulins are excreted in breast milk and the potential for adverse reactions in the nursing infant exists, the manufacturer recommends a decision be made to discontinue nursing or to discontinue the drug, taking into account the importance of treatment to the mother.

Warnings/Precautions Discontinue infusion immediately (and permanently) if signs of anaphylaxis occur; do not reinitiate therapy. Discontinue in patients with severe infusion reaction, severe allergic reactions, or cytokine release syndromes. If a mild to moderate infusion reaction develops, temporarily discontinue the infusion; if the reaction resolves, may reinitiate at a lower infusion rate. Consider premedication with acetaminophen, antihistamines, and corticosteroids. If infusion-related reactions recur despite appropriate premedication and infusion rate reduction, discontinue therapy. Administer in a setting equipped to provide resuscitation equipment; medications for the treatment of hypersensitivity reactions (eg, bronchodilators, epinephrine, antihistamines, and corticosteroids) should be readily available. Siltuximab may mask signs and symptoms of infection, including signs of acute inflammation (eg, fever, C-reactive protein elevation). Do not administer to patients with severe infections (until infection resolves); monitor closely for infections and initiate appropriate anti-infective therapy if needed. If infection develops, withhold therapy until resolved. Siltuximab administration may result in elevated hemoglobin levels in patients with multicentric Castleman disease; monitor blood counts prior to each dose for the first 12 months and every 3 dosing cycles thereafter, or as clinically necessary. May require therapy interruption. Gastrointestinal perforation has been observed in clinical trials. Use with caution in patients at risk for perforation; promptly evaluate concerning symptoms. Do not administer live vaccines to patients receiving siltuximab; IL-6 inhibition may interfere with immune response to vaccination. Approved for use only in patients who are HIV negative and HHV-8 negative. Siltuximab was not studied in patients positive for these disease states due to the lack of drug binding to virally produced IL-6 in a nonclinical study. Potentially significant drug-drug interactions may exist, requiring dose or frequency adjustment, additional monitoring, and/or selection of alternative therapy.

Adverse Reactions

>10%:

Cardiovascular: Peripheral edema (16%)

Central nervous system: Fatigue (21%; long-term exposure)

Dermatologic: Pruritus (28%), skin rash (28%)

Endocrine & metabolic: Weight gain (19%), hyperuricemia (11%)

Gastrointestinal: Diarrhea (32%; long-term exposure), abdominal pain (12%)

Neuromuscular & skeletal: Arthralgia (21%; long-term exposure), limb pain (21%; long-term exposure)

Respiratory: Upper respiratory tract infection (26%; long-term exposure: 63%)

1% to 10%:

Cardiovascular: Hypotension (4% to 6%; grades 3/4: 2% [anaphylactic reaction])

Central nervous system: Headache (8%)

Dermatologic: Eczema (4%), psoriasis (4%), skin hyperpigmentation (4%), xeroderma (4%)

Endocrine & metabolic: Hypertriglyceridemia (8%), dehydration (4%), hyper-cholesterolemia (4%)

Gastrointestinal: Constipation (8%), decreased appetite (4%)

Hematologic & oncologic: Thrombocytopenia (9%)

Renal: Renal insufficiency (8%)

Respiratory: Lower respiratory tract infection (8%), oropharyngeal pain (8%)

Miscellaneous: Infusion related reaction (5%)

<1%: Anaphylaxis, antibody development (non-neutralizing)

Drug Interactions

Metabolism/Transport Effects None known.

Avoid Concomitant Use

Avoid concomitant use of Siltuximab with any of the following: BCG (Intravesical); Belimumab; Natalizumab; Pimecrolimus; Tacrolimus (Topical); Vaccines (Live)

Increased Effect/Toxicity

Siltuximab may increase the levels/effects of: Belimumab; Fingolimod; Leflunomide; Natalizumab; Tofacitinib; Vaccines (Live)

The levels/effects of Siltuximab may be increased by: Denosumab; Ocrelizumab; Pimecrolimus; Roflumilast; Tacrolimus (Topical); Trastuzumab

Decreased Effect

Siltuximab may decrease the levels/effects of: BCG (Intravesical); Coccidioides immitis Skin Test; CYP3A4 Substrates; Nivolumab; Sipuleucel-T; Tertomotide; Vaccines (Inactivated); Vaccines (Live)

The levels/effects of Siltuximab may be decreased by: Echinacea

Storage/Stability Store intact vials at 2°C to 8°C (36°F to 46°F); protect from light. Reconstituted solution should be further diluted in D5W for infusion within 2 hours; complete infusion within 4 hours of dilution of the reconstituted solution to the infusion container. Discard any unused portion of the reconstituted solution or solution diluted for infusion.

Preparation for Administration Allow intact vials to come to room temperature (~30 minutes) and remain at room temperature for the duration of preparation. Reconstitute with 5.2 mL (100 mg vial) or 20 mL (400 mg vial) SWFI to a final concentration of 20 mg/mL; gently swirl to fully dissolve powder (usually takes <60 minutes). Do not shake or swirl vigorously. Must further dilute within 2 hours to 250 mL with D5W (infusion bag must be made of polyvinyl chloride [PVC], polyolefin [PO], polypropylene [PP], or polyethylene [PE], or PE bottles may be used. After all solids are completely dissolved, remove a volume equal to the total calculated dose volume of reconstituted siltuximab from the bag of D5W; slowly add the appropriate volume of reconstituted siltuximab solution to the infusion bag and gently invert to mix. Complete infusion within 4 hours of dilution of the reconstituted solution to the infusion bag.

Mechanism of Action Chimeric monoclonal antibody which binds with high affinity and specificity to IL-6; prevents IL-6 from binding to both soluble and membrane-bound IL-6 receptors. Overproduction of IL-6 may lead to systemic manifestations in multicentric Castleman disease (MCD) patients by inducing C-reactive protein (CRP) synthesis (Kurzrock, 2010). Lowering serum IL-6 levels may improve systemic symptoms of Castleman disease.

Pharmacodynamics/Kinetics

Distribution: 4.5 L

Half-life elimination: ~21 days (range: 14.2 to 29.7 days)

Dosing

Adult & Geriatric Note: Consider delaying first dose if ANC <1000/mm^3, platelets <75,000/mm^3, and hemoglobin ≥17 g/dL; subsequent doses may be delayed if ANC <1000/mm^3, platelets <50,000/mm^3, and hemoglobin ≥17 g/dL. Do not reduce dose.

Castleman disease, multicentric (in patients who are HIV negative and HHV-8 negative): IV: 11 mg/kg over 1 hour every 3 weeks until treatment failure

Renal Impairment

CrCl ≥15 mL/minute: No initial dosage adjustment is necessary.

CrCl <15 mL/minute: There are no dosage adjustments provided in the manufacturer's labeling (has not been studied).

End-stage renal disease (ESRD): There are no dosage adjustments provided in the manufacturer's labeling (has not been studied).

Hepatic Impairment

Mild to moderate impairment (Child Pugh class A or B): No initial dosage adjustment is necessary.

Severe impairment (Child Pugh class C): There are no dosage adjustments provided in the manufacturer's labeling (has not been studied).

Adjustment for Toxicity

Hematologic toxicity: ANC <1000/mm^3, platelets <50,000/mm^3, and hemoglobin ≥17 g/dL: Consider delaying treatment until ANC ≥1000/mm^3, platelets ≥50,000/mm^3, and hemoglobin <17 g/dL

Anaphylaxis, cytokine release syndromes, and/or severe infusion-related or allergic reactions: Discontinue permanently.

Infection, severe: Withhold treatment until infection resolves.

Administration Administer IV over 1 hour using administration sets lined with polyvinyl chloride (PVC), polyurethane (PU), or polyethylene (PE), which contain a 0.2 micron inline polyethersulfone (PES) filter. Do not infuse in the same line with other medications. Complete infusion within 4 hours of dilution of the reconstituted solution to the infusion container.

Emetic Potential Minimal (<10%)

◀ **Monitoring Parameters** Monitor complete blood count with differential prior to each dose for the first 12 months and every 3 dosing cycles thereafter, or as clinically necessary; monitor for anaphylaxis and signs/symptoms of infusion-related, allergic, or cytokine release reactions; monitor for infection and signs/symptoms of gastrointestinal perforation.

Dosage Forms Excipient information presented when available (limited, particularly for generics); consult specific product labeling.

Solution Reconstituted, Intravenous [preservative free]:

Sylvant: 100 mg (1 ea); 400 mg (1 ea) [contains mouse (murine) and/or hamster protein, polysorbate 80]

◆ **Simulect** *see* Basiliximab *on page* 215

Sipuleucel-T (si pu LOO sel tee)

Brand Names: US Provenge

Index Terms APC8015; Prostate Cancer Vaccine, Cell-Based

Pharmacologic Category Cellular Immunotherapy, Autologous

Use Prostate cancer, metastatic: Treatment of asymptomatic or minimally symptomatic metastatic castrate-resistant (hormone-refractory) prostate cancer.

Labeled Contraindications There are no contraindications listed in the manufacturer's labeling.

Pregnancy Considerations Animal reproduction studies have not been conducted. Not indicated for use in women.

Breastfeeding Considerations Not indicated for use in women.

Warnings/Precautions For autologous use only; patient identity must be matched to the patient identifiers on the infusion bag and on the Final Product Disposition Notification (provided by manufacturer) prior to infusion; confirmation of product release must be received from the manufacturer prior to infusion.

Acute infusion reactions may occur within 1 day of infusion and are usually mild or moderate for most patients; the incidence of severe reaction may be higher with the second infusion, while the third infusion is associated with a decrease in the incidence of severe reactions. Premedication with oral acetaminophen and diphenhydramine is recommended. Depending on the severity of infusion reaction, interrupt or slow infusion rate; in clinical trials, acetaminophen, intravenous (IV) H_1 and/or H_2 antagonists, and low-dose meperidine were used to manage acute symptoms. Symptoms of acute infusion reaction may include chills, rigor, fever, bronchospasm, dyspnea, hypoxia, hypertension, tachycardia, syncope, hypotension, joint or muscle aches, nausea, vomiting, dizziness, fatigue, headache, and weakness; fever and chills usually resolved within 2 days. Observe patient for at least 30 minutes after infusion.

Cerebrovascular (hemorrhagic and ischemic stroke) and cardiovascular events (myocardial infarction [MI]) have occurred; transient ischemic attacks have been reported following infusion (postmarketing reports). Such events usually occurred in patients with multiple risk factors for cerebrovascular or cardiovascular incidents. Deep venous thrombosis (DVT) and pulmonary embolism occurred following sipuleucel-T infusion (postmarketing reports), usually in patients with multiple risk factors for thromboembolism. Use with caution in patients at risk for thromboembolic events. Closely monitor during infusion in patients with cardiac or pulmonary conditions. Concurrent use with immunosuppressives (eg, corticosteroids) has not been studied; may alter the efficacy and/or safety of sipuleucel-T. Carefully evaluate patients for appropriateness of reducing or discontinuing immunosuppressive agents prior to treatment. Concurrent use with chemotherapy has not been studied. In clinical trials, patients who had androgen deprivation therapy without prior bilateral orchiectomy were continued on gonadal suppression with a luteinizing hormone-releasing hormone (LHRH) agonist (Higano, 2009).

Apply universal precautions for product handling; sipuleucel-T is not routinely tested for transmissible infectious diseases; patient specific leukapheresis collection and activated product may have a risk for infectious disease transmission. Preliminary sterility testing is done based on a 2-day incubation period; final (7-day incubation) testing is not available until after administration; physicians will be notified if 7-day sterility tests are positive for microbial contamination. If unable to receive a scheduled reinfusion, an additional leukapheresis procedure may be required; advise patients of this possibility before treatment initiation.

Adverse Reactions Note: Initial infusion-related events usually present within the first 24 hours after administration.

>10%:

Central nervous system: Chills (53%; grades ≥3: 2%), fatigue (41%; grades ≥3: 1%), headache (18%; grades ≥3: <1%), dizziness (12%; grades ≥3: <1%), pain (12%)

Gastrointestinal: Nausea (22%; grades ≥3: <1%), vomiting (13% grades ≥3: <1%), constipation (12%; grades ≥3: <1%)

Hematologic: Anemia (13%)

Hypersensitivity: Severe infusion related reaction (71%; grade 3: 4%)

Neuromuscular & skeletal: Back pain (30%; grades ≥3: 3%), myalgia (12%; grades ≥3: <1%), weakness (11%; grades ≥3: 1%)

Miscellaneous: Fever (31%; grades ≥3: 1%), citrate toxicity (15%)

1% to 10%:

Cardiovascular: Hypertension (8% grades ≥3: <1%), hemorrhagic stroke (4%)

Dermatologic: Diaphoresis (5%; grades ≥3: <1%), skin rash (5%)

Gastrointestinal: Anorexia (7%), acute ischemic stroke (4%)

Genitourinary: Hematuria (8%)

Neuromuscular & skeletal: Musculoskeletal pain (9%; grades ≥3: <1%), muscle spasm (8%; grades ≥3: <1%), neck pain (6%), tremor (5%)

Renal: Hematuria (8%)

Respiratory: Flu-like symptoms (10%), dyspnea (9%; grades ≥3: 2%)

<1%, postmarketing, and/or case reports: Cerebrovascular accident, eosinophilia, hypotension, myasthenia gravis, myocardial infarction, myositis, paresthesia (grades ≥3), pulmonary embolism, rhabdomyolysis, sepsis, syncope, transient ischemic attacks, tumor flare, venous thrombosis

Drug Interactions

Metabolism/Transport Effects None known.

Avoid Concomitant Use There are no known interactions where it is recommended to avoid concomitant use.

Increased Effect/Toxicity There are no known significant interactions involving an increase in effect.

Decreased Effect

The levels/effects of Sipuleucel-T may be decreased by: Immunosuppressants

◄ **Storage/Stability** Do not remove the infusion bag from the insulated polyurethane container within the shipping box until administration (do not remove the insulated container from the shipping box, or open the lid of the insulated container, until administration). Product may only remain at room temperature for ≤3 hours once removed from shipping container; after removal from shipping container, do not return product to container. Infusion must begin prior to product expiration.

Preparation for Administration Sipuleucel-T will arrive as a prepared patient-specific 250 mL suspension in lactated Ringer's injection. Contents may appear clear to opaque and will be a white to red color, including shades of off-white, cream, light yellow, and orange. If clumps or clots are present, gently mix to resuspend. Do not administer if the bag leaks during handling, is damaged, or if clumps remain.

Mechanism of Action Autologous cellular immunotherapy which stimulates an immune response against an antigen (PAP) expressed in most prostate cancer tissues. Peripheral blood is collected (~3 days prior to infusion) from the patient via leukapheresis, from which peripheral blood mononuclear cells (PBMCs) are isolated. Antigen presenting cell (APC) precursors, consisting of CD54-positive cells that include dendritic cells, are isolated from the PBMCs. The APCs are then activated (*in vitro*) with a recombinant human fusion protein, PAP-GM-CSF (also termed PA2024), composed of an antigen specific for prostate cancer, prostatic acid phosphatase (PAP) linked to granulocyte-macrophage colony-stimulating factor (GM-CSF) and cultured for ~40 hours. The final product, sipuleucel-T, is reinfused into the patient, inducing T-cell immunity to tumors that express PAP.

Dosing

Adult & Geriatric Note: Premedicate with oral acetaminophen 650 mg and an antihistamine (eg, diphenhydramine 50 mg) ~30 minutes prior to infusion. For autologous use only. Do not infuse until confirmation of product release has been received from the company.

Prostate cancer, metastatic: IV: Each dose contains ≥50 million autologous CD54+ cells (obtained through leukapheresis) activated with PAP-GM-CSF; administer doses at ~2-week intervals for a total of 3 doses (Kantoff, 2010). If unable to receive a scheduled infusion, an additional leukapheresis procedure will be necessary prior to continuing a course of treatment.

Renal Impairment There are no dosage adjustments provided in the manufacturer's labeling.

Hepatic Impairment There are no dosage adjustments provided in the manufacturer's labeling.

Adjustment for Toxicity Acute infusion reaction: Interrupt or slow infusion rate (depending on the severity of infusion reaction); may require acetaminophen, IV H$_1$ and/or H$_2$ antagonists, or low-dose meperidine to manage acute symptoms.

Administration For autologous use only; the identity of the patient must be matched to the patient identifiers on the infusion bag and on the "Final Product Disposition Notification" prior to infusion. Do not infuse until confirmation of product release is received from the company. Keep the sealed infusion bag in the insulated polyurethane container inside the shipping box until ready for administration. Prior to infusion, inspect bag for signs of leaks (do not administer if leaking) or damage. Gently mix to resuspend contents; inspect for clumps or clotting; small clumps should disperse with the gentle mixing; do not administer if clumps remain. Infusion must begin prior to the expiration date and time; do **NOT** infuse if expired.

For IV infusion only. Infuse over ~60 minutes; infuse the entire contents of the bag. Do **NOT** use a cell filter for infusion. For acute infusion reaction, interrupt or slow infusion rate (depending on the severity of infusion reaction); may require acetaminophen, IV H$_1$ and/or H$_2$ antagonists, or low-dose meperidine to manage acute symptoms. If infusion is interrupted, keep infusion bag at room temperature; do not resume if bag is retained at room temperature for >3 hours. Observe patient for at least 30 minutes after infusion.

Monitoring Parameters Monitor for infusion reaction during and for at least 30 minutes after infusion; monitor closely during infusion for patients with cardiovascular and pulmonary disease; monitor for thromboembolic and vascular events.

Prescribing and Access Restrictions Patients may receive Sipuleucel-T at a participating site. Physicians must go through an inservice and register to prescribe the treatment; patients must also complete an enrollment form. Information on registration and enrollment is available at 1-877-336-3736.

Dosage Forms Excipient information presented when available (limited, particularly for generics); consult specific product labeling.

Suspension, Intravenous [preservative free]:

Provenge: (250 mL)

Sirolimus (sir OH li mus)

Related Information

Hematopoietic Cell Transplantation *on page* 2365
Safe Handling of Hazardous Drugs *on page* 2379

Brand Names: US Rapamune

Brand Names: Canada Rapamune

Index Terms Rapamycin

Pharmacologic Category Immunosuppressant Agent; mTOR Kinase Inhibitor

Use

Lymphangioleiomyomatosis: Treatment of lymphangioleiomyomatosis. Therapeutic drug monitoring is recommended for all patients receiving sirolimus.

Renal transplantation (rejection prophylaxis): Prophylaxis of organ rejection in patients receiving renal transplants (in low-to-moderate immunologic risk patients in combination with cyclosporine and corticosteroids with cyclosporine withdrawn 2 to 4 months after transplant, and in high immunologic risk patients in combination with cyclosporine and corticosteroids for the first year after transplant). Therapeutic drug monitoring is recommended for all patients receiving sirolimus. High immunologic risk renal transplant patients are defined (per the manufacturer's labeling) as Black transplant recipients and/or repeat renal transplant recipients who lost a previous allograft based on an immunologic process and/or patients with high PRA (panel-reactive antibodies; peak PRA level >80%).

Limitations of use (renal transplantation): Cyclosporine withdrawal has not been studied in patients with Banff grade 3 acute rejection or vascular rejection prior to cyclosporine withdrawal, patients who are dialysis-dependent, patients with serum creatinine >4.5 mg/dL, Black patients, patients with multiorgan transplants or secondary transplants, or those with high levels of PRA. In patients at high immunologic risk, the safety and efficacy of sirolimus used in combination with cyclosporine and cortico-steroids have not been studied beyond 1 year; therefore, after the first 12 months following transplantation, consider any adjustments to the immu-nosuppressive regimen on the basis of the clinical status of the patient. The safety and efficacy of sirolimus have not been established in patients younger than 13 years or in pediatric renal transplant patients younger than 18 years who are considered at high immunologic risk. The Kidney Disease: Improving Global Outcomes (KDIGO) guidelines for the care of renal transplant recipients recommend not initiating sirolimus until graft function has been established and surgical wounds have healed (KDIGO 2009). Avoid the use of sirolimus in combination with calcineurin inhibitors, particularly in the early post transplant period due to an increased risk of nephrotoxicity (KDIGO 2009; Webster 2006).

Labeled Contraindications Hypersensitivity to sirolimus or any component of the formulation

Pregnancy Considerations Adverse events have been observed in animal reproduction studies. Effective contraception must be initiated before therapy with sirolimus and continued for 12 weeks after discontinuation.

The National Transplantation Pregnancy Registry (NTPR) is a registry which follows pregnancies which occur in maternal transplant recipients or those fathered by male transplant recipients. The NTPR encourages reporting of pregnancies following solid organ transplant by contacting them at 877-955-6877 or NTPR@giftoflifeinstitute.org.

Breastfeeding Considerations It is not known if sirolimus is excreted in breast milk. Due to the potential for serious adverse reactions in the nursing infant, the manufacturer recommends a decision be made whether to dis-continue nursing or to discontinue the drug, taking into account the importance of treatment to the mother.

Warnings/Precautions [US Boxed Warning]: Immunosuppressive agents, including sirolimus, increase the risk of infection and may be associated with the development of lymphoma. Immune suppression may also increase the risk of opportunistic infections including activation of latent viral infections (including BK virus-associated nephropathy), fatal infections, and sepsis. Prophylactic treatment for *Pneumocystis jirovecii* pneumonia (PCP) should be administered for 1 year post-transplant; prophylaxis for cytomegalovirus (CMV) should be taken for 3 months post-transplant in patients at risk for CMV. Progressive multifocal leukoencephalopathy (PML), an opportunistic CNS infection caused by reactivation of the JC virus, has been reported in patients receiving immunosuppressive therapy, including sirolimus. Clinical findings of PML include apathy, ataxia, cognitive deficiency, confusion, and hemiparesis; promptly evaluate any patient presenting with neurological changes; consider decreasing the degree of immunosuppression with consideration to the risk of organ rejection in transplant patients.

[US Boxed Warning]: Sirolimus is not recommended for use in liver or lung transplantation. Bronchial anastomotic dehiscence cases have been reported in lung transplant patients when sirolimus was used as part of an immunosuppressive regimen; most of these reactions were fatal. Studies indicate an association with an increased risk of hepatic artery thrombosis (HAT), graft failure, and increased mortality (with evidence of infection) in liver transplant patients when sirolimus is used in combination with cyclosporine and/or tacrolimus. Most cases of HAT occurred within 30 days of transplant.

In renal transplant patients, *de novo* use without cyclosporine has been associated with higher rates of acute rejection. Sirolimus should be used in combination with cyclosporine (and corticosteroids) initially when used in renal transplant patients. Cyclosporine may be withdrawn in low-to-moderate immunologic risk patients after 2 to 4 months, in conjunction with an increase in sirolimus dosage. In high immunologic risk patients, use in combination with cyclosporine and corticosteroids is recommended for the first year. Safety and efficacy of combination therapy with cyclosporine in high immunologic risk patients has not been studied beyond 12 months of treatment; adjustment of immunosuppressive therapy beyond 12 months should be considered based on clinical judgment. Monitor renal function closely when combined with cyclosporine; consider dosage adjustment or discontinue in patients with increasing serum creatinine.

May increase serum creatinine and decrease GFR. Use caution when used concurrently with medications which may alter renal function. May delay recovery of renal function in patients with delayed allograft function. Increased urinary protein excretion has been observed when converting renal transplant patients from calcineurin inhibitors to sirolimus during maintenance therapy. A higher level of proteinuria prior to sirolimus conversion correlates with a higher degree of proteinuria after conversion. In some patients, proteinuria may reach nephrotic levels; nephrotic syndrome (new onset) has been reported. Increased risk of BK viral-associated nephropathy which may impair renal function and cause graft loss; consider decreasing immunosuppressive burden if evidence of deteriorating renal function.

Use caution with hepatic impairment; a reduction in the maintenance dose is recommended. Has been associated with an increased risk of fluid accumulation and lymphocele; peripheral edema, lymphedema, ascites, and pleural and pericardial effusions (including significant effusions and tamponade) were reported; use with caution in patients in whom fluid accumulation may be poorly tolerated, such as in cardiovascular disease (heart failure or hypertension) and pulmonary disease. Cases of interstitial lung disease (ILD) (eg, pneumonitis, bronchiolitis obliterans organizing pneumonia [BOOP], pulmonary fibrosis) have been observed (some fatal); may be associated with pulmonary hypertension (including pulmonary arterial hypertension) and risk may be increased with higher trough levels. ILD may resolve with dose reduction or discontinuation of therapy. Potentially significant drug-drug interactions may exist, requiring dose or frequency adjustment, additional monitoring, and/or selection of alternative therapy. Concurrent use with a calcineurin inhibitor (cyclosporine, tacrolimus) may increase the risk of calcineurin inhibitor-induced hemolytic uremic syndrome/thrombotic thrombocytopenic purpura/thrombotic microangiopathy (HUS/TTP/TMA). Immunosuppressants may affect response to vaccination. Therefore, during treatment with sirolimus, vaccination may be less effective. The use of live vaccines should be avoided.

Hypersensitivity reactions, including anaphylactic/anaphylactoid reactions, angioedema, exfoliative dermatitis, and hypersensitivity vasculitis have been reported. Angioedema risk is increased in patients with elevated sirolimus levels and/or concurrent use with other drugs known to cause angioedema (eg, ACE inhibitors). Angioedema resolved following discontinuation or dose reduction in some cases. Immunosuppressant therapy is associated with an increased risk of skin cancer; limit sun and ultraviolet light exposure; use appropriate sun protection. May increase serum lipids (cholesterol and

◀ triglycerides); use with caution in patients with hyperlipidemia; monitor cholesterol/lipids; if hyperlipidemia occurs, follow current guidelines for management (diet, exercise, lipid lowering agents); antihyperlipidemic therapy may not be effective in normalizing levels. May be associated with wound dehiscence and impaired healing; use caution in the perioperative period. Patients with a body mass index (BMI) >30 kg/m^2 are at increased risk for abnormal wound healing.

Sirolimus tablets and oral solution are not bioequivalent, due to differences in absorption. Clinical equivalence was seen using 2 mg tablet and 2 mg solution. It is not known if higher doses are also clinically equivalent. Monitor sirolimus levels if changes in dosage forms are made. Some dosage forms may contain propylene glycol; large amounts are potentially toxic and have been associated hyperosmolality, lactic acidosis, seizures, and respiratory depression; use caution (AAP, 1997; Zar 2007). **[US Boxed Warning]: Should only be used by physicians experienced in immunosuppressive therapy and management of transplant patients. Adequate laboratory and supportive medical resources must be readily available.** Sirolimus concentrations are dependent on the assay method (eg, chromatographic and immunoassay) used; assay methods are not interchangeable. Variations in methods to determine sirolimus whole blood concentrations, as well as interlaboratory variations, may result in improper dosage adjustments, which may lead to subtherapeutic or toxic levels. Determine the assay method used to assure consistency (or accommodations if changes occur), and for monitoring purposes, be aware of alterations to assay method or reference range and that values from different assays may not be interchangeable.

Adverse Reactions Incidence of many adverse effects is dose related. Reported events exclusive to renal transplant patients unless otherwise noted. Frequency not always defined.

Cardiovascular: Peripheral edema (≥20% to 58%, LAM and renal transplants), hypertension (49%), edema (18% to 20%), chest pain (LAM), deep vein thrombosis, pulmonary embolism, tachycardia

Central nervous system: Headache (≥20% to 34%, LAM and renal transplants), pain (29% to 33%), dizziness (LAM)

Dermatologic: Acne vulgaris (≥20% to 22%, LAM and renal transplants), skin rash (10% to 20%)

Endocrine & metabolic: Hypertriglyceridemia (45% to 57%), hypercholesterolemia (≥20% to 46%, LAM and renal transplants), amenorrhea, diabetes mellitus, hypermenorrhea, hypervolemia, hypokalemia, increased lactate dehydrogenase, menstrual disease, ovarian cyst

Gastrointestinal: Constipation (36% to 38%), abdominal pain (≥20% to 36%, LAM and renal transplants), diarrhea (≥20% to 35%, LAM and renal transplants), nausea (≥20% to 31%, LAM and renal transplants), stomatitis (3% to >20%)

Genitourinary: Urinary tract infection (33%)

Hematologic & oncologic: Anemia (23% to 33%), thrombocytopenia (14% to 30%), lymphoproliferative disorder (≤3%; including lymphoma), skin carcinoma (≤3%; includes basal cell carcinoma, squamous cell carcinoma, melanoma), hemolytic-uremic syndrome, leukopenia, lymphocele, thrombotic thrombocytopenic purpura

Infection: Herpes simplex infection, herpes zoster, sepsis

Neuromuscular & skeletal: Arthralgia (25% to 31%), myalgia (LAM), osteonecrosis

Renal: Increased serum creatinine (39% to 40%), pyelonephritis

Respiratory: Nasopharyngitis (LAM), epistaxis, pneumonia, upper respiratory tract infection (LAM)

Miscellaneous: Wound healing impairment

<3%, postmarketing, and/or case reports: Abnormal hepatic function tests, anaphylactoid reaction, anaphylaxis, angioedema, ascites, azoospermia, cardiac tamponade, cytomegalovirus, dehiscence (fascial), Epstein-Barr infection, exfoliative dermatitis, fluid retention, focal segmental glomerulosclerosis, gingival hyperplasia, hepatic necrosis, hepatotoxicity, hyperglycemia, hypersensitivity angiitis, hypersensitivity reaction, hypophosphatemia, incisional hernia, increased serum ALT, increased serum AST, increased susceptibility to infection (including opportunistic), interstitial pulmonary disease (dose related; includes pneumonitis, pulmonary fibrosis, and bronchiolitis obliterans organizing pneumonia with no identified infectious etiology), joint disorders, lymphedema, Merkel cell carcinoma, mycobacterium infection, nephrotic syndrome, neutropenia, pancreatitis, pancytopenia, pericardial effusion, pleural effusion, pneumonia due to *Pneumocystis carinii*, progressive multifocal leukoencephalopathy, proteinuria, pseudomembranous colitis, pulmonary alveolitis, pulmonary hemorrhage, renal disease (BK virus-associated), reversible posterior leukoencephalopathy syndrome, tuberculosis, weight loss, wound dehiscence

Drug Interactions

Metabolism/Transport Effects Substrate of CYP3A4 (major), P-glycoprotein; **Note:** Assignment of Major/Minor substrate status based on clinically relevant drug interaction potential

Avoid Concomitant Use

Avoid concomitant use of Sirolimus with any of the following: Antihepaciviral Combination Products; BCG (Intravesical); Conivaptan; Crizotinib; Deferiprone; Dipyrone; Enzalutamide; Fusidic Acid (Systemic); Grapefruit Juice; Idelalisib; MiFEPRIStone; Natalizumab; Pimecrolimus; Posaconazole; Tacrolimus (Systemic); Tacrolimus (Topical); Vaccines (Live); Voriconazole

Increased Effect/Toxicity

Sirolimus may increase the levels/effects of: ACE Inhibitors; CloZAPine; CycloSPORINE (Systemic); Deferiprone; Fingolimod; Leflunomide; Natalizumab; Tacrolimus (Systemic); Tacrolimus (Topical); Tofacitinib; Vaccines (Live); Verapamil

The levels/effects of Sirolimus may be increased by: Antihepaciviral Combination Products; Aprepitant; Boceprevir; Clotrimazole (Topical); Conivaptan; Crizotinib; CycloSPORINE (Systemic); CYP3A4 Inhibitors (Moderate); CYP3A4 Inhibitors (Strong); Dasatinib; Denosumab; DilTIAZem; Dipyrone; Fluconazole; Fosaprepitant; Fusidic Acid (Systemic); Grapefruit Juice; Idelalisib; Isavuconazonium Sulfate; Itraconazole; Ketoconazole (Systemic); Macrolide Antibiotics; Micafungin; MiFEPRIStone; Nelfinavir; Netupitant; Ocrelizumab; Palbociclib; P-glycoprotein/ABCB1 Inhibitors; Pimecrolimus; Posaconazole; Promazine; Ranolazine; Roflumilast; Stiripentol; Tacrolimus (Systemic); Tacrolimus (Topical); Telaprevir; Trastuzumab; Venetoclax; Verapamil; Voriconazole

Decreased Effect

Sirolimus may decrease the levels/effects of: Antidiabetic Agents; BCG (Intravesical); Coccidioides immitis Skin Test; Nivolumab; Sipuleucel-T; Tacrolimus (Systemic); Tertomotide; Vaccines (Inactivated); Vaccines (Live)

◀ *The levels/effects of Sirolimus may be decreased by:* Bosentan; CYP3A4 Inducers (Moderate); CYP3A4 Inducers (Strong); Dabrafenib; Deferasirox; Echinacea; Efavirenz; Enzalutamide; Mitotane; Sarilumab; Siltuximab; St John's Wort; Tocilizumab

Food Interactions Grapefruit juice may decrease clearance of sirolimus. Ingestion with high-fat meals decreases peak concentrations but increases AUC by 23% to 35%. Management: Avoid grapefruit juice. Take consistently (either with or without food) to minimize variability.

Hazardous Drugs Handling Considerations

Hazardous agent (NIOSH 2016 [group 2]).

Use appropriate precautions for receiving, handling, administration, and disposal. Gloves (single) should be worn during receiving, unpacking, and placing in storage. NIOSH recommends single gloving for administration of intact tablets or capsules. NIOSH recommends double gloving, a protective gown, and (if there is a potential for vomit or spit up) eye/face protection for administration of an oral liquid/feeding tube administration (NIOSH 2016).

Storage/Stability

Oral solution: Store at 2°C to 8°C (36°F to 46°F). Protect from light. A slight haze may develop in refrigerated solutions, but the quality of the product is not affected. After opening, solution should be used within 1 month. If necessary, may be stored at temperatures up to 25°C (77°F) for ≤15 days after opening. Product may be stored in amber syringe for a maximum of 24 hours (at room temperature or refrigerated). Discard syringe after single use. Solution should be used immediately following dilution.

Tablet: Store at 20°C to 25°C (68°F to 77°F). Protect from light.

Mechanism of Action Sirolimus inhibits T-lymphocyte activation and proliferation in response to antigenic and cytokine stimulation and inhibits antibody production. Its mechanism differs from other immunosuppressants. Sirolimus binds to FKBP-12, an intracellular protein, to form an immunosuppressive complex which inhibits the regulatory kinase, mTOR (mechanistic target of rapamycin). This inhibition suppresses cytokine mediated T-cell proliferation, halting progression from the G1 to the S phase of the cell cycle. It inhibits acute rejection of allografts and prolongs graft survival.

In lymphangioleiomyomatosis, the mTOR signaling pathway is activated through the loss of the tuberous sclerosis complex (TSC) gene function (resulting in cellular proliferation and release of lymphangiogenic growth factors). By inhibiting the mTOR pathway, sirolimus prevents the proliferation of lymphangioleiomyomatosis cells.

Pharmacodynamics/Kinetics

Absorption: Rapid

Distribution: 12 L/kg (range: 4 to 20 L/kg)

Protein binding: ~92%, primarily to albumin

Metabolism: Extensive; in intestinal wall via P-glycoprotein and hepatic via CYP3A4 to 7 major metabolites

Bioavailability: Oral solution: 14%; Oral tablet: 27% higher relative to the oral solution; oral solution and tablets are not bioequivalent however, clinical equivalence shown at 2 mg dose

Half-life elimination:

Children: 13.7 ± 6.2 hours

Adults: Mean: 62 hours (range: 46 to 78 hours); extended in hepatic impairment (Child-Pugh class A or B) to 113 hours

Time to peak: Oral solution: 1 to 3 hours; Tablet: 1 to 6 hours

Excretion: Feces (91% due to P-glycoprotein-mediated efflux into gut lumen); urine (2%)

Dosing

Adult & Geriatric

Lymphangioleiomyomatosis: Adults: Oral: Initial: 2 mg once daily. Obtain trough concentration in 10 to 20 days; adjust dose to maintain a target concentration of 5 to 15 ng/mL.

Dosage adjustment for lymphangioleiomyomatosis: Once the maintenance dose is adjusted, further adjustments should be made at 7- to 14-day intervals to account for the long half-life of sirolimus. In general, dose proportionality may be assumed. New sirolimus dose **equals** current dose **multiplied by** (target concentration **divided by** current concentration). Once a stable dose is achieved, trough concentrations should be assessed at least every 3 months.

Renal transplant (rejection prophylaxis): Oral:

Low-to-moderate immunologic risk:

<40 kg: Loading dose: 3 mg/m^2 on day 1, followed by maintenance dosing of 1 mg/m^2 once daily

≥40 kg: Loading dose: 6 mg on day 1; maintenance: 2 mg once daily

High immunologic risk: Loading dose: Up to 15 mg on day 1; maintenance: 5 mg/day; obtain trough concentration between days 5 to 7 and adjust accordingly. Continue concurrent cyclosporine/sirolimus/corticosteroid therapy for 1 year following transplantation. Further adjustment of the regimen must be based on clinical status.

Dosage adjustment for renal transplantation: Sirolimus dosages should be adjusted in small increments to maintain 24-hour trough concentrations within desired range based on risk and concomitant therapy. Dosage should be adjusted at intervals of 7 to 14 days to account for the long half-life of sirolimus. Maximum loading dose: 40 mg/day (although typical loading doses are not generally this high). Whole blood concentrations should not be used as the sole basis for dosage adjustment (monitor clinical signs/symptoms, tissue biopsy, and laboratory parameters).

Maintenance therapy after withdrawal of cyclosporine: According to the manufacturer, cyclosporine withdrawal is not recommended in high immunological risk renal transplant patients. Following 2 to 4 months of combined therapy, withdrawal of cyclosporine may be considered in low-to-moderate immunologic risk patients. Cyclosporine should be discontinued over 4 to 8 weeks, and a necessary increase in the dosage of sirolimus (up to fourfold) should be anticipated due to removal of metabolic inhibition by cyclosporine and to maintain adequate immunosuppressive effects. Dose-adjusted trough target concentrations are typically 16 to 24 ng/mL for the first year post-transplant and 12 to 20 ng/mL thereafter (per the manufacturer; measured by chromatographic methodology). Target trough concentrations of ~5 to 15 ng/mL are often used in clinical practice (Kahan 2000; Stenton 2005); refer to specific institutional protocol for target sirolimus trough concentrations.

Graft-versus-host disease (GVHD) (off-label use): Oral:

GVHD (prevention): 12 mg loading dose on day -3, followed by 4 mg daily (target trough level: 3 to 12 ng/mL); taper off after 6 to 9 months (Armand 2008; Cutler 2007). Additional trials may be necessary to further define the role of sirolimus in this condition.

◀ **Treatment of refractory acute GVHD:** 4 to 5 mg/m^2 for 14 days (no loading dose) (Benito 2001). Additional trials may be necessary to further define the role of sirolimus in this condition.

Treatment of chronic GVHD: 6 mg loading dose, followed by 2 mg daily (target trough level: 7 to 12 ng/mL) for 6 to 9 months (Couriel 2005). Additional trials may be necessary to further define the role of sirolimus in this condition.

Heart transplantation (prophylaxis of organ rejection and allograft vasculopathy) (off-label use): Oral: **Note:** The use of sirolimus in the immediate post-cardiac transplant period (ie, *de novo* heart transplant) as a primary immunosuppressant has fallen out of favor due to adverse effects (eg, impaired wound healing and infection); however, patients may be converted to sirolimus from a calcineurin inhibitor (after at least 6 months from time of transplant [Costanzo 2010]).

Conversion from a calcineurin inhibitor (CNI) (ie, cyclosporine, tacrolimus): Reduce cyclosporine by 25 mg twice daily or tacrolimus by 1 mg twice daily followed by initiation of sirolimus 1 mg once daily; adjust sirolimus dose to target trough level of 8 to 14 ng/mL, withdraw CNI, repeat biopsy 2 weeks after CNI withdrawal (Topilsky 2012). Alternatively, maintain CNI concentrations and initiate sirolimus 1 mg once daily for 1 week; adjust sirolimus to target trough levels of 10 to 15 ng/mL over 2 weeks, then reduce CNI to target 50% of therapeutic concentrations and after 2 weeks evaluate for rejection. If no rejection, continue same regimen for an additional month, then reduce CNI to 25% of therapeutic concentrations with repeat biopsy 2 weeks later; if no rejection, may discontinue CNI after 2 weeks and continue to maintain sirolimus trough levels of 10 to 15 ng/mL (usual doses required to maintain target levels: 1 to 8 mg daily) (Kushwaha 2005). Refer to specific institutional protocol for target sirolimus trough concentrations; trough will vary based on time from transplant, assay method, and concurrent or transitioning therapies.

Conversion from antiproliferative immunosuppressive drug (ie, azathioprine or mycophenolate) while maintaining calcineurin inhibitor: Upon discontinuation of antiproliferative, administer sirolimus 6 mg loading dose followed by 2 mg once daily titrated to a target trough level of 4 to 15 ng/mL (Mancini 2003) or 4 to 12 ng/mL per ISHLT recommendations (Costanzo 2010).

Lung transplantation (rejection prophylaxis) (off-label use): Oral: Initial loading dose: 5 mg once, followed by a maintenance dose of 3 mg once daily; titrate to a target trough level of 5 to 13 ng/mL (Snell 2002). Do not initiate sirolimus until after the bronchial anastomosis has completely healed (approximately 90 days) due to potential fatal airway dehiscence with earlier initiation (King-Biggs 2003). Additional trials may be necessary to further define the role of sirolimus in this condition.

Renal angiomyolipoma (off-label use): Oral: Initial: 0.5 mg/m^2 once daily titrated to a target trough level of 3 to 6 ng/mL (may increase to target trough level of 6 to 10 ng/mL if <10% reduction in lesion diameters at 2 months) for 2 years (Davies 2011)

Pediatric Renal transplant (rejection prophylaxis): Low-to-moderate immunologic risk: Adolescents ≥13 years: Oral: Refer to adult dosing.

Renal Impairment No dosage adjustment is necessary. However, adjustment of regimen (including discontinuation of therapy) should be considered when used concurrently with cyclosporine and elevated or increasing serum creatinine is noted.

Hepatic Impairment

Loading dose: No dosage adjustment is necessary.

Maintenance dose:

Mild to moderate impairment (Child-Pugh classes A and B): Reduce maintenance dose by ~33%.

Severe impairment (Child-Pugh class C): Reduce maintenance dose by ~50%.

Administration Administer consistently (either with or without food). *Renal transplant:* Sirolimus should be taken 4 hours after oral cyclosporine (Neoral or Gengraf).

Solution: Mix (by stirring vigorously) with at least 60 mL of water or orange juice. No other liquids should be used for dilution. Patient should drink diluted solution immediately. The cup should then be refilled with an additional 120 mL of water or orange juice, stirred vigorously, and the patient should drink the contents at once.

Tablet: Do not crush, split, or chew.

Monitoring Parameters Monitor LFTs and CBC during treatment. Monitor sirolimus levels in all patients (especially in pediatric patients, patients ≥13 years of age weighing <40 kg, patients with hepatic impairment, or on concurrent potent inhibitors or inducers of CYP3A4 or P-gp, and/or if cyclosporine dosing is markedly reduced or discontinued), and when changing dosage forms of sirolimus. Also monitor serum cholesterol and triglycerides, blood pressure, serum creatinine, and urinary protein. Serum drug concentrations should be determined 3 to 4 days after loading doses and 7 to 14 days after dosage adjustments for renal transplant patients; however, these concentrations should not be used as the sole basis for dosage adjustment, especially during withdrawal of cyclosporine (monitor clinical signs/symptoms, tissue biopsy, and laboratory parameters). Monitor serum trough concentration 10 to 20 days after initiating therapy for lymphangioleiomyomatosis and 7 to 14 days after dosage adjustments. Once a stable dose is achieved, trough concentrations should be assessed at least every 3 months. **Note:** Concentrations and ranges are dependent on and will vary with assay methodology (chromatographic or immunoassay); assay methods are not interchangeable.

Medication Guide Available Yes

Dosage Forms Excipient information presented when available (limited, particularly for generics); consult specific product labeling.

Solution, Oral:

Rapamune: 1 mg/mL (60 mL) [contains alcohol, usp]

Tablet, Oral:

Rapamune: 0.5 mg, 1 mg, 2 mg

Generic: 0.5 mg, 1 mg, 2 mg

Dosage Forms: Canada Information with regard to form, strength, and availability of products uniquely available in Canada but currently not available in the US. Refer also to Dosage Forms.

Excipient information presented when available (limited, particularly for generics); consult specific product labeling.

Tablet, Oral:

Rapamune: 5 mg

◆ **Sitavig** *see* Acyclovir (Topical) *on page 56*

◆ **SKF 104864** *see* Topotecan *on page 1790*

◆ **SKF 104864-A** *see* Topotecan *on page 1790*

◆ **SKI-606** *see* Bosutinib *on page 281*

Sodium Thiosulfate (SOW dee um thye oh SUL fate)

Related Information

Management of Drug Extravasations *on page 2271*

Index Terms Disodium Thiosulfate Pentahydrate; Pentahydrate; Sodium Hyposulfate; Sodium Thiosulphate; Thiosulfuric Acid Disodium Salt

Pharmacologic Category Antidote; Antidote, Extravasation

Use Cyanide poisoning: Treatment of acute, life-threatening cyanide poisoning in combination with sodium nitrite. Consider consultation with a poison control center at 1-800-222-1222.

Labeled Contraindications There are no contraindications listed within the manufacturer's labeling.

Pregnancy Considerations Teratogenic effects were not observed in animal reproduction studies of sodium thiosulfate. In general, medications used as antidotes should take into consideration the health and prognosis of the mother; antidotes should be administered to pregnant women if there is a clear indication for use and should not be withheld because of fears of teratogenicity (Bailey 2003).

Breastfeeding Considerations It is not known if sodium thiosulfate is excreted in breast milk. Because sodium thiosulfate may be used as an antidote in life-threatening situations, breastfeeding is not a contraindication to use. It is not known when breastfeeding may safely be restarted following administration; the manufacturer recommends caution be used following administration to nursing women.

Warnings/Precautions Due to the risk for serious adverse effects, use with caution in patients where the diagnosis of cyanide poisoning is uncertain. However, if clinical suspicion of cyanide poisoning is high, treatment should not be delayed. Treatment of cyanide poisoning should include external decontamination and supportive therapy. Collection of pretreatment blood cyanide concentrations does not preclude administration and should not delay administration in the emergency management of highly suspected or confirmed cyanide toxicity. Pretreatment levels may be useful as postinfusion levels may be inaccurate. Monitor patients for return of symptoms for 24-48 hours; repeat treatment (one-half the original dose) should be administered if symptoms return. Fire victims may present with both cyanide and carbon monoxide poisoning. In these patients, the induction of methemoglobinemia with amyl nitrite or sodium nitrite is contraindicated until carbon monoxide levels return to normal due to the risk of tissue hypoxia. Methemoglobinemia decreases the oxygen-carrying capacity of hemoglobin and the presence of carbon monoxide prevents hemoglobin from releasing oxygen to the tissues. In this scenario, sodium thiosulfate may be used alone to promote the clearance of cyanide. Hydroxocobalamin, however, should be considered to avoid the nitrite-related problems and because sodium thiosulfate has a slow onset of action. Hydroxocobalamin, however, should be considered to avoid the nitrite-related problems and because sodium thiosulfate has a slow onset of action. Consider consultation with a poison control center at 1-800-222-1222.

The presence of sulfite hypersensitivity should not preclude the use of this medication.

Adverse Reactions Frequency not defined

Cardiovascular: Hypotension

Central nervous system: Disorientation, flushing sensation, headache, salty taste

Gastrointestinal: Nausea, vomiting

Hematologic & oncologic: Prolonged bleeding time

Drug Interactions

Metabolism/Transport Effects None known.

Avoid Concomitant Use There are no known interactions where it is recommended to avoid concomitant use.

Increased Effect/Toxicity There are no known significant interactions involving an increase in effect.

Decreased Effect There are no known significant interactions involving a decrease in effect.

Storage/Stability Store at 20°C to 25°C (68°F to 77°F); excursions permitted to 15°C to 30°C (59°F to 86°F). Protect from light. Do not freeze.

Extravasation management (off-label use/route): Store the 1/6 M solution for SubQ administration at 15°C to 30°C (59°F to 86°F) (Polovich 2009).

Preparation for Administration

Calciphylaxis (off-label use): May dilute dose in 100 mL of NS (Nigwekar 2013)

Extravasation management (off-label use/route): To prepare a 1/6 M solution for SubQ administration (off-label route), add 4 mL of a 10% sodium thiosulfate solution to 6 mL SWFI or 1.6 mL of a 25% sodium thiosulfate solution to 8.4 mL SWFI (Polovich 2009).

Mechanism of Action

Cyanide toxicity: Serves as a sulfur donor in rhodanese-catalyzed formation of thiocyanate (much less toxic than cyanide)

Extravasation management: Neutralizes the reactive species of mechlorethamine; reduces the formation of hydroxyl radicals which cause tissue injury

Pharmacodynamics/Kinetics

Half-life elimination: Thiosulfate: ~3 hours (Howland 2011); Thiocyanate: ~3 days; Renal impairment: ≤9 days

Excretion: Urine (~20% to 50% as unchanged drug)

Dosing

Adult

Cyanide poisoning: IV: **Note:** Administer in conjunction with sodium nitrite. Administer sodium nitrite first, followed immediately by the administration of sodium thiosulfate: 12.5 g (50 mL of a 25% solution); may repeat at one-half the original dose if symptoms of cyanide toxicity return

Note: Monitor the patient for 24 to 48 hours; if symptoms return, repeat both sodium nitrite and sodium thiosulfate at one-half the original doses.

Calciphylaxis (off-label use): IV: **Note:** Optimal dose is not established.

◀

> *Dialysis patients:* 25 g administered 3 times per week during the last hour of or after the hemodialysis session. Therapy should continue until there is complete resolution of symptoms (Ackermann 2007; Auriemma 2011; Cicone 2004; Nigwekar 2013; Subramaniam 2008).
>
> *Patients not on dialysis (normal renal function or mildly reduced GFR):* 25 g administered 3 times per week (Baker 2007; Hackett 2011).

Extravasation management (off-label use):

Mechlorethamine: SubQ (off-label route): Inject 2 mL of a 1/6 M (~4%) sodium thiosulfate solution (into the extravasation site) for each mg of mechlorethamine suspected to have extravasated (Pérez Fidalgo 2012; Polovich 2009)

Cisplatin, concentrated: Inject 2 mL of a 1/6 M (~4%) sodium thiosulfate solution into existing IV line for each 100 mg of cisplatin extravasated; consider also injecting 1 mL of a 1/6 M (~4%) sodium thiosulfate solution as 0.1 mL subcutaneous injections (clockwise) into the area around the extravasation, may repeat subcutaneous injections several times over the next 3-4 hours (Ener 2004)

Bendamustine: SubQ: Bendamustine extravasation may be managed with 1/6 M (~4%) sodium thiosulfate solution in the same manner as mechlorethamine extravasation (Schulmeister 2011)

Management of delayed calcium extravasation (calcinosis cutis) (off-label use): IV: 12.5 g over 30 minutes; may increase gradually to 25 g 3 times per week; monitor for non-anion gap acidosis, hypocalcemia, severe nausea (Reynolds 2014). Additional data may be necessary to further define the role of sodium thiosulfate for this condition.

Geriatric Refer to adult dosing; use with caution due to likelihood of decreased renal function.

Pediatric Cyanide poisoning: IV: **Note:** Administer in conjunction with sodium nitrite. Administer sodium nitrite first, followed immediately by the administration of sodium thiosulfate. 250 mg/kg (1 mL/kg or ~30 to 40 mL/m^2 of a 25% solution) or 500 mg/kg (2 mL/kg of a 25% solution) (Howland 2011); maximum dose: 12.5 g (50 mL of a 25% solution) (Mintegi 2013); may repeat at one-half the original dose if symptoms of cyanide toxicity return

Note: Monitor the patient for 24-48 hours; if symptoms return, repeat both sodium nitrite and sodium thiosulfate at one-half the original doses.

Renal Impairment

No dosage adjustment provided in manufacturer's labeling; however, renal elimination is significant and risk of adverse effects may be increased in patients with renal impairment.

Calciphylaxis (off-label use): No dosage adjustment necessary. When used for patients not on dialysis (normal renal function or mildly reduced GFR), because sodium thiosulfate is cleared by the kidney, dose may be adjusted based on appearance of adverse effects (eg, metabolic acidosis, hypotension) (Hackett 2011; Nigwekar 2013).

Hepatic Impairment No dosage adjustment provided in the manufacturer's labeling (has not been studied).

Administration

IV: Cyanide poisoning: Administer by IV infusion over 10 to 30 minutes immediately after the administration of sodium nitrite (Howland 2011). Decrease rate of infusion in the event of significant hypotension.

Calciphylaxis (off-label use): Administer by IV infusion over 30 to 60 minutes (Cicone 2004; Nigwekar 2013).

Extravasation management (off-label use): Stop vesicant infusion immediately and disconnect IV line (leave needle/cannula in place); gently aspirate extravasated solution from the IV line (do **NOT** flush the line); remove needle/cannula (temporarily keep in place for cisplatin extravasation to allow for sodium thiosulfate administration through the needle/cannula); elevate extremity.

Mechlorethamine: Inject subcutaneously (off-label route) into the extravasation site using ≤25-gauge needle; change needle with each injection (Pérez Fidalgo 2012; Polovich 2009).

Cisplatin, concentrated: Inject into the existing IV line; consider also injecting 1 mL as 0.1 mL subcutaneous injections (clockwise) into the area around the extravasation using a new 25- or 27-gauge needle for each injection (Ener 2004).

Bendamustine: SubQ: Bendamustine extravasation may be managed with sodium thiosulfate in the same manner as mechlorethamine extravasation (Schulmeister 2011).

Monitoring Parameters

Cyanide poisoning: Monitor for at least 24-48 hours after administration; blood pressure and heart rate during and after infusion; hemoglobin/hematocrit; co-oximetry; serum lactate levels; venous-arterial PO_2 gradient; serum methemoglobin and oxyhemoglobin. Pretreatment cyanide levels may be useful diagnostically.

Extravasation management: Monitor and document extravasation site for pain, blister formation, skin sloughing, arm/hand swelling/stiffness; monitor for fever, chills, or worsening pain

When used in the management of delayed calcium extravasation (calcinosis cutis), monitor for non-anion gap acidosis, hypocalcemia, severe nausea (Reynolds 2014).

Dosage Forms Excipient information presented when available (limited, particularly for generics); consult specific product labeling. [DSC] = Discontinued product

Solution, Intravenous:

Generic: 10% [100 mg/mL] (10 mL [DSC]); 25% [250 mg/mL] (50 mL)

Sonidegib (soe ni DEG ib)

Related Information
Common Toxicity Criteria *on page 2242*

Management of Chemotherapy-Induced Nausea and Vomiting in Adults *on page 2253*

Safe Handling of Hazardous Drugs *on page 2379*

Brand Names: US Odomzo

Index Terms Erismodegib; LDE225; NVP-LDE225; Sonidegib Phosphate

Pharmacologic Category Antineoplastic Agent, Hedgehog Pathway Inhibitor

Use Basal cell carcinoma, locally advanced: Treatment of adult patients with locally advanced basal cell carcinoma (BCC) that has recurred following surgery or radiation therapy, or those who are not candidates for surgery or radiation therapy.

Labeled Contraindications There are no contraindications listed in the manufacturer's labeling.

Pregnancy Considerations [US Boxed Warning]: Sonidegib can cause embryo-fetal death or severe birth defects when administered to a pregnant woman. Sonidegib is embryotoxic, fetotoxic, and teratogenic in animals. Verify the pregnancy status of females of reproductive potential prior to initiating therapy. Advise females of reproductive potential to use effective contraception during treatment with sonidegib and for at least 20 months after the last dose. Advise males of the potential risk of exposure through semen and to use condoms with a pregnant partner or a female partner of reproductive potential during treatment with sonidegib and for at least 8 months after the last dose. It is not known if sonidegib is present in semen. Males with female partners of reproductive potential should use condoms even following a vasectomy. Advise male patients not to donate sperm during sonidegib treatment and for at least 8 months after the last sonidegib dose.

Health care providers should notify the manufacturer of pregnancies which may occur following exposure to sonidegib (888-669-6682).

Breastfeeding Considerations It is not known if sonidegib is excreted in breast milk. Due to the potential for serious adverse reactions in the breastfeeding infant, breastfeeding is not recommended by the manufacturer during therapy and for at least 20 months after treatment.

Warnings/Precautions [US Boxed Warning]: Sonidegib can cause embryo-fetal death or severe birth defects when administered to a pregnant woman. Sonidegib is embryotoxic, fetotoxic, and teratogenic in animals. Verify the pregnancy status of females of reproductive potential prior to initiating therapy. Advise females of reproductive potential to use effective contraception during treatment with sonidegib and for at least 20 months after the last dose. Advise males of the potential risk of exposure through semen and to use condoms with a pregnant partner or a female partner of reproductive potential during treatment with sonidegib and for at least 8 months after the last dose. It is not known if sonidegib is present in semen. Advise patients not to donate sperm during sonidegib treatment and for at least 8 months after the last sonidegib dose. Amenorrhea lasting for at least 18 months was observed in women of reproductive potential. Advise patients not to donate blood or blood products during sonidegib treatment and for at least 20 months after the last sonidegib dose.

Musculoskeletal toxicity occurred in more than two-thirds of patients treated with sonidegib (including grade 3 and 4 events). Muscle spasms, musculoskeletal pain, and myalgia were the most frequently reported musculoskeletal adverse reactions. Increased serum creatine kinase (CK) levels were also commonly observed (some events were grade 3 or 4); CK elevations were usually preceded by musculoskeletal pain and myalgia. When CK elevations were grade 2 or higher, the median time to symptom onset was ~13 weeks (range: 2 to 39 weeks), and the median time to resolution (to ≤ grade 1) was 12 days. More than one-quarter of patients required medical management for musculoskeletal toxicity (eg, magnesium supplementation, muscle relaxants, and analgesics/opioids); several patients required intravenous hydration or hospitalization. Rhabdomyolysis was observed in 1 patient in clinical trials (at a dose higher than the FDA-approved dose). Monitor serum CK levels and serum creatinine at baseline and periodically during therapy (more frequently if muscle symptoms are reported or if clinically indicated). Advise patients to promptly report new unexplained muscle pain, tenderness, or weakness (either occurring during therapy or persisting after discontinuation). May require therapy interruption or discontinuation. Increased serum creatinine was observed in the majority of patients receiving sonidegib, although the measurement remained within the normal range in more than 75% of patients. While dosage adjustment is not required in patients with renal impairment, monitor serum creatinine at baseline and periodically, particularly if patients present with musculoskeletal toxicity. Potentially significant interactions may exist, requiring dose or frequency adjustment, additional monitoring, and/or selection of alternative therapy. One 200 mg sonidegib capsule is equivalent to 281 mg of the diphosphate salt of sonidegib.

Adverse Reactions

>10%:

Central nervous system: Fatigue (41%), headache (15%), pain (14%)

Dermatologic: Alopecia (53%)

Endocrine & metabolic: Hyperglycemia (51%), weight loss (30%), increased serum ALT (19%), increased serum AST (19%), increased amylase (16%)

Gastrointestinal: Dysgeusia (46%), increased serum lipase (43%), nausea (39%), diarrhea (32%), decreased appetite (23%), abdominal pain (18%), vomiting (11%)

Hematologic & oncologic: Anemia (32%), lymphocytopenia (28%, grades 3/4: 3%)

Neuromuscular & skeletal: Increased creatine phosphokinase (61%, grades 3/4: 8%), muscle spasm (54%; grade 3: 3%), musculoskeletal pain (32%, grade 3: 1%), myalgia (19%)

Renal: Increased serum creatinine (92%)

1% to 10%:

Dermatologic: Pruritus (10%)

<1%, postmarketing, and/or case reports: Amenorrhea, rhabdomyolysis

Drug Interactions

Metabolism/Transport Effects Substrate of CYP3A4 (major); **Note:** Assignment of Major/Minor substrate status based on clinically relevant drug interaction potential; **Inhibits** BCRP

Avoid Concomitant Use

Avoid concomitant use of Sonidegib with any of the following: Conivaptan; CYP3A4 Inducers (Moderate); CYP3A4 Inducers (Strong); CYP3A4 Inhibitors (Strong); Fusidic Acid (Systemic); Idelalisib

Increased Effect/Toxicity

The levels/effects of Sonidegib may be increased by: Conivaptan; CYP3A4 Inhibitors (Moderate); CYP3A4 Inhibitors (Strong); Dasatinib; Fosaprepitant; Fusidic Acid (Systemic); Idelalisib; Palbociclib; Simeprevir; Stiripentol

Decreased Effect

The levels/effects of Sonidegib may be decreased by: CYP3A4 Inducers (Moderate); CYP3A4 Inducers (Strong); Deferasirox; Sarilumab; Siltuximab; Tocilizumab

Food Interactions Taking sonidegib with a high-fat meal (~1,000 calories with 50% fat content) will increase systemic exposure (7- to 8-fold). Management: Do not administer with food; must be taken on an empty stomach, at least 1 hour before and 2 hours after food.

Hazardous Drugs Handling Considerations

Hazardous agent (meets NIOSH 2016 criteria). This medication is not on the NIOSH (2016) list; however, it meets the criteria for a hazardous drug. Drugs are classified as hazardous based on their properties; the properties of a hazardous drug include one or more of the following characteristics: carcinogenic, teratogenic (or other developmental toxicity), reproductive toxicity, organotoxic at low doses, genotoxic, and/or new agents with structural or toxicity profiles similar to existing hazardous agents.

Use appropriate precautions for receiving, handling, administration, and disposal. Gloves (single) should be worn during receiving, unpacking, and placing in storage. NIOSH recommends single gloving for administration of intact tablets or capsules (NIOSH 2016).

Storage/Stability Store at 25°C (77°F); excursions permitted to 15°C to 30°C (59°F to 86°F).

Mechanism of Action Basal cell cancer is associated with mutations in Hedgehog pathway components. Hedgehog regulates cell growth and differentiation in embryogenesis; while generally not active in adult tissue, Hedgehog mutations associated with basal cell cancer can activate the pathway resulting in unrestricted proliferation of skin basal cells (Von Hoff, 2009). Sonidegib is a selective Hedgehog pathway inhibitor which binds to and inhibits Smoothened homologue (SMO), the transmembrane protein involved in Hedgehog signal transduction.

Pharmacodynamics/Kinetics

Absorption: AUC_{inf} and C_{max} are increased by 7.4- to 7.8-fold, respectively, when administered with a high-fat meal (~1,000 calories with 50% fat content)

Distribution: 9,166 L

Protein binding: >97%

Metabolism: Primarily hepatic through CYP3A

Bioavailability: <10% of an oral dose is absorbed

Half-life elimination: ~28 days

Time to peak: 2 to 4 hours

Excretion: Feces (~70%); urine (30%)

Dosing

Adult & Geriatric Note: Verify pregnancy status of females of reproductive potential prior to therapy initiation. Measure serum creatine kinase (CK) levels and renal function tests in all patients prior to starting treatment.

Basal cell carcinoma, locally advanced: Oral: 200 mg once daily until disease progression or unacceptable toxicity (Migden, 2015)

Missed doses: If a dose is missed, skip the missed dose and resume dosing with the next scheduled dose.

Renal Impairment

CrCl 30 to 89 mL/minute: There are no dosage adjustments provided in the manufacturer's labeling; however, mild or moderate impairment had no clinically meaningful effect on sonidegib exposure (compared to patients with normal renal function).

CrCl <30 mL/minute: There are no dosage adjustments provided in the manufacturer's labeling.

Hepatic Impairment Mild, moderate, or severe impairment (Child-Pugh classes A, B, and C): There are no dosage adjustments provided in the manufacturer's labeling; however, hepatic impairment had no clinically meaningful effect on sonidegib exposure (compared to patients with normal hepatic function).

Adjustment for Toxicity

Withhold treatment for any of the following (may resume at 200 mg daily upon resolution of toxicity):

Creatine kinase (CK) serum elevation between 2.5 and 10 times ULN (first occurrence) or between 2.5 and 5 times ULN (recurrent)

Musculoskeletal toxicity, severe or intolerable

Permanently discontinue therapy for:

CK serum elevation >2.5 times ULN with worsening renal function

CK serum elevation >10 times ULN

CK serum elevation >5 times ULN (recurrent)

Musculoskeletal toxicity, severe or intolerable (recurrent)

Administration Oral: Administer on an empty stomach at least 1 hour before or 2 hours after a meal.

Emetic Potential Minimal (<10%)

Monitoring Parameters Serum creatine kinase (CK) and serum creatinine (baseline, periodically during treatment, and at least weekly with musculoskeletal toxicity and CK elevations >2.5 times ULN until resolution), liver function, pregnancy status, signs/symptoms of musculoskeletal toxicity.

Medication Guide Available Yes

Dosage Forms Excipient information presented when available (limited, particularly for generics); consult specific product labeling.

Capsule, Oral:

Odomzo: 200 mg

◆ **Sonidegib Phosphate** *see* Sonidegib *on page 1682*

SORAfenib (sor AF e nib)

Related Information

Common Toxicity Criteria *on page 2242*

Management of Chemotherapy-Induced Nausea and Vomiting in Adults *on page 2253*

Prevention of Chemotherapy-Induced Nausea and Vomiting in Children *on page 2310*

Safe Handling of Hazardous Drugs *on page 2379*

Brand Names: US NexAVAR

Brand Names: Canada Nexavar

Index Terms BAY 43-9006; Sorafenib Tosylate

Pharmacologic Category Antineoplastic Agent, Tyrosine Kinase Inhibitor; Antineoplastic Agent, Vascular Endothelial Growth Factor (VEGF) Inhibitor

◀ **Use**

Hepatocellular cancer: Treatment of unresectable hepatocellular cancer (HCC)

Renal cell cancer, advanced: Treatment of advanced renal cell cancer (RCC)

Thyroid cancer, differentiated: Treatment of locally recurrent or metastatic, progressive, differentiated thyroid cancer (refractory to radioactive iodine treatment)

Labeled Contraindications Known severe hypersensitivity to sorafenib or any component of the formulation; use in combination with carboplatin and paclitaxel in patients with squamous cell lung cancer

Pregnancy Considerations Animal reproduction studies have demonstrated teratogenicity and fetal loss. Based on its mechanism of action and because sorafenib inhibits angiogenesis, a critical component of fetal development, adverse effects on pregnancy would be expected. Women of childbearing potential should be advised to avoid pregnancy. Men and women of reproductive potential should use effective birth control during treatment and for at least 2 weeks after treatment is discontinued.

Breastfeeding Considerations It is not known if sorafenib is present in breast milk. Due to the potential for serious adverse reactions in the breastfed infant, a decision should be made to discontinue sorafenib or to discontinue breastfeeding during therapy, taking into account the importance of treatment to the mother.

Warnings/Precautions May cause hypertension (generally mild-to-moderate), especially in the first 6 weeks of treatment; monitor; use caution in patients with underlying or poorly-controlled hypertension; consider discontinuing (temporary or permanent) in patients who develop severe or persistent hypertension while on appropriate antihypertensive therapy. May cause cardiac ischemia or infarction; consider discontinuing (temporarily or permanently) in patients who develop these conditions; use in patients with unstable coronary artery disease or recent myocardial infarction has not been studied. QT prolongation has been observed; may increase the risk for ventricular arrhythmia. Avoid use in patients with congenital long QT syndrome; monitor electrolytes and ECG in patients with heart failure, bradyarrhythmias, and concurrent medications known to prolong the QT interval; correct electrolyte (calcium, magnesium, potassium) imbalances; interrupt treatment for QTc interval >500 msec or for ≥60 msec increase from baseline. In a scientific statement from the American Heart Association, sorafenib has been determined to be an agent that may exacerbate underlying myocardial dysfunction (magnitude: minor) (AHA [Page 2016]).

Serious bleeding events may occur (consider permanently discontinuing if serious); monitor PT/INR in patients on warfarin therapy. Fatal bleeding events have been reported. Thyroid cancer patients with tracheal, bronchial, and esophageal infiltration should be treated with local therapy prior to administering sorafenib due to the potential bleeding risk. May complicate wound healing; temporarily withhold treatment for patients undergoing major surgical procedures (the appropriate timing for reinitiation after surgical procedures has not been determined). Gastrointestinal perforation has been reported (rare); monitor patients for signs/symptoms (abdominal pain, constipation, or vomiting); discontinue treatment if gastrointestinal perforation occurs. Potentially significant drug-drug interactions may exist, requiring dose or frequency adjustment, additional monitoring, and/or selection of alternative therapy. Avoid concurrent use with strong CYP3A4 inducers (eg, carbamazepine, dexamethasone, phenobarbital, phenytoin, rifampin, St John's wort); may decrease sorafenib levels/effects. Use caution when administering sorafenib with compounds that are metabolized predominantly via UGT1A1 (eg, irinotecan). Use in combination with carboplatin and paclitaxel in patients with squamous cell lung cancer is contraindicated.

Hand-foot skin reaction and rash (generally grades 1 or 2) are the most common drug-related adverse events, and typically appear within the first 6 weeks of treatment; usually managed with topical treatment, treatment delays, and/or dose reductions. Consider permanently discontinuing with severe or persistent dermatological toxicities. The risk for hand-foot skin reaction increased with cumulative doses of sorafenib (Azad 2009). The incidence of hand-foot syndrome is also increased in patients treated with sorafenib plus bevacizumab in comparison to those treated with sorafenib monotherapy (Azad 2009). The following treatments may be used to manage hand-foot skin reaction in addition to the recommended dosage modifications (Lacouture 2008): Prior to treatment initiation, a pedicure is recommended to remove hyperkeratotic areas/calluses, which may predispose to HFSR; avoid vigorous exercise/activities which may stress hands or feet. During therapy, patients should reduce exposure to hot water (may exacerbate hand-foot symptoms); avoid constrictive footwear and excessive skin friction. Patients may also wear thick cotton gloves or socks and should wear shoes with padded insoles. Grade 1 HFSR may be relieved with moisturizing creams, cotton gloves and socks (at night) and/or keratolytic creams such as urea (20% to 40%) or salicylic acid (6%). Apply topical steroid (eg, clobetasol ointment) twice daily to erythematous areas of grade 2 HFSR; topical anesthetics (eg, lidocaine 2%) and then systemic analgesics (if appropriate) may be used for pain control. Resolution of acute erythema may result in keratotic areas which may be softened with keratolytic agents. Severe dermatologic toxicities, including Stevens-Johnson syndrome (SJS) and toxic epidermal necrolysis (TEN) have been reported; may be life-threatening; discontinue sorafenib for suspected SJS or TEN.

Sorafenib impairs exogenous thyroid suppression; TSH level elevations were commonly observed in the thyroid cancer study; monitor TSH levels monthly and as clinically necessary, and adjust thyroid replacement as needed. Sorafenib levels in patients with mild-to-moderate hepatic impairment (Child-Pugh classes A and B) were similar to levels observed in patients without hepatic impairment; has not been studied in patients with severe hepatic impairment. In a small study of Asian patients with advanced HCC, sorafenib demonstrated efficacy with adequate tolerability in a hepatitis B-endemic area (Yau 2009). There have been reports of sorafenib-induced hepatitis (including hepatic failure and death) which is characterized by hepatocellular liver damage and transaminase increases (significant); increased bilirubin and INR may also occur. Monitor hepatic function regularly; discontinue sorafenib for unexplained significant transaminase increases.

Adverse Reactions

>10%:

Cardiovascular: Hypertension (9% to 41%; grade 3: 3% to 4%; grade 4: <1%; grades 3/4: 10%, onset: ~3 weeks)

Central nervous system: Fatigue (37% to 46%), headache (≤10% to 17%), mouth pain (14%), voice disorder (13%), peripheral sensory neuropathy (≤13%), pain (11%)

◄

Dermatologic: Palmar-plantar erythrodysesthesia (21% to 69%; grade 3: 6% to 8%; grades 3/4: 19%), alopecia (14% to 67%), skin rash (including desquamation; 19% to 40%; grade 3: ≤1%; grades 3/4: 5%), pruritus (14% to 20%), xeroderma (10% to 13%), erythema (≥10%)

Endocrine & metabolic: Hypoalbuminemia (≤59%), weight loss (10% to 49%), hypophosphatemia (35% to 45%; grade 3: 11% to 13%; grade 4: <1%), increased thyroid stimulating hormone level (>0.5 mU/L: 41%; due to impairment of exogenous thyroid suppression), hypocalcemia (12% to 36%), increased amylase (30% to 34% [usually transient])

Gastrointestinal: Diarrhea (43% to 68%; grade 3: 2% to 10%; grade 4: <1%), increased serum lipase (40% to 41% [usually transient]), abdominal pain (11% to 31%), decreased appetite (30%), anorexia (16% to 29%), stomatitis (24%), nausea (21% to 24%), constipation (14% to 16%), vomiting (11% to 16%)

Hematologic & oncologic: Lymphocytopenia (23% to 47%; grades 3/4: ≤13%), thrombocytopenia (12% to 46%; grades 3/4: 1% to 4%), increased INR (≤42%), neutropenia (≤18%; grades 3/4: ≤5%), hemorrhage (15% to 17%; grade 3: 2%), leukopenia

Hepatic: Increased serum ALT (59%; grades 3/4: 4%), increased serum AST (54%; grades 3/4: 2%), hepatic insufficiency (≤11%; grade 3: 2%; grade 4: 1%)

Infection: Infection

Neuromuscular & skeletal: Limb pain (15%), weakness (12%), myalgia

Respiratory: Dyspnea (≤14%), cough (≤13%)

Miscellaneous: Fever (11%)

1% to 10%:

Cardiovascular: Ischemic heart disease (including myocardial infarction; ≤3%), cardiac failure (2%, congestive), flushing

Central nervous system: Depression, glossalgia

Dermatologic: Hyperkeratosis (7%), acne vulgaris, exfoliative dermatitis, folliculitis

Endocrine & metabolic: Hypokalemia (5% to 10%), hyponatremia, hypothyroidism

Gastrointestinal: Dysgeusia (6%), dyspepsia, dysphagia, gastroesophageal reflux disease, mucositis, xerostomia

Genitourinary: Erectile dysfunction, proteinuria

Hematologic & oncologic: Squamous cell carcinoma of skin (3%; grades 3/4: 3%), anemia

Hepatic: Increased serum transaminases (transient)

Neuromuscular & skeletal: Muscle spasm (10%), arthralgia (≤10%), myalgia

Renal: Renal failure

Respiratory: Epistaxis (7%), flu-like symptoms, hoarseness, rhinorrhea

<1%, postmarketing, and/or case reports: Acute renal failure, anaphylaxis, angioedema, aortic dissection, amyotrophy, cardiac arrhythmia, cardiac failure, cerebral hemorrhage, cholangitis, cholecystitis, dehydration, eczema, erythema multiforme, gastritis, gastrointestinal hemorrhage, gastrointestinal perforation, gynecomastia, hepatic failure, hepatitis, hypersensitivity reaction (skin reaction, urticaria), hypertensive crisis, hyperthyroidism, increased serum alkaline phosphatase, increased serum bilirubin, interstitial pulmonary disease (acute respiratory distress, interstitial pneumonia, lung inflammation, pneumonitis, pulmonitis, radiation pneumonitis), jaundice, malignant neoplasm of skin (keratoacanthomas), nephrotic syndrome, ostealgia, osteonecrosis of the jaw, pancreatitis, pleural effusion, prolonged QT interval on ECG, respiratory tract hemorrhage, reversible posterior leukoencephalopathy

syndrome, rhabdomyolysis, Stevens-Johnson syndrome, thromboembolism, tinnitus, toxic epidermal necrolysis, transient ischemic attacks, tumor lysis syndrome, tumor pain

Drug Interactions

Metabolism/Transport Effects Substrate of CYP3A4 (minor), UGT1A9; **Note:** Assignment of Major/Minor substrate status based on clinically relevant drug interaction potential; **Inhibits** BCRP, BSEP, CYP2C8 (weak), CYP2C9 (moderate), UGT1A9

Avoid Concomitant Use

Avoid concomitant use of SORAfenib with any of the following: Amodiaquine; BCG (Intravesical); CARBOplatin; Cholic Acid; CYP3A4 Inducers (Strong); Deferiprone; Dipyrone; Natalizumab; PACLitaxel (Conventional); Pimecrolimus; St John's Wort; Tacrolimus (Topical); Vaccines (Live)

Increased Effect/Toxicity

SORAfenib may increase the levels/effects of: Acetaminophen; Amodiaquine; Bisphosphonate Derivatives; Bosentan; Cannabis; CARBOplatin; Carvedilol; Cholic Acid; CloZAPine; CYP2C9 Substrates; Deferiprone; DOCEtaxel; DOXOrubicin (Conventional); Dronabinol; Fingolimod; Fluorouracil (Systemic); Fluorouracil (Topical); Highest Risk QTc-Prolonging Agents; Irinotecan Products; Leflunomide; Moderate Risk QTc-Prolonging Agents; Natalizumab; PACLitaxel (Conventional); Propacetamol; Tetrahydrocannabinol; Tofacitinib; Vaccines (Live); Warfarin

The levels/effects of SORAfenib may be increased by: Acetaminophen; Bevacizumab; CYP3A4 Inhibitors (Strong); Denosumab; Dipyrone; MiFEPRIStone; Ocrelizumab; Pimecrolimus; Promazine; Roflumilast; Tacrolimus (Topical); Trastuzumab

Decreased Effect

SORAfenib may decrease the levels/effects of: BCG (Intravesical); Coccidioides immitis Skin Test; Dacarbazine; Fluorouracil (Systemic); Fluorouracil (Topical); Nivolumab; Sipuleucel-T; Tertomotide; Vaccines (Inactivated); Vaccines (Live)

The levels/effects of SORAfenib may be decreased by: CYP3A4 Inducers (Strong); Echinacea; Neomycin; St John's Wort

Food Interactions Bioavailability is decreased 29% with a high-fat meal (bioavailability is similar to fasting state when administered with a moderate-fat meal). Management: Administer on an empty stomach 1 hour before or 2 hours after eating.

Hazardous Drugs Handling Considerations

Hazardous agent (NIOSH 2016 [group 1]).

Use appropriate precautions for receiving, handling, administration, and disposal. Gloves (single) should be worn during receiving, unpacking, and placing in storage.

NIOSH recommends single gloving for administration of intact tablets or capsules. If manipulating tablets/capsules (eg, to prepare an oral suspension), NIOSH recommends double gloving, a protective gown, and preparation in a controlled device; if not prepared in a controlled device, respiratory and eye/face protection as well as ventilated engineering controls are recommended. NIOSH recommends double gloving, a protective gown, and (if there is a potential for vomit or spit up) eye/face protection for administration of an oral liquid/feeding tube administration (NIOSH 2016).

◀ **Storage/Stability** Store at 25°C (77°F); excursions are permitted between 15°C and 30°C (59°F and 86°F). Protect from moisture.

Mechanism of Action Multikinase inhibitor; inhibits tumor growth and angiogenesis by inhibiting intracellular Raf kinases (CRAF, BRAF, and mutant BRAF), and cell surface kinase receptors (VEGFR-1, VEGFR-2, VEGFR-3, PDGFR-beta, cKIT, FLT-3, RET, and RET/PTC)

Pharmacodynamics/Kinetics

Protein binding: 99.5%

Metabolism: Hepatic, via CYP3A4 (primarily oxidated to the pyridine N-oxide; active, minor) and UGT1A9 (glucuronidation)

Bioavailability: 38% to 49%; reduced by 29% when administered with a high-fat meal

Half-life elimination: 25 to 48 hours

Time to peak, plasma: ~3 hours

Excretion: Feces (77%, 51% of dose as unchanged drug); urine (19%, as metabolites)

Dosing

Adult & Geriatric Note: Interrupt treatment (temporarily) in patients undergoing major surgical procedures.

Hepatocellular cancer (HCC): Oral: 400 mg twice daily; continue until no longer clinically benefiting or until unacceptable toxicity occurs (Llovet 2008)

Renal cell cancer (RCC), advanced: Oral: 400 mg twice daily; continue until no longer clinically benefiting or until unacceptable toxicity occurs (Escudier 2007; Escudier 2009)

Thyroid cancer, differentiated: Oral: 400 mg twice daily; continue until no longer clinically benefiting or until unacceptable toxicity occurs (Brose 2013)

Angiosarcoma (off-label use): Oral: 400 mg twice daily (Maki 2009)

Gastrointestinal stromal tumor (GIST) (off-label use): Oral: 400 mg twice daily (Wiebe 2008)

Renal Impairment

Manufacturer's labeling: No dosage adjustment is necessary for mild, moderate, or severe impairment (not dependent on dialysis); has not been studied in dialysis patients.

A pharmacokinetic study evaluated sorafenib dosing to determine an initial tolerable dose in patients with varying degrees of renal dysfunction. The following empiric starting doses were identified based on patient tolerance (Miller 2009):

CrCl 40 to 59 mL/minute: 400 mg twice daily

CrCl 20 to 39 mL/minute: 200 mg twice daily

CrCl <20 mL/minute: Data inadequate to define dose

Hemodialysis (any CrCl): 200 mg once daily

Hepatic Impairment

Hepatic impairment at baseline:

Manufacturer's labeling:

Mild to moderate (Child-Pugh class A and B) impairment: No dosage adjustment is necessary.

Severe impairment (Child-Pugh class C): There are no dosage adjustments provided in the manufacturer's labeling (has not been studied).

A pharmacokinetic study evaluated sorafenib dosing to determine an initial tolerable dose in patients with varying degrees of hepatic dysfunction. The following empiric starting doses were identified based on patient tolerance (Miller 2009):

Mild hepatic dysfunction (bilirubin >1 to ≤1.5 times ULN and/or AST >ULN): 400 mg twice daily

Moderate hepatic dysfunction (bilirubin >1.5 to ≤3 times ULN; any AST): 200 mg twice daily

Severe hepatic dysfunction:

Albumin <2.5 g/dL (any bilirubin and any AST): 200 mg once daily

Bilirubin >3 to 10 x ULN (any AST): A dose of 200 mg every 3 days was **not** tolerated, therefore no dosage was identified in this pharmacokinetic study for patients meeting these parameters.

Drug-induced liver injury during treatment: Unexplained (eg, not due to viral hepatitis or progressive underlying malignancy) significantly increased transaminases: Discontinue treatment.

Adjustment for Toxicity Temporary interruption and/or dosage reduction may be necessary for management of adverse drug reactions.

Cardiovascular toxicity:

Cardiac ischemia or infarction: Consider temporary interruption or permanent discontinuation.

Hypertension, severe or persistent (despite antihypertensive therapy): Consider temporary interruption or permanent discontinuation.

QT prolongation (QTc interval >500 msec or ≥60 msec increase from baseline): Interrupt treatment.

Gastrointestinal perforation: Permanently discontinue.

Hemorrhage requiring medical intervention: Consider permanent discontinuation.

Dermatologic toxicity: If Stevens-Johnson syndrome or toxic epidermal necrolysis is suspected, discontinue therapy.

US labeling:

RCC and HCC: If dosage reductions are necessary, decrease dose to 400 mg once daily. If further reductions are needed, decrease dose to 400 mg every other day.

Grade 1 (numbness, dysesthesia, paresthesia, tingling, painless swelling, erythema, or discomfort of the hands or feet which do not disrupt normal activities): Continue sorafenib and consider symptomatic treatment with topical therapy.

Grade 2 (painful erythema and swelling of the hands or feet and/or discomfort affecting normal activities):

First occurrence: Continue sorafenib and consider symptomatic treatment with topical therapy. **Note:** If no improvement within 7 days, see dosing for second or third occurrence.

Second or third occurrence (or no improvement after 7 days of 1st occurrence): Hold treatment until resolves to grade 0-1; resume treatment with dose reduced by one dose level (400 mg daily or 400 mg every other day).

Fourth occurrence: Discontinue treatment.

◀

Grade 3 (moist desquamation, ulceration, blistering, or severe pain of the hands or feet or severe discomfort that prevents working or performing daily activities):

First or second occurrence: Hold treatment until resolves to grade 0-1; resume treatment with dose reduced by one dose level (400 mg daily or 400 mg every other day).

Third occurrence: Discontinue treatment.

Thyroid cancer:

First dose level reduction: Reduce to 600 mg daily (in 2 divided doses, as 400 mg and 200 mg, separated by 12 hours).

Second dose level reduction: Reduce dose to 200 mg twice daily.

Third dose level reduction: Reduce dose to 200 mg once daily.

Grade 1 (numbness, dysesthesia, paresthesia, tingling, painless swelling, erythema, or discomfort of the hands or feet which do not disrupt normal activities): Continue sorafenib treatment.

Grade 2 (painful erythema and swelling of the hands or feet and/or discomfort affecting normal activities):

First occurrence: Decrease dose to 600 mg daily (in divided doses). **Note:** If no improvement within 7 days, see dosing for second occurrence.

Second occurrence (or no improvement after 7 days of the reduced dose after 1st occurrence): Hold treatment until resolved or improved to grade 1; if resumed, decrease the dose by 1 dose level.

Third occurrence: Hold treatment until resolved or improved to grade 1; if resumed, decrease the dose by 1 dose level.

Fourth occurrence: Permanently discontinue.

Grade 3 (moist desquamation, ulceration, blistering, or severe pain of the hands or feet or severe discomfort that prevents working or performing daily activities):

First occurrence: Hold treatment until resolved or improved to grade 1; if resumed, decrease by 1 dose level.

Second occurrence: Hold treatment until resolved or improved to grade 1; if resumed, decrease by 2 dose levels.

Third occurrence: Permanently discontinue.

Following improvement of grade 2 or 3 dermatologic toxicity to grade 0 or 1 after at least 28 days of a reduced dose, the sorafenib dose may be increased 1 dose level from the reduced dose (~50% of patients requiring dose reduction for dermatologic toxicity may meet the criteria for increased dosing; and half of those patients may tolerate the increased dose without recurrent grade 2 or higher dermatologic toxicity).

Canadian labeling: RCC and HCC:

Grade 1 (any occurrence): Initiate supportive treatment immediately and continue sorafenib.

Grade 2:

First occurrence: Initiate supportive treatment immediately and consider a dose reduction to 400 mg daily for 28 days. If toxicity resolves to ≤ grade 1 after 28 days with dose reduction, increase dose to 400 mg twice daily. If toxicity does not resolve to ≤ grade 1 despite dose reduction, withhold treatment for a minimum of 7 days until toxicity resolves to ≤ grade 1, then resume treatment at reduced dose of 400 mg daily for 28 days. If toxicity remains ≤ grade 1 at the reduced dose for 28 days, increase dose to 400 mg twice daily.

Second or third occurrence: Follow procedure for first occurrence; however, when resuming treatment, decrease dose to 400 mg daily (indefinitely).

Fourth occurrence: Treatment discontinuation should be considered based on clinical assessment and patient preference.

Grade 3:

First occurrence: Initiate supportive measures immediately and withhold treatment for a minimum of 7 days and until toxicity ≤ grade 1. Resume at reduced dose of 400 mg daily for 28 days. If toxicity remains ≤ grade 1 at the reduced dose for 28 days, increase dose to 400 mg twice daily.

Second occurrence: Follow procedure for first occurrence; however, when resuming treatment, decrease dose to 400 mg daily (indefinitely).

Third occurrence: Treatment discontinuation should be considered based on clinical assessment and patient preference.

Administration Administer on an empty stomach (1 hour before or 2 hours after eating).

Emetic Potential Children and Adults: Minimal (<10%)

Extemporaneous Preparations An oral suspension may be prepared with tablets. Place two 200 mg tablets into a glass containing 60 mL (2 oz) water; let stand 5 minutes before stirring. Stir until tablets are completely disintegrated, forming a uniform suspension. Administer within 1 hour after preparation. Stir suspension again immediately before administration. To ensure the full dose is administered, rinse glass several times with a total of 180 mL (6 oz) water and administer residue. **Note:** Brown tablet coating may initially form a thin film but has no effect on the dosing accuracy.

Nexavar data on file, Bayer Healthcare Pharmaceuticals.

Monitoring Parameters

CBC with differential, electrolytes (magnesium, potassium, calcium), phosphorus, lipase and amylase levels; liver function tests; blood pressure (baseline, weekly for the first 6 weeks, then periodic); monitor for hand-foot skin reaction and other dermatologic toxicities; monitor ECG in patients at risk for prolonged QT interval; signs/symptoms of bleeding, GI perforation, and heart failure.

Thyroid function testing:

Patients with differentiated thyroid cancer: Monitor TSH monthly.

Patients with RCC and HCC (Hamnvik 2011):

Preexisting levothyroxine therapy: Obtain baseline TSH levels, then monitor every 4 weeks until levels and levothyroxine dose are stable, then monitor every 2 months

Without preexisting thyroid hormone replacement: TSH at baseline, then every 4 weeks for 4 months, then every 2 to 3 months

Prescribing and Access Restrictions Available from specialty pharmacies. Further information may be obtained at 1-866-639-2827 or www.nexavar-us.com.

Dosage Forms Excipient information presented when available (limited, particularly for generics); consult specific product labeling.

Tablet, Oral:

NexAVAR: 200 mg

◀ **Hazardous Drugs Handling Considerations**
Hazardous agent (NIOSH 2016 [group 1]).

Use appropriate precautions for receiving, handling, administration, and disposal. Gloves (single) should be worn during receiving, unpacking, and placing in storage.

NIOSH recommends double gloving, a protective gown, ventilated engineering controls (a class II biological safety cabinet or a compounding aseptic containment isolator), and closed system transfer devices (CSTDs) for preparation. Double gloving, a gown, and (if dosage form allows) CSTDs are required during administration (NIOSH 2016).

Storage/Stability Store intact vials refrigerated at 2°C to 8°C (36°F to 46°F). Protect from light. The manufacturer recommends use within 12 hours of reconstitution; vial does not contain a preservative.

Preparation for Administration Reconstitute powder with 9.5 mL D5W or NS to a concentration of 100 mg/mL. May further dilute for infusion in D5W or NS.

Mechanism of Action Inhibits DNA synthesis by alkylation and cross-linking the strands of DNA, and by possible protein modification; cell cycle nonspecific

Pharmacodynamics/Kinetics
Onset: 1500 mg/m^2 once weekly: Onset of response: 17 days; median time to maximum response: 35 days
Distribution: Concentrates in liver, kidney, and pancreatic beta cells
Metabolism: Rapid; primarily hepatic
Half-life elimination: <1 hour
Excretion: Urine (primarily; as parent drug and metabolites)

Dosing
Adult Note: Streptozocin is associated with a high emetic potential; antiemetics are recommended to prevent nausea and vomiting (Basch, 2011; Roila, 2010).

Pancreatic islet cell carcinoma, metastatic: IV:
Daily schedule: 500 mg/m^2/day for 5 consecutive days every 6 weeks until maximum benefit or until unacceptable toxicity
Weekly schedule: 1000 mg/m^2 once weekly; if therapeutic response not achieved after 2 weeks, may escalate dose to a maximum of 1500 mg/m^2 weekly
Off-label dosing: 1000 mg/m^2 once every 3 weeks for up to 6 cycles (in combination with leucovorin, fluorouracil and cisplatin) (Turner, 2010) **or** 400 mg/m^2 days 1 to 5 every 4 weeks (in combination with fluorouracil and doxorubicin) until disease progression or unacceptable toxicity (Kouvaraki, 2004)

Adrenal carcinoma, metastatic (off-label use): IV: 1000 mg once daily for 5 days (cycle 1) followed by 2000 mg on day 1 (subsequent cycles) every 3 weeks (in combination with mitotane) (Fassnacht, 2012; Khan 2000)

Geriatric Refer to adult dosing. Select dose cautiously, beginning at the lower end of dosing range.

Renal Impairment No dosage adjustment provided in the manufacturer's labeling; however, it is recommended to use clinical judgment weighing benefit vs risk of renal toxicity in patients with preexisting renal impairment. The following dosing adjustments have been recommended (Aronoff, 2007):
Adults (based on a usual dose of 500 mg/m^2):
CrCl >50 mL/minute: No dosage adjustment necessary.

CrCl 10-50 mL/minute: Administer 75% of dose

CrCl <10 mL/minute: Administer 50% of dose

Hepatic Impairment No dosage adjustment provided in the manufacturer's labeling. However, streptozocin is rapidly hepatically metabolized; dose should be decreased in patients with severe liver disease.

Obesity *ASCO Guidelines for appropriate chemotherapy dosing in obese adults with cancer:* Utilize patient's actual body weight (full weight) for calculation of body surface area- or weight-based dosing, particularly when the intent of therapy is curative; manage regimen-related toxicities in the same manner as for nonobese patients; if a dose reduction is utilized due to toxicity, consider resumption of full weight-based dosing with subsequent cycles, especially if cause of toxicity (eg, hepatic or renal impairment) is resolved (Griggs, 2012).

Adjustment for Toxicity *Bone marrow suppression or hepatic dysfunction:* May require dosage reduction or discontinuation.

Administration Streptozocin is associated with a high emetic potential; antiemetics are recommended to prevent nausea and vomiting (Basch, 2011; Dupuis, 2011; Roila, 2010).

Administer as either a rapid IV injection **or** as short or prolonged infusion.

Irritant with vesicant-like properties; ensure proper needle or catheter placement prior to and during infusion; avoid extravasation.

Extravasation management: If extravasation occurs, stop infusion immediately and disconnect (leave cannula/needle in place); gently aspirate extravasated solution (do **NOT** flush the line); remove needle/cannula; elevate extremity.

Vesicant/Extravasation Risk Irritant with vesicant-like properties

Emetic Potential Children and Adults: High (>90%)

Monitoring Parameters Renal function tests, including BUN, serum creatinine, and serial urinalysis, and serum electrolytes (at baseline, weekly during, and for 4 weeks after treatment); 24-hour urine collection if proteinuria is detected on urinalysis; liver function tests (weekly), CBC with differential and platelets (weekly), blood glucose; monitor infusion site

Dosage Forms Excipient information presented when available (limited, particularly for generics); consult specific product labeling.

Solution Reconstituted, Intravenous:

Zanosar: 1 g (1 ea)

◆ **Streptozotocin** see Streptozocin on page 1694

◆ **Strontium-89 Chloride** see Strontium-89 on page 1697

Strontium-89 (STRON shee um atey nine)

Brand Names: US Metastron

Brand Names: Canada Metastron

Index Terms SR-89; Sr89; Strontium Chloride SR 89; Strontium-89 Chloride

Pharmacologic Category Radiopharmaceutical

Use

Skeletal metastases (bone pain): Relief of bone pain in patients with skeletal metastases.

Limitation of use: Confirm the presence of bone metastases prior to therapy.

Pregnancy Risk Factor D

◀ **Dosing**

Adult & Geriatric Skeletal metastases (bone pain): IV: 148 megabecquerel (MBq; 4 millicurie [mCi]) **or** 1.5 to 2.2 MBq (40 to 60 microCi)/kg; repeat doses should be based on individual response, symptoms, and blood counts and are generally not recommended at intervals <90 days. Measure dose by a suitable radioactivity calibration system immediately prior to administration.

Renal Impairment There are no dosage adjustments provided in the manufacturer's labeling. However, consider benefit versus risk due to extensive renal excretion.

Hepatic Impairment There are no dosage adjustments provided in the manufacturer's labeling.

Additional Information Complete prescribing information should be consulted for additional detail.

Dosage Forms Excipient information presented when available (limited, particularly for generics); consult specific product labeling.

Solution, Intravenous, as chloride [preservative free]:

Metastron: 1 mCi/mL (4 mL) [pyrogen free]

♦ **Strontium Chloride SR 89** *see* Strontium-89 *on page 1697*
♦ **SU011248** *see* SUNItinib *on page 1707*
♦ **Suberoylanilide Hydroxamic Acid** *see* Vorinostat *on page 1935*
♦ **Sucralfate Paste (Orafate, ProThelial)** *see* Mucosal Coating Agent *on page 1280*

Sulfamethoxazole and Trimethoprim
(sul fa meth OKS a zole & trye METH oh prim)

Brand Names: US Bactrim; Bactrim DS; Sulfatrim Pediatric

Brand Names: Canada Apo-Sulfatrim; Apo-Sulfatrim DS; Apo-Sulfatrim Pediatric; Protrin DF; Septra Injection; Teva-Trimel; Teva-Trimel DS; Trisulfa; Trisulfa DS; Trisulfa S

Index Terms Co-Trimoxazole; Septra; SMX-TMP; SMZ-TMP; Sulfamethoxazole/Trimethoprim; Sulfatrim; TMP-SMX; TMP-SMZ; Trimethoprim and Sulfamethoxazole

Pharmacologic Category Antibiotic, Miscellaneous; Antibiotic, Sulfonamide Derivative

Use

Oral: Treatment of urinary tract infections due to *Escherichia coli*, *Klebsiella* and *Enterobacter* sp, *Morganella morganii*, *Proteus mirabilis* and *Proteus vulgaris*; acute otitis media; acute exacerbations of chronic bronchitis due to susceptible strains of *Haemophilus influenzae* or *Streptococcus pneumoniae*; treatment and prophylaxis of *Pneumocystis* pneumonia (PCP); traveler's diarrhea due to enterotoxigenic *E. coli*; treatment of Shigellosis caused by *Shigella flexneri* or *Shigella sonnei*

IV: Treatment of *Pneumocystis* pneumonia (PCP); treatment of Shigellosis caused by *Shigella flexneri* or *Shigella sonnei*; treatment of severe or complicated urinary tract infections due to *E. coli*, *Klebsiella* and *Enterobacter* spp, *M. morganii*, *P. mirabilis*, and *P. vulgaris*

Pregnancy Risk Factor D

Dosing

Adult & Geriatric Dosage recommendations are based on the trimethoprim component. Double-strength tablets are equivalent to sulfamethoxazole 800 mg and trimethoprim 160 mg.

General dosing guidelines:

Oral: 1 to 2 double-strength tablets (sulfamethoxazole 800 mg; trimethoprim 160 mg) every 12 to 24 hours

IV: 8 to 20 mg TMP/kg/day divided every 6 to 12 hours

Acne vulgaris (alternate therapy) (off-label use): Oral: One single-strength tablet (sulfamethoxazole 400 mg; trimethoprim 80 mg) or one double-strength tablet (sulfamethoxazole 800 mg; trimethoprim 160 mg) once or twice daily (Amin 2007; Tan 2005) **or** one double-strength tablet (sulfamethoxazole 800 mg; trimethoprim 160 mg) twice daily initially followed by one double-strength tablet (sulfamethoxazole 800 mg; trimethoprim 160 mg) once daily as maintenance (Tan 2003). The shortest possible duration should be used to minimize development of bacterial resistance; re-evaluate at 3 to 4 months (AAD [Zaenglein 2016])

Bacterial meningitis (off-label use): IV: 10 to 20 mg TMP/kg/day in divided doses every 6 to 12 hours (IDSA [Tunkel 2004])

Bite wounds (animal) (off-label use) (IDSA [Stevens 2014]):

Oral: One double-strength tablet twice daily; in combination with clindamycin or metronidazole

IV: 5 to 10 mg TMP/kg/day in divided doses every 6 to 12 hours in combination with clindamycin or metronidazole

Brain abscess, empyema, and epidural abscess (MRSA) (off-label use): IV: 5 mg TMP/kg/**dose** every 8 to 12 hours for 4 to 6 weeks (IDSA [Liu 2011])

Chronic bronchitis (acute): Oral: One double-strength tablet every 12 hours for 10 to 14 days

Cyclosporiasis (off-label use): Oral, IV: 160 mg TMP twice daily for 7 to 10 days. **Note:** AIDS patients: Oral: One double-strength tablet 2 to 4 times/day for 10 days, then 1 double-strength tablet 3 times/week for 10 weeks (Pape 1994; Verdier 2000).

Diabetic foot infection, mild (off-label use): Oral: One double-strength tablet 1 or 2 times/day. Continue therapy until resolution of infection (usually 1 to 2 weeks), but not through complete wound healing (Eleftheriadou 2010; IDSA [Lipsky 2012]; Lipsky 2004)

Granuloma inguinale (donovanosis) (off-label use): Oral: One double-strength tablet every 12 hours for at least 3 weeks and until lesions have healed (CDC [Workowski 2015]). **Note:** If symptoms do not improve within the first few days of therapy, the addition of gentamicin may be considered (CDC [Workowski 2015]).

Isosporiasis (*Isospora belli* infection) in HIV-infected patients (off-label use; HHS [OI adult 2015]):

Treatment: Oral, IV: 160 mg TMP 4 times/day for 10 days **or** 160 mg TMP 2 times/day for 7 to 10 days. May start with twice daily regimen and increase dose and/or duration up to 3 to 4 weeks if symptoms worsen or persist.

Chronic maintenance therapy (secondary prophylaxis) in patients with CD4 count <200 cells/mm^3: Oral: 160 mg TMP 3 times/week (preferred) or alternatively, 160 mg TMP daily or 320 mg TMP 3 times/week.

Melioidosis (*Burkholderia pseudomallei*) (off-label use) (Lipsitz 2012): Oral, IV:

Severe, acute phase involving brain, prostate, bone, or joint: Administer as 2 divided doses; given with ceftazidime or a carbapenem for ≥10 days followed by eradication therapy:

Adults <40 kg: 320 mg TMP daily

Adults 40 to 60 kg: 480 mg TMP daily

Adults >60 kg: 640 mg TMP daily

Eradication therapy: Administer as 2 divided doses for ≥12 weeks:

Adults <40 kg: 320 mg TMP daily

Adults 40 to 60 kg: 480 mg TMP daily

Adults >60 kg: 640 mg TMP daily

Postexposure prophylaxis: Administer as 2 divided doses for 21 days:

Adults <40 kg: 320 mg TMP daily

Adults 40 to 60 kg: 480 mg TMP daily

Adults >60 kg: 640 mg TMP daily

***Nocardia* (off-label use):** Oral, IV:

Cutaneous infections: 5 to 10 mg TMP/kg/day in 2 to 4 divided doses

Severe infections (pulmonary/cerebral): 15 mg TMP/kg/day in 2 to 4 divided doses for 3 to 4 weeks, then 10 mg TMP/kg/day in 2 to 4 divided doses. Treatment duration is controversial; an average of 7 months has been reported.

Note: Therapy for severe infection may be initiated IV and converted to oral therapy (frequently converted to approximate dosages of oral solid dosage forms: 2 DS tablets every 8 to 12 hours). Although not widely available, sulfonamide levels should be considered in patients with questionable absorption, at risk for dose-related toxicity, or those with poor therapeutic response.

Osteomyelitis due to MRSA (off-label use): Oral, IV: 3.5 to 4 mg TMP/kg/dose every 8 to 12 hours for a minimum of 8 weeks with rifampin 600 mg once daily (IDSA [Liu 2011])

***Pneumocystis* pneumonia:** HIV-infected patients (off-label dose; HHS [OI adult 2017]):

Primary or secondary prophylaxis: Oral: 80 or 160 mg TMP daily **or** alternatively, 160 mg TMP 3 times/week

Duration of prophylaxis: May discontinue primary or secondary prophylaxis if CD4 count increases from <200 cells/mm^3 to ≥200 cells/mm^3 for at least 3 months in response to ART; therapy must be restarted if CD4 count <200 cells/mm^3

Treatment:

Mild to moderate: Oral: 15 to 20 mg TMP/kg/day in 3 divided doses for 21 days **or** alternatively, 320 mg TMP 3 times daily for 21 days

Moderate to severe: Initial: IV: 15 to 20 mg TMP/kg/day in 3 to 4 divided doses for 21 days; may switch to oral therapy after clinical improvement

Prosthetic joint infection (off-label use): Oral phase treatment (after completion of pathogen-specific IV therapy) following debridement and prosthesis retention or 1-stage exchange:

Total ankle, elbow, hip, or shoulder arthroplasty: 160 mg TMP 2 times daily for 3 months. **Note:** Must be used in combination with rifampin (Cordero-Ampuero 2007; Osmon 2013).

Total knee arthroplasty: Adults: 160 mg TMP 2 times daily for 6 months. **Note:** Must be used in combination with rifampin (Cordero-Ampuero 2007; Osmon 2013).

Q fever (off-label use): Oral:

Acute (in pregnant women) (CDC 2013): 160 mg TMP twice daily throughout pregnancy but not beyond 32 weeks' gestation. **Note:** Discontinue therapy for the final 8 weeks of pregnancy due to hyperbilirubinemia risk

Chronic: Infectious Disease consult recommended for treatment of chronic Q fever

Septic arthritis due to MRSA (off-label use): Oral, IV: 3.5 to 4 mg TMP/kg/**dose** every 8 to 12 hours for 3 to 4 weeks (some experts combine with rifampin) (IDSA [Liu 2011])

Shigellosis: Note: Due to reported widespread resistance, empiric therapy with sulfamethoxazole and trimethoprim is not recommended (CDC-NARMS 2010; WHO 2005).

Oral: One double-strength tablet every 12 hours for 5 days

IV: 8 to 10 mg TMP/kg/day in divided doses every 6, 8, or 12 hours for 5 days

Skin/soft tissue infection due to MSSA or MRSA (off-label use): Oral: 1 to 2 double-strength tablets every 12 hours for 5 to 10 days (IDSA [Liu 2011]) or 7 to 14 days (IDSA [Stevens 2014]); **Note:** If beta-hemolytic *Streptococcus* spp are also suspected, a beta-lactam antibiotic should be added to the regimen (IDSA [Liu 2011])

Spontaneous bacterial peritonitis (prevention) (off-label use): Oral: Long-term prophylaxis: One double-strength (trimethoprim 160 mg/sulfamethoxazole 800 mg) tablet once daily (preferred) (Lontos 2014). Daily dosing for 5 days per week has been studied (Alvarez 2005; Singh 1995), but concerns regarding bacterial resistance with intermittent dosing limit use (AASLD [Runyon 2012]). American Association for the Study of Liver Diseases (AASLD) guidelines note that intermittent dosing (ie, 5 days/week, once weekly) of antibiotics, although shown to be effective in SBP prevention, may be inferior to daily dosing due to development of bacterial resistance. Daily dosing regimens are preferred (AASLD [Runyon 2012]).

Stenotrophomonas maltophilia **(ventilator-associated pneumonia) (off-label use):** IV: Most clinicians have utilized 12 to 15 mg TMP/kg/day for the treatment of VAP caused by *Stenotrophomonas maltophilia*. Higher doses (up to 20 mg TMP/kg/day) have been mentioned for treatment of severe infection in patients with normal renal function (Looney 2009; Vartivarian 1989; Wood 2010)

Surgical-site infections (trunk or extremity [away from axilla or perineum]) (off-label use): Oral: One double-strength tablet every 6 hours (IDSA [Stevens 2014])

Toxoplasma gondii **encephalitis in HIV-infected patients (off-label use; HHS [OI adult 2016]:**

Primary prophylaxis: Oral: 160 mg TMP daily (preferred) **or** 160 mg TMP 3 times/week **or** 80 mg TMP daily; primary prophylaxis is indicated for Toxoplasma IgG-positive patients with CD4 count <100 cells/mm^3

Treatment (alternative to preferred therapy): Oral, IV: 5 mg/kg TMP twice daily for at least 6 weeks; longer duration may be needed if clinical or radiologic disease is extensive or response is incomplete at 6 weeks.

Chronic maintenance therapy (alternative to preferred therapy): Oral: 160 mg TMP once or twice daily; may discontinue when asymptomatic and CD4 count >200 cells/mm^3 for >6 months in response to ART. **Note:** Once-daily dosing may be associated with an increased risk of relapse; if used, a gradual transition (eg, follow acute treatment with 4 to 6 weeks of 160 mg TMP twice daily before lowering to once-daily dosing) may be beneficial.

Travelers' diarrhea: Oral: One double-strength tablet every 12 hours for 5 days

Urinary tract infection:

Oral: One double-strength tablet every 12 hours

Duration of therapy: Uncomplicated: 3 to 5 days; Complicated: 7 to 10 days

Pyelonephritis: 14 days

Prostatitis: Acute: 2 weeks; Chronic: 2 to 3 months

IV: 8 to 10 mg TMP/kg/day in divided doses every 6, 8, or 12 hours for 14 days with severe infections

Pediatric Recommendations are based on the trimethoprim component.

General dosing guidelines: Children >2 months: Manufacturer's labeling:

Mild to moderate infections: Oral: 8 mg TMP/kg/day in divided doses every 12 hours

Serious infection:

Oral: 15 to 20 mg TMP/kg/day in divided doses every 6 hours

IV: 8 to 12 mg TMP/kg/day in divided doses every 6 to 12 hours

Indication-specific dosing:

Acute otitis media: Infants >2 months and Children: Oral: 8 mg TMP/kg/day in divided doses every 12 hours for 10 days. **Note:** Recommended by the American Academy of Pediatrics as an alternative agent in penicillin allergic patients at a dose of 6 to 10mg TMP/kg/day (AOM guidelines 2004).

Cyclosporiasis (off-label use): Infants >2 months and Children: Oral, IV: 5 mg TMP/kg twice daily for 7 to 10 days (*Red Book* 2009)

Head lice (*Pediculosis capitis*) (off-label use): Children ≥2 years: Oral: 10 mg TMP/kg/day in 2 divided doses for 7 to 10 days **or** 8 mg TMP/kg/day in 2 divided doses for 12 days with lindane shampoo also applied on day one (Hipolito 2001; Sim 2003).

Isosporiasis (*Isospora belli* infection) in HIV-infected patients (off-label use): Adolescents: Refer to adult dosing.

Melioidosis (*Burkholderia pseudomallei*) (off-label use; Lipsitz 2012): Oral, IV:

Severe, acute phase involving brain, prostate, bone, or joint: Administer as 2 divided doses; given with ceftazidime or a carbapenem for ≥10 days followed by eradication therapy:

Children: 16 mg TMP/kg/day (maximum: 640 mg TMP daily)

Adolescents: Refer to adult dosing

Eradication therapy: Administer as 2 divided doses for ≥12 weeks:

Children: 16 mg TMP/kg/day (maximum: 640 mg TMP daily)

Adolescents: Refer to adult dosing.

Postexposure prophylaxis: Administer as 2 divided doses for 21 days:

Children: 16 mg TMP/kg/day (maximum: 640 mg TMP daily)

Adolescents: Refer to adult dosing.

***Pneumocystis* pneumonia (PCP) (HIV-exposed/-positive) (off-label dose):**

Prophylaxis:

Infants (at least 4 weeks of age) and Children: Oral: 150 mg TMP/m^2/day or 5 mg TMP/kg/day for 3 to 7 days of every week; total daily dose may be given in divided doses every 12 hours for 3 consecutive or alternating days, in divided doses every 12 hours every day or as a single daily dose for 3 consecutive days; maximum daily dose: TMP 320 mg/day (HHS [OI pediatric 2016])

Adolescents: Oral: 80 to 160 mg TMP daily or alternatively, 160 mg TMP 3 times weekly (HHS [OI adult 2016]):

Treatment:

Infants ≥2 months and Children: Initial: IV: 15 to 20 mg TMP/kg/day in divided doses every 6 hours for 21 days; as acute pneumonitis subsides in patients with mild to moderate disease and no malabsorption issues nor diarrhea, may transition to oral therapy of same daily dose (15 to 20 mg/kg/day TMP) administered in divided doses 3 or 4 times daily (HHS [OI pediatric 2016])

Adolescents (HHS [OI adult 2017]):

Mild to moderate: Oral: 15 to 20 mg TMP/kg/day in 3 divided doses for 21 days **or** alternatively, 320 mg TMP 3 times daily for 21 days

Moderate to severe: Initial: IV: 15 to 20 mg TMP/kg/day in 3 to 4 divided doses for 21 days; may switch to oral after clinical improvement

Q fever (off-label use): Oral:

Acute: Infants ≥2 months and Children <8 years with mild or uncomplicated illness (if patient remains febrile past 5 days of doxycycline treatment): 4 to 20 mg TMP/kg/day in divided doses every 12 hours (maximum: trimethoprim 320 mg daily) (CDC 2013). **Note:** Some clinicians may recommend initial treatment with sulfamethoxazole and trimethoprim for children <8 years with mild or uncomplicated illness (CDC 2013; Hartzell 2008).

Chronic: Infectious Disease consult recommended for treatment of chronic Q fever (CDC 2013)

Shigellosis: Infants ≥2 months, Children, and Adolescents: Note: Due to reported widespread resistance, empiric therapy with sulfamethoxazole and trimethoprim is not recommended (CDC-NARMS 2010; WHO 2005). Oral:

Manufacturer's labeling: 8 mg TMP/kg/day in divided doses every 12 hours for 5 days

Alternate recommendations (off-label dose): 10 mg TMP/kg/day in divided doses every 12 hours for 5 days (Ashkenazi 1993)

IV: 8 to 10 mg TMP/kg/day in divided doses every 6, 8, or 12 hours for 5 days

Skin/soft tissue infection due to MSSA or MRSA (off-label use): Note: If beta-hemolytic *Streptococcus* spp are also suspected, a beta-lactam antibiotic should be added to the regimen (IDSA [Liu 2011])

Oral: 8 to 12 mg TMP/kg/day in divided doses every 12 hours for 5 to 10 days (IDSA [Liu 2011] or 7 to 14 days (IDSA [Stevens 2014])

IV: 8 to 12 mg TMP/kg/day in divided doses every 6 hours for 7 to 14 days (IDSA [Stevens 2014])

***Toxoplasma gondii* encephalitis in HIV-exposed/-infected patients (off-label use):**

Primary prophylaxis:

Infants ≥2 months and Children: Oral: 150 mg TMP/m^2/day for 3 to 7 days of every week; total daily dose may be given in divided doses every 12 hours for 3 consecutive or alternating days, in divided doses every 12 hours every day or as a single daily dose for 3 consecutive days (HHS [OI pediatric 2013])

Adolescents: Oral: Refer to adult dosing.

Treatment (alternative to preferred therapy): Adolescents: Oral, IV: Refer to adult dosing.

Chronic maintenance therapy (alternative to preferred therapy): Adolescents: Oral: Refer to adult dosing.

Urinary tract infection: Infants >2 months and Children:

Treatment:

Oral: Manufacturer's labeling: 8 mg TMP/kg/day in divided doses every 12 hours for 10 days

IV: Manufacturer's labeling: 8 to 10 mg TMP/kg/day in divided doses every 6, 8, or 12 hours for 14 days with serious infections

Prophylaxis: Oral: 2 mg TMP/kg/**dose** daily or 5 mg TMP/kg/**dose** twice weekly

Renal Impairment

Adults:

Manufacturer's labeling: Oral, IV:

CrCl >30 mL/minute: No dosage adjustment necessary.

CrCl 15 to 30 mL/minute: Administer 50% of recommended dose.

CrCl <15 mL/minute: Use is not recommended and is contraindicated per the manufacturer's labeling in severe renal disease if renal function cannot be monitored.

Alternate recommendations:

Aronoff 2007: Oral, IV: **Note:** The following dosage adjustments are based on a usual recommended dose of 5 to 20 mg TMP/kg/day in divided doses every 6 to 12 hours.

GFR 30 to 50 mL/minute/1.73m^2: 5 to 7.5 mg TMP/kg every 8 hours

GFR 10 to 29 mL/minute/1.73m^2: 5 to 10 mg TMP/kg every 12 hours

GFR <10 mL/minute/1.73m^2: Not recommended; if used, 5 to 10 mg TMP/kg every 24 hours

Intermittent hemodialysis (IHD): Not recommended; if used, 5 to 10 mg TMP/kg every 24 hours (dose after hemodialysis on dialysis days)

Peritoneal dialysis: Not recommended; if used, 5 to 10 mg TMP/kg every 24 hours

Golightly 2013:

Oral: **Note:** The following dosage adjustments are based on a usual maintenance dose of 1 double-strength tablet every 12 hours.

GFR 10 to 50 mL/minute: One double-strength tablet once, followed by 1 single-strength tablet every 12 hours.

GFR <10 mL/minute: Avoid use; if necessary, 1 double-strength tablet once, followed by 1 single-strength tablet every 24 hours.

Hemodialysis: One double-strength tablet once, followed by 1 single-strength tablet every 24 hours (dose after hemodialysis on dialysis days)

IV: **Note:** The following dosage adjustments are based on a usual maintenance dose of 4 to 5 mg TMP/kg every 6 hours.

GFR 10 to 50 mL/minute: 4 to 5 mg TMP/kg every 12 hours.

GFR <10 mL/minute: Avoid use; if necessary, 2.5 to 5 mg TMP/kg every 24 hours.

Hemodialysis: 2.5 to 5 mg TMP/kg every 24 hours (dose after hemodialysis on dialysis days)

HHS (OI adult 2016) *Pneumocystis* pneumonia (PCP), treatment: **Note:** Renal function may be estimated using the Cockcroft-Gault formula for dosage adjustment purposes.

Oral: **Note:** The following dosage adjustments are based on a usual maintenance dose of 2 double-strength tablets every 8 hours.

CrCl 10 to 30 mL/minute: Two double-strength tablets every 12 hours

CrCl <10 mL/minute: One double-strength tablet every 12 hours **or** 2 double-strength tablets every 24 hours

Hemodialysis: 2 double-strength tablets once daily (dose after hemodialysis on dialysis days); consider therapeutic drug monitoring to optimize therapy

IV: **Note:** The following dosage adjustments are based on a usual maintenance dose of 5 mg TMP/kg every 8 hours.

CrCl 10 to 30 mL/minute: 5 mg TMP/kg every 12 hours

CrCl <10 mL/minute: 5 mg TMP/kg every 24 hours

Hemodialysis: 5 mg TMP/kg once daily (dose after hemodialysis on dialysis days); consider therapeutic drug monitoring to optimize therapy

Continuous renal replacement therapy (CRRT) (Heintz 2009; Trotman 2005): Drug clearance is highly dependent on the method of renal replacement, filter type, and flow rate. Appropriate dosing requires close monitoring of pharmacologic response, signs of adverse reactions due to drug accumulation, as well as drug concentrations in relation to target trough (if appropriate). The following are general recommendations only (based on dialysate flow/ultrafiltration rates of 1 to 2 L/hour and minimal residual renal function) and should not supersede clinical judgment:

CVVH/CVVHD/CVVHDF: Oral, IV: 2.5 to 7.5 mg/kg of TMP every 12 hours. **Note:** Dosing regimen dependent on clinical indication. Critically ill patients with *P. jirovecii* pneumonia receiving CVVHDF may require up to 10 mg/kg every 12 hours (Heintz 2009).

Pediatric:

Manufacturer's labeling: Infants ≥2 months, Children, and Adolescents: Oral, IV:

CrCl >30 mL/minute: No dosage adjustment necessary

CrCl 15 to 30 mL/minute: Administer 50% of recommended dose

CrCl <15 mL/minute: Use is not recommended and is contraindicated per the manufacturer's labeling in severe renal disease if renal function cannot be monitored.

Alternate recommendations:

Children and Adolescents (Veltri 2004): Oral, IV: **Note:** Renally adjusted dose recommendations are based on doses of 3 to 5 mg/kg/**dose** every 12 hours.

CrCl 10 to 50 mL/minute/1.73 m^2: 3 to 5 mg TMP/kg/**dose** every 18 hours

CrCl <10 mL/minute/1.73 m^2: 3 to 5 mg TMP/kg/**dose** every 24 hours

Hemodialysis: 3 to 5 mg TMP/kg/**dose** every 24 hours; administer 2.5 mg TMP/kg/**dose** after each dialysis session

CRRT (CAVH/CVVH/CAVHD/CVVHD):

Combined dialysis flow + ultrafiltration rate <1,500 mL/m^2/hour: 3 to 5 mg TMP/kg/**dose** every 18 hours

Combined dialysis flow + ultrafiltration rate ≥1,500 mL/m^2/hour: 4 to 5 mg TMP/kg/**dose** every 18 hours

Pneumocystis pneumonia (PCP), treatment: Oral, IV:

Children (Veltri 2004): **Note:** Renally adjusted dose recommendations are based on doses of 5 mg/kg/**dose** every 6 hours.

CrCl 10 to 50 mL/minute/1.73 m^2: 5 mg TMP/kg/**dose** every 8 hours

CrCl <10 mL/minute/1.73 m^2: 5 mg TMP/kg/**dose** every 12 hours

Hemodialysis: 5 mg TMP/kg/**dose** every 12 hours; administer 2.5 mg TMP/kg/**dose** after each dialysis session

CRRT: CAVH/CVVH/CAVHD/CVVHD: 5 mg TMP/kg/**dose** every 8 hours

Adolescents: Refer to adult dosing.

Hepatic Impairment There are no dosage adjustments provided in manufacturer's labeling. Use with caution; use is contraindicated in cases of marked hepatic damage.

Additional Information Complete prescribing information should be consulted for additional detail.

Dosage Forms Considerations The 5:1 ratio (SMX:TMP) remains constant in all dosage forms.

Dosage Forms Excipient information presented when available (limited, particularly for generics); consult specific product labeling.

Solution, Intravenous:

Generic: Sulfamethoxazole 80 mg and trimethoprim 16 mg per mL (5 mL, 10 mL, 30 mL)

Suspension, Oral:

Sulfatrim Pediatric: Sulfamethoxazole 200 mg and trimethoprim 40 mg per 5 mL (473 mL) [contains alcohol, usp, fd&c red #40, fd&c yellow #6 (sunset yellow), methylparaben, polysorbate 80, propylene glycol, propylparaben, saccharin sodium; cherry flavor]

Generic: Sulfamethoxazole 200 mg and trimethoprim 40 mg per 5 mL (20 mL, 473 mL)

Tablet, Oral:

Bactrim: Sulfamethoxazole 400 mg and trimethoprim 80 mg [scored; contains sodium benzoate]

Bactrim DS: Sulfamethoxazole 800 mg and trimethoprim 160 mg [scored; contains sodium benzoate]

Generic: Sulfamethoxazole 400 mg and trimethoprim 80 mg, Sulfamethoxazole 800 mg and trimethoprim 160 mg

Dosage Forms: Canada Information with regard to form, strength, and availability of products uniquely available in Canada but currently not available in the US. Refer also to Dosage Forms.

Excipient information presented when available (limited, particularly for generics); consult specific product labeling.

Tablet, Oral: Sulfamethoxazole 100 mg and trimethoprim 20 mg

SUNItinib (su NIT e nib)

Related Information

Management of Chemotherapy-Induced Nausea and Vomiting in Adults *on page 2253*

Prevention of Chemotherapy-Induced Nausea and Vomiting in Children *on page 2310*

Safe Handling of Hazardous Drugs *on page 2379*

Brand Names: US Sutent

Brand Names: Canada Sutent

Index Terms SU011248; SU11248; Sunitinib Malate

Pharmacologic Category Antineoplastic Agent, Tyrosine Kinase Inhibitor; Antineoplastic Agent, Vascular Endothelial Growth Factor (VEGF) Inhibitor; Vascular Endothelial Growth Factor (VEGF) Inhibitor

Use

Gastrointestinal stromal tumor: Treatment of gastrointestinal stromal tumor (GIST) after disease progression on or intolerance to imatinib

Pancreatic neuroendocrine tumors, advanced: Treatment of progressive, well-differentiated pancreatic neuroendocrine tumors in patients with unresectable locally advanced or metastatic disease

Renal cell carcinoma, advanced: Treatment of advanced renal cell carcinoma

Labeled Contraindications There are no contraindications listed in the manufacturer's US labeling.

Canadian labeling: Hypersensitivity to sunitinib or any component of the formulation; pregnancy

Pregnancy Considerations Animal reproduction studies have demonstrated teratogenicity, embryotoxicity, and fetal loss. Because sunitinib inhibits angiogenesis, a critical component of fetal development, adverse effects on pregnancy would be expected. Women of childbearing potential should be advised to avoid pregnancy if receiving sunitinib.

Breastfeeding Considerations It is not known if sunitinib is excreted in human milk. Due to the potential for serious adverse reactions in the nursing infant, the decision to discontinue breastfeeding or discontinue sunitinib should take into account the benefits of treatment to the mother.

Warnings/Precautions [US Boxed Warning]: Hepatotoxicity, which may be severe and/or fatal, has been observed in clinical trials and in postmarketing surveillance. Signs of liver failure include jaundice, elevated transaminases, and/or hyperbilirubinemia, in conjunction with encephalopathy, coagulopathy and/or renal failure. Monitor liver function tests at baseline, with each treatment cycle, and if clinically indicated. Withhold treatment for grade 3 or 4 hepatotoxicity; discontinue if hepatotoxicity does not resolve. Do not reinitiate in patients with severe changes in liver function tests or other signs/symptoms of liver failure. Sunitinib has not been studied in patients with ALT or AST >2.5 times ULN (or >5 times ULN if due to liver metastases).

Cardiovascular events (some fatal), including heart failure, cardiomyopathy, myocardial ischemia and myocardial infarction (MI) have been reported. Use with caution in patients at risk for cardiovascular events. May cause a decrease in left ventricular ejection fraction (LVEF), including some grade 3 reductions. Obtain LVEF evaluation prior to treatment. Discontinue with clinical signs and symptoms of heart failure. Interrupt therapy and/or decrease dose with LVEF <50% and >20% reduction from baseline in patients without clinical heart failure signs/symptoms. Patients with cardiac events (MI, bypass ▶

◀ grafts, symptomatic heart failure, cerebrovascular accident, transient ischemic attack, and pulmonary embolism) within the previous 12 months were excluded from clinical trials and it is not known if the risk for left ventricular dysfunction is increased in patient with these conditions; assess risks versus benefits; monitor for clinical signs/symptoms of heart failure, in addition to baseline, also obtain periodic LVEF evaluation.

May cause hypertension; monitor and control with antihypertensives if needed; interrupt therapy until hypertension is controlled for severe hypertension. Use caution and closely monitor in patients with underlying or poorly controlled hypertension. Potentially significant drug-drug interactions may exist, requiring dose or frequency adjustment, additional monitoring, and/or selection of alternative therapy.

Hemorrhagic events have been reported including epistaxis, rectal, gingival, upper GI, urinary tract, genital, brain, wound bleeding, tumor-related, and hemoptysis/pulmonary hemorrhage; may be serious and/or fatal. Proteinuria and nephrotic syndrome have been reported; some cases have led to renal failure and fatal outcomes. Monitor for new onset or worsening proteinuria with baseline and periodic urinalysis and follow up with 24-hour urine protein if clinically indicated. If urine protein is ≥3 g/24 hours, interrupt treatment and reduce the dose. Discontinue treatment in patients with nephrotic syndrome or persistent urine protein ≥3 g/24 hours despite dose reductions. The safety of continuing treatment with sunitinib in patients with moderate to severe proteinuria has not been evaluated. Thrombotic microangiopathy (including thrombotic thrombocytopenic purpura and hemolytic uremic syndrome), sometimes leading to renal failure or fatality, has been reported with sunitinib, both as monotherapy and in combination with bevacizumab. Discontinue if thrombotic microangiopathy develops; effects may be reversible after discontinuation. Impaired wound healing has been reported with sunitinib; temporarily withhold treatment for patients undergoing major surgical procedures; the optimal time to resume treatment after a procedure has not been determined. Serious and fatal GI complications, including GI perforation, have occurred (rarely). Pancreatitis has been observed in RCC patients; discontinue sunitinib if symptoms are present. Thyroid dysfunction (eg, hypothyroidism, hyperthyroidism, and thyroiditis) may occur; the risk for hypothyroidism appears to increase with therapy duration; hyperthyroidism, sometimes followed by hypothyroidism has also been reported; monitor thyroid function at baseline. Patients not receiving thyroid hormone replacement therapy at sunitinib initiation should be monitored (TSH) every 4 weeks for 4 months and then every 2 to 3 months; those already receiving levothyroxine prior to initiating sunitinib should have TSH monitored every 4 weeks until levels and levothyroxine dose are stable, then monitor every 2 months (Hamnvik, 2011). Adrenal function abnormalities have been reported; monitor for adrenal insufficiency in patients with stress such as trauma, severe infection, or who are undergoing surgery. Symptomatic hypoglycemia has been associated with sunitinib; may result in loss of consciousness or require hospitalization. Hypoglycemia occurred infrequently in patients with renal cell cancer and gastrointestinal stromal tumors (GIST); however, the incidence is higher (~10%) in patients with pancreatic neuroendocrine tumors (PNET); preexisting glucose homeostasis abnormalities were not always present in hypoglycemic patients with PNET. Blood glucose decreases may be worse in patients with diabetes. Monitor blood glucose levels regularly during and following discontinuation of treatment. Dose modifications of antidiabetic medications may be necessary to minimize the risk of hypoglycemia.

Severe cutaneous reactions, including erythema multiforme (EM), Stevens-Johnson syndrome (SJS), and toxic epidermal necrolysis (TEN) have been reported (some fatal); if signs/symptoms of EM, SJS, or TEN (progressive skin rash, often with blisters or mucosal lesions) are present, discontinue sunitinib. Do not restart treatment if SJS or TEN are suspected. Necrotizing fasciitis (with fatalities) has been reported, including perineum necrotizing fasciitis and fasciitis secondary to fistula formation. Discontinue sunitinib in patients who develop necrotizing fasciitis. Sunitinib may cause skin and/or hair depigmentation or discoloration. Hand-foot skin reaction (HFSR) observed with tyrosine kinase inhibitors (TKIs) is distinct from hand-foot syndrome (palmar-plantar erythrodysesthesia) associated with traditional chemotherapy agents; HFSR due to TKIs is localized with defined hyperkeratotic lesions; symptoms include burning, dysesthesia, paresthesia, or tingling on the palms/soles, and generally occur within the first 2 to 4 weeks of treatment; pressure and flexor areas may develop blisters (callus-like), dry/cracked skin, edema, erythema, desquamation, or hyperkeratosis (Appleby, 2011). The following treatments may be used in addition to the recommended dosage modifications (Lacouture, 2008). Prior to treatment initiation, a pedicure is recommended to remove hyperkeratotic areas/calluses, which may predispose to HFSR; avoid vigorous exercise/activities that may stress hands or feet. During therapy, patients should reduce exposure to hot water (may exacerbate hand-foot symptoms); avoid constrictive footwear and excessive skin friction. Patients may also wear thick cotton gloves or socks and should wear shoes with padded insoles. Grade 1 HFSR may be relieved with moisturizing creams, cotton gloves and socks (at night) and/or keratolytic creams such as urea (20% to 40%) or salicylic acid (6%). Apply topical steroid (eg, clobetasol ointment) twice daily to erythematous areas of grade 2 HFSR; topical anesthetics (eg, lidocaine 2%) and then systemic analgesics (if appropriate) may be used for pain control. Resolution of acute erythema may result in keratotic areas which may be softened with keratolytic agents. Reversible posterior leukoencephalopathy syndrome (RPLS) has been reported (rarely, some fatal); symptoms include confusion, headache, hypertension, lethargy, seizure, blindness and/or other vision, or neurologic disturbances; interrupt treatment and begin hypertension management. Tumor lysis syndrome (TLS), including fatalities, has been reported, predominantly in patients with RCC or GIST; risk for TLS is higher in patients with a high tumor burden prior to treatment; monitor closely; correct clinically significant dehydration and treat high uric acid levels prior to initiation of treatment. An increased incidence of fatigue, thyroid dysfunction and treatment-induced hypertension was reported in patients with renal insufficiency (CrCl ≤60 mL/minute) who received sunitinib for the treatment of renal cell cancer (Gupta, 2011).

Osteonecrosis of the jaw (ONJ), also referred to as medication-related osteonecrosis of the jaw (MRONJ) has been reported with sunitinib. Concurrent bisphosphonate use or dental disease may increase the risk for ONJ. According to a position paper by the American Association of Maxillofacial Surgeons (AAOMS), MRONJ has been associated with bisphosphonates and other antiresorptive agents (denosumab), and antiangiogenic agents (eg, bevacizumab, sunitinib) used for the treatment of osteoporosis or malignancy. Antiangiogenic agents, when given concomitantly with antiresorptive agents, are associated with an increased risk of ONJ. Other risk factors for MRONJ include dentoalveolar surgery (eg, tooth extraction, dental implants), preexisting inflammatory dental disease, and concomitant corticosteroid use. Consider a dental examination and preventive dentistry prior to initiation of sunitinib (and during therapy); if possible, avoid invasive dental procedures in patients with current or prior bisphosphonate use. The AAOMS suggests that if medically permissible, initiation of antiangiogenic agents for cancer therapy should be delayed until optimal dental health is attained (if extractions are required, antiangiogenesis therapy should delayed until the extraction site has mucosalized or until after adequate osseous healing). Once antiangiogenic therapy for oncologic disease is initiated, procedures that involve direct osseous injury and placement of dental implants should be avoided. Patients developing ONJ during therapy should receive care by an oral surgeon (AAOMS [Ruggiero 2014]).

Dosing schedules vary by indication; some treatment regimens are continuous daily dosing; other treatment schedules are daily dosing for 4 weeks of a 6-week cycle (4 weeks on, 2 weeks off).

Adverse Reactions

>10%:

Cardiovascular: Hypertension (27% to 34%, GIST: 8% to 15%; grade 3: 10% to 13%, GIST: 4%), decreased left ventricular ejection fraction (RCC: 16% to 27%, grade 3: 3% to 7%; GIST: 11%, grade 3: 1%), peripheral edema (RCC: 24%), chest pain (RCC: 13%), severe hypertension (4% to 10%; >200 mmHg systolic or 110 mmHg diastolic)

Central nervous system: Fatigue (RCC: 62%, pNET: 33%), glossalgia (pNET: ≤48%; RCC: 11%), mouth pain (pNET: ≤48%; RCC: 6% to 14%), headache (18% to 23%), insomnia (15% to 18%), chills (RCC: 14%), depression (RCC: 11%), dizziness (RCC: 11%)

Dermatologic: Skin discoloration (≤25% to 30%; yellow color), hair discoloration (20% to 29%; GIST: 7%), palmar-plantar erythrodysesthesia (23% to 29%, GIST: 14%; grades 3/4: 4% to 8%), xeroderma (15% to 23%), skin rash (14% to 18%; RCC: 29%), alopecia (5% to 14%), erythema (RCC: 12%), pruritus (RCC: 12%)

Endocrine & metabolic: Increased uric acid (RCC: 46%), decreased serum calcium (34% to 42%), decreased serum albumin (pNET: 41%, RCC: 28%), decreased serum phosphate (31% to 36%), increased serum glucose (RCC: 23%), decreased serum potassium (12% to 21%), decreased serum sodium (RCC: 20%), decreased serum magnesium (pNET: 19%), increased serum potassium (16% to 18%), hypothyroidism (4% to 7%; RCC: 16%), increased serum calcium (RCC: 13%), increased serum sodium (10% to 13%)

Gastrointestinal: Diarrhea (59% to 66%; GIST: 40%), nausea (RCC: 58%; pNET: 45%), increased serum lipase (17% to 25%; RCC: 56%; grades 3/4: 5% to 18%), anorexia (RCC: 48%; GIST: 33%), mucositis (47% to 48%, GIST: 29%; includes aphthous stomatitis, dry mucous membranes, gingival pain, gingivitis, glossitis, oral discomfort, oral mucosal ulcer, stomatitis, tongue ulceration), dysgeusia (21%; RCC: 47%), vomiting (34% to 39%), abdominal pain (30% to 39%), increased serum amylase (17% to 20%; RCC: 35%; grades 3/4: 4% to 6%), dyspepsia (34%; pNET: 15%), constipation (20% to 23%), weight loss (16%), flatulence (RCC: 14%), xerostomia (RCC: 13%), gastroesophageal reflux disease (RCC: 12%)

Hematologic & oncologic: Decreased hemoglobin (RCC: 79%, pNET: 65%, GIST: 26%; grades 3/4: ≤8%), leukocyte disorder (decreased leukocytes; RCC: 78%; grades 3/4: 8%), decreased neutrophils (71% to 77%, GIST: 53%; grades 3/4: 10% to 17%), abnormal absolute lymphocyte count (decreased; RCC: 68%, pNET: 56%, GIST: 38%; grades 3/4: RCC: 18%, pNET: 7%), decreased platelet count (60% to 68%, GIST: 38%, GIST and RCC: grades 3/4: 5% to 9%), hemorrhage (18% to 22%; RCC: 37%; RCC and GIST, grades 3/4: 3% to 4%; includes hematemesis, hematochezia, hematoma, hemoptysis, melena, metrorrhagia)

Hepatic: Increased serum AST (pNET: 72%, RCC: 56%, GIST: ≤39%; grades 3/4: ≤2% to 5%), increased serum ALT (pNET: 61%; RCC: 51%; GIST: ≤39%; grades 3/4: ≤2% to 4%), increased serum alkaline phosphatase (RCC: 46%; GIST: 24%; grades 3/4: 2% to 4%), increased serum bilirubin (16% to 20%; pNET: 37%; RCC and GIST, grades 3/4: 1%), increased indirect serum bilirubin (RCC and GIST: 10% to 13%; grades 3/4: ≤1%)

Neuromuscular & skeletal: Increased creatine phosphokinase (RCC: 49%), limb pain (RCC: 40%; GIST: ≤14%), weakness (22% to 34%), arthralgia (RCC: 30%; pNET: 15%), back pain (RCC: 28%), myalgia (GIST: ≤14%)

Renal: Increased serum creatinine (RCC: 70%; GIST: 12%)

Respiratory: Cough (RCC: 27%), dyspnea (RCC: 26%), epistaxis (pNET: 20%), nasopharyngitis (RCC: 14%), oropharyngeal pain (RCC: 14%), upper respiratory tract infection (RCC: 11%)

Miscellaneous: Fever (RCC: 22%)

1% to 10%:

Cardiovascular: Deep vein thrombosis (≤3%), pulmonary embolism (≤3%)

Endocrine & metabolic: Hypoglycemia (2%; pNET: 10%)

Gastrointestinal: Hemorrhoids (RCC: 10%), pancreatitis (1%)

Respiratory: Flu-like symptoms (RCC: 5%)

<1%, postmarketing, and/or case reports: Acute renal failure, adrenocortical insufficiency, arterial thrombosis (includes cerebral infarction, cerebrovascular accident, transient ischemic attack), cardiac failure, cardiomyopathy, cerebral hemorrhage, cholecystitis (particularly acalculous), erythema multiforme, esophagitis, fistula (sometimes associated with tumor necrosis and/or regression), fulminant necrotizing fasciitis (including of the perineum), gastrointestinal hemorrhage, gastrointestinal perforation, hemolytic uremic syndrome, hepatic failure, hepatotoxicity, hypersensitivity (includes angioedema), hyperthyroidism, ischemic heart disease, myocardial infarction, myopathy (with/without acute renal failure), nephrotic syndrome, neutropenic infection, osteonecrosis of the jaw, preeclampsia (like syndrome with proteinuria and reversible hypertension) (Gallucci 2013; Patel 2008), prolonged Q-T interval on ECG (dose dependent), proteinuria, pulmonary hemorrhage, pyoderma gangrenosum (including positive dechallenges), renal insufficiency, respiratory tract hemorrhage, respiratory tract infection (may be serious), reversible posterior leukoencephalopathy syndrome, rhabdomyolysis (with/without acute renal failure), seizure, sepsis, septic shock, skin infection (may be serious), Stevens-Johnson syndrome, thrombotic thrombocytopenic purpura, thyroiditis (Feldt 2012), torsades de pointes, toxic epidermal necrolysis, tumor hemorrhage, tumor lysis syndrome, urinary tract hemorrhage, urinary tract infection (may be serious), ventricular arrhythmia, wound healing impairment

Drug Interactions

Metabolism/Transport Effects Substrate of CYP3A4 (major); **Note:** Assignment of Major/Minor substrate status based on clinically relevant drug interaction potential; **Inhibits** BCRP

Avoid Concomitant Use

Avoid concomitant use of SUNItinib with any of the following: BCG (Intravesical); Bevacizumab; Conivaptan; Fusidic Acid (Systemic); Idelalisib; Natalizumab; Pimecrolimus; St John's Wort; Tacrolimus (Topical); Temsirolimus; Vaccines (Live)

Increased Effect/Toxicity

SUNItinib may increase the levels/effects of: Bevacizumab; Bisphosphonate Derivatives; Fingolimod; Highest Risk QTc-Prolonging Agents; Hypoglycemia-Associated Agents; Leflunomide; Moderate Risk QTc-Prolonging Agents; Natalizumab; Tofacitinib; Vaccines (Live)

The levels/effects of SUNItinib may be increased by: Androgens; Antidiabetic Agents; Antifungal Agents (Azole Derivatives, Systemic); Aprepitant; Bevacizumab; Conivaptan; CYP3A4 Inhibitors (Moderate); CYP3A4 Inhibitors (Strong); Dasatinib; Denosumab; Fosaprepitant; Fusidic Acid (Systemic); Grapefruit Juice; Herbs (Hypoglycemic Properties); Idelalisib; MAO Inhibitors; MiFEPRIStone; Netupitant; NiCARdipine; Ocrelizumab; Palbociclib; Pegvisomant; Pimecrolimus; Prothionamide; Quinolone Antibiotics; Roflumilast; Salicylates; Selective Serotonin Reuptake Inhibitors; Simeprevir; Stiripentol; Tacrolimus (Topical); Temsirolimus; Trastuzumab

Decreased Effect

SUNItinib may decrease the levels/effects of: BCG (Intravesical); Coccidioides immitis Skin Test; Nivolumab; Sipuleucel-T; Tertomotide; Vaccines (Inactivated); Vaccines (Live)

The levels/effects of SUNItinib may be decreased by: Bosentan; CYP3A4 Inducers (Moderate); CYP3A4 Inducers (Strong); Dabrafenib; Deferasirox; Dexamethasone (Systemic); Echinacea; Enzalutamide; Mitotane; Quinolone Antibiotics; Sarilumab; Siltuximab; St John's Wort; Tocilizumab

Food Interactions Grapefruit juice may increase the levels/effects of sunitinib. Food has no effect on the bioavailability of sunitinib. Management: Avoid grapefruit juice.

Hazardous Drugs Handling Considerations

Hazardous agent (NIOSH 2016 [group 1]).

Use appropriate precautions for receiving, handling, administration, and disposal. Gloves (single) should be worn during receiving, unpacking, and placing in storage.

NIOSH recommends single gloving for administration of intact tablets or capsules. If manipulating tablets/capsules (eg, to prepare an oral suspension), NIOSH recommends double gloving, a protective gown, and preparation in a controlled device; if not prepared in a controlled device, respiratory and eye/face protection as well as ventilated engineering controls are recommended. NIOSH recommends double gloving, a protective gown, and (if there is a potential for vomit or spit up) eye/face protection for administration of an oral liquid/feeding tube administration (NIOSH 2016).

Storage/Stability Store at 25°C (77°F); excursions are permitted between 15°C to 30°C (59°F to 86°F).

Mechanism of Action Exhibits antitumor and antiangiogenic properties by inhibiting multiple receptor tyrosine kinases, including platelet-derived growth factors (PDGFRα and PDGFRβ), vascular endothelial growth factors (VEGFR1, VEGFR2, and VEGFR3), FMS-like tyrosine kinase-3 (FLT3), colony-stimulating factor type 1 (CSF-1R), and glial cell-line-derived neurotrophic factor receptor (RET).

Pharmacodynamics/Kinetics

Distribution: V_d/F: 2230 L

Protein binding: Sunitinib: 95%; SU12662: 90%

Metabolism: Hepatic; primarily metabolized by CYP3A4 to the N-desethyl metabolite SU12662 (active)

Half-life elimination: Terminal: Sunitinib: 40 to 60 hours; SU12662: 80 to 110 hours

Time to peak, plasma: 6 to 12 hours

Excretion: Feces (61%); urine (16%)

Dosing

Adult & Geriatric Note: Dosage modifications should be done in increments or decrements of 12.5 mg; individualize based on safety and tolerability.

Gastrointestinal stromal tumor (GIST): Oral: 50 mg once daily for 4 weeks of a 6-week treatment cycle (4 weeks on, 2 weeks off)

GIST off-label dosing: Oral: 37.5 mg once daily, continuous daily dosing (George, 2009, *EJC*)

Pancreatic neuroendocrine tumors, advanced (PNET): Oral: 37.5 mg once daily, continuous daily dosing (maximum daily dose used in clinical trials: 50 mg)

Renal cell cancer, advanced (RCC): Oral: 50 mg once daily for 4 weeks of a 6-week treatment cycle (4 weeks on, 2 weeks off)

Soft tissue sarcoma, non-GIST (off-label use): Oral: 37.5 mg once daily, continuous daily dosing (George, 2009, *JCO*)

Thyroid cancer, refractory (off-label use): Oral: 50 mg once daily for 4 weeks of a 6-week treatment cycle (4 weeks on, 2 weeks off) (Cohen, 2008; Ravaud, 2008)

Dosage adjustment with concurrent CYP3A4 inhibitor: Avoid concomitant administration with strong CYP3A4 inhibitors (eg, clarithromycin, erythromycin, itraconazole, ketoconazole, nefazodone, protease inhibitors, telithromycin, voriconazole); if concomitant administration with a strong CYP3A4 inhibitor cannot be avoided, consider a dose reduction to a minimum of 37.5 mg/day (GIST, RCC) or 25 mg/day (PNET).

Dosage adjustment with concurrent CYP3A4 inducer: Avoid concomitant administration with strong CYP3A4 inducers (eg, carbamazepine, dexamethasone, phenobarbital, phenytoin, rifampin, St John's wort); if concomitant administration with a strong CYP3A4 inducer cannot be avoided, consider a dosage increase (with careful monitoring for toxicity) to a maximum of 87.5 mg/day (GIST, RCC) or 62.5 mg/day (PNET).

Renal Impairment

Mild, moderate, or severe impairment: No initial adjustment required; subsequent adjustments may be needed based on safety and tolerance.

ESRD on hemodialysis: No initial adjustment required; subsequent dosage **increases** (up to twofold) may be required due to reduced (47%) exposure

Hepatic Impairment

Preexisting hepatic impairment: No adjustment is necessary with mild-to-moderate (Child-Pugh class A or B) hepatic impairment; not studied in patients with severe (Child-Pugh class C) hepatic impairment. Studies excluded patients with ALT or AST >2.5 x ULN, or if due to liver metastases, ALT or AST >5 x ULN.

Hepatotoxicity during treatment: Hepatic adverse events ≥ grade 3 or 4: Withhold treatment; discontinue if hepatotoxicity does not resolve. Do not reinitiate in patients with severe changes in liver function tests or other signs/symptoms of liver failure.

Adjustment for Toxicity Dosage modifications should be done in increments or decrements of 12.5 mg; individualize based on safety and tolerability.

Cardiac toxicity:

Ejection fraction <50% and >20% below baseline without evidence of CHF: Interrupt treatment and/or reduce dose.

LV dysfunction with CHF clinical manifestations: Discontinue treatment.

Dermatologic toxicity:

Signs/symptoms of erythema multiforme (EM), Stevens-Johnson syndrome (SJS), and toxic epidermal necrolysis (TEN), including progressive skin rash, often with blisters or mucosal lesions: Discontinue sunitinib; do not restart treatment if SJS or TEN are suspected.

Necrotizing fasciitis: Discontinue sunitinib.

Hypertension, severe: Temporarily interrupt treatment until hypertension is controlled.

Nephrotic syndrome: Discontinue treatment.

Pancreatitis: Discontinue treatment.

Proteinuria:

Urine protein ≥3 g/24 hours: Interrupt treatment and reduce the dose.

Persistent urine protein ≥3 g/24 hours despite dose reductions: Discontinue treatment.

Reversible posterior leukoencephalopathy (RPLS): Temporarily withhold treatment; after resolution, may resume with discretion.

Thrombotic microangiopathy: Discontinue treatment.

Administration Avoid contact with broken or leaking capsules; if contact occurs, wash immediately with soap and water.

Emetic Potential

Children: Minimal (<10%)

Adults: Low (10% to 30%)

Extemporaneous Preparations A 10 mg/mL sunitinib oral suspension may be made with capsules and a 1:1 mixture of Ora-Sweet and Ora-Plus. Empty the contents of three 50 mg sunitinib capsules into a mortar; add small portions of vehicle and mix to a uniform paste. Mix while adding vehicle in incremental proportions to 15 mL. Transfer to amber plastic bottle and label "shake well". This suspension maintains an average concentration of 96% to 106% (of the original concentration) at room temperature or refrigerated for up to 60 days in plastic amber prescription bottles.

Navid F, Christensen R, Minkin P, et al, "Stability of Sunitinib in Oral Suspension," *Ann Pharmacother*, 2008, 42(7):962-6.

Monitoring Parameters LVEF, baseline (and periodic with cardiac risk factors), ECG (12-lead; baseline and periodic), blood pressure; adrenal function CBC with differential and platelets (prior to each treatment cycle), liver function tests (baseline, with each cycle and if clinically indicated), serum chemistries including magnesium, phosphate, and potassium (prior to each treatment cycle), blood glucose levels (regularly during and following discontinuation of treatment), urinalysis (for proteinuria development or worsening); consider dental exam prior to treatment initiation; symptoms of hypothyroidism, hyperthyroidism, or thyroiditis; signs/symptoms of hypoglycemia

Thyroid function testing (Hamnvik, 2011):

Preexisting levothyroxine therapy: Obtain baseline TSH levels, then monitor every 4 weeks until levels and levothyroxine dose are stable, then monitor every 2 months

Without preexisting thyroid hormone replacement: TSH at baseline, then every 4 weeks for 4 months, then every 2-3 months

Dietary Considerations Avoid grapefruit juice.

Medication Guide Available Yes

Dosage Forms Excipient information presented when available (limited, particularly for generics); consult specific product labeling.

Capsule, Oral:

Sutent: 12.5 mg, 25 mg, 37.5 mg, 50 mg

- ◆ **Sunitinib Malate** see SUNItinib on page 1707
- ◆ **Supprelin LA** see Histrelin on page 912
- ◆ **Sustol** see Granisetron on page 895
- ◆ **Sutent** see SUNItinib on page 1707
- ◆ **Sylatron** see Peginterferon Alfa-2b on page 1473
- ◆ **Sylvant** see Siltuximab on page 1663
- ◆ **Symproic** see Naldemedine on page 1297
- ◆ **Sympt-X [OTC]** see Glutamine on page 886
- ◆ **Syndros** see Dronabinol on page 647
- ◆ **Synribo** see Omacetaxine on page 1375
- ◆ **Tabloid** see Thioguanine on page 1774

Tacrolimus (Systemic) (ta KROE li mus)

Related Information

Hematopoietic Cell Transplantation on page 2365

Management of EGFR Inhibitor Toxicities: Dermatologic, Ocular, and Gastrointestinal on page 2291

Safe Handling of Hazardous Drugs on page 2379

Brand Names: US Astagraf XL; Envarsus XR; Hecoria [DSC]; Prograf

Brand Names: Canada Advagraf; Prograf; Sandoz-Tacrolimus

Index Terms FK506

Pharmacologic Category Calcineurin Inhibitor; Immunosuppressant Agent

Use Organ rejection prophylaxis:

Astagraf XL: Prevention of organ rejection in kidney transplant recipients in combination with other immunosuppressants.

Envarsus XR: Prevention of organ rejection in kidney transplant recipients converted from tacrolimus immediate-release formulation, in combination with other immunosuppressants.

Hecoria and Prograf: Prevention of organ rejection in heart, kidney, and liver transplant recipients

◀ **Note:** Extended-release products (Astagraf XL and Envarsus XR) are not interchangeable or substitutable with immediate release tacrolimus. In addition, the once-daily formulations (Astagraf XL and Envarsus XR) are not interchangeable with each other due to significantly different pharmacokinetic properties.

Labeled Contraindications Hypersensitivity to tacrolimus, polyoxyl 60 hydrogenated castor oil (HCO-60), or any other component of the formulation.

Pregnancy Considerations Adverse events were observed in animal reproduction studies. Tacrolimus crosses the human placenta and is measurable in the cord blood, amniotic fluid, and newborn serum. Tacrolimus concentrations in the placenta may be higher than the maternal serum (Jain 1997). Infants with lower birth weights have been found to have higher tacrolimus concentrations (Bramham 2013). Transient neonatal hyperkalemia and renal dysfunction have been reported.

Tacrolimus pharmacokinetics are altered during pregnancy. Whole blood concentrations decrease as pregnancy progresses; however, unbound concentrations increase. Measuring unbound concentrations may be preferred, especially in women with anemia or hypoalbuminemia. If unbound concentration measurement is not available, interpretation of whole blood concentrations should account for RBC count and serum albumin concentration (Hebert 2013; Zheng 2012).

In general, women who have had a kidney transplant should be instructed that fertility will be restored following the transplant but that pregnancy should be avoided for ~2 years. Tacrolimus may be used as an immunosuppressant during pregnancy. The risk of infection, hypertension, and pre-eclampsia may be increased in pregnant women who have had a kidney transplant (EPBG 2002).

The National Transplantation Pregnancy Registry (NTPR) is a registry which follows pregnancies which occur in maternal transplant recipients or those fathered by male transplant recipients. The NTPR encourages reporting of pregnancies following solid organ transplant by contacting them at 877-955-6877 or NTPR@giftoflifeinstitute.org.

Breastfeeding Considerations Tacrolimus is excreted into breast milk; concentrations are variable and lower than that of the maternal serum. The low bioavailability of tacrolimus following oral absorption may also decrease the amount of exposure to a nursing infant (Bramham 2013; French 2003; Gardiner 2006). In one study, tacrolimus serum concentrations in the infants did not differ between those who were bottle fed or breast-fed (all infants were exposed to tacrolimus throughout pregnancy) (Bramham 2013). Available information suggests that tacrolimus exposure to the nursing infant is ≤0.5% of the weight-adjusted maternal dose (Bramham 2013; French 2003; Gardiner 2006). The manufacturer recommends that nursing be discontinued, taking into consideration the importance of the drug to the mother.

Warnings/Precautions [US Boxed Warning]: **Risk of developing infections (including bacterial, viral [including CMV], fungal, and protozoal infections [including opportunistic infections]) is increased.** Latent viral infections may be activated, including BK virus (associated with polyoma virus-associated nephropathy [PVAN]) and JC virus (associated with progressive multifocal leukoencephalopathy [PML]); may result in serious adverse effects. Immunosuppression increases the risk for CMV viremia and/or CMV disease; the risk of CMV disease is increased for patients who are CMV-seronegative prior to transplant and receive a graft from a CMV-seropositive donor. Monitor for development of infection; consider reduction in immuno-suppression if PVAN, PML, CMV viremia and/or CMV disease occurs. **[US Boxed Warning]: Immunosuppressive therapy may result in the development of lymphoma and other malignancies (predominantly skin malignancies)**. The risk for new-onset diabetes and insulin-dependent post-transplant diabetes mellitus (PTDM) is increased with tacrolimus use after transplantation, including in patients without pretransplant history of diabetes mellitus; insulin dependence may be reversible; monitor blood glucose frequently; risk is increased in African-American and Hispanic kidney transplant patients. Nephrotoxicity (acute or chronic) may occur when used in high doses, in patients with impaired renal function, or with other nephrotoxic drugs (eg, sirolimus, cyclosporine) or when administered concomitantly with CYP3A inhibitors (due to increased tacrolimus concentrations). Monitor renal function and consider dosage reduction in nephrotoxicity occurs. Neurotoxicity may occur especially when used in high doses; tremor headache, coma and delirium have been reported and are associated with serum concentrations. Seizures may also occur. Posterior reversible encephalopathy syndrome (PRES) has been reported; symptoms (altered mental status, headache, hypertension, seizures, and visual disturbances) are reversible with dose reduction or discontinuation of therapy; stabilize blood pressure and reduce dose with suspected or confirmed PRES diagnosis.

Pure red cell aplasia (PRCA) has been reported in patients receiving tacrolimus. Use with caution in patients with risk factors for PRCA including parvovirus B19 infection, underlying disease, or use of concomitant medications associated with PRCA (eg, mycophenolate). Discontinuation of therapy should be considered with diagnosis of PRCA. Monitoring of serum concentrations (trough for oral therapy) is essential to prevent organ rejection and reduce drug-related toxicity. Use caution in renal or hepatic dysfunction, dosing adjustments may be required. Delay initiation of therapy in kidney transplant patients if postoperative oliguria occurs; begin therapy no sooner than 6 hours and within 24 hours post-transplant, but may be delayed until renal function has recovered. Mild-to-severe hyperkalemia may occur; monitor serum potassium levels. Hypertension may commonly occur; antihypertensive treatment may be necessary; avoid use of potassium-sparing diuretics due to risk of hyperkalemia; concurrent use of calcium channel blockers may require tacrolimus dosage adjustment. Gastrointestinal perforation may occur; all reported cases were considered to be a complication of transplant surgery or accompanied by infection, diverticulum, or malignant neoplasm. Myocardial hypertrophy has been reported (rare). Prolongation of the QT/QTc and torsade de pointes may occur; avoid use in patients with congenital long QT syndrome. Consider obtaining electrocardiograms and monitoring electrolytes (magnesium, potassium, calcium) periodically during treatment in patients with congestive heart failure, bradyarrhythmias, those taking certain antiarrhythmic medications or other medicinal products that lead to QT prolongation, and those with electrolyte disturbances such as hypokalemia, hypocalcemia, or hypomagnesemia. Potentially significant drug-drug/drug-food interactions may exist, requiring dose or frequency adjustment, additional monitoring, and/or selection of alternative therapy. Concomitant use with strong CYP3A inducers and/or inhibitors may alter tacrolimus whole blood concentrations, potentially leading to rejection and/or increased toxicity, respectively. Monitor tacrolimus whole blood trough concentrations closely. In liver transplantation, the tacrolimus dose and target range should be reduced to minimize the risk of nephrotoxicity when used in combination with everolimus. Extended release

Respiratory: Allergic rhinitis, asthma, atelectasis, cough, flu-like symptoms, pleural effusion, pneumothorax, pulmonary edema, respiratory tract infection

Miscellaneous: Fever, postoperative pain, postoperative wound complication, wound healing impairment

1% to 10%: Gastrointestinal: Gastroenteritis (2% to 7%)

<1%, postmarketing, and/or case reports: Adult respiratory distress syndrome, agranulocytosis, anaphylactoid reaction, anaphylaxis, angioedema, basal cell carcinoma, biliary tract disease (stenosis), blindness, cerebrovascular accident, coma, deafness, decreased serum fibrinogen, delirium, disseminated intravascular coagulation, dysarthria, graft versus host disease (acute and chronic), hemiparesis, hemolytic-uremic syndrome, hemorrhagic cystitis, hepatic cirrhosis, hepatic failure, hepatic necrosis, hepatic sinusoidal obstruction syndrome (formerly known as hepatic veno-occlusive disease), hepatosplenic T-cell lymphomas, hepatotoxicity, hyperpigmentation, immune thrombocytopenia, interstitial pulmonary disease, leukemia, leukoencephalopathy, liver steatosis, lymphoproliferative disorder (post-transplant or related to Epstein-Barr virus), malignant lymphoma, malignant melanoma, multi-organ failure, mutism, optic atrophy, osteomyelitis, photophobia, polyarthritis, progressive multifocal leukoencephalopathy (PML), prolonged partial thromboplastin time, prolonged Q-T interval on ECG, pulmonary hypertension, pure red cell aplasia, quadriplegia, reversible posterior leukoencephalopathy syndrome, rhabdomyolysis, septicemia, squamous cell carcinoma, status epilepticus, Stevens-Johnson syndrome, supraventricular extrasystole, supraventricular tachycardia, thrombotic thrombocytopenic purpura, torsades de pointes, toxic epidermal necrolysis, urticaria, venous thrombosis, ventricular fibrillation

Drug Interactions

Metabolism/Transport Effects Substrate of CYP3A4 (major), P-glycoprotein; **Note:** Assignment of Major/Minor substrate status based on clinically relevant drug interaction potential

Avoid Concomitant Use

Avoid concomitant use of Tacrolimus (Systemic) with any of the following: BCG (Intravesical); Conivaptan; Crizotinib; CycloSPORINE (Systemic); Deferiprone; Dipyrone; Enzalutamide; Eplerenone; Foscarnet; Fusidic Acid (Systemic); Grapefruit Juice; Idelalisib; MiFEPRIStone; Natalizumab; Nelfinavir; Ombitasvir, Paritaprevir, and Ritonavir; Ombitasvir, Paritaprevir, Ritonavir, and Dasabuvir; Pimecrolimus; Potassium-Sparing Diuretics; Sirolimus; Tacrolimus (Topical); Temsirolimus; Vaccines (Live)

Increased Effect/Toxicity

Tacrolimus (Systemic) may increase the levels/effects of: Afatinib; CloZAPine; Colchicine; CycloSPORINE (Systemic); Deferiprone; Dronedarone; Fenofibrate and Derivatives; Fingolimod; Fosphenytoin; Highest Risk QTc-Prolonging Agents; Leflunomide; Moderate Risk QTc-Prolonging Agents; Natalizumab; Phenytoin; Sirolimus; Temsirolimus; Tofacitinib; Vaccines (Live)

The levels/effects of Tacrolimus (Systemic) may be increased by: Alcohol (Ethyl); Antidepressants (Serotonin Reuptake Inhibitor/Antagonist); Aprepitant; Asunaprevir; Azithromycin (Systemic); Boceprevir; Calcium Channel Blockers (Dihydropyridine); Calcium Channel Blockers (Nondihydropyridine); Chloramphenicol; Clotrimazole (Oral); Clotrimazole (Topical); Conivaptan; Crizotinib; CycloSPORINE (Systemic); CYP3A4 Inhibitors (Moderate); CYP3A4 Inhibitors (Strong); Daclatasvir; Danazol; Dasatinib;

Denosumab; Dipyrone; Dronedarone; Efonidipine; Eplerenone; Ertapenem; Erythromycin (Systemic); Fluconazole; Fosaprepitant; Foscarnet; Fusidic Acid (Systemic); Glecaprevir and Pibrentasvir; Grapefruit Juice; Grazoprevir; Idelalisib; Isavuconazonium Sulfate; Itraconazole; Ketoconazole (Systemic); LevoFLOXacin (Systemic); MiFEPRIStone; Nelfinavir; Netupitant; Nonsteroidal Anti-Inflammatory Agents; Ocrelizumab; Ombitasvir, Paritaprevir, and Ritonavir; Ombitasvir, Paritaprevir, Ritonavir, and Dasabuvir; Palbociclib; P-glycoprotein/ABCB1 Inhibitors; Pimecrolimus; Posaconazole; Potassium-Sparing Diuretics; Promazine; Protease Inhibitors; Proton Pump Inhibitors; Ranolazine; Ritonavir; Roflumilast; Schisandra; Sirolimus; Stiripentol; Tacrolimus (Topical); Telaprevir; Temsirolimus; Tofisopam; Trastuzumab; Voriconazole

Decreased Effect

Tacrolimus (Systemic) may decrease the levels/effects of: Antidiabetic Agents; BCG (Intravesical); Coccidioides immitis Skin Test; Nivolumab; Sipuleucel-T; Tertomotide; Vaccines (Inactivated); Vaccines (Live)

The levels/effects of Tacrolimus (Systemic) may be decreased by: Asunaprevir; Bosentan; Caspofungin; Cinacalcet; CYP3A4 Inducers (Moderate); CYP3A4 Inducers (Strong); Dabrafenib; Daclatasvir; Deferasirox; Echinacea; Efavirenz; Enzalutamide; Fosphenytoin; Ledipasvir; Mitotane; Phenytoin; Rifamycin Derivatives; Sarilumab; Sevelamer; Siltuximab; Sirolimus; St John's Wort; Temsirolimus; Tocilizumab

Food Interactions

Ethanol: Alcohol may increase the rate of release of extended-release tacrolimus and adversely affect tacrolimus safety and/or efficacy. Management: Avoid alcohol.

Food: Food decreases rate and extent of absorption. High-fat meals have most pronounced effect (37% and 25% decrease in AUC, respectively, and 77% and 25% decrease in C_{max}, respectively, for immediately release and extended release formulations). Grapefruit juice, a CYP3A4 inhibitor, may increase serum level and/or toxicity of tacrolimus. Management: Administer with or without food (immediate release), but be consistent. Administer extended release on an empty stomach. Avoid concurrent use of grapefruit juice.

Hazardous Drugs Handling Considerations

Hazardous agent (NIOSH 2016 [group 2]).

Use appropriate precautions for receiving, handling, administration, and disposal. Gloves (single) should be worn during receiving, unpacking, and placing in storage.

NIOSH recommends single gloving for administration of intact tablets or capsules. If manipulating tablets/capsules (eg, to prepare an oral suspension), NIOSH recommends double gloving, a protective gown, and preparation in a controlled device; if not prepared in a controlled device, respiratory and eye/face protection as well as ventilated engineering controls are recommended. NIOSH recommends double gloving, a protective gown, and (if there is a potential for vomit or spit up) eye/face protection for administration of an oral liquid/feeding tube administration. For IV preparation, double gloves, a protective gown, ventilated engineering controls (a class II biological safety cabinet or a compounding aseptic containment isolator), and closed system transfer devices (CSTDs) are recommended. Double gloving, a gown, and (if dosage form allows) CSTDs are required during IV administration (NIOSH 2016).

◀ **Storage/Stability**

Injection: Prior to dilution, store at 5°C to 25°C (41°F to 77°F). Following dilution, stable for 24 hours in D5W or NS in glass or polyethylene containers. Do not store in polyvinyl chloride containers since the polyoxyl 60 hydrogenated castor oil injectable vehicle may leach phthalates from polyvinyl chloride containers.

Capsule, tablet:

Astagraf XL, Envarsus XR, Prograf: Store at 25°C (77°F); excursions permitted between 15°C and 30°C (59°F and 86°F).

Hecoria: Store at 20°C to 25°C (68°F to 77°F).

Preparation for Administration Injection: Dilute with 5% dextrose injection or 0.9% sodium chloride injection to a final concentration between 0.004 mg/mL and 0.02 mg/mL.

Mechanism of Action Suppresses cellular immunity (inhibits T-lymphocyte activation), by binding to an intracellular protein, FKBP-12 and complexes with calcineurin dependent proteins to inhibit calcineurin phosphatase activity

Pharmacodynamics/Kinetics

Absorption: Better in resected patients with a closed stoma; unlike cyclosporine, clamping of the T-tube in liver transplant patients does not alter trough concentrations or AUC; Oral: Incomplete and variable (5% to 67%); the rate and extent of absorption is decreased (27%) by food (particularly a high-fat meal). Oral absorption may be variable in stem cell transplant patients with mucositis due to the conditioning regimen.

Distribution: Distributes to erythrocytes, lung, kidneys, pancreas, liver, heart, and spleen; V_d: Children: 2.6 L/kg (mean); Adults: 0.85 to 1.41 L/kg (mean) in liver and renal transplant patients

Protein binding: ~99% primarily to albumin and alpha-1 acid glycoprotein

Metabolism: Extensively hepatic via CYP3A4 to eight possible metabolites (major metabolite, 31-demethyl tacrolimus, shows same activity as tacrolimus in vitro)

Bioavailability: Oral: Children: 7% to 55%, Adults: 7% to 32%; Absolute: Unknown

Half-life elimination:

Children: 7.7 to 15.3 hours

Adults: Immediate release: Variable, 23 to 46 hours in healthy volunteers; 2.1 to 36 hours in transplant patients; prolonged in patients with severe impairment

Adults: Extended release: 38 ± 3 hours; prolonged in patients with severe hepatic impairment

Time to peak: Oral: 0.5 to 6 hours

Excretion: Feces (~93%); urine (<1% as unchanged drug)

Clearance: 7 to 103 mL/minute/kg (average: 30 mL/minute/kg); clearance higher in children

Dosing

Adult Note: Hecoria has been discontinued in the US for more than 1 year.

Immunosuppression after solid-organ transplant, sublingual administration: Sublingual (off-label route): Immediate release: Optimal dosing has not been determined. In dosing regimens using sublingual administration of the contents of immediate release tacrolimus capsules, the sublingual to oral dosing ratio has ranged from 1:3 to 1:1 (Collin 2010; Nasiri-Toosi 2012). However, most studies suggest a dosing ratio of 1:2 (or 50% of the oral dose given sublingually), and most centers use this approach in practice (Doligalski 2014; Watkins 2012). Adjust dose based on serum trough concentrations. Lower doses of sublingual tacrolimus may be required during coadministration of drugs that inhibit tacrolimus metabolism (Collin 2010; Reams 2002).

Prevention of organ rejection in transplant recipients: Note: While recommendations for initial doses exist, drug interactions should be considered. After initial dose, titrate to achieve target trough concentrations. Adjunctive therapy with other immunosuppressants including but not limited to corticosteroids is recommended early post-transplant. IV route should only be used in patients not able to take oral medications and continued only until oral medication can be tolerated; anaphylaxis has been reported with IV administration. If switching from IV to oral, the oral dose should be started 8 to 12 hours after stopping the infusion. Sublingual administration should be considered in those unable to take oral.

Liver transplant:
Oral:
Immediate release: Initial: 0.1 to 0.15 mg/kg/day in 2 divided doses, given every 12 hours (titrate to target trough concentrations), consider lower dose in liver transplant recipients with graft dysfunction.
Extended release: 0.1 to 0.2 mg/kg once daily in combination with corticosteroids; initiate within 12 to 18 hours of transplantation; titrate to target trough concentrations (Advagraf Canadian product labeling 2015). **Note:** In the US, Astagraf XL is not approved for use in liver transplantation due to an increase in mortality in female liver transplant recipients receiving Astagraf XL.
Conversion from immediate release to extended release (Advagraf [Canadian product]): Patients stable on immediate release tacrolimus may be converted to extended release by initiating extended-release treatment in a 1:1 ratio (mg:mg) using previously established total daily dose of immediate-release product. Administer once daily.
IV: Initial: 0.03 to 0.05 mg/kg/day as a continuous infusion

Heart transplant: Use in combination with an antimetabolite agent (eg, azathioprine or mycophenolate mofetil) is recommended. Instead of an antimetabolite, may also use in combination with an mTOR kinase inhibitor (eg, everolimus, sirolimus) (Fuchs 2014; Guethoff 2015).
Oral: Immediate release: Initial: 0.075 mg/kg/day in 2 divided doses, given every 12 hours (titrate to target trough concentrations)
IV: Initial: 0.01 mg/kg/day as a continuous infusion
Conversion from oral to continuous IV infusion: According to the ISHLT guidelines for the care of heart transplant recipients, convert from oral to IV by administering one-fifth (1/5th) of the oral daily dose as a continuous infusion over 24 hours (ISHLT [Costanzo 2010]).

Kidney transplant: Use in combination with azathioprine or mycophenolate mofetil is recommended. **Note:** African-American patients may require larger doses to attain trough concentration.
Oral:
Immediate release (Hecoria, Prograf): Initial: 0.2 mg/kg/day in combination with azathioprine or 0.1 mg/kg/day in combination with mycophenolate mofetil; titrate to target trough concentrations. Administer in 2 divided doses, given every 12 hours.
Conversion from immediate release oral to IV: Administer one-third (1/3rd) of the oral dose as a continuous infusion over 24 hours.

Extended release (Advagraf [Canadian product], Astagraf XL):

With basiliximab induction (prior to reperfusion or within 48 hours of transplant completion): 0.15 to 0.2 mg/kg once daily (in combination with corticosteroids and mycophenolate); titrate to target trough concentrations

Without basiliximab induction: Preoperative dose (administer within 12 hours prior to reperfusion): 0.1 mg/kg (in combination with corticosteroids and mycophenolate)

Without basiliximab induction: Postoperative dosing (administer at least 4 hours after preoperative dose and within 12 hours of reperfusion): 0.2 mg/kg once daily (in combination with corticosteroids and mycophenolate); titrate to target trough concentrations

Conversion from IV to extended release (Astagraf XL, Envarsus XR): Administer the first oral extended release dose 8 to 12 hours after discontinuation of IV tacrolimus

Conversion from immediate release to extended release (Advagraf [Canadian product], Astagraf XL): Initiate extended release treatment in a 1:1 ratio (mg:mg) using previously established total daily dose of immediate release (Advagraf Canadian product labeling 2015; Van Hooff 2012). Administer once daily.

Conversion from immediate release to extended release (Envarsus XR): Initiate extended-release treatment with a once-daily dose that is 70% to 80% of the total daily dose of the immediate-release tacrolimus

IV: Initial: 0.03 to 0.05 mg/kg/day as a continuous infusion

Graft-versus-host disease (GVHD) (off-label use):

Prevention:

Oral: Convert from IV to immediate release oral dose (1:4 ratio): Multiply total daily IV dose times 4 and administer in 2 divided oral doses per day, every 12 hours (Uberti 1999; Yanik 2000).

IV: Initial: 0.03 mg/kg/day (based on lean body weight) as continuous infusion. Treatment should begin at least 24 hours prior to stem cell infusion and continued only until oral medication can be tolerated (Przepiorka 1999; Yanik 2000).

Treatment:

Oral: Immediate release: 0.06 mg/kg twice daily (Furlong 2000; Przepiorka 1999)

IV: Initial: 0.03 mg/kg/day (based on lean body weight) as continuous infusion (Furlong 2000; Przepiorka 1999)

Lung transplant (off-label use): Usually used in a combination regimen that contains a corticosteroid and either azathioprine or mycophenolate (Snell 2013).

Oral, nasogastric: Immediate release: 0.05 to 0.3 mg/kg/day in 2 divided doses, given every 12 hours (usual dose: 0.05 mg/kg every 12 hours); titrate to target trough concentrations (Treede 2001; Treede 2012; Zuckermann 2003). May also be administered sublingually at ~50% of the oral/NG dose (Doligalski 2014; Watkins 2012).

Note: May convert from twice-daily dosing to once-daily dosing (on a mg per mg basis) using the extended-release formulation (Astagraf XL [US] or Advagraf [Canada]) in stable lung transplant recipients (Mendez 2014). May convert to extended-release Envarsus with a once-daily dose that is 70% to 80% of the total daily dose of immediate-release tacrolimus although clinical trial data is lacking.

IV: 0.01 to 0.05 mg/kg over 24 hours as a continuous IV infusion; titrate to target trough concentrations (Treede 2001; Treede 2012; Zuckermann 2003). For patients receiving the initial dose of tacrolimus intravenously, may begin immediately after transplantation, or up to 2 days postoperatively depending on renal function and hemodynamic stability (Treede 2001; Treede 2012; Witt 2013; Zuckermann 2003). When patient is able to take oral medication, may switch to an oral maintenance regimen (typically transitioned after extubation).

Rheumatoid arthritis (refractory) (off-label use): Oral: Immediate release: 2 to 3 mg once daily in combination with NSAID and/or oral corticosteroid therapy; 3 mg once daily resulted in better ACR response rates (Yocum 2003). In patients not responsive to methotrexate alone, may add tacrolimus at a lower dose (ie, 1.5 mg once daily) in combination with methotrexate (Lee 2016). Carefully monitor serum creatinine during therapy.

Geriatric Refer to adult dosing. Use with caution; begin at the low end of dosing range.

Pediatric Note: Hecoria has been discontinued in the US for more than 1 year.

Liver transplant:
Oral: Immediate release: Initial: 0.15 to 0.20 mg/kg/day in 2 divided doses, given every 12 hours (titrate to target trough concentrations)
IV: Initial: 0.03 to 0.05 mg/kg/day as a continuous infusion
Note: The initial postoperative dose of tacrolimus should begin no sooner than 6 hours after liver and heart transplant and within 24 hours of kidney transplant (but may be delayed until renal function has recovered). Adjunctive therapy with corticosteroids is recommended early post-transplant. IV route should only be used in patients not able to take oral medications and continued only until oral medication can be tolerated; anaphylaxis has been reported with IV administration. If switching from IV to oral, the oral dose should be started 8-12 hours after stopping the infusion. Patients without preexisting renal or hepatic dysfunction have required (and tolerated) higher doses than adults to achieve similar blood concentrations. It is recommended that therapy be initiated at the **high end** of the recommended adult IV and oral dosing ranges; dosage adjustments may be required.

Prevention of graft-vs-host disease (GVHD) (off-label use): Oral, IV: Refer to adult dosing.

Renal Impairment Renal impairment does not affect the elimination or serum concentrations of tacrolimus; however, tacrolimus may cause nephrotoxicity requiring dose reduction. Evidence suggests that lower doses should be used; patients should receive doses at the lowest amount of the recommended IV and oral dosing ranges; further reductions in dose below these ranges may be required.
Hemodialysis: Not removed by hemodialysis; supplemental dose is not necessary.
Peritoneal dialysis: Significant drug removal is unlikely based on physiochemical characteristics.

Hepatic Impairment Use of tacrolimus in liver transplant recipients experiencing post-transplant hepatic impairment may be associated with increased risk of developing renal insufficiency related to high whole blood levels of tacrolimus. The presence of moderate-to-severe hepatic dysfunction (serum bilirubin >2 mg/dL; Child-Pugh score ≥10) appears to affect the metabolism of tacrolimus. The half-life of the drug was prolonged and the

◄ clearance reduced after IV administration. The bioavailability of tacrolimus was also increased after oral administration. The higher plasma concentrations as determined by ELISA, in patients with severe hepatic dysfunction are probably due to the accumulation of metabolites of lower activity. These patients should be monitored closely and dosage adjustments should be considered. Some evidence indicates that lower doses could be used in these patients.

Administration

IV: If IV administration is necessary, administer by continuous infusion (generally, over 24 hours). Do not use PVC tubing when administering diluted solutions. Do not mix with solutions with a pH ≥9 (eg, acyclovir or ganciclovir) due to chemical degradation of tacrolimus (use different ports in multilumen lines). Do not alter dose with concurrent T-tube clamping. Adsorption of the drug to PVC tubing may become clinically significant with low concentrations.

Oral:

Immediate release: Administer with or without food; be consistent with timing and composition of meals if GI intolerance occurs and administration with food becomes necessary (per manufacturer). If dosed once daily, administer in the morning. If dosed twice daily, doses should be 12 hours apart. If the morning and evening doses differ, the larger dose (differences are never >0.5 to 1 mg) should be given in the morning. Some data suggests that the larger dose should be given in the evening since tacrolimus exposure may be reduced in the evening (Iwahori 2005; Min 1997; Park 2007). If dosed 3 times daily, separate doses by 8 hours.

Combination therapy with everolimus for liver transplantation: Administer tacrolimus at the same time as everolimus.

Extended release: For all US preparations, administer on an empty stomach at least 1 hour before or 2 hours after a meal. Advagraf [Canadian product] labeling suggests that the capsule may be taken with food if necessary but should be administered consistently with or without food. Swallow whole, do not chew, crush, or divide. Take once daily in the morning at a consistent time each day. Missed doses may be taken up to 14 hours (15 hours for Envarsus XR) after scheduled time; if >14 hours (>15 hours for Envarsus XR), resume at next regularly scheduled time; do not double a dose to make up for a missed dose.

Nasogastric tube: If unable to swallow capsules, contents of immediate release capsule(s) may be mixed with water and flushed through a nasogastric tube; clamp nasogastric tube for 30 to 60 minutes after administration (Taylor 2001). **Note:** Dosing for immediate release capsules is not equivalent to dosing of Envarsus XR. When switching from Envarsus XR to immediate release capsules for nasogastric administration, consider administering a 20% to 30% higher total daily dose of immediate release tacrolimus.

Sublingual: If unable to swallow capsules, tacrolimus may be administered sublingually (at a reduced dose) by opening the immediate-release capsules and placing the contents of the capsule(s) under the tongue, allowing contents to completely dissolve. The patient should avoid swallowing for 5 to 15 minutes and avoid oral intake for 15 to 30 minutes; also avoid mechanical suctioning for at least 30 minutes after administration (Doligalski 2014; Pennington 2015; Watkins 2012). **Note:** Absorption of a single dose of tacrolimus suspension given by the sublingual route was inadequate. (Snell 2013b)

Extemporaneous Preparations A 0.5 mg/mL tacrolimus oral suspension may be made with immediate release capsules and a 1:1 mixture of Ora-Plus and Simple Syrup, N.F. Mix the contents of six 5 mg tacrolimus capsules with quantity of vehicle sufficient to make 60 mL. Store in glass or plastic amber prescription bottles; label "shake well". Stable for 56 days at room temperature (Esquivel 1996; Foster 1996).

A 1 mg/mL tacrolimus oral suspension may be made with immediate release capsules, sterile water, Ora-Plus, and Ora-Sweet. Pour the contents of six 5 mg capsules into a plastic amber prescription bottle. Add ~5 mL of sterile water and agitate bottle until drug disperses into a slurry. Add equal parts Ora-Plus and Ora-Sweet in sufficient quantity to make 30 mL. Store in plastic amber prescription bottles; label "shake well". Stable for 4 months at room temperature (Elefante 2006).

Elefante A, Muindi J, West K, et al, "Long-Term Stability of a Patient-Convenient 1 mg/mL Suspension of Tacrolimus for Accurate Maintenance of Stable Therapeutic Levels," *Bone Marrow Transplant.* 2006, 37(8):781-4.

Esquivel C, So S, McDiarmid S, Andrews W, and Colombani PM, "Suggested Guidelines for the Use of Tacrolimus in Pediatric Liver Transplant Patients," *Transplantation*, 1996, 61(5):847-8.

Foster JA, Jacobson PA, Johnson CE, et al, "Stability of Tacrolimus in an Extemporaneously Compounded Oral Liquid (Abstract of Meeting Presentation)," *American Society of Health-System Pharmacists Annual Meeting*, 1996, 53:P-52(E).

Monitoring Parameters Renal function, hepatic function, serum electrolytes (magnesium, phosphorus, potassium), glucose and blood pressure, measure 3 times/week for first few weeks, then gradually decrease frequency as patient stabilizes. Signs/symptoms of anaphylactic reactions during IV infusion should also be monitored. Patients should be monitored for hypersensitivity during the first 30 minutes of the infusion, and frequently thereafter. Monitor for QT prolongation, consider echocardiographic evaluation in patients who develop renal failure, electrolyte abnormalities, or clinical manifestations of ventricular dysfunction.

Whole blood concentrations should be used for monitoring (trough for oral therapy drawn typically within 30 minutes prior to the next dose); frequency varies depending on transplant type, time since transplantation, and clinical situation. Tacrolimus serum levels may be falsely elevated in infected liver transplant patients due to interference from beta-galactosidase antibodies.

Dietary Considerations Capsule: Administer immediate release with or without food; be consistent with timing and composition of meals, food decreases bioavailability. Administer extended release on an empty stomach 1 hour before or 2 hours after a meal. Avoid grapefruit and grapefruit juice. Avoid alcohol.

Product Availability Hecoria has been discontinued in the US for more than 1 year.

Medication Guide Available Yes

Dosage Forms Considerations Prograf injection contains polyoxyl 60 hydrogenated castor oil (HCO-60)

Dosage Forms Excipient information presented when available (limited, particularly for generics); consult specific product labeling. [DSC] = Discontinued product

Capsule, Oral:

Hecoria: 0.5 mg [DSC], 1 mg [DSC], 5 mg [DSC]

Prograf: 0.5 mg, 1 mg, 5 mg

Generic: 0.5 mg, 1 mg, 5 mg

Capsule Extended Release 24 Hour, Oral:
  Astagraf XL: 0.5 mg, 1 mg, 5 mg
Solution, Intravenous:
  Prograf: 5 mg/mL (1 mL) [contains alcohol, usp, cremophor el]
Tablet Extended Release 24 Hour, Oral:
  Envarsus XR: 0.75 mg, 1 mg, 4 mg

Dosage Forms: Canada Information with regard to form, strength, and availability of products uniquely available in Canada but currently not available in the US. Refer also to Dosage Forms.

Excipient information presented when available (limited, particularly for generics); consult specific product labeling.
Capsule Extended Release 24 Hour, Oral:
  Advagraf: 0.5 mg, 1 mg, 3 mg, 5 mg

◆ **Tafinlar** *see* Dabrafenib *on page 486*
◆ **Tagrisso** *see* Osimertinib *on page 1389*
◆ **Talc** *see* Talc (Sterile) *on page 1728*
◆ **Talc for Pleurodesis** *see* Talc (Sterile) *on page 1728*

Talc (Sterile) (talk STARE il)

Brand Names: US Sclerosol Intrapleural; Sterile Talc Powder
Index Terms Intrapleural Talc; Sterile Talc; Steritalc; Talc; Talc for Pleurodesis
Pharmacologic Category Sclerosing Agent
Use
  Pleural effusion, malignant: Sclerosing agent to decrease or prevent the recurrence of malignant pleural effusion in symptomatic patients (following maximal drainage of pleural effusion).
  Pneumothorax: Sclerosing agent to decrease the recurrence of pneumothorax.
Pregnancy Risk Factor B (manufacturer specific)
Dosing
  Adult
    Pleural effusion, malignant:
      Intrapleural aerosol: 4 to 8 g (1 to 2 cans) as a single dose
      Intrapleural suspension:
        Sterile Talc Powder: 5 g
        Steritalc: 2 to 5 g (based on patient condition other doses may be used); maximum cumulative dose: 10 g
    Pneumothorax: Intrapleural: Steritalc: 2 g (based on patient condition other doses may be used); maximum cumulative dose: 10 g
  Renal Impairment There are no dosage adjustments provided in the manufacturer's labeling.
  Hepatic Impairment There are no dosage adjustments provided in the manufacturer's labeling.
Additional Information Complete prescribing information should be consulted for additional detail.
Dosage Forms Excipient information presented when available (limited, particularly for generics); consult specific product labeling.
Aerosol Powder, Intrapleural:
  Sclerosol Intrapleural: 4 g (30 g) [contains dichlorodifluoromethane]
Suspension Reconstituted, Intrapleural:
  Sterile Talc Powder: 5 g (1 ea)

Talimogene Laherparepvec (tal IM oh jeen la her pa REP vek)

Related Information

Management of Chemotherapy-Induced Nausea and Vomiting in Adults *on page 2253*

Safe Handling of Hazardous Drugs *on page 2379*

Brand Names: US Imlygic

Index Terms GM-CSF-Encoding Oncolytic Herpes Simplex Virus; Imlygic; OncoVEX GM-CSF; T-VEC; Talminogene Laherparepvec

Pharmacologic Category Antineoplastic Agent, Oncolytic Virus

Use

Melanoma, unresectable: Treatment (local) of unresectable cutaneous, subcutaneous, and nodal lesions in patients with melanoma recurrent after initial surgery

Limitations of use: Has not been shown to improve overall survival or have an effect on visceral metastases.

Labeled Contraindications Immunocompromised patients, including those with a history of primary or acquired immunodeficient states, leukemia, lymphoma, AIDS or other clinical manifestations of infection with human immunodeficiency viruses, and those on immunosuppressive therapy; pregnancy

Pregnancy Considerations Use is contraindicated in pregnant women. Women of reproductive potential should use effective contraception during therapy. Talimogene laherparepvec is a live, attenuated, genetically modified herpes simplex virus type 1 (HSV-1). HSV-1 is known to cross the placenta, can be transmitted during birth, and produce infections in the fetus or neonate. It is not known if this can occur following exposure to talimogene laherparepvec. Pregnant women should not prepare or administer this medication. Pregnant women who are in close contact of patients treated with talimogene laherparepvec should not change dressings or clean injection sites, and should avoid direct contact with the injection site, dressings, or body fluids of patients.

Breastfeeding Considerations It is not known if talimogene laherparepvec is present in breast milk. The manufacturer recommends a decision be made to discontinue breastfeeding or to discontinue the drug, taking into account the importance of treatment to the mother.

Warnings/Precautions Health care providers who are immunocompromised or pregnant should not prepare or administer talimogene laherparepvec. Accidental talimogene laherparepvec exposure may lead to herpetic infection. Health care providers, close contacts (eg, household members, caregivers, sex partners, or persons sharing the same bed), pregnant women, and newborns should avoid direct contact with injected lesions, dressings, or body fluids of patients treated with talimogene laherparepvec. Protective gloves should be worn when assisting patients with dressing changes; safely dispose of used dressings, gloves, and cleaning materials. Needle stick and/or splash-back to the eyes have been reported during talimogene laherparepvec preparation and administration. If accidently exposed to talimogene laherparepvec, clean the affected area thoroughly with soap and water and/or a disinfectant. Contact a health care provider if signs/symptoms of herpetic infection develop. Counsel patients to avoid touching or scratching injection site(s) or the dressings (may lead to inadvertent transfer of drug to other parts of the body).

◄ Herpetic infections (eg, cold sores and herpetic keratitis) have been reported; disseminated herpetic infection may occur in immunocompromised patients. If herpes-like lesions develop, follow standard practice to prevent viral transmission; contact a health care provider for evaluation. Suspected herpetic lesions should be reported to Amgen at 1-855-465-9442. Talimogene laherparepvec is sensitive to acyclovir. Acyclovir (or other antiviral medications) may interfere with the efficacy of talimogene laherparepvec; consider the risks and benefits of treatment prior to administering antiviral agents. Immune-mediated events (eg, glomerulonephritis, pneumonitis, vasculitis, vitiligo, and worsening psoriasis) have been reported in clinical studies. Consider risk/benefit ratio of initiating treatment in patients with underlying autoimmune disease or prior to continuing talimogene laherparepvec treatment in patients who develop immune-mediated events. Obstructive airway disorder has been observed following talimogene laherparepvec therapy; use caution when injecting lesions close to major airways.

Injection-site complications, such as necrosis, tumor tissue ulceration, and impaired healing may occur during treatment with talimogene laherparepvec. Cellulitis and systemic bacterial infection have been observed. Monitor wounds carefully; infection precautions are recommended, particularly if tissue necrosis results in open wounds. Patients with underlying risk factors for impaired wound healing (eg, previous radiation at the injection site or lesions in poorly vascularized areas) may be at risk for complications. One patient had a lower extremity amputation 6 months after talimogene laherparepvec administration due to an infected non-healing wound. Monitor closely. Consider risk/benefit of continued treatment in patients with persistent infection or impaired wound healing at injection site(s). In one clinical study, a patient with smoldering multiple myeloma developed a plasmacytoma near the talimogene laherparepvec injection site. Consider the risks/benefits of talimogene laherparepvec therapy in patients with multiple myeloma or in those who develop plasmacytoma during treatment. Potentially significant interactions may exist, requiring dose or frequency adjustment, additional monitoring, and/or selection of alternative therapy. Talimogene laherparepvec is available in two different dose strengths: 10^6 (1 million) plaque-forming units (PFU) per mL (initial dose only), and 10^8 (100 million) PFU per mL (all subsequent doses). Verify appropriate dose and vial prior to preparation and administration.

Adverse Reactions Most reactions resolved within 72 hours.
>10%:
  Central nervous system: Fatigue (50%), chills (49%), headache (19%)
  Gastrointestinal: Nausea (36%), vomiting (21%), diarrhea (19%), constipation (12%)
  Local: Pain at injection site (28%)
  Neuromuscular & skeletal: Myalgia (18%), arthralgia (17%), limb pain (16%)
  Respiratory: Flu-like symptoms (31%)
  Miscellaneous: Fever (43%)
1% to 10%:
  Central nervous system: Dizziness (10%)
  Endocrine & metabolic: Weight loss (6%)
  Gastrointestinal: Abdominal pain (9%)
  Respiratory: Oropharyngeal pain (6%)
Frequency not defined:
  Cardiovascular: Deep vein thrombosis, vasculitis

Dermatologic: Cellulitis, dermatitis, exacerbation of psoriasis, skin rash, vitiligo

Gastrointestinal: Oral herpes

Infection: Bacterial infection (systemic), herpes virus infection

Ophthalmic: Herpes simplex keratitis

Renal: Glomerulonephritis

Respiratory: Acute asthma, pneumonitis

Drug Interactions

Metabolism/Transport Effects None known.

Avoid Concomitant Use There are no known interactions where it is recommended to avoid concomitant use.

Increased Effect/Toxicity There are no known significant interactions involving an increase in effect.

Decreased Effect

The levels/effects of Talimogene Laherparepvec may be decreased by: Antiherpetic Antivirals

Hazardous Drugs Handling Considerations

Hazardous agent (meets NIOSH 2016 criteria). This medication is not on the NIOSH (2016) list; however, it meets the criteria for a hazardous drug. Drugs are classified as hazardous based on their properties; the properties of a hazardous drug include one or more of the following characteristics: carcinogenic, teratogenic (or other developmental toxicity), reproductive toxicity, organotoxic at low doses, genotoxic, and/or new agents with structural or toxicity profiles similar to existing hazardous agents.

Use appropriate precautions for receiving, handling, administration, and disposal. Gloves (single) should be worn during receiving, unpacking, and placing in storage.

NIOSH recommends double gloving, a protective gown, and ventilated engineering controls (a class II biological safety cabinet or a compounding aseptic containment isolator) for preparation. Double gloving and a protective gown are required during administration (NIOSH 2016).

Storage/Stability Store intact vials at -90°C to -70°C (-130°F to -94°F); protect from light. Store vials in the carton until use. Thaw vials immediately prior to administration. If not used immediately, may store (in the original vial and carton) refrigerated at 2°C to 8°C (36°F to 46°F) for up to 12 hours (for the 10^6 [1 million] PFU per mL strength) or up to 48 hours (for the 10^8 [100 million] PFU per mL strength). Do not refreeze vials after thawing; discard any vial left in the refrigerator if longer than the specified times. After thawed, do not shake.

Preparation for Administration Health care providers who are immunocompromised or pregnant should not prepare or administer talimogene laherparepvec and should not handle injection sites, dressings, or body fluids of treated patients. Personal protective equipment (eg, gown or laboratory coat, safety glasses or face shield, and gloves) should be worn during preparation or administration. Cover any exposed wounds prior to handling talimogene laherparepvec. If accidental exposure occurs through an eye splash or a splash to mucous membranes, flush the area with clean water for at least 15 minutes. If exposure to broken skin or a needle stick occurs, clean the affected area thoroughly with soap and water and/or a disinfectant. Clean all surfaces that may have come in contact with talimogene laherparepvec and treat spills with virucidal agents such as sodium hypochlorite 1% or 70% isopropyl alcohol and blot using absorbent materials. Dispose of all materials that may have come into contact with talimogene laherparepvec as biohazardous waste.

Thaw vials at room temperature until talimogene laherparepvec is liquid (~30 minutes); do not thaw at higher temperatures. Keep vial in the original carton during thawing. Swirl gently; do not shake. Administer immediately after thawing or store in the refrigerator for 12 to 48 hours (vial strength dependent; see Storage/Stability for details). Do not refreeze after thawing. Withdraw the vial contents (using a detachable needle of 18 to 26 gauge) into the syringe (note the total volume). Avoid generating aerosols; use a biologic safety cabinet if available.

Mechanism of Action Talimogene laherparepvec is a genetically modified attenuated herpes simplex virus 1 (HSV) oncolytic virus which selectively replicates in and lyses tumor cells (Andtbacka 2015). Talimogene laherparepvec is modified through deletion of two nonessential viral genes. Deletion of the herpes virus neurovirulence factor gene ICP34.5 diminishes viral pathogenicity and increases tumor-selective replication; deletion of the ICP47 gene reduces virally mediated suppression of antigen presentation and increases the expression of the HSV US11 gene (Andtback 2015). Virally derived GM-CSF recruits and activates antigen-presenting cells, leading to an antitumor immune response.

Pharmacodynamics/Kinetics Time to peak: Peak levels of talimogene laherparepvec were detected in the urine on the day of treatment

Dosing

Adult & Geriatric Note: Administer by intralesional injection into cutaneous, subcutaneous, and/or nodal lesions that are visible, palpable, or detectable by ultrasound. It may not be possible to inject all lesions at each treatment visit or over the full course of treatment. Previously injected and/or uninjected lesion(s) may be treated at subsequent visits.

Melanoma, unresectable: Intralesional: Maximum volume (per treatment visit, for all injected lesions combined): 4 mL. Continue treatment for at least 6 months unless other therapy is necessary or until there are no injectable lesions to treat. Reinitiate treatment if new unresectable lesions appear after a previous complete response.

Use the following to determine the volume of talimogene laherparepvec to be injected (lesion size is based on longest dimension; when lesions are clustered together, inject them as a single lesion):
- If the lesion size is >5 cm, inject up to 4 mL
- If the lesion size is >2.5 cm to 5 cm, inject up to 2 mL
- If the lesion size is >1.5 cm to 2.5 cm, inject up to 1 mL
- If the lesion size is >0.5 cm to 1.5 cm, inject up to 0.5 mL
- If the lesion size is ≤0.5 cm, inject up to 0.1 mL

Initial treatment visit: Inject up to 4 mL at a concentration of 10^6 (1 million) PFU/mL. Inject largest lesion(s) first; inject remaining lesion(s) based on lesion size until maximum injection volume is reached or all lesions have been treated.

Second treatment visit (3 weeks after initial treatment): Inject up to 4 mL at a concentration of 10^8 (100 million) PFU/mL. Inject any new lesion(s) that have developed since initial treatment first; inject remaining lesion(s) based on lesion size until maximum injection volume is reached or all lesions have been treated.

All subsequent treatment visits, including reinitiation (2 weeks after previous treatment): Inject up to 4 mL at a concentration of 10^8 (100 million) PFU/mL. Inject any new lesion(s) that have developed since previous treatment first; inject remaining lesion(s) based on lesion size until maximum injection volume is reached or all lesions have been treated.

Renal Impairment Dosage adjustment for renal impairment: There are no dosage adjustments provided in the manufacturer's labeling (has not been studied).

Hepatic Impairment Dosage adjustment for hepatic impairment: There are no dosage adjustments provided in the manufacturer's labeling (has not been studied).

Administration Administer by intralesional injection into cutaneous, subcutaneous, and/or nodal lesions that are visible, palpable, or detectable by ultrasound. Clean the lesion and surrounding areas with alcohol and allow to dry. If necessary, treat the injection site with a topical or local anesthetic agent (but do not inject the anesthetic directly into the lesion [inject around periphery of lesion]). Using a single insertion point, inject talimogene laherparepvec (using a 22 to 26 gauge needle) along multiple tracks as far as the needle allows within the lesion to achieve dispersion; multiple lesion points may be used if a lesion is larger than the radial reach of the needle.

Inject talimogene laherparepvec evenly and completely within the lesion by pulling the needle back without removing it from the lesion. Redirect the needle as necessary while injecting the remainder of the dose; continue until the full dose is evenly and completely dispersed. Remove the needle from the lesion slowly to avoid leakage. Repeat steps for other lesions to be treated. Use a new needle if the needle is completely removed from a lesion and each time a different lesion is injected. Apply pressure with sterile gauze for at least 30 seconds after the injection is completed; swab the injection site(s) and surrounding areas with alcohol. Change gloves, then cover lesion(s) with an absorbent pad and dry occlusive dressing, and wipe the exterior of the dressing with alcohol. The injection site should be covered for at least the first week after each treatment or longer if the injection site is weeping or oozing (replace dressing if it falls off).

Immunocompromised or pregnant health care providers should not prepare or administer talimogene laherparepvec and should not have direct contact with injection sites, dressings, or body fluids of treated patients. Avoid accidental exposure; follow biohazard precautions (personal protective equipment) for administration. Patients should place used dressings and cleaning materials in a sealed plastic bag and dispose of with household waste.

Emetic Potential Low (10% to 30%)

Monitoring Parameters Monitor for signs/symptoms of herpetic infections (eg, cold sores and herpetic keratitis), injection-site complications, obstructive airway disease, and immune-mediated events

Medication Guide Available Yes

Dosage Forms Excipient information presented when available (limited, particularly for generics); consult specific product labeling.

Suspension, Intralesional [preservative free]:

Imlygic: 10^6 (1 million) PFU/mL (1 mL); 10^8 (100 million) PFU/mL (1 mL) [contains bovine serum]

◆ **Talminogene Laherparepvec** *see* Talimogene Laherparepvec
on page 1729

Tamoxifen (ta MOKS i fen)

Related Information

Hypercalcemia of Malignancy *on page 2341*

Safe Handling of Hazardous Drugs *on page 2379*

Brand Names: US Soltamox

Brand Names: Canada Apo-Tamox; Mylan-Tamoxifen; Nolvadex-D; PMS-Tamoxifen; Teva-Tamoxifen

Index Terms ICI-46474; Nolvadex; Tamoxifen Citras; Tamoxifen Citrate

Pharmacologic Category Antineoplastic Agent, Estrogen Receptor Antagonist; Selective Estrogen Receptor Modulator (SERM)

Use Treatment of metastatic (female and male) breast cancer; adjuvant treatment of breast cancer after primary treatment with surgery and radiation; reduce risk of invasive breast cancer in women with ductal carcinoma *in situ* (DCIS) after surgery and radiation; reduce the incidence of breast cancer in women at high risk

Labeled Contraindications Hypersensitivity to tamoxifen or any component of the formulation; concurrent warfarin therapy or history of deep vein thrombosis or pulmonary embolism (when tamoxifen is used for breast cancer risk reduction in women at high risk for breast cancer or with ductal carcinoma *in situ* [DCIS])

Pregnancy Considerations Animal reproduction studies have demonstrated fetal adverse effects and fetal loss. There have been reports of vaginal bleeding, birth defects and fetal loss in pregnant women. Tamoxifen use during pregnancy may have a potential long term risk to the fetus of a DES-like syndrome. For sexually-active women of childbearing age, initiate during menstruation (negative β-hCG immediately prior to initiation in women with irregular cycles). Tamoxifen may induce ovulation. Barrier or nonhormonal contraceptives are recommended. Pregnancy should be avoided during treatment and for 2 months after treatment has been discontinued.

Breastfeeding Considerations It is not known if tamoxifen is excreted in breast milk, however, it has been shown to inhibit lactation. Due to the potential for adverse reactions, women taking tamoxifen should not breastfeed.

Warnings/Precautions **[U.S. Boxed Warning]: Serious and life-threatening events (some fatal), including stroke, pulmonary emboli, and uterine or endometrial malignancies, have occurred at an incidence greater than placebo during use for breast cancer risk reduction in women at high-risk for breast cancer and in women with ductal carcinoma *in situ* (DCIS). In women already diagnosed with breast cancer, the benefits of tamoxifen treatment outweigh risks; evaluate risks versus benefits (and discuss with patients) when used for breast cancer risk reduction.** An increased incidence of thromboembolic events, including DVT and pulmonary embolism, has been associated with use for breast cancer; risk is increased with concomitant chemotherapy; use with caution in individuals with a history of thromboembolic events. Thrombocytopenia and/or leukopenia may occur; neutropenia and pancytopenia have been reported rarely. Although the relationship to tamoxifen therapy is uncertain, rare hemorrhagic episodes have occurred in patients with significant thrombocytopenia. Use with caution in patients with hyperlipidemias; infrequent postmarketing cases of hyperlipidemias have been reported. Decreased visual acuity, retinal vein thrombosis, retinopathy, corneal changes, color perception changes, and increased incidence of cataracts (and the need for cataract surgery), have been reported. Hypercalcemia has occurred in some patients with bone metastasis, usually within a few weeks of therapy initiation; institute appropriate hypercalcemia management; discontinue if severe. Local disease flare and increased bone and tumor pain may occur in patients with metastatic breast cancer; may be associated with (good) tumor response.

Potentially significant drug-drug interactions may exist, requiring dose or frequency adjustment, additional monitoring, and/or selection of alternative therapy. Decreased efficacy and an increased risk of breast cancer recurrence has been reported with concurrent moderate or strong CYP2D6 inhibitors (Aubert, 2009; Dezentje, 2009). Concomitant use with select SSRIs may result in decreased tamoxifen efficacy. Strong CYP2D6 inhibitors (eg, fluoxetine, paroxetine) and moderate CYP2D6 inhibitors (eg, sertraline) are reported to interfere with transformation to the active metabolite endoxifen; when possible, select alternative medications with minimal or no impact on endoxifen levels (NCCN Breast Cancer Risk Reduction Guidelines v.1.2013; Sideras, 2010). Weak CYP2D6 inhibitors (eg, venlafaxine, citalopram) have minimal effect on the conversion to endoxifen (Jin, 2005; NCCN Breast Cancer Risk Reduction Guidelines v.1.2013); escitalopram is also a weak CYP2D6 inhibitor. In a retrospective analysis of breast cancer patients taking tamoxifen and SSRIs, concomitant use of paroxetine and tamoxifen was associated with an increased risk of death due to breast cancer (Kelly, 2010). Lower plasma concentrations of endoxifen have been observed in patients associated with reduced CYP2D6 activity (Jin, 2005; Schroth, 2009) and may be associated with reduced efficacy, although data is conflicting. Routine CYP2D6 testing is not recommended at this time in order to determine optimal endocrine therapy (NCCN Breast Cancer Guidelines v.2.2013; Visvanathan, 2009).

Tamoxifen use may be associated with changes in bone mineral density (BMD) and the effects may be dependent upon menstrual status. In post-menopausal women, tamoxifen use is associated with a protective effect on bone mineral density (BMD), preventing loss of BMD which lasts over the 5-year treatment period. In premenopausal women, a decline (from baseline) in BMD mineral density has been observed in women who continued to menstruate; may be associated with an increased risk of fractures. Liver abnormalities such as cholestasis, fatty liver, hepatitis, and hepatic necrosis have occurred. Hepatocellular carcinomas have been reported in some studies; relationship to treatment is unclear. Tamoxifen is associated with an increased incidence of uterine or endometrial cancers. Endometrial hyperplasia, polyps, endometriosis, uterine fibroids, and ovarian cysts have occurred. Monitor and promptly evaluate any report of abnormal vaginal bleeding. Amenorrhea and menstrual irregularities have been reported with tamoxifen use.

Adverse Reactions

>10%:

Cardiovascular: Vasodilatation (41%), flushing (33%), hypertension (11%), peripheral edema (11%)

Central nervous system: Mood changes (12% to 18%), pain (3% to 16%), depression (2% to 12%)

Dermatologic: Skin changes (6% to 19%), skin rash (13%)

Endocrine & metabolic: Hot flash (3% to 80%), fluid retention (32%), menstrual disease (6% to 25%), weight loss (23%), amenorrhea (16%)

Gastrointestinal: Nausea (5% to 26%), vomiting (12%)

Genitourinary: Vaginal discharge (13% to 55%), vaginal hemorrhage (2% to 23%)
Hematologic & oncologic: Lymphedema (11%)
Neuromuscular & skeletal: Weakness (18%), arthritis (14%), arthralgia (11%)
Respiratory: Pharyngitis (14%)

1% to 10%:
Cardiovascular: Chest pain (5%), venous thrombosis (5%), edema (4%), ischemic heart disease (3%), angina pectoris (2%), deep vein thrombosis (≤2%), myocardial infarction (1%)
Central nervous system: Insomnia (9%), dizziness (8%), headache (8%), anxiety (6%), paresthesia (5%), fatigue (4%)
Dermatologic: Diaphoresis (6%), alopecia (≤5%)
Endocrine & metabolic: Oligomenorrhea (9%), weight gain (9%), hyper-cholesterolemia (4%), ovarian cyst (3%)
Gastrointestinal: Abdominal pain (9%), constipation (4% to 8%), diarrhea (7%), dyspepsia (6%), abdominal cramps (1%), anorexia (1%)
Genitourinary: Urinary tract infection (10%), leukorrhea (9%), mastalgia (6%), vaginitis (5%), vulvovaginitis (5%)
Hematologic & oncologic: Thrombocytopenia (≤10%), anemia (5%), breast neoplasm (5%), neoplasm (5%; second primary)
Hepatic: Increased serum AST (5%), increased serum bilirubin (2%)
Hypersensitivity: Hypersensitivity reaction (3%)
Infection: Infection (≤9%), sepsis (≤9%)
Neuromuscular & skeletal: Back pain (10%), ostealgia (6% to 10%), bone fracture (7%), osteoporosis (7%), arthropathy (5%), myalgia (5%), muscu-loskeletal pain (3%)
Ophthalmic: Cataract (7%)
Renal: Increased serum creatinine (≤2%)
Respiratory: Cough (4% to 9%), dyspnea (8%), flu-like symptoms (6%), bronchitis (5%), sinusitis (5%), throat irritation (oral solution: 5%)
Miscellaneous: Cyst (5%)

Frequency not defined:
Cardiovascular: Cerebrovascular accident, phlebitis (including superficial), pulmonary embolism, thrombosis (retinal vein)
Central nervous system: Tumor pain (during treatment of metastatic breast cancer; generally resolves with continuation)
Dermatologic: Pruritus vulvae
Endocrine & metabolic: Hypercalcemia, hyperlipidemia
Gastrointestinal: Cholestasis, dysgeusia
Genitourinary: Endometrial hyperplasia, endometrial polyps, endometriosis, vaginal dryness
Hematologic & oncologic: Endometrial carcinoma, tumor flare (during treat-ment of metastatic breast cancer; generally resolves with continuation; includes increased lesion size and erythema), uterine fibroids
Hepatic: Hepatic necrosis, hepatitis, liver steatosis
Ophthalmic: Corneal changes, retinopathy

<1%, postmarketing, and/or case reports: Angioedema, bullous pemphigoid, erythema multiforme, hypertriglyceridemia, impotence, interstitial pneumo-nitis, loss of libido (males), pancreatitis, Stevens-Johnson syndrome, vision color changes

Drug Interactions

Metabolism/Transport Effects Substrate of CYP2A6 (minor), CYP2B6 (minor), CYP2C9 (major), CYP2D6 (major), CYP2E1 (minor), CYP3A4 (major); **Note:** Assignment of Major/Minor substrate status based on clinically relevant drug interaction potential; **Inhibits** CYP2C8 (moderate), CYP2C9 (weak)

Avoid Concomitant Use

Avoid concomitant use of Tamoxifen with any of the following: Amodiaquine; Conivaptan; CYP2D6 Inhibitors (Strong); Fusidic Acid (Systemic); Idelalisib; Ospemifene; Vitamin K Antagonists

Increased Effect/Toxicity

Tamoxifen may increase the levels/effects of: Amodiaquine; Chloroquine; CYP2C8 Substrates; Highest Risk QTc-Prolonging Agents; Hydroxychloroquine; Mipomersen; Moderate Risk QTc-Prolonging Agents; Ospemifene; Selexipag; Vitamin K Antagonists

The levels/effects of Tamoxifen may be increased by: Abiraterone Acetate; Asunaprevir; Conivaptan; CYP2C9 Inhibitors (Moderate); CYP2C9 Inhibitors (Strong); CYP3A4 Inhibitors (Moderate); CYP3A4 Inhibitors (Strong); Dasatinib; Fosaprepitant; Fusidic Acid (Systemic); Idelalisib; Imatinib; MiFEPRIStone; Netupitant; Palbociclib; Panobinostat; Peginterferon Alfa-2b; Simeprevir; Stiripentol

Decreased Effect

Tamoxifen may decrease the levels/effects of: Anastrozole; Letrozole; Ospemifene

The levels/effects of Tamoxifen may be decreased by: Bexarotene (Systemic); Bosentan; CYP2C9 Inducers (Strong); CYP2D6 Inhibitors (Moderate); CYP2D6 Inhibitors (Strong); CYP3A4 Inducers (Moderate); CYP3A4 Inducers (Strong); Dabrafenib; Deferasirox; Enzalutamide; Mitotane; Peginterferon Alfa-2b; Rifamycin Derivatives; Sarilumab; Siltuximab; St John's Wort; Tocilizumab

Food Interactions Grapefruit juice may decrease the metabolism of tamoxifen. Management: Avoid grapefruit juice.

Hazardous Drugs Handling Considerations

Hazardous agent (NIOSH 2016 [group 1]).

Use appropriate precautions for receiving, handling, administration, and disposal. Gloves (single) should be worn during receiving, unpacking, and placing in storage.

NIOSH recommends single gloving for administration of intact tablets or capsules. If manipulating tablets/capsules (eg, to prepare an oral suspension), NIOSH recommends double gloving, a protective gown, and preparation in a controlled device; if not prepared in a controlled device, respiratory and eye/face protection as well as ventilated engineering controls are recommended. NIOSH recommends double gloving, a protective gown, and (if there is a potential for vomit or spit up) eye/face protection for administration of an oral liquid/feeding tube administration (NIOSH 2016).

Storage/Stability

Oral solution: Store at ≤25°C (77°F); do not freeze or refrigerate. Protect from light. Discard opened bottle after 3 months.

Tablets: Store at 20°C to 25°C (68°F to 77°F). Protect from light.

◄ **Mechanism of Action** Competitively binds to estrogen receptors on tumors and other tissue targets, producing a nuclear complex that decreases DNA synthesis and inhibits estrogen effects; nonsteroidal agent with potent anti-estrogenic properties which compete with estrogen for binding sites in breast and other tissues; cells accumulate in the G_0 and G_1 phases; therefore, tamoxifen is cytostatic rather than cytocidal.

Pharmacodynamics/Kinetics

Absorption: Well absorbed

Distribution: High concentrations found in uterus, endometrial and breast tissue

Protein binding: 99%

Metabolism: Hepatic; via CYP2D6 to 4-hydroxytamoxifen and via CYP3A4/5 to N-desmethyl-tamoxifen. Each is then further metabolized into endoxifen (4-hydroxy-tamoxifen via CYP3A4/5 and N-desmethyl-tamoxifen via CYP2D6); both 4-hydroxy-tamoxifen and endoxifen are 30- to 100-fold more potent than tamoxifen

Half-life elimination: Tamoxifen: ~5 to 7 days; N-desmethyl tamoxifen: ~14 days

Time to peak, serum:

Children 2 to 10 years (female): ~8 hours

Adults: ~5 hours

Excretion: Feces (26% to 51%); urine (9% to 13%)

Clearance: Higher (~2.3 fold) in female pediatric patients (2 to 10 years) compared to adult breast cancer patients; within pediatric population, clearance faster in children 2 to 6 years compared to older children

Dosing

Adult & Geriatric Note: For the treatment of breast cancer, patients receiving both tamoxifen and chemotherapy should receive treatment sequentially, with tamoxifen following completion of chemotherapy.

Breast cancer treatment: Oral:

Adjuvant therapy (females): 20 mg once daily for 5 years

Premenopausal women: Duration of treatment is 5 years (Burstein 2010; NCCN Breast Cancer guidelines v.2.2013)

Postmenopausal women: Duration of tamoxifen treatment is 2-3 years followed by an aromatase inhibitor (AI) to complete 5 years; may take tamoxifen for the full 5 years (if contraindications or intolerance to AI) or extended therapy: 4.5 to 6 years of tamoxifen followed by 5 years of an AI (Burstein 2010; NCCN Breast Cancer guidelines v.2.2013)

ER-positive early breast cancer: Extended duration: Duration of treatment of 10 years demonstrated a reduced risk of recurrence and mortality (Davies 2012)

Metastatic (males and females): 20-40 mg daily (doses >20 mg should be given in 2 divided doses). **Note:** Although the FDA-approved labeling recommends dosing up to 40 mg daily, clinical benefit has not been demonstrated with doses above 20 mg daily (Bratherton 1984).

Ductal carcinoma in situ (DCIS) (females), to reduce the risk for invasive breast cancer: 20 mg once daily for 5 years

Breast cancer risk reduction (pre- and postmenopausal high-risk females): Oral: 20 mg once daily for 5 years

Endometrial carcinoma, recurrent, metastatic, or high-risk (endometrioid histologies only) (off-label use): Oral:

Monotherapy: 20 mg twice daily until disease progression or unacceptable toxicity (Thigpen 2001)

Combination therapy: 20 mg twice daily for 3 weeks (alternating with megestrol acetate every 3 weeks); continue alternating until disease progression or unacceptable toxicity) (Fiorica 2004)

Gynecomastia (off-label use): Oral: 20 mg once daily for up to 12 months (Boccardo 2005; Fradet 2007). The majority of published experiences have been in adult men with prostate cancer receiving bicalutamide. Use has also been reported in patients with idiopathic gynecomastia.

Induction of ovulation (off-label use): Oral: 20 mg once daily (range: 20-80 mg once daily) for 5 days (Steiner 2005)

Oligospermia (off-label use): Oral: 10 mg twice daily (Adamopoulos 1995; Adamopoulos 1997; Adamopoulos 2003; Buvat 1987); most effective when used in combination with testosterone (Adamopoulos 2003). The treatment period in clinical trials was up to 18 months (Buvat 1987). Although doses of 10 to 40 mg/day have been used, increasing dose after 6 months from 10 mg twice daily to 20 mg twice daily did not increase sperm count (Buvat 1987).

Ovarian cancer, advanced and/or recurrent (off-label use): Oral: 20 mg twice daily (Hatch 1991; Markman 1996)

Paget's disease of the breast (risk reduction; with DCIS or without associated cancer): Oral: 20 mg once daily for 5 years (NCCN Breast Cancer Guidelines v.2.2013)

Dosage adjustment for DVT, pulmonary embolism, cerebrovascular accident, or prolonged immobilization: Discontinue tamoxifen (NCCN Breast Cancer Risk Reduction Guidelines v.1.2013)

Pediatric Females: Precocious puberty secondary to McCune-Albright syndrome (off-label use): Oral: A dose of 20 mg daily has been reported in patients 2-10 years of age; safety and efficacy have not been established for treatment of longer than 1 year duration (Eugster, 2003)

Renal Impairment No dosage adjustment provided in manufacturer's labeling.

Chronic dialysis: No dosage adjustment necessary (Janus, 2013).

Hepatic Impairment No dosage adjustment provided in manufacturer's labeling (has not been studied).

Administration Administer tablets or oral solution orally with or without food. Use supplied dosing cup for oral solution.

Extemporaneous Preparations A 0.5 mg/mL oral suspension may be prepared with tablets. Place two 10 mg tablets into 40 mL purified water and let stand ~2-5 minutes. Stir until tablets are completely disintegrated (dispersion time for each 10 mg tablet is ~2-5 minutes). Administer immediately after preparation. To ensure the full dose is administered, rinse glass several times with water and administer residue.

Lam MS, "Extemporaneous Compounding of Oral Liquid Dosage Formulations and Alternative Drug Delivery Methods for Anticancer Drugs," *Pharmacotherapy,* 2011, 31(2):164-92.

Monitoring Parameters CBC with platelets, serum calcium, LFTs; triglycerides and cholesterol (in patients with preexisting hyperlipidemias); INR and PT (in patients on vitamin K antagonists); abnormal vaginal bleeding; breast and gynecologic exams (baseline and routine), mammogram (baseline and routine); signs/symptoms of DVT (leg swelling, tenderness) or PE (shortness of breath); ophthalmic exam (if vision problem or cataracts); bone mineral density (premenopausal women)

Test Interactions T_4 elevations (which may be explained by increases in thyroid-binding globulin) have been reported; not accompanied by clinical hyperthyroidism

◀ **Dietary Considerations** Tablets and oral solution may be taken with or without food. Avoid grapefruit and grapefruit juice.

Additional Information Estrogen receptor status may predict if adjuvant treatment with tamoxifen is of benefit. In metastatic breast cancer, patients with estrogen receptor positive tumors are more likely to benefit from tamoxifen treatment. With tamoxifen use to reduce the incidence of breast cancer in high risk-women, high risk is defined as women ≥35 years of age with a 5 year NCI Gail model predicted risk of breast cancer ≥1.67%.

Oncology Comment: The American Society of Clinical Oncology (ASCO) guidelines for adjuvant endocrine therapy in postmenopausal women with HR-positive breast cancer (Burstein, 2010) recommend considering aromatase inhibitor (AI) therapy at some point in the treatment course (primary, sequentially, or extended). Optimal duration at this time is not known; however, treatment with an AI should not exceed 5 years in primary and extended therapies, and 2-3 years if followed by tamoxifen in sequential therapy (total of 5 years). If initial therapy with AI has been discontinued before the 5 years, consideration should be taken to receive tamoxifen for a total of 5 years. The optimal time to switch to an AI is also not known; but data supports switching after 2-3 years of tamoxifen (sequential) or after 5 years of tamoxifen (extended). If patient becomes intolerant or has poor adherence, consideration should be made to switch to another AI or initiate tamoxifen.

Recent data suggest that continuing tamoxifen for 10 years (rather than stopping after 5 years of therapy) may provide a further reduction in breast cancer recurrence and mortality in women with early stage disease (Davies, 2012). The Adjuvant Tamoxifen: Longer Against Shorter (ATLAS) trial randomized 6846 patients with estrogen receptor positive disease to continue tamoxifen for a total of 10 years of treatment or to stop after 5 years. Breast cancer recurrence was observed in 617 patients in the 10-year arm versus 711 recurrences in the 5-year arm (p=0.002). Breast cancer mortality was significantly reduced with 10 years of tamoxifen therapy versus 5 years (331 deaths vs 397 deaths, respectively; p=0.01) (Davies, 2012).

The adjuvant endocrine therapy of choice is tamoxifen for men with breast cancer and for pre- or perimenopausal women at diagnosis. CYP2D6 genotyping is not recommended, however, due to the potential for drug-drug interactions use caution and consider avoiding concomitant therapy with tamoxifen and known CYP2D6 inhibitors.

Medication Guide Available Yes

Dosage Forms Excipient information presented when available (limited, particularly for generics); consult specific product labeling.
Solution, Oral:
  Soltamox: 10 mg/5 mL (150 mL) [sugar free; contains alcohol, usp, propylene glycol; licorice-aniseed flavor]
Tablet, Oral:
  Generic: 10 mg, 20 mg

◆ **Tamoxifen Citras** see Tamoxifen on page 1734
◆ **Tamoxifen Citrate** see Tamoxifen on page 1734
◆ **TAP-144** see Leuprolide on page 1131
◆ **Tarceva** see Erlotinib on page 716
◆ **Targretin** see Bexarotene (Systemic) on page 246
◆ **Targretin** see Bexarotene (Topical) on page 251

- **Taro-Anastrozole (Can)** *see* Anastrozole *on page 135*
- **Taro-Ciprofloxacin (Can)** *see* Ciprofloxacin (Systemic) *on page 393*
- **Taro-Fluconazole (Can)** *see* Fluconazole *on page 807*
- **Taro-Zoledronic Acid (Can)** *see* Zoledronic Acid *on page 1945*
- **Taro-Zoledronic Acid Concentrate (Can)** *see* Zoledronic Acid *on page 1945*
- **TAS-102** *see* Trifluridine and Tipiracil *on page 1837*
- **Tasigna** *see* Nilotinib *on page 1314*
- **Taxol** *see* PACLitaxel (Conventional) *on page 1402*
- **Taxotere** *see* DOCEtaxel *on page 606*
- **Tazicef** *see* CefTAZidime *on page 360*
- **Tazidime** *see* CefTAZidime *on page 360*
- **Tazobactam and Piperacillin** *see* Piperacillin and Tazobactam *on page 1513*
- **Tazocin (Can)** *see* Piperacillin and Tazobactam *on page 1513*
- **Tbo-Filgrastim** *see* Filgrastim *on page 792*
- **Tc99m Sestamibi** *see* Technetium Tc 99m Sestamibi *on page 1741*
- **Tc99m-Sulfur Colloid** *see* Technetium Tc 99m Sulfur Colloid *on page 1742*
- **Tc99m Tilmanocept** *see* Technetium Tc 99m Tilmanocept *on page 1743*
- **T-Cell Growth Factor** *see* Aldesleukin *on page 71*
- **TCGF** *see* Aldesleukin *on page 71*
- **T-DM1** *see* Ado-Trastuzumab Emtansine *on page 57*
- **TDX** *see* Raltitrexed *on page 1572*
- **Tecentriq** *see* Atezolizumab *on page 188*
- **Technetium (99mTc) Sestamibi** *see* Technetium Tc 99m Sestamibi *on page 1741*
- **Technetium (99mTc) Sulfur Colloid** *see* Technetium Tc 99m Sulfur Colloid *on page 1742*
- **Technetium (99mTc) Tilmanocept** *see* Technetium Tc 99m Tilmanocept *on page 1743*
- **Technetium Sestamibi (99mTc)** *see* Technetium Tc 99m Sestamibi *on page 1741*
- **Technetium Sulfur Colloid (99mTc)** *see* Technetium Tc 99m Sulfur Colloid *on page 1742*

Technetium Tc 99m Sestamibi

(tek NEE shee um tee see nyne tee nyne em ses ta MIB ee)

Brand Names: US Cardiolite

Index Terms 99m Technetium Sestamibi; 99mTc-Sestamibi; Tc99m Sestamibi; Technetium (99mTc) Sestamibi; Technetium Sestamibi (99mTc)

Pharmacologic Category Radiopharmaceutical

Use Imaging agent: Myocardial perfusion agent used in detection of coronary artery disease in conjunction with exercise stress testing or pharmacologic stress testing to identify reversible myocardial ischemia with or without myocardial infarction; planar breast imaging after mammography to assist in

◀ evaluation of breast lesions in patients with abnormal mammogram or palpable breast mass (second-line)

Pregnancy Risk Factor C

Dosing

Adult

Breast imaging: IV (based on 70 kg patient): 20 to 30 mCi (740 to 1,110 MBq)

Myocardial imaging: IV (based on 70 kg patient): 10 to 30 mCi (370 to 1,110 MBq)

Geriatric Refer to adult dosing.

Renal Impairment There are no dosage adjustments provided in the manufacturer's labeling.

Hepatic Impairment There are no dosage adjustments provided in the manufacturer's labeling.

Additional Information Complete prescribing information should be consulted for additional detail.

Dosage Forms Excipient information presented when available (limited, particularly for generics); consult specific product labeling.

Kit, Intravenous:

Cardiolite: 2-methoxyisobutyl isonitrile (MIBI) copper tetrafluoroborate 1 mg (5s, 20s) [pyrogen free; vial contents to be combined with Technetium Tc 99m pertechnetate sodium (not included)]

Generic: 2-methoxyisobutyl isonitrile (MIBI) copper tetrafluoroborate 1 mg (5s, 20s, 30s) [vial contents to be combined with Technetium Tc 99m pertechnetate sodium (not included)]

Technetium Tc 99m Sulfur Colloid

(tek NEE shee um tee see nyne tee nyne em SUL fyoor ko LOYD)

Index Terms 99mTc-Sulfur Colloid; Sulfur Colloid; Tc99m-Sulfur Colloid; Technetium (99mTc) Sulfur Colloid; Technetium (^{99m}Tc) Sulfur Colloid; Technetium Sulfur Colloid (^{99m}Tc)

Pharmacologic Category Radiopharmaceutical

Use Imaging agent: Localization of lymph nodes draining a primary tumor in patients with breast cancer or malignant melanoma (when used with a handheld gamma counter); reticuloendothelial cell imaging agent (liver, spleen, bone marrow); evaluation of peritoneovenous shunt patency; esophageal transit studies, gastroesophageal reflux scintigraphy, detection of pulmonary aspiration of gastric contents

Pregnancy Risk Factor C

Dosing

Adult & Geriatric

Breast cancer or malignant melanoma, lymph node localization: SubQ: 3.7-37 MBq (0.1-1 mCi) in volumes ranging from 0.1 to 1 mL

Peritoneovenous shunt patency evaluation:

Intraperitoneal injection: 37-111 MBq (1-3 mCi)

Percutaneous transtubal (efferent limb) injection: 12-37 MBq (0.3-1 mCi) in a maximum volume of 0.5 mL

Reticuloendothelial cell imaging:

Bone marrow: IV: 111-444 MBq (3-12 mCi)

Liver/spleen: IV: 37-296 MBq (1-8 mCi)

Esophageal transit studies, gastroesophageal reflux scintigraphy, pulmonary aspiration imaging:
Gastroesophageal studies: Oral: 5.55-11.1 MBq (0.15-0.3 mCi)
Pulmonary aspiration studies: Oral: 11.1-18.5 MBq (0.3-0.5 mCi)

Pediatric
Reticuloendothelial cell imaging:
Bone marrow: Pediatrics: IV: 1.11-5.55 MBq/**kg** (0.03-0.15 mCi/**kg**)
Liver/spleen:
Newborns: IV: 7.4-18.5 MBq (0.2-0.5 mCi)
Children: IV: 0.56-2.78 MBq/**kg** (0.015-0.075 mCi/**kg**)

Esophageal transit studies, gastroesophageal reflux scintigraphy, pulmonary aspiration imaging: *Gastroesophageal studies or pulmonary aspiration studies:* Pediatrics: Oral or nasogastric tube: 3.7-11.1 MBq (0.1-0.3 mCi)

Renal Impairment No dosage adjustment provided in manufacturer's labeling.

Hepatic Impairment No dosage adjustment provided in manufacturer's labeling.

Additional Information Complete prescribing information should be consulted for additional detail.

Dosage Forms Excipient information presented when available (limited, particularly for generics); consult specific product labeling.
Kit, Injection:
Generic: Contents to be combined with Technetium Tc 99m pertechnetate sodium (not included)]

Technetium Tc 99m Tilmanocept
(tek NEE shee um tee see nyne tee nyne em til MAN oh sept)

Brand Names: US Lymphoseek

Index Terms 99mTc-Tilmanocept; Tc99m Tilmanocept; Technetium (99mTc) Tilmanocept; Technetium Tilmanocept (99mTc)

Pharmacologic Category Radiopharmaceutical

Use
Diagnostic imaging: Radioactive diagnostic agent indicated with or without scintigraphic imaging (using a handheld gamma counter) for:
- Lymphatic mapping to locate lymph nodes draining a primary tumor site in patients with solid tumors for which this procedure is a component of intraoperative management.
- Guiding sentinel lymph node biopsy in patients with clinically node negative squamous cell carcinoma of the oral cavity, breast cancer, or melanoma.

Pregnancy Risk Factor C

Dosing
Adult & Geriatric Note: The route of administration, number of injections, and total injection volume per patient will vary depending on cancer and planned injection technique.
Breast cancer lymphatic mapping: Intradermal, SubQ, subareolar, or peritumoral: 18.5 MBq (0.5 mCi) as radioactivity dose and 50 mcg as a mass dose at least 15 minutes prior to intraoperative lymphatic mapping
Melanoma lymphatic mapping: Intradermal or SubQ: 18.5 MBq (0.5 mCi) as radioactivity dose and 50 mcg as a mass dose at least 15 minutes prior to intraoperative lymphatic mapping

◄ **Oral cavity squamous cell carcinoma sentinel lymph node biopsy:**
Peritumoral: 18.5 MBq (0.5 mCi) as radioactivity dose and 50 mcg as a
mass dose at least 15 minutes prior to intraoperative sentinel node biopsy

Renal Impairment There are no dosage adjustments provided in the
manufacturer's labeling.

Hepatic Impairment There are no dosage adjustments provided in the
manufacturer's labeling.

Additional Information Complete prescribing information should be consulted for additional detail.

Prescribing and Access Restrictions Lymphoseek may only be obtained
through Cardinal Health's Nuclear Pharmacy Services.

Dosage Forms Excipient information presented when available (limited,
particularly for generics); consult specific product labeling.
Injection, powder for reconstitution [kit]:
Lymphoseek: Tilmanocept 250 mcg (5s) [vial contents to be combined with
Technetium Tc 99m pertechnetate sodium (not included)]

◆ **Technetium Tilmanocept (99mTc)** *see* Technetium Tc 99m Tilmanocept
on page 1743

Telotristat Ethyl (tel OH tri state ETH il)

Brand Names: US Xermelo

Index Terms LX1032; LX1606; Telotristat Etiprate; Xermelo

Pharmacologic Category Tryptophan Hydroxylase Inhibitor

Use Carcinoid syndrome diarrhea: Treatment of carcinoid syndrome diarrhea (in combination with somatostatin analog therapy) in adults with symptoms inadequately controlled by somatostatin analog therapy

Labeled Contraindications There are no contraindications listed within the
manufacturer's labeling.

Pregnancy Considerations Adverse events were observed in some animal
reproduction studies.

Breastfeeding Considerations It is not known if telotristat ethyl is present in
breast milk. According to the manufacturer, the decision to continue or
discontinue breastfeeding during therapy should take into account the risk
of infant exposure, the benefits of breastfeeding to the infant, and benefits of
treatment to the mother. Breastfed infants should be monitored for constipation.

Warnings/Precautions Constipation has been reported in clinical trials.
Although rarely serious, some events resulted in hospitalization, intestinal
perforation or bowel obstruction (these events occurred at a dose higher than
the recommended dose). Patients with advanced carcinoid tumors may be at
risk for altered gastrointestinal tract wall integrity; monitor closely for constipation and/or severe, persistent, or worsening abdominal pain. Discontinue
for severe constipation and/or the development of severe persistent or
worsening abdominal pain.

Adverse Reactions
>10%:
Central nervous system: Headache (11%)
Gastrointestinal: Nausea (13%)
1% to 10%:
Cardiovascular: Peripheral edema (7%)
Central nervous system: Depression (9%)
Endocrine & metabolic: Increased gamma-glutamyl transferase (9%)

Gastrointestinal: Decreased appetite (7%), flatulence (7%), abdominal pain (≥5%), constipation (≥5%)

Hepatic: Increased serum alkaline phosphatase (<5%), increased serum ALT (<5%), increased serum AST (<5%)

Miscellaneous: Fever (7%)

Drug Interactions

Metabolism/Transport Effects Induces CYP3A4 (weak)

Avoid Concomitant Use There are no known interactions where it is recommended to avoid concomitant use.

Increased Effect/Toxicity There are no known significant interactions involving an increase in effect.

Decreased Effect

Telotristat Ethyl may decrease the levels/effects of: CloZAPine; HYDRO-codone; NiMODipine

The levels/effects of Telotristat Ethyl may be decreased by: Octreotide

Food Interactions Administration with food results in higher exposure to telotristat ethyl and telotristat.

Storage/Stability Store at 25°C (77°F); excursions permitted to 15°C to 30°C (59°F to 86°F).

Mechanism of Action Telotristat ethyl is a small molecule inhibitor of tryptophan hydroxylase (TPH). TPH converts tryptophan to 5-hydroxytryptophan and ultimately to serotonin, and is the rate-limiting enzyme in serotonin synthesis (Kulke 2017). Decreased production of peripheral serotonin by telotristat ethyl results in a reduction in the frequency of carcinoid syndrome diarrhea.

Pharmacodynamics/Kinetics

Distribution: The high molecular weight and acidic moieties of telotristat ethyl inhibit the compound from crossing the blood brain barrier (Kulke 2017).

Protein binding: >99%

Metabolism: Telotristat ethyl is hydrolyzed via carboxylesterases to the metabolite telotristat (active); telotristat is further metabolized.

Half-life elimination: Telotristat ethyl: ~0.6 hours; Telotristat: ~5 hours

Time to peak: Telotristat ethyl: 0.5 to 2 hours; Telotristat: 1 to 3 hours

Excretion: Feces (~93%); urine (<1%)

Dosing

Adult & Geriatric Carcinoid syndrome diarrhea: Oral: 250 mg 3 times daily

Missed dose: If a dose is missed, administer the next dose at the regularly scheduled time; do not take 2 doses at the same time.

Renal Impairment

CrCl >20 mL/minute: There are no dosage adjustments provided in the manufacturer's labeling; however, population pharmacokinetic analysis suggests that CrCl 20 to 89 mL/minute does not affect telotristat pharmacokinetics.

End-stage renal disease (ESRD) requiring dialysis: There are no dosage adjustment provided in the manufacturer's labeling (has not been studied).

Hepatic Impairment

Mild impairment (total bilirubin >1 to 1.5 times ULN or AST > ULN): There are no dosage adjustments provided in the manufacturer's labeling; however, population pharmacokinetic analysis suggests that mild hepatic impairment does not affect telotristat pharmacokinetics.

◄ Moderate or severe impairment (total bilirubin >1.5 times ULN and any AST): There are no dosage adjustments provided in the manufacturer's labeling (has not been studied).

Adjustment for Toxicity Gastrointestinal toxicity: Discontinue for severe constipation or for development of severe, persistent or worsening abdominal pain

Administration Administer with food. If used in combination with short-acting octreotide, administer octreotide at least 30 minutes after telotristat ethyl. Rescue octreotide (short-acting) and antidiarrheals were allowed and unrestricted in a clinical study (Kulke 2017).

Monitoring Parameters Monitor for symptoms of constipation and/or severe, persistent, or worsening abdominal pain

Dosage Forms Excipient information presented when available (limited, particularly for generics); consult specific product labeling.

Tablet, Oral:

Xermelo: 250 mg

♦ **Telotristat Etiprate** *see* Telotristat Ethyl *on page 1744*
♦ **Temodal (Can)** *see* Temozolomide *on page 1746*
♦ **Temodar** *see* Temozolomide *on page 1746*

Temozolomide (te moe ZOE loe mide)

Related Information

Common Toxicity Criteria *on page 2242*

Management of Chemotherapy-Induced Nausea and Vomiting in Adults *on page 2253*

Prevention of Chemotherapy-Induced Nausea and Vomiting in Children *on page 2310*

Safe Handling of Hazardous Drugs *on page 2379*

Brand Names: US Temodar

Brand Names: Canada ACH-Temozolomide; ACT Temozolomide; Temodal

Index Terms SCH 52365; TMZ

Pharmacologic Category Antineoplastic Agent, Alkylating Agent (Triazene)

Use

Anaplastic astrocytoma: Treatment of refractory anaplastic astrocytoma (refractory to a regimen containing a nitrosourea and procarbazine)

Glioblastoma multiforme: Treatment of newly-diagnosed glioblastoma multiforme (initially in combination with radiotherapy, then as maintenance treatment)

Labeled Contraindications

Hypersensitivity (eg, allergic reaction, anaphylaxis, urticaria, Stevens-Johnson syndrome, toxic epidermal necrolysis) to temozolomide or any component of the formulation; hypersensitivity to dacarbazine (both drugs are metabolized to MTIC)

Canadian labeling: Additional contraindications (not in U.S. labeling): Not recommended in patients with severe myelosuppression

Pregnancy Considerations Adverse events were observed in animal reproduction studies. May cause fetal harm when administered to pregnant women. Male and female patients should avoid pregnancy while receiving temozolomide.

Breastfeeding Considerations It is not known if temozolomide is excreted in breast milk. Due to the potential for serious adverse reactions in the nursing infant, the manufacturer recommends a decision be made whether to discontinue nursing or to discontinue the drug, taking into account the importance of treatment to the mother.

Warnings/Precautions *Pneumocystis jirovecii* pneumonia (PCP) may occur; risk is increased in those receiving steroids or longer dosing regimens; monitor all patients for development of PCP (particularly if also receiving corticosteroids); PCP prophylaxis is required in patients receiving radiotherapy in combination with the 42-day temozolomide regimen. Myelosuppression may occur; may require treatment interruption, dose reduction, and/or discontinuation; monitor blood counts; an increased incidence has been reported in geriatric and female patients. Prolonged pancytopenia resulting in aplastic anemia has been reported (may be fatal); concurrent use of temozolomide with medications associated with aplastic anemia (eg, carbamazepine, cotrimoxazole, phenytoin) may obscure assessment for development of aplastic anemia. ANC should be ≥1,500/mm^3 and platelets ≥100,000/mm^3 prior to treatment. Rare cases of myelodysplastic syndrome and secondary malignancies, including acute myeloid leukemia, have been reported. Use caution in patients with severe hepatic or renal impairment; has not been studied in dialysis patients. Hepatotoxicity has been reported; may be severe or fatal. Monitor liver function tests at baseline, halfway through the first cycle, prior to each subsequent cycle, and at ~2 to 4 weeks after the last dose. Postmarketing reports of hepatotoxicity have included liver function abnormalities, hepatitis, hepatic failure, cholestasis, hepatitis cholestasis, jaundice, cholelithiasis, hepatic steatosis, hepatic necrosis, hepatic lesion, and hepatic encephalopathy (Sarganas 2012).

Temozolomide is associated with a moderate emetic potential (Dupuis 2011; Roila 2010); antiemetics are recommended to prevent nausea and vomiting. Increased MGMT (O-6-methylguanine-DNA methyltransferase) activity/levels within tumor tissue is associated with temozolomide resistance. Glioblastoma patients with decreased levels (due to methylated MGMT promoter) may be more likely to benefit from the combination of radiation therapy and temozolomide (Hegi 2008; Stupp 2009). Determination of MGMT status may be predictive for response to alkylating agents. Potentially significant drug-drug interactions may exist, requiring dose or frequency adjustment, additional monitoring, and/or selection of alternative therapy. Bioequivalence has only been established when IV temozolomide is administered over 90 minutes; shorter or longer infusion times may result in suboptimal dosing.

Polysorbate 80: Some dosage forms may contain polysorbate 80 (also known as Tweens). Hypersensitivity reactions, usually a delayed reaction, have been reported following exposure to pharmaceutical products containing polysorbate 80 in certain individuals (Isaksson 2002; Lucente 2000; Shelley 1995). Thrombocytopenia, ascites, pulmonary deterioration, and renal and hepatic failure have been reported in premature neonates after receiving parenteral products containing polysorbate 80 (Alade 1986; CDC 1984). See manufacturer's labeling.

Adverse Reactions With CNS malignancies, it may be difficult to distinguish between CNS adverse events caused by temozolomide versus the effects of progressive disease.

>10%:

Cardiovascular: Peripheral edema (11%)

Central nervous system: Fatigue (34% to 61%), headache (23% to 41%), seizure (6% to 23%), hemiparesis (18%), dizziness (5% to 12%), ataxia (8% to 11%)

Dermatologic: Alopecia (55%), skin rash (8% to 13%)

Gastrointestinal: Nausea (49% to 53%; grades 3/4: 1% to 10%), vomiting (29% to 42%; grades 3/4: 2% to 6%), constipation (22% to 33%), anorexia (9% to 27%), diarrhea (10% to 16%)

Hematologic & oncologic: Lymphocytopenia (grades 3/4: 55%), thrombocytopenia (grades 3/4: adults: 4% to 19%; children: 25%), neutropenia (grades 3/4: adults: 8% to 14%; children: 20%), leukopenia (grades 3/4: 11%)

Infection: Viral infection (11%)

Neuromuscular & skeletal: Weakness (7% to 13%)

Miscellaneous: Fever (13%)

1% to 10%:

Central nervous system: Amnesia (10%), insomnia (4% to 10%), drowsiness (9%), paresthesia (9%), paresis (8%), anxiety (7%), memory impairment (7%), abnormal gait (6%), depression (6%), confusion (5%)

Dermatologic: Pruritus (5% to 8%), xeroderma (5%), erythema (1%)

Endocrine & metabolic: Hypercorticoidism (8%), weight gain (5%)

Gastrointestinal: Stomatitis (9%), abdominal pain (5% to 9%), dysphagia (7%), dysgeusia (5%)

Genitourinary: Urinary incontinence (8%), urinary tract infection (8%), mastalgia (females 6%), urinary frequency (6%)

Hematologic & oncologic: Anemia (grades 3/4: 4%)

Hypersensitivity: Hypersensitivity reaction (≤3%)

Neuromuscular & skeletal: Back pain (8%), arthralgia (6%), myalgia (5%)

Ophthalmic: Blurred vision (5% to 8%), diplopia (5%), visual disturbance (visual deficit/vision changes 5%)

Respiratory: Pharyngitis (8%), upper respiratory tract infection (8%), cough (5% to 8%), sinusitis (6%), dyspnea (5%)

Miscellaneous: Radiation injury (2% maintenance phase after radiotherapy)

<1%, postmarketing, and/or case reports (limited to important or life-threatening): Agitation, anaphylaxis, apathy, aplastic anemia, cholestasis, cytomegalovirus disease (primary and reactivation), diabetes insipidus, emotional lability, erythema multiforme, febrile neutropenia, flu-like symptoms, hallucination, hematoma, hemorrhage, hepatitis, hepatitis B (reactivation), hepatotoxicity, herpes simplex encephalitis, herpes simplex infection, herpes zoster, hyperbilirubinemia, hyperglycemia, hypersensitivity pneumonitis, hypokalemia, increased serum alkaline phosphatase, increased serum transaminases, injection site reaction (erythema, irritation, pain, pruritus, swelling, warmth), interstitial pneumonitis, metastases (including myeloid leukemia), myelodysplastic syndrome, neuropathy, opportunistic infection (including pneumocystosis), oral candidiasis, pancytopenia (may be prolonged), peripheral neuropathy, petechia, pneumonitis, pulmonary fibrosis, Stevens-Johnson syndrome, toxic epidermal necrolysis, weight loss

Drug Interactions

Metabolism/Transport Effects None known.

Avoid Concomitant Use

Avoid concomitant use of Temozolomide with any of the following: BCG (Intravesical); Deferiprone; Dipyrone; Natalizumab; Pimecrolimus; Tacrolimus (Topical); Vaccines (Live)

Increased Effect/Toxicity

Temozolomide may increase the levels/effects of: CloZAPine; Deferiprone; Fingolimod; Leflunomide; Natalizumab; Tofacitinib; Vaccines (Live)

The levels/effects of Temozolomide may be increased by: Denosumab; Dipyrone; Ocrelizumab; Palifermin; Pimecrolimus; Promazine; Roflumilast; Tacrolimus (Topical); Trastuzumab; Valproate Products

Decreased Effect

Temozolomide may decrease the levels/effects of: BCG (Intravesical); Coccidioides immitis Skin Test; Lenograstim; Nivolumab; Sipuleucel-T; Vaccines (Inactivated); Vaccines (Live)

The levels/effects of Temozolomide may be decreased by: Echinacea

Food Interactions Food reduces rate and extent of absorption. Management: Administer consistently either with food or without food (was administered in studies under fasting and nonfasting conditions).

Hazardous Drugs Handling Considerations

Hazardous agent (NIOSH 2016 [group 1]).

Use appropriate precautions for receiving, handling, administration, and disposal. Gloves (single) should be worn during receiving, unpacking, and placing in storage.

NIOSH recommends single gloving for administration of intact tabloto or capsules. It manipulating tablets/capsules (eg, to prepare an oral suspension), NIOSH recommends double gloving, a protective gown, and preparation in a controlled device; if not prepared in a controlled device, respiratory and eye/face protection as well as ventilated engineering controls are recommended. NIOSH recommends double gloving, a protective gown, and (if there is a potential for vomit or spit up) eye/face protection for administration of an oral liquid/feeding tube administration. For IV preparation, double gloves, a protective gown, ventilated engineering controls (a class II biological safety cabinet or a compounding aseptic containment isolator), and closed system transfer devices (CSTDs) are recommended. Double gloving, a gown, and (if dosage form allows) CSTDs are required during IV administration (NIOSH 2016).

Storage/Stability

Capsule: Store at room temperature of 25°C (77°F); excursions permitted to 15°C to 30°C (59°F to 86°F).

Injection: Store intact vials refrigerated at 2°C to 8°C (36°F to 46°F). Reconstituted vials may be stored for up to 14 hours at room temperature of 25°C (77°F); infusion must be completed within 14 hours of reconstitution.

Preparation for Administration Bring to room temperature prior to reconstitution. Reconstitute each 100 mg vial with 41 mL sterile water for injection to a final concentration of 2.5 mg/mL. Swirl gently; do not shake. Place dose without further dilution into a 250 mL empty sterile infusion bag. Infusion must be completed within 14 hours of reconstitution.

Mechanism of Action Temozolomide is a prodrug which is rapidly and nonenzymatically converted to the active alkylating metabolite MTIC [(methyl-triazene-1-yl)-imidazole-4-carboxamide]; this conversion is spontaneous, nonenzymatic, and occurs under physiologic conditions in all tissues to which it distributes. The cytotoxic effects of MTIC are manifested through alkylation (methylation) of DNA at the O^6, N^7 guanine positions which lead to DNA double strand breaks and apoptosis. Non-cell cycle specific.

◀ **Pharmacodynamics/Kinetics**

Absorption: Oral: Rapid and complete

Distribution: V_d: Parent drug: 0.4 L/kg; penetrates blood-brain barrier; CSF levels are ~35% to 39% of plasma levels (Yung 1999)

Protein binding: 15%

Metabolism: Prodrug, hydrolyzed to the active form, MTIC; MTIC is eventually eliminated as CO_2 and 5-aminoimidazole-4-carboxamide (AIC), a natural constituent in urine; CYP isoenzymes play only a minor role in metabolism (of temozolomide and MTIC)

Bioavailability: Oral: 100% (on a mg-per-mg basis, IV temozolomide, infused over 90 minutes, is bioequivalent to an oral dose)

Half-life elimination: Mean: Parent drug: Children: 1.7 hours; Adults: 1.6-1.8 hours

Time to peak: Oral: Empty stomach: 1 hour; with food (high-fat meal): 2.25 hours

Excretion: Urine (~38%; parent drug 6%); feces <1%

Clearance: 5.5 L/hour/m^2; women have a ~5% lower clearance than men (adjusted for body surface area); children 3-17 years have similar temozolomide clearance as adults

Dosing

Adult Note: Temozolomide is associated with a moderate emetic potential (Roila 2010); antiemetics are recommended to prevent nausea and vomiting. Prior to dosing, ANC should be ≥1,500/mm^3 and platelets ≥100,000/mm^3.

Anaplastic astrocytoma (refractory): Oral, IV: Initial dose: 150 mg/m^2 once daily for 5 consecutive days of a 28-day treatment cycle. If ANC ≥1,500/mm^3 and platelets ≥100,000/mm^3, on day 1 of subsequent cycles, may increase to 200 mg/m^2 once daily for 5 consecutive days of a 28-day treatment cycle. May continue until disease progression.

Dosage modification for toxicity:

ANC <1,000/mm^3 or platelets <50,000/mm^3 on day 22 or day 29 (day 1 of next cycle): Postpone therapy until ANC >1,500/mm^3 and platelets >100,000/mm^3; reduce dose by 50 mg/m^2/day (but not below 100 mg/m^2) for subsequent cycle

ANC 1,000 to 1,500/mm^3 or platelets 50,000-100,000/mm^3 on day 22 or day 29 (day 1 of next cycle): Postpone therapy until ANC >1,500/mm^3 and platelets >100,000/mm^3; maintain initial dose

Glioblastoma multiforme (newly diagnosed, high-grade glioma): Oral, IV:

Concomitant phase: 75 mg/m^2 once daily for 42 days with focal radiotherapy (60 Gy administered in 30 fractions). **Note:** PCP prophylaxis is required during concomitant phase and should continue in patients who develop lymphocytopenia until lymphocyte recovery to ≤ grade 1. Obtain weekly CBC.

Continue at 75 mg/m^2 once daily throughout the 42-day concomitant phase (up to 49 days) as long as ANC ≥1,500/mm^3, platelet count ≥100,000/mm^3, and nonhematologic toxicity ≤ grade 1 (excludes alopecia, nausea/vomiting)

Dosage modification for toxicity:

ANC ≥500/mm^3 but <1,500/mm^3 **or** platelet count ≥10,000/mm^3 but <100,000/mm^3 **or** grade 2 nonhematologic toxicity (excludes alopecia, nausea/vomiting): Interrupt therapy

ANC <500/mm^3 **or** platelet count <10,000/mm^3 **or** grade 3/4 nonhematologic toxicity (excludes alopecia, nausea/vomiting): Discontinue therapy

Maintenance phase (consists of 6 treatment cycles): Begin 4 weeks after concomitant phase completion. **Note:** Each subsequent cycle is 28 days (consisting of 5 days of drug treatment followed by 23 days without treatment). Draw CBC on day 22 (or within 48 hours of day 22); hold next cycle and do weekly CBC until ANC >1,500/mm^3 and platelet count >100,000/mm^3; dosing modification should be based on lowest blood counts and worst nonhematologic toxicity during the previous cycle.

Cycle 1: 150 mg/m^2 once daily for 5 days of a 28-day treatment cycle

Cycles 2 to 6: May increase to 200 mg/m^2 once daily for 5 days; repeat every 28 days (if ANC ≥1,500/mm^3, platelets ≥100,000/mm^3 and nonhematologic toxicities for cycle 1 are ≤ grade 2 [excludes alopecia, nausea/vomiting]); **Note:** If dose was not escalated at the onset of cycle 2, do not increase for cycles 3 to 6)

Dosage modification (during maintenance phase) for toxicity:

ANC <1,000/mm^3, platelet count <50,000/mm^3, or grade 3 nonhematologic toxicity (excludes alopecia, nausea/vomiting) during previous cycle: Decrease dose by 1 dose level (by 50 mg/m^2/day for 5 days), unless dose has already been lowered to 100 mg/m^2/day, then discontinue therapy.

If dose reduction <100 mg/m^2/day is required or grade 4 nonhematologic toxicity (excludes alopecia, nausea/vomiting), or if the same grade 3 nonhematologic toxicity occurs after dose reduction: Discontinue therapy

Cutaneous T-cell lymphoma, advanced (mycosis fungoides [MF] and Sézary syndrome [SS]; off-label use): Oral: 200 mg/m^2 once daily for 5 days every 28 days for up to 1 year (Querfeld 2011)

Ewing's sarcoma, recurrent or progressive (off-label use): Oral: 100 mg/m^2/dose days 1 to 5 every 21 days (in combination with irinotecan) (Casey 2009). Additional data may be necessary to further define the role of temozolomide in this condition

Glioblastoma multiforme (recurrent glioma) (off-label use): Oral: 200 mg/m^2 once daily for 5 days every 28 days; if previously treated with chemotherapy, initiate at 150 mg/m^2 once daily for 5 days every 28 days and increase to 200 mg/m^2 once daily for 5 days every 28 days with cycle 2 if no hematologic toxicity (Brada 2001; Yung 2000)

Melanoma, advanced or metastatic (off-label use): Oral: 200 mg/m^2 once daily for 5 days every 28 days (for up to 12 cycles). For subsequent cycles reduce dose to 75% of the original dose for grade 3/4 hematologic toxicity and reduce the dose to 50% of the original dose for grade 3/4 nonhematologic toxicity (Middleton 2000).

Neuroendocrine tumors, advanced (off-label use): Oral: 150 mg/m^2 once daily for 7 days every 14 days (in combination with thalidomide) until disease progression (Kulke 2006) **or** 200 mg/m^2 once daily (at bedtime) days 10 to 14 of a 28-day treatment cycle (in combination with capecitabine) (Strosberg 2011)

Primary CNS lymphoma, refractory (off-label use): Oral: 150 mg/m^2 once daily for 5 days every 28 days, initially in combination with rituximab (for 4 cycles), followed by temozolomide monotherapy: 150 mg/m^2 once daily for 5 days every 28 days for 8 cycles (Wong 2004) **or** 150 mg/m^2 once daily on days 1 to 7 and 15 to 21 every 28 days (initially in combination with rituximab for 1 or 2 cycles), followed by temozolomide maintenance

◀ monotherapy: 150 mg/m² once daily for 5 days every 28 days (Enting 2004). However, additional data may be necessary to further define the role of temozolomide in this condition.

Soft tissue sarcoma (off-label use): Oral:

Soft tissue sarcoma, metastatic or unresectable: 75 mg/m² once daily for 6 weeks (Garcia del Muro 2005)

Hemangiopericytoma/solitary fibrous tumor: 150 mg/m² once daily days 1 to 7 and days 15 to 21 of a 28-day treatment cycle (in combination with bevacizumab) (Park 2011). Additional data may be necessary to further define the role of temozolomide in this condition

Geriatric Refer to adult dosing. **Note:** Patients ≥70 years of age in the anaplastic astrocytoma study had a higher incidence of grade 4 neutropenia and thrombocytopenia in the first cycle of therapy than patients <70 years of age.

Pediatric Note: Temozolomide is associated with a moderate emetic potential (Dupuis 2011); antiemetics are recommended to prevent nausea and vomiting.

Ewing's sarcoma, recurrent or progressive (off-label use): Children and Adolescents: Oral: Refer to adult dosing.

Neuroblastoma, relapsed or refractory (off-label use):

Children and Adolescents: Oral: 100 mg/m²/dose days 1 to 5 every 21 days (in combination with irinotecan) for up to 6 cycles (Bagatell 2011)

Children ≥6 months and Adolescents: Oral: 150 mg/m²/dose days 1 to 5 every 28 days (in combination with topotecan) until disease progression or unacceptable toxicity (Di Giannatale 2014)

Renal Impairment Oral:

CrCl ≥36 mL/minute/m²: There are no dosage adjustments provided in the manufacturer's labeling; however, dosage adjustment is not likely needed as no effect on temozolomide clearance was demonstrated.

Severe renal impairment (CrCl <36 mL/minute/m²): There are no dosage adjustments provided in the manufacturer's labeling; use with caution (has not been studied).

Dialysis patients: There are no dosage adjustments provided in the manufacturer's labeling (has not been studied).

Hepatic Impairment

Mild to moderate impairment: There are no dosage adjustments provided in the manufacturer's labeling; however, pharmacokinetics are similar to patients with normal hepatic function.

Severe hepatic impairment: There are no dosage adjustments provided in the manufacturer's labeling; use with caution (has not been studied).

Obesity *ASCO Guidelines for appropriate chemotherapy dosing in obese adults with cancer:* Utilize patient's actual body weight (full weight) for calculation of body surface area- or weight-based dosing, particularly when the intent of therapy is curative; manage regimen-related toxicities in the same manner as for nonobese patients; if a dose reduction is utilized due to toxicity, consider resumption of full weight-based dosing with subsequent cycles, especially if cause of toxicity (eg, hepatic or renal impairment) is resolved (Griggs 2012).

Combination Regimens

Bone sarcoma (Ewing sarcoma): Irinotecan-Temozolomide (Ewing Sarcoma) on page 2161

Primary CNS Lymphoma: Temozolomide-Rituximab (CNS Lymphoma) on page 2212

Administration

Temozolomide is associated with a moderate emetic potential (Dupuis 2011; Roila 2010); antiemetics are recommended to prevent nausea and vomiting.

Oral: Swallow capsules whole with a glass of water. Absorption is affected by food; therefore, administer consistently either with food or without food (was administered in studies under fasting and nonfasting conditions). May administer on an empty stomach and/or at bedtime to reduce nausea and vomiting. Do not repeat dose if vomiting occurs after dose is administered; wait until the next scheduled dose. Do not open or chew capsules; avoid contact with skin or mucous membranes if capsules are accidentally opened or damaged.

IV: Infuse over 90 minutes. Flush line before and after administration. May be administered through the same IV line as sodium chloride 0.9%; do not administer other medications through the same IV line.

Emetic Potential Children and Adults: IV and Oral: Moderate (30% to 90%)

Extemporaneous Preparations A 10 mg/mL temozolomide oral suspension may be compounded in a vertical flow hood. Mix the contents of ten 100 mg capsules and 500 mg of povidone K-30 powder in a glass mortar; add 25 mg anhydrous citric acid dissolved in 1.5 mL purified water and mix to a uniform paste; mix while adding 50 mL Ora-Plus in incremental proportions. Transfer to an amber plastic bottle, rinse mortar 4 times with small portions of either Ora-Sweet or Ora-Sweet SF, and add quantity of Ora-Sweet or Ora-Sweet SF sufficient to make 100 mL. Store in plastic amber prescription bottles; label "shake well" and "refrigerate"; include the beyond-use date. Stable for 7 days at room temperature or 60 days refrigerated (preferred).

Trissel LA, Yanping Z, and Koontz SE, "Temozolomide Stability in Extemporaneously Compounded Oral Suspension," *Int J Pharm Compound*, 2006, 10(5):396-9.

Monitoring Parameters CBC with differential and platelets (prior to each cycle; weekly during glioma concomitant phase treatment; at or within 48 hours of day 22 and weekly until ANC >1,500/mm^3 and platelets >100,000/mm^3 for glioma maintenance and astrocytoma treatment). Monitor liver function tests at baseline, halfway through the first cycle, prior to each subsequent cycle, and at ~2 to 4 weeks after the last dose.

Dietary Considerations The incidence of nausea/vomiting is decreased when taken on an empty stomach. Take capsules consistently either with food or without food (absorption is affected by food).

Dosage Forms Excipient information presented when available (limited, particularly for generics); consult specific product labeling.

Capsule, Oral:

Temodar: 5 mg [contains fd&c blue #2 (indigotine)]

Temodar: 20 mg, 100 mg

Temodar: 140 mg [contains fd&c blue #2 (indigotine)]

Temodar: 180 mg, 250 mg

Generic: 5 mg, 20 mg, 100 mg, 140 mg, 180 mg, 250 mg

Solution Reconstituted, Intravenous:

Temodar: 100 mg (1 ea) [pyrogen free; contains polysorbate 80]

Temsirolimus (tem sir OH li mus)

Related Information

Common Toxicity Criteria *on page 2242*

Management of Chemotherapy-Induced Nausea and Vomiting in Adults *on page 2253*

Prevention of Chemotherapy-Induced Nausea and Vomiting in Children *on page 2310*

Safe Handling of Hazardous Drugs *on page 2379*

Brand Names: US Torisel

Brand Names: Canada Torisel

Index Terms CCI-779

Pharmacologic Category Antineoplastic Agent, mTOR Kinase Inhibitor

Use Renal cell carcinoma, advanced: Treatment of advanced renal cell carcinoma (RCC)

Labeled Contraindications

Bilirubin >1.5 times the upper limit of normal (ULN)

Canadian labeling: Additional contraindications (not in the US labeling): History of anaphylaxis after exposure to temsirolimus, sirolimus, or any component of the formulation

Pregnancy Considerations Adverse events have been observed in animal reproduction studies. Based on its mechanism of action, temsirolimus may cause fetal harm if administered to a pregnant woman. Women of childbearing potential should be advised to avoid pregnancy. Men and women should use effective birth control during temsirolimus treatment, and continue for 3 months after temsirolimus discontinuation.

Breastfeeding Considerations It is not known if temsirolimus is excreted in breast milk. Due to the potential for serious adverse reactions in the nursing infant, a decision should be made to discontinue breastfeeding or to discontinue temsirolimus, taking into account the importance of treatment to the mother.

Warnings/Precautions Hypersensitivity/infusion reactions (eg, anaphylaxis, apnea, dyspnea, flushing, loss of consciousness, hypotension, and/or chest pain) have been reported. Infusion reaction may occur during the initial infusion (early in infusion) or with subsequent infusions. Premedicate with an antihistamine (H_1 antagonist) prior to infusion; monitor throughout infusion (appropriate supportive care should be available); interrupt infusion for hypersensitivity reaction and observe patient for 30-60 minutes. With discretion, treatment may be resumed at a slower infusion rate; administer an H_1 antagonist (if not given as premedication) and/or an IV H_2 antagonist ~30 minutes prior to resuming infusion. For severe infusion reactions, assess risk versus benefit of continued treatment. Use with caution in patients with hypersensitivity temsirolimus, sirolimus (a metabolite), or polysorbate 80. Angioneurotic edema has been reported; concurrent use with other drugs known to cause angioedema (eg, ACE inhibitors) may increase risk.

Temsirolimus is predominantly cleared by the liver; use with caution and reduce dose in patients with mild hepatic impairment (bilirubin >1 to 1.5 x ULN or AST >ULN with bilirubin ≤ULN). Toxicities were increased in patients with baseline bilirubin >1.5 x ULN. Use is contraindicated in patients with moderate-to-severe hepatic impairment (bilirubin >1.5 x ULN).

Potentially significant interactions may exist, requiring dose or frequency adjustment, additional monitoring, and/or selection of alternative therapy.

Avoid concomitant use with strong CYP3A4 inhibitors and strong CYP3A4 inducers; consider alternative agents that avoid or lessen the potential for CYP-mediated interactions. Patients should not be immunized with live, viral vaccines during or shortly after treatment and should avoid close contact with recently vaccinated (live vaccine) individuals. Patients who are receiving anticoagulant therapy or those with CNS tumors/metastases may be at increased risk for developing intracerebral bleeding (may be fatal). Combination therapy with temsirolimus and sunitinib has resulted in dose-limiting toxicities, including grade 3 or 4 rash, gout, and/or cellulitis.

Some dosage forms may contain polysorbate 80 (also known as Tweens). Hypersensitivity reactions, usually a delayed reaction, have been reported following exposure to pharmaceutical products containing polysorbate 80 in certain individuals (Isaksson, 2002; Lucente 2000; Shelley, 1995). Thrombocytopenia, ascites, pulmonary deterioration, and renal and hepatic failure have been reported in premature neonates after receiving parenteral products containing polysorbate 80 (Alade, 1986; CDC, 1984). See manufacturer's labeling.

Increases in serum glucose commonly occur during treatment; initiation or alteration of insulin and/or oral hypoglycemic therapy may be required; monitor serum glucose before and during treatment; use with caution in patients with diabetes. Use with caution in patients with hyperlipidemia; may increase serum lipids (cholesterol and triglycerides); initiation or dosage adjustment of antihyperlipidemic agents may be required; monitor cholesterol/triglyceride panel at baseline and periodically during treatment. Treatment may result in immunosuppression, may increase risk of opportunistic infections and/or sepsis. *Pneumocystis jiroveci* pneumonia (PCP) has been reported; some cases were fatal. Development of PCP may be associated with the use of concomitant corticosteroids or other immunosuppressive agents; consider PCP prophylaxis in patients receiving concomitant immunosuppressive or corticosteroid therapy. Interstitial lung disease (ILD), sometimes fatal, has been reported; symptoms include dyspnea, cough, hypoxia, and/or fever, although asymptomatic or mild cases may present; promptly evaluate worsening respiratory symptoms. If symptoms develop, consider withholding temsirolimus until symptom recovery and radiographic improvement occur. Consider empiric treatment with corticosteroids and/or antibiotic therapy; baseline chest radiographic assessment (CT scan or x-ray) is recommended; follow periodically, even in the absence of clinical pulmonary symptoms. Cases of bowel perforation (fatal) have occurred (usually presenting with abdominal pain, bloody stools, diarrhea, fever, or metabolic acidosis); promptly evaluate any new or worsening abdominal pain or bloody stools. Temsirolimus may be associated with impaired wound healing; use caution in the perioperative period. Cases of acute renal failure with rapid progression have been reported (unrelated to disease progression), including cases unresponsive to dialysis. An increased incidence of rash, infection and dose interruptions have been reported in patients with renal insufficiency (CrCl ≤60 mL/minute) who received mTOR inhibitors for the treatment of renal cell cancer (Gupta, 2011). Elderly patients may be more likely to experience adverse reactions, including diarrhea, edema, and pneumonia.

Adverse Reactions

>10%:

Cardiovascular: Edema (35%), chest pain (16%)

Central nervous system: Pain (28%), headache (15%), insomnia (12%)

◀

Dermatologic: Skin rash (47%), pruritus (19%), nail disease (14%), xeroderma (11%)

Endocrine & metabolic: Increased serum glucose (89%; grades 3/4: 16%), increased serum cholesterol (87%; grades 3/4: 2%), hypertriglyceridemia (83%; grades 3/4: 44%), hypophosphatemia (49%; grades 3/4: 18%), hyperglycemia (26%), hyperlipidemia (≥30%), hypokalemia (21%; grades 3/4: 5%), weight loss (19%)

Gastrointestinal: Mucositis (41%), nausea (37%), anorexia (32%), diarrhea (27%), abdominal pain (21%; grades 3/4: 4%), constipation (20%), dysgeusia (20%), stomatitis (20%), vomiting (19%)

Genitourinary: Urinary tract infection (15%)

Hematologic & oncologic: Decreased hemoglobin (94%; grades 3/4: 20%), lymphocytopenia (53%; grades 3/4: 16%), thrombocytopenia (40%; grades 3/4: 1%; dose-limiting toxicity), decreased white blood cell count (32%; grades 3/4: 1%), anemia (≥30%), decreased neutrophils (19%; grades 3/4: 5%)

Hepatic: Increased serum alkaline phosphatase (68%; grades 3/4: 3%), increased serum AST (38%; grades 3/4: 2%)

Infection: Infection (20%; grades 3/4: 3%; includes abscess, bronchitis, cellulitis, herpes simplex, herpes zoster)

Neuromuscular & skeletal: Weakness (51%), back pain (20%), arthralgia (18%)

Renal: Increased serum creatinine (57%; grades 3/4: 3%)

Respiratory: Dyspnea (28%), cough (26%), epistaxis (12%), pharyngitis (12%)

Miscellaneous: Fever (24%; grades 3/4: 1%)

1% to 10%:

Cardiovascular: Hypertension (7%), venous thromboembolism (2%; includes deep vein thrombosis and pulmonary embolism), pericardial effusion (1%), thrombophlebitis (1%)

Central nervous system: Chills (8%), depression (4%), convulsions (1%)

Dermatologic: Acne vulgaris (10%)

Endocrine & metabolic: Diabetes mellitus (5%)

Gastrointestinal: Gastrointestinal hemorrhage (1%)

Hematologic & oncologic: Rectal hemorrhage (1%)

Hepatic: Hyperbilirubinemia (8%)

Infection: Sepsis (1%), wound infection (1%)

Neuromuscular & skeletal: Myalgia (8%)

Ophthalmic: Conjunctivitis (8%; including lacrimation disorder)

Respiratory: Rhinitis (10%), pneumonia (8%), upper respiratory tract infection (7%), pleural effusion (4%)

Miscellaneous: Wound healing impairment (1%)

<1%, postmarketing, and/or case reports: Acute renal failure, angioedema, causalgia, cholecystitis, cholelithiasis, decreased glucose tolerance, extravasation reactions (with pain, swelling, warmth, erythema), hypersensitivity reaction, interstitial pulmonary disease, intestinal perforation, pancreatitis, pneumonitis, rhabdomyolysis, seizure, Stevens-Johnson syndrome

Drug Interactions

Metabolism/Transport Effects Substrate of CYP3A4 (major), P-glycoprotein; **Note:** Assignment of Major/Minor substrate status based on clinically relevant drug interaction potential

Avoid Concomitant Use

Avoid concomitant use of Temsirolimus with any of the following: BCG (Intravesical); Conivaptan; Deferiprone; Dipyrone; Fusidic Acid (Systemic); Grapefruit Juice; Idelalisib; Itraconazole; Natalizumab; Pimecrolimus; SUNItinib; Tacrolimus (Systemic); Tacrolimus (Topical); Vaccines (Live)

Increased Effect/Toxicity

Temsirolimus may increase the levels/effects of: ACE Inhibitors; CloZAPine; CycloSPORINE (Systemic); Deferiprone; Fingolimod; Leflunomide; Natalizumab; SUNItinib; Tacrolimus (Systemic); Tacrolimus (Topical); Tofacitinib; Vaccines (Live)

The levels/effects of Temsirolimus may be increased by: Aprepitant; Conivaptan; CYP3A4 Inhibitors (Moderate); CYP3A4 Inhibitors (Strong); Dasatinib; Denosumab; Dipyrone; Fluconazole; Fosaprepitant; Fusidic Acid (Systemic); Grapefruit Juice; Idelalisib; Itraconazole; Ketoconazole (Systemic); Macrolide Antibiotics; MiFEPRIStone; Netupitant; Ocrelizumab; Palbociclib; P-glycoprotein/ABCB1 Inhibitors; Pimecrolimus; Posaconazole; Promazine; Protease Inhibitors; Ranolazine; Roflumilast; Simeprevir; Stiripentol; Tacrolimus (Systemic); Tacrolimus (Topical); Trastuzumab

Decreased Effect

Temsirolimus may decrease the levels/effects of: Antidiabetic Agents; BCG (Intravesical); Coccidioides immitis Skin Test; Nivolumab; Sipuleucel-T; Tacrolimus (Systemic); Tertomotide; Vaccines (Inactivated); Vaccines (Live)

The levels/effects of Temsirolimus may be decreased by: Bosentan; CarBAMazepine; CYP3A4 Inducers (Moderate); CYP3A4 Inducers (Strong); Dabrafenib; Deferasirox; Dexamethasone (Systemic); Echinacea; Enzalutamide; Fosphenytoin; Mitotane; Phenytoin; Rifamycin Derivatives; Sarilumab; Siltuximab; St John's Wort; Tocilizumab

Food Interactions Grapefruit and grapefruit juice may increase the levels/effects of sirolimus. Management: Avoid grapefruit and grapefruit juice.

Hazardous Drugs Handling Considerations

Hazardous agent (NIOSH 2016 [group 1]).

Use appropriate precautions for receiving, handling, administration, and disposal. Gloves (single) should be worn during receiving, unpacking, and placing in storage.

NIOSH recommends double gloving, a protective gown, ventilated engineering controls (a class II biological safety cabinet or a compounding aseptic containment isolator), and closed system transfer devices (CSTDs) for preparation. Double gloving, a gown, and (if dosage form allows) CSTDs are required during administration (NIOSH 2016).

Storage/Stability Store intact vials refrigerated at 2°C to 8°C (36°F to 46°F). Diluted solution in the vial (10 mg/mL) is stable for 24 hours at room temperature (below 25°C [77°F]). Solutions diluted for infusion (in NS) must be infused within 6 hours of preparation. Protect from light during storage, preparation, and handling.

Preparation for Administration Preparation requires a two-step dilution process (do not add undiluted temsirolimus to aqueous solution; addition to aqueous solution prior to step 1 will result in precipitation). *Step 1:* Total amount in undiluted vial is 30 mg/1.2 mL (25 mg/mL concentration); contains overfill. Vials should initially be diluted with 1.8 mL of provided diluent to a concentration of 10 mg/mL. Once diluted with provided diluent, mix by inverting vial. *Step 2:* After allowing air bubbles to subside, the intended dose should be withdrawn from the 10 mg/mL diluted vial (ie, 2.5 mL for a 25 mg dose) and further diluted in 250 mL of NS in a non-DEHP/non-PVC container (glass, polyolefin, or polypropylene). Mix by inverting bottle or bag; avoid excessive shaking (may result in foaming).

Mechanism of Action Temsirolimus and its active metabolite, sirolimus, are targeted inhibitors of mTOR (mechanistic target of rapamycin) kinase activity. Temsirolimus (and sirolimus) bind to FKBP-12, an intracellular protein, to form a complex which inhibits mTOR signaling, halting the cell cycle at the G1 phase in tumor cells. Inhibition of mTOR blocks downstream phosphorylation of p70S6k and S6 ribosomal proteins. In renal cell carcinoma, mTOR inhibition also exhibits anti-angiogenesis activity by reducing levels of HIF-1 and HIF-2 alpha (hypoxia inducible factors) and vascular endothelial growth factor (VEGF).

Pharmacodynamics/Kinetics

Distribution: V_{dss}: 172 L

Metabolism: Hepatic; via CYP3A4 to sirolimus (primary active metabolite) and 4 minor metabolites

Half-life elimination: Temsirolimus: ~17 hours; Sirolimus: ~55 hours

Time to peak, plasma: Temsirolimus: At end of infusion; Sirolimus: 0.5 to 2 hours after temsirolimus infusion

Excretion: Feces (78%); urine (<5%)

Dosing

Adult & Geriatric Note: For infusion reaction prophylaxis, premedicate with an H_1 antagonist (eg, diphenhydramine 25 to 50 mg IV) ~30 minutes prior to infusion.

Renal cell cancer (RCC), advanced: IV: 25 mg once weekly; continue until disease progression or unacceptable toxicity

Dosage adjustment for concomitant CYP3A4 inhibitors/inducers:

CYP3A4 inhibitors: Avoid concomitant administration with strong CYP3A4 inhibitors (eg, clarithromycin, itraconazole, ketoconazole, nefazodone, protease inhibitors, telithromycin, voriconazole); if concomitant administration with a strong CYP3A4 inhibitor cannot be avoided, consider a dose reduction to 12.5 mg once weekly. When a strong CYP3A4 inhibitor is discontinued; allow ~1 week to elapse prior to adjusting the temsirolimus upward to the dose used prior to initiation of the CYP3A4 inhibitor.

CYP3A4 inducers: Avoid concomitant administration with strong CYP3A4 inducers (eg, carbamazepine, dexamethasone, phenobarbital, phenytoin, rifabutin, rifampin, St John's wort); if concomitant administration with a strong CYP3A4 inducer cannot be avoided, consider adjusting temsirolimus dose up to 50 mg once weekly. If the strong CYP3A4 enzyme inducer is discontinued, reduce the temsirolimus to the dose used prior to initiation of the CYP3A4 inducer.

Endometrial cancer (locally advanced, recurrent, and/or metastatic) (off-label use): IV: 25 mg once weekly; continue until disease progression or unacceptable toxicity (Oza 2011). Additional trials may be necessary to further define the role of temsirolimus in this condition.

Renal Impairment No dosage adjustment necessary.

Hemodialysis: There are no dosage adjustments provided in the manufacturer's labeling (has not been studied).

Hepatic Impairment

Mild hepatic impairment (bilirubin >1 to 1.5 x ULN or AST >ULN with bilirubin ≤ULN): Reduce dose to 15 mg once weekly.

Moderate-to-severe hepatic impairment (bilirubin >1.5 x ULN): Use is contra-indicated.

Adjustment for Toxicity

Hematologic toxicity: ANC <1000/mm^3 or platelets <75,000/mm^3: Withhold treatment until resolves and reinitiate treatment with the dose reduced by 5 mg weekly; minimum dose: 15 mg weekly if adjustment for toxicity is needed.

Nonhematologic toxicity: Any toxicity ≥ grade 3: Withhold treatment until resolves to ≤ grade 2; reinitiate treatment with the dose reduced by 5 mg weekly; minimum dose: 15 mg weekly if adjustment for toxicity is needed.

Infusion/hypersensitivity reaction: Interrupt infusion and observe for 30 to 60 minutes; treatment may be resumed with discretion at a slower infusion rate (up to 60 minutes); administer an H$_1$ antagonist (if not given as premed-ication) and/or an IV H$_2$ antagonist 30 minutes prior to resuming infusion.

Interstitial lung disease: Consider withholding treatment for clinically signifi-cant respiratory symptoms until after recovery of symptoms or radiographic improvement.

Administration Infuse over 30 to 60 minutes via an infusion pump (preferred). Use polyethylene-lined non-DEHP administration tubing. Administer through an inline polyethersulfone filter ≤5 micron; if set does not contain an inline filter, a polyethersulfone end filter (0.2 to 5 micron) should be added (do not use both an inline and an end filter). Premedicate with an H$_1$ antagonist (eg, diphenhydramine 25 to 50 mg IV) ~30 minutes prior to infusion. Monitor during infusion; interrupt infusion for hypersensitivity/infusion reaction; monitor for 30 to 60 minutes; may reinitiate at a reduced infusion rate (over 60 minutes) with discretion, 30 minutes after administration of a histamine H$_1$ antagonist and/or a histamine H$_2$ antagonist (eg, famotidine or ranitidine). Administration should be completed within 6 hours of admixture.

Emetic Potential

Children: Minimal (<10%)

Adults: Low (10% to 30%)

Monitoring Parameters CBC with differential and platelets (weekly), serum chemistries including glucose (baseline and every other week), serum choles-terol and triglycerides (baseline and periodic), liver function (baseline and periodic), renal function tests (baseline and periodic)

Monitor for infusion reactions; infection; symptoms of ILD (or radiographic changes), symptoms of hyperglycemia (excessive thirst, polyuria); symptoms of bowel perforation

Dietary Considerations Avoid grapefruit juice (may increase the levels of the major metabolite, sirolimus).

Dosage Forms Excipient information presented when available (limited, particularly for generics); consult specific product labeling.

Solution, Intravenous:

Torisel: 25 mg/mL (1 mL) [contains alcohol, usp, polyethylene glycol, poly-sorbate 80, propylene glycol]

Teniposide (ten i POE side)

Related Information

Management of Chemotherapy-Induced Nausea and Vomiting in Adults *on page 2253*

Management of Drug Extravasations *on page 2271*

Prevention of Chemotherapy-Induced Nausea and Vomiting in Children *on page 2310*

Safe Handling of Hazardous Drugs *on page 2379*

Brand Names: Canada Vumon

Index Terms EPT; PTG; VM-26

Pharmacologic Category Antineoplastic Agent, Podophyllotoxin Derivative; Antineoplastic Agent, Topoisomerase II Inhibitor

Use Acute lymphoblastic leukemia, refractory: Treatment of refractory childhood acute lymphoblastic leukemia (ALL) in combination with other chemotherapy

Labeled Contraindications Hypersensitivity to teniposide, polyoxyl 35/poly-oxyethylated castor oil (Cremophor EL), or any component of the formulation

Pregnancy Considerations Adverse effects were observed in animal reproduction studies. May cause fetal harm if administered during pregnancy. Women of childbearing potential should avoid becoming pregnant during teniposide treatment.

Breastfeeding Considerations It is not known if teniposide is excreted in breast milk. Due to the potential for serious adverse reactions in the nursing infant, a decision should be made to discontinue teniposide or to discontinue breastfeeding, taking into account the importance of treatment to the mother.

Warnings/Precautions [US Boxed Warning]: Severe myelosuppression resulting in infection or bleeding may occur; may be dose-limiting; monitor blood counts. Patients with Down syndrome and leukemia may be more sensitive to the myelosuppressive effects; reduced initial doses are recommended. Contains polyoxyl 35/polyoxyethylated castor oil (Cremophor EL), which is associated with hypersensitivity reactions. **[US Boxed Warning]: Hypersensitivity reactions, including anaphylaxis-like reactions, have been reported; may occur with initial dosing or with repeated exposure to teniposide. Epinephrine, with or without corticosteroids and antihistamines, has been employed to alleviate hypersensitivity reaction symptoms.** Hypersensitivity reactions may include bronchospasm, dyspnea, hypertension, hypotension, tachycardia, flushing, chills, fever, or urticaria. Monitor closely during infusion (observe continuously for first 60 minutes, frequently thereafter). Stop infusion for signs of anaphylaxis; immediate treatment for anaphylactic reaction should be available during administration (may require treatment with epinephrine, corticosteroids, antihistamines, pressors, or volume expanders). Patients experiencing prior hypersensitivity are at risk for recurrence; re-treat only if the potential benefit outweighs the risk of hypersensitivity; premedication (with corticosteroids and antihistamines) is recommended for re-treatment. Hypotension may occur with rapid infusion; infuse slowly over at least 30 to 60 minutes; discontinue for clinically significant hypotension; if infusion is restarted after being withheld for hypotension, reinitiate at a slower infusion rate.

Use with caution in patients with renal or hepatic impairment; may require dosage reduction in patients with significant impairment. Teniposide is considered an irritant (Perez Fidalgo, 2012). For IV use only; ensure proper catheter/needle position prior to infusion; monitor infusion site; may cause local tissue necrosis and/or thrombophlebitis if extravasation occurs. Since teniposide is highly bound to plasma proteins, carefully monitor patients with hypoalbuminemia. Product contains about 43% alcohol. Acute CNS depression, hypotension and metabolic acidosis have been reported; these events occurred in patients who received high-dose teniposide (investigation protocol) and were premedicated with antiemetics, which along with the alcohol content of teniposide, may have contributed to the CNS depression. **[US Boxed Warning]: Should be administered under the supervision of an experienced cancer chemotherapy physician. Appropriate management of therapy and complications is possible only when adequate treatment facilities are readily available.** Potentially significant drug-drug interactions may exist, requiring dose or frequency adjustment, additional monitoring, and/or selection of alternative therapy.

Benzyl alcohol and derivatives: Some dosage forms may contain benzyl alcohol; large amounts of benzyl alcohol (≥99 mg/kg/day) have been associated with a potentially fatal toxicity ("gasping syndrome") in neonates; the "gasping syndrome" consists of metabolic acidosis, respiratory distress, gasping respirations, CNS dysfunction (including convulsions, intracranial hemorrhage), hypotension, and cardiovascular collapse (AAP ["Inactive" 1997]; CDC, 1982); some data suggests that benzoate displaces bilirubin from protein binding sites (Ahlfors, 2001); avoid or use dosage forms containing benzyl alcohol with caution in neonates. See manufacturer's labeling.

N,N-dimethylacetamide: Teniposide contains N,N-dimethylacetamide, which is incompatible with many closed system transfer devices (CSTDs); the plastic components of CSTDs may dissolve and result in subsequent leakage and potential infusion of dissolved plastic into the patient (ISMP [Smetzer 2015]).

Adverse Reactions

>10%:

Gastrointestinal: Mucositis (76%), diarrhea (33%), nausea and vomiting (29%; mild to moderate)

Hematologic & oncologic: Neutropenia (95%), leukopenia (89%), anemia (88%), thrombocytopenia (85%), bone marrow depression (75%)

Infection: Infection (12%)

1% to 10%:

Cardiovascular: Hypotension (2%; may be intractable; associated with rapid [<30 minutes] infusions)

Dermatologic: Alopecia (9%; usually reversible), skin rash (3%)

Hematologic & oncologic: Hemorrhage (5%)

Hypersensitivity: Hypersensitivity reaction (5%; includes bronchospasm, chills, dyspnea, fever, flushing, hypertension, hypotension, tachycardia, or urticaria)

Miscellaneous: Fever (3%)

<1%, postmarketing, and/or case reports: Cardiac arrhythmia, central nervous system depression, confusion, fluid and electrolyte disturbance, headache, hepatic insufficiency, metabolic acidosis, neuropathy (severe), neurotoxicity, renal insufficiency, thrombophlebitis, weakness

Drug Interactions

Metabolism/Transport Effects Substrate of CYP3A4 (major), P-glycoprotein; **Note:** Assignment of Major/Minor substrate status based on clinically relevant drug interaction potential; **Inhibits** CYP2C9 (weak)

◀ **Avoid Concomitant Use**

Avoid concomitant use of Teniposide with any of the following: BCG (Intravesical); Conivaptan; Deferiprone; Dipyrone; Fusidic Acid (Systemic); Idelalisib; Natalizumab; Pimecrolimus; Tacrolimus (Topical); Vaccines (Live)

Increased Effect/Toxicity

Teniposide may increase the levels/effects of: CloZAPine; Deferiprone; Fingolimod; Leflunomide; Natalizumab; Tofacitinib; Vaccines (Live); VinCRIStine; VinCRIStine (Liposomal)

The levels/effects of Teniposide may be increased by: Aprepitant; Conivaptan; CYP3A4 Inhibitors (Moderate); CYP3A4 Inhibitors (Strong); Dasatinib; Denosumab; Dipyrone; Fosaprepitant; Fusidic Acid (Systemic); Idelalisib; MiFEPRIStone; Netupitant; Ocrelizumab; Palbociclib; Palifermin; P-glycoprotein/ABCB1 Inhibitors; Pimecrolimus; Promazine; Ranolazine; Roflumilast; Simeprevir; Stiripentol; Tacrolimus (Topical); Trastuzumab

Decreased Effect

Teniposide may decrease the levels/effects of: BCG (Intravesical); Coccidioides immitis Skin Test; Lenograstim; Nivolumab; Sipuleucel-T; Tertomotide; Vaccines (Inactivated); Vaccines (Live)

The levels/effects of Teniposide may be decreased by: Barbiturates; Bosentan; CYP3A4 Inducers (Moderate); CYP3A4 Inducers (Strong); Dabrafenib; Deferasirox; Echinacea; Enzalutamide; Fosphenytoin; Mitotane; Phenytoin; Sarilumab; Siltuximab; St John's Wort; Tocilizumab

Hazardous Drugs Handling Considerations

Hazardous agent (NIOSH 2016 [group 1]).

Use appropriate precautions for receiving, handling, administration, and disposal. Gloves (single) should be worn during receiving, unpacking, and placing in storage.

NIOSH recommends double gloving, a protective gown, ventilated engineering controls (a class II biological safety cabinet or a compounding aseptic containment isolator), and (if compatible) closed system transfer devices (CSTDs) for preparation. Double gloving, a gown, and (if compatible and dosage form allows) CSTDs are required during administration (NIOSH 2016).

Storage/Stability Store ampuls in refrigerator at 2°C to 8°C (36°F to 46°F). Protect from light. Solutions diluted for infusion in D5W or NS to a concentration of 0.1, 0.2, or 0.4 mg/mL are stable at room temperature for up to 24 hours after preparation; solutions diluted to 1 mg/mL should be used within 4 hours of preparation. Because precipitation may occur at any concentration, the manufacturer recommends administrating as soon as possible after preparation. Use appropriate precautions for handling and disposal. Do not refrigerate solutions prepared for infusion.

Preparation for Administration Precipitation may occur at any concentration. Teniposide must be diluted with either D5W or NS solutions to a final concentration of 0.1, 0.2, 0.4, or 1 mg/mL. **Solutions should be prepared in non-DEHP-containing containers such as glass or polyolefin containers.** The use of polyvinyl chloride (PVC) containers is not recommended. Because precipitation may occur at any concentration, the manufacturer recommends administrating as soon as possible after preparation. Teniposide contains N,N-dimethylacetamide, which is incompatible with many closed system transfer devices (CSTDs); the plastic components of CSTDs may dissolve and result in subsequent leakage and potential infusion of dissolved plastic into the patient (ISMP [Smetzer 2015]).

Mechanism of Action Teniposide does not inhibit microtubular assembly; it has been shown to delay transit of cells through the S phase and arrest cells in late S or early G_2 phase, preventing cells from entering mitosis. Teniposide is a topoisomerase II inhibitor, and appears to cause DNA strand breaks by inhibition of strand-passing and DNA ligase action.

Pharmacodynamics/Kinetics

Distribution: V_{dss}: Children: 3 to 11 L/m^2; Adults: 8 to 44 L/m^2; mainly into liver, kidneys, small intestine, and adrenals; limited distribution into CSF <1%

Protein binding: >99%; primarily albumin

Metabolism: Extensively hepatic

Half-life elimination: Children: 5 hours

Excretion: Urine (44%, 4% to 12% as unchanged drug); feces (≤10%)

Clearance: Renal: 10% of total body clearance

Dosing

Adult Note: Patients with Down syndrome and leukemia may be more sensitive to the myelosuppressive effects; administer the first course at half the usual dose and adjust dose in subsequent cycles upward based on degree of toxicities (myelosuppression and mucositis) in the previous course(s).

Acute lymphoblastic leukemia (ALL) consolidation treatment (off-label use; combination chemotherapy): IV: 165 mg/m^2/dose days 1, 4, 8, and 11 of alternating consolidation cycles (Linker, 1991)

Pediatric Note: Patients with Down syndrome and leukemia may be more sensitive to the myelosuppressive effects; administer the first course at half the usual dose and adjust dose in subsequent cycles upward based on degree of toxicities (myelosuppression and mucositis) in the previous course(s).

Acute lymphoblastic leukemia (ALL), refractory (combination chemotherapy): IV: 165 mg/m^2 twice weekly for 8 to 9 doses (in combination with cytarabine) **or** 250 mg/m^2 weekly for 4 to 8 weeks (in combination with vincristine and prednisone)

Renal Impairment There are no specific dosage adjustments provided in the manufacturer's labeling (has not been studied). However, dosage adjustment may be necessary in patients with significant renal impairment.

Hepatic Impairment There are no specific dosage adjustments provided in the manufacturer's labeling (has not been studied). However, dosage adjustment may be necessary in patients with significant hepatic impairment.

Combination Regimens

Leukemia, acute lymphocytic: Linker Protocol (ALL) on page 2167

Administration IV; must be administered slowly (over at least 30-60 minutes); do not administer by rapid IV injection. Administer through non-DEHP-containing administration sets. Incompatible with heparin; flush infusion line with D5W or NS before and after infusion. Precipitation may occur at any concentration; administer as soon as possible after preparation; inspect solution prior to administration. Observe patient continuously for at least the first 60 minutes after the start of the infusion, observe frequently thereafter. Stop infusion for signs of anaphylaxis (may require treatment with epinephrine, corticosteroids, antihistamines, pressors, or volume expanders); discontinue for clinically significant hypotension during infusion; if infusion is restarted after being withheld for hypotension, reinitiate at a slower infusion rate.

◀   Teniposide contains N, N-dimethylacetamide, which is incompatible with many closed system transfer devices (CSTDs); the plastic components of CSTDs may dissolve and result in subsequent leakage and potential infusion of dissolved plastic into the patient (ISMP [Smetzer 2015]).

Vesicant/Extravasation Risk Irritant

Emetic Potential Children: Low (10% to 30%)

Monitoring Parameters CBC with differential and platelet count, renal and hepatic function tests; blood pressure; monitor for hypersensitivity reaction (observe continuously for first 60 minutes of infusion, frequently thereafter)

Dosage Forms Considerations Injectable solution may contain alcohol, benzyl alcohol, or polyoxyl 35/polyoxyethylated castor oil (Cremophor EL)

Dosage Forms Excipient information presented when available (limited, particularly for generics); consult specific product labeling.

Solution, Intravenous:

  Generic: 10 mg/mL (5 mL)

- **Teva-Valacyclovir (Can)** *see* ValACYclovir *on page* 1852
- **Teva-Voriconazole (Can)** *see* Voriconazole *on page* 1925
- **TG** *see* Thioguanine *on page* 1774
- **6-TG (error-prone abbreviation)** *see* Thioguanine *on page* 1774

Thalidomide (tha LI doe mide)

Related Information

Chemotherapy-Induced Peripheral Neuropathy *on page* 2236

Common Toxicity Criteria *on page* 2242

Hematopoietic Cell Transplantation *on page* 2365

Management of Chemotherapy-Induced Nausea and Vomiting in Adults *on page* 2253

Prevention of Chemotherapy-Induced Nausea and Vomiting in Children *on page* 2310

Safe Handling of Hazardous Drugs *on page* 2379

Brand Names: US Thalomid

Brand Names: Canada Thalomid

Pharmacologic Category Angiogenesis Inhibitor; Antineoplastic Agent; Immunomodulator, Systemic

Use

Erythema nodosum leprosum: Acute treatment of cutaneous manifestations of moderate to severe erythema nodosum leprosum; maintenance treatment for prevention and suppression of cutaneous manifestations of erythema nodosum leprosum recurrence

Limitation of use: Thalidomide is not indicated as monotherapy for erythema nodosum leprosum treatment in the presence of moderate to severe neuritis.

Multiple myeloma: Treatment of newly diagnosed multiple myeloma (in combination with dexamethasone)

Labeled Contraindications

Hypersensitivity to thalidomide or any component of the formulation; pregnancy

Canadian labeling: Additional contraindications (not in the US labeling): Hypersensitivity to lenalidomide or pomalidomide; females at risk of becoming pregnant and male patients who are unable to follow or comply with conditions for use (refer to manufacturer labeling); breastfeeding

Pregnancy Considerations [US Boxed Warning]: Thalidomide is contraindicated in pregnant women. Thalidomide may cause severe birth defects or embryo-fetal death if taken during pregnancy. Thalidomide cannot be used in women who are pregnant or may become pregnant during therapy as even a single dose may cause severe birth defects. In order to decrease the risk of fetal exposure, thalidomide is available only through a special restricted distribution program (Thalomid REMS). Reproduction studies in animals and data from pregnant women have shown evidence of fetal abnormalities; use is contraindicated in women who are or may become pregnant. Anomalies observed in humans include amelia, phocomelia, bone defects, ear and eye abnormalities, facial palsy, congenital heart defects, urinary and genital tract malformations; mortality in ~40% of infants at or shortly after birth has also been reported.

Women of reproductive potential must avoid pregnancy beginning 4 weeks prior to therapy, during therapy, during therapy interruptions, and for at least 4 weeks after therapy is discontinued. Two forms of effective/reliable contraception or total abstinence from heterosexual intercourse must be used by females who are not infertile or who have not had a hysterectomy. A negative pregnancy test (sensitivity of at least 50 milliunits/mL) 10 to 14 days prior to therapy, within 24 hours prior to beginning therapy, weekly during the first 4 weeks, and every 4 weeks (every 2 weeks for women with irregular menstrual cycles) thereafter is required for women of childbearing potential. Thalidomide must be immediately discontinued for a missed period, abnormal pregnancy test or abnormal menstrual bleeding; refer patient to a reproductive toxicity specialist if pregnancy occurs during treatment.

Females of reproductive potential (including health care workers and care-givers) must also avoid contact with thalidomide capsules.

Thalidomide is also present in the semen of males. Males (even those vasectomized) must use a latex or synthetic condom during any sexual contact with women of childbearing potential and for up to 28 days following discontinuation of therapy. Males taking thalidomide must not donate sperm.

The parent or legal guardian for patients between 12 to 18 years of age must agree to ensure compliance with the required guidelines.

A pregnancy exposure registry has been created to monitor outcomes in females exposed to thalidomide during pregnancy and female partners of male patients and to understand the root cause for the pregnancy. The pregnancy exposure registry may be contacted at 1-888-423-5436. If pregnancy occurs during treatment, thalidomide must be immediately discontinued and the patient referred to a reproductive toxicity specialist. Any suspected fetal exposure to thalidomide must be reported to the FDA via the MedWatch program (1-800-FDA-1088) and to Celgene Corporation (1-888-423-5436).

Breastfeeding Considerations It is not known if thalidomide is present in breast milk. Due to the potential for serious adverse reactions in the breastfed infant, breastfeeding is not recommended by the manufacturer.

Warnings/Precautions [US Boxed Warning]: Thalidomide use for the treatment of multiple myeloma is associated with an increased risk for venous thromboembolism (VTE), including deep vein thrombosis (DVT) and pulmonary embolism (PE); the risk is increased when used in combination with standard chemotherapy agents, including dexamethasone. In one controlled study, the incidence of VTE was 22.5% in patients receiving thalidomide in combination with dexamethasone, compared to 4.9% for dexamethasone alone. Monitor for signs and symptoms of thromboembolism (shortness of breath, chest pain, or arm or leg swelling) and instruct patients to seek prompt medical attention with development of these symptoms. Consider thromboprophylaxis based on risk factors. Ischemic heart disease, including MI and stroke, also occurred at a higher rate (compared to placebo) in myeloma patients receiving thalidomide plus dexamethasone who had not received prior treatment. Assess individual risk factors for thromboembolism and consider thromboprophylaxis. The American Society of Clinical Oncology guidelines for VTE prophylaxis and treatment recommend thromboprophylaxis for patients receiving thalidomide in combination with chemotherapy and/or dexamethasone; either aspirin or low molecular weight heparin (LMWH) are recommended for lower risk patient and LMWH is recommended for higher risk patients (Lyman 2013). Anticoagulant prophylaxis should be individualized and selected based on the venous thromboembolism risk of the combination treatment regimen, using the safest and easiest to administer (Palumbo 2008). Monitor for signs/symptoms of thromboembolism and advise patients to seek immediate care if symptoms (shortness of breath, chest pain, arm/leg swelling) develop. Other medications that are also associated with thromboembolism should be used with caution. In a scientific statement from the American Heart Association, thalidomide has been determined to be an agent that may exacerbate underlying myocardial dysfunction (magnitude: minor) (AHA [Page 2016]).

May cause leukopenia and neutropenia; avoid initiating therapy if ANC <750/mm^3. Persistent neutropenia may require treatment interruption. Thrombocytopenia (including grades 3 and 4) has been reported; may require dose reduction, treatment delay, or discontinuation. Monitor for signs and symptoms of bleeding (including petechiae, epistaxis, and gastrointestinal bleeding), especially if concomitant medication may increase the risk of bleeding. Monitor CBC with differential and platelets. Anemia has also been observed. May cause bradycardia; use with caution when administering concomitantly with medications that may also decrease heart rate. May require thalidomide dose reduction or discontinuation. Stevens-Johnson syndrome (SJS) and toxic epidermal necrolysis (TEN) have been reported (may be fatal); withhold therapy and evaluate if skin rash occurs; permanently discontinue if rash is exfoliative, purpuric, bullous or if SJS or TEN is suspected. Hypersensitivity, including erythematous macular rash, possibly associated with fever, tachycardia and hypotension has been reported. May require treatment interruption for severe reactions; discontinue if recurs with rechallenge. Abnormal liver function tests, hepatitis and cholestatic jaundice have been reported. Hepatotoxicity (including hepatocellular and cholestatic injury) has been observed rarely (case reports), with a mean time to development of 46 days; most events resolved after discontinuing thalidomide (Vilas-Boas 2012).

Increased incidence of second primary malignancies (SPMs), including acute myeloid leukemia (AML) and myelodysplastic syndrome (MDS), has been observed in previously untreated multiple myeloma patients receiving thalidomide in combination with melphalan, and prednisone. In addition to AML and MDS, solid tumors have been reported with thalidomide maintenance treatment for multiple myeloma (Usmani 2012). Carefully evaluate patients for SPMs prior to and during treatment and manage as clinically indicated.

Thalidomide is commonly associated with peripheral neuropathy; may be irreversible. Neuropathy generally occurs following chronic use (over months), but may occur with short-term use; onset may be delayed. Use caution with other medications that may also cause peripheral neuropathy. Monitor for signs/symptoms of neuropathy monthly for the first 3 months of therapy and regularly thereafter. Electrophysiological testing may be considered at baseline and every 6 months to detect asymptomatic neuropathy. To limit further damage, immediately discontinue (if clinically appropriate) in patients who develop neuropathy. Reinitiate therapy only if neuropathy returns to baseline; may require dosage reduction or permanent discontinuation. Seizures (including grand mal convulsions) have been reported in postmarketing data; monitor closely for clinical changes indicating potential seizure activity in patients with a history of seizures, concurrent therapy with drugs that alter seizure threshold, or conditions that predispose to seizures. May cause dizziness, drowsiness, and/or somnolence; caution patients about performing tasks that require

◀ mental alertness (eg, operating machinery or driving). Avoid ethanol and concomitant medications that may exacerbate these symptoms; dose reductions may be necessary for excessive drowsiness or somnolence. May cause orthostatic hypotension; use with caution in patients who would not tolerate transient hypotensive episodes. When arising from a recumbent position, advise patients to sit upright for a few minutes prior to standing. Constipation may commonly occur. May require treatment interruption or dosage reduction. Certain adverse reactions (constipation, fatigue, weakness, nausea, hypokalemia, hyperglycemia, DVT, pulmonary embolism, atrial fibrillation) are more likely in elderly patients. In studies conducted prior to the use of antiretroviral therapy, thalidomide use was associated with increased viral loads in HIV infected patients. Monitor viral load after the 1st and 3rd months of therapy and every 3 months thereafter. Patients with a high tumor burden may be at risk for tumor lysis syndrome; monitor closely; institute appropriate management for hyperuricemia.

Potentially significant drug-drug interactions may exist, requiring dose or frequency adjustment, additional monitoring, and/or selection of alternative therapy. Patients should not donate blood during thalidomide treatment and for 4 weeks after therapy discontinuation.

[US Boxed Warning]: Thalidomide is contraindicated in pregnant women. Thalidomide may cause severe birth defects or embryo-fetal death if taken during pregnancy. Thalidomide cannot be used in women who are pregnant or may become pregnant during therapy as even a single dose may cause severe birth defects. In order to decrease the risk of fetal exposure, thalidomide is available only through a special restricted distribution program (Thalomid REMS). Use is also contraindicated in women who may become pregnant. Pregnancy must be excluded prior to therapy initiation with 2 negative pregnancy tests. Women of reproductive potential must avoid pregnancy beginning 4 weeks prior to therapy, during therapy, during therapy interruptions, and for ≥4 weeks after therapy is discontinued; two reliable methods of birth control, or abstinence from heterosexual intercourse, must be used. Males taking thalidomide (even those vasectomized) must use a latex or synthetic condom during any sexual contact with women of childbearing potential and for up to 28 days following discontinuation of therapy. Males taking thalidomide must not donate sperm. Some forms of contraception may not be appropriate in certain patients. An intrauterine device (IUD) or implantable contraceptive may increase the risk of infection or bleeding; estrogen containing products may increase the risk of thromboembolism.

Due to the embryo-fetal risk, thalidomide is only available through a restricted program under the Thalomid REMS program. Prescribers and pharmacies must be certified with the program to prescribe or dispense thalidomide. Patients must sign an agreement and comply with the REMS program requirements.

Adverse Reactions

>10%:

Cardiovascular: Edema (57%), embolism (≤23%), thrombosis (≤23%), hypotension (16%)

Central nervous system: Fatigue (79%), neuropathy (8%; sensory: 54%; motor: 22%), myasthenia (40%), drowsiness (36% to 38%), dizziness (4% to 20%), confusion (28%), agitation (≤26%), anxiety (≤26%), headache (13% to 19%), paresthesia (6% to 16%)

Dermatologic: Desquamation (≤30%), skin rash (≤30%), xeroderma (21%), maculopapular rash (4% to 19%), diaphoresis (13%), acne vulgaris (3% to 11%)

Endocrine & metabolic: Hypocalcemia (72%), weight loss (23%), weight gain (22%)

Gastrointestinal: Constipation (3% to 55%), nausea (4% to 28%), anorexia (3% to 28%), diarrhea (4% to 19%), oral candidiasis (4% to 11%)

Genitourinary: Hematuria (11%)

Hematologic & oncologic: Leukopenia (17% to 35%), neutropenia (31%), anemia (13%), lymphadenopathy (13%)

Hepatic: Increased serum AST (3% to 25%), increased serum bilirubin (14%)

Neuromuscular & skeletal: Tremor (4% to 26%), weakness (6% to 22%), myalgia (17%), arthralgia (13%)

Respiratory: Dyspnea (42%)

Miscellaneous: Fever (19% to 23%)

1% to 10%:
Cardiovascular: Peripheral edema (3% to 8%), facial edema (4%)

Central nervous system: Insomnia (9%), nervousness (3% to 9%), malaise (8%), vertigo (8%), pain (3% to 8%)

Dermatologic: Fungal dermatitis (4% to 9%), pruritus (3% to 8%), nail disease (3% to 4%)

Endocrine & metabolic: Hyperlipidemia (6% to 9%), albuminuria (3% to 8%)

Gastrointestinal: Xerostomia (8% to 9%), flatulence (8%), toothache (4%)

Genitourinary: Impotence (3% to 8%)

Hepatic: Abnormal hepatic function tests (9%)

Infection: Infection (6% to 8%)

Neuromuscular & skeletal: Back pain (4% to 6%), neck pain (4%), neck stiffness (4%)

Respiratory: Pharyngitis (4% to 8%), sinusitis (3% to 8%), rhinitis (4%)

<1%, postmarketing, and/or case reports: Acute renal failure, amenorrhea, angioedema, aphthous stomatitis, atrial fibrillation, biliary obstruction, bradycardia, cardiac arrhythmia, carpal tunnel syndrome, cerebrovascular accident, change in prothrombin time, chronic myelocytic leukemia, deafness, decreased creatinine clearance, depression, diplopia, dysesthesia, ECG abnormality, eosinophilia, epistaxis, erythema multiforme, erythema nodosum, erythroleukemia, exfoliative dermatitis, febrile neutropenia, footdrop, galactorrhea, gastric ulcer, granulocytopenia, gynecomastia, hangover effect, hearing loss, hepatomegaly, Hodgkin's lymphoma, hypercalcemia, hyperkalemia, hypersensitivity reaction, hypertension, hyperthyroidism, hyperuricemia, hypokalemia, hypomagnesemia, hyponatremia, hypoproteinemia, hypothyroidism, increased blood urea nitrogen, increased lactate dehydrogenase, increased serum alkaline phosphatase, increased serum ALT, increased serum creatinine, intestinal obstruction, intestinal perforation, interstitial pneumonitis, interstitial pulmonary disease, lethargy, leukocytosis, loss of consciousness, lymphedema, lymphocytopenia, mental status changes, metastases (AML, MDS, solid tumors), migraine, myocardial infarction, myxedema, nystagmus, oliguria, orthostatic hypotension, pancytopenia, petechia, peripheral neuritis, pleural effusion, psychosis, pulmonary embolism, pulmonary hypertension, purpura, Raynaud's phenomenon, renal failure, seizure, sepsis, septic shock, sexual disorder, sick sinus syndrome, skin photosensitivity, status epilepticus, Stevens-Johnson syndrome, stupor, syncope, tachycardia, thrombocytopenia, toxic epidermal necrolysis, transient ischemic attacks, tumor lysis syndrome, urinary incontinence, urticaria,

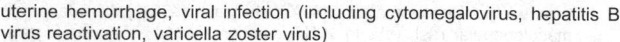

uterine hemorrhage, viral infection (including cytomegalovirus, hepatitis B virus reactivation, varicella zoster virus)

Drug Interactions

Metabolism/Transport Effects None known.

Avoid Concomitant Use

Avoid concomitant use of Thalidomide with any of the following: Abatacept; Anakinra; Azelastine (Nasal); BCG (Intravesical); Canakinumab; Certolizumab Pegol; CNS Depressants; Deferiprone; Dipyrone; Natalizumab; Orphenadrine; Oxomemazine; Paraldehyde; Pimecrolimus; Rilonacept; Tacrolimus (Topical); Tocilizumab; Tofacitinib; Vaccines (Live); Vedolizumab

Increased Effect/Toxicity

Thalidomide may increase the levels/effects of: Abatacept; Amifostine; Anakinra; Azelastine (Nasal); Bisphosphonate Derivatives; Canakinumab; Certolizumab Pegol; Deferiprone; DULoxetine; Fingolimod; Hypotension-Associated Agents; Leflunomide; Levodopa; MetyroSINE; Natalizumab; Nitroprusside; Orphenadrine; Pamidronate; Paraldehyde; Piribedil; Pramipexole; Rilonacept; ROPINIRole; Rotigotine; Selective Serotonin Reuptake Inhibitors; Tofacitinib; Vaccines (Live); Vedolizumab; Zoledronic Acid

The levels/effects of Thalidomide may be increased by: Alfuzosin; Blood Pressure Lowering Agents; Brimonidine (Topical); Cannabis; Chlorphenesin Carbamate; CNS Depressants; Contraceptives (Estrogens); Contraceptives (Progestins); Denosumab; Dexamethasone (Systemic); Diazoxide; Dimethindene (Topical); Dipyrone; Dronabinol; Erythropoiesis-Stimulating Agents; Estrogen Derivatives; Herbs (Hypotensive Properties); Kava Kava; Lofexidine; Magnesium Sulfate; Minocycline; Molsidomine; Nabilone; Naftopidil; Nicergoline; Nicorandil; Obinutuzumab; Ocrelizumab; Oxomemazine; Pentoxifylline; Phosphodiesterase 5 Inhibitors; Pimecrolimus; Prostacyclin Analogues; Quinagolide; Roflumilast; Rufinamide; Tacrolimus (Topical); Tetrahydrocannabinol; Tocilizumab; Trastuzumab

Decreased Effect

Thalidomide may decrease the levels/effects of: BCG (Intravesical); Coccidioides immitis Skin Test; Nivolumab; Sipuleucel-T; Tertomotide; Vaccines (Inactivated); Vaccines (Live)

The levels/effects of Thalidomide may be decreased by: Echinacea

Hazardous Drugs Handling Considerations

Hazardous agent (NIOSH 2016 [group 2]).

Use appropriate precautions for receiving, handling, administration, and disposal. Gloves (single) should be worn during receiving, unpacking, and placing in storage.

NIOSH recommends single gloving for administration of intact tablets or capsules. If manipulating tablets/capsules (eg, to prepare an oral suspension), NIOSH recommends double gloving, a protective gown, and preparation in a controlled device; if not prepared in a controlled device, respiratory and eye/face protection as well as ventilated engineering controls are recommended. NIOSH recommends double gloving, a protective gown, and (if there is a potential for vomit or spit up) eye/face protection for administration of an oral liquid/feeding tube administration (NIOSH 2016).

Storage/Stability Store at 20°C to 25°C (68°F to 77°F); excursions are permitted between 15°C and 30°C (59°F and 86°F). Protect from light. Keep in original package.

Mechanism of Action Immunomodulatory and antiangiogenic characteristics; immunologic effects may vary based on conditions; may suppress excessive tumor necrosis factor-alpha production in patients with ENL, yet may increase plasma tumor necrosis factor-alpha levels in HIV-positive patients. In multiple myeloma, thalidomide is associated with an increase in natural killer cells and increased levels of interleukin-2 and interferon gamma. Other proposed mechanisms of action include suppression of angiogenesis, prevention of free-radical-mediated DNA damage, increased cell mediated cytotoxic effects, and altered expression of cellular adhesion molecules.

Pharmacodynamics/Kinetics

Absorption: Slow, good

Distribution: V_d: 1.1 L/kg

Protein binding: 55% to 66%

Metabolism: Minimal (unchanged drug is the predominant circulating component)

Half-life elimination: 5.5 to 7.3 hours

Time to peak, plasma: ~2 to 5 hours

Excretion: Urine (~92%; <4% of the dose as unchanged drug); feces (<2%)

Dosing

Adult

Erythema nodosum leprosum, acute cutaneous: Oral: Initial: 100 to 300 mg once daily at bedtime, continue until signs/symptoms subside (usually ~2 weeks), then taper off in 50 mg decrements every 2 to 4 weeks. For severe cases with moderate to severe neuritis, corticosteroids may be initiated with thalidomide (taper off and discontinue corticosteroids when neuritis improves).

Patients weighing <50 kg: Initiate at lower end of the dosing range

Severe cutaneous reaction or patients previously requiring high doses: May be initiated at up to 400 mg once daily at bedtime or in divided doses

Erythema nodosum leprosum, maintenance (prevention/suppression, or with flares during tapering attempts): Oral: Maintain on the minimum dosage necessary to control the reaction; efforts to taper off should be attempted every 3 to 6 months, in decrements of 50 mg every 2 to 4 weeks.

Multiple myeloma, newly diagnosed: Oral: 200 mg once daily at bedtime (in combination with dexamethasone)

Multiple myeloma (off-label dosing or combinations):

In combination with bortezomib and dexamethasone (off-label combination): Induction therapy: 100 mg once daily for the first 14 days, then 200 mg once daily for 3 (21-day) cycles (Cavo 2010) **or** 100 mg once daily for up to 8 (21-day) cycles (Kaufman 2010)

In combination with melphalan and prednisone (off-label combination): 200 to 400 mg once daily (Facon 2007) **or** 100 mg once daily (Palumbo 2008) **or** 50 to 100 mg once daily, depending on patient tolerance (Hulin 2009)

Multiple myeloma, maintenance (following autologous stem cell transplant; off-label use): Oral: 200 mg once daily starting 3 to 6 months after transplant; continue until disease progression or unacceptable toxicity (Brinker 2006) **or** 100 mg once daily starting 42 to 60 days following transplant; increase to 200 mg once daily after 2 weeks if tolerated; continue for up to 12 months (in combination with prednisolone) (Spencer 2009)

Multiple myeloma, salvage therapy: Initial: 200 mg once daily at bedtime; may increase daily dose by 200 mg every 2 weeks (if tolerated) to a maximum of 800 mg once daily at bedtime (Singhal, 1999) **or** 100 mg once daily (in combination with dexamethasone) (Palumbo 2001) **or** 200 mg once daily (in combination with bortezomib and dexamethasone) for 1 year (Garderet 2012) **or** 400 mg once daily at bedtime (in combination with dexamethasone, cisplatin, doxorubicin, cyclophosphamide and etoposide) (Lee 2003)

AIDS-related aphthous stomatitis (off-label use): Oral: 200 mg once daily at bedtime for up to 8 weeks, if no response, then 200 mg twice daily for 4 weeks (Jacobson, 1997)

Chronic graft-versus-host disease (refractory), treatment (off-label second-line use; optimum dose not determined): Oral: Initial: 100 mg once daily at bedtime, with dose escalation up to 400 mg daily in 3 to 4 divided doses (Wolff 2010) **or** Initial: 50 to 100 mg 3 times daily; maximum dose: 600 to 1,200 mg daily (Kulkarni 2003) **or** 200 mg 4 times daily (dose adjusted to goal thalidomide concentration of ≥5 mcg/mL 2 hours postdose) (Vogelsang, 1992) **or** 100 to 300 mg 4 times daily (Parker, 1995)

Systemic light chain amyloidosis (off-label use): Oral: 200 mg once daily (starting dose 50 to 100 mg once daily; titrate at 4-week intervals) in combination with cyclophosphamide and dexamethasone (Wechalekar 2007)

Uremic pruritus, refractory (off-label use): Oral: 100 mg once daily at bedtime (Silva 1994). Additional data is necessary to further define the role of thalidomide in this condition; several other treatment modalities with more benign safety profiles are available.

Waldenström macroglobulinemia (off-label use): Oral: ≤200 mg once daily for up to 52 weeks (in combination with rituximab) (Treon 2008)

Geriatric Refer to adult dosing. A reduced initial dose may be appropriate (depending on patient tolerance) in patients ≥75 years (Hulin 2009).

Pediatric

Erythema nodosum leprosum, acute cutaneous: Children ≥12 years: Oral: Refer to adult dosing.

Erythema nodosum leprosum, maintenance (prevention/suppression, or with flares during tapering attempts): Children ≥12 years: Oral: Refer to adult dosing.

Chronic graft-versus-host disease (refractory), treatment (off-label second-line use; limited data): Children ≥3 years: Oral: 3 mg/kg 4 times daily (dose adjusted to goal thalidomide concentration of ≥5 mcg/mL 2 hours postdose) (Vogelsang 1992) **or** Initial: 3 to 6 mg/kg/day in 2 to 4 divided doses; target dose 12 mg/kg/day; Maximum daily dose: 800 mg (Rovelli, 1998)

Renal Impairment No dosage adjustment necessary for patients with renal impairment and on dialysis (per manufacturer). In a study of 6 patients with end-stage renal disease on dialysis, although clearance was increased by dialysis, a supplemental dose was not needed (Eriksson 2003).

Multiple myeloma: An evaluation of 29 newly diagnosed myeloma patients with renal failure (serum creatinine ≥2 mg/dL) treated with thalidomide and dexamethasone (some also received cyclophosphamide) found that toxicities and efficacy were similar to patients with normal renal function (Seol 2010). A study evaluating induction therapy with thalidomide and dexamethasone in 31 newly diagnosed myeloma patients with renal failure (CrCl <50 mL/minute), including 16 patients with severe renal impairment (CrCl

<30 mL/minute) and 7 patients on chronic hemodialysis found that toxicities were similar to patients without renal impairment and that thalidomide and dexamethasone could be administered safely (Tosi 2009). The International Myeloma Working Group (IMWG) suggests that thalidomide may be safely administered to patients with renal impairment, including those on dialysis (Dimopoulos 2016). The IMWG recommends the use of the Chronic Kidney Disease Epidemiology Collaboration (CKD-EPI) equation (preferred) or the Modification of Diet in Renal Disease (MDRD) formula to evaluate renal function estimation in multiple myeloma patients with a stable serum creatinine.

Hepatic Impairment There are no dosage adjustments provided in the manufacturer's labeling (has not been studied). However, thalidomide does not appear to undergo significant hepatic metabolism.

Adjustment for Toxicity

ANC ≤750/mm³: Withhold treatment if clinically appropriate

Grade 3 or 4 adverse reactions: Consider dose reduction, delay or discontinuation (based on clinical judgment).

Multiple myeloma:

Constipation, oversedation: Temporarily withhold or continue with a reduced dose

Peripheral neuropathy:

The manufacturer recommends to temporarily withhold or continue with a reduced dose.

The follow adjustments have also been recommended (Richardson 2012):

Grade 1: Reduce dose by 50%

Grade 2: Temporarily interrupt therapy; once resolved to ≤ grade 1, resume therapy with a 50% dosage reduction (if clinically appropriate)

Grade 3 or higher: Discontinue therapy

Combination Regimens

Multiple myeloma:

Bortezomib-Thalidomide-Dexamethasone (Multiple Myeloma) on page 2000

DTPACE (Multiple Myeloma) on page 2098

Melphalan-Prednisone-Thalidomide (Multiple Myeloma) on page 2172

Thalidomide-Dexamethasone (MM) on page 2212

VDT-PACE (Multiple Myeloma) on page 2229

Administration

Administer orally, preferably at bedtime once daily, at least 1 hour after the evening meal. Doses >400 mg/day may be given in divided doses at least 1 hour after meals. Swallow capsules whole with water. Capsules should not be opened or crushed.

Capsules should remain in blister pack until ingestion. If exposed to the powder content from broken capsules or body fluids from patients receiving thalidomide, the exposed area should be washed immediately and thoroughly with soap and water.

Missed doses: For missed doses, if <12 hours patient may receive dose; if >12 hours wait until next dose due.

Emetic Potential

Children: Minimal (<10%)

Adults: Low (10% to 30%)

◀ **Extemporaneous Preparations** A 20 mg/mL oral suspension may be prepared with capsules and a 1:1 mixture of Ora-Sweet and Ora-Plus. Empty the contents of twelve 100 mg capsules into a glass mortar. Add small portions of the vehicle and mix to a uniform paste; mix while adding the vehicle in incremental proportions to almost 60 mL; transfer to an amber calibrated bottle, rinse mortar with vehicle, and add quantity of vehicle sufficient to make 60 mL. Label "shake well," "protect from light," and "refrigerate". Stable for 35 days refrigerated.

Kraft S, Johnson CE, and Tyler RP, "Stability of an Extemporaneously Prepared Thalidomide Suspension," *Am J Health Syst Pharm*, 2011, 69(1):56-8.

Monitoring Parameters CBC with differential, platelets; thyroid function tests (TSH at baseline then every 2 to 3 months during thalidomide treatment [Hamnvik 2011]). Hepatic function tests (periodic; particularly with preexisting hepatic dysfunction or concomitant use of drugs associated with hepatotoxicity). In HIV-seropositive patients: viral load after 1 and 3 months, then every 3 months. Pregnancy testing (sensitivity of at least 50 milliunits/mL) is required 10 to 14 days prior to therapy, within 24 hours prior to initiation of therapy, weekly during the first 4 weeks, then every 4 weeks in women with regular menstrual cycles or every 2 weeks in women with irregular menstrual cycles. Signs of neuropathy monthly for the first 3 months, then periodically during treatment; consider monitoring of sensory nerve application potential amplitudes (at baseline and every 6 months) to detect asymptomatic neuropathy. Monitor for signs and symptoms of thromboembolism (shortness of breath, chest pain, arm/leg swelling), tumor lysis syndrome, bradycardia and syncope; monitor for clinical changes indicating potential seizure activity (in patients with a history of seizure).

Prescribing and Access Restrictions Canada: Access to thalidomide is restricted through a controlled distribution program called RevAid. Only physicians and pharmacists enrolled in this program are authorized to prescribe or dispense thalidomide. Patients must be enrolled in the program by their physicians. Further information is available at www.RevAid.ca or by calling 1-888-738-2431.

Medication Guide Available Yes

Dosage Forms Excipient information presented when available (limited, particularly for generics); consult specific product labeling.

Capsule, Oral:

Thalomid: 50 mg, 100 mg

Thalomid: 150 mg, 200 mg [contains fd&c blue #2 (indigotine)]

◆ **Thalomid** see Thalidomide on page 1765

◆ **THC** see Dronabinol on page 647

◆ **TheraCys** see BCG (Intravesical) on page 219

Thioguanine (thye oh GWAH neen)

Related Information

Management of Chemotherapy-Induced Nausea and Vomiting in Adults on page 2253

Prevention of Chemotherapy-Induced Nausea and Vomiting in Children on page 2310

Safe Handling of Hazardous Drugs on page 2379

Brand Names: US Tabloid

Brand Names: Canada Lanvis

Index Terms 2-Amino-6-Mercaptopurine; 6-TG (error-prone abbreviation); 6-Thioguanine (error-prone abbreviation); TG; Tioguanine

Pharmacologic Category Antineoplastic Agent, Antimetabolite; Antineoplastic Agent, Antimetabolite (Purine Analog)

Use

Acute myeloid leukemia: Treatment (remission induction and consolidation) of acute myeloid (nonlymphocytic) leukemia (AML)

Limitations of use: The use of thioguanine for AML maintenance therapy or other similar long-term continuous treatments is not recommended due to the high risk of hepatotoxicity.

Labeled Contraindications Prior resistance to thioguanine (or mercaptopurine)

Canadian labeling: Additional contraindications (not in US labeling): Hypersensitivity to thioguanine or any component of the formulation

Pregnancy Considerations Adverse effects have been observed in animal reproduction studies. May cause fetal harm if administered during pregnancy. Women of childbearing potential should avoid becoming pregnant during treatment.

Breastfeeding Considerations Due to the potential for serious adverse reactions in the nursing infant, the manufacturer recommends a decision be made to discontinue thioguanine or to discontinue breastfeeding during treatment, taking into account the importance of treatment to the mother.

Warnings/Precautions Not recommended for maintenance therapy or long-term continuous treatment; long-term continuous therapy or maintenance treatment is associated with a high risk for hepatotoxicity, hepatic sinusoidal obstruction syndrome (SOS; formerly called veno-occlusive disease), or portal hypertension; monitor liver function carefully for liver toxicity and discontinue in patients with evidence of hepatotoxicity, hepatic SOS (eg, hyperbilirubinemia, hepatomegaly [tender], and weight gain due to ascites and fluid retention) or portal hypertension (eg, splenomegaly, thrombocytopenia, esophageal varices); hepatotoxicity with or without transaminase elevations may occur; pathologic findings of hepatotoxicity include hepatoportal sclerosis, idiopathic noncirrhotic portal hypertension (including nodular regenerative hyperplasia), peliosis hepatitis, and periportal fibrosis. Hepatotoxicity may be more prevalent in male patients. Advise patients to avoid alcohol; may increase the risk for hepatotoxicity.

Myelosuppression (anemia, leukopenia, and/or thrombocytopenia) is a common dose-related toxicity (may be delayed); monitor for infection (due to leukopenia) or bleeding (due to thrombocytopenia); withhold treatment with abnormally significant drop in blood counts. Patients with genetic enzyme deficiency of thiopurine methyltransferase (TPMT) or who are receiving drugs which inhibit this enzyme (mesalazine, olsalazine, sulfasalazine) may be highly sensitive to myelosuppressive effects and may require substantial dose reductions.

Hyperuricemia occurs commonly with treatment; institute adequate hydration and prophylactic allopurinol. Thioguanine is potentially carcinogenic. Cross resistance with mercaptopurine generally occurs. Avoid vaccination with live vaccines during treatment. Potentially significant drug-drug interactions may exist, requiring dose or frequency adjustment, additional monitoring, and/or selection of alternative therapy.

Adverse Reactions Frequency not defined.

Cardiovascular: Esophageal varices, hepatic sinusoidal obstruction syndrome (formerly known as hepatic veno-occlusive disease), portal hypertension

Endocrine & metabolic: Fluid retention, hyperuricemia (common), weight gain

Gastrointestinal: Anorexia, intestinal necrosis, intestinal perforation, nausea, stomatitis, vomiting

Hematologic & oncologic: Anemia (may be delayed), bone marrow hypoplasia, granulocytopenia, hemorrhage, leukopenia (common; may be delayed), pancytopenia, splenomegaly, thrombocytopenia (common; may be delayed)

Hepatic: Ascites, hepatic necrosis (centrilobular), hepatitis, hepatomegaly (tender), hepatotoxicity, hyperbilirubinemia, increased liver enzymes, jaundice

Infection: Infection

Drug Interactions

Metabolism/Transport Effects None known.

Avoid Concomitant Use

Avoid concomitant use of Thioguanine with any of the following: BCG (Intravesical); Deferiprone; Dipyrone; Natalizumab; Pimecrolimus; Tacrolimus (Topical); Vaccines (Live)

Increased Effect/Toxicity

Thioguanine may increase the levels/effects of: CloZAPine; Deferiprone; Fingolimod; Leflunomide; Natalizumab; Tofacitinib; Vaccines (Live)

The levels/effects of Thioguanine may be increased by: 5-ASA Derivatives; Denosumab; Dipyrone; Ocrelizumab; Palifermin; Pimecrolimus; Promazine; Roflumilast; Tacrolimus (Topical); Trastuzumab

Decreased Effect

Thioguanine may decrease the levels/effects of: BCG (Intravesical); Coccidioides immitis Skin Test; Lenograstim; Nivolumab; Sipuleucel-T; Tertomotide; Vaccines (Inactivated); Vaccines (Live)

The levels/effects of Thioguanine may be decreased by: Echinacea

Hazardous Drugs Handling Considerations

Hazardous agent (NIOSH 2016 [group 1]).

Use appropriate precautions for receiving, handling, administration, and disposal. Gloves (single) should be worn during receiving, unpacking, and placing in storage.

NIOSH recommends single gloving for administration of intact tablets or capsules. If manipulating tablets/capsules (eg, to prepare an oral suspension), NIOSH recommends double gloving, a protective gown, and preparation in a controlled device; if not prepared in a controlled device, respiratory and eye/face protection as well as ventilated engineering controls are recommended. NIOSH recommends double gloving, a protective gown, and (if there is a potential for vomit or spit up) eye/face protection for administration of an oral liquid/feeding tube administration (NIOSH 2016).

Storage/Stability Store at 15°C to 25°C (59°F to 77°F). Protect from moisture.

Mechanism of Action Purine analog that is incorporated into DNA and RNA resulting in the blockage of synthesis and metabolism of purine nucleotides

Pharmacodynamics/Kinetics

Absorption: ~30% (range: 14% to 46%; highly variable)

Distribution: Does not reach therapeutic concentrations in the CSF

Metabolism: Hepatic; rapidly and extensively via thiopurine methyltransferase (TPMT) to 2-amino-6-methylthioguanine (MTG; active) and inactive compounds

Half-life elimination: Terminal: 5 to 9 hours

Time to peak, serum: Within 8 hours; predominantly metabolite(s)

Excretion: Urine, primarily as metabolites

Dosing

Adult

Acute myeloid leukemia (AML): Oral: 2 mg/kg once daily for 4 weeks; if no clinical improvement after 4 weeks and ANC and platelet counts are not depressed, may increase dose to 3 mg/kg once daily with careful monitoring.

Acute lymphoblastic leukemia (ALL) (off-label use): Oral: Late intensification treatment phase: 60 mg/m^2 once daily on days 29 to 42 (in combination with doxorubicin, vincristine, dexamethasone, cyclophosphamide and cytarabine) (Larson 1995; Larson 1998)

Pediatric

Acute myeloid leukemia (AML): Oral: 2 mg/kg once daily for 4 weeks; if no clinical improvement after 4 weeks and ANC and platelet counts are not depressed, may increase dose to 3 mg/kg once daily with careful monitoring.

Acute lymphoblastic leukemia (ALL) (off-label use): Oral:

Children ≥1 year and Adolescents: Delayed Intensification treatment phase: 60 mg/m^2/day for 14 days on days 28 to 41 (in combination with vincristine, dexamethasone, doxorubicin, cyclophosphamide, cytarabine, asparaginase, and methotrexate) (Lange 2002; Nachman 1998)

Adolescents ≥15 years: Late intensification treatment phase: 60 mg/m^2 once daily on days 29 to 42 (in combination with doxorubicin, vincristine, dexamethasone, cyclophosphamide, and cytarabine) (Larson 1995; Larson 1998)

Renal Impairment

Adults: There are no dosage adjustments provided in the manufacturer's labeling.

Children: No dosage adjustment required (Aronoff 2007).

Hepatic Impairment

Hepatic impairment prior to treatment: There are no dosage adjustments provided in the manufacturer's labeling.

Hepatotoxicity during treatment: Deterioration in transaminases, alkaline phosphatase or bilirubin, toxic hepatitis, biliary stasis, clinical jaundice, evidence of hepatic sinusoidal obstruction syndrome (veno-occlusive disease), or evidence of portal hypertension: Discontinue treatment.

Combination Regimens

Leukemia, acute lymphocytic:

CALGB 8811 Regimen (ALL) on page 2003

CALGB 9111 Regimen (ALL) on page 2004

Administration Administer orally; total daily dose can be given at one time.

Emetic Potential Children and Adults: Minimal (<10%)

Extemporaneous Preparations 20 mg/mL (ASHP Standard Concentration) (ASHP 2017)

A 20 mg/mL oral suspension may be prepared in a vertical flow hood with tablets and Ora-Plus and Ora-Sweet **or** methylcellulose 1% and simple syrup (Aliabadi 2011).

Ora-Plus and Ora-Sweet: Crush fifteen 40 mg thioguanine tablets in a mortar and reduce to a fine powder. Add 5 mL of Ora-Plus in incremental proportions and mix to a uniform paste. Transfer to a graduated amber glass bottle, rinse mortar with Ora-Sweet and add sufficient quantity to make 30 mL. Label "shake well." Stable for 63 days at room temperature.

Methylcellulose and simple syrup: Crush fifteen 40 mg thioguanine tablets in a mortar and reduce to a fine powder. Add 3.33 mL of methylcellulose 1% in incremental proportions and mix to a uniform paste. Transfer to a graduated amber glass bottle, rinse mortar with simple syrup and add sufficient quantity to make 30 mL. Label "shake well." Stable for 63 days at room temperature.
Aliabadi HM, Romanick M, Somayaji V, Mahdipoor P, Lavasanifar A. Stability of compounded thioguanine oral suspensions [published correction appears in *Am J Health Syst Pharm.* 2011;68 (14):1278.]. *Am J Health Syst Pharm.* 2011;68(10):900-908.

Monitoring Parameters CBC with differential and platelet count (frequently); liver function tests (weekly when beginning therapy then monthly, more frequently in patients with liver disease or concurrent hepatotoxic drugs); serum uric acid; some laboratories offer testing for TPMT deficiency

Monitor for signs/symptoms of hepatotoxicity, portal hypertension (splenomegaly, esophageal varices, thrombocytopenia), or sinusoidal obstruction syndrome (veno-occlusive disease; fluid retention, ascites, hepatomegaly with tenderness, or hyperbilirubinemia); monitor for tumor lysis syndrome

Dosage Forms Excipient information presented when available (limited, particularly for generics); consult specific product labeling.
Tablet, Oral:
Tabloid: 40 mg

◆ **6-Thioguanine (error-prone abbreviation)** *see* Thioguanine *on page 1774*

◆ **Thiophosphoramide** *see* Thiotepa *on page 1778*

◆ **Thioplex** *see* Thiotepa *on page 1778*

◆ **Thiosulfuric Acid Disodium Salt** *see* Sodium Thiosulfate *on page 1678*

Thiotepa (thye oh TEP a)

Related Information
Common Toxicity Criteria *on page 2242*
Management of Chemotherapy-Induced Nausea and Vomiting in Adults *on page 2253*
Management of Drug Extravasations *on page 2271*
Prevention of Chemotherapy-Induced Nausea and Vomiting in Children *on page 2310*
Safe Handling of Hazardous Drugs *on page 2379*

Brand Names: US Tepadina

Index Terms TESPA; Thiophosphoramide; Thioplex; Triethylenethiophosphoramide; TSPA

Pharmacologic Category Antineoplastic Agent, Alkylating Agent

Use Beta-thalassemia, class 3: To reduce the risk of graft rejection when used in conjunction with high-dose busulfan and cyclophosphamide as a preparative regimen for allogeneic hematopoietic progenitor (stem) cell transplantation in pediatric patients with class 3 beta-thalassemia.

Labeled Contraindications Known hypersensitivity (allergy) to thiotepa or any component of the formulation; concomitant use with live or attenuated vaccines (Tepadina)

Pregnancy Considerations Adverse events were observed in animal reproduction studies. Based on the mechanism of action, thiotepa may cause fetal harm if used in pregnant women. Verify pregnancy status in women of reproductive potential prior to therapy initiation. Effective contraception should be used during treatment and for at least 6 months after the final dose. Males with female partners of reproductive potential should use effective contraception during therapy and for at least 1 year after the final dose. Both male and female fertility may be affected by thiotepa administration.

Breastfeeding Considerations It is not known if thiotepa is present in breast milk. Due to the potential for serious adverse reactions in the breastfeeding infant, breastfeeding is not recommended by the manufacturer.

Warnings/Precautions Myelosuppression (leukopenia, thrombocytopenia, and anemia) may commonly occur, particularly when used as part of the preparative regimen for hematopoietic stem cell transplantation (HSCT) or in patients with compromised bone marrow function. Do not initiate the HSCT conditioning regimen if a stem cell donor is not available. Monitor blood counts closely. Monitor for infection or bleeding; death due to septicemia and hemorrhage has occurred. Myelosuppression (including fatal cases) has also been reported with intravesicular administration (due to systemic absorption). Fatal encephalopathy has been reported in patients receiving high-dose thiotepa. Headache, apathy, psychomotor retardation, disorientation, confusion, amnesia, hallucinations, drowsiness, somnolence, seizures, coma, inappropriate behavior, and forgetfulness have also been reported (may be dose dependent). If severe or life-threatening central nervous system toxicity occurs, discontinue treatment and manage as necessary. CNS toxicity, including seizures and intracranial hemorrhage was reported in pediatric patients who receive the recommended dose in combination with busulfan and cyclophosphamide as a stem cell conditioning regimen for beta thalassemia; do not exceed the recommended dose.

In patients receiving high-dose thiotepa, the parent drug and/or its active metabolites may be partially excreted through the skin. Thiotepa may cause skin discoloration, pruritus, blistering, desquamation, and peeling (may be more severe in skin folds, groin, axillae, and neck areas, and under dressings). Change occlusive dressing and clean covered skin at least twice daily during and for 48 hours after thiotepa administration (when used as a component of the HSCT preparative regimen). Patients should shower/bathe in water twice daily through 48 hours after receiving thiotepa. Change bed sheets daily. Accidental thiotepa exposure is also associated with skin reactions; wash skin thoroughly with soap and water and flush mucous membranes if skin and/or mucous membrane contact occurs.

Thiotepa may be carcinogenic; myelodysplastic syndrome and acute myeloid leukemia (AML) have been reported. There is an increased risk of secondary malignancies with thiotepa use. Hepatic sinusoidal obstruction syndrome (SOS, also called veno-occlusive disease [VOD]) may occur in patients receiving thiotepa in combination with busulfan and cyclophosphamide as a preparative regimen prior to HSCT. Monitor serum transaminases, bilirubin and for signs/symptoms of hepatic SOS through day +28 of stem cell transplant; provide supportive care if SOS develops. Use with caution in patients with hepatic impairment; thiotepa is extensively hepatically metabolized; moderate (bilirubin >1.5 to 3 times ULN and any AST) or severe (bilirubin >3 times ULN and any AST) impairment may result in increased plasma concentrations and increased toxicity. Use with caution in patients with renal impairment; decreased renal excretion may result in increased thiotepa and TEPA plasma concentrations and increased toxicity. Monitor closely. In children, thiotepa is associated with a high emetic potential at doses ≥300 mg/m² (Dupuis 2011) and is associated with a moderate emetic potential (depending on dose/indication) in adults (Roila 2016); antiemetics are recommended to prevent nausea and vomiting. Thiotepa is also associated with mucositis.

When used for intrathecal administration (off-label route), should not be prepared during the preparation of any other agents; after preparation, keep intrathecal medications in an isolated location or container clearly marked with a label identifying as "intrathecal" use only; delivery of intrathecal medications to the patient should only be with other medications also intended for administration into the central nervous system (Jacobson 2009). Potentially significant drug-drug interactions may exist, requiring dose or frequency adjustment, additional monitoring, and/or selection of alternative therapy. Do not administer live or attenuated viral or bacterial vaccines until the immunosuppressive effects of thiotepa have resolved.

Adverse Reactions Frequency not defined.

Central nervous system: Chills, dizziness, fatigue, headache

Dermatologic: Alopecia, contact dermatitis, dermatitis, skin depigmentation (with topical treatment), skin rash, urticaria

Endocrine & metabolic: Amenorrhea

Gastrointestinal: Abdominal pain, anorexia, nausea, vomiting

Genitourinary: Dysuria, hematuria, inhibition of spermatogenesis, urinary retention

Hematologic & oncologic: Anemia, hemorrhage, leukopenia, thrombocytopenia

Hypersensitivity: Anaphylactic shock, hypersensitivity reaction

Infection: Infection

Local: Pain at injection site

Neuromuscular & skeletal: Weakness

Ophthalmic: Blurred vision, conjunctivitis

Respiratory: Asthma, epistaxis, laryngeal edema, wheezing

Miscellaneous: Fever

<1%, postmarketing, and/or case reports: Acute myelocytic leukemia (AML), cystitis (chemical; bladder instillation), hemorrhagic cystitis (bladder instillation), myelodysplastic syndrome

Drug Interactions

Metabolism/Transport Effects None known.

Avoid Concomitant Use

Avoid concomitant use of Thiotepa with any of the following: BCG (Intravesical); Deferiprone; Dipyrone; Natalizumab; Pimecrolimus; Tacrolimus (Topical); Vaccines (Live)

Increased Effect/Toxicity

Thiotepa may increase the levels/effects of: CloZAPine; CYP2B6 Substrates; Deferiprone; Fingolimod; Leflunomide; Natalizumab; Tofacitinib; Vaccines (Live)

The levels/effects of Thiotepa may be increased by: Denosumab; Dipyrone; Ocrelizumab; Palifermin; Pimecrolimus; Promazine; Roflumilast; Tacrolimus (Topical); Trastuzumab

Decreased Effect

Thiotepa may decrease the levels/effects of: BCG (Intravesical); Coccidioides immitis Skin Test; Lenograstim; Nivolumab; Sipuleucel-T; Tertomotide; Vaccines (Inactivated); Vaccines (Live)

The levels/effects of Thiotepa may be decreased by: Echinacea

Hazardous Drugs Handling Considerations

Hazardous agent (NIOSH 2016 [group 1]).

Use appropriate precautions for receiving, handling, administration, and disposal. Gloves (single) should be worn during receiving, unpacking, and placing in storage.

NIOSH recommends double gloving, a protective gown, ventilated engineering controls (a class II biological safety cabinet or a compounding aseptic containment isolator), and closed system transfer devices (CSTDs) for preparation. Double gloving, a gown, and (if dosage form allows) CSTDs are required during administration (NIOSH 2016).

Storage/Stability

Tepadina: Store intact vials at 2°C to 8°C (36°F to 46°F). Protect from light; do not freeze. Reconstituted solution (10 mg/mL) is stable for 8 hours when stored at 2°C to 8°C (36°F to 46°F). Solution further diluted for infusion in NS is stable for 24 hours when stored at 2°C to 8°C (36°F to 46°F), or for 4 hours when stored at 25°C (77°F).

Generic product labeling: Store intact vials at 2°C to 8°C (36°F to 46°F). Protect from light. Reconstituted solutions (10 mg/mL) are stable for up to 8 hours when stored under refrigeration. Solutions further diluted for infusion in NS should be used immediately.

Intrathecal thiotepa (off-label use/route): After preparation, keep intrathecal medications in an isolated location or container clearly marked with a label identifying as "intrathecal" use only.

Preparation for Administration

Tepadina: Reconstitute each 15 mg vial with 1.5 mL SWFI, or each 100 mg vial with 10 mL SWFI, to a concentration of 10 mg/mL. Gently mix by repeated inversions. Solution may be clear or opalescent; do not use if particulate matter is present. Further dilute reconstituted solution for IV infusion in 500 mL NS (1,000 mL NS if dose >500 mg). If dose is <250 mg, dilute in an appropriate volume of NS to achieve a final concentration of 0.5 to 1 mg/mL.

Generic product labeling: Reconstitute each 15 mg vial with 1.5 mL SWFI to a concentration of ~10 mg/mL. Solutions for IV use should be further diluted in NS injection prior to infusion. Filter through a 0.22 micron filter (polysulfone membrane [eg, Sterile Aerodisc] or triton-free cellulose mixed ester [eg, Millex-GS]) prior to administration; do not use solutions which precipitate or remain opaque after filtering. Solutions for intravesicular administration should be diluted in 30 to 60 mL NS.

Intrathecal administration (off-label use/route): Dilute to a concentration of 1 mg/mL in preservative-free buffered solution (Grossman 1993). Intrathecal medications should not be prepared during the preparation of any other agents.

Mechanism of Action Thiotepa is an alkylating agent which produces cross-linking of DNA strands leading to inhibition of DNA, RNA, and protein synthesis; thiotepa is cell-cycle independent (Perry 2012)

◀ **Pharmacodynamics/Kinetics**

Distribution: V_{dss}: 0.3 to 1.6 L/kg; penetrates into CSF (Maanen 2000); the mean volume of distribution following a single IV dose in pediatric patients receiving a 5 mg/kg dose was 1.2 L/kg or 30 L/m^2

Protein binding: ~10% to 20%

Metabolism: Extensively hepatic via cytochrome P450 system, primarily to the major (active) metabolite TEPA (Maanen 2000; Perry 2012)

Half-life elimination: Terminal:

Pediatrics (5 mg/kg IV dose): Thiotepa: 1.7 hours; TEPA: 4 hours

Adults (20 mg to 250 mg/m^2 IV dose): Thiotepa: 1.4 to 3.7 hours; TEPA: 4.9 to 17.6 hours

Excretion: Urine (<2% of thiotepa dose; <11% of TEPA)

Dosing

Adult & Geriatric Note: Thiotepa is associated with a moderate emetic potential in adults (depending on dose/indication); antiemetics may be recommended to prevent nausea and vomiting (Roila 2016). Although included in the manufacturer's labeling as approved uses, other contemporary therapies have replaced the use of thiotepa for the treatment of papillary bladder, ovarian, and breast cancers, as well as malignant intracavitary effusions.

Hematopoietic stem cell transplant (HSCT) for CNS malignancy (off-label use): IV: 250 mg/m^2/day for 3 days beginning 9 days prior to transplant (in combination with busulfan and cyclophosphamide) (Soussain 2008) **or** 150 mg/m^2/dose every 12 hours for 6 doses, followed by stem cell reinfusion 96 hours after completion of thiotepa (Abrey 2006)

Leptomeningeal metastases (off-label use/route): Intrathecal: 10 mg twice a week (on days 1 and 4 each week) for 8 weeks (Grossman 1993)

Pediatric Note: In children, thiotepa is associated with a high emetic potential at doses ≥300 mg/m^2; antiemetics are recommended to prevent nausea and vomiting (Dupuis 2011).

Beta-thalassemia, class 3 (Tepadina): Infants, Children, and Adolescents: IV: 5 mg/kg every 12 hours for 2 doses on the sixth day prior to allogeneic hematopoietic stem cell transplantation (in combination with high-dose busulfan and cyclophosphamide)

Hematopoietic stem cell transplant (HSCT) for CNS malignancy (off-label use): IV: 300 mg/m^2/day for 3 days beginning 8 days prior to transplant (in combination with topotecan and carboplatin) (Gilheeney 2010) **or** 300 mg/m^2/day for 3 days beginning 5 days prior to transplant (in combination with carboplatin and etoposide) (Dunkel 2010; Grodman 2009)

Renal Impairment

There are no dosage adjustments provided in the manufacturer's labeling. Use with caution; decreased renal excretion may result in increased thiotepa and TEPA plasma concentrations and increased toxicity. Monitor patients with moderate (CrCl 30 to 59 mL/minute) to severe (CrCl <30 mL/minute) impairment for toxicity.

Hemodialysis: Thiotepa is dialyzable.

Hepatic Impairment There are no dosage adjustments provided in the manufacturer's labeling. Use with caution; thiotepa is extensively hepatically metabolized. Moderate (bilirubin >1.5 to 3 times ULN and any AST) or severe (bilirubin >3 times ULN and any AST) impairment may result in increased plasma concentrations and increased toxicity. Monitor closely.

Obesity

American Society for Blood and Marrow Transplantation (ASBMT) practice guideline committee position statement on chemotherapy dosing in obesity: Utilize actual body weight (full weight) for calculation of body surface area in thiotepa dosing for hematopoietic stem cell transplant conditioning regimens in adult patients weighing ≤120% of their ideal body weight (IBW). In patients weighing >120% IBW, utilize adjusted body weight 40% (ABW40) to calculate BSA (Bubalo 2014).

ABW40: Adjusted wt (kg) = Ideal body weight (kg) + 0.4 [actual wt (kg) - ideal body weight (kg)]

Adjustment for Toxicity

Central nervous system toxicity, severe or life-threatening: Discontinue thiotepa and provide supportive care.

Hypersensitivity reactions (eg, anaphylaxis or other clinically significant reaction): Discontinue thiotepa and manage as appropriate; monitor until signs/symptoms resolve.

Administration

In children, thiotepa is associated with a high emetic potential at doses ≥300 mg/m² (Dupuis 2011) and is associated with a moderate emetic potential (depending on dose/indication) in adults (Roila 2016); antiemetics may be recommended to prevent nausea and vomiting.

IV: Administer over 3 hours via a central line (when administering as part of the preparative regimen for hematopoietic stem cell transplantation in class 3 beta-thalassemia). Infusion times may vary by protocol or dose for off-label uses; refer to specific protocols. Filtering does not alter thiotepa potency. *Tepadina:* Administer using a 0.2 micron in-line filter; flush line prior to and after infusion with ~5 mL NS.

Intrathecal route (off-label use/route): Was administered in 10 mL (preserva-tive free) buffered solutions (Grossman 1993)

Vesicant/Extravasation Risk May be an irritant

Emetic Potential

Children:

≥300 mg/m²: High (>90%)

<300 mg/m²: Low (10% to 30%)

Adults: Moderate (30% to 90%)

Monitoring Parameters CBC with differential and platelet count frequently throughout therapy; renal and liver function tests; signs/symptoms of hyper-sensitivity reactions, dermatologic toxicity, hepatic sinusoidal obstruction syndrome, and CNS toxicity

Dosage Forms Excipient information presented when available (limited, particularly for generics); consult specific product labeling.

Solution Reconstituted, Injection:

Tepadina: 15 mg (1 ea); 100 mg (1 ea)

Solution Reconstituted, Injection [preservative free]:

Generic: 15 mg (1 ea)

- ◆ **Thorazine** *see* ChlorproMAZINE *on page 388*
- ◆ **Three-Factor PCC** *see* Factor IX Complex (Human) [(Factors II, IX, X)] *on page 767*
- ◆ **Thrombate III** *see* Antithrombin *on page 152*
- ◆ **Thrombate III® (Can)** *see* Antithrombin *on page 152*
- ◆ **Thymocyte Stimulating Factor** *see* Aldesleukin *on page 71*

♦ **Thymoglobulin** *see* Antithymocyte Globulin (Rabbit) *on page 159*
♦ **Thyrogen** *see* Thyrotropin Alfa *on page 1784*

Thyrotropin Alfa (thye roe TROH pin AL fa)

Brand Names: US Thyrogen
Brand Names: Canada Thyrogen
Index Terms Human Thyroid Stimulating Hormone; Recombinant Human Thyrotropin; Rh-TSH; Thyrotropin Alpha; TSH
Pharmacologic Category Diagnostic Agent
Use

Diagnostic imaging: Adjunctive diagnostic tool for serum thyroglobulin (Tg) testing (with or without radioiodine imaging) in follow up of patients with well-differentiated thyroid cancer who have previously undergone thyroidectomy. Limitations of use: Thyrotropin alfa-stimulated Tg levels are generally lower than and do not correlate with Tg levels after thyroid hormone withdrawal; even when thyrotropin alfa-stimulated Tg testing is performed in combination with radioiodine imaging, there is a risk of missing a thyroid cancer diagnosis or of underestimating disease extent; anti-Tg antibodies may confound Tg assay and render Tg levels uninterpretable, in such cases, even with a negative or low-stage thyrotropin alfa radioiodine scan, consider further patient evaluation.

Thyroid tissue remnant ablation: Adjunctive treatment for radioiodine ablation of thyroid tissue remnants after total or near-total thyroidectomy in patients with well-differentiated thyroid cancer without evidence of metastatic disease
Limitations of use: The effect of thyrotropin alfa on long-term thyroid cancer outcomes has not been determined. Due to relatively small clinical experience, it is not possible to conclude if long-term thyroid cancer outcomes would be equivalent after thyrotropin alfa use or withholding thyroid hormone for TSH elevation prior to remnant ablation.

Labeled Contraindications
U.S. labeling: There are no contraindications listed in the manufacturer's labeling.
Canadian labeling: Hypersensitivity to thyrotropin alfa or any component of the formulation.

Pregnancy Considerations Animal reproduction studies have not been conducted. Effects on the fetus or pregnant woman are unknown.

Breastfeeding Considerations It is not known if thyrotropin alfa is excreted in breast milk. The manufacturer recommends that caution be exercised when administering thyrotropin alfa to nursing women.

Warnings/Precautions Thyrotropin alfa use may cause a transient (over 7 to 14 days) and significant rise in serum thyroid hormone concentration in patients with substantial *in situ* thyroid tissue or with functional thyroid cancer metastases. Thyrotropin alfa-induced hyperthyroidism may result in serious complications in patients with certain risk factors (heart disease, extensive metastatic disease or with underlying serious illness); consider hospitalization for administration and subsequent observation. Deaths within 24 hours of thyrotropin alfa administration have been reported. Elderly patients with residual thyroid disease and patients with a known history of heart disease in the presence of significant residual thyroid tissue are at increased risk for thyrotropin alfa-induced hyperthyroidism.

Postmarketing reports of stroke or symptoms suggestive of stroke (eg, unilateral weakness) have occurred within 3 days of administration in patients without known central nervous system metastases. A majority of these patients had risk factors for stroke (eg, smokers or history of migraine) or were young women taking oral contraceptives. Patients should be well hydrated prior to administration. Sudden, rapid, and painful growth of residual thyroid tissue or distant metastases may occur following thyrotropin alfa administration. Symptoms are associated with tissue location and include acute hemiplegia, hemiparesis, and vision loss 1 to 3 days after administration. Laryngeal edema, pain at site of distant metastases, and respiratory distress requiring tracheotomy have also been reported. Consider glucocorticoid premedication in patients where local tumor enlargement may compromise vital structures (trachea, CNS, or extensive macroscopic lung metastases). Thyrotropin alfa elimination is significantly reduced in dialysis-dependent end-stage renal impairment, leading to prolonged elevation of TSH levels.

Adverse Reactions

>10%: Gastrointestinal: Nausea (11%)

1% to 10%:
  Central nervous system: Headache (6%), dizziness (2%), fatigue (2%)
  Gastrointestinal: Vomiting (2%)
  Neuromuscular & skeletal: Weakness (1%)

Frequency not defined: Endocrine & metabolic: Altered thyroid hormone levels (increased)

<1%, postmarketing, and/or case reports: Cerebrovascular accident (with and without physiologic symptoms like unilateral weakness), flu-like symptoms (transient; including arthralgia, chills, fever, malaise, myalgia, shivering), hypersensitivity reaction (including dyspnea, flushing, pruritus, skin rash, urticaria), injection site reaction (including bruising, erythema, pain, and pruritus)

Drug Interactions

Metabolism/Transport Effects None known.

Avoid Concomitant Use There are no known interactions where it is recommended to avoid concomitant use.

Increased Effect/Toxicity There are no known significant interactions involving an increase in effect.

Decreased Effect There are no known significant interactions involving a decrease in effect.

Storage/Stability Store intact vials at 2°C to 8°C (36°F to 46°F). Protect from light. May store reconstituted solution for up to 24 hours between 2°C and 8°C (36°F and 46°F); avoid microbial contamination. If reconstituted solution is not refrigerated, use within 3 hours. Discard unused portion of the vial.

Preparation for Administration Reconstitute each vial with 1.2 mL of sterile water for injection to a concentration of 0.9 mg/mL. Gently swirl vial until dissolved; do not shake. Reconstituted solution should be clear and colorless; do not use if cloudy or discolored.

Mechanism of Action Thyrotropin alfa, derived from a recombinant DNA source, has the identical amino acid sequence as endogenous human thyroid stimulating hormone (TSH). As a diagnostic tool in conjunction with serum thyroglobulin (Tg) testing, thyrotropin alfa stimulates the secretion of Tg from any remaining thyroid tissues (remnants). Under conditions of successful thyroidectomy and complete ablation, very little serum Tg should be detected under TSH stimulatory conditions; conversely, elevated Tg levels suggest the presence of remnant thyroid tissues. Since the source of TSH is exogenous, stimulation of Tg synthesis can be achieved in euthyroid patients, avoiding the need for thyroid hormone withdrawal.

As an adjunctive agent for radioiodine ablation treatment of thyroid cancer tissue remnants, thyrotropin alfa binds to TSH receptors on these tissues, stimulating the uptake and organification of iodine, including radiolabeled iodine (I^{131}). Cancerous tissue is destroyed via gamma emission from the radioiodine concentrated in these tissues.

Pharmacodynamics/Kinetics

Half-life elimination: 25 ± 10 hours

Time to peak: Median: 10 hours (range: 3-24 hours)

Dosing

Adult & Geriatric Note: Consider pretreatment with glucocorticoids for patients in whom local tumor expansion may compromise vital anatomic structures (such as trachea, CNS, or extensive macroscopic lung metastases).

Diagnostic imaging: IM: 0.9 mg, followed 24 hours later by a second 0.9 mg dose; obtain serum Tg sample 72 hours after the second thyrotropin alfa injection

Thyroid tissue remnant ablation: IM: 0.9 mg, followed 24 hours later by a second 0.9 mg dose.

Radioiodine administration should be given 24 hours following the second thyrotropin alfa injection (for diagnostic scanning and remnant ablation). Perform diagnostic scanning 48 hours after radioiodine administration (72 hours after the second thyrotropin alfa injection). Post-therapy scanning may be delayed (additional days) to allow decline of background activity.

Renal Impairment There are no dosage adjustments provided in the manufacturer's labeling; however, elimination is significantly slower in dialysis-dependent end-stage renal impairment and TSH level elevation may be prolonged.

Hepatic Impairment There are no dosage adjustments provided in the manufacturer's labeling (has not been studied).

Administration Administer only by IM injection into the buttock. Do **not** administer intravenously.

Monitoring Parameters Neurologic adverse events (hemiplegia, hemiparesis, stroke, weakness); dyspnea, dysphonia, stridor or other symptoms of local tumor growth

Test Interactions Thyroglobulin assay may be confounded by thyroglobulin antibodies, possibly leading to misinterpreted or difficult to interpret thyroglobulin levels. Routine measurement of TSH levels after thyrotropin alfa use is not recommended.

Dosage Forms Excipient information presented when available (limited, particularly for generics); consult specific product labeling.

Solution Reconstituted, Intramuscular:

Thyrogen: 1.1 mg (1 ea)

Tisagenlecleucel (tis a jen lek LOO sel)

Brand Names: US Kymriah

Index Terms CTL019; Kymriah

Pharmacologic Category Antineoplastic Agent, Anti-CD19; Antineoplastic Agent, CAR-T Immunotherapy; CAR-T Cell Immunotherapy; Cellular Immunotherapy, Autologous; Chimeric Antigen Receptor T-Cell Immunotherapy

Use Acute lymphoblastic leukemia: Treatment of B-cell precursor acute lymphoblastic leukemia (ALL) that is refractory or in second or later relapse in patients up to 25 years of age.

Labeled Contraindications There are no contraindications listed in the manufacturer's labeling.

Product Availability Kymriah: FDA approved August 2017; anticipated availability is currently undetermined

Dosage Forms Excipient information presented when available (limited, particularly for generics); consult specific product labeling.

Suspension, Intravenous:

Kymriah: (1 ea) [contains albumin human, dextran 40, dimethyl sulfoxide]

♦ **TMP-SMX** see Sulfamethoxazole and Trimethoprim on page 1698

♦ **TMP-SMZ** see Sulfamethoxazole and Trimethoprim on page 1698

♦ **TMZ** see Temozolomide on page 1746

Tobramycin (Systemic) (toe bra MYE sin)

Brand Names: Canada JAMP-Tobramycin; Tobramycin For Injection; Tobramycin For Injection, USP; Tobramycin Injection; Tobramycin Injection, USP

Index Terms Tobramycin Sulfate

Pharmacologic Category Antibiotic, Aminoglycoside

Use Treatment of documented or suspected infections caused by susceptible gram-negative bacilli, including *Pseudomonas aeruginosa*.

Pregnancy Risk Factor D

Dosing

Adult Note: Individualization is **critical** because of the low therapeutic index.

In underweight and nonobese patients, use of total body weight (TBW) instead of ideal body weight for determining the initial mg/kg/dose is widely accepted (Nicolau 1995). Ideal body weight (IBW) also may be used to determine doses for patients who are neither underweight nor obese (Gilbert 2009).

Initial and periodic plasma drug levels (eg, peak and trough with conventional dosing, post dose level at a prespecified time with extended-interval dosing) should be determined, particularly in critically-ill patients with serious infections or in disease states known to significantly alter aminoglycoside pharmacokinetics (eg, cystic fibrosis, burns, or major surgery).

Severe life-threatening infections: IM, IV:

Conventional: 1 to 2.5 mg/kg/dose every 8 to 12 hours; to ensure adequate peak concentrations early in therapy, higher initial dosage may be considered in selected patients when extracellular water is increased (edema, septic shock, postsurgical, and/or trauma)

Once-daily: 4 to 7 mg/kg/dose once daily; some clinicians recommend this approach for all patients with normal renal function; this dose is at least as efficacious with similar, if not less, toxicity than conventional dosing.

◄

Brucellosis: IM, IV: 240 mg (IM) daily or 5 mg/kg (IV) daily for 7 days; either regimen recommended in combination with doxycycline

Cholangitis: IM, IV: 4 to 6 mg/kg once daily with ampicillin

CNS shunt infection: Intrathecal (off-label route): 5 to 20 mg/day (Tunkel, 2004)

Diverticulitis, complicated: IM, IV: 1.5 to 2 mg/kg every 8 hours (with ampicillin and metronidazole)

Meningitis *(Enterococcus or Pseudomonas aeruginosa)*: IV: 5 mg/kg/day in divided doses every 8 hours (administered with another bacteriocidal drug)

Pelvic inflammatory disease: IM, IV: Loading dose: 2 mg/kg, then 1.5 mg/kg every 8 hours **or** 4.5 mg/kg once daily

Plague *(Yersinia pestis):* IM, IV: Treatment: 5 mg/kg/day, followed by postexposure prophylaxis with doxycycline

Pneumonia, hospital-acquired or ventilator-associated: IV: 5 to 7 mg/kg/day once daily for 7 days; may consider shorter or longer duration depending on rate of clinical improvement. When used as empiric therapy, use in combination with an agent active against *S. aureus* and an additional antipseudomonal agent. **Note:** Aminoglycosides are not recommended as monotherapy in patients with hospital-acquired or ventilator-associated pneumonia due to *P. aeruginosa* (Kalil 2016).

Prophylaxis against endocarditis (dental, oral, upper respiratory procedures, GI/GU procedures): IM, IV: 1.5 mg/kg with ampicillin (50 mg/kg) 30 minutes prior to procedure. **Note:** AHA guidelines now recommend prophylaxis only in patients undergoing invasive procedures and in whom underlying cardiac conditions may predispose to a higher risk of adverse outcomes should infection occur. As of April 2007, routine prophylaxis no longer recommended by the AHA.

Tularemia: IM, IV: 5 mg/kg/day divided every 8 hours for 1 to 2 weeks

Urinary tract infection: IM, IV: 1.5 mg/kg/dose every 8 hours

Geriatric Dosage should be based on an estimate of ideal body weight.

IM, IV: 1.5 to 5 mg/kg/day in 1 to 2 divided doses

IV: Once daily or extended interval: 5 to 7 mg/kg/dose given every 24, 36, or 48 hours based on creatinine clearance

Pediatric Individualization is **critical** because of the low therapeutic index

Use of ideal body weight (IBW) for determining the mg/kg/dose appears to be more accurate than dosing on the basis of total body weight (TBW).

Usual dosage range: IM, IV:

Infants and Children <5 years: 2.5 mg/kg/dose every 8 hours

Children >5 years: 2 to 2.5 mg/kg/dose every 8 hours

CNS shunt infection: Intrathecal (off-label route): Refer to adult dosing.

Cystic fibrosis: IM, IV: 2.5 to 3.3 mg/kg every 6 to 8 hours. **Note:** Some patients may require larger or more frequent doses if serum levels document the need (eg, cystic fibrosis or febrile granulocytopenic patients).

Renal Impairment IM, IV:

Conventional dosing:

CrCl >60 mL/minute: Administer every 8 hours.

CrCl 40 to 60 mL/minute: Administer every 12 hours.

CrCl 20 to 39 mL/minute: Administer every 24 hours.

CrCl <20 mL/minute: Loading dose, then monitor levels.

High-dose therapy: Interval may be extended (eg, every 48 hours) in patients with moderate renal impairment (CrCl 30 to 59 mL/minute) and/or adjusted based on serum level determinations.

Intermittent hemodialysis (IHD) (administer after hemodialysis on dialysis days) (Heintz 2009): Dialyzable (25% to 70%; variable; dependent on filter, duration, and type of HD): IV:

Loading dose of 2 to 3 mg/kg, followed by:

Mild UTI or synergy: 1 mg/kg/dose every 48 to 72 hours; consider redosing for pre-HD or post-HD serum concentrations <1 mg/L

Moderate to severe UTI: 1 to 1.5 mg/kg/dose every 48 to 72 hours; consider redosing for pre-HD serum concentrations <1.5 to 2 mg/L or post-HD concentrations <1 mg/L

Systemic gram-negative infection: 1.5 to 2 mg/kg/dose every 48 to 72 hours; consider redosing for pre-HD serum concentrations <3 to 5 mg/L or post-HD serum concentrations <2 mg/L

Note: Dosing dependent on the assumption of 3 times/week, complete IHD sessions.

Peritoneal dialysis (PD):

Administration via peritoneal dialysis (PD) fluid:

Gram-negative infection: 4 to 8 mg/L (4 to 8 mcg/mL) of PD fluid

Gram-positive infection (ie, synergy): 3 to 4 mg/L (3 to 4 mcg/mL) of PD fluid

Administration IVPB/IM: Dose as for CrCl <10 mL/minute and follow levels

Continuous renal replacement therapy (CRRT) (Heintz 2009; Trotman 2005): Drug clearance is highly dependent on the method of renal replacement, filter type, and flow rate. Appropriate dosing requires close monitoring of pharmacologic response, signs of adverse reactions due to drug accumulation, as well as target drug concentrations (if appropriate). **Note:** The following are general recommendations only (based on dialysate flow/ultrafiltration rates of 1 to 2 L/hour and minimal residual renal function) and should not supersede clinical judgment:

CVVH/CVVHD/CVVHDF: IV:

Mild UTI or synergy: Loading dose of 2 to 3 mg/kg, followed by 1 mg/kg/dose every 24 to 36 hours (redose when serum concentration <1 mg/L [Heintz 2009])

Moderate-severe UTI: Loading dose of 2 to 3 mg/kg, followed by 1 to 1.5 mg/kg/dose every 24 to 36 hours (redose when serum concentration <1.5 to 2 mg/L [Heintz 2009])

Systemic gram-negative infection: Loading dose of 2 to 3 mg/kg, followed by 1.5 to 2.5 mg/kg/dose every 24 to 48 hours (generally accepted to redose when serum concentration <2 mg/L; one reference suggests redosing when <3 mg/L [Heintz 2009])

Hepatic Impairment No dosage adjustment necessary; does not undergo hepatic metabolism.

Obesity In moderate obesity (TBW/IBW ≥1.25) or greater, (eg, morbid obesity [TBW/IBW >2]), initial dosage requirement may be estimated using a dosing weight of IBW + 0.4 (TBW - IBW) (Traynor 1995).

Additional Information Complete prescribing information should be consulted for additional detail.

◀ **Dosage Forms** Excipient information presented when available (limited, particularly for generics); consult specific product labeling. [DSC] = Discontinued product

Solution, Injection:
  Generic: 10 mg/mL (2 mL); 80 mg/2 mL (2 mL); 1.2 g/30 mL (30 mL); 2 g/50 mL (50 mL)
Solution, Intravenous:
  Generic: 80 mg (100 mL [DSC])
Solution Reconstituted, Injection:
  Generic: 1.2 g (1 ea)
Solution Reconstituted, Injection [preservative free]:
  Generic: 1.2 g (1 ea)

- ◆ **Tobramycin For Injection (Can)** see Tobramycin (Systemic) on page 1787
- ◆ **Tobramycin For Injection, USP (Can)** see Tobramycin (Systemic) on page 1787
- ◆ **Tobramycin Injection (Can)** see Tobramycin (Systemic) on page 1787
- ◆ **Tobramycin Injection, USP (Can)** see Tobramycin (Systemic) on page 1787
- ◆ **Tobramycin Sulfate** see Tobramycin (Systemic) on page 1787
- ◆ **Tolak** see Fluorouracil (Topical) on page 835
- ◆ **Tomudex (Can)** see Raltitrexed on page 1572
- ◆ **Topical Fluorouracil** see Fluorouracil (Topical) on page 835
- ◆ **Toposar** see Etoposide on page 729

Topotecan (toe poe TEE kan)

Related Information

Management of Chemotherapy-Induced Nausea and Vomiting in Adults on page 2253

Management of Drug Extravasations on page 2271

Prevention of Chemotherapy-Induced Nausea and Vomiting in Children on page 2310

Safe Handling of Hazardous Drugs on page 2379

Brand Names: US Hycamtin

Brand Names: Canada Hycamtin; Topotecan For Injection; Topotecan Hydrochloride For Injection

Index Terms Hycamptamine; SKF 104864; SKF 104864-A; Topotecan HCl; Topotecan Hydrochloride

Pharmacologic Category Antineoplastic Agent, Camptothecin; Antineoplastic Agent, Topoisomerase I Inhibitor

Use

Cervical cancer, recurrent or resistant: Treatment of recurrent or resistant (stage IVB) cervical cancer (in combination with cisplatin) which is not amenable to curative treatment

Ovarian cancer, metastatic: Treatment of metastatic ovarian cancer (as a single agent) after disease progression on or after initial or subsequent chemotherapy

Small cell lung cancer, relapsed:
  Injection: Treatment of small cell lung cancer (as a single agent) in patients with platinum-sensitive disease which has progressed at least 60 days after initiation of first-line chemotherapy

Oral: Treatment of relapsed small cell lung cancer in patients with a prior complete or partial response and who are at least 45 days from the end of first-line chemotherapy

Labeled Contraindications

Hypersensitivity to topotecan or any component of the formulation

Canadian labeling: Additional contraindications (not in U.S. labeling): Severe renal impairment (CrCl <20 mL/minute); pregnancy; breastfeeding; severe bone marrow depression

Pregnancy Considerations Adverse effects were observed in animal reproduction studies. May cause fetal harm in pregnant women. Women of childbearing potential should use highly effective contraception to prevent pregnancy during treatment and for at least 1 month after therapy discontinuation. Males with female partners of childbearing potential should use highly effective contraception during treatment and for 3 months after therapy discontinuation. Topotecan may have both acute and long-term effects on fertility in women; fertility in males may be impaired due to effects on spermatogenesis.

Breastfeeding Considerations It is not known if topotecan is excreted in breast milk. Due to the potential for serious adverse reactions in the nursing infant, the manufacturer recommends to discontinue breastfeeding in women who are receiving topotecan.

Warnings/Precautions [US Boxed Warning]: May cause severe myelosuppression. Monitor blood counts frequently. Do NOT administer to patients with baseline neutrophils <1500/mm^3 and platelets <100,000/mm^3. The dose-limiting toxicity is bone marrow suppression (primarily neutropenia); may also cause thrombocytopenia and anemia. Grade 3 and 4 events were common. Severe myelotoxicity has also been reported when used in combination with cisplatin. Neutropenia is not cumulative overtime. The median duration of neutropenia and thrombocytopenia was 7 days and 5 days, respectively. Nadir neutrophil and platelet counts occurred at a median of 15 days (when administered orally). In a clinical study comparing IV to oral topotecan, G-CSF support was administered in a higher percentage of patients receiving oral topotecan (Eckardt 2007). Bone marrow suppression may require dosage reduction and/or growth factor support. Topotecan-induced neutropenia may lead to typhlitis (neutropenic enterocolitis), including fatalities; should be considered in patients presenting with neutropenia, fever, and abdominal pain.

Diarrhea has been reported with oral topotecan; may be severe (requiring hospitalization); incidence may be higher in the elderly; educate patients on early recognition and proper management, including diet changes, increase in fluid intake, antidiarrheals, and antibiotics. The median time to onset of diarrhea (grade 2 or worse) was 9 days. The incidence of diarrhea may be higher in the elderly. Do not administer in patients with grade 3 or 4 diarrhea; reduce dose upon recovery to ≤ grade 1 toxicity. Interstitial lung disease (ILD) (with fatalities) has been reported; discontinue use in patients with confirmed ILD diagnosis; risk factors for ILD include a history of ILD, pulmonary fibrosis, lung cancer, thoracic radiation, and the use of colony-stimulating factors or medication with pulmonary toxicity; monitor pulmonary symptoms (cough, fever, dyspnea, and/or hypoxia). Use caution in renal impairment; may require dose adjustment (use in severe renal impairment is contraindicated in the Canadian labeling). Potentially significant drug-drug interactions may exist, requiring dose or frequency adjustment, additional monitoring, and/or selection of alternative therapy. Topotecan exposure is increased when oral topotecan is used concurrently with P-glycoprotein inhibitors; avoid concurrent use. Topotecan overdoses have been reported; potential causes include omission of the leading zero and missing the decimal point when prescribing, preparing, and administering. Recommended intravenous doses should generally not exceed 4 mg in adults; verify dose prior to administration. Extravasation injuries have been reported (some severe); if extravasation occurs, discontinue infusion immediately and manage appropriately. Ensure proper needle or catheter placement prior to and during infusion. Avoid extravasation.

Adverse Reactions

>10%:

Central nervous system: Fatigue (oral: 11% to 19%)

Dermatologic: Alopecia (oral: 10% to 20%)

Gastrointestinal: Nausea (oral: 27% to 33%), anorexia (intravenous: 32%; oral: 7% to 14%), diarrhea (oral: 14% to 22%, grade 3: 4%, grade 4: ≤1%; intravenous: grades 3/4: 6%), vomiting (oral: 19% to 21%)

Hematologic & oncologic: Anemia (oral: 94% to 98%; grades 3/4: 25%; grade 3: 15% to 18%; grade 4: 7% to 10%; intravenous: grades 3/4: 37% to 42%), neutropenia (oral: 83% to 91%; grade 3: 24% to 28%; grade 4: 32% to 33%; intravenous: grade 4: 70% to 80%; nadir 12 to 15 days; duration: 7 days), thrombocytopenia (oral: 81%; grade 3: 29% to 30%; grade 4: 6% to 7%; intravenous: grade 4: 27% to 29%; nadir: 15 days; duration: 3 to 5 days), febrile neutropenia (intravenous: grade 3/4: 23% to 28%; oral: grade 4: 4%), neutropenic infection (13% to 17%)

1% to 10%:

Gastrointestinal: Abdominal pain (intravenous: grades 3/4: 5% to 6%)

Hepatic: Increased liver enzymes (intravenous: 8%; transient)

Neuromuscular & skeletal: Weakness (3% to 7%)

Respiratory: Dyspnea (intravenous: 6% to 9%)

Miscellaneous: Fever (oral: 5% to 7%), sepsis (intravenous: grades 3/4: 5%; oral: 2%)

<1%, postmarketing, and/or case reports: Anaphylactoid reactions, angioedema, arthralgia, chest pain, cough, dermatitis (severe), extravasation, headache, hemorrhage (severe, associated with thrombocytopenia), hypersensitivity reaction, interstitial pulmonary disease, leukopenia, myalgia, neutropenic enterocolitis, pancytopenia, paresthesia, pruritus (severe), skin rash, stomatitis, typhlitis

Drug Interactions

Metabolism/Transport Effects Substrate of BCRP

Avoid Concomitant Use

Avoid concomitant use of Topotecan with any of the following: BCG (Intravesical); Deferiprone; Dipyrone; Natalizumab; P-glycoprotein/ABCB1 Inhibitors; Pimecrolimus; Tacrolimus (Topical); Vaccines (Live); Velpatasvir; Voxilaprevir

Increased Effect/Toxicity

Topotecan may increase the levels/effects of: CloZAPine; Deferiprone; Fingolimod; Leflunomide; Natalizumab; Tofacitinib; Vaccines (Live)

The levels/effects of Topotecan may be increased by: BCRP/ABCG2 Inhibitors; Denosumab; Dipyrone; Granulocyte Colony-Stimulating Factors; Ocrelizumab; Palifermin; P-glycoprotein/ABCB1 Inhibitors; Pimecrolimus; Platinum Derivatives; Promazine; Roflumilast; Tacrolimus (Topical); Trastuzumab; Velpatasvir; Voxilaprevir

Decreased Effect

Topotecan may decrease the levels/effects of: BCG (Intravesical); Coccidioides immitis Skin Test; Lenograstim; Nivolumab; Sipuleucel-T; Tertomotide; Vaccines (Inactivated); Vaccines (Live)

The levels/effects of Topotecan may be decreased by: Echinacea; Fosphenytoin-Phenytoin

Hazardous Drugs Handling Considerations

Hazardous agent (NIOSH 2016 [group 1]).

Use appropriate precautions for receiving, handling, administration, and disposal. Gloves (single) should be worn during receiving, unpacking, and placing in storage.

NIOSH recommends double gloving, a protective gown, ventilated engineering controls (a class II biological safety cabinet or a compounding aseptic containment isolator), and closed system transfer devices (CSTDs) for IV preparation. Double gloving, a gown, and (if dosage form allows) CSTDs are required during IV administration. NIOSH recommends single gloving for administration of an intact tablet/capsule (NIOSH 2016). If manipulating tablets/capsules (eg, to prepare an oral suspension), NIOSH recommends double gloving, a protective gown, and preparation in a controlled device; if not prepared in a controlled device, respiratory and eye/face protection as well as ventilated engineering controls are recommended. NIOSH recommends double gloving, a protective gown, and (if there is a potential for vomit or spit up) eye/face protection for administration of an oral liquid/feeding tube administration.

Storage/Stability

IV:

Solution for injection: Store intact vials at 2°C to 8°C (36°F to 45°F). Protect from light. Single-use vials should be discarded after initial vial entry. Stability of solutions diluted for infusion is variable; refer to specific product information for details.

Lyophilized powder: Store intact vials at 20°C to 25°C (68°F to 77°F). Protect from light. Reconstituted solution is stable for up to 28 days at 20°C to 25°C (68°F to 77°F), although the manufacturer recommends use immediately after reconstitution. Solutions diluted in D5W or NS are stable for 24 hours at room temperature (manufacturer's labeling) or up to 7 days under refrigeration (Craig 1997). Reconstituted solution for injection (reconstituted with bacteriostatic SWFI to 1 mg/mL) for oral administration is stable for 14 days at 4°C in plastic syringes (Daw 2004).

Oral: Store at 2°C to 8°C (36°F to 46°F). Protect from light.

Preparation for Administration Reconstitute lyophilized powder with 4 mL SWFI. Reconstituted lyophilized powder and solution for injection should be further diluted in D5W or NS for infusion.

Mechanism of Action Binds to topoisomerase I and stabilizes the cleavable complex so that religation of the cleaved DNA strand cannot occur. This results in the accumulation of cleavable complexes and single-strand DNA breaks. Topotecan acts in S phase of the cell cycle.

Pharmacodynamics/Kinetics Note: Pharmacokinetic data in pediatric patients and young adults (0.4-22 years) demonstrated a high level of interpatient variability (43% to 57% dependent upon parameter evaluated) as well as intrapatient variability (20% to 22% dependent upon parameter evaluated) (Schaiquevich 2007)

Absorption: Oral: Rapid

Distribution: V_d:

Pediatric patients and young adults (0.4-22 years): Mean range: 32.2-32.7 L/m^2 (Schaiquevich, 2007)

Adults: 25 to 75 L/m^2 (Hartmann 2006)

Protein binding: ~35%

Metabolism: Undergoes a rapid, pH-dependent hydrolysis of the lactone ring to yield a relatively inactive hydroxy acid in plasma; metabolized in the liver to N-demethylated metabolite

Bioavailability: Oral: Capsule: Adults: ~40%; data from pediatric patients (1-18 years) showed that, while highly variable, the reported median oral bioavailability with oral administration of the reconstituted parenteral solution is similar to adults (Daw 2004; Zamboni 1999)

Half-life elimination:

Pediatric patients (0-18 years): Lactone moiety: 2.58 hours ± 0.15 (range: 0.2-7.1 hours) (Santana 2005)

Adults: IV: 2 to 3 hours; renal impairment: ~5 hours; Oral: 3 to 6 hours

Time to peak, plasma:

Pediatric patients (1-18 years): Parenteral formulation (reconstituted lyophilized formulation): 0.75-2 hours (Zamboni 1999)

Adults: Oral: 1 to 2 hours; delayed with high-fat meal (3 to 4 hours)

Excretion:

IV: Urine (51%; ~3% as N-desmethyl topotecan); feces (18%; ~2% as N-desmethyl topotecan)

Oral: Urine (20%; 2% as N-desmethyl topotecan); feces (33%; <2% as N-desmethyl topotecan)

Clearance:

Pediatric patients (0.4-18 years): GFR most significant determinant of clearance; a linear model with GFR has been observed; BSA is also a significant determinant of clearance and AUC more so than patient weight; infants <6 months have decreased clearance (Schaiquevich 2007). However, pharmacokinetic data from six pediatric patients with severe renal impairment (n=5: Unilateral nephrectomy; n=1: Anephric on hemodialysis) suggests that other mechanisms than GFR may assist with renal clearance; in these patients, overall systemic clearance was shown to be similar to matched controls (age, BSA, and Scr) despite decreased GFR (Iacono 2003; Iacono 2004)

Adults: Topotecan plasma clearance is 24% higher in males than in female patients

Dosing

Adult & Geriatric Note: Baseline neutrophil count should be ≥1500/mm^3 and platelets should be ≥100,000/mm^3 prior to treatment; for re-treatment, neutrophil count should be >1000/mm^3; platelets >100,000/mm^3 and hemoglobin ≥9 g/dL. Intravenous doses should generally not exceed 4 mg; verify dose prior to administration.

Cervical cancer, recurrent or resistant: IV: 0.75 mg/m^2/day for 3 days (in combination with cisplatin on day 1 only, [with hydration]) every 21 days

Ovarian cancer, metastatic: IV: 1.5 mg/m^2/day for 5 consecutive days every 21 days **or** (off-label dosing) 1.25 mg/m^2/day for 5 days every 21 days until disease progression or unacceptable toxicity or a maximum of 12 months (Sehouli 2011) **or** (weekly administration; off-label dosing) 4 mg/m^2 on days 1, 8, and 15 every 28 days until disease progression or unacceptable toxicity or a maximum of 12 months (Sehouli 2011)

Small cell lung cancer (SCLC), relapsed:
IV: 1.5 mg/m^2/day for 5 consecutive days every 21 days
Oral: 2.3 mg/m^2/day for 5 consecutive days every 21 days (round dose to the nearest 0.25 mg); if patient vomits after dose is administered, do not give a replacement dose.

Ewing's sarcoma, relapsed/refractory or metastatic (off-label use): IV: 0.75 mg/m^2/day for 5 consecutive days every 21 days (in combination with cyclophosphamide) (Hunold 2006; Saylors 2001)

Primary CNS lymphoma, relapsed or refractory (off-label use): IV: 1.5 mg/m^2 for 5 days every 21 days for a maximum of 10 cycles or until disease progression or unacceptable toxicity (Voloschin 2008). Additional data may be necessary to further define the role of topotecan in this condition.

Rhabdomyosarcoma, metastatic (off-label use): Adults <21 years: IV: 0.75 mg/m^2/day for 5 consecutive days every 21 days for 2 cycles (window therapy; in combination with cyclophosphamide); if objective response occurred by week 6, follow with alternating cycles of vincristine, topotecan, and cyclophosphamide (VTC) with vincristine, dactinomycin, and cyclophosphamide (VAC) (Walterhouse 2004)

Pediatric Note: Baseline neutrophil count should be ≥1500/mm^3 and platelets should be ≥100,000/mm^3 prior to treatment; for re treatment, neutrophil count should be >1000/mm^3; platelets >100,000/mm^3 and hemoglobin ≥9 g/dL. Intravenous doses should generally not exceed 4 mg; verify dose prior to administration.

CNS malignancy, relapsed/refractory (off-label use; based on limited data): Oral: 0.8 mg/m^2/day for 21 consecutive days every 4 weeks for ≥12 cycles (Minturn 2011); additional data may be necessary to further define the role of topotecan in this condition

Ewing's sarcoma, relapsed/refractory or metastatic (off-label use): IV: 0.75 mg/m^2/day for 5 consecutive days every 21 days (in combination with cyclophosphamide) (Hunold 2006; Saylors 2001)

Neuroblastoma, relapsed/refractory (off-label use): IV: 0.75 mg/m^2/day for 5 days every 21 days (in combination with cyclophosphamide) (Ashraf 2013; London 2010) **or** 2 mg/m^2/day for 5 days every 21 days (monotherapy) (London 2010)

Rhabdomyosarcoma, metastatic (off-label use): IV: 0.75 mg/m^2/day for 5 consecutive days every 21 days for 2 cycles (window therapy; in combination with cyclophosphamide); if objective response occurred by week 6, follow with alternating cycles of vincristine, topotecan, and cyclophosphamide (VTC) with vincristine, dactinomycin, and cyclophosphamide (VAC) (Walterhouse 2004)

Renal Impairment
Manufacturer's labeling:
IV (single agent topotecan):
CrCl ≥40 mL/minute: No dosage adjustment necessary.
CrCl 20 to 39 mL/minute: Reduce dose to 0.75 mg/m^2/dose
CrCl <20 mL/minute: There are no dosage adjustments provided in manufacturer's U.S. labeling (insufficient data available for dosing recommendation); use is contraindicated in the Canadian labeling.

◀

Oral:

CrCl ≥50 mL/minute: No dosage adjustment necessary.

CrCl 30 to 49 mL/minute: Reduce dose to 1.5 mg/m²/day; may increase after the 1st cycle by 0.4 mg/m²/day if no severe hematologic or gastrointestinal toxicities occur.

CrCl <30 mL/minute: Reduce dose to 0.6 mg/m²/day; may increase after the 1st cycle by 0.4 mg/m²/day if no severe hematologic or gastrointestinal toxicities occur.

Alternate recommendations:

Aronoff 2007: IV:

Adults:

CrCl >50 mL/minute: Administer 75% of dose

CrCl 10 to 50 mL/minute: Administer 50% of dose

CrCl <10 mL/minute: Administer 25% of dose

Hemodialysis: Avoid use

Continuous ambulatory peritoneal dialysis (CAPD): Avoid use

Continuous renal replacement therapy (CRRT): 0.75 mg/m²

Children:

CrCl 30 to 50 mL/minute: Administer 75% of dose

CrCl 10 to 29 mL/minute: Administer 50% of dose

CrCl <10 mL/minute: Administer 25% of dose

Continuous renal replacement therapy (CRRT): Administer 50% of dose

Kintzel 1995: IV:

CrCl 46 to 60 mL/minute: Administer 80% of dose

CrCl 31 to 45 mL/minute: Administer 75% of dose

CrCl ≤30 mL/minute: Administer 70% of dose

Hepatic Impairment Manufacturer's labeling:

IV:

US labeling: Bilirubin 1.7 to 15 mg/dL: There are no dosage adjustments provided in the manufacturer's labeling, although clearance is reduced up to 33%.

Canadian labeling: Bilirubin >1.5 to <10 mg/dL: No dosage adjustment is necessary (the half-life is increased slightly; usual doses are generally tolerated).

Oral: There is no dosage adjustment provided in the manufacturer's labeling; however, dosage adjustment is likely not necessary as the pharmacokinetics of topotecan do not differ significantly based on serum bilirubin, ALT, or AST.

Obesity *ASCO Guidelines for appropriate chemotherapy dosing in obese adults with cancer:* Utilize patient's actual body weight (full weight) for calculation of body surface area- or weight-based dosing, particularly when the intent of therapy is curative; manage regimen-related toxicities in the same manner as for nonobese patients; if a dose reduction is utilized due to toxicity, consider resumption of full weight-based dosing with subsequent cycles, especially if cause of toxicity (eg, hepatic or renal impairment) is resolved (Griggs 2012).

Adjustment for Toxicity

Cervical cancer (cisplatin may also require dosage adjustment): IV: Severe febrile neutropenia (<1000/mm³ with temperature of ≥38°C) or platelet count <25,000/mm³: Reduce topotecan to 0.6 mg/m²/day for subsequent cycles (may consider G-CSF support [beginning on day 4] prior to instituting dose reduction for neutropenic fever).

If necessary, may further reduce dose to 0.45 mg/m²/day for subsequent cycles.

Ovarian cancer: IV: Dosage adjustment for hematological effects: Severe neutropenia (<500/mm³) or platelet count <25,000/mm³: Reduce dose to 1.25 mg/m²/day for subsequent cycles (may consider G-CSF support [beginning on day 6] prior to instituting dose reduction for severe neutropenia). **Note:** The Canadian labeling states that the dose may be further reduced to 1 mg/m²/day if necessary.

Small cell lung cancer (SCLC):

IV: Dosage adjustment for hematological effects: Severe neutropenia (<500/mm³) or platelet count <25,000/mm³: Reduce dose to 1.25 mg/m²/day for subsequent cycles (may consider G-CSF support [beginning on day 6] prior to instituting dose reduction for severe neutropenia). **Note:** The Canadian labeling states that the dose may be further reduced to 1 mg/m²/day if necessary.

Oral:

Severe neutropenia (neutrophils <500/mm³ associated with fever or infection or lasting ≥7 days) or prolonged neutropenia (neutrophils 500/mm³ to 1000/mm³ lasting beyond day 21) or platelets <25,000/mm³: Reduce dose by 0.4 mg/m²/day for subsequent cycles.

Diarrhea (grade 3 or 4): Do not administer to patients with grade 3 or 4 diarrhea. Upon recovery to ≤ grade 1 toxicity, reduce dose by 0.4 mg/m²/day for subsequent cycles.

Combination Regimens

Bone sarcoma (Ewing sarcoma): Cyclophosphamide-Topotecan (Ewing Sarcoma) on page 2078

Cervical cancer:

Bevacizumab-Paclitaxel-Topotecan (Cervical) on page 1995

Cisplatin-Topotecan (Cervical Cancer) on page 2060

Neuroblastoma: Cyclophosphamide-Topotecan (Neuroblastoma) on page 2078

Ovarian cancer:

Bevacizumab-Topotecan Daily (Ovarian) on page 1995

Bevacizumab-Topotecan Weekly (Ovarian) on page 1996

Soft tissue sarcoma (rhabdomyosarcoma): Cyclophosphamide-Topotecan (Rhabdomyosarcoma) on page 2079

Administration

IV: Administer IVPB over 30 minutes. For combination chemotherapy with cisplatin, administer pretreatment hydration.

Oral: Administer without regard to meals. Swallow whole; do not open, crush, chew, or divide capsule. If vomiting occurs after dose, do not take replacement dose. For patients unable to swallow capsules whole, reconstituted topotecan solution for injection (1 mg/mL concentration) may be mixed with up to 30 mL of acidic fruit juice (eg, apple, orange, grape) immediately prior to oral administration (Daw 2004).

Vesicant/Extravasation Risk Irritant

Emetic Potential Children and Adults: Low (10% to 30%)

Extemporaneous Preparations For patients unable to swallow capsules whole, reconstituted topotecan solution for injection (1 mg/mL concentration) may be mixed with up to 30 mL of acidic fruit juice (eg, apple, orange, grape) immediately prior to oral administration.

Daw NC, Santana VM, Iacono LC, et al. Phase I and pharmacokinetic study of topotecan administered orally once daily for 5 days for 2 consecutive weeks to pediatric patients with refractory solid tumors. J Clin Oncol. 2004;22(5):829-837.

◀ **Monitoring Parameters** CBC with differential and platelet count, renal function tests, bilirubin; monitor for symptoms of interstitial lung disease; diarrhea symptoms/hydration status

Dosage Forms Excipient information presented when available (limited, particularly for generics); consult specific product labeling. [DSC] = Discontinued product

Capsule, Oral:
  Hycamtin: 0.25 mg, 1 mg
Solution, Intravenous [preservative free]:
  Generic: 4 mg/4 mL (4 mL)
Solution Reconstituted, Intravenous:
  Generic: 4 mg (1 ea [DSC])
Solution Reconstituted, Intravenous [preservative free]:
  Hycamtin: 4 mg (1 ea)
  Generic: 4 mg (1 ea)

◆ **Topotecan For Injection (Can)** see Topotecan on page 1790

◆ **Topotecan HCl** see Topotecan on page 1790

◆ **Topotecan Hydrochloride** see Topotecan on page 1790

◆ **Topotecan Hydrochloride For Injection (Can)** see Topotecan on page 1790

Toremifene (tore EM i feen)

Related Information
Safe Handling of Hazardous Drugs on page 2379

Brand Names: US Fareston

Brand Names: Canada Fareston

Index Terms FC1157a; Toremifene Citrate

Pharmacologic Category Antineoplastic Agent, Estrogen Receptor Antagonist; Selective Estrogen Receptor Modulator (SERM)

Use Breast cancer, metastatic: Treatment of metastatic breast cancer in postmenopausal women with estrogen receptor-positive or unknown tumors

Labeled Contraindications Known hypersensitivity to toremifene or any component of the formulation; congenital/acquired QT prolongation (long QT syndrome), uncorrected hypokalemia, uncorrected hypomagnesemia

Pregnancy Considerations Adverse events were observed in animal reproduction studies. Based on the mechanism of action, may cause fetal harm if administered during pregnancy. Toremifene is only approved for use in postmenopausal women; however, if prescribed in premenopausal women, effective non-hormonal contraception should be used.

Breastfeeding Considerations It is not known if toremifene is present in breast milk. Due to the potential for serious adverse reactions in the breastfed infant, the manufacturer recommends a decision be made to discontinue breastfeeding or to discontinue the drug, taking into account the importance of treatment to the mother.

Warnings/Precautions [US Boxed Warning]: May prolong the QT interval; QT$_c$ prolongation is dose-dependent and concentration-dependent. QT prolongation may lead to a form of ventricular tachycardia called torsades de pointes, which may result in syncope, seizure and/or sudden death. Use is contraindicated in patients with congenital or acquired QT prolongation (long QT syndrome), uncorrected hypokalemia, or uncorrected hypomagnesemia. Avoid use with other medications

known to prolong the QT interval and with strong CYP3A4 inhibitors. Use with caution in patients with heart failure, hepatic impairment, or electrolyte abnormalities. Monitor electrolytes; correct hypokalemia and hypomagnesemia prior to treatment. Obtain ECG at baseline and as clinically indicated in patients at risk for QT prolongation.

Hypercalcemia and tumor flare have been reported during the first weeks of treatment in some breast cancer patients with bone metastases; monitor closely for hypercalcemia. Institute appropriate measures if hypercalcemia occurs, and if severe, discontinue treatment. Medications that decrease renal calcium excretion (eg, thiazide diuretics) may increase the risk of hypercalcemia in patients receiving toremifene. Tumor flare consists of diffuse musculoskeletal pain and erythema with initial increased size of tumor lesions that later regress; is often accompanied by hypercalcemia. Tumor flare does not imply treatment failure or represent tumor progression. Leukopenia and thrombocytopenia have been reported rarely; monitor leukocyte and platelet counts in patients with leukopenia and thrombocytopenia. Endometrial cancer, hypertrophy, hyperplasia, and uterine polyps have been reported. Long-term use of toremifene in patients with preexisting endometrial hyperplasia has not been established. Baseline and annual gynecological exams are recommended in all patients; closely monitor patients who are at high risk for endometrial cancer. Use with caution in patients with hepatic failure. Grades 3 and 4 transaminase increases and hyperbilirubinemia have been reported, including jaundice, hepatitis, and non-alcoholic fatty liver disease. Monitor liver function tests periodically. Avoid use in patients with a history of thromboembolic disease. Potentially significant drug-drug/drug-food interactions may exist, requiring dose or frequency adjustment, additional monitoring, and/or selection of alternative therapy.

Adverse Reactions

>10%:
  Dermatologic: Diaphoresis (20%)
  Endocrine & metabolic: Hot flash (35%)
  Gastrointestinal: Nausea (14%)
  Genitourinary: Vaginal discharge (13%)
  Hepatic: Increased serum alkaline phosphatase (8% to 19%), increased serum AST (5% to 19%)
1% to 10%:
  Cardiovascular: Edema (5%), cardiac arrhythmia (≤2%), cerebrovascular accident (≤2%), local thrombophlebitis (≤2%), pulmonary embolism (≤2%), thrombosis (≤2%), transient ischemic attacks (≤2%), cardiac failure (≤1%), myocardial infarction (≤1%)
  Central nervous system: Dizziness (9%)
  Endocrine & metabolic: Hypercalcemia (≤3%)
  Gastrointestinal: Vomiting (4%)
  Genitourinary: Vaginal hemorrhage (2%)
  Hepatic: Increased serum bilirubin (1% to 2%)
  Ophthalmic: Cataract (≤10%), xerophthalmia (≤9%), visual field defect (≤4%), corneal disease (≤2%), glaucoma (≤2%), visual disturbance (≤2%), diplopia (≤2%)
<1%, postmarketing, and/or case reports: Alopecia, angina pectoris, anorexia, arthritis, ataxia, blurred vision, constipation, corneal opacity (reversible; including corneal verticulata), depression, dermatitis, dyspnea, endometrial carcinoma, endometrial hyperplasia, fatigue, hepatotoxicity (including hepatitis, nonalcoholic fatty liver disease), jaundice, lethargy, leukopenia,

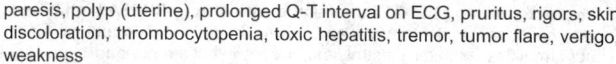

paresis, polyp (uterine), prolonged Q-T interval on ECG, pruritus, rigors, skin discoloration, thrombocytopenia, toxic hepatitis, tremor, tumor flare, vertigo, weakness

Drug Interactions

Metabolism/Transport Effects Substrate of CYP1A2 (minor), CYP3A4 (major); **Note:** Assignment of Major/Minor substrate status based on clinically relevant drug interaction potential

Avoid Concomitant Use

Avoid concomitant use of Toremifene with any of the following: Amifampridine; CYP3A4 Inducers (Strong); CYP3A4 Inhibitors (Strong); Grapefruit Juice; Highest Risk QTc-Prolonging Agents; Hydroxychloroquine; MiFEPRIStone; Mizolastine; Moderate Risk QTc-Prolonging Agents; Ospemifene; Probucol; Promazine; Vinflunine

Increased Effect/Toxicity

Toremifene may increase the levels/effects of: Highest Risk QTc-Prolonging Agents; Ospemifene; Vitamin K Antagonists

The levels/effects of Toremifene may be increased by: Amifampridine; Bilastine; Buprenorphine; CYP3A4 Inhibitors (Strong); Grapefruit Juice; Hydroxychloroquine; Indapamide; MiFEPRIStone; Mizolastine; Moderate Risk QTc-Prolonging Agents; Probucol; Promazine; QTc-Prolonging Agents (Indeterminate Risk and Risk Modifying); Teneligliptin; Thiazide and Thiazide-Like Diuretics; Vinflunine; Xipamide

Decreased Effect

Toremifene may decrease the levels/effects of: Ospemifene; Sugammadex

The levels/effects of Toremifene may be decreased by: Bosentan; CYP3A4 Inducers (Moderate); CYP3A4 Inducers (Strong); Dabrafenib; Deferasirox; Sarilumab; Siltuximab; St John's Wort; Tocilizumab

Food Interactions Grapefruit juice may increase toremifene levels. Management: Avoid grapefruit juice.

Hazardous Drugs Handling Considerations

Hazardous agent (NIOSH 2016 [group 1]).

Use appropriate precautions for receiving, handling, administration, and disposal. Gloves (single) should be worn during receiving, unpacking, and placing in storage. NIOSH recommends single gloving for administration of intact tablets or capsules (NIOSH 2016).

Storage/Stability Store at 25°C (77°F); excursions permitted to 15°C to 30°C (59°F to 86°F); protect from heat. Protect from light.

Mechanism of Action Nonsteroidal, triphenylethylene derivative with potent antiestrogenic properties (also has estrogenic effects). Competitively binds to estrogen receptors on tumors and inhibits the growth stimulating effects of estrogen.

Pharmacodynamics/Kinetics

Absorption: Well absorbed

Distribution: V_d: 580 L

Protein binding, plasma: >99.5%, primarily to albumin

Metabolism: Extensively hepatic, principally by CYP3A4 to N-demethyltoremifene (a weak antiestrogen)

Bioavailability: Not affected by food

Half-life elimination: Toremifene: ~5 days, ~7 days (females >60 years); N-demethyltoremifene: 6 days

Time to peak, serum: ≤3 hours

Excretion: Primarily feces; urine (~10%) during a 1-week period

Dosing

Adult & Geriatric

Breast cancer, metastatic: Postmenopausal women: Oral: 60 mg once daily, continue until disease progression.

Desmoid tumors (aggressive fibromatosis) (off-label use): Oral: 180 mg once daily until disease progression or unacceptable toxicity (Fiore 2015). Additional data may be necessary to further define the role of toremifene in this condition.

Renal Impairment There are no dosage adjustments listed in the manufacturer's labeling. However, pharmacokinetics in patients with renal impairment are similar to those in patients with normal renal function and dosage adjustment is unlikely to be necessary.

Hepatic Impairment There are no dosage adjustments provided in the manufacturer's labeling. However, hepatic impairment increases the half-life of toremifene.

Administration Administer with or without food.

Monitoring Parameters CBC with differential (periodically), electrolytes (magnesium and potassium prior to and periodically during treatment; calcium periodically), hepatic function tests (periodically). Obtain ECG (baseline and periodically during treatment) in patients at risk for QT prolongation. In patients with bone metastases, monitor closely for hypercalcemia during the first few weeks of treatment. Baseline and annual gynecological exams (patients at high risk for endometrial cancer should be closely monitored). Signs/symptoms of uterine disorders (bleeding, discharge, pelvic pain/pressure).

Dietary Considerations Avoid grapefruit juice.

Dosage Forms Excipient information presented when available (limited, particularly for generics); consult specific product labeling.

Tablet, Oral:

Fareston: 60 mg

◆ **Toremifene Citrate** see Toremifene on page 1798

◆ **Torisel** see Temsirolimus on page 1754

◆ **Tositumomab I-131** see Tositumomab and Iodine I 131 Tositumomab on page 1801

Tositumomab and Iodine I 131 Tositumomab

(toe si TYOO mo mab & EYE oh dyne eye one THUR tee one toe si TYOO mo mab)

Brand Names: US Bexxar [DSC]

Brand Names: Canada Bexxar

Index Terms 131 I Anti-B1 Antibody; 131 I-Anti-B1 Monoclonal Antibody; Anti-CD20-Murine Monoclonal Antibody I-131; Iodine I 131 Tositumomab and Tositumomab; Tositumomab I-131

Pharmacologic Category Antineoplastic Agent, Anti-CD20; Antineoplastic Agent, Monoclonal Antibody; Radiopharmaceutical

Use

Non-Hodgkin lymphoma: Treatment of relapsed or refractory CD20 positive, low-grade, follicular, or transformed non-Hodgkin lymphoma (NHL), with progression during or after rituximab treatment

Limitations of use: Tositumomab and iodine I 131 tositumomab is only indicated for a single course of treatment; safety/efficacy of additional courses have not been established. Not indicated for first-line treatment of CD20-positive NHL.

Pregnancy Risk Factor D

Dosing

Adult & Geriatric Non-Hodgkin lymphoma (NHL), relapsed or refractory: IV: Dosing consists of four components administered in 2 steps. Refer to manufacturer's labeling for additional details. Indicated for a single treatment course. Thyroid protective agents (SSKI, Lugol solution or potassium iodide) should be administered beginning at least 24 hours prior to step 1. Premedicate with acetaminophen 650 mg and diphenhydramine 50 mg orally 30 minutes prior to step 1 and step 2.

Step 1: Dosimetric step (Day 0):
Tositumomab 450 mg administered over 60 minutes
Iodine I 131 tositumomab (containing I-131 5 mCi and tositumomab 35 mg) administered over 20 minutes

Note: Whole body dosimetry and biodistribution should be determined on Day 0; days 2, 3, or 4; and day 6 or 7 prior to administration of Step 2. If biodistribution is not acceptable, do not administer the therapeutic step. On day 6 or 7, calculate the patient specific activity of iodine I 131 tositumomab to deliver 75 cGy total body dose (TBD) or 65 cGy TBD (in mCi).

Step 2: Therapeutic step (one dose administered 7 to 14 days after step 1):
Tositumomab 450 mg administered over 60 minutes
Iodine I 131 tositumomab:
Platelets ≥150,000/mm^3: Iodine I 131 calculated to deliver 75 cGy total body irradiation and tositumomab 35 mg over 20 minutes
Platelets ≥100,000/mm^3 and <150,000/mm^3: Iodine I 131 calculated to deliver 65 cGy total body irradiation and tositumomab 35 mg over 20 minutes

Renal Impairment There are no specific dosage adjustments provided in the manufacturer's labeling (has not been studied). However, greater exposure to I-131 tositumomab may occur in patients with renal impairment.

Hepatic Impairment There are no dosage adjustments provided in the manufacturer's labeling.

Adjustment for Toxicity
Infusion-related toxicity (with tositumomab or iodine I-131 tositumomab):
Mild-to-moderate: Reduce infusion rate by 50%
Severe: Interrupt infusion; after complete resolution, resume with previous infusion rate reduced by 50%
Serious allergic reaction: Discontinue infusion.

Additional Information Complete prescribing information should be consulted for additional detail.

Product Availability Bexxar: Manufacturing and sales discontinued (in the US and Canada) February 2014. In the United States, the last day to schedule dosing is February 11, 2014; the final day for patient availability is February 20, 2014.

Dosage Forms Excipient information presented when available (limited, particularly for generics); consult specific product labeling. [DSC] = Discontinued product

Note: Not all components are shipped from the same facility. When ordering, ensure that all will arrive on the same day.

Kit [dosimetric package]: Tositumomab 225 mg/16.1 mL [2 vials], tositumomab 35 mg/2.5 mL [1 vial], and iodine I 131 tositumomab 0.1 mg/mL and 0.61mCi/mL (20 mL) [1 vial] [DSC]

Kit [therapeutic package]: Tositumomab 225 mg/16.1 mL [2 vials], tositumomab 35 mg/2.5 mL [1 vial], and iodine I 131 tositumomab 1.1 mg/mL and 5.6 mCi/mL (20 mL) [1 or 2 vials] [DSC]

◆ **Totect** *see Dexrazoxane on page 593*

◆ **tPA** *see Alteplase on page 97*

◆ **tRA** *see Tretinoin (Systemic) on page 1830*

Trabectedin (tra BEK te din)

Related Information
Common Toxicity Criteria *on page 2242*

Management of Chemotherapy-Induced Nausea and Vomiting in Adults *on page 2253*

Management of Drug Extravasations *on page 2271*

Safe Handling of Hazardous Drugs *on page 2379*

Brand Names: US Yondelis

Brand Names: Canada Yondelis

Index Terms Ecteinascidin; Ecteinascidin 743; ET-743

Pharmacologic Category Antineoplastic Agent, Miscellaneous

Use Soft tissue sarcoma: Treatment of unresectable or metastatic soft tissue sarcoma (liposarcoma or leiomyosarcoma) in patients who have received a prior anthracycline-containing regimen.

Labeled Contraindications

Known, severe hypersensitivity (including anaphylaxis) to trabectedin or any component of the formulation

Canadian labeling: Additional contraindications (not in the US labeling): Active serious or uncontrolled infection; breastfeeding

Pregnancy Considerations Animal reproduction studies have not been conducted. Based on the mechanism of action, trabectedin may cause fetal harm if administered during pregnancy. Women of reproductive potential should use effective contraception during and for at least 2 months after treatment. Males with partners of reproductive potential should use effective contraception during and for at least 5 months following treatment. Trabectedin may cause decreased fertility in males and females.

Breastfeeding Considerations It is not known if trabectedin is present in breast milk. Due to the potential for serious adverse reactions in the breastfed infant, the manufacturer recommends discontinuing breastfeeding during trabectedin treatment.

Warnings/Precautions Anemia, neutropenia, and thrombocytopenia commonly occur; neutropenic fever and neutropenic sepsis (with fatalities) have been reported. The median onset for first occurrence of grade 3/4 neutropenia was 16 days (range: 8 days to ~10 months) and median time to recovery was 13 days (range: 3 days to ~2 months). Monitor blood counts prior to each dose and periodically throughout treatment cycle. Withhold treatment for neutrophil count <1,500/mm^3. Reduce dose (permanently) for life-threatening or prolonged severe neutropenia in the preceding cycle.

Trabectedin may cause rhabdomyolysis and musculoskeletal toxicity (some fatal). CPK elevations occurred in nearly one-third of patients receiving trabectedin; grade 3 and 4 CPK elevations, some complicated by renal failure, occurred. The median time to first occurrence of grade 3 or 4 CPK elevation was 2 months (range: 1 to 11.5 months) and the median time to complete resolution was 14 days (range: 5 to 30 days). Monitor CPK levels prior to each dose; withhold treatment for CPK levels >2.5 times ULN; discontinue permanently if rhabdomyolysis occurs. Capillary leak syndrome (CLS) has been reported, including serious cases resulting in death. Symptoms include hypotension, edema, and hypoalbuminemia; monitor for signs/symptoms of CLS. Discontinue if CLS develops and manage as appropriate.

Cardiomyopathy, including HF, decreased ejection fraction, diastolic dysfunction, or right ventricular dysfunction, has been observed; some events were grades 3 and 4. The median time to development of grades 3 and 4 cardiomyopathy was ~5 months (range: 1 to 15 months). Monitor left ventricular ejection fraction (LVEF) by echocardiogram or MUGA scan prior to treatment initiation and every 2 to 3 months until trabectedin is discontinued. Withhold treatment if LVEF is below the lower limit of normal (LLN); permanently discontinue for symptomatic cardiomyopathy or persistent ventricular dysfunction that does not recover to LLN within 3 weeks. Patients with a history of New York Heart Association class II, III, or IV heart failure or abnormal LVEF were excluded from the sarcoma study. Pulmonary embolism has been reported.

Hepatotoxicity (including hepatic failure) may occur with trabectedin. Grade 3 and 4 LFT elevations (AST, ALT, total bilirubin, or alkaline phosphatase) occurred in over one-third of patients. The median onset for grade 3/4 ALT or AST elevations was 29 days (range: 3 days to 11.5 months) and the median time to resolution was 13 days (range: 4 days to ~4 months). Drug-induced liver injury (ALT or AST elevation >3 times ULN, alkaline phosphatase <2 times ULN, and total bilirubin ≥2 times ULN) and ALT or AST elevations >8 times ULN have been reported. Monitor LFTs prior to each dose; elevated LFTs may require treatment interruption, dose reduction, and/or discontinuation (based on severity and duration). Premedication with dexamethasone (4 mg twice daily the day prior to administration) has been reported to reduce the incidence of hepatotoxicity (Grosso 2006). Patients with bilirubin above the ULN or AST or ALT >2.5 times the ULN were excluded from the sarcoma clinical trial. Symptoms of hypersensitivity reactions have been reported.

Vesicant; ensure proper needle or catheter placement prior to and during infusion. Infuse through a central line. Avoid extravasation. Extravasation of trabectedin with subsequent tissue necrosis requiring debridement has been reported; evidence of necrosis may be delayed up to 1 week after extravasation. Trabectedin is associated with a moderate emetic potential; antiemetics are recommended to prevent nausea and vomiting (Roila 2016). Nausea and vomiting are common; corticosteroid premedication (eg, dexamethasone) is recommended; other antiemetics may also be needed. Constipation and diarrhea (generally mild) also commonly occur. Potentially significant drug-drug interactions may exist, requiring dose or frequency adjustment, additional monitoring, and/or selection of alternative therapy.

Adverse Reactions

>10%:

Cardiovascular: Peripheral edema (28%)

Central nervous system: Fatigue (69%), headache (25%), insomnia (15%)

Endocrine & metabolic: Hypoalbuminemia (63%)

Gastrointestinal: Nausea (75%), vomiting (46%), constipation (37%), decreased appetite (37%), diarrhea (35%)

Hematologic & oncologic: Anemia (96%; grades 3/4: 19%), neutropenia (66%; grades 3/4: 43%), thrombocytopenia (59%; grades 3/4: 21%)

Hepatic: Increased serum ALT (90%), increased serum AST (84%), increased serum alkaline phosphokinase (70%), hyperbilirubinemia (13%)

Neuromuscular & skeletal: Increased creatine phosphokinase (32% to 33%), arthralgia (15%), myalgia (12%)

Renal: Increased serum creatinine (46%)

Respiratory: Dyspnea (25%)

1% to 10%:

Cardiovascular: Pulmonary embolism (<10%), cardiomyopathy (6%)

Central nervous system: Hypoesthesia (<10%), paresthesia (<10%), peripheral neuropathy (<10%)

Frequency not defined:

Hepatic: Hepatic failure

Hypersensitivity: Anaphylaxis

<1%, postmarketing, and/or case reports: Capillary leak syndrome, hepatotoxicity, rhabdomyolysis

Drug Interactions

Metabolism/Transport Effects Substrate of CYP3A4 (major), P-glycoprotein; **Note:** Assignment of Major/Minor substrate status based on clinically relevant drug interaction potential

Avoid Concomitant Use

Avoid concomitant use of Trabectedin with any of the following: Alcohol (Ethyl); BCG (Intravesical); Conivaptan; CYP3A4 Inducers (Strong); CYP3A4 Inhibitors (Moderate); CYP3A4 Inhibitors (Strong); Deferiprone; Dipyrone; Fusidic Acid (Systemic); Idelalisib; Natalizumab; Pimecrolimus; St John's Wort; Tacrolimus (Topical); Vaccines (Live)

Increased Effect/Toxicity

Trabectedin may increase the levels/effects of: CloZAPine; Deferiprone; Fingolimod; Leflunomide; Natalizumab; Tofacitinib; Vaccines (Live)

The levels/effects of Trabectedin may be increased by: Alcohol (Ethyl); Conivaptan; CYP3A4 Inhibitors (Moderate); CYP3A4 Inhibitors (Strong); Dasatinib; Denosumab; Dipyrone; Fosaprepitant; Fusidic Acid (Systemic); HMG-CoA Reductase Inhibitors; Idelalisib; Ocrelizumab; Palbociclib; Palifermin; P-glycoprotein/ABCB1 Inhibitors; Pimecrolimus; Promazine; Ranolazine; Roflumilast; Simeprevir; Stiripentol; Tacrolimus (Topical); Trastuzumab

Decreased Effect

Trabectedin may decrease the levels/effects of: BCG (Intravesical); Coccidioides immitis Skin Test; Lenograstim; Nivolumab; Sipuleucel-T; Tertomotide; Vaccines (Inactivated); Vaccines (Live)

The levels/effects of Trabectedin may be decreased by: Bosentan; CYP3A4 Inducers (Moderate); CYP3A4 Inducers (Strong); Dabrafenib; Deferasirox; Echinacea; Sarilumab; Siltuximab; St John's Wort; Tocilizumab

◄ **Food Interactions** Coadministration with grapefruit or grapefruit juice may increase trabectedin plasma concentrations. Management: Avoid concomitant administration with grapefruit or grapefruit juice.

Hazardous Drugs Handling Considerations

Hazardous agent (NIOSH 2016 [group 1] criteria).

Use appropriate precautions for receiving, handling, administration, and disposal. Gloves (single) should be worn during receiving, unpacking, and placing in storage.

NIOSH recommends double gloving, a protective gown, ventilated engineering controls (a class II biological safety cabinet or a compounding aseptic containment isolator), and closed system transfer devices (CSTDs) for preparation. Double gloving, a gown, and (if dosage form allows) CSTDs are required during administration (NIOSH 2016).

Storage/Stability Store intact vials at 2°C to 8°C (36°F to 46°F). Solutions diluted for infusion in NS or D5W should be used within 30 hours of reconstitution (infusion should be completed within that 30 hours).

Preparation for Administration Reconstitute the 1 mg vial with 20 mL SWFI resulting in a reconstituted concentration of 0.05 mg/mL. Shake until completely dissolved. Immediately after reconstitution, further dilute for infusion in 500 mL NS or D5W. Diluted solution is compatible in type I glass, polyvinyl chloride (PVC) and polyethylene (PE) bags and tubing, PE and polypropylene (PP) mixture bags, polyethersulfone (PES) inline filters, titanium, platinum, or plastic ports, silicone and polyurethane catheters, and pumps with PVC, PE, or PE/PP contact surfaces. Do not mix with other medications.

Mechanism of Action Trabectedin is a marine-derived compound (alkylating agent) which blocks the cell cycle at the G_2/M phase by covalently binding to the minor DNA groove, bending the helix toward the major groove and altering DNA transcription (Garcia-Carbonero 2005). Affects activity of DNA binding proteins, transcription factors and DNA repair mechanism, leading to cell death.

Pharmacodynamics/Kinetics

Distribution: V_{dss}: >5,000 L

Protein binding: ~97%; to plasma proteins

Metabolism: Extensively hepatic; via CYP3A4

Half-life elimination: ~175 hours

Excretion: Feces (58%; only negligible amounts as unchanged drug); urine (6%; only negligible amounts as unchanged drug)

Dosing

Adult & Geriatric Note: Prior to each treatment cycle, ANC should be ≥1,500/mm³, platelets ≥100,000/mm³ total bilirubin ≤ ULN, and alkaline phosphatase, ALT, AST, and CPK ≤2.5 times ULN.

Premedications: Administer dexamethasone 20 mg IV 30 minutes prior to each infusion. Trabectedin is associated with a moderate emetic potential (Roila 2016); additional antiemetics may be considered.

Soft tissue sarcoma, unresectable/metastatic: IV: 1.5 mg/m² continuous infusion over 24 hours once every 3 weeks; continue until disease progression or unacceptable toxicity (Demetri 2016).

Ovarian cancer, relapsed, platinum sensitive (off-label use): IV: 1.1 mg/m² over 3 hours every 3 weeks (in combination with doxorubicin liposomal), continue as long as clinical benefit is demonstrated or until disease progression or confirmed complete response or for 2 or more cycles beyond complete response (Monk 2010; Monk 2012; Poveda 2011). Delay treatment and/or reduce the trabectedin dose (to 0.9 mg/m^2, then to 0.75 mg/m^2) for toxicities (doxorubicin liposomal may also require modification), consider discontinuing if a second dose reduction is not tolerated (Monk 2010).

Renal Impairment

CrCl ≥30 mL/minute: No dosage adjustment is necessary.

CrCl <30 mL/minute or ESRD: There is no dosage adjustment provided in the manufacturer's labeling (has not been studied).

Hemodialysis: Hemodialysis is not expected to enhance elimination of trabectedin.

Hepatic Impairment

Hepatic impairment prior to treatment:

Mild impairment (bilirubin 1 to 1.5 times ULN and any AST or ALT): No initial dosage adjustment necessary.

Moderate impairment (bilirubin 1.5 to 3 times ULN and AST or ALT <8 times ULN: Reduce dose from 1.5 mg/m^2 to 0.9 mg/m^2.

Severe impairment: (bilirubin >3 to 10 times ULN and any AST or ALT): Do not administer.

Hepatotoxicity during treatment:

Recommended dose reduction levels in patients with mild or moderate hepatic impairment at baseline (once a dose is reduced it should not be increased in subsequent cycles):

Mild impairment:

First dose reduction: 1.2 mg/m^2 once every 3 weeks.

Second dose reduction: 1 mg/m^2 once every 3 weeks.

Moderate impairment:

First dose reduction: 0.6 mg/m^2 once every 3 weeks.

Second dose reduction: 0.3 mg/m^2 once every 3 weeks.

Total bilirubin >ULN: Delay dose for up to 3 weeks and reduce the next dose by one dose level

AST or ALT >2.5 times ULN: Delay dose for up to 3 weeks

AST or ALT >5 times ULN during prior cycle: Delay dose for up to 3 weeks and reduce the next dose by one dose level

Alkaline phosphatase >2.5 times ULN: Delay dose for up to 3 weeks and reduce the next dose by one dose level

Severe liver dysfunction (bilirubin 2 times ULN and AST or ALT 3 times ULN with alkaline phosphatase <2 times ULN in prior treatment cycle in patients with normal hepatic function at baseline): Permanently discontinue.

Exacerbation of hepatic dysfunction in patients with preexisting moderate impairment: Permanently discontinue.

Adverse reactions with trabectedin administered at 0.3 mg/m^2 (in patients with preexisting moderate hepatic impairment) and requiring further dose reduction: Permanently discontinue.

Obesity *ASCO Guidelines for appropriate chemotherapy dosing in obese adults with cancer:* Utilize patient's actual body weight (full weight) for calculation of body surface area- or weight-based dosing, particularly when the intent of therapy is curative; manage regimen-related toxicities in the same manner as for nonobese patients; if a dose reduction is utilized due to toxicity, consider resumption of full weight-based dosing with subsequent cycles, especially if cause of toxicity (eg, hepatic or renal impairment) is resolved (Griggs 2012).

Adjustment for Toxicity

Soft tissue sarcoma:

Recommended dose reduction levels (once a dose is reduced it should not be increased in subsequent cycles):

First dose reduction: 1.2 mg/m^2 once every 3 weeks

Second dose reduction: 1 mg/m^2 once every 3 weeks

Hematologic toxicity:

ANC <1,500/mm^3: Delay dose for up to 3 weeks

ANC <1,000/mm^3 with fever or infection or <500/mm^3 lasting >5 days during prior cycle: Delay dose for up to 3 weeks and reduce the next dose by one dose level

Platelets <100,000/mm^3: Delay dose for up to 3 weeks

Platelets <25,000/mm^3 during prior cycle: Delay dose for up to 3 weeks and reduce the next dose by one dose level

Nonhematologic toxicity:

Creatine phosphokinase >2.5 times ULN: Delay dose for up to 3 weeks

Creatine phosphokinase >5 times ULN during prior cycle: Delay dose for up to 3 weeks and reduce the next dose by one dose level

Decreased left ventricular ejection fraction (LVEF): Less than the lower limit of normal (LLN) or clinical evidence of cardiomyopathy: Delay dose for up to 3 weeks

Decreased LVEF: Absolute decrease of 10% or more from baseline and less than the LLN or clinical evidence of cardiomyopathy during prior cycle: Delay dose for up to 3 weeks and reduce the next dose by one dose level

Other nonhematologic toxicity: Grade 3 or 4: Delay dose for up to 3 weeks and reduce the next dose by one dose level

Adverse reactions with trabectedin administered at 1 mg/m^2 (in patients with normal hepatic function) or 0.3 mg/m^2 (in patients with preexisting moderate hepatic impairment; refer to Dosing: Hepatic Impairment) and requiring further dose reduction: Permanently discontinue.

Capillary leak syndrome: Discontinue treatment.

Persistent adverse events requiring a delay of more than 3 weeks: Permanently discontinue.

Combination Regimens

Ovarian cancer: Trabectedin-Doxorubicin (Liposomal) (Ovarian) on page 2215

Administration Trabectedin is associated with a moderate emetic potential; antiemetics are recommended to prevent nausea and vomiting (Roila 2016).

Infuse through a central line with a 0.2 micron polyethersulfone filter. Infusion must be completed within 30 hours of reconstitution. Premedicate with a corticosteroid (eg, dexamethasone 20 mg IV) 30 minutes prior to treatment; additional antiemetics may be needed.

Soft tissue sarcoma: Single-agent therapy: Infuse as a continuous infusion over 24 hours

Ovarian cancer (off-label use): Combination therapy with doxorubicin liposomal: Administer doxorubicin liposomal first (flush line with D5W) then follow with trabectedin infusion over 3 hours (Monk 2010).

Vesicant; ensure proper needle or catheter placement prior to and during infusion; avoid extravasation.

Extravasation management: If extravasation occurs, stop infusion immediately and disconnect (leave cannula/needle in place); gently aspirate extravasated solution (do **NOT** flush the line); remove needle/cannula; elevate extremity.

Vesicant/Extravasation Risk Vesicant

Emetic Potential Moderate (30% to 90%)

Monitoring Parameters CBC with differential (baseline, prior to each dose, and periodically throughout treatment cycles); total bilirubin (prior to each cycle; more frequently if clinically indicated), ALT, AST, and alkaline phosphatase (prior to each cycle; more frequently if clinically indicated); renal function (baseline and during treatment); CPK (prior to each treatment cycle), evaluate LVEF via MUGA or echocardiogram (baseline and every 2 to 3 months); monitor for signs/symptoms of capillary leak syndrome; monitor infusion site for signs/symptoms of extravasation

Dietary Considerations Avoid grapefruit and grapefruit juice.

Dosage Forms Excipient information presented when available (limited, particularly for generics); consult specific product labeling.

Solution Reconstituted, Intravenous:

Yondelis: 1 mg (1 ea)

Trametinib (tra ME ti nib)

Related Information

Management of Chemotherapy-Induced Nausea and Vomiting in Adults on page 2253

Brand Names: US Mekinist

Brand Names: Canada Mekinist

Index Terms GSK1120212; Trametinib Dimethyl Sulfoxide

Pharmacologic Category Antineoplastic Agent, MEK Inhibitor

Use

Melanoma (metastatic or unresectable): Treatment of unresectable or metastatic melanoma in patients with a BRAF V600E or BRAF V600K mutation (as detected by an approved test), either as a single-agent or in combination with dabrafenib.

Limitations of use: Trametinib is not indicated for use in melanoma patients who have received prior BRAF-inhibitor therapy.

Non-small cell lung cancer (metastatic): Treatment of metastatic non-small cell lung cancer (NSCLC) in patients with BRAF V600E mutation as detected by an approved test (in combination with dabrafenib).

Labeled Contraindications

There are no contraindications listed in the manufacturer's US labeling.

Canadian labeling: Hypersensitivity to trametinib or any component of the formulation.

Pregnancy Considerations Adverse effects were observed in animal reproduction studies. Based on its mechanism of action, trametinib would be expected to cause fetal harm if administered to a pregnant woman. Females of reproductive potential should use a highly effective contraceptive during therapy and for 4 months after treatment is complete. When trametinib is used in combination with dabrafenib, a highly effective nonhormonal contraceptive method should be used (dabrafenib may diminish efficacy of hormonal contraceptives). Fertility may also be impaired in females. Due to a risk for impaired spermatogenesis, males who may want to father a child should seek fertility/family planning counseling prior to initiating combination therapy with dabrafenib.

◀ **Breastfeeding Considerations** It is not known if trametinib is present in breast milk. Due to the potential for serious adverse reactions in the breastfed infant, breastfeeding is not recommended by the manufacturer during treatment and for 4 months after the last dose.

Warnings/Precautions Cardiac events such as heart failure, left ventricular dysfunction, or decreased left ventricular ejection fraction (LVEF) were observed in clinical trials (for single-agent trametinib and when used in combination with dabrafenib). The median time to onset of cardiomyopathy in melanoma patients for single-agent trametinib was ~2 months (range: 16 to 156 days) and ~8 months (range: ~1 to 25 months) when used in combination with dabrafenib. The median time of onset of cardiomyopathy in patients with NSCLC was 6.7 months (range: 1.4 to 14.1 months). In some patients, cardiomyopathy developed within the first month of treatment. Assess LVEF (by echocardiogram or MUGA scan) prior to therapy initiation, at one month, and then at 2- to 3-month intervals while on therapy. Cardiac dysfunction may require treatment interruption, dosage reduction, or discontinuation; such measures resulted in resolution of cardiomyopathy in some patients. May cause hypertension; monitor blood pressure. Venous thromboembolism events (some fatal) may occur (was observed when used in combination with dabrafenib). DVT and PE occurred at an increased incidence with combination therapy. Patients should seek immediate medical attention with symptoms of DVT or PE (shortness of breath, chest pain, arm/leg swelling). Withhold trametinib for uncomplicated DVT or PE; may resume at a lower dose if improves within 3 weeks; permanently discontinue trametinib for life-threatening PE. Interstitial lung disease (ILD) and pneumonitis were observed in clinical trials; the median time to initial presentation in melanoma patients was ~5 months (range: 2 to ~6 months). Monitor for new or progressive pulmonary symptoms (eg, cough, dyspnea, hypoxia, pleural effusion, infiltrates); withhold treatment if symptoms occur; permanently discontinue with diagnosis of ILD or pneumonitis. Neutropenia (including grade 3 and 4 events) has been observed when used in combination with dabrafenib. Monitor complete blood counts at baseline and as clinically needed during therapy. Elevated liver function tests have been reported with trametinib, including grade 3 and 4 events. Monitor hepatic function as clinically necessary.

Dermatologic toxicity (eg, rash, dermatitis, acneiform rash, palmar-plantar erythrodysesthesia syndrome, and erythema) was commonly observed in trametinib-treated patients (either as a single-agent or when used in combination with dabrafenib); some patients required hospitalization for severe toxicity or for secondary skin infections. In melanoma studies, the median time to onset and resolution of skin toxicity for single-agent trametinib was 15 days (range: 1 to 221 days) and 48 days (range: 1 to 282 days), respectively. The median time to onset and resolution of skin toxicity for combination therapy was 2 months (range: 1 day to 22 months) and 1.2 months (range: 1 day to ~24 months), respectively in melanoma studies. Monitor for dermatologic toxicity and signs/symptoms of secondary infections. Treatment interruption, dose reductions, and/or therapy discontinuation may be necessary. New primary cutaneous malignancies (which are associated with dabrafenib as single-agent therapy) may occur when trametinib is given in combination with dabrafenib. The incidence of basal cell carcinoma (BCC) in melanoma patients is ~3% for combination therapy versus 6% for single-agent dabrafenib. The median time to BCC diagnosis ranged from ~3 to 24 months for patients receiving combination therapy for the treatment of melanoma. Cutaneous squamous cell carcinomas (cuSCC), including keratoacanthoma, occurred at a lower rate for combination therapy in melanoma patients compared to single-agent dabrafenib (3% vs 10%, respectively), with a median time to diagnosis ranging from ~2 to 17 months for combination therapy. Cases of cuSCC also occurred in patients with NSCLC, with a first occurrence onset ranging from 25 days to ~12 months. New primary melanoma occurred rarely in patients receiving trametinib. Dermatologic exams should be performed prior to initiation of combination therapy, every 2 months while receiving combination treatment, and for up to 6 months following discontinuation.

Retinal pigment epithelial detachments (RPED) and retinal vein occlusion were seen in clinical trials (rare). Detachments were typically bilateral and multifocal and occurred in the central macular area of the retina. Retinal vein occlusion may lead to macular edema, degeneration, decreased visual function, neovascularization, and glaucoma. Promptly (within 24 hours) refer patients for ophthalmological evaluations if loss of vision or other visual disturbances occur. Ophthalmic exams (including retinal evaluation) should be performed periodically during treatment and with visual disturbances. Interrupt trametinib therapy for RPED; may resume if resolves within 3 weeks; reduce the dose or discontinue if not resolved within 3 weeks. Permanently discontinue if retinal vein occlusion develops. Uveitis and iritis have been reported when trametinib is used in combination with dabrafenib and are managed symptomatically with ophthalmic steroid and mydriatic drops (does not require alteration in trametinib therapy).

Serious febrile reactions and fever (any severity) accompanied by hypotension, rigors/chills, dehydration, or renal failure may occur when trametinib is used in combination with dabrafenib. The incidence and severity were higher with combination therapy than with single-agent dabrafenib; the median time to onset of fever was 1.2 months (range: 1 to 23 days) and duration was 3 days (range: 1 day to 1.7 months) for patients receiving combination therapy for the treatment of melanoma. Withhold trametinib for fever >104°F (if using in combination, withhold dabrafenib for fever ≥101.3°F) or for any fever with rigors/chills, hypotension, dehydration, or renal failure (evaluate for infection); may require prophylactic antipyretics as secondary prophylaxis upon therapy resumption. Administer corticosteroids (eg, prednisone 10 mg daily or equivalent) for at least 5 days for second or subsequent episodes of pyrexia if temperature does not return to baseline within 3 days of fever onset, or for pyrexia associated with complications (eg, dehydration, hypotension, severe chills/rigors with no evidence of active infection). Hemorrhage, including symptomatic bleeding in a critical area/organ, may occur with trametinib, either as a single agent or in combination with dabrafenib. Major bleeding events (some fatal) included intracranial or gastrointestinal hemorrhage; may require treatment interruption and dosage reduction; permanently discontinue trametinib (and dabrafenib) for all grade 4 hemorrhagic events and any grade 3 event that does not improve with therapy interruption. Colitis and GI perforation, including fatal cases, have been reported with monotherapy and when administered concomitantly with dabrafenib; monitor closely for development of colitis and GI perforations. While not reported with single-agent trametinib, hyperglycemia may occur while on combination therapy with dabrafenib; may require initiation of insulin or oral hypoglycemic agent therapy (or an increased dose if already taking); monitor serum glucose at baseline and as clinically necessary in patients with preexisting diabetes or hyperglycemia. Instruct patients to report symptoms of severe hyperglycemia (eg, polydipsia, polyuria).

Trametinib is not indicated for treatment of patients with melanoma who have progressed on prior BRAF-inhibitor therapy. Prior to initiating therapy, confirm BRAF mutation status with an approved test; approved for use in melanoma patients with BRAF V600K and BRAF V600E mutations and NSCLC patients with BRAF V600E mutation. Data regarding use in melanoma patients with BRAF V600K mutation is limited; compared to BRAF V600E mutation, lower response rates have been observed with BRAF V600K mutation. Data regarding other less common BRAF V600 mutations in melanoma is lacking. There are case reports of noncutaneous malignancies, including pancreatic cancer (KRAS mutation-positive), colorectal cancer (recurrent NRAS mutation-positive), hand and neck cancer, and glioblastoma, with combination therapy; monitor for signs/symptoms of noncutaneous malignancies. No trametinib dosage modification is necessary for new primary cutaneous and noncutaneous malignancies; dabrafenib should be permanently discontinued if RAS mutation-positive noncutaneous malignancies develop. Serious adverse reactions (tumor promotion, hemolytic anemia), which occur with single-agent dabrafenib, may also occur when trametinib is administered in combination with dabrafenib. Potentially significant drug-drug interactions may exist, requiring dose or frequency adjustment, additional monitoring, and/or selection of alternative therapy.

Adverse Reactions
Adverse reactions reported with monotherapy:
>10%:

Cardiovascular: Hypertension (15%), cardiomyopathy (7% to 11%; defined as cardiac failure, decreased left ventricular ejection fraction, or left ventricular dysfunction)

Dermatologic: Skin toxicity (87%, most commonly dermatitis acneiform rash, palmar-plantar erythrodysesthesia, erythema, skin rash; severe: 12%; severe toxicity and secondary skin infection requiring hospitalization: 6%; skin rash (57%; grades 3/4: 8%), acneiform eruption (19%; grades 3/4: <1%), xeroderma (11%)

Endocrine & metabolic: Hypoalbuminemia (42%)

Gastrointestinal: Diarrhea (43%), stomatitis (15%), abdominal pain (13%)

Hematologic & oncologic: Anemia (38%; grades 3/4: 2%), lymphedema (32%; includes edema, peripheral edema; grades 3/4: 1%), hemorrhage (13%; includes epistaxis, gingival bleeding, hematochezia, rectal hemorrhage, melena, vaginal hemorrhage, hemorrhoidal hemorrhage, hematuria, conjunctival hemorrhage; grades 3/4: <1%)

Hepatic: Increased serum AST (60%), increased serum ALT (39%), increased serum alkaline phosphatase (24%)

1% to 10%:

Cardiovascular: Decreased left ventricular ejection fraction (5%, ≥20% below baseline), bradycardia

Central nervous system: Dizziness

Dermatologic: Paronychia (10%), pruritus (10%; grades 3/4: 2%), cellulitis, folliculitis, pustular rash

Gastrointestinal: Dysgeusia, xerostomia

Neuromuscular & skeletal: Rhabdomyolysis

Ophthalmic: Blurred vision, dry eye syndrome

Respiratory: Interstitial pulmonary disease (≤2%), pneumonitis (≤2%)

<1%, postmarketing, and/or case reports: Retinal detachment, retinal vein occlusion

Adverse reactions reported with dual therapy (trametinib plus dabrafenib):

>10%:

Cardiovascular: Hypertension (25% to 26%), peripheral edema (21% to 25%; includes edema and lymphedema; grades 3/4: ≤1%), prolonged Q-T Interval on ECG (4% QTcF increased >60 msec; <1% QTcF prolongation to >500 msec)

Central nervous system: Headache (30% to 33%), chills (31%; grades 3/4: <1%), dizziness (11% to 14%)

Dermatologic: Skin toxicity (55% any skin toxicity; severe toxicity: <1%), skin rash (32% to 42%; includes generalized rash, pruritic rash, erythematous rash, papular rash, vesicular rash, macular rash, maculopapular rash, folliculitis rash; grades 3/4: ≤1%), xeroderma (10% to 12%)

Endocrine & metabolic: Hyperglycemia (60% to 65%; grades 3/4: 5% to 6%), hypoalbuminemia (48% to 53%), hypophosphatemia (38%), exacerbation of diabetes mellitus (27%), hyponatremia (24% to 25%)

Gastrointestinal: Nausea (34% to 35%), diarrhea (30% to 31%), vomiting (25% to 27%), abdominal pain (18% to 26%), constipation (13%)

Hematologic & oncologic: Neutropenia (46% to 50%; grades 3/4: 6% to 7%), anemia (43%; grades 3/4: 2%), lymphocytopenia (32% to 38%; grades 3/4: 8% to 9%), thrombocytopenia (19% to 21%; grades 3/4: <1%), hemorrhage (18% to 19%; includes epistaxis, hematochezia, decreased hemoglobin, purpura, rectal hemorrhage; grades 3/4: 2%; includes hepatic hematoma, duodenal ulcer hemorrhage)

Hepatic: Increased serum AST (59% to 60%), increased serum alkaline phosphatase (49% to 50%), increased serum ALT (44% to 48%)

Neuromuscular & skeletal: Arthralgia (25% to 26%), myalgia (13% to 15%)

Respiratory: Cough (20% to 21%)

Miscellaneous: Fever (54% to 57%; grades 3/4: 5% to 7%), febrile reaction (complicated with dehydration: 2%, complicated with severe chills/rigors: <1%, complicated with renal failure: <1%, complicated with syncope: <1%)

1% to 10%:

Cardiovascular: Bradycardia (<10%), cardiomyopathy (6%), venous thromboembolism (3%; deep vein thrombosis, pulmonary embolism), hypertension

Central nervous system: Intracranial hemorrhage (1%)

Gastrointestinal: Gastrointestinal hemorrhage (6%), pancreatitis

Hematologic & oncologic: Basal cell carcinoma (3%), squamous cell carcinoma of skin (3%; including keratoacanthoma)

Neuromuscular & skeletal: Rhabdomyolysis (<10%)

Respiratory: Pneumonitis (1%)

<1%, postmarketing, and/or case reports: Malignant melanoma

Drug Interactions

Metabolism/Transport Effects Inhibits CYP2C8 (weak)

Avoid Concomitant Use

Avoid concomitant use of Trametinib with any of the following: Amodiaquine

Increased Effect/Toxicity

Trametinib may increase the levels/effects of: Amodiaquine; Dabrafenib

Decreased Effect There are no known significant interactions involving a decrease in effect.

◀ **Food Interactions** Administration with a high-fat, high-calorie meal decreased AUC by 24%, C_{max} by 70%, and delayed T_{max} by ~4 hours. Management: Administer 1 hour before or 2 hours after a meal.

Hazardous Drugs Handling Considerations

Hazardous agent (NIOSH 2016 [group 1]).

Use appropriate precautions for receiving, handling, administration, and disposal. Gloves (single) should be worn during receiving, unpacking, and placing in storage. NIOSH recommends single gloving for administration of intact tablets or capsules (NIOSH 2016).

Storage/Stability Store refrigerated at 2°C to 8°C (36°F to 46°F); do not freeze. Dispense in original bottle; do not remove desiccant. Protect from light and moisture. Do not transfer to pill boxes.

Mechanism of Action Trametinib reversibly and selectively inhibits mitogen-activated extracellular kinase (MEK) 1 and 2 activation and kinase activity. MEK is a downstream effector of the protein kinase B-raf (BRAF); BRAF V600 mutations result in constitutive activation of the BRAF pathway (including MEK1 and MEK2). Through inhibition of MEK 1 and 2 kinase activity, trametinib causes decreased cellular proliferation, cell cycle arrest, and increased apoptosis (Kim 2013). The combination of trametinib and dabrafenib allows for greater inhibition of the MAPK pathway, resulting in BRAF V600 melanoma cell death (Flaherty 2012). Trametinib plus dabrafenib has been reported to synergistically inhibit cell growth in lung cancer cell lines which are BRAF V600E-mutant (Planchard 2016).

Pharmacodynamics/Kinetics

Absorption: Rapid; decreased with a high-fat, high-calorie meal

Distribution: 214 L

Protein binding: ~97% to plasma proteins

Metabolism: Predominantly deacetylation (via hydrolytic enzymes) alone or with mono-oxygenation or in combination with glucuronidation

Bioavailability: 72%

Half-life elimination: 4 to 5 days

Time to peak: 1.5 hours; delayed with a high-fat, high-calorie meal

Excretion: Feces (>80%); urine (<20% with <0.1% as unchanged drug)

Dosing

Adult Note: Confirm BRAF V600 mutation status prior to treatment initiation.

> **Melanoma (metastatic or unresectable) (with BRAF V600E or BRAF V600K mutations):** Oral: 2 mg once daily (either as a single-agent or in combination with dabrafenib), continue until disease progression or unacceptable toxicity.

> **Non-small cell lung cancer (metastatic) (with BRAF V600E mutation):** Oral: 2 mg once daily (in combination with dabrafenib); continue until disease progression or unacceptable toxicity (Planchard 2016).

Missed doses: Do not take a missed dose within 12 hours of the next dose.

Renal Impairment

Mild to moderate impairment (GFR ≥30 mL/minute/1.73 m²): No dosage adjustment necessary.

Severe impairment (GFR <30 mL/minute/1.73 m²): There are no dosage adjustments provided in the manufacturer's labeling (has not been studied); however, renal excretion is low and is unlikely to affect drug exposure.

Hepatic Impairment

Mild impairment (total bilirubin ≤ ULN and AST > ULN **or** total bilirubin >1 to 1.5 times ULN with any AST): No dosage adjustment necessary.

Moderate to severe impairment: There are no dosage adjustments provided in the manufacturer's labeling (has not been studied).

Adjustment for Toxicity

Recommended trametinib dose reductions for toxicity:

First dose reduction: 1.5 mg once daily

Second dose reduction: 1 mg once daily

Subsequent modification (if unable to tolerate 1 mg once daily): Permanently discontinue

Note: If using combination therapy, refer to dabrafenib monograph for recommended dabrafenib dose reductions

Cardiac:

Asymptomatic, 10% or greater absolute decrease in LVEF from baseline and LVEF is below institutional lower limits of normal (LLN) from pretreatment value: Interrupt trametinib therapy for up to 4 weeks. If LVEF improves to normal within 4 weeks following therapy interruption, resume at a lower dose level. If LVEF does not improve to normal within 4 weeks following therapy interruption, permanently discontinue trametinib.

>20% absolute decrease in LVEF from baseline and LVEF is below institutional LLN: Permanently discontinue trametinib.

Symptomatic heart failure: Permanently discontinue trametinib.

Dermatologic:

Intolerable Grade 2 skin toxicity or Grade 3 or 4 skin toxicity: Interrupt trametinib therapy for up to 3 weeks. If toxicity improves within 3 weeks, resume at a lower dose level. If toxicity does not improve within 3 weeks following therapy interruption, permanently discontinue trametinib.

New primary cutaneous malignancies: No trametinib dosage modification is necessary.

Fever: Fever >40°C (104°F) or fever (any severity) complicated by rigors, hypotension, dehydration, or renal failure: Interrupt trametinib therapy until fever resolves, then resume at the same or a lower dose level. May require prophylactic antipyretics (secondary prophylaxis) upon resumption. Administer corticosteroids (eg, prednisone 10 mg daily or equivalent) for at least 5 days for second or subsequent pyrexia if temperature does not return to baseline within 3 days of onset of fever, or for fever associated with complications (eg, dehydration, hypotension, severe chills/rigors with no evidence of active infection).

Hemorrhage:

Grade 3 hemorrhage: Interrupt trametinib therapy. If hemorrhage improves, resume at a lower dose level. If hemorrhage does not improve following therapy interruption, permanently discontinue trametinib.

Grade 4 hemorrhage: Permanently discontinue trametinib.

Ocular:

Uveitis and iritis: No trametinib dosage modification necessary.

Retinal pigment epithelial detachments (RPED): Interrupt trametinib therapy for up to 3 weeks. If improves within 3 weeks following therapy interruption, resume at the same or lower dose level. If RPED does not improve within 3 weeks following therapy interruption, reduce dose or permanently discontinue trametinib.

Retinal vein occlusion: Permanently discontinue trametinib.

Pulmonary: Interstitial lung disease or pneumonitis: Permanently discontinue trametinib.

Venous thromboembolism:

Uncomplicated DVT or PE: Interrupt trametinib therapy for up to 3 weeks. If improves to ≤ grade 1 within 3 weeks following therapy interruption, resume at a lower dose level. If toxicity does not improve within 3 weeks following therapy interruption, permanently discontinue trametinib.

Life-threatening PE: Permanently discontinue trametinib.

Other toxicity:

Intolerable Grade 2 adverse reaction or any Grade 3 adverse reaction: Interrupt therapy. If toxicity improves to ≤ grade 1 following therapy interruption, resume at a lower dose level. If toxicity does not improve following therapy interruption, permanently discontinue trametinib.

Grade 4 adverse reaction:

First occurrence: Interrupt trametinib therapy until improves to ≤ grade 1, then resume at a lower dose level **or** permanently discontinue trametinib.

Recurrence: Permanently discontinue trametinib.

New primary noncutaneous malignancy: No trametinib dosage modification is necessary.

Combination Regimens

Lung cancer (non-small cell): Dabrafenib-Trametinib (NSCLC) on page 2083
Melanoma: Dabrafenib-Trametinib (Melanoma) on page 2082

Administration Oral: Administer at least 1 hour before or 2 hours after a meal. Administer dose at the same time each day, whether administered as a single agent or in combination with dabrafenib (when administered in combination with dabrafenib, take the once daily trametinib dose either with the morning or with the evening dabrafenib dose).

Emetic Potential Minimal (<10%)

Monitoring Parameters BRAF V600K or V600E mutation status (prior to treatment); CBC and liver function tests at baseline and periodically; assess LVEF (by echocardiogram or MUGA scan) at baseline, 1 month after therapy initiation, and then at 2- to 3-month intervals; ophthalmological evaluation periodically during treatment and with visual disturbances; monitor for signs/symptoms of pulmonary toxicity (eg, cough dyspnea, hypoxia, pleural effusion, or infiltrates); monitor for dermatologic toxicity and secondary skin infections; blood pressure; diarrhea; signs/symptoms of bleeding, colitis, and GI perforations.

For patients receiving combination therapy with dabrafenib: Blood glucose (baseline and periodically in patients with preexisting diabetes or hyperglycemia); dermatologic exams should be performed prior to treatment initiation, every 2 months while receiving combination treatment, and for up to 6 months following therapy discontinuation. Monitor for signs/symptoms of cutaneous and noncutaneous malignancies and uveitis/iritis.

Monitor adherence.

Dosage Forms Excipient information presented when available (limited, particularly for generics); consult specific product labeling.

Tablet, Oral:

Mekinist: 0.5 mg, 2 mg

◆ **Trametinib Dimethyl Sulfoxide** *see* Trametinib *on page* 1809

Tranexamic Acid (tran eks AM ik AS id)

Brand Names: US Cyklokapron; Lysteda

Brand Names: Canada Cyklokapron; GD-Tranexamic Acid; Tranexamic Acid Injection; Tranexamic Acid Injection BP

Index Terms Cyklokapron

Pharmacologic Category Antifibrinolytic Agent; Antihemophilic Agent; Hemostatic Agent; Lysine Analog

Use

Cyclic heavy menstrual bleeding (oral): Treatment of cyclic heavy menstrual bleeding.

Tooth extraction in patients with hemophilia (injection, oral [Cyklokapron; Canadian product]): Short-term use in hemophilia patients to reduce or prevent hemorrhage and reduce need for replacement therapy during and following tooth extraction

Pregnancy Risk Factor B

Dosing

Adult & Geriatric

Cyclic heavy menstrual bleeding: Oral:

Lysteda: 1,300 mg 3 times daily (3,900 mg/day) for up to 5 days during monthly menstruation

Cyklokapron [Canadian product]: 1,000 to 1,500 mg 3 to 4 times daily

Tooth extraction in patients with hemophilia (in combination with appropriate factor replacement therapy): IV: 10 mg/kg immediately before surgery, then 10 mg/kg 3 to 4 times daily; may be used for 2 to 8 days

IV: 10 mg /kg as a single dose 2 hours prior to procedure (in conjunction with Factor VIII and IX); following procedure, administer oral tranexamic acid for 6 to 8 days

Oral: Cyklokapron [Canadian product]: 25 mg/kg as a single dose 2 hours prior to procedure, then 25 mg/kg 3 to 4 times daily for 6 to 8 days

Off-label uses:

Elective cesarean section, blood loss reduction (off-label use): IV: 1,000 mg over 5 minutes at least 10 minutes prior to skin incision (Gungorduk 2011)

Hereditary angioedema (HAE) (off-label use):

Long-term prophylaxis: Oral: 1,000 to 1,500 mg 2 to 3 times daily; reduce to 500 mg/dose once or twice daily when frequency of attacks reduces (Gompels 2005; Levy 2010) **or** 25 mg/kg/dose administered 2 to 3 times daily (Bowen 2004)

Short-term prophylaxis (eg, for dental work): Oral: 75 mg/kg/day divided 2 to 3 times daily for 5 days before and 2 days after the event (Bowen 2004) **or** 1,000 mg 4 times daily for 48 hours before and after procedure (Gompels 2005)

Treatment of acute HAE attack: Oral, IV: 25 mg/kg/dose (maximum single dose: 1,000 mg) every 3 to 4 hours (maximum: 75 mg/kg/day) (Bowen 2004) **or** 1,000 mg 4 times daily for 48 hours (Gompels 2005)

Hip fracture surgery, blood conservation (off-label use): IV: 15 mg/kg administered at the time of skin incision followed by a second dose (15 mg/kg) 3 hours later (Zufferey 2010). Additional data may be necessary to further define the role of tranexamic acid in this setting.

◀ **Intracranial hemorrhage associated with thrombolytics (plasminogen-activator) (eg, alteplase, reteplase, or tenecteplase) (off-label use):** IV: 10 to 15 mg/kg over 20 minutes (as an alternative to cryoprecipitate); check fibrinogen levels after administration, if fibrinogen <150 mg/dL, cryoprecipitate is recommended (NCS/SCCM [Frontera 2016]).

Orthognathic surgery, blood loss reduction (off-label use): IV: 20 mg/kg over 15 minutes prior to incision (Choi 2009)

Perioperative blood loss reduction in *bilateral* total knee arthroplasty (off-label use): IV:

Three-dose regimen: 10 mg/kg administered as a slow IV infusion 30 minutes before tourniquet deflation for the first operation, 30 minutes before tourniquet deflation for the second operation, and 3 hours after commencement of the second dose (Kim 2014).

Two-dose regimen: 10 or 15 mg/kg administered over 10 minutes before deflation of the first tourniquet, with the second dose administered 3 hours after the first dose (MacGillivray 2011).

Perioperative blood loss reduction in *unilateral* total knee arthroplasty (off-label use): IV:

Intra- and postoperative regimen: 10 mg/kg at least 10 to 30 minutes prior to tourniquet release (deflation) and 10 mg/kg at 3 hours after the first dose (Alvarez 2008; Camarasa 2006; Maniar 2012). Instead of the second dose, a postoperative infusion may be administered at 1 mg/kg/hour for 6 hours (Alvarez 2008).

Pre- and intraoperative regimen: 10 mg/kg at least 20 minutes or immediately before tourniquet inflation and repeated at least 15 minutes prior to deflation or immediately after release of tourniquet (Lozano 2008; Maniar 2012).

Pre-, intra-, and postoperative regimen: 10 mg/kg at least 20 minutes before tourniquet inflation, repeated at least 15 minutes prior to deflation and postoperatively at 3 hours after the second dose (Maniar 2012).

Post-operative bleeding associated with cervical conization (prevention/reduction) (off-label use):

IV/Oral: Intra- and postoperative regimen: 1 g IV infusion during procedure followed by oral therapy 1 g 3 times daily for 14 days, beginning the day after procedure (Grunsdell 1984).

Oral: Postoperative regimen: 1500 mg every 8 hours beginning the evening following the procedure and continuing for 12 days (Rybo 1972).

Postpartum hemorrhage (off-label use): IV: 1,000 mg over 10 minutes given within 3 hours of vaginal birth or cesarean section; if bleeding continues after 30 minutes or stops and restarts within 24 hours after the first dose, a second dose of 1,000 mg may be given (WOMAN Trial Collaborators 2017).

Prevention of dental procedure bleeding in patients on oral anticoagulant therapy (off-label use): Oral rinse: 4.8% solution: Hold 10 mL in mouth and rinse for 2 minutes then spit out. Repeat 4 times daily for 2 days after procedure. **Note:** Patient should not eat or drink for 1 hour after using oral rinse (Carter 2003).

Prevention of perioperative bleeding associated with cardiac surgery (off-label use): IV: Loading dose of 30 mg/kg over 30 minutes (total loading dose includes a test dose administered over the first 10 minutes followed by the remainder of dose) prior to incision, followed by 16 mg/kg/hour until sternal closure; add an additional 2 mg/kg to cardiopulmonary bypass circuit (Fergusson 2008)

or

Loading dose of 10 mg/kg over 20 minutes prior to incision followed by 2 mg/kg/hour continued for 2 hours after transfer to ICU; add a prime dose of 50 mg for a 2.5 L cardiopulmonary bypass circuit; maintenance infusion adjusted for renal insufficiency (Nuttall 2008)

or

Loading dose of 10-15 mg/kg over 10 to 15 minutes, followed by 1 to 1.5 mg/kg/hour. The authors suggest adding 2 to 2.5 mg/kg to cardiopulmonary bypass circuit; however, amounts have varied widely in clinical trials (Gravlee 2008).

Prevention of perioperative bleeding associated with spinal surgery (eg, spinal fusion) (off-label use): IV: 2,000 mg over 20 minutes prior to incision followed by 100 mg/hour during surgery and for 5 hours postoperatively (Elwatidy 2008) **or** 10 mg/kg prior to incision followed by 1 mg/kg/hour for the remainder of the surgery; discontinue at time of wound closure (Wong 2008)

Total hip replacement surgery, blood conservation (off-label use): IV: 10 to 15 mg/kg (or 1,000 mg) administered over 5 to 10 minutes immediately before the operation or 15 minutes before skin incision; the preoperative dose may be followed by 10 mg/kg administered 3 to 12 hours after the operation. Postoperative doses ranged from a 10 mg/kg IV bolus (or 1,000 mg) to a 1 mg/kg/hour infusion over 10 hours (Gandhi 2013; Oremus 2014).

Note: Multiple regimens have been evaluated in varying degrees of evidence quality. The regimen listed here reflects the more commonly used dosing based on a number of prospective randomized controlled trials (Johansson 2005; McConnell 2011; Niskanen 2005; Oremus 2014). Metaanalyses have also been conducted demonstrating significant reduction in blood loss perioperatively without an increased risk of thromboembolic events (Gandhi 2013; Sukeik 2011; Zhou 2013). The use of *intra-articular* tranexamic acid (ie, 1,000 mg/50 mL of NaCl 0.9% sprayed into the wound at the end of the procedure) has also been evaluated demonstrating effectiveness (Alshryda 2014a; Alshryda 2014b).

Transurethral prostatectomy, blood loss reduction (off-label use): Oral: 2,000 mg 3 times daily on the operative and first postoperative day (Rannikko 2004)

Trauma-associated hemorrhage (off-label use): IV: Loading dose: 1,000 mg over 10 minutes, followed by 1,000 mg over the next 8 hours. **Note:** Clinical trial included patients with significant hemorrhage (SBP <90 mm Hg, heart rate >110 bpm, or both) or those at risk of significant hemorrhage. Treatment began within 8 hours of injury; however, every effort should be made to give as soon as possible (ideally within 3 hours of injury since treatment beyond 3 hours has been shown to be significantly less effective and may be associated with harm) (CRASH-2 Trial Collaborators 2010; CRASH-2 Trial Collaborators 2011).

◄   **Traumatic hyphema (off-label use):** Oral: 25 mg/kg administered 3 times daily for 5 to 7 days (Rahmani, 1999; Vangsted, 1983; Varnek, 1980). **Note:** This same regimen may also be used for secondary hemorrhage after an initial traumatic hyphema event.

Pediatric

Cyclic heavy menstrual bleeding: Children ≥12 years (postmenarche) and Adolescents: Oral: Refer to adult dosing.

Hereditary angioedema (HAE) (off-label use): Oral:

Long-term prophylaxis: 20 to 40 mg/kg/day in 2 to 3 divided doses (maximum dose: 3,000 mg daily) (Farkas 2007) **or** 50 mg/kg/day (or 1,000 to 2,000 mg daily; depending on age and size of patient); may consider alternate-day regimen or twice-weekly regimen when frequency of attacks reduces; diarrhea may be a dose-limiting side effect (Gompels 2005)

Short-term prophylaxis: 20 to 40 mg/kg/day in 2 to 3 divided doses (maximum dose: 3,000 mg daily) (Farkas 2007) **or** 500 mg 4 times daily (Gompels 2005). **Note:** For short-term prophylaxis (eg, dental work), initiate 2-5 days before and continue for 2 days after the procedure (Bowen 2004; Gompels 2005).

Prevention of perioperative bleeding associated with cardiac surgery (off-label use): IV: 10 mg/kg given over 30 minutes prior to incision, 10 mg/kg while on cardiopulmonary bypass, and 10 mg/kg administered after protamine reversal (Chauhan 2004a; Chauhan 2004b)

or

Loading dose of 100 mg/kg over 15 minutes prior to incision, followed by 10 mg/kg/hour infusion (continued until ICU transport); add 100 mg/kg to pump reservoir when cardiopulmonary bypass initiated (Reid, 1997)

Prevention of perioperative bleeding associated with craniosynostosis surgery (off-label use): IV: Loading dose of 50 mg/kg over 15 minutes prior to incision, followed by 5 mg/kg/hour (Goobie 2011) **or** 15 mg/kg over 15 minutes prior to incision, followed by 10 mg/kg/hour until skin closure (Dadure 2011)

Prevention of perioperative bleeding associated with spinal surgery (eg, spinal fusion) (off-label use): Children and Adolescents: IV: 10 mg/kg given over 15 minutes prior to incision followed by 1 mg/kg/hour for the remainder of the surgery; discontinue at time of wound closure (Neilipovitz 2001; Verma 2010)

or

100 mg/kg over 15 minutes prior to incision followed by 10 mg/kg/hour until skin closure (Sethna 2005)

or

30 mg/kg over 20 minutes prior to incision followed by 1 mg/kg/hour during surgery and for 5 hours postoperatively (Elwatidy 2008)

Tooth extraction in patients with hemophilia (in combination with appropriate factor replacement therapy): Children and Adolescents: IV: Refer to adult dosing.

Traumatic hyphema (off-label use): Oral: Refer to adult dosing.

Renal Impairment

IV formulation:

Tooth extraction in patients with hemophilia:

Serum creatinine 1.36 to 2.83 mg/dL: Maintenance dose of 10 mg/kg/dose twice daily

Serum creatinine 2.83 to 5.66 mg/dL: Maintenance dose of 10 mg/kg/dose once daily

Serum creatinine >5.66 mg/dL: Maintenance dose of 10 mg/kg/dose every 48 hours **or** 5 mg/kg/dose once daily

Cardiac surgery (the following dose adjustments have been recommended [Nuttall 2008]):

Serum creatinine 1.6 to 3.3 mg/dL: Reduce maintenance infusion to 1.5 mg/kg/hour (based on a 25% reduction from 2 mg/kg/hour)

Serum creatinine 3.3 to 6.6 mg/dL: Reduce maintenance infusion to 1 mg/kg/hour (based on a 50% reduction from 2 mg/kg/hour)

Serum creatinine >6.6 mg/dL: Reduce maintenance infusion to 0.5 mg/kg/hour (based on a 75% reduction from 2 mg/kg/hour)

Oral formulation:

Lysteda:

Serum creatinine >1.4 to 2.8 mg/dL: 1,300 mg twice daily (2,600 mg/day) for up to 5 days

Serum creatinine 2.9 to 5.7 mg/dL: 1,300 mg once daily for up to 5 days

Serum creatinine >5.7 mg/dL: 650 mg once daily for up to 5 days

Cyklokapron [Canadian product]:

Serum creatinine 1.4 to 2.8 mg/dL (120 to 250 micromol/L): 15 mg/kg twice daily

Serum creatinine 2.8 to 5.7 mg/dL (250 to 500 micromol/L): 15 mg/kg every 24 hours

Serum creatinine ≥5.7 mg/dL (≥500 micromol/L): 15 mg/kg every 48 hours

Hepatic Impairment No dosage adjustment is necessary.

Additional Information Complete prescribing information should be consulted for additional detail.

Dosage Forms Excipient information presented when available (limited, particularly for generics); consult specific product labeling.

Solution, Intravenous:

Cyklokapron: 1000 mg/10 mL (10 mL)

Generic: 1000 mg/10 mL (10 mL)

Solution, Intravenous [preservative free]:

Generic: 1000 mg/10 mL (10 mL)

Tablet, Oral:

Lysteda: 650 mg

Generic: 650 mg

Dosage Forms: Canada Information with regard to form, strength, and availability of products uniquely available in Canada but currently not available in the US. Refer also to Dosage Forms.

Excipient information presented when available (limited, particularly for generics); consult specific product labeling.

Tablet, Oral:

Cyklokapron: 500 mg

◆ **Tranexamic Acid Injection (Can)** *see* Tranexamic Acid *on page 1816*

◆ **Tranexamic Acid Injection BP (Can)** *see* Tranexamic Acid *on page 1816*

◆ **trans-Retinoic Acid** *see* Tretinoin (Systemic) *on page 1830*

◆ **trans Vitamin A Acid** *see* Tretinoin (Systemic) *on page 1830*

◄ Some patients tolerated re-treatment, while others experienced a second severe reaction. When used in combination with myelosuppressive chemotherapy, trastuzumab may increase the incidence of neutropenia (moderate-to-severe) and febrile neutropenia; the incidence of anemia may be higher when trastuzumab is added to chemotherapy. Rare cases of nephrotic syndrome with evidence of glomerulopathy have been reported, with an onset of 4 to 18 months from trastuzumab initiation; complications may include volume overload and HF. The incidence of renal impairment was increased in metastatic gastric cancer patients when trastuzumab is added to chemotherapy.

May cause serious pulmonary toxicity (dyspnea, hypoxia, interstitial pneumonitis, pulmonary infiltrates, pleural effusion, noncardiogenic pulmonary edema, pulmonary insufficiency, acute respiratory distress syndrome, and/or pulmonary fibrosis); use caution in patients with preexisting pulmonary disease or patients with extensive pulmonary tumor involvement. Establish HER2 status prior to treatment with an approved test, either HER2 protein overexpression by validated immunohistochemistry (IHC) assay or gene amplification by fluorescence in situ hybridization (FISH) assay. Due to differences in disease histopathology (eg, incomplete membrane staining and more frequent heterogeneous HER2 expression in gastric cancer), tests appropriate for the specific tumor type (breast or gastric) should be used to assess HER2 status. Unreliable results may occur from improper assay performance, such as use of suboptimally fixed tissue, failure to utilize specified reagents or to include appropriate controls for assay validation, or incorrectly following specific assay instructions. Information regarding HER2 diagnostic testing may be found at http://www.fda.gov/CompanionDiagnostics. **[US Boxed Warning]: Trastuzumab exposure during pregnancy may result in oligohydramnios and oligohydramnios sequence (pulmonary hypoplasia, skeletal malformations and neonatal death). Advise patients of these risks and the need for effective contraception.** Effective contraception is recommended in women of childbearing potential during treatment and for at least 7 months after the last trastuzumab dose. Conventional trastuzumab and ado-trastuzumab emtansine are **not** interchangeable; verify product label prior to reconstitution and administration to prevent medication errors. Dosing and treatment schedules between conventional trastuzumab (Herceptin) and ado-trastuzumab emtansine (Kadcyla) are different; confusion between the products may potentially cause harm to the patient. Potentially significant drug-drug interactions may exist, requiring dose or frequency adjustment, additional monitoring, and/or selection of alternative therapy.

Adverse Reactions Percentages reported with single-agent therapy.

>10%:

Cardiovascular: Decreased left ventricular ejection fraction (4% to 22%)

Central nervous system: Pain (47%), chills (5% to 32%), headache (10% to 26%), insomnia (14%), dizziness (4% to 13%)

Dermatologic: Skin rash (4% to 18%)

Gastrointestinal: Nausea (6% to 33%), diarrhea (7% to 25%), vomiting (4% to 23%), abdominal pain (2% to 22%), anorexia (14%)

Infection: Infection (20%)

Neuromuscular & skeletal: Weakness (4% to 42%), back pain (5% to 22%)

Respiratory: Cough (5% to 26%), dyspnea (3% to 22%), rhinitis (2% to 14%), pharyngitis (2% to 12%)

Miscellaneous: Infusion related reaction (21% to 40%, chills and fever most common; severe: 1%), fever (6% to 36%)

1% to 10%:

Cardiovascular: Peripheral edema (5% to 10%), edema (8%), cardiac failure (2% to 7%; severe: <1%), tachycardia (5%), hypertension (4%), arrhythmia (3%), palpitations (3%)

Central nervous system: Paresthesia (2% to 9%), depression (6%), peripheral neuritis (2%), neuropathy (1%)

Dermatologic: Acne vulgaris (2%), nail disease (2%), pruritus (2%)

Gastrointestinal: Constipation (2%), dyspepsia (2%)

Genitourinary: Urinary tract infection (3% to 5%)

Hematologic & oncologic: Anemia (4%; grade 3: <1%), leukopenia (3%)

Hypersensitivity: Hypersensitivity reaction (3%)

Infection: Influenza (4%), herpes simplex infection (2%)

Neuromuscular & skeletal: Arthralgia (6% to 8%), ostealgia (3% to 7%), myalgia (4%), muscle spasm (3%)

Respiratory: Flu-like symptoms (2% to 10%), sinusitis (2% to 9%), nasopharyngitis (8%), upper respiratory tract infection (3%), epistaxis (2%), pharyngolaryngeal pain (2%)

Miscellaneous: Accidental injury (6%)

<1%, postmarketing, and/or case reports (as a single-agent or with combination chemotherapy): Abnormality in thinking, adult respiratory distress syndrome, amblyopia, anaphylactic shock, anaphylactoid reaction, anaphylaxis, angioedema, apnea, ascites, asthma, ataxia, blood coagulation disorder, bradycardia, bronchitis, bronchospasm, cardiogenic shock, cardiomyopathy, cellulitis, cerebral edema, cerebrovascular accident, cerebrovascular disease, chest discomfort, colitis, coma, confusion, cystitis, deafness, dermal ulcer, dermatitis, dyspnea on exertion, dysuria, erysipelas, esophageal ulcer, febrile neutropenia, focal segmental glomerulosclerosis, gastritis, gastroenteritis, glomerulonephritis (membranous, focal and fibrillary), glomerulopathy, hematemesis, hemorrhage, hemorrhagic cystitis, hepatic failure, hepatic injury, hepatitis, herpes zoster, hiccups, hydrocephalus, hydronephrosis, hypercalcemia, hypervolemia, hypoprothrombinemia, hypotension, hypothyroidism, hypoxia, immune thrombocytopenia, intestinal obstruction, interstitial pneumonitis, interstitial pulmonary disease, jaundice, laryngeal edema, laryngitis, lethargy, leukemia (acute), limb pain, lymphangitis, madarosis, mania, mastalgia, meningitis, musculoskeletal pain, myopathy, nephrotic syndrome, neutropenia, neutropenic sepsis, oligohydramnios, onychoclasis, osteonecrosis, oxygen desaturation, pancreatitis, pancytopenia, paresis, paroxysmal nocturnal dyspnea, pathological fracture, pericardial effusion, pericarditis, pleural effusion, pneumonitis, pneumothorax, pulmonary edema (noncardiogenic), pulmonary fibrosis, pulmonary hypertension, pulmonary infiltrates, pyelonephritis, radiation injury, renal failure, respiratory distress, respiratory failure, seizure, sepsis, shock, syncope, stomatitis, thrombosis (including mural), thyroiditis (autoimmune), urticaria, vertigo, ventricular dysfunction, wheezing

Drug Interactions

Metabolism/Transport Effects None known.

Avoid Concomitant Use

Avoid concomitant use of Trastuzumab with any of the following: Belimumab

Increased Effect/Toxicity

Trastuzumab may increase the levels/effects of: Antineoplastic Agents (Anthracycline, Systemic); Belimumab; Immunosuppressants

The levels/effects of Trastuzumab may be increased by: PACLitaxel (Conventional)

◄ **Decreased Effect**
Trastuzumab may decrease the levels/effects of: PACLitaxel (Conventional)

Hazardous Drugs Handling Considerations
Hazardous agent (meets NIOSH 2016 criteria). This medication is not on the NIOSH (2016) list; however, it meets the criteria for a hazardous drug. Drugs are classified as hazardous based on their properties; the properties of a hazardous drug include one or more of the following characteristics: carcinogenic, teratogenic (or other developmental toxicity), reproductive toxicity, organotoxic at low doses, genotoxic, and/or new agents with structural or toxicity profiles similar to existing hazardous agents.

Use appropriate precautions for receiving, handling, administration, and disposal. Gloves (single) should be worn during receiving, unpacking, and placing in storage.

NIOSH recommends double gloving, a protective gown, ventilated engineering controls (a class II biological safety cabinet or a compounding aseptic containment isolator), and closed system transfer devices (CSTDs) for preparation. Double gloving, a gown, and (if dosage form allows) CSTDs are required during administration (NIOSH 2016).

Storage/Stability Prior to reconstitution, store intact vials at 2°C to 8°C (36°F to 46°F). Following reconstitution with bacteriostatic SWFI, the solution in the vial is stable refrigerated for 28 days from the date of reconstitution; do not freeze. Solutions reconstituted with sterile water for injection without preservatives must be used immediately. The solution diluted in polyvinylchloride or polyethylene bags containing 250 mL NS for infusion may be stored refrigerated for up to 24 hours prior to use; do not freeze.

Preparation for Administration Check vial labels to assure appropriate product is being reconstituted (conventional trastuzumab and ado-trastuzumab emtansine are different products and are **NOT** interchangeable).

Reconstitute each 420 mg vial (multidose vial) with 20 mL of **bacteriostatic sterile water for injection** (**sterile water for injection** may be used if a patient has a known hypersensitivity to benzyl alcohol). Reconstitute each 150 mg vial (single use vial) with 7.4 mL of **sterile water for injection**. Direct the stream of diluent into the lyophilized cake. The reconstituted solutions (in the vial) will have a concentration of 21 mg/mL. Swirl gently; do not shake. Slight foaming may occur during reconstitution. Allow vial to rest undisturbed for ~5 minutes. Solutions reconstituted with sterile water for injection must be used immediately. Further dilute the appropriate volume for the trastuzumab dose in 250 mL NS prior to administration; **do not use D5W**. Gently invert bag to mix.

440 mg vial [Canadian product]: Reconstitute each 440 mg vial with 20 mL **bacteriostatic sterile water for injection** (**sterile water for injection** may be used if a patient has a known hypersensitivity to benzyl alcohol) to a concentration of 21 mg/mL, then follow above for further instructions.

Mechanism of Action Trastuzumab is a monoclonal antibody which binds to the extracellular domain of the human epidermal growth factor receptor 2 protein (HER-2); it mediates antibody-dependent cellular cytotoxicity by inhibiting proliferation of cells which overexpress HER-2 protein.

Pharmacodynamics/Kinetics Note: In most patients, trastuzumab concentrations will decrease to ~3% (~97% washout) by 7 months following discontinuation.

Dosing

Adult & Geriatric Note: Do **NOT** substitute conventional trastuzumab for or with ado-trastuzumab emtansine; products are different and are **NOT** interchangeable.

Breast cancer, adjuvant treatment, HER2+: IV: **Note:** Extending adjuvant treatment beyond 1 year is not recommended

With concurrent paclitaxel or docetaxel:

Initial loading dose: 4 mg/kg infused over 90 minutes, followed by

Maintenance dose: 2 mg/kg infused over 30 minutes weekly for total of 12 weeks, followed 1 week later (when concurrent chemotherapy completed) by 6 mg/kg infused over 30 to 90 minutes every 3 weeks for total therapy duration of 52 weeks

With concurrent docetaxel/carboplatin:

Initial loading dose: 4 mg/kg infused over 90 minutes, followed by

Maintenance dose: 2 mg/kg infused over 30 minutes weekly for total of 18 weeks, followed 1 week later (when concurrent chemotherapy completed) by 6 mg/kg infused over 30 to 90 minutes every 3 weeks for total therapy duration of 52 weeks

Following completion of multi-modality anthracycline-based chemotherapy:

Initial loading dose: 8 mg/kg infused over 90 minutes, followed by

Maintenance dose: 6 mg/kg infused over 30 to 90 minutes every 3 weeks for total therapy duration of 52 weeks

Breast cancer, metastatic, HER2+ (either as a single agent or in combination with paclitaxel): IV:

Initial loading dose: 4 mg/kg infused over 90 minutes, followed by

Maintenance dose: 2 mg/kg infused over 30 minutes weekly until disease progression

Gastric cancer, metastatic, HER2+ (in combination with cisplatin and either capecitabine or fluorouracil for 6 cycles followed by trastuzumab monotherapy; Bang 2010): IV:

Initial loading dose: 8 mg/kg infused over 90 minutes, followed by

Maintenance dose: 6 mg/kg infused over 30 to 90 minutes every 3 weeks until disease progression

Missed doses: If a dose is missed by ≤1 week, the usual maintenance dose should be administered as soon as possible (do not wait until the next planned cycle) and subsequent maintenance doses should be administered 7 or 21 days later (based on patient's maintenance dose/schedule); if a dose is missed by >1 week, then a re-loading dose (4 mg/kg if patient receives trastuzumab weekly; 8 mg/kg if on an every-3-week schedule) should be administered, followed by the usual maintenance dose administered 7 or 21 days later (based on patient's maintenance dose/schedule).

Breast cancer (early stage, locally advanced, or inflammatory), neoadjuvant treatment, HER2+ (off-label use): IV: Trastuzumab, pertuzumab, and docetaxel (in patients with operable disease who had received no prior chemotherapy): Initial: 8 mg/kg (cycle 1) followed by 6 mg/kg every 3 weeks for a total of 4 neoadjuvant cycles; postoperatively, administer 3 cycles of adjuvant FEC [fluorouracil, epirubicin, and cyclophosphamide] chemotherapy and continue trastuzumab to complete 1 year of treatment (Gianni 2012)

◄   **Breast cancer, metastatic, HER2+ (off-label combinations):** IV: **Note:** There are multiple trastuzumab-containing regimens for the treatment of HER2+ metastatic breast cancer; commonly used regimens are listed below:

Trastuzumab, pertuzumab, and docetaxel (in patients with no prior anti-HER2 therapy or chemotherapy to treat metastatic disease): Initial: 8 mg/kg followed by a maintenance dose of 6 mg/kg every 3 weeks until disease progression or unacceptable toxicity (Baselga 2012)

Trastuzumab, pertuzumab, and weekly paclitaxel: Initial: 8 mg/kg followed by a maintenance dose of 6 mg/kg every 3 weeks until disease progression (Dang 2015)

Trastuzumab and lapatinib (in patients with progression on prior trastuzumab containing therapy): Initial: 4 mg/kg followed by a maintenance dose of 2 mg/kg every week (Blackwell 2010; Blackwell 2012)

Other trastuzumab combinations: Initial: 8 mg/kg followed by a maintenance dose of 6 mg/kg every 3 weeks until disease progression or unacceptable toxicity (in combination with docetaxel **or** vinorelbine) (Andersson 2011) **or** 4 mg/kg loading dose followed by a maintenance dose of 2 mg/kg weekly until disease progression (in combination with docetaxel) (Marty 2005)

Renal Impairment

CrCl 30 to 90 mL/minute: There are no dosage adjustments provided in the manufacturer's labeling, although no clinically significant pharmacokinetic differences have been observed.

CrCl <30 mL/minute: There are no dosage adjustments provided in the manufacturer's labeling (has not been studied).

End-stage renal disease (ESRD) (with or without hemodialysis): There are no dosage adjustments provided in the manufacturer's labeling (has not been studied).

Hepatic Impairment There are no dosage adjustments provided in the manufacturer's labeling (has not been studied).

Adjustment for Toxicity

Cardiotoxicity: LVEF ≥16% decrease from baseline or LVEF below normal limits and ≥10% decrease from baseline: Withhold treatment for at least 4 weeks and repeat LVEF every 4 weeks. May resume trastuzumab treatment if LVEF returns to normal limits within 4 to 8 weeks and remains at ≤15% decrease from baseline value. Discontinue permanently for persistent (>8 weeks) LVEF decline or for >3 incidents of treatment interruptions for cardiomyopathy.

Infusion-related events:

Mild-moderate infusion reactions: Decrease infusion rate.

Dyspnea, clinically significant hypotension: Interrupt infusion.

Severe or life-threatening infusion reactions: Discontinue.

Combination Regimens

Breast cancer:

AC (Dose-Dense) followed by Paclitaxel (Dose-Dense)-Trastuzumab (Breast) on page 1977

AC followed by Paclitaxel-Trastuzumab (Breast) on page 1979

Capecitabine-Trastuzumab (Breast) on page 2010

Carboplatin-Docetaxel-Trastuzumab (Breast) on page 2012

Carboplatin-Paclitaxel-Trastuzumab (Breast) on page 2022

Docetaxel Every 3 Weeks-Trastuzumab (Breast) on page 2090

Docetaxel-Trastuzumab followed by FEC (Breast) on page 2095

Administration Check label to ensure appropriate product is being administered (conventional trastuzumab and ado-trastuzumab emtansine are different
products and are **NOT** interchangeable).

Administered by IV infusion; loading doses are infused over 90 minutes;
maintenance doses may be infused over 30 minutes if tolerated. Do not
administer with D5W. **Do not administer IV push or by rapid bolus. Do
not mix with any other medications.**

Observe patients closely during the infusion for fever, chills, or other infusion-
related symptoms. Treatment with acetaminophen, diphenhydramine, and/or
meperidine is usually effective for managing infusion-related events.

Emetic Potential Children and Adults: Minimal (<10%)

Monitoring Parameters Assessment for HER2 overexpression and HER2
gene amplification by validated immunohistochemistry (IHC) or fluorescence
in situ hybridization (FISH) methodology (pretherapy); test should be specific
for cancer type (breast vs gastric cancer). Pregnancy test (prior to treatment in
women of reproductive potential). Monitor vital signs during infusion; signs
and symptoms of cardiac dysfunction; LVEF (baseline, every 3 months during
treatment, upon therapy completion and if component of adjuvant therapy,
every 6 months for at least 2 years; if treatment is withheld for significant LVEF
dysfunction, monitor LVEF at 4-week intervals); signs and symptoms of
infusion reaction or pulmonary toxicity; if pregnancy inadvertently occurs
during treatment, monitor amniotic fluid volume

Dosage Forms Excipient information presented when available (limited,
particularly for generics); consult specific product labeling.
Solution Reconstituted, Intravenous:
Herceptin: 440 mg (1 ea) [contains benzyl alcohol, mouse (murine) and/or
hamster protein]
Solution Reconstituted, Intravenous [preservative free]:
Herceptin: 150 mg (1 ea)

Tretinoin (Systemic) (TRET i noyn)

Related Information

Management of Chemotherapy-Induced Nausea and Vomiting in Adults *on page 2253*

Management of EGFR Inhibitor Toxicities: Dermatologic, Ocular, and Gastrointestinal *on page 2291*

Prevention of Chemotherapy-Induced Nausea and Vomiting in Children *on page 2310*

Safe Handling of Hazardous Drugs *on page 2379*

Brand Names: Canada Vesanoid

Index Terms All trans Retinoic Acid; All-trans Retinoic Acid; All-trans Vitamin A Acid; ATRA; Ro 5488; tRA; trans Vitamin A Acid; trans-Retinoic Acid; Tretinoinum; Vesanoid

Pharmacologic Category Antineoplastic Agent, Retinoic Acid Derivative; Retinoic Acid Derivative

Use Acute promyelocytic leukemia (remission induction): Induction of remission in patients with acute promyelocytic leukemia, French American British (FAB) classification M3 (including the M3 variant) characterized by t (15;17) translocation and/or PML/RARα gene presence

Labeled Contraindications Hypersensitivity to tretinoin, other retinoids, parabens, or any component of the formulation

Pregnancy Considerations Adverse events were observed in animal reproduction studies. **[US Boxed Warning]: High risk of teratogenicity; if treatment with tretinoin is required in women of childbearing potential, two reliable forms of contraception should be used simultaneously during and for 1 month after discontinuation of treatment, unless abstinence is the chosen method. Within 1 week prior to starting therapy, serum or urine pregnancy test (sensitivity at least 50 milliunits/mL) should be collected. If possible, delay therapy until results are available. Repeat pregnancy testing and contraception counseling monthly throughout the period of treatment.** Contraception must be used even when there is a history of infertility or menopause, unless a hysterectomy has been performed. Tretinoin was detected in the serum of a neonate at birth following maternal use of standard doses during pregnancy (Takitani 2005). Use in humans for the treatment of acute promyelocytic leukemia (APL) is limited and exposure occurred after the first trimester in most cases (Valappil 2007). However, major fetal abnormalities and spontaneous abortions have been reported with other retinoids; some of these abnormalities were fatal. If the clinical condition of a patient presenting with APL during pregnancy warrants immediate treatment, tretinoin use should be avoided in the first trimester; treatment with tretinoin may be considered in the second and third trimester with careful fetal monitoring, including cardiac monitoring (Sanz 2009).

Breastfeeding Considerations It is not known if tretinoin is excreted in breast milk. Due to the potential for serious adverse reactions in the nursing infant, breastfeeding should be discontinued prior to treatment initiation.

Warnings/Precautions [US Boxed Warning]: About 25% of patients with APL treated with tretinoin have experienced APL differentiation syndrome (DS) (formerly called retinoic-acid-APL [RA-APL] syndrome), which is characterized by fever, dyspnea, acute respiratory distress, weight gain, radiographic pulmonary infiltrates and pleural or pericardial effusions, edema, and hepatic, renal, and/or multiorgan failure. The

syndrome may be accompanied by impaired myocardial contractility and episodic hypotension. It has been observed with or without concomitant leukocytosis. Intubation and mechanical ventilation have been required in some cases due to progressive hypoxemia; fatalities due to multiorgan failure have occurred. The syndrome generally occurs during the first month of treatment, with some cases reported following the first dose. Management has not been defined, although high-dose steroids given at the first suspicion appear to reduce morbidity and mortality. Regardless of the leukocyte count, at the first signs suggestive of APL differentiation syndrome (eg, unexplained fever, dyspnea and/or weight gain, abnormal chest auscultatory findings, radiographic abnormalities), immediately initiate corticosteroid therapy with dexamethasone 10 mg IV every 12 hours for 3 to 5 days (or until the symptoms resolve); taper off over 2 weeks. Most patients do not require termination of tretinoin therapy during treatment of the APL differentiation syndrome.

[US Boxed Warning]: During treatment, ~40% of patients will develop rapidly evolving leukocytosis. Patients who present with a high WBC at diagnosis (>5,000/mm^3) are at increased risk of further rapid increase in WBC counts. Rapidly evolving leukocytosis is associated with a higher risk of life-threatening complications. Initiate treatment with high-dose corticosteroids immediately if signs and symptoms of APL differentiation syndrome are present with leukocytosis. Chemotherapy may be added to tretinoin treatment in patients presenting with a WBC count >5,000/mm^3 or for a rapid WBC increase in patients leukopenic at start of treatment (may result in a lower incidence of APL differentiation syndrome). Consider adding full-dose chemotherapy (including an anthracycline if not contraindicated) to tretinoin therapy on day 1 or 2 for patients presenting with a WBC count >5,000/mm^3; immediately add for patients presenting with a WBC count <5,000/mm^3 if the WBC count reaches ≥6,000/mm^3 by day 5, ≥10,000/mm^3 by day 10, or ≥15,000/mm^3 by day 28.

[US Boxed Warning]: High risk of teratogenicity; if treatment with tretinoin is required in women of childbearing potential, two reliable forms of contraception should be used during and for 1 month after discontinuation of treatment, unless abstinence is the chosen method. Within 1 week prior to starting therapy, serum or urine pregnancy test (sensitivity at least 50 milliunits/mL) should be collected. If possible, delay therapy until results are available. Repeat pregnancy testing and contraception counseling monthly throughout the period of treatment. Microdosed progesterone products ("minipill") may provide inadequate pregnancy protection. Repeat pregnancy testing and contraception counseling monthly throughout the period of treatment. If possible, initiation of treatment with tretinoin should be delayed until negative pregnancy test result is confirmed.

Retinoids have been associated with pseudotumor cerebri (benign intracranial hypertension), especially in children. Concurrent use of other drugs associated with this effect (eg, tetracyclines) may increase risk. Early signs and symptoms include papilledema, headache, nausea, vomiting, visual disturbances, intracranial noises, or pulsate tinnitus.

Up to 60% of patients experienced hypercholesterolemia or hypertriglyceridemia, which were reversible upon completion of treatment. Venous thrombosis and MI have been reported in patient without risk factors for thrombosis or MI; the risk for thrombosis (arterial and venous) is increased during the first month of treatment. Use with caution with antifibrinolytic agents; thrombotic complications have been reported (rarely) with concomitant use. Elevated liver function test results occur in 50% to 60% of patients during treatment. Carefully monitor liver function test results during treatment and give consideration to a temporary withdrawal of tretinoin if test results reach >5 times the upper limit of normal. Most liver function test abnormalities will resolve without interruption of treatment or after therapy completion. May cause headache, malaise, and/or dizziness; caution patients about performing tasks which require mental alertness (eg, operating machinery or driving). Effects may be potentiated when used with other sedative drugs or ethanol. **[US Boxed Warning]: Should be administered under the supervision of an experienced cancer chemotherapy physician. Patients with APL are at high risk and can have severe adverse reactions to tretinoin. Administer tretinoin only to patients with APL under the close supervision of a provider who is experienced in the management of patients with acute leukemia, and in a facility with laboratory and supportive services for appropriate monitoring.** Tretinoin treatment for APL should be initiated early, discontinue if pending cytogenetic analysis does not confirm APL by t(15;17) translocation or the presence of the PML/RARα fusion protein (caused by translocation of the promyelocytic [PML] gene on chromosome 15 and retinoic acid receptor [RAR] alpha gene on chromosome 17). Potentially significant drug-drug interactions may exist, requiring dose or frequency adjustment, additional monitoring, and/or selection of alternative therapy.

Tretinoin (which is also known as all-*trans* retinoic acid, or ATRA) and isotretinoin may be confused, while both products may be used in cancer treatment, they are **not** interchangeable; verify product prior to dispensing and administration to prevent medication errors.

Adverse Reactions Most patients will experience drug-related toxicity, especially headache, fever, weakness and fatigue. These are seldom permanent or irreversible and do not typically require therapy interruption.

>10%:

Cardiovascular: Peripheral edema (52%), chest discomfort (32%), edema (29%), cardiac arrhythmia (23%), flushing (23%), hypotension (14%), hypertension (11%), localized phlebitis (11%)

Central nervous system: Headache (86%), malaise (66%), shivering (63%), pain (37%), dizziness (20%), anxiety (17%), paresthesia (17%), depression (14%), insomnia (14%), confusion (11%)

Dermatologic: Xeroderma (≤77%), skin rash (54%), diaphoresis (20%), pruritus (20%), alopecia (14%), skin changes (14%)

Endocrine & metabolic: Hypercholesterolemia (≤60%), hypertriglyceridemia (≤60%), weight gain (23%), weight loss (17%)

Gastrointestinal: Dry mucous membranes (≤77%), nausea (≤57%), vomiting (≤57%), gastrointestinal hemorrhage (34%), abdominal pain (31%), mucositis (26%), diarrhea (23%), anorexia (17%), constipation (17%), dyspepsia (14%), abdominal distention (11%)

Hematologic & oncologic: Hemorrhage (60%), leukocytosis (40%), disseminated intravascular coagulation (26%)

Hepatic: Increased liver enzymes (50% to 60%)

Infection: Infection (58%)

Neuromuscular & skeletal: Ostealgia (77%), APL differentiation syndrome (≤25%), myalgia (14%)

Ophthalmic: Eye disease (17%), visual disturbance (17%)

Otic: Otalgia (23%; ear fullness)

Renal: Renal insufficiency (11%)

Respiratory: Upper respiratory complaint (63%), dyspnea (60%), respiratory insufficiency (26%), pleural effusion (20%), pneumonia (14%), rales (14%), wheezing (expiratory: 14%)

Miscellaneous: Fever (83%)

1% to 10%:

Cardiovascular: Cardiac failure (6%), facial edema (6%), cardiomegaly (3%), cardiomyopathy (3%), cerebrovascular accident (3%), heart murmur (3%), ischemia (3%), myocardial infarction (3%), myocarditis (3%), pericarditis (3%)

Central nervous system: Agitation (9%), cerebral hemorrhage (9%), flank pain (9%), intracranial hypertension (9%), hallucination (6%), abnormal gait (3%), agnosia (3%), aphasia (3%), asterixis (3%), ataxia (3%), brain disease (3%), cerebral edema (cerebellar: 3%), central nervous system depression (3%), coma (3%), dementia (3%), drowsiness (3%), dysarthria (3%), facial paralysis (3%), forgetfulness (3%), hemiplegia (3%), hyporeflexia (3%), hypothermia (3%), loss of consciousness (3%), seizure (3%), speech disturbance (3%)

Dermatologic: Cellulitis (8%), pallor (6%)

Endocrine & metabolic: Disturbance in fluid balance (6%), acidosis (3%)

Gastrointestinal: Gastrointestinal ulcer (3%)

Genitourinary: Dysuria (9%), benign prostatic hypertrophy (3%), urinary frequency (3%)

Hematologic & oncologic: Lymphatic disease (6%)

Hepatic: Hepatosplenomegaly (9%), ascites (3%), hepatitis (3%)

Local: Local inflammation (bone: 3%)

Neuromuscular & skeletal: Lower extremity weakness (3%), myelopathy (3%), tremor (3%)

Ophthalmic: Decreased visual acuity (6%), decreased pupillary reflex (3%), visual field defect (3%)

Otic: Hearing loss (6%; may be irreversible)

Renal: Acute renal failure (3%), renal tubular necrosis (3%)

Respiratory: Lower respiratory signs and symptoms (9%), pulmonary infiltrates (6%), asthma (3%), laryngeal edema (3%), pulmonary hypertension (3%)

<1%, postmarketing, and/or case reports: Arterial thrombosis, basophilia, erythema nodosum, histamine release (hyperhistaminemia), hypercalcemia, hypersensitivity angiitis, myositis, pancreatitis, pseudotumor cerebri, renal infarction, Sweet's syndrome, thrombocythemia, ulcer (genital), venous thrombosis

Drug Interactions

Metabolism/Transport Effects Substrate of CYP2A6 (minor), CYP2B6 (minor), CYP2C8 (major), CYP2C9 (minor); **Note:** Assignment of Major/Minor substrate status based on clinically relevant drug interaction potential; **Inhibits** CYP2C9 (weak); **Induces** CYP2E1 (weak/moderate)

◄ **Avoid Concomitant Use**

Avoid concomitant use of Tretinoin (Systemic) with any of the following: Aminolevulinic Acid (Systemic); BCG (Intravesical); Multivitamins/Fluoride (with ADE); Multivitamins/Minerals (with ADEK, Folate, Iron); Multivitamins/Minerals (with AE, No Iron); Natalizumab; Pimecrolimus; Tacrolimus (Topical); Tetracycline Derivatives; Vaccines (Live); Vitamin A

Increased Effect/Toxicity

Tretinoin (Systemic) may increase the levels/effects of: Amifostine; Aminolevulinic Acid (Systemic); Aminolevulinic Acid (Topical); Antifibrinolytic Agents; Antipsychotic Agents (Second Generation [Atypical]); DULoxetine; Fingolimod; Hypotension-Associated Agents; Leflunomide; Levodopa; Natalizumab; Nitroprusside; Pholcodine; Porfimer; Tofacitinib; Vaccines (Live); Verteporfin

The levels/effects of Tretinoin (Systemic) may be increased by: Abiraterone Acetate; Alfuzosin; Barbiturates; Benperidol; Blood Pressure Lowering Agents; Brimonidine (Topical); CYP2C8 Inhibitors (Moderate); CYP2C8 Inhibitors (Strong); Deferasirox; Denosumab; Diazoxide; Herbs (Hypotensive Properties); Lormetazepam; Lumacaftor; MiFEPRIStone; Molsidomine; Multivitamins/Fluoride (with ADE); Multivitamins/Minerals (with ADEK, Folate, Iron); Multivitamins/Minerals (with AE, No Iron); Naftopidil; Nicergoline; Nicorandil; Obinutuzumab; Ocrelizumab; Pentoxifylline; Phosphodiesterase 5 Inhibitors; Pimecrolimus; Prostacyclin Analogues; Quinagolide; Roflumilast; Tacrolimus (Topical); Tetracycline Derivatives; Trastuzumab; Vitamin A

Decreased Effect

Tretinoin (Systemic) may decrease the levels/effects of: BCG (Intravesical); Coccidioides immitis Skin Test; Contraceptives (Estrogens); Contraceptives (Progestins); Nivolumab; Sipuleucel-T; Tertomotide; Vaccines (Inactivated); Vaccines (Live)

The levels/effects of Tretinoin (Systemic) may be decreased by: CYP2C8 Inducers (Strong); Dabrafenib; Echinacea; Lumacaftor

Food Interactions Absorption of retinoids has been shown to be enhanced when taken with food. Management: Administer with a meal.

Hazardous Drugs Handling Considerations

Hazardous agent (NIOSH 2016 [group 3]).

Use appropriate precautions for receiving, handling, administration, and disposal. Gloves (single) should be worn during receiving, unpacking, and placing in storage.

NIOSH recommends single gloving for administration of intact tablets or capsules. If manipulating tablets/capsules (eg, to prepare an oral suspension), NIOSH recommends double gloving, a protective gown, and preparation in a controlled device; if not prepared in a controlled device, respiratory and eye/face protection as well as ventilated engineering controls are recommended. NIOSH recommends double gloving, a protective gown, and (if there is a potential for vomit or spit up) eye/face protection for administration of an oral liquid/feeding tube administration (NIOSH 2016).

Storage/Stability Store capsule at 20°C to 25°C (68°F to 77°F). Protect from light.

Mechanism of Action Tretinoin appears to bind one or more nuclear receptors and decreases proliferation and induces differentiation of APL cells; initially produces maturation of primitive promyelocytes and repopulates the marrow and peripheral blood with normal hematopoietic cells to achieve complete remission

Pharmacodynamics/Kinetics Note: Reported pediatric values similar to adult (Smith 1992; Takitani 2004)

Absorption: Well absorbed

Protein binding: >95%, predominantly to albumin

Metabolism: Hepatic via CYP; primary metabolite: 4-oxo-all-*trans*-retinoic acid; displays autometabolism

Half-life elimination: Terminal: Parent drug: 0.5 to 2 hours

Time to peak, serum: 1 to 2 hours

Excretion: Urine (63%); feces (30%)

Dosing

Adult & Geriatric Note: Induction treatment of APL with tretinoin should be initiated early; discontinue if pending cytogenetic analysis does not confirm t (15;17) translocation or the presence of the PML/RARα fusion protein.

Acute promyelocytic leukemia (APL): Oral:

Remission induction (manufacturer's labeling): 45 mg/m^2/day in 2 equally divided doses until documentation of complete remission (CR); discontinue 30 days after CR or after 90 days of treatment, whichever occurs first

Remission induction (in combination with an anthracycline ± cytarabine): 45 mg/m^2/day in 2 equally divided doses until complete remission or 90 days (Powell 2010) or until complete hematologic remission (Ades 2008; Sanz 2008; Sanz 2010)

Remission induction (in combination with arsenic trioxide; off-label combination): 45 mg/m^2/day in 2 equally divided doses until <5% blasts in marrow and no abnormal promyelocytes or up to 85 days (Estey 2006; Ravandi 2009)

Consolidation therapy (off-label use): 45 mg/m^2/day in 2 equally divided doses for 15 days each month for 3 months (in combination with chemotherapy) (Lo-Coco 2010; Sanz 2010) **or** 45 mg/m^2/day for 14 days every 4 weeks for 7 cycles (in combination with arsenic trioxide) (Ravandi 2009)

Maintenance therapy, intermediate- and high-risk patients (off-label use): 45 mg/m^2/day in 2 equally divided doses for 15 days every 3 months for 2 years (Ades 2008; Sanz 2004) **or** 45 mg/m^2/day in 2 equally divided doses for 7 days every other week for 1 year (Powell 2010)

Pediatric Note: Induction treatment of APL with tretinoin should be initiated early; discontinue if pending cytogenetic analysis does not confirm t(15;17) translocation or the presence of the PML/RARα fusion protein.

Acute promyelocytic leukemia (APL): Oral:

Remission induction (manufacturer's labeling): 45 mg/m^2/day in 2 equally divided doses until documentation of complete remission (CR); discontinue 30 days after CR or after 90 days of treatment, whichever occurs first

Remission induction (in combination with an anthracycline; off-label dose): 25 mg/m^2/day in 2 equally divided doses until complete remission or 90 days (Ortega 2005)

Consolidation therapy, intermediate- and high-risk patients (off-label use): 25 mg/m^2/day in 2 equally divided doses for 15 days each month for 3 months (Ortega 2005)

Maintenance therapy, intermediate- and high-risk patients (off-label use): 25 mg/m^2/day in 2 equally divided doses for 15 days every 3 months for 2 years (Ortega 2005)

Renal Impairment There are no dosage adjustments provided in the manufacturer's labeling (has not been studied).

Hepatic Impairment There are no dosage adjustments provided in the manufacturer's labeling (has not been studied).

Adjustment for Toxicity

APL differentiation syndrome: Initiate dexamethasone 10 mg IV every 12 hours for 3 to 5 days; consider interrupting tretinoin until resolution of hypoxia

Liver function tests >5 times the upper limit of normal: Consider temporarily withholding treatment

Combination Regimens

Leukemia, acute promyelocytic:

Tretinoin-Arsenic Trioxide (APL) on page 2218

Tretinoin-Daunorubicin-Cytarabine Induction, Consolidation, Maintenance (APL) on page 2218

Tretinoin-Idarubicin (APL) on page 2221

Administration

Administer orally with a meal; do not crush capsules.

Tretinoin has also been administered sublingually by squeezing the capsule contents beneath the tongue (Kueh 1999).

Low plasma concentrations have been reported when tretinoin has been administered through a feeding tube, although patient-specific impaired absorption or a lack of excipient (eg, soybean oil) may have been a contributing factor (Takitani 2004).

Emetic Potential Children and Adults: Low (10% to 30%)

Extemporaneous Preparations Although the manufacturer does not recommend the use of the capsule contents to extemporaneously prepare a suspension of tretinoin (due to reports of low plasma levels) (Vesanoid data on file), there are limited case reports of use in patients who are unable to swallow the capsules whole. In a patient with a nasogastric (NG) tube, tretinoin capsules were cut open, with partial aspiration of the contents aspirated into a glass syringe. The residual capsule contents were mixed with soybean oil, aspirated into the syringe, and administered (Shaw 1995). Tretinoin capsules have also been mixed with sterile water (~20 mL) and heated in a water bath to melt the capsules and create an oily suspension for NG tube administration (Bargetzi 1996). Tretinoin has also been administered sublingually by squeezing the capsule contents beneath the tongue (Kueh 1999).

Bargetzi MJ, Tichelli A, Gratwohl A, et al, "Oral All-Transretinoic Acid Administration in Intubated Patients With Acute Promyelocytic Leukemia," *Schweiz Med Wochenschr*, 1996, 126 (45):1944-5.

Kueh YK, Liew PP, Ho PC, et al, "Sublingual Administration of All-*Trans*-Retinoic Acid to a Comatose Patient With Acute Promyelocytic Leukemia," *Ann Pharmacother*, 1999, 33(4):503-5.

Shaw PJ, Atkins MC, Nath CE, et al, "ATRA Administration in the Critically Ill Patient," *Leukemia*, 1995, 9(7):1288.

Vesanoid data on file, Roche Pharmaceuticals

Monitoring Parameters Bone marrow cytology to confirm t(15;17) translocation or the presence of the PML/RARα fusion protein (do not withhold treatment initiation for results); monitor CBC with differential, coagulation profile, liver function test results, and triglyceride and cholesterol levels frequently; monitor closely for signs of APL differentiation syndrome (eg, monitor volume status, pulmonary status, temperature, respiration)

Dietary Considerations The absorption of retinoids (as a class) is enhanced when taken with food. Capsule contains soybean oil.

Dosage Forms Excipient information presented when available (limited, particularly for generics); consult specific product labeling.

Capsule, Oral:

Generic: 10 mg

♦ **Tretinoinum** see Tretinoin (Systemic) on page 1830
♦ **Tretten** see Factor XIII A-Subunit (Recombinant) on page 781
♦ **Trexall** see Methotrexate on page 1205
♦ **Triacetyluridine** see Uridine Triacetate on page 1847
♦ **Triethylenethiophosphoramide** see Thiotepa on page 1778

Trifluridine and Tipiracil (trye FLURE i deen & tye PIR a sil)

Related Information

Common Toxicity Criteria on page 2242
Safe Handling of Hazardous Drugs on page 2379

Brand Names: US Lonsurf

Index Terms TAS-102; Tipiracil and Trifluridine; Trifluridine and Tipiracil Hydrochloride; Trifluridine/Tipiracil HCl

Pharmacologic Category Antineoplastic Agent, Antimetabolite; Antineoplastic Agent, Antimetabolite (Pyrimidine Analog); Thymidine Phosphorylase Inhibitor

Use Colorectal cancer, metastatic: Treatment of metastatic colorectal cancer in patients who have been previously treated with fluoropyrimidine-, oxaliplatin- and irinotecan-based chemotherapy, an anti-VEGF biological therapy, and if RAS wild-type, an anti-EGFR therapy.

Labeled Contraindications There are no contraindications listed in the manufacturer's labeling.

Pregnancy Considerations Based on animal studies and on the mechanism of action, use of trifluridine/tipiracil would be expected to cause fetal harm when used during pregnancy. Females of reproductive potential should use effective contraception during therapy. Males who have female partners of reproductive potential should use condoms during therapy and for at least 3 months following the final dose.

Breastfeeding Considerations It is not known if trifluridine or tipiracil are present in breast milk. Due to the potential for serious adverse reactions in the breastfed infant, breastfeeding is not recommended by the manufacturer during therapy and for one day following the last dose.

Warnings/Precautions Severe and life-threatening bone marrow suppression (anemia, neutropenia, thrombocytopenia) has occurred, including a fatality related to neutropenic infection. In one clinical trial, close to 10% of patients received growth factor support. Monitor blood counts prior to the start of each cycle as well as on day 15, or more frequently if clinically necessary. May require therapy interruption and/or dose reduction. Trifluridine/tipiracil is associated with a moderate emetic potential; antiemetics are recommended ▶

to prevent nausea and vomiting. Nausea, vomiting, diarrhea, and abdominal pain have been commonly reported. Stomatitis may also occur. Advise patients to report severe gastrointestinal toxicity to their health care provider. Patients with severe hepatic impairment (total bilirubin >3 times ULN and any AST) were not included in studies; do not initiate in patients with baseline moderate or severe hepatic impairment. In a pharmacokinetic study in patients with hepatic impairment, several patients with moderate impairment experienced grade 3 or 4 bilirubin elevations. Use with caution in patients with renal impairment; dosage adjustments due to toxicities may be necessary in patients with moderate impairment. Patients with severe renal impairment (CrCl <30 mL/minute) or end-stage renal disease (ESRD) were excluded from the clinical trial. Patients ≥65 years experienced a higher incidence of grade 3 and grade 4 neutropenia and thrombocytopenia, as well as increased grade 3 anemia compared to younger patients. Trifluridine/tipiracil is available in two tablet strengths (trifluridine 15 mg/tipiracil 6.14 mg and trifluridine 20 mg/tipiracil 8.19 mg); both tablet strengths may be necessary to provide the correct dose. Read labels carefully in order to ensure the appropriate dose is administered. Dosing is based on the trifluridine component. The manufacturer recommends rounding doses to the nearest 5 mg increment. Potentially significant drug-drug interactions may exist, requiring dose or frequency adjustment, additional monitoring, and/or selection of alternative therapy.

Adverse Reactions

>10%:

Central nervous system: Fatigue (≤52%)

Gastrointestinal: Nausea (48%), decreased appetite (39%), diarrhea (32%), vomiting (28%), abdominal pain (21%)

Hematologic & oncologic: Anemia (77%; grade 3: 18%), neutropenia (67%; grade 3: 27%; grade 4: 11%), thrombocytopenia (42%; grade 3: 5%; grade 4: 1%)

Neuromuscular & skeletal: Weakness (≤52%)

Miscellaneous: Fever (19%)

1% to 10%:

Cardiovascular: Pulmonary embolism (2%)

Dermatologic: Alopecia (7%)

Gastrointestinal: Stomatitis (8%), dysgeusia (7%)

Genitourinary: Urinary tract infection (4%)

Respiratory: Nasopharyngitis (4%)

<1%, postmarketing, and/or case reports: Lung disease

Drug Interactions

Metabolism/Transport Effects None known.

Avoid Concomitant Use

Avoid concomitant use of Trifluridine and Tipiracil with any of the following: BCG (Intravesical); Deferiprone; Dipyrone; Natalizumab; Pimecrolimus; Tacrolimus (Topical); Vaccines (Live)

Increased Effect/Toxicity

Trifluridine and Tipiracil may increase the levels/effects of: CloZAPine; Deferiprone; Fingolimod; Highest Risk QTc-Prolonging Agents; Leflunomide; Moderate Risk QTc-Prolonging Agents; Natalizumab; Tofacitinib; Vaccines (Live)

The levels/effects of Trifluridine and Tipiracil may be increased by: Denosumab; Dipyrone; MiFEPRIStone; Ocrelizumab; Pimecrolimus; Promazine; Roflumilast; Tacrolimus (Topical); Trastuzumab

Decreased Effect

Trifluridine and Tipiracil may decrease the levels/effects of: BCG (Intravesical); Coccidioides immitis Skin Test; Nivolumab; Sipuleucel-T; Tertomotide; Vaccines (Inactivated); Vaccines (Live)

The levels/effects of Trifluridine and Tipiracil may be decreased by: Echinacea

Hazardous Drugs Handling Considerations

Hazardous agent (NIOSH 2016 [group 1]).

Use appropriate precautions for receiving, handling, administration, and disposal. Gloves (single) should be worn during receiving, unpacking, and placing in storage. NIOSH recommends single gloving for administration of intact tablets or capsules (NIOSH 2016).

Storage/Stability
Store at 20°C to 25°C (68°F to 77°F); excursions are permitted to 15°C to 30°C (59°F to 86°F). If stored outside the original bottle, discard tablets after 30 days.

Mechanism of Action
Trifluridine, the active cytotoxic component of trifluridine/tipiracil, is a thymidine-based nucleic acid analogue; the triphosphate form of trifluridine is incorporated into DNA which interferes with DNA synthesis and inhibits cell proliferation. Tipiracil is a potent thymidine phosphorylase inhibitor which prevents the rapid degradation of trifluridine, allowing for increased trifluridine exposure (Mayer 2015).

Pharmacodynamics/Kinetics

Protein binding: Trifluridine: >96% (primarily to albumin); Tipiracil: <8%

Metabolism: Trifluridine and tipiracil are not metabolized by cytochrome P450 (CYP) enzymes. Trifluridine is mainly eliminated by metabolism via thymidine phosphorylase to form an inactive metabolite, 5-(trifluoromethyl) uracil (FTY)

Half-life elimination: Trifluridine: 2.1 hours (at steady state); Tipiracil: 2.4 hours (at steady state)

Time to peak, plasma: ~2 hours

Excretion:
  Trifluridine: Urine (55% [as inactive metabolite FTY and trifluridine glucuronide isomers]; <3% [as unchanged drug]); feces (<3% [as unchanged drug]); expired air (<3%)
  Tipiracil: Urine (27% [as tipiracil and 6-HMU]); feces (50% [as tipiracil and 6-HMU])

Dosing

Adult & Geriatric Note: Obtain blood counts prior to starting each cycle and on day 15 of each cycle. Do not initiate a cycle until ANC ≥1,500/mm³ or febrile neutropenia is resolved, platelets are ≥75,000/mm³, and/or grade 3 or 4 nonhematologic reactions are ≤ grade 1. Trifluridine/tipiracil is associated with a moderate emetic potential; antiemetics are recommended to prevent nausea and vomiting.

Colorectal cancer, metastatic: Oral: 35 mg/m² (based on the trifluridine component) twice daily on days 1 to 5 and days 8 to 12 of a 28-day cycle (maximum per dose: trifluridine 80 mg); continue until disease progression or unacceptable toxicity (Mayer 2015). The manufacturer recommends rounding each dose to the nearest 5 mg increment.
Missed dose: Do not take additional doses to make up for missed or held doses.

Renal Impairment

CrCl ≥30 mL/minute: No initial dosage adjustment is necessary. Monitor closely; patients with moderate impairment (CrCl 30 to 59 mL/minute) may experience greater toxicity and may require dose reduction during treatment.

CrCl <30 mL/minute and ESRD: There are no dosage adjustments provided in the manufacturer's labeling (has not been studied).

Hepatic Impairment

Mild impairment (total bilirubin ≤ ULN and AST >ULN or total bilirubin <1 to 1.5 times ULN and any AST): No dosage adjustment necessary.

Moderate impairment (total bilirubin >1.5 to 3 times ULN and any AST) or severe impairment (total bilirubin >3 times ULN and any AST): Do not initiate therapy.

Adjustment for Toxicity A maximum of 3 dose reductions are allowed (to a minimum dose of 20 mg/m^2). Do not re-escalate dose after it has been reduced.

Hematologic toxicity:

ANC <500/mm^3 (uncomplicated or resulting in >1 week delay in the start of the next cycle) or febrile neutropenia: Interrupt therapy; following recovery to ANC ≥1,500/mm^3 or resolution of febrile neutropenia, may resume therapy with the dose reduced by 5 mg/m^2/dose from the previous dose

Platelets <50,000/mm^3 (or resulting in >1 week delay in the start of the next cycle): Interrupt therapy; following recovery to platelets ≥75,000/mm^3, may resume therapy with the dose reduced by 5 mg/m^2/dose from the previous dose

Nonhematologic toxicity: Grade 3 or 4 toxicity: Interrupt therapy until recovery to ≤ grade 1; following recovery, may resume with the dose reduced by 5 mg/m^2/dose from the previous dose (excludes dose reduction for grade 3 nausea and/or vomiting controlled by antiemetic therapy or grade 3 diarrhea responsive to antidiarrheal treatment).

Combination Regimens

Colorectal cancer: Trifluridine and Tipiracil (Colorectal Regimen) on page 2224

Administration

Trifluridine/tipiracil is associated with a moderate emetic potential; antiemetics are recommended to prevent nausea and vomiting.

Administer orally twice daily within 1 hour of completion of morning and evening meals.

Emetic Potential Moderate (30% to 90%)

Monitoring Parameters Complete blood counts prior to each cycle and on day 15 of each cycle (or more frequently if clinically necessary); signs/symptoms of gastrointestinal toxicity.

Dosage Forms Excipient information presented when available (limited, particularly for generics); consult specific product labeling.

Tablet, Oral:

Lonsurf: Trifluridine 15 mg and tipiracil 6.14 mg, Trifluridine 20 mg and tipiracil 8.19 mg

◆ **Trifluridine and Tipiracil Hydrochloride** *see* Trifluridine and Tipiracil *on page 1837*

◆ **Trifluridine/Tipiracil HCl** *see* Trifluridine and Tipiracil *on page 1837*

Trimethobenzamide (trye meth oh BEN za mide)

Brand Names: US Tigan

Brand Names: Canada Tigan

Index Terms Trimethobenzamide HCl; Trimethobenzamide Hydrochloride

Pharmacologic Category Antiemetic

Use Nausea/vomiting: Treatment of postoperative nausea and vomiting; treatment of nausea associated with gastroenteritis

Dosing

Adult

Nausea/vomiting: Note: Use the lowest effective dosage based on response and tolerability.

Oral: 300 mg 3 or 4 times daily

IM: 200 mg 3 or 4 times daily

Geriatric Refer to adult dosing; increase the dosing interval and adjust as needed based on patient response.

Renal Impairment

CrCl >70 mL/minute/1.73 m²: There are no dosage adjustments provided in the manufacturer's labeling.

CrCl ≤70 mL/minute/1.73 m²: Increase the dosing interval and adjust as needed based on patient response; monitor renal function closely.

Hepatic Impairment Avoid use in patients with hepatic impairment (due to potential risk of hepatotoxicity).

Additional Information Complete prescribing information should be consulted for additional detail.

Dosage Forms Excipient information presented when available (limited, particularly for generics); consult specific product labeling. [DSC] = Discontinued product

Capsule, Oral, as hydrochloride:

Tigan: 300 mg

Generic: 300 mg

Solution, Intramuscular, as hydrochloride:

Tigan: 100 mg/mL (2 mL)

Tigan: 100 mg/mL (20 mL) [contains phenol]

Generic: 100 mg/mL (2 mL [DSC], 20 mL [DSC])

◆ **Trimethobenzamide HCl** see Trimethobenzamide on page 1841

◆ **Trimethobenzamide Hydrochloride** see Trimethobenzamide on page 1841

◆ **Trimethoprim and Sulfamethoxazole** see Sulfamethoxazole and Trimethoprim on page 1698

◆ **Triptodur** see Triptorelin on page 1841

Triptorelin (trip toe REL in)

Related Information

Safe Handling of Hazardous Drugs on page 2379

Brand Names: US Trelstar Mixject; Trelstar [DSC]; Triptodur

Brand Names: Canada Decapeptyl; Trelstar

Index Terms AY-25650; CL-118,532; D-Trp(6)-LHRH; Detryptoreline; Triptodur; Triptorelin Embonate; Triptorelin Pamoate; Tryptoreline

Pharmacologic Category Gonadotropin Releasing Hormone Agonist

◀ **Use**

Advanced prostate cancer: Palliative treatment of advanced prostate cancer

Assisted reproductive technologies: Decapeptyl [Canadian product]: Adjunctive therapy in women undergoing controlled ovarian hyperstimulation for assisted reproductive technologies (ART)

Labeled Contraindications

Hypersensitivity to triptorelin or any component of the formulation, other GnRH agonists or GnRH; pregnancy

Canadian labeling: Additional contraindications (not in US labeling): Breast-feeding women

Pregnancy Considerations Use is contraindicated in pregnant women. When used for ART, pregnancy must be ruled out prior to therapy and nonhormonal contraception should be used until menses occurs. Due to the short half-life of triptorelin (formulations used for ART), it is not expected to be present in the maternal serum at the time of embryo transfer. In case reports, spontaneous abortion, congenital anomalies, and other adverse events have been reported following triptorelin (Decapeptyl) exposure during pregnancy.

Breastfeeding Considerations It is not known if triptorelin is excreted in breast milk. Trelstar is not indicated for use in women.

Warnings/Precautions Transient increases in testosterone can lead to worsening symptoms (bone pain, hematuria, bladder outlet obstruction, neuropathy) of prostate cancer during the first few weeks of therapy. Androgen-deprivation therapy (ADT) may increase the risk for decreased bone mineral density. Hyperglycemia and an increased risk of developing diabetes has been reported with therapy and may manifest as diabetes or worsening of glycemic control in patients with diabetes; monitor blood glucose and/or glycosylated hemoglobin (HbA_{1c}) as clinically necessary. Cases of spinal cord compression, which may contribute to weakness or paralysis (possible fatal complications), have been reported. Closely observe (during the first 2 weeks of treatment) patients with metastatic vertebral lesions or urinary tract obstruction. Hypersensitivity reactions including angioedema and anaphylactic shock have occurred; discontinue if severe reaction occurs. Rare cases of pituitary apoplexy (frequently secondary to pituitary adenoma) have been observed with GnRH agonist administration (onset from 1 hour to usually <2 weeks); may present as sudden headache, vomiting, visual or mental status changes, and infrequently cardiovascular collapse; immediate medical attention required.

ADT may increase the risk for cardiovascular disease (Levine, 2010). Myocardial infarction, sudden cardiac death and stroke have been reported in men receiving GnRH agonists. ADT may prolong the QT/QTc interval; consider the benefits of ADT versus the risk for QT prolongation in patients with a history of QTc prolongation, congenital long QT syndrome, heart failure, frequent electrolyte abnormalities, and in patients with medications known to prolong the QT interval. Consider periodic monitoring of electrocardiograms and electrolytes in at-risk patients.

Decapeptyl [Canadian product]: Ovarian hyperstimulation syndrome (OHSS) is a rare exaggerated response to ovulation induction therapy (Corbett 2014; Fiedler 2012). This syndrome may begin within 24 hours of treatment but may become most severe 7 to 10 days after therapy (Corbett 2014). Symptoms of mild/moderate OHSS may include abdominal distention/discomfort, diarrhea, nausea, and/or vomiting. Severe OHSS symptoms may include severe abdominal pain, anuria/oliguria, ascites, severe dyspnea, hypotension, or nausea/vomiting (intractable). Decreased creatinine clearance, hemoconcentration, hypoproteinemia, elevated liver enzymes, elevated WBC, and electrolyte imbalances may also be present (ASRM 2016; Corbett 2014; Fiedler 2012). Treatment is primarily symptomatic and includes fluid and electrolyte management, analgesics, and prevention of thromboembolic complications (ASRM 2016; SOGC-CFAS 2011). Therapy with gonadotropins should be stopped.

Adverse Reactions Prostate cancer: As reported with all strengths; frequency of effect may vary by strength:

>10%:

Endocrine & metabolic: Hot flash (59% to 72%), increased serum glucose, increased testosterone (peak: days 2-4; decline to low levels by weeks 3-4)

Hematologic & oncologic: Decreased hemoglobin, decreased red blood cells

Hepatic: Increased serum alkaline phosphatase (2% to >10%), increased serum ALT, increased serum AST

Neuromuscular & skeletal: Musculoskeletal pain (12% to 13%)

Renal: Increased blood urea nitrogen

1% to 10%:

Cardiovascular: Lower extremity edema (6%), hypertension (≤4%), chest pain (2%), dependent edema (2%), peripheral edema (≤1%)

Central nervous system: Headache (2% to 7%), pain (2% to 3%), dizziness (1% to 3%), fatigue (2%), insomnia (1% to ≤2%), emotional lability (1%)

Dermatologic: Skin rash (2%), pruritus (1%)

Endocrine & metabolic: Decreased libido (2%), gynecomastia (2%)

Gastrointestinal: Nausea (3%), anorexia (2%), constipation (2%), dyspepsia (2%), mastalgia (2%), vomiting (2%), abdominal pain (1%), diarrhea (1%)

Genitourinary: Erectile dysfunction (10%), testicular atrophy (8%), impotence (2% to 7%), dysuria (5%), urinary retention (≤1%), urinary tract infection (≤1%)

Hematologic & oncologic: Anemia (1%)

Local: Pain at injection site (4%)

Neuromuscular & skeletal: Leg pain (2% to 5%), back pain (≤3%), leg cramps (2%), arthralgia (≤2%), myalgia (1%), weakness (1%)

Ophthalmic: Conjunctivitis (1%), eye pain (1%)

Respiratory: Cough (2%), dyspnea (1%), pharyngitis (1%)

Reproductive studies:

>10%:

Central nervous system: Headache (4% to 27%)

Gastrointestinal: Abdominal pain (9% to 15%)

Genitourinary: Vaginal hemorrhage (2% to 24%)

Local: Inflammation at injection site (10% to 12%)

1% to 10%:

Cardiovascular: Flushing (4%)

Central nervous system: Dizziness (4% to 5%), fatigue (3% to 4%), malaise (2%)

Endocrine & metabolic: Spontaneous abortion (7%), dysmenorrhea (2% to 6%), ovarian hyperstimulation syndrome (3%), hot flash (2%), ovarian cyst (1%)

Gastrointestinal: Nausea (3% to 10%), vomiting (3%), abdominal distension (2%), diarrhea (2%)

Genitourinary: Pelvic pain (6%), gynecological pain (adnexa uteri, 2%), leukorrhea (2%)

◄

      Local: Pain at injection site (4% to 7%), bruising at injection site (3%), injection site reaction (2% to 3%)

      Neuromuscular & skeletal: Postoperative pain (3% to 4%), back pain (3%)

      Respiratory: Upper respiratory tract infection (4%), flu-like symptoms (3%), pharyngitis (3%), dyspnea (2%), rhinitis (2%)

Postmarketing and/or case reports (all indications): Anaphylactic shock, anaphylaxis, angioedema, bladder outflow obstruction, blurred vision, cerebrovascular accident, circulatory shock, deep vein thrombosis, dyspareunia, exacerbation of depression, hematuria, hypersensitivity reaction, increased appetite, limb pain, myocardial infarction, neuropathy, ostealgia, pituitary apoplexy, prolonged Q-T interval on ECG, pulmonary embolism, renal insufficiency, seizure, sleep disorder, spinal cord compression, thrombophlebitis, tissue necrosis at injection site, transient ischemic attacks, tumor flare, urethral obstruction, vaginal dryness

Drug Interactions

Metabolism/Transport Effects None known.

Avoid Concomitant Use

Avoid concomitant use of Triptorelin with any of the following: Corifollitropin Alfa; Indium 111 Capromab Pendetide

Increased Effect/Toxicity

Triptorelin may increase the levels/effects of: Corifollitropin Alfa; Highest Risk QTc-Prolonging Agents; Moderate Risk QTc-Prolonging Agents

The levels/effects of Triptorelin may be increased by: MiFEPRIStone

Decreased Effect

Triptorelin may decrease the levels/effects of: Antidiabetic Agents; Choline C 11; Indium 111 Capromab Pendetide

Hazardous Drugs Handling Considerations

Hazardous agent (NIOSH 2016 [group 1]).

Use appropriate precautions for receiving, handling, administration, and disposal. Gloves (single) should be worn during receiving, unpacking, and placing in storage.

For IM preparation, double gloves, a protective gown, and ventilated engineering controls (a class II biological safety cabinet or a compounding aseptic containment isolator) are recommended. Double gloving and a protective gown are required during IM administration (NIOSH 2016).

Storage/Stability

Trelstar: Store at 20°C to 25°C (68°F to 77°F). Do not freeze MIXJECT system. Administer immediately after reconstitution.

Decapeptyl [Canadian product]: Store at 2°C to 8°C (36°F to 46°F); do not freeze. Protect from light.

Preparation for Administration

Trelstar: Reconstitute with 2 mL sterile water for injection. Shake well to obtain a uniform suspension. Solution will appear milky. Administer immediately after reconstitution.

MIXJECT System: Follow manufacturer's instructions for mixing prior to use.

Mechanism of Action Triptorelin is an agonist analog of gonadotropin releasing hormone (GnRH) and causes suppression of ovarian and testicular steroidogenesis due to decreased levels of LH and FSH with subsequent decrease in testosterone (male) and estrogen (female) levels. After chronic and continuous administration, usually 2 to 4 weeks after initiation, a sustained decrease in LH and FSH secretion occurs. When used for ART, prevents premature LH surge in women undergoing controlled ovarian hyperstimulation.

Pharmacodynamics/Kinetics

Distribution: V_d: 30 to 33 L

Protein binding: None

Metabolism: Unknown; unlikely to involve CYP; no known metabolites

Half-life elimination: 2.8 ± 1.2 hours

  Moderate-to-severe renal impairment: 6.6 to 7.7 hours

  Hepatic impairment: 7.6 hours

Time to peak: 1 to 3 hours

Excretion: Urine (42% as intact peptide); hepatic

Dosing

Adult & Geriatric

Advanced prostate carcinoma: IM:

3.75 mg once every 4 weeks **or**

11.25 mg once every 12 weeks **or**

22.5 mg once every 24 weeks

Controlled ovarian hyperstimulation for assisted reproductive technologies (ART) (adjunctive therapy): *Decapeptyl [Canadian product]):* Females: SubQ: Usual dose: 0.1 mg once daily initiated on day 2 or 3 or days 21 to 23 of menstrual cycle (or 5 to 7 days prior to expected onset of menses). Dose may be adjusted according to ovarian response as measured by ovarian ultrasound with or without serum estradiol levels. Treatment is continued until follicles achieve suitable size (typically 4 to 7 weeks).

Treatment of paraphilia/hypersexuality (off-label use; Guay, 2009; Thibaut, 1993): Males:

Note: May cause an initial increase in androgen concentrations which may be treated with an antiandrogen (eg, flutamide, cyproterone) for 1 to 2 months (Guay, 2009). Avoid use in patients with osteoporosis or active pituitary pathology.

SubQ: Test dose: 1 mg (observe for hypersensitivity)

IM: 3.75 mg monthly

Renal Impairment There are no dosage adjustments provided in the manufacturer's labeling. However, renal impairment increases systemic exposure to triptorelin.

Hepatic Impairment There are no dosage adjustments provided in the manufacturer's labeling. However, hepatic impairment increases systemic exposure to triptorelin.

Administration

Administer by IM injection into the buttock; alternate injection sites. Administer immediately after reconstitution.

Decapeptyl [Canadian product] is administered by subcutaneous injection into the lower abdomen; alternate injection sites. If a dose is missed, it can be administered on the same day; however, do not double doses.

Monitoring Parameters

Serum testosterone levels, prostate-specific antigen, glucose and HbA_{1c} (periodically), bone density, signs and symptoms of emerging cardiovascular disease; consider periodic monitoring of electrocardiograms and electrolytes.

Decapeptyl [Canadian product]: Negative pregnancy test prior to initiation of therapy; signs/symptoms of allergic reaction for 30 minutes after administration; ultrasound and/or estradiol levels to assess follicle development; ultrasound to assess number and size of follicles

OHSS: Monitoring of hospitalized patients should include abdominal circumference, albumin, cardiorespiratory status, electrolytes, fluid balance, hematocrit, hemoglobin, serum creatinine, urine output, urine specific gravity, vital signs, weight (daily or as necessary) and liver enzymes (weekly) (SOGC-CFAS 2011).

Treatment of paraphilia/hypersexuality (off-label use): The following monitoring has been recommended for other GnRH agonists: CBC (baseline, monthly for 4 months then every 6 months); serum testosterone (baseline, monthly for 4 months then every 6 months); serum LH (baseline and every 6 months), FSH (baseline), serum BUN and creatinine (baseline and every 6 months); bone density (baseline and yearly); ECG (baseline) (Reilly 2000)

Test Interactions Pituitary-gonadal function may be suppressed with chronic administration and for up to 8 weeks after triptorelin therapy has been discontinued.

Product Availability

Triptodur: FDA approved June 2017; anticipated availability during fourth quarter of 2017.

Triptodur is an extended release IM injection approved for the treatment of pediatric patients 2 years and older with central precocious puberty.

Dosage Forms Excipient information presented when available (limited, particularly for generics); consult specific product labeling. [DSC] = Discontinued product

Suspension Reconstituted, Intramuscular:

Trelstar: 3.75 mg (1 ea [DSC]); 11.25 mg (1 ea [DSC]) [contains polysorbate 80]

Trelstar Mixject: 3.75 mg (1 ea); 11.25 mg (1 ea); 22.5 mg (1 ea) [contains polysorbate 80]

Suspension Reconstituted ER, Intramuscular:

Triptodur: 22.5 mg (1 ea) [contains polysorbate 80]

Dosage Forms: Canada Information with regard to form, strength, and availability of products uniquely available in Canada but currently not available in the US. Refer also to Dosage Forms.

Excipient information presented when available (limited, particularly for generics); consult specific product labeling.

Injection, solution, as acetate [preservative free]:

Decapeptyl: 100 mcg/mL (equivalent to 95.6 mcg triptorelin free base) (1 mL) [prefilled syringe]

Uridine Triacetate (URE i deen trye AS e tate)

Related Information

Mucositis and Stomatitis *on page* 2299

Brand Names: US Vistogard; Xuriden

Index Terms PN401; Triacetyluridine; Vistonuridine

Pharmacologic Category Antidote; Endocrine and Metabolic Agent, Miscellaneous

Use

Hereditary orotic aciduria: Treatment of hereditary orotic aciduria

Fluoropyrimidine overdose/overexposure: Emergency treatment of fluorouracil or capecitabine overdose (regardless of the presence of symptoms) or early-onset severe or life-threatening cardiac or CNS toxicity and/or early-onset unusually severe adverse reactions (eg, GI toxicity and/or neutropenia) within 96 hours following the end of fluorouracil or capecitabine administration (in pediatrics and adults).

Limitations of use: Uridine triacetate is not recommended for nonemergent treatment of adverse reactions associated with fluorouracil or capecitabine (because it may diminish efficacy of these medications). Safety and efficacy of uridine triacetate initiated more than 96 hours following the end of fluorouracil or capecitabine administration have not been established.

Labeled Contraindications There are no contraindications listed in the manufacturer's labeling.

Pregnancy Considerations Adverse events were not observed in animal reproduction studies. Information related to the use of uridine triacetate for the treatment of hereditary orotic aciduria and fluoropyrimidine overdose/severe (life-threatening) toxicity during pregnancy is limited; monitor closely, dose adjustments may be required (Bensen 1991). In general, medications used as antidotes should take into consideration the health and prognosis of the mother; antidotes should be administered to pregnant women if there is a clear indication for use and should not be withheld because of fears of teratogenicity (Bailey 2003).

Breastfeeding Considerations It is not known if uridine triacetate is excreted into breast milk. According to the manufacturer, the decision to breast-feed during therapy should take into account the risk of exposure to the infant and the benefits of treatment to the mother.

Warnings/Precautions There are no warnings listed in the manufacturer's labeling.

◀ **Adverse Reactions**
1% to 10%:
Gastrointestinal: Vomiting (10%), nausea (5%), diarrhea (3%)

Drug Interactions

Metabolism/Transport Effects None known.

Avoid Concomitant Use There are no known interactions where it is recommended to avoid concomitant use.

Increased Effect/Toxicity There are no known significant interactions involving an increase in effect.

Decreased Effect There are no known significant interactions involving a decrease in effect.

Storage/Stability Store at 25°C (77°F); excursions permitted to 15°C to 30°C (59°F to 86°F).

Fluoropyrimidine overdose/overexposure: Use within 30 minutes of preparation in soft food.

Hereditary orotic aciduria: If administering in food (applesauce, pudding, or yogurt), use immediately after preparation.

Preparation for Administration Measure the dose using either a scale accurate to at least 0.1 g, or a graduated teaspoon, accurate to the fraction of the dose to be administered; discard the unused portion of granule packet (do not use granules left in the open packet).

Fluoropyrimidine overdose/overexposure:

Oral administration: Mix each dose with 3 to 4 ounces of soft food (applesauce, pudding, or yogurt).

Nasogastric (NG) or gastrostomy tube administration: Prepare ~100 mL of a food starch-based thickening product in water and stir briskly until thickener has dissolved. Crush contents of one full 10 g packet to a fine powder. Add the crushed powder to ~100 mL of reconstituted thickening product. For pediatric patients receiving less than 10 g, prepare the mixture at a ratio of no more than 1 g/10 mL of reconstituted thickening product and mix thoroughly.

Hereditary orotic aciduria:

Administration with food: Place 3 to 4 ounces of applesauce, pudding or yogurt in a small clean container. Mix the measured amount of granules in the applesauce, pudding or yogurt.

Administration in milk or infant formula: May be mixed with milk or infant formula for patients receiving a dose of up to 2 g (3/4 teaspoon). After weighing/measuring the dose, pour 5 mL of milk or infant formula into a 30 mL medicine cup. Insert the tip of an oral syringe into medicine cup and draw up 5 mL of milk/infant formula into syringe. Hold the syringe with the tip pointing upward, pull down on the plunger until the plunger reaches 10 mL (this will add air to the syringe). Place the cap over the tip of the syringe. Then invert the syringe so the syringe tip is pointing down, and remove the plunger. Pour the measured amount of uridine triacetate granules into the syringe barrel and reinsert the syringe plunger. Do not push up on the plunger. Gently swirl the syringe to mix the uridine triacetate granules with the liquid. Turn the syringe so the syringe tip is pointing up. Then remove the syringe cap and push up on the plunger until plunger reaches the 5 mL mark to remove air from the syringe. Place the tip of the syringe in the patient's mouth between the cheek and gum at the back of the mouth.

Gently push the plunger all the way down. Refill the syringe with another 5 mL of milk/infant formula. Gently swirl the syringe to rinse remaining uridine triacetate granules from the syringe barrel. Place the tip of the syringe in the patient's mouth between the cheek and gum at the back of the mouth. Gently push the plunger all the way down. May follow with a bottle of milk or infant formula.

Mechanism of Action Uridine triacetate is an acetylated form of uridine which is deacetylated following administration to provide circulating uridine in patients with hereditary orotic aciduria. In patients with fluorouracil overdose or overexposure, uridine triacetate is a direct chemical antagonist against fluorouracil toxicity (Bamat 2013). Uridine reduces incorporation of fluorouridine triphosphate (FUTP; a fluorouracil metabolite) into RNA of hematopoietic progenitor cells and gastrointestinal mucosal cells to reduce fluorouracil toxicity in normal tissues (Hidalgo 2000).

Pharmacodynamics/Kinetics

Onset: Hereditary orotic aciduria: Oral exogenous uridine improves hematologic abnormalities within 2 to 3 weeks; urinary orotic acid reduced within 1 to 2 weeks of initiating therapy.

Duration of action: Hereditary orotic aciduria: Hematologic abnormalities and orotic aciduria return within days up to 2 to 3 weeks after discontinuation or dose reduction.

Distribution: Distributes into cells; crosses the blood brain barrier

Metabolism: Deacetylated (by nonspecific esterases) to uridine and free acetate (Hidalgo 2000)

Half-life elimination: 2 to 2.5 hours

Time to peak: 2 to 3 hours

Excretion: Urine; also catabolic metabolism in tissues.

Dosing

Adult & Geriatric

Fluoropyrimidine overdose/overexposure: Oral: 10 g every 6 hours for 20 doses beginning as soon as possible after overdose or early-onset toxicity within 96 hours after the end of fluorouracil or capecitabine administration (Bamat 2013; von Borstel 2009). Administer the full course of 20 doses, even if the patient appears or feels well.

Hereditary orotic aciduria: Oral: Initial: 60 mg/kg once daily; increase to 120 mg/kg (maximum: 8 g) for insufficient efficacy (eg, urine orotic acid levels remaining above normal or increasing above the usual/expected range for the patient; lab values affected by orotic acid [red or white blood cell indices] worsening; worsening disease signs/symptoms).

◄

Uridine Triacetate Daily Dose for Hereditary Orotic Aciduria Based on Weight (kg)

Patient weight	60 mg/kg[1] dose Dose in grams (dose in teaspoons[2])	120 mg/kg[1] dose Dose in grams (dose in teaspoons[2])
≤5 kg	0.4 g (1/8 tsp)	0.8 g (1/4 tsp)
6 to 10 kg	0.4 to 0.6 g (1/4 tsp)	0.8 to 1.2 g (1/2 tsp)
11 to 15 kg	0.7 to 0.9 g (1/2 tsp)	1.4 to 1.8 g (3/4 tsp or 1 entire packet)
16 to 20 kg	1 to 1.2 g (1/2 tsp)	2 to 2.4 g (1 tsp)
21 to 25 kg	1.3 to 1.5 g (1/2 tsp)	2.6 to 3 g (1 tsp)
26 to 30 kg	1.6 to 1.8 g (3/4 tsp or 1 entire packet)	3.2 to 3.6 g (1 1/4 tsp)
31 to 35 kg	1.9 to 2.1 g (3/4 tsp or 1 entire packet)	3.8 to 4.2 g (1 1/2 tsp or 2 entire packets)
36 to 40 kg	2.2 to 2.4 g (1 tsp)	4.4 to 4.8 g (1 3/4 tsp)
41 to 45 kg	2.5 to 2.7 g (1 tsp)	5 to 5.4 g (2 tsp or 3 entire packets)
46 to 50 kg	2.8 to 3 g (1 tsp)	5.6 to 6 g (2 tsp or 3 entire packets)
51 to 55 kg	3.1 to 3.3 g (1 1/4 tsp)	6.2 to 6.6 g (2 1/4 tsp)
56 to 60 kg	3.4 to 3.6 g (1 1/4 tsp)	6.8 to 7.2 g (2 1/2 tsp)
61 to 65 kg	3.7 to 3.9 g (1 1/2 tsp or 2 entire packets)	7.4 to 7.8 g (2 1/2 tsp)
66 to 70 kg	4 to 4.2 g (1 1/2 tsp or 2 entire packets)	8 g (2 3/4 tsp or 4 entire packets)
71 to 75 kg	4.3 to 4.5 g (1 1/2 tsp or 2 entire packets)	8 g (2 3/4 tsp or 4 entire packets)
>75 kg	6 g (2 tsp or 3 entire packets)	8 g (2 3/4 tsp or 4 entire packets)

Note: One packet contains uridine triacetate 2 g.
[1]Doses rounded (by the manufacturer) by weight category to achieve approximate dose level
[2]A 2 gram uridine triacetate (Xuriden) packet contains approximately 3/4 tsp

Pediatric

Fluoropyrimidine overdose/overexposure: Oral: 6.2 g/m^2 (maximum: 10 g/dose) every 6 hours for 20 doses beginning as soon as possible after overdose or early-onset toxicity within 96 hours after the end of fluorouracil or capecitabine administration. Administer the full course of 20 doses, even if the patient appears or feels well.

Uridine Triacetate Pediatric Dose for Fluoropyrimidine Overdose/Overexposure Based on Body Surface Area (BSA; m²)

Patient BSA	Uridine Triacetate 6.2 g/m²/dose[a]	
	Dose in grams	Dose in graduated teaspoons
0.34 to 0.44 m²	2.1 to 2.7 g	1 tsp
0.45 to 0.55 m²	2.8 to 3.4 g	1 1/4 tsp
0.56 to 0.66 m²	3.5 to 4.1 g	1 1/2 tsp
0.67 to 0.77 m²	4.2 to 4.8 g	1 3/4 tsp
0.78 to 0.88 m²	4.9 to 5.4 g	2 tsp
0.89 to 0.99 m²	5.5 to 6.1 g	2 1/4 tsp
1 to 1.1 m²	6.2 to 6.8 g	2 1/2 tsp
1.11 to 1.21 m²	6.9 to 7.5 g	2 3/4 tsp
1.22 to 1.32 m²	7.6 to 8.1 g	3 tsp
1.33 to 1.43 m²	8.2 to 8.8 g	3 1/4 tsp
≥1.44 m²	10 g	1 full packet

Note: One Vistogard packet contains uridine triacetate 10 g.

[a]Doses rounded by BSA to achieve approximate dose; each dose is administered every 6 hours for 20 doses.

Hereditary orotic aciduria: Infants, Children, and Adolescents: Oral: Refer to adult dosing.

Renal Impairment There are no dosage adjustments provided in the manufacturer's labeling.

Hepatic Impairment There are no dosage adjustments provided in the manufacturer's labeling.

Administration

Granules: Measure the prescribed dose using either a scale accurate to at least 0.1 gram, or a graduated teaspoon, accurate to the fraction of the dose to be administered (accurate to 1/4 teaspoonful). Discard the unused portion of granule packet after measuring out the dose. Do not chew granules. May be administered without regard to meals (food does not have an effect on uridine exposure).

Fluoropyrimidine overdose/overexposure: Administer orally; begin as soon as possible after overdose or early-onset toxicity within 96 hours following the end of fluorouracil or capecitabine overdose/overexposure (Bamat 2013; von Borstel 2009). Administer within 30 minutes of preparation (in soft food such as applesauce, pudding, or yogurt), followed by at least 120 mL water. If patient vomits within 2 hours of taking dose, administer another complete dose as soon as possible after vomiting episode. If a dose is missed, administer the missed dose as soon as possible and then administer the next dose at the regularly scheduled time. If necessary to administer through a nasogastric or gastrostomy tube (due to stomatitis or mucositis), mix with thickening agent (see Preparation for Administration); following administration, flush tube with water. Administer the full treatment course (all 20 doses), even if the patient appears or feels well.

◀ Hereditary orotic aciduria:

Administration with food: May be mixed in food (ie, 3 to 4 ounces of applesauce, pudding, or yogurt) and administered immediately, followed by drinking at least 120 mL water. Do not chew the granules. Do not save for later use.

Administration in milk or infant formula: May be mixed with milk or infant formula for patients receiving a dose of up to 2 grams (3/4 teaspoon). See Preparation for Administration for oral syringe preparation instructions. Place the tip of the oral syringe in the patient's mouth between the cheek and gum at the back of the mouth. Gently push the plunger all the way down. Refill the syringe with another 5 mL of milk/infant formula. Gently swirl the syringe to rinse remaining uridine triacetate granules from the syringe barrel. Place the tip of the oral syringe in the patient's mouth between the cheek and gum at the back of the mouth. Gently push the plunger all the way down. May follow with a bottle of milk or infant formula.

Monitoring Parameters Fluoropyrimidine overdose/overexposure: CBC with differential; gastrointestinal toxicity (Hidalgo 2000).

Prescribing and Access Restrictions Fluorouracil accidental overdose/overexposure: Uridine triacetate (formerly called vistonuridine) is available through select specialty pharmacies. Procurement information is available from BTG Specialty Solutions at 1-844-293-0007; information on case management for transitioning from inpatient to outpatient care is available at 1-844-374-0604.

Dosage Forms Excipient information presented when available (limited, particularly for generics); consult specific product labeling.

Packet, Oral:

Vistogard: 10 g (4 ea, 20 ea) [orange flavor]

Xuriden: 2 g (1 ea, 30 ea) [orange flavor]

◆ **Uromitexan (Can)** *see* Mesna *on page 1199*

ValACYclovir (val ay SYE kloe veer)

Brand Names: US Valtrex

Brand Names: Canada Apo-Valacyclovir; Auro-Valacyclovir; CO Valacyclovir; DOM-Valacyclovir; JAMP-Valacyclovir; Mar-Valacyclovir; Mylan-Valacyclovir; PHL-Valacyclovir; PMS-Valacyclovir; Priva-Valacyclovir; PRO-Valacyclovir; Riva-Valacyclovir; Sandoz-Valacyclovir; Teva-Valacyclovir; Valtrex

Index Terms Valacyclovir HCl; Valacyclovir Hydrochloride

Pharmacologic Category Antiviral Agent; Antiviral Agent, Oral

Use Treatment of herpes zoster (shingles) in immunocompetent patients; treatment of first-episode and recurrent genital herpes in immunocompetent patients; suppression of recurrent genital herpes and reduction of transmission of genital herpes in immunocompetent patients; suppression of genital herpes in HIV-infected individuals; treatment of herpes labialis (cold sores); chickenpox in immunocompetent children

Pregnancy Risk Factor B

Dosing

Adult & Geriatric

Herpes labialis (cold sores): Oral: 2 g every 12 hours for 1 day

Herpes labialis (cold sores) in HIV-infected patients (off-label use): Oral: 1 g twice daily for 5 to 10 days (HHS [OI adult 2016])

Herpes zoster (shingles): Oral:

Immunocompetent patients: 1 g 3 times daily for 7 days

HIV-infected patients, acute localized dermatomal (off-label use): 1 g 3 times daily for 7 to 10 days; consider longer duration if lesions resolve slowly (HHS [OI adult 2016])

Herpes simplex virus (HSV), genital infection: Oral:

Manufacturer's labeling:

Initial episode: Immunocompetent patients: 1 g twice daily for 10 days. **Note:** CDC STD guidelines recommend a treatment duration of 7 to 10 days (CDC [Workowski 2015]).

Recurrent episode: Immunocompetent patients: 500 mg twice daily for 3 days or alternatively (off-label dose), 1,000 mg once daily for 5 days (CDC [Workowski 2015])

Reduction of transmission: 500 mg once daily (source partner)

Suppressive therapy:

Immunocompetent patients: 1 g once daily (500 mg once daily in patients with ≤9 recurrences per year). **Note:** Safety and efficacy have been documented for up to 1 year (CDC [Workowski 2015]).

HIV-infected patients (CD4 ≥100 cells/mm^3): 500 mg twice daily

Alternate dosing: HIV-infected patients:

Initial or recurrent episodes (off-label use): 1 g twice daily for 5 to 10 days (HHS [OI adult 2016])

Chronic suppressive therapy: 500 mg twice daily; continue indefinitely regardless of CD4 count in patients with severe recurrences or in patients who want to minimize frequency of recurrences (HHS [OI adult 2016])

B virus, postexposure prophylaxis (off-label use): Oral: 1 g 3 times daily for 14 days (Tunkel 2008)

CMV reactivation (prevention in allogeneic HSCT recipients) (off-label use): Oral: 2 g 3 to 4 times daily; in combination with screening for CMV reactivation; begin at engraftment and continue to day 100 (Tomblyn 2009)

HSV keratitis (off-label use) (White 2014): Oral

Epithelial keratitis, dendritic: 500 mg twice daily for 7 to 10 days

Epithelial keratitis, geographic: 1 g 3 times daily for 14 to 21 days

Stromal keratitis, without epithelial ulceration: 500 mg once daily; use in combination with therapeutic dose of topical corticosteroid, for the duration of corticosteroid treatment

Stromal keratitis, with epithelial ulceration: 1 g 3 times daily for 7 to 10 days, then reduce to 500 mg once daily; use in combination with therapeutic dose of topical corticosteroid, for the duration of corticosteroid treatment

Endothelial keratitis: 500 mg twice daily for 7 to 10 days, then reduce to 500 mg once daily; use in combination with therapeutic dose of topical corticosteroid, for the duration of corticosteroid treatment.

HSV reactivation (prevention in seropositive HSCT recipients) (off-label use) (Tomblyn 2009): Oral:

Early reactivation: 500 mg once daily **or** 500 mg twice daily in highly immune-suppressed patients (eg, T cell depletion, anti-T cell antibodies, high-dose steroids). Initiate at the beginning of conditioning therapy and continue until engraftment or until mucositis resolves

Late reactivation: 500 mg twice daily

Varicella (chickenpox) in HIV-infected patients (off-label use): 1 g 3 times daily for 5 to 7 days in uncomplicated cases (HHS [OI adult 2016])

Varicella zoster virus (VZV) acute retinal necrosis (ARN) in HIV-infected patients (off-label use): Oral: 1 g 3 times daily for 6 weeks following initial treatment with acyclovir IV and intravitreal ganciclovir (HHS [OI adult 2016])

VZV, postexposure prophylaxis (HSCT recipients) (off-label use): Oral: 1 g 3 times daily; initiate within 96 hours (preferably, 48 hours) of exposure and continue until 22 days after exposure (Tomblyn 2009)

VZV reactivation (prevention in HSCT recipients) (off-label use): Oral: 500 mg twice daily for 1 year after HSCT (Tomblyn 2009)

Pediatric

Herpes labialis (cold sores): Children ≥12 years and Adolescents: Oral: Refer to adult dosing.

Herpes labialis (cold sores) in HIV-infected patients (off-label use): Adolescents: Oral: Refer to adult dosing.

Herpes simplex virus, genital infection in HIV-infected patients: Adolescents (off-label population): Oral:

Initial or recurrent episodes (off-label use): 1 g twice daily for 5 to 14 days (HHS [OI adult 2015])

Chronic suppressive therapy (off-label dose): 500 mg twice daily; continue indefinitely regardless of CD4 count in patients with severe recurrences or in patients who want to minimize frequency of recurrences (HHS [OI adult 2015])

Herpes zoster (shingles) in HIV-infected patients (off-label use): Adolescents: Oral: Refer to adult dosing.

Varicella (chickenpox):

Immunocompetent patients: Children ≥2 years and Adolescents: Oral: 20 mg/kg/dose 3 times daily for 5 days (maximum: 1 g 3 times daily)

HIV-infected patients (off-label use): Adolescents: Oral: Refer to adult dosing.

Renal Impairment

Herpes zoster: Adults:

CrCl 30 to 49 mL/minute: 1 g every 12 hours

CrCl 10 to 29 mL/minute: 1 g every 24 hours

CrCl <10 mL/minute: 500 mg every 24 hours

Genital herpes: Adults:

US labeling:

Initial episode:

CrCl 10 to 29 mL/minute: 1 g every 24 hours

CrCl <10 mL/minute: 500 mg every 24 hours

Recurrent episode: CrCl <29 mL/minute: 500 mg every 24 hours

Suppressive therapy: CrCl <29 mL/minute:

For usual dose of 1 g every 24 hours or 500 mg every 12 hours, decrease dose to 500 mg every 24 hours

For usual dose of 500 mg every 24 hours, decrease dose to 500 mg every 48 hours

Canadian labeling:

Initial episode:

CrCl 10 to 29 mL/minute: 1 g every 24 hours

CrCl <10 mL/minute: 500 mg every 24 hours

Recurrent episode:

CrCl 10 to 29 mL/minute: 500 mg every 24 hours

CrCl <10 mL/minute: 500 mg every 24 hours

Suppressive therapy:
CrCl 10 to 29 mL/minute:
Immunocompetent or HIV-infected patients: 500 mg every 24 hours
Immunocompetent patients with ≤9 recurrences/year: 500 mg every 48 hours
CrCl <10 mL/minute:
Immunocompetent or HIV-infected patients: 500 mg every 24 hours
Immunocompetent patients with ≤9 recurrences/year: 500 mg every 48 hours

Herpes labialis (cold sores): Adolescents and Adults *(US labeling)* or Adults *(Canadian labeling)*:
CrCl 30 to 49 mL/minute: 1 g every 12 hours for 2 doses
CrCl 10 to 29 mL/minute: 500 mg every 12 hours for 2 doses
CrCl <10 mL/minute: 500 mg as a single dose

Hemodialysis: Dialyzable (~33% removed during 4-hour session); administer dose postdialysis

Chronic ambulatory peritoneal dialysis/continuous arteriovenous hemofiltration dialysis: Pharmacokinetic parameters are similar to those in patients with ESRD; supplemental dose not needed following dialysis

Hepatic Impairment No dosage adjustment necessary.

Additional Information Complete prescribing information should be consulted for additional detail.

Dosage Forms Excipient information presented when available (limited, particularly for generics); consult specific product labeling.
Tablet, Oral:
Valtrex: 500 mg [contains fd&c blue #2 aluminum lake]
Valtrex: 1 g [scored; contains fd&c blue #2 aluminum lake]
Generic: 500 mg, 1 g

◆ **Valacyclovir HCl** *see* ValACYclovir *on page 1852*

◆ **Valacyclovir Hydrochloride** *see* ValACYclovir *on page 1852*

◆ **Valchlor** *see* Mechlorethamine (Topical) *on page 1173*

◆ **Valcyte** *see* ValGANciclovir *on page 1855*

◆ **9-Valent HPV** *see* Papillomavirus (9-Valent) Vaccine (Human, Recombinant) *on page 1452*

ValGANciclovir (val gan SYE kloh veer)

Brand Names: US Valcyte
Brand Names: Canada Apo-Valganciclovir; Valcyte
Index Terms Valganciclovir HCl; Valganciclovir Hydrochloride
Pharmacologic Category Antiviral Agent
Use
Cytomegalovirus, prophylaxis (solid organ transplant recipients):
Prevention of cytomegalovirus (CMV) in high-risk adult patients (donor CMV seropositive/recipient CMV seronegative) undergoing kidney, heart, or kidney/pancreas transplantation
Prevention of CMV in high risk pediatric patients undergoing kidney transplant (age 4 months to 16 years) or heart transplant (age 1 month to 16 years)
CMV retinitis, treatment (AIDS-related): Treatment of cytomegalovirus (CMV) retinitis in patients with acquired immunodeficiency syndrome (AIDS)

CrCl 25 to 39 mL/minute: 450 mg every 2 days

CrCl 10 to 24 mL/minute: 450 mg twice weekly

CrCl <10 mL/minute:

Manufacturer labeling: Use not recommended; ganciclovir (with appropriately specified renal dosage adjustment) should be used instead of valganciclovir

Alternate dosing: HIV infected persons: Consider valganciclovir solution 100 mg 3 times weekly (Lucas, 2014)

End stage renal disease (ESRD) on intermittent hemodialysis (IHD):

Manufacturer labeling: Use not recommended; ganciclovir (with appropriately specified renal dosage adjustment) should be used instead of valganciclovir.

Alternate dosing: HIV-1 infected persons: Consider valganciclovir solution: 100 mg 3 times weekly (Lucas, 2014); valganciclovir is dialyzable and should be administered following dialysis.

Hepatic Impairment There are no dosage adjustments provided in the manufacturer labeling (has not been studied).

Additional Information Complete prescribing information should be consulted for additional detail.

Dosage Forms Excipient information presented when available (limited, particularly for generics); consult specific product labeling.

Solution Reconstituted, Oral:

Valcyte: 50 mg/mL (88 mL) [contains saccharin sodium, sodium benzoate; tutti-frutti flavor]

Generic: 50 mg/mL (88 mL)

Tablet, Oral:

Valcyte: 450 mg

Generic: 450 mg

◆ **Valganciclovir HCl** *see* ValGANciclovir *on page 1855*

◆ **Valganciclovir Hydrochloride** *see* ValGANciclovir *on page 1855*

Valrubicin (val ROO bi sin)

Related Information

Management of Chemotherapy-Induced Nausea and Vomiting in Adults *on page 2253*

Prevention of Chemotherapy-Induced Nausea and Vomiting in Children *on page 2310*

Safe Handling of Hazardous Drugs *on page 2379*

Brand Names: US Valstar

Brand Names: Canada Valtaxin

Index Terms *N*-trifluoroacetyladriamycin-14-valerate; AD32

Pharmacologic Category Antineoplastic Agent, Anthracycline; Antineoplastic Agent, Topoisomerase II Inhibitor

Use Bladder cancer: Intravesical treatment of BCG-refractory bladder carcinoma in situ of the urinary bladder when cystectomy would be associated with unacceptable morbidity or mortality.

Labeled Contraindications Known hypersensitivity to anthracyclines, polyoxyl castor oil, or any component of the formulation; perforated bladder; concurrent urinary tract infection; small bladder capacity (unable to tolerate a 75 mL instillation)

Pregnancy Considerations Adverse effects were observed in animal reproduction studies. Systemic exposure (eg, with bladder perforation) during human pregnancy may result in fetal harm. Women of childbearing potential should avoid becoming pregnant during treatment. All patients of reproductive age should use an effective method of contraception during the treatment period.

Breastfeeding Considerations It is not known if valrubicin is excreted in breast milk. Due to the potential for serious adverse reactions in the nursing infant, breastfeeding should be discontinued prior to initiation of therapy.

Warnings/Precautions Delay valrubicin therapy for at least 2 weeks after transurethral resection and/or fulguration. Evaluate bladder status prior to instillation; do not administer if mucosal integrity of bladder has been compromised or bladder perforation is present (delay treatment until restoration of bladder integrity). Use aseptic technique to prevent urinary tract infection or traumatizing urinary mucosa. Although clamping of the urinary catheter after administration is not recommended, use caution and appropriate medical supervision if performed. Irritable bladder symptoms may occur during instillation and retention, and for a brief time after voiding. Use caution in patients with severe irritable bladder symptoms. Red-tinged urine is typical for the first 24 hours after instillation. Prolonged symptoms or discoloration should prompt contact with the physician.

Contains polyoxyl castor oil which may be associated with hypersensitivity reactions; use is contraindicated in patients with hypersensitivity to polyoxyl castor oil. Delaying cystectomy for intravesical treatment may lead to metastatic bladder cancer; the risk for metastatic disease increases with delay duration; reconsider cystectomy for recurrence or if complete response to treatment does not occur within 3 months.

Adverse Reactions In general, local adverse reactions occur during or shortly after instillation and resolve within 1 to 7 days.

>10%: Genitourinary: Irritable bladder (88%), urinary frequency (61%), urinary urgency (57%), dysuria (56%), bladder spasm (31%), hematuria (29%; microscopic: 3%; gross hematuria: 1%), bladder pain (28%), urinary incontinence (22%), cystitis (15%), urinary tract infection (15%), red urine discoloration

1% to 10%:
Cardiovascular: Chest pain (3%), vasodilatation (2%), peripheral edema (1%)
Central nervous system: Localized burning (5%), headache (4%), malaise (4%), dizziness (3%)
Dermatologic: Skin rash (3%)
Endocrine & metabolic: Hyperglycemia (1%)
Gastrointestinal: Abdominal pain (5%), nausea (5%), diarrhea (3%), vomiting (2%), flatulence (1%)
Genitourinary: Nocturia (7%), urinary retention (4%), urethral pain (3%), pelvic pain (1%)
Hematologic & oncologic: Anemia (2%)
Neuromuscular & skeletal: Weakness (4%), back pain (3%), myalgia (1%)
Respiratory: Pneumonia (1%)
Miscellaneous: Fever (2%)
<1%, postmarketing, and/or case reports: Ageusia, increased nonprotein nitrogen, pruritus, reduced urine flow, skin irritation (local), tenesmus, urethritis

◀ **Drug Interactions**

Metabolism/Transport Effects None known.

Avoid Concomitant Use There are no known interactions where it is recommended to avoid concomitant use.

Increased Effect/Toxicity There are no known significant interactions involving an increase in effect.

Decreased Effect There are no known significant interactions involving a decrease in effect.

Hazardous Drugs Handling Considerations

Hazardous agent (NIOSH 2016 [group 1]).

Use appropriate precautions for receiving, handling, administration, and disposal. Gloves (single) should be worn during receiving, unpacking, and placing in storage.

NIOSH recommends double gloving, a protective gown, and preparation in a controlled device or use of ventilated engineering controls (a class II biological safety cabinet or a compounding aseptic containment isolator) for preparation; if not prepared in a controlled device, respiratory and eye/face protection as well as ventilated engineering controls are recommended. NIOSH recommends double gloving, a protective gown, and eye/face and respiratory protection for intravesical administration (NIOSH 2016).

Storage/Stability Store intact vials at 2°C to 8°C (36°F to 48°F). Do not freeze. Solutions diluted in 0.9% sodium chloride are stable for 12 hours at room temperature.

Preparation for Administration Allow vials to slowly warm to room temperature (do not heat) prior to use. A waxy precipitate (due to polyoxyl castor oil) may form at temperatures <4°C, warm vial in the hand until solution is clear (do not use vial if particulate still present). Dilute 800 mg (20 mL) with 55 mL NS (total volume of 75 mL). Use non-PVC containers (glass, polyolefin, or polypropylene) and administration sets to avoid leaching of DEHP plasticizers. Stable for 12 hours at room temperature when diluted in 0.9% sodium chloride. Do not mix with other drugs.

Mechanism of Action Blocks function of DNA topoisomerase II; inhibits DNA synthesis, causes extensive chromosomal damage, and arrests cell development (G_2 phase); unlike other anthracyclines, does not appear to intercalate DNA; readily penetrates cells.

Pharmacodynamics/Kinetics

Absorption: Intravesical: Penetrates into bladder wall; negligible systemic absorption (dependent on bladder wall condition; trauma to mucosa may increase absorption, bladder wall perforation may significantly increase absorption and systemic myelotoxicity).

Metabolism: Negligible after intravesical instillation and 2-hour retention

Excretion: Urine (post 2-hour retention): 98.6% as intact drug; 0.4% as N-trifluoroacetyladriamycin)

Dosing

Adult & Geriatric Note: Delay for at least 2 weeks after transurethral resection and/or fulguration.

Bladder cancer: Intravesical: 800 mg once weekly (retain for 2 hours) for 6 weeks

Renal Impairment There are no dosage adjustments provided in the manufacturer's labeling. However, dosage adjustment unlikely due to low systemic absorption.

Hepatic Impairment There are no dosage adjustments provided in the manufacturer's labeling. However, dosage adjustment unlikely due to low systemic absorption.

Adjustment for Toxicity In clinical trials (Steinberg 2000), treatment was delayed for 1 week for the following adverse events: Grade 3 dysuria (not controlled with phenazopyridine), frequency/urgency lasting >24 hours, grade 2 gross hematuria (without clots) lasting >48 hours, grade 3 hematuria (with clots) lasting >48 hours. For local toxicities <grade 4 (eg, dysuria [not controlled with phenazopyridine] or severe bladder spasm), anticholinergic therapy (systemic or topical) or topical anesthesia was administered prior to subsequent instillations.

Administration For intravesical use only; not for IV or IM use.

Intravesicular bladder instillation: Insert urinary catheter, empty bladder prior to instillation, slowly by gravity flow, instill 800 mg/75 mL (in 0.9% sodium chloride injection), remove catheter. Retain in the bladder for 2 hours, then void. Administer through non-PVC tubing due to the polyoxyl castor oil component. Maintain adequate hydration following treatment.

Emetic Potential Children and Adults: Minimal (<10%)

Monitoring Parameters Cystoscopy, biopsy, and urine cytology every 3 months for recurrence or progression

Dosage Forms Excipient information presented when available (limited, particularly for generics); consult specific product labeling.

Solution, Intravesical [preservative free]:

Valstar: 40 mg/mL (5 mL) [contains alcohol, usp, cremophor el]

◆ **Valstar** see Valrubicin on page 1858

◆ **Valtaxin (Can)** see Valrubicin on page 1858

◆ **Valtrex** see ValACYclovir on page 1852

◆ **Val-Vancomycin (Can)** see Vancomycin on page 1861

◆ **Vanc-Mycophenolate (Can)** see Mycophenolate on page 1283

◆ **Vancocin** see Vancomycin on page 1861

◆ **Vancocin HCl** see Vancomycin on page 1861

Vancomycin (van koe MYE sin)

Brand Names: US First-Vancomycin 25; First-Vancomycin 50; Vancocin HCl; Vancomycin+SyrSpend SF PH4

Brand Names: Canada JAMP-Vancomycin; PMS-Vancomycin; Sterile Vancomycin Hydrochloride, USP; Val-Vancomycin; Vancocin; Vancomycin Hydrochloride for Injection; Vancomycin Hydrochloride for Injection, USP

Index Terms Vancocin; Vancomycin HCl; Vancomycin Hydrochloride

Pharmacologic Category Glycopeptide

Use

Clostridium difficile **infection (oral):** Treatment of *C. difficile* infection (CDI)

Endocarditis (injection):

Corynebacteria (diphtheroids): Treatment of diphtheroid endocarditis in combination with either rifampin, an aminoglycoside, or both in early-onset prosthetic valve endocarditis caused by diphtheroids

Enterococcal: Treatment of endocarditis caused by enterococci (eg, *Enterococcus faecalis*), in combination with an aminoglycoside

Staphylococcal: Treatment of staphylococcal endocarditis

◀

Streptococcal: Treatment of endocarditis due to *Streptococcus viridans* or *Streptococcus bovis,* as monotherapy or in combination with an aminoglycoside

Staphylococcal infections (injection): Treatment of serious or severe infections (eg, septicemia, bone infections, lower respiratory tract infections, skin and skin structure infections) caused by susceptible strains of methicillin-resistant (beta-lactam-resistant) staphylococci; empiric therapy of infections when methicillin-resistant staphylococci are suspected

Pregnancy Risk Factor B (oral); C (injection)

Dosing

Adult & Geriatric

Usual dosage range: Note: Initial IV dosing in nonobese patients should be based on actual body weight; subsequent dosing should generally be adjusted based on serum trough vancomycin concentrations and renal function. Patient-specific pharmacokinetic calculations may be needed to determine appropriate dose and interval in patients expected to have altered pharmacokinetics (eg, morbid obesity, burns, critical illness, unstable renal function, pregnancy, cystic fibrosis). For patients with uncomplicated skin and soft tissue infections who are not obese and have normal renal function, serum trough monitoring is generally not needed (IDSA [Liu 2011]).

IV: **Note:** Ineffective for treating *C. difficile* infections (CDIs): 15 to 20 mg/kg/dose (rounded to the nearest 250 mg; usual maximum: 2 g/dose initially) every 8 to 12 hours (ASHP/IDSA/SIDP [Rybak 2009]). **Note:** 15 mg/kg/dose (usual maximum: 2 g/dose initially) every 12 hours is a usual starting dose in most nonobese patients with normal renal function; refer to infection-specific dosing (Drew 2017; IDSA [Liu 2011]; Murray 2015).

Loading dose: Complicated infections in seriously ill patients: A loading dose of 25 to 30 mg/kg (based on actual body weight) may be used to rapidly achieve target concentrations (ASHP/IDSA/SIDP [Rybak 2009]; Reardon 2015).

Oral: **Note:** Ineffective for treating systemic infections: 125 to 500 mg 4 times daily

Indication-specific dosing:

Bacteremia (off-label dose):

Empiric therapy or pathogen-specific therapy for methicillin-resistant S. aureus: IV: 15 to 20 mg/kg/dose (usual maximum: 2 g/dose initially) every 8 to 12 hours; adjust dose to obtain a trough concentration of 15 to 20 mcg/mL. A loading dose may be considered in seriously ill patients (ASHP/IDSA/SIDP [Rybak 2009]; IDSA [Liu 2011]). For catheter-related bloodstream infections, consider antibiotic lock therapy for catheter salvage, in addition to systemic therapy (IDSA [Mermel 2009]).

Empiric therapy or pathogen-specific therapy for methicillin-resistant coagulase-negative staphylococci: IV: 15 to 20 mg/kg/dose (usual maximum: 2 g/dose initially) every 8 to 12 hours (most patients with normal renal function can be started with 15 mg/kg/dose every 12 hours); adjust dose to obtain a trough concentration of 15 to 20 mcg/mL (Drew 2017). For catheter-related bloodstream infections, consider antibiotic lock therapy for catheter salvage, in addition to systemic therapy (IDSA [Mermel 2009]).

Antibiotic lock technique (catheter salvage strategy (off-label use): Prepare lock solution to final concentration of vancomycin 5 mg/mL (may be combined with heparin 5,000 units/mL). Instill into each lumen of the catheter access port using a volume sufficient to fill the catheter (2 to 5 mL) with a dwell time of 48 to 72 hours. Dwell times will depend on frequency of catheter use. Withdraw lock solution prior to catheter use; replace with fresh vancomycin lock solution after catheter use. For catheter-related bloodstream infections consider antibiotic lock technique, in addition to systemic antibiotics. Duration of lock therapy should be 10 to 14 days (IDSA [Mermel 2009]; LaPlante 2007).

Brain abscess, intracranial or spinal epidural abscess (off-label dose): As a component of empiric therapy or pathogen specific therapy for methicillin-resistant *S. aureus*: IV: 15 to 20 mg/kg/dose (usual maximum: 2 g/dose initially) every 8 to 12 hours; adjust dose to obtain a trough concentration of 15 to 20 mcg/mL. A loading dose may be considered in seriously ill patients (ASHP/IDSA/SIDP [Rybak 2009]; IDSA [Liu 2011]).

Cerebrospinal fluid (CSF) shunt infection (off-label use): As a component of empiric therapy or pathogen-specific therapy (eg, methicillin-resistant *S. aureus* or coagulase-negative staphylococci):

IV: 15 to 20 mg/kg/dose (usual maximum: 2 g/dose initially) every 8 to 12 hours; adjust dose to obtain a trough concentration of 15 to 20 mcg/mL (IDSA [Tunkel 2017]). A loading dose may be considered in seriously ill patients (ASHP/IDSA/SIDP [Rybak 2009]).

Intraventricular (adjunct to systemic therapy, use a preservative-free preparation): 5 to 20 mg; adjust dosage and administration interval based on CSF vancomycin concentrations (goal: 10 to 20 times MIC of causative organism), ventricular size, and daily output from ventricular drain. When intraventricular vancomycin is administered via a ventricular drain, clamp drain for 15 to 60 minutes after administration (allows solution to equilibrate in CSF) (IDSA [Tunkel 2004; Tunkel 2017]). **Note:** Intraventricular administration is generally reserved for use in patients who fail parenteral therapy despite removal of CSF shunt or when CSF shunt cannot be removed (Baddour 2017).

***Clostridium difficile* infection (CDI):**

Oral:

Mild or moderate CDI:

Initial episode or first relapse: 125 mg 4 times daily for 10 to 14 days (AHRQ [Butler 2016]; Kelly 2017)

Second relapse: Pulsed and/or tapered therapy over 6 to 7 weeks (Kelly 2017; SHEA/IDSA [Cohen 2010])

Severe, complicated CDI: 125 to 500 mg 4 times daily (ACG [Surawicz 2013]; ESCMID [Debast 2014]; SHEA/IDSA [Cohen 2010])); with or without IV metronidazole (Rokas 2015). Vancomycin retention enema may be added if there is concern that orally administered vancomycin may not reach colon (ACG [Surawicz 2013]).

Rectal (intracolonic) (off-label route): Retention enema: **Note:** Institution-specific protocols vary; optimal regimen not established. Consider assessing serum concentration as absorption may occur through inflamed mucosa (SHEA/IDSA [Cohen 2010]).

Severe, complicated infection in patients with a condition that may prevent oral vancomycin from reaching the colon (eg, ileus, megacolon, ileostomy) or unable to tolerate oral therapy: 500 mg every 6 hours (in 100 mL NS) (SHEA/IDSA [Cohen 2010]) retained for 1 hour (Apisarntha-narak 2002), with oral vancomycin (if tolerated) with or without concurrent IV metronidazole; dose adjustment and/or altered volume (eg, up to 500 mL NS) may be needed based upon extent of disease and patient weight (ACG [Surawicz 2013]; SHEA/IDSA [Cohen 2010]).

Endocarditis, treatment (off-label dose):

Enterococcus (native or prosthetic valve; penicillin-resistant strains or patients unable to tolerate beta-lactams): IV: 15 mg/kg/dose (usual maximum: 2 g/dose initially) every 12 hours in combination with gentamicin for 6 weeks; adjust dose to obtain a trough concentration of 10 to 20 mcg/mL (AHA [Baddour 2015]); some experts favor a trough of 15 to 20 mcg/mL (BSAC [Gould 2012]; ESC [Habib 2015]).

S. aureus, methicillin-resistant or methicillin-susceptible (severe-beta lactam hypersensitivity; alternative agent): IV:

Native valve: 15 mg/kg/dose (usual maximum: 2 g/dose initially) every 12 hours for 6 weeks; dose adjusted to obtain a serum trough concentration of 10 to 20 mcg/mL (AHA [Baddour 2015]) **or** 15 to 20 mg/kg/dose (usual maximum dose: 2 g/dose initially) every 8 to 12 hours for 6 weeks; adjust dose to obtain a trough concentration of 15 to 20 mcg/mL (IDSA [Lui 2011]).

Prosthetic valve: 15 mg/kg/dose (usual maximum: 2 g/dose initially) every 12 hours; adjust dose to obtain a trough concentration of 10 to 20 mcg/mL (AHA [Baddour 2015]) **or** 15 to 20 mg/kg/dose (usual maximum: 2 g/dose initially) every 8 to 12 hours; adjust dose to obtain a trough concentration of 15 to 20 mcg/mL (IDSA [Lui 2011]). Duration of therapy: At least 6 weeks (combine with rifampin for the entire duration of therapy and gentamicin for the first 2 weeks) (AHA [Baddour 2015]; IDSA [Lui 2011]).

Viridans group Streptococcus and S. bovis (native or prosthetic valve; penicillin or ceftriaxone intolerance): IV: 15 mg/kg/dose (usual maximum dose: 2 g/dose initially) every 12 hours for 4 weeks (native valve) or 6 weeks (prosthetic valve); adjust dose to obtain a trough concentration of 10 to 15 mcg/mL (AHA [Baddour 2015]).

Endophthalmitis (off-label use): Intravitreal: Usual dose: 1 mg/0.1 mL NS or sterile water injected into vitreum, usually in combination with ceftazidime (Durand 2017; Kelsey 1995). May repeat after 48 hours if needed based on culture result (Durand 2017).

Group B streptococcus (neonatal prophylaxis) (off-label use; alternative agent): IV: 20 mg/kg (maximum: 2 g/dose) every 8 hours from onset of labor until delivery (Onwuchuruba 2014). **Note:** Reserved for penicillin allergic patients at high risk for anaphylaxis and if organism is resistant to clindamycin or when no susceptibility data are available (CDC 2010).

Intra-abdominal infection (off-label use): As a component of empiric therapy or pathogen-specific therapy (eg, methicillin-resistant *S. aureus*): IV: 15 to 20 mg/kg/dose (usual maximum: 2 g/dose initially) every 8 to 12 hours; adjust dose to obtain a trough concentration of 15 to 20 mcg/mL (ASHP/IDSA/SIDP [Rybak 2009]; IDSA [Solomkin 2010]).

Meningitis, bacterial (off-label use): As a component of empiric therapy or pathogen-specific therapy (eg, methicillin-resistant *S. aureus* or penicillin- and cephalosporin-resistant *S. pneumoniae*): IV: 15 to 20 mg/kg/dose (usual maximum: 2 g/dose initially) every 8 to 12 hours; adjust dose to obtain a trough concentration of 15 to 20 mcg/mL (IDSA [Tunkel 2004; 2017]) A loading dose may be considered in seriously ill patients (ASHP/IDSA/SIDP [Rybak 2009]; IDSA [Liu 2011]).

Osteomyelitis (off-label dose): As a component of empiric therapy or pathogen-specific therapy (eg, methicillin-resistant *S. aureus*): IV: 15 to 20 mg/kg/dose (usual maximum: 2 g/dose initially) every 8 to 12 hours (IDSA [Liu 2011]) **or** 15 to 20 mg/kg/dose (usual maximum: 2 g/dose initially) every 12 hours (IDSA [Berbari 2015]); adjust dose to obtain a trough concentration of 15 to 20 mcg/mL. A loading dose may be considered in seriously ill patients (ASHP/IDSA/SIDP [Rybak 2009]).

Perioperative prophylaxis (in combination with other appropriate agents when coverage for methicillin-resistant *S. aureus* is indicated or for gram-positive coverage in patients unable to tolerate beta-lactams) (off-label use): IV: 15 mg/kg (usual maximum: 2 g/dose initially) started within 60 to 120 minutes prior to initial surgical incision. Vancomycin doses may be repeated intraoperatively in 2 half-lives (approximately 8 to 12 hours in patients with normal renal function) if procedure is lengthy or if there is excessive blood loss (ASHP/IDSA/SIS/SHEA [Bratzler 2013]). In cases where an extension of prophylaxis is warranted post-operatively, total duration should be ≤24 hours (Anderson 2014). **Postoperative** prophylaxis is not recommended in clean and clean-contaminated surgeries (CDC [Berrios-Torres 2017]).

Peritonitis, treatment (continuous ambulatory dialysis [CAPD] patients) (off-label use): Intraperitoneal: **Note:** Intraperitoneal administration is preferred to IV administration. Adjust dose to obtain a trough concentration between 15 and 20 mcg/mL (ISPD [Li 2016])

Intermittent (preferred): 15 to 30 mg/kg added to one exchange of CAPD solution every 5 to 7 days (allow to dwell for ≥6 hours); supplemental doses and more frequent monitoring of serum levels may be needed for patients receiving automated peritoneal dialysis (APD) or with significant residual renal function (ISPD [Li 2016]).

Continuous (all exchanges): Loading dose: 30 mg/kg added to first exchange of CAPD solution; maintenance dose: 1.5 mg/kg/bag for each subsequent exchange of CAPD solution (Bunke 1983; ISPD [Li 2016])

Pneumonia, *S. aureus* (methicillin-resistant): IV:

Community-acquired pneumonia (CAP) (hospitalized patient): As a component of empiric therapy or pathogen-specific therapy for community-acquired methicillin-resistant S. aureus: 15 to 20 mg/kg/dose (usual maximum: 2 g/dose initially) every 8 to 12 hours (ASHP/IDSA/SIDP [Rybak 2009]; IDSA [Liu 2011]; IDSA [Mandell 2007]); most patients with normal renal function can be started with 15 mg/kg/dose (usual maximum: 2 g/dose initially) every 12 hours. Adjust dose to obtain a trough concentration of 15 to 20 mcg/mL (File 2017). A loading dose may be considered in seriously ill patients (ASHP/IDSA/SIDP [Rybak 2009]; IDSA [Liu 2011]; IDSA [Mandell 2007]).

Hospital-acquired pneumonia (HAP) or ventilator-associated pneumonia (VAP): As a component of empiric therapy or pathogen-specific therapy for methicillin-resistant *S. aureus*: 15 to 20 mg/kg/dose (usual maximum: 2 g/dose initially) every 8 to 12 hours; adjust dose to obtain a trough concentration of 15 to 20 mcg/mL. A loading dose may be considered in seriously ill patients (ASHP/IDSA/SIDP [Rybak 2009]; ATS/IDSA [Kalil 2016]).

Prosthetic joint infection (off-label use): IV:

Pathogen-specific therapy for methicillin-resistant or susceptible S. aureus (alternative agent in beta-lactam intolerance): IV: 15 to 20 mg/kg/dose (usual maximum: 2 g/dose initially) every 8 to 12 hours (Berbari 2017; IDSA [Liu 2011]) **or** 15 mg/kg/dose (usual maximum: 2 g/dose initially) every 12 hours (IDSA [Osmon 2013]); adjust dose to obtain a trough concentration of 15 to 20 mcg/mL (ASHP/IDSA/SIDP [Rybak 2009]). **Note:** May be combined with oral rifampin in selected cases (eg, debridement and retention of prosthesis or one-stage arthroplasty).

Pathogen-specific therapy for Enterococcus spp (penicillin susceptible [alternative agent] or penicillin resistant): 15 mg/kg/dose (usual maximum: 2 g/dose initially) every 12 hours (Berbari 2017; IDSA [Osmon 2013]).

Sepsis/septic shock (off-label dose): As a component of empiric therapy or pathogen-specific therapy of methicillin-resistant *S. aureus*: IV: 15 to 20 mg/kg/dose (usual maximum: 2 g/dose initially) every 8 to 12 hours; adjust dose to obtain a trough concentration of 15 to 20 mcg/mL (ASHP/IDSA/SIDP [Rybak 2009]). Administer within 1 hour of identifying sepsis (Rhodes 2017). A loading dose may be considered in seriously ill patients (ASHP/IDSA/SIDP [Rybak 2009]; Rhodes 2017). A duration of therapy of 7 to 10 days is generally adequate for serious infections; a variety of factors play a role in determining optimal duration of therapy (Rhodes 2017).

Septic arthritis, without prosthetic material (off-label dose): As a component of empiric therapy or pathogen-specific therapy of methicillin-resistant *S. aureus* or coagulase-negative staphylococci: IV: 15 to 20 mg/kg/dose (usual maximum: 2 g/dose initially) every 8 to 12 hours; adjust dose to obtain a trough concentration of 15 to 20 mcg/mL (ASHP/IDSA/SIDP [Rybak 2009]; IDSA [Liu 2011]). Most patients with normal renal function can be started with 15 mg/kg/dose (usual maximum: 2 g/dose initially) every 12 hours (Goldenberg 2017).

Skin and soft tissue infections (hospitalized patient) (off-label dose): As a component of empiric therapy or pathogen-specific therapy of methicillin-resistant *S. aureus*: IV: 15 mg/kg/dose (usual maximum: 2 g/dose initially) every 12 hours (IDSA [Stevens 2014]); adjust dose to obtain a trough concentration of 10 to 15 mcg/mL (uncomplicated infection) or 15 to 20 mcg/mL (complicated infection or seriously ill) (ASHP/IDSA/SIDP [Rybak 2009]; IDSA [Liu 2011]; IDSA [Stevens 2014]). **Note:** For empiric therapy of necrotizing infection, must be used in combination with other agents (IDSA [Stevens 2014]).

Surgical site infections (off-label use): As a component of empiric therapy or pathogen-specific therapy of methicillin-resistant *S. aureus*: IV: 15 mg/kg/dose (usual maximum: 2 g/dose initially) every 12 hours; adjust dose to obtain trough concentrations of 10 to 15 mcg/mL (uncomplicated infection) or 15 to 20 mcg/mL (complicated infections or seriously ill) (ASHP/IDSA/SIDP [Rybak 2009]; IDSA [Stevens 2014]).

Pediatric

Usual dosage range: Note: Initial IV dosing should be based on actual body weight; subsequent dosing adjusted based on serum trough vancomycin concentrations.

Infants >2 months (60 days), Children, and Adolescents (Red Book [AAP 2015]): **Note:** Every 6 hour dosing recommended as initial dosage regimen if targeting trough serum concentrations >10 mcg/mL (Benner 2009; Frymoyer 2009) in patients with normal renal function. Close monitoring of serum concentrations and assurance of adequate hydration status is recommended; utilize local antibiogram and protocols for further guidance.

Mild to moderate infection: IV: 40 to 45 mg/kg/**day** divided every 6 to 8 hours; dose and frequency should be individualized based on serum concentrations; usual maximum daily dose: 2,000 mg/**day**

Severe infection: IV: 45 to 60 mg/kg/**day** divided every 6 to 8 hours; dose and frequency should be individualized based on serum concentrations; usual maximum daily dose: 4,000 mg/**day**

Indication-specific dosing:

Bacteremia (off-label use): Empiric therapy or pathogen-specific therapy (eg, methicillin-resistant *S. aureus*): Children and Adolescents: IV: 15 mg/kg/dose every 6 hours for 2 to 6 weeks depending on severity (IDSA [Liu 2011])

Brain abscess, intracranial epidural abscess, spinal epidural abscess (*S. aureus* [methicillin-resistant]) (off-label use): As a component of empiric therapy or pathogen specific therapy for methicillin-resistant *S. aureus*: Children and Adolescents: IV: 15 mg/kg/dose every 6 hours for 4 to 6 weeks (with or without rifampin) (IDSA [Liu 2011])

***C. difficile* infection (CDI):** Infants >1 month, Children, and Adolescents:

Manufacturer's labeling: Oral: 40 mg/kg/day in 3 to 4 divided doses for 7 to 10 days (maximum: 2,000 mg/day)

HIV-exposed/-positive patients: Adolescents: Oral: 125 mg 4 times daily for 10 to 14 days (HHS [OI adult 2017])

Endocarditis, treatment (off-label dose):

S. aureus (methicillin-resistant):

Native valve: Children and Adolescents: IV: 15 mg/kg/dose every 6 hours for 6 weeks (IDSA [Liu 2011])

Prosthetic valve: Children and Adolescents: IV: 15 mg/kg/dose every 6 hours for at least 6 weeks (combine with rifampin for the entire duration of therapy and gentamicin for the first 2 weeks) (IDSA [Liu 2011]).

Meningitis, bacterial: Infants >1 month, Children, and Adolescents: IV: 15 mg/kg/dose every 6 hours (for empiric therapy, use in combination with a third-generation cephalosporin); duration of therapy should be individualized based upon clinical response (in general, 10 to 21 days) (IDSA [Tunkel 2004]). For methicillin-resistant *S. aureus*, treat for 2 weeks (with or without rifampin) (IDSA [Liu 2011]).

Osteomyelitis (off-label use): As a component of empiric therapy or pathogen-specific therapy (eg, methicillin-resistant *S. aureus*): Children and Adolescents: IV: 15 mg/kg/dose every 6 hours for 4 to 6 weeks (IDSA [Liu 2011]).

Perioperative prophylaxis (off-label use): Children and Adolescents: IV: 15 mg/kg/dose within 120 minutes prior to surgical incision. May be administered in combination with other antibiotics depending upon the surgical procedure (ASHP/IDSA/SIS/SHEA [Bratzler 2013]).

Note: For patients known to be colonized with methicillin-resistant *S. aureus*, a single 15 mg/kg preoperative dose may be added to other recommended agents for the specific procedure (ASHP/IDSA/SIS/SHEA [Bratzler 2013]).

Pneumonia:

Community-acquired pneumonia (CAP) (IDSA/PIDS, 2011): Infants >3 months, Children, and Adolescents: IV: **Note:** In children ≥5 years, a macrolide antibiotic should be added if atypical pneumonia cannot be ruled out. Also consider if community-acquired MRSA suspected.

◄

Group A *Streptococcus* (alternative to ampicillin or penicillin in beta-lactam allergic patients): 40 to 60 mg/kg/day divided every 6 to 8 hours

Presumed bacterial (in addition to recommended antibiotic therapy), *S. pneumoniae*, moderate to severe infection (MICs to penicillin ≤2.0 mcg/mL) (alternative to ampicillin or penicillin): 40 to 60 mg/kg/day divided every 6 to 8 hours

S. aureus (methicillin-susceptible) (alternative to cefazolin/oxacillin): 40 to 60 mg/kg/day divided every 6 to 8 hours

S. aureus, moderate to severe infection (methicillin-resistant +/- clinda-mycin susceptible) (preferred): 40 to 60 mg/kg/day divided every 6 to 8 hours **or** dosing to achieve AUC/MIC >400

Alternate regimen: 60 mg/kg/day divided every 6 hours for 7 to 21 days, depending on severity (Liu 2011)

S. pneumoniae, moderate to severe infection (MICs to penicillin ≥4.0 mcg/mL) (alternative to ceftriaxone in beta-lactam allergic patients): 40 to 60 mg/kg/day divided every 6 to 8 hours

Health care-associated pneumonia (HAP): As a component of empiric therapy or pathogen-specific therapy for methicillin-resistant *S. aureus:* Infants, Children, and Adolescents: IV: 60 mg/kg/day divided every 6 hours for 7 to 21 days depending on severity (IDSA [Liu 2011])

Prophylaxis against infective endocarditis: Children and Adolescents: IV: Dental, oral, or upper respiratory tract surgery: 20 mg/kg/dose administered 1 hour prior to the procedure. **Note:** American Heart Association (AHA) guidelines recommend prophylaxis only in patients undergoing invasive procedures and in whom underlying cardiac conditions may predispose to a higher risk of adverse outcomes should infection occur.

GI/GU procedure: 20 mg/kg (plus gentamicin 1.5 mg/kg) administered 1 hour prior to surgery. **Note:** Routine prophylaxis no longer recommended by the AHA.

Septic arthritis (off-label use): As a component of empiric therapy or pathogen-specific therapy of methicillin-resistant *S. aureus*: Children and Adolescents: IV: 15 mg/kg/dose every 6 hours for minimum of 3 to 4 weeks (IDSA [Liu 2011])

Skin and soft tissue infections, complicated (off-label use): As a component of empiric therapy or pathogen-specific therapy of methi-cillin-resistant *S. aureus*: Infants, Children, and Adolescents: IV:

Non-necrotizing infection: 10 mg/kg/dose every 6 hours (IDSA [Stevens 2014])

Necrotizing infection: 15 mg/kg/dose every 6 hours (IDSA [Stevens 2014])

Alternate dosing: *S. aureus* (methicillin-resistant): 60 mg/kg/day divided every 6 hours for 7 to 14 days (IDSA [Liu 2011])

Renal Impairment

Oral: There are no dosage adjustments provided in the manufacturer's labeling. However, dosage adjustment unlikely due to low systemic absorption.

IV: Note: Vancomycin levels should be monitored in patients with any renal impairment: In critically ill patients with renal insufficiency, the initial loading dose (~25 mg/kg) should not be reduced. However, subsequent dosage adjustments should be made based on renal function and trough serum concentrations (Wang 2001).

Vancomycin Initial Dosage Regimens for Patients With Impaired Renal Function (Golightly 2013)

eGFR (mL/minute per 1.73 m²)	Actual Body Weight			
	<60 kg	60 to 80 kg	81 to 100 kg	>100 kg
>90	750 mg every 8 hours	1,000 mg every 8 hours	1,250 mg every 8 hours	1,500 mg every 8 hours
50 to 90	750 mg every 12 hours	1,000 mg every 12 hours	1,250 mg every 12 hours	1,000 mg every 8 hours
15 to 49	750 mg every 24 hours	1,000 mg every 24 hours	1,250 mg every 24 hours	1,500 mg every 24 hours
<15[a]	750 mg	1,000 mg	1,250 mg	1,500 mg

[a]Check a random vancomycin level in 24 hours after the dose. If random level is ≤20 mcg/mL, repeat the dose. If random level is >20 mcg/mL, do not re-dose; repeat random level in 12 hours.

Dialysis: Poorly dialyzable by intermittent hemodialysis; however, use of high-flux membranes and continuous renal replacement therapy (CRRT) increases vancomycin clearance, and generally requires replacement dosing (Launay-Vacher 2002).

End stage renal disease (ESRD) on intermittent hemodialysis (IHD) (administer after hemodialysis on dialysis days): Following loading dose of 15 to 25 mg/kg, give either 500 to 1,000 mg **or** 5 to 10 mg/kg after each dialysis session (Heintz 2009). **Note:** Dosing dependent on the assumption of 3 times/week, complete IHD sessions.

Redosing based on pre-HD concentrations:
<10 mg/L: Administer 1,000 mg after HD
10 to 25 mg/L: Administer 500 to 750 mg after HD
>25 mg/L: Hold vancomycin

Redosing based on post-HD concentrations: <10 to 15 mg/L: Administer 500 to 1,000 mg

Peritoneal dialysis (PD): 1 g every 4 to 7 days (Aronoff 2007)

Continuous renal replacement therapy (CRRT) (Heintz 2009; Trotman 2005): Drug clearance is highly dependent on the method of renal replacement, filter type, and flow rate. Appropriate dosing requires close monitoring of pharmacologic response, signs of adverse reactions due to drug accumulation, as well as drug concentrations in relation to target trough (if appropriate). The following are general recommendations only (based on dialysate flow/ultrafiltration rates of 1 to 2 L/hour and minimal residual renal function) and should not supersede clinical judgment:

CVVH: Loading dose of 15 to 25 mg/kg, followed by either 1,000 mg every 48 hours **or** 10 to 15 mg/kg every 24 to 48 hours

CVVHD: Loading dose of 15 to 25 mg/kg, followed by either 1,000 mg every 24 hours **or** 10 to 15 mg/kg every 24 hours

CVVHDF: Loading dose of 15 to 25 mg/kg, followed by either 1,000 mg every 24 hours **or** 7.5 to 10 mg/kg every 12 hours

Note: Consider redosing patients receiving CRRT for vancomycin concentrations <10 to 15 mg/L.

Hepatic Impairment

Oral: There are no dosage adjustments provided in the manufacturer's labeling. However, dosage adjustment unlikely due to low systemic absorption.

IV: There are no dosage adjustments provided in the manufacturer's labeling. However, degrees of hepatic dysfunction do not affect the pharmacokinetics of vancomycin (Marti, 1996).

◀ **Additional Information** Complete prescribing information should be consulted for additional detail.

Dosage Forms Considerations First-Vancomycin oral solution and Vancomycin+SyrSpend SF oral suspension are compounding kits. Refer to manufacturer's labeling for compounding instructions.

Dosage Forms Excipient information presented when available (limited, particularly for generics); consult specific product labeling. [DSC] = Discontinued product

Capsule, Oral:

Vancocin HCl: 125 mg, 250 mg [contains fd&c blue #2 (indigotine)]

Generic: 125 mg, 250 mg

Solution, Intravenous:

Generic: 1000 mg/100 mL in Dextrose 5% (100 mL); 1000 mg/200 mL in Dextrose 5% (200 mL); 1000 mg/200 mL in NaCl 0.9% (200 mL); 1000 mg/250 mL in Dextrose 5% (250 mL); 1000 mg/250 mL in NaCl 0.9% (250 mL); 1250 mg/250 mL in Dextrose 5% (250 mL); 1250 mg/250 mL in NaCl 0.9% (250 mL); 1500 mg/150 mL in NaCl 0.9% (150 mL); 1500 mg/250 mL in Dextrose 5% (250 mL); 1500 mg/250 mL in NaCl 0.9% (250 mL); 1500 mg/500 mL in Dextrose 5% (500 mL); 1500 mg/500 mL in NaCl 0.9% (500 mL); 1750 mg/250 mL in NaCl 0.9% (250 mL); 1750 mg/300 mL in NaCl 0.9% (300 mL); 1750 mg/500 mL in Dextrose 5% (500 mL); 1750 mg/500 mL in NaCl 0.9% (500 mL); 2000 mg/250 mL in NaCl 0.9% (250 mL); 2000 mg/500 mL in Dextrose 5% (500 mL); 2000 mg/500 mL in NaCl 0.9% (500 mL); 2500 mg/500 mL in NaCl 0.9% (500 mL); 500 mg/100 mL in Dextrose 5% (100 mL); 750 mg/150 mL in Dextrose 5% (150 mL); 750 mg/250 mL in NaCl 0.9% (250 mL)

Solution, Intravenous [preservative free]:

Generic: 750 mg/250 mL in NaCl 0.9% (250 mL)

Solution, Oral:

First-Vancomycin 25: 25 mg/mL (150 mL, 300 mL) [contains fd&c red #40, fd&c yellow #10 (quinoline yellow), sodium benzoate; white grape flavor]

First-Vancomycin 50: 50 mg/mL (150 mL, 210 mL, 300 mL) [contains fd&c red #40, fd&c yellow #10 (quinoline yellow), sodium benzoate; white grape flavor]

Solution Reconstituted, Intravenous:

Generic: 500 mg (1 ea [DSC]); 1000 mg (1 ea [DSC]); 5000 mg (1 ea)

Solution Reconstituted, Intravenous [preservative free]:

Generic: 500 mg (1 ea); 750 mg (1 ea); 1000 mg (1 ea); 5000 mg (1 ea); 10 g (1 ea)

Suspension, Oral:

Vancomycin+SyrSpend SF PH4: 50 mg/mL (120 mL, 240 mL)

♦ **Vancomycin HCl** see Vancomycin on page 1861

♦ **Vancomycin Hydrochloride** see Vancomycin on page 1861

♦ **Vancomycin Hydrochloride for Injection (Can)** see Vancomycin on page 1861

♦ **Vancomycin Hydrochloride for Injection, USP (Can)** see Vancomycin on page 1861

♦ **Vancomycin+SyrSpend SF PH4** see Vancomycin on page 1861

♦ **Vanc-Ondansetron (Can)** see Ondansetron on page 1380

Vandetanib (van DET a nib)

Related Information

Common Toxicity Criteria *on page* 2242
Management of Chemotherapy-Induced Nausea and Vomiting in Adults *on page* 2253
Management of EGFR Inhibitor Toxicities: Dermatologic, Ocular, and Gastro-intestinal *on page* 2291
Safe Handling of Hazardous Drugs *on page* 2379

Brand Names: US Caprelsa

Brand Names: Canada Caprelsa

Index Terms AZD6474; Zactima; ZD6474; Zictifa

Pharmacologic Category Antineoplastic Agent, Epidermal Growth Factor Receptor (EGFR) Inhibitor; Antineoplastic Agent, Tyrosine Kinase Inhibitor; Antineoplastic Agent, Vascular Endothelial Growth Factor (VEGF) Inhibitor

Use Thyroid cancer, medullary (locally advanced or metastatic): Treatment of metastatic or unresectable locally-advanced medullary thyroid cancer (symptomatic or progressive)

Labeled Contraindications Congenital long QT syndrome

Canadian labeling: Additional contraindications (not in the US labeling): Known hypersensitivity to vandetanib or any component of the formulation; persistent Fridericia-corrected QT interval (QTcF) ≥500 msec; uncorrected hypokalemia, hypomagnesemia, or hypocalcemia; uncontrolled hypertension

Pregnancy Considerations Adverse events have been observed in animal reproduction studies. Because vandetanib inhibits angiogenesis, a critical component of fetal development, adverse effects on pregnancy would be expected. Women of childbearing potential should be advised to avoid pregnancy and use effective contraception during and for 4 months following treatment with vandetanib.

Breastfeeding Considerations It is not known if vandetanib is excreted in human breast milk. Due to the potential for serious adverse reactions in the nursing infant, a decision should be made to discontinue vandetanib or to discontinue breastfeeding, taking into account the importance of treatment to the mother.

Warnings/Precautions [US Boxed Warning]: May prolong the QT interval; torsade de pointes and sudden death have been reported. Do not use in patients with hypocalcemia, hypokalemia, hypomagnesemia, or long QT syndrome. Correct electrolyte imbalance (hypocalcemia, hypokalemia, and/or hypomagnesemia) prior to initiating therapy. Monitor electrolytes periodically. Avoid the use of QT-prolonging agents. If concomitant use with QT-prolonging agents cannot be avoided, monitor ECG more frequently. Monitor electrolytes, TSH, and ECG at baseline, 2 to 4 weeks, and 8 to 12 weeks after therapy initiation, and then every 3 months or as clinically necessary (more frequently if clinically indicated). Vandetanib has a long half-life (19 days), therefore, adverse reactions (including QT prolongation) may resolve slowly; monitor appropriately. Ventricular tachycardia has also been reported. The potential for QT prolongation is dose dependent. Do not initiate treatment unless QT interval, Fridericia-corrected QT interval (QTcF) is <450 msec. During treatment, if QTcF >500 msec, withhold vandetanib and resume at a reduced dose when QTcF is <450 msec. Do not use in patients with a history of torsade de pointes, congenital long QT syndrome, bradyarrhythmias, or uncompensated heart failure. Patients with ventricular arrhythmias or recent MI were excluded from clinical trials. To reduce the risk of QT prolongation, maintain serum calcium and magnesium within normal limits and maintain serum potassium ≥4 mEq/L. Heart failure (HF) has been reported; monitor for signs and symptoms of HF; may require discontinuation (HF may not be reversible upon discontinuation). Hypertension and hypertensive crisis have been observed with vandetanib; monitor blood pressure and initiate or adjust antihypertensive therapy as needed; may require vandetanib dosage adjustment or treatment interruption; discontinue vandetanib (permanently) if blood pressure cannot be adequately controlled.

Diarrhea may commonly occur. May cause electrolyte imbalance (closely monitor electrolytes and ECGs to detect QT prolongation resulting from dehydration). Withhold vandetanib treatment until resolution for severe diarrhea; dose reduction is recommended when treatment is resumed. Antidiarrheal medication and/or other routine diarrhea management may be indicated. Stevens-Johnson syndrome (SJS), toxic epidermal necrolysis (TEN), and other serious skin reactions (including fatal reactions) have been reported. Mild to moderate skin reactions, including acne, dermatitis, dry skin, palmar-plantar erythrodysesthesia syndrome, pruritus, and rash have also been reported. Withhold treatment for dermatologic toxicity of grade 3 or higher; consider a reduced dose or permanent discontinuation upon improvement in symptoms. Discontinue permanently for severe dermatologic toxicity and refer patient for immediate evaluation. Grade 1 acneiform rash may be managed with topical corticosteroids and topical antibiotics; grade 2 may be managed with topical corticosteroids and systemic (oral) antibiotics; grade 3 or intolerable grade 2 acneiform rash may be managed with treatment interruption, topical corticosteroids and systemic (oral) antibiotics and systemic corticosteroids (Lacouture 2014). Increased risk of photosensitivity is associated with use; effective sunscreen and protective clothing are recommended during and for at least 4 months after treatment discontinuation.

Reversible posterior leukoencephalopathy syndrome (RPLS) been observed with vandetanib; symptoms of RPLS include altered mental function, confusion, headache, seizure, or visual disturbances; generally associated with hypertension; consider discontinuing treatment if RPLS occurs. Serious and sometimes fatal hemorrhagic events have been reported with use; discontinue in patients with severe hemorrhage; do not administer in patients with a recent history of hemoptysis with ≥2.5 mL of red blood. Ischemic cerebrovascular events (some fatal) have been observed with vandetanib; discontinue treatment in patients with severe ischemic events (the safety of resuming treatment after an ischemic event has not been studied). Interstitial lung disease (ILD) or pneumonitis (including fatalities) has been reported with vandetanib. Patients should be advised to report any new or worsening respiratory symptoms; ILD should be suspected with nonspecific respiratory symptoms such as hypoxia, pleural effusion, cough, or dyspnea. Interrupt therapy for acute or worsening pulmonary symptoms; discontinue if ILD diagnosis is confirmed.

Increased doses of thyroid replacement therapy have been required in patients with prior thyroidectomy; obtain TSH at baseline, at 2-4 weeks, 8-12 weeks, and every 3 months after vandetanib initiation; if signs and symptoms of hypothyroidism occur during treatment, evaluate thyroid hormone levels and adjust replacement therapy if needed. Dosage reduction is recommended in patients with moderate-to-severe renal impairment. Exposure is increased in patients with impaired renal function; closely monitor QT interval; has not been studied in patients with end stage renal disease requiring dialysis. Not recommended for use in patients with moderate-to-severe hepatic impairment. Potentially significant drug-drug interactions may exist, requiring dose or frequency adjustment, additional monitoring, and/or selection of alternative therapy. Due to the risk for serious treatment-related adverse events, use in patients whose disease is not progressive or symptomatic should be only be undertaken after careful consideration. **[US Boxed Warning]: Vandetanib is only available through a restricted access program; prescribers and pharmacies must be certified with the restricted distribution program to prescribe and dispense vandetanib.**

Adverse Reactions

>10%:

Cardiovascular: Hypertension (33%; grades 3/4: 9%), prolonged Q-T interval on ECG (14%; grades 3/4: 8%)

Central nervous system: Headache (26%), fatigue (24%)

Dermatologic: Skin rash (53%), acne vulgaris (35%), xeroderma (15%), skin photosensitivity (13%), pruritus (11%)

Endocrine & metabolic: Hypocalcemia (11% to 57%), hypoglycemia (24%)

Gastrointestinal: Colitis (≤57%; grades 3/4: ≤11%), diarrhea (≤57%; grades 3/4: ≤11%), nausea (33%), abdominal pain (21%), decreased appetite (21%), vomiting (15%), dyspepsia (11%)

Hematologic & oncologic: Hemorrhage (grades ≤2: 14%)

Hepatic: Increased serum ALT (51%)

Ophthalmic: Corneal changes (13%)

Renal: Increased serum creatinine (16%)

Respiratory: Upper respiratory tract infection (23%)

1% to 10%:

Cardiovascular: Cerebral ischemia (1%)

Central nervous system: Depression (10%)

Dermatologic: Nail disease (9%), alopecia (8%)

Endocrine & metabolic: Hypomagnesemia (7%), hypothyroidism (6%)

Gastrointestinal: Xerostomia (9%), dysgeusia (8%)

Genitourinary: Proteinuria (10%)

Hematologic & oncologic: Neutropenia (10%), thrombocytopenia (9%)

Neuromuscular & skeletal: Muscle spasm (6%)

Ophthalmic: Blurred vision (9%)

Frequency not defined:

Cardiovascular: Torsades de pointes, ventricular tachycardia

Central nervous system: Reversible posterior leukoencephalopathy syndrome

Dermatologic: Stevens-Johnson syndrome, toxic epidermal necrolysis

Respiratory: Interstitial pulmonary disease, pneumonitis

<1%, postmarketing, and/or case reports: Intestinal perforation, pancreatitis

Drug Interactions

Metabolism/Transport Effects Substrate of CYP3A4 (major); **Note:** Assignment of Major/Minor substrate status based on clinically relevant drug interaction potential; **Inhibits** BCRP

Avoid Concomitant Use

Avoid concomitant use of Vandetanib with any of the following: Amifampridine; CYP3A4 Inducers (Strong); Highest Risk QTc-Prolonging Agents; Hydroxychloroquine; MiFEPRIStone; Mizolastine; Moderate Risk QTc-Prolonging Agents; Probucol; Promazine; St John's Wort; Vinflunine

◄ **Increased Effect/Toxicity**

Vandetanib may increase the levels/effects of: Bisphosphonate Derivatives; Digoxin; Highest Risk QTc-Prolonging Agents; MetFORMIN

The levels/effects of Vandetanib may be increased by: Amifampridine; Bilastine; Buprenorphine; Hydroxychloroquine; Indapamide; MiFEPRIStone; Mizolastine; Moderate Risk QTc-Prolonging Agents; Probucol; Promazine; QTc-Prolonging Agents (Indeterminate Risk and Risk Modifying); Teneligliptin; Vinflunine; Xipamide

Decreased Effect

The levels/effects of Vandetanib may be decreased by: Bosentan; CYP3A4 Inducers (Moderate); CYP3A4 Inducers (Strong); Dabrafenib; Deferasirox; Sarilumab; Siltuximab; St John's Wort; Tocilizumab

Hazardous Drugs Handling Considerations

Hazardous agent (NIOSH 2016 [group 1]).

Use appropriate precautions for receiving, handling, administration, and disposal. Gloves (single) should be worn during receiving, unpacking, and placing in storage.

NIOSH recommends single gloving for administration of intact tablets or capsules. If manipulating tablets/capsules (eg, to prepare an oral suspension), NIOSH recommends double gloving, a protective gown, and preparation in a controlled device; if not prepared in a controlled device, respiratory and eye/face protection as well as ventilated engineering controls are recommended. NIOSH recommends double gloving, a protective gown, and (if there is a potential for vomit or spit up) eye/face protection for administration of an oral liquid/feeding tube administration (NIOSH 2016).

Storage/Stability Store at 25°C (77°F); excursions permitted to 15°C to 30°C (59°F to 86°F).

Mechanism of Action Multikinase inhibitor; inhibits tyrosine kinases including epidermal growth factor reception (EGFR), vascular endothelial growth factor (VEGF), rearranged during transfection (RET), protein tyrosine kinase 6 (BRK), TIE2, EPH kinase receptors and SRC kinase receptors, selectively blocking intracellular signaling, angiogenesis and cellular proliferation

Pharmacodynamics/Kinetics

Absorption: Slow

Protein binding: ~90%; to albumin and alpha 1-acid-glycoprotein

Distribution: V_d: ~7450 L

Metabolism: Hepatic, via CYP3A4 to N-desmethyl vandetanib and via flavin-containing monooxygenase enzymes to vandetanib-N-oxide

Bioavailability: Not affected by food

Half-life, elimination: 19 days

Time to peak: 6 hours (range: 4 to 10 hours)

Excretion: Feces (~44%); urine (~25%)

Dosing

Adult & Geriatric Note: Do not initiate treatment unless QTcF <450 msec. Avoid concomitant use of QT-prolonging agents and strong CYP3A4 inducers. To reduce the risk of QT prolongation, maintain serum calcium and magnesium within normal limits and maintain serum potassium ≥4 mEq/L.

Thyroid cancer, medullary (locally advanced or metastatic): Oral: 300 mg once daily, continue until disease progression or unacceptable toxicity.

Missed dose: Missed doses should be omitted if within 12 hours of the next scheduled dose.

Renal Impairment

CrCl ≥50 mL/minute: No dosage adjustment necessary.

CrCl <50 mL/minute: Reduce initial dose to 200 mg once daily; closely monitor QT interval.

ESRD requiring dialysis: There are no dosage adjustments provided in the manufacturer's labeling (has not been studied).

Hepatic Impairment

Mild impairment (Child-Pugh class A): There are no dosage adjustments provided in the manufacturer's labeling.

Moderate and severe impairment (Child-Pugh class B or C): Use is not recommended.

Adjustment for Toxicity

Toxicity ≥ grade 3: Interrupt dose until resolves or improves to grade 1, then resume at a reduced dose

Dosage reduction: Reduce from 300 mg once daily to 200 mg once daily, further reduce if needed to 100 mg once daily. For recurrent toxicities, reduce dose to 100 mg once daily after symptom improvement to ≤ grade 1 toxicity, if continued treatment is warranted.

Management of specific toxicities:

Cardiac: QTcF >500 msec: Withhold dose until QTcF returns to <450 msec, then resume at a reduced dose

Dermatologic toxicity: Withhold treatment for dermatologic toxicity of grade 3 or higher. Consider a reduced dose or permanent discontinuation upon improvement in symptoms. Permanently discontinue for severe dermatologic toxicity; may require systemic corticosteroid therapy.

Diarrhea (severe): Withhold treatment until resolution. Dose reduction is recommended when treatment is resumed. Closely monitor electrolytes and ECGs to detect QT prolongation resulting from dehydration.

Heart failure: May require discontinuation.

Hemorrhage (severe): Discontinue.

Hypertension: Initiate or adjust antihypertensive therapy as needed; may require vandetanib dosage adjustment or treatment interruption; discontinue permanently if blood pressure cannot be adequately controlled.

Interstitial lung disease (ILD)/pneumonitis: Interrupt therapy for acute or worsening pulmonary symptoms. Discontinue if ILD diagnosis is confirmed.

Ischemic cerebrovascular events (severe): Discontinue treatment (safety of resuming treatment after an ischemic event has not been studied).

Reversible posterior leukoencephalopathy syndrome (RPLS): Discontinue treatment.

Administration May be administered with or without food. Do not crush tablet. If unable to swallow tablet whole or if nasogastric or gastrostomy tube administration is necessary, disperse one tablet in 2 ounces of water (noncarbonated only) and stir for 10 minutes to disperse (will not dissolve completely) and administer immediately. Rinse residue in glass with additional 4 ounces of water (noncarbonated only) and administer.

Emetic Potential Low (10% to 30%)

Extemporaneous Preparations An oral solution may be prepared using the tablet. Disperse one tablet in 2 ounces of water (noncarbonated only) and stir for 10 minutes to disperse (will not dissolve completely) and administer immediately. Rinse residue in glass with additional 4 ounces of water (noncarbonated only) and administer.

Monitoring Parameters Monitor electrolytes (calcium, magnesium, potassium), TSH, and ECG (QT interval) at baseline, at 2 to 4 weeks, at 8 to 12 weeks, and every 3 months thereafter; also monitor QT interval at same frequency for dose reduction due to QT interval or treatment delays >2 weeks (monitor electrolytes and ECG more frequently if diarrhea occurs). Monitor renal function, hepatic function, blood pressure; monitor for signs and symptoms of heart failure, reversible posterior leukoencephalopathy syndrome (RPLS), pulmonary and skin toxicities

Prescribing and Access Restrictions In Canada, vandetanib is available only through the CAPRELSA Restricted Distribution Program. Prescribers and pharmacies must be certified with the program to prescribe or dispense vandetanib. Further information may be obtained at 1-800-589-6215 or visit www.caprelsa.ca/rdp

Medication Guide Available Yes

Dosage Forms Excipient information presented when available (limited, particularly for generics); consult specific product labeling.
Tablet, Oral:
Caprelsa: 100 mg, 300 mg

Vemurafenib (vem ue RAF e nib)

Related Information

Management of Chemotherapy-Induced Nausea and Vomiting in Adults on page 2253

Safe Handling of Hazardous Drugs on page 2379

Brand Names: US Zelboraf

Brand Names: Canada Zelboraf

Index Terms BRAF(V600E) Kinase Inhibitor RO5185426; PLX4032; RG7204; RO5185426

Pharmacologic Category Antineoplastic Agent, BRAF Kinase Inhibitor

Use Melanoma, unresectable or metastatic: Treatment of unresectable or metastatic melanoma in patients with a BRAFV600E mutation (as detected by an approved test).

Labeled Contraindications

There are no contraindications listed in the manufacturer's US labeling.
Canadian labeling: Hypersensitivity to vemurafenib or any component of the formulation.

Pregnancy Considerations Adverse effects were not demonstrated in animal reproduction studies. However, based on the mechanism of action, vemurafenib may cause fetal harm if administered during pregnancy or in patients who become pregnant during treatment. Women of reproductive potential should use effective contraception methods during treatment and for at least 2 weeks after the last dose.

Breastfeeding Considerations It is not known if vemurafenib is present in breast milk. Due to the potential for serious adverse reactions in the breastfed infant, breastfeeding is not recommended by the manufacturer during treatment and for 2 weeks after the last dose.

Warnings/Precautions Only patients with a BRAFV600 mutation-positive melanoma (including BRAFV600E) will benefit from treatment; mutation must be detected and confirmed by an approved test prior to treatment. The cobas 4800 BRAF V600 Mutation Test was used in clinical trials and is FDA-approved to detect BRAFV600E mutation.

Cutaneous squamous cell carcinomas (cuSCC), keratoacanthomas, and melanoma have been reported (at a higher rate in patients receiving vemurafenib compared to control). Cutaneous SCC generally occurs early in the treatment course (median onset: 7 to 8 weeks) and is managed with excision (while continuing vemurafenib treatment). Approximately one-third of patients experienced >1 cuSCC occurrence and the median time between occurrences was 6 weeks. Potential risk factors for cuSCC include age ≥65 years, history of skin cancer, or chronic sun exposure. Monitor for skin lesions (with dermatology evaluation) at baseline and every 2 months during treatment; consider continued monitoring for 6 months after treatment. Noncutaneous squamous cell carcinomas (non-cuSCC) of the head and neck have also been observed; monitor closely for signs/symptoms. Vemurafenib may promote malignancies correlated with RAS activation; monitor for signs/symptoms of other malignancies.

Dermatologic reactions have been observed, including case reports of Stevens-Johnson syndrome and toxic epidermal necrolysis; discontinue (permanently) for severe dermatologic toxicity. Photosensitivity ranging from mild to severe has been reported. Advise patients to avoid sun exposure and wear protective clothing and use effective UVA/UVB sunscreen and lip balm (SPF ≥30) when outdoors. Dosage modifications are recommended for intolerable photosensitivity consisting of erythema ≥10% to 30% of body surface area. Uveitis (including iritis), blurred vision, and photophobia may occur; monitor for signs and symptoms. Uveitis may be managed with corticosteroid and mydriatic eye drops. Retinal vein occlusion has been reported in clinical trials. Radiation sensitization and recall (some cases may be severe or involve cutaneous and visceral organs) have been reported in patients treated with radiation prior to, during, or after treatment with vemurafenib; fatal cases have been reported in patients with visceral organ involvement. Monitor closely when vemurafenib is administered concomitantly or sequentially with radiation treatment.

QT prolongation (dose-dependent) has been observed; may lead to increased risk for ventricular arrhythmia, including torsade de pointes. Monitor electrolytes (calcium, magnesium and potassium) at baseline and with dosage adjustments. Monitor ECG at baseline, 15 days after initiation, then monthly for 3 months, then every 3 months thereafter (more frequently if clinically appropriate); also monitor with dosage adjustments. Do not initiate treatment if baseline QTc >500 msec. During treatment, if QTc >500 msec, temporarily interrupt treatment; correct electrolytes and control other risk factors for QT prolongation. May reinitiate with a dose reduction once QTc falls to <500 msec. Discontinue (permanently), if after correction of risk factors, both the QTc continues to increase >500 msec and there is >60 msec change above baseline. Do not initiate treatment in patients with electrolyte abnormalities which are not correctable, long QT syndrome, or taking concomitant medication known to prolong the QT interval.

Cases of Dupuytren contracture and plantar fascial fibromatosis have been reported with vemurafenib use (Chan 2015; Perez 2017; Vandersleyen 2016). In June of 2017, the vemurafenib manufacturer issued a "Dear Healthcare Provider" letter stating that the majority of cases reported were mild to moderate, although disabling Dupuytren contracture cases have been observed. The median time to onset was 224 days from therapy initiation; the majority of patients experienced symptom resolution or improvement with interruption or discontinuation of vemurafenib (Perez 2017). Per the manufacturer, fibromatoses may require therapy interruption or treatment discontinuation.

Acute kidney injury, including interstitial nephritis, acute tubular necrosis, and serum creatinine elevations have been reported; monitor serum creatinine. Liver injury has been reported with use, and may cause functional impairment such as coagulopathy or other organ dysfunction. Monitor transaminases, alkaline phosphatase and bilirubin at baseline and monthly during therapy, or as clinically necessary. May require dosage reduction, therapy interruption, or discontinuation. Anaphylaxis and severe hypersensitivity may occur during treatment or upon reinitiation. Serious reactions have included generalized rash, erythema, hypotension, and drug rash with eosinophilia and systemic symptoms (DRESS syndrome). Discontinue (permanently) with severe hypersensitivity reaction. Pancreatitis has been reported (rare). Onset occurs within 2 weeks of initiation, with exacerbation occurring upon rechallenge at a reduced dose (Muluneh 2013). Consider evaluating unexplained abdominal pain for pancreatitis (eg, serum lipase and amylase; abdominal CT) as clinically indicated. Elderly patients may be at increased risk for adverse effects; in clinical trials, there was an increased incidence of cuSCC and keratoacanthoma, atrial fibrillation, peripheral edema, and nausea/decreased appetite in patients ≥65 years of age. Potentially significant drug-drug interactions may exist, requiring dose or frequency adjustment, additional monitoring, and/or selection of alternative therapy.

Adverse Reactions

>10%:

Cardiovascular: Peripheral edema (17% to 23%)

Central nervous system: Fatigue (38% to 54%), headache (23% to 27%)

Dermatologic: Skin rash (37% to 52%; grade 3: 7% to 8%), skin photosensitivity (33% to 49%; grade 3: 3%), alopecia (36% to 45%), pruritus (23% to 30%), hyperkeratosis (24% to 28%; actinic: 8% to 17%; seborrheic: 10% to 14%; pilaris: ≤10%), maculopapular rash (9% to 21%), xeroderma (16% to 19%), sunburn (10% to 14%), erythema (8% to 14%), papular rash (5% to 13%)

Gastrointestinal: Nausea (35% to 37%; grade 3: 2%), diarrhea (28% to 29%; grade 3: <1%), vomiting (18% to 26%; grade 3: 1% to 2%), decreased appetite (18% to 21%), constipation (12% to 16%), dysgeusia (11% to 14%)

Hematologic & oncologic: Cutaneous papilloma (21% to 30%), squamous cell carcinoma of skin (24%; grade 3: 22% to 24%)

Hepatic: Increased gamma-glutamyl transferase (5% to 15%)

Neuromuscular & skeletal: Arthralgia (53% to 67%), myalgia (13% to 24%), limb pain (9% to 18%), back pain (8% to 11%), musculoskeletal pain (8% to 11%), weakness (2% to 11%)

Renal: Increased serum creatinine (up to 3x ULN: 26%; greater than 3x ULN: 1%)

Respiratory: Cough (8% to 12%)

Miscellaneous: Fever (17% to 19%)

1% to 10%:

Cardiovascular: Atrial fibrillation, hypotension, prolonged Q-T interval on ECG, retinal vein occlusion, vasculitis

Central nervous system: Cranial nerve palsy (facial), dizziness, peripheral neuropathy

Dermatologic: Erythema nodosum, folliculitis, palmar-plantar erythrodysesthesia, Stevens-Johnson syndrome, toxic epidermal necrolysis

Endocrine & metabolic: Weight loss

Hematologic & oncologic: Basal cell carcinoma, malignant melanoma (new primary), squamous cell carcinoma (oropharyngeal)

Hepatic: Increased serum alkaline phosphatase, increased serum ALT, increased serum AST, increased serum bilirubin

Hypersensitivity: Anaphylaxis, hypersensitivity

Neuromuscular & skeletal: Arthritis, panniculitis

Ophthalmic: Blurred vision, iritis, photophobia, uveitis

<1%, postmarketing, and/or case reports: Acute interstitial nephritis, acute renal failure, acute tubular necrosis, chronic myelomonocytic leukemia with NRAS mutation (progression of preexisting condition), drug reaction with eosinophilia and systemic symptoms (DRESS syndrome), febrile neutropenia, fibrosis (Dupuytren contracture), hepatic injury, local acneiform eruptions (Ansai 2016), neutropenia, pancreatitis, plantar fasciitis, recall skin sensitization

Drug Interactions

Metabolism/Transport Effects Substrate of BCRP, CYP3A4 (major), P-glycoprotein; **Note:** Assignment of Major/Minor substrate status based on clinically relevant drug interaction potential; **Inhibits** BCRP, CYP1A2 (moderate), CYP2D6 (weak), P-glycoprotein; **Induces** CYP3A4 (weak)

Avoid Concomitant Use

Avoid concomitant use of Vemurafenib with any of the following: Alosetron; Amifampridine; Aminolevulinic Acid (Systemic); Conivaptan; CYP3A4 Inhibitors (Strong); Fusidic Acid (Systemic); Highest Risk QTc-Prolonging Agents; Hydroxychloroquine; Idelalisib; MiFEPRIStone; Mizolastine; Moderate Risk QTc-Prolonging Agents; PAZOPanib; Probucol; Promazine; Silodosin; Topotecan; VinCRIStine (Liposomal); Vinflunine

Increased Effect/Toxicity

Vemurafenib may increase the levels/effects of: Afatinib; Alosetron; Aminolevulinic Acid (Systemic); Aminolevulinic Acid (Topical); Betrixaban; Bilastine; Brentuximab Vedotin; Celiprolol; Colchicine; CYP1A2 Substrates; Dabigatran Etexilate; Digoxin; DOXOrubicin (Conventional); Edoxaban; Everolimus; Highest Risk QTc-Prolonging Agents; Naldemedine; Naloxegol;

PAZOPanib; Perhexiline; P-glycoprotein/ABCB1 Substrates; Pirfenidone; Porfimer; Prucalopride; Rasagiline; RifAXIMin; Silodosin; TiZANidine; Topotecan; Venetoclax; Verteporfin; VinCRIStine (Liposomal); Warfarin

The levels/effects of Vemurafenib may be increased by: Amifampridine; Aprepitant; Buprenorphine; Conivaptan; CYP3A4 Inhibitors (Moderate); CYP3A4 Inhibitors (Strong); Fosaprepitant; Fusidic Acid (Systemic); Hydroxychloroquine; Idelalisib; Indapamide; Ipilimumab; MiFEPRIStone; Mizolastine; Moderate Risk QTc-Prolonging Agents; Netupitant; Palbociclib; P-glycoprotein/ABCB1 Inhibitors; Probucol; Promazine; QTc-Prolonging Agents (Indeterminate Risk and Risk Modifying); Simeprevir; Stiripentol; Teneligliptin; Vinflunine; Xipamide

Decreased Effect

Vemurafenib may decrease the levels/effects of: HYDROcodone; NiMODipine

The levels/effects of Vemurafenib may be decreased by: Bosentan; CYP3A4 Inducers (Moderate); CYP3A4 Inducers (Strong); Dabrafenib; Deferasirox; Enzalutamide; Mitotane; Sarilumab; Siltuximab; St John's Wort; Tocilizumab

Food Interactions Grapefruit and grapefruit juice may inhibit CYP3A4-mediated metabolism of vemurafenib. Management: Avoid concurrent use.

Hazardous Drugs Handling Considerations

Hazardous agent (NIOSH 2016 [group 1]).

Use appropriate precautions for receiving, handling, administration, and disposal. Gloves (single) should be worn during receiving, unpacking, and placing in storage. NIOSH recommends single gloving for administration of intact tablets or capsules. Although the manufacturer does not recommend crushing the tablets, if manipulating tablets/capsules (eg, to prepare an oral suspension), NIOSH recommends double-gloving, a protective gown, and preparation in a controlled device; if not prepared in a controlled device, respiratory and eye/face protection as well as ventilated engineering controls are recommended. NIOSH recommends double-gloving, a protective gown, and (if there is a potential for vomit or spit up) eye/face protection for administration of an oral liquid/feeding tube administration (NIOSH 2016).

Storage/Stability Store at 20°C to 25°C (68°F to 77°F); excursions permitted to 15°C and 30°C (59°F and 86°F). Store in the original container with the lid tightly closed.

Mechanism of Action Vemurafenib is a low molecular weight oral BRAF kinase inhibitor (potent) which inhibits tumor growth in melanomas by inhibiting kinase activity of certain mutated forms of BRAF, including BRAF with V600E mutation, thereby blocking cellular proliferation in melanoma cells with the mutation. Does not have activity against cells with wild-type BRAF. BRAFV600E activating mutations are present in ~50% of melanomas; V600E mutation involves the substitution of glutamic acid for valine at amino acid 600.

Pharmacodynamics/Kinetics

Distribution: V_d: ~106 L

Protein binding: >99%, to albumin and α_1-acid glycoprotein

Half-life, elimination: 57 hours (range: 30 to 120 hours)

Time to peak: ~3 hours

Excretion: Feces (~94%); urine (~1%)

Dosing
Adult & Geriatric
Melanoma, metastatic or unresectable (with BRAFV600E mutation): Oral: 960 mg every 12 hours; continue until disease progression or unacceptable toxicity.

Missed doses: A missed dose may be taken up to 4 hours prior to the next scheduled dose. If it is within 4 hours of the next scheduled dose, administer the next dose at the regular schedule. If vomiting occurs after a dose is taken, do not take an additional dose; continue with the next scheduled dose.

Erdheim-Chester disease, refractory (with BRAF V600E mutation) (off-label use): Oral: 480 or 960 mg twice daily (Haroche 2014; Hyman 2015).

Melanoma, metastatic or unresectable (with BRAFV600K mutation) (off-label use): Oral: 960 mg every 12 hours; continue until disease progression or unacceptable toxicity (Chapman 2011; Sosman 2012).

Melanoma, metastatic or unresectable (with BRAFV600E or V600K mutations) (off-label combination): Oral: 960 mg every 12 hours (in combination with cobimetinib); continue until disease progression or unacceptable toxicity (Larkin 2014).

Non-small cell lung cancer, refractory (with BRAF V600 mutation) (off-label use): Oral: 960 mg twice daily (Hyman 2015). Additional data may be necessary to further define the role of vemurafenib in this condition.

Dosage adjustment for concomitant strong CYP3A4 inducers: Avoid concomitant use of strong CYP3A4 inducers. If concurrent use of a strong CYP3A4 inducer (eg, carbamazepine, phenytoin, rifampin) cannot be avoided, increase the vemurafenib dose by 240 mg as tolerated. After the strong CYP3A4 inducer has been discontinued for 2 weeks, resume the vemurafenib dose that was used prior to initiating the CYP3A4 inducer.

Renal Impairment
Mild to moderate impairment (preexisting): No dosage adjustment necessary.

Severe impairment (preexisting): There are no dosage adjustments provided in the manufacturer's labeling (data are insufficient to determine if dosage adjustment is necessary); use with caution.

Nephrotoxicity/creatinine abnormalities during treatment: Refer to Dosing: Adjustment for Toxicity and manage with dose reduction, treatment interruption, or discontinuation.

Hepatic Impairment
Mild to moderate impairment (preexisting): No dosage adjustment necessary.

Severe impairment (preexisting): There are no dosage adjustments provided in manufacturer's labeling (data are insufficient to determine if dosage adjustment is necessary); use with caution.

Hepatotoxicity/lab abnormalities during treatment: Refer to Dosing: Adjustment for Toxicity and manage with dose reduction, treatment interruption, or discontinuation.

Adjustment for Toxicity Note: Do not dose reduce below 480 mg twice daily. NCI Common Terminology Criteria for Adverse Events (CTC-AE) version 4.0 used for adverse event grades.

Grade 1 or grade 2 (tolerable) toxicity: No dosage adjustment recommended.

◄ **Grade 2 (intolerable) or grade 3 toxicity:**
First incident: Interrupt treatment until toxicity returns to grade 0 or 1, then resume at 720 mg twice daily
Second incident: Interrupt treatment until toxicity returns to grade 0 or 1, then resume at 480 mg twice daily
Third incident: Discontinue permanently.

Grade 4 toxicity:
First incident: Interrupt treatment until toxicity returns to grade 0 or 1, then resume at 480 mg twice daily **or** discontinue permanently
Second incident: Discontinue permanently.

Specific toxicities:
New primary cutaneous malignancies: No dosage adjustment recommended.
Severe hypersensitivity or severe dermatologic toxicity: Discontinue permanently.
QTc interval changes:
QTc >500 msec (grade ≥3): Temporarily withhold treatment, correct electrolytes and control risk factors for QT prolongation; may reinitiate with a dose reduction once QTc ≤500 msec (≤ grade 2).
QTc persistently >500 msec and >60 msec above baseline: Discontinue permanently.

Combination Regimens
Melanoma: Cobimetinib-Vemurafenib (Melanoma) on page 2068

Administration Doses should be administered orally in the morning and evening, ~12 hours apart. May be taken with or without a meal. If vomiting occurs after a dose is taken, do not take an additional dose; continue with the next scheduled dose.

Swallow whole with a glass of water; do not crush or chew. There are case reports of vemurafenib administration after crushing (Janson 2013; Khimani 2014), however vemurafenib is nearly insoluble in water and is manufactured as a microprecipitated bulk powder core (to improve solubility/bioavailability) within a film coated tablet (Shah 2013). Pharmacokinetics and efficacy of administration other than swallowing tablets whole have not been determined.

Emetic Potential Minimal (<10%)

Monitoring Parameters Liver transaminases, alkaline phosphatase and bilirubin at baseline and monthly during treatment (or as clinically appropriate). Serum creatinine at baseline and periodically during treatment. Electrolytes (calcium, magnesium and potassium) at baseline and after dosage modification. ECG at baseline, 15 days after initiation, then monthly for 3 months, then every 3 months thereafter (more frequently if clinically appropriate) and with dosage adjustments. Dermatology evaluation (for new skin lesions) at baseline and every 2 months during treatment; also consider continued monitoring for 6 months after completion of treatment. Signs/symptoms of hypersensitivity reactions, uveitis, and malignancies; signs of radiation sensitization and recall. Monitor adherence.

Dietary Considerations Avoid grapefruit and grapefruit juice.

Prescribing and Access Restrictions Available through specialty pharmacies. Further information may be obtained from the manufacturer, Genentech, at 1-888-249-4918, or at http://www.zelboraf.com.

Medication Guide Available Yes

Dosage Forms Excipient information presented when available (limited, particularly for generics); consult specific product labeling.
Tablet, Oral:
Zelboraf: 240 mg

♦ **Venclexta** see Venetoclax on page 1883

♦ **Venclexta Starting Pack** see Venetoclax on page 1883

Venetoclax (ven ET oh klax)

Related Information

Common Toxicity Criteria on page 2242

Management of Chemotherapy-Induced Nausea and Vomiting in Adults on page 2253

Safe Handling of Hazardous Drugs on page 2379

Brand Names: US Venclexta; Venclexta Starting Pack

Brand Names: Canada Venclexta

Index Terms ABT-0199; ABT-199; BCL-2 Inhibitor GDC-0199; GDC-0199; RG7601

Pharmacologic Category Antineoplastic Agent; Antineoplastic Agent, BCL-2 Inhibitor

Use Chronic lymphocytic leukemia: Treatment of chronic lymphocytic leukemia (CLL) in patients with 17p deletion (as detected by an approved test) who have received at least one prior therapy.

Labeled Contraindications

Concomitant use with strong CYP3A inhibitors at initiation and during ramp-up phase

Canadian labeling: Additional contraindications (not in the US labeling): Hypersensitivity to venetoclax or any component of the formulation

Pregnancy Considerations Based on the mechanism of action and data from animal reproduction studies, venetoclax is expected to cause fetal harm if administered during pregnancy. Females of reproductive potential should have a pregnancy test prior to therapy, and use effective contraception during treatment and for at least 30 days after the final dose. Based on animal data, venetoclax may compromise fertility in males.

Breastfeeding Considerations It is not known if venetoclax is excreted in breast milk. Due to the potential for serious adverse reactions in the breast-feeding infant, breastfeeding is not recommended by the manufacturer.

Warnings/Precautions Venetoclax may cause a rapid reduction in tumor volume and therefore a risk for tumor lysis syndrome (TLS) is present during the initial 5-week dose escalation phase of treatment. TLS has occurred with venetoclax in previously treated chronic lymphocytic leukemia (CLL) patients with high tumor burden; renal failure (requiring dialysis) and fatalities have been reported. Changes in blood chemistries consistent with TLS may occur as early as 6 to 8 hours after the first dose and with dose increases, and require prompt management. The risk for TLS is increased with high tumor burden and comorbidities; creatinine clearance <80 mL/minute further increases TLS risk. Assess risk for TLS; initiate appropriate TLS prophylactic management (eg, hydration and antihyperuricemic therapy); monitor blood chemistries closely and manage abnormalities promptly. May require treatment interruption and dose reduction. The risk for TLS may decrease as tumor burden decreases. Patients at high risk for TLS may require hospitalization at treatment initiation. Concomitant use of CYP3A or P-gp inhibitors at initiation or during dose escalation may increase the risk for TLS. Patients with decreased renal function (CrCl <80 mL/minute) are at increased risk for TLS and may require more intensive TLS prophylaxis and monitoring during treatment initiation and dose escalation.

Neutropenia, thrombocytopenia and anemia may occur. Grade 3 and 4 neutropenia occurred in almost half of patients receiving venetoclax. Neutropenic fever has been reported. Monitor CBC with differential throughout treatment. May require treatment interruption and/or dose reduction. Consider antimicrobials and WBC growth factor support as clinically indicated. Adverse events may be increased in patients with moderate hepatic impairment; monitor closely for toxicity.

Select patients for treatment (of relapsed or refractory chronic lymphocytic leukemia) based on the presence of a 17p deletion. Patients without a 17p deletion at diagnosis should be re-tested at relapse as acquisition of 17p deletion may occur. Information on approved tests for 17p deletion detection may be found at http://www.fda.gov/CompanionDiagnostics. Potentially significant drug-drug interactions may exist, requiring dose or frequency adjustment, additional monitoring, and/or selection of alternative therapy. Live vaccinations should not be administered prior to, during, or after venetoclax treatment until B-cell recovery occurs. Vaccines may be less effective.

Adverse Reactions

>10%:

Cardiovascular: Peripheral edema (11%; grades 3/4: <1%)

Central nervous system: Fatigue (21%; grades 3/4: 2%), headache (15%; grades 3/4: <1%)

Endocrine & metabolic: Hyperkalemia (20%; ≥ grade 3: 2%), hyperphosphatemia (15%; ≥ grade 3: 3%), hypokalemia (12%; grades 3/4: 4%)

Gastrointestinal: Diarrhea (35%; grades 3/4: <1%), nausea (33%; grades 3/4: <1%), vomiting (15%; grades 3/4: <1%), constipation (14%)

Hematologic & oncologic: Neutropenia (45%; grades 3/4: 41%), anemia (29%; grades 3/4: 18%), thrombocytopenia (22%; grades 3/4: 15%)

Respiratory: Upper respiratory tract infection (22%; grades 3/4: 1%), cough (13%)

Miscellaneous: Fever (16%; grades 3/4: <1%)

1% to 10%:

Endocrine & metabolic: Hypocalcemia (9%; ≥ grade 3: 3%), hyperuricemia (6%; ≥ grade 3: 2%)

Hematologic & oncologic: Tumor lysis syndrome (2 to 3 week ramp-up phase: 12%; 5 week ramp-up phase: 6%; ≥ grade 3: 6%), febrile neutropenia (5%; grades 3/4: 5%)

Neuromuscular & skeletal: Back pain (10%; grades 3/4: <1%)

Respiratory: Pneumonia (8%; grades 3/4: 5%)

Drug Interactions

Metabolism/Transport Effects Substrate of CYP3A4 (major), P-glycoprotein; **Note:** Assignment of Major/Minor substrate status based on clinically relevant drug interaction potential

Avoid Concomitant Use

Avoid concomitant use of Venetoclax with any of the following: BCG (Intravesical); Bitter Orange; Conivaptan; CYP3A4 Inducers (Moderate); CYP3A4 Inducers (Strong); Deferiprone; Dipyrone; Fusidic Acid (Systemic); Grapefruit Juice; Idelalisib; Star Fruit; Vaccines (Live)

Increased Effect/Toxicity

Venetoclax may increase the levels/effects of: CloZAPine; Deferiprone; Digoxin; Everolimus; Sirolimus; Vaccines (Live); Warfarin

The levels/effects of Venetoclax may be increased by: Bitter Orange; Conivaptan; CYP3A4 Inhibitors (Moderate); CYP3A4 Inhibitors (Strong); Dasatinib; Dipyrone; Fosaprepitant; Fusidic Acid (Systemic); Grapefruit Juice; Idelalisib; MiFEPRIStone; Palbociclib; P-glycoprotein/ABCB1 Inhibitors; Promazine; Star Fruit; Stiripentol

Decreased Effect

Venetoclax may decrease the levels/effects of: BCG (Intravesical); Vaccines (Inactivated); Vaccines (Live)

The levels/effects of Venetoclax may be decreased by: CYP3A4 Inducers (Moderate); CYP3A4 Inducers (Strong); Deferasirox; Sarilumab; Siltuximab; Tocilizumab

Food Interactions Coadministration with grapefruit products, Seville oranges, and/or Star Fruit may increase venetoclax plasma concentrations. Management: Avoid concomitant administration with grapefruit products, Seville oranges, and Star Fruit.

Hazardous Drugs Handling Considerations

Hazardous agent (meets NIOSH 2016 criteria). This medication is not on the NIOSH (2016) list; however, it meets the criteria for a hazardous drug. Drugs are classified as hazardous based on their properties; the properties of a hazardous drug include one or more of the following characteristics: carcinogenic, teratogenic (or other developmental toxicity), reproductive toxicity, organotoxic at low doses, genotoxic, and/or new agents with structural or toxicity profiles similar to existing hazardous agents.

Use appropriate precautions for receiving, handling, administration, and disposal. Gloves (single) should be worn during receiving, unpacking, and placing in storage. NIOSH recommends single gloving for administration of intact tablets or capsules (NIOSH 2016).

Storage/Stability Store at or below 30°C (86°F).

Mechanism of Action Venetoclax has cytotoxic activity in tumor cells which overexpress BCL-2. Venetoclax selectively inhibits the anti-apoptotic protein BCL-2, which is overexpressed in chronic lymphocytic leukemia (CLL) cells. BCL-2 mediates tumor cell survival and has been associated with chemotherapy resistance. Venetoclax binds directly to the BCL-2 protein, displacing pro-apoptotic proteins and restoring the apoptotic process.

Pharmacodynamics/Kinetics

Distribution: V_{dss}: 256 to 321 L

Protein binding: Highly bound to plasma proteins

Metabolism: Hepatic, predominantly via CYP3A4/5; the major metabolite is M27 (has BCL-2 inhibitory activity)

Half-life, elimination: ~26 hours

Time to peak: 5 to 8 hours

Excretion: Feces (>99.9%; ~21% as unchanged drug); Urine (<0.1%)

Dosing

Adult & Geriatric Note: Assess risk for tumor lysis syndrome (TLS); administer prophylactic hydration and antihyperuricemics.

◄ **Chronic lymphocytic leukemia, relapsed/refractory, 17p deletion:** Oral: Escalate dose in weekly increments over 5 weeks to gradually debulk and reduce the risk of TLS:

Week 1: 20 mg once daily

Week 2: 50 mg once daily

Week 3: 100 mg once daily

Week 4: 200 mg once daily

Week 5 and thereafter: 400 mg once daily; continue until disease progression or unacceptable toxicity.

Premedications: Hydration and antihyperuricemic therapy based on TLS risk:

Low tumor burden (all lymph nodes <5 cm and absolute lymphocyte count [ALC] <25,000/mm^3): Outpatient: Hydrate with 1.5 to 2 L of oral hydration and administer allopurinol (beginning 2 to 3 days prior to venetoclax initiation). Administer IV hydration for patients unable to tolerate oral hydration.

Medium tumor burden (any lymph node 5 to <10 cm or ALC ≥25,000/mm^3): Outpatient: Hydrate with 1.5 to 2 L of oral hydration (administer IV hydration for patients unable to tolerate oral hydration; consider additional IV hydration) and administer allopurinol (beginning 2 to 3 days prior to venetoclax initiation).

High tumor burden (any lymph node ≥10 cm OR ALC ≥25,000/mm^3 and any lymph node ≥5 cm): Inpatient: Hydrate with 1.5 to 2 L of oral hydration (administer IV hydration for patients unable to tolerate oral hydration) and 150 to 200 mL/hour IV hydration as tolerated; administer allopurinol (beginning 2 to 3 days prior to venetoclax initiation); consider rasburicase if baseline uric acid is elevated.

Dosage adjustment for concomitant CYP3A and P-glycoprotein (P-gp) inhibitors:

Strong CYP3A inhibitors: The use of strong CYP3A inhibitors is contraindicated at initiation of venetoclax and during dose escalation. For patients who have completed dose escalation and are on a steady daily venetoclax dose, reduce the venetoclax dose by at least 75% when a strong CYP3A inhibitor must be used concurrently.

Moderate CYP3A inhibitors and P-gp inhibitors: Avoid concomitant use of venetoclax with moderate CYP3A and P-gp inhibitors (consider alternative treatments); if concurrent use cannot be avoided, reduce the venetoclax dose by at least 50%.

Following discontinuation of the CYP3A or P-gp inhibitor: 2 to 3 days after the inhibitor is discontinued, resume the venetoclax dose that was used prior to initiating the CYP3A or P-gp inhibitor.

Renal Impairment

CrCl ≥30 mL/minute: No dosage adjustment necessary; use with caution due to increased risk for TLS.

CrCl <30 mL/minute: There are no dosage adjustments provided in the manufacturer's labeling (has not been studied).

End-stage renal disease (ESRD) requiring dialysis: There are no dosage adjustments provided in the manufacturer's labeling (has not been studied). Dialysis is unlikely to significantly remove venetoclax (due to large volume of distribution and extensive protein binding).

Hepatic Impairment

Mild impairment (normal total bilirubin and AST > upper limit of normal [ULN] or total bilirubin >1 to 1.5 times ULN): No dosage adjustment necessary.

Moderate impairment (total bilirubin >1.5 to 3 times ULN): No dosage adjustment necessary; monitor closely for signs of toxicity.

Severe impairment (total bilirubin >3 times ULN): There are no dosage adjustments provided in the manufacturer's labeling (has not been studied).

Adjustment for Toxicity Interrupt or reduce dose for toxicities. Reassess risk for tumor lysis syndrome in patients who have had an interruption in dosing of >1 week during the first 5 weeks or >2 weeks at 400 mg once daily (to determine if re-initiation with a reduced dose is necessary).

Dose Reduction Levels for Venetoclax Toxicity

Dose at interruption	Restart dose[a]
400 mg	300 mg
300 mg	200 mg
200 mg	100 mg
100 mg	50 mg
50 mg	20 mg
20 mg	10 mg

Consider discontinuation for patients who require dose reductions to less than 100 mg for more than 2 weeks.

[a]During dose escalation phase, continue the reduced dose for 1 week prior to increasing the dose.

Tumor lysis syndrome (TLS):

Blood chemistry changes or symptoms suggestive of TLS: Withhold the next day's dose.

If resolved within 24 to 48 hours of the last dose: Resume at the same dose.

If blood chemistry changes require more than 48 hours to resolve: Resume at a reduced dose.

Clinical TLS (laboratory TLS with clinical consequences such as acute renal failure, cardiac arrhythmias, sudden death, and/or seizure): Withhold dose; following resolution, resume at a reduced dose.

Hematologic toxicity:

Grade 3 or 4 neutropenia with infection or fever or grade 4 hematologic toxicities (except lymphopenia):

First occurrence: Interrupt treatment. May administer granulocyte-colony stimulating factors (G-CSFs) with venetoclax to reduce infection risk associated with neutropenia. May resume at the same dose once toxicity is resolved to grade 1 or baseline.

Second and subsequent occurrences: Interrupt treatment. Consider G-CSFs as clinically indicated. Resume at a lower dose level once toxicity is resolved (see dosage reduction levels in above table; a larger dose reduction may be necessary based on clinical discretion).

Nonhematologic toxicities, Grade 3 or 4 toxicity:

First occurrence: Interrupt treatment. May resume at the same dose once toxicity is resolved to grade 1 or baseline (no dosage adjustment is necessary).

Second and subsequent occurrences: Interrupt treatment. Resume at a lower dose level once toxicity is resolved (see dosage reduction levels in above table; a larger dose reduction may be necessary based on clinical discretion).

Administration

Oral: Administer with a meal and water at approximately the same time each day. Swallow whole; do not crush, chew, or break.

Missed or vomited doses: If a dose is missed and it is within 8 hours of the missed usual dosing time, administer the missed dose as soon as possible and resume the normal daily dosing schedule. If it is more than 8 hours, do not administer the missed dose and resume the usual dosing schedule the next day. If the patient vomits following administration of a dose, no additional doses should be administered that day; the next prescribed dose should be taken at the usual time.

Emetic Potential Low (10% to 30%)

Monitoring Parameters 17p deletion status (prior to treatment initiation or at relapse); pregnancy test (prior to treatment in females of reproductive potential); CBC with differential (throughout treatment); blood chemistries (potassium, uric acid, phosphorus, calcium, and creatinine); assess tumor burden, including radiographic evaluation (eg, CT scan) for tumor lysis syndrome (TLS) risk evaluation.

Blood chemistry monitoring based on tumor burden/TLS risk:

Low risk (all lymph node <5 cm and absolute lymphocyte count [ALC] <25,000/mm^3) or medium risk (any lymph node 5 to <10 cm or ALC ≥25,000/mm^3): Prior to first dose, 6 to 8 hours, and 24 hours after first 20 mg and 50 mg dose, and prior to each subsequent initial ramp up dose.

High risk (any lymph node ≥10 cm OR ALC ≥25,000/mm^3 and any lymph node ≥5 cm): Prior to first dose, 4, 8, 12, and 24 hours after first 20 mg and 50 mg dose, and prior to plus 6 to 8 hours and 24 hours after each subsequent initial ramp up dose.

Dietary Considerations Administration with a low-fat meal increased exposure by ~3.4 fold and administration with a high-fat meal increased exposure by ~5.1 to 5.3 fold, compared to fasting. Avoid grapefruit products, Seville oranges, and Star Fruit.

Prescribing and Access Restrictions Available through specialty pharmacies and distributors. Further information may be obtained from the manufacturer.

Medication Guide Available Yes

Dosage Forms Excipient information presented when available (limited, particularly for generics); consult specific product labeling.

Tablet, Oral:

Venclexta: 10 mg, 50 mg, 100 mg

Tablet Therapy Pack, Oral:

Venclexta Starting Pack: Week 1: 10 mg (14); Week 2: 50 mg (7); Week 3: 100 mg (7); Week 4: 100 mg (14) (42 ea)

◆ **Venipuncture CPI** see Lidocaine and Prilocaine on page 1150

◆ **Venofer** see Iron Sucrose on page 1057

◆ **VePesid** see Etoposide on page 729

◆ **Vepesid (Can)** see Etoposide on page 729

◆ **Vesanoid** see Tretinoin (Systemic) on page 1830

◆ **Vfend** see Voriconazole on page 1925

◆ **VFEND (Can)** see Voriconazole on page 1925

◆ **Vfend IV** see Voriconazole on page 1925

◆ **VFEND For Injection (Can)** see Voriconazole on page 1925

◆ **9vHPV** *see* Papillomavirus (9-Valent) Vaccine (Human, Recombinant) *on page 1452*

◆ **Vidaza** *see* AzaCITIDine *on page 206*

VinBLAStine (vin BLAS teen)

Related Information

Management of Chemotherapy-Induced Nausea and Vomiting in Adults *on page 2253*

Management of Drug Extravasations *on page 2271*

Prevention of Chemotherapy-Induced Nausea and Vomiting in Children *on page 2310*

Safe Handling of Hazardous Drugs *on page 2379*

Brand Names: Canada Vinblastine Sulphate Injection

Index Terms Velban; Vinblastine Sulfate; Vincaleukoblastine; VLB

Pharmacologic Category Antineoplastic Agent, Antimicrotubular; Antineoplastic Agent, Vinca Alkaloid

Use Treatment of Hodgkin lymphoma; lymphocytic lymphoma; histiocytic lymphoma; mycosis fungoides; testicular cancer; Kaposi sarcoma; histiocytosis X (Letterer-Siwe disease); has also been used for the treatment of refractory/resistant breast cancer and choriocarcinoma

Labeled Contraindications Significant granulocytopenia (unless as a result of condition being treated); presence of bacterial infection

Pregnancy Considerations Adverse effects were observed in animal reproduction studies. May cause fetal harm if administered during pregnancy. Women of childbearing potential should avoid becoming pregnant during vinblastine treatment. Aspermia has been reported in males who have received treatment with vinblastine.

Breastfeeding Considerations It is not known if vinblastine is excreted in breast milk. Due to the potential for serious adverse reactions in the nursing infant, a decision should be made whether to discontinue vinblastine or to discontinue breastfeeding, taking into account the importance of treatment to the mother.

Warnings/Precautions Avoid eye contamination (exposure may cause severe irritation). **[US Boxed Warning]: For IV use only. Intrathecal administration may result in death.** To prevent administration errors, the Institute for Safe Medication Practices (ISMP) Targeted Medication Safety Best Practices for Hospitals initiative strongly recommends dispensing vinblastine diluted in a minibag (ISMP, 2014). **If not dispensed in a minibag, affix an auxiliary label stating "For intravenous use only - fatal if given by other routes" and also place in an overwrap labeled "Do not remove covering until moment of injection."** Vinblastine should **NOT** be prepared during the preparation of any intrathecal medications. After preparation, keep vinblastine in a location **away** from the separate storage location recommended for intrathecal medications. Vinblastine should **NOT** be delivered to the patient at the same time with any medications intended for central nervous system administration.

[US Boxed Warning]: Vinblastine is a vesicant; ensure proper needle or catheter placement prior to and during infusion. Avoid extravasation. Extravasation may cause significant irritation. Individuals administering should be experienced in vinblastine administration. If extravasation occurs, discontinue immediately and initiate appropriate extravasation management, including local injection of hyaluronidase and moderate

◄ **heat application to the affected area. Use a separate vein to complete administration.**

Leukopenia commonly occurs; granulocytopenia may be severe with higher doses. The leukocyte nadir generally occurs 5 to 10 days after administration; recovery typically occurs 7 to 14 days later. Monitor for infections if WBC <2,000/mm^3. Leukopenia may be more pronounced in cachectic patients and patients with skin ulceration and may be less pronounced with lower doses used for maintenance therapy. Leukocytes and platelets may fall considerably with moderate doses when marrow is infiltrated with malignant cells (further use in this situation is not recommended). Thrombocytopenia and anemia may occur rarely.

May rarely cause disabling neurotoxicity; usually reversible. Seizures and severe and permanent CNS damage has occurred with higher then recommended doses and/or when administered more frequently than recommended. Acute shortness of breath and severe bronchospasm have been reported, most often in association with concurrent administration of mitomycin; may occur within minutes to several hours following vinblastine administration or up to 14 days following mitomycin administration; use caution in patients with preexisting pulmonary disease. Use with caution in patients with hepatic impairment; toxicity may be increased; may require dosage modification. Use with caution in patients with ischemic heart disease. Stomatitis may occur (rare); may be disabling, but is usually reversible.

Potentially significant drug-drug interactions may exist, requiring dose or frequency adjustment, additional monitoring, and/or selection of alternative therapy. **[US Boxed Warning]: Should be administered under the supervision of an experienced cancer chemotherapy physician.**

Benzyl alcohol and derivatives: Some dosage forms may contain benzyl alcohol; large amounts of benzyl alcohol (≥99 mg/kg/day) have been associated with a potentially fatal toxicity ("gasping syndrome") in neonates; the "gasping syndrome" consists of metabolic acidosis, respiratory distress, gasping respirations, CNS dysfunction (including convulsions, intracranial hemorrhage), hypotension, and cardiovascular collapse (AAP ["Inactive" 1997]; CDC, 1982); some data suggests that benzoate displaces bilirubin from protein binding sites (Ahlfors, 2001); avoid or use dosage forms containing benzyl alcohol with caution in neonates. See manufacturer's labeling.

Adverse Reactions Frequency not defined.

Cardiovascular: Angina pectoris, cerebrovascular accident, ECG abnormality, hypertension (common), ischemic heart disease, limb ischemia, myocardial infarction, Raynaud's phenomenon

Central nervous system: Decreased deep tendon reflex, depression, dizziness, headache, malaise (common), metallic taste, neurotoxicity (duration: >24 hours), paresthesia, peripheral neuritis, seizure, tumor pain (common), vertigo

Dermatologic: Alopecia (common), dermatitis, skin blister, skin photosensitivity (rare), skin rash

Endocrine & metabolic: Hyperuricemia, SIADH (syndrome of inappropriate antidiuretic hormone secretion)

Gastrointestinal: Abdominal pain, anorexia, constipation (common), diarrhea, enterocolitis (hemorrhagic), gastrointestinal hemorrhage, intestinal obstruction, nausea (mild), paralytic ileus, stomatitis, toxic megacolon, vomiting (mild)

Genitourinary: Azoospermia, urinary retention

Hematologic & oncologic: Anemia, bone marrow depression (common), granulocytopenia (common; nadir: 5 to 10 days; recovery: 7 to 14 days; dose-limiting toxicity), hemolytic uremic syndrome, leukopenia (common; nadir: 5 to 10 days; recovery: 7 to 14 days; dose-limiting toxicity), rectal hemorrhage, thrombocytopenia (recovery within a few days), thrombotic thrombocytopenic purpura

Local: Local irritation

Neuromuscular & skeletal: Jaw pain (common), myalgia, ostealgia (common), weakness

Ophthalmic: Nystagmus

Otic: Auditory disturbance, deafness, vestibular disturbance

Respiratory: Bronchospasm, dyspnea, pharyngitis

Miscellaneous: Radiation recall phenomenon

Drug Interactions

Metabolism/Transport Effects Substrate of CYP2D6 (minor), CYP3A4 (major), P-glycoprotein; **Note:** Assignment of Major/Minor substrate status based on clinically relevant drug interaction potential

Avoid Concomitant Use

Avoid concomitant use of VinBLAStine with any of the following: BCG (Intravesical); Conivaptan; Deferiprone; Dipyrone; Fusidic Acid (Systemic); Idelalisib; Natalizumab; Pimecrolimus; Tacrolimus (Topical); Vaccines (Live)

Increased Effect/Toxicity

VinBLAStine may increase the levels/effects of: CloZAPine; Deferiprone; Fingolimod; Leflunomide; MitoMYcin (Systemic); Natalizumab; Tofacitinib; Tolterodine; Vaccines (Live)

The levels/effects of VinBLAStine may be increased by: Aprepitant; Conivaptan; CYP3A4 Inhibitors (Moderate); CYP3A4 Inhibitors (Strong); Dasatinib; Denosumab; Dipyrone; Fosaprepitant; Fusidic Acid (Systemic); Idelalisib; Itraconazole; Lopinavir; Macrolide Antibiotics; MiFEPRIStone; Netupitant; Ocrelizumab; Palbociclib; Palifermin; P-glycoprotein/ABCB1 Inhibitors; Pimecrolimus; Posaconazole; Promazine; Ranolazine; Ritonavir; Roflumilast; Simeprevir; Stiripentol; Tacrolimus (Topical); Trastuzumab; Voriconazole

Decreased Effect

VinBLAStine may decrease the levels/effects of: BCG (Intravesical); Coccidioides immitis Skin Test; Lenograstim; Nivolumab; Sipuleucel-T; Tertomotide; Vaccines (Inactivated); Vaccines (Live)

The levels/effects of VinBLAStine may be decreased by: Bosentan; CYP3A4 Inducers (Moderate); CYP3A4 Inducers (Strong); Dabrafenib; Deferasirox; Echinacea; Enzalutamide; Mitotane; Sarilumab; Siltuximab; St John's Wort; Tocilizumab

Hazardous Drugs Handling Considerations

Hazardous agent (NIOSH 2016 [group 1]).

Use appropriate precautions for receiving, handling, administration, and disposal. Gloves (single) should be worn during receiving, unpacking, and placing in storage.

NIOSH recommends double gloving, a protective gown, ventilated engineering controls (a class II biological safety cabinet or a compounding aseptic containment isolator), and closed system transfer devices (CSTDs) for preparation. Double gloving, a gown, and (if dosage form allows) CSTDs are required during administration (NIOSH 2016).

Storage/Stability

Note: Vinblastine should be dispensed in a minibag (ISMP 2014). Although not recommended, if prepared in a syringe, the syringe must be dispensed in an overwrap which bears the statement "Do not remove covering until the moment of injection. Fatal if given intrathecally. For IV use only."

Store intact vials at 2°C to 8°C (36°F to 46°F). Protect from light. Solutions diluted for infusion in NS, D5W, or LR (20 mcg/mL concentration) are stable for up to 21 days if protected from light (Beijnen 1989). The formulation of vinblastine may have changed since this stability study was conducted; consult the manufacturer's prescribing information for further information. Follow USP 797 recommendations for beyond use dates based on the level of risk for preparation.

Preparation for Administration Note: In order to prevent inadvertent intrathecal administration, the Institute for Safe Medication Practices (ISMP) strongly recommends dispensing vinblastine in a minibag (**NOT** in a syringe).

For infusion, dilute in 25 to 50 mL NS, D5W, or LR; dilution in larger volumes (≥100 mL) of IV fluids is not recommended.

Mechanism of Action Vinblastine binds to tubulin and inhibits microtubule formation, therefore, arresting the cell at metaphase by disrupting the formation of the mitotic spindle; it is specific for the M and S phases. Vinblastine may also interfere with nucleic acid and protein synthesis by blocking glutamic acid utilization.

Pharmacodynamics/Kinetics

Metabolism: Hepatic (via CYP3A) to active metabolite

Half-life elimination: Terminal: ~25 hours

Excretion: Feces (10%); urine (14%)

Dosing

Adult & Geriatric Note: Frequency and duration of therapy may vary by indication, concomitant combination chemotherapy and hematologic response. **For IV use only.** In order to prevent inadvertent intrathecal administration, the Institute for Safe Medication Practices (ISMP) strongly recommends dispensing vinblastine in a minibag (**NOT** a syringe).

Hodgkin lymphoma, lymphocytic lymphoma, histiocytic lymphoma, mycosis fungoides, testicular cancer, Kaposi sarcoma, histiocytosis X (Letterer-Siwe disease): *Manufacturer's labeling:* IV: 3.7 mg/m^2; adjust dose every 7 days (based on white blood cell response) up to 5.5 mg/m^2 (second dose); 7.4 mg/m^2 (third dose); 9.25 mg/m^2 (fourth dose); and 11.1 mg/m^2 (fifth dose); do not administer more frequently than every 7 days. Usual dosage range: 5.5 to 7.4 mg/m^2 every 7 days; Maximum dose: 18.5 mg/m^2; dosage adjustment goal is to reduce white blood cell count to ~3,000/mm^3

Off-label and/or indication-specific dosing:

Hodgkin lymphoma (off-label dosing): IV:

ABVD regimen: 6 mg/m^2 days 1 and 15 of a 28-day cycle (in combination with doxorubicin, bleomycin, dacarbazine, and radiation therapy) for 2 cycles (early/favorable disease) or for 4 cycles (early/unfavorable disease) (Eich 2010; Engert 2007)

Stanford V regimen: 6 mg/m^2 weeks 1, 3, 5, 7, 9, and 11 (in combination with doxorubicin, mechlorethamine, vincristine, bleomycin, etoposide, and prednisone) (Bartlett 1995; Gordon 2013; Horning 2002)

Testicular cancer (off-label dosing): VeIP regimen: IV: 0.11 mg/kg daily for 2 days every 21 days (in combination with ifosfamide, cisplatin, and mesna) for 4 cycles (Loehrer 1988; Loehrer 1988 [correction]; Loehrer 1998)

Bladder cancer (off-label use): IV:

Metastatic disease:

Dose-dense MVAC regimen: 3 mg/m^2 day 2 every 14 days (in combination with methotrexate, doxorubicin, cisplatin, and filgrastim) until disease progression or unacceptable toxicity (Sternberg 2001; Sternberg 2006)

MVAC regimen: 3 mg/m^2 days 2, 15, and 22 every 28 days (in combination with methotrexate, doxorubicin, and cisplatin) for up to 6 cycles (von der Maase 2000) **or** 3 mg/m^2 days 2, 15, and 22 every 28 days (in combination with methotrexate, doxorubicin, and cisplatin) until disease progression or unacceptable toxicity (Sternberg 2001; Sternberg 2006) **or** 3 mg/m^2 days 1, 15, and 22 every 28 days (in combination with methotrexate, doxorubicin, cisplatin, and filgrastim) for up to 6 cycles (Bamias 2004)

Neoadjuvant treatment:

MVAC regimen: 3 mg/m^2 days 2, 15, and 22 every 28 days (in combination with methotrexate, doxorubicin, and cisplatin) for 3 cycles (Grossman 2003)

CMV regimen: 4 mg/m^2 days 1 and 8 every 21 days (in combination with methotrexate, cisplatin, and leucovorin) for 3 cycles (Griffiths 2011)

Melanoma, metastatic (off-label use): IV:

CVD regimen: 2 mg/m^2 days 1 to 4 and 22 to 25 of a 6-week treatment cycle (in combination with cisplatin and dacarbazine); may repeat if tumor response (Eton 2002)

CVD + immunotherapy regimen: 1.5 mg/m^2 days 1 to 4 and 22 to 25 of a 6-week treatment cycle (in combination with cisplatin, dacarbazine, aldesleukin, and interferon alfa-2b); may repeat if tumor response (Eton 2002)

Non-small cell lung cancer (off-label use): IV:

Adjuvant treatment after complete resection: 4 mg/m^2 days 1, 8, 15, 22, and 29, then every 2 weeks (in combination with cisplatin) until last cisplatin dose (Arriagada 2004)

Concurrent radiation: 5 mg/m^2 days 1, 8, 15, 22, and 29 (in combination with cisplatin and concurrent radiation therapy) (Curran 2011)

Soft tissue sarcoma (desmoid tumors, aggressive fibromatosis), advanced (off-label use): IV: 6 mg/m^2 every 7 to 10 days (dose usually rounded to 10 mg) in combination with methotrexate for 1 year (Azzarelli 2001)

Pediatric Note: Frequency and duration of therapy may vary by indication, concomitant combination chemotherapy and hematologic response. **For IV use only.** In order to prevent inadvertent intrathecal administration, the Institute for Safe Medication Practices (ISMP) strongly recommends dispensing vinblastine in a minibag (**NOT** a syringe).

Hodgkin lymphoma: IV: Initial dose: 6 mg/m^2; do not administer more frequently than every 7 days **or** ABVD regimen (off-label dosing; advanced disease): IV: 6 mg/m^2 days 1 and 15 of a 28-day cycle (in combination with doxorubicin, bleomycin, dacarbazine, and radiation therapy) for 6 cycles (Hutchinson 1998)

◄ **Letterer-Siwe disease:** IV: Initial dose: 6.5 mg/m^2; do not administer more frequently than every 7 days

Testicular cancer: IV: Initial dose: 3 mg/m^2; do not administer more frequently than every 7 days

Renal Impairment No dosage adjustment necessary.

Hepatic Impairment

The manufacturer's labeling recommends the following adjustment: Serum bilirubin >3 mg/dL: Administer 50% of dose

The following adjustments have also been recommended (Floyd 2006; Superfin 2007):

Serum bilirubin 1.5 to 3 mg/dL or transaminases 2 to 3 times ULN: Administer 50% of dose

Serum bilirubin >3 times ULN: Avoid use.

Obesity *ASCO Guidelines for appropriate chemotherapy dosing in obese adults with cancer:* Utilize patient's actual body weight (full weight) for calculation of body surface area- or weight-based dosing, particularly when the intent of therapy is curative; manage regimen-related toxicities in the same manner as for nonobese patients; if a dose reduction is utilized due to toxicity, consider resumption of full weight-based dosing with subsequent cycles, especially if cause of toxicity (eg, hepatic or renal impairment) is resolved (Griggs 2012).

Combination Regimens

Bladder cancer:
CMV (Bladder) on page 2068
Dose Dense MVAC (Bladder Cancer) on page 2096
MVAC (Bladder) on page 2179
Lung cancer (non-small cell): Cisplatin-Vinblastine (NSCLC) on page 2061
Lymphoma, Hodgkin:
ABVD Early Stage (Hodgkin) on page 1974
ABVD (Hodgkin) on page 1975
ChlVPP (Hodgkin) on page 2033
C-MOPP/ABV Hybrid (Hodgkin) on page 2067
MOPP/ABVD (Hodgkin) on page 2176
MOPP/ABV Hybrid (Hodgkin) on page 2177
Stanford V (Hodgkin) on page 2209
VAMP (Hodgkin) on page 2226
Melanoma:
Cisplatin-Vinblastine-Dacarbazine (Melanoma) on page 2061
CVD-Interleukin-Interferon (Melanoma) on page 2075
Soft tissue sarcoma: Methotrexate-Vinblastine (Soft Tissue Sarcoma) on page 2173
Testicular cancer: VeIP (Testicular) on page 2231

Administration In order to prevent inadvertent intrathecal administration, the Institute for Safe Medication Practices (ISMP) strongly recommends dispensing vinblastine in a minibag (NOT in a syringe). For IV administration only. **Fatal if given intrathecally.** The preferred administration is as a short infusion in a 25 to 50 mL minibag. If administration via a minibag is not possible, may also be administered as an undiluted 1-minute infusion into a free flowing IV line to prevent venous irritation/extravasation. Prolonged administration times (≥30 to 60 minutes) and/or increased administration volumes may increase the risk of vein irritation and extravasation.

Vesicant; ensure proper needle or catheter placement prior to and during infusion. Avoid extravasation.

Extravasation management: If extravasation occurs, stop infusion immediately and disconnect (leave cannula/needle in place); gently aspirate extravasated solution (do **NOT** flush the line); initiate hyaluronidase antidote; remove needle/cannula; apply dry warm compresses for 20 minutes 4 times a day for 1 to 2 days; elevate extremity (Perez Fidalgo 2012). Remaining portion of the vinblastine dose should be infused through a separate vein.

Hyaluronidase: If needle/cannula still in place, administer 1 to 6 mL hyaluronidase (150 units/mL) into the existing IV line; the usual dose is 1 mL hyaluronidase for each 1 mL of extravasated drug (Perez Fidalgo 2012; Schulmeister 2011). If needle/cannula was removed, inject 1 to 6 mL (150 units/mL) subcutaneously in a clockwise manner using 1 mL for each 1 mL of drug extravasated (Schulmeister 2011) **or** administer 1 mL (150 units/mL) as 5 separate 0.2 mL injections (using a 25-gauge needle) subcutaneously into the extravasation site (Polovich 2009).

Vesicant/Extravasation Risk Vesicant

Emetic Potential Children and Adults: Minimal (<10%)

Monitoring Parameters CBC with differential and platelet count, serum uric acid, hepatic function tests

Dosage Forms Excipient information presented when available (limited, particularly for generics); consult specific product labeling. [DSC] = Discontinued product

Solution, Intravenous, as sulfate:
  Generic: 1 mg/mL (10 mL)
Solution Reconstituted, Intravenous, as sulfate:
  Generic: 10 mg (1 ea [DSC])

VinCRIStine (vin KRIS teen)

Related Information

Brand Names: US Vincasar PFS

Brand Names: Canada Vincristine Sulfate Injection; Vincristine Sulfate Injection USP

Index Terms Conventional Vincristine; Leurocristine Sulfate; Oncovin; Vincristine (Conventional); Vincristine Sulfate

Pharmacologic Category Antineoplastic Agent, Antimicrotubular; Antineoplastic Agent, Vinca Alkaloid

Use Treatment of acute lymphocytic leukemia (ALL), Hodgkin lymphoma, non-Hodgkin lymphomas, Wilms' tumor, neuroblastoma, rhabdomyosarcoma

◄ **Labeled Contraindications**

Patients with the demyelinating form of Charcot-Marie-Tooth syndrome

Documentation of allergenic cross-reactivity for drugs in this class is limited. However, because of similarities in chemical structure and/or pharmacologic actions, the possibility of cross-sensitivity cannot be ruled out with certainty.

Pregnancy Considerations Animal reproduction studies have demonstrated teratogenicity and fetal loss. May cause fetal harm if administered during pregnancy. Women of childbearing potential should avoid becoming pregnant during treatment.

Breastfeeding Considerations It is not known if vincristine is present in breast milk. Due to the potential for serious adverse reactions in the breastfed infant, the decision to discontinue vincristine or to discontinue breastfeeding should take into account the benefits of treatment to the mother.

Warnings/Precautions Avoid eye contamination. **[US Boxed Warning]: For IV administration only; inadvertent intrathecal administration usually results in death.** To prevent administration errors, the Institute for Safe Medication Practices (ISMP) Targeted Medication Safety Best Practices for Hospitals initiative and the World Health Organization strongly recommend dispensing vincristine diluted in a minibag (ISMP 2014, WHO 2007), **if not dispensed in a minibag, affix an auxiliary label stating "For intravenous use only - fatal if given by other routes" and also place in an overwrap labeled "Do not remove covering until moment of injection."** Vincristine should **NOT** be prepared during the preparation of any intrathecal medications. After preparation, keep vincristine in a location **away** from the separate storage location recommended for intrathecal medications. Vincristine should **NOT** be delivered to the patient at the same time with any medications intended for central nervous system administration.

[US Boxed Warning]: Vincristine is a vesicant; ensure proper needle or catheter placement prior to and during infusion. Avoid extravasation. Individuals administering should be experienced in vincristine administration. Extravasation may cause significant irritation. If extravasation occurs, discontinue immediately and initiate appropriate extravasation management, including local injection of hyaluronidase and moderate heat application to the affected area. Use a separate vein to complete administration.

Neurotoxicity, including alterations in mental status such as depression, confusion, or insomnia may occur; neurologic effects are dose-limiting (may require dosage reduction) and may be additive with those of other neurotoxic agents and spinal cord irradiation. Use with caution in patients with preexisting neuromuscular disease and/or with concomitant neurotoxic agents. Constipation, paralytic ileus, intestinal necrosis and/or perforation may occur; constipation may present as upper colon impaction with an empty rectum (may require flat film of abdomen for diagnosis); generally responds to high enemas and laxatives. All patients should be on a prophylactic bowel management regimen.

Potentially significant drug-drug interactions may exist, requiring dose or frequency adjustment, additional monitoring, and/or selection of alternative therapy. Acute shortness of breath and severe bronchospasm have been reported with vinca alkaloids, usually when used in combination with mitomycin. Onset may be several minutes to hours after vincristine administration and up to 2 weeks after mitomycin. Progressive dyspnea may occur. Permanently discontinue vincristine if pulmonary dysfunction occurs.

Use with caution in patients with hepatic impairment; dosage modification required. May be associated with hepatic sinusoidal obstruction syndrome (SOS; formerly called veno-occlusive disease), increased risk in children <3 years of age; use with caution in hepatobiliary dysfunction. Monitor for signs or symptoms of hepatic SOS, including bilirubin >1.4 mg/dL, unexplained weight gain, ascites, hepatomegaly, or unexplained right upper quadrant pain (Arndt, 2004). Acute uric acid nephropathy has been reported with vincristine.

Adverse Reactions Frequency not defined.

Cardiovascular: Edema, hepatic sinusoidal obstruction syndrome (formerly known as hepatic veno-occlusive disease), hypertension, hypotension, ischemic heart disease, myocardial infarction, phlebitis

Central nervous system: Abnormal gait, ataxia, coma, cranial nerve dysfunction (auditory impairment, extraocular muscle impairment, laryngeal muscle impairment, motor dysfunction, paralysis, paresis, vestibular damage, vocal cord paralysis), decreased deep tendon reflex, dizziness, headache, neuralgia (common), neurotoxicity (dose-related), paralysis, paresthesia, parotid pain, peripheral neuropathy (common), seizure, sensorimotor neuropathy, sensory disturbance, vertigo

Dermatologic: Alopecia (common), skin rash

Endocrine & metabolic: Hyperuricemia, uric acid nephropathy (acute), weight loss

Gastrointestinal: Abdominal cramps, abdominal pain, anorexia, constipation (common), diarrhea, intestinal necrosis, intestinal perforation, nausea, oral mucosa ulcer, paralytic ileus, sore throat, vomiting

Genitourinary: Bladder dysfunction (atony), dysuria, urinary retention

Hematologic & oncologic: Anemia (mild), hemolytic uremic syndrome, leukopenia (mild), thrombocytopenia (mild), thrombotic thrombocytopenic purpura

Local: Local irritation (if infiltrated)

Neuromuscular & skeletal: Amyotrophy, back pain, foot-drop, jaw pain, limb pain, myalgia, ostealgia

Ophthalmic: Cortical blindness (transient), nystagmus, optic atrophy with blindness

Otic: Deafness

Renal: Polyuria

Respiratory: Bronchospasm, dyspnea

Miscellaneous: Fever, tissue necrosis (if infiltrated)

<1%, postmarketing, and/or case reports: Anaphylaxis, hypersensitivity reaction, SIADH (syndrome of inappropriate antidiuretic hormone secretion)

Drug Interactions

Metabolism/Transport Effects Substrate of CYP3A4 (major), P-glycoprotein; **Note:** Assignment of Major/Minor substrate status based on clinically relevant drug interaction potential

Avoid Concomitant Use

Avoid concomitant use of VinCRIStine with any of the following: BCG (Intravesical); Conivaptan; Fusidic Acid (Systemic); Idelalisib; Natalizumab; Pimecrolimus; Tacrolimus (Topical); Vaccines (Live)

Increased Effect/Toxicity

VinCRIStine may increase the levels/effects of: Fingolimod; Leflunomide; MitoMYcin (Systemic); Natalizumab; Tofacitinib; Vaccines (Live)

The levels/effects of VinCRIStine may be increased by: Aprepitant; Conivaptan; CYP3A4 Inhibitors (Moderate); CYP3A4 Inhibitors (Strong); Dasatinib; Denosumab; Fosaprepitant; Fusidic Acid (Systemic); Idelalisib; Itraconazole; Lopinavir; Macrolide Antibiotics; MiFEPRIStone; Netupitant;

NIFEdipine; Ocrelizumab; Palbociclib; Palifermin; P-glycoprotein/ABCB1 Inhibitors; Pimecrolimus; Posaconazole; Ranolazine; Ritonavir; Roflumilast; Simeprevir; Stiripentol; Tacrolimus (Topical); Teniposide; Trastuzumab; Voriconazole

Decreased Effect

VinCRIStine may decrease the levels/effects of: BCG (Intravesical); Coccidioides immitis Skin Test; Fosphenytoin; Lenograstim; Nivolumab; Phenytoin; Sipuleucel-T; Tertomotide; Vaccines (Inactivated); Vaccines (Live)

The levels/effects of VinCRIStine may be decreased by: Bosentan; CYP3A4 Inducers (Moderate); CYP3A4 Inducers (Strong); Dabrafenib; Deferasirox; Echinacea; Enzalutamide; Fosphenytoin; Mitotane; Phenytoin; Sarilumab; Siltuximab; St John's Wort; Tocilizumab

Hazardous Drugs Handling Considerations

Hazardous agent (NIOSH 2016 [group 1]).

Use appropriate precautions for receiving, handling, administration, and disposal. Gloves (single) should be worn during receiving, unpacking, and placing in storage.

NIOSH recommends double gloving, a protective gown, ventilated engineering controls (a class II biological safety cabinet or a compounding aseptic containment isolator), and closed system transfer devices (CSTDs) for preparation. Double gloving, a gown, and (if dosage form allows) CSTDs are required during administration (NIOSH 2016).

Storage/Stability Store intact vials refrigerated at 2°C to 8°C (36°F to 46°F). Protect from light.

IV solution: Diluted in 25 to 50 mL NS or D5W, stable for 7 days under refrigeration, or 2 days at room temperature. In ambulatory pumps, solution is stable for 7 days at room temperature. After preparation, keep vincristine in a location away from the separate storage location recommended for intrathecal medications. **Note:** Vincristine should be dispensed in a minibag (ISMP 2014). While dispensing vincristine in a syringe is NOT recommended, if prepared in a syringe, affix an auxiliary label stating **"For intravenous use only - fatal if given by other routes"** to the syringe, and the syringe must be dispensed in the manufacturer-provided overwrap which bears the statement **"Do not remove covering until the moment of injection. For intravenous use only. Fatal if given intrathecally."**

Preparation for Administration Solutions for IV infusion may be mixed in NS or D5W. **Note:** In order to prevent inadvertent intrathecal administration the World Health Organization (WHO) and the Institute for Safe Medication Practices (ISMP) strongly recommend dispensing vincristine in a minibag (**NOT** in a syringe). Vincristine should **NOT** be prepared during the preparation of any intrathecal medications.

Mechanism of Action Binds to tubulin and inhibits microtubule formation, therefore, arresting the cell at metaphase by disrupting the formation of the mitotic spindle; it is specific for the M and S phases. Vincristine may also interfere with nucleic acid and protein synthesis by blocking glutamic acid utilization.

Pharmacodynamics/Kinetics Note: In pediatric patients, significant intrapatient and interpatient variability has been reported (Gidding 1999).

Distribution: Rapidly removed from bloodstream and tightly bound to tissues; penetrates blood-brain barrier poorly

Metabolism: Extensively hepatic, via CYP3A4

Half-life elimination: Terminal: 85 hours (range: 19-155 hours)

Excretion: Feces (~80%); urine (10% to 20%; <1% as unchanged drug)

Clearance: In pediatric patients, correlation with diagnosis has been reported; clearance in patients with ALL and non-Hodgkin lymphoma higher than Wilms' tumor (Gidding 1999):

Infants: Vincristine clearance is lower compared to children; more closely related to body weight than to body surface area (Crom1994)

Children and Adolescents 2 to 18 years: Reported means: 357 to 482 mL/minute/m^2; some suggest faster clearance in children <10 years of age than in adolescents (Crom 1994); however, more recent data does not support this finding nor a dosage reduction in adolescent patients (Frost 2003; Gidding 1999)

Dosing

Adult & Geriatric Note: Doses may be capped at a maximum of 2 mg/dose. Dosing and frequency may vary by protocol and/or treatment phase; refer to specific protocol. In order to prevent inadvertent intrathecal administration, the World Health Organization (WHO) and the Institute for Safe Medication Practices (ISMP) strongly recommend dispensing vincristine in a minibag (**NOT** a syringe).

Dosing in the manufacturer's labeling: IV: 1.4 mg/m^2/dose; frequency may vary based on protocol

Additional dosing in combination therapy; indication-specific and/or off-label dosing:

Acute lymphocytic leukemia (ALL): IV:

Hyper-CVAD regimen: 2 mg/dose days 4 and 11 during odd-numbered cycles (cycles 1, 3, 5, 7) of an 8-cycle phase, followed by maintenance treatment (if needed) of 2 mg monthly for 2 years (Kantarjian, 2004)

CALBG 8811 regimen: Induction phase: 2 mg/dose days 1, 8, 15, and 22 (4-week treatment cycle); Early intensification phase: 2 mg/dose days 15, and 22 (4-week treatment cycle, repeat once); Late intensification phase: 2 mg/dose days 1, 8, 15 (8-week treatment cycle); Maintenance phase: 2 mg/dose day 1 every 4 weeks until 24 months from diagnosis (Larson, 1995)

Central nervous system tumors: IV: PCV regimen: 1.4 mg/m^2/dose (maximum dose: 2 mg) on days 8 and 29 of a 6-week treatment cycle for a total of 6 cycles (van de Bent, 2006) **or** 1.4 mg/m^2/dose (no maximum dose) on days 8 and 29 of a 6-week treatment cycle for up to 4 cycles (Cairncross, 2006)

Hodgkin lymphoma: IV:

BEACOPP regimen: 1.4 mg/m^2/dose (maximum dose: 2 mg) on day 8 of a 21-day treatment cycle (Diehl, 2003)

Stanford-V regimen: 1.4 mg/m^2/dose (maximum dose: 2 mg) in weeks 2, 4, 6, 8, 10, and 12 (Horning, 2000; Horning, 2002)

Non-Hodgkin lymphoma: IV:

Burkitt lymphoma:

CODOX-M/IVAC: Cycles 1 and 3 (CODOX-M): 1.5 mg/m^2 (no maximum dose) days 1 and 8 of cycle 1 and days 1, 8, and 15 of cycle 3 (Magrath, 1996) **or** 1.5 mg/m^2 (maximum dose: 2 mg) days 1 and 8 of cycles 1 and 3 (Mead 2002; Mead 2008); CODOX-M is in combination with cyclophosphamide, doxorubicin, methotrexate, and CNS prophylaxis and alternates with IVAC (etoposide, ifosfamide, mesna, cytarabine, and CNS prophylaxis) for a total of 4 cycles

Hyper-CVAD: 2 mg (flat dose) days 4 and 11 of courses 1, 3, 5, and 7 (in combination with cyclophosphamide, doxorubicin, and dexamethasone) and alternates with even courses 2, 4, 6, and 8 (methotrexate and cytarabine) (Thomas, 2006)

Follicular lymphoma: CVP regimen: 1.4 mg/m^2/dose (maximum dose: 2 mg) on day 1 of a 21-day treatment cycle (in combination with cyclophosphamide and prednisone) for 8 cycles (Marcus, 2005)

Large B-cell lymphoma:

CHOP regimen: 1.4 mg/m^2/dose (maximum dose: 2 mg) on day 1 of a 21-day treatment cycle for 8 cycles (Coiffier, 2002)

EPOCH regimen: 0.4 mg/m^2/day continuous infusion for 4 days (over 96 hours) (total 1.6 mg/m^2/cycle; dose not usually capped) of a 21-day treatment cycle (Wilson, 2002)

Ewing's sarcoma (off-label use): IV: VAC/IE regimen: VAC: 2 mg/m^2 (maximum dose: 2 mg) on day 1 of a 21-day treatment cycle (in combination with doxorubicin and cyclophosphamide), alternates with IE (ifosfamide and etoposide) for a total of 17 cycles (Grier, 2003)

Gestational trophoblastic tumors, high-risk (off-label use): IV: EMA/CO regimen: 1 mg/m^2 on day 8 of 2-week treatment cycle (in combination with etoposide methotrexate, dactinomycin, and cyclophosphamide), continue for at least 2 treatment cycles after a normal hCG level (Escobar 2003; Lurain 2006)

Multiple myeloma (off-label use): IV:

DVD regimen: 1.4 mg/m^2/dose (maximum dose: 2 mg) on day 1 of a 28-day treatment cycle (Rifkin, 2006)

VAD regimen: 0.4 mg/day continuous infusion for 4 days (over 96 hours) (total 1.6 mg/cycle) of a 28-day treatment cycle (Rifkin, 2006)

Ovarian cancer (off-label use): IV: VAC regimen: 1.5 mg/m^2/dose (maximum dose: 2 mg) weekly for 8-12 weeks (Slayton, 1985)

Small cell lung cancer (off-label use): IV: CAV regimen: 1.4 mg/m^2/dose day 1 of a 21-day treatment cycle (Hong, 1989) **or** 2 mg/dose on day 1 of a 21-day treatment cycle (von Pawel, 1999)

Thymoma, advanced (off-label use): IV: ADOC regimen: 0.6 mg/m^2 on day 3 every 3 weeks (in combination with cisplatin, doxorubicin, and cyclophosphamide) (Fornasiero, 1991)

Pediatric Note: Doses may be capped at a maximum of 2 mg/dose. Dosing and frequency may vary by protocol and/or treatment phase; refer to specific protocol. In order to prevent inadvertent intrathecal administration, the World Health Organization (WHO) and the Institute for Safe Medication Practices (ISMP) strongly recommend dispensing vincristine in a minibag (**NOT** in a syringe).

Dosing in the manufacturer's labeling: IV:

Children ≤10 kg: 0.05 mg/kg/dose once weekly

Children >10 kg: 1.5 to 2 mg/m^2/dose; frequency may vary based on protocol

Additional dosing in combination therapy; indication-specific and/or off-label dosing:

Acute lymphocytic lymphoma (ALL): IV: Induction phase: 1.5 mg/m^2/dose days 0, 7, 14, and 21; Consolidation phase: 1.5 mg/m^2/dose days 0, 28, and 56; Delayed intensification phase: 1.5 mg/m^2/dose days 0, 7, and 14; Maintenance phase: 1.5 mg/m^2/dose days 0, 28, and 56 (Bostrom, 2003) **or** Induction phase: 1.5 mg/m^2/dose days 0, 7, 14, and 21; Consolidation phase: 1.5 mg/m^2/dose days 0, 28, and 56; Interim maintenance phases: 1.5 mg/m^2/dose days 0 and 28; Delayed intensification phase: 1.5 mg/m^2/dose days 0, 7, and 14; Maintenance phase: 1.5 mg/m^2/dose every 4 weeks (Avramis, 2002)

Burkitt lymphoma and B-cell ALL: IV: 1.5 mg/m^2 (maximum dose: 2 mg) on days 4 and 11 of initial phase cycle (initial phase is in combination with cyclophosphamide, doxorubicin, and CNS prophylaxis; alternates with secondary phase) for a total of 4 cycles of each phase (Bowman, 1996) **or** 1.5 mg/m^2 (maximum dose: 2 mg) on day 1 of cycle AA (in combination with dexamethasone, ifosfamide, methotrexate, cytarabine, etoposide and CNS prophylaxis) and on day 1 of cycle BB (in combination with dexamethasone, cyclophosphamide, methotrexate, doxorubicin, and CNS prophylaxis) (Reiter, 1999)

Ewing's sarcoma (off-label use): IV: 2 mg/m^2/dose (maximum dose: 2 mg) on day 1 of a 21-day cycle, administer either every cycle or during odd-numbered cycles (Grier, 2003) **or** 0.67 mg/m^2/day continuous infusion days 1, 2, and 3 (total 2 mg/m^2/cycle; maximum dose/cycle: 2 mg) during cycles 1, 2, 3, and 6 (Kolb, 2003)

Hodgkin lymphoma: IV: BEACOPP regimen: 2 mg/m^2/dose (maximum dose: 2 mg) on day 7 of a 21-day treatment cycle (Kelly, 2002)

Neuroblastoma: IV:

CE-CAdO regimen: 1.5 mg/m^2 (maximum dose: 2 mg) days 1 and 5 every 21 days for 2 cycles (Rubie, 1998) **or** 0.05 mg/kg days 1 and 5 for 2 cycles (Rubie, 2001)

CAV-P/VP regimen (off-label dosing): 0.033 mg/kg/day continuous infusion days 1, 2, and 3, then 1.5 mg/m^2 bolus day 9 of courses 1, 2, 4, and 6 (Kushner, 1994)

Retinoblastoma (off-label use): IV:

Children: 0.05 mg/kg on day 1 every 21 days (in combination with carboplatin) for 8 cycles (Rodriguez-Galindo, 2003)

or

Children ≤36 months: 0.05 mg/kg on day 0 every 28 days (in combination with carboplatin and etoposide) for 6 cycles (Freidman, 2000)

or

Children >36 months: 1.5 mg/m^2 (maximum dose: 2 mg) on day 0 every 28 days (in combination with carboplatin and etoposide) for 6 cycles (Friedman, 2000)

Rhabdomyosarcoma: IV:

VA regimen: 1.5 mg/m^2/dose (maximum dose: 2 mg) weeks 1-8, weeks 13-20, and weeks 25-32 (Crist, 2001)

VAC regimen: 1.5 mg/m^2/dose (maximum dose: 2 mg) weeks 0-12, week 16, weeks 20-25; Continuation therapy: Weeks 29-34, and weeks 38-43 (Crist, 2001)

Wilms' tumor: IV:

Children <1 year: 0.75 mg/m^2/dose weekly for 10-11 weeks, then every 3 weeks for 15 additional weeks (total 25-26 weeks) (Pritchard, 1995)

Children ≥1 year: 1.5 mg/m^2/dose weekly for 10-11 weeks, then every 3 weeks for 15 additional weeks (total 25-26 weeks) (Pritchard, 1995)

or

Children ≤30 kg: 0.05 mg/kg/dose (maximum dose: 2 mg) weeks 1, 2, 4, 5, 6, 7, 8, 10, and 11, followed by 0.067 mg/kg/dose (maximum dose: 2 mg) weeks 12, 13, 18, and 24 (Green, 2007)

Children >30 kg: 1.5 mg/m^2/dose (maximum dose: 2 mg) weeks 1, 2, 4, 5, 6, 7, 8, 10, and 11, followed by 2 mg/m^2/dose (maximum dose: 2 mg) weeks 12, 13, 18, and 24 (Green, 2007)

◄ **Renal Impairment** No dosage adjustment necessary (Kintzel 1995).
Hepatic Impairment The manufacturer's labeling recommends the following adjustment: Serum bilirubin >3 mg/dL: Administer 50% of normal dose. The following adjustments have also been recommended:

Floyd 2006: Serum bilirubin 1.5 to 3 mg/dL or transaminases 2 to 3 times ULN or alkaline phosphatase increased: Administer 50% of dose.

Superfin 2007:

Serum bilirubin 1.5 to 3 mg/dL: Administer 50% of dose.

Serum bilirubin >3 mg/dL: Avoid use.

Obesity *ASCO Guidelines for appropriate chemotherapy dosing in obese adults with cancer:* Dose should be capped at a maximum of 2 mg due to neurotoxicity concerns (Griggs 2012)

Combination Regimens

Bone sarcoma (Ewing Sarcoma): VAC Alternating With IE (Ewing Sarcoma) on page 2224

Brain tumors:

COPE on page 2074

PCV (Brain Tumor Regimen) on page 2191

POC on page 2196

Gestational trophoblastic tumor: EMA/CO (Gestational Trophoblastic Tumor) on page 2101

Leukemia, acute lymphocytic:

CALGB 8811 Regimen (ALL) on page 2003

CALGB 9111 Regimen (ALL) on page 2004

DVP on page 2099

Hyper-CVAD + Imatinib on page 2145

Hyper-CVAD (Leukemia, Acute Lymphocytic) on page 2146

Linker Protocol (ALL) on page 2167

MTX/6-MP/VP (Maintenance) on page 2178

POMP on page 2197

PVA (POG 8602) on page 2197

PVDA on page 2199

VAD/CVAD on page 2226

Lung cancer (small cell): CAV (Small Cell Lung Cancer) on page 2027

Lymphoma, Hodgkin:

BEACOPP-14 (Hodgkin) on page 1981

BEACOPP Escalated (Hodgkin) on page 1982

BEACOPP Escalated Plus Standard (Hodgkin) on page 1983

BEACOPP Standard (Hodgkin) on page 1984

C-MOPP/ABV Hybrid (Hodgkin) on page 2067

MOPP/ABVD (Hodgkin) on page 2176

MOPP/ABV Hybrid (Hodgkin) on page 2177

MOPP (Hodgkin) on page 2178

Stanford V (Hodgkin) on page 2209

Lymphoma, non-Hodgkin:

EPOCH Dose-Adjusted (NHL) on page 2105

EPOCH (Dose-Adjusted)-Rituximab (NHL) on page 2106

Lymphoma, non-Hodgkin (AIDS-Related):

CHOP (NHL-AIDS-Related) on page 2035

EPOCH Dose-Adjusted (NHL-AIDS-Related) on page 2106

EPOCH Dose-Adjusted-Rituximab (NHL-AIDS-Related) on page 2107

Lymphoma, non-Hodgkin (Burkitt):
Lymphoma, non-Hodgkin (Follicular):
Multiple myeloma:
Neuroblastoma:
Retinoblastoma:
Soft tissue sarcoma (rhabdomyosarcoma):
Wilms' tumor:

Administration For IV administration only. **FATAL IF GIVEN INTRATHE-
CALLY.**

**In order to prevent inadvertent intrathecal administration, the World
Health Organization (WHO) and the Institute for Safe Medication Practices (ISMP) strongly recommend dispensing vincristine in a minibag
(NOT in a syringe).** Vincristine should **NOT** be delivered to the patient at the
same time with any medications intended for central nervous system
administration.

IV: Preferred administration is as a short 5- to 10-minute infusion in a 25 to 50
mL minibag. If administration via minibag is not possible, may also be
administered as a slow (1-minute) push. Some protocols utilize a 24-hour
continuous infusion.

Vesicant; ensure proper needle or catheter placement prior to and during
infusion. Avoid extravasation.

◀ **Extravasation management:** If extravasation occurs, stop infusion immediately and disconnect (leave cannula/needle in place); gently aspirate extravasated solution (do **NOT** flush the line); initiate hyaluronidase antidote; remove needle/cannula; apply dry warm compresses for 20 minutes 4 times a day for 1 to 2 days; elevate (Perez Fidalgo 2012). Remaining portion of the vincristine dose should be infused through a separate vein.

Hyaluronidase: If needle/cannula still in place, administer 1 to 6 mL hyaluronidase (150 units/mL) into the existing IV line; the usual dose is 1 mL hyaluronidase for each 1 mL of extravasated drug (Perez Fidalgo 2012, Schulmeister 2011). If needle/cannula was removed, inject 1 to 6 mL (150 units/mL) subcutaneously in a clockwise manner using 1 mL for each 1 mL of drug extravasated (Schulmeister 2011) **or** administer 1 mL (150 units/mL) as 5 separate 0.2 mL injections (using a 25-gauge needle) subcutaneously into the extravasation site (Polovich 2009).

Vesicant/Extravasation Risk Vesicant

Emetic Potential Children and Adults: Minimal (<10%)

Monitoring Parameters Serum electrolytes (sodium), hepatic function tests, CBC with differential, serum uric acid; monitor infusion site; neurologic examination, monitor for constipation/ileus and for signs/symptoms of peripheral neuropathy

Dosage Forms Excipient information presented when available (limited, particularly for generics); consult specific product labeling.

Solution, Intravenous, as sulfate:
  Vincasar PFS: 1 mg/mL (1 mL, 2 mL)
Solution, Intravenous, as sulfate [preservative free]:
  Generic: 1 mg/mL (1 mL, 2 mL)

VinCRIStine (Liposomal) (vin KRIS teen lye po SO mal)

Related Information

Common Toxicity Criteria *on page 2242*

Management of Chemotherapy-Induced Nausea and Vomiting in Adults *on page 2253*

Safe Handling of Hazardous Drugs *on page 2379*

Brand Names: US Marqibo

Index Terms Liposomal Vincristine; Liposome Vincristine; Vincristine Liposomal Sulfate; Vincristine Liposome; Vincristine Sulfate Liposome; VSLI

Pharmacologic Category Antineoplastic Agent, Antimicrotubular; Antineoplastic Agent, Vinca Alkaloid

Use Acute lymphoblastic leukemia (relapsed): Treatment of relapsed Philadelphia chromosome-negative (Ph-) acute lymphoblastic leukemia (ALL) in adult patients in second or greater relapse or whose disease has progressed after two or more antileukemic therapies.

Labeled Contraindications Hypersensitivity to vincristine, liposomal vincristine, or any component of the formulation; patients with Charcot-Marie-Tooth syndrome or other demyelinating conditions; administration via the intrathecal route

Pregnancy Considerations Adverse events (fetal malformations, decreased fetal weight, and fetal loss) were observed in animal reproduction studies at doses less than the recommended human dose. Based on the mechanism of action, adverse fetal events would be expected to occur with use in pregnant women. Women of reproductive potential should avoid becoming pregnant during therapy.

Breastfeeding Considerations It is not known if liposomal vincristine is present in breast milk. Due to the potential for adverse reactions in the breastfed infant, the decision to discontinue breastfeeding or to discontinue liposomal vincristine should take into account the benefits of treatment to the mother.

Warnings/Precautions [US Boxed Warning]: For IV administration only. Intrathecal administration is contraindicated; inadvertent intrathecal administration has resulted in death. Liposomal vincristine should **NOT** be prepared during the preparation of any intrathecal medications. After preparation, keep liposomal vincristine in a location **away** from the separate storage location recommended for intrathecal medications. Liposomal vincristine should **NOT** be delivered to the patient at the same time with any medications intended for central nervous system administration.

[US Boxed Warning]: Vincristine LIPOSOME and conventional vincristine are NOT interchangeable. Dosing differs between formulations; verify intended product and dose prior to preparation and administration to avoid overdoses. Avoid extravasation of liposomal vincristine (conventional vincristine is a vesicant). Only individuals experienced with vesicant administration should administer liposomal vincristine. Check for proper needle placement; if extravasation occurs, discontinue liposomal vincristine infusion immediately and institute appropriate extravasation management procedures.

Grade 3 and greater neutropenia, anemia, and thrombocytopenia were observed in clinical trials. Monitor blood counts closely and adjust dose or withhold therapy if necessary. Constipation, ileus, bowel obstruction, and colonic pseudo-obstruction have occurred with liposomal vincristine. Patients should be initiated on a prophylactic bowel regimen including a stool softener, dietary fiber, and hydration; laxative treatments may be considered. Severe fatigue was noted in clinical trials; treatment delay, dosage adjustment, or discontinuation may be necessary.

Neuropathies (sensory and motor) are common and cumulative. Neuropathy symptoms may include paresthesia, hyper-/hypoesthesia, hyporeflexia or areflexia, neuralgia, jaw pain, cranial neuropathy, ileus, arthralgia, myalgia, muscle spasm, and/or weakness. Evaluate neurologic status of patients closely prior to liposomal vincristine administration; neurologic toxicity risk is greater when given to patients with preexisting neuromuscular conditions or when used concomitantly with other neurotoxic agents. Treatment delay, dosage adjustment, and/or discontinuation may be necessary. Tumor lysis syndrome may occur as a consequence of therapy; monitor closely for signs and symptoms and manage accordingly.

Hepatotoxicity (including fatal cases) and increased AST have been reported. Monitor hepatic function tests; reduce dose or interrupt therapy if necessary. Use caution in patients with hepatic impairment; liposomal vincristine has not been studied in patients with severe hepatic impairment. In a study in a limited number of melanoma patients with moderate (Child-Pugh class B) hepatic impairment secondary to liver metastases, C_{max} and AUC were comparable to those in patients with normal hepatic function; patients with hepatic impairment received a liposomal vincristine dose of 1 mg/m^2 every 2 weeks versus 2 mg/m^2 in subjects with normal hepatic function (Bedikian 2011). Potentially significant drug-drug interactions may exist, requiring dose or frequency adjustment, additional monitoring, and/or selection of alternative therapy.

Avoid concomitant therapy with strong CYP3A4 or P-glycoprotein (P-gp) inducers or inhibitors. Use with caution in the elderly patient population; conventional vincristine may cause or exacerbate hyponatremia or syndrome of inappropriate antidiuretic hormone secretion; monitor sodium closely with therapy initiation or dosage adjustments (Beers Criteria).

Adverse Reactions

>10%:

Central nervous system: Fatigue (41%), peripheral neuropathy (39%; grades 3/4: 17%), insomnia (32%)

Gastrointestinal: Constipation (57%), nausea (52%), diarrhea (37%), decreased appetite (33%)

Hematologic & oncologic: Febrile neutropenia (38%; grades 3/4: 31%), anemia (34%; grades 3/4: 17%), neutropenia (grades 3/4: 18%), thrombocytopenia (grades 3/4: 17%)

Hepatic: Increased serum AST (grades 3/4: 6% to 11%)

Miscellaneous: Fever (43%)

1% to 10%:

Cardiovascular: Hypotension (grades 3/4: 6%), septic shock (grades 3/4: 6%)

Central nervous system: Pain (grades 3/4: 8%), mental status changes (grades 3/4: 4%), myasthenia (grades 3/4: 1%)

Gastrointestinal: Abdominal pain (grades 3/4: 8%), intestinal obstruction (grades 3/4: 6%)

Infection: Staphylococcal bacteremia (grades 3/4: 6%)

Neuromuscular & skeletal: Weakness (grades 3/4: 5%)

Respiratory: Pneumonia (grades 3/4: 8%), respiratory distress (grades 3/4: 6%), respiratory failure (grades 3/4: 5%)

Drug Interactions

Metabolism/Transport Effects Substrate of CYP3A4 (major), P-glycoprotein; **Note:** Assignment of Major/Minor substrate status based on clinically relevant drug interaction potential

Avoid Concomitant Use

Avoid concomitant use of VinCRIStine (Liposomal) with any of the following: BCG (Intravesical); Conivaptan; CYP3A4 Inducers (Strong); CYP3A4 Inhibitors (Strong); Deferiprone; Dexamethasone (Systemic); Dipyrone; Fusidic Acid (Systemic); Idelalisib; Natalizumab; P-glycoprotein/ABCB1 Inducers; P-glycoprotein/ABCB1 Inhibitors; Pimecrolimus; St John's Wort; Tacrolimus (Topical); Vaccines (Live)

Increased Effect/Toxicity

VinCRIStine (Liposomal) may increase the levels/effects of: CloZAPine; Deferiprone; Fingolimod; Leflunomide; MitoMYcin (Systemic); Natalizumab; Tofacitinib; Vaccines (Live)

The levels/effects of VinCRIStine (Liposomal) may be increased by: Aprepitant; Conivaptan; CYP3A4 Inhibitors (Moderate); CYP3A4 Inhibitors (Strong); Dasatinib; Denosumab; Dipyrone; Fosaprepitant; Fusidic Acid (Systemic); Idelalisib; Netupitant; NIFEdipine; Ocrelizumab; Palbociclib; Palifermin; P-glycoprotein/ABCB1 Inhibitors; Pimecrolimus; Promazine; Roflumilast; Stiripentol; Tacrolimus (Topical); Teniposide; Trastuzumab

Decreased Effect

VinCRIStine (Liposomal) may decrease the levels/effects of: BCG (Intravesical); Coccidioides immitis Skin Test; Lenograstim; Nivolumab; Sipuleucel-T; Tertomotide; Vaccines (Inactivated); Vaccines (Live)

The levels/effects of VinCRIStine (Liposomal) may be decreased by: Bosentan; CYP3A4 Inducers (Moderate); CYP3A4 Inducers (Strong); Dabrafenib; Deferasirox; Dexamethasone (Systemic); Echinacea; P-glycoprotein/ABCB1 Inducers; Sarilumab; Siltuximab; St John's Wort; Tocilizumab

Hazardous Drugs Handling Considerations

Hazardous agent (NIOSH 2016 [group 1]).

Use appropriate precautions for receiving, handling, administration, and disposal. Gloves (single) should be worn during receiving, unpacking, and placing in storage.

NIOSH recommends double gloving, a protective gown, ventilated engineering controls (a class II biological safety cabinet or a compounding aseptic containment isolator), and closed system transfer devices (CSTDs) for preparation. Double gloving, a gown, and (if dosage form allows) CSTDs are required during administration (NIOSH 2016).

Storage/Stability

Store intact kit (containing vincristine vial, sphingomyelin/cholesterol liposome vial, and sodium phosphate vial) at 2°C to 8°C (36°F to 46°F); do not freeze. Use appropriate precautions for handling and disposal. Once prepared and diluted in D5W or NS, liposomal vincristine is stable for no more than 12 hours at room temperature. After preparation, keep liposomal vincristine in a location away from the separate storage location recommended for intrathecal medications.

Preparation for Administration

Vincristine liposome preparation requires 60 to 90 minutes of dedicated time utilizing the manufacturer supplied kit. Do not reuse kit components with future doses.

Water bath process:

1). Outside the sterile area, fill a water bath to a depth of at least 8 cm (3.2 inches); water should be heated to and maintained at **63°C to 67°C** (145.4°F to 152.6°F) for the entire procedure (use calibrated thermometer to monitor temperature). Maintain water depth of at least 8 cm (3.2 inches) throughout process. Water bath must remain outside the sterile area.

2). In a biological safety cabinet, vent the sodium phosphate vial with a sterile venting needle (with a 0.2 micron filter or other suitable venting device). Venting needle should always be kept above liquid level. Remove 1 mL of sphingomyelin/cholesterol liposome injection and inject into the sodium phosphate vial. Withdraw 5 mL of vincristine sulfate injection and inject into the sodium phosphate vial. Remove the venting needle and gently invert the sodium phosphate vial 5 times to mix (do **not** shake). Place flotation ring on the sodium phosphate vial.

3). Confirm the water bath is maintained between **63°C to 67°C** (145.4°F to 152.6°F). Outside the sterile area, place constituted sodium phosphate vial in the water bath for 10 minutes. Record constitution start and stop time, as well as starting and ending water temperature. After 10 minutes, remove the vial (with tongs), remove flotation ring, then dry the vial, affix vial overlabel, and gently invert 5 times to mix (do **not** shake).

◀ **Block heater process (do NOT use water):**

1). Arrange the 3 heater blocks in the block heater; the block holding the constitution vial is centered between the 2 other blank heater blocks (refer to manufacturer labeling for further information). Place a calibrated thermometer in the block opening adjacent to the vial well; thermometer should remain in the block opening through preparation. Turn on block heater and set to 75°C (167°F); verify block temperature (temperature should be 75°C ± 2°C). Equilibrate at this temperature for 15 minutes; maintain block temperature throughout procedure. The flotation ring included in the kit is not required with the block heater process.

2). In a biological safety cabinet, vent the sodium phosphate vial with a sterile venting needle (with a 0.2-micron filter or other suitable venting device). Venting needle should always be kept above liquid level. Remove 1 mL of sphingomyelin/cholesterol liposome injection and inject into the sodium phosphate vial. Withdraw 5 mL of vincristine sulfate injection and inject into the sodium phosphate vial. Remove the venting needle and gently invert the sodium phosphate vial 5 times to mix (do **not** shake).

3). Confirm the block heater temperature is **73°C to 77°C** (163.4°F to 170.6°F). Outside the sterile area, place constituted sodium phosphate vial into the block heater for 18 minutes. Record constitution start and stop time, as well as starting and ending block heater temperature. After 18 minutes, remove the vial (with tongs), affix vial overlabel, and gently invert 5 times to mix (do **not** shake).

Following water or block heater process: Allow the vial to equilibrate for at least 30 minutes at room temperature (15°C to 30°C [59°F to 86°F]), but for no longer than 12 hours. Once prepared, vincristine sulfate liposome concentration is 5 mg per 31 mL (0.16 mg/mL). Return vial to biologic safety cabinet. Calculate patient's vincristine liposome dose (based on actual BSA); remove corresponding volume from 100 mL NS or D5W infusion bag. Inject vincristine liposome dose into the infusion bag (final volume of 100 mL). Do not use if a precipitate or other foreign matter is present in the vial or infusion bag. The amount contained in each vial may exceed the prescribed dose; use care with dosage and volume calculations. Discard unused portion of the vial. After preparation, keep liposomal vincristine in a location away from the separate storage location recommended for intrathecal medications.

Mechanism of Action The vincristine liposomal formulation increases the half-life, allowing for enhanced cytotoxic activity in tumor cells. The liposomal formulation of vincristine consists of vincristine encapsulated in sphingosomes, which are composed of sphingomyelin and cholesterol (Bedikian 2006).

Pharmacodynamics/Kinetics

Distribution: V_{dss}: 2.7 L (Bedikian 2006)

Metabolism: Primarily hepatic

Half-life elimination: 45 hours (urinary half-life); dependent on rate of vincristine release from sphingosome (Bedikian 2006)

Excretion: Feces (69%); urine (<8%)

Dosing

Adult & Geriatric Note: Vincristine liposomal and conventional vincristine are **NOT** interchangeable. Dosing differs between formulations; verify intended product and dose prior to preparation and administration. The liposomal vincristine dose is based on actual body surface area (BSA) and was not capped in studies (O'Brien 2009; Rodriguez 2009; Silverman, 2010).

Acute lymphoblastic leukemia (relapsed; Philadelphia chromosome-negative): IV: 2.25 mg/m^2 once every 7 days

Renal Impairment There are no dosage adjustments provided in the manufacturer's labeling (has not been studied); however, liposomal vincristine is minimally excreted by the kidney and like the conventional formulation, likely does not require dosage adjustment in renal impairment.

Hepatic Impairment

Hepatic impairment prior to treatment initiation:

Moderate impairment (Child-Pugh class B): In a study in a limited number of melanoma patients with moderate (Child-Pugh class B) hepatic impairment secondary to liver metastases, C_{max} and AUC were comparable to those in patients with normal hepatic function; patients with hepatic impairment received a dose of 1 mg/m^2 every 2 weeks versus 2 mg/m^2 in subjects with normal hepatic function (Bedikian 2011).

Severe impairment (Child-Pugh class C): There are no dosage adjustments provided in the manufacturer's labeling (has not been studied).

Hepatotoxicity during treatment: Reduce dose or interrupt treatment.

Adjustment for Toxicity

Demyelinating conditions (including Charcot-Marie-Tooth syndrome): Use is contraindicated.

Fatigue, severe: Consider dose delay, reduction, or therapy discontinuation.

Hematologic toxicity: Grade 3 or 4 neutropenia, thrombocytopenia, or anemia: Consider dose reduction or modification.

Peripheral neuropathy:

Grade 3 or persistent grade 2 toxicity: Interrupt therapy until recovery to grade 1 or 2, then reduce dose to 2 mg/m^2. If grade 3 toxicity persists or if grade 4 toxicity occurs, discontinue liposomal vincristine.

Persistent grade 2 toxicity after first dose reduction to 2 mg/m^2: Interrupt therapy for up to 7 days until recovery to grade 1, then reduce dose to 1.825 mg/m^2. If neuropathy increases to grade 3 or 4, discontinue liposomal vincristine.

Persistent grade 2 toxicity after second dose reduction to 1.825 mg/m^2: Interrupt therapy for up to 7 days until recovery to grade 1, then reduce dose to 1.5 mg/m^2. If neuropathy increases to grade 3 or 4, discontinue liposomal vincristine.

Preexisting neuropathy, severe: Assess treatment benefit versus risk.

Administration For IV administration only. **FATAL IF GIVEN INTRATHECALLY.** Liposomal vincristine should **NOT** be delivered to the patient at the same time as any medications intended for central nervous system administration.

IV: Infuse over 1 hour. Do not administer IV push or bolus; do not use with in-line filters. Do not administer with other medications. Infusion must be completed within 12 hours of preparation.

Conventional vincristine is a vesicant. Limited information is available regarding liposomal vincristine extravasation, but may cause inflammation if extravasated; avoid extravasation.

Emetic Potential Minimal (<10%)

Monitoring Parameters CBC with differential and platelets; hepatic function; signs/symptoms of peripheral neuropathy or other neurologic toxicities; sodium (in elderly patients; conventional vincristine may cause or exacerbate hyponatremia or syndrome of inappropriate antidiuretic hormone secretion); signs/symptoms of tumor lysis syndrome; symptoms of constipation; monitor infusion site for extravasation

Dosage Forms Excipient information presented when available (limited, particularly for generics); consult specific product labeling.
Suspension, Intravenous, as sulfate:
Marqibo: 5 mg/31 mL (1 ea)

Vindesine (VIN de seen)

Related Information
Index Terms DAVA; Deacetyl Vinblastine Carboxamide; Desacetyl Vinblastine Amide; DVA; Eldisine; Lilly CT-3231; VDS; Vindesine Sulfate
Pharmacologic Category Antineoplastic Agent, Antimicrotubular; Antineoplastic Agent, Vinca Alkaloid
Use Note: Not approved in the US and/or Canada
Acute lymphoblastic leukemia: Treatment of resistant childhood acute lymphoblastic leukemia
Breast cancer: Treatment of advanced breast cancer unresponsive to appropriate endocrine surgery and/or hormonal therapy (if indicated)
Chronic myeloid leukemia: Treatment of blast crisis of chronic myeloid leukemia
Melanoma, malignant: Treatment of unresponsive malignant melanoma
Labeled Contraindications Hypersensitivity to vindesine sulphate or any component of the formulation; intrathecal administration (fatal); demyelinating form of Charcot-Marie-Tooth syndrome; severe granulocytopenia (<1500/mm^3) or severe thrombocytopenia; severe bacterial infection
Pregnancy Considerations Animal reproduction studies suggest teratogenic effects. Women of childbearing potential and men with female partners of childbearing potential should use effective contraception to prevent pregnancy during treatment.
Breastfeeding Considerations Use during breastfeeding is not recommended.
Warnings/Precautions Avoid eye contamination; severe irritation or corneal ulceration may occur. **For IV use only. Intrathecal administration may be fatal.** To prevent administration errors, the World Health Organization strongly recommends dispensing vinca alkaloids diluted in a minibag (WHO 2007), **if not dispensed in a minibag, affix an auxiliary label stating "For intravenous use only - fatal if given by other routes" and also place in an overwrap labeled "Do not remove covering until moment of injection."** Vindesine should be administered by individuals experienced in administering vinca alkaloids. Vinca alkaloids should **NOT** be prepared during the preparation of any intrathecal medications. After preparation, keep vindesine in a location **away** from the separate storage location recommended for intrathecal medications. Vindesine should **NOT** be delivered to the patient at the

same time with any medications intended for central nervous system administration (Jacobson 2009).

Vindesine is a vesicant; ensure proper needle or catheter placement prior to and during infusion. Avoid extravasation. Extravasation may cause significant irritation. If extravasation occurs, discontinue immediately and initiate appropriate extravasation management, including local injection of hyaluronidase and moderate heat application to the affected area. Use a separate vein to complete administration.

Vindesine has been reported to have cross-resistance with vincristine. Neurotoxicity (eg, paresthesias, jaw pain, loss of deep tendon reflexes, foot drop, headache, and convulsions) may occur; may require dose reduction. Use with caution in patients with neuromuscular disease; neurotoxicity may be additive. Neurotoxicity associated with vindesine may typically be less severe/progressive than that seen with other vinca alkaloids. Nausea, vomiting, constipation, ileus, stomatitis, diarrhea, and/or abdominal pain may occur. Monitor for acute abdominal pain (paralytic ileus may be a risk if further doses are administered). Patients should be on a prophylactic bowel regimen to prevent obstipation. Granulocytopenia is the dose-limiting toxicity; the nadir is generally 3 to 5 days after administration and recovery is rapid and usually complete within 7 to 10 days after the dose. Monitor for infection if granulocytes are <1,000/mm^3. Thrombocytopenia may occur if administered more frequently than once weekly, although platelets are usually unaffected or may increase when vindesine is administered weekly; thrombocytopenia is more likely when platelets are already low prior to treatment. Mild anemia may occur (rare). Acute shortness of breath and severe bronchospasm have been reported with vinca alkaloids, usually when used in combination with mitomycin (may be severe in patients with preexisting pulmonary toxicity). Onset may be several minutes to hours after vinca administration and up to 2 weeks after mitomycin. Progressive dyspnea may occur. Permanently discontinue vindesine if pulmonary dysfunction occurs.

Use with caution (if at all) in patients with hepatic impairment. Dosage reduction may be necessary for significant hepatic or biliary impairment. If radiation therapy is through portals which include the liver, delay the use of vindesine until after completion of radiation therapy. Potentially significant drug-drug interactions may exist, requiring dose or frequency adjustment, additional monitoring, and/or selection of alternative therapy.

Adverse Reactions Frequency not defined.

Central nervous system: Chills, convulsions, decreased deep tendon reflex, depression, headache, malaise, neurotoxicity, peripheral neuritis, tingling sensation of hands or feet

Dermatologic: Alopecia, cellulitis (with extravasation), localized vesiculation mouth, maculopapular rash

Gastrointestinal: Abdominal pain, anorexia, constipation, diarrhea, dyspepsia, dysphagia, intestinal obstruction, nausea, paralytic ileus, perforated duodenal ulcer, stomatitis, vomiting

Hematologic & oncologic: Granulocytopenia (nadir: 3 to 5 days; recovery: 7 to 10 days), mild anemia, thrombocythemia, thrombocytopenia

Local: Injection site reaction

Neuromuscular & skeletal: Foot-drop, jaw pain, musculoskeletal pain, weakness

Respiratory: Bronchospasm, dyspnea

Miscellaneous: Fever

◀ **Drug Interactions**

Metabolism/Transport Effects Substrate of CYP3A4 (minor); **Note:** Assignment of Major/Minor substrate status based on clinically relevant drug interaction potential

Avoid Concomitant Use

Avoid concomitant use of Vindesine with any of the following: BCG (Intravesical); Deferiprone; Dipyrone; Natalizumab; Pimecrolimus; Tacrolimus (Topical); Vaccines (Live)

Increased Effect/Toxicity

Vindesine may increase the levels/effects of: CloZAPine; Deferiprone; Fingolimod; Leflunomide; MitoMYcin (Systemic); Natalizumab; Tofacitinib; Vaccines (Live)

The levels/effects of Vindesine may be increased by: CYP3A4 Inhibitors (Moderate); CYP3A4 Inhibitors (Strong); Denosumab; Dipyrone; Macrolide Antibiotics; Ocrelizumab; Palifermin; Pimecrolimus; Posaconazole; Promazine; Roflumilast; Tacrolimus (Topical); Trastuzumab; Voriconazole

Decreased Effect

Vindesine may decrease the levels/effects of: BCG (Intravesical); Coccidioides immitis Skin Test; Lenograstim; Nivolumab; Phenytoin; Sipuleucel-T; Tertomotide; Vaccines (Inactivated); Vaccines (Live)

The levels/effects of Vindesine may be decreased by: Echinacea

Hazardous Drugs Handling Considerations

Hazardous agent (meets NIOSH 2016 criteria). This medication is not on the NIOSH (2016) list; however, it meets the criteria for a hazardous drug. Drugs are classified as hazardous based on their properties; the properties of a hazardous drug include one or more of the following characteristics: carcinogenic, teratogenic (or other developmental toxicity), reproductive toxicity, organotoxic at low doses, genotoxic, and/or new agents with structural or toxicity profiles similar to existing hazardous agents.

Use appropriate precautions for receiving, handling, administration, and disposal. Gloves (single) should be worn during receiving, unpacking, and placing in storage.

NIOSH recommends double gloving, a protective gown, ventilated engineering controls (a class II biological safety cabinet or a compounding aseptic containment isolator), and closed system transfer devices (CSTDs) for preparation. Double gloving, a gown, and (if dosage form allows) CSTDs are required during administration (NIOSH 2016).

Storage/Stability Store intact vials at 2°C to 8°C (36°F to 46°F). Solutions reconstituted in preservative-free sodium chloride 0.9% (NS) may be stored for up to 24 hours refrigerated. Solutions reconstituted with NS containing 2% benzyl alcohol may be stored for up to 28 days refrigerated.

Preparation for Administration Reconstitute powder with 5 mL sodium chloride 0.9% (NS) to a concentration of 1 mg/mL. Reconstitute with NS preserved with 2% benzyl alcohol if planning to retain reconstituted vindesine beyond 24 hours. May further dilute for infusion with dextrose 5% in water or sodium chloride. Dispensing in a mini bag is preferred (WHO 2007). Do not mix with other medications.

Mechanism of Action Vindesine is a semisynthetic vinca alkaloid derived from vinblastine; works by binding to and stabilizing tubulin disrupting the formation of the mitotic spindle to arrest the cell cycle at metaphase.

Pharmacodynamics/Kinetics
Metabolism: Hepatic

Excretion: Feces; urine

Dosing

Adult & Geriatric

Breast cancer, advanced: Adults: IV: Initial: 3 mg/m^2; if no toxicity and granulocyte count is acceptable (avoid sustained granulocyte counts <2,500/mm^3), may increase dose in 0.5 mg/m^2 increments at weekly intervals (do not increase dose if granulocyte count <1,500/mm^3, platelet count <100,000/mm^3, or if acute abdominal pain is present). Usual range: 3 to 4 mg/m^2; maximum dose/week: 4 mg/m^2.

Chronic myeloid leukemia (blast crisis): Adults: IV: Initial: 3 mg/m^2; if no toxicity and granulocyte count is acceptable (avoid sustained granulocyte counts <2,500/mm^3), may increase dose in 0.5 mg/m^2 increments at weekly intervals (do not increase dose if granulocyte count <1,500/mm^3, platelet count <100,000/mm^3, or if acute abdominal pain is present). Usual range: 3 to 4 mg/m^2; maximum dose/week: 4 mg/m^2.

Melanoma, malignant, unresponsive: Adults: IV: Initial: 3 mg/m^2; if no toxicity and granulocyte count is acceptable (avoid sustained granulocyte counts <2,500/mm^3), may increase dose in 0.5 mg/m^2 increments at weekly intervals (do not increase dose if granulocyte count <1,500/mm^3, platelet count <100,000/mm^3, or if acute abdominal pain is present). Usual range: 3 to 4 mg/m^2; maximum dose/week: 4 mg/m^2.

Non-Hodgkin lymphoma, diffuse large B-cell (off-label use):

Adults ≤59 years: IV: 2 mg/m^2 on days 1 and 5 every 2 weeks (in combination with doxorubicin, cyclophosphamide, bleomycin, prednisone, and rituximab [R-ACVBP regimen]) for 4 cycles (with growth factor support), followed by sequential consolidation therapy (Molina 2014; Recher 2011).

Adults <61 years: IV: 2 mg/m^2 on days 1 and 5 every 2 weeks (in combination with doxorubicin, cyclophosphamide, bleomycin, and predni-sone [ACVBP regimen]) for 3 cycles, followed by sequential consolidation therapy (Reyes 2005).

T-cell leukemia/lymphoma (off-label use): Adults: IV: 2.4 mg/m^2 on day 15 (as part of the VCAP-AMP-VECP multi-agent chemotherapy regimen) (Tsukasaki 2007).

Pediatric

Acute lymphoblastic leukemia, resistant: Children: IV: Initial: 4 mg/m^2; if no toxicity and granulocyte count is acceptable (avoid sustained granulo-cyte counts <2,500/mm^3), may increase dose in 0.5 mg/m^2 increments at weekly intervals (do not increase dose if granulocyte count <1,500/mm^3, platelet count <100,000/mm^3, or if acute abdominal pain is present). Usual range: 4 to 5 mg/m^2.

Renal Impairment There are no dosage adjustments provided in the manufacturer's labeling.

Hepatic Impairment Dosage reductions may be necessary for significant hepatic or biliary impairment, however the manufacturer's labeling does not provide specific adjustment recommendations.

Obesity *ASCO Guidelines for appropriate chemotherapy dosing in obese adults with cancer:* Utilize patient's actual body weight (full weight) for calculation of body surface area- or weight-based dosing, particularly when the intent of therapy is curative; manage regimen-related toxicities in the same manner as for nonobese patients; if a dose reduction is utilized due to toxicity, consider resumption of full weight-based dosing with subsequent cycles, especially if cause of toxicity (eg, hepatic or renal impairment) is resolved (Griggs 2012).

Adjustment for Toxicity

Gastrointestinal toxicity (acute abdominal pain): Withhold dose. After treatment is resumed, do not increase dose above the dose where acute abdominal pain occurred.

Neurotoxicity: May require dose reduction or temporary discontinuation.

Pulmonary toxicity (progressive dyspnea requiring chronic therapy): Discontinue (do not readminister).

Administration For IV administration only. **Fatal if given intrathecally. In order to prevent inadvertent intrathecal administration, the World Health Organization (WHO) strongly recommends dispensing vinca alkaloids in a minibag (NOT in a syringe).** Vindesine should **NOT** be delivered to the patient at the same time with any medications intended for central nervous system administration.

Administer as a rapid IV push over 1 to 3 minutes into a free flowing IV line.

Vesicant; ensure proper needle or catheter placement prior to and during infusion; avoid extravasation.

Extravasation management: If extravasation occurs, stop infusion immediately and disconnect (leave cannula/needle in place); gently aspirate extravasated solution (do **NOT** flush the line); initiate hyaluronidase antidote; remove needle/cannula; apply dry warm compresses for 20 minutes 4 times a day for 1 to 2 days; elevate extremity (Perez Fidalgo 2012). Remaining portion of the vindesine dose should be infused through a separate vein.

Hyaluronidase: If needle/cannula still in place, administer 1 to 6 mL hyaluronidase (150 units/mL) into the existing IV line; the usual dose is 1 mL hyaluronidase for each 1 mL of extravasated drug (Perez Fidalgo 2012; Schulmeister 2011). If needle/cannula was removed, inject 1 to 6 mL (150 units/mL) subcutaneously in a clockwise manner using 1 mL for each 1 mL of drug extravasated (Schulmeister 2011) **or** administer 1 mL (150 units/mL) as 5 separate 0.2 mL injections (using a 25-gauge needle) subcutaneously into the extravasation site (Polovich 2009).

Vesicant/Extravasation Risk Vesicant

Monitoring Parameters CBC with differential, liver function tests; monitor infusion site, monitor for infection, neurotoxicity, or pulmonary toxicity.

Product Availability Not available in the US.

Dosage Forms Excipient information presented when available (limited, particularly for generics); consult specific product labeling.

Solution Reconstituted, Injection, as sulphate: Eldisine: 5 mg [contains mannitol]

◆ **Vindesine Sulfate** *see* Vindesine *on page 1910*

Vinorelbine (vi NOR el been)

Related Information

Management of Chemotherapy-Induced Nausea and Vomiting in Adults *on page 2253*

Management of Drug Extravasations *on page 2271*

Prevention of Chemotherapy-Induced Nausea and Vomiting in Children *on page 2310*

Safe Handling of Hazardous Drugs *on page 2379*

Brand Names: US Navelbine

Brand Names: Canada Navelbine; Vinorelbine Injection, USP; Vinorelbine Tartrate for Injection

Index Terms Dihydroxydeoxynorvinkaleukoblastine; Vinorelbine Tartrate; Vinorelbine, inj

Pharmacologic Category Antineoplastic Agent, Antimicrotubular; Antineoplastic Agent, Vinca Alkaloid

Use Treatment of non-small cell lung cancer (NSCLC)

Labeled Contraindications Pretreatment granulocyte counts <1000/mm^3

Pregnancy Considerations Animal reproduction studies have demonstrated embryotoxicity, fetotoxicity, decreased fetal weight, and delayed ossification. May cause fetal harm if administered during pregnancy. Women of childbearing potential should avoid becoming pregnant during vinorelbine treatment.

Breastfeeding Considerations It is not known if vinorelbine is excreted in breast milk. Due to the potential for serious adverse reactions in the nursing infant, breastfeeding should be discontinued during treatment.

Warnings/Precautions [U.S. Boxed Warning]: **For IV use only; intrathecal administration of other vinca alkaloids has resulted in death. If dispensed in a syringe, should be labeled "for intravenous use only - fatal if given intrathecally".** [U.S. Boxed Warning]: **Vesicant; ensure proper needle or catheter placement prior to and during infusion. Avoid extravasation. Extravasation may cause local tissue necrosis and/or thrombophlebitis.** [U.S. Boxed Warning]: **Severe granulocytopenia may occur with treatment (may lead to infection); granulocyte counts should be ≥1000 cells/mm^3 prior to treatment initiation; dosage adjustment may be required based on blood counts (monitor blood counts prior to each dose).** Granulocytopenia is a dose-limiting toxicity; nadir is generally 7-10 days after administration and recovery occurs within the following 7-14 days. Monitor closely for infections and/or fever in patients with severe granulocytopenia. Use with extreme caution in patients with compromised marrow reserve due to prior chemotherapy or radiation therapy.

Fatal cases of interstitial pulmonary changes and ARDS have been reported (with single-agent therapy (mean onset of symptoms: 1 week); promptly evaluate changes in baseline pulmonary symptoms or any new onset pulmonary symptoms (eg, dyspnea, cough, hypoxia). Acute shortness of breath and severe bronchospasm have been reported with vinca alkaloids; usually associated with the concurrent administration of mitomycin.

Vinorelbine should **NOT** be prepared during the preparation of any intrathecal medications. After preparation, keep vinorelbine in a location **away** from the separate storage location recommended for intrathecal medications. Elimination is predominantly hepatic; while there is no evidence that toxicity is enhanced in patients with elevated transaminases, use with caution in

◀ patients with severe hepatic injury or impairment; dosage modification required for elevated total bilirubin. May cause new onset or worsening of preexisting neuropathy; use with caution in patients with neuropathy; monitor for new or worsening sign/symptoms of neuropathy; dosage adjustment required. May cause severe constipation (grade 3-4), paralytic ileus, intestinal obstruction, necrosis, and/or perforation; some events were fatal. Oral vinorelbine (not available in the U.S.) is associated with a moderate antiemetic potential; antiemetics are recommended to prevent nausea/vomiting (Dupuis, 2011; Roila, 2010); IV vinorelbine has a minimal emetic potential (Dupuis, 2011; Roila, 2010). Potentially significant drug-drug interactions may exist, requiring dose or frequency adjustment, additional monitoring, and/or selection of alternative therapy. May have radiosensitizing effects with prior or concurrent radiation therapy; radiation recall reactions may occur in patients who have received prior radiation therapy. Avoid eye contamination (exposure may cause severe irritation). **[U.S. Boxed Warning]: Should be administered under the supervision of an experienced cancer chemotherapy physician.**

Adverse Reactions Reported with single-agent therapy.

>10%:

Central nervous system: Fatigue (27%), peripheral neuropathy (25%; grade 3: 1%; grade 4: <1%)

Dermatologic: Alopecia (12% to 30%)

Gastrointestinal: Nausea (31% to 44%; grade 3: 1% to 2%), constipation (35%; grade 3: 3%), vomiting (20% to 31%; grade 3: 1% to 2%), diarrhea (12% to 17%)

Hematologic & oncologic: Leukopenia (83% to 92%; grade 4: 6% to 15%), granulocytopenia (90%; grade 4: 36%; nadir: 7 to 10 days; recovery 14 to 21 days), neutropenia (85%; grade 4: 28%), anemia (83%; grades 3/4: 9%)

Hepatic: Increased serum AST (67%; grade 3: 5%; grade 4: 1%), increased serum bilirubin (total bilirubin: 5% to 13%; grade 3: 4%; grade 4: 3%)

Local: Injection site reaction (22% to 28%; includes erythema at injection site, vein discoloration), pain at injection site (16%)

Neuromuscular & skeletal: Weakness (36%)

Renal: Increased serum creatinine (13%)

1% to 10%:

Cardiovascular: Localized phlebitis (7% to 10%), chest pain (5%)

Central nervous system: Decreased deep tendon reflex (<5%)

Dermatologic: Skin rash (<5%)

Gastrointestinal: Paralytic ileus (1%)

Hematologic & oncologic: Febrile neutropenia (≤8%; grade 4: ≤4%), thrombocytopenia (3% to 5%; grades 3/4: 1%)

Infection: Sepsis (≤8%; grade 4: ≤4%)

Neuromuscular & skeletal: Arthralgia (<5%), myalgia (<5%), jaw pain (<5%)

Otic: Ototoxicity (≤1%)

Respiratory: Dyspnea (7%)

<1%, postmarketing, and/or case reports: Abdominal pain, anaphylaxis, angioedema, back pain, deep vein thrombosis, dysphagia, esophagitis, flushing, headache, hemolytic-uremic syndrome, hemorrhagic cystitis, hypersensitivity reaction, hypertension, hyponatremia, hypotension, intestinal necrosis, intestinal obstruction, intestinal perforation, interstitial pulmonary disease, ischemic heart disease, localized rash, mucositis, myasthenia, myocardial infarction (rare), pancreatitis, pneumonia, pruritus, pulmonary edema, pulmonary embolism, radiation recall phenomenon (dermatitis,

esophagitis), skin blister, SIADH (syndrome of inappropriate antidiuretic hormone secretion), tachycardia, thromboembolism, thrombotic thrombocytopenic purpura, tumor pain, unsteady gait, urticaria, urticaria at injection site, vasodilatation

Drug Interactions

Metabolism/Transport Effects Substrate of CYP2D6 (minor), CYP3A4 (major); **Note:** Assignment of Major/Minor substrate status based on clinically relevant drug interaction potential

Avoid Concomitant Use

Avoid concomitant use of Vinorelbine with any of the following: BCG (Intravesical); Conivaptan; Deferiprone; Dipyrone; Fusidic Acid (Systemic); Idelalisib; Natalizumab; Pimecrolimus; Tacrolimus (Topical); Vaccines (Live)

Increased Effect/Toxicity

Vinorelbine may increase the levels/effects of: CloZAPine; Deferiprone; Fingolimod; Leflunomide; MitoMYcin (Systemic); Natalizumab; Tofacitinib; Vaccines (Live)

The levels/effects of Vinorelbine may be increased by: Aprepitant; Ceritinib; CISplatin; Conivaptan; CYP3A4 Inhibitors (Strong); Dasatinib; Denosumab; Dipyrone; Fosaprepitant; Fusidic Acid (Systemic); Gefitinib; Idelalisib; Macrolide Antibiotics; MiFEPRIStone; Netupitant; Ocrelizumab; PACLitaxel (Conventional); PACLitaxel (Protein Bound); Palbociclib; Palifermin; Pimecrolimus; Posaconazole; Promazine; Roflumilast; Simeprevir; Stiripentol; Tacrolimus (Topical); Trastuzumab; Voriconazole

Decreased Effect

Vinorelbine may decrease the levels/effects of: BCG (Intravesical); Coccidioides immitis Skin Test; Lenograstim; Nivolumab; Sipuleucel-T; Tertomotide; Vaccines (Inactivated); Vaccines (Live)

The levels/effects of Vinorelbine may be decreased by: Echinacea

Hazardous Drugs Handling Considerations

Hazardous agent (NIOSH 2016 [group 1]).

Use appropriate precautions for receiving, handling, administration, and disposal. Gloves (single) should be worn during receiving, unpacking, and placing in storage.

NIOSH recommends double gloving, a protective gown, ventilated engineering controls (a class II biological safety cabinet or a compounding aseptic containment isolator), and closed system transfer devices (CSTDs) for preparation. Double gloving, a gown, and (if dosage form allows) CSTDs are required during administration (NIOSH 2016).

Storage/Stability Store intact vials refrigerated at 2°C to 8°C (36°F to 46°F); do not freeze. Protect from light. Intact vials are stable at room temperature of 25°C (77°F) for up to 72 hours. Solutions diluted for infusion in polypropylene syringes (D5W or NS) or polyvinyl chloride bags (D5W, NS, 1/2NS, D51/2NS, LR, or Ringer's) are stable for 24 hours at 5°C to 30°C (41°F to 86°F). After preparation, keep vinorelbine in a location **away** from the separate storage location recommended for intrathecal medications.

Preparation for Administration Dilute in D5W or NS to a final concentration of 1.5-3 mg/mL (for syringe) or D5W, NS, 1/2NS, D51/2NS, LR, or Ringer's to a final concentration of 0.5 to 2 mg/mL (for IV bag). Vinorelbine should **NOT** be prepared during the preparation of any intrathecal medications.

◄ **Mechanism of Action** Semisynthetic vinca alkaloid which binds to tubulin and inhibits microtubule formation, therefore, arresting the cell at metaphase by disrupting the formation of the mitotic spindle; it is specific for the M and S phases. Vinorelbine may also interfere with nucleic acid and protein synthesis by blocking glutamic acid utilization.

Pharmacodynamics/Kinetics

Distribution: V_d: binds extensively to human platelets and lymphocytes (80% to 91%)

Children and Adolescents 2 to 17 years: 21.1 ± 12.2 L/kg (Johansen 2006)

Adults: 25 to 40 L/kg

Protein binding: 80% to 91%

Metabolism: Extensively hepatic, via CYP3A4, to two metabolites, deacetylvinorelbine (active) and vinorelbine N-oxide

Half-life elimination: Triphasic:

Children and Adolescents 2 to 17 years: Terminal: 16.5 ± 9.7 hours (Johansen 2006)

Adults: Terminal: 28 to 44 hours

Excretion: Feces (46%); urine (18%, 10% to 12% as unchanged drug)

Dosing

Adult & Geriatric

Non-small cell lung cancer (NSCLC): IV:

Single-agent therapy: 30 mg/m² every 7 days until disease progression or unacceptable toxicity

Combination therapy: 25-30 mg/m² every 7 days (in combination with cisplatin)

Off-label dosing: 25 mg/m² days 1 and 8 every 21 days (in combination with cisplatin and cetuximab) for up to 6 cycles (Pirker, 2009) **or** 25-30 mg/m² days 1, 8, and 15 every 28 days (in combination with gemcitabine) for 6 cycles **or** until disease progression or unacceptable toxicity (Herbst, 2002; Greco, 2007)

Breast cancer, metastatic (off-label use): IV: 25 mg/m² every 7 days (as a single agent) until disease progression or unacceptable toxicity (Zelek, 2001) **or** 30 mg/m² every 7 days (as a single agent); after 13 weeks, may administer every 14 days for patient convenience, continue until disease progression or unacceptable toxicity (Vogel, 1999) **or** 25 mg/m² every 7 days (in combination with trastuzumab) until disease progression or unacceptable toxicity (Burstein, 2001; Burstein 2007) **or** 30 or 35 mg/m² days 1 and 8 every 21 days (in combination with trastuzumab) until disease progression or unacceptable toxicity (Andersson, 2011)

Cervical cancer (off-label use): IV: 30 mg/m² days 1 and 8 of a of a 21-day treatment cycle (Muggia, 2004; Muggia, 2005)

Hodgkin lymphoma, relapsed or refractory (off-label use): IV:

GVD regimen: 15 mg/m² (post-transplant patients) or 20 mg/m² (transplant-naïve patients) on days 1 and 8 of a 21-day cycle (in combination with gemcitabine and doxorubicin liposomal) for 2 to 6 cycles (Bartlett, 2007)

IGEV regimen: 20 mg/m² on day 1 of a 21-day cycle (in combination with ifosfamide, mesna, gemcitabine, and prednisolone) for 4 cycles (Santoro, 2007)

Malignant pleural mesothelioma (off-label use): IV: 30 mg/m^2 (maximum dose: 60 mg) every 7 days per 6-week treatment cycle, continue until disease progression (Stebbing, 2009) **or** 30 mg/m^2 (maximum dose: 60 mg) every 7 days for 6 weeks, off 2 weeks, then repeat cycle (Muers, 2008)

Ovarian cancer, relapsed (off-label use): IV: 25 mg/m^2 every 7 days (Bajetta, 1996) **or** 30 mg/m^2 days 1 and 8 of a 21-day treatment cycle (Rothenberg, 2004) until disease progression or unacceptable toxicity

Salivary gland cancer, recurrent (off-label use): IV: 25 mg/m^2 on days 1 and 8 of a 21-day cycle (in combination with cisplatin) for a minimum of 3 cycles and for up to 6 cycles (Airoldi, 2001) **or** 30 mg/m^2 every 7 days (monotherapy) for a minimum of 9 weeks and for up to 6 cycles (Airoldi, 2001)

Small cell lung cancer, refractory (off-label use): IV: 25 or 30 mg/m^2 every 7 days until disease progression or unacceptable toxicity (Furuse, 1996; Jessem, 1993)

Soft tissue sarcoma, advanced (off-label use): IV: 25 mg/m^2 days 1 and 8 of a 21-day treatment cycle (in combination with gemcitabine) until disease progression or unacceptable toxicity (Dileo, 2007)

Renal Impairment

Renal insufficiency: No dosage adjustment necessary.

Hemodialysis: Initial: IV: Reduce dose to 20 mg/m^2/week; administer either after dialysis (on dialysis days) or on nondialysis days (Janus, 2010)

Hepatic Impairment Note: In patients with concurrent hematologic toxicity and hepatic impairment, administer the lower of the doses determined from the adjustment recommendations.

Administer with caution in patients with hepatic insufficiency. In patients who develop hyperbilirubinemia during treatment with vinorelbine, the dose should be adjusted for total bilirubin as follows:

Serum bilirubin ≤2 mg/dL: Administer 100% of dose

Serum bilirubin 2.1-3 mg/dL: Administer 50% of dose (Ecklund, 2005; Floyd, 2006; Superfin, 2006)

Serum bilirubin >3 mg/dL: Administer 25% of dose (Ecklund, 2005; Floyd, 2006; Superfin, 2006)

Patients (breast cancer) with extensive liver metastases (>75% of liver volume): Administer 50% of dose (Ecklund, 2005; Superfin, 2006)

Obesity ASCO Guidelines for appropriate chemotherapy dosing in obese adults with cancer: Utilize patient's actual body weight (full weight) for calculation of body surface area- or weight-based dosing, particularly when the intent of therapy is curative; manage regimen-related toxicities in the same manner as for nonobese patients; if a dose reduction is utilized due to toxicity, consider resumption of full weight-based dosing with subsequent cycles, especially if cause of toxicity (eg, hepatic or renal impairment) is resolved (Griggs, 2012).

Adjustment for Toxicity Note: In patients with concurrent hematologic toxicity and hepatic impairment, administer the lower of the doses determined from the adjustment recommendations.

Dosage adjustment in hematological toxicity (based on granulocyte counts):

Granulocytes ≥1500 cells/mm^3 on day of treatment: Administer 100% of starting dose.

Granulocytes 1000-1499 cells/mm^3 on day of treatment: Administer 50% of starting dose.

Granulocytes <1000 cells/mm³ on day of treatment: Do not administer. Repeat granulocyte count in 1 week. If 3 consecutive doses are held because granulocyte count is <1000 cells/mm³, discontinue vinorelbine.

Adjustment: For patients who, during treatment, have experienced fever or sepsis while granulocytopenic or had 2 consecutive weekly doses held due to granulocytopenia, subsequent doses of vinorelbine should be:

75% of starting dose for granulocytes ≥1500 cells/mm³

37.5% of starting dose for granulocytes 1000-1499 cells/mm³

Dosage adjustment for neurotoxicity: Neurotoxicity ≥ grade 2: Discontinue treatment

Dosage adjustment for other adverse events: Severe adverse events: Reduce dose or discontinue treatment

Combination Regimens

Breast cancer: Trastuzumab-Vinorelbine (Breast) on page 2217

Cervical cancer: Cisplatin-Vinorelbine (Cervical Cancer) on page 2063

Head and neck cancer: Gemcitabine-Vinorelbine (Head and Neck) on page 2140

Lung cancer (non-small cell):

Cetuximab-Cisplatin-Vinorelbine (NSCLC) on page 2031

Cisplatin-Vinorelbine (Adjuvant NSCLC) on page 2062

Cisplatin-Vinorelbine (Metastatic NSCLC) on page 2063

Gemcitabine-Vinorelbine (NSCLC) on page 2140

Lymphoma, Hodgkin:

GVD (Hodgkin) on page 2143

IGEV (Hodgkin) on page 2155

Soft tissue sarcoma: Gemcitabine-Vinorelbine (Soft Tissue Sarcoma) on page 2141

Administration For IV use only; **FATAL IF GIVEN INTRATHECALLY.** Administer as a direct intravenous push or rapid bolus, over 6-10 minutes (up to 30 minutes). Longer infusions may increase the risk of pain and phlebitis. Intravenous doses should be followed by at least 75-125 mL of saline or D5W to reduce the incidence of phlebitis and inflammation.

Vesicant; ensure proper needle or catheter position prior to administration. Avoid extravasation.

Extravasation management: If extravasation occurs, stop infusion immediately and disconnect (leave cannula/needle in place); gently aspirate extravasated solution (do **NOT** flush the line); initiate hyaluronidase antidote; remove needle/cannula; apply dry warm compresses for 20 minutes 4 times a day for 1-2 days; elevate extremity (Perez Fidalgo, 2012). Remaining portion of the vinorelbine dose should be infused through a separate vein.

Hyaluronidase: If needle/cannula still in place, administer 1-6 mL hyaluronidase (150 units/mL) into the existing IV line; the usual dose is 1 mL hyaluronidase for each 1 mL of extravasated drug (Perez Fidalgo, 2012; Schulmeister, 2011). If needle/cannula was removed, inject 1-6 mL (150 units/mL) subcutaneously in a clockwise manner using 1mL for each 1 mL of drug extravasated (Schulmeister, 2011) **or** administer 1 mL (150 units/mL) as 5 separate 0.2 mL injections (using a 25-gauge needle) subcutaneously into the extravasation site (Polovich, 2009).

Vesicant/Extravasation Risk Vesicant.

Emetic Potential
Children and Adults:
IV: Minimal (<10%)
Oral (not available in the U.S.): Moderate (30% to 90%)

Monitoring Parameters CBC with differential and platelet count (prior to each dose, and after treatment); hepatic function tests; monitor for new-onset pulmonary symptoms (or worsening from baseline); monitor for neuropathy (new or worsening symptoms; monitor infusion site; monitor for signs symptoms of constipation/ileus

Dosage Forms Excipient information presented when available (limited, particularly for generics); consult specific product labeling.
Solution, Intravenous:
Navelbine: 10 mg/mL (1 mL); 50 mg/5 mL (5 mL)
Generic: 10 mg/mL (1 mL); 50 mg/5 mL (5 mL)
Solution, Intravenous [preservative free]:
Generic: 10 mg/mL (1 mL); 50 mg/5 mL (5 mL)

♦ **Vinorelbine, inj** see Vinorelbine on page 1915
♦ **Vinorelbine Injection, USP (Can)** see Vinorelbine on page 1915
♦ **Vinorelbine Tartrate** see Vinorelbine on page 1915
♦ **Vinorelbine Tartrate for Injection (Can)** see Vinorelbine on page 1915

Vismodegib (vis moe DEG ib)

Related Information
Common Toxicity Criteria on page 2242
Management of Chemotherapy-Induced Nausea and Vomiting in Adults on page 2253
Safe Handling of Hazardous Drugs on page 2379

Brand Names: US Erivedge
Brand Names: Canada Erivedge
Index Terms GDC-0449; Hedgehog Antagonist GDC-0449
Pharmacologic Category Antineoplastic Agent, Hedgehog Pathway Inhibitor

Use Basal cell carcinoma, metastatic or locally advanced: Treatment of metastatic basal cell carcinoma, or locally-advanced basal cell carcinoma that has recurred following surgery or in patients who are not candidates for surgery, and not candidates for radiation therapy

Labeled Contraindications
There are no contraindications listed in the manufacturer's US labeling.
Canadian labeling: Hypersensitivity to vismodegib or any component of the formulation; pregnancy or females at risk of becoming pregnant; breastfeeding; male patients or female patients of childbearing potential who do not comply with the Erivedge Pregnancy Prevention Program; children and adolescents <18 years of age.

Pregnancy Considerations [US Boxed Warning]: May result in severe birth defects or embryo-fetal death. Teratogenic effects (severe midline defects, missing digits, and other irreversible malformations), embryotoxic, and fetotoxic events were observed in animal reproduction studies when administered in doses less than the normal human dose. Based on its mechanism of action adverse effects on pregnancy would be expected. **[US Boxed Warning]: Verify pregnancy status (in females of reproductive potential) within 7 days prior to initiating treatment and advise patients** ▶

(female and male) of the risk of birth defects, the need for contraception and risk of exposure through semen and to use condoms with a pregnant partner or a female partner of childbearing potential. In females of childbearing potential, obtain pregnancy test within 7 days prior to treatment initiation; after the negative pregnancy test, initiate highly effective contraception prior to the first vismodegib dose and continue during treatment and for 24 months after the final dose. During treatment (including treatment interruptions) and for 3 months after treatment, male patients should not donate sperm and should use condoms with spermicide (even after vasectomy) if their partner is of childbearing potential.

Women exposed to vismodegib during pregnancy (directly or via seminal fluid) are encouraged to participate in the Erivedge Pregnancy Pharmacovigilance program by contacting the Genentech Adverse Event Line (1-888-835-2555). Pregnancies occurring during or within 7 months after treatment should be reported to the Genentech Adverse Event Line.

In Canada, vismodegib is available only through a controlled distribution program (Erivedge Pregnancy Prevention Program). Female and male patients of reproductive potential must be registered with the program and comply with all requirements. Females of childbearing potential should use 2 simultaneous forms of effective contraception beginning at least 4 weeks prior to treatment initiation, during treatment (including treatment interruptions), and for 24 months after discontinuation. Pregnancy testing should be performed within 7 days prior to treatment initiation, monthly during treatment (including treatment interruptions), and for 24 months after discontinuation. For females of child bearing potential, a new prescription is required each month to allow for monthly pregnancy testing. During treatment (including treatment interruptions) and for 2 months after treatment, male patients should not donate sperm and should use condoms with spermicide (even after vasectomy) if their partner is of childbearing potential. Any suspected exposure (directly or via seminal fluid) during pregnancy should be immediately reported to the Erivedge Pregnancy Prevention Program at 1-888-748-8926.

Breastfeeding Considerations It is not known if vismodegib is excreted in breast milk. Due to the potential for serious adverse reactions in the breast-feeding infant, breastfeeding is not recommended by the manufacturer during therapy and for 24 months after the last vismodegib dose.

Warnings/Precautions [US Boxed Warnings]: May result in severe birth defects or embryo-fetal death. Teratogenic effects (severe midline defects, missing digits, and other irreversible malformations), embryotoxic, and fetotoxic events were observed in animal reproduction studies. Verify pregnancy status (in females of reproductive potential) within 7 days prior to initiating treatment and advise patients (female and male) of the risk of birth defects, the need for contraception and risk of exposure through semen and to use condoms with a pregnant partner or a female partner of childbearing potential. Amenorrhea was observed in women of reproductive potential; it is unknown if this is reversible.

Nausea, vomiting, diarrhea, constipation, abdominal pain, and decreased appetite may occur (usually grade 1 or 2). Advise patients not to donate blood or blood products during vismodegib treatment and for at least 24 months after the last vismodegib dose. Vismodegib is present in semen, although the amount of drug in semen that may cause embryotoxicity and/or fetotoxicity is not known. Advise patients not to donate sperm during vismodegib treatment and for 3 months after the last vismodegib dose. Premature fusion of the epiphyses has been reported in pediatric patients exposed to vismodegib; the fusion progressed after vismodegib discontinuation in some cases. In a study of vismodegib in patients with basal cell nevus syndrome (not an approved use), with discontinuation of vismodegib treatment, taste alteration and muscle cramps abated within 1 month, and scalp and body hair began to regrow within 3 months (Tang 2012). Potentially significant drug-drug interactions may exist, requiring dose or frequency adjustment, additional monitoring, and/or selection of alternative therapy.

Adverse Reactions

>10%:

Central nervous system: Fatigue (40%)

Dermatologic: Alopecia (64%)

Endocrine & metabolic: Amenorrhea (≤30%)

Gastrointestinal: Dysgeusia (55%), weight loss (45%), nausea (30%), diarrhea (29%), decreased appetite (25%), constipation (21%), vomiting (14%), ageusia (11%)

Neuromuscular & skeletal: Muscle spasm (72%), arthralgia (16%)

1% to 10%:

Endocrine & metabolic: Hypokalemia, hyponatremia

Neuromuscular & skeletal: Increased creatine phosphokinase

Renal: Azotemia

Drug Interactions

Metabolism/Transport Effects Substrate of CYP2C9 (minor), CYP3A4 (minor), P-glycoprotein; **Note:** Assignment of Major/Minor substrate status based on clinically relevant drug interaction potential; **Inhibits** BCRP, CYP2C9 (weak)

Avoid Concomitant Use There are no known interactions where it is recommended to avoid concomitant use.

Increased Effect/Toxicity There are no known significant interactions involving an increase in effect.

Decreased Effect There are no known significant interactions involving a decrease in effect.

Hazardous Drugs Handling Considerations

Hazardous agent (NIOSH 2016 [group 1]).

Use appropriate precautions for receiving, handling, administration, and disposal. Gloves (single) should be worn during receiving, unpacking, and placing in storage. NIOSH recommends single gloving for administration of intact tablets or capsules (NIOSH 2016).

Storage/Stability Store at 20°C to 25°C (68°F to 77°F); excursions permitted to 15°C to 30°C (59°F to 86°F). Keep bottle closed tightly to protect from moisture.

Mechanism of Action Basal cell cancer is associated with mutations in Hedgehog pathway components. Hedgehog regulates cell growth and differentiation in embryogenesis; while generally not active in adult tissue, Hedgehog mutations associated with basal cell cancer can activate the pathway resulting in unrestricted proliferation of skin basal cells. Vismodegib is a selective Hedgehog pathway inhibitor which binds to and inhibits Smoothened homologue (SMO), the transmembrane protein involved in Hedgehog signal transduction.

Pharmacodynamics/Kinetics

Distribution: V_d: 16.4 to 26.6 L

◀ Males: In a small pharmacokinetic study, the average vismodegib concentration in semen was 6.5% of the average steady state plasma concentration on day 8

Protein binding: >99%; primarily to serum albumin and alpha₁ acid glycoprotein (AAG)

Metabolism: Metabolized by oxidation, glucuronidation, and pyridine ring cleavage, although >98% of circulating components are as the parent drug

Bioavailability: ~32%

Half-life, elimination: Continuous daily dosing: ~4 days; Single dose: ~12 days

Time to peak: ~2.4 days (Graham 2011)

Excretion: Feces (82%); urine (4%)

Dosing

Adult

Basal cell carcinoma, metastatic or locally advanced: Oral: 150 mg once daily until disease progression or unacceptable toxicity.

Missed doses: If a dose is missed, do not make up; resume dosing with the next scheduled dose.

Renal Impairment No dosage adjustment necessary.

Hepatic Impairment No dosage adjustment necessary.

Adjustment for Toxicity In clinical trials, no dosage reductions were allowed for toxicities, however, treatment interruptions up to 4 to 8 weeks were allowed for toxicity recovery (Basset-Seguin 2015; Sekulic 2012).

Administration Oral: May be taken with or without food. Swallow capsules whole; do not open or crush.

Emetic Potential Minimal (<10%)

Monitoring Parameters Pregnancy test within 1 week prior to treatment initiation.

Prescribing and Access Restrictions

US: Available at specialty pharmacies through the Erivedge Access Solutions program. Further information may be obtained from the manufacturer, Genentech, at 1-888-249-4918, or at www.ErivedgeAccessSolutions.com

Canada: Available through a controlled distribution program called Erivedge Pregnancy Prevention Program (EPPP). Registration with the program is required for participating prescribers and pharmacies. Patients must also be registered with the program and meet all necessary requirements to receive vismodegib. Consult product monograph for detailed information regarding program requirements. Further information may also be obtained at 1-888-748-8926 or at www.erivedge.ca.

Medication Guide Available Yes

Dosage Forms Excipient information presented when available (limited, particularly for generics); consult specific product labeling.

Capsule, Oral:

Erivedge: 150 mg

von Willebrand Factor (Recombinant)
(von WILL le brand FAK tor ree KOM be nant)
Brand Names: US Vonvendi
Index Terms rVWF
Pharmacologic Category Antihemophilic Agent; Blood Product Derivative
Use von Willebrand disease: Treatment (on demand) and control of bleeding episodes in adults with von Willebrand disease (VWD).
Dosing
Adult & Geriatric
von Willebrand disease: IV: **Note:** If baseline factor VIII coagulation (FVIII: C) activity is <40% or is unknown, administer factor VIII (recombinant) with the first infusion of VWF (recombinant). If factor VIII (recombinant) is required to control bleeding, the VWF (recombinant) dose should be ≥30% than the factor VIII (recombinant) dose (VWF [recombinant] to factor VIII [recombinant] ratio of 1.3:1). The initial dose of VWF (recombinant) should achieve >60% of VWF levels (based on VWF:RCo >0.6 units/mL, and a factor VIII (recombinant) infusion should achieve factor VIII levels >40% (FVIII:C >0.4 units/mL). If an immediate rise in FVIII:C is not necessary or if baseline FVIII:C is sufficient to ensure hemostasis, VWF (recombinant) may be administered without factor VIII (recombinant).
Minor hemorrhage (eg, epistaxis [readily managed], menorrhagia, oral bleeding): Initial: 40 to 50 units/kg; maintenance dose: 40 to 50 units/kg every 8 to 24 hours (as clinically required); adjust dose based on location and extent of bleeding.
Major hemorrhage (eg, CNS trauma, epistaxis [severe or refractory], GI bleeding, hemarthrosis, menorrhagia, traumatic hemorrhage): Initial: 50 to 80 units/kg; maintenance dose: 40 to 60 units/kg every 8 to 24 hours for ~2 to 3 days (as clinically required); adjust dose based on location and extent of bleeding. Maintain trough levels of VWF:RCo >50%.
Renal Impairment There are no dosage adjustments provided in the manufacturer's labeling.
Hepatic Impairment There are no dosage adjustments provided in the manufacturer's labeling.
Additional Information Complete prescribing information should be consulted for additional detail.
Dosage Forms Excipient information presented when available (limited, particularly for generics); consult specific product labeling.
Solution Reconstituted, Intravenous [preservative free]:
Vonvendi: 650 units (1 ea); 1300 units (1 ea) [contains mouse (murine) and/or hamster protein, polysorbate 80]

◆ **Voraxaze** see Glucarpidase *on page 883*

Voriconazole (vor i KOE na zole)
Brand Names: US Vfend; Vfend IV
Brand Names: Canada Apo-Voriconazole; Sandoz-Voriconazole; Teva-Voriconazole; VFEND; VFEND For Injection; Voriconazole For Injection
Index Terms UK109496
Pharmacologic Category Antifungal Agent, Oral; Antifungal Agent, Parenteral
Use Treatment of fungal infections: Treatment of invasive aspergillosis; treatment of esophageal candidiasis; treatment of candidemia (in non-neutropenic patients); treatment of disseminated *Candida* infections of the skin

◄ and abdomen, kidney, bladder wall, and wounds; treatment of serious fungal infections caused by *Scedosporium apiospermum* and *Fusarium* spp. (including *Fusarium solani*) in patients intolerant of, or refractory to, other therapy

Hazardous Drugs Handling Considerations

Hazardous agent (NIOSH 2016 [group 3]).

Use appropriate precautions for receiving, handling, administration, and disposal. Gloves (single) should be worn during receiving, unpacking, and placing in storage.

NIOSH recommends single gloving for administration of intact tablets or capsules. NIOSH recommends double gloving, a protective gown, and (if there is a potential for vomit or spit up) eye/face protection for administration of an oral liquid/feeding tube administration. For IV preparation, double gloves, a protective gown, ventilated engineering controls (a class II biological safety cabinet or a compounding aseptic containment isolator), and closed system transfer devices (CSTDs) are recommended. Double gloving, a gown, and (if dosage form allows) CSTDs are required during IV administration (NIOSH 2016).

Dosing

Adult & Geriatric

Aspergillosis, invasive, including disseminated and extrapulmonary infection; treatment:

IV:

Initial: 6 mg/kg every 12 hours for 2 doses

Maintenance dose: 4 mg/kg every 12 hours

Oral: Maintenance dose:

Manufacturer's labeling: **Note:** If patient has inadequate clinical response, titrate in 50 mg/dose increments for weight <40 kg and 100 mg/dose increments for weight ≥40 kg.

Weight <40 kg: 100 mg every 12 hours

Weight ≥40 kg: 200 mg every 12 hours

Alternate recommendations: Oral: 200 to 300 mg every 12 hours **or** weight-based dosing (3 to 4 mg/kg) every 12 hours. **Note:** In patients able to tolerate oral administration, may consider oral in place of IV; however, IV administration is recommended in seriously ill patients (IDSA [Patterson 2016]).

Duration of therapy: Minimum of 6 to 12 weeks, although duration is highly dependent on degree/duration of immunosuppression, disease site, and evidence of disease improvement (IDSA [Patterson 2016]).

Aspergillosis, invasive (prophylaxis during prolonged neutropenia) (alternative therapy) (off-label use): Oral: 200 mg twice daily (IDSA [Patterson 2016])

Aspergillosis, ocular (off-label use):

Endophthalmitis: Intravitreal: 100 mcg/0.1 mL of an extemporaneously prepared solution administered intravitreally (need for a repeat dose is at physician discretion); concomitant systemic (IV or oral) voriconazole therapy is also recommended (Hariprasad 2008; Hoenigl 2013; Kramer 2006; IDSA [Patterson 2016]; Riddell 2011).

Keratitis: Ophthalmic: Dosing may vary; the following dosing regimen has been used in trials: 1 drop of an extemporaneously prepared 1% ophthalmic solution applied topically to the cornea of the affected eye every 1 hour while awake for 1 week, then every 2 hours while awake for 2 weeks;

further continuation was at physician discretion (IDSA [Patterson 2016]; Prajna 2010; Prajna 2013)

Candidemia in non-neutropenic patients and disseminated *Candida* infections in skin, and infections in abdomen, kidney, bladder wall and wounds: Treatment should continue for a minimum of 14 days following resolution of symptoms or following last positive culture, whichever is longer.

IV:

Initial: 6 mg/kg every 12 hours for 2 doses

Maintenance: 3 to 4 mg/kg every 12 hours

Oral:

Manufacturer's labeling: Maintenance dose: **Note:** If patient has inadequate clinical response, titrate in 50 mg/dose increments for weight <40 kg and 100 mg/dose increments for weight ≥40 kg

Weight <40 kg: 100 mg every 12 hours

Weight ≥40 kg: 200 mg every 12 hours

Alternate recommendations (IDSA [Pappas 2016]): Candidemia in non-neutropenic patients:

Initial therapy: 400 mg (6 mg/kg) IV every 12 hours for 2 doses, followed by 200 mg (3 mg/kg) IV or orally every 12 hours. **Note:** Voriconazole is considered alternative therapy and offers little advantage over fluconazole as first-line therapy of candidemia.

Step-down therapy (after patient has responded to initial therapy): Oral: Isolates of C. glabrata (voriconazole-susceptible isolates): 200 to 300 mg (3 to 4 mg/kg) twice daily

Isolates of C. krusei (selected cases): 200 mg every 12 hours

Duration: Continue for 14 days **after** first negative blood culture and resolution of signs/symptoms; step-down therapy to voriconazole (eg, after 5 to 7 days in nonneutropenic patients) is recommended only in select clinically stable patients with certain voriconazole-susceptible isolates and negative repeat cultures.

Candidiasis, endophthalmitis (with or without vitritis) (off-label use) (IDSA [Pappas 2016]): Voriconazole-susceptible isolates:

Systemic therapy: Loading dose: 400 mg (6 mg/kg) IV twice daily for 2 doses, then 300 mg (4 mg/kg) IV or orally twice daily for at least 4 to 6 weeks until examination indicates resolution; for patients with vitritis or with macular involvement (with or without vitritis), an intravitreal injection of voriconazole or amphotericin B deoxycholate is also recommended.

Intravitreal therapy: Patients with vitritis or with macular involvement (with or without vitritis): Intravitreal: 100 mcg of an extemporaneously prepared solution in 0.1 mL sterile water or NS; concomitant antifungal systemic therapy is also recommended.

Candidiasis, esophageal:

US labeling: Oral: Treatment should continue for a minimum of 14 days, and for at least 7 days following resolution of symptoms. **Note:** If patient has inadequate clinical response, titrate in 50 mg/dose increments for weight <40 kg and 100 mg/dose increments for weight ≥40 kg

Weight <40 kg: 100 mg every 12 hours; maximum: 300 mg daily

Weight ≥40 kg: 200 mg every 12 hours; maximum: 600 mg daily

Alternative dosing:

Fluconazole-refractory: Oral, IV (off-label route): 200 mg (3 mg/kg) twice daily for 14 to 21 days (IDSA [Pappas 2016])

HIV-positive patients (alternative to preferred therapy): Oral, IV (off-label route): 200 mg twice daily for 14 to 21 days (HHS [OI adult 2015])

◀ **Dosage adjustment in patients with inadequate response:**
IV: Maintenance dose may be increased from 3 mg/kg every 12 hours to 4 mg/kg every 12 hours, depending upon condition.

Oral: Maintenance dose may be increased from 200 mg every 12 hours to 300 mg every 12 hours in patients weighing ≥40 kg (or to 150 mg every 12 hours in patients <40 kg), depending upon condition.

Dosage adjustment in patients unable to tolerate treatment:
IV: Maintenance dose may be reduced from 4 mg/kg every 12 hours to 3 mg/kg every 12 hours, depending upon condition.

Oral: Maintenance dose may be reduced in 50 mg decrements to a minimum dosage of 200 mg every 12 hours in patients weighing ≥40 kg (or to 100 mg every 12 hours in patients <40 kg), depending upon condition.

Dosage adjustment in patients receiving concomitant CYP450 enzyme inducers or substrates:
Efavirenz: Oral: Increase maintenance dose of voriconazole to 400 mg every 12 hours and reduce efavirenz dose to 300 mg once daily; upon discontinuation of voriconazole, return to the initial dose of efavirenz.

Phenytoin:
IV: Increase voriconazole maintenance dose to 5 mg/kg every 12 hours.
Oral: Increase voriconazole maintenance dose to 400 mg every 12 hours in patients ≥40 kg (200 mg every 12 hours in patients <40 kg).

Pediatric
Pediatric: **Note:** In pediatric patients <12 years, bioequivalence between the oral tablet and suspension has not been determined; due to possible shortened gastric transit time in infants and children, absorption of tablets may be different than adults; it is recommended that infants and children <12 years only receive oral suspension formulation [Vfend prescribing information (Europe Medicines Agency) 2013]. Data suggest higher doses (mg/kg) than adults are required in patients <15 years and weighing <50 kg. Although FDA approved for treatment of certain fungal infections in patients ≥12 years, the manufacturer's dosing may not achieve necessary therapeutic targets and possible suboptimal response in patients <15 years may occur (Friberg 2012).

General dosing, susceptible infection:
Infants and Children <2 years (off-label): IV, Oral (oral suspension): Initial: 9 mg/kg/dose every 12 hours followed by monitoring of serum trough concentrations typically initiated after 3 to 5 days; adjust dose to achieve target trough (>1 mcg/mL); median final dosage: 31.5 mg/kg/**day** (range: 12 to 71 mg/kg/**day**) divided every 12 hours; dosing based on 2 pharmacokinetic studies that included a total of 17 patients <2 years (Bartenlink 2013; Gerin 2011)

Children 2 to <12 years (off-label; *Red Book* [AAP 2015]):
Loading dose: IV: 9 mg/kg/dose every 12 hours for 2 doses on day 1
Maintenance:
IV: 8 mg/kg/dose every 12 hours; monitor serum concentrations to maintain trough >2 mcg/mL
Oral (oral suspension): 9 mg/kg/dose every 12 hours; maximum initial dose: 350 mg/dose; **Note:** In most patients, oral therapy has not been recommended as initial therapy for treatment; it has been recommended to convert from parenteral to oral therapy only after significant clinical improvement has been observed [Vfend prescribing information (Europe Medicines Agency) 2013].

Children ≥12 years and Adolescents ≤14 years (off-label; Friberg 2012): **Note:** In this age group, body weight is more important than age in predicting pharmacokinetics

IV:

<50 kg: Loading dose: 9 mg/kg/dose every 12 hours for 2 doses; followed by maintenance dose of 4 to 8 mg/kg/dose every 12 hours

≥50 kg: Loading dose: 6 mg/kg/dose every 12 hours for 2 doses; followed by maintenance dose of 3 to 4 mg/kg/dose every 12 hours

Oral: **Note:** Higher doses may be required if adequate trough concentrations are not achieved; monitor trough concentrations closely

<50 kg: 9 mg/kg/dose every 12 hours; maximum dose: 350 mg/dose

≥50 kg: 200 mg every 12 hours

Adolescents ≥15 years:

IV: Loading dose: 6 mg/kg/dose every 12 hours for 2 doses; followed by a maintenance dose of 3 to 4 mg/kg/dose every 12 hours

Oral: 200 mg every 12 hours

Aspergillosis, invasive, including disseminated and extrapulmonary infection; treatment: Note: Duration of therapy should be a minimum of 6 to 12 weeks, although duration is highly dependent on degree/duration of immunosuppression, disease site, and evidence of disease improvement. Monitor trough concentrations in patients with invasive aspergillosis; in pediatric patients <50 kg, therapeutic drug monitoring is critical to ensure efficacy and minimize toxicity; may consider switching to oral therapy once patient is stable and able to tolerate (IDSA [Patterson 2016]).

Children 2 to <12 years (off-label):

IV: Loading dose: 9 mg/kg/dose every 12 hours for 2 doses on day 1, followed by a maintenance dose of 8 mg/kg/dose every 12 hours (Friberg 2012; IDSA [Patterson 2016]; *Red Book* [AAP 2015])

Oral (oral suspension): 9 mg/kg/dose every 12 hours; maximum dose: 350 mg/dose; higher doses may be required if adequate trough concentrations are not achieved; monitor trough concentrations closely (Friberg 2012; IDSA [Patterson 2016])

Children ≥12 years and Adolescents ≤14 years (off-label): **Note:** In this age group, body weight is more important than age in predicting pharmacokinetics (Friberg 2012; IDSA [Patterson 2016]); monitor trough concentrations closely; higher doses may be required if adequate trough concentrations are not achieved.

<50 kg:

IV: Loading dose: 9 mg/kg/dose every 12 hours for 2 doses; followed by maintenance dose of 8 mg/kg/dose every 12 hours

Oral: 9 mg/kg/dose every 12 hours

≥50 kg:

IV: Loading dose: 6 mg/kg/dose every 12 hours for 2 doses; followed by maintenance dose of 4 mg/kg/dose every 12 hours

Oral: 200 to 300 mg every 12 hours **or** 3 to 4 mg/kg/dose every 12 hours

Adolescents ≥15 years (off-label; IDSA [Patterson 2016]):

IV: Loading dose: 6 mg/kg/dose every 12 hours for 2 doses; followed by maintenance dose of 4 mg/kg/dose every 12 hours

Oral: 200 to 300 mg every 12 hours **or** 3 to 4 mg/kg/dose every 12 hours

Candidiasis, prophylaxis for patients at high risk of invasive candidiasis (eg, AML, recurrent ALL, allogeneic HSCT) (off-label use):
Children 2 to <12 years (Dvorak 2012; ESCMID [Hope 2012]; Friberg 2012):
  IV: Loading dose: 9 mg/kg/dose every 12 hours for 2 doses on day 1, followed by a maintenance dose of 8 mg/kg/dose every 12 hours
  Oral (oral suspension): 9 mg/kg/dose every 12 hours; maximum dose: 350 mg/dose
Children ≥12 years and Adolescents ≤14 years: **Note:** In this age group, body weight is more important than age in predicting pharmacokinetics (Friberg 2012)
  <50 kg:
    IV: Loading dose: 9 mg/kg/dose every 12 hours for 2 doses; followed by maintenance dose of 8 mg/kg/dose every 12 hours (Dvorak 2012; ESCMID [Hope 2012]; Friberg 2012)
    Oral: 9 mg/kg/dose every 12 hours; maximum dose: 350 mg/dose (ESCMID [Hope 2012]; Friberg 2012)
  ≥50 kg:
    IV: 4 mg/kg/dose every 12 hours (Tomblyn 2009)
    Oral: 200 mg every 12 hours (Tomblyn 2009; Wingard 2010)
Adolescents ≥15 years:
  IV: 4 mg/kg/dose every 12 hours (Tomblyn 2009)
  Oral: 200 mg every 12 hours (Tomblyn 2009; Wingard 2010)
Candidiasis, invasive; treatment: Note: Voriconazole is considered an alternative therapy and offers little advantage over fluconazole as first-line therapy of candidemia. Step-down therapy to oral voriconazole is recommended only in select clinically stable patients with certain voriconazole-susceptible isolates (eg, *C. krusei*) and negative repeat cultures (IDSA [Pappas 2016]).
Children 2 to <12 years (off-label; ESCMID [Hope 2012]; IDSA [Pappas 2016]):
  IV: Loading dose: 9 mg/kg/dose every 12 hours for 2 doses on day 1, followed by a maintenance dose of 8 mg/kg/dose every 12 hours
  Oral (oral suspension): 9 mg/kg/dose every 12 hours; maximum dose: 350 mg/dose
Children ≥12 years and Adolescents ≤14 years (off label): **Note:** In this age group, body weight is more important than age in predicting pharmacokinetics (Friberg 2012)
  <50 kg:
    IV: Loading dose: 9 mg/kg/dose every 12 hours for 2 doses; followed by maintenance dose of 8 mg/kg/dose every 12 hours (ESCMID [Hope 2012]; Friberg 2012; IDSA [Pappas 2016])
    Oral: 9 mg/kg/dose every 12 hours; maximum dose: 350 mg/dose (ESCMID [Hope 2012]; Friberg 2012; IDSA [Pappas 2016])
  ≥50 kg:
    IV: Loading dose: 400 mg (6 mg/kg/dose) every 12 hours for 2 doses, followed by 200 mg (3 mg/kg/dose) every 12 hours (ESCMID [Hope 2012]; Friberg 2012; IDSA [Pappas 2016])
    Oral: 200 mg (3 mg/kg/dose) every 12 hours (ESCMID [Hope 2012]; Friberg 2012; IDSA [Pappas 2016])
Adolescents ≥15 years (off-label):
  IV: Loading dose: 400 mg (6 mg/kg/dose) every 12 hours for 2 doses, followed by 200 mg (3 mg/kg/dose) every 12 hours (IDSA [Pappas 2016])

Oral: 200 mg (3 mg/kg/dose) every 12 hours (IDSA [Pappas 2016])

Candidiasis, esophageal (fluconazole-refractory); treatment: Treatment should continue for 14 to 21 days (IDSA [Pappas 2016])

Children 2 to <12 years:

IV (off-label): Loading dose: 9 mg/kg/dose every 12 hours for 2 doses; followed by maintenance dose of 8 mg/kg/dose every 12 hours (IDSA [Pappas 2016])

Oral (oral suspension): 9 mg/kg/dose every 12 hours; maximum dose: 350 mg/dose (IDSA [Pappas 2016])

Children ≥12 years and Adolescents ≤14 years: **Note:** In this age group, body weight is more important than age in predicting pharmacokinetics (Friberg 2012)

<50 kg:

IV (off-label): Loading dose: 9 mg/kg/dose every 12 hours for 2 doses; followed by maintenance dose of 8 mg/kg/dose every 12 hours (Friberg 2012; IDSA [Pappas 2016])

Oral: 9 mg/kg/dose every 12 hours; maximum dose: 350 mg/dose (Friberg 2012; IDSA [Pappas 2016])

≥50 kg: IV (off-label), Oral: 200 mg (3 mg/kg/dose) twice daily (IDSA [Pappas 2016])

Adolescents ≥15 years: IV (off-label), Oral: 200 mg (3 mg/kg/dose) twice daily (IDSA [Pappas 2016])

Candidiasis, intravascular infections (endocarditis/implantable cardiac devices [eg, pacemaker, ICD, VAD]); treatment (off-label use): Note: Voriconazole should only be used as step-down therapy in clinically stable, culture-negative patients following initial therapy

Children 2 to <12 years: Oral (oral suspension): 9 mg/kg/dose every 12 hours; maximum dose: 350 mg/dose (IDSA [Pappas 2016])

Children ≥12 years and Adolescents ≤14 years: **Note:** In this age group, body weight is more important than age in predicting pharmacokinetics (Friberg 2012)

<50 kg: Oral: 9 mg/kg/dose every 12 hours; maximum dose: 350 mg/dose (Friberg 2012; IDSA [Pappas 2016])

≥50 kg: Oral: 200 to 300 mg (3 to 4 mg/kg/dose) twice daily (Friberg 2012; IDSA [Pappas 2016])

Adolescents ≥15 years: Oral: 200 to 300 mg (3 to 4 mg/kg/dose) twice daily (IDSA [Pappas 2016])

Candidiasis, oropharyngeal (fluconazole-refractory); treatment (off-label use): Treatment should continue for up to 28 days (IDSA [Pappas 2016])

Children 2 to <12 years: Oral (oral suspension): 9 mg/kg/dose every 12 hours; maximum dose: 350 mg/dose (IDSA [Pappas 2016])

Children ≥12 years and Adolescents ≤14 years: **Note:** In this age group, body weight is more important than age in predicting pharmacokinetics (Friberg 2012)

<50 kg: Oral: 9 mg/kg/dose every 12 hours; maximum dose: 350 mg/dose (Friberg 2012; IDSA [Pappas 2016])

≥50 kg: Oral: 200 mg twice daily (Friberg 2012; IDSA [Pappas 2016])

Adolescents ≥15 years: Oral: 200 mg twice daily (IDSA [Pappas 2016])

◀ **Candidiasis, endophthalmitis (with or without vitritis):** Voriconazole-susceptible isolates (off-label use):

Systemic therapy: **Note:** For patients with vitritis or with macular involvement (with or without vitritis), an intravitreal injection of voriconazole or amphotericin B deoxycholate is also recommended (IDSA [Pappas 2016]).

Children 2 to <12 years:

IV: Loading dose: 9 mg/kg/dose every 12 hours for 2 doses; followed by maintenance dose of 8 mg/kg/dose every 12 hours (IDSA [Pappas 2016])

Oral (oral suspension): 9 mg/kg/dose every 12 hours; maximum dose: 350 mg/dose (IDSA [Pappas 2016])

Children ≥12 years and Adolescents ≤14 years: **Note:** In this age group, body weight is more important than age in predicting pharmacokinetics (Friberg 2012)

<50 kg:

IV: Loading dose: 9 mg/kg/dose every 12 hours for 2 doses; followed by maintenance dose of 8 mg/kg/dose every 12 hours (Friberg 2012; IDSA [Pappas 2016])

Oral: 9 mg/kg/dose every 12 hours; maximum dose: 350 mg/dose (Friberg 2012; IDSA [Pappas 2016])

≥50 kg:

IV: Loading dose: 400 mg (6 mg/kg/dose) every 12 hours for 2 doses, followed by 300 mg (4 mg/kg/dose) twice daily (Friberg 2012; IDSA [Pappas 2016])

Oral: 300 mg (4 mg/kg/dose) twice daily (Friberg 2012; IDSA [Pappas 2016])

Adolescents ≥15 years:

IV: Loading dose: 400 mg (6 mg/kg/dose) every 12 hours for 2 doses, followed by 300 mg (4 mg/kg/dose) twice daily (IDSA [Pappas 2016])

Oral: 300 mg (4 mg/kg/dose) twice daily (IDSA [Pappas 2016])

Intravitreal therapy: Patients with vitritis or with macular involvement (with or without vitritis): Children ≥2 years and Adolescents: Intravitreal: 100 **mcg** of an extemporaneously prepared solution in 0.1 mL sterile water or NS; concomitant systemic antifungal therapy is also recommended.

Renal Impairment

IV:

CrCl ≥50 mL/minute: There are no dosage adjustments provided in the manufacturer's labeling.

CrCl <50 mL/minute: There are no specific dosage adjustments provided in the manufacturer's labeling. Due to accumulation of the intravenous vehicle (cyclodextrin), the manufacturer recommends the use of oral voriconazole in these patients unless an assessment of the benefit:risk justifies the use of IV voriconazole; if IV therapy is used, closely monitor serum creatinine and change to oral voriconazole when possible. IV therapy has been used in select patients with CrCl <50 mL/minute using varying doses (median duration of treatment 7 to 10 days) (Neofytos 2012; Oude Lashof 2012).

Oral:

Mild to severe impairment: No dosage adjustment necessary.

Dialysis: Poorly dialyzed; no supplemental dose or dosage adjustment necessary, including patients on intermittent hemodialysis (IHD) with thrice weekly sessions or peritoneal dialysis.

Continuous renal replacement therapy (CRRT) (Heintz 2009): Drug clearance is highly dependent on the method of renal replacement, filter type, and flow rate. Appropriate dosing requires close monitoring of pharmacologic response, signs of adverse reactions due to drug accumulation, as well as drug concentrations in relation to target trough (if appropriate). The following are general recommendations only (based on dialysate flow/ultrafiltration rates of 1 to 2 L/hour and minimal residual renal function) and should not supersede clinical judgment:

CVVH, CVVHD, and CVVHDF: Loading dose of 400 mg every 12 hours for 2 doses, followed by 200 mg every 12 hours.

Hepatic Impairment

Mild to moderate impairment (Child-Pugh class A or B): Following standard loading dose, reduce maintenance dosage by 50%

Severe impairment (Child-Pugh class C): There are no dosage adjustments provided in the manufacturer's labeling (has not been studied). Should only be used if benefit outweighs risk; monitor closely for toxicity

Obesity Use ideal body weight (IBW) for most obese patients in weight-based dosing calculations; consider using an adjusted body weight (adjusted body weight=0.4 [total body weight – IBW] + IBW) in obese patients with life-threatening invasive fungal infections. Confirm selection of an appropriate dose with therapeutic drug monitoring (Eljaaly 2016).

Additional Information Complete prescribing information should be consulted for additional detail.

Dosage Forms Excipient information presented when available (limited, particularly for generics); consult specific product labeling.

Solution Reconstituted, Intravenous:
Generic: 200 mg (1 ea)
Solution Reconstituted, Intravenous [preservative free]:
Vfend IV: 200 mg (1 ea) [latex free]
Vfend IV: 200 mg (1 ea)
Generic: 200 mg (1 ea)
Suspension Reconstituted, Oral:
Vfend: 40 mg/mL (75 mL) [contains sodium benzoate; orange flavor]
Generic: 40 mg/mL (75 mL)
Tablet, Oral:
Vfend: 50 mg, 200 mg
Generic: 50 mg, 200 mg

◆ **Voriconazole For Injection (Can)** see Voriconazole on page 1925

Vorinostat (vor IN oh stat)

Related Information

Hematopoietic Cell Transplantation on page 2365

Management of Chemotherapy-Induced Nausea and Vomiting in Adults on page 2253

Prevention of Chemotherapy-Induced Nausea and Vomiting in Children on page 2310

Safe Handling of Hazardous Drugs on page 2379

Brand Names: US Zolinza

Brand Names: Canada Zolinza

Index Terms SAHA; Suberoylanilide Hydroxamic Acid

Pharmacologic Category Antineoplastic Agent, Histone Deacetylase (HDAC) Inhibitor

◀ **Use Cutaneous T-cell lymphoma:** Treatment of cutaneous manifestations of cutaneous T-cell lymphoma (CTCL) with progressive, persistent, or recurrent disease on or following 2 systemic treatments

Labeled Contraindications There are no contraindications in the manufacturer's U.S. labeling.

Canadian labeling: Hypersensitivity to vorinostat or any component of the formulation; severe hepatic impairment (total bilirubin ≥3 times ULN)

Pregnancy Considerations Adverse events were observed in animal reproduction studies. Based on the mechanism of action, may cause fetal harm if administered during pregnancy. Inform patient of potential hazard if used during pregnancy or if pregnancy occurs during treatment.

Breastfeeding Considerations It is not known if vorinostat is excreted in breast milk. Due to the potential for serious adverse reactions in the nursing infant, the decision to discontinue vorinostat or to discontinue breastfeeding should take into account the benefits of treatment to the mother.

Warnings/Precautions Pulmonary embolism and deep vein thrombosis (DVT) have been reported; monitor for signs/symptoms; use caution in patients with a history of thrombotic events. Dose-related thrombocytopenia and/or anemia may occur; may require dosage adjustments or discontinuation; monitor blood counts (every 2 weeks for 2 months, then monthly). Gastrointestinal bleeding due to severe thrombocytopenia has been reported in patients receiving vorinostat in combination with other histone deacetylase inhibitors (eg, valproic acid); monitor platelet counts more frequently in patients receiving concomitant histone deacetylase inhibitor therapy. QT_c prolongation has been observed; baseline and periodic ECGs were done in clinical trials (Duvic, 2007; Olsen, 2007). Correct electrolyte abnormalities prior to treatment and monitor and correct potassium, calcium, and magnesium levels during therapy. Use caution in patients with a history of QT_c prolongation or with medications known to prolong the QT interval. May cause hyperglycemia (may be severe); monitor serum glucose and use with caution in diabetics; may require diet and/or therapy modifications. Nausea, vomiting, and diarrhea may occur; antiemetics and antidiarrheals may be required; control preexisting nausea, vomiting, and diarrhea prior to treatment initiation; replace fluids and electrolytes to avoid dehydration. Adverse anastomotic healing events have occurred in patients recovering from bowel surgery; use with caution in the perioperative period in patients requiring bowel surgery. May cause dizziness or fatigue; caution patients about performing tasks which require mental alertness (eg, operating machinery or driving). Use with caution in patients with hepatic impairment; dose reductions are recommended (elimination is predominantly hepatic). The Canadian labeling does not recommend use in patients with moderate hepatic impairment (total bilirubin 1.5 to 3 times ULN) and contraindicates use in severe hepatic impairment (bilirubin ≥3 times ULN). Potentially significant drug-drug interactions may exist, requiring dose or frequency adjustment, additional monitoring, and/or selection of alternative therapy.

Adverse Reactions

>10%:

Cardiovascular: Peripheral edema (13%)

Central nervous system: Fatigue (52%), chills (16%), dizziness (15%), headache (12%)

Dermatologic: Alopecia (19%), pruritus (12%)

Endocrine & metabolic: Hyperglycemia (8% to 69%; grade 3: 5%), weight loss (21%), dehydration (1% to 16%)

Gastrointestinal: Diarrhea (52%), nausea (41%), dysgeusia (28%), anorexia (24%), xerostomia (16%), constipation (15%), vomiting (15%), decreased appetite (14%)

Genitourinary: Proteinuria (51%)

Hematologic & oncologic: Thrombocytopenia (26%; grades 3/4: 6%), anemia (14%; grades 3/4: 2%)

Neuromuscular & skeletal: Muscle spasm (20%)

Renal: Increased serum creatinine (16% to 47%)

Respiratory: Cough (11%), upper respiratory tract infection (11%)

Miscellaneous: Fever (11%)

1% to 10%:

Cardiovascular: Pulmonary embolism (5%), prolonged Q-T interval on ECG (3% to 4%)

Hematologic & oncologic: Squamous cell carcinoma of skin (4%)

<1%, postmarketing, and/or case reports: Abdominal pain, acute ischemic stroke, angioedema, bacteremia (streptococcal), blurred vision, chest pain, cholecystitis, deafness, deep vein thrombosis, diverticulitis, dysphagia, exfoliative dermatitis, gastrointestinal hemorrhage, Guillain-Barre syndrome, hemoptysis, hypertension, hypokalemia, hyponatremia, infection, infection due to enterococcus, lethargy, leukopenia, myocardial infarction, neutropenia, pneumonia, renal failure, sepsis, spinal cord injury, syncope, T-cell lymphoma, tumor hemorrhage, ureteral obstruction, obstructive uropathy (ureteropelvic junction), urinary retention, vasculitis, weakness

Drug Interactions

Metabolism/Transport Effects None known.

Avoid Concomitant Use

Avoid concomitant use of Vorinostat with any of the following: BCG (Intravesical); Deferiprone; Dipyrone

Increased Effect/Toxicity

Vorinostat may increase the levels/effects of: CloZAPine; Deferiprone; Highest Risk QTc-Prolonging Agents; Moderate Risk QTc-Prolonging Agents; Vitamin K Antagonists

The levels/effects of Vorinostat may be increased by: Dipyrone; MiFEPRIStone; Promazine; Valproate Products

Decreased Effect

Vorinostat may decrease the levels/effects of: Antidiabetic Agents; BCG (Intravesical)

Hazardous Drugs Handling Considerations

Hazardous agent (NIOSH 2016 [group 1]).

Use appropriate precautions for receiving, handling, administration, and disposal. Gloves (single) should be worn during receiving, unpacking, and placing in storage.

NIOSH recommends single gloving for administration of intact tablets or capsules. If manipulating tablets/capsules (eg, to prepare an oral suspension), NIOSH recommends double gloving, a protective gown, and preparation in a controlled device; if not prepared in a controlled device, respiratory and eye/face protection as well as ventilated engineering controls are recommended. NIOSH recommends double gloving, a protective gown, and (if there is a potential for vomit or spit up) eye/face protection for administration of an oral liquid/feeding tube administration (NIOSH 2016).

◄ **Storage/Stability** Store at 20°C to 25°C (68°F to 77°F); excursions permitted to 15°C to 30°C (59°F to 86°F).

Mechanism of Action Inhibits histone deacetylase enzymes, HDAC1, HDAC2, HDAC3, and HDAC6, which catalyze acetyl group removal from protein lysine residues (including histones and transcription factors). Histone deacetylase inhibition results in accumulation of acetyl groups, which alters chromatin structure and transcription factor activation; cell growth is terminated and apoptosis occurs.

Pharmacodynamics/Kinetics

Protein binding: ~71%

Metabolism: Glucuronidated and hydrolyzed (followed by beta-oxidation) to inactive metabolites

Bioavailability: Fasting: ~43%

Half-life elimination: ~2 hours

Time to peak, plasma: With high-fat meal: ~4 hours (range: 2 to 10 hours)

Excretion: Urine: 52% (~52% as inactive metabolites; <1% as unchanged drug)

Dosing

Adult & Geriatric Cutaneous T-cell lymphoma (CTCL): Oral: 400 mg once daily until disease progression or unacceptable toxicity

Renal Impairment There are no dosage adjustments provided in the manufacturer's labeling (has not been studied). However, based on the minimal renal elimination, adjustment not expected. Use with caution.

Hepatic Impairment

U.S. labeling: Initial:

Mild-to-moderate impairment (total bilirubin 1-3 times ULN **or** AST >ULN): 300 mg once daily

Severe impairment (total bilirubin >3 times ULN): There are no dosage adjustments provided in the manufacturer's labeling (evidence is insufficient for a starting dose recommendation). Doses of 100 to 200 mg once daily were studied in a limited number of patients with severe impairment (Ramalingam, 2010); according to the manufacturer, the maximum dose used was 200 mg once daily.

Canadian labeling:

Mild impairment (total bilirubin >1 to 1.5 times ULN or total bilirubin ≤ULN and AST >ULN): 300 mg once daily

Moderate impairment (total bilirubin 1.5-3 times ULN): Use is not recommended

Severe impairment (total bilirubin ≥3 times ULN): Use is contraindicated

Adjustment for Toxicity

U.S. labeling: Intolerance: Reduce dose to 300 mg once daily; if needed, may further reduce to 300 mg daily for 5 consecutive days per week

Canadian labeling: Grade 3 or 4 toxicity: Interrupt therapy until resolves to ≤ grade 1 (excluding grade 3 anemia and thrombocytopenia). Upon recovery, may reduce dose to 300 mg once daily. If necessary, may further reduce dose to 300 mg once daily for 5 consecutive days per week.

Additionally, in clinical trials, **dose reductions** were instituted for the following adverse events: Increased serum creatinine, decreased appetite, hypokalemia, leukopenia, nausea, neutropenia, thrombocytopenia, and vomiting. Vorinostat was **discontinued** for the following adverse events: Anemia, angioneurotic edema, weakness, chest pain, exfoliative dermatitis, DVT, ischemic stroke, lethargy, pulmonary embolism, and spinal cord injury.

Treatment was withheld in clinical trials for grade 4 anemia or thrombocytopenia or other grade 3 or 4 drug related toxicity, until resolved to ≤ grade 1. Treatment was reinitiated with dose reduction (Olsen, 2007).

Administration Administer with food. Do not open, crush, break, or chew capsules. Avoid direct skin or mucous membrane contact with crushed or broken capsules and/or capsule contents. Maintain adequate hydration (≥2 L/day fluids) during treatment.

Emetic Potential Children and Adults: Low (10% to 30%)

Extemporaneous Preparations Although not recommended by the manufacturer, a 50 mg/mL oral suspension may be prepared with capsules. Add 20 mL Ora-Plus® into a glass bottle (≥4 oz). Add the contents of twenty 100 mg capsules and shake thoroughly to disperse (may take up to 3 minutes). Add 20 mL Ora-Sweet® and shake to disperse. Label "shake well". Stable for 14 days at room temperature.

Fouladi M, Park JR, Stewart CF, et al, "Pediatric Phase I Trial and Pharmacokinetic Study of Vorinostat: A Children's Oncology Group Phase I Consortium Report," *J Clin Oncol*, 2010, 28 (22):3623-9.

Monitoring Parameters CBC with differential and serum chemistries, including calcium, magnesium, potassium, glucose and creatinine (baseline, then every 2 weeks for 2 months, then monthly, or as clinically necessary), hepatic function, INR (if on concomitant warfarin therapy), fluid status, signs/symptoms of thromboembolism. Baseline and periodic ECGs were done in clinical trials (and are recommended in the Canadian labeling).

Dosage Forms Excipient information presented when available (limited, particularly for generics); consult specific product labeling.

Capsule, Oral:

Zolinza: 100 mg

Ziv-Aflibercept (Systemic) (ziv a FLIB er sept)

Brand Names: US Zaltrap

Index Terms Aflibercept I.V.; Vascular Endothelial Growth Factor Trap; VEGF Trap; VEGF Trap R1R2

Pharmacologic Category Antineoplastic Agent; Vascular Endothelial Growth Factor (VEGF) Inhibitor

Use Colorectal cancer, metastatic: Treatment of metastatic colorectal cancer (in combination with fluorouracil, leucovorin, and irinotecan [FOLFIRI]) in patients who are resistant to or have progressed on an oxaliplatin-based regimen

Labeled Contraindications There are no contraindications listed in the manufacturer's labeling.

Pregnancy Considerations Adverse events were observed in animal reproduction studies with doses providing systemic exposure equivalent to ~30% of a human dose. The incidence of fetal malformations increased with increasing doses. Patients (male and female) should use effective contraception during therapy and for at least 3 months following treatment.

Breastfeeding Considerations It is not known if ziv-aflibercept is excreted into breast milk. Due to the potential for serious adverse reactions in the nursing infant, the manufacturer recommends a decision to be made whether to discontinue nursing or to discontinue aflibercept, taking into account the importance of treatment to the mother.

Warnings/Precautions The risk for hemorrhage is increased with ziv-aflibercept. **[U.S. Boxed Warning]: Severe and occasionally fatal hemorrhage, including gastrointestinal (GI) bleeding, has been reported with ziv-aflibercept/FOLFIRI. Monitor for signs and symptoms of GI and other severe bleeding events; do not administer to patients with severe hemorrhage;** discontinue if severe hemorrhage develops. Hemorrhagic events have also included hematuria, postprocedural hemorrhage, intracranial hemorrhage, and pulmonary hemorrhage/hemoptysis.

[U.S. Boxed Warning]: Severe or fatal GI perforation is a possibility; discontinue ziv-aflibercept if GI perforation occurs; monitor for signs/symptoms of GI perforation. The risk for GI and non-GI fistulas is increased with ziv-aflibercept; fistula sites have included anal, enterovesical, enterocutaneous, colovaginal and intestinal; discontinue in patients who develop fistula. Severe diarrhea and dehydration have been reported; the incidence of diarrhea is increased in patients ≥65 years of age; monitor elderly patients closely for diarrhea.

Proteinuria, nephrotic syndrome, and thrombotic microangiopathy (TMA) have been associated with ziv-aflibercept. Evaluate for proteinuria during treatment with urine dipstick and/or urinary protein creatinine ratio (UPCR); if dipstick ≥2+ for protein or UPCR >1, obtain 24-hour urine collection. Withhold ziv-aflibercept for proteinuria ≥2 g per 24 hours; for recurrent proteinuria, withhold treatment until <2 g per 24 hours and then resume with permanent dose reduction. Discontinue treatment for nephrotic syndrome or TMA.

The risk for grades 3/4 hypertension is increased; onset is generally within the first 2 treatment cycles. Monitor blood pressure every 2 weeks (more frequently if clinically indicated); treat with appropriate antihypertensive therapy (may require adjustment of existing antihypertensives); temporarily withhold treatment with uncontrolled hypertension; may reinitiate with permanent dose reduction when controlled. Discontinue for hypertensive crisis or encephalopathy. Patients with NYHA class III or IV heart failure were excluded from clinical trials.

[U.S. Boxed Warning]: Severely compromised wound healing may occur with ziv-aflibercept/FOLFIRI. Discontinue ziv-aflibercept with compromised wound healing. Withhold ziv-aflibercept at least 4 weeks prior to elective surgery. Do not resume ziv-aflibercept treatment until at least 4 weeks after major surgery AND until the surgical wound is completely healed. For minor surgeries (eg, central venous access port placement, biopsy, or tooth extraction), ziv-aflibercept may be resumed or initiated as soon as the surgical wound is fully healed.

◀ A higher incidence of neutropenia and complications due to neutropenia (neutropenic fever and infection) occurred in patients receiving ziv-aflibercept; leukopenia and thrombocytopenia were also observed in clinical trials; monitor CBC with differential (baseline and prior to each cycle); delay treatment until ANC is ≥1,500/mm^3. Cases of reversible posterior leukoencephalopathy syndrome (RPLS) have been reported; confirm diagnosis with MRI; discontinue ziv-aflibercept if verified; symptoms generally resolve or improve within days, although persistent neurologic symptoms and death have been reported. Arterial thrombotic events (ATE), including transient ischemic attack, cerebrovascular accidents, and angina have occurred. Discontinue ziv-aflibercept in patients who experience ATEs. Certain adverse events, such as diarrhea, dizziness, weakness, weight loss, and dehydration, occurred at a higher incidence in elderly compared to younger adults; monitor closely during treatment.

Adverse Reactions Note: Reactions reported in combination therapy with fluorouracil, leucovorin, and irinotecan (FOLFIRI).

>10%:

Cardiovascular: Hypertension (41%; grade 3: 19%; grade 4: <1%)

Central nervous system: Fatigue (48%), voice disorder (25%; grades 3/4: <1%), headache (22%)

Dermatologic: Palmar-plantar erythrodysesthesia (11%)

Endocrine & metabolic: Weight loss (32%)

Gastrointestinal: Diarrhea (69%; grades 3/4: 19%), stomatitis (50%), decreased appetite (32%), abdominal pain (27%), upper abdominal pain (11%)

Genitourinary: Proteinuria (62%, grades 3/4: 8%)

Hematologic: Leukopenia (78%; grades 3/4: 16%), neutropenia (67%; grades 3/4: 37%), thrombocytopenia (48%; grades 3/4: 3%), hemorrhage (38%; grades 3/4: 3%)

Hepatic: Increased serum AST (62%), increased serum ALT (50%)

Infection: Infection (46%, grades 3/4: 12%)

Neuromuscular & skeletal: Weakness (18%; grades 3/4: 5%)

Renal: Increased serum creatinine (23%)

Respiratory: Epistaxis (28%; grades 3/4: <1%), dyspnea (12%)

1% to 10%:

Cardiovascular: Venous thromboembolic events (9%), pulmonary embolism (5%), arterial thromboembolism (3%; grades 3/4: 2%)

Central nervous system: Reversible posterior encephalopathy syndrome (1%)

Dermatologic: Hyperpigmentation (8%)

Endocrine & metabolic: Dehydration (9%; grades 3/4: 4%)

Gastrointestinal: Hemorrhoids (6%), proctalgia (5%), rectal hemorrhage (5%; grades 3/4: <1%), rectal pain (5%)

Genitourinary: Urinary tract infection (9%), nephrotic syndrome (1%)

Hematologic: Febrile neutropenia (grades 3/4: 4%)

Immunologic: Immunogenicity (3%)

Infection: Neutropenic sepsis

Respiratory: Oropharyngeal pain (8%), rhinorrhea (6%)

Miscellaneous: Fistula formation (2%; grades 3/4: <1%)

Frequency not defined:

Central nervous system: Intracranial hemorrhage (severe)

Hematologic & oncologic: Pulmonary hemorrhage

<1%, postmarketing, and/or case reports: Osteonecrosis of the jaw, reduced ejection fracture, thrombotic thrombocytopenic purpura, wound healing impairment

Drug Interactions

Metabolism/Transport Effects None known.

Avoid Concomitant Use

Avoid concomitant use of Ziv-Aflibercept (Systemic) with any of the following: BCG (Intravesical); Deferiprone; Dipyrone

Increased Effect/Toxicity

Ziv-Aflibercept (Systemic) may increase the levels/effects of: Bisphosphonate Derivatives; CloZAPine; Deferiprone

The levels/effects of Ziv-Aflibercept (Systemic) may be increased by: Dipyrone; Promazine

Decreased Effect

Ziv-Aflibercept (Systemic) may decrease the levels/effects of: BCG (Intravesical)

Hazardous Drugs Handling Considerations

Hazardous agent (NIOSH 2016 [group 1]).

Use appropriate precautions for receiving, handling, administration, and disposal. Gloves (single) should be worn during receiving, unpacking, and placing in storage.

NIOSH recommends double gloving, a protective gown, ventilated engineering controls (a class II biological safety cabinet or a compounding aseptic containment isolator), and closed system transfer devices (CSTDs) for preparation. Double gloving, a gown, and (if dosage form allows) CSTDs are required during administration (NIOSH 2016).

Storage/Stability Store intact vials refrigerated at 2°C to 8°C (36°F to 46°F). Protect from light (store in original outer carton).

Solutions diluted for infusion in D5W or NS may be stored in refrigerator for up to 24 hours, or at 20°C to 25°C (68°F to 77°F) for up to 8 hours.

Preparation for Administration Prior to infusion, dilute in D5W or NS to a final concentration of 0.6 to 8 mg/mL. Use polyvinyl chloride (PVC) infusion bags containing DEHP or polyolefin bags. After initial vial puncture, do not re-enter; discard any unused portion of the vial. Do not mix with other medications.

Mechanism of Action Also known as VEGF-trap, ziv-aflibercept is a recombinant fusion protein which is comprised of portions of binding domains for vascular endothelial growth factor (VEGF) receptors 1 and 2, attached to the Fc portion of human IgG1. Ziv-aflibercept acts as a decoy receptor for VEGF-A, VEGF-B, and placental growth factor (PIGF) which prevent VEGF receptor binding/activation to their receptors (an action critical to angiogenesis), thus leading to antiangiogenesis and tumor regression.

Pharmacodynamics/Kinetics Half-life elimination: ~6 days (range: 4 to 7 days)

Dosing

Adult & Geriatric Colorectal cancer, metastatic: IV: 4 mg/kg every 2 weeks (in combination with fluorouracil, leucovorin, and irinotecan [FOLFIRI]), continue until disease progression or unacceptable toxicity

Renal Impairment There are no dosage adjustments provided in the manufacturer's labeling; however, need for adjustment is not likely because exposure in patients with mild, moderate, and severe impairment was similar to that of patients with normal renal function.

Hepatic Impairment

Mild (total bilirubin >1 to 1.5 times ULN) to moderate (total bilirubin >1.5 to 3 times ULN) impairment: There are no dosage adjustments provided in the manufacturer's labeling; however, need for adjustment is not likely because exposure was similar to that of patients with normal hepatic function.

Severe impairment (total bilirubin >3 times ULN): There are no dosage adjustments provided in the manufacturer's labeling (no data available).

Adjustment for Toxicity

Arterial thrombotic events: Discontinue treatment.

Fistula formation: Discontinue treatment.

Gastrointestinal perforation: Discontinue treatment.

Hemorrhage, severe: Discontinue treatment.

Hypertension:

Recurrent or severe hypertension: Temporarily withhold treatment until controlled and then resume with a permanent dose reduction to 2 mg/kg every 2 weeks.

Hypertensive crisis or hypertensive encephalopathy: Discontinue treatment.

Neutropenia: Temporarily withhold treatment until ANC is ≥1500/mm^3.

Renal effects:

Proteinuria (≥2 g/24 hours): Temporarily withhold treatment until proteinuria <2 g/24 hours and then resume at previous dose.

Recurrent proteinuria: Temporarily withhold treatment until proteinuria <2 g/24 hours and then resume with a permanent dose reduction to 2 mg/kg every 2 weeks.

Nephrotic syndrome or thrombotic microangiopathy: Discontinue treatment

Reversible posterior leukoencephalopathy syndrome (RPLS): Discontinue treatment.

Surgery/wound healing impairment:

Elective surgery: Temporarily withhold treatment for at least 4 weeks prior to elective surgery; do not resume until at least 4 weeks after major surgery AND until wound is fully healed; for minor surgery (eg, biopsy, central venous port placement, tooth extraction), may be resumed after wound is fully healed.

Wound healing impaired: Discontinue treatment.

Note: For toxicities related to FOLFIRI, refer to individual Fluorouracil (Systemic) or Irinotecan monographs.

Combination Regimens

Colorectal cancer: Ziv-Aflibercept + FOLFIRI (Colorectal) on page 2234

Administration IV: Infuse over 1 hour. Do not administer as an IV push or bolus. Administer prior to any FOLFIRI component. Do not administer other medications through the same intravenous line.

Infuse via a 0.2 micron polyethersulfone filter; do not use filters made of polyvinylidene fluoride (PVDF) or nylon. Administer with one of the following types of infusion sets: Polyvinyl chloride (PVC) containing DEHP, DEHP-free PVC containing trioctyl-trimellitate (TOTM), polypropylene, polyethylene lined PVC, or polyurethane.

Emetic Potential Low (10% to 30%)

Monitoring Parameters CBC with differential (baseline and prior to each cycle); urine protein (dipstick analysis and/or urinary protein creatinine ratio [UPCR], obtain 24-hour urine collection if dipstick ≥2+ for protein or UPCR >1); blood pressure (every 2 weeks; more frequently if clinically indicated); monitor for signs/symptoms of hemorrhage or GI perforation; monitor elderly patients closely for diarrhea and/or dehydration. Monitor wounds for healing impairment.

Dosage Forms Excipient information presented when available (limited, particularly for generics); consult specific product labeling.
Solution, Intravenous [preservative free]:
  Zaltrap: 100 mg/4 mL (4 mL); 200 mg/8 mL (8 mL)

Zoledronic Acid (zoe le DRON ik AS id)

Related Information

Brand Names: US Reclast; Zometa

Brand Names: Canada Aclasta; Taro-Zoledronic Acid; Taro-Zoledronic Acid Concentrate; Zoledronic Acid Injection; Zoledronic Acid for Injection; Zoledronic Acid Z; Zometa Concentrate

Index Terms CGP-42446; Zol 446; Zoledronate

Pharmacologic Category Bisphosphonate Derivative

Use

Bone metastases from solid tumors (Zometa): Treatment of documented bone metastases from solid tumors (in conjunction with standard antineoplastic therapy); prostate cancer should have progressed following treatment with at least one hormonal therapy.

Glucocorticoid-induced osteoporosis (Reclast, Aclasta [Canadian product]): Treatment and prevention of glucocorticoid-induced osteoporosis in men and women who are initiating or continuing systemic glucocorticoids in a daily dose equivalent to 7.5 mg or more of prednisone and who are expected to remain on glucocorticoids for at least 12 months.

Hypercalcemia of malignancy (Zometa): Treatment of hypercalcemia (albumin-corrected serum calcium ≥12 mg/dL) of malignancy.

Multiple myeloma (Zometa): Treatment of osteolytic lesions of multiple myeloma.

Osteoporosis in men (Reclast, Aclasta [Canadian product]): To increase bone mass in men with osteoporosis.

Paget disease of bone (Reclast, Aclasta [Canadian product]): Treatment of Paget disease of bone in men and women. **Note:** In patients without contraindications, zoledronic acid is recommended as the treatment of choice per Endocrine Society guidelines (Singer 2014).

Postmenopausal osteoporosis (Reclast, Aclasta [Canadian product]): Treatment and prevention of osteoporosis in postmenopausal women.

Limitations of use: Safety and efficacy for treatment of hypercalcemia associated with hyperparathyroidism or with other non-tumor-related conditions have not been established. Safety and efficacy for osteoporosis treatment is based on clinical data of 3 years duration; the optimal duration has not been determined. All patients on bisphosphonate therapy for the treatment of osteoporosis should be re-evaluated periodically for the need to continue therapy; consider discontinuing after 3 to 5 years in patients at low-risk for fracture; re-evaluate fracture risk periodically in patients who discontinue therapy.

Labeled Contraindications

US labeling:

Hypersensitivity to zoledronic acid or any component of the formulation; hypocalcemia (Reclast only); CrCl <35 mL/minute and in those with evidence of acute renal impairment (Reclast only).

Canadian labeling:

All indications: Hypersensitivity to zoledronic acid or other bisphosphonates, or any component of the formulation; uncorrected hypocalcemia at the time of infusion; pregnancy, breastfeeding

Nononcology uses: Additional contraindications: Use in patients with CrCl <35 mL/minute and use in patients with evidence of acute renal impairment due to an increased risk of renal failure

Documentation of allergenic cross-reactivity for bisphosphonates is limited. However, because of similarities in chemical structure and/or pharmacologic actions, the possibility of cross-sensitivity cannot be ruled out with certainty.

Pregnancy Considerations Adverse events were observed in animal reproduction studies. It is not known if bisphosphonates cross the placenta, but fetal exposure is expected (Djokanovic, 2008; Stathopoulos, 2011). Bisphosphonates are incorporated into the bone matrix and gradually released over time. The amount available in the systemic circulation varies by dose and duration of therapy. Theoretically, there may be a risk of fetal harm when pregnancy follows the completion of therapy; however, available data have not shown that exposure to bisphosphonates during pregnancy significantly increases the risk of adverse fetal events (Djokanovic, 2008; Levy, 2009; Stathopoulos, 2011). Until additional data is available, most sources recommend discontinuing bisphosphonate therapy in women of reproductive potential as early as possible prior to a planned pregnancy; use in premenopausal women should be reserved for special circumstances when rapid bone loss is occurring (Bhalla, 2010; Pereira, 2012; Stathopoulos, 2011). Because hypocalcemia has been described following *in utero* bisphosphonate exposure, exposed infants should be monitored for hypocalcemia after birth (Djokanovic, 2008; Stathopoulos, 2011).

Breastfeeding Considerations It is not known if zoledronic acid is excreted into breast milk. Due to the potential for serious adverse reactions in the nursing infant, the manufacturer recommends a decision be made to discontinue nursing or to discontinue the drug, taking into account the importance of treatment to the mother.

Warnings/Precautions Osteonecrosis of the jaw (ONJ), also referred to as medication-related osteonecrosis of the jaw (MRONJ), has been reported in patients receiving bisphosphonates. Known risk factors for MRONJ include invasive dental procedures (eg, tooth extraction, dental implants, bony surgery), cancer diagnosis, concomitant therapy (eg, chemotherapy, corticosteroids, angiogenesis inhibitors), poor oral hygiene, ill-fitting dentures, and comorbid disorders (anemia, coagulopathy, infection, preexisting dental disease). Risk may increase with duration of bisphosphonate use and/or may be reported at a greater frequency based on tumor type (eg, advanced breast cancer or multiple myeloma). According to a position paper by the American Association of Maxillofacial Surgeons (AAOMS), MRONJ has been associated with bisphosphonates and other antiresorptive agents (denosumab), and antiangiogenic agents (eg, bevacizumab, sunitinib) used for the treatment of osteoporosis or malignancy; risk is significantly higher in cancer patients receiving antiresorptive therapy compared to patients receiving osteoporosis treatment (regardless of medication used or dosing schedule). MRONJ risk is also increased with monthly IV antiresorptive therapy compared to the minimal risk associated with oral bisphosphonate use, although risk appears to increase with oral bisphosphonates when duration of therapy exceeds 4 years. The manufacturer's labeling states that there are no data to suggest whether discontinuing bisphosphonates in patients requiring invasive dental procedures reduces the risk of ONJ. The manufacturer recommends a dental exam and preventive dentistry be performed prior to placing patients with risk factors on chronic bisphosphonate therapy and that during therapy, invasive dental procedures be avoided, if possible. The AAOMS suggests that if medically permissible, initiation of IV bisphosphonates for cancer therapy should be delayed until optimal dental health is attained (if extractions are required, antiresorptive therapy should delayed until the extraction site has mucosalized or until after adequate osseous healing). Once IV bisphosphonate therapy is initiated for oncologic disease, procedures that involve direct osseous injury and placement of dental implants be avoided. Patients developing ONJ during therapy should receive care by an oral surgeon (AAOMS [Ruggiero 2014]).

Atypical, low-energy, or low-trauma femur fractures have been reported in patients receiving bisphosphonates. The fractures include subtrochanteric femur (bone just below the hip joint) and diaphyseal femur (long segment of the thigh bone). Some patients experience prodromal pain weeks or months before the fracture occurs. It is unclear if bisphosphonate therapy is the cause for these fractures; atypical femur fractures have also been reported in patients not taking bisphosphonates, and in patients receiving glucocorticoids. Patients receiving long-term (>3 to 5 years) bisphosphonate therapy may be at an increased risk. Patients presenting with thigh or groin pain with a history of receiving bisphosphonates should be evaluated for femur fracture. Consider interrupting bisphosphonate therapy in patients who develop a femoral shaft fracture; assess for fracture in the contralateral limb.

Infrequently, severe (and occasionally debilitating) musculoskeletal (bone, joint, and/or muscle) pain have been reported during bisphosphonate treatment. The onset of pain ranged from a single day to several months. Consider discontinuing therapy in patients who experience severe symptoms; symptoms usually resolve upon discontinuation. Some patients experienced recurrence when rechallenged with same drug or another bisphosphonate; avoid use in patients with a history of these symptoms in association with bisphosphonate therapy.

Hypocalcemia (including severe and life-threatening cases) has been reported with use; patients with Paget disease may be at significant risk for hypocalcemia after treatment with zoledronic acid (because pretreatment rate of bone turnover may be elevated); severe and life-threatening hypocalcemia has also been reported with oncology-related uses. Measure serum calcium prior to treatment initiation. Correct preexisting hypocalcemia before initiation of therapy in patients with Paget disease, osteoporosis, or oncology indications. Use with caution with other medications known to cause hypocalcemia (severe hypocalcemia may develop). Ensure adequate calcium and vitamin D supplementation during therapy. Use caution in patients with disturbances of calcium and mineral metabolism (eg, hypoparathyroidism, thyroid/parathyroid, surgery, malabsorption syndromes, excision of small intestine).

Nononcology indications: Use is contraindicated in patients with CrCl <35 mL/minute and in patients with evidence of acute renal impairment due to an increased risk of renal failure. Do not use single doses >5 mg and do not infuse over less than 15 minutes. Obtain serum creatinine and calculate creatinine clearance (using actual body weight) with the Cockcroft-Gault formula prior to each administration. In the management of osteoporosis, reevaluate the need for continued therapy periodically; the optimal duration of treatment has not yet been determined. Consider discontinuing after 3 to 5 years of use in patients at low risk for fracture; following discontinuation, reevaluate fracture risk periodically.

Oncology indications: Use caution in mild to moderate renal dysfunction; dosage adjustment required. In cancer patients, do not use single doses >4 mg and do not infuse over less than 15 minutes (renal toxicity has been reported with doses >4 mg or infusions administered over less than 15 minutes). Risk factors for renal deterioration include preexisting renal insufficiency and repeated doses of zoledronic acid and other bisphosphonates. Dehydration and the use of other nephrotoxic drugs which may contribute to renal deterioration should be identified and managed. Use is not recommended in patients with severe renal impairment (serum creatinine >3 mg/dL or CrCl <30 mL/minute) and bone metastases (limited data); use in patients with hypercalcemia of malignancy and severe renal impairment (serum creatinine >4.5 mg/dL for hypercalcemia of malignancy) should only be done if the benefits outweigh the risks. Diuretics should not be used before correcting hypovolemia. Renal deterioration, resulting in renal failure and dialysis has occurred in patients treated with zoledronic acid after single and multiple infusions at recommended doses of 4 mg over 15 minutes. Assess renal function (eg, serum creatinine) prior to each dose and withhold for renal deterioration [increase in serum creatinine of 0.5 mg/dL (if baseline level normal) or increase of 1 mg/dL (if baseline level abnormal)]; treatment should be withheld until renal function returns to within 10% of baseline.

Adequate hydration is required during treatment (urine output ~2 L/day); avoid overhydration, especially in patients with heart failure. Preexisting renal compromise, severe dehydration, and concurrent use with diuretics or other nephrotoxic drugs may increase the risk for renal impairment. Single and multiple infusions in patients with both normal and impaired renal function have been associated with renal deterioration, resulting in renal failure and dialysis or death (rare). Patients with underlying moderate to severe renal impairment, increased age, concurrent use of nephrotoxic or diuretic medications, or severe dehydration prior to or after zoledronic acid administration may have an increased risk of acute renal impairment or renal failure. Others with increased risk include patients with renal impairment or dehydration secondary to fever, sepsis, gastrointestinal losses, or diuretic use. If history or physical exam suggests dehydration, treatment should not be given until the patient is normovolemic. Transient increases in serum creatinine may be more pronounced in patients with impaired renal function; consider monitoring creatinine clearance in at-risk patients taking other renally eliminated drugs.

Conjunctivitis, uveitis, episcleritis, iritis, scleritis, and orbital inflammation have been reported (infrequently) with use; further ophthalmic evaluation (and possibly therapy discontinuation) may be necessary in patients with complicated infection. Use caution in patients with aspirin-sensitive asthma (may cause bronchoconstriction) and elderly patients (because decreased renal function occurs more commonly in elderly patients). Rare cases of urticaria and angioedema and very rare cases of anaphylactic reactions/shock have been reported. Do not administer Zometa and Reclast (Aclasta [Canadian product]) to the same patient for different indications.

Breast cancer (metastatic): The American Society of Clinical Oncology (ASCO) updated guidelines on the role of bone-modifying agents (BMAs) in the prevention and treatment of skeletal-related events for metastatic breast cancer patients (Van Poznak 2011). The guidelines recommend initiating a BMA (denosumab, pamidronate, zoledronic acid) in patients with metastatic breast cancer to the bone. There is currently no literature indicating the superiority of one particular BMA. Optimal duration is not yet defined; however, the guidelines recommend continuing therapy until substantial decline in patient's performance status. The ASCO guidelines are in alignment with prescribing information for dosing, renal dose adjustments, infusion times, prevention and management of osteonecrosis of the jaw, and monitoring of laboratory parameter recommendations. BMAs are not the first-line therapy for pain. BMAs are to be used as adjunctive therapy for cancer-related bone pain associated with bone metastasis, demonstrating a modest pain control benefit. BMAs should be used in conjunction with agents such as NSAIDS, opioid and nonopioid analgesics, corticosteroids, radiation/surgery, and interventional procedures.

Multiple myeloma: The American Society of Clinical Oncology (ASCO) has published guidelines on bisphosphonate use for prevention and treatment of bone disease in multiple myeloma (Kyle, 2007). Bisphosphonate (pamidronate or zoledronic acid) use is recommended in multiple myeloma patients with lytic bone destruction or compression spine fracture from osteopenia. Bisphosphonates may also be considered in patients with pain secondary to osteolytic disease, adjunct therapy to stabilize fractures or impending fractures, and for multiple myeloma patients with osteopenia but no radiographic evidence of lytic bone disease. Bisphosphonates are not recommended in patients with solitary plasmacytoma, smoldering (asymptomatic) or indolent myeloma, or monoclonal gammopathy of undetermined significance. The guidelines recommend monthly treatment for a period of 2 years. At that time, consider discontinuing in responsive and stable patients, and reinitiate if a new-onset skeletal-related event occurs. The ASCO guidelines are in alignment with prescribing information for dosing, renal dose adjustments, infusion times, prevention and management of osteonecrosis of the jaw, and monitoring of laboratory parameter recommendations. According to the guidelines, in patients with a serum creatinine >3 mg/dL or CrCl <30 mL/minute or extensive bone disease, an alternative bisphosphonate (pamidronate) should be used. Monitor for albuminuria every 3 to 6 months; in patients with unexplained albuminuria >500 mg/24 hours, withhold the dose until level returns to baseline, then recheck every 3 to 4 weeks. Upon reinitiation, the guidelines recommend considering increasing the zoledronic acid infusion time to at least 30 minutes; however, one study has demonstrated that extending the infusion to 30 minutes did not change the safety profile (Berenson, 2011).

◄ **Adverse Reactions**
  Oncology indications:
  >10%:
    Cardiovascular: Lower extremity edema (5% to 21%), hypotension (11%)
    Central nervous system: Fatigue (39%), headache (5% to 19%), dizziness (18%), insomnia (15% to 16%), depression (14%), anxiety (11% to 14%), agitation (13%), confusion (7% to 13%), hypoesthesia (12%), rigors (11%)
    Dermatologic: Alopecia (12%), dermatitis (11%)
    Endocrine & metabolic: Dehydration (5% to 14%), hypophosphatemia (13%), hypokalemia (12%), hypomagnesemia (11%)
    Gastrointestinal: Nausea (29% to 46%), vomiting (14% to 32%), constipation (27% to 31%), diarrhea (17% to 24%), anorexia (9% to 22%), weight loss (16%), abdominal pain (14% to 16%), decreased appetite (13%)
    Genitourinary: Urinary tract infection (12% to 14%)
    Hematologic & oncologic: Anemia (22% to 33%), progression of cancer (16% to 20%), neutropenia (12%)
    Infection: Candidiasis (12%)
    Neuromuscular & skeletal: Ostealgia (55%), weakness (5% to 24%), myalgia (23%), arthralgia (5% to 21%), back pain (15%), paresthesia (15%), limb pain (14%), skeletal pain (12%)
    Renal: Renal insufficiency (8% to 17%; up to 40% in patients with abnormal baseline creatinine)
    Respiratory: Dyspnea (22% to 27%), cough (12% to 22%)
    Miscellaneous: Fever (32% to 44%; most common symptom of acute phase reaction)
  1% to 10%:
    Cardiovascular: Chest pain (5% to 10%)
    Central nervous system: Somnolence (5% to 10%)
    Endocrine & metabolic: Hypocalcemia (5% to 10%; grades 3/4: ≤1%), hypermagnesemia (grade 3: 2%)
    Gastrointestinal: Dyspepsia (10%), dysphagia (5% to 10%), mucositis (5% to 10%), sore throat (8%), stomatitis (8%)
    Hematologic & oncologic: Granulocytopenia (5% to 10%), pancytopenia (5% to 10%), thrombocytopenia (5% to 10%)
    Infection: Infection (nonspecific; 5% to 10%)
    Renal: Increased serum creatinine (grades 3/4: ≤2%)
    Respiratory: Upper respiratory tract infection (10%)
  Nononcology indications:
  >10%:
    Cardiovascular: Hypertension (5% to 13%)
    Central nervous system: Pain (2% to 24%), fever (9% to 22%), headache (4% to 20%), chills (2% to 18%), fatigue (2% to 18%), flank pain (≤2%)
    Endocrine & metabolic: Hypocalcemia (≤3%; Paget disease 21%), dehydration (3%)
    Gastrointestinal: Nausea (5% to 18%), upper abdominal pain (5%), abdominal distension (≤2%)
    Immunologic: Infusion-related reaction (4% to 25%)
    Neuromuscular & skeletal: Arthralgia (9% to 27%), myalgia (5% to 23%), back pain (4% to 18%), limb pain (3% to 16%), musculoskeletal pain (≤12%), osteoarthritis (6%)
    Respiratory: Flu-like symptoms (1% to 11%)

1% to 10%:

Cardiovascular: Chest pain (1% to 8%), peripheral edema (3% to 6%), atrial fibrillation (1% to 3%), palpitations (≤3%)

Central nervous system: Dizziness (2% to 9%), rigors (8%), malaise (1% to 7%), hypoesthesia (≤6%), lethargy (3% to 5%), vertigo (1% to 4%), paresthesia (2%), hyperthermia (≤2%)

Dermatologic: Skin rash (2% to 3%), hyperhidrosis (≤3%)

Gastrointestinal: Abdominal pain (1% to 9%), diarrhea (5% to 8%), vomiting (2% to 8%), constipation (6% to 7%), dyspepsia (2% to 7%), abdominal discomfort (1% to 2%), anorexia (1% to 2%)

Hematologic & oncologic: Change in serum protein (C-reactive protein increased; ≤5%)

Neuromuscular & skeletal: Ostealgia (3% to 9%), arthritis (2% to 9%), neck pain (1% to 7%), shoulder pain (≤7%), muscle spasm (2% to 6%), weakness (2% to 6%), stiffness (1% to 5%), jaw pain (2% to 4%), joint swelling (≤3%)

Ophthalmic: Eye pain (≤2%)

Renal: Increased serum creatinine (2%)

Respiratory: Dyspnea (5% to 7%)

All indications: <1%, postmarketing, and/or case reports: Acute phase reaction-like symptoms (including pyrexia, fatigue, bone pain, arthralgia, myalgia, chills, influenza-like illness; usually resolves within 3 to 4 days of onset, although may take up to 14 days to resolve), acute renal failure (requiring hospitalization/dialysis), acute renal tubular necrosis (toxic), anaphylactic shock, anaphylaxis, angioedema, arthralgia (sometimes severe and/or incapacitating), blurred vision, bradycardia, bronchoconstriction, bronchospasm, cardiac arrhythmia, cerebrovascular accident, conjunctivitis, diaphoresis, drowsiness, dysgeusia, episcleritis, exacerbation of asthma, Fanconi syndrome (acquired), femur fracture (diaphyseal or subtrochanteric), hematuria, hyperesthesia, hyperkalemia, hypernatremia, hyperparathyroidism, hypersensitivity reaction, hypertension, injection site reaction (eg, itching, pain, redness), interstitial pulmonary disease, iridocyclitis, iritis, muscle cramps, myalgia (sometimes severe and/or incapacitating), numbness, osteonecrosis (including external auditory canal, femur, and hip), osteonecrosis of the jaw, periorbital edema, periorbital swelling, prolonged QT interval on ECG, proteinuria, pruritus, renal insufficiency, scleritis, seizure, skin rash, Stevens-Johnson syndrome, tetany, toxic epidermal necrolysis, tremor, urticaria, uveitis, weight gain, xerostomia

Drug Interactions

Metabolism/Transport Effects None known.

Avoid Concomitant Use There are no known interactions where it is recommended to avoid concomitant use.

Increased Effect/Toxicity

Zoledronic Acid may increase the levels/effects of: Deferasirox

The levels/effects of Zoledronic Acid may be increased by: Aminoglycosides; Calcitonin; Nonsteroidal Anti-Inflammatory Agents; Systemic Angiogenesis Inhibitors; Thalidomide

Decreased Effect

The levels/effects of Zoledronic Acid may be decreased by: Proton Pump Inhibitors

Hazardous Drugs Handling Considerations
Hazardous agent (NIOSH 2016 [group 3]).

Use appropriate precautions for receiving, handling, administration, and disposal. Gloves (single) should be worn during receiving, unpacking, and placing in storage.

NIOSH recommends double gloving, a protective gown, ventilated engineering controls (a class II biological safety cabinet or a compounding aseptic containment isolator), and closed system transfer devices (CSTDs) if compounding. Double gloving and a gown are required during administration (NIOSH 2016). Premixed solutions may be excluded from some hazardous drug handling requirements; assess risk to determine appropriate containment strategy (USP-NF 2017).

Storage/Stability Solution for injection:
Aclasta [Canadian product]: Store at room temperature of 15°C to 30°C (59°F to 86°F). Keep sealed in original package until administration.

Reclast: Store at room temperature of 25°C (77°F); excursions permitted to 15°C to 30°C (59°F to 86°F). After opening, stable for 24 hours at 2°C to 8°C (36°F to 46°F). If refrigerated, allow the refrigerated solution to reach room temperature before administration.

Zometa: Store concentrate vials and ready-to-use bottles at 25°C (77°F); excursions permitted to 15°C to 30°C (59°F to 86°F). Diluted solutions for infusion in D5W or NS which are not used immediately after preparation should be refrigerated at 2°C to 8°C (36°F to 46°F). Infusion of solution must be completed within 24 hours of preparation. The ready-to-use bottles are for single use only; if any preparation is necessary (preparing reduced dosage for patients with renal impairment), the prepared, diluted solution may be refrigerated at 2°C to 8°C (36°F to 46°F) if not used immediately. Infusion of solution must be completed within 24 hours of preparation. The previously withdrawn volume from the ready-to-use solution should be discarded; do not store or reuse.

Preparation for Administration
Solution for injection:
Concentrate vials (4 mg/5 mL): Further dilute in 100 mL NS or D5W prior to administration.

Ready-to-use bottles (4 mg/100 mL and 5 mg/100 mL): No further preparation is necessary. If reduced doses are required for patients with renal impairment, withdraw the appropriate volume of solution and replace with an equal amount of NS or D5W.

Mechanism of Action A bisphosphonate which inhibits bone resorption via actions on osteoclasts or on osteoclast precursors; inhibits osteoclastic activity and skeletal calcium release induced by tumors. Decreases serum calcium and phosphorus, and increases their elimination. In osteoporosis, zoledronic acid inhibits osteoclast-mediated resorption, therefore reducing bone turnover.

Pharmacodynamics/Kinetics
Distribution: Binds to bone
Protein binding: 23% to 53%
Metabolism: Primarily eliminated intact via the kidney; metabolism not likely
Half-life elimination: Triphasic; Terminal: 146 hours
Excretion: Urine (39% ± 16% as unchanged drug) within 24 hours; feces (<3%)

Dosing

Adult & Geriatric Note: Acetaminophen administration after the infusion may reduce symptoms of acute-phase reactions. Patients treated for bone metastases from solid tumors, multiple myeloma, and Paget disease should receive a daily calcium and vitamin D supplement, and patients with osteoporosis should receive calcium and vitamin D supplementation if dietary intake is inadequate.

Bone metastases from solid tumors (Zometa): IV: 4 mg once every 3 to 4 weeks

Bone metastases due to breast cancer or prostate cancer (off-label dosing): IV: 4 mg once every 12 weeks; dosing once every 12 weeks (compared to once every 4 weeks) did not result in an increased risk of skeletal events within 2 years in patients with at least 1 site of bone involvement (Himmelstein 2017).

Hypercalcemia of malignancy (albumin-corrected serum calcium ≥12 mg/dL) (Zometa): IV: 4 mg (maximum) given as a single dose. Wait at least 7 days before considering re-treatment.

Multiple myeloma osteolytic lesions (Zometa): IV: 4 mg once every 3 to 4 weeks

Multiple myeloma (off-label dosing): IV: 4 mg once every 12 weeks; dosing once every 12 weeks (compared to once every 4 weeks) did not result in an increased risk of skeletal events within 2 years in patients with at least 1 site of bone involvement (Himmelstein 2017).

Osteoporosis, glucocorticoid-induced, treatment and prevention (Reclast, Aclasta [Canadian product]): IV: 5 mg once a year

Osteoporosis, prevention (Reclast): IV: 5 mg once every 2 years
Canadian labeling (Aclasta): 5 mg as a single (one-time) dose

Osteoporosis, treatment (Reclast, Aclasta [Canadian product]): IV: 5 mg once a year; consider discontinuing after 3 to 5 years of use in patients at low risk for fracture

Paget disease (Reclast, Aclasta [Canadian product]): IV: 5 mg as a single dose.

Re-treatment: Data concerning retreatment is not available; retreatment may be considered for relapse (increase in alkaline phosphatase) if appropriate, for inadequate response, or in patients who are symptomatic. *Canadian labeling (Aclasta):* Data concerning retreatment is limited; retreatment with 5 mg (single dose) may be considered for relapse after an interval of at least 1 year from initial treatment.

The Endocrine Society guidelines suggest re-treatment is seldom required within 5 years (Singer 2014).

Postrenal transplant bone loss (prevention) (off-label use): IV: 4 mg at week 2 and month 3 after engraftment (Haas 2003; Schwarz 2004). Additional data may be necessary to further define the role of zoledronic acid in this condition.

Bone loss associated with androgen deprivation therapy in prostate cancer, prevention (off-label use): IV: 4 mg once every 3 months for 1 year (Smith, 2003) or 4 mg every 12 months (Michaelson 2007)

Bone loss associated with aromatase inhibitor therapy in women with breast cancer, prevention (off-label use): IV: 4 mg once every 6 months for 5 years (Brufsky 2012)

Renal Impairment Note: Prior to each dose, obtain serum creatinine and calculate the creatinine clearance using the Cockcroft-Gault formula.

◀ *Nononcology uses:* **Note:** Use actual body weight in the Cockcroft-Gault formula when calculating clearance for nononcology uses.

CrCl ≥35 mL/minute: No dosage adjustment is necessary.

CrCl <35 mL/minute: Use is contraindicated.

Oncology uses:

Multiple myeloma and bone metastases:

CrCl >60 mL/minute: 4 mg (no dosage adjustment is necessary)

CrCl 50 to 60 mL/minute: Reduce dose to 3.5 mg

CrCl 40 to 49 mL/minute: Reduce dose to 3.3 mg

CrCl 30 to 39 mL/minute: Reduce dose to 3 mg

CrCl <30 mL/minute: Use is not recommended.

Hypercalcemia of malignancy:

Mild to moderate impairment: No dosage adjustment is necessary.

Severe impairment (serum creatinine >4.5 mg/dL): Evaluate risk versus benefit

Dosage adjustment for renal toxicity (during treatment):

Hypercalcemia of malignancy: Evidence of renal deterioration: Evaluate risk versus benefit.

Multiple myeloma and bone metastases: Evidence of renal deterioration: Withhold dose until renal function returns to within 10% of baseline; renal deterioration defined as follows:

Normal baseline creatinine: Increase of 0.5 mg/dL

Abnormal baseline creatinine: Increase of 1 mg/dL

Reinitiate therapy at the same dose administered prior to treatment interruption.

Multiple myeloma: Albuminuria >500 mg/24 hours (unexplained): Withhold dose until return to baseline, then reevaluate every 3 to 4 weeks; consider reinitiating with a longer infusion time of at least 30 minutes (Kyle 2007).

Hepatic Impairment There are no dosage adjustments provided in the manufacturer's labeling (has not been studied); however, zoledronic acid is not metabolized hepatically.

Administration

If refrigerated, allow solution to reach room temperature before administration. Infuse over at least 15 minutes. Flush IV line with 10 mL NS flush following infusion. Infuse in a line separate from other medications. Patients must be appropriately hydrated prior to treatment. Acetaminophen after administration may reduce the incidence of acute reaction (eg, arthralgia, fever, flu-like symptoms, myalgia).

Multiple myeloma: If treatment is withheld for unexplained albuminuria, consider increasing the infusion time to at least 30 minutes upon reinitiation (Kyle 2007).

Monitoring Parameters Prior to initiation of therapy, dental exam and preventive dentistry for patients at risk for osteonecrosis, including all cancer patients

Nononcology uses: Serum creatinine prior to each dose, especially in patients with risk factors, calculate creatinine clearance before each treatment (consider interim monitoring in patients at risk for acute renal failure), evaluate fluid status and adequately hydrate patients prior to and following administration.

Osteoporosis: Bone mineral density (BMD) should be evaluated 1 to 2 years after initiating therapy and every 2 years thereafter (NOF [Cosman 2014]); in patients with combined zoledronic acid and glucocorticoid treatment, BMD should be made at initiation of therapy and repeated after 6 to 12 months; serum calcium and 25(OH)D; annual measurements of height and weight, assessment of chronic back pain; serum calcium and 25(OH)D; phosphorus and magnesium; may consider monitoring biochemical markers of bone turnover

Paget disease: Alkaline phosphatase at 6 to 12 weeks for initial response to treatment (when bone turnover will have shown a substantial decline) and potentially at 6 months (maximal suppression of high bone turnover); following treatment completion, monitor at ~1- to 2-year intervals (Singer, 2014); monitoring more specific biochemical markers of bone turnover (eg, serum P1NP, NTX, serum beta-CTx) is generally only warranted in patients with Paget disease who have abnormal liver or biliary tract function or when early assessment of response to treatment is needed (eg, spinal compression, very active disease) (Singer, 2014); serum calcium and 25(OH)D; phosphorus and magnesium; symptoms of hypocalcemia, pain

Oncology uses: Serum creatinine prior to each dose; serum electrolytes, phosphate, magnesium, and hemoglobin/hematocrit should be evaluated regularly. Monitor serum calcium to assess response and avoid overtreatment. In patients with multiple myeloma, monitor urine every 3 to 6 months for albuminuria.

Test Interactions Bisphosphonates may interfere with diagnostic imaging agents such as technetium-99m-diphosphonate in bone scans.

Dietary Considerations

Multiple myeloma or metastatic bone lesions from solid tumors: Take daily calcium supplement (500 mg) and daily multivitamin (with 400 units vitamin D).

Osteoporosis: Ensure adequate calcium and vitamin D intake; if dietary intake is inadequate, dietary supplementation is recommended. Women and men should consume:

Calcium: 1,000 mg/day (men: 50 to 70 years) **or** 1200 mg/day (women ≥51 years and men ≥71 years) (IOM 2011; NOF [Cosman 2014])

Vitamin D: 800 to 1,000 int. units/day (men and women ≥50 years) (NOF 2014). Recommended Dietary Allowance (RDA): 600 int. units/day (men and women ≤70 years) **or** 800 int. units/day (men and women ≥71 years) (IOM 2011).

Paget disease: Take elemental calcium 1500 mg/day (750 mg twice daily or 500 mg 3 times/day) and vitamin D 800 units/day, particularly during the first 2 weeks after administration.

Medication Guide Available Yes

Dosage Forms Excipient information presented when available (limited, particularly for generics); consult specific product labeling. [DSC] = Discontinued product

Concentrate, Intravenous:

Zometa: 4 mg/5 mL (5 mL)

Generic: 4 mg/5 mL (5 mL)

Concentrate, Intravenous [preservative free]:

Generic: 4 mg/5 mL (5 mL)

◄ Solution, Intravenous:
  Reclast: 5 mg/100 mL (100 mL)
  Zometa: 4 mg/100 mL (100 mL)
  Generic: 4 mg/100 mL (100 mL); 5 mg/100 mL (100 mL)
Solution, Intravenous [preservative free]:
  Generic: 4 mg/100 mL (100 mL); 5 mg/100 mL (100 mL)
Solution Reconstituted, Intravenous:
  Generic: 4 mg (1 ea [DSC])
Dosage Forms: Canada Information with regard to form, strength, and availability of products uniquely available in Canada but currently not available in the US. Refer also to Dosage Forms.

Excipient information presented when available (limited, particularly for generics); consult specific product labeling.
Concentrate, Intravenous:
  Zometa: 4 mg/5 mL (5 mL)
Infusion, Solution [premixed]:
  Aclasta: 5 mg/100 mL (100 mL)

CHEMOTHERAPY REGIMEN
INDEX

CHEMOTHERAPY REGIMEN INDEX

GASTROINTESTINAL

Anal Cancer

Biliary Adenocarcinoma

Colorectal Cancer

Esophageal Cancer

Gastric Cancer

LUNG CANCER

LYMPHOMA

MALIGNANT PLEURAL MESOTHELIOMA

MULTIPLE MYELOMA

ALPHABETICAL LISTING OF CHEMOTHERAPY REGIMENS

5 + 2 (Cytarabine-Daunorubicin) (AML Induction)
Index Terms Cytarabine-Daunorubicin (5 + 2) (AML); Daunorubicin-Cytarabine (5 + 2) (AML)

Use Leukemia, acute myeloid

Regimen

Cytarabine: IV: 100 mg/m^2/day continuous infusion days 1 to 5
  [total dose/cycle = 500 mg/m^2]
Daunorubicin: IV: 45 mg/m^2/day IV bolus days 1 and 2
  [total dose/cycle = 90 mg/m^2]
May administer a second induction cycle if needed

References

Rai KR, Holland JF, Glidewell OJ, et al, "Treatment of Acute Myelocytic Leukemia: A Study by Cancer and Leukemia Group B," *Blood*, 1981, 58(6):1203-12.

5 + 2 (Cytarabine-Daunorubicin) (AML Postremission)
Index Terms Cytarabine-Daunorubicin (5 + 2) (AML); Daunorubicin-Cytarabine (5 + 2) (AML)

Use Leukemia, acute myeloid

Regimen

Cytarabine: IV: 100 mg/m^2/day continuous infusion days 1 to 5
  [total dose/cycle = 500 mg/m^2]
Daunorubicin: IV: 45 mg/m^2/day IV bolus days 1 and 2
  [total dose/cycle = 90 mg/m^2]
Administer 2 courses

References

Wiernik PH, Banks P, Case Jr DC, et al, "Cytarabine Plus Idarubicin or Daunorubicin as Induction and Consolidation Therapy for Previously Untreated Adult Patients With Acute Myeloid Leukemia," *Blood*, 1992, 79(2):313-9.

5 + 2 (Cytarabine-Idarubicin) (AML Consolidation)
Index Terms Cytarabine-Idarubicin (5 + 2) (AML Consolidation); Idarubicin-Cytarabine (5 + 2) (AML Consolidation)

Use Leukemia, acute myeloid

Regimen

Cytarabine: IV: 100 mg/m^2/day continuous infusion days 1 to 5
  [total dose/cycle = 500 mg/m^2]
Idarubicin: IV: 13 mg/m^2/day IV bolus days 1 and 2
  [total dose/cycle = 26 mg/m^2]
Administer 2 courses

References

Wiernik PH, Banks P, Case Jr DC, et al, "Cytarabine Plus Idarubicin or Daunorubicin as Induction and Consolidation Therapy for Previously Untreated Adult Patients With Acute Myeloid Leukemia," *Blood*, 1992, 79(2):313-9.

5 + 2 (Cytarabine-Mitoxantrone) (AML Consolidation)
Index Terms Cytarabine-Mitoxantrone (5 + 2) (AML Consolidation)

Use Leukemia, acute myeloid

Regimen

Cytarabine: IV: 100 mg/m^2/day continuous infusion days 1 to 5
  [total dose/cycle = 500 mg/m^2]
Mitoxantrone: IV: 12 mg/m^2/day days 1 and 2
  [total dose/cycle = 24 mg/m^2]
Administered every 28 days for a total of 2 cycles

References

Arlin Z, Case DC Jr, Moore J, et al, "Randomized Multicenter Trial of Cytosine Arabinoside With Mitoxantrone or Daunorubicin in Previously Untreated Adult Patients With Acute Nonlympho-cytic Leukemia (ANLL). Lederle Cooperative Group," *Leukemia*, 1990, 4(3):177-83.

5 + 2 + 5 (Cytarabine-Daunorubicin-Etoposide) (AML Consolidation)

Index Terms Cytarabine-Daunorubicin-Etoposide (5 + 2 + 5) (AML Consolidation)

Use Leukemia, acute myeloid

Regimen

Cytarabine: IV: 100 mg/m^2/day continuous infusion days 1 to 5
  [total dose/cycle = 500 mg/m^2]
Daunorubicin: IV: 50 mg/m^2/day IV bolus days 1 and 2
  [total dose/cycle = 100 mg/m^2]
Etoposide: IV: 75 mg/m^2/day over 1 hour days 1 to 5
  [total dose/cycle = 375 mg/m^2]
Administer 2 courses

References

Bishop JF, Lowenthal RM, Joshua D, et al, "Etoposide In Acute Nonlymphocytic Leukemia, Australian Leukemia Study Group," *Blood*, 1990, 75(1):27-32.
Bishop JF, Matthews JP, Young GA, et al, "A Randomized Study of High-Dose Cytarabine in Induction in Acute Myeloid Leukemia," *Blood*, 1996, 87(5):1710-7.

7 + 3 (Cytarabine-Daunorubicin) (AML Induction)

Index Terms Cytarabine-Daunorubicin (7 + 3) (AML Induction)

Use Leukemia, acute myeloid

Regimen NOTE: Multiple variations are listed.

Variation 1:
  Cytarabine: IV: 100 mg/m^2/day continuous infusion days 1 to 7
    [total dose/cycle = 700 mg/m^2]
  Daunorubicin: IV: 45 mg/m^2/day IV bolus days 1, 2, and 3
    [total dose/cycle = 135 mg/m^2]
  May administer a second induction cycle if needed
Variation 2 (≥60 years of age):
  Cytarabine: IV: 100 mg/m^2/day continuous infusion days 1 to 7
    [total dose/cycle = 700 mg/m^2]
  Daunorubicin: IV: 30 mg/m^2/day days 1, 2, and 3
    [total dose/cycle = 90 mg/m^2]
  May administer a second induction cycle if needed (at a reduced dose of
    daunorubicin [45 mg/m^2])
Variation 3 (between 17 and 60 years of age):
  Cytarabine: IV: 100 mg/m^2/day continuous infusion days 1 to 7
    [total dose/cycle = 700 mg/m^2]
  Daunorubicin: IV: 90 mg/m^2/day IV bolus days 1, 2, and 3
    [total dose/cycle = 270 mg/m^2]
  May administer a second induction cycle if needed
Variation 4 (<60 years of age):
  Cytarabine: IV: 200 mg/m^2/day continuous infusion days 1 to 7
    [total dose/cycle = 1400 mg/m^2]
  Daunorubicin: IV: 45 mg/m^2/day IV bolus days 1, 2, and 3
    [total dose/cycle = 135 mg/m^2]
  May administer a second induction cycle if needed

References

Variation 1:

Dillman RO, Davis RB, Green MR, et al, "A Comparative Study of Two Different Doses of Cytarabine for Acute Myeloid Leukemia: A Phase III Trial of Cancer and Leukemia Group B," *Blood*, 1991, 78(10):2520-6.

Rai KR, Holland JF, Glidewell OJ, et al, "Treatment of Acute Myelocytic Leukemia: A Study by Cancer and Leukemia Group B," *Blood*, 1981, 58(6):1203-12.

Yates J, Glidewell O, Wiernik P, et al, "Cytosine Arabinoside With Daunorubicin or Adriamycin® for Therapy of Acute Myelocytic Leukemia: A CALGB Study," *Blood*, 1982, 60(2):454-62.

Variation 2:

Dillman RO, Davis RB, Green MR, et al, "A Comparative Study of Two Different Doses of Cytarabine for Acute Myeloid Leukemia: A Phase III Trial of Cancer and Leukemia Group B," *Blood*, 1991, 78(10):2520-6.

Variation 3:

Fernandez HF, Sun Z, Yao X, et al, "Anthracycline Dose Intensification in Acute Myeloid Leukemia," *N Engl J Med*, 2009, 361(13):1249-59.

Variation 4:

Dillman RO, Davis RB, Green MR, et al, "A Comparative Study of Two Different Doses of Cytarabine for Acute Myeloid Leukemia: A Phase III Trial of Cancer and Leukemia Group B," *Blood*, 1991, 78(10):2520-6.

7 + 3 (Cytarabine-Idarubicin) (AML Induction)

Index Terms Cytarabine-Idarubicin (7 + 3) (AML Induction)

Use Leukemia, acute myeloid

Regimen NOTE: Multiple variations are listed.

Variation 1:

Cytarabine: IV: 100 mg/m^2/day continuous infusion days 1 to 7
  [total dose/cycle = 700 mg/m^2]

Idarubicin: IV: 12 mg/m^2/day slow IV infusion days 1, 2, and 3
  [total dose/cycle = 36 mg/m^2]

May administer a second induction cycle if needed

Variation 2:

Cytarabine: IV: 100 mg/m^2/day continuous infusion days 1 to 7
  [total dose/cycle = 700 mg/m^2]

Idarubicin: IV: 13 mg/m^2/day slow IV infusion days 1, 2, and 3
  [total dose/cycle = 39 mg/m^2]

May administer a second induction cycle if needed

References

Variation 1:

Vogler WR, Velez-Garcia E, Weiner RS, et al, "A Phase III Trial Comparing Idarubicin and Daunorubicin in Combination With Cytarabine in Acute Myelogenous Leukemia: A Southeastern Cancer Study Group Study," *J Clin Oncol*, 1992, 10(7):1103-11.

Variation 2:

Wiernik PH, Banks P, Case Jr DC, et al, "Cytarabine Plus Idarubicin or Daunorubicin as Induction and Consolidation Therapy for Previously Untreated Adult Patients With Acute Myeloid Leukemia," *Blood*, 1992, 79(2):313-9.

7 + 3 (Cytarabine-Mitoxantrone) (AML Induction)

Index Terms Cytarabine-Mitoxantrone (7 + 3) (AML Induction)

Use Leukemia, acute myeloid

Regimen

Induction:

Cytarabine: IV: 100 mg/m^2/day continuous infusion days 1 to 7
  [total dose/cycle = 700 mg/m^2]

Mitoxantrone: IV: 12 mg/m^2/day days 1, 2, and 3
  [total dose/cycle = 36 mg/m^2]

Reinduction if needed:
  Cytarabine: IV: 100 mg/m²/day continuous infusion days 1 to 5
    [total dose/cycle = 500 mg/m²]
  Mitoxantrone: IV: 12 mg/m²/day days 1 and 2
    [total dose/cycle = 24 mg/m²]

References

Arlin Z, Case DC Jr, Moore J, et al, "Randomized Multicenter Trial of Cytosine Arabinoside With Mitoxantrone or Daunorubicin in Previously Untreated Adult Patients With Acute Nonlymphocytic Leukemia (ANLL). Lederle Cooperative Group," *Leukemia*, 1990, 4(3):177-83.

7 + 3 + 7 (Cytarabine-Daunorubicin-Etoposide) (AML Induction)

Index Terms Cytarabine-Daunorubicin-Etoposide (7 + 3 + 7) (AML Induction)
Use Leukemia, acute myeloid
Regimen
  Cytarabine: IV: 100 mg/m²/day continuous infusion days 1 to 7
    [total dose/cycle = 700 mg/m²]
  Daunorubicin: IV: 50 mg/m²/day days 1, 2, and 3
    [total dose/cycle = 150 mg/m²]
  Etoposide: IV: 75 mg/m²/day over 1 hour days 1 to 7
    [total dose/cycle = 525 mg/m²]
  Up to 3 induction cycles may be given based on individual response

References

Bishop JF, Lowenthal RM, Joshua D, et al, "Etoposide in Acute Nonlymphocytic Leukemia, Australian Leukemia Study Group," *Blood*, 1990, 75(1):27-32.

Bishop JF, Matthews JP, Young GA, et al, "A Randomized Study of High-Dose Cytarabine in Induction in Acute Myeloid Leukemia," *Blood*, 1996, 87(5):1710-7.

Bishop JF, Matthews JP, Young GA, et al, "Intensified Induction Chemotherapy With High Dose Cytarabine and Etoposide for Acute Myeloid Leukemia: A Review and Updated Results of the Australian Leukemia Study Group," *Leuk Lymphoma*, 1998, 28(3-4):315-27.

◆ A1 (NEW) (Neuroblastoma) *see* New A1 (Neuroblastoma) *on page* 2180

A3 (Neuroblastoma)

Index Terms Cyclophosphamide, Doxorubicin, Etoposide, Cisplatin (Neuroblastoma); Regimen A3 (Neuroblastoma)
Use Neuroblastoma
Regimen
  Cycle 1 (New A1):
    Cyclophosphamide: IV: 1200 mg/m² over 6 hours day 1
      [total dose/cycle = 1200 mg/m²]
    Doxorubicin: IV: 40 mg/m² day 3
      [total dose/cycle = 40 mg/m²]
    Etoposide: IV: 100 mg/m²/day days 1 to 5
      [total dose/cycle = 500 mg/m²]
    Cisplatin: IV: 90 mg/m² day 5
      [total dose/cycle = 90 mg/m²]
    Treatment cycle is 28 days
  Cycles 2-5 (A3):
    Cyclophosphamide: IV: 1200 mg/m²/day over 6 hours days 1 and 2
      [total dose/cycle = 2400 mg/m²]
    Doxorubicin: IV: 40 mg/m² day 3
      [total dose/cycle = 40 mg/m²]
    Etoposide: IV: 100 mg/m²/day days 1 to 5
      [total dose/cycle = 500 mg/m²]

Cisplatin: IV: 25 mg/m^2/day continuous infusion days 1 to 5
[total dose/cycle = 125 mg/m^2]
Repeat cycle every 28 days for 5 cycles (total of 6 cycles, cycle 1 administer
New A1, cycles 2 to 5 administer A3)

References

Kaneko M, Nishihira H, Mugishima H, et al, "Stratification of Treatment of Stage 4 Neuroblastoma Patients Based on N-myc Amplification Status. Study Group of Japan for Treatment of Advanced Neuroblastoma, Tokyo, Japan," *Med Pediatr Oncol*, 1998, 31(1):1-7.

Kaneko M, Tsuchida Y, Mugishima H, et al, "Intensified Chemotherapy Increases the Survival Rates in Patients With Stage 4 Neuroblastoma With MYCN Amplification," *J Pediatr Hematol Oncol*, 2002, 24(8):613-21.

Abiraterone-Prednisone (Prostate)

Index Terms Prednisone-Abiraterone (Prostate)

Use Prostate cancer

Regimen

Abiraterone acetate: Oral: 1000 mg once daily days 1 to 28
[total dose/cycle = 28,000 mg]
Prednisone: Oral: 5 mg twice a day days 1 to 28
[total dose/cycle = 280 mg]
Repeat cycle every 28 days until disease progression or unacceptable toxicity

References

de Bono JS, Logothetis CJ, Molina A, et al, "Abiraterone and Increased Survival in Metastatic Prostate Cancer," *New Engl J Med*, 2011, 364(21):1995-2005.

Ryan CJ, Smith MR, de Bone JS, et al, "Interim Analysis (IA) Results of COU-AA-302, A Randomized, Phase III Study of Abiraterone Acetate (AA) in Chemotherapy-Naïve Patients (pts) With Metastatic Castration-Resistant Prostate Cancer (mCRPC)," *J Clin Oncol*, 2012, 30 (18):LBA4518 [abstract LBA4518 from 2012 ASCO Annual Meeting].

ABVD Early Stage (Hodgkin)

Index Terms Doxorubicin, Bleomycin, Vinblastine, Dacarbazine (Hodgkin)

Use Lymphoma, Hodgkin

Regimen NOTE: Multiple variations are listed.

Variation 1 (newly diagnosed, stage I or II, favorable prognosis with no clinical risk factors):
Doxorubicin: IV: 25 mg/m^2/day days 1 and 15
[total dose/cycle = 50 mg/m^2]
Bleomycin: IV: 10 units/m^2/day days 1 and 15
[total dose/cycle = 20 units/m^2]
Vinblastine: IV: 6 mg/m^2/day days 1 and 15
[total dose/cycle = 12 mg/m^2]
Dacarbazine: IV: 375 mg/m^2/day days 1 and 15
[total dose/cycle = 750 mg/m^2]
Repeat cycle every 28 days for a total of 2 cycles followed by 20 Gy of radiation therapy

Variation 2 (newly diagnosed, stage IA or IIA non-bulky, favorable and unfavorable):
Doxorubicin: IV: 25 mg/m^2/day days 1 and 15
[total dose/cycle = 50 mg/m^2]
Bleomycin: IV: 10 units/m^2/day days 1 and 15
[total dose/cycle = 20 units/m^2]
Vinblastine: IV: 6 mg/m^2/day days 1 and 15
[total dose/cycle = 12 mg/m^2]
Dacarbazine: IV: 375 mg/m^2/day days 1 and 15
[total dose/cycle = 750 mg/m^2]

Repeat cycle every 28 days for a total of 4 to 6 cycles. Patient who had complete remission after 2 cycles received a total of 4 cycles, and if the patient did not have a complete remission after 2 cycles received a total of 6 cycles.

Variation 3 (newly diagnosed, stage I and II with certain risk factors, unfavorable prognosis):

Doxorubicin: IV: 25 mg/m^2/day days 1 and 15
 [total dose/cycle = 50 mg/m^2]

Bleomycin: IV: 10 units/m^2/day days 1 and 15
 [total dose/cycle = 20 units/m^2]

Vinblastine: IV: 6 mg/m^2/day days 1 and 15
 [total dose/cycle = 12 mg/m^2]

Dacarbazine: IV: 375 mg/m^2/day days 1 and 15
 [total dose/cycle = 750 mg/m^2]

Repeat cycle every 28 days for a total of 4 cycles followed by 30 Gy of radiation therapy

Variation 4 (newly diagnosed, stage I, II, IIIA, non-bulky):

Doxorubicin: IV: 25 mg/m^2/day days 1 and 15
 [total dose/cycle = 50 mg/m^2]

Bleomycin: IV: 10 units/m^2/day days 1 and 15
 [total dose/cycle = 20 units/m^2]

Vinblastine: IV: 6 mg/m^2/day days 1 and 15
 [total dose/cycle = 12 mg/m^2]

Dacarbazine: IV: 375 mg/m^2/day days 1 and 15
 [total dose/cycle = 750 mg/m^2]

Repeat cycle every 28 days for a total of 6 cycles followed by radiation therapy

References

Variation 1:

Engert A, Plütschow A, Eich HT, et al. Reduced treatment intensity in patients with early-stage Hodgkin's lymphoma. N Engl J Med. 2010;363(7):640-652.

Variation 2:

Meyer RM, Gospodarowicz MK, Connors JM, et al. ABVD alone versus radiation-based therapy in limited-stage Hodgkin's lymphoma. N Engl J Med. 2012;366(5):399-408.

Variation 3:

Eich HT, Diehl V, Görgen H, et al. Intensified chemotherapy and dose-reduced involved-field radiotherapy in patients with early unfavorable Hodgkin's lymphoma: final analysis of the German Hodgkin Study Group HD11 trial. J Clin Oncol. 2010;28(27):4199-4206.

Variation 4:

Straus DJ, Portlock CS, Qin J, et al. Results of a prospective randomized clinical trial of doxorubicin, bleomycin, vinblastine, and dacarbazine (ABVD) followed by radiation therapy (RT) versus ABVD alone for stages I, II, and IIIA nonbulky Hodgkin disease. Blood. 2004;104 (12):3483-3489.

ABVD (Hodgkin)

Index Terms Doxorubicin-Bleomycin-Vinblastine-Dacarbazine (Hodgkin)

Use Lymphoma, Hodgkin

Regimen

Doxorubicin: IV: 25 mg/m^2/day days 1 and 15
 [total dose/cycle = 50 mg/m^2]

Bleomycin: IV: 10 units/m^2/day days 1 and 15
 [total dose/cycle = 20 units/m^2]

Vinblastine: IV: 6 mg/m^2/day days 1 and 15
[total dose/cycle = 12 mg/m^2]
Dacarbazine: IV: 375 mg/m^2/day days 1 and 15
[total dose/cycle = 750 mg/m^2]
Repeat cycle every 28 days for 6-8 cycles

References

Bonadonna G and Santoro A, "ABVD Chemotherapy in the Treatment of Hodgkin's Disease," *Cancer Treat Rev*, 1982, 9(1):21-35.

Canellos GP, Anderson JR, Propert KJ, et al, "Chemotherapy of Advanced Hodgkin's Disease With MOPP, ABVD, or MOPP Alternating With ABVD," *N Engl J Med*, 1992, 327(21):1478-84.

Viviani S, Zinzani PL, Rambaldi A, et al, "ABVD Versus BEACOPP for Hodgkin's Lymphoma When High-Dose Salvage Is Planned," *N Engl J Med*, 2011, 365(3):203-12.

AC (Breast)

Index Terms Cyclophosphamide-Doxorubicin (Breast); Doxorubicin-Cyclophosphamide (Breast)

Use Breast cancer

Regimen NOTE: Multiple variations are listed.
Variation 1 (adjuvant):
Doxorubicin: IV: 60 mg/m^2 day 1
[total dose/cycle = 60 mg/m^2]
Cyclophosphamide: IV: 600 mg/m^2 day 1
[total dose/cycle = 600 mg/m^2]
Repeat cycle every 21 days for 4 cycles
Variation 2 (metastatic):
Doxorubicin: IV: 60 mg/m^2 day 1
[total dose/cycle = 60 mg/m^2]
Cyclophosphamide: IV: 600 mg/m^2 day 1
[total dose/cycle = 600 mg/m^2]
Repeat cycle every 21 days for up to 8 cycles

References

Variation 1:

Fisher B, Brown AM, Dimitrov NV, et al, "Two Months of Doxorubicin-Cyclophosphamide With and Without Interval Reinduction Therapy Compared With 6 Months of Cyclophosphamide, Methotrexate, and Fluorouracil in Positive-Node Breast Cancer Patients With Tamoxifen-Nonresponsive Tumors: Results From the National Surgical Adjuvant Breast and Bowel Project B-15," *J Clin Oncol*, 1990, 8(9):1483-96.

Variation 2:

Nabholtz JM, Falkson C, Campos D, et al. Docetaxel and doxorubicin compared with doxorubicin and cyclophosphamide as first-line chemotherapy for metastatic breast cancer: results of a randomized, multicenter, phase III trial. *J Clin Oncol*. 2003;21(6):968-75.

AC (Dose-Dense) followed by Paclitaxel (Dose-Dense) (Breast)

Index Terms Doxorubicin, Cyclophosphamide, Paclitaxel Dose Dense (Breast)

Use Breast cancer

Regimen
Cycles 1-4:
Doxorubicin: IV: 60 mg/m^2 day 1
[total dose/cycle = 60 mg/m^2]
Cyclophosphamide: IV: 600 mg/m^2 day 1
[total dose/cycle = 600 mg/m^2]

Filgrastim: SubQ: 5 mcg/kg/day days 3 to 10, rounded to either 300 or 480 mcg/day

[total dose/cycle = 40 mcg/kg, 2400-3840 mcg/cycle]

Repeat cycle every 14 days for 4 cycles

followed by

Cycles 5-8:

Paclitaxel: IV: 175 mg/m^2 day 1

[total dose/cycle = 175 mg/m^2]

Filgrastim: SubQ: 5 mcg/kg/day days 3 to 10, rounded to either 300 or 480 mcg/day

[total dose/cycle = 40 mcg/kg, 2400-3840 mcg/cycle]

Repeat cycle every 14 days for 4 cycles

References

Citron ML, Berry DA, Cirrincione C, et al, "Randomized Trial of Dose-Dense Versus Convention-ally Scheduled and Sequential Versus Concurrent Combination Chemotherapy as Postoperative Adjuvant Treatment of Node-Positive Primary Breast Cancer: First Report of Intergroup Trial C9741/Cancer Leukemia Group B Trial 9741," *J Clin Oncol*, 2003, 21(8):1431-9.

AC (Dose-Dense) followed by Paclitaxel (Dose-Dense)-Trastuzumab (Breast)

Index Terms Doxorubicin, Cyclophosphamide, Paclitaxel (Dose-Dense), Trastuzumab (Breast)

Use Breast cancer

Regimen

Cycles 1-4 of AC (dose-dense):

Doxorubicin: IV: 60 mg/m^2 day 1

[total dose/cycle = 60 mg/m^2]

Cyclophosphamide: IV: 600 mg/m^2 day 1

[total dose/cycle = 600 mg/m^2]

Pegfilgrastim: SubQ: 6 mg day 2

[total dose/cycle = 6 mg]

Repeat cycle every 14 days for 4 cycles

followed by

Cycle 1 of Paclitaxel (dose-dense)-Trastuzumab:

Paclitaxel: IV: 175 mg/m^2 day 1

[total dose/cycle 1 = 175 mg/m^2]

Pegfilgrastim: SubQ: 6 mg day 2

[total dose/cycle = 6 mg]

Trastuzumab: IV: 4 mg/kg (loading dose) day 1 cycle 1 only

followed by

Trastuzumab: IV: 2 mg/kg day 8

[total dose/cycle 1 = 6 mg/kg]

Treatment cycle is 14 days

followed by

Cycles 2-4 of Paclitaxel (dose-dense)-Trastuzumab:

Paclitaxel: IV: 175 mg/m^2 day 1

[total dose/cycle 1 = 175 mg/m^2]

Pegfilgrastim: SubQ: 6 mg day 2

[total dose/cycle = 6 mg]

Trastuzumab: IV: 2 mg/kg days 1 and 8
[total dose/cycle = 4 mg/kg]
Repeat cycle every 14 days for 3 cycles
followed by
Trastuzumab: IV: 6 mg/kg day 1
[total dose/cycle = 6 mg/kg]
Repeat cycle every 21 days to complete one year of Trastuzumab

References

Dang C, Fornier M, Sugarman S, et al. The safety of dose-dense doxorubicin and cyclo-phosphamide followed by paclitaxel with trastuzumab in HER-2/neu overexpressed/amplified breast cancer. *J Clin Oncol*. 2008;26(8):1216-22.

AC (Dose-Dense) followed by Paclitaxel Weekly (Breast)

Index Terms Doxorubicin, Cyclophosphamide, Paclitaxel (Breast)

Use Breast cancer

Regimen

Cycles 1-4 (Citron, 2003):
Doxorubicin: IV: 60 mg/m^2 day 1
[total dose/cycle = 60 mg/m^2]
Cyclophosphamide: IV: 600 mg/m^2 day 1
[total dose/cycle = 600 mg/m^2]
Filgrastim: SubQ: ~5 mcg/kg/day days 3 to 10 (rounded to either 300 or 480 mcg/day)
[total dose/cycle = ~40 mcg/kg, 2400-3840 mcg/cycle]
Repeat cycle every 14 days for 4 cycles
followed by (Sparano, 2008):
Paclitaxel: IV: 80 mg/m^2 over 1 hour day 1
[total dose/cycle = 80 mg/m^2]
Repeat cycle every 7 days for 12 cycles

References

Citron ML, Berry DA, Cirrincione C, et al, "Randomized Trial of Dose-Dense Versus Convention-ally Scheduled and Sequential Versus Concurrent Combination Chemotherapy as Postoperative Adjuvant Treatment of Node-Positive Primary Breast Cancer: First Report of Intergroup Trial C9741/Cancer Leukemia Group B Trial 9741," *J Clin Oncol*, 2003, 21(8):1431-9.

Sparano JA, Wang M, Martino S, et al, "Weekly Paclitaxel in the Adjuvant Treatment of Breast Cancer," *N Engl J Med*, 2008, 358(16):1663-71.

AC followed by Docetaxel Every 3 Weeks (Breast)

Index Terms Doxorubicin, Cyclophosphamide, Docetaxel (Breast)

Use Breast cancer

Regimen

Doxorubicin: IV: 60 mg/m^2 over 5-15 minutes day 1
[total dose/cycle = 60 mg/m^2]
Cyclophosphamide: IV: 600 mg/m^2 over 30-60 minutes day 1
[total dose/cycle = 600 mg/m^2]
Repeat cycle every 21 days for 4 cycles
followed by
Docetaxel: IV: 100 mg/m^2 over 1 hour day 1
[total dose/cycle = 100 mg/m^2]
Repeat cycle every 21 days for 4 cycles

References

Sparano JA, Wang M, Martino S, et al, "Weekly Paclitaxel in the Adjuvant Treatment of Breast Cancer," *N Engl J Med*, 2008, 358(16):1663-71.

Swain SM, Jeong JH, Geyer CE, et al, "Longer Therapy, Iatrogenic Amenorrhea, and Survival in Early Breast Cancer, *N Engl J Med*, 2010, 362(22):2053-65.

AC followed by Paclitaxel-Trastuzumab (Breast)

Index Terms Doxorubicin, Cyclophosphamide, Paclitaxel, Trastuzumab (Breast)

Use Breast cancer

Regimen

Cycles 1-4 of AC:

Doxorubicin: IV: 60 mg/m^2 day 1

[total dose/cycle = 60 mg/m^2]

Cyclophosphamide: IV: 600 mg/m^2 day 1

[total dose/cycle = 600 mg/m^2]

Repeat cycle every 21 days for 4 cycles

followed by

Cycle 1 of Paclitaxel-Trastuzumab:

Paclitaxel: IV: 80 mg/m^2 day 1

[total dose/cycle = 80 mg/m^2]

Trastuzumab: IV: 4 mg/kg (loading dose) day 1

[total dose/cycle = 4 mg/kg]

Treatment cycle is 7 days for 1 cycle

followed by

Weekly Paclitaxel-Trastuzumab:

Paclitaxel: IV: 80 mg/m^2 day 1

[total dose/cycle = 80 mg/m^2]

Trastuzumab: IV: 2 mg/kg day 1

[total dose/cycle = 2 mg/kg]

Repeat cycle every 7 days for 11 cycles

followed by

Weekly Trastuzumab:

Trastuzumab: IV: 2 mg/kg day 1

[total dose/cycle = 2 mg/kg]

Repeat cycle every 7 days for 40 cycles (total of 52 weeks of trastuzumab)

References

Romond EH, Perez EA, Bryant J, et al, "Trastuzumab Plus Adjuvant Chemotherapy for Operable HER2-Positive Breast Cancer," *N Engl J Med*, 2005, 353(16):1673-84.

AC followed by Paclitaxel Weekly (Breast)

Index Terms Doxorubicin, Cyclophosphamide, Paclitaxel (Breast)

Use Breast cancer

Regimen

Doxorubicin: IV: 60 mg/m^2 over 5-15 minutes day 1

[total dose/cycle = 60 mg/m^2]

Cyclophosphamide: IV: 600 mg/m^2 over 30-60 minutes day 1

[total dose/cycle = 600 mg/m^2]

Repeat cycle every 21 days for 4 cycles

followed by

Paclitaxel: IV: 80 mg/m^2 over 1 hour day 1

[total dose/cycle = 80 mg/m^2]

Repeat cycle every 7 days for 12 cycles

References

Sparano JA, Wang M, Martino S, et al, "Weekly Paclitaxel in the Adjuvant Treatment of Breast Cancer, *N Engl J Med*, 2008, 358(16):1663-71.

AD (Soft Tissue Sarcoma)

Index Terms Doxorubicin-Dacarbazine (Soft Tissue Sarcoma)

Use Soft tissue sarcoma

Regimen NOTE: Multiple variations are listed.

Variation 1 (metastatic):

Doxorubicin: IV: 15 mg/m^2/day continuous infusion days 1 to 4
[total dose/cycle = 60 mg/m^2]

Dacarbazine: IV: 187.5 mg/m^2/day continuous infusion days 1 to 4
[total dose/cycle = 750 mg/m^2]

Repeat cycle every 21 days; maximum lifetime doxorubicin dose of 450 mg/m^2

Variation 2 (metastatic):

Doxorubicin: IV: 60 mg/m^2 IV bolus day 1
[total dose/cycle = 60 mg/m^2]

Dacarbazine: IV: 750 mg/m^2/day IV bolus day 1
[total dose/cycle = 750 mg/m^2]

Repeat cycle every 21 days; maximum lifetime doxorubicin dose of 450 mg/m^2

Variation 3 (metastatic):

Doxorubicin: IV: 15 mg/m^2/day continuous infusion days 1 to 4
[total dose/cycle = 60 mg/m^2]

Dacarbazine: IV: 250 mg/m^2/day continuous infusion days 1 to 4
[total dose/cycle = 1000 mg/m^2]

Repeat cycle every 21 days

Variation 4 (metastatic):

Doxorubicin: IV: 60 mg/m^2 day 1
[total dose/cycle = 60 mg/m^2]

Dacarbazine: IV: 250 mg/m^2/day days 1 to 5
[total dose/cycle = 1250 mg/m^2]

Repeat cycle every 21 days until disease progression; when maximum lifetime doxorubicin dose received, continue with single agent dacarbazine

References

Variations 1 and 2:

Zalupski M, Metch B, Fletcher WS, et al, "Phase III Comparison of Doxorubicin and Dacarbazine Given by Bolus Versus Infusion in Patients With Soft-Tissue Sarcomas: A Southwest Oncology Group Study," *J Natl Cancer Inst*, 1991, 83(13):926-32.

Variation 3:

Antman K, Crowley J, Balcerzak SP, et al, "An Intergroup Phase III Randomized Study of Doxorubicin and Dacarbazine With or Without Ifosfamide and Mesna in Advanced Soft Tissue and Bone Sarcomas," *J Clin Oncol*, 1993, 11(7):1276-85.

Variation 4:

Borden EC, Amato DA, Rosenbaum C, et al, "Randomized Comparison of Three Adriamycin Regimens for Metastatic Soft Tissue Sarcomas," *J Clin Oncol*, 1987, 5(6):840-50.

AIM (Soft Tissue Sarcoma)

Index Terms Doxorubicin-Ifosfamide (Soft Tissue Sarcoma); Ifosfamide-Doxorubicin (Soft Tissue Sarcoma)

Use Soft tissue sarcoma

Regimen NOTE: Mesna uroprotection should be administered before and 4 and 8 hours after ifosfamide days 1 to 4.
Ifosfamide: IV: 1,500 mg/m^2/day over 2 hours days 1 to 4
[total dose/cycle = 6,000 mg/m^2]
Doxorubicin: IV: 20 mg/m^2/day continuous infusion days 1, 2, and 3
[total dose/cycle = 60 mg/m^2]
Filgrastim: SubQ: 5 mcg/kg/day for 10 days, starting 24 hours after last dose of mesna
[total dose/cycle = 50 mcg/kg]
Repeat cycle every 21 days for a total of 4 cycles for localized disease and 6 cycles for metastatic disease

References

Worden FP, Taylor JM, Biermann JS, et al. Randomized phase II evaluation of 6 g/m^2 of ifosfamide plus doxorubicin and granulocyte colony-stimulating factor (G-CSF) compared with 12 g/m^2 of ifosfamide plus doxorubicin and G-CSF in the treatment of poor-prognosis soft tissue sarcoma. *J Clin Oncol.* 2005;23(1):105-112.

BEACOPP-14 (Hodgkin)

Index Terms Bleomycin, Etoposide, Doxorubicin, Cyclophosphamide, Vincristine, Procarbazine, Prednisone (Hodgkin)
Use Lymphoma, Hodgkin
Regimen
Bleomycin: IV: 10 units/m^2 day 8
[total dose/cycle = 10 units/m^2]
Etoposide: IV: 100 mg/m^2/day days 1, 2, and 3
[total dose/cycle = 300 mg/m^2]
Doxorubicin: IV: 25 mg/m^2 day 1
[total dose/cycle = 25 mg/m^2]

Cyclophosphamide: IV: 650 mg/m^2 day 1
[total dose/cycle = 650 mg/m^2]
Vincristine: IV: 1.4 mg/m^2 (maximum dose: 2 mg) day 8
[total dose/cycle = 1.4 mg/m^2; maximum: 2 mg]
Procarbazine: Oral: 100 mg/m^2/day days 1 to 7
[total dose/cycle = 700 mg/m^2]
Prednisone: Oral: 80 mg/m^2/day days 1 to 7
[total dose/cycle = 560 mg/m^2]
Filgrastim: SubQ: 300 mcg/day (patients <75 kg) or 480 mcg/day (patients ≥75 kg) days 8 to13
Repeat cycle every 14 days for a total of 8 cycles

References

Sieber M, Bredenfeld H, Josting A, et al, "14-Day Variant of the Bleomycin, Etoposide, Doxorubicin, Cyclophosphamide, Vincristine, Procarbazine, and Prednisone Regimen in Advanced-Stage Hodgkin's Lymphoma: Results of a Pilot Study of the German Hodgkin's Lymphoma Study Group," *J Clin Oncol*, 2003, 21(9):1734-9.

◆ **BEACOPP Baseline (Hodgkin)** *see* BEACOPP Standard (Hodgkin)
on page 1984

BEACOPP Escalated (Hodgkin)

Index Terms Bleomycin, Etoposide, Doxorubicin, Cyclophosphamide, Vincristine, Procarbazine, Prednisone (Hodgkin)

Use Lymphoma, Hodgkin

Regimen

Bleomycin: IV: 10 units/m^2 day 8
[total dose/cycle = 10 units/m^2]
Etoposide: IV: 200 mg/m^2/day days 1, 2, and 3
[total dose/cycle = 600 mg/m^2]
Doxorubicin: IV: 35 mg/m^2 day 1
[total dose/cycle = 35 mg/m^2]
Cyclophosphamide: IV: 1200 mg/m^2 day 1
[total dose/cycle = 1200 mg/m^2]
Vincristine: IV: 1.4 mg/m^2 (maximum dose: 2 mg) day 8
[total dose/cycle = 1.4 mg/m^2: maximum: 2 mg]
Procarbazine: Oral: 100 mg/m^2/day days 1 to 7
[total dose/cycle = 700 mg/m^2]
Prednisone: Oral: 40 mg/m^2/day days 1 to 14
[total dose/cycle = 560 mg/m^2]
Filgrastim: SubQ: 300 or 480 mcg/day (depending on weight of 75 kg) day 8 until leukocyte recovery (3 days at >1000/mm^3)
Repeat cycle every 21 days for a total of 8 cycles

References

Diehl V, Franklin J, Hasenclever D, et al, "BEACOPP, A New Dose-Escalated and Accelerated Regimen, Is at Least as Effective as COPP/ABVD in Patients With Advanced-Stage Hodgkin's Lymphoma: Interim Report From a Trial of the German Hodgkin's Lymphoma Study Group," *J Clin Oncol*, 1998, 16(12):3810-21.

Diehl V, Franklin J, Pfreundschuh M, et al, "Standard and Increased-Dose BEACOPP Chemotherapy Compared With COPP-ABVD for Advanced Hodgkin's disease," *N Engl J Med*, 2003, 348(24):2386-95.

Engert A, Diehl V, Franklin J, et al, "Escalated-Dose BEACOPP in the Treatment of Patients With Advanced-Stage Hodgkin's Lymphoma: 10 Years of Follow-Up of the GHSG HD9 Study," *J Clin Oncol*, 2009, 27(27):4548-54.

BEACOPP Escalated Plus Standard (Hodgkin)

Index Terms Bleomycin, Etoposide, Doxorubicin, Cyclophosphamide, Vincristine, Procarbazine, Prednisone (Hodgkin)

Use Lymphoma, Hodgkin

Regimen NOTE: Multiple variations are listed.

Variation 1: BEACOPP Escalated for 4 cycles **followed by** 2 cycles of BEACOPP Standard

BEACOPP Escalated for 4 cycles:

Bleomycin: IV: 10 units/m^2 day 8
[total dose/cycle = 10 units/m^2]

Etoposide: IV: 200 mg/m^2/day days 1, 2, and 3
[total dose/cycle = 600 mg/m^2]

Doxorubicin: IV: 35 mg/m^2 day 1
[total dose/cycle = 35 mg/m^2]

Cyclophosphamide: IV: 1250 mg/m^2 day 1
[total dose/cycle = 1250 mg/m^2]

Vincristine: IV: 1.4 mg/m^2 (maximum dose: 2 mg) day 8
[total dose/cycle = 1.4 mg/m^2: maximum: 2 mg]

Procarbazine: Oral: 100 mg/m^2/day days 1 to 7
[total dose/cycle = 700 mg/m^2]

Prednisone: Oral: 40 mg/m^2/day days 1 to 14
[total dose/cycle = 560 mg/m^2]

Filgrastim: SubQ: 300 mcg/day day 8 until neutrophil recovery (>500/mm^3)

Repeat cycle every 21 days for a total of 4 cycles

Followed by BEACOPP Standard for 2 cycles:

Bleomycin: IV: 10 units/m^2 day 8
[total dose/cycle = 10 units/m^2]

Etoposide: IV: 100 mg/m^2/day days 1, 2, and 3
[total dose/cycle = 300 mg/m^2]

Doxorubicin: IV: 25 mg/m^2 day 1
[total dose/cycle = 25 mg/m^2]

Cyclophosphamide: IV: 650 mg/m^2 day 1
[total dose/cycle = 650 mg/m^2]

Vincristine: IV: 1.4 mg/m^2 (maximum dose: 2 mg) day 8
[total dose/cycle = 1.4 mg/m^2: maximum: 2 mg]

Procarbazine: Oral: 100 mg/m^2/day days 1 to 7
[total dose/cycle = 700 mg/m^2]

Prednisone: Oral: 40 mg/m^2/day days 1 to 14
[total dose/cycle = 560 mg/m^2]

Filgrastim: SubQ: 300 mcg/day day 8 until neutrophil recovery (>500/mm^3)

Repeat cycle every 21 days for a total of 2 cycles

Variation 2: BEACOPP Escalated for 4 cycles **followed by** 4 cycles of BEACOPP Standard

BEACOPP Escalated for 4 cycles:

Bleomycin: IV: 10 units/m^2 day 8
[total dose/cycle = 10 units/m^2]

Etoposide: IV: 200 mg/m^2/day days 1, 2, and 3
[total dose/cycle = 600 mg/m^2]

Doxorubicin: IV: 35 mg/m^2 day 1
[total dose/cycle = 35 mg/m^2]

Cyclophosphamide: IV: 1250 mg/m^2 day 1
[total dose/cycle = 1250 mg/m^2]

Vincristine: IV: 1.4 mg/m^2 (maximum dose: 2 mg) day 8
[total dose/cycle = 1.4 mg/m^2: maximum: 2 mg]
Procarbazine: Oral: 100 mg/m^2/day days 1 to 7
[total dose/cycle = 700 mg/m^2]
Prednisone: Oral: 40 mg/m^2/day days 1 to 14
[total dose/cycle = 560 mg/m^2]
Filgrastim: SubQ: 300 mcg/day day 8 until neutrophil count >1000/mm^3 for 3 consecutive days)
Repeat cycle every 21 days for a total of 4 cycles
Followed by BEACOPP Standard for 4 cycles:
Bleomycin: IV: 10 units/m^2 day 8
[total dose/cycle = 10 units/m^2]
Etoposide: IV: 100 mg/m^2/day days 1, 2, and 3
[total dose/cycle = 300 mg/m^2]
Doxorubicin: IV: 25 mg/m^2 day 1
[total dose/cycle = 25 mg/m^2]
Cyclophosphamide: IV: 650 mg/m^2 day 1
[total dose/cycle = 650 mg/m^2]
Vincristine: IV: 1.4 mg/m^2 (maximum dose: 2 mg) day 8
[total dose/cycle = 1.4 mg/m^2: maximum: 2 mg]
Procarbazine: Oral: 100 mg/m^2/day days 1 to 7
[total dose/cycle = 700 mg/m^2]
Prednisone: Oral: 40 mg/m^2/day days 1 to 14
[total dose/cycle = 560 mg/m^2]
Filgrastim: SubQ: 300 mcg/day day 8 until neutrophil count >1000/mm^3 for 3 consecutive days)
Repeat cycle every 21 days for a total of 4 cycles

References

Variation 1:
Federico M, Luminari S, Iannitto E, et al, "ABVD Compared With BEACOPP Compared With CEC for the Initial Treatment of Patients With Advanced Hodgkin's Lymphoma: Results From the HD2000 Gruppo Italiano per lo Studio dei Linfomi Trial," *J Clin Oncol*, 2009, 27(5):805-11.
Variation 2:
Viviani S, Zinzani PL, Rambaldi A, et al, "ABVD Versus BEACOPP for Hodgkin's Lymphoma When High-Dose Salvage Is Planned," *N Engl J Med*, 2011, 365(3):203-12.

BEACOPP Standard (Hodgkin)

Index Terms BEACOPP Baseline (Hodgkin); Bleomycin, Etoposide, Doxorubicin, Cyclophosphamide, Vincristine, Procarbazine, Prednisone (Hodgkin)
Use Lymphoma, Hodgkin
Regimen
Bleomycin: IV: 10 units/m^2 day 8
[total dose/cycle = 10 units/m^2]
Etoposide: IV: 100 mg/m^2/day days 1, 2, and 3
[total dose/cycle = 300 mg/m^2]
Doxorubicin: IV: 25 mg/m^2 day 1
[total dose/cycle = 25 mg/m^2]
Cyclophosphamide: IV: 650 mg/m^2 day 1
[total dose/cycle = 650 mg/m^2]
Vincristine: IV: 1.4 mg/m^2 (maximum dose: 2 mg) day 8
[total dose/cycle = 1.4 mg/m^2; maximum: 2 mg]
Procarbazine: Oral: 100 mg/m^2/day days 1 to 7
[total dose/cycle = 700 mg/m^2]

Prednisone: Oral: 40 mg/m^2/day days 1 to 14

[total dose/cycle = 560 mg/m^2]

Repeat cycle every 21 days for a total of 8 cycles

References

Diehl V, Franklin J, Hasenclever D, et al, "BEACOPP, a New Dose-Escalated and Accelerated Regimen, Is at Least as Effective as COPP/ABVD in Patients With Advanced-Stage Hodgkin's Lymphoma: Interim Report From a Trial of the German Hodgkin's Lymphoma Study Group," *J Clin Oncol*, 1998, 16(12):3810-21.

Diehl V, Sieber M, Rüffer U, et al, "BEACOPP: An Intensified Chemotherapy Regimen in Advanced Hodgkin's Disease. The German Hodgkin's Lymphoma Study Group," *Ann Oncol*, 1997, 8(2):143-8.

Bendamustine-Bortezomib-Rituximab (NHL-Follicular)

Index Terms Bortezomib-Bendamustine-Rituximab (NHL-Follicular); Rituximab-Bortezomib-Bendamustine (NHL-Follicular); VBR (NHL-Follicular)

Use Lymphoma, non-Hodgkin (relapsed/refractory follicular NHL)

Regimen NOTE: Multiple variations are listed.

Variation 1:

Bortezomib: IV: 1.3 mg/m^2/day days 1, 4, 8, and 11

[total dose/cycle = 5.2 mg/m^2]

Rituximab: IV: 375 mg/m^2 day 1

[total dose/cycle = 375 mg/m^7]

Bendamustine: IV: 90 mg/m^2/day over 30 to 60 minutes days 1 and 4

[total dose/cycle = 180 mg/m^2]

Repeat cycle every 28 days for 6 cycles

Variation 2:

Cycle 1:

Bortezomib: IV: 1.6 mg/m^2/day days 1, 8, 15, and 22

[total dose/cycle = 6.4 mg/m^2]

Bendamustine: IV: 90 mg/m^2/day over 60 minutes days 1 and 2

[total dose/cycle = 180 mg/m^2]

Rituximab: IV: 375 mg/m^2/day days 1, 8, 15, and 22 cycle 1 only

[total dose/cycle 1 = 1,500 mg/m^2]

Treatment duration for cycle 1 is 35 days

Cycles 2 to 5:

Bortezomib: IV: 1.6 mg/m^2/day days 1, 8, 15, and 22

[total dose/cycle = 6.4 mg/m^2]

Bendamustine: IV: 90 mg/m^2/day over 60 minutes days 1 and 2

[total dose/cycle = 180 mg/m^2]

Rituximab: IV: 375 mg/m^2 day 1

[total dose/cycle = 375 mg/m^2]

Repeat cycle every 35 days for a total of 5 cycles

References

Variation 1:

Friedberg JW, Vose JM, Kelly JL, et al. The combination of bendamustine, bortezomib, and rituximab for patients with relapsed/refractory indolent and mantle cell non-Hodgkin lymphoma. *Blood*. 2011;117(10):2807-2812.

Variation 2:

Fowler N, Kahl BS, Lee P, et al. Bortezomib, bendamustine, and rituximab in patients with relapsed or refractory follicular lymphoma: the phase II VERTICAL study. *J Clin Oncol*. 2011;29(25):3389-3395.

Bendamustine-Lenalidomide-Dexamethasone (Multiple Myeloma)

Index Terms BLD (Multiple Myeloma); Lenalidomide-Bendamustine-Dexamethasone (Multiple Myeloma)

Use Multiple myeloma

Regimen

Bendamustine: IV: 75 mg/m^2/day days 1 and 2
[total dose/cycle = 150 mg/m^2]

Lenalidomide: Oral: 10 mg once daily days 1 to 21
[total dose/cycle = 210 mg]

Dexamethasone: Oral: 40 mg once daily on days 1, 8, 15, and 22
[total dose/cycle = 160 mg]

Repeat cycle every 28 days for up to a maximum of 8 cycles

References

Lentzsch S, O'Sullivan A, Kennedy RC, et al. Combination of bendamustine, lenalidomide, and dexamethasone (BLD) in patients with relapsed or refractory multiple myeloma is feasible and highly effective: results of phase 1/2 open-label, dose escalation study. *Blood*. 2012;119 (20):4608-4613.

Bendamustine-Obinutuzumab (NHL-Follicular)

Index Terms Obinutuzumab-Bendamustine (NHL-Follicular)

Use Lymphoma, non-Hodgkin (rituximab-refractory follicular NHL)

Regimen

Cycle 1:

Obinutuzumab: IV: 1,000 mg/day days 1, 8, and 15
[total dose/cycle = 3,000 mg]

Bendamustine: IV: 90 mg/m^2/day days 1 and 2
[total dose/cycle = 180 mg/m^2]

Treatment cycle is 28 days

Cycles 2 to 6:

Obinutuzumab: IV: 1,000 mg day 1
[total dose/cycle = 1,000 mg]

Bendamustine: IV: 90 mg/m^2/day days 1 and 2
[total dose/cycle = 180 mg/m^2]

Repeat cycle every 28 days for a total of 6 cycles

Maintenance (in patients who achieve stable disease, complete response, or partial response):

Obinutuzumab: IV: 1,000 mg day 1
[total dose/cycle = 1,000 mg]

Repeat cycle every 2 months for a total of 2 years

References

Sehn LH, Chua NS, Mayer J, et al. GADOLIN: Primary results from a phase III study of obinutuzumab plus bendamustine compared with bendamustine alone in patients with rituximab-refractory indolent non-Hodgkin lymphoma. *J Clin Oncol*. 2015;33(18s):LBA8502 (abstract LBA8502 from 2015 ASCO annual meeting].

Bendamustine-Rituximab (CLL)

Index Terms B-R (CLL); BR (CLL); Rituximab-Bendamustine (CLL)

Use Leukemia, chronic lymphocytic

Regimen NOTE: Multiple variations are listed.
 Variation 1 (relapsed/refractory):
  Cycle 1:
   Rituximab: IV: 375 mg/m^2 day 0 cycle 1 only
    [total dose/cycle 1 = 375 mg/m^2]
   Bendamustine: IV: 70 mg/m^2/day days 1 and 2
    [total dose/cycle = 140 mg/m^2]
  Cycle 2 to 6:
   Rituximab: IV: 500 mg/m^2 day 1
    [total dose/cycle = 500 mg/m^2]
   Bendamustine: IV: 70 mg/m^2/day days 1 and 2
    [total dose/cycle = 140 mg/m^2]
  Repeat cycle every 28 days for up to 6 cycles
 Variation 2 (first-line):
  Cycle 1:
   Rituximab: IV: 375 mg/m^2 day 0 cycle 1 only
    [total dose/cycle 1 = 375 mg/m^2]
   Bendamustine: IV: 90 mg/m^2/day days 1 and 2
    [total dose/cycle = 180 mg/m^2]
  Cycles 2 to 6:
   Rituximab: IV: 500 mg/m^2 day 1
    [total dose/cycle = 500 mg/m^2]
   Bendamustine: IV: 90 mg/m^2/day days 1 and 2
    [total dose/cycle = 180 mg/m^2]
  Repeat cycle every 28 days for up to 6 cycles

References
Variation 1:
Fischer K, Cramer P, Busch R, et al. Bendamustine combined with rituximab in patients with relapsed and/or refractory chronic lymphocytic leukemia: a multicenter phase II trial of the German Chronic Lymphocytic Leukemia Study Group. *J Clin Oncol.* 2011;29(26):3559-3566.
Variation 2:
Fischer K, Cramer P, Busch R, et al. Bendamustine in combination with rituximab for previously untreated patients with chronic lymphocytic leukemia: a multicenter phase II trial of the German Chronic Lymphocytic Leukemia Study Group. *J Clin Oncol.* 2012;30(26):3209-3216.

Bendamustine-Rituximab (NHL-Follicular)

Index Terms B-R (NHL-Follicular); BR (NHL-Follicular); Rituximab-Bendamustine (NHL-Follicular)
Use Lymphoma, non-Hodgkin (grade 1 and grade 2 follicular)
Regimen
 Rituximab: IV: 375 mg/m^2 day 1
  [total dose/cycle = 375 mg/m^2]
 Bendamustine: IV: 90 mg/m^2/day over 30 to 60 minutes days 1 and 2
  [total dose/cycle = 180 mg/m^2]
 Repeat cycle every 28 days for 6 to 8 cycles

References
Flinn IW, van der Jagt R, Kahl BS, et al. Randomized trial of bendamustine-rituximab or R-CHOP/R-CVP in first-line treatment of indolent NHL or MCL: the BRIGHT study. *Blood.* 2014;123 (19):2944-2952.
Rummel MJ, Niederle N, Maschmeyer G, et al. Bendamustine plus rituximab versus CHOP plus rituximab as first-line treatment for patients with indolent and mantle-cell lymphomas: an open-label, multicentre, randomised, phase 3 non-inferiority trial. *Lancet.* 2013;381(9873):1203-1210.

Bendamustine-Rituximab (NHL-Mantle Cell)

Index Terms B-R (NHL-Mantle Cell); BR (NHL-Mantle Cell); Rituximab-Bendamustine (NHL-Mantle Cell)

◀ **Use** Lymphoma, non-Hodgkin (Mantle cell)
Regimen NOTE: Multiple variations are listed.
Variation 1 (first-line):
Rituximab: IV: 375 mg/m² day 1
[total dose/cycle = 375 mg/m²]
Bendamustine: IV: 90 mg/m²/day over 30 to 60 minutes days 1 and 2
[total dose/cycle = 180 mg/m²]
Repeat cycle every 28 days for 6 to 8 cycles
Variation 2 (refractory):
Rituximab: IV: 375 mg/m² day 1
[total dose/cycle = 375 mg/m²]
Bendamustine: IV: 90 mg/m²/day over 30 minutes days 1 and 2
[total dose/cycle = 180 mg/m²]
Repeat cycle every 28 days for up to 6 cycles

References

Variation 1:
Flinn IW, van der Jagt R, Kahl BS, et al. Randomized trial of bendamustine-rituximab or R-CHOP/
R-CVP in first-line treatment of indolent NHL or MCL: the BRIGHT study. *Blood*. 2014;123
(19):2944-2952.
Rummel MJ, Niederle N, Maschmeyer G, et al. Bendamustine plus rituximab versus CHOP plus
rituximab as first-line treatment for patients with indolent and mantle-cell lymphomas: an open-
label, multicentre, randomised, phase 3 non-inferiority trial. *Lancet*. 2013;381(9873):1203-1210.
Variation 2:
Rummel M, Kaiser U, Balser C, et al. Bendamustine plus rituximab versus fludarabine plus
rituximab for patients with relapsed indolent and mantle-cell lymphomas: a multicentre, randomised, open-label, non-inferiority phase 3 trial. *Lancet Oncol*. 2016;17(1):57-66.

Bendamustine-Rituximab (Waldenstrom Macroglobulinemia)

Index Terms BR (Waldenstrom Macroglobulinemia); Rituximab-Bendamustine (Waldenstrom Macroglobulinemia)
Use Waldenstrom macroglobulinemia
Regimen NOTE: Multiple variations are listed.
Variation 1:
Rituximab: IV: 375 mg/m² day 1 or day 2
[total dose/cycle = 375 mg/m²]
Bendamustine: IV: 90 mg/m²/day days 1 and 2
[total dose/cycle = 180 mg/m²]
Repeat cycle every 28 days for 6 cycles
Variation 2:
Rituximab: IV: 375 mg/m²/day days 1, 7, 35, 63, 91, 120
[total dose = 2250 mg/m²]
Bendamustine: IV: 90 mg/m²/day over 30 minutes days 8 and 9, 36 and 37,
64 and 65, and 92 and 93
[total dose = 720 mg/m²]

References

Variation 1:
Treon SP, Hanzis C, Tripsas C, et al. Bendamustine therapy in patients with relapsed or refractory
Waldenström's macroglobulinemia. *Clin Lymphoma Myeloma Leuk*. 2011; 11(1):133-135.
Variation 2:
Rummel MJ, Al-Batran SE, Kim SZ, et al. Bendamustine plus rituximab is effective and has a
favorable toxicity profile in the treatment of mantle cell and low-grade non-Hodgkin's lymphoma.
J Clin Oncol. 2005;23(15):3383-3389.

BEP (Ovarian)

Index Terms Bleomycin-Etoposide-Cisplatin (Ovarian)

Use Ovarian cancer (germ cell tumors)
Regimen
Bleomycin: IV: 30 units once weekly
[total dose/cycle = 90 units]
Etoposide: IV: 100 mg/m^2/day days 1 to 5
[total dose/cycle = 500 mg/m^2]
Cisplatin: IV: 20 mg/m^2/day days 1 to 5
[total dose/cycle = 100 mg/m^2]
Repeat cycle every 21 days for 3 cycles
References
Williams S, Blessing JA, Liao SY, Ball H, Hanjani P. Adjuvant therapy of ovarian germ cell tumors with cisplatin, etoposide, and bleomycin: a trial of the Gynecologic Oncology Group. *J Clin Oncol.* 1994;12(4):701-706.

BEP (Testicular)

Index Terms Bleomycin-Etoposide-Cisplatin (Testicular)
Use Testicular cancer
Regimen NOTE: Multiple variations are listed.
Variation 1 (good risk):
Bleomycin: IV: 30 units/day days 1, 8, and 15
[total dose/cycle = 90 units]
Etoposide: IV: 100 mg/m^2/day days 1 to 5
[total dose/cycle = 500 mg/m^2]
Cisplatin: IV: 20 mg/m^2/day days 1 to 5
[total dose/cycle = 100 mg/m^2]
Repeat cycle every 21 days for 3 cycles
Variation 2 (intermediate/poor risk):
Bleomycin: IV: 30 units/day days 1, 8, and 15
[total dose/cycle = 90 units]
Etoposide: IV: 100 mg/m^2/day days 1 to 5
[total dose/cycle = 500 mg/m^2]
Cisplatin: IV: 20 mg/m^2/day days 1 to 5
[total dose/cycle = 100 mg/m^2]
Repeat cycle every 21 days for 4 cycles
References
Variation 1:
Einhorn LH, Williams SD, Loehrer PJ, Birch R, Drasga R, Omura G, et al. Evaluation of optimal duration of chemotherapy in favorable-prognosis disseminated germ cell tumors: a Southeastern Cancer Study Group protocol. *J Clin Oncol.* 1989;7(3):387-391.
Garcia-del-Muro X, Maroto P, Gumà J, et al. Chemotherapy as an alternative to radiotherapy in the treatment of stage IIA and IIB testicular seminoma: a Spanish Germ Cell Cancer Group Study. *J Clin Oncol.* 2008;26(33):5416-5421.
Saxman SB, Finch D, Gonin R, Einhorn LH. Long-term follow-up of a phase III study of three versus four cycles of bleomycin, etoposide, and cisplatin in favorable-prognosis germ-cell tumors: the Indian University experience. *J Clin Oncol.* 1998;16(2):702-706.
Variation 2:
Culine S, Kramar A, Théodore C, et al. Randomized trial comparing bleomycin/etoposide/cisplatin with alternating cisplatin/cyclophosphamide/doxorubicin and vinblastine/bleomycin regimens of chemotherapy for patients with intermediate- and poor-risk metastatic nonseminomatous germ cell tumors: Genito-Urinary Group of the French Federation of Cancer Centers Trial T93MP. *J Clin Oncol.* 2008;26(3):421-427.
Nichols CR, Catalano PJ, Crawford ED, Vogelzang NJ, Einhorn LH, Loehrer PJ. Randomized comparison of cisplatin and etoposide and either bleomycin or ifosfamide in treatment of advanced disseminated germ cell tumors: an Eastern Cooperative Oncology Group, Southwest Oncology Group, and Cancer and Leukemia Group B Study. *J Clin Oncol.* 1998;16(4):1287-1293.

Bevacizumab-Carboplatin-Gemcitabine (Ovarian)

Index Terms Bevacizumab-Gemcitabine-Carboplatin (Ovarian); Carboplatin-Gemcitabine-Bevacizumab (Ovarian); GC-Bevacizumab (Ovarian)

Use Ovarian cancer

Regimen

Bevacizumab: IV: 15 mg/kg day 1
[total dose/cycle = 15 mg/kg]
Gemcitabine: IV: 1000 mg/m^2/day days 1 and 8
[total dose/cycle = 2000 mg/m^2]
Carboplatin: IV: AUC 4 day 1
[total dose/cycle = AUC = 4]
Repeat cycle every 21 days for 6-10 cycles
followed by
Bevacizumab: IV: 15 mg/kg day 1
[total dose/cycle = 15 mg/kg]
Repeat cycle every 21 days until disease progression or unacceptable toxicity

References

Aghajanian C, Blank SV, Goff BA, et al, "OCEANS: A Randomized, Double-Blind, Placebo-Controlled Phase III Trial of Chemotherapy With or Without Bevacizumab in Patients With Platinum-Sensitive Recurrent Epithelial Ovarian, Primary Peritoneal, or Fallopian Tube Cancer," *J Clin Oncol*, 2012, 30(17):2039-45.

Bevacizumab-Carboplatin-Paclitaxel (NSCLC)

Index Terms Bevacizumab-Paclitaxel-Carboplatin (NSCLC); Carboplatin-Paclitaxel-Bevacizumab (NSCLC)

Use Lung cancer, non-small cell (nonsquamous cell histology)

Regimen

Paclitaxel: IV: 200 mg/m^2 day 1
[total dose/cycle = 200 mg/m^2]
Carboplatin: IV: AUC 6 day 1
[total dose/cycle = AUC = 6]
Bevacizumab: IV: 15 mg/kg day 1
[total dose/cycle = 15 mg/kg]
Repeat cycle every 21 days for 6 cycles
followed by
Bevacizumab: IV: 15 mg/kg day 1
[total dose/cycle = 15 mg/kg]
Repeat cycle every 21 days until disease progression or unacceptable toxicity

References

Sandler A, Gray R, Perry MC, et al, "Paclitaxel-Carboplatin Alone or With Bevacizumab for Nonsmall-Cell Lung Cancer," *N Engl J Med*, 2006, 355(24):2542-50.

Bevacizumab-Carboplatin-Pemetrexed (NSCLC)

Index Terms Carboplatin-Pemetrexed-Bevacizumab (NSCLC); Pemetrexed-Carboplatin-Bevacizumab (NSCLC)

Use Lung cancer, non-small cell

Regimen

Pemetrexed: IV: 500 mg/m^2 over 10 minutes day 1
[total dose/cycle = 500 mg/m^2]
Carboplatin: IV: AUC 6 day 1
[total dose/cycle = AUC = 6]

Bevacizumab: IV: 15 mg/kg day 1
  [total dose/cycle = 15 mg/kg]
Repeat cycle every 21 days for 6 cycles
followed by
Pemetrexed: IV: 500 mg/m^2 over 10 minutes day 1
  [total dose/cycle = 500 mg/m^2]
Bevacizumab: IV: 15 mg/kg day 1
  [total dose/cycle = 15 mg/kg]
Repeat cycle every 21 days until disease progression or unacceptable toxicity
References
Patel JD, Hensing TA, Rademaker A, et al, "Phase II Study of Pemetrexed and Carboplatin Plus Bevacizumab With Maintenance Pemetrexed and Bevacizumab as First-Line Therapy for Nonsquamous Non-Small-Cell Lung Cancer," *J Clin Oncol*, 2009, 27(20):3284-9.

Bevacizumab-Cisplatin-Gemcitabine (NSCLC)

Index Terms Cisplatin-Gemcitabine-Bevacizumab (NSCLC)
Use Lung cancer, non-small cell
Regimen
Cisplatin: IV: 80 mg/m^2 day 1
  [total dose/cycle = 80 mg/m^2]
Gemcitabine: IV: 1250 mg/m^2/day days 1 and 8
  [total dose/cycle = 2500 mg/m^2]
Bevacizumab: IV: 7.5 or 15 mg/kg day 1
  [total dose/cycle = 7.5 or 15 mg/kg]
Repeat cycle every 21 days for up to 6 cycles
followed by
Bevacizumab: IV: 7.5 or 15 mg/kg day 1
  [total dose/cycle = 7.5 or 15 mg/kg]
Repeat cycle every 21 days until disease progression or unacceptable toxicity
References
Reck M, von Pawel J, Zatloukal P, et al, "Overall Survival With Cisplatin-Gemcitabine and Bevacizumab or Placebo as First-Line Therapy for Nonsquamous Non-Small-Cell Lung Cancer: Results From a Randomised Phase III Trial AVAiL," *Ann Oncol*, 2010, 21(9):1804-9.
Reck M, von Pawel J, Zatloukal P, et al, "Phase III Trial of Cisplatin Plus Gemcitabine With Either Placebo or Bevacizumab as First-Line Therapy for Nonsquamous Non-Small-Cell Lung Cancer: AVAiL," *J Clin Oncol*, 2009, 27(8):1227-34.

Bevacizumab-Cisplatin-Paclitaxel (Cervical)

Index Terms Bevacizumab-Paclitaxel-Cisplatin (Cervical); Cisplatin-Paclitaxel-Bevacizumab (Cervical)
Use Cervical cancer
Regimen
Bevacizumab: IV: 15 mg/kg day 1
  [total dose/cycle = 15 mg/kg]
Paclitaxel: IV: 135-175 mg/m^2 day 1
  [total dose/cycle = 135-175 mg/m^2]
Cisplatin: IV: 50 mg/m^2 day 1
  [total dose/cycle = 50 mg/m^2]
Repeat cycle every 21 days until disease progression or unacceptable toxicity
References
Tewari KS, Sill MW, Long HJ 3rd, et al. Improved survival with bevacizumab in advanced cervical cancer. *N Engl J Med.* 2014;370(8):734-743.

◆ **Bevacizumab-Doxil (Ovarian)** *see* Bevacizumab-Doxorubicin (Liposomal) (Ovarian) *on page 1992*

Bevacizumab-Doxorubicin (Liposomal) (Ovarian)

Index Terms Bevacizumab-Doxil (Ovarian); Doxorubicin (Liposomal)-Bevacizumab (Ovarian)

Use Ovarian cancer

Regimen

Bevacizumab: IV: 10 mg/kg days 1 and 15
  [total dose/cycle = 20 mg/kg]
Doxorubicin (liposomal): IV: 40 mg/m^2 day 1
  [total dose/cycle = 40 mg/m^2]
Repeat cycle every 28 days until disease progression or unacceptable toxicity

References

Pujade-Lauraine E, Hilpert F, Weber B, et al. Bevacizumab combined with chemotherapy for platinum-resistant recurrent ovarian cancer: the AURELIA open-label randomized phase III trial. J Clin Oncol. 2014;32(13):1302-1308.

Bevacizumab-Fluorouracil-Leucovorin (Colorectal)

Index Terms Fluorouracil-Leucovorin-Bevacizumab (Colorectal)

Use Colorectal cancer (metastatic)

Regimen

Bevacizumab: IV: 5 mg/kg/day days 1, 15, 29, and 43
  [total dose/cycle = 20 mg/kg]
Leucovorin Calcium: IV: 500 mg/m^2/day over 2 hours days 1, 8, 15, 22, 29, and 36
  [total dose/cycle = 3,000 mg/m^2]
Fluorouracil: IV bolus: 500 mg/m^2/day days 1, 8, 15, 22, 29, and 36 (administer midway through leucovorin infusion)
  [total dose/cycle = 3,000 mg/m^2]
Repeat cycle every 56 days through 96 weeks or until disease progression (bevacizumab monotherapy may continue after confirmed complete response or unacceptable toxicity to fluorouracil/leucovorin)

References

Kabbinavar FF, Schulz J, McCleod M, et al. Addition of bevacizumab to bolus fluorouracil and leucovorin in first-line metastatic colorectal cancer: results of a randomized phase II trial. J Clin Oncol. 2005;23(16):3697-3705.

Bevacizumab + FOLFIRI (Colorectal)

Index Terms Bevacizumab, Irinotecan, Leucovorin, Fluorouracil (Colorectal)

Use Colorectal cancer

Regimen

Bevacizumab: IV: 5 mg/kg day 1
  [total dose/cycle = 5 mg/kg]
Irinotecan: IV: 180 mg/m^2 over 90 minutes day 1
  [total dose/cycle = 180 mg/m^2]
Leucovorin Calcium: IV: 400 mg/m^2 over 2 hours day 1
  [total dose/cycle = 400 mg/m^2]
Fluorouracil: IV bolus: 400 mg/m^2 day 1
  followed by IV: 2400 mg/m^2 continuous infusion (CI) over 46 hours beginning day 1
    [total fluorouracil dose/cycle (bolus and CI) = 2800 mg/m^2]
Repeat cycle every 14 days until disease progression or unacceptable toxicity

References

Fuchs CS, Marshall J, Mitchell E, et al, "Randomized, Controlled Trial of Irinotecan Plus Infusional, Bolus, or Oral Fluoropyrimidines in First-Line Treatment of Metastatic Colorectal Cancer: Results From the BICC-C Study," J Clin Oncol, 2007, 25(30):4779-86.

Bevacizumab FOLFOX (Colorectal)

Index Terms Bevacizumab-Oxaliplatin-Leucovorin-Fluorouracil (Colorectal);
Oxaliplatin-Fluorouracil-Leucovorin-Bevacizumab (Colorectal)

Use Colorectal cancer

Regimen NOTE: Multiple variations are listed.

Variation 1:

Bevacizumab: IV: 5 mg/kg day 1
[total dose/cycle = 5 mg/kg]

Oxaliplatin: IV: 85 mg/m^2 over 2 hours day 1
[total dose/cycle = 85 mg/m^2]

Leucovorin Calcium: IV: 350 mg over 2 hours day 1
[total dose/cycle = 350 mg]

Fluorouracil: IV bolus: 400 mg/m^2 day 1
followed by IV: 2400 mg/m^2 continuous infusion over 46 hours beginning day 1
[total dose/cycle (bolus and continuous infusion) = 2800 mg/m^2]

Repeat cycle every 14 days until disease progression or unacceptable toxicity

Variation 2:

Bevacizumab: IV: 5 mg/kg over 30 to 90 minutes day 1
[total dose/cycle = 5 mg/kg]

Oxaliplatin: IV: 85 mg/m^2 over 2 hours day 1
[total dose/cycle = 85 mg/m^2]

Leucovorin Calcium: IV: 200 mg/m^2/day over 2 hours days 1 and 2
[total dose/cycle = 400 mg/m^2]

Fluorouracil: IV bolus: 400 mg/m^2/day days 1 and 2
followed by IV: 600 mg/m^2/day continuous infusion over 22 hours days 1 and 2
[total dose/cycle (bolus and continuous infusion) = 2000 mg/m^2]

Repeat cycle every 14 days; up to a maximum of 24 cycles

Variation 3:

Bevacizumab: IV: 10 mg/kg over 30 to 90 minutes day 1
[total dose/cycle = 10 mg/kg]

Oxaliplatin: IV: 85 mg/m^2 over 2 hours day 1
[total dose/cycle = 85 mg/m^2]

Leucovorin Calcium: IV: 200 mg/m^2/day over 2 hours days 1 and 2
[total dose/cycle = 400 mg/m^2]

Fluorouracil: IV bolus: 400 mg/m^2/day days 1 and 2
followed by IV: 600 mg/m^2/day continuous infusion over 22 hours days 1 and 2
[total dose/cycle (bolus and continuous infusion) = 2000 mg/m^2]

Repeat cycle every 14 days

References

Variation 1:

Hochster HS, Hart LL, Ramanathan RK, et al. Safety and efficacy of oxaliplatin and fluoropyrimidine regimens with or without bevacizumab as first-line treatment of metastatic colorectal cancer: results of the TREE Study. *J Clin Oncol.* 2008;26(21):3523-3529.

Variation 2:

Saltz LB, Clarke S, Díaz-Rubio E, et al. Bevacizumab in combination with oxaliplatin-based chemotherapy as first-line therapy in metastatic colorectal cancer: a randomized phase III study. *J Clin Oncol.* 2008;26(12):2013-2019.

Variation 3:

Giantonio BJ, Catalano PJ, Meropol NJ, et al. Bevacizumab in combination with oxaliplatin, fluorouracil, and leucovorin (FOLFOX4) for previously treated metastatic colorectal cancer: results from the Eastern Cooperative Oncology Group Study E3200. *J Clin Oncol*. 2007; 25 (12):1539-1544.

♦ **Bevacizumab-Gemcitabine-Carboplatin (Ovarian)** *see* Bevacizumab-Carboplatin-Gemcitabine (Ovarian) *on page 1990*

♦ **Bevacizumab-Interferon Alfa 2b (RCC)** *see* Bevacizumab-Interferon Alfa (RCC) *on page 1994*

Bevacizumab-Interferon Alfa (RCC)

Index Terms Bevacizumab-Interferon Alfa 2b (RCC); Interferon Alfa 2b-Bevacizumab (RCC); Interferon Alfa-Bevacizumab (RCC)

Use Renal cell cancer

Regimen

Interferon Alfa-2b: SubQ: 9 million units on 3 nonconsecutive days per week

[total dose/cycle = 108 million units]

Bevacizumab: IV: 10 mg/kg days 1 and 15

[total dose/cycle = 20 mg/kg]

Repeat cycle every 28 days until disease progression or unacceptable toxicity

References

Rini BI, Halabi S, Rosenberg JE, et al, "Bevacizumab Plus Interferon Alfa Compared With Interferon Alfa Monotherapy in Patients With Metastatic Renal Cell Carcinoma: CALGB 90206," *J Clin Oncol*, 2008, 26(33):5422-8.

Rini BI, Halabi S, Rosenberg JE, et al, "Phase III Trial of Bevacizumab Plus Interferon Alfa Versus Interferon Alfa Monotherapy in Patients With Metastatic Renal Cell Carcinoma: Final Results of CALGB 90206," *J Clin Oncol*, 2010, 28(13):2137-43.

Bevacizumab-Irinotecan (Glioblastoma)

Index Terms Irinotecan-Bevacizumab (Glioblastoma)

Use Brain tumors

Regimen NOTE: Patients receiving concurrent antiepileptic enzyme-inducing drugs received an increased dose of irinotecan (340 mg/m^2/dose).

Bevacizumab: IV: 10 mg/kg day 1

[total dose/cycle = 10 mg/kg]

Irinotecan: IV: 125 mg/m^2 day 1

[total dose/cycle = 125 mg/m^2]

Repeat cycle every 14 days

References

Vredenburgh JJ, Desjardins A, Herndon JE 2nd, et al, "Bevacizumab Plus Irinotecan in Recurrent Glioblastoma Multiforme," *J Clin Oncol*, 2007, 25(30):4722-9.

♦ **Bevacizumab, Irinotecan, Leucovorin, Fluorouracil (Colorectal)** *see* Bevacizumab + FOLFIRI (Colorectal) *on page 1992*

♦ **Bevacizumab-Oxaliplatin-Leucovorin-Fluorouracil (Colorectal)** *see* Bevacizumab FOLFOX (Colorectal) *on page 1993*

Bevacizumab-Paclitaxel (Breast)

Index Terms Paclitaxel-Bevacizumab (Breast)

Use Breast cancer

Regimen
Paclitaxel: IV: 90 mg/m^2/day days 1, 8, and 15
[total dose/cycle = 270 mg/m^2]
Bevacizumab: IV: 10 mg/kg/day days 1 and 15
[total dose/cycle = 20 mg/kg]
Repeat cycle every 28 days until disease progression or unacceptable toxicity

References
Brufsky AM, Hurvitz S, Perez E, et al, "RIBBON-2 A Randomized, Double-Blind, Placebo-Controlled, Phase III Trial Evaluating the Efficacy and Safety of Bevacizumab in Combination With Chemotherapy for Second-Line Treatment of Human Epidermal Growth Factor 2-Negative Metastatic Breast Cancer," *J Clin Oncol*, 2011, 29(32):4286-93.

Miller K, Wang M, Cralow J, et al, "Paclitaxel Plus Bevacizumab Versus Paclitaxel Alone for Metastatic Breast Cancer," *N Engl J Med*, 2007, 357(26):2666-76.

♦ **Bevacizumab-Paclitaxel-Carboplatin (NSCLC)** *see* Bevacizumab-Carboplatin-Paclitaxel (NSCLC) *on page 1990*

♦ **Bevacizumab-Paclitaxel-Cisplatin (Cervical)** *see* Bevacizumab-Cisplatin-Paclitaxel (Cervical) *on page 1991*

Bevacizumab-Paclitaxel (Ovarian)
Index Terms Paclitaxel-Bevacizumab (Ovarian)
Use Ovarian cancer
Regimen
Bevacizumab: IV: 10 mg/kg days 1 and 15
[total dose/cycle = 20 mg/kg]
Paclitaxel: IV: 80 mg/m^2/day days 1, 8, 15, and 22
[total dose/cycle = 320 mg/m^2]
Repeat cycle every 28 days until disease progression or unacceptable toxicity

References
Pujade-Lauraine E, Hilpert F, Weber B, et al. Bevacizumab combined with chemotherapy for platinum-resistant recurrent ovarian cancer: the AURELIA open-label randomized phase III trial. *J Clin Oncol*. 2014;32(13):1302-1308.

Bevacizumab-Paclitaxel-Topotecan (Cervical)
Index Terms Bevacizumab-Topotecan-Paclitaxel (Cervical); Paclitaxel-Topotecan-Bevacizumab (Cervical)
Use Cervical cancer
Regimen
Bevacizumab: IV: 15 mg/kg day 1
[total dose/cycle = 15 mg/kg]
Topotecan: IV: 0.75 mg/m^2 days 1 to 3
[total dose/cycle = 2.25 mg/m^2]
Paclitaxel: IV: 175 mg/m^2 day 1
[total dose/cycle = 175 mg/m^2]
Repeat cycle every 21 days until disease progression or unacceptable toxicity

References
Tewari KS, Sill MW, Long HJ 3rd, et al. Improved survival with bevacizumab in advanced cervical cancer. *N Engl J Med*. 2014;370(8):734-743.

Bevacizumab-Topotecan Daily (Ovarian)
Index Terms Topotecan Daily-Bevacizumab (Ovarian)
Use Ovarian cancer

◄ **Regimen**
Bevacizumab: IV: 15 mg/kg day 1
[total dose/cycle = 15 mg/kg]
Topotecan: IV: 1.25 mg/m²/day days 1, 2, 3, 4, and 5
[total dose/cycle = 6.25 mg/m²]
Repeat cycle every 21 days until disease progression or unacceptable toxicity

References

Pujade-Lauraine E, Hilpert F, Weber B, et al. Bevacizumab combined with chemotherapy for platinum-resistant recurrent ovarian cancer: the AURELIA open-label randomized phase III trial. *J Clin Oncol.* 2014;32(13):1302-1308.

◆ **Bevacizumab-Topotecan-Paclitaxel (Cervical)** *see* Bevacizumab-Paclitaxel-Topotecan (Cervical) *on page 1995*

Bevacizumab-Topotecan Weekly (Ovarian)

Index Terms Topotecan Weekly-Bevacizumab (Ovarian)
Use Ovarian cancer
Regimen
Bevacizumab: IV: 10 mg/kg days 1 and 15
[total dose/cycle = 20 mg/kg]
Topotecan: IV: 4 mg/m²/day days 1, 8, and 15
[total dose/cycle = 12 mg/m²]
Repeat cycle every 28 days until disease progression or unacceptable toxicity

References

Pujade-Lauraine E, Hilpert F, Weber B, et al. Bevacizumab combined with chemotherapy for platinum-resistant recurrent ovarian cancer: the AURELIA open-label randomized phase III trial. *J Clin Oncol.* 2014;32(13):1302-1308.

Bevacizumab + XELOX (Colorectal)

Index Terms Bevacizumb-Capecitabine-Oxaliplatin (Colorectal Cancer); Bevacizumb-CapeOx (Colorectal Cancer); Bevacizumb-CAPOX (Colorectal Cancer); Bevacizumb-Oxaliplatin-Capecitabine (Colorectal Cancer)
Use Colorectal cancer
Regimen NOTE: Multiple variations are listed.
Variation 1:
Bevacizumab: IV: 7.5 mg/kg day 1
[total dose/cycle = 7.5 mg/kg]
Oxaliplatin: IV: 130 mg/m² day 1
[total dose/cycle = 130 mg/m²]
Capecitabine: Oral: 850 mg/m² twice daily days 1 (beginning with evening dose) to 15 (ending with morning dose)
[total dose/cycle = 23,800 mg/m²]
Repeat cycle every 21 days
Variation 2:
Bevacizumab: IV: 7.5 mg/kg over 30-90 minutes day 1
[total dose/cycle = 7.5 mg/kg]
Oxaliplatin: IV: 130 mg/m² over 2 hours day 1
[total dose/cycle = 130 mg/m²]
Capecitabine: Oral: 1000 mg/m² twice daily days 1 to 14
[total dose/cycle = 28,000 mg/m²]
Repeat cycle every 21 days

References
Variation 1:
Hochster HS, Hart LL, Ramanathan RK, et al, "Safety and Efficacy of Oxaliplatin and Fluoropyrimidine Regimens With or Without Bevacizumab as First-Line Treatment of Metastatic Colorectal Cancer: Results of the TREE Study," *J Clin Oncol*, 2008, 26(21):3523-9.
Variation 2:
Saltz LB, Clarke S, Díaz-Rubio E, et al, "Bevacizumab in Combination With Oxaliplatin-Based Chemotherapy as First-Line Therapy in Metastatic Colorectal Cancer: A Randomized Phase III Study," *J Clin Oncol*, 2008, 26(12):2013-9.

◆ **Bevacizumb-Capecitabine-Oxaliplatin (Colorectal Cancer)** see Bevacizumab + XELOX (Colorectal) *on page 1996*

◆ **Bevacizumb-CapeOx (Colorectal Cancer)** see Bevacizumab + XELOX (Colorectal) *on page 1996*

◆ **Bevacizumb-CAPOX (Colorectal Cancer)** see Bevacizumab + XELOX (Colorectal) *on page 1996*

◆ **Bevacizumb-Oxaliplatin-Capecitabine (Colorectal Cancer)** see Bevacizumab + XELOX (Colorectal) *on page 1996*

◆ **Biweekly Cetlri (Colorectal)** see Cetuximab (Biweekly)-Irinotecan (Colorectal) *on page 2029*

◆ **BLD (Multiple Myeloma)** see Bendamustine-Lenalidomide-Dexamethasone (Multiple Myeloma) *on page 1986*

◆ **Bleomycin-Etoposide-Cisplatin (Ovarian)** see BEP (Ovarian) *on page 1988*

◆ **Bleomycin, Etoposide, Doxorubicin, Cyclophosphamide, Vincristine, Procarbazine, Prednisone (Hodgkin)** see BEACOPP-14 (Hodgkin) *on page 1981*

◆ **Bleomycin, Etoposide, Doxorubicin, Cyclophosphamide, Vincristine, Procarbazine, Prednisone (Hodgkin)** see BEACOPP Escalated (Hodgkin) *on page 1982*

◆ **Bleomycin, Etoposide, Doxorubicin, Cyclophosphamide, Vincristine, Procarbazine, Prednisone (Hodgkin)** see BEACOPP Escalated Plus Standard (Hodgkin) *on page 1983*

◆ **Bleomycin, Etoposide, Doxorubicin, Cyclophosphamide, Vincristine, Procarbazine, Prednisone (Hodgkin)** see BEACOPP Standard (Hodgkin) *on page 1984*

◆ **Bleomycin-Etoposide-Cisplatin (Testicular)** see BEP (Testicular) *on page 1989*

◆ **Bortezomib-Bendamustine-Rituximab (NHL-Follicular)** see Bendamustine-Bortezomib-Rituximab (NHL-Follicular) *on page 1985*

◆ **Bortezomib-Cyclophosphamide-Dexamethasone (Multiple Myeloma)** see Cyclophosphamide-Bortezomib-Dexamethasone (Multiple Myeloma) *on page 2076*

◆ **Bortezomib-Daratumumab-Dexamethasone (Multiple Myeloma)** see Daratumumab-Bortezomib-Dexamethasone (Multiple Myeloma) *on page 2083*

Bortezomib-Dexamethasone (Amyloidosis)
Index Terms Dexamethasone-Bortezomib (Amyloidosis)
Use Systemic light chain amyloidosis

Regimen

Bortezomib: IV: 1.3 mg/m^2/dose days 1, 4, 8, and 11
[total dose/cycle = 5.2 mg/m^2]
Dexamethasone: Oral: 40 mg/day days 1 to 4
[total dose/cycle = 160 mg]
Repeat cycle every 21 days

References

Kastritis E, Wechalekar AD, Dimopoulos MA, et al, "Bortezomib With or Without Dexamethasone in Primary Systemic (Light Chain) Amyloidosis," *J Clin Oncol*, 2010, 28(6):1031-7.

Bortezomib-Dexamethasone (Multiple Myeloma)

Index Terms Dexamethasone-Bortezomib (Multiple Myeloma); VD (Multiple Myeloma)

Use Multiple myeloma

Regimen

Cycles 1 and 2:
Bortezomib: IV: 1.3 mg/m^2/day days 1, 4, 8, and 11
[total dose/cycle = 5.2 mg/m^2]
Dexamethasone: Oral: 40 mg/day days 1 to 4 and days 9 to 12
[total dose/cycle = 320 mg]
Repeat cycle every 21 days for cycles 1 and 2
Cycles 3 and 4:
Bortezomib: IV: 1.3 mg/m^2/day days 1, 4, 8, and 11
[total dose/cycle = 5.2 mg/m^2]
Dexamethasone: Oral: 40 mg/day days 1 to 4
[total dose/cycle = 160 mg]
Repeat cycle every 21 days for cycles 3 and 4

References

Harousseau JL, Attal M, Avet-Loiseau H, et al. Bortezomib plus dexamethasone is superior to vincristine plus doxorubicin plus dexamethasone as induction treatment prior to autologous stem-cell transplantation in newly diagnosed multiple myeloma: results of the IFM 2005-01 phase III trial. *J Clin Oncol*. 2010;28(30):4621-4629.

♦ **Bortezomib-Dexamethasone-Panobinostat (Multiple Myeloma)** *see* Panobinostat-Bortezomib-Dexamethasone (Multiple Myeloma) *on page 2190*

Bortezomib-Dexamethasone-Rituximab (Waldenstrom Macroglobulinemia)

Index Terms BDR (Waldenstrom Macroglobulinemia)

Use Waldenstrom Macroglobulinemia

Regimen

Bortezomib: IV: 1.3 mg/m^2 days 1, 4, 8, and 11
[total dose/cycle = 5.2 mg/m^2]
Dexamethasone: IV: 40 mg days 1, 4, 8, and 11
[total dose/cycle = 160 mg]
Rituximab: IV: 375 mg/m^2 day 11
[total dose/cycle = 375 mg/m^2]
Repeat cycle every 21 days for 4 cycles, followed by a 12 week interruption, then repeat cycle every 12 weeks for 4 cycles

References

Treon SP, Ioakimidis L, Soumerai JD, et al, "Primary Treatment of Waldenstrom Macroglobulinemia With Bortezomib, Dexamethasone, and Rituximab: WMCTG Clinical Trial 05-180," *J Clin Oncol*, 2009, 27(23):3830-5.

◆ **Bortezomib-Dexamethasone-Thalidomide-Cisplatin-Doxorubicin-Cyclo-phosphamide-Etoposide (Multiple Myeloma)** *see* VDT-PACE (Multiple Myeloma) *on page 2229*

◆ **Bortezomib-Doxil (Multiple Myeloma)** *see* Bortezomib-Doxorubicin (Liposomal) (Multiple Myeloma) *on page 1999*

Bortezomib-Doxorubicin-Dexamethasone (Multiple Myeloma)

Index Terms Dexamethasone-Bortezomib-Doxorubicin (Multiple Myeloma); Doxorubicin-Dexamethasone-Bortezomib (Multiple Myeloma); PAD (Multiple Myeloma)

Use Multiple myeloma (first-line)

Regimen

Induction:

Bortezomib: IV: 1.3 mg/m^2/day days 1, 4, 8, and 11
[total dose/cycle = 5.2 mg/m^2]
Doxorubicin: IV: 9 mg/m^2/day days 1 to 4
[total dose/cycle = 36 mg/m^2]
Dexamethasone: Oral: 40 mg/day days 1 to 4, 9 to 12, and 17 to 20
[total dose/cycle = 480 mg]
Repeat cycle every 28 days for 3 cycles, followed by high-dose melphalan and autologous stem-cell transplantation

Maintenance:

Bortezomib: IV: 1.3 mg/m^2/day day 1 (starting 4 weeks after high-dose melphalan)
[total dose/cycle = 1.3 mg/m^2]
Repeat cycle every 14 days for 2 years

References

Sonneveld P, Schmidt-Wolf IG, van der Holt B, et al. Bortezomib induction and maintenance treatment in patients with newly diagnosed multiple myeloma: results of the randomized phase III HOVON-65/ GMMG-HD4 trial. *J Clin Oncol.* 2012;30(24):2946-2955.

Bortezomib-Doxorubicin (Liposomal) (Multiple Myeloma)

Index Terms Bortezomib-Doxil (Multiple Myeloma); Doxorubicin (Liposomal)-Bortezomib (Multiple Myeloma)

Use Multiple myeloma (relapsed, refractory)

Regimen

Bortezomib: IV: 1.3 mg/m^2/day days 1, 4, 8, and 11
[total dose/cycle = 5.2 mg/m^2]
Doxorubicin (liposomal): IV: 30 mg/m^2 over 1 hour day 4
[total dose/cycle = 30 mg/m^2]
Repeat cycle every 21 days for at least 8 cycles or until disease progression or unacceptable toxicity

References

Orlowski RZ, Nagler A, Sonneveld P, et al. Randomized phase III study of pegylated liposomal doxorubicin plus bortezomib compared with bortezomib alone in relapsed or refractory multiple myeloma: combination therapy improves time to progression. *J Clin Oncol.* 2007;25 (25):3892-3901.

◆ **Bortezomib-Lenalidomide-Dexamethasone (Multiple Myeloma)** *see* Lenalidomide-Bortezomib-Dexamethasone (Multiple Myeloma) *on page 2163*

Bortezomib-Rituximab (Waldenstrom Macroglobulinemia)

Index Terms Rituximab-Bortezomib (Waldenstrom Macroglobulinemia)

Use Waldenstrom Macroglobulinemia

Regimen

Bortezomib: IV: 1.6 mg/m^2/day days 1, 8, and 15 (cycles 1 to 6)
[total dose/cycle = 4.8 mg/m^2]

Rituximab: IV: 375 mg/m^2/day days 1, 8, 15, and 22 (cycles 1 and 4 only)
[total dose/cycle (cycles 1 and 4 only) = 1500 mg/m^2]

Repeat cycle every 28 days for a total of 6 cycles; bortezomib administered for all 6 cycles and rituximab administered cycles 1 and 4 only

References

Ghobrial IM, Hong F, Padmanabhan S, et al, "Phase II Trial of Weekly Bortezomib in Combination With Rituximab in Relapsed or Refractory and Refractory Waldenstrom Macroglobulinemia," *J Clin Oncol*, 2010, 28(8):1422-8.

Bortezomib-Thalidomide-Dexamethasone (Multiple Myeloma)

Index Terms Dexamethasone-Bortezomib-Thalidomide (Multiple Myeloma); Thalidomide-Dexamethasone-Bortezomib (Multiple Myeloma); VTd (Multiple Myeloma); vtD (Multiple Myeloma); VTD (Multiple Myeloma)

Use Multiple myeloma (first-line and relapsed/refractory)

Regimen NOTE: Multiple variations are listed.

Variation 1 (first-line):

Induction Cycle 1:

Bortezomib: IV: 1.3 mg/m^2/day days 1, 4, 8, and 11
[total dose/cycle = 5.2 mg/m^2]

Thalidomide: Oral: 100 mg daily days 1 to 14, then 200 mg daily days 15 to 21
[total dose/cycle = 2,800 mg]

Dexamethasone: Oral: 40 mg/day days 1, 2, 4, 5, 8, 9, 11, and 12
[total dose/cycle = 320 mg]

Treatment cycle is 21 days

Induction Cycles 2 and 3:

Bortezomib: IV: 1.3 mg/m^2/day days 1, 4, 8, and 11
[total dose/cycle = 5.2 mg/m^2]

Thalidomide: Oral: 200 mg daily days 1 to 21
[total dose/cycle = 4,200 mg]

Dexamethasone: Oral: 40 mg/day days 1, 2, 4, 5, 8, 9, 11, and 12
[total dose/cycle = 320 mg]

Repeat cycle every 21 days for a total of 3 induction cycles. Patients may then proceed to double autologous stem-cell transplant. Transplants were done 3 to 6 months apart; once haemopoiesis after first transplant, patients were given thalidomide 100 mg daily and dexamethasone 40 mg days 1 to 4 every 28 days until the day before the second transplant.

Consolidation Cycles 1 and 2 (beginning 3 months after second transplant):

Bortezomib: IV: 1.3 mg/m^2/day days 1, 8, 15, and 22
[total dose/cycle = 5.2 mg/m^2]

Thalidomide: Oral: 100 mg daily days 1 to 35
[total dose/cycle = 3,500 mg]

Dexamethasone: Oral: 40 mg/day days 1, 2, 8, 9, 15, 16, 22, and 23
[total dose/cycle = 320 mg]
Repeat cycle every 35 days for a total of 2 consolidation cycles
Maintenance:
Dexamethasone: Oral: 40 mg/day days 1 to 4
[total dose/cycle = 160 mg]
Repeat cycle every 28 days until disease progression or unacceptable toxicity

Variation 2 (first-line):
Cycles 1 and 2:
Bortezomib: IV: 1 mg/m^2/day days 1, 4, 8, and 11
[total dose/cycle = 4 mg/m^2]
Thalidomide: Oral: 100 mg daily days 1 to 21
[total dose/cycle = 2,100 mg]
Dexamethasone: Oral: 40 mg/day days 1 to 4 and 9 to 12
[total dose/cycle = 320 mg]
Treatment cycle is 21 days

Cycles 3 and 4:
Bortezomib: IV: 1 mg/m^2/day days 1, 4, 8, and 11; if less than partial response after cycle 2, may increase to 1.3 mg/m^2 for cycles 3 and 4)
[total dose/cycle = 4 to 5.2 mg/m^2]
Thalidomide: Oral: 100 mg daily days 1 to 21; if less than partial response after cycle 2 may increase to 200 mg/day for cycles 3 and 4
[total dose/cycle = 2,100 to 4,200 mg]
Dexamethasone: Oral: 40 mg/day days 1 to 4
[total dose/cycle = 160 mg]
Repeat cycle every 21 days for a total of 4 cycles. Patients may then proceed to transplantation.

Variation 3 (first-line and relapsed):
Bortezomib: IV: 1.3 mg/m^2/day days 1, 4, 8, and 11
[total dose/cycle = 5.2 mg/m^2]
Thalidomide: Oral: 100 mg daily days 1 to 21
[total dose/cycle = 2,100 mg]
Dexamethasone: Oral: 40 mg/day days 1 to 4 and 9 to 12
[total dose/cycle = 320 mg]
Repeat cycle every 21 days for up to 8 cycles. Patients may proceed to stem cell transplantation after 3 to 4 cycles.

References
Variation 1:
Cavo M, Pantani L, Petrucci MT, et al. Bortezomib-thalidomide-dexamethasone is superior to thalidomide-dexamethasone as consolidation therapy after autologous hematopoietic stem cell transplantation in patients with newly diagnosed multiple myeloma. *Blood*. 2012;120(1):9-19.
Cavo M, Tacchetti P, Patriarca F, et al. Bortezomib with thalidomide plus dexamethasone compared with thalidomide plus dexamethasone as induction therapy before, and consolidation therapy after, double autologous stem-cell transplantation in newly diagnosed multiple myeloma: a randomised phase 3 study. *Lancet*. 2010;376(9758):2075-2085.
Variation 2:
Moreau P, Avet-Loiseau H, Facon T, et al. Bortezomib plus dexamethasone versus reduced-dose bortezomib, thalidomide plus dexamethasone as induction treatment before autologous stem cell transplantation in newly diagnosed multiple myeloma. *Blood*. 2011;118(22):5752-5758.
Variation 3:
Kaufman JI, Nooka A, Vrana M, Gleason C, Heffner LT, and Lonial S. Bortezomib, thalidomide, and dexamethasone as induction therapy for patients with symptomatic multiple myeloma: a retrospective study. *Cancer*. 2010;116(13):3143-3151.

◆ **Botezomib-Rituximab-Cyclophosphamide-Doxorubicin-Prednisone (NHL-Mantle Cell)** *see* VcR-CAP (NHL-Mantle Cell) *on page 2228*

- ◆ **B-R (CLL)** *see* Bendamustine-Rituximab (CLL) *on page 1986*
- ◆ **B-R (NHL-Follicular)** *see* Bendamustine-Rituximab (NHL-Follicular) *on page 1987*
- ◆ **B-R (NHL-Mantle Cell)** *see* Bendamustine-Rituximab (NHL-Mantle Cell) *on page 1987*
- ◆ **BR (Waldenstrom Macroglobulinemia)** *see* Bendamustine-Rituximab (Waldenstrom Macroglobulinemia) *on page 1988*

Cabazitaxel-Prednisone (Prostate)

Index Terms Prednisone-Cabazitaxel (Prostate)

Use Prostate cancer

Regimen

Cabazitaxel: IV: 25 mg/m^2 over 1 hour day 1
[total dose/cycle = 25 mg/m^2]
Prednisone: Oral: 10 mg once daily days 1 to 21
[total dose/cycle = 210 mg]
Repeat cycle every 21 days

References

De Bono JS, Oudard S, Ozguroglu M, et al, "Prednisone Plus Cabazitaxel or Mitoxantrone for Metastatic Castration-Resistant Prostate Cancer Progressing After Docetaxel Treatment: A Randomised Open-Label Trial," *Lancet,* 2010, 376(9747):1147-54.

CAF IV (Breast)

Index Terms Cyclophosphamide, Doxorubicin, Fluorouracil IV (Breast); FAC IV (Breast)

Use Breast cancer

Regimen NOTE: Multiple variations are listed.

Variation 1:
Fluorouracil: IV: 500 mg/m^2/day days 1 and 8
[total dose/cycle = 1000 mg/m^2]
Doxorubicin: IV: 50 mg/m^2 over 72 hours days 1-3
[total dose/cycle = 50 mg/m^2]
Cyclophosphamide: IV: 500 mg/m^2 day 1
[total dose/cycle = 500 mg/m^2]
Repeat cycle every 21-28 days for up to 6 cycles
Variation 2:
Fluorouracil: IV: 500 mg/m^2/day days 1 and 8
[total dose/cycle = 1000 mg/m^2]
Doxorubicin: IV: 50 mg/m^2 day 1
[total dose/cycle = 50 mg/m^2]
Cyclophosphamide: IV: 500 mg/m^2 day 1
[total dose/cycle = 500 mg/m^2]
Repeat cycle every 21 days for up to 9 cycles

References

Variation 1:

Assikis V, Buzdar A, Yang Y, et al, "A Phase III Trial of Sequential Adjuvant Chemotherapy for Operable Breast Carcinoma: Final Analysis With 10-Year Follow-Up," *Cancer,* 2003, 97 (11):2716-23.

Variation 2:

Hortobagyi GN, Gutterman JU, Blumenschein GR, et al, "Combination Chemoimmunotherapy of Metastatic Breast Cancer With 5-Fluorouracil, Adriamycin, Cyclophosphamide, and BCG," *Cancer,* 1979, 43(4):1225-33.

CAF Oral (Breast)

Index Terms Cyclophosphamide, Doxorubicin, Fluorouracil Oral (Breast); FAC Oral (Breast)

Use Breast cancer

Regimen

Cyclophosphamide: Oral: 100 mg/m^2/day days 1 to 14
[total dose/cycle = 1400 mg/m^2]

Doxorubicin: IV: 30 mg/m^2/day days 1 and 8
[total dose/cycle = 60 mg/m^2]

Fluorouracil: IV: 500 mg/m^2/day days 1 and 8
[total dose/cycle = 1000 mg/m^2]

Repeat cycle every 28 days, until a cumulative doxorubicin dose of 450 mg/m^2 in the metastatic setting (Bull, 1978), and for a total of 6 cycles in the adjuvant setting (Hutchins, 2005)

References

Bull JM, Tormey DC, Li SH, et al, "A Randomized Comparative Trial of Adriamycin® Versus Methotrexate in Combination Drug Therapy," *Cancer,* 1978, 41(5):1649-57.

Hutchins LF, Green SJ, Ravdin PM, et al, "Randomized, Controlled Trial of Cyclophosphamide, Methotrexate, and Fluorouracil Versus Cyclophosphamide, Doxorubicin, and Fluorouracil With and Without Tamoxifen for High-Risk, Node-Negative Breast Cancer: Treatment Results of Intergroup Protocol INT-0102," *J Clin Oncol,* 2005, 23(33):8313-21.

CALGB 8811 Regimen (ALL)

Index Terms Larson 8811 Regimen (ALL); Larson Regimen 8811 (ALL)

Use Leukemia, acute lymphocytic

Regimen

Induction, patients <60 years of age (4-week cycle):

Cyclophosphamide: IV: 1200 mg/m^2 day 1
[total dose/cycle = 1200 mg/m^2]

Daunorubicin: IV: 45 mg/m^2/dose days 1, 2, and 3
[total dose/cycle – 135 mg/m^2]

Vincristine: IV: 2 mg/dose days 1, 8, 15, and 22
[total dose/cycle = 8 mg]

Prednisone: Oral: 60 mg/m^2/dose days 1 to 21
[total dose/cycle = 1260 mg/m^2]

Asparaginase *(E. coli)*: SubQ: 6000 units/m^2/dose days 5, 8, 11, 15, 18, and 22
[total dose/cycle = 36,000 units/m^2]

Induction, patients ≥60 years of age (4-week cycle):

Cyclophosphamide: IV: 800 mg/m^2 day 1
[total dose/cycle = 800 mg/m^2]

Daunorubicin: IV: 30 mg/m^2/dose days 1, 2, and 3
[total dose/cycle = 90 mg/m^2]

Vincristine: IV: 2 mg/dose days 1, 8, 15, and 22
[total dose/cycle = 8 mg]

Prednisone: Oral: 60 mg/m^2/dose days 1 to 7
[total dose/cycle = 420 mg/m^2]

Asparaginase *(E. coli)*: SubQ: 6000 units/m^2/dose days 5, 8, 11, 15, 18, and 22
[total dose/cycle = 36,000 units/m^2]

Early intensification (4-week cycle; repeat cycle once):

Methotrexate: Intrathecal: 15 mg/dose day 1
[total dose/cycle = 15 mg]

Cyclophosphamide: IV: 1000 mg/m² day 1
[total dose/cycle = 1000 mg/m²]

Mercaptopurine: Oral: 60 mg/m²/dose days 1 to 14
[total dose/cycle = 840 mg/m²]

Cytarabine: SubQ: 75 mg/m²/dose days 1 to 4 and 8 to 11
[total dose/cycle = 600 mg/m²]

Vincristine: IV: 2 mg/dose days 15 and 22
[total dose/cycle = 4 mg]

Asparaginase *(E. coli)*: SubQ: 6000 units/m²/dose days 15, 18, 22, and 25
[total dose/cycle = 24,000 units/m²]

CNS prophylaxis/interim maintenance (12-week duration; with cranial irradiation days 1 to 12):

Methotrexate: Intrathecal: 15 mg/dose days 1, 8, 15, 22, and 29
[total dose/cycle = 75 mg]

Mercaptopurine: Oral: 60 mg/m²/dose days 1 to 70
[total dose/cycle = 4200 mg/m²]

Methotrexate: Oral: 20 mg/m²/dose days 36, 43, 50, 57, and 64
[total dose/cycle = 100 mg/m²]

Late intensification (8-week cycle):

Doxorubicin: IV: 30 mg/m²/dose days 1, 8, and 15
[total dose/cycle = 90 mg/m²]

Vincristine: IV: 2 mg/dose days 1, 8, and 15
[total dose/cycle = 6 mg]

Dexamethasone: Oral: 10 mg/m²/dose days 1 to 14
[total dose/cycle = 140 mg/m²]

Cyclophosphamide: IV: 1000 mg/m² day 29
[total dose/cycle = 1000 mg/m²]

Thioguanine: Oral: 60 mg/m²/dose days 29 to 42
[total dose/cycle = 840 mg/m²]

Cytarabine: SubQ: 75 mg/m²/dose days 29 to 32 and 36 to 39
[total dose/cycle = 600 mg/m²]

Maintenance (continue until 24 months from diagnosis):

Vincristine: IV: 2 mg/dose day 1 every 4 weeks
[total dose/4 weeks = 2 mg]

Prednisone: Oral: 60 mg/m²/dose days 1 to 5 every 4 weeks
[total dose/4 weeks = 300 mg/m²]

Methotrexate: Oral: 20 mg/m²/dose days 1, 8, 15, and 22
[total dose/phase = 80 mg/m²]

Mercaptopurine: Oral: 60 mg/m²/dose days 1 to 28
[total dose/phase = 1680 mg/m²]

References

Larson RA, Dodge RK, Burns CP, et al. A five-drug remission induction regimen with intensive consolidation for adults with acute lymphoblastic leukemia: Cancer and Leukemia Group B Study 8811. *Blood.* 1995;85(8):2025-2037.

CALGB 9111 Regimen (ALL)

Index Terms Larson 9111 Regimen (ALL); Larson Regimen 9111 (ALL)

Use Leukemia, acute lymphocytic

Regimen

Induction, patients <60 years of age (4-week cycle):

Cyclophosphamide: IV: 1200 mg/m^2 day 1
[total dose/cycle = 1200 mg/m^2]

Daunorubicin: IV: 45 mg/m^2/dose days 1, 2, and 3
[total dose/cycle = 135 mg/m^2]

Vincristine: IV: 2 mg/dose days 1, 8, 15, and 22
[total dose/cycle = 8 mg]

Prednisone: Oral: 60 mg/m^2/dose days 1 to 21
[total dose/cycle = 1260 mg/m^2]

Asparaginase *(E. coli)*: SubQ, IM: 6000 units/m^2/dose days 5, 8, 11, 15, 18, and 22
[total dose/cycle = 36,000 units/m^2]

Filgrastim: SubQ: 5 mcg/kg/day starting day 4; continue for at least 7 days and until ANC ≥1000/mm^3 on two draws, 24 hours apart

Induction, patients ≥60 years of age (4-week cycle):

Cyclophosphamide: IV: 800 mg/m^2 day 1
[total dose/cycle = 800 mg/m^2]

Daunorubicin: IV: 30 mg/m^2/dose days 1, 2, and 3
[total dose/cycle = 90 mg/m^2]

Vincristine: IV: 2 mg/dose days 1, 8, 15, and 22
[total dose/cycle = 8 mg]

Prednisone: Oral: 60 mg/m^2/dose days 1 to 7
[total dose/cycle = 420 mg/m^2]

Asparaginase *(E. coli)*: SubQ, IM: 6000 units/m^2/dose days 5, 8, 11, 15, 18, and 22
[total dose/cycle = 36,000 units/m^2]

Filgrastim: SubQ: 5 mcg/kg/day starting day 4; continue for at least 7 days and until ANC ≥1000/mm^3 on two draws, 24 hours apart

Early intensification (4-week cycle; repeat cycle once):

Methotrexate: Intrathecal: 15 mg/dose day 1
[total dose/cycle = 15 mg]

Cyclophosphamide: IV: 1000 mg/m^2 day 1
[total dose/cycle = 1000 mg/m^2]

Mercaptopurine: Oral: 60 mg/m^2/dose days 1 to 14
[total dose/cycle = 840 mg/m^2]

Cytarabine: SubQ: 75 mg/m^2/dose days 1 to 4 and 8 to 11
[total dose/cycle = 600 mg/m^2]

Vincristine: IV: 2 mg/dose days 15 and 22
[total dose/cycle = 4 mg]

Asparaginase *(E. coli)*: SubQ, IM: 6000 units/m^2/dose days 15, 18, 22, and 25
[total dose/cycle = 24,000 units/m^2]

Filgrastim: SubQ: 5 mcg/kg/day starting day 2; continue at least 14 days and until ANC ≥5000/mm^3 on two draws, 24 hours apart

CNS prophylaxis/interim maintenance (12-week duration; with cranial irradiation days 1 to 12):

Methotrexate: Intrathecal: 15 mg/dose days 1, 8, 15, 22, and 29
[total dose/cycle = 75 mg]

Mercaptopurine: Oral: 60 mg/m^2/dose days 1 to 70
[total dose/cycle = 4200 mg/m^2]

Methotrexate: Oral: 20 mg/m^2/dose days 36, 43, 50, 57, and 64
[total dose/cycle = 100 mg/m^2]

Late intensification (8-week cycle):
Doxorubicin: IV: 30 mg/m^2/dose days 1, 8, and 15
[total dose/cycle = 90 mg/m^2]
Vincristine: IV: 2 mg/dose days 1, 8, and 15
[total dose/cycle = 6 mg]
Dexamethasone: Oral: 10 mg/m^2/dose days 1 to 14
[total dose/cycle = 140 mg/m^2]
Cyclophosphamide: IV: 1000 mg/m^2 day 29
[total dose/cycle = 1000 mg/m^2]
Thioguanine: Oral: 60 mg/m^2/dose days 29 to 42
[total dose/cycle = 840 mg/m^2]
Cytarabine: SubQ: 75 mg/m^2/dose days 29 to 32 and 36 to 39
[total dose/cycle = 600 mg/m^2]
Maintenance (continue until 24 months from diagnosis):
Vincristine: IV: 2 mg/dose day 1 every 4 weeks
[total dose/4 weeks = 2 mg]
Prednisone: Oral: 60 mg/m^2/dose days 1 to 5 every 4 weeks
[total dose/4 weeks = 300 mg/m^2]
Mercaptopurine: Oral: 60 mg/m^2/dose days 1 to 28
[total dose/phase = 1680 mg/m^2]
Methotrexate: Oral: 20 mg/m^2/dose days 1, 8, 15, and 22
[total dose/phase = 80 mg/m^2]

References

Larson RA, Dodge RK, Linker CA, et al. A randomized controlled trial of filgrastim during remission induction and consolidation chemotherapy for adults with acute lymphoblastic leukemia: CALGB Study 9111. *Blood*. 1998;92(5):1556-1564.

- ♦ **Capecitabine-Cisplatin-Epirubicin (Gastric/Esophageal)** *see* Epirubicin-Cisplatin-Capecitabine (Gastric/Esophageal) *on page 2103*
- ♦ **Capecitabine-Cisplatin (Esophageal Cancer)** *see* Cisplatin-Capecitabine (Esophageal Cancer) *on page 2036*
- ♦ **Capecitabine-Cisplatin (Gastric Cancer)** *see* Cisplatin-Capecitabine (Gastric Cancer) *on page 2036*
- ♦ **Capecitabine-Cisplatin-Trastuzumab (Gastric Cancer)** *see* Trastuzumab-Cisplatin-Capecitabine (Gastric Cancer) *on page 2215*

Capecitabine-Docetaxel (Breast)

Index Terms Docetaxel-Capecitabine (Breast)
Use Breast cancer
Regimen
Capecitabine: Oral: 1250 mg/m^2 twice daily days 1 to 14
[total dose/cycle = 35,000 mg/m^2]
Docetaxel: IV: 75 mg/m^2 over 1 hour day 1
[total dose/cycle = 75 mg/m^2]
Repeat cycle every 21 days until disease progression or unacceptable toxicity
References

O'Shaughnessy J, Miles D, Vukelja S, et al, "Superior Survival With Capecitabine Plus Docetaxel Combination Therapy in Anthracycline-Pretreated Patients With Advanced Breast Cancer: Phase III Trial Results," *J Clin Oncol*, 2002, 20(12):2812-23.

Capecitabine-Docetaxel (Gastric Cancer)

Index Terms Docetaxel-Capecitabine (Gastric Cancer)
Use Gastric cancer

Regimen NOTE: Multiple variations are listed.

Variation 1:

Capecitabine: Oral: 1000 mg/m^2 twice daily days 1 to 14
[total dose/cycle = 28,000 mg/m^2]

Docetaxel: IV: 75 mg/m^2 day 1
[total dose/cycle = 75 mg/m^2]

Repeat cycle every 3 weeks for up to 9 cycles or until disease progression or unacceptable toxicity

Variation 2:

Capecitabine: Oral: 1000 mg/m^2 twice daily days 1 to 14
[total dose/cycle = 28,000 mg/m^2]

Docetaxel: IV: 36 mg/m^2 days 1 and 8
[total dose/cycle = 72 mg/m^2]

Repeat cycle every 3 weeks until disease progression or unacceptable toxicity

Variation 3:

Capecitabine: Oral: 825 mg/m^2 twice daily days 1 to 14
[total dose/cycle = 23,100 mg/m^2]

Docetaxel: IV: 75 mg/m^2 day 1
[total dose/cycle = 75 mg/m^2]

Repeat cycle every 3 weeks until disease progression

Variation 4:

Capecitabine: Oral: 1250 mg/m^2 twice daily days 1 to 14
[total dose/cycle = 35,000 mg/m^2]

Docetaxel: IV: 75 mg/m^2 day 1
[total dose/cycle = 75 mg/m^2]

Repeat cycle every 3 weeks until disease progression for up to a maximum of 6 cycles

References

Variation 1:
Kim JG, Sohn SK, Kim DH, et al, "Phase II Study of Docetaxel and Capecitabine in Patients With Metastatic or Recurrent Gastric Cancer," *Oncology*, 2005, 68(2-3):190-5.
Variation 2:
Chun JH, Kim HK, Lee JS, et al, "Weekly Docetaxel in Combination With Capecitabine in Patients With Metastatic Gastric Cancer," *Am J Clin Oncol*, 2005, 28(2):188-94.
Variation 3:
Giordano KF, Jatoi A, Stella PJ, et al, "Docetaxel and Capecitabine in Patients With Metastatic Adenocarcinoma of the Stomach and Gastroesophageal Junction: A Phase II Study From the North Central Cancer Treatment Group," *Ann Oncol*, 2006, 17(4):652-6.
Variation 4:
Park YH, Ryoo BY, Choi SJ, et al, "A Phase II Study of Capecitabine and Docetaxel Combination Chemotherapy in Patients With Advanced Gastric Cancer," *Br J Cancer*, 2004, 90(7):1329-33.

◆ **Capecitabine-Gemcitabine (Biliary Cancer)** *see* Gemcitabine-Capecitabine (Biliary Cancer) on page 2134

Capecitabine-Gemcitabine (Pancreatic)

Index Terms Gemcitabine-Capecitabine (Pancreatic)

Use Pancreatic cancer

Regimen NOTE: Multiple variations are listed.

Variation 1 (adjuvant therapy):

Gemcitabine: IV: 1,000 mg/m^2/day days 1, 8, and 15
[total dose/cycle = 3,000 mg/m^2]

Capecitabine: Oral: 830 mg/m^2/dose twice daily on days 1 to 21
[total dose/cycle = 34,860 mg/m^2]

Repeat cycle every 28 days for a total of 6 cycles, beginning within 12 weeks of resection (Neoptolemos 2017); American Society of Clinical Oncology guidelines recommend initiating within 8 weeks of resection (Khorana 2017)

Variation 2 (advanced or metastatic disease):

Gemcitabine: IV: 1,000 mg/m²/day over 30 minutes days 1, 8, and 15
[total dose/cycle = 3,000 mg/m²]

Capecitabine: Oral: 830 mg/m²/dose twice daily on days 1 to 21
[total dose/cycle = 34,860 mg/m²]

Repeat cycle every 28 days until disease progression or unacceptable toxicity

References

Variation 1:

Neoptolemos JP, Palmer DH, Ghaneh P, et al. Comparison of adjuvant gemcitabine and capecitabine with gemcitabine monotherapy in patients with resected pancreatic cancer (ESPAC-4): a multicentre, open-label, randomised, phase 3 trial. *Lancet*. 2017;389 (10073):1011-1024.

Khorana AA, Mangu PB, Berlin J, et al. Potentially curable pancreatic cancer: American Society of Clinical Oncology clinical practice guideline update. *J Clin Oncol*. 2017;35(20):2324-2328.

Variation 2:

Cunningham D, Chau I, Stocken DD, et al, "Phase III Randomized Comparison of Gemcitabine Versus Gemcitabine Plus Capecitabine in Patients With Advanced Pancreatic Cancer," *J Clin Oncol*, 2009, 27(33):5513-8.

♦ **Capecitabine-Irinotecan (Esophageal Cancer)** *see* Irinotecan-Capecitabine (Esophageal Cancer) *on page* 2157

♦ **Capecitabine-Irinotecan (Gastric Cancer)** *see* Irinotecan-Capecitabine (Gastric Cancer) *on page* 2158

Capecitabine-Ixabepilone (Breast)

Index Terms Ixabepilone-Capecitabine (Breast)

Use Breast cancer

Regimen

Capecitabine: Oral: 1000 mg/m² twice daily days 1 to 14
[total dose/cycle = 28,000 mg/m²]

Ixabepilone: IV: 40 mg/m² over 3 hours day 1
[total dose/cycle = 40 mg/m²]

Repeat cycle every 21 days until disease progression or unacceptable toxicity

References

Sparano JA, Vrdoljak E, Rixe O, et al, "Randomized Phase III Trial of Ixabepilone Plus Capecitabine Versus Capecitabine in Patients With Metastatic Breast Cancer Previously Treated With an Anthracycline and a Taxane," *J Clin Oncol*, 2010, 28(20):3256-63.

Thomas ES, Gomez HL, Li RK, et al, "Ixabepilone Plus Capecitabine for Metastatic Breast Cancer Progressing After Anthracycline and Taxane Treatment," *J Clin Oncol*, 2007, 25(33):5210-7.

Capecitabine + Lapatinib (Breast)

Index Terms Lapatinib-Capecitabine (Breast)

Use Breast cancer

Regimen

Capecitabine: Oral: 1000 mg/m² twice daily days 1 to 14 within 30 minutes after a meal
[total dose/cycle = 28,000 mg/m²]

Lapatinib: Oral: 1250 mg/day days 1 to 21 one hour before or one hour after a meal
[total dose/cycle = 26,250 mg]

Repeat cycle every 21 days until disease progression or unacceptable toxicity

References

Bachelot T, Romieu G, Campone M, et al, "Lapatinib Plus Capecitabine in Patients With Previously Untreated Brain Metastases From HER2-Positive Metastatic Breast Cancer (LAND-SCAPE): A Single-Group Phase 2 Study," *Lancet Oncol*, 2013, 14(1):64-71.

Cameron D, Casey M, Oliva C, et al, "Lapatinib Plus Capecitabine in Woman With HER-2-Positive Advanced Breast Cancer: Final Survival Analysis of a Phase III Randomized Trial," *Oncologist*, 2010, 15(9):924-34.

Geyer CE, Forster J, Lindquist D, et al, "Lapatinib Plus Capecitabine for HER2-Positive Advanced Breast Cancer," *N Engl J Med*, 2006, 355(26):2733-43.

◆ **Capecitabine-Oxaliplatin (Biliary Cancer)** *see* CAPOX (Biliary Cancer) *on page 2010*

◆ **Capecitabine-Oxaliplatin (Colorectal)** *see* XELOX (Colorectal) *on page 2233*

◆ **Capecitabine-Oxaliplatin-Epirubicin (Gastric/Esophageal)** *see* Epirubicin-Oxaliplatin-Capecitabine (Gastric/Esophageal) *on page 2104*

Capecitabine-Oxaliplatin (Gastric)

Index Terms CAPOX (Gastric); Oxaliplatin-Capecitabine (Gastric); XELOX (Gastric)

Use Gastric cancer

Regimen

Capecitabine: Oral: 1000 mg/m^2 twice daily days 1 to 14, taken with water within 30 minutes after a meal
[total dose/cycle = 28,000 mg/m^2]
Oxaliplatin: IV: 130 mg/m^2 day 1
[total dose/cycle = 130 mg/m^2]
Repeat cycle every 21 days for 8 cycles

References

Bang YJ, Kim YW, Yang HK, et al. Adjuvant capecitabine and oxaliplatin for gastric cancer after D2 gastrectomy (CLASSIC): a phase 3 open-label, randomised controlled trial. *Lancet*. 2012;379(9813):315-321.

◆ **Capecitabine-Oxaliplatin (Pancreatic)** *see* CAPOX (Pancreatic) *on page 2011*

Capecitabine-Oxaliplatin (Unknown Primary, Adenocarcinoma)

Index Terms CAPOX (Unknown Primary, Adenocarcinoma); Oxaliplatin-Capecitabine (Unknown Primary, Adenocarcinoma)

Use Unknown primary (adenocarcinoma)

Regimen

Capecitabine: Oral: 1,000 mg/m^2 twice daily days 1 to 14, taken with water within 30 minutes after a meal
[total dose/cycle = 28,000 mg/m^2]
Oxaliplatin: IV: 130 mg/m^2 day 1
[total dose/cycle = 130 mg/m^2]
Repeat cycle every 21 days for 6 cycles or may continue until clinical benefit no longer realized

References

Hainsworth JD, Spigel DR, Burris HA 3rd, et al. Oxaliplatin and capecitabine in the treatment of patients with recurrent or refractory carcinoma of unknown primary site: a phase 2 trial of the Sarah Cannon Oncology Research Consortium. *Cancer*. 2010;116(10):2448-2454.

Capecitabine-Trastuzumab (Breast)

Index Terms Trastuzumab-Capecitabine (Breast)

Use Breast cancer

Regimen NOTE: Multiple variations are listed.

Variation 1:

Cycle 1:

Capecitabine: Oral: 1250 mg/m^2 twice daily days 1 to 14
[total dose/cycle 1 = 35,000 mg/m^2]

Trastuzumab: IV: 4 mg/kg (loading dose) over 90 minutes day 1 cycle 1
followed by IV: 2 mg/kg/day over 30 minute days 8 and 15 cycle 1
[total dose/cycle 1 = 8 mg/kg]

Treatment cycle is 21 days

Subsequent cycles:

Capecitabine: Oral: 1250 mg/m^2 twice daily days 1 to 14
[total dose/cycle = 35,000 mg/m^2]

Trastuzumab: IV: 2 mg/kg/day over 30 minutes days 1, 8, and 15
[total dose/cycle = 6 mg/kg]

Repeat cycle every 21 days until disease progression or unacceptable toxicity

Variation 2:

Cycle 1:

Capecitabine: Oral: 1250 mg/m^2 twice daily days 1 to 14
[total dose/cycle 1 = 35,000 mg/m^2]

Trastuzumab: IV: 8 mg/kg (loading dose) day 1 cycle 1
[total dose/cycle 1 = 8 mg/kg]

Treatment cycle is 21 days

Subsequent cycles:

Capecitabine: Oral: 1250 mg/m^2 twice daily days 1 to 14
[total dose/cycle = 35,000 mg/m^2]

Trastuzumab: IV: 6 mg/kg day 1
[total dose/cycle = 6 mg/kg]

Repeat cycle every 21 days

References

Variation 1:

Schaller G, Fuchs I, Gonsch T, et al, "Phase II Study of Capecitabine Plus Trastuzumab in Human Epidermal Growth Factor Receptor 2 Overexpressing Metastatic Breast Cancer Pretreated With Anthracyclines or Taxanes," *J Clin Oncol*, 2007, 25(22):3246-50.

Variation 2:

Bartsch R, Wenzel C, Altorjai G, et al, "Capecitabine and Trastuzumab in Heavily Pretreated Metastatic Breast Cancer," *J Clin Oncol*, 2007, 25(25):3853-8.

◆ **CapeOx (Colorectal)** *see* XELOX (Colorectal) *on page 2233*

CAPOX (Biliary Cancer)

Index Terms Capecitabine-Oxaliplatin (Biliary Cancer); Oxaliplatin-Capecitabine (Biliary Cancer)

Use Biliary adenocarcinoma

Regimen

Capecitabine: Oral: 1000 mg/m^2/dose twice daily days 1 to 14
[total dose/cycle = 28,000 mg/m^2]

Oxaliplatin: IV: 130 mg/m^2 over 2 hours day 1
[total dose/cycle = 130 mg/m^2]

Repeat cycle every 3 weeks

References

Nehls O, Oettle H, Hartmann JT, et al, "Capecitabine Plus Oxaliplatin as First-Line Treatment in Patients With Advanced Biliary System Adenocarcinoma: A Prospective Multicentre Phase II Trial," *Br J Cancer*, 2008, 98(2):309-15.

◆ **CAPOX (Colorectal)** *see* XELOX (Colorectal) *on page 2233*

◆ **CAPOX (Gastric)** *see* Capecitabine-Oxaliplatin (Gastric) *on page 2009*

CAPOX (Pancreatic)

Index Terms Capecitabine-Oxaliplatin (Pancreatic); Oxaliplatin-Capecitabine (Pancreatic); XELOX (Pancreatic)

Use Pancreatic cancer

Regimen NOTE: Multiple variations are listed.

Variation 1 (patients <65 years of age and ECOG PS <2):

Capecitabine: Oral: 1000 mg/m^2 twice daily days 1 to 14

[total dose/cycle = 28,000 mg/m^2]

Oxaliplatin: IV: 130 mg/m^2 over 2 hours day 1

[total dose/cycle = 130 mg/m^2]

Repeat cycle every 21 days until disease progression or unacceptable toxicity

Variation 2 (patients >65 years of age, ECOG PS of 2, or significant comorbidities):

Capecitabine: Oral: 750 mg/m^2 twice daily days 1 to 14

[total dose/cycle = 21,000 mg/m^2]

Oxaliplatin: IV: 110 mg/m^2 over 2 hours day 1

[total dose/cycle = 110 mg/m^2]

Repeat cycle every 21 days until disease progression or unacceptable toxicity

References

Variations 1 and 2:
Xiong HQ, Varadhachary GR, Blais JC, et al, "Phase 2 Trial of Oxaliplatin Plus Capecitabine (XELOX) as Second-Line Therapy for Patients With Advanced Pancreatic Cancer," *Cancer*, 2008, 113(8):2046-52.

◆ **CAPOX (Unknown Primary, Adenocarcinoma)** *see* Capecitabine-Oxaliplatin (Unknown Primary, Adenocarcinoma) *on page 2009*

◆ **Carboplatin-Abraxane (NSCLC)** *see* Carboplatin-Paclitaxel (Protein Bound) (NSCLC) *on page 2022*

Carboplatin-Cetuximab (Head and Neck Cancer)

Index Terms Cetuximab-Carboplatin (Head and Neck Cancer)

Use Head and neck cancer

Regimen

Cycle 1:

Cetuximab: IV: 400 mg/m^2 (loading dose) day 1 (week 1, cycle 1 only)

[total loading dose = 400 mg/m^2]

followed by IV: 250 mg/m^2/day days 8 and 15

[total dose/cycle 1 = 900 mg/m^2]

Carboplatin: IV: AUC 5 day 1

[total dose/cycle = AUC = 5]

Treatment cycle is 3 weeks

Subsequent cycles:

Cetuximab: IV: 250 mg/m^2/day days 1, 8, and 15

[total dose/cycle = 750 mg/m^2]

Carboplatin: IV: AUC 5 day 1

[total dose/cycle = AUC = 5]

Repeat cycle every 3 weeks until disease progression or unacceptable toxicity for up to a maximum of 8 cycles

References

Chan AT, Hsu MM, Goh BC, et al, "Multicenter, Phase II Study of Cetuximab in Combination With Carboplatin in Patients With Recurrent or Metastatic Nasopharyngeal Carcinoma," *J Clin Oncol*, 2005, 23(15):3568-76.

Carboplatin-Docetaxel (Ovarian)

Index Terms Docetaxel-Carboplatin (Ovarian)

Use Ovarian cancer

Regimen NOTE: Multiple variations are listed.

Variation 1:

Docetaxel: IV: 60 mg/m^2 over 60 minutes day 1

[total dose/cycle = 60 mg/m^2]

Carboplatin: IV: AUC 6 over 30 minutes day 1

[total dose/cycle = AUC = 6]

Repeat cycle every 21 days for 6 cycles

Variation 2:

Docetaxel: IV: 75 mg/m^2 over 60 minutes day 1

[total dose/cycle = 75 mg/m^2]

Carboplatin: IV: AUC 5 over 30-60 minutes day 1

[total dose/cycle = AUC = 5]

Repeat cycle every 21 days for 6 cycles

Variation 3:

Docetaxel: IV: 35 mg/m^2 (maximum dose: 70 mg) over 60 minutes days 1, 8, and 15

[total dose/cycle = 105 mg/m^2, maximum dose/cycle = 210 mg]

Carboplatin: IV: AUC 2 over 30 minutes days 1, 8, and 15

[total dose/cycle = AUC = 6]

Repeat cycle every 28 days until disease progression or unacceptable toxicity or 2 cycles post complete response

References

Variation 1:

Markman M, Kennedy A, Webster K, et al, "Combination Chemotherapy With Carboplatin and Docetaxel in the Treatment of Cancers of the Ovary and Fallopian Tube and Primary Carcinoma of the Peritoneum," *J Clin Oncol*, 2001, 19(7):1901-5.

Variation 2:

Strauss HG, Henze A, Teichmann A, et al, "Phase II Trial of Docetaxel and Carboplatin in Recurrent Platinum-Sensitive Ovarian, Peritoneal, and Tubal Cancer," *Gynecol Oncol*, 2007, 104(3):612-6.

Vasey PA, Jayson GC, Gordon A, et al, "Phase III Randomized Trial of Docetaxel-Carboplatin Versus Paclitaxel-Carboplatin as First-line Chemotherapy for Ovarian Carcinoma," *J Natl Cancer Inst*, 2004, 96(22):1682-91.

Variation 3:

Kushner DM, Connor JP, Sanchez F, et al, "Weekly Docetaxel and Carboplatin for Recurrent Ovarian and Peritoneal Cancer," *Gynecol Oncol*, 2007, 105(2):358-64.

Carboplatin-Docetaxel-Trastuzumab (Breast)

Index Terms TCH (Breast); Trastuzumab-Docetaxel-Carboplatin (Breast)

Use Breast cancer

Regimen

Cycle 1:

Trastuzumab: IV: 4 mg/kg (loading dose) day 1 cycle 1

followed by IV: 2 mg/kg/day days 8 and 15 cycle 1

[total dose/cycle 1 = 8 mg/kg]

Docetaxel: IV: 75 mg/m^2 day 1

[total dose/cycle 1 = 75 mg/m^2]

Carboplatin: IV: AUC 6 day 1

[total dose/cycle 1 = AUC = 6]

Treatment cycle is 21 days

Cycles 2-6:

Trastuzumab: IV: 2 mg/kg/day days 1, 8, and 15

[total dose/cycle = 6 mg/kg]

Docetaxel: IV: 75 mg/m^2 day 1

[total dose/cycle = 75 mg/m^2]

Carboplatin: IV: AUC 6 day 1

[total dose/cycle = AUC = 6]

Repeat cycle every 21 days for a total of 6 cycles

Followed by:

Trastuzumab: IV: 6 mg/kg/day day 1

[total dose/cycle = 6 mg/kg]

Repeat cycle every 21 days for 11 cycles (to complete 1 year of Trastuzumab)

References

Slamon D, Eiermann W, Robert N, et al, "Adjuvant Trastuzumab in HER2-Positive Breast Cancer," *N Engl J Med*, 2011, 365(14):1273-83.

Carboplatin-Docetaxel (Unknown Primary, Adenocarcinoma)

Index Terms Docetaxel-Carboplatin (Unknown Primary, Adenocarcinoma)

Use Unknown primary (adenocarcinoma)

Regimen

Docetaxel: IV: 65 mg/m^2 over 1 hour day 1

[total dose/cycle = 65 mg/m^2]

Carboplatin: IV: AUC 6 over 20 minutes day 1

[total dose/cycle = AUC = 6]

Repeat cycle every 21 days for up to a maximum of 8 cycles

References

Greco FA, Erland JB, Morrissey LH, et al, "Carcinoma of Unknown Primary Site: Phase II Trials With Docetaxel Plus Cisplatin or Carboplatin," *Ann Oncol*, 2000, 11(2):211-5.

Carboplatin-Docetaxel (Unknown Primary, Squamous Cell)

Index Terms Docetaxel-Carboplatin (Unknown Primary, Squamous Cell)

Use Unknown primary (squamous cell)

Regimen

Docetaxel: IV: 75 mg/m^2 over 30 minutes day 1

[total dose/cycle = 75 mg/m^2]

Carboplatin: IV: AUC 5 over 30 minutes day 1

[total dose/cycle = AUC = 5]

Repeat cycle every 21 days for up to a maximum of 8 cycles

References
Pentheroudakis G, Briasoulis E, Kalofonos HP, et al, "Docetaxel and Carboplatin Combination Chemotherapy as Outpatient Palliative Therapy in Carinoma of Unknown Primary: A Multicentre Hellenic Cooperative Oncology Group Phase II Study," *Acta Oncol*, 2008, 47(6):1148-55.

Carboplatin-Doxorubicin (Liposomal) (Ovarian)

Index Terms Doxorubicin (Liposomal)-Carboplatin (Ovarian)

Use Ovarian cancer

Regimen NOTE: Multiple variations are listed.

Variation 1:

Doxorubicin (liposomal): IV: 30 mg/m^2 day 1

[total dose/cycle = 30 mg/m^2]

Carboplatin: IV: AUC 5 day 1

[total dose/cycle = AUC = 5]

Repeat cycle every 28 days until disease progression or unacceptable toxicity

Variation 2:

Doxorubicin (liposomal): IV: 30 mg/m^2 over 60 minutes day 1

[total dose/cycle = 30 mg/m^2]

Carboplatin: IV: AUC 5 over 30 minutes day 1

[total dose/cycle = AUC = 5]

Repeat cycle every 21 days for 6 cycles

References

Variation 1:

Pujade-Lauraine E, Wagner U, Aavall-Lundqvist E, et al, "Pegylated Liposomal Doxorubicin and Carboplatin Compared With Paclitaxel and Carboplatin for Patients With Platinum-Sensitive Ovarian Cancer in Late Relapse," *J Clin Oncol*, 2010, 28(20):3323-9.

Variation 2:

Pignata S, Scambia G, Ferrandina G, et al, "Carboplatin Plus Paclitaxel Versus Carboplatin Plus Pegylated Liposomal Doxorubicin as First-Line Treatment for Patients With Ovarian Cancer: The MITO-2 Randomized Phase III Trial," *J Clin Oncol*, 2011, 29(27):3628-35.

◆ **Carboplatin, Etoposide, Cyclophosphamide, Doxorubicin, Vincristine (Neuroblastoma)** see CE-CAdO (Neuroblastoma) *on page 2028*

Carboplatin-Etoposide (Ovarian Germ Cell Tumor)

Index Terms Etoposide-Carboplatin (Ovarian Germ Cell Tumor)

Use Ovarian cancer (adjuvant therapy in completely resected stage IB-III dysgerminoma)

Regimen

Etoposide: IV: 120 mg/m^2/day days 1, 2, and 3

[total dose/cycle = 360 mg/m^2]

Carboplatin: IV: 400 mg/m^2 day 1

[total dose/cycle = 400 mg/m^2]

Repeat cycle every 28 days for a total of 3 cycles

References

Williams SD, Kauderer J, Burnett AF, et al. Adjuvant therapy of completely resected dysgerminoma with carboplatin and etoposide: a trial of the Gynecologic Oncology Group. *Gynecol Oncol*. 2004;95(3):496-499.

Carboplatin-Etoposide-Paclitaxel (Unknown Primary, Adenocarcinoma)

Index Terms Paclitaxel-Carboplatin-Etoposide (Unknown Primary)

Use Unknown primary, adenocarcinoma

Regimen
Paclitaxel: IV: 200 mg/m^2 over 1 hour day 1
  [total dose/cycle = 200 mg/m^2]
Carboplatin: IV: AUC 6 over 20-30 minutes day 1
  [total dose/cycle = AUC = 6]
Etoposide: Oral: 50 mg/day days 1, 3, 5, 7, and 9
  and Oral: 100 mg/day days 2, 4, 6, 8, and 10
    [total dose/cycle = 750 mg]
Repeat cycle every 21 days for a total of 4-8 cycles

References
Greco FA, Burris HA 3rd, Erland JB, et al, "Carcinoma of Unknown Primary Site," *Cancer*, 2000, 89(12):2655-60.

Carboplatin-Etoposide (Retinoblastoma)
Index Terms Etoposide-Carboplatin (Retinoblastoma)
Use Retinoblastoma
Regimen
Etoposide: IV: 100 mg/m^2/day over 1 hour days 1 to 5
  [total dose/cycle = 500 mg/m^2]
Carboplatin: IV: 160 mg/m^2/day over 1 hour days 1 to 5
  [total dose/cycle = 800 mg/m^2]
Repeat cycle in 21 to 28 days for a total of 2 cycles

References
Doz F, Neuenschwander S, Plantaz D, et al, "Etoposide and Carboplatin in Extraocular Retino-blastoma: A Study by the Societe Francaise d'Oncologie Pediatrique," *J Clin Oncol*, 1995, 13 (4):902-9.

Carboplatin-Etoposide (Small Cell Lung Cancer)
Index Terms EC (Small Cell Lung Cancer); Etoposide-Carboplatin (Small Cell Lung Cancer)
Use Lung cancer, small cell
Regimen NOTE: Multiple variations are listed.
Variation 1 (limited stage with thoracic radiotherapy):
  Carboplatin: IV: AUC 6 over 1 hour day 1
    [total dose/cycle = AUC = 6]
  Etoposide: IV: 100 mg/m^2/day over 2 hours days 1, 2, and 3
    [total dose/cycle = 300 mg/m^2]
  Repeat cycle every 21 days for 6 cycles
Variation 2 (extensive):
  Carboplatin: IV: AUC 5 day 1
    [total dose/cycle = AUC = 5]
  Etoposide: IV: 100 mg/m^2/day days 1, 2, and 3
    [total dose/cycle = 300 mg/m^2]
  Repeat cycle every 21 days for 6 cycles
Variation 3 (elderly, limited, and extensive):
  Carboplatin: IV: AUC 5 over 1 hour day 1
    [total dose/cycle = AUC = 5]
  Etoposide: IV: 100 mg/m^2/day over 1 hour days 1, 2, and 3
    [total dose/cycle = 300 mg/m^2]
  Repeat cycle every 28 days for 4 cycles

References

Variation 1:

Skarlos DV, Samantas E, Briassoulis E, et al, "Randomized Comparison of Early Versus Late Hyperfractionated Thoracic Irradiation Concurrently With Chemotherapy in Limited Disease Small-Cell Lung Cancer: A Randomized Phase II Study of the Hellenic Cooperative Oncology Group (HeCOG)," *Ann Oncol*, 2001, 12(9):1231-8.

Variation 2:

Socinski MA, Smit EF, Lorigan P, et al, "Phase III Study of Pemetrexed Plus Carboplatin Compared With Etoposide Plus Carboplatin in Chemotherapy-Naïve Patients With Extensive-Stage Small Cell-Cell Lung Cancer," *J Clin Oncol*, 2009, 27(28):4787-92.

Variation 3:

Okamoto H, Watanabe K, Nishiwaki Y, et al, "Phase II Study of Area Under the Plasma-Concentration-Versus-Time Curve-Based Carboplatin Plus Standard-Dose Intravenous Etoposide in Elderly Patients With Small-Cell Lung Cancer," *J Clin Oncol*, 1999, 17(11):3540-5.

Carboplatin-Etoposide-Vincristine (Retinoblastoma)

Index Terms Etoposide-Carboplatin-Vincristine (Retinoblastoma); Vincristine-Carboplatin-Etoposide (Retinoblastoma)

Use Retinoblastoma

Regimen NOTE: Multiple variations are listed.

Variation 1 (<1 year of age):

Carboplatin: IV: 20 mg/kg day 1

[total dose/cycle = 20 mg/kg]

Etoposide Phosphate: IV: 5 mg/kg day 1

[total dose/cycle = 5 mg/kg]

Vincristine: IV: 0.05 mg/kg day 1

[total dose/cycle = 0.05 mg/kg]

Variation 2 (age >1 year):

Carboplatin: IV: 550-600 mg/m^2 day 1

[total dose/cycle = 550-600 mg/m^2]

Etoposide Phosphate: IV: 150 mg/m^2 day 1

[total dose/cycle = 150 mg/m^2]

Vincristine: IV: 1.5-2 mg/m^2 day 1

[total dose/cycle = 1.5-2 mg/m^2]

Variation 3 (≤36 months of age):

Carboplatin: IV: 18.6 mg/kg day 1

[total dose/cycle = 18.6 mg/kg]

Etoposide: IV: 5 mg/kg days 1 and 2

[total dose/cycle = 10 mg/kg]

Vincristine: IV: 0.05 mg/kg day 1 (maximum dose: 2 mg)

[total dose/cycle = 0.05 mg/kg; maximum dose: 2 mg]

Repeat cycle every 28 days for a total of 6 cycles

Variation 4 (>36 months of age):

Carboplatin: IV: 560 mg/m^2 day 1

[total dose/cycle = 560 mg/m^2]

Etoposide: IV: 150 mg/m^2 days 1 and 2

[total dose/cycle = 300 mg/m^2]

Vincristine: IV: 1.5 mg/m^2 day 1 (maximum dose: 2 mg)

[total dose/cycle = 1.5 mg/m^2; maximum dose: 2 mg]

Repeat cycle every 28 days for a total of 6 cycles

References

Variations 1 and 2:

Sussman DA, Escalona-Benz E, Benz MS, et al, "Comparison of Retinoblastoma Reduction for Chemotherapy vs External Beam Radiotherapy," *Arch Ophthalmol*, 2003, 121(7):979-84.

Variations 3 and 4:
Friedman DL, Himelstein B, Shields CL, et al, "Chemoreduction and Local Ophthalmic Therapy for Intraocular Retinoblastoma," *J Clin Oncol*, 2000, 18(1):12-7.
Shields CL, Honavar SG, Meadows AT, et al, "Chemoreduction for Unilateral Retinoblastoma," *Arch Ophthalmol*, 2002, 120(12):1653-8.

◆ **Carboplatin-Fluorouracil-Cetuximab (Head and Neck Cancer)** *see* Cetuximab-Carboplatin-Fluorouracil (Head and Neck Cancer) *on page 2030*

◆ **Carboplatin-Fluorouracil (Head and Neck Cancer)** *see* Fluorouracil-Carboplatin (Head and Neck Cancer) *on page 2123*

◆ **Carboplatin-Gemcitabine-Bevacizumab (Ovarian)** *see* Bevacizumab-Carboplatin-Gemcitabine (Ovarian) *on page 1990*

Carboplatin-Gemcitabine (Bladder)

Index Terms GC (Bladder); Gemcitabine-Carboplatin (Bladder)

Use Bladder cancer

Regimen

Gemcitabine: IV: 1000 mg/m^2/day over 30 minutes days 1 and 8
[total dose/cycle = 2000 mg/m^2]
Carboplatin: IV: AUC 4.5 over 60 minutes day 1
[total dose/cycle = AUC = 4.5]
Repeat cycle every 21 days until disease progression or unacceptable toxicity

References

De Santis M, Bellmunt J, Mead G, et al. Randomized phase II/III trial assessing gemcitabine/carboplatin and methotrexate/carboplatin/vinblastine in patients with advanced urothelial cancer who are unfit for cisplatin-based chemotherapy: EORTC study 30986. *J Clin Oncol*. 2012;30 (2):191-199.

Carboplatin-Gemcitabine (NSCLC)

Index Terms GC (NSCLC); Gemcitabine-Carboplatin (NSCLC)

Use Lung cancer, non-small cell

Regimen NOTE: Multiple variations are listed.

Variation 1:
Gemcitabine: IV: 1000 mg/m^2/day over 30 minutes days 1, 8, and 15
[total dose/cycle = 3000 mg/m^2]
Carboplatin: IV: AUC 5 day 1
[total dose/cycle = AUC = 5]
Repeat cycle every 28 days for up to 4 cycles

Variation 2:
Gemcitabine: IV: 1000 mg/m^2/day days 1 and 8
[total dose/cycle = 2000 mg/m^2]
Carboplatin: IV: AUC 5 day 1
[total dose/cycle = AUC = 5]
Repeat cycle every 21 days for up to 4 cycles

References

Variation 1:
Danson S, Middleton MR, O'Byrne KJ, et al, "Phase III Trial of Gemcitabine and Carboplatin Versus Mitomycin, Ifosfamide, and Cisplatin or Mitomycin, Vinblastine, and Cisplatin in Patients With Advanced Nonsmall Cell Lung Carcinoma," *Cancer*, 2003, 98(3):542-53.
Variation 2:
Grønberg BH, Bremnes RM, Fløtten O, et al, "Phase III Study by the Norwegian Lung Cancer Study Group: Pemetrexed Plus Carboplatin Compared With Gemcitabine Plus Carboplatin as First-Line Chemotherapy in Advanced Non-Small-Cell Lung Cancer," *J Clin Oncol*, 2009, 27 (19):3217-24

Carboplatin-Gemcitabine (Ovarian)

Index Terms Gemcitabine-Carboplatin (Ovarian)

Use Ovarian cancer

Regimen

Gemcitabine: IV: 1000 mg/m^2/day days 1 and 8

[total dose/cycle = 2000 mg/m^2]

Carboplatin: IV: AUC 4 day 1

[total dose/cycle = AUC = 4]

Repeat cycle every 21 days for 6-10 cycles

References

Pfisterer J, Plante M, Vergote I, et al, "Gemcitabine Plus Carboplatin Compared With Carboplatin in Patients With Platinum-Sensitive Recurrent Ovarian Cancer: An Intergroup Trial of the AGO-OVAR, the NCIC CTG, and the EORTC GCG," *J Clin Oncol*, 2006, 24(29):4699-707.

Carboplatin-Irinotecan (Small Cell Lung Cancer)

Index Terms IC (Small Cell Lung Cancer); IP (Small Cell Lung Cancer); Irinotecan-Carboplatin (Small Cell Lung Cancer)

Use Lung cancer, small cell

Regimen NOTE: Multiple variations are listed.

Variation 1:

Carboplatin: IV: AUC 5 (Calvert formula) day 1

[total dose/cycle = AUC = 5]

Irinotecan: IV: 175 mg/m^2 day 1

[total dose/cycle = 175 mg/m^2]

Repeat cycle every 21 days for a total of 4 cycles

Variation 2:

Carboplatin: IV: AUC 5 (Calvert formula) over 1 hour day 1

[total dose/cycle = AUC = 5]

Irinotecan: IV: 50 mg/m^2/day over 30 minutes days 1, 8, and 15

[total dose/cycle = 150 mg/m^2]

Repeat cycle every 28 days

References

Variation 1:

Hermes A, Bergman B, Bremnes R, et al, "Irinotecan Plus Carboplatin Versus Oral Etoposide Plus Carboplatin in Extensive Small-Cell Lung Cancer: A Randomized Phase III Trial," *J Clin Oncol*, 2008, 26(26):4261-7.

Variation 2:

Schmittel A, Fischer von Weikersthal L, Sebastian M, et al, "A Randomized Phase II Trial of Irinotecan Plus Carboplatin Versus Etoposide Plus Carboplatin Treatment in Patients With Extended Disease Small-Cell Lung Cancer," *Ann Oncol*, 2006, 17(4):663-7.

Schmittel A, Sebastian M, Fischer von Weikersthal L, et al, "A German Multicenter, Randomized Phase III Trial Comparing Irinotecan-Carboplatin With Etoposide-Carboplatin as First-Line Therapy for Extensive-Disease Small-Cell Lung Cancer," *Ann Oncol*, 2011, 22(8):1798-804.

◆ **Carboplatin-nab Paclitaxel (NSCLC)** *see* Carboplatin-Paclitaxel (Protein Bound) (NSCLC) *on page 2022*

◆ **Carboplatin-Paclitaxel-Bevacizumab (NSCLC)** *see* Bevacizumab-Carboplatin-Paclitaxel (NSCLC) *on page 1990*

Carboplatin-Paclitaxel (Cervical Cancer)

Index Terms Paclitaxel-Carboplatin (Cervical Cancer)

Use Cervical cancer

Regimen NOTE: Multiple variations are listed.

Variation 1:

Paclitaxel: IV: 175 mg/m^2 over 3 hours day 1 (reduce to 155 mg/m^2 over 3 hours day 1 if prior pelvic irradiation)

[total dose/cycle = 175 (or 155) mg/m^2]

Carboplatin: IV: AUC 5 or 6 day 1

[total dose/cycle = AUC = 5 or 6]

Repeat cycle every 28 days for up to a total of 6-9 cycles

Variation 2:

Paclitaxel: IV: 175 mg/m^2 over 3 hours day 1

[total dose/cycle = 175 mg/m^2]

Carboplatin: IV: AUC 5 day 1

[total dose/cycle = AUC = 5]

Repeat cycle every 21 days for 6-9 cycles

References

Variation 1:

Tinker AV, Bhagat K, Swenerton KD, et al, "Carboplatin and Paclitaxel for Advanced and Recurrent Cervical Carcinoma: The British Columbia Cancer Agency Experience," *Gynecol Oncol*, 2005, 98(1):54-8.

Variation 2:

Pectasides D, Fountzilas G, Papaxoinis G, et al, "Carboplatin and Paclitaxel in Metastatic or Recurrent Cervical Cancer," *Int J Gynecol Cancer*, 2009, 19(4):777-81.

Carboplatin-Paclitaxel (Endometrial)

Index Terms Paclitaxel-Carboplatin (Endometrial); TC (Endometrial)

Use Endometrial cancer

Regimen NOTE: Multiple variations are listed.

Variation 1:

Paclitaxel: IV: 175 mg/m^2 day 1

[total dose/cycle = 175 mg/m^2]

Carboplatin: IV: AUC 6 day 1

[total dose/cycle = AUC = 6]

Repeat cycle every 21 days for a total for 7 cycles

Variation 2:

Paclitaxel: IV: 175 mg/m^2 over 3 hours day 1

[total dose/cycle = 175 mg/m^2]

Carboplatin: IV: AUC 5 over 1 hour day 1

[total dose/cycle = AUC = 5]

Repeat cycle every 21 days for a total of 6 to 9 cycles

Variation 3:

Paclitaxel: IV: 80 mg/m^2 over 60 minutes days 1, 8, and 15

[total dose/cycle = 240 mg/m^2]

Carboplatin: IV: AUC 2 over 30 minutes days 1, 8, and 15

[total dose/cycle = AUC = 6]

Repeat cycle every 28 days until disease progression or unacceptable toxicity

References

Variation 1:

Miller DS, Filiaci G, Fleming G, et al. Randomized phase III noninferiority trial of first line chemotherapy for metastatic or recurrent endometrial carcinoma: A Gynecologic Oncology Group Study. *Gynecol Oncol.* 2012;125(3):771.

Variation 2:

Pectasides D, Xiros N, Papaxoinis G, et al. Carboplatin and paclitaxel in advanced or metastatic endometrial cancer. *Gynecol Oncol.* 2008;109(2):250-254.

Variation 3:
Secord AA, Havrilesky LJ, Carney ME, et al. Weekly low-dose paclitaxel and carboplatin in the treatment of advanced or recurrent cervical and endometrial cancer. *Int J Clin Oncol.* 2007;12 (1):31-36.

♦ **Carboplatin-Paclitaxel (Esophageal Cancer)** *see* Paclitaxel-Carboplatin (Esophageal Cancer) *on page* 2183

Carboplatin-Paclitaxel (NSCLC)

Index Terms Paclitaxel-Carboplatin (NSCLC); PC (NSCLC); TC (NSCLC)

Use Lung cancer, non-small cell

Regimen NOTE: Multiple variations are listed.

Variation 1:
Paclitaxel: IV: 225 mg/m^2 over 3 hours day 1
[total dose/cycle = 225 mg/m^2]
Carboplatin: IV: AUC 6 day 1
[total dose/cycle = AUC = 6]
Repeat cycle every 21 days

Variation 2:
Paclitaxel: IV: 200 mg/m^2 over 3 hours day 1
[total dose/cycle = 200 mg/m^2]
Carboplatin: IV: AUC 6 day 1
[total dose/cycle = AUC = 6]
Repeat cycle every 21 days

Variation 3:
Paclitaxel: IV: 100 mg/m^2/week over 3 hours for 6 weeks
[total dose/cycle = 600 mg/m^2]
Carboplatin: IV: AUC 2 weekly over 30 to 60 minutes for 6 weeks
[total dose/cycle = AUC = 12]
Repeat cycle every 8 weeks

Variation 4:
Paclitaxel: IV: 100 mg/m^2/day days 1, 8, and 15
[total dose/cycle = 300 mg/m^2]
Carboplatin: IV: AUC 6 day 1
[total dose/cycle = AUC = 6]
Repeat cycle every 28 days

References

Variation 1:
Belani CP, Ramalingam S, Perry MC, et al. Randomized, phase III study of weekly paclitaxel in combination with carboplatin versus standard every-3-weeks administration of carboplatin and paclitaxel for patients with previously untreated advanced non-small-cell lung cancer. *J Clin Oncol.* 2008;26(3):468-473.

Schiller JH, Harrington D, Belani CP, et al. Comparison of four chemotherapy regimens for advanced non-small-cell lung cancer. *N Engl J Med*, 2002;346(2):92-98.

Variation 2:
Ohe Y, Ohashi Y, Kubota K, et al. Randomized phase III study of cisplatin plus irinotecan versus carboplatin plus paclitaxel, cisplatin plus gemcitabine, and cisplatin plus vinorelbine for advanced non-small-cell lung cancer: Four-Arm Cooperative Study in Japan. *Ann Oncol.* 2007;18(2):317-323.

Schuette W, Blankenburg T, Guschall W, et al. Multicenter randomized trial for stage IIIB/IV non-small-cell lung cancer using every-3-week versus weekly paclitaxel/carboplatin. *Clin Lung Cancer.* 2006;7(5):338-343.

Variation 3:
Schuette W, Blankenburg T, Guschall W, et al. Multicenter randomized trial for stage IIIB/IV non-small-cell lung cancer using every-3-week versus weekly paclitaxel/carboplatin. *Clin Lung Cancer.* 2006;7(5):338-343.

Variation 4:
Belani CP, Ramalingam S, Perry MC, et al. Randomized, phase III study of weekly paclitaxel in combination with carboplatin versus standard every-3-weeks administration of carboplatin and paclitaxel for patients with previously untreated advanced non-small-cell lung cancer. *J Clin Oncol.* 2008;26(3):468-473.

Carboplatin-Paclitaxel (Ovarian)

Index Terms Paclitaxel-Carboplatin (Ovarian)

Use Ovarian cancer

Regimen NOTE: Multiple variations are listed.

Variation 1:
Paclitaxel: IV: 175 mg/m^2 over 3 hours day 1
[total dose/cycle = 175 mg/m^2]
Carboplatin: IV: AUC 7.5 day 1
[total dose/cycle = AUC = 7.5]
Repeat cycle every 21 days for a total of 6 cycles

Variation 2:
Paclitaxel: IV: 175-185 mg/m^2 over 3 hours day 1
[total dose/cycle = 175-185 mg/m^2]
Carboplatin: IV: AUC 5-6 day 1
[total dose/cycle = AUC = 5-6]
Repeat cycle every 21 days

Variation 3:
Paclitaxel: IV: 175 mg/m^2 over 3 hours day 1
[total dose/cycle = 175 mg/m^2]
Carboplatin: IV: AUC 5 day 1
[total dose/cycle = AUC = 5]
Repeat cycle every 21 days

Variation 4:
Paclitaxel: IV: 175 mg/m^2 over 3 hours day 1
[total dose/cycle = 175 mg/m^2]
Carboplatin: IV: AUC 7.5 over 30 minutes day 1
[total dose/cycle = AUC = 7.5]
Repeat cycle every 21 days for 3-6 cycles

Variation 5:
Paclitaxel: IV: 80 mg/m^2 over 1 hour days 1, 8, and 15
[total dose/cycle = 240 mg/m^2]
Carboplatin: IV: AUC 6 over 1 hour day 1
[total dose/cycle = AUC = 6]
Repeat cycle every 21 days for a total of 6 cycles

References

Variation 1:
Ozols RF, Bundy BN, Greer BE, et al, "Phase III Trial of Carboplatin and Paclitaxel Compared With Cisplatin and Paclitaxel in Patients With Optimally Resected Stage III Ovarian Cancer: A Gynecologic Oncology Group Study," *J Clin Oncol*, 2003, 21(17):3194-200.
Variation 2:
Parmar MK, Ledermann JA, Colombo N, et al, "Paclitaxel Plus Platinum-Based Chemotherapy Versus Conventional Platinum-Based Chemotherapy in Women With Relapsed Ovarian Cancer: The ICON4/AGO-OVAR-2.2 Trial," *Lancet*, 2003, 361(9375):2099-106.
Variation 3:
Neijt JP, Engelholm SA, Tuxen MK, et al, "Exploratory Phase III Study of Paclitaxel and Cisplatin Versus Paclitaxel and Carboplatin in Advanced Ovarian Cancer," *J Clin Oncol*, 2000, 18 (17):3084-92.
Vasey PA, Jayson GC, Gordon A, et al, "Phase III Randomized Trial of Docetaxel-Carboplatin Versus Paclitaxel-Carboplatin as First-Line Chemotherapy for Ovarian Carcinoma," *J Natl Cancer Inst*, 2004, 96(22):1682-91.

◄ Variation 4:
Bell J, Brady MF, Young RC, et al, "Randomized Phase III Trial of Three Versus Six Cycles of Adjuvant Carboplatin and Paclitaxel in Early Stage Epithelial Ovarian Carcinoma: A Gynecologic Oncology Group Study," *Gynecol Oncol*, 2006, 102(3):432-9.
Variation 5:
Katsumata N, Yasuda M, Takahashi F, et al, "Dose-Dense Paclitaxel Once a Week in Combination With Carboplatin Every 3 Weeks for Advanced Ovarian Cancer: A Phase III, Open-Label, Randomised Trial," *Lancet*, 2009, 374(9698):1331-8.

Carboplatin-Paclitaxel (Protein Bound) (NSCLC)

Index Terms Carboplatin-Abraxane (NSCLC); Carboplatin-nab Paclitaxel (NSCLC); nab Paclitaxel-Carboplatin (NSCLC); nab-PC (NSCLC); Paclitaxel (Protein Bound)-Carboplatin (NSCLC)

Use Lung cancer, non-small cell

Regimen

Paclitaxel (Protein Bound): IV: 100 mg/m^2/day over 30 minutes days 1, 8, and 15

[total dose/cycle = 300 mg/m^2]

Carboplatin: IV: AUC 6 day 1

[total dose/cycle = AUC = 6]

Repeat cycle every 21 days for at least 6 cycles or until disease progression or unacceptable toxicity

References

Socinski MA, Bondarenko I, Karaseva NA, et al, "Weekly nab-Paclitaxel in Combination With Carboplatin Versus Solvent-Based Paclitaxel Plus Carboplatin as First-Line Therapy in Patients With Advanced Non-Small-Cell Lung Cancer: Final Results of a Phase III Trial," *J Clin Oncol*, 2012, 30(17):2055-62.

Carboplatin-Paclitaxel (Thymoma/Thymic)

Use Thymoma/thymic carcinoma (advanced previously untreated)

Regimen

Paclitaxel: IV: 225 mg/m^2 over 3 hours day 1

[total dose/cycle = 225 mg/m^2]

Carboplatin: IV: AUC 6 over 30 minutes day 1

[total dose/cycle = AUC = 6]

Repeat cycle every 21 days for up to 6 cycles

References

Lemma GL, Lee JW, Aisner SC, et al. Phase II study of carboplatin and paclitaxel in advanced thymoma and thymic carcinoma. *J Clin Oncol*. 2011;29(15):2060-2065.

Carboplatin-Paclitaxel-Trastuzumab (Breast)

Index Terms Paclitaxel-Carboplatin-Trastuzumab (Breast); TCH (Breast); TPC (Breast); Trastuzumab-Paclitaxel-Carboplatin (Breast)

Use Breast cancer

Regimen

Variation 1:

Cycle 1:

Trastuzumab: IV: 4 mg/kg (loading dose) cycle 1 day 1

followed by IV: 2 mg/kg days 8 and 15

[total dose/cycle 1 = 8 mg/kg]

Paclitaxel: IV: 175 mg/m^2 day 2

[total dose/cycle = 175 mg/m^2]

Carboplatin: IV: AUC 6 day 2

[total dose/cycle = AUC = 6]

Treatment cycle is 21 days

Subsequent cycles:

Trastuzumab: IV: 2 mg/kg days 1, 8, and 15

[total dose/cycle = 6 mg/kg]

Paclitaxel: IV: 175 mg/m^2 day 2

[total dose/cycle = 175 mg/m^2]

Carboplatin: IV: AUC 6 day 2

[total dose/cycle = AUC = 6]

Repeat cycle every 21 days for a total of at least 6 cycles

followed by:

Trastuzumab: IV: 2 mg/kg once weekly until disease progression or unacceptable toxicity

Variation 2:

Cycle 1:

Paclitaxel: IV: 80 mg/m^2 over 1 hour days 1, 8, and 15

[total dose/cycle 1 = 240 mg/m^2]

Carboplatin: IV: AUC 2 over 15 minutes days 1, 8, and 15

[total dose/cycle 1 = AUC = 6]

Trastuzumab: IV: 4 mg/kg (loading dose) over 90 minutes cycle 1 day 1

followed by IV: 2 mg/kg over 30 minutes days 8, 15, and 22

[total dose/cycle 1 = 10 mg/kg]

Treatment cycle is 28 days

Subsequent cycles:

Paclitaxel: IV: 80 mg/m^2 over 1 hour days 1, 8, and 15

[total dose/cycle = 240 mg/m^2]

Carboplatin: IV: AUC 2 over 15 minutes days 1, 8, and 15

[total dose/cycle = AUC = 6]

Trastuzumab: IV: 2 mg/kg over 30 minutes days 1, 8, 15, and 22

[total dose/cycle = 8 mg/kg]

Repeat cycle every 28 days for a maximum of 6 cycles

followed by:

Trastuzumab: IV: 6 mg/kg every 21 days until disease progression or unacceptable toxicity

References

Variation 1:

Robert N, Leyland Jones B, Asmar L, et al, "Randomized Phase III Study of Trastuzumab, Paclitaxel, and Carboplatin Compared With Trastuzumab and Paclitaxel in Women With HER-2-Overexpressing Metastatic Breast Cancer," *J Clin Oncol*, 2006, 24(18):2786-92.

Variation 2:

Perez EA, Suman VJ, Rowland KM, et al, "Two Concurrent Phase II Trials of Paclitaxel/ Carboplatin/Trastuzumab (Weekly or Every-3-Week Schedule) as First-Line Therapy in Women With HER2-Overexpressing Metastatic Breast Cancer: NCCTG Study 983252," *Clin Breast Cancer*, 2005, 6(5):425-32.

Carboplatin-Paclitaxel (Unknown Primary, Adenocarcinoma)

Index Terms Carbo-Tax (Unknown Primary); Paclitaxel-Carboplatin (Unknown Primary)

Use Unknown primary (adenocarcinoma)

Regimen

Carboplatin: IV: Target AUC 6 day 1

[total dose/cycle = AUC = 6]

followed by

Paclitaxel: IV: 200 mg/m^2 infused over 3 hours day 1

[total dose/cycle = 200 mg/m^2]

Filgrastim: SubQ: 300 mcg/day days 5 to 12
[total dose/cycle = 2400 mcg]
Repeat cycle every 21 days for a total of 6 or 8 cycles

References

Briasoulis E, Kalofonos H, Bafaloukos D, et al, "Carboplatin Plus Paclitaxel in Unknown Primary Carcinoma: A Phase II Hellenic Cooperative Oncology Group Study," *J Clin Oncol*, 2000, 18 (17):3101-7.

◆ **Carboplatin-Pemetrexed-Bevacizumab (NSCLC)** *see* Bevacizumab-Carboplatin-Pemetrexed (NSCLC) *on page 1990*

Carboplatin-Pemetrexed (Mesothelioma)

Index Terms Pemetrexed-Carboplatin (Mesothelioma)
Use Malignant pleural mesothelioma
Regimen

Pemetrexed: IV: 500 mg/m^2 over 10 minutes day 1
[total dose/cycle = 500 mg/m^2]
Carboplatin: IV: AUC 5 over 30 minutes day 1 (start 30 minutes after pemetrexed)
[total dose/cycle = AUC = 5]
Repeat cycle every 21 days

References

Ceresoli GL, Zucali PA, Favaretto AG, et al, "Phase II Study of Pemetrexed Plus Carboplatin in Malignant Pleural Mesothelioma," *J Clin Oncol*, 2006, 24(9):1443-8.

Santoro A, O'Brien ME, Stahel RA, et al, "Pemetrexed Plus Cisplatin or Pemetrexed Plus Carboplatin for Chemonaïve Patients With Malignant Pleural Mesothelioma: Results of the International Expanded Access Program," *J Thorac Oncol*, 2008, 3(7):756-63.

Carboplatin-Pemetrexed (NSCLC)

Index Terms Pemetrexed-Carboplatin (NSCLC)
Use Lung cancer, non-small cell
Regimen

Pemetrexed: IV: 500 mg/m^2 day 1
[total dose/cycle = 500 mg/m^2]
Carboplatin: IV: AUC 5 day 1
[total dose/cycle = AUC = 5]
Repeat cycle every 21 days for a maximum of 4 cycles

References

Gronberg BH, Bremnes RM, Flotten O, et al, "Phase III Study by the Norwegian Lung Cancer Study Group: Pemetrexed Plus Carboplatin Compared With Gemcitabine Plus Carboplatin as First-Line Chemotherapy in Advanced Non-Small-Cell Lung Cancer," *J Clin Oncol*, 2009, 27 (19):3217-24.

Carboplatin-Pemetrexed-Pembrolizumab (NSCLC)

Index Terms Pembrolizumab-Pemetrexed-Carboplatin (NSCLC)
Use Lung cancer, non-small cell (metastatic nonsquamous)
Regimen

Induction:
Pembrolizumab: IV: 200 mg over 30 minutes day 1
[total dose/cycle = 200 mg]
Pemetrexed: IV: 500 mg/m^2 over 10 minutes day 1
[total dose/cycle = 500 mg/m^2]
Carboplatin: IV: AUC 5 over 15 to 60 minutes day 1
[total dose/cycle = AUC = 5]
Repeat cycle every 21 days for up to 4 cycles

Maintenance:
Pembrolizumab: IV: 200 mg over 30 minutes day 1
[total dose/cycle = 200 mg]
Repeat cycle every 21 days (with or without optional indefinite pemetrexed maintenance) until disease progression, unacceptable toxicity, or for up to 24 months

References

Langer CJ, Gadgeel SM, Borghaei H, et al. Carboplatin and pemetrexed with or without pembrolizumab for advanced, non-squamous non-small-cell lung cancer: a randomised, phase 2 cohort of the open-label KEYNOTE-021 study. *Lancet Oncol.* 2016;17(11):1497-1508.

Carboplatin-Vincristine (Retinoblastoma)

Index Terms Vincristine-Carboplatin (Retinoblastoma)

Use Retinoblastoma

Regimen NOTE: Multiple variations are listed.
Variation 1 (GFR ≥50 mL/minute/m^2):
Carboplatin: IV: 560 mg/m^2 day 1
[total dose/cycle = 560 mg/m^2]
Vincristine: IV: 0.05 mg/kg day 1
[total dose/cycle = 0.05 mg/kg]
Repeat cycle every 21 days for up to a total of 8 cycles
Variation 2 (GFR <50 mL/minute/m^2):
Carboplatin: IV: AUC 6.5 day 1
[total dose/cycle = AUC 6.5]
Vincristine: IV: 0.05 mg/kg day 1
[total dose/cycle = 0.05 mg/kg]
Repeat cycle every 21 days for up to a total of 8 cycles

References

Rodriguez-Galindo C, Wilson MW, Haik BG, et al. Treatment of intraocular retinoblastoma with vincristine and carboplatin. *J Clin Oncol.* 2003;21(10):2019-2025.

◆ **Carbo-Tax (Unknown Primary)** *see* Carboplatin-Paclitaxel (Unknown Primary, Adenocarcinoma) *on page 2023*

Carfilzomib-Dexamethasone (Multiple Myeloma)

Index Terms Dexamethasone-Carfilzomib (Multiple Myeloma)

Use Multiple myeloma (relapsed/refractory patients that have received 1 to 3 prior lines of therapy)

Regimen NOTE: Hydrate with oral fluids (30 mL/kg) at least 48 hours prior to initiating cycle 1, as well as with 250 to 500 mL normal saline (or other appropriate IV fluid) before dosing (recommended) and after (if needed) administration during cycle 1 (continue oral and/or IV hydration in subsequent cycles if necessary); dosed based upon a maximum BSA of 2.2 m^2
Cycle 1:
Carfilzomib: IV: 20 mg/m^2 over 30 minutes days 1 and 2 (cycle 1)
followed by: 56 mg/m^2 over 30 minutes days 8, 9, 15, and 16 (cycle 1)
[total dose/cycle = 264 mg/m^2]
Dexamethasone: Oral or IV: 20 mg once daily on days 1, 2, 8, 9, 15, 16, 22, and 23
[total dose/cycle = 160 mg]
Treatment cycle duration is 28 days

◀ Subsequent Cycles:

Carfilzomib: IV: 56 mg/m^2 over 30 minutes days 1, 2, 8, 9, 15, and 16

[total dose/cycle = 336 mg/m^2]

Dexamethasone: Oral or IV: 20 mg once daily on days 1, 2, 8, 9, 15, 16, 22, and 23

[total dose/cycle = 160 mg]

Repeat cycle every 28 days until disease progression or unacceptable toxicity

References

Dimopoulos MA, Moreau P, Palumbo A, et al. Carfilzomib and dexamethasone versus bortezomib and dexamethasone for patients with relapsed or refractory multiple myeloma (ENDEAVOR): a randomised, phase 3, open-label, multicentre study. *Lancet Oncol.* 2016;17(1):27-38.

Kyprolis (carfilzomib) [prescribing information]. Thousand Oaks, CA: Onyx Pharmaceuticals Inc; May 2017.

Carfilzomib, Lenalidomide, Dexamethasone (Multiple Myeloma)

Index Terms CRd (Multiple Myeloma); Lenalidomide, Carfilzomib, Dexamethasone (Multiple Myeloma)

Use Multiple myeloma (relapsed)

Regimen

Cycle 1:

Carfilzomib: IV: 20 mg/m^2/day over 10 minutes days 1 and 2 (cycle 1)

followed by: 27 mg/m^2/day over 10 minutes days 8, 9, 15, and 16 (cycle 1)

[total dose/cycle = 148 mg/m^2]

Lenalidomide: Oral: 25 mg once daily days 1 to 21

[total dose/cycle = 525 mg]

Dexamethasone: Oral: 40 mg once daily on days 1, 8, 15, and 22

[total dose/cycle = 160 mg]

Treatment cycle duration is 28 days

Cycles 2 to 12:

Carfilzomib: IV: 27 mg/m^2/day over 10 minutes days 1, 2, 8, 9, 15, and 16

[total dose/cycle = 162 mg/m^2]

Lenalidomide: Oral: 25 mg once daily days 1 to 21

[total dose/cycle = 525 mg]

Dexamethasone: Oral: 40 mg once daily on days 1, 8, 15, and 22

[total dose/cycle = 160 mg]

Treatment cycle duration is 28 days

Cycles 13 to 18:

Carfilzomib: IV: 27 mg/m^2/day over 10 minutes days 1, 2, 15, and 16

[total dose/cycle = 108 mg/m^2]

Lenalidomide: Oral: 25 mg once daily days 1 to 21

[total dose/cycle = 525 mg]

Dexamethasone: Oral: 40 mg once daily on days 1, 8, 15, and 22

[total dose/cycle = 160 mg]

Treatment cycle duration is 28 days

Subsequent Cycles:
Lenalidomide: Oral: 25 mg once daily days 1 to 21
[total dose/cycle = 525 mg]
Dexamethasone: Oral: 40 mg once daily on days 1, 8, 15, and 22
[total dose/cycle = 160 mg]
Repeat cycle every 28 days until disease progression or unacceptable toxicity

References
Stewart AK, Rajkumar SV, Dimopoulos MA, et al. Carfilzomib, lenalidomide, and dexamethasone for relapsed multiple myeloma. *N Engl J Med*. 2015;372(2):142-152.

♦ **Carmustine-Etoposide-Cytarabine-Melphalan (Hodgkin)** *see* mini-BEAM (Hodgkin) *on page 2174*

CAV-P/VP (Neuroblastoma)

Index Terms Cyclophosphamide, Doxorubicin, Vincristine, Etoposide, Cisplatin (Neuroblastoma); N6 Protocol (Neuroblastoma)

Use Neuroblastoma

Regimen NOTE: The interval between courses is not fixed; the next course to begin upon hematologic recovery (ANC ≥500/mm^3 and platelets ≥100,000/mm^3)

Course 1, 2, 4, and 6 (CAV):
Cyclophosphamide: IV: 70 mg/kg/day over 6 hours days 1 and 2
[total dose/cycle = 140 mg/kg]
Doxorubicin: IV: 25 mg/m^2/day continuous infusion days 1, 2, and 3
[total dose/cycle = 75 mg/m^2]
Vincristine: IV: 0.033 mg/kg/day continuous infusion days 1, 2, and 3
[total dose/cycle = 0.099 mg/kg]
Vincristine: IV: 1.5 mg/m^2 bolus day 9
[total dose/cycle = 1.5 mg/m^2]
Course 3, 5, and 7 (P/VP):
Etoposide: IV: 200 mg/m^2/day over 2 hours days 1, 2, and 3
[total dose/cycle = 600 mg/m^2]
Cisplatin: IV: 50 mg/m^2/day over 1 hour days 1 to 4
[total dose/cycle = 200 mg/m^2]

References
Kushner BH, LaQuaglia MP, Bonilla MA, et al, "Highly Effective Induction Therapy for Stage 4 Neuroblastoma in Children Over 1 Year of Age," *J Clin Oncol*, 1994, 12(12):2607-13.

CAV (Small Cell Lung Cancer)

Index Terms Cyclophosphamide, Doxorubicin, Vincristine (Small Cell Lung Cancer)

Use Lung cancer, small cell

Regimen
Cyclophosphamide: IV: 1000 mg/m^2 day 1
[total dose/cycle = 1000 mg/m^2; maximum: 2000 mg]
Doxorubicin: IV: 45 mg/m^2 day 1
[total dose/cycle = 45 mg/m^2; maximum: 100 mg]
Vincristine: IV: 2 mg day 1
[total dose/cycle = 2 mg]
Repeat cycle every 21 days

References
von Pawel J, Schiller JH, Shephard FA, et al, "Topotecan Versus Cyclophosphamide, Doxorubicin, and Vincristine for the Treatment of Recurrent Small-Cell Lung Cancer," *J Clin Oncol*, 1999, 17 (2):658-67.

◆ **2-CDA-Rituximab (NHL-Mantle Cell)** *see* Cladribine-Rituximab (NHL-Mantle Cell) *on page 2064*

CDDP/VP-16
Use Brain tumors
Regimen
Cisplatin: IV: 90 mg/m^2 day 1
 [total dose/cycle = 90 mg/m^2]
Etoposide: IV: 150 mg/m^2/day days 3 and 4
 [total dose/cycle = 300 mg/m^2]
Repeat cycle every 21 days
References
Kovnar EH, Kellie SJ, Horowitz ME, et al, "Preirradiation Cisplatin and Etoposide in the Treatment of High-Risk Medulloblastoma and Other Malignant Embryonal Tumors of the Central Nervous System: A Phase II Study," *J Clin Oncol*, 1990, 8(2):330-6.

CE-CAdO (Neuroblastoma)
Index Terms Carboplatin, Etoposide, Cyclophosphamide, Doxorubicin, Vincristine (Neuroblastoma)
Use Neuroblastoma
Regimen
Variation 1:
 Cycles 1 and 2 (CE):
  Carboplatin: IV: 200 mg/m^2/day days 1, 2, and 3
   [total dose/cycle = 600 mg/m^2]
  Etoposide: IV: 150 mg/m^2/day days 1, 2, and 3
   [total dose/cycle = 450 mg/m^2]
 Repeat CE cycle once at 21 days, then follow with
 Cycles 3 and 4 (CAdO):
  Cyclophosphamide: IV: 300 mg/m^2/day days 1 to 5
   [total dose/cycle = 1500 mg/m^2]
  Doxorubicin: IV: 60 mg/m^2 day 5
   [total dose/cycle = 60 mg/m^2]
  Vincristine: IV: 1.5 mg/m^2 (maximum dose: 2 mg) days 1 and 5
   [total dose/cycle = 3 mg/m^2 (maximum: 2 mg/dose)]
 Repeat CAdO cycle once at 21 days
Variation 2:
 Cycles 1 and 2 (CE):
  Carboplatin: IV: 6.6 mg/kg/day days 1, 2, and 3
   [total dose/cycle = 19.8 mg/kg]
  Etoposide: IV: 5 mg/kg/day days 1, 2, and 3
   [total dose/cycle = 15 mg/kg]
 Repeat CE cycle once, then follow with
 Cycles 3 and 4 (CAdO):
  Cyclophosphamide: IV: 10 mg/kg/day days 1 to 5
   [total dose/cycle = 50 mg/kg]
  Doxorubicin: IV: 2 mg/kg day 5
   [total dose/cycle = 2 mg/kg]

Vincristine: IV: 0.05 mg/kg days 1 and 5
[total dose/cycle = 0.1 mg/kg]
Repeat CAdO cycle once

References

Variation 1:
Rubie H, Michon J, Plantaz D, et al, "Unresectable Localized Neuroblastoma: Improved Survival After Primary Chemotherapy Including Carboplatin-Etoposide. Neuroblastoma Study Group of the Societe Francaise d'Oncologie Pediatrique (SFOP)," *Br J Cancer*, 1998, 77(12):2310-7.
Variation 2:
Rubie H, Plantaz D, Coze C, et al, "Localised and Unresectable Neuroblastoma in Infants: Excellent Outcome With Primary Chemotherapy. Neuroblastoma Study Group, Société Française d'Oncologie Pédiatrique," *Med Pediatr Oncol*, 2001, 36(1):247-50.

CEPP (NHL-DLBCL)

Index Terms Cyclophosphamide-Etoposide-Procarbazine-Prednisone (NHL-DLBCL)

Use Lymphoma, non-Hodgkin (DLBCL)

Regimen

Cyclophosphamide: IV: 600 to 650 mg/m^2/day days 1 and 8
[total dose/cycle = 1,200 to 1,300 mg/m^2]
Etoposide: IV: 70 to 85 mg/m^2/day days 1, 2, and 3
[total dose/cycle = 210 to 255 mg/m^2]
Procarbazine: Oral: 60 mg/m^2/day days 1 to 10
[total dose/cycle = 600 mg/m^2]
Prednisone: Oral: 60 mg/m^2/day days 1 to 10
[total dose/cycle = 600 mg/m^2]
Repeat cycle every 28 days

References

Chao NJ, Rosenberg SA, Horning SJ. CEPP(B): an effective and well-tolerated regimen in poor-risk, aggressive non-Hodgkin's lymphoma. *Blood*. 1990;76(7):1293-1298.

Cetuximab (Biweekly)-Irinotecan (Colorectal)

Index Terms Biweekly CetIri (Colorectal); Every 2 Weeks Cetuximab-Irinotecan (Colorectal); Irinotecan-Biweekly Cetuximab (Colorectal)

Use Colorectal cancer

Regimen

Cycle 1:
Cetuximab: IV: 500 mg/m^2 over 120 minutes day 1 cycle 1
[total dose/cycle 1 = 500 mg/m^2]
Irinotecan: IV: 180 mg/m^2 over 30 minutes day 1 cycle 1
[total dose/cycle 1 = 180 mg/m^2]
Treatment cycle is 14 days
Subsequent cycles:
Cetuximab: IV: 500 mg/m^2 over 60 minutes day 1
[total dose/cycle = 500 mg/m^2]
Irinotecan: IV: 180 mg/m^2 over 30 minutes day 1
[total dose/cycle = 180 mg/m^2]
Repeat cycle every 14 days until disease progression or unacceptable toxicity

References

Martín-Martorell P, Roselló S, Rodríguez-Braun E, et al, "Biweekly Cetuximab and Irinotecan in Advanced Colorectal Cancer Patients Progressing After at Least One Previous Line of Chemotherapy: Results of a Phase II Single Institution Trial," *Br J Cancer*, 2008, 99(3):455-8.
Pfeiffer P, Nielsen D, Bjerregaard J, et al, "Biweekly Cetuximab and Irinotecan as Third-Line Therapy in Patients With Advanced Colorectal Cancer After Failure to Irinotecan, Oxaliplatin and 5-Fluorouracil," *Ann Oncol*, 2008, 19(6):1141-5.

Cetuximab-Carboplatin-Fluorouracil (Head and Neck Cancer)

Index Terms Carboplatin-Fluorouracil-Cetuximab (Head and Neck Cancer)
Use Head and neck cancer
Regimen
Cycle 1:
Cetuximab: IV: 400 mg/m^2 (loading dose) day 1 (week 1, cycle 1 only)
[total loading dose = 400 mg/m^2]
followed by IV: 250 mg/m^2/day days 8 and 15
[total dose/cycle 1 = 900 mg/m^2]
Carboplatin: IV: AUC 5 day 1
[total dose/cycle = AUC = 5]
Fluorouracil: IV: 1000 mg/m^2/day continuous infusion days 1 to 4
[total dose/cycle = 4000 mg/m^2]
Treatment cycle is 3 weeks
Subsequent cycles:
Cetuximab: IV: 250 mg/m^2/day days 1, 8, and 15
[total dose/cycle = 750 mg/m^2]
Carboplatin: IV: AUC 5 day 1
[total dose/cycle = AUC = 5]
Fluorouracil: IV: 1000 mg/m^2/day continuous infusion days 1 to 4
[total dose/cycle = 4000 mg/m^2]
Repeat cycle every 3 weeks for a total of up to 6 cycles (cetuximab monotherapy may be continued thereafter until disease progression or unacceptable toxicity)

References
Vermorken JB, Mesia R, Rivera F, et al, "Platinum-Based Chemotherapy Plus Cetuximab in Head and Neck Cancer," *N Engl J Med*, 2008, 359(11):1116-27.

◆ **Cetuximab-Carboplatin (Head and Neck Cancer)** *see* Carboplatin-Cetuximab (Head and Neck Cancer) *on page* 2011

Cetuximab-Cisplatin-Fluorouracil (Head and Neck Cancer)

Index Terms Cisplatin-Fluorouracil-Cetuximab (Head and Neck Cancer)
Use Head and neck cancer
Regimen
Cycle 1:
Cetuximab: IV: 400 mg/m^2 (loading dose) day 1 (week 1, cycle 1 only)
[total loading dose = 400 mg/m^2]
followed by IV: 250 mg/m^2/day days 8 and 15
[total dose/cycle 1 = 900 mg/m^2]
Cisplatin: IV: 100 mg/m^2 day 1
[total dose/cycle = 100 mg/m^2]
Fluorouracil: IV: 1000 mg/m^2/day continuous infusion days 1 to 4
[total dose/cycle = 4000 mg/m^2]
Treatment cycle is 3 weeks
Subsequent cycles:
Cetuximab: IV: 250 mg/m^2/day days 1, 8, and 15
[total dose/cycle = 750 mg/m^2]
Cisplatin: IV: 100 mg/m^2 day 1
[total dose/cycle = 100 mg/m^2]

Fluorouracil: IV: 1000 mg/m²/day continuous infusion days 1 to 4
[total dose/cycle = 4000 mg/m²]

Repeat cycle every 3 weeks for a total of up to 6 cycles (cetuximab monotherapy may be continued thereafter until disease progression or unacceptable toxicity)

References

Vermorken JB, Mesia R, Rivera F, et al, "Platinum-Based Chemotherapy Plus Cetuximab in Head and Neck Cancer," *N Engl J Med*, 2008, 359(11):1116-27.

◆ **Cetuximab-Cisplatin (Head and Neck Cancer)** *see* Cisplatin-Cetuximab (Head and Neck Cancer) *on page 2037*

Cetuximab-Cisplatin-Vinorelbine (NSCLC)

Index Terms Cisplatin-Vinorelbine-Cetuximab (NSCLC)

Use Lung cancer, non-small cell

Regimen

Cycle 1:

Cetuximab: IV: 400 mg/m² (loading dose) over 2 hours day 1 (week 1, cycle 1 only)
[total loading dose = 400 mg/m²]
 followed by IV: 250 mg/m²/day over 1 hour days 8 and 15
 [total dose/cycle 1 = 900 mg/m²]

Cisplatin: IV: 80 mg/m² day 1
[total dose/cycle = 80 mg/m²]

Vinorelbine: IV: 25 mg/m²/day days 1 and 8
[total dose/cycle = 50 mg/m²]

Treatment cycle is 21 days

Cycles 2-6:

Cetuximab: IV: 250 mg/m²/day over 1 hour days 1, 8, and 15
[total dose/cycle = 750 mg/m²]

Cisplatin: IV: 80 mg/m² day 1
[total dose/cycle = 80 mg/m²]

Vinorelbine: IV: 25 mg/m²/day days 1 and 8
[total dose/cycle = 50 mg/m²]

Repeat cycle every 21 days for a maximum of 6 cycles
 followed by
Cetuximab: IV: 250 mg/m²/day over 1 hour days 1, 8, and 15
[total dose/cycle = 750 mg/m²]

Repeat cycle every 21 days until disease progression or unacceptable toxicity

References

Pirker R, Pereira JR, Szczesna A, et al, "Cetuximab Plus Chemotherapy in Patients With Advanced Non-Small-Cell Lung Cancer (FLEX): An Open-Label Randomised Phase III Trial," Lancet, 2009, 373(9674):1525-31.

Pirker R, Pereira JR, von Pawel J, et al, "EGFR Expression as a Predictor of Survival for First-Line Chemotherapy Plus Cetuximab in Patients With Advanced Non-Small-Cell Lung Cancer: Analysis of Data From the Phase 3 FLEX Study," *Lancet Oncol*, 2012, 13(1):33-42.

Cetuximab + FOLFIRI (Colorectal)

Index Terms Cetuximab, Irinotecan, Leucovorin, Fluorouracil (Colorectal)

Use Colorectal cancer

◀ **Regimen**
Cycle 1:
Cetuximab: IV: 400 mg/m^2 (loading dose) over 120 minutes day 1 (week 1, cycle 1 only)
followed by IV: 250 mg/m^2/day over 60 minutes day 8
[total dose/cycle 1 = 650 mg/m^2]
Irinotecan: IV: 180 mg/m^2 over 30-90 minutes day 1
[total dose/cycle = 180 mg/m^2]
Leucovorin (racemic): IV: 400 mg/m^2 over 120 minutes day 1
[total dose/cycle = 400 mg/m^2]
Fluorouracil: IV bolus: 400 mg/m^2 day 1
followed by IV: 2400 mg/m^2 continuous infusion (CI) over 46 hours beginning day 1
[total fluorouracil dose/cycle (bolus and CI) = 2800 mg/m^2]
Treatment cycle is 14 days
Subsequent cycles:
Cetuximab: IV: 250 mg/m^2/day over 60 minutes days 1 and 8
[total dose/cycle = 500 mg/m^2]
Irinotecan: IV: 180 mg/m^2 over 30-90 minutes day 1
[total dose/cycle = 180 mg/m^2]
Leucovorin (racemic): IV: 400 mg/m^2 over 120 minutes day 1
[total dose/cycle = 400 mg/m^2]
Fluorouracil: IV bolus: 400 mg/m^2 day 1
followed by IV: 2400 mg/m^2 CI over 46 hours beginning day 1
[total fluorouracil dose/cycle (bolus and CI) = 2800 mg/m^2]
Repeat cycle every 14 days until disease progression or unacceptable toxicity

References

Van Custem E, Köhne CH, Hitre E, et al, "Cetuximab and Chemotherapy as Initial Treatment for Metastatic Colorectal Cancer," *N Engl J Med*, 2009, 360(14):1408-17.
Van Custem E, Köhne CH, Láng I, et al, "Cetuximab Plus Irinotecan, Fluorouracil, and Leucovorin as First-Line Treatment for Metastatic Colorectal Cancer: Updated Analysis of Overall Survival According to Tumor KRAS and BRAF Mutation Status," *J Clin Oncol*, 2011, 29(15):2011-9.

Cetuximab-Irinotecan (Colorectal)

Index Terms Irinotecan-Cetuximab
Use Colorectal cancer
Regimen NOTE: Multiple variations are listed.
Variation 1:
Cycle 1:
Cetuximab: IV: 400 mg/m^2 (loading dose) day 1 (week 1, cycle 1 only)
followed by IV: 250 mg/m^2/day days 8, 15, 22, 29, and 36
[total dose/cycle 1 = 1650 mg/m^2]
Irinotecan: IV: 125 mg/m^2/day days 1, 8, 15, and 22
[total dose/cycle = 500 mg/m^2]
Treatment cycle is 42 days (6 weeks)
Subsequent cycles:
Cetuximab: IV: 250 mg/m^2/day days 1, 8, 15, 22, 29, and 36
[total dose/cycle = 1500 mg/m^2]
Irinotecan: IV: 125 mg/m^2/day days 1, 8, 15, and 22
[total dose/cycle = 500 mg/m^2]
Repeat cycle every 42 days (6 weeks) until disease progression or unacceptable toxicity

Variation 2:
Cycle 1:
Cetuximab: IV: 400 mg/m^2 (loading dose) day 1 (week 1, cycle 1 only)
followed by IV: 250 mg/m^2/day days 8 and 15
[total dose/cycle 1 = 900 mg/m^2]
Irinotecan: IV: 350 mg/m^2 day 1
[total dose/cycle = 350 mg/m^2]
Treatment cycle is 21 days
Subsequent cycles:
Cetuximab: IV: 250 mg/m^2/day days 1, 8, and 15
[total dose/cycle = 750 mg/m^2]
Irinotecan: IV: 350 mg/m^2 day 1
[total dose/cycle = 350 mg/m^2]
Repeat cycle every 21 days until disease progression or unacceptable toxicity

References

Variation 1 and 2:
Cunningham D, Humblet Y, Siena S, et al, "Cetuximab Monotherapy and Cetuximab Plus Irinotecan in Irinotecan-Refractory Metastatic Colorectal Cancer," *N Engl J Med*, 2004, 351 (4):337-45.
Variation 2:
Sobrero AF, Maurel J, Fehrenbacher L, et al, "EPIC: Phase III Trial of Cetuximab Plus Irinotecan After Fluoropyrimidine and Oxaliplatin Failure in Patients With Metastatic Colorectal Cancer," *J Clin Oncol*, 2008, 26(14):2311-9.

◆ **Cetuximab, Irinotecan, Leucovorin, Fluorouracil (Colorectal)** see Cetuximab + FOLFIRI (Colorectal) on page 2031

◆ **Cetuximab-Paclitaxel** see Paclitaxel-Cetuximab on page 2183

◆ **CF (Esophageal Cancer)** see Cisplatin-Fluorouracil (Esophageal Cancer) on page 2045

◆ **CF (Gastric Cancer)** see Cisplatin-Fluorouracil (Gastric Cancer) on page 2047

◆ **CF (Head and Neck Cancer)** see Cisplatin-Fluorouracil (Head and Neck Cancer) on page 2048

◆ **CF (NHL-Mantle Cell)** see Fludarabine-Cyclophosphamide (NHL-Mantle Cell) on page 2110

ChIVPP (Hodgkin)

Index Terms Chlorambucil, Vinblastine, Procarbazine, Prednisolone (Hodgkin); Chlorambucil, Vinblastine, Procarbazine, Prednisone (Hodgkin); CHLVPP (Hodgkin)

Use Lymphoma, Hodgkin

Regimen NOTE: Multiple variations are listed.
Variation 1:
Chlorambucil: Oral: 6 mg/m^2/day (maximum dose: 10 mg/day) days 1 to 14
[total dose/cycle = 84 mg/m^2; maximum: 140 mg/cycle]
Vinblastine: IV: 6 mg/m^2/day (maximum dose: 10 mg/dose) days 1 and 8
[total dose/cycle = 12 mg/m^2; maximum: 20 mg/cycle]
Procarbazine: Oral: 100 mg/m^2/day (maximum dose: 150 mg/day) days 1 to 14
[total dose/cycle = 1400 mg/m^2; maximum: 2100 mg/cycle]
Prednisone or Prednisolone: Oral: 40 mg/day days 1 to 14
[total dose/cycle = 560 mg]

◀ Repeat cycle every 28 days to complete remission plus 2 cycles; minimum of 6 cycles, maximum of 8 cycles

Variation 2:

Chlorambucil: Oral: 6 mg/m^2/day days 1 to 14

[total dose/cycle = 84 mg/m^2]

Vinblastine: IV: 6 mg/m^2/day days 1 and 8

[total dose/cycle = 12 mg/m^2]

Procarbazine: Oral: 100 mg/m^2/day days 1 to 14

[total dose/cycle = 1400 mg/m^2]

Prednisone: Oral: 40 mg/day days 1 to 14

[total dose/cycle = 560 mg]

Repeat cycle every 28 days for 6 cycles

References

Variation 1:

The International ChIVPP Treatment Group, "ChIVPP Therapy for Hodgkin's Disease: Experience of 960 Patients," *Ann Oncol*, 1995, 6(2):167-72.

Selby P, Patel P, Milan S, et al, "ChIVPP Combination Chemotherapy for Hodgkin's Disease: Long-Term Results," *Br J Cancer*, 1990, 62(2):279-85.

Variation 2:

Vose JM, Bierman PJ, Anderson JR, et al, "CHLVPP Chemotherapy With Involved-Field Irradiation for Hodgkin's Disease: Favorable Results With Acceptable Toxicity," *J Clin Oncol*, 1991, 9 (8):1421-5.

Chlorambucil-Obinutuzumab (CLL)

Index Terms Obinutuzumab-Chlorambucil (CLL)

Use Leukemia, chronic lymphocytic

Regimen

Cycle 1:

Obinutuzumab: IV: 100 mg day 1, followed by 900 mg day 2, followed by 1,000 mg days 8 and 15

[total dose/cycle = 3,000 mg]

Chlorambucil: Oral: 0.5 mg/kg/day days 1 and 15

[total dose/cycle = 1 mg/kg]

Treatment cycle duration is 28 days

Cycles 2 to 6:

Obinutuzumab: IV: 1,000 mg day 1

[total dose/cycle = 1,000 mg]

Chlorambucil: Oral: 0.5 mg/kg/day days 1 and 15

[total dose/cycle = 1 mg/kg]

Repeat cycle every 28 days for a total of 6 cycles

References

Gazyva (obinutuzumab) [prescribing information]. South San Francisco, CA: Genentech Inc; December 2014.

Goede V, Fischer K, Busch R, et al. Obinutuzumab plus chlorambucil in patients with CLL and coexisting conditions. *N Engl J Med*. 2014;370(12):1101-1110.

Chlorambucil-Ofatumumab (CLL)

Index Terms Ofatumumab-Chlorambucil (CLL)

Use Leukemia, chronic lymphocytic (previously untreated)

Regimen

Cycle 1:

Chlorambucil: Oral: 10 mg/m^2/day days 1 to 7
[total dose/cycle = 70 mg/m^2]

Ofatumumab: IV: 300 mg day 1

followed by:

Ofatumumab: IV: 1,000 mg day 8
[total dose/cycle 1 = 1,300 mg]

Treatment cycle is 28 days

Cycle 2 to 12:

Chlorambucil: Oral: 10 mg/m^2/day days 1 to 7
[total dose/cycle = 70 mg/m^2]

Ofatumumab: IV: 1,000 mg day 1
[total dose/cycle = 1,000 mg]

Repeat cycle every 28 days for at least 3 cycles until best response or a maximum of 12 cycles

References

Hillmen P, Robak T, Janssens A, et al. Chlorambucil plus ofatumumab versus chlorambucil alone in previously untreated patients with chronic lymphocytic leukaemia (COMPLEMENT 1): a randomised, multicentre, open-label phase 3 trial. *Lancet.* 2015;385(9980):1873-1883.

Chlorambucil-Prednisone (CLL)

Index Terms Prednisone-Chlorambucil (CLL)

Use Leukemia, chronic lymphocytic

Regimen

Chlorambucil: Oral: 30 mg/m^2 day 1
[total dose/cycle = 30 mg/m^2]

Prednisone: Oral: 80 mg/day days 1 to 5
[total dose/cycle = 400 mg]

Repeat cycle every 14 days until disease progression for a maximum duration of 9 months (if no response at 9 months), 15 months (if complete response at 9 months), or 18 months (if partial response at 9 months)

References

Raphael B, Anderson JW, Silber R, et al, "Comparison of Chlorambucil and Prednisone Versus Cyclophosphamide, Vincristine, and Prednisone as Initial Treatment for Chronic Lymphocytic Leukemia: Long-Term Follow-up of an Eastern Cooperative Oncology Group Randomized Clinical Trial," *J Clin Oncol*, 1991, 9(5):770-6.

- ◆ **Chlorambucil, Vinblastine, Procarbazine, Prednisolone (Hodgkin)** *see* ChlVPP (Hodgkin) *on page* 2033

- ◆ **Chlorambucil, Vinblastine, Procarbazine, Prednisone (Hodgkin)** *see* ChlVPP (Hodgkin) *on page* 2033

- ◆ **2-chloro-2'-deoxyadenosine-Rituximab (Waldenstrom Macroglobulinemia)** *see* Cladribine-Rituximab (Waldenstrom Macroglobulinemia) *on page* 2064

- ◆ **CHLVPP (Hodgkin)** *see* ChlVPP (Hodgkin) *on page* 2033

CHOP (NHL-AIDS-Related)

Index Terms Cyclophosphamide-Vincristine-Doxorubicin-Prednisone (NHL-AIDS-Related); Doxorubicin-Prednisone-Cyclophosphamide-Vincristine (NHL-AIDS-Related); Vincristine-Doxorubicin-Prednisone-Cyclophosphamide (NHL-AIDS-Related)

Use Lymphoma, non-Hodgkin (AIDS-related)

◄ **Regimen** NOTE: CNS prophylaxis was administered according to each investigators discretion. Cytarabine 50 mg intrathecally (IT) weekly for the first 4 weeks of treatment was recommended.

Cyclophosphamide: IV: 750 mg/m^2 day 1
  [total dose/cycle = 750 mg/m^2]
Doxorubicin: IV: 50 mg/m^2 day 1
  [total dose/cycle = 50 mg/m^2]
Vincristine: IV: 1.4 mg/m^2 (maximum dose: 2 mg) day 1
  [total dose/cycle = 1.4 mg/m^2; maximum: 2 mg]
Prednisone: Oral: 100 mg once daily days 1 to 5
  [total dose/cycle = 500 mg]
Filgrastim: SubQ: 300 mcg/day (<70 kg patient) or 480 mcg/day (>70 kg patient) days 4 to 13

Repeat cycle every 21 days; at least 4 cycles were administered or 2 cycles beyond complete response

References

Ratner L, Lee J, Tang S, et al. Chemotherapy for human immunodeficiency virus-associated non-Hodgkin's lymphoma in combination with highly active antiretroviral therapy. *J Clin Oncol.* 2001;19(8):2171-2178.

♦ **CHOP-Rituximab (NHL-DLBCL)** *see* R-CHOP (NHL-DLBCL) *on page 2200*
♦ **CHOP-Rituximab (NHL-Follicular)** *see* R-CHOP (NHL-Follicular) *on page 2201*
♦ **Cisplatin-5FU (Cervical Cancer)** *see* Cisplatin-Fluorouracil (Cervical Cancer) *on page 2044*
♦ **Cisplatin-Capecitabine-Epirubicin (Gastric/Esophageal)** *see* Epirubicin-Cisplatin-Capecitabine (Gastric/Esophageal) *on page 2103*

Cisplatin-Capecitabine (Esophageal Cancer)

Index Terms Capecitabine-Cisplatin (Esophageal Cancer)
Use Esophageal cancer
Regimen

Cisplatin: IV: 80 mg/m^2 over 2 hours day 1
  [total dose/cycle = 80 mg/m^2]
Capecitabine: Oral: 1000 mg/m^2/dose twice daily, days 1 to 14
  [total dose/cycle = 28,000 mg/m^2]

Repeat cycle every 3 weeks until disease progression or unacceptable toxicity

References

Kang YK, Kang WK, Shin DB, et al, "Capecitabine/Cisplatin Versus 5-Fluorouracil/Cisplatin as First-Line Therapy in Patients With Advanced Gastric Cancer: A Randomised Phase III Non-inferiority Trial," *Ann Oncol,* 2009, 20(4):666-73.

Cisplatin-Capecitabine (Gastric Cancer)

Index Terms Capecitabine-Cisplatin (Gastric Cancer)
Use Gastric cancer
Regimen

Cisplatin: IV: 80 mg/m^2 over 2 hours day 1
  [total dose/cycle = 80 mg/m^2]
Capecitabine: Oral: 1000 mg/m^2/dose twice daily, days 1 to 14
  [total dose/cycle = 28,000 mg/m^2]

Repeat cycle every 3 weeks until disease progression or unacceptable toxicity

References

Kang YK, Kang WK, Shin DB, et al, "Capecitabine/Cisplatin Versus 5-Fluorouracil/Cisplatin as First-Line Therapy in Patients With Advanced Gastric Cancer: A Randomised Phase III Non-inferiority Trial," *Ann Oncol*, 2009, 20(4):666-73.

◆ **Cisplatin-Capecitabine-Trastuzumab (Gastric Cancer)** *see* Trastuzumab-Cisplatin-Capecitabine (Gastric Cancer) *on page 2215*

Cisplatin-Cetuximab (Head and Neck Cancer)

Index Terms Cetuximab-Cisplatin (Head and Neck Cancer)

Use Head and neck cancer

Regimen NOTE: Multiple variations are listed.

Variation 1:

Cycle 1:

Cetuximab: IV: 400 mg/m^2 (loading dose) day 1 (week 1, cycle 1 only)
[total loading dose = 400 mg/m^2]
 followed by IV: 250 mg/m^2/day days 8, 15, and 22
 [total dose/cycle 1 = 1150 mg/m^2]
Cisplatin: IV: 100 mg/m^2 day 1
[total dose/cycle = 100 mg/m^2]
Treatment cycle is 4 weeks

Subsequent cycles:

Cetuximab: IV: 250 mg/m^2/day days 1, 8, 15, and 22
[total dose/cycle = 1000 mg/m^2]
Cisplatin: IV: 100 mg/m^2 day 1
[total dose/cycle = 100 mg/m^2]
Repeat cycle every 4 weeks

Variation 2:

Cycle 1:

Cetuximab: IV: 400 mg/m^2 (loading dose) day 1 (week 1, cycle 1 only)
[total loading dose = 400 mg/m^2]
 followed by IV: 250 mg/m^2/day days 8 and 15
 [total dose/cycle 1 = 900 mg/m^2]
Cisplatin: IV: 75-100 mg/m^2 day 1
[total dose/cycle = 75-100 mg/m^2]
Treatment cycle is 3 weeks

Subsequent cycles:

Cetuximab: IV: 250 mg/m^2/day days 1, 8, and 15
[total dose/cycle = 750 mg/m^2]
Cisplatin: IV: 75-100 mg/m^2 day 1
[total dose/cycle = 75-100 mg/m^2]
Repeat cycle every 3 weeks

References

Variation 1:
Burtness B, Goldwasser MA, Flood W, et al, "Phase III Randomized Trial of Cisplatin Plus Placebo Compared With Cisplatin Plus Cetuximab in Metastatic/Recurrent Head and Neck Cancer: An Eastern Cooperative Oncology Group Study," *J Clin Oncol*, 2005, 23(34):8646-54.
Variation 2:
Herbst RS, Arquette M, Shin DM, et al, "Phase II Multicenter Study of the Epidermal Growth Factor Receptor Antibody Cetuximab and Cisplatin for Recurrent and Refractory Aquamous Cell Carcinoma of the Head and Neck," *J Clin Oncol*, 2005, 23(24):5578-87.

◆ **Cisplatin-Cytarabine-Dexamethasone (NHL-DLBCL)** *see* DHAP (NHL-DLBCL) *on page 2087*

◆ **Cisplatin-Cytarabine-Dexamethasone-Rituximab (NHL-DLBCL)** *see* R-DHAP (NHL-DLBCL) *on page 2202*

Cisplatin-Docetaxel-Fluorouracil (Unknown Primary, Squamous Cell)

Index Terms Fluorouracil-Cisplatin-Docetaxel (Unknown Primary); TPF (Unknown Primary)

Use Unknown primary (squamous cell)

Regimen

Docetaxel: IV: 75 mg/m^2 day 1

[total dose/cycle = 75 mg/m^2]

Cisplatin: IV: 75 mg/m^2 day 1

[total dose/cycle = 75 mg/m^2]

Fluorouracil: IV: 750 mg/m^2/day continuous infusion days 1 to 5

[total dose/cycle = 3750 mg/m^2]

Repeat cycle every 21 days for a total of 3 cycles

References

Pointreau Y, Garaud P, Chapet S, et al, "Randomized Trial of Induction Chemotherapy With Cisplatin and 5-Fluorouracil With or Without Docetaxel for Larynx Preservation," *J Natl Cancer Inst*, 2009, 101(7):498-506.

Cisplatin-Docetaxel-Gemcitabine (Bladder)

Index Terms Gemcitabine-Cisplatin-Docetaxel (Bladder)

Use Bladder cancer

Regimen

Docetaxel: IV: 35 mg/m^2/day over 30 minutes days 1 and 8

[total dose/cycle = 70 mg/m^2]

Gemcitabine: IV: 800 mg/m^2/day over 30 minutes days 1 and 8

[total dose/cycle = 1600 mg/m^2]

Cisplatin: IV: 35 mg/m^2/day over 1 hour days 1 and 8

[total dose/cycle = 70 mg/m^2]

Filgrastim: SubQ: 150 mcg/m^2/day days 3 to 6 and days 10 to 15

[total dose/cycle = 1500 mcg/m^2]

Repeat cycle every 21 days for at least 6 cycles, maximum of 8 cycles

References

Pectasides D, Glotsos J, Bountouroglou N, et al, "Weekly Chemotherapy With Docetaxel, Gemcitabine and Cisplatin in Advanced Transitional Cell Urothelial Cancer: A Phase II Trial," *Ann Oncol*, 2002, 13(2):243-50.

Cisplatin-Docetaxel (NSCLC)

Index Terms DC (NSCLC); Docetaxel-Cisplatin (NSCLC)

Use Lung cancer, non-small cell

Regimen

Docetaxel: IV: 75 mg/m^2 day 1

[total dose/cycle = 75 mg/m^2]

Cisplatin: IV: 75 mg/m^2 day 1

[total dose/cycle = 75 mg/m^2]

Repeat cycle every 21 days

References

Fossella F, Pereira JR, von Pawel J, et al. Randomized, multinational, phase III study of docetaxel plus platinum combinations versus vinorelbine plus cisplatin for advanced non-small-cell lung cancer: the TAX 326 study group. *J Clin Oncol*. 2003;21(16):3016-3024.

Schiller JH, Harrington D, Belani CP, et al. Comparison of four chemotherapy regimens for advanced non-small-cell lung cancer. *N Engl J Med*, 2002;346(2):92-98.

Cisplatin-Docetaxel (Unknown Primary, Adenocarcinoma)

Index Terms Docetaxel-Cisplatin (Unknown Primary, Adenocarcinoma)

Use Unknown primary (adenocarcinoma)

Regimen NOTE: Multiple variations are listed.

Variation 1:

Docetaxel: IV: 75 mg/m^2 over 1 hour day 1

[total dose/cycle = 75 mg/m^2]

Cisplatin: IV: 75 mg/m^2 over 1 hour day 1

[total dose/cycle = 75 mg/m^2]

Repeat cycle every 21 days for up to a total of 8 cycles

Variation 2:

Docetaxel: IV: 60 mg/m^2 over 1 hour day 1

[total dose/cycle = 60 mg/m^2]

Cisplatin: IV: 80 mg/m^2 over 2 hours day 1

[total dose/cycle = 80 mg/m^2]

Repeat cycle every 21 days

References

Variation 1:

Greco FA, Erland JB, Morrissey LH, et al, "Carcinoma of Unknown Primary Site: Phase II Trials With Docetaxel Plus Cisplatin or Carboplatin," *Ann Oncol*, 2000, 11(2):211-5.

Variation 2:

Mukai H, Katsumata N, Ando M, et al, "Safety and Efficacy of a Combination of Docetaxel and Cisplatin in Patients With Unknown Primary Cancer," *Am J Clin Oncol*, 2010, 33(1):32-5.

Cisplatin-Docetaxel (Unknown Primary, Squamous Cell)

Index Terms Docetaxel-Cisplatin (Unknown Primary, Squamous Cell)

Use Unknown primary (squamous cell)

Regimen

Docetaxel: IV: 60 mg/m^2 over 1 hour day 1

[total dose/cycle = 60 mg/m^2]

Cisplatin: IV: 80 mg/m^2 over 2 hours day 1

[total dose/cycle = 80 mg/m^2]

Repeat cycle every 21 days for up to 6 cycles

References

Mukai H, Katsumata N, Ando M, et al, "Safety and Efficacy of a Combination of Docetaxel and Cisplatin in Patients With Unknown Primary Cancer," *Am J Clin Oncol*, 2010, 33(1):32-5.

Cisplatin-Doxorubicin Continuous Infusion (Hepatoblastoma)

Index Terms Doxorubicin continuous infusion-Cisplatin (Hepatoblastoma)

Use Hepatoblastoma

Regimen

Cisplatin: IV: 90 mg/m^2 over 6 hours day 1

[total dose/cycle = 90 mg/m^2]

Doxorubicin: IV: 20 mg/m^2/day continuous infusion for 96 hours (begin 4 hours after completion of cisplatin)

[total dose/cycle = 80 mg/m^2]

Repeat cycle every 21 days for a total of 4 to 8 cycles

References

Ortega JA, Douglass EC, Feusner JH, et al. Randomized comparison of cisplatin/vincristine/fluorouracil and cisplatin/continuous infusion doxorubicin for treatment of pediatric hepatoblastoma: a report from the children's cancer group and the pediatric oncology group. *J Clin Oncol.* 2000;18(14):2665-2675.

◆ **Cisplatin-Doxorubicin-Cyclophosphamide-Etoposide-Bortezomib-Dexamethasone-Thalidomide (Multiple Myeloma)** *see* VDT-PACE (Multiple Myeloma) *on page* 2229

◆ **Cisplatin-Doxorubicin-Cyclophosphamide-Etoposide-Dexamethasone-Thalidomide (Multiple Myeloma)** *see* DTPACE (Multiple Myeloma) *on page* 2098

Cisplatin-Doxorubicin (Endometrial)

Index Terms AP (Endometrial); DC (Endometrial); Doxorubicin-Cisplatin (Endometrial)

Use Endometrial cancer

Regimen NOTE: Multiple variations are listed.

Variation 1 (<65 years old with no prior external radiation):
   Doxorubicin: IV: 60 mg/m² day 1
   [total dose/cycle = 60 mg/m²]
   Cisplatin: IV: 50 mg/m² day 1
   [total dose/cycle = 50 mg/m²]
   Repeat cycle every 21 days; maximum cumulative dose of doxorubicin 500 mg/m²

Variation 2 (>65 years old and/or prior external radiation):
   Doxorubicin: IV: 45 mg/m² day 1, may be escalated to 60 mg/m² on cycle 2 if no > grade 1 toxicity)
   [total dose/cycle = 45 to 60 mg/m²]
   Cisplatin: IV: 50 mg/m² day 1
   [total dose/cycle = 50 mg/m²]
   Repeat cycle every 21 days; maximum cumulative dose of doxorubicin 500 mg/m²

Variation 3 (≤65 years old with no prior pelvic radiation):
   Doxorubicin: IV: 60 mg/m² day 1
   [total dose/cycle = 60 mg/m²]
   Cisplatin: IV: 50 mg/m² over 1 hour day 1
   [total dose/cycle = 50 mg/m²]
   Repeat cycle every 21 days up to a maximum of 7 cycles

Variation 4 (>65 years old or prior pelvic radiation):
   Doxorubicin: IV: 45 mg/m² day 1
   [total dose/cycle = 45 mg/m²]
   Cisplatin: IV: 50 mg/m² over 1 hour day 1
   [total dose/cycle = 50 mg/m²]
   Repeat cycle every 21 days up to a maximum of 7 cycles

References

Variations 1 and 2:
Thigpen JT, Brady MF, Homesley HD, et al. Phase III trial of doxorubicin with or without cisplatin in advanced endometrial carcinoma: a Gynecologic Oncology Group Study. *J Clin Oncol.* 2004;22 (19):3902-3908.
Variations 3 and 4:
Fleming GF, Brunetto VL, Cella D, et al. Phase III trial of doxorubicin plus cisplatin with or without paclitaxel plus filgrastim in advanced endometrial carcinoma: a Gynecologic Oncology Group Study. *J Clin Oncol.* 2004;22(11):2159-2166.

Cisplatin-Doxorubicin-Etoposide-Cyclophosphamide (Neuroblastoma)

Use Neuroblastoma

Regimen

Cisplatin: IV: 60 mg/m^2 over 6 hours day 0
[total dose/cycle = 60 mg/m^2]
Doxorubicin: IV: 30 mg/m^2 day 2
[total dose/cycle = 30 mg/m^2]
Etoposide: IV: 100 mg/m^2/day days 2 and 5
[total dose/cycle = 200 mg/m^2]
Cyclophosphamide: IV: 1000 mg/m^2/day days 3 and 4
[total dose/cycle = 2000 mg/m^2]
Repeat cycle every 28 days for a total of 5 cycles

References

Matthay KK, Villablanca JG, Seeger RC, et al, "Treatment of High-Risk Neuroblastoma With Intensive Chemotherapy, Radiotherapy, Autologous Bone Marrow Transplantation, and 13-*cis*-Retinoic Acid. Children's Cancer Group," *N Engl J Med*, 1999, 341(16):1165-73.

Cisplatin-Doxorubicin-Paclitaxel (Endometrial)

Index Terms Paclitaxel-Doxorubicin-Cisplatin (Endometrial); TAP (Endometrial)

Use Endometrial cancer

Regimen

Doxorubicin: IV: 45 mg/m^2 day 1
[total dose/cycle = 45 mg/m^2]
Cisplatin: IV: 50 mg/m^2 day 1
[total dose/cycle = 50 mg/m^2]
Paclitaxel: IV: 160 mg/m^2 over 3 hours day 2
[total dose/cycle = 160 mg/m^2]

Growth Factor:

Filgrastim: SubQ: 5 mcg/kg/day days 3 to 12

or

Pegfilgrastim: SubQ: 6 mg day 3

Repeat cycle every 21 days; maximum of 6 cycles (Homesley, 2009) or a maximum of 7 cycles (Fleming, 2004; Miller, 2012)

References

Fleming GF, Brunetto VL, Cella D, et al. Phase III trial of doxorubicin plus cisplatin with or without paclitaxel plus filgrastim in advanced endometrial carcinoma: a Gynecologic Oncology Group Study. *J Clin Oncol*. 2004;22(11):2159-2166.

Homesley HD, Filiaci V, Gibbons SK, et al. A randomized phase III trial in advanced endometrial carcinoma of surgery and volume directed radiation followed by cisplatin and doxorubicin with or without paclitaxel: A Gynecologic Oncology Group study. *Gynecol Oncol*. 2009;112(3):543-552.

Miller DS, Filiaci G, Fleming G, et al. Randomized phase III noninferiority trial of first line chemotherapy for metastatic or recurrent endometrial carcinoma: A Gynecologic Oncology Group Study. *Gynecol Oncol*. 2012;125(3):771.

Cisplatin-Etoposide (NSCLC)

Index Terms Etoposide-Cisplatin (NSCLC); PE (NSCLC)

Use Lung cancer, non-small cell

◄ **Regimen** NOTE: Multiple variations are listed.
  Variation 1 (adjuvant):
    Cisplatin: IV: 80 mg/m² day 1
      [total dose/cycle = 80 mg/m²]
    Etoposide: IV: 100 mg/m²/day days 1, 2, and 3
      [total dose/cycle = 300 mg/m²]
    Repeat cycle every 21 days for a total of 4 cycles
  Variation 2 (adjuvant):
    Cisplatin: IV: 100 mg/m² day 1
      [total dose/cycle = 100 mg/m²]
    Etoposide: IV: 100 mg/m²/day days 1, 2, and 3
      [total dose/cycle = 300 mg/m²]
    Repeat cycle every 28 days for a total of 3 cycles
  Variation 3 (adjuvant):
    Cisplatin: IV: 100 mg/m² day 1
      [total dose/cycle = 100 mg/m²]
    Etoposide: IV: 100 mg/m²/day days 1, 2, and 3
      [total dose/cycle = 300 mg/m²]
    Repeat cycle every 28 days for a total of 4 cycles
  Variation 4 (adjuvant):
    Cisplatin: IV: 120 mg/m²/day days 1, 29, and 71
      [total dose/treatment = 360 mg/m²]
    Etoposide: IV: 100 mg/m²/day days 1, 2, 3, 29, 30, 31, 71, 72, and 73
      [total dose/treatment = 900 mg/m²]
  Variation 5 (concurrent radiation):
    Cisplatin: IV: 50 mg/m²/day days 1 and 8
      [total dose/cycle = 100 mg/m²]
    Etoposide: IV: 50 mg/m²/day days 1 to 5
      [total dose/cycle = 250 mg/m²]
    Repeat cycle every 28 days for a total of 2 cycles

References
Variations 1 to 4:
Arriagada R, Bergman B, Dunant A, et al. Cisplatin-based adjuvant chemotherapy in patients with completely resected non-small-cell lung cancer. *N Engl J Med.* 2004;350(4):351-360.
Arriagada R, Dunant A, Pignon JP, et al. Long-term results of the international adjuvant lung cancer trial evaluating adjuvant Cisplatin-based chemotherapy in resected lung cancer. *J Clin Oncol.* 2010;28(1):35-42.
Variation 5:
Albain KS, Crowley JJ, Turrisi AT 3rd, et al. Concurrent cisplatin, etoposide, and chest radiotherapy in pathologic stage IIIB non-small-cell lung cancer: a Southwest Oncology Group phase II study, SWOG 9019. *J Clin Oncol.* 2002;20(16):3454-3460.
Albain KS, Swann RS, Rusch VW, et al. Radiotherapy plus chemotherapy with or without surgical resection for stage III non-small-cell lung cancer: a phase III randomised controlled trial. *Lancet.* 2009;374(9687):379-386.

Cisplatin-Etoposide (Small Cell Lung Cancer)
Index Terms EP (Small Cell Lung Cancer); Etoposide-Cisplatin (Small Cell Lung Cancer); PE (Small Cell Lung Cancer)
Use Lung cancer, small cell
Regimen NOTE: Multiple variations are listed.
  Variation 1 (limited stage with concurrent thoracic radiotherapy):
    Etoposide: IV: 120 mg/m²/day days 1, 2, and 3
      [total dose/cycle = 360 mg/m²]

Cisplatin: IV: 60 mg/m^2 day 1
[total dose/cycle = 60 mg/m^2]
Repeat cycle every 21 days for 4 cycles
Variation 2 (limited stage with concurrent thoracic radiotherapy):
Etoposide: IV: 100 mg/m^2/day days 1, 2, and 3
[total dose/cycle = 300 mg/m^2]
Cisplatin: IV: 80 mg/m^2 day 1
[total dose/cycle = 80 mg/m^2]
Repeat cycle every 28 days for 4 cycles
Variation 3 (extensive stage):
Etoposide: IV: 100 mg/m^2/day days 1, 2, and 3
[total dose/cycle = 300 mg/m^2]
Cisplatin: IV: 80 mg/m^2 day 1
[total dose/cycle = 80 mg/m^2]
Repeat cycle every 21 days for 4 cycles
Variation 4 (extensive stage):
Etoposide: IV: 100 mg/m^2 day 1
[total IV dose/cycle = 100 mg/m^2]
followed by: Etoposide: Oral: 200 mg/m^2/day days 2, 3, and 4
[total oral dose/cycle = 600 mg/m^2]
Cisplatin: IV: 75 mg/m^2 day 1
[total dose/cycle = 75 mg/m^2]
Repeat cycle every 21 days for a maximum of 5 cycles
Variation 5 (extensive stage):
Etoposide: IV: 80 mg/m^2/day days 1, 2, and 3
[total dose/cycle = 240 mg/m^2]
Cisplatin: IV: 80 mg/m^2 day 1
[total dose/cycle = 80 mg/m^2]
Repeat cycle every 21 days for maximum of 8 cycles
Variation 6 (extensive stage):
Etoposide: IV: 100 mg/m^2/day days 1, 2, and 3
[total dose/cycle = 300 mg/m^2]
Cisplatin: IV: 25 mg/m^2/day days 1, 2, and 3
[total dose/cycle = 75 mg/m^2]
Repeat cycle every 21 to 28 days for 6 cycles
Variation 7 (extensive stage):
Etoposide: IV: 80 mg/m^2/day days 1 to 5
[total dose/cycle = 400 mg/m^2]
Cisplatin: IV: 20 mg/m^2/day days 1 to 5
[total dose/cycle = 100 mg/m^2]
Repeat cycle every 21 days for 4 cycles

References

Variation 1:
Turrisi AT, Kyungmann K, Blum R, et al, "Twice-Daily Compared With Once-Daily Thoracic Radiotherapy in Limited Small-Cell Lung Cancer Treated Concurrently With Cisplatin and Etoposide," *N Engl J Med*, 1999, 340(4):265-71.
Variation 2:
Takada M, Fukuoka M, Kawahara M, et al, "Phase III Study of Concurrent Verses Sequential Thoracic Radiotherapy in Combination With Cisplatin and Etoposide for Limited-Stage Small-Cell Lung Cancer: Results of the Japan Clinical Oncology Group Study 9104," *J Clin Oncol*, 2002, 20(14):3054-60.
Variation 3:
Lara Jr PN, Natale R, Crowley J, et al, "Phase III Trial of Irinotecan/Cisplatin Compared With Etoposide/Cisplatin in Extensive-Stage Small-Cell Lung Cancer: Clinical and Pharmacogenomic Results From SWOG S0124," *J Clin Oncol*, 2009, 27(15):2530-5.

◀

Variation 4:

Sundstrom S, Bremnes RM, Kaasa S, et al, "Cisplatin and Etoposide Regimen Is Superior to Cyclophosphamide, Epirubicin, and Vincristine Regimen in Small-Cell Lung Cancer: Results From a Randomized Phase III Trial With 5 Years' Follow-Up," *J Clin Oncol*, 2002, 20 (24):4665-72.

Variation 5:

Ihde DC, Mulshine JL, Kramer BS, et al, "Prospective Randomized Comparison of High-Dose and Standard-Dose Etoposide and Cisplatin Chemotherapy in Patients With Extensive-Stage Small-Cell Lung Cancer," *J Clin Oncol*, 1994, 12(10):2022-34.

Variation 6:

Evans WK, Shepherd FA, Feld R, et al, "VP-16 and Cisplatin as First-Line Therapy for Small-Cell Lung Cancer," *J Clin Oncol*, 1985, 3(11):1471-7.

Variation 7:

Roth BJ, Johnson DH, Einhorn LH, et al, "Randomized Study of Cyclophosphamide, Doxorubicin, and Vincristine Versus Etoposide and Cisplatin Versus Alternation of These Two Regimens in Extensive Small-Cell Lung Cancer: A Phase III Trial of the Southeastern Cancer Study Group," *J Clin Oncol*, 1992, 10(2):281-91.

◆ **Cisplatin-Etoposide (Testicular)** *see* EP (Testicular) *on page* 2108

Cisplatin-Fluorouracil (Bladder Cancer)

Index Terms Fluorouracil-Cisplatin (Bladder Cancer)

Use Bladder cancer

Regimen In combination with radiation therapy

Note: Begin infusion(s) 2 hours before radiation therapy on days 1, 3, 15, and 17:

Cisplatin: IV: 15 mg/m^2/day over 2 hours days 1, 2, 3, 15, 16, and 17
[total dose/cycle = 90 mg/m^2]

Fluorouracil: IV: 400 mg/m^2/day over 2 hours days 1, 2, 3, 15, 16, and 17
[total dose/cycle = 2400 mg/m^2]

References

Housset M, Maulard C, Chretien Y, et al, "Combined Radiation and Chemotherapy for Invasive Transitional-Cell Carcinoma of the Bladder: A Prospective Study," *J Clin Oncol*, 1993, 11 (11):2150-7.

Cisplatin-Fluorouracil (Cervical Cancer)

Index Terms 5FU-Cisplatin (Cervical Cancer); Cisplatin-5FU (Cervical Cancer); Fluorouracil-Cisplatin (Cervical Cancer)

Use Cervical cancer

Regimen NOTE: Multiple variations are listed.

Variation 1 (with concurrent radiation therapy):

Cisplatin: IV: 75 mg/m^2 day 1
[total dose/cycle = 75 mg/m^2]

Fluorouracil: IV: 1000 mg/m^2/day continuous infusion days 1 to 4 (96 hours)
[total dose/cycle = 4000 mg/m^2]

Repeat cycle every 21 days for a total 3 cycles

Variation 2 (with concurrent radiation therapy):

Cisplatin: IV: 50 mg/m^2 day 1 starting 4 hours before radiotherapy
[total dose/cycle = 50 mg/m^2]

Fluorouracil: IV: 1000 mg/m^2/day continuous infusion days 2 to 5 (96 hours)
[total dose/cycle = 4000 mg/m^2]

Repeat cycle every 28 days for a total of 2 cycles

Variation 3 (cycles 1 and 2 are with concurrent radiation therapy):

Cisplatin: IV: 70 mg/m^2 day 1
[total dose/cycle = 70 mg/m^2]

Fluorouracil: IV: 1000 mg/m^2/day continuous infusion days 1 to 4 (96 hours)
[total dose/cycle = 4000 mg/m^2]

Repeat cycle every 21 days for a total of 4 cycles

References

Variation 1:

Morris M, Eifel PJ, Lu J, et al, "Pelvic Radiation With Concurrent Chemotherapy Compared With Pelvic and Para-aortic Radiation for High-Risk Cervical Cancer," *N Engl J Med*, 1999, 340 (15):1137-43.

Variation 2:

Whitney CW, Sause W, Bundy BN, et al, "Randomized Comparison of Fluorouracil Plus Cisplatin Versus Hydroxyurea as an Adjunct to Radiation Therapy in Stage IIB-IVA Carcinoma of the Cervix With Negative Para-aortic Lymph Nodes: A Gynecologic Oncology Group and Southwest Oncology Group Study," *J Clin Oncol*, 1999, 17(5):1339-48.

Variation 3:

Peters WA 3rd, Liu PY, Barrett RJ 2nd, et al, "Concurrent Chemotherapy and Pelvic Radiation Therapy Compared With Pelvic Radiation Therapy Alone as Adjuvant Therapy After Radical Surgery in High-Risk Early-Stage Cancer of the Cervix," *J Clin Oncol*, 2000, 18(8):1606-13.

◆ **Cisplatin-Fluorouracil-Cetuximab (Head and Neck Cancer)** *see* Cetuximab-Cisplatin-Fluorouracil (Head and Neck Cancer) *on page 2030*

◆ **Cisplatin-Fluorouracil-Epirubicin (Gastric/Esophageal)** *see* Epirubicin-Cisplatin-Fluorouracil (Gastric/Esophageal) *on page 2103*

Cisplatin-Fluorouracil (Esophageal Cancer)

Index Terms CF (Esophageal Cancer); Fluorouracil-Cisplatin (Esophageal Cancer)

Use Esophageal cancer

Regimen NOTE: Multiple variations are listed.

Variation 1:

Cisplatin: IV: 100 mg/m^2/dose day 1

[total dose/cycle = 100 mg/m^2]

Fluorouracil: IV: 1000 mg/m^2/day continuous infusion days 1 to 5

[total dose/cycle = 5000 mg/m^2]

Repeat cycle every 28 days until disease progression or unacceptable toxicity.

Variation 2:

Cycles 1 to 3 (prior to surgery):

Cisplatin: IV: 100 mg/m^2/dose day 1

[total dose/cycle = 100 mg/m^2]

Fluorouracil: IV: 1000 mg/m^2/day continuous infusion days 1 to 5

[total dose/cycle = 5000 mg/m^2]

Treatment cycles 1-3 are 28 days each

Cycles 4 and 5 (postoperative):

Cisplatin: IV: 75 mg/m^2/dose day 1

[total dose/cycle = 75 mg/m^2]

Fluorouracil: IV: 1000 mg/m^2/day continuous infusion days 1 to 5

[total dose/cycle = 5000 mg/m^2]

Treatment cycles 4 and 5 are 28 days each

Variation 3 (in combination with radiation therapy):

Cycle 1:

Cisplatin: IV: 75 mg/m^2/dose day 1

[total dose/cycle = 75 mg/m^2]

Fluorouracil: IV: 1000 mg/m^2/day continuous infusion days 1 to 4

[total dose/cycle = 4000 mg/m^2]

Treatment cycle is 28 days

◀

Cycles 2 to 4:
  Cisplatin: IV: 75 mg/m^2/dose day 1
    [total dose/cycle = 75 mg/m^2]
  Fluorouracil: IV: 1000 mg/m^2/day continuous infusion days 1 to 4
    [total dose/cycle = 4000 mg/m^2]
  Repeat cycle every 21 days for 3 more cycles (total of 4 cycles)
Variation 4 (in combination with radiation therapy):
  Cisplatin: IV: 100 mg/m^2/dose day 1
    [total dose/cycle = 100 mg/m^2]
  Fluorouracil: IV: 1000 mg/m^2/day continuous infusion days 1 to 4
    [total dose/cycle = 4000 mg/m^2]
  Repeat cycle every 28 days for total of 2 cycles
Variation 5 (in combination with radiation therapy):
  Cisplatin: IV: 75 mg/m^2/dose day 1
    [total dose/cycle = 75 mg/m^2]
  Fluorouracil: IV: 1000 mg/m^2/day continuous infusion days 1 to 4
    [total dose/cycle = 4000 mg/m^2]
  Repeat cycle every 28 days for 4 cycles
Variation 6 (in combination with radiation therapy):
  Cycles 1 and 2:
    Cisplatin: IV: 75 mg/m^2/dose day 1
      [total dose/cycle = 75 mg/m^2]
    Fluorouracil: IV: 1000 mg/m^2/day continuous infusion days 1 to 4
      [total dose/cycle = 4000 mg/m^2]
    Treatment cycles 1 and 2 are 28 days each; cycle 2 is followed by a 2-week rest
  Cycles 3 and 4 (begin cycle 3 at week 11):
    Cisplatin: IV: 75 mg/m^2/dose day 1
      [total dose/cycle = 75 mg/m^2]
    Fluorouracil: IV: 1000 mg/m^2/day continuous infusion days 1 to 4
      [total dose/cycle = 4000 mg/m^2]
    Treatment cycles 3 and 4 are 28 days each
Variation 7 (in combination with radiation therapy):
  Cycles 1 to 4:
    Cisplatin: IV: 15 mg/m^2/day days 1 to 5
      [total dose/cycle = 75 mg/m^2]
    Fluorouracil: IV: 800 mg/m^2/day continuous infusion days 1 to 5
      [total dose/cycle = 4000 mg/m^2]
    Repeat cycles 1-4 every 21 days; cycle 4 is followed by a 1-week rest
  Cycles 5 (begin cycle 5 at week 14):
    Cisplatin: IV: 15 mg/m^2/day days 1 to 5
      [total dose/cycle = 75 mg/m^2]
    Fluorouracil: IV: 800 mg/m^2/day continuous infusion days 1 to 5
      [total dose/cycle = 4000 mg/m^2]
Variation 8:
  Cisplatin: IV: 80 mg/m^2/dose day 1
    [total dose/cycle = 80 mg/m^2]
  Fluorouracil: IV: 800 mg/m^2/day continuous infusion days 1 to 5
    [total dose/cycle = 4000 mg/m^2]
  Repeat cycle every 21 days until disease progression or unacceptable toxicity.

References

Variation 1:

Ajani JA, Moiseyenko VM, Tjulandin S, et al, "Quality of Life With Docetaxel Plus Cisplatin and Fluorouracil Compared With Cisplatin and Fluorouracil From a Phase III Trial for Advanced Gastric or Gastroesophageal Adenocarcinoma: The V-325 Study Group," *J Clin Oncol*, 2007, 25 (22):3210-6.

Dank M, Zaluski J, Barone C, et al, "Randomized Phase III Study Comparing Irinotecan Combined With 5-Fluorouracil and Folinic Acid to Cisplatin Combined With 5-Fluorouracil in Chemotherapy Naive Patients With Advanced Adenocarcinoma of the Stomach or Esophagogastric Junction," *Ann Oncol*, 2008, 19(8):1450-7.

Van Cutsem E, Moiseyenko VM, Tjulandin S, et al, "Phase III Study of Docetaxel and Cisplatin Plus Fluorouracil Compared With Cisplatin and Fluorouracil As First-Line Therapy for Advanced Gastric Cancer: A Report of the V325 Study Group," *J Clin Oncol*, 2006, 24(31):4991-7.

Variation 2:

Kelsen DP, Ginsberg R, Pajak TF, et al, "Chemotherapy Followed by Surgery Compared With Surgery Alone for Localized Esophageal Cancer," *N Engl J Med*, 1998, 339(27):1979-84.

Variation 3:

Cooper JS, Guo MD, Herskovic A, et al, "Chemoradiotherapy of Locally Advanced Esophageal Cancer: Long-Term Follow-Up of a Prospective Randomized Trial (RTOG 85-01). Radiation Therapy Oncology Group," *JAMA*, 1999, 281(17):1623-7.

Variation 4:

Tepper J, Krasna MJ, Niedzwiecki D, et al, "Phase III Trial of Trimodality Therapy With Cisplatin, Fluorouracil, Radiotherapy, and Surgery Compared With Surgery Alone for Esophageal Cancer: CALGB 9781," *J Clin Oncol*, 2008, 26(7):1086-92.

Variation 5 and 6:

Minsky BD, Pajak TF, Ginsberg RJ, et al, "INT 0123 (Radiation Therapy Oncology Group 94-05) Phase III Trial of Combined-Modality Therapy for Esophageal Cancer: High-Dose Versus Standard-Dose Radiation Therapy," *J Clin Oncol*, 2002, 20(5):1167-74.

Variation 7:

Bedenne L, Michel P, Bouché O, et al, "Chemoradiation Followed by Surgery Compared With Chemoradiation Alone in Squamous Cancer of the Esophagus: FFCD 9102," *J Clin Oncol*, 2007, 25(10):1160-8.

Variation 8:

Kang YK, Kang WK, Shin DB, et al, "Capecitabine/Cisplatin Versus 5-Fluorouracil/Cisplatin as First-Line Therapy in Patients With Advanced Gastric Cancer: A Randomised Phase III Non-inferiority Trial," *Ann Oncol*, 2009, 20(4):666-73.

Cisplatin-Fluorouracil (Gastric Cancer)

Index Terms CF (Gastric Cancer); Fluorouracil-Cisplatin (Gastric Cancer)

Use Gastric cancer

Regimen NOTE: Multiple variations are listed.

Variation 1:

Cisplatin: IV: 100 mg/m^2 day 1

[total dose/cycle = 100 mg/m^2]

Fluorouracil: IV: 1000 mg/m^2/day continuous infusion days 1 to 5

[total dose/cycle = 5000 mg/m^2]

Repeat cycle every 4 weeks until disease progression or unacceptable toxicity

Variation 2:

Cisplatin: IV: 80 mg/m^2 over 2 hours day 1

[total dose/cycle = 80 mg/m^2]

Fluorouracil: IV: 800 mg/m^2/day continuous infusion days 1 to 5

[total dose/cycle = 4000 mg/m^2]

Repeat cycle every 21 days until disease progression or unacceptable toxicity

◀ Variation 3:
Fluorouracil: IV: 1000 mg/m^2/day continuous infusion days 1 to 5
[total dose/cycle = 5000 mg/m^2]
Cisplatin: IV: 100 mg/m^2 day 2
[total dose/cycle = 100 mg/m^2]
Repeat cycle every 4 weeks

References

Variation 1:

Ajani JA, Moiseyenko VM, Tjulandin S, et al, "Clinical Benefit With Docetaxel Plus Fluorouracil and Cisplatin Compared With Cisplatin and Fluorouracil in a Phase III Trial of Advanced Gastric or Gastroesophageal Cancer Adenocarcinoma: The V-325 Study Group," *J Clin Oncol*, 2007, 25 (22):3205-9.

Dank M, Zaluski J, Barone C, et al, "Randomized Phase III Study Comparing Irinotecan Combined With 5-Fluorouracil and Folinic Acid to Cisplatin Combined With 5-Fluorouracil in Chemotherapy Naive Patients With Advanced Adenocarcinoma of the Stomach or Esophagogastric Junction," *Ann Oncol*, 2008, 19(8):1450-7.

Van Cutsem E, Moiseyenko VM, Tjulandin S, "Phase III Study of Docetaxel and Cisplatin Plus Fluorouracil Compared With Cisplatin and Fluorouracil as First-Line Therapy for Advanced Gastric Cancer: A Report of the V325 Study Group," *J Clin Oncol*, 2006, 24(31):4991-7.

Variation 2:

Kang YK, Kang WK, Shin DB, "Capecitabine/Cisplatin Versus 5-Fluorouracil/Cisplatin as First-Line Therapy in Patients With Advanced Gastric Cancer: A Randomised Phase III Noninferiority Trial," *Ann Oncol*, 2009, 20(4):666-73.

Variation 3:

Vanhoefer U, Rougier P, Wilke H, et al, "Final Results of a Randomized Phase III Trial of Sequential High-Dose Methotrexate, Fluorouracil, and Doxorubicin Versus Etoposide, Leucovorin, and Fluorouracil Versus Infusional Fluorouracil and Cisplatin in Advanced Gastric Cancer: A Trial of the European Organization for Research and Treatment of Cancer Gastrointestinal Tract Cancer Cooperative Group," *J Clin Oncol*, 2000, 18(14):2648-57.

Cisplatin-Fluorouracil (Head and Neck Cancer)

Index Terms CF (Head and Neck Cancer); Fluorouracil-Cisplatin (Head and Neck Cancer)

Use Head and neck cancer

Regimen NOTE: Multiple variations are listed.

Variation 1:
Cisplatin: IV: 100 mg/m^2 day 1
[total dose/cycle = 100 mg/m^2]
Fluorouracil: IV: 1000 mg/m^2/day continuous infusion days 1 to 4
[total dose/cycle = 4000 mg/m^2]
Repeat cycle every 3 weeks

Variation 2:
Cisplatin: IV: 100 mg/m^2 day 1
[total dose/cycle = 100 mg/m^2]
Fluorouracil: IV: 1000 mg/m^2/day continuous infusion days 1 to 4
[total dose/cycle = 4000 mg/m^2]
Repeat cycle every 3 or 4 weeks

Variation 3:
Cisplatin: IV: 100 mg/m^2 day 1
[total dose/cycle = 100 mg/m^2]
Fluorouracil: IV: 1000 mg/m^2/day continuous infusion days 1 to 5
[total dose/cycle = 5000 mg/m^2]
Repeat cycle every 3 or 4 weeks

Variation 4:
  Cisplatin: IV: 60 mg/m^2 day 1
    [total dose/cycle = 60 mg/m^2]
  Fluorouracil: IV: 800 mg/m^2/day continuous infusion days 1 to 5
    [total dose/cycle = 4000 mg/m^2]
  Repeat cycle every 14 days
Variation 5:
  Cisplatin: IV: 20 mg/m^2/day days 1 to 5
    [total dose/cycle = 100 mg/m^2]
  Fluorouracil: IV: 200 mg/m^2/day days 1 to 5
    [total dose/cycle = 1000 mg/m^2]
  Repeat cycle every 3 weeks
Variation 6:
  Cisplatin: IV: 80 mg/m^2 continuous infusion day 1
    [total dose/cycle = 80 mg/m^2]
  Fluorouracil: IV: 800 mg/m^2/day continuous infusion days 2 to 6
    [total dose/cycle = 4000 mg/m^2]
  Repeat cycle every 3 weeks
Variation 7:
  Cisplatin: IV: 75 mg/m^2 day 1
    [total dose/cycle = 75 mg/m^2]
  Fluorouracil: IV: 1000 mg/m^2/day continuous infusion days 1 to 4
    [total dose/cycle = 4000 mg/m^2]
  Repeat cycle every 4 weeks
Variation 8:
  Cisplatin: IV: 120 mg/m^2 day 1
    [total dose/cycle = 120 mg/m^2]
  Fluorouracil: IV: 1000 mg/m^2/day continuous infusion days 1 to 5
    [total dose/cycle = 5000 mg/m^2]
  Repeat cycle every 3 weeks
Variation 9:
  Cisplatin: IV: 25 mg/m^2/day continuous infusion days 1 to 4
    [total dose/cycle = 100 mg/m^2]
  Fluorouracil: IV: 1000 mg/m^2/day days 1 to 4
    [total dose/cycle = 4000 mg/m^2]
  Repeat cycle every 3 weeks
Variation 10:
  Fluorouracil: IV: 350 mg/m^2/day continuous infusion days 1 to 5
    [total dose/cycle = 1750 mg/m^2]
  Cisplatin: IV: 50 mg/m^2 day 6
    [total dose/cycle = 50 mg/m^2]
  Repeat cycle every 3 weeks
Variation 11:
  Cisplatin: IV: 5 mg/m^2/day continuous infusion days 1 to 14
    [total dose/cycle = 70 mg/m^2]
  Fluorouracil: IV: 200 mg/m^2/day continuous infusion days 1 to 14
    [total dose/cycle = 2800 mg/m^2]
  With concurrent radiation therapy, cycle does not repeat
Variation 12 (administer during the final 2 weeks of radiation therapy; weeks 6 and 7):
  Cisplatin: IV: 10 mg/m^2/day days 1 to 5 beginning week 6
    [total dose/week = 50 mg/m^2]

Fluorouracil: IV: 400 mg/m^2/day continuous infusion days 1 to 5 beginning week 6

[total dose/week = 2000 mg/m^2]

Repeat cycle one time in week 7

Variation 13:

Cisplatin: IV: 100 mg/m^2/day day 1 (concurrent with radiation therapy)

[total dose/cycle = 100 mg/m^2]

Repeat cycle every 3 weeks for a total of 3 cycles

Followed by (postradiation chemotherapy; begin 4 weeks after radiotherapy or the last cisplatin dose):

Cisplatin: IV: 80 mg/m^2 day 1

[total dose/cycle = 80 mg/m^2]

Fluorouracil: IV: 1000 mg/m^2/day continuous infusion days 1 to 4

[total dose/cycle = 4000 mg/m^2]

Repeat cycle every 4 weeks for a total of 3 cycles

References

Variation 1:

Forastiere AA, Metch B, Schuller DE, et al, "Randomized Comparison of Cisplatin Plus Fluorouracil and Carboplatin Plus Fluorouracil Versus Methotrexate in Advanced Squamous-Cell Carcinoma of the Head and Neck: A Southwest Oncology Group Study," *J Clin Oncol*, 1992, 10(8):1245-51.

Gibson MK, Li Y, Murphy B, et al, "Randomized Phase III Evaluation of Cisplatin Plus Fluorouracil Versus Cisplatin Plus Paclitaxel in Advanced Head and Neck Cancer (E1395): An Intergroup Trial of the Eastern Cooperative Oncology Group," *J Clin Oncol*, 2005, 23(15):3562-7.

Variation 2:

Kish J, Drelichman A, Jacobs J, et al, "Clinical Trial of Cisplatin and 5-FU Infusion as Initial Treatment for Advanced Squamous Cell Carcinoma of the Head and Neck," *Cancer Treat Rep*, 1982, 66(3):471-4.

Mercier RJ, Neal GD, Mattox DE, et al, "Cisplatin and 5-Fluorouracil Chemotherapy in Advanced or Recurrent Squamous Cell Carcinoma of the Head and Neck," *Cancer*, 1987, 60(11):2609-12.

Variation 3:

Dasmahapatra KS, Citrin P, Hill GJ, et al, "A Prospective Evaluation of 5-Fluorouracil Plus Cisplatin in Advanced Squamous-Cell Cancer of the Head and Neck," *J Clin Oncol*, 1985, 3 (11):1486-9.

Rooney M, Kish J, Jacobs J, et al, "Improved Complete Response Rate and Survival in Advanced Head and Neck Cancer After Three-Course Induction Therapy With 120-Hour 5-FU Infusion and Cisplatin," *Cancer*, 1985, 55(5):1123-8.

Variation 4:

Taylor SG 4th, Murthy AK, Showel JL, et al, "Improved Control in Advanced Head and Neck Cancer With Simultaneous Radiation and Cisplatin/5-FU Chemotherapy," *Cancer Treat Rep*, 1985, 69(9):933-9.

Variation 5:

Merlano M, Tatarek R, Grimaldi A, et al, "Phase I-II Trial With Cisplatin and 5-FU in Recurrent Head and Neck Cancer: An Effective Outpatient Schedule," *Cancer Treat Rep*, 1985, 69 (9):961-4.

Variation 6:

Amrein PC and Weitzman SA, "Treatment of Squamous-Cell Carcinoma of the Head and Neck With Cisplatin and 5-Fluorouracil," *J Clin Oncol*, 1985, 3(12):1632-9.

Variation 7:

Adelstein DJ, Li Y, Adams GL, et al, "An Intergroup Phase III Comparison of Standard Radiation and Two Schedules of Concurrent Chemoradiotherapy in Patients With Unresectable Squamous Cell Head and Neck Cancer," *J Clin Oncol*, 2003, 21(1):92-8.

Adelstein DJ, Sharan VM, Earle AS, et al, "Chemoradiotherapy as Initial Management in Patients With Squamous Cell Carcinoma of the Head and Neck," *Cancer Treat Rep*, 1986, 70(6):761-7.

Variation 8:

Paredes J, Hong WK, Felder TB, et al, "Prospective Randomized Trial of High-Dose Cisplatin and Fluorouracil Infusion With or Without Sodium Diethyldithiocarbamate in Recurrent and/or Metastatic Squamous Cell Carcinoma of the Head and Neck," *J Clin Oncol*, 1988, 6(6):955-62.

Variation 9:

Bernal AG, Cruz JJ, Sanchez P, et al, "Four-Day Continuous Infusion of Cisplatin and 5-Fluorouracil in Head and Neck Cancer," *Cancer*, 1989, 63(10):1927-30.

Variation 10:

Denham JW and Abbott RL, "Concurrent Cisplatin, Infusional Fluorouracil, and Conventionally Fractionated Radiation Therapy in Head and Neck Cancer: Dose-Limiting Mucosal Toxicity," *J Clin Oncol*, 1991, 9(3):458-63.

Variation 11:

Arcangeli G, Saracino B, Danesi DT, et al, "Accelerated Hyperfractionated Radiotherapy and Concurrent Protracted Venous Infusion Chemotherapy in Locally-Advanced Head and Neck Cancer," *Am J Clin Oncol*, 2002, 25(5):431-7.

Variation 12:

Garden AS, Harris J, Vokes EE, et al, "Preliminary Results of Radiation Therapy Oncology Group 97-03: A Randomized Phase II Trial of Concurrent Radiation and Chemotherapy for Advanced Squamous Cell Carcinomas of the Head and Neck," *J Clin Oncol*, 2004, 22(14):2856-64.

Variation 13:

Al-Sarraf M, LeBlanc M, Giri PG, et al, "Chemoradiotherapy Versus Radiotherapy in Patients With Advanced Nasopharyngeal Cancer: Phase III Randomized Intergroup Study 0099," *J Clin Oncol*, 1998, 16(4):1310-7.

Cisplatin-Fluorouracil-Paclitaxel (Unknown Primary, Squamous Cell)

Index Terms Cisplatin-Paclitaxel-Fluorouracil (Unknown Primary); PCF (Unknown Primary)

Use Unknown primary (squamous cell)

Regimen

Paclitaxel: IV: 175 mg/m^2 over 3 hours day 1
   [total dose/cycle = 175 mg/m^2]
Cisplatin: IV: 100 mg/m^2 day 2
   [total dose/cycle = 100 mg/m^2]
Fluorouracil: IV: 500 mg/m^2/day continuous infusion days 2 to 6
   [total dose/cycle = 2500 mg/m^2]
Repeat cycle every 21 days for a total of 3 cycles

References

Hitt R, López-Pousa A, Martínez-Trufero J, et al, "Phase III Study Comparing Cisplatin Plus Fluorouracil to Paclitaxel, Cisplatin, and Fluorouracil Induction Chemotherapy Followed by Chemoradiotherapy in Locally Advanced Head and Neck Cancer," *J Clin Oncol*, 2005, 23 (34):8636-45.

♦ **Cisplatin-Fluorouracil-Trastuzumab (Gastric Cancer)** *see* Trastuzumab-Cisplatin-Fluorouracil (Gastric Cancer) *on page 2216*

♦ **Cisplatin-Gemcitabine-Bevacizumab (NSCLC)** *see* Bevacizumab-Cisplatin-Gemcitabine (NSCLC) *on page 1991*

♦ **Cisplatin-Gemcitabine (Biliary Cancer)** *see* Gemcitabine-Cisplatin (Biliary Cancer) *on page 2135*

Cisplatin-Gemcitabine (Bladder)

Index Terms GC (Bladder); Gemcitabine-Cisplatin (Bladder); GP (Bladder)

Use Bladder cancer

Regimen NOTE: Multiple variations are listed.

Variation 1 (metastatic):
Gemcitabine: IV: 1000 mg/m^2/day days 1, 8, and 15
   [total dose/cycle = 3000 mg/m^2]
Cisplatin: IV: 70 mg/m^2 day 2
   [total dose/cycle = 70 mg/m^2]
Repeat cycle every 28 days for a maximum of 6 cycles

Variation 2 (neoadjuvant):
Cisplatin: IV: 70 mg/m^2 day 1
[total dose/cycle = 70 mg/m^2]
Gemcitabine: IV: 1000 mg/m^2/day days 1 and 8
[total dose/cycle = 2000 mg/m^2]
Repeat cycle every 21 days for 4 cycles
Variation 3 (neoadjuvant):
Cisplatin: IV: 35 mg/m^2/day days 1 and 8
[total dose/cycle = 70 mg/m^2]
Gemcitabine: IV: 1000 mg/m^2/day days 1 and 8
[total dose/cycle = 2000 mg/m^2]
Repeat cycle every 21 days for 4 cycles

References

Variation 1:

von der Maase H, Hansen SW, Roberts JT, et al. Gemcitabine and cisplatin versus methotrexate, vinblastine, doxorubicin, and cisplatin in advanced or metastatic bladder cancer: results of a large, randomized, multinational, multicenter, phase III study. *J Clin Oncol.* 2000;18 (17):3068-3077.

Variations 2 and 3:

Dash A, Pettus JA 4th, Herr HW, et al. A role for neoadjuvant gemcitabine plus cisplatin in muscle-invasive urothelial carcinoma of the bladder: a retrospective experience. *Cancer.* 2008;113 (9):2471-2477.

Cisplatin-Gemcitabine (Cervical)

Index Terms Gemcitabine-Cisplatin (Cervical)

Use Cervical cancer

Regimen NOTE: Multiple variations are listed.

Variation 1:
Gemcitabine: IV: 1250 mg/m^2/day over 30 minutes days 1 and 8
[total dose/cycle = 2500 mg/m^2]
Cisplatin: IV: 50 mg/m^2 over 60 minutes day 1
[total dose/cycle = 50 mg/m^2]
Repeat cycle every 21 days for up to a total of 6 cycles
Variation 2:
Gemcitabine: IV: 1000 mg/m^2/day days 1 and 8
[total dose/cycle = 2000 mg/m^2]
Cisplatin: IV: 50 mg/m^2 day 1
[total dose/cycle = 50 mg/m^2]
Repeat cycle every 21 days for up to a total of 6 cycles; responders may continue beyond 6 cycles
Variation 3:
Cisplatin: IV: 30 mg/m^2/day days 1 and 8
[total dose/cycle = 60 mg/m^2]
Gemcitabine: IV: 800 mg/m^2/day days 1 and 8
[total dose/cycle = 1600 mg/m^2]
Repeat cycle every 28 days until disease progression or unacceptable toxicity

References

Variation 1:

Burnett AF, Roman LD, Garcia AA, Muderspach LI, Brader KR, Morrow CP. A phase II study of gemcitabine and cisplatin in patients with advanced, persistent, or recurrent squamous cell carcinoma of the cervix. *Gynecol Oncol.* 2000;76(1):63-66.

Variation 2:

Monk BJ, Sill MW, McMeekin DS, et al. Phase III trial of four cisplatin-containing doublet combinations in stage IVB, recurrent, or persistent cervical carcinoma: a Gynecologic Oncology Group study. *J Clin Oncol.* 2009;27(28):4649-4655.

Variation 3:
Brewer CA, Blessing JA, Nagourney RA, McMeekin DS, Lele S, Zweizig SL. Cisplatin plus gemcitabine in previously treated squamous cell carcinoma of the cervix: a phase II study of the Gynecologic Oncology Group. *Gynecol Oncol*. 2006;100(2):385-388.

Cisplatin-Gemcitabine (Mesothelioma)

Index Terms Gemcitabine-Cisplatin (Mesothelioma)

Use Malignant pleural mesothelioma

Regimen NOTE: Multiple variations are listed.

Variation 1:

Cisplatin: IV: 100 mg/m^2 over 1 hour day 1

[total dose/cycle = 100 mg/m^2]

Gemcitabine: IV: 1000 mg/m^2/day over 30 minutes days 1, 8, and 15

[total dose/cycle = 3000 mg/m^2]

Repeat cycle every 28 days for up to a total of 6 cycles

Variation 2:

Gemcitabine: IV: 1250 mg/m^2/day over 30 minutes days 1 and 8

[total dose/cycle = 2500 mg/m^2]

Cisplatin: IV: 80 mg/m^2 over 3 hours day 1

[total dose/cycle = 80 mg/m^2]

Repeat cycle every 21 days for up to a total of 6 cycles

Variation 3:

Gemcitabine: IV: 1000 mg/m^2/day over 30 minutes days 1, 8, and 15

[total dose/cycle = 3000 mg/m^2]

Cisplatin: IV: 30 mg/m^2/day over 30 minutes days 1, 8, and 15

[total dose/cycle = 90 mg/m^2]

Repeat cycle every 28 days

References

Variation 1:
Nowak AK, Byrne MJ, Williamson R, et al, "A Multicentre Phase II Study of Cisplatin and Gemcitabine for Malignant Mesothelioma," *Br J Cancer*, 2002, 87(5):491-6.
Variation 2:
van Haarst JM, Baas P, Manegold Ch, et al, "Multicentre Phase II Study of Gemcitabine and Cisplatin in Malignant Pleural Mesothelioma," *Br J Cancer*, 2002, 86(3):342-5.
Variation 3:
Kalmadi SR, Rankin C, Kraut MJ, et al, "Gemcitabine and Cisplatin in Unresectable Malignant Mesothelioma of the Pleura: A Phase II Study of the Southwest Oncology Group (SWOG 9810)," *Lung Cancer*, 2008, 60:259-63.

Cisplatin-Gemcitabine-Necitumumab (NSCLC)

Index Terms Gemcitabine-Cisplatin-Necitumumab (NSCLC); Necitumumab-Cisplatin-Gemcitabine (NSCLC)

Use Lung cancer, non-small cell (first-line metastatic squamous non-small cell)

Regimen

Necitumumab: IV: 800 mg over 60 minutes days 1 and 8

[total dose/cycle = 1,600 mg]

Gemcitabine: IV: 1,250 mg/m^2 over 30 minutes days 1 and 8

[total dose/cycle = 2,500 mg/m^2]

Cisplatin: IV: 75 mg/m^2 over 2 hours day 1

[total dose/cycle = 75 mg/m^2]

Repeat cycle every 21 days for a total of 6 cycles. Single agent necitumumab (at the dose and schedule listed above) may be continued after the completion of 6 cycles of combination chemotherapy in patients without disease progression.

References

Thatcher N, Hirsch FR, Luft AV, et al. Necitumumab plus gemcitabine and cisplatin versus gemcitabine and cisplatin alone as first-line therapy in patients with stage IV squamous non-small-cell lung cancer (SQUIRE): an open-label, randomised, controlled phase 3 trial. *Lancet Oncol*. 2015;16(7):763-774.

Cisplatin-Gemcitabine (NSCLC)

Index Terms GC (NSCLC); Gemcitabine-Cisplatin (NSCLC)

Use Lung cancer, non-small cell

Regimen NOTE: Multiple variations are listed.

Variation 1:

Gemcitabine: IV: 1,000 mg/m^2/day over 30 minutes days 1, 8, and 15
[total dose/cycle = 3,000 mg/m^2]

Cisplatin: IV: 100 mg/m^2 day 1
[total dose/cycle = 100 mg/m^2]

Repeat cycle every 28 days (for up to 6 cycles Sandler 2000)

Variation 2:

Cisplatin: IV: 100 mg/m^2 over 60 minutes day 1
[total dose/cycle = 100 mg/m^2]

Gemcitabine: IV: 1,250 mg/m^2/day over 30 minutes days 1 and 8
[total dose/cycle = 2,500 mg/m^2]

Repeat cycle every 21 days for up to 6 cycles

Variation 3:

Gemcitabine: IV: 1,250 mg/m^2/day over 30 minutes days 1 and 8
[total dose/cycle = 2,500 mg/m^2]

Cisplatin: IV: 80 mg/m^2 day 1
[total dose/cycle = 80 mg/m^2]

Repeat cycle every 21 days for up to 6 cycles

Variation 4:

Gemcitabine: IV: 1,000 mg/m^2/day over 30 minutes days 1 and 8
[total dose/cycle = 2,000 mg/m^2]

Cisplatin: IV: 80 mg/m^2 day 1
[total dose/cycle = 80 mg/m^2]

Repeat cycle every 21 days until disease progression or unacceptable toxicity

References

Variation 1:

Comella P, Frasci G, Panza N, et al. Randomized trial comparing cisplatin, gemcitabine, and vinorelbine with either cisplatin and gemcitabine or cisplatin and vinorelbine in advanced non-small-cell lung cancer: interim analysis of a phase III trial of the Southern Italy Cooperative Oncology Group. *J Clin Oncol*. 2000;18(7):1451-1457.

Sandler AB, Nemunaitis J, Denham C, et al. Phase III trial of gemcitabine plus cisplatin versus cisplatin alone in patients with locally advanced or metastatic non-small-cell lung cancer. *J Clin Oncol*. 2000;18(1):122-130.

Schiller JH, Harrington D, Belani CP, et al. Comparison of four chemotherapy regimens for advanced non-small-cell lung cancer. *N Engl J Med*. 2002;346(2):92-98.

Variation 2:

Cardenal F, López-Cabrerizo MP, Antón A, et al. Randomized phase III study of gemcitabine-cisplatin versus etoposide-cisplatin in the treatment of locally advanced or metastatic non-small-cell lung cancer. *J Clin Oncol*. 1999;17(1):12-18.

Variation 3:

Smit EF, van Meerbeeck JP, Lianes P, et al. Three-arm randomized study of two cisplatin-based regimens and paclitaxel plus gemcitabine in advanced non-small-cell lung cancer: a phase III trial of the European Organization for Research and Treatment of Cancer Lung Cancer Group–EORTC 08975. *J Clin Oncol*. 2003;21(21):3909-3917.

Variation 4:
Ohe Y, Ohashi Y, Kubota K, et al. Randomized phase III study of cisplatin plus irinotecan versus carboplatin plus paclitaxel, cisplatin plus gemcitabine, and cisplatin plus vinorelbine for advanced non-small-cell lung cancer: Four-Arm Cooperative Study in Japan. *Ann Oncol*. 2007;18(2):317-323.

Cisplatin-Gemcitabine (Pancreatic)

Index Terms GemCis (Pancreatic); Gemcitabine-Cisplatin (Pancreatic)

Use Pancreatic cancer

Regimen NOTE: Multiple variations are listed.

Variation 1:

Cisplatin: IV: 50 mg/m^2/day over 1 hour days 1 and 15
 [total dose/cycle = 100 mg/m^2]

Gemcitabine: IV: 1000 mg/m^2/day over 30 minutes days 1 and 15
 [total dose/cycle = 2000 mg/m^2]

Repeat cycle every 28 days

Variation 2:

Cycle 1:

Cisplatin: IV: 25 mg/m^2/day days 1, 8, 15, 29, 36, and 43 (cycle 1 only)
 [total dose/cycle 1 = 150 mg/m^2]

Gemcitabine: IV: 1000 mg/m^2/day over 30 minutes days 1, 8, 15, 22, 29, 36, and 43 (cycle 1 only), 1 hour after cisplatin
 [total dose/cycle 1 = 7000 mg/m^2]

Treatment cycle is 56 days

Subsequent cycles:

Cisplatin: IV: 25 mg/m^2/day days 1, 8, and 15
 [total dose/cycle = 75 mg/m^2]

Gemcitabine: IV: 1000 mg/m^2/day over 30 minutes days 1, 8, and 15, 1 hour after cisplatin
 [total dose/cycle = 3000 mg/m^2]

Repeat cycle every 28 days until disease progression or unacceptable toxicity

References

Variation 1:
Heinemann V, Quietzsch D, Gieseler F, et al, "Randomized Phase III Trial of Gemcitabine Plus Cisplatin Compared With Gemcitabine Alone in Advanced Pancreatic Cancer," *J Clin Oncol*, 2006, 24(24):3946-52.

Variation 2:
Colucci G, Labianca R, Di Costanzo F, et al, "Randomized Phase III Trial of Gemcitabine Plus Cisplatin Compared With Single-Agent Gemcitabine As First-Line Treatment of Patients With Advanced Pancreatic Cancer: The GIP-1 Study," *J Clin Oncol*, 2010, 28(10):1645-51.

Cisplatin-Gemcitabine (Unknown Primary, Adenocarcinoma)

Index Terms Gemcitabine-Cisplatin (Unknown Primary)

Use Unknown primary (adenocarcinoma)

Regimen

Gemcitabine: IV: 1250 mg/m^2/day days 1 and 8
 [total dose/cycle = 2500 mg/m^2]

Cisplatin: IV: 100 mg/m^2 day 1
 [total dose/cycle = 100 mg/m^2]

Repeat cycle every 21 days

References

Culine S, Lortholary A, Voigt JJ, et al, "Cisplatin in Combination With Either Gemcitabine or Irinotecan in Carcinomas of Unknown Primary Site: Results of a Randomized Phase II Study - Trial for the French Study Group on Carcinomas of Unknown Primary (GEFCAPI 01)," *J Clin Oncol*, 2003, 21(18):3479-82.

- **Cisplatin-Ifosfamide-Epirubicin (Osteosarcoma)** *see* Ifosfamide-Cisplatin-Epirubicin (Osteosarcoma) *on page 2155*
- **Cisplatin-Ifosfamide-Paclitaxel (Penile)** *see* Paclitaxel-Ifosfamide-Cisplatin (Penile) *on page 2186*
- **Cisplatin-Ifosfamide-Paclitaxel (Testicular)** *see* TIP (Testicular) *on page 2214*
- **Cisplatin-Irinotecan (Esophageal Cancer)** *see* Irinotecan-Cisplatin (Esophageal Cancer) *on page 2159*

Cisplatin-Irinotecan (Gastric)

Index Terms Irinotecan-Cisplatin (Gastric)

Use Gastric cancer

Regimen NOTE: Multiple variations are listed.

Variation 1:

Irinotecan: IV: 65 mg/m^2/day over 90 minutes days 1, 8, 15, and 22
[total dose/cycle = 260 mg/m^2]

Cisplatin: IV: 30 mg/m^2/day over 60 minutes days 1, 8, 15, and 22
[total dose/cycle = 120 mg/m^2]

Repeat cycle every 6 weeks until disease progression or unacceptable toxicity

Variation 2:

Irinotecan: IV: 70 mg/m^2/day over 90 minutes days 1 and 15
[total dose/cycle = 140 mg/m^2]

Cisplatin: IV: 70 mg/m^2 over 2 hours day 1
[total dose/cycle = 70 mg/m^2]

Repeat cycle every 28 days for up to 6 cycles

References

Variation 1:

Ajani JA, Baker J, Pisters PW, et al.CPT-11 plus cisplatin in patients with advanced, untreated gastric or gastroesophageal junction carcinoma: results of a phase II study. *Cancer.* 2002;94 (3):641-646.

Variation 2:

Park SH, Choi EY, Bang SM, et al. Salvage chemotherapy with irinotecan and cisplatin in patients with metastatic gastric cancer failing both 5-fluorouracil and taxanes. *Anticancer Drugs.* 2005;16 (6):621-625.

Cisplatin-Irinotecan (NSCLC)

Index Terms Irinotecan-Cisplatin (NSCLC)

Use Lung cancer, non-small cell

Regimen

Cisplatin: IV: 80 mg/m^2 day 1
[total dose/cycle = 80 mg/m^2]

Irinotecan: IV: 60 mg/m^2/dose days 1, 8, and 15
[total dose/cycle = 180 mg/m^2]

Repeat cycle every 28 days for at least 3 more cycles or until disease progression or unacceptable toxicity

References

Ohe Y, Ohashi Y, Kubota K, et al, "Randomized Phase III Study of Cisplatin Plus Irinotecan Versus Carboplatin Plus Paclitaxel, Cisplatin Plus Gemcitabine, and Cisplatin Plus Vinorelbine for Advanced Non-Small-Cell Lung Cancer: Four-Arm Cooperative Study in Japan," *Ann Oncol*, 2007, 18(2):317-23.

Cisplatin-Irinotecan (Small Cell Lung Cancer)

Index Terms IP (Small Cell Lung Cancer); Irinotecan-Cisplatin (Small Cell Lung Cancer)

Use Lung cancer, small cell

Regimen NOTE: Multiple variations are listed.

Variation 1:

Cisplatin: IV: 60 mg/m^2 day 1

[total dose/cycle = 60 mg/m^2]

Irinotecan: IV: 60 mg/m^2/day days 1, 8, and 15

[total dose/cycle = 180 mg/m^2]

Repeat cycle every 28 days for 4 cycles

Variation 2:

Cisplatin: IV: 30 mg/m^2/day days 1 and 8

[total dose/cycle = 60 mg/m^2]

Irinotecan: IV: 65 mg/m^2/day days 1 and 8

[total dose/cycle = 130 mg/m^2]

Repeat cycle every 21 days for at least 4 cycles

References

Variation 1:

Lara PN Jr, Natale R, Crowley J, et al, "Phase III Trial of Irinotecan/Cisplatin Compared With Etoposide/Cisplatin in Extensive-Stage Small-Cell Lung Cancer: Clinical and Pharmacogenomic Results from SWOG S0124," *J Clin Oncol*, 2009, 27(15):2530-5.

Noda K, Nishiwaki Y, Kawahara M, et al, "Irinotecan Plus Cisplatin Compared With Etoposide Plus Cisplatin for Extensive Small-Cell Lung Cancer," *N Engl J Med*, 2002, 346(2):85-91.

Variation 2:

Hanna N, Bunn PA Jr, Langer C, et al, "Randomized Phase III Trial Comparing Irinotecan/Cisplatin With Etoposide/Cisplatin in Patients With Previously Untreated Extensive-Stage Disease Small-Cell Lung Cancer," *J Clin Oncol*, 2006, 24(13):2038-43.

◆ **Cisplatin-Methotrexate-Doxorubicin (Osteosarcoma)** *see* MAP (Osteosarcoma) *on page* 2170

◆ **Cisplatin-Paclitaxel-Bevacizumab (Cervical)** *see* Bevacizumab-Cisplatin-Paclitaxel (Cervical) *on page* 1991

Cisplatin-Paclitaxel (Cervical Cancer)

Index Terms Paclitaxel-Cisplatin (Cervical Cancer)

Use Cervical cancer

Regimen

Paclitaxel: IV: 135 mg/m^2 continuous infusion over 24 hours day 1

[total dose/cycle = 135 mg/m^2]

Cisplatin: IV: 50 mg/m^2 day 2

[total dose/cycle = 50 mg/m^2]

Repeat cycle every 21 days for up to a total of 6 cycles; responders may continue beyond 6 cycles

References

Monk BJ, Sill MW, McMeekin DS, et al, "Phase III Trial of Four Cisplatin-Containing Doublet Combinations in Stage IVB, Recurrent, or Persistent Cervical Carcinoma: A Gynecologic Oncology Group Study," *J Clin Oncol*, 2009, 27(28):4649-55.

Moore DH, Blessing JA, McQuellon RP, et al, "Phase III Study of Cisplatin With or Without Paclitaxel in Stage IVB, Recurrent, or Persistent Squamous Cell Carcinoma of the Cervix: A Gynecologic Oncology Group Study," *J Clin Oncol*, 2004, 22(15):3113-9.

+ **Cisplatin-Paclitaxel (Esophageal Cancer)** *see* Paclitaxel-Cisplatin (Esophageal Cancer) *on page 2184*
+ **Cisplatin-Paclitaxel-Fluorouracil (Unknown Primary)** *see* Cisplatin-Fluorouracil-Paclitaxel (Unknown Primary, Squamous Cell) *on page 2051*

Cisplatin-Paclitaxel (Head and Neck Cancer)

Index Terms Paclitaxel-Cisplatin (Head and Neck Cancer)

Use Head and neck cancer

Regimen NOTE: Multiple variations are listed.

Variation 1 (with concurrent radiation therapy):
Paclitaxel: IV: 30 mg/m^2 day 1
[total dose/week = 30 mg/m^2]
Cisplatin: IV: 20 mg/m^2 day 2
[total dose/week = 20 mg/m^2]
Repeat every week for a total of 7 weeks

Variation 2:
Paclitaxel: IV: 175 mg/m^2 dose over 3 hours day 1
[total dose/cycle = 175 mg/m^2]
Cisplatin: IV: 75 mg/m^2/dose day 1
[total dose/cycle = 75 mg/m^2]
Repeat cycle every 3 weeks

References

Variation 1:

Garden AS, Harris J, Vokes EE, et al, "Preliminary Results of Radiation Therapy Oncology Group 97-03: A Randomized Phase II Trial of Concurrent Radiation and Chemotherapy for Advanced Squamous Cell Carcinomas of the Head and Neck," *J Clin Oncol*, 2004, 22(14):2856-64.

Variation 2:

Gibson MK, Li Y, Murphy B, et al, "Randomized Phase III Evaluation of Cisplatin Plus Fluorouracil Versus Cisplatin Plus Paclitaxel in Advanced Head and Neck Cancer (E1395): An Intergroup Trial of the Eastern Cooperative Oncology Group," *J Clin Oncol*, 2005, 23(15):3562-7.

Cisplatin-Paclitaxel Intraperitoneal (Ovarian)

Index Terms Paclitaxel-Cisplatin Intraperitoneal (Ovarian)

Use Ovarian cancer

Regimen Note: I.P. therapies administered in 2 liters warmed saline

Paclitaxel: IV: 135 mg/m^2 continuous infusion over 24 hours day 1
[total IV dose/cycle = 135 mg/m^2]
Cisplatin: I.P.: 100 mg/m^2 day 2
[total I.P. dose/cycle = 100 mg/m^2]
Paclitaxel: I.P.: 60 mg/m^2 day 8
[total I.P. dose/cycle = 60 mg/m^2]
Repeat cycle every 21 days for 6 cycles

References

Armstrong DK, Bundy B, Wenzel L, et al, "Intraperitoneal Cisplatin and Paclitaxel in Ovarian Cancer," *N Engl J Med*, 2006, 354(1):34-43.

Cisplatin-Paclitaxel (NSCLC)

Index Terms Paclitaxel-Cisplatin (NSCLC)

Use Lung cancer, non-small cell

Regimen

Paclitaxel: IV: 135 mg/m^2 continuous infusion over 24 hours day 1

[total dose/cycle = 135 mg/m^2]

Cisplatin: IV: 75 mg/m^2 day 2

[total dose/cycle = 75 mg/m^2]

Repeat cycle every 21 days

References

Schiller JH, Harrington D, Belani CP, et al. Comparison of four chemotherapy regimens for advanced non-small-cell lung cancer. *N Engl J Med*, 2002;346(2):92-98.

Cisplatin-Paclitaxel (Ovarian)

Index Terms Paclitaxel-Cisplatin (Ovarian)

Use Ovarian cancer

Regimen

Paclitaxel: IV: 135 mg/m^2 continuous infusion over 24 hours day 1

[total dose/cycle = 135 mg/m^2]

Cisplatin: IV: 75 mg/m^2 day 2

[total dose/cycle = 75 mg/m^2]

Repeat cycle every 21 days for a total of 6 cycles

References

McGuire WP, Hoskins WJ, Brady MF, et al, "Cyclophosphamide and Cisplatin Compared With Paclitaxel and Cisplatin in Patients With Stage III and Stage IV Ovarian Cancer," *N Engl J Med*, 1996, 334(1):1-6.

Muggia FM, Braly PS, Brady MF, et al, "Phase III Randomized Study of Cisplatin Versus Paclitaxel Versus Cisplatin and Paclitaxel in Patients With Suboptimal Stage III or IV Ovarian Cancer: A Gynecologic Oncology Group Study," *J Clin Oncol*, 2000, 18(1):106-15.

Cisplatin-Pemetrexed (Mesothelioma)

Index Terms Pemetrexed-Cisplatin (Mesothelioma)

Use Malignant pleural mesothelioma

Regimen

Pemetrexed: IV: 500 mg/m^2 over 10 minutes day 1

[total dose/cycle = 500 mg/m^2]

Cisplatin: IV: 75 mg/m^2 over 2 hours day 1 (start 30 minutes after pemetrexed)

[total dose/cycle = 75 mg/m^2]

Repeat cycle every 21 days

References

Santoro A, O'Brien ME, Stahel RA, et al, "Pemetrexed Plus Cisplatin or Pemetrexed Plus Carboplatin for Chemonaïve Patients With Malignant Pleural Mesothelioma: Results of the International Expanded Access Program," *J Thorac Oncol*, 2008, 3(7):756-63.

Vogelzang NJ, Rusthoven JJ, Symanowski J, et al, "Phase III Study of Pemetrexed in Combination With Cisplatin Versus Cisplatin Alone in Patients With Malignant Pleural Mesothelioma," *J Clin Oncol*, 2003, 21(14):2636-44.

Cisplatin-Pemetrexed (NSCLC)

Index Terms Pemetrexed-Cisplatin (NSCLC)

Use Lung cancer, non-small cell

Regimen

Pemetrexed: IV: 500 mg/m^2 day 1

[total dose/cycle = 500 mg/m^2]

Cisplatin: IV: 75 mg/m^2 day 1

[total dose/cycle = 75 mg/m^2]

Repeat cycle every 21 days for up to 6 cycles

References

Scagliotti GV, Parikh P, von Pawel J, et al, "Phase III Study Comparing Cisplatin Plus Gemcitabine With Cisplatin Plus Pemetrexed in Chemotherapy-Naive Patients With Advanced-Stage Non-Small-Cell Lung Cancer," *J Clin Oncol*, 2008, 26(21):3543-51.

Cisplatin-Raltitrexed (Mesothelioma)

Index Terms Raltitrexed-Cisplatin (Mesothelioma)

Use Malignant pleural mesothelioma

Regimen

Raltitrexed: IV: 3 mg/m^2 over 15 minutes day 1

[total dose/cycle = 3 mg/m^2]

Cisplatin: IV: 80 mg/m^2 over 1-2 hours day 1

[total dose/cycle = 80 mg/m^2]

Repeat cycle every 21 days until disease progression or unacceptable toxicity.

References

Bottomley A, Coens C, Efficace F, et al, "Symptoms and Patient-Reported Well-Being: Do They Predict Survival in Malignant Pleural Mesothelioma? A Prognostic Factor Analysis of EORTC-NCIC 08983: Randomized Phase III Study of Cisplatin With or Without Raltitrexed in Patients With Malignant Pleural Mesothelioma," *J Clin Oncol*, 2007, 25(36):5770-6.

van Meerbeeck JP, Gaafar R, Manegold C, et al, "Randomized Phase III Study of Cisplatin With or Without Raltitrexed in Patients With Malignant Pleural Mesothelioma: An Intergroup Study of the European Organisation for Research and Treatment of Cancer Lung Cancer Group and the National Cancer Institute of Canada," *J Clin Oncol*, 2005, 23(28):6881-9.

Cisplatin-Topotecan (Cervical Cancer)

Index Terms Topotecan-Cisplatin (Cervical Cancer)

Use Cervical cancer

Regimen NOTE: Multiple variations are listed.

Variation 1 (Body surface area capped at 2 m^2 maximum):

Topotecan: IV: 0.75 mg/m^2/day days 1, 2, and 3

[total dose/cycle = 2.25 mg/m^2]

Cisplatin: IV: 50 mg/m^2 day 1 only

[total dose/cycle = 50 mg/m^2]

Repeat cycle every 21 days for up to a total of 6 cycles; responders may continue beyond 6 cycles

Variation 2:

Topotecan: IV: 0.75 mg/m^2/day days 1, 2, and 3

[total dose/cycle = 2.25 mg/m^2]

Cisplatin: IV: 50 mg/m^2 day 1 only

[total dose/cycle = 50 mg/m^2]

Repeat cycle every 21 days for up to a total of 6 cycles; responders may continue beyond 6 cycles

References

Variation 1:

Long HJ 3rd, Bundy BN, Grendys EC Jr, et al, "Randomized Phase III Trial of Cisplatin With or Without Topotecan in Carcinoma of the Uterine Cervix: A Gynecologic Oncology Group Study," *J Clin Oncol*, 2005, 23(21):4626-33.

Variation 2:

Monk BJ, Sill MW, McMeekin DS, et al, "Phase III Trial of Four Cisplatin-Containing Doublet Combinations in Stage IVB, Recurrent, or Persistent Cervical Carcinoma: A Gynecologic Oncology Group Study," *J Clin Oncol*, 2009, 27(28):4649-55.

◆ **Cisplatin-Vinblastine-Dacarbazine-Interleukin-Interferon (Melanoma)**
see CVD-Interleukin-Interferon (Melanoma) *on page* 2075

Cisplatin-Vinblastine-Dacarbazine (Melanoma)

Index Terms CVD; Dacarbazine-Cisplatin-Vinblastine; Vinblastine-Cisplatin-Dacarbazine

Use Melanoma

Regimen NOTE: Multiple variations are listed.

Variation 1:

Cisplatin: IV: 20 mg/m^2/day days 2 to 5

[total dose/cycle = 80 mg/m^2]

Vinblastine: IV: 1.6 mg/m^2/day days 1 to 5

[total dose/cycle = 8 mg/m^2]

Dacarbazine: IV: 800 mg/m^2 day 1

[total dose/cycle = 800 mg/m^2]

Repeat cycle every 21 days

Variation 2:

Cisplatin: IV: 20 mg/m^2/day days 1 to 4

[total dose/cycle = 80 mg/m^2]

Vinblastine: IV: 2 mg/m^2/day days 1 to 4

[total dose/cycle = 8 mg/m^2]

Dacarbazine: IV: 800 mg/m^2 day 1

[total dose/cycle = 800 mg/m^2]

Repeat cycle every 21 days

References

Variation 1:

Legha SS, Ring S, Papadopoulos N, et al, "A Prospective Evaluation of a Triple-Drug Regimen Containing Cisplatin, Vinblastine, and Dacarbazine (CVD) for Metastatic Melanoma," *Cancer*, 1989, 64(10):2024-9.

Variation 2:

Eton O, Legha SS, Bedikian AY, et al, "Sequential Biochemotherapy Versus Chemotherapy for Metastatic Melanoma: Results From a Phase III Randomized Trial," *J Clin Oncol*, 2002, 20 (8):2045-52.

Cisplatin-Vinblastine (NSCLC)

Index Terms Vinblastine-Cisplatin (NSCLC)

Use Lung cancer, non-small cell

Regimen NOTE: Multiple variations are listed.

Variation 1 (concurrent radiation preferred):

Cisplatin: IV: 100 mg/m^2/day days 1 and 29

[total dose/treatment = 200 mg/m^2]

Vinblastine: IV: 5 mg/m^2/week days 1, 8, 15, 22, and 29

[total dose/treatment = 25 mg/m^2]

Variation 2 (sequential radiation):

Cisplatin: IV: 100 mg/m^2/day days 1 and 29

[total dose/treatment = 200 mg/m^2]

Vinblastine: IV: 5 mg/m^2/week days 1, 8, 15, 22, and 29

[total dose/treatment = 25 mg/m^2]

Variation 3 (adjuvant therapy):

Cisplatin: IV: 80 mg/m^2/day days 1, 22, 43, and 64

[total dose/treatment = 320 mg/m^2]

Vinblastine: IV: 4 mg/m^2/day days 1, 8, 15, 22, 29, 43, and 57

[total dose/treatment = 28 mg/m^2]

Variation 4 (adjuvant therapy):

Cisplatin: IV: 100 mg/m^2/day days 1, 29, and 57

[total dose/treatment = 300 mg/m^2]

◀

Vinblastine: IV: 4 mg/m^2/day days 1, 8, 15, 22, 29, 43, and 57
[total dose/treatment = 28 mg/m^2]
Variation 5 (adjuvant therapy):
Cisplatin: IV: 100 mg/m^2/day days 1, 29, 57, and 85
[total dose/treatment = 400 mg/m^2]
Vinblastine: IV: 4 mg/m^2/day days 1, 8, 15, 22, 29, 43, 57, 71, and 85
[total dose/treatment = 36 mg/m^2]

References

Variations 1 and 2:
Curran WJ Jr, Paulus R, Langer CJ, et al. Sequential vs. concurrent chemoradiation for stage III non-small cell lung cancer: randomized phase III trial RTOG 9410. J Natl Cancer Inst. 2011;103 (19):1452-1460.
Variations 3, 4, and 5:
Arriagada R, Bergman B, Dunant A, et al. Cisplatin-based adjuvant chemotherapy in patients with completely resected non-small-cell lung cancer. N Engl J Med. 2004;350(4):351-360.

Cisplatin-Vinorelbine (Adjuvant NSCLC)

Index Terms VC (Adjuvant NSCLC); Vinorelbine-Cisplatin (Adjuvant NSCLC)
Use Lung cancer, non-small cell (adjuvant)
Regimen NOTE: Multiple variations are listed.
Variation 1:
Cisplatin: IV: 50 mg/m^2/day days 1 and 8
[total dose/cycle = 100 mg/m^2]
Vinorelbine: IV: 25 mg/m^2/day days 1, 8, 15, and 22
[total dose/cycle = 100 mg/m^2]
Repeat cycle every 28 days for total of 4 cycles
Variation 2:
Vinorelbine: IV: 30 mg/m^2/day days 1, 8, 15, and 22
[total dose/cycle = 120 mg/m^2]
Cisplatin: IV: 100 mg/m^2 day 1
[total dose/cycle = 100 mg/m^2]
Repeat cycle every 28 days for total of 4 cycles
Variation 3:
Cisplatin: IV: 80 mg/m^2 day 1
[total dose/cycle = 80 mg/m^2]
Vinorelbine: IV: 30 mg/m^2/day days 1, 8, and 15
[total dose/cycle = 90 mg/m^2]
Repeat cycle every 21 days for total of 4 cycles
Note: Vinorelbine treatment is discontinued after day 1 of the final treatment cycle
Variation 4:
Cisplatin: IV: 100 mg/m^2 day 1
[total dose/cycle = 100 mg/m^2]
Vinorelbine: IV: 30 mg/m^2/day days 1, 8, 15, and 22
[total dose/cycle = 120 mg/m^2]
Repeat cycle every 28 days for total of 3 or 4 cycles
Note: Vinorelbine treatment is discontinued after day 1 of the final treatment cycle

References

Variation 1:
Butts CA, Ding K, Seymour L, et al. Randomized phase III trial of vinorelbine plus cisplatin compared with observation in completely resected stage IB and II non-small-cell lung cancer: updated survival analysis of JBR.10. J Clin Oncol. 2010;28(1):29-34.
Winton T, Livingston R, Johnson D, et al. Vinorelbine plus cisplatin vs. observation in resected non-small-cell lung cancer. N Engl J Med. 2005;352(25):2589-2597.

Variation 2:

Douillard JY, Rosell R, De Lena M, et al. Adjuvant vinorelbine plus cisplatin versus observation in patients with completely resected stage IB-IIIA non-small-cell lung cancer (Adjuvant Navelbine International Trialist Association [ANITA]): a randomised controlled trial. *Lancet Oncol.* 2006;7 (9):719-727.

Variations 3 and 4:

Arriagada R, Bergman B, Dunant A, et al. Cisplatin-based adjuvant chemotherapy in patients with completely resected non-small-cell lung cancer. *N Engl J Med.* 2004;350(4):351-360.

Arriagada R, Dunant A, Pignon JP, et al. Long-term results of the international adjuvant lung cancer trial evaluating adjuvant cisplatin-based chemotherapy in resected lung cancer. *J Clin Oncol.* 2010;28(1):35-42.

Cisplatin-Vinorelbine (Cervical Cancer)

Index Terms Vinorelbine-Cisplatin (Cervical Cancer)

Use Cervical cancer

Regimen NOTE: Multiple variations are listed.

Variation 1:

Cisplatin: IV: 50 mg/m^2 day 1
[total dose/cycle = 50 mg/m^2]
Vinorelbine: IV: 30 mg/m^2/day days 1 and 8
[total dose/cycle = 60 mg/m^2]
Repeat cycle every 21 days for up to a total of 6 cycles; responders may continue beyond 6 cycles

Variation 2:

Cisplatin: IV: 80 mg/m^2 day 1
[total dose/cycle = 80 mg/m^2]
Vinorelbine: IV: 25 mg/m^2/day days 1 and 8
[total dose/cycle = 50 mg/m^2]
Repeat cycle every 21 days for a total of 3-6 cycles

References

Variation 1:

Monk BJ, Sill MW, McMeekin DS, et al, "Phase III Trial of Four Cisplatin-Containing Doublet Combinations in Stage IVB, Recurrent, or Persistent Cervical Carcinoma: A Gynecologic Oncology Group Study," *J Clin Oncol*, 2009, 27(28):4649-55.

Variation 2:

Gebbia V, Caruso M, Testa A, et al, "Vinorelbine and Cisplatin for the Treatment of Recurrent and/or Metastatic Carcinoma of the Uterine Cervix," *Oncology*, 2002, 63(1):31-7.

Pignata S, Silvestro G, Ferrari E, et al, "Phase II Study of Cisplatin and Vinorelbine as First-Line Chemotherapy in Patients With Carcinoma of the Uterine Cervix," *J Clin Oncol*, 1999, 17 (3):756-60.

◆ **Cisplatin-Vinorelbine-Cetuximab (NSCLC)** *see* Cetuximab-Cisplatin-Vinorelbine (NSCLC) *on page 2031*

Cisplatin-Vinorelbine (Metastatic NSCLC)

Index Terms VC (Metastatic NSCLC); Vinorelbine-Cisplatin (Metastatic NSCLC)

Use Lung cancer, non-small cell (metastatic)

Regimen NOTE: Multiple variations are listed.

Variation 1:

Cisplatin: IV: 100 mg/m^2 day 1
[total dose/cycle = 100 mg/m^2]
Vinorelbine: IV: 25 mg/m^2/day days 1, 8, 15, and 22
[total dose/cycle = 100 mg/m^2]
Repeat cycle every 28 days for up to 10 cycles

Variation 2:
Cisplatin: IV: 80 mg/m^2 day 1
[total dose/cycle = 80 mg/m^2]
Vinorelbine: IV: 25 mg/m^2/day days 1 and 8
[total dose/cycle = 50 mg/m^2]
Repeat cycle every 21 days

References

Variation 1:
Kelly K, Crowley J, Bunn PA Jr, et al. Randomized phase III trial of paclitaxel plus carboplatin versus vinorelbine plus cisplatin in the treatment of patients with advanced non-small-cell lung cancer: a Southwest Oncology Group trial. *J Clin Oncol*. 2001;19(13):3210-3218.
Variation 2:
Ohe Y, Ohashi Y, Kubota K, et al. Randomized phase III study of cisplatin plus irinotecan versus carboplatin plus paclitaxel, cisplatin plus gemcitabine, and cisplatin plus vinorelbine for advanced non-small-cell lung cancer: Four-Arm Cooperative Study in Japan. *Ann Oncol*. 2007;18(2):317-323.

♦ **Cladribine-Cytarabine-G-CSF** *see* CLAG (AML Induction) *on page* 2065

♦ **Cladribine-Cytarabine-Mitoxantrone-G-CS** *see* CLAG-M (AML Induction) *on page* 2065

Cladribine-Rituximab (NHL-Mantle Cell)

Index Terms 2-CDA-Rituximab (NHL-Mantle Cell); Rituximab-Cladribine (NHL-Mantle Cell)

Use Lymphoma, non-Hodgkin (Mantle cell)

Regimen
Rituximab: IV: 375 mg/m^2 day 1
[total dose/cycle = 375 mg/m^2]
Cladribine: IV: 5 mg/m^2/day over 2 hours days 1 to 5
[total dose/cycle = 25 mg/m^2]
Growth Factor:
Pegfilgrastim: SubQ: 6 mg day 6
or
Filgrastim: SubQ: Days 6 to 15 (no dose specified)
Repeat cycle every 28 days for a total of 2 to 6 cycles

References

Inwards DJ, Fishkin PA, Hillman DW, et al. Long-term results of the treatment of patients with mantle cell lymphoma with cladribine (2-CDA) alone (95-80-53) or 2-CDA and rituximab (N0189) in the North Central Cancer Treatment Group. *Cancer*. 2008;113(1):108-116.

Cladribine-Rituximab (Waldenstrom Macroglobulinemia)

Index Terms 2-chloro-2'-deoxyadenosine-Rituximab (Waldenstrom Macroglobulinemia); Rituximab-Cladribine (Waldenstrom Macroglobulinemia)

Use Waldenstrom macroglobulinemia

Regimen
Rituximab: IV: 375 mg/m^2 day 1
[total dose/cycle = 375 mg/m^2]
Cladribine: SubQ: 0.1 mg/kg/day once daily days 1 to 5
[total dose/cycle = 0.5 mg/kg]
Repeat cycle every 28 days for 4 cycles

References

Laszlo D, Andreola G, Rigacci L, et al. Rituximab and subcutaneous 2-chloro-2'-deoxyadenosine combination treatment for patients with Waldenstrom macroglobulinemia: clinical and biologic results of a phase II multicenter study. *J Clin Oncol*. 2010;28(13):2233-2238.

CLAG (AML Induction)

Index Terms Cladribine-Cytarabine-G-CSF

Use Leukemia, acute myeloid

Regimen

Cladribine: IV: 5 mg/m^2/day over 2 hours days 1 to 5
  [total dose/cycle = 25 mg/m^2]
Cytarabine: IV: 2 g/m^2/day over 4 hours days 1 to 5 (begin 2 hours after cladribine)
  [total dose/cycle = 10 g/m^2]
Filgrastim: SubQ: 300 mcg daily days 0 to 5 (start 24 hours prior to chemotherapy; for a total of 6 days)
  [total dose/cycle = 1800 mcg]
May administer a second induction cycle if needed

References

Robak T, Wrzesień-Kuś A, Lech-Marańda E, et al, "Combination Regimen of Cladribine (2-Chlorodeoxyadenosine), Cytarabine and G-CSF (CLAG) as Induction Therapy for Patients With Relapsed or Refractory Acute Myeloid Leukemia," *Leuk Lymphoma*, 2000, 39(1-2):121-9.

Wrzesień-Kuś A, Robak T, Lech-Marańda E, et al, "A Multicenter, Open, Non-Comparative Phase II Study of the Combination of Cladribine (2-Chlorodeoxyadenosine), Cytarabine, and G-CSF as Induction Therapy in Refractory Acute Myeloid Leukemia – A Report of the Polish Adult Leukemia Group (PALG)," *Eur J Haematol*, 2003;71(3):155–62.

CLAG-M (AML Induction)

Index Terms Cladribine-Cytarabine-Mitoxantrone-G-CS

Use Leukemia, acute myeloid

Regimen

Cladribine: IV: 5 mg/m^2/day over 2 hour days 1 to 5
  [total dose/cycle = 25 mg/m^2]
Cytarabine: IV: 2 g/m^2/day over 4 hours days 1 to 5 (begin 2 hours after cladribine)
  [total dose/cycle = 10 g/m^2]
Mitoxantrone: IV: 10 mg/m^2/day days 1 to 3
  [total dose/cycle = 30 mg/m^2]
Filgrastim: SubQ: 300 mcg daily days 0 to 5 (start 24 hours prior to chemotherapy; for a total of 6 days)
  [total dose/cycle = 1800 mcg]
May administer a second induction cycle if needed

References

Wierzbowska A, Robak T, Pluta A, et al, "Cladribine Combined With High Doses of Arabinoside Cytosine, Mitoxantrone, and G-CSF (CLAG-M) is a Highly Effective Salvage Regimen in Patients With Refractory and Relapsed Acute Myeloid Leukemia of the Poor Risk: A Final Report of the Polish Adult Leukemia Group," *Eur J Haematol* 2008; 80(2):115-26.

Clofarabine-Cyclophosphamide-Etoposide (ALL)

Index Terms CLOVE Regimen (ALL); Cyclophosphamide-Clofarabine-Etoposide (ALL); Etoposide-Cyclophosphamide-Clofarabine (ALL)

Use Leukemia, acute lymphocytic (relapsed/refractory; persistent minimal residual disease; bridging regimen to hematopoietic stem cell transplant; ≤21 years of age)

Regimen

Clofarabine: IV: 20 to 30 mg/m^2/day days 1 to 5
  [total dose/cycle = 100 to 150 mg/m^2]
Cyclophosphamide: IV: 300 to 340 mg/m^2/day days 1 to 5
  [total dose/cycle = 1,500 to 1,700 mg/m^2]

◀   Etoposide: IV: 100 mg/m^2/day days 1 to 5
    [total dose/cycle = 500 mg/m^2]

References

Gossai N, Verneris NR, Karras NA, Gorman MF, Patel NS, Burke MJ. A clofarabine-based bridging regimen in patients with relapsed ALL and persistent minimal residual disease (MRD). *Bone Marrow Transplant*. 2014;49(3):440-442.

Clofarabine-Cytarabine (AML)

Index Terms Cytarabine-Clofarabine (AML); GCLAC (AML)
Use Leukemia, acute myeloid (relapsed/refractory, 18 to 70 years of age)
Regimen
  Induction:
    Filgrastim: SubQ: 5 mcg/kg (round to nearest vial size) once daily beginning
      day 0 and continuing until the ANC ≥2,000/mm^3 for 2 consecutive days
    Clofarabine: IV: 25 mg/m^2/day over 1 hour days 1 to 5
      [total dose/cycle = 125 mg/m^2]
    Cytarabine: IV: 2,000 mg/m^2/day over 2 hours days 1 to 5 (beginning 4 hours
      after start of clofarabine)
      [total dose/cycle = 10,000 mg/m^2]
    A second induction cycle may be administered after day 21 if needed, up to a
      maximum of 2 induction cycles
  Consolidation:
    Filgrastim: SubQ: 5 mcg/kg (round to nearest vial size) once daily beginning
      day 0 and continuing until the ANC ≥2,000/mm^3 for 2 consecutive days
    Clofarabine: IV: 20 mg/m^2/day over 1 hour days 1 to 5
      [total dose/cycle = 100 mg/m^2]
    Cytarabine: IV: 1,000 mg/m^2/day over 2 hours days 1 to 5 (beginning 4 hours
      after start of clofarabine)
      [total dose/cycle = 5,000 mg/m^2]
    Repeat consolidation every 21 days for 1 or 2 cycles, up to a maximum of 2
      consolidation cycles

References

Becker PS, Kantarjian HM, Appelbaum FR, et al. Clofarabine with high dose cytarabine and granulocyte colony-stimulating factor (G-CSF) priming for relapsed and refractory acute myeloid leukaemia. *Br J Haematol*. 2011;155(2):182-189.

◆ **CLOVE Regimen (ALL)** *see* Clofarabine-Cyclophosphamide-Etoposide
  (ALL) on page 2065

CMF Oral (Breast)

Index Terms Cyclophosphamide, Methotrexate, Fluorouracil (Breast)
Use Breast cancer
Regimen NOTE: Multiple variations are listed.
  Variation 1 (patients ≤60 years of age):
    Methotrexate: IV: 40 mg/m^2/day days 1 and 8
      [total dose/cycle = 80 mg/m^2]
    Fluorouracil: IV: 600 mg/m^2/day days 1 and 8
      [total dose/cycle = 1200 mg/m^2]
    Cyclophosphamide: Oral: 100 mg/m^2/day days 1 to 14
      [total dose/cycle = 1400 mg/m^2]
    Repeat cycle every 28 days for 12 cycles
  Variation 1 (patients >60 years of age):
    Methotrexate: IV: 30 mg/m^2/day days 1 and 8
      [total dose/cycle = 60 mg/m^2]

Fluorouracil: IV: 400 mg/m²/day days 1 and 8
  [total dose/cycle = 800 mg/m²]
Cyclophosphamide: Oral: 100 mg/m²/day days 1 to 14
  [total dose/cycle = 1400 mg/m²]
Repeat cycle every 28 days for 12 cycles

Variation 2 (adjuvant treatment):
Methotrexate: IV: 40 mg/m²/day days 1 and 8
  [total dose/cycle = 80 mg/m²]
Fluorouracil: IV: 600 mg/m²/day days 1 and 8
  [total dose/cycle = 1200 mg/m²]
Cyclophosphamide: Oral: 100 mg/m²/day days 1 to 14
  [total dose/cycle = 1400 mg/m²]
Repeat cycle every 28 days for a total of 6 cycles

Variation 3 (metastatic disease):
Methotrexate: IV: 40 mg/m²/day days 1 and 8
  [total dose/cycle = 80 mg/m²]
Fluorouracil: IV: 600 mg/m²/day days 1 and 8
  [total dose/cycle = 1200 mg/m²]
Cyclophosphamide: Oral: 100 mg/m²/day days 1 to 14
  [total dose/cycle = 1400 mg/m²]
Repeat cycle every 28 days until disease progression or unacceptable toxicity

References

Early Breast Cancer Trialists' Collaborative Group (EBCTCG), Peto R, Davies C, et al, "Comparisons Between Different Polychemotherapy Regimens for Early Breast Cancer: Meta-Analysis of Long-Term Outcome Among 100,000 Women in 123 Randomised Trials," *Lancet*, 2012, 379 (9814):432-44.

Goldhirsch A, Colleoni M, Coates AS, et al, "Adding Adjuvant CMF Chemotherapy to Either Radiotherapy or Tamoxifen: Are All CMFs Alike? The International Breast Cancer Study Group (IBCSG)" *Ann Oncol*, 1998, 9(5):489-93.

Variation 1:
Bonadonna G, Brusamolino E, Valagussa P, et al, "Combination Chemotherapy as an Adjuvant Treatment in Operable Breast Cancer," *N Engl J Med*, 1976, 294(8):405-10.

Bonadonna G, Valagussa P, Moliterni A, et al, "Adjuvant Cyclophosphamide, Methotrexate, and Fluorouracil in Node-Positive Breast Cancer: The Results of 20 Years of Follow-Up," *N Engl J Med*, 1995, 332(14):901-6.

Canellos GP, Pocock SJ, Taylor SG III, et al, "Combination Chemotherapy for Metastatic Breast Carcinoma, Prospective Comparison of Multiple Drug Therapy With L-Phonylalanine Mustard," *Cancer*, 1976, 38(5):1002-0.

Variation 2:
Hutchins LF, Green SJ, Ravdin PM, et al, "Randomized, Controlled Trial of Cyclophosphamide, Methotrexate, and Fluorouracil Versus Cyclophosphamide, Doxorubicin, and Fluorouracil With and Without Tamoxifen for High-Risk, Node-Negative Breast Cancer: Treatment Results of Intergroup Protocol INT-0102," *J Clin Oncol*, 2005, 23(33):8313-21.

Variation 3:
Engelsman E, Klijn JC, Rubens RD, et al, "'Classical' CMF Versus a 3-Weekly Intravenous CMF Schedule in Postmenopausal Patients With Advanced Breast Cancer: An EORTC Breast Cancer Co-Operative Group Phase III Trial (10808)," *Eur J Cancer*, 1991, 27(8):966-70.

C-MOPP/ABV Hybrid (Hodgkin)

Index Terms Cyclophosphamide-Vincristine-Procarbazine-Prednisone-Doxorubicin-Bleomycin-Vinblastine (Hodgkin)

Use Lymphoma, Hodgkin

Regimen

Cyclophosphamide: IV: 650 mg/m²/day day 1
  [total dose/cycle = 650 mg/m²]
Vincristine: IV: 1.4 mg/m²/day (maximum dose: 3 mg) day 1
  [total dose/cycle = 1.4 mg/m²; maximum dose/cycle: 3 mg]

◄ Procarbazine: Oral: 100 mg/m^2/day days 1 to 7
[total dose/cycle = 700 mg/m^2]
Prednisone: Oral: 40 mg/m^2/day days 1 to 14
[total dose/cycle = 560 mg/m^2]
Doxorubicin: IV: 35 mg/m^2/day day 8
[total dose/cycle = 35 mg/m^2]
Bleomycin: IV: 10 units/m^2/day day 8
[total dose/cycle = 10 units/m^2]
Vinblastine: IV: 6 mg/m^2/day day 8
[total dose/cycle = 6 mg/m^2]
Repeat cycles every 28 days for a total of 8 cycles

References

Montoto S, Camós M, López-Guillermo A, et al, "Hybrid Chemotherapy Consisting of Cyclo-phosphamide, Vincristine, Procarbazine, Prednisone, Doxorubicin, Bleomycin, and Vinblastine (C-MOPP/ABV) as First-Line Treatment for Patients With Advanced Hodgkin Disease," *Cancer*, 2000;88(9):2142-8.

CMV (Bladder)

Use Bladder cancer, neoadjuvant
Regimen
Methotrexate: IV: 30 mg/m^2/day days 1 and 8
[total dose/cycle = 60 mg/m^2]
Vinblastine: IV: 4 mg/m^2/day days 1 and 8
[total dose/cycle = 8 mg/m^2]
Cisplatin: IV: 100 mg/m^2 day 2
[total dose/cycle = 100 mg/m^2]
Leucovorin Calcium: Oral or IV: 15 mg every 6 hours for 4 doses days 2 and 9, starting 24 hours after day 1 and day 8 methotrexate
[total dose/cycle = 120 mg]
Repeat cycle every 21 days for 3 cycles

References

Griffiths G, Hall R, Sylvester R, et al. International phase III trial assessing neoadjuvant cisplatin, methotrexate, and vinblastine chemotherapy for muscle-invasive bladder cancer: long-term results of the BA06 30894 trial. *J Clin Oncol.* 2011;29(16):2171-2177.

Neoadjuvant cisplatin, methotrexate, and vinblastine chemotherapy for muscle-invasive bladder cancer: a randomised controlled trial. International collaboration of trialists. *Lancet.* 1999;354 (9178):533-540.

Cobimetinib-Vemurafenib (Melanoma)

Use Melanoma (first-line, unresectable locally advanced or metastatic BRAF V600E or V600K mutation-positive melanoma)
Regimen
Cobimetinib: Oral: 60 mg once daily, taken with or without food, days 1 to 21
[total dose/cycle = 1,260 mg]
Vemurafenib: Oral: 960 mg every 12 hours, taken with or without food, days 1 to 28
[total dose/cycle = 53,760 mg]
Repeat cycle every 28 days until disease progression or unacceptable toxicity

References

Larkin J, Ascierto PA, Dréno B, et al. Combined vemurafenib and cobimetinib in BRAF-mutated melanoma. *N Engl J Med.* 2014;371(20):1867-1876.

CODOX-M/IVAC (NHL-Burkitt)

Index Terms Cyclophosphamide-Doxorubicin-Vincristine-Methotrexate-Cytar-abine-Ifosfamide-Etoposide (NHL-Burkitt)

Use Lymphoma, non-Hodgkin (Burkitt)

Regimen NOTE: Multiple variations are listed.

Variation 1:

CODOX-M (Cycles 1 and 3; cycles begin when ANC >1,000/mm^3):

Cyclophosphamide: IV: 800 mg/m^2 day 1

followed by IV: 200 mg/m^2/day days 2 to 5

[total dose/cycle = 1,600 mg/m^2]

Vincristine: IV: 1.5 mg/m^2/day (no maximum dose) days 1 and 8 (cycle 1) and days 1, 8, and 15 (cycle 3; day 15 in cycle 3 only if no neuropathy)

[total dose/cycle = 3 to 4.5 mg/m^2]

Doxorubicin: IV: 40 mg/m^2 day 1

[total dose/cycle = 40 mg/m^2]

Methotrexate: IV: 1,200 mg/m^2 (loading dose) over 1 hour day 10

followed by IV: 240 mg/m^2/hour for 23 hours day 10

[total dose/cycle = 6,720 mg/m^2]

Leucovorin Calcium: IV: 192 mg/m^2 day 11 (begin 36 hours after the start of methotrexate infusion)

followed by IV: 12 mg/m^2 every 6 hours until methotrexate level <5 x 10^{-8} micromolar

Cytarabine: Intrathecal: 70 mg/day (adjust to age-appropriate dose if ≤3 years of age) days 1 and 3

[total dose/cycle = 140 mg]

Methotrexate: Intrathecal: 12 mg (adjust to age-appropriate dose if ≤3 years of age) day 15

[total dose/cycle = 12 mg]

Sargramostim: SubQ: 7.5 mcg/kg/day beginning day 13, continue until ANC >1,000/mm^3

Note: If CNS disease present, administer additional intrathecal treatment in cycle 1: Cytarabine 70 mg (adjust to age-appropriate dose if ≤3 years of age) day 5 and methotrexate 12 mg (adjust to age-appropriate dose if ≤3 years of age) day 17

IVAC (Cycles 2 and 4; cycles begin when ANC >1,000/mm^3):

Ifosfamide: IV: 1,500 mg/m^2/day days 1 to 5

[total dose/cycle = 7,500 mg/m^2]

Mesna: IV: 360 mg/m^2 every 3 hours days 1 to 5

[total dose/cycle = 14,400 mg/m^2]

Etoposide: IV: 60 mg/m^2/day days 1 to 5

[total dose/cycle = 300 mg/m^2]

Cytarabine: IV: 2,000 mg/m^2 every 12 hours, for 4 doses, days 1 and 2

[total dose/cycle = 8,000 mg/m^2]

Methotrexate: Intrathecal: 12 mg day 5

[total dose/cycle = 12 mg]

Sargramostim: SubQ: 7.5 mcg/kg/day beginning day 7, continue until ANC >1000/mm^3

Note: If CNS disease present, administer additional intrathecal treatment in cycle 2: Cytarabine 70 mg/day (adjust to age-appropriate dose if ≤3 years of age) days 7 and 9

Variation 2:

CODOX-M (Cycles 1 and 3; cycles begin when ANC >1,000/mm^3 without growth factor support and an unsupported platelet count >75,000/mm^3):

Cyclophosphamide: IV: 800 mg/m^2 day 1

followed by IV: 200 mg/m^2/day days 2 to 5

[total dose/cycle = 1,600 mg/m^2]

Vincristine: IV: 1.5 mg/m^2/day (maximum dose: 2 mg) days 1 and 8
[total dose/cycle = 3 mg/m^2; maximum: 4 mg/cycle]

Doxorubicin: IV: 40 mg/m^2 day 1
[total dose/cycle = 40 mg/m^2]

Methotrexate: IV: 300 mg/m^2 (100 mg/m^2 if >65 years of age) (loading dose) over 1 hour day 10
followed by IV: 2,700 mg/m^2 (900 mg/m^2 if >65 years of age) over 23 hours day 10
[total dose/cycle = 3,000 mg/m^2 (1,000 mg/m^2 if >65 years of age)]

Leucovorin Calcium: IV: 15 mg/m^2 every 3 hours day 11 (begin 36 hours after the start of methotrexate infusion) for 5 doses
followed by IV: 15 mg/m^2 every 6 hours until methotrexate level <5 x 10^{-8} micromolar

Cytarabine: Intrathecal: 70 mg/day days 1 and 3
[total dose/cycle = 140 mg]

Methotrexate: Intrathecal: 12 mg day 15
[total dose/cycle = 12 mg]

Leucovorin Calcium: Oral: 15 mg day 16 (24 hours after intrathecal methotrexate)

Filgrastim: SubQ: 5 mcg/kg/day beginning day 13, continue until ANC >1,000/mm^3

Note: If CNS disease present, administer additional intrathecal treatment: Cytarabine 70 mg day 5 and methotrexate 12 mg (with leucovorin rescue) day 17

IVAC (Cycles 2 and 4; cycles begin when ANC >1,000/mm^3 without growth factor support and an unsupported platelet count >75,000/mm^3):

Ifosfamide: IV: 1,500 mg/m^2/day (1,000 mg/m^2/day if >65 years of age) over 1 hour days 1 to 5
[total dose/cycle = 7,500 mg/m^2 (5,000 mg/m^2 if >65 years of age)]

Mesna: IV: 300 mg/m^2/day (200 mg/m^2/day if >65 years of age) over 1 hour mixed with each ifosfamide dose days 1 to 5
followed by IV: 300 mg/m^2 (200 mg/m^2 if >65 years of age) every 4 hours for 2 doses/day days 1 to 5
[total dose/cycle = 4,500 mg/m^2 (3,000 mg/m^2 if >65 years of age)]

Etoposide: IV: 60 mg/m^2/day over 1 hour days 1 to 5
[total dose/cycle = 300 mg/m^2]

Cytarabine: IV: 2,000 mg/m^2 (1,000 mg/m^2 if >65 years of age) over 3 hours every 12 hours, for 4 doses, days 1 and 2
[total dose/cycle = 8,000 mg/m^2 (4,000 mg/m^2 if >65 years of age)]

Methotrexate: Intrathecal: 12 mg day 5
[total dose/cycle = 12 mg]

Leucovorin Calcium: Oral: 15 mg day 6 (24 hours after intrathecal methotrexate)

Filgrastim: SubQ: 5 mcg/kg/day beginning day 7, continue until ANC >1,000/mm^3

Note: If CNS disease present, administer additional intrathecal treatment: Cytarabine 70 mg/day on days 7 and 9

Variation 3:

CODOX-M (Cycles 1 and 3; cycles begin when ANC >1,000/mm^3 without growth factor support and an unsupported platelet count >75,000/mm^3):

Cyclophosphamide: IV: 800 mg/m^2 day 1
followed by IV: 200 mg/m^2/day days 2 to 5
[total dose/cycle = 1,600 mg/m^2]

Vincristine: IV: 1.5 mg/m^2/day (maximum dose: 2 mg) days 1 and 8
[total dose/cycle = 3 mg/m^2; maximum: 4 mg/cycle]

Doxorubicin: IV: 40 mg/m^2 day 1
[total dose/cycle = 40 mg/m^2]

Methotrexate: IV: 1,200 mg/m^2 (loading dose) over 1 hour day 10
followed by IV: 240 mg/m^2/hour for 23 hours day 10
[total dose/cycle = 6,720 mg/m^2]

Leucovorin Calcium: IV: 192 mg/m^2 day 11 (begin 36 hours after the start of methotrexate infusion)
followed by IV: 12 mg/m^2 every 6 hours until methotrexate level <5 x 10^{-8} micromolar

Cytarabine: Intrathecal: 70 mg/day days 1 and 3
[total dose/cycle = 140 mg]

Methotrexate: Intrathecal: 12 mg day 15
[total dose/cycle = 12 mg]

Leucovorin Calcium: Oral: 15 mg day 16 (24 hours after intrathecal methotrexate)

Filgrastim: SubQ: 5 mcg/kg/day beginning day 13, continue until ANC >1,000/mm^3

Note: If CNS disease present, administer additional intrathecal treatment in cycle 1: Cytarabine 70 mg (15 mg if via Ommaya reservoir) day 5 and methotrexate 12.5 mg (2 mg if via Ommaya reservoir) day 17

IVAC (Cycles 2 and 4; cycles begin when ANC >1,000/mm^3 without growth factor support and an unsupported platelet count >75,000/mm^3):

Ifosfamide: IV: 1,500 mg/m^2/day over 1 hour days 1 to 5
[total dose/cycle = 7,500 mg/m^2]

Mesna: IV: 360 mg/m^2 mixed with each ifosfamide dose over 1 hour days 1 to 5
followed by IV: 360 mg/m^2 every 3 hours for 7 doses/day days 1 to 5
[total dose/cycle = 14,400 mg/m^2]

Etoposide: IV: 60 mg/m^2/day over 1 hour days 1 to 5
[total dose/cycle = 300 mg/m^2]

Cytarabine: IV: 2,000 mg/m^2 over 3 hours every 12 hours, for 4 doses, days 1 and 2
[total dose/cycle = 8,000 mg/m^2]

Methotrexate: Intrathecal: 12 mg day 5
[total dose/cycle = 12 mg]

Leucovorin Calcium: Oral: 15 mg day 6 (24 hours after intrathecal methotrexate)

Filgrastim: SubQ: 5 mcg/kg/day beginning day 7, continue until ANC >1,000/mm^3

Note: If CNS disease present, administer additional intrathecal treatment in cycle 2: Cytarabine 70 mg/day (15 mg if via Ommaya reservoir) days 7 and 9

Variation 4:

CODOX-M (Cycles 1 and 3; cycles begin when ANC >1,000/mm^3):

Cyclophosphamide: IV: 800 mg/m^2/day days 1 and 2
[total dose/cycle = 1,600 mg/m^2]

Vincristine: IV: 1.4 mg/m^2/day (maximum dose: 2 mg) days 1 and 10
[total dose/cycle = 2.8 mg/m^2; maximum: 4 mg/cycle]

Doxorubicin: IV: 50 mg/m^2 day 1
[total dose/cycle = 50 mg/m^2]

Methotrexate: IV: 3,000 mg/m^2 day 10
[total dose/cycle = 3,000 mg/m^2]

Leucovorin Calcium: IV: 200 mg/m² day 11 (24 hours after methotrexate infusion)

followed by Oral, IV: 15 mg/m² every 6 hours until methotrexate level <0.1 micromolar

Cytarabine: Intrathecal: 50 mg/day days 1 and 3
[total dose/cycle = 100 mg]

Hydrocortisone: Intrathecal: 50 mg/day days 1 and 3
[total dose/cycle = 100 mg]

Methotrexate: Intrathecal: 12 mg day 1
[total dose/cycle = 12 mg]

Filgrastim: SubQ: Dose not specified, days 3 to 8 and day 12 until ANC >1,000 mm³

Note: If CNS disease present, administer additional intrathecal treatment in cycle 1: Cytarabine 50 mg day 5 and methotrexate 12 mg day 10

IVAC (Cycles 2 and 4; cycles begin when ANC >1,000/mm³):

Ifosfamide: IV: 1,500 mg/m²/day days 1 to 5
[total dose/cycle = 7,500 mg/m²]

Mesna: IV: 1,500 mg/m²/day (in divided doses) days 1 to 5
[total dose/cycle = 7,500 mg/m²]

Etoposide: IV: 60 mg/m²/day days 1 to 5
[total dose/cycle = 300 mg/m²]

Cytarabine: IV: 2,000 mg/m² every 12 hours, for 4 doses, days 1 and 2
[total dose/cycle = 8,000 mg/m²]

Methotrexate: Intrathecal: 12 mg day 5
[total dose/cycle = 12 mg]

Hydrocortisone: Intrathecal: 50 mg day 5
[total dose/cycle = 50 mg]

Filgrastim: SubQ: Dose not specified, daily beginning day 6 until ANC >1,000/mm³

Note: If CNS disease present, administer additional intrathecal treatment in cycle 2: Cytarabine 50 mg/day days 3 and 5

References

Variation 1:

Magrath I, Adde M, Shad A, et al, "Adults and Children With Small Non-Cleaved-Cell Lymphoma Have a Similar Excellent Outcome When Treated With the Same Chemotherapy Regimen," *J Clin Oncol*, 1996, 14(3):925-34.

Variation 2:

Mead GM, Barrans SL, Qian W, et al, "A Prospective Clinicopathologic Study of Dose-Modified CODOX-M/IVAC in Patients With Sporadic Burkitt Lymphoma Defined Using Cytogenetic and Immunophenotypic Criteria (MRC/NCRI LY10 Trial)," *Blood*, 2008, 112(6):2248-60.

Variation 3:

Mead GM, Sydes MR, Walewski J, et al, "An International Evaluation of CODOX-M and CODOX-M Alternating With IVAC in Adult Burkitt's Lymphoma: Results of United Kingdom Lymphoma Group LY06 Study," *Ann Oncol*, 2002, 13(8):1264-74.

Variation 4:

Lacasce A, Howard O, Lib S, et al, "Modified Magrath Regimens for Adults With Burkitt and Burkitt-Like Lymphomas: Preserved Efficacy With Decreased Toxicity," *Leuk Lymphoma*, 2004, 45(4):761-7.

CODOX-M (NHL-Burkitt)

Index Terms Cyclophosphamide-Doxorubicin-Vincristine-Methotrexate-Cytarabine (NHL-Burkitt)

Use Lymphoma, non-Hodgkin (Burkitt)

Regimen NOTE: Multiple variations are listed.
Variation 1:
  Cyclophosphamide: IV: 800 mg/m^2 day 1
    followed by IV: 200 mg/m^2/day days 2 to 5
      [total dose/cycle = 1,600 mg/m^2]
  Vincristine: IV: 1.5 mg/m^2/day (no maximum dose) days 1 and 8
    [total dose/cycle = 3 mg/m^2]
  Doxorubicin: IV: 40 mg/m^2 day 1
    [total dose/cycle = 40 mg/m^2]
  Methotrexate: IV: 1,200 mg/m^2 (loading dose) over 1 hour day 10
    followed by IV: 240 mg/m^2/hour for 23 hours day 10
      [total dose/cycle = 6,720 mg/m^2]
  Leucovorin Calcium: IV: 192 mg/m^2 day 11 (begin 36 hours after the start of
    methotrexate infusion)
    followed by IV: 12 mg/m^2 every 6 hours until methotrexate level <5 x 10^{-8}
    micromolar
  Cytarabine: Intrathecal: 70 mg (adjust to age-appropriate dose if ≤3 years of
    age) day 1
    [total dose/cycle = 70 mg]
  Methotrexate: Intrathecal: 12 mg (adjust to age-appropriate dose if ≤3 years
    of age) day 3
    [total dose/cycle = 12 mg]
  Repeat cycle when ANC >1,000/mm^3 for a total of 3 cycles
Variation 2:
  Cyclophosphamide: IV: 800 mg/m^2 day 1
    followed by IV: 200 mg/m^2/day days 2 to 5
      [total dose/cycle = 1,600 mg/m^2]
  Vincristine: IV: 1.5 mg/m^2/day (maximum dose: 2 mg) days 1 and 8
    [total dose/cycle = 3 mg/m^2; maximum: 4 mg/cycle]
  Doxorubicin: IV: 40 mg/m^2 day 1
    [total dose/cycle = 40 mg/m^2]
  Methotrexate: IV: 1,200 mg/m^2 (loading dose) over 1 hour day 10
    followed by IV: 240 mg/m^2/hour for 23 hours day 10
      [total dose/cycle = 6,720 mg/m^2]
  Leucovorin Calcium: IV: 192 mg/m^2 day 11 (begin 36 hours after the start of
    methotrexate infusion)
    followed by IV: 12 mg/m^2 every 6 hours until methotrexate level <5 x 10^{-8}
    micromolar
  Cytarabine: Intrathecal: 70 mg/day days 1 and 3
    [total dose/cycle = 140 mg]
  Methotrexate: Intrathecal: 12 mg day 15
    [total dose/cycle = 12 mg]
  Leucovorin Calcium: Oral: 15 mg day 16 (24 hours after intrathecal metho-
    trexate)
  Filgrastim: SubQ: 5 mcg/kg/day beginning day 13, continue until ANC
    >1,000/mm^3
  Repeat cycle when ANC >1,000/mm^3 without growth factor support and an
    unsupported platelet count of >75,000/mm^3 for a total of 3 cycles
Variation 3:
  Cyclophosphamide: IV: 800 mg/m^2/day days 1 and 2
    [total dose/cycle = 1,600 mg/m^2]
  Vincristine: IV: 1.4 mg/m^2/day (maximum dose: 2 mg) days 1 and 10
    [total dose/cycle = 2.8 mg/m^2; maximum: 4 mg/cycle]

◄

Doxorubicin: IV: 50 mg/m^2 day 1
   [total dose/cycle = 50 mg/m^2]
Methotrexate: IV: 3,000 mg/m^2 day 10
   [total dose/cycle = 3,000 mg/m^2]
Leucovorin Calcium: IV: 200 mg/m^2 day 11 (24 hours after methotrexate infusion)
   followed by Oral, IV: 15 mg/m^2 every 6 hours until methotrexate level <0.1 micromolar
Cytarabine: Intrathecal: 50 mg day 1
   [total dose/cycle = 50 mg]
Hydrocortisone: Intrathecal: 50 mg day 1
   [total dose/cycle = 50 mg]
Methotrexate: Intrathecal: 12 mg day 1
   [total dose/cycle = 12 mg]
Filgrastim: SubQ: Dose not specified; days 3 to 8 and day 12 if ANC <1,000/mm^3; administer until ANC >1,000/mm^3
Repeat cycle when ANC >1,000/mm^3 for a total of 3 cycles

References

Variation 1:
Magrath I, Adde M, Shad A, et al. Adults and children with small non-cleaved-cell lymphoma have a similar excellent outcome when treated with the same chemotherapy regimen. *J Clin Oncol.* 1996;14(3):925-934.
Variation 2:
Mead GM, Sydes MR, Walewski J, et al. An international evaluation of CODOX-M and CODOX-M alternating with IVAC in adult Burkitt's Lymphoma: results of United Kingdom Lymphoma Group LY06 Study. *Ann Oncol.* 2002;13(8):1264-1274.
Variation 3:
Lacasce A, Howard O, Lib S, et al. Modified magrath regimens for adults with burkitt and burkitt-like lymphomas: preserved efficacy with decreased toxicity. *Leuk Lymphoma.* 2004;45 (4):761-767.

COPE

Index Terms Baby Brain I
Use Brain tumors
Regimen
Cycle A:
Vincristine: IV: 0.065 mg/kg/day (maximum dose: 1.5 mg) days 1 and 8
   [total dose/cycle = 0.13 mg/kg]
Cyclophosphamide: IV: 65 mg/kg day 1
   [total dose/cycle = 65 mg/kg]
Cycle B:
Cisplatin: IV: 4 mg/kg day 1
   [total dose/cycle = 4 mg/kg]
Etoposide: IV: 6.5 mg/kg/day days 3 and 4
   [total dose/cycle = 13 mg/kg]
Repeat cycle every 28 days in the following sequence: AABAAB

References

Duffner PK, Horowitz ME, Krischer JP, et al "Postoperative Chemotherapy and Delayed Radiation in Children Less Than Three Years of Age With Malignant Brain Tumors," *N Engl J Med*, 1993, 328(24):1725-31.

◆ **CRd (Multiple Myeloma)** *see* Carfilzomib, Lenalidomide, Dexamethasone (Multiple Myeloma) *on page 2026*

◆ **CVD** *see* Cisplatin-Vinblastine-Dacarbazine (Melanoma) *on page 2061*

◆ **CVD-IL-2-IFN (Melanoma)** *see* CVD-Interleukin-Interferon (Melanoma) *on page 2075*

CVD-Interleukin-Interferon (Melanoma)

Index Terms Cisplatin-Vinblastine-Dacarbazine-Interleukin-Interferon (Melanoma); CVD-IL-2-IFN (Melanoma)

Use Melanoma

Regimen NOTE: Multiple variations are listed.

Variation 1:

Cisplatin: IV: 20 mg/m²/day days 1 to 4 and 22 to 25
[total dose/cycle = 160 mg/m²]

Vinblastine: IV: 1.5 mg/m²/day days 1 to 4 and 22 to 25
[total dose/cycle = 12 mg/m²]

Dacarbazine: IV: 800 mg/m²/day days 1 and 22
[total dose/cycle = 1600 mg/m²]

Aldesleukin: IV: 9 million units/m²/day continuous infusion days 5 to 8, 17 to 20, and 26 to 29
[total dose/cycle = 108 million units/m²]

Interferon alfa-2b: SubQ: 5 million units/m²/day days 5 to 9, 17 to 21, and 26 to 30
[total dose/cycle = 75 million units/m²]

Repeat every 42 days (maximum of five 21-day cycles for cytokine [interleukin and interferon] component)

Variation 2:

Cisplatin: IV: 20 mg/m²/day days 1 to 4
[total dose/cycle = 80 mg/m²]

Vinblastine: IV: 1.6 mg/m²/day days 1 to 4
[total dose/cycle = 6.4 mg/m²]

Dacarbazine: IV: 800 mg/m² day 1
[total dose/cycle = 800 mg/m²]

Aldesleukin: IV: 9 million units/m²/day continuous infusion days 1 to 4
[total dose/cycle = 36 million units/m²]

Interferon alfa: SubQ: 5 million units/m²/day days 1 to 5, 7, 9, 11, and 13
[total dose/cycle = 45 million units/m²]

Repeat cycle every 21 days for a total of 6 cycles

Variation 3:

Cisplatin: IV: 20 mg/m²/day days 1 to 4
[total dose/cycle = 80 mg/m²]

Vinblastine: IV: 1.2 mg/m²/day days 1 to 4
[total dose/cycle = 4.8 mg/m²]

Dacarbazine: IV: 800 mg/m² day 1
[total dose/cycle = 800 mg/m²]

Aldesleukin: IV: 9 million units/m²/day continuous infusion days 1 to 4
[total dose/cycle = 36 million units/m²]

Interferon alfa-2b: SubQ: 5 million units/m²/day days 1 to 5, 8, 10, and 12
[total dose/cycle = 40 million units/m²]

Repeat cycle every 21 days (maximum: 4 cycles)

References

Variation 1:
Eton O, Legha SS, Bedikian AY, et al, "Sequential Biochemotherapy Versus Chemotherapy for Metastatic Melanoma: Results From a Phase III Randomized Trial," *J Clin Oncol*, 2002, 20 (8):2045-52.
Variation 2:
Legha SS, Ring S, Eton O, et al, "Development of a Biochemotherapy Regimen With Concurrent Administration of Cisplatin, Vinblastine, Dacarbazine, Interferon Alfa, and Interleukin-2 for Patients With Metastatic Melanoma," *J Clin Oncol*, 1998, 16(5):1752-9.

◀

Variation 3:
McDermott DF, Mier JW, Lawrence DP, et al, "A Phase II Pilot Trial of Concurrent Biochemotherapy With Cisplatin, Vinblastine, Dacarbazine, Interleukin 2, and Interferon Alpha-2B in Patients With Metastatic Melanoma," *Clin Cancer Res*, 2000, 6(6):2201-8.

◆ **CVP-R (NHL-Follicular)** *see* R-CVP (NHL-Follicular) *on page* 2202

◆ **CyBorD (Multiple Myeloma)** *see* Cyclophosphamide-Bortezomib-Dexamethasone (Multiple Myeloma) *on page* 2076

Cyclophosphamide-Bortezomib-Dexamethasone (Multiple Myeloma)

Index Terms Bortezomib-Cyclophosphamide-Dexamethasone (Multiple Myeloma); CyBorD (Multiple Myeloma); Cyclophosphamide-Bortezomib-Dexamethasone (Multiple Myeloma); VCD (Multiple Myeloma)

Use Multiple myeloma

Regimen NOTE: Multiple variations are listed.

Variation 1:

Cycles 1 and 2:
Cyclophosphamide: Oral: 300 mg/m^2/day on days 1, 8, 15, and 22
[total dose/cycle = 1,200 mg/m^2]
Bortezomib: IV: 1.5 mg/m^2/day on days 1, 8, 15, and 22
[total dose/cycle = 6 mg/m^2]
Dexamethasone: Oral: 40 mg/day on days 1 to 4, 9 to 12, and 17 to 20
[total dose/cycle = 480 mg]
Repeat cycle every 28 days for 2 cycles

Cycles 3 and 4:
Cyclophosphamide: Oral: 300 mg/m^2/day on days 1, 8, 15, and 22
[total dose/cycle = 1,200 mg/m^2]
Bortezomib: IV: 1.5 mg/m^2/day on days 1, 8, 15, and 22
[total dose/cycle = 6 mg/m^2]
Dexamethasone: Oral: 40 mg/day on days 1, 8, 15, and 22
[total dose/cycle = 160 mg]
Repeat cycle every 28 days for 2 cycles

Variation 2:
Cyclophosphamide: Oral: 300 mg/m^2/day on days 1, 8, 15, and 22
[total dose/cycle = 1,200 mg/m^2]
Bortezomib: IV: 1.3 mg/m^2/day on days 1, 4, 8, and 11
[total dose/cycle = 5.2 mg/m^2]
Dexamethasone: Oral: 40 mg/day on days 1 to 4, 9 to 12, and 17 to 20
[total dose/cycle = 480 mg]
Repeat cycle every 28 days for a total of 4 cycles

References

Variation 1:
Reeder CB, Reece DE, Kukreti V, et al. Once- versus twice-weekly bortezomib induction therapy with CyBorD in newly diagnosed multiple myeloma. *Blood*. 2010;115(16):3416-3417.
Khan ML, Reeder CB, Kumar SK, et al. A comparison of lenalidomide/dexamethasone versus cyclophosphamide/lenalidomide/dexamethasone versus cyclophosphamide/bortezomib/dexamethasone in newly diagnosed multiple myeloma. *Br J Haematol*. 2012;156(3):326-333.
Variation 2:
Reeder CB, Reece DE, Kukrati V, et al. Cyclophosphamide, bortezomib and dexamethasone induction for newly diagnosed multiple myeloma: high response rates in a phase II clinical trial. *Leukemia*. 2009;23(7):1337-1341.

◆ **Cyclophosphamide-Clofarabine-Etoposide (ALL)** *see* Clofarabine-Cyclophosphamide-Etoposide (ALL) *on page 2065*

◆ **Cyclophosphamide-Docetaxel (Breast)** *see* TC (Breast) *on page 2211*

◆ **Cyclophosphamide-Doxorubicin (Breast)** *see* AC (Breast) *on page 1976*

◆ **Cyclophosphamide, Doxorubicin, Etoposide, Cisplatin (Neuroblastoma)** *see* A3 (Neuroblastoma) *on page 1973*

◆ **Cyclophosphamide, Doxorubicin, Etoposide, Cisplatin (Neuroblastoma)** *see* New A1 (Neuroblastoma) *on page 2180*

◆ **Cyclophosphamide-Doxorubicin-Etoposide-Prednisone-Vincristine (Dose-Adjusted) (NHL-AIDS-Related)** *see* EPOCH Dose-Adjusted (NHL-AIDS-Related) *on page 2106*

◆ **Cyclophosphamide, Doxorubicin, Fluorouracil IV (Breast)** *see* CAF IV (Breast) *on page 2002*

◆ **Cyclophosphamide, Doxorubicin, Fluorouracil Oral (Breast)** *see* CAF Oral (Breast) *on page 2003*

◆ **Cyclophosphamide-Doxorubicin-Rituximab-Etoposide-Prednisone-Vincristine (Dose-Adjusted) (NHL-AIDS-Related)** *see* EPOCH Dose-Adjusted-Rituximab (NHL-AIDS-Related) *on page 2107*

◆ **Cyclophosphamide, Doxorubicin, Vincristine, Etoposide, Cisplatin (Neuroblastoma)** *see* CAV-P/VP (Neuroblastoma) *on page 2027*

◆ **Cyclophosphamide-Doxorubicin-Vincristine-Methotrexate-Cytarabine-Ifosfamide-Etoposide (NHL-Burkitt)** *see* CODOX-M/IVAC (NHL-Burkitt) *on page 2068*

◆ **Cyclophosphamide-Doxorubicin-Vincristine-Methotrexate-Cytarabine (NHL-Burkitt)** *see* CODOX-M (NHL-Burkitt) *on page 2072*

◆ **Cyclophosphamide-Doxorubicin-Vincristine-Prednisone-Rituximab (NHL-DLBCL** *see* R-CHOP (NHL-DLBCL) *on page 2200*

◆ **Cyclophosphamide, Doxorubicin, Vincristine (Small Cell Lung Cancer)** *see* CAV (Small Cell Lung Cancer) *on page 2027*

Cyclophosphamide-Epirubicin (Breast)

Index Terms EC (Breast); Epirubicin-Cyclophosphamide (Breast)

Use Breast cancer

Regimen NOTE: Multiple variations are listed.

Variation 1 (metastatic):
Epirubicin: IV: 75 mg/m^2 day 1
[total dose/cycle = 75 mg/m^2]
Cyclophosphamide: IV: 600 mg/m^2 day 1
[total dose/cycle = 600 mg/m^2]
Repeat cycle every 21 days for up to 6 cycles

Variation 2 (adjuvant):
Epirubicin: IV: 100 mg/m^2 day 1
[total dose/cycle = 100 mg/m^2]
Cyclophosphamide: IV: 830 mg/m^2 day 1
[total dose/cycle = 830 mg/m^2]
Repeat cycle every 21 days for up to 8 cycles

◄ **References**
Variation 1:
Langley RE, Carmichael J, Jones AL, et al, "Phase III Trial of Epirubicin Plus Paclitaxel Compared With Epirubicin Plus Cyclophosphamide As First-Line Therapy for Metastatic Breast Cancer: United Kingdom National Cancer Research Institute Trial AB01," *J Clin Oncol*, 2005, 23 (33):8322-30.
Variation 2:
Piccart MJ, Di Leo A, Beauduin M, et al, "Phase III Trial Comparing Two Dose Levels of Epirubicin Combined With Cyclophosphamide With Cyclophosphamide, Methotrexate, and Fluorouracil in Node-Positive Breast Cancer," *J Clin Oncol*, 2001, 19(12):3103-10.

Cyclophosphamide-Topotecan (Ewing Sarcoma)

Index Terms TOPO/CYC (Ewing Sarcoma); Topotecan-Cyclophosphamide (Ewing Sarcoma)

Use Ewing sarcoma

Regimen

Cyclophosphamide: IV: 250 mg/m^2/day over 30 minutes days 1 to 5
[total dose/cycle = 1,250 mg/m^2]

Topotecan: IV: 0.75 mg/m^2/day over 30 minutes days 1 to 5
[total dose/cycle = 3.75 mg/m^2]

Filgrastim: SubQ: 5 mcg/kg daily beginning on day 6 until ANC ≥1,500/mm^3 after time of expected nadir

Repeat cycle every 21 days until disease progression or unacceptable toxicity

References
Hunold A, Weddeling N, Paulussen M, Ranft A, Liebscher C, Jürgens H. Topotecan and cyclophosphamide in patients with refractory or relapsed Ewing tumors. *Pediatr Blood Cancer.* 2006;47(6):795-800.
Saylors RL 3rd, Stine KC, Sullivan J, et al. Cyclophosphamide plus topotecan in children with recurrent or refractory solid tumors: a Pediatric Oncology Group phase II study. *J Clin Oncol.* 2001;19(15):3463-3469.

Cyclophosphamide-Topotecan (Neuroblastoma)

Index Terms TOPO/CTX (Neuroblastoma); Topotecan-Cyclophosphamide (Neuroblastoma)

Use Neuroblastoma

Regimen

Cyclophosphamide: IV: 250 mg/m^2/day over 30 minutes days 1 to 5
[total dose/cycle = 1,250 mg/m^2]

Topotecan: IV: 0.75 mg/m^2/day over 30 minutes days 1 to 5
[total dose/cycle = 3.75 mg/m^2]

Filgrastim: SubQ: 5 mcg/kg daily beginning on day 6 until ANC recovery as defined per study

Repeat cycle every 21 days until disease progression or unacceptable toxicity (up to 1 year [London 2010])

References

Ashraf K, Shaikh F, Gibson P, Baruchel S, Irwin MS. Treatment with topotecan plus cyclophosphamide in children with first relapse of neuroblastoma. *Pediatr Blood Cancer*. 2013;60 (10):1636-1641.

London WB, Frantz CN, Campbell LA, et al. Phase II randomized comparison of topotecan plus cyclophosphamide versus topotecan alone in children with recurrent or refractory neuroblastoma: a Children's Oncology Group study. *J Clin Oncol*. 2010;28(24):3808-3815.

Saylors RL 3rd, Stine KC, Sullivan J, et al. Cyclophosphamide plus topotecan in children with recurrent or refractory solid tumors: a Pediatric Oncology Group phase II study. *J Clin Oncol*. 2001;19(15):3463-3469.

Cyclophosphamide-Topotecan (Rhabdomyosarcoma)

Index Terms Topotecan Cyclophosphamide (Rhabdomyosarcoma)

Use Soft tissue sarcoma (rhabdomyosarcoma)

Regimen

Cyclophosphamide: IV: 250 mg/m^2/day over 30 minutes days 1 to 5
[total dose/cycle = 1,250 mg/m^2]

Topotecan: IV: 0.75 mg/m^2/day over 30 minutes days 1 to 5
[total dose/cycle = 3.75 mg/m^2]

Filgrastim: SubQ: 5 mcg/kg daily beginning on day 6 until ANC ≥1,500/mm^3 after time of expected nadir

Repeat cycle every 21 days until disease progression and unacceptable toxicity

References

Saylors RL 3rd, Stine KC, Sullivan J, et al. Cyclophosphamide plus topotecan in children with recurrent or refractory solid tumors: a Pediatric Oncology Group phase II study. *J Clin Oncol*. 2001;19(15):3463-3469.

- **Cytarabine-Daunorubicin-Etoposide (5 + 2 + 5) (AML Consolidation)** see 5 + 2 + 5 (Cytarabine-Daunorubicin-Etoposide) (AML Consolidation) on page 1971
- **Cytarabine-Daunorubicin-Etoposide (7 + 3 + 7) (AML Induction)** see 7 + 3 + 7 (Cytarabine-Daunorubicin-Etoposide) (AML Induction) on page 1973
- **Cytarabine-Etoposide-Mitoxantrone-CSF (AML Induction)** see MEC-G (AML Induction) on page 2170

Cytarabine (High Dose)-Daunorubicin (AML Induction)

Index Terms HDAC-Daunorubicin (AML Induction); HIDAC-Daunorubicin (AML Induction)

Use Leukemia, acute myeloid

Regimen
Cytarabine: IV: 2 g/m^2/day over 1 hour every 12 hours days 1 to 6 (12 total doses)
[total dose/cycle = 24 g/m^2]
Daunorubicin: IV: 45 mg/m^2/day IV bolus days 7 to 9
[total dose/cycle = 135 mg/m^2]

References
Weick JK, Kopecky KJ, Appelbaum FR, et al, "A Randomized Investigation of High-Dose Versus Standard-Dose Cytosine Arabinoside With Daunorubicin in Patients With Previously Untreated Acute Myeloid Leukemia: A Southwest Oncology Group Study," Blood, 1996, 88(8):2841-51.

Cytarabine (High Dose)-Daunorubicin-Etoposide (AML Induction)

Index Terms HIDAC-3-7 (AML Induction)

Use Leukemia, acute myeloid

Regimen
Daunorubicin: IV: 50 mg/m^2/day days 1, 2, and 3
[total dose/cycle = 150 mg/m^2]
Cytarabine: IV: 3 g/m^2/dose over 3 hours every 12 hours days 1, 3, 5, and 7 (8 total doses)
[total dose/cycle = 24 g/m^2]
Etoposide: IV: 75 mg/m^2/day days 1 to 7
[total dose/cycle = 525 mg/m^2]
Up to 3 induction cycles may be given based on individual response

References
Bishop JF, Matthews JP, Young GA, et al, "A Randomized Study of High-Dose Cytarabine in Induction in Acute Myeloid Leukemia," Blood, 1996, 87(5):1710-7.

Cytarabine (High-Dose Single-Agent AML Induction Regimen)

Index Terms HD Cytarabine (Single Agent AML Induction); HIDAC (Single Agent AML Induction)

Use Leukemia, acute myeloid

Regimen NOTE: Multiple variations are listed.
Variation 1 (ages 14 to 50 years):
Cytarabine: IV: 3 g/m^2 over 2 hours every 12 hours days 1 to 6 (total of 12 doses)
[total dose/cycle = 36 g/m^2]
May administer a second induction cycle if needed

Variation 2 (ages >50 years):
  Cytarabine: IV: 2 g/m^2 over 2 hours every 12 hours days 1 to 6 (total of 12 doses)
  [total dose/cycle = 24 g/m^2]
May administer a second induction cycle if needed

References
Karanes C, Kopecky K.J, Head DR, et al "A Phase III Comparison of High Dose ARA-C (HIDAC) Versus HIDAC Plus Mitoxantrone in the Treatment of First Relapsed or Refractory Acute Myeloid Leukemia - Southwest Oncology Group Study," *Leuk Res*, 1999, 23(9): 787-94.

◆ **Cytarabine-Idarubicin (5 + 2) (AML Consolidation)** *see* 5 + 2 (Cytarabine-Idarubicin) (AML Consolidation) *on page 1970*

◆ **Cytarabine-Idarubicin (7 + 3) (AML Induction)** *see* 7 + 3 (Cytarabine-Idarubicin) (AML Induction) *on page 1972*

◆ **Cytarabine-Mitoxantrone (5 + 2) (AML Consolidation)** *see* 5 + 2 (Cytarabine-Mitoxantrone) (AML Consolidation) *on page 1970*

◆ **Cytarabine-Mitoxantrone (7 + 3) (AML Induction)** *see* 7 + 3 (Cytarabine-Mitoxantrone) (AML Induction) *on page 1972*

Cytarabine (Single-Agent AML Consolidation Regimen)

Use Leukemia, acute myeloid

Regimen NOTE: Multiple variations are listed.
  Variation 1:
    Cytarabine: IV: 3 g/m^2 over 3 hours every 12 hours on days 1, 3, and 5 (total of 6 doses)
    [total dose/cycle = 18 g/m^2]
    Repeat cycle every 4 to 5 weeks (depending on marrow recovery) for a total of 4 postremission cycles
  Variation 2:
    Cytarabine: IV: 400 mg/m^2/day continuous Infusion on days 1 to 5
    [total dose/cycle = 2000 mg/m^2]
    Repeat cycle every 4 to 5 weeks (depending on marrow recovery) for a total of 4 postremission cycles
  Variation 3:
    Cytarabine: IV: 100 mg/m^2/day continuous infusion on days 1 to 5
    [total dose/cycle = 500 mg/m^2]
    Repeat cycle every 4 to 5 weeks (depending on marrow recovery) for a total of 4 postremission cycles
  Variation 4 (≥60 years of age):
    Cytarabine: IV: 100 mg/m^2/day continuous infusion on days 1 to 5
    [total dose/cycle = 500 mg/m^2]
    Repeat cycle every 28 days for a total of 4 consolidation cycles
  Variation 5 (≤50 years of age):
    Cytarabine: IV: 3 g/m^2 every 12 hours on days 1 to 3 (total of 6 doses)
    [total dose/cycle = 18 g/m^2]
    Administer a total of 3 consolidation cycles
  Variation 6 (>50 years of age):
    Cytarabine: IV: 2 g/m^2 every 12 hours on days 1 to 3 (total of 6 doses)
    [total dose/cycle = 12 g/m^2]
    Administer a total of 3 consolidation cycles

◄ Variation 7 (>65 years of age):

Cytarabine: SubQ: 10 mg/m^2/dose every 12 hours days 1 to 14

[total dose/cycle = 280 mg/m^2]

Repeat cycle every 6 weeks for 18 months

References

Variations 1, 2, and 3:

Mayer RJ, Davis RB, Schiffer CA, et al, "Intensive Postremission Chemotherapy in Adults With Acute Myeloid Leukemia, Cancer and Leukemia Group B," *N Engl J Med*, 1994, 331 (14):896-903.

Variation 4:

Stone RM, Berg DT, George SL, et al, "Postremission Therapy in Older Patients With *de novo* Acute Myeloid Leukemia: A Randomized Trial Comparing Mitoxantrone and Intermediate-Dose Cytarabine With Standard-Dose Cytarabine," *Blood*, 2001, 98(3):548-53.

Variations 5 and 6.

Karanes C, Kopecky KJ, Head DR, et al "A Phase III Comparison of High Dose ARA-C (HIDAC) Versus HIDAC Plus Mitoxantrone in the Treatment of First Relapsed or Refractory Acute Myeloid Leukemia - Southwest Oncology Group Study," *Leuk Res*, 1999, 23(9):787-94.

Variation 7:

Tilly H, Castaigne S, Bordessoule D, et al, "Low-Dose Cytarabine Versus Intensive Chemotherapy in the Treatment of Acute Nonlymphocytic Leukemia in the Elderly," *J Clin Oncol*, 1990, 8 (2):272-9.

Cytarabine (SubQ Single-Agent AML Induction Regimen)

Use Leukemia, acute myeloid

Regimen NOTE: Multiple variations are listed.

Variation 1 (>50 years of age):

Cytarabine: SubQ: 20 mg/m^2/day days 1 to 14

[total dose/cycle = 280 mg/m^2]

Repeat cycle every 28 days for at least 4 cycles

Variation 2 (>65 years of age):

Cytarabine: SubQ: 10 mg/m^2/day every 12 hours days 1 to 21

[total dose/cycle = 420 mg/m^2]

After 15 days, a second induction course may be administered if needed

References

Variation 1:

Fenaux P, Mufti GJ, Hellstrom-Lindberg E, et al, "Azacitidine Prolongs Overall Survival Compared With Conventional Care Regimens in Elderly Patients With Low Bone Marrow Blast Count Acute Myeloid Leukemia, *J Clin Oncol*, 2010, 28(4):562-9.

Variation 2:

Tilly H, Castaigne S, Bordessoule D, et al, "Low-Dose Cytarabine Versus Intensive Chemotherapy in the Treatment of Acute Nonlymphocytic Leukemia in the Elderly," *J Clin Oncol*, 1990, 8 (2):272-9.

Dabrafenib-Trametinib (Melanoma)

Use Melanoma

Regimen

Dabrafenib: Oral: 150 mg twice daily days 1 to 28

[total dose/cycle = 8400 mg]

Trametinib: Oral: 2 mg once daily days 1 to 28

[total dose/cycle = 56 mg]

Repeat cycle every 28 days

References

Flaherty KT, Infante JR, Daud A, et al. Combined BRAF and MEK inhibition in melanoma with BRAF V600 mutations. *N Engl J Med*. 2012;367(18):1694-1703.

Dabrafenib-Trametinib (NSCLC)

Index Terms Trametinib-Dabrafenib (NSCLC)

Use Lung cancer, non-small cell (relapsed or refractory, metastatic with BRAF V600E mutation)

Regimen

Dabrafenib: Oral: 150 mg twice daily at least 1 hour before or 2 hours after a meal days 1 to 21

[total dose/cycle = 6,300 mg]

Trametinib: Oral: 2 mg once daily at least 1 hour before or 2 hours after a meal days 1 to 21

[total dose/cycle = 42 mg]

Repeat cycle every 21 days until disease progression or unacceptable toxicity

References

Planchard D, Besse B, Groen HJ, et al. Dabrafenib plus trametinib in patients with previously treated BRAF(V600E)-mutant metastatic non-small cell lung cancer: an open-label, multicentre phase 2 trial. *Lancet Oncol.* 2016;17(7):984-993.

◆ **Dacarbazine-Cisplatin-Vinblastine** *see* Cisplatin-Vinblastine-Dacarbazine (Melanoma) *on page 2061*

◆ **Dactinomycin-Vincristine (Rhabdomyosarcoma)** *see* VA (Rhabdomyosarcoma) *on page 2227*

◆ **Dactinomycin-Vincristine (Wilms' Tumor)** *see* EE-4A (Wilms' Tumor) *on page 2100*

◆ **Dactinomycin-Doxorubicin-Vincristine (Wilms' Tumor)** *see* DD-4A (Wilms' Tumor) *on page 2086*

◆ **DA EPOCH (NHL-AIDS-Related)** *see* EPOCH Dose-Adjusted (NHL-AIDS-Related) *on page 2106*

Daratumumab-Bortezomib-Dexamethasone (Multiple Myeloma)

Index Terms Bortezomib-Daratumumab-Dexamethasone (Multiple Myeloma)

Use Multiple myeloma (relapsed/refractory to at least 1 prior therapy)

Regimen NOTE: Premedicate approximately 1 hour prior to daratumumab infusion with dexamethasone, an oral antipyretic, and an oral or IV antihistamine. Dexamethasone is administered IV prior to the first daratumumab infusion; oral administration may be considered prior to subsequent infusions. Consider administering low-dose oral methylprednisolone (20 mg or less) or equivalent on the first day after the daratumumab infusion. If dexamethasone is administered the day after the daratumumab infusion as part of combination chemotherapy, additional post-infusion corticosteroid therapy may not be necessary. To prevent herpes zoster reactivation, initiate antiviral prophylaxis within 1 week after starting daratumumab and continue for 3 months following completion of treatment. Per the manufacturer, daratumumab dosing should be based on actual body weight.

Daratumumab: IV: 16 mg/kg once weekly for 9 doses (weeks 1 to 9), then 16 mg/kg once every 3 weeks for 5 doses (weeks 10 to 24), then 16 mg/kg once every 4 weeks (weeks 25 and beyond) until disease progression or unacceptable toxicity

Bortezomib: SubQ: 1.3 mg/m^2/day on days 1, 4, 8, and 11 of a 21 day cycle for a total of 8 cycles

Dexamethasone: Oral or IV: Patients ≤75 years: 20 mg/day on days 1, 2, 4, 5, 8, 9, 11, and 12 (20 mg once weekly in patients >75 years, BMI <18.5, poorly controlled diabetes, or corticosteroid intolerance). Per the daratumumab manufacturer, dexamethasone 20 mg is administered prior to each daratumumab infusion; post-infusion dexamethasone may not be necessary if regimen specific dexamethasone is administered the day after the daratumumab infusion. Dexamethasone doses may vary (particularly if methylprednisolone is also administered); refer to references and/or institutional protocols for additional details

References

Darzalex (daratumumab) [prescribing information]. Horsham, PA: Janssen Biotech, Inc; June 2017.

Palumbo A, Chanan-Khan A, Weisel K, et al. Daratumumab, bortezomib, and dexamethasone for multiple myeloma. N Engl J Med. 2016;375(8):754-766.

Daratumumab-Lenalidomide-Dexamethasone (Multiple Myeloma)

Index Terms Lenalidomide-Daratumumab-Dexamethasone (Multiple Myeloma)

Use Multiple myeloma (received at least 1 prior line of therapy)

Regimen NOTE: Premedicate approximately 1 hour prior to daratumumab infusion with dexamethasone, an oral antipyretic, and an oral or IV antihistamine. Dexamethasone is administered IV prior to the first daratumumab infusion; oral administration may be considered prior to subsequent infusions. To prevent herpes zoster reactivation, initiate antiviral prophylaxis within 1 week after starting daratumumab and continue for 3 months following completion of treatment. Per the manufacturer, daratumumab dosing should be based on actual body weight. Consider reducing the dexamethasone dose to a total of 20 mg/**week** in patients >75 years or with a BMI <18.5.

Cycles 1 and 2 (weeks 1 to 8):
  Daratumumab: IV: 16 mg/kg weekly on days 1, 8, 15, and 22
    [total dose/cycle = 64 mg/kg]
  Lenalidomide: Oral: 25 mg daily days 1 to 21
    [total dose/cycle = 525 mg]
  Dexamethasone: IV or Oral: 20 mg days 1, 2, 8, 9, 15, 16, 22, and 23 (administer prior to daratumumab on days 1, 8, 15, and 22)
    [total dose/cycle = 160 mg]
  Repeat cycle every 28 days for a total of 2 cycles

Cycles 3 to 6 (weeks 9 to 24):
  Daratumumab: IV: 16 mg/kg every 2 weeks on days 1 and 15
    [total dose/cycle = 32 mg/kg]
  Lenalidomide: Oral: 25 mg daily days 1 to 21
    [total dose/cycle = 525 mg]
  Dexamethasone: IV or Oral: 20 mg days 1, 2, 15, and 16 (administer prior to daratumumab on days 1 and 15) and 40 mg on days 8 and 22
    [total dose/cycle = 160 mg]
  Repeat cycle every 28 days for a total of 4 cycles

Subsequent Cycles (week 25 onwards):
  Daratumumab: IV: 16 mg/kg day 1
    [total dose/cycle = 16 mg/kg]
  Lenalidomide: Oral: 25 mg daily days 1 to 21
    [total dose/cycle = 525 mg]

Dexamethasone: IV or Oral: 20 mg days 1 and 2 (administer prior to daratumumab on day 1) and 40 mg on days 8, 15, and 22
[total dose/cycle = 160 mg]
Repeat cycle every 28 days until disease progression or unacceptable toxicity

References

Dimopoulos MA, Oriol A, Nahi H, et al. Daratumumab, lenalidomide, and dexamethasone for multiple myeloma. N Engl J Med. 2016;375(14):1319-1331.

Daratumumab-Pomalidomide-Dexamethasone (Multiple Myeloma)

Index Terms Pomalidomide-Daratumumab-Dexamethasone (Multiple Myeloma)

Use Multiple myeloma (relapsed/refractory)

Regimen NOTE: Premedicate approximately 1 hour prior to daratumumab infusion with dexamethasone, an oral antipyretic, and an oral or IV antihistamine. Dexamethasone is administered IV prior to the first daratumumab infusion; oral administration may be considered prior to subsequent infusions. Consider administering low-dose oral methylprednisolone (20 mg or less) or equivalent on the first day after the daratumumab infusion. If dexamethasone is administered the day after the daratumumab infusion as part of combination chemotherapy, additional post infusion corticosteroid therapy may not be necessary. To prevent herpes zoster reactivation, initiate antiviral prophylaxis within 1 week after starting daratumumab and continue for 3 months following completion of treatment. Per the manufacturer, daratumumab dosing should be based on actual body weight.
Daratumumab: IV: 16 mg/kg once weekly for 8 doses (weeks 1 to 8), then 16 mg/kg once every 2 weeks for 8 doses (weeks 9 to 24), then 16 mg/kg once every 4 weeks (weeks 25 and beyond) until disease progression or unacceptable toxicity
Pomalidomide: Oral: 4 mg daily on days 1 to 21 of a 28 day cycle
Dexamethasone: Oral or IV: Patients ≤75 years: 40 mg weekly (20 mg weekly in patients >75 years). Per the daratumumab manufacturer, 20 mg of the dexamethasone is administered prior to the daratumumab infusion (on daratumumab days) and the remainder of the dexamethasone dose (if >20 mg) is administered following the daratumumab infusion; post infusion dexamethasone may not be necessary if regimen-specific dexamethasone is administered the day after the daratumumab infusion. Dexamethasone doses may vary (particularly if methylprednisolone is also administered); refer to references and/or institutional protocols for additional details.

References

Chari A, Suvannasankha A, Fay JW, et al. Daratumumab plus pomalidomide and dexamethasone in relapsed and/or refractory multiple myeloma [published online ahead of print July 21, 2017]. Blood. 2017.

Darzalex (daratumumab) [prescribing information]. Horsham, PA: Janssen Biotech, Inc; June 2017.

♦ **DC (NSCLC)** see Cisplatin-Docetaxel (NSCLC) on page 2038

♦ **DD4A (Wilms' Tumor)** see DD-4A (Wilms' Tumor) on page 2086

DD-4A (Wilms' Tumor)

Index Terms Dactinomycin-Doxorubicin-Vincristine (Wilms' Tumor); DD4A (Wilms' Tumor); Regimen DD-4A (Wilms' Tumor)

Use Wilms' tumor

Regimen

Dactinomycin: IV: 45 mcg/kg day 1 of weeks 0, 6, 12, 18, 24, 30, 36, 42, 48, and 54

[total dose = 450 mcg/kg]

Doxorubicin: IV: 45 mg/m^2 days 1 of weeks 3 and 9

Followed by

Doxorubicin: IV: 30 mg/m^2 days 1 of weeks 15, 21, 27, 33, 39, 45, and 51

[total dose = 300 mg/m^2]

Vincristine: IV: 1.5 mg/m^2 day 1 of weeks 1 to 10

Followed by

Vincristine: IV: 2 mg/m^2 day 1 of weeks 12, 15, 18, 21, 24, 27, 30, 33, 36, 39, 42, 45, 48, 51, and 54

[total dose = 45 mg/m^2]

Treatment course duration is week 0 through week 54

References

Green DM, Breslow NE, Beckwith JB, et al, "Effect of Duration of Treatment on Treatment Outcome and Cost of Treatment for Wilms' Tumor: A Report From the National Wilms' Tumor Study Group," *J Clin Oncol*, 1998, 16(12):3744-51.

♦ **DDM-VAC (Bladder Cancer)** see Dose Dense MVAC (Bladder Cancer) on page 2096

Dexa-BEAM (Hodgkin)

Index Terms Dexamethasone, Carmustine, Etoposide, Cytarabine, Melphalan (Hodgkin)

Use Lymphoma, Hodgkin

Regimen

Dexamethasone: Oral: 8 mg every 8 hours days 1 to 10

[total dose/cycle = 240 mg]

Carmustine: IV: 60 mg/m^2 day 2

[total dose/cycle = 60 mg/m^2]

Etoposide: IV: 75 mg/m^2/day days 4 to 7

[total dose/cycle = 300 mg/m^2]

Cytarabine: IV: 100 mg/m^2/dose every 12 hours days 4 to 7 (total of 8 doses)

[total dose/cycle = 800 mg/m^2]

Melphalan: IV: 20 mg/m^2 day 3

[total dose/cycle = 20 mg/m^2]

Repeat cycle every 28 days; consider stem cell transplantation after 2 cycles in responding patients and a maximum of 4 cycles (total) in nontransplant candidates

References

Pfreundschuh MG, Rueffer U, Lathan B, et al, "Dexa-BEAM in Patients With Hodgkin's Disease Refractory to Multidrug Chemotherapy Regimens: A Trial of the German Hodgkin's Disease Study Group," *J Clin Oncol*, 1994, 12(3):580-6.

♦ **Dexamethasone-Bortezomib (Amyloidosis)** see Bortezomib-Dexamethasone (Amyloidosis) on page 1997

- **Dexamethasone-Bortezomib-Doxorubicin (Multiple Myeloma)** *see* Bortezomib-Doxorubicin-Dexamethasone (Multiple Myeloma) *on page 1999*

- **Dexamethasone-Bortezomib (Multiple Myeloma)** *see* Bortezomib-Dexamethasone (Multiple Myeloma) *on page 1998*

- **Dexamethasone-Bortezomib-Panobinostat (Multiple Myeloma)** *see* Panobinostat-Bortezomib-Dexamethasone (Multiple Myeloma) *on page 2190*

- **Dexamethasone-Bortezomib-Thalidomide (Multiple Myeloma)** *see* Bortezomib-Thalidomide-Dexamethasone (Multiple Myeloma) *on page 2000*

- **Dexamethasone-Carfilzomib (Multiple Myeloma)** *see* Carfilzomib-Dexamethasone (Multiple Myeloma) *on page 2025*

- **Dexamethasone, Carmustine, Etoposide, Cytarabine, Melphalan (Hodgkin)** *see* Dexa-BEAM (Hodgkin) *on page 2086*

- **Dexamethasone-Cisplatin-Cytarabine (Hodgkin)** *see* DHAP (Hodgkin) *on page 2087*

- **Dexamethasone-Cisplatin-Cytarabine (NHL-DLBCL)** *see* DHAP (NHL-DLBCL) *on page 2087*

- **Dexamethasone-Lenalidomide (Multiple Myeloma)** *see* Lenalidomide-Dexamethasone (Multiple Myeloma) *on page 2166*

- **Dexamethasone (Low-Dose)-Lenalidomide (Multiple Myeloma)** *see* Lenalidomide-Dexamethasone (Multiple Myeloma) *on page 2166*

- **Dexamethasone-Thalidomide (MM)** *see* Thalidomide-Dexamethasone (MM) *on page 2212*

- **Dexamethasone-Thalidomide-Cisplatin-Doxorubicin-Cyclophosphamide-Etoposide (Multiple Myeloma)** *see* DTPACE (Multiple Myeloma) *on page 2098*

DHAP (Hodgkin)

Index Terms Dexamethasone-Cisplatin-Cytarabine (Hodgkin)

Use Lymphoma, Hodgkin

Regimen

Salvage treatment:

Dexamethasone: IV: 40 mg/day days 1 to 4

[total dose/cycle = 160 mg]

Cisplatin: IV: 100 mg/m^2 continuous infusion for 24 hours day 1

[total dose/cycle = 100 mg/m^2]

Cytarabine: IV: 2000 mg/m^2 over 3 hours every 12 hours day 2 (total of 2 doses)

[total dose/cycle = 4000 mg/m^2]

Filgrastim: SubQ: 5 mcg/kg/day beginning 24 hours after last dose of cytarabine, continue until leukocytes ≥2500/mm^3 for 3 days

Administer 2 cycles

References

Josting A, Rudolph C, Reiser M, et al, "Time-Intensified Dexamethasone/Cisplatin/Cytarabine: An Effective Salvage Therapy With Low Toxicity in Patients With Relapsed and Refractory Hodgkin's Disease," *Ann Oncol*, 2002, 13(10):1628-35.

DHAP (NHL-DLBCL)

Index Terms Cisplatin-Cytarabine-Dexamethasone (NHL-DLBCL); Dexamethasone-Cisplatin-Cytarabine (NHL-DLBCL)

Use Lymphoma, non-Hodgkin (DLBCL relapsed/refractory)

Regimen NOTE: Multiple variations are listed.
Variation 1 (patients ≤70 years of age):
Dexamethasone: IV or Oral: 40 mg daily days 1 to 4
[total dose/cycle = 160 mg]
Cisplatin: IV: 100 mg/m^2 continuous infusion over 24 hours day 1
[total dose/cycle = 100 mg/m^2]
Cytarabine: IV: 2,000 mg/m^2 over 3 hours every 12 hours for 2 doses day 2
(begins at the end of the cisplatin infusion)
[total dose/cycle = 4,000 mg/m^2]
Repeat cycle every 21 to 28 days for 6 to 10 cycles (usually for 4 cycles
beyond maximum response)
Variation 2 (patients >70 years of age):
Dexamethasone: IV or Oral: 40 mg daily days 1 to 4
[total dose/cycle = 160 mg]
Cisplatin: IV: 100 mg/m^2 continuous infusion over 24 hours day 1
[total dose/cycle = 100 mg/m^2]
Cytarabine: IV: 1,000 mg/m^2 over 3 hours every 12 hours for 2 doses day 2
(begins at the end of the cisplatin infusion)
[total dose/cycle = 2,000 mg/m^2]
Repeat cycle every 21 to 28 days for 6 to 10 cycles (usually for 4 cycles
beyond maximum response)

References

Variation 1 and 2:
Velasquez WS, Cabanillas F, Salvador P, et al. Effective salvage therapy for lymphoma with
cisplatin in combination with high-dose Ara-C and dexamethasone (DHAP). *Blood.* 1988;71
(1):117-122.

♦ **Docetaxel-Capecitabine (Breast)** *see* Capecitabine-Docetaxel (Breast)
on page 2006

♦ **Docetaxel-Capecitabine (Gastric Cancer)** *see* Capecitabine-Docetaxel
(Gastric Cancer) *on page 2006*

♦ **Docetaxel-Carboplatin (Ovarian)** *see* Carboplatin-Docetaxel (Ovarian)
on page 2012

♦ **Docetaxel-Carboplatin (Unknown Primary, Adenocarcinoma)** *see* Carboplatin-Docetaxel (Unknown Primary, Adenocarcinoma) *on page 2013*

♦ **Docetaxel-Carboplatin (Unknown Primary, Squamous Cell)** *see* Carboplatin-Docetaxel (Unknown Primary, Squamous Cell) *on page 2013*

♦ **Docetaxel-Cisplatin-Fluorouracil-Carboplatin (Head and Neck)** *see*
Docetaxel-Cisplatin-Fluorouracil (Head and Neck) *on page 2089*

♦ **Docetaxel-Cisplatin-Fluorouracil-ChemoXRT (Head and Neck)** *see* Docetaxel-Cisplatin-Fluorouracil (Head and Neck) *on page 2089*

Docetaxel-Cisplatin-Fluorouracil (Gastric/Esophageal Cancer)

Index Terms DCF (Gastric/Esophageal Cancer); TCF (Gastric/Esophageal
Cancer)
Use Esophageal cancer; Gastric cancer
Regimen NOTE: Multiple variations are listed.
Variation 1:
Docetaxel: IV: 75 mg/m^2 day 1
[total dose/cycle = 75 mg/m^2]

Cisplatin: IV: 75 mg/m^2 day 1
[total dose/cycle = 75 mg/m^2]

Fluorouracil: IV: 750 mg/m^2/day continuous infusion days 1 to 5
[total dose/cycle = 3750 mg/m^2]

Repeat cycle every 21 days until disease progression or unacceptable toxicity

Variation 2:

Docetaxel: IV: 75 mg/m^2 day 1
[total dose/cycle = 75 mg/m^2]

Cisplatin: IV: 75 mg/m^2 over 4 hours day 1
[total dose/cycle = 75 mg/m^2]

Fluorouracil: IV: 300 mg/m^2/day continuous infusion days 1 to 14
[total dose/cycle = 4200 mg/m^2]

Repeat cycle every 21 days until disease progression or unacceptable toxicity for up to a maximum of 8 cycles

References

Variation 1:

Ajani JA, Fodor MB, Tjulandin SA, et al, "Phase II Multi-Institutional Randomized Trial of Docetaxel Plus Cisplatin With or Without Fluorouracil in Patients With Untreated, Advanced Gastric, or Gastroesophageal Adenocarcinoma," *J Clin Oncol*, 2005, 23(24):5660-7.

Ajani JA, Moiseyenko VM, Tjulandin S, et al, "Quality of Life With Docetaxel Plus Cisplatin and Fluorouracil Compared With Cisplatin and Fluorouracil From a Phase III Trial for Advanced Gastric or Gastroesophageal Adenocarcinoma: The V-325 Study Group," *J Clin Oncol*, 2007, 25(22):3210-6.

Van Cutsem E, Moiseyenko VM, Tjulandin S, et al, "Phase III Study of Docetaxel and Cisplatin Plus Fluorouracil Compared With Cisplatin and Fluorouracil as First-Line Therapy for Advanced Gastric Cancer: A Report of the V325 Study Group," *J Clin Oncol*, 2006, 24(31):4991-7.

Variation 2:

Roth AD, Fazio N, Stupp R, et al, "Docetaxel, Cisplatin, and Fluorouracil; Docetaxel and Cisplatin; and Epirubicin, Cisplatin, and Fluorouracil as Systemic Treatment for Advanced Gastric Carcinoma: A Randomized Phase II Trial of the Swiss Group for Clinical Cancer Research," *J Clin Oncol*, 2007, 25(22):3217-23.

Docetaxel-Cisplatin-Fluorouracil (Head and Neck)

Index Terms Docetaxel-Cisplatin-Fluorouracil (Head and Neck); Docetaxel-Cisplatin-Fluorouracil-Carboplatin (Head and Neck); Docetaxel-Cisplatin-Fluorouracil-ChemoXRT (Head and Neck); TPF (Head and Neck); TPF-Chemoradiation Therapy (Head and Neck)

Use Head and neck cancer

Regimen NOTE: Multiple variations are listed.

Variation 1:

Docetaxel: IV: 75 mg/m^2 over 1 hour day 1
[total dose/cycle = 75 mg/m^2]

Cisplatin: IV: 75 mg/m^2 over 1 hour day 1
[total dose/cycle = 75 mg/m^2]

Fluorouracil: IV: 750 mg/m^2/day continuous infusion days 1 to 5
[total dose/cycle = 3,750 mg/m^2]

Repeat cycle every 21 days for up to a total of 4 cycles (after 4 to 7 weeks, follow with radiation therapy)

Variation 2:

Induction Chemotherapy:

Docetaxel: IV: 75 mg/m^2 over 1 hour day 1
[total dose/cycle = 75 mg/m^2]

Cisplatin: IV: 100 mg/m^2 over 30 minutes to 3 hours day 1
[total dose/cycle = 100 mg/m^2]

Fluorouracil: IV: 1,000 mg/m^2/day continuous infusion days 1 to 4
[total dose/cycle = 4,000 mg/m^2]
Repeat cycle every 21 days for total of 3 cycles
Chemoradiation therapy (begin 3 to 8 weeks after the start of the third induction therapy cycle):
Carboplatin: IV: AUC 1.5 over 1 hour day 1
[total dose/cycle = AUC 1.5]
Repeat cycle every 7 days for up to a total of 7 weekly doses during radiation therapy

References

Variation 1:

Vermorken JB, Remenar E, van Herpen C, et al. Cisplatin, fluorouracil, and docetaxel in unresectable head and neck cancer. *N Engl J Med.* 2007;357(17):1695-1704.

Variation 2:

Haddad R, O'Neill A, Rabinowits G, et al. Induction chemotherapy followed by concurrent chemoradiotherapy (sequential chemoradiotherapy) versus concurrent chemoradiotherapy alone in locally advanced head and neck cancer (PARADIGM): a randomised phase 3 trial. *Lancet Oncol.* 2013;14(3):257-264.

Posner MR, Hershock DM, Blajman CR, et al. Cisplatin and fluorouracil alone or with docetaxel in head and neck cancer. *N Engl J Med.* 2007;357(17):1705-1715.

Docetaxel Every 3 Weeks-Trastuzumab (Breast)

Index Terms Trastuzumab-Docetaxel Every 3 Weeks (Breast)

Use Breast cancer

Regimen

Cycle 1:

Docetaxel: IV: 100 mg/m^2 day 1
[total dose/cycle 1 = 100 mg/m^2]
Trastuzumab: IV: 4 mg/kg (loading dose) day 1 cycle 1
followed by IV: 2 mg/kg/day days 8 and 15 cycle 1
[total dose/cycle 1 = 8 mg/kg]
Treatment cycle is 21 days
Subsequent cycles:
Docetaxel: IV: 100 mg/m^2 day 1
[total dose/cycle = 100 mg/m^2]

Trastuzumab: IV: 2 mg/kg/day days 1, 8, and 15
[total dose/cycle = 6 mg/kg]
Repeat cycle every 21 days for a total of at least 6 cycles
followed by
Trastuzumab: IV: 2 mg/kg/day days 1, 8, and 15
[total dose/cycle = 6 mg/kg]
Repeat cycle every 21 days until disease progression or unacceptable toxicity

References

Marty M, Cognetti F, Maraninchi D, et al, "Randomized Phase II Trial of the Efficacy and Safety of Trastuzumab Combined With Docetaxel in Patients With Human Epidermal Growth Factor Receptor 2-Positive Metastatic Breast Cancer Administered as First-Line Treatment: The M77001 Study Group," *J Clin Oncol*, 2005, 23(19):4265-74.

Docetaxel-Gemcitabine (Ewing Sarcoma)

Index Terms Gemcitabine-Docetaxel (Ewing Sarcoma)

Use Ewing sarcoma

Regimen

Gemcitabine: IV: 675 mg/m^2/day over 90 minutes days 1 and 8
[total dose/cycle = 1,350 mg/m^2]
Docetaxel: IV: 100 mg/m^2 over 60 minutes day 8
[total dose/cycle = 100 mg/m^2]
Growth Factor:
Filgrastim: SubQ: 300 mcg once daily days 9 to 15
or
Pegfilgrastim: SubQ: 6 mg administered day 9
Repeat cycle every 21 days

References

Leu KM, Ostruszka LJ, Shewach D, et al. Laboratory and clinical evidence of synergistic cytotoxicity of sequential treatment with gemcitabine followed by docetaxel in the treatment of sarcoma. *J Clin Oncol*. 2004;22(9):1706-1712.

Navid F, Willert JR, McCarville MB, et al. Combination of gemcitabine and docetaxel in the treatment of children and young adults with refractory bone sarcoma. *Cancer*. 2008;113(2):419-425.

Docetaxel-Gemcitabine (NSCLC)

Index Terms GD (NSCLC); Gemcitabine-Docetaxel (NSCLC)

Use Lung cancer, non-small cell

Regimen

Gemcitabine: IV: 1000 mg/m^2 over 30 minutes days 1 and 8
[total dose/cycle = 2000 mg/m^2]
Docetaxel: IV: 85 mg/m^2 over 60 minutes day 8 (prior to gemcitabine)
[total dose/cycle = 85 mg/m^2]
Repeat cycle every 21 days for a total of 8 cycles

References

Pujol JL, Breton JL, Gervais R, et al. Gemcitabine-docetaxel versus cisplatin-vinorelbine in advanced or metastatic non-small-cell lung cancer: a phase III study addressing the case for cisplatin. *Ann Oncol*. 2005;16(4):602-610.

Docetaxel-Gemcitabine (Osteosarcoma)

Index Terms Gemcitabine-Docetaxel (Osteosarcoma)

Use Osteosarcoma

Regimen

Gemcitabine: IV: 675 mg/m^2/day over 90 minutes days 1 and 8
[total dose/cycle = 1,350 mg/m^2]
Docetaxel: IV: 100 mg/m^2 over 60 minutes day 8
[total dose/cycle = 100 mg/m^2]

Growth Factor:

Filgrastim: SubQ: 300 mcg once daily days 9 to 15

or

Pegfilgrastim: SubQ: 6 mg administered day 9

Repeat cycle every 21 days

References

Leu KM, Ostruszka LJ, Shewach D, et al. Laboratory and clinical evidence of synergistic cytotoxicity of sequential treatment with gemcitabine followed by docetaxel in the treatment of sarcoma. *J Clin Oncol.* 2004;22(9):1706-1712.

Navid F, Willert JR, McCarville MB, et al. Combination of gemcitabine and docetaxel in the treatment of children and young adults with refractory bone sarcoma. *Cancer.* 2008;113 (2):419-425.

Docetaxel-Gemcitabine (Soft Tissue Sarcoma)

Index Terms Gemcitabine-Docetaxel (Soft Tissue Sarcoma)

Use Soft tissue sarcoma

Regimen NOTE: Multiple variations are listed.

Variation 1:

Gemcitabine: IV: 675 mg/m^2/day over 90 minutes days 1 and 8
[total dose/cycle = 1350 mg/m^2]
Docetaxel: IV: 100 mg/m^2 over 60 minutes day 8
[total dose/cycle = 100 mg/m^2]

Growth factor:

Filgrastim: SubQ: 300 mcg once daily days 9 to 15

or

Pegfilgrastim: SubQ: 6 mg administered day 9

Repeat cycle every 21 days

Variation 2:

Gemcitabine: IV: 900 mg/m^2/day over 90 minutes days 1 and 8
[total dose/cycle = 1800 mg/m^2]
Docetaxel: IV: 100 mg/m^2 over 60 minutes day 8
[total dose/cycle = 100 mg/m^2]

Growth factor:

Filgrastim: SubQ: 5 mcg/kg once daily, starting day 9 or 10, for 7 to 10 days

or

Pegfilgrastim: SubQ: 6 mg administered day 9 or 10

Repeat cycle every 21 days

References

Variation 1:

Leu KM, Ostruszka LJ, Shewach D, et al. Laboratory and clinical evidence of synergistic cytotoxicity of sequential treatment with gemcitabine followed by docetaxel in the treatment of sarcoma. *J Clin Oncol.* 2004;22(9):1706-1712.

Variation 2:

Maki RG, Wathen JK, Patel SR, et al. Randomized phase II study of gemcitabine and docetaxel compared with gemcitabine alone in patients with metastatic soft tissue sarcomas: results of sarcoma alliance for research through collaboration study 002 [corrected]. *J Clin Oncol.* 2007;25 (19):2755-2763.

Docetaxel-Gemcitabine (Unknown Primary, Adenocarcinoma)

Index Terms Gemcitabine-Docetaxel (Unknown Primary)

Use Unknown primary (adenocarcinoma)

Regimen

Gemcitabine: IV: 1000 mg/m^2/day over 30 minutes days 1 and 8
[total dose/cycle = 2000 mg/m^2]
Docetaxel: IV: 75 mg/m^2 over 1 hour day 8
[total dose/cycle = 75 mg/m^2]
Repeat cycle every 21 days for up to a total of 6 cycles

References

Pouessel D, Culine S, Becht C, et al, "Gemcitabine and Docetaxel as Front-Line Chemotherapy in Patients With Carcinoma of an Unknown Primary Site," *Cancer*, 2004, 100(6):1257-61.

Docetaxel-Gemcitabine (Uterine Leiomyosarcoma)

Index Terms Gemcitabine-Docetaxel (Uterine Leiomyosarcoma)

Use Uterine sarcoma (uterine leiomyosarcoma)

Regimen

Variation 1 (no history of pelvic radiation):
Gemcitabine: IV: 900 mg/m^2/day over 90 minutes days 1 and 8
[total dose/cycle = 1800 mg/m^2]
Docetaxel: IV: 100 mg/m^2 over 60 minutes day 8
[total dose/cycle = 100 mg/m^2]
Growth factor:
Filgrastim: SubQ: 150 mcg/m^2 days 9 to 15
or
Pegfilgrastim: SubQ: 6 mg day 9 or 10
Repeat cycle every 21 days until disease progression or unacceptable toxicity

Variation 2 (prior pelvic radiation):
Gemcitabine: IV: 675 mg/m^2/day over 90 minutes days 1 and 8
[total dose/cycle = 1350 mg/m^2]
Docetaxel: IV: 75 mg/m^2 over 60 minutes day 8
[total dose/cycle = 75 mg/m^2]
Growth factor:
Filgrastim: SubQ: 150 mcg/m^2 days 9 to 15
or
Pegfilgrastim: SubQ: 6 mg day 9 or 10
Repeat cycle every 21 days until disease progression or unacceptable toxicity

References

Variations 1 and 2:
Hensley ML, Blessing JA, Degeest K, Abulafia O, Rose PG, Homesley HD. Fixed-dose rate gemcitabine plus docetaxel as second-line therapy for metastatic uterine leiomyosarcoma: a Gynecologic Oncology Group phase II study. *Gynecol Oncol*. 2008;109(3):323-328.
Hensley ML, Blessing JA, Mannel R, Rose PG. Fixed-dose rate gemcitabine plus docetaxel as first-line therapy for metastatic uterine leiomyosarcoma: a Gynecologic Oncology Group phase II trial. *Gynecol Oncol*. 2008;109(3):329-334.

Docetaxel-Oxaliplatin-Leucovorin-Fluorouracil (Esophageal Cancer)

Index Terms FLOT (Esophageal Cancer); Oxaliplatin-Docetaxel-Leucovorin-Fluorouracil (Esophageal Cancer)

◄ **Use** Esophageal cancer
Regimen
Docetaxel: IV: 50 mg/m^2 day 1
  [total dose/cycle = 50 mg/m^2]
Oxaliplatin: IV: 85 mg/m^2 day 1
  [total dose/cycle = 85 mg/m^2]
Leucovorin Calcium: IV: 200 mg/m^2 day 1
  [total dose/cycle = 200 mg/m^2]
Fluorouracil: IV: 2600 mg/m^2/day continuous infusion over 24 hours day 1
  [total dose/cycle = 2600 mg/m^2]
Repeat cycle every 14 days until disease progression or unacceptable toxicity
  for up to a total of 8 cycles.

References

Al-Batran SE, Hartmann JT, Hofheinz R, et al, "Biweekly Fluorouracil, Leucovorin, Oxaliplatin, and Docetaxel (FLOT) for Patients With Metastatic Adenocarcinoma of the Stomach or Esophago-gastric Junction: A Phase II Trial of the Arbeitsgemeinschaft Internistische Onkologie," *Ann Oncol*, 2008, 19(11):1882-7.

♦ **Docetaxel-Pertuzumab-Trastuzumab (Metastatic Breast)** *see* Pertuzumab-Trastuzumab-Docetaxel (Metastatic Breast) *on page 2195*

♦ **Docetaxel-Pertuzumab-Trastuzumab (Neoadjuvant Breast)** *see* Pertuzumab-Trastuzumab-Docetaxel (Neoadjuvant Breast) *on page 2195*

Docetaxel-Prednisone (Prostate)

Index Terms Prednisone-Docetaxel (Prostate)
Use Prostate cancer
Regimen
Docetaxel: IV: 75 mg/m^2 over 1 hour day 1
  [total dose/cycle = 75 mg/m^2]
Prednisone: Oral: 5 mg twice daily days 1 to 21
  [total dose/cycle = 210 mg]
Repeat cycle every 21 days, for a maximum 10 cycles

References

Berthold DR, Pond GR, Soban F, et al, "Docetaxel Plus Prednisone or Mitoxantrone Plus Prednisone for Advanced Prostate Cancer: Updated Survival in the TAX 327 Study," *J Clin Oncol*, 2008, 26(2):242-5.

Tannock IF, de Wit R, Berry WR, et al, "Docetaxel Plus Prednisone or Mitoxantrone Plus Prednisone for Advanced Prostate Cancer," *N Engl J Med*, 2004, 351(15):1502-12.

Docetaxel-Ramucirumab (NSCLC)

Index Terms Ramucirumab-Docetaxel (NSCLC)
Use Lung cancer, non-small cell (second-line, stage IV, disease progression on platinum-based chemotherapy)
Regimen
Ramucirumab: IV: 10 mg/kg over 1 hour day 1
  [total dose/cycle = 10 mg/kg]
Docetaxel: IV: 75 mg/m^2 day 1
  [total dose/cycle = 75 mg/m^2]
Repeat cycle every 21 days until disease progression or unacceptable toxicity
References

Garon EB, Ciuleanu TE, Arrieta O, et al. Ramucirumab plus docetaxel versus placebo plus docetaxel for second-line treatment of stage IV non-small-cell lung cancer after disease progression on platinum-based therapy (REVEL): a multicentre, double-blind, randomised phase 3 trial. *Lancet*. 2014;384(9944):665-673.

◆ **Docetaxel-Trastuzumab-Fluorouracil-Epirubicin-Cyclophosphamide (Breast)** see Docetaxel-Trastuzumab followed by FEC (Breast) on page 2095

Docetaxel-Trastuzumab followed by FEC (Breast)

Index Terms Docetaxel-Trastuzumab-Fluorouracil-Epirubicin-Cyclophosphamide (Breast); Trastuzumab-Docetaxel-FEC (Breast)

Use Breast cancer

Regimen

Cycle 1:

Trastuzumab: IV: 4 mg/kg (loading dose) over 90 minutes day 1 cycle 1

followed by IV: 2 mg/kg/day over 30 minutes days 8 and 15 cycle 1

[total dose/cycle 1 = 8 mg/kg]

Docetaxel: IV: 80-100 mg/m^2 over 1 hour day 1

[total dose/cycle 1 = 80-100 mg/m^2]

Treatment cycle is 21 days

Cycles 2 and 3:

Trastuzumab: IV: 2 mg/kg/day days 1, 8, and 15

[total dose/cycle = 6 mg/kg]

Docetaxel: IV: 80-100 mg/m^2 over 1 hour day 1

[total dose/cycle = 80-100 mg/m^2]

Repeat docetaxel-trastuzumab cycle every 21 days for a total of 3 cycles

Cycles 4, 5, and 6 (FEC):

Fluorouracil: IV: 600 mg/m^2 day 1

[total dose/cycle = 600 mg/m^2]

Epirubicin: IV: 60 mg/m^2 day 1

[total dose/cycle = 60 mg/m^2]

Cyclophosphamide: IV: 600 mg/m^2 day 1

[total dose/cycle = 600 mg/m^2]

Repeat FEC cycle every 21 days for total of 3 cycles

References

Joesnuu H, Bono P, Kataja V, et al, "Fluorouracil, Epirubicin, and Cyclophosphamide With Either Docetaxel or Vinorelbine, With or Without Trastuzumab, As Adjuvant Treatments of Breast Cancer: Final Results of the FinHer Trial," J Clin Oncol, 2009, 27(34):5685-92.

Joensuu H, Kellokumpu-Lehtinen PL, Bono P, et al, "Adjuvant Docetaxel or Vinorelbine With or Without Trastuzumab for Breast Cancer," N Engl J Med, 2006, 354(8):809-20.

Docetaxel Weekly-Trastuzumab (Breast)

Index Terms Trastuzumab-Docetaxel Weekly (Breast)

Use Breast cancer

Regimen

Cycle 1:

Docetaxel: IV: 35 mg/m^2/day over 30 minutes days 1, 8, and 15

[total dose/cycle 1 = 105 mg/m^2]

Trastuzumab: IV: 4 mg/kg (loading dose) over 90 minutes day 0 cycle 1

followed by IV: 2 mg/kg/day over 30 minutes days 8, 15, and 22 cycle 1

[total dose/cycle 1 = 10 mg/kg]

Treatment cycle is 28 days

◀ Subsequent cycles:
Docetaxel: IV: 35 mg/m^2/day over 30 minutes days 1, 8, and 15
[total dose/cycle = 105 mg/m^2]
Trastuzumab: IV: 2 mg/kg/day over 30 minutes days 1, 8, 15, and 22
[total dose/cycle = 8 mg/kg]
Repeat cycle every 28 days until disease progression or unacceptable
toxicity

References

Esteva FJ, Valero V, Booser D, et al, "Phase II Study of Weekly Docetaxel and Trastuzumab for Patients With HER-2-Overexpressing Metastatic Breast Cancer," *J Clin Oncol*, 2002, 20 (7):1800-8.

- ◆ **Dose-Adjusted EPOCH (NHL)** *see* EPOCH Dose-Adjusted (NHL)
  on page 2105
- ◆ **Dose-Adjusted EPOCH (NHL-AIDS-Related)** *see* EPOCH Dose-Adjusted
  (NHL-AIDS-Related) *on page 2106*
- ◆ **Dose-Adjusted Etoposide-Vincristine-Doxorubicin-Cyclophosphamide-
  Prednisone (NHL)** *see* EPOCH Dose-Adjusted (NHL) *on page 2105*
- ◆ **Dose Dense M-VAC** *see* Dose Dense MVAC (Bladder Cancer)
  on page 2096

Dose Dense MVAC (Bladder Cancer)

Index Terms DDM-VAC (Bladder Cancer); DDMVAC (Bladder Cancer); Dose
Dense M-VAC; HD-MVAC (Bladder Cancer); High-Dose-Intensity M-VAC
(Bladder Cancer); MVAC (Bladder Cancer)

Use Bladder cancer

Regimen NOTE: Multiple variations are listed.

Variation 1:
Methotrexate: IV: 30 mg/m^2 day 1
[total dose/cycle = 30 mg/m^2]
Vinblastine: IV: 3 mg/m^2 day 2
[total dose/cycle = 3 mg/m^2]
Doxorubicin: IV: 30 mg/m^2 day 2
[total dose/cycle = 30 mg/m^2]
Cisplatin: IV: 70 mg/m^2 day 2
[total dose/cycle = 70 mg/m^2]
Filgrastim: SubQ: 240 mcg/m^2 days 4 to 10 (discontinue if ANC
>30,000/mm^3 or may extend up to a total of 14 days if needed)
Repeat cycle every 14 days until disease progression or unacceptable
toxicity

Variation 2:
Methotrexate: IV: 30 mg/m^2 day 1
[total dose/cycle = 30 mg/m^2]
Vinblastine: IV: 3 mg/m^2 day 2
[total dose/cycle = 3 mg/m^2]
Doxorubicin: IV: 30 mg/m^2 day 2
[total dose/cycle = 30 mg/m^2]
Cisplatin: IV: 70 mg/m^2 day 2
[total dose/cycle = 70 mg/m^2]
Filgrastim: SubQ: Days 3 to 7 (dose not specified)
Repeat cycle every 14 days until disease progression or unacceptable
toxicity

References

Variation 1:
Sternberg CN, de Mulder PH, Schornagel JH, et al. Randomized phase III trial of high-dose-intensity methotrexate, vinblastine, doxorubicin, and cisplatin (MVAC) chemotherapy and recombinant human granulocyte colony-stimulating factor versus classic MVAC in advanced urothelial tract tumors: European Organization for Research and Treatment of Cancer Protocol no. 30924. *J Clin Oncol.* 2001;19(10):2638-2646.

Variation 2:
Sternberg CN, de Mulder P, Schornagel JH, et al. Seven year update of an EORTC phase III trial of high-dose intensity M-VAC chemotherapy and G-CSF versus classic M-VAC in advanced urothelial tract tumours. *Eur J Cancer.* 2006;42(1):50-54.

◆ **Doxil-Vincristine-Dexamethasone (Multiple Myeloma)** *see* Doxorubicin (Liposomal)-Vincristine-Dexamethasone (Multiple Myeloma) *on page 2098*

◆ **Doxorubicin, Bleomycin, Vinblastine, Dacarbazine (Hodgkin)** *see* ABVD Early Stage (Hodgkin) *on page 1974*

◆ **Doxorubicin-Bleomycin-Vinblastine-Dacarbazine (Hodgkin)** *see* ABVD (Hodgkin) *on page 1975*

◆ **Doxorubicin-Cisplatin (Endometrial)** *see* Cisplatin-Doxorubicin (Endometrial) *on page 2040*

◆ **Doxorubicin continuous infusion-Cisplatin (Hepatoblastoma)** *see* Cisplatin-Doxorubicin Continuous Infusion (Hepatoblastoma) *on page 2039*

◆ **Doxorubicin-Cyclophosphamide (Breast)** *see* AC (Breast) *on page 1976*

◆ **Doxorubicin, Cyclophosphamide, Docetaxel (Breast)** *see* AC followed by Docetaxel Every 3 Weeks (Breast) *on page 1978*

◆ **Doxorubicin, Cyclophosphamide, Docetaxel (Breast)** *see* TAC (Breast) *on page 2211*

◆ **Doxorubicin-Cyclophosphamide-Etoposide-Bortezomib-Dexamethasone-Thalidomide-Cisplatin (Multiple Myeloma)** *see* VDT-PACE (Multiple Myeloma) *on page 2229*

◆ **Doxorubicin-Cyclophosphamide-Etoposide-Dexamethasone-Thalidomide-Cisplatin (Multiple Myeloma)** *see* DTPACE (Multiple Myeloma) *on page 2098*

◆ **Doxorubicin, Cyclophosphamide, Paclitaxel (Breast)** *see* AC (Dose-Dense) followed by Paclitaxel Weekly (Breast) *on page 1978*

◆ **Doxorubicin, Cyclophosphamide, Paclitaxel (Breast)** *see* AC followed by Paclitaxel Weekly (Breast) *on page 1979*

◆ **Doxorubicin, Cyclophosphamide, Paclitaxel Dose Dense (Breast)** *see* AC (Dose-Dense) followed by Paclitaxel (Dose-Dense) (Breast) *on page 1976*

◆ **Doxorubicin, Cyclophosphamide, Paclitaxel (Dose-Dense), Trastuzumab (Breast)** *see* AC (Dose-Dense) followed by Paclitaxel (Dose-Dense)-Trastuzumab (Breast) *on page 1977*

◆ **Doxorubicin, Cyclophosphamide, Paclitaxel, Trastuzumab (Breast)** *see* AC followed by Paclitaxel-Trastuzumab (Breast) *on page 1979*

◆ **Doxorubicin-Dacarbazine-Ifosfamide-Mesna (Soft Tissue Sarcoma)** *see* MAID (Soft Tissue Sarcoma) *on page 2169*

◆ **Doxorubicin-Dacarbazine (Soft Tissue Sarcoma)** *see* AD (Soft Tissue Sarcoma) *on page 1980*

◆ **Doxorubicin-Dexamethasone-Bortezomib (Multiple Myeloma)** *see* Bortezomib-Doxorubicin-Dexamethasone (Multiple Myeloma) *on page 1999*

- **Doxorubicin-Etoposide-Prednisone-Vincristine-Cyclophosphamide (Dose-Adjusted) (NHL-AIDS-Related)** *see* EPOCH Dose-Adjusted (NHL-AIDS-Related) *on page 2106*

- **Doxorubicin-Ifosfamide (Soft Tissue Sarcoma)** *see* AIM (Soft Tissue Sarcoma) *on page 1980*

- **Doxorubicin (Liposomal)-Bevacizumab (Ovarian)** *see* Bevacizumab-Doxorubicin (Liposomal) (Ovarian) *on page 1992*

- **Doxorubicin (Liposomal)-Bortezomib (Multiple Myeloma)** *see* Bortezomib-Doxorubicin (Liposomal) (Multiple Myeloma) *on page 1999*

- **Doxorubicin (Liposomal)-Carboplatin (Ovarian)** *see* Carboplatin-Doxorubicin (Liposomal) (Ovarian) *on page 2014*

- **Doxorubicin Liposomal-Trabectedin (Ovarian)** *see* Trabectedin-Doxorubicin (Liposomal) (Ovarian) *on page 2215*

Doxorubicin (Liposomal)-Vincristine-Dexamethasone (Multiple Myeloma)

Index Terms Doxil-Vincristine-Dexamethasone (Multiple Myeloma); DVD (Multiple Myeloma); DVd (Multiple Myeloma)

Use Multiple myeloma

Regimen

Doxorubicin (liposomal): IV: 40 mg/m^2 over 1 hour day 1
[total dose/cycle = 40 mg/m^2]

Vincristine: IV: 1.4 mg/m^2 (maximum dose: 2 mg) day 1
[total dose/cycle = 1.4 mg/m^2; maximum = 2 mg]

Dexamethasone: Oral: 40 mg once daily days 1 to 4
[total dose/cycle = 160 mg]

Repeat cycle every 28 days for at least four cycles in patients who are responding and proceeding to transplant or until maximal response, disease progression, or unacceptable toxicity

References

Rifkin RM, Gregory SA, Mohrbacher A, Hussein MA. Pegylated liposomal doxorubicin, vincristine, and dexamethasone provide significant reduction in toxicity compared with doxorubicin, vincristine, and dexamethasone in patients with newly diagnosed multiple myeloma: a phase III multicenter randomized trial. *Cancer.* 2006;106(4):848-858.

- **Doxorubicin-Methotrexate-Cisplatin (Osteosarcoma)** *see* MAP (Osteosarcoma) *on page 2170*

- **Doxorubicin-Olaratumab (Soft Tissue Sarcoma)** *see* Olaratumab-Doxorubicin (Soft Tissue Sarcoma) *on page 2181*

- **Doxorubicin-Prednisone-Cyclophosphamide-Vincristine (NHL-AIDS-Related)** *see* CHOP (NHL-AIDS-Related) *on page 2035*

- **Doxorubicin-Rituximab-Etoposide-Prednisone-Vincristine-Cyclophosphamide (Dose-Adjusted) (NHL-AIDS-Related)** *see* EPOCH Dose-Adjusted-Rituximab (NHL-AIDS-Related) *on page 2107*

- **Doxorubicin-Vincristine-Prednisone-Rituximab-Cyclophosphamide (NHL-DLBCL)** *see* R-CHOP (NHL-DLBCL) *on page 2200*

DTPACE (Multiple Myeloma)

Index Terms Cisplatin-Doxorubicin-Cyclophosphamide-Etoposide-Dexamethasone-Thalidomide (Multiple Myeloma); Cyclophosphamide-Etoposide-Dexamethasone-Thalidomide-Cisplatin-Doxorubicin (Multiple Myeloma);

Dexamethasone-Thalidomide-Cisplatin-Doxorubicin-Cyclophosphamide-Etoposide (Multiple Myeloma); Doxorubicin-Cyclophosphamide-Etoposide-Dexamethasone-Thalidomide-Cisplatin (Multiple Myeloma); Etoposide-Dexamethasone-Thalidomide-Cisplatin-Doxorubicin-Cyclophosphamide (Multiple Myeloma); Thalidomide-Dexamethasone-Cisplatin-Doxorubicin-Cyclophosphamide-Etoposide (Multiple Myeloma)

Use Multiple myeloma

Regimen

Dexamethasone: Oral: 40 mg daily days 1 to 4
[total dose/cycle = 160 mg]

Thalidomide: Oral: 400 mg daily at night
[total dose/cycle = 11,200 to 16,800 mg]

Cisplatin: IV: 10 mg/m^2/day continuous infusion days 1 to 4
[total dose/cycle = 40 mg/m^2]

Doxorubicin: IV: 10 mg/m^2/day continuous infusion days 1 to 4
[total dose/cycle = 40 mg/m^2]

Cyclophosphamide: IV: 400 mg^2/day continuous infusion days 1 to 4
[total dose/cycle = 1,600 mg/m^2]

Etoposide: IV: 40 mg/m^2/day continuous infusion days 1 to 4
[total dose/cycle = 160 mg/m^2]

Filgrastim: SubQ: Initiate 10 mcg/kg once daily on day +5 after the first cycle of DTPACE; continue until completion of stem cell collection. In subsequent cycles, initiate filgrastim 300 mcg (or per institutional policy) once daily on day +5 of chemotherapy; continue until ANC is >1,000/mm^3 for 2 consecutive days

Repeat cycle every 4 to 6 weeks

References

Lee CK, Barlogie B, Munshi N, et al. DTPACE: an effective, novel combination chemotherapy with thalidomide for previously treated patients with myeloma. *J Clin Oncol.* 2003;21(14):2732-2739.

◆ **DVD (Multiple Myeloma)** see Doxorubicin (Liposomal)-Vincristine-Dexamethasone (Multiple Myeloma) on page 2098

DVP

Use Leukemia, acute lymphocytic

Regimen Induction:

Daunorubicin: IV: 25 mg/m^2/day days 1, 8, and 15
[total dose/cycle = 75 mg/m^2]

Vincristine: IV: 1.5 mg/m^2/day (maximum dose: 2 mg) days 1, 8, 15, and 22
[total dose/cycle = 6 mg/m^2]

Prednisone: Oral: 60 mg/m^2/day days 1 to 28 then taper over next 14 days
[total dose/cycle = 1680 mg/m^2 + taper over next 14 days]

Administer single cycle; used in conjunction with intrathecal chemotherapy

References

Belasco JB, Luery N, and Scher C, "Multiagent Chemotherapy in Relapsed Acute Lymphoblastic Leukemia in Children," *Cancer*, 1990, 66(12):2492-7.

◆ **EC (Breast)** see Cyclophosphamide-Epirubicin (Breast) on page 2077

◆ **ECF (Gastric/Esophageal)** see Epirubicin-Cisplatin-Fluorouracil (Gastric/Esophageal) on page 2103

EC (NSCLC)

Use Lung cancer, non-small cell

Regimen

Etoposide: IV: 120 mg/m^2/day days 1, 2, and 3
[total dose/cycle = 360 mg/m^2]
Carboplatin: IV: AUC 6 day 1
[total dose/cycle = AUC = 6]
Repeat cycle every 21-28 days

References

Birch R, Weaver CH, Hainsworth JD, et al, "A Randomized Study of Etoposide and Carboplatin With or Without Paclitaxel in the Treatment of Small Cell Lung Cancer," *Semin Oncol*, 1997, 24(4 Suppl 12):S12-135, 137.

- ◆ **EC (Small Cell Lung Cancer)** *see* Carboplatin-Etoposide (Small Cell Lung Cancer) *on page 2015*

- ◆ **ECX (Gastric/Esophageal)** *see* Epirubicin-Cisplatin-Capecitabine (Gastric/ Esophageal) *on page 2103*

- ◆ **EE4A (Wilms' Tumor)** *see* EE-4A (Wilms' Tumor) *on page 2100*

EE-4A (Wilms' Tumor)

Index Terms Dactinomycin-Vincristine (Wilms' Tumor); EE4A (Wilms' Tumor); Regimen EE-4A (Wilms' Tumor); Vincristine-Dactinomycin (Wilms' Tumor)

Use Wilms' tumor

Regimen

Dactinomycin: IV: 45 mcg/kg day 1 of weeks 0, 3, 6, 9, 12, 15, and 18
[total dose = 315 mcg/kg]
Vincristine: IV: 1.5 mg/m^2 day 1 of weeks 1 to 10

Followed by

Vincristine: IV: 2 mg/m^2 day 1 of weeks 12, 15, and 18
[total dose = 21 mg/m^2]
Treatment course duration is week 0 through week 18

References

Green DM, Breslow NE, Beckwith JB, et al, "Effect of Duration of Treatment on Treatment Outcome and Cost of Treatment for Wilms' Tumor: A Report From the National Wilms' Tumor Study Group," *J Clin Oncol*, 1998, 16(12):3744-51.

Elotuzumab-Lenalidomide-Dexamethasone (Multiple Myeloma)

Index Terms Lenalidomide-Dexamethasone-Elotuzumab (Multiple Myeloma)

Use Multiple myeloma (relapsed and/or refractory in patients who have received 1 to 3 prior therapies)

Regimen Note: Premedicate with dexamethasone, an H1-blocker, an H2-blocker, and acetaminophen ~45 to 90 minutes prior to elotuzumab infusion to prevent infusion reaction.

Cycles 1 and 2:

Elotuzumab: IV: 10 mg/kg/day days 1, 8, 15, and 22
[total dose/cycle = 40 mg/kg]
Lenalidomide: Oral: 25 mg/day days 1 to 21
[total dose/cycle = 525 mg]
Dexamethasone: Oral and IV: On days that elotuzumab is administered, give dexamethasone 28 mg orally 3 to 24 hours before elotuzumab infusion **plus** dexamethasone 8 mg IV 45 to 90 minutes prior to infusion.
[total oral dose/cycle = 112 mg; total IV dose/cycle = 32 mg]
Repeat cycle every 28 days for a total of 2 cycles

Cycle 3 and subsequent cycles:
Elotuzumab: IV: 10 mg/kg/day days 1 and 15
[total dose/cycle = 20 mg/kg]
Lenalidomide: Oral: 25 mg/day days 1 to 21
[total dose/cycle = 525 mg]
Dexamethasone: Oral and IV: On days that elotuzumab is administered (eg, days 1 and 15 of cycle 3 and beyond), give dexamethasone 28 mg orally 3 to 24 hours before elotuzumab infusion **plus** dexamethasone 8 mg IV 45 to 90 minutes prior to infusion. On days that elotuzumab is **not** administered but dexamethasone is due (eg, days 8 and 22 of cycle 3 and beyond), administer dexamethasone 40 mg orally.
[total oral dose/cycle = 136 mg; total IV dose/cycle = 16 mg]
Repeat cycle every 28 days until disease progression or unacceptable toxicity

References

Lonial S, Dimopoulos M, Palumbo A, et al. Elotuzumab therapy for relapsed or refractory multiple myeloma. *N Engl J Med.* 2015;373(7):621-631.

◆ **EMA (AML)** see Mitoxantrone-Etoposide-Cytarabine (AML) on page 2175

EMA/CO (Gestational Trophoblastic Tumor)

Index Terms Etoposide-Methotrexate-Dactinomycin-Leucovorin-Cyclophosphamide-Vincristine (Gestational Trophoblastic Tumor)

Use Gestational trophoblastic tumor

Regimen

Dactinomycin: IV: 0.5 mg/day days 1 and 2
[total dose/cycle = 1 mg]
Etoposide: IV: 100 mg/m^2/day over 30 minutes days 1 and 2
[total dose/cycle = 200 mg/m^2]
Methotrexate: IV bolus: 100 mg/m^2 day 1
followed by
Methotrexate: IV: 200 mg/m^2 continuous infusion over 12 hours day 1
[total dose/cycle = 300 mg/m^2]
Leucovorin Calcium: Oral, IM: 15 mg every 12 hours for 4 doses (begin 24 hours after start of methotrexate) days 2 and 3
[total dose/cycle = 60 mg]
Vincristine: IV: 1 mg/m^2 day 8
[total dose/cycle = 1 mg/m^2]
Cyclophosphamide: IV: 600 mg/m^2 day 8
[total dose/cycle = 600 mg/m^2]
Repeat cycle every 14 days, continue for at least 2 treatment cycles after a normal hCG level

References

Escobar PF, Lurain JR, Singh DK, Bozorgi K, Fishman DA. Treatment of high-risk gestational trophoblastic neoplasia with etoposide, methotrexate, actinomycin D, cyclophosphamide, and vincristine chemotherapy. *Gynecol Oncol.* 2003;91(3):552-557.

Lurain JR, Singh DK, Schink JC. Primary treatment of metastatic high-risk gestational trophoblastic neoplasia with EMA-CO chemotherapy. *J Reprod Med.* 2006;51(10):767-772.

EMA/EP (Gestational Trophoblastic Tumor)

Index Terms EP/EMA (Gestational Trophoblastic Tumor); Etoposide-Cisplatin-Methotrexate-Dactinomycin (Gestational Trophoblastic Tumor); Etoposide-Methotrexate-Leucovorin-Dactinomycin-Cisplatin (Gestational Trophoblastic Tumor)

Use Gestational trophoblastic tumor

◀ **Regimen**
Etoposide: IV: 150 mg/m² over 30 minutes day 1
[total dose/cycle = 150 mg/m²]
Cisplatin: IV: 25 mg/m² over 4 hours each for 3 consecutive doses day 1
[total dose/cycle = 75 mg/m²]
Alternate weekly with:
Etoposide: IV: 100 mg/m² over 30 minutes day 1
[total dose/cycle = 100 mg/m²]
Methotrexate: IV: 300 mg/m² over 12 hours day 1
[total dose/cycle = 300 mg/m²]
Dactinomycin: IV: 0.5 mg (IV bolus) day 1
[total dose/cycle = 0.5 mg]
Leucovorin Calcium: Oral, IM: 15 mg twice daily for 4 doses days 2 and 3
(begin 24 hours after the start of methotrexate)
[total dose/cycle = 60 mg]
Alternate weekly EP and EMA

References
Newlands ES, Bower M, Holden L, et al. Management of resistant gestational trophoblastic tumors. *J Reprod Med.* 1998;43(2):111-118.

Newlands ES, Mulholland PJ, Holden L, Seckl MJ, Rustin GJ. Etoposide and cisplatin/etoposide, methotrexate, and actinomycin D (EMA) chemotherapy for patients with high-risk gestational trophoblastic tumors refractory to EMA/cyclophosphamide and vincristine chemotherapy and patients presenting with metastatic placental site trophoblastic tumors. *J Clin Oncol.* 2000;18 (4):854-859.

◆ **EMA-G (AML Induction)** see MEC-G (AML Induction) on page 2170

EMA (Gestational Trophoblastic Tumor)

Index Terms Etoposide-Methotrexate-Dactinomycin-Leucovorin (Gestational Trophoblastic Tumor); MEA (Gestational Trophoblastic Tumor)
Use Gestational trophoblastic tumor
Regimen
Dactinomycin: IV bolus: 0.5 mg/day days 1 to 5
[total dose/cycle = 2.5 mg]
Etoposide: IV: 100 mg/day over 1 hour days 1 to 5
[total dose/cycle = 500 mg]
Methotrexate: IV bolus: 150 mg day 1
followed by: IV: 300 mg over 4 hours day 1
[total dose/cycle = 450 mg]
Leucovorin Calcium: IM: 15 mg every 12 hours for 3 doses beginning on day 2
(24 hours after start of methotrexate)
[total dose/cycle = 45 mg]
Repeat cycle every 14 to 21 days, continue until hCG level decreases to within
normal range (<1 mIU/mL)

References
Matsui H, Suzuka K, Iitsuka Y, Seki K, Sekiya S. Combination chemotherapy with methotrexate, etoposide, and actinomycin D for high-risk gestational trophoblastic tumors. *Gynecol Oncol.* 2000;78(1):28-31.

◆ **EOF (Gastric/Esophageal)** see Epirubicin-Oxaliplatin-Fluorouracil (Gastric/Esophageal) on page 2105

◆ **EOX (Gastric/Esophageal)** see Epirubicin-Oxaliplatin-Capecitabine (Gastric/Esophageal) on page 2104

◆ **EP/EMA (Gestational Trophoblastic Tumor)** see EMA/EP (Gestational Trophoblastic Tumor) on page 2101

Epirubicin-Cisplatin-Capecitabine (Gastric/Esophageal)

Index Terms Capecitabine-Cisplatin-Epirubicin (Gastric/Esophageal); Cisplatin-Capecitabine-Epirubicin (Gastric/Esophageal); ECX (Gastric/Esophageal)

Use Esophageal cancer; Gastric cancer

Regimen

Epirubicin: IV: 50 mg/m² day 1
[total dose/cycle = 50 mg/m²]
Cisplatin: IV: 60 mg/m² day 1
[total dose/cycle = 60 mg/m²]
Capecitabine: Oral: 625 mg/m² twice daily days 1 to 21; administer within 30 minutes after a meal
[total dose/cycle = 26,250 mg/m²]
Repeat cycle every 21 days for up to 8 cycles

References

Cunningham D, Starling N, Rao S, et al. Capecitabine and oxaliplatin for advanced esophago-gastric cancer. *N Engl J Med.* 2008;358(1):36-46.

Epirubicin-Cisplatin-Fluorouracil (Gastric/Esophageal)

Index Terms Cisplatin-Fluorouracil-Epirubicin (Gastric/Esophageal); ECF (Gastric/Esophageal); Fluorouracil-Cisplatin-Epirubicin (Gastric/Esophageal)

Use Esophageal cancer; Gastric cancer

Regimen NOTE: Multiple variations are listed.

Variation 1:
Epirubicin: IV: 50 mg/m² day 1
[total dose/cycle = 50 mg/m²]
Cisplatin: IV: 60 mg/m² day 1
[total dose/cycle = 60 mg/m²]
Fluorouracil: IV: 200 mg/m²/day continuous infusion days 1 to 21
[total dose/cycle = 4,200 mg/m²]
Repeat cycle every 21 days for up to a maximum of 8 cycles
Variation 2:
Epirubicin: IV: 50 mg/m² day 1
[total dose/cycle = 50 mg/m²]
Cisplatin: IV: 60 mg/m² day 1
[total dose/cycle = 60 mg/m²]
Fluorouracil: IV: 200 mg/m²/day continuous infusion days 1 to 21
[total dose/cycle = 4,200 mg/m²]
Repeat cycle every 21 days for 6 cycles (3 cycles preoperatively and 3 cycles postoperatively)

References

Variation 1:
Cunningham D, Starling N, Rao S, et al. Capecitabine and oxaliplatin for advanced esophago-gastric cancer. *N Engl J Med.* 2008;358(1):36-46.
Variation 2:
Cunningham D, Allum WH, Stenning SP, et al. Perioperative chemotherapy versus surgery alone for resectable gastroesophageal cancer. *N Engl J Med.* 2006;355(1):11-20.

◆ **Epirubicin-Cyclophosphamide (Breast)** *see* Cyclophosphamide-Epirubicin (Breast) *on page 2077*

Epirubicin-Ifosfamide (Soft Tissue Sarcoma)

Index Terms Ifosfamide-Epirubicin (Soft Tissue Sarcoma)

Use Soft tissue sarcoma (adjuvant)

Regimen NOTE: Multiple variations are listed.

Variation 1 (begin no later than 4 weeks after surgery):

Epirubicin: IV: 25 mg/m^2/day days 1, 2, and 3

[total dose/cycle = 75 mg/m^2]

Ifosfamide: IV: 1,200 mg/m^2/day days 1 to 5

[total dose/cycle = 6,000 mg/m^2]

Mesna: IV: 240 mg/m^2 administer before and 4 and 8 hours after ifosfamide (total of 3 doses/day) days 1 to 5

[total dose/cycle = 3,600 mg/m^2]

Repeat cycle every 28 days for a total of 4 cycles

Variation 2:

Epirubicin: IV: 60 mg/m^2/day days 1 and 2

[total dose/cycle = 120 mg/m^2]

Ifosfamide: IV: 1,800 mg/m^2/day over 1 hour days 1 to 5

[total dose/cycle = 9,000 mg/m^2]

Mesna: IV bolus: 360 mg/m^2 administer before and 4 and 8 hours after ifosfamide (total of 3 doses/day) days 1 to 5

[total dose/cycle = 5,400 mg/m^2]

Filgrastim: SubQ: 300 mcg/day days 8 to 15

[total dose/cycle = 2,400 mg/m^2]

Repeat cycle every 21 days for a total of 5 cycles

References

Variation 1:

Petrioli R, Coratti A, Correale P, et al. Adjuvant epirubicin with or without Ifosfamide for adult soft-tissue sarcoma. *Am J Clin Oncol.* 2002;25(5):468-473.

Variation 2:

Frustaci S, Gherlinzoni F, De Paoli A, et al. Adjuvant chemotherapy for adult soft tissue sarcomas of the extremities and girdles: results of the Italian randomized cooperative trial. *J Clin Oncol.* 2001;19(5):1238-1247.

Epirubicin-Oxaliplatin-Capecitabine (Gastric/Esophageal)

Index Terms Capecitabine-Oxaliplatin-Epirubicin (Gastric/Esophageal); EOX (Gastric/Esophageal); Oxaliplatin-Capecitabine-Epirubicin (Gastric/Esophageal)

Use Esophageal cancer; Gastric cancer

Regimen

Epirubicin: IV: 50 mg/m^2 day 1

[total dose/cycle = 50 mg/m^2]

Oxaliplatin: IV: 130 mg/m^2 over 2 hours day 1

[total dose/cycle = 130 mg/m^2]

Capecitabine: Oral: 625 mg/m^2 twice daily days 1 to 21; administer within 30 minutes after a meal

[total dose/cycle = 26,250 mg/m^2]

Repeat cycle every 21 days for up to 8 cycles

References

Cunningham D, Starling N, Rao S, et al. Capecitabine and oxaliplatin for advanced esophago-gastric cancer. *N Engl J Med.* 2008;358(1):36-46.

Epirubicin-Oxaliplatin-Fluorouracil (Gastric/Esophageal)

Index Terms EOF (Gastric/Esophageal); Fluorouracil-Oxaliplatin-Epirubicin (Gastric/Esophageal); Oxaliplatin-Fluorouracil-Epirubicin (Gastric/Esophageal)

Use Esophageal cancer; Gastric cancer

Regimen

Epirubicin: IV: 50 mg/m^2 day 1
[total dose/cycle = 50 mg/m^2]
Oxaliplatin: IV: 130 mg/m^2 over 2 hours day 1
[total dose/cycle = 130 mg/m^2]
Fluorouracil: IV: 200 mg/m^2/day continuous infusion days 1 to 21
[total dose/cycle = 4,200 mg/m^2]
Repeat cycle every 21 days for up to 8 cycles

References

Cunningham D, Starling N, Rao S, et al. Capecitabine and oxaliplatin for advanced esophago-gastric cancer. *N Engl J Med*. 2008;358(1):36-46.

EPOCH Dose-Adjusted (NHL)

Index Terms Dose-Adjusted EPOCH (NHL); Dose-Adjusted Etoposide-Vincristine-Doxorubicin-Cyclophosphamide-Prednisone (NHL)

Use Lymphoma, non-Hodgkin

Regimen

Etoposide: IV: 50 mg/m^2/day continuous infusion days 1 to 4
[total dose/cycle = 200 mg/m^2]
Vincristine: IV: 0.4 mg/m^2/day continuous infusion days 1 to 4
[total dose/cycle = 1.6 mg/m^2]
Doxorubicin: IV: 10 mg/m^2/day continuous infusion days 1 to 4
[total dose/cycle = 40 mg/m^2]
Cyclophosphamide: IV: 750 mg/m^2 day 5
[total dose/cycle = 750 mg/m^2]
Prednisone: Oral: 60 mg/m^2/day (given once daily or in 2 divided doses) days 1 to 5 or days 1 to 6 (some centers may use 60 mg/m^2 twice daily days 1 to 5)
[total dose/cycle = 300 to 360 mg/m^2 or 600 mg/m^2]
Filgrastim: SubQ: 5 mcg/kg/day beginning day 6 or 8; continue until ANC recovery

Repeat cycle every 21 days with etoposide, doxorubicin, and cyclophosphamide dose adjustments (based on CBC 2 times/week) according to the following schedule:
Nadir ANC ≥500/mm^3: 20% to 25% increase (above previous cycle) for etoposide, doxorubicin, and cyclophosphamide
Nadir ANC <500/mm^3 (on 1 or 2 measurements): Same doses as previous cycle
Nadir ANC <500/mm^3 (on ≥3 measurements) or nadir platelet <25,000/mm^3 (on 1 measurement): 20% to 25% decrease below previous cycle for etoposide, doxorubicin, and cyclophosphamide (dosing adjustments below starting dose levels only apply to cyclophosphamide)

References

Gutierrez M, Chabner BA, Pearson D, et al, "Role of a Doxorubicin-Containing Regimen in Relapsed and Resistant Lymphomas: An 8-Year Follow-Up Study of EPOCH," *J Clin Oncol*, 2000, 18(21):3633-42.

Wilson WH, Bryant G, Bates S, et al, "EPOCH Chemotherapy: Toxicity and Efficacy in Relapsed and Refractory Non-Hodgkin's Lymphoma," *J Clin Oncol*, 1993, 11(8):1573-82.
Wilson WH, Grossbard ML, Pittaluga S, et al, "Dose-Adjusted EPOCH Chemotherapy for Untreated Large B-Cell Lymphomas: A Pharmacodynamic Approach With High Efficacy," *Blood*, 2002, 99(8):2685-93.

EPOCH Dose-Adjusted (NHL-AIDS-Related)

Index Terms Cyclophosphamide-Doxorubicin-Etoposide-Prednisone-Vincristine (Dose-Adjusted) (NHL-AIDS-Related); DA EPOCH (NHL-AIDS-Related); Dose-Adjusted EPOCH (NHL-AIDS-Related); Doxorubicin-Etoposide-Prednisone-Vincristine-Cyclophosphamide (Dose-Adjusted) (NHL-AIDS-Related); Etoposide-Prednisone-Vincristine-Cyclophosphamide-Doxorubicin (Dose-Adjusted) (NHL-AIDS-Related); Vincristine-Cyclophosphamide-Doxorubicin-Etoposide-Prednisone (Dose-Adjusted) (NHL-AIDS-Related)

Use Lymphoma, AIDS-related

Regimen

Etoposide: IV: 50 mg/m^2/day continuous infusion days 1 to 4
[total dose/cycle = 200 mg/m^2]
Vincristine: IV: 0.4 mg/m^2/day continuous infusion days 1 to 4
[total dose/cycle = 1.6 mg/m^2]
Doxorubicin: IV: 10 mg/m^2/day continuous infusion days 1 to 4
[total dose/cycle = 40 mg/m^2]
Cyclophosphamide: IV: 375 mg/m^2 day 5 for CD4+ cells ≥100/mm^3 **or** 187 mg/m^2 day 5 for CD4+ cells <100/mm^3
[total dose/cycle = 187 **or** 375 mg/m^2]
Prednisone: Oral: 60 mg/m^2/day days 1 to 5
[total dose/cycle = 300 mg/m^2]
Filgrastim: SubQ: 5 mcg/kg/day beginning day 6; continue until ANC >5000/mm^3 (past nadir)
Repeat cycle every 21 days for 6 cycles with cyclophosphamide dose adjusted based on previous cycle nadir according to the following schedule:
Nadir ANC >500/mm^3: Increase cyclophosphamide dose by 187 mg/m^2 above previous cycle dose (maximum dose: 750 mg/m^2)
Nadir ANC <500/mm^3 or platelet <25,000/mm^3: Decrease cyclophosphamide dose by 187 mg/m^2 below previous cycle dose

References

Little RF, Pittaluga S, Grant N, et al. Highly effective treatment of acquired immunodeficiency syndrome-related lymphoma with dose-adjusted EPOCH: impact of antiretroviral therapy suspension and tumor biology. *Blood*. 2003;101(12):4653-4659.

EPOCH (Dose-Adjusted)-Rituximab (NHL)

Index Terms EPOCH (Dose-Adjusted)-R (NHL); R-EPOCH Dose Adjusted (NHL); Rituxan-Etoposide-Prednisone-Vincristine-Cyclophosphamide-Doxorubicin (Dose-Adjusted) (NHL); Rituximab-EPOCH Dose Adjusted (NHL)

Use Lymphoma, non-Hodgkin

Regimen

Rituximab: IV: 375 mg/m^2 day 1
[total dose/cycle = 375 mg/m^2]
Etoposide: IV: 50 mg/m^2/day continuous infusion days 1 to 4
[total dose/cycle = 200 mg/m^2]
Vincristine: IV: 0.4 mg/m^2/day continuous infusion days 1 to 4
[total dose/cycle = 1.6 mg/m^2]
Doxorubicin: IV: 10 mg/m^2/day continuous infusion days 1 to 4
[total dose/cycle = 40 mg/m^2]

Cyclophosphamide: IV: 750 mg/m² day 5
 [total dose/cycle = 750 mg/m²]
Prednisone: Oral: 60 mg/m²/day (given once daily or in 2 divided doses) days 1 to 5 (some centers may use 60 mg/m² twice daily days 1 to 5)
 [total dose/cycle = 300 mg/m² or 600 mg/m²]
Filgrastim: SubQ: 5 mcg/kg/day beginning day 6; continue until ANC recovery
Repeat cycle every 21 days (for at least 2 cycles beyond best response; minimum of 6 cycles and maximum of 8 cycles) with etoposide, doxorubicin, and cyclophosphamide dose adjustments (based on CBC 2 times/week) according to the following schedule:
Nadir ANC ≥500/mm³: 20% increase (above previous cycle) for etoposide, doxorubicin, and cyclophosphamide
Nadir ANC <500/mm³ (on 1 or 2 measurements): Same doses as previous cycle
Nadir ANC <500/mm³ (on ≥3 measurements): 20% decrease below previous cycle for etoposide, doxorubicin, and cyclophosphamide (dosing adjustments below starting dose levels only apply to cyclophosphamide)

References

García-Suárez J, Bañas H, Arribas I, et al, "Dose-Adjusted EPOCH Plus Rituximab Is an Effective Regimen in Patients With Poor-Prognostic Untreated Diffuse Large B-Cell Lymphoma: Results From a Prospective Observational Study," *Br J Haematol*, 2007, 136(2):276-85.

Wilson WH, Gutierrez M, O'Connor P, et al, "The Role of Rituximab and Chemotherapy in Aggressive B-Cell Lymphoma: A Preliminary Report of Dose-Adjusted EPOCH-R," *Semin Oncol*, 2002, 29(1 Suppl 2):41-7.

EPOCH Dose-Adjusted-Rituximab (NHL-AIDS-Related)

Index Terms Cyclophosphamide-Doxorubicin-Rituximab-Etoposide-Prednisone-Vincristine (Dose-Adjusted) (NHL-AIDS-Related); Doxorubicin-Rituximab-Etoposide-Prednisone-Vincristine-Cyclophosphamide (Dose-Adjusted) (NHL-AIDS-Related); EPOCH (Dose-Adjusted)-R (NHL-AIDS-Related); Etoposide-Prednisone-Vincristine-Cyclophosphamide-Doxorubicin-Rituximab (Dose-Adjusted) (NHL-AIDS-Related); R-DA-EPOCH (NHL-AIDS-Related); R-EPOCH Dose-Adjusted (NHL-AIDS-Related); Rituximab-EPOCH (Dose-Adjusted) (NHL-AIDS-Related); Rituximab-Etoposide-Prednisone-Vincristine-Cyclophosphamide-Doxorubicin (Dose-Adjusted) (NHL-AIDS-Related); Vincristine-Cyclophosphamide-Doxorubicin-Rituximab-Etoposide-Prednisone (Dose-Adjusted) (NHL-AIDS-Related)

Use Lymphoma, non-Hodgkin (AIDS-related)

Regimen

Rituximab: IV: 375 mg/m² over 2 to 6 hours day 1
 [total dose/cycle = 375 mg/m²]
Etoposide: IV: 50 mg/m²/day continuous infusion days 1 to 4
 [total dose/cycle = 200 mg/m²]
Vincristine: IV: 0.4 mg/m²/day continuous infusion days 1 to 4
 [total dose/cycle = 1.6 mg/m²]
Doxorubicin: IV: 10 mg/m²/day continuous infusion days 1 to 4
 [total dose/cycle = 40 mg/m²]
Cyclophosphamide: IV: 375 mg/m² day 5 for CD4+ cells ≥100/mm³ **or** 187 mg/m² day 5 for CD4+ cells <100/mm³
 [total dose/cycle = 187 **or** 375 mg/m²]
Prednisone: Oral: 60 mg/m²/day days 1 to 5
 [total dose/cycle = 300 mg/m²]

◀ Filgrastim: SubQ: 5 mcg/kg/day beginning day 6 (24 hours after chemotherapy); continue until neutrophil recovery
or
   Pegfilgrastim: SubQ: 6 mg day 6 (24 hours after chemotherapy) for 1 dose
Repeat cycle every 21 days for 2 cycles beyond complete response (minimum of 4 cycles and maximum of 6 cycles) with cyclophosphamide dose adjusted based on previous cycle nadir according to the following schedule:
Nadir ANC >500/mm^3 and platelet >25,000/mm^3: Increase cyclophosphamide dose by 187 mg/m^2 above previous cycle dose (maximum dose: 750 mg/m^2)
Nadir ANC <500/mm^3 or platelet <25,000/mm^3: Decrease cyclophosphamide dose by 187 mg/m^2 below previous cycle dose

References
Little RF, Pittaluga S, Grant N, et al. Highly effective treatment of acquired immunodeficiency syndrome-related lymphoma with dose-adjusted EPOCH: impact of antiretroviral therapy suspension and tumor biology. *Blood*. 2003;101(12):4653-4659.

Sparano JA, Lee JY, Kaplan LD, et al. Rituximab plus concurrent infusional EPOCH chemotherapy is highly effective in HIV-associated B-cell non-Hodgkin lymphoma. *Blood*. 2010;115 (15):3008-3016.

◆ **EPOCH (Dose-Adjusted)-R (NHL)** *see* EPOCH (Dose-Adjusted)-Rituximab (NHL) *on page 2106*

◆ **EPOCH (Dose-Adjusted)-R (NHL-AIDS-Related)** *see* EPOCH Dose-Adjusted-Rituximab (NHL-AIDS-Related) *on page 2107*

◆ **EP (Small Cell Lung Cancer)** *see* Cisplatin-Etoposide (Small Cell Lung Cancer) *on page 2042*

EP (Testicular)
Index Terms Cisplatin-Etoposide (Testicular); Etoposide-Cisplatin (Testicular)
Use Testicular cancer
Regimen
Etoposide: IV: 100 mg/m^2/day days 1 to 5
   [total dose/cycle = 500 mg/m^2]
Cisplatin: IV: 20 mg/m^2/day days 1 to 5
   [total dose/cycle = 100 mg/m^2]
Repeat cycle every 21 days for 4 cycles
References
Culine S, Kerbrat P, Kramar A. et al. Refining the optimal chemotherapy regimen for good-risk metastatic nonseminomatous germ-cell tumors: a randomized trial of the Genito-Urinary Group of the French Federation of Cancer Centers (GETUG T93BP). *Ann Oncol*. 2007;18(5):917-924.

Xiao H, Mazumdar M, Bajorin DF, et al. Long-term follow-up of patients with good-risk germ cell tumors treated with etoposide and cisplatin. *J Clin Oncol*. 1997;15(7):2553-2558.

Erlotinib-Gemcitabine (Pancreatic)
Index Terms Gemcitabine-Erlotinib (Pancreatic)
Use Pancreatic cancer
Regimen
Cycle 1:
Gemcitabine: IV: 1000 mg/m^2/day over 30 minutes days 1, 8, 15, 22, 29, 36, and 43 (cycle 1 only)
   [total dose/cycle 1 = 7000 mg/m^2]
Erlotinib: Oral: 100 mg once daily days 1 to 56
   [total dose/cycle 1 = 5600 mg]
Treatment cycle is 56 days

Subsequent cycles:
  Gemcitabine: IV: 1000 mg/m^2/day over 30 minutes days 1, 8, and 15
    [total dose/cycle = 3000 mg/m^2]
  Erlotinib: Oral: 100 mg once daily days 1 to 28
    [total dose/cycle = 2800 mg]
  Repeat cycle every 28 days

References

Moore MJ, Goldstein D, Hamm J, et al, "Erlotinib Plus Gemcitabine Compared With Gemcitabine Alone in Patients With Advanced Pancreatic Cancer: A Phase III Trial of the National Cancer Institute of Canada Clinical Trials Group," *J Clin Oncol*, 2007, 25(15):1960-6.

ESHAP

Use Lymphoma, non-Hodgkin

Regimen NOTE: Multiple variations are listed.
  Variation 1:
    Etoposide: IV: 40 mg/m^2/day days 1 to 4
      [total dose/cycle = 160 mg/m^2]
    Methylprednisolone: IV: 250-500 mg/day days 1 to 5
      [total dose/cycle = 1250-2500 mg]
    Cytarabine: IV: 2000 mg/m^2 day 5
      [total dose/cycle = 2000 mg/m^2]
    Cisplatin: IV: 25 mg/m^2/day continuous infusion days 1 to 4
      [total dose/cycle = 100 mg/m^2]
    Repeat cycle every 21-28 days
  Variation 2:
    Etoposide: IV: 40 mg/m^2/day days 1 to 4
      [total dose/cycle = 160 mg/m^2]
    Methylprednisolone: IV: 500 mg/day days 1 to 5
      [total dose/cycle = 2500 mg]
    Cytarabine: IV: 2000 mg/m^2 day 5
      [total dose/cycle = 2000 mg/m^2]
    Cisplatin: IV: 25 mg/m^2/day continuous infusion days 1 to 4
      [total dose/cycle = 100 mg/m^2]
    Repeat cycle every 21-28 days
  Variation 3:
    Etoposide: IV: 60 mg/m^2/day days 1 to 4
      [total dose/cycle = 240 mg/m^2]
    Methylprednisolone: IV: 500 mg/day days 1 to 4
      [total dose/cycle = 2000 mg]
    Cytarabine: IV: 2000 mg/m^2 day 5
      [total dose/cycle = 2000 mg/m^2]
    Cisplatin: IV: 25 mg/m^2/day continuous infusion days 1 to 4
      [total dose/cycle = 100 mg/m^2]
    Repeat cycle every 21 days

References

Variation 1:
Velasquez WF, McLaughlin P, Tucker S, et al, "ESHAP - An Effective Chemotherapy Regimen in Refractory and Relapsing Lymphoma: A 4-Year Follow-up Study," *J Clin Oncol*, 1994, 12 (6):1169-76.
Variation 2:
Wang WS, Chiou TJ, Liu JH, et al, "ESHAP as Salvage Therapy for Refractory Non-Hodgkin's Lymphoma: Taiwan Experience," *Jpn J Clin Oncol*, 1999, 29(1):33-7.
Variation 3:
Rodriguez MA, Cabanillas FC, Velasquez W, et al, "Results of a Salvage Treatment Program for Relapsing Lymphoma: MINE Consolidated With ESHAP," *J Clin Oncol*, 1995, 13(7):1734-41.

ESHAP (Hodgkin)
Index Terms Etoposide-Methylprednisolone-Cytarabine-Cisplatin (Hodgkin)
Use Lymphoma, Hodgkin
Regimen
Etoposide: IV: 40 mg/m^2/day days 1 to 4
[total dose/cycle = 160 mg/m^2]
Methylprednisolone: IV: 500 mg/day days 1 to 4
[total dose/cycle = 2000 mg]
Cisplatin: IV: 25 mg/m^2/day days 1 to 4
[total dose/cycle = 100 mg/m^2]
Cytarabine: IV: 2000 mg/m^2 day 5
[total dose/cycle = 2000 mg/m^2]
Filgrastim: SubQ: 5 mcg/kg/day days 6 to 18
Repeat cycle every 21 to 28 days for 3 cycles (if transplant candidate) or 6 cycles (nontransplant candidate)

References
Aparicio J, Segura A, Garcerá S, et al, "ESHAP is an Active Regimen for Relapsing Hodgkin's Disease," *Ann Oncol*, 1999, 10(5):593-5.

- ◆ **Etoposide-Methotrexate-Dactinomycin-Leucovorin (Gestational Trophoblastic Tumor)** *see* EMA (Gestational Trophoblastic Tumor) *on page 2102*

- ◆ **Etoposide-Methotrexate-Leucovorin-Dactinomycin-Cisplatin (Gestational Trophoblastic Tumor)** *see* EMA/EP (Gestational Trophoblastic Tumor) *on page 2101*

- ◆ **Etoposide-Methylprednisolone-Cytarabine-Cisplatin (Hodgkin)** *see* ESHAP (Hodgkin) *on page 2110*

- ◆ **Etoposide-Prednisone-Vincristine-Cyclophosphamide-Doxorubicin (Dose-Adjusted) (NHL-AIDS-Related)** *see* EPOCH Dose-Adjusted (NHL-AIDS-Related) *on page 2106*

- ◆ **Etoposide-Prednisone-Vincristine-Cyclophosphamide-Doxorubicin-Rituximab (Dose-Adjusted) (NHL-AIDS-Related)** *see* EPOCH Dose-Adjusted-Rituximab (NHL-AIDS-Related) *on page 2107*

Everolimus-Exemestane (Breast)

Index Terms Exemestane-Everolimus (Breast)

Use Breast cancer

Regimen

Everolimus: Oral: 10 mg once daily

Exemestane: Oral: 25 mg once daily

Continue until disease progression or unacceptable toxicity

References

Baselga J, Campone M, Piccart M, et al, "Everolimus in Postmenopausal Hormone-Receptor-Positive Advanced Breast Cancer," *N Engl J Med*, 2012, 366(6):520-9.

Everolimus-Lenvatinib (RCC)

Index Terms Lenvatinib-Everolimus (RCC)

Use Renal cell cancer (advanced, refractory to one prior anti-angiogenic therapy)

Regimen NOTE: Administer together at the same time each day with or without food

Everolimus: Oral: 5 mg once daily

[total dose/cycle = 140 mg]

Lenvatinib: Oral: 18 mg once daily

[total dose/cycle = 504 mg]

Repeat cycle every 28 days until disease progression or unacceptable toxicity

References

Motzer RJ, Hutson TE, Glen H, et al. Lenvatinib, everolimus, and the combination in patients with metastatic renal cell carcinoma: a randomised, phase 2, open-label, multicentre trial. *Lancet Oncol*. 2015;16(15):1473-1482.

- ◆ **Every 2 Weeks Cetuximab-Irinotecan (Colorectal)** *see* Cetuximab (Biweekly)-Irinotecan (Colorectal) *on page 2029*

- ◆ **Exemestane-Everolimus (Breast)** *see* Everolimus-Exemestane (Breast) *on page 2111*

- ◆ **FAC IV (Breast)** *see* CAF IV (Breast) *on page 2002*

- ◆ **FAC Oral (Breast)** *see* CAF Oral (Breast) *on page 2003*

- ◆ **FC (CLL)** *see* Fludarabine-Cyclophosphamide (CLL) *on page 2116*

- ◆ **FCMR (NHL-Follicular Cell)** *see* Fludarabine-Cyclophosphamide-Mitoxantrone-Rituximab (NHL-Follicular) *on page 2117*

- ◆ **FC (NHL-Mantle Cell)** *see* Fludarabine-Cyclophosphamide (NHL-Mantle Cell) *on page* 2118
- ◆ **FCR (CLL)** *see* Fludarabine-Cyclophosphamide-Rituximab (CLL) *on page* 2119
- ◆ **FCR (NHL-Follicular)** *see* Fludarabine-Cyclophosphamide-Rituximab (NHL-Follicular) *on page* 2120

FEC followed by Docetaxel Every 3 Weeks (Breast)

Index Terms Fluorouracil, Epirubicin, Cyclophosphamide, Docetaxel (Breast)
Use Breast cancer
Regimen
Fluorouracil: IV: 500 mg/m^2 day 1
 [total dose/cycle = 500 mg/m^2]
Epirubicin: IV: 100 mg/m^2 day 1
 [total dose/cycle = 100 mg/m^2]
Cyclophosphamide: IV: 500 mg/m^2 day 1
 [total dose/cycle = 500 mg/m^2]
Repeat cycle every 21 days for 3 cycles
followed by
Docetaxel: IV: 100 mg/m^2 day 1
 [total dose/cycle = 100 mg/m^2]
Repeat cycle every 21 days for 3 cycles
References
Roche H, Fumoleau P, Spielmann M, et al, "Sequential Adjuvant Epirubicin-Based and Docetaxel Chemotherapy For Node-Positive Breast Cancer Patients: The FNCLCC PACS 01 Trial," *J Clin Oncol*, 2006, 24(36):5664-71.

FEC followed by Paclitaxel Weekly (Breast)

Index Terms FEC-P (Breast); Fluorouracil, Epirubicin, Cyclophosphamide, Paclitaxel (Breast)
Use Breast cancer
Regimen
Fluorouracil: IV: 600 mg/m^2 day 1
 [total dose/cycle = 600 mg/m^2]
Epirubicin: IV: 90 mg/m^2 day 1
 [total dose/cycle = 90 mg/m^2]
Cyclophosphamide: IV: 600 mg/m^2 day 1
 [total dose/cycle = 600 mg/m^2]
Repeat cycle every 21 days for 4 cycles
followed by 3 weeks no treatment, then
Paclitaxel: IV: 100 mg/m^2 over 1 hour day 1
 [total dose/cycle = 100 mg/m^2]
Repeat cycle every 7 days for 8 cycles
References
Martín Miguel, Rodríguez-Lescure A, Ruiz A, et al, "Randomized Phase 3 Trial of Fluorouracil, Epirubicin, and Cyclophosphamide Alone or Followed by Paclitaxel for Early Breast Cancer," *J Natl Cancer Inst*, 2008, 100(11):805-814.

FEC IV (Breast)

Index Terms Fluorouracil, Epirubicin, Cyclophosphamide (Breast)
Use Breast cancer

Regimen NOTE: Multiple variations are listed.
Variation 1 (adjuvant):
Fluorouracil: IV: 500 mg/m^2 day 1
[total dose/cycle = 500 mg/m^2]
Cyclophosphamide: IV: 500 mg/m^2 day 1
[total dose/cycle = 500 mg/m^2]
Epirubicin: IV: 100 mg/m^2 day 1
[total dose/cycle = 100 mg/m^2]
Repeat cycle every 21 days for 6 cycles
Variation 2 (metastatic):
Fluorouracil: IV: 500 mg/m^2 days 1 and 8
[total dose/cycle = 1000 mg/m^2]
Cyclophosphamide: IV: 400 mg/m^2 days 1 and 8
[total dose/cycle = 800 mg/m^2]
Epirubicin: IV: 50 mg/m^2 days 1 and 8
[total dose/cycle = 100 mg/m^2]
Repeat cycle every 21-28 days for 6 to 9 cycles

References

Variation 1:
Bonneterre J, Roché H, Kerbrat P, et al, "Epirubicin Increases Long-Term Survival in Adjuvant Chemotherapy of Patients With Poor-Prognosis, Node-Positive, Early Breast Cancer: 10-Year Follow-Up Results of the French Adjuvant Study Group 05 Randomized Trial," *J Clin Oncol*, 2005, 23(12):2686-93.

French Adjuvant Study Group. Benefit of a high-dose epirubicin regimen in adjuvant chemotherapy for node-positive breast cancer patients with poor prognostic factors: 5-year follow-up results of French Adjuvant Study Group 05 randomized trial. *J Clin Oncol*. 2001;19(3):602-11.

Variation 2:
Ackland SP, Anton A, Breitbach GP, et al, "Dose-Intensive Epirubicin-Based Chemotherapy is Superior to an Intensive Intravenous Cyclophosphamide, Methotrexate, and Fluorouracil Regimen in Metastatic Breast Cancer: A Randomized Multinational Study," *J Clin Oncol*, 2001, 19 (4):943-53.

FEC Oral (Breast)

Index Terms Fluorouracil, Epirubicin, Cyclophosphamide (Breast)

Use Breast cancer

Regimen NOTE: Multiple variations are listed.
Variation 1 (adjuvant):
Cyclophosphamide: Oral: 75 mg/m^2/day days 1 to 14
[total dose/cycle = 1050 mg/m^2]
Epirubicin: IV: 60 mg/m^2/day days 1 and 8
[total dose/cycle = 120 mg/m^2]
Fluorouracil: IV: 500 mg/m^2/day days 1 and 8
[total dose/cycle = 1000 mg/m^2]
Repeat cycle every 28 days for 6 cycles
Variation 1 (metastatic):
Cyclophosphamide: Oral: 100 mg/m^2/day days 1 to 14
[total dose/cycle = 1400 mg/m^2]
Epirubicin: IV: 30 mg/m^2/day days 1 and 8
[total dose/cycle = 60 mg/m^2]
Fluorouracil: IV: 500 mg/m^2/day days 1 and 8
[total dose/cycle = 1000 mg/m^2]
Repeat cycle every 28 days

References

Variation 1:

Levine MN, Bramwell VH, Pritchard KI, et al, "Randomized Trial of Intensive Cyclophosphamide, Epirubicin, and Fluorouracil Chemotherapy Compared With Cyclophosphamide, Methotrexate, and Fluorouracil in Premenopausal Women With Node-Positive Breast Cancer, National Cancer Institute of Canada Clinical Trials Group," *J Clin Oncol*, 1998, 16(8):2651-8.

Variation 2:

Estaban E, Lacave AJ, Fernández JL. Phase III trial of cyclophosphamide, epirubicin, fluorouracil (CEF) versus cyclophosphamide, mitoxantrone, fluorouracil (CNF) in women with metastatic breast cancer. *Breast Cancer Res Treat*. 1999;58(2):141-50.

◆ **FEC-P (Breast)** *see* FEC followed by Paclitaxel Weekly (Breast) on page 2112

FLAG (AML Induction)

Index Terms Fludarabine-ARAC-GCSF (AML Induction); Fludarabine-Cytarabine-Filgrastim (AML Induction)

Use Leukemia, acute myeloid

Regimen NOTE: Multiple variations are listed.

Variation 1:

Fludarabine: IV: 30 mg/m^2/day over 30 minutes days 1 to 5

[total dose/cycle = 150 mg/m^2]

Cytarabine: IV: 2 g/m^2/day over 4 hours days 1 to 5 (begin 4 hours after fludarabine infusion)

[total dose/cycle = 10 g/m^2]

Filgrastim: SubQ: 300 mcg 12 hours prior to start of fludarabine then 300 mcg/day days 2 through 5

[total dose/cycle = 1500 mcg]

followed by Filgrastim: SubQ: 300 mcg/day beginning one week after the end of treatment and continuing until complete neutrophil recovery

Variation 2:

Fludarabine: IV: 30 mg/m^2/day over 30 minutes days 1 to 5

[total dose/cycle = 150 mg/m^2]

Cytarabine: IV: 2 g/m^2/day over 4 hours days 1 to 5 (begin 3.5 hours after end of fludarabine infusion)

[total dose/cycle = 10 g/m^2]

Filgrastim: SubQ: 5 mcg/kg/day beginning 24 hours prior to start of fludarabine and continuing until ANC >500 mm^3

May repeat cycle one time for partial remission

Variation 3:

Fludarabine: IV: 30 mg/m^2/day over 30 minutes days 1 to 5

[total dose/cycle = 150 mg/m^2]

Cytarabine: IV: 2 g/m^2/day over 2 hours days 1 to 5 (begin 4 hours after the start of fludarabine infusion)

[total dose/cycle = 10 g/m^2]

Filgrastim: SubQ or IV: 300 mcg/day beginning the day prior to start of chemotherapy and continuing during chemotherapy and until ANC >1000 mm^3

May receive a second cycle

Variation 4:

Fludarabine: IV: 25 mg/m^2/day over 30 minutes days 1 to 5

[total dose/cycle = 125 mg/m^2]

Cytarabine: IV: 2 g/m^2/day over 4 hours days 1 to 5 (begin 4 hours after start of fludarabine infusion)

[total dose/cycle = 10 g/m^2]

Filgrastim: SubQ: 5 mcg/kg/day beginning 24 hours prior to start of cytarabine and continuing until ANC >500 mm^3

May repeat cycle in patients with complete remission and partial remission

References

Variation 1:
Clavio M, Carrara P, Miglino M, et al, "High Efficacy of Fludarabine-Containing Therapy (FLAG-FLANG) in Poor Risk Acute Myeloid Leukemia," *Haematologica*, 1996, 81(6):513-20.

Variation 2:
Montillo M, Mirto S, Petti MC, et al, "Fludarabine, Cytarabine, and G-CSF (FLAG) for the Treatment of Poor Risk Acute Myeloid Leukemia," *Am J Hematol*, 1998, 58(2):105-9.

Variation 3:
Virchis A, Koh M, Rankin P, et al, "Fludarabine, Cytosine Arabinoside, Granulocyte-Colony Stimulating Factor With or Without Idarubicin in the Treatment of High Risk Acute Leukaemia or Myelodysplastic Syndromes," *Br J Haematol*, 2004, 124(1):26-32.

Variation 4:
Ossenkoppele GJ, Graveland WJ, Sonneveld P, et al, "The Value of Fludarabine in Addition to ARA-C and G-CSF in the Treatment of Patients With High-Risk Myelodysplastic Syndromes and AML in Elderly Patients," *Blood*, 2004, 103(8):2908-13.

FLAG-IDA (AML Induction)

Use Leukemia, acute myeloid

Regimen NOTE: Multiple variations are listed.

Variation 1:

Fludarabine: IV: 30 mg/m^2/day over 30 minutes days 1 to 5
[total dose/cycle = 150 mg/m^2]

Cytarabine: IV: 2 g/m^2/day over 4 hours days 1 to 5 (begin 4 hours after the start of fludarabine)
[total dose/cycle = 10 g/m^2]

Idarubicin: IV: 10 mg/m^2/day days 1, 2, and 3
[total dose/cycle = 30 mg/m^2]

Filgrastim: SubQ: 5 mcg/kg from day 6 until ANC >500/mm^3

Variation 2:

Fludarabine: IV: 30 mg/m^2/day over 30 minutes days 1 to 5
[total dose/cycle = 150 mg/m^2]

Cytarabine: IV: 2 g/m^2/day over 2 hours days 1 to 5 (begin 4 hours after the start of fludarabine infusion)
[total dose/cycle = 10 g/m^2]

Idarubicin: IV: 8 mg/m^2/day over 30 minutes days 1, 2, and 3
[total dose/cycle = 24 mg/m^2]

Filgrastim: SubQ or IV: 300 mcg/day beginning the day prior to start of chemotherapy and continuing during chemotherapy and until ANC >1000/mm^3

May receive up to 2 cycles

Variation 3:

Fludarabine: IV: 30 mg/m^2/day over 30 minutes days 1 to 4
[total dose/cycle = 120 mg/m^2]

Cytarabine: IV: 2 g/m^2/day over 4 hours days 1 to 4 (begin 4 hours after fludarabine treatment)
[total dose/cycle = 8 g/m^2]

Idarubicin: IV: 10 mg/m^2/day days 1, 2, and 3
[total dose/cycle = 30 mg/m^2]

Filgrastim: Sub Q: see article for dose and frequency

References

Variation 1:
Pastore D, Specchia G, Carluccio P, et al, "FLAG-IDA in the Treatment of Refractory/Relapsed Acute Myeloid Leukemia: Single-Center Experience," *Ann Hematol*, 2003, 82(4):231-5.

◄

Variation 2:

Virchis A, Koh M, Rankin P, et al, "Fludarabine, Cytosine Arabinoside, Granulocyte-Colony Stimulating Factor With or Without Idarubicin in the Treatment of High Risk Acute Leukaemia or Myelodysplastic Syndromes," *Br J Haematol*, 2004, 124(1):26-32.

Variation 3:

De la Rubia J, Regadera AI, Martin G, et al, "FLAG-IDA Regimen in the Treatment of Patients With High-Risk Myeloid Malignancies," *Leuk Res*, 2002, 26(8):725-30.

♦ **FLO (Gastric/Esophageal)** *see* Fluorouracil-Leucovorin-Oxaliplatin (Gastric/Esophageal) *on page 2127*

♦ **FLOT (Esophageal Cancer)** *see* Docetaxel-Oxaliplatin-Leucovorin-Fluorouracil (Esophageal Cancer) *on page 2093*

FLOX (Colorectal)

Index Terms Oxaliplatin-Leucovorin-Fluorouracil (Colorectal)

Use Colorectal cancer

Regimen

Oxaliplatin: IV: 85 mg/m^2 over 2 hours days 1, 15, and 29

[total dose/cycle = 255 mg/m^2]

Leucovorin Calcium: IV: 500 mg/m^2/day over 2 hours weekly for 6 weeks on days 1, 8, 15, 22, 29, and 36

[total dose/cycle = 3000 mg/m^2]

Fluorouracil: IV: 500 mg/m^2/day bolus (1 hour after beginning the leucovorin infusion) weekly for 6 weeks on days 1, 8, 15, 22, 29, and 36

[total dose/cycle = 3000 mg/m^2]

Repeat cycle every 8 weeks for a total of 3 cycles

References

Kuebler JP, Wieand HS, O'Connell MJ, et al, "Oxaliplatin Combined With Weekly Bolus Fluorouracil and Leucovorin as Surgical Adjuvant Chemotherapy for Stage II and III Colon Cancer: Results From NSABP C-07," *J Clin Oncol*, 2007, 25(16):2198-204.

♦ **Fludarabine-ARAC-GCSF (AML Induction)** *see* FLAG (AML Induction) *on page 2114*

Fludarabine-Cyclophosphamide (CLL)

Index Terms Cyclophosphamide-Fludarabine (CLL); FC (CLL)

Use Leukemia, chronic lymphocytic

Regimen NOTE: Multiple variations are listed.

Variation 1:

Fludarabine: IV: 25 mg/m^2/day days 1, 2, and 3

[total dose/cycle = 75 mg/m^2]

Cyclophosphamide: IV: 250 mg/m^2/day days 1, 2, and 3

[total dose/cycle = 750 mg/m^2]

Repeat cycle every 4 weeks for up to 6 cycles

Variation 2:

Fludarabine: IV: 30 mg/m^2/day days 1, 2, and 3

[total dose/cycle = 90 mg/m^2]

Cyclophosphamide: IV: 250 mg/m^2/day days 1, 2, and 3

[total dose/cycle = 750 mg/m^2]

Repeat cycle every 4 weeks for up to 6 cycles

Variation 3:

Cyclophosphamide: IV: 600 mg/m^2 day 1

[total dose/cycle = 600 mg/m^2]

Fludarabine: IV: 20 mg/m²/day days 1 to 5
  [total dose/cycle = 100 mg/m²]
Repeat cycle every 4 weeks for up to 6 cycles
Variation 4:
  Fludarabine: IV: 30 mg/m²/day days 1, 2, and 3
    [total dose/cycle = 90 mg/m²]
  Cyclophosphamide: IV: 300 mg/m²/day days 1, 2, and 3
    [total dose/cycle = 900 mg/m²]
Repeat cycle every 4 weeks for up to 6 cycles
Variation 5:
  Fludarabine: IV: 30 mg/m²/day days 1, 2, and 3
    [total dose/cycle = 90 mg/m²]
  Cyclophosphamide: IV: 300 mg/m²/day days 1, 2, and 3
    [total dose/cycle = 900 mg/m²]
Repeat cycle every 4-6 weeks for up to 6 cycles

References

Variation 1:
Catovsky D, Richards S, Matutes E, et al, "Assessment of Fludarabine Plus Cyclophosphamide for Patients With Chronic Lymphocytic Leukaemia (The LRF CLL4 Trial): A Randomised Controlled Trial," *Lancet*, 2007, 370(9583):230-9.
O'Brien S, Moore JO, Boyd TE, et al, "Randomized Phase III Trial of Fludarabine Plus Cyclophosphamide With or Without Oblimersen Sodium (Bcl-2 Antisense) in Patients With Relapsed or Refractory Chronic Lymphocytic Leukemia," *J Clin Oncol*, 2007, 25(9):1114-20.
Variation 2:
Eichhorst BF, Busch R, Obwandner T, et al, "Health-Related Quality of Life in Younger Patients With Chronic Lymphocytic Leukemia Treated With Fludarabine Plus Cyclophosphamide or Fludarabine Alone for First-Line Therapy: A Study by the German CLL Study Group," *J Clin Oncol*, 2007, 25(13):1722-31.
Variation 3:
Flinn IW, Neuberg DS, Grever MR, et al, "Phase III Trial of Fludarabine Plus Cyclophosphamide Compared With Fludarabine for Patients With Previously Untreated Chronic Lymphocytic Leukemia: US Intergroup Trial E2997," *J Clin Oncol*, 2007, 25(7):793-8.
Variation 4:
Wierda W, O'Brien S, Faderl S, et al, "A Retrospective Comparison of Three Sequential Groups of Patients With Recurrent/Refractory Chronic Lymphocytic Leukemia Treated With Fludarabine-Based Regimens," *Cancer*, 2006, 106(2):337-45.
Variation 5:
O'Brien SM, Kantarjian HM, Cortes J, et al, "Results of the Fludarabine and Cyclophosphamide Combination Regimen in Chronic Lymphocytic Leukemia," *J Clin Oncol*, 2001, 19(5):1414-20.

Fludarabine-Cyclophosphamide-Mitoxantrone-Rituximab (NHL-Follicular)

Index Terms FCMR (NHL-Follicular Cell); R-FCM (NHL-Follicular Cell); Rituximab-Fludarabine-Cyclophosphamide-Mitoxantrone (NHL-Follicular Cell)

Use Lymphoma, non-Hodgkin (follicular cell relapsed, refractory)

Regimen NOTE: Multiple variations are listed.

Consider pretherapy cytoreduction with cyclophosphamide 200 mg/m²/day over 1 hour for 3 to 5 days for patients with high tumor burden (bulky disease >10 cm) and/or lymphocytes >20,000/mm³ for both variations below.

Variation 1:
  Rituximab: IV: 375 mg/m² day 1
    [total dose/cycle = 375 mg/m²]
  Fludarabine: IV: 25 mg/m²/day over 30 minutes days 2, 3, and 4
    [total dose/cycle = 75 mg/m²]
  Cyclophosphamide: IV: 200 mg/m²/day over 4 hours days 2, 3, and 4
    [total dose/cycle = 600 mg/m²]

Mitoxantrone: IV: 8 mg/m^2 over 30 minutes day 2
[total dose/cycle = 8 mg/m^2]
Repeat cycle every 28 days for total of 4 cycles
followed by (in patients with complete or partial remission):
Maintenance rituximab (begin 3 months after completion of induction cycle 4):
Rituximab: IV: 375 mg/m^2/day days 1, 8, 15, and 22
[total dose/cycle = 1,500 mg/m^2]
Repeat maintenance cycle once after 3 months (6 months after completion of induction cycle 4) for a total of 2 maintenance cycles.
Variation 2:
Rituximab: IV: 375 mg/m^2 day 1
[total dose/cycle = 375 mg/m^2]
Fludarabine: IV: 25 mg/m^2/day over 30 minutes days 2, 3, and 4
[total dose/cycle = 75 mg/m^2]
Cyclophosphamide: IV: 200 mg/m^2/day over 4 hours days 2, 3, and 4
[total dose/cycle = 600 mg/m^2]
Mitoxantrone: IV: 8 mg/m^2 over 30 minutes day 2
[total dose/cycle = 8 mg/m^2]
Repeat cycle every 28 days for total of 4 cycles
followed by (in patients with complete or partial remission):
Maintenance rituximab (begin 3 months after completion of induction cycle 4):
Rituximab: IV: 375 mg/m^2/day days 1, 8, 15, and 22
[total dose/cycle = 1,500 mg/m^2]
Repeat maintenance cycle once after 6 months (9 months after completion of induction cycle 4) for a total of 2 maintenance cycles.

References

Variation 1:
Forstpointner R, Dreyling M, Repp R, et al. The addition of rituximab to a combination of fludarabine, cyclophosphamide, mitoxantrone (FCM) significantly increases the response rate and prolongs survival as compared with FCM alone in patients with relapsed and refractory follicular and mantle cell lymphomas: results of a prospective randomized study of the German Low-Grade Lymphoma Study Group. *Blood.* 2004;104(10):3064-3071.
Variation 2:
Forstpointner R, Unterhalt M, Dreyling M, et al. Maintenance therapy with rituximab leads to a significant prolongation of response duration after salvage therapy with a combination of rituximab, fludarabine, cyclophosphamide, and mitoxantrone (R-FCM) in patients with recurring and refractory follicular and mantle cell lymphomas: results of a prospective randomized study of the German Low Grade Lymphoma Study Group (GLSG). *Blood.* 2006;108(13):4003-4008.

Fludarabine-Cyclophosphamide (NHL-Mantle Cell)

Index Terms CF (NHL-Mantle Cell); Cyclophosphamide-Fludarabine (NHL-Mantle Cell); FC (NHL-Mantle Cell)
Use Lymphoma, non-Hodgkin (Mantle cell)
Regimen NOTE: Multiple variations are listed.
Variation 1:
Fludarabine: IV: 20 mg/m^2/day days 1 to 5
[total dose/cycle = 100 mg/m^2]
Cyclophosphamide: IV: 800 mg/m^2/dose day 1
[total dose/cycle = 800 mg/m^2]
Repeat cycle every 3-4 weeks for up to a total of 5 cycles
Variation 2:
Fludarabine: IV: 20 mg/m^2/day days 1 to 5
[total dose/cycle = 100 mg/m^2]

Cyclophosphamide: IV: 1000 mg/m^2/dose day 1
[total dose/cycle = 1000 mg/m^2]
Repeat cycle every 3-4 weeks for up to a total of 5 cycles
Variation 3:
Fludarabine: IV: 25 mg/m^2/day days 1 to 4
[total dose/cycle = 100 mg/m^2]
Cyclophosphamide: IV: 1000 mg/m^2/dose day 1
[total dose/cycle = 1000 mg/m^2]
Repeat cycle every 3-4 weeks for up to a total of 5 cycles

References
Variations 1-3:
Cohen BJ, Moskowitz C, Straus D, et al, "Cyclophosphamide/Fludarabine (CF) Is Active in the Treatment of Mantle Cell Lymphoma," *Leuk Lymphoma*, 2001, 42(5):1015-22.

Fludarabine-Cyclophosphamide-Ofatumumab (CLL)

Index Terms OFA-FC (CLL); Ofatumumab-Fludarabine-Cyclophosphamide (CLL)

Use Leukemia, chronic lymphocytic (relapsed)

Regimen
Cycle 1:
Ofatumumab: IV: 300 mg day 1
followed by:
Ofatumumab: IV: 1,000 mg day 8
[total dose/cycle 1 = 1,300 mg]
Fludarabine: IV: 25 mg/m^2/day days 1, 2, and 3
[total dose/cycle = 75 mg/m^2]
Cyclophosphamide: IV: 250 mg/m^2/day days 1, 2, and 3
[total dose/cycle = 750 mg/m^2]
Treatment cycle duration is 28 days
Cycles 2 to 6:
Ofatumumab: IV: 1,000 mg day 1
[total dose/cycle = 1,000 mg]
Fludarabine: IV: 25 mg/m^2/day days 1, 2, and 3
[total dose/cycle = 75 mg/m^2]
Cyclophosphamide: IV: 250 mg/m^2/day days 1, 2, and 3
[total dose/cycle = 750 mg/m^2]
Repeat cycle every 28 days for a total of 6 cycles

References
Robak T, Warzocha K, Govind Babu K, et al. Ofatumumab plus fludarabine and cyclophosphamide in relapsed chronic lymphocytic leukemia: results from the COMPLEMENT 2 trial. *Leuk Lymphoma*. 2017;58(5):1084-1093.

Fludarabine-Cyclophosphamide-Rituximab (CLL)

Index Terms FCR (CLL); R-FC (CLL); Rituximab-Fludarabine-Cyclophosphamide (CLL)

Use Leukemia, chronic lymphocytic (first-line and refractory)

Regimen
Cycle 1:
Rituximab: IV: 375 mg/m^2 day 1
[total dose/cycle = 375 mg/m^2]
Fludarabine: IV: 25 mg/m^2/day days 2, 3, and 4
[total dose/cycle = 75 mg/m^2]

Cyclophosphamide: IV: 250 mg/m^2/day days 2, 3, and 4
[total dose/cycle = 750 mg/m^2]
Treatment cycle duration is 28 days
Cycles 2 to 6:
Rituximab: IV: 500 mg/m^2 day 1
[total dose/cycle = 500 mg/m^2]
Fludarabine: IV: 25 mg/m^2/day days 1, 2, and 3
[total dose/cycle = 75 mg/m^2]
Cyclophosphamide: IV: 250 mg/m^2/day days 1, 2, and 3
[total dose/cycle = 750 mg/m^2]
Repeat cycle every 28 days for a total of 6 cycles

References
Robak T, Dmoszynska A, Solal-Céligny P, et al. Rituximab plus fludarabine and cyclophosphamide prolongs progression-free survival compared with fludarabine and cyclophosphamide alone in previously treated chronic lymphocytic leukemia. *J Clin Oncol.* 2010;28(10):1756-1765.

Hallek M, Fischer K, Fingerle-Rowson G, et al. Addition of rituximab to fludarabine and cyclophosphamide in patients with chronic lymphocytic leukaemia: a randomised, open-label, phase 3 trial. *Lancet.* 2010;376(9747):1164-1174.

Fludarabine-Cyclophosphamide-Rituximab (NHL-Follicular)

Index Terms FCR (NHL-Follicular); Rituximab-Fludarabine-Cyclophospha-mide (NHL-Follicular)
Use Lymphoma, non-Hodgkin (Follicular lymphoma)
Regimen
Cycle 1:
Rituximab: IV: 375 mg/m^2 day 15
[total dose/cycle = 375 mg/m^2]
Fludarabine: IV: 25 mg/m^2/day days 1, 2, and 3
[total dose/cycle = 75 mg/m^2]
Cyclophosphamide: IV: 300 mg/m^2/day days 1, 2, and 3
[total dose/cycle = 900 mg/m^2]
Treatment cycle is 3 weeks
Cycles 2-4:
Rituximab: IV: 375 mg/m^2 day 1
[total dose/cycle = 375 mg/m^2]
Fludarabine: IV: 25 mg/m^2/day days 1, 2, and 3
[total dose/cycle = 75 mg/m^2]
Cyclophosphamide: IV: 300 mg/m^2/day days 1, 2, and 3
[total dose/cycle = 900 mg/m^2]
Each treatment cycle is 3 weeks

References
Sacchi S, Pozzi S, Marcheselli R, et al, "Rituximab in Combination With Fludarabine and Cyclophosphamide in the Treatment of Patients With Recurrent Follicular Lymphoma," *Cancer,* 2007, 110(1):121-8.

♦ **Fludarabine-Cytarabine-Filgrastim (AML Induction)** *see* FLAG (AML Induction) *on page* 2114

Fludarabine-Mitoxantrone-Dexamethasone-Rituximab

Index Terms FNDR (NHL); Rituximab-Fludarabine-Mitoxantrone-Dexametha-sone
Use Lymphoma, non-Hodgkin

Regimen
Cycle 1:
  Rituximab: IV: 375 mg/m²/day days 1 and 8
    [total dose/cycle = 750 mg/m²]
  Fludarabine: IV: 25 mg/m²/day days 1, 2, and 3
    [total dose/cycle = 75 mg/m²]
  Mitoxantrone: IV: 10 mg/m²/dose day 1
    [total dose/cycle = 10 mg/m²]
  Dexamethasone: IV or Oral: 20 mg/m²/day days 1 to 5
    [total dose/cycle = 100 mg/m²]
  Treatment cycle is 28 days
Cycles 2-5:
  Rituximab: IV: 375 mg/m² day 1
    [total dose/cycle = 375 mg/m²]
  Fludarabine: IV: 25 mg/m²/day days 2, 3, and 4
    [total dose/cycle = 75 mg/m²]
  Mitoxantrone: IV: 10 mg/m²/dose day 2
    [total dose/cycle = 10 mg/m²]
  Dexamethasone: IV or Oral: 20 mg/m²/day days 1 to 5
    [total dose/cycle = 100 mg/m²]
  Repeat cycle every 28 days
Cycles 6-8:
  Fludarabine: IV: 25 mg/m²/day days 1, 2, and 3
    [total dose/cycle = 75 mg/m²]
  Mitoxantrone: IV: 10 mg/m²/dose day 1
    [total dose/cycle = 10 mg/m²]
  Dexamethasone: IV or Oral: 20 mg/m²/day days 1 to 5
    [total dose/cycle = 100 mg/m²]
  Repeat cycle every 28 days
  followed by:
    Interferon maintenance:
      Interferon alfa-2b: SubQ: 3 million units/m² days 1 to 14
        [total dose/cycle = 42 million units/m²]
      Dexamethasone: Oral: 8 mg/day days 1, 2, and 3
        [total dose/cycle = 24 mg]
      Repeat cycle every month for 1 year

References
McLaughlin P, Hagemeister FB, Rodriguez MA, et al, "Safety of Fludarabine, Mitoxantrone, and Dexamethasone Combined With Rituximab in the Treatment of Stage IV Indolent Lymphoma," *Semin Oncol*, 2000, 27(6 Suppl 12):37-41.

Fludarabine-Rituximab (CLL)
Index Terms Rituximab-Fludarabine (CLL)
Use Leukemia, chronic lymphocytic
Regimen
Cycle 1:
  Rituximab: IV: 375 mg/m²/day days 1 and 4 (or 50 mg/m² day 1, followed by 325 mg/m² day 3, and then 375 mg/m² day 5)
    [total dose/cycle = 750 mg/m²]
  Fludarabine: IV: 25 mg/m²/day over 20 to 30 minutes days 1 to 5
    [total dose/cycle = 125 mg/m²]
  Treatment cycle is 28 days

◀ Cycle 2 to 6:
Rituximab: IV: 375 mg/m^2 day 1
[total dose/cycle = 375 mg/m^2]
Fludarabine: IV: 25 mg/m^2/day over 20 to 30 minutes days 1 to 5
[total dose/cycle = 125 mg/m^2]
Repeat cycle every 28 days for a total of 6 cycles

References

Byrd JC, Peterson BL, Morrison VA, et al. Randomized phase 2 study of fludarabine with concurrent vs sequential treatment with rituximab in symptomatic, untreated patients with B-cell chronic lymphocytic leukemia: results from cancer and leukemia group B 9712 (CALGB 9712). *Blood.* 2003;101(1):6-14.

Woyach JA, Ruppert AS, Heerema NA, et al. Chemoimmunotherapy with fludarabine and rituximab produces extended overall survival and progression-free survival in chronic lympho-cytic leukemia: long-term follow-up of CALGB study 9712. *J Clin Oncol.* 2011;29(10):1349-1355.

Fludarabine-Rituximab (NHL-Follicular)

Index Terms Rituximab-Fludarabine (NHL-Follicular)
Use Lymphoma, non-Hodgkin (Follicular lymphoma)
Regimen
Week 1:
Rituximab: IV: 375 mg/m^2/dose for 2 doses 4 days apart
[total dose/week = 750 mg/m^2]
Week 2:
Fludarabine: IV: 25 mg/m^2/day days 1 to 5
[total dose/week = 125 mg/m^2]
Week 5:
Rituximab: IV: 375 mg/m^2/dose day 5
[total dose/week = 375 mg/m^2]
Week 6:
Fludarabine: IV: 25 mg/m^2/day days 1 to 5
[total dose/week = 125 mg/m^2]
Week 10:
Fludarabine: IV: 25 mg/m^2/day days 1 to 5
[total dose/week = 125 mg/m^2]
Week 13:
Rituximab: IV: 375 mg/m^2/dose day 5
[total dose/week = 375 mg/m^2]
Week 14:
Fludarabine: IV: 25 mg/m^2/day days 1 to 5
[total dose/week = 125 mg/m^2]
Week 18:
Fludarabine: IV: 25 mg/m^2/day days 1 to 5
[total dose/week = 125 mg/m^2]
Week 21:
Rituximab: IV: 375 mg/m^2/dose day 5
[total dose/week = 375 mg/m^2]
Week 22:
Fludarabine: IV: 25 mg/m^2/day days 1 to 5
[total dose/week = 125 mg/m^2]
Week 26:
Rituximab: IV: 375 mg/m^2/dose for 2 doses 4 days apart
[total dose/week = 750 mg/m^2]

References

Czuczman MS, Koryzna A, Mohr A, et al, "Rituximab in Combination With Fludarabine Chemo-therapy in Low-Grade or Follicular Lymphoma," *J Clin Oncol*, 2005, 23(4):694-704.

Fluorouracil-Carboplatin (Head and Neck Cancer)

Index Terms Carboplatin-Fluorouracil (Head and Neck Cancer)

Use Head and neck cancer

Regimen NOTE: Multiple variations are listed.

Variation 1:

Fluorouracil: IV: 600 mg/m^2/day continuous infusion days 1 to 4
[total dose/cycle = 2400 mg/m^2]
Carboplatin: IV: 70 mg/m^2/day days 1 to 4
[total dose/cycle = 280 mg/m^2]
Repeat cycle every 3 weeks for 3 cycles

Variation 2:

Fluorouracil: IV: 1000 mg/m^2/day continuous infusion days 1 to 4
[total dose/cycle = 4000 mg/m^2]
Carboplatin: IV: 300 mg/m^2/dose day 1 (may escalate to 360 mg/m^2/dose in
future cycles for grade 0 or 1 hematologic toxicity)
[total dose/cycle = 300-360 mg/m^2]
Repeat cycle every 28 weeks

Variation 3:

Carboplatin: IV: 400 mg/m^2 day 1
[total dose/cycle = 400 mg/m^2]
Fluorouracil: IV: 1000 mg/m^2/day continuous infusion days 1 to 4
[total dose/cycle = 4000 mg/m^2]
Repeat cycle every 28 days for a total of 2 or 3 cycles

References

Variation 1:

Denis F, Garaud P, Bardet E, et al, "Final Results of the 94-01 French Head and Neck Oncology
and Radiotherapy Group Randomized Trial Comparing Radiotherapy Alone With Concomitant
Radiochemotherapy in Advanced-Stage Oropharynx Carcinoma," *J Clin Oncol*, 2004, 22
(1):69-76.

Variation 2:

Forastiere AA, Metch B, Schuller DE, et al, "Randomized Comparison of Cisplatin Plus Fluorouracil and Carboplatin Plus Fluorouracil Versus Methotrexate in Advanced Squamous-Cell
Carcinoma of the Head and Neck: A Southwest Oncology Group Study," *J Clin Oncol*, 1992,
10(8):1245-51.

Gregoire V, Beauduin M, Humblet Y, et al, "A Phase I-II Trial of Induction Chemotherapy With
Carboplatin and Fluorouracil in Locally Advanced Head and Neck Squamous Cell Carcinoma: A
Report From the UCL-Oncology Group, Belgium," *J Clin Oncol*, 1991, 9(8):1385-02.

- **Fluorouracil, Epirubicin, Cyclophosphamide (Breast)** *see* FEC IV (Breast) *on page 2112*
- **Fluorouracil, Epirubicin, Cyclophosphamide (Breast)** *see* FEC Oral (Breast) *on page 2113*
- **Fluorouracil, Epirubicin, Cyclophosphamide, Docetaxel (Breast)** *see* FEC followed by Docetaxel Every 3 Weeks (Breast) *on page 2112*
- **Fluorouracil, Epirubicin, Cyclophosphamide, Paclitaxel (Breast)** *see* FEC followed by Paclitaxel Weekly (Breast) *on page 2112*

Fluorouracil-Hydroxyurea (Head and Neck Cancer)

Index Terms Hydroxyurea-Fluorouracil (Head and Neck Cancer)

Use Head and neck cancer

Regimen NOTE: Administered with concurrent radiation therapy

Fluorouracil: IV: 800 mg/m^2/day continuous infusion days 1 to 5
[total dose/cycle = 4000 mg/m^2]

Hydroxyurea: Oral: 1000 mg/dose every 12 hours for 11 doses beginning day 1
[total dose/cycle = 11,000 mg]

Repeat cycle every other week for a total therapy duration of 13 weeks

References

Garden AS, Harris J, Vokes EE, et al, "Preliminary Results of Radiation Therapy Oncology Group 97-03: A Randomized Phase II Trial of Concurrent Radiation and Chemotherapy for Advanced Squamous Cell Carcinomas of the Head and Neck," *J Clin Oncol*, 2004, 22(14):2856-64.

- **Fluorouracil-Leucovorin-Bevacizumab (Colorectal)** *see* Bevacizumab-Fluorouracil-Leucovorin (Colorectal) *on page 1992*

Fluorouracil-Leucovorin Bolus (Colorectal)

Index Terms 5FU-Leucovorin Bolus (Colorectal); 5FU-LV Bolus (Colorectal); FU-LV Bolus (Colorectal); Leucovorin-Fluorouracil (Colorectal)

Use Colorectal cancer (adjuvant and metastatic)

Regimen NOTE: Multiple variations are listed.

Variation 1 (Mayo Regimen; adjuvant treatment):

Leucovorin Calcium: IV push: 20 mg/m^2/day days 1 to 5
[total dose/cycle = 100 mg/m^2]

Fluorouracil: IV push: 425 mg/m^2/day days 1 to 5
[total dose/cycle = 2,125 mg/m^2]

Repeat cycle at 4 weeks, 8 weeks, and every 5 weeks thereafter for a total of 6 cycles

Variation 2 (Mayo Regimen; metastatic treatment):

Leucovorin Calcium: IV push: 20 mg/m^2/day days 1 to 5
[total dose/cycle = 100 mg/m^2]

Fluorouracil: IV push: 425 mg/m^2/day days 1 to 5
[total dose/cycle = 2,125 mg/m^2]

Repeat cycle at 4 weeks, 8 weeks, and every 5 weeks thereafter

Variation 3 (Roswell Regimen; adjuvant treatment):

Leucovorin Calcium: IV: 500 mg/m^2 over 2 hours days 1, 8, 15, 22, 29, and 36
[total dose/cycle = 3,000 mg/m^2]

Fluorouracil: IV push: 500 mg/m^2 days 1, 8, 15, 22, 29, and 36; start 1 hour after start of leucovorin infusion
[total dose/cycle = 3,000 mg/m^2]

Repeat cycle every 8 weeks for a total of 4 cycles

Variation 4 (Roswell Regimen):
  Leucovorin Calcium: IV: 500 mg/m² over 2 hours days 1, 8, 15, 22, 29, and 36
  [total dose/cycle = 3,000 mg/m²]
  Fluorouracil: IV push: 500 mg/m² days 1, 8, 15, 22, 29, and 36; start 1 hour after start of leucovorin infusion
  [total dose/cycle = 3,000 mg/m²]
  Repeat cycle every 8 weeks until disease progression or unacceptable toxicity
Variation 5 (metastatic disease):
  Leucovorin Calcium: IV: 20 mg/m² over 2 hours day 1
  [total dose/cycle = 20 mg/m²]
  Fluorouracil: IV push: 500 mg/m² day 1; start 1 hour after start of leucovorin infusion
  [total dose/cycle = 500 mg/m²]
  Repeat cycle weekly (may require treatment delay or dose reduction for toxicity) until disease progression or unacceptable toxicity

References

Variations 1 and 3:
Haller DG, Catalano PJ, Macdonald JS, et al. Phase III study of fluorouracil, leucovorin, and levamisole in high-risk stage II and III colon cancer: final report of Intergroup 0089. J Clin Oncol. 2005;23(34):8671-8678.
O'Connell MJ, Mailliard JA, Kahn MJ, et al. Controlled trial of fluorouracil and low-dose leucovorin given for 6 months as postoperative adjuvant therapy for colon cancer. J Clin Oncol. 1997;15 (1):246-250.
Variation 2:
Poon MA, O'Connell MJ, Moertel CG, et al. Biochemical modulation of fluorouracil: evidence of significant improvement of survival and quality of life in patients with advanced colorectal carcinoma. J Clin Oncol. 1989;7(10):1407-1418.
Variation 4:
Haller DG, Catalano PJ, Macdonald JS, et al. Phase III study of fluorouracil, leucovorin, and levamisole in high-risk stage II and III colon cancer: final report of Intergroup 0089. J Clin Oncol. 2005;23(34):8671-8678.
Jäger E, Heike M, Bernhard H, et al. Weekly high-dose leucovorin versus low-dose leucovorin combined with fluorouracil in advanced colorectal cancer: results of a randomized multicenter trial. Study Group for Palliative Treatment of Metastatic Colorectal Cancer Study Protocol 1. J Clin Oncol. 1996;14(8):2274-2279.
Variation 5:
Jäger E, Heike M, Bernhard H, et al. Weekly high-dose leucovorin versus low-dose leucovorin combined with fluorouracil in advanced colorectal cancer: results of a randomized multicenter trial. Study Group for Palliative Treatment of Metastatic Colorectal Cancer Study Protocol 1. J Clin Oncol. 1996;14(8):2274-2279.

Fluorouracil-Leucovorin Infusional (Colorectal)

Index Terms 5FU-LV Infusional (Colorectal); FU-Leucovorin Infusional (Colorectal); FU-LV Infusional (Colorectal)

Use Colorectal cancer (adjuvant and metastatic)

Regimen NOTE: Multiple variations are listed.

Variation 1 (adjuvant):
  Leucovorin Calcium: IV: 200 mg/m²/day over 2 hours days 1 and 2
  [total dose/cycle = 400 mg/m²]
  Fluorouracil: IV bolus: 400 mg/m²/day days 1 and 2
  followed by IV: 600 mg/m²/day continuous infusion (CI) over 22 hours days 1 and 2
  [total fluorouracil dose/cycle (bolus and CI) = 2,000 mg/m²]
  Repeat cycle 14 days for a total of 12 cycles

◀ Variation 2 (metastatic):
Leucovorin Calcium: IV: 200 mg/m^2/day over 2 hours days 1 and 2
[total dose/cycle = 400 mg/m^2]
Fluorouracil: IV bolus: 400 mg/m^2/day days 1 and 2
followed by IV: 600 mg/m^2/day CI over 22 hours days 1 and 2
[total fluorouracil dose/cycle (bolus and CI) = 2,000 mg/m^2]
Repeat cycle 14 days until disease progression or unacceptable toxicity

References

Variation 1:
André T, Quinaux E, Louvet C, et al. Phase III study comparing a semimonthly with a monthly regimen of fluorouracil and leucovorin as adjuvant treatment for stage II and III colon cancer patients: final results of GERCOR C96.1. *J Clin Oncol.* 2007;25(24):3732-3738.
Variation 2:
de Gramont A, Bosset JF, Milan C, et al. Randomized trial comparing monthly low-dose leucovorin and fluorouracil bolus with bimonthly high-dose leucovorin and fluorouracil bolus plus continuous infusion for advanced colorectal cancer: a French intergroup study. *J Clin Oncol.* 1997;15 (2):808-815.

◆ **Fluorouracil-Leucovorin-Irinotecan (Esophageal Cancer)** *see* Irinotecan-Fluorouracil-Leucovorin (Esophageal Cancer) *on page 2160*

◆ **Fluorouracil-Leucovorin-Irinotecan (Gastric Cancer)** *see* Irinotecan-Leucovorin-Fluorouracil (Gastric Cancer) *on page 2160*

Fluorouracil-Leucovorin-Irinotecan (Liposomal) (Pancreatic)

Use Pancreatic cancer (metastatic, gemcitabine-refractory)

Regimen

Irinotecan (Liposomal): IV: 70 mg/m^2 over 90 minutes day 1 (reduce initial starting dose to 50 mg/m^2 in patients known to be homozygous for the UGT1A1*28 allele, dose may be increased to 70 mg/m^2 as tolerated in subsequent cycles)
[total dose/cycle = 70 mg/m^2]
Leucovorin Calcium: IV: 400 mg/m^2 over 30 minutes, given after irinotecan (liposomal) infusion, day 1
[total dose/cycle = 400 mg/m^2]
Fluorouracil: IV: 2,400 mg/m^2 continuous infusion over 46 hours beginning day 1
[total fluorouracil dose/cycle = 2,400 mg/m^2]
Repeat cycle every 14 days until disease progression or unacceptable toxicity

References

Wang-Gillam A, Li CP, Bodoky G, et al. Nanoliposomal irinotecan with fluorouracil and folinic acid in metastatic pancreatic cancer after previous gemcitabine-based therapy (NAPOLI-1): a global, randomised, open-label, phase 3 trial. *Lancet.* 2016;387(10018):545-557.

Fluorouracil-Leucovorin-Irinotecan (Saltz Regimen) (Colorectal)

Index Terms 5FU-LV-CPT-11 (Saltz Regimen) (Colorectal); Irinotecan-Fluorouracil-Leucovorin (Saltz Regimen) (Colorectal); Saltz Regimen (Colorectal)

Use Colorectal cancer

Regimen

Irinotecan: IV: 125 mg/m^2/day over 90 minutes days 1, 8, 15, and 22
[total dose/cycle = 500 mg/m^2]
Leucovorin Calcium: IV bolus: 20 mg/m^2/day days 1, 8, 15, and 22
[total dose/cycle = 80 mg/m^2]

Fluorouracil: IV bolus: 500 mg/m^2/day days 1, 8, 15, and 22
[total dose/cycle = 2000 mg/m^2]
Repeat cycle every 42 days until disease progression or unacceptable toxicity

References

Saltz LB, Cox JV, Blanke C, et al. Irinotecan plus fluorouracil and leucovorin for metastatic colorectal cancer. Irinotecan study group. N Engl J Med. 2000;343(13):905-914.

◆ **Fluorouracil, Leucovorin, Oxaliplatin (Colorectal)** *see* FOLFOX4 (Colorectal) *on page 2130*

◆ **Fluorouracil-Leucovorin-Oxaliplatin (Colorectal)** *see* FOLFOX6 and mFOLFOX6 (Colorectal) *on page 2131*

Fluorouracil-Leucovorin-Oxaliplatin (Gastric/Esophageal)

Index Terms FLO (Gastric/Esophageal); FOLFOX (Gastric/Esophageal); Oxaliplatin–Leucovorin–Fluorouracil (Gastric/Esophageal)

Use Esophageal cancer; Gastric cancer

Regimen NOTE: Multiple variations are listed.

Variation 1:
Oxaliplatin: IV: 85 mg/m^2 over 2 hours day 1
[total dose/cycle = 85 mg/m^2]
Leucovorin Calcium: IV: 200 mg/m^2 over 2 hours day 1
[total dose/cycle = 200 mg/m^2]
Fluorouracil: IV: 2,600 mg/m^2 continuous infusion over 24 hours day 1
[total dose/cycle = 2,600 mg/m^2]
Repeat cycle every 14 days until disease progression or unacceptable toxicity

Variation 2:
Oxaliplatin: IV: 85 mg/m^2 over 2 hours day 1
[total dose/cycle = 85 mg/m^2]
Leucovorin Calcium: IV: 200 mg/m^2 over 2 hours day 1
[total dose/cycle = 200 mg/m^2]
Fluorouracil: IV bolus: 400 mg/m^2 over 10 minutes day 1
followed by IV: 1,600 mg/m^2 continuous infusion over 48 hours beginning day 1
[total dose/cycle = 2,000 mg/m^2]
Repeat cycle every 14 days for a total of 6 cycles; cycles 1 to 3 were administered with radiation therapy and cycles 4 to 6 were administered after completion of radiation therapy

References

Variation 1:
Al-Batran SE, Hartmann JT, Probst S, et al. Phase III trial in metastatic gastroesophageal adenocarcinoma with fluorouracil, leucovorin plus either oxaliplatin or cisplatin: a study of the arbeitsgemeinschaft internistische onkologie. J Clin Oncol. 2008;26(9):1435-1442.
Variation 2:
Conroy T, Galais MP, Raoul JL, et al. Definitive chemoradiotherapy with FOLFOX versus fluorouracil and cisplatin in patients with oesophageal cancer (PRODIGE5/ACCORD17): final results of a randomised, phase 2/3 trial. Lancet Oncol. 2014;15(3):305-314.

◆ **Fluorouracil, Leucovorin, Oxaliplatin (Pancreatic)** *see* FOLFOX (Pancreatic) *on page 2133*

Fluorouracil-Leucovorin (Pancreatic)

Index Terms 5FU-Folinic Acid (Pancreatic); 5FU-Leucovorin (Pancreatic); 5FU-LV (Pancreatic)

◄ **Use** 5FU-Folinic Acid (Pancreatic)
Regimen
Leucovorin Calcium: IV: 20 mg/m^2/day bolus days 1 to 5
[total dose/cycle = 100 mg/m^2]
Fluorouracil: IV: 425 mg/m^2/day bolus days 1 to 5
[total dose/cycle = 2125 mg/m^2]
Repeat cycle every 28 days for 6 cycles

References

Neoptolemos JP, Stocken DD, Bassi C, et al, "Adjuvant Chemotherapy With Fluorouracil Plus Folinic Acid Vs Gemcitabine Following Pancreatic Cancer Resection: A Randomized Controlled Trial," *JAMA*, 2010, 304(10):1073-81.

Neoptolemos JP, Stocken DD, Friess H, et al, "A Randomized Trial of Chemoradiotherapy and Chemotherapy After Resection of Pancreatic Cancer," *N Engl J Med*, 2004, 350(12):1200-10.

Neoptolemos JP, Stocken DD, Smith CT, et al, "Adjuvant 5-Fluorouracil and Folinic Acid Vs Observation for Pancreatic Cancer: Composite Data From the ESPAC-1 and -3 (v1) Trials," *Br J Cancer*, 2009, 100(2):246-50.

Fluorouracil-Mitomycin (Anal Cancer)

Index Terms Mitomycin-Fluorouracil (Anal Cancer)
Use Anal cancer
Regimen NOTE: Multiple variations are listed.
Variation 1 (in combination with radiotherapy):
Fluorouracil: IV: 1000 mg/m^2/day continuous infusion days 1 to 4 and days 29 to 32
[total dose/cycle = 8000 mg/m^2]
Mitomycin: IV: 10 mg/m^2/day (maximum dose: 20 mg) days 1 and 29
[total dose/cycle = 20 mg/m^2; maximum: 40 mg]
Variation 2 (in combination with radiotherapy):
Fluorouracil: IV: 1000 mg/m^2/day continuous infusion days 1 to 4
[total dose/cycle = 4000 mg/m^2]
Mitomycin: IV: 10 mg/m^2/dose (maximum dose: 20 mg) day 1
[total dose/cycle = 10 mg/m^2; maximum: 20 mg]
Repeat cycle in 28 days (total of 2 cycles)

References

Variation 1:
Ajani JA, Winter KA, Gunderson LL, et al, "Fluorouracil, Mitomycin, and Radiotherapy vs Fluorouracil, Cisplatin, and Radiotherapy for Carcinoma of the Anal Canal: A Randomized Controlled Trial," *JAMA*, 2008, 299(16):1914-21.

Variation 2:
Flam M, John M, Pajak TF, et al, "Role of Mitomycin in Combination With Fluorouracil and Radiotherapy, and of Salvage Chemoradiation in the Definitive Nonsurgical Treatment of Epidermoid Carcinoma of the Anal Canal: Results of a Phase III Randomized Intergroup Study," *J Clin Oncol*, 1996, 14(9):2527-39.

◆ **Fluorouracil-Oxaliplatin-Epirubicin (Gastric/Esophageal)** *see* Epirubicin-Oxaliplatin-Fluorouracil (Gastric/Esophageal) *on page 2105*

◆ **Fluorouracil-Paclitaxel (Esophageal Cancer)** *see* Paclitaxel-Fluorouracil (Esophageal Cancer) *on page 2185*

◆ **FNDR (NHL)** *see* Fludarabine-Mitoxantrone-Dexamethasone-Rituximab *on page 2120*

FOLFIRI (Colorectal)

Use Colorectal cancer
Regimen
Irinotecan: IV: 180 mg/m^2 over 90 minutes day 1
[total dose/cycle = 180 mg/m^2]

Leucovorin Calcium: IV: 400 mg/m^2 over 2 hours day 1

[total dose/cycle = 400 mg/m^2]

Fluorouracil: IV bolus: 400 mg/m^2 day 1

followed by IV: 2400 mg/m^2 continuous infusion over 46 hours beginning day 1

[total fluorouracil dose/cycle (bolus and continuous infusion) = 2800 mg/m^2]

Repeat cycle every 14 days until disease progression or unacceptable toxicity

References

Fuchs CS, Marshall J, Mitchell E, et al. Randomized, controlled trial of irinotecan plus infusional, bolus, or oral fluoropyrimidines in first-line treatment of metastatic colorectal cancer: results from the BICC-C study. *J Clin Oncol.* 2007;25(30):4779-4786.

FOLFIRINOX (Pancreatic)

Index Terms Irinotecan-Oxaliplatin-Fluorouracil-Leucovorin (Pancreatic); Oxaliplatin-Irinotecan-Fluorouracil-Leucovorin (Pancreatic)

Use Pancreatic cancer

Regimen

Oxaliplatin: IV: 85 mg/m^2 over 2 hours day 1

[total dose/cycle = 85 mg/m^2]

Leucovorin Calcium: IV: 400 mg/m^2 over 2 hours day 1

[total dose/cycle = 400 mg/m^2]

Irinotecan: IV: 180 mg/m^2 over 90 minutes day 1

[total dose/cycle = 180 mg/m^2]

Fluorouracil: IV bolus: 400 mg/m^2 day 1

followed by IV: 2400 mg/m^2 continuous infusion (CI) over 46 hours beginning day 1

[total fluorouracil dose/cycle (bolus and CI) = 2800 mg/m^2]

Note: Bolus and CI fluorouracil are both given on day 1

Repeat cycle every 14 days until disease progression or unacceptable toxicity, 12 cycles recommended

References

Conroy T, Desseigne F, Ychou M, et al, "FOLFIRINOX Versus Gemcitabine for Metastatic Pancreatic Cancer," *N Engl J Med*, 2011, 364(19):1817-25.

Conroy T, Paillot B, François E, et al, "Irinotecan Plus Oxaliplatin and Leucovorin-Modulated Fluorouracil in Advanced Pancreatic Cancer-A Groupe Tumeurs Digestives of the Federation Nationale des Centres de Lutte Contre le Cancer Study," *J Clin Oncol*, 2005, 23(6):1228-36.

◆ **FOLFOX 6 (Pancreatic)** see FOLFOX (Pancreatic) on page 2133

FOLFOX1 (Colorectal)

Index Terms Oxaliplatin-Leucovorin-Fluorouracil (Colorectal)

Use Colorectal cancer

Regimen

Oxaliplatin: IV: 130 mg/m^2 over 2 hours day 1 (every other cycle)

[total dose/cycle = 130 mg/m^2]

Leucovorin Calcium: IV: 500 mg/m^2/day over 2 hours days 1 and 2

[total dose/cycle = 1000 mg/m^2]

Fluorouracil: IV: 1500-2000 mg/m^2/day continuous infusion over 22 hours days 1 and 2

[total dose/cycle = 3000-4000 mg/m^2]

Repeat cycle every 14 days until disease progression or unacceptable toxicity

References

de Gramont A, Tournigand C, Louvet C, et al, "Oxaliplatin, Folinic Acid, and 5-Fluorouracil (FOLFOX) in Pretreated Patients With Metastatic Advanced Cancer, The GERCOD," *Rev Med Interne*, 1997, 18(10):769-75.

FOLFOX2 (Colorectal)

Index Terms Oxaliplatin-Leucovorin-Fluorouracil (Colorectal)

Use Colorectal cancer

Regimen

Oxaliplatin: IV: 100 mg/m^2 over 2 hours day 1

[total dose/cycle = 100 mg/m^2]

Leucovorin Calcium: IV: 500 mg/m^2/day over 2 hours days 1 and 2

[total dose/cycle = 1000 mg/m^2]

Fluorouracil: IV: 1500-2000 mg/m^2/day continuous infusion over 22 hours days 1 and 2

[total dose/cycle = 3000-4000 mg/m^2]

Repeat cycle every 14 days until disease progression or unacceptable toxicity

References

de Gramont A, Tournigand C, Louvet C, et al, "Oxaliplatin, Folinic Acid and 5-Fluorouracil (Folfox) in Pretreated Patients With Metastatic Advanced Cancer. The GERCOD," *Rev Med Interne*, 1997, 18(10):769-75.

de Gramont A, Vignoud J, Tournigand C, et al, "Oxaliplatin With High-Dose Leucovorin and 5-Fluorouracil 48-Hour Continuous Infusion in Pretreated Metastatic Colorectal Cancer," *Eur J Cancer*, 1997, 33(2):214-9.

FOLFOX3 (Colorectal)

Index Terms Oxaliplatin-Leucovorin-Fluorouracil (Colorectal)

Use Colorectal cancer

Regimen

Oxaliplatin: IV: 85 mg/m^2 over 2 hours day 1

[total dose/cycle = 85 mg/m^2]

Leucovorin Calcium: IV: 500 mg/m^2/day over 2 hours days 1 and 2

[total dose/cycle = 1000 mg/m^2]

Fluorouracil: IV: 1500-2000 mg/m^2/day continuous infusion over 22 hours days 1 and 2

[total dose/cycle = 3000-4000 mg/m^2]

Repeat cycle every 14 days until disease progression or unacceptable toxicity

References

de Gramont A, Tournigand C, Louvet C, et al, "Oxaliplatin, Folinic Acid, and 5-Fluorouracil (FOLFOX) in Pretreated Patients With Metastatic Advanced Cancer, The GERCOD," *Rev Med Interne*, 1997, 18(10):769-75.

FOLFOX4 (Colorectal)

Index Terms Fluorouracil, Leucovorin, Oxaliplatin (Colorectal); Oxaliplatin, Leucovorin, Fluorouracil (Colorectal)

Use Colorectal cancer

Regimen NOTE: Multiple variations are listed.

Variation 1:

Oxaliplatin: IV: 85 mg/m^2 over 2 hours day 1

[total dose/cycle = 85 mg/m^2]

Leucovorin: IV: 200 mg/m^2/day over 2 hours days 1 and 2

[total dose/cycle = 400 mg/m^2]

Fluorouracil: IV bolus: 400 mg/m^2/day days 1 and 2

followed by IV: 600 mg/m^2/day continuous infusion (CI) over 22 hours days 1 and 2

[total dose/cycle (bolus and CI) = 2000 mg/m^2]

Repeat cycle every 14 days for a total of 12 cycles in the adjuvant setting; and until disease progression or unacceptable toxicity in the metastatic setting.

Variation 2:

Oxaliplatin: IV: 85 mg/m^2 over 2 hours day 1

[total dose/cycle = 85 mg/m^2]

Leucovorin (L-isomer): IV: 100 mg/m^2/day over 2 hours days 1 and 2

[total dose/cycle = 200 mg/m^2]

Fluorouracil: IV bolus: 400 mg/m^2/day days 1 and 2

followed by IV: 600 mg/m^2/day continuous infusion (CI) over 22 hours days 1 and 2

[total dose/cycle (bolus and CI) = 2000 mg/m^2]

Repeat cycle every 14 days

References

Variation 1:

Andre T, Boni C, Mounedji-Boudiaf L, et al, "Oxaliplatin, Fluorouracil, and Leucovorin as Adjuvant Treatment for Colon Cancer," *N Engl J Med*, 2004, 350(23):2343-51.

Andre T, Boni C, Navarro M, et al, "Improved Overall Survival With Oxaliplatin, Fluorouracil, and Leucovorin as Adjuvant Treatment in Stage II or III Colon Cancer in the MOSAIC Trial," *J Clin Oncol*, 2009, 27(19):3109-16.

de Gramont A, Figer A, Seymour M, et al, "Leucovorin and Fluorouracil With or Without Oxaliplatin as First-Line Treatment in Advanced Colorectal Cancer," *J Clin Oncol*, 2000, 18(16):2938-47.

Variation 2:

Colucci G, Gebbia V, Paoletti G, et al, "Phase III Randomized Trial of FOLFIRI Versus FOLFOX4 in the Treatment of Advanced Colorectal Cancer: A Multicenter Study Gruppo Oncologico Dell'Italia Meridionale," *J Clin Oncol*, 2005, 23(22):4866-75.

FOLFOX6 and mFOLFOX6 (Colorectal)

Index Terms Fluorouracil-Leucovorin-Oxaliplatin (Colorectal); mFOLFOX6 and FOLFOX6 (Colorectal); Modified Fluorouracil-Leucovorin-Oxaliplatin (Colorectal); Modified FOLFOX6 (Colorectal); Oxaliplatin-Leucovorin-Fluorouracil (Colorectal)

Use Colorectal cancer

Regimen NOTE: Multiple variations are listed.

Variation 1:

Cycles 1 and 2:

Oxaliplatin: IV: 100 mg/m^2 over 2 hours day 1

[total dose/cycle = 100 mg/m^2]

Leucovorin Calcium: IV: 400 mg/m^2 over 2 hours day 1

[total dose/cycle = 400 mg/m^2]

Fluorouracil: IV bolus: 400 mg/m^2 day 1

followed by IV: 2400 mg/m^2 continuous infusion (CI) over 46 hours beginning day 1

[total fluorouracil dose/cycle (bolus and CI) = 2800 mg/m^2]

Repeat cycle every 14 days for 2 cycles

Subsequent Cycles:

Oxaliplatin: IV: 100 mg/m^2 over 2 hours day 1

[total dose/cycle = 100 mg/m^2]

Leucovorin Calcium: IV: 400 mg/m^2 over 2 hours day 1

[total dose/cycle = 400 mg/m^2]

Fluorouracil: IV bolus: 400 mg/m^2 day 1

followed by IV: 3000 mg/m^2 continuous infusion (CI) over 46 hours beginning day 1

[total fluorouracil dose/cycle (bolus and CI) = 3400 mg/m^2]

Repeat cycle every 14 days until disease progression or unacceptable toxicity

Variation 2:

Oxaliplatin: IV: 85 mg/m^2 over 2 hours day 1

[total dose/cycle = 85 mg/m^2]

Leucovorin Calcium: IV: 350 mg over 2 hours day 1

[total dose/cycle = 350 mg]

Fluorouracil: IV bolus: 400 mg/m^2 day 1

followed by IV: 2400 mg/m^2 continuous infusion (CI) over 46 hours beginning day 1

[total fluorouracil dose/cycle (bolus and CI) = 2800 mg/m^2]

Repeat cycle every 14 days until disease progression or unacceptable toxicity

References

Variation 1:

Maindrault-Goebel F, Louvet C, Andre T, et al, "Oxaliplatin Added to the Simplified Bimonthly Leucovorin and 5-Fluorouracil Regimen as Second-Line Therapy for Metastatic Colorectal Cancer (FOLFOX6), GERCOR," *Eur J Cancer*, 1999, 35(9):1338-42.

Tournigand C, André T, Achille E, et al, "FOLFIRI Followed by FOLFOX6 or the Reverse Sequence in Advanced Colorectal Cancer: A Randomized GERCOR Study," *J Clin Oncol*, 2004, 22(2):229-37.

Variation 2:

Cheeseman SL, Joel SP, Chester JD, et al, "A 'Modified de Gramont' Regimen of Fluorouracil, Alone and With Oxaliplatin, for Advanced Colorectal Cancer," *Br J Cancer*, 2002, 87(4): 393-9.

Hochster HS, Hart LL, Ramanathan RK, et al, "Safety and Efficacy of Oxaliplatin and Fluoropyrimidine Regimens With or Without Bevacizumab as First-Line Treatment of Metastatic Colorectal Cancer: Results of the TREE Study," *J Clin Oncol*, 2008, 26(21):3523-9.

FOLFOX7 (Colorectal)

Use Colorectal cancer

Regimen

Oxaliplatin: IV: 130 mg/m^2 over 2 hours day 1

[total dose/cycle = 130 mg/m^2]

Leucovorin Calcium: IV: 400 mg/m^2 over 2 hours day 1

[total dose/cycle = 400 mg/m^2]

Fluorouracil: IV bolus: 400 mg/m^2 day 1

followed by IV: 2400 mg/m^2 continuous infusion (CI) over 46 hours beginning on day 1

total fluorouracil dose/cycle (bolus and CI) = 2800 mg/m^2

Repeat cycle every 14 days for a total of 8 cycles; evaluate every 2 months; may resume if disease progression

References

Maindrault-Goebel F, de Gramont A, Louvet C, et al, "High-Dose Intensity Oxaliplatin Added to the Simplified Bimonthly Leucovorin and 5-Fluorouracil Regimen as Second-Line Therapy for Metastatic Colorectal Cancer (FOLFOX 7)," *Eur J Cancer*, 2001, 37(8):1000-5.

◆ **FOLFOX (Gastric/Esophageal)** *see* Fluorouracil-Leucovorin-Oxaliplatin (Gastric/Esophageal) *on page 2127*

FOLFOXIRI (Colorectal)

Index Terms Irinotecan, Oxaliplatin, Leucovorin, Fluorouracil (Colorectal)

Use Colorectal cancer

Regimen
Irinotecan: IV: 165 mg/m² over 1 hour day 1
  [total dose/cycle = 165 mg/m²]
Oxaliplatin: IV: 85 mg/m² over 2 hours day 1
  [total dose/cycle = 85 mg/m²]
Leucovorin Calcium: IV: 200 mg/m² over 2 hours day 1
  [total dose/cycle = 200 mg/m²]
Fluorouracil: IV: 3200 mg/m² continuous infusion over 48 hours beginning day 1
  [total dose/cycle = 3200 mg/m²]
Repeat cycle every 14 days for a maximum of 12 cycles

References
Falcone A, Ricci S, Brunetti I, et al, "Phase III Trial of Infusional Fluorouracil, Leucovorin, Oxaliplatin, and Irinotecan (FOLFOXIRI) Compared With Infusional Fluorouracil, Leucovorin, and Irinotecan (FOLFIRI) as First-Line Treatment for Metastatic Colorectal Cancer: The Gruppo Oncologico Nord Ovest," J Clin Oncol, 2007, 25(13):1670-6.

FOLFOX (Pancreatic)
Index Terms Fluorouracil, Leucovorin, Oxaliplatin (Pancreatic); FOLFOX 6 (Pancreatic); Oxaliplatin, Fluorouracil, Leucovorin (Pancreatic)

Use Pancreatic cancer

Regimen
Oxaliplatin: IV: 100 mg/m² day 1
  [total dose/cycle = 100 mg/m²]
Leucovorin Calcium: IV: 400 mg/m² day 1
  [total dose/cycle = 400 mg/m²]
Fluorouracil: IV bolus: 400 mg/m² day 1
  followed by IV: 3000 mg/m² continuous infusion (CI) over 46 hours beginning day 1
  [total fluorouracil dose/cycle (bolus and CI) = 3400 mg/m²]
Repeat cycle every 14 days until disease progression or unacceptable toxicity

References
Ghosn M, Farhat N, Kattan J, et al, "FOLFOX-6 Combination as the First-Line Treatment of Locally Advanced and/or Metastatic Pancreatic Cancer," Am J Clin Oncol, 2007, 30(1):15-20.

GDP (Hodgkin)

Index Terms Gemcitabine-Dexamethasone-Cisplatin (Hodgkin)
Use Lymphoma, Hodgkin
Regimen

Gemcitabine: IV: 1000 mg/m^2 over 30 minutes days 1 and 8
[total dose/cycle = 2000 mg/m^2]
Dexamethasone: Oral: 40 mg/day (divided doses) days 1 to 4
[total dose/cycle = 160 mg]
Cisplatin: IV: 75 mg/m^2 over 1 hour day 1, administer after gemcitabine
[total dose/cycle = 75 mg/m^2]
Repeat cycle every 21 days; consider stem cell transplantation after 2 cycles in responding patients; and a maximum of 6 cycles in nontransplant candidates

References

Baetz T, Belch A, Couban S, et al, "Gemcitabine, Dexamethasone and Cisplatin is an Active and Non-Toxic Chemotherapy Regimen in Relapsed or Refractory Hodgkin's Disease: A Phase II Study by the National Cancer Institute of Canada Clinical Trials," *Ann Oncol*, 2003, 14 (12):1762-7.

Gemcitabine-Capecitabine (Biliary Cancer)

Index Terms Capecitabine-Gemcitabine (Biliary Cancer)
Use Biliary adenocarcinoma

Regimen

Gemcitabine: IV: 1000 mg/m^2/day over 30 minutes days 1 and 8
[total dose/cycle = 2000 mg/m^2]
Capecitabine: Oral: 650 mg/m^2 twice daily days 1 to 14
[total dose/cycle = 18,200 mg/m^2]
Repeat cycle every 21 days until disease progression or unacceptable toxicity

References

Knox JJ, Hedley D, Oza A, et al, "Combining Gemcitabine and Capecitabine in Patients With Advanced Biliary Cancer: A Phase II Trial," *J Clin Oncol*, 2005, 23(10):2332-8.

- ◆ **Gemcitabine-Capecitabine (Pancreatic)** *see* Capecitabine-Gemcitabine (Pancreatic) *on page 2007*

- ◆ **Gemcitabine-Carboplatin (Bladder)** *see* Carboplatin-Gemcitabine (Bladder) *on page 2017*

- ◆ **Gemcitabine-Carboplatin (NSCLC)** *see* Carboplatin-Gemcitabine (NSCLC) *on page 2017*

- ◆ **Gemcitabine-Carboplatin (Ovarian)** *see* Carboplatin-Gemcitabine (Ovarian) *on page 2018*

Gemcitabine-Cisplatin (Biliary Cancer)

Index Terms Cisplatin-Gemcitabine (Biliary Cancer)
Use Biliary adenocarcinoma
Regimen NOTE: Multiple variations are listed.

Variation 1:
Gemcitabine: IV: 1250 mg/m^2/dose days 1 and 8
[total dose/cycle = 2500 mg/m^2]
Cisplatin: IV: 75 mg/m^2/dose day 1
[total dose/cycle = 75 mg/m^2]
Repeat cycle every 3 weeks

Variation 2:
Gemcitabine: IV: 1000 mg/m^2/dose days 1 and 8
[total dose/cycle = 2000 mg/m^2]
Cisplatin: IV: 70 mg/m^2/dose day 1
[total dose/cycle = 70 mg/m^2]
Repeat cycle every 3 weeks (maximum: 6 cycles)

References

Variation 1:
Thongprasert S, Napapan S, Charoentum C, et al, "Phase II Study of Gemcitabine and Cisplatin as First-Line Chemotherapy in Inoperable Biliary Tract Carcinoma," *Ann Oncol*, 2005, 16 (2):279-81.
Variation 2:
Doval DC, Sekhon JS, Gupta SK, et al, "A Phase II Study of Gemcitabine and Cisplatin in Chemotherapy-Naive, Unresectable Gall Bladder Cancer," *Br J Cancer*, 2004, 90(8):1516-20.

- ◆ **Gemcitabine-Cisplatin (Bladder)** *see* Cisplatin-Gemcitabine (Bladder) *on page 2051*

- ◆ **Gemcitabine-Cisplatin (Cervical)** *see* Cisplatin-Gemcitabine (Cervical) *on page 2052*

- ◆ **Gemcitabine-Cisplatin-Dexamethasone (NHL-DLBCL)** *see* Gemcitabine-Dexamethasone-Cisplatin (NHL-DLBCL) *on page 2136*

- ◆ **Gemcitabine-Cisplatin-Dexamethasone-Rituximab (NHL-DLBCL)** *see* Rituximab-Gemcitabine-Dexamethasone-Cisplatin (NHL-DLBCL) *on page 2208*

♦ **Gemcitabine-Cisplatin-Docetaxel (Bladder)** *see* Cisplatin-Docetaxel-Gemcitabine (Bladder) *on page 2038*

♦ **Gemcitabine-Cisplatin (Mesothelioma)** *see* Cisplatin-Gemcitabine (Mesothelioma) *on page 2053*

♦ **Gemcitabine-Cisplatin-Necitumumab (NSCLC)** *see* Cisplatin-Gemcitabine-Necitumumab (NSCLC) *on page 2053*

♦ **Gemcitabine-Cisplatin (NSCLC)** *see* Cisplatin-Gemcitabine (NSCLC) *on page 2054*

♦ **Gemcitabine-Cisplatin (Pancreatic)** *see* Cisplatin-Gemcitabine (Pancreatic) *on page 2055*

♦ **Gemcitabine-Cisplatin (Unknown Primary)** *see* Cisplatin-Gemcitabine (Unknown Primary, Adenocarcinoma) *on page 2055*

Gemcitabine-Dexamethasone-Carboplatin (Hodgkin)

Index Terms GCD (Hodgkin); GDC (Hodgkin); Gemcitabine-Dexamethasone-Carboplatin (Hodgkin)

Use Lymphoma, Hodgkin (relapsed refractory)

Regimen

Gemcitabine: IV: 1,000 mg/m^2/day over 30 minutes days 1 and 8
[total dose/cycle = 2,000 mg/m^2]
Dexamethasone: Oral: 40 mg/day days 1 to 4
[total dose/cycle = 160 mg]
Carboplatin: IV: AUC 5 over 30 minutes day 1
[total dose/cycle = AUC = 5]
Repeat cycle every 21 days for up to 4 cycles

References

Gopal AK, Press OW, Shustov AR, et al. Efficacy and safety of gemcitabine, carboplatin, dexamethasone, and rituximab in patients with relapsed/refractory lymphoma: a prospective multi-center phase II study by the Puget Sound Oncology Consortium. *Leuk Lymphoma.* 2010;51(8):1523-1529.

♦ **Gemcitabine-Dexamethasone-Carboplatin (Hodgkin)** *see* Gemcitabine-Dexamethasone-Carboplatin (Hodgkin) *on page 2136*

♦ **Gemcitabine-Dexamethasone-Carboplatin-Rituximab (NHL-DLBCL)** *see* Rituximab-Gemcitabine-Dexamethasone-Carboplatin (NHL-DLBCL) *on page 2207*

♦ **Gemcitabine-Dexamethasone-Cisplatin (Hodgkin)** *see* GDP (Hodgkin) *on page 2134*

Gemcitabine-Dexamethasone-Cisplatin (NHL-DLBCL)

Index Terms GDP (NHL-DLBCL); Gemcitabine-Cisplatin-Dexamethasone (NHL-DLBCL)

Use Lymphoma, non-Hodgkin (DLBCL recurrent/refractory)

Regimen

Gemcitabine: IV: 1,000 mg/m^2 over 30 minutes days 1 and 8
[total dose/cycle = 2,000 mg/m^2]
Dexamethasone: IV or Oral: 40 mg/day in divided doses days 1 to 4
[total dose/cycle = 160 mg]
Cisplatin: IV: 75 mg/m^2 over 1 hour day 1
[total dose/cycle = 75 mg/m^2]

Repeat cycle every 21 days for 2 to 6 cycles; eligible patients proceeding to transplant received 2 cycles and nontransplant eligible patients received up to 6 cycles

References

Crump M, Baetz T, Couban S, et al. Gemcitabine, dexamethasone, and cisplatin in patients with recurrent or refractory aggressive histology B-cell non-Hodgkin lymphoma: a Phase II study by the National Cancer Institute of Canada Clinical Trials Group (NCIC-CTG). *Cancer.* 2004;101 (8):1835-1842.

♦ **Gemcitabine-Dexamethasone-Cisplatin-Rituximab (NHL-DLBCL)** *see* Rituximab-Gemcitabine-Dexamethasone-Cisplatin (NHL-DLBCL) *on page 2208*

♦ **Gemcitabine-Docetaxel-Capecitabine (Pancreatic)** *see* GTX (Pancreatic) *on page 2142*

♦ **Gemcitabine-Docetaxel (Ewing Sarcoma)** *see* Docetaxel-Gemcitabine (Ewing Sarcoma) *on page 2091*

♦ **Gemcitabine-Docetaxel (NSCLC)** *see* Docetaxel-Gemcitabine (NSCLC) *on page 2091*

♦ **Gemcitabine-Docetaxel (Osteosarcoma)** *see* Docetaxel-Gemcitabine (Osteosarcoma) *on page 2091*

♦ **Gemcitabine-Docetaxel (Soft Tissue Sarcoma)** *see* Docetaxel-Gemcitabine (Soft Tissue Sarcoma) *on page 2092*

♦ **Gemcitabine-Docetaxel (Unknown Primary)** *see* Docetaxel-Gemcitabine (Unknown Primary, Adenocarcinoma) *on page 2093*

♦ **Gemcitabine-Docetaxel (Uterine Leiomyosarcoma)** *see* Docetaxel-Gemcitabine (Uterine Leiomyosarcoma) *on page 2093*

♦ **Gemcitabine-Erlotinib (Pancreatic)** *see* Erlotinib-Gemcitabine (Pancreatic) *on page 2108*

♦ **Gemcitabine-nab Paclitaxel (Pancreatic)** *see* Gemcitabine-Paclitaxel (Protein Bound) (Pancreatic) *on page 2139*

Gemcitabine-Oxaliplatin-Paclitaxel (Testicular)

Index Terms GOP (Testicular); Oxaliplatin-Gemcitabine-Paclitaxel (Testicular); Paclitaxel-Gemcitabine-Oxaliplatin (Testicular)

Use Testicular cancer

Regimen

Gemcitabine: IV: 800 mg/m^2/day over 30 minutes days 1 and 8
  [total dose/cycle = 1600 mg/m^2]
Paclitaxel: IV: 80 mg/m^2/day over 1 hour days 1 and 8
  [total dose/cycle = 160 mg/m^2]
Oxaliplatin: IV: 130 mg/m^2 over 2 hours day 1
  [total dose/cycle = 130 mg/m^2]
Repeat cycle every 21 days for 2 cycles beyond best response, maximum of 8 cycles

References

Bokemeyer C, Oechsle K, Honecker F, et al, "Combination Chemotherapy With Gemcitabine, Oxaliplatin, and Paclitaxel in Patients With Cisplatin-Refractory or Multiply Relapsed Germ-Cell Tumors: A Study of the German Testicular Cancer Study Group," *Ann Oncol*, 2008, 19 (3):448-53.

♦ **Gemcitabine-Oxaliplatin-Rituximab (NHL-DLBCL)** *see* GEMOX-R (NHL-DLBCL) *on page 2141*

♦ **Gemcitabine-Oxaliplatin-Rituximab (NHL-Mantle Cell)** *see* GEMOX-R (NHL-Mantle Cell) *on page* 2141

♦ **Gemcitabine-Oxaliplatin (Testicular)** *see* GEMOX (Testicular) *on page* 2142

Gemcitabine-Paclitaxel (Bladder)

Index Terms Paclitaxel-Gemcitabine (Bladder)

Use Bladder cancer

Regimen NOTE: Multiple variations are listed.

Variation 1:

Paclitaxel: IV: 200 mg/m^2 over 1 hour day 1

[total dose/cycle = 200 mg/m^2]

Gemcitabine: IV: 1000 mg/m^2/day over 30 minutes days 1, 8, and 15

[total dose/cycle = 3000 mg/m^2]

Repeat cycle every 21 days for 6 cycles

Variation 2:

Gemcitabine: IV: 2500 to 3000 mg/m^2 day 1

[total dose/cycle = 2500 to 3000 mg/m^2]

Paclitaxel: IV: 150 mg/m^2 day 1

[total dose/cycle = 150 mg/m^2]

Repeat cycle every 14 days

Variation 3:

Paclitaxel: IV: 150 mg/m^2 over 3 hours day 1

[total dose/cycle = 150 mg/m^2]

Gemcitabine: IV: 2500 mg/m^2 over 30 minutes day 1

[total dose/cycle = 2500 mg/m^2]

Repeat cycle every 14 days up to a maximum of 12 cycles

References

Variation 1:

Meluch AA, Greco FA, Burris HA 3rd, et al. Paclitaxel and gemcitabine chemotherapy for advanced transitional-cell carcinoma of the urothelial tract: a phase II trial of the Minnie pearl cancer research network. *J Clin Oncol.* 2001;19(12):3018-3024.

Variation 2:

Sternberg CN, Calabrò F, Pizzocaro G, Marini L, Schnetzer S, Sella A. Chemotherapy with an every-2-week regimen of gemcitabine and paclitaxel in patients with transitional cell carcinoma who have received prior cisplatin-based therapy. *Cancer.* 2001;92(12):2993-2998.

Variation 3:

Calabrò F, Lorusso V, Rosati G, et al. Gemcitabine and paclitaxel every 2 weeks in patients with previously untreated urothelial carcinoma. *Cancer.* 2009;115(12):2652-2659.

Gemcitabine-Paclitaxel (Breast)

Index Terms GT (Breast); Paclitaxel-Gemcitabine (Breast)

Use Breast cancer

Regimen

Paclitaxel: IV: 175 mg/m^2 over 3 hours day 1

[total dose/cycle = 175 mg/m^2]

Gemcitabine: IV: 1250 mg/m^2 over 30 minutes days 1 and 8

[total dose/cycle = 2500 mg/m^2]

Repeat cycle every 21 days until disease progression or unacceptable toxicity

References

Albain KS, Nag SM, Calderillo-Ruiz G, et al, "Gemcitabine Plus Paclitaxel Versus Paclitaxel Monotherapy in Patients With Metastatic Breast Cancer and Prior Anthracycline Treatment," *J Clin Oncol,* 2008, 26(24):3950-7.

◆ **Gemcitabine-Paclitaxel (nanoparticle albumin bound) (Pancreatic)** *see* Gemcitabine-Paclitaxel (Protein Bound) (Pancreatic) *on page 2139*

Gemcitabine-Paclitaxel (Protein Bound) (Pancreatic)

Index Terms Gemcitabine-Abraxane (Pancreatic); Gemcitabine-nab Paclitaxel (Pancreatic); Gemcitabine-Paclitaxel (nanoparticle albumin bound) (Pancreatic); Paclitaxel (Protein Bound)-Gemcitabine (Pancreatic)

Use Pancreatic cancer

Regimen NOTE: Multiple variations are listed.

Variation 1:

Cycle 1:

Paclitaxel (protein bound): IV: 125 mg/m^2/day days 1, 8, 15, 29, 36, and 43
[total dose/cycle = 750 mg/m^2]
Gemcitabine: IV: 1000 mg/m^2/day days 1, 8, 15, 29, 36, and 43
[total dose/cycle = 6000 mg/m^2]
Cycle 1 duration is 8 weeks

Subsequent cycles:

Paclitaxel (protein bound): IV: 125 mg/m^2/day days 1, 8, and 15
[total dose/cycle = 375 mg/m^2]
Gemcitabine: IV: 1000 mg/m^2/day days 1, 8, and 15
[total dose/cycle = 3000 mg/m^2]
Repeat cycle every 28 days until disease progression or unacceptable toxicity

Variation 2:

Gemcitabine: IV: 1000 mg/m^2/day days 1, 8, and 15
[total dose/cycle = 3000 mg/m^2]
Paclitaxel (protein bound): IV: 125 mg/m^2/day days 1, 8, and 15
[total dose/cycle = 375 mg/m^2]
Repeat cycle every 28 days until disease progression or unacceptable toxicity

References

Variation 1:
Von Hoff DD, Ervin T, Arena FP, et al. Increased Survival in Pancreatic Cancer with nab-Paclitaxel plus Gemcitabine. *N Engl J Med*. 2013 [epub ahead of print].
Variation 2:
Von Hoff DD, Ramanathan RK, Borad MJ, et al, "Gemcitabine Plus Nab-Paclitaxel Is an Active Regimen in Patients With Advanced Pancreatic Cancer: A Phase I/II Trial," *J Clin Oncol*, 2011, 29(34):4548-54.

Gemcitabine-Paclitaxel (Testicular)

Index Terms Paclitaxel-Gemcitabine (Testicular)

Use Testicular cancer

Regimen

Paclitaxel: IV: 100 mg/m^2/day over 1 hour days 1, 8, and 15
[total dose/cycle = 300 mg/m^2]
Gemcitabine: IV: 1000 mg/m^2/day over 30 minutes days 1, 8, and 15
[total dose/cycle = 3000 mg/m^2]
Repeat cycle every 28 days for a maximum of 6 cycles

References

Einhorn LH, Brames MJ, Juliar B, et al, "Phase II Study of Paclitaxel Plus Gemcitabine Salvage Chemotherapy for Germ Cell Tumors After Progression Following High-Dose Chemotherapy With Tandem Transplant," *J Clin Oncol*, 2007, 25(5):513-6.
Mulherin BP, Brames MJ, Einhorn LH, at el, "Long-Term Survival With Paclitaxel and Gemcitabine for Germ Cell Tumors After Progression Following High-Dose Chemotherapy With Tandem Transplants," *J Clin Oncol*, 2011, 29:4562 [abstract 4562 from 2011 ASCO Annual Meeting].

◆ **Gemcitabine-Vinorelbine-Doxorubicin (Liposomal) (Hodgkin)** see GVD (Hodgkin) *on page 2143*

Gemcitabine-Vinorelbine (Head and Neck)

Index Terms GV (Head and Neck); Vinorelbine-Gemcitabine (Head and Neck)

Use Head and neck cancer (nasopharyngeal)

Regimen

Vinorelbine: IV: 25 mg/m^2/day days 1 and 8
[total dose/cycle = 50 mg/m^2]
Gemcitabine: IV: 1000 mg/m^2/day over 30 minutes days 1 and 8
[total dose/cycle = 2000 mg/m^2]
Repeat cycle every 21 days for 6 cycles

References

Chen C, Wang FH, Wang ZQ, et al. Salvage gemcitabine-vinorelbine chemotherapy in patients with metastatic nasopharyngeal carcinoma pretreated with platinum-based chemotherapy. *Oral Oncol.* 2012;48(11):1146-1151.

Gemcitabine-Vinorelbine (NSCLC)

Index Terms GemVin (NSCLC); GV (NSCLC); Vinorelbine-Gemcitabine (NSCLC)

Use Lung cancer, non-small cell

Regimen NOTE: Multiple variations are listed.

Variation 1:
Gemcitabine: IV: 1000 mg/m^2/day days 1, 8, and 15
[total dose/cycle = 3000 mg/m^2]
Vinorelbine: IV: 25 mg/m^2/day days 1, 8, and 15
[total dose/cycle = 75 mg/m^2]
Repeat cycle every 28 days for up to 6 cycles

Variation 2:
Vinorelbine: IV: 25 mg/m^2/day over 10 minutes days 1, 8, and 15
[total dose/cycle = 75 mg/m^2]
Gemcitabine: IV: 900 mg/m^2/day over 30 minutes days 1, 8, and 15
[total dose/cycle = 2700 mg/m^2]
Repeat cycle every 28 days for a recommended 6 cycles, further treatment could be administered until disease progression or unacceptable toxicity

Variation 3:
Gemcitabine: IV: 1000 mg/m^2/day over 30 minutes days 1 and 8
[total dose/cycle = 2000 mg/m^2]
Vinorelbine: IV: 25 mg/m^2/day over 15 minutes days 1 and 8, one hour after completion of gemcitabine
[total dose/cycle = 50 mg/m^2]
Repeat cycle every 21 days for up to 6 cycles

References

Variation 1:
Greco FA, Spigel DR, Kuzur ME, et al. Paclitaxel/carboplatin/gemcitabine versus gemcitabine/vinorelbine in advanced non-small-cell lung cancer: a phase II/III study of the Minnie Pearl Cancer Research Network. *Clin Lung Cancer.* 2007;8(8):483-487.
Variation 2:
Herbst RS, Khuri FR, Lu C, et al. The novel and effective nonplatinum, nontaxane combination of gemcitabine and vinorelbine in advanced non-small cell lung carcinoma: potential for decreased toxicity and combination with biological therapy. *Cancer.* 2002;95(2):340-353.
Variation 3:
Gridelli C, Gallo C, Shepherd FA, et al. Gemcitabine plus vinorelbine compared with cisplatin plus vinorelbine or cisplatin plus gemcitabine for advanced non-small-cell lung cancer: a phase III trial of the Italian GEMVIN Investigators and the National Cancer Institute of Canada Clinical Trials Group. *J Clin Oncol.* 2003;21(16):3025-3034.

Laack E, Dickgreber N, Müller T, et al. Randomized phase III study of gemcitabine and vinorelbine versus gemcitabine, vinorelbine, and cisplatin in the treatment of advanced non-small-cell lung cancer: from the German and Swiss Lung Cancer Study Group. *J Clin Oncol.* 2004;22 (12):2348-2356.

Gemcitabine-Vinorelbine (Soft Tissue Sarcoma)

Index Terms Vinorelbine-Gemcitabine (Soft Tissue Sarcoma)

Use Soft tissue sarcoma

Regimen

Vinorelbine: IV: 25 mg/m^2/day over 10 minutes days 1 and 8

[total dose/cycle = 50 mg/m^2]

Gemcitabine: IV: 800 mg/m^2/day over 90 minutes days 1 and 8

[total dose/cycle = 1600 mg/m^2]

Repeat cycle every 21 days until disease progression or unacceptable toxicity

References

Dileo P, Morgan JA, Zahrieh D, et al. Gemcitabine and vinorelbine combination chemotherapy for patients with advanced soft tissue sarcomas: results of a phase II trial. *Cancer.* 2007;109 (9):1863-1869.

GEMOX (Biliary Cancer)

Use Biliary adenocarcinoma

Regimen

Gemcitabine: IV: 1000 mg/m^2 day 1

[total dose/cycle = 1000 mg/m^2]

Oxaliplatin: IV: 100 mg/m^2 day 2

[total dose/cycle = 100 mg/m^2]

Repeat cycle every 2 weeks

References

Andre T, Tournigand C, Rosmorduc O, et al, "Gemcitabine Combined With Oxaliplatin (GEMOX) in Advanced Biliary Tract Adenocarcinoma: A GERCOR Study," *Ann Oncol,* 2004, 15(9):1339-43.

GEMOX-R (NHL-DLBCL)

Index Terms Gemcitabine-Oxaliplatin-Rituximab (NHL-DLBCL); Oxaliplatin-Gemcitabine-Rituximab (NHL-DLBCL); Rituximab-Gemcitabine-Oxaliplatin (NHL-DLBCL)

Use Lymphoma, non-Hodgkin (DLBCL)

Regimen

Rituximab: IV: 375 mg/m^2 day 1

[total dose/cycle = 375 mg/m^2]

Gemcitabine: IV: 1000 mg/m^2 day 1

[total dose/cycle = 1000 mg/m^2]

Oxaliplatin: IV: 100 mg/m^2 day 1

[total dose/cycle = 100 mg/m^2]

Repeat cycle every 21 days for a total of 6 to 8 cycles

References

López A, Gutiérrez A, Palacios A, et al, "GEMOX-R Regimen is a Highly Effective Salvage Regimen in Patients With Refractory/Relapsing Diffuse Large-Cell Lymphoma: A Phase II Study," *Eur J Haematol,* 2008, 80(2):127-32.

GEMOX-R (NHL-Mantle Cell)

Index Terms Gemcitabine-Oxaliplatin-Rituximab (NHL-Mantle Cell); Oxaliplatin-Gemcitabine-Rituximab (NHL-Mantle Cell); Rituximab-Gemcitabine-Oxaliplatin (NHL-Mantle Cell)

Use Lymphoma, non-Hodgkin (Mantle cell)

Regimen
Rituximab: IV: 375 mg/m^2 day 1
[total dose/cycle = 375 mg/m^2]
Gemcitabine: IV: 1000 mg/m^2 day 1
[total dose/cycle = 1000 mg/m^2]
Oxaliplatin: IV: 100 mg/m^2 day 1
[total dose/cycle = 100 mg/m^2]
Repeat cycle every 21 days for a maximum of 8 cycles

References
Rodríguez J, Gutierrez A, Palacios A, et al, "Rituximab, Gemcitabine and Oxaliplatin: An Effective Regimen in Patients With Refractory and Relapsing Mantle Cell Lymphoma," *Leuk Lymphoma*, 2007, 48(11):2172-8.

GEMOX (Testicular)

Index Terms Gemcitabine-Oxaliplatin (Testicular); Oxaliplatin-Gemcitabine (Testicular)

Use Testicular cancer

Regimen NOTE: Multiple variations are listed.

Variation 1:
Gemcitabine: IV: 1000 mg/m^2/day over 30 minutes days 1 and 8
[total dose/cycle = 2000 mg/m^2]
Oxaliplatin: IV: 130 mg/m^2 over 2 hours day 1
[total dose/cycle = 130 mg/m^2]
Repeat cycle every 21 days for a total of at least 2 cycles (maximum: 6 cycles)

Variation 2:
Gemcitabine: IV: 1250 mg/m^2/day over 30 minutes days 1 and 8
[total dose/cycle = 2500 mg/m^2]
Oxaliplatin: IV: 130 mg/m^2 over 2 hours day 1
[total dose/cycle = 130 mg/m^2]
Repeat cycle every 21 days for a maximum of 6 cycles

References
Variation 1:
Kollmannsberger C, Beyer J, Liersch R, et al, "Combination Chemotherapy With Gemcitabine Plus Oxaliplatin in Patients With Intensively Pretreated or Refractory Germ Cell Cancer: A Study of the German Testicular Cancer Study Group," *J Clin Oncol*, 2004, 22(1):108-14.
Pectasides D, Pectasides M, Farmakis D, et al, "Gemcitabine and Oxaliplatin (GEMOX) in Patients With Cisplatin-Refractory Germ Cell Tumors: A Phase II Study," *Ann Oncol*, 2004, 15 (3):493-7.
Variation 2:
De Giorgi U, Rosti G, Aieta M, et al, "Phase II Study of Oxaliplatin and Gemcitabine Salvage Chemotherapy in Patients With Cisplatin-Refractory Nonseminomatous Germ Cell Tumor," *Eur Urol*, 2006, 50(5):1032-8.

♦ **GemVin (NSCLC)** *see* Gemcitabine-Vinorelbine (NSCLC) *on page 2140*

♦ **GOP (Testicular)** *see* Gemcitabine-Oxaliplatin-Paclitaxel (Testicular) *on page 2137*

♦ **GP (Bladder)** *see* Cisplatin-Gemcitabine (Bladder) *on page 2051*

♦ **GT (Breast)** *see* Gemcitabine-Paclitaxel (Breast) *on page 2138*

GTX (Pancreatic)

Index Terms Gemcitabine-Docetaxel-Capecitabine (Pancreatic)

Use Pancreatic cancer

Regimen NOTE: Multiple variations are listed.
  Variation 1:
    Gemcitabine: IV: 750 mg/m^2/day over 75 minutes days 4 and 11
      [total dose/cycle = 1500 mg/m^2]
    Docetaxel: IV: 30 mg/m^2/day over 60 minutes days 4 and 11
      [total dose/cycle = 60 mg/m^2]
    Capecitabine: Oral: 750 mg/m^2/dose twice daily days 1 to 14
      [total dose/cycle = 21,000 mg/m^2]
    Repeat cycle every 21 days
  Variation 2:
    Gemcitabine: IV: 600 mg/m^2/day over 60 minutes days 4 and 11
      [total dose/cycle = 1200 mg/m^2]
    Docetaxel: IV: 30 mg/m^2/day over 60 minutes days 4 and 11
      [total dose/cycle = 60 mg/m^2]
    Capecitabine: Oral: 500 mg/m^2/dose twice daily days 1 to 14
      [total dose/cycle = 14,000 mg/m^2]
    Repeat cycle every 21 days until disease progression or unacceptable
    toxicities

References

Variation 1:
Fine RL, Fogelman DR, Schreibman SM, et al, "The Gemcitabine, Docetaxel, and Capecitabine (CTX) Regimen for Metastatic Pancreatic Cancer. A Retrospective Analysis," *Cancer Chemother Pharmacol*, 2008, 61(1):167-75.
Variation 2:
Dakik HK, Moskovic DJ, Carlson PJ, et al. The use of GTX as second-line and later chemotherapy for metastatic pancreatic cancer: a retrospective analysis. *Cancer Chemother Pharmacol*. 2012;69(2):425-30.

GVD (Hodgkin)

Index Terms Gemcitabine-Vinorelbine-Doxorubicin (Liposomal) (Hodgkin)
Use Lymphoma, Hodgkin
Regimen NOTE: Multiple variations are listed.
  Variation 1 (for transplant-naive patients):
    Vinorelbine: IV: 20 mg/m^2/day over 6-10 minutes days 1 and 8
      [total dose/cycle = 40 mg/m^2]
    Gemcitabine: IV: 1000 mg/m^2/day over 30 minutes days 1 and 8
      [total dose/cycle = 2000 mg/m^2]
    Doxorubicin liposomal: IV: 15 mg/m^2/day over 30-60 minutes days 1 and 8
      [total dose/cycle = 30 mg/m^2]
    Repeat cycle every 21 days for a total of 2 to 6 cycles
  Variation 2 (for patients with prior transplant):
    Vinorelbine: IV: 15 mg/m^2/day over 6-10 minutes days 1 and 8
      [total dose/cycle = 30 mg/m^2]
    Gemcitabine: IV: 800 mg/m^2/day over 30 minutes days 1 and 8
      [total dose/cycle = 1600 mg/m^2]
    Doxorubicin liposomal: IV: 10 mg/m^2/day over 30-60 minutes days 1 and 8
      [total dose/cycle = 20 mg/m^2]
    Repeat cycle every 21 days for a total of 2 to 6 cycles

References

Variations 1 and 2:
Bartlett NL, Niedzwiecki D, Johnson JL, et al, "Gemcitabine, Vinorelbine, and Pegylated Liposomal Doxorubicin (GVD), A Salvage Regimen in Relapsed Hodgkin's Lymphoma: CALGB 59804," *Ann Oncol*, 2007, 18(6):1071-9.

◆ **GV (Head and Neck)** *see* Gemcitabine-Vinorelbine (Head and Neck)
  on page 2140

- ◆ **GV (NSCLC)** *see* Gemcitabine-Vinorelbine (NSCLC) *on page 2140*
- ◆ **HDAC-Daunorubicin (AML Induction)** *see* Cytarabine (High Dose)-Daunorubicin (AML Induction) *on page 2080*
- ◆ **HD Cytarabine (Single Agent AML Induction)** *see* Cytarabine (High-Dose Single-Agent AML Induction Regimen) *on page 2080*

HDMTX

Use Osteosarcoma

Regimen

Methotrexate: IV: 12 g/m²/week for 2-12 weeks
[total dose/cycle = 24-144 g/m²]

Leucovorin calcium rescue: Oral, IV: 15 mg/m² every 6 hours (beginning 30 hours after the beginning of the 4-hour methotrexate infusion) for 10 doses; **serum methotrexate levels must be monitored**
[total dose/cycle = 150 mg/m²]

References

Camitta BM and Holcenberg JS, "Safety of Delayed Leucovorin 'Rescue' Following High-Dose Methotrexate in Children," *Med Pediatr Oncol*, 1978, 5(1):55-9.

- ◆ **HD-MVAC (Bladder Cancer)** *see* Dose Dense MVAC (Bladder Cancer) *on page 2096*
- ◆ **HIDAC-3-7 (AML Induction)** *see* Cytarabine (High Dose)-Daunorubicin-Etoposide (AML Induction) *on page 2080*
- ◆ **HIDAC-Daunorubicin (AML Induction)** *see* Cytarabine (High Dose)-Daunorubicin (AML Induction) *on page 2080*
- ◆ **HIDAC (Single Agent AML Induction)** *see* Cytarabine (High-Dose Single-Agent AML Induction Regimen) *on page 2080*
- ◆ **High-Dose-Intensity M-VAC (Bladder Cancer)** *see* Dose Dense MVAC (Bladder Cancer) *on page 2096*
- ◆ **Hydroxyurea-Fluorouracil (Head and Neck Cancer)** *see* Fluorouracil-Hydroxyurea (Head and Neck Cancer) *on page 2124*

Hyper-CVAD Alternating With High-Dose Methotrexate-Cytarabine + Rituximab + CNS Prophylaxis (NHL-Burkitt)

Index Terms Rituximab, Cyclophosphamide, Vincristine, Doxorubicin, Dexamethasone, Methotrexate, Cytarabine (NHL-Burkitt); Rituximab-Hyper-CVAD Alternating With High-Dose Methotrexate-Cytarabine (NHL-Burkitt)

Use Lymphoma, non-Hodgkin (Burkitt)

Regimen

Cycle A (Cycles 1, 3, 5, and 7):

Rituximab: IV: 375 mg/m²/day over 2 to 6 hours days 1 and 11 cycles 1 and 3 only
[total dose/cycle = 750 mg/m²]

Cyclophosphamide: IV: 300 mg/m² every 12 hours, for 6 doses, days 1, 2, and 3
[total dose/cycle = 1800 mg/m²]

Mesna: IV: 600 mg/m² continuous infusion days 1, 2, and 3
[total dose/cycle = 1800 mg/m²]

Vincristine: IV: 2 mg/day days 4 and 11
[total dose/cycle = 4 mg]

Doxorubicin: IV: 50 mg/m^2 continuous infusion over 24 hours day 4
[total dose/cycle = 50 mg/m^2]

Dexamethasone: Oral, IV: 40 mg/day days 1 to 4 and 11 to 14
[total dose/cycle = 320 mg]

CNS Prophylaxis

Methotrexate: Intrathecal: 12 mg (6 mg by Ommaya reservoir) day 2

Cytarabine: Intrathecal: 100 mg day 7

CNS prophylaxis to be given with each course (total of 16 Intrathecal treatments)

Filgrastim: SubQ: 10 mcg/kg daily, starting 24 hours after completion of chemotherapy and continuing until WBC ≥3000/mm^3

Cycle B (Cycles 2, 4, 6, and 8):

Rituximab: IV: 375 mg/m^2/day over 2 to 6 hours days 2 and 8 on cycles 2 and 4 only
[total dose/cycle = 750 mg/m^2]

Methotrexate: IV: 1000 mg/m^2 continuous infusion over 24 hours day 1
[total dose/cycle = 1000 mg/m^2]

Leucovorin: IV: 50 mg (start 12 hours after the end of the methotrexate infusion)

followed by IV: 15 mg every 6 hours, for 8 doses or until methotrexate level ≤0.1 mmol/L
[total dose/cycle = 170 mg]

Cytarabine: IV: 3000 mg/m^2 every 12 hours, for 4 doses, day 2 and 3
[total dose/cycle = 12,000 mg/m^2]

CNS Prophylaxis

Methotrexate: Intrathecal: 12 mg (6 mg by Ommaya reservoir) day 2

Cytarabine: Intrathecal: 100 mg day 7

CNS prophylaxis to be given with each course (total of 16 Intrathecal treatments)

Filgrastim: SubQ: 10 mcg/kg daily, starting 24 hours after completion of chemotherapy and continuing until WBC ≥3000/mm^3

Repeat every 14 to 21 days (depending on count recovery) in the following sequence: ABABABAB

References

Thomas DA, Faderl S, O'Brien S, et al. Chemoimmunotherapy with hyper-CVAD plus rituximab for the treatment of adult Burkitt and Burkitt-type lymphoma or acute lymphoblastic leukemia. *Cancer.* 2006;106(7):1569-1580.

Thomas DA, Kantarjian HM, Cortes J, et al. Long-Term Outcome after Hyper-CVAD and Rituximab Chemoimmunotherapy for Burkitt (BL) or Burkitt-Like (BLL) Leukemia/Lymphoma and Mature B-Cell Acute Lymphocytic Leukemia (ALL). *Blood.* 2008;112:1929 [abstract 1929 from 2008 ASH Annual Meeting].

Hyper-CVAD + Imatinib

Use Leukemia, acute lymphocytic

Regimen

Cycle A: (Cycles 1, 3, 5, and 7)

Imatinib: Oral: 400 mg/day days 1 to 14
[total dose/cycle = 5600 mg]

Cyclophosphamide: IV: 300 mg/m^2 every 12 hours, for 6 doses, days 1, 2, and 3
[total dose/cycle = 1800 mg/m^2]

Mesna: IV 600 mg/m^2/day continuous infusion days 1, 2, and 3
[total dose/cycle = 1800 mg/m^2]

Vincristine: IV: 2 mg/day days 4 and 11
[total dose/cycle = 4 mg]

◀

    Doxorubicin: IV: 50 mg/m^2/day continuous infusion day 4
      [total dose/cycle = 50 mg/m^2]
    Dexamethasone: Oral, IV: 40 mg/day days 1 to 4 and 11 to 14
      [total dose/cycle = 320 mg]
    Cycle B: (Cycles 2, 4, 6, and 8)
    Imatinib: Oral: 400 mg/day days 1 to 14
      [total dose/cycle = 5600 mg]
    Methotrexate: IV: 1 g/m^2/day continuous infusion day 1
      [total dose/cycle = 1 g/m^2]
    Leucovorin: IV: 50 mg then 15 mg every 6 hours, for 8 doses (start 12 hours
    after the end of the methotrexate infusion)
      [total dose/cycle = 170 mg]
    Cytarabine: IV: 3 g/m^2 every 12 hours for 4 doses, days 2 and 3
      [total dose/cycle = 12 g/m^2]
Repeat every 6 weeks in the following sequence: ABABABAB

CNS Prophylaxis
    Methotrexate: Intrathecal: 12 mg/day day 2
      [total dose/cycle = 12 mg/day]
    or 6 mg Into Ommaya day 2
      [total dose/cycle = 6 mg/day]
    Cytarabine: Intrathecal: 100 mg/day day 7 or 8
      [total dose/cycle = 100 mg/day]
Repeat cycle every 3 weeks for 3 or 4 cycles

Maintenance (POMP)
    Imatinib: Oral: 600 mg/day
      [total dose/cycle = 18,000 mg]
    Vincristine: IV: 2 mg/day day 1
      [total dose/cycle = 2 mg]
    Prednisone: Oral: 200 mg/day days 1 to 5
      [total dose/cycle = 1000 mg/m^2]
Repeat cycle every month (except months 6 and 13) for 13 months

Intensification
    Imatinib: Oral: 400 mg/day days 1 to 14
      [total dose/cycle = 5600 mg]
    Cyclophosphamide: IV: 300 mg/m^2 every 12 hours, for 6 doses, days 1, 2,
    and 3
      [total dose/cycle = 1800 mg/m^2]
    Mesna: IV: 600 mg/m^2/day continuous infusion days 1, 2, and 3
      [total dose/cycle = 1800 mg/m^2]
    Vincristine: IV: 2 mg/day days 4 and 11
      [total dose/cycle = 4 mg]
    Doxorubicin: 50 mg/m^2/day continuous infusion day 4
      [total dose/cycle = 50 mg/m^2]
    Dexamethasone: IV or Oral: 40 mg/day days 1 to 4 and 11 to 14
      [total dose/cycle = 320 mg]
    Cycle is given in months 6 and 13 during maintenance

References
Thomas DA, Faderl S, Cortes J, et al, "Treatment of Philadelphia Chromosome-Positive Acute
    Lymphocytic Leukemia With Hyper-CVAD and Imatinib Mesylate," *Blood*, 2004, 103
    (12):4396-407.

Hyper-CVAD (Leukemia, Acute Lymphocytic)

Use Leukemia, acute lymphocytic

Regimen NOTE: Multiple variations are listed.
Variation 1:
  Cycle A (Cycles 1, 3, 5, and 7):
    Cyclophosphamide: IV: 300 mg/m^2 every 12 hours, for 6 doses, days 1, 2, and 3
      [total dose/cycle = 1800 mg/m^2]
    Mesna: IV: 1200 mg/m^2/day continuous infusion days 1, 2, and 3
      [total dose/cycle = 3600 mg/m^2]
    Vincristine: IV: 2 mg/day days 4 and 11
      [total dose/cycle = 4 mg]
    Doxorubicin: IV: 50 mg/m^2 day 4
      [total dose/cycle = 50 mg/m^2]
    Dexamethasone: (route not specified): 40 mg/day days 1 to 4 and 11 to 14
      [total dose/cycle = 320 mg]
  Cycle B (Cycles 2, 4, 6, and 8):
    Methotrexate: IV: 1 g/m^2 continuous infusion day 1
      [total dose/cycle = 1g/m^2]
    Leucovorin: (route not specified): 15 mg every 6 hours, for 8 doses (start 12 hours after end of methotrexate infusion)
      [total dose/cycle = 120 mg]
    Cytarabine: IV: 3 g/m^2 every 12 hours, for 4 doses, days 2 and 3
      [total dose/cycle = 12 g/m^2]
    Methylprednisolone: IV: 50 mg twice daily, for 6 doses, days 1, 2, and 3
      [total dose/cycle = 300 mg/m^2]
  Repeat every 6 weeks in the following sequence: ABABABAB
CNS Prophylaxis
  Methotrexate: Intrathecal: 12 mg/day day 2
    [total dose/cycle = 12 mg]
  or 6 mg/day into Ommaya day 2
    [total dose/cycle = 6 mg]
  Cytarabine: Intrathecal: 100 mg day 8
    [total dose/cycle = 100 mg]
  Repeat cycle every 3 weeks
Maintenance (POMP)
  Mercaptopurine: Oral: 50 mg 3 times/day
    [total dose/cycle = 4200-4650 mg]
  Vincristine: IV: 2 mg day 1
    [total dose/cycle = 2 mg]
  Methotrexate: Oral: 20 mg/m^2/day days 1, 8, 15, and 22
    [total dose/cycle = 80 mg/m^2]
  Prednisone: Oral: 200 mg/day days 1 to 5
    [total dose/cycle = 1000 mg/m^2]
  or
  Mercaptopurine: IV: 1 g/m^2/day days 1 to 5
    [total dose/cycle = 5 g/m^2]
  Vincristine: IV: 2 mg day 1
    [total dose/cycle = 2 mg]
  Methotrexate: IV: 10 mg/m^2/day days 1 to 5
    [total dose/cycle = 50 mg/m^2]
  Prednisone: Oral: 200 mg/day days 1 to 5
    [total dose/cycle = 1000 mg/m^2]
  Repeat cycles every month for 2 years

Variation 2:
Cycle A (Cycles 1, 3, 5, and 7):
Cyclophosphamide: IV: 300 mg/m^2 every 12 hours, for 6 doses, days 1, 2, and 3
[total dose/cycle = 1800 mg/m^2]
Mesna: IV: 600 mg/m^2/day continuous infusion days 1, 2, and 3
[total dose/cycle = 1800 mg/m^2]
Vincristine: IV: 2 mg/day days 4 and 11
[total dose/cycle = 4 mg]
Doxorubicin: IV: 50 mg/m^2 day 4
[total dose/cycle = 50 mg/m^2]
Dexamethasone: Oral, IV: 40 mg/day days 1 to 4 and 11 to 14
[total dose/cycle = 320 mg]
Cycle B (Cycles 2, 4, 6, and 8):
Methotrexate: IV: 1 g/m^2 continuous infusion day 1
[total dose/cycle = 1 g/m^2]
Leucovorin: IV: 50 mg (start 12 hours after end of methotrexate infusion)
followed by IV: 15 mg every 6 hours, for 8 doses
[total dose/cycle = 170 mg]
Cytarabine: IV: 3 g/m^2 every 12 hours, for 4 doses, days 2 and 3
[total dose/cycle = 12 g/m^2]
Repeat every 6 weeks in the following sequence: ABABABAB
CNS Prophylaxis
Methotrexate: Intrathecal: 12 mg day 2
[total dose/cycle = 12 mg]
or 6 mg into Ommaya day 2
[total dose/cycle = 6 mg]
Cytarabine: Intrathecal: 100 mg day 7
[total dose/cycle = 100 mg]
Repeat cycle every 3 weeks
Variation 3:
Cycle A (Cycles 1, 3, 5, and 7):
Cyclophosphamide: IV: 300 mg/m^2 every 12 hours, for 6 doses, days 1, 2, and 3
[total dose/cycle = 1800 mg/m^2]
Mesna: IV: 600 mg/m^2/day continuous infusion days 1, 2, and 3
[total dose/cycle = 1800 mg/m^2]
Vincristine: IV: 2 mg/day days 4 and 11
[total dose/cycle = 4 mg]
Doxorubicin: IV: 50 mg/m^2 continuous infusion day 4
[total dose/cycle = 50 mg/m^2]
Dexamethasone: Oral, IV: 40 mg/day days 1 to 4 and 11 to 14
[total dose/cycle = 320 mg]
Cycle B (Cycles 2, 4, 6, and 8):
Methotrexate: IV: 200 mg/m^2 day 1
followed by IV: 800 mg/m^2 continuous infusion day 1
[total dose/cycle = 1 g/m^2]
Leucovorin: IV: 50 mg (start 12 hours after end of methotrexate infusion)
followed by IV: 15 mg every 6 hours, for 8 doses
[total dose/cycle = 170 mg/m^2]
Cytarabine: IV: 3 g/m^2 every 12 hours, for 4 doses, days 2 and 3
[total dose/cycle = 12 g/m^2]
Repeat every 6 weeks in the following sequence: ABABABAB

CNS Prophylaxis
Methotrexate: Intrathecal: 12 mg day 2
  [total dose/cycle = 12 mg]
or 6 mg into Ommaya day 2
  [total dose/cycle = 6 mg]
Cytarabine: Intrathecal: 100 mg day 7 **or** 8
  [total dose/cycle = 100 mg]
Repeat cycles every 3 weeks for 6 or 8 cycles
Maintenance (POMP)
Mercaptopurine: Oral: 50 mg 3 times/day
  [total dose/cycle = 4200-4650 mg]
Vincristine: IV: 2 mg day 1
  [total dose/cycle = 2 mg]
Methotrexate: Oral, I V: 20 mg/m^2/ day days 1, 8, 15, and 22
  [total dose/cycle = 80 mg/m^2]
Prednisone: Oral: 200 mg/day days 1 to 5
  [total dose/cycle = 1000 mg/m^2]
or
Mercaptopurine: IV: 1 g/m^2/day days 1 to 5
  [total dose/cycle = 5 g/m^2]
Vincristine: IV: 2 mg day 1
  [total dose/cycle = 2 mg]
Methotrexate: IV: 10 mg/m^2/day days 1 to 5
  [total dose/cycle = 50 mg/m^2]
Prednisone: Oral: 200 mg/day days 1 to 5
  [total dose/cycle = 1000 mg]
Repeat cycles every month (except months 7 and 11 or 9 and 12) for 2 years
Intensification
Etoposide: IV: 100 mg/m^2/day days 1 to 5
  [total dose/cycle = 500 mg/m^2]
Pegaspargase: IV: 2500 units/m^2 day 1
  [total dose/cycle = 2500 units/m^2]
Given during months 9 and 12 of maintenance
or
Methotrexate: IV: 100 mg/m^2/day days 1, 8, 15, and 22
  [total dose/cycle = 400 mg/m^2]
Asparaginase: IV: 20,000 units/day days 2, 9, 16, and 23
  [total dose/cycle = 80,000 units]
Given during months 7 and 11 of maintenance
Variation 4:
  Cycle A (Cycles 1, 3, 5, and 7):
  Cyclophosphamide: IV: 300 mg/m^2 every 12 hours, for 6 doses, days 1, 2, and 3
    [total dose/cycle = 1800 mg/m^2]
  Mesna: IV: 600 mg/m^2/day continuous infusion days 1, 2, and 3
    [total dose/cycle = 1800 mg/m^2]
  Vincristine: IV: 2 mg/day days 4 and 11
    [total dose/cycle = 4 mg]
  Doxorubicin: IV: 50 mg/m^{2}day 4
    [total dose/cycle = 50 mg/m^2]
  Dexamethasone: (route not specified): 40 mg/day days 1 to 4 and 11 to 14
    [total dose/cycle = 320 mg]

◄ Cycle B (Cycles 2, 4, 6, and 8):
  Methotrexate: IV: 200 mg/m^2 day 1
    followed by IV: 800 mg/m^2 continuous infusion day 1
    [total dose/cycle = 1 g/m^2]
  Leucovorin: (route not specified): 15 mg every 6 hours, for 8 doses (start 24 hours after end of methotrexate infusion)
    [total dose/cycle = 120 mg]
  Cytarabine: IV: 3 g/m^2 every 12 hours, for 4 doses, days 2 and 3
    [total dose/cycle = 12 g/m^2]
  Repeat every 6 weeks in the following sequence: ABABABAB
CNS Prophylaxis
  Methotrexate: Intrathecal: 12 mg day 2
    [total dose/cycle = 12 mg]
  Cytarabine: Intrathecal: 100 mg day 8
    [total dose/cycle = 100 mg]
  Repeat cycle every 3 weeks for 4 or 8 cycles
Maintenance (POMP)
  Mercaptopurine: Oral: 50 mg 3 times/day
    [total dose/cycle = 4200-4650 mg]
  Vincristine: IV: 2 mg day 1
    [total dose/cycle = 2 mg]
  Methotrexate: Oral: 20 mg/m^2/day days 1, 8, 15, and 22
    [total dose/cycle = 80 mg/m^2]
  Prednisone: Oral: 200 mg/day days 1 to 5
    [total dose/cycle = 1000 mg/m^2]
  or
  Mercaptopurine: IV: 1 g/m^2/day days 1 to 5
    [total dose/cycle = 5 g/m^2]
  Vincristine: IV: 2 mg day 1
    [total dose/cycle = 2 mg]
  Methotrexate: IV: 10 mg/m^2/day days 1 to 5
    [total dose/cycle = 50 mg/m^2]
  Prednisone: Oral: 200 mg/day days 1 to 5
    [total dose/cycle = 1000 mg/m^2]
  or
  Interferon alfa: SubQ: 5 million units/m^2 daily
    [total dose/cycle = 140-155 million units/m^2]
  Cytarabine: SubQ: 10 mg daily
    [total dose/cycle = 280-310 mg]
  Repeat cycles every month for 2 years
Variation 5:
  Cycle A (Cycles 1, 4, 6, and 8):
  Cyclophosphamide: IV: 300 mg/m^2 every 12 hours, for 6 doses, days 1, 2, and 3
    [total dose/cycle = 1800 mg/m^2]
  Mesna: IV: 600 mg/m^2/day continuous infusion days 1, 2, and 3
    [total dose/cycle = 1800 mg/m^2]
  Vincristine: IV: 2 mg/day days 4 and 11
    [total dose/cycle = 4 mg]
  Doxorubicin: IV: 50 mg/m^2 continuous infusion day 4
    [total dose/cycle = 50 mg/m^2]
  Dexamethasone: Oral, IV: 40 mg/day days 1 to 4 and 11 to 14
    [total dose/cycle = 320 mg]

Cycle B (Cycles 3, 5, 7, and 9):
  Methotrexate: IV: 200 mg/m^2 day 1
    followed by IV: 800 mg/m^2 continuous infusion day 1
    [total dose/cycle = 1 g/m^2]
  Leucovorin: IV: 50 mg (start 12 hours after end of methotrexate infusion)
    followed by IV: 15 mg every 6 hours, for 8 doses
    [total dose/cycle = 170 mg]
  Cytarabine: IV: 3 g/m^2 every 12 hours, for 4 doses, days 2 and 3
    [total dose/cycle = 12 g/m^2]
Cycle C: Liposomal Daunorubicin/Cytarabine (Cycle 2):
  Daunorubicin, liposomal: IV: 150 mg/m^2/day days 1 and 2
    [total dose/cycle = 300 mg/m^2]
  Cytarabine: IV: 1.5 g/m^2/day continuous infusion days 1 and 2
    [total dose/cycle = 3 g/m^2]
  Prednisone: Oral: 200 mg/day days 1 to 5
    [total dose/cycle = 1000 mg]
  Administer in the following sequence: ACBABABA (Cycle C does not repeat)
CNS Prophylaxis
  Methotrexate: Intrathecal: 12 mg day 2
    [total dose/cycle = 12 mg]
  or 6 mg into Ommaya day 2
    [total dose/cycle = 6 mg]
  Cytarabine: Intrathecal: 100 mg day 7 **or** 8
    [total dose/cycle = 100 mg]
  Repeat cycle every 3 weeks for 6 or 8 cycles
Maintenance (POMP)
  Mercaptopurine: IV: 1 g/m^2/day days 1 to 5
    [total dose/cycle = 5 g/m^2]
  Vincristine: IV: 2 mg day 1
    [total dose/cycle = 2 mg]
  Methotrexate: IV: 10 mg/m^2/day days 1 to 5
    [total dose/cycle = 50 mg/m^2]
  Prednisone: Oral: 200 mg/day days 1 to 5
    [total dose/cycle = 1000 mg]
  Repeat cycles monthly, except months 6, 7, 18, and 19 for 3 years
Intensification
  Methotrexate: IV: 100 mg/m^2/day days 1, 8, 15, and 22
    [total dose/cycle = 400 mg/m^2]
  Asparaginase: IV: 20,000 units/day days 2, 9, 16, and 23
    [total dose/cycle = 80,000 units]
  Given during months 6 and 18 of maintenance
  Cyclophosphamide: IV: 300 mg/m^2 every 12 hours, for 6 doses, days 1, 2, and 3
    [total dose/cycle = 1800 mg/m^2]
  Mesna: IV: 600 mg/m^2/day continuous infusion days 1, 2, and 3
    [total dose/cycle = 1800 mg/m^2]
  Vincristine: IV: 2 mg/day days 4 and 11
    [total dose/cycle = 4 mg]
  Doxorubicin: IV: 50 mg/m^2/day continuous infusion day 4
    [total dose/cycle = 50 mg/m^2]
  Dexamethasone: Oral, IV: 40 mg/day days 1 to 4 and 11 to 14
    [total dose/cycle = 320 mg]
  Given during months 7 and 19 of maintenance

◄
References
Variation 1:

Kantarjian H, Thomas D, O'Brien S, et al, "Long-Term Follow-Up Results of Hyperfractionated Cyclophosphamide, Vincristine, Doxorubicin, and Dexamethasone (Hyper-CVAD), A Dose-Intensive Regimen, in Adult Acute Lymphocytic Leukemia," *Cancer*, 2004, 101(12):2788-2801.

Variation 2:

Thomas DA, Cortes J, O'Brien S, et al, "Hyper-CVAD Program in Burkitt's-Type Adult Acute Lymphoblastic Leukemia," *J Clin Oncol*, 1999, 17(8):2461-70.

Variation 3:

Thomas DA, O'Brien S, Cortes J, et al, "Outcome With the Hyper-CVAD Regimens in Lymphoblastic Lymphoma," *Blood*, 2004, 104(6):1624-30.

Variation 4:

Kantarjian HM, O'Brien S, Smith TL, et al, "Results of Treatment With Hyper-CVAD, A Dose-Intensive Regimen, in Adult Acute Lymphocytic Leukemia," *J Clin Oncol*, 2000, 18(3): 547-61.

Variation 5:

Thomas DA, O'Brien S, Cortes J, et al, "Outcome With the Hyper-CVAD Regimens in Lymphoblastic Lymphoma," *Blood*, 2004, 104(6):1624-30.

Hyper-CVAD (Multiple Myeloma)
Use Multiple myeloma
Regimen
Cyclophosphamide: IV: 300 mg/m^2 every 12 hours, for 6 doses, days 1, 2, and 3

[total dose/cycle = 1800 mg/m^2]

Mesna: IV: 600 mg/m^2/day continuous infusion days 1, 2, and 3

[total dose/cycle = 1800 mg/m^2]

Doxorubicin: IV: 25 mg/m^2/day continuous infusion days 4 and 5

[total dose/cycle = 50 mg/m^2]

Vincristine: IV: 1 mg/day continuous infusion days 4 and 5

followed by IV: 2 mg day 11

[total dose/cycle = 4 mg]

Dexamethasone: Oral, IV: 20 mg/m^2/day days 1 to 5 and 11 to 14

[total dose/cycle = 180 mg/m^2]

Repeat cycle once if ≥50% reduction in myeloma protein

Maintenance
Cyclophosphamide: Oral: 125 mg/m^2 every 12 hours, for 10 doses, days 1 to 5

[total dose/cycle = 1250 mg/m^2]

Dexamethasone: Oral: 20 mg/m^2/day days 1 to 5

[total dose/cycle = 100 mg/m^2]

Repeat maintenance cycle every 5 weeks

References
Dimopoulos MA, Weber D, Kantarjian H, et al, "HyperCVAD for VAD-Resistant Multiple Myeloma," *Am J Hematol*, 1996, 52(2):77-81.

Ibrutinib-Bendamustine-Rituximab (CLL)
Index Terms Ibrutinib-BR (CLL); Rituximab-Bendamustine-Ibrutinib (CLL)
Use Leukemia, chronic lymphocytic (relapsed/refractory)
Regimen NOTE: Patients with deletion 17p are known to respond poorly to bendamustine plus rituximab and were excluded from this study.

Cycle 1:

Ibrutinib: Oral: 420 mg once daily days 1 to 28

[total dose/cycle = 11,760 mg]

Rituximab: IV: 375 mg/m^2 day 1 cycle 1 only

[total dose/cycle 1 = 375 mg/m^2]

Bendamustine: IV: 70 mg/m^2/day days 2 and 3
[total dose/cycle = 140 mg/m^2]
Cycles 2 to 6:
Ibrutinib: Oral: 420 mg once daily days 1 to 28
[total dose/cycle = 11,760 mg]
Rituximab: IV: 500 mg/m^2 day 1
[total dose/cycle = 500 mg/m^2]
Bendamustine: IV: 70 mg/m^2/day days 1 and 2
[total dose/cycle = 140 mg/m^2]
Repeat cycle every 28 days for up to 6 cycles
Subsequent cycles:
Ibrutinib: Oral: 420 mg once daily days 1 to 28
[total dose/cycle = 11,760 mg]
Repeat cycle every 28 days until disease progression or unacceptable toxicity

References

Chanan-Khan A, Cramer P, Demirkan F, et al. Ibrutinib combined with bendamustine and rituximab compared with placebo, bendamustine, and rituximab for previously treated chronic lymphocytic leukaemia or small lymphocytic lymphoma (HELIOS): a randomised, double-blind, phase 3 study. *Lancet Oncol.* 2016;17(2):200-211.

◆ **Ibrutinib-BR (CLL)** *see* Ibrutinib-Bendamustine-Rituximab (CLL) *on page 2152*

◆ **ICE (Ewing Sarcoma)** *see* Ifosfamide-Carboplatin-Etoposide (Ewing Sarcoma) *on page 2154*

ICE (Hodgkin)

Index Terms Ifosfamide-Carboplatin-Etoposide (Hodgkin)

Use Lymphoma, Hodgkin

Regimen

Etoposide: IV: 100 mg/m^2/day days 1 to 3
[total dose/cycle = 300 mg/m^2]
Carboplatin: IV: AUC 5 day 2 (maximum dose: 800 mg)
[total dose/cycle = AUC 5, maximum dose: 800 mg]
Ifosfamide: IV: 5 g/m^2/day continuous infusion for 24 hours day 2
[total dose/cycle = 5 g/m^2]
Mesna: IV: 5 g/m^2/day continuous infusion for 24 hours day 2
[total dose/cycle = 5 g/m^2]
Filgrastim: 5 mcg/kg/day days 5 to 12 (except during PBPC mobilization)
Repeat cycle every 14 days for 2 cycles

References

Moskowitz CH, Nimer SD, Zelenetz AD, et al, "A 2-Step Comprehensive High-Dose Chemoradiotherapy Second-Line Program for Relapsed and Refractory Hodgkin Disease: Analysis by Intent to Treat and Development of a Prognostic Model," *Blood*, 2001, 97(3):616-23.

◆ **ICE (Osteosarcoma)** *see* Ifosfamide-Carboplatin-Etoposide (Osteosarcoma) *on page 2154*

◆ **IC (Small Cell Lung Cancer)** *see* Carboplatin-Irinotecan (Small Cell Lung Cancer) *on page 2018*

◆ **Idarubicin-ATRA (APL)** *see* Tretinoin-Idarubicin (APL) *on page 2221*

◆ **Idarubicin-Cytarabine (5 + 2) (AML Consolidation)** *see* 5 + 2 (Cytarabine-Idarubicin) (AML Consolidation) *on page 1970*

◆ **Idarubicin-Tretinoin (APL)** *see* Tretinoin-Idarubicin (APL) *on page 2221*

Idelalisib-Rituximab (CLL)

Index Terms Rituximab-Idelalisib (CLL)
Use Leukemia, chronic lymphocytic
Regimen
Idelalisib: Oral: 150 mg twice daily starting day 1, continue until disease progression or unacceptable toxicity
Rituximab: IV: 375 mg/m^2 day 1
  followed by: IV: 500 mg/m^2 every 2 weeks for 4 doses
    followed by: IV: 500 mg/m^2 every 4 weeks for 3 doses
Total of 8 Rituximab infusions.

References
Furman RR, Sharman JP, Coutre SE, et al. Idelalisib and rituximab in relapsed chronic lymphocytic leukemia. New Engl J Med. 2014;370(11):997-1007.

Ifosfamide-Carboplatin-Etoposide (Ewing Sarcoma)

Index Terms ICE (Ewing Sarcoma)
Use Ewing sarcoma (recurrent, refractory)
Regimen NOTE: Mesna uroprotection should be administered.
Ifosfamide: IV: 1,800 mg/m^2/day days 1 to 5
  [total dose/cycle = 9,000 mg/m^2]
Carboplatin: IV: 400 mg/m^2/day days 1 and 2
  [total dose/cycle = 800 mg/m^2]
Etoposide: IV: 100 mg/m^2/day days 1 to 5
  [total dose/cycle = 500 mg/m^2]
Filgrastim: SubQ: 5 to 10 mcg/kg/day days 6 to 18 if ANC ≥1,000/mm^3 or until post nadir ANC ≥1,000/mm^3
  [total dose/cycle = up to 65 to 130 mcg/kg]
Repeat cycle every 21 days for up to 12 cycles

References
Van Winkle P, Angiolillo A, Krailo M, et al. Ifosfamide, carboplatin, and etoposide (ICE) reinduction chemotherapy in a large cohort of children and adolescents with recurrent/refractory sarcoma: the Children's Cancer Group (CCG) experience. Pediatr Blood Cancer. 2005;44(4):338-347.

♦ **Ifosfamide-Carboplatin-Etoposide (Hodgkin)** *see* ICE (Hodgkin)
  on page 2153

Ifosfamide-Carboplatin-Etoposide (Osteosarcoma)

Index Terms ICE (Osteosarcoma)
Use Osteosarcoma (recurrent, refractory)
Regimen NOTE: Mesna uroprotection should be administered.
Ifosfamide: IV: 1,800 mg/m^2/day days 1 to 5
  [total dose/cycle = 9,000 mg/m^2]
Carboplatin: IV: 400 mg/m^2/day days 1 and 2
  [total dose/cycle = 800 mg/m^2]
Etoposide: IV: 100 mg/m^2/day days 1 to 5
  [total dose/cycle = 500 mg/m^2]
Filgrastim: SubQ: 5 to 10 mcg/kg/day days 6 to 18 if ANC ≥1,000/mm^3 or until post nadir ANC ≥1,000/mm^3
  [total dose/cycle = up to 65 to 130 mcg/kg]
Repeat cycle every 21 days for up to 12 cycles

References
Van Winkle P, Angiolillo A, Krailo M, et al. Ifosfamide, carboplatin, and etoposide (ICE) reinduction chemotherapy in a large cohort of children and adolescents with recurrent/refractory sarcoma: the Children's Cancer Group (CCG) experience. Pediatr Blood Cancer. 2005;44(4):338-347.

Ifosfamide-Cisplatin-Epirubicin (Osteosarcoma)

Index Terms Cisplatin-Ifosfamide-Epirubicin (Osteosarcoma)
Use Bone sarcoma (osteosarcoma, pre and postoperative)
Regimen

Cycles 1 to 3 (prior to surgery):
Epirubicin: IV: 90 mg/m^2 over 15 minutes day 1
[total dose/cycle = 90 mg/m^2]
Cisplatin: IV: 100 mg/m^2 over 2 hours day 1
[total dose/cycle = 100 mg/m^2]
Ifosfamide: IV: 2,000 mg/m^2/day over 4 hours days 2, 3, and 4
[total dose/cycle = 6,000 mg/m^2]
Mesna: IV: 2,000 mg/m^2/day over 4 hours days 2, 3, and 4
[total dose/cycle = 6,000 mg/m^2]
Repeat cycle every 21 days for 3 cycles
Cycles 4 to 6 (after surgery):
Epirubicin: IV: 90 mg/m^2 over 15 minutes day 1
[total dose/cycle = 90 mg/m^2]
Cisplatin: IV: 100 mg/m^2 over 2 hours day 1
[total dose/cycle = 100 mg/m^2]
Ifosfamide: IV: 2,000 mg/m^2/day over 4 hours days 2, 3, and 4
[total dose/cycle = 6,000 mg/m^2]
Mesna: IV: 2,000 mg/m^2/day over 4 hours days 2, 3, and 4
[total dose/cycle = 6,000 mg/m^2]
Repeat cycle every 28 days for 3 cycles

References

Basaran M, Bavbek ES, Saglam S, et al. A phase II study of cisplatin, ifosfamide and epirubicin combination chemotherapy in adults with nonmetastatic and extremity osteosarcomas. *Oncology.* 2007;72(3-4):255-260.

◆ **Ifosfamide-Doxorubicin (Soft Tissue Sarcoma)** *see* AIM (Soft Tissue Sarcoma) *on page 1980*

◆ **Ifosfamide-Epirubicin (Soft Tissue Sarcoma)** *see* Epirubicin-Ifosfamide (Soft Tissue Sarcoma) *on page 2103*

Ifosfamide-Etoposide (Ewing Sarcoma)

Use Bone sarcoma (Ewing sarcoma)
Regimen NOTE: Mesna uroprotection should be administered.

Etoposide: IV: 100 mg/m^2/day over 1 hour days 1 to 5
[total dose/cycle = 500 mg/m^2]
Ifosfamide: IV: 1,800 mg/m^2/day days 1 to 5
[total dose/cycle = 9,000 mg/m^2]
Repeat cycle every 21 days for a total of 12 cycles

References

Miser JS, Kinsella TJ, Triche TJ, et al. Ifosfamide with mesna uroprotection and etoposide: an effective regimen in the treatment of recurrent sarcomas and other tumors of children and young adults. *J Clin Oncol.* 1987;5(8):1191-1198.

◆ **Ifosfamide, Gemcitabine, Vinorelbine, Prednisolone (Hodgkin)** *see* IGEV (Hodgkin) *on page 2155*

IGEV (Hodgkin)

Index Terms Ifosfamide, Gemcitabine, Vinorelbine, Prednisolone (Hodgkin)
Use Lymphoma, Hodgkin

◀ **Regimen**
Ifosfamide: IV: 2000 mg/m^2/day over 2 hours days 1 to 4
[total dose/cycle = 8000 mg/m^2]
Mesna: IV: 2600 mg/m^2/day days 1 to 4
[total dose/cycle = 10,400 mg/m^2]
Gemcitabine: IV: 800 mg/m^2 days 1 and 4
[total dose/cycle = 1600 mg/m^2]
Vinorelbine: IV: 20 mg/m^2 day 1
[total dose/cycle = 20 mg/m^2]
Prednisolone: IV: 100 mg days 1 to 4
[total dose/cycle = 400 mg/m^2]
Filgrastim: Days 7 to 12 of each course or up to apheresis in the course of mobilization
Repeat cycle every 21 days for a total of 4 cycles

References
Santoro A, Magagnoli M, Spina M, et al, "Ifosfamide, Gemcitabine, and Vinorelbine: A New Induction Regimen for Refractory and Relapsed Hodgkin's Lymphoma," *Haematologica*, 2007, 92(1):35-41.

◆ **IL-2-Interferon Alfa 2 (RCC)** *see* Interleukin 2-Interferon Alfa-2 (RCC) *on page 2156*

◆ **Interferon Alfa 2b-Bevacizumab (RCC)** *see* Bevacizumab-Interferon Alfa (RCC) *on page 1994*

◆ **Interferon Alfa 2-Interleukin (RCC)** *see* Interleukin 2-Interferon Alfa-2 (RCC) *on page 2156*

◆ **Interferon Alfa-Bevacizumab (RCC)** *see* Bevacizumab-Interferon Alfa (RCC) *on page 1994*

Interleukin 2-Interferon Alfa-2 (RCC)

Index Terms Aldesleukin-Interferon Alfa-2 (RCC); IL-2-Interferon Alfa 2 (RCC); Interferon Alfa 2-Interleukin (RCC)
Use Renal cell cancer
Regimen
Induction (2 cycles):
Aldesleukin: IV: 18 million units/m^2/day continuous infusion days 1 to 5 and days 12 to 16
[total dose/cycle = 180 million units/m^2]
Repeat aldesleukin induction cycle one time (total of 2 cycles) after a 3-week rest between cycles
Interferon Alfa-2: SubQ: 6 million units/dose 3 times weekly continuously (no rest break) during induction cycles
[total dose/week = 18 million units/week]
Maintenance (begin after a 3-week aldesleukin rest):
Aldesleukin: IV: 18 million units/m^2/day continuous infusion days 1 to 5
[total dose/cycle = 90 million units/m^2]
Repeat aldesleukin maintenance cycle 3 times (total of 4 maintenance cycles) after 3-week rest between cycles
Interferon Alfa-2: SubQ: 6 million units/dose 3 times weekly continuously (no rest break) during maintenance cycles
[total dose/week = 18 million units/week]
References
Negrier S, Escudier B, Lasset C, et al, "Recombinant Human Interleukin-2, Recombinant Human Interferon Alfa-2a, or Both in Metastatic Renal-Cell Carcinoma. Groupe Français d'Immunothérapie," *N Engl J Med*, 1998, 338(18):1272-8.

Ipilimumab-Nivolumab (Melanoma)

Index Terms Nivolumab-Ipilimumab (Melanoma)

Use Melanoma (unresectable, metastatic, first-line)

Regimen NOTE: Multiple variations are listed.

Variation 1:

Cycles 1 to 4:

Nivolumab: IV: 1 mg/kg over 60 minutes day 1
  [total dose/cycle = 1 mg/kg]

Ipilimumab: IV: 3 mg/kg over 90 minutes day 1
  [total dose/cycle = 3 mg/kg]

Repeat cycle every 21 days for a total of 4 cycles

Subsequent Cycles:

Nivolumab: IV: 240 mg (flat dose) over 60 minutes day 1
  [total dose/cycle = 240 mg]

Repeat cycle every 14 days until disease progression or unacceptable
  toxicity

Variation 2:

Cycles 1 to 4:

Nivolumab: IV: 1 mg/kg over 60 minutes 1 day
  [total dose/cycle = 1 mg/kg]

Ipilimumab: IV: 3 mg/kg over 90 minutes day 1
  [total dose/cycle = 3 mg/kg]

Repeat cycle every 21 days for a total of 4 cycles

Subsequent Cycles:

Nivolumab: IV: 3 mg/kg over 60 minutes day 1
  [total dose/cycle = 3 mg/kg]

Repeat cycle every 14 days until disease progression or unacceptable
  toxicity; treatment beyond progression was allowed in patients tolerating
  drug and experiencing clinical benefit

References

Variation 1:
Opdivo (nivolumab) [prescribing information]. Princeton, NJ: Bristol-Myers Squibb; November 2016.
Variation 2:
Larkin J, Chiarion-Sileni V, Gonzalez R, et al. Combined Nivolumab and Ipilimumab or Mono-therapy in Untreated Melanoma. *N Engl J Med*. 2015;373(1):23-34.

- ◆ **IP (Small Cell Lung Cancer)** *see* Carboplatin-Irinotecan (Small Cell Lung Cancer) *on page 2018*

- ◆ **IP (Small Cell Lung Cancer)** *see* Cisplatin-Irinotecan (Small Cell Lung Cancer) *on page 2057*

- ◆ **IRd (Multiple Myeloma)** *see* Ixazomib-Lenalidomide-Dexamethasone (Multiple Myeloma) *on page 2162*

- ◆ **Irinotecan-Bevacizumab (Glioblastoma)** *see* Bevacizumab-Irinotecan (Glioblastoma) *on page 1994*

- ◆ **Irinotecan-Biweekly Cetuximab (Colorectal)** *see* Cetuximab (Biweekly)-Irinotecan (Colorectal) *on page 2029*

Irinotecan-Capecitabine (Esophageal Cancer)

Index Terms Capecitabine-Irinotecan (Esophageal Cancer)

Use Esophageal cancer

◀ **Regimen** NOTE: Multiple variations are listed.

Variation 1:

Irinotecan: IV: 250 mg/m^2/dose day 1

[total dose/cycle = 250 mg/m^2]

Capecitabine: Oral: 1000 mg/m^2/dose twice daily days 1 to 14

[total dose/cycle = 28000 mg/m^2]

Repeat cycle every 21 days until disease progression or unacceptable toxicity

Variation 2:

Irinotecan: IV: 250 mg/m^2/dose day 1

[total dose/cycle = 250 mg/m^2]

Capecitabine: Oral: 1000 mg/m^2/dose twice daily days 1 to 14

[total dose/cycle = 28000 mg/m^2]

Repeat cycle every 21 days for up to 24 weeks

References

Variation 1:

Moehler M, Kanzler S, Geissler M, et al, "A Randomized Multicenter Phase II Study Comparing Capecitabine With Irinotecan or Cisplatin in Metastatic Adenocarcinoma of the Stomach or Esophagogastric Junction," *Ann Oncol*, 2010, 21(1):71-7.

Variation 2:

Leary A, Assersohn L, Cunningham D, et al, "A Phase II Trial Evaluating Capecitabine and Irinotecan as Second Line Treatment in Patients With Oesophago-Gastric Cancer Who Have Progressed on, or Within 3 Months of Platinum-Based Chemotherapy," *Cancer Chemother Pharmacol*, 2009, 64(3):455-62.

Irinotecan-Capecitabine (Gastric Cancer)

Index Terms Capecitabine-Irinotecan (Gastric Cancer)

Use Gastric cancer

Regimen NOTE: Multiple variations are listed.

Variation 1:

Irinotecan: IV: 250 mg/m^2/dose day 1

[total dose/cycle = 250 mg/m^2]

Capecitabine: Oral: 1000 mg/m^2/dose twice daily days 1 to 14

[total dose/cycle = 28000 mg/m^2]

Repeat cycle every 21 days until disease progression or unacceptable toxicity

Variation 2:

Irinotecan: IV: 250 mg/m^2/dose day 1

[total dose/cycle = 250 mg/m^2]

Capecitabine: Oral: 1000 mg/m^2/dose twice daily days 1 to 14

[total dose/cycle = 28000 mg/m^2]

Repeat cycle every 21 days for up to 24 weeks

References

Variation 1:

Moehler M, Kanzler S, Geissler M, et al, "A Randomized Multicenter Phase II Study Comparing Capecitabine With Irinotecan or Cisplatin in Metastatic Adenocarcinoma of the Stomach or Esophagogastric Junction," *Ann Oncol*, 2010, 21(1):71-7.

Variation 2:

Leary A, Assersohn L, Cunningham D, et al, "A Phase II Trial Evaluating Capecitabine and Irinotecan as Second Line Treatment in Patients With Oesophago-Gastric Cancer Who Have Progressed on, or Within 3 Months of Platinum-Based Chemotherapy," *Cancer Chemother Pharmacol*, 2009, 64(3):455-62.

◆ **Irinotecan-Carboplatin (Small Cell Lung Cancer)** *see* Carboplatin-Irinotecan (Small Cell Lung Cancer) *on page 2018*

◆ **Irinotecan-Cetuximab** *see* Cetuximab-Irinotecan (Colorectal) *on page 2032*

Irinotecan-Cisplatin (Esophageal Cancer)

Index Terms Cisplatin-Irinotecan (Esophageal Cancer)

Use Esophageal cancer

Regimen NOTE: Multiple variations are listed.

Variation 1:

Cisplatin: IV: 30 mg/m^2/dose days 1, 8, 15, and 22
  [total dose/cycle = 120 mg/m^2]

Irinotecan: IV: 65 mg/m^2/dose days 1, 8, 15, and 22
  [total dose/cycle = 260 mg/m^2]

Repeat cycle every 6 weeks until disease progression.

Variation 2 (with concurrent radiation therapy):

Cisplatin: IV: 30 mg/m^2/dose on day 1 and 8
  [total dose/cycle = 60 mg/m^2]

Irinotecan: IV: 65 mg/m^2/dose day 1 and 8
  [total dose/cycle = 130 mg/m^2]

Treatment cycle is 21 days; cycle is not repeated.

Variation 3:

Cisplatin: IV: 30 mg/m^2/dose on days 1, 8, 22, and 29
  [total dose/cycle = 120 mg/m^2]

Irinotecan: IV: 50 mg/m^2/dose on days 1, 8, 22, and 29
  [total dose/cycle = 200 mg/m^2]

Administered (with concurrent radiation therapy) over one 5-week treatment
  cycle.

Followed by: Postoperative therapy:

Cisplatin: IV: 30 mg/m^2/dose on days 1 and 8
  [total dose/cycle = 60 mg/m^2]

Irinotecan: IV: 65 mg/m^2/dose on days 1 and 8
  [total dose/cycle = 130 mg/m^2]

Repeat postop cycle every 21 days for a total of 3 cycles.

Variation 4:

Cisplatin: IV: 30 mg/m^2/dose on day 1 and 8
  [total dose/cycle = 60 mg/m^2]

Irinotecan: IV: 65 mg/m^2/dose day 1 and 8
  [total dose/cycle = 130 mg/m^2]

Repeat cycle every 21 days.

References

Variation 1:
Ilson DH, Saltz L, Enzinger P, et al, "Phase II Trial of Weekly Irinotecan Plus Cisplatin in Advanced Esophageal Cancer," *J Clin Oncol*, 1999, 17(10):3270-5.

Variation 2:
Sharma R, Yang GY, Nava HR, et al, "A Single Institution Experience With Neoadjuvant Chemoradiation (CRT) With Irinotecan (I) and Cisplatin (C) in Locally Advanced Esophageal Carcinoma (LAEC)," *J Clin Oncol*, 2009, 27(15S):e15619 [abstract e15619 from 2009 annual ASCO meeting].

Variation 3:
Kleinberg L, Powell ME, Forastiere AA, et al, "Survival Outcome of E1201: An Eastern Cooperative Oncology Group (ECOG) Randomized Phase II Trial of Neoadjuvant Preoperative Paclitaxel/Cisplatin/Radiotherapy (RT) or Irinotecan/Cisplatin/RT in Endoscopy With Ultrasound (EUS) Staged Esophageal Adenocarcinoma," *J Clin Oncol*, 2008, 26(15S):4532 [abstract 4532 from 2008 annual ASCO meeting].

Variation 4:
Ilson DH, "Phase II Trial of Weekly Irinotecan/Cisplatin in Advanced Esophageal Cancer," *Oncology (Williston Park)*, 2004, 18(14 Suppl14):22-5.

◆ **Irinotecan-Cisplatin (Gastric)** *see* Cisplatin-Irinotecan (Gastric)
  on page 2056

◆ **Irinotecan-Cisplatin (NSCLC)** *see* Cisplatin-Irinotecan (NSCLC) *on page 2056*

◆ **Irinotecan-Cisplatin (Small Cell Lung Cancer)** *see* Cisplatin-Irinotecan (Small Cell Lung Cancer) *on page 2057*

Irinotecan-Fluorouracil-Leucovorin (Esophageal Cancer)

Index Terms Fluorouracil-Leucovorin-Irinotecan (Esophageal Cancer); Irinotecan-Leucovorin-Fluorouracil (Esophageal cancer)

Use Esophageal cancer

Regimen NOTE: Multiple variations are listed.

Variation 1:

Irinotecan: IV: 80 mg/m^2/dose days 1, 8, 15, 22, 29, and 36
[total dose/week = 480 mg/m^2]

Fluorouracil: IV: 2000 mg/m^2/dose continuous infusion over 24 hours days 1, 8, 15, 22, 29, and 36
[total dose/cycle = 12,000 mg/m^2]

Leucovorin Calcium: IV: 500 mg/m^2/dose continuous infusion over 24 hours days 1, 8, 15, 22, 29, and 36
[total dose/week = 3000 mg/m^2]

Repeat cycle every 8 weeks until disease progression or unacceptable toxicity.

Variation 2:

Irinotecan: IV: 80 mg/m^2/dose day 1
[total dose/cycle = 80 mg/m^2]

Leucovorin Calcium: IV: 500 mg/m^2/dose over 2 hours day 1
[total dose/cycle = 500 mg/m^2]

Fluorouracil: IV: 2000 mg/m^2/dose continuous infusion over 22 hours day 1 (begin immediately after leucovorin)
[total dose/cycle = 2000 mg/m^2]

Repeat every week for 6 weeks followed by a 1-week rest, continue until disease progression or unacceptable toxicity.

References

Variation 1:

Wolff K, Wein A, Reulbach U, et al, "Weekly High-Dose 5-Fluorouracil as a 24-h Infusion and Sodium Folinic Acid (AIO Regimen) Plus Irinotecan in Patients With Locally Advanced Nonresectable and Metastatic Adenocarcinoma or Squamous Cell Carcinoma of the Oesophagus: A Phase II Trial," *Anticancer Drugs*, 2009, 20(3):165-73.

Variation 2:

Dank M, Zaluski J, Barone C, et al, "Randomized Phase III Study Comparing Irinotecan Combined With 5-Fluorouracil and Folinic Acid to Cisplatin Combined With 5-Fluorouracil in Chemotherapy Naive Patients With Advanced Adenocarcinoma of the Stomach or Esophagogastric Junction," *Ann Oncol*, 2008, 19(8):1450-7.

◆ **Irinotecan-Fluorouracil-Leucovorin (Saltz Regimen) (Colorectal)** *see* Fluorouracil-Leucovorin-Irinotecan (Saltz Regimen) (Colorectal) *on page 2126*

◆ **Irinotecan-Leucovorin-Fluorouracil (Esophageal cancer)** *see* Irinotecan-Fluorouracil-Leucovorin (Esophageal Cancer) *on page 2160*

Irinotecan-Leucovorin-Fluorouracil (Gastric Cancer)

Index Terms Fluorouracil-Leucovorin-Irinotecan (Gastric Cancer)

Use Gastric cancer

Regimen NOTE: Multiple variations are listed.

Variation 1:

Irinotecan: IV: 80 mg/m²/dose day 1

[total dose/week = 80 mg/m²]

Leucovorin Calcium: IV: 500 mg/m²/dose over 2 hours day 1

[total dose/week = 500 mg/m²]

Fluorouracil: IV: 2000 mg/m²/dose continuous infusion over 22 hours day 1

[total dose/week = 2000 mg/m²]

Repeat cycle weekly for 6 weeks followed by a 1-week rest; repeat until disease progression or unacceptable toxicity

Variation 2:

Irinotecan: IV: 180 mg/m²/dose day 1

[total dose/cycle = 180 mg/m²]

Leucovorin Calcium: IV: 200 mg/m²/dose over 2 hours days 1 and 2

[total dose/cycle = 400 mg/m²]

Fluorouracil: IV bolus: 400 mg/m² days 1 and 2

followed by IV: 600 mg/m²/dose continuous infusion over 22 hours days 1 and 2

[total dose/cycle = 2000 mg/m²]

Repeat cycle every 14 days for at least 4 cycles or until disease progression or unacceptable toxicity

References

Variation 1:

Dank M, Zaluski J, Barone C, et al, "Randomized Phase III Study Comparing Irinotecan Combined With 5-Fluorouracil and Folinic Acid to Cisplatin Combined With 5-Fluorouracil in Chemotherapy Naive Patients With Advanced Adenocarcinoma of the Stomach or Esophagogastric Junction," *Ann Oncol*, 2008, 19(8):1450-7.

Variation 2:

Bouché O, Raoul JL, Bonnetain F, et al, "Randomized Multicenter Phase II Trial of a Biweekly Regimen of Fluorouracil and Leucovorin (LV5FU2), LV5FU2 Plus Cisplatin, or LV5FU2 Plus Irinotecan in Patients With Previously Untreated Metastatic Gastric Cancer: A Federation Francophone de Cancerologie Digestive Group Study–FFCD 9803," *J Clin Oncol*, 2004, 22 (21):4319-28.

◆ **Irinotecan-Oxaliplatin-Fluorouracil-Leucovorin (Pancreatic)** *see* FOL-FIRINOX (Pancreatic) *on page* 2129

◆ **Irinotecan, Oxaliplatin, Leucovorin, Fluorouracil (Colorectal)** *see* FOL-FOXIRI (Colorectal) *on page* 2132

Irinotecan-Temozolomide (Ewing Sarcoma)

Index Terms Temozolomide-Irinotecan (Ewing Sarcoma)

Use Ewing sarcoma

Regimen

Irinotecan: IV: 20 mg/m²/dose days 1 to 5 and days 8 to 12

[total dose/cycle = 200 mg/m²]

Temozolomide: Oral: 100 mg/m²/dose days 1 to 5

[total dose/cycle = 500 mg/m²]

Repeat cycle every 21 days

References

Casey DA, Wexler LH, Merchant MS, et al, "Irinotecan and Temozolomide for Ewing Sarcoma: The Memorial Sloan-Kettering Experience," *Pediatr Blood Cancer*, 2009, 53(6):1029-34.

◆ **Ixabepilone-Capecitabine (Breast)** *see* Capecitabine-Ixabepilone (Breast) *on page* 2008

Ixazomib-Lenalidomide-Dexamethasone (Multiple Myeloma)

Index Terms IRd (Multiple Myeloma); Lenalidomide-Dexamethasone-Ixazomib (Multiple Myeloma)

Use Multiple myeloma (relapsed and/or refractory)

Regimen

Ixazomib: Oral: 4 mg once weekly on days 1, 8, and 15; at least 1 hour before or 2 hours after food

[total dose/cycle = 12 mg]

Lenalidomide: Oral: 25 mg daily on days 1 to 21

[total dose/cycle = 525 mg]

Dexamethasone: Oral: 40 mg once weekly on days 1, 8, 15, and 22

[total dose/cycle = 160 mg]

Repeat cycle every 28 days until disease progression or unacceptable toxicity

References

Moreau P, Masszi T, Grzasko N, et al. Oral ixazomib, lenalidomide, and dexamethasone for multiple myeloma. *N Engl J Med.* 2016;374(17):1621-1634.

◆ **Lapatinib-Capecitabine (Breast)** *see* Capecitabine + Lapatinib (Breast) *on page 2008*

Lapatinib-Letrozole (Breast)

Index Terms Letrozole-Lapatinib (Breast)

Use Breast cancer

Regimen

Lapatinib: Oral: 1500 mg once daily days 1 to 28

[total dose/cycle = 42,000 mg]

Letrozole: Oral: 2.5 mg once daily days 1 to 28

[total dose/cycle = 70 mg]

Repeat cycle every 28 days until disease progression or unacceptable toxicity

References

Johnston S, Pippen J Jr, Pivot X, et al, "Lapatinib Combined With Letrozole Versus Letrozole and Placebo as First-Line Therapy for Postmenopausal Hormone Receptor-Positive Metastatic Breast Cancer," *J Clin Oncol*, 2009, 27(33):5538-46.

Lapatinib-Trastuzumab (Breast)

Index Terms Trastuzumab-Lapatinib (Breast)

Use Breast cancer

Regimen

Cycle 1:

Trastuzumab: IV: 4 mg/kg (loading dose) day 1 cycle 1 only

[total dose/cycle 1 = 4 mg/kg]

Lapatinib: Oral: 1000 mg/day days 1 to 7, take on an empty stomach 1 hour before or 1 hour after a meal

[total dose/cycle = 7000 mg]

Treatment cycle is 7 days

Subsequent cycles:

Trastuzumab: IV: 2 mg/kg day 1

[total dose/cycle = 2 mg/kg]

Lapatinib: Oral: 1000 mg/day days 1 to 7, take on an empty stomach 1 hour before or 1 hour after a meal

[total dose/cycle = 7000 mg]

Repeat cycle every 7 days

References

Blackwell KL, Burstein HJ, Storniolo AM, et al. Overall survival benefit with lapatinib in combination with trastuzumab for patients with human epidermal growth factor receptor 2-positive metastatic breast cancer: final results from the EGF104900 Study. *J Clin Oncol.* 2012;30 (21):2585-2592.

Blackwell KL, Burstein HJ, Storniolo AM, et al. Randomized study of lapatinib alone or in combination with trastuzumab in women with ErbB2-positive, trastuzumab-refractory metastatic breast cancer. *J Clin Oncol.* 2010;28(7):1124-1130.

Lenalidomide-Bortezomib-Dexamethasone (Multiple Myeloma)

Index Terms Bortezomib-Lenalidomide-Dexamethasone (Multiple Myeloma); RVD (Multiple Myeloma); VDR (Multiple Myeloma); VRd (Multiple Myeloma)

Use Multiple myeloma (first-line, transplant eligible or relapsed/refractory)

Regimen NOTE: Multiple variations are listed.

Variation 1 (first-line, transplant eligible):

Induction cycles 1 to 4:

Lenalidomide: Oral: 25 mg daily days 1 to 14
  [total dose/cycle = 350 mg]
Bortezomib: IV: 1.3 mg/m^2/day days 1, 4, 8, and 11
  [total dose/cycle = 5.2 mg/m^2]
Dexamethasone: Oral: 20 mg daily days 1, 2, 4, 5, 8, 9, 11, and 12
  [total dose/cycle = 160 mg]

Repeat cycle every 21 days for 4 cycles; patients with at least a partial response could proceed to autologous stem cell transplantation (after at least 4 cycles) or continue 4 more cycles of induction

Induction cycles 5 to 8:

Lenalidomide: Oral: 25 mg daily days 1 to 14
  [total dose/cycle = 350 mg]
Bortezomib: IV: 1.3 mg/m^2/day days 1, 4, 8, and 11
  [total dose/cycle = 5.2 mg/m^2]
Dexamethasone: Oral: 10 mg daily days 1, 2, 4, 5, 8, 9, 11, and 12
  [total dose/cycle = 80 mg]

Repeat cycle every 21 days for 4 cycles (total of 8 induction cycles); patients with at least a partial response could proceed to autologous stem cell transplantation or proceed to maintenance therapy

Maintenance:

Lenalidomide: Oral: 25 mg daily days 1 to 14 (or dose tolerated at end of cycle 8 induction)

[total dose/cycle = 350 mg]

Bortezomib: IV: 1.3 mg/m^2/day days 1 and 8 (or dose tolerated at end of cycle 8 induction)

[total dose/cycle = 2.6 mg/m^2]

Dexamethasone: Oral: 10 mg daily days 1, 2, 8, and 9

[total dose/cycle = 40 mg]

Repeat cycle every 21 days

Variation 2 (first-line, transplant eligible):

Induction:

Lenalidomide: Oral: 25 mg daily days 1 to 14

[total dose/cycle = 350 mg]

Bortezomib: IV: 1.3 mg/m^2/day days 1, 4, 8, and 11

[total dose/cycle = 5.2 mg/m^2]

Dexamethasone: Oral: 40 mg daily days 1, 8, and 15

[total dose/cycle = 120 mg]

Repeat cycle every 21 days for up to 8 cycles then proceed to maintenance therapy. Alternatively, patients could undergo autologous stem cell transplantation any time after 4 cycles.

Maintenance:

Bortezomib: IV: 1.3 mg/m^2/day days 1, 8, 15, and 22

[total dose/cycle = 5.2 mg/m^2]

Repeat cycle every 42 days for a total of 4 cycles

Variation 3 (first-line, transplant eligible):

Induction:

Lenalidomide: Oral: 25 mg daily days 1 to 14

[total dose/cycle = 350 mg]

Bortezomib: IV: 1.3 mg/m^2/day days 1, 8, and 15

[total dose/cycle = 3.9 mg/m^2]

Dexamethasone: Oral: 40 mg daily days 1, 8, and 15

[total dose/cycle = 120 mg]

or

Dexamethasone: Oral: 20 mg daily days 1, 2, 8, 9, 15, and 16

[total dose/cycle = 120 mg]

Repeat cycle every 21 days

Variation 4 (newly diagnosed and no intent for immediate transplant):

Induction:

Lenalidomide: Oral: 25 mg daily days 1 to 14

[total dose/cycle = 350 mg]

Bortezomib: IV: 1.3 mg/m^2/day days days 1, 4, 8, and 11

[total dose/cycle = 5.2 mg/m^2]

Dexamethasone: Oral: 20 mg daily days 1, 2, 4, 5, 8, 9, 11, and 12

[total dose/cycle = 160 mg]

Repeat cycle every 21 days for 8 cycles

Maintenance:

Lenalidomide: Oral: 25 mg daily days 1 to 21

[total dose/cycle = 525 mg]

Dexamethasone: Oral: 40 mg daily days 1, 8, 15, and 22

[total dose/cycle = 160 mg]

Repeat cycle every 28 days until disease progression or unacceptable toxicity

Variation 5 (relapsed or relapsed/refractory):
Induction cycles 1 to 4:
Lenalidomide: Oral: 15 mg daily days 1 to 14
[total dose/cycle = 210 mg]
Bortezomib: IV: 1 mg/m^2/day days 1, 4, 8, and 11
[total dose/cycle = 4 mg/m^2]
Dexamethasone: Oral: 20 mg daily days 1, 2, 4, 5, 8, 9, 11, and 12
[total dose/cycle = 160 mg]
Repeat cycle every 21 days for 4 cycles
Induction cycles 5 to 8:
Lenalidomide: Oral: 15 mg daily days 1 to 14
[total dose/cycle = 210 mg]
Bortezomib: IV: 1 mg/m^2/day days 1, 4, 8, and 11
[total dose/cycle = 4 mg/m^2]
Dexamethasone: Oral: 10 mg daily days 1, 2, 4, 5, 8, 9, 11, and 12
[total dose/cycle = 80 mg]
Repeat cycle every 21 days for 4 cycles (total of 8 induction cycles); patients with response or stable disease could proceed to maintenance therapy
Maintenance:
Lenalidomide: Oral: 15 mg daily days 1 to 14 (or dose tolerated at end of cycle 8 induction)
[total dose/cycle = 210 mg]
Bortezomib: IV: 1 mg/m^2/day days 1 and 8 (or dose tolerated at end of cycle 8 induction)
[total dose/cycle = 2 mg/m^2]
Dexamethasone: Oral: 10 mg daily days 1, 2, 8, and 9
[total dose/cycle = 40 mg]
Repeat cycle every 21 days until disease progression or unacceptable toxicity (may selectively discontinue any component while continuing the balance of maintenance therapy)

References

Variation 1:
Richardson PG, Weller E, Lonial S, et al. Lenalidomide, bortezomib, and dexamethasone combination therapy in patients with Newly diagnosed multiple myeloma. *Blood.* 2010;116 (5):679-686.
Variation 2:
Kumar S, Flinn I, Richardson PG, et al. Randomized, multicenter, phase 2 study (EVOLUTION) of combinations of bortezomib, dexamethasone, cyclophosphamide, and lenalidomide in previously untreated multiple myeloma. *Blood.* 2012;119(19):4375-4382.
Variation 3:
Rajkumar SV. Multiple myeloma: 2011 update on diagnosis, risk-stratification, and management. *Am J Hematol.* 2011;86(1):57-65.
Variation 4:
Durie BG, Hoering A, Abidi MH, et al. Bortezomib with lenalidomide and dexamethasone versus lenalidomide and dexamethasone alone in patients with newly diagnosed myeloma without intent for immediate autologous stem-cell transplant (SWOG S0777): a randomised, open-label, phase 3 trial. *Lancet.* 2017;389(10068):519-527.
Variation 5:
Richardson PG, Xie W, Jagannath S, et al. A phase 2 trial of lenalidomide, bortezomib, and dexamethasone in patients with relapsed and relapsed/refractory myeloma. *Blood.* 2014;123 (10):1461-1469.

◆ **Lenalidomide, Carfilzomib, Dexamethasone (Multiple Myeloma)** *see* Carfilzomib, Lenalidomide, Dexamethasone (Multiple Myeloma) *on page 2026*

◆ **Lenalidomide-Daratumumab-Dexamethasone (Multiple Myeloma)** *see* Daratumumab-Lenalidomide-Dexamethasone (Multiple Myeloma) on page 2084

◆ **Lenalidomide-Dexamethasone-Elotuzumab (Multiple Myeloma)** *see* Elotuzumab-Lenalidomide-Dexamethasone (Multiple Myeloma) on page 2100

◆ **Lenalidomide-Dexamethasone-Ixazomib (Multiple Myeloma)** *see* Ixazomib-Lenalidomide-Dexamethasone (Multiple Myeloma) on page 2162

Lenalidomide-Dexamethasone (Multiple Myeloma)

Index Terms Dexamethasone (Low-Dose)-Lenalidomide (Multiple Myeloma); Dexamethasone-Lenalidomide (Multiple Myeloma); Rd (Multiple Myeloma)

Use Multiple myeloma

Regimen NOTE: Multiple variations are listed.

Variation 1 (low dose dexamethasone):

Lenalidomide: Oral: 25 mg/day days 1 to 21
[total dose/cycle = 525 mg]

Dexamethasone: Oral: 40 mg/day days 1, 8, 15, and 22
[total dose/cycle = 160 mg]

Repeat cycle every 28 days

Variation 2:

Cycles 1 to 4:

Lenalidomide: Oral: 25 mg/day days 1 to 21
[total dose/cycle = 525 mg]

Dexamethasone: Oral: 40 mg/day days 1 to 4, 9 to 12, and 17 to 20 (cycles 1 to 4)
[total dose/cycle = 480 mg]

Repeat cycle every 28 days for 4 cycles

Subsequent cycles:

Lenalidomide: Oral: 25 mg/day days 1 to 21
[total dose/cycle = 525 mg]

Dexamethasone: Oral: 40 mg/day days 1 to 4
[total dose/cycle = 160 mg]

Repeat cycle every 28 days until disease progression or unacceptable toxicity

References

Variation 1:

Rajkumar SV, Jacobus S, Callander NS, et al. Lenalidomide plus high-dose dexamethasone versus lenalidomide plus low-dose dexamethasone as initial therapy for newly diagnosed multiple myeloma: an open-label randomised controlled trial. *Lancet Oncol.* 2010;11(1):29-37.

Variation 2:

Dimopoulos MA, Chen C, Spencer A, et al. Long-term follow-up on overall survival from the MM-009 and MM-010 phase III trials of lenalidomide plus dexamethasone in patients with relapsed or refractory multiple myeloma. *Leukemia.* 2009;23(11):2147-2152.

Dimopoulos M, Spencer A, Attal M, et al. Lenalidomide plus dexamethasone for relapsed or refractory multiple myeloma. *N Engl J Med.* 2007;357(21):2123-2132.

Weber DM, Chen C, Niesvizky R, et al. Lenalidomide plus dexamethasone for relapsed multiple myeloma in North America. *N Engl J Med.* 2007;357(21):2133-2142.

Lenalidomide-Rituximab (CLL)

Index Terms Rituximab-Lenalidomide (CLL)

Use Leukemia, chronic lymphocytic (relapsed/refractory)

Regimen

Cycle 1:

Rituximab: IV: 375 mg/m^2/day days 1, 8, 15, and 22
[total dose/cycle = 1,500 mg/m^2]

Lenalidomide: Oral: 10 mg daily starting on day 9 of cycle 1
[total dose/cycle = 200 mg]

Treatment duration of cycle 1 is 28 days

Cycle 2:

Lenalidomide: Oral: 10 mg daily days 1 to 28
[total dose/cycle = 280 mg]

Treatment duration of cycle 2 is 28 days

Cycles 3 to 12:

Rituximab: IV: 375 mg/m^2 day 1
[total dose/cycle = 375 mg/m^2]

Lenalidomide: Oral: 10 mg daily days 1 to 28
[total dose/cycle = 280 mg]

Repeat cycle every 28 days for a total of 12 cycles; if patients experienced ongoing partial or complete response lenalidomide could be continued beyond 12 cycles

References

Badoux XC, Keating MJ, Wen S, et al. Phase II study of lenalidomide and rituximab as salvage therapy for patients with relapsed or refractory chronic lymphocytic leukemia. *J Clin Oncol.* 2013;31(5):584-591.

◆ **Lenvatinib-Everolimus (RCC)** *see* Everolimus-Lenvatinib (RCC) on page 2111

◆ **Letrozole-Lapatinib (Breast)** *see* Lapatinib-Letrozole (Breast) on page 2162

◆ **Letrozole-Palbociclib (Breast)** *see* Palbociclib-Letrozole (Breast) on page 2189

Letrozole-Ribociclib (Breast Cancer Regimen)

Index Terms Ribociclib-Letrozole (Breast Cancer Regimen)

Use Breast cancer, advanced (HR-Positive, HER2-Negative)

Regimen

Ribociclib: Oral: 600 mg once daily days 1 to 21
[total dose/cycle = 12,600 mg]

Letrozole: Oral: 2.5 mg once daily days 1 to 28
[total dose/cycle = 70 mg]

Repeat cycle every 28 days until disease progression or unacceptable toxicity

References

Hortobagyi GN, Stemmer SM, Burris HA, et al. Ribociclib as first-line therapy for HR-positive, advanced breast cancer. *N Engl J Med.* 2016;375(18):1738-1748.

◆ **Leucovorin-Fluorouracil (Colorectal)** *see* Fluorouracil-Leucovorin Bolus (Colorectal) on page 2124

Linker Protocol (ALL)

Use Leukemia, acute lymphocytic

Regimen

Remission induction:

Daunorubicin: IV: 50 mg/m^2/day days 1, 2, and 3
[total dose/cycle = 150 mg/m^2]

◀

Vincristine: IV: 2 mg/day days 1, 8, 15, and 22
[total dose/cycle = 8 mg]
Prednisone: Oral: 60 mg/m²/day days 1 to 28
[total dose/cycle = 1680 mg/m²]
Asparaginase: IM: 6000 units/m²/day days 17 to 28
[total dose/cycle = 72,000 units/m²]
If residual leukemia in bone marrow on day 14:
Daunorubicin: IV: 50 mg/m² day 15
[total dose/cycle = 50 mg/m²]
If residual leukemia in bone marrow on day 28:
Daunorubicin: IV: 50 mg/m²/day days 29 and 30
[total dose/cycle = 100 mg/m²]
Vincristine: IV: 2 mg/day days 29 and 36
[total dose/cycle = 4 mg]
Prednisone: Oral: 60 mg/m²/day days 29 to 42
[total dose/cycle = 840 mg/m²]
Asparaginase: IM: 6000 units/m²/day days 29 to 35
[total dose/cycle = 42,000 units/m²]

Consolidation therapy:
Treatment A (cycles 1, 3, 5, and 7):
Daunorubicin: IV: 50 mg/m²/day days 1 and 2
[total dose/cycle = 100 mg/m²]
Vincristine: IV: 2 mg/day days 1 and 8
[total dose/cycle = 4 mg]
Prednisone: Oral: 60 mg/m²/day days 1 to 14
[total dose/cycle = 840 mg/m²]
Asparaginase: IM: 12,000 units/m²/day days 2, 4, 7, 9, 11, and 14
[total dose/cycle = 72,000 units/m²]
Treatment B (cycles 2, 4, 6, and 8):
Teniposide: IV: 165 mg/m²/day days 1, 4, 8, and 11
[total dose/cycle = 660 mg/m²]
Cytarabine: IV: 300 mg/m²/day days 1, 4, 8, and 11
[total dose/cycle = 1200 mg/m²]
Treatment C (cycle 9):
Methotrexate: IV: 690 mg/m² continuous infusion over 42 hours day 1
[total dose/cycle = 690 mg/m²]
Leucovorin: IV: 15 mg/m² every 6 hours for 12 doses (start at end of
methotrexate infusion)
[total dose/cycle = 180 mg/m²]
Administer remission induction regimen for one cycle only. Repeat consolidation cycle every 28 days.

References
Linker CA, Levitt LJ, O'Donnell M, et al, "Treatment of Adult Acute Lymphoblastic Leukemia With
Intensive Cyclical Chemotherapy: A Follow-up Report," *Blood*, 1991 78(11):2814-22.

◆ **Lonsurf (Colorectal Regimen)** *see* Trifluridine and Tipiracil (Colorectal
Regimen) *on page* 2224

MAC (Gestational Trophoblastic Tumor)
Index Terms Methotrexate-Leucovorin-Cyclophosphamide-Dactinomycin
(Gestational Trophoblastic Tumor)
Use Gestational trophoblastic tumor

Regimen

Methotrexate: IM: 1 mg/kg/day days 1, 3, 5, and 7
[total dose/cycle = 4 mg/kg]

Leucovorin Calcium: IM: 0.1 mg/kg/day (begin 24 hours after each methotrexate injection) days 2, 4, 6, and 8
[total dose/cycle = 0.4 mg/kg]

Dactinomycin: IV: 12 mcg/kg/day days 1 to 5
[total dose/cycle = 60 mcg/kg]

Cyclophosphamide: IV: 3 mg/kg/day days 1 to 5
[total dose/cycle = 15 mg/kg]

Repeat cycle every 21 days, continue until 3 consecutive normal hCG levels and then 1 more cycle

References

Berkowitz RS, Goldstein DP, Bernstein MR. Modified triple chemotherapy in the management of high-risk metastatic gestational trophoblastic tumors. *Gynecol Oncol*. 1984;19(2):173-181.

MAID (Soft Tissue Sarcoma)

Index Terms Doxorubicin-Dacarbazine-Ifosfamide-Mesna (Soft Tissue Sarcoma); Mesna-Doxorubicin-Ifosfamide-Dacarbazine (Soft Tissue Sarcoma)

Use Soft tissue sarcoma (metastatic, unresectable)

Regimen NOTE: Multiple variations are listed. Mesna uroprotection should be administered.

Variation 1 (no prior radiation):

Doxorubicin: IV: 20 mg/m^2/day continuous infusion days 1, 2, and 3
[total dose/cycle = 60 mg/m^2]

Ifosfamide: IV: 2,500 mg/m^2/day continuous infusion days 1, 2, and 3
[total dose/cycle = 7,500 mg/m^2]

Dacarbazine: IV: 300 mg/m^2/day continuous infusion days 1, 2, and 3
[total dose/cycle = 900 mg/m^2]

Repeat cycle every 21 days (delay 1 week if WBC <3,000/mm^3 or platelets <100,000/mm^3)

Variation 2 (if prior pelvic irradiation):

Doxorubicin: IV: 20 mg/m^2/day continuous infusion days 1, 2, and 3
[total dose/cycle = 60 mg/m^2]

Ifosfamide: IV: 1,500 mg/m^2/day continuous infusion days 1, 2, and 3
[total dose/cycle = 4,500 mg/m^2]

Dacarbazine: IV: 300 mg/m^2/day continuous infusion days 1, 2, and 3
[total dose/cycle = 900 mg/m^2]

Repeat cycle every 21 days (delay 1 week if WBC <3,000/mm^3 or platelets <100,000/mm^3)

Variation 3:

Doxorubicin: IV: 15 mg/m^2/day continuous infusion days 1 to 4
[total dose/cycle = 60 mg/m^2]

Ifosfamide: IV: 2,000 mg/m^2/day continuous infusion days 1, 2, and 3
[total dose/cycle = 6,000 mg/m^2]

Dacarbazine: IV: 250 mg/m^2/day continuous infusion days 1 to 4
[total dose/cycle = 1,000 mg/m^2]

Repeat cycle every 21 days (or when WBC ≥3,000/mm^3 and platelets ≥100,000/mm^3)

References

Variations 1 and 2:
Elias A, Ryan L, Sulkes A, et al. Response to mesna, doxorubicin, ifosfamide, and dacarbazine in 108 patients with metastatic or unresectable sarcoma and no prior chemotherapy. *J Clin Oncol*. 1989;7(9):1208-1216.

Variation 3:

Antman K, Crowley J, Balcerzak SP, et al. An intergroup phase III randomized study of doxorubicin and dacarbazine with or without ifosfamide and mesna in advanced soft tissue and bone sarcomas. *J Clin Oncol.* 1993;11(7):1276-1285.

MAP (Osteosarcoma)

Index Terms Cisplatin-Methotrexate-Doxorubicin (Osteosarcoma); Doxorubicin-Methotrexate-Cisplatin (Osteosarcoma); Methotrexate-Doxorubicin-Cisplatin (Osteosarcoma)

Use Osteosarcoma (resectable, high grade)

Regimen

Neoadjuvant (induction) therapy: Weeks 1 to 10:

Cisplatin: IV: 60 mg/m^2/day over 4 hours days 1 and 2 of weeks 1 and 6
[total dose/neoadjuvant (induction) therapy = 240 mg/m^2]

Doxorubicin: IV: 37.5 mg/m^2/day continuous infusion over 24 hours days 1 and 2 of weeks 1 and 6
[total dose/neoadjuvant (induction) therapy = 150 mg/m^2]

Methotrexate: IV: 12 g/m^2 (maximum dose: 20 g/dose) over 4 hours day 1 of weeks 4, 5, 9, and 10 for a total of 4 neoadjuvant (induction) doses
[total dose/neoadjuvant (induction) therapy = 48 g/m^2; maximum: 80 g]

Leucovorin calcium rescue: IV: (Dose not specified) beginning 24 to 28 hours after start of methotrexate infusion and continued until serum methotrexate level <0.1 micromolar

Surgery of the primary tumor: Week 11

Adjuvant (maintenance) therapy: Weeks 12 to 29:

Cisplatin: IV: 60 mg/m^2/day over 4 hours days 1 and 2 of weeks 12 and 17
[total dose/adjuvant (maintenance) therapy = 240 mg/m^2]

Doxorubicin: IV: 37.5 mg/m^2/day continuous infusion over 24 hours days 1 and 2 of weeks 12, 17, 22, and 26
[total dose/adjuvant (maintenance) therapy = 300 mg/m^2]

Methotrexate: IV: 12 g/m^2 (maximum dose: 20 g/dose) over 4 hours day 1 of weeks 15, 16, 20, 21, 24, 25, 28, and 29 for a total of 8 adjuvant (maintenance) doses
total dose/adjuvant (maintenance) therapy = 96 g/m^2: maximum: 160 g]

Leucovorin calcium rescue: IV: (Dose not specified) beginning 24 to 28 hours after start of methotrexate infusion and continued until serum methotrexate level <0.1 micromolar

References

Bielack SS, Smeland S, Whelan JS, et al. Methotrexate, doxorubicin, and cisplatin (MAP) plus maintenance pegylated interferon alfa-2b versus MAP alone in patients with resectable high-grade osteosarcoma and good histologic response to preoperative MAP: first results of the EURAMOS-1 good response randomized controlled trial. *J Clin Oncol.* 2015;33(20):2279-2287.
Whelan JS, Bielack SS, Marina N, et al. EURAMOS-1, an international randomised study for osteosarcoma: results from pre-randomisation treatment. *Ann Oncol.* 2015;26(2):407-414.

◆ **MEA (Gestational Trophoblastic Tumor)** *see* EMA (Gestational Trophoblastic Tumor) *on page* 2102

◆ **MEC (AML)** *see* Mitoxantrone-Etoposide-Cytarabine (AML) *on page* 2175

MEC-G (AML Induction)

Index Terms Cytarabine-Etoposide-Mitoxantrone-CSF (AML Induction); EMA-G (AML Induction)

Use Leukemia, acute myeloid

Regimen
Variation 1:
Mitoxantrone: IV: 12 mg/m²/day days 1, 2, and 3
[total dose/cycle = 36 mg/m²]
Cytarabine: IV: 500 mg/m²/day continuous infusion days 1, 2, and 3 and days 8, 9, and 10
[total dose/cycle = 3000 mg/m²]
Etoposide: IV: 200 mg/m²/day continuous infusion days 8, 9, and 10
[total dose/cycle = 600 mg/m²]
Sargramostim: IV: 5 mcg/kg/day over 6 hours days 4 to 8
Variation 2:
Mitoxantrone: IV: 12 mg/m²/day IV bolus days 1, 2, and 3
[total dose/cycle = 36 mg/m²]
Cytarabine: IV: 500 mg/m²/day continuous infusion days 1, 2, and 3 and days 8, 9, and 10
[total dose/cycle = 3000 mg/m²]
Etoposide: IV: 200 mg/m²/day continuous infusion days 8, 9, and 10
[total dose/cycle = 600 mg/m²]
Filgrastim: SubQ: 5 mcg/kg/day starting on day 4 til ANC >500/mm³ for 2 consecutive days
Administer one cycle only

References
Variation 1:
Archimbaud E, Fenaux P, Reiffers J, et al, "Granulocyte-Macrophage Colony-Stimulating Factor in Association to Timed-Sequential Chemotherapy With Mitoxantrone, Etoposide, and Cytarabine for Refractory Acute Myelogenous Leukemia," *Leukemia*, 1993, 7(3):372-7.
Variation 2:
He XY, Elson P, Pohlman B, et al, "Timed Sequential Chemotherapy With Concomitant Granulocyte Colony-Stimulating Factor for High-Risk Acute Myelogenous Leukemia: A Single Arm Clinical Trial," *BMC Cancer*, 2002, 2:12.
He XY, Pohlman B, Lichtin A, et al, "Timed-Sequential Chemotherapy With Concomitant Granulocyte Colony-Stimulating Factor for Newly Diagnosed De Novo Acute Myelogenous Leukemia," *Leukemia*, 2003, 17(6):1078-84.

◆ **Mechlorethamine, Doxorubicin, Vinblastine, Vincristine, Bleomycin, Etoposide, Prednisone (Hodgkin)** *see* Stanford V (Hodgkin) *on page 2209*

◆ **Mechlorethamine, Vincristine, Procarbazine, Prednisone, Doxorubicin, Bleomycin, Vinblastine, Dacarbazine (Hodgkin)** *see* MOPP/ABVD (Hodgkin) *on page 2176*

◆ **Mechlorethamine, Vincristine, Procarbazine, Prednisone, Doxorubicin, Bleomycin, Vinblastine (Hodgkin)** *see* MOPP/ABV Hybrid (Hodgkin) *on page 2177*

◆ **Mechlorethamine, Vincristine, Procarbazine, Prednisone (Hodgkin)** *see* MOPP (Hodgkin) *on page 2178*

Melphalan-Prednisone (Multiple Myeloma)
Index Terms MP (Multiple Myeloma)
Use Multiple myeloma
Regimen NOTE: Multiple variations are listed.
Variation 1:
Melphalan: Oral: 0.25 mg/kg/dose days 1 to 4
[total dose/cycle = 1 mg/kg]
Prednisone: Oral: 2 mg/kg/dose days 1 to 4
[total dose/cycle = 8 mg/kg]
Repeat cycle every 6 weeks for a total of 12 cycles

◄ Variation 2:
Melphalan: Oral: 4 mg/m^2/dose days 1 to 7
[total dose/cycle = 28 mg/m^2]
Prednisone: Oral: 40 mg/m^2/dose days 1 to 7
[total dose/cycle = 280 mg/m^2]
Repeat cycle every 4 weeks for a total of 6 cycles
Variation 3:
Melphalan: Oral: 9 mg/m^2/dose days 1 to 4
[total dose/cycle = 36 mg/m^2]
Prednisone: Oral: 60 mg/m^2/dose days 1 to 4
[total dose/cycle = 240 mg/m^2]
Repeat cycle every 6 weeks for a total of 9 cycles
Variation 4:
Melphalan: Oral: 6 mg/m^2/dose days 1 to 7
[total dose/cycle = 42 mg/m^2]
Prednisone: Oral: 60 mg/m^2/dose days 1 to 7
[total dose/cycle = 420 mg/m^2]
Repeat cycle every 4 weeks for a total of 6 cycles
Followed by (in responders):
Interferon alfa: SubQ: 3 million units/dose 3 times/week until relapse
Dexamethasone: Oral: 40 mg/dose days 1 to 4 every 2 months until relapse

References

Variation 1:
Facon T, Mary JY, Hulin C, et al, "Melphalan and Prednisone Plus Thalidomide Versus Melphalan and Prednisone Alone or Reduced-Intensity Autologous Stem Cell Transplantation in Elderly Patients With Multiple Myeloma (IFM 99-06): A Randomised Trial," *Lancet*, 2007, 370 (9594):1209-18.
Facon T, Mary JY, Pégourie B, et al, "Dexamethasone-Based Regimens Versus Melphalan-Prednisone for Elderly Multiple Myeloma Patients Ineligible for High-Dose Therapy," *Blood*, 2006, 107(4):1292-8.
Variation 2:
Palumbo A, Bringhen S, Caravita T, et al, "Oral Melphalan and Prednisone Chemotherapy Plus Thalidomide Compared With Melphalan and Prednisone Alone in Elderly Patients With Multiple Myeloma: Randomised Controlled Trial," *Lancet*, 2006, 367(9513):825-31.
Palumbo A, Bringhen S, Liberati AM, et al, "Oral Melphalan, Prednisone, and Thalidomide in Elderly Patients With Multiple Myeloma: Updated Results of a Randomized Controlled Trial," *Blood*, 2008, 112(8):3107-14.
Variation 3:
San Miguel JF, Schlag R, Khuageva NK, et al, "Bortezomib Plus Melphalan and Prednisone for Initial Treatment of Multiple Myeloma," *N Engl J Med*, 2008, 359(9):906-17.
Variation 4:
Palumbo A, Bringhen S, Petrucci MT, et al, "Intermediate-Dose Melphalan Improves Survival of Myeloma Patients Aged 50 to 70: Results of a Randomized Controlled Trial," *Blood*, 2004, 104 (10):3052-7.

Melphalan-Prednisone-Thalidomide (Multiple Myeloma)

Index Terms MPT (Multiple Myeloma)

Use Multiple myeloma

Regimen NOTE: Multiple variations are listed.
Variation 1:
Melphalan: Oral: 4 mg/m^2/day days 1 to 7
[total dose/cycle = 28 mg/m^2]
Prednisone: Oral: 40 mg/m^2/day days 1 to 7
[total dose/cycle = 280 mg/m^2]

Thalidomide: Oral: 100 mg/day days 1 to 28
  [total dose/cycle = 2800 mg]
Repeat cycle every 28 days for 6 cycles
followed by
Thalidomide: Oral: 100 mg daily (as maintenance)
Variation 2:
  Melphalan: Oral: 0.25 mg/kg/dose days 1 to 4
    [total dose/cycle = 1 mg/kg]
  Prednisone: Oral: 2 mg/kg/dose days 1 to 4
    [total dose/cycle = 8 mg/kg]
  Thalidomide: Oral: 100-400 mg/day days 1 to 42
    [total dose/cycle = 4200-16,800 mg]
  Repeat cycle every 6 weeks for a total of 12 cycles (discontinue thalidomide
  on day 4 of the last cycle)

References

Variation 1:
Palumbo A, Bertola A, Musto P, et al, "Oral Melphalan, Prednisone, and Thalidomide for Newly
  Diagnosed Patients With Myeloma," *Cancer* , 2005, 104(7):1428-33.
Palumbo A, Bringhen S, Caravita T, et al, "Oral Melphalan and Prednisone Chemotherapy Plus
  Thalidomide Compared With Melphalan and Prednisone Alone in Elderly Patients With Multiple
  Myeloma: Randomised Controlled Trial," *Lancet*, 2006, 367(9513):825-31.
Palumbo A, Bringhen S, Liberati AM, et al, "Oral Melphalan, Prednisone, and Thalidomide in
  Elderly Patients With Multiple Myeloma: Updated Results of a Randomized Controlled Trial,"
  Blood, 2008, 112(8):3107-14.
Variation 2:
Facon T, Mary JY, Hulin C, et al, "Melphalan and Prednisone Plus Thalidomide Versus Melphalan
  and Prednisone Alone or Reduced-Intensity Autologous Stem Cell Transplantation in Elderly
  Patients With Multiple Myeloma (IFM 99-06): A Randomised Trial," *Lancet*, 2007, 370
  (9594):1209-18.

◆ **Mesna-Doxorubicin-Ifosfamide-Dacarbazine (Soft Tissue Sarcoma)** *see*
  MAID (Soft Tissue Sarcoma) *on page 2169*

◆ **Mesna-Ifosfamide-Mitoxantrone-Etoposide and Etoposide-Methylprednisolone-Cytarabine-Cisplatin (Hodgkin)** *see* MINE-ESHAP (Hodgkin)
  on page 2174

◆ **Methotrexate-Doxorubicin-Cisplatin (Osteosarcoma)** *see* MAP (Osteosarcoma) *on page 2170*

◆ **Methotrexate-Leucovorin-Cyclophosphamide-Dactinomycin (Gestational Trophoblastic Tumor)** *see* MAC (Gestational Trophoblastic Tumor)
  on page 2168

◆ **Methotrexate-Vinblastine-Doxorubicin-Cisplatin (Bladder)** *see* MVAC
  (Bladder) *on page 2179*

Methotrexate-Vinblastine (Soft Tissue Sarcoma)

Index Terms Vinblastine-Methotrexate (Soft Tissue Sarcoma)
Use Soft tissue sarcoma (desmoid tumor, aggressive fibromatosis)
Regimen
  Methotrexate: IV: 30 mg/m² day 1 (dose usually rounded to 50 mg)
    [total dose/cycle = 30 mg/m²]
  Vinblastine: IV: 6 mg/m² day 1 (dose usually rounded to 10 mg)
    [total dose/cycle = 6 mg/m²]
  Repeat cycle every 7 to 10 days for 1 year (52 treatments)
References
Azzarelli A, Gronchi A, Bertulli R, et al. Low-dose chemotherapy with methotrexate and vinblastine
  for patients with advanced aggressive fibromatosis. *Cancer.* 2001;92(5):1259-1264.

♦ **mFOLFOX6 and FOLFOX6 (Colorectal)** *see* FOLFOX6 and mFOLFOX6 (Colorectal) *on page 2131*

MINE-ESHAP (Hodgkin)

Index Terms Mesna-Ifosfamide-Mitoxantrone-Etoposide and Etoposide-Methylprednisolone-Cytarabine-Cisplatin (Hodgkin)

Use Lymphoma, Hodgkin

Regimen

Refractory disease (alternate MINE regimen with ESHAP regimen for a total of 2 MINE cycles and 2 ESHAP cycles):

MINE Regimen:

Mesna: IV: 2250 mg/m^2/day days 1, 2, and 3
[total dose/cycle = 6750 mg/m^2]

Ifosfamide: IV: 1500 mg/m^2/day days 1, 2, and 3
[total dose/cycle = 4500 mg/m^2]

Mitoxantrone: IV: 10 mg/m^2 day 1
[total dose/cycle = 10 mg/m^2]

Etoposide: IV: 80 mg/m^2/day days 1, 2, and 3
[total dose/cycle = 240 mg/m^2]

Treatment cycle is 28 days

ESHAP Regimen:

Etoposide: IV: 40 mg/m^2/day days 1 to 4
[total dose/cycle = 160 mg/m^2]

Methylprednisolone: IV: 250 mg/day days 1 to 4
[total dose/cycle = 1000 mg]

Cisplatin: IV: 25 mg/m^2/day continuous infusion over 21 hours days 1 to 4
[total dose/cycle = 100 mg/m^2]

Cytarabine: IV: 2000 mg/m^2 day 5
[total dose/cycle = 2000 mg/m^2]

Treatment cycle is 28 days

References

Fernandex de Larrea C, Martinez C, Gaya A, et al, "Salvage Chemotherapy With Alternating MINE-ESHAP Regimen in Relapsed or Refractory Hodgkin's Lymphoma Followed By Autologous Stem-Cell Transplantation," *Ann Oncol*, 2010, 21(6):1211-6.

mini-BEAM (Hodgkin)

Index Terms Carmustine-Etoposide-Cytarabine-Melphalan (Hodgkin)

Use Lymphoma, Hodgkin

Regimen

Carmustine: IV: 60 mg/m^2 over 30 minutes day 1
[total dose/cycle = 60 mg/m^2]

Etoposide: IV: 75 mg/m^2/day over 30 minutes days 2 to 5
[total dose/cycle = 300 mg/m^2]

Cytarabine: IV: 100 mg/m^2 every 12 hours days 2 to 5 (total of 8 doses)
[total dose/cycle = 800 mg/m^2]

Melphalan: IV: 30 mg/m^2 over 15 minutes day 6
[total dose/cycle = 30 mg/m^2]

Repeat cycle every 4 to 6 weeks

References

Colwill R, Crump M, Couture F, et al, "Mini-BEAM as Salvage Therapy for Relapsed or Refractory Hodgkin's Disease Before Intensive Therapy and Autologous Bone Marrow Transplantation," *J Clin Oncol*, 1995, 13(2):396-402.

Martín A, Fernández-Jiménez MC, Caballero MD, et al. "Long-Term Follow-Up in Patients Treated With Mini-BEAM as Salvage Therapy for Relapsed or Refractory Hodgkin's Disease," *Br J Haematol*, 2001, 113(1):161-71.

◆ **Mitomycin-Fluorouracil (Anal Cancer)** *see* Fluorouracil-Mitomycin (Anal Cancer) *on page 2128*

Mitoxantrone-Etoposide (AML Induction)

Index Terms MV (AML Induction)

Use Leukemia, acute myeloid

Regimen

Mitoxantrone: IV: 10 mg/m^2/day over ≤15 minutes days 1 to 5

   [total dose/cycle = 50 mg/m^2]

Etoposide: IV: 100 mg/m^2/day over 30 minutes days 1 to 5

   [total dose/cycle = 500 mg/m^2]

May administer a second induction cycle if needed

References

Ho AD, Lipp T, Ehninger G, et al, "Combination of Mitoxantrone and Etoposide in Refractory Acute Myelogenous Leukemia an Active and Well-Tolerated Regimen," *J Clin Oncol*, 1988, 6 (2):213-17.

Mitoxantrone-Etoposide-Cytarabine (AML)

Index Terms EMA (AML); MEC (AML)

Use Leukemia, acute myeloid (relapsed, refractory)

Regimen NOTE: Multiple variations are listed.

Variation 1 (induction):

Etoposide: IV: 80 mg/m^2/day over 1 hour days 1 to 6

   [total dose/cycle = 480 mg/m^2]

Cytarabine: IV: 1,000 mg/m^2/day over 6 hours days 1 to 6

   [total dose/cycle = 6,000 mg/m^2]

Mitoxantrone: IV: 6 mg/m^2/day days 1 to 6 (3 hours after the end of the cytarabine infusion)

   [total dose/cycle = 36 mg/m^2]

Patients in complete remission proceeded to consolidation therapy

Variation 2:

Etoposide: IV: 100 mg/m^2/day over 2 hours days 1 to 5

   [total dose/cycle = 500 mg/m^2]

Cytarabine: IV: 1,000 mg/m^2/day days 1 to 5

   [total dose/cycle = 5,000 mg/m^2]

Mitoxantrone: IV: 8 mg/m^2/day days 1 to 5

   [total dose/cycle = 40 mg/m^2]

References

Variation 1:

Amadori S, Arcese W, Isacchi G, et al. Mitoxantrone, etoposide, and intermediate-dose cytarabine: an effective and tolerable regimen for the treatment of refractory acute myeloid leukemia. *J Clin Oncol*. 1991;9(7):1210-1214.

Variation 2:

Döhner H, Weisdorf DJ, Bloomfield CD. Acute myeloid leukemia. *N Engl J Med*. 2015;373 (12):1136-1152.

Kohrt HE, Patel S, Ho M, et al. Second-line mitoxantrone, etoposide, and cytarabine for acute myeloid leukemia: a single-center experience. *Am J Hematol*. 2010;85(11):877-881.

Mitoxantrone-Prednisone (Prostate)

Index Terms MP (Prostate); Prednisone-Mitoxantrone (Prostate)

Use Prostate cancer

Regimen NOTE: Multiple variations are listed.

Variation 1:

Mitoxantrone: IV: 12 mg/m^2 day 1

   [total dose/cycle = 12 mg/m^2]

◄ Prednisone: Oral: 5 mg twice daily
[total dose/cycle = 210 mg]
Repeat cycle every 21 days, for up to a cumulative mitoxantrone dose of
140 mg/m^2 (Tannock, 1996); or for a total of 6 cycles (Berry, 2002); or for up
to a total of 10 cycles (Tannock, 2004)
Variation 2:
Cycle 1:
Mitoxantrone: IV: 12 mg/m^2 day 1
[total dose/cycle = 12 mg/m^2]
Prednisone: Oral: 5 mg twice daily
[total dose/cycle = 210 mg]
Treatment cycle is 21 days
Cycles 2-8:
Mitoxantrone: IV: 12-14 mg/m^2 day 1 (increase to 14 mg/m^2 if granulocyte
nadir is >1000/mm^3 and platelet nadir >50,000/mm^3)
[total dose/cycle = 12-14 mg/m^2]
Prednisone: Oral: 5 mg twice daily
[total dose/cycle = 210 mg]
Repeat cycle every 21 days for a maximum of 8 cycles

References

Variation 1:
Berry W, Dakhil S, Modiano M, et al, "Phase III Study of Mitoxantrone Plus Low Dose Prednisone
Versus Low Dose Prednisone Alone in Patients With Asymptomatic Hormone Refractory
Prostate Cancer," *J Urol*, 2002, 168(6):2439-43.
Tannock IF, de Wit R, Berry WR, et al, "Docetaxel Plus Prednisone or Mitoxantrone Plus
Prednisone for Advanced Prostate Cancer," *N Engl J Med*, 2004, 351(15):1502-12.
Tannock IF, Osoba D, Stockler MR, et al, "Chemotherapy With Mitoxantrone Plus Prednisone or
Prednisone Alone For Symptomatic Hormone-Resistant Prostate Cancer: A Canadian Random-
ized Trial With Palliative End Points," *J Clin Oncol*, 1996, 14(6):1756-64.
Variation 2:
Moore MJ, Osoba D, Murphy K, et al, "Use of Palliative Endpoints to Evaluate the Effects of
Mitoxantrone and Low-Dose Prednisone in Patients With Hormonally Resistant Prostate
Cancer," *J Clin Oncol*, 1994, 12(4):689-94.

♦ **Modified Fluorouracil-Leucovorin-Oxaliplatin (Colorectal)** *see* FOLFOX6
and mFOLFOX6 (Colorectal) *on page* 2131

♦ **Modified FOLFOX6 (Colorectal)** *see* FOLFOX6 and mFOLFOX6 (Colorectal) *on page* 2131

MOPP/ABVD (Hodgkin)

Index Terms Mechlorethamine, Vincristine, Procarbazine, Prednisone, Dox-
orubicin, Bleomycin, Vinblastine, Dacarbazine (Hodgkin)
Use Lymphoma, Hodgkin
Regimen NOTE: Multiple variations are listed.
Variation 1:
Mechlorethamine: IV: 6 mg/m^2/day days 1 and 8
[total dose/cycle = 12 mg/m^2]
Vincristine: IV: 1.4 mg/m^2/day days 1 and 8
[total dose/cycle = 2.8 mg/m^2]
Procarbazine: Oral: 100 mg/m^2/day days 1 to 14
[total dose/cycle = 1400 mg/m^2]
Prednisone: Oral: 40 mg/m^2/day days 1 to 14 (during cycles 1, 4, 7, and
10 **only**)
[total dose/cycle = 560 mg/m^2]
Doxorubicin: IV: 25 mg/m^2/day days 29 and 43
[total dose/cycle = 50 mg/m^2]

Bleomycin: IV: 10 units/m^2/day days 29 and 43
  [total dose/cycle = 20 units/m^2]
Vinblastine: IV: 6 mg/m^2/day days 29 and 43
  [total dose/cycle = 12 mg/m^2]
Dacarbazine: IV: 375 mg/m^2/day days 29 and 43
  [total dose/cycle = 750 mg/m^2]
Repeat cycle every 56 days for a total of 6 cycles.
Variation 2:
  Mechlorethamine: IV: 6 mg/m^2/day days 1 and 8
    [total dose/cycle = 12 mg/m^2]
  Vincristine: IV: 1.4 mg/m^2/day (maximum dose: 2 mg) days 1 and 8
    [total dose/cycle = 2.8 mg/m^2; maximum dose/cycle: 4 mg]
  Procarbazine: Oral: 100 mg/m^2/day days 1 to 14
    [total dose/cycle = 1400 mg/m^2]
  Prednisone: Oral: 40 mg/m^2/day days 1 to 14 (during cycles 1 and 7 **only**)
    [total dose/cycle = 560 mg/m^2]
  Doxorubicin: IV: 25 mg/m^2/day days 29 and 43
    [total dose/cycle = 50 mg/m^2]
  Bleomycin: IV: 10 units/m^2/day days 29 and 43
    [total dose/cycle = 20 units/m^2]
  Vinblastine: IV: 6 mg/m^2/day days 29 and 43
    [total dose/cycle = 12 mg/m^2]
  Dacarbazine: IV: 375 mg/m^2/day days 29 and 43
    [total dose/cycle = 750 mg/m^2]
  Repeat cycle every 56 days for a total of 6 cycles.

References

Variation 1:
Bonadonna G, Valagussa P, and Santoro A, "Alternating Noncross-Resistant Combination Chemotherapy or MOPP in State IV Hodgkin's Disease. A Report of 8-Year Results," *Ann Int Med*, 1986, 104(6):739-46.
Variation 2:
Canellos, GP, Anderson JR, Propert KJ, et al, "Chemotherapy of Advanced Hodgkin's Disease With MOPP, ABVD, or MOPP Alternating With ABVD," *N Engl J Med*, 1992, 327(21):1478-84.

MOPP/ABV Hybrid (Hodgkin)

Index Terms Mechlorethamine, Vincristine, Procarbazine, Prednisone, Doxorubicin, Bleomycin, Vinblastine (Hodgkin)

Use Lymphoma, Hodgkin

Regimen

Mechlorethamine: IV: 6 mg/m^2 day 1
  [total dose/cycle = 6 mg/m^2]
Vincristine: IV: 1.4 mg/m^2 (maximum dose: 2 mg) day 1
  [total dose/cycle = 1.4 mg/m^2; maximum: 2 mg/cycle]
Procarbazine: Oral: 100 mg/m^2/day days 1 to 7
  [total dose/cycle = 700 mg/m^2]
Prednisone: Oral: 40 mg/m^2/day days 1 to 14
  [total dose/cycle = 560 mg/m^2]
Doxorubicin: IV: 35 mg/m^2 day 8
  [total dose/cycle = 35 mg/m^2]
Bleomycin: IV: 10 units/m^2 day 8
  [total dose/cycle = 10 units/m^2]
Vinblastine: IV: 6 mg/m^2 day 8
  [total dose/cycle = 6 mg/m^2]
Repeat cycle every 28 days for a maximum of 8 cycles

◀ **References**
Conners JM, Klimo P, Adams G, et al, "Treatment of Advanced Hodgkin's Disease With Chemotherapy – Comparison of MOPP/ABV Hybrid Regimen With Alternating Courses of MOPP and
ABVD: A Report From the National Cancer Institute of Canada Clinical Trials," *J Clin Oncol*,
1997, 15(4):1638-45.

Klimo P and Connors JM, "MOPP/ABV Hybrid Program: Combination Chemotherapy Based on
Early Introduction of Seven Effective Drugs for Advanced Hodgkin's Disease," *J Clin Oncol*,
1985, 3(9):1174-82.

MOPP (Hodgkin)

Index Terms Mechlorethamine, Vincristine, Procarbazine, Prednisone (Hodgkin)

Use Lymphoma, Hodgkin

Regimen NOTE: Multiple variations are listed.

Variation 1:

Mechlorethamine: IV: 6 mg/m^2/day days 1 and 8
[total dose/cycle = 12 mg/m^2]

Vincristine: IV: 1.4 mg/m^2/day days 1 and 8
[total dose/cycle = 2.8 mg/m^2]

Procarbazine: Oral: 100 mg/m^2/day days 1 to 14
[total dose/cycle = 1400 mg/m^2]

Prednisone: Oral: 40 mg/m^2/day days 1 to 14 (cycles 1 and 4)
[total dose/cycle = 560 mg/m^2]

Repeat cycle every 28 days for 6 cycles

Variation 2:

Mechlorethamine: IV: 6 mg/m^2/day days 1 and 8
[total dose/cycle = 12 mg/m^2]

Vincristine: IV: 1.4 mg/m^2/day (maximum dose: 2 mg) days 1 and 8
[total dose/cycle = 2.8 mg/m^2; maximum dose/cycle = 4 mg]

Procarbazine: Oral: 100 mg/m^2/day days 1 to 14
[total dose/cycle = 1400 mg/m^2]

Prednisone: Oral: 40 mg/m^2/day days 1 to 14 (cycles 1 and 4)
[total dose/cycle = 560 mg/m^2]

Repeat cycle every 28 days for 6-8 cycles

References
Variation 1:
Devita VT Jr, Serpick AA, and Carbone PP, "Combination Chemotherapy in the Treatment of
Advanced Hodgkin's Disease," *Ann Intern Med*, 1970, 73(6):881-95.
Variation 2:
Canellos GP, Anderson JR, Propert KJ, et al, "Chemotherapy of Advanced Hodgkin's Disease
With MOPP, ABVD, or MOPP Alternating With ABVD," *N Engl J Med*, 1992, 327(21):1478-84.

◆ **MP (Multiple Myeloma)** *see* Melphalan-Prednisone (Multiple Myeloma) *on page 2171*

◆ **MP (Prostate)** *see* Mitoxantrone-Prednisone (Prostate) *on page 2175*

◆ **MPT (Multiple Myeloma)** *see* Melphalan-Prednisone-Thalidomide (Multiple Myeloma) *on page 2172*

MTX/6-MP/VP (Maintenance)

Use Leukemia, acute lymphocytic

Regimen

Methotrexate: Oral: 20 mg/m^2 weekly
[total dose/cycle = 80 mg/m^2]

Mercaptopurine: Oral: 75 mg/m^2/day
[total dose/cycle = 2250 mg/m^2]

Vincristine: IV: 1.5 mg/m^2 day 1
[total dose/cycle = 1.5 mg/m^2]
Prednisone: Oral: 40 mg/m^2/day days 1 to 5
[total dose/cycle = 200 mg/m^2]
Repeat monthly for 2-3 years

References

Bleyer WA, Sather HN, Nickerson HJ, et al, "Monthly Pulses of Vincristine and Prednisone Prevent Bone Marrow and Testicular Relapse in Low-Risk Childhood Acute Lymphoblastic Leukemia: A Report of the CCG-161 Study by the Childrens Cancer Study Group," *J Clin Oncol*, 1991, 9 (6):1012-21.

MVAC (Bladder)

Index Terms M-VAC (Bladder); Methotrexate-Vinblastine-Doxorubicin-Cisplatin (Bladder)

Use Bladder cancer

Regimen NOTE: Multiple variations are listed.
Variation 1 (neoadjuvant):
Methotrexate: IV: 30 mg/m^2/day days 1, 15, and 22
[total dose/cycle = 90 mg/m^2]
Vinblastine: IV: 3 mg/m^2/day days 2, 15, and 22
[total dose/cycle = 9 mg/m^2]
Doxorubicin: IV: 30 mg/m^2 day 2
[total dose/cycle = 30 mg/m^2]
Cisplatin: IV: 70 mg/m^2 day 2
[total dose/cycle = 70 mg/m^2]
Repeat cycle every 28 days for a total of 3 cycles
Variation 2 (metastatic):
Methotrexate: IV: 30 mg/m^2/day days 1, 15, and 22
[total dose/cycle = 90 mg/m^2]
Vinblastine: IV: 3 mg/m^2/day days 2, 15, and 22
[total dose/cycle = 9 mg/m^2]
Doxorubicin: IV: 30 mg/m^2 day 2
[total dose/cycle = 30 mg/m^2]
Cisplatin: IV: 70 mg/m^2 day 2
[total dose/cycle = 70 mg/m^2]
Repeat cycle every 28 days; for up to a total of 6 cycles (von der Maase 2000) or until disease progression or unacceptable toxicity (Sternberg 2001)
Variation 3 (metastatic):
Methotrexate: IV: 30 mg/m^2/day days 1, 15, and 22
[total dose/cycle = 90 mg/m^2]
Vinblastine: IV: 3 mg/m^2/day days 1, 15, and 22
[total dose/cycle = 9 mg/m^2]
Doxorubicin: IV: 30 mg/m^2 day 1
[total dose/cycle = 30 mg/m^2]
Cisplatin: IV: 70 mg/m^2 day 1
[total dose/cycle = 70 mg/m^2]
Filgrastim was administered on days 7, 8, 9, 25, and 26
Repeat cycle every 28 days for a total of 6 cycles

References

Variation 1:
Grossman HB, Natale RB, Tangen CM, et al. Neoadjuvant chemotherapy plus cystectomy compared with cystectomy alone for locally advanced bladder cancer. *N Engl J Med*. 2003;349(9):859-866.

Variation 2:

Sternberg CN, de Mulder PH, Schornagel JH, et al. Randomized phase III trial of high-dose-intensity methotrexate, vinblastine, doxorubicin, and cisplatin (MVAC) chemotherapy and recombinant human granulocyte colony-stimulating factor versus classic MVAC in advanced urothelial tract tumors: European Organization for Research and Treatment of Cancer Protocol no. 30924. *J Clin Oncol.* 2001;19(10):2638-2646.

Sternberg CN, de Mulder P, Schornagel JH, et al. Seven year update of an EORTC phase III trial of high-dose intensity M-VAC chemotherapy and G-CSF versus classic M-VAC in advanced urothelial tract tumours. *Eur J Cancer.* 2006;42(1):50-54.

von der Maase H, Hansen SW, Roberts JT, et al. Gemcitabine and cisplatin versus methotrexate, vinblastine, doxorubicin, and cisplatin in advanced or metastatic bladder cancer: results of a large, randomized, multinational, multicenter, phase III study. *J Clin Oncol.* 2000;17 (17):3068-3077.

Variation 3:

Bamias A, Aravantinos G, Deliveliotis C, et al. Docetaxel and cisplatin with granulocyte colony-stimulating factor (C CSF) versus MVAC with G-CSF in advanced urothelial carcinoma: a multicenter, randomized, phase III study from the Hellenic Cooperative Oncology Group. *J Clin Oncol.* 2004;22(2):220-228.

New A1 (Neuroblastoma)

Index Terms A1 (NEW) (Neuroblastoma); Cyclophosphamide, Doxorubicin, Etoposide, Cisplatin (Neuroblastoma); NEW A1 (Neuroblastoma); Regimen new A1 (Neuroblastoma)

Use Neuroblastoma

Regimen

Cyclophosphamide: IV: 1200 mg/m^2 over 6 hours day 1
[total dose/cycle = 1200 mg/m^2]
Doxorubicin: IV: 40 mg/m^2 day 3
[total dose/cycle = 40 mg/m^2]
Etoposide: IV: 100 mg/m^2/day days 1 to 5
[total dose/cycle = 500 mg/m^2]
Cisplatin: IV: 90 mg/m^2 day 5
[total dose/cycle = 90 mg/m^2]
Repeat cycle every 28 days for up to a total of 6 cycles

References

Kaneko M, Nishihira H, Mugishima H, et al, "Stratification of Treatment of Stage 4 Neuroblastoma Patients Based on N-myc Amplification Status. Study Group of Japan for Treatment of Advanced Neuroblastoma, Tokyo, Japan," *Med Pediatr Oncol*, 1998, 31(1):1-7.

Kaneko M, Tsuchida Y, Mugishima H, et al, "Intensified Chemotherapy Increases the Survival Rates in Patients With Stage 4 Neuroblastoma With MYCN Amplification," *J Pediatr Hematol Oncol*, 2002, 24(8):613-21.

◆ **Nivolumab-Ipilimumab (Melanoma)** *see* Ipilimumab-Nivolumab (Melanoma) *on page 2157*

◆ **Obinutuzumab-Bendamustine (NHL-Follicular)** *see* Bendamustine-Obinutuzumab (NHL-Follicular) *on page 1986*

◆ **Obinutuzumab-Chlorambucil (CLL)** *see* Chlorambucil-Obinutuzumab (CLL) *on page 2034*

◆ **OFA-FC (CLL)** *see* Fludarabine-Cyclophosphamide-Ofatumumab (CLL) *on page 2119*

OFAR (CLL)

Index Terms Oxaliplatin-Fludarabine-Cytarabine-Rituximab (CLL)

Use Leukemia, chronic lymphocytic

Regimen

Cycle 1:

Oxaliplatin: IV: 25 mg/m^2/dose day 1 to 4

[total dose/cycle = 100 mg/m^2]

Fludarabine: IV: 30 mg/m^2/dose days 2 and 3

[total dose/cycle = 60 mg/m^2]

Cytarabine: IV: 1000 mg/m^2/dose over 2 hours days 2 and 3

[total dose/cycle = 2000 mg/m^2]

Rituximab: IV: 375 mg/m^2 day 3

[total dose/cycle = 375 mg/m^2]

Treatment cycle is 4 weeks

Cycles 2-6:

Oxaliplatin: IV: 25 mg/m^2/dose day 1 to 4

[total dose/cycle = 100 mg/m^2]

Fludarabine: IV: 30 mg/m^2/dose days 2 and 3

[total dose/cycle = 60 mg/m^2]

Cytarabine: IV: 1000 mg/m^2/dose over 2 hours days 2 and 3

[total dose/cycle = 2000 mg/m^2]

Rituximab: IV: 375 mg/m^2 day 1

[total dose/cycle = 375 mg/m^2]

Repeat cycle every 4 weeks (maximum: 6 cycles)

References

Tsimberidou AM, Wierda WG, Plunkett W, et al, "Phase I-II Study of Oxaliplatin, Fludarabine, Cytarabine, and Rituximab Combination Therapy in Patients With Richter's Syndrome or Fludarabine-Refractory Chronic Lymphocytic Leukemia," *J Clin Oncol*, 2008, 26(2):196-203.

◆ **Ofatumumab-Chlorambucil (CLL)** *see* Chlorambucil-Ofatumumab (CLL) *on page 2034*

◆ **Ofatumumab-Fludarabine-Cyclophosphamide (CLL)** *see* Fludarabine-Cyclophosphamide-Ofatumumab (CLL) *on page 2119*

Olaratumab-Doxorubicin (Soft Tissue Sarcoma)

Index Terms Doxorubicin-Olaratumab (Soft Tissue Sarcoma)

Use Soft tissue sarcoma (unresectable or metastatic)

Regimen NOTE: Patients were permitted to receive dexrazoxane in cycles 5 to 8

Cycles 1 to 8:

Olaratumab: IV: 15 mg/kg over 60 minutes days 1 and 8

[total dose/cycle = 30 mg/kg]

◀

Doxorubicin: IV: 75 mg/m^2 day 1
[total dose/cycle = 75 mg/m^2]
Repeat cycle every 21 days for a total of 8 cycles
Followed by (in the absence of disease progression or unacceptable toxicity)
Olaratumab: IV: 15 mg/kg/day over 60 minutes days 1 and 8
[total dose/cycle = 30 mg/kg]
Repeat cycle every 21 days until disease progression or unacceptable toxicity

References

Tap WD, Jones RL, Van Tine BA, et al. Olaratumab and doxorubicin versus doxorubicin alone for treatment of soft-tissue sarcoma: an open-label phase 1b and randomised phase 2 trial. *Lancet.* 2016;388(10043):488-497.

- ◆ **Oxaliplatin-Leucovorin-Fluorouracil (Colorectal)** *see* FOLFOX1 (Colorectal) *on page 2129*

- ◆ **Oxaliplatin-Leucovorin-Fluorouracil (Colorectal)** *see* FOLFOX2 (Colorectal) *on page 2130*

- ◆ **Oxaliplatin-Leucovorin-Fluorouracil (Colorectal)** *see* FOLFOX3 (Colorectal) *on page 2130*

- ◆ **Oxaliplatin, Leucovorin, Fluorouracil (Colorectal)** *see* FOLFOX4 (Colorectal) *on page 2130*

- ◆ **Oxaliplatin-Leucovorin-Fluorouracil (Colorectal)** *see* FOLFOX6 and mFOLFOX6 (Colorectal) *on page 2131*

- ◆ **Oxaliplatin-Leucovorin-Fluorouracil (Gastric/Esophageal)** *see* Fluorouracil-Leucovorin-Oxaliplatin (Gastric/Esophageal) *on page 2127*

- ◆ **Paclitaxel-Bevacizumab (Breast)** *see* Bevacizumab-Paclitaxel (Breast) *on page 1994*

- ◆ **Paclitaxel-Bevacizumab (Ovarian)** *see* Bevacizumab-Paclitaxel (Ovarian) *on page 1995*

- ◆ **Paclitaxel-Carboplatin (Cervical Cancer)** *see* Carboplatin-Paclitaxel (Cervical Cancer) *on page 2018*

- ◆ **Paclitaxel-Carboplatin (Endometrial)** *see* Carboplatin-Paclitaxel (Endometrial) *on page 2019*

Paclitaxel-Carboplatin (Esophageal Cancer)

Index Terms Carboplatin-Paclitaxel (Esophageal Cancer)

Use Esophageal cancer

Regimen

Paclitaxel: IV: 50 mg/m^2/dose over 1 hour days 1, 8, 15, 22, and 29
[total dose/cycle = 250 mg/m^2]
Carboplatin: IV: AUC = 2 days 1, 8, 15, 22, and 29
[total dose/cycle = AUC = 10]
Administer with concurrent radiation therapy; cycle does not repeat.

References

van Meerten E, Muller K, Tilanus HW, et al ""Neoadjuvant Concurrent Chemoradiation With Weekly Paclitaxel and Carboplatin for Patients With Oesophageal Cancer: A Phase II Study," *Br J Cancer*, 2006, 94(10):1389-94.

- ◆ **Paclitaxel-Carboplatin-Etoposide (Unknown Primary)** *see* Carboplatin-Etoposide-Paclitaxel (Unknown Primary, Adenocarcinoma) *on page 2014*

- ◆ **Paclitaxel-Carboplatin (Ovarian)** *see* Carboplatin-Paclitaxel (Ovarian) *on page 2021*

- ◆ **Paclitaxel-Carboplatin-Trastuzumab (Breast)** *see* Carboplatin-Paclitaxel-Trastuzumab (Breast) *on page 2022*

- ◆ **Paclitaxel-Carboplatin (Unknown Primary)** *see* Carboplatin-Paclitaxel (Unknown Primary, Adenocarcinoma) *on page 2023*

Paclitaxel-Cetuximab

Index Terms Cetuximab-Paclitaxel

Use Head and neck cancer

Regimen
Week 1:
Paclitaxel: IV: 80 mg/m² day 1
[total dose/week 1 = 80 mg/m²]
Cetuximab: IV: 400 mg/m² (loading dose) day 1 (week 1 only)
[total loading dose (week 1) = 400 mg/m²]
Subsequent weeks:
Paclitaxel: IV: 80 mg/m² day 1
[total dose/week = 80 mg/m²]
Cetuximab: IV: 250 mg/m² day 1
[total dose/week = 250 mg/m²]

References
Hitt R, Irigoyen H, Nunez J, et al, "Phase II Study of Combination Cetuximab and Weekly Paclitaxel in Patients With Metastatic/Recurrent Squamous Cell Carcinama of Head and Neck (SCCHN): Spanish Head and Neck Cancer Group (TTCC)," *J Clin Oncol*, 2007, 25(18S) [abstract 6012 from 2007 ASCO Annual Meeting].

◆ Paclitaxel-Cisplatin (Cervical Cancer) *see* Cisplatin-Paclitaxel (Cervical Cancer) *on page 2057*

Paclitaxel-Cisplatin (Esophageal Cancer)
Index Terms Cisplatin-Paclitaxel (Esophageal Cancer)
Use Esophageal cancer
Regimen NOTE: Multiple variations are listed.
Variation 1:
Paclitaxel: IV: 50 mg/m²/dose over 1 hour days 1, 8, 15, 22, and 29
[total dose/cycle = 250 mg/m²]
Cisplatin: IV: 30 mg/m²/dose days 1, 8, 15, 22, and 29
[total dose/cycle = 150 mg/m²]
Administered (with concurrent radiation therapy) over one 5-week treatment cycle.
Followed by: Postoperative therapy:
Paclitaxel: IV: 175 mg/m²/dose day 1
[total dose/cycle = 175 mg/m²]
Cisplatin: IV: 75 mg/m²/dose day 1
[total dose/cycle = 75 mg/m²]
Repeat postop cycle every 21 days for a total of 3 cycles.
Variation 2:
Paclitaxel: IV: 60 mg/m²/dose over 3 hours days 1, 8, 15, and 22
[total dose/cycle = 240 mg/m²]
Cisplatin: IV: 75 mg/m²/dose over 2 hours day 1
[total dose/cycle = 75 mg/m²]
Filgrastim: SubQ: 5 mcg/kg/day starting day 23; continue until ANC >10,000/mm³
Administer with concurrent radiation therapy; cycle does not repeat.
Variation 3:
Paclitaxel: IV: 90 mg/m²/dose over 3 hours day 1
[total dose/cycle = 90 mg/m²]
Cisplatin: IV: 50 mg/m²/dose over 1 hour day 1
[total dose/cycle = 50 mg/m²]
Repeat cycle every 14 days until disease progression or unacceptable toxicity.

References

Variation 1:

Kleinberg L, Powell ME, Forastiere AA, et al, "Survival Outcome of E1201: An Eastern Cooperative Oncology Group (ECOG) Randomized Phase II Trial of Neoadjuvant Preoperative Paclitaxel/Cisplatin/Radiotherapy (RT) or Irinotecan/Cisplatin/RT in Endoscopy With Ultrasound (EUS) Staged Esophageal Adenocarcinoma," *J Clin Oncol*, 2008, 26(15S):4532 [abstract 4532 from 2008 annual ASCO meeting].

Variation 2:

Urba SG, Orringer MB, Ianettonni M, et al, "Concurrent Cisplatin, Paclitaxel, and Radiotherapy as Preoperative Treatment for Patients With Locoregional Esophageal Carcinoma," *Cancer*, 2003, 98(10):2177-83.

Variation 3:

Petrasch S, Welt A, Reinacher A, et al, "Chemotherapy With Cisplatin and Paclitaxel in Patients With Locally Advanced, Recurrent or Metastatic Oesophageal Cancer," *Br J Cancer*, 1998, 78 (4):511-4.

Paclitaxel-Cisplatin-Fluorouracil (Esophageal Cancer)

Index Terms Paclitaxel-Fluorouracil-Cisplatin (Esophageal Cancer); TCF (Esophageal Cancer)

Use Esophageal cancer

Regimen

Paclitaxel: IV: 175 mg/m^2 over 3 hours day 1

[total dose/cycle = 175 mg/m^2]

Cisplatin: IV: 20 mg/m^2/day days 1 to 5 for cycles 1, 2, and 3

[total dose/cycle = 100 mg/m^2]

then 15 mg/m^2/day days 1 to 5

[total dose/cycle = 75 mg/m^2]

Fluorouracil: IV: 750 mg/m^2/day continuous infusion days 1 to 5

[total dose/cycle = 3750 mg/m^2]

Repeat cycle every 28 days

References

Ilson DH, Ajani J, Bhalla K, et al, "Phase II Trial of Paclitaxel, Fluorouracil, and Cisplatin in Patients With Advanced Carcinoma of the Esophagus," *J Clin Oncol*, 1998, 16(5):1826-34.

◆ **Paclitaxel-Cisplatin-Gemcitabine (Bladder)** *see* PCG (Bladder) *on page 2191*

◆ **Paclitaxel-Cisplatin (Head and Neck Cancer)** *see* Cisplatin-Paclitaxel (Head and Neck Cancer) *on page 2058*

◆ **Paclitaxel-Cisplatin Intraperitoneal (Ovarian)** *see* Cisplatin-Paclitaxel Intraperitoneal (Ovarian) *on page 2058*

◆ **Paclitaxel-Cisplatin (NSCLC)** *see* Cisplatin-Paclitaxel (NSCLC) *on page 2058*

◆ **Paclitaxel-Cisplatin (Ovarian)** *see* Cisplatin-Paclitaxel (Ovarian) *on page 2059*

◆ **Paclitaxel-Doxorubicin-Cisplatin (Endometrial)** *see* Cisplatin-Doxorubicin-Paclitaxel (Endometrial) *on page 2041*

◆ **Paclitaxel-Fluorouracil-Cisplatin (Esophageal Cancer)** *see* Paclitaxel-Cisplatin-Fluorouracil (Esophageal Cancer) *on page 2185*

Paclitaxel-Fluorouracil (Esophageal Cancer)

Index Terms Fluorouracil-Paclitaxel (Esophageal Cancer)

Use Esophageal cancer

Regimen

Paclitaxel: IV: 45 mg/m^2/dose over 3 hours day 1

[total dose/cycle = 45 mg/m^2]

Fluorouracil: IV: 300 mg/m^2/day continuous infusion days 1 to 5
[total dose/cycle = 1500 mg/m^2]

Repeat cycle weekly for 5 weeks; administer concurrent with radiation therapy; cycle does not repeat.

References

Schnirer II, Komaki R, Yao JC, et al, "Pilot Study of Concurrent 5-Fluorouracil/Paclitaxel Plus Radiotherapy in Patients With Carcinoma of the Esophagus and Gastroesophageal Junction," *Am J Clin Oncol*, 2001, 24(1):91-5.

♦ **Paclitaxel-Gemcitabine (Bladder)** see Gemcitabine-Paclitaxel (Bladder) on page 2138

♦ **Paclitaxel-Gemcitabine (Breast)** see Gemcitabine-Paclitaxel (Breast) on page 2138

♦ **Paclitaxel-Gemcitabine-Oxaliplatin (Testicular)** see Gemcitabine-Oxaliplatin-Paclitaxel (Testicular) on page 2137

♦ **Paclitaxel-Gemcitabine (Testicular)** see Gemcitabine-Paclitaxel (Testicular) on page 2139

Paclitaxel-Ifosfamide-Cisplatin (Penile)

Index Terms Cisplatin-Ifosfamide-Paclitaxel (Penile)

Use Penile cancer (squamous cell, neoadjuvant)

Regimen

Paclitaxel: IV: 175 mg/m^2 over 3 hours day 1
[total dose/cycle = 175 mg/m^2]

Ifosfamide: IV: 1,200 mg/m^2/day over 2 hours days 1, 2, and 3
[total dose/cycle = 3,600 mg/m^2]

Cisplatin: IV: 25 mg/m^2/day over 2 hours days 1, 2, and 3
[total dose/cycle = 75 mg/m^2]

Mesna: IV: 400 mg/m^2 prior to each ifosfamide dose and 200 mg/m^2 at 4 and 8 hours after each ifosfamide dose, days 1, 2, and 3
[total dose/cycle = 2,400 mg/m^2]

Repeat cycle every 21 to 28 days for 4 cycles. **Note:** The cycle was repeated on day 22 if the patient's absolute neutrophil count was at least 1,400/mm^3 and platelet count was at least 100,000/mm^3).

References

Pagliaro LC, Williams DL, Daliani D, et al. Neoadjuvant paclitaxel, ifosfamide, and cisplatin chemotherapy for metastatic penile cancer: a phase II study. *J Clin Oncol*. 2010;28 (24):3851-3857.

♦ **Paclitaxel-Ifosfamide-Cisplatin (Testicular)** see TIP (Testicular) on page 2214

Paclitaxel-Pertuzumab-Trastuzumab (Breast)

Index Terms Pertuzumab-Trastuzumab-Paclitaxel (Breast); Trastuzumab-Pertuzumab-Paclitaxel (Breast)

Use Breast cancer (metastatic, HER-2 positive)

Regimen NOTE: No mandate on the order of administration.

Cycle 1:

Trastuzumab: IV: 8 mg/kg (loading dose) day 1 cycle 1
[total dose/cycle 1 = 8 mg/kg]

Paclitaxel: IV: 80 mg/m^2 days 1, 8, and 15
[total dose/cycle 1 = 240 mg/m^2]

Pertuzumab: IV: 840 mg (loading dose) day 1 cycle 1
[total dose/cycle 1 = 840 mg]
Treatment cycle is 21 days
Subsequent cycles:
Trastuzumab: IV: 6 mg/kg day 1
[total dose/cycle = 6 mg/kg]
Paclitaxel: IV: 80 mg/m^2 days 1, 8, and 15
[total dose/cycle = 240 mg/m^2]
Pertuzumab: IV: 420 mg day 1
[total dose/cycle = 420 mg]
Repeat cycle every 21 days (if progression-free after 6 months, paclitaxel may be stopped while trastuzumab and pertuzumab are continued)

References

Dang C, Iyengar N, Datko F, et al. Phase II study of paclitaxel given once per week along with trastuzumab and pertuzumab in patients with human epidermal growth factor receptor 2-positive metastatic breast cancer. *J Clin Oncol*. 2015;33(5):442-447.

◆ **Paclitaxel (Protein Bound)-Carboplatin (NSCLC)** *see* Carboplatin-Paclitaxel (Protein Bound) (NSCLC) *on page* 2022

◆ **Paclitaxel (Protein Bound)-Gemcitabine (Pancreatic)** *see* Gemcitabine-Paclitaxel (Protein Bound) (Pancreatic) *on page* 2139

Paclitaxel-Ramucirumab (Gastric)

Index Terms Ramucirumab-Paclitaxel (Gastric)
Use Gastric cancer
Regimen
Ramucirumab: IV: 8 mg/kg days 1 and 15
[total dose/cycle = 16 mg/kg]
Paclitaxel: IV: 80 mg/m^2 days 1, 8, and 15
[total dose/cycle = 240 mg/m^2]
Repeat cycle every 28 days until disease progression or unacceptable toxicity

References

Wilke H, Muro K, Van Cutsem E, et al. Ramucirumab plus paclitaxel versus placebo plus paclitaxel in patients with previously treated advanced gastric or gastro-oesophageal junction adenocarcinoma (RAINBOW): a double-blind, randomised phase 3 trial. *Lancet Oncol*. 2014;15 (11):1224-1235.

◆ **Paclitaxel-Topotecan-Bevacizumab (Cervical)** *see* Bevacizumab-Paclitaxel-Topotecan (Cervical) *on page* 1995

Paclitaxel-Trastuzumab (Breast)

Index Terms Trastuzumab-Paclitaxel (Breast)
Use Breast cancer
Regimen NOTE: Multiple variations are listed.
Variation 1 (weekly [preferred]):
Cycle 1:
Trastuzumab: IV: 4 mg/kg (loading dose) over 90 minutes day 0 cycle 1 only
[total dose/cycle 1 = 4 mg/kg]
Paclitaxel: IV: 90 mg/m^2 over 1 hour day 1
[total dose/cycle 1 = 90 mg/m^2]
Treatment cycle 1 is 7 days

Subsequent cycles:

Paclitaxel: IV: 90 mg/m^2 over 1 hour day 1

[total dose/cycle = 90 mg/m^2]

Trastuzumab: IV: 2 mg/kg over 30 minutes day 1

[total dose/cycle = 2 mg/kg]

Repeat cycle every 7 days until disease progression or unacceptable toxicity

Variation 2 (weekly [preferred]):

Cycle 1:

Trastuzumab: IV: 4 mg/kg (loading dose) over 90 minutes day 1 cycle 1 only

[total dose/cycle 1 = 4 mg/kg]

Paclitaxel: IV: 80 mg/m^2 over 1 hour day 1

[total dose/cycle 1 = 80 mg/m^2]

Treatment cycle 1 is 7 days

Subsequent cycles:

Trastuzumab: IV: 2 mg/kg over 30 minutes day 1

[total dose/cycle = 2 mg/kg]

Paclitaxel: IV: 80 mg/m^2 over 1 hour day 1

[total dose/cycle = 80 mg/m^2]

Repeat cycle every 7 days

Variation 3 (every 3 weeks):

Cycle 1:

Trastuzumab: IV: 4 mg/kg (loading dose) over 90 minutes day 1 cycle 1 only

followed by:

Trastuzumab: IV: 2 mg/kg/day over 30 minutes days 8, 15

[total dose/cycle 1 = 8 mg/kg]

Paclitaxel: IV: 175 mg/m^2 over 3 hours day 1

[total dose/cycle 1 = 175 mg/m^2]

Treatment cycle 1 is 21 days

Subsequent cycles:

Trastuzumab: IV: 2 mg/kg/day over 30 minutes days 1, 8, 15

[total dose/cycle = 6 mg/kg]

Paclitaxel: IV: 175 mg/m^2 over 3 hours day 1

[total dose/cycle = 175 mg/m^2]

Repeat cycle every 21 days

References

Variation 1:

Seidman AD, Fornier MN, Esteva FJ, et al, "Weekly Trastuzumab and Paclitaxel Therapy for Metastatic Breast Cancer With Analysis of Efficacy by HER2 Immunophenotype and Gene Amplification," *J Clin Oncol*, 2001, 19(10):2587-95.

Variation 2 and 3:

Seidman AD, Berry D, Cirrincione C, et al, "Randomized Phase III Trial of Weekly Compared With Every-3-Weeks Paclitaxel for Metastatic Breast Cancer, With Trastuzumab for all HER-2 Overexpressors and Random Assignment to Trastuzumab or Not in HER-2 Nonoverexpressors: Final Results of Cancer and Leukemia Group B Protocol 9840," *J Clin Oncol*, 2008, 26 (10):1642-9.

◆ **Paclitaxel-Carboplatin (NSCLC)** *see* Carboplatin-Paclitaxel (NSCLC) *on page 2020*

◆ **PAD (Multiple Myeloma)** *see* Bortezomib-Doxorubicin-Dexamethasone (Multiple Myeloma) *on page 1999*

Palbociclib-Fulvestrant (Breast)

Index Terms Fulvestrant-Palbociclib (Breast)

Use Breast cancer, advanced second-line endocrine-based therapy (ER-Positive, HER2-Negative, relapsed or progressed during prior endocrine therapy)

Regimen NOTE: In the study, premenopausal and perimenopausal patients also received goserelin (starting at least 4 weeks prior to randomization and then every 28 days) for the duration of therapy.

Cycle 1:

Palbociclib: Oral: 125 mg once daily (with food) for 21 days, followed by 7 days off treatment

[total dose/cycle = 2,625 mg]

Fulvestrant: IM: 500 mg days 1 and 15

[total dose/cycle = 1,000 mg]

Treatment cycle is 28 days

Subsequent Cycles:

Palbociclib: Oral: 125 mg once daily (with food) for 21 days, followed by 7 days off treatment

[total dose/cycle = 2,625 mg]

Fulvestrant: IM: 500 mg day 1

[total dose/cycle = 500 mg]

Repeat cycle every 28 days until disease progression or unacceptable toxicity

References

Turner NC, Ro J, André F, et al. Palbociclib in Hormone-Receptor-Positive Advanced Breast Cancer. *N Engl J Med.* 2015;373(3):209-219.

Palbociclib-Letrozole (Breast)

Index Terms Letrozole-Palbociclib (Breast)

Use Breast cancer, advanced (ER-Positive, HER2-Negative)

Regimen

Palbociclib: Oral: 125 mg once daily (with food) for 21 days, followed by 7 days off treatment

[total dose/cycle = 2,625 mg]

Letrozole: Oral: 2.5 mg once daily days 1 to 28

[total dose/cycle = 70 mg]

Repeat cycle every 28 days until disease progression or unacceptable toxicity

References

Finn RS, Crown JP, Lang I, et al. The cyclin-dependent kinase 4/6 inhibitor palbociclib in combination with letrozole versus letrozole alone as first-line treatment of oestrogen receptor-positive, HER2-negative, advanced breast cancer (PALOMA-1/TRIO-18): a randomised phase 2 study. *Lancet Oncol.* 2015;16(1):25-35.

Panitumumab + FOLFIRI (Colorectal)

Use Colorectal cancer

Regimen

Panitumumab: IV: 6 mg/kg over 30-60 minutes day 1

[total dose/cycle = 6 mg/kg]

Irinotecan: IV: 180 mg/m^2 day 1

[total dose/cycle = 180 mg/m^2]

Leucovorin (racemic): IV: 400 mg/m^2 day 1

[total dose/cycle = 400 mg/m^2]

◄

Fluorouracil: IV bolus: 400 mg/m^2 day 1
  followed by IV: 2400 mg/m^2 continuous infusion (CI) over 46 hours beginning day 1
  [total fluorouracil dose/cycle (bolus and CI) = 2800 mg/m^2]
Repeat cycle every 14 days until disease progression or unacceptable toxicity

References

Peeters M, Price TJ, Cervantes A, et al, "Randomized Phase III Study of Panitumumab With Fluorouracil, Leucovorin, and Irinotecan (FOLFIRI) Compared With FOLFIRI Alone as Second-Line Treatment in Patients With Metastatic Colorectal Cancer," *J Clin Oncol*, 2010, 28 (31):4706-13.

Panitumumab + FOLFOX4 (Colorectal)

Use Colorectal cancer

Regimen

Panitumumab: IV: 6 mg/kg over 30-60 minutes day 1
  [total dose/cycle = 6 mg/kg]
Oxaliplatin: IV: 85 mg/m^2 day 1
  [total dose/cycle = 85 mg/m^2]
Leucovorin: IV: 200 mg/m^2/day days 1 and 2
  [total dose/cycle = 400 mg/m^2]
Fluorouracil: IV bolus: 400 mg/m^2/day days 1 and 2
  followed by IV: 600 mg/m^2 continuous infusion (CI) over 22 hours days 1 and 2
  [total fluorouracil dose/cycle (bolus and CI) = 2000 mg/m^2]
Note: Bolus fluorouracil and continuous infusion fluorouracil are both given on each day
Repeat cycle every 14 days until disease progression or unacceptable toxicity

References

Douillard JY, Siena S, Cassidy J, et al, "Randomized, Phase III Trial of Panitumumab With Infusional Fluorouracil, Leucovorin, and Oxaliplatin (FOLFOX4) Versus FOLFOX4 Alone as First-Line Treatment in Patients With Previously Untreated Metastatic Colorectal Cancer: The PRIME Study," *J Clin Oncol*, 2010, 28(31):4697-705.

Panobinostat-Bortezomib-Dexamethasone (Multiple Myeloma)

Index Terms Bortezomib-Dexamethasone-Panobinostat (Multiple Myeloma); Dexamethasone-Bortezomib-Panobinostat (Multiple Myeloma)

Use Multiple myeloma (relapsed/refractory)

Regimen

Phase I: Cycles 1 to 8:
  Panobinostat: Oral: 20 mg days 1, 3, 5, 8, 10, and 12
    [total dose/cycle = 120 mg]
  Bortezomib: IV: 1.3 mg/m^2/day days 1, 4, 8, and 11
    [total dose/cycle = 5.2 mg/m^2]
  Dexamethasone: Oral: 20 mg daily days 1, 2, 4, 5, 8, 9, 11, and 12
    [total dose/cycle = 160 mg]
  Repeat cycle every 21 days for 8 cycles; if patient derives clinical benefit then proceed to phase II
Phase II: Cycles 9 to 12:
  Panobinostat: Oral: 20 mg days 1, 3, 5, 8, 10, 12, 22, 24, 26, 29, 31, and 33
    [total dose/cycle = 240 mg]
  Bortezomib: IV: 1.3 mg/m^2/day days 1, 8, 22, and 29
    [total dose/cycle = 5.2 mg/m^2]

Dexamethasone: Oral: 20 mg daily days 1, 2, 8, 9, 22, 23, 29, and 30
[total dose/cycle = 160 mg]
Repeat cycle every 42 days for 4 cycles

References

San-Miguel JF, Hungria VT, Yoon SS, et al. Panobinostat plus bortezomib and dexamethasone versus placebo plus bortezomib and dexamethasone in patients with relapsed or relapsed and refractory multiple myeloma: a multicentre, randomised, double-blind phase 3 trial. *Lancet Oncol.* 2014;15(11):1195-1206.

◆ **PCF (Unknown Primary)** *see* Cisplatin-Fluorouracil-Paclitaxel (Unknown Primary, Squamous Cell) *on page* 2051

PCG (Bladder)

Index Terms Paclitaxel-Cisplatin-Gemcitabine (Bladder)
Use Bladder cancer (locally advanced, metastatic)
Regimen
Paclitaxel: IV: 80 mg/m^2/day days 1 and 8
[total dose/cycle = 160 mg/m^2]
Cisplatin: IV: 70 mg/m^2 day 1
[total dose/cycle = 70 mg/m^2]
Gemcitabine: IV: 1,000 mg/m^2/day days 1 and 8
[total dose/cycle = 2,000 mg/m^2]
Repeat cycle every 21 days until disease progression, unacceptable toxicity, or a maximum of up to 6 cycles

References

Bellmunt J, von der Maase H, Mead GM, et al. Randomized phase III study comparing paclitaxel/cisplatin/gemcitabine (PCG) and gemcitabine/cisplatin (GC) in patients with locally advanced (LA) or metastatic (M) urothelial cancer without prior systemic therapy; EORTC30987/Intergroup Study. *J Clin Oncol.* 2007;25(suppl 18):LBA5030.

Bellmunt J, von der Maase H, Mead GM, et al. Randomized phase III study comparing paclitaxel/cisplatin/gemcitabine and gemcitabine/cisplatin in patients with locally advanced or metastatic urothelial cancer without prior systemic therapy: EORTC Intergroup Study 30987. *J Clin Oncol.* 2012;30(10):1107-1113.

◆ **PC (NSCLC)** *see* Carboplatin-Paclitaxel (NSCLC) *on page* 2020

◆ **PCR (CLL)** *see* Pentostatin-Cyclophosphamide-Rituximab (CLL) *on page* 2193

PCV (Brain Tumor Regimen)

Index Terms Procarbazine-CCNU-Vincristine; Procarbazine-Lomustine-Vincristine
Use Brain tumors
Regimen NOTE: Multiple variations are listed.
Variation 1:
Lomustine: Oral: 110 mg/m^2 day 1
[total dose/cycle = 110 mg/m^2]
Procarbazine: Oral: 60 mg/m^2/day days 8 to 21
[total dose/cycle = 840 mg/m^2]
Vincristine: IV: 1.4 mg/m^2/day (maximum dose: 2 mg) days 8 and 29
[total dose/cycle = 2.8 mg/m^2; maximum: 4 mg]
Repeat cycle every 6 weeks for a total of 6 cycles
Variation 2:
Lomustine: Oral: 110 mg/m^2 day 1
[total dose/cycle = 110 mg/m^2]
Procarbazine: Oral: 60 mg/m^2/day days 8 to 21
[total dose/cycle = 840 mg/m^2]

◄   Vincristine: IV: 1.4 mg/m^2/day (maximum dose: 2 mg) days 8 and 29
    [total dose/cycle = 2.8 mg/m^2; maximum: 4 mg]
  Repeat cycle every 6 weeks for a total of 7 cycles
Variation 3:
  Procarbazine: Oral: 75 mg/m^2/day days 8 to 21
    [total dose/cycle = 1050 mg/m^2]
  Lomustine: Oral: 130 mg/m^2 day 1
    [total dose/cycle = 130 mg/m^2]
  Vincristine: IV: 1.4 mg/m^2/day (no maximum) days 8 and 29
    [total dose/cycle = 2.8 mg/m^2; no maximum]
  Repeat cycle every 6 weeks for a total of 6 cycles
Variation 4:
  Procarbazine: Oral: 75 mg/m^2/day days 8 to 21
    [total dose/cycle = 1050 mg/m^2]
  Lomustine: Oral: 130 mg/m^2 day 1
    [total dose/cycle = 130 mg/m^2]
  Vincristine: IV: 1.4 mg/m^2/day (no maximum) days 8 and 29
    [total dose/cycle = 2.8 mg/m^2; no maximum]
  Repeat cycle every 6 weeks for up to a total of 4 cycles
Variation 5:
  Lomustine: Oral: 110 mg/m^2 day 1
    [total dose/cycle = 110 mg/m^2]
  Procarbazine: Oral: 60 mg/m^2/day days 8 to 21
    [total dose/cycle = 840 mg/m^2]
  Vincristine: IV: 1.4 mg/m^2/day days 8 and 29
    [total dose/cycle = 2.8 mg/m^2]
  Repeat cycle every 6-8 weeks for 1 year

References

Variation 1:
van den Bent MJ, Carpentier AF, Brandes AA, et al, "Adjuvant Procarbazine, Lomustine, and Vincristine Improves Progression-Free Survival But Not Overall Survival in Newly Diagnosed Anaplastic Oligodendrogliomas and Oligoastrocytomas: A Randomized European Organisation for Research and Treatment of Cancer Phase III Trial," *J Clin Oncol*, 2006, 24(18):2715-22.
Variation 2:
Levin VA, Uhm JH, Jaeckle KA, et al, "Phase III Randomized Study of Postradiotherapy Chemotherapy With Alpha-Difluoromethylornithine-Procarbazine, N-(2-Chloroethyl)-N'-Cyclohexyl-N-Nitrosurea, Vincristine (DFMO-PCV) Versus PCV for Glioblastoma Multiforme," *Clin Cancer Res*, 2000, 6(10):3878-84.
Variation 3:
Cairncross G, Macdonald D, Ludwin S, et al, "Chemotherapy for Anaplastic Oligodendroglioma. National Cancer Institute of Canada Clinical Trials Group," *J Clin Oncol*, 1994, 12(10):2013-21.
Variation 4:
Intergroup Radiation Therapy Oncology Group Trial 9402, Cairncross G, Berkey B, et al, "Phase III Trial of Chemotherapy Plus Radiotherapy Compared With Radiotherapy Alone for Pure and Mixed Anaplastic Oligodendroglioma: Intergroup Radiation Therapy Oncology Group Trial 9402," *J Clin Oncol*, 2006, 24(18):2707-14.
Variation 5:
Levin VA, Silver P, Hannigan J, et al, "Superiority of Post-Radiotherapy Adjuvant Chemotherapy With CCNU, Procarbazine, and Vincristine (PCV) Over BCNU for Anaplastic Gliomas: NCOG 6G61 Final Report," *Int J Radiat Oncol Biol Phys*, 1990, 18(2):321-4.

◆ **Pembrolizumab-Pemetrexed-Carboplatin (NSCLC)** *see* Carboplatin-Pemetrexed-Pembrolizumab (NSCLC) *on page 2024*

◆ **Pemetrexed-Carboplatin-Bevacizumab (NSCLC)** *see* Bevacizumab-Carboplatin-Pemetrexed (NSCLC) *on page 1990*

◆ **Pemetrexed-Carboplatin (Mesothelioma)** *see* Carboplatin-Pemetrexed (Mesothelioma) *on page 2024*

- ◆ **Pemetrexed-Carboplatin (NSCLC)** *see* Carboplatin-Pemetrexed (NSCLC) on page 2024
- ◆ **Pemetrexed-Cisplatin (Mesothelioma)** *see* Cisplatin-Pemetrexed (Mesothelioma) on page 2059
- ◆ **Pemetrexed-Cisplatin (NSCLC)** *see* Cisplatin-Pemetrexed (NSCLC) on page 2059
- ◆ **PE (NSCLC)** *see* Cisplatin-Etoposide (NSCLC) on page 2041

Pentostatin-Cyclophosphamide-Rituximab (CLL)

Index Terms Cyclophosphamide-Pentostatin-Rituximab (CLL); PCR (CLL)

Use Leukemia, chronic lymphocytic

Regimen NOTE: Multiple variations are listed.

Variation 1 (refractory):

Cycle 1:

Cyclophosphamide: IV: 600 mg/m^2 day 1
[total dose/cycle = 600 mg/m^2]

Pentostatin: IV: 4 mg/m^2 day 1
[total dose/cycle = 4 mg/m^2]

Filgrastim: SubQ: 300 mcg (patients ≤70 kg) or 480 mcg (patients >70 kg) daily beginning 2 days after each treatment and continued until ANC >5,000/mm^3 or >1,500/mm^3 for 2 days

Treatment cycle duration is 21 days

Cycles 2 to 6:

Cyclophosphamide: IV: 600 mg/m^2 day 1
[total dose/cycle = 600 mg/m^2]

Pentostatin: IV: 4 mg/m^2 day 1
[total dose/cycle = 4 mg/m^2]

Rituximab: IV: 375 mg/m^2 day 1
[total dose/cycle = 375 mg/m^2]

Filgrastim: SubQ: 300 mcg (patients ≤70 kg) or 480 mcg (patients >70 kg) daily beginning 2 days after each treatment and continued until ANC >5,000/mm^3 or >1,500/mm^3 for 2 days

Repeat cycle every 21 days for total of 3 cycles, if at least partial response, continue for a total of 6 cycles

Variation 2 (first-line):

Cycle 1:

Cyclophosphamide: IV: 600 mg/m^2 day 1
[total dose/cycle = 600 mg/m^2]

Pentostatin: IV: 2 mg/m^2 day 1
[total dose/cycle = 2 mg/m^2]

Rituximab: IV: 100 mg/m^2 day 1 cycle 1 only
followed by IV: 375 mg/m^2/day days 3 and 5 cycle 1 only
[total dose/cycle 1 = 850 mg/m^2]

Filgrastim: SubQ: Daily (dose not specified) beginning day 3 and continued for 10 consecutive days or until ANC >1,000/mm^3 for 2 consecutive days

Treatment cycle duration is 21 days

Cycles 2 to 6:

Cyclophosphamide: IV: 600 mg/m^2 day 1
[total dose/cycle = 600 mg/m^2]

Pentostatin: IV: 2 mg/m^2 day 1
[total dose/cycle = 2 mg/m^2]

Rituximab: IV: 375 mg/m^2 day 1
[total dose/cycle = 375 mg/m^2]
Filgrastim: SubQ: Daily (dose not specified) beginning day 3 and continued
for 10 consecutive days or until ANC >1,000/mm^3 for 2 consecutive days
Repeat cycle every 21 days for a total of 6 cycles

References

Variation 1:

Lamanna N, Kalaycio M, Maslak P, et al. Pentostatin, cyclophosphamide, and rituximab is an active, well-tolerated regimen for patients with previously treated chronic lymphocytic leukemia. *J Clin Oncol.* 2006;24(10):1575-1581.

Variation 2:

Kay NE, Geyer SM, Call TG, et al. Combination chemoimmunotherapy with pentostatin, cyclophosphamide, and rituximab shows significant clinical activity with low accompanying toxicity in previously untreated B chronic lymphocytic leukemia. *Blood.* 2007;109(2):405-411.

Shanafelt TD, Lin T, Geyer SM, et al. Pentostatin, cyclophosphamide, and rituximab regimen in older patients with chronic lymphocytic leukemia. *Cancer.* 2007;109(11):2291-2298.

PEP-C (NHL)

Index Terms Prednisone, Etoposide, Procarbazine, Cyclophosphamide (NHL)

Use Lymphoma, non-Hodgkin (refractory, recurrent follicular, marginal zone, small lymphocytic, diffuse large cell)

Regimen

Prednisone: Oral: 20 mg once daily after breakfast (morning dose)
Cyclophosphamide: Oral: 50 mg once daily after lunch (afternoon dose)
Etoposide: Oral: 50 mg once daily after dinner (evening dose)
Procarbazine: Oral: 50 mg once daily at bedtime (night dose)
Length of cycle and frequency vary. Patients are treated daily in the induction phase until leukocyte count <3,000/mm^3. Hold treatment and when leukocyte count >3,000/mm^3 patients were then treated in a maintenance phase. In the maintenance phase the doses were the same but the frequency was adjusted to maintain a white blood count of at least 3,000/mm^3.

References

Coleman M, Martin P, Ruan J, et al. Prednisone, etoposide, probarbazine, and cyclophosphamide (PEP-C) oral combination chemotherapy regimen for recurring/refractory lymphoma: low-dose metronomic, multidrug therapy. *Cancer.* 2008;112(10):2228-2232.

PEP-C (NHL-Mantle Cell)

Index Terms Prednisone, Etoposide, Procarbazine, Cyclophosphamide (NHL-Mantle)

Use Lymphoma, non-Hodgkin (relapsed, refractory Mantle cell)

Regimen

Prednisone: Oral: 20 mg once daily after breakfast (morning dose)
Cyclophosphamide: Oral: 50 mg once daily after lunch (afternoon dose)
Etoposide: Oral: 50 mg once daily after dinner (evening dose)
Procarbazine: Oral: 50 mg once daily at bedtime (night dose)
Length of cycle and frequency vary. Patients are treated daily in the induction phase until leukocyte count <3,000/mm^3. Hold treatment and when leukocyte count >3,000/mm^3 patients were then treated in a maintenance phase. In the maintenance phase the doses were the same but the frequency was adjusted to maintain a white blood count of at least 3,000/mm^3.

References

Coleman M, Martin P, Ruan J, et al. Low-dose metronomic, multidrug therapy with the PEP-C oral combination chemotherapy regimen for mantle cell lymphoma. *Leuk Lymphoma.* 2008;49(3):447-450.

Pertuzumab-Trastuzumab-Docetaxel (Metastatic Breast)

Index Terms Docetaxel-Pertuzumab-Trastuzumab (Metastatic Breast); Trastuzumab-Pertuzumab-Docetaxel (Metastatic Breast)

Use Breast cancer, metastatic (HER2-positive, first-line treatment)

Regimen

Cycle 1:

Pertuzumab: IV: 840 mg (loading dose) day 1 cycle 1

[total dose/cycle 1 = 840 mg]

Trastuzumab: IV: 8 mg/kg (loading dose) day 2 cycle 1

[total dose/cycle 1 = 8 mg/kg]

Docetaxel: IV: 75 mg/m^2 day 2 (administer after trastuzumab on day 2)

[total dose/cycle 1 = 75 mg/m^2]

Treatment cycle duration is 21 days

Subsequent cycles:

Pertuzumab: IV: 420 mg day 1

[total dose/cycle = 420 mg]

Trastuzumab: IV: 6 mg/kg day 1

[total dose/cycle = 6 mg/kg]

Docetaxel: IV: 75 mg/m^2 day 1 (may escalate to 100 mg/m^2 if tolerated; administer after trastuzumab and pertuzumab)

[total dose/cycle = 75 to 100 mg/m^2]

Repeat cycle every 21 days until disease progression or unacceptable toxicity (minimum of 6 cycles of docetaxel). In the case of discontinuation of chemotherapy owing to toxic effects, antibody therapy may be continued until disease progression.

References

Baselga J, Cortés J, Kim SB, et al. Pertuzumab plus trastuzumab plus docetaxel for metastatic breast cancer. *N Engl J Med.* 2012;366(2):109-119.

Swain SM, Baselga J, Kim SB, et al. Pertuzumab, trastuzumab, and docetaxel in HER2-positive metastatic breast cancer. *N Engl J Med.* 2015;372(8):724-734.

Pertuzumab-Trastuzumab-Docetaxel (Neoadjuvant Breast)

Index Terms Docetaxel-Pertuzumab-Trastuzumab (Neoadjuvant Breast); Trastuzumab-Pertuzumab-Docetaxel (Neoadjuvant Breast)

Use Breast cancer, neoadjuvant

Regimen

Cycle 1:

Trastuzumab: IV: 8 mg/kg (loading dose) day 1 cycle 1

[total dose/cycle 1 = 8 mg/kg]

Pertuzumab: IV: 840 mg (loading dose) day 1 cycle 1

[total dose/cycle 1 = 840 mg]

Docetaxel: IV: 75 mg/m^2 day 1 (administer after trastuzumab and pertuzumab)

[total dose/cycle 1 = 75 mg/m^2]

Treatment cycle is 21 days

Cycles 2-4:

Trastuzumab: IV: 6 mg/kg day 1

[total dose/cycle = 6 mg/kg]

Pertuzumab: IV: 420 mg day 1

[total dose/cycle = 420 mg]

Docetaxel: IV: 75 mg/m^2 day 1 (may escalate to 100 mg/m^2 if tolerated; administer after trastuzumab and pertuzumab)
[total dose/cycle = 75-100 mg/m^2]
Repeat cycle every 21 days for a total of 4 cycles

References

Gianni L, Pienkowski T, Im YH, et al. Efficacy and safety of neoadjuvant pertuzumab and trastuzumab in women with locally advanced, inflammatory, or early HER2-positive breast cancer (NeoSphere): a randomised multicentre, open-label, phase 2 trial. *Lancet Oncol.* 2012;13(1):25-32.

◆ **Pertuzumab-Trastuzumab-Paclitaxel (Breast)** *see* Paclitaxel-Pertuzumab-Trastuzumab (Breast) *on page 2186*

◆ **PE (Small Cell Lung Cancer)** *see* Cisplatin-Etoposide (Small Cell Lung Cancer) *on page 2042*

POC

Use Brain tumors
Regimen

Prednisone: Oral: 40 mg/m^2/day days 1 to 14
[total dose/cycle = 560 mg/m^2]
Vincristine: IV: 1.5 mg/m^2/day (maximum dose: 2 mg) days 1, 8, and 15
[total dose/cycle = 4.5 mg/m^2]
Lomustine: Oral: 100 mg/m^2 day 1
[total dose/cycle = 100 mg/m^2]
Repeat cycle every 6 weeks

References

Finlay JL, Boyett JM, Yates AJ, et al, "Randomized Phase III Trial in Childhood High-Grade Astrocytoma Comparing Vincristine, Lomustine, and Prednisone With the Eight-Drugs-In-1-Day Regimen. Childrens Cancer Group," *J Clin Oncol,* 1995, 13(1):112-23.

◆ **Pomalidomide-Daratumumab-Dexamethasone (Multiple Myeloma)** *see* Daratumumab-Pomalidomide-Dexamethasone (Multiple Myeloma) *on page 2085*

Pomalidomide-Dexamethasone (Multiple Myeloma)

Index Terms POM-LoDEX (Multiple Myeloma); Pomalidomide-Low-Dose Dexamethasone (Multiple Myeloma)
Use Multiple myeloma
Regimen

Pomalidomide: Oral: 4 mg once daily days 1 to 21
[total dose/cycle = 84 mg]
Dexamethasone: Oral: 40 mg once daily on days 1, 8, 15, and 22
[total dose/cycle = 160 mg]
Repeat cycle every 28 days until disease progression or unacceptable toxicity

References

Richardson PG, Siegel DS, Vij R, et al. Pomalidomide alone or in combination with low-dose dexamethasone in relapsed and refractory multiple myeloma: a randomized phase 2 study. *Blood.* 2014;123(12):1826-1832.

San Miguel J, Weisel K, Moreau P, et al. Pomalidomide plus low-dose dexamethasone versus high-dose dexamethasone alone for patients with relapsed and refractory multiple myeloma (MM-003): a randomised, open-label, phase 3 trial. *Lancet Oncol.* 2013;14(11):1055-1066.

◆ **Pomalidomide-Low-Dose Dexamethasone (Multiple Myeloma)** *see* Pomalidomide-Dexamethasone (Multiple Myeloma) *on page 2196*

◆ **POM-LoDEX (Multiple Myeloma)** *see* Pomalidomide-Dexamethasone (Multiple Myeloma) *on page 2196*

POMP

Use Leukemia, acute lymphocytic

Regimen Maintenance:

Mercaptopurine: Oral: 50 mg 3 times/day

[total dose/cycle = 4200-4650 mg]

Methotrexate: Oral: 20 mg/m^2 once weekly

[total dose/cycle = 80 mg/m^2]

Vincristine: IV: 2 mg day 1

[total dose/cycle = 2 mg]

Prednisone: Oral: 200 mg/day days 1 to 5

[total dose/cycle = 1000 mg]

Repeat cycle monthly for 2 years

References

Kantarjian HM, O'Brien S, Smith TL, et al, "Results of Treatment With Hyper-CVAD, a Dose-Intensive Regimen, in Adult Acute Lymphocytic Leukemia," *J Clin Oncol*, 2000, 18(3):547-61.

PVA (POG 8602)

Index Terms AlinC 14

Use Leukemia, acute lymphocytic

Regimen

Induction:

Prednisone: Oral: 40 mg/m^2/day (maximum dose: 60 mg) given in 3 divided doses days 0 to 28

[total dose/cycle = 1160 mg/m^2]

Vincristine: IV: 1.5 mg/m^2/day (maximum dose: 2 mg) days 0, 7, 14, and 21

[total dose/cycle = 6 mg/m^2; maximum: 8 mg]

Asparaginase: IM: 6000 units/m^2 3 times per week for 2 weeks

[total dose/cycle = 36,000 units/m^2]

Intrathecal therapy (triple): Days 0 and 22

Leucovorin: Route and dose not specified: Single dose 24 hours after every intrathecal treatment days 1 and 23

Administer one cycle only

◀ **CNS consolidation:**
Mercaptopurine: Oral: 75 mg/m^2/day days 29 to 43
[total dose/cycle = 1125 mg/m^2]
Intrathecal therapy (triple): Days 29 and 36
Leucovorin: Route and dose not specified: Single dose 24 hours after every
intrathecal treatment days 30 and 37
Administer one cycle only

Intensification:
Regimen A:
Methotrexate: IV: 1000 mg/m^2 continuous infusion over 24 hours day 1
[total dose/cycle = 1000 mg/m^2]
Cytarabine: IV: 1000 mg/m^2 continuous infusion over 24 hours day 1 (start
12 hours after start of methotrexate)
[total dose/cycle = 1000 mg/m^2]
Leucovorin: IM, IV, or Oral: 30 mg/m^2 at 24 and 36 hours after the start of
methotrexate
[total dose/cycle = 60 mg/m^2]
followed by IM, IV, or Oral: 3 mg/m^2 at 48, 60, and 72 hours after the start
of methotrexate
[total dose/cycle = 9 mg/m^2]
Repeat cycle every 3 weeks for 6 cycles (administered weeks 7, 10, 13, 16,
19, and 22)
Intrathecal therapy (triple): Weeks 9, 12, 15, and 18
Leucovorin: Route and dose not specified: Single dose 24 hours after every
intrathecal treatment weeks 9, 12, 15, and 18
or
Regimen B:
Methotrexate: IV: 1000 mg/m^2 continuous infusion over 24 hours day 1
[total dose/cycle = 1000 mg/m^2]
Cytarabine: IV: 1000 mg/m^2 continuous infusion over 24 hours day 1 (start
12 hours after methotrexate)
[total dose/cycle = 1000 mg/m^2]
Leucovorin: IM, IV, or Oral: 30 mg/m^2 at 24 and 36 hours after the start of
methotrexate
[total dose/cycle = 60 mg/m^2]
followed by IM, IV, or Oral: 3 mg/m^2 at 48, 60, and 72 hours after the start
of methotrexate
[total dose/cycle = 9 mg/m^2]
Repeat cycle every 12 weeks for 6 cycles (administer weeks 7, 19, 31, 43,
55, and 67)
Intrathecal therapy (triple): Weeks 9, 12, 15, and 18
Leucovorin: Route and dose not specified: Single dose 24 hours after every
intrathecal treatment weeks 9, 12, 15, and 18

Maintenance:
Regimen A:
Methotrexate: IM: 20 mg/m^2 weekly, weeks 25 to 156
[total dose/cycle = 2640 mg/m^2]
Mercaptopurine: Oral: 75 mg/m^2 daily, weeks 25 to 156
[total dose/cycle = 69,300 mg/m^2]
Intrathecal therapy (triple): Every 8 weeks, weeks 26 through 105
Leucovorin: Route and dose not specified: Single dose 24 hours after every
intrathecal treatment weeks 26 through 105

Prednisone: Oral: 40 mg/m^2/day (maximum dose: 60 mg) days 1 to 7 (given in 3 divided doses), weeks 8, 17, 25, 41, 57, 73, 89, and 105
[total dose/cycle = 2240 mg/m^2; maximum: 3360 mg]

Vincristine: IV: 1.5 mg/m^2/day (maximum dose: 2 mg) day 1, weeks 8, 9, 17, 18, 25, 26, 41, 42, 57, 58, 73, 74, 89, 90, 105, and 106
[total dose/cycle = 24 mg/m^2; maximum: 32 mg]

or

Regimen B:

Methotrexate: IM: 20 mg/m^2 weekly, weeks 22-28, 34-40, 46-52, and 58-64
[total dose/cycle = 560 mg/m^2]

Mercaptopurine: Oral: 75 mg/m^2 daily for 7 weeks, weeks 22-28, 34-40, 46-52, and 58-64
[total dose/cycle = 14700 mg/m^2]

followed by

Methotrexate: IM: 20 mg/m^2 weekly, weeks 70 to 156
[total dose/cycle = 1720 mg/m^2]

Mercaptopurine: Oral: 75 mg/m^2 daily, weeks 70 to 156
[total dose/cycle = 45,150 mg/m^2]

Intrathecal therapy (triple): Every 8 weeks, weeks 26 through 105

Leucovorin: Route and dose not specified: Single dose 24 hours after every intrathecal treatment weeks 26 through 105

Prednisone: Oral: 40 mg/m^2/day (maximum dose: 60 mg) days 1 to 7 (given in 3 divided doses), weeks 0, 17, 25, 41, 57, 73, 89, and 105
[total dose/cycle = 2240 mg/m^2]

Vincristine: IV: 1.5 mg/m^2/day (maximum dose: 2 mg) day 1, weeks 8, 9, 17, 18, 25, 26, 41, 42, 57, 58, 73, 74, 89, 90, 105, and 106
[total dose/cycle = 24 mg/m^2; maximum dose: 32 mg]

References

Land VJ, Shuster JJ, Crist WM, et al, "Comparison of Two Schedules of Intermediate-Dose Methotrexate and Cytarabine Consolidation Therapy for Childhood B-Precursor Cell Acute Lymphoblastic Leukemia: A Pediatric Oncology Group Study," *J Clin Oncol*, 1994, 12 (9):1939-45.

PVDA

Use Leukemia, acute lymphocytic

Regimen Induction:

Prednisone: Oral: 60 mg/m^2/day days 1 to 28
[total dose/cycle = 1680 mg/m^2]

Vincristine: IV: 1.5 mg/m^2/day days 1, 8, 15, and 22
[total dose/cycle = 6 mg/m^2]

Daunorubicin: IV: 25 mg/m^2/day days 1, 8, 15, and 22
[total dose/cycle = 100 mg/m^2]

Asparaginase: IM, SubQ, or IV: 5000 units/m^2/day days 1 to 14
[total dose/cycle = 70,000 units/m^2]

Administer one cycle only; used in conjunction with intrathecal chemotherapy

References

Hoelzer D, Thiel E, Loffler H, et al, "Intensified Therapy in Acute Lymphoblastic and Acute Undifferentiated Leukemia in Adults," *Blood*, 1984, 64(1):38-47.

◆ **Raltitrexed-Cisplatin (Mesothelioma)** *see* Cisplatin-Raltitrexed (Mesothelioma) *on page 2060*

◆ **Ramucirumab-Docetaxel (NSCLC)** *see* Docetaxel-Ramucirumab (NSCLC) *on page 2094*

Ramucirumab-FOLFIRI (Colorectal)

Index Terms Ramucirumab-Irinotecan-Leucovorin-Fluorouracil (Colorectal Cancer)

Use Colorectal cancer (relapsed, refractory)

Regimen

Ramucirumab: IV: 8 mg/kg over 60 minutes day 1
[total dose/cycle = 8 mg/kg]

Irinotecan: IV: 180 mg/m^2 over 90 minutes day 1
[total dose/cycle = 180 mg/m^2]

Leucovorin Calcium: IV: 400 mg/m^2 over 2 hours day 1
[total dose/cycle = 400 mg/m^2]

Fluorouracil: IV bolus: 400 mg/m^2 day 1
followed by IV: 2,400 mg/m^2 continuous infusion over 48 hours beginning day 1
[total fluorouracil dose/cycle (bolus and continuous infusion) = 2,800 mg/m^2]

Repeat cycle every 14 days until disease progression or unacceptable toxicity

References

Tabernero J, Yoshino T, Cohn AL, et al. Ramucirumab versus placebo in combination with second-line FOLFIRI in patients with metastatic colorectal carcinoma that progressed during or after first-line therapy with bevacizumab, oxaliplatin, and a fluoropyrimidine (RAISE): a randomised, double-blind, multicentre, phase 3 study. *Lancet Oncol.* 2015;16(5):499-508.

♦ **Ramucirumab-Irinotecan-Leucovorin-Fluorouracil (Colorectal Cancer)** *see* Ramucirumab-FOLFIRI (Colorectal) *on page 2200*

♦ **Ramucirumab-Paclitaxel (Gastric)** *see* Paclitaxel-Ramucirumab (Gastric) *on page 2187*

R-CHOP (NHL-DLBCL)

Index Terms CHOP-Rituximab (NHL-DLBCL); Cyclophosphamide-Doxorubicin-Vincristine-Prednisone-Rituximab (NHL-DLBCL; Doxorubicin-Vincristine-Prednisone-Rituximab-Cyclophosphamide (NHL-DLBCL); RCHOP (NHL-DLBCL); Rituximab-CHOP (NHL-DLBCL); Vincristine-Prednisone-Rituximab-Cyclophosphamide-Doxorubicin (NHL-DLBCL)

Use Lymphoma, non-Hodgkin

Regimen NOTE: Multiple variations are listed.

Variation 1:

Rituximab: IV: 375 mg/m^2 day 1
[total dose/cycle = 375 mg/m^2]

Cyclophosphamide: IV: 750 mg/m^2 day 1
[total dose/cycle = 750 mg/m^2]

Doxorubicin: IV: 50 mg/m^2 day 1
[total dose/cycle = 50 mg/m^2]

Vincristine: IV: 1.4 mg/m^2 (maximum dose: 2 mg) day 1
[total dose/cycle = 1.4 mg/m^2; maximum: 2 mg]

Prednisone: Oral: 100 mg daily on days 1 to 5
[total dose/cycle = 500 mg]

Repeat cycle every 21 days for a total of 6 cycles

Variation 2 (non-bulky limited stage):

Rituximab: IV: 375 mg/m^2 days -7, 1, 22, and 43
[total dose/cycle = 1,500 mg/m^2]

Cyclophosphamide: IV: 750 mg/m^2 days 3, 24, and 45
[total dose/cycle = 2,250 mg/m^2]

Doxorubicin: IV: 50 mg/m^2 days 3, 24, and 45
[total dose/cycle = 150 mg/m^2]

Vincristine: IV: 1.4 mg/m^2 (maximum dose: 2 mg) days 3, 24, and 45
[total dose/cycle = 4.2 mg/m^2; maximum: 6 mg/cycle]

Prednisone: Oral: 100 mg/day for 5 days on days 3 to 7, 24 to 28, and 45 to 49
[total dose/cycle = 1,500 mg]

Cycle does not repeat; followed by radiation therapy beginning on day 66

References

Variation 1:

Pfreundschuh M, Trümper L, Osterborg A et al. CHOP-like chemotherapy plus rituximab versus CHOP-like chemotherapy alone in young patients with good-prognosis diffuse large-B-cell lymphoma: a randomised controlled trial by the MabThera International Trial (MInT) Group. *Lancet Oncol.* 2006;7(5):379-391.

Pfreundschuh M, Kuhnt E, Trümper L, et al. CHOP-like chemotherapy with or without rituximab in young patients with good-prognosis diffuse large-B-cell lymphoma: 6-year results of an open-label randomised study of the MabThera International Trial (MInT) Group. *Lancet Oncol.* 2011;12 (11):1013-1022.

Variation 2:

Persky DO, Unger JM, Spier CM, et al. Phase II study of rituximab plus three cycles of CHOP and involved-field radiotherapy for patients with limited-stage aggressive B-cell lymphoma: Southwest Oncology Group study 0014. *J Clin Oncol.* 2008;26(14):2258-2263.

◆ RCHOP (NHL-DLBCL) *see* R-CHOP (NHL-DLBCL) *on page 2200*

R-CHOP (NHL-Follicular)

Index Terms CHOP-Rituximab (NHL-Follicular); RCHOP (NHL-Follicular); Rituximab-CHOP (NHL-Follicular)

Use Lymphoma, non-Hodgkin (first-line treatment for advanced follicular lymphoma)

Regimen

Rituximab: IV: 375 mg/m^2 day 1
[total dose/cycle = 375 mg/m^2]

Cyclophosphamide: IV: 750 mg/m^2 day 1
[total dose/cycle = 750 mg/m^2]

Doxorubicin: IV: 50 mg/m^2 day 1
[total dose/cycle = 50 mg/m^2]

Vincristine: IV: 1.4 mg/m^2 (maximum dose: 2 mg) day 1
[total dose/cycle = 1.4 mg/m^2; maximum: 2 mg]

Prednisone: Oral: 100 mg/day days 1 to 5
[total dose/cycle = 500 mg]

Repeat cycle every 21 days for up to 6 cycles

References

Rummel MJ, Niederle N, Maschmeyer G, et al. Bendamustine plus rituximab versus CHOP plus rituximab as first-line treatment for patients with indolent and mantle-cell lymphomas: an open-label, multicentre, randomised, phase 3 non-inferiority trial. *Lancet.* 2013;381(9873):1203-1210.

◆ RCHOP (NHL-Follicular) *see* R-CHOP (NHL-Follicular) *on page 2201*

R-CHOP (Waldenstrom Macroglobulinemia)

Index Terms Rituximab-Cyclophosphamide-Doxorubicin-Vincristine-Prednisone (Waldenstrom Macroglobulinemia)

Use Waldenstrom Macroglobulinemia

◄ **Regimen**

Rituximab: IV: 375 mg/m² day 1
[total dose/cycle = 375 mg/m²]
Cyclophosphamide: IV: 750 mg/m² day 1
[total dose/cycle = 750 mg/m²]
Doxorubicin: IV: 50 mg/m² day 1
[total dose/cycle = 50 mg/m²]
Vincristine: IV: 1.4 mg/m² (maximum dose: 2 mg) day 1
[total dose/cycle = 1.4 mg/m²; maximum: 2 mg]
Prednisone: Oral: 100 mg/day days 1 to 5
[total dose/cycle = 500 mg]
Repeat cycle every 21 days for 6 cycles

References

Ioakimidis L, Patterson CJ, Hunter ZR, et al. Comparative outcomes following CP-R, CVP-R, and CHOP-R in Waldenström's macroglobulinemia. *Clin Lymphoma Myeloma*. 2009;9(1):62-6.

R-CVP (NHL-Follicular)

Index Terms CVP-R (NHL-Follicular); RCVP (NHL-Follicular); Rituximab-CVP (NHL-Follicular); Rituximab-Cyclophosphamide-Vincristine-Prednisone (NHL-Follicular)

Use Lymphoma, non-Hodgkin (first-line therapy for advanced follicular lymphoma)

Regimen

Rituximab: IV: 375 mg/m² day 1
[total dose/cycle = 375 mg/m²]
Cyclophosphamide: IV: 750 mg/m² day 1
[total dose/cycle = 750 mg/m²]
Vincristine: IV: 1.4 mg/m² (maximum dose: 2 mg) day 1
[total dose/cycle = 1.4 mg/m² (maximum: 2 mg/cycle)]
Prednisone: Oral: 40 mg/m²/day days 1 to 5
[total dose/cycle = 200 mg/m²]
Repeat cycle every 21 days for up to 8 cycles

References

Federico M, Luminari S, Dondi A, et al. R-CVP versus R-CHOP versus R-FM for the initial treatment of patients with advanced-stage follicular lymphoma: results of the FOLL05 trial conducted by the Fondazione Italiana Linfomi. *J Clin Oncol*. 2013;31(12):1506-1513.

Marcus R, Imrie K, Belch A, et al. CVP chemotherapy plus rituximab compared with CVP as first-line treatment for advanced follicular lymphoma. *Blood*. 2005;105(4):1417-1423.

♦ **RCVP (NHL-Follicular)** *see* R-CVP (NHL-Follicular) *on page 2202*

♦ **R-DA-EPOCH (NHL-AIDS-Related)** *see* EPOCH Dose-Adjusted-Rituximab (NHL-AIDS-Related) *on page 2107*

R-DHAP (NHL-DLBCL)

Index Terms Cisplatin-Cytarabine-Dexamethasone-Rituximab (NHL-DLBCL); Rituximab-Dexamethasone-Cisplatin-Cytarabine (NHL-DLBCL)

Use Lymphoma, non-Hodgkin (DLBCL relapsed/refractory transplant eligible)

Regimen

Rituximab: IV: 375 mg/m² day 1
[total dose/cycle = 375 mg/m²]
Dexamethasone: Oral: 40 mg daily days 1 to 4
[total dose/cycle = 160 mg]
Cisplatin: IV: 100 mg/m² continuous infusion over 24 hours day 1
[total dose/cycle = 100 mg/m²]

Cytarabine: IV: 2,000 mg/m² over 3 hours every 12 hours for 2 doses day 2 (begins at the end of the cisplatin infusion)
[total dose/cycle = 4,000 mg/m²]

Repeat cycle every 21 days for 2 cycles followed by autologous stem-cell transplant; patients without complete or partial response were allowed 1 additional cycle

References

Crump M, Kuruvilla J, Couban S, et al. Randomized comparison of gemcitabine, dexamethasone, and cisplatin versus dexamethasone, cytarabine, and cisplatin chemotherapy before autologous stem-cell transplantation for relapsed and refractory aggressive lymphomas: NCIC-CTG LY.12. *J Clin Oncol*. 2014;32(31):3490-3496.

◆ **Rd (Multiple Myeloma)** *see* Lenalidomide-Dexamethasone (Multiple Myeloma) *on page 2166*

◆ **Regimen A3 (Neuroblastoma)** *see* A3 (Neuroblastoma) *on page 1973*

◆ **Regimen DD-4A (Wilms' Tumor)** *see* DD-4A (Wilms' Tumor) *on page 2086*

◆ **Regimen EE-4A (Wilms' Tumor)** *see* EE-4A (Wilms' Tumor) *on page 2100*

Regimen I (Wilms' Tumor)

Index Terms Vincristine, Doxorubicin, Cyclophosphamide, Mesna, Etoposide

Use Wilms' tumor

Regimen NOTE: Multiple variations are listed.

Variation 1 (patients ≤30 kg):

Vincristine: IV: 0.05 mg/kg (maximum dose: 2 mg) IV push day 1 of weeks 1, 2, 4 to 8, 10 and 11

Followed by

Vincristine 0.067 mg/kg (maximum dose: 2 mg) IV push day 1 of weeks 12, 13, 18, and 24
[total dose = 0.718 mg/kg; maximum: 26 mg]

Doxorubicin: IV: 1.5 mg/kg IV push day 1 of weeks 0, 6, 12, 18, and 24
[total dose = 7.5 mg/kg]

Cyclophosphamide: IV: 14.7 mg/kg/day days 1 to 5 of weeks 3, 9, 15, and 21
[total dose = 294 mg/kg]

Mesna: IV: 3 mg/kg/dose 4 doses/day (after cyclophosphamide) days 1 to 5 of weeks 3, 9, 15, and 21
[total dose = 240 mg/kg]

Cyclophosphamide: IV: 14.7 mg/kg/day days 1 to 3 of weeks 6, 12, 18, and 24
[total dose = 176.4 mg/kg]

Mesna: IV: 3 mg/kg/dose 4 doses/day (after cyclophosphamide) days 1 to 3 of weeks 6, 12, 18, and 24
[total dose = 144 mg/kg]

Etoposide: IV: 3.3 mg/kg/day days 1 to 5 of weeks 3, 9, 15, and 21
[total dose = 66 mg/kg]

Filgrastim: SubQ: 5 mcg/kg/day beginning 24 hours after last dose of chemotherapy and continued until ANC ≥10,000/mm³ or for a minimum of 1 week

Treatment course duration is week 0 through week 24

Variation 2 (patients >30 kg):
Vincristine: IV: 1.5 mg/m^2 (maximum dose: 2 mg) IV push day 1 of weeks 1, 2, 4 to 8, 10 and 11
Followed by
Vincristine 2 mg/m^2 (maximum dose: 2 mg) IV push days 1 of weeks 12, 13, 18, and 24
[total dose = 21.5 mg/m^2; maximum: 26 mg]
Doxorubicin: IV: 45 mg/m^2 IV push day 1 of weeks 0, 6, 12, 18, and 24
[total dose = 225 mg/m^2]
Cyclophosphamide: IV: 440 mg/m^2/day days 1 to 5 of weeks 3, 9, 15, and 21
[total dose = 8800 mg/m^2]
Mesna: IV: 90 mg/m^2/dose 4 doses/day (after cyclophosphamide) days 1 to 5 of weeks 3, 9, 15, and 21
[total dose = 7200 mg/m^2]
Cyclophosphamide: IV: 440 mg/m^2/day days 1 to 3 of weeks 6, 12, 18, and 24
[total dose = 5280 mg/m^2]
Mesna: IV: 90 mg/m^2/dose 4 doses/day (after cyclophosphamide) days 1 to 3 of weeks 6, 12, 18, and 24
[total dose = 4320 mg/m^2]
Etoposide: IV: 100 mg/m^2/day days 1 to 5 of weeks 3, 9, 15, and 21
[total dose = 2000 mg/m^2]
Filgrastim: SubQ: 5 mcg/kg/day beginning 24 hours after last dose of chemotherapy and continued until ANC ≥10,000/mm^3 or for a minimum of 1 week
Treatment course duration is week 0 through week 24

References
Variations 1 and 2:
Green DM, Cotton CA, Malogolowkin M, et al, "Treatment of Wilms Tumor Relapsing After Initial Treatment With Vincristine and Actinomycin D: A Report From the National Wilms Tumor Study Group," *Pediatr Blood Cancer*, 2007, 48(5):493-9.

♦ **Regimen new A1 (Neuroblastoma)** *see* New A1 (Neuroblastoma) on page 2180

♦ **R-EPOCH Dose Adjusted (NHL)** *see* EPOCH (Dose-Adjusted)-Rituximab (NHL) *on page 2106*

♦ **R-EPOCH Dose-Adjusted (NHL-AIDS-Related)** *see* EPOCH Dose-Adjusted-Rituximab (NHL-AIDS-Related) *on page 2107*

R-ESHAP (NHL-DLBCL)

Index Terms Cytarabine-Cisplatin-Etoposide-Methylprednisolone-Rituximab (NHL-DLBCL); Rituximab-Etoposide-Methylprednisolone-Cytarabine-Cisplatin (NHL-DLBCL)

Use Lymphoma, non-Hodgkin (DLBCL relapsed/refractory)

Regimen
Rituximab: IV: 375 mg/m^2 day 1 or day 5
[total dose/cycle = 375 mg/m^2]
Etoposide: IV: 40 to 60 mg/m^2/day over 1 hour days 1 to 4
[total dose/cycle = 160 to 240 mg/m^2]
Methylprednisolone: IV: 250 to 500 mg/day over 15 minutes days 1 to 4 or days 1 to 5
[total dose/cycle = 1,000 to 2,500 mg]
Cisplatin: IV: 25 mg/m^2/day continuous infusion days 1 to 4
[total dose/cycle = 100 mg/m^2]

Cytarabine: IV: 2,000 mg/m^2 over 2 hours day 5
  [total dose/cycle = 2,000 mg/m^2]
Repeat cycle every 21 to 28 days for up to a total of 6 cycles

References

Martin A, Conde E, Arnan M, et al. R-ESHAP as salvage therapy for patients with relapsed or refractory diffuse large B-cell lymphoma: the influence of prior exposure to rituximab on outcome. A GEL/TAMO study. *Haematologica.* 2008;93(12):1829-1836.

◆ **R-FC (CLL)** *see* Fludarabine-Cyclophosphamide-Rituximab (CLL) on page 2119

◆ **R-FCM (NHL- Follicular Cell)** *see* Fludarabine-Cyclophosphamide-Mitoxantrone-Rituximab (NHL-Follicular) on page 2117

◆ **R-GCD (NHL-DLBCL)** *see* Rituximab-Gemcitabine-Dexamethasone-Carboplatin (NHL-DLBCL) on page 2207

◆ **R-GDC (NHL-DLBCL)** *see* Rituximab-Gemcitabine-Dexamethasone-Carboplatin (NHL-DLBCL) on page 2207

◆ **R-GDP (NHL-DLBCL)** *see* Rituximab-Gemcitabine-Dexamethasone-Cisplatin (NHL-DLBCL) on page 2208

◆ **Ribociclib-Letrozole (Breast Cancer Regimen)** *see* Letrozole-Ribociclib (Breast Cancer Regimen) on page 2167

R-ICE (NHL-DLBCL)

Index Terms R-ICE (NHL-DLBCL); RICE (NHL-DLBCL); Rituximab-ICE (NHL-DLBCL); Rituximab-Ifosfamide-Carboplatin-Etoposide (NHL-DLBCL)

Use Lymphoma, non-Hodgkin (before autologous stem cell transplantation for relapsed or primary refractory DLBCL)

Regimen

Forty-eight hours prior to cycle 1:
  Rituximab: IV: 375 mg/m^2 48 hours prior to initiation of cycle 1
    [total dose/cycle = 375 mg/m^2]
Cycles 1 and 2:
  Rituximab: IV: 375 mg/m^2 day 1
    [total dose/cycle = 375 mg/m^2]
  Etoposide: IV: 100 mg/m^2/day days 3, 4, and 5
    [total dose/cycle = 300 mg/m^2]
  Carboplatin: IV: AUC = 5 (maximum dose: 800 mg) day 4
    [total dose/cycle = AUC = 5 (maximum dose/cycle: 800 mg)]
  Ifosfamide: IV: 5,000 mg/m^2 continuous infusion over 24 hours beginning on day 4
    [total dose/cycle = 5,000 mg/m^2]
  Mesna: IV: 5,000 mg/m^2 continuous infusion over 24 hours beginning on day 4
    [total dose/cycle = 5,000 mg/m^2]
  Filgrastim: SubQ: 5 mcg/kg/day days 7 to 14
    [total dose/cycle = 40 mcg/kg]
  Repeat cycle every 14 days for 2 cycles
Cycle 3:
  Rituximab: IV: 375 mg/m^2 day 1
    [total dose/cycle = 375 mg/m^2]
  Etoposide: IV: 100 mg/m^2/day days 3, 4, and 5
    [total dose/cycle = 300 mg/m^2]
  Carboplatin: IV: AUC = 5 (maximum dose: 800 mg) day 4
    [total dose/cycle = AUC = 5 (maximum dose/cycle: 800 mg)]

◀ Ifosfamide: IV: 5,000 mg/m^2 continuous infusion over 24 hours beginning on day 4

[total dose/cycle = 5,000 mg/m^2]

Mesna: IV: 5,000 mg/m^2 continuous infusion over 24 hours beginning on day 4

[total dose/cycle = 5,000 mg/m^2]

Filgrastim: SubQ: 10 mcg/kg/day days 7 until end of leukapheresis

Treatment cycle is 14 days

References

Kewalramani T, Zelenetz AD, Nimer SD, et al. Rituximab and ICE as second-line therapy before autologous stem cell transplantation for relapsed or primary refractory diffuse large B-cell lymphoma. *Blood.* 2004;103(10):3684-3688.

Rituximab-Gemcitabine-Dexamethasone-Carboplatin (NHL-DLBCL)

Index Terms Gemcitabine-Dexamethasone-Carboplatin-Rituximab (NHL-DLBCL); R-GCD (NHL-DLBCL); R-GDC (NHL-DLBCL)

Use Lymphoma, non-Hodgkin (DLBCL relapsed refractory)

Regimen

Gemcitabine: IV: 1,000 mg/m^2/day over 30 minutes days 1 and 8
  [total dose/cycle = 2,000 mg/m^2]
Dexamethasone: Oral: 40 mg/day days 1 to 4
  [total dose/cycle = 160 mg]
Carboplatin: IV: AUC 5 over 30 minutes day 1
  [total dose/cycle = AUC = 5]
Rituximab: IV: 375 mg/m^2 day 8
  [total dose/cycle = 375 mg/m^2]
Repeat cycle every 21 days for up to 4 cycles

References

Gopal AK, Press OW, Shustov AR, et al. Efficacy and safety of gemcitabine, carboplatin, dexamethasone, and rituximab in patients with relapsed/refractory lymphoma: a prospective multi-center phase II study by the Puget Sound Oncology Consortium. *Leuk Lymphoma.* 2010;51(8):1523-1529.

Rituximab-Gemcitabine-Dexamethasone-Cisplatin (NHL-DLBCL)

Index Terms Gemcitabine-Cisplatin-Dexamethasone-Rituximab (NHL-DLBCL); Gemcitabine-Dexamethasone-Cisplatin-Rituximab (NHL-DLBCL); R-GDP (NHL-DLBCL)

Use Lymphoma, non-Hodgkin (DLBCL recurrent/refractory, transplant eligible patients)

Regimen

Rituximab: IV: 375 mg/m^2 day 1
[total dose/cycle = 375 mg/m^2]

Gemcitabine: IV: 1,000 mg/m^2/day over 30 minutes days 1 and 8
[total dose/cycle = 2,000 mg/m^2]

Dexamethasone: Oral: 40 mg/day days 1 to 4
[total dose/cycle = 160 mg]

Cisplatin: IV: 75 mg/m^2 day 1
[total dose/cycle = 75 mg/m^2]

Repeat cycle every 21 days for 2 cycles followed by autologous stem-cell transplant; patients without complete or partial response were allowed 1 additional cycle

References

Crump M, Kuruvilla J, Couban S, et al. Randomized comparison of gemcitabine, dexamethasone, and cisplatin versus dexamethasone, cytarabine, and cisplatin chemotherapy before autologous stem-cell transplantation for relapsed and refractory aggressive lymphomas: NCIC-CTG LY.12. *J Clin Oncol*. 2014;32(31):3490-3496.

◆ **Rituximab-Gemcitabine-Oxaliplatin (NHL-DLBCL)** *see* GEMOX-R (NHL-DLBCL) *on page 2141*

◆ **Rituximab-Gemcitabine-Oxaliplatin (NHL-Mantle Cell)** *see* GEMOX-R (NHL-Mantle Cell) *on page 2141*

◆ **Rituximab-Hyper-CVAD Alternating With High-Dose Methotrexate-Cytarabine (NHL-Burkitt)** *see* Hyper-CVAD Alternating With High-Dose Methotrexate-Cytarabine + Rituximab + CNS Prophylaxis (NHL-Burkitt) *on page 2144*

Rituximab-Hyper-CVAD (NHL-Mantle Cell)

Index Terms Rituximab-Cyclophosphamide-Vincristine-Doxorubicin-Methotrexate-Cytarabine (NHL-Mantle Cell)

Use Lymphoma, non-Hodgkin (Mantle cell)

Regimen

Cycle A (Cycles 1, 3, 5 [and 7, if needed]):

Rituximab: IV: 375 mg/m^2 day 1
[total dose/cycle = 375 mg/m^2]

Cyclophosphamide: IV: 300 mg/m^2 over 3 hours every 12 hours for 6 doses days 2, 3, and 4
[total dose/cycle = 1,800 mg/m^2]

Mesna: IV: 600 mg/m^2/day continuous infusion over 24 hours days 2, 3, and 4, beginning 1 hour prior to start of cyclophosphamide and finishing 12 hours after last dose of cyclophosphamide
[total dose/cycle = 1,800 mg/m^2]

Vincristine: IV: 1.4 mg/m^2/day (maximum dose: 2 mg) days 5 (12 hours after last dose of cyclophosphamide) and 12
[total dose/cycle = 2.8 mg/m^2; maximum: 4 mg]

Doxorubicin: IV: 16.7 mg/m^2/day continuous infusion over 24 hours days 5, 6, and 7 (12 hours after last dose of cyclophosphamide)
[total dose/cycle = 50.1 mg/m^2]

Dexamethasone: Oral, IV: 40 mg/day days 2 to 5 and days 12 to 15
[total dose/cycle = 320 mg]

Filgrastim: SubQ: 5 mcg/kg daily starting 24 to 36 hours after completion of doxorubicin infusion and continuing for 10 days

Treatment cycle is 21 days

Cycle B (Cycles 2, 4, 6 [and 8, if needed]):

Rituximab: IV: 375 mg/m^2 day 1
[total dose/cycle = 375 mg/m^2]

Methotrexate: IV: 200 mg/m^2 over 2 hours day 2 (50% dose reduction for patients with serum creatinine >1.5 mg/dL)
followed by IV: 800 mg/m^2 continuous infusion over 22 hours day 2
[total dose/cycle = 1,000 mg/m^2]

Leucovorin: Oral: 50 mg (start 12 hours after the end of the methotrexate infusion)
followed by Oral: 15 mg every 6 hours for 8 doses
[total dose/cycle = 170 mg]

Cytarabine: IV: 3,000 mg/m^2 over 2 hours every 12 hours for 4 doses days 3 and 4 (or 1,000 mg/m^2 in patients >60 years old and in patients with serum creatinine >1.5 mg/dL)
[total dose/cycle = 12,000 mg/m^2]

Filgrastim: SubQ: 5 mcg/kg daily starting 24 to 36 hours after completion of cytarabine infusion and continuing for 10 days

Treatment cycle is 21 days

Alternate cycles A and B every 21 days in the following sequence: ABABA-BAB. Patients who achieved a complete remission after 2 cycles (AB) received a total of 6 cycles (ABABAB). Patients who achieved a partial response after 2 cycles and a complete remission after 6 cycles received a total of 8 cycles.

References

Romaguera JE, Fayad L, Rodriguez MA, et al. High rate of durable remissions after treatment of newly diagnosed aggressive mantle cell lymphoma with rituximab plus hyper-CVAD alternating with rituximab plus high-dose methotrexate and cytarabine. *J Clin Oncol.* 2005;23 (28):7013-7023.

- ◆ **Rituximab-ICE (NHL-DLBCL)** *see* R-ICE (NHL-DLBCL) *on page 2205*

- ◆ **Rituximab-Idelalisib (CLL)** *see* Idelalisib-Rituximab (CLL) *on page 2154*

- ◆ **Rituximab-Ifosfamide-Carboplatin-Etoposide (NHL-DLBCL)** *see* R-ICE (NHL-DLBCL) *on page 2205*

- ◆ **Rituximab-Lenalidomide (CLL)** *see* Lenalidomide-Rituximab (CLL) *on page 2166*

- ◆ **Rituximab-Temozolomide (CNS Lymphoma)** *see* Temozolomide-Rituximab (CNS Lymphoma) *on page 2212*

- ◆ **RVD (Multiple Myeloma)** *see* Lenalidomide-Bortezomib-Dexamethasone (Multiple Myeloma) *on page 2163*

- ◆ **Saltz Regimen (Colorectal)** *see* Fluorouracil-Leucovorin-Irinotecan (Saltz Regimen) (Colorectal) *on page 2126*

Stanford V (Hodgkin)

Index Terms Mechlorethamine, Doxorubicin, Vinblastine, Vincristine, Bleomycin, Etoposide, Prednisone (Hodgkin)

◀ **Use** Lymphoma, Hodgkin

Regimen NOTE: Multiple variations are listed.

Variation 1 (advanced or locally extensive disease with bulky mediastinal adenopathy):

Mechlorethamine: IV: 6 mg/m^2 day 1 on weeks 1, 5, and 9
[total dose/cycle = 18 mg/m^2]

Doxorubicin: IV: 25 mg/m^2 day 1 on weeks 1, 3, 5, 7, 9, and 11
[total dose/cycle = 150 mg/m^2]

Vinblastine: IV: 6 mg/m^2 day 1 on weeks 1, 3, 5, 7, 9, and 11
[total dose/cycle = 36 mg/m^2]

Vincristine: IV: 1.4 mg/m^2 (maximum dose: 2 mg) day 1 on weeks 2, 4, 6, 8, 10, and 12
[total dose/cycle = 8.4 mg/m^2; maximum: 12 mg]

Bleomycin: IV: 5 units/m^2 day 1 on weeks 2, 4, 6, 8, 10, and 12
[total dose/cycle = 30 units/m^2]

Etoposide: IV: 60 mg/m^2/day days 1 and 2 on weeks 3, 7, and 11
[total dose/cycle = 360 mg/m^2]

Prednisone: Oral: 40 mg/m^2 every other day for 10 weeks
[total dose prior to taper = 1,400 mg/m^2]

 followed by tapering of prednisone dose during weeks 11 and 12

Treatment cycle is 12 weeks, followed by radiation 2 to 3 weeks after completion of chemotherapy

Variation 2 (stage I to IIA nonbulky):

Mechlorethamine: IV: 6 mg/m^2 day 1 on weeks 1 and 5
[total dose/cycle = 12 mg/m^2]

Doxorubicin: IV: 25 mg/m^2 day 1 on weeks 1, 3, 5, and 7
[total dose/cycle = 100 mg/m^2]

Vinblastine: IV: 6 mg/m^2 day 1 on weeks 1, 3, 5, and 7
[total dose/cycle = 24 mg/m^2]

Vincristine: IV: 1.4 mg/m^2 (maximum dose: 2 mg) day 1 on weeks 2, 4, 6, and 8
[total dose/cycle = 5.6 mg/m^2; maximum: 8 mg]

Bleomycin: IV: 5 units/m^2 day 1 on weeks 2, 4, 6, and 8
[total dose/cycle = 20 units/m^2]

Etoposide: IV: 60 mg/m^2/day days 1 and 2 on weeks 3 and 7
[total dose/cycle = 240 mg/m^2]

Prednisone: Oral: 40 mg/m^2 every other day for 6 weeks
[total dose prior to taper = 840 mg/m^2]

 followed by tapering of prednisone 10 mg/day during weeks 7 and 8

Treatment cycle is 8 weeks, followed by radiation 1 to 3 weeks after completion of chemotherapy

References

Variation 1:

Gordon LI, Hong F, Fisher RI, et al. Randomized phase III trial of ABVD versus Stanford V with or without radiation therapy in locally extensive and advanced-stage Hodgkin lymphoma: an intergroup study coordinated by the Eastern Cooperative Oncology Group (E2496). *J Clin Oncol.* 2013;31(6):684-691.

Horning SJ, Hoppe RT, Breslin S, et al. Stanford V and radiotherapy for locally extensive and advanced Hodgkin's disease: mature results of a prospective clinical trial. *J Clin Oncol.* 2002;20 (3):630-637.

Variation 2:

Advani RH, Hoppe RT, Baer D, et al. Efficacy of abbreviated Stanford V chemotherapy and involved-field radiotherapy in early-stage Hodgkin lymphoma: mature results of the G4 trial. *Ann Oncol.* 2013;24(4):1044-1048.

TAC (Breast)

Index Terms Docetaxel, Doxorubicin, Cyclophosphamide (Breast); Doxorubicin, Cyclophosphamide, Docetaxel (Breast)

Use Breast cancer

Regimen

Doxorubicin: IV: 50 mg/m^2 over 15 minutes day 1
[total dose/cycle = 50 mg/m^2]
Cyclophosphamide: IV: 500 mg/m^2 day 1
[total dose/cycle = 500 mg/m^2]
Docetaxel: IV: 75 mg/m^2 over 1 hour day 1, administered 1 hour after cyclophosphamide
[total dose/cycle = 75 mg/m^2]
Repeat cycle every 21 days for 6 cycles

References

Mackey JR, Martin M, Pienkowski T, et al, "Adjuvant Docetaxel, Doxorubicin, and Cyclophosphamide in Node-Positive Breast Cancer: 10-Year Follow Up of the Phase III Randomised BCIRG 001 Trial," *Lancet Oncol*, 2013, 14(1):72-80.

Martin M, Pienkowski T, Mackey J, et al, "Adjuvant Docetaxel for Node-Positive Breast Cancer," *N Engl J Med*, 2005, 352(22):2302-13.

◆ **TAP (Endometrial)** *see* Cisplatin-Doxorubicin-Paclitaxel (Endometrial) on page 2041

TC (Breast)

Index Terms Cyclophosphamide-Docetaxel (Breast); Docetaxel-Cyclophosphamide (Breast)

Use Breast cancer

Regimen

Docetaxel: IV: 75 mg/m^2 day 1
[total dose/cycle = 75 mg/m^2]
Cyclophosphamide: IV: 600 mg/m^2 day 1
[total dose/cycle = 600 mg/m^2]
Repeat cycle every 21 days for 4 cycles

References

Jones SE, Savin MA, Holmes FA, et al, "Phase III Trial Comparing Doxorubicin Plus Cyclophosphamide With Docetaxel Plus Cyclophosphamide as Adjuvant Therapy for Operable Breast Cancer," *J Clin Oncol*, 2006, 24(34):5381-7.

Jones S, Holmes FA, O'Shaughnessy JO, et al, "Docetaxel With Cyclophosphamide Is Associated With an Overall Survival Benefit Compared With Doxorubicin and Cyclophophosphamide: 7-Year Follow-Up of US Oncology Research Trial 9735," *J Clin Oncol*, 2009, 27(8):1177-83.

◆ **TC (Endometrial)** *see* Carboplatin-Paclitaxel (Endometrial) on page 2019

◆ **TCF (Esophageal Cancer)** *see* Paclitaxel-Cisplatin-Fluorouracil (Esophageal Cancer) on page 2185

◆ **TCF (Gastric/Esophageal Cancer)** *see* Docetaxel-Cisplatin-Fluorouracil (Gastric/Esophageal Cancer) on page 2088

◆ **TCH (Breast)** *see* Carboplatin-Docetaxel-Trastuzumab (Breast) on page 2012

◆ **TCH (Breast)** *see* Carboplatin-Paclitaxel-Trastuzumab (Breast) on page 2022

◆ **TC (NSCLC)** *see* Carboplatin-Paclitaxel (NSCLC) on page 2020

◆ **Temozolomide-Irinotecan (Ewing Sarcoma)** *see* Irinotecan-Temozolomide (Ewing Sarcoma) on page 2161

Temozolomide-Rituximab (CNS Lymphoma)

Index Terms Rituximab-Temozolomide (CNS Lymphoma)

Use Primary CNS lymphoma

Regimen NOTE: Multiple variations are listed.

Variation 1:

Induction therapy (cycles 1 to 4):

Rituximab: IV: 375 mg/m^2 day 1

[total dose/cycle = 375 mg/m^2]

Temozolomide: Oral: 150 mg/m^2/day days 1 to 5

[total dose/cycle = 750 mg/m^2]

Repeat cycle every 28 days for a total of 4 cycles

followed by

Maintenance therapy:

Temozolomide: Oral: 150 mg/m^2/day days 1 to 5

[total dose/cycle = 750 mg/m^2]

Repeat cycle every 28 days for a total of 8 cycles

Variation 2:

Induction therapy (cycles 1 and 2):

Rituximab: IV: 750 mg/m^2 days 1, 8, 15, and 22

[total dose/cycle = 3000 mg/m^2]

Temozolomide: Oral: 150 mg/m^2/day days 1 to 7 and days 15 to 21

[total dose/cycle = 2100 mg/m^2]

Administer cycle every 28 days for a total of 1 or 2 cycles

followed by

Maintenance therapy:

Temozolomide: Oral: 150 mg/m^2/day days 1 to 5

[total dose/cycle = 750 mg/m^2]

Repeat cycle every 28 days

References

Variation 1:

Wong ET, Tishler R, Barron L, Wu JK. Immunochemotherapy with rituximab and temozolomide for central nervous system lymphomas. *Cancer.* 2004;101(1):139-145.

Variation 2:

Enting RH, Demopoulos A, DeAngelis LM, Abrey LE. Salvage therapy for primary CNS lymphoma with a combination of rituximab and temozolomide. *Neurology.* 2004;63(5):901-903.

- ◆ **Thalidomide-Cisplatin-Doxorubicin-Cyclophosphamide-Etoposide-Bortezomib-Dexamethasone (Multiple Myeloma)** *see* VDT-PACE (Multiple Myeloma) *on page 2229*

- ◆ **Thalidomide-Dexamethasone-Bortezomib (Multiple Myeloma)** *see* Bortezomib-Thalidomide-Dexamethasone (Multiple Myeloma) *on page 2000*

- ◆ **Thalidomide-Dexamethasone-Cisplatin-Doxorubicin-Cyclophosphamide-Etoposide (Multiple Myeloma)** *see* DTPACE (Multiple Myeloma) *on page 2098*

Thalidomide-Dexamethasone (MM)

Index Terms Dexamethasone-Thalidomide (MM)

Use Multiple myeloma

Regimen NOTE: Multiple variations are listed.

Variation 1 (refractory):

Thalidomide: Oral: 100 mg/day days 1 to 28

[total dose/cycle = 2800 mg]

Dexamethasone: Oral: 40 mg/day days 1 to 4
[total dose/cycle = 160 mg]
Repeat cycle every 28 days
Variation 2 (refractory):
 Thalidomide: Oral: 200 mg/day days 1 to 14 (cycle 1)
  followed by Oral: 400 mg/day days 15 to 28 (cycle 1)
  [total dose/cycle = 8400 mg]
 Thalidomide: Oral: 400 mg/day days 1 to 28 (subsequent cycles)
  [total dose/cycle = 11,200 mg]
 Dexamethasone: Oral: 20 mg/m^2/day days 1 to 4, 9 to 12, and 17 to 20
 (cycle 1)
  [total dose/cycle = 240 mg/m^2]
   followed by Oral: 20 mg/m^2/day days 1 to 4 (subsequent cycles)
   [total dose/cycle = 80 mg/m^2]
 Repeat cycle every 28 days
Variation 3 (newly diagnosed):
 Thalidomide: Oral: 200 mg/day days 1 to 28
  [total dose/cycle = 5600 mg]
 Dexamethasone: Oral: 40 mg/day days 1 to 4, 9 to 12, and 17 to 20
  [total dose/cycle = 480 mg]
 Repeat cycle every 28 days
Variation 4 (newly diagnosed):
 Thalidomide: Oral: 50 mg/day days 1 to 14
  followed by Oral: 100 mg/day days 15 to 28 (cycle 1)
  [total dose/cycle 1 = 2100 mg]
   followed by Oral: 200 mg/day days 1 to 28 (starting with cycle 2 and
   subsequent cycles)
   [total dose/cycle = 5600 mg]
 Dexamethasone: Oral: 40 mg/day days 1 to 4, 9 to 12, and 17 to 20 (cycles 1
 to 4)
  [total dose/cycle 1 to 4 = 480 mg]
   followed by Oral: 40 mg/day days 1 to 4 (starting with cycle 5 and
   subsequent cycles)
   [total dose/cycle = 160 mg]
 Repeat cycle every 28 days until disease progression or unacceptable
 toxicity
Variation 5 (newly diagnosed):
 Thalidomide: Oral: 100 mg/day days 1 to 14
  followed by Oral: 200 mg/day days 15 to 28 (cycle 1)
  [total dose/cycle = 4200 mg]
   followed by Oral: 200 mg/day days 1 to 28 (starting with cycle 2 and
   subsequent cycles)
   [total dose/cycle = 5600 mg]
 Dexamethasone: Oral: 40 mg/day days 1 to 4, 9 to 12, and 17 to 20 (odd
 cycles)
  [total dose/cycle = 480 mg]
 Dexamethasone: Oral: 40 mg/day days 1 to 4 (even cycles)
  [total dose/cycle = 160 mg]
 Repeat cycle every 28 days for a total of 4 cycles
Variation 6 (newly diagnosed induction):
 Thalidomide: Oral: 50 mg/day; may escalate by 50 mg per week to a
 maximum dose of 400 mg/day
 [total dose/cycle = up to 14,000 mg]

Dexamethasone: Oral: 40 mg/day days 1 to 4, 9 to 12, and 17 to 20
[total dose/cycle = 480 mg]
Repeat cycle every 35 days for a total of 3 cycles

References

Variation 1:

Palumbo A, Giaccone L, Bertola A, et al, "Low-Dose Thalidomide Plus Dexamethasone Is an Effective Salvage Therapy for Advanced Myeloma," *Haematologica*, 2001, 86(4):399-403.

Variation 2:

Dimopoulos MA, Zervas K, Kouvatseas G, et al, "Thalidomide and Dexamethasone Combination for Refractory Multiple Myeloma," *Ann Oncol*, 2001, 12(7):991-5.

Variation 3:

Rajkumar SV, Blood E, Vesole D, et al, "Phase III Clinical Trial of Thalidomide Plus Dexamethasone Compared With Dexamethasone Alone in Newly Diagnosed Multiple Myeloma: A Clinical Trial Coordinated by the Eastern Cooperative Oncology Group," *J Clin Oncol*, 2006, 24(3):431-6.

Variation 4:

Rajkumar SV, Rosiñol L, Hussein M, et al, "Multicenter, Randomized, Double-Blind, Placebo-Controlled Study of Thalidomide Plus Dexamethasone Compared With Dexamethasone as Initial Therapy for Newly Diagnosed Multiple Myeloma," *J Clin Oncol*, 2008, 26(13):2171-7.

Variation 5:

Cavo M, Zamagni E, Tosi P, et al, "Superiority of Thalidomide and Dexamethasone Over Vincristine-Doxorubicin Dexamethasone (VAD) as Primary Therapy in Preparation for Autologous Transplantation for Multiple Myeloma," *Blood*, 2005, 106(1):35-9.

Variation 6:

Hussein MA, Bolejack V, Zonder JA, et al, "Phase II Study of Thalidomide Plus Dexamethasone Induction Followed by Tandem Melphalan-Based Autotransplantation and Thalidomide-Plus-Prednisone Maintenance for Untreated Multiple Myeloma: A Southwest Oncology Group Trial (S0204)," *J Clin Oncol*, 2009, 27(21):3510-7.

TIP (Testicular)

Index Terms Cisplatin-Ifosfamide-Paclitaxel (Testicular); Paclitaxel-Ifosfamide-Cisplatin (Testicular)

Use Testicular cancer

Regimen

Paclitaxel: IV: 250 mg/m^2 continuous infusion day 1
[total dose/cycle = 250 mg/m^2]
Ifosfamide: IV: 1500 mg/m^2/day over 60 minutes days 2 to 5
[total dose/cycle = 6000 mg/m^2]
Cisplatin: IV: 25 mg/m^2/day over 30 minutes days 2 to 5
[total dose/cycle = 100 mg/m^2]
Mesna: IV: 500 mg/m^2 prior to ifosfamide and every 4 hours for 2 doses, days 2 to 5
[total dose/cycle = 6000 mg/m^2]
Filgrastim SubQ: 5 mcg/kg daily days 7 to 18 (discontinue if WBC >10,000/mm^3 for 2 days)
Repeat cycle every 21 days for 4 cycles

References

Kondagunta GV, Bacik J, Donadio A. et al. Combination of paclitaxel, ifosfamide, and cisplatin is an effective second-line therapy for patients with relapsed testicular germ cell tumors. *J Clin Oncol.* 2005;23(27):6549-6555.

◆ **TOPO/CTX (Neuroblastoma)** *see* Cyclophosphamide-Topotecan (Neuroblastoma) *on page 2078*

◆ **TOPO/CYC (Ewing Sarcoma)** *see* Cyclophosphamide-Topotecan (Ewing Sarcoma) *on page 2078*

◆ **Topotecan-Cisplatin (Cervical Cancer)** *see* Cisplatin-Topotecan (Cervical Cancer) *on page 2060*

Trabectedin-Doxorubicin (Liposomal) (Ovarian)

Index Terms Doxorubicin Liposomal-Trabectedin (Ovarian); Trabectedin-Doxil (Ovarian)

Use Ovarian cancer (relapsed, platinum-sensitive)

Regimen

Doxorubicin (liposomal): IV: 30 mg/m^2 over 90 minutes day 1
[total dose/cycle = 30 mg/m^2]

Trabectedin: IV: 1.1 mg/m^2 over 3 hours (via central line) day 1
[total dose/cycle = 1.1 mg/m^2]

Repeat cycle every 21 days until disease progression or unacceptable toxicity, or two or more cycles beyond confirmed complete response

References

Monk BJ, Herzog TJ, Kaye SB, et al. Trabectedin plus pegylated liposomal doxorubicin in recurrent ovarian cancer. *J Clin Oncol.* 2010;28(19):3107-3114.

Monk BJ, Herzog TJ, Kaye SB, et al. Trabectedin plus pegylated liposomal doxorubicin (PLD) versus PLD in recurrent ovarian cancer: overall survival analysis. *Eur J Cancer.* 2012;48 (15):2361-2368.

Poveda A, Vergote I, Tjulandin S, et al. Trabectedin plus pegylated liposomal doxorubicin in relapsed ovarian cancer: outcomes in the partially platinum-sensitive (platinum-free interval 6-12 months) subpopulation of OVA-301 phase III randomized trial. *Ann Oncol.* 2011;22(1):39-48.

Trastuzumab-Cisplatin-Capecitabine (Gastric Cancer)

Index Terms Capecitabine-Cisplatin-Trastuzumab (Gastric Cancer); Cisplatin-Capecitabine-Trastuzumab (Gastric Cancer)

Use Gastric cancer

Regimen
Cycle 1:
Capecitabine: Oral: 1000 mg/m^2/dose twice daily days 1 to 14
[total dose/cycle = 28,000 mg/m^2]
Cisplatin: IV: 80 mg/m^2/dose day 1
[total dose/cycle = 80 mg/m^2]
Trastuzumab: IV: 8 mg/kg/dose (loading dose) day 1
[total dose/cycle 1 = 8 mg/kg]
Treatment cycle is 21 days
Cycles 2-6:
Capecitabine: Oral: 1000 mg/m^2/dose twice daily days 1 to 14
[total dose/cycle = 28,000 mg/m^2]
Cisplatin: IV: 80 mg/m^2/dose day 1
[total dose/cycle = 80 mg/m^2]
Trastuzumab: IV: 6 mg/kg/dose day 1
[total dose/cycle = 6 mg/kg]
Treatment cycle is 21 days
Subsequent cycles:
Trastuzumab: IV: 6 mg/kg/dose day 1
[total dose/cycle = 6 mg/kg]
Repeat cycle every 3 weeks until disease progression or unacceptable
toxicity

References
Bang YJ, Van Cutsem E, Feyereislova A, et al, "Trastuzumab in Combination With Chemotherapy Versus Chemotherapy Alone for Treatment of HER2-Positive Advanced Gastric or Gastro-Oesophageal Junction Cancer (ToGA): A Phase 3, Open-Label, Randomised Controlled Trial," Lancet, 2010, 376(9742):687-97.

Trastuzumab-Cisplatin-Fluorouracil (Gastric Cancer)
Index Terms Cisplatin-Fluorouracil-Trastuzumab (Gastric Cancer); Fluorouracil-Cisplatin-Trastuzumab (Gastric Cancer)
Use Gastric cancer
Regimen
Cycle 1:
Fluorouracil: IV: 800 mg/m^2/day continuous infusion days 1 to 5
[total dose/cycle = 4000 mg/m^2]
Cisplatin: IV: 80 mg/m^2/dose day 1
[total dose/cycle = 80 mg/m^2]
Trastuzumab: IV: 8 mg/kg/dose (loading dose) day 1
[total dose/cycle 1 = 8 mg/kg]
Treatment cycle is 21 days
Cycles 2-6:
Fluorouracil: IV: 800 mg/m^2/day continuous infusion days 1 to 5
[total dose/cycle = 4000 mg/m^2]
Cisplatin: IV: 80 mg/m^2/dose day 1
[total dose/cycle = 80 mg/m^2]
Trastuzumab: IV: 6 mg/kg/dose day 1
[total dose/cycle = 6 mg/kg]
Treatment cycle is 21 days
Subsequent cycles:
Trastuzumab: IV: 6 mg/kg/dose day 1
[total dose/cycle = 6 mg/kg]
Repeat cycle every 3 weeks until disease progression or unacceptable
toxicity

References
Bang YJ, Van Cutsem E, Feyereislova A, et al, "Trastuzumab in Combination With Chemotherapy Versus Chemotherapy Alone for Treatment of HER2-Positive Advanced Gastric or Gastro-Oesophageal Junction Cancer (ToGA): A Phase 3, Open-Label, Randomised Controlled Trial," *Lancet*, 2010, 376(9742):687-97.

Trastuzumab-Vinorelbine (Breast)

Index Terms Vinorelbine-Trastuzumab (Breast)

Use Breast cancer

Regimen NOTE: Multiple variations are listed.

Variation 1:

Cycle 1:

Trastuzumab: IV: 4 mg/kg (loading dose) over 90 minutes day 1 cycle 1

[total dose/cycle 1 = 4 mg/kg]

Vinorelbine: IV: 25 mg/m^2 over 6-10 minutes day 1

[total dose/cycle 1 = 25 mg/m^2]

Treatment cycle is 7 days

Subsequent cycles:

Trastuzumab: IV: 2 mg/kg over 30 minutes day 1

[total dose/cycle = 2 mg/kg]

Vinorelbine: IV: 25 mg/m^2 over 6-10 minutes day 1

[total dose/cycle = 25 mg/m^2]

Repeat cycle every 7 days until disease progression or unacceptable toxicity

Variation 2:

Cycle 1:

Trastuzumab: IV: 8 mg/kg (loading dose) over 90 minutes day 1 cycle 1

[total dose/cycle 1 = 8 mg/kg]

Vinorelbine: IV: 30-35 mg/m^2/day days 1 and 8

[total dose/cycle 1 = 60-70 mg/m^2]

Treatment cycle is 21 days

◀

Subsequent cycles:

Trastuzumab: IV: 6 mg/kg over 30 minutes day 1

[total dose/cycle = 6 mg/kg]

Vinorelbine: IV: 30-35 mg/m²/day days 1 and 8

[total dose/cycle = 60-70 mg/m²]

Repeat cycle every 21 days until disease progression or unacceptable toxicity

References

Variation 1:

Burstein HJ, Keshaviah A, Baron AD, et al, "Trastuzumab Plus Vinorelbine or Taxane Chemotherapy for HER2-Overesxpressing Metastatic Breast Cancer: The Trastuzumab and Vinorelbine or Taxane Study," *Cancer*, 2007, 110(5):965-72.

Burstein HJ, Kuter I, Campos SM, et al, "Clinical Activity of Trastuzumab and Vinorelbine in Women With HER2-Overexpressing Metastatic Breast Cancer," *J Clin Oncol*, 2001, 19 (10):2722-30.

Variation 2:

Andersson M, Lidbrink E, Bjerre K, et al, "Phase III Randomized Study Comparing Docetaxel Plus Trastuzumab With Vinorelbine Plus Trastuzumab as First-Line Therapy of Metastatic or Locally Advanced Human Epidermal Growth Factor Receptor 2-Positive Breast Cancer: The HERNATA Study," *J Clin Oncol*, 2011, 29(3):264-71.

Tretinoin-Arsenic Trioxide (APL)

Index Terms Arsenic Trioxide-ATRA (APL); ATRA-Arsenic Trixoide (APL)

Use Leukemia, acute promyelocytic

Regimen

Induction (continue until <5% blasts in marrow and no abnormal promyelocytes):

Tretinoin: Oral: 45 mg/m²/day (in 2 divided doses) day 1 up to day 85

[total induction dose = up to 3825 mg/m²]

Arsenic Trioxide: IV: 0.15 mg/kg/day over 1 hour beginning day 10 up to day 85

[total induction dose = up to 11.25 mg/kg]

Postremission therapy (beginning with complete remission):

Tretinoin: Oral: 45 mg/m²/day weeks 1, 2, 5, 6, 9, 10, 13, 14, 17, 18, 21, 22, 25, 26

[total postremission dose = 4410 mg/m²]

Arsenic Trioxide: IV: 0.15 mg/kg/day Monday through Friday weeks 1 to 4, 9 to 12, 17 to 20, and 25 to 28

[total postremission dose = 12 mg/kg]

References

Estey E, Garcia-Manero G, Ferrajoli A, et al, "Use of All-*Trans* Retinoic Acid Plus Arsenic Trioxide as an Alternative to Chemotherapy in Untreated Acute Promyelocytic Leukemia," *Blood*, 2006, 107(9):3469-73.

Ravandi F, Estey E, Jones D, et al, "Effective Treatment of Acute Promyelocytic Leukemia With All-*Trans*-Retinoic Acid, Arsenic Trioxide, and Gemtuzumab Ozogamicin," *J Clin Oncol*, 2009, 27 (4):504-10.

Tretinoin-Daunorubicin-Cytarabine Induction, Consolidation, Maintenance (APL)

Index Terms Arsenic Trioxide-ATRA-Daunorubicin-Cytarabine (APL); ATRA-Daunorubicin-AraC (APL); ATRA-Daunorubicin-Cytarabine (APL); ATRA-Daunorubicin-Cytarabine-Arsensic Trioxide (APL)

Use Leukemia, acute promyelocytic

Regimen NOTE: Multiple variations are listed.

Variation 1:

Induction:

Tretinoin: Oral: 45 mg/m^2/day (in 2 divided doses) day 1 until complete remission or day 90

Daunorubicin: IV: 50 mg/m^2/day days 3, 4, 5, and 6

[total dose/cycle = 200 mg/m^2]

Cytarabine: IV: 200 mg/m^2/day continuous infusion for 7 days beginning on day 3

[total dose/cycle = 1,400 mg/m^2]

Consolidation (begin within 2 to 4 weeks of hematologic remission):

Cycles 1 and 2:

Arsenic Trioxide: IV: 0.15 mg/kg/day over 1 hour days 1 to 5 for 5 weeks followed by 2 weeks off

[total dose/cycle = 3.75 mg/kg]

Repeat cycle in 49 days (7 weeks) for a total of 2 cycles

Cycles 3 and 4:

Tretinoin: Oral: 45 mg/m^2/day (in 2 divided doses) days 1 to 7

[total dose/cycle = 315 mg/m^2]

Daunorubicin: IV: 50 mg/m^2/day days 1, 2, and 3

[total dose/cycle = 150 mg/m^2]

Repeat for a total of 2 cycles

Maintenance (if patient remains in complete remission, begin 2 to 4 weeks after recovery from consolidation):

Mercaptopurine: Oral: 60 mg/m^2 daily for 1 year

[total dose/maintenance = 21,900 mg/m^2]

Methotrexate: Oral: 20 mg/m^2 weekly for 1 year

[total dose/maintenance = 1,040 mg/m^2]

Tretinoin: Oral: 45 mg/m^2/day (in 2 divided doses) days 1 to 7, every other week for 1 year

[total dose/maintenance = 8,190 mg/m^2]

or maintenance with:

Tretinoin: Oral: 45 mg/m^2/day (in 2 divided doses) days 1 to 7, every other week for 1 year

[total dose/maintenance = 8,190 mg/m^2]

Variation 2 (patients ≤60 years of age and WBC <10,000/mm^3):

Induction:

Tretinoin: Oral: 45 mg/m^2/day (in 2 divided doses) day 1 until hematologic complete remission

Daunorubicin: IV: 60 mg/m^2/day days 3, 4, and 5

[total dose/cycle = 180 mg/m^2]

Cytarabine: IV: 200 mg/m^2/day continuous infusion for 7 days beginning on day 3

[total dose/cycle = 1,400 mg/m^2]

Consolidation:

Course 1:

Daunorubicin: IV: 60 mg/m^2/day days 1, 2, and 3

[total dose/cycle = 180 mg/m^2]

Cytarabine: IV: 200 mg/m^2/day days 1 to 7

[total dose/cycle = 1,400 mg/m^2]

Course 2:
Daunorubicin: IV: 45 mg/m^2/day days 1, 2, and 3
[total dose/cycle = 135 mg/m^2]
Cytarabine: IV: 1,000 mg/m^2 every 12 hours for 8 doses days 1 to 4
[total dose/cycle = 8,000 mg/m^2]

Maintenance:
Mercaptopurine: Oral: 50 or 90 mg/m^2 daily
[total dose/12 week maintenance cycle = 4,200 or 7,560 mg/m^2 (84 days)]
Methotrexate: Oral: 15 mg/m^2 weekly
[total dose/12 week maintenance cycle = 180 mg/m^2]
Tretinoin: Oral: 45 mg/m^2/day (in 2 divided doses) days 1 to 15
[total dose/12 week maintenance cycle = 675 mg/m^2]
Repeat cycle every 12 weeks for 2 years

Variation 3 (patients ≤60 years of age and WBC ≥10,000/mm^3):
Induction:
Tretinoin: Oral: 45 mg/m^2/day (in 2 divided doses) day 1 until hematologic complete remission
Daunorubicin: IV: 60 mg/m^2/day days 3, 4, and 5
[total dose/cycle = 180 mg/m^2]
Cytarabine: IV: 200 mg/m^2/day continuous infusion for 7 days beginning on day 3
[total dose/cycle = 1,400 mg/m^2]

Consolidation:
Course 1:
Daunorubicin: IV: 60 mg/m^2/day days 1, 2, and 3
[total dose/cycle = 180 mg/m^2]
Cytarabine: IV: 200 mg/m^2/day days 1 to 7
[total dose/cycle = 1,400 mg/m^2]
Course 2:
Daunorubicin: IV: 45 mg/m^2/day days 1, 2, and 3
[total dose/cycle = 135 mg/m^2]
Cytarabine: IV: 2,000 mg/m^2 every 12 hours for 10 doses days 1 to 5
(Ades 2006; patients <50 years; Ades 2008) or 1,500 mg/m^2 every 12 hours for 10 doses days 1 to 5 (patients 50 to 60 years; Ades 2008)
[total dose/cycle = 15,000 mg/m^2 to 20,000 mg/m^2]

Intrathecal prophylaxis: Five intrathecal injections: First dose in between induction and consolidation and 2 doses during each consolidation phase:
Methotrexate (preservative free): Intrathecal: 15 mg
Cytarabine (preservative free): Intrathecal: 50 mg
Corticosteroids (preservative free): Intrathecal: Dose unspecified

Maintenance:
Mercaptopurine: Oral: 50 or 90 mg/m^2 daily
[total dose/12 week maintenance cycle = 4,200 or 7,560 mg/m^2 (84 days)]
Methotrexate: Oral: 15 mg/m^2 weekly
[total dose/12 week maintenance cycle = 180 mg/m^2]
Tretinoin: Oral: 45 mg/m^2/day (in 2 divided doses) days 1 to 15
[total dose/12 week maintenance cycle = 675 mg/m^2]
Repeat cycle every 12 weeks for 2 years

Variation 4 (patients >60 years of age and WBC >10,000/mm^3):
Induction:
Tretinoin: Oral: 45 mg/m^2/day (in 2 divided doses) day 1 until hematologic complete remission
Daunorubicin: IV: 60 mg/m^2/day days 3, 4, and 5
[total dose/cycle = 180 mg/m^2]

Cytarabine: IV: 200 mg/m^2/day continuous infusion for 7 days beginning on day 3

[total dose/cycle = 1,400 mg/m^2]

Consolidation:

Course 1:

Daunorubicin: IV: 60 mg/m^2/day days 1, 2, and 3

[total dose/cycle = 180 mg/m^2]

Cytarabine: IV: 200 mg/m^2/day days 1 to 7

[total dose/cycle = 1,400 mg/m^2]

Course 2:

Daunorubicin: IV: 45 mg/m^2/day days 1, 2, and 3

[total dose/cycle = 135 mg/m^2]

Cytarabine: IV: 1,000 mg/m^2 every 12 hours for 8 doses days 1 to 4

[total dose/cycle = 8,000 mg/m^2]

Intrathecal prophylaxis: Five intrathecal injections: First dose in between induction and consolidation and 2 doses during each consolidation phase:

Methotrexate (preservative free): Intrathecal: 15 mg

Cytarabine (preservative free): Intrathecal: 50 mg

Corticosteroids (preservative free): Intrathecal: Dose unspecified

Maintenance:

Mercaptopurine: Oral: 50 or 90 mg/m^2 daily

[total dose/12 week maintenance cycle = 4,200 or 7,560 mg/m^2 (84 days)]

Methotrexate: Oral: 15 mg/m^2 weekly

[total dose/12 week maintenance cycle = 180 mg/m^2]

Tretinoin: Oral: 45 mg/m^2/day (in 2 divided doses) days 1 to 15

[total dose/12 week maintenance cycle = 675 mg/m^2]

Repeat cycle every 12 weeks for 2 years

References

Variation 1:

Powell BL, Moser B, Stock W, et al. Arsenic trioxide improves event-free and overall survival for adults with acute promyelocytic leukemia: North American Leukemia Intergroup Study C9710. *Blood*. 2010;116(19):3751-3757.

Variations 2, 3, and 4:

Adès L, Chevret S, Raffoux E, et al, "Is Cytarabine Useful in the Treatment of Acute Promyelocytic Leukemia? Results of a Randomized Trial From the European Acute Promyelocytic Leukemia Group," *J Clin Oncol*, 2006, 24(36):5703-10.

Adès L, Sanz MA, Chevret S, et al. Treatment of newly diagnosed acute promyelocytic leukemia (APL): a comparison of French-Belgian-Swiss and PETHEMA results. *Blood*. 2008;111 (3):1078-1084.

Tretinoin-Idarubicin (APL)

Index Terms ATRA-Idarubicin (APL); Idarubicin-ATRA (APL); Idarubicin-Tretinoin (APL)

Use Leukemia, acute promyelocytic

Regimen NOTE: Multiple variations are listed.

Variation 1 (high-risk and ≤60 years of age):

Induction:

Tretinoin: Oral: 45 mg/m^2/day (in 2 divided doses) day 1 until complete hematologic remission

≤20 years: Oral: 25 mg/m^2/day (in 2 divided doses) day 1 until complete hematologic remission

Idarubicin: IV: 12 mg/m^2/day days 2, 4, 6, and 8 (omit day 8 for patients >70 years of age)

[total dose/cycle = 36 to 48 mg/m^2]

◀ **Consolidation** (administer courses sequentially at 1-month intervals for 3 months):

Course 1:

Idarubicin: IV: 5 mg/m^2/day days 1 to 4
  [total dose/cycle = 20 mg/m^2]

Cytarabine: IV: 1,000 mg/m^2/day days 1 to 4
  [total dose/cycle = 4,000 mg^2]

Tretinoin: Oral: 45 mg/m^2/day (in 2 divided doses) days 1 to 15
  [total dose/cycle = 675 mg/m^2]

Course 2:

Mitoxantrone: IV: 10 mg/m^2/day days 1 to 5
  [total dose/cycle = 50 mg/m^2]

Tretinoin: Oral: 45 mg/m^2/day (in 2 divided doses) days 1 to 15
  [total dose/cycle = 675 mg/m^2]

Course 3:

Idarubicin: IV: 12 mg/m^2 day 1
  [total dose/cycle = 12 mg/m^2]

Cytarabine: IV: 150 mg/m^2 every 8 hours days 1 to 4
  [total dose/cycle = 1,800 mg^2]

Tretinoin: Oral: 45 mg/m^2/day (in 2 divided doses) days 1 to 15
  [total dose/cycle = 675 mg/m^2]

Maintenance:

Mercaptopurine: Oral: 50 mg/m^2 daily
  [total dose/cycle = 4,500 mg/m^2 (90 days)]

Methotrexate: IM: 15 mg/m^2 weekly
  [total dose/cycle = 180 mg/m^2]

Tretinoin: Oral: 45 mg/m^2/day (in 2 divided doses) days 1 to 15
  [total dose/cycle = 675 mg/m^2]

Repeat cycle every 3 months for 2 years

Variation 2 (intermediate risk and high risk patients >60 years of age):

Induction:

Tretinoin: Oral: 45 mg/m^2/day (in 2 divided doses) day 1 until complete hematologic remission
  ≤20 years: Oral: 25 mg/m^2/day (in 2 divided doses) day 1 until complete hematologic remission

Idarubicin: IV: 12 mg/m^2/day days 2, 4, 6, and 8 (omit day 8 for patients >70 years of age)
  [total dose/cycle = 36 to 48 mg/m^2]

Consolidation (administer courses sequentially at 1-month intervals for 3 months):

Course 1:

Idarubicin: IV: 7 mg/m^2/day days 1 to 4
  [total dose/cycle = 28 mg/m^2]

Tretinoin: Oral: 45 mg/m^2/day (in 2 divided doses) days 1 to 15
  [total dose/cycle = 675 mg/m^2]

Course 2:

Mitoxantrone: IV: 10 mg/m^2/day days 1 to 3
  [total dose/cycle = 30 mg/m^2]

Tretinoin: Oral: 45 mg/m^2/day (in 2 divided doses) days 1 to 15
  [total dose/cycle = 675 mg/m^2]

Course 3:
  Idarubicin: IV: 12 mg/m^2 days 1 and 2
    [total dose/cycle = 24 mg/m^2]
  Tretinoin: Oral: 45 mg/m^2/day (in 2 divided doses) days 1 to 15
    [total dose/cycle = 675 mg/m^2]
Maintenance:
  Mercaptopurine: Oral: 50 mg/m^2 daily
    [total dose/cycle = 4,500 mg/m^2 (90 days)]
  Methotrexate: IM: 15 mg/m^2 weekly
    [total dose/cycle = 180 mg/m^2]
  Tretinoin: Oral: 45 mg/m^2/day (in 2 divided doses) days 1 to 15
    [total dose/cycle = 675 mg/m^2]
  Repeat cycle every 3 months for 2 years
Variation 3 (low risk):
Induction:
  Tretinoin: Oral: 45 mg/m^2/day (in 2 divided doses) day 1 until complete
    hematologic remission
    ≤20 years: Oral: 25 mg/m^2/day (in 2 divided doses) day 1 until complete
    hematologic remission
  Idarubicin: IV: 12 mg/m^2/day days 2, 4, 6, and 8 (omit day 8 for patients >70
    years of age)
    [total dose/cycle = 36 to 48 mg/m^2]
Consolidation (administer courses sequentially at 1-month intervals for 3
months):
Course 1:
  Idarubicin: IV: 5 mg/m^2/day days 1 to 4
    [total dose/cycle = 20 mg/m^2]
  Tretinoin: Oral: 45 mg/m^2/day (in 2 divided doses) days 1 to 15
    [total dose/cycle = 675 mg/m^2]
Course 2:
  Mitoxantrone: IV: 10 mg/m^2/day days 1 to 3
    [total dose/cycle = 30 mg/m^2]
  Tretinoin: Oral: 45 mg/m^2/day (in 2 divided doses) days 1 to 15
    [total dose/cycle = 675 mg/m^2]
Course 3:
  Idarubicin: IV: 12 mg/m^2 day 1
    [total dose/cycle = 12 mg/m^2]
  Tretinoin: Oral: 45 mg/m^2/day (in 2 divided doses) days 1 to 15
    [total dose/cycle = 675 mg/m^2]
Maintenance:
  Mercaptopurine: Oral: 50 mg/m^2 daily
    [total dose/cycle = 4,500 mg/m^2 (90 days)]
  Methotrexate: IM: 15 mg/m^2 weekly
    [total dose/cycle = 180 mg/m^2]
  Tretinoin: Oral: 45 mg/m^2/day (in 2 divided doses) days 1 to 15
    [total dose/cycle = 675 mg/m^2]
  Repeat cycle every 3 months for 2 years

References

Variations 1, 2, and 3:
Sanz MA, Montesinos P, Rayón C, et al. Risk-adapted treatment of acute promyelocytic leukemia based on all-trans retinoic acid and anthracycline with addition of cytarabine in consolidation therapy for high-risk patients: further improvements in treatment outcome. *Blood.* 2010;115 (25):5137-5146.

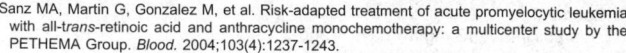

Sanz MA, Martin G, Gonzalez M, et al. Risk-adapted treatment of acute promyelocytic leukemia with all-*trans*-retinoic acid and anthracycline monochemotherapy: a multicenter study by the PETHEMA Group. *Blood*. 2004;103(4):1237-1243.

Trifluridine and Tipiracil (Colorectal Regimen)

Index Terms Lonsurf (Colorectal Regimen)

Use Colorectal cancer (metastatic, previously treated with fluoropyrimidine, oxaliplatin, irinotecan, anti-VEGF, and anti-EGFR if RAS wild-type)

Regimen NOTE: Dose based on trifluridine component.

Trifluridine and Tipiracil: Oral: 35 mg/m^2 (maximum trifluridine dose: 80 mg) twice daily on days 1 to 5 and days 8 to 12; within 1 hour of completion of morning and evening meals

[total dose/cycle = 700 mg/m^2 (maximum trifluridine dose/cycle: 1,600 mg]

Repeat cycle every 28 days until disease progression or unacceptable toxicity

References

Mayer RJ, Van Cutsem E, Falcone A, et al. Randomized trial of TAS-102 for refractory metastatic colorectal cancer. *N Engl J Med*. 2015;372(20):1909-1919.

VAC Alternating With IE (Ewing Sarcoma)

Use Ewing sarcoma

Regimen

Cycle A (Odd numbered cycles):

Cyclophosphamide: IV: 1200 mg/m^2 day 1 (followed by mesna; dose not specified)

[total dose/cycle = 1200 mg/m^2]

Vincristine: IV: 2 mg/m^2 (maximum dose: 2 mg) day 1

[total dose/cycle = 2 mg/m^2; maximum: 2 mg]

Doxorubicin: IV: 75 mg/m^2 day 1, for 5 cycles (maximum cumulative dose: 375 mg/m^2)

[total dose/cycle = 75 mg/m^2; maximum cumulative dose: 375 mg/m^2]

Dactinomycin: IV: 1.25 mg/m^2 day 1, begin cycle 11 (after reaching maximum cumulative doxorubicin dose)

[total dose/cycle = 1.25 mg/m^2]

Cycle B (Even numbered cycles):

Ifosfamide: IV: 1800 mg/m^2/day days 1 to 5 (given with mesna)

[total dose/cycle = 9000 mg/m^2]

Etoposide: IV: 100 mg/m^2/day days 1 to 5

[total dose/cycle = 500 mg/m^2]

Alternate Cycles A and B, administering a cycle every 3 weeks (alternating in the following sequence: ABABAB) for 17 cycles

References

Grier HE, Krailo MD, Tarbell NJ, et al, "Addition of Ifosfamide and Etoposide to Standard Chemotherapy for Ewing's Sarcoma and Primitive Neuroectodermal Tumor of Bone," *N Engl J Med*, 2003, 348(8):694-701.

VAC (Ovarian)

Index Terms Vincristine, Dactinomycin, Cyclophosphamide (Ovarian)

Use Ovarian cancer (germ cell tumor)

Regimen

Vincristine: IV: 1.5 mg/m^2/day (maximum dose: 2 mg) days 1, 8, 15, and 22 for 2-3 cycles

[total dose/cycle = 6 mg/m^2 (maximum: 8 mg)] for 2-3 cycles

Dactinomycin: IV: 300 mcg/m^2/day days 1 to 5

[total dose/cycle = 1500 mcg/m^2]

Cyclophosphamide: IV: 150 mg/m^2/day days 1 to 5
[total dose/cycle = 750 mg/m^2]
Repeat cycle every 28 days for at least 10 cycles; vincristine is only administered for 2-3 cycles

References

Slayton RE, Park RC, Silverberg SG, et al, "Vincristine, Dactinomycin, and Cyclophosphamide in the Treatment of Malignant Germ Cell Tumors of the Ovary. A Gynecologic Oncology Group Study (A Final Report)," *Cancer*, 1985, 56(2):243-8.

VAC Pulse

Use Soft tissue sarcoma (rhabdomyosarcoma)

Regimen

Vincristine: IV: 2 mg/m^2/dose (maximum dose: 2 mg/dose) every 7 days, for 12 weeks

Dactinomycin: IV: 0.015 mg/kg/day (maximum dose: 0.5 mg/day) days 1 to 5, every 3 months for 5 courses

Cyclophosphamide: Oral, IV: 10 mg/kg/day for 7 days, repeat every 6 weeks

References

Wilbur JR, Sutow WW, Sullivan MP, et al, "Chemotherapy of Sarcomas," *Cancer*, 1975, 36 (2):765-9.

VAC (Rhabdomyosarcoma)

Use Soft tissue sarcoma (rhabdomyosarcoma)

Regimen

Induction (weeks 1 to 17):

Vincristine: IV push: 1.5 mg/m^2 (maximum dose: 2 mg) day 1 of weeks 1 to 13, then one dose at week 17

Dactinomycin: IV push: 0.015 mg/kg/day (maximum dose: 0.5 mg) days 1 to 5 of weeks 1, 4, 7, and 17

Cyclophosphamide: IV: 2.2 g/m^2 day 1 of weeks 1, 4, 7, 10, 13, and 17

Continuation (weeks 21 to 44):

Vincristine: IV push: 1.5 mg/m^2 (maximum dose: 2 mg) day 1 of weeks 21 to 26, 30 to 35, and 39 to 44

Dactinomycin: IV push: 0.015 mg/kg/day (maximum dose: 0.5 mg) days 1 to 5 of weeks 21, 24, 30, 33, 39, and 42

Cyclophosphamide: IV: 2.2 g/m^2 day 1 of weeks 21, 24, 30, 33, 39, and 42

References

Baker KS, Anderson JR, Link MP, et al, "Benefit of Intensified Therapy for Patients With Local or Regional Embryonal Rhabdomyosarcoma: Results From the Intergroup Rhabdomyosarcoma Study IV," *J Clin Oncol*, 2000, 18(12):2427-34.

VAD

Use Multiple myeloma

Regimen

Vincristine: IV: 0.4 mg/day continuous infusion days 1 to 4
[total dose/cycle = 1.6 mg]

Doxorubicin: IV: 9 mg/m^2/day continuous infusion days 1 to 4
[total dose/cycle = 36 mg/m^2]

Dexamethasone: Oral: 40 mg/day days 1 to 4, 9 to 12, and 17 to 20
[total dose/cycle = 480 mg]

Repeat cycle every 28-35 days

References

Barlogie B, Smith L, and Alexanian R, "Effective Treatment of Advanced Multiple Myeloma Refractory to Alkylating Agents," *N Engl J Med*, 1984, 310(21):1353-6.

VAD/CVAD

Use Leukemia, acute lymphocytic

Regimen Induction cycle:

Vincristine: IV: 0.4 mg/day continuous infusion days 1 to 4 and 24 to 27
   [total dose/cycle = 3.2 mg]

Doxorubicin: IV: 12 mg/m^2/day continuous infusion days 1 to 4 and 24 to 27
   [total dose/cycle = 96 mg/m^2]

Dexamethasone: Oral: 40 mg/day days 1 to 4, 9 to 12, 17 to 20, 24 to 27, 32 to 35, and 40 to 43
   [total dose/cycle = 960 mg]

Cyclophosphamide: IV: 1 g/m^2 day 24
   [total dose/cycle = 1 g/m^2]

Administer one cycle only

References

Kantarjian H, Walters RS, Keating MJ, et al, "Results of the Vincristine, Doxorubicin, and Dexamethasone Regimen in Adults With Standard and High-Risk Acute Lymphocytic Leukemia," *J Clin Oncol*, 1990, 8(6):994-1004.

VAD (Wilms' Tumor)

Index Terms Vincristine, Dactinomycin, Doxorubicin (Wilms' Tumor)

Use Wilms' tumor

Regimen NOTE: Multiple variations are listed.

Variation 1 (Stage III favorable disease; children ≥1 year):

Vincristine: IV: 1.5 mg/m^2 weekly for 10 to 11 weeks

Followed by:

Vincristine: IV: 1.5 mg/m^2 every 3 weeks

Dactinomycin: IV: 1.5 mg/m^2 every 6 weeks

Doxorubicin: IV: 40 mg/m^2 every 6 weeks

NOTE: Alternate dactinomycin and doxorubicin; administer dactinomycin at 3 weeks and doxorubicin in 3 weeks

Treatment continued for 1 year

Variation 2 (Stage III favorable disease; children <1 year):

Vincristine: IV: 0.75 mg/m^2 weekly for 10 to 11 weeks

Followed by:

Vincristine: IV: 0.75 mg/m^2 every 3 weeks

Dactinomycin: IV: 0.75 mg/m^2 every 6 weeks

Doxorubicin: IV: 20 mg/m^2 every 6 weeks

NOTE: Alternate dactinomycin and doxorubicin; administer dactinomycin at 3 weeks and doxorubicin in 3 weeks

Treatment continued for 1 year

References

Variations 1 and 2:

Pritchard J, Imeson J, Barnes J, et al, "Results of the United Kingdom Children's Cancer Study Group First Wilms' Tumor Study," *J Clin Oncol*, 1995, 13(1):124-33.

VAMP (Hodgkin)

Index Terms Vinblastine, Doxorubicin, Methotrexate, Prednisone (Hodgkin)

Use Lymphoma, Hodgkin

Regimen NOTE: Patients <21 years of age

Vinblastine: IV: 6 mg/m^2/day days 1 and 15
   [total dose/cycle = 12 mg/m^2]

Doxorubicin: IV: 25 mg/m^2/day days 1 and 15
   [total dose/cycle = 50 mg/m^2]

Methotrexate: IV: 20 mg/m^2/day days 1 and 15
   [total dose/cycle = 40 mg/m^2]
Prednisone: Oral: 40 mg/m^2/day days 1 to 14 (omit after mediastinal radiation)
   [total dose/cycle = 560 mg/m^2]
Repeat cycle every 28 days for a total of 4 cycles

References

Donaldson SS, Link MP, Weinstein HJ, et al, "Final Results of a Prospective Clinical Trial With VAMP and Low-Dose Involved Radiation for Children With Low-Risk Hodgkin's Disease," *J Clin Oncol*, 2007, 25(3):332-7.

VA (Rhabdomyosarcoma)

Index Terms Dactinomycin-Vincristine (Rhabdomyosarcoma); Vincristine-Dactinomycin (Rhabdomyosarcoma)

Use Soft tissue sarcoma (rhabdomyosarcoma, newly diagnosed low risk)

Regimen NOTE: Dosing based on age and/or weight. Omit dactinomycin at week 6 in patients beginning radiation at week 3, weeks 15 and 18 in patients beginning radiation at week 12, and weeks 30 and 33 in patients beginning radiation at week 28.

Variation 1 (patients <1 year):
   Vincristine: IV: 0.025 mg/kg; (maximum dose: 2 mg) weekly for weeks 0 to 8, 12 to 20, 24 to 32, and 36 to 44
      [total dose/year = 0.9 mg/kg (maximum dose/year: 72 mg)]
   Dactinomycin: IV: 0.025 mg/kg; (maximum dose: 2.5 mg) every 3 weeks during weeks 0 through 45
      [total dose/year = 0.4 mg/kg (maximum dose/year: 40 mg)]
   Treatment is 1 year

Variation 2 (patients ≥1 year to <3 years):
   Vincristine: IV: 0.05 mg/kg (maximum dose: 2 mg) weekly for weeks 0 to 8, 12 to 20, 24 to 32, and 36 to 44
      [total dose/year = 1.8 mg/kg (maximum dose/year: 72 mg)]
   Dactinomycin: IV: 0.045 mg/kg (maximum dose: 2.5 mg) every 3 weeks during weeks 0 through 45
      [total dose/year = 0.72 mg/kg (maximum dose/year: 40 mg)]
   Treatment is 1 year

Variation 3 (patients ≥3 years):
   Vincristine: IV: 1.5 mg/m^2 (maximum dose: 2 mg) weekly for weeks 0 to 8, 12 to 20, 24 to 32, and 36 to 44
      [total dose/year = 54 mg/m^2 (maximum dose/year: 72 mg)]
   Dactinomycin: IV: 0.045 mg/kg (maximum dose: 2.5 mg) every 3 weeks during weeks 0 through 45
      [total dose/year = 0.72 mg/kg (maximum dose/year: 40 mg)]
   Treatment is 1 year

References

Raney RB, Walterhouse DO, Meza JL, et al. Results of the Intergroup Rhabdomyosarcoma Study Group D9602 protocol, using vincristine and dactinomycin with or without cyclophosphamide and radiation therapy, for newly diagnosed patients with low-risk embryonal rhabdomyosarcoma: a report from the Soft Tissue Sarcoma Committee of the Children's Oncology Group. *J Clin Oncol*. 2011;29(10):1312-1318.

VBMCP (Multiple Myeloma)

Use Multiple myeloma

Regimen NOTE: Multiple variations are listed.

Variation 1:

Vincristine: IV: 1.2 mg/m^2 day 1
[total dose/cycle = 1.2 mg/m^2]

Carmustine: IV: 20 mg/m^2 day 1
[total dose/cycle = 20 mg/m^2]

Melphalan: Oral: 8 mg/m^2/day days 1 to 4
[total dose/cycle = 32 mg/m^2]

Cyclophosphamide: IV: 400 mg/m^2 day 1
[total dose/cycle = 400 mg/m^2]

Prednisone: Oral: 40 mg/m^2/day days 1 to 7
[total dose/cycle = 280 mg/m^2]

Repeat cycle every 35 days for up to 2 years or until disease progression

Variation 2:

Vincristine: IV: 1.2 mg/m^2 (maximum dose: 2 mg) day 1
[total dose/cycle = 1.2 mg/m^2; maximum: 2 mg]

Carmustine: IV: 20 mg/m^2 day 1
[total dose/cycle = 20 mg/m^2]

Melphalan: Oral: 8 mg/m^2/day days 1 to 4
[total dose/cycle = 32 mg/m^2]

Cyclophosphamide: IV: 400 mg/m^2 day 1
[total dose/cycle = 400 mg/m^2]

Prednisone: Oral: 40 mg/m^2/day days 1 to 7 (all cycles)
[total dose/cycle = 280 mg/m^2]
followed by Oral: 20 mg/m^2/day days 8 to 14 (first 3 cycles only)
[total dose/cycle = 140 mg/m^2]

Repeat cycle every 35 days

References

Variation 1:

Kyle RA, Leong T, Li S, et al, "Complete Response in Multiple Myeloma: Clinical Trial E9486, an Eastern Cooperative Oncology Group Study Not Involving Stem Cell Transplantation," *Cancer*, 2006, 106(9):1958-66.

Variation 2:

Oken MM, Harrington DP, Abramson N, et al, "Comparison of Melphalan and Prednisone With Vincristine, Carmustine, Melphalan, Cyclophosphamide, and Prednisone in the Treatment of Multiple Myeloma: Results of Eastern Cooperative Oncology Group Study E2479," *Cancer*, 1997, 79(8):1561-7.

◆ **VBR (NHL-Follicular)** *see* Bendamustine-Bortezomib-Rituximab (NHL-Follicular) *on page 1985*

◆ **VC (Adjuvant NSCLC)** *see* Cisplatin-Vinorelbine (Adjuvant NSCLC) *on page 2062*

◆ **VCD (Multiple Myeloma)** *see* Cyclophosphamide-Bortezomib-Dexamethasone (Multiple Myeloma) *on page 2076*

◆ **VC (Metastatic NSCLC)** *see* Cisplatin-Vinorelbine (Metastatic NSCLC) *on page 2063*

VcR-CAP (NHL-Mantle Cell)

Index Terms Botezomib-Rituximab-Cyclophosphamide-Doxorubicin-Prednisone (NHL-Mantle Cell); Rituximab-Bortezomib-Cyclophosphamide-Doxorubicin-Prednisone (NHL-Mantle Cell); VR-CAP (NHL-Mantle Cell)

Use Lymphoma, non-Hodgkin (first-line, transplant ineligible, stage 2 to 4 mantle cell)

Regimen
Bortezomib: IV: 1.3 mg/m²/day days 1, 4, 8, and 11
  [total dose/cycle = 5.2 mg/m²]
Rituximab: IV: 375 mg/m² day 1
  [total dose/cycle = 375 mg/m²]
Cyclophosphamide: IV: 750 mg/m² day 1
  [total dose/cycle = 750 mg/m²]
Doxorubicin: IV: 50 mg/m² day 1
  [total dose/cycle = 50 mg/m²]
Prednisone: Oral: 100 mg/m²/day days 1 to 5
  [total dose/cycle = 500 mg/m²]
Repeat cycle every 21 days for 6 to 8 cycles. If response first documented at cycle 6, treatment could continue for an additional 2 more cycles.

References
Robak T, Huang H, Jin J, et al. Bortezomib-based therapy for newly diagnosed mantle-cell lymphoma. *N Engl J Med.* 2015;372(10):944-953.

◆ **VD (Multiple Myeloma)** *see* Bortezomib-Dexamethasone (Multiple Myeloma) *on page 1998*

◆ **VDR (Multiple Myeloma)** *see* Lenalidomide-Bortezomib-Dexamethasone (Multiple Myeloma) *on page 2163*

VDT-PACE (Multiple Myeloma)

Index Terms Bortezomib-Dexamethasone-Thalidomide-Cisplatin-Doxorubicin-Cyclophosphamide-Etoposide (Multiple Myeloma); Cisplatin-Doxorubicin-Cyclophosphamide-Etoposide-Bortezomib-Dexamethasone-Thalidomide (Multiple Myeloma); Cyclophosphamide-Etoposide-Bortezomib-Dexamethasone-Thalidomide-Cisplatin-Doxorubicin (Multiple Myeloma); Doxorubicin-Cyclophosphamide-Etoposide-Bortezomib-Dexamethasone-Thalidomide-Cisplatin (Multiple Myeloma); Etoposide-Bortezomib-Dexamethasone-Thalidomide-Cisplatin-Doxorubicin-Cyclophosphamide (Multiple Myeloma); Thalidomide-Cisplatin-Doxorubicin-Cyclophosphamide-Etoposide-Bortezomib-Dexamethasone (Multiple Myeloma); VTD-PACE (Multiple Myeloma)

Use Multiple myeloma

Regimen NOTE: VDT-PACE is given for 2 cycles prior to and after completion of tandem transplants. Interim therapy with thalidomide and dexamethasone is administered between induction cycles, between transplants, and between consolidation therapies when platelets recover to ≥50,000/mm³.
Induction cycles 1 and 2 (initiate second induction cycle within 8 weeks of cycle 1):
Bortezomib: SubQ: 1 mg/m² on days 1, 4, 8, and 11
  [total dose/cycle = 4 mg/m²]
Dexamethasone: Oral: 40 mg once daily on days 4 to 7 (cycle 1) and days 1 to 4 (cycle 2)
  [total dose/cycle = 160 mg]
Thalidomide: Oral: 200 mg once daily on days 4 to 7 (cycle 1) and days 1 to 4 (cycle 2)
  [total dose/cycle = 800 mg]
Cisplatin: IV: 10 mg/m²/day continuous infusion days 4 to 7 (cycle 1) and days 1 to 4 (cycle 2)
  [total dose/cycle = 40 mg/m²]
Doxorubicin: IV: 10 mg/m²/day continuous infusion days 4 to 7 (cycle 1) and days 1 to 4 (cycle 2)
  [total dose/cycle = 40 mg/m²]

◄ Cyclophosphamide: IV: 400 mg/m²/day continuous infusion days 4 to 7 (cycle 1) and days 1 to 4 (cycle 2)
[total dose/cycle = 1,600 mg/m²]

Etoposide: IV: 40 mg/m²/day continuous infusion days 4 to 7 (cycle 1) and days 1 to 4 (cycle 2)
[total dose/cycle = 160 mg/m²]

Consolidation cycles 1 and 2 (initiate the first cycle 6 weeks to 4 months after last transplant and initiate the second cycle 2 to 4 months after cycle 1):

Bortezomib: SubQ: 1 mg/m² days 1, 4, 8, and 11
[total dose/cycle = 4 mg/m²]

Dexamethasone: Oral: 40 mg once daily days 1 to 4
[total dose/cycle = 160 mg]

Thalidomide: Oral: 200 mg once daily days 1 to 4
[total dose/cycle = 800 mg]

Cisplatin: IV: 7.5 mg/m²/day continuous infusion days 1 to 4 (cycle 1) and days 4 to 7 (cycle 2)
[total dose/cycle = 30 mg/m²]

Doxorubicin: IV: 7.5 mg/m²/day continuous infusion days 1 to 4 (cycle 1) and days 4 to 7 (cycle 2)
[total dose/cycle = 30 mg/m²]

Cyclophosphamide: IV: 300 mg/m²/day continuous infusion days 1 to 4 (cycle 1) and days 4 to 7 (cycle 2)
[total dose/cycle = 1,200 mg/m²]

Etoposide: IV: 30 mg/m²/day continuous infusion days 1 to 4 (cycle 1) and days 4 to 7 (cycle 2)
[total dose/cycle = 120 mg/m²]

Interim Therapy (administer between induction cycles, between transplants, and between consolidation therapies when platelets recover to ≥50,000/mm³):

Thalidomide: Oral: 50 mg once daily (between induction cycles and transplants) **or** 100 mg once daily (between consolidation cycles)
[total dose/cycle = 1,050 to 2,100 mg]

Dexamethasone: Oral: 20 mg once daily on days 1 to 4
[total dose/cycle = 80 mg]

Repeat cycle every 21 days (refer to protocol for further information)

Maintenance:

Year 1 (initiate 1 to 4 months after consolidation cycle 2):

Bortezomib: SubQ: 1 mg/m² on days 1, 4, 8, and 11
[total dose/cycle = 4 mg/m²]

Dexamethasone: Oral: 20 mg once daily days 1 to 4 and days 8 to 11
[total dose/cycle = 160 mg]

Thalidomide: Oral: 100 mg once daily
[total dose/cycle = 2,800 mg]

Repeat cycle every 28 days for 1 year

Years 2 and 3:

Dexamethasone: Oral: 20 mg once daily days 1 to 4
[total dose/cycle = 80 mg]

Thalidomide: Oral: 100 mg every other day
[total dose/cycle = 1,400 mg]

Repeat cycle every 28 days for 2 years

References
Barlogie B, Anaissie E, van Rhee F, et al. Incorporating bortezomib into upfront treatment for multiple myeloma: early results of totaltherapy 3. *Br J Haematol*. 2007;138(2):176-185.

Pineda-Roman M, Zangari M, Haessler J, et al. Sustained complete remissions in multiple myeloma linked to bortezomib in total therapy 3: comparison with total therapy 2. *Br J Haematol*. 2008;140(6):625-634.

VeIP (Testicular)

Index Terms Vinblastine-Ifosfamide-Cisplatin (Testicular); VIP (Vinblastine) (Testicular)

Use Testicular cancer

Regimen

Vinblastine: IV: 0.11 mg/kg/day days 1 and 2
[total dose/cycle = 0.22 mg/kg]

Ifosfamide: IV: 1200 mg/m^2/day days 1 to 5
[total dose/cycle = 6000 mg/m^2]

Cisplatin: IV: 20 mg/m^2/day days 1 to 5
[total dose/cycle = 100 mg/m^2]

Mesna: IV: 400 mg/m^2 prior to ifosfamide day 1
followed by IV: 1200 mg/m^2/day continuous infusion days 1 to 5
[total dose/cycle = 6400 mg/m^2]

Repeat cycle every 21 days for 4 cycles

References
Loehrer PJ Sr, Gonin R, Nichols CR, Weathers T, Einhorn LH. Vinblastine plus ifosfamide plus cisplatin as initial salvage therapy in recurrent germ cell tumor. *J Clin Oncol*. 1998;16 (7):2500-2504.

Loehrer PJ Sr, Lauer R, Roth BJ, Williams SD, Kalasinski LA, Einhorn LH. Salvage therapy in recurrent germ cell cancer: ifosfamide and cisplatin plus either vinblastine or etoposide. *Ann Intern Med*. 1988;109(7):540-546.

Correction: Incomplete dosage information in article on germ cell cancer. *Ann Intern Med*. 1988;109(10):846.

VIM-D (Hodgkin)

Index Terms Etoposide-Ifosfamide-Mitoxantrone-Dexamethasone (Hodgkin)

Use Lymphoma, Hodgkin

Regimen

Etoposide: IV: 100 mg/m^2 over 30 minutes day 1
[total dose/cycle = 100 mg/m^2]

Ifosfamide: IV: 4 g/m^2 continuous infusion over 24 hours day 1
[total dose/cycle = 4 g/m^2]

Mesna: IV: 1 g/m^2 IV bolus day 1
followed by: Mesna: IV: 6 g/m^2 continuous infusion over 36 hours
[total dose/cycle = 7 g/m^2]

Mitoxantrone: IV: 10 mg/m^2 IV bolus day 1
[total dose/cycle = 10 mg/m^2]

Dexamethasone: Oral: 40 mg/day days 1 to 5
[total dose/cycle = 200 mg]

Repeat cycle every 28 days; treat 3 cycles post remission

References
Phillips JK, Spearing RL, Davies JM, et al, "VIM-D Salvage Chemotherapy in Hodgkin's Disease," *Cancer Chemother Pharmacol*, 1990, 27(2):161-3.

♦ **Vinblastine-Cisplatin-Dacarbazine** *see* Cisplatin-Vinblastine-Dacarbazine (Melanoma) *on page* 2061

♦ **Vinblastine-Cisplatin (NSCLC)** *see* Cisplatin-Vinblastine (NSCLC) *on page* 2061

VIP (Testicular)

Index Terms Etoposide-Ifosfamide-Cisplatin (Testicular); VIP (Etoposide) (Testicular)

Use Testicular cancer

Regimen

Etoposide: IV: 75 mg/m^2/day days 1 to 5
  [total dose/cycle = 375 mg/m^2]
Ifosfamide: IV: 1200 mg/m^2/day days 1 to 5
  [total dose/cycle = 6000 mg/m^2]
Cisplatin: IV: 20 mg/m^2/day days 1 to 5
  [total dose/cycle = 100 mg/m^2]
Mesna: IV: 120 mg/m^2 prior to ifosfamide day 1
  followed by IV: 1200 mg/m^2/day continuous infusion days 1 to 5
  [total dose/cycle = 6120 mg/m^2]
Filgrastim: SubQ: 5 mcg/kg daily days 7 to 16
Repeat cycle every 21 days for 4 cycles

References

Nichols CR, Catalano PJ, Crawford ED, Vogelzang NJ, Einhorn LH, Loehrer PJ. Randomized comparison of cisplatin and etoposide and either bleomycin or ifosfamide in treatment of advanced disseminated germ cell tumors: an Eastern Cooperative Oncology Group, Southwest Oncology Group, and Cancer and Leukemia Group B Study. *J Clin Oncol.* 1998;16 (4):1287-1293.

◆ **VIP (Vinblastine) (Testicular)** *see* VeIP (Testicular) *on page 2231*

◆ **VR-CAP (NHL-Mantle Cell)** *see* VcR-CAP (NHL-Mantle Cell) *on page 2228*

◆ **VRd (Multiple Myeloma)** *see* Lenalidomide-Bortezomib-Dexamethasone (Multiple Myeloma) *on page 2163*

◆ **VTd (Multiple Myeloma)** *see* Bortezomib-Thalidomide-Dexamethasone (Multiple Myeloma) *on page 2000*

◆ **VTD-PACE (Multiple Myeloma)** *see* VDT-PACE (Multiple Myeloma) *on page 2229*

XELOX (Colorectal)

Index Terms Capecitabine-Oxaliplatin (Colorectal); CapeOx (Colorectal); CAPOX (Colorectal); Oxaliplatin-Capecitabine (Colorectal)

Use Colorectal cancer

Regimen NOTE: Multiple variations are listed.

Variation 1 (adjuvant):
  Oxaliplatin: IV: 130 mg/m^2 over 2 hours day 1
    [total dose/cycle = 130 mg/m^2]
  Capecitabine: Oral: 1000 mg/m^2 twice daily days 1 to 14
    [total dose/cycle = 28,000 mg/m^2]
  Repeat cycle every 21 days for 8 cycles
Variation 2 (metastatic):
  Oxaliplatin: IV: 130 mg/m^2 over 2 hours day 1
    [total dose/cycle = 130 mg/m^2]
  Capecitabine: Oral: 1000 mg/m^2 twice daily days 1 (beginning with evening dose) to 15 (ending with morning dose)
    [total dose/cycle = 28,000 mg/m^2]
  Repeat cycle every 21 days

◀

Variation 3 (metastatic):
Oxaliplatin: IV: 130 mg/m^2 day 1
[total dose/cycle = 130 mg/m^2]
Capecitabine: Oral: 850 mg/m^2 twice daily days 1 (beginning with evening dose) to 15 (ending with morning dose)
[total dose/cycle = 23,800 mg/m^2]
Repeat cycle every 21 days

References

Variation 1:
Haller DG, Tabernero J, Maroun J, et al, "Capecitabine Plus Oxaliplatin Compared With Fluorouracil and Folinic Acid as Adjuvant Therapy for Stage III Colon Cancer," *J Clin Oncol*, 2011, 29(11):1465-71.
Variation 2:
Cassidy J, Clarke S, Díaz-Rubio E, et al, "Randomized Phase III Study of Capecitabine Plus Oxaliplatin Compared With Fluorouracil/Folinic Acid Plus Oxaliplatin as First-Line Therapy for Metastatic Colorectal Cancer," *J Clin Oncol*, 2008, 26(12):2006-12.
Cassidy J, Tabernero J, Twelves C, et al, "XELOX (Capecitabine Plus Oxaliplatin): Active First-Line Therapy for Patients With Metastatic Colorectal Cancer," *J Clin Oncol*, 2004, 22 (11):2084-91.
Variation 3:
Hochster HS, Hart LL, Ramanathan RK, et al, "Safety and Efficacy of Oxaliplatin and Fluoropyrimidine Regimens With or Without Bevacizumab as First-Line Treatment of Metastatic Colorectal Cancer: Results of the TREE Study," *J Clin Oncol*, 2008, 26(21):3523-9.

◆ **XELOX (Gastric)** see Capecitabine-Oxaliplatin (Gastric) on page 2009

◆ **XELOX (Pancreatic)** see CAPOX (Pancreatic) on page 2011

Ziv-Aflibercept + FOLFIRI (Colorectal)

Index Terms Ziv-Aflibercept, Irinotecan, Leucovorin, Fluorouracil (Colorectal)
Use Colorectal cancer
Regimen

Ziv-Aflibercept: IV: 4 mg/kg over 1 hour day 1
[total dose/cycle = 4 mg/kg]
Irinotecan: IV: 180 mg/m^2 over 90 minutes day 1
[total dose/cycle = 180 mg/m^2]
Leucovorin Calcium: IV: 400 mg/m^2 over 2 hours day 1
[total dose/cycle = 400 mg/m^2]
Fluorouracil: IV bolus: 400 mg/m^2 day 1
followed by IV: 2400 mg/m^2 continuous infusion (CI) over 46 hours beginning day 1
[total fluorouracil dose/cycle (bolus and CI) = 2800 mg/m^2]
Repeat cycle every 14 days until disease progression or unacceptable toxicity

References

Van Cutsem E, Tabernero J, Lakomy R, et al, "Addition of Aflibercept to Fluorouracil, Leucovorin, and Irinotecan Improves Survival in a Phase III Randomized Trial in Patients With Metastatic Colorectal Cancer Previously Treated With an Oxaliplatin-Based Regimen," *J Clin Oncol*, 2012 [epub ahead of print].

◆ **Ziv-Aflibercept, Irinotecan, Leucovorin, Fluorouracil (Colorectal)** see Ziv-Aflibercept + FOLFIRI (Colorectal) on page 2234

SPECIAL TOPICS

CHEMOTHERAPY-INDUCED PERIPHERAL NEUROPATHY

INTRODUCTION

Chemotherapy-induced peripheral neuropathy (CIPN) is a common dose-related cumulative toxicity associated with many chemotherapeutic agents. CIPN occurs in close to 40% of patients receiving cancer therapy, although the actual incidence rate and severity varies depending on the chemotherapy regimen and dosing, duration of exposure, concomitant use of other neurotoxic drugs, and assessment methodology (Hershman 2014; Piccolo 2014). CIPN may adversely affect patient quality of life (QOL) and toxicity may necessitate chemotherapy dose reduction or therapy cessation, possibly compromising cancer outcomes. In addition, persistent CIPN in cancer survivors may lead to physical functional decline and an increased risk of falls. A secondary data analysis of a pooled sample of women after cancer treatment who self-reported symptoms of CIPN showed decreased walking speed, altered gait pattern, increased disability, and increased fall risk (all statistically significant) as compared to women who did not report symptoms of CIPN (Winters-Stone 2017). In many instances, CIPN may be partially or wholly reversible after therapy discontinuation; however, if it is not identified early and managed appropriately, permanent toxicity may occur. It is crucial that health care providers alert patients of the signs and symptoms of this condition in order to promptly identify its development and treat accordingly.

Chemotherapy agents frequently associated with CIPN include the platinum agents, taxanes, vinca alkaloids, bortezomib (route-specific), thalidomide, ixabepilone, and dinutuximab. Neuropathy symptoms in patients receiving chemotherapy are primarily sensory in nature and may include numbness, tingling/burning, paresthesias, hyperalgesia, and loss of tendon reflexes. The distribution of symptoms is mostly symmetric and distal and the condition spreads to the extremities in a "stocking and glove" pattern as it worsens (Hershman 2014; Piccolo 2014). Motor nerve function generally remains intact in patients with CIPN.

In addition to CIPN, taxanes and oxaliplatin may cause an acute neuropathy syndrome that is clinically separate from CIPN. Oxaliplatin-induced acute neuropathy occurs in the hours to days following administration; manifestations include throat discomfort, muscle cramps, discomfort swallowing cold liquids, and sensitivity to touching cold items or being exposed to cool temperatures. Patients receiving paclitaxel, particularly those administered higher individual doses, may develop an acute pain syndrome consisting of arthralgia/myalgia symptoms. This acute syndrome typically develops 1 to 3 days after administration and mostly resolves within a week.

While prevention and treatment of CIPN are often managed similarly to other neuropathic conditions such as diabetic peripheral neuropathy or postherpetic neuralgia, high-quality data with consistent evidence that supports such therapy is limited in the cancer patient population. Further research needs to be conducted to provide guidance on the management of this serious and potentially debilitating toxicity.

PREVENTION

Many agents have been investigated for the prevention of CIPN, but minimal efficacy and lack of consistent evidence supporting these options limits their use. A recently published guideline by the American Society of Clinical Oncology (ASCO) does not support the use of acetyl-L-carnitine (ALC), amifostine, amitriptyline, calcium/magnesium infusions (for oxaliplatin-induced neuropathy), diethyldithio-carbamate (DDTC), glutathione, nimodipine, Org 2766, all-*trans*-retinoic acid, rhuLIF, or vitamin E for CIPN prevention (Hershman 2014). No recommendations can be made on the use of N-acetylcysteine, carbamazepine, glutamate, goshajinkigan, omega-3 fatty acids, or oxcarbazepine for CIPN prevention at this time (Hershman 2014). The following discussion is a brief summary of the data for CIPN prevention of select agents.

Venlafaxine

Venlafaxine, a serotonin and norepinephrine reuptake inhibitor (SNRI), was studied in a randomized, double-blind, placebo-controlled phase 3 trial in 48 patients with oxaliplatin-induced acute neurotoxicity (EFFOX trial). Eligible patients included those who experienced acute neuropathy after oxaliplatin therapy; patients with preexisting neuropathy or diabetes were excluded. Patients were randomized to receive venlafaxine 50 mg orally 1 hour prior to oxaliplatin on day 1 and extended release venlafaxine 37.5 mg orally twice daily on days 2 through 11 or placebo; oxaliplatin was administered every 14 days. The primary end point was the percentage of patients with complete relief of acute neuropathy; secondary endpoints included percentage of patients with ≥50% pain relief, mean Neuropathic Pain Symptom Inventory (NPSI) and numeric rating scale (NRS) score variations during treatment, and percentage of patients with grade 0 and grade 3 neuropathy at 3 months (Durand 2012).

Venlafaxine-treated patients were significantly more likely than placebo-treated patients to achieve complete symptom relief (31.3% vs 5.3%, respectively; p=0.03). At 3 months after conclusion of oxaliplatin treatment, 38.5% of venlafaxine-treated patients reported no neuropathy compared with 5.6% of patients in the placebo group (p=0.06). In addition, significantly fewer patients with grade 3 neuropathy were observed in the venlafaxine group (0% vs 33.3%; p=0.03) at 3 months after treatment (Durand 2012).

While these data suggest that venlafaxine may be beneficial in the prevention of oxaliplatin-associated CIPN, its routine use in clinical practice is not currently recommended until additional data becomes available (Hershman 2014).

Calcium/Magnesium Infusions

Many clinical trials have been performed to evaluate the use of calcium and magnesium infusions for the prevention of oxaliplatin-associated neuropathy. Calcium and magnesium infusions are thought to prevent neuropathy by increasing the extracellular concentrations of these electrolytes, thereby decreasing the hyperexcitability of oxaliplatin-subjected neurons (Piccolo 2014). Its use is controversial; while some data support the efficacy of calcium and magnesium infusions for this indication, questions regarding its effect on tumor control remain.

The CONcePT trial (Combined Oxaliplatin Neurotoxicity Prevention Trial) evaluated whether patients receiving FOLFOX/bevacizumab for the treatment of metastatic colorectal cancer allowed patients to remain on therapy longer with intermittent oxaliplatin administration compared to a conventional oxaliplatin schedule (Hochster 2014). Patients were also randomized to calcium/magnesium infusion (administered at a dose of 1 g each, given pre- and post-oxaliplatin) or placebo for neurotoxicity prophylaxis. Randomization was conducted in a 2x2 factorial design (intermittent vs conventional oxaliplatin; calcium/magnesium vs placebo). The study was terminated early due to a decreased tumor response rate in patients receiving calcium and magnesium; however, retrospective review of computed tomography scans collected during the study did not demonstrate an inferior response in patients receiving calcium and magnesium (Hochster 2014).

Subsequent to the CONcePT trial, several other prospective clinical trials studying calcium/magnesium for prevention of oxaliplatin-associated neuropathy were closed. Grothey and colleagues studied 102 patients with colon cancer receiving adjuvant therapy with FOLFOX; patients were randomly assigned to receive calcium/magnesium infusions pre- and post-oxaliplatin or placebo (Grothey 2011). Calcium and magnesium significantly decreased the incidence of chronic, cumulative, $\geq$ grade 2 sensory neuropathy (p=0.018). Acute muscle spasms attributed to oxaliplatin were also reduced (p=0.01), but calcium/magnesium infusions did not appear to decrease cold sensitivity toxicities (Grothey 2011). Additionally, a large, randomized trial in 353 patients receiving FOLFOX as adjuvant therapy for colon cancer failed to show statistically significant differences in neuropathy scores in patients who received calcium and magnesium pre- and post-oxaliplatin compared to placebo (Loprinzi 2014).

Until further data is available to confirm that administering calcium and magnesium does not decrease tumor response rates, the use of this strategy to prevent oxaliplatin-induced peripheral neuropathy is not recommended (Hershman 2014).

Amifostine

The chemoprotective effects of amifostine are thought to be due to its binding of toxic chemotherapy metabolites, thus preventing damage to normal tissue. To investigate its chemoprotective benefits, 242 patients with stage III or IV ovarian cancer were randomized to receive amifostine 910 mg/m^2 or placebo prior to cyclophosphamide and cisplatin administration (Kemp 1996). After six cycles of therapy, severity of cisplatin-associated peripheral neuropathy was significantly decreased in the amifostine arm as compared to placebo (p=0.029). Amifostine was also studied in ovarian cancer patients receiving carboplatin and paclitaxel (Lorusso 2003). Similar to the previous trial, patients were randomly assigned to receive amifostine at 910 mg/m^2 prior to chemotherapy. The incidence of grade 3 or 4 neurotoxicity was significantly reduced in the amifostine arm as compared to placebo (3.7% vs 7.2%, respectively; p=0.02); however, other studies utilizing amifostine have not demonstrated significant efficacy for prevention of CIPN (Hilpert 2005; Openshaw 2004). Given the adverse effect profile of amifostine (including cardiovascular, dermatologic, and gastrointestinal toxicities), as well as conflicting and limited efficacy data, this agent is not recommended for CIPN prevention (Hershman 2014).

Vitamin E

Vitamin E has been studied in CIPN prevention for its antioxidant and free radical scavenging properties. A phase 3, randomized, double-blind, placebo-controlled study was performed in 189 patients receiving neurotoxic chemotherapy (taxanes, platinum agents, or a combination of agents) (Kottschade 2011). Patients were randomized to receive vitamin E 400 mg twice daily or placebo; the primary study objective was the incidence of ≥ grade 2 sensory neuropathy. The results did not show a statistically significant difference between the groups; the incidence of ≥ grade 2 sensory neuropathy was 34% in the vitamin E arm vs 29% in the placebo group (p=0.43). In addition, no significant differences were seen in time to neuropathy onset or chemotherapy dose reductions due to neuropathy (Kottschade 2011).

Other small studies have shown a positive benefit of using vitamin E for CIPN prevention, but limited patient numbers and methodological concerns reduce their applicability (Pace 2003; Pace 2010). Further research is needed to recommend vitamin E for CIPN prevention.

TREATMENT

Treatment options for CIPN include therapy interruption or discontinuation, chemotherapy dose reduction, alteration of the route of administration (bortezomib) or use of an adjuvant medication to provide symptomatic pain relief. Reducing, interrupting, or discontinuing chemotherapy is not an ideal management option (particularly in the curative setting), as patient outcomes could be adversely affected by decreasing chemotherapy dose intensity. Identifying viable CIPN treatment options is crucial in order to optimize cancer-related care. While data for management of other neuropathic conditions is plentiful, data for treatment of CIPN remains limited. Currently, the ASCO guidelines recommend duloxetine for CIPN treatment; tricyclic antidepressants (eg, nortriptyline or desipramine), gabapentin or pregabalin, or a topical gel containing baclofen, amitriptyline, and ketamine may be offered to select patients if the risk/benefit ratio is acceptable (Hershman 2014). The following discussion provides a brief summary of the data for CIPN treatment of select agents.

DULoxetine

Duloxetine was evaluated in a randomized, double-blind, placebo-controlled, crossover trial of patients with a diagnosis of ≥ grade 1 sensory neuropathy and a pain score of ≥4 on a Brief Pain Inventory-Short Form scale of 1 to 10 after receiving therapy with paclitaxel, another taxane, cisplatin, or oxaliplatin (Smith 2013). Patients received either placebo for 5 weeks or duloxetine 30 mg daily for the first week, followed by duloxetine 60 mg daily for 4 additional weeks; the crossover study design also included a 2 week washout between treatment periods. After 5 weeks of therapy, patients receiving duloxetine reported a mean decrease in pain score of 1.06 (95% CI, 0.72 to 1.40) vs 0.34 (95% CI, 0.01 to 0.66) in patients receiving placebo (p=0.003) (Smith 2013). Analysis of secondary outcomes showed that duloxetine-treated patients experienced a greater decrease in pain interfering with daily activities and an increased quality of life as compared to patients who received placebo.

A subgroup analysis of the interaction between treatment group and chemotherapy class suggests that duloxetine may be of most benefit in patients receiving oxaliplatin therapy compared to those who received taxanes, although the results were not statistically significant (p=0.13). Overall, duloxetine was well tolerated, with fatigue, nausea, and insomnia being the most commonly reported adverse events (Smith 2013).

Gabapentin

Gabapentin is commonly used to treat diabetic neuropathy and postherpetic pain, and due to its largely favorable side effect profile, it has been used frequently for CIPN management despite limited trial data for this indication.

Rao et al conducted a multicenter, double-blind, randomized, crossover trial in 115 patients with symptomatic CIPN to evaluate the effect of gabapentin on CIPN pain (Rao 2007). Eligible patients were those with an average daily reported pain score of ≥4 on a scale of 1 to 10 or those with a score of ≥1 on the Eastern Cooperative Oncology Group Neuropathy scale (ENS). Patients were stratified according to the class of neurotoxic chemotherapy regimen received and then randomized to either gabapentin (target dose of 2,700 mg daily) or placebo. After taking the maximum tolerated dose for 3 weeks, gabapentin was weaned off and patients crossed over to the opposite arm. The primary efficacy measure was the self-reported average daily pain score, measured by the numeric rating scale and the ENS. While gabapentin was well-tolerated, no statistically significantly change in the pain score was observed as compared to placebo (Rao 2007).

Despite a lack of data demonstrating a benefit of using gabapentin for CIPN treatment, the current ASCO guidelines suggest that it may still be a reasonable option to offer patients suffering from this condition. Given its acceptable side effect profile, its efficacy in treating other types of neuropathic pain, and limited options for CIPN management, gabapentin (or the mechanistically similar pre-gabalin) may provide benefit to select patients (Hershman 2014).

Tricyclic Antidepressants

Tricyclic antidepressants such as amitriptyline and nortriptyline have shown efficacy in the management of other neuropathic conditions. While amitriptyline has been studied in small trials for CIPN, efficacy was not seen due to insufficient statistical power (Kautio 2008; Kautio 2009). Nortriptyline was studied in a randomized, double-blind, placebo-controlled, crossover trial to evaluate its efficacy in treating cisplatin-induced neuropathy (Hammack 2002). Eligible patients had evidence of sensory peripheral neuropathy due to cisplatin on exam and had painful paresthesiae for at least 1 month. Fifty-one patients were randomly assigned to receive either nortriptyline (starting dose of 25 mg daily, titrated at weekly intervals to a target dose of 100 mg daily) or placebo for 4 weeks, after which they were crossed over to the opposite arm. No significant differences between nortriptyline and placebo was observed with respect to paresthesiae (mean scores of 49 and 55, respectively, on a 100-point visual analog scale; p=0.78), nor was quality of life improved with nortriptyline use (Hammack 2002).

Given the lack of efficacy data and significant adverse event profile, tricyclic antidepressants are not considered first-line therapy for treatment of CIPN (Piccolo 2014). However, the ASCO guidelines state that they may still be considered in select patients if the possible benefit outweighs the toxicity risk (Hershman 2014).

REFERENCES

Durand JP, Deplanque G, Montheil V, et al. Efficacy of venlafaxine for the prevention and relief of oxaliplatin-induced acute neurotoxicity: results of EFFOX, a randomized, double-blind, placebo-controlled phase III trial. *Ann Oncol.* 2012;23(1):200-205.

Grothey A, Nikcevich DA, Sloan JA, et al. Intravenous calcium and magnesium for oxaliplatin-induced sensory neurotoxicity in adjuvant colon cancer: NCCTG N04C7. *J Clin Oncol.* 2011;29 (4):421-427.

Hammack JE, Michalak JC, Loprinzi CL, et al. Phase III evaluation of nortriptyline for alleviation of symptoms of cis-platinum-induced peripheral neuropathy. *Pain.* 2002;98(1-2):195-203.

Hershman DL, Lacchetti C, Dworkin RH, et al. Prevention and management of chemotherapy-induced peripheral neuropathy in survivors of adult cancers: American Society of Clinical Oncology clinical practice guideline. *J Clin Oncol.* 2014;32(18):1941-1967.

Hilpert F, Stähle A, Tomé O, et al. Neuroprotection with amifostine in the first-line treatment of advanced ovarian cancer with carboplatin/paclitaxel-based chemotherapy – a double-blind, placebo-controlled, randomized phase II study from the Arbeitsgemeinschaft Gynäkologische Onkologoie (AGO) Ovarian Cancer Study Group. *Support Care Cancer.* 2005;13(10):797-805.

Hochster HS, Grothey A, Hart L, et al. Improved time to treatment failure with an intermittent oxaliplatin strategy: results of CONcePT. *Ann Oncol.* 2014;25(6):1172-1178.

Kautio AL, Haanpää M, Leminen A, Kalso E, Kautiainen H, Saarto T. Amitriptyline in the prevention of chemotherapy-induced neuropathic symptoms. *Anticancer Res.* 2009;29 (7):2601-2606.

Kautio AL, Haanpää M, Saarto T, Kalso E. Amitriptyline in the treatment of chemotherapy-induced neuropathic symptoms. *J Pain Symptom Manage.* 2008;35(1):31-39.

Kemp G, Rose P, Lurain J, et al. Amifostine pretreatment for protection against cyclophospha-mide-induced and cisplatin-induced toxicities: results of a randomized control trial in patients with advanced ovarian cancer. *J Clin Oncol.* 1996;14(7):2101-2112.

Kottschade LA, Sloan JA, Mazurczak MA, et al. The use of vitamin E for the prevention of chemotherapy-induced peripheral neuropathy: results of a randomized phase III clinical trial. *Support Care Cancer.* 2011;19(11):1769-1777.

Loprinzi CL, Qin R, Dakhil SR, et al. Phase III randomized, placebo-controlled, double-blind study of intravenous calcium and magnesium to prevent oxaliplatin-induced sensory neurotoxicity (N08CB/Alliance). *J Clin Oncol.* 2014;32(10):997-1005.

Lorusso D, Ferrandina G, Greggi S, et al. Phase III multicenter randomized trial of amifostine as cytoprotectant in first-line chemotherapy in ovarian cancer patients. *Ann Oncol.* 2003;14 (7):1086-1093.

Openshaw H, Beamon K, Synold TW, et al. Neurophysiological study of peripheral neuropathy after high-dose Paclitaxel: lack of neuroprotective effect of amifostine. *Clin Cancer Res.* 2004;10 (2):461-467.

Pace A, Giannarelli D, Galiè E, et al. Vitamin E neuroprotection for cisplatin neuropathy: a randomized, placebo-controlled trial. *Neurology.* 2010;74(9):762-766.

Pace A, Savarese A, Picardo M, et al. Neuroprotective effect of vitamin E supplementation in patients treated with cisplatin chemotherapy. *J Clin Oncol.* 2003;21(5):927-931.

Piccolo J, Kolesar JM. Prevention and treatment of chemotherapy-induced peripheral neuropathy. *Am J Health Syst Pharm.* 2014;71(1):19-25.

Rao RD, Michalak JC, Sloan JA, et al. Efficacy of gabapentin in the management of chemo-therapy-induced peripheral neuropathy: a phase 3 randomized, double-blind, placebo con-trolled, crossover trial (N00C3). *Cancer.* 2007;110(9):2110-2118.

Smith EM, Pang H, Cirrincione C, et al. Effect of duloxetine on pain, function, and quality of life among patients with chemotherapy-induced painful peripheral neuropathy: a randomized clinical trial. *JAMA.* 2013;309(13):1359-1367.

Winters-Stone KM, Horak F, Jacobs PG, et al. Falls, functioning, and disability among women with persistent symptoms of chemotherapy-induced peripheral neuropathy. *J Clin Oncol.* 2017: JCO2016713552.

COMMON TOXICITY CRITERIA

Selected Common Toxicity Criteria[a]

Toxicity	Grade 0	Grade 1	Grade 2	Grade 3	Grade 4
Hematologic					
Leukocytes (WBC)	WNL	3,000/mm³ to <LLN	2,000 to <3,000/mm³	1,000 to <2,000/mm³	<1,000/mm³
Neutrophils (ANC)	WNL	1,500/mm³ to <LLN	1,000 to <1,500/mm³	500 to <1,000/mm³	<500/mm³
Lymphocytes	WNL	800/mm³ to <LLN	500 to <800/mm³	200 to <500/mm³	<200/mm³
Anemia (Hgb)	WNL	10 g/dL to <LLN	8 to <10 g/dL	v3: 6.5 to <8 g/dL v4: <8 g/dL	v3: <6.5 g/dL v4: Life-threatening
Platelets	WNL	75,000/mm³ to <LLN	50,000 to <75,000/mm³	25,000 to <50,000/mm³	<25,000/mm³
Hemorrhage	None	Mild, no intervention indicated	Intervention indicated (symptomatic or medical)	Transfusion (and/or other intervention) indicated	Life-threatening; major intervention indicated
Cardiovascular					
Acute coronary syndrome	None		Symptomatic, progressive angina / normal cardiac enzymes; hemodynamically stable	Symptomatic, unstable angina and/or acute MI; abnormal cardiac enzymes; hemodynamically stable	Symptomatic, unstable angina and/or acute MI; abnormal cardiac enzymes; hemodynamically unstable
Atrial fibrillation	None	Asymptomatic; intervention not indicated	Medical intervention indicated (nonurgent)	Symptomatic; incomplete medical control or controlled with device or ablation	Life-threatening; urgent intervention required
Chest pain (cardiac)	None	Mild pain	Moderate pain; limits instrumental ADL	Pain at rest; limits self-care ADL	
Heart failure	None	Asymptomatic with laboratory (eg, B-Natriuretic Peptide [BNP]) or cardiac imaging abnormalities	Symptoms with mild to moderate activity or exertion	Symptoms (severe) at rest or with minimal activity/exertion; intervention indicated	Life-threatening; urgent intervention indicated
Hypotension	None	v3: Changes v4: Asymptomatic; no treatment required	v3: Brief (<24 hours) treatment (eg, fluid replacement or other therapy) required v4: Nonurgent medical intervention indicated	v3: Sustained (>24 hours) treatment required; resolves without persisting physiologic consequences v4: Medical intervention indicated	v3: Shock v4: Life-threatening; urgent intervention indicated

Selected Common Toxicity Criteria[a] (continued)

Toxicity	Grade 0	Grade 1	Grade 2	Grade 3	Grade 4
Hypertension	None	v3: Increase of DBP >20 mm Hg or to >150/100; treatment not required v4: Prehypertension (SBP 120 to 139 mm Hg or DBP 80 to 89 mm Hg)	v3: Recurrent or persistent grade 1 level; may require monotherapy treatment v4: Stage 1 (SBP 140 to 159 mm Hg or DBP 90 to 99 mm Hg); medical intervention indicated; recurrent or persistent (≥24 hours); symptomatic increase of >20 mm Hg (DBP) or to >140/90; monotherapy indicated	v3: More intensive treatment or >1 drug required v4: Stage 2 (SBP ≥160 mm Hg or DBP ≥100 mm Hg); medical intervention indicated; >1 drug or more intensive therapy indicated	v3: Life-threatening (eg, hypertensive crisis) v4: Life-threatening (eg, malignant hypertension, hypertensive crisis); urgent intervention indicated
Left ventricular systolic dysfunction	None	v3: Asymptomatic; resting ejection fraction (EF) >50% to <60%; shortening fraction (SF) >24% to <30%	v3: Asymptomatic; resting EF >40% to <50%; SF >15% to <24%	v3: Symptomatic heart failure (HF) responsive to intervention; EF >20% to <50%; SF <15% v4: Symptomatic due to decreased ejection fraction; responsive to intervention	v3: Refractory or poorly controlled HF: EF <20%; intervention indicated v4: Refractory or poorly controlled HF due to decreased ejection fraction; intervention indicated
Myocardial infarction (MI)	None	v3: Asymptomatic arterial narrowing without ischemia	v3: Asymptomatic; testing suggestive of ischemia; stable angina v4: Asymptomatic cardiac enzymes minimally abnormal; no evidence of ischemic ECG changes	v3: Symptomatic; testing consistent with ischemia; unstable angina; intervention indicated v4: Severely symptomatic; abnormal cardiac enzymes; hemodynamically stable; ECG changes consistent with infarction	v3: Acute MI v4: Life-threatening; hemodynamically unstable
Pericardial effusion	None	v3: Asymptomatic effusion	v4: Small- to moderate-sized asymptomatic effusion	Physiologic consequences	Life-threatening consequences; urgent intervention indicated
Pericarditis	None	Asymptomatic; ECG or physical findings consistent with diagnosis	Symptomatic (eg, chest pain)	Physiologic consequences (eg, pericardial constriction)	Life-threatening; urgent intervention indicated

Selected Common Toxicity Criteria[a] (continued)

Toxicity	Grade 0	Grade 1	Grade 2	Grade 3	Grade 4
QTc prolongation	WNL	v3: QTc >450 to 470 msec v4: QTc >450 to 480 msec	v3: QTc >470 to 500 msec; ≥60 msec increase from baseline v4: QTc 481 to 500 msec	v3: QTc >500 msec v4: QTc ≥501 msec (on 2 separate ECGs)	v3: QTc >500 msec with life-threatening signs or symptoms (eg, arrhythmia, CHF, hypotension, shock, syncope); Torsades de pointes v4: QTc ≥501 msec or >60 msec change from baseline and Torsades de pointes or polymorphic ventricular tachycardia or signs/symptoms or serious arrhythmia
Sinus bradycardia	None	Asymptomatic; intervention not indicated	v3: Medical intervention indicated (nonurgent) v4: Symptomatic; medical intervention indicated	v3: Symptomatic; incomplete medical control or controlled with device v4: Severe, medically significant; medical intervention indicated	v3: Life-threatening v4: Life-threatening; urgent intervention indicated
Sinus tachycardia	None	Asymptomatic; intervention not indicated	Symptomatic; medical intervention indicated (nonurgent)	v3: Symptomatic; incomplete medical control or controlled with device v4: Urgent medical intervention indicated	v3: Life-threatening
Supraventricular tachycardia	None	Asymptomatic; intervention not indicated	Symptomatic; medical intervention indicated (nonurgent)	v3: Symptomatic; incomplete medical control or controlled with device v4: Medical intervention indicated	v3: Life-threatening v4: Life-threatening; urgent intervention indicated
Syncope	Absent			v3: Present v4: Fainting; orthostatic collapse	Life-threatening consequences

Selected Common Toxicity Criteria[a] (continued)

Toxicity	Grade 0	Grade 1	Grade 2	Grade 3	Grade 4
Thrombosis/embolism	None	v4: Superficial	v3: DVT or cardiac thrombosis; intervention not indicated v4: Venous thrombosis (uncomplicated DVT); medical intervention indicated	v3: DVT or cardiac thrombosis; intervention indicated v4: Thrombosis (eg, uncomplicated pulmonary embolism, nonembolic cardiac mural thrombus); medical intervention indicated	v3: Pulmonary embolism/life threatening thrombus v4: Life-threatening (eg, pulmonary embolism, cerebrovascular event, arterial insufficiency); hemodynamic or neurologic instability; urgent intervention indicated
Dermatologic					
Rash (acne/acneiform)	None	v3: Intervention not indicated v4: Papules and/or pustules covering <10% of BSA	v3: Intervention indicated v4: Papules and/or pustules covering 10% to 30% of BSA; limits ADL	v3: Pain, disfigurement, ulceration, desquamation v4: Papules and/or pustules covering >30% of BSA; limits self-care ADL; local superinfection requiring oral antibiotics	v4: Papules or pustules associated with extensive superinfection with IV antibiotics indicated; life-threatening consequences
Rash	None	v3: Macular or papular eruption v4: Macules or papules covering <10% of BSA	v3: Macular or papular eruption or erythema w/pruritus affecting <50% of BSA v4: Macules or papules covering 10% to 30% of BSA; limits ADL	v3: Severe erythema/desquamation/macular, papular, or vesicular eruption covering ≥50% of BSA v4: Macules or papules covering >30% of BSA; limits self-care ADL	v3: Generalized exfoliative, ulcerative, or bullous dermatitis
Rash (erythema multiforme)	None	v4: Lesions covering <10% of BSA	v3: Scattered eruption v4: Lesions covering 10% to 30% of BSA, associated with skin tenderness	v3: Severe eruption; IV fluids, tube feeding, or TPN indicated v4: Lesions covering >30% of BSA, associated with oral or genital erosions	v3: Life-threatening eruption; disabling v4: Lesions covering >30% of BSA, associated with fluid or electrolyte abnormality; ICU or burn unit indicated
Hand-foot syndrome	None	Minimal skin changes or dermatitis without pain	v3: Skin changes or pain not interfering with ADL v4: Skin changes with pain; limits ADL	v3: Ulcerative dermatitis or skin changes with pain; interferes with ADL v4: Severe skin changes (peeling, blisters, bleeding, edema, hyperkeratosis) with pain; limits self-care ADL	

Selected Common Toxicity Criteria[a] *(continued)*

Toxicity	Grade 0	Grade 1	Grade 2	Grade 3	Grade 4
Alopecia	None	v3: Thinning or patchy v4: Hair loss ≥50% (of normal)	v3: Complete v4: Hair loss ≥50% (of normal)		v3: Life-threatening; disabling v4: Life-threatening; urgent intervention indicated
Photosensitivity	None	v3: Painless erythema v4: Painless erythema covering <10% of BSA	v3: Painful erythema v4: Tender erythema covering 10% to 30% of BSA	v3: Erythema with desquamation v4: Erythema covering >30% of BSA and erythema with blistering; systemic corticosteroid and pain therapy indicated	Life-threatening consequences
Gastrointestinal					
Nausea	None	Loss of appetite/able to eat	v3: Oral intake decreased, no significant weight loss, dehydration, or malnutrition; IV fluids indicated <24 hours v4: Oral intake decreased, no significant weight loss, dehydration, or malnutrition	v3: Inadequate oral caloric or fluid intake/IV fluids required ≥24 hours v4: Inadequate oral caloric or fluid intake; tube feeding, TPN, or hospitalization indicated	Life-threatening consequences
Vomiting	None	v3: 1 episode per 24 hours v4: 1 to 2 episodes per 24 hours	v3: 2 to 5 episodes per 24 hours; IV fluids indicated <24 hours v4: 3 to 5 episodes per 24 hours	v3: ≥6 episodes per 24 hours, IV fluids, or TPN required ≥24 hours v4: ≥6 episodes per 24 hours, IV fluids, tube feeding, or TPN required	Life-threatening consequences
Diarrhea	None	<4 stools/day increase over baseline	v3: 4 to 6 stools/day increase over baseline; IV fluids indicated <24 hours; does not limit ADL v4: 4 to 6 stools/day increase over baseline	v3: ≥7 stools/day increase over baseline; IV fluids required ≥24 hours; hospitalization; interferes with ADL v4: ≥7 stools/day increase over baseline; incontinence; hospitalization; limits self-care ADL	v3: Life-threatening consequences; urgent intervention indicated v4: Life-threatening consequences; urgent intervention indicated
Constipation	None	Occasional or intermittent symptoms; occasional use of stool softeners, laxatives, dietary modification, or enemas	Persistent symptoms; regular use of laxatives or enemas indicated	Obstipation with manual evacuation indicated; limits self-care ADL	Life-threatening consequences (eg, obstruction, toxic megacolon); urgent intervention indicated

Selected Common Toxicity Criteria[a] (continued)

Toxicity	Grade 0	Grade 1	Grade 2	Grade 3	Grade 4
Mucositis/stomatitis	None	v3: Mucosal erythema v4: Asymptomatic or mild	v3: Patchy ulcerations v4: Moderate pain; does not interfere with oral intake; modified diet needed	v3: Confluent ulceration, bleeding with minor trauma v4: Severe pain, interferes with oral intake	v3: Tissue necrosis/bleeding; life-threatening v4: Life-threatening; urgent intervention indicated
GI bleeding	None	Mild; intervention not indicated	Symptomatic; mild intervention indicated	Transfusion required; intervention indicated	Life-threatening consequences; urgent intervention indicated
Amylase elevation	None	>ULN to 1.5 x ULN	>1.5 to 2 x ULN	>2 to 5 x ULN	>5 x ULN
Lipase elevation	None	>ULN to 1.5 x ULN	>1.5 to 2 x ULN	>2 to 5 x ULN	>5 x ULN
Ascites	None	Asymptomatic	Symptomatic; intervention indicated	Symptomatic; invasive intervention indicated	v3: Life-threatening consequences v4: Life-threatening consequences; urgent operative intervention indicated
Hepatic					
Alkaline phosphatase elevation	WNL	>ULN to 2.5 x ULN	>2.5 to 5 x ULN	>5 to 20 x ULN	>20 x ULN
AST elevation	WNL	v3: >ULN to 2.5 x ULN v4: >ULN to 3 x ULN	v3: >2.5 to 5 x ULN v4: >3 to 5 x ULN	>5 to 20 x ULN	>20 x ULN
ALT elevation	WNL	v3: >ULN to 2.5 x ULN v4: >ULN to 3 x ULN	v3: >2.5 to 5 x ULN v4: >3 to 5 x ULN	>5 to 20 x ULN	>20 x ULN
Hyperbilirubinemia	WNL	>ULN to 1.5 x ULN	>1.5 to 3 x ULN	>3 to 10 x ULN	>10 x ULN
Metabolic					
CPK (creatine phosphokinase)	WNL	>LLN to 2.5 x ULN	>2.5 to 5 x ULN	>5 to 10 x ULN	>10 x ULN
Dehydration	None	Increased oral fluids indicated; dry mucous membranes, diminished skin turgor	IV fluids indicated <24 hours	v3: IV fluids indicated ≥24 hours v4: IV fluids or hospitalization indicated	v3: Life-threatening (eg, hemodynamic collapse) v4: Life-threatening; urgent intervention indicated

Selected Common Toxicity Criteria[a] (continued)

Toxicity	Grade 0	Grade 1	Grade 2	Grade 3	Grade 4
Hypoalbuminemia	WNL	3 g/dL to <LLN	2 to <3 g/dL	<2 g/dL	v4: Life-threatening; urgent intervention indicated
Hypercholesteremia	None	>ULN to 300 mg/dL	>300 to 400 mg/dL	>400 to 500 mg/dL	>500 mg/dL
Hyperglycemia	WNL	>ULN to 160 mg/dL	>160 to 250 mg/dL	>250 to 500 mg/dL	>500 mg/dL
Hypertriglyceridemia	None	v3: >ULN to 2.5 x ULN v4: 150 to 300 mg/dL	v3: >2.5 to 5 x ULN v4: >300 to 500 mg/dL	v3: >5 to 10 x ULN v4: >500 to 1000 mg/dL	v3: >10 x ULN v4: >1000 mg/dL; life-threatening
Hyperuricemia	WNL	>ULN to 10 mg/dL (without physiologic consequences)	>ULN to 10 mg/dL (without physiologic consequences)	>ULN to 10 mg/dL (with physiologic consequences)	>10 mg/dL; life-threatening
Hypoglycemia	WNL	55 mg/dL to <LLN	40 to <55 mg/dL	30 to <40 mg/dL	<30 mg/dL
Hypocalcemia	WNL	Corrected calcium: 8 mg/dL to <LLN	Corrected calcium: 7 to <8 mg/dL	v3: Corrected calcium: 6 to <7 mg/dL v4: Corrected calcium: 6 to <7 mg/dL; hospitalization indicated	v3: Corrected calcium: <6 mg/dL v4: Corrected calcium: <6 mg/dL; life-threatening
Hypokalemia	WNL	3 mmol/L to <LLN	v3: 3 mmol/L to <LLN v4: 3 mmol/L to <LLN; symptomatic; intervention indicated	v3: 2.5 to <3 mmol/L v4: 2.5 to <3 mmol/L; hospitalization indicated	v3: <2.5 mmol/L v4: <2.5 mmol/L; life-threatening
Hypomagnesemia	WNL	1.2 mg/dL to <LLN	0.9 to <1.2 mg/dL	0.7 to <0.9 mg/dL	v3: <0.7 mg/dL v4: <0.7 mg/dL; life-threatening
Hypophosphatemia	WNL	2.5 mg/dL to <LLN	2 to <2.5 mg/dL	1 to <2 mg/dL	v3: <1 mg/dL v4: <1 mg/dL; life-threatening

Selected Common Toxicity Criteria[a] *(continued)*

Toxicity	Grade 0	Grade 1	Grade 2	Grade 3	Grade 4
Ocular					
Cataract		Asymptomatic; detected on exam only	Symptomatic with moderate decrease in visual acuity (20/40 or better); decreased visual function (correctable with glasses)	Symptomatic with marked decrease in visual acuity (worse than 20/40 but better than 20/200); operative intervention indicated (cataract surgery) indicated	v4: Blindness (20/200 or worse) in affected eye
Conjunctivitis		Mild symptoms or asymptomatic; intervention not indicated	v3: Symptomatic; topical intervention (eg, antibiotics or other topical intervention) indicated; interferes with function but not ADL v4: Symptomatic; topical intervention (eg, antibiotics) indicated; limits instrumental ADL	v3: Symptomatic; interferes with ADL; operative intervention indicated v4: Limits self-care ADL	
Corneal ulceration			v3: Symptomatic; interferes with function but not ADL v4: Symptomatic; intervention indicated (eg, topical agents); limits instrumental ADL	v3: Symptomatic; interferes with ADL; operative intervention indicated v4: Limits self-care ADL; declining vision (worse than 20/40 but better than 20/200)	Perforation or blindness (worse than 20/200) in the affected eye
Eye dryness		v3: Mild; intervention not indicated v4: Asymptomatic; clinical or diagnostic observations only; mild symptoms relieved by lubricants	v3: Symptomatic; interferes with function but not ADL; medical intervention indicated v4: Symptomatic; multiple agents indicated; limits instrumental ADL	v3: Symptomatic or decrease in visual acuity; interferes with ADL; operative intervention indicated v4: Decrease in visual acuity (worse than 20/40); limits self-care ADL	
Eye pain		Mild pain	Moderate pain; limits instrumental ADL	Severe pain; limits self-care ADL	
Glaucoma		Elevated intraocular pressure (EIOP); intervention indicated (single topical agent); no visual field deficit	EIOP causing early visual field deficits; intervention indicated (multiple topical/oral agents); limits instrumental ADL	EIOP causing marked visual field defects (eg, involving both superior and inferior visual fields); operative intervention indicated; limits self-care ADL	v3: Blindness (20/200 or worse); enucleation indicated v4: Blindness (20/200 or worse) in affected eye

Selected Common Toxicity Criteria[a] *(continued)*

Toxicity	Grade 0	Grade 1	Grade 2	Grade 3	Grade 4
Keratitis			v3: Symptomatic and interferes with function but does not interfere with ADL	v3: Symptomatic; interferes with ADL; operative intervention indicated	Perforation or blindness (20/200 or worse) in affected eye
			v4: Symptomatic; medical intervention indicated (eg, topical agents); limits instrumental ADL	v4: Decline in vision (worse than 20/40 but better than 20/200); limits self-care ADL	
Photophobia		Symptomatic; does not limit ADL	v3: Symptomatic and interferes with function but does not interfere with ADL	v3: Symptomatic; limits ADL	
			v4: Symptomatic; limits instrumental ADL	v4: Limits self-care ADL	
Retinal detachment		Asymptomatic	Exudative and visual acuity 20/40 or better	Rhegmatogenous or exudative detachment; operative intervention indicated; decline in vision (worse than 20/40 but better than 20/200)	Blindness (20/200 or worse) in affected eye
Retinopathy		Asymptomatic; clinical or diagnostic observations only	Symptomatic with moderate decrease in visual acuity (20/40 or better); limits instrumental ADL	Symptomatic with marked decrease in visual acuity (worse than 20/40 but better than 20/200); disabling; limits self-care ADL	Blindness (20/200 or worse) in affected eye
Uveitis		Asymptomatic; clinical or diagnostic observations only	Anterior uveitis; medical intervention indicated	Posterior or pan-uveitis	Blindness (20/200 or worse) in affected eye
Watering eyes		Intervention not indicated	v4: Intervention indicated	v4: Operative intervention indicated	
Renal/Genitourinary					
Hematuria	None	v3: Minimal or microscopic; intervention not indicated	v3: Gross bleeding; intervention or irrigation required	v3: Transfusion or intervention indicated	Life-threatening consequences; urgent intervention indicated
		v4: Asymptomatic; intervention not indicated	v4: Symptomatic; catheter or irrigation indicated; limits ADL	v4: Gross hematuria, transfusion, IV medications, or hospitalization indicated; limits self-care ADL	
Serum creatinine elevation	WNL	v3: >ULN to 1.5 x ULN	v3: >1.5 to 3 x ULN	v3: >3 to 6 x ULN	>6 x ULN
		v4: >1 to 1.5 x baseline; >ULN to 1.5 x ULN	v4: >1.5 to 3 x baseline; >1.5 to 3 x ULN	v4: >3 x baseline; >3 to 6 x ULN	

Selected Common Toxicity Criteria[a] *(continued)*

Toxicity	Grade 0	Grade 1	Grade 2	Grade 3	Grade 4
			Respiratory		
Dyspnea	None	v3: Dyspnea on exertion (can walk 1 flight of stairs without stopping) v4: Dyspnea with moderate exertion	v3: Dyspnea on exertion (cannot walk 1 flight of stairs or 1 city block without stopping) v4: Dyspnea with minimal exertion; limits ADL	v3: Dyspnea with ADL v4: Dyspnea at rest; limits self-care ADL	v3: Dyspnea at rest; intubation/ventilator support indicated v4: Life-threatening; urgent intervention indicated
Epistaxis	None	Mild; no intervention indicated	Symptomatic; intervention indicated	Transfusion required; intervention indicated	Life-threatening consequences; urgent intervention indicated
Pleural effusion	None	Asymptomatic	v3: Symptomatic; intervention required (diuretics or up to 2 thoracenteses) v4: Symptomatic; intervention required (thoracentesis or tube drainage)	v3: Symptomatic, oxygen, thoracentesis, tube drainage, or pleurodesis required v4: Severe symptoms; intervention indicated	v3: Life-threatening; intubation or urgent intervention required
Pneumonitis/pulmonary infiltrates	None	Asymptomatic; radiographic findings only	Symptomatic but does not interfere with ADL	Symptomatic; interferes with ADL; oxygen indicated	Life-threatening; ventilator support indicated
			CNS/Neurologic		
Fatigue/weakness	None	v3: Mild fatigue over baseline v4: Fatigue relieved by rest	v3: Moderate; some difficulty with ADL v4: Fatigue not relieved by rest; limits ADL	v3: Severe; interferes with ADL v4: Fatigue not relieved by rest; limits self-care ADL	Disabling
Neuropathy, motor	Normal	Asymptomatic; weakness on exam	Symptomatic weakness; mild difficulty with function	Weakness; interferes with ADL	Life-threatening/disabling
Neuropathy, sensory	Normal	Asymptomatic paresthesia/ deep tendor reflex loss	v3: Paresthesia/sensory loss; interferes with function but not ADL v4: Moderate symptoms; limits ADL	v3: Sensory loss/paresthesia; interferes w/ADL v4: Severe symptoms; limits self-care ADL	v3: Disabling v4: Life-threatening/ disabling

Selected Common Toxicity Criteria[a] (continued)

Toxicity	Grade 0	Grade 1	Grade 2	Grade 3	Grade 4
			Miscellaneous		
Allergic reaction	None	Transient flushing or rash, drug fever <38°C	v3: Rash, flushing, urticaria, dyspnea, drug fever ≥38°C; v4: Intervention or interruption of infusion indicated	v3: Symptomatic bronchospasm; parenteral medications indicated; v4: Prolonged recurrence of symptoms after initial improvement	Life-threatening; urgent intervention indicated
Anaphylaxis	None			Symptomatic bronchospasm; parenteral treatment required; allergy-related edema, angioedema, hypotension	Life-threatening; urgent intervention indicated
Infusion-related reaction	None	Mild, transient; infusion interruption or intervention not indicated	Interruption indicated; responds promptly to symptomatic treatment; prophylactic medications indicated ≤24 hours	Prolonged reaction (not initially responding to symptomatic treatment); symptoms recur following initial improvement; hospitalization indicated	Life-threatening; urgent intervention indicated
Fever	None	38°C to 39°C (100.4°F to 102.2°F)	>39°C to 40°C (102.3°F to 104°F)	>40°C (104°F) for ≤24 hours	>40°C (104°F) for >24 hours
Neutropenic fever	None			v3: ANC <1,000/mm³ with temperature ≥38.3°C (101.3°F); v4: ANC <1,000/mm³ with single temperature >38.3°C (101.3°F) or sustained temperature ≥38°C (100.4°F) for >1 hour	Life-threatening; urgent intervention indicated

DBP = diastolic blood pressure, SBP = systolic blood pressure, BSA = body surface area, ADL = activities of daily living, WNL = within normal limits, LLN = lower limits of normal, ULN = upper limits of normal

[a]The National Cancer Institute (NCI) Cancer Therapy Evaluation Program (CTEP) has developed version 4 of the Common Terminology Criteria for Adverse Events (CTCAE). While version 4 is transitioning into practice, protocols and/or dosage reduction recommendations may be based on version 3. When version 4 differs from version 3, the differences are noted. Adapted from the NCI Common Terminology Criteria for Adverse Events (CTCAE) versions 3.0 and 4.0. http://ctep.cancer.gov/protocolDevelopment/electronic_applications/ctc.htm#ctc_40_conversion. Accessed May 2013 and November 2015.

MANAGEMENT OF CHEMOTHERAPY-INDUCED NAUSEA AND VOMITING IN ADULTS

Nausea: The feeling or sensation of an imminent desire to vomit.

Vomiting: The forceful upward expulsion of gastric contents.

Retching: Rhythmic, labored, spasmodic respiratory movements involving the diaphragm, chest wall, and abdominal muscles.

Nausea and vomiting are common side effects of many antineoplastic agents. Studies, both prior to the advent of serotonin antagonists and after their introduction, have been conducted asking chemotherapy patients to rank the five most distressing symptoms in order from most to least severe. Nausea and vomiting remained among the top three most distressing symptoms, despite the use of serotonin antagonists for prevention or management of acute chemotherapy-induced nausea and vomiting. Uncontrolled nausea and vomiting can have a significant impact on a patient's overall attitude, quality of life, compliance, and response to treatment. Uncontrolled nausea and vomiting can result in dehydration, electrolyte imbalances, weight loss, and malnutrition. Prolonged vomiting and retching can cause esophageal and/or gastric ruptures (Mallory-Weiss tears, Boerhaave syndrome) and bleeding. Even in the absence of actual emesis, patients may experience varying degrees of nausea, often accompanied by anorexia.

Table 1. Other Causes of Nausea or Vomiting

Abdominal Emergencies
Appendicitis
Cholecystitis
GI obstruction
Peritonitis
Acute Systemic Infections
Bacterial
Parasitic
Viral
Cardiovascular Disorders
Congestive heart failure
Hypotension
Myocardial infarction
Syncope
Neurologic
Increased intracranial pressure
Mènière's disease
Otitis interna
Severe or chronic pain
Anticipatory nausea and vomiting
Vestibular dysfunction
Drugs
Anesthetics
Antibiotics
Antineoplastics
Aspirin
Cardiac glycosides
Ethanol

Levodopa
Nonsteroidal anti-inflammatory agents
Opioids
QuiNIDine
Steroids
Theophylline
Endocrine Disorders
Adrenal insufficiency
Diabetes mellitus
Gastrointestinal Disorders
Dyspepsia
Gastric outlet obstruction
Gastroparesis
Heartburn
Partial or complete bowel obstruction
Constipation
Hepatic metastases
Metabolic
Hypercalcemia
Hyperglycemia
Hyponatremia
Uremia
Pregnancy
Psychogenic Stimuli
Therapy-Related
Postsurgical
Radiation Therapy

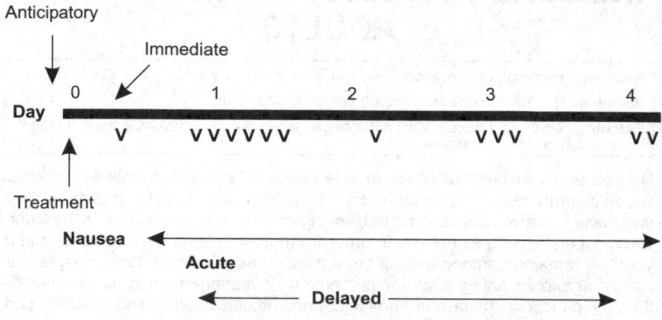

Patterns of Drug-Induced Nausea / Vomiting

Table 2 describes the emetogenic potential of many of the antineoplastic agents. This table has been developed based on various guidelines and publications including: American Society of Clinical Oncology (ASCO), Multinational Association of Supportive Care in Cancer (MASCC)/European Society of Medical Oncology (ESMO), and National Comprehensive Cancer Network (NCCN). Several factors affect the emetic potential of these agents. For some drugs, such as cyclophosphamide or methotrexate, the dose administered has a significant effect on the drug's emetogenicity. Higher doses of these agents are much more emetogenic than low doses. The method of administration can also affect the incidence of nausea. Cytarabine, when given as a continuous infusion, is generally moderately emetogenic; however, higher cytarabine doses with short infusion times can produce a much higher incidence and severity of nausea and vomiting. Patient-related risk factors for nausea and vomiting include: Age (<50 years), female gender, prior experiences with chemotherapy, psychosocial factors (anxiety, depression), history of morning sickness with pregnancies, and history of motion sickness.

Table 2. Emetogenic Potential of Antineoplastic Agents

Highly Emetogenic Chemotherapy (Frequency of Emesis: >90%)

AC (either DOXOrubicin or epiRUBicin in combination with cyclophosphamide)	Dacarbazine
	DACTINomycin
Altretamine	DOXOrubicin ≥60 mg/m^2
Carboplatin AUC ≥4	EpiRUBicin >90 mg/m^2
Carmustine >250 mg/m^2	Mechlorethamine
CISplatin	Procarbazine (oral)
Cyclophosphamide ≥1,500 mg/m^2	Streptozocin

Moderately Emetogenic Chemotherapy
(Frequency of Emesis: 30% to 90%)

Aldesleukin >12 to 15 million units/m^2
Alemtuzumab
Amifostine >300 mg/m^2
Arsenic trioxide
AzaCITIDine
Bendamustine
Bosutinib
Busulfan (IV) or ≥4 mg/day (oral)
Cabozantinib
CARBOplatin AUC <4
Carmustine ≤250 mg/m^2
Ceritinib
Clofarabine
Crizotinib
Cyclophosphamide <1,500 mg/m^2 (IV)
Cyclophosphamide ≥100 mg/m^2/day
  (oral)
Cytarabine >1,000 mg/m^2
DAUNOrubicin
DInutuximab
DOXOrubicin <60 mg/m^2
EpiRUBicin ≤90 mg/m^2

Estramustine
IDArubicin
Ifosfamide
Imatinib
Interferon alfa ≥10 million units/m^2
Irinotecan
Irinotecan (liposomal)
Lenvatinib
Lomustine
Melphalan (IV)
Methotrexate ≥250 mg/m^2 (IV)
Mitotane
Oxaliplatin
RomiDEPsin
Rucaparib
Temozolomide (IV)
Temozolomide (oral)
ThIotepa
Trabectedin
Trifluridine and tipiracil
Vinorelbine (oral [not available in the
  US])

Low Emetogenic Chemotherapy (Frequency of Emesis: 10% to 30%)

Ado-trastuzumab emtansine
Afatinib
Aldesleukin ≤12 million units/m^2
Alectinib
Amifostine ≤300 mg
Atezolizumab
Axitinib
Belinostat
Bexarotene (oral)
Blinatumomab
Bortezomib
Brentuximab vedotin
Cabazitaxel
Capecitabine
Carfilzomib
Cetuximab
Cobimetinib
Cytarabine ≤1,000 mg/m^2
Dabrafenib
Dasatinib
DAUNOrubicin (liposomal)
DOCEtaxel
DOXOrubicin (liposomal)
Elotuzumab
EriBULin
Etoposide (IV)
Etoposide (oral)
Everolimus

Floxuridine
Fludarabine (oral [not available in the
  US])
Fluorouracil
Gemcitabine
Ibrutinib
Idelalisib
Interferon alfa >5 million to <10 million
  units/m^2
Ipilimumab
Ixabepilone
Ixazomib
Lapatinib
Lenalidomide
Methotrexate >50 to <250 mg/m^2 (IV)
MitoMYcin
MitoXANTRONE
Necitumumab
Nilotinib
Olaparib
Omacetaxine
Osimertinib
PACLitaxel
PACLitaxel protein bound
Palbociclib
Panitumumab
Panobinostat
PAZOpanib

PEMEtrexed
Pentostatin
Pertuzumab
PONATinib
Regorafenib
Sonidegib
SUNItinib
Talimogene laherparepvec
Tegafur and Uracil (not available in the US)
Temsirolimus

Teniposide
Thalidomide
Topotecan
Trametinib
Tretinoin
Vandetanib
Venetoclax
Vinflunine (not available in the US)
Vorinostat
Ziv-aflibercept

Minimal Emetogenic Chemotherapy (Frequency of Emesis: <10%)

Asparaginase
Bevacizumab
Bleomycin
Busulfan <4 mg/day
Chlorambucil
Cladribine
Cyclophosphamide <100 mg/m^2/day (oral)
Cytarabine <100 mg/m^2
Daratumumab
Decitabine
Denileukin diftitox
Dexrazoxane
Erlotinib
Fludarabine (IV)
Gefitinib
Gemtuzumab ozogamicin
Hydroxyurea
Interferon alfa <5 million units/m^2
Melphalan (oral)
Mercaptopurine
Methotrexate ≤50 mg/m^2 (IV)
Methotrexate (oral)

Nelarabine
Nivolumab
Obinutuzumab
Ofatumumab
Pegaspargase
Peginterferons
Pembrolizumab
Pomalidomide
PRALAtrexate
Ramucirumab
RiTUXimab
Ruxolitinib
Siltuximab
SORAfenib
Thioguanine (oral)
Trastuzumab
Valrubicin
Vemurafenib
VinBLAStine
VinCRIStine
VinCRIStine (liposomal)
Vinorelbine (IV)
Vismodegib

Types of Chemotherapy-Associated Nausea and Vomiting

Nausea and vomiting caused by cytotoxic therapy generally falls into one of five categories: Acute, delayed, anticipatory, breakthrough, or refractory.

Acute nausea or vomiting is seen within the first 18 to 24 hours of drug administration, with the peak incidence seen at 4 to 6 hours. Acute nausea and vomiting tends to be responsive to drug therapy. Guidelines support the use of a neurokinin-1 receptor antagonist, serotonin antagonist, and dexamethasone combination for the prevention of acute nausea and vomiting in a patient receiving a highly emetogenic regimen. Patients receiving regimens classified as moderately emetogenic are recommended to be given a serotonin antagonist and dexamethasone. For multi-day chemotherapy regimens, antiemetics should be administered for each day of chemotherapy and for 2 days after (Basch 2011).

Delayed nausea or vomiting usually begins after the first 18 to 24 hours of drug administration but may occur up to 7 days after chemotherapy, with the peak incidence in 2 to 3 days. The classic causative agent for delayed nausea and vomiting is cisplatin; however the phenomenon has also been described with cyclophosphamide, doxorubicin, carboplatin, and ifosfamide administration. The exact cause of this side effect is not clear; however, it is believed to have a separate mechanism from acute nausea or vomiting. Gastritis, tissue destruction, electrolyte fluctuations, or effects on the central or peripheral nervous system have all been postulated as possible mechanisms for delayed nausea and vomiting.

Delayed nausea and vomiting is not as responsive to drug therapy when compared to acute nausea and vomiting. The MASCC/ESMO guidelines recommend the use of dexamethasone and aprepitant (or fosaprepitant) for the prevention of delayed emesis associated with high emetic risk chemotherapy (MASCC/ESMO [Roila 2016]).

While not drug-induced *per se*, anticipatory nausea and vomiting is also a relatively common complication of antineoplastic therapy. Anticipatory nausea and vomiting occurs due to inadequate control of nausea and vomiting in the past. Sights, smells, or sounds can also trigger anticipatory nausea and vomiting. This type of nausea and vomiting occurs before the administration of chemotherapy and has a variable response to drug therapy. The most active antiemetic regimen appropriate for the chemotherapy treatment is recommended; these antiemetics should be administered with the initial chemotherapy, as opposed to retrospective assessment of response with a less active antiemetic regimen (Basch 2011).

Breakthrough nausea and vomiting is defined as nausea and/or vomiting despite adequate prophylaxis therapy and requires rescue therapy. Refractory nausea and vomiting on the other hand occurs during subsequent cycles of chemotherapy when antiemetic prophylaxis or rescue therapy (or both) has failed in earlier cycles.

Before changing a patient's antiemetic regimen, it is important to determine when the patient experienced the nausea and vomiting. Basing the decision on the timing of the episode(s) will help guide the change(s) in the regimen. If the patient experienced nausea and vomiting within the first 24 hours, it would be appropriate to change the patient's prophylactic acute regimen. If the patient had no episodes until day 2, it would be more appropriate to change the delayed regimen for the patient.

A number of possible alternatives exist when changing a patient's acute regimen, including switching to another serotonin antagonist, adding a neurokinin receptor antagonist (eg, aprepitant, fosaprepitant) to the previous serotonin antagonist/ steroid regimen, switching to a nonserotonin modulating antiemetic, or adding an benzodiazepine prophylactically. When changing the delayed regimen, there are numerous possibilities including: Adding a neurokinin receptor antagonist, dopamine antagonists, benzodiazepines, or cannabinoids, depending on the specific patient situation. Olanzapine is a thienobenzodiazepine antipsychotic that blocks multiple receptors associated with nausea or vomiting, including dopamine, histamine, muscarinic, and serotonin receptors. A few small trials have reported olanzapine effective (in combination with a steroid and serotonin antagonist) for prevention of delayed nausea and vomiting.

◀

Table 3. Classification of Antiemetic Agents

Antihistamines	DiphenhydrAMINE, hydrOXYzine, promethazine
Anticholinergics	Scopolamine
Benzodiazepines	DiazePAM, LORazepam
Butyrophenones	Droperidol, haloperidol
Cannabinoids	Dronabinol, nabilone
Corticosteroids	Dexamethasone, methylPREDNISolone
Neurokinin antagonists	Aprepitant, fosaprepitant, netupitant[a]
Phenothiazines	ChlorproMAZINE, perphenazine, prochlorperazine, thiethylperazine, triflupromazine[b], (promethazine)
Serotonin antagonists	Dolasetron, granisetron, ondansetron, palonosetron, tropisetron[b]
Substituted benzamides	Metoclopramide, trimethobenzamide
Thienobenzodiazepines	OLANZapine

[a]Netupitant and palonosetron (oral) available as a fixed combination oral agent
[b]Not commercially available in the United States

Table 4. Site of Action of Antiemetic Agents

Emetic center	Antihistamines, anticholinergics, serotonin antagonists, thienobenzodiazepines(?)
Chemoreceptor trigger zone (CTZ)	Benzamides, butyrophenones, phenothiazines, thienobenzodiazepines(?)
Cerebral cortex	Antihistamines, benzodiazepines, cannabinoids, (corticosteroids), neurokinin antagonists(?), thienobenzodiazepines(?)
Peripheral	Metoclopramide, neurokinin antagonists, serotonin antagonists, thienobenzodiazepines(?)
Unknown	Corticosteroids

Table 5. Neurokinin (NK$_1$) Receptor Doses

Drug	Dose
Aprepitant	125 mg orally on day 1 of chemotherapy, followed by 80 mg orally on days 2 and 3
Fosaprepitant	150 mg IV on day 1 of chemotherapy
Rolapitant	180 mg orally on day 1 of chemotherapy
Netupitant	300 mg netupitant/0.5 mg palonosetron orally on day 1 of chemotherapy

Table 6. Typical Serotonin Antagonist Doses

Drug	Oral	IV	SubQ	Transdermal
Dolasetron	100 mg	(contraindicated)		
Granisetron	1 or 2 mg	0.01 mg/kg or 1 mg (maximum: 1 mg)	10 mg per 7 days (extended release)	3.1 mg per 24 hours
Ondansetron	16 to 24 mg (or 8 mg twice daily)	8 mg or 0.15 mg/kg (maximum: 16 mg)		
Palonosetron	0.5 mg[a]	0.25 mg		
Tropisetron[b]	5 mg	5 mg		

[a]Netupitant and palonosetron (oral) available as a fixed combination oral agent
[b]Not commercially available in the United States

Receptors for a large number of different neurotransmitters, including dopamine, serotonin, substance P, endocannabinoids, acetylcholine, histamine, opioids, and benzodiazepines, are involved in the vomiting reflex. Blockade of one or more of these receptors is the basic mechanism of action of most antiemetic agents.

Anticholinergics. Alkaloids (eg, atropine and scopolamine) exhibit some antiemetic activity, primarily postoperative nausea and vomiting, and motion sickness. The apparent mechanism of action is blockage of central muscarinic receptors. Toxicities, such as sedation, restlessness, blurred vision, and dry mouth, limit the systemic use of these agents. Although evidence for use in chemotherapy-induced nausea and vomiting is limited, transdermal scopolamine may be useful in patients whose nausea is positional or due to motion.

Antihistamines. The antihistamines block H_1 receptors both centrally and in the middle ear. A number of drugs in this class are effective against motion sickness and labyrinth disorders, but only diphenhydramine, hydroxyzine, and promethazine seem to have any activity against chemotherapy-induced nausea or vomiting. The major toxicities seen with these drugs are drowsiness, sedation, and dry mouth. These agents are most commonly used to enhance the efficacy of combination antiemetic regimens, although hydroxyzine or promethazine are occasionally used to treat mild to moderate nausea in patients who cannot tolerate, or are refractory to, other antiemetics. Diphenhydramine can be used in combination with dopamine antagonists to prevent extrapyramidal reactions seen with these agents at high doses.

Benzodiazepines. The exact antiemetic mechanism or location of action of the benzodiazepines is unclear. An inhibitory effect on the vomiting center, anxiolytic activity, and general CNS depression have all been postulated. Possible sites of action include the limbic system, vomiting center, cerebrum, and brain stem. The most common side effects include sedation, drowsiness, disinhibition, motor incoordination, and amnesia. In this setting, the anterograde amnesia induced by the benzodiazepine is usually considered a desired therapeutic effect rather than an adverse reaction. Benzodiazepines are commonly used as adjuncts to conventional antiemetics in the prophylaxis and treatment of chemotherapy-induced acute, breakthrough, and refractory nausea and vomiting. The benzodiazepines are also highly effective in the prevention of anticipatory nausea and vomiting. As single agents, the benzodiazepines have only mild antiemetic activity. Lorazepam is the most commonly used benzodiazepine for chemotherapy induced nausea and vomiting, but midazolam and diazepam have also been used. Lorazepam is a useful adjunct but is not recommended as a single-agent antiemetic (ASCO [Hesketh 2017]).

Butyrophenones. A group of dopamine antagonists that can be effective in treating chemotherapy-induced nausea and vomiting are the butyrophenones. Both haloperidol and droperidol have been reported to have antiemetic activity against highly, moderately, and mild emetogenic chemotherapy, although their use may be reserved for management of breakthrough nausea and vomiting. Droperidol has been associated with cardiovascular toxicities, particularly QT prolongation and torsade de points. These toxicities, some fatal, occurred in patients receiving recommended doses or lower and also in patients with no known risk factors, which has ultimately limited the use of this agent. However, one trial comparing ondansetron and droperidol found no difference in the incidence or severity of QTc interval changes between the two drugs. As with most other antiemetics, the optimum response to the butyrophenones is seen in multidrug regimens. Like other dopamine blockers, extrapyramidal reactions, restlessness, sedation, and hypotension are relatively common side effects.

Cannabinoids. Proper evaluation of the antiemetic activity of cannabinoid derivatives has been hindered by social and political stigmas associated with marijuana use. Evidence is currently insufficient to recommend treatment with medical marijuana for nausea/vomiting prevention in cancer patients receiving chemotherapy or radiation therapy (ASCO [Hesketh 2017]). Tetrahydrocannabinol, levonantradol, and nabilone may be effective in treating chemotherapy-induced nausea and vomiting. The specific site and mechanism of activity is unclear. Inhibition of endorphins in the emetic center, suppression of prostaglandin synthesis, and inhibition of medullary activity through an unspecified cortical action have all been postulated. Cannabinoids can inhibit buildup of cyclic adenosine monophosphate and cannabinoid receptors have been identified in the hippocampus, hypothalamus, and cortex. Cannabinoids used by the oral route seem to be most effective against mild to moderately emetogenic chemotherapy. Blurred vision, hypotension, and tachycardia, and a number of CNS complications, including euphoria, dysphoria, hallucinations, and sedation can be seen with cannabinoid therapy. Cannabinoids offer an alternative in patients unable to tolerate, or who are refractory to, other antiemetic agents.

Corticosteroids. The mechanism of antiemetic activity for the steroids is unknown, although alterations of cell permeability and inhibition of prostaglandin activity have been postulated. In spite of this uncertainty, corticosteroids, particularly dexamethasone, are frequent components of combination antiemetic regimens for high to moderately emetogenic chemotherapy. Studies have demonstrated a synergistic activity with metoclopramide and serotonin antagonists resulting in a 20% increase in effectiveness. For delayed nausea and vomiting, monotherapy dexamethasone appears to be more effective than serotonin antagonists for delayed nausea and vomiting. Side effects from single or short term dosing of dexamethasone are infrequent, but may include euphoria, anxiety, insomnia, increased appetite, and hyperglycemia. For patients in whom a corticosteroid is not clearly contraindicated, these agents are an important component of antiemetic therapy. The use of a dexamethasone-containing antiemetic regimen may not be appropriate in certain immunotherapies and cellular therapies.

Neurokinin-1 (NK$_1$) Receptor Antagonists. Neurokinin, or substance P, antagonists are the latest class of antiemetics. Substance P is a tachykinin (neurokinin) located in neurons of the central and peripheral nervous system. It is associated with a variety of functions, including emesis, depression, inflammatory pain and inflammatory/immune responses in asthma, and other diseases. Substance P's activity is mediated by the NK$_1$ receptor, a G-protein receptor coupled to the inositol phosphate signal pathway. Blocking this receptor is a mechanism to treat conditions mediated at least in part by substance P. Several neurokinin receptor antagonists, including aprepitant (MK-869, L-754030), its prodrug L-758298, ezlopitant (CJ-11974), fosaprepitant, rolapitant (SCH-619734), vofopitant (GR-205171), and CP-122721 have been studied. Aprepitant, fosaprepitant, and rolapitant are approved for marketing; netupitant is approved as a combination product with palonosetron (oral fixed combination containing netupitant 300 mg and palonosetron 0.5 mg).

NK$_1$ antagonists are effective in preventing cisplatin-induced nausea and vomiting, when used in conjunction with a serotonin antagonist and steroid. Addition of a neurokinin antagonist to a serotonin antagonist and steroid combination increases control of acute nausea by 10% to 15%, and control of delayed nausea by 20% to 30%. Most studies indicate the neurokinin receptors are less effective than serotonin antagonists, particularly for prevention of acute nausea within the first 8 to 12 hours. However, the neurokinin antagonists appear to be more effective than serotonin antagonists in preventing delayed nausea (days 2 to 5). Aprepitant has a very complex metabolism. Aprepitant is a substrate of 3A4 and when administered for 3 days is an inhibitor of 3A4, and an inducer of 3A4 and 2C9 if administered for more than 14 days. Caution should be used when administering with oral contraceptives, warfarin, dexamethasone, midazolam, and 3A4 inhibitors and inducers. Side effects, although similar to placebo, may include asthenia/fatigue, dizziness, hiccups, gastritis/heartburn, diarrhea, and mild and transient increase in LFTs. Aprepitant is available in capsules and a suspension (for adults unable to swallow capsules). Rolapitant is a moderate inhibitor of CYP2D6; due to the long half-life, the inhibitory effect may persist for at least 7 days (concurrent use of rolapitant with thioridazine is contraindicated due to a significant increase in plasma concentrations of thioridizine). Current guidelines recommend aprepitant, fosaprepitant, or rolapitant as initial therapy for highly emetogenic regimens (including high dose cisplatin) or moderately emetogenic regimens that contain both doxorubicin and cyclophosphamide.

Phenothiazines. Phenothiazines were the first class of drugs accepted as antiemetic therapy for antineoplastic chemotherapy. Blockade of dopamine (D$_2$) receptors in the area postrema (chemoreceptor trigger zone and vomiting center) appears to be their primary mechanism of action. A number of different drugs, including chlorpromazine, perphenazine, prochlorperazine, promethazine, and thiethylperazine (no longer marketed in the United States), have antiemetic activity. Common toxicities such as extrapyramidal reactions, restlessness, sedation, and hypotension limit the use of these drugs. Phenothiazines are most effective against mild to moderate nausea or vomiting, but have little impact on emesis from highly emetogenic agents such as dacarbazine or cisplatin. Higher doses of these agents may have increased activity, but the increased incidence and severity of side effects prohibits their use. Since the serotonin antagonists became available, use of the phenothiazines generally has been limited to prevention of nausea from mildly emetogenic chemotherapy, treatment of breakthrough nausea or vomiting in patients refractory to a serotonin blocker, or in association with dexamethasone to treat delayed nausea.

Serotonin (5-HT$_3$) Antagonists. A major advance in antiemetic therapy was the introduction of the serotonin (5-HT$_3$) antagonists. These agents have been shown to block serotonin in two ways: Peripheral antagonism by blocking release from enterochromaffin cells in the GI tract and central antagonism of receptors in the medulla. The high efficacy rate of these agents in preventing acute nausea and vomiting for highly and moderately emetogenic agents, coupled with their low incidence of side effects, has made them the standard of care in these settings.

Studies comparing serotonin antagonist plus dexamethasone with dexamethasone monotherapy or serotonin antagonist monotherapy have demonstrated that the combination regimen is significantly better than either agent alone. The addition of corticosteroids is synergistic and results in an increase in response of approximately 20%. Conversely, serotonin antagonists are not as efficacious as corticosteroids for delayed nausea and vomiting.

In addition to IV and oral formulations, the serotonin antagonist granisetron is available in a transdermal patch formulation and an extended release subcutaneous injection. The patch contains 34.3 mg of granisetron and releases 3.1 mg/day. The patch was approved based on a noninferiority study compared to oral granisetron in the setting of highly and moderately emetogenic chemotherapy. The patch is recommended to be applied 24 to 48 hours prior to chemotherapy. The extended release subcutaneous injection should be administered as a single 10 mg injection at least 30 minutes prior to chemotherapy on day 1 and administered no more frequently than once every 7 days (avoid use in patients with CrCl <30 mL/minute and extend the interval to no more frequently than every 14 days for CrCl 30 to 59 mL/minute).

The currently available serotonin antagonists have relatively flat dose/response curves. Dose response studies have demonstrated that granisetron's efficacy seems to reach a plateau at 0.01 mg/kg. There appears to be no difference in efficacy between granisetron doses of 0.01 mg/kg and 0.04 mg/kg. A few small studies suggest higher doses of granisetron (3 mg IV or 0.04 to 0.24 mg/kg) may be effective in treating breakthrough nausea; however, none of these reports found the improvement to be statistically significant. A similar limitation exists for dolasetron, ondansetron, and palonosetron. Data are also lacking on the value of using a different serotonin antagonist to treat nausea or vomiting resulting from the failure of the initial serotonin antagonist regimen.

Toxicities with these agents, including headache, constipation or diarrhea, and elevated transaminases, have been minimal. QTc prolongation and/or ECG abnormalities have been observed with dolasetron, granisetron, ondansetron, and palonosetron. Due to the risk for torsade de points, the use of the IV formulation of dolesetron is contraindicated in the prevention of chemotherapy-induced nausea and vomiting and the maximum recommended single IV ondansetron dose is 16 mg.

Tropisetron is not available in the US; however, oral and IV formulations are marketed internationally.

Substituted Benzamides. Metoclopramide is the most commonly used antiemetic drug in this category. Prior to introduction of the serotonin antagonists, high-dose (1 to 3 mg/kg) metoclopramide was the preferred drug for prevention of nausea or vomiting from highly emetogenic chemotherapy. Metoclopramide's ability to block central and peripheral dopamine receptors was believed to be the mechanism of its antiemetic activity. Recognition that high doses also blocked peripheral serotonin receptors in the intestines led to the identification of the role serotonin inhibition has in preventing nausea or vomiting, and, ultimately, to development of the serotonin antagonists. Like the phenothiazines, use of metoclopramide is complicated by extrapyramidal reactions, restlessness, sedation, and hypotension. Diarrhea is also a significant side effect, especially with the high doses used for antiemetic therapy. Also like the phenothiazines, the current use of metoclopramide is generally limited, although may be for prevention of nausea from mild to moderately emetogenic chemotherapy, prophylaxis of delayed nausea or vomiting, or treatment of breakthrough nausea and vomiting.

Olanzapine is a thienobenzodiazepine antipsychotic that blocks multiple receptors associated with nausea or vomiting, including dopamine, histamine, muscarinic, and serotonin receptors. A randomized trial comparing the combination of a neurokinin 1 antagonist, 5-HT$_3$-antagonist, and a steroid with or without olanzapine in patients receiving highly emetogenic chemotherapy showed that the proportion of patients with no nausea was significantly greater in the olanzapine group compared to the placebo group (Navari 2016). Other trials have reported olanzapine effective (in combination with a steroid and 5-HT$_3$-antagonist) for prevention of delayed nausea and vomiting. Olanzapine may also be utilized for breakthrough nausea and vomiting in adults who experience nausea and vomiting despite optimal prophylaxis with a regimen that did not include olanzapine. Consider a reduced olanzapine dose (reduce dose to 5 mg) in elderly or over-sedated patients.

REPRESENTATIVE ANTIEMETIC REGIMENS

HIGHLY EMETOGENIC CHEMOTHERAPY

Neurokinin 1 antagonist- *and* olanzapine-containing regimen:

Aprepitant 125 mg orally day 1, followed by aprepitant 80 mg orally days 2 and 3 **or** fosaprepitant 150 mg IV on day 1 only **plus**

Dexamethasone 12 mg orally or IV day 1, followed by 8 mg orally or IV once daily days 2 to 4 **plus**

OLANZapine 10 mg orally once daily days 1 to 4 **plus**

Serotonin antagonist as follows:

- Dolasetron 100 mg orally day 1 **or**

- Granisetron 1 or 2 mg daily or 1 mg twice daily orally **or** 1 mg or 0.01 mg/kg (maximum: 1 mg) IV day 1 or 10 mg SubQ day 1 or 34.3 mg transdermal patch (3.1 mg per 24 hours; maximum duration: 7 days) applied 24 to 48 hours prior to first chemotherapy dose **or**

- Ondansetron 16 to 24 mg orally or 8 to 16 mg IV or 0.15 mg/kg (maximum dose: 16 mg) IV day 1 **or**

◄ • Palonosetron 0.25 mg IV day 1

or

Neurokinin 1 antagonist-containing regimen:

Aprepitant 125 mg orally day 1, followed by aprepitant 80 mg orally days 2 and 3 **or** fosaprepitant 150 mg IV on day 1 only **or** rolapitant 180 mg orally ~1 to 2 hours prior to chemotherapy on day 1 only **plus**

Dexamethasone 12 mg orally or IV day 1, followed by 8 mg orally or IV once daily days 2 to 4 (with aprepitant) or dexamethasone 12 mg orally or IV day 1, followed by 8 mg orally or IV day 2, followed by 8 mg orally or IV twice daily days 3 and 4 (with fosaprepitant 150 mg) **or** dexamethasone 12 mg orally or IV day 1, followed by 8 mg orally or IV twice daily days 2 to 4 (with rolapitant) **plus**

Serotonin antagonist as follows:

- Dolasetron 100 mg orally day 1 **or**

- Granisetron 1 or 2 mg daily or 1 mg twice daily orally **or** 1 mg or 0.01 mg/kg (maximum: 1 mg) IV day 1 or 10 mg SubQ day 1 or 34.3 mg transdermal patch (3.1 mg per 24 hours; maximum duration: 7 days) applied 24 to 48 hours prior to first chemotherapy dose **or**

- Ondansetron 16 to 24 mg orally or 8 to 16 mg IV or 0.15 mg/kg (maximum dose: 16 mg) IV day 1 **or**

- Palonosetron 0.25 mg IV day 1

NK_1 *fixed combination:* Netupitant 300 mg/palonosetron 0.5 mg orally 1 hour prior to chemotherapy on day 1 plus dexamethasone 12 mg orally or IV 30 minutes prior to chemotherapy day 1, followed by dexamethasone 8 mg orally once daily days 2 to 4

± LORazepam 0.5 to 2 mg orally, IV, or sublingual every 6 hours days 1 to 4, if needed

± H_2-blocker or proton pump inhibitor (PPI)

or

OLANZapine-containing regimen:

OLANZapine 10 mg orally once daily days 1 to 4 **plus** palonosetron 0.25 mg IV day 1 **plus** dexamethasone 20 mg IV day 1

± LORazepam 0.5 to 2 mg orally, IV, or sublingual every 6 hours days 1 to 4, if needed

± H_2-blocker or proton pump inhibitor (PPI)

or

Granisetron extended release subcutaneous antiemetic regimen (for antiemetic prophylaxis with anthracycline/cyclophosphamide):

Granisetron extneded release injection 10 mg subcutaneously on day 1 **plus** dexamethasone 20 mg IV, followed by dexamethasone 8 mg orally twice a day on days 2, 3, and 4 (a neurokinin-1 antagonist may be included in the antiemetic regimen if needed (with appropriate dexamethasone dosage adjustment)

MODERATELY EMETOGENIC CHEMOTHERAPY

Palonosetron 0.25 mg IV day 1 (may substitute granisetron or ondansetron if palonosetron not available), **plus** dexamethasone days 1 to 3, ± aprepitant **or**:

Day 1:

Aprepitant 125 mg orally **or** fosaprepitant 150 mg IV (in selected patients) **or** rolapitant 180 mg orally ~1 to 2 hours prior to chemotherapy **plus**

Dexamethasone 8 to 12 mg orally (or 4 mg twice daily) or IV **or** dexamethasone 20 mg orally or IV (with rolapitant) **plus**

Serotonin antagonist as follows:

- Dolasetron 100 mg orally **or**
- Granisetron 1 or 2 mg daily or 1 mg twice daily orally **or** 1 mg or 0.01 mg/kg (maximum: 1 mg) IV or 10 mg SubQ day 1 or 34.3 mg transdermal patch (3.1 mg per 24 hours; maximum duration: 7 days) applied 24 to 48 hours prior to first chemotherapy dose **or**
- Ondansetron 16 to 24 mg orally or 8 to 16 mg IV or 0.15 mg/kg IV (maximum dose: 16 mg IV) **or**
- Palonosetron 0.25 mg IV

± LORazepam 0.5 to 2 mg orally, IV, or sublingual every 6 hours, if needed

± H_2 blocker or PPI

Day 2 (and beyond):

Aprepitant 80 mg orally days 2 and 3 (if oral aprepitant included day 1) **or**

± Dexamethasone 8 mg daily (or 4 mg twice daily) orally or IV for 2 days or 8 mg daily or 4 mg twice daily for 2 to 3 days **or**

Serotonin antagonist as follows (only if did not receive long-acting serotonin antagonist on day 1):

- Dolasetron 100 mg daily orally **or**
- Granisetron 1 to 2 mg daily or 1 mg twice daily orally **or** 1 mg or 0.01 mg/kg (maximum: 1 mg) IV **or**
- Ondansetron 8 mg twice daily or 16 mg daily orally or 8 to 16 mg IV or 0.15 mg/kg (maximum dose: 16 mg) IV

± LORazepam 0.5 to 2 mg orally, IV, or sublingual every 6 hours, if needed

± H_2 blocker or PPI

or

OLANZapine-containing regimen:

Day 1:

OLANZapine 10 mg orally **plus** dexamethasone 20 mg IV **plus** palonosetron 0.25 mg IV

± LORazepam 0.5 to 2 mg orally, IV, or sublingual every 6 hours, if needed

± H_2 blocker or PPI

Day 2 (and beyond):

OLANZapine 10 mg orally days 2 and 3 (if given day 1)

± LORazepam 0.5 to 2 mg orally, IV, or sublingual every 6 hours, if needed

± H_2 blocker or PPI

LOW EMETOGENIC CHEMOTHERAPY

Dexamethasone 12 mg orally or IV daily or 4 to 8 mg orally or IV daily prior to chemotherapy **or**

Prochlorperazine 10 mg orally or IV prior to chemotherapy and then every 6 hours if needed (maximum: 40 mg/day) **or**

Serotonin antagonists (oral): Dolasetron 100 mg daily or granisetron 2 mg daily or 1 mg twice daily or ondansetron 8 to 16 mg daily

± LORazepam 0.5 to 2 mg orally, IV, or sublingual every 6 hours if needed

± H_2 blocker or PPI

MINIMAL EMETOGENIC CHEMOTHERAPY

No routine prophylaxis is necessary.

ORAL CHEMOTHERAPY

High to moderate emetogenic risk:

Serotonin antagonists (oral): Dolasetron 100 mg daily or granisetron 1 to 2 mg daily or 1 mg twice daily or granisetron 34.3 mg transdermal patch (3.1 mg per 24 hours; maximum duration: 7 days) applied 24 to 48 hours prior to first chemotherapy dose or ondansetron 8 to 16 mg daily

± LORazepam 0.5 to 2 mg orally or sublingual every 6 hours, if needed

± H_2 blocker or PPI

Low to minimal emetogenic risk:

Prochlorperazine 10 mg orally prior to chemotherapy and then every 6 hours (maximum: 40 mg/day) as needed **or**

Serotonin antagonists (oral): Dolasetron 100 mg daily (if needed) or granisetron 1 to 2 mg daily (if needed) or 1 mg twice daily (if needed) or ondansetron 8 to 16 mg daily (if needed)

± LORazepam 0.5 to 2 mg orally every 6 hours, if needed

± H_2 blocker or PPI

BREAKTHROUGH TREATMENT OPTIONS

Prochlorperazine 25 mg rectally every 12 hours or 10 mg orally or IV every 6 hours **or**

Promethazine 12.5 to 25 mg orally or IV every 4 to 6 hours **or**

Haloperidol 0.5 to 1 mg orally every 6 hours as needed **or**

LORazepam 0.5 to 2 mg orally every 6 hours **or**

Dolasetron 100 mg orally **or**

Granisetron 1 to 2 mg daily or 1 mg twice daily orally or 0.01 mg/kg (maximum: 1 mg) IV or 34.3 mg transdermal patch (3.1 mg per 24 hours; maximum duration: 7 days) **or**

Ondansetron 16 mg daily orally or IV **or**

Dronabinol:

Capsule: 5 mg 3 to 4 times daily **or** 5 to 10 mg orally every 6 to 8 hours **or** 2.5 to 10 mg 3 or 4 times daily **or** (manufacturer labeling) 5 mg/m^2 to 15 mg/m^2 orally 1 to 3 hours prior to chemotherapy, then every 2 to 4 hours after chemotherapy (for a total of 4 to 6 doses per day)

Oral solution: Initial: 4.2 mg/m^2 (rounded to the nearest 0.1 mg increment [or to the nearest 0.1 mL measurable increment on the calibrated oral dosing syringe]) 1 to 3 hours prior to chemotherapy and then every 2 to 4 hours after chemotherapy for a total of 4 to 6 doses/day. Titrate dose in 2.1 mg/m^2 increments (during a cycle or in subsequent cycles) to clinical response. Maximum: 12.6 mg/m^2/dose and 4 to 6 doses/day **or**

Titrate dose in 2.1 mg/m^2 increments (during a cycle or in subsequent cycles) to clinical response. Maximum: 12.6 mg/m^2/dose and 4 to 6 doses/day **or**

Nabilone 1 to 2 mg orally twice a day **or**

Dexamethasone 12 mg orally or IV daily **or**

OLANZapine 10 mg daily for 3 days **or**

Scopolamine transdermal one patch every 72 hours **or**

Metoclopramide:

Low dose: 10 to 20 mg orally or IV every 6 hours

High dose: 1 to 2 mg/kg/dose IV before chemotherapy and repeat 2 hours after chemotherapy (for nausea and vomiting refractory or intolerant to antiemetics with a higher therapeutic index) or 0.5 mg/kg orally every 6 hours on days 2 to 4

General Principles for Managing Nausea and Vomiting

Key to prevention is aggressively prescribing the most effective antiemetic regimen during initial therapy.

A. **Prevention**

  a. **Antiemetics are most effective when given prophylactically.**

  b. Depending on the antiemetic agent(s) and route(s) of administration, pretreatment may range from 1 hour to 5 minutes prior to administration of the antineoplastic agent(s).

  c. **Emetogenic potential is additive and may be different on different days of the regimen.**

  d. **Provide patient with delayed nausea regimen for 2 to 3 days and PRN antiemetics while at home.**

    e.   In most cases, **combination antiemetics are required for optimum control of nausea.** Two or more agents, from *different pharmacologic categories*, may be required to achieve optimal results.

    f.   **Avoid duplication of agents from the same pharmacologic category.**

    g.   **Doses and intervals of the antiemetic regimen need to be individualized for each patient.** "PRN" regimens should not be used for highly and moderately emetogenic chemotherapy. A fixed schedule of drug administration is preferable.

    h.   **If a patient has had no nausea for 24 hours** while on their scheduled antiemetic regimen, **it is usually possible to switch to a "PRN" regimen.** The patient should be advised to resume the fixed schedule *at the FIRST sign of recurrent nausea*, and continue it until they have had at least 24 hours without nausea.

    i.   **Titrate antiemetic dose to patient tolerance.**

    j.   **Anticipatory nausea and vomiting can often be minimized if the patient receives effective prophylaxis against nausea from the first cycle of therapy.**

    k.   **If anticipatory nausea does develop, an anxiolytic agent is usually the drug of choice.**

    l.   **"If it's not broken – DON'T fix it!"** Regardless of your own preferences, if the patient's current antiemetic regimen is working, don't change it.

B.   Antiemetics

    a.   **The serotonin antagonists have a "ceiling" dose,** above which there is little or no added antiemetic effect.

    b.   **Serotonin antagonists are most effective within the first 24 hours.** Most studies of multiple day dosing show a sharp decline in the efficacy of the serotonin antagonists after the second or third day.

    c.   **Neurokinin antagonists are not very effective as single agents,** and should only be used in combination with a serotonin antagonist and steroid.

    d.   **Serotonin and neurokinin blockers are most effective in scheduled prophylactic regimens;** rather than in "PRN" regimens to chase existing vomiting.

    e.   **Serotonin and neurokinin antagonists have limited efficacy in stopping nausea or vomiting once it has begun.** A dopamine blocker may be more effective.

   f.   **Other antiemetics, such as cannabinoids, antihistamines, or anticholinergics, have limited use as initial therapy.** They are best used in combination with more effective agents (steroids, dopamine, or serotonin blockers); or, as second- or third-line therapy.

SELECTED READINGS

Aapro M. 5-HT$_3$-receptor antagonists in the management of nausea and vomiting in cancer and cancer treatment. *Oncology.* 2005;69(2):97-109.

Basch E, Prestrud AA, Hesketh PJ, et al. Antiemetics: American Society of Clinical Oncology clinical practice guideline update. *J Clin Oncol.* 2011;29(31):4189-4198.

Dupuis LL, Boodhan S, Sung L, et al. Guideline for the classification of the acute emetogenic potential of antineoplastic medication in pediatric cancer patients. *Pediatr Blood Cancer.* 2011;57(2):191-198.

Geling O, Eichler HG. Should 5-hydroxytryptamine-3 receptor antagonists be administered beyond 24 hours after chemotherapy to prevent delayed emesis? Systematic re-evaluation of clinical evidence and drug cost implications. *J Clin Oncol.* 2005;23(6):1289-1294.

Gralla RJ, Bosnjak SM, Hontsa A, et al. A phase III study evaluating the safety and efficacy of NEPA, a fixed-dose combination of netupitant and palonosetron, for prevention of chemotherapy-induced nausea and vomiting over repeated cycles of chemotherapy. *Ann Oncol.* 2014;25(7):1333-1339.

Graves T. Emesis as a complication of cancer chemotherapy: pathophysiology, importance, and treatment. *Pharmacotherapy.* 1992;12(4):337-345.

Grunberg SM, Hesketh PJ. Control of chemotherapy-induced emesis. *N Engl J Med.* 1993;329 (24):1790-1796.

Grunberg SM, Warr D, Gralla RJ, et al. Evaluation of new antiemetic agents and definition of antineoplastic agent emetogenicity – state of the art. *Support Care Cancer.* 2011;19(Suppl 1): S43-S47.

Hesketh PJ, Bohlke K, Lyman GH, et al. Antiemetics: American Society of Clinical Oncology focused guideline update. *J Clin Oncol. J Clin Oncol.* 2016;34(4):381-386.

Hesketh PJ. Chemotherapy-induced nausea and vomiting. *N Engl J Med.* 2008;358 (23):2482-2494.

Hesketh PJ, Kris MG, Basch E, et al. Antiemetics: American Society of Clinical Oncology clinical practice guideline update. *J Clin Oncol.* 2017:JCO2017744789.

Hesketh PJ, Kris MG, Grunberg SM, et al. Proposal for classifying the acute emetogenicity of cancer chemotherapy. *J Clin Oncol.* 1997;15(1):103-109.

Hesketh PJ, Van Belle S, Aapro M, et al. Differential involvement of neurotransmitters through the time course of cisplatin-induced emesis as revealed by therapy with specific receptor antagonists. *Eur J Cancer.* 2003;39(8):1074-1080.

Holdsworth MT. Ethical issues regarding study designs used in serotonin-antagonist drug development. *Ann Pharmacother.* 1996;30(10):1182-1184.

Horiot JC. Antiemetic therapy in cancer: an update. *Expert Opin Pharmacother.* 2005;6 (10):1713-1723.

Jordan K, Schmoll HJ, Aapro MS. Comparative activity of antiemetic drugs. *Crit Rev Oncol Hematol.* 2007;61(2):162-175.

Kris MG, Hesketh PJ, Somerfield MR, et al. American Society of Clinical Oncology guideline for antiemetics in oncology: update 2006. *J Clin Oncol.* 2006;24(18):2932-2947.

Lohr L. Chemotherapy-induced nausea and vomiting. *Cancer J.* 2008;14(2):85-93.

National Comprehensive Cancer Network (NCCN). NCCN clinical practice guidelines in oncology: antiemesis. v.2.2017. http://www.nccn.org/professionals/physician_gls/PDF/antiemesis.pdf

Navari RM, Aapro M. Antiemetic prophylaxis for chemotherapy-induced nausea and vomiting. *N Engl J Med.* 2016;374(14):1356-1367.

Navari RM, Gray SE, Kerr AC. Olanzapine versus aprepitant for the prevention of chemotherapy-induced nausea and vomiting: a randomized phase III trial. *J Support Oncol.* 2011;9(5):188-195.

Navari RM, Nagy CK, Gray SE. The use of olanzapine versus metoclopramide for the treatment of breakthrough chemotherapy-induced nausea and vomiting in patients receiving highly emetogenic chemotherapy. *Support Care Cancer.* 2013;21(6):1655-1663.

Navari RM. Prevention of emesis from multiple-day and high-dose chemotherapy regimens. *J Natl Compr Canc Netw.* 2007;5(1):51-59.

Navari RM, Qin R, Ruddy KJ, et al. Olanzapine for the prevention of chemotherapy-induced nausea and vomiting. *N Engl J Med.* 2016;375(2):134-142.

Oo TH, Hesketh PJ. Drug insight: new antiemetics in the management of chemotherapy-induced nausea and vomiting. *Nat Clin Pract Oncol.* 2005;2(4):196-201.

Rapoport BL, Chasen MR, Gridelli C, et al. Safety and efficacy of rolapitant for prevention of chemotherapy-induced nausea and vomiting after administration of cisplatin-based highly emetogenic chemotherapy in patients with cancer: two randomised, active-controlled, double-blind, phase 3 trials. *Lancet Oncol.* 2015;16(9):1079-1089.

Roila F, Molassiotis A, Herrstedt J, et al. 2016 MASCC and ESMO guideline update for the prevention of chemotherapy- and radiotherapy-induced nausea and vomiting and of nausea and vomiting in advanced cancer patients. *Ann Oncol.* 2016;27(suppl 5):v119-v133.

Roscoe JA, Heckler CE, Morrow GR, et al. Prevention of delayed nausea: a University of Rochester Cancer Center Community Clinical Oncology Program study of patients receiving chemotherapy. *J Clin Oncol.* 2012;30(27):3389-3395.

Schwartzberg LS, Modiano MR, Rapoport BL, et al. Safety and efficacy of rolapitant for prevention of chemotherapy-induced nausea and vomiting after administration of moderately emetogenic chemotherapy or anthracycline and cyclophosphamide regimens in patients with cancer: a randomised, active-controlled, double-blind, phase 3 trial. *Lancet Oncol.* 2015;16(9):1071-1078.

Trigg ME, Higa GM. Chemotherapy-induced nausea and vomiting: antiemetic trials that impacted clinical practice. *J Oncol Pharm Pract.* 2010;16(4):233-244.

Weinstein C, Jordan K, Green SA, et al. Single-dose fosaprepitant for the prevention of chemotherapy-induced nausea and vomiting associated with moderately emetogenic chemotherapy: results of a randomized, double-blind phase III trial. *Ann Oncol.* 2016;27(1):172-178.

MANAGEMENT OF DRUG EXTRAVASATIONS

A potential complication of drug therapy is extravasation. A variety of symptoms, including erythema, ulceration, pain, tissue sloughing, and necrosis, are possible. A variety of drugs have been reported to cause tissue damage if extravasated.

DEFINITIONS

- **Extravasation:** Unintentional or inadvertent leakage (or instillation) of fluid out of a blood vessel into surrounding tissue

- **Irritant:** An agent that causes aching, tightness, and phlebitis with or without inflammation, but does not typically cause tissue necrosis. Irritants can cause necrosis if the extravasation is severe or left untreated.

- **Vesicant:** An agent that has the potential to cause blistering, severe tissue injury, or tissue necrosis when extravasated

- **Flare:** Local, nonpainful, possibly allergic reaction often accompanied by reddening along the vein

PREVENTING EXTRAVASATIONS

Although it is not possible to prevent all extravasations, a few precautions can minimize the risk to the patient. The vein used should be a large, intact vessel with good blood flow. Veins in the forearm (ie, basilic, cephalic, and median antebrachial) are usually good options for peripheral infusions. To minimize the risk of dislodging the catheter, avoid using veins in the hands, dorsum of the foot, and any joint space (eg, antecubital). It is important to remember to not administer chemotherapy distal to a recent venipuncture.

A frequently recommended precaution against drug extravasation is the use of a central venous catheter. Use of a central venous line has several advantages, including high patient satisfaction, reliable venous access, high flow rates, and rapid dilution of the drug. Many institutions encourage or require use of a vascular access device for administration of vesicant agents. Despite their benefit, central lines are not an absolute solution. Vascular access devices are subject to a number of complications. Misplacement/migration of the catheter or improper placement of the needle in accessing injection ports, and cuts, punctures, infections, or rupture of the catheter itself have all been reported.

Education of both the patient and practitioner is imperative. Educate the patient to immediately report any signs of pain, itching, tingling, burning, redness, swelling, or discomfort, all of which could be early signs of extravasation. Symptoms of extravasation which may appear later include blistering, ulceration, and necrosis. Ensure the health care team is informed of the risks and management strategies for both prevention and treatment of extravasations. Absence of blood return, resistance upon administration, or interruption of the IV flow should raise suspicion of potential extravasation.

INITIAL EXTRAVASATION MANAGEMENT

1. **Stop the infusion:** At the first suspicion of extravasation, the drug infusion and IV fluids should be stopped.

2. **Do NOT remove the catheter/needle:** The IV tubing should be disconnected, but the catheter/needle should be left in place to facilitate aspiration of fluid from the extravasation site and, if appropriate, administration of an antidote.

3. **Aspirate fluid:** To the extent possible, the extravasated drug solution should gently be removed from the subcutaneous tissues. It is important to avoid any friction or pressure to the area.

4. **Do NOT flush the line:** Flooding the infiltration site with saline or dextrose in an attempt to dilute the drug solution is not recommended.

5. **Remove the catheter/needle:** If an antidote is not going to be administered into the extravasation site, the catheter/needle should be removed. If an antidote is to be injected into the area, it should be injected through the catheter to ensure delivery of the antidote to the extravasation site. When this has been accomplished, the catheter should then be removed.

6. **Elevate:** The affected extremity should be elevated.

7. **Compresses:** If indicated, apply dry compress to area of extravasation (either cold or warm, depending on vesicant extravasated).

8. **Monitor and document:** Mark the extravasation site (using a surgical felt pen, gently draw an outline on the skin of the extravasation area) and photograph if possible. Monitor and document the event and follow-up activities according to institutional policy.

Table 1: Vesicant Agents and Extravasation Management

Extravasated Medication	Preferred Antidote	Antidote Administration	Supportive Management	Comments
Ado-Trastuzumab Emtansine	No known antidote	No recommendation	No recommendation	May be a vesicant; delayed skin necrosis has been observed (case report) following extravasation (Shafaee 2017)
Amino Acids (4.25%)/parenteral nutrition	Hyaluronidase	Hyaluronidase: Intradermal or SubQ: Inject a total of 1 to 1.7 mL (15 units/mL) as five separate 0.2 to 0.3 mL injections (using a 25-gauge needle) into area of extravasation at the leading edge in a clockwise manner (MacCara 1983; Reynolds 2014; Zenk 1981)	Apply dry cold compresses (Hurst 2004)	
Aminophylline	Hyaluronidase	Hyaluronidase: Intradermal or SubQ: Inject a total of 1 to 1.7 mL (15 units/mL) as five separate 0.2 to 0.3 mL injections (using a 25-gauge needle) into area of extravasation at the leading edge in a clockwise manner (MacCara 1983; Reynolds 2014; Zenk 1981)	Apply dry cold compresses (Hurst 2004; Reynolds 2014)	
Amsacrine	No known antidote	No known antidote	Apply dry warm compresses (Schulmeister 2011)	Not commercially available in the US
Bendamustine	Sodium Thiosulfate	May be managed in the same manner as mechlorethamine extravasation (Schulmeister 2011): Sodium thiosulfate ¹⁄₆ M solution: Inject subcutaneously into extravasation area using 2 mL for each mg of mechlorethamine suspected to have extravasated (Pérez Fidalgo 2012; Polcvich 2009)	Apply dry cold compresses for 20 minutes 4 times/day for 1 to 2 days (Pérez Fidalgo 2012)	Irritant with vesicant-like properties (reports of both irritant and vesicant reactions)
Calcium Chloride (≥10%)	Hyaluronidase	Hyaluronidase: Intradermal or SubQ: Inject a total of 1 to 1.7 mL (15 units/mL) as five separate 0.2 to 0.3 mL injections (using a 25-gauge needle) into area of extravasation at the leading edge in a clockwise manner (MacCara 1983; Reynolds 2014; Zenk 1981)	Apply dry cold compresses (Hurst 2004; Reynolds 2014)	
Calcium Gluconate	Hyaluronidase	Hyaluronidase: Intradermal or SubQ: Inject a total of 1 to 1.7 mL (15 units/mL) as five separate 0.2 to 0.3 mL injections (using a 25-gauge needle) into area of extravasation at the leading edge in a clockwise manner (MacCara 1983; Reynolds 2014; Zenk 1981)	Apply dry cold compresses (Hurst 2004; Reynolds 2014)	

Table 1: Vesicant Agents and Extravasation Management *(continued)*

Extravasated Medication	Preferred Antidote	Antidote Administration	Supportive Management	Comments
CISplatin (>0.4 mg/mL)	Sodium Thiosulfate	Sodium thiosulfate 1/6 M solution: Inject 2 mL into existing IV line for each 100 mg of cisplatin extravasated; then consider also injecting 1 mL as 0.1 mL subcutaneous injections (clockwise) around the area of extravasation; may repeat subcutaneous injections several times over the next 3 to 4 hours (Ener 2004) Dimethyl sulfoxide (DMSO) may also be considered an option. Apply topically to a region covering twice the affected area every 8 hours for 7 days; begin within 10 minutes of extravasation; do not cover with a dressing (Pérez Fidalgo 2012).	Information conflicts regarding use of warm or cold compresses	
Contrast Media	Hyaluronidase	Hyaluronidase: Intradermal or SubQ: Inject a total of 1 to 1.7 mL (15 units/mL) as five separate 0.2 to 0.3 mL injections (using a 25-gauge needle) into area of extravasation at the leading edge in a clockwise manner (MacCara 1983; Reynolds 2014; Zenk 1981) The injection of a total of 5 mL (150 units/mL) as five separate 1 mL injections around the extravasation site has been also used successfully (Rowlett 2012)	Information conflicts regarding use of dry warm or dry cold compresses	
DACTINomycin	No known antidote	No known antidote	Apply dry cold compress for 20 minutes 4 times/day for 1 to 2 days (Pérez Fidalgo 2012)	
Dantrolene	No known antidote	No known antidote	No recommendation	

Table 1: Vesicant Agents and Extravasation Management *(continued)*

Extravasated Medication	Preferred Antidote	Antidote Administration	Supportive Management	Comments
DAUNOrubicin (Conventional)	Dexrazoxane or topical Dimethyl Sulfoxide (DMSO)	**Adults:** Dexrazoxane 1,000 mg/m^2 (maximum dose: 2,000 mg) IV (administer in a large vein remote from site of extravasation) over 1 to 2 hours days 1 and 2, then 500 mg/m^2 (maximum dose: 1,000 mg) IV over 1 to 2 hours day 3; begin within 6 hours after extravasation (Mouridsen 2007; Pérez Fidalgo 2012). **Note:** Reduce dexrazoxane dose by 50% in patients with moderate to severe renal impairment (CrCl <40 mL/min). **Pediatrics and Adults:** DMSO: Apply topically to a region covering twice the affected area every 8 hours for 7 days; begin within 10 minutes of extravasation; do not cover with a dressing (Pérez Fidalgo 2012)	Apply dry cold compress for 20 minutes 4 times/day for 1 to 2 days (Pérez Fidalgo 2012). Withhold cooling for 15 minutes before and after dexrazoxane.	If using dexrazoxane, do not use DMSO. Administer dexrazoxane through a large vein remote from area of the extravasation.
Dextrose (≥10%)	Hyaluronidase	Hyaluronidase: **Dextrose 10%:** Intradermal or SubQ: Inject a total of 1 to 1.7 mL (15 units/mL) as five separate 0.2 to 0.3 mL injections (using a 25-gauge needle) into area of extravasation at the leading edge in a clockwise manner (MacCara 1983 Reynolds 2014; Zenk 1981) **Dextrose 50%:** Injection of a total of 1 mL (150 units/mL) as five separate 0.2 mL injections administered along the leading edge of erythema has been used successfully (Wiegand 2010)	Apply dry cold compresses (Hurst 2014; Reynolds 2014)	
DiazePAM	No known antidote	No known antidote	Apply dry cold compresses (Hurst 2004; Reynolds 2014)	
Digoxin	No known antidote	No known antidote	No recommendation	
DOCEtaxel	No known antidote	No known antidote	Information conflicts regarding use of warm or cold compresses	Irritant with vesicant-like properties (reports of both irritant and vesicant reactions)

Table 1: Vesicant Agents and Extravasation Management *(continued)*

Extravasated Medication	Preferred Antidote	Antidote Administration	Supportive Management	Comments
DOPamine	Phentolamine	Phentolamine: Dilute 5 to 10 mg in 10 to 20 mL NS and administer into extravasation site as soon as possible after extravasation; may readminister if patient remains symptomatic (Reynolds 2014) *Alternatives to phentolamine (due to shortage):* Nitroglycerin topical 2% ointment (based on limited data) Adults: Apply a 1-inch strip to the site of ischemia; may repeat every 8 hours as necessary (Reynolds 2014) Pediatrics: Apply 4 mm/kg as a thin ribbon to the site of ischemia; may repeat after 8 hours if needed (Wong 1992) **or** apply a 1-inch strip to the site of ischemia; may repeat every 8 hours as necessary (Denkler 1989; Reynolds 2014) Terbutaline (based on limited case reports): Infiltrate extravasation area using a solution of terbutaline 1 mg diluted in 10 mL in NS (large extravasation site; administration volume varied from 3 to 10 mL) **or** 1 mg diluted in 1 mL 0.9% NS (small/distal extravasation site; administration volume varied from 0.5 to 1 mL) (Stier 1999)	Apply dry warm compresses (Hurst 2004)	
DOXOrubicin (Conventional)	Dexrazoxane or topical DMSO	Adults: Dexrazoxane 1,000 mg/m² (maximum dose: 2,000 mg) IV (administer in a large vein remote from site of extravasation) over 1 to 2 hours days 1 and 2, then 500 mg/m² (maximum dose: 1,000 mg) IV over 1 to 2 hours day 3; begin within 6 hours after extravasation (Mouridsen 2007; Pérez Fidalgo 2012). **Note:** Reduce dexrazoxane dose by 50% in patients with moderate to severe renal impairment (CrCl <40 mL/min). Pediatrics and Adults: DMSO: Apply topically to a region covering twice the affected area every 8 hours for 7 days; begin within 10 minutes of extravasation; do not cover with a dressing (Pérez Fidalgo 2012)	Apply dry cold compress for 20 minutes 4 times/day for 1 to 2 days (Pérez Fidalgo 2012). Withhold cooling for 15 minutes before and after dexrazoxane.	If using dexrazoxane, do not use DMSO. Administer dexrazoxane through a large vein remote from area of the extravasation.

Table 1: Vesicant Agents and Extravasation Management *(continued)*

Extravasated Medication	Preferred Antidote	Antidote Administration	Supportive Management	Comments
EPINEPHrine	Phentolamine	Phentolamine: Dilute 5 to 10 mg in 10 to 20 mL NS and administer into extravasation site as soon as possible after extravasation; may readminister if patient remains symptomatic (Reynolds 2014) *Alternatives to phentolamine (due to shortage):* Nitroglycerin topical 2% ointment (based on limited data): Adults: Apply a 1-inch strip to the site of ischemia; may repeat every 8 hours as necessary (Reynolds 2014) Pediatrics: Apply 4 mm/kg as a thin ribbon to the site of ischemia; may repeat after 8 hours if needed (Wong 1992) or apply a 1-inch strip to the site of ischemia; may repeat every 8 hours as necessary (Denkler 1989; Reynolds 2014) Terbutaline (based on limited case reports): Infiltrate extravasation area using a solution of terbutaline 1 mg diluted in 10 mL in NS (large extravasation site; administration volume varied from 3 to 10 mL) or 1 mg diluted in 1 mL NS (small/distal extravasation site; administration volume varied from 0.5 to 1 mL) (Reynolds 2014; Siler 1999)	Apply dry warm compresses (Hurst 2004)	
EpiRUBicin	Dexrazoxane or topical DMSO	Adults: Dexrazoxane 1,000 mg/m² (maximum dose: 2,000 mg) IV (administer in a large vein remote from site of extravasation) over 1 to 2 hours days 1 and 2, then 500 mg/m² (maximum dose: 1,000 mg) IV over 1 to 2 hours day 3; begin within 6 hours after extravasation (Mouridsen 2007; Pérez Fidalgo 2012). Note: Reduce dexrazoxane dose by 50% in patients with moderate to severe renal impairment (CrCl <40 mL/min). Pediatrics and Adults: DMSO: Apply topically to a region covering twice the affected area every 8 hours for 7 days; begin within 10 minutes of extravasation; do not cover with a dressing (Pérez Fidalgo 2012)	Apply dry cold compress for 20 minutes 4 times/day for 1 to 2 days (Pérez Fidalgo 2012). Withhold cooling for 15 minutes before and after dexrazoxane.	If using dexrazoxane, do not use DMSO. Administer dexrazoxane through a large vein remote from area of the extravasation.
Esmolol	No known antidote	No known antidote	No recommendation	

Table 1: Vesicant Agents and Extravasation Management (continued)

Extravasated Medication	Preferred Antidote	Antidote Administration	Supportive Management	Comments
HydrOXYzine	No known antidote	No known antidote	No recommendation	**Note:** Labeled route of administration for parenteral hydroxyzine is by IM injection only; IV administration is contraindicated.
IDArubicin	Dexrazoxane or topical DMSO	Adults: Dexrazoxane 1,000 mg/m^2 (maximum dose: 2,000 mg) IV (administer in a large vein remote from site of extravasation) over 1 to 2 hours days 1 and 2, then 500 mg/m^2 (maximum dose: 1,000 mg) IV over 1 to 2 hours day 3; begin within 6 hours after extravasation (Mouridsen 2007; Pérez Fidalgo 2012). **Note:** Reduce dexrazoxane dose by 50% in patients with moderate to severe renal impairment (CrCl <40 mL/min). Pediatrics and Adults: DMSO: Apply topically to a region covering twice the affected area every 8 hours for 7 days; begin within 10 minutes of extravasation; do not cover with a dressing (Pérez Fidalgo 2012)	Apply dry cold compress for 20 minutes 4 times/day for 1 to 2 days (Pérez Fidalgo 2012). Withhold cooling for 15 minutes before and after dexrazoxane.	If using dexrazoxane, do not use DMSO. Administer dexrazoxane through a large vein remote from area of the extravasation.
Mannitol (>5%)	Hyaluronidase	Hyaluronidase: Intradermal or SubQ: Inject a total of 1 to 1.7 mL (15 units/mL) as five separate 0.2 to 0.3 mL injections (using a 25-gauge needle) into area of extravasation at the leading edge in a clockwise manner (Reynolds 2014) or SubQ: Administer multiple 0.5 to 1 mL injections of a 15 units/mL solution around the periphery of the extravasation (Kumar 2003)	Apply dry cold compresses (Reynolds 2014)	

Table 1: Vesicant Agents and Extravasation Management *(continued)*

Extravasated Medication	Preferred Antidote	Antidote Administration	Supportive Management	Comments
Mechlorethamine	Sodium Thiosulfate	Sodium thiosulfate ⅙ M solution: Inject subcutaneously into extravasation area using 2 mL for each mg of mechlorethamine suspected to have extravasated (Pérez Fidalgo 2012; Polovich 2009)	Apply ice for 6 to 12 hours after sodium thiosulfate administration (Mustargen prescribing information 2012; Polovich 2009) **or** may apply dry cold compresses for 20 minutes 4 times/day for 1 to 2 days (Pérez Fidalgo 2012)	
Metaraminol	Phentolamine	Phentolamine: Dilute 5 to 10 mg in 10 to 20 mL NS and administer into extravasation site as soon as possible after extravasation; may readminister if patient remains symptomatic (Reynolds 2014) *Alternative to phentolamine (due to shortage):* Nitroglycerin topical 2% ointment (based on limited data for other vesicants): Apply a 1-inch strip to the site of ischemia; may repeat every 8 hours as necessary (Reynolds 2014)	Apply dry warm compresses (Hurst 2004)	Not commercially available in the US
Methylene Blue	Nitroglycerin topical 2% ointment	Nitroglycerin topical 2% ointment (based on mechanism of extravasation injury): Apply a 1-inch strip on the site of ischemia; may redose every 8 hours as necessary (Reynolds 2014)	Apply dry, warm compresses (based on mechanism of extravasation injury) proximal to the injection site (Reynolds 2014)	
MitoMYcin	Topical DMSO	DMSO: Apply topically to a region covering twice the affected area every 8 hours for 7 days; begin within 10 minutes of extravasation; do not cover with a dressing (Pérez Fidalgo 2012)	Apply dry cold compress for 20 minutes 4 times/day for 1 to 2 days (Pérez Fidalgo 2012)	

Table 1: Vesicant Agents and Extravasation Management *(continued)*

Extravasated Medication	Preferred Antidote	Antidote Administration	Supportive Management	Comments
MitoXANTRONE	Dexrazoxane or topical DMSO	Adults: Dexrazoxane 1,000 mg/m² (maximum dose: 2,000 mg) IV (administer in a large vein remote from site of extravasation) over 1 to 2 hours days 1 and 2, then 500 mg/m² (maximum dose: 1,000 mg) IV over 1 to 2 hours day 3; begin within 6 hours after extravasation (Mouridsen 2007; Pérez Fidalgo 2012). **Note:** Reduce dexrazoxane dose by 50% in patients with moderate to severe renal impairment (CrCl <40 mL/min). Pediatrics and Adults: DMSO: Apply topically to a region covering the affected area every 8 hours for 7 days; begin within 10 minutes of extravasation; do not cover with a dressing (Pérez Fidalgo 2012)	Apply dry cold compress for 20 minutes 4 times/day for 1 to 2 days (Pérez Fidalgo 2012)	Irritant with vesicant-like properties (reports of both irritant and vesicant reactions). Administer dexrazoxane through a large vein remote from area of the extravasation.
Nafamostat	No known antidote	No known antidote	No recommendation	Not commercially available in the US
Nafcillin	Hyaluronidase	Hyaluronidase: Intradermal or SubQ: Inject a total of 1 to 1.7 mL (15 units/mL) as five separate 0.2 to 0.3 mL injections (using a 25-gauge needle) into area of extravasation at the leading edge in a clockwise manner (MacCara 1983; Reynolds 2014; Zenk 1981)	Apply dry cold compresses (Hurst 2004; Reynolds 2014)	

Table 1: Vesicant Agents and Extravasation Management *(continued)*

Extravasated Medication	Preferred Antidote	Antidote Administration	Supportive Management	Comments
Norepinephrine	Phentolamine	Phentolamine: Dilute 5 to 10 mg in 10 to 20 mL NS and administer into extravasation site as soon as possible after extravasation; may readminister if patient remains symptomatic (Reynolds 2014); **or** dilute 5 to 10 mg in 10 mL NS and administer into extravasation area (within 12 hours of extravasation) (Phentolamine prescribing information 2015) *Alternatives to phentolamine (due to shortage):* Nitroglycerin topical 2% ointment (based on limited data): Adults: Apply a 1-inch strip to the site of ischemia; may repeat every 8 hours as necessary (Reynolds 2014) Pediatrics: Apply 4 mm/kg as a thin ribbon to the site of ischemia; may repeat after 8 hours if needed (Wong 1992) **or** apply a 1-inch strip to the site of ischemia; may repeat every 8 hours as necessary (Denkler 1989; Reynolds 2014) Terbutaline (based on limited case reports): Infiltrate extravasation area using a solution of terbutaline 1 mg diluted in 10 mL in NS (large extravasation site; administration volume varied from 3 to 10 mL), **or** 1 mg diluted in 1 mL NS (small/distal extravasation site; administration volume varied from 0.5 to 1 mL) (Reynolds 2014; Siler 1999)	Apply dry warm compresses (Hurst 2004)	
Oxaliplatin	No known antidote	No known antidote	Information conflicts regarding use of warm or cold compresses Cold compresses could potentially precipitate or exacerbate peripheral neuropathy (de Lemos 2005)	Irritant with vesicant-like properties (reports of both irritant and vesicant reactions)

Table 1: Vesicant Agents and Extravasation Management *(continued)*

Extravasated Medication	Preferred Antidote	Antidote Administration	Supportive Management	Comments
PACLitaxel	Hyaluronidase	Hyaluronidase: *If needle/cannula still in place:* Administer 1 to 6 mL (150 units/mL) into existing IV line; usual dose is 1 mL for each 1 mL of extravasated drug; if needle/cannula has been removed, inject subcutaneously in a clockwise manner around area of extravasation; may repeat severa times over the next 3 to 4 hours (Ener 2004)	Information conflicts regarding use of warm or cold compresses	Irritant with vesicant-like properties (reports of both irritant and vesicant reactions)
Pentamidine	No known antidote	No known antidote	Dry warm compresses (Reynolds 2014)	Irritant with vesicant-like properties (reports of both irritant and vesicant reactions)
Phenylephrine	Phentolamine	Phentolamine: Dilute 5 to 10 mg in 10 to 20 mL NS and administer into extravasation site as soon as possible after extravasation; may readminister if patient remains symptomatic (Reynolds 2014) *Alternative to phentolamine (due to shortage):* Nitroglycerin topical 2% ointment (based on limited data): Adults: Apply a 1-inch strip to the site of ischemia; may repeat every 8 hours as necessary (Reynolds 2014) Pediatrics: Apply 4 mm/kg as a thin ribbon to the site of ischemia; rr ay repeat after 8 hours if needed (Wong 1992) **or** apply a 1-inch strip to the site of ischemia; may repeat every 8 hours as necessary (Denkler 1989; Reynolds 2014)	Apply dry warm compresses (Hurst 2004)	
Phenytoin	No antidote **or** Hyaluronidase	Conflicting information: Do not use antidotes (pediatrics) (Montgomery 1999) Hyaluronidase: SubQ: Inject four separate 0.2 mL injections of 15 units/mL (using a 25-gauge needle) into area of extravasation (Sokol 1998); may consider for refractory cases (Reynolds 2014)	Apply dry cold compresses (Reynolds 2014)	
Potassium Acetate (>0.1 mEq/mL)	Hyaluronidase	Hyaluronidase: Intradermal or SubQ: Inject a total of 1 to 1.7 mL (15 units/mL) as five separate 0.2 to 0.3 mL injections (using a 25-gauge needle) into area of extravasation at the leading edge in a clockwise manner (MacCara 1983; Zenk 1981)	Apply dry cold compresses (Hurst 2004; Reynolds 2014)	Reports of both irritant and vesicant reactions

Table 1: Vesicant Agents and Extravasation Management *(continued)*

Extravasated Medication	Preferred Antidote	Antidote Administration	Supportive Management	Comments
Potassium Chloride (>0.1 mEq/mL)	Hyaluronidase	Hyaluronidase: Intradermal or SubQ: Inject a total of 1 to 1.7 mL (15 units/mL) as five separate 0.2 to 0.3 mL injections (using a 25-gauge needle) into area of extravasation at the leading edge in a clockwise manner (MacCara 1983; Reynolds 2014; Zenk 1981)	Apply dry cold compresses (Hurst 2004; Reynolds 2014)	Reports of both irritant and vesicant reactions
Potassium Phosphate (may depend on concentration)	Hyaluronidase	Hyaluronidase: Intradermal or SubQ: Inject a total of 1 to 1.7 mL (15 units/mL) as five separate 0.2 to 0.3 mL injections (using a 25-gauge needle) into area of extravasation at the leading edge in a clockwise manner (MacCara 1983; Reynolds 2014; Zenk 1981)	Apply dry cold compresses (Hurst 2004; Reynolds 2014)	May be an irritant
Promethazine	No known antidote	No known antidote	Information conflicts: Apply dry cold (Hurst 2004) or dry warm compresses (Reynolds 2014)	**Note:** Preferred route of administration for promethazine is by deep intramuscular (IM) injection. If IV route is used, discontinue infusion immediately with onset of burning/pain; evaluate for inadvertent arterial injection or extravasation.
Sodium Bicarbonate (≥8.4%)	Hyaluronidase	Hyaluronidase: Intradermal or SubQ: Inject a total of 1 to 1.7 mL (15 units/mL) as five separate 0.2 to 0.3 mL injections (using a 25-gauge needle) into area of extravasation at the leading edge in a clockwise manner (Reynolds 2014)	Apply dry cold compresses (Hurst 2004; Reynolds 2014)	
Sodium Chloride (>1%)	Hyaluronidase	Hyaluronidase: Intradermal or SubQ: Inject a total of 1 to 1.7 mL (15 units/mL) as five separate 0.2 to 0.3 mL injections (using a 25-gauge needle) into area of extravasation at the leading edge in a clockwise manner (Reynolds 2014)	Apply dry cold compresses (Reynolds 2014)	
Streptozocin	No known antidote	No known antidote	No recommendation	Irritant with vesicant-like properties (reports of both irritant and vesicant reactions)

Table 1: Vesicant Agents and Extravasation Management *(continued)*

Extravasated Medication	Preferred Antidote	Antidote Administration	Supportive Management	Comments
Total Parenteral Nutrition (TPN)	Hyaluronidase	Hyaluronidase: Intradermal or SubQ: Inject a total of 1 to 1.7 mL (15 units/mL) as five separate 0.2 to 0.3 mL injections (using a 25-gauge needle) into area of extravasation at the leading edge in a clockwise manner (MacCara 1983; Reynolds 2014; Zenk 1981). May also inject hyaluronidase through catheter that caused the infiltration (Reynolds 2014) *Alternative to hyaluronidase:* Nitroglycerin topical 2% ointment: Apply a 1-inch strip on the site of ischemia; may repeat every 8 hours as necessary (Reynolds 2014)	Apply dry cold compresses (Hurst 2004; Reynolds 2014)	
Trabectedin	No known antidote	No known antidote	No recommendation	
Tromethamine	No known antidote	No known antidote	No recommendation	
Vasopressin	Nitroglycerin topical 2% ointment	Nitroglycerin topical 2% ointment (based on mechanism of extravasation injury): Adults: Apply a 1-inch strip on the site of ischemia; may repeat every 8 hours as necessary (Reynolds 2014) Pediatrics: Apply 4 mm/kg as a thin ribbon to the site of ischemia; may repeat after 8 hours if needed (Wong 1992) or apply a 1-inch strip to the site of ischemia; may repeat every 8 hours as necessary (Denkler 1989; Reynolds 2014)	Apply warm compresses (based on mechanism of extravasation injury proximal to the injection site (Reynolds 2014)	
VinBLAStine	Hyaluronidase	Hyaluronidase: *If needle/cannula still in place:* Administer 1 to 6 mL (150 units/mL) into existing IV line; usual dose is 1 mL for each 1 mL of extravasated drug (Pérez Fidalgo 2012; Schulmeister 2011) *If needle/cannula was removed:* Inject 1 to 6 mL (150 units/mL) subcutaneously in a clockwise manner using 1 mL for each 1 mL of drug extravasated (Schulmeister 2011) or administer 1 mL (150 units/mL) as five separate 0.2 mL injections (using a 25-gauge needle) into the extravasation site (Polovich 2009)	Apply dry warm compress for 20 minutes 4 times/day for 1 to 2 days (Pérez Fidalgo 2012)	

Table 1: Vesicant Agents and Extravasation Management *(continued)*

Extravasated Medication	Preferred Antidote	Antidote Administration	Supportive Management	Comments
VinCRIStine	Hyaluronidase	Hyaluronidase: *If needle/cannula still in place:* Administer 1 to 6 mL (150 units/mL) into existing IV line; usual dose is 1 mL for each 1 mL of extravasated drug (Pérez Fidalgo 2012; Schulmeister 2011) *If needle/cannula was removed:* Inject 1 to 6 mL (150 units/mL) subcutaneously in a clockwise manner using 1 mL for each 1 mL of drug extravasated (Schulmeister 2011) **or** administer 1 mL (150 units/mL) as five separate 0.2 mL injections (using a 25-gauge needle) into the extravasation site (Polovich 2009)	Apply dry warm compress for 20 minutes 4 times/day for 1 to 2 days (Pérez Fidalgo 2012)	
Vindesine	Hyaluronidase	Hyaluronidase: *If needle/cannula still in place:* Administer 1 to 6 mL (150 units/mL) into existing IV line; usual dose is 1 mL for each 1 mL of extravasated drug (Pérez Fidalgo 2012; Schulmeister 2011) *If needle/cannula was removed:* Inject 1 to 6 mL (150 units/mL) subcutaneously in a clockwise manner using 1 mL for each 1 mL of drug extravasated (Schulmeister 2011) **or** administer 1 mL (150 units/mL) as five separate 0.2 mL injections (using a 25-gauge needle) into the extravasation site (Polovich 2009)	Apply dry warm compress for 20 minutes 4 times/day for 1 to 2 days (Pérez Fidalgo 2012)	Not commercially available in the US
Vinorelbine	Hyaluronidase	Hyaluronidase: *If needle/cannula still in place:* Administer 1 to 6 mL (150 units/mL) into existing IV line; usual dose is 1 mL for each 1 mL of extravasated drug (Pérez Fidalgo 2012; Schulmeister 2011) *If needle/cannula was removed:* Inject 1 to 6 mL (150 units/mL) subcutaneously in a clockwise manner using 1 mL for each 1 mL of drug extravasated (Schulmeister 2011) **or** administer 1 mL (150 units/mL) as five separate 0.2 mL injections (using a 25-gauge needle) into the extravasation site (Polovich 2009)	Apply dry warm compress for 20 minutes 4 times/day for 1 to 2 days (Pérez Fidalgo 2012)	

◀ **SUPPORTIVE MANAGEMENT**

Compresses: Two issues for which there is less consensus are the application of warm or cold compresses and the use of various antidotes for extravasation management. A variety of recommendations exists for each of these concerns; however, there is no consensus concerning the proper approach.

Cold: Intermittent cooling of the area of extravasation results in vasoconstriction, potentially restricting the spread of the drug and decreasing the pain and inflammation in the area. Application of dry cold compresses for 20 minutes 4 times/day for 1 to 2 days is usually recommended as immediate treatment for most drug extravasations, including anthracycline, antibiotic (eg, mitomycin or dactinomycin), or alkylating agent extravasation (Pérez Fidalgo 2012). Cold dry compresses may also be utilized in the management of nonvesicant extravasations.

Warm: Application of dry warm compresses results in a localized vasodilation and increased blood flow. Increased circulation is believed to facilitate removal of the drug from the area of extravasation. Application of dry warm compresses for 20 minutes 4 times/day for 1 to 2 days is generally recommended for extravasation of vinca alkaloid, taxane, and platinum derivatives (Pérez Fidalgo 2012). Avoid moist heat. Most data are from animal studies with relatively few human case reports. Animal models indicate application of heat exacerbates the damage from anthracycline extravasations.

For some agents, such as oxaliplatin and taxanes, there are conflicting recommendations. Some reports recommend application of cold; others recommend warm.

For most vasopressors (dopamine, ephedrine, norepinephrine, and phenylephrine), dry, warm compresses may be applied (Hurst 2004). Cool compresses should be avoided with vasopressor extravasation as cooling may exacerbate vasoconstrictive effects (Reynolds 2014).

Table 2: Agents Associated With Irritation or Occasional Extravasation Reactions[a]

Acyclovir (>7 mg/mL)	Gabexate[b,c]
Arginine	Gemcitabine
Arsenic Trioxide	Ibritumomab
Bendamustine[b]	Ifosfamide
Bleomycin	Irinotecan (Conventional)
Bortezomib	Ixabepilone
Busulfan	Melphalan
CARBOplatin	MitoXANTRONE[b]
Carmustine	Oxaliplatin[b]
CISplatin (≤0.4 mg/mL)	PACLitaxel (Conventional)[b]
Cladribine	PACLitaxel (Protein Bound)
Cyclophosphamide	Pentamidine[b]
Dacarbazine	Sodium Phenylacetate and Sodium Benzoate[b]
DAUNOrubicin Citrate (Liposomal)	Streptozocin[b]

Table 2: Agents Associated With Irritation or Occasional Extravasation Reactions[a] *(continued)*

DOCEtaxel[b]	Teniposide
DOXOrubicin (Liposomal)	Thiopental[b,c]
Etoposide	Thiotepa
Etoposide Phosphate	Topotecan
Fluorouracil	Treosulfan[b,c]

[a]List may not be all-inclusive.
[b]Irritant with vesicant-like properties (there have been reports of both irritant and vesicant reactions)
[c]Not available in the US

The nurse administering the vesicant agent should monitor the patient and IV site frequently. Prior to drug administration, verify the patency of the IV line. The line should be flushed with 5 to 10 mL of a saline or dextrose solution (depending on compatibility) and the drug(s) infused through the side of a free-flowing IV line over 2 to 5 minutes. If an extravasation occurs, it is important to monitor the site closely at 24 hours, 1 week, 2 weeks, and as necessary for any signs and symptoms of extravasation.

EXTRAVASATION-SPECIFIC ANTIDOTES

Dexrazoxane: Dexrazoxane, a derivative of EDTA, is an intracellular chelating agent initially approved as a cardioprotective agent in patients receiving anthracycline therapy. It is believed that the cardioprotective effect of dexrazoxane is a result of chelating iron following intracellular hydrolysis. Dexrazoxane is not an effective chelator itself but is hydrolyzed intracellularly to an open-ring chelator form, which complexes with iron, other heavy metals, and doxorubicin complexes to inhibit the generation of free radicals. In the management of anthracycline-induced extravasation, dexrazoxane may act by reversibly inhibiting topoisomerase II, protecting tissue from anthracycline cytotoxicity, thereby decreasing tissue damage.

Dexrazoxane is administered as 3 IV infusions over 1 to 2 hours through a different venous access location: 1,000 mg/m^2 within 6 hours, 1,000 mg/m^2 after 24 hours, and 500 mg/m^2 after 48 hours of the actual extravasation up to a maximum total dose of 2,000 mg on days 1 and 2 and 1,000 mg on day 3, respectively (Mouridsen 2007). Localized cooling was permitted (except within 15 minutes before and after dexrazoxane infusion). Prior to administering dexrazoxane, discontinue DMSO as studies suggest the single agent is more effective than when used in combination with DMSO. **Note:** Reduce dexrazoxane dose by 50% in patients with moderate to severe renal impairment (CrCl <40 mL/minute).

Dimethyl sulfoxide (DMSO): Case reports and small studies have suggested that DMSO is an effective treatment for certain chemotherapy extravasations (anthracyclines, mitomycin, and mitoxantrone). DMSO has free-radical scavenger properties, which increases removal of vesicant drugs from tissues to minimize tissue damage in extravasation management (Pérez Fidalgo 2012). Common dosing is to apply topically by gently painting DMSO 50% solution onto an area twice the size of the extravasation with a saturated gauze pad or cotton swab every 8 hours for 7 days (Pérez Fidalgo 2012). Allow the site to dry. Do not cover with a dressing, as severe blistering may result. During application, DMSO may cause local erythema. Clinical reports of DMSO use are difficult to interpret due to variations in DMSO concentration (50% to 99%); the product is only commercially available in the United States at a concentration of 50% (vol/vol) solution in water.

Hyaluronidase: Hyaluronidase is an enzyme that destroys hyaluronic acid, an essential component of connective tissue. This results in increased permeability of the tissue, facilitating diffusion and absorption of fluids. It is postulated that increasing the diffusion of extravasated fluids results in more rapid absorption, thereby limiting tissue damage. In individual case reports, hyaluronidase has been reported effective in preventing tissue damage from a wide variety of agents, including vinca alkaloids, epipodophyllotoxins, and taxanes. The ESMO/EONS guidelines suggest that 150 to 900 units may be administered subcutaneously around the area of chemotherapy extravasation (Pérez Fidalgo 2012). Administration as 5 separate 0.2 mL (15 units/mL) SubQ or intradermal injections into the extravasation site has been reported (MacCara 1983). A 24-gauge or smaller needle should be used. It is recommended to use a new syringe for each injection site. If needle/cannula still in place, administration of a 1 to 6 mL hyaluronidase (150 units/mL) has been reported in the management of plant alkaloid extravasation (Pérez Fidalgo 2012; Schulmeister 2011) and paclitaxel extravasation (Ener 2004). Refer to Table 1 for vesicant-specific management.

Phentolamine: Phentolamine minimizes tissue injury due to extravasation of norepinephrine and other sympathomimetic vasoconstrictors. Inject 5 to 10 mg diluted in 10 to 20 mL normal saline and inject/infiltrate into the extravasation area; begin as soon as possible after extravasation but within 12 hours. May readminister if patient remains symptomatic.

Topical nitroglycerin or terbutaline (alternatives to phentolamine): Terbutaline and topical nitroglycerin have been used (case reports) as alternatives to phentolamine in the event of phentolamine supply shortages. Topical nitroglycerin (2% ointment) is reported to reverse the vasoconstriction at the extravasation site caused by infiltration of sympathomimetic vasoconstrictors; case reports for use in neonates/infants suggest resolution of ischemia (Denkler 1989; Wong 1992).

Sodium thiosulfate: Sodium thiosulfate ($^1/_6$ molar) has been recommended for treatment of mechlorethamine, concentrated cisplatin, and bendamustine extravasations. Sodium thiosulfate provides a substrate for alkylation by mechlorethamine, preventing the alkylation and subsequent destruction in subcutaneous tissue.

Preparation of a $^1/_6$ molar solution of sodium thiosulfate:

- Dilute 4 mL of a sodium thiosulfate 10% solution into a syringe with 6 mL of sterile water for injection, resulting in 10 mL of $^1/_6$ molar solution

  or

- Dilute 1.6 mL of a sodium thiosulfate 25% solution with 8.4 mL of sterile water for injection, resulting in 10 mL of $^1/_6$ molar solution

Inject the $^1/_6$ molar sodium thiosulfate solution either into the existing needle/cannula or subcutaneously around the edge of the extravasation site using a tuberculin syringe, using a new syringe for each injection site. The dose of sodium thiosulfate and route of administration depend on the amount of drug extravasated. Refer to Table 1 for vesicant-specific dosing.

REFERENCES

Albanell J, Baselga J. Systemic therapy emergencies. *Semin Oncol*. 2000;27(3):347-361.

Bellin MF, Jakobsen JA, Tomassin I, et al. Contrast medium extravasation injury: guidelines for prevention and management. *Eur Radiol*. 2002;12(11):2807-2812.

Bertelli G. Prevention and management of extravasation of cytotoxic drugs. *Drug Saf*. 1995;12 (4):245-255.

Boyle DM, Engelking C. Vesicant extravasation: myths and realities. *Oncol Nurs Forum*. 1995;22 (1):57-67.

de Lemos ML. Role of dimethylsulfoxide for mangement of chemotherapy extravasation. *J Oncol Pharm Practice*. 2004;10(4):197-200.

de Lemos ML, Walisser S. Management of extravasation of oxaliplatin. *J Oncol Pharm Pract*. 2005;11(4):159-162.

Denkler KA, Cohen BE. Reversal of dopamine extravasation injury with topical nitroglycerin ointment. *Plast Reconstr Surg*. 1989;84(5):811-813.

Doellman D, Hadaway L, Bowe-Geddes LA, et al. Infiltration and extravasation: update on prevention and management. *J Infus Nurs*. 2009;32(4):203-211.

Dorr RT. Antidotes to vesicant chemotherapy extravasations. *Blood Rev*. 1990;4(1):41-60.

Dorr RT, Soble M, Alberts DS. Efficacy of sodium thiosulfate as a local antidote to mechlorethamine skin toxicity in the mouse. *Cancer Chemother Pharmacol*. 1988;22(4):299-302.

Dumbarton TC, Gorman SK, Minor S, Loubani O, White F, Green R. Local cutaneous necrosis secondary to a prolonged peripheral infusion of methylene blue in vasodilatory shock. *Ann Pharmacother*. 2012;46(3):e6.

Ener RA, Meglathery SB, Styler M. Extravasation of systemic hemato-oncological therapies. *Ann Oncol*. 2004;15(6):858-862.

Hadaway L. Infiltration and extravasation. *Am J Nurs*. 2007;107(8):64-72.

Hastings-Tolsma MT, Yucha CB, Tompkins J, Robson L, Szeverenyi N. Effect of warm and cold applications on the resolution of IV infiltrations. *Res Nurs Health*. 1993;16(3):171-178.

Hurst S, McMillan M. Innovative solutions in critical care units: extravasation guidelines. *Dimens Crit Care Nurs*. 2004;23(3):125-128.

Kumar MM, Sprung J. The use of hyaluronidase to treat mannitol extravasation. *Anesth Analg*. 2003;97(4):1199-1200.

Kurul S, Saip P, Aydin T. Totally implantable venous-access ports: local problems and extravasation injury. *Lancet Oncol*. 2002;3(11):684-692.

Larson DL. Alterations in wound healing secondary to infusion injury. *Clin Plast Surg*. 1990;17 (3):509-517.

Larson DL. Treatment of tissue extravasation by antitumor agents. *Cancer*. 1982;49 (9):1796-1799.

Larson DL. What is the appropriate management of tissue extravasation by antitumor agents? *Plast Reconstr Surg*. 1985;75(3):397-405.

MacCara ME. Extravasation: a hazard of intravenous therapy. *Drug Intell Clin Pharm*. 1983;17 (10):713-717.

Montgomery LA, Hanrahan K, Kottman K, Otto A, Barrett T, Hermiston B. Guideline for IV infiltrations in pediatric patients. *Pediatr Nurs*. 1999;25(2):167-169, 173-180.

Mouridsen HT, Langer SW, Buter J, et al. Treatment of anthracycline extravasation with savene (dexrazoxane): results from two prospective clinical multicentre studies. *Ann Oncol*. 2007;18 (3):546-550.

Mustargen product information, Lundbeck, 2012

Peberdy MA, Callaway CW, Neumar RW, et al. Part 9: post-cardiac arrest care: 2010 American Heart Association guidelines for cardiopulmonary resuscitation and emergency cardiovascular care. *Circulation*. 2010;122(18 Suppl 3):S768-S786.

Pérez Fidalgo JA, García Fabregat L, Cervantes A, et al. Management of chemotherapy extravasation: ESMO-EONS clinical practice guidelines. *Ann Oncol*. 2012;23(Suppl 7): vii167-173.

Perry MC. Extravasation. *The Chemotherapy Source Book*. 4th ed. Philadelphia, PA; 2008.

Phentolamine [prescribing information]. Eatontown, NJ: West-Ward Pharmaceuticals; September 2015.

Polovich M, Whitford JN, Olsen M. *Chemotherapy and Biotherapy Guidelines and Recommendations for Practice*. 3rd ed. Pittsburgh, PA: Oncology Nursing Society; 2009.

Reynolds PM, Maclaren R, Mueller SW, Fish DN, Kiser TH. Management of extravasation injuries: a focused evaluation of noncytotoxic medications. *Pharmacotherapy*. 2014;34(6):617-632.

Rowlett J. Extravasation of contrast media managed with recombinant human hyaluronidase. *Am J Emerg Med*. 2012;30(9):2102.

Schrijvers DL. Extravasation: a dreaded complication of chemotherapy. *Ann Oncol*. 2003;14 (Suppl 3):iii26-iii30.

Schulmeister L, Camp-Sorrell D. Chemotherapy extravasation from implanted ports. *Oncol Nurs Forum*. 2000;27(3):531-538.

Schulmeister L. Extravasation management: clinical update. *Semin Oncol Nurs*. 2011;27(1):82-90.

Schulmeister L. Preventing and managing vesicant chemotherapy extravasations. *J Support Oncol*. 2010;8(5):212-215.

Shafaee MN, Salahudeen AA, Valero V. Skin necrosis after ado-trastuzumab emtansine extravasation. *J Oncol Pract*. 2017:JOP2016020198.

Sokol DK, Dahlmann A, Dunn DW. Hyaluronidase treatment for intravenous phenytoin extravasation. *J Child Neurol*. 1998;13(5):246-247.

Stanford BL, Hardwicke F. A review of clinical experience with paclitaxel extravasations. *Support Care Cancer*. 2003;11(5):270-277.

Stier PA, Bogner MP, Webster K, Leikin JB, Burda A. Use of subcutaneous terbutaline to reverse peripheral ischemia. *Am J Emerg Med*. 1999;17(1):91-94.

Wang CL, Cohan RH, Ellis JH, Adusumilli S, Dunnick NR. Frequency, management, and outcome of extravasation of nonionic iodinated contrast medium in 69,657 intravenous injections. *Radiology*. 2007;243(1):80-87.

Wiegand R, Brown J. Hyaluronidase for the management of dextrose extravasation. *Am J Emerg Med*. 2010;28(2):257.

Wong AF, McCulloch LM, Sola A. Treatment of peripheral tissue ischemia with topical nitroglycerin ointment in neonates. *J Pediatr*. 1992;121(6):980-983.

Zenk KE. Management of intravenous extravasations. *Infusion*. 1981;5(4):77-79.

MANAGEMENT OF EGFR INHIBITOR TOXICITIES: DERMATOLOGIC, OCULAR, AND GASTROINTESTINAL

BACKGROUND

Epidermal growth factor receptor inhibitor (EGFRI) therapy is used in the treatment of advanced and metastatic malignant diseases arising from epithelial tissue, such as non-small cell lung cancer, colorectal cancer, squamous cell cancer of the head and neck, pancreatic cancer, and breast cancer. The epidermal growth factor receptor (EGFR) is found on the surface of most human cells. The EGFR is a transmembrane protein belonging to the ErbB-2 (avian erythroblastosis oncogene B-like) family of membrane-bound receptor protein tyrosine kinases (EGFR/ErbB1, Her2/ErbB2, Her3/ErbB3, and Her4/ErbB4). Receptor activation is preceded by ligand binding to the extracellular domain of EGFR which facilitates dimerization of the EGFR-ligand and another EGFR or ErbB family monomer. Following dimerization, the internal tyrosine kinase domain becomes activated which generates molecular second messaging within the cell (Berlanga-Acosta 2009; Ciardiello 2008). Receptor activation yields intracellular signaling that promotes cell proliferation and inhibits apoptosis. Cellular motility is also modulated by EGFR functionality. EGFR is overexpressed and activated in many cancers that arise from epithelial tissue, making it an attractive target for anticancer therapy.

Common adverse effects from pharmacologic inhibition of EGFR generally represent perturbation of this molecule's role in the homeostasis of epithelial tissue, including skin, mucosa, hair, nails, and various other epithelial surfaces (Agero 2006; Berlanga-Acosta 2009). Effective management of adverse effects with EGFRI therapy is important to maintain optimal dose intensity of anticancer therapy and improve patient quality of life (Baas 2012). Most adverse effects attributed to EGFRI administration are mild to moderate in severity; however, the chronic nature of these side effects can become unbearable to the patient.

Commercially available EGFRI therapy includes small molecules that inhibit the EGFR intracellular protein tyrosine kinase domain (afatinib, erlotinib, gefitinib, lapatinib, neratinib, osimertinib, vandetanib) and monoclonal antibodies (cetuximab, necitumumab, panitumumab) that bind and block the external ligand binding domain.

DERMATOLOGIC TOXICITIES

Rash

Rash is the most common dermatologic adverse effect reported with EGFRI therapy. Patients may experience physical and psychosocial discomfort with EGFRI rash due to its distribution in cosmetically sensitive anatomic locations (Lacouture 2011). Dermatologic descriptions of EGFRI rash include monomorphous erythematous maculopapules, acneiform, acneiform-follicular, acne-like, sterile form of suppurative folliculitis, inflammatory follicular papules and pustules, and rosacea-like reaction (Agero 2006). The rash appearance often resembles acne vulgaris; however, it is important to recognize that the ▶

◀ pathophysiology and etiology of EGFRI rash is not the same as acne vulgaris (Agero 2006; Pérez-Soler 2005). Rash description based on anatomic location and using the phenotypic terms pustular papular rash, pustular eruption, or follicular and intrafollicular pustular eruption is recommended by experts in the field (Pérez-Soler 2005). Dry skin generally accompanies rash with EGFRI therapy (Agero 2006; Lacouture 2011). Rash severity is graded using the National Cancer Institute Common Toxicity Criteria for Adverse Events. Most cases of rash are mild to moderate in severity and cause some pain, burning, and itching (Agero 2006; Lacouture 2011). The face (specifically nose, cheeks, nasolabial folds, chin, and forehead) and areas of the upper torso are the most commonly affected locations; additional anatomic sites affected by EGFRI rash include the scalp, abdomen, buttocks, arms, and legs (Agero 2006). Rash onset is generally 7 to 21 days following initiation of therapy with maximal rash severity generally noted by weeks 3 to 5. Rash from EGFRI therapy is considered reversible; resolution generally occurs within 4 weeks following discontinuation of the causative agent (Agero 2006). Hyperpigmentation and erythema may persist for months to years in some cases (Lacouture 2011). Rash recurrence may occur with medication rechallenge. In some cases, rash resolves or waxes and wanes with continued EGFRI administration. The occurrence and severity of follicular rash is proposed as a surrogate marker for response to EGFRI therapy; findings from pharmacokinetic studies suggest that rash may be an indicator of pharmacologic activity that correlates with EGFR occupancy and blockage (Agero 2006).

A unique presentation of delayed skin toxicity attributed to EGFRI therapy is reported in 3 patients treated with erlotinib and one patient treated with vandetanib. Rash onset was several months after completion of therapy. All patients demonstrated an acneiform rash affecting the limbs and sparing the face. Severe pruritis and *Staphylococcus aureus* super infection accompanied the skin toxicity (Sibaud 2016).

Skin toxicity occurs more commonly with EGFRI monoclonal antibody administration than with the small molecule TKIs (Baas 2012; Lacouture 2011). Severe skin toxicity occurs more frequently with addition of radiotherapy (Niyazi 2011). EGFRI rash is a dose-related adverse effect, for both incidence and severity (Balagula 2011). Age may be a factor for risk of dermatologic toxicity with EGFRI therapy. Age over 70 years is a reported risk factor for skin toxicity with erlotinib therapy in patients with non-small cell lung cancer. Age under 70 years is a reported risk factor for skin toxicity with cetuximab therapy in patients with colorectal cancer (Lacouture 2011). Risk of rash with erlotinib therapy is greater in nonsmokers, which probably corresponds to increased bioavailability in this group (Balagula 2011; Lacouture 2011). Skin phenotype may modulate the severity of EGFRI rash. One retrospective analysis reported the greatest rate of serious rash with erlotinib therapy occurred in fair-skinned patients with a lower rate in medium-skinned patients and the lowest rate noted in dark-skinned patients. This study also reported similar rate of rash development throughout all four seasons with a trend towards more frequent grade 3 to 4 rashes during the winter months (Luu 2011). One study identified an increased density of *Demodex folliculorum* (DF) in skin biopsies taken from patients treated with EGFRI therapy. DF is a transparent mite that colonizes human hair follicles; increased concentrations of DF are implicated in the pathogenesis of various dermatologic diseases, including papulopustular rosacea and related conditions, pityriasis folliculorum, and blepharitis (Gerber 2011). Dermatologic toxicity with EGFRI therapy may affect the scalp and yield hair loss. Hair loss is considered a transient effect; resolution is generally expected following discontinuation of therapy. In cases of severe scalp inflammation, known as scarring alopecia, hair may not grow back. Management of scalp toxicity follows the same recommendations as general rash management (Lacouture 2011). EGFRI therapy may yield changes in hair texture, such as making it curlier, finer, or brittle.

Secondary infections at affected anatomic sites were noted in 38% of 221 patients receiving treatment for EGFRI skin toxicity. The most frequently isolated organisms were *Staphylococcus aureus* (60% of infectious diagnoses) and methicillin-resistant *Staphylococcus aureus* (14% of infectious diagnoses); less frequent infectious diagnoses included dermatophytes, *Herpes simplex*, and *Herpes zoster* (Eilers 2010). Another study isolated *Staphylococcus aureus* in 55% of cultures taken from papulopustular eruptions in patients treated with erlotinib (17 patients) or cetuximab (12 patients) (Amitay-Laish 2010). Additional serious complications attributed to dermatologic toxicity with EGFRI therapy include exfoliative dermatitis, bullous dermatitis, and rash covering >50% of the patient's body surface area (Agero 2006).

Pre-emptive therapy beginning with EGFRI initiation may be recommended due to the predictable occurrence of rash in most patients (Lacouture 2011). The Pan Canadian Rash Trial may support the use of minocycline prophylactically or as treatment at time of rash onset (Melosky 2016). The usual constituents of preventive therapy are orally administered minocycline 100 mg once daily or doxycycline 100 mg twice daily in combination with twice daily application of a topical moisturizing agent (alcohol-free, thick emollient cream), hydrocortisone 1% cream, and sunscreen (para-aminobenzoic acid-free, sun protection factor ≤15, UVA and UVB protective) (Balagula 2011; Lacouture 2011). The recommended duration of preventive therapy is 4 to 8 weeks (Lacouture 2011; Melosky 2016). The Pan Canadian Rash Trial was a randomized open-label study comparing prophylactic minocycline 100 mg twice daily for 4 weeks versus beginning treatment with minocycline at rash onset versus no treatment (until appearance of grade 3 rash) in 150 patients receiving erlotinib for non-small cell lung cancer. While the overall incidence of all grade rashes was similar in all treatment groups, the incidence of grade 3 rashes was reduced in the treatments providing minocycline therapy prophylactically or at the initial time of rash appearance. In addition, prophylactic minocycline significantly prolonged the time to the most severe grade of rash. Patients receiving prophylactic or reactive minocycline had a longer overall survival than patients receiving no treatment, but the difference was not statistically significant (Melosky 2016). Administration of oral doxycycline 100 mg twice daily in combination with the aforementioned topical therapy reduced the rate of grade 2 or greater skin toxicity by 50% during weeks 1 to 6 of panitumumab therapy relative to observation and reactive treatment. Quality of life scores were better in the group receiving preemptive skin care (Lacouture 2011). Administration of minocycline 100 mg daily during weeks 1 to 8 of cetuximab therapy reduced moderate to severe facial rash and significantly reduced moderate to severe itching (p=0.05) relative to placebo (Scope 2007). Doxycycline is preferred for patients with impaired renal function. Minocycline is considered to be less photosensitizing than other tetracyclines (Lacouture 2011). Tetracycline is not recommended for EGFRI rash prevention; a placebo-controlled trial conducted by the North Central Cancer Treatment Group demonstrated overall efficacy for this intervention to be similar to placebo (Jatoi 2008). Topical administration of tazarotene 0.05% cream did not improve skin tolerance to panitumumab therapy in a placebo-controlled trial. Moreover, one-third of patients treated with tazarotene discontinued therapy due to local irritation (Scope 2007). The topical calcineurin inhibitor pimecrolimus did not improve the severity of facial rash or patient perception of symptomatology when tested as a preventive measure with cetuximab therapy (Scope 2009). Lifestyle modifications to support skin health during EGFRI therapy include avoiding the sun, bathing with tepid water, and avoiding prolonged showering in hot water (Balagula 2011).

Treatment of EGFRI rash is based primarily on anecdotal information. The MASCC Skin Study Group recommendations include application of a moderate- to high-potency topical corticosteroid and clindamycin 1% to affected areas (Lacouture 2011). The MASCC Skin Study Group guidelines also discuss the use of systemic isotretinoin. One small noncomparative study evaluated the use of oral clindamycin (450 mg daily days 1 to 10, 300 mg daily days 11 to 20) in combination with oral isotretinoin (20 mg daily on days 11 to 20) for treatment of grade 2 to 3 rash with erlotinib therapy. Rash resolution within 14 days of beginning the intervention was reported for 6 of 7 patients (Bidoli 2010). The use of oral tretinoin (20 to 30 mg daily for 20 days; 30 to 40 mg daily) for management of EGFRI skin toxicity is also described in case reports (Gutzmer 2005; Vezzoli 2008). Systemically administered retinoids must be used cautiously because they are associated with dermatologic toxicities (mucocutaneous xerosis, desquamation, paronychia, photosensitization) and liver dysfunction (Balagula 2011). Routine use of systemic corticosteroids is discouraged due to the toxicity associated with repeated administration. Additional ancillary treatments, such as antimicrobials, should be utilized as warranted by the patient's clinical history and symptomatology.

Pruritus

Pruritus occurring with EGFRI therapy often accompanies other dermatologic adverse effects. Pruritus may develop during the first 2 weeks of treatment, although the onset of pruritus correlates with the onset of acneiform rash (Fischer 2013). Effective management of the underlying dermatologic pathology is an essential aspect of managing pruritus in these patients. Recommendations from the MASCC Skin Study Group (Lacouture 2011) include application of topical products, such as moderate- to high-potency corticosteroids, menthol 0.5%, pramoxine 1%, or doxepin creams. Topical lidocaine and topical antihistamine creams are not recommended due to the systemic absorption that occurs with these products. Systemic antihistamines can be used as warranted for symptom control; nonsedating products are preferable for patient safety. Additional agents to consider when systemic antihistamines do not provide adequate relief from pruritus include gabapentin, pregabalin, or oral doxepin. A correspondence describes two cases of refractory erlotinib-associated pruritus that were managed with oral aprepitant therapy (Vincenzi 2010). However, the use of aprepitant for EGFRI pruritus is not recommended by the MASCC Skin Study Group due to the risks of drug-drug interactions and lack of safety data for continuous administration. Patients should be instructed to treat their skin gently and wear comfortable, loose-fitting clothing.

Miscellaneous Dermatologic Adverse Effects

Other dermatologic adverse effects attributed to EGFRI administration include brittle hair, facial hirsutism, onycholysis or onychodystrophy, paronychia (nail fold inflammation), skin fissures, and tympanic membrane rupture (Garden 2012; Lee 2008). These side effects are managed as appropriate for the severity, symptomatology, and patient's clinical condition.

Ocular Adverse Effects

Ocular adverse effects attributed to EGFRI therapy are reported. The most common ocular symptoms in 45 patients presenting to an ophthalmology clinic were foreign body sensation (38%), dryness (32%), itchiness (28%), rash (22%), redness (14%), eyelash changes (12%), blurry vision (7%), tearing (6%), burning (3%), and photophobia (3%) (Borkar 2013). Many reports of ocular adverse effects were associated with cetuximab or erlotinib therapy (Borkar 2013; Cohen 2011). These are presumably an extension of the pharmacologic effect of EGFRI because EGFR is normally expressed in basal epithelial cells of the cornea and conjunctiva. EGFRI therapy can weaken the cornea, which is evidenced by corneal thinning, ulceration, melting, perforation, punctate keratitis (pinpoint distribution of epithelial damage), blepharitis, dysfunctional tear syndrome (symptoms from tear film with abnormal composition) (Borkar 2013; Saint-Jean 2012). Lower lid ectropion (outward lid orientation due to tissue weakening) is reported with erlotinib therapy (Saint-Jean 2012). Infectious keratitis with *Staphylococcus epidermidis* is attributed to a nonhealing corneal ulcer arising during chronic erlotinib administration (Johnson 2009). Corneal damage with EGFRI therapy can also be due to direct abrasion secondary to irregular eyelash growth, resulting from trichomegaly (elongation of the eyelashes) and misdirected eyelash growth (Saif 2010; Saint-Jean 2012). The median onset to trichomegaly is 12 weeks after starting therapy; however, onset may occur as early as 3 weeks to as long as 8 months after therapy initiation. Trichomegaly and other eyelash abnormalities are transient effects that resolve with discontinuation of EGFRI administration (Cohen 2011). Hypertrichosis can also affect the eyebrows; however, medical sequelae to this side effect have not been reported (Cohen 2011). Symptoms warranting prompt referral to an ophthalmologist include sustained ocular pain or loss of vision; severe eye redness or light sensitivity; lack of response within 1 week of beginning therapy for blepharitis, meibomitis, or dysfunctional tear syndrome; and misdirected eyelash growth. In addition, ophthalmologic management is indicated to rule out infection and monitor intraocular pressure when corticosteroid eye drops are utilized. Approaches to the management of EGFRI ocular toxicity are presented in the table below (Borkar 2013).

Management of EGFRI-Associated Ocular Adverse Effects (Borkar 2013)

Adverse Effect	Recommendation
Dry eyes	Mild symptoms: Supplemental ophthalmic artificial tears solution
	Moderate to severe or persistent symptoms: Refer to ophthalmologist for evaluation of tear film or concomitant contributing conditions, and for ocular anti-inflammatory medications
Blepharitis (eyelid margin inflammation); meibomitis (eyelid margin sebaceous gland inflammation)	Gentle lid scrubs and warm compress (5-minute application duration) twice daily
	Hyperemia or crust formation: Ocular neomycin-polymyxin B-dexamethasone ointment applied at bedtime for 2 weeks
	Severe or persistent hyperemia or crust formation: Oral doxycycline 50 mg twice daily for 2 weeks, followed by 50 mg once daily for 4 weeks
Trichomegaly	Refer patient to ophthalmologist for trimming and removal of excessively curled, misdirected, or irritating eyelashes

(continued)

Management of EGFRI-Associated Ocular Adverse Effects (Borkar 2013)
(continued)

Adverse Effect	Recommendation
Eyelid skin rash/hyperemia	Acute reactions: Fluorometholone 0.1% ointment applied to affected eyelid skin and margin 1 to 3 times daily for 1 week (maximum duration of 2 weeks). Ophthalmologist evaluation of intraocular pressure recommended within 4 weeks of treatment initiation.
	Chronic reactions: Tacrolimus 0.03% ointment or pimecrolimus 1% cream applied to external eyelid skin twice daily. Tacrolimus 0.1% may be used for insufficient response to lower concentration. Topical calcineurin products should be applied to the skin only; they are not formulated for administration to the eyelid margin. Maximum duration of therapy is 6 months.

Gastrointestinal Toxicities

Gastrointestinal adverse effects may arise with EGFRI therapy. Diarrhea frequently occurs and may be dose-limiting, either due to secondary complications such as dehydration or to patient intolerance. Other common side effects include stomatitis, mucositis, xerostomia, pharyngitis, dysphagia, and taste alteration (Watters 2011). Gastrointestinal perforation is an infrequent but potentially life-threatening adverse event reported with some EGFRI therapy.

Diarrhea may alter gastrointestinal integrity and affect the pharmacokinetics of oral medications, nutritional agents, and fluids. The onset of diarrhea with EGFRI administration is generally within 1 week of beginning therapy and the severity is usually mild to moderate. The duration of diarrhea may be 1 to 2 weeks or this adverse effect may persist for the duration of therapy (Loriot 2008). Diarrhea is a common dose-limiting side effect for erlotinib, gefitinib, and lapatinib (Cherny 2008; Loriot 2008). In general, diarrhea occurs more frequently with orally administered therapy than with monoclonal antibody administration (Loriot 2008). Coadministration of capecitabine, fluorouracil, or irinotecan can increase the risk and severity of diarrhea (Cherny 2008). Diarrhea associated with EGFRI therapy is presumably secretory in nature (Loriot 2008).

Loperamide is recommended as initial therapy for treatment-related diarrhea; EGFRI dose reduction may also be instituted, if appropriate (Loriot 2008). The usual dose of loperamide is 4 mg to initiate therapy, followed by 2 mg every 2 to 4 hours or following each unformed stool. Loperamide is the preferred medication for use in management of diarrhea because it is minimally absorbed from the gastrointestinal tract; however, other opioids, such as tincture of opium, codeine, and morphine, can also be used (Cherny 2008). Octreotide is useful for the management of severe or refractory diarrhea occurring with cytotoxic chemotherapy; however, the utility of this product has not been tested in the management of diarrhea from molecularly targeted anticancer therapy (Loriot 2008). Medications (eg, laxatives, antacids, stool softeners, antimicrobials) and dietary habits (eg, high fiber content, lactose-containing) that may be contributing to diarrhea should be modified whenever possible (Loriot 2008). Oral or parenteral hydration and rehydration with electrolyte repletion are essential for prevention of medical consequences of diarrhea, including dehydration and major organ dysfunction (Benson 2004; Cherny 2008). Medical conditions, such as infection or partial bowel obstruction, that may promote diarrhea should be identified and managed.

Stomatitis associated with EGFRI therapy is characterized by erythema and pain without extensive ulceration to nonkeratinized tissue. Oral ulceration becomes more prominent when EGFRI therapy is used in combination with radiotherapy or cytotoxic therapy (Watters 2011). Refer to Mucositis and Stomatitis on page 2299 for additional information about the management of stomatitis. Anorexia is common with oral EGFRI therapy; the rate of grade 3 or greater anorexia for erlotinib and gefitinib is 2% to 9%.

REFERENCES

Agero AL, Dusza SW, Benvenuto-Andrade C, Busam KJ, Myskowski P, Halpern AC. Dermatologic side effects associated with the epidermal growth factor receptor inhibitors. *J Am Acad Dermatol.* 2006;55(4):657-670.

Amitay-Laish I, David M, Stemmer SM. Staphylococcus coagulase-positive skin inflammation associated with epidermal growth factor receptor-targeted therapy: an early and a late phase of papulopustular eruptions. *Oncologist.* 2010;15(9):1002-1008.

Baas JM, Krens LL, Guchelaar HJ, et al. Recommendations on management of EGFR inhibitor-induced skin toxicity: a systematic review. *Cancer Treat Rev.* 2012;38(5):505-514.

Balagula Y, Garbe C, Myskowski PL, et al. Clinical presentation and management of dermatological toxicities of epidermal growth factor receptor inhibitors. *Int J Dermatol.* 2011;50(2):129-146.

Benson AB 3rd, Ajani JA, Catalano RB, et al. Recommended guidelines for the treatment of cancer treatment-induced diarrhea. *J Clin Oncol.* 2004;22(14):2918-2926.

Bidoli P, Cortinovis DL, Colombo I, et al. Isotretinoin plus clindamycin seem highly effective against severe erlotinib-induced skin rash in advanced non-small cell lung cancer. *J Thorac Oncol.* 2010;5(10):1662-1663.

Borkar DS, Lacouture ME, Basti S. Spectrum of ocular toxicities from epidermal growth factor receptor inhibitors and their intermediate-term follow-up: a five-year review. *Support Care Cancer.* 2013;21(4):1167-1174.

Cherny NI. Evaluation and management of treatment-related diarrhea in patients with advanced cancer: a review. *J Pain Symptom Manage.* 2008;36(4):413-423.

Ciardiello F, Tortora G. EGFR antagonists in cancer treatment. *N Engl J Med.* 2008;358(11):1160-1174.

Cohen PR, Escudier SM, Kurzrock R. Cetuximab-associated elongation of the eyelashes: case report and review of eyelash trichomegaly secondary to epidermal growth factor receptor inhibitors. *Am J Clin Dermatol.* 2011;12(1):63-67.

Eilers RE Jr, Gandhi M, Patel JD, et al. Dermatologic infections in cancer patients treated with epidermal growth factor receptor inhibitor therapy. *J Natl Cancer Inst.* 2010;102(1):47-53.

Fischer A, Rosen AC, Ensslin CJ, Wu S, Lacouture ME. Pruritus to anticancer agents targeting the EGFR, BRAF, and CTLA-4. *Dermatol Ther.* 2013;26(2):135-148.

Garden BC, Wu S, Lacouture ME. The risk of nail changes with epidermal growth factor inhibitors: a systematic review of the literature and meta-analysis. *J Am Acad Dermatol.* 2012;67(3):400-408.

Gerber PA, Kukova G, Buhren BA, Homey B. Density of *Demodex folliculorum* in patients receiving epidermal growth factor receptor inhibitors. *Dermatology.* 2011;222(2):144-147.

Gutzmer R, Werfel T, Mao R, Kapp A, Elsner J. Successful treatment with oral isotretinoin of acneiform skin lesions associated with cetuximab therapy. *Br J Dermatol.* 2005;153(4):849-851.

Jatoi A, Rowland K, Sloan JA, et al. Tetracycline to prevent epidermal growth factor receptor inhibitor-induced skin rashes: results of a placebo-controlled trial from the North Central Cancer Treatment Group (N03CB). *Cancer.* 2008;113(4):847-853.

Johnson KS, Levin F, Chu DS. Persistent corneal epithelial defect associated with erlotinib treatment. *Cornea.* 2009;28(6):706-707.

Lacouture ME, Anadkat MJ, Bensadoun RJ, et al. Clinical practice guidelines for the prevention and treatment of EGFR inhibitor-associated dermatologic toxicities. *Support Care Cancer.* 2011;19(8):1079-1095.

Lee SM, Buchler T, Joseph T, Lai C. Bilateral eardrum perforation after long-term treatment with erlotinib. *J Clin Oncol.* 2008;26(15):2582-2584.

Loriot Y, Perlemuter G, Malka D, et al. Drug insight: gastrointestinal and hepatic adverse effects of molecular-targeted agents in cancer therapy. *Nat Clin Pract Oncol.* 2008;5(5):268-278.

Luu W, Boone SL, Patel J, et al. Higher severity grade of erlotinib-induced rash is associated with lower skin phototype. *Clin Exp Dermatol.* 2011;36(7):733-738.

Melosky B, Anderson H, Burkes RL, et al. Pan Canadian Rash Trial: a randomized phase III trial evaluating the impact of a prophylactic skin treatment regimen on epidermal growth factor receptor-tyrosine kinase inhibitor-induced skin toxicities in patients with metastatic lung cancer. *J Clin Oncol.* 2016;34(8):810-815.

MANAGEMENT OF EGFR INHIBITOR TOXICITIES: DERMATOLOGIC, OCULAR, AND GASTROINTESTINAL

Niyazi M, Maihoefer C, Krause M, Rödel C, Budach W, Belka C. Radiotherapy and "new" drugs-new side effects? *Radiat Oncol*. 2011;6:177.

Pastore S, Lulli D, Girolomoni G. Epidermal growth factor receptor signalling in keratinocyte biology: implications for skin toxicity of tyrosine kinase inhibitors. *Arch Toxicol*. 2014;88(6):1189-1203.

Pérez-Soler R, Delord JP, Halpern A, et al. HER1/EGFR inhibitor-associated rash: future directions for management and investigation outcomes from the HER1/EGFR inhibitor rash management forum. *Oncologist*. 2005;10(5):345-356.

Saif MW, Gnanaraj J. Erlotinib-induced trichomegaly in a male patient with pancreatic cancer. *Cutan Ocul Toxicol*. 2010;29(1):62-66.

Saint-Jean A, Sainz de la Maza M, Morral M, et al. Ocular adverse events of systemic inhibitors of the epidermal growth factor receptor: report of 5 cases. *Ophthalmology*. 2012;119(9):1798-1802.

Scope A, Agero AL, Dusza SW, et al. Randomized double-blind trial of prophylactic oral minocycline and topical tazarotene for cetuximab-associated acne-like eruption. *J Clin Oncol*. 2007;25(34):5390-5396.

Scope A, Lieb JA, Dusza SW, et al. A prospective randomized trial of topical pimecrolimus for cetuximab-associated acnelike eruption. *J Am Acad Dermatol*. 2009;61(4):614-620.

Sibaud V, Tournier E, Roché H, Del Giudice P, Delord JP, Hubiche T. Late epidermal growth factor receptor inhibitor-related papulopustular rash: a distinct clinical entity. *Clin Exp Dermatol*. 2016;41(1):34-37.

Vezzoli P, Marzano AV, Onida F, et al. Cetuximab-induced acneiform eruption and the response to isotretinoin. *Acta Derm Venereol*. 2008;88(1):84-86.

Vincenzi B, Tonini G, Santini D. Aprepitant for erlotinib induced pruritus. *N Engl J Med*. 2010;363(4):397-398.

Voigt M, Braig F, Göthel M, et al. Functional dissection of the epidermal growth factor receptor epitopes targeted by panitumumab and cetuximab. *Neoplasia*. 2009;14(11):1023-1031.

Watters AL, Epstein JB, Agulnik M. Oral complications of targeted cancer therapies: a narrative literature review. *Oral Oncol*. 2011;47(6):441-448.

MUCOSITIS AND STOMATITIS

Mucositis and stomatitis (also known as mucosal barrier injury) are general terms for the erythema, edema, desquamation, and ulceration of the gastrointestinal tract caused by many antineoplastic drugs and external beam radiation therapy (radiotherapy). Stomatitis refers to the finding of mucositis in the mouth or oropharynx. Gastrointestinal complications of mucositis include pain, xerostomia, bloating, diarrhea, malabsorption, and dysmotility. Airway compromise can develop from severe tissue damage and inflammation. Mucositis is defined as severe (grade 3 to 4) when the pain and anatomic damage prevent adequate oral hydration and oral nutrition, or airway compromise is evident (Table 1). Severe mucositis increases the risk of infectious complications. Moreover, some opportunistic infections, such as herpesvirus, cause and exacerbate mucositis. In addition, severe and prolonged mucositis contributes to anticancer treatment dosage reductions and delays, and increases the cost of therapy.

Table 1. National Cancer Institute (NCI) Common Toxicity Criteria Grading for Mucositis and Associated Adverse Events

Grade 0	Grade 1	Grade 2	Grade 3	Grade 4
No signs or symptoms	v3: Mucosal erythema v4: Asymptomatic or mild symptoms; intervention not indicated	v3: Patchy ulcerations v4: Moderate pain; not interfering with oral intake; modified diet indicated	v3: Confluent ulceration, bleeding with minor trauma v4: Severe pain; interfering with oral intake	v3: Tissue necrosis/ bleeding; life-threatening v4: Life-threatening consequences; urgent intervention indicated

The severity of chemotherapy-associated mucositis is related to drug selection, increased dose amount, combination versus single agent chemotherapy, administration rate (eg, extended infusion of cell cycle-specific chemotherapy drugs), route of administration, concurrent radiotherapy, and female gender. A survey of 696 patients with advanced cancer determined that the diagnoses most associated with mucositis were head and neck cancer, lung cancer, brain cancer, gastrointestinal cancer, and prostate cancer (Mercadante 2015). Genetic polymorphisms and comorbidities (eg, malnutrition) may also contribute to the risk for mucositis. The frequency of severe mucositis for patients undergoing standard dose therapy and high dose therapy is 5% to 40% and 60% to 100%, respectively. Major organ impairment that prolongs the clearance of anticancer treatments can increase the likelihood and severity of mucositis. Patients with Down syndrome or carriers of the methylenetetrahydrofolate reductase *677 TT* genotype have an increased risk of severe mucositis following methotrexate administration. The severity of mucositis secondary to radiotherapy is related to the anatomic site of radiation exposure, radiation dose, and dosage fractionation. Grade 3 to 4 mucositis occurs in more than 50% of patients undergoing radiotherapy to the head and neck, abdomen, or pelvis. Table 2 lists various anticancer treatments associated with severe mucositis. The duration and severity of regimen-related mucositis can be increased by concurrent infections from opportunistic bacterial or viral pathogens affecting the gastrointestinal tract. Moreover, graft-versus-host disease can worsen regimen-related mucositis following allogeneic hematopoietic stem cell transplantation.

Table 2. Standard Dose Regimens Associated With Grade 3 to 4 Mucositis

Occurring in ≥30% of Patients	Occurring in ≥10% of Patients
Anthracycline + docetaxel + fluorouracil	Anthracycline + cyclophosphamide
Taxane + radiotherapy	Anthracycline + taxane
Docetaxel + fluorouracil	Anthracycline + cyclophosphamide +
Paclitaxel + fluorouracil + radiotherapy	docetaxel
Taxane + platinum + radiotherapy	Anthracycline + cyclophosphamide +
Taxane + platinum + fluorouracil	paclitaxel
Oxaliplatin + radiotherapy	Anthracycline + docetaxel + platinum
Platinum + taxane + radiotherapy	Capecitabine + docetaxel
Fluorouracil CIV[a] + platinum + radiotherapy	Docetaxel
Fluorouracil + leucovorin + taxane	Platinum + radiotherapy
Irinotecan	Platinum + gemcitabine + taxane
Irinotecan + fluorouracil + radiotherapy	Platinum + taxane + irinotecan
Irinotecan + fluorouracil + leucovorin	Platinum + methotrexate + leucovorin
Irinotecan + fluorouracil + leucovorin +	Fluorouracil CIV[a]
platinum	Fluorouracil CIV[a] + radiotherapy
	Fluorouracil CIV[a] + platinum
	Fluorouracil + leucovorin
	Fluorouracil + leucovorin + mitomycin
	Irinotecan + taxane
	PRALAtrexate

[a]CIV, continuous intravenous infusion; adapted from Sonis ST, Elting LS, Keefe D, et al. Perspectives on cancer therapy-induced mucosal injury: pathogenesis, measurement, epidemiology, and consequences for patients. *Cancer.* 2004;100(9 Suppl):1995-2025.

MUCOSITIS PREVENTION AND TREATMENT

Evidence-based clinical practice guidelines for management of regimen-related mucositis have been published by the Mucositis Study Group of the Multinational Association of Supportive Care in Cancer and International Society of Oral Oncology (MASCC/ISOO). Recommendations and suggestions from the Mucositis Study Group for and against specific interventions in the management of oral mucositis are presented in Table 3 and Table 4, respectively (Lalla 2014). Recommendations and suggestions for and against specific interventions in the management of gastrointestinal mucositis are presented in Table 7 and Table 8, respectively (Lalla 2014).

Table 3. MASCC/ISOO Oral Mucositis Recommended Interventions

Recommendations supported by level I and II evidence
1. Oral cryotherapy (30 minutes) for prevention of oral mucositis in patients receiving bolus fluorouracil chemotherapy
2. Palifermin to prevent oral mucositis for patients receiving high-dose chemotherapy and total body irradiation, followed by autologous hematopoietic stem cell transplantation (HSCT) for a hematological malignancy
3. Low-level laser therapy to prevent oral mucositis for patients receiving high-dose chemotherapy, (with or without total body irradiation) for HSCT
4. Patient-controlled analgesia using morphine for management of pain due to oral mucositis in patients undergoing HSCT
5. Benzydamine mouthwash to prevent oral mucositis for patients with head and neck cancer receiving moderate-dose radiation therapy (up to 50 Gy) without concomitant chemotherapy (benzydamine is available in Canada; not approved in the US)

(continued)

Table 3. MASCC/ISOO Oral Mucositis Recommended Interventions
(continued)

Suggestions supported by level III and IV evidence
1. Oral care procedures for prevention of oral mucositis in all age groups and across all cancer treatment settings
2. Oral cryotherapy to prevent oral mucositis for patients receiving high-dose melphalan, with or without total body irradiation, prior to HSCT
3. Low-level laser therapy to prevent oral mucositis for patients undergoing radiotherapy, without concomitant chemotherapy, for head and neck cancer
4. Transdermal fentanyl may be effective to treat pain due to oral mucositis in patients receiving conventional or high-dose chemotherapy, with or without total body irradiation   * The patient's opioid tolerance and expected duration of moderate to severe pain must be considered prior to use of transdermal fentanyl.
5. Morphine 2% mouthwash may be effective to treat pain due to oral mucositis in patients receiving chemoradiation for head and neck cancer.
6. Doxepin 0.5% mouthwash may be effective to treat pain due to oral mucositis.
7. Systemic zinc supplements administered orally may be used to prevent oral mucositis in oral cancer patients receiving radiation therapy or chemoradiation.

Good oral hygiene is an essential constituent of routine supportive care for stomatitis and mucositis. Regular, gentle brushing with a soft toothbrush or cotton swab several times a day is helpful in removing dental plaque. Rinsing the mouth with water rinses or a saline/bicarbonate solution helps remove debris and increases the pH, slowing the growth of oral flora. Use of mouthwashes containing alcohol may be painful or may dry the oral mucosa; phenol may promote mucosal ulceration.

Guidelines from the European Society of Medical Oncology (ESMO) on management of oral and gastrointestinal mucosal injury (Peterson 2015) also recommend eliminating sources of oral mucosal trauma (eg, sharp edges or ill-fitting dentures), avoiding hot foods and drinks, and avoiding hard, sharp/crusty, or spicy foods. The ESMO guidelines also recommend regular dental examinations, daily oral mucosa inspections, adequate hydration, and lip balm. Smoking and alcohol should be avoided.

Palifermin is a recombinant human keratinocyte growth factor that works in a receptor-mediated manner to reduce the duration and severity of mucositis by promoting epithelial cell proliferation, differentiation, and migration. Palifermin is indicated to decrease the incidence and duration of severe oral mucositis in patients with hematologic malignancies receiving myelotoxic therapy requiring hematopoietic stem cell support. The 2008 American Society of Clinical Oncology (ASCO) guidelines for the use of chemotherapy and radiotherapy protectants recommend palifermin to decrease the incidence of severe mucositis in patients undergoing autologous stem-cell transplantation with a total body irradiation (TBI) conditioning regimen. Additionally, palifermin may be considered in patients undergoing myeloablative allogeneic stem-cell transplantation with a TBI conditioning regimen. (Goldberg 2013; Hensley 2009). Data are insufficient however, for autologous and allogeneic transplant, to recommend palifermin when the conditioning regimen is chemotherapy only (Hensley 2009). The manufacturer instructs against use of palifermin in patients receiving melphalan 200 mg/m² as a conditioning regimen prior to autologous hematopoietic stem cell transplantation due to a lack of efficacy demonstrated in a placebo-controlled trial. The labeled dose for palifermin is 60 mcg/kg/day IV for 3 doses prior to myelotoxic therapy, with the third dose given at least 24 hours before the chemotherapy and then 60 mcg/kg/day for 3 doses after myelotoxic therapy beginning on the same day as hematopoietic stem cell infusion.

Weekly administration of palifermin for reduction of mucositis secondary to chemoradiotherapy for head and neck cancer was tested in two randomized, double-blind, placebo-controlled clinical trials (Henke 2011; Le 2011). In both studies, palifermin administration reduced the incidence, time to onset, and duration of severe mucositis. However, in both studies, patient reported mouth soreness scores and interruptions in therapy were similar for palifermin- and placebo-treated cohorts. Overall survival and disease response were similar for the palifermin- and placebo-treated patients. An exploratory phase II trial testing weekly palifermin versus placebo to reduce dysphagia with chemoradiotherapy for stage III non-small cell lung cancer suggests decreased regimen-related toxicity and improved dose intensity with palifermin administration (Schuette 2012). Single-dose palifermin prior to doxorubicin-based chemotherapy for the treatment of soft tissue sarcoma reduced patient-reported symptoms of oral mucositis (Vandhan-Raj 2010).

Administration of palifermin concurrently with chemotherapy can cause increased severity of mucositis because epithelial cells are stimulated to proliferate when exposed to the systemic cytotoxic therapy. Precautions from the manufacturer include the lack of safety and efficacy data in patients with solid tumors. The effect of palifermin on tumor growth in patients has not been established; however, palifermin promotes in vitro and in vivo epithelial tumor growth in experimental models.

Amifostine has been studied for reduction of chemotherapy-associated mucositis; however, the findings are equivocal. Due to insufficient data, the ASCO guidelines for the use of chemotherapy and radiotherapy protectants do not recommend amifostine to reduce the incidence of radiation therapy-induced mucositis associated with head and neck cancer or to prevent esophagitis due to concurrent chemoradiotherapy in patients with non-small cell lung cancer. Amifostine use to prevent xerostomia in patients with head and neck cancer receiving concurrent platinum-based chemotherapy is not supported; however, the guidelines suggest that the use of amifostine may be considered to reduce the incidence of xerostomia in patients with head and neck cancer undergoing radiation therapy alone (Hensley 2009).

Uridine triacetate is an orally administered antidote for fluorouracil- or capecitabine-induced early onset severe or life-threatening adverse effects or overdosage. It is important to acknowledge that uridine triacetate has not been tested for modulation of fluorouracil or capecitabine toxicity for patients receiving standard chemotherapy doses who do not exhibit early onset severe or life-threatening adverse effects. The side effect profile of uridine triacetate is favorable (generally mild to moderate vomiting [10%], nausea [5%], diarrhea [3%]); however, the product acquisition cost is noteworthy. Uridine triacetate was approved for commercial use based on a 96% survival rate for 135 patients receiving treatment for fluorouracil and capecitebine early onset severe or life-threatening adverse effects (n=117) or overdosage (n=18). The mortality rate in 25 historical controls who received best supportive care following a fluorouracil overdose was 84%. A published study presenting the same population expanded to 147 patients (plus the same 25 historical controls) reports a similar rate of survival and prevention of mucositis and leukopenia (Ma 2017). The product labeling instructs initiation of uridine triacetate therapy within 96 hours of fluorouracil or capecitabine overdose/overexposure. Antidote efficacy is reduced when uridine triacetate is initiated more than 96 hours following the last fluoropyrimidine dose (Ma 2017).

Some clinical trials report reduced mucositis with prophylactic administration of oral glutamine. A common dosage of glutamine is 10 g three times daily (30 g/day) using powdered glutamine mixed with food or beverage. Oral glutamine appears to be generally well tolerated. It should be noted that most clinical trials evaluating the efficacy of oral glutamine for reduction in regimen-related mucositis were small in numbers of patients evaluated and did not use a placebo control; additional data is necessary to further define the role of oral glutamine for mucositis (Sayles 2016).

Regular gum chewing by pediatric patients to promote salivation as a means for preventing chemotherapy-induced mucositis did not reduce the rate of severe stomatitis following administration of intensive treatment regimens. However, the frequency of grades 1 to 4 stomatitis was significantly reduced with gum chewing five times daily with lower intensity chemotherapy regimens. In the multivariate analysis, the risk of oral mucositis was related only to the type of chemotherapy regimen used. There is lack of sufficient evidence to support routine use of celecoxib, vitamin E, or allopurinol rinse for prevention of mucositis.

Cryotherapy reduces oral mucositis associated with intravenous bolus administration of fluorouracil, methotrexate, and high-dose melphalan. Cryotherapy requires that the patient hold ice in their mouth for 30 to 60 minutes before and following chemotherapy administration. Cryotherapy purportedly reduces local oromucosal blood flow and consequently reduces chemotherapy exposure to the affected area. Patient tolerance limits the duration of cryotherapy treatments and reduces the utility of cryotherapy for chemotherapy with prolonged systemic clearance or drugs administered by protracted continuous infusion.

MUCOSITIS OR STOMATITIS DUE TO TARGETED AGENTS

Oral care for patients taking targeted agents should align with basic oral care for mucositis due to standard chemotherapy. Due to the risk for infections, saline mouth rinses are recommended for these patients (Peterson 2015).

Table 4. Interventions NOT Recommended by MASCC/ISOO for Oral Mucositis

Lack of efficacy supported by level I and II evidence
1. PTA (polymyxin, tobramycin, amphotericin B) and BCoG (bacitracin, clotrimazole, gentamicin) antimicrobial lozenges and PTA paste are not recommended in patients receiving radiation therapy for head and neck cancer.
2. Iseganan antimicrobial mouthwash is not recommended in patients receiving high-dose chemotherapy (with or without total body irradiation) for HSCT or in patients receiving radiation therapy or concomitant chemoradiation for head and neck cancer.
3. Sucralfate mouthwash is not recommended for prevention of oral mucositis in patients receiving chemotherapy for cancer or in patients receiving radiation therapy or chemoradiotherapy for head and neck cancer.
4. Sucralfate mouthwash is not recommended for treatment of oral mucositis in patients receiving chemotherapy for cancer or in patients receiving radiation therapy for head and neck cancer.
5. Intravenous glutamine is not recommended for prevention of oral mucositis in patients receiving high-dose chemotherapy (with or without total body irradiation) for HSCT.

(continued)

◄ **Table 4. Interventions NOT Recommended by MASCC/ISOO for Oral Mucositis** *(continued)*

Lack of efficacy supported by level III and IV evidence
1. Chlorhexidine mouthwash is not recommended for prevention of oral mucositis in patients receiving radiation therapy for head and neck cancer.
2. Sargramostim (GM-CSF) mouthwash is not recommended for prevention of oral mucositis in patients receiving high-dose chemotherapy for autologous or allogeneic HSCT.
3. Misoprostol mouthwash is not recommended for prevention of oral mucositis in patients receiving radiation therapy for head and neck cancer.
4. Systemic pentoxifylline, administered orally, is not recommended for prevention of oral mucositis in patients undergoing bone marrow transplantation.
5. Systemic pilocarpine, administered orally, is not recommended for prevention of oral mucositis in patients receiving radiation therapy for head and neck cancer or in patients receiving high-dose chemotherapy (with or without total body irradiation) for HSCT.

Therapy of stomatitis consists primarily of symptomatic support.

Pain control is a crucial part of stomatitis therapy. In addition to making the patient more comfortable, adequate pain control allows the patient to communicate and eat normally, thereby improving quality of life and reducing nutritional complications. Opioid analgesia is frequently required for management of moderate to severe pain from mucositis. Gabapentin may be useful as an adjunct to opioid therapy when additional analgesia is warranted (Bar 2010). Topical application of local anesthetics is the most common approach to management of mild to moderate pain from stomatitis. Local application of cold sometimes provides adequate relief. Diphenhydramine has been used, but may cause drying of local tissues and sedation. Most products also contain significant amounts of alcohol which can exacerbate symptomatology. Local anesthetics (eg, benzocaine, lidocaine, tetracaine) are more potent than diphenhydramine, and are not associated with significant drying of local tissues. However, the numbing effect of these agents can impair swallowing. In addition, most of these products are unpalatable, and some are relatively expensive. The following table lists some of the commonly used agents.

Table 5. Various Mouth Care Products

Product	Concentration(s)	Dosage
<u>Anesthetics</u>		
Benzocaine	5% to 20%	1 to 5 mL; swish and expectorate every 4 to 6 hours
DiphenhydrAMINE	12.5 mg per 5 mL	5 mL; swish and expectorate (or swallow) every 4 to 6 hours
Lidocaine	1%	5 mL; swish and expectorate (or swallow) every 2 to 3 hours
<u>Antimicrobials</u>		
Amphotericin B	100 mg/mL	1 mL qid; swish in mouth as long as possible; swallow or expectorate
Clotrimazole	10 mg	1 troche tid (prophylaxis)
		One 5 times/day for 14 days (treatment)
Nystatin	100,000 units/mL	5 mL; swish and expectorate (or swallow) every 4 to 6 hours
	100,000 units (vaginal tablet)	1 every 4 to 6 hours (dissolve in mouth)

(continued)

Table 5. Various Mouth Care Products *(continued)*

Product	Concentration(s)	Dosage
Mouth Rinses		
Sodium bicarbonate (8.4 g per 50 mEq per 0.9% NaCl [1,000 mL] mixture)	0.5 mEq per 10 mL	5 to 15 mL every 3 to 4 hours
Sodium chloride	0.9%	5 to 15 mL every 3 to 4 hours

Many institutions and prescribers use locally compounded anesthetic formulations for treatment of stomatitis pain. Although the exact formulae may vary tremendously, the general rubric includes a local anesthetic to which one or more of the following are added: A second anesthetic, aluminum hydroxide/magnesium hydroxide suspension, diphenhydramine, hydrocortisone, kaolin/pectin suspension, sucralfate suspension, nystatin, tetracycline, and/or water. Controlled trials comparing various formulations with each other, or with the various individual ingredients are not available. However, these products often form the mainstay of symptomatic treatment for stomatitis. Examples of recipes for a few such formulations are found in Table 6.

A number of groups have studied sucralfate as a therapy for various oral ulcerative conditions with equivocal results. Although the results published to date do not demonstrate a real advantage to sucralfate therapy, some patients may experience subjective benefit from its use. Sucralfate is commercially available as a tablet (1 g) or suspension (1 g per 10 mL). When placed into water, the tablet readily absorbs the fluid and forms a gelatinous suspension.

Table 6. Examples of Extemporaneously Compounded Oral Stomatitis Products

Anesthetics

Diphenhydramine syrup 5 mL + lidocaine 2% 5 to 10 mL + aluminum/magnesium hydroxide suspension 5 to 15 mL (Maalox/Mylanta) (may also be referred to as "BMX"). **Note:** Avoid diphenhydramine products containing alcohol.

Lidocaine 2% 45 mL + diphenhydramine elixir 30 mL + sodium bicarbonate 8.4 g + 0.9% sodium chloride qs 1,000 mL

Intubation: Nondepolarizing neuromuscular blockade should be used for the patient with severe mucositis requiring intubation to support the airway. One case report describes succinylcholine-induced hyperkalemia in a patient with severe mucositis following treatment chemotherapy.

Xerostomia

Xerostomia often accompanies stomatitis, particularly in patients who have received radiation to the neck and lower jaw. The condition can result in severe pain, dysphagia, malnutrition, and secondary infections. Subcutaneous or intravenous push administration of amifostine 200 mg/m^2 15 to 30 minutes prior to radiotherapy of the head and neck reduces acute and chronic xerostomia. The dose of amifostine for reduction of radiation-associated xerostomia and mucositis can be standardized to 500 mg in 0.9% sodium chloride 2.5 mL. Benzydamine oral rinse (not available in the United States), which has local anesthetic and anti-inflammatory properties, may be used for the prevention of radiation-induced mucositis in head and neck cancer patients. Artificial saliva substitutes can provide symptomatic relief from dry mouth and throat discomfort following chemotherapy and radiotherapy. Saliva substitutes, which generally contain a mixture of electrolytes, sugar(s), and carboxymethylcellulose, are available without a prescription.

Infections

In spite of good oral hygiene, some patients develop oral infections. This is particularly common in the patient with additional sources of immunosuppression, such as severe neutropenia, treatment with exogenous immunosuppressants, or disease-related immune impairment. One organism most commonly seen in such infections is *Candida albicans*. Topical treatment with nystatin or clotrimazole is usually sufficient to control these infections. Such treatments are usually well tolerated and produce minimal systemic effects. Nystatin 400,000 to 600,000 units (4 to 6 mL) four times a day, swished in the mouth for at least 2 minutes, then swallowed is recommended. Alternatively, nystatin vaginal tablets can be used orally. Clotrimazole 10 mg five times a day is another effective treatment for these infections. Troches are placed under the tongue or in a buccal cavity and allowed to dissolve. In some patients, clotrimazole used three times a day is an effective prophylaxis against oral *Candida* infections. Patients with significant xerostomia may have trouble dissolving the nystatin or clotrimazole tablets, and may require an artificial saliva product to moisten the mouth. Oral or intravenous administration of fluconazole 100 to 200 mg daily may be necessary for treatment of microbiologically documented or presumed oromucosal candidiasis in the patient with moderate to severe mucositis extending proximally beyond the mouth or the patient with additional sources of immune suppression. Fluconazole should be continued for at least 2 weeks, and until microbiologic and clinical evidence of infectious disease have resolved and the patient's immune recovery is considered adequate. Alternative systemic antifungal agents that can be considered for treatment of oromucosal and esophageal candidiasis include anidulafungin, caspofungin, itraconazole, micafungin, posaconazole, voriconazole, and amphotericin B products. Mean absorption and area under the curve are reduced ~10% when isavuconazole is administered orally to patients with mucositis; however, this effect is not expected to negatively impact the efficacy or safety of antifungal therapy (Kovanda 2017). Based on a pharmacokinetic study, the use of oral tablets is preferred to oral suspension for posaconazole treatment in patients with mucositis due to the demonstrated degree of difference in systemic absorption (Vanstraelen 2016).

Herpes simplex virus is another common pathogen causing oral and other gastrointestinal infections in the patient with moderate to severe mucositis. The risk for oral Herpes simplex infection is greatest in patients with an additional source of immune compromise. Systemic treatment with acyclovir, famciclovir, or valacyclovir is required for oromucosal or gastrointestinal Herpes simplex infection. Alternative systemic antiviral agents for treatment of resistant Herpes simplex infections include ganciclovir, valganciclovir, and foscarnet.

Gastrointestinal Mucositis

Symptoms of gastrointestinal mucositis include pain, nausea, vomiting, and diarrhea. The following are recommendations/suggestions for and against specific interventions in the management of gastrointestinal mucositis (Lalla 2014).

Table 7. MASCC/ISOO Gastrointestinal Mucositis (Not Including the Oral Cavity) Recommended Interventions

Recommendations supported by level I and II evidence
1. Intravenous amifostine ($\geq$340 mg/m^2) is recommended to prevent proctitis in patients receiving radiation treatment
2. Subcutaneous octreotide ($\geq$100 mcg twice daily) is recommended to treat chemotherapy-induced diarrhea associated with HSCT (if loperamide is ineffective)

Suggestions supported by level III and IV evidence
1. Intravenous amifostine may be used to prevent esophagitis due to concomitant chemotherapy and radiation therapy in patients with non-small cell lung cancer
2. Sucralfate enemas may be used to treat chronic radiation-induced proctitis in patients with rectal bleeding
3. Systemic sulfasalazine (500 mg orally twice daily) may be used to prevent radiation-induced enteropathy in patients receiving radiation therapy to the pelvis
4. Probiotics containing *Lactobacillus* species may be used to prevent diarrhea in patients receiving chemotherapy and/or radiation therapy for a pelvic malignancy
5. Hyperbaric oxygen may be used to treat radiation-induced proctitis in patients receiving radiation therapy for solid tumors

Table 8. Interventions NOT Recommended by MASCC/ISOO for Gastrointestinal Mucositis

Lack of efficacy supported by level I and II evidence
1. Systemic oral sucralfate is not recommended to treat gastrointestinal mucositis in patients receiving radiation therapy for a solid tumor
2. Oral aspirin (ASA), mesalazine, and olsalazine are not recommended to prevent acute radiation-induced diarrhea in patients receiving radiation therapy for a pelvic malignancy
3. Misoprostol suppositories are not recommended to prevent acute radiation-induced proctitis in patients receiving radiation therapy for prostate cancer

REFERENCES AND SELECTED READINGS

Aisa Y, Mori T, Kudo M, et al. Oral cryotherapy for the prevention of high-dose melphalan-induced stomatitis in allogeneic hematopoietic stem cell transplant recipients. *Support Care Cancer.* 2005;13(4):266-269.

Al-Khafaji AH, Dewhirst WE, Cornell CJ Jr, Quill TJ. Succinylcholine-induced hyperkalemia in a patient with mucositis secondary to chemotherapy. *Crit Care Med.* 2001;29(6):1274-1276.

Alterio D, Jereczek-Fossa BA, Zuccotti GF, et al. Tetracaine oral gel in patients treated with radiotherapy for head-and-neck cancer: final results of a phase II study. *Int J Radiat Oncol Biol Phys.* 2006;64(2):392-395.

Bar Ad V, Weinstein G, Dutta PR, Chalian A, Both S, Quon H. Gabapentin for the treatment of pain related to radiation-induced mucositis in patients with head and neck tumors treated with intensity-modulated radiation therapy. *Head Neck.* 2010;32(2):173-177.

Chan A, Ignoffo RJ. Survey of topical oral solutions for the treatment of chemo-induced oral mucositis. *J Oncol Pharm Pract.* 2005;11(4):139-143.

El-Housseiny AA, Saleh SM, El-Masry AA, Allam AA. The effectiveness of vitamin "E" in the treatment of oral mucositis in children receiving chemotherapy. *J Clin Pediatr Dent.* 2007;31(3):167-170.

Gandemer V, Le Deley MC, Dollfus C, et al. Multicenter randomized trial of chewing gum for preventing oral mucositis in children receiving chemotherapy. *J Pediatr Hematol Oncol.* 2007;29(2):86-94.

Garre ML, Relling MV, Kalwinsky D, et al. Pharmacokinetics and toxicity of methotrexate in children with down syndrome and acute lymphocytic leukemia. *J Pediatr.* 1987;111(4):606-612.

Goldberg JD, Zheng J, Castro-Malaspina H, et al. Palifermin is efficacious in recipients of TBI-based but not chemotherapy-based allogeneic hematopoietic stem cell transplants. *Bone Marrow Transplant.* 2013;48(1):99-104.

Gori E, Arpinati M, Bonifazi F, et al. Cryotherapy in the prevention of oral mucositis in patients receiving low-dose methotrexate following myeloablative allogeneic stem cell transplantation: a prospective randomized study of the Gruppo Italiano Trapianto Di Midollo Osseo Nurses group. *Bone Marrow Transplant.* 2007;39(6):347-352.

Henke M, Alfonsi M, Foa P, et al. Palifermin decreases severe oral mucositis of patients undergoing postoperative radiochemotherapy for head and neck cancer: a randomized, placebo-controlled trial. *J Clin Oncol.* 2011;29(20):2815-2820.

Hensley ML, Hagerty KL, Kewalramani T, et al. American Society of Clinical Oncology 2008 clinical practice guideline update: use of chemotherapy and radiotherapy protectants. *J Clin Oncol.* 2009;27(1):127-145.

Javle MM, Cao S, Durrani FA, et al. Celecoxib and mucosal protection: translation from an animal model to a phase I clinical trial of celecoxib, irinotecan, and 5-fluorouracil. *Clin Cancer Res.* 2007;13(3):965-971.

Kepivance (palifermin) [prescribing information]. Stockholm, Sweden: Swedish Orphan Biovitrum; May 2013.

Kovanda LL, Marty FM, Maertens J, et al. Impact of mucositis on absorption and systemic drug exposure of isavuconazole. *Antimicrob Agents Chemother.* 2017;61(6).

Lalla RV, Bowen J, Barasch A, et al. MASCC/ISOO clinical practice guidelines for the management of mucositis secondary to cancer therapy. *Cancer.* 2014;120(10):1453-1461.

Le QT, Kim HE, Schneider CJ, et al. Palifermin reduces severe mucositis in definitive chemo-radiotherapy of locally advanced head and neck cancer: a randomized, placebo-controlled study. *J Clin Oncol.* 2011;29(20):2808-2814.

Lilleby K, Garcia P, Gooley T, et al. A prospective, randomized study of cryotherapy during administration of high-dose melphalan to decrease the severity and duration of oral mucositis in patients with multiple myeloma undergoing autologous peripheral blood stem cell transplantation. *Bone Marrow Transplant.* 2006;37(11):1031-1035.

Ma WW, Saif MW, El-Rayes BF, et al. Emergency use of uridine triacetate for the prevention and treatment of life-threatening 5-fluorouracil and capecitabine toxicity. *Cancer.* 2017;123 (2):345-356.

Mercadante S, Aielli F, Adile C, et al. Prevalence of oral mucositis, dry mouth, and dysphagia in advanced cancer patients. *Support Care Cancer.* 2015;23(11):3249-3255.

Mori T, Yamazaki R, Aisa Y, et al. Brief oral cryotherapy for the prevention of high-dose melphalan-induced stomatitis in allogeneic hematopoietic stem cell transplant recipients. *Support Care Cancer.* 2006;14(4):392-396.

National Cancer Institute common terminology criteria for adverse events (CTCAE) version 3. Available at http://ctep.cancer.gov/protocolDevelopment/electronic_applications/docs/ctcaev3.pdf. Accessed October 13, 2014.

National Cancer Institute common terminology criteria for adverse events (CTCAE) version 4.03. Available at http://evs.nci.nih.gov/ftp1/CTCAE/CTCAE_4.03_2010-06-14_QuickReference_8.5x11.pdf. Accessed September 29, 2014.

Peterson DE, Boers-Doets CB, Bensadoun RJ, Herrstedt J; ESMO Guidelines Committee. Management of oral and gastrointestinal mucosal injury: ESMO Clinical Practice Guidelines for diagnosis, treatment, and follow-up. *Ann Oncol.* 2015;26(Suppl 5):v139-v151.

Potting CM, Uitterhoeve R, Op Reimer WS, Van Achterberg T. The effectiveness of commonly used mouthwashes for the prevention of chemotherapy-induced oral mucositis: a systematic review. *Eur J Cancer Care (Engl).* 2006;15(5):431-439.

Quintiliani R, Owens NJ, Quercia RA, Klimek JJ, Nightingale CH. Treatment and prevention of oropharyngeal candidiasis. *Am J Med.* 1984;77(4D):44-48.

Sayles C, Hickerson SC, Bhat RR, Hall J, Garey KW, Trivedi MV. Oral glutamine in preventing treatment-related mucositis in adult patients with cancer: a systematic review. *Nutr Clin Pract.* 2016;31(2):171-179.

Schuette W, Krzakowski MJ, Massuti B, et al. Randomized phase II study of palifermin for reducing dysphagia in patients receiving concurrent chemoradiotherapy for locally advanced unresectable non-small cell lung cancer. *J Thorac Oncol.* 2012;7(1):157-164.

Sonis ST, Elting LS, Keefe D, et al. Perspectives on cancer therapy-induced mucosal injury: pathogenesis, measurement, epidemiology, and consequences for patients. *Cancer.* 2004;100(9 Suppl):1995-2025.

Stokman MA, Wachters FM, Koopmans P, et al. Outcome of local application of amifostine (WR-1065) on epirubicin-induced oral mucositis. A phase II study. *Anticancer Res.* 2004;24 (5B):3263-3267.

Sung L, Tomlinson GA, Greenberg ML, et al. Serial controlled N-of-1 trials of topical vitamin E as prophylaxis for chemotherapy-induced oral mucositis in paediatric patients. *Eur J Cancer.* 2007;43(8):1269-1275.

Vadhan-Raj S, Trent J, Patel S, et al. Single-dose palifermin prevents severe oral mucositis during multicycle chemotherapy in patients with cancer: a randomized trial. *Ann Intern Med.* 2010;153 (6):358-367.

Vanstraelen K, Prattes J, Maertens J, et al. Posaconazole plasma exposure correlated to intestinal mucositis in allogeneic stem cell transplant patients. *Eur J Clin Pharmacol.* 2016;72(8):953-63.

Vokurka S, Bystricka E, Koza V, et al. Higher incidence of chemotherapy induced oral mucositis in females: a supplement of multivariate analysis to a randomized multicentre study. *Support Care Cancer.* 2006;14(9):974-976.

Yokomizo H, Yoshimatsu K, Hashimoto M, et al. Prophylactic efficacy of allopurinol ice ball for leucovorin/5-fluorouracil therapy-induced stomatitis. *Anticancer Res.* 2004;24(2C):1131-1134.

PREVENTION OF CHEMOTHERAPY-INDUCED NAUSEA AND VOMITING IN CHILDREN

Note: Unless otherwise specified, emetogenic potential listed is for single agent treatment. For multi-agent regimens, if not otherwise specified, emetogenic potential should be based on the component with the higher emetic potential.

Highly Emetogenic Chemotherapy (Frequency of Emesis: >90%)

Altretamine
CARBOplatin
Carmustine >250 mg/m^2
CISplatin
Cyclophosphamide ≥1,000 mg/m^2
Cytarabine 3,000 mg/m^2
Dacarbazine
DACTINomycin
Mechlorethamine
Methotrexate ≥12 g/m^2
Procarbazine (oral)
Streptozocin

Thiotepa ≥300 mg/m^2
Multi-agent regimens:
   Cyclophosphamide + Anthracycline
     (DOXOrubicin or epiRUBicin)
   Cyclophosphamide + Etoposide
   Cytarabine 150 to 200 mg/m^2 +
     DAUNOrubicin
   Cytarabine 300 mg/m^2 + Etoposide
   Cytarabine 300 mg/m^2 + Teniposide
   DOXOrubicin + Ifosfamide
   DOXOrubicin + Methotrexate 5 g/m^2
   Etoposide + Ifosfamide

Moderately Emetogenic Chemotherapy (Frequency of Emesis: 30% to 90%)

Aldesleukin >12 to 15 million units/m^2
Amifostine >300 mg/m^2
Arsenic trioxide
AzaCITIDine
Bendamustine
Busulfan (IV)
Carmustine ≤250 mg/m^2
Clofarabine
Cyclophosphamide <1,000 mg/m^2 (IV)
Cyclophosphamide (oral)
Cytarabine >200 mg/m^2 to
   <3,000 mg/m^2
DAUNOrubicin
Dinutuximab
DOXOrubicin

EpiRUBicin
Etoposide (oral)
IDArubicin
Ifosfamide
Imatinib
Intrathecal treatment (methotrexate
   and/or cytarabine ± hydrocortisone)
Irinotecan
Lomustine
Melphalan >50 mg/m^2
Methotrexate ≥250 **mg**/m^2 to <12 **g**/m^2
Mitotane
Oxaliplatin ≥75 mg/m^2
Temozolomide (IV)
Temozolomide (oral)

Low Emetogenic Chemotherapy (Frequency of Emesis: 10% to <30%)

Aldesleukin ≤12 million units/m^2
Amifostine ≤300 mg/m^2
Bexarotene (oral)
Busulfan (oral)
Capecitabine
Cytarabine ≤200 mg/m^2
DOCEtaxel
DOXOrubicin (liposomal)
Etoposide (IV)
Everolimus
Fludarabine (oral)
Fluorouracil
Gemcitabine

Ixabepilone
Methotrexate >50 to <250 mg/m^2
MitoMYcin
MitoXANTRONE
Nilotinib
PACLitaxel
PACLitaxel (protein bound)
PEMEtrexed
Teniposide
Thiotepa <300 mg/m^2
Topotecan
Tretinoin
Vorinostat

Minimal Emetogenic Chemotherapy (Frequency of Emesis: <10%)

Alemtuzumab
Asparaginase
Bevacizumab
Bleomycin
Bortezomib
Cetuximab
Chlorambucil
Cladribine
Dasatinib
Decitabine
Denileukin diftitox
Dexrazoxane
Erlotinib
Fludarabine (IV)
Gefitinib
Gemtuzumab ozogamicin
Hydroxyurea
Interferon alfa
Lapatinib
Lenalidomide

Melphalan (oral, low dose)
Mercaptopurine (oral)
Methotrexate ≤50 mg/m^2
Methotrexate (oral)
Nelarabine
Panitumumab
Pegaspargase
Peginterferon alfa
Pentostatin
RiTUXimab
SORAfenib
SUNItinib
Temsirolimus
Thalidomide
Thioguanine (oral)
Trastuzumab
Valrubicin
VinBLAStine
VinCRIStine
Vinorelbine (IV)

Prevention of Acute Nausea and Vomiting

Acute nausea and vomiting includes vomiting, retching, or nausea which occurs within 24 hours of administration of chemotherapeutic agents. Guidelines for prevention of acute nausea and vomiting from the Pediatric Oncology Group of Ontario (POGO) recommend the following for pediatric patients ages 1 month to 18 years (Dupuis 2013; Patel 2017):

For prevention of acute nausea and vomiting due to chemotherapy with **highly** emetogenic risk:

Infants ≥6 months, Children, and Adolescents receiving chemotherapy agents that do **not** potentially interact with aprepitant: Ondansetron or granisetron or palonosetron plus dexamethasone plus aprepitant

Infants ≥6 months, Children, and Adolescents receiving chemotherapy agents that **potentially** interact with aprepitant: Ondansetron or granisetron or palonosetron plus dexamethasone

Infants ≥6 months, Children, and Adolescents receiving highly emetogenic chemotherapeutic agents that do **not** potentially interact with aprepitant **and** who cannot receive corticosteroids (due to contraindications): Palonosetron plus aprepitant

Infants <6 months: Ondansetron or granisetron or palonosetron plus dexamethasone

Infants, Children, and Adolescents who cannot receive corticosteroids (due to contraindications): Palonosetron

PREVENTION OF CHEMOTHERAPY-INDUCED NAUSEA AND VOMITING IN CHILDREN

◀ For prevention of acute nausea and vomiting due to chemotherapy with **moderately** emetogenic risk:

Infants, Children, and Adolescents: Ondansetron or granisetron or palonosetron plus dexamethasone

Infants ≥6 months, Children, and Adolescents receiving moderately emetogenic chemotherapeutic agents that do **not** potentially interact with aprepitant **and** who cannot receive corticosteroids (due to contraindications): Ondansetron or granisetron or palonosetron plus aprepitant

Infants ≥6 months, Children, and Adolescents receiving chemotherapy agents that **potentially** interact with aprepitant **and** who cannot receive corticosteroids (due to contraindications): Palonosetron

Infants <6 months who cannot receive corticosteroids (due to contraindications): Palonosetron

For prevention of acute nausea and vomiting due to chemotherapy with **low** emetogenic risk: Infants, Children, and Adolescents: Ondansetron or granisetron

For prevention of acute nausea and vomiting due to chemotherapy with **minimal** emetogenic risk: No routine prophylaxis

Pediatric Antiemetic Dosing Based on Emetogenic Potential

Name	Chemotherapy Emetogenic Potential	Route/Dose
Serotonin Antagonists		
Granisetron	High	IV: 40 mcg/kg/dose as a single daily dose
	Moderate or low	IV: 40 mcg/kg/dose as a single daily dose
		Oral: 40 mcg/kg/dose every 12 hours
Ondansetron	High	IV, Oral: 0.15 mg/kg/dose (5 mg/m^2/dose); prior to chemotherapy and then every 8 hours (maximum recommended IV dose: 16 mg)
	Moderate	IV, Oral: 0.15 mg/kg/dose (5 mg/m^2/dose); prior to chemotherapy and then every 12 hours (maximum: 8 mg/dose)
	Low	IV, Oral: 0.3 mg/kg/dose (10 mg/m^2/dose); prior to chemotherapy (maximum IV dose: 16 mg)
Palonosetron	High or moderate	Infants 1 month to <17 years: IV: 0.02 mg/kg once prior to chemotherapy (maximum: 1.5 mg/dose)
		Adolescents ≥17 years: IV: 0.25 mg once prior to chemotherapy
Substance P/Neurokinin 1 Receptor Antagonist		
Aprepitant	High or moderate	Infants ≥6 months, Children, and Adolescents: Oral: 3 mg/kg (maximum dose: 125 mg) on day 1 prior to chemotherapy, followed by 2 mg/kg (maximum dose: 80 mg) once daily on days 2 and 3

(continued)

Pediatric Antiemetic Dosing Based on Emetogenic Potential *(continued)*

Name	Chemotherapy Emetogenic Potential	Route/Dose
Corticosteroid		
Dexamethasone	High	IV, Oral: 6 mg/m^2/dose every 6 hours **Note:** If administering with aprepitant, reduce dexamethasone dose by 50%
	Moderate	IV, Oral: ≤0.6 m^2: 2 mg every 12 hours >0.6 m^2 4 mg every 12 hours **Note:** If administering with aprepitant, reduce dexamethasone dose by 50%
DOPamine Receptor Antagonist		
Metoclopramide		IV, Oral: 1 mg/kg/dose IV prior to chemotherapy, then 0.0375 mg/kg/dose orally every 6 hours (administer concomitantly with diphenhydramine or benztropine)
Cannabinoid		
Nabilone		Oral: <18 kg: 0.5 mg twice daily 18 to 30 kg: 1 mg twice daily >30 kg: 1 mg 3 times daily Maximum daily dose: 0.06 mg/kg/**day**

Management of Breakthrough or Refractory Nausea and Vomiting

Breakthrough nausea and vomiting is defined as nausea and/or vomiting that occurs despite adequate prophylactic therapy and requires rescue treatment. Refractory nausea and vomiting occurs during subsequent cycles of chemotherapy when the antiemetic prophylaxis or changes to the antiemetic regimen (or both) have failed in earlier cycles. If breakthrough or refractory nausea and vomiting occurs, POGO guidelines for the treatment of breakthrough and prevention of refractory nausea and vomiting (Flank 2016) recommend escalating the antiemetic regimen for children who received acute prophylaxis for minimal, low, or moderate emetogenic chemotherapy. For children who received acute prophylaxis for highly emetogenic chemotherapy and are experiencing breakthrough nausea or vomiting, the POGO guidelines recommend the addition of oral olanzapine (0.1 mg/kg/dose once daily [maximum 10 mg/dose]; if necessary, may increase to 0.14 mg/kg/dose once daily [maximum 10 mg/dose]) to the antiemetic regimen. If olanzapine cannot be added, methotrimeprazine (not available in the US) or metoclopramide (in children >1 year of age) may be added. Patients should be monitored for extrapyramidal symptoms if olanzapine or metoclopramide are added. If refractory nausea or vomiting occurs despite the use of antiemetic prophylaxis for highly emetogenic chemotherapy, the guidelines recommend changing the 5HT$_3$ antagonist from ondansetron or granisetron to palonosetron; if palonosetron is not available, the 5HT$_3$ antagonist should be changed from ondansetron to granisetron. If this intervention is not successful, consider adding aprepitant (if not already received and there are no contraindications [eg, drug interactions]). If refractory nausea and vomiting persists, then olanzapine, methotrimeprazine (not available in the US), or metoclopramide (if >1 year of age) may be added or acupressure or electroacupuncture may be employed.

◀ **Prevention and Treatment of Anticipatory Nausea and Vomiting**

The risk for anticipatory nausea and vomiting will be minimized if acute and delayed nausea and vomiting associated with chemotherapy are optimally managed. If anticipatory nausea and vomiting develop, interventions including hypnosis and/or systematic desensitization (eg, deep muscle relaxation with imagery) may be offered to help manage symptoms (Dupuis 2014; Roila 2010). Guidelines for prevention and treatment of anticipatory nausea and vomiting from POGO recommend the following for pediatric patients ages 1 month to 18 years (Dupuis 2014): Lorazepam 0.04 to 0.08 mg/kg/dose (maximum dose: 2 mg) administered orally once at bedtime the evening prior to chemotherapy and once prior to chemotherapy the next day may be used to prevent or treat anticipatory nausea and vomiting.

REFERENCES

Basch E, Prestrud AA, Hesketh PJ, et al. Antiemetics: American Society of Clinical Oncology clinical practice guideline update. *J Clin Oncol.* 2011;29(31):4189-4198.

Dupuis LL, Boodhan S, Holdsworth M, et al. Guideline for the prevention of acute nausea and vomiting due to antineoplastic medication in pediatric cancer patients. *Pediatr Blood Cancer.* 2013;60(7):1073-1082.

Dupuis LL, Boodhan S, Sung L, et al. Guideline for the classification of the acute emetogenic potential of antineoplastic medication in pediatric cancer patients. *Pediatr Blood Cancer.* 2011;57(2):191-198.

Dupuis LL, Robinson PD, Boodhan S, et al. Guideline for the prevention and treatment of anticipatory nausea and vomiting due to chemotherapy in pediatric cancer patients. *Pediatr Blood Cancer.* 2014;61(8):1506-1512.

Emend (aprepitant) [prescribing information]. Whitehouse Station, NJ: Merck & Co; August 2015.

Flank J, Robinson PD, Holdsworth M, et al. Guideline for the treatment of breakthrough and the prevention of refractory chemotherapy-induced nausea and vomiting in children with cancer. *Pediatr Blood Cancer.* 2016;63(7):1144-1151.

Kang HJ, Loftus S, Taylor A, DiCristina C, Green S, Zwaan CM. Aprepitant for the prevention of chemotherapy-induced nausea and vomiting in children: a randomised, double-blind, phase 3 trial. *Lancet Oncol.* 2015;16(4):385-394.

Multinational Association of Supportive Care in Cancer. MASCC/ESMO antiemetic guideline 2016. Available at http://www.mascc.org/antiemetic-guidelines. Accessed June 15, 2016.

National Comprehensive Cancer Network (NCCN). Clinical practice guidelines in oncology: antiemesis. v.2.2017. Available at http://www.nccn.org/professionals/physician_gls/PDF/antiemesis.pdf

Patel P, Robinson PD, Thackray J, et al. Guideline for the prevention of acute chemotherapy-induced nausea and vomiting in pediatric cancer patients: A focused update [published online April 28, 2017]. *Pediatr Blood Cancer.*

Roila F, Molassiotis A, Herrstedt J, et al. 2016 MASCC and ESMO guideline update for the prevention of chemotherapy- and radiotherapy-induced nausea and vomiting and of nausea and vomiting in advanced cancer patients. *Ann Oncol.* 2016;27(suppl 5):v119-v133.

TUMOR LYSIS SYNDROME

INTRODUCTION

Tumor lysis syndrome (TLS) is a potentially life-threatening disorder that is characterized as an acute metabolic disturbance resulting from the rapid destruction of tumor cells. Cellular destruction releases intracellular constituents (nucleic acids, anions, cations, peptides) that overwhelm the body's normal mechanisms for their utilization, excretion, and elimination. Signs and symptoms of TLS often develop within 72 hours of beginning cytotoxic chemotherapy in patients with newly diagnosed acute leukemias (acute lymphoblastic leukemia [ALL] and acute myeloid leukemia [AML]) or lymphoproliferative malignancies (Burkitt and non-Burkitt's lymphomas). Moreover, TLS can occur spontaneously in malignant diseases with vigorous cell turnover. Although most commonly reported in patients with hematologic and lymphoid malignancies, TLS has also been reported with solid tumors such as breast cancer, colon cancer, melanoma, ovarian cancer, prostate cancer, small cell lung cancer, and testicular cancer. Acute TLS attributed to administration of a corticosteroid, imatinib, rituximab, sorafenib, and zoledronic acid in patients with treatment-sensitive tumors have been reported in the medical literature. Additional treatment and diagnostic procedures attributed with causing tumor lysis syndrome include total body irradiation, splenic irradiation, staging laparotomy, laparoscopic splenectomy preceded by splenic artery embolization, and radiofrequency interstitial thermal ablation of metastatic hepatic lesions. Metabolic abnormalities associated with acute TLS include hyperphosphatemia, hyperkalemia, hyperuricemia, azotemia, hypocalcemia, and metabolic acidosis. Cardiac arrhythmias, seizures, and major organ failure can occur in severe cases of TLS. Hyperkalemia, hyperuricemia, and hypocalcemia can produce cardiac arrhythmias, tetany, and sudden death. Acute renal failure can occur due to precipitation of uric acid and calcium phosphate in the renal tubules.

PREDISPOSING FACTORS

1. Leukemia with high white blood cell count (see Risk Stratification Table) or rapidly increasing peripheral blast count

2. Solid tumors with bulky disease (>10 cm), high tumor cell proliferation rate, wide metastatic dispersal, and/or bone marrow involvement

3. Acute myeloid leukemia

4. Marked sensitivity of the tumor to a particular treatment modality

5. Renal impairment, including preexisting volume depletion

6. Elevated pretreatment lactic dehydrogenase (LDH) serum concentrations (>2 times ULN)

7. Elevated pretreatment uric acid (>7.5 mg/dL), potassium, and/or phosphate serum concentrations independent of renal impairment

◀ CLINICAL FEATURES AND TREATMENT

Classification and Risk Stratification

TLS can be described according to laboratory abnormalities (LTLS) or clinical complications (CTLS). LTLS is the presence of 2 or more abnormal lab values or a 25% change in lab values within 3 days before or 7 days after chemotherapy. Laboratory values to monitor include uric acid, potassium, phosphorus, and calcium. CTLS is defined as LTLS with at least one clinical manifestation such as renal insufficiency, seizures, cardiac arrhythmias, or sudden death.

Certain patients have greater risk for developing LTLS and/or CTLS and should be treated more aggressively to reduce its occurrence and severity. Risk stratification guides what type of prophylaxis and management therapies should be used for which patients. Recommendations for patients classified as high risk include aggressive prophylactic treatment with hydration and rasburicase while being monitored closely in an ICU or similarly monitored setting. Intermediate risk patients should receive prophylactic treatment with hydration and allopurinol; if hyperuricemia does develop in these patients, consider rasburicase. Initial management of pediatric patients at intermediate risk may include rasburicase. Patients at low risk for developing TLS require no prophylactic therapy but should be monitored closely and treated as necessary.

Risk Stratification

Type of Cancer	High Risk	Intermediate Risk	Low Risk
Non-Hodgkin lymphoma (NHL)	Burkitt, Burkitt-ALL (B-ALL), lymphoblastic lymphoma	Diffuse large B-cell lymphoma (DLBCL)	Indolent NHL
Acute lymphoblastic leukemia (ALL)	WBC ≥100,000 cells/mm^3	WBC 50,000 to 100,000 cells/mm^3	WBC ≤50,000 cells/mm^3
Acute myeloid leukemia (AML)	WBC ≥50,000 cells/mm^3; monoblastic; higher or rapidly increasing peripheral blast count	WBC 10,000 to 50,000 cells/mm^3	WBC ≤10,000 cells/mm^3
Chronic lymphocytic leukemia (CLL)		WBC 10,000 to 100,000 cells/mm^3; treatment with fludarabine	WBC ≤10,000 cells/mm^3
Other hematologic malignancies (chronic myeloid leukemia [CML], multiple myeloma) and solid tumors		Rapid proliferation with expected rapid response to therapy	Remainder of patients

LDH ≥2 x ULN, renal impairment, or elevated uric acid, potassium, or phosphate serum concentrations increases risk level (Sarno 2013)

Monitoring

Patients presenting with TLS and high-risk patients receiving anticancer therapy should have laboratory and clinical parameters (serum uric acid, phosphate, calcium, creatinine, LDH, and fluid input and output) monitored frequently to track the severity and trajectory of the pathologic effects. Frequent assessment of serum chemistries and fluid balance is necessary to avert pathophysiologic adverse events and guide the duration of rasburicase therapy. For all patients treated with rasburicase, wait at least 4 hours to check serum uric acid after drug administration, then every 6 to 8 hours until LDH normalization (Coiffier 2008) and then at least once daily thereafter. Electrolyte and fluid abnormalities must be addressed at the time that they are identified. However, rasburicase is administered no more frequently than once daily to achieve uric acid control for 5 doses or once daily based on serum uric acid levels.

Intermediate risk patients should be monitored throughout and for at least 24 hours after completion of chemotherapy. If rasburicase is not used, laboratory parameters should be monitored 8 hours after initiation of chemotherapy and regularly thereafter according to the patient's clinical condition and institutional practice.

Low risk patients should be monitored as determined by the institution and patient factors. If TLS has not occurred within 2 days, development is very unlikely.

General Principles

Prevention and early management of TLS are aimed at decreasing the risk of morbidity and mortality from cardiac arrhythmias, seizures, and organ failure. In patients with high or intermediate risk, vigorous hydration is the cornerstone of the initial management for acute or potential TLS. Patients should be hydrated with 2 to 3 L/m^2/day (200 mL/kg/day if ≤10 kg) intravenous fluid (Children: D5W^1/$_4$NS, Adults: Not specified) to maintain urine output of 80 to 100 mL/m^2/hour (4 to 6 mL/kg/hour if ≤10 kg), with diuretic use if necessary (avoid or minimize diuretic use in patients with hypovolemia or obstructive uropathy). Due to the tendency for calcium phosphate nephrocalcinosis and the potential for metabolic alkalosis, urinary alkalinization with sodium bicarbonate is no longer universally recommended for the treatment and prevention of TLS (Coiffier 2008).

Allopurinol should be administered to intermediate risk patients to decrease endogenous uric acid production and reduce associated urinary obstruction; dose reductions may be required for renal dysfunction (Coiffier 2008). In adult or pediatric patients, give 150 to 300 mg/m^2/day (or 10 mg/kg/day in pediatric patients) divided every 8 hours (maximum: 800 mg/day) orally or 200 to 400 mg/m^2/day IV (in 1 to 3 divided doses; maximum: 600 mg/day). The median time to plasma uric acid control with allopurinol is 27 hours (Cortes 2010). While allopurinol decreases uric acid production, it is ineffective in reducing markedly elevated uric acid concentrations which may allow renotubular crystal formation and obstruction despite its administration. In addition, allopurinol impedes the clearance of purine analogues such as mercaptopurine and azathioprine. One randomized double-blind phase III study compared febuxostat 120 mg daily vs oral allopurinol 200 mg, 300 mg, or 600 mg daily for control of serum uric acid levels in 346 patients at moderate or high risk for TLS receiving chemotherapy. The primary endpoints were serum uric acid area under the curve (AUC) and creatinine value change after 7 days of treatment. Eligibility criteria included serum uric acid <10 mg/dL. At enrollment, ~88% of patients had a serum uric acid ≤7.5 mg/dL in febuxostat and allopurinol treatment arms. The study reported a statistically significant difference (favoring febuxostat) in treatment arm mean serum uric acid AUCs (p<0.0001). However, it should be noted that for both treatment arms, the mean serum uric acid level remained <7.5 mg/dL throughout the treatment period. Changes in creatinine and adverse event rates were similar between the two treatment groups (Spina 2016). The study did not report what proportion of allopurinol-treated patients received the 200 mg, 300 mg, or

600 mg dose amounts (Spina 2015). The labeled dose for febuxostat for management of hyperuricemia with gout is 40 to 80 mg once daily; febuxostat is not approved for use in TLS.

Rasburicase is administered to rapidly reduce uric acid concentrations; significant reduction in plasma uric acid concentrations is measurable four hours following drug administration. Rasburicase, which is a recombinant form of urate oxidase produced in *Saccharomyces cerevisiae*, catalyzes the degradation of uric acid to allantoin, which is more soluble and readily excreted by the kidneys. Rasburicase is reserved for patients at high risk for TLS (or considered in intermediate risk pediatric patients), patients with elevated uric acid concentrations, or patients with signs of moderate to severe renal impairment or other major organ dysfunction. The major risks associated with administration of rasburicase include anaphylaxis, hypersensitivity reactions, methemoglobinemia, and hemolysis. Rasburicase is contraindicated in patients with glucose-6-phosphate dehydrogenase deficiency due to an increased risk of methemoglobinemia and hemolytic anemia. An additional concern with rasburicase administration is the development of neutralizing antibodies. This phenomenon was observed in 64% of 28 normal, healthy volunteers studied; the effect of neutralizing antibodies on the efficacy of this product with repeated usage is unknown. Rasburicase appears to be less immunogenic in patients with hematologic or lymphoid malignancies receiving chemotherapy. One study reported detection of neutralizing antibodies in 2% of 184 patients with hematologic or lymphoid malignancies treated with rasburicase before and throughout chemotherapy (Cortes 2010).

Rasburicase is approved for use in pediatric and adult patients, with the labeled dose of 0.2 mg/kg/dose daily for up to five days. Due to the costs and risks of therapy plus the immediate and measurable effects of rasburicase administration on plasma uric acid levels, some centers administer a single dose which is repeated daily as warranted by plasma uric acid concentrations. A meta-analysis of 10 studies (2 prospective and 8 retrospective) evaluating plasma uric acid levels following administration of single dose rasburicase in 269 patients reported similar reductions in plasma uric acid levels from single dose in comparison to repeated daily dose administrations. In addition, the study reported that plasma uric acid was effectively controlled (<4.5 mg/dL) at 24, 48, and 72 hours following single-dose rasburicase administration (Feng 2013). The following doses (based on risk for TLS) and duration of treatment based on plasma uric acid concentrations have been recommended for children: 0.2 mg/kg once daily (duration based on plasma uric acid concentrations) for high risk patients, 0.15 mg/kg once daily (duration based on plasma uric acid concentrations) for intermediate risk, and 0.05 to 0.1 mg/kg once daily (duration based on clinical judgment) if used for low-risk patients (Coiffier 2008). Weight- and risk-based dosing as detailed above has been reported in adults. Fixed-dose rasburicase, ranging from 3 to 7.5 mg as a single dose (Hutcherson 2006; McDonnell 2006; Reeves 2008; Trifilio 2006) with doses (1.5 to 6 mg) repeated if needed (based on serum uric acid concentrations) has also been reported in adults. The optimal timing of rasburicase administration (with respect to chemotherapy administration) is not specified in the manufacter's labeling. In some studies, including the clinical trials used for product approval, chemotherapy was administered 4 to 48 hours after the first rasburicase dose (Cortes 2010; Kikuchi 2009; Vadhan-Raj 2012) in order to provide a window of time for demonstration of plasma uric acid reduction independent of anticancer treatment effects. In the absence of confounding clinical variables, such as moderate to severe adverse events, rasburicase can be administered irrespective of chemotherapy timing.

Upon rasburicase administration, serum uric acid levels generally decrease within 4 hours. In order to allow for appropriate therapeutic effect and to accurately assess the need for a repeat dose, repeat uric acid levels should be drawn no earlier than 4 hours post-rasburicase dose. Rasburicase will degrade uric acid in vitro when the blood sample is stored at room temperature. Consequently, to prevent artifactually reduced uric acid concentrations, plasma samples must be collected in prechilled tubes, then immediately placed in an ice water bath until centrifuged at 4°C. Plasma must be analyzed within four hours of collection.

Clinical features and treatment for specific metabolic disorders are discussed in the following sections.

Hyperuricemia

Cytolysis during TLS releases purine and pyrimidine nucleotides into the blood-stream and extracellular tissues. Oxidation of the purines hypoxanthine and xanthine yields uric acid, which can precipitate in the renal tubules and cause oliguric renal failure. A high concentration of uric acid and an acidic urine pH promote uric acid crystallization and renotubular precipitation. Maintenance of urine flow is utilized to reduce purine precipitation and preserve renal function. Allopurinol blocks the endogenous production of uric acid by inhibiting the enzyme xanthine oxidase, which oxidizes hypoxanthine and xanthine to uric acid. Allopurinol is used prophylactically during the early management of TLS in intermediate risk patients. Rasburicase decreases existing uric acid concentrations by conversion of this molecule to the inactive and soluble metabolite allantoin, which is readily excreted by the kidneys. Rasburicase should be used prophylactically in high risk patients or in patients with preexisting hyperuricemia or acute renal impairment.

Hyperkalemia

Potassium is primarily an intracellular ion that is released during massive cellular breakdown. Increasing concentrations of serum potassium can be dangerous, leading to cardiac arrhythmias or sudden death, especially in the presence of hypocalcemia (see following discussion). Standard treatments to remove potassium from the blood stream and extracellular fluids should be initiated as warranted by the patient's serum potassium concentration and electrocardiographic abnormalities. Other sources of potassium intake (including nutritional sources, medications, and intravenous solutions) should be eliminated in patients at risk for or with TLS. Pharmaceutical measures routinely used to manage hyperkalemia in patients with TLS include volume expansion with forced diuresis, administration of insulin with glucose, and the cation exchange product sodium polystyrene sulfonate. Sodium bicarbonate can be administered IV push to induce influx of potassium into cells. Textbook algorithms for management of hyperkalemia include instructions for administration of calcium as a cardioprotective measure; however, this is **not** a standard intervention in the setting of TLS. Calcium gluconate administration must be done judiciously in the patient with TLS as it can precipitate as calcium phosphate in highly perfused tissues. Monitor patient ECG and cardiac rhythm closely for arrhythmias.

Hyperphosphatemia

The release of intracellular inorganic phosphate following massive cellular breakdown sets into motion several important clinical features. Serum phosphate concentrations will quickly exceed the threshold for normal renal excretion, with phosphate excretion becoming limited by the glomerular filtration rate. Any azotemia that develops during therapy will hinder phosphate excretion. Treatment includes the use of phosphate binders such as aluminum hydroxide, sevelamer, calcium carbonate (avoid use in patients with hypercalcemia and limit use to pediatric patients), or lanthanum carbonate (avoid use in pediatric patients). In severe cases of hyperphosphatemia, hemodialysis or hemofiltration may be necessary.

Hypocalcemia

High phosphate concentrations will also cause reciprocal hypocalcemia. Although generally asymptomatic, hypocalcemia may cause neuromuscular irritation, tetany, and cardiac dysrhythmias. Symptomatic patients may receive calcium gluconate intravenously (slowly, with ECG monitoring) to increase serum calcium concentrations. Unfortunately, despite hypocalcemia, the solubility product of calcium and phosphate may be exceeded in acute TLS due to high concentrations of phosphate, resulting in tissue calcification and organ failure. For this reason, calcium gluconate should be administered cautiously and only if necessary.

Hemodialysis/Hemofiltration

Due to the unpredictability of TLS, renal replacement therapy may be needed and can be lifesaving. Hemodialysis or hemofiltration may be used to control and maintain fluid volume and/or to remove uric acid, phosphate, and potassium from serum. Intermittent hemodialysis, continuous arteriovenous hemodialysis, or continuous veno-venous hemodiafiltration should be considered as warranted by the severity of serum chemistry abnormalities, major organ dysfunction, and the patient's response to pharmaceutical treatments.

Leukoreduction/Plasmapheresis

Leukoreduction, which utilizes plasmapheresis and hydroxyurea to rapidly decrease the peripheral white blood cell count, is performed in some cases of acute myeloid leukemia. The primary goal of leukoreduction is to reduce the risk of complications from serum hyperviscosity syndrome consequent to a very high white blood cell count. However, leukoreduction can indirectly reduce the risk of TLS as removal of circulating blasts diminishes the primary source of cells undergoing lysis in patients with acute myeloid leukemia. Plasmapheresis is used infrequently and very cautiously in patients with acute promyelocytic leukemia due to the inherent disease-related risks of coagulopathy, hemorrhage, and hypotension in this population. Plasmapheresis is rarely used for leukoreduction in patients with lymphocytic or lymphoblastic leukemias as these patients are at lower risk for hyperviscosity syndrome despite a high white blood cell count. This is because lymphocytes do not have the same 'sticky' quality as myeloid cells. Hydroxyurea can be used without plasmapheresis to achieve leukoreduction.

REFERENCES

Abu-Alfa AK, Younes A. Tumor lysis syndrome and acute kidney injury: evaluation, prevention, and management. *Am J Kidney Dis.* 2010;55(5 Suppl 3):S1-S13.

Al-Kali A, Farooq S, Tfayli A. Tumor lysis syndrome after starting treatment with gleevec in a patient with chronic myelogenous leukemia. *J Clin Pharm Ther.* 2009;34(5):607-610.

Arnold TM, Reuter JP, Delman BS, Shanholtz CB. Use of single-dose rasburicase in an obese female. *Ann Pharmacother.* 2004;38(9):1428-1431.

Barry BD, Kell MR, Redmond HP. Tumor lysis syndrome following endoscopic radiofrequency interstitial thermal ablation of colorectal liver metastases. *Surg Endosc.* 2002;16(7):1109.

Cairo MS, Bishop M. Tumour lysis syndrome: new therapeutic strategies and classification. *Br J Haematol.* 2004;127(1):3-11.

Cairo MS, Coiffier B, Reiter A, Younes A; TLS Expert Panel. Recommendations for the evaluation of risk and prophylaxis of tumour lysis syndrome (TLS) in adults and children with malignant diseases: an expert TLS panel consensus. *Br J Haematol.* 2010;149(4):578-586.

Chen SW, Hwang WS, Tsao CJ, Liu HS, Huang GC. Hydroxyurea and splenic irradiation-induced tumour lysis syndrome: a case report and review of the literature. *J Clin Pharm Ther.* 2005;30(6):623-625.

Coiffier B, Altman A, Pui CH, Younes A, Cairo MS. Guidelines for the management of pediatric and adult tumor lysis syndrome: an evidence-based review. *J Clin Oncol.* 2008;26(16):2767-2778.

Coiffier B, Mounier N, Bologna S, et al. Efficacy and safety of rasburicase (recombinant urate oxidase) for the prevention and treatment of hyperuricemia during induction chemotherapy of aggressive non-hodgkin's lymphoma: results of the GRAAL1 (Groupe d'Etude Des Lymphomes De l'Adulte trial on rasburicase activity in adult lymphoma) study. *J Clin Oncol.* 2003;21(23):4402-4406.

Cortes J, Moore JO, Maziarz RT, et al. Control of plasma uria acid in adults at risk for tumor lysis syndrome: efficacy and safety of rasburicase alone and rasburicase followed by allopurinol compared with allopurinol alone – results of a multicenter phase III study. *J Clin Oncol.* 2010;28(27):4207-4213.

Duzova A, Cetin M, Gümrük F, Yetgin S. Acute tumour lysis syndrome following a single-dose corticosteroid in children with acute lymphoblastic leukaemia. *Eur J Haematol.* 2001;66(6):404-407.

Feng X, Dong K, Pham D, Pence S, Inciardi J, Bhutada NS. Efficacy and cost of single-dose rasburicase in prevention and treatment of adult tumour lysis syndrome: a meta-analysis. *J Clin Pharm Ther.* 2013;38(4):301-308.

Gemici C. Tumour lysis syndrome in solid tumours. *Clin Oncol (R Coll Radiol).* 2006;18(10):773-780.

Habib GS, Saliba WR. Tumor lysis syndrome after hydrocortisone treatment in metastatic melanoma: a case report and review of the literature. *Am J Med Sci.* 2002;323(3):155-157.

Huang WS, Yang CH. Sorafenib induced tumor lysis syndrome in an advanced hepatocellular carcinoma patient. *World J Gastroenterol.* 2009;15(35):4464-4466.

Hutcherson DA, Gammon DC, Bhatt MS, Faneuf M. Reduced-dose rasburicase in the treatment of adults with hyperuricemia associated with malignancy. *Pharmacotherapy.* 2006;26(2):242-247.

Jabr FI. Acute tumor lysis syndrome induced by rituximab in diffuse large B-cell lymphoma. *Int J Hematol.* 2005;82(4):312-314.

Kikuchi A, Kigasawa H, Tsurusawa M, et al. A study of rasburicase for the management of hyperuricemia in pediatric patients with newly diagnosed hematologic malignancies at high risk for tumor lysis syndrome. *Int J Hematol.* 2009;90(4):492-500.

Kurt M, Onal IK, Elkiran T, Altun B, Altundag K, Gullu I. Acute tumor lysis syndrome triggered by zoledronic acid in patient with metastatic lung adenocarcinoma. *Med Oncol.* 2005;22(2):203-206.

Lee AC, Li CK, So KT, Chan R. Treatment of impending tumor lysis with single-dose rasburicase. *Ann Pharmacother.* 2003;37(11):1614-1617.

Lee MH, Cheng KI, Jang RC, Hsu JH, Dai ZK, Wu JR. Tumour lysis syndrome developing during an operation. *Anaesthesia.* 2007;62(1):85-87.

Leibowitz AB, Adamsky C, Gabrilove J, Labow DM. Intraoperative acute tumor lysis syndrome during laparoscopic splenectomy preceded by splenic artery embolization. *Surg Laparosc Endosc Percutan Tech.* 2007;17(3):210-211.

Lerza R, Botta M, Barsotti B, et al. Dexamethasone-induced acute tumor lysis syndrome in a T-cell malignant lymphoma. *Leuk Lymphoma.* 2002;43(5):1129-1132.

Linck D, Basara N, Tran V, et al. Peracute onset of severe tumor lysis syndrome immediately after 4 Gy fractionated TBI as part of reduced intensity preparative regimen in a patient with T-ALL with high tumor burden. *Bone Marrow Transplant.* 2003;31(10):935-937.

Liu CY, Sims-McCallum RP, Schiffer CA. A single dose of rasburicase is sufficient for the treatment of hyperuricemia in patients receiving chemotherapy. *Leuk Res.* 2005;29(4):463-465.

Mato AR, Riccio BE, Qin L, et al. A predictive model for the detection of tumor lysis syndrome during AML induction therapy. *Leuk Lymphoma*. 2006;47(5):877-883.

McBride A, Westervelt P. Recognizing and managing the expanded risk of tumor lysis syndrome in hematologic and solid malignancies. *J Hematol Oncol*. 2012;5:75.

McDonnell AM, Lenz KL, Frei-Lahr DA, Hayslip J, Hall PD. Single-dose rasburicase 6 mg in the management of tumor lysis syndrome in adults. *Pharmacotherapy*. 2006;26(6):806-812.

Oztop I, Demirkan B, Yaren A, et al. Rapid tumor lysis syndrome in a patient with metastatic colon cancer as a complication of treatment with 5-fluorouracil/leucoverin and irinotecan. *Tumori*. 2004;90(5):514-516.

Reeves DJ, Bestul DJ. Evaluation of a single fixed dose of rasburicase 7.5 mg for the treatment of hyperuricemia in adults with cancer. *Pharmacother*. 2008;28(6):685-690.

Riccio B, Mato A, Olson EM, Berns JS, Luger S. Spontaneous tumor lysis syndrome in acute myeloid leukemia: two cases and a review of the literature. *Cancer Biol Ther*. 2006;5 (12):1614-1617.

Rostom AY, El-Hussainy G, Kandil A, Allam A. Tumor lysis syndrome following hemi-body irradiation for metastatic breast cancer. *Ann Oncol*. 2000;11(10):1349-1351.

Sarno J. Prevention and management of tumor lysis syndrome in adults with malignancy. *J Adv Pract Oncol*. 2013;4(2):101-106.

Sorscher SM. Tumor lysis syndrome following docetaxel therapy for extensive metastatic prostate cancer. *Cancer Chemother Pharmacol*. 2004;54(2):191-192.

Spina M, Nagy Z, Ribera JM, et al. FLORENCE: a randomized, double-blind, phase III pivotal study of febuxostat versus allopurinol for theprevention of tumor lysis syndrome (TLS) in patients with hematologic malignancies at intermediate tohigh TLS risk. *Ann Oncol*. 2015;26 (10):2155-2161.

Theodorou D, Lagoudianakis E, Pattas M, et al. Pretreatment tumor lysis syndrome associated with bulky retroperitoneal tumors. Recognition is the mainstay of therapy. *Tumori*. 2006;92 (6):540-541.

Trifilio S, Gordon L, Singhal S, et al. Reduced-dose rasburicase (recombinant xanthine oxidase) in adult cancer patients with hyperuricemia. *Bone Marrow Transplant*. 2006;37(11):997-1001.

Vadhan-Raj S, Fayad LE, Fanale MA, et al. A randomized trial of a single-dose rasburicase versus five-daily doses in patients at risk for tumor lysis syndrome. *Ann Oncol*. 2012;23(6):1640-1645.

Wagner J, Arora S. Oncologic metabolic emergencies. *Emerg Med Clin North Am*. 2014;32 (3):509-525.

Yahata T, Nishikawa N, Aoki Y, Tanaka K. Tumor lysis syndrome associated with weekly paclitaxel treatment in a case with ovarian cancer. *Gynecol Oncol*. 2006;103(2):752-754.

Zigrossi P, Brustia M, Bobbio F, Campanini M. Flare and tumor lysis syndrome with atypical features after letrozole therapy in advanced breast cancer. A case report. *Ann Ital Med Int*. 2001;16(2):112-117.

OPIOID CONVERSION TABLE AND MORPHINE EQUIVALENT DOSE TABLE

Opioid Conversion Table

This table serves as a general guide to opioid conversion. Utilization of a direct conversion without a detailed patient and medication assessment is not recommended and may result in over- or underdosing. Chronic administration may alter pharmacokinetics and change the parenteral:oral ratio.

Opioid Analgesics – Initial Oral Dosing Commonly Used for Severe Pain

Drug	Equianalgesic Dose (mg)		Initial Oral Dose	
	Oral	Parenteral[a]	Children[b]	Adults[b]
Buprenorphine	—	0.4	IM/IV: Children 2 to 12 years: 2 to 6 mcg/kg every 4 to 6 hours	IM/IV: 0.3 mg every 6 to 8 hours Transdermal: 5 mcg/hour
Butorphanol	—	2	—	IM: 1 to 4 mg every 3 to 4 hours IV: 0.5 to 2 mg every 3 to 4 hours Intranasal: 1 mg (1 spray) every 3 to 4 hours
Codeine	200	100	0.5 to 1 mg/kg	30 to 60 mg
FentaNYL	—	0.1	—	—
HYDROmorphone	7.5	1.5	0.06 mg/kg	Opioid-naïve: 2 to 4 mg
Levorphanol	2	—	0.04 mg/kg	2 to 4 mg
Meperidine[c]	300	100	Not recommended	
Methadone[d]	See Guidelines for Conversion to Oral Methadone in Adults	Variable	See detailed Methadone monograph	See detailed Methadone monograph
Morphine	30	10	0.3 mg/kg	15 to 30 mg
Nalbuphine	—	10	0.1 to 0.2 mg/kg every 3 to 4 hours	10 mg every 3 to 6 hours
OxyCODONE	20	—	0.2 mg/kg	10 to 20 mg
OxyMORphone	10	1	—	5 to 10 mg

(continued)

◀ **Opioid Analgesics – Initial Oral Dosing Commonly Used for Severe Pain**
(continued)

Drug	Equianalgesic Dose (mg)		Initial Oral Dose	
	Oral	Parenteral[a]	Children[b]	Adults[b]
Pentazocine	—	—	IM: Children 5 to 8 years: 15 mg/kg Children and Adolescents 9 to 14 years: 30 mg/kg	Oral: 50 mg every 3 to 4 hours IM: 30 to 60 mg every 3 to 4 hours IV: 30 mg every 3 to 4 hours
Tramadol	120	100	—	50 to 100 mg every 4 to 6 hours
Tapentadol	100	—	—	50 to 100 mg every 4 to 6 hours

Guidelines for Conversion to Oral Methadone in Adults[d]	
Oral Morphine Dose or Equivalent (mg/day)	Oral Morphine:Oral Methadone (Conversion Ratio)
<100	3:1
100 to 300	5:1
300 to 600	8:1
600 to 1,000	10:1
>1,000	15:1

[a]Standard parenteral doses (IM) for acute pain in adults; can be used to convert doses for IV infusions and repeated small IV boluses. For single IV boluses, use half the IM dose.

[b]For patients at the extremes of age (eg, <6 months of age and >70 years of age), consider lowering the starting doses by 25% to 75%, then titrating the dose upward or downward as indicated.

[c]Not recommended for routine use

[d]Conversion of higher doses may be guided by the following (consult a pain or palliative care specialist if unfamiliar with methadone prescribing): As the total daily chronic dose of morphine increases, the equianalgesic dose ratio (morphine:methadone) changes (American Pain Society 2016). Total daily dose should be divided by 3; delivered every 8 hours. Methadone is significantly more potent with repetitive dosing (due to its active metabolite). Begin methadone at lower doses and gradually titrate. Applicability to pediatric patients is unknown.

Morphine Equivalent Dose Table

This table should only be used for analytic purposes when prescription data are used to determine the morphine equivalent dose and **should NOT be used to determine doses when converting a patient from one opioid to another**. Use of this table for the purposes of any clinical decision-making warrants caution.

Drug	Morphine Equivalent Dose (MED) Conversion Factor
Buprenorphine patch (mcg/hour)[a]	12.6
Buprenorphine tablet or film (mg)[b]	30
Buprenorphine film (mcg)	0.03
Butorphanol (mg)	7
Codeine (mg)	0.15
Dihydrocodeine (mg)	0.25

(continued)

(continued)

Drug	Morphine Equivalent Dose (MED) Conversion Factor
FentaNYL buccal or sublingual tablet, lozenge, or troche (mcg)[c]	0.13
FentaNYL film or oral spray (mcg)[d]	0.18
FentaNYL nasal spray (mcg)[e]	0.16
FentaNYL patch (mcg)[f]	7.2
HYDROcodone (mg)	1
HYDROmorphone (mg)	4
Levorphanol tartrate (mg)	11
Meperidine hydrochloride (mg)	0.1
Methadone (mg)[g]	
>0 to ≤20	4
>20 to ≤40	8
>40 to ≤60	10
>60	12
Morphine (mg)	1
Opium (mg)	1
OxyCODONE (mg)	1.5
OxyMORphone (mg)	3
Pentazocine (mg)	0.37
Tapentadol (mg)[h]	0.4
TraMADol (mg)	0.1

[a]The MED conversion factor for buprenorphine patches is based on the assumption that 1 mg of parenteral buprenorphine is equivalent to 75 mg of oral morphine, that one patch delivers the dispensed mcg/hour over a 24-hour day, and that the patch remains in place for 7 days. For example, 5 mcg/hour buprenorphine patch x 24 hours = 120 mcg/day buprenorphine = 9 mg/day oral morphine milligram equivalent. The conversion factor *not* accounting for days would be 9/5 or 1.8. However, since the patch remains in place for 7 days, the conversion factor was multiplied by 7 (1.8 x 7 = 12.6).

[b]Buprenorphine formulations with an FDA-approved indication for Medication Assisted Treatment (MAT) are excluded from Medicare's Overutilization Monitoring System's opioid overutilization reporting.

[c]The MED conversion factor for fentanyl buccal tablets, sublingual tablets, lozenges, and troches is 0.13. This conversion factor should be multiplied by the number of mcg in a given lozenge/troche.

[d]The MED conversion factor for fentanyl film and oral spray is 0.18. This reflects a 40% greater bioavailability for films compared to lozenges and tablets and 38% greater bioavailability for oral sprays compared to lozenges and tablets.

[e]The MED conversion factor for fentanyl nasal spray is 0.16, which reflects a 20% greater bioavailability for sprays compared to lozenges and tablets.

[f]The MED conversion factor for fentanyl patches is based on the assumption that 1 mg of parenteral fentanyl is equivalent to 100 mg of oral morphine, that one patch delivers the dispensed mcg/hour over a 24-hour day, and that the patch remains in place for 3 days. For example: 25 mcg/hour fentanyl patch x 24 hours = 600 mcg/day fentanyl = 60 mg/day oral morphine milligram equivalent. The conversion factor *not* accounting for days would be 60/25 or 2.4. However, since the patch remains in place for 3 days, the conversion factor was multiplied by 3 (2.4 x 3 = 7.2).

[g]https://www.cdc.gov/drugoverdose/pdf/calculating_total_daily_dose-a.pdf

This table is derived from the Department of Health and Human Services (DHHS) Centers for Medicare and Medicaid Services (CMS) "Opioid Morphine Milligram Equivalent (MME) Conversion Factors" table. Available at https://www.cms.gov/Medicare/Prescription-Drug-Coverage/PrescriptionDrugCovContra/Downloads/Opioid-Morphine-EQ-Conversion-Factors-April-2017.pdf

REFERENCES

Department of Health and Human Services (DHHS) Centers for Medicare and Medicaid Services (CMS). Opioid morphine milligram equivalent (MME) conversion factors. April 2017. Available at https://www.cms.gov/Medicare/Prescription-Drug-Coverage/PrescriptionDrugCovContra/Downloads/Opioid-Morphine-EQ-Conversion-Factors-April-2017.pdf

National Cancer Institute. Pain (PDQ). Last modified May 7, 2009. Available at http://www.cancer.gov/cancertopics/pdq/supportivecare/pain/HealthProfessional/page1

National Comprehensive Cancer Network (NCCN). Clinical practice guidelines in oncology: adult cancer pain. Version 1, 2009. Available at http://www.nccn.org/professionals/physician_gls/PDF/pain.pdf

Patanwala AE, Duby J, Waters D, Erstad BL. Opioid conversions in acute care. *Ann Pharmacother.* 2007;41(2):255-266.

Principles of Analgesic Use in the Treatment of Acute Pain and Cancer Pain. 7th ed. Chicago, IL: American Pain Society; 2016.

CHRONIC PAIN MANAGEMENT (CANCER)

DEFINITION AND INCIDENCE

Pain is defined by the International Society for the Study of Pain as "an unpleasant sensory and emotional experience associated with actual or potential tissue damage, or described in terms of such damage." The reported incidence of pain in cancer patients varies with the method used to determine the presence of pain, and the type and stage of cancer. It is estimated that 51% of patients with various stages of cancer experience pain, and patients with advanced disease are more likely to have severe pain. Pain in cancer patients may be due to the disease itself (eg, metastatic bone disease, visceral involvement); it may be secondary to some treatments (eg, painful neuropathy from vincristine or paclitaxel, or postoperative pain); it may result from complications associated with cancer (eg, postherpetic neuralgia); or it may have been present prior to the diagnosis of cancer and be unrelated to cancer (eg, arthritis). Most often, treatment guidelines and discussions focus on the management of chronic pain associated with progressive disease.

PAIN MEASUREMENT

The severity of pain is generally measured using a visual analogue scale (VAS), a numeric rating scale (NRS), or a verbal rating scale (VRS). A similar scale that uses facial expressions representing pain severity instead of numerals can be used for pediatric or cognitively impaired patients (faces pain scale [FPS]). The aforementioned pain scales are all considered to be valid and reliable measures of pain severity and changes in pain severity.

The VAS uses a 100 millimeter line to represent the range of pain severity from no pain to worst imaginable pain. Patients are instructed to mark a spot on the line that best correlates with their perceived pain severity. The NRS uses a numeric scale of 0 (no pain) to 10 (worst imaginable pain) for patients to select which number best represents their perceived pain severity. Numerical ratings of 1 to -3, 4 to -6, and 7 to -10 are generally considered mild, moderate, and severe, respectively. The VRS offers 5 phrases representing pain severity ratings as a measurement tool. The FPS consists of 6 facial expressions representing pain severity from no pain to very high pain.

Visual Analogue Scale (VAS)

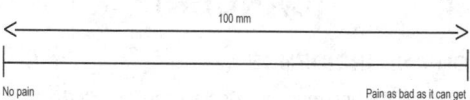

Numeric Rating Scale (NRS)

1 2 3 4 5 6 7 8 9 10

No pain   Pain as bad as it can get

Verbal Rating Scale (VRS)

[ ] No pain
[ ] Mild pain
[ ] Moderate pain
[ ] Intense pain
[ ] Maximum pain

NONOPIOID ANALGESICS

The World Health Organization recommends a stepwise approach to the management of cancer pain (see figure).

WHO Three-Step Analgesic Ladder

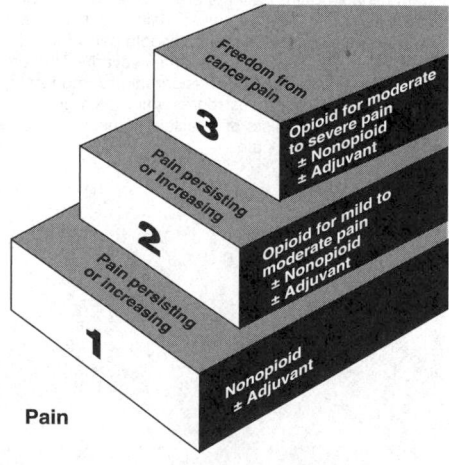

This approach recommends that the choice of therapy match the severity of pain (ie, strong opioids for moderate to severe pain). Nonopioids for (mild) cancer pain include acetaminophen, nonsteroidal anti-inflammatory drugs (NSAIDs), and aspirin. All of these have a ceiling above which increasing the dose will not enhance pain relief and will increase the likelihood of side effects. Although nonopioid analgesics are traditionally WHO step 1 products, they do have a role in the management of moderate to severe cancer pain. One blinded, placebo-controlled study reports that acetaminophen added to a strong opioid regimen in cancer patients improves pain control and well-being.

Acetaminophen is commonly used for the management of mild to moderate pain. Use (including amounts contained in combination products) should be limited to a maximum daily dose of acetaminophen 4,000 mg per 24 hours (acute use) or 3,000 mg per 24 hours (chronic use) to reduce the risk of hepatotoxicity. Concerns regarding the use of NSAIDs in chronic cancer pain include the reversible inhibition of platelet aggregation, and the potential for gastropathy and nephrotoxicity. Aspirin is frequently avoided because of the potential for gastropathy and inhibition of platelet aggregation. Platelets exposed to aspirin become acetylated and permanently impaired. Celecoxib and nonacetylated salicylates, such as choline salicylate and magnesium salicylate, do not inhibit platelet aggregation.

OPIOID ANALGESICS

Opioid analgesic therapy should be initiated when adequate doses of nonopioid analgesics provide inadequate pain control or they are poorly tolerated.

Opioid analgesics for severe, persistent pain should be given "around-the-clock", not on an "as needed" or "PRN" basis. It is easier to prevent pain from recurring than to treat it once it has recurred. Titration of opioids to pain relief is easiest and safest using short-acting drugs (average duration of pain relief of 4 hours) or a continuous parenteral infusion. Once adequate pain relief is achieved, the 24-hour opioid dose can be given as a long-acting preparation (eg, sustained release morphine or oxycodone, transdermal fentanyl). In fact, opioid requirements can be increased in a similar manner for patients with worsening chronic pain daily. Short-acting medication for breakthrough pain, which is a transient worsening of otherwise stable pain in a patient taking an opioid, should always be available. Doses for breakthrough pain (ie, rescue doses) are commonly 5% to 15% of the 24-hour opioid dose, and may be administered every 1 to 2 hours as needed.

The oral route of administration for opioid analgesics is preferred whenever possible. All opioids undergo a high first-pass effect, which must be considered when converting from one route of administration to another. The parenteral to oral ratios for effectiveness of the different opioids vary from 1:2 to 1:6. The parenteral to oral dose ratio for morphine is 1:3 and 1:6 for the treatment of chronic pain and acute pain, respectively. Opioid equianalgesic doses are listed in the table that follows. Dose titration of opioid analgesics is based on pain control and patient tolerance; there is no maximum dosage for administration of opioid analgesics. Tolerance develops to most of the medication-related adverse effects, except constipation and myoclonus.

Table 1. Opioid Analgesics

Drug	Route of Administration	Approximate Equianalgesic Dose (mg)	Approximate Duration[a] (hours)
Codeine	IM, IV	100 to 130	4 to 6
	Oral	200	
FentaNYL[b]	IV	0.1	0.5 to 2
HYDROcodone	Oral	30 to 45	4 to 6
HYDROmorphone	IM, IV, SubQ	1.5	2 to 5
	Oral, rectal	7.5	
Meperidine	IM, IV, SubQ	75	2 to 4
	Oral	300	
Methadone	IM, IV, SubQ	Variable	6 to 12
	Oral	See Guidelines for Conversion to Oral Methadone in Adults	
Morphine	IM, IV, SubQ	10	3 to 4[c]
	Oral, rectal	30	
OxyCODONE	Oral	20	4 to 6[c]
OxyMORphone	Oral	10	3 to 6[c]

Guidelines for Conversion to Oral Methadone in Adults[d]	
Oral Morphine Dose or Equivalent (mg/day)	Oral Morphine:Oral Methadone (Conversion Ratio)
<90	4:1
90 to 300	8:1
>300	12:1

[a]Parenteral or immediate-release products

[b]Transdermal fentanyl conversion presented in separate table that follows

[c]Duration for sustained release dosage forms is 8 to 12 hours (MS Contin, Oramorph SR), 24 hours (Kadian), 12 hours (Opana ER, OxyCONTIN)

[d]Conversion of higher doses may be guided by the following (consult a pain or palliative care specialist if unfamiliar with methadone prescribing): As the total daily chronic dose of morphine increases, the equianalgesic dose ratio (morphine:methadone) changes (American Pain Society 2008). Total daily dose should be divided by 3; delivered every 8 hours. Methadone is significantly more potent with repetitive dosing (due to its active metabolite). Begin methadone at lower doses and gradually titrate. Applicability to pediatric patients is unknown.

Meperidine is not recommended for chronic use. This is because of the potential for accumulation of a neurotoxic metabolite, normeperidine (see following information). Meperidine administration is best reserved for incident pain (ie, before a painful manipulation or procedure).

Tolerance is characterized by the requirement for a higher dose of opioid in order to produce the same effect previously seen with a lower dose. Tolerance develops to many side effects of opioids: respiratory depression, sedation, nausea, and vomiting. Tolerance does not usually develop to constipation or myoclonus. When a given dose of opioid is not effective, for whatever reason, and if side effects are tolerable, the dose can be increased. Physical dependence occurs with regular use of opioids, but is only of clinical importance if the opioid is abruptly discontinued or an opioid antagonist (eg, naloxone) is administered, in which cases a withdrawal syndrome can be seen. Opioids should be tapered in patients whose pain improves. Signs and symptoms of withdrawal can be reduced by maintaining at least 25% of the previous day's opioid dose. The opioid can be discontinued when the total daily dose is the equivalent of 10 to 15 mg of intramuscular morphine. Psychological dependence is defined as a "pattern of compulsive drug use characterized by a continued craving for an opioid and the need to use the opioid for effects other than pain relief." Unlike tolerance and physical dependence, psychological dependence is a characteristic of the patient, and is a function of environmental, social, economic, and personality factors. Psychological dependence or addiction, can develop in patients requiring management of chronic pain; however, this is **not** a valid reason to undertreat pain.

The most troublesome side effect associated with chronic opioid use is constipation, and, as noted above, tolerance to constipation does not occur. Regular use of stimulant laxatives is often required.

Tolerance does develop to opioid-induced respiratory depression, allowing safe dose escalation. In the event of an acute overdose, or in the case of respiratory depression not responding to supportive measures, naloxone can be used. Naloxone administration is reserved for serious situations because it precipitates withdrawal symptoms and the prompt return of pain in patients physically dependent on opioids. Other side effects of naloxone administration include nausea, vomiting, sedation, sweating, itching, dry mouth, and tremulousness. Initiate naloxone therapy with low doses (0.1 to 0.2 mg) repeated and increased as warranted by respiratory rate and patient comfort. Naltrexone is only available as an oral formulation, which limits its utility for acute reversal of opioid toxicity. Tolerance develops to nausea and vomiting, and these effects are more likely to occur when opioid therapy is initiated. Phenothiazines can be used to treat nausea and vomiting. Dimenhydrinate or meclizine can also be used to treat this side effect. Tolerance usually develops to sedation. For those patients in whom persistent or profound sedation limits opioid dose escalation and therefore pain relief, the use of stimulants (eg, dextroamphetamine, methylphenidate) should be considered. Sweating and itching are thought to be due to histamine release. Morphine and meperidine are notable for causing histamine release. Switching to another opioid should be considered for patients with intolerable sweating or itching. Seizures associated with opioids are generally attributed to accumulation of neurotoxic metabolites or large overdoses that presumably cause hypoxia. Normeperidine, a metabolite of meperidine that can accumulate with frequent repeated doses or in patients with renal insufficiency, is the most well-known of these neurotoxic metabolites. Distinct from seizures, myoclonic jerks may be seen with the use of high doses of opioids. Occasional reports indicate that they may also be seen with relatively lower doses. Benzodiazepines have been suggested to control this side effect as tolerance does not typically develop to this adverse event.

Opioid-induced hyperalgesia (OIH) should be suspected when analgesic efficacy is inexplicably lost or when generalized or worsening pain develops during aggressive opioid titration. OIH is a rare consequence of opioid therapy in cancer patients, and most often seen with aggressive morphine titration. The underlying mechanism is thought to be related to inhibition of glycinergic activity at the level of the spinal cord by phenanthrene-type opioids that promotes a strychnine-like excitatory effect. Additional biochemical mechanisms implicated in OIH include upregulation of intracellular phosphokinase C which activates the NMDA receptor system, and intraspinal dynorphin-mediated substance P and glutamate release. In the scenario of OIH, continued dose escalation aggravates pain which then improves with dose reduction. Management of OIH includes dose reduction or interruption of treatment with the offending agent. Replacing a phenanthrene derivative to a piperidine-type opioid, such as fentanyl or methadone, is recommended. The addition of low-dose methadone to chronically administered phenanthrene derivative opioid analgesia has been suggested as a strategy to mitigate OIH.

As previously noted, the oral route of administration for opioids is generally preferred. When oral administration is not possible, several other routes are available (see Table 1). Morphine and hydromorphone are also available in rectal suppositories. The recommended rectal dose is the same as the oral dose. Continuous subcutaneous or intravenous infusions administered with an infusion control device are useful when oral administration is impossible. Continuous parenteral infusion of opioids provides more consistent pain relief and patient tolerance compared to intermittent injections which result in peaks and valleys of pain relief or side effects. Continuous infusions also allow for quick titration of opioid in patients with uncontrolled pain. Patient-controlled analgesia provides a continuous infusion of opioid with a capacity for patient-administered bolus injections for breakthrough pain. This is not unlike the concept of regularly scheduled sustained release oral opioid with immediate release tablets for breakthrough, as previously discussed. Assessment of the use of breakthrough doses, whether oral or parenteral, provides a basis for adjusting the dose/rate of the underlying opioid. Transdermal fentanyl is another alternative, long-acting, analgesic for patients unable to take oral opioids. Transdermal fentanyl should be avoided when initiating chronic analgesia in opioid-naïve patients to reduce the risk of profound respiratory depression. As is the case with sustained release oral opioids, it is preferable to titrate to pain relief using short-acting drugs, and then switch to transdermal fentanyl. The manufacturer recommends equianalgesic conversion to the fentanyl patch as presented in Table 2. This schema represents a conservative conversion from an oral or parenteral opioid to the fentanyl transdermal system, so the tabulated information should **not** be used to convert from fentanyl transdermal to an oral or parenteral opioid analgesic.

Table 2. Dosing Guidelines for Conversion to FentaNYL Transdermal Systems

Current Analgesic	Daily Dosage (mg/day)			
Morphine (oral)	60 to 134	135 to 224	225 to 314	315 to 404
Morphine (parenteral)	10 to 22	23 to 37	38 to 52	53 to 67
HYDROmorphone (oral)	8 to 17	17.1 to 28	28.1 to 39	39.1 to 51
HYDROmorphone (parenteral)	1.5 to 3.4	3.5 to 5.6	5.7 to 7.9	8 to 10
OxyCODONE (oral)	30 to 67	67.5 to 112	112.5 to 157	157.5 to 202
Meperidine (parenteral)	75 to 165	166 to 278	279 to 390	391 to 503
FentaNYL transdermal recommended dose[a]	25 mcg/hour	50 mcg/hour	75 mcg/hour	100 mcg/hour

[a]Recommendations are based on US product labeling and differ from Canadian transdermal product labeling; see current Canadian product label.

One method for switching transdermal fentanyl and oral methadone is described by using the transdermal fentanyl:oral methadone conversion factor of 1:20 (daily dose:daily dose) to change patients (n=31) with inadequate pain control from one product to another (Mercandante 2005). Oral methadone was administered in divided doses every eight hours. Fentanyl patches were removed when the first dose of methadone was administered. Conversely, for patients transitioning to transdermal fentanyl, the patch was applied with administration of the last methadone dose. This method was used successfully in 24 of 31 patients (78%) with improved pain control reported within 24 hours of product conversion and acceptable patient tolerance. Inadequate symptom control (6 patients) and adverse effects (1 patient) were the reasons for unsuccessful switching in seven patients. Using this conversion ratio, treatment with transdermal fentanyl 200 mcg/hour is switched to oral methadone 96 mg daily administered in divided doses as 30 mg every eight hours.

A similar method has been described which calculates the appropriate methadone dose using two steps (Benitez-Rosario 2004). First, the patient's daily transdermal fentanyl dose is converted to the equivalent oral morphine dose using a ratio of fentanyl:oral morphine of 1:100. The resultant value is converted to the equivalent daily dose of oral methadone using the ratio of oral morphine:oral methadone ratio of 5:1 or 10:1. The calculated methadone dose is divided for administration every 8 to 12 hours beginning 8 to 24 hours following removal of the transdermal fentanyl system. Using this method, a patient with adequate pain control from transdermal fentanyl 100 mcg/hour would be receiving a daily dose of fentanyl 2.4 mg every 24 hours, which converts to oral morphine 240 mg per 24-hour, which converts to oral methadone 24 to 48 mg per 24 hours. So, 8 to 24 hours after removing the fentanyl patch, a dosage of oral methadone 15 mg administered every 8 or 12 hours can be started.

Intraspinal administration of opioids should be reserved for patients in whom systemic administration of opioids results in unacceptable or unmanageable toxicity. Epidural morphine is 5 to 10 times more potent than parenteral morphine, and intrathecal morphine is 10 times more potent than epidural morphine. Bupivacaine, clonidine, and ketamine have been added to epidural morphine infusions to enhance effectiveness.

Partial opioid agonists (eg, buprenorphine) or agonist-antagonists (eg, pentazocine, butorphanol, dezocine, nalbuphine) are generally not recommended for use in chronic cancer pain management. They have a ceiling for analgesic effectiveness, above which side effects are much more likely to increase, and they may precipitate withdrawal in patients receiving opioid agonists (eg, morphine). Naloxone may not be effective in reversing respiratory depression caused by buprenorphine.

Tramadol is a synthetic opioid that inhibits the neuronal reuptake of norepinephrine and serotonin. This product is indicated for the management of moderate pain and it has been tested in the management of mild to moderate cancer pain. Its use is limited by the risk of seizures which have occurred in patients taking the usual and recommended dosage. One comparative study reported that the rate of vomiting, dizziness, anorexia, and weakness was greater with tramadol than codeine or hydrocodone when used for cancer pain (Rodriguez, 2007). Abrupt discontinuation of tramadol can precipitate withdrawal symptoms, such as tremors, sweating, diarrhea, upper respiratory symptoms, and rarely, hallucinations. The dosage of tramadol must be adjusted for impaired renal function.

ADJUVANT ANALGESICS

Adjuvant analgesics are frequently used in addition to, rather than instead of, opioid analgesics. Adjuvants are often drugs that have primary indications other than pain, but may provide pain relief in certain situations. NSAIDs are commonly used for pain due to bone metastases (see individual NSAID monographs). Anticonvulsants like gabapentin and pregabalin are commonly used as adjunctive therapy for neuropathic pain. Additional drugs that have been used for this purpose include SNRI antidepressants (eg, duloxetine, venlafaxine), tricyclic antidepressants (eg, amitriptyline, nortriptyline), other anticonvulsants (eg, carbamazepine), corticosteroids (not used solely for pain), and antiarrhythmics (eg, topical lidocaine). Methadone and ketamine are thought to improve neuropathic pain through blockade of the N-methyl-D-aspartate (NMDA) receptor. Medicinal cannabis and cannabinoids have been shown to offer modest pain relief in their various forms, although they should be reserved for adjuvant use and not as first-line management of chronic pain due to cancer (Paice 2016); laws regarding medicinal application vary by individual states. Neuropathic pain, often characterized by sharp, shooting, lancinating sensations, may result from nerve compression, infiltration, or destruction by tumor or from other associated conditions (eg, postherpetic neuralgia). Pain relief is usually not complete and, as is the case with NSAIDs in bone pain, these drugs are generally used in addition to opioids. Baclofen has also been used as an adjuvant analgesic for various types of neuropathic pain. Strontium-89 is a radiopharmaceutical that is reported to decrease the need for analgesics in patients with osteoblastic bone metastases. Prostate cancer is the most frequent malignancy associated with painful osteoblastic lesions. The bisphosphonates pamidronate and zoledronic acid are used to decrease pain and adverse skeletal events in patients with multiple myeloma and breast cancer. Capsaicin is a topically applied adjuvant analgesic that depletes substance P, a "painful" neurotransmitter. Capsaicin is recommended for use in postherpetic neuralgia and other painful neuropathies.

RECOMMENDATIONS

Guidelines from the American Society of Clinical Oncology (ASCO) for the management of chronic pain in adult cancer survivors (Paice 2016) recommend screening for pain at each encounter. Patients with complex needs may require additional resources for comprehensive chronic pain management. In patients without contraindications or potentially serious drug interactions, systemic non-opioid analgesics (acetaminophen, NSAIDs), adjuvant analgesics (antidepressants, anticonvulsants), and/or topical analgesics may be utilized to relieve pain and help improve function. In carefully selected patients who do not respond to conservative management, a trial of opioids may be initiated. New onset pain in patients with recurrent disease, secondary malignancy, or late-onset treatment effects should be evaluated, managed, and monitored, and the risks of adverse effects of opioids should be assessed. While balancing the need for access to opioids for adequate pain relief in patients with cancer, clinicians should also have a comprehensive understanding of the potential for tolerance, dependence, abuse, and addiction. Precautions should be employed to minimize abuse, addiction, and adverse consequences; if opioids are no longer needed to control pain, doses should be tapered off in order to avoid abstinence syndrome. Proper education of patients and family members/caretakers regarding safe storage, use, and disposal of controlled substances should be provided.

REFERENCES

Axelrod DJ, Reville B. Using methadone to treat opioid-induced hyperalgesia and refractory pain. *J Opioid Manag.* 2007;3(2):113-114.

Benítez-Rosario MA, Feria M, Salinas-Martín A, Martínez-Castillo LP, Martín-Ortega JJ. Opioid switching from transdermal fentanyl to oral methadone in patients with cancer pain. *Cancer.* 2004;101(12):2866-2873.

Benrath J, Scharbert G, Gustorff B, Adams HA, Kress HG. Long-term intrathecal S(+)-ketamine in a patient with cancer-related neuropathic pain. *Br J Anaesth.* 2005;95(2):247-249.

Berenson JR, Lichtenstein A, Porter L, et al. Efficacy of pamidronate in reducing skeletal events in patients with advanced multiple myeloma. Myeloma aredia study group. *N Engl J Med.* 1996;334 (8):488-493.

Cordell GA, Araujo OE. Capsaicin: identification, nomenclature, and pharmacotherapy. *Ann Pharmacother.* 1993;27(3):330-336.

Davis MP, Shaiova LA, Angst MS. When opioids cause pain. *J Clin Oncol.* 2007;25 (28):4497-4498.

Elsner F, Radbruch L, Loick G, Gaertner J, Sabatowski R. Intravenous versus subcutaneous morphine titration in patients with persisting exacerbation of cancer pain. *J Palliat Med.* 2005;8 (4):743-750.

Ferreira-Valente MA, Pais-Ribeiro JL, Jensen MP. Validity of four pain intensity rating scales. *Pain.* 2011;152(10):2399-2404.

Fromm GH. Baclofen as an adjuvant analgesic. *J Pain Symptom Manage.* 1994;9(8):500-509.

Højsted J, Sjøgren P. Addiction to opioids in chronic pain patients: a literature review. *Eur J Pain.* 2007;11(5):490-518.

Holdsworth MT, Adams VR, Chavez CM, Vaughan LJ, Duncan MH. Continuous midazolam infusion for the management of morphine-induced myoclonus. *Ann Pharmacother.* 1995;29 (1):25-29.

Jackson KC 2nd. Pharmacotherapy for neuropathic pain. *Pain Pract.* 2006;6(1):27-33.

Jacox A, Carr DB, Payne R, et al. Management of cancer pain. *Clinical Practice Guideline No. 9, AHCPR Publication No. 94-0592.* Rockville, MD: Agency for Health Care Policy and Research, U.S. Department of Health and Human Services, Public Health Service; 1994.

Laizure SC. Considerations in morphine therapy. *Am J Hosp Pharm.* 1994;51(16):2042-2043.

Levy MH, Chwistek M, Mehta RS. Management of chronic pain in cancer survivors. *Cancer J.* 2008;14(6):401-409.

Levy MH. Pharmacologic treatment of cancer pain. *N Engl J Med.* 1996;335(15):1124-1132.

Lossignol DA, Obiols-Portis M, Body JJ. Successful use of ketamine for intractable cancer pain. *Support Care Cancer.* 2005;13(3):188-193.

Mercadante SL, Berchovich M, Casuccio A, Fulfaro F, Mangione S. A prospective randomized study of corticosteroids as adjuvant drugs to opioids in advanced cancer patients. *Am J Hosp Palliat Care.* 2007;24(1):13-19.

Mercadante S, Ferrera P, Villari P, Casuccio A.. Rapid switching between transdermal fentanyl and methadone in cancer patients. *J Clin Oncol.* 2005;23(22):5229-5234.

Paice JA, Portenoy R, Lacchetti C, et al. Management of chronic pain in survivors of adult cancers: American Society of Clinical Oncology clinical practice guideline. *J Clin Oncol.* 2016;34 (27):3325-3345.

Potter JM, Reid DB, Shaw RJ, Hackett P, Hickman PE. Myoclonus associated with treatment with high doses of morphine: the role of supplemental drugs. *BMJ.* 1989;299(6692):150-153.

Principles of analgesic use in the treatment of acute pain and cancer pain. 6th ed. Glenview, IL: American Cancer Pain Society; 2008.

Robinson RG, Preston DF, Baxter KG, Dusing RW, Spicer JA. Clinical experience with strontium-89 in prostatic and breast cancer patients. *Semin Oncol.* 1993;20(3 Suppl 2):44-48.

Rodriguez RF, Bravo LE, Castro F, et al. Incidence of weak opioids adverse events in the management of cancer pain: a double-blind comparative trial. *J Palliat Med.* 2007;10(1):56-60.

Rodriguez RF, Castillo JM, Del Pilar Castillo M, et al. Codeine/acetaminophen and hydrocodone/ acetaminophen combination tablets for the management of chronic cancer pain in adults: a 23-day, prospective, double-blind, randomized, parallel-group study. *Clin Ther.* 2007;29(4):581-587.

Salpeter SR, Buckley JS, Bruera E. The use of very-low-dose methadone for palliative pain control and the prevention of opioid hyperalgesia. *J Palliat Med.* 2013;16(6):616-622.

Stearns L, Boortz-Marx R, Du Pen S, et al. Intrathecal drug delivery for the management of cancer pain: a multidisciplinary consensus of best clinical practices. *J Support Oncol.* 2005;3 (6):399-408.

Stockler M, Vardy J, Pillai A, Warr D. Acetaminophen (paracetamol) improves pain and well-being in people with advanced cancer already receiving a strong opioid regimen: a randomized, double-blind, placebo-controlled cross-over trial. *J Clin Oncol.* 2004;22(16):3389-3394.

Svendsen KB, Andersen S, Arnason S, et al. Breakthrough pain in malignant and non-malignant diseases: a review of prevalence, characteristics and mechanisms. *Eur J Pain.* 2005;9 (2):195-206.

Szeto HH, Inturrisi CE, Houde R, Saal S, Cheigh J, Reidenberg MM. Accumulation of normeperidine, an active metabolite of meperidine in patients with renal failure of cancer. *Ann Intern Med.* 1977;86(6):738-741.

Tsavaris N, Kopterides P, Kosmas C, et al. Analgesic activity of high-dose intravenous calcitonin in cancer patients with bone metastases. *Oncol Rep.* 2006;16(4):871-875.

Vranken JH, van der Vegt MH, Kal JE, Kruis MR. Treatment of neuropathic cancer pain with continuous intrathecal administration of S +-ketamine. *Acta Anaesthesiol Scand.* 2004;48 (2):249-252.

Wallace E, Ridley J, Bryson J, Mak E, Zimmermann C. Addition of methadone to another opioid in the management of moderate to severe cancer pain: a case series. *J Palliat Med.* 2013;16 (3):305-309.

Wellington K, Goa KL. Zoledronic acid: a review of its use in the management of bone metastases and hypercalcaemia of malignancy. *Drugs.* 2003;63(4):417-437.

Yucel A, Ozyalcin S, Koknel Talu G, et al. The effect of venlafaxine on ongoing and experimentally induced pain in neuropathic pain patients: a double blind, placebo controlled study. *Eur J Pain.* 2005;9(4):407-416.

HOSPICE (END OF LIFE) CARE

Hospice care is provided to maintain comfort and control symptoms in the dying patient. Most patients receiving hospice care have a life expectancy of 6 months or less. The pharmaceutical component of hospice care is one aspect pertaining to the quality of dying and death. The quality of dying and death entails the physical experience, psychological experience, social and cultural comprehension, spiritual or existential understanding, life closure and death preparation, and the circumstances of death. For cancer patients, the type and stage of malignant disease and their health care experience impact the quality of dying and death.

Important communications between the patient and loved one or the patient and health care professional is best conducted early during hospice care rather than later. Many people are unable to effectively communicate within hours to days before death occurs. The percentage of patients who are awake, drowsy, or comatose one week prior to death is 56%, 44%, and zero, respectively. In comparison, 24 hours before death 26% of patients are awake, 62% of patients are drowsy, and 12% are comatose. And within 6 hours of death 8% of patients are awake, 42% of patients are drowsy, and 50% are comatose.

Pharmacists provide medication therapy management at admission and periodic intervals to ensure the patients' palliative needs are being met. Drug therapy is reviewed for necessity, benefit duration, and relation to "terminal diagnosis." Patients receiving medications which provide potential long-term health benefits with a risk of short-term adverse events can have their current medication profile evaluated and potentially modified.

It is difficult to predict the expected time of impending death. Some patients become progressively less responsive until they die; whereas, other experience symptomatology portending death. Noisy respirations (also known as death rattle) occur when patients are obtunded or too weak to expectorate secretions. The noise is generated by secretions that accumulate in the hypopharynx and bronchial tree and oscillate with the movement of air during inspiration and exhalation. Noisy respirations generally develop within 2 to 3 days of death. Respiration with involuntary mandibular movement, cyanosis of the extremities, and loss of radial pulse occur approximately eight hours, five hours, and three hours, respectively, prior to death. Interestingly, the time from respiration with mandibular movement or cyanosis to death is markedly prolonged in patients with primary lung cancer or metastatic malignant disease affecting the lungs. Additional adverse events associated with dying include agitation or restlessness, delirium, dyspnea, incontinence of urine or stool, irregular breathing including gasping or 20- to 30-second interruptions in respiration, nausea, and swelling of the extremities.

It is important to provide safe and appropriate therapy relative to the expected outcome of therapy. Medications utilized in hospice care are often for off-label uses and are administered outside of the usual dosage range. In addition, many medications used for symptom control are prone to diversion for recreational use. In order to effectively deliver pharmacologic medication therapy for hospice care, it is important for institutions to develop policies and procedures governing the management and use of drugs for end of life care.

◄ Noisy respirations are generally managed by placement of the patient in a semiprone position, reduction of parenteral hydration, explanation of the situation to family members and visitors, gentle nasopharyngeal or tracheal suctioning, and administration of anticholinergic medications. Transdermal scopolamine and parenteral glycopyrrolate are used in the management of noisy respirations. The commercially available patch delivers scopolamine 1 mg over 72 hours. A single patch may be sufficient for reduction of noisy respirations; however, additional patches can be applied without exceeding the daily dose of subcutaneous scopolamine administered to European hospice patients. Administration of scopolamine 1.2 mg per 24 hours by continuous subcutaneous infusion for reduction of noisy respirations is reported in the medical literature. Application of four patches is expected to deliver scopolamine 1.3 mg per 24 hours. Parenteral scopolamine is not licensed for use in the United States. Glycopyrrolate 0.2 mg can be administered by subcutaneous or intravenous bolus. Administration of glycopyrrolate 0.6 mg per 24 hours by continuous subcutaneous infusion for management of noisy respirations is reported in the medical literature. Administration of parenteral medications can be difficult for patients who are dying at home or outside of a hospital. In such circumstances, ipratropium bromide 0.03% nasal solution may provide an alternative to glycopyrrolate. Sublingual administration of ipratropium bromide 0.03% nasal solution two sprays 1 to 3 times daily is reportedly effective for reduction of drug induced sialorrhea. One drawback to sublingual administration may be erratic absorption for patients with excess secretions in the oral cavity. Atropine 1% ophthalmic drops are a suboptimal selection because each drop of solution delivers 0.5 mg of atropine, which is a pharmacologic dose that can modulate heart rate.

Opioid therapy is the cornerstone of treatment for pain and dyspnea in hospice care. Opioid requirements tend to increase in the dying patient. The proportion of dying patients requiring opioids expands from 42% one week before death to 78% during the final 48 hours of life. In addition, the daily opioid dose increases 2- to 3-fold during the same time frame. Increased opioid requirements are thought to be due to progression of the patient's underlying pathophysiologic problems instead of the development of tolerance. Refer to Chronic Pain Management (Cancer) on page 2327 and Palliative Care Medicine (Cancer) on page 2352

Delirium can present at the end of life, with or without agitation. The etiology can be multifactorial and treatment should begin with removing causative factor(s). In some instances, however, no cause is ever determined and symptom management is the goal. Typical or conventional antipsychotics (eg, haloperidol [preferred] or chlorpromazine) have been shown to be effective in both hypoactive and hyperactive delirium but should not be used in patients with Lewy Body Dementia or Parkinson disease. If typical antipsychotics are not tolerated well, atypical antipsychotics (eg, aripiprazole, olanzapine, quetiapine, risperidone, ziprasidone) are also used in delirium and can be used in patients with Lewy Body Dementia, Parkinson disease, or a history of extrapyramidal symptoms (EPS) from typical (conventional) antipsychotics. Usual dosing for both types of dementia is on the lower end of the dosing range or below the labeled use dosing ranges (Protus 2015).

Pharmacologic sedation is often required for end of life delirium, restlessness, and agitation. This type of palliative sedation is used for refractory symptoms and to relieve intolerable suffering. Normally the goal of sedation is to manage symptoms without appreciably reducing the patient's level of consciousness. End of life sedation has not been shown to shorten survival. Sedation during hospice care can include proportional palliative sedation (PPS) or, less commonly, palliative sedation to achieve unconsciousness (PSU). The goal of PPS is to provide an adequate amount of sedation for symptom control and maintain consciousness, as much as possible. Gradual titration of a benzodiazepine is commonly used for PPS. Two of the most commonly studied benzodiazepines for end of life sedation are midazolam and lorazepam. Additional drugs that have been utilized for end of life sedation are propofol and phenobarbital. Respiratory depression caused by phenobarbital should be considered when this product is administered. Haloperidol (preferred) and chlorpromazine may be utilized for patients with concurrent delirium and/or restlessness. The potential for QTc interval prolongation with haloperidol and chlorpromazine should be considered. The goal of PSU is to induce unconsciousness. This is reserved for refractory cases with unbearable symptoms. PSU is generally accomplished by rapid titration of a benzodiazepine to the state of unconsciousness, with continuation of adequate doses to maintain unconsciousness.

Medication administration can be problematic in the hospice setting. Oral administration, which is the preferred route whenever possible, can be ineffective and dangerous for the obtunded, delirious, or actively dying patient. Intravenous medication administration is often problematic for patients who choose to die outside of the hospital. Moreover, venous access can become difficult in all care environments with reduced peripheral blood circulation in the dying patient. Intramuscular administration is too painful for repeated use. Subcutaneous administration of medications is feasible if it can be accomplished without causing undue discomfort for the patient. Repeated subcutaneous bolus of medications can cause discomfort for some patients. Certain opioids, such as morphine, hydromorphone, and fentanyl, can be administered by continuous subcutaneous infusion. The utility of continuous subcutaneous infusion of medications is generally limited by the rate of fluid volume administration required for drug delivery. Rectal administration of medications can be used in the hospice setting. The Macy Catheter is a device that facilitates discreet and hygienic rectal administration. This device consists of two lumens, one for medication administration and the other for inflation of a retention balloon. The retention balloon can be deflated for device removal or left in place for device expulsion by defecation. Transdermal administration is an option for selected medications, such as scopolamine and fentanyl.

SELECTED READINGS

Back IN, Jenkins K, Blower A, Beckhelling J. A study comparing hyoscine hydrobromide and glycopyrrolate in the treatment of death rattle. *Palliat Med.* 2001;15(4):329-336.

Hales S, Zimmermann C, Rodin G. The quality of dying and death. *Arch Intern Med.* 2008;168 (9):912-918.

Hugel H, Ellershaw J, Gambles M. Respiratory tract secretions in the dying patient: a comparison between glycopyrronium and hyoscine hydrobromide. *J Palliat Med.* 2006;9(2):279-284.

Kåss RM, Ellershaw J. Respiratory tract secretions in the dying patient: a retrospective study. *J Pain Symptom Manage.* 2003;26(4):897-902.

Kehl KA. Treatment of terminal restlessness: a review of the evidence. *J Pain Palliat Care Pharmacother.* 2004;18(1):5-30.

Kintzel PE, Chase SL, Thomas W, Vancamp DM, Clements EA. Anticholinergic medications for managing noisy respirations in adult hospice patients. *Am J Health Syst Pharm.* 2009;66 (5):458-464.

Maltoni M, Scarpi E, Rosati M, et al. Palliative sedation in end-of-life care and survival: a systematic review. *J Clin Oncol.* 2012;30(12):1378-1383.

Morita T, Ichiki T, Tsunoda J, Inoue S, Chihara S. A prospective study on the dying process in terminally ill cancer patients. *Am J Hosp Palliat Care.* 1998;15(4):217-222.

Pantilat SZ, Isaac M. End-of-life care for the hospitalized patient. *Med Clin North Am.* 2008;92 (2):349-370.

Protus BM, Kimbrel JM, Grauer PA. *Palliative Care Consultant: a reference guide for palliative care. Guidelines for effective management of symptoms.* 4th ed. Montgomery, AL; 2015.

Quill TE, Lo B, Brock DW, Meisel A. Last-resort options for palliative sedation. *Ann Intern Med.* 2009;151(6):421-424.

HYPERCALCEMIA OF MALIGNANCY

INTRODUCTION

Hypercalcemia of malignancy (HCM) affects 20% to 30% of patients with advanced cancer. It is the most frequently occurring life-threatening metabolic disorder in this patient population. The highest incidence is seen in patients with lung, breast, and renal cell cancers. In addition to these solid tumors, HCM is also commonly observed in patients with the hematologic malignancies multiple myeloma and human T-cell lymphotropic virus type I (HTLV-1)-associated T-cell lymphoma. Even with appropriate treatment, 30-day mortality rates following the HCM diagnosis approach 50% (Stewart 2005). Poor prognostic indicators include corrected serum calcium exceeding 11.3 mg/dL (hazard ratio [HR]: 2.21), serum albumin <3.6 g/dL (HR: 2.41), squamous cell carcinoma (HR: 2.64), and metastatic disease affecting the bone (HR: 1.44) or liver (HR: 2.22) (Penel 2008).

PATHOPHYSIOLOGY

The primary cause of HCM is increased bone resorption secondary to osteoclast activation which is mediated by proteins and cytokines released by tumor cells or their microenvironment. HCM can be classified into 4 types (local humoral, osteolytic, calcitriol secreting lymphomas, and ectopic hyperparathyroidism). Parathyroid-hormone-related protein (PTHrP)-mediated hypercalcemia (or humoral HCM) is the most common cause in solid tumors without bone metastasis. PTHrP released by the tumor initially stimulates osteoblasts to secrete receptor activator of nuclear factor-kappa ligand (RANKL). RANKL activates osteoclasts, resulting in increased bone resorption. PTHrP also promotes calcium renal tubular reabsorption. In patients with bone metastasis, local osteoclastic bone resorption is increased in the areas surrounding the tumor within the marrow space. Some lymphomas produce calcitriol (1,25[OH]$_2$D3), leading to hypercalcemia due to increased osteoclastic bone resorption and enhanced intestinal absorption of calcium. Lastly, a very rare cause of HCM is ectopic secretion of parathyroid hormone (PTH).

SYMPTOMS AND DIAGNOSIS

One early sign of hypercalcemia is polyuria, which develops as the body tries to eliminate excess ionized calcium from the serum. Polyuria causes intravascular volume depletion and dehydration, which signals the body to retain sodium. The ensuing renotubular reabsorption of sodium promotes concurrent reabsorption of calcium that fuels the hypercalcemia. Acute renal impairment may occur due to intravascular volume depletion and calcium-phosphate precipitation in the renal tubules. Neurologic adverse effects are generally the most serious sequelae of hypercalcemia. Confusion is common and patients can progress to somnolence and coma. Malaise and muscle weakness occur. Gastrointestinal adverse effects include anorexia, constipation, ileus, nausea, and vomiting. Cardiac effects include bradycardia and other dysrhythmias. Symptom severity is related to the degree of hypercalcemia and the rate at which the serum calcium increased.

Diagnosis of HCM is confirmed with laboratory measurement of serum calcium levels. As total calcium levels are associated with patients' albumin stores, it is important to calculate the serum ionized calcium level using the equation [corrected Ca++ (mg/dL) = measured serum Ca++ (mg/dL) + 0.8 x (4 - measured serum albumin in g/dL)]. However, this equation may not always accurately reflect true ionized calcium levels; in such cases, directly measuring serum ionized calcium is prudent. PTH and PTHrP may be measured in the occasional cases in which the cause of hypercalcemia is not clear. Likewise, $1,25(OH)_2D3$ levels may be assessed if sarcoidosis or other granulomatous conditions, or the $1,25(OH)_2D3$ lymphoma syndrome, is in the differential diagnosis.

Body System	Symptoms
General	Dehydration, weight loss, pruritis, polydipsia
Neuromuscular	Fatigue, lethargy, muscle weakness, hyporeflexia, confusion, psychosis, seizure, obtundation, coma
Gastrointestinal	Anorexia, nausea, vomiting, constipation, ileus
Renal	Polyuria, renal insufficiency
Cardiac	Bradycardia, prolonged PR, shortened QT, wide T wave, arrhythmias

MANAGEMENT

The first treatment priority of HCM is reversal of dehydration to reduce the serum calcium concentration and preserve renal function. Once normovolemia is restored, furosemide is often added; however, the primary role of a loop diuretic in this situation is to prevent volume overload. First-line therapies to reduce bone resorption include bisphosphonates and calcitonin. Second-line therapies include corticosteroids for multiple myeloma and lymphoid malignancies. Denosmuab is approved for treatment of HCM after an adequate trial of bisphosphonate therapy. Hemodialysis may be necessary in severe cases of hypercalcemia. Treatment of the underlying malignancy is also an option for reducing HCM for some patients. However, the metabolic benefits of effective anticancer treatment may not be clinically evident for a period of weeks to months. Unfortunately, many patients with HCM have cancer that has progressed despite the standard anticancer therapies.

Treatment is based on symptomatology and the serum calcium level. The criteria for initiation of treatment are generally hypercalcemia with signs of toxicity (polyuria, mental status changes, renal dysfunction, cardiac dysrhythmias) attributed to hypercalcemia. A total calcium level exceeding 13 mg/dL is cited as criteria for initiation of therapy; although, it is unusual for HCM to present without related symptomatology.

0.9% Sodium Chloride

The intravenous fluid used for rehydration is 0.9% sodium chloride because it effectively improves intravascular volume and promotes renal excretion of calcium. The rate of administration of sodium chloride depends on the degree of dehydration, the severity of hypercalcemia, and the cardiopulmonary status of the patient. Ideally, patients should receive 0.9% sodium chloride at a rate of 2 to 3 L/m^2 per 24 hours; however, this often must be attenuated relative to what the patient's cardiopulmonary status can accommodate. Hydration rates as high as 5 L/m^2 per 24 hours have been used in severe cases. Following rehydration, proximal tubular reabsorption of sodium, and therefore calcium, will decrease. Further, other treatments for hypercalcemia require prior volume replacement in order to minimize toxicities. Sodium chloride can lower serum calcium by approximately 2 mg/dL. Saline hydration has an immediate but transient effect. Even if normocalcemia is achieved, serum calcium will increase again unless additional treatments aimed at reducing bone resorption or treating the under-lying malignancy are administered.

Furosemide

The major use of furosemide in the management of cancer-associated hyper-calcemia is to prevent and manage fluid overload in order to facilitate the administration of sodium chloride for volume replacement. A usual starting dose of furosemide is 10 to 20 mg by intravenous push every 6 to 12 hours around the clock or as needed to maintain an acceptable rate of urine output. Loop diuretics are not effective agents for enhancing renal excretion of calcium. Loop diuretics should be used with caution to avoid intravascular volume depletion with exacerbation of hypercalcemia and renal impairment.

Bisphosphonates

Bisphosphonates bind to hydroxyapatite in bone and inhibit osteoclastic bone resorption. Pamidronate and zoledronic acid are the most commonly used bisphosphonates for management of HCM. Intravenous ibandronate is also a treatment option for this condition. The dose of intravenous ibandronate used for HCM in clinical trials is 2 mg or 4 mg. In an analysis of two randomized, double-blind comparison trials with 275 of 287 subjects evaluable for efficacy, zoledronic acid was superior to pamidronate for normalization of serum calcium by day 4 (50% vs 33% of patients) and day 10 (88% vs 70% of patients) of therapy (Major 2001). The median duration of normocalcemia was 32 days for zoledronic acid 4 mg and 18 days for pamidronate 90 mg. However, the frequency of renal impairment was greater in the zoledronic acid treatment arm.

Bisphosphonates should be used with caution in patients with severe renal impairment because these products are eliminated by the kidneys and can cause nephrotoxicity. Pamidronate has not been studied in patients with serum creatinine exceeding 3 mg/dL or creatinine clearance <30 mL/minute. Renal dosage adjustment of zoledronic acid administered for the treatment of HCM is not warranted when the serum creatinine is <4.5 mg/dL. The manufacturer of intravenous ibandronate recommends against use of this product for serum creatinine exceeding 2.3 mg/dL or creatinine clearance <30 mL/min.

Common side effects of bisphosphonates are mild and include fever and infusion site reactions, such as phlebitis. Avascular osteonecrosis of the jaw (ONJ) is an infrequent but serious adverse effect of bisphosphonate therapy. ONJ can be an extremely painful condition. Most reported cases of ONJ involve cancer patients receiving intravenous bisphosphonate therapy while undergoing dental proce-dures. Risk factors for ONJ during bisphosphonate therapy include cancer, chemotherapy, radiotherapy, corticosteroids, poor oral hygiene, preexisting dental disease or infection, anemia, and coagulopathy. Patients should maintain good oral hygiene and have a dental examination with preventive dentistry prior to treatment with bisphosphonates. Another adverse effect identified in women receiving bisphosphonate therapy for postmenopausal osteoporosis is severe musculoskeletal pain that develops within days, weeks or months of beginning treatment. This condition may become debilitating and necessitate discontinua-tion of bisphosphonate therapy.

Denosumab

Denosumab, a monoclonal antibody which binds to RANKL and inhibits osteo-clast formation, function, and survival, is approved for hypercalcemia of malignancy that is refractory to bisphosphonate therapy. The relatively slower time to onset of serum calcium reduction limits the utility of this agent for first- or second-line therapy. In a single arm study, denosumab was effective in reducing the serum calcium in nearly two-thirds of bisphosphonate-refractory (corrected serum calcium remaining ≥11.5 mg/dL 7 to 30 days after IV bisphosphonate treatment) patients (n=33); the median time to response was 9 days, the median duration of response was 104 days, and the median duration of complete response was 34 days (Hu 2014).

Denosumab may play a role in deterrence of HCM. An analysis of data from two double-blind, placebo-controlled phase III studies evaluating denosumab (n=1,912) and zoledronic acid (n=1,910) for prevention of skeletal-related adverse events in patients with metastatic cancer or multiple myeloma reported longer time to an episode of HCM in patients treated with denosumab (HR 0.63, 95% confidence interval 0.41, 0.98, p=0.042) (Diel 2015). The divergence in rate of hypercalcemic episodes was noted at 6 months of therapy and continued throughout the duration of study analysis. However, according to the product labeling, denosumab is not indicated for the prevention of skeletal-related events in patients with multiple myeloma; in multiple myeloma trials, denosumab was noninferior to zoledronic acid in delaying time to first skeletal-related event and mortality was increased in a subset of the denosumab-treated group.

Hypocalcemia has been reported with denosumab use; monitor serum calcium levels accordingly.

Practitioners should inquire about denosumab administration in patents presenting for management of HCM. Recent administration of densoumab may influence the approach to management of HCM.

Calcitonin

Calcitonin works in a receptor-mediated manner to inhibit bone resorption and enhance urinary excretion of calcium. It is the fastest acting of the agents used to treat hypercalcemia and may be given safely before rehydration is complete. The usual starting dose of calcitonin is 4 units/kg by subcutaneous injection every 12 hours. Side effects are mild and infrequent and include nausea, abdominal cramps, and flushing. Calcitonin lowers serum calcium by ~2 mg/dL. Resistance to the pharmacologic effects of calcitonin generally develops with a few days of therapy. In fact, this can become apparent clinically as rebound hypercalcemia.

Corticosteroids

Corticosteroid administration is added to therapy when the underlying malignancy is a steroid-responsive disease, such as multiple myeloma, and lymphoma.

Other

Bortezomib has a dual anticancer and bone stabilizing effect. This medication, which is used in the treatment of multiple myeloma and mantle cell lymphoma, stimulates osteoblast differentiation, and inhibits osteoclast formation and bone resorption independently of its anticancer effect.

Drug	Usual Dose	Onset of Effect (hours)	Duration of Effect
Bisphosphonates (IV)			
Pamidronate	60 or 90 mg	24 to 48	Median: 10 days (1 to 30)
Zoledronic acid	4 mg	24 to 48	Median: 10 days (1 to 30)
Calcitonin (SubQ)	4 units/kg q12h	4	Median: 2 day (1 to 6)
Denosumab (SubQ)	120 mg every 4 weeks; during the first month, give an additional 120 mg on days 8 and 15	Median: 9 days; time to complete response: 23 days	Median: 104 days; duration of complete response: 34 days
0.9% sodium chloride (IV)	2 to 3 L/m^2 per 24 hours	12 to 48	Transient

Treatments are listed in alphabetical order. See text for guidance on priority and order of use.

REFERENCES

Diel IJ, Body JJ, Stopeck AT, et al. The role of denosumab in the prevention of hypercalcaemia of malignancy in cancer patients with metastatic bone disease. *Eur J Cancer.* 2015;51 (11):1467-1475.

Hu MI, Glezerman IG, Leboulleux S, et al. Denosumab for treatment of hypercalcemia of malignancy. *J Clin Endocrinol Metab.* 2014;99(9):3144-3152.

LeGrand SB, Leskuski D, Zama I. Narrative review: furosemide for hypercalcemia: an unproven yet common practice. *Ann Intern Med.* 2008;149(4):259-263.

Major P, Lortholary A, Hon J, et al. Zoledronic acid is superior to pamidronate in the treatment of hypercalcemia of malignancy: a pooled analysis of two randomized, controlled clinical trials. *J Clin Oncol.* 2001;19(2):558-567.

Nussbaum SR, Younger J, Vandepol CJ, et al. Single-dose intravenous therapy with pamidronate for the treatment of hypercalcemia of malignancy: comparison of 30-, 60-, and 90-mg dosages. *Am J Med.* 1993;95(3):297-304.

Penel N, Dewas S, Doutrelant P, Clisant S, Yazdanpanah Y, Adenis A. Cancer-associated hypercalcemia treated with intravenous diphosphonates: a survival and prognostic factor analysis. *Support Care Cancer.* 2008;16(4):387-392.

Perlia CP, Gubisch NJ, Wolter J, Edelberg D, Dederick MM, Taylor SG 3rd. Mithramycin treatment of hypercalcemia. *Cancer.* 1970;25:389-394.

Rosner MH, Dalkin AC. Onco-nephrology: the pathophysiology and treatment of malignancy-associated hypercalcemia. *Clin J Am Soc Nephrol.* 2012;7(10):1722-1729.

Shemerdiak WP, Kukreja SC, Lad TE, York PA, Henderson WJ. Evaluation of routine ionized calcium determination in cancer patients. *Clin Chem.* 1981;27:1621-1622.

Stewart AF. Clinical practice. Hypercalcemia associated with cancer. *N Engl J Med.* 2005;352 (4):373-379.

MALIGNANT PLEURAL EFFUSIONS

Malignant pleural effusion is an accumulation of fluid in the pleural space separating the lung and chest wall. It may be attributed to primary tumor growth, direct extension of tumor from an adjacent anatomic structure, or metastatic dissemination to the affected area. By definition, malignant pleural effusion must contain cancer cells. Lung (particularly adenocarcinoma), breast, and lymphoid malignancies account for two-thirds of malignant pleural effusions, but they are also found in cancer with unknown primary, gastric cancer, ovarian carcinomas, and mesothelioma. Case reports describe malignant pleural effusions with multiple myeloma, juvenile granulose cell tumor, pulmonary leiomyosarcoma, pleural liposarcoma, malignant melanoma, primitive neuroendocrine tumor, renal medullary carcinoma, and salivary gland cancer. A malignant pleural effusion may be the presenting sign of cancer, but most often it is a complication of a previously diagnosed malignancy. The median duration of survival following the diagnosis of malignant pleural effusion is 5 months; however, prolonged survival is possible in some cases. Predictors of less favorable outcome include high-risk tumors, poor performance status, lower pleural fluid glucose levels, leukocytosis, anemia, and hypoxemia.

PATHOPHYSIOLOGY

The pleura is a thin membrane that covers the lungs and chest wall. It is composed of the visceral pleura (covering the surface of the lungs) and the parietal pleura (covering the thoracic cavity). The interface between the two surfaces is the pleural space. Normally, pleural fluid production is <100 mL/day. Movement of fluid within the pleural space is governed by hydrostatic and oncotic pressures that follow Starling's law of transcapillary exchange. Hydrostatic pressure in the parietal capillaries is higher, causing a net movement into the pleural space. Reabsorption of the fluid occurs primarily through lymphatics on the parietal surface and less prominently via lymphatics on the visceral surface. Changes in pleural fluid production, reabsorption, or both produce a pleural effusion.

Malignancies can cause a fluid imbalance within the pleural space in several ways. Malignant cells in the pleural space can cause an inflammatory response that increases both capillary permeability and the net filtration of fluid, proteins, and cells into the pleural space. In addition, malignant obstruction of lymphatic channels and changes in pleural fluid protein content can impair reabsorption and drainage of fluid from the pleural space. The resulting fluid accumulation is exudative and is characterized by an increased concentration of protein and cells, decreased glucose levels compared to the serum, and an absence of eosinophils.

CLINICAL SYMPTOMS AND DIAGNOSIS

The most common symptom is dyspnea, often in conjunction with cough, chest pain, tachypnea, and reduced exercise tolerance. Symptoms are often related not to the amount of pleural fluid present, but to the rate of fluid accumulation. Patients with pleural effusions may be asymptomatic. A diagnosis often begins with a chest x-ray, which will demonstrate fluid accumulation on the posteroanterior (PA) and lateral decubitus film. Physical findings include dullness to percussion, decreased breath sounds, decreased diaphragmatic excursion, and possible contralateral tracheal deviation. In asymptomatic patients, malignant pleural effusion is generally diagnosed incidentally from radiographic imaging performed for other reasons.

TREATMENT PRINCIPLES

The goal of treatment is to effectively provide symptomatic relief with the least amount of risk and discomfort to the patient. Mainstays of therapy include fluid drainage (thoracentesis) with prevention of fluid reaccumulation by way of pleurodesis or an implanted pleural catheter. Successful palliation of dyspnea is possible with either pleurodesis or chronic drainage. Not all patients benefit from treatment. Some patients with effusions are asymptomatic and may not require treatment until symptoms develop. Individuals with a life expectancy of <1 month may benefit from oxygen, opioids, and possibly thoracentesis.

SYSTEMIC AND RADIATION THERAPY

Malignant pleural effusions arising from treatment-sensitive cancers are managed with systemic or radiation therapy intended to reduce the effusion by treating the underlying malignant cause. Improvement of malignant pleural effusions with systemic or radiation therapy is most likely to occur when the underlying cause is lymphoma, small cell lung cancer, germ cell tumor, breast cancer, ovarian cancer, prostate cancer, or thyroid cancer. Systemic therapy may be administered in addition to local therapy (effusion drainage) and pleurodesis (local instillation of treatment).

LOCAL THERAPY

Thoracentesis is the process of removing fluid from the pleural space using a specialized catheter and syringe under local anesthetic. This procedure can be done at the bedside and is utilized frequently for symptomatic patients. Thoracentesis is ineffective for long-term control of the malignant pleural effusion. Recurrence is frequent and repeated procedures carry a risk of increased complications, such as pneumothorax; ultrasound-guided thoracentesis can be performed to reduce this risk.

Tube thoracostomy (chest tube) is effective in controlling a malignant pleural effusion for a short period of time. Its 30-day success rate is ~70%. However, it is ineffective in the long-term control of effusions. Tubal thoracostomy is most useful in draining the fluid from the pleural space prior to instilling a sclerosing agent.

Indwelling pleural catheters with small bore tubing can be placed subcutaneously to provide long-term drainage of malignant pleural effusions. Patients can be educated to drain the catheters on a routine basis or as needed for symptom relief. The most common complication is pain or other symptoms due to intrapleural loculations, which occur in ~8% of cases. Additional complications reported in <5% of cases include unsuccessful insertion, asymptomatic loculations, cellulitis, empyema, and pneumothorax. Pleuroperitoneal shunts represent another tool that can be used for management of malignant pleural effusion.

PLEURODESIS

Pleurodesis, or sclerosis, should be considered in patients who experience symptomatic relief from thoracentesis with complete lung re-expansion and who have a life expectancy of at least weeks to months. The primary goals of pleurodesis are prevention of effusion reaccumulation and reduced hospitalizations for thoracentesis. Sclerosing agents act by promoting an inflammatory response in the pleura that causes fibrin adhesions of the visceral and parietal pleura. This results in fixed obliteration of the pleural space, which is prohibitive to recurrent effusion accumulation. Sclerosing agents are administered via a thoracostomy tube following demonstration of adequate effusate drainage (<200 mL/day).

The efficacy of pleurodesis is categorized as complete success, partial success, or failure. Criteria for complete success are long-term symptom relief and absence of fluid reaccumulation. Criteria for partial success are improved symptomatology with <50% of fluid reaccumulation without additional thoracentesis. Any less of a response is categorized as pleurodesis failure.

Successful use of a sclerosing agent depends on its uniform distribution in the pleural space and the dose of selected drug. The presence of loculations within the pleural space can interfere with distribution of the sclerosing agent. Immediate and complete lung expansion is desirable for pleurodesis. However, the clinical outcome for patients experiencing partial lung expansion is similar with respect to quality of life, procedure-related complications, extent of effusion drainage, hospital stay duration, and overall survival. Effective lung expansion and durable prevention of effusion reaccumulation may be related to tumor type. Patients with lung cancer and mesothelioma tend to have a less favorable response to pleurodesis in comparison to patients with breast or other cancers. Another factor that influences the efficacy of pleurodesis is the extent of tumor involving the pleural space.

SCLEROSING AGENTS

Sterile talc is one of the oldest and most effective sclerosing agents for treatment of malignant pleural effusions. Successful talc pleurodesis is achieved in 70% to 96% of patients. Meta-analysis infers that talc is a more effective sclerosing agent than bleomycin or tetracycline and tetracycline analogues. Pharmaceutical grade sterile asbestos-free talc is commercially available for use as a sclerosing agent. Talc powder is prepared as a sterile suspension for bedside administration through a chest tube. The usual dose of talc suspension is 2 to 5 g in 100 mL of 0.9% sodium chloride, with a maximum recommended cumulative dose of 10 g. Powdered talc is also available in a pressurized spray canister for administration under video-assisted thoracic surgery (VATS, thoracoscopy) or open thoracotomy. Aerosolized talc is available in single-use 4 g canisters; the usual dose is 4 to 8 g. Pain and fever are the most common acute side effects of pleurodesis. Rare serious adverse effects of talc pleurodesis include adult respiratory distress syndrome (ARDS), pneumonia, empyema, hemoptysis, bronchopleural fistula, tachycardia, hypotension, and infection. Cases of ARDS have usually occurred in patients receiving instillations of talc suspension at doses of 10 g. Some sterile talc formulations contain lead as an impurity and are therefore contraindicated in pregnancy; breastfeeding should be avoided.

The TIME2 study compared symptom control with talc pleurodesis vs an indwelling pleural catheter in 106 cases of previously untreated malignant pleural effusion. A 100 mm visual analogue scale (VAS) was used to measure dyspnea; a score of 0 mm indicated no dyspnea and a score of 100 mm indicated maximal dyspnea. Dyspnea was similarly improved in both groups for the initial 6 weeks of therapy (p=0.96). Assessment at 6 months identified a mean VAS score difference of 14 mm favoring symptom palliation in the group with implanted pleural catheters. This finding was statistically significant (p=0.01); however, it did not translate into a difference in quality of life between the two groups (p=0.14). More patients treated with talc pleurodesis (22%) required additional pleural procedures for symptom control compared to those with implanted pleural catheters (6%) (p=0.03). In addition, pleurodesis required hospitalization for a median 4 days (interquartile range: 2 to 6 days); whereas, catheter implantation was generally an entirely outpatient procedure (initial hospitalization for median 0 days [interquartile range: 0 to 1 days]). Treatment-related adverse events were more common in patients with implanted pleural catheters (40%) than in patients treated with pleurodesis (13%) (p=0.002) (Davies 2012).

Bleomycin 1 mg/kg (1 unit/kg) in 100 mL of 0.9% sodium chloride is an effective agent for controlling malignant pleural effusions. The range of intrapleural bleomycin doses reported in the literature is 24 to 240 mg. However, due to a lack of increased efficacy at doses >60 mg, some authors have recommended limiting the dose to 60 mg or 1 mg/kg body weight. Bleomycin has not demonstrated an efficacy advantage over talc and the acquisition cost of bleomycin is substantially greater than that of talc (Haddad 2004). Common toxicities associated with intrapleural bleomycin include pain, fever, and gastrointestinal adverse effects (nausea, vomiting, diarrhea). Serious adverse effects are more common in patients with elderly age or reduced renal function.

Parenteral tetracycline was one of the most widely used sclerosing agents prior to its removal from the market in the mid-1990s. Doxycycline 500 mg injection mixed in 50 to 100 mL of 0.9% sodium chloride effectively treats pleural effusions in 50% to 75% of patients; however, repeated instillations are generally required to achieve results similar to tetracycline. Intrapleural minocycline following VATS for spontaneous pneumothorax reduced prolonged postoperative air leaks, chest drainage, and hospital days for 313 patients relative to 51 consecutive historical controls (Chen 2004). The author reported administration of minocycline 300 to 400 mg injection in 20 mL of 0.9% sodium chloride through a chest tube. Due to a lack of stability information, this dose of minocycline should be prepared immediately before use. Chest pain was a common complaint after pleurodesis with minocycline.

Additional products that have been used as sclerosing agents for pleurodesis are povidone iodine, silver nitrate, and hyperthermic distilled water.

OTHER

Intrapleural administration of cytotoxic chemotherapy is reported. Its use is based on the premise that cytotoxic chemotherapy can exert anticancer and proinflammatory actions. In addition, intrapleural administration of chemotherapy may yield a regional advantage with intrapleural drug levels greatly exceeding drug levels in the plasma (Heffner 2008; Lombardi 2010). Vascular endothelial growth factor (VEGF) is believed to be a mediator in malignant pleural effusion formation and accumulation (Kitamura 2013). Inhibition of VEGF using bevacizumab in combination with chemotherapy for the management of malignant pleural effusion in patients with non-small cell lung cancer has been reported (Kitamura 2013). The reader is cautioned that the safety and efficacy of intrapleural administration of cytotoxic and biologic chemotherapy is not extensively tested.

A phase II study tested intrapleural administration of paclitaxel 120 mg/m^2 for the treatment of malignant pleural effusion in 18 patients with ovarian cancer (11 patients) or breast cancer (7 patients). Paclitaxel was infused after thoracentesis. The catheter used for paclitaxel administration was clamped for a period of 24 hours, after which it remained in place until drainage was <200 mL over 24 hours. Objective response (complete plus partial success rate) at 1 month and 2 months following treatment was reported in 78% and 89% of patients, respectively.

Common side effects included chest pain, fever, and dyspnea. Pleural fluid paclitaxel concentrations were approximately 10,000-fold greater than those measured in the plasma. The half-life of intrapleural paclitaxel was approximately 68 hours (Lombardi 2012). A phase I study with pharmacokinetic analysis of intrapleural docetaxel 50 to 125 mg/m^2 reported a 1,000-fold difference in concurrent drug concentrations measured in the pleural fluid relative to those in the plasma. This relative AUC from 0 to 36 hours for docetaxel in pleural fluid was 2,000 to 7,000 times greater than the corresponding plasma AUC (Jones 2010).

GENERAL PLEURODESIS PROCEDURE

Effusate is drained via a chest tube until the fluid production is <200 mL/day. The patient is premedicated with systemic analgesia (usually a parenteral opioid), sedation, and intrapleural administration of a topical anesthetic (typically lidocaine 1%). The sclerosing agent is instilled through the chest tube and the tube is clamped for 1 to 2 hours; the tube is then unclamped to drain the pleural fluid. The chest tube can be removed when drainage is <100 to 150 mL per 24 hours (Dresler 2005; Kvale 2007). Some procedures include frequent repositioning of the patient during the time that the chest tube is clamped to facilitate uniform distribution of the sclerosing agent, although the efficacy of repositioning is untested and its use is controversial.

COMPLICATIONS

Management of malignant pleural effusions is associated with several complications. Pain from insertion of the chest tube or instillation of the sclerosing agent should be pretreated with parenteral opioids. Traction pneumothorax results from repeated attempts to re-expand the lung. Cough is caused by lung re-expansion and is self-limiting. Fluid loculation is associated with drainage and pleurodesis. Lysis of adhesions may be necessary prior to pleurodesis. Empyema (purulent fluid) formation from contamination or bronchopulmonary communication should be treated with appropriate antibiotics.

REFERENCES

Antonangelo L, Rosa AG, Corá AP, Acencio MM, Moreira LC, Suso FV. Uncommon pleural effusion: pleuropulmonary metastasis from primitive neuroectodermal tumor. *J Bras Pneumol.* 2009;35(6):606-609.

Chen JS, Hsu HH, Kuo SW, et al. Effects of additional minocycline pleurodesis after thoracoscopic procedures for primary spontaneous pneumothorax. *Chest.* 2004;125(1):50-55.

Dagli AF, Pehlivan S, Ozercan MR. Pleural liposarcoma mimicking carcinoma in pleural effusion cytology: a case report. *Acta Cytol.* 2010;54(4):601-604.

Davies HE, Mishra EK, Kahan BC, et al. Effect of an indwelling pleural catheter vs chest tube and talc pleurodesis for relieving dyspnea in patients with malignant pleural effusion: the TIME2 randomized controlled trial. *JAMA.* 2012;307(22):2383-2389.

Dresler CM, Olak J, Herndon JE 2nd, et al. Phase III intergroup study of talc poudrage vs talc slurry sclerosis for malignant pleural effusion. *Chest.* 2005;127(3):909-915.

Ellis CL, Burroughs F, Michael CW, Li QK. Cytology of metastatic renal medullary carcinoma in pleural effusion: a study of two cases. *Diagn Cytopathol.* 2009;37(11):843-848.

Haddad FJ, Younes RN, Gross JL, Deheinzelin D. Pleurodesis in patients with malignant pleural effusions: talc slurry or bleomycin? Results of a prospective randomized trial. *World J Surg.* 2004;28(8):749-753.

Heffner JE, Klein JS. Recent advances in the diagnosis and management of malignant pleural effusions. *Mayo Clin Proc.* 2008;83(2):235-250.

Hirata T, Yonemori K, Hirakawa A, et al. Efficacy of pleurodesis for malignant pleural effusions in breast cancer patients. *Eur Respir J.* 2011;38(6):1425-1430.

Jones DR, Taylor MD, Petroni GR, et al. Phase I trial of intrapleural docetaxel administered through an implantable catheter in subjects with a malignant pleural effusion. *J Thorac Oncol.* 2010;5(1):75-81.

Kaur H, Bagga R, Saha SC, et al. Juvenile granulosa cell tumor of the ovary presenting with pleural effusion and ascites. *Int J Clin Oncol*. 2009;14(1):78-81.

Kitamura K, Kubota K, Ando M, et al. Bevacizumab plus chemotherapy for advanced non-squamous non-small-cell lung cancer with malignant pleural effusion. *Cancer Chemother Pharmacol*. 2013;71(2):457-461.

Kriegel I, Daniel C, Falcou MC, et al. Use of a subcutaneous implantable pleural port in the management of recurrent malignant pleurisy: five-year experience based on 168 subcutaneous implantable pleural ports. *J Palliat Med*. 2011;14(7):829-834.

Kubo A, Koh Y, Kawaguchi T, et al. Malignant pleural effusion from lung adenocarcinoma treated by gefitinib. *Intern Med*. 2011;50(7):745-748.

Kvale PA, Selecky PA, Prakash UB; American College of Chest Physicians. Palliative care in lung cancer: ACCP evidence-based clinical practice guidelines (2nd edition). *Chest*. 2007;132(3 Suppl):368S-403S.

Lombardi G, Nicoletto MO, Gusella M, et al. Intrapleural paclitaxel for malignant pleural effusion from ovarian and breast cancer: a phase II study with pharmacokinetic analysis. *Cancer Chemother Pharmacol*. 2012;69(3):781-787.

Lombardi G, Zustovich F, Nicoletto MO, Donach M, Artioli G, Pastorelli D. Diagnosis and treatment of malignant pleural effusion: a systematic literature review and new approaches. *Am J Clin Oncol*. 2010;33(4):420-423.

Mitra S, Kundu S, Pattari SK, Ghosal AG. Metastatic pleural effusion: a rare presentation of salivary gland adenoid cystic carcinoma. *Indian J Chest Dis Allied Sci*. 2011;53(2):107-110.

Passamonte PM, Luger AM. Primary pulmonary leiomyosarcoma with digital clubbing and pleural effusion. Case report. *Mo Med*. 1984;81(10):667-668.

Ryu JS, Ryu HJ, Lee SN, et al. Prognostic impact of minimal pleural effusion in non-small-cell lung cancer. *J Clin Oncol*. 2014;32(9):960-967.

Shameem M, Akhtar J, Baneen U, et al. Malignant melanoma presenting as an isolated pleural effusion. *Monaldi Arch Chest Dis*. 2011;75(2).138-140.

Suzuki K, Servais EL, Rizk NP, et al. Palliation and pleurodesis in malignant pleural effusion: the role for tunneled pleural catheters. *J Thorac Oncol*. 2011;6(4):702-707.

Terra RM, Junqueira JJ, Teixeira LR, Vargas FS, Pégo-Fernandes PM, Jatene FB. Is full postpleurodesis lung expansion a determinant of a successful outcome after talc pleurodesis? *Chest*. 2009;136(2):361-368.

Wang Z, Xia G, Lan L, et al. Pleural effusion in multiple myeloma. *Intern Med*. 2016;55(4):339-345.

Zamboni MM, da Silva CT Jr, Baretta R, Cunha ET, Cardoso GP. Important prognostic factors for survival in patients with malignant pleural effusion. *BMC Pulm Med*. 2015;15:29.

PALLIATIVE CARE MEDICINE (CANCER)

SCOPE OF PALLIATIVE CARE MEDICINE

The primary objective of palliative care is to improve quality of life through prevention of and relief from suffering (Herman 2013). Palliative care addresses symptoms arising from serious, life-threatening diseases and intractable symptoms caused by benign conditions that depreciate quality of life. Palliative care is often used in the management of patients with life expectancies extending months, years, or decades; however, it can also be an essential part of end-of-life (hospice) care. The scope of palliative care embraces improving quality of life for patients and their significant others. In addition to traditional disease-based medical treatments, comprehensive provision of palliative care strives to optimize functional capabilities, facilitate decision-making, and extend opportunities for personal growth. Elements of effective palliative care include an appropriate philosophy of care plus a well-organized infrastructure to address physical, psychological, social, cultural, and spiritual aspects of health.

The American Society of Clinical Oncology (ASCO) published a clinical practice guideline update in January of 2017 to provide evidence-based recommendations to the 2012 provisional clinical opinion (PCO). The 2012 PCO stated that palliative care should be offered in addition to standard anticancer therapy at the time of initial diagnosis of metastatic non-small cell lung cancer (NSCLC) (Smith 2012). The updated ASCO guideline recommendations now state that all patients (inpatient and outpatient) with any advanced cancer should receive dedicated palliative care services early in the disease course, concurrent with active treatment (Ferrel 2017). In several randomized controlled trials, demonstration of improved patient and caregiver outcomes with the addition of palliative care to standard therapy provided the impetus for the ASCO PCO. Advantages conferred with palliative care in the management of metastatic NSCLC include improvement in symptom control, mood, patient satisfaction, and reduced caregiver burden (Pirl 2012; Smith 2012). In addition, appropriate utilization of hospice services and reduced futile intensive terminal care were substantiated with early initiation of palliative care. Longer median survival, despite less aggressive end-of-life care, was reported for 77 patients with metastatic NSCLC randomized to receive palliative care (in addition to standard anticancer therapy) at the time of initial diagnosis vs a cohort of 74 patients randomized to receive standard anticancer therapy alone (p=0.02) (Temel 2010). Palliative care achieves these benefits without causing harm to the patient or caregiver, and without increasing the overall cost of care (Smith 2012). In fact, a prospective, observational study that examined 969 patient cases in five hospitals determined that direct health care costs are reduced with earlier palliative care consultation for hospitalized patients with advanced cancers. The cost of hospitalization was reduced 14% and 24% when the consultation was placed within six days and two days, respectively, of hospital admission in comparison to patients not receiving palliative care consultations (May 2015). Despite these positive findings, the ASCO provisional clinical opinion acknowledges that stringently performed palliative care research is in its infancy. To facilitate the integration of palliative care into standard oncology practice, ASCO recommends the following investigative priorities: Optimal timing and venue (inpatient, outpatient/community) for palliative care, reimbursement models, interventions providing greatest benefit,

benefit in diseases other than lung cancer, and impact of palliative care across the continuum of care (especially during the delivery of anticancer therapy).

Medication Safety and Administration

Palliative care is provided most effectively by an interdisciplinary team specializing in this area of medicine. One central aspect of palliative care is symptom control for intractable situations following an adequate trial of the therapeutic standard of care. Subsequently, medications may be prescribed for off-label indications at doses outside of the norm and for administration by atypical routes. Due to this unique practice approach, clinical and regulatory challenges related to the delivery of pharmaceutical products for palliative care directly impact the pharmacy department. Moreover, since palliative care medicine is an evolving field, medical literature supporting the safety and efficacy of certain interventions may be scant. Some medications used for symptom management are controlled substances or medications prone to diversion, so the pharmacy department and all members of the palliative care team must adhere to stringent methods of drug accountability. To address these challenges, pharmacy departments should formalize policies and procedures that support the legitimate and uniform delivery of palliative pharmaceutical care.

Subcutaneous administration of palliative care medications may replace other standard routes of administration for patient comfort, patient functional ability (eg, dysphagia), inadequate venous access, and to support delivery of care in the home setting. Case series and case reports describe off-label subcutaneous administration of parenteral medications. Local adverse effects can occur with subcutaneous administration of pharmaceutical products. Common localized adverse effects include injection site pain, swelling, redness, and irritation. One observational study monitored 120 patients who received subcutaneous injections in the thighs (39%) and upper arms (29%); 3,957 injections via 243 needles were administered. Most local adverse effects were noted on the third or fourth day following needle placement and generally occurred in the fully active patients (Bartz 2014). The volume of subcutaneous administration and product characteristics (eg, pH, irritant potential) may affect the suitability for this route of administration. Due to risk of malabsorption or patient discomfort, avoid edematous limbs, indurated (hard) skin, painful areas, irradiated skin, and areas overlaying bone when injecting subcutaneously. Continuous subcutaneous infusion of morphine or hydromorphone (diluted in 5% dextrose solution) at a rate of 0.5 to 10 mL/hour is described (Bruera 1988). Parenteral fentanyl, haloperidol, infusional lidocaine, methadone, metoclopramide, midazolam, and oxymorphone have also been administered subcutaneously for use in the palliative care setting (Bartz 2014; Brose 1991; Protus 2015).

SYMPTOM MANAGEMENT

Pain

The management of pain, including both opioid and nonopioid analgesic therapy, should be optimized as per standard clinical practice; for more information, refer to Chronic Pain Management (Cancer) on page 2327. Nonopioid analgesic therapy for cancer-related pain may include both pharmaceutical and non-pharmacological interventions. Nonsteroidal anti-inflammatory drugs (NSAIDs), bisphosphonates, and radiotherapy should be used as appropriate for bone pain. External beam radiation may be helpful for tumor size reduction with pain relief in some cases. NSAIDs or corticosteroids should be used as warranted for inflammatory pain. Gabapentin, pregabalin, and antidepressants (TCAs, including nortriptyline and desipramine, or SNRIs, including duloxetine and venlafaxine) may improve neuropathic pain.

In cases of intractable pain, high doses of opioid analgesia may be required for adequate pain management. The oral route of administration is preferred whenever possible. Opioid administration by continuous subcutaneous or intravenous infusion (with or without patient-controlled PRN boluses) is also an option; however, subcutaneous infusion of methadone should be avoided due to local irritation. Some patients may require intraspinal opioid administration to achieve and tolerate adequate pain control.

Methadone can be administered by continuous intravenous infusion and patient-controlled analgesia; however, this intervention is often reserved for select patients as a bridge to intraspinal therapy because methadone prolongs the QTc interval and exhibits discordance between its pharmacokinetics and pharmacodynamics. The risk of torsade de pointes is increased when the QTc interval exceeds 500 milliseconds. Consensus guidelines (Shaiova 2008) pertaining to intravenous administration of methadone recommend assessment of the QTc interval at baseline, 24 hours, and 4 days after initiation of methadone, as well as assessment following any significant dose increase or at the discretion of the practitioner. More frequent monitoring of the QTc interval should be considered for patients with a QTc interval exceeding 450 milliseconds. Patients should be advised of the risk of dysrhythmias with methadone so that they may make an informed decision about their therapy. Since the half-life of methadone exceeds the duration of analgesia, the consensus guidelines state that the initial rate titration must be performed at least 12 hours after initiation of the infusion to allow evolution of side effects prior to increasing systemic drug concentrations. Subsequent rate titrations should be executed once daily. The consensus guidelines also recommend liberal use of PRN boluses before and between rate titration of methadone by continuous intravenous infusion. Due to incomplete cross-tolerance between methadone and high-dose morphine, a 25% to 50% reduction in the calculated methadone dose at infusion initiation is recommended for patients requiring >50 mg/hour of morphine. In addition, the consensus guidelines recommend the following conversion factors (Shaiova 2008):

| Opioid | Basal Rate (mg/hour) | Methadone | |
		Basal Rate (mg/hour)	PRN Bolus Available Every 15 Minutes
Morphine	10	1	1
HYDROmorphone	1.5	0.3	0.3
FentaNYL	0.25	1.25	1.25

Intravenous lidocaine is used for severe intractable neuropathic pain. The efficacy of lidocaine is greater in the treatment of peripheral sensory neuropathy vs symptoms caused by a central pain syndrome. Small studies report administration of intravenous lidocaine 1 to 5 mg/kg over a period of 30 minutes to 6 hours. Alternatively, some centers use a set dose of 100 to 150 mg infused intravenously over a period of 30 to 60 minutes. Analgesia superior to placebo is reported in crossover design trials. The reported time to maximum analgesia is 1 to 6 hours, with the reported duration of analgesia ranging from hours to days to weeks. Common adverse effects include lightheadedness, vertical nystagmus, feeling drunk, and sedation. Administration of intravenous lidocaine 1 to 5 mg/kg over a period of 30 minutes to 6 hours without demonstration of cardiac or central nervous system toxicity is reported; the lack of serious side effects is probably explained by the rapid metabolism of systemic lidocaine. Caution should be exercised when using intravenous lidocaine in patients who are elderly, debilitated, or have poor hepatic function. Instead of intravenous lidocaine infusion, one case series of three patients with neuropathic cancer pain describes chronic administration of lidocaine 100 to 160 mg/hour by continuous subcutaneous infusion (Brose 1991). With administration by continuous infusion via any route, periodic assessment of serum lidocaine levels should be considered.

Ketamine is used as an adjunct to opioid therapy for intractable cancer pain and neuropathic pain. Ketamine can be administered orally, intravenously, and subcutaneously. Ketamine can also be administered intramuscularly; however, this route is rarely used for repeated administration. The recommended dose of oral ketamine is 20 to 60 mg 3 to 4 times daily plus PRN administration of ketamine 20 mg every 3 hours. When ketamine is being discontinued, tapering the dose at a rate of 25% per 24 hours may reduce the likelihood of dysphoria. Ketamine is commercially available as a parenteral formulation and the oral dose can be mixed in cola immediately prior to ingestion. To reduce the risk of drug diversion or inadvertent ingestion by a family member, some institutions have the nurse squirt the dose of ketamine from an oral syringe into the patient's mouth with cola or another beverage to follow. Intravenous ketamine is generally given as a continuous infusion starting at 1 to 2 mg/hour; administration as an intravenous bolus of 0.1 to 0.4 mg/kg is also reported in the literature. Ketamine may cause hallucinations, drowsiness, and confusion. At anesthetic doses (1 to 4.5 mg/kg via intravenous bolus), ketamine causes hypertension and tachycardia. Common adverse effects described with infusional ketamine for palliative care include nausea (63%), vomiting (47%), and central nervous system effects (93%) (psychomimetic effects, hallucinations, dizziness, feeling of inebriation). Cystitis attributed to ketamine administration is primarily reported with repeated oral administration. A case of markedly elevated blood pressure is also described following repeated oral administration of ketamine (Van Hecke 2014). Cases of hepatotoxicity, which are common with ketamine-based substance abuse, are reported with ketamine administered by continuous intravenous infusion to manage chronic regional pain syndrome.

Dyspnea

The sensation of dyspnea is a complex disorder that is influenced by many pathophysiologic changes within and outside of the cardiopulmonary system. Opioid (usually morphine) administration is the cornerstone of medication therapy for reducing the sensation of chronic dyspnea in advanced cancer patients. Opioid medications should always be used cautiously; however, medical literature supports the safety and efficacy of opioid administration for the management of chronic dyspnea in this patient population. Morphine (or an equivalent opioid) can be administered to cancer patients with mild to severe dyspnea for symptom control without having a deleterious effect on SaO_2, $PaCO_2$, or heart rate. These findings are consistent when evaluated relative to whether the patient was opioid-naïve or hypoxic (SaO_2 <90%) at baseline. For opioid-naïve patients, morphine doses in the range of 1 to 3 mg by intravenous push or 5 to 10 mg orally PRN every 4 hours may be sufficient to improve dyspnea; opioid-tolerant patients will need higher doses to relieve dyspnea. There is no advantage to morphine administration by nebulization vs use of the subcutaneous, intravenous, or oral routes.

The identification and management of comorbid conditions also contributes to the relief of dyspnea symptoms. Treatment of anxiety using lorazepam or another suitable product may improve the sensation of dyspnea. The addition of furosemide to therapy should be considered when heart failure may be a contributing factor. For patients with chronic obstructive pulmonary disease, long acting beta-agonists improve dyspnea. The use of oxygen therapy in all patients with dyspnea is controversial due to conflicting information about its efficacy in the medical literature; patients with chronic obstructive pulmonary disease are most likely to benefit from oxygen therapy.

Other nonpharmacological therapies are also helpful in the management of dyspnea. Slow, deep breathing or breathing into a paper bag, along with increasing air flow and air quality in the patient's room, are helpful. This can be accomplished with an open window or a fan to create a draft (ribbons on the fan can aid in creating a visual effect of air movement). Encourage relaxation with a quiet and calm environment with music and/or with light massage. Reduce exposure to possible triggers, such as strong odors, perfumes, and smoke. Provide support and companionship, as isolation and spiritual issues may worsen dyspnea symptoms (Protus 2015).

Cough/Hiccups

Initial symptomatic treatment of persistent cough due to chronic disease affecting the lungs includes guaifenesin, dextromethorphan, and benzonatate. Nebulized saline can help thin secretions and aid in expectoration. For intractable cough despite usual therapies, nebulized lidocaine may provide relief. Symptomatic relief from nebulized lidocaine occurs rapidly for responding patients. Common adverse effects of this therapy include oropharyngeal numbness and an unpleasant taste. It is also important to note that nebulized lidocaine causes a transient loss of gag reflex. Nebulized lidocaine for intractable cough is often administered as follows:

Nebulized Lidocaine for Intractable Cough Administration

Lidocaine 4% preservative-free 2.5 mL
Administer by nebulization every 4 hours as needed.
Note: Patient should have nothing by mouth for 30 minutes before and 2 hours after each dose.

Intractable hiccups, which are generally defined as hiccups lasting more than 1 month, impair the quality and activities of daily life. Hiccups are caused by repeated, involuntary, spasmodic contractions of the diaphragm, followed by a sudden closure of the glottis, which blocks incoming air to produce the characteristic sounds. Hiccups can present secondary to gastric extension and diaphragmatic irritation. Drugs credited with causing intractable hiccups include aprepitant, dexamethasone, doxycycline, etoposide, megestrol acetate, and perphenazine. When hiccups are thought to be medication-related, interruption of therapy should be tried. Nonpharmacologic methods for hiccup cessation should be attempted prior to drug therapy. Examples of nonpharmacologic therapy include holding one's breath, breathing inside of a paper (nonplastic) grocery bag, gasping with sudden fright, the Valsalva maneuver, hyperventilation, slowly drinking water, and drinking water from the "wrong side" of a glass. Gastric distention relief (eg, fasting, lavage, vomiting) or vagal maneuvers (eg, digital rectal massage, ocular compression, or carotid massage) may also provide hiccup relief (Protus 2015).

Medications used to manage intractable hiccups include chlorpromazine, haloperidol, metoclopramide, baclofen, and gabapentin. Chlorpromazine may be administered orally or intravenously at a dosage of 25 to 50 mg 3 to 4 times daily as needed or around the clock. Chlorpromazine may also be administered intramuscularly; however, this route is seldom utilized for repeated administration. Haloperidol 0.5 mg has been given orally every six hours as needed for hiccups (Protus 2015). Haloperidol is less sedating than chlorpromazine, has more versatile dosing, and has other indications in relation to palliative care, including treatment of nausea and vomiting via oral or subcutaneous delivery (Hardy 2010; Protus 2015). Metoclopramide, baclofen, and gabapentin are administered on a scheduled basis around the clock (instead of PRN) for this indication. Metoclopramide 10 mg is generally administered 4 times daily (orally or intravenously) for control of hiccups. The dosage of baclofen for intractable hiccups is 5 to 10 mg by mouth 3 to 4 times daily. Gabapentin administered 300 to 400 mg 3 times daily by mouth for control of hiccups is reported in the medical literature, but gabapentin has a wide margin of safety and doses up to 3,600 mg/day are well-tolerated in patients with adequate renal function. Combination therapy using drugs with different pharmacologic mechanisms of action and nonoverlapping toxicity may be tried for patients not responding to single-agent therapy.

Hiccups that continue despite an adequate trial of chlorpromazine, metoclopramide, and baclofen may respond to nebulized lidocaine. The dosage, time to effect, and safety of nebulized lidocaine is described in the preceding section pertaining to management of intractable cough.

Fatigue

Cancer-related fatigue (CRF) is a persistent sensation of physical, emotional, or cognitive tiredness or exhaustion attributed to oncologic disease or its treatment that exceeds the usual severity for associated actions and hinders normal activities. ASCO released a clinical practice guideline adaptation in 2014 to outline screening, assessment, and management of fatigue in adult cancer survivors. The recommendation includes quantitative screening for fatigue at least annually (and as clinically indicated). Laboratory evaluation can be considered based on severity and presence of other symptoms. Contributing factors must be addressed and treated first (eg, activity level, anemia, anxiety, depression, emotional distress, medication adverse effects, nutritional deficit, pain, sleep disturbances, other comorbidities). Patients should be educated and counseled in fatigue management strategies, including increasing physical activity, cognitive behavioral therapy, and other psychosocial interventions, along with mind-body approaches (eg, yoga, reiki, massage, and music therapy) (Bower 2014).

Pharmacological interventions include methylphenidate and modafinil and can be used in patients with advanced disease and even during active therapy. There is, however, limited evidence of their effectiveness in reducing fatigue in patients who are currently disease-free after active treatment (Bower 2014). Small pilot studies evaluating supplements (eg, ginseng, vitamin D) have found no consistent evidence of their effectiveness.

Other psychostimulants, such as dextroamphetamine, may also be considered (Protus 2015). The use of corticosteroids, progestational steroids, antidepressants, and vitamins for the management of CRF has also been reported (Campos 2011). It is important to note, fatigue may be a protective response against suffering at the end of life. Avoid treatment with worsening physical or existential discomfort (Protus 2015).

REFERENCES

Attal N, Rouaud J, Brasseur L, Chauvin M, Bouhassira D. Systemic lidocaine in pain due to peripheral nerve injury and predictors of response. *Neurology.* 2004;62(2):218-225.

Bartz L, Klein C, Seifert A, Herget I, Ostgathe C, Stiel S. Subcutaneous administration of drugs in palliative care: results of a systematic observational study. *J Pain Symptom Manage.* 2014;48 (4):540-547.

Bower JE, Bak K, Berger A, et al. Screening, assessment, and management of fatigue in adult survivors of cancer: an American Society of Clinical oncology clinical practice guideline adaptation. *J Clin Oncol.* 2014;32(17):1840-1850.

Brose WG, Cousins MJ. Subcutaneous lidocaine for treatment of neuropathic cancer pain. *Pain.* 1991;45(2):145-148.

Bruera E, Brenneis C, Michaud M, et al. Use of the subcutaneous route for the administration of narcotics in patients with cancer pain. *Cancer.* 1988;62(2):407-411.

Campos MP, Hassan BJ, Riechelmann R, Del Giglio A. Cancer-related fatigue: a practical review. *Ann Oncol.* 2011;22(6):1273-1279.

Clemens KE, Quednau I, Klaschik E. Use of oxygen and opioids in the palliation of dyspnoea in hypoxic and nonhypoxic palliative care patients: a prospective study. *Support Care Cancer.* 2009;17(4):367-377.

Clinical Practice Guidelines for Quality Palliative Care. 2nd ed. Pittsburgh, PA: National Consensus Project for Quality Palliative Care; 2009. http://www.nationalconsensusproject.org/guideline.pdf

Dy SM, Lorenz KA, Naeim A, Sanati H, Walling A, Asch SM. Evidence-based recommendations for cancer fatigue, anorexia, depression, and dyspnea. *J Clin Oncol.* 2008;26(23):3886-3895.

Enarson MC, Hays H, Woodroffe MA. Clinical experience with oral ketamine. *J Pain Symptom Manage.* 1999;17(5):384-386.

Escalante CP, Meyers C, Reuben JM, et al. A randomized, double-blind, 2-period, placebo-controlled crossover trial of a sustained-release methylphenidate in the treatment of fatigue in cancer patients. *Cancer J.* 2014;20(1):8-14.

Ferrell BR, Temel JS, Temin S, et al. Integration of palliative care into standard oncology care: American Society of Clinical Oncology clinical practice guideline update. *J Clin Oncol.* 2017;35 (1):96-112.

Gong S, Sheng P2, Jin H, et al. Effect of methylphenidate in patients with cancer-related fatigue: a systematic review and meta-analysis. *PLoS One.* 2014;9(1):e84391.

Hardy JR, O'Shea A, White C, Gilshenan K, Welch L, Douglas C. The efficacy of haloperidol in the management of nausea and vomiting in patients with cancer. *J Pain Symptom Manage.* 2010;40 (1):111-116.

Herman C. National Consensus Project Updates Palliative Care Guidelines. *Aging Today Online.* September 26, 2013. Available at http://asaging.org/blog/national-consensus-project-updates-palliative-care-guidelines

Hovey E, de Souza P, Marx G, et al. Phase III, randomized, double-blind, placebo-controlled study of modafinil for fatigue in patients treated with docetaxel-based chemotherapy. *Support Care Cancer.* 2014;22(5):1233-1242.

Jean-Pierre P, Morrow GR, Roscoe JA, et al. A phase 3 randomized, placebo-controlled, double-blind, clinical trial of the effect of modafinil on cancer-related fatigue among 631 patients receiving chemotherapy: a University of Rochester Cancer Center community clinical oncology program research base study. *Cancer.* 2010;116(14):3513-3520.

Kannan TR, Saxena A, Bhatnagar S, Barry A. Oral ketamine as an adjuvant to oral morphine for neuropathic pain in cancer patients. *J Pain Symptom Manage.* 2002;23(1):60-65.

Kerr CW, Drake J, Milch RA, et al. Effects of methylphenidate on fatigue and depression: a randomized, double-blind, placebo-controlled trial. *J Pain Symptom Manage.* 2012;43(1):68-77.

Lower EE, Fleishman S, Cooper A, et al. Efficacy of dexmethylphenidate for the treatment of fatigue after cancer chemotherapy: a randomized clinical trial. *J Pain Symptom Manage.* 2009;38(5):650-662.

May P, Garrido MM, Cassel JB, et al. Prospective cohort study of hospital palliative care teams for inpatients with advanced cancer: earlier consultation is associated with larger cost-saving effect. *J Clin Oncol.* 2015;33(25):2745-2752.

Midgren B, Hansson L, Karlsson JA, Simonsson BG, Persson CG. Capsaicin-induced cough in humans. *Am Rev Respir Dis.* 1992;146(2):347-351.

Neeno TA, Rosenow EC 3rd. Intractable hiccups. Consider nebulized lidocaine. *Chest.* 1996;110 (4):1129-1130.

Paulsen O, Klepstad P, Rosland JH, et al. Efficacy of methylprednisolone on pain, fatigue, and appetite loss in patients with advanced cancer using opioids: a randomized, placebo-controlled, double-blind trial. *J Clin Oncol.* 2014;32(29):3221-3228.

Pirl WF, Greer JA, Traeger L, et al. Depression and survival in metastatic non-small-cell lung cancer: effects of early palliative care. *J Clin Oncol.* 2012;30(12):1310-1315.

Protus BM, Kimbrel JM, Grauer PA. *Palliative Care Consultant: a reference guide for palliative care. Guidelines for effective management of symptoms.* 4th ed. Montgomery, AL; 2015.

Qaseem A, Snow V, Shekelle P, et al. Evidence-based interventions to improve the palliative care of pain, dyspnea, and depression at the end of life: a clinical practice guideline from the American College of Physicians. *Ann Intern Med.* 2008;148(2):141-146.

Rizzo JD, Brouwers M, Hurley P, et al. American Society of Clinical Oncology/American Society of Hematology clinical practice guideline update on the use of epoetin and darbepoetin in adult patients with cancer. *J Clin Oncol.* 2010;28(33):4996-5010.

Shaiova L, Berger A, Blinderman CD, et al. Consensus guideline on parenteral methadone use in pain and palliative care. *Palliat Support Care.* 2008;6(2):165-176.

Smith TJ, Temin S, Alesi ER, et al. American Society of Clinical Oncology provisional clinical opinion: the integration of palliative care into standard oncology care. *J Clin Oncol.* 2012;30 (8):880-887.

Spathis A, Fife K, Blackhall F, et al. Modafinil for the treatment of fatigue in lung cancer: results of a placebo-controlled, double-blind, randomized trial. *J Clin Oncol.* 2014;32(18):1882-1888.

Sternberg CN, Molina A, North S, et al. Effect of abiraterone acetate on fatigue in patients with metastatic castration-resistant prostate cancer after docetaxel chemotherapy. *Ann Oncol.* 2013;24(4):1017-1025.

Temel JS, Greer JA, Muzikansky A, et al. Early palliative care for patients with metastatic non-small-cell lung cancer. *N Engl J Med.* 2010;363(8):733-742.

Tremont-Lukats IW, Hutson PR, Backonja MM. A randomized, double-masked, placebo-controlled pilot trial of extended IV lidocaine infusion for relief of ongoing neuropathic pain. *Clin J Pain.* 2006;22(3):266-271.

van Hecke O, Guthrie B. Oral ketamine analgesia in chronic pain and problematic rise in blood pressure. *BMJ Case Rep.* 2014;2014.

Yennurajalingam S, Frisbee-Hume S, Palmer JL, et al. Reduction of cancer-related fatigue with dexamethasone: a double-blind, randomized, placebo-controlled trial in patients with advanced cancer. *J Clin Oncol.* 2013;31(25):3076-3082.

VENOUS THROMBOEMBOLISM IN THE CANCER PATIENT

INTRODUCTION

Venous thromboembolism (VTE) is a common and life-threatening complication in cancer patients. Overall, ~500,000 new cases of VTE are diagnosed annually, 1 in 5 of which are diagnosed in cancer patients. Patients with active cancer have at least a 6- to 7-fold increased risk of VTE. Development of VTE is a major cause of mortality in this population; it may increase the likelihood of death by up to 47-fold in certain patients (Khorana 2007). Diagnosis of VTE or superficial venous thrombosis in a young or middle-aged person without an identifiable cause raises suspicion for underlying malignancy. VTE is generally diagnosed in cancer patients within the first few months of malignant disease and may be related to a number of intrinsic (eg, tumor aggressiveness) or extrinsic (eg, surgery, radiation) factors. Pathophysiologic causes for VTE in cancer patients include hypercoagulability, vessel wall damage, and vessel stasis from direct compression by tumors. Given the significant morbidity and mortality caused by VTE, it is important for the clinician to recognize patients at risk for VTE and to offer appropriate prophylactic and treatment strategies. In addition, clinicians should provide patients with proper education regarding signs and symptoms of VTE.

VTE RISK ASSESSMENT

VTE risk should be assessed in all cancer patients at the time of chemotherapy initiation and periodically thereafter. VTE risk factors in this patient population can be separated into three categories: patient-related (ie, intrinsic and extrinsic factors), cancer-related, and treatment-related. Patient-related factors include an active cancer diagnosis, previous VTE, hypercoagulable state (eg, factor V Leiden, lupus anticoagulant, anticardiolipin antibodies), >70 years of age, obesity (BMI ≥30 kg/m^2), hospitalization, and bed rest/immobility (for at least 3 days). Increased comorbid burden defined by coexisting conditions, such as pulmonary disease, kidney disease, and infections, is also associated with a greater risk of VTE.

The type of cancer also influences VTE risk. A diagnosis of metastatic cancer arising from the pancreas, stomach, bladder, uterus, kidney, and lung confers a greater risk for VTE, as do diagnoses of acute leukemia, multiple myeloma, and non-Hodgkin lymphoma. Lower risk for VTE is associated with breast cancer, prostate cancer, and head and neck cancers. In addition, histologic subtype also plays a role in VTE prevalence, with adenocarcinomas having a higher risk compared to squamous cell cancers. Advanced stage of disease, poor patient performance status, and the finding of leukocytosis or thrombocytosis (platelet count >350,000/microliter) at presentation all may put patients at risk for thrombosis. Lastly, VTE risk factors specific to multiple myeloma include M-spike >1.6 g/dL, progressive disease, and hyperviscosity syndrome.

Treatment-related and iatrogenic factors, such as surgery, the presence of a central venous access device (CVAD), and chemotherapy and/or radiotherapy administration, place cancer patients in jeopardy of developing VTE. The reported incidence of ultrasound-detected upper extremity deep venous thrombosis (DVT) is variable (2% to 67%) (Rooden 2005) and the incidence of pulmonary embolism (PE) on autopsy reports was up to 50% (Verso 2003) in cancer patients with CVADs. The 3 main classes of cancer drugs which may lead to VTE include cytotoxic chemotherapy, hormonal therapy with estrogenic properties, and anti-angiogenic medications. Administration of cytotoxic chemotherapy is associated with a 2- to 6-fold increased risk of VTE. Selective estrogen receptor modulator (tamoxifen) administration is associated with 2- to 5-fold increased risk of VTE among women with breast cancer (Kahn 2012). The findings of one meta-analysis indicate that the incidence of VTE (all grades) is ~11% with bevacizumab (in combination with chemotherapy or immunotherapy) administration (Hurwitz 2011). The immune modulating products lenalidomide and thalidomide are thrombogenic, especially when administered in combination with a corticosteroid or cytotoxic chemotherapy. Treatment of multiple myeloma and lymphoid malignancies often involves chronic or episodic corticosteroid administration, which further increases the risk of VTE. Ancillary therapies used to prevent and manage disease and treatment-related adverse events can also increase the likelihood of VTE. Two such examples are erythopoietin-stimulating agents (ESA) administered for anemia and corticosteroids, which may be administered for antiemesis, as well as other indications.

VTE PROPHYLAXIS

Due to the high risk of VTE in hospitalized patients with cancer, prophylactic anticoagulation using a low molecular weight heparin (LMWH), fondaparinux, or unfractionated heparin should be administered to all hospitalized patients with active cancer and acute medical illness or reduced mobility (in the absence of bleeding or other contraindications) according to standard guidelines. Prophylaxis with LMWH or unfractionated heparin is also recommended in patients with cancer prior to undergoing major surgery and continuing for at least 7 to 10 days postoperatively (unless contraindicated). In patients for whom anticoagulation is absolutely or relatively contraindicated (eg, recent central nervous system bleeding, major active bleeding, recent lumbar puncture, low platelet count), intermittent pneumatic venous compression devices (IPCs) may be considered for VTE prophylaxis. There is not enough evidence to support or oppose routine thromboprophylaxis in patients hospitalized for short chemotherapy courses, minor procedures, or for hematopoietic stem cell transplantation.

Criteria for VTE prophylaxis in the outpatient cancer setting are not clearly delineated. Routine pharmacologic thromboprophylaxis is not recommended for most ambulatory cancer patients; however, some surgical and medical oncology patients are at high risk for VTE and may benefit from extended outpatient prophylaxis. For surgical oncology patients (particularly high-risk patients undergoing abdominal or pelvic surgery), continued administration of VTE prophylaxis after hospital discharge for a period of up to 4 weeks following major surgery may be recommended. Multiple myeloma patients receiving thrombotic anticancer therapy (lenalidomide or thalidomide in combination with dexamethasone >480 mg monthly or doxorubicin or multiagent chemotherapy) also may require outpatient VTE prophylaxis. LMWHs, unfractionated heparin, and warfarin are the primary agents used for VTE prophylaxis in cancer patients. Aspirin can be considered for VTE prophylaxis in patients with multiple myeloma at relatively low-risk for VTE (no more than one VTE risk factor). Risk stratification criteria based on tumor site, prechemotherapy platelet count, prechemotherapy leukocyte count, anemia and ESA administration, and body size have been proposed (Dutia 2012). Overall, primary pharmacologic prophylaxis for VTE in ambulatory cancer patients remains controversial because it increases the risk of bleeding with indeterminate efficacy for prevention of VTE.

VTE TREATMENT

Initial treatment of VTE in cancer patients is similar to that of noncancer patients, with unfractionated heparin, LMWHs, and warfarin (vitamin K antagonist [VKA]) providing the cornerstone of anticoagulant therapy. Initial assessment and management of VTE in cancer patients is conducted according to clinical practice guidelines and institutional policy. According to the American College of Chest Physicians (CHEST) guidelines, the use of LMWH is preferred over a VKA or a novel oral anticoagulant (eg, dabigatran, rivaroxaban, apixaban) for the first 3 months of treatment in cancer patients who develop DVT of the leg or PE. If initial therapy with LMWH is not feasible, the use of VKAs or novel anticoagulants is an acceptable alternative. In patients who do not have a high bleeding risk and continue to have active cancer, patients may receive extended anticoagulants with no scheduled stop date using the same anticoagulant chosen during the initial 3 months of therapy (ACCP [Kearon 2016]). For treatment of a catheter-related DVT, the recommended duration of treatment is at least 3 months and for as long as the catheter remains in place.

Special situations related to cancer and its treatments may complicate delivery of safe and effective therapeutic anticoagulation. Low platelet counts due to hematologic malignancies or cytotoxic treatments may be present in cancer patients requiring anticoagulation. Unfortunately, limited options exist for patients with an active clotting process, despite a low platelet count, so management of therapeutic anticoagulation in the setting of thrombocytopenia must be handled judiciously on a case-by-case basis. Inferior vena cava (IVC) filter placement is one method for reducing the risk of PE in patients with DVT who have contra-indications to anticoagulant therapy. Drawbacks to IVC filter placement include lack of systemic anticoagulant effect and increased risk of recurrent DVT. Cancer patients requiring anticoagulation may also need intrathecal administration of chemotherapy. Anticoagulation must be interrupted for spinal injection and intra-thecal medication administration. The American Society of Regional Anesthesia and Pain Medicine (ASRA) recommends withholding LMWH for at least 24 hours and unfractionated heparin for at least 1 hour before spinal injection for the delivery of analgesia. Warfarin should be held for 4 to 5 days prior to spinal injection.

ANTICOAGULANT SELECTION

Anticoagulant selection may be influenced by cancer and its treatments. The anticoagulant activity of warfarin is readily affected by diet, drug interactions, liver function, and certain physiologic stressors. Food intake in the cancer patient can vary relative to disease- and treatment-related factors that alter taste sensation, reduce appetite, and cause adverse gastrointestinal events. Numerous thera-peutic and ancillary medications used in the management of cancer interact with the anticoagulant intensity of warfarin. Due to the extensive and expanding list of medications that interact with warfarin, the reader should refer to specific drug monographs for detailed information about particular medications. Hepatic function in the cancer patient can be impaired due to primary or metastatic tumor growth in the liver. In addition, any physiologic stressor, such as infection, can alter the anticoagulant effect of warfarin in this patient population.

LMWHs are not prone to altered anticoagulant intensity by the myriad of dietary, drug, and physiologic factors affecting warfarin therapy. However, all commer-cially available LMWHs are excreted renally and may require dosage adjust-ments in patients with renal dysfunction; anti-Xa monitoring may facilitate appropriate administration in this clinical scenario. Unfractionated heparin should be considered as an alternative to LMWH for use in patients with severely impaired renal function.

The use of novel oral anticoagulants is not currently recommended as first-line therapy for either prevention or treatment of VTE in cancer patients (Kearon 2016). In patients with cancer who cannot take LMWHs, expert opinion does not prefer a VKA over a novel oral anticoagulant (Kearon 2016). While some oral anticoagulants are approved for selected VTE prevention/treatment indications, trials using these agents included few patients with malignancies. There is growing data that support the efficacy of these agents in cancer patients (Vedovati 2015); however, it is important to note that most trials in cancer patients have used UFH or warfarin as a comparator and trials comparing oral agents to LMWH are lacking. Unpredictable absorption, potential for increased adverse events, alterations in metabolism, and potential drug interactions are among concerns with the use of novel oral anticoagulants in patients with malignancies (Lyman 2013). Further data from randomized controlled trials including patients with malignancies are needed to confirm the safety and efficacy of these agents in cancer patients.

Anticoagulant Comparison Table

Name	Use	DVT and PE Dose	Adjust Dose for Renal Impairment?
Low Molecular Weight Heparins			
Dalteparin	Prophylaxis	SubQ: 2,500 to 5,000 units once daily	Yes
	Treatment	SubQ: Month 1: 200 units/kg once daily (maximum dose: 18,000 units) Months 2 to 6: 150 units/kg once daily (maximum dose: 18,000 units)	
Enoxaparin	Prophylaxis	SubQ: 30 mg q12h or 40 mg once daily	Yes
	Treatment	SubQ: 1 mg/kg q12h	
Heparin			
Heparin	Prophylaxis	SubQ: 5,000 units q8 to 12h	No
	Treatment	IV: 80 units/kg (bolus), then 18 units/kg/ hour	
Selective Anti-Xa Inhibitor			
Fondaparinux	Prophylaxis	SubQ: ≥50 kg: 2.5 mg once daily (prophylactic use is contraindicated in patients <50 kg)	Yes
	Treatment	SubQ: <50 kg: 5 mg once daily 50 to 100 kg: 7.5 mg once daily >100 kg: 10 mg once daily	
Vitamin K Antagonists			
Warfarin	Prophylaxis	Oral: Variable	No
	Treatment	Oral: Variable; adjust dose to maintain INR 2 to 3	

(continued)

Anticoagulant Comparison Table (continued)

Name	Use	DVT and PE Dose	Adjust Dose for Renal Impairment?
Novel Oral Anticoagulants			
Apixaban	Treatment	10 mg twice daily for 7 days, followed by 5 mg twice daily (for long-term treatment) or 2.5 mg twice daily (for extended therapy)	Yes
Betrixaban	Prophylaxis	160 mg single dose on day 1, followed by 80 mg once daily for 35 to 42 days	Yes
Dabigatran	Treatment	150 mg twice daily	Yes
Rivaroxaban	Treatment	15 mg twice daily for 21 days, followed by 20 mg once daily	Yes

REFERENCES

Battinelli EM, Murphy DL, Connors JM. Venous thromboembolism overview. *Hematol Oncol Clin North Am*. 2012;26(2):345-367.

Dutia M, White RH, Wun T. Risk assessment models for cancer-associated venous thromboembolism. *Cancer*. 2012;118(14):3468-3476.

Horlocker TT, Wedel DJ, Rowlinson JC, et al. Regional anesthesia in the patient receiving antithrombotic or thrombolytic therapy: American Society of Regional Anesthesia and Pain Medicine evidence-based guidelines (third edition). *Reg Anesth Pain Med*. 2010;35(1):64-101.

Hurwitz HI, Saltz LB, Van Cutsem E, et al. Venous thromboembolic events with chemotherapy plus bevacizumab: a pooled analysis of patients in randomized phase II and III studies. *J Clin Oncol*. 2011;29(13):1757-1764.

Kahn SR, Lim W, Dunn AS, et al. Prevention of VTE in nonsurgical patients: antithrombotic therapy and prevention of thrombosis, 9th ed: American College of Chest Physicians evidence-based clinical practice guidelines. *Chest*. 2012;141(2 Suppl):e195S-e226S.

Kearon C, Akl EA, Ornelas J, et al. Antithrombotic therapy for VTE disease: CHEST guideline and expert panel report. *Chest*. 2016;149(2):315-352.

Khorana AA, Francis CW, Culakova E, Kuderer NM, Lyman GH. Thromboembolism is a leading cause of death in cancer patients receiving outpatient chemotherapy. *J Thromb Haemost*. 2007;5(3):632-634.

Lyman GH, Bohlke K, Khorana AA, et al. Venous thromboembolism prophylaxis and treatment in patients with cancer: american society of clinical oncology clinical practice guideline update 2014. *J Clin Oncol*. 2015;33(6):654-656.

Lyman GH, Khorana AA, Kuderer NM, et al. Venous thromboembolism prophylaxis and treatment in patients with cancer: American Society of Clinical Oncology clinical practice guideline update. *J Clin Oncol*. 2013;31(17):2189-2204.

Palumbo A, Cavo M, Bringhen S, et al. Aspirin, warfarin, or enoxaparin thromboprophylaxis in patients with multiple myeloma treated with thalidomide: a phase III, open-label, randomized trial. *J Clin Oncol*. 2011;29(8):986-993.

Rooden CJ, Tesselaar ME, Osanto S, Rosendaal FR, Huisman MV. Deep vein thrombosis associated with central venous catheters – a review. *J Thromb Haemost*. 2005;3(11):2409-2419.

Sørensen HT, Sværke C, Farkas DK, et al. Superficial and deep venous thrombosis, pulmonary embolism and subsequent risk of cancer. *Eur J Cancer*. 2012;48(4):586-593.

Vedovati MC, Germini F, Agnelli G, Becattini C. Direct oral anticoagulants in patients with VTE and cancer: a systematic review and meta-analysis. *Chest*. 2015;147(2):475-483.

Verso M, Agnelli G. Venous thromboembolism associated with long-term use of central venous catheters in cancer patients. *J Clin Oncol*. 2003;21(19):3665-3675.

HEMATOPOIETIC CELL TRANSPLANTATION

INTRODUCTION

Hematopoietic cell transplantation (HCT) involves the infusion of hematopoietic stem and progenitor cells into a patient in order to treat malignant disease and nonmalignant hematologic, lymphopoietic, congenital, and other disorders. Hematopoietic cells are immature cells that mature and differentiate into the various functional myeloid (eg, neutrophils, monocytes, macrophages, megakaryocytes, erythrocytes) and lymphoid cells (eg, T lymphocytes, B lymphocytes, natural killer cells) of the hematopoietic system. Hematopoietic cells are transplanted in order to replace diseased hematopoietic cells, reduce the duration of pancytopenia following administration of high dose chemotherapy, or to generate antitumor immunity in cancer patients. Allogeneic hematopoietic cell transplants require donation of hematopoietic cells from a healthy donor; whereas, autologous transplantation uses hematopoietic cells previously collected from the patient undergoing treatment. Allogeneic hematopoietic cell transplants are further classified as related transplants (donor and recipient are siblings or first-degree relatives), unrelated transplants (donor and recipient are not related by pedigree), syngeneic transplants (donor and recipient are identical twins), or umbilical cord blood transplants (donated product is harvested from placental-umbilical cord source). Immunologic likeness of the donor and recipient is determined by comparison of the genotype of donor and recipient class I and class II major histocompatibility (MHC) antigens. MHC Class I antigens (HLA-A, HLA-B, HLA-C) are present on all nucleated cells in the body and provide a means for the immune system to differentiate self vs nonself. MHC Class II proteins (HLA-D) are present on antigen presenting cells, such as macrophages, dendritic cells, B lymphocytes, and activated endothelial cells, and are critical in initiation and maintenance of long-lasting immunity and tolerance.

Hematopoietic cell transplants are classified according to the intensity of the pretransplant preparative regimen. Myeloablative chemotherapy regimens administer the highest possible dose of chemotherapy, with the doses limited by regimen-related nonhematologic toxicity. The goal of the myeloablative regimen is to achieve the maximum anticancer effect and complete immunosuppression through the effects of the high dose cytotoxic agents. The goal of the nonmyeloablative preparative or reduced intensity conditioning (RIC) regimen is to inhibit the recipient immune system adequately to allow engraftment of the donated hematopoietic cells. Complete donor engraftment following nonmyeloablative transplantation typically occurs after a period of mixed chimerism (coexistence of donor and recipient hematologic cells) and is associated with antitumor effect mediated by donor immune cells.

Terms that are synonymous with hematopoietic cell transplantation include bone marrow transplantation, peripheral blood cell transplantation, and peripheral blood cell rescue. The following table lists clinical uses for allogeneic and autologous myeloablative hematopoietic cell transplantation.

Condition	Allogeneic	Autologous
Acute lymphocytic leukemia (ALL)	+	+
Acute myelogenous leukemia (AML)	+	+
Acute promyelocytic leukemia	+	+
Myelodysplastic syndromes	+	-
Myelofibrosis and myeloproliferative diseases	+	-
Chronic lymphocytic leukemia (CLL)	+	+
Chronic myelogenous leukemia (CML)	+	-
Non-Hodgkin lymphomas (NHL)	+	+
Hodgkin lymphoma	+	+
Multiple myeloma (MM)	+	+
Severe aplastic anemia (SAA)	+	-
Sickle cell disease (SCD)	+	-
Congenital immunodeficiency syndromes	+	-
Germ cell/testicular cancer	-	+
Ewing sarcoma	-	+
Congenital hematopoietic disorders	+	-
Inborn errors of metabolism	+	-
Paroxysmal nocturnal hemoglobinuria	+	-
Wiskott-Aldrich syndrome	+	-

SOURCES, COLLECTION, AND PROCESSING OF HEMATOPOIETIC PROGENITOR CELLS

Hematopoietic progenitor cells used for transplantation are generally gathered from the peripheral blood. The hematopoietic stem and progenitor cells are removed via leukapheresis, which is routinely done in an ambulatory setting. Cells collected for autologous transplantation are processed and cryopreserved for future use. Cells collected for allogeneic transplantation are processed and infused immediately (within 24 hours). Leukapheresis involves the processing of ~10 L of peripheral blood over a 2- to 6-hour period. The usual goal is a product containing at least 2×10^6/kg and ideally 5×10^6/kg of recipient weight of CD34$^+$ cells, which closely correlate with the content of stem and progenitor cells collected. This may be accomplished by 1 or several leukaphereses. Donors may require calcium supplementation during leukapheresis due to the citrate anticoagulant used during the procedure. Common medical risks to the allogeneic donor of peripheral hematopoietic cells include adverse effects from treatment with a colony-stimulating factor (bone pain) and adverse events associated with leukapheresis (acute hypocalcemia, catheter-related discomfort). Although no long-term toxicity has been reported in donors treated with colony-stimulating factors, rare serious toxicity such as splenic rupture can occur and the donor must be screened carefully prior to donation.

The peripheral blood concentration of hematopoietic cells and progenitor cells must be increased to facilitate successful collection. This process is known as peripheral progenitor cell mobilization. After administration of chemotherapy, colony-stimulating factors, or a combination of the two agents, the numbers of circulating early and late progenitor cells expands. A colony-stimulating factor, such as filgrastim or sargramostim, is used for this purpose in the healthy allogeneic donor. For the autologous donor, a colony-stimulating factor is administered alone or prescribed following chemotherapy. Mobilization of hematopoietic progenitor cells can be more difficult in patients with hematologic malignancies or a history of extensive treatment with chemotherapy and radiation. Plerixafor can be used in combination with filgrastim to enhance hematopoietic cell mobilization in heavily pretreated autologous donors. The following table provides the dosage and schedule for some of the more commonly used mobilization regimens. Selection of the chemotherapy for mobilization in the autologous donor is primarily based on the type of cancer being treated.

Mobilization Agent	Dosage and Duration
Filgrastim (G-CSF)	10 mcg/kg/day SubQ for 5 to 7 days or until target WBC; dose escalation to 16 to 32 mcg/kg/day has been used to improve inadequate mobilization
Sargramostim (GM-CSF)	250 mg/m^2/day SubQ for 5 to 7 days or until target WBC
Etoposide (VP-16)	2 g/m^2 IV over 2 hours, followed in 24 hours by filgrastim or sargramostim until target WBC
Cyclophosphamide	4 g/m^2 (range of 1.5 to 7 g/m^2) IV over 2 hours followed at 24 hours by filgrastim 5 to 10 mcg/kg/day until target WBC; higher doses are also used (7 g/m^2)
Cytarabine plus etoposide	Cytarabine 2 g/m^2 IV q12h x 8 doses + etoposide 40 mg/kg over 4 days, then filgrastim 10 mcg/kg/day from day 14 until cells collected
Plerixafor (in combination with filgrastim)	0.24 mg/kg SubQ once daily for up to 4 consecutive days beginning ~11 hours prior to apheresis; maximum dose: 40 mg/day

Abbreviations: SubQ = subcutaneous, WBC = white blood cell count

Historically, the bone marrow was the primary source of hematopoietic cells for transplantation and it still represents an equivalent, hematopoietic cell source in the setting of allogeneic transplantation. The bone marrow contains populations of hematopoietic cells ranging from the pluripotent stem cell, early progenitor cells, and later, more differentiated progenitor cells that all exist within and are supported by the bone marrow stroma (matrix composed of connective tissue, reticuloendothelial cells, adipose cells). Compared to blood, the concentration of T lymphocytes is significantly lower in the marrow. Bone marrow can be harvested by removing an adequate volume of marrow (~10 mL/kg) from the posterior iliac crests of the donor or patient. This is generally done in an operating room and requires general or local anesthesia. Common medical risks to the donor of bone marrow include the risks of undergoing anesthesia, and transient moderate pain in the area of cell harvesting. Severe anemia can also develop. The frequency of life-threatening complications, which have included thromboembolic disorders, aspiration pneumonia, and cardiac dysrhythmias, is ≤0.3%. Hematopoietic engraftment (normalization of the peripheral white blood cell count) occurs earlier following peripheral hematopoietic cell transplantation than following bone marrow transplantation. However, chronic graft-versus-host disease (GVHD) risk is lower with the bone marrow source.

Umbilical cord blood (UCB) is another source of hematopoietic progenitor cells. The product, which is harvested from the placenta and umbilical cord immediately after birth, can be processed and transplanted or frozen for future use. The product obtained from UCB contains a high proportion of pluripotent stem cells and natural killer cells, and a low proportion of mature lymphocytes. The time to engraftment is generally longer following UCB transplantation than following peripheral blood or bone marrow hematopoietic cell transplantation. Moreover, UCB transplantation is generally reserved for children and small adults because the number of stem cells that can be collected from cord blood may be inadequate to support timely engraftment for larger patients. The risk for severe GVHD is lower with UCB even when HLA matching is not perfect. The process of harvesting UCB does not present a medical risk to the donor, because the actual collection of cells is done after the placenta is extruded as part of the birthing process. One investigational strategy for expanding the pool of UCB is to transplant UCB from two donors instead of a single donor. Preliminary data (in children and adolescents) demonstrates similar survival rates between cohorts receiving 2-unit vs 1-unit UCB transplantation with increased grade III to IV GVHD and longer time to platelet recovery with infusion of the 2-unit product (Wagner 2014).

The hematopoietic progenitor cells may be treated prior to transplantation to eradicate tumor cell contamination in the product following autologous donation or reduce the number of T lymphocytes that may promote graft-versus-host disease in an allogeneic recipient. The term purging refers to the removal of tumor cells by various techniques such as binding to specific monoclonal antibodies or incubation with cytotoxic drugs, such as 4-hydroperoxycyclophosphamide, that spare the immature stem cells. *Ex vivo* T lymphocyte reduction, also known as T cell depletion, is generally achieved using monoclonal antibodies directed against surface proteins expressed on T lymphocytes. Engraftment is generally delayed following transplantation of hematopoietic progenitor cells that have undergone *ex vivo* purging or T cell depletion.

AUTOLOGOUS MYELOABLATIVE TRANSPLANTATION

Chemotherapy and dosage selection for autologous myeloablative HSCT is based on three important principles:

1. Certain drugs such as alkylating agents and etoposide exhibit steep dose-response curves when used to treat susceptible malignancies. Therefore, when the dose-limiting adverse effect of these drugs is myelosuppression, high doses can be administered with hematopoietic cell rescue to achieve high response rates.

2. High doses of chemotherapy with nonoverlapping nonhematologic major organ toxicity can be combined without compromising lives.

3. Cryopreserved bone marrow and/or blood progenitor cells can rescue the patient from the myeloablative effects of the high-dose chemotherapy.

Administration of filgrastim or sargramostim following reinfusion of the autologous hematopoietic progenitor cells significantly shortens the duration of neutropenia associated with myeloablative chemotherapy (refer to filgrastim or sargramostim monographs for dosing, etc). The hematopoietic recovery period following HCT is generally 1 to 2 weeks, which is shorter than that for bone marrow or UCB transplants which require 2 to 4 weeks. The monocytes and neutrophils engraft first followed by the platelets about a week later. The most common complications associated with autologous HSCT are febrile neutropenia, serum electrolyte abnormalities, infection, bleeding, gastrointestinal toxicities (mucositis, nausea, vomiting, and diarrhea), and less commonly, other organ toxicities that are related to the specific chemotherapy administered. The following table lists commonly used chemotherapy agents with their dose-limiting toxicities in SCT.

Chemotherapy	Standard Dose[a]	Maximum HCT Dose as Single Agent[b]	Maximum HCT Dose in Combination[b]	Dose-Limiting Toxicity
Busulfan (oral)	4 mg/day	16 mg/kg	16 mg/kg	GI, liver (SOS[c]), CNS (seizure), pulmonary
Busulfan (IV)		12 mg/kg	12 mg/kg	GI, liver (SOS[c]), CNS (seizure), pulmonary
CARBOplatin	400 mg/m²	2,000 mg/m²	1,800 mg/m²	Liver, renal
Carmustine	200 mg/m²	800 mg/m²	600 mg/m²	Liver, pulmonary
CISplatin	50 to 100 mg/m²	180 to 200 mg/m²	165 to 200 (in BEP) mg/m²	Renal, neuropathy
Cyclophosphamide	600 to 1,875 mc/m²	200 mg/kg or 7.5 g/m²	200 mg/kg or 7.5 g/m²	Cardiac, hemorrhagic cystitis, liver (SOS[c])
Etoposide	100 mg/m²/dose x 1 to 5 days	2,400 mg/m²	2,400 mg/m²	GI, hypotension
Melphalan	40 mg/m²	220 mg/m²	140 to 180 mg/m²	GI
MitoXANTRONE	12 mg/m²/day x 3	90 mg/m²	60 to 80 mg/m²	GI, cardiac

[a]Usual dose for therapy that does not include HCT
[b]Maximum dose is divided for administration ove⁻ 2 or more days
[c]SOS = sinusoidal obstructive syndrome

ALLOGENEIC MYELOABLATIVE TRANSPLANTATION

The principle behind allogeneic myeloablative hematopoietic cell transplantation is that hematological disease can be cured by complete marrow ablation with profound immunosuppression so that the donor cells can engraft and successfully replace the patient's diseased hematopoietic system. Post-transplant immunosuppressive therapy is essential for successful engraftment of donor cells and prevention of GVHD. Preparative regimens for allogeneic transplantation are based on the need for both marrow ablation and immunosuppression. Commonly used regimens are listed below.

Acronym	Chemotherapy Drugs (Total Dose)	Dosages and Scheduling
BuCy	Busulfan (12 to 16 mg/kg); dose determined using patient-specific pharmacokinetics	0.875 to 1 mg/kg/dose PO q6h x 16 doses; or 1 mg/kg/dose PO q6h x 12 doses; or 0.8 mg/kg IV q6h x 16 doses
	Cyclophosphamide (120 mg/kg)	60 mg/kg/dose IV q24h x 2 doses
FTBI/Cy or CyTBI	Fractionated total body irradiation	1,200 to 1,500 cGy divided bid over 3 to 5 days
	Cyclophosphamide (120 to 200 mg/kg)	50 mg/kg/dose IV q24h x 4 doses or 60 mg/kg/dose IV q24h x 2 doses
TBI-VP16-Cy	Fractionated total body irradiation	1,200 to 1,400 cGy divided bid over 3 to 5 days
	Etoposide (30 mg/kg)	30 mg/kg/dose IV x 1 dose
	Cyclophosphamide (120 mg/kg)	60 mg/kg/dose IV q24h x 2 doses
Bu/Mel	Busulfan (16 mg/kg); dose determined using patient-specific pharmacokinetics	1 mg/kg/dose PO q6h x 16 doses
	Melphalan (135 to 140 mg/m^2)	45 mg/m^2/dose IV q24h x 3, or 140 mg/m^2 once
FTBI/Mel	Fractionated total body irradiation	1,200 to 1,500 cGy divided bid over 3 to 5 days
	Melphalan (135 to 140 mg/m^2)	45 mg/m^2/dose IV q24h x 2, 70 mg/m^2 IV q24h x 2, or 140 mg/m^2 once
CyATG	Cyclophosphamide (200 mg/kg)	50 mg/kg/dose IV q24h x 4
	Lymphocyte immune globulin (90 to 160 mg/kg)	30 to 40 mg/kg/dose IV q24 to 48h x 3 to 4 doses

The systemic exposure to busulfan correlates with safety and efficacy of therapy. Busulfan area under the plasma concentration versus time curve (AUC) exceeding 1,500 micromole/minutes per dose (24,000 micromole/minutes per total course of therapy) is associated with an increased risk of regimen-related toxicity, including sinusoidal obstruction syndrome (SOS) and seizures. Busulfan AUC lower than 900 micromole/minutes per dose (14,400 micromole/minutes per total course of therapy) correlates with graft failure and disease recurrence (Ciurea 2009). Use of patient-specific pharmacokinetics to determine the optimal dose of oral busulfan is warranted due to the extreme interpatient variability of oral absorption and pharmacokinetic parameters. Pharmacokinetics can also be used to optimize the delivery of intravenous busulfan therapy (Ciurea 2009).

Lymphocyte immune globulin or antithymocyte globulin is included in the preparative regimen for patients with severe aplastic anemia. Lymphocyte immune globulin or antithymocyte globulin is often added to the preparative regimen for allogeneic transplants when the donor and recipient are immunologically mismatched or unrelated, and for umbilical cord blood transplants. This added immunosuppression improves engraftment and may decrease acute GVHD.

Hematopoietic growth factors (filgrastim or sargramostim) are usually administered after infusion of allogeneic donor blood cells. The doses range from 5 to 10 mcg/kg/day and administration is begun either on day 0 or +1 or may be delayed up to 6 days post-cell infusion. The colony stimulating factors are discontinued when the absolute neutrophil count reaches a designated target, which is often in the range of 5,000 to 10,000/mm^3.

Allogeneic HSCT recipients are at risk for all of the common complications associated with administration of high-dose chemotherapy, including febrile neutropenia, serum electrolyte abnormalities, infection, bleeding, gastrointestinal toxicities (mucositis, nausea, vomiting, and diarrhea), and less commonly, other organ toxicities that are related to the specific chemotherapy administered. The risk of posttransplant complications is greater in allogeneic transplant recipients due to the chronic immunosuppression required to prevent GVHD.

NONMYELOABLATIVE TRANSPLANTS

Nonmyeloablative or RIC HSCT is achieved by administration of immunosuppressive conditioning regimens that are less directly cytotoxic to bone marrow and nonhematopoietic tissue(s). Nonmyeloablative transplantation utilizes the graft-versus-leukemia effect as part of the overall treatment. The safety impetus for use of RIC is to allow allogeneic HSCT in patients unable to tolerate the myeloablative preparative regimens, such as elderly patients, or patients with an extensive history of chemotherapy treatment, impaired major organ function, or comorbid conditions. Clinical trials and case series describe use of nonmyeloablative hematopoietic cell transplantation for the following diseases: Congenital immunodeficiency syndromes, acute myelogenous leukemia, myelodysplastic syndrome, acute lymphocytic leukemia, multiple myeloma, non-Hodgkin lymphoma, Hodgkin disease, sickle cell disease, renal cell carcinoma, and various advanced solid tumors. Most of the published studies and case series report use of this procedure in patients with relapsed or refractory disease, elderly patients, or those unable to tolerate myeloablative preparative regimens.

The premise supporting nonmyeloablative transplantation is that nonmyeloablative, but sufficiently immunosuppressive conditioning regimens, yield a state of mixed chimerism in the recipient, which gradually converts to full donor chimerism. The chimeric engraftment supports a graft-versus-malignancy effect. Complete donor engraftment, also known as 100% donor chimerism, occurs when all of the detectable hematopoietic cells are of donor origin. Complete donor chimerism occurring within 30 to 90 days following transplantation is generally associated with disease response. Because antitumor effects of nonmyeloablative allogeneic transplants appear somewhat late (2 to 3 months after the procedure), patients with active or poorly controlled malignancies do not appear to be optimal candidates for this type of transplantation.

Examples of reduced-intensity preparative regimens are listed in the following table.

Acronym	Chemotherapy Drugs (Total Dose)	Dosages and Scheduling
Flu/ATG	Lymphocyte immune globulin 40 mg/kg (Atgam)	10 mg/kg/day IV on 4 consecutive days
	Antithymoglobulin 10 mg/kg (Thymoglobulin)	2.5 mg/kg/day IV on 4 consecutive days
	Fludarabine 125 mg/m^2	25 mg/m^2/day IV on 5 consecutive days
FC-ATG	Fludarabine 125 mg/m^2	25 mg/m^2/day IV on days -6 to -2
	Cyclophosphamide 120 mg/kg	60 mg/kg/day IV on days -3 and -2
	Lymphocyte immune globulin 60 mg/kg (Atgam)	20 mg/kg/day IV on 3 consecutive days
TBI/Flu	Total body irradiation 4 Gy	2 Gy/day on days -8 and -7
	Fludarabine 125 mg/m^2	25 mg/m^2/day IV on days -6 to -2
Flu/Mel/ATG	Fludarabine 125 mg/m^2	25 mg/m^2/day IV on days -6 to -2
	Melphalan 140 to 180 mg/m^2	70 to 90 mg/m^2/day IV on days -3 and -2
	Lymphocyte immune globulin 120 mg/kg (Atgam)	30 mg/kg/day IV on days -4 to -1
Bu/Flu/ATG	Busulfan 8 mg/kg	1 mg/kg/dose PO q6h X8 doses on days -6 and -5
	Fludarabine 125 mg/m^2	25 mg/m^2/day IV on days -6 to -2
	Antithymocyte globulin (Fresnius) 10 mg/kg	2.5 mg/kg/day IV on 4 consecutive days
Cy/Flu/TBI	Cyclophosphamide 50 mg/kg	50 mg/kg IV on day -6
	Fludarabine 200 mg/m^2	40 mg/m^2/day IV on days -6 to -2
	TBI 200 cGy	TBI 200 cGy on day -1

Most complications following nonmyeloablative hematopoietic cell transplantation are related to GVHD and the immunosuppression required for treatment of GVHD. Infectious complications from cytomegalovirus, herpes virus, candidiasis, aspergillosis, and other opportunistic microbes are common. Treatment of moderate to severe GVHD is similar to the approach taken for that of GVHD following myeloablative allogeneic hematopoietic cell transplantation (see Post-transplant Complications).

Less regimen-related toxicity occurs with RIC, so it is considered as an alternative therapeutic modality for patients unable to tolerate the adverse effects inherent to myeloablative therapy. However, patients undergoing nonmyeloablative transplantation must have adequate organ function and physiologic reserve for chronic administration of immunosuppressive therapy and management of opportunistic infections that may arise.

DONOR LYMPHOCYTE INFUSION

Donor lymphocyte infusion (DLI) is a technique that involves transfusion of lymphocytes from the original HSCT donor in order to treat relapsed or refractory hematologic cancers following allogeneic HSCT. The donor lymphocytes are contained within a white blood cell product obtained by apheresis (leukapheresis) from the donor. The anticancer effect of DLI is secondary to a graft-versus-tumor effect triggered when the donor lymphocytes recognize antigens on the malignant cells as nonself. A surrogate marker for graft-versus-leukemia is clinical evidence of GVHD. The efficacy of DLI is related to the type of cancer being treated, the dose of infused lymphocytes, and the demonstration of a graft-versus-host response. Durable responses to DLI are reported with chronic myeloid leukemia; lesser responses are reported with lymphomas, multiple myeloma, and acute myeloid leukemia.

POST-TRANSPLANT COMPLICATIONS

Graft-Versus-Host Disease

GVHD is an immune-mediated reaction initiated by donor T-cell recognition of recipient tissues as nonself. GVHD which occurs before 100 days post-transplant is classified as acute GVHD, and after 100 days, it is classified as chronic GVHD. Acute GVHD primarily affects the skin, gastrointestinal tract, and liver. It is graded based on extent of organ involvement from grade I (mild) to grade IV (life-threatening). Chronic GVHD affects the skin, gastrointestinal tract, liver, and other organs and tissues, including the lungs, lacrimal glands, and connective tissue. Chronic GVHD is generally graded as limited or extensive disease. Mortality ranges from 10% to 30%. There is a strong positive correlation between development of acute or chronic GVHD and decreased risk of malignancy recurrence due to associated graft vs malignancy effect.

Given the high morbidity and mortality associated with severe GVHD, post-transplant care is directed to prevent this complication. A combination of 2 to 3 immunosuppressants is used to prevent GVHD. The selection of prophylactic immunosuppressants used is based on the degree of risk for GVHD and the risk of malignant relapse. In general, as the depth and duration of immunosuppression increase, so does the risk of malignant relapse, and infectious disease. Commonly used prophylactic immunosuppressants include cyclosporine or tacrolimus plus methotrexate, with addition of a methylprednisolone for patients at high risk for GVHD.

GVHD Prophylactic Agents	Usual Dose and Schedule
CycloSPORINE	2.5 to 4 mg/kg/day IV continuous infusion or divided q12h over 2 to 6 hours. Adjust dose according to toxicity and blood concentrations. Convert to oral dose when appropriate. Start day -4 to -1.
Tacrolimus	0.02 to 0.03 mg/kg/day IV continuous infusion. Adjust dose according to toxicity and blood concentrations. Transition (using appropriate conversion) to oral dose when appropriate. Start day -1.
Methotrexate	15 mg/m^2/dose on day +1, 10 mg/m^2/dose on days +3, +6, and +11; give IV push.
MethylPREDNISolone	Variable; 0.5 to 1 mg/kg/day divided q6 to 12h then taper. May start day +1 up to +7; increase dose for acute GVHD reactions.
Mycophenolate mofetil	1 g/dose IV or PO q12h; or 15 mg/kg/dose IV or PO q12h. Start day +1.
Sirolimus	12 mg PO on day -3, then 4 mg PO daily

Cyclosporine and tacrolimus administration are initiated intravenously for patient tolerance and to assure optimal systemic exposure. Initiation of oral administration is generally done for clinically well patients following resolution of regimen-related mucositis and recovery of blood counts. Conversion of cyclosporine from continuous intravenous infusion to twice daily oral administration of modified cyclosporine may be done in HST patients using a 1 mg (IV):2 mg (PO) ratio for the daily doses of the parenteral and enteral products (Inoue 2014). Conversion of tacrolimus from continuous intravenous infusion to twice daily oral administration may be done using approximately a 1 mg (IV):4 mg (PO) ratio for the daily doses of the parenteral and enteral products (Uberti 1999; Yanik 2000). Based on therapeutic drug monitoring, the oral dose of cyclosporine or tacrolimus is often ultimately reduced ~50% or more in patients receiving triazole antifungal (posaconazole, voriconazole, itraconazole) prophylaxis or treatment. Cyclosporine and tacrolimus are major substrates for CYP3A4 and prone to effects of enzyme inducers and inhibitors. Monitor trough blood concentrations closely.

Initial treatment of acute GVHD includes addition of a corticosteroid or a dosage increase of ongoing corticosteroid treatment. Other agents used for the treatment of steroid-refractory acute GVHD include lymphocyte immune globulin or antithymocyte globulin, interleukin-2 receptor antagonists (basiliximab), tumor necrosis factor antagonists (etanercept, infliximab), sirolimus, and pentostatin. Thalidomide, pentostatin, PUVA (8-methoxypsoralen plus UV-A radiation), rituximab, and ruxolitinib also have been utilized in the setting of steroid-refractory GVHD. Addition of a corticosteroid or a dosage increase of ongoing corticosteroid treatment and optimization of calcineurin inhibitor therapy are also the cornerstone of initial management for chronic GVHD (Wolff 2011). The Bruton kinase inhibitor ibrutinib is approved for second-line therapy of chronic GVHD. Other treatments used for chronic GVHD include photophoresis, m-TOR inhibitors, thalidomide, hydroxychloroquine, imatinib, rituximab, alemtuzumab, mycophenylate, and cytotoxic immunosuppressants.

Infection

Allogeneic hematopoietic cell transplantation is associated with a wide range of infectious complications that occur during identifiable time periods after the transplant. The early period of neutropenia is most commonly associated with bacterial infections, fungal infections (*Candida* species), and herpes simplex virus (HSV) reactivation. *Pneumocystis jirovecii* pneumonia (PCP) risk increases with duration of immunosuppressive therapy. Other life-threatening opportunistic infections typically occurring 2 to 3 months post-transplant include aspergillosis and CMV (disseminated or pneumonitis). Other serious atypical viral and fungal infections can also be seen at this later time. Infections with rhinovirus and coronavirus are common during the first 100 days following allogeneic HSCT and tend to present as symptoms of rhinorrhea, congestion, postnasal drip, sputum production, and cough. Lower respiratory tract infections attributed to rhinovirus or coronavirus occur in ~2% of infected patients.

Prophylaxis for certain infections is routine while others are treated when they are diagnosed. Trimethoprim-sulfamethoxazole or a fluoroquinolone is given during the preparative regimen for selective gut decontamination. Trimethoprim-sulfamethoxazole is also administered after hematopoietic recovery on a 2 to 3 times weekly schedule as PCP prophylaxis. The major concern with trimethoprim-sulfamethoxazole is the myelosuppressive effect. Alternative antimicrobials for patients allergic to sulfonamide antimicrobials include inhaled pentamidine, oral dapsone, or oral atovaquone. Fungal prophylaxis is routinely given as well. This generally consists of posaconazole or voriconazole. Other antifungal agents used prophylactically include fluconazole, micafungin, itraconazole, or an amphotericin B product. Inhalational amphotericin B can also be used to decrease risk of pulmonary aspergillosis. Acyclovir is routinely used to prevent HSV reinfection. The role of acyclovir for prevention of CMV infection is controversial. Some centers routinely prescribe acyclovir immediately following the transplant for prevention of CMV or HSV infection. After cellular recovery, the patient may be switched to ganciclovir or valganciclovir therapy. The hematologic toxicity of ganciclovir and valganciclovir precludes its routine use at an earlier point in the transplant; however, CMV therapy is started preemptively before engraftment with the finding of CMV DNA by polymerase chain reaction in the peripheral white blood cells. The role of antibacterial prophylaxis or continued gut decontamination varies with transplant centers but is often used in some form. Prophylactic antimicrobials are generally administered throughout the duration of exogenous immunosuppression following allogeneic hematopoietic cell transplantation. The American Society of Clinical Oncology (ASCO) provisional clinical opinion update on hepatitis B virus (HBV) screening recommends screening patients for HBV prior to HSCT or initiation of anti-CD20 antibody therapy to identify patients with chronic or clinically resolved HBV infection. Serologic tests to detect HBV virus include hepatitis B surface antigen (HBsAg) and hepatitis B core antibody (anti-HBc) measurements; either a total anti-HBc (with both IgG and IgM) or anti-HBc IgG test should be used to screen for chronic or unresolved HBV infection (do not use anti-HBc IgM as it may only confirm acute HBV infection). In addition, clinical and laboratory signs of hepatitis or HBV should be monitored until patients are considered immunocompetent following HSCT. The ASCO provisional clinical opinion recommends initiation of prophylactic antiviral treatment for patients with chronic HBV infection (HBsAg-positive/anti-HBc-positive) without delaying anticancer therapy. Selection of antiviral therapy should be based on products with low rates of viral resistance. Antiviral therapy should be continued for 6 to 12 months following completion of cancer therapy. Providers should monitor patients with a clinically resolved HBV infection (HBsAg-negative/anti-HBc-positive) by serial analysis of serum alanine aminotransferase or HBV DNA approximately every 3 months with prompt initiation of antiviral therapy as warranted by laboratory findings. In addition, patients with risk factors for HBV infection (eg, residence in a geographic location with ≥2% HBV prevalence, household or sexual contact with HBV-infected patients, high-risk behaviors [eg, intravenous drug use], HIV infection) should also be screened and monitored for HBV infection or reactivation prior to beginning immunosuppressive therapy. The American Society for Blood and Marrow Transplantation (ASBMT) recommends screening for hepatitis C virus (HCV) prior to transplantation (Torres 2015). Completion of HCV treatment for seropositive patients with direct acting antivirals (DAAs) prior to initiation of the conditioning regimen is recommended whenever possible. Otherwise, initiation of DDAs promptly following posttransplant immune reconstitution is recommended. The effect of immune dysregulation on the efficacy of DAAs is not fully elucidated. GVHD flare secondary to reduction in immunotherapy may cloud the diagnostic evaluation of HCV disease. According to ASBMT recommendations, initiation of DAA should not be delayed for HST patients meeting any of the following criteria: development of fibrosing cholestatic HCV, cirrhosis with deteriorating condition, or hematopoietic cell transplant for treatment of HCV-related lymphoproliferative disorder (Torres 2015). Long-term survivors infected with HCV should be offered antiviral therapy with DAAs. Interruption of therapy is not recommended as it is associated with treatment failure. Antiviral treatment with interferon-based therapy is not recommended due to suboptimal efficacy and treatment-related immunomodulatory effects (Torres 2015). Patient monitoring can be complicated by posttransplant loss of HCV seropositivity, which was observed in 13% of 434 HCV-infected patients treated at a single center (Kyvernitakis 2016).

◀ **Mucositis**

Mucositis is a common cause of morbidity following HCT. The incidence and severity is related to the intensity of the conditioning regimen. An analysis of 395 patients in 8 studies receiving myeloablative conditioning and 245 patients in 6 studies receiving RIC reported the incidence and severity of oral mucositis in allogeneic transplant recipients (Chaudhry 2016). The overall incidence of oral mucositis was 73% and 87% following myeloablative and RIC transplants, respectively. For patients experiencing oral mucositis the incidence of grades 2 to 4 toxicity was 80% and 72% for myeloablative and RIC transplant recipients, respectively. Administration of methotrexate as part of the GVHD prophylaxis regimen increased the rate of mucositis compared to procedures without methotrexate (83% vs 55%; p<0.0001) (Chaudhry 2016). The keratinocyte growth factor palifermin is approved for reduction of oral mucositis in autologous hematopoietic cell transplantation. The cornerstones of therapy for mucositis tend to be analgesia, oral hygiene, and supportive care.

Sinusoidal Obstruction Syndrome

Hepatic sinusoidal obstruction syndrome (SOS), formerly known as hepatic veno-occlusive disease (VOD), can occur as a result of the pretransplant conditioning regimen. Risk factors for hepatic SOS include preexisting liver disease, malignant involvement of the liver, serum ferritin level exceeding 1,000 ng/mL, malnutrition, prior extensive chemotherapy treatment, and previous treatment with busulfan, imatinib, or gemtuzumab ozogamicin. SOS, which usually presents within the first 3 weeks after transplant, results from obstruction of blood flow in the small hepatic veins. Signs and symptoms include right upper quadrant pain or tenderness, hepatomegaly, weight gain, ascites, hyperbilirubinemia, and thrombocytopenia. Treatment options include supportive care and defibrotide (which has antithrombotic, thrombolytic, and anti-ischemic properties). Low-dose heparin and ursodiol have also been used for SOS prophylaxis; defibrotide may be considered for prevention of SOS in pediatric patients with at least 1 risk factor for SOS.

ABNORMAL PAPANICOLAOU SMEAR RESULTS

One analysis of Papanicolaou (Pap) smears following hematopoietic cell transplantation reported 6 of 44 (14%) and 2 of 18 (11%) tests with abnormal results in allogeneic and autologous recipients, respectively. For allogeneic HCT recipients, 5 of 44 (11%) specimens had therapy-related atypical cellular changes mimicking precancerous results. The pathologic findings were described as enlarged hyperchromatic nuclei, vacuolated cytoplasm, and occasional tadpole-like cells. Atypical Pap-smear results were most common prior to day +100 (p=0.0002). Resolution of atypical cells was demonstrated with repeat Pap-smears performed after day +100 (Yu 2017).

FUTURE DIRECTIONS

Improved methods for prevention of GVHD following allogeneic HSCT will benefit posttransplant quality of life and promote prolonged survival. Preliminary clinical trials demonstrate efficacy for prevention of severe acute and chronic GVHD with posttransplant administration of high-dose cyclophosphamide as the only GVHD prophylaxis or with a short course of sirolimus following HLA-matched allogeneic HSCT with a myeloablative conditioning regimen (Kanakry 2014; Solomon 2014). Clinical trials are evaluating the immunomodulatory and anti-inflammatory effects of atorvastatin as a modulator of GVHD (Choi 2014). The proteasome inhibitor bortezomib demonstrated clinical efficacy for reduction of GVHD; however, the outcome may not be improved with this agent due to toxicity (Choi 2014). Histone deacetylase inhibitors, such as vorinostat, are being tested for immunoregulatory and anti-inflammatory effects that may reduce the severity of GVHD (Choi 2014).

REFERENCES

Anasetti C, Logan BR, Lee SJ, et al. Peripheral-blood stem cells versus bone marrow from unrelated donors. *N Engl J Med.* 2012;367(16):1487-1496.

Bacigalupo A. Second EBMT workshop on reduced intensity allogeneic hemopoietic stem cell transplants (RI-HSCT). *Bone Marrow Transplant.* 2002;29:191-195.

Ballen KK, Gluckman E, Broxmeyer HE. Umbilical cord blood transplantation: the first 25 years and beyond. *Blood.* 2013;122(4):491-498.

Carreras E. How I manage sinusoidal obstruction syndrome after haematopoietic cell transplantation. *Br J Haematol.* 2015;168(4):481-491.

Chang YJ, Huang XJ. Donor lymphocyte infusions for relapse after allogeneic transplantation: when, if and for whom? *Blood Rev.* 2013;27(1):55-62.

Chaudhry HM, Bruce AJ, Wolf RC, et al. The incidence and severity of oral mucositis among allogeneic hematopoietic stem cell transplantation patients: a systematic review. *Biol Blood Marrow Transplant.* 2016;22(4):605-616.

Choi SW, Reddy P. Current and emerging strategies for the prevention of graft-versus-host disease. *Nat Rev Clin Oncol.* 2014;11(9):536-547.

Ciurea SO, Andersson BS. Busulfan in hematopoietic stem cell transplantation. *Biol Blood Marrow Transplant.* 2009;15(5):523-536.

Copelan EA. Hematopoietic stem-cell transplantation. *N Engl J Med.* 2006;354(17):1813-1826.

Cutler C, Logan B, Nakamura R, et al. Tacrolimus/sirolimus vs tacrolimus/methotrexate as GVHD prophylaxis after matched, related donor allogeneic HCT. *Blood.* 2014;124(8):1372-1377.

Deol A, Lum LG. Role of donor lymphocyte infusions in relapsed hematological malignancies after stem cell transplantation revisited. *Cancer Treat Rev.* 2010;36(7):528-538.

Ho VT, Soiffer RJ. The history and future of T-cell depletion as graft-versus-host disease prophylaxis for allogeneic hematopoietic cell transplantation. *Blood.* 2001;98:3192-3204.

Hwang JP, Somerfield MR, Alston-Johnson DE, et al. Hepatitis B virus screening for patients with cancer before therapy: American Society of Clinical Oncology provisional clinical opinion update. *J Clin Oncol.* 2015;33(19):2212-2220.

Inoue Y, Saito T, Ogawa K, et al. Pharmacokinetics of cyclosporine a conversion from twice-daily infusion to oral administration in allogeneic hematopoietic stem cell transplantation. *Am J Ther.* 2014;21(5):377-384.

Kanakry CG, Tsai HL, Bolaños-Meade J, et al. Single-agent GVHD prophylaxis with posttransplantation cyclophosphamide after myeloablative, HLA-matched BMT for AML, ALL, and MDS. *Blood.* 2014;124(25):3817-3827.

Kedmi M, Dray L, Grisariu S, et al. The effect of cyclosporine initiation time on the outcome of matched allogeneic stem-cell transplantation following fludarabine-based conditioning. *Transpl Int.* 2012;25(12):1241-1247.

Klingebiel T, Schlegel PG. GVHD: overview on pathophysiology, incidence, clinical and biological features. *Bone Marrow Transplant.* 1998;21(Suppl 2):S45-S49.

Kyvernitakis A, Mahale P, Popat UR, et al. Hepatitis C virus infection in patients undergoing hematopoietic cell transplantation in the era of direct-acting antiviral agents. *Biol Blood Marrow Transplant.* 2016;22(4):717-722.

Majhail NS, Farnia SH, Carpenter PA, et al. Indications for autologous and allogeneic hematopoietic cell transplantation: guidelines from the American Society for Blood and Marrow Transplantation. *Biol Blood Marrow Transplant.* 2015;21(11):1863-1869.

Maradei SC, Maiolino A, de Azevedo AM, Colares M, Bouzas LF, Nucci M. Serum ferritin as risk factor for sinusoidal obstruction syndrome of the liver in patients undergoing hematopoietic stem cell transplantation. *Blood.* 2009;114(6):1270-1275.

Martin PJ, Rizzo JD, Wingard JR, et al. First- and second-line systemic treatment of acute graft-versus-host disease: recommendations of the American Society of Blood and Marrow Transplantation. *Biol Blood Marrow Transplant.* 2012;18(8):1150-1163.

McClune BL, Weisdorf DJ, Pedersen TL, et al. Effect of age on outcome of reduced-intensity hematopoietic cell transplantation for older patients with acute myeloid leukemia in first complete remission or with myelodysplastic syndrome. *J Clin Oncol.* 2010;28(11):1878-1887.

Milano F, Campbell AP, Guthrie KA, et al. Human rhinovirus and coronavirus detection among allogeneic hematopoietic stem cell transplantation recipients. *Blood.* 2010;115(10):2088-2094.

Mogul MJ. Unrelated cord blood transplantation vs matched unrelated donor bone marrow transplantation: the risks and benefits of each choice. *Bone Marrow Transplant.* 2000;25(Suppl 2):S58-S60.

Richardson PG, Riches ML, Kernan NA, et al. Phase 3 trial of defibrotide for the treatment of severe veno-occlusive disease and multi-organ failure. *Blood.* 2016;127(13):1656-1665.

Richardson PG, Smith AR, Triplett BM, et al. Defibrotide for patients with hepatic veno-occlusive disease/sinusoidal obstruction syndrome: interim results from a treatment IND study. *Biol Blood Marrow Transplant.* 2017;23(6):997-1004.

Ringdén O, Labopin M, Ehninger G, et al. Reduced intensity conditioning compared with myeloablative conditioning using unrelated donor transplants in patients with acute myeloid leukemia. *J Clin Oncol.* 2009;27(27):4570-4577.

Rowe JM, Ciobanu N, Ascensao J, et al. Recommended guidelines for the management of autologous and allogeneic bone marrow transplantation. A report from the Eastern Cooperative Oncology Group (ECOG). *Ann Intern Med.* 1994;120:143-158.

Ruutu T, Gratwohl A, de Witte T, et al. Prophylaxis and treatment of GVHD: EBMT-ELN working group recommendations for a standardized practice. *Bone Marrow Transplant.* 2014;49(2):168-173.

Solomon SR, Sanacore M, Zhang X, et al. Calcineurin inhibitor – free graft-versus-host disease prophylaxis with post-transplantation cyclophosphamide and brief-course sirolimus following reduced-intensity peripheral blood stem cell transplantation. *Biol Blood Marrow Transplant.* 2014;20(11):1828-1834.

Storb R, Gyurkocza B, Storer BE, et al. Allogeneic hematopoietic cell transplantation following minimal intensity conditioning: predicting acute graft-versus-host disease and graft-versus-tumor effects. *Biol Blood Marrow Transplant.* 2013;19(5):792-798.

Torres HA, Chong PP, De Lima M, et al. Hepatitis C virus infection among hematopoietic cell transplant donors and recipients: American Society for Blood and Marrow Transplant Task Force recommendations. *Biol Blood Marrow Transplant.* 2015;21(11):1870-1882.

Uberti JP, Cronin S, Ratanatharathorn V. Optimum use of tacrolimus in the prophylaxis of graft versus host disease. *BioDrugs.* 1999;11(5):343-358.

Vogelsang GB, Arai S. Mycophenolate mofetil for the prevention and treatment of graft-versus-host disease following stem cell transplantation: preliminary findings. *Bone Marrow Transplant.* 2001;27:1255-1262.

Wagner JE Jr, Eapen M, Carter S, et al. One-unit versus two-unit cord-blood transplantation for hematologic cancers. *N Engl J Med.* 2014;371(18):1685-1694.

Wolff D, Schleuning M, von Harsdorf S, et al. Consensus conference on clinical practice in chronic GVHD: second-line treatment of chronic graft-versus-host disease. *Biol Blood Marrow Transplant.* 2011;17(1):1-17.

Yanik G, Levine JE, Ratanatharathorn V, Dunn R, Ferrara J, Hutchinson RJ. Tacrolimus (FK506) and methotrexate as prophylaxis for acute graft-versus-host disease in pediatric allogeneic stem cell transplantation. *Bone Marrow Transplant.* 2000;26(2):161-167.

Yu SC, Huang HH, Li CC, et al. Cervical papanicolaou smears in hematopoietic stem cell transplant recipients: high prevalence of therapy-related atypia during the acute phase. *Biol Blood Marrow Transplant.* 2017;23(8):1367-1373.

Zeiser R, Burchert A, Lengerke C, et al. Ruxolitinib in corticosteroid-refractory graft-versus-host disease after allogeneic stem cell transplantation: a multicenter survey. *Leukemia.* 2015;29(10):2062-2068.

SAFE HANDLING OF HAZARDOUS DRUGS

Early concerns regarding the identification and exposure risk of hazardous drugs in health care setting were primarily focused on antineoplastic medications, but now have expanded to numerous other agents (eg, antivirals, hormones, bioengineered medications). The criteria for a hazardous drug include one or more of the following characteristics:

- Carcinogenic
- Teratogenic (or other developmental toxicity)
- Causing reproductive toxicity
- Organotoxic at low doses
- Genotoxic
- New agents with structural or toxicity profiles similar to existing hazardous agents

Agencies and/or organizations have developed definitions, created lists, and generated guidelines to minimize risk of exposure to products considered hazardous. The Environmental Protection Agency (EPA), National Institute for Occupational Safety and Health (NIOSH), and American Society of Health-System Pharmacists (ASHP) have created definitions of hazardous agents (table 1) which may be useful. Based on their definitions, these agencies developed lists of agents which are identified as hazardous drugs or should be handled as hazardous (table 2).

Table 1. Criteria for Defining Hazardous Agents

EPA	NIOSH	ASHP
Meets one of the following criteria: Ignitability: Create fire (under certain conditions) or are spontaneously combustible and have a flash point <60°C (140°F) Corrosivity: Acids or bases (pH ≤2 or ≥12.5) capable of corroding metal containers Reactivity: Unstable under "normal" conditions; may cause explosions, toxic fumes, gases, or vapors if heated, compressed, or mixed with water Toxicity: Harmful or fatal if ingested or absorbed; may leach from the waste and pollute ground water when disposed of on land **OR**	Carcinogenic Teratogenic or other developmental toxicity Reproductive toxicity Organotoxic at low doses Genotoxic **and/or** New drugs with structural and toxicity profiles similar to existing hazardous agents	Genotoxic Carcinogenic Teratogenic or impairs fertility Causes serious organ or other toxicity at low doses
Appears on one of the following lists: F: Wastes (nonspecific) from common or industrial manufacturing processes from nonspecific sources K: Specific (source) wastes from specific industries (eg, petroleum or pesticides) P (acutely toxic) or U (toxic): Wastes (unused form) from certain discarded commercial chemical products		

When considering the effects of agents on reproductive and developmental toxicity and carcinogenicity, NIOSH evaluated the dose at which adverse effects occurred. If observed at, near, or below the maximum recommended dose for humans, it was considered relevant; if occurred at doses well above the maximum human dose, then NIOSH did not consider it in the hazardous drug evaluation.

NIOSH updated its list of antineoplastic and hazardous drugs in 2016. Medications with special handling precautions in the product labeling and medications with hazardous characteristics or with structural/toxicity profiles similar to agents on the NIOSH list are also listed in Table 2. In order to account for hazardous nonantineoplastic medications, as well as varying dosage forms, the 2014 update categorized hazardous drugs into three groups to account for the diversity of potential exposures:

- NIOSH Group 1: Antineoplastic drugs (may also pose a reproductive risk)

- NIOSH Group 2: Nonantineoplastic drugs that meet at least one of the NIOSH criteria (may also pose a reproductive risk)

- NIOSH Group 3: Nonantineoplastic drugs with adverse reproductive effects; pose a reproductive risk to men and/or women who are actively attempting conception and to women who are pregnant or breastfeeding

According to NIOSH, to prevent improper handling, all hazardous drugs (regardless of the formulation) should be labeled as hazardous. Medications listed in group 3 may not pose as serious a risk to personnel not at risk for reproductive toxicity due to age or infertility, although they should still be handled as hazardous. Reproductive risks for group 3 are generally higher in females; however, may also apply to males. Regardless of reproductive risk, all hazardous drugs should be handled according to procedures. It is important to note that for medications in groups 1 and 2, in addition to meeting the NIOSH hazardous drug criteria, some may also pose a reproductive risk in susceptible populations.

Some hazardous drug dosage forms, such as coated tablets or capsules, may not present as substantial a risk for occupational exposure; however, if these formulations are altered outside of a ventilated cabinet (eg, by crushing tablets or compounding solutions), the exposure risk is increased. Uncoated tablets may also create a risk of dust absorption via skin absorption or inhalation when counting tablets. Automated counting machines should not be utilized when counting hazardous tablets and capsules due to the potential to introduce powders or dust into the air. Dedicated counting and pouring equipment should be allocated for hazardous drugs and should be cleaned thoroughly after use. Liquid preparations should be used whenever possible in lieu of compounding oral solutions; if compounding is necessary, appropriate protective measures should be utilized.

According to NIOSH, each organization should create a list of drugs considered to be hazardous, based on medications within their formulary. Using the organization's criteria, newly approved/added drugs should be evaluated and, if deemed hazardous, added to the list. Medications which include guidance for hazardous drug handling within the manufacturer's prescribing information should automatically be added to the NIOSH list of hazardous drugs.

Table 2 Drugs Listed as or Considered Hazardous

	NIOSH List[a]			EPA List[b,c]	Product Labeling[d]	Structure or Toxicity Profile Similar to Existing Hazardous Agents	Not on NIOSH List, but Meets NIOSH Criteria[e]
	Group 1	Group 2	Group 3				
Abacavir		X					
Abiraterone	X						
Acitretin			X				
Ado-Trastuzumab Emtansine	X				X		
Afatinib	X						
Aflibercept						X	X
Alectinib						X	X
Alefacept		X					
Alitretinoin			X				
Altretamine	X				X		
Ambrisentan			X		X		
Amsacrine	X				X		
Anastrozole	X						
Apomorphine		X					
Arsenic Trioxide	X			P-listed	X		
Axitinib	X				X		
AzaCITIDine	X				X		
AzaTHIOprine		X			X		X
Bazedoxifene					X	X	
BCG Vaccine	X				X		
Belinostat	X				X		
Belotecan					X	X	X
Bendamustine	X				X		

◀

Table 2. Drugs Listed as or Considered Hazardous *(continued)*

	NIOSH List[a]			EPA List[b,c]	Product Labeling[d]	Structure or Toxicity Profile Similar to Existing Hazardous Agents	Not on NIOSH List, but Meets NIOSH Criteria[e]
	Group 1	Group 2	Group 3				
Bexarotene	X						
Bicalutamide	X						
Bleomycin	X				X		
Bortezomib	X				X		
Bosentan			X				
Bosutinib	X				X		
Brentuximab Vedotin	X				X		
Brigatinib						X	X
Buserelin						X	X
Busulfan	X				X		
Cabazitaxel	X				X		
Cabergoline			X				
Cabozantinib	X						
Capecitabine	X				X		
CarBAMazepine		X					
CARBOplatin	X				X		
Carfilzomib	X						
Carmustine	X				X		
Ceritinib						X	
Cetrorelix			X				X
Chlorambucil	X			U-listed	X		
Chloramphenicol		X					
Choriogonadotropin Alfa			X				

Table 2. Drugs Listed as or Considered Hazardous *(continued)*

	NIOSH List[a]			EPA List[b,c]	Product Labeling[d]	Structure or Toxicity Profile Similar to Existing Hazardous Agents	Not on NIOSH List, but Meets NIOSH Criteria[e]
	Group 1	Group 2	Group 3				
Cidofovir					X		
CISplatin	X				X		
Cladribine	X				X		
Clofarabine	X				X		
ClomiPHENE			X				
ClonazePAM			X				
Cobimetinib						X	
Colchicine			X				X
Crizotinib	X						
Cyclophosphamide	X			U-listed	X		
CycloSPORINE		X					
Cyproterone						X	X
Cytarabine	X				X		
Cytarabine (Liposomal)	X				X		
Dabrafenib	X						
Dacarbazine	X				X		
DACTINomycin	X				X		
Dasatinib	X				X		
DAUNOrubicin	X			U-listed	X		
DAUNOrubicin (Liposomal)	X			U-listed	X		
Decitabine	X				X		
Deferiprone		X					
Degarelix	X				X		

2383

Table 2. Drugs Listed as or Considered Hazardous (continued)

	NIOSH List[a]			EPA List[b,c]	Product Labeling[d]	Structure or Toxicity Profile Similar to Existing Hazardous Agents	Not on NIOSH List, but Meets NIOSH Criteria[e]
	Group 1	Group 2	Group 3				
Desogestrel		X					
Dexrazoxane		X			X		
Dichlorodifluoromethane				U-listed			
Diethylstilbestrol		X		U-listed			
Dinoprostone			X				
Divalproex		X					
DOCEtaxel	X				X		
DOXOrubicin	X				X		
DOXOrubicin (Liposomal)	X				X		
Dronedarone			X				
Dutasteride			X		X		
Dydrogesterone		X					
Enasidenib							X
Entecavir		X					
Enzalutamide	X						
EPINEPHrine (does not include EPINEPHrine salts)				P-listed			
EpiRUBicin	X				X		
Ergonovine/Methylergonovine			X				
EriBULin	X						
Erlotinib	X						
Eslicarbazepine			X				
Estradiol		X					

Table 2. Drugs Listed as or Considered Hazardous (continued)

	NIOSH List[a]			EPA List[b,c]	Product Labeling[d]	Structure or Toxicity Profile Similar to Existing Hazardous Agents	Not on NIOSH List, but Meets NIOSH Criteria[e]
	Group 1	Group 2	Group 3				
Estramustine	X			X			
Estriol						X	X
Estrogen-Progestin Combinations							
Estrogens (Conjugated)		X					
Estrogens (Esterified)		X					
Estropipate		X					
Etoposide	X				X		
Etoposide Phosphate	X				X		
Everolimus	X				X		
Exemestane	X						
Finasteride			X		X		
Fingolimod		X					
Floxuridine	X				X		
Fluconazole			X				
Fludarabine	X				X		
Fluorouracil	X				X		
Fluoxymesterone		X					
Flutamide	X						
Formaldehyde				U-listed			
Fosphenytoin		X					
Fulvestrant	X						
Ganciclovir		X			X		

Table 2. Drugs Listed as or Considered Hazardous (continued)

| | NIOSH List[a] | | | EPA List[b,c] | Product Labeling[d] | Structure or Toxicity Profile Similar to Existing Hazardous Agents | Not on NIOSH List, but Meets NIOSH Criteria[e] |
	Group 1	Group 2	Group 3				
Ganirelix			X				
Gefitinib						X	X
Gemcitabine	X				X		
Gemtuzumab Ozogamicin	X				X		
Gonadotropin, Chorionic			X				
Goserelin	X						
Hexachlorophene				U-listed			
Histrelin	X						
Hydroxyurea	X				X		
Ibrutinib						X	X
Icatibant			X				
IDArubicin	X				X		
Idelalisib							X
Ifosfamide	X				X		
Imatinib	X				X		
Inotuzumab Ozogamicin					X	X	X
Irinotecan	X				X		
Irinotecan (Liposomal)	X				X		
ISOtretinoin					X	X	X
Ixabepilone	X				X		
Ixazomib	X				X		
Lapatinib						X	X
Leflunomide		X					

Table 2. Drugs Listed as or Considered Hazardous (continued)

	NICSH List[a]			EPA List[b,c]	Product Labeling[d]	Structure or Toxicity Profile Similar to Existing Hazardous Agents	Not on NIOSH List, but Meets NIOSH Criteria[e]
	Group 1	Group 2	Group 3				
Lenalidomide					X		
Lenvatinib		X				X	X
Letrozole	X						
Leuprolide	X						
Lindane				U-listed			
Liraglutide		X					
Lomitapide			X				
Lomustine	X				X		
Macitentan			X		X		
Mechlorethamine	X				X		
MedroxyPROGESTERone		X					
Megestrol	X						
Melphalan	X			U-listed	X		
Menotropins			X				
Mercaptopurine	X				X		
Mercury				U-listed			
MethIMAzole		X					
Methotrexate	X				X		
MethylTESTOSTERone			X				
Midostaurin							X
MiFEPRIStone			X				
Mipomersen		X					
MiSOPROStol			X				

Table 2. Drugs Listed as or Considered Hazardous *(continued)*

	NIOSH List[a]			EPA List[b,c]	Product Labeling[d]	Structure or Toxicity Profile Similar to Existing Hazardous Agents	Not on NIOSH List, but Meets NIOSH Criteria[e]
	Group 1	Group 2	Group 3				
MitoMYcin	X			U-listed	X		
Mitotane	X			U-listed	X		
MitoXANTRONE	X				X		
Mycophenolate		X			X		
Nafarelin	X				X		
Nelarabine			X				
Neratinib						X	X
Nevirapine		X					
Nicotine				P-listed			
Nilotinib	X						
Nilutamide						X	X
Nintedanib						X	X
Niraparib							X
Nitroglycerin (doses in "finished form" are excluded)				P-listed			
Olaparib							X
Olaratumab							X
Olmutinib						X	X
Omacetaxine	X				X		
Osimertinib						X	X
Ospemifene		X					
Oxaliplatin	X				X		
OXcarbazepine		X					

Table 2. Drugs Listed as or Considered Hazardous *(continued)*

	NIOSH List[a]			EPA List[b,c]	Product Labeling[d]	Structure or Toxicity Profile Similar to Existing Hazardous Agents	Not on NIOSH List, but Meets NIOSH Criteria[e]
	Group 1	Group 2	Group 3				
Oxytocin			X				
PACLitaxel	X				X		
PACLitaxel (Protein Bound)	X				X		
Palbociclib							X
Palifermin		X					
Paliperidone		X					
Pamidronate			X				
Panobinostat	X				X		
Paraldehyde				U-listed			
PARoxetine			X				
Pasireotide			X				
PAZOPanib	X						
Peginesatide			X		X		
PEMEtrexed	X				X		
Pentetate Calcium Trisodium			X				
Pentostatin	X						
Pertuzumab	X				X		
Phenacetin				U-listed			
Phenol				U-listed			
Phenoxybenzamine		X					
Physostigmine				P-listed			
Phenytoin		X					
Pimecrolimus						X	X

Table 2. Drugs Listed as or Considered Hazardous *(continued)*

| | NIOSH List[a] | | | EPA List[b,c] | Product Labeling[d] | Structure or Toxicity Profile Similar to Existing Hazardous Agents | Not on NIOSH List, but Meets NIOSH Criteria[e] |
	Group 1	Group 2	Group 3				
Pipobroman		X					
Plerixafor			X				
Pomalidomide	X				X		
PONATinib	X						
PRALAtrexate	X				X		
Prasterone							X
Procarbazine	X				X	X	
Progesterone		X					
Progestins		X					
Propylthiouracil		X					
Radotinib						X	X
Raloxifene		X					
Raltitrexed		X			X	X	
Rasagiline							X
Regorafenib	X						
Reserpine				U-listed			
Resorcinol				U-listed			
Ribavirin			X				
Ribociclib							X
Riociguat			X				
RisperiDONE		X					
RomiDEPsin	X				X		
Rucaparib							X

Table 2. Drugs Listed as or Considered Hazardous (continued)

	NIOSH List[a]			EPA List[b,c]	Product Labeling[d]	Structure or Toxicity Profile Similar to Existing Hazardous Agents	Not on NIOSH List, but Meets NIOSH Criteria[e]
	Group 1	Group 2	Group 3				
Ruxolitinib						X	X
Saccharin				U-listed			
Selenium Sulfide				U-listed			
Sirolimus		X					
Sonidegib						X	X
SORAfenib	X						
Spironolactone		X					
Streptozocin	X			U-listed	X		
SUNitinib	X						
Tacrolimus		X					
Talimogene Laherparepvec					X		X
Tamoxifen	X						
Tegafur and Uracil					X	X	X
Tegafur, Gimeracil, and Oteracil					X	X	X
Temazepam			X				
Temozolomide	X				X		
Temsirolimus	X				X		
Teniposide	X				X		
Teriflunamide		X					
Testosterone			X				
Thalidomide		X			X		
Thioguanine	X				X		

Table 2. Drugs Listed as or Considered Hazardous *(continued)*

	NIOSH List[a]			EPA List[b,c]	Product Labeling[d]	Structure or Toxicity Profile Similar to Existing Hazardous Agents	Not on NIOSH List, but Meets NIOSH Criteria[e]
	Group 1	Group 2	Group 3				
Thiotepa	X				X		
Tibolone		X					
Tofacitinib		X					
Topiramate			X				
Topotecan	X				X		
Toremifene	X						
Trabectedin	X				X		
Trametinib	X						
Trastuzumab							X
Treosulfan					X	X	X
Tretinoin			X				
Trichloromonofluoromethane				U-listed			
Trifluridine and Tipiracil	X				X		
Triptorelin	X						
Ulipristal			X				
Uracil Mustard				U-listed			
ValGANciclovir		X			X		
Valproic Acid		X	X				
Valrubicin	X				X		
Vandetanib	X				X		
Vemurafenib	X						
Venetoclax							X
Vigabatrin			X				

Table 2. Drugs Listed as or Considered Hazardous *(continued)*

| | NIOSH List[a] | | | EPA List[b,c] | Product Labeling[d] | Structure or Toxicity Profile Similar to Existing Hazardous Agents | Not on NIOSH List, but Meets NIOSH Criteria[e] |
	Group 1	Group 2	Group 3				
VinBLAStine	X				X		
VinCRIStine	X				X		
VinCRIStine (Liposomal)	X				X		
Vindesine					X	X	X
Vinflunine					X	X	X
Vinorelbine	X				X		
Vismodegib	X				X		
Voriconazole			X				
Vorinostat	X				X		
Warfarin			X	<0.3%: U-listed; >0.3%: P-listed	X		
Zidovudine		X					
Ziprasidone			X				
Ziv-aflibercept	X						
Zoledronic Acid			X				
Zonisamide			X				

[a]US Department of Health and Human Services; Centers for Disease Control and Prevention; National Institute for Occupational Safety and Health. NIOSH list of antineoplastic and other hazardous drugs in healthcare settings, 2016. Available http://www.cdc.gov/niosh/topics/antineoplastic/pdf/hazardous-drugs-list_2016-161.pdf. Updated September 2016. Accessed November 8, 2016.

[b]Healthcare Environmental Resource Center (HERC). Pharmaceutical wastes in healthcare facilities. Available at http://www.hercenter.org/hazmat/pharma.cfm#listed. Accessed November 8, 2016.

[c]Healthcare Environmental Resource Center (HERC). Hazardous waste determination. http://www.hercenter.org/hazmat/hazdeterm.cfm. Accessed November 8, 2016.

[d]Product labeling (prescribing information) indicates precautions for safe handling and disposal should be followed.

[e]Meets one or more of the NIOSH characteristics for defining hazardous agents: Carcinogenicity, Teratogenicity (or other developmental toxicity), Reproductive toxicity, Organ toxicity (at low doses), Genotoxicity, and/or New drugs with structural and/or toxicity profiles similar to existing hazardous agents (http://www.cdc.gov/niosh/topics/antineoplastic/pdf/hazardous-drugs-list_2016-161.pdf)

NIOSH has developed guidance on personal protective equipment when working with various dosage forms of hazardous drugs within the health care setting. These recommendations are listed in Table 3.

Table 3. Personal Protection for Handling Hazardous Drugs

Formulation	Activity	Gloving	Protective Gown	Eye/Face Protection	Respiratory Protection	Ventilation Controls
All formulations	Receiving, unpacking, and storing	Single	Only for spills	No	Only for spills	No
Intact tablet or capsule	Administration from a unit dose package	Single	No	No	No	N/A
Tablets or capsules	Cutting, crushing, or manipulating	Double	Yes	No	Yes (if not done in a controlled device)	Yes
Tablets or capsules	Administration	Single	No	Yes (if vomit or potential for spit up)	No	N/A
Oral liquid (or feeding tube)	Compounding	Double	Yes	Yes (if not done in a controlled device)	Yes (if not done in a controlled device)	Yes
Oral liquid (or feeding tube)	Administration	Double	Yes	Yes (if vomit or potential for spit up)	No	N/A
Topical product	Compounding	Double	Yes	Yes	Yes (if not done in a controlled device)	Yes
Topical product	Administration	Double	Yes	Yes (if liquid could splash)	Yes (if potential inhalation)	N/A
SubQ or IM injection from a vial	Preparation for administration	Double	Yes	Yes (if not done in a controlled device)	Yes (if not done in a controlled device)	Yes (BSC or CACI)
SubQ or IM injection from a vial	Administration	Double	Yes	Yes (if liquid could splash)	No	N/A
Withdrawing and/or mixing IV or IM solutions from a vial or ampule	Compounding	Double	Yes	No	No	Yes (BSC or CACI; CSTD recommended)
Withdrawing and/or mixing IV or IM solutions from a vial or ampule	Administration	Double	Yes	Yes (if liquid could splash)	No	N/A (CSTD required)

Table 3. Personal Protection for Handling Hazardous Drugs *(continued)*

Formulation	Activity	Gloving	Protective Gown	Eye/Face Protection	Respiratory Protection	Ventilation Controls
Irrigation solutions	Compounding	Double	Yes	Yes (if not done in a controlled device)	Yes (if not done in a controlled device)	Yes (BSC or CACI; CSTD recommended)
	Administration	Double	Yes	Yes	Yes	N/A
Inhalation powder or solution/ aerosol treatment	Compounding	Double	Yes	Yes (if not done in a controlled device)	Yes (if not done in a controlled device)	Yes (BSC or CACI)
	Aerosol treatment	Double	Yes	Yes	Yes	Yes (if applicable)
	Administration	Double	Yes	Yes (if liquid could splash)	Yes (if inhalation potential)	N/A
Drug and metabolites in body fluids	Disposal and cleaning	Double	Yes	Yes (if liquid could splash)	Yes (if inhalation potential)	N/A
Drug-contaminated waste	Disposal and cleaning	Double	Yes	Yes (if liquid could splash)	Yes (if inhalation potential)	N/A
Spills	Cleaning	Double	Yes	Yes	Yes	N/A

BSC = biologic safety cabinet (class II), CACI = compounding aseptic containment isolator, CSTD = closed system transfer device

US Department of Health and Human Services; Centers for Disease Control and Prevention; National Institute for Occupational Safety and Health. NIOSH list of antineoplastic and other hazardous drugs in the healthcare settings. 2016. Available at http://www.cdc.gov/niosh/topics/antineoplastic/pdf/hazardous-drugs-list_2016-161.pdf. Updated September 2013. Accessed November 8, 2016.

Hazardous drugs must be stored, transported, prepared, administered, and disposed of under conditions that protect the health care worker from acute and chronic/low level exposure.

Each institution or facility must create its own policy or guideline, including the facility-specific list of drugs deemed hazardous. According to the Joint Commission standards, organizations should minimize risks associated with handling hazardous medications. Orientation and routine training related to safe handling of hazardous drugs is recommended. Until proven otherwise, most institutions consider investigational drugs to be hazardous and to be handled accordingly, particularly if the mechanism of action suggests a potential for concern. Hazardous drug procedures must include all possible routes of administration.

Additional information regarding development and implementation of an institutional policy/guideline, areas at risk, personnel at risk, risk management, spill management, personnel training, surveillance, and medicine disposal may be found at:

ASHP Guidelines on Handling Hazardous Drugs:
http://www.ashp.org/DocLibrary/BestPractices/PrepGdlHazDrugs.aspx

Environmental Protection Agency Recommendations:
http://hercenter.org/hazmat/hazdeterm.cfm
http://hercenter.org/hazmat/pharma.cfm

Food and Drug Administration Safe Medicine Disposal Options:
http://www.fda.gov/Drugs/NewsEvents/ucm464197.htm

NIOSH List of Antineoplastic and Other Hazardous Drugs in Health Care Settings:
http://www.cdc.gov/niosh/topics/antineoplastic/pdf/hazardous-drugs-list_2016-161.pdf

Identification of Personnel and Locations in the Facility at Risk for Occupational Exposure to Hazardous Drugs

- Pharmacy
    - Receiving storage and inventory
    - Dose preparation and dispensing
    - Drug waste disposal
- Nursing Unit
    - Drug administration
    - Drug waste disposal
    - Patient waste disposal
- Other areas
    - Laboratory
    - Operating/procedure rooms
    - Veterinary department
    - Facility shipping/receiving
    - Environmental/laundry services
    - Maintenance services

While the greatest risk of occupational exposure to hazardous drugs occurs during preparation and administration of these agents, it is important to recognize that a risk of exposure can occur throughout the facility from the moment of delivery through the disposal of product and contaminated human waste. Drug preparation and administration may occur in nontraditional areas of the institution including the operating room and in veterinary facilities. Procedures should address the importance of proper labeling and packaging and separation of hazardous vs nonhazardous inventories throughout the facility. Drug containers should be examined upon their arrival at the pharmacy. Containers that show signs of damage should be handled carefully and may require quarantine and decontamination before being placed in stock. Give consideration to routinely quarantining and decontaminating all hazardous drug containers as part of the inspection process before placing in stock.

Mechanisms/Routes of Occupational Exposure

- Inhalation of dust or aerosolized droplets (most common)

- Absorption through skin (most common)

- Ingestion from contaminated food/drink

- Accidental injection during preparation/administration/disposal

Potential Adverse Effects of Hazardous Exposure

- Skin disorders

- Reproductive effects (eg, spontaneous abortion, stillbirth, congenital malformation)

- Leukemia and other cancers

Risk Management

- Use and maintenance of equipment designed to minimize exposure during handling

  - Buffer/Ante transition area

  - Biological safety cabinets, isolators

  - Closed system drug-transfer devices

  - Personal protective equipment

  - Deactivation, decontamination, and cleaning procedures

Barrier protection through the use of ventilation controls and personal protective equipment is the current standard to minimize exposure when handling hazardous drugs. NIOSH and ASHP recommend the use of a containment device such as a Class II biological safety cabinet or a compounding aseptic containment isolator. Closed system transfer devices (CSTDs) minimize workplace contamination by preventing escape of drug or vapor out of the device. Gloves, gowns, respiratory protection, hair and shoe covers, and eye protection represent the core of personal protective equipment. Guidelines for choice of gowns and gloving and the circumstances to employ this protection are published by ASHP, NIOSH, and in USP 800.

- Hazardous drug spill management

  - Size and location

  - Spill kit use

  - Worker contamination

Procedures for handling spills throughout a facility are described by ASHP and NIOSH. Institutional procedures should focus on location and size of the spill, how to handle a spill when a spill kit is not available, and how to respond to a worker contamination (emergent treatment, follow-up care).

- Personnel training in the handling of hazardous drugs

  - Prior to handling hazardous drugs

  - Periodic and ongoing testing

Personnel throughout a facility must have training in the handling of hazardous drugs that are relevant to their job description. Pharmacy personnel who compound and dispense hazardous drugs must be fully trained in the storing, preparation, dispensing, and disposal of these agents. Such training should include didactic, as well as demonstrating hands-on technique, and such validation should be repeated on a regular schedule. Special training may be necessary for hazardous drugs administered by routes outside of traditional administration routes and when administered in settings outside of traditional settings (eg, at home).

- Environmental and medical surveillance

  - Components of a comprehensive medical surveillance program

  - Reproductive and health questionnaires (at time of hire and periodically)

  - Drug handling history (to estimate current and prior exposure)

  - Baseline clinical evaluation plan (including related medical history, physical exam, lab work)

  - Follow-up plan (for those with health changes suggestive of toxicity or acute exposure)

  - Potential use of environmental sampling techniques

  - Use of common marker hazardous drugs for assay purposes

The goal of medical surveillance is to minimize adverse effects on the health of workers exposed to hazardous drugs. NIOSH recommends that medical surveillance be employed by the facility, and may include the basic observation of employee symptom complaints or monitoring for changes in health status as part of routine checkups. Some programs follow the employee more closely and procedures may include periodic lab studies (eg, blood cell counts), physical exam, detailed medical history and occupational exposure history, and/or biologic studies. Environmental sampling to look for surface contamination in hazardous drug preparation and administration areas may be considered, particularly in institutions with high volumes. Certain hazardous drugs serve as markers which allow for assay for measurable contamination, and can alert the facility for proper follow-up.

- Work practices regarding reproductive risks to health care workers

  - Alternative duty options

    Since hazardous drugs are associated with reproductive risks, policies and guidelines should address health care workers whom are pregnant, attempting to conceive or father a child, and whom are breastfeeding. Workers of reproductive capability should acknowledge in writing that they understand the risk of handling hazardous drugs and be given the opportunity for reassignment or alternate work duty.

USP <800>

USP <800> is a chapter of the United States Pharmacopeia (USP) Compounding Compendium. USP <800> was published February 1, 2016 and will be effective (and enforceable) on July 1, 2018. The standards outlined in USP <800> apply to areas where hazardous drugs are stored, transported, compounded, and administered.

REFERENCES

American Society of Hospital Pharmacists. ASHP guidelines on handling hazardous drugs. 2006;63(12):1172-1193.

Baker ES, Connor TH. Monitoring occupational exposure to cancer chemotherapy drugs. Am J Health Syst Pharm. 1996;53(22):2713-2723.

Bos RP, Sessink PJ. Biomonitoring of occupational exposures to cytostatic anticancer drugs. Rev Environ Health. 1997;12(1):43-58.

Connor TH, Anderson RW, Sessink PJ, Broadfield L, Power LA. Surface contamination with antineoplastic agents in six cancer treatment centers in Canada and the United States. Am J Health Syst Pharm. 1999;56(14):1427-1432.

Connor TH, DeBord DG, Pretty JR, et al. Evaluation of antineoplastic drug exposure of health care workers at three university-based US cancer centers. J Occup Environ Med. 2010;52 (10):1019-1027.

Connor TH, McDiarmid MA. Preventing occupational exposures to antineoplastic drugs in health care settings. CA Cancer J Clin. 2006;56(6):354-365.

Connor TH. Permeability of nitrile rubber, latex, polyurethane, and neoprene gloves to 18 antineoplastic drugs. Am J Health Syst Pharm. 1999;56(23):2450-2453.

Connor TH, Sessink PJ, Harrison BR, et al. Surface contamination of chemotherapy drug vials and evaluation of new vial-cleaning techniques: results of three studies. Am J Health Syst Pharm. 2005;62(5):475-484.

Healthcare Environmental Resource Center (HERC). Hazardous waste determination. http://www.hercenter.org/hazmat/hazdeterm.cfm. Accessed November 8, 2016.

Healthcare Environmental Resource Center (HERC). Pharmaceutical wastes in healthcare facilities. http://www.hercenter.org/hazmat/pharma.cfm#listed. Accessed November 8, 2016.

Lawson CC, Rocheleau CM, Whelan EA, et al. Occupational exposures among nurses and risk of spontaneous abortion. Am J Obstet Gynecol. 2012;206(4):327.

McDiarmid MA, Oliver MS, Roth TS, Rogers B, Escalante C. Chromosome 5 and 7 abnormalities in oncology personnel handling anticancer drugs. J Occup Environ Med. 2010;52 (10):1028-1034.

National Institute for Occupational Safety and Health (NIOSH). Medical surveillance for healthcare workers exposed to hazardous drugs. 2012. http://www.cdc.gov/niosh/docs/wp-solutions/2013-103/. Accessed January 22, 2013.

National Institute for Occupational Safety and Health (NIOSH). Preventing occupational exposure to antineoplastic and other hazardous drugs in health care settings. http://www.cdc.gov/niosh/docs/2004-165/2004-165d.html#o. Accessed October 1, 2007.

Polovich M. Safe Handling of Hazardous Drugs. 2nd ed. Pittsburgh, PA: Oncology Nursing Society; 2011.

Sessink PJ, Bos RP. Drugs hazardous to healthcare workers. Evaluation of methods for monitoring occupational exposure to cytostatic drugs. Drug Saf. 1999;20(4):347-359.

Sessink PJ, Anzion RB, Van den Broek PH, Bos RP. Detection of contamination with antineoplastic agents in a hospital pharmacy department. Pharm Weekbl Sci. 1992;14(1):16-22.

Sessink PJ, Boer KA, Scheefhals AP, Anzion RB, Bos RP. Occupational exposure to antineoplastic agents at several departments in a hospital. Environmental contamination and excretion of cyclophosphamide and ifosfamide in urine of exposed workers. *Int Arch Occup Environ Health*. 1992;64(2):105-112.

Sorsa M, Anderson D. Monitoring of occupational exposure to cytostatic anticancer agents. *Mutat Res*. 1996;355(1-2):253-261.

US Department of Health and Human Services; Centers for Disease Control and Prevention; National Institute for Occupational Safety and Health. NIOSH list of antineoplastic and other hazardous drugs in healthcare settings, 2016. Available at http://www.cdc.gov/niosh/topics/antineoplastic/pdf/hazardous-drugs-list_2016-161.pdf. Updated September 2016. Accessed May 27, 2017.

APPENDIX TABLE OF CONTENTS

MILLIEQUIVALENT AND MILLIMOLE CALCULATIONS AND CONVERSIONS

DEFINITIONS AND CALCULATIONS

Definitions

mole	=	gram molecular weight of a substance (aka molar weight)
millimole (mM)	=	milligram molecular weight of a substance (a millimole is 1/1,000 of a mole)
equivalent weight	=	gram weight of a substance which will combine with or replace 1 gram (1 mole) of hydrogen; an equivalent weight can be determined by dividing the molar weight of a substance by its ionic valence
milliequivalent (mEq)	=	milligram weight of a substance which will combine with or replace 1 milligram (1 millimole) of hydrogen (a milliequivalent is 1/1,000 of an equivalent)

Calculations

moles	=	$\dfrac{\text{weight of a substance (grams)}}{\text{molecular weight of that substance (grams)}}$
millimoles	=	$\dfrac{\text{weight of a substance (grams) x 1,000}}{\text{molecular weight of that substance (grams)}}$
equivalents	=	moles x valence of ion
milliequivalents	=	millimoles x valence of ion
moles	=	$\dfrac{\text{equivalents}}{\text{valence of ion}}$
millimoles	=	$\dfrac{\text{milliequivalents}}{\text{valence of ion}}$
millimoles	=	moles x 1,000
milliequivalents	=	equivalents x 1,000

Note: Use of equivalents and milliequivalents is valid only for those substances which have fixed ionic valences (eg, sodium, potassium, calcium, chlorine, magnesium, bromine, etc). For substances with variable ionic valences (eg, phosphorous), a reliable equivalent value cannot be determined. In these instances, one should calculate millimoles (which are fixed and reliable) rather than milliequivalents.

MILLIEQUIVALENT CONVERSIONS

To convert mg/100 mL to mEq/L the following formula may be used:

$$\frac{\text{(mg per 100 mL) x 10 x valence}}{\text{atomic weight}} = \text{mEq/L}$$

To convert mEq/L to mg/100 mL the following formula may be used:

$$\frac{\text{(mEq/L) x atomic weight}}{\text{10 x valence}} = \text{mg per 100 mL}$$

To convert mEq/L to volume of percent of a gas the following formula may be used:

$$\frac{(mEq/L) \times 22.4}{10} = \text{volume percent}$$

Valences and Atomic Weights of Selected Ions

Substance	Electrolyte	Valence	Molecular Wt
Calcium	Ca^{++}	2	40
Chloride	Cl^-	1	35.5
Magnesium	Mg^{++}	2	24
Phosphate	HPO_4^{--} (80%)	1.8	96[a]
pH = 7.4	$H_2PO_4^-$ (20%)	1.8	96[a]
Potassium	K^+	1	39
Sodium	Na^+	1	23
Sulfate	SO_4^{--}	2	96[a]

[a]The molecular weight of phosphorus only is 31 and sulfur only is 32.

Approximate Milliequivalents — Weights of Selected Ions

Salt	mEq/g Salt	mg Salt/mEq
Calcium carbonate [$CaCO_3$]	20	50
Calcium chloride [$CaCl_2 \cdot 2H_2O$]	14	74
Calcium gluceptate [$Ca(C_7H_{13}O_8)_2$]	4	245
Calcium gluconate [$Ca(C_6H_{11}O_7)_2 \cdot H_2O$]	5	224
Calcium lactate [$Ca(C_3H_5O_3)_2 \cdot 5H_2O$]	7	154
Magnesium gluconate [$Mg(C_6H_{11}O_7)_2 \cdot H_2O$]	5	216
Magnesium oxide [MgO]	50	20
Magnesium sulfate [$MgSO_4$]	17	60
Magnesium sulfate [$MgSO_4 \cdot 7H_2O$]	8	123
Potassium acetate [$K(C_2H_3O_2)$]	10	98
Potassium chloride [KCl]	13	75
Potassium citrate [$K_3(C_6H_5O_7) \cdot H_2O$]	9	108
Potassium iodide [KI]	6	166
Sodium acetate [$Na(C_2H_3O_2)$]	12	82
Sodium acetate [$Na(C_2H_3O_2) \cdot 3H_2O$]	7	136
Sodium bicarbonate [$NaHCO_3$]	12	84
Sodium chloride [$NaCl$]	17	58
Sodium citrate [$Na_3(C_6H_5O_7) \cdot 2H_2O$]	10	98
Sodium iodine [NaI]	7	150
Sodium lactate [$Na(C_3H_5O_3)$]	9	112
Zinc sulfate [$ZnSO_4 \cdot 7H_2O$]	7	144

ACID-BASE ASSESSMENT

Henderson-Hasselbalch Equation

$$pH = 6.1 + \log ([HCO_3^-] / (0.03) [PaCO_2])$$

Normal arterial blood pH: 7.4 (normal range: 7.35 to 7.45)

Where:

$[HCO_3^-]$ = Serum bicarbonate concentration

$PaCO_2$ = Arterial carbon dioxide partial pressure

Alveolar Gas Equation

$$P_iO_2 \quad = \quad F_iO_2 \times (\text{total atmospheric pressure} - \text{vapor pressure of } H_2O \text{ at } 37°C)$$

$$= \quad F_iO_2 \times (760 \text{ mm Hg} - 47 \text{ mm Hg})$$

$$PAO_2 \quad = \quad P_iO_2 - (PaCO_2/ R)$$

Alveolar-arterial oxygen (A-a) gradient = $PAO_2 - PaO_2$

or

A-a gradient = $[(F_iO_2 \times 713) - (PaCO_2/0.8)] - PaO_2$

A-a gradient normal ranges:

Children	15 to 20 mm Hg
Adults	20 to 25 mm Hg

where:

P_iO_2 = Oxygen partial pressure of inspired gas (mm Hg) (150 mm Hg in room air at sea level)

F_iO_2 = Fractional pressure of oxygen in inspired gas (0.21 in room air)

PAO_2 = Alveolar oxygen partial pressure

PaO_2 = Arterial oxygen partial pressure

$PaCO_2$ = Arterial carbon dioxide partial pressure

R = Respiratory exchange quotient (typically 0.8, increases with high carbohydrate diet, decreases with high fat diet)

Acid-Base Disorders

Acute metabolic acidosis:
$PaCO_2$ expected = 1.5 $([HCO_3^-])$ + 8 ± 2 **or**
Expected decrease in $PaCO_2$ = 1.3 (1-1.5) x decrease in $[HCO_3^-]$

Acute metabolic alkalosis:
Expected increase in $PaCO_2$ = 0.6 (0.5-1) x increase in $[HCO_3^-]$

Acute respiratory acidosis (<6 h duration):
For every $PaCO_2$ increase of 10 mm Hg, $[HCO_3^-]$ increases by 1 mEq/L

Chronic respiratory acidosis (>6 h duration):
  For every $PaCO_2$ increase of 10 mm Hg, $[HCO_3^-]$ increases by 4 mEq/L

Acute respiratory alkalosis (<6 h duration):
  For every $PaCO_2$ decrease of 10 mm Hg, $[HCO_3^-]$ decreases by 2 mEq/L

Chronic respiratory alkalosis (>6 h duration):
  For every $PaCO_2$ decrease of 10 mm Hg, $[HCO_3^-]$ increases by 5 mEq/L

SELECTED CLINICAL EQUATIONS

CORRECTED SODIUM

Corrected Na^+ = measured Na^+ + [1.5 x (glucose − 150 divided by 100)]

Note: Do not correct for glucose <150.

WATER DEFICIT

Water deficit = 0.6 x body weight [1 − (140 divided by Na^+)]

Note: Body weight is estimated weight in kg when fully hydrated; **Na^+** is serum or plasma sodium. Use corrected Na^+ if necessary. Consult medical references for recommendations for replacement of deficit.

TOTAL SERUM CALCIUM CORRECTED FOR ALBUMIN LEVEL

[(Normal albumin − patient's albumin) x 0.8] + patient's measured total calcium

OSMOLALITY

Definition: The summed concentrations of all osmotically active solute particles.

Predicted serum osmolality =

$$mOsm/L = (2 \text{ x serum } Na^{++}) + \frac{\text{serum glucose}}{18} + \frac{BUN}{2.8}$$

The normal range of serum osmolality is 285 to 295 mOsm/L.

Calculated Osm

Note: Osm is a term used to reconcile osmolality and osmolarity

Osmol gap = measured Osm − calculated Osm

0 to +10: Normal
>10: Abnormal
<0: Probable lab or calculation error

Drugs Causing Osmolar Gap
(by freezing-point depression, gap is >10 mOsm)
Ethanol
Ethylene glycol
Glycerol
Iodine (questionable)
Isopropanol (acetone)
Mannitol
Methanol
Sorbitol

BICARBONATE DEFICIT

HCO_3^- deficit = (0.4 x wt in kg) x (HCO_3^- desired − HCO_3^- measured)

Note: In clinical practice, the calculated quantity may differ markedly from the actual amount of bicarbonate needed or that which may be safely administered.

ANION GAP

Definition: The difference in concentration between unmeasured cation and anion equivalents in serum.

Anion gap = $Na^+ - (Cl^- + HCO_3^-)$
  (The normal anion gap is 10 to 14 mEq/L)

Differential Diagnosis of Increased Anion Gap Acidosis

Organic anions
  Lactate (sepsis, hypovolemia, seizures, large tumor burden)
  Pyruvate
  Uremia
  Ketoacidosis (β-hydroxybutyrate and acetoacetate)
  Amino acids and their metabolites
  Other organic acids

Inorganic anions
  Hyperphosphatemia
  Sulfates
  Nitrates

Differential Diagnosis of Decreased Anion Gap

Organic cations
  Hypergammaglobulinemia

Inorganic cations
  Hyperkalemia
  Hypercalcemia
  Hypermagnesemia

Medications and toxins
  Lithium

Hypoalbuminemia

RETICULOCYTE INDEX

(% retic divided by 2) x (patient's Hct divided by normal Hct) **or**
(% retic divided by 2) x (patient's Hgb divided by normal Hgb)

Normal index: 1
Good marrow response: 2 to 6

CORRECTED QT INTERVAL EQUATIONS

Bazett (B) Formula:

QTcB: $QTc = QT/(R - R \text{ interval}^{0.5})$

or

QTcB: $QTc = QT/\text{Square root of } (R - R \text{ interval})$

Frederica (F) Formula:

QTcF: $QTc = QT/(R - R \text{ interval}^{0.33})$

BODY SURFACE AREA

Body Surface Area (BSA) – Adults and Pediatric

$$\text{BSA (m}^2) = \frac{kg^{0.425} \times cm^{0.725} \times 71.84}{10,000}$$

or

$$\log \text{BSA (m}^2) = \frac{(\log kg \times 0.425) + (\log cm \times 0.725) + 1.8564}{10,000}$$

DuBois D, DuBois EF. A formula to estimate the approximate surface area if height and weight be known. *Arch Intern Med.* 1916;17:863-871.

$$\text{BSA (m}^2) = \sqrt{\frac{ht \text{ (in)} \times wt \text{ (lb)}}{3131}} \quad \textbf{or} \quad \text{BSA (m}^2) = \sqrt{\frac{ht \text{ (cm)} \times wt \text{ (kg)}}{3600}}$$

Lam TK, Leung DT. More on simplified calculation of body-surface area. *N Engl J Med.* 1988;318 (17):1130 (letter).
Mostellor RD. Simplified calculation of body surface area. *N Engl J Med.* 1987;317:1098 (letter).

Ideal Body Weight

Men: 50 kg + 2.3 kg/inch >5 feet
Women: 45 kg + 2.3 kg/inch >5 feet

Devine BJ. Gentamicin therapy. *Drug Intelligence and Clinical Pharmacy.* 1974;8:650-655.

or

Men: 51.65 kg + 1.85 kg/inch >5 feet
Women: 48.67 kg + 1.7 kg/inch >5 feet

Robinson JD, Lupkiewicz SM, Palenik L, Lopez LM, Ariet M. Determination of ideal body weight for drug dosage calculations. *Am J Hosp Pharm.* 1983;40(6):1016-1019.

Adjusted Body Weight

Adjusted wt (kg) = ideal body weight (kg) + 0.25 [actual wt (kg) - ideal body weight (kg)]

Adjusted wt (kg) = ideal body weight (kg) + 0.4 [actual wt (kg) – ideal body weight (kg)]

Bubalo J, Carpenter PA, Majhail N, et al. Conditioning chemotherapy dose adjustment in obese patients: a review and position statement by the American Society for Blood and Marrow Transplantation practice guideline committee. *Biol Blood Marrow Transplant.* 2014;20 (5):600-616.

Area Under the Curve (AUC) for CARBOplatin Dosing

CARBOplatin (mg) = desired AUC x (25 + GFR)

GFR = creatinine clearance (measured or estimated)

Calvert AH, Newell DR, Gumbrell LA, et al. Carboplatin dosage: prospective evaluation of a simple formula based on renal function. *J Clin Oncol.* 1989;7(11):1748-1756.

RENAL FUNCTION ESTIMATION IN ADULT PATIENTS

Evaluation of a patient's renal function often includes the use of equations to estimate glomerular filtration rate (GFR) (eg, estimated GFR [eGFR] creatinine clearance [CrCl]) using an endogenous filtration marker (eg, serum creatinine) and other patient variables. For example, the Cockcroft-Gault equation estimates renal function by calculating CrCl and is typically used to steer medication dosing. Equations which calculate eGFR are primarily used to categorize chronic kidney disease (CKD) staging and monitor progression. The rate of creatinine clearance does not always accurately represent GFR; creatinine may be cleared by other renal mechanisms in addition to glomerular filtration and serum creatinine concentrations may be affected by nonrenal factors (eg, age, gender, race, body habitus, illness, diet). In addition, these equations were developed based on studies in limited populations and may either over- or underestimate the renal function of a specific patient.

Nevertheless, most clinicians estimate renal function using CrCl as an indicator of actual renal function for the purpose of adjusting medication doses. For medications that require dose adjustment for renal impairment, utilization of eGFR (ie, Modification of Diet in Renal Disease [MDRD]) may overestimate renal function by up to 40% which may result in supratherapeutic medication doses (Hermsen 2009). These equations should only be used in the clinical context of patient-specific factors noted during the physical exam/work-up. The 2012 National Kidney Foundation (NKF)-Kidney Disease Improving Global Outcomes (KDIGO) CKD guidelines state that drug dosing should be based on an e-GFR which is **not** adjusted for body surface area (BSA) (ie, reported in units of mL/minute per 1.73 m^2) since the effect of eGFR adjusted for BSA compared to eGFR without adjustments for BSA has not been extensively studied. **Decisions regarding drug therapy and doses must be based on clinical judgment.**

RENAL FUNCTION ESTIMATION EQUATIONS

Commonly used equations to estimate renal function utilizing the endogenous filtration marker serum creatinine include the Cockcroft-Gault, Jelliffe, four-variable Modification of Diet in Renal Disease (MDRD), six-variable MDRD (aka, MDRD extended), and Chronic Kidney Disease Epidemiology Collaboration (CKD-EPI). All of these equations, except for the CKD-EPI, were originally developed using a serum creatinine assay measured by the alkaline picrate-based (Jaffe) method. Many substances, including proteins, can interfere with the accuracy of this assay and overestimate serum creatinine concentration. The NKF and The National Kidney Disease Education Program (NDKEP) advocated for a universal creatinine assay, in order to ensure an accurate estimate of renal function in patients. As a result, a more specific enzymatic assay with an isotope dilution mass spectrometry (IDMS)-traceable international standard was developed. Compared to the older methods, IDMS-traceable assays may report lower serum creatinine values and may, therefore, overestimate renal function when used in the original equations not re-expressed for use with a standardized serum creatinine assay (eg, Cockcroft-Gault, Jelliffe, original MDRD). Updated four-variable MDRD and six-variable MDRD equations based on serum creatinine measured by the IDMS-traceable method has been proposed for adults (Levey 2006); the Cockcroft-Gault and Jelliffe equations have not been re-expressed and may overestimate renal function when used with a serum creatinine measured by the IDMS-traceable method. However, at this point, all laboratories should be using creatinine methods calibrated to be IDMS traceable.

The CKD-EPI creatinine equation, published in 2009, uses the same four variables as the four-variable MDRD (serum creatinine, age, sex, and race), but allows for more precision when estimating higher GFR values (eg, eGFR >60 mL/minute per 1.73 m^2) as compared to the MDRD equation. The NKDEP has not made a recommendation on the general implementation of the CKD-EPI equation but does suggest that laboratories which report numeric values for eGFR >60 mL/minute per 1.73 m^2 should consider the use of CKD-EPI. The NKD-KDIGO 2012 CKD guidelines recommend that clinicians use a creatinine-derived equation for the evaluation and management of CKD and specifically recommend that clinical laboratories use the 2009 CKD-EPI equation when reporting eGFR in adults.

The following factors may contribute to an inaccurate estimation of renal function (Stevens 2006):

- Increased creatinine generation (may underestimate renal function):

    - Black patients

    - Muscular body habitus

    - Ingestion of cooked meats

- Decreased creatinine generation (may overestimate renal function):

    - Increased age

    - Female patients

    - Hispanic patients

    - Asian patients

    - Amputees

    - Malnutrition, inflammation, or deconditioning (eg, cancer, severe cardiovascular disease, hospitalized patients)

    - Neuromuscular disease

    - Vegetarian diet

- Rapidly changing serum creatinine (either up or down): In patients with rapidly rising serum creatinines (ie, increasing by >0.5 to 0.7 mg/dL/day), it is best to assume that the patient's renal function is severely impaired

Use extreme caution when estimating renal function in the following patient populations:

- Low body weight (actual body weight < ideal body weight)

- Liver transplant

- Elderly patients (>90 years of age)

- Dehydration

- Recent kidney transplantation (serum creatinine values may decrease rapidly and can lead to renal function underestimation; conversely, delayed graft function may be present)

Note: In most situations, the use of the patient's ideal body weight (IBW) is recommended for estimating renal function, except when the patient's actual body weight (ABW) is less than ideal. Use of actual body weight (ABW) in obese patients (and possibly patients with ascites) may significantly overestimate renal function. Some clinicians prefer to use an adjusted body weight in such cases [eg, IBW + 0.4 (ABW - IBW)]; the adjustment factor may vary based on practitioner and/or institutional preference.

IDMS-traceable methods

Method 1: MDRD equation[a]:

$$eGFR = 175 \times (Creatinine)^{-1.154} \times (Age)^{-0.203} \times (Gender) \times (Race)$$

where:

eGFR = estimated GFR; calculated in mL/minute per 1.73 m^2

Creatinine is input in mg/dL

Age is input in years

Gender: Females: Gender = 0.742; Males: Gender = 1

Race: Black: Race = 1.212; White or other: Race = 1

Method 2: MDRD Extended equation:

$$eGFR = 161.5 \times (Creatinine)^{-0.999} \times (Age)^{-0.176} \times (SUN)^{-0.170} \times (Albumin)^{0.318} \times (Gender) \times (Race)$$

where:

eGFR = estimated GFR; calculated in mL/minute per 1.73 m^2

Creatinine is input in mg/dL

Age is input in years

SUN = Serum Urea Nitrogen; input in mg/dL

Albumin = Serum Albumin; input in g/dL

Gender: Females: Gender = 0.762; Males: Gender = 1

Race: Black: Race = 1.18; White or other: Race = 1

Method 3: CKD-EPI equation[b]:

$$eGFR = 141 \times (Creatinine/k)^{Exp} \times (0.993)^{Age} \times (Gender) \times (Race)$$

where:

eGFR = estimated GFR; calculated in mL/minute per 1.73 m^2

(Creatinine/k):

Creatinine is input in mg/dL

k: Females: k = 0.7; Males: k = 0.9

Exp:

When (Creatinine/k) is ≤1: Females: Exp = -0.329; Males: Exp = -0.411

When (Creatinine/k) is >1: Exp = -1.209

Age is input in years

Gender: Females: Gender = 1.018; Males: Gender = 1

Race: Black: Race = 1.159; White or other: Race = 1

◀ **Alkaline picrate-based (Jaffe) methods**

Note: These equations have not been updated for use with serum creatinine methods traceable to IDMS. Use with IDMS-traceable serum creatinine methods may overestimate renal function; use with caution.

Method 1: MDRD equation:

$$eGFR = 186 \times (Creatinine)^{-1.154} \times (Age)^{-0.203} \times (Gender) \times (Race)$$

where:

eGFR = estimated GFR; calculated in mL/minute per 1.73 m^2

Creatinine is input in mg/dL

Age is input in years

Gender: Females: Gender = 0.742; Males: Gender = 1

Race: Black: Race = 1.212; White or other: Race = 1

Method 2: MDRD Extended equation:

$$eGFR = 170 \times (Creatinine)^{-0.999} \times (Age)^{-0.176} \times (SUN)^{-0.170} \times (Albumin)^{0.318} \times (Gender) \times (Race)$$

where:

eGFR = estimated GFR; calculated in mL/minute per 1.73 m^2

Creatinine is input in mg/dL

Age is input in years

SUN = Serum Urea Nitrogen; input in mg/dL

Albumin = Serum Albumin; input in g/dL

Gender: Females: Gender = 0.762; Males: Gender = 1

Race: Black: Race = 1.18; White or other: Race = 1

Method 3: Cockcroft-Gault equation[c]

Males: $CrCl = [(140 - Age) \times Weight] / (72 \times Creatinine)$

Females: $CrCl = \{[(140 - Age) \times Weight] / (72 \times Creatinine)\} \times 0.85$

where:

CrCl = creatinine clearance; calculated in mL/minute

Age is input in years

Weight is input in kg

Creatinine is input in mg/dL

Method 4: Jelliffe equation

Males: $CrCl = \{98 - [0.8 \times (Age - 20)]\} / (Creatinine)$

Females: CrCl = Use above equation, then multiply result by 0.9

where:

CrCl = creatinine clearance; calculated in mL/minute per 1.73 m^2

Age is input in years

Creatinine is input in mg/dL

FOOTNOTES

[a]Preferred equation for CKD staging National Kidney Disease Education Program

[b]Recommended equation for the reporting of eGFR by the NKD-KDIGO guidelines

[c]Equation typically used for adjusting medication doses

REFERENCES

Cockcroft DW, Gault MH. Prediction of creatinine clearance from serum creatinine. *Nephron*. 1976;16(1):31-41.

Dowling TC, Matzke GR, Murphy JE, Burckart GJ. Evaluation of renal drug dosing: prescribing information and clinical pharmacist approaches. *Pharmacotherapy*. 2010;30(8):776-786.

Hermsen ED, Maiefski M, Florescu MC, Qiu F, Rupp ME. Comparison of the modification of diet in renal disease and Cockcroft-Gault equations for dosing antimicrobials. *Pharmacotherapy*. 2009;29(6):649-655.

Jelliffe RW. Letter: creatinine clearance: bedside estimate. *Ann Intern Med*. 1973;79(4):604-605.

Kidney disease: improving global outcomes (KDIGO) CKD work group. KDIGO 2012 clinical practice guidelines for the evaluation and management of chronic kidney disease. *Kidney Inter*. 2013;3:1-150. http://www.kdigo.org/clinical_practice_guidelines/pdf/CKD/KDIGO_2012_CKD_GL.pdf

Levey AS, Bosch JP, Lewis JB, Greene T, Rogers N, Roth D. A more accurate method to estimate glomerular filtration rate from serum creatinine: a new prediction equation. Modification of diet in renal disease study group. *Ann Intern Med*. 1999;16;130(6):461-470.

Levey AS, Coresh J, Greene T, et al. Using standardized serum creatinine values in the modification of diet in renal disease study equation for estimating glomerular filtration rate. *Ann Intern Med*. 2006;145(4):247-254.

Levey AS, Stevens LA, Schmid CH, et al. A new equation to estimate glomerular filtration rate. *Ann Intern Med*. 2009;150(9):604-612.

National Kidney Disease Education Program. GFR calculators. http://www.nkdep.nih.gov/professionals/gfr_calculators. Accessed April 24, 2013.

Stevens LA, Coresh J, Greene T, Levey AS. Assessing kidney function – measured and estimated glomerular filtration rate. *N Engl J Med*. 2006;354(23):2473-2483.

RENAL FUNCTION ESTIMATION IN PEDIATRIC PATIENTS

Evaluation of a patient's renal function often includes the use of equations to estimate glomerular filtration rate (GFR) (eg, estimated GFR [eGFR] creatinine clearance [CrCl]) using an endogenous filtration marker (eg, serum creatinine) and other patient variables. For example, the Schwartz equation estimates renal function by calculating eGFR and is typically used to steer medication dosing or categorize chronic kidney disease (CKD) staging and monitor progression. The rate of creatinine clearance does not always accurately represent GFR; creatinine may be cleared by other renal mechanisms in addition to glomerular filtration and serum creatinine concentrations may be affected by nonrenal factors (eg, age, gender, race, body habitus, illness, diet). In addition, these equations were developed based on studies in limited populations and may either over- or underestimate the renal function of a specific patient.

Nevertheless, most clinicians use an eGFR or CrCl as an indicator of renal function in pediatric patients for the purposes of adjusting medication doses. These equations should be used in the clinical context of patient-specific factors noted during the physical exam/work-up. **Decisions regarding drug therapy and doses must be made on clinical judgment.**

RENAL FUNCTION ESTIMATION EQUATIONS

Commonly used equations to estimate renal function utilizing the endogenous filtration marker serum creatinine include the Schwartz and Traub-Johnson equations. Both equations were originally developed using a serum creatinine assay measured by the alkaline picrate-based (Jaffe) method. Many substances, including proteins, can interfere with the accuracy of this assay and overestimate serum creatinine concentration. The National Kidney Foundation and The National Kidney Disease Education Program advocated for a universal creatinine assay, in order to ensure an accurate estimate of GFR in patients. As a result, a more specific enzymatic assay with an isotope dilution mass spectrometry (IDMS)-traceable international standard was developed. Compared to the older methods, IDMS-traceable assays may report lower serum creatinine values and may, therefore, overestimate renal function when used in the original equations. An updated Schwartz equation (eg, Bedside Schwartz) based on serum creatinine measured by the IDMS-traceable method has been proposed for pediatrics (Schwartz 2009); the Traub-Johnson equation has not been re-expressed. The original Schwartz and Traub-Johnson equations may overestimate renal function when used with a serum creatinine measured by the IDMS-traceable method. However, at this point, all laboratories should be using creatinine methods calibrated to be IDMS traceable.

The following factors may contribute to an inaccurate estimation of renal function (Stevens 2006):

- Increased creatinine generation (may underestimate renal function):
    - Black patients
    - Muscular body habitus
    - Ingestion of cooked meats

- Decreased creatinine generation (may overestimate renal function):

    - Increased age

    - Female patients

    - Asian patients

    - Amputees

    - Malnutrition, inflammation, or deconditioning (eg, cancer, severe cardiovascular disease, hospitalized patients)

    - Neuromuscular disease

    - Vegetarian diet

- Rapidly changing serum creatinine (either up or down):

    - In patients with rapidly rising serum creatinines (ie, increasing by >0.5 to 0.7 mg/dL/day), it is best to assume that the patient's renal function is severely impaired

Use extreme caution when estimating renal function in the following patient populations:

- Low body weight (actual body weight < ideal body weight)

- Liver transplant

- Prematurity (especially very low birth weight)

- Dehydration

- Recent kidney transplantation (serum creatinine values may decrease rapidly and can lead to renal function underestimation; conversely, delayed graft function may be present)

IDMS-traceable method: Bedside Schwartz[a]

Note: This equation is for use in ages 1 to 16 years.

eGFR = (0.413 X Height) / Creatinine

where:

eGFR = estimated GFR; calculated in mL/minute per 1.73 m^2

Height (length) is input in cm

Creatinine = Sr_{Cr} input in mg/dL

Alkaline picrate-based (Jaffe) methods

Note: These equations have not been updated for use with serum creatinine methods traceable to IDMS. Use with IDMS-traceable serum creatinine methods may overestimate renal function; use with caution.

Method 1: Schwartz equation

Note: This equation may not provide an accurate estimation of creatinine clearance for infants <6 months of age or for patients with severe starvation or muscle wasting.

eGFR = (k X Height) / Creatinine

where:

eGFR = estimated GFR; calculated in mL/minute per 1.73 m^2

Height (length) is input in cm

k = constant of proportionality that is age-specific

<1 year preterm: 0.33

<1 year full-term: 0.45

1 to 12 years: 0.55

>12 years female: 0.55

>12 years male: 0.7

Creatinine is input in mg/dL

Method 2: Traub-Johnson equation

Note: This equation is for use in ages 1 to 18 years.

CrCl = (0.48 X Height) / Creatinine

where:

CrCl = estimated creatinine clearance; calculated in mL/minute per 1.73 m^2

Height (length) is input in cm

Creatinine = Sr_{Cr} input in mg/dL

FOOTNOTES

[a]National Kidney Disease Education Program preferred equation

REFERENCES

Dowling TC, Matzke GR, Murphy JE, Burckart GJ. Evaluation of renal drug dosing: prescribing information and clinical pharmacist approaches. *Pharmacotherapy.* 2010;30(8):776-786.

Myers GL, Miller WG, Coresh J, et al. Recommendations for improving serum creatinine measurement: a report from the laboratory working group of the National Kidney Disease Education Program. *Clin Chem.* 2006;52(1):5-18.

National Kidney Disease Education Program. GFR calculators. http://www.nkdep.nih.gov/profes-sionals/gfr_calculators. Accessed April 24, 2013.

Pottel H, Mottaghy FM, Zaman Z, Martens F. On the relationship between glomerular filtration rate and serum creatinine in children. *Pediatr Nephrol.* 2010;25(5):927-934.

Schwartz GJ, Brion LP, Spitzer A. The use of plasma creatinine concentration for estimating glomerular filtration rate in infants, children, and adolescents. *Pediatr Clin North Am.* 1987;34 (3):571-590.

Schwartz GJ, Haycock GB, Edelmann CM Jr, Spitzer A. A simple estimate of glomerular filtration rate in children derived from body length and plasma creatinine. *Pediatrics.* 1976;58(2):259-263.

Schwartz GJ, Muñoz A, Schneider MF, et al. New equations to estimate GFR in children with CKD. *J Am Soc Nephrol.* 2009;20(3):629-637.

Staples A, LeBlond R, Watkins S, Wong C, Brandt J. Validation of the revised Schwartz estimating equation in a predominantly non-CKD population. *Pediatr Nephrol.* 2010;25(11):2321-2326.

Stevens LA, Coresh J, Greene T, Levey AS. Assessing kidney function – measured and estimated glomerular filtration rate. *N Engl J Med.* 2006;354(23):2473-2483.

Traub SL, Johnson CE. Comparison of methods of estimating creatinine clearance in children. *Am J Hosp Pharm.* 1980;37(2):195-201.

CORTICOSTEROIDS SYSTEMIC EQUIVALENCIES

Glucocorticoid	Approximate Equivalent Dose (mg)	Routes of Administration	Relative Anti-inflammatory Potency	Relative Mineralocorticoid Potency	Protein Binding (%)	Half-life Plasma (minutes)
Short-Acting						
Cortisone	25	PO, IM	0.8	0.8	90	30
Hydrocortisone	20	IM, IV	1	1	90	90
Intermediate-Acting						
MethylPREDNISolone[a]	4	PO, IM, IV	5	0	—	180
PrednisoLONE	5	PO, IM, IV, intra-articular, intradermal, soft tissue injection	4	0.8	90 to 95	200
PredniSONE	5	PO	4	0.8	<50	120 to 180
Triamcinolone[a]	4	IM, intra-articular, intradermal, intrasynovial, soft tissue injection	5	0	—	300
Long-Acting						
Betamethasone	0.75	PO, IM, intra-articular, intradermal, intrasynovial, soft tissue injection	25	0	64	100 to 300
Dexamethasone	0.75	PO, IM, IV, intra-articular, intradermal, soft tissue injection	25 to 30	0	—	100 to 300
Mineralocorticoids						
Fludrocortisone	—	PO	10	125	42	200

[a]May contain propylene glycol as an excipient in injectable forms
Asare K. Diagnosis and treatment of adrenal insufficiency in the critically ill patient. *Pharmacotherapy.* 2007;27(11):1512-1528.
Frey BM, Frey FJ. Clinical pharmacokinetics of prednisone and prednisolone. *Clin Pharmacokinet.* 1990;19(2):126-146.

IMMUNE GLOBULIN PRODUCT COMPARISON

Brand Name	Concentration	pH	Initial Rate IV	Initial Rate SubQ[a]	Max Rate IV[b]	Max Rate SubQ[a]	IgA Content (mcg/mL)	Osmolarity/ Osmolality (mOsmol/kg)[a]	Comments
Bivigam	10%	4 to 4.6	0.3 mL/kg/hour	–	3.6 mL/kg/hour	–	≤200	Not available	Contains polysorbate 80
Carimune NF[c]	3%	6.4 to 6.8	1 mL/kg/hour	–	6 mL/kg/hour	–	Trace[d]	192 to 498[e]	Contains sucrose
	12%		0.24 mL/kg/hour		1.5 mL/kg/hour			768 to 1,074[e]	
Flebogamma DIF	5%	5 to 6	0.6 mL/kg/hour	–	6 mL/kg/hour	–	<50	240 to 370	
	10%		0.6 mL/kg/hour		4.8 mL/kg/hour		<100		
GamaSTAN S/D	15% to 18%	6.4 to 7.2	–	–	–	–	Not available	Not available	For IM use
Gammagard S/D	5%	6.4 to 7.2	0.5 mL/kg/hour	–	4 mL/kg/hour	–	≤1[f]	636	Contains polysorbate 80
	10%		0.5 mL/kg/hour		8 mL/kg/hour		≤2[f]	1,250	
Gammagard Liquid	10%	4.6 to 5.1	0.5 mL/kg/hour	<40 kg: 15 mL/hour/site with a maximum of 8 sites; ≥40 kg: 20 mL/hour/site with a maximum of 8 sites	5 mL/kg/hour; 5.4 mL/kg/hour (MMN only)	<40 kg: 20 mL/hour/site with a maximum of 8 sites; rate: 160 mL/hour; ≥40 kg: 30 mL/hour/site with a maximum of 8 sites; rate: 240 mL/hour	37	240 to 300	
Gammaked	10%	4 to 4.5	0.6 mL/kg/hour; 1.2 mL/kg/hour (CIDP only)	20 mL/hour/site with a maximum of 8 sites	4.8 mL/kg/hour	Not determined	46	258	

(continued)

Brand Name	Concentration	pH	Initial Rate		Max Rate		IgA Content (mcg/mL)	Osmolarity/ Osmolality (mOsmol/kg)	Comments
			IV	SubQ[a]	IV[b]	SubQ[a]			
Gammaplex	5%	4.8 to 5	0.6 mL/kg/ hour	–	4.8 mL/kg/ hour	–	<10	420 to 500	Contains polysorbate 80
Gamunex-C	10%	4 to 4.5	0.6 mL/kg/ hour 1.2 mL/kg/ hour (CIDP only)	20 mL/hour/site with a maximum of 8 sites	4.8 mL/kg/ hour	Not determined	46	258	
Hizentra	20%	4.6 to 5.2	–	15 mL/hour/site with a maximum of 4 sites	–	Up to 25 mL/hour/ site with a maximum of 4 sites; maximum **total** rate: 50 mL/hour	≤50	380	Contains L-proline and polysorbate 80

IMMUNE GLOBULIN PRODUCT COMPARISON

(continued)

Brand Name	Concentration	pH	Initial Rate IV	Initial Rate SubQ[a]	Max Rate IV[b]	Max Rate SubQ[a]	IgA Content (mcg/mL)	Osmolarity/Osmolality (mOsmol/kg)	Comments
HyQvia	10%	4.6 to 5.1	—	*First 2 infusions:* <40 kg: 5 mL/hour for 5 to 15 minutes; 10 mL/hour for 5 to 15 minutes; 20 mL/hour for 5 to 15 minutes; 40 mL/hour for 5 to 15 minutes; then 80 mL/hour for remainder of infusion ≥40 kg: 10 mL/hour for 5 to 15 minutes; 30 mL/hour for 5 to 15 minutes; 60 mL/hour for 5 to 15 minutes; 120 mL/hour for 5 to 15 minutes; then 240 mL/hour for remainder of infusion *Next 2 or 3 infusions:* <40 kg: 10 mL/hour for 5 to 15 minutes; 20 mL/hour for 5 to 15 minutes; 40 mL/hour for 5 to 15 minutes; 80 mL/hour for 5 to 15 minutes; then 160 mL/hour for remainder of infusion ≥40 kg: 10 mL/hour for 5 to 15 minutes; 30 mL/hour for 5 to 15 minutes; 120 mL/hour for 5 to 15 minutes; 240 mL/hour for 5 to 15 minutes; then 300 mL/hour for remainder of infusion	—	<40 kg: 160 mL/hour ≥40 kg: 300 mL/hour	37	240 to 300	Supplied with hyaluronidase (human recombinant)
Octagam	5%	5.1 to 6	0.6 mL/kg/hour	—	4 mL/kg/hour	—	≤200	310 to 380	Contains maltose

2420

(continued)

Brand Name	Concentration	pH	Initial Rate		Max Rate		IgA Content (mcg/mL)	Osmolarity/ Osmolality (mOsmol/kg)	Comments
			IV	SubQ[a]	IV[b]	SubQ[a]			
Octagam	10%	4.5 to 5	0.6 mL/kg/ hour	–	7.2 mL/kg/ hour	–	106	310 to 380	Sucrose-free
Privigen	10%	4.6 to 5	0.3 mL/kg/ hour	–	2.4 mL/kg/ hour (ITP) 4.8 mL/kg/ hour	–	≤25	240 to 440	Contains L-proline

CIDP = chronic inflammatory demyelinating polyneuropathy, ITP = immune thrombocytopenia (formerly known as idiopathic thrombocytopenic purpura), MMN = multifocal motor neuropathy

[a] Subcutaneous administration **only** for the treatment of primary humoral immunodeficiency (PI)

[b] Lower infusion rates should be used in patients at risk for renal dysfunction or thrombotic complications; see specific product information for details.

[c] Other concentrations may be prepared; see product information for additional details.

[d] Per product information; other sources list IgA content as 1,000 to 2,000 mcg/mL for 6% solution (Siegel J. Immune globulins: therapeutic, pharmaceutical, cost, and administration considerations. *Pharm Prac News*. 2013).

[e] Osmolarity depends on concentration and diluent used; see product information for details.

[f] Data presented is based on the maximum concentration that can be prepared. The 5% solution with IgA content <2.2 mcg/mL has been discontinued. The lower IgA product (ie, IgA <1 mcg/mL for the 5% prepared solution) is available by special request; contact manufacturer or see specific product information for details.

ORAL ANTICOAGULANT COMPARISON CHART

Medication	Mechanism of Action	Metabolism	Monitoring Parameters	Pharmacotherapy Pearls	Reversal Strategies[a]	Preoperative/Preprocedure Management (General Guide)
Warfarin	Inhibits formation of vitamin K-dependent clotting factors II, VII, IX, X, and proteins C and S	CYP2C9 CYP1A2 CYP3A4 CYP2C19	PT/INR (individualized; depends on INR stability)	CYP1A2, 3A4, 2C9, and 2C19 drug interactions and vitamin K-containing food interactions Full therapeutic effect usually seen within 5 to 7 days Half-life is ~40 hours	Vitamin K (route and dose will depend on clinical situation and INR) For major bleeding at any INR): Consider PCC with vitamin K ± FFP	Hold at least 5 days before surgery, depending on urgency of surgery/procedure, may administer low-dose IV or oral vitamin K Minor dental and minor dermatological procedures or cataract surgery: Continue warfarin (with hemostatic agent [dental] or local hemostasis [dermatological]); may also discontinue use 2 to 3 days prior to dental procedures. Patients with prior stroke undergoing dental procedures should routinely continue warfarin.
Dabigatran (Pradaxa)	Directly inhibits thrombin	Hepatic glucuronidation P-gp substrate	Routine lab monitoring not required; aPTT, ECT (if available), TT (most sensitive) may be used to detect presence of dabigatran Renal function	Compliance issues (BID dosing) Specific conversions to/from warfarin, parenteral anticoagulants Renal dosing adjustment required; per ACCP, contraindicated with CrCl ≤30 mL/minute Use with caution in patients ≥80 years of age Dose reduction or avoidance required if used with dronedarone, ketoconazole, P-gp inhibitors P-gp drug interactions Half-life is 12 to 17 hours; considerably prolonged with severe renal impairment	IdaruCIZUmab Dabigatran is ~60% dialyzable Activated charcoal may be used if ingestion occurred <2 hours prior to presentation	CrCl ≥50 mL/minute: Hold 1 to 2 days before surgery CrCl <50 mL/minute: Hold 3 to 5 days before surgery May consider holding for >5 days in patients undergoing major surgery, spinal puncture, or insertion of a spinal or epidural catheter or port

(continued)

Medication	Mechanism of Action	Metabolism	Monitoring Parameters	Pharmacotherapy Pearls	Reversal Strategies[a]	Preoperative/Preprocedure Management (General Guide)
Apixaban (Eliquis)	Directly inhibits factor Xa	CYP3A4 P-gp substrate	Routine lab monitoring not required; PT, INR, and aPTT may be used to detect presence of apixaban	Compliance issues (BID dosing)	No specific antidote; for major bleeding, may consider PCC, activated PCC (ie, FEIBA NF), or recombinant factor VIIa	Hold at least 24 to 48 hours, depending on risk or location of bleeding, before elective surgery or invasive procedures.
				Specific conversions to/from warfarin, parenteral anticoagulants		
				Renal dosing adjustment required (NVAF); the AHA/ASA recommends to avoid use with CrCl <25 mL/minute	Apixaban is **not** dialyzable	
				Not recommended in patients with severe liver impairment	Activated charcoal may be used if ingestion occurred within 2 to 5 hours of presentation	
				CYP3A4 and P-gp drug interactions		
				Half-life is ~8 to 15 hours; slightly prolonged with renal impairment		
Betrixaban (Bevyxxa)	Directly inhibits factor Xa	Minimal CYP-independent hydrolysis P-gp substrate	Routine lab monitoring not required Renal function	Renal dosing adjustment required	No specific antidote	Caution: Half-life is 19 to 27 hours; anticoagulant effect expected to persist for ≥72 hours.
				P-gp drug interactions; dose reduction required if used with P-gp inhibitors		

(continued)

Medication	Mechanism of Action	Metabolism	Monitoring Parameters	Pharmacotherapy Pearls	Reversal Strategies[a]	Preoperative/Preprocedure Management (General Guide)
Edoxaban (Savaysa)	Directly inhibits factor Xa	CYP3A4 (minor) Hydrolysis (minimal) P-gp substrate	Routine lab monitoring not required	Specific conversions to/from warfarin, parenteral anticoagulants DVT/PE: Dose reduction necessary for patients <60 kg, concomitant P-gp inhibitor, or if CrCl 15 to 50 mL/minute. Not recommended if CrCl <15 mL/minute NVAF: **Do not use if CrCl >95 mL/minute.** Dose reduction necessary if CrCl 15 to 50 mL/minute. Not recommended if CrCl <15 mL/minute	No specific antidote Edoxaban is **not** dialyzable	Discontinue at least 24 hours prior to elective surgery or invasive procedures
Rivaroxaban (Xarelto)	Directly inhibits factor Xa	CYP3A4 CYP3A5 CYP2J2 P-gp substrate	Routine lab monitoring not required; may use PTT to detect presence of rivaroxaban Renal and hepatic function	Administer doses ≥15 mg/day with food Dosing frequency depends on indication Specific conversions to/from warfarin, parenteral anticoagulants Renal dosing adjustment required Avoid in moderate or severe hepatic impairment CYP3A4 and P-gp drug interactions Half-life is 5 to 9 hours; slightly prolonged with renal impairment	No specific antidote; for major bleeding, may consider PCC, activated PCC (ie, FEIBA NF), or recombinant factor VIIa[b] Rivaroxaban is **not** dialyzable	Hold at least 24 hours before surgery; longer duration of treatment cessation may be necessary based on individual patient situation and physician clinical judgment

Abbreviations: ACCP = American College of Chest Physicians, AHA/ASA = American Heart Association/American Stroke Association, aPTT = activated partial thromboplastin time, BID = twice daily, DVT = deep venous thrombosis, ECT = ecarin clotting time, FFP = fresh frozen plasma, INR = international normalized ratio, NVAF = nonvalvular atrial fibrillation, PCC = prothrombin complex concentrate, PE = pulmonary embolism, P-gp = P-glycoprotein, PT = prothrombin time, TT = thrombin time.

Note: Recommendations listed reflect only the US labeling or US clinical practice guidelines.

[a] Management of anticoagulant-associated bleeding requires careful consideration of the indication for anticoagulant therapy, and bleeding extent (eg, epistaxis vs intracranial hemorrhage); minor bleeding may only require local hemostasis.

[b] The evidence in support of these reversal strategies is limited; an exception to this may be the use of a 4-factor PCC for rivaroxaban reversal. The only available 4-factor PCC currently in the US is Kcentra. Other 4-factor PCCs **not** available in the US include Beriplex P/N, Cofact, and Octaplex. Betulin VH and Profilnine SD **do not** contain adequate levels of factor VII and are considered 3-factor PCCs. **See References on next page.**

Oral Anticoagulant comparison chart *(continued)*

References:

Armstrong MJ, Gronseth G, Anderson DC, et al. Summary of evidence-based guideline: periprocedural management of antithrombotic medications in patients with ischemic cerebrovascular disease: report of the Guideline Development Subcommittee of the American Academy of Neurology. *Neurology.* 2013;80 (22):2065-2069.

Furie KL, Goldstein LB, Albers GW, et al. Oral antithrombotic agents for the prevention of stroke in nonvalvular atrial fibrillation: a science advisory for health care professionals from the American Heart Association/American Stroke Association. *Stroke.* 2012;43(12):3442-3453.

Guyatt GH, Akl EA, Crowther M, et al. Executive summary: antithrombotic therapy and prevention of thrombosis, 9th ed: American College of Chest Physicians evidence-based clinical practice guidelines. *Chest* 2012;141(2 Suppl):7S-47S.

Kaatz S, Kouides PA, Garcia DA, et al Guidance on the emergent reversal of oral thrombin and factor Xa inhibitors. *Am J Hematol.* 2012;87(Suppl 1):S141-S145.

Levi M, Eerenberg E, Kamphuisen PW. Bleeding risk and reversal strategies for old and new anticoagulants and antiplatelet agents. *J Thromb Haemost.* 2011;9(9):1705-1712.

Poulsen BK, Grove EL, Husted SE. New oral anticoagulants: a review of the literature with particular emphasis on patients with impaired renal function. *Drugs.* 2012;72(13):1739-1753.

Wolzt M, Levi M, Sarich TC, et al. Effect of recombinant factor VIIa on melagatran-induced inhibition of thrombin generation and platelet activation in healthy volunteers. *Thromb Haemost.* 2004;5(6):1090-1096.

ORAL ANTIPLATELET COMPARISON CHART

Medication	Mechanism of Action	Reversible Platelet Inhibition	Prodrug	Metabolism	Pharmacotherapy Pearls	Reversal Strategies[a]	Preoperative/Preprocedure Management (General Guide)
Aspirin	Inhibits cyclooxygenase-1 and 2	No		CYP2C9	Chronic NSAID use can compromise antiplatelet effects Monitor for GI ulceration	No specific antidote Consider platelet transfusion ± DDAVP Normal platelet function returns within 7 to 10 days after discontinuation	Hold 7 to 10 days before surgery May be continued through surgery for CABG or noncardiac surgery in patients with moderate to high cardiac risk Minor dental or dermatological procedures or cataract surgery: Continue through procedure. AAN recommends continuation when undergoing any dental procedure for patients taking aspirin for ischemic stroke prevention.
Cilostazol (Pletal)	Inhibits platelet phosphodiesterase III	Yes	No	CYP3A4 CYP2C19 CYP1A2 CYP2D6	Administer before or 2 hours after meals Contraindicated in patients with heart failure of any severity CYP3A4 and 2C19 drug interactions	No specific antidote Normal platelet function returns within 4 days after discontinuation	Hold 2 to 3 days before surgery
Clopidogrel (Plavix)	Inhibits P2Y$_{12}$ component of ADP receptors	No	Yes	CYP2C19 CYP3A4	CYP2C19 inhibitors may reduce concentrations of active metabolite CYP2C19 polymorphisms may affect clopidogrel efficacy	No specific antidote Consider platelet transfusion ± DDAVP Normal platelet function returns within 7 to 10 days after discontinuation	Hold 5 to 10 days before surgery[b]

(continued)

Medication	Mechanism of Action	Reversible Platelet Inhibition	Prodrug	Metabolism	Pharmacotherapy Pearls	Reversal Strategies[a]	Preoperative/Preprocedure Management (General Guide)
Prasugrel (Effient)	Inhibits P2Y$_{12}$ component of ADP receptors	No	Yes	CYP3A4 CYP2B6	Reduce maintenance dose to 5 mg in patients <60 kg Contraindicated in patients with history of stroke, TIA Not recommended in patients ≥75 years of age	No specific antidote Consider platelet transfusion ± DDAVP Normal platelet function returns within 5 to 9 days after discontinuation	Hold 5 to 7 days before surgery[b]
Ticagrelor (Brilinta)	Inhibits P2Y$_{12}$ component of ADP receptors	Yes	No	CYP3A4 CYP3A5	Used in combination with aspirin; daily maintenance aspirin dose should not exceed 81 mg CYP3A4 drug interactions BID dosing Monitor closely for dyspnea, bradyarrhythmia (including ventricular pauses)	No specific antidote Consider aminocaproic acid, tranexamic acid, recombinant factor VIIa Normal platelet function returns within 3 to 5 days after discontinuation	Hold at least 5 days before surgery[b]

(continued)

Medication	Mechanism of Action	Reversible Platelet Inhibition	Prodrug	Metabolism	Pharmacotherapy Pearls	Reversal Strategies[a]	Preoperative/Preprocedure Management (General Guide)
Ticlopidine	Inhibits $P2Y_{12}$ component of ADP receptors	No	Yes	CYP3A4	Black Box warning on hematologic toxicities (aplastic anemia, TTP) Frequent CBC monitoring required BID dosing	No specific antidote Consider platelet transfusion ± DDAVP Normal platelet function returns within 5 to 10 days after discontinuation	Hold 10 to 14 days before surgery
Vorapaxar	Inhibits PAR-1	Yes[c]	No	CYP3A4 CYP2J2	Use in combination with aspirin and/or clopidogrel Contraindicated in patients with history of stroke, TIA, or ICH Extremely long effective half-life of 3 to 5 days	No specific antidote Significant inhibition of platelet aggregation remains 4 weeks after discontinuation	No recommendation can be made

[a]Management of antiplatelet-associated bleeding requires careful consideration of the indication for antiplatelet therapy and bleeding extent (eg, epistaxis vs intracranial hemorrhage); minor bleeding may only require local hemostasis.

[b]When urgent CABG is necessary, the ACCF/AHA CABG guidelines recommend discontinuation for at least 24 hours prior to surgery (Hillis 2011).

[c]Due to the very long half-life, vorapaxar is effectively irreversible.

Armstrong MJ, Gronseth G, Anderson DC, et al. Summary of evidence-based guideline: periprocedural management of antithrombotic medications in patients with ischemic cerebrovascular disease: report of the Guideline Development Subcommittee of the American Academy of Neurology. *Neurology.* 2013;80(22):2065-2069.

Hillis LD, Smith PK, Anderson JL, et al. 2011 ACCF/AHA guideline for coronary artery bypass graft surgery: executive summary: a report of the American College of Cardiology Foundation/American Heart Association task force on practice guidelines. *Circulation.* 2011;124(23):2610-2642.

Levi M, Eerenberg E, Kamphuisen PW. Bleeding risk and reversal strategies for old and new anticoagulants and antiplatelet agents. *J Thromb Haemost.* 2011;9(9):1705-1712.

Patrono C, Andreotti F, Arnesen H, et al. Antiplatelet agents for the treatment and prevention of atherothrombosis. *Eur Heart J.* 2011;32(23):2922-2932.

REFERENCE VALUES FOR ADULTS

CHEMISTRY

Test	Values	Remarks
Serum/Plasma		
Acetone	Negative	
Albumin	3.2 to 5 g/dL	
Alcohol, ethyl	Negative	
Aldolase	1.2 to 7.6 IU/L	
Ammonia	20 to 70 mcg/dL	Specimen to be placed on ice as soon as collected.
Amylase	30 to 110 units/L	
Bilirubin, direct	0 to 0.3 mg/dL	
Bilirubin, total	0.1 to 1.2 mg/dL	
Calcium	8.6 to 10.3 mg/dL	
Calcium, ionized	2.24 to 2.46 mEq/L	
Chloride	95 to 108 mEq/L	
Cholesterol, total	≤200 mg/dL	Fasted blood required – normal value affected by dietary habits. This reference range is for a general adult population.
HDL cholesterol	40 to 60 mg/dL	Fasted blood required – normal value affected by dietary habits
LDL cholesterol	<160 mg/dL	If triglyceride is >400 mg/dL, LDL cannot be calculated accurately (Friedewald equation). Target LDL-C depends on patient's risk factors.
CO_2	23 to 30 mEq/L	
Creatine kinase (CK) isoenzymes		
CK-BB	0%	
CK-MB (cardiac)	0% to 3.9%	
CK-MM (muscle)	96% to 100%	
CK-MB levels must be both ≥4% and 10 IU/L to meet diagnostic criteria for CK-MB positive result consistent with myocardial injury.		
Creatine phosphokinase (CPK)	8 to 150 IU/L	
Creatinine	0.5 to 1.4 mg/dL	
Ferritin	13 to 300 ng/mL	
Folate	3.6 to 20 ng/dL	
GGT (gamma-glutamyltranspeptidase)		
male	11 to 63 IU/L	
female	8 to 35 IU/L	
GLDH	To be determined	
Glucose (preprandial)	<115 mg/dL	Goals different for diabetics

CHEMISTRY (continued)

Test	Values	Remarks
Glucose, fasting	60 to 110 mg/dL	Goals different for diabetics
Glucose, nonfasting (2 hours postprandial)	<120 mg/dL	Goals different for diabetics
Hemoglobin A_{1c}	<8	
Hemoglobin, plasma free	<2.5 mg per 100 mL	
Hemoglobin, total glycosolated (HbA_1)	4% to 8%	
Iron	65 to 150 mcg/dL	
Iron binding capacity, total (TIBC)	250 to 420 mcg/dL	
Lactic acid	0.7 to 2.1 mEq/L	Specimen to be kept on ice and sent to lab as soon as possible
Lactate dehydrogenase (LDH)	56 to 194 IU/L	
Lactate dehydrogenase (LDH) isoenzymes		
LD_1	20% to 34%	
LD_2	29% to 41%	
LD_3	15% to 25%	
LD_4	1% to 12%	
LD_5	1% to 15%	

Flipped LD_1/LD_2 ratios (>1 may be consistent with myocardial injury) particularly when considered in combination with a recent CK-MB positive result.

Test	Values	Remarks
Lipase	23 to 208 units/L	
Magnesium	1.6 to 2.5 mg/dL	Increased by slight hemolysis
Osmolality	289 to 308 mOsm/kg	
Phosphatase, alkaline		
Adults 25 to 60 years	33 to 131 IU/L	
Adults ≥61 years	51 to 153 IU/L	
Infancts to adolescents	Values range up to 3 to 5 times higher than adults	
Phosphate, inorganic	2.8 to 4.2 mg/dL	
Potassium	3.5 to 5.2 mEq/L	Increased by slight hemolysis
Prealbumin	>15 mg/dL	
Protein, total	6.5 to 7.9 g/dL	
AST	<35 IU/L (20 to 48)	
ALT (10 to 35)	<35 IU/L	
Sodium	134 to 149 mEq/L	
Thyroid stimulating hormone (TSH)		
Adults ≤20 years	0.7 to 6.4 milliunits/L	
21 to 54 years	0.4 to 4.2 milliunits/L	
55 to 87 years	0.5 to 8.9 milliunits/L	
Transferrin	>200 mg/dL	
Triglycerides	45 to 155 mg/dL	Fasted blood required

CHEMISTRY (continued)

Test	Values	Remarks
Troponin I	<1.5 ng/mL	
Urea nitrogen (BUN)	7 to 20 mg/dL	
Uric acid		
Male	2 to 8 mg/dL	
Female	2 to 7.5 mg/dL	
Cerebrospinal Fluid		
Glucose	50 to 70 mg/dL	
Protein	15 to 45 mg/dL	CSF obtained by lumbar puncture

Note: Bloody specimen gives erroneously high value due to contamination with blood proteins

Urine
(24-hour specimen is required for all these tests unless specified)

Test	Values	Remarks
Amylase	32 to 641 units/L	The value is in units/L and **not** calculated for total volume.
Amylase, fluid (random samples)		Interpretation of value left for physician, depends on the nature of fluid
Calcium	Depends upon dietary intake	
Creatine		
Male	150 mg per 24 hours	Higher value on children and during pregnancy
Female	250 mg per 24 hours	
Creatinine	1,000 to 2,000 mg per 24 hours	
Creatinine clearance (endogenous)		
Male	85 to 125 mL/minute	A blood sample must accompany urine specimen.
Female	75 to 115 mL/minute	
Glucose	1 g per 24 hours	
5-hydroxyindoleacetic acid	2 to 8 mg per 24 hours	
Iron	0.15 mg per 24 hours	Acid washed container required
Magnesium	146 to 209 mg per 24 hours	
Osmolality	500 to 800 mOsm/kg	With normal fluid intake
Oxalate	10 to 40 mg per 24 hours	
Phosphate	400 to 1,300 mg per 24 hours	
Potassium	25 to 120 mEq per 24 hours	Varies with diet; the interpretation of urine electrolytes and osmolality should be left for the physician
Sodium	40 to 220 mEq per 24 hours	

◀ **CHEMISTRY** (continued)

Test	Values	Remarks
Porphobilinogen, qualitative	Negative	
Porphyrins, qualitative	Negative	
Proteins	0.05 to 0.1 g per 24 hours	
Salicylate	Negative	
Urea clearance	60 to 95 mL/minute	A blood sample must accompany specimen.
Urea N	10 to 40 g per 24 hours	Dependent on protein intake
Uric acid	250 to 750 mg per 24 hours	Dependent on diet and therapy
Urobilinogen	0.5 to 3.5 mg per 24 hours	For qualitative determination on random urine, send sample to urinalysis section in Hematology Lab.
Xylose absorption test		
Children	16% to 33% of ingested xylose	
Feces		
Fat, 3-day collection	<5 g/day	Value depends on fat intake of 100 g/d for 3 days preceding and during collection
Gastric Acidity		
Acidity, total, 12 hours	10 to 60 mEq/L	Titrated at pH 7

Blood Gases

	Arterial	Capillary	Venous
pH	7.35 to 7.45	7.35 to 7.45	7.32 to 7.42
pCO_2 (mm Hg)	35 to 45	35 to 45	38 to 52
pO_2 (mm Hg)	70 to 100	60 to 80	24 to 48
HCO_3 (mEq/L)	19 to 25	19 to 25	19 to 25
TCO_2 (mEq/L)	19 to 29	19 to 29	23 to 33
O_2 saturation (%)	90 to 95	90 to 95	40 to 70
Base excess (mEq/L)	-5 to +5	-5 to +5	-5 to +5

HEMATOLOGY

Complete Blood Cell Count

Age	Hgb (g/dL)	Hct (%)	RBC (mill/mm^3)	RDW
0 to 3 days	15 to 20	45 to 61	4 to 5.9	<18
1 to 2 weeks	12.5 to 18.5	39 to 57	3.6 to 5.5	<17
1 to 6 months	10 to 13	29 to 42	3.1 to 4.3	<16.5
7 months to 2 years	10.5 to 13	33 to 38	3.7 to 4.9	<16
2 to 5 years	11.5 to 13	34 to 39	3.9 to 5	<15
5 to 8 years	11.5 to 14.5	35 to 42	4 to 4.9	<15
13 to 18 years	12 to 15.2	36 to 47	4.5 to 5.1	<14.5
Adult male	13.5 to 16.5	41 to 50	4.5 to 5.5	<14.5
Adult female	12 to 15	36 to 44	4 to 4.9	<14.5

Age	MCV (fL)	MCH (pg)	MCHC (%)	Plts (x 10^3/mm^3)
0 to 3 days	95 to 115	31 to 37	29 to 37	250 to 450
1 to 2 weeks	86 to 110	28 to 36	28 to 38	250 to 450
1 to 6 months	74 to 96	25 to 35	30 to 36	300 to 700
7 mo to 2 years	70 to 84	23 to 30	31 to 37	250 to 600
2 to 5 years	75 to 87	24 to 30	31 to 37	250 to 550
5 to 8 years	77 to 95	25 to 33	31 to 37	250 to 550
13 to 18 years	78 to 96	25 to 35	31 to 37	150 to 450
Adult male	80 to 100	26 to 34	31 to 37	150 to 450
Adult female	80 to 100	26 to 34	31 to 37	150 to 450

WBC and Differential

Age	WBC (x 10^3/mm^3)	Segs	Bands	Lymphs	Monos
0 to 3 days	9 to 35	32 to 62	<18	19 to 29	5 to 7
1 to 2 weeks	5 to 20	14 to 34	<14	36 to 45	6 to 10
1 to 6 months	6 to 17.5	13 to 33	<12	41 to 71	4 to 7
7 months to 2 years	6 to 17	15 to 35	<11	45 to 76	3 to 6
2 to 5 years	5.5 to 15.5	23 to 45	<11	35 to 65	3 to 6
5 to 8 years	5 to 14.5	32 to 54	<11	28 to 48	3 to 6
13 to 18 years	4.5 to 13	34 to 64	<11	25 to 45	3 to 6
Adults	4.5 to 11	35 to 66	<11	24 to 44	3 to 6

Age	Eosinophils	Basophils	Atypical Lymphs	No. of NRBCs
0 to 3 days	0 to 2	0 to 1	0 to 8	0 to 2
1 to 2 weeks	0 to 2	0 to 1	0 to 8	0
1 to 6 months	0 to 3	0 to 1	0 to 8	0
7 months to 2 years	0 to 3	0 to 1	0 to 8	0
2 to 5 years	0 to 3	0 to 1	0 to 8	0
5 to 8 years	0 to 3	0 to 1	0 to 8	0
13 to 18 years	0 to 3	0 to 1	0 to 8	0
Adults	0 to 3	0 to 1	0 to 8	0

Bands = band neutrophils, lymphs = lymphocytes, monos = monocytes, segs = segmented neutrophils

Erythrocyte Sedimentation Rates and Reticulocyte Counts

Sedimentation rate, Westergren

Children 0 to 20 mm/h
Adult male 0 to 15 mm/hour
Adult female 0 to 20 mm/hour

Sedimentation rate, Wintrobe

Children 0 to 13 mm/hour
Adult male 0 to 10 mm/hour
Adult female 0 to 15 mm/hour

Reticulocyte count

Newborns 2% to 6%
1 to 6 months 0% to 2.8%
Adults 0.5% to 1.5%

PHARMACOLOGIC CATEGORY INDEX

Antineoplastic Agent, Alkylating Agent (Nitrogen Mustard)

Antineoplastic Agent, Alkylating Agent (Nitrosourea)

Antineoplastic Agent, Alkylating Agent (Triazene)

Antineoplastic Agent, Anaplastic Lymphoma Kinase Inhibitor

Antineoplastic Agent, Anthracenedione

Antineoplastic Agent, Anthracycline

Antineoplastic Agent, Antiandrogen

Antineoplastic Agent, Antibiotic

Antineoplastic Agent, Antibody Drug Conjugate

Antineoplastic Agent, Anti-CD19

Antineoplastic Agent, Anti-CD19/CD3

Antineoplastic Agent, Anti-CD20

Antineoplastic Agent, Anti-CD22

Antineoplastic Agent, Anti-CD30

Antineoplastic Agent, Anti-CD33

NOTES

NOTES

NOTES

NOTES

NOTES

Other Lexicomp Offerings

Drug Information Handbook

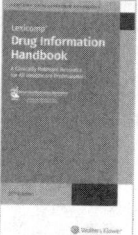

An easy-to-use reference for pharmacists, physicians and other healthcare professionals requiring fast access to relevant drug information, this handbook presents over 1,650 drug monographs, each with up to 45 fields of information. A valuable appendix includes hundreds of charts and reviews of special topics such as guidelines for treatment and therapy recommendations. A pharmacologic category index is also provided.

Pediatric & Neonatal Dosage Handbook

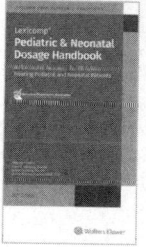

This book is designed for healthcare professionals requiring quick access to relevant pediatric drug information. Each monograph contains multiple fields of content, including usual dosage by age group, indication, and route of administration. Drug interactions, adverse reactions, extemporaneous preparations, pharmacodynamics/pharmacokinetics data and medication safety issues are also covered.

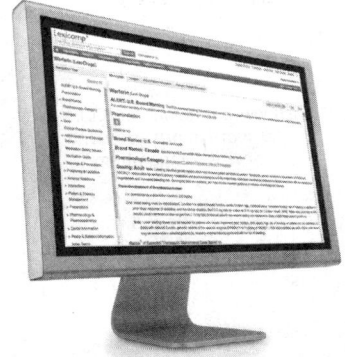
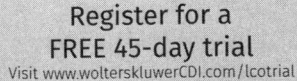

Lexicomp® Mobile Apps

Available for tablets and smartphones

At Wolters Kluwer Clinical Drug Information, we take pride in creating quality drug information for use at the point of care. Our Lexicomp content is not subject to third-party recommendations, but based on the contributions of our respected authors and editors, internal clinical team and thousands of professionals within the healthcare industry who continually review and validate our data.

With Lexicomp Mobile Apps, you have access to timely drug information anytime, anywhere on your mobile devices. All updates are included with your annual subscription.

Lexicomp Mobile Apps databases include:

- Adult Drug Information
- Pediatric and Neonatal Drug Information
- Drug Interactions
- Natural Products
- Toxicology
- Household Products
- Infectious Diseases
- Lab and Diagnostic Procedures
- Nursing Drug Information
- Dental Drug Information
- Pharmacogenomics
- Patient Education
- Drug Identification
- Medical Calculators

- IV Compatibility*
- Drug Allergy and Idiosyncratic Reactions
- Pregnancy and Lactation
- The 5-Minute Clinical Consult
- The 5-Minute Pediatric Consult
- AHFS Essentials
- Stedman's Medical Dictionary for the Health Professions and Nursing
- Stedman's Medical Abbreviations

* IV compatibility information © Trissel's™2 Clinical Pharmaceutics Database by Lawrence A. Trissel

Visit www.wolterskluwerCDI.com for more information and device compatability!

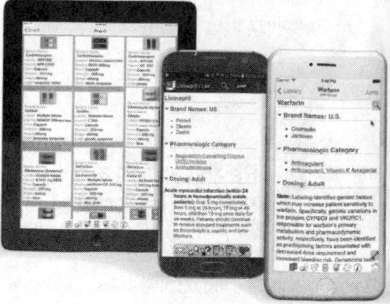